VOLUME 2

Therapeutic DRUGS

EDITED BY

SIR COLIN DOLLERY

EDITORIAL BOARD

ALAN R. BOOBIS
DENIS BURLEY
DAVID MARGERISON DAVIES
DONALD S. DAVIES
PETER IAN HARRISON
MICHAEL L' E. ORME
B. KEVIN PARK
LEON I. GOLDBERG

Churchill Livingstone

EDINBURGH LONDON MELBOURNE NEW YORK TOKYO AND MADRID 1991

CHILL LIVINGSTONE
cal Division of Longman Group UK
mited

Distributed in the United States of America by Churchill Livingstone Inc., 1560 Broadway, New York, N.Y. 10036, and by associated companies, branches and representatives throughout the world.

First published 1991

ISBN 0-443-02846-X

British Library Cataloguing in Publication Data
CIP catalogue record for this book is available from the British Library.

Library of Congress-in-Publication Data
Therapeutic drugs/edited by Sir Colin Dollery; editorial board,
Alan R. Boobis ... [et al.].
p. cm.
Includes bibliographical references and indexes.
1. Drugs—Handbooks, manuals, etc. 2. Pharmacology—Handbooks, manuals, etc. I. Dollery, Colin T.
[DNLM: 1. Drug Therapy—handbooks. 2. Drugs—handbooks. QV 39 T398]
RM301.12.T44 1991
615.5′8—dc20
DNLM/DLC
for Library of Congress

Printed and bound in Great Britain by
William Clowes Limited, Beccles and London

ACKNOWLEDGEMENTS

Publishing manager: Timothy Horne
Project coordinator: Julia Merrick
Design: Design Resource Unit
Production: I Macaulay Hunter, Lesley W Small
Computer Services: Janet Mundy and User Friendly Computer Services
Copy editors: Susan Boobis PhD, Jolyon Phillips PhD, Anne Russell
Proof readers: Pauline Cairns, Angus Macdonald, Paul Morgan, David Swinden, Jane Ward PhD
Editorial Assistant: Patricia Aubertel
Sales promotion: Hilary Brown

The publishers also gratefully acknowledge the help given by many others, particularly the coordinators in the early stages of the project: Susan Faulding and Helen Orpe.

Preface

Therapeutic drugs are the principal output of modern biology designed for the relief of human suffering. The modern era began with the advent of the organic chemistry industry in the early years of this century but underwent a remarkable acceleration during and after the 1939–45 war. Medicinal chemists have always played a central role but the advance of quantitative pharmacology has been a vital influence because it permitted precise structure–activity work within a chemical series once a new lead had been discovered. In the last 5–10 years molecular biology and biotechnology have become increasingly important, as the presence in this book of interferons, colony-stimulating factors and epoetin testifies.

As late as the 1950s the investigation of drugs in man was poorly organized. Senior scientists and physicians at the sponsoring company often tried the drug on themselves before it was given to patients, but the background knowledge, about kinetics, metabolism and toxicity in animals, was often quite limited. A series of disasters, of which thalidomide was the most dramatic, focused attention on the need for much more systematic investigation of toxic effects before first administration to man. Meanwhile, biochemists and clinical pharmacologists were beginning to understand the pharmacokinetic basis of the wide interindividual variation in response of patients given the same dose of a drug. Often the explanation turned out to be differences in the rate of metabolism of the drug and investigators realized that it was commonplace to have a five-fold range of concentrations for the same dose in different people. Many examples of much wider ranges were discovered; the most extreme examples often proved to be due to genetic polymorphisms of drug-metabolizing enzymes.

In parallel, methods of measuring drug action in man underwent a radical improvement. Uncontrolled, poorly performed and optimistically published studies began to be replaced by soundly designed, well controlled experiments yielding data of similar (and sometimes higher) quality to that obtained in animal experiments. These studies proved to be remarkably safe in competent hands and were seen as a crucial step in measuring drug action in man, establishing a dose–response curve and laying the first foundations of a safety profile. Often, combined studies of drug action and metabolism were particularly illuminating. In a few instances, most notably with some antiepileptic drugs, it proved possible to establish a range of plasma concentrations at which an optimal therapeutic effect occurred and to use this in the routine control of treatment in difficult cases. In others, active metabolites were identified and a few of these became new drugs in their own right.

Kinetic studies also led to a greater understanding of optimal dosage intervals. With drugs mainly excreted via the kidneys, means of avoiding toxicity by adjusting the dose or dosage interval were devised.

Clinical trials emerged from the testimonial era to be seen as the precise clinical experiments they really are. Undoubtedly, the pressure of a small number of high quality national drug control agencies played a crucial part in raising standards, as did the remarkable scientific resources of the leading research-based pharmaceutical companies. Each clinical indication now had to be validated by a properly designed clinical trial containing a control or comparison group, and with sufficient numbers to permit a valid statistical conclusion. One consequence was to make clear that many useful treatments were not quite as effective as uncontrolled observations had led physicians to believe.

Public interest in safety has often surpassed interest in efficacy and here too standards of data collection and evaluation have risen sharply. Adverse effects are now usually evaluated systematically during premarketing clinical studies by use of questionnaires or check lists. Patients who drop out of studies or die are very carefully followed up to assess causality. However, patients included in clinical trials are so carefully screened that few die or suffer serious adverse effects. Once on the market drugs are often not used with the same care and patient selection is less rigid. Serious untoward effects may then appear. Careful monitoring of drugs after release on to the market by spontaneous reporting systems, such as the 'Yellow Card' of the UK Medicines Control Agency or 'Pharmacovigilance' in France, has detected a number of new adverse effects. Close monitoring of defined patient groups using systems such as Prescription Event Monitoring in the UK or the Boston Collaborative Drug Surveillance Program in the USA gives useful incidence data, as well as serving as a detection system. **Despite these safeguards, constant vigilance for new adverse effects is a duty for all prescribers.** Vulnerable groups of people such as children, pregnant or lactating women, the elderly or individuals with renal failure need special consideration.

There has been an explosion of knowledge accompanying the therapeutic revolution. Although there are many excellent publications about drugs, it is our belief that none gives a comprehensive picture of the breadth of information that an intelligent and careful prescriber needs. Our aim in this book is to bring together that information in a form that is easy to use. The editors and contributors hope you will find it useful.

I am already preparing for the first supplement to this edition which will be published towards the end of 1992. This will contain about 25 new monographs and approximately the same number of major revisions for drugs where new indications have been established, major new trials have been published, or serious toxicity has been revealed. Suggestions about new chemical entities that should be included or monographs that ought to be revised will be most welcome from readers in all parts of the world. Please write to me with your proposals and give as much detail as you can about the reasons for making the suggestion.

We are grateful to the many drug information officers and medical directors in the pharmaceutical industry who gave us much valuable assistance, although the content of each monograph has been decided by the contributors and editors alone. Our contributors, from around the world, deserve special thanks for their patience as the editors made more and yet more demands on them.

It is a great sadness that one member of our editorial team did not live to see the book published. Dr Leon Goldberg, who was head of clinical pharmacology at Emory University in Atlanta and later at the University of Chicago, was a friend of all of us and made many useful suggestions in the early stages of the project. Sadly he was not well enough to take part fully in the editorial process but we hope that our efforts may serve to honour his memory.

1991 C.T.D.

Contributors

Mrs F M Abbott
Suva, Fiji

Dr Darrell Abernethy
Director, Program in Clinical Pharmacology, Brown University, Rhode Island, New York, USA

Professor H Erdal Akalin
Hacettepe University School of Medicine, Ankara, Turkey

Dr S G Allan
Formerly Senior Registrar, Western General Hospital, Edinburgh

Dr K D Allen
Consultant Microbiologist, Whiston Hospital, Merseyside

Dr A Amdisen
Formerly Aarhus University, Denmark

Dr Michael G Anderson
Consultant Physician, West Middlesex University Hospital, Middlesex

Dr B M Ansell
Head of Division of Rheumatology, Clinical Research Centre, London

Professor Marian Apfelbaum
Laboratory of Human Nutrition, Hopital Bichat, Paris, France

Dr Ann E Arnold
Consultant Psychiatrist, Central Middlesex Hospital, London

Dr Leonard Arnolda
Department of Medicine, Flinders Medical Centre, South Australia

Dr J K Aronson
Clinical Reader in Clinical Pharmacology, Radcliffe Infirmary, Oxford

Dr Charles Ashton
Senior Registrar, Department of Geriatric Medicine, Guy's Hospital, London

Dr Nigel S Baber
Director, Clinical Pharmacology, Glaxo Group Research Ltd, Middlesex

Dr D J Back
Reader in Pharmacology & Therapeutics, University of Liverpool, Liverpool

Dr G Bakris
Assistant Professor of Medicine, Ochsner Clinic, New Orleans, USA

Professor S G Ball
BHF Professor of the Chair of Cardiovascular Studies, University of Leeds, Leeds

Professor T A Ban
Department of Psychiatry, Vanderbilt University, Nashville, USA

Dr Paul Barczak
Consultant Psychiatrist, Lincoln County Hospital, Lincoln

Dr J N W N Barker
Senior Registrar, Guy's Hospital, London

Dr R J Barlow
Research Registrar, St John's Skin Centre, St Thomas's Hospital, London

Dr S Barnass
Senior Registrar in Medical Microbiology, St Bartholomew's Hospital, London

Dr T R E Barnes
Senior Lecturer in Psychiatry, Horton Hospital, Epsom

Professor Peter J Barnes
Professor of Thoracic Medicine, National Heart & Lung Institute, London

Dr J H Baron
Senior Lecturer & Consultant, Royal Postgraduate Medical School, London

Dr C A Bartzokas
Consultant in Medical Microbiology, Clatterbridge General Hospital, Merseyside

Dr D N Bateman
Consultant Physician and Reader in Therapeutics, Wolfson Unit of Clinical Pharmacology, Newcastle upon Tyne

Dr Peter Baylis
Reader in Endocrinology, Royal Victoria Infirmary, Newcastle upon Tyne

Dr K F Bayston
Honorary Senior Registrar in Infectious Diseases, Hammersmith Hospital, London

Professor R W Beard
Head of Department of Obstetrics & Gynaecology, St Mary's Hospital Medical School, London

Mrs C Beer
Drug Information Manager, Plymouth Health Authority, Plymouth

Dr R A V Benn
Microbiology Department, Fairfax Institute of Pathology, Royal Prince Albert Hospital, Camperdown, Australia

Dr D K Benn
Senior Registrar in Psychiatry, St George's Hospital, Morpeth

Dr P Bennett
Reader in Clinical Pharmacology, School of Postgraduate Medicine, University of Bath

Dr R S Bexton
Consultant Cardiologist, Freeman Hospital, Newcastle upon Tyne

Dr H A Bird
Senior Lecturer in Rheumatology, University of Leeds, Leeds

Professor Don Birkett
Department of Clinical Pharmacology, Flinders Medical Centre, South Australia

Professor I Blair
Director, Mass Spectrometry Resource, Vanderbilt University, Nashville, USA

Dr Peter Bliss
Lecturer, Medical Oncology, Western General Hospital, Edinburgh

Mr T H Bloomfield
Consultant Obstetrician & Gynaecologist, West Wales General Hospital, Dyfed, Wales

Professor D P de Bono
Professor of Cardiology, British Heart Foundation, University of Leicester, Leicester

Dr Susan Boobis
South Harrow, London

Dr Nicholas A Boon
Consultant Cardiologist & Honorary Senior Lecturer, Royal Infirmary, Edinburgh

Professor David Botero
Professor of Parasitology, Universidad Pontificia Bolivatiana, Columbia

Professor I A D Bouchier
Professor of Medicine, University of Edinburgh, Edinburgh

Professor Jean Bousquet
Service des Maladies Respiratoires, Centre Hospitalier Universitaire, Montpellier, France

Dr C Brass
Assistant Clinical Professor, SUNY at Buffalo, New York, USA

Dr Craig Brater
Director of Clinical Pharmacology, Indiana University School of Medicine, Indiana, USA

Professor D D Breimer
Division of Pharmacology, University of Leiden, The Netherlands

Dr M J Brodie
Consultant Clinical Pharmacologist, Western Infirmary, Glasgow

Professor R V Brooks
Former Professor of Chemical Endocrinology, Guy's and St Thomas's Hospitals, London

Professor P Brooks
Professor of Rheumatology, Royal North Shore Hospital, Sydney, Australia

Mr A Brown
Department of Pharmacy, Fazakerley Hospital, Liverpool

Professor M J Brown
Professor of Clinical Pharmacology, University of Cambridge, Cambridge

Dr K A Bryett
Commercial Development Manager, Merieux Ltd, Maidenhead

Dr Charles R Buchanan
Clinical Lecturer/Honorary Senior Registrar, Institute of Child Health, London

Dr R E S Bullingham
Director of European Clinical Studies, Syntex Research, Maidenhead

Dr M D Burley
Director, Centre for Pharmaceutical Medicine, Woking

Mr I Burn
Honorary Consulting Surgeon, Charing Cross Hospital, London

Dr Silvio Caccia
Istituto Di Ricerche Farmacologiche 'Mario Negri', Milan, Italy

Dr J Calam
Senior Lecturer in Medicine, Royal Postgraduate Medical School, London

Dr G Caldwell
Senior Registrar in Medicine & Endocrinology, Newcastle General Hospital, Newcastle upon Tyne

Professor D B Calne
Head, Division of Neurology, University Hospital, British Columbia, Canada

Dr Giles V Campion
Clinical Lecturer, Department Rheumatology, Bristol Royal Infirmary, Bristol

Dr R Canetta
Bristol-Myers Squibb, Connecticut, USA

Ms Linda Cardozo
Consultant Obstetrician & Gynaecologist, King's College Hospital, London

Dr Stuart Carne
Senior Tutor in General Practice, Royal Postgraduate Medical School, London

Professor R Y Cartwright
Consultant Microbiologist, St Luke's Hospital, Guildford

Dr R Cerio
Senior Registrar & Tutor in Dermatology, Institute of Dermatology, London

Dr J Chakraborty
Senior Lecturer in Clinical Biochemistry, University of Surrey, Guildford

Dr Douglas A Chamberlain
Consultant Cardiologist, Brighton Health Authority, Brighton

Professor G V P Chamberlain
Head, Department of Obstetrics & Gynaecology, St George's Hospital Medical School, London

Dr Kelvin Chan
Reader in Pharmacology, The Chinese University of Hong Kong, Hong Kong

Dr Israel Chanarin
Head, Haematology Section, MRC Clinical Research Centre, Middlesex

Dr W Chapman
Oklahoma, USA

Dr D M Chaput de Saintonge
Senior Lecturer in Clinical Pharmacology & Therapeutics, Royal London Hospital Medical College, London

Mr Clive R Charig
Senior Registrar in Urology, St George's Hospital, London

Dr Stuart Checkley
Dean, Institute of Psychiatry, De Crespigny Park, London,

Dr D A Cherry
Director & Senior Lecturer, Flinders Medical Centre, South Australia

Dr Peter L Chiodini
Consultant Parasitologist, The Hospital for Tropical Diseases, London

Dr J Christenson
Pediatrics & Infectious Diseases, University of Utah Medical Center, Salt Lake City, USA

Dr A C Chu
Consultant Dermatologist, Hammersmith Hospital, London

Professor R S J Clarke
Professor of Anaesthesia, The Queen's University of Belfast, Belfast

Dr John G F Cleland
Senior Lecturer in Medicine, Hammersmith Hospital, London

Dr Neil Clendeninn
Head, Chemotherapy Section, Cancer Therapy Department, North Carolina, USA

Dr Diana Cody
Consultant Psychiatrist, Tyrone & Fermanagh Hospital, Northern Ireland

Dr Robert E Coleman
Senior Lecturer in Medical Oncology, Weston Park Hospital, Sheffield

Dr A D Toft
Consultant Physician, Royal Infirmary, Edinburgh

Dr G Tognoni
Chief, Clinical Pharmacology, Istituto de Ricerche 'Mario Negri', Italy

Dr Edward G Tuddenham
Director, Haemostasis Research Group, Northwick Park Hospital, Middlesex

Dr W M G Tunbridge
Consultant Physician, Newcastle General Hospital, Newcastle upon Tyne

Dr H Uderman
Assistant Professor, University of Massachusetts Medical Center, Worcester, USA

Dr R J Unwin
Senior Lecturer, Department of Clinical Pharmacology, Royal Postgraduate Medical School, London

Dr James Upward
Lecturer in Clinical Pharmacology, Southampton University, Southampton

Dr S J Urbaniak
Regional Director, Transfusion Centre, Aberdeen Royal Infirmary, Aberdeen

Dr J A Vale
Director & Physician, West Midlands Poisons Unit, Dudley Road Hospital, Birmingham

Dr Malcolm Vanden Burg
Chairman, Medical & Clinical Management Ltd, Romford, Essex

Professor Dr Alex Vermeulen
Department of Endocrinology, University Hospital Ghent, Belgium

Professor M Verstraete
Professor of Medicine, University of Leuven, Leuven, Belgium

Dr J P Vestey
Lecturer/Honorary Senior Registrar, Royal Infirmary of Edinburgh, Edinburgh

Professor C F H Vickers
Emeritus Professor, Dept of Dermatology, University of Liverpool, Liverpool

Dr Glyn N Volans
Director, National Poisons Unit, New Cross Hospital, London

Professor Denis N Wade
Chairman, Johnson & Johnson Research Pty Ltd, Australia

Dr D G Waller
Senior Lecturer in Clinical Pharmacology, Southampton General Hospital, Southampton

Dr S C Wallis
Senior Lecturer, Endocrinology & Metabolism, Royal Postgraduate Medical School, London

Dr M J Walport
Reader in Rheumatological Medicine, Royal Postgraduate Medical School, London

Dr R P Walt
Senior Lecturer in Medicine, University of Birmingham, Birmingham

Dr Julian R F Walters
Senior Lecturer, Department of Medicine, Royal Postgraduate Medical School, London

Dr T D Wardle
Research Fellow, Hope Hospital, Manchester

Dr D W Warnock
Head Mycologist, Bristol Royal Infirmary, Bristol

Mrs P S Warrington
Unit Pharmacist, Western General Hospital, Edinburgh

Professor J A H Wass
Professor of Clinical Endocrinology, St Bartholomew's Hospital Medical College, London

Dr Michael F R Waters
Consultant Leprologist and Physician, Hospital for Tropical Diseases, London

Dr J Waxman
Senior Lecturer and Honorary Consultant, Royal Postgraduate Medical School, London

Professor Wendell W Weber
Department of Pharmacology, University of Michigan, Michigan, USA

Mr A Webster
Clinical Psychology Trainee, Newham District Psychology Department, London

Dr John Webster
Consultant Physician, Aberdeen Royal Infirmary, Aberdeen

Dr D H G Wegner
formerly Senior Clinical Monitor, Bayer AG Pharmaceutical Research Centre, Germany

Dr S L Weinstein
Director, Clinical Psychopharmacology, New York Psychiatric Institute, New York, USA

Professor W H Wernsdorfer
Visiting Professor, National Centre Drug Research, Universiti Sains Malaysia, Malaysia

Dr Lawrence J Whalley
Senior Lecturer, University Department of Psychiatry, Edinburgh University, Edinburgh

Dr Andrew White
Senior Registrar, Wessex Regional Health Authority, Hampshire

Dr Albert T White Jnr
Associate/Fellow, Department of Medicine, University of Alabama, USA

Professor J M A Whitehouse
Director, Wessex Medical Oncology Unit, Southampton General Hospital, Southampton

Professor B Whiting
Head of Division of Clinical Pharmacology, University of Glasgow, Glasgow

Professor T L Whitsett
Director of Clinical Pharmacology, University of Oklahoma, Oklahoma City, USA

Professor J G Whitwam
Director & Professor of Anaesthetics, Royal Postgraduate Medical School, London

Mrs Lynda Wight
Managing Director, Medical & Clinical Research Consultants, Romford, Essex

Dr J A W Wildsmith
Consultant/Senior Lecturer, Royal Infirmary, Edinburgh

Dr Martin Wilkins
Senior Lecturer in Medicine & Clinical Pharmacology, Royal Postgraduate Medical School, London

Dr P M Wilkinson
Consultant Physician/Clinical Pharmacologist, Christie Hospital & Holt Radium Institute, Manchester

Dr Marcia Wilkinson
Honorary Medical Director, City of London Migraine Clinic, London

Mr G Williams
Consultant Urologist, Hammersmith Hospital, London

Professor J D Williams
Professor of Medical Microbiology, The London Hospital Medical College, London

Dr Christopher Williams
Senior Lecturer, CRC Medical Oncology Unit, Southampton General Hospital, Southampton

Mrs Katherine Willson
Head of Drug Information, St George's Hospital, London

Dr Sunil J Wimalawansa
Senior Lecturer in Medicine, Royal Postgraduate Medical School, London

Dr Christopher G Winearls
Consultant Nephrologist, Churchill Hospital, Oxford

Dr L M H Wing
Department of Clinical Pharmacology, Flinders Medical Centre, South Australia

Professor Robert M L Winston
Professor of Fertility Studies, Royal Postgraduate Medical School, London

Dr R Wise
Consultant Medical Microbiologist, Dudley Road Hospital, Birmingham

Professor Joseph A Witkowski
Clinical Professor of Dermatology, University of Pennsylvania, Philadelphia, USA

Dr E Ch Wolters
Neurology Department, Vrije Universiteit, Amsterdam, The Netherlands

Dr J C L Wong
Senior Lecturer in Pharmacology, The Chinese University of Hong Kong, Hong Kong

Dr M J Wood
Consultant Physician, East Birmingham Hospital, Birmingham

Professor H Frank Woods
Sir George Franklin Professor of Medicine, Royal Hallamshire Hospital, Sheffield

Dr Anthony D Woolf
Consultant Rheumatologist, Royal Cornwall Hospital, Truro

Dr Stephen G Wright
Senior Lecturer, Department of Clinical Sciences, London School of Hygiene & Tropical Medicine, London

Dr A L Wright
Consultant Dermatologist, Bradford Royal Infirmary, Bradford

Dr D A Yardumian
Consultant Haematologist, The North Middlesex Hospital, London

Dr K Yau
Senior Registrar in Anaesthetics, Hammersmith Hospital, London

Dr John H K Yeung
Lecturer in Pharmacology, Faculty of Medicine, The Chinese University of Hong Kong, Hong Kong

Professor A Zanchetti
Professor of Medicine, University of Milan, Italy

Dr D A Zideman
Consultant Anaesthetist, Hammersmith Hospital, London

Dr Thom J Zimmerman
Professor & Chairman, Deptartment of Ophthalmology & Visual Science, University of Louisville, Kentucky, USA

Introduction

NOTE TO READERS

The monographs in this book do not indicate the terms of licences granted by national regulatory agencies. These can vary widely and it is imperative that readers satisfy themselves as to the current legal requirements in their own location. Indications, contraindications and dosages must be checked with appropriate official national formularies and local hospital or other guidelines.

How to read a monograph

A doctor, a pharmacist or a nurse who needs information about a drug wants to find it quickly, clearly and unambiguously. This book is organized to meet that objective and yet satisfy the demand for the immense amount of new knowledge that is available about drugs used in therapy. Each monograph is organized under the same set of headings in a logical order, so once you have become used to the layout it is very easy to find any particular piece of information, whether it is the mechanism of action, the effect of an overdose or the results of major clinical trials. Each monograph is self-sufficient, so cross-references have been kept to a minimum, even if that means some repetition. With older drugs there is often less information available, because standards of investigation have risen steadily over the last 25 or more years. Even with modern drugs it can be difficult to find important items of information which may lie hidden in un-indexed conference proceedings or the vaults of national drug regulatory agencies.

The name of the drug

The monograph is headed by the non-proprietary or generic name which is the same in almost all countries. Drugs are listed in alphabetical order of this name. The name is followed by a very brief statement about the therapeutic use of the drug.

Chemistry

The first entry in this section is the accepted name for the drug, followed, in parentheses, by the more common proprietary names. Under this will be found the molecular formula, of the salt if this is the preparation normally available. The molecular formula can be utilized in searches of a number of chemical data bases. This is followed by the full chemical name, again of the salt if appropriate. In most cases the structure of the compound is also provided.

The following information is provided in a table offset from the body of the text: the molecular weight of the form normally used therapeutically, with that of the free acid or base in parentheses if appropriate. In such cases the nature of the compound is indicated, i.e. whether it is an acid or a base in the free state. This is followed by the pKa, an indication of the tendency of the compound to ionize. The two entries following this, on solubility in alcohol and in water, indicate the number of parts of the respective solvent in which one part of the drug in the form normally available (i.e. as the salt if this is the form normally available) is soluble at room temperature. The final entry in this table is the octanol/water partition coefficient of the free form of the drug, which provides a measure of the lipid solubility of the compound.

The table is followed by a description of the normal physical state, appearance and odour of the drug, together with information on whether the drug is a natural compound or prepared by chemical synthesis. Finally, in this section there is an indication of whether the drug occurs in any combination preparations, together with the proprietary names of the more common of these.

Pharmacology

Most drugs have relatively specific actions as agonists or antagonists at receptors, as enzyme inhibitors, antimetabolites, alkylating agents, etc. The pharmacology section of each monograph deals with the main pharmacological actions of the drug in question, usually defined from animal studies — both in isolated organ studies and in vivo. Drugs are not always as specific as their inventors might wish, and improved understanding of the molecular structure of receptors and enzymes has provided an explanation. Receptors for entirely different ligands may show considerable homology, which makes it easier to understand why a drug may have some effect upon apparently dissimilar receptors, e.g. α-adrenergic, histaminic, dopaminergic.

It is usual nowadays to express pharmacological activity in terms of the molar concentration of the drug which produces the effect. Most dose–response curves for agonists are 'S' shaped if the effect is plotted against the logarithm of the concentration. The activity of the drug can be expressed as the molar concentration which causes 50% of the maximum effect (EC_{50}). The lower the concentration, the more active the drug. For competitive antagonists the log dose–response curve to the agonist is shifted in a parallel fashion to the right.

This section includes dose–response relationships for the various actions of the drug, where these are known, but for many older drugs this aspect of their pharmacology is not always well studied. The section deals primarily with the mechanism of action of the drug concerned.

Toxicology

Drugs undergo rigorous safety tests in animals and with isolated cells in vitro before being administered to man. The schedules of tests required by different regulatory authorities are broadly similar but there are some differences, particularly in the duration of some tests. Whilst it is true that tests in animals are not infallible predictors of safety in use in man (see practolol), it is nevertheless true that the vast majority of drugs, when used within the normal range of doses, do not produce serious adverse effects. This demonstrates the value of tests conducted in animals and with isolated cells in protecting man from toxic drugs.

General toxicology

Acute toxicity tests are conducted in two species in which a single dose is administered by the proposed route of use in man and intravenously to ensure adequate systemic exposure. Animals are observed for not less than 7 days, at which time an autopsy is performed. The purpose of this test is to document the signs of acute toxicity and the mode of death. Semi-quantitative data on the dose–effect relationship are also obtained.

Repeated dose toxicity tests are conducted for six months (longer for some authorities) in two species. The animals are closely monitored for signs of toxicity and there is full autopsy at the end of the study. The drug is administered by the route or routes proposed for administration to man. Three dose levels, ranging from the proposed human dose up to one that produces target organ toxicity, are employed. The purpose of the test is to obtain information on toxic effects which may arise from repeated dosing and to determine the margin of safety between therapeutic and toxic doses. For highly metabolized drugs, safety margins are better related to systemic exposure (plasma concentration–time profiles) than to dose/body weight because of very rapid metabolism in test animals compared to man. Thus pharmacokinetic data are an important part of repeated-dose toxicity tests.

Mutagenic potential

This is evaluated early in drug development by a battery of tests conducted in vitro and in vivo. These tests are designed to detect changes in genetic material in cells or animals which may present a genetic hazard to future generations and/or a risk of cancer to the present generation.

Carcinogenic potential

This is assessed for drugs to be used for long periods in man. The tests may also be required for drugs whose chemical structure suggests carcinogenic potential or those that are positive in the tests for mutagenesis, irrespective of their proposed use. Studies of carcinogenic potential are conducted in two species and require dosing for a substantial period of the animal's life-span at three dose levels. The top dose should produce a systemic exposure which is a significant multiple of the likely human exposure. At the end of the study a comparison of the incidence of tumours in control and treated animals is made to assess carcinogenic potential. Many drugs (e.g. cyclophosphamide) are thought to produce tumours because of their genotoxic effects, but others such as clofibrate do not directly damage genetic material but are said to be non-genotoxic carcinogens.

Reproductive toxicology

This seeks to reveal any effects of drugs which may cause loss of or damage to the fetus or which cause harm to the offspring in later life. Effects may range from damage to male or female gametes or effects on embryogenesis to abnormalities in uterine growth. Tests are conducted in two species, one of which is not a rodent. Three dose levels are used and the top dose should produce some evidence of maternal toxicity. Different dosing schedules are used to test for teratogenesis, effect on fertility and in pre- and post-natal studies.

The section under 'Toxicology' will usually give the acute toxicity of the drug, the prominent features of toxicity in animals, and point out where serious toxic effects observed in man were not predicted by tests in animals (e.g. practolol).

Clinical pharmacology

This section covers the data available concerning the pharmacological effect of the drug in man, for example on blood pressure and heart rate and CNS effects such as sedation or EEG changes. Data about the dose–response relationship and duration of action are included when available. Undesired pharmacological effects are mentioned and these are relevant to the section on adverse reactions. In the case of antimicrobial drugs this section gives the main groups of organisms affected by the drug. Precise information about clinical pharmacology is often lacking for older drugs.

There have been considerable advances in recent years in the methods used to measure drug action in man and the results may show important differences from animal studies. Pharmacologists working with animals may be able to detect a range of different effects over a wide span of concentrations. However, human studies may show that only some of these occur at the lower concentrations that often prevail after therapeutic doses. Another important difference between animal and human pharmacology is the lack of a satisfactory animal model for many human diseases. The difference is most obvious for CNS disorders such as depression and schizophrenia, but it applies to many other conditions.

There is often a wide gap between the pharmacological action and its therapeutic application and a number of important effects have been discovered by chance when a drug has been given for another purpose, for example the diuretic and hypoglycaemic effects of sulphonamides.

Pharmacokinetics

Information on the quantification, absorption, distribution, extent of metabolism and excretion of the drug is provided in this section. At the beginning of the section will be found an indication of the currently preferred method for the quantification of the drug serum or plasma, together with a source reference and the limits of detection of the method.

The remainder of the section systematically covers the fate of the drug in the body. Whilst information is incomplete for some drugs, each monograph follows the same overall layout. The extent of absorption of the drug following its normal route of administration is indicated, together with the time that it takes the plasma concentration to reach a peak and any influence that eating might have on this. The bioavailability, a measure of systemic exposure to the parent drug following administration by the route indicated, depends upon the extent of absorption and presystemic metabolism, usually in the intestinal wall or liver. The difference between the extent of absorption and the bioavailability indicates the extent of extraction across the small intestine and/or liver. Where the fraction of the dose extracted by these organs has been determined, this is indicated. Where relevant, the degree of inter-individual variation in absorption or presystemic metabolism is indicated, together with those factors known to influence these processes, for example concurrent exposure to an enzyme inducing agent. The half life of elimination of the drug in plasma is given, both the mean value for a group of healthy volunteers, and the range of values that will be encountered within the normal population. The half life, together with the frequency of dosing, gives an indication of whether, and to what extent, accumulation of the drug will occur during chronic treatment.

Information on the distribution of the drug now follows. An indication of how widely the compound is distributed throughout the body, together with the speed of this distribution, is given. This is followed by the apparent volume of distribution and some indication of any tissues in which the drug is known to be localized. The extent of plasma protein binding and the identity of the protein involved, if known, are provided. If available, information on the concentration of the drug achieved in the CSF and the tendency of the compound to penetrate to the CNS are given, together with the ratio of the CSF to plasma and brain to plasma concentrations. This information is available only for a limited number of compounds and is often obtained from autopsy or from animal studies. The extent and likelihood of the drug being excreted in breast milk and undergoing placental transfer will usually be found at this point in the monograph. The significance of any such distribution will be found in the sections on 'High risk groups'.

Basic pharmacokinetic data are provided in a box offset from the body of the text. These include the following:

Oral absorption. This is the percentage of the dose absorbed from the gastro-intestinal tract following oral administration. This is not necessarily the same as the amount of drug reaching the systemic circulation, as there may be some presystemic metabolism (*q.v.*).

Presystemic metabolism. This is the metabolism which takes place between the site of administration of the drug and entry into the systemic circulation. If presystemic metabolism occurs following oral administration, it will be in the small intestine and/or in the liver. The extent of absorption and presystemic metabolism determine the bioavailability of the drug, a measure of total systemic exposure. It is calculated from the ratio of the area under the plasma concentration–time curve following an oral dose to that after an intravenous dose, the assumption being that the intravenous dose is 100% bioavailable. Whereas both incomplete absorption and high presystemic metabolism will reduce the amount of parent drug reaching the systemic circulation, with high presystemic metabolism (and good absorption) the intestinal and/or hepatic cells are exposed to high concentrations of the compound, and although the parent drug may not reach the systemic circulation, the products of such metabolism may be present at high concentrations. Although frequently inactive, in some instances these can contribute to the pharmacological effect of the drug, e.g. terfenadine.

The plasma half life. The plasma half life is the time taken for the plasma concentration of the drug to decline by 50%. For drugs eliminated by first-order processes, i.e. where the rate of elimination is proportional to the concentration of the drug, the half life is a constant term, as a constant fraction of the dose is eliminated in unit time. For some drugs several half lives are described. These are named alphabetically using lower case Greek letters in order of ascending duration of the half life. Thus the shortest is the α half life, the next the β half life, and the third the γ half life. The α-phase usually reflects distribution of the drug into the tissues, and is often seen only after intravenous administration; following oral administration the distribution phase is usually obscured by the absorption phase, during which time the concentration of the drug in plasma is increasing. For many drugs only two half lives are discernible after intravenous administration, the α and β half lives. Where there is a long, γ half life this is due to the slow equilibration of the drug from a so-called 'deep compartment', i.e. the time taken for the drug to diffuse from some tissues back into the plasma is slow relative to its rate of elimination. The half life for the slowest component of the plasma decay curve measurable for a drug is usually termed the elimination or terminal half life. The half life of most importance clinically is that which determines accumulation to steady state during chronic dosing, usually the elimination half life. The *range* quoted for the half life will be the extremes of the values found, usually in studies of normal volunteers, whilst the *mean* will be the average of the averages of several studies in healthy subjects.

The volume of distribution. This is a proportionality constant that relates the amount of drug in the body to the plasma concentration. The volume of distribution, more properly the apparent or virtual volume of distribution, rarely corresponds to a physiological compartment, because of selective tissue binding of the drug. Thus, it may range from 70 000 litres for a tricyclic antidepressant that is highly bound to tissue proteins to less than 5 litres for a drug with a high molecular weight, such as a plasma expander.

Plasma protein binding. This is the percentage of the drug present in plasma that is bound reversibly to plasma proteins. For most drugs it is constant over the range of concentrations encountered in the therapeutic use of the compound. However, for a few such as aspirin, there is saturation of binding as the concentration of the drug increases within the normal therapeutic range. Many drugs bind to albumin, but a number of basic drugs such as propranolol bind to α_1-acid glycoprotein. Change in the percentage of a drug bound to plasma proteins rarely has clinical consequences in itself. However, there is often a corresponding change in the total concentration of the drug so that attempts to restore total drug levels to those prior to the alteration in protein binding will result in excessively high or low free concentrations of the compound, and it is the free concentration that determines pharmacological effect. The precept here is to treat the patient, not the plasma concentration.

If an active metabolite of a drug contributes substantially to its effect, pharmacokinetic information for the metabolite will also be provided, if possible.

The kinetics box is followed by basic information on the metabolism and excretion of the drug. This includes the extent to which the drug is metabolized and the major site of such metabolism, the amount of the drug eliminated unchanged and the main routes of excretion. Together, this information provides some indication of the likely effect of hepatic and renal disease on the pharmacokinetics of the drug. Where appropriate studies have been performed, the specific effects of liver disease, renal disease and old age on the pharmacokinetics of the compound are provided, together with some indication as to whether these are likely to be of therapeutic importance.

Where the kinetics of the drug are markedly influenced by other factors, such as enzyme-inducing agents or inhibitors, this information is provided here.

Concentration–effect relationship

In in vitro studies it is common to show a correlation between the concentration of drug present and the pharmacological action of the drug. However, in in vivo studies, particularly in man, it is much more difficult to show such a relationship. Sometimes there may be a correlation between the free (unbound) concentration in plasma or between CSF concentrations and the therapeutic effect, but making these measurements may be difficult. In a few instances, there is a sufficiently close correlation between the effect (which may be difficult to measure in an individual patient) and the total plasma concentration for this measurement to be a useful guide to clinical dosage. This section gives data about this topic where it is known. If the drug is known to have an active metabolite this will also be discussed in this section. For many drugs no such relationship has been studied. In the case of antibiotics the concentration usually quoted will be the minimum inhibitory concentration (MIC) affecting 50% or 90% of strains of the organism in question. However, these data are usually acquired from in vitro studies and may not always be of direct relevance to the clinical situation. For drugs that act locally, e.g. on the skin, many laxatives and constipating agents, these data will not usually be given.

Metabolism

Most drugs are low molecular weight (typically 200–300 daltons), lipid-soluble compounds. Their lipid solubility is necessary for diffusion to their site of action. As a consequence of this, although they are readily filtered at the glomerulus they will be extensively reabsorbed from the proximal tubule, so that only a small fraction of the dose can be eliminated by urinary excretion. However, the enzymes of drug metabolism can convert lipid-soluble compounds into more water-soluble products that can be excreted in the urine or faeces. The major organ of such metabolism is the liver, but other tissues that can contribute include the small intestine, kidney and the plasma.

The reactions of drug metabolism can conveniently be divided into two phases: phase I, which involves functionalization by oxidation, reduction or hydrolysis, and phase II, which involves conjugation or synthetic reactions with endogenous donor molecules such as glucuronic acid, sulphate and acetate. Products of phase I metabolism frequently serve as substrates for phase II reactions, although any drug with a suitable functional group, such as an amino or hydroxyl group, may be conjugated directly, e.g. paracetamol, oxazepam, morphine.

The phase I reactions are the more important in reducing or terminating biological effect, altering the drug in such a way that it is no longer able to interact with its specific target site. Of the phase I reactions, those catalysed by the cytochrome P450-dependent mixed-function oxidase system predominate. There are multiple forms of cytochrome P450, subject to influence by a wide variety of genetic, environmental, physiological and pathological factors. The most important of these effects include induction, in which there is increased synthesis or decreased breakdown of P450, which occurs with compounds as diverse as anticonvulsant drugs, hydrocarbons in cigarette smoke, alcohol (ethanol) and macrolide antibiotics such as rifampicin. Induction often results in increased elimination of the drug, with a concomitant reduction in its intensity and duration of action. Inhibition of cytochrome P450 may also be important, reducing the elimination of the compound and increasing the intensity and duration of its action. There are several mechanisms of inhibition. Some drugs act as highly specific, competitive inhibitors of a single form of P450, in which case only when a drug depends largely upon that form of P450 for its elimination will such inhibition be relevant. Examples include the inhibition of desmethylimipramine oxidation by quinidine and of cyclosporin A by ketoconazole. For most drugs, their elimination depends upon several enzymes. Some compounds act as relatively non-specific inhibitors of P450, for example cimetidine. Genetic variation in the activity or amount of a form of P450 may also contribute to interindividual differences in response to a drug. There are at least two genetic polymorphisms of P450, one of the debrisoquine/sparteine oxidizing form and one of the mephenytoin oxidizing form.

Although the phase II enzymes are less commonly responsible for termination of drug effect than the phase I enzymes, the metabolites finally eliminated in the urine or faeces are most frequently their products, due to the sequential action of phase I and phase II enzymes. Quantitatively, the most important phase II reactions are glucuronidation and sulphation, many compounds often forming both conjugates. Although there are several forms of the enzymes catalysing these reactions, they appear to be less specific, at least towards drugs, than the phase I enzymes. Variation in their activity has not been as well studied as for the P450 enzymes. Some of the enzymes of glucuronidation are inducible, but not to the same extent as the oxidizing enzymes. The acetylation of some amine-containing drugs, such as sulphadimidine, dapsone, isoniazid and hydralazine, is subject to genetic polymorphism.

Whilst the liver is the major organ of biotransformation, other tissues may contribute. Establishing which organ is responsible for the metabolism of a drug in vivo can be extremely difficult, and sometimes no clear answer is forthcoming. Certainly, the small intestine is an important site of sulphation of drugs such as isoprenaline, when these are given orally, and of the deamination of some biogenic amines which are ingested, such as tyramine. The plasma can catalyse a number of hydrolytic reactions, such as the conversion of aspirin to salicylic acid and the inactivation of succinylcholine. Drugs that are close structural analogues of endogenous compounds may serve as substrates for highly specific enzymes such as catechol *O*-methyltransferase and monoamine oxidase A. These are more the exceptions than the rule, and most drugs are metabolized by the so-called 'xenobiotic' metabolizing enzymes. However, an increasing number of peptides are being developed for therapeutic use, and these are usually metabolized by enzymes normally involved in the degradation of endogenous proteins and peptides.

Although the products of drug metabolism are often less active than the parent compound, this is not always so. In some instances, the compound administered is a pro-drug, and has no biological activity until metabolized, e.g. cyclophosphamide, enalapril. Some of the products of metabolism have sufficient biological activity to contribute to the therapeutic effect of the parent compound, e.g. some of the oxidation products of tricyclic antidepressants and of benzodiazepines. Finally, some metabolites are chemically reactive and may be responsible for toxic injury to cells, e.g. paracetamol, isoniazid. In such instances the toxic pathway is usually a minor route of metabolism, and it is only when the other pathways are compromised, such as by saturating them in overdose, that toxicity ensues.

The details of the routes and extent of metabolism of the drug are provided in this section. The overall extent to which the drug is metabolized is indicated, together with the organ primarily responsible for such metabolism. The percentage of the dose excreted unchanged is given and the major routes of excretion are indicated. This should provide some indication of the likely effects of impaired hepatic and renal function on the pharmacokinetics of the drug. This is followed by a description of the major routes of metabolism, accompanied for some drugs by a structural diagram. Some indication of the fraction of the dose excreted as each of the major identified metabolites is provided. Such knowledge may help in interpreting or anticipating drug–drug interactions. Where metabolites have been shown to be pharmacologically active, this is indicated, together with an evaluation of whether such metabolites contribute to the therapeutic effect of the parent drug. This section also includes information on any pharmacogenetic or environmental factors known to have a major influence on the metabolism of the drug.

Pharmaceutics

Drugs are rarely suitable for administration to patients as the unadulterated pure chemical in a capsule or solution. The complex science of pharmaceutics has sprung up to convert drugs with unpromising physical properties, instability in moisture or oxygen, unsuitably short half lives, etc., into products which can be used easily and with confidence by patients and doctors. This often involves close control of powder form (amorphous or crystalline), particle size, tablet compression forces and use of inactive excipients. These last include binding agents, solubilizing agents, antioxidants, preservatives and coatings to ensure the stability and release of the basic drug and the absence of microbial contamination. Newer dosage forms may utilize microencapsulation, special matrices or osmotic pump technology. Esterification and flavouring additives are employed to increase palatability.

The monographs include details of the appropriate sterilization method if the drug is used in eye drop or injection formulations. If there are potentially allergenic components such as tartrazine in the formulation, these are mentioned, but it should be noted formulations may vary from country to country, even from the same manufacturer. Identification codes are given for the main solid dose forms used in the United Kingdom and the United States of America. It has not been practical, for reasons of space, to list all the generic equivalents of drugs whose patents have expired. Neither have combination products of many drugs been included. Shelf-life is derived from rigorous stability studies over a wide range of temperatures. These are included in the text where known. It is inevitable in a dynamic research-driven market that improvements will be made in many formulations during a product's life. Current formulations should be selected from national or local formularies and manufacturers' data sheet compendia.

Therapeutic use

Indications

Indications are given initially as a list, and amplified later in the text. Few drugs have only a single use and for some the list is very long. Under this heading are listed generally approved indications. As national drug control authorities usually approve therapeutic claims for each condition separately, the permitted indications may vary in different countries. Consult your national formulary or drug compendium to check whether a particular indication is approved in your country.

Contraindications

Contraindications are also presented as a list, with later discussion in the text. Some contraindications are absolute, such as a previous anaphylactic reaction to benzylpenicillin. Others represent sensible advice about appropriate precautions in special groups of patients. Both are listed under this heading. Adverse reactions that occur because physicians have overlooked or forgotten known contraindications are indefensible.

Mode of use

In this section more details are given about how the drug is used, with advice about the dosage regimen, duration of treatment, efficacy, etc.

Adverse reactions

Virtually all drugs have the capacity to cause harm, even death, in some patients under some circumstances. The sub-headings used reflect a gradation of severity.

Potentially life-threatening effects
This section deals with the most serious adverse reactions that have either caused death or could do so. Some indication of frequency is given, but for very serious but very low frequency events it may not be possible to give a reliable quantitative estimate.

Acute overdosage
Taking a deliberate overdose of a drug is common, accidental overdosage due to medical, nursing or pharmaceutical error is not vanishingly rare. It is useful to know what doses are likely to cause serious or fatal toxicity, the clinical manifestations and any specific or general measures that can be used in treatment. Kinetic data are often useful in overdose cases, either as a guide to the need for treatment (e.g. in paracetamol overdose), or to the rate of recovery. Drug half lives after therapeutic doses are an unreliable guide to the duration of action of a very large dose which may saturate drug metabolizing enzymes so that elimination becomes zero order (a constant amount per unit time rather than a constant fraction).

Severe or irreversible adverse effects
The distinction between this category and potentially life-threatening effects is often one of degree, but there are many adverse actions, such as neurotoxicity, which are not often fatal but may be irreversible.

Symptomatic adverse effrects
Symptomatic adverse effects of drugs, such as nausea, headaches, fatigue, are extremely common, but it helps to have an idea of their frequency and pattern so that patients can be warned in advance.

Interference with clinical pathology tests
The chemical methods used in clinical pathology are often chosen for their simplicity and ease of automation. Such methods may lack specificity and the presence of therapeutic drugs may interfere with the assay and produce a misleading result. Information about known technical interference with clinical pathology tests is listed here. Improved methods, using separation techniques such as HPLC, often overcome these problems, and you should consult your laboratory about any apparent problems which may only apply to one particular method.

High risk groups

Some patient groups are more vulnerable than others. Contributors of monographs were asked to review a standard list of headings.

Neonates
In the first few hours of life both renal excretion and hepatic metabolism are abnormal and normal doses, adjusted for body weight, can lead to prolonged effects.

Breast milk
With some drugs, concentrations in human milk have been studied and a clear statement can be made. Often we have to give a warning, not because we know that there is a problem but because we cannot say for certain that there is not.

Children
Drugs are quite often used in children but rarely tested or systematically studied in them. This is understandable (for legal and ethical reasons) but unsatisfactory. In many instances we have had to warn that there is no evidence about safety or efficacy of use in children.

Pregnancy
Concern about teratogenic effects has, understandably, made physicians and manufacturers very conservative about studying drugs in pregnancy. This can give rise to problems with drugs such as antihypertensives and antibiotics which may need to be used in pregnancy. Such evidence as there is tends to be compilations of case reports.

The elderly
The elderly are more often ill, so they receive more prescriptions and are therefore prone to more drug interactions. Organs such as the brain, heart and kidney have a diminished reserve which may predispose to adverse effects. Repair of injured tissues is slow. All these factors enjoin caution about the number and dose of drugs prescribed to older patients.

Concurrent disease
Some disorders predispose to adverse reactions. Examples include:

Renal disease. While only a few drugs are predominantly excreted unchanged in the urine, some of these, e.g. aminoglycoside antibiotics and digoxin, are very important because of their toxicity in overdose.

Hepatic disease. Surprisingly, because so many drugs are metabolized in the liver, quite severe chronic hepatic disease often has only a modest effect in prolonging drug half lives. Acute hepatic necrosis is another matter and may cause very marked reduction in the speed of drug elimination. The presence of portocaval shunts may increase the systemic bioavailability of drugs with a high presystemic metabolism.

Heart disease. Diseased hearts are more vulnerable to pro-arrhythmic effects of drugs, including inotropic agents and antiarrhythmics. Heart failure makes the heart vulnerable to drugs with negative inotropic actions and may prolong the half life of drugs (e.g. lignocaine) whose rate of elimination is dependent on liver blood flow.

Drug interactions

The multiplicity of drugs prescribed to acutely ill patients, especially the elderly with diseases of several systems, gives rise to a rich field of potential interactions. The most common is the additive effects of drugs which share a common action, especially CNS depressants. Interactions have been divided into three categories.

Potentially hazardous interactions
The most serious problem is when one drug that has to be closely regulated, such as a coumarin anticoagulant, has its half life radically changed by another drug that induces (e.g. rifampicin) or inhibits (e.g. cimetidine) the enzymes that metabolize it. Although the belief is deeply embedded in textbooks, displacement of one drug from protein binding by another is much less important. Most of the widely quoted examples are due to inhibition of metabolism not to displacement from binding.

Other significant interactions
This heading is for items that do not fit into the other two categories, such as less important changes in kinetics.

Potentially useful interactions
Although regulatory bodies discourage combined products, drugs are often administered together to achieve a greater combined effect (e.g. a β-adrenergic blocking drug and diuretic in hypertension), or to minimize an unwanted effect (e.g. combining a penicillin with a β-lactamase inhibitor).

Clinical trials

Clinical trials are listed individually, with a paragraph describing the design and a summary of the main results. Major outcome trials are listed as such. Trials that do not deal with outcome but which are properly controlled are listed as randomized controlled trials. Trials that do not fulfil either of these criteria are listed as other trials.

Drug efficacy is what really matters and the ultimate evidence of efficacy rests upon properly designed clinical experiments in patients who have been allocated by a random procedure to two or more different treatments, one of which is often with an inactive placebo. The largest and longest clinical trials deal with *outcome*, i.e. cure or death. Randomized controlled trials are still extremely valuable even if they do not deal with outcome of the disease. In well designed clinical trials, very careful thought is given to inclusion and exclusion criteria and to the calculation of the numbers required to achieve a stated significance and power. The meaning of significance is well understood (the probability that an observed difference might have arisen by chance). When designing a trial or when a trial fails to show a significant difference between groups the power of the trial is an important issue. Simply stated power is a confidence (or probability) that a difference of a stated magnitude between the groups would have been detected if it existed. In practice, clinical trials are often too small, excessive emphasis is placed upon findings in sub-groups which were not defined in advance, and the working of exclusion criteria may make the patients included untypical of patients to whom the results are generalized.

References

An important objective of the book is to provide the reader with a substantial number of references which can be used to study the evidence upon which statements are based and provide a starting point for an enquiry in depth. In many cases the reference list begins with a small number of general review articles and then lists 20–50 (or even more) original sources. A few long-established but still useful remedies have very few high quality publications about them, but with some modern drugs the reverse applies.

To find a monograph

Monographs appear in alphabetical order of the drug's non-proprietary or generic name. There are three indexes that will identify this.

(1) The **Name Index** lists all variants of the non-proprietary or generic name, proprietary names and chemical names that are included in the chemistry section of the monograph. In this and the other indexes, the reference is to the generic name under which the monograph is to be found in the alphabetical listing.
(2) The **Therapeutic Use Index** lists the monographs under major divisions of therapeutic use (e.g. cardiovascular system). All the main body systems and/or organs are included, along with major functional groups (e.g. anaesthesia).
(3) The **Pharmacological Action Index** lists the monographs under the pharmacological mechanism of action of the drug. Inevitably this can vary from the very precise (e.g. enzyme inhibitors) to the general (e.g. disinfectants):

Selection of drug monographs

Selecting the drugs for inclusion in the book was difficult. Originality, therapeutic value, extent of use and inclusion in the WHO list of essential drugs were the main criteria. Unique drugs such as octreotide or granulocyte colony stimulating factor were included even if the clinical indications were limited. Among drug groups for which many representatives have been marketed the lead compound and the most widely used analogues were chosen. For a class with very extensive clinical use such as the neuroleptic D2 receptor antagonists or the dihydropyridine, calcium L-channel blocking drugs, many representatives are to be found in the book but in drugs classes that are less widely used or where use is declining e.g. histamine H1 receptor antagonists there are fewer.

K

Kanamycin (acid sulphate)

Kanamycin, the first aminoglycoside antibiotic after streptomycin to have an acceptably low incidence of neurotoxicity, gained widespread acceptance in the treatment of systemic Gram-negative infections. Resistance amongst the Enterobacteriaeceae eventually became widespread and newer aminoglycosides, especially gentamicin, have largely replaced its use for this purpose.

Chemistry

Kanamycin is a complex of three antibiotics produced by *Streptomyces kanamyceticus*. The major component is kanamycin A, usually known as kanamycin, and the minor components are kanamycin B and kanamycin C.
Kanamycin acid sulphate (Kannasyn)
$C_{18}H_{36}N_4O_47H_2SO_4$
Kanamycin sulphate (Cantrex, Cristalomicina, Kamycin, Kamynex, Kantrex, Otokalixin, Resistomycin, Ophthalmokalixan, Kantrexil, Kano, Kanescin, Kanaqua).
$C_{18}H_{36}N_4O_{11}.H_2SO_4$

Kanamycin A acid sulphate
6-O-(3-Amino-3-deoxy-α-D-glucopyranosyl)-4-O-(6-amino-6-deoxy-α-D-glucopyranosyl)-2-deoxy-D-streptamine acid sulphate

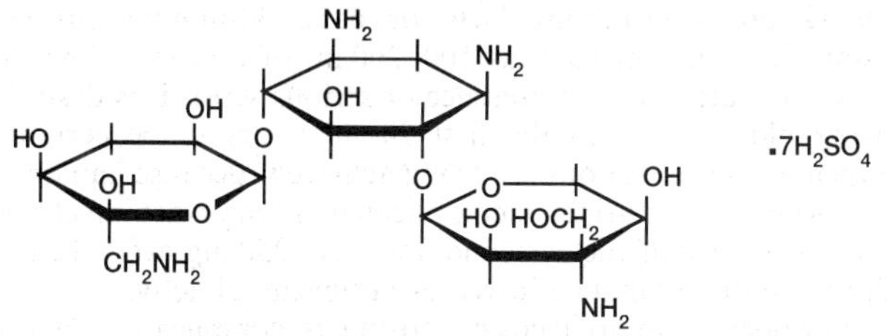

	Acid sulphate	Sulphate
Molecular weight (free base)	[illegible] (484.5)	582.6
pKa	7.2	
Solubility		
in alcohol	<1 in 10 000	<1 in 10 000
in water	1 in 1	1 in 8
Octanol/water partition coefficient	low	

Kanamycin is an aminoglycoside antibiotic complex derived from *Streptomyces kanamyceticus*, discovered by Okami and Umezawa[1] in Japanese soil. Of its three components, kanamycin A dominates in the preparation usually known as kanamycin. The acid sulphate is a white or almost white, hygroscopic odourless crystalline powder, readily soluble in water, cationic and highly polar. Kanamycin is an ingredient of a number of proprietary ointments in combination with antifungals and steroids.

Pharmacology

Like other aminoglycosides, kanamycin is first actively transported across the bacterial cell membrane by an oxygen-dependent system. Factors determining the rate of intracellular accumulation include the concentration of divalent cations (Mg^{++} and Ca^{++}), environmental pH and oxygen tension. Aminoglycosides are inactive under anaerobic conditions.

Aminoglycosides bind irreversibly to the 30S subunit of the bacterial ribosome, blocking protein synthesis by inhibiting the movement of peptidyl-tRNA associated with translocation, as well as increasing the frequency of misreading of the genetic code due to incorrect codon–anticodon interaction. The effect is bactericidal.

Toxicology

Doses of 280–300 $mg.kg^{-1}$ of kanamycin A and 140–150 $mg.kg^{-1}$ of kanamycin B are acutely lethal for mice, causing respiratory paralysis due to neuromuscular blockade.[2]

Clinical pharmacology

Most strains of *Enterobacteriaceae* are sensitive to kanamycin, being inhibited by concentrations of 3–6 $mg.l^{-1}$. *Pseudomonas aeruginosa* is only inhibited by 64–128 $mg.l^{-1}$ so that kanamycin is not useful for treatment of systemic pseudomonas infections. Streptococci and *Listeria monocytogenes* are usually resistant to kanamycin and staphylococci, although often sensitive in vitro, are usually resistant in vivo. This is because kanamycin does not enter macrophages and because of the development of resistant small-colony variants during therapy. Kanamycin is also active in vitro against diphtheroids, gonococci, meningococci, *Haemophilus* spp., *Mycoplasma*, *Brucella* spp., *Campylobacter jejuni* and *Mycobacterium tuberculosis*, although the clinical significance of these findings remains to be determined.

Kanamycin has no activity against anaerobes.

Resistance

Resistance to aminoglycosides is the consequence of bacterial inactivating enzymes, cell wall impermeability or changes in the 30S ribosomal proteins. Epidemic resistance amongst the Enterobacteriaceae results from plasmid-determined inactivating enzymes which acetylate, adenylate or phosphorylate the aminoglycoside substrate. Following widespread use of kanamycin in the 1960s, resistance in Gram-negative bacteria has become endemic and is often linked to plasmid-determined resistance to sulphonamide, streptomycin, chloramphenicol and tetracycline.

Synergy

Variable degrees of antibacterial synergy can be demonstrated in vitro when aminoglycosides are combined with either β-lactam antibiotics (penicillins and cephalosporins) or vancomycin. Although this is rarely used clinically, kanamycin and penicillins are synergistic against *Streptococcus faecalis* and kanamycin and cephalosporins are synergistic against Enterobacteriaceae.

Pharmacokinetics

The numerous methods which exist for measurement of plasma levels include bioassay, high pressure liquid chromatography, substrate-labelled fluorescent immunoassay (SLFIA), radioimmunoassay and enzyme-multiplied immunoassay technique (EMIT). Commercial systems for immunoassays are highly accurate and specific.[3] The limit of detection by the most sensitive of these techniques is 50 $\mu g.l^{-1}$.

Absorption from the gastrointestinal tract is negligible except in the presence of extensive mucosal damage. Following intramuscular injection the drug is rapidly and completely absorbed, peak serum levels being achieved in 60–90 minutes. In adults, intravenous infusion of 500 mg of kanamycin over 20–30 minutes yields peak levels of about 25–30 $mg.l^{-1}$ in a distribution volume which approximates that of the extracellular space, 0.3 $l.kg^{-1}$. Due to its polarity kanamycin does not diffuse into cells.

After distribution within extracellular tissues the serum level of kanamycin, like other aminoglycosides, falls exponentially. The elimination half life is a little more than 2 h in healthy individuals but because excretion is related only to renal function, it may be very much longer in chronic renal failure.

Aminoglycosides are well absorbed from the peritoneal cavity. In anephric patients, peritoneal lavage with aminoglycoside solutions leads to blood levels which, over a period of days, approach that of the lavaging fluid. In the presence of skin loss (burns, trauma, dermatitis), topically applied aminoglycosides can reach significant levels in the blood. There is minimal absorption following instillation into the bladder, cerebrospinal fluid or bronchial tree.

K

Oral absorption	negligible
Presystemic metabolism	nil
Plasma half life	
range	2.2–2.5 h
mean	2.3 h
Volume of distribution	~0.3 $l.kg^{-1}$
Plasma protein binding	<5%

Levels of aminoglycosides in interstitial fluid are 17–30% of those in the serum and therapeutic levels are achieved in ascitic, peritoneal, pleural and synovial fluids.

Penetration into the brain, cerebrospinal fluid and eye is poor and adequate therapy of infection in these sites usually requires direct instillation of the drug. Penetration of bronchial secretions seems to be barely above the minimal inhibitory concentration of most Gram-negative respiratory pathogens. Although kanamycin achieves poor levels in bile, Hansbrough et al[4] found therapeutic levels of kanamycin in the wall of the gall bladder in specimens collected at cholecystectomy.

With the exception of the proximal tubular cells of the kidney, aminoglycosides do not accumulate in, or even enter, cells. Absence from polymorphs accounts for failure to kill intraleukocytic staphylococci in vitro and probably accounts for the poor therapeutic performance of aminoglycosides in staphylococcal infections.

Although specific information is not available it is very unlikely that kanamycin would be excreted in breast milk. It does cross the placenta to a small extent, fetal concentrations achieving 16% of those in the maternal blood.

Kanamycin is excreted by glomerular filtration so that the concentration in urine vastly exceeds that of plasma unless renal dysfunction is present. The total body clearance is 75–100 $ml.min^{-1}$ per 1.73 m^2, which is slightly less than that of endogenous creatinine due to the partial reabsorption of the drug by proximal tubular cells by absorptive pinocytosis. Aminoglycosides are then transferred to and accumulate in lysosomes, being unable to diffuse across cell membranes or be metabolized. At high concentrations of the drug there is inhibition of lysosomal lipid metabolism, which results in the accumulation of phospholipids, lysosome leakage and eventually the formation of myeloid bodies. Up to 95% of the dose is excreted in the urine unchanged, with trace amounts in the bile.

Kanamycin is minimally bound to plasma proteins.

The elimination of the drug is reduced in patients with impaired renal function and in the elderly where renal function has deteriorated. In such patients the dosage will require adjustment. Hepatic disease is unlikely to affect the elimination of the drug.

Kanamycin has a relatively narrow therapeutic index. As a consequence, changes in its kinetics, most likely due to an alteration in renal function, will usually require some adjustment in dose.

Concentration–effect relationship

After administration of kanamycin in the usual dose (7.5 $mg.kg^{-1}$), peak plasma levels are about six-fold and interstitial fluid levels one to two-fold that required to inhibit susceptible *Enterobacteriaceae* (about 4 $mg.l^{-1}$). Unlike penicillins, high peak levels of aminoglycosides increase the killing rate and slow the regrowth of bacteria, i.e. the postantibiotic effect is prolonged.

Metabolism

There is no evidence to suggest that aminoglycosides are metabolized. Up to 90% of the dose is recovered unchanged in the urine over 24 h, most being excreted in the first 6 h. Small amounts of the drug are excreted in bile.

Pharmaceutics

Kanamycin is available in parenteral, oral and topical forms. Kanamycin sulphate for injection is marketed as a powder (kanamycin acid sulphate) to be dissolved in Water for Injection or as a sterile solution containing sulphuric acid, stabilizers and preservatives at a pH of 4 to 6. Formulations include 75 mg per 2 ml, 250 mg per 2 ml, 500 mg per 2 ml and 1 g per 3 ml (Kantrex, Bristol, USA) and 1 g per 4 ml (Kannasyn, Winthrop, UK).

Kanamycin (acid sulphate)

The reconstituted injection may be diluted with glucose 5% or sodium chloride 0.9% for slow intermittent infusion.

Oral formulations include Kantrex capsules (Bristol, USA) 500 mg white capsules coded '3506', for the short-term suppression of normal bowel flora.

Proprietary ointments contain kanamycin (0.5%), often together with antifungals and steroids.

Like other aminoglycosides, kanamycin is stable with a long shelf-life. Kanamycin should not be mixed with heparin, amphotericin nor the salts of weak acids, including penicillins and cephalosporins.

Therapeutic use

Indications

1. Gram-negative sepsis
2. Urinary tract infection
3. Gonorrhoea
4. Enteritis, hepatic encephalopathy, bowel 'sterilization'
5. Tuberculosis
6. Meningitis
7. Topical use.

Contraindications

1. Renal failure, old age
2. Neuromuscular blocking agents
3. Hypersensitivity to aminoglycosides.

Mode of use

Parenterally administered kanamycin is used mostly for the treatment of suspected or proven infections due to Gram-negative organisms. The drug is given intramuscularly or intravenously, the latter being preferred if there is circulatory collapse associated with septicaemia. The recommended dose is 15 $mg.kg^{-1}$ daily, divided into two equal doses. This is usually achieved in adults of 60–70 kg by giving 500 mg every 12 hours intramuscularly or as a 30-minute intravenous infusion (in a diluent such as 100–200 ml of normal saline or 5% dextrose in water). In the presence of serious sepsis it is desirable to measure blood levels in the first 24–48 hours to be certain that therapeutic concentrations are being achieved. Because kanamycin is well concentrated in urine, uncomplicated urinary tract infections can be treated with half the systemic dose (i.e. 250 mg every 12 hours). Making the urine alkaline increases antibacterial activity.

In newborns, aminoglycoside dosing is complicated by rapidly changing renal function and volume of distribution. Because the extracellular fluid space of newborns is approximately 40–44% of body weight, decreasing to 26% at six months, it has been suggested that aminoglycoside doses might be better related to surface area rather than weight in this age group. At less than one week of age, McCracken recommends 7.5 $mg.kg^{-1}$ 12-hourly for low birth weight (<2000 g) and 10 $mg.kg^{-1}$ 12-hourly for full birth weight babies, and after one week of age, 10 $mg.kg^{-1}$ 12-hourly and 10 $mg.kg^{-1}$ 8-hourly, respectively.[5,6] Despite these guidelines, serum concentrations need to be measured frequently and doses adjusted accordingly.

The use of kanamycin in patients with renal insufficiency requires careful attention to dose and duration of therapy. The initial dose should be determined only by an estimate of the extracellular fluid volume (in adults, usually the body weight) but subsequent dosing must be determined by estimates of glomerular filtration rate. Using the serum creatinine as a measure of renal function, nomograms have been created[7] which can be used to determine doses which prevent the accumulation of the drug by reducing the size of the 12-hourly dose or by increasing the time intervals between repeated doses. A simple scheme for an adult of 60–70 kg is given in Table 1.

Table 1

Renal function	Dose schedule
Normal	500 mg every 12 hours
Mild impairment	500 mg every 18 hours
Moderate impairment	500 mg every 24 hours
Severe impairment	250 mg every 24 hours

Kanamycin (acid sulphate)

Regardless of how the dosing is adjusted when renal function is compromised, serum levels should be monitored to keep peak levels (measured 1 h after an intramuscular dose or 30 min after an intravenous dose) below 30 mg.l^{-1} and trough levels below 10 mg.l^{-1}.

Indications

1. Gram-negative sepsis
The use of kanamycin for the treatment of hospital-associated Gram-negative sepsis, the cornerstone of the management of this condition in the 1960s, has been largely replaced by gentamicin. The latter has the advantage of antipseudomonal activity, is inactivated by fewer epidemic strains of Gram-negative rods and is no more expensive. Nevertheless, provided the organism is susceptible to kanamycin, there is no reason to believe that the therapeutic response is inferior to that expected of the newer aminoglycosides.

Kanamycin has long been favoured for the treatment of suspected or proven neonatal sepsis and there is an extensive literature on the subject,[8] including pharmacokinetic studies which revealed the need to use doses of up to 30 mg.kg^{-1} per day in older neonates.[5,6]

2. Urinary tract infection
Like other aminoglycosides, kanamycin is an effective agent for the treatment of urinary tract infection. Bladder infections are cured by a single intramuscular dose of 0.5 g.

3. Gonorrhoea
Kanamycin given as a single intramuscular dose of 2 g cures more than 90% of uncomplicated gonorrhoea in males and females.[9,10]

4. Enteritis, hepatic encephalopathy, bowel 'sterilization', neonatal necrotizing enterocolitis
Kanamycin, like neomycin, has been used orally to treat a variety of disorders associated with enteric bacteria. Mucosal invasive infections such as shigellosis and salmonellosis certainly do not respond to aminoglycosides. While the evidence for efficacy in neonatal enteropathogenic *Escherichia coli* diarrhoea is dubious, aminoglycosides such as neomycin or kanamycin are still used in the hope of reducing cross-infection.

Reduction in the colonic content of aerobic bacteria can be achieved using oral kanamycin although, like neomycin, prolonged use can cause malabsorption.

Alimentary kanamycin given in a dose of 15 mg.kg^{-1} daily has been advocated as prophylaxis for neonatal necrotizing enterocolitis[11] but the results of controlled trials using oral aminoglycosides have been conflicting with more recent evidence suggesting that these drugs neither prevent intestinal perforation nor alter the course of the disease.

5. Tuberculosis
Kanamycin was once a useful second line alternative to streptomycin for the treatment of disease due to resistant *Mycobacterium tuberculosis*. However, such prolonged treatment led to frequent ototoxicity and it is fortunate that there are now safer and better drugs available. In *M. tuberculosis*, there is partial cross-resistance between kanamycin, capreomycin and viomycin and complete cross-resistance between kanamycin and amikacin.[12]

6. Meningitis
Aminoglycoside levels in cerebrospinal fluid do not usually reach therapeutic levels during systemic therapy. Meningeal inflammation increases CSF kanamycin levels with peaks averaging 43% of serum levels, a concentration which is likely to be subtherapeutic for many Gram-negative bacteria unless potentially toxic systemic doses are used.

Intraventricular or intrathecal kanamycin in doses of 5–25 mg daily has been used with some success to treat Gram-negative meningitis.[13]

7. Topical use
Like neomycin and framycetin, kanamycin may be used in topical formulations for the treatment of superficial skin infections. Hypersensitivity to aminoglycosides is much more frequent when they are used this way, as is the development of resistance. Aminoglycosides applied to the external auditory canal can be ototoxic if the tympanic membrane is perforated.

Contraindications

Provided drug levels can be measured during the course of therapy, there are no absolute contraindications to the use of kanamycin at any age. The drug should be used cautiously in the elderly and preferably for less than two weeks or in a total dose not exceeding 14 g. Patients with myasthenia gravis should only receive aminoglycosides in an intensive care setting. In patients with critically compromised renal function, it is preferable to use antibiotics other than aminoglycosides whenever possible.

Adverse reactions

Potentially life-threatening effects
Large doses of aminoglycosides cause neuromuscular blockade, the effect being potentiated by anaesthesia, muscle relaxants and myasthenia gravis and antagonized by calcium and neostigmine.

Most accounts of this adverse effect were recorded when large doses of kanamycin were used to lavage the peritoneal cavity before the rapid absorption of aminoglycosides from such sites was appreciated.

Acute overdosage
Accidental parenteral use of large doses of aminoglycosides can cause eighth nerve damage as well as neuromuscular blockade. Haemodialysis or peritoneal dialysis may be used to hasten removal of the drug, while intravenous calcium and neostigmine may reverse neuromuscular blockade.

Severe or irreversible adverse effects

Ototoxicity
Aminoglycoside uptake by the endolymph and perilymph of the inner ear is dose-dependent. Because these drugs are only slowly released from these sites, they are capable of prolonged damaging exposure to the hair cells of the cochlea, the ampullar cristae of the semicircular canals and the maculae of the utricle and saccule. Histological changes in the cochlea are most obvious in the basal turns so that the hearing loss, which often goes unrecognized, is most marked in the higher frequencies.

Initial and potentially reversible symptoms include tinnitus, mild high frequency hearing loss detected by audiogram, vertigo and ataxia. Overt deafness, should it occur, usually appears suddenly during therapy but occasionally it may appear and progress after its cessation. It may be unilateral and although it may improve with time, it is usually permanently incapacitating.

Amikacin and kanamycin are more likely to cause auditory (cochlear) than vestibular damage; the reverse is true of streptomycin and gentamicin.

The risk factors most commonly thought to be associated with aminoglycoside ototoxicity are impaired renal function and large total dose. Other factors include concurrent administration of other ototoxic agents (other aminoglycosides, 'loop' diuretics, vancomycin), prior exposure to aminoglycosides or intense noise, hereditary tendency and old age. Although evaluations of ototoxicity are less frequently performed in infants, the overall impression is that it is rare at this age. Kanamycin was introduced before the advent of phased clinical trials of new drugs so that only limited prospective data on the incidence of ototoxicity are available. The Boston Collaborative Drug Surveillance Program prospectively looked for deafness in 243 in-patients given kanamycin and found four (1.6%) who developed clinical deafness while in hospital.[14]

Nephrotoxicity
Nephrotoxicity due to aminoglycosides is associated with the gradual accumulation of these drugs in proximal tubular cells and the excretion of brush border enzymes, lysosomal enzymes, β-2-microglobulin and cellular debris in the form of casts. Tubular dysfunction is manifest as defective concentrating ability but over two to three weeks of administration, glomerular filtration rate gradually falls and serum creatinine rises. Risk factors for nephrotoxicity include prolonged administration, sodium and water depletion (including sepsis), prior aminoglycoside administration, prior renal disease and combination with other nephrotoxic drugs such as cisplatin and cyclosporin.[15] The few clinical trials that have compared the nephrotoxicity of kanamycin with that of other aminoglycosides have found no differences. In the rat, kanamycin and amikacin are somewhat less nephrotoxic than gentamicin.

Symptomatic adverse effects
Tinnitus and a sense of fullness in the ears may follow bolus injection of aminoglycosides and are an occasional prelude to serious ototoxicity. Circumoral paraesthesia may occur.

Kanamycin given orally in doses of 12 g daily causes diarrhoea and malabsorption of 2–30% of ingested fat (cf. neomycin, 13–42%), apparently because of the precipitation of bile salts.[16]

Other effects
Transient elevations of serum aminotransferases are occasionally reported.

Interference with clinical pathology tests
No interference with clinical pathology tests has been reported.

High risk groups

Neonates
Doses of kanamycin should take into account gestational age at birth (as an estimate of renal function) and body surface area (as an estimate of extracellular fluid volume) but frequent monitoring of blood levels is imperative.

Breast milk. Information concerning the concentration of kanamycin in breast milk does not seem to be available but there are no reports of adverse effects in neonates fed by mothers receiving kanamycin.

Children
At this age, kanamycin is well tolerated. Unless treatment is prolonged, the incidence of ototoxicity and nephrotoxicity is low.

Pregnant women
Kanamycin crosses the placental barrier, yielding peak fetal levels of about 16% of the maternal level and a half life of about 3.7 h. Aminoglycosides are not known to be teratogenic in man or animals, but prolonged use in pregnancy should be avoided because of the risk of fetal ototoxicity.

The elderly
Special care is required when using kanamycin in the elderly in whom renal function and blood levels should be measured frequently and the drug given no longer than is necessary.

Drug interactions

Potentially hazardous interactions
Neuromuscular blocking agents may be potentiated by the aminoglycosides, the effect being reversed by the use of intravenous calcium salts.

Other significant interactions
Kanamycin, like other aminoglycosides, may be inactivated by β-lactam antibiotics, especially when mixed in the same syringe or intravenous giving set. This interaction may continue in specimens of body fluids collected for serum sampling of peak and trough levels; hence, unless properly handled (that is, assayed promptly, frozen, etc.) falsely low serum levels may be read, resulting in an increased risk of excessively high doses being given and of toxicity to the patient.

Potentially useful interactions
Synergy can frequently be demonstrated between aminoglycosides and β-lactam antibiotics in vitro.

Major outcome trials

1. Murdoch T McC, Gray J A, Geddes A M, Wallace E T 1966 Clinical experience with kanamycin in septicaemia caused by Gram-negative organisms. Annals of the New York Academy of Science 132: part 2: 842–849

49 patients septicaemic on clinical grounds (temperature > 101°F, blood pressure < 110/60, diminished urine output) were given kanamycin, 250 mg every six hours, for 14 days. 21 patients were bacteraemic with organisms all inhibited by 4 mg.l^{-1} of the drug. Maximum recorded serum levels ranged from 1 to 8 mg.l^{-1}. 9.5% of bacteraemic patients died but none in whom only bacilluria was detected. There was no eighth nerve damage recorded.

2. Fischnaller J E, Pedersen A H B, Ronald A R, Bonin P, Tronca E L 1968 Kanamycin sulphate in the treatment of acute gonococcal urethritis in men. Journal of the American Medical Association 203: 107–110

A single intramuscular dose of 2 g of kanamycin was given to 155 men with acute gonococcal urethritis. When examined three days later, 144 patients (93%) were asymptomatic. *Neisseria gonorrhoeae* was still present in urethral swabs of five of the 11 patients with persistent symptoms but all of these isolates were still inhibited by 10 mg.l^{-1} of the kanamycin. Three patients reported slight unsteadiness or dizziness for a few hours and five reported various degrees of malaise.

3. Cantey J R 1974 Plague in Vietnam: clinical observations and treatment with kanamycin. Archives of Internal Medicine 133: 280–283

18 Vietnamese villagers with mostly culture-proven plague were treated with kanamycin, 15 mg.kg^{-1} per day intramuscularly, for 10 days. There were three deaths, all in patients who were hypotensive at the time of admission. The author concluded that the cure rate was comparable to that of streptomycin, variously reported as 4% to 29%.

General review articles

Bunn P A 1970 Kanamycin. Medical Clinics of North American 54: 1245–1256

Finegold S M 1959 Kanamycin. Archives of Internal Medicine 104: 15

Garrod L P, Lewis A A G, King A J, Morton O (eds) 1967 The clinical aspects of kanamycin. Postgraduate Medical Journal suppl, May

Giusti D L 1973 Drug Intelligence and Clinical Pharmacy 540

Mann C H (ed) 1966 Kanamycin: appraisal after eight years of clinical application. Annals of the New York Academy of Science 132, Art 2: 771–1090

Monograph 1958 Annals of the New York Academy of Science 76, Art 2: 17–408

Whelton A, Neu H C (eds) 1982 The aminoglycosides: microbiology, clinical use and toxicology. Marcel Dekker, New York

References

1. Umezawa H, Ueda M, Maeda K et al 1957 Production and isolation of a new antibiotic, kanamycin. Journal of Antibiotics (Japan) 10A: 181
2. Price K E 1986 Aminoglycoside research 1975–1985: prospects for development of improved agents. Antimicrobial Agents and Chemotherapy 29: 543–548
3. Edberg S C, Barry A L, Young L S 1984 Therapeutic drug monitoring: antimicrobial agents. Cumitech 20, American Society for Microbiology, Washington, DC
4. Hansbrough J F, Clark J E, Reimer L G 1981 Concentrations of kanamycin and amikacin in human gallbladder bile and wall. Antimicrobial Agents and Chemotherapy 20: 515–517
5. Howard J B, McCracken G H 1975 Reappraisal of kanamycin usage in neonates. Journal of Pediatrics 86: 949–956
6. McCracken G H, Threlkeld N 1976 Kanamycin dosage in neonates. Journal of Pediatrics 89: 313–314
7. Mawer G E, Lucas S B, McGough J G 1972 Nomogram for kanamycin dosage. Lancet 2: 45
8. Siegal J D, McCracken G H 1982 Aminoglycosides in pediatrics. In: Whelton A, Neu H C (eds) The aminoglycosides: microbiology, clinical use and toxicology. Marcel Dekker, New York, pp 527–555
9. Hooten W F, Nicol C S 1967 Kanamycin in the treatment of gonorrhoea in females. Postgraduate Medical Journal (suppl) May: 68–69
10. Fischnaller J E, Pedersen A H B, Ronald A R, Bonin P, Tronca E L 1968 Kanamycin sulphate in the treatment of acute gonorrheal urethritis in men. Journal of the American Medical Association 203: 909–912
11. Egan E A, Mantilla G, Nelson R M, Eitzman D V A prospective controlled trial of oral kanamycin in the prevention of neonatal necrotizing enterocolitis. Journal of Pediatrics 89: 467–470
12. Mitchison D A 1984 Drug resistance in Mycobacteria. British Medical Bulletin 40: 84–90
13. Lorber J 1967 Intrathecal and intraventricular kanamycin in the treatment of meningitis and ventriculitis in infants. Postgraduate Medical Journal (May suppl): 52–54
14. Boston Collaborative Drug Surveillance Program 1973 Drug-induced deafness. Journal of the American Medical Association 224: 515–516
15. Moore R D, Smith C R, Lipsky J J 1984 Risk factors for nephrotoxicity in patients treated with aminoglycosides. Annals of Internal Medicine 100: 352–357
16. Faloon W W, Paes I C, Woolfolk D, Nankin H, Wallace K, Naro E N 1966 Effect of neomycin and kanamycin upon intestinal absorption. Annals of the New York Academy of Science 76 art 2: 879–887

Kaolin

Kaolin is a purified hydrated aluminium silicate. The native clay is derived from the decomposition of the felspar of granite rocks. It contains about 47% of silica, 40% of alumina and 13% of water. It is mined in large quantities in Cornwall, UK, amongst other places.

Chemistry

Light kaolin BP, light kaolin (natural) BP, heavy kaolin BPC (Kaopectate, Kaylene, Kaylene-ol, KLN Suspension, One minute Kaolin poultice, Kaodene, Kaonorm, Kao-C)
Chemically kaolin is almost pure aluminium silicate having the formula $Al_2O_3.2SiO_2.2H_2O$ together with a number of trace elements

Table 1

Composition	Light kaolin wt (%)	Light kaolin (natural) wt (%)	Heavy kaolin wt (%)
SiO_2	47.00	47.00	48.00
Al_2O_3	37.80	37.80	37.00
Fe_2O_3	0.60	0.60	0.80
TiO_2	0.04	0.04	0.05
CaO	0.06	0.06	0.07
MgO	0.20	0.20	0.20
K_2O	1.10	1.10	1.80
Na_2O	0.10	0.10	0.08
Loss on ignition	13.10	13.10	12.00

Kaolin is a light, fine white (light kaolin) or greyish white (heavy kaolin) unctuous powder; odourless, almost tasteless, when mixed with hot water it has an odour of clay. It is china clay, freed from gritty particles by elutriation.

Kaolin conforms in physical and chemical properties to the purity required by the British Pharmacopoeia 1988 and is determined by the test methods defined in that specification. Heavy kaolin also conforms to those requirements laid down by the European Pharmacopoeia 1989.

Table 2

	Light kaolin	Light kaolin (natural)	Heavy kaolin
pH	7.5 ± 0.5	5.0 ± 0.5	5.0 ± 0.5
Colour—ISO	84.5 ± 1.0	84.5 ± 1.0	82.5
Specific gravity	2.6	2.6	2.6
Particulate size			
53 μm	0.01 wt. % max.	0.01 wt. % max.	0.05 wt. % max.
10 μm	0.5 wt. % max.	0.5 wt. % max.	12.00 wt. % max.
2 μm	75.0 ± 3.0 wt. %	75.0 ± 3.0 wt. %	45.0 wt. % max.

Light kaolin also includes a suitable dispersing agent. The kaolins are insoluble in water, organic solvents, mineral acids and solutions of alkali hydroxides.

Pharmacology

Light kaolin has good absorbent properties and when given by mouth adsorbs toxic and other substances from the gastrointestinal tract.[1] It increases stool bulk and is also used in the symptomatic treatment of conditions associated with diarrhoea.[1]

Kaolin adsorbs by means of electrostatic charges. The overall charge on the kaolin particle is always negative and hence the adsorption of cations is favoured. However, as pH is reduced, positively charged sites develop and so the overall charge becomes less negative and cationic adsorption capacity falls. It thus follows that adsorption by kaolin is dependent on environmental pH, which may also have an effect on the ionic state of the adsorbate.[2,3]

Heavy kaolin is used externally to reduce local inflammation of the skin and alleviate pain. Light kaolin is also applied topically in a variety of dusting powders and as a basis of disinfectant powders. Kaolin is not absorbed from the gastrointestinal tract.

Toxicology

In experimental animals, intravenous injection of kaolin resulted in hypercoagulability of blood.[4]

Clinical pharmacology

When treating cases of diarrhoea of non-specific origin, the essential consequence is dehydration and the fundamental treatment is one of fluid and electrolyte rehydration.[5] Kaolin administration is probably of only secondary importance. Constipation may ensue but other systemic effects are not expected since kaolin is not absorbed.

Pharmacokinetics

When taken orally or applied topically kaolin is not absorbed.

Concentration–effect relationship

Not applicable.

Metabolism

When taken orally it remains unchanged throughout transit of the gastrointestinal tract.

Pharmaceutics

Kaolin powder is liable to be heavily contaminated with bacteria, including *Bacillus anthracis*, *Clostridium tetani*, and *Clostridium welchii*. Prior to incorporation into pharmaceutical formulations, kaolin powder must be sterilized by dry heat.

All oral formulations containing kaolin should be freshly prepared. Mixtures containing kaolin settle out very quickly because of the dense nature of kaolin particles. This may be overcome by incorporating a suitable suspending agent such as a xanthan gum[6] into the formulation. Donnagel-PG (Robins, UAS) contains kaolin, opium and belladonna alkaloids. Carboxymethylcellulose is used as the suspending agent. The formulation also includes sodium benzoate, alcohol, citric acid and fructose syrup. Parapectolin (Rorer, USA) contains kaolin, opium and camphorated opium tincture (paregoric) together with carboxymethylcellulose, benzoic acid, parabens and saccharin sodium. Vigorous shaking of the mixture should always occur immediately prior to withdrawing a dose.

Dusting powders and poultices containing kaolin should be subjected to dry heat sterilization if the kaolin powder used in these formulations has not been previously sterilized.

Preparations should be stored in suitable coloured glass or plastic jars.

Kaolin is used in the following official formulations:-

Kaolin Mixture BP
Kaolin and Morphine Mixture (BP)
Paediatric Kaolin Mixture (BP)
Kaolin and Opium Mixture (APF)
Liquid Paraffin and Kaolin Emulsion (BPC 1949)
Calcium Carbonate Powder Co. (BPC)
Magnesium Carbonate Powder Co. (BPC)
Magnesium Carbonate Tabs. Co. (BPC)
Compound Kaolin Dusting Powder (APF)
Compound Kaolin Powder (BPC 1963)
Kaolin Poultice

Light kaolin BP is also used for clarification purposes. In a study[7] to investigate the stability of morphine in Kaolin and Morphine mixture BP, the authors found that 25% of the total morphine content of the mixture is bound to the kaolin and as such is not freely available for absorption when administered orally.

K

Kaolin is also a component of a number of laboratory haematological clotting tests.[8]

Therapeutic use

Indications

1. Symptomatic treatment of diarrhoea
2. Absorbent for some toxic substances taken orally, although it is not the first choice
3. Topical application for reducing inflammation
4. As a diluent and dispersant for topically applied drugs.

Contraindications

1. Patients with intestinal obstruction
2. Concurrent administration of atropine, digoxin, lincomycin or promazine.

Mode of use

Kaolin is administered orally, as a mixture formulated according to the particular indication.

For paediatric use the range is as follows:

Up to 1 year — 1 g every 4 hours
1–5 years — 2 g every 4 hours
6–12 years — adult dose
For adult use — 2–4 g every 4 hours.

No information is available to suggest that a change in dosage is warranted in elderly patients.

Recommended range of dose is 15 to 75 g although routine use should not exceed that outlined above.

When used as a constituent of dusting powders or as a poultice, kaolin should not be applied to open wounds or to large raw surface areas.

Indications

1. Diarrhoea
The use of kaolin in treating non-specific diarrhoea is a traditional remedy but is of only secondary importance. If, however, fluid and electrolyte balance is normal, its use may help to bring symptomatic relief. This concept, however, is not supported by a study of 204 patients suffering from acute non-specific diarrhoea.[9] Similar conclusions were drawn by the authors in a study of kaolin used in infantile gastroenteritis.[10]

2. Adsorbence of toxic preparations
The adsorbent properties of kaolin have been used to reduce the body's rate of absorption of toxic chemicals and poisons although better alternative preparations are now available such as attapulgite[11] and Fuller's Earth.[12]

3. Topical application
Kaolin has been used externally as a poultice and as a component of dusting powders and pastes.[13] Its use in these formulations is well established although its efficacy remains clinically unproven.

Contraindications

1. Intestinal obstruction
Administration of kaolin should be avoided in patients suffering from intestinal obstruction caused by a pre-existing disease state. There is also a reported fatality of a patient dependent on kaolin and morphine, due to intestinal obstruction caused by the kaolin content.

2. Concurrent drug administration
There is evidence suggesting that when either atropine, digoxin, lincomycin or promazine are taken concurrently with kaolin-containing preparations, the drug is adsorbed onto the kaolin thereby decreasing the amount of drug available for absorption. In these circumstances kaolin administration should be avoided.

Adverse reactions

Potentially life-threatening effects
No reports of toxic or adverse effects in man have been reported as a result of either oral or topical use of pharmaceutical preparations containing kaolin when used within the recommended dose range. There are, however, a number of reports of toxic or adverse effects in man when excessive amounts of kaolin have been self-administered in the form of kaolin and morphine mixture.

Two reports[14,15] have identified the ingested kaolin as the cause of hypokalaemia in patients dependent on the mixture. The probable mechanism is by potassium binding to kaolin in the gut thereby preventing absorption. This hypothesis is supported by other reports[16,17] of clay ingestion impairing absorption of various cations including potassium, iron, zinc and mercury.

Acute overdosage
One case has been reported[18] of a 34-year-old man who injected himself with 30 ml of a preparation containing kaolin. The patient developed defibrination syndrome. Severe bronchial cellulitis was secondary to extravasation of the injected suspension.

Severe or irreversible adverse effects
Kaolinosis has been reported in many patients due to inhalation of kaolin dust. Many of these patients were men engaged in extraction of the material and some were women working with the purified powder in a chemical factory. This condition was the subject of two recent review articles.[19,20]

Symptomatic adverse effects
Constipation may occur.

High risk groups

As long as administration or application of kaolin is performed according to the dosage regimen and/or recommended method of application, no risk exists for any particular patient group.

Drug interactions

Potentially hazardous interactions

Atropine. There was significant adsorption of atropine when it was added to an aqueous suspension of light kaolin. This occurred at the rate of 18.8 mg of atropine per g of kaolin.[21]

Digoxin. Concurrent administration with kaolin-containing mixtures should be avoided. A severe reduction in the rate and extent of digoxin absorption was noted in two studies.[22,23] This interaction could be virtually eliminated by having a dosing interval of at least two hours between the two drugs.

Other significant reactions
The absorption of lincomycin[24] and promazine[25] may also be affected in the presence of kaolin although good clinical evidence in support of this appears to be lacking.

Potentially useful interactions
Absorption of some poisons and toxic chemicals from the gastrointestinal tract may be reduced by the adsorption of these toxins onto kaolin.[26] However, better alternative adsorbents are now available for use in this field.

References

1. Reynolds A 1982 Antacids and some other gastrointestinal agents. Martindale, the extra pharmacopoeia, 28th edn. The Pharmaceutical Press, London, p 81
2. Clarke C D, Armstrong N A 1972 The influence of pH on the adsorption of benzoic acid by kaolin. The Pharmaceutical Journal 209: 44–46
3. Armstrong N A, Clarke C D 1971 The adsorption of crystal violet by kaolin. Journal of Pharmacy and Pharmacology 23: 95S–100S
4. Gurewich V, Thomas D P 1965 Pathogenesis of venous thrombosis in relation to its prevention by dextran and heparin. Journal of Laboratory and Clinical Medicine 66: 604–612
5. Cutting W A M, Marshal W C 1979 Loperamide and acute infective diarrhoea in children. Lancet 2: 1022
6. Evans B K, Fenton-May V 1986 Keltrol. The Pharmaceutical Journal 237: 736–737
7. Helliwell K, Game P 1981 Stability of morphine in kaolin and morphine mixture BP. The Pharmaceutical Journal 227: 128–129
8. Welsh P N 1972 The effect of collagen and kaolin on the intrinsic coagulant activity of platelets. British Journal of Haematology 22: 393–405
9. Alestig K, Trallfoss B, Stenquist K 1979 Acute non-specific diarrhoea: studies on the use of charcoal, kaolin, pectin and diphenoxylate. The Practitioner 222: 859–862
10. Holdaway M D 1977 Management of gastroenteritis in early childhood. Drugs 14: 383
11. Barr M, Arista E S 1957 Adsorption studies on clays. The adsorption of two alkaloids by activated attalpulgite, challoysite and kaolin. Journal of American Pharmaceutical Association Scientific Edition 46: 493

12. Spoerke D G, Smolinske S C, Wruk K M, Rumock B H 1986 Infrequently used antidotes: indications and availability. Veterinary and Human Toxicology 28: 69–75
13. Pashly D H, Leiback J G, Horner J A 1987 The effects of burnishing NaF/kaolin/glycerine paste on dentine permeability. Journal of Periodontology 56: 19–23
14. Barragry J M, Morris D V 1980 Fatal dependence on kaolin and morphine mixture. Postgraduate Medical Journal 56: 180–181
15. Todd G R G, Blair A L T, McElnay J C, Reddell J G 1985 Dependence on kaolin and morphine mixture, hypokalaemia and hypertension. Irish Journal of Medical Sciences 154: 409–410
16. Gonzales J J, Owens W, Ungaro P C, Werk E E, Wentz P W 1982 Clay ingestion: a rare cause of hypokalaemia. Annals of Internal Medicine 97: 65–66
17. Halstead J A 1968 Geophagia in man: its nature and nutritional effects. American Journal of Clinical Nutrition 21: 1384–1393
18. Lanse S B, Farzan S 1979 Defibrination syndrome due to intravenous kaolin injection. Archives of Internal Medicine 139: 251
19. Wells I P, Bhatt R C V, Flanagan M 1985 Kaolinosis: a radiological review. Clinical Radiology 36: 579–582
20. Wagner J C, Pooley F D, Gibbs A, Lyons J, Sheers G, Moncrieff C B 1986 Inhalation of china stone and china clay dusts: relationships between the mineralogy of dust retained in the lungs and pathological changes. Thorax 41: 190–196
21. Ridout C W 1968 The adsorption of atropine from aqueous solution by kaolin. Pharmaceutica Acta Helvetica 43: 42
22. Brown D D, Juhl R P 1976 Decreased bioavailability of digoxin due to antacids and kaolin–pectin. New England Journal of Medicine 295: 1034
23. Albert K S, Ayres J W, DiSanto A R et al 1978 Influence of kaolin–pectin suspension on digoxin bioavailability. Journal of Pharmaceutical Sciences 67: 1582
24. George C F 1987 Drug interactions. In: Prasad A B (ed) British National Formulary, No 14. The Pharmaceutical Press, London, p 429
25. Sorby D L, Liu G 1966 Effects of adsorbents on drug absorption II. Journal of Pharmaceutical Sciences 55: 504
26. Meredith T J, Vale J A 1987 Treatment of paraquat poisoning in man: methods to prevent absorption. Human Toxicology 6: 49–55

Ketamine (hydrochloride)

Ketamine is a non-barbiturate general anaesthetic agent which may be given intravenously or intramuscularly.

Chemistry

Ketamine (Ketalar, Ketaject, Ketanest)
$C_{13}H_{16}ClNO.HCl$
(dl)-2-(2-Chlorophenyl)-2-(methylamino)cyclohexanone hydrochloride

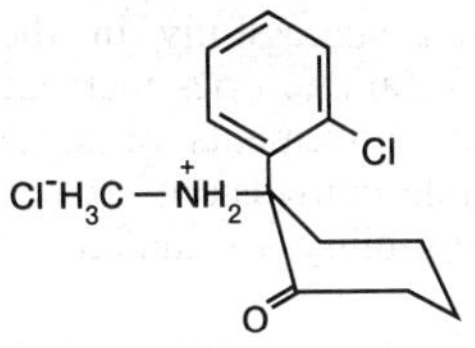

S (d)–Ketamine hydrochloride

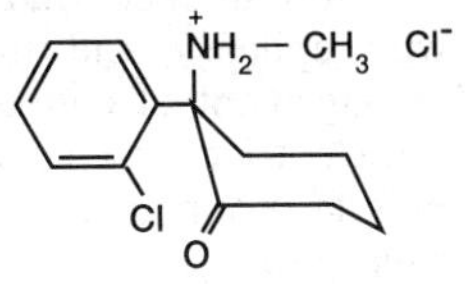

R (l)–Ketamine hydrochloride

Molecular weight (free base)	274.2 (237.7)
pKa	7.5
Solubility	
in alcohol	1 in 14
in water	1 in 4
Octanol/water partition coefficient	—

Ketamine hydrochloride is a white, crystalline powder prepared by chemical synthesis. It is supplied as a colourless solution, pH 3.5–5.5, in concentrations of 1%, 5% and 10%, the latter two containing 0.01% benzethonium as preservative. The currently available preparation is a 50:50 racemic mixture of the two isomers. Volunteer studies indicate that S(d)-ketamine is three to five times more potent in terms of anaesthetic effect than the R(l) form, but with a similar degree of cardiovascular stimulation and duration of action.[1]

Ketamine is not available in any combined preparations.

Pharmacology

Ketamine is a general anaesthetic agent which may be used intravenously or intramuscularly to induce anaesthesia and also to maintain anaesthesia as the sole agent. The mechanism of action of ketamine is unclear.

Toxicology

No adverse effects were found when pregnant bitches were given 25 $mg.kg^{-1}$ ketamine intramuscularly twice a week for 3 weeks during pregnancy. The breeding performance and condition of litters of rats were not affected when 20 $mg.kg^{-1}$ ketamine was given intravenously or intramuscularly during the premating or perinatal period. No effects were observed on rabbit litters when 20 $mg.kg^{-1}$ intramuscularly was given daily during the period of organogenesis.

Rats given 2.5–10.0 $mg.kg^{-1}$ daily intravenously for 6 weeks showed no drug-related toxic effects on autopsy. There were no consistent haematological or haemopoietic alterations.

Clinical pharmacology

Ketamine is a unique general anaesthetic in that it produces a state of 'dissociative anaesthesia' in which there is a functional and electrophysiological dissociation between the thalamoneocortical and limbic systems.[2] It is devoid of hypnotic properties, but causes amnesia and prolonged analgesia. A feeling of dissociation becomes apparent some 15 seconds after an intravenous injection of 1.5–2.0 $mg.kg^{-1}$, with unconsciousness occurring after about 30 seconds. Following a single intravenous dose the anaesthetic state will last 8–10 min with analgesia persisting for 30–40 min. An intramuscular dose of 10 $mg.kg^{-1}$ will take 3–5 min for full effect with a duration of 10–20 min.

Administration of ketamine intravenously results in consistent and marked changes in the electroencephalogram, with an initial shift from dominant alpha frequencies to fast theta activity and then to less rhythmic slow theta frequencies. Delta wave amplitude is increased, but beta waves are unchanged. On recovery, theta waves are replaced by low-voltage, fast-frequency activity; alpha activity does not reappear for at least 0.5–1 h after drug injection even though the subject is in full contact with the environment. The burst suppression pattern or EEG fast waves characteristic of barbiturates and other sedative-hypnotics are not seen.[2] Onset of unconsciousness cannot be assigned to a specific EEG pattern.[3]

Further work has indicated epileptiform activity in both the thalamus and limbic systems following ketamine, but there is no evidence that this seizure activity spreads to the cerebral cortex.[4] It is therefore unlikely that ketamine would cause convulsions in patients with epilepsy and indeed it has been used successfully in the management of convulsions.[5] Nevertheless, ketamine does increase muscle tone and sudden, involuntary, jerky movements of large muscle groups can occur, which may resemble convulsions. It has been used safely in patients with a susceptibility to malignant hyperthermia.[6,7]

In contrast to other intravenous anaesthetics, ketamine causes an increase in both cerebral blood flow and cerebral oxygen uptake.[8] This also accounts for the concomitant rise in intracranial and cerebrospinal fluid pressure, which may be dangerous in patients with intracranial pathology where rises in pressure tend to be more marked.

In animals, ketamine anaesthesia has been shown to reduce acetylcholine turnover rates in the caudate nucleus and hippocampus,[9] and this might be related to the electrophysiological changes in subcortical structures. Increasing central acetylcholine concentrations with physostigmine has been shown to antagonize the sedative and anaesthetic actions of ketamine, but not its analgesic effects.[10,11] Ketamine has been shown to decrease the average lifetime of single-channel currents activated by acetylcholine in a dose-dependent fashion and at concentrations that are clinically relevant.[12] However, the effects were not consistent with a sequential blocking model in which molecules of drug bind to an open channel to occlude it. In human cortical cells, ketamine induced rapid opening and closing of sodium channels at a rate greater than 50 Hz.[13] This fast flickering led to a voltage-independent reduction in the fractional channel opening time. Long complete closures (>4 s) were also observed.

Analgesic effects. The intense analgesia that follows ketamine administration outlasts its full anaesthetic effect and can also be produced by subanaesthetic doses. The exact mechanism of its analgesic action is unknown. Ketamine blocks conduction of impulses associated with pain perception in the spinoreticular tracts, whilst having no effect on spinothalamic transmission.[14] It also has a depressant effect on medial thalamic nuclei[15] and the nuclei involved in impulse transmission in the medial medullary reticular formation.[16] The above work suggests that the analgesic effect of ketamine is due to blockage of the motivational affective dimension rather than the somatic component of pain perception. Other work suggests that analgesia is due to suppression of impulse transmission in the dorsal horn of grey matter of the spinal cord.[17]

The concept that ketamine binds stereospecifically to opiate receptors is no longer tenable. Fratta and colleagues[18] found that ketamine was unable to displace ^{3}H-dihydromorphone or ^{3}H-methionine enkephalin from opiate receptors in rat brain. They were also unable to antagonize ketamine-induced analgesia with naloxone.

The analgesia might be related to an effect on the N-methyl-D-aspartate (NMDA) subclass of receptor, which are involved in the hyperexcitable state, or wind-up, in dorsal horn neurones and in the hippocampus, where a short burst of activity can induce prolonged increased excitability of pathways, or long-term potentiation.[19,20] Ketamine has marked NMDA antagonist properties; it does not block the receptor, but rather the ionic channels opened by NMDA receptor activation.[21]

Emergence phenomena. Recovery from ketamine anaesthesia may be accompanied by psychotomimetic activity (emergence reactions). Some patients are completely orientated in time and space, whilst others may show marked alterations in mood and report alterations in body image, floating sensations, vivid and sometimes terrifying dreams and occasional frank delirium.[22] Some patients become aggressive, whilst others are withdrawn; most feel completely numb. These effects can be minimized by concomitant use of central depressant drugs such as opioids and benzodiazepines (see Adverse effects).

Cardiovascular effects. In contrast to all other intravenous induction agents, ketamine stimulates rather than depresses the cardiovascular system. Following an induction dose of 1.5–2.0 mg intravenously in unpremedicated patients, the arterial pressure increases by about 20–40 mmHg over a period of 3–5 min and then decreases to baseline over the next 10–20 min. This is accompanied by increases in heart rate and in cardiac output, which is mainly due to the tachycardia rather than an increase in stroke volume; these changes are smaller in well sedated patients. There is, however, a large interindividual variation and on occasion the increase in blood pressure can be alarming. Cardiac arrhythmias are very uncommon following ketamine. There is also an increase in pulmonary artery pressure and pulmonary vascular resistance. Myocardial oxygen consumption is increased and the drug is contraindicated when myocardial blood flow is compromised.

Although ketamine administration is accompanied by a marked increase in circulating noradrenaline,[23] the circulatory effects are primarily due to direct central nervous system stimulation with an increase in efferent sympathetic activity. Injection of ketamine directly into the cerebral circulation of animals results in an immediate increase in arterial blood pressure, heart rate and cardiac output.[24]

Respiratory effects. Respiratory depression is not a feature of clinical doses of ketamine given to unpremedicated patients, but may accompany rapid administration. The laryngeal and pharyngeal reflexes are depressed, but to a much lesser degree than with other anaesthetic agents, and self-maintenance of a patent airway is a feature of ketamine anaesthesia. Salivary secretions are increased and an antisialogogue is usually necessary before ketamine is given. Bronchial relaxation is also a feature of ketamine administration.

Ketamine isomers. The individual enantiomers of ketamine have been tested in surgical patients and volunteers and their effects compared with the racemic mixture.[25,26] The duration of action and the anaesthetic state do not differ between the three preparations. The (d) isomer is about four times more potent than the (l) form, but the latter is associated with more agitated behaviour postoperatively than d-ketamine and the racemic mixture. Patients found the (d) form more acceptable than the (l) form and the racemic mixture. In volunteers,[26] the anaesthetic state did not differ significantly between the three types, but recovery times were shorter following the individual isomers. Recovery of psychomotor skills was more rapid following d-ketamine than the racemic compound. The pharmacokinetic profiles did not differ between the three types and hence the difference must be due to pharmacodynamic factors. Despite the apparent superiority of d-ketamine over the racemic mixture, it has never been made commercially available.

Although ketamine is a general anaesthetic, it differs in several respects from the conventional intravenous and inhalational agents: the eyes remain open and often show a slow nystagmus, while light and corneal reflexes may remain intact; muscle tone is not reduced and may be increased and spontaneous, purposeless movements may occur during surgical anaesthesia; laryngeal reflexes tend to be maintained; the cardiovascular system is stimulated, not depressed; respiratory depression is not a feature.

Pharmacokinetics

The preferred analytical method for detection of ketamine, norketamine (metabolite I) and dehydronorketamine (metabolite II) as their heptafluorabutyryl derivatives is gas–liquid chromatography with electron-capture detection,[27] although nitrogen detection can be used, with a limit of detection of 10 $\mu g.l^{-1}$.

Following oral administration of ketamine 0.5 $mg.kg^{-1}$ to volunteers, mean peak plasma ketamine concentration are 45.0±10.0 (mean±SEM) μg.l⁻¹ occurring after 30±5 min. Mean bioavailability is 16.5%.[28] In plasma, the drug is about 20–50% protein bound. Ketamine has been given orally for short painful procedures,[29] but reports on this route of administration are limited.

Ketamine is rapidly and extensively distributed throughout the body. Following bolus intravenous injection, the plasma ketamine concentration–time data satisfactorily fit a two-compartment open model.[28,30] The redistribution half life of a single bolus is 11–17 min and the terminal plasma half life is 151–186 min.[30,31] The plasma half life following an infusion of ketamine at a rate of 41.0±21 (mean±SD) μg.kg⁻¹.min⁻¹ has been found to be 79 min.[32] The apparent volume of distribution ranges from 214 to 347 l and total body clearance[30,31] from 1.23 to 1.32 l.min⁻¹. Plasma half life, clearance and volume of distribution (relative to body weight) are not significantly different in adults and children, although absorption following intramuscular injection is more rapid in the latter.[33]

Ketamine is likely to be excreted in breast milk, but this would be of no clinical relevance. It crosses the placenta in induction doses but in amounts that have no adverse effects on the neonate.

Ketamine undergoes extensive biotransformation in the liver. About 90% of the dose is excreted in the urine, with only 2% as the unchanged drug.

Renal disease is unlikely to affect the kinetics of the drug, but it is rarely used in these cases because of the associated hypertension. Although specific information is not available, it is likely that bioavailability will be increased and elimination reduced in hepatic disease.

Bioavailability	~16.5%
Plasma half life range	2–4 h
Volume of distribution	~4 l.kg⁻¹
Plasma protein binding	20–50%

Concentration–effect relationship

Plasma concentrations on awakening following 2.2 mg.kg⁻¹ ketamine intravenously in adults have been measured in the range[34] 700–1200 μg.l⁻¹. In children, the plasma levels on awakening vary very widely, being between 870 and 3780 μg.l⁻¹, which might be related to the difficulty in determining the exact point of awakening.[33]

Following an infusion of ketamine to supplement nitrous oxide anaesthesia, consciousness returned at plasma concentrations[32] less than 640 μg.l⁻¹.

Plasma ketamine levels greater than 100–150 μg.l⁻¹ in volunteers are associated with analgesia without impairment of consciousness.[28] Maintenance of such levels by a continuous infusion of 4 μg.kg⁻¹.min⁻¹ resulted in poor analgesia in postoperative patients.[35]

Metabolism

Ketamine undergoes extensive hepatic metabolism with only 2% of the dose recovered unchanged in the urine. 88% of the dose can be recovered as metabolites in the urine over 72 h.

The biodegradation of ketamine is relatively complicated (Fig. 1). Demethylation occurs to norketamine (metabolite I). This in turn can undergo hydroxylation in two different positions to form metabolites III and IV. These can be excreted as conjugates, or more likely be converted into metabolite II by dehydration. Ketamine itself may also undergo hydroxylation of its cyclohexylamine ring at two different sites, resulting in metabolites V and VI. Similarly, these may be conjugated and excreted, or may undergo dehydration to form ketamine metabolite VII. This in turn can be demethylated to form metabolite II. Most of the material in urine is present as conjugates of hydroxylated metabolites (80%). Only 16% of the dose can be recovered in urine as hydroxylated ketamine or norketamine. Metabolites I (norketamine) and II (dehydronorketamine) are easily measured in the same assay as for ketamine. Norketamine has about one-sixth of the potency of ketamine and is formed at concentrations in the plasma similar to those of the parent compound.

Pharmaceutics

Ketamine (Ketalar; Parke-Davis, UK/USA) is supplied as a colourless solution in strengths of 1%, 5% and 10% with pH ranging from 3.5 to 5.5. Solutions should not therefore be mixed with barbiturates (alkaline). The stronger two solutions contain 0.01% benzethonium chloride as a preservative. Solutions should be protected from light. Ketamine is clinically compatible with all common anaesthetic agents when adequate respiratory exchange is maintained.

Fig. 1 Metabolism of ketamine

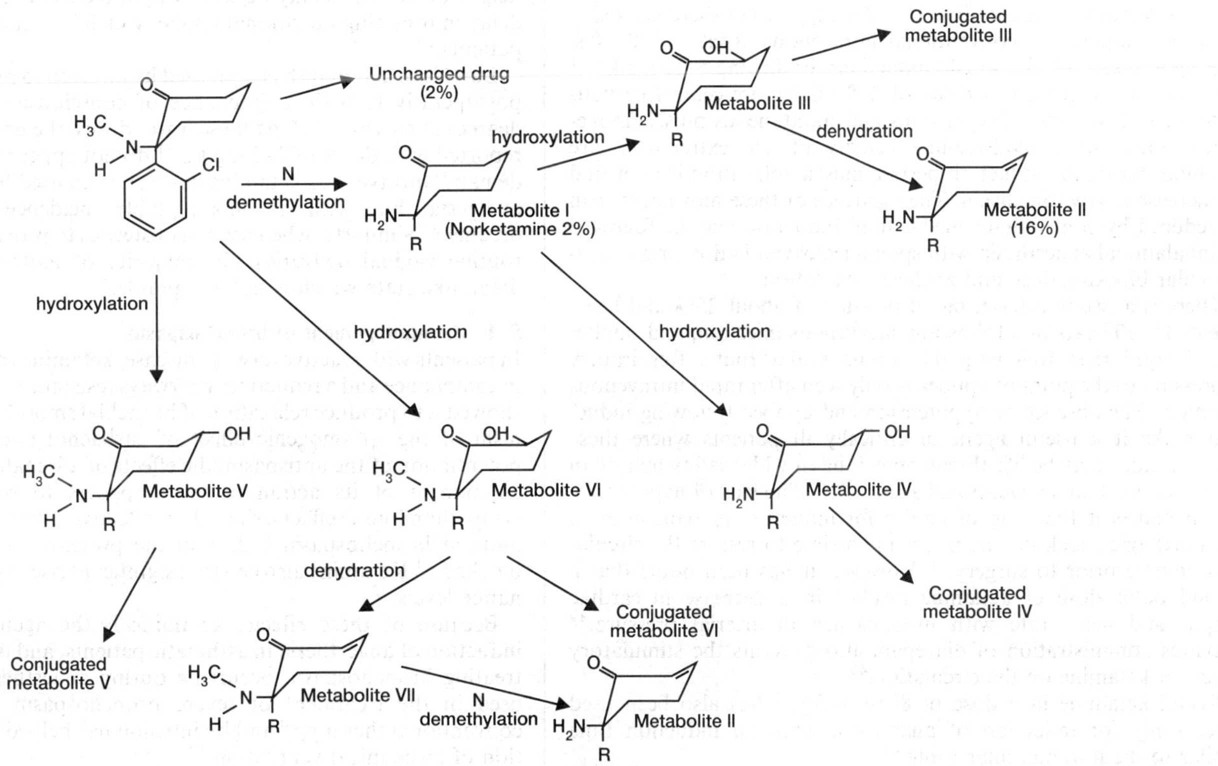

Therapeutic use

Indications

1. Induction of general anaesthesia, particularly in neonates and high risk patients
2. As sole anaesthetic agent for short, painful procedures not requiring muscle relaxation, and for surgery under adverse circumstances
3. As a method of sedation for diagnostic and therapeutic procedures in children, such as cardiac catheterization, neuroradiological investigations, ophthalmological investigation, repeat radiotherapy
4. Painful procedures such as burns dressings
5. In the management of intractable bronchospasm and as an induction agent in patients with pulmonary disease
6. Miscellaneous, such as an anticonvulsant and for intravenous regional analgesia.

Contraindications

1. General precautions for all intravenous anaesthetic agents
2. Hypertension
3. Severe angina and recent myocardial infarction
4. Raised intracranial pressure
5. Raised intraocular pressure
6. History of psychiatric disorders
7. Operations on the pharynx, larynx and tracheobronchial tree.

Mode of use

To induce general anaesthesia prior to maintenance with inhalational agents, ketamine is given intravenously (1.0–2.0 mg.kg^{-1}) or intramuscularly as simple injections (5.0–10.0 mg.kg^{-1} in children and adults; 12.5 mg.kg^{-1} in neonates). If used as a sole agent, half the intravenous or intramuscular dose is given when there are signs of purposeful response to painful stimuli. It may also be given by intravenous infusion to maintain anaesthesia (40 μg.kg^{-1}.min^{-1}) following an induction dose of 2 mg.kg^{-1}, to supplement nitrous oxide (25 μg.kg^{-1}.min^{-1}), provide postoperative analgesia or in the management of severe bronchospasm (40 μg.kg^{-1}.min^{-1}). Hypertension and psychotomimetic effects are common when used alone, thus severely limiting its use, and other drugs are required to control these effects.

Indications

1. Induction of anaesthesia

The intravenous induction dose is 1–2 mg.kg^{-1}, but there is a delay in onset compared to conventional intravenous agents of 30–90 s, making it unsuitable for 'crash' inductions. Following 5–10 mg.kg^{-1} intramuscularly, there is a delay of 2–8 min before central nervous system effects are seen. Hypertonus and spontaneous muscle movements, including convulsive-like activity of the extremities, are common during the induction period; muscle relaxation is poor and an increase in jaw tone usual. The incidence of these movements can be reduced by concomitant medication. Induction may be followed by inhalational anaesthesia with spontaneous ventilation or a neuromuscular blocking drug and artificial ventilation.

There is a rise in arterial blood pressure of about 25% and heart rate of 15–20 beats/min following intravenous injection, and smaller and delayed rises following the intramuscular route. Respiratory depression to the point of apnoea is only seen after rapid intravenous injection. The absence of hypotension and apnoea following induction make it a useful agent in critically ill patients where these complications may be life-threatening; it has a wider safety margin in these patients than conventional agents.[36,37] The lack of hypotensive action makes it the drug of choice for induction in patients with haemorrhagic shock in whom it is impossible to restore the circulation volume prior to surgery.[38] However, it has been noted that a second bolus dose of ketamine resulted in a decrease in cardiac output and heart rate with little change in arterial pressure.[39] Previous administration of diazepam also prevents the stimulatory effects of ketamine on the circulation.[40]

Rectal ketamine in a dose of 8–10 mg.kg^{-1} has also been used successfully for induction of anaesthesia with an induction time similar to the intramuscular route.[41]

2. As sole anaesthetic agent

It may be used intravenously or intramuscularly as the sole anaesthetic agent in operations not requiring muscular relaxation.[42,43] It is particularly useful for surgeons working alone because of the ease of administration and self-maintenance of a patient airway. It is very valuable in situations of mass casualties such as wars and civil disturbances, where it can be used for extensive surgical toilet, amputations, insertion of chest drains, etc., under adverse circumstances and where there is limited access to the airway.[44,45] It has also been used successfully intrathecally under field conditions to provide analgesia for surgery of the lower limbs.[46]

3. As a sedative for diagnostic and therapeutic procedures

Ketamine is highly effective as a method of sedation for cardiac catheterization in children when given intramuscularly.[47] It is widely used for ophthalmological examinations in children,[48] although reports of its effects on intraocular pressure vary.[49,50] Intramuscular ketamine is the agent of choice for sedation of young children undergoing repeated radiotherapy, where the child must be kept completely immobile during the procedure and maintain an airway without any personnel in the room during the period of treatment.[51] It has also been used for neurodiagnostic procedures such as pneuomoencephalograms and ventriculograms.

During performance of painful nerve blocks and positioning of patients with fractures prior to such blocks, the ideal premedicant would produce analgesia, sedation and amnesia without cardiorespiratory depression. Ketamine has been successfully used intravenously for the purpose,[52] and is usually combined with a benzodiazepine to reduce the incidence of adverse psychotomimetic effects.

The reason that ketamine is so useful in situations where the airway is compromised or where the patient has to be left unattended is the fact that muscle tone is not depressed as with other agents, both intravenous and inhalational. Laryngeal reflexes are not depressed to the same degree as with other anaesthetics, but some degree of laryngeal incompetence does occur.[53] Ketamine also evokes marked salivation which can interfere with airway maintenance, and an anticholinergic drug is essential prior to its use.

4. Painful procedures

Ketamine has been used extensively for changing burns dressings, debridement and skin grafting in children and adults.[54] Low doses (1.5–2.0 mg.kg^{-1} intramuscularly) have a rapid onset, provide good analgesia and rapid recovery. Ketamine is free from the problems of repeated anaesthetics associated with other agents, although some degree of tolerance may be seen. Rapid recovery results in minimal delay in resuming nutritional intake, which is so important in burnt patients.[55]

Low-dose ketamine has been used by infusion to produce analgesia postoperatively with maintenance of consciousness, with varying degrees of success.[35,56] At these lower doses, the unpleasant dreams reported with doses of 2–3 mg.kg^{-1} do not appear to occur.[56] 'On-demand' intravenous ketamine has also been used for postoperative analgesia, but with an unacceptable incidence of frightening dreams.[57] Similarly, when used in obstetrics to provide analgesia for routine vaginal deliveries, the majority of mothers experience a dreamlike state which is not acceptable.[1]

5. In the management of bronchospasm

In patients with reactive airways disease, ketamine causes an increase in compliance and a reduction in airways resistance.[58] In vitro studies showed it to produce relaxation of bronchial smooth muscle, antagonism of the spasmogenic effect of carbachol and histamine and potentiation of the antispasmodic effects of adrenaline.[59] The major component of its action in vitro appears to be related to its sympathomimetic effects, since the protective action against antigen-induced bronchospasm is lost in the presence of β-adrenoceptor blockade.[1] Ketamine also causes a significant rise in plasma noradrenaline levels.[23]

Because of these effects, ketamine is the agent of choice for induction of anaesthesia in asthmatic patients, and is also effective in treating bronchospasm occurring during anaesthesia. It has been used in the treatment of severe bronchospasm after failure of conventional therapy,[60] and by infusion has helped to avoid institution of mechanical ventilation.[61]

Ketamine (hydrochloride)

6. Miscellaneous
Despite the fact that ketamine produces an increase in muscle tone and occasionally convulsive-like activity it has been used successfully as an anticonvulsant.[5] It has been used in the technique of intravenous regional analgesia, but consciousness is lost following tourniquet release, thus limiting its use.[62] It has been used safely in patients with a history compatible with malignant hyperthermia,[6,7] and also in patients with acute intermittent porphyria,[63] even though it induces ALA synthetase activity in animals.[64]

Contraindications

1. General precautions for all intravenous anaesthetic agents
Despite the fact that ketamine is easy to use, it is a general anaesthetic agent and should only be administered by those who are skilled in resuscitation and tracheal intubation. Full resuscitative apparatus and a means of ventilating the lungs must always be present when ketamine is used.

2. Hypertension
A rise in arterial blood pressure is invariable following ketamine and on occasion can be considerable. It is thus contraindicated in patients with sustained or poorly controlled hypertension.

3. Severe angina and recent myocardial infarction
Ketamine produces a dose-related rise in the rate pressure product, which is often in excess of 100%, and thus a marked increase in myocardial work.

4. Raised intracranial pressure
Ketamine will further raise intracranial pressure, with the possibility of coning.

5. Raised intraocular pressure
The rise in intraocular pressure produced by ketamine could be dangerous in patients with glaucoma, and in penetrating eye injuries may result in extrusion of intraocular contents.

6. Psychiatric disorders
Because of the known psychotomimetic effects of ketamine, it is not recommended for patients with psychiatric disorders. Neither should it be used in those with a high alcohol intake.

7. Operations on the larynx, pharynx and tracheobronchial tree
Ketamine cannot be used as the sole agent for operations in these areas as active reflexes are maintained.

Adverse reactions

Potentially life-threatening effects
Unlike conventional general anaesthetic agents, both inhalational and intravenous, ketamine does not cause a dose-related depression of the cardiovascular and respiratory systems. It is thus a very safe agent in this respect, even in critically ill and elderly patients.

Acute overdosage
There have been no reports of deliberate overdose.

Severe or irreversible adverse effects
Following injection of 1–2 $mg.kg^{-1}$ intravenously, a rise in arterial systolic pressure of 20–40 mmHg can be expected, but there is a wide variation in individual response. The systolic arterial pressure rises over 3–5 min and then declines to normal over the next 10–20 min. The rise in diastolic pressure is slightly less. There is little evidence of a dose-related response with amounts greater than 1 $mg.kg^{-1}$. There is also a tachycardia and a rise in cardiac output mainly due to the tachycardia rather than to an increase in stroke volume. These cardiostimulatory effects can produce serious sequelae in patients with cardiac disease. Most premedicant drugs will decrease the rise in arterial pressure, but pancuronium must be avoided as a muscle relaxant as this too causes cardiovascular stimulation. A significant increase in plasma noradrenaline levels accompanies ketamine anaesthesia.[23] Labetalol is the most effective drug in attenuating ketamine-induced tachycardia and hypertension.[65]

Symptomatic adverse effects
Psychomimetic reactions. The emergence reactions are the main drawback to ketamine anaesthesia. They occur during the recovery period and can be extremely unpleasant to the patient and disturbing to other patients and personnel in the recovery area. The psychic sensations consist of alteration in body image, extracorporeal experiences, floating sensations, vivid dreams, 'weird trips' and frank delirium. It is thought that recovery of consciousness begins while there is still loss of skin and musculoskeletal sensation so that the ability to feel gravity is lost, producing a sensation of body detachment or floating in space.[66] The vivid dreams usually disappear on awakening, but there are reports of prolonged psychic phenomena occurring for periods up to one year, and symptoms have been likened to the effects of LSD 25.[67]

The reported incidence of these psychic disturbances varies from less than 5% to more than 30%. Factors associated with a higher incidence of emergence reactions include age (more than 16 years old); sex (females greater than males); patients who frequently dream; large doses (>2 $mg.kg^{-1}$ intravenously); rapid administration; a history of personality problems.[1] Allowing patients to recover in a quiet area with their eyes covered does not reduce the incidence of reactions.[68]

Many central sedative drugs have been used in an attempt to prevent these emergence reactions. The most effective of these are the benzodiazepines, diazepam being the most widely used, and they may be given at the start or at the end of the procedure.[69]

Cardiovascular effects. In children with congenital heart disease, ketamine 2 $mg.kg^{-1}$ intravenously increases pulmonary arterial pressure and the ratio between pulmonary and systemic vascular resistance, but no change in the ratio of pulmonary to systemic blood flow or the amount or direction of intracardiac shunting.[70] It has been used successfully in patients with Eisenmenger's syndrome,[71] where the combination of a fall in systemic vascular resistance with an increase in pulmonary vascular resistance would prove disastrous.

Other effects
Ketamine causes a slight elevation in blood glucose and slight decrease in free fatty acids.[72] It activates the pituitary–adrenal axis with adrenal release of catecholamines[73] and cortisol.[74] The metabolic and endocrine responses to surgery during ketamine anaesthesia do not differ from those of patients anaesthetized with thiopentone and halothane.[75]

Interference with clinical pathology tests
Ketamine is not known to interfere with any clinical pathological measurements.

High risk groups

Neonates
Due to the fact that it can be administered intramuscularly, ketamine has been used extensively in neonates both to induce anaesthesia and as the sole agent. The dose may have to be increased up to 12.5 $mg.kg^{-1}$ intramuscularly in order to achieve satisfactory operating conditions.[43]

Breast milk. Ketamine is likely to be excreted in breast milk, but the amounts are unlikely to be of clinical relevance.

Children
There is no specific contraindication to its use, although resistance to its effects may be found in children with retarded cerebral development.[42]

Pregnant women
Ketamine has been used successfully as an induction agent with the usual precautions and contraindications. It crosses the placenta in induction doses but in amounts that have no adverse effects on the neonate when used for anaesthesia for Caesarean section.

The elderly
Apart from the usual contraindications, ketamine can be safely used in the elderly.

Drug interactions

Potentially hazardous interactions
Drugs with an action on the cardiovascular system similar to that of ketamine should be avoided. This includes the neuromuscular relaxant pancuronium and the oxytocic, ergometrine. Sustained rises in arterial pressure have been reported in a patient receiving thyroxine therapy. Concurrent administration of ketamine and aminophylline may decrease the seizure threshold.[76]

Other significant interactions

Alcoholics tend to be resistant to ketamine anaesthesia, as to other anaesthetics. Exaggerated psychotomimetic effects may be seen in the recovery period in these patients.

Potentially useful interactions

Combination with central sedative drugs, particularly benzodiazepines, will reduce the occurrence of psychotomimetic reactions and also the severity of the cardiovascular response.

Clinical trials

1. Corssen G, Miyasaka M, Domino E F 1968 Changing concepts in pain control during surgery: dissociative anaesthesia with CI-581. Anesthesia and Analgesia 47: 746–759

This study describes the use of ketamine as the sole anaesthetic agent in 900 patients, aged 5 days to 86 years, for a total of 1508 diagnostic and surgical procedures, of which 217 were out-patients. It was used intramuscularly for 210 of the procedures. Anaesthesia was adequate on 1333 occasions. Disadvantages included occasional excessive vasopressor activity, excess salivation in the absence of an antisialogogue, a 2.8% incidence of vivid dreaming and 3.3% incidence of emergence delirium. The authors concluded that ketamine was a safe, effective and easily administered short-acting anaesthetic with minor complications, when proper criteria and methods were followed.

Other trials

1. Coppel D L, Dundee J W 1972 Ketamine anaesthesia for cardiac catheterization. Anaesthesia 27: 25–31

Ketamine was used intramuscularly, with supplementary doses intravenously, in 40 children aged from 2 months to 13 years (mean 4 years) undergoing cardiac catheterization. Satisfactory operating conditions were provided in 37 children, tracheal intubation only being required on one occasion. The authors concluded that ketamine was a suitable agent for use in a dark X-ray room and seemed to be a safe agent in these poor risk patients.

2. Edge W G, Morgan M 1977 Ketamine and paediatric radiotherapy. Anaesthesia and Intensive Care 5: 153–156

This study describes the administration of 272 ketamine anaesthetics to 16 children aged from 3 months to 7 years (mean 3 years) undergoing radiotherapy. Satisfactory conditions were provided in every case with a low incidence of complications. The authors concluded that ketamine was the most satisfactory available agent for repeated sedation in these children where personnel cannot remain in the same room during the periods of treatment.

General review articles

White P F, Way W L, Trevor A J 1982 Ketamine — its pharmacology and therapeutic uses. Anesthesiology 56: 119–136

Zsigmond E K, Domino E F 1980 Ketamine. Clinical pharmacology, pharmacokinetics and current clinical uses. Anesthesiology Review 7: 13–33

References

1. White P F 1985 Ketamine — its use as an intravenous anaesthetic. In: Clinics in Anaesthesiology 2. Intravenous Anaesthesiology, pp 43–64
2. Domino E G, Chodoff P, Corssen G 1985 Pharmacological effects of CI-581, a new dissociative anaesthetic in man. Clinical Pharmacology and Therapeutics 6: 279–290
3. Virtue R W, Alamis J M, Mari M, Lafargna R T, Vogel J H K, Metcalf D R 1967 An anaesthetic agent: 2-ortho-chlorophenyl-2-methylamino cyclohexanone HCl (CI-581). Anesthesiology 28: 823–833
4. Corsenn G, Little S G, Tavakoli M 1974 Ketamine and epilepsy. Anesthesia and Analgesia 53: 319–335
5. Sybert J W, Kyff J V 1983 Ketamine treatment of status epilepticus. Anesthesiology 58: 203
6. Zsigmond E K 1971 Malignant hyperthermia with subsequent uneventful general anaesthesia. Anesthesia and Analgesia 50: 1111–1112
7. Wadhwa R K, Tantisira B 1974 Parotidectomy in a patient with malignant hyperthermia. Anesthesiology 40: 191
8. Takeshita H, Okuda Y, Sari A 1972 The effects of ketamine anesthesia on cerebral circulation and metabolism in man. Anesthesiology 36: 69
9. Ngai S H, Cheney D L, Finck A D 1978 Acetylcholine concentrations and turnover in rat brain structures during anesthesia with halothane, enflurane and ketamine. Anesthesiology 48: 4–10
10. Balmer H G R, Wyte S R 1977 Antagonism of ketamine by physostigmine. British Journal of Anaesthesia 49: 510
11. Lawrence D, Livingston A 1979 The effect of physostigmine and neostigmine on ketamine anaesthesia and analgesia. British Journal of Pharmacology 67: 426
12. Wachtel R E 1988 Ketamine decreases open time of single channel currents activated by acetycholine. Anesthesiology 68: 563–570
13. Frenkel C, Urban B W 1989 Molecular actions of racemic ketamine on single sodium channels from human brain cortex. Anesthesia and Analgesia 68: 591
14. Sparks D L, Corssen G, Sides J, Black J, Kholeif A 1973 Ketamine-induced anesthesia: neural mechanisms in the Rhesus monkey. Anesthesia and Analgesia 54: 189–195
15. Massopust L C Jr, Wolin L R, Alkin M S 1972 Electrophysiologic and behavioural responses to ketamine hydrochloride in the Rhesus monkey. Anesthesia and Analgesia 51: 329–341
16. Ohtami M, Kikuchi H, Kitahata L M et al 1979 Effects of ketamine on nociceptive cells in the medial medullary reticular formation of the cat. Anesthesiology 51: 414–417
17. Kitahata L M, Taub A, Kosaka Y 1973 Lamina-specific suppression of dorsal-horn unit activity by ketamine-hydrochloride. Anesthesiology 38: 4–11
18. Fratta W, Casu M, Balestrieri A, Lovisella A, Biggio G, Gessa G L 1980 Failure of ketamine to interact with opiate receptors. European Journal of Pharmacology 61: 389–391
19. Dickensen A H, Sullivan A F 1987 Evidence for a role of the NMDA receptor in the frequency dependent potentiation of deep rat dorsal horn nociceptive neurones following C fibre stimulation. Neuropharmacology 26: 1235–1238
20. McQuay H J, Dickensen A H 1990 Implications of nervous system plasticity for pain management. Anaesthesia 45: 101–102
21. Stone T W, Burton N R 1988 NMDA receptors and ligands in the vertebrate CNS. Progress in Neurobiology 30: 333
22. White P F, Way W L, Travers A J 1982 Ketamine — its pharmacology and therapeutic uses. Anesthesiology 56: 119–136
23. Zsigmond E K, Kelsch R C 1974 Elevated plasma norepinephrine concentration during ketamine anesthesia. Clinical Pharmacology and Therapeutics 14: 149
24. Ivankovich A D, Miletich D J, Reimann C, Albrecht R F, Zahed B 1974 Cardiovascular effects of centrally administered ketamine in goats. Anesthesia and Analgesia 53: 924–933
25. White P F, Ham J, Way W L, Trevor A J 1980 Pharmacology of ketamine isomers in surgical patients. Anesthesiology 52: 231–239
26. White P F, Schüttler J, Shafer A, Stanski D R, Horai Y, Trevor A J 1985 Comparative pharmacology of ketamine isomers. Studies in volunteers. British Journal of Anaesthesia 57: 197–203
27. Chang T, Glazko A J 1972 Biotransformation and metabolism of ketamine. International Anesthesiology Clinics 19: 157–177
28. Grant I S, Nimmo W S, Clements J A 1981 Pharmacokinetics and analgesic effects of I.M. and oral ketamine. British Journal of Anaesthesia 53: 805–810
29. Morgan A J, Dutkiewicz T W S 1983 Oral ketamine. Anaesthesia 33: 293
30. Wieber J, Gryler Rd, Hengstmann J H, Dengler H J 1975 Pharmacokinetics of ketamine in man. Anaesthesist 24: 260–266
31. Clements J A, Nimmo W S 1981 Pharmacokinetics and analgesic effects of ketamine in man. British Journal of Anaesthesia 53: 27–30
32. Idvall J, Ahlgren I, Aronsen K F, Stenberg P 1979 Ketamine infusions: pharmacokinetics and clinical effects. British Journal of Anaesthesia 51: 1167–1173
33. Grant I S, Nimmo W S, McNicol I R, Clements J A 1983 Ketamine disposition in adults and children. British Journal of Anaesthesia 55: 1107–1111
34. Little B, Chang T, Chucot L et al 1972 A study of ketamine as an obstetrical anesthetic. American Journal of Obstetrics and Gynecology 113: 247–258
35. Owen H, Reekie R M, Clements A J, Watson Rd, Nimmo W S 1987 Analgesia from morphine and ketamine. Anaesthesia 42: 1051–1056
36. Lorham P H, Lipperman M 1971 A clinical appraisal of the use of ketamine hydrochloride in the aged. Anesthesia and Analgesia 50: 448–451
37. Vaughan R W, Stephen C R 1974. Abdominal and thoracic surgery in adults with ketamine, nitrous oxide and d-tubocurarine. Anesthesia and Analgesia 52: 271–280
38. Bond A C, Davies C K 1974 Ketamine amd pancuronium for the shocked patient. Anaesthesia 29: 59–62
39. Savege T M, Colvin M P, Weaver E J M, Bond C, Drake J, Inniss R 1976 A comparison of some cardiorespiratory effects of Althesin and ketamine when used for induction of anesthesia in patients with cardiac disease. British Journal of Anaesthesia 48: 1071–1081
40. Jackson A P F, Dhadphale P R, Callaghan M L, Alseri S 1978 Haemodynamic studies during induction of anaesthesia for open-heart surgery using diazepam and ketamine. British Journal of Anaesthesia 50: 375–378
41. Saint-Maurice C, Laguenie G, Conturier C, Gontail-Fland F 1979 Rectal ketamine in paediatric anaesthesia. British Journal of Anaesthesia 51: 573–574
42. Morgan M, Loh L, Singer L, Moore P H 1971 Ketamine as the sole anaesthetic agent for minor surgical procedures. Anaesthesia 26: 158–165
43. Phillips L A, Seruvatu S G, Rika P N, Tirikula U 1970 Anaesthesia for the surgeon–anaesthetist in difficult situations. The use of intramuscular 2(0-chlorophenyl)-2 methylamino cyclohexanone HCl (Parke Davis CI-581, Ketamine). Anaesthesia 25: 36–45
44. Dundee J W, Wyant G M 1974 Intravenous anaesthesia, 1st edn. Churchill Livingstone, Edinburgh
45. Bion J F 1984 Infusion analgesia for acute war injuries. A comparison of pentazocine and ketamine. Anaesthesia 39: 560–564
46. Bion J F 1984 Intrathecal ketamine for war surgery. A preliminary study under field conditions. Anaesthesia 39: 1023–1028
47. Dillon J B 1971 Rational use of ketamine as an anaesthetic. Proceedings of the Royal Society of Medicine 64: 1153–1156
48. Falls H F, Hoy J E, Corssen G 1966 CI-581: an intravenous or intramuscular anesthetic for office ophthalmic surgery. American Journal of Ophthalmology 61: 1093–1095

49. AplIvor D 1973 Ketamine in paediatric ophthalmological surgery. An evaluation of its efficacy and postoperative effects. Anaesthesia 28: 501–508
50. Reuler M, Glass D D, Arens J F 1975 Ketamine and intraocular pressure. Anaesthesia 43: 575–578
51. Bennett J A, Bullimore J A 1973 The use of ketamine hydrochloride for radiotherapy in young children. British Journal of Anaesthesia 45: 197–201
52. Thompson G E, Moore D C 1971 Ketamine, diazepam and Innovar: a computerized comparative study. Anesthesia and Analgesia 50: 458–463
53. Taylor P A, Towey R M 1971 Depression of laryngeal reflexes during ketamine anaesthesia. British Medical Journal 2: 688–689
54. Brown J M 1985 Aspects of thermal injury. Recent Advances in Anaesthesia and Analgesia 15: 155–172
55. Demline R H, Ellerbee S, Jarrett F 1978 Ketamine anaesthesia for tangential excision of burn eschar: a burn unit procedure. Journal of Trauma 18: 269–270
56. Ito Y, Ichiyanagi K 1974 Post-operative pain relief with ketamine infusion. Anaesthesia 29: 222–229
57. Austin T R 1981 Ketamine on demand for postoperative analgesia. Anaesthesia 36: 214
58. Corssen G, Gutierrez J, Reves J G, Huber F C 1972 Ketamine in the anesthetic management of asthmatic patients. Anesthesia and Analgesia 51: 588–596
59. Lundy P M, Gowdey C W, Colhoun P M 1974 Tracheal smooth muscle relaxant effect of ketamine. British Journal of Anaesthesia 46: 333–336
60. Fisher M M 1977 Ketamine hydrochloride in severe brochospasm. Anaesthesia 32: 771–772
61. Strube P J, Hallam P L 1986 Ketamine by continuous infusion in status asthmaticus. Anaesthesia 41: 1017–1019
62. Amiot J F, Bouhji P, Palacci J H, Balliner E 1985 Intravenous regional analgesia with ketamine. Anaesthesia 40: 899–901
63. Bancroft G H, Lanria J I 1983 Ketamine infusion for Cesarean section in a patient with acute intermittent porphyria and achondroplastic dwarfism. Anesthesiology 53: 143–144
64. Kostrewski E, Gregor A 1978 Ketamine in acute intermittent porphyria — dangerous or safe. Anesthesiology 49: 376–377
65. Dundee J W, Lilburn J K, Moore J 1978 Attempted reduction of the cardiostimulatory effects of ketamine by labetalol. Anaesthesia 33: 506–511
66. Collier B B 1972 Ketamine and the conscious mind. Anaesthesia 27: 120–134
67. Schorn T O F, Whitwam J G 1980 Are there long term effects of ketamine on the central nervous system? British Journal of Anaesthesia 52: 967–968
68. Hejja P, Galloon S 1975 A consideration of ketamine dreams. Canadian Anaesthestists Society Journal 22: 100–105
69. Knox J W D, Bovill J G, Clarke R S J, Dundee J W 1970 Clinical study of induction agents. XXXVI: Ketamine. British Journal of Anaesthesia 42: 875–885
70. Morray J P, Lynn A M, Stamm S J, Herndon P S, Kawabori I, Stevenson J G 1984 Hemodynamic effects of ketamine in children with congenital heart disease. Anesthesia and Analgesia 63: 895–899
71. Lumley J, Whitwan J G, Morgan M 1977 General anesthesia in the presence of Eisenmenger's syndrome. Anesthesia and Analgesia 56: 543–547
72. Kaniaris P, Lekakis D, Kykomiatis M, Kastanas E 1975 Serum free fatty acid and blood sugar levels in children under halothane, thiopentone and ketamine anaesthesia. Canadian Anaesthestists' Society Journal 22: 509–518
73. Takki S, Nikki P, Jaattela A, Tammisto T 1972 Ketamine and plasma catecholamines. British Journal of Anaesthesia 44: 1318–1322
74. Oyama T, Matsumoto F, Kudo T 1970 Effects of ketamine on adrenocortical function in man. Anesthesia and Analgesia 49: 697–700
75. Lacoumenta S, Walsh E S, Waterman A E, Ward I, Patterson J L, Hall G M 1984 Effects of ketamine anaesthesia on the metabolic response to pelvic surgery. British Journal of Anaesthesia 56: 493–497
76. Hirshman C A, Krieger W, Littlejohn G, Lee R, Julien R 1982 Ketamine–aminophylline induced decrease in seizure threshold. Anesthesiology 56: 464–467

Ketanserin (tartrate)

Ketanserin is a serotonin $5\text{-}HT_2$ receptor blocking drug that has been developed for hypertension and peripheral vascular disorders.

Chemistry

Ketanserin tartrate (Sufrexal, Serefrex)
$C_{22}H_{22}FN_3O_3.C_4H_6O_6$
(d)-3-[2-[4-(4-Flurobenzoyl)piperidino]ethyl-2,4(1H,3H)-quinazolinedione [R-(R*,R*)]-2,3-dihydroxybutanedioate(1:1)

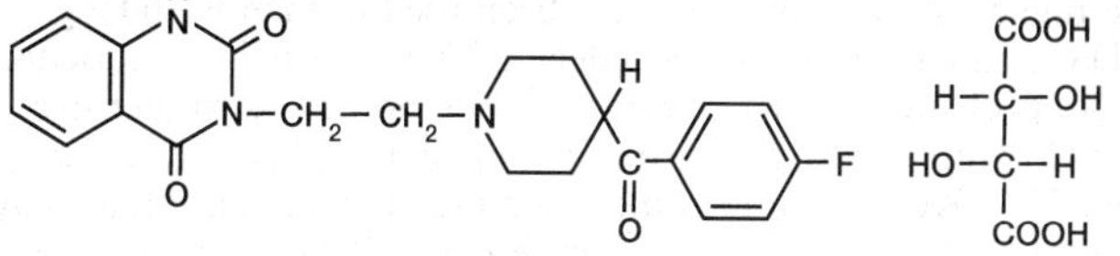

Molecular weight (free base)	545.52 (395.47)
pKa (free base)	7.5
Solubility (tartrate)	
in alcohol	1 in 417
in water	1 in 42
Octanol/water partition coefficient	—

The drug is prepared by chemical synthesis. The dextrorotary stereoisomer is used chemically. It is not available in combination preparations.

Pharmacology

Ketanserin is a competitive antagonist at 5-hydroxytryptamine (5-HT) or serotonin (S) receptors of the $5\text{-}HT_2$ (or S_2) subtype. Ketanserin also possesses α_1-adrenergic and H_1-histaminergic antagonistic properties.[1,2] It has weak dopamine-blocking effects. The main pharmacological actions of the drug are:

1. Selective inhibition of serotonin-induced vasoconstriction but not vasodilation, and inhibition of serotonin-induced amplification of vasoconstriction caused by other agents.[3,4]
2. Selective inhibition of serotonin-induced platelet aggregation and serotonin-induced amplification of platelet aggregation caused by other agents.[3,4]
3. At concentrations higher than those needed to be an antagonist at $5\text{-}HT_2$-receptors, α_1-adrenergic blockade occurs.[5,6]

Toxicology

Ketanserin does not induce any histopathological changes in specific target organs at doses close to those used in man. The major target organ for toxic overdosing of functional nature is the central nervous system. There is no primary embryotoxic or teratogenic potential in rats or rabbits, except at maternally toxic doses in rats where secondarily increased embryonal resorption or decreased litter survival was noted. In a battery of mutagenicity tests, including the Ames test in *Salmonella*, ketanserin showed no mutagenic activity. In carcinogenicity tests lasting up to 24 months in rats no carcinogenic potential has been observed. In 18 month tests in mice, a slight prolactin-mediated mammary gland stimulation and subsequently increased incidence of mammary gland tumours was observed at high dose levels in female mice. Since at therapeutic dose levels in man, ketanserin does not elevate prolactin levels, the effects seen in mice are probably irrelevant. It is unlikely that ketanserin has genotoxic potential.

Clinical pharmacology

Serotonin S_2 antagonistic effects on ex vivo platelet aggregation have been demonstrated in man. Some studies in man have also demonstrated a shift of the dose–response curve for the pressor effects of α_1-adrenergic agonists like phenylephrine and methoxamine. While ketanserin lowers blood pressure in hypertensive patients,[7,8] the more selective 5-HT_2 antagonist ritanserin (and other investigational drugs with specific 5-HT_2 blocking properties) has no antihypertensive effects in dose ranges where the 5-HT_2 antagonistic properties are similar or more pronounced than for ketanserin. This indicates that the 5-HT_2 blocking properties of ketanserin are not solely responsible for its antihypertensive effects,[9] but other mechanisms contribute.[10,11] There has been considerable disagreement as to what these mechanisms may be and the relative importance of α-adrenergic blockade.[12] Daily doses of ketanserin in the range of 20–80 mg produce reductions in systolic and diastolic blood pressures. The dose–response curve is relatively flat. Ketanserin causes a slight reduction of heart rate, which may be due to its sympatho-inhibitory actions. The antihypertensive effects of ketanserin are well documented during single as well as multiple dosing.

In clinical practice, the dose starts at 20 mg, twice daily and after 2 to 4 weeks the dose is increased (if necessary) to 40 mg, twice daily. The highest dose known to have been used in man is 160 mg.

The main haemodynamic effect of ketanserin is a reduction of blood pressure in hypertensive,[7,8] but not in normotensive subjects,[13,14] primarily by the reduction of peripheral vascular resistance.[15,16] Ketanserin also increases muscle and skin blood flow in patients with peripheral vascular disease (PVD),[17,18] and has thus proved useful in the treatment of Reynaud's phenomenon.[19–21]

In therapeutic doses ketanserin induces an inhibition of serotonin-induced platelet aggregation ex vivo.[22–24]

Ketanserin also induces haemorrheological effects, demonstrated as improvement of red blood cell deformability in patients with cardiovascular diseases[25–28] and improvement of whole blood viscosity and white blood cell clogging, although the importance of these actions is not clear. It prolongs the QTc interval of the ECG.[33–35]

Pharmacokinetics

Plasma levels of ketanserin are measured by high performance liquid chromatography (HPLC) with UV[36] or fluorescence[37] detection. The methods are specific and the limits of sensitivity are 1–10 $\mu g.l^{-1}$ (UV) and 0.1–0.2 $\mu g.l^{-1}$ (fluorescence), respectively. Following oral administration, ketanserin is almost completely absorbed and peak plasma levels are reached within 0.5–2 hours.[13,38–41] Ketanserin is subject to considerable presystemic metabolism in the liver and the absolute bioavailability is around 50%.[38,39,41] The compound is extensively distributed to tissues (99%) and the volume of distribution is in the order of 3–6 $l.kg^{-1}$. Plasma protein binding, mainly to albumin, is in the order of 95%.[42] Ketanserin is extensively metabolized and less than 2% is excreted in urine as the parent compound.[38,45] Only 0.2% of the dose is excreted in the faeces. The major metabolic pathway is ketone reduction, leading to ketanserinol which is excreted mainly in the urine.[38,45] Ketanserinol, which by itself does not contribute to the overall pharmacological effect of ketanserin is partly reoxidized into ketanserin and it is likely that the terminal half life of ketanserin is related to the slow ketanserin regeneration from the metabolite.[38,39,43] Following single intravenous or oral administration, the terminal half life is around 15 hours.[13,39,40] Following chronic oral dosing (20–40 mg twice daily) the kinetics of the drug remain linear and steady state levels are reached within 4 days[40,44] consistent with the single dose half life. During chronic treatment with the usual dosage of 40 mg twice daily steady state levels fluctuate between 40 (trough levels) and 100–140 (peak levels) $\mu g.l^{-1}$.[38] The pharmacokinetic properties are predictable in a wide group of patients and there is no influence of duration of treatment, age, sex or body weight[29,30] of patients, or concomitant treatment with β-blockers and diuretics.[45] In patients with severe hepatocellular insufficiency the plasma protein binding is reduced (to around 93%) and the bioavailability of ketanserin is markedly higher due to reduced hepatic elimination.[46] In patients with renal insufficiency, elimination of the metabolite ketanserinol is prolonged but the plasma levels of ketanserin are similar to those observed in patients with normal renal function,[30–32,47–49] Ketanserin is not removed by haemodialysis.[50]

Ketanserin crosses the blood–brain barrier to a small extent, with brain levels similar to the free concentration in plasma. No information is available on the excretion of the drug in breast milk, although in dogs, breast milk levels are twice those in plasma. No information is available on the placental transfer of ketanserin.

Oral absorption	~100%
Presystemic metabolism	50%
Plasma half life	
range	—
mean	15 h
Volume of distribution	3–6 $l.kg^{-1}$
Plasma protein binding	95%

Concentration–effect relationship

Several studies in groups of patients have been unable to identify a clear relationship between plasma concentrations of ketanserin and the blood pressure reduction.[38,51,52] However, there may be a correlation between plasma concentrations and the decrease in blood pressure in the individual patients.[35] There are no data on the direct relationship between side effects and plasma concentrations of ketanserin. However, the side effects are clearly dose-related and at least in the individual patient coincide with the peak plasma concentrations 1–2 hours after tablet intake.[53] Furthermore, several reports have indicated that the prolongation of the QTc-interval is related to the plasma concentrations.[35,48]

Metabolism

Ketanserin is extensively metabolized in the liver, with less than 20% of the dose excreted in the urine. Three major pathways of metabolism of ketanserin have been described: (1) ketone reduction to ketanserinol and 6-hydroxyketanserinol, (2) oxidative N-dealkylation to the quinazoline acetic acid derivative, and (3) aromatic hydroxylation to 6-hydroxyketanserin and its reduced form (Fig. 1).

Of the metabolites formed, none has significant pharmacological activity. Ketanserinol is the major metabolite in man and is present in higher concentrations than ketanserin at steady state. However, it is 1000 times less biologically active than ketanserin. 6-Hydroxyketanserin has a pharmacological profile and potency similar to that of ketanserin, but this metabolite is not detectable in plasma and represents only a small overall contribution in ketanserin metabolism (<2.3% of dose).[45,46]

Pharmaceutics

Ketanserin (Serefrex; Janssen, UK) is available in oral and parenteral forms.

1. Ampoules containing 5 mg ketanserin per ml (2 ml and 10 ml ampoules).
2. Tablets containing 20 mg or 40 mg ketanserin: oblong, white, scored and film-coated; inscribed with 'Ke 20' or 'Ke 40' on one side, 'JANSSEN' on the other side. The 20 mg tablets contain 27.6 mg ketanserin tartrate (equivalent to 20 mg ketanserin). The 40 mg tablets contain 55.2 mg ketanserin tartrate (equivalent to 40 mg ketanserin).
3. Ketanserin for parenteral use is supplied in colourless siliconed glass ampoules. Ampoules contain 6.9 mg ketanserin tartrate per ml (equivalent to 5 mg ketanserin).

None of the formulations contains known potentially allergenic substances.

Ketanserin tablet formulations are stable and require no special storage conditions. The ampoules should be protected from light. The maximum shelf-life of the tablet and ampoule formulations is 5 years, when stored at room temperature.

Therapeutic use

Indications

1. Essential hypertension (mild, moderate and severe)
2. Acute hypertensive episodes.

Ketanserin (tartrate)

Contraindications

There are no absolute contraindications but caution should be observed in giving the drug to patients with hypokalaemia (spontaneous or induced by diuretics), concomitant treatment with antiarrhythmics or in patients with second or third degree heart block.

Mode of use

The usual parenteral therapeutic dose is 10 mg (range 5–30 mg) and should be titrated individually based on the degree of hypertension. When administered intravenously, an infusion of 3 mg.min^{-1} is given until a response is obtained up to a maximum of 30 mg. Alternatively, repeated injections of 5 mg every few minutes can be given until the patient responds (to a maximum of 30 mg). If administered intramuscularly, 10 mg is injected and this may be repeated after 15–30 min, if necessary. A continuous intravenous infusion may also be used: 2–6 mg.h^{-1} of ketanserin added to ordinary infusion fluids. An infusion is, however, always to be preceded by a loading injection.

Oral therapy with ketanserin starts with 20 mg twice daily. After 2 to 4 weeks, the dose is increased to 40 mg twice daily unless blood pressure is adequately controlled with the initial dose. Doses larger than 40 mg per intake are not recommended, since they are less well tolerated and do not usually provide additional blood pressure reduction.[54,55] In patients with hepatic insufficiency doses higher than 20 mg twice daily are not recommended.

Indications

1. Essential hypertension
Ketanserin is indicated in the management of mild, moderate or severe hypertension.[56–60] It lowers blood pressure to approximately the same extent as other antihypertensives to which it has been compared (diuretics,[61] β-blockers,[61,62] nifedipine,[63] methyldopa,[63] prazosin,[64] captopril[65]). It has been claimed to have particular advantages in older patients[61] (>60 years of age) although this claim has also been made for other antihypertensives. In older patients, ketanserin seems to be better tolerated, as the initial subjective effects often seen in younger patients (lightheadedness, drowsiness) are less frequent. Most of the antihypertensive effect occurs with the first dose, but a small further reduction is usually seen following 3–4 weeks of treatment. The resting pressure is controlled by twice daily therapy,[67] but once daily treatment has been successful in some patients. The antihypertensive efficacy is maintained during long-term therapy[68] and tolerance is not reported. When treatment is stopped, there is no rebound hypertension,[59,60] but a gradual return to pretreatment levels. Ketanserin can be combined with diuretics (provided patients are normokalaemic) or β-blockers in patients who do not adequately respond to either drug alone.[66]

2. Acute hypertensive episodes
In hypertensive episodes of various aetiologies (severe uncontrolled hypertension,[69,70] intra- and postoperative hypertension,[71] carcinoid syndrome,[72] pre-eclampsia or eclampsia[73]), a dose of 10–20 mg of ketanserin is given intravenously, which usually controls high blood pressure. The decrease in blood pressure can be maintained by a continuous infusion of ketanserin at a rate of 2–6 mg.h^{-1}.

Life-threatening ventricular arrhythmias (Torsades de Pointe) have been induced by the drug in patients with severe hypokalaemia.

Adverse reactions

Potentially life-threatening effects
Deaths caused by ketanserin are rare and the frequency cannot be accurately calculated. Deaths or life-threatening events seem to be related to ventricular arrhythmias (Torsades de Pointe) which most likely occur where there is diuretic-induced hypokalaemia or a drug-induced QT prolongation.[12,74,75]

Acute overdosage
Data on deliberate overdosage are limited. The most likely manifestations of overdosage would be sleepiness, drowsiness, visual disturbances, and possibly syncope.

Severe or irreversible adverse effects
Eight cases of ventricular tachycardia were reported among 18 000 patients treated up to 1986. All 8 cases had other factors possibly contributing to the development of arrhythmia.[12,34]

Symptomatic adverse effects
Parenteral treatment with ketanserin may induce transient hypotension in volume-depleted patients, after a slow intravenous injection of a 10 mg dose. At higher doses (28–38 mg) drowsiness and sleepiness are frequent.[12,76]

Oral treatment with therapeutic doses (20–40 mg) of ketanserin may cause lightheadedness, drowsiness and lack of concentration, especially in young patients. These effects which are dose-dependent, usually disappear within a few days. During chronic treatment in placebo-controlled trials somnolence was present slightly more often with ketanserin treatment (7% vs 4%).[12,53]

Other effects
After intravenous administration of ketanserin modest and inconsistent increases in plasma renin, angiotensin II and catecholamines have been reported.[14,77] However, no effect was observed followed chronic oral treatment[64,67] Ketanserin treatment did not effect the basal release of pituitary hormones, thyroid function or plasma cortisol levels.[78,79] There are no known adverse effects on routine haematology or biochemistry.[80] Several studies report no changes in serum cholesterol or triglycerides.[62,67,81] Other long-term studies

Fig. 1 The metabolism of ketanserin

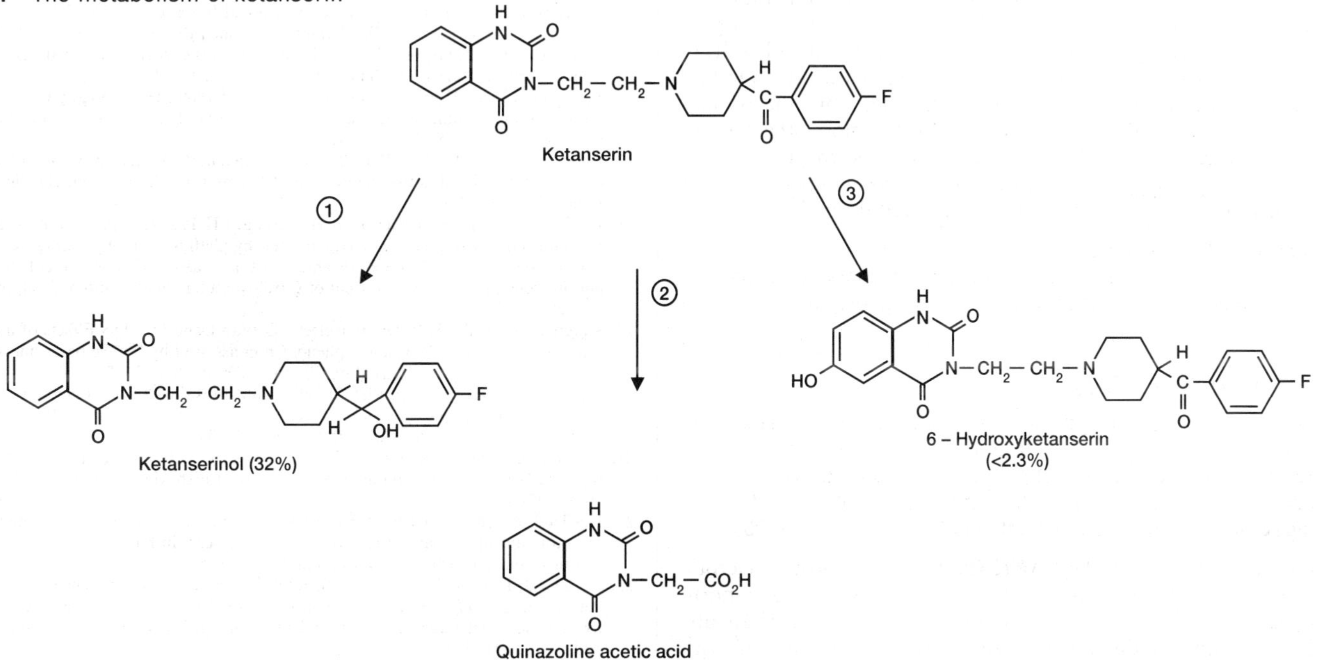

K

indicated a fall in total cholesterol and low density lipoproteins and a rise in high density lipoproteins.[82,83] Ketanserin does not interfere with carbohydrate metabolism or antidiabetic treatment.[83,84]

Interference with clinical pathology tests
There are no reports of ketanserin interfering with biochemical tests.

High risk groups

Neonates
Little or no information is yet available on ketanserin therapy in neonates.

Breast milk. Excretion in human breast milk has not yet been studied, but in dogs the levels of ketanserin in milk are twice those in plasma. Consequently, it is best that mothers taking the drug should not breast-feed.

Children
Ketanserin dose should be reduced in relation to body surface area or weight. Otherwise no special precautions are needed.

Pregnant women
Ketanserin has been used in pre-eclampsia or eclampsia. As for all new drugs, potential benefits should clearly outweigh the potential risk. There are few studies on the use of ketanserin in pregnant women. However, in one study there was a tendency for increased morbidity among infants born to mothers treated with ketanserin compared to those treated with α-methyldopa.[85]

The elderly
No special precautions are required. Ketanserin has been claimed to have special benefits in this age group although more evidence is needed.

Concurrent disease
In patients with severe liver disease the ketanserin dose should not exceed 20 mg twice daily due to reduced elimination. In patients with severe renal insufficiency undergoing haemodialysis, steady-state levels of ketanserin were similar to those in patients with normal kidney function. Ketanserin is not removed by haemodialysis.

Drug interactions

Potentially hazardous interactions

Potassium-losing diuretics. Combination with potassium-losing diuretics should be avoided since this can exacerbate ventricular arrhythmias.

Antiarrhythmics of classes Ia, Ic and III. Concomitant treatment with drugs which prolong repolarization or markedly depress conduction and affect repolarization differentially should be avoided.[74,75]

Other significant interactions
Specific interaction studies have revealed that co-administration of ketanserin with digoxin,[38] digitoxin,[86] propranolol[87] and metoprolol[51] does not meaningfully alter the pharmacokinetics of either drug. In vitro experiments have indicated that the plasma protein binding of ketanserin does not influence (or is influenced by) the protein binding of other highly bound drugs.[42] Furthermore, there is no evidence that ketanserin induces or reduces hepatic enzyme systems and it is unlikely that ketanserin treatment will have important effect on the metabolism of concurrently administered drugs.[88]

Potentially useful interactions
The effects of ketanserin and β-blockers or (potassium-sparing) diuretics are additive in patients who respond poorly to either drug alone.

Major outcome trials

1. Prevention of Artherosclerotic Complications with Ketanserin (PACK) Trial Group 1989 Platelet function during long term treatment with ketanserin of claudication patients with peripheral artherosclerosis. A multicenter, double-blind, placebo-controlled trial. Thrombosis Research 55: 13–23

A large prospective trial, the PACK (Prevention of Atherosclerotic Complications with Ketanserin) trial,[75] was set up to confirm retrospective pooled findings of studies in claudication patients, which suggested a reduction in major cardiovascular events with ketanserin as compared to placebo.[89] A total of 3899 patients with claudication were included; 1930 received ketanserin 40 mg three times daily and 1969 received placebo for at least one year. The incidence (intention to treat analysis) of primary endpoints (definite myocardial infarction, major stroke, amputation above the ankle, excision of ischaemic viscera, death from vascular causes and secondary vascular complications) was similar in both groups (436 ketanserin vs 474 placebo) and the overall mortality in ketanserin group was 117% of that in placebo group. Secondary analysis revealed an adverse interaction between ketanserin and potassium wasting diuretics resulting in cardiac events. Subgroup analysis when patients taking diuretics and/or antiarrhythmics were excluded indicated that total number of cardiovascular events were less frequent during ketanserin treatment ($p = 0.02$) and that multiple events was reduced by 51% in ketanserin group ($p = 0.006$). The number of primary events, however, was not significantly less common (25%) in the ketanserin group.

References

1. Leysen J E, Awouters F, Kennis L, Laduron P M 1981 Receptor binding profile of R 41 468, a novel antagonist at 5-HT_2 receptors. Life Science 28: 1015–1022
2. Van Nueten J M, Janssen P A J, Van Beek J, Xhonneaux R, Verbeuren T J, Vanhoutte P M 1981 Vascular effects of ketanserin (R41 468), a novel antagonist of 5-HT_2 receptors. Journal of Pharmacology and Experimental Therapeutics 218: 217–230
3. DeClerck F, David J-L, Janssen P A J 1982 Inhibition of 5-hydroxytryptamine-induced and -amplified human platelet aggregation by ketanserin (R41 468), a selective 5-HT_2 receptor antagonist. Agents and Actions 12: 388–397
4. DeClerck F 1986 Review: blood platelets in human essential hypertension. Agents and Actions 18: 563–580
5. Pettersson A, Gradin K, Hedner T, Persson B 1985 Antihypertensive mechanism of action of ketanserin and some ketanserin analogues in the spontaneously hypertensive rat. Naunyn Schmiedeberg's Archives of Pharmacology 329: 394–397
6. Fozard J R 1982 Mechanism of the hypotensive effect of ketanserin. Journal of Cardiovascular Pharmacology 4: 829–838
7. Wenting G J, Man in't Veld A J, Woittiez A J J, Bommsma F, Schalekamp M A D H 1982 5-HT, alpha-adrenoceptors, and blood pressure: effects of ketanserin in essential hypertension and autonomic insufficiency. Hypertension 6: 100–109
8. Zabludowski J R, Zoccali C, Isles C G et al 1984 Effect of the 5-hydroxytryptamine type 2 receptor antagonist, ketansein, on blood pressure, the renin–angiotensin system and the sympatho-adrenal function in patients with essential hypertension. British Journal of Clinical Pharmacology 17: 309–316
9. Hedner T, Persson B 1988 Experience with ketanserin and ritanserin in hypertensive patients. Journal of Cardiovascular Pharmacology 11 (suppl 1): S44–S48
10. Ramage A G The effects of ketanserin, methysergide and LY 53 857 on sympathetic nerve activity. European Journal of Pharmacology 113: 295–303
11. Gradin K, Pettersson A, Hedner T, Persson B 1989 Central sympathoinhibitory effect of ketanserin in the spontaneously hypertensive rat. Pharmacology and Toxicology 64: 352–355
12. Vanhoutte P, Amery A, Birkenhager W et al 1988 Serotonergic mechanisms in hypertension. Focus on the effects of ketanserin. Hypertension 11: 111–133
13. Reimann I W, Okonkwo P O, Klotz U 1983 Pharmacokinetics of ketanserin in man. European Journal of Clinical Pharmacology 25: 73–76
14. Degli Uberti E C, Trasforini G, Margutti A R, Rotola C A, Pansini R 1982 Effect of ketanserin, a new inhibitor of 5-HT_2 receptors, on plasma renin activity and aldosterone levels in normal subjects. Hormonal Research 16: 244–248
15. Blauw G J, van Brummelen P, Chang P C, Vermeij P, Van Zweiten P A 1987 Effects of 5-hydroxytryptamine and ketanserin on the forearm vascular resistance in man. British Journal of Clinical Pharmacology 23: 631P
16. Jageneau A H M, Horig C, Loots W, Symoens J 1980 Plethysmographic registration of volume changes in hand vein: effects of serotonin and of a specific antagonist. Angiology 31: 828–832
17. Bounameaux H, Holditch T, Hellermans H, Berent A, Verhagen R 1985 Placebo controlled double-blind two-centre trial of ketanserin in intermittent claudication. Lancet 2: 1268–1271
18. De Cree J, Leempoels J, Geuskens H, Verhagen H 1985 Comparison of blood pressure ratio by doppler velocitymetry and by plethysmography during treatment with ketanserin, a 5-HT_2-receptor antagonist: a measure of improved collateral and microcirculatory flow. Journal of Cardiovascular Pharmacology 7 (suppl 7): 592–594
19. Kunnen J J, Dahler H P, Doorenspleet J G, Van Oene J C 1988 Effects of intra-arterial ketanserin in Raynaud's phenomenon assessed by ^{99m}Tc-pertechnetate scintigraphy. European Journal of Clinical Pharmacology 34: 267–271
20. Seibolt J R, Terregino C A 1986 Selective antagonism of S_2-serotonergic receptors relieves but do not prevent cold induced vasoconstriction in primary Raynaud's phenomenon. Journal of Rheumatology 13: 337–340
21. Stranden E, Roald O K, Krogh K 1982 Treatment of Raynaud's phenomenon with the 5-HT_2-receptor antagonist ketanserin. British Medical Journal 285: 1069–1071
22. DeClerck F, Xhonneaux B 1985 Continuous inhibition of platelet S_2-serotonergic receptors during chronic administration of ketanserin in humans. Journal of Cardiovascular Pharmacology 7 (suppl 7): S23–S25
23. De Cree J, Leempoels J, Demoen B, Roels V, Verhagen H 1985 The effect of ketanserin, a 5-HT_2-receptor antagonist, on 5-hydroxytryptamine-induced irreversible platelet aggregation in patients with cardiovascular diseases. Agents and Actions 16: 313–317

Ketanserin (tartrate)

24. Vermylen J, Arnout J, Deckmyn H, Xhonneaux B, DeClerck F 1986 Continuous inhibition of the platelet S_2-serotonergic receptors during the long term administration of ketanserin. Thrombotic Research 42: 721–723
25. Zannad F, Voisin P, Pointel J P, Schmitt C, Fraitag B, Stoltz J F 1985 Effects of ketanserin on platelet function and red cell filterability in hypertension and peripheral vascular disease. Journal of Cardiovascular Pharmacology 7 (suppl 7): S32–S34
26. Bogar L, Matrai A, Walker R T, Flute P T, Dormandy J A 1985 Haemorheological effects of a 5-HT_2-receptor antagonist (ketanserin). Clinical Hemorheology 5: 115–121
27. Walker R T, Matrai A, Bogar L, Dormandy J A 1985 Serotonin and the flow properties of blood. Journal of Cardiovascular Pharmacology 7 (suppl 7): S35–S37
28. De Cree J, Geukens H, Leempoels J, Demoen B, Verhagen H 1985 The effects of ketanserin, a 5-HT_2-receptor antagonist on the impaired blood cell filtration in patients with acute myocardial infarction. Clinical Hemorrheology 5: 115–121
29. Omvik P, Lund-Johansen P 1983 Long-term effects on central hemodynamics and body fluid volumes of ketanserin in essential hypertension: studies at rest and during dynamic exercise. Journal of Hypertension 1: 405–412
30. De Leeuw P W, Van Es P N, Van Soest D A W, Tchang P T, Birkanhäger W H 1983 Effects of chronic oral treatment with ketanserin, a new 5-HT_2-antagonist in essential hypertension. Journal of Hypertension 4 (suppl 2): 379–380
31. Wenting G J, Man in't Veld A J, Woittiez A J J, Boomsma F, Schalekamp M A D H 1982 Treatment of hypertension with ketanserin, a new selective 5-HT_2 receptor antagonist. British Medical Journal 284: 537–539
32. Navis G, De Jong P E, Van Der Hem G K, De Zeuw D 1986 Renal effects of ketanserin in essential hypertension. Journal of Hypertension 4 (suppl 1): S95–S98
33. Cameron H C, Waller P C, Ramsay L E 1987 The effect of ketanserin on the QT interval. British Journal of Clinical Pharmacology 23: 630P
34. Stott D J, McLenachan J M, Ball S G 1986 Ketanserin, the QT interval and autonomic function testing in normal subjects. British Journal of Clinical Pharmacology 21: 84P
35. Donnelly R, Elliot H L, Meredith P A, Hughes D M A, Reid J L 1988 Ketanserin concentration–effect relationships in individual hypertensive patients. British Journal of Clinical Pharmacology 26: 61–64
36. Lindelauf F 1983 Determination of ketanserin and its major metabolite (reduced ketanserin) in human plasma by high performance liquid chromatography. Journal of Chromatography 277: 396–400
37. Okonkwo P O, Reimann I W, Woestenborghs R, Klotz U 1983 High-performance liquid chromatography assay with fluorimetric detection of ketanserin, a new antihypertensive agent and serotonin S_2 antagonist in human plasma. Journal of Chromatography 272: 411–416
38. Person B, Heykants J, Hedner T 1990 Clinical pharmacokinetics of ketanserin. Clinical Pharmacokinetics (in press)
39. Heykants J, van Peer A, Woestenborghs R, Gould S, Mills J 1986 Pharmacokinetics of ketanserin and its metabolite ketanserin-ol in man after intravenous, intramuscular and oral administration. European Journal of Clinical Pharmacology 31: 343–350
40. Trenk D, Mosler A, Kirch W, Meinertz T, Jänchen E 1983 Pharmacokinetics and pharmacodynamics of the 5-HT_2-receptor antagonist ketanserin in man. Journal of Cardiovascular Pharmacology 5: 1034–1039
41. Persson B, Pettersson A, Hedner T 1987 Pharmacokinetics of ketanserin in patients with essential hypertension. European Journal of Clinical Pharmacology 32: 259–265
42. Meuldermans W, van Houdt J, Mostmans E, Knaeps F, Verluyten W, Heykants J 1988 Plasma protein binding of ketanserin and its distribution in blood. Arzneimittel-Forschung 38(I): 794–800
43. Van Peer A, Woestenborghs R, Embrechts L, Heykants J 1986 Pharmacokinetic approach to equilibrium between ketanserin and ketanserin-ol. European Journal of Clinical Pharmacology 31: 339–342
44. Uji Y, Ikeda M, Deguchi T, Sugimoto T, Kobayashi S 1988 Phase I study of KJK-945 (ketanserin-tartrate). Journal of Clinical Therapeutical Medicine 4 (suppl 1): 3–20
45. Meuldermans W, Hendrickx J, Woestenborghs R et al 1988 Absorption, metabolism and excretion of ketanserin in man after oral administration. Arzneimittel-Forschung 38 (I): 789–794
46. Lebrec D, Hadengue A, Gaudin C, Levron J C, Fraitag B, Berhelot P, Benhamon J P 1990 Pharmacokinetics of ketanserin in patients with cirrhosis. Clinical Pharmacokinetics (in press)
47. Barendregt J N M, van Peer A, van den Hoeven J G, Oene J C, Tjandra Y I 1990 Ketanserin pharmacokinetics in patients with renal failure. British Journal of Clinical Pharmacology
48. Proppe D, Manthei P 1989 Effect von Ketanserin bei Langzeitbehandlung von Hypertonikern mit eingeschrankter Nierenfunktion. Tagund der deutschen Gesellschaft fur Innere Medizin, Weisbaden, Germany, April 2–6, Nr 95
49. Onoyama K, Oochi N, Ando T, Fujishima M, Uji Y, Kobayashi S 1988 Pharmacokinetic properties of ketanserin in patients with chronic renal failure after single-dose oral administration. Current Therapeutic Research 43: 1099–1108
50. Zazgornik J, Scholz N, Kuska J, Minar E 1986 Plasma concentrations of ketanserin in chronic hemodialyzed patients. Internal Journal of Clinical Pharmacology and Therapeutical Toxicity 24: 674–676
51. Hedner T, Pettersson A, Persson B 1986 Blood pressure reduction and pharmacokinetics of ketanserin in hypertensive patients. Journal of Hypertension 4 (suppl 1): S91–S93
52. Donnelly R, Elliot H L, Meredith P A, Reid J L 1987 Acute and chronic ketanserin in essential hypertension: antihypertensive mechanisms and pharmacokinetics. British Journal of Clinical Pharmacology 24: 599–606
53. Breckenridge A 1986 Ketanserin — a new antihypertensive agent. Journal of Hypertension 4 (suppl 1): S13–S16
54. Andrén L, Svensson A, Dahlöf B, Eggertsen R, Hansson L 1983 Ketanserin in hypertension, early clinical evaluation and dose finding study of a new 5-HT2 receptor antagonist. Acta Medica Scandinavica 214: 125–130
55. Hedner T, Persson B, Berglund G 1985 A comparative and long-term evaluation of ketanserin in the treatment of essential hypertension. Journal of Cardiovascular Pharmacology 7 (suppl 7): S148–S153
56. Fagard R, Fiochi R, Lijnen P et al 1984 Haemodynamic and humoral responses to chronic ketanserin treatment in essential hypertension. British Heart Journal 51: 149–156
57. Cameron H A, Ramsay L E 1985 Ketanserin in essential hypertension: a double-blind, placebo-controlled study. Postgraduate Medical Journal 61: 583–586
58. DeCree J, Leempoels J, Geukens H, De Cock W, Verhaegen H 1981 the antihypertensive effects of ketanserin (R41 468), a novel 5-hydroxytryptamine-blocking agent, in patients with essential hypertension. Clinical Science 61: 473S–476S
59. McGourty J C, Silas J H, Cowen K J 1985 Controlled trial of ketanserin in hypertension. British Journal of Clinical Pharmacology 20: 37–40
60. Wellens D, Peeters G, Baeten B, Sieben G, Symoens J 1986 Double-blind comparison of ketanserin with placebo in patients with essential hypertension
61. Rosendorff C, Murray G D 1986 Ketanserin versus metoprolol and hydrochlorothiazide in essential hypertension: only ketanserin's hypotensive effect is age-related. Journal of Hypertension 4 (suppl 6): S109–S111
62. Sheps S G, Schirger A, Zachariah P K et al 1987 Comparison of ketanserin and metoprolol in the treatment of essential hypertension. Archives of Internal Medicine 147: 291–296
63. Janssens M, Symoens J 1986 Ketanserin compared to nifedipine and methyldopa in patients aged above 50 years: two international multicenter studies. Journal of Hypertension 4 (suppl 6): S115–S118
64. Stokes G S, Mennie B A, Marwood J F 1986 Ketanserin and prazosin: a comparison of antihypertensive and biochemical effects. Clinical Pharmacology and Therapeutics 40: 56–63
65. Meyer P, Safar M 1988 Comparison of ketanserin and captopril in older hypertensives. A double-blind randomized trial. Drugs 36 (suppl 1): 144–147
66. Hedner T, Persson B 1984 Ketanserin in combination with beta-adrenergic receptor blocking agents in the treatment of essential hypertension. British Journal of Clinical Pharmacology 18: 765–771
67. Woittiez A J J, Wenting G J, Van Den Meiracker A H et al 1986 Chronic effect of ketanserin in mild to moderate essential hypertension. Hypertension 8: 167–173
68. Hedner T, Persson B, Berglund G 1984 Experience with ketanserin, a serotonin (S2) antagonist, in longterm treatment of essential hypertension. Clinical and Experimental Hypertension (A) 6: 743–751
69. Murphy B F, Witworth J A, Kincaid-Smith P 1985 Ketanserin in the acute management of severe hypertension. Journal of Cardiovascular Pharmacology 7 (suppl 7): S168–S171
70. Milei J, Lemus J, Schiavone M, Lucioni M C 1987 Ketanserin in parental treatment of acute essential hypertension: a dose response curve. Journal of Cardiovascular Pharmacology 10 (suppl 3): 120–124
71. Griffiths H B A, Whitwam J G 1986 Ketanserin and the cardiovascular system: II. A study of its effect in patients undergoing myocardial revascularization. Anaesthesia 41: 712–716
72. Houghton K, Carter J A 1986 Peri-operative management of carcinoid syndrome using ketanserin. Anaesthesia 41: 596–599
73. Weiner C P, Socol M L, Vaisrab N 1984 Control of pre-eclamptic hypertension by ketanserin, a new serotonin receptor antagonist. American Journal of Obstetrics and Gynecology 149: 496–500
74. Singh B n, Nademanee K, Symoens J, Janssens M 1987 Ketanserin and QT_c prolongation. European Heart Journal 8: 667–668
75. Prevention of Artherosclerotic Complications with Ketanserin (PACK) Trial Group 1989 Platelet function during log term treatment with ketanserin of claudication patients with peripheral artherosclerosis. A multicenter, double-blind, placebo-controlled trial. Thrombosis Research 55: 13–23
76. Jennings A A, Opie L H 1987 Effects of intravenous ketanserin on severely hypertensive patients with double-blind crossover assessment of central side effects. Journal of Cardiovascular Pharmacology 9: 120–124
77. Zoccali C, Zabludowski J R, Isles C G et al 1983 The effect of a 5-HT antagonist, ketanerin, on blood pressure, the renin–angiotensin system and sympatho-adrenal function in normal man. British Journal of Clinical Pharmacology 16: 305–311
78. Gordin A, Mustajoki P, Pelkonen R 1985 Ketanserin without effect of basal anterior pituitary hormone secretion in healthy subjects. Journal of Endocrinological Investigations 8: 73–75
79. O'Malley B P, Jennings P E, Cook N, Barnett D B, Rosenthal F D 1984 The role of serotonin (5-HT) in the control of TSH and prolactin release in euthyroid subjects assessed by administration of ketanserin (5-HT_2 antagonist) and zimelidine (5-HT) reuptake inhibitor). Psychoneuroendocrinology 9: 13–19
80. Symoens J, Janssens M 1986 Ketanserin: a novel cardiovascular drug. Drug Development Research 8: 159–172
81. Rosenthal J, Koehle W, Gruebel B, Fisher R 1986 Moderate essential hypertension control: a double blind crossover study between a serotonin antagonist and a post-synaptic alpha-blocker. Journal of Hypertension 4 (suppl 1): S85–S87
82. Amery A, Fagard R, Fiocchi R, Lijnen P, Staessen J, Vanhees L 1985 Ketanserin: new hypotensive drug? Journal of Cardiovascular Pharmacology 7 (suppl 7): S176–S182
83. Nakamura H, Hirata F, Yasugi T, Mizuno M, Saito E et al 1988 Effects of ketanserin tartrate on serum lipids in patients with essential hypertension. Drugs 36 (suppl 1): 25–34
84. Janka H U, Mehnert H, Fisher R, Seiler K-U 1988 Influence of ketanserin on glucose and lipid metabolism in diabetic patients with hypertension. Drugs 36 (suppl 1): 123–125
85. Voto L S, Zin C, Neira J, Lapidus A M, Marguiles M Ketanserin versus alpha-methyldopa in the treatment of hypertension of pregnancy (in press)
86. Ochs H R, Verburg-Ochs B, Holler M, Greenblatt H D J 1985 Effect of ketanserin on the kinetics of digoxin and digitoxin. Journal of Cardiovascular Pharmacology 7: 205–207

87. Ochs H R, Greenblatt D J, Holer M, Labedzky 1987 The interactions of propranolol and ketanserin. Clinical Pharmacology and Therapeutics 41: 55–60
88. Waller P C, Tucker G T, Ramsay L E 1987 Lack of effect of ketanserin on indices of hepatic enzyme induction. British Journal of Clinical Pharmacology 24: 118–119
89. Clement D L, Duprez D 1990 Effect of ketanserin in the treatment of patients with intermittent claudication. Results from 13 placebo-controlled parallel group studies. Journal of Cardiovascular Pharmacology (in press)

Ketazolam

Ketazolam is a long-acting benzodiazepine that is used in the treatment of anxiety and spasticity.

Chemistry

Ketazolam (Anxon, Contamex, Loftran, Solatran)
$C_{20}H_{17}ClN_2O_3$
11-Chloro-(8,12b-dihydro)-2,8-dimethyl-12b-phenyl-4H-[1,3]oxazino[3,2-d][1,4]benzodiazepine-4,7(6H)-dione

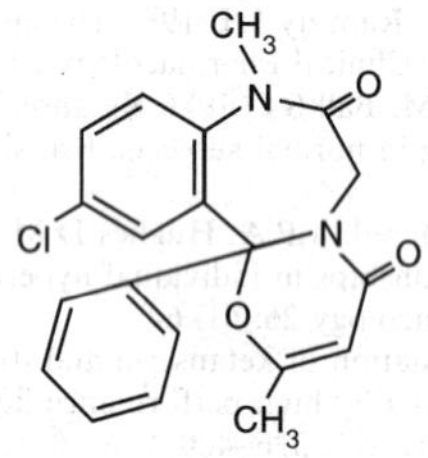

Molecular weight	368.8
pKa	—
Solubility	
in alcohol	1 in 100
in water	<1 in 1000
Octanol/water partition coefficient	—

The drug is a white monomorphic crystalline powder prepared by chemical synthesis.

Pharmacology

Benzodiazepine compounds exhibit specific and high affinity binding to sites within the central nervous system, leading to profound but reversible alterations in the kinetics of a GABA-dependent transmembrane chloride channel and enhancement of GABA-ergic synaptic inhibition within the CNS. It is likely that binding of benzodiazepine compounds to such receptors is at least partly responsible for their clinical effects since there is broad agreement between the relative binding affinities of different benzodiazepines in vitro and their pharmacological potency in vivo. Ketazolam is bound with high affinity to the benzodiazepine binding sites. It is metabolised rapidly and its metabolites have major biological effects.

In common with other benzodiazepine compounds, ketazolam exhibits hypnotic, antianxiety, anticonvulsant and muscle relaxant effects when administered to laboratory animals.

Toxicology

The oral LD_{50} in the rat is greater than 5000 $mg.kg^{-1}$ and greater than 2500 $mg.kg^{-1}$ in the mouse when administered intraperitoneally.[1] Subacute and chronic toxicity testing in animals has revealed no clinically relevant adverse effects. Animal testing has not revealed any teratogenicity.

Clinical pharmacology

Ketazolam is an effective anxiolytic drug in clinical practice. Early open studies suggested that ketazolam provides useful anxiolytic activity in the treatment of severe anxiety,[2,3] though high doses (up to 300 mg daily) were used.[2] Subsequent short-term (four weeks), placebo-controlled, double-blind, crossover studies have confirmed that once daily oral ketazolam is an effective treatment for moderate to severe anxiety, with the optimum dose being approximately 50 mg:[4–7] An improvement in symptoms was consistently observed after one week of continuous administration, and this improvement was generally sustained. Several double-blind studies have compared the anxiolytic efficacy and side-effect profile of ketazolam with that of diazepam,[8–12] and have shown that ketazolam has an anxiolytic potency that is approximately half that of diazepam. Several of these studies reported a higher incidence of adverse effects, particularly drowsiness, in diazepam-treated patients. This observation is probably attributable to poor study design, since these studies compared the effects of ketazolam administered at bedtime with diazepam given three times daily. Despite this, these data have been used to suggest that ketazolam has a side-effect profile that is superior to that of diazepam.[1] Generally similar results were obtained in studies comparing ketazolam with clorazepate[13,14] and lorazepam.[15] Ketazolam remains effective in the longer term;[16] continued usage may necessitate an increase in dose,[16] but there are no good data on the development of pharmacological tolerance. Anxiety symptoms may recur following cessation of treatment,[16] but systematic studies are unavailable.

Ketazolam appears as effective as diazepam in the treatment of spasticity associated with multiple sclerosis and previous cerebrovascular accident.[17]

Pharmacokinetics

Many analytical methods have been applied to the measurement of benzodiazepine compounds in plasma.[18] High performance liquid chromatography (HPLC) to compare samples with internal standards has performance characteristics that are adequate for routine use.[19]

Ketazolam is well absorbed following oral administration, and peak plasma concentrations of the parent compound are reached after two hours. After a single dose of radiolabelled ketazolam, peak plasma concentrations of approximately 4 μg.l^{-1} of ketazolam and 17 μg.l^{-1} of diazepam were measured at 2 h and 10 h respectively.[19]

In common with other benzodiazepine compounds, ketazolam is highly protein-bound. Ketazolam is extensively metabolized to compounds with important biological activity (see below). The elimination half life of unchanged ketazolam is very short, being approximately 1.5 h. After a single 30 mg oral dose of ^{14}C-ketazolam, 80% of the radioactivity is excreted in the urine and 20% in the faeces.[20] The major urinary metabolite is oxazepam, primarily in a conjugated form.

Oral absorption	~100%
Presystemic metabolism	—
Plasma half life	
range	1–5 h
Volume of distribution	—
Plasma protein binding	—

Concentration–effect relationship

Gottschalk and others found no significant correlation between ketazolam/N-desmethylketazolam levels and anxiety or hostility parameters in chronic alcoholics undergoing alcohol withdrawal after 21 days treatment.[21] Studies with other benzodiazepine compounds have yielded inconsistent results.[18] Knowledge of plasma levels does not influence the management of benzodiazepine overdosage, but may occasionally be helpful in the diagnosis of poor compliance with medication.

Metabolism

Ketazolam is rapidly metabolized by the liver to desmethyl metabolites, particularly N-desmethylketazolam and N-desmethyldiazepam, each with a plasma half life of 50 h.[20] High levels of these metabolites appear in the plasma, together with a low level of the unchanged drug and a small amount of diazepam (Fig. 1). Since these compounds have major biological effects, it is likely that the desmethyl metabolites account for the anxiolytic effects of ketazolam when administered once daily. Diazepam is also metabolized to desmethyldiazepam, which explains why the pharmacodynamic and side-effect profile of ketazolam is so similar to that of diazepam. The major urinary metabolite is oxazepam which is excreted primarily in the glucuronide form.

Fig. 1 The metabolism of ketazolam

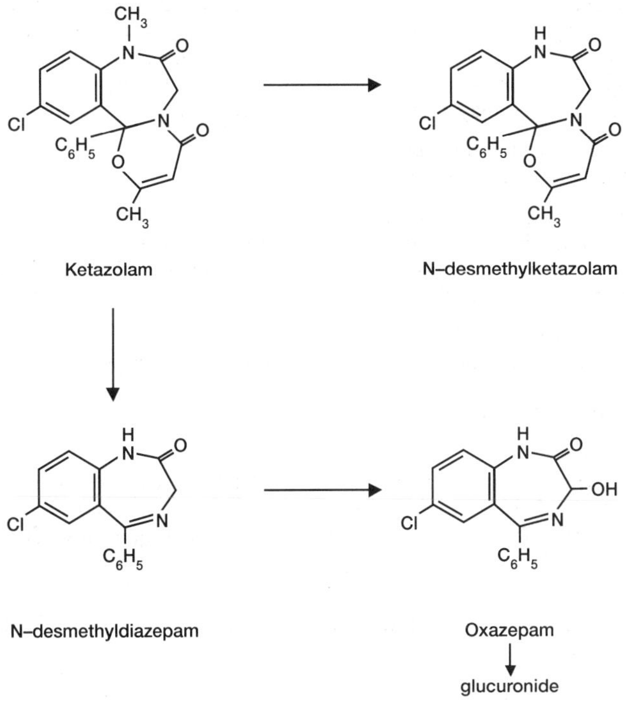

Pharmaceutics

Ketazolam (Anxon; Smith Kline Beecham, UK) is available as dark pink/light pink capsules, in two sizes containing 15 mg or 30 mg ketazolam, overprinted with the product name 'Anxon' and the strength.

Therapeutic use

Indications

1. Treatment of anxiety, tension, irritability and similar stress-related symptoms
2. Management of spasticity associated with conditions such as spinal cord trauma, cerebrovascular accident and multiple sclerosis.

Contraindications

1. Known hypersensitivity to benzodiazepine compounds
2. Phobic or obsessional states
3. Chronic psychosis.

Mode of use

For all indications, treatment is begun with a single oral dose of 30 mg, taken before retiring. The effective dose range is usually 15–60 mg, taken either as a single dose before retiring or in divided doses.

Doses as high as 200 mg daily may be required in the treatment of spasticity. Though there are no data concerning rebound anxiety following sudden withdrawal of therapy, nor concerning dependence, it should be assumed to occur,[22] and therefore therapy should be tailed off gradually.

Adverse reactions

As with other benzodiazepine compounds, most reported adverse effects are related to the primary pharmacological action of this group of compounds. Virtually all such adverse effects are dose-related.[23]

Potentially life-threatening effects

None has been reported.

K

Acute overdosage
It is extremely difficult for physically healthy individuals to commit suicide by deliberate overdosage of any benzodiazepine taken alone. Symptoms of overdosage may include drowsiness and ataxia, with coma in severe cases. Symptomatic treatment only is required. Gastric lavage may be useful if performed soon after ingestion.

Severe or irreversible adverse effects
None has been reported.

Symptomatic adverse effects
Other than drowsiness and lightheadedness, the incidence of symptomatic side effects is no greater than that which is observed during treatment with placebo.

Interference with clinical pathology tests
No interferences of this kind appear to have been reported.

High risk groups

Neonates
According to the Anxon data sheet, there are insufficient data to recommend the administration of ketazolam to children of any age.

Breast milk. It is recommended that the drug be avoided by breast-feeding mothers.

Children
What has been said above about neonates also applies to older children.

Pregnant women
Studies in humans have not been performed but it is recommended that ketazolam should not be administered during pregnancy.

The elderly
There are no specific data on the pharmacokinetics of ketazolam in the elderly. Bresolin et al found that ketazolam 15 mg was an effective anxiolytic agent in more than 80% of elderly patients,[23] though 43% of the placebo patients also responded to treatment. The data sheet recommends that a reduced dosage be used initially in elderly patients.

Drug interactions

Potentially hazardous interactions
There are no reports of adverse drug reactions specific to ketazolam, but in common with the other benzodiazepines, ketazolam may potentiate other centrally acting agents such as alcohol, tranquillisers, antidepressants, hypnotics, analgesics and anaesthetics.

Potentially useful interactions
None has been reported.

General review articles

Owen R T 1980 Ketazolam. Drugs of Today 16: 295–297

References

1. Anxon product booklet. Beecham Research Laboratories.
2. Gallant D M, Guerrero-Figueroa R, Swanson W C 1973 U-28,774 (Ketazolam): an early evaluation of a new antianxiety agent. Current Therapeutic Research 15: 123–126
3. Fabre L F, Harris R T 1974 Pilot open-label study on U-29,774 in anxious patients. Current Therapeutic Research 16: 848–852
4. Fabre L F, Harris R T, Stubbs D F 1976 Double-blind controlled efficacy study of ketazolam (U-28,774). Journal of International Medical Research 4: 50–54
5. Bowden C L 1978 Double-blind placebo-controlled trial of ketazolam in anxiety. Current Therapeutic Research 24: 170–178
6. Cohn J B, Gottschalk L A 1980 Double-blind comparison of ketazolam and placebo using once-a-day dosing. Journal of Clinical Pharmacology 20: 676–680
7. Owieczka J, Van Meerbeeck P, Nystrom C, Lens F 1981 Double-blind comparison of ketazolam and placebo administered once a day in the treatment of anxiety. Acta Therapeutica 7: 159–174
8. Fabre L F, McLendon D M, Gainey A 1978 Double-blind comparison of ketazolam administered once a day with diazepam and placebo in anxious out-patients. Current Therapeutic Research 24: 875–882
9. Multi-centre Study 1980 A double blind comparison of ketazolam given once each day with diazepam given in divided doses and placebo in the treatment of anxiety. British Journal of Clinical Practice 34: 117–123
10. Feighner J P 1980 Ketazolam once-a-day in the treatment of anxiety: a double blind comparison with diazepam and placebo. Current Therapeutic Research 28: 425–431
11. Kim K K, Sirman A, Trainor F S, Lee B Y 1980 Anxiolytic efficacy and safety of ketazolam compared with diazepam and placebo. Clinical Therapeutics 3: 9–14

Ketazolam

12. Davies J G, Rose A J 1980 A double-blind comparison of ketazolam given once each day with diazepam given in divided doses and placebo in the treatment of anxiety. Multicentre study. British Journal of Clinical Practice 37: 107–113
13. Fabre L F, McLendon D M 1979 Ketazolam administered once-a-day compared to clorazepate t.i.d. and placebo in a double-blind study to anxious out-patients. Current Therapeutic Research 25: 710–720
14. Nair N P V, Singh A N 1982 Ketazolam in the treatment of anxiety: a standard- and placebo-controlled study. Current Therapeutic Research 31: 679–691
15. Perez-Rincon H, Alvarez-Rueda J M, Trujillo A 1981 A comparative double-blind study between ketazolam and lorazepam in the treatment of anxiety. Current Therapeutic Research 29: 936–942
16. Fabre L F, McLendon D M, Stephens A G 1981 Comparison of the therapeutic effect, tolerance and safety of ketazolam and diazepam administered for six months with chronic anxiety neurosis. Journal of International Medical Research 9: 191–198
17. Basmajian J V, Shankardass K, Russell D 1984 Ketazolam treatment for spasticity: double-blind study of a new drug. Archives of Physical Medicine and Rehabilitation 65: 698–701
18. Norman T R, Burrows G D 1984 Plasma concentrations of benzodiazepines — a review of clinical findings and implications. Progress in Neuro-Psychopharmacology and Biological Psychiatry 8: 115–126
19. Kabra P M, Stevens G L, Marian L J 1978 High pressure liquid chromatographic analysis of diazepam, oxazepam and N-desmethyldiazepam in human blood. Journal of Chromatography 150: 355–360
20. Eberts F S, Philopoulos Y, Reineke L M, Vliek R W, Metxler C N 1977 Disposition of ketazolam, a new anxiolytic agent. Pharmacologist 19: 165
21. Gottschalk L A, Cohn J B 1978 The relationship of diazepam and ketazolam blood levels to anxiety and hostility in chronic alcoholics. Psychopharmacology Bulletin 14: 39–43
22. Edwards J G 1981 Adverse effects of antianxiety drugs. Drugs 22: 495–514
23. Bresolin N, Monza G, Scarpini E et al 1988 Treatment of anxiety with ketazolam in elderly patients. Clinical Therapeutics 10: 536–542

Ketoconazole

Ketoconazole is an orally absorbed imidazole, active against a broad spectrum of pathogenic fungi.

Chemistry

Ketoconazole (Nizoral)
$C_{26}H_{28}Cl_2N_4O_4$
1-Acetyl -4-(4-(2-(2,4-dichlorophenyl) r-2-(1H-imidazol-1ylmethyl)-1,3-dioxolan-4-yl)methoxy)phenyl)piperazine

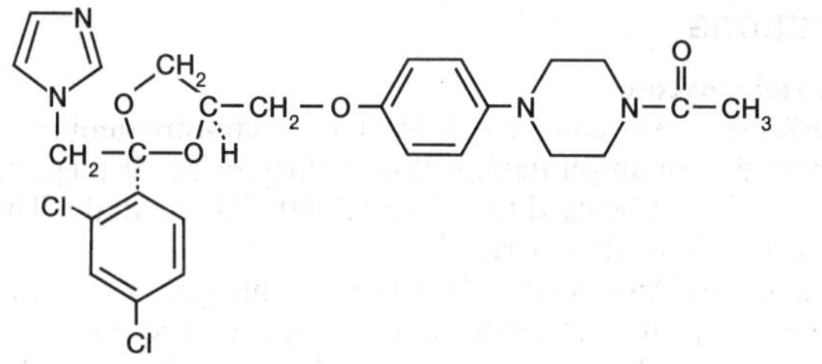

Molecular weight	531.4
pKa	6.51, 2.94
Solubility	
in alcohol	1 in 54
in water	almost insoluble
Octanol/water partition coefficient	5400 (pH 11.8)

Ketoconazole is an off-white or beige odourless powder prepared by chemical synthesis. It is not available in any combination preparation.

Pharmacology

Ketoconazole alters the permeability of yeast and fungal cell membranes. Inhibition of ergosterol biosynthesis, the major sterol of these cell membranes, is accompanied by accumulation of 14α-methylsterol.[1] A concentration of 0.01 μg.ml^{-1} inhibited the growth of *C. albicans* after 7 days culture, but toxic effects on human fibroblasts in vitro were only seen with concentrations over 100 μg.ml^{-1}.[2] The drug has also been shown to inhibit testosterone synthesis in humans and in isolated rat Leydig cells.[3] Serum and saliva testosterone concentrations fell to 30% of basal levels 4 to 6 hours after oral administration of the drug.[4] A fall in plasma levels of androstenedione during treatment with ketoconazole occurs in parallel with the fall in testosterone levels, and is accompanied by a rise in levels of 17α-hydroxyprogesterone suggesting that ketoconazole affects the enzyme C17–20 lyase.[5] The pharmacological effectiveness of the drug can be assessed in vitro by measurement of the minimal inhibitory concentration (MIC) of the fungal species being treated. However, this will depend on the individual organism, the size of innoculum and the culture medium.[6]

Toxicology

The LD_{50} for ketoconazole has been determined 7 days after a single dose in animal studies as follows[7] (all values are mg.kg^{-1} for male and female animals respectively): (a) intravenous administration: mice 47 and 42; rats 86 and 86; guinea pigs 23 and 33; dogs 42 and 56; (b) oral administration: mice 786 and 618; rats 287 and 166; guinea pigs 178 and 226; dogs 937 and 640.

Long-term treatment (20–52 weeks) in beagle dogs caused reversible anorexia, emesis, and rise in serum levels of hepatic enzymes at doses of 20–40 mg.kg^{-1} body weight. Higher doses (80 mg.kg^{-1}) caused jaundice and death within 4 weeks.

Histological changes were seen in liver, kidney, adrenals and ovaries of rats treated with 20–160 mg.kg^{-1}. Fertility was reduced in male rats treated with about 80 mg.kg^{-1} and in female rats treated with 40 mg.kg^{-1}.

Teratogenicity (oligodactylia and syndactylia) occurred in offspring of female rats treated with approximately 80 mg.kg^{-1} or more.[7]

No mutagenicity has been demonstrated (Ames test and others)[6] and no carcinogenic effects have been reported. Reports of hepatotoxicity in humans will be discussed later.

Clinical pharmacology

Ketoconazole is a broad-spectrum orally absorbed antifungal agent active against a wide variety of fungi and yeasts. In humans it suppresses testosterone[3] and adrenal steroid[8] levels.

The recommended daily dose is 200 mg daily as a single dose taken with a meal, usually for 14 days. In some infections where the response is poor 400 mg daily can be given.

The risk of hepatotoxicity increases with longer duration of treatment, but is particularly prominent in the first few months. Courses of greater than 14 days should only be given after due consideration of the risks; liver function should be monitored in such cases.

The incidence of reported symptomatic hepatic reactions is in the order of 1/10 000 to 1/15 000 and is usually reversible if treatment is stopped.[9–11]

In man, higher doses of up to 2 g daily have been used to treat serious coccidioidomycoccal meningitis.

Ketoconazole is also available as a topical formulation in a cream base for the treatment of superficial fungal and yeast infections; a shampoo formulation is used for pityriasis capitis.

Pharmacokinetics

The concentration of the drug in plasma can be measured by gas chromatography[12] which has a sensitivity of 10 μg.l^{-1} or by high performance liquid chromatography (HPLC)[13] which, using UV absorbance detection at 254 nm, has a detection limit of 2 μg.l^{-1} of plasma.[14]

Ketoconazole is readily but incompletely absorbed after oral dosing. Although the manufacturers recommend that the drug should be taken with a meal, there are conflicting reports regarding the effect of food on drug absorption.[15–19] Ketoconazole is lipophilic with poor water solubility except at low pH,[15] and absorption should therefore be increased in the presence of a meal. However, the demonstration that cimetidine,[16] antacids[16] and, in some studies, food[17] impair absorption can be explained by the basic nature of the drug. Although administration of ketoconazole with food is unlikely to be a cause of therapeutic failure,[18] patients requiring antacids or H_2 antagonists should take these at least 2 hours after ketoconazole.[16]

Peak serum concentrations of ketoconazole occur within 3 hours of administration and are proportional to dose.[15] In animals the drug is rapidly and widely distributed throughout the body[20] and it is likely that the same is true in man.

Although the volume of distribution is only 0.36 l.kg^{-1} (assuming an average weight of 70 kg)[21] ketoconazole is extensively bound in human whole blood (99%), with 84% to proteins and 15% to erythrocytes.[22] Distribution is not significantly altered by obesity.[19] Penetration into saliva is high[19] but detectable penetration into CSF occurs only in the presence of inflamed meninges[19] and concentrations attainable are inadequate for treatment of fungal meningitis.[23]

Although placental transfer is low the drug has been shown to be teratogenic when used in high dosage in rats,[7] and its use in pregnancy is therefore contraindicated. In dogs, the drug has been detected in breast milk at 22% of peak plasma values and it is therefore contraindicated in nursing mothers, although no human data are available.

Ketoconazole is extensively metabolized in the liver. It has been suggested that the elimination of ketoconazole is impaired in liver disease. Renal impairment has little effect on the kinetics of the drug.

The pharmacokinetics of ketoconazole have recently been extensively reviewed.[24]

Oral absorption	incomplete
Presystemic metabolism	significant
Plasma half life	
range	6–10 h
mean	
Volume of distribution	0.36 l.kg^{-1}
Plasma protein binding	99%

Concentration–effect relationship

Ketoconazole therapy is appropriate for a wide variety of organisms which have differing MICs:[6] concentration–effect relationship will therefore vary in each case.

Metabolism

Ketoconazole undergoes extensive hepatic metabolism, the major route of elimination being as metabolites in bile. In three human volunteers given ^{3}H-ketoconazole 2.5 mg.kg^{-1}, about 70% of the administered dose was excreted within 4 days (57% in faeces and 13% in urine). Of the faecal radioactivity 20–65% was due to unchanged drug, and 2–4% of urinary radioactivity.[25,26] First-pass presystemic elimination, which may be saturable, has been reported in some studies.[19,21,25] Double peaks in the serum concentration have been reported, suggesting that there may be enterohepatic circulation.[19] The major metabolic reactions in man are:

1. Oxidation of the imidazole ring followed by degradation of the oxidized imidazole (although the main metabolite has not been conclusively identified, this seems to be the most important of the metabolic pathways)
2. Oxidative degradation of the piperazine ring
3. Aromatic hydroxylation.

The precise identification of the major metabolites has not yet been determined[27] but they are thought not to be pharmacologically active. Ketoconazole inhibits the metabolism of many substates of P450-dependent oxidation, particularly P450 IIIA. Ketoconazole itself appears to be oxidised by P450 IIIA and inducers of this isoenzyme, such as rifampicin, reduce the plasma levels of the drug.

Pharmaceutics

Ketoconazole (Nizoral; Janssen, UK/US) is available as oral and topical formulations. None requires any special storage conditions.
Tablets: ketoconazole 200 mg. White, flat, half-scored, uncoated tablets marked 'JANSSEN' on one side and 'K/200' on the reverse. They also contain lactose and corn starch. Shelf-life is 5 years.
Suspension: ketoconazole 20 mg.ml^{-1}. Pink, cherry flavoured suspension in amber glass bottles of 100 ml. Also contains sodium benzoate and cherry cream flavour. Shelf-life is 3 years.
Topical: ketoconazole 2% w/w. White, non-staining, water-miscible cream. Contains propylene glycol, cetyl alcohol, stearyl alcohol, sorbitan monostearate, polysorbates 60 and 80, sodium bisulphite, isopropyl myristate. None of these is a notable contact sensitizer. Shelf-life is 3 years.
Shampoo: ketoconazole 2%. Contains sodium lauryl sulphate, disodium monolauryl sulphosuccinate, coconut fatty acid diethanolamide, laurdimonium hydrolysed animal collagen, macrogol 120 methyl glucose dioleate, imidurea, erythrosin, perfume and hydrochloric acid to pH 6.0.

Therapeutic use

Indications

Oral

1. Systemic mycoses: paracoccidioidomycosis, coccidioidomycosis, candidosis and histoplasmosis
2. Severe chronic mucocutaneous candidiasis
3. Disabling candidal chronic paronychia
4. Serious mycoses of the gastrointestinal tract not responsive, or resistant, to other therapy
5. Chronic vaginal candidosis not responsive to other therapy
6. Prophylaxis in immunosuppressed patients
7. Culturally determined dermatophyte infections (excluding toenails and toeclefts) unresponsive to other therapy.

Topical

1. Dermatophyte (ringworm) infections
2. Cutaneous candidosis
3. Pityriasis versicolor
4. Seborrhoeic dermatitis and pityriasis capitis (dandruff) due to *Pityrosporum* spp.

Contraindications

1. Pre-existing liver disease
2. Pregnancy
3. Nursing mothers
4. Hypersensitivity to imidazole drugs.

Mode of use

The treatment for systemic mycosis and dermatophyte infections is normally 200 mg ketoconazole daily for 14 days, or longer if clinical response is poor. The dose may be increased to 400 mg daily if response to 200 mg daily is poor. However it may be wise to measure plasma levels before increasing the dose (maximum 8 mg.kg^{-1}.day^{-1}).

Indications

1. Systemic mycoses

Candidosis. Systemic candidosis is a life-threatening condition best treated with amphotericin B or 5-flucytosine. If these drugs fail, ketoconazole can be used in a dose of 200–400 mg daily. This regime was effective in a small series.[28]

Paracoccidioidomycosis. This is a chronic granulomatous disease affecting skin, mucous membranes, lymph nodes, and occasionally internal organs. Ketoconazole, in a dose of 200 mg daily, is now considered drug of first choice for this condition,[29] and should be continued for 6 months.

Coccidioidomycosis. This disease is endemic in the western USA and varies from a benign respiratory infection to a disseminated fatal disease. In a review of 46 patients treated with ketoconazole, improvement was seen in the majority of cases during treatment although it was not possible to state that the drug was curative.[30] Doses used depended upon site and severity of infection. An initial dose of 200 mg daily is recommended.

Histoplasmosis. This is a pulmonary disease found worldwide, and endemic to the Mississippi and Ohio valleys in the USA. Ketoconazole 200 mg daily appears to be effective in patients who are not immunocompromised.[31,32]

2. Chronic mucocutaneous candidiasis

Ketoconazole is a major advance in the treatment of this chronic and often disabling disease which is due to cellular immunodeficiency.[33,34] The dose is 200–400 mg daily. Because of the underlying abnormality, relapses are common and repeated courses of ketoconazole may be required.

3. Disabling candidal chronic paronychia

Paronychia due to candida spp. is a fairly common condition but usually responds to topical treatments; systemic therapy is rarely required.

4. Mycoses of the gastrointestinal tract

Severe oral and oesophageal candidal infections, not responding to 'topical' treatment with antifungal lozenges, have been shown to respond to ketoconazole.[35]

5. Chronic vaginal candidosis

Ketoconazole is only indicated in the rare cases where topical treatment with pessaries has failed. It has been shown to be effective in almost 90% of cases.[36] The recommended dose is 400 mg once daily for five days.

6. Prophylaxis in immunosuppressed patients

Ketoconazole has been shown to be superior to oral amphotericin B and nystatin (neither of which is absorbed from the gastrointestinal tract) in the prophylactic treatment of patients immunocompromised due to haematological malignancies or their treatment.[37] Ketoconazole 400 mg daily (200 mg daily in children) was continued during therapy until patients had neutrophil counts of over $1.0 \times 10^9 l^{-1}$.

Ketoconazole

7. Resistant dermatophyte infections
Patients with *Trichophyton rubrum* infection of trunk and distal limbs who failed to respond to griseofulvin responded well to ketoconazole 200–400 mg daily.[33]

Topical treatment
Ketoconazole cream can be used, like other topical imidazoles, for the treatment of dermatophyte (ringworm) infection, cutaneous candidosis, or pityriasis versicolor (a yeast infection due to *Pityrosporum orbiculare*). It may either be used alone or in conjunction with a systemic agent.

Ketoconazole is recognized to be effective in treatment of seborrhoeic dermatitis,[38] but the cream and shampoo preparations have only recently been approved for treatment of seborrhoeic dermatitis and pityriasis capitis (dandruff). Evidence for the role of *Pityrosporum* spp. in the pathogenesis of these disorders and details of the effects of ketoconazole in their treatment, have been summarized by Shuster and colleagues.[39]

Contraindications

1. Pre-existing liver disease
Both biochemical and symptomatic hepatic reactions have occurred during ketoconazole treatment.[9] It has been suggested that ketoconazole metabolism is altered in the presence of hepatic insufficiency[19] although this is not supported by all studies.[32] It is suggested that ketoconazole should be given only when there is no alternative in the presence of previous hepatic injury.

2. Pregnancy
Teratogenicity in rats[7] is discussed above. The drug is therefore contraindicated in pregnancy.

3. Nursing mothers
Ketoconazole can be demonstrated in breast milk in dogs.[21] It is therefore contraindicated in women who are breast-feeding.

Adverse reactions

Potentially life-threatening effects

Hepatitis. Asymptomatic elevation of hepatic enzymes (ALT, AST, gamma GT, alkaline phosphatase) to 50% above normal levels were found in 14% of over 1000 patients.[9] Jaundice has been reported to occur in 1/10 000 patients worldwide,[9] and more recently 1/15 000 patients in the USA.[10] A small number of fatalities have been reported but the majority of these probably occurred in patients in whom therapy was continued despite clinical evidence of hepatic damage. A recent review of hepatic reactions in patients taking ketoconazole in the UK demonstrated that hepatitis was usually reversible if treatment was stopped, and identified continuation of therapy after onset of jaundice and other symptoms of hepatitis as a risk factor for more serious reactions.[11] The absence of the usual hallmarks of hypersensitivity, and the wide range of treatment duration before any manifestation of toxicity (0.5–26 weeks) suggests that idiosyncratic hepatic damage has a metabolic rather than hypersensitivity basis.[10,40] Positive responses to rechallenge have been reported[9,41] but none had an immediate response within 48 hours. Although most cases of hepatic damage have been reversible, and in patients taking standard therapeutic doses (200–400 mg daily), this risk is probably not justifiable for treatment of relatively trivial disease.

In patients with severe hepatic reactions a variety of histological changes have been reported. The most consistent have been acinar necrosis, mononuclear or mixed inflammatory infiltrate, proliferation of bile ductules, and canalicular cholestasis.

Anaphylaxis. Rare cases of anaphylaxis after the fiirst dose have been reported.

Acute overdosage
No cases of accidental or deliberate overdose have been reported. Should they occur then gastric lavage with sodium bicarbonate is recommended to prevent further absorption of the drug.

Severe or irreversible adverse effects

Androgen suppression. Ketoconazole causes rapid depression of serum testosterone, to about 25% of baseline levels at 4 hours after ingestion, with recovery at 24 hours after each single daily dose.[3] In most patients this has no effect on libido or secondary sexual characteristics. In a few patients, gynaecomastia has been reported with therapeutic doses of ketoconazole. Higher or more frequent doses may cause oligospermia and adrenal suppression which appear to be dose-related.[42]

Symptomatic adverse effects
Nausea, vomiting, pruritus, abdominal pain, diarrhoea, headache, urticaria and dizziness have all been reported but are all uncommon with the exception of nausea (3–10%).[21]

Interference with clinical pathology tests
It has been suggested that ketoconazole may interfere with measurement of serum triglycerides, as raised triglyceride levels were found in patients with normal levels of cholesterol.[43]

High risk groups

Neonates
There is no information available in neonates.

Breast milk. Breast-feeding is contraindicated in patients taking this drug.

Children
The dose should be reduced in children in whom 3 $mg.kg^{-1}$ body weight is the recommended dose.

Pregnant women
Ketoconazole is contraindicated in pregnancy.

The elderly
Normal doses are used in elderly patients.

Concurrent disease

Renal impairment. Very little ketoconazole is excreted renally, hence renal impairment is not a contraindication. Studies in patients continuing ambulatory peritoneal dialysis showed negligible penetration into the CAPD fluid and concluded that the drug is unlikely to be of value in treatment of fungal peritonitis in such patients.[44]

Drug interactions

Absorption
Absorption of ketoconazole is reduced by drugs which reduce gastric acidity.[16] Such drugs should therefore be taken 2 hours after ketoconazole.

Metabolic
All imidazole drugs interfere with hepatic microsomal enzymes[21] and interactions have been reported with the following drugs:

Warfarin. Although not supported by all studies,[19] ketoconazole has been demonstrated to interact with warfarin,[45] to cause reduction of anticoagulant activity.

Antituberculous therapy. Both rifampicin,[19,46,47] and isoniazid[47] cause reduction in ketoconazole levels. Rifampicin levels are also reduced by concomitant ketoconazole therapy but this effect appears to be due to decreased absorption of rifampicin as it is maximal when the drugs are taken simultaneously and avoided completely by separating the doses.[47,48]

Phenytoin. Low, and late, peak levels of ketoconazole have been reported in a patient taking phenytoin,[19] although this patient was known to have low peak ketoconazole levels before phenytoin was introduced.

Alcohol. Acute facial flushing and nausea have been reported following concomitant ingestion of alcohol and ketoconazole.[49]

Cyclosporin A. The simultaneous administration of ketoconazole and cyclosporin A leads to an increase in blood levels of cyclosporin A,[50–52] and therefore a risk of nephrotoxicity due to cyclosporin. Cyclosporin A levels should be monitored carefully and the dose adjusted accordingly. This effect may be due to competitive inhibition of the cytochrome P450 system[51] which is important in the disposition of ketoconazole.[19]

General review articles

1. Graybill J R (ed) 1983 American Journal of Medicine 74 (1B): 1–90
2. Restrepo A, Stevens D A, Utz J P (eds) 1980 First international symposium on ketoconazole. Reviews of Infectious Diseases 2 (4): 519–699
3. Refs 21,22,39,53,54

Ketoconazole

References

1. Borgers M, Van den Bossche H, De Brabander M 1983 The mechanism of action of the new anti-mycotic ketoconazole. American Journal of Medicine 74 (1B): 2–8
2. Borgers M 1980 Mechanism of action of antifungal drugs, with special reference to the imidazole derivatives. Reviews of Infectious Diseases 2: 520–534
3. Pont A, Williams P L, Azhar S, Reitz R E, Bochra C, Stevens D A 1982 Ketoconazole blocks testosterone synthesis. Archives of Internal Medicine 142: 2137–2140
4. Schurmeyer T, Nieschiag E 1982 Ketoconazole-induced drop in serum and saliva testosterone. Lancet 2: 1098
5. Santen R J, Van den Bossche H, Symoens J, Brugmans J, DeCoster R 1983 Site of action of low dose ketoconazole on androgen biosynthesis in men. Journal of Clinical Endocrinology and Metabolism 57: 732–736
6. Odds F C 1980 Laboratory evaluation of antifungal agents: a comparative study of five imidazole derivatives of clinical importance. Journal of Antimicrobial Chemotherapy 6: 749–761
7. Heel R C 1982 Toxicology and safety studies. In: Levine H B (ed) Ketoconazole in the management of fungal disease. ADIS Press, New York ch 7, pp 74–76
8. Pont A, Williams P L, Loose D S et al 1982 Ketoconazole blocks adrenal steroid synthesis. Annals of Internal Medicine 97: 370–372
9. Janssen P A J, Symoens J E 1983 Hepatic reactions during ketoconazole treatment. American Journal of Medicine 74 (1B): 80–85
10. Lewis J H, Zimmerman H J, Benson G D, Ishak K G 1984 Hepatic injury associated with ketoconazole therapy. Analysis of 33 cases. Gastroenterology 86: 503–513
11. Lake-Bakaar G, Scheuer P J, Sherlock S 1987 Hepatic reactions associated with ketoconazole in the United Kingdom. British Medical Journal 294: 419–422
12. Woestenborghs R, Michielsen L, Michiels M, Heykants J 1978 Gas chromatographic determination of R 41 400 in plasma, urine, faeces and tissues. Janssen Pharmaceutica Preclinical Research Report R 41 400/18 (unpublished)
13. Warnock D W, Richardson M D, Turner A 1982 HPLC and other non-biological methods for quantitation of antifungal drugs. Journal of Antimicrobial Chemotherapy 10: 467–478
14. Ene M D, Williamson P J, Daneshmend T K, Blatchford N R 1984 Systemic absorption of ketoconazole from vaginal pessaries. British Journal of Clinical Pharmacology 17: 173–175
15. Daneshmend T K, Warnock D W, Turner A, Roberts C J C 1981 Pharmacokinetics of ketoconazole in normal subjects. Journal of Antimicrobial Chemotherapy 8: 299–304
16. Van Der Meer J W M, Keuning J J, Scheijgrond H W, Heykants J, Van Cutsen J, Brugmans J 1980 The influence of gastric acidity on the bioavailability of ketoconazole. Journal of Antimicrobial Chemotherapy 6: 552–554
17. Männistö P T, Mäntylä R, Nykänen S, Lamminsivu U, Ottoila P 1982 Impairing effect of food on ketoconazole absorption. Antimicrobial Agents and Chemotherapy 21: 730–733
18. Daneshmend T K, Warnock D W, Ene M D et al 1984 Influence of food on the pharmacokinetics of ketoconazole. Antimicrobial Agents and Chemotherapy 25: 1–3
19. Brass C, Galgiani J N, Blaschke T F, DeFelice R, O'Reilly R A, Stevens D A 1982 Disposition of ketoconazole, an oral antifungal, in humans. Antimicrobial Agents and Chemotherapy 21: 151–158
20. Michiels M, Michielsen L, Woestenborghs R, Hendrixks R, Heykants J 1979 Absorption and distribution of $_3$H-ketoconazole following oral administration to the male and female Wistar rat. Janssen Pharmaceutica Preclinical Research Report R 41 400/30 (unpublished)
21. Van Tyle J H 1984 Ketoconazole. Mechanism of action, spectrum of activity, pharmacokinetics, drug interactions, adverse reactions and therapeutic use. Pharmacotherapy 4: 343–373
22. Heel R C, Brogden R N, Carmine A, Morley P A, Speight T M, Avery G S 1982 Ketoconazole: a review of its therapeutic efficacy in superficial and systemic fungal infections. Drugs 23: 1–36
23. Graybill J R, Lundberg D, Donovan W, Levine H B, Rodriguez M D, Drutz D J 1980 Treatment of coccidioidomycosis with ketoconazole: clinical and laboratory studies of 18 patients. Reviews of Infectious Diseases 2: 661–673
24. Daneshmend T K, Warnock D W 1988 Clinical pharmacokinetics of ketoconazole, Clinical Pharmacokinetics 14: 13–34
25. Gascoine E W, Barton G J, Michaels M, Meuldermans W, Heykants J 1981 The kinetics of ketoconazole in animals and man. Clinical Research Reviews 1: 177–187
26. Heel R C 1982 Pharmacokinetic properties. In: Levine H B (ed) Ketoconazole in the management of fungal disease. ADIS Press, New York, ch 6, pp 67–73
27. Meuldermans W, Hurkmans R, Hendrickx J, Lenoir H, Lauwers W, Heykants J 1979 Absorption, excretion and biotransformation of ketoconazole in man. Janssen Clinical Research Report R41 400/23
28. Cucé L C, Wroclawski E L, Sampaia S A P 1980 Treatment of paracoccidioidomycosis, candidiasis, chromomycosis, lobomycosis, and mycetoma with ketoconazole. International Journal of Dermatology 19: 405–408
29. Repestro A, Gomez I, Cano L E et al 1983 Treatment of paracoccidioidomycosis with ketoconazole: a three-year experience. American Journal of Medicine 74 (1B): 48–52
30. Stevens D A, Stiller R L, Williams P L, Sugar A M 1983 Experience with ketoconazole in three major manifestations of progressive coccidioidomycosis. American Journal of Medicine 74 (1B): 58–63
31. Slama T G 1983 Treatment of disseminated and progressive cavitary histoplasmosis with ketoconazole. American Journal of Medicine 74 (1B): 70–73
32. Hawkins S S, Gregory D W, Alford R H 1981 Progressive disseminated histoplasmosis: favourable response to ketoconazole. Annals of Internal Medicine 95: 446–449
33. Hay R J 1983 Ketoconazole in the treatment of fungal infection. Clinical and laboratory studies. American Journal of Medicine 74 (1B): 16–19
34. Rosenblatt H M, Stiehm E R 1983 Therapy of chronic mucocutaneous candidiasis. American Journal of Medicine 74 (1B): 20–22
35. Ferrant A, Michaux J L 1978 The treatment of oral thrush with ketoconazole in patients with malignancies. Janssen Pharmaceutica Preclinical Research Report R 41 400/17 (unpublished)
36. Bisschop M P J M, Merkus J M W M, Scheygrond H, Van Cutsen J, van de Kuy A 1979 Treatment of vaginal candidiasis with ketoconazole, a new, orally active, antimycotic. European Journal of Obstetrics, Gynecology, and Reproductive Biology 9: 253–259
37. Hann I M, Prentice H G, Corringham R et al 1982 Ketoconazole versus nystatin plus amphotericin B for fungal prophylaxis in severely immunocompromised patients. Lancet 1: 826–829
38. Ford G P, Farr P M, Ive F A, Shuster S 1984 The response of seborrhoeic dermatitis to ketoconazole. British Journal of Dermatology 111: 603–607
39. Shuster S, Blatchford N (eds) 1988 Seborrhoeic dermatitis and dandruff — a fungal disease. International Congress and Symposium Series, Number 132. Royal Society of Medicine Services, London
40. Zimmerman H J 1978 Classification of hepatotoxins and mechanisms of toxicity. In: Hepatotoxicity: the adverse effects of drugs and other chemicals on the liver. Appleton-Century-Crofts, New York, pp 91–121
41. Heiberg J K, Svejgaard E 1981 Toxic hepatitis during ketoconazole treatment. British Medical Journal 283: 825–826
42. Pont A, Graybill J R, Craven P C et al 1984 High dose ketoconazole therapy and adrenal and testicular function in humans. Archives of Internal Medicine 144: 2150–2153
43. Dismukes W E, Stamm M, Graybill J R et al 1983 Treatment of systemic mycoses with ketoconazole: emphasis on toxicity and clinical response in fifty-two patients. Annals of Internal Medicine 98: 13–20
44. Chapman J R, Warnock D W 1983 Ketoconazole and fungal CAPD peritonitis. Lancet 2: 510–511
45. Smith A G 1984 Potentiation of oral anticoagulants by ketoconazole. British Medical Journal 288: 188–189
46. Drouhet E, Dupont B 1983 Laboratory and clinical assessment of ketoconazole in deep-seated mycoses. American Journal of Medicine 74 (1B): 30–47
47. Engelhard D, Stutman H R, Marks M I 1984 Interaction of ketoconazole with rifampicin and isoniazid. New England Journal of Medicine 311: 1681–1683
48. Doble N, Hykin P, Shaw R, Keal E E 1985 Pulmonary *Mycobacterium tuberculosis* in acquired immune deficiency syndrome. British Medical Journal 291: 849–850
49. Fazio R A, Wickremesinghe P C, Arsura E L 1983 Ketoconazole therapy of candida esophagitis — a prospective study of twelve cases. American Journal of Gastroenterology 79: 261–264
50. Ferguson R M, Sutherland D E, Simmons R L, Najarian J S 1982 Ketoconazole, cyclosporin metabolism, and renal transplantation. Lancet 2: 882–883
51. Dieperink H, Moller J 1982 Ketoconazole and cyclosporin A. Lancet 2: 1217
52. Cunningham C, Burke M D, Whiting P H, Simpson J G, Wheatley D N 1982 Ketoconazole, cyclosporin, and the kidney. Lancet 2: 1464–1465
53. Symoens J, Cauwenbergh G 1983 Ketoconazole, a new step in the management of fungal disease. Progress in Drug Research 27: 63–84
54. Levine H B 1982 Ketoconazole in the management of fungal disease. ADIS Press, New York

Ketoprofen

Ketoprofen is a derivative of propionic acid which is widely used in the treatment of patients with rheumatic diseases. In controlled clinical trials ketoprofen was found to be comparable in therapeutic efficacy to other non-steroidal anti-inflammatory drugs including aspirin, ibuprofen and indomethacin.

Chemistry

Ketoprofen
(Orudis, Oruvail (sustained-release presentation), Alrheumat, Alreumat, Alreumin, Alrheumun, Alrhumat, Anaus, Atrosilene (as lysinate), Capisten, Fastum, Flexen, ISO-K, Kefenid, Ketalgin, Keto, Kevadon, Lertus, Profenid, Remauric, Rofenid, Salient, Sinketol)
$C_{16}H_{14}O_3$
(RS)-2-(3-Benzoylphenyl)propionic acid

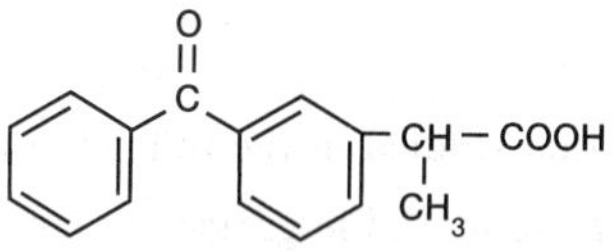

Molecular weight	254.3
pKa (-COOH)	4.55
Solubility	
in alcohol	~1 in 5
in water	<1 in 10 000
Octanol/water partition coefficient (pH 7:4)	1.0

White or off-white odourless powder with a sharp bitter taste. It is prepared by chemical synthesis as a racemate. Ketoprofen is not available in any combination preparations.

Pharmacology

Ketoprofen is a non-steroidal anti-inflammatory drug (NSAID) with analgesic and antipyretic actions. It inhibits cyclo-oxygenase activity with a reduction in the tissue production of prostaglandins such as $PgF_{2}\alpha$ and PgE_2. The anti-inflammatory activity is greater than that of aspirin but in animal studies is less than that of indomethacin or phenylbutazone.[1] Ketoprofen causes gastric erosions and prolongs the bleeding time by its effects on platelet function. Ketoprofen inhibits bradykinin-induced bronchoconstriction in guinea pigs.[1] It also inhibits leucocyte migration, though its effects in this regard are less marked than those of naproxen.

Toxicology

Acute studies have been performed in mice, rats, guinea-pigs and dogs; and oral chronic studies in rats, dogs and monkeys. The main target organ was the gastrointestinal mucosa, mainly ulceration, particularly at higher doses in dogs. Other possible target organs (effects seen at high dosage) were the kidneys (changes in renal tubules in rats and pyelonephritic changes in dogs, but no changes in baboons) and the testes (effect on spermatogenesis, probably reversible in dogs, not seen in rats or baboons). No carcinogenic effects have been observed in mice or rats. Similarly, no teratogenic effects have been observed in mice, rats or rabbits. In rabbits there was slight embryotoxicity at 12 $mg.kg^{-1}$ given orally.

Clinical pharmacology

Ketoprofen is an effective anti-inflammatory and analgesic drug in clinical practice and is used in the treatment of rheumatoid and osteoarthritis. It is as effective in clinical trials as other NSAIDs such as naproxen from both the efficacy and side effect point of view. Ketoprofen relieves joint swelling and pain in patients with rheumatoid arthritis but has no long term effect on the disease process. Ketoprofen inhibits platelet adhesiveness and prolongs bleeding time. By inhibiting prostaglandin synthesis in the uterus ketoprofen may delay the onset of labour.

Ketoprofen has no effect on renal function in normal individuals but like other NSAIDs may worsen renal function in patients whose renal function depends on the production of prostaglandin E_2 (e.g. in hypertension, diabetes, cirrhosis of the liver). This interference with prostaglandin synthesis may explain the loss of hypotensive control or diuretic effect of many drugs when a NSAID is co-administered. Ketoprofen may cause gastric erosions partly by directly irritating the gastric mucosa and partly by inhibiting the synthesis of cytoprotective prostaglandins. The usual daily dose of 100-200 mg offers mild to moderate analgesia in both inflammatory and non-inflammatory conditions.

Pharmacokinetics

Concentrations of the parent drug are measured by high pressure liquid chromatography with UV detection. The limit of detection[2] in plasma is 0.05 $mg.l^{-1}$
Ketoprofen is well absorbed after oral administration with peak plasma concentrations occurring at 1 to 2 hours. The bioavailability of ketoprofen may be reduced by the concomitant taking of food, although the amount of unchanged ketoprofen in urine collected for 48 hours following single and multiple-dose administration did not change with food intake.[3] The plasma half life is 1–3 hours for ketoprofen[4,5] and 5–12 hours for the slow release preparation, Oruvail.[6] There is little presystemic metabolism. Ketoprofen is highly bound to plasma proteins (95%) and concentrations of free ketoprofen may be elevated in disease states associated with hypoproteinaemia. The volume of distribution is 0.11 $l.kg^{-1}$. The pharmacokinetics of ketoprofen uptake into synovial fluid has been studied. The area under the curve for total ketoprofen was greater in serum than synovial fluid but the free fraction area under the curve was similar at both sites. Thereafter, residence time in synovial fluid was approximately 6 hours compared with 2 hours in serum.[7] Excretion of ketoprofen into breast milk is low, due to high plasma protein binding. For the same reason, placenta transfer is likely to be low.

Elimination of the drug is reduced in the elderly.

Ketoprofen is extensively metabolized in the liver, largely by conjugation. Most of the drug is excreted in the urine, with 10-20% in the bile. Only 1% of the dose is excreted unchanged.

Oral absorption	>90%
Presystemic metabolism	minimal
Plasma half life	
range	1–3 h
Volume of distribution	0.11 $l.kg^{-1}$
Plasma protein binding	95%

Concentration–effect relationship

Most investigators have used ketoprofen at between 50 and 150 mg in acute studies of pain relief and between 75 and 200 mg daily for long-term administration. The manufacturer's recommended dose is 100–200 mg daily. The range of plasma concentrations[4] has been estimated to lie between 1–5 $mg.l^{-1}$ in every day use, but there is no evidence of any correlation between the plasma concentration of ketoprofen and its therapeutic effect. It has been suggested that the prolonged residence time of the drug in synovial fluid compared with plasma may explain the longer duration of therapeutic effect than would be predicted from the short plasma half life.[7]

Metabolism

Ketoprofen is extensively metabolized in the liver. Only approximately 1% of the dose is excreted unchanged in the urine. The main pathway of metabolism is glucuronic acid conjugation, with hydroxylation as a minor pathway. The metabolites are excreted mainly in the urine with 80% of the dose as the glucuronide.[8]

10–20% of the dose is excreted in bile. Some enterohepatic circulation is probable. The metabolic products of ketoprofen appear to be pharmacologically inert.

Pharmaceutics

Ketoprofen is available in the following forms:

Orudis (Rhone-Poulenc UK), an opaque green/opaque purple capsule containing 50 mg ketoprofen with each half printed 'Orudis 50' in white.

Orudis 100 (Rhone-Poulenc UK), a pink coloured opaque capsule containing 100 mg ketoprofen printed 'Orudis 100' in black.

Orudis (Wyeth US), an opaque dark green/light green capsule containing 50 mg ketoprofen. One half marked 'WYETH 4181' and the other half marked 'ORUDIS 50'.

A dark green/white capsule containing 75 mg ketoprofen. One half marked 'WYETH 4187' and the other half marked 'ORUDIS 75'. The shelf-life of the above capsules is 5 years. The following are available in the UK:

Orudis suppositories each containing 100 mg ketoprofen. Shelf-life 3 years.

The base is Witepsol.

Orudis should be stored in a dry place below 20°C.

Two sustained release preparations:

A transparent pink capsule with opaque purple cap, holding white pellets, with each half printed 'Oruvail 100' in white. Each capsule contains 100 mg ketoprofen in a pH-sensitive controlled-release preparation. Shelf-life 3 years in the UK, but varies according to territory and climate.

A transparent pink capsule with opaque white cap, holding white pellets, with each half printed 'Oruvail 200' in blue. Each capsule contains 200 mg ketoprofen in a pH-sensitive controlled-release preparation. Shelf-life 2 years in calendar packs and Securitainers.

Oruvail capsules contain ketoprofen in the form of free-flowing controlled-release pellets. The individual pellets are white spheres about 1 mm in diameter, each consisting of an inert core of starch and sucrose on to which ketoprofen is deposited and then surround by a semi-permeable pH-sensitive membrane. There is no release of drug in the stomach.

None of the formulations contains tartrazine and no special storage conditions are needed.

Therapeutic use

Indications

1. Rheumatic disease — for anti-inflammatory and analgesic use in rheumatoid arthritis, osteoarthritis, ankylosing spondylitis, gout
2. Periarticular and musculoskeletal indications — for analgesia in bursitis, tendinitis, synovitis, tenosynovitis, lumbago

Other uses

3. Prophylaxis and treatment of migraine headache
4. Surgical and traumatic uses — for analgesic action after sports injuries, orthopaedic manipulations, dental extractions, surgery
5. Infectious diseases — for analgesic, anti-inflammatory and antipyretic purposes
6. Gynaecological uses — in dysmenorrhoea, following IUCD insertion and for uterine relaxation and analgesia in the postpartum, non-nursing mother.

Contraindications

1. Bronchospasm
   Patients with rhinitis, nasal polyps and asthma associated with aspirin may show cross-sensitivity with other nonsteroidal anti-inflammatory drugs including ketoprofen.
2. Peptic ulceration
   Ketoprofen should not be administered to patients with active peptic ulceration or with a history of recurrent peptic ulceration or chronic dyspepsia.
3. Severe renal insufficiency.

Mode of use

Oral treatment with ketoprofen is 50–100 mg twice daily, taken with food to minimize gastrointestinal disturbance. Rectal dosage is with one suppository (100 mg) late at night, supplemented with the day time use of ketoprofen capsules, as necessary. The sustained-release preparation, Oruvail, is administered orally, usually with food. Dosage is 100–200 mg once daily, depending on patient weight and severity of symptoms. For most indications the maximum benefit of the drug is seen within a few days. The drug may be stopped suddenly or substituted with an equivalent dose of an alternative non-steroidal anti-inflammatory drug without adverse effects.

Indications

1. Rheumatic diseases

Ketoprofen performed better than placebo in trials in rheumatoid arthritis, ankylosing spondylitis and osteoarthritis. It is comparable in activity to other non-steroidal anti-inflammatory drugs including aspirin, ibuprofen and indomethacin (reviewed in[9]). Several double-blind multicentre studies have shown ketoprofen to be comparable in effect with ibuprofen and indomethacin.[9,11] There is no evidence that it modifies the long-term course of any of the above diseases. It is an effective agent in the relief of acute attacks of gout.[9] 100 mg ketoprofen three times daily was comparable in efficacy to 50 mg indomethacin three times daily in a double-blind trial of the treatment of acute gout in 59 patients.[12]

2. Periarticular and musculoskeletal indications

Ketoprofen has proved effective in symptomatic relief of a wide variety of periarticular conditions including frozen shoulder, epicondylitis and tendonitis.[9]

Other uses

The drug has also been studied in the following conditions.

3. Prophylaxis and treatment of migraine headache

Ketoprofen administration was associated with a significant reduction in an index of headache activity in a 12 week, double-blind, cross-over comparison with placebo.[13]

4. Surgical and traumatic uses

50–100 mg of ketoprofen has shown roughly equivalent analgesic activity to 90 mg of codeine amongst patients with postoperative dental pain[14] and amongst postpartum women.[15,16]

5. Antipyretic uses

Ketoprofen was effective in controlling rises in temperature following major surgery.[17]

6. Gynaecological uses

Ketoprofen has similar activity to other non-steroidal inflammatory drugs in relieving dysmenorrhoea. It has been shown to have greater activity than placebo[18] and roughly equivalent activity to indomethacin.[19]

Adverse reactions

Potentially life-threatening effects

Deaths caused by ketoprofen are very rare and are probably mainly due to idiosyncrasy such as anaphylaxis rather than to the pharmacological effects of the drug, though very occasionally gastrointestinal haemorrhage may have a fatal outcome.

Acute overdosage

13 cases of overdosage have been reported worldwide with non-serious adverse effects, which were reversible. Features of poisoning with other members of the propionic acid group are drowsiness, gastrointestinal pain, vomiting and hypotension due to bronchospasm. Gastrointestinal haemorrhage is a possibility. Gastric lavage may be performed if large quantities have been taken, but otherwise treatment is supportive.

Severe or irreversible adverse effects

Acute interstitial nephritis has been associated with the administration of many non-steroidal anti-inflammatory drugs including ketoprofen.[20] Patients with renal impairment, cardiac failure or hepatic cirrhosis may show a reversible decline in renal function due to a reduction in glomerular blood flow secondary to a reduction in intrarenal vasodilatory prostaglandin synthesis.[21]

Ketoprofen

Symptomatic adverse effects

Gastrointestinal disturbance is common and comparable in incidence to that produced by other propionic acid derivatives such a naproxen. In the United Kingdom 33.2 serious gastrointestinal reactions were reported to the Committee of Safety of Medicines per million prescriptions, a rate comparable to that of the majority of non-steroidal anti-inflammatory drugs.[22]

Other effects

Non-steroidal anti-inflammatory drugs have been associated with a fall in creatinine clearance. This is discussed above. No evidence of systematic changes of basic serum biochemical parameters has been noted.

Interference with clinical pathology tests

No technical interference of this kind is known.

High risk groups

Neonates

The drug is unlikely to be used in this age-group and the appropriate dosage has not been established.

Breast milk. Trace amounts of the drug appear in breast milk, and the manufacturers advise against its use during breast feeding unless unavoidable.

Children

There appears to be no contraindication to the use of the drug in children, but the appropriate dosage has not yet been established.

Pregnant women

Embryopathic effects have not been recorded with ketoprofen, but it is recommended to avoid medication during pregnancy. Most non-steroidal anti-inflammatory drugs have an adverse effect on the fetus through their pharmacological properties, including possible premature closure of ductus arteriosus and pulmonary hypertension.

The elderly

A single dose of 150 mg of ketoprofen was given to a group of elderly patients; the maximum plasma concentration was 50% higher and the rate of clearance 50% slower in these subjects compared with a control group of young subjects.[23] Plasma profiles of ketoprofen concentrations were measured in 9 elderly patients after 1 day and 10 days of treatment with a controlled-release preparation of ketoprofen, and were found to be virtually superimposable.[6]

Drug interactions

Potentially hazardous interactions

Warfarin, sulphonylureas, and hydantoins. Ketoprofen is highly protein-bound. In theory, interaction is possible following concomitant use of other protein bound drugs, for example, anticoagulants, sulphonamides, and hydantoins. In practice, such interactions seem extremely rare, and there is just a single report of prolongation of the prothrombin time and gastrointestinal bleeding occurring in a patient, taking several drugs, following the addition of ketoprofen, 75 mg daily.[24]

Methotrexate. In common with other non-steroidal anti-inflammatory drugs, a hazardous interaction of ketoprofen with methotrexate has been reported.[25] The mode of action of non-steroidal anti-inflammatory drugs in causing this effect is not certain, but may be via inhibition of the tubular secretion of methotrexate.

Frusemide. Like other non-steroidal anti-inflammatory drugs, ketoprofen slightly inhibits the sodium diuresis induced by frusemide.

β-blockers. Ketoprofen may reduce the antihypertensive effect of β-blockers.

Lithium. Lithium intoxication has been reported as a result of concurrent administration of ketoprofen.[26]

Potentially useful interactions

Probenecid. The effects of probenecid on ketoprofen pharmacokinetics were investigated. Increases in the concentration of ketoprofen and of ketoprofen conjugates were observed.[27]

References

1. Julour L, Guyonnet J C, Ducrot R, Fournel J, Pasquet 1976 Ketoprofen (19.583 R.P.)(2-(3 benzoylphenyl)-propionic acid). Main pharmacological properties — outline of toxicological and pharmacokinetic date. Scandinavian Journal of Rheumatology 5 (suppl 14): 33–44
2. Kay C M, Sankey M G, Holt J E 1981 A high pressure liquid chromatographic method for the assay of ketoprofen in plasma and urine and its application to determining the urinary excretion of free and conjugated ketoprofen following oral administration to man. British Journal of Clinical Pharmacology 11: 395–398
3. Caillé G, Du Sovich P, Besner J G, Gervais P, Vezina M 1989 Effects of food and sucralfate on the pharmacokinetics of naproxen and ketoprofen in humans. American Journal of Medicine 86 (suppl 6A): 38–44
4. Lewellen O R W, Templeton R 1976 The pharmacokinetics of ketoprofen in man during and after repeated oral dosing (50 mg qid) with 'Orudis'. Scandinavian Journal of Rheumatology (suppl 14): 53–62
5. Ishizaki T, Sasaki T, Suganuma T, Horai Y, Chiba K, Watanabe M, Asuke W, Hoshi H 1980 Pharmacokinetics of ketoprofen following single oral, intramuscular and rectal doses and after repeated oral administration. European Journal of Clinical Pharmacology, 18: 407–414
6. Dennis H J, French P C, Crome P, Babiker M, Shillingford J, Hopkins R 1985 Pharmacokinetic profile of controlled release ketoprofen in elderly patients. British Journal of Clinical Pharmacology 20: 567–573
7. Netter P, Bannwarth B, Lapicque F et al 1987 Total and free ketoprofen in serum and synovial fluid after intramuscular injection. Clinical Pharmacology and Therapeutics 42: 555–561
8. Delbarre F, Roucayrol J C, Amor B, Ingrand J, Bourat G, Fournel J, Courjaret J 1976 Pharmacokinetic study of ketoprofen (19 583 RP) in man using the tritiated compound. Scandinavian Journal of Rheumatology (suppl 14): 45–52
9. Fossgreen J 1976 Ketoprofen: a survey of current publications. Scandinavian Journal of Rheumatology 5 (suppl 14): 7–32
10. Colin A, Bennett R M, Sukhpunyaraka S, Goldman A L et al 1977 Double-blind, multi-centre parallel trial of ketoprofen and ibuprofen in the treatment of rheumatoid arthritis. Journal of Rheumatology 4: 153–157
11. Caldwell J R, Germain B F, Lourie S H et al 1988 Ketoprofen versus indomethacin in patients with rheumatoid arthritis: a multicenter double blind comparative study. Journal of Rheumatology 15: 1476–1479
12. Altman R D, Honig S, Levin J M, Lightfoot R W 1988 Ketoprofen versus indomethacin in patients with acute gouty arthritis: a multicenter double-blind comparative study. Journal of Rheumatology 15: 1422–1430
13. Stensrud P, Sjaastad O 1974 Clinical trial of a new antibradykinin, anti-inflammatory drug, ketoprofen (19.583 R.P.) in migraine prophylaxis. Headache 14: 96
14. Mehlisch D Frakes L, Cavaliere M B, Felman M 1984 A double-blind parallel comparison of ketoprofen, codeine, and placebo in patients with moderate to severe dental pain. Journal of Clinical Pharmacology 24: 486–492
15. Kantor T, Cavaliere M B, Hopper M, Roepke S 1984 A double-blind parallel comparison of ketoprofen, codeine and placebo in patients with moderate to severe postpartum pain. Journal of Clinical Pharmacology 24: 228–234
16. Sunshine A, Zighelboim I, Laska E, Siegel C, Olson N Z, De Castro A 1986 A double-blind, parallel comparison of ketoprofen, aspirin, and placebo in patients with postpartum pain. Journal of Clinical Pharmacology 26: 706–711
17. Keinnannen-Kiukaanniemi S, Simila S, Kouvalainen K 1980 Oral anti-pyretic therapy evaluation of the propionic acid derivatives, ibuprofen, ketoprofen, fenoprofen and naproxen. Pediatrics and Pediologie 15: 239–244
18. Gleeson S, Sobie J 1983 Efficacy of ketoprofen in treating primary dysmenorrhoea. Canadian Medical Association Journal 129: 842–843
19. Kaupilla A, Puolakka J, Ulikorkala O 1979 The relief of primary dysmenorrhoea by ketoprofen and indomethacin. Prostaglandins 18: 647–653
20. Ducret F, Pointet P, Martin D, Villermet B 1982 Insuffisance renale aigue induite par le ketoprofene. Nephrologie 3: 105–106
21. Toto R D, Anderson S A, Brown-Cartwright D, Kokko J P, Brater D C 1986 Effects of acute and chronic dosing of NSAIDs in patients with renal insufficiency. Kidney International 30: 760–768
22. Anon CSM update: Non-steroidal anti-inflammatory drugs and serious gastrointestinal adverse reactions. British Medical Journal 292: 1190–1191
23. Advenier C, Roux A, Gobert C, Massias P, Varoquaux O, Flouvat B 1983 Pharmacokinetics of ketoprofen in the elderly. British Journal of Clinical Pharmacology 16: 65–70
24. Flessner M F, Knight H 1988 Prolongation of the prothrombin time and severe gastrointestinal bleeding associated with combined use of warfarin and ketoprofen. Journal of the American Medical Association 259: 353
25. Thyss A, Milano G, Kubar J, Namer M, Schneider M 1986 Clinical and pharmacokinetic evidence of a life threatening interaction between methotrexate and ketoprofen. Lancet 1: 256–258
26. Singer L, Imbs J L, Danion J M, Singer P, Krieger-Finance F, Schmidt M, Schwartz J 1981 Risque d'intoxication par le lithium en cas de traitment associe par les anti-inflammatoires non-steroidiens. Therapie 36: 323–326
27. Upton R A, Williams R L, Buskin J N 1982 Effects of probenecid on ketoprofen. Clinical Pharmacology and Therapeutics 31: 705–712

K

Ketotifen (fumarate)

Recently introduced for the prophylaxis of asthma, the mode of action of ketotifen is similar to that of sodium cromoglycate, but it can be given orally. It is also an antihistamine.

Chemistry

Ketotifen fumarate (Zaditen)
$C_{19}H_{19}NOS.C_4H_4O_4$
4-(1-Methyl-4-piperidylidene)-4H-benzo[4,5]cyclohepta [1,2-b]-thiophen-10(9H)-one hydrogen fumarate

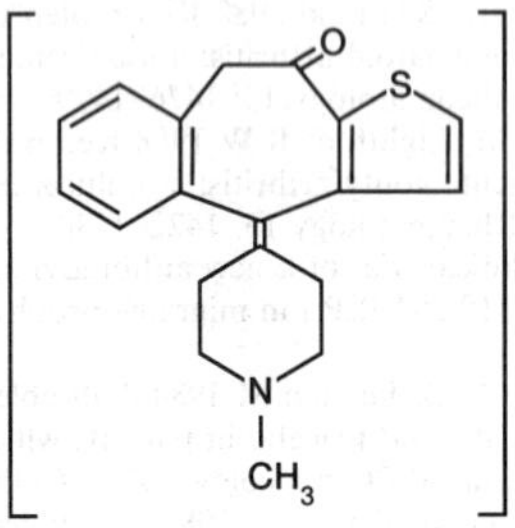

Molecular weight (free base)	425.5 (309.4)
pKa (amino group)	8.43
Solubility	
in alcohol	soluble
in water	slight
Octanol/water partition coefficient	0.7

Ketotifen hydrogenfumarate is a white to yellowish, or brown-tinged yellowish, finely crystalline powder which is either odourless or has a weak but characteristic odour. It is prepared synthetically. It is not available in any compound preparations.

Pharmacology

Ketotifen is a potent antihistamine which exhibits strong H_1-receptor blocking activity. In addition it has been shown to possess anti-anaphylactic properties and is effective in preventing asthmatic attacks.

Laboratory experiments[1,2] suggest that this activity of the drug may be mainly due to the inhibition of release of chemical mediators from tissue mast cells and basophils, in particular histamine and the leukotrienes, and to calcium antagonistic properties. On the basis of their studies Martin and Roemer suggested that ketotifen, although chemically unrelated, had similar actions to sodium cromoglycate (SCG). However, histamine release from rat peritoneal mast cells was not inhibited by ketotifen although SCG produced a dose-dependent inhibition. Additionally, ketotifen does not display cross tachyphylaxis, a phenomenon used to identify drugs with actions similar to SCG. Phillips[3] and co-workers have also suggested a different mode of action for the two drugs since ketotifen, but not SCG, has potent inhibitory effects on histamine and allergen-induced weals in human skin. Thus, it seems probable that the antihistamine action is more important.

Ketotifen has been shown to inhibit platelet activating factor (PAF)-induced hyperreactivity in guinea pig airways as well as preventing eosinophilic infiltration. However, there is no evidence that ketotifen influences the level of hyper-responsiveness in asthmatic patients[4] nor influences eosinophilic infiltration in the human lung.

Toxicology

Single-dose studies of ketotifen in rodents have shown that there is a relatively low level of acute toxicity. LD_{50} values are above 300 mg.kg^{-1} orally and between 5 and 20 mg.kg^{-1} intravenously in the mouse, rat and rabbit.

Prolonged toxicity has been studied in the rat. Rats were treated for 13 weeks with ketotifen, 10, 33 or 157 mg.kg^{-1} daily. The two high doses led to an enlargement of the liver with hepatocyte swelling. The highest dose also induced degenerative changes in the β-cells of the endocrine pancreas and a loss in body weight. All changes were reversible after a recovery period of four weeks. No toxic symptoms were observed at the daily dose of 10 mg.kg^{-1}.

Carcinogenicity
Studies performed in mice have examined the possible carcinogenic potential of ketotifen. No increase in tumour frequency was seen over a study period of 74 weeks using doses of 1.7, 13.5 and 18.8 mg.kg^{-1} daily.

Fertility and teratology
Ketotifen administered to male and female rats in doses up to 10 mg.kg^{-1} daily over 10 weeks does not affect breeding performance or fertility.

Teratology studies in the rat and rabbits have revealed no evidence of adverse effects on organogenesis when administered from day 6–15 and day 6–18 post-coitum respectively. In the rat a daily oral dose of 100 mg.kg^{-1} caused increased mortality of the dams, whilst in the rabbit a daily oral dose of 45 mg.kg^{-1} resulted in increased average fetal weight.

Perinatal and postnatal studies in female rats revealed no adverse effects up to weaning at doses of up to 10 mg.kg^{-1} daily.

Clinical pharmacology

Ketotifen has been shown in vitro to possess both antihistaminic and 'anti-allergic' properties. In addition it is capable of blocking in vitro release of mediators from rat peritoneal mast cells.[1]

The exact mode of action of ketotifen in vivo is unclear. It has been shown to be extremely effective in protecting patients against histamine-induced bronchospasm both in single doses and when administered long term.[5–7] The effectiveness of a single dose of ketotifen in this situation suggests that any effect of ketotifen on histamine inhalation is almost certainly attributable to its antihistaminic properties rather than to a more fundamental effect on bronchial hyperreactivity.

Ketotifen lacks significant anticholinergic activity in vitro[1] and fails to protect individuals against acetylcholine- induced bronchoconstriction. However, differing results have been obtained when ketotifen is administered for long periods and provocation testing with acetylcholine or methacholine is repeated at intervals. Mattson[8] found that ketotifen had no effect in preventing the methacholine-induced decrease in lung volumes following challenge whereas Sotier[9] was able to find a decrease in the intensity of methacholine-induced bronchospasm after five weeks treatment with ketotifen.

Since no anticholinergic properties were evident in vitro these latter results suggest that ketotifen may decrease bronchial hyperreactivity.

The efficacy of ketotifen against allergen-induced bronchoconstriction in man was demonstrated by Girard[10] in 1977. However, other investigators[5] have shown that it does not differ from clemastine in this respect and therefore this action of ketotifen probably depends upon blocking the histaminic component of the early reaction.

Ketotifen has also been shown to prevent aspirin-induced asthma in many susceptible patients, when administered for 3–7 days prior to challenge.[11] Since aspirin inhibits prostaglandin synthesis, this type of asthma could result from an increase of lipoxygenase products as a consequence of aspirin-induced inhibition of the cyclo-oxygenase pathway of arachidonic acid metabolism. However, the mechanism of aspirin-induced asthma is still unclear and this action of ketotifen cannot be taken as evidence of an inhibitory action upon the release of leuokotrienes.

Pharmacokinetics

The preferred analytical method is mass spectrometry after gas chromatographic separation,[12] with a limit of sensitivity of 50 ng.l^{-1}. Gastrointestinal absorption of ketotifen following oral administration is rapid, with an absorption half life of less than one hour.[13] Peak plasma concentrations are achieved at 2 h after dosing. Studies with tritium-labelled drug show two elimination half lives, of 3 and 22 hours. 30–50% of radioactivity is excreted in the urine and the remainder in the faeces. The route of elimination is independent of the route of administration. Most activity is eliminated during the first 24 hours with no indication of possible retention of the parent compound or metabolites. Biliary excretion is quantitatively important and appears to be mainly responsible for faecal elimination.

Plasma levels of ketotifen and its N-glucuronide derivative in plasma during twice daily oral dosage with 1 mg of ketotifen are similar in adults and children. Minimum concentrations of ketotifen in plasma of children following four days treatment are 0.89 ± 0.12 mg.l^{-1}, maximum concentrations being up to 50% higher at 1.29 ± 0.15 mg.l^{-1}. Plasma concentrations of the N-glucuronide derivative follow a similar pattern but are, on average, 3.5 times higher.

Protein binding studies show that, within a plasma concentration range of 1–200 mg.l^{-1} at least 75% of ketotifen is protein bound. Binding affinity, however, is low.

It has been difficult to obtain an exact value for the volume of distribution of ketotifen. All single-dose studies in man have employed an analytical procedure that is unable to distinguish between the parent drug and its metabolites.

Distribution studies in the rat have shown that radioactivity declines rapidly in all tissues in parallel with blood levels. The highest drug levels were found in excretory organs, the liver and kidney, and in the lung. No retention of radioactivity was observed in any tissue.

Oral absorption	>90%
Presystemic metabolism	low
Plasma half life	22 h
Volume of distribution	
Plasma protein binding	⩾75%

Ketotifen is extensively metabolized in the liver, the drug and its products being excreted in both urine and faeces, with slightly more eliminated by the latter route.

The effects of hepatic disease on the pharmacokinetics of ketotifen are not known, but it is likely that biotransformation will be impaired, with consequent increases in the plasma concentrations of the drug and prolonged half life. It is unlikely that old age alters the pharmacokinetics of the drug to any significant extent. The amount of drug, if any, that is excreted in breast milk is not known. It is not known whether or not the drug crosses the placenta.

Concentration–effect relationship

Little or no data is available on dose–response effects related to clinically relevant modes of action in humans.

Metabolism

Ketotifen is subject to extensive biotransformation in the liver. The two major metabolites of the drug in man are:

1. two isomeric forms of a quaternary N-glucuronic acid conjugate of the parent compound.
2. the demethylated product, nor-ketotifen.

There is also 10-hydroxylation to 10-hydroxyketotifen. The polar glucuronide is the major metabolite in human plasma and is also present in the urine and, possibly, in the bile. The non-polar desmethyl derivative occurs principally in the urine. The glucuronide metabolite is readily hydrolysed back to the active ketotifen and the demethylated product has pharmacological activity similar to that of ketotifen (Fig. 1).

Pharmaceutics

1. Zaditen ketotifen 1 mg capsules (Sandoz, UK): white, opaque, gelatine capsules containing 1.38 mg of ketotifen hydrogen fumarate equivalent to 1 mg of ketotifen base. Coded 'CS'.
2. Zaditen ketotifen 1 mg tablets (Sandoz, UK): off-white, uncoated, round, flat, bevel-edged tablets 7 mm in diameter. Scored on one side and marked 'ZADITEN 1' on the reverse. Each tablet contains 1.38 mg of ketotifen hydrogen fumarate equivalent to 1 mg of ketotifen base.

Fig. 1

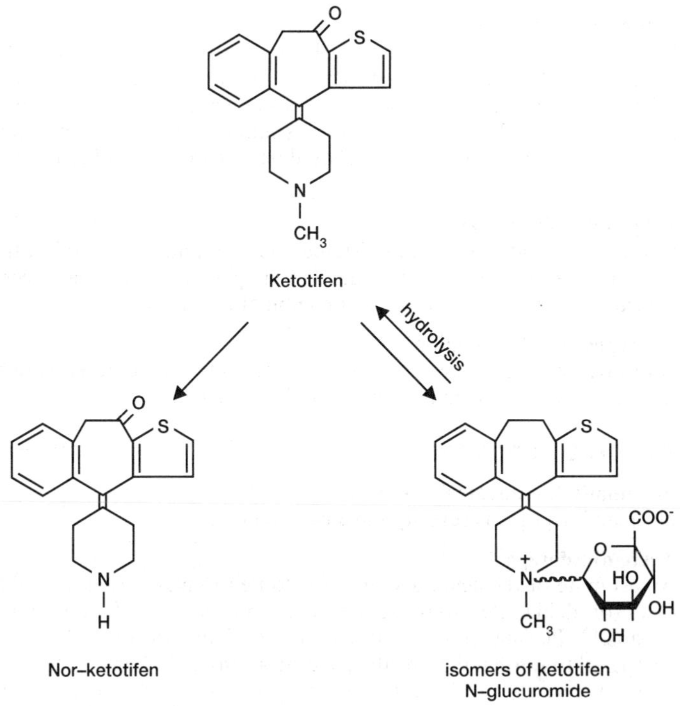

3. Zaditen ketotifen elixir (Sandoz, UK): clear, colourless, strawberry-flavoured elixir. Each 5 ml spoonful contains 1.38 mg of ketotifen hydrogen fumarate, equivalent to 1 mg of ketotifen base, and 1.5 g of sucrose. Zaditen elixir may be diluted with Syrup BP containing parahydroxybenzoate preservatives.

Capsules and tablets should be protected from heat and moisture. Diluted elixir should be used within 14 days.
In some countries Zaditen 2 mg modified release tablets and Zaditen oral drop solution 1 mg.ml^{-1} are available.

Therapeutic use

The drug is of value in patients who suffer from more than one atopic disease, e.g. asthma and rhinitis, when one formulation benefits both conditions.

Indications

1. Prophylaxis of bronchial asthma
2. Allergic rhinitis (seasonal and perennial)
3. Allergic conjunctivitis.

Contraindications

1. When drowsiness could be a hazard
2. Concomitantly with oral antidiabetic agents
3. Pregnancy and breast-feeding.

Mode of use

Recommended dosage for adults is 1–2 mg twice daily with food. The modified release tablet is taken once a day after dinner. Ketotifen is not recommended for use in children under two years of age. Recommended dosage for children over two years of age is 1 mg twice daily with food.

Indications

1. Bronchial asthma
Ketotifen is indicated for the treatment of mild asthma, particularly in children and in adults who find inhaled treatment unacceptable.

2, 3. Allergic rhinitis and conjunctivitis
Recommended dosage schedules as for bronchial asthma.

Ketotifen (fumarate)

K

Contraindications and precautions

1. Impaired alertness
Drowsiness may occur, particularly during the first days of treatment. Patients should be warned not to drive or operate machinery until the effect of treatment on the individual is known. Ketotifen may also potentiate the effects of sedatives, hypnotics, antihistamines and alcohol. For this reason patients should be advised to avoid alcoholic drinks.

2. Oral antidiabetic agents
Ketotifen should not be administered concomitantly with oral antidiabetic agents since a reversible fall in platelet count has been recorded in a few patients on this combination of therapy.

3. Pregnancy and lactation
Although there is no evidence of teratogenic effects, ketotifen is not recommended in pregnancy or during breast feeding.

Adverse reactions

Potentially life-threatening effects
No reactions of this severity have been reported.

Acute overdosage
An estimate of the acute toxicity of ketotifen in man based on eight cases of deliberate overdose has been reported by Jefferys and Volans.[15] Plasma concentrations ranged from 16 to 122 $\mu g.l^{-1}$ compared to normal therapeutic concentrations of 1–4 $\mu g.l^{-1}$. Symptoms observed were those suggested by toxicity studies in animals and included drowsiness, confusion, dyspnoea, cyanosis, tachycardia, hyperexcitability and convulsions. In most cases gastric lavage was performed following which patients made a full recovery with only supportive treatment.

Severe or irreversible adverse effects
No reactions of this kind have been encountered.

Symptomatic adverse effects
Postmarketing surveillance has shown that the symptomatic adverse effects of ketotifen are few and relatively minor.[14] In common with other preparations with antihistaminic activity, the most common side effects reported are those of drowsiness and lethargy. The incidence of drowsiness appears to decline during extended periods of treatment, being 14% after three months and only 2% after 12 months. Fewer adverse effects are reported in children, again the most common being drowsiness or sedation.

Interference with clinical pathology tests
No technical interferences of this kind have been reported.

High risk groups

Neonates
Ketotifen is not recommended for the treatment of neonates or children under the age of two years.

Breast milk. There is no information on whether or not the drug enters breast milk, so mothers taking the drug should not breast-feed their infants.

Children
In children aged 2–12 years no special precautions are necessary. Indeed the incidence of adverse events recorded in children is slightly lower than that in adults.[14]

Pregnant women
Although there is no evidence of any teratogenic effect, ketotifen is not recommended during pregnancy.

The elderly
Ketotifen may be administered safely to the elderly. The incidence of side effects in over 900 patients of 70 years and over is identical to that in the adult population as a whole (27.5% after three months treatment).[14]

Drug interactions

Potentially hazardous interactions
A reversible fall in platelet counts has been reported in a few patients receiving ketotifen concomitantly with oral antidiabetic agents. The mechanism of this interaction is unknown and therefore ketotifen should not be used when oral hypoglycaemics are being administered.

The sedative effects of ketotifen may be potentiated by alcohol and other CNS depressants, e.g. hypnotics, antihistamines and alcohol.

Potentially useful interactions
No potentially useful drug interactions are known.

Major outcome trials

Asthma

1. Dyson A S, Mackay A D 1980 Ketotifen in adult asthma. British Medical Journal 280: 360–361

In this large scale study of the effect of ketotifen. 1 mg or 2 mg twice daily, and placebo in 50 patients with atopic asthma, subjective assessments of daytime breathlessness were significantly improved on ketotifen 2 mg twice daily. This effect was seen only in patients whose concomitant medication did not include inhaled corticosteroids. In this group of patients consumption of inhaled salbutamol was also significantly reduced.

2. Lane D J 1980 A steroid sparing effect of ketotifen in steroid dependent asthmatics. Clinical Allergy 10: 519–525

A comparison of the steroid-sparing effect of ketotifen and placebo was studied in 81 patients. Mean daily prednisolone dosage was reduced by 4 mg in patients on active therapy compared to only 1.7 mg in the placebo group.

3. Guibout P, Choffel C, Constans P, Fabre C, Robillard M 1984 Efficacy of ketotifen in adult asthmatic patients: a six month double-blind versus placebo study. Respiration 46 (suppl 1): 20–21

It has been suggested that ketotifen does not achieve its maximum effect on symptoms or requirements for additional medication until it has been regularly administered for at least one month. This has been confirmed by Guibout and co-workers in a six-month study of the effect of ketotifen and placebo on symptoms and drug consumption in 41 adult asthmatics. A significant reduction in both asthmatic symptoms and attack frequency was reported, compared to baseline values, in the group treated with ketotifen. This effect began one month after the start of treatment and became more pronounced at the end of six months. Comparisons with placebo also confirmed this effect, benefits from active treatment becoming evident after one month and increasing during continuous long-term treatment.

4. Tinkelman D G, Moss B A, Bukantz S C et al 1985 A multi centre trial of the prophylactic effect of ketotifen, theophylline, and placebo in atopic asthma. Journal of Allergy and Clinical Immunology 76: 487–497

This multi-centre trial which included 229 patients treated with ketotifen, 73 treated with theophylline and 72 treated with placebo showed no difference in efficacy between ketotifen and theophylline. The authors concluded that ketotifen was at least as effective as theophylline in controlling asthma.

5. Leupold Von W, Generlich H, Klöditz E et al 1984 Erfahrunge mit ketotifen beim Kindlichen Asthma bronchiale. Deutsch Gesundheit Wes 39: 430–434

Studies of the clinical efficacy of ketotifen in children have produced varying results. However, this may be due to the fact that, in many cases, the drug was used short-term.

In a study of 40 asthmatic children between the ages of one and six years over a longer period of three months, Leupold and co-workers were able to show that 60% of the children showed clinical benefit. In a further study the same investigators reported the effect of ketotifen and SCG in 60 patients aged 7–18 years. Over a three-month period ketotifen was as effective as SCG in improving asthmatic symptoms. The rate of improvement was slightly slower on ketotifen therapy, highlighting the slow onset of action of ketotifen therapy and the need for continuing long-term treatment.

6. Rackham A, Brown C A, Chandra R K et al 1989 A Canadian multi center study with Zaditen (ketotifen) in the treatment of bronchial asthma in children aged 5–17 years. Journal of Allergy Clinical Immunology 84: 286–295

This placebo-controlled study involving 138 asthmatic children with a mean age of 10 years showed that, after 26 weeks of treatment with ketotifen, 60% of the children stopped their additional theophylline treatment compared to only 34% of children in the placebo group who stopped theophylline.

Rhinitis

7. Blainey A D, Ollier S, Gould C, Davies R J 1983
Antihistamines in seasonal allergic rhinitis: a double-blind study of ketotifen and clemastine. Thorax 38: 70

There are very few large-scale controlled studies of ketotifen in the management of rhinitis. One controlled study of the effects of ketotifen in seasonal allergic rhinitis in 48 patients was reported by Blainey in 1983. Symptom records for rhinorrhoea, sneezing and nasal blockage were kept throughout the summer. In addition, nasal hyperreactivity was assessed at three-weekly intervals by histamine provocation testing. After six weeks of therapy both symptom scores and nasal responsiveness to histamine were significantly reduced in patients receiving ketotifen therapy in comparison with placebo. The authors conclude that ketotifen is an effective treatment of seasonal allergic rhinitis in adults.

References

1. Martin U L, Römer D 1978 The pharmacological properties of a new, orally active anti-anaphylactic compound: ketotifen a benzocycloheptathiophene. Drug Research 28: 770–782
2. Ney U M, Bretz U, Martin U 1982 Pharmacology of ketotifen. Research and Clinical Forums 4: 9–16
3. Phillips M J, Meyrick Thomas R J, Moodley I, Davies R J 1983 A comparison of the in vivo effects of ketotifen, clemastine, chlorpheniramine and sodium cromoglycate on histamine and allergen induced weals in human skin. British Journal of Clinical Pharmacology 15: 277–286
4. Graff-Lonnevig V, Hedlin G 1985 The effect of ketotifen on bronchial hyperreactivity in childhood asthma. Journal of Allergy and Clinical Immunology 76: 59–63
5. Phillips M J, Ollier S, Gould C A L, Davies R J 1984 Effect of antihistamines and anti-allergic drugs on responses to allergen and histamine provocation tests in man. Thorax 39: 345–351
6. Mattson K, Poppins H, Nikander-Hurme R 1979 Preventive effect of ketotifen, a new antiallergic agent, on histamine-induced bronchoconstriction in asthmatics. Clinical Allergy 9: 411–416
7. Gozalo-Reques F, Calas Sanz C, Senent Sanchez C, Rubio Sates K, Herrero Lopez T, de Barrio Fernandez M 1985 Long-term modification on histamine-induced bronchoconstriction by disodium cromoglycate and ketotifen versus placebo. Allergy 40: 242–249
8. Mattson K, Poppins H, Hurme R 1979 A controlled study on the preventive effects of ketotifen, an antiallergic agent, on methacholine-induced bronchoconstriction in asthmatics. Clinical Allergy 9: 495–501
9. Sotier M, Stein D 1980 The modification of non-specific bronchial hyperreactivity with anti-allergic drugs. Excerpta Medica 18: 25
10. Girard J P, Cuevas M 1977 Anti-asthmatic properties of a new peroral drug (HC20-511). Acta Allergolica 32: 27–34
11. Wuethrich B 1979 Protective effect of ketotifen and disodium cromoglycate against bronchoconstriction induced by aspirin, benzoic acid or tartrazine in intolerant asthmatics. Respiration 37: 224–231
12. Perhaj Z, Laplanche R 1979 Documenta Sandoz, Sandoz, Basel
13. Kennedy G R 1982 Metabolism and pharmacokinetics of ketotifen in children. Research and Clinical Forums 4: 17–20
14. Maclay W P, Crowder D 1982 Post-marketing surveillance of ketotifen (Zaditen): an interim report. Research and Clinical Forums 4: 51–57
15. Jefferys D B, Volans G N 1981 Ketotifen overdose: surveillance of the toxicity of a new drug. British Medical Journal 282: 1755–1756

Labetalol (hydrochloride)

Labetalol was first synthesized by Glaxo Group Research Limited in the UK and patented in September 1967. It has both α- and β-adrenoceptor blocking activity.

Chemistry

Labetalol hydrochloride (ibidomide hydrochloride, Trandate, Normodyne, Labrocol)
$C_{19}H_{24}N_2O_3$.HCl
5-{(RS)-1-Hydroxy-2-[(RS)-1-methyl-3-phenylpropyl)amino]ethyl}-salicylamide hydrochloride

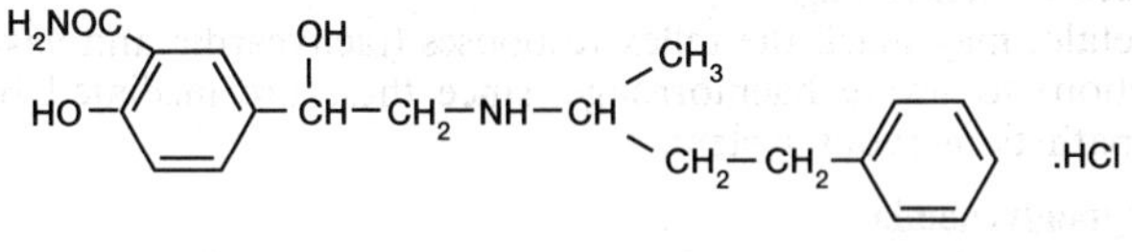

Molecular weight (free base)	364.9 (328.4)
pKa (phenol; NH_2)	7.4, 8.7
Solubility	
in alcohol	1 in 60
in water	>1 in 30
Octanol/water partition coefficient	7.08

Labetalol hydrochloride is a white or off-white odourless crystalline powder. It has two optical centres and, therefore, four optical isomers. Clinical preparations consist of equal proportions of all four isomers.

Pharmacology

Labetalol is a competitive antagonist at β_1- and β_2-adrenoceptors and has some intrinsic activity at β_2-adrenoceptors. It has membrane stabilizing activity but is approximately 4.5 times less potent than propranolol in this respect.[1] Labetalol has, in addition to its β-blocking action, a competitive antagonist action at postsynaptic α-adrenoceptors.[2] In isolated tissues labetalol is 4–8 times more potent at β- than α-adrenoceptors.[3]

Toxicology

When given to rats in doses up to 200 mg.kg^{-1} daily and dogs in doses up to 100 mg.kg^{-1} daily for periods of 3 months, labetalol produced no evidence of drug-related toxicity.[4] Similar doses administered over a 1-year period again produced no toxic effects.[4] In rats and rabbits no teratological effects were found when labetalol was administered during pregnancy.[4]

Labetalol has been shown to bind reversibly to ocular melanin,[4] but no changes attributable to the drug have been found in the eyes of rabbit fetuses or weanling rabbits, or in dogs and cats treated with maximum tolerated doses for several months.[4]

Clinical pharmacology

Competitive β-adrenoceptor blockade has been demonstrated in man by the parallel shift (to the right) in the log dose–heart rate response curve for isoprenaline[5] and antagonism of exercise-induced tachycardia. Competitive α-adrenoceptor blockade has been demonstrated in man by the parallel shift (to the right) in the log dose–pressor response curve to phenylephrine.[5] The potency ratio of α:β-adrenoceptor antagonism is approximately 7:1 when given intravenously and 3:1 following oral dosing.[5]

After intravenous administration in doses ranging from 0.5 to 2.0 mg.kg^{-1}, labetalol produced an almost immediate fall in blood pressure[5–7] accompanied by either a small increase[5,7] or a decrease[6,8] in heart rate. The effect on cardiac output was generally minor and peripheral resistance was usually reduced.[6,7] Labetalol produced significant blunting of the heart rate and blood pressure responses to exercise[5] and blocked the pressor and heart rate responses to parenteral adrenaline.[9]

Pharmacokinetics

The preferred analytical method uses high performance liquid chromatography with UV detection. The limit of sensitivity is 10 μg.l^{-1}.[10]

Labetalol is absorbed rapidly after oral administration. In fasting subjects, the peak plasma concentration occurred 20–60 minutes after a 100 mg dose and 40–90 minutes after a 200 mg dose.[11] Systemic bioavailability ranged from 11 to 86% after a 100 mg dose and 19 to 49% after a 200 mg dose.[11] The wide variation among individuals in total plasma labetalol concentrations is due to extensive presystemic metabolism. Enzyme inhibition, for example by concurrent cimetidine therapy, may cause a reduction in presystemic metabolism with a consequent increase in bioavailability.[12]

In man, the distribution volume is high, indicating drug accumulation in the tissues.[11] However, labetalol is less lipid soluble than propranolol, so little enters the brain.[13] Studies in which radiolabelled labetalol was given to animals showed accumulation of radioactivity in the lungs, liver and kidneys.[13] Labetalol crosses the placenta but the concentration in fetal plasma is less than that in the maternal blood (1.2–5.3:1).[14] Labetalol enters breast milk but its concentration is still only 25–50% of that found in maternal plasma. This does not appear to be sufficient to have any effect on the breast-feeding infant.[15]

Oral absorption	Well absorbed
Presystemic metabolism	14–89%
Plasma half life	
range	1.7–6.1 h
mean	3.3 h
Volume of distribution	3.4–10.7 l.kg^{-1}
Plasma protein binding	50%

Labetalol undergoes hepatic biotransformation, and less than 5% of the drug is recovered unchanged in the urine.[13] In elderly patients the bioavailability of labetalol tends to be increased[16] presumably due to a decrease in presystemic metabolism. The bioavailability is considerably increased in patients with hepatic cirrhosis.[17] By contrast, in patients with severe renal impairment (creatinine clearance 6 ml.min^{-1}) neither the half life nor plasma clearance are affected.[10]

Concentration–effect relationship

Plasma concentrations in the range 30–165 μg.l^{-1} produce increasing blockade of an exercise-induced tachycardia. However, there are interindividual differences in the response to a particular plasma concentration.[18] As with most β-adrenoceptor antagonists there is no clear relationship between the plasma concentration of labetalol and its antihypertensive action.[18]

Metabolism

Elimination of labetalol is mainly by hepatic biotransformation to glucuronides. Less than 5% of labetalol is excreted unchanged in urine. Its metabolites are mainly excreted in urine (55–60%) but 12–27% are excreted in the faeces.[13] Smaller amounts of the O-phenylglucuronide have been identified.[13]

Pharmaceutics

Labetalol (Normodyne, Schering USA/Trandate, Allen and Hanburys, UK) is available in oral and parenteral preparations. Tablets contain 50, 100, 200 or 400 mg of labetalol hydrochloride. These are circular and biconvex, orange in colour, and marked on one face with the proprietary name: tablet dosage is followed by the letters AH (for example, Trandate 100 AH).

An aqueous solution of labetalol hydrochloride is available for parenteral administration in a concentration of 5 g.l^{-1}. The solution, which is colourless, is prepared in ampoules which contain 20 ml.

No special storage precautions are required for tablets but solutions of labetalol should be protected from the light.

Therapeutic use

Indications

1. The control of all grades of hypertension including pregnancy-induced hypertension
2. The treatment of angina in patients with hypertension
3. The management of catecholamine excess and patients with phaeochromocytoma.

Contraindications

1. Bronchospasm
2. Untreated heart failure or low cardiac output
3. Bradycardia and 2nd or 3rd degree heart block
4. Severe haemorrhage
5. Hypoglycaemia.

Mode of use

Both the α- and β-adrenoceptor blocking actions of labetalol contribute to its clinical usefulness.

Oral treatment is usually started with 100 mg twice daily (50 mg twice daily in elderly) and increased at intervals of 1–2 weeks until adequate blood pressure control is achieved or a maximum of 2.4 g daily is reached. At higher doses, postural hypotension (the drug's major dose-limiting side effect) is likely to occur.[19]

Intravenous labetalol should be used with great care as it is intended for use in emergencies where rapid control of the blood pressure is thought to be desirable. Because the intravenous route avoids presystemic metabolism the dose should be proportionately lower than the oral one.

Sudden withdrawal of labetalol therapy should be avoided in patients with angina pectoris because an exacerbation of anginal symptoms (and even myocardial infarction) may follow.

Indications

1. Hypertension

Labetalol is used for the treatment of all grades of hypertension, either alone or in combination with a benzothiadiazine (thiazide) diuretic.[20] It reduces the systolic and diastolic blood pressure at rest and attenuates the rise in pressure induced by exercise.[21] A starting dose of 100 mg twice daily may be increased at weekly intervals according to the response.[21]

The antihypertensive action of labetalol is probably due in large part to β-adrenoceptor antagonism (the mode of action of β-adrenoceptor antagonists in reducing blood pressure has not been determined). However, the α-adrenoceptor blocking action (which causes a reduction in peripheral vascular resistance) is also important.

2. Angina pectoris

In patients with both hypertension and angina pectoris, amelioration of anginal symptoms has been observed when labetalol has been used in daily doses ranging from 300 to 1200 mg to control the blood pressure.[21] In normotensive patients, labetalol has also been shown to have antianginal properties.[22,23] However, at present labetalol is not licensed for the latter purpose.

3. Phaeochromocytoma

Labetalol inhibits both the chronotropic and pressor effects of circulating catecholamines.[9] It has been found to be effective both pre- and perioperatively in the management of patients with phaeochromocytoma. In one study[24] satisfactory blood pressure control was achieved in four patients with adrenal tumours. However, another patient could not tolerate high doses of labetalol and was treated with a combination of propranolol and phenoxybenzamine. One case has been reported in which labetalol provoked a hypertensive response in a patient with a phaeochromocytoma that secreted mainly adrenaline.

Contraindications

1. Bronchospasm

Labetalol has a lesser tendency to cause bronchoconstriction than propranolol[25] but has been reported to cause severe bronchospasm in patients with asthma.[26] It may render such patients unresponsive to normal doses of bronchodilators such as salbutamol.

2. Untreated cardiac failure and low cardiac output

The adverse effects of β-adrenoceptor blockade on myocardial contractility are counteracted by the α-adrenoceptor blocking actions of labetalol which cause a reduction in afterload.[27] Labetalol may, therefore, be of value in situations where pure β-adrenoceptor antagonists cannot be used. Thus, Timmis and associates administered an infusion of labetalol to four patients who had hypertension and pulmonary oedema following acute myocardial infarction and observed a fall in both systolic and diastolic blood pressure which was accompanied by a reduction in pulmonary artery diastolic pressure.[8] Similar results have been reported by others[28] but such therapy should be limited to an intensive care unit where invasive monitoring and resuscitation equipment are available. Labetalol causes a reduction in myocardial contractility in animals[3] and, in patients with impaired left ventricular function, may cause a reduction in cardiac output[8] and/or precipitate cardiac failure.[22,29]

3. Bradycardia

Labetalol has a variable effect on the heart rate and can depress conduction in the A-V node.[30] In patients with high grade atrioventricular block or severe sinus bradycardia its use may be hazardous.

4. Severe haemorrhage

Labetalol may mask the reflex responses (tachycardia and vasoconstriction) to severe haemorrhage, since these are mediated by the sympathetic nervous system.

5. Hypoglycaemia

The metabolic response to hypoglycaemia is achieved, in part, through stimulation of β-adrenoceptors. Thus, labetalol may enhance any tendency to hypoglycaemia and will mask some of the symptomatic responses, e.g. tremor. However, unlike propranolol its additional α-adrenoceptor blocking effects will prevent the rise in diastolic pressure which occurs in response to hypoglycaemia.

Adverse reactions

Potentially life-threatening effects

Deaths caused by labetalol are rare. One case has been reported in which an asthmatic died after receiving labetalol (400 mg) which had been intended for another patient.[26] Sudden withdrawal of β-adrenoceptor blockade in patients with ischaemic heart disease has been reported to cause worsening of symptoms and even fatal myocardial infarction. Sudden withdrawal of labetalol should, therefore, be avoided in patients with angina pectoris.

Acute overdosage

Bradycardia and cardiogenic shock may follow a large overdose of labetalol. Therapy with atropine (up to 3 mg intravenously) and noradrenaline has been suggested to combat these problems.[31] As with other β-blockers, glucagen is likely to be a useful antidote. One case has been reported in which 7.2 g of labetalol were taken together with 9.6 g of acebutolol and 625 mg of trimipramine.[32] On admission to hospital, the patient was unconscious with an unrecordable blood pressure and a pulse rate of 60 beats.min^{-1}. She was given 1 mg of atropine intravenously followed by intravenous infusions of dopamine and isoprenaline plus fluid replacement and bolus doses of glucagon and calcium chloride. Initially, isoprenaline and dopamine doses of 1.6 mg.min^{-1} and 200 μg.kg^{-1}.min^{-1} respectively were required to maintain the systolic blood pressure above 100 mmHg and the pulse rate above 100 beats.min^{-1}. These two agents were gradually withdrawn and the patient was well enough to be discharged home after 5 days.

Severe or irreversible adverse effects

Labetalol may cause postural hypotension and precipitate heart failure.[19,22,29] It has been reported to cause bronchospasm in susceptible patients. In addition, there are reports of licheniform skin rashes, retention of urine, systemic lupus erythematosus (two cases) and toxic myopathy (one case). Disturbances of liver function tcsts nine cases of frank jaundice[33] and liver necrosis have also been recorded.

Symptomatic adverse effects

Labetalol is generally well tolerated but may cause postural hypoten-

Labetalol (hydrochloride)

sion, headache, nasal stuffiness, scalp tingling, diarrhoea, ejaculatory failure and worsening of intermittent claudication. Other unwanted effects include dyspepsia, nausea and vomiting and nightmares.[20,29,33]

Interference with clinical pathology tests
Labetalol interferes with fluorimetric methods of analysis of catecholamines.[34]

High risk groups

Neonates
No information is available on the use of labetalol in the neonate.

Breast milk. Labetalol is excreted in breast milk with an average milk to plasma ratio of 1.5. However the small amount of drug ingested by the nursing infant is unlikely to produce any adverse effects.[35]

Children
Little information is available on the use of labetalol in children. However, Jones used it in nine children aged 1–14 years for the control of hypertension during surgical correction of post-ductal coarctation of the aorta.[36] Labetalol was administered intravenously in a dose of 0.5–1 $mg.kg^{-1}$ while anaesthesia was maintained with nitrous oxide and 1% halothane. The immediate fall in blood pressure was felt to be excessive in six patients, but rapid recovery followed when the halothane concentration was reduced. Overall, blood pressure control was thought to be satisfactory.

Bailey used labetalol preoperatively to treat an 8-year-old girl with hypertensive encephalopathy secondary to a phaeochromocytoma. The initial response to oral labetalol (100 mg twice daily) was satisfactory. However, additional intravenous bolus doses (0.08–0.17 $mg.kg^{-1}$) were required to maintain control of the blood pressure.[37]

Pregnant women
Although no teratogenic effects have been demonstrated in animals, the routine use of labetalol during the first trimester of pregnancy is not recommended. Labetalol crosses the placenta and adverse effects on the fetus and neonate are possible. However, in practice bradycardia, hypotension and hypoglycaemia are uncommon.[14]

The elderly
Provided the starting dose is small (50 mg twice daily) there should be no particular problems in elderly patients. The dosage can then be increased as necessary at intervals of 1–2 weeks.

Drug interactions

Potentially hazardous interactions

Anaesthetic agents. The heart rate may fall during general anaesthesia in patients treated with labetalol. This tendency can be minimized by the intravenous administration of atropine, either before or during the operation. The hypotensive effects of halothane are enhanced by labetalol.

Class 1 anticarrhythmic agents. Care should be taken if labetalol is used concomitantly with these drugs or calcium antagonists of the rerapamil type.

Other significant reactions

Cimetidine. The bioavailability of labetalol can be increased by concurrent administration of cimetidine (which inhibits the metabolism of the former).[12]

Hypoglycaemic agents. Labetalol may increase the incidence and severity of hypoglycaemic episodes in some diabetic patients as well as delaying their recovery from hypoglycaemia.

Tricyclic antidepressants. It has been suggested that there may be an increased incidence of tremor during therapy with a combination of labetalol and tricyclic antidepressants:[38] the mechanism of this action is not known.

Other effects. The bioavailability of labetalol is increased when it is administered with food.[39]

Clinical trials

Labetalol has been shown to be effective in the treatment of mild, moderate and severe hypertension and the published experience of its use for these indications has been summarized in several authoritative reviews.[40–42] In this context labetalol has been shown to have an effect which is superior to placebo[40] and to diuretic therapy[40] and at least comparable to that of conventional β-adrenoceptor antagonists,[40–45] methyldopa,[40,42] clonidine[40] and nifedipine.[47]

References

1. Farmer J B, Kennedy I, Levy G P, Marshall R J 1972 Pharmacology of AH 5158; a drug which blocks both α and β-adrenoceptors. British Journal of Pharmacology 45: 660–675
2. Blakeley A G H, Summers R J 1977 The effects of labetalol (AH 5158) on adrenergic transmission in the cat spleen. British Journal of Pharmacology 59: 643–650
3. Brittain R T, Levy G P 1976 A review of the animal pharmacology of labetalol, a combined α- and β-adrenoceptor blocking drug. British Journal of Clinical Pharmacology (suppl): 681–694
4. Poynter D, Martin L E, Harrison C, Cook J 1976 Affinity of labetalol for ocular melanin. British Journal of Clinical Pharmacology 3: 711–721
5. Richards D A, Prichard B N C, Boakes A J, Tuckman J, Knight E J 1977 Pharmacological basis for antihypertensive effects of intravenous labetalol. British Heart Journal 39: 99–106
6. Gagnon R-M, Morissette M, Présant S, Savard D, Lemire J 1982 Hemodynamic and coronary effects of intravenous labetalol in coronary artery disease. American Journal of Cardiology 49: 1267–1269
7. Joekes A M, Thompson F D 1976 Acute haemodynamic effects of labetalol and its subsequent use as an oral hypotensive agent. British Journal of Clinical Pharmacology 3: 789S–793S
8. Timmis A D, Fowler M B, Jaggarao N S V, Chamberlain D A 1980 Labetalol infusion for the treatment of hypertension in acute myocardial infarction. European Heart Journal 1: 413–416
9. Struthers A D, Whitesmith R, Reid J L 1983 Metabolic and haemodynamic effects of increased circulating adrenaline in man. Effect of labetalol, an alpha and beta blocker. British Heart Journal 50: 277–281
10. Wood A J, Ferry D G, Bailey R R 1982 Elimination kinetics of labetalol in severe renal failure. British Journal of Clinical Pharmacology 13: 81S–86S
11. McNeil J J, Anderson A E, Louis W J, Morgan D J 1979 Pharmacokinetics and pharmacodynamic studies of labetalol in hypertensive subjects. British Journal of Clinical Pharmacology 8: 157S–161S
12. Daneshmend T K, Roberts C J C 1981 Cimetidine and bioavailability of labetalol. Lancet 1: 565
13. Martin L E, Hopkins R, Bland R 1976 Metabolism of labetalol by animals and man. British Journal of Clinical Pharmacology 3 (suppl 3): 695–710
14. Michael C A 1979 Use of labetalol in the treatment of severe hypertension during pregnancy. British Journal of Clinical Pharmacology 8: 211S–215S
15. Leitz F, Bariletto S, Gural R, Jaworsky L, Patrick J, Symchowicz S 1983 Secretion of labetalol in breast milk of lactating women. Federation Proceedings 42 (3): 500
16. Kelly J G, McGarry K, O'Malley K, O'Brien E T 1982 Bioavailability of labetalol increases with age. British Journal of Clinical Pharmacology 14: 304–305
17. Homeida M, Jackson L, Roberts C J C 1978 Decreased first-pass metabolism of labetalol in chronic liver disease. British Medical Journal 2: 1048–1050
18. Richards D A, Maconochie J G, Bland R E, Hopkins R, Woodings E P, Martin L E 1977 Relationship between plasma concentrations and pharmacological effects of labetalol. European Journal of Clinical Pharmacology 11: 85–90
19. Dargie H J, Dollery C T, Daniel J 1976 Labetalol in resistant hypertension. British Journal of Clinical Pharmacology 3: 751S–755S
20. Michelson E L, Frishman W H, Lewis J E et al 1983 Multicenter clinical evaluation of longterm efficacy and safety of labetalol in treatment of hypertension. American Journal of Medicine 75(4A): 68–80
21. Halprin S, Frishman W, Kirschner M, Strom J 1980 Clinical pharmacology of the new beta-adrenergic blocking drugs. Part II. Effects of oral labetalol in patients with both angina pectoris and hypertension: a preliminary experience. American Heart Journal 99: 388–396
22. Upward J W, Akhras F, Jackson G 1985 Oral labetalol in the management of stable angina pectoris in normotensive patients. British Heart Journal 53: 53–57
23. Quyyumi A A, Wright C, Mockus L, Shackell M, Sutton G C, Fox K M 1985 Effects of combined alpha and beta adrenoceptor blockade in patients with angina pectoris. A double blind study comparing labetalol with placebo. British Heart Journal 53: 47–52
24. Rosei E A, Brown J J, Lever A F, Robertson A S, Robertson J I S, Trust P M 1976 Treatment of phaeochromocytoma and of clonidine withdrawal hypertension with labetalol. British Journal of Clinical Pharmacology 3 (suppl 3): 809–815
25. Skinner C, Gaddie J, Palmer K N V 1975 Comparison of intravenous AH 5158 (ibidomide) and propranolol in asthma. British Medical Journal 2: 59–61
26. Editorial 1977 Inquests. Pharmaceutical Journal 219: 139
27. Taylor S H, Silke B, Nelson G I C, Okoli R C, Ahuja R C 1982 Haemodynamic advantages of combined alpha-blockade and beta-blockade over beta-blockade alone in patients with coronary heart disease. British Medical Journal 285: 325–327
28. Marx P G, Reid D S 1979 Labetalol infusion in acute myocardial infarction with systemic hypertension. British Journal of Clinical Pharmacology 8: 233S–238S
29. New Zealand Hypertension Study Group 1981 A multicentre study of labetalol in hypertension. New Zealand Medical Journal 93: 215–218
30. Upward J W, McLeod A A, Daly K, Jackson G 1983 The electrophysical effects of intravenous labetalol in man. Circulation 68 (suppl III): 274
31. Richards D A, Prichard B N C 1978 Self-poisoning with beta-blockers. British Medical Journal 1: 1623–1624
32. Lewis M, Kallenbach J, Germond C et al 1983 Survival following massive overdose of adrenergic blocking agents (acebutolol and labetalol). Europea Journal 4: 328–332
33. Feldschreiber P 1984 The clinical profiles of long term labetalol therapy. N in Clinical Pharmacology 5: 45–50

L

34. Richards D A, Harris D M, Martin L E 1979 Labetalol and urinary catecholamines. British Medical Journal 1: 685
35. Lunell N-O, Kulas J, Rane A 1985 Transfer of labetalol into amniotic fluid and breast milk in the human. European Journal of Clinical Pharmacology 28: 597–599
36. Jones S E F 1979 Coarctation in children. Controlled hypotension using labetalol and halothane. Anaesthesia 34: 1052–1055
37. Bailey R R 1979 Labetalol in the treatment of a patient with phaeochromocytoma: a case report. British Journal of Clinical Pharmacology 8: 1415S–1425S
38. Personal communication (Duncan, Flockhart and Co Ltd)
39. Melander A, McLean A 1983 Influence of food on presystemic clearance of drugs. Clinical Pharmacokinetics 8: 286–296
40. MacCarthy E P, Bloomfield S S 1983 Labetalol: a review of its pharmacology, pharmacokinetics, clinical use and adverse effects. Pharmacotherapy 3: 193–219
41. Kanto J H 1985 Current status of labetalol, the first α- and β-blocking agent. International Journal of Clinical Pharmacology, Therapy and Toxicology 23: 617–628
42. Brogden R N, Heel R C, Speight T M, Avery G S 1978 Labetalol: a review of its pharmacology and therapeutic use in hypertension. Drugs 15: 251–270
43. Pandhi P, Aslam S, Sharma B K, Sharma P L, Wahi P L 1985 A double-blind crossover clinical trial of labetalol and propranolol in patients with essential hypertension. International Journal of Clinical Pharmacology, Therapy and Toxicology 23: 101–104
44. Jee L D, Opie L H 1985 Double-blind trial comparing labetalol with atenolol in the treatment of systemic hypertension with angina pectoris. American Journal of Cardiology 56: 551–554
45. Pandhi P, Sharma P L, Sharma B K, Wahi P L 1986 Comparative effect of propranolol and labetalol on isometric exercise and cold stress induced increase in arterial blood pressure. International Journal of Clinical Pharmacology, Therapy and Toxicology 24: 249–253
46. McNeil J J, Louis W J 1979 A double-blind crossover comparison of pindolol, metoprolol, atenolol and labetalol in mild to moderate hypertension. British Journal of Clinical Pharmacology 8: 163S–166S
47. Ohman K P, Weiner L, von Schenk H, Karlberg B E 1985 Antihypertensive and metabolic effects of nifedipine and labetalol alone and in combination in primary hypertension. European Journal of Clinical Pharmacology 29: 149–154

Lactulose

Lactulose is a disaccharide consisting of two monosaccharides, galactose and fructose, joined by an oxygen bond. Unlike lactose, which it resembles in structure, lactulose has no corresponding disaccharidase on the brush border of human intestinal mucosal cells. Thus ingested lactulose is not split into its component monosaccharides in the human gut and travels intact to the colon. There it is metabolized by the local flora into acetic and lactic acids. The result is increased osmolality and decreased pH. It is these actions which led to its introduction, first for the treatment of portal–systemic encephalopathy, and later for the treatment of constipation, especially in the young and old.

Chemistry

Lactulose (Duphalac, Bifiteral, Cephulac, Monilac, Chronulac Portalac)
$C_{12}H_{22}O_{11}$
4-O-β-d-Galactopyranosyl-d-fructose

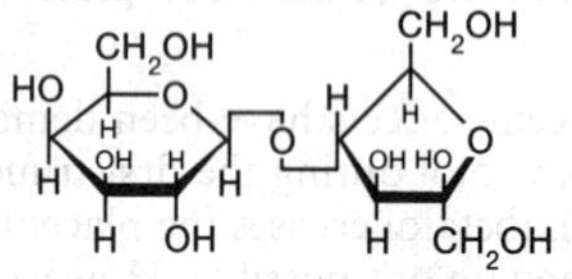

Molecular weight	343.3
pKa	—
Solubility	
in alcohol	—
in water	high
Octanol/water partition coefficient	—

Lactulose is manufactured from lactose by incubating it with lime-water at 35°C for several days.[1] It is a colourless to pale yellow syrup with a slightly sweet taste and is very soluble in water.

Pharmacology

There is no disaccharidase in the brush border of the human intestinal mucosa cell capable of splitting lactulose into its constituent monosaccharides. Thus little absorption occurs in the small intestine and the lactulose reaches the colon intact. In the ascending colon, the lactulose is degraded by the local flora and there is evidence that this process is virtually complete 20–30 minutes after the disaccharide reaches the colon.[2] There Gram-positive cocci and bacilli, especially lactobacilli and streptococci, metabolize lactulose to produce principally lactic and acetic acid.[3] The result is a sharp drop in faecal pH.[4–7] This occurs with no demonstrable change in the faecal flora.[4,8]

Toxicology

The manufacturer states that no teratogenic effects could be found at doses up to 20 times the expected human dose. Other animal studies show remarkably little acute or chronic toxicity.[1]

Clinical pharmacology

Lactulose appears to be well tolerated even in large amounts. A recommended dose for constipation is 2.5 ml twice daily for infants and 15 ml twice daily for adults. 15 ml contains 10 g lactulose (see Pharmaceutics section). For portal–systemic encephalopathy, doses of 50 ml three times a day and higher have been used.[9]

Lactulose consistently acidifies the stool,[6,10,11,12] but there is no detectable change in the faecal flora.[8] In dogs, lactulose lowers the pH of colon content and blood levels of ammonia.[11] The colon/blood ammonia ratio correlates with pH.[11] On the other hand, other sugars such as mannitol and sorbitol cause an acid stool but faecal ammonia remains the same.[10] Lactulose increases stool nitrogen. Therefore the effect of lactulose may be due to purging protein substrates before the ammonia can be produced. However, the exact sequence of events that lead to the reduction in blood ammonia in portal–systemic encephalopathy remains unknown.

The diarrhoea caused by lactulose appears on slim evidence to result from the osmotic effect of the unabsorbed carbohydrates rather than from the production of volatile fatty acids in the colon.[13]

Orally administered lactulose is fermented in the caecum and hydrogen is released.[14] This is the basis of a test used to measure small intestinal transit.[15] The interval between the ingestion and the appearance of H_2 in the breath averages 72 minutes in normal individuals and is apparently reproducible. However, some patients do not produce H_2.[16] Antibiotics and vigorous bowel preparations may greatly alter the gut flora and interfere with H_2 production.

Pharmacokinetics

Plasma levels of lactulose are insignificant since less than 1% of the drug is absorbed. In the colon, lactulose is hydrolysed to galactose and fructose which in turn lead to the production of lactic acid, formic acid, acetic acid, carbon dioxide and hydrogen.[16,17]

Concentration–effect relationship

Lactulose is minimally absorbed and plasma levels play no therapeutic role.

Metabolism

The extremely small amount of absorbed drug is excreted in the urine. There is no evidence for an enterohepatic circulation.

The important metabolic reactions of lactulose occur in the gut and are discussed above. Gut metabolites include organic acids which may contribute to the osmotic catharsis and reduce the faecal pH.[16]

Pharmaceutics

Lactulose is a pale yellow syrup.[1] A 15 ml dose of Chronulac (Merrell Dow, USA) or Duphalac (Duphar, UK) contains 10 g of lactulose, 2.2 g of galactose, 1.2 g of lactose and 1.8 g of other sugars.[17] This makes the syrup very sweet so that some patients tolerate it poorly. Cephulac (Merrell Dow, USA) is an equivalent formulation, but is also marketed as a rectal enema.

Lacticol (β-galactosido-sorbital) is a disaccharide analogue of lactulose.[18] It is chemically pure. Thus it is less sweet and available as a powder; a feature which may make it more acceptable than lactulose in the future.

The manufacturer states that the shelf-life is 3 years.[1] Lactulose should be stored below 20°C but not allowed to freeze.

Therapeutic use

Indications

1. Constipation
2. Portal–systemic encephalopathy
3. Transit time studies.

Contraindications

1. Galactosaemia.

Mode of use

1. Constipation: adults should begin with 15 ml of lactulose daily and increase or decrease the dose as necessary to achieve the desired effect. Children need much less.
2. Portal–systemic encephalopathy: the initial dose is 30 to 50 ml of lactulose three times per day. In severe cases, 50 ml may be given every 2 to 3 hours until the first soft stool appears.
3. For transit time studies, 5, 10 or 20 g of lactulose are given. The syrup is rendered isotonic by the addition of 50, 100 or 200 ml of water respectively.[15]

Indications

1. Constipation

Lactulose increases the stool frequency, weight, volume and water content in normal individuals and the effect is greater with 60 g than with 30 g per day.[19] In a double-blind study of constipated laxative users, 80% improved on lactulose even when the other laxatives were discontinued.[20] Only 33% improved on placebo. The drug appears to be a suitable laxative for children and in an optimal dose is as effective as senna with fewer side effects.[21,22]

Lactulose appears to be particularly useful in the elderly. One controlled trial compared lactulose with glucose.[23] The group receiving lactulose had less faecal impaction, required fewer enemas and suffered less cramps, bloating, flatulence and tenesmus. The drug has been found to be useful in elderly long-stay,[24,25,25a] incontinent,[26] barium impacted,[27] terminally ill[28] and vincristine-treated patients.[29]

2. Portal–systemic encephalopathy

In a double-blind trial, lactulose was superior to sorbitol in improving portal–systemic encephalopathy symptoms and the electroencephalogram.[4] It also reduced stool pH and arterial ammonia. A dose of 30 ml of lactulose four times a day (80 g daily) appears to be as effective as 1.5 g of neomycin four times a day.[9] Neomycin might be expected to destroy some lactulose-metabolizing colon bacteria, thus interfering with the suggested action of the drug.[16] However, one small study demonstrated that the beneficial effect of lactulose plus neomycin in portal–systemic encephalopathy is greater than that of either drug alone.[30]

Since faecal fermentation of lactulose occurs rapidly,[2] lactulose enemas have been used with apparent success.[31]

3. Transit time studies

Estimating the breath H_2 at intervals after ingestion of lactulose has been used to determine mouth–caecum transit time.[15] In normal individuals, the average transit is 72 minutes. The results are reproducible and compare well with a method whereby ingested polyethylene glycol is collected via a peroral ileal tube.

Adverse reactions

Potentially life-threatening effects

Aggressive treatment may result in dehydration and hypernatraemia.[32]

Acute overdosage

No cases of this kind appear to have been reported.

Severe or irreversible adverse effects

Apart from those mentioned above, none has been described.

Symptomatic adverse effects

An overdose will cause diarrhoea which in many instances is the desired effect. The effect of lactulose on the looseness, consistency and frequency of stool is dose-related. The absence of untoward hepatic, liver or cardiac effects makes the drug ideally suited to patients with portal–systemic encephalopathy or elderly patients with constipation. The very sweet taste may be nauseating and interfere with compliance. Some patients experience bloating and abdominal cramps.

High risk groups

None.

Drug interactions

An interaction with asacol is theoretically possible as it has been suggested that reduced colonic pH may prevent release of mesalazine.

References

1. Information provided by the manufacturer
2. Peled Y, Gilat T 1979 The metabolism of lactulose by the fecal flora. Gastroenterology 77: 821–823
3. Elkington S G 1970 Lactulose. Gut 11: 1043–1048
4. Elkington S G, Floch M H, Conn H O 1969 Lactulose in the treatment of portal–systemic encephalopathy. New England Journal of Medicine 281: 408–412
5. Fessel J M, Conn H O 1973 Lactulose in the treatment of acute hepatic encephalopathy. American Journal of the Medical Sciences 266: 103–110

6. Bown R L, Gibson J A, Sladen G E et al 1970 Effects of lactulose and other laxatives on ileal and colonic pH as measured by a radiotelemetry device. Gut 11: 1043–1048
7. Avery G S, Davies E F, Brogden R N 1972 Lactulose: a review. Drugs 4: 7–48
8. Conn H O, Floch M H Effects of lactulose and lactobacillus acidophilus on the fecal flora. American Journal of Clinical Nutrition 23: 1588–1594
9. Conn H O, Leevy C M, Vlahcevic Z R et al 1977 Comparison of lactulose and neomycin in the treatment of chronic portal–systemic encephalopathy. Gastroenterology 72: 573–583
10. Agostini L, Down P F, Murison J, Wrong O M 1972 Faecal ammonia and pH during lactulose administration in man: comparison with other. Gut 13: 859–866
11. Bircher J, Haemmerli U P, Trabert E et al 1971. The mechanism of action in portal–systemic encephalopathy. Rev Eur Etu Clin et Biol 16: 352–357
12. Vince A, Killingley M, Wrong O M 1978 Effect of lactulose on ammonia production in a fecal incubation system. Gastroenterology 74: 544–549
13. Saunders D R, Wiggins H S 1981 How do single doses of carbohydrates such as lactulose cause diarrhea? Gastroenterology 81: 1272
14. Levitt M D, Donaldson R M 1970 Use of respiratory hydrogen (H_2) excretion to detect carbohydrate malabsorption. Journal of Laboratory and Clinical Medicine 75: 937–945
15. Bond J H, Levitt M D 1975 Investigation of small bowel transit time in man utilizing pulmonary hydrogen (H_2). Journal of Laboratory and Clinical Medicine 85: 546–555
16. Gilat T, Ben Hur H, Gelman-Malachi E et al 1978 Alterations of the colonic flora and their effect on the hydrogen breath test. Gut 19: 602–605
17. Review. Lactulose (Chronulac) for constipation. 1980 Medical Letter on Drugs and Therapeutics 22: 2–4
18. Lanthier P L, Morgan M Y 1985 Lacticol in the treatment of chronic hepatic encephalopathy: an open comparison with lactulose. Gut 26: 415–420
19. Bass P, Dennis S 1981 The laxative effects of lactulose in normal and constipated subjects. Journal of Clinical Gastroenterology 3: 23–28
20. Wesselius de C A, Sparis A, Braadbaart G E, Bergh-Bohlken G E 1968 Treatment of chronic constipation with lactulose syrup: results of a double-blind study. Gut 9: 84–86
21. Bush R T 1972 Lactulose: an ideal laxative for children. New Zealand Medical Journal 71: 364–365
22. Perkin J M 1977 Constipation in childhood: a controlled comparison between lactulose and standardized Senna. Current Medical Research and Opinion 4: 540–543
23. Saunders J F 1978 Lactulose syrup assessed in a double-blind study of elderly constipated patients. Journal of the American Geriatrics Society 26: 236–239
24. Brocklehurst J C, Kirkland J L, Martin J, Ashford J 1983 Constipation in long-stay elderly patients: its treatment and prevention by lactulose. Gastroenterology 29: 181–184
25. Kahanpaa A 1975 Some observations of the use of lactulose in the treatment of constipation in the elderly. Gerontology 20: 79–85
25a. Champion M C, Thompson W G, Kilgour J A et al. 1986 Efficacy and cost-effectiveness of lactulose in the treatment of constipation in elderly psychiatric patients. American Journal of Gastroenterology 81: 872
26. Ryan D, Wilson A, Muir T S, Judge T G 1974 The reduction of faecal incontinence by the use of 'Dulphalac' in geriatric patients. Current Medical Research and Opinion 2: 329–333
27. Prout B J, Datta S B, Wilson T S 1972 Colonic retention of barium in the elderly after barium meal examination and its treatment. British Medical Journal 2: 550–553
28. Crowther A G O 1978 Management of constipation in terminally ill patients. Journal of International Medical Research 6: 348–353
29. Harris A C 1977 Lactulose in vincristine induced constipation. Medical Journal of Australia 22: 273–274
30. Pirotte J, Guffens J M, Devos J 1974 Comparative study of basal arterial ammonemia and of orally-induced hyperammonemia in chronic portal systemic encephalopathy treated with neomycin and lactulose. Digestion 10: 435–444
31. Kersh E S, Rifkin H 1973 Lactulose enemas. Annals of Internal Medicine 78: 81–84
32. Kaupke C, Sprague T, Gitnick G L 1977 Hypernatremia after the administration of the lactulose. Annals of Internal Medicine 86: 745–746

Latamoxef disodium

Latamoxef disodium is a novel β-lactam antibiotic, with a sulphur atom substituted for the oxygen atom in the cephem nucleus. It was introduced in Britain in 1983. It was originally marketed as Moxalactam but renamed latamoxef to make the chemical structure of the antibiotic clearer. Moxalactam has been retained as the trade name. Latamoxef was originally seen as a useful agent for the prophylaxis and therapy of surgical patients but the high incidence of postoperative bleeding associated with its use means that it now has a very limited role.

Chemistry

Latamoxef disodium (Moxalactam)
$C_{20}H_{18}N_6O_9SNa_2$
Disodium salt of (6R,7R)-7-[Carboxy(4-hydroxyphenyl)acetyl]-amino-7-methoxy-3-[(1-methyl-1*H*-tetrazol-5-yl)thio]methyl]-8-oxo-5-oxa-1-azabicyclo[4.2.0]oct-2-ene-2-carboxylic acid

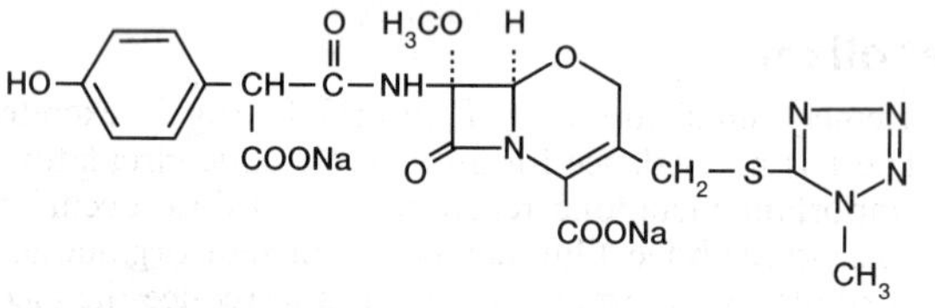

Molecular weight (free acid)	564.5 (520.5)
pKa (carboxyl)	3.7
Solubility	
in alcohol	insoluble
in water	high
Octanol/water partition coefficient	low

Latamoxef is insoluble in most organic solvents. It is a white crystalline powder, freely soluble in normal saline and available for parenteral use only.

It is prepared by chemical synthesis. In addition to the carbon 6 and carbon 7, the carbon 1 of the phenyl ring is optically active. The commercial preparation is a mixture of the R(–) and S(–) epimers.

Pharmacology

Latamoxef is a bactericidal antibiotic active against most aerobic Gram-negative bacteria and the commonly occurring anaerobic Gram-negative bacteria.[1,2,3]

Latamoxef kills bacteria by interfering in the synthesis of the bacterial cell wall. Peptidoglycan is a heteropolymeric structure that provides the cell wall with mechanical stability. The final stage in the synthesis of peptidoglycan involves the completion of the cross-linking and the terminal glycine residue of the pentaglycine bridge is linked to the fourth residue of the pentapeptide (d-alanine). The transpeptidase enzyme that performs this step is inhibited by penicillins and cephalosporins. As a result the bacterial cell wall is weakened, the cell swells and then ruptures.

Toxicology

There are no reports of toxicological results in animals that are of potential clinical relevance. There was no evidence of carcinogenicity or teratogenicity in tests lasting up to six months in mice and rabbits.

Latamoxef disodium

Clinical pharmacology

Latamoxef has good activity against *Escherichia coli* and *Klebsiella pneumoniae* but poor activity against *Staphylococcus aureus* and *Pseudomonas aeruginosa*.[4,5] Studies on colonic microflora after parenteral administration of latamoxef showed a significant reduction in both aerobic and anaerobic bacteria.[6] It has no activity against *Streptococcus faecalis*. Colonic overgrowth with latamoxef-resistant *Pseudomonas* spp. and yeasts occurred in patients given three doses but not in patients given a single dose. Therapy with latamoxef has resulted in the overgrowth of *Clostridium difficile* and its toxin: cases of pseudomembranous colitis may occur with latamoxef, as with any antibiotic.[7] Bacteria resistant to latamoxef have emerged during therapy: the majority of these isolates have been *Pseudomonas* spp. against which latamoxef has low intrinsic activity.[8] It has been suggested that prior therapy with other cephalosporins such as cefoxitin may induce resistance to latamoxef (and other third generation cephalosporins) so that sensitivity testing is mandatory before therapy and again if there is a poor response to initial therapy.[9]

Latamoxef is resistant to destruction by many β-lactamases.[10]

Single and multiple intramuscular and intravenous injections of latamoxef showed that serum levels achieved were well in excess of the minimum inhibitory concentration (MIC) of the pathogens listed as sensitive to latamoxef[11] The only side effect noted was some discomfort at the site of injection.

Pharmacokinetics

Latamoxef is usually assayed by bioassay, using agar diffusion with a Gram-negative organism as indicator. There is no significant absorption from the gastrointestinal tract, and no presystemic metabolism. The plasma half life is approximately 1.6 hours, and the volume of distribution, is 8.5 l. Latamoxef is 40% protein bound. Latamoxef, in common with other third generation cephalosporins, achieves far greater penetration into cerebrospinal fluid than earlier agents. In neonates, CSF levels were approximately 20% of simultaneous serum levels, which is considerably in excess of the MIC of many Gram-negative organisms causing meningitis, including *Haemophilus influenzae* and *Neisseria meningitidis*.[12] Tissue samples of colonic intestinal mucosa taken after administration of 2 g of latamoxef before colorectal surgery showed good penetration, with tissue samples showing mean levels of 22 $\mu g.g^{-1}$, with a simultaneous serum level of 29 $mg.l^{-1}$.[8] Tissue samples of latamoxef after 1 g preoperative dose in patients undergoing arterial surgery were above the MIC required for common Gram-negative pathogens, but were barely adequate for *Staph. aureus*.[13] A study comparing the penetration of latamoxef and cephazolin into cancerous bone showed that the two agents achieved similar bone levels, although in the case of latamoxef this would not be sufficient for treatment of the commonest pathogen, *Staph. aureus*.[14]

Oral absorption	negligible
Presystemic metabolism	none
Plasma half life	
range	1.3–2.6 h
mean	1.6 h
Volume of distribution	8.5 l
Plasma protein binding	40%

The effects of hepatic disease on the kinetics of the drug are not known, though they are unlikely to be very marked. In renal dysfunction and are-related change in renal function the elimination of the drug is reduced, which may require adjustment of the dose.

Concentration–effect relationship

Antibiotic concentration in serum or tissues in excess of the minimum inhibitory concentration (MIC) of the organism responsible for the infection are required for effective therapy with any antibiotic. Latamoxef achieves serum levels well in excess of MIC for pathogens such as *E. coli* and *Klebsiella* spp., but not for organisms such as *Staph. aureus* or *Pseudomonas* spp., and this is reflected in the higher number of therapeutic failures when latamoxef alone is used to treat these pathogens.[7] Tissue levels are invariably lower than simultaneous serum levels, and a combination of surgical drainage of pus and antibiotic therapy is usually necessary for resolution of abscesses. Difficult infections such as osteomyelitis and deep-seated kidney infections with stones often require prolonged therapy lasting up to 6 weeks or more with a high antibiotic dose.

Metabolism

Latamoxef is excreted primarily by the kidneys. Approximately 75% of a first dose of latamoxef was detected in urine samples within 12 hours, with virtually all the dose given recovered in the urine within 24 hours.[11] Small amounts of latamoxef can be detected in the stools after parenteral administration, presumably reflecting biliary excretion, but non-renal clearance is low.

Concentrations of latamoxef in serum with and without probenecid show no significant difference.[11] This suggests that latamoxef is excreted mainly by glomerular filtration, with only a small amount excreted through the renal tubules. There is no evidence of any hepatic metabolism of latamoxef: chromatographic studies show that the 1% of decarboxylated latamoxef present from the time of manufacture can be detected in the urine after administration of latamoxef, and that there are no other metabolites or breakdown products.

Pharmaceutics

Latamoxef (Moxalactam — Lilly, no longer available in the UK) is available in vials of powder for intramuscular or intravenous injection of 500 mg, 1 g and 2 g. There is no oral preparation, and no potentially allergenic substance in the preparation.

The unreconstituted vials can be stored at room temperature, and after reconstitution may be stored in a refrigerator for up to 96 hours or at room temperature for a maximum of 12 hours. The maximum shelf-life of the unreconstituted vials is 2 years.

Therapeutic use

Indications

1. Lower respiratory tract infections
2. Urinary tract infections
3. Intra-abdominal infections
4. Gynaecological infections
5. Septicaemia
6. Skin and soft tissue infections
7. Bone and joint infections
8. Meningitis.

In all these infections, latamoxef will give reliable cover against Gram-negative organisms. It has poor activity against Gram-positive organisms such as *Staph. aureus* and, if infection with these organisms is likely, a combination of latamoxef and penicillin or flucloxacillin should be used. In neonatal Gram-negative meningitis, for example, latamoxef alone would provide inadequate therapy if *Streptococcus agalactiae* was an actual or potential pathogen pending microbiological results, and a combination of latamoxef and penicillin should be used. Latamoxef, as a parenteral preparation, is intended for use in hospitals only: it is highly active against Gram-negative organisms including *Bacteroides* spp. and provides useful cover against the range of pathogens expected after lower abdominal or gynaecological surgery. Latamoxef has also been recommended for use as prophylaxis in large bowel and abdominal surgery.

Contraindications

1. Allergy to penicillins or cephalosporins
2. Concomitant high-dose heparin or anticoagulants.

Mode of use

Latamoxef is the first member of the new oxalactam group of antibiotics. It has a broad spectrum of activity against Gram-negative organisms, and good stability to β-lactamases. A leader in the Lancet in 1981 concluded that latamoxef was not 'that greater sought after commodity the safe and reliable broad-spectrum antibiotic which may be used in almost any serious infection, but ... will prove useful in the management of coliform and Haemophilus meningitis, and in infections caused by Gram-negative bacilli resistant to other antibiotics.'

Latamoxef disodium

L

Serious side effects due to latamoxef had not been seen in large numbers then (although hypoprothrombinaemia was noted in 29 patients out of 3558 reviewed) and this complication has reduced even the limited indications listed above.[32] The serious complication of postoperative bleeding seen since then, particularly in the elderly and in more recent studies, mean that latamoxef should be used with great caution in surgical patients. There are many other effective antibiotics available for both the prophylaxis of large bowel surgery, and the therapy of postoperative complications, and there should be no need for the routine use of latamoxef in these patients. Similarly while latamoxef appears appropriate therapy for neonatal Gram-negative meningitis, other agents such as cefotaxime are also available. It is difficult to recommend a specific role for latamoxef: many clinicians and microbiologists feel that the new generation of cephalosporins should be reserved for use in specific cases where the causative organism is known to be resistant to first line agents and this, combined with the known bleeding problems associated with latamoxef, mean that there are now very few indications for the first-line use of latamoxef.

The recommended range of dose in adults is 500 mg to 4 g per day, rising to a maximum of 12 g a day in divided doses in patients with life-threatening infections. For children the recommended dose schedule is:

0–1 week of age 25 $mg.kg^{-1}$ 12-hourly
1–4 weeks of age 25 $mg.kg^{-1}$ 8-hourly
Infants and children 50 $mg.kg^{-1}$ 12-hourly

The highest dose known to be used is 16 g daily.

The daily dose should be determined by the severity and site of infection, and the sensitivity to the causative organisms if known. Higher doses of up to 12 g a day are recommended for meningitis in adults with *Enterobacteriaecaea*, or for septicaemia secondary to deep-seated infection. Intravenous rather than intramuscular injection is recommended for life-threatening infections such as septicaemia or meningitis.

When renal function is impaired a reduced dose must be employed (see 'Concurrent disease').

Indications

1. Lower respiratory tract infections
Latamoxef should not be used for respiratory infections due to standard pathogens such as *Streptococcus pneumoniae* or *Haemophilus influenzae*, but should be considered for proven Gram-negative bacterial pneumonia, particularly in patients needing mechanical ventilation or in intensive care. Latamoxef was effective in 84 out of 119 patients with non-*Haemophilus* Gram-negative pneumonia, with most treatment failures occurring in patients with infection due to *Pseudomonas* spp.[15]

2. Urinary tract infection
There are many effective oral agents available to treat uncomplicated urinary tract infections, and latamoxef should be considered only for complicated urinary tract infections requiring parenteral therapy. Latamoxef was as effective as gentamicin in this group of patients, although, disappointingly, only 4 out of 10 patients with gentamicin-resistant latamoxef-sensitive isolates were cured with latamoxef.[16]

3. Intra-abdominal infections
Surgical drainage as well as antibiotic therapy is usually necessary here. Latamoxef penetrates peritoneal fluid well, and has a broad spectrum of aerobic and anaerobic activity. It was effective in 38 out of 48 patients with intra-abdominal infections, although there was super-infection with latamoxef-resistant isolates in 18 patients.[17] There are currently several other antibiotics effective in the therapy of intra-abdominal infections. Combinations of penicillin, gentamicin and metronidazole or an established cephalosporin such as cefuroxime plus metronidazole are well tried. A study of latamoxef in intra-abdominal infections from Birmingham[18] showed an unacceptably high incidence of side effects (see 'Adverse effects') and, faced with well established and non-toxic combinations, it is difficult to recommend the routine use of latamoxef.

4. Gynaecological infections
The range of pathogens in postoperative gynaecological or obstetric infections is similar to that in abdominal surgery. Latamoxef is a useful reserve antibiotic here, but there is no evidence that it is more effective than the current standard therapy of metronidazole and ampicillin or cephradine.

5. Septicaemia
Latamoxef has been used to treat septicaemia in neutropenic patients[19] and those with a normal immune system.[20,21] It should not be used alone if there is any chance of infection with Gram-positive organisms, and it should not be used for proven *Pseudomonas* infections. In addition, for neutropenic patients it is common practice to use a combination of antibiotics such as mezlocillin or cefuroxime and gentamicin. There is no evidence that latamoxef alone or in combination is more effective than these established regimes.

6. Skin and soft tissue infections
The majority of these infections are caused by Gram-positive organisms such as *Staph. aureus* and *Streptococcus pyogenes* for which latamoxef is inappropriate therapy. For Gram-negative soft tissue infections or wound infections, latamoxef provides adequate cover against aerobes and anaerobes. There is no evidence that it is more effective than a combination of another cephalosporin and metronidazole, however.

7. Bone and joint infections
Latamoxef achieves levels in bone sufficient to inhibit virtually all potential Gram-negative pathogens including *H. influenzae*. The majority of bone and joint infections are caused by Gram-positive infections, however, so latamoxef should only be considered for proven Gram-negative infections. Therapy of bone and joint infections usually lasts for several weeks and the risk of side effects is probably too high for the routine use of latamoxef here.

8. Meningitis
Latamoxef penetrated cerebrospinal fluid well, with CSF levels ranging from 10% to 30% of serum levels in neonates.[12] It is very active against the coliforms predominating in neonatal meningitis and against *H. influenzae*. Its modest activity against other pathogens causing meningitis mean that it should not be used alone unless the pathogen is known. Both neonatal and Gram-negative meningitis in children has been shown to respond well to latamoxef,[12,22] and this is one of the few conditions where latamoxef remains a first-line agent, although even here other new cephalosporins such as cefotaxime or ceftizoxime will be as effective.

Contraindications

1. Hypersensitivity
Use of latamoxef is specifically contraindicated in patients who have shown a previous hypersensitivity reaction to latamoxef.

Latamoxef may be given, with caution, to patients with a previous history of allergy to penicillins.

2. Concomitant heparin or anticoagulants
There is a high risk of prolonged bleeding time in patients who are receiving concomitant high-dose heparin or oral anticoagulants if latamoxef is used as well (see below).

Adverse reactions

Potentially life-threatening effects
The most serious adverse effect that has been reported after therapy with latamoxef is bleeding, which has a high incidence.[18] Hypothrombinaemia or drug-induced platelet dysfunction may occur after therapy with latamoxef.[23,24] A report from Birmingham[18] comparing latamoxef alone with latamoxef and metronidazole for the prophylaxis of elective colorectal surgery showed a high rate of postoperative bleeding in both groups. Of the first 97 patients given latamoxef, alone or in combination with metronidazole, there were 12 cases of postoperative bleeding. The next 13 patients were given vitamin K with latamoxef, but there were 5 further cases of postoperative bleeding, and the trial was discontinued because of the unacceptably high incidence of bleeding. The authors noted that postoperative bleeding with a prolonged prothrombin time was a greater problem if therapy was continued for 5 days, but felt that the risk of postoperative bleeding was too great for them to recommend latamoxef, even for short-term prophylaxis, with or without covering vitamin K. The problem of hypoprothrombinaemia and platelet

Latamoxef disodium

dysfunction secondary to treatment with cephalosporin and oxalactam antibiotics was reviewed in 1983.[25] Patients treated with cefamandole, latamoxef or cefoperazone have developed this condition,[26] but latamoxef has been the drug most commonly implicated. Postoperative bleeding secondary to hypoprothrombinaemia and/or platelet dysfunction is most likely to occur in the elderly and malnourished although the problem has been noted in patients as young as 36, or in patients with a degree of renal failure. Bleeding associated with latamoxef therapy has been noted by several authors:[18,23,24,26,27,28] there appear to be two mechanisms involved. In the first, the N-methyltetrazolethiol side-chains present in latamoxef (and cefamandole and cefoperazone) may impair vitamin K production from the gastrointestinal tract. Abnormalities of platelet function after latamoxef therapy have also been seen. A comparison of bleeding times and platelet function in patients randomized to receive latamoxef or cefotaxime found minimal abnormalities in the cefotaxime group, but a significant increase in the bleeding time in patients receiving latamoxef, particularly in those with impaired renal function. In addition, in the latamoxef group, the increased bleeding time was accompanied by decreased ADP-induced platelet aggregation.[29] It has been suggested that latamoxef should be combined with vitamin K, but this will not always be effective,[18] and until more is known about the mechanism of bleeding after the administration of latamoxef, it would seem safest to restrict the use of the drug. Anaphylaxis due to allergy to latamoxef is an uncommon occurrence, but a previous history of allergy, particularly to cephalosporins, should always be sought.

Acute overdosage
No cases of deliberate overdose are known.

Severe or irreversible adverse effects
There are no irreversible side effects.

Symptomatic adverse effects
Gastrointestinal adverse effects such as diarrhoea occur in approximately 2% of patients, but nausea and vomiting are rare. Pseudomembranous colitis may occur during or after therapy. Minor hypersensitivity reactions such as skin rashes and drug fever may occur in 1 to 2% of patients given latamoxef, but these disappear when the drug is stopped. Anaphylaxis has been reported.

Other effects
Transient hepatic enzyme elevation has been detected in about 4% of patients given latamoxef, but this is usually of no clinical significance. A transient deterioration of renal function, with increases in serum creatinine and urea and sometimes haematuria and pyuria have been reported in less than 1% of patients given latamoxef. There is no evidence of significant deterioration in renal function associated with any of the newer cephalosporins, and clinical experience has shown that it is safe to use cephalosporins such as latamoxef with gentamicin and frusemide if necessary. The dose of latamoxef should be reduced in renal failure in line with the manufacturer's recommendations, to reduce the risk of the adverse effects, such as encephalopathy, common to all β-lactam antibiotics. There have been reports of patients developing a positive Coombs' test during latamoxef therapy.

Interference with clinical pathology tests
None is known.

High risk groups

Neonates
If latamoxef is used in neonates, care should be taken not to exceed the recommended dose, particularly in premature neonates where there may be a degree of renal immaturity. Studies on the use of latamoxef in neonates and children have shown that it is effective in a variety of infections, including meningitis, septicaemia and urinary infections.[12,30]

Breast milk. Latamoxef enters breast milk in small but significant amounts and, because of effects on the gut flora of the infants, latamoxef should not be given to nursing mothers.[31]

Children
What has been said about neonates applies also to children.

Pregnant women
There is no information on the use of the drug in pregnant women, but animal studies show little evidence of toxicity or teratogenicity.

The elderly
The dose may have to be reduced or the dose interval increased in the elderly if there is evidence of renal impairment, and particular attention should be paid to the possibility of bleeding in this group.

Concurrent disease
When the renal function is impaired a reduced dose must be employed, depending on the degree of renal impairment, the severity of the infection and the susceptibility of the causative organism.

Drug interactions

The potentially hazardous interaction between latamoxef and heparin or anticoagulants has been mentioned. In addition, an antabuse effect has been noted if alcohol is taken after administration of latamoxef.

Major outcome trials

There have been many open and comparative studies of latamoxef and also of all the other new cephalosporins. No one trial or trials stand out as pre-eminent, and many clinicians and microbiologists feel that the newer cephalosporins should not be used routinely, but should be kept in reserve for specific infections or specific clinical problems. The new agents are all markedly more active than their predecessors, but it is feared that overuse of the new agents will lead to rapid development of bacterial resistance. The new agents are also more expensive than the earlier ones and, in addition, it has been difficult to establish greater in vivo success with the new agents in comparison with those used previously despite the marked in vitro differences. The three studies detailed below highlight specific areas where latamoxef has been useful.

1. Ribner B S, Raeder R, Becher T M, Freimer E H 1983 Treatment of serious infections with moxalactam. American Journal of Medicine 74: 396–400

In 93 hospital patients, 111 bacterial infections, including meningitis, pneumonia, septicaemia and urinary tract infections, were treated with latamoxef alone. 75% of the infections responded. The authors measured latamoxef levels in blood, cerebrospinal fluid, peritoneal fluid and abscess fluid and found that the great majority of isolates had mean inhibitory concentrations below those achieved in the fluids measured.

2. Stambaugh J E, MacAdams J 1982 The efficacy and safety of Moxalactam in the treatment of acute bacterial infections in immunosuppressed patients with cancer. Current Therapeutic Research 31: 864–71

In 89 immunosuppressed patients treated with latamoxef alone for 109 infections, 80% of the infections responded, with most treatment failures with infections due to Gram-positive organisms. There were no serious side effects, although four patients developed superinfection with *Strep. faecalis* and three with latamoxef-resistant *Pseudomonas aeruginosa*.

3. Kammer R B 1982 Moxalactam: clinical efficacy and safety. Reviews of Infectious Diseases 4 (suppl): 712–720

A review of 2234 patients from studies in many different American centres treated with Moxalactam showed that the overall response rate was 89%. This ranged from 94% in septicaemias (where patients with Gram-positive and Gram-negative infections responded well) to 83% in urinary tract infections. This relatively low figure was probably due to the number of complicated infections treated and the low doses used. There was a low incidence of side effects, with hypersensitivity in 3% and gastrointestinal upset in 2%. Hypoprothrombinaemia occurred in 25 patients, and clinically apparent bleeding in 3 patients only. This is a much lower figure than in the trial by Morris et al,[18] but there have been several reports of bleeding in more recent trials.

General review article

A major review of latamoxef based on a symposium held in London in 1981 was published by the Infectious Diseases Society of America: Reviews of Infectious Diseases 1982 4 (suppl 1): 726

References

1. Barza M, Tally F P, Jacobus N V, Gorbach S L 1979 In vitro activity of LY127 935. Antimicrobial Agents and Chemotherapy 16: 287–292
2. Wise R, Andrews J M, Bedford K A 1979 LY127 935, a novel oxa-beta lactam: an in vitro comparison with other β-lactam antibiotics. Antimicrobial Agents and Chemotherapy 16: 341–345
3. Gilchrist M J R, Washington J A 1982 In vitro activity of moxalactam against anaerobic bacteria. Reviews of Infections Diseases 4 (suppl): 511–515
4. Jones R N, Fuchs P C, Sanmers M, Gavan L, Barry A L, Gerhlach E H 1980 Moxalactam (LY127 935), a new semi-synthetic 1-oxa-β-lactam antibiotic with remarkable in vitro antimicrobial activity: in vitro comparison with cefamandole and tobramycin. Antimicrobial Agents and Chemotherapy 17: 750–756
5. McNamee W, Drusano G L, Takem B A, Standiford H C 1984 The serum bactericidal activity of latamoxef (Moxalactam), cefoperazone and cefotaxime. Journal of Antimicrobial Chemotherapy 14: 491–498
6. Kager L, Malmborg A S, Nord C E, Sjostedt S 1984 Impact of single dose as compared to three dose prophylaxis with latamoxef (Moxalactam) on the colonic microflora in patients undergoing colorectal surgery. Journal of Antimicrobial Chemotherapy 14: 171–178
7. Gunner-Deevy H, Jones P G, Kauffman C A et al 1984 Effect of therapy with latamoxef (Moxalactam) on carriage of Clostridium difficile. Journal of Antimicrobial Chemotherapy 13: 521–524
8. Kammer R B 1982 Moxalactam: clinical summary of efficacy and safety. Reviews of Infectious Diseases 4 (suppl): 712–719
9. Levin M H, Weinstein R A, Kalins S A 1983 Cefoxitin disc induction of latamoxef (Moxalactam) resistance. Journal of Antimicrobial Chemotherapy 12: 524
10. Richmond M H 1980 The β-lactamase stability of a novel lactam antibiotic containing a 7 β-methoxyoxacephem nucleus. Journal of Antimicrobial Chemotherapy 6: 445–454
11. Shimada J, Ueda Y 1982 Moxalactam absorption, excretion, distribution and metabolism. Reviews of Infectious Diseases 4 (suppl): 569–580
12. Schaad U B, McCraken Jr G H, Threlkeld N, Thomas M L 1981 Clinical evaluation of a new broad spectrum oxa-beta-lactam antibiotic, Moxalactam, in neonates and infants. Journal of Paediatrics 98: 129–136
13. Stewart J, Courtney D F, Fowler B, Ramsden C H, Kester R C 1984 The penetration of latamoxef disodium (Moxalactam) into the subcutaneous fat and skeletal muscle of ischaemic lower limbs with atherosclerotic disease. Journal of Antimicrobial Chemotherapy 13: 377–382
14. Hume A L, Polk R, Kline B, Cardea J 1983 Comparative penetration of latamoxef (Moxalactam) and cefazolin into human knees following simultaneous administration. Journal of Antimicrobial Chemotherapy 12: 623–628
15. Saito A 1982 Clinical evaluation of Moxalactam in the treatment of respiratory tract infections, hepatobiliary infections and septicaemias. Reviews of Infectious Diseases 4 (suppl): 623–628
16. Penn R E, Preheim L C, Sanders C C, Giger D K 1983 Comparison of Moxalactam and gentamicin in the treatment of complicated urinary tract infections. Antimicrobial Agents and Chemotherapy 24: 494–499
17. Murphy T F, Barja M 1982 Treatment of intra-abdominal infection with Moxalactam. Review of Infectious Diseases 4 (suppl): 670–675
18. Morris D L, Fabricius P J, Ambrose N S, Scammell B, Burdon D W, Keighley M R B 1984 A high incidence of bleeding is observed in a trial to determine whether addition of metronidazole is needed with latamoxef for prophylaxis of colorectal surgery. Journal of Hospital Infection 5: 398–409
19. Mavier R L, Faro S, Sanders C V et al 1982 Moxalactam in the therapy of serious infections. Antimicrobial Agents and Chemotherapy 21: 650–654
20. Wilson W R, Henry R K, Keys T F et al 1984 Empiric therapy with Moxalactam alone in patients with bacteraemia. Mayo Clinic Proceedings 59: 318–326
21. Rilner B S, Raeder R, Becke T M, Freimer E H 1983 Treatment of serious infections with Moxalactam. American Journal of Medicine 74: 396–400
22. Rahal J 1982 Moxalactam therapy for Gram-negative bacillary meningitis. Reviews of Infectious Diseases 4 (suppl): 606–609
23. Panwalker A D, Rosenfeld J 1983 Haemorrhage, diarrhoea and superinfection associated with the use of Moxalactam. Journal of Infectious Diseases 147: 171–172
24. Weitekamp R M, Aber R C 1983 Prolonged bleeding times and bleeding diathesis associated with moxalactam administration. Journal of the American Medical Association 249: 69–71
25. Smith C R, Lipsky J J 1983 Hypoprothrombinaemia and platelet dysfunction caused by cephalosporin and oxalactam antibiotics. Journal of Antimicrobial Chemotherapy 11: 496–497
26. Neu H C 1983 Adverse effects of new cephalosporins. Annals of Internal Medicine 98: 415–416
27. Bruck K 1983 Hypoprothrombinaemia and cephalosporins. Lancet 1: 535–536
28. Hackman R, Clark J, Rolla A, Thomas S, Kaldany A, D'Elia J A 1982 Bleeding in patients with infections; are cephalosporins helping or hurting. Archives of Internal Medicine 142: 1440
29. Andrasy K, Kodevisch J, Fritz S, Ritz E 1983 New betalactam antibiotics and haemorrhagic diathesis: comparison of Moxalactam and cefotaxime. Clinical Therapeutics 6: 34–42
30. De Louvois J, James J, Mulhall A 1984 Latamoxef and the new born. Archives of Disease in Childhood 59: 346–350
31. Miller R D, Keegan K A, Thrupp L D, Brann J 1984 Human breast milk concentration of Moxalactam. American Journal of Obstetrics and Gynecology 148: 348–349
32. Anonymous 1981 Moxalactam. Lancet 2: 23–4

Levodopa

Levodopa is a natural intermediary in the enzymatic synthesis of dopamine from L-tyrosine. Exogenous levodopa is rapidly decarboxylated by L-aromatic amino acid decarboxylase (LAAD). About 1% of orally administered levodopa will pass the blood–brain barrier (BBB) to be converted to dopamine, mostly in the basal ganglia. In combination with a peripheral LAAD inhibitor, e.g. benserazide or carbidopa, this amount will increase significantly.

Chemistry

Levodopa (dihydroxyphenylalanine, dopa, L-dopa, laevodopa, Bendopa, Biodopa, Brocadopa, Cerepar, Deadopa, Dopaflex, Dopal, Dopaidan, Dopalina, Dopar, Doparkine, Doparl, Dopasol, Dopastom, Dopastral, Cilandopa, Doprin, Eldopal, Eldopar, Eldopatec, Eurodopa, Helfo-dopa, Larodopa, Ledopa, Parda, Levopa, Sobiodopa, Veldopa)
$C_9H_{11}NO_4$
(L)-3-(3,4-Dihydroxyphenyl)-L-alanine

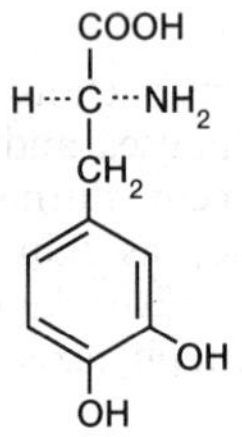

Molecular weight	197.2
pKa	2.3, 8.7, 9.7, 13.4
Solubility	
in alcohol	<1 in 10 000
in water	1 in 300
Octanol/water partition coefficient	low

Levodopa is a white to off-white, odourless, crystalline powder. It is freely soluble in dilute aqueous solutions of mineral acids and alkali carbonates.

Levodopa is available in combination with carbidopa (Sinemet, Sinemet-Plus) and with benserazide (Madopar).

Levodopa can be extracted from naturally occurring ground velvet beans, with acetic acid.[1,2] Levodopa is the (L)-isomer of dopa.

Pharmacology

Levodopa is the aromatic amino acid precursor of the natural neurotransmitter dopamine. Unlike dopamine, levodopa can cross the BBB and is subject to carboxylation by LAAD, both peripherally and centrally, into dopamine. Oral levodopa will reach the basal ganglia where it will enhance dopaminergic transmission, after decarboxylation. In the periphery oral levodopa will, after decarboxylation, stimulate the peripheral dopamine receptors (e.g. in the area postrema) and the β-adrenergic receptors (e.g. in the cardiovascular system).

Toxicology

The LD_{50} of levodopa is about 3650 $mg.kg^{-1}$ in mice, over 4000 $mg.kg^{-1}$ in rats and about 600 $mg.kg^{-1}$ in rabbits.[3] In oral subacute toxicity studies with doses up to 1000 $mg.kg^{-1}$ daily for 13 weeks in monkeys, no treatment-related effects were evident. In rats, treatment-related morphologic changes occurred in salivary glands

Levodopa

(hypertrophy of acinar cells) and adrenals (cytoplasmal rarefaction of the zona glomerulosa) at all dosage levels, while in kidneys of rats receiving 500–1000 $mg.kg^{-1}$ daily tubular necrosis was noticed next in frequency to necrosis of superficial epithelium in the stomach. Clinical signs of toxicity included hyperventilation and decreased activity. Administration of 125 and 250 $mg.kg^{-1}$ levodopa in pregnant rabbits induced a dose-dependent teratogenic effect. Anomalies included septal defects, missing ductus arteriosus, fused aortas and pulmonary arches, and transpositions. The same types of malformations were also seen in one mouse after chronic 500 $mg.kg^{-1}$ daily. Other effects on reproduction as seen after treatment with levodopa in combination with carbidopa included skeletal anomalies, especially of vertebral and skull bones.[4] Visceral and skeletal malformations were found in chronic experiments with 100 and 200 $mg.kg^{-1}$ daily in rats and 40–50 $mg.kg^{-1}$ daily in dogs.[3]

Clinical pharmacology

Levodopa is a precursor of dopamine and noradrenaline in the pathway of catecholamine synthesis. Decarboxylation of levodopa by LAAD into dopamine will take place extra- as well as intra-cerebrally.

Dopamine is an important neurotransmitter that regulates functions in brain, heart, vascular system, kidney and gut. The most relevant clinical syndrome of dopamine imbalance in the brain is parkinsonism, caused either by toxic factors, e.g. reserpine or methylphenyltetrahydropyridine (MPTP), or by yet unknown causes, resulting in degeneration of dopaminergic nigral neurones (with possible abiotrophic interaction[5]) — as is the case in Parkinson's disease.

Oral levodopa, especially in company with a peripheral decarboxylase inhibitor, can modify symptoms of parkinsonism in most cases.[6] On the other hand, a relative surplus of intracerebral dopamine, which can result from overdosage with levodopa in Parkinson patients or hypersensitivity of the dopaminergic receptors, will induce involuntary movements such as chorea, dystonia and myoclonus.[7] Other centrally mediated effects of modifying intracerebral levels of amines by the administration of oral levodopa are psychiatric symptoms (agitation, confusion, anxiety states, delirium, hypomania, hallucinations and overt psychosis).[8]

The main extracerebral action of dopamine is on the adrenergic receptors in the vascular system. Dopamine has the ability to increase cardiac output and to affect vascular resistance of selected vascular beds. These cardiovascular effects contribute to the dopaminergic action on the kidneys together with its direct diuretic effects on nephrons.[9] Dopamine is used in doses above 3.0 $mg.kg^{-1}.min^{-1}$ because of its inotropic and vasoconstrictive properties, while in lower dosages it has diuretic properties and increases blood flow to certain vascular beds, including the renal vasculature.[10] Other peripheral dopaminergic effects are its actions on the extra-BBB-situated dopamine receptors in the chemoreceptor trigger zone in the area postrema within the fourth ventricle, resulting in nausea and vomiting, and on hypothalamic dopamine systems, lowering the plasma concentration of prolactin. Dopamine receptors have also been identified in the stomach, the retina, the carotid body and the superior cervical ganglion. In clinical usage of levodopa postural hypotension is the most common cardiovascular problem.

Pharmacokinetics

The preferred analytical method for levodopa and dopamine in biological fluids is high performance liquid chromatography with electrochemical detection.[11] The limit of sensitivity is 1 $\mu g.l^{-1}$. Dopamine can also be measured radioenzymatically after sulphatase-catalysed hydrolysis of any sulphate conjugates.[12]

Levodopa is rapidly and extensively absorbed from the small intestine. Most of a dose is subject to presystemic metabolism, principally by decarboxylation by LAAD, in the intestinal mucosa. Bioavailability is normally about 33% but this can be increased by inhibiting decarboxylase activity with carbidopa or benserazide.

Oral levodopa is absorbed mainly in the jejunum, and is transported across the membrane by a saturable, facilitated carrier system.[13] The first major variable to affect the rate of levodopa absorption is the gastric emptying time and the amount of natural amino acids present, which compete for the same system; the longer levodopa stays in the stomach and jejunum, the more will be biotransformed, e.g. by LAAD. There is an inverse relationship between gastric acidity and gastric emptying: antacids will thus increase, and anticholinergics decrease, the rate of levodopa absorption. When levodopa is taken without any food there is a very fast, but also brief, increase in plasma levels of the drug. Low protein diets enhance the transport of levodopa from the small intestine into the portal vein.

Following oral administration, peak plasma concentrations of levodopa are achieved within 1–2 h. Peak concentrations show 10-fold variation amongst individuals.

As with most drugs, the clearance of levodopa from plasma is biphasic.[14] Levodopa is not significantly bound to plasma proteins. During the distribution phase, levodopa is widely distributed to the tissues, including red blood cells, liver, kidney, muscle and across the BBB into the central nervous system. Levodopa crosses the BBB via a saturable stereospecific, bidirectional transport system. As in the gut, transport into the brain is specific for neutral amino acids. Ingestion of high-protein meals during an intravenous levodopa infusion causes transient clinical deterioration in Parkinson patients, without altering levodopa plasma levels.[15] Normally, less than 1% of an oral dose of levodopa reaches the brain.

Another variable that affects levodopa plasma levels, and thus distribution in tissues like the nervous system, is the activity of LAAD. Dopamine, produced by the decarboxylation of levodopa by LAAD, does not cross the BBB, and is subject to further metabolism, particularly by monoamine oxidase in endothelial cells. Studies in dogs suggest that over half of orally administered levodopa is decarboxylated in the gut before entering the systemic circulation. Because of the widespread presence of this enzyme, about two-thirds of the urinary metabolites of an oral dose of levodopa occur as dopamine or its metabolites.[16] Other peripheral enzymatic pathways for levodopa biotransformation are O-methylation by catechol-O-methyltransferase (COMT), especially in the liver but also in other tissues, which accounts for 10% of the dose, and to a relatively minor extent, oxidation to melanin and transamination. The clearance of levodopa from plasma is very rapid, the plasma half life averaging 1.3 h.[14] Urinary excretion of levodopa is fast: about 75% will appear within 24 h, primarily in the form of metabolites (dihydroxyphenylacetic acid (DOPAC) and homovanillic acid (HVA)). Less than 1% of an oral dose is recovered unchanged. Faecal excretion of levodopa accounts for only a small fraction (<1%).

Oral absorption	extensive
Presystemic metabolism	>50%
Plasma half life	
mean	1.3 h
Volume of distribution	—
Plasma protein binding	minimal

Levodopa is excreted in breast milk. The drug may cross the placenta but specific data in man are lacking.

Concentration–effect relationship

There is no evidence for a direct relationship between the plasma concentration of levodopa and its effects in parkinsonism.

Metabolism

Both exogenously and naturally synthesized levodopa are converted to the active constituent dopamine by the action of the enzyme LAAD, sometimes referred to as dopa decarboxylase. This enzyme is ubiquitous, present not only in neurones that produce dopamine and other catecholamines and indoleamines, but also in gastrointestinal cells, liver, kidney, pancreas, adrenal glands, blood and the capillary endothelium of the brain.

Another route of metabolism of levodopa is by O-methylation, catalysed by catechol-O-methyltransferase. This enzyme is present in high concentrations in the red blood cells and in the liver; a significant proportion of oral levodopa is metabolized to 3-O-methyldopa in these tissues. The enzymatic inactivation of dopamine in the brain is catalysed by two enzymes, monoamine oxidase (MAO) and COMT. In the monkey, MAO type A is localized in nigrostriatal dopamine-containing neurones and glial cells,[17] has high substrate specificity for serotonin and is inhibited by clorgyline, while type B is distributed primarily in serotoninergic neurones and glial cells,[13] has high substrate specificity for catecholamines and is inhibited by deprenyl.[18] MAO A oxidizes both noradrenaline and dopamine while MAO B oxidizes dopamine without concomitant effects on noradrenaline. Brain COMT is localized extraneuronally in glial cells.[19] MAO oxidizes dopamine to dihydroxyphenylacetic acid, COMT methylates dopamine to 3-methoxytyramine and together they convert dopamine to 3-methoxy-4-hydroxyphenylacetic acid (HVA, homovanillic acid).

Dopamine, synthesized from exogenous levodopa in the cytoplasm of dopaminergic neurones, is stored in vesicles which are released by depolarization of the cell. It also diffuses into the extracellular space where it may come into contact with dopaminergic receptors and produce a pharmacological effect.[20] There are two types of dopamine receptors: the D-1 receptor, linked to adenylate cyclase and D-2, not dependent on adenylate cyclase.[21] As yet, the relative roles of these two receptors are not fully understood. Once dopamine leaves the receptor site, most of it will re-enter the dopaminergic neurones via a high-affinity, carrier-mediated reuptake system. It will then be stored again, or oxidized by MAO to dihydroxyphenylacetic acid. Some will escape from the synaptic cleft, and will be O-methylated by COMT to 3-methoxytyramine.

Levodopa and its metabolites are excreted primarily in the urine, 70–80% of a dose being recovered within 24 h, with $<1\%$ as the unchanged drug. Approximately 50% of the material present in the urine is accounted for by DOPAC and HVA, 10% as dopamine and $\leqslant 30\%$ as 3-O-methyldopa.

Pharmaceutics

Levodopa is available in oral form.

1. Larodopa (Roche, UK) is a 500 mg white hexagonal tablet with quarter scoring.
2. Brocadopa (Brocades, UK): clear capsules in 125 mg, 250 mg and 500 mg strengths They are marked with both the trade name and strength.
3. Larodopa (Roche, USA): capsules, containing 100 mg (pink and scarlet), 250 mg (pink and beige) and 500 mg (pink). There are also pink, scored tablets containing 100, 250 or 500 mg of levodopa embossed 'Larodopa' and with the tablet strength.

   Levodopa in combination with LAAD inhibitors are available as:

4. Madopar (Roche) capsules or tablets in a levodopa/benserazide 1:4 ratio (50/12.5, 100/25 and 200/50 mg), and as Sinemet (MSD, UK) tablets in a levodopa/carbidopa 1:10 and 1:4 ratio (100/10, 250/25 and 50/12.5, 100/25 mg).

Dopar capsules contain tartrazine; Sinemet 100/10 and 250/25 contain FD&C Blue no. 2; and the 50/12.5 and 100/25 capsules contain D&C Yellow no. 10 and FD&C Yellow no. 6. These dyes are potentially allergenic substances.

Therapeutic use

Indications

1. Levodopa is employed for the treatment of idiopathic and postencephalitic parkinsonism, and symptomatic parkinsonism caused, for example, by carbon monoxide, manganese or MPTP.

Contraindications

Levodopa, or levodopa in combination with benserazide or carbidopa, is contraindicated in narrow-angle glaucoma, psychosis and other conditions in which sympathomimetic amines are contraindicated: severely decompensated endocrine, renal, hepatic and cardiac disorders. Because levodopa may activate melanoma, it should not be administered in the case of suspicious skin lesions or in a patient with a history of melanoma.

Mode of use

Based on a wide range of clinical experience and controlled therapeutic studies, it can be concluded that the combination of levodopa with a peripheral LAAD inhibitor is at least as effective as levodopa alone in the treatment of parkinsonism. This combination will permit administration of lower doses of levodopa, provide more rapid dosage titration, reduce unwanted peripheral effects of levodopa as caused by stimulation of dopamine receptors in the area postrema (nausea, vomiting) or adrenergic receptors in the cardiovascular system (arrhythmias).

Dopamine, the major intermediary metabolite of levodopa, is administered in doses of $3\ mg.kg^{-1}.min^{-1}$ or more to support the cardiovascular system of critically ill patients because of its inotropic and vasoconstrictive properties; in lower dosage dopamine has diuretic properties and increases blood flow in the renal vascular bed.[10]

It is unusual to prescribe levodopa without a peripheral decarboxylase inhibitor, but the following information is provided in case such an inhibitor is unavailable.

The optimal daily dose should be determined by careful individual titration. The initial recommended intake is 0.25–1 g daily, divided into two or more doses. The daily intake should be increased by maximal 0.5 g every 3–7 days, as tolerated. Total dose should not exceed 8 g per day; the optimal therapeutic response may not be obtained for 6 months.

Levodopa/benserazide or levodopa/carbidopa combinations, as currently taken by most patients with parkinsonism, decrease the daily levodopa requirements by 75–80%.[22] The major consequence of this combination is to reduce the total amount of circulating dopamine resulting from levodopa decarboxylation, thereby reducing the peripheral side effects which include nausea, vomiting and cardiac arrhythmias.

In order to obtain an optimal effect dietary instructions are helpful: not only does food produce a physical barrier to gastric emptying, but large molecular amino acids like phenylalanine and leucine compete with levodopa for the intestinal as well as BBB active transport mechanism.[23] Levodopa should therefore be taken after light meals during the day. Taken without food, it achieves a fast, but only very brief, therapeutic response.[23]

When intolerable side effects occur during the initial stage of treatment, the dosage should not be increased further, rather it should be decreased; interruption of treatment is seldom necessary. Other standard antiparkinsonian treatment may be continued while levodopa, or levodopa/LAAD inhibitor combination, is administered.

Recently some studies have been performed with sustained-release levodopa/carbidopa (CR-3 or CR-4, both containing 200 mg levodopa and 50 mg carbidopa), in order to achieve stable plasma levodopa levels and avoid 'wearing-off' reactions.[24] Only limited improvement has been reported so far.[25–27]

Fig. 1 Metabolism of levodopa

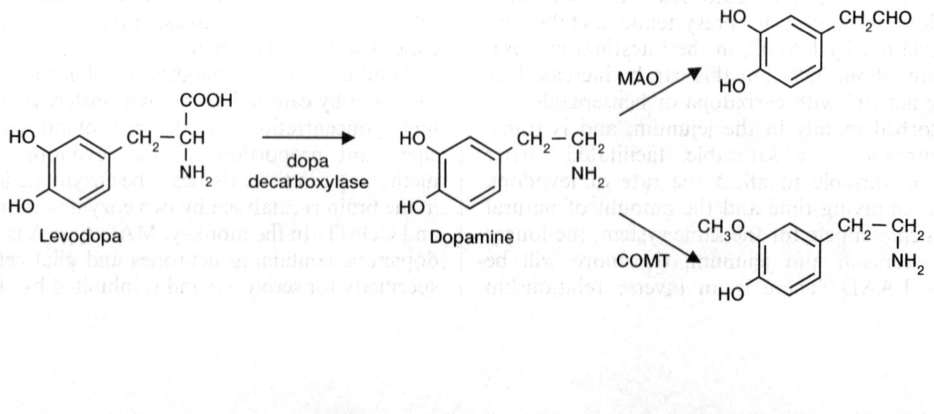

Levodopa

Patients should be monitored carefully when the dosage of levodopa is reduced abruptly or discontinued. A symptom complex resembling the neuroleptic malignant syndrome can occur, including muscular rigidity, elevated body temperature, mental changes and increased plasma creatinine phosphokinase.[28]

If general anaesthesia is required, levodopa therapy should be stopped some 12 hours before surgery and it should be started again immediately after. Whenever treatment with levodopa is interrupted for longer periods, dosage should be adjusted gradually; in most cases, the patient can be titrated to his previous therapeutic dosage.

Adverse reactions

Potentially life-threatening effects

Severe postural hypotension (described below) may occasionally be a danger to life, particularly in the elderly. The possibility of inducing a condition resembling the neuroleptic malignant syndrome, on rapid reduction of dose or drug withdrawal, has been mentioned already.

Acute overdosage

In overdosage pyridoxine HCl (vitamin B_6), acting as a co-enzyme for LAAD in the gut,[29] rapidly reverses the CNS toxic and therapeutic effects of levodopa by increasing peripheral decarboxylation. When peripheral decarboxylase inhibitor is administered together with levodopa, the antagonistic effect of pyridoxine is lost. In acute overdosage, general supportive measures are employed, along with immediate gastric lavage. ECG monitoring and careful observation should be undertaken for the possible development of arrhythmias; if required antiarrhythmic (β-blockade) therapy should be given.

Severe or irreversible adverse effects

During levodopa therapy, peripheral adverse effects, caused by its decarboxylated derivative dopamine, are frequent. These comprise nausea, vomiting, anorexia, abdominal pain, diarrhoea and constipation, which when severe may be regarded as serious. Cardiac irregularities or palpitations are less frequent. These peripheral adverse effects often disappear or diminish with the combination of levodopa and an LAAD inhibitor.[30] Orthostatic hypotension results from a combination of central and peripheral actions of dopamine.

During the course of chronic treatment of parkinsonism with levodopa, whether or not in combination with LAAD inhibitors, several types of central adverse effects frequently occur. The two most common are dyskinesias and mental disturbances.

Levodopa-induced involuntary movements seem to occur only in patients with degeneration of the nigrostriatal dopaminergic system.[31] These movements appear at critical, high (most commonly) or low plasma levodopa levels,[32] particularly in patients with severe akinesia, responding dramatically to levodopa;[33] they are provoked by medications which stimulate dopamine transmission and reduced by dopamine receptor antagonists.[34] These observations give evidence for the hypothesis that these involuntary movements result from stimulation of hypersensitive (compensating) dopamine receptors. The topography of these movements is related to brain structures with impaired dopaminergic transmission. It has been suggested that choreic, dystonic or ballistic patterns result from selective dysfunction in, respectively, the caudate nucleus, the putaminopallidal complex or the subthalamic area.[7]

Mid-dose dyskinesias can be improved by diminution and fractionating of the daily dose of levodopa; onset and end-of-dose dyskinesias sometimes benefit from increasing and fractionating this daily dose.[35]

The occurrence of inconsistent or erratic responses to individual levodopa doses is generally a consequence of the dose failing to reach its site of action[36] because of compromised absorption, distribution or metabolism of levodopa. So the content and quantity of the meals, changes in gastric acidity, and accumulation of 3-O-methyldopa must always be considered. Often judicious changes in levodopa dose and dosing interval can give some relief. The progressive global failure to respond, usually seen in elderly patients, may result from pharmacokinetic or pharmacodynamic changes or loss of dopamine receptors in ageing.[37]

Mental disturbances, in particular delirium or hallucinations, are most frequently observed in older patients after prolonged treatment with high daily doses of levodopa.[38] The cause of these psychiatric symptoms remains unclear. Dysfunction of the dopaminergic system, as well as the noradrenergic, serotoninergic and cholinergic systems, may be involved. It has been postulated that bradyphrenia, often seen in chronically treated parkinsonian patients, results from deficient striatal and corticolimbic dopaminergic transmission. Stimulation of hypersensitive (compensating) receptors may cause the various psychiatric adverse effects.[7]

Degeneration of the noradrenergic ceruleocortical neurones may be implicated in the intellectual deterioration. The depressive states observed in about 50% of the parkinsonian population[39] may also be related to the central noradrenergic deficiency.[7]

The response to levodopa treatment is usually stable for 2–5 years; subsequently more than 50% of patients begin to develop fluctuations.[40] The initial long-duration response to each dose changes through the years to a short-duration response; from four hours to as little as one hour, though plasma levodopa levels do not alter over the year. Potential mechanisms to explain the delayed onset of fluctuations in response are: (1) the accumulating 3-O-methyldopa plasma levels compete with more success for the levodopa BBB transport mechanism (also an explanation for any beneficial effect of drug holidays).[41] (2) The consequence of the progressive loss of dopaminergic nigrostriatal neurones is a drastic reduction in LAAD activity and dopamine formation. (3) There is a diminishing storage capacity for dopamine in nerve endings as the disease progresses. Fluctuations are most likely the consequence of recurring striatal dopamine deficiency, for any of the above reasons, after the initial response to levodopa treatment.[42] This last hypothesis is strengthened by experiences with MPTP.[43,44]

Symptomatic adverse effects

Gastrointestinal upsets and palpitations occur and range from trivial to severe.

Other effects

Levodopa treatment can lead to slight elevations of transaminase, alkaline phosphatase and protein-bound iodine levels. There may also be mild transient leucopenia and thrombocytopenia.

Interference with clinical pathology tests

Levodopa has been reported to interfere with serum tests for bilirubin, catecholamines, creatinine, glucose and uric acid; and urine tests for amino acids, creatinine, creatinine clearance, oestrogens, glucose, homogentisic acid, uric acid, ketones, vanillylmandelic acid and 5-hydroxyindoleacetic acid.

High risk groups

Neonates

The drug is not used in neonates.

Breast milk. Levodopa may enter breast milk, so women taking the drug should not breast feed.

Children

Experience with levodopa and levodopa/LAAD inhibitor in patients under 18 years of age is limited, though they have been given to young rigid patients with Huntington's disease, and to children with the Segawa variant of dystonia.

Pregnant women

Experience of the effects of levodopa, and combinations of levodopa with LAAD inhibitors, on human pregnancy is limited.[45] However, these drugs have caused visceral and skeletal malformations in animal studies. At dosages in excess of 200 $mg.kg^{-1}$ daily, levodopa has an adverse effect on fetal and postnatal growth and viability. Therefore, the use of these drugs in women of child-bearing potential requires that the anticipated benefits of the drug be weighed against possible hazards to the mother and the fetus.

The elderly

The drug may be used in the elderly, though the possibility of orthostatic hypotension should be borne in mind.

Drug interactions

Potentially hazardous interactions

Antihypertensive drugs. When levodopa is given with antihypertensive drugs there may be postural hypotension, so doses may require adjustment.

Levodopa

L

MAO inhibitors. Levodopa should not be given with, or within 2 weeks after, non-specific or type A MAO inhibitors; type B inhibitors produce a useful interaction with levodopa.[46]

Papaverine. Since this antispasmodic and vasodilator compound has been reported to have dopamine-receptor-blocking activity it is advisable not to prescribe it to patients who are being treated with levodopa, since recurrence of extrapyramidal symptomatology would probably ensue.

Sympathomimetic drugs. Levodopa may potentiate the effects of sympathomimetic drugs such as ephedrine, amphetamine, adrenaline and isoproterenol.

Other significant interactions

Pyridoxine reverses the therapeutic (and toxic) effects of oral levodopa; however, this problem is less likely if an LAAD inhibitor is included in the regimen.

Potentially useful interactions

Type B monoamine oxidase inhibitors have a synergistic effect.

Concomitant administration of levodopa with anticholinergic drugs may result in a mild degree of increased efficacy. Gradual reduction in anticholinergic dosage may be necessary, both during initiation of levodopa therapy and after optimum dosage is obtained. Large doses of anticholinergics, by delaying gastric emptying, may increase gastric degradation of levodopa.

Clinical trials

1. Friedman J 1985 'Drug holidays' in the treatment of Parkinson's disease. Archives of Internal Medicine 145: 913–915
2. Albani C, Asper R, Hacisalihzade S S, Baumgartner G 1986 Individual levodopa therapy in Parkinson's disease. Advances in Neurology 45: 497–501
3. Bermejo F P, Calandre L H, Molina J A, Martinez P, De Yebenes J G 1986 Long-lasting drug holiday in Parkinson's disease. Advances in Neurology 45: 503-506
4. Bozek C, Suchowersky O, Purves S, Calne S, Calne D B 1986 Sinemet in Parkinson's disease: efficacy with and without food. Clinical Neuropharmacology 9: 196–199
5. Cedarbaum J M, McDowell F H 1986 Sixteen-year follow-up of 100 patients begun on levodopa in 1968: emerging problems. Advances in Neurology 45: 469–472
6. Chase T N, Juncos J, Serrati C, Fabbrini G, Bruno G 1986 Fluctuation in response to chronic levodopa therapy: pathogenetic and therapeutic considerations. Advances in Neurology 45: 477–480
7. Hardie R J, Andrew J L, Stern G M 1986 Pharmacokinetics of levodopa and motor fluctuations. Advances in Neurology 45: 487–492
8. Kaye J A, Feldman R G 1986 The role of l-dopa holiday in the long-term management of Parkinson's disease. Clinical Neuropharmacology 9: 1–13
9. Lees A J 1986 L-dopa treatment and Parkinson's disease. Quartery Journal of Medicine 59: 535–547
10. Marion M H, Stocchi F, Quinn N P, Jenner P, Marsden C D 1986 Repeated levodopa infusions in fluctuating Parkinson's disease: clinical and pharmacokinetic data. Clinical Neuropharmacology 9: 165–181
11. Mena M A, Muradas V, Bazan E, Reiriz J, de Yebenes J G 1986 Pharmacokinetics of l-dopa in patients with Parkinson's disease. Advances in Neurology 45: 481–486
12. Nutt J G, Woodward W R 1986 Levodopa pharmacokinetics and pharmacodynamics in fluctuating parkinsonian patients. Neurology 36: 739–744
13. Poewe W H, Lees A J, Stern G M 1986 Low-dose l-dopa therapy in Parkinson's disease: a 6-year follow-up study. Neurology 36: 1528–1530
14. Gancher S T, Nutt J G, Woodward W R 1987 Peripheral pharmacokinetics of levodopa in untreated, stable, and fluctuating parkinsonian patients. Neurology 37: 940–944
15. Fabbrini G, Juncos J, Mouradian M M, Serrati C, Chase T N 1987 Levodopa pharmacokinetic mechanisms and motor fluctuations in Parkinson's disease. Annals of Neurology 21: 370–376
16. Mouradian M M, Juncos J L, Serrati C, Fabbrini G, Palmeri S, Chase T N 1987 Exercise and the antiparkinsonian response to levodopa. Clinical Neuropharmacology 10: 351–355

General review articles

Agid Y, Javoy-Agid F, Ruberg M 1987 Biochemistry of neurotransmitters in Parkinson's disease. In: Marsden C D, Fahn S (eds) Movement disorders 2. Butterworths, London, pp 166–230

Wooten G F 1987 Pharmacokinetics of levodopa. In: Marsden C D, Fahn S (eds) Movement disorders 2. Butterworths, London, pp 231-248

Jankovic J, Calne D B 1987 Parkinson's disease: etiology and treatment. Current Neurology 7: 193–234

Calne D B 1984 Long-term complications of levodopa therapy. In: Winlow W, Markstein R (eds) The neurobiology of dopamine systems. Manchester University Press, Manchester, England, pp 341–349

Pinder R M, Brogden R N, Sawyer P R, Speight T M, Avery G S 1976 Levodopa and decarboxylase inhibitors: a review of their clinical pharmacology and use in the treatment of parkinsonism. Drugs 11: 329–377

References

1. Wysong D V 1966 U.S.A. Patent 3 253 023 Assigned to Dow Chemical Comp, 24-05 1966
2. Krieger K H, Lago J, Zwantuck J A 1968 U.S.A. Patent 3 405 159 Assigned to Merck & Co, 08-10 1968
3. Theiss E G, Scharer K 1971 Toxicity of l-dopa and a decarboxylase inhibitor in animal experiments. In: Ajuria-guerra J de, Gauthier G (eds) Monoamines noyaux gris centraux et syndrome de Parkinson. Georg & Cie, Geneva, pp 497–504
4. Merck, Sharp & Dohme 1984 Sinemet. Canadian product monograph, MS&D, Kirkland, Quebec, Canada, 27–11 1984
5. Calne D B, McGeer E, Eisen A, Spencer P 1986 Alzheimer's disease, Parkinson's disease, and motor neurone disease: abiotropic interaction between ageing and environment? Lancet 2: 1067–1070
6. Barbeau A 1981 The l-dopa story 1958–1979. In: Rose F C, Capildeo R (eds) Research progress in Parkinson's disease, Pitman Medical, Kent, England, pp 221–225
7. Agid Y, Javoy-Agid F, Ruberg M 1987 Biochemistry of neurotransmitters in Parkinson's disease. In: Marsden C D, Fahn S (eds) Movement disorders 2. Butterworths, London, ch 10, pp 166–230
8. Rondot P, Recondo J de, Coignet A, Ziegler M 1984 Mental disorders in Parkinson's disease after treatment with l-dopa. Advances in Neurology 40: 259–269
9. Chernow B, Rainey T G, Lake C R 1982 Endogenous and exogenous catecholamines in critical care medicine. Critical Care Medicine 409–416
10. Dasta J F, Kirby M G 1986 Pharmacology and therapeutic use of low-dose dopamine. Pharmacotherapy 6: 304–310
11. Wagner J, Vitali P, Palfreyman M G 1982 Simultaneous determination of 3,4-dihydroxyphenylalanine, 5-hydroxy-tryptophan, dopamine, 4-hydroxy-3-methoxyphenylalanine, nor-epinephrine, 3,4-dihydroxyphenyl-acetic acid, homovanillic acid, serotonin, and 5-hydroxyindoleacetic acid in rat cerebrospinal fluid and brain by high-performance liquid chromatography with electrochemical detection. Journal of Neurochemistry 38: 1241–1254
12. Johnson G A, Baker C A, Smith R T 1980 Radioenzymatic assay of sulphate conjugates of catecholamines and dopa in plasma. Life Sciences 26: 1591–1598
13. Nutt J G, Fellman J H 1984 Pharmacokinetics of levodopa. Clinical Neuropharmacology 7: 35–49
14. Nutt J G, Woodward W R, Anderson J L 1985 Effect of carbidopa on pharmacokinetics of intravenously administered levodopa; implications for mechanism of action of carbidopa in the treatment of parkinsonism. Annals of Neurology 18: 537–543
15. Nutt J G, Woodward W R, Hammerstad J P, Carter J H, Anderson J L 1984 'On-off' phenomenon in Parkinson's disease: relationship to l-dopa absorption and transport. New England Journal of Medicine 310: 483–488
16. Morgan J P, Bianchine J R, Spiegel H E, Rivera-Calimlim L, Hersey R M 1971 Metabolism of levodopa in patients with Parkinson's disease. Archives of Neurology 25: 39–44
17. Denny R M, Fritz R R, Patel N T, Abell C 1982 Human liver MAO-A and MAO-B separated by immunoaffinity chromatography with MAO-B-specific monoclonal antibody. Science 215: 1400–1403
18. Pearce L B, Roth J A 1984 Monoamine oxidase: separation of the type A and B activities. Biochemical Pharmacology 33: 1809–1811
19. Kaplan G P, Hartman B K, Creveling C R 1979 Immunohistochemical demonstration of catechol-O-methyltransferase in mammalian brain. Brain Research 167: 241–250
20. Melamed E, Globus M, Uzzan A, Rosenthal J 1985 Is dopamine formed from exogenous l-dopa stored within vesicles in striatal dopaminergic nerve terminals? Implications for l-dopa's mechanism for action in Parkinson's disease. Neurology 35 (suppl 1): 118
21. Stoof J C, Kebabian J W 1984 Two dopamine receptors: biochemistry, physiology, and pharmacology. Life Sciences 35: 2281–2296

22. Reid J L, Calne D B, Vakil S D, Allen J G, Davies C A 1972 Plasma concentration of levodopa in parkinsonism before and after inhibition of peripheral decarboxylase. Journal of Neurological Sciences 17: 45–51
23. Jankovic J, Calne D B 1987 Parkinson's disease: etiology and treatment. Current Neurology 7: 193–234
24. Hardie R J, Lees A J, Stern G M 1984 On-off fluctuations in Parkinson's disease: a clinical and neuropharmacological study. Brain 107: 487–506
25. Nutt J G, Woodward W R, Carter J H 1986 Clinical and biochemical studies with controlled-release levodopa/carbidopa. Neurology 36: 1206–1211
26. Cedarbaum J M, Breck L, Kutt H, McDowell F H 1987 Controlled-release levodopa/carbidopa. Neurology 37: 233–241
27. Goetz C G, Tanner C M, Klawans H L, Shannon K L, Carroll V S 1987 Parkinson's disease and motor fluctuations: long acting carbidopa/levodopa (CR-4-Sinemet). Neurology 37: 875–878
28. Gibb W R G, Griffith D N W 1986 Levodopa withdrawal syndrome identical to neuroleptic malignant syndrome. Postgraduate Medical Journal 62: 59–60
29. Klawans H L, Ringel S P, Shenker D M 1971 Failure of vitamin B6 to reverse the l-dopa effect in patients on a dopa decarboxylase inhibitor. Journal of Neurology, Neurosurgery and Psychiatry 34: 682–686
30. Marsden C D, Parkes J D, Rees J E 1973 Long term treatment of Parkinson's disease with an extracerebral dopa decarboxylase inhibitor (MK 486) and levodopa. Advances in Neurology 3: 79–96
31. Agid Y, Bonnet A M, Signoret J L, L'Hermitte F 1979 Clinical, pharmacological and biochemical approach of 'onset' and 'end of dose' dyskinesias. Advances in Neurology 24: 401–409
32. Muenter M D, Sharpless N S, Tyce G M, Darley F L 1977 Patterns of dystonia ('I-D-I' and 'D-I-D') in response to l-dopa therapy for Parkinson's disease. Mayo Clinic Proceedings 52: 163–174
33. Agid Y, Bonnet A M, Ruberg M, Javoy-Agid F 1985 Pathophysiology of levodopa induced abnormal involuntary movements. In: Casey D, Chase T N, Christensen V, Gerlach J (eds) Dyskinesia, Research and Treatment. Psychopharmacology. Springer Verlag, Berlin (suppl 2), pp 145–159
34. Klawans H L, Weiner W J 1974 Attempted use of haloperidol in the treatment of l-dopa induced dyskinesias. Journal of Neurology, Neurosurgery and Psychiatry 37: 427–430
35. H'Hermitte F, Agid Y, Signoret J L 1978 Onset and end-of-dose levodopa-induced dyskinesias, possible treatment by increasing the daily doses of levodopa. Archives of Neurology 35: 261–263
36. Quinn N, Marsden C D, Parkes J D 1982 Complicated response fluctuations in Parkinson's disease: response to intravenous infusion of levodopa. Lancet 2: 412–415
37. Wong D F, Wagner H N, Dannals R F, Links J M, Frost J J, Ravert H T 1984 Effects of age on dopamine and serotonin receptors measured by positron tomography in the living human brain. Science 226: 1393–1396
38. Calne D B 1984 Long-term complications of levodopa therapy. In: Winlow W, Markstein R (eds) The neurobiology of dopamine systems. Manchester University Press, Manchester, pp 341–349
39. Mayeux R, Williams J B W, Stern Y, Cote L 1984 Depression and Parkinson's disease. Advances in Neurology 40: 241–250
40. Marsden C D, Schachter M 1981 Assessment of extrapyramidal disorders. British Journal of Clinical Pharmacology 11: 129–151
41. Kaye J A, Feldman R G 1986 The role of l-dopa holiday in the long-term management of Parkinson's disease. Clinical Neuropharmacology 9: 1–13
42. Spencer S E, Wooten G F 1984 Altered pharmacokinetics of l-dopa metabolism in rat striatum deprived of dopaminergic innervation. Neurology 34: 1105–1108
43. Langston J W, Ballard P 1984 Parkinsonism induced by 1-methyl-4-phenyl-1,2,3,6 tetrahydropyridine (MTPT): implications for treatment and the pathogenesis of Parkinson's disease. Canadian Journal of Neurological Science 11 (suppl 1): 160–165
44. Wooten G F 1987 Pharmacokinetics of levodopa. In: Marsden C D, Fahn S (eds) Movement disorders 2. Butterworths, London, England, ch 11, pp 231–248
45. Cook D G, Klawans H L 1985 Levodopa during pregnancy. Clinical Neuropharmacology 8: 93–95
46. Birkmayer W, Riederer P 1984 Deprenyl prolongs the therapeutic efficacy of combined l-dopa. Advances in Neurology 40: 475–481

Levonorgestrel

Levonorgestrel is an orally active progestational agent which is principally used in combination with the synthetic oestrogen ethinyloestradiol for contraception or for the control of menstrual disorders and endometriosis and in conjunction with 'natural' oestrogens as hormone replacement therapy (HRT). It is also given as a 'progestogen only' contraceptive. A number of delivery systems for contraceptive steroids have been tried.

Chemistry

Levonorgestrel; (d)-norgestrel

$C_{21}H_{28}O_2$

13-Ethyl-17β-hydroxy-18,19-dinor-17α-pregn-4-en-20-yn-3-one

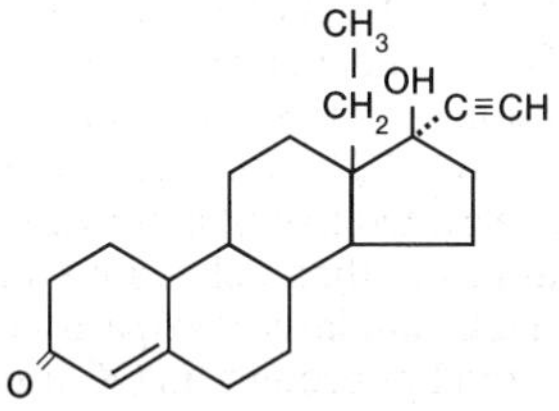

Molecular weight	312.5
pKa	—
Solubility	
in alcohol	1 in 120
in water	insoluble
Octanol/water partition coefficient	—

Levonorgestrel is a white, or almost white, almost odourless crystalline powder which is obtained by chemical synthesis. The (l) isomer is used clinically. Eugynon 50 and Neogest contain (d)-norgestrel.

It is available in combination with oestradiol in a variety of preparations (Microgynon 30, Ovranette 30, Eugynon 30, Ovran 30, Ovran, Logynon, Trinordiol, Microval, Norgeston)

Pharmacology

Levonorgestrel is a progestational steroid which is more potent as an inhibitor of ovulation than norethisterone with similar androgenic activity. Both inhibition of ovulation and inhibition of sperm migration through the cervical mucus have been demonstrated.

Toxicology

A carcinogenic effect can be produced in certain strains of mice and rats when progestogens, oestrogens and combinations of the hormones are given in high doses throughout their life span. The susceptibility to tumour induction by hormonal contraceptives is not consistent in different strains of mice and rats and such studies have not provided useful predictive information of the potential carcinogenicity in women.

Risks to a baby born due to failure of oral contraceptives appear to be slight. A mild feminizing action on a male fetus or a virilizing action on a female fetus are possibilities.

Clinical pharmacology

Combined contraceptives (progestogen and oestrogen) exert their effects largely through inhibition of ovulation. There is a consistent suppression of the mid-cycle peak of LH.[1] On the basis of endometrial and ovarian biopsies, length of cycle and endocrine assays, it has been concluded that progestogen-only preparations produce their antifertility effect without completely inhibiting ovulation.[2–4] Levonorgestrel (30 μg) causes variable suppression of FSH, LH and ovulation with the major effect on changes in the cervical mucus so that sperm migration is impeded. Alteration of endometrial structure and the induction of a defective functioning of the corpus luteum have also been postulated.

A number of metabolic effects of levonorgestrel, either alone or in combination with ethinyloestradiol, have been evaluated over the last decade. In an earlier study it was reported that in women given 75 μg levonorgestrel daily for one year there was no significant increase in weight or triglyceride or cholesterol concentrations; however, blood glucose and plasma insulin concentrations were significantly elevated.[5] Wynn and Niththyananthan[6] concluded from a large study involving a number of different oral contraceptive preparations that levonorgestrel either alone or in combination with ethinyloestradiol caused a significant reduction in HDL_2. However, other studies have failed to show significant suppression of HDL cholesterol or the HDL_2 subfraction by low dose combined oral contraceptives.[7–9] For example, in a comprehensive study by März et al[7] the effects of a triphasic combination of ethinyloestradiol and levonorgestrel on serum lipids and lipoproteins were assessed. It was found that total triglycerides, phospholipids, HDL triglycerides, HDL_3-C, apolipoprotein A, A-1, A-11 and LDL phospholipids were increased whereas HDL phospholipids, HDL_2 and HDL_3 phospholipids, HDL_2-C, VLDL phospholipids, VLDL cholesterol, pre-β-lipoprotein cholesterol, LDL triglycerides, LDL cholesterol, β-lipoprotein cholesterol and apolipoprotein B were unchanged. The authors concluded that provided the assumption is correct that high LDL cholesterol and apolipoprotein B and low HDL subfractions and apolipoprotein A are associated with an elevated risk of atherosclerosis the results seem to represent beneficial rather than deleterious side effects of the low-dose oral contraceptives. Similarly, Gaspard et al[8] concluded their study on serum lipids and lipoproteins in OC users by stating that the triphasic OC containing low doses of levonorgestrel does not induce obvious clinically significant alterations of lipid metabolism. This has been an area of some controversy. In the judgement of some[10] the changes in HDL cholesterol in relation to oral contraceptives have been over-emphasized.

Norgestrel is a more potent suppressor of the oestrogen-induced increase of sex hormone binding globulin (SHBG) than either norethisterone or desogestrel.[10] The oestrogen-induced effect upon caeruloplasmin is much less affected by concurrent administration of a progestogen.

Most changes in metabolism occur during the first three months of use and after this time there is little, if any, further change. The relationship of metabolic changes to clinical side effects is obscure.

Pharmacokinetics

As for other contraceptive steroids the analytical method is radioimmunoassay[11,12] which has a sensitivity of 25 $ng.l^{-1}$.

In combined oral contraceptives

After a single oral dose, levonorgestrel is rapidly absorbed with peak concentrations between 30 min and 2 h.[12,13] The plasma concentration of the drug declines in a biexponential fashion with an α-phase half life of between 50 and 180 min and a β-phase half life varying from 10 to 26 hours.[13] Plasma clearance was estimated to be 105 ± 16 $ml.h^{-1}.kg^{-1}$ following a 150 μg dose and 113 ± 14 $ml.h^{-1}.kg^{-1}$ after a 250 μg dose. The apparent volume of distribution[12] is approximately 1.9 $l.kg^{-1}$. Peak plasma concentrations are 2–7 $\mu g.l^{-1}$ after a 250 μg dose.

During long-term treatment with levonorgestrel there is considerable variation in the plasma concentrations between individuals. Back et al[14] found that the steady state plasma concentration in women taking 150 μg daily varied seven-fold. During the first cycle of treatment with combined oral contraceptives, plasma concentrations of levonorgestrel rose to higher levels than expected from simple pharmacological considerations. There was a close correlation between plasma levonorgestrel concentrations and the SHBG capacity in plasma.[15] The increase in SHBG capacity is due to the effect of co-administered ethinyloestradiol. Levonorgestrel alone will suppress SHBG capacity[15] so that the overall effect seen depends on the doses present. In women recently pregnant, SHBG capacities may be very high. Using equilibrium dialysis techniques, the binding of levonorgestrel in plasma is 93–95%;[13] binding is to both SHBG and albumin.

Oral absorption	100%
Presystemic metabolism	nil
Plasma half-life	
range	10.26 h
mean	—
Volume of distribution	1.9 $l.kg^{-1}$
Plasma protein binding	93–95%

In progestogen-only preparations

Peak plasma levels (around 1 $\mu g.l^{-1}$) occur at 1–2 hours after the administration of 30 μg levonorgestrel.[16] Plasma levels after 24 hours are similar to those seen after the intake of 300 μg norethisterone.

Other delivery systems

A number of levonorgestrel-containing delivery systems have been developed with the aim of avoiding the fluctuations in plasma concentrations associated with daily oral administration of either the combined or progestogen-only contraceptive. Three different types of delivery system have been tried, viz. subdermal implants, intravaginal rings and steroid releasing IUDs.

Plasma concentrations of 0.15–0.25 $\mu g.l^{-1}$ and 0.3–0.6 $\mu g.l^{-1}$ have been measured after insertion of either a 30 mg or 40 mg silastic rod.[16] The daily release rate of levonorgestrel was estimated to be about 75–100 μg daily from the latter implant and provided contraceptive protection for approximately 1 year. In a long-term study levonorgestrel concentrations were measured for up to 7 years following insertion of 4 rods each containing about 52 mg of steroid. The mean plasma concentration was 0.49 ± 0.13 $\mu g.l^{-1}$ in the first year and decreased to 0.34 ± 0.06 $\mu g.l^{-1}$ in the fifth year of treatment.[17]

Intravaginal rings containing 50 mg levonorgestrel were found to release up to 300 μg daily with mean plasma levels[16] varying between 1.7 and 4 $\mu g.l^{-1}$. A much smaller release rate of 25 μg daily from a different type of levonorgestrel impregnated vaginal device gave a peak concentration of 0.5 $\mu g.l^{-1}$ 3–4 days after insertion, after which the plasma levels declined in a linear fashion to 60% of the initial level in 90 days.[18]

A number of different levonorgestrel-releasing intrauterine contraceptive devices have been tested. In one study two different devices releasing either 10 or 30 μg daily were shown to give plasma concentrations of 207 ± 64 and 235 ± 87 $ng.l^{-1}$ respectively over a 12 week period.[19] By measuring the steroid in breast milk it was also shown that approximately 0.1% of the daily dose passed into breast milk.

Concentration–effect relationship

There is no information available on the relationship of plasma

Fig. 1 Metabolism of levonorgestrel

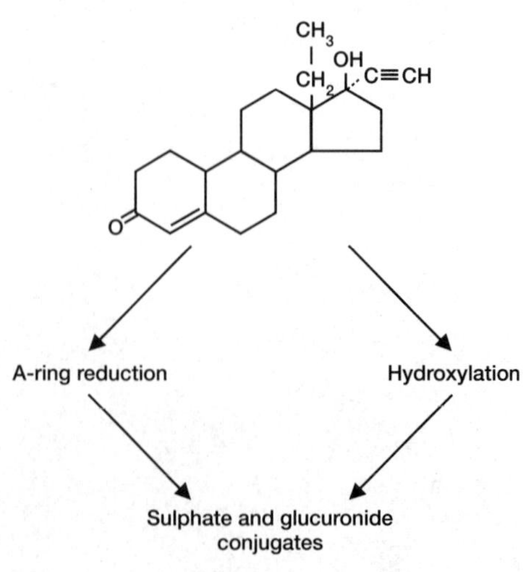

concentrations of the steroid to the inhibition of hypothalamic pituitary function. Daily administration of 75 µg causes an inhibition or suppression of LH and FSH.

Metabolism

Levonorgestrel is extensively metabolized in the liver with very little of the unchanged drug excreted. The main metabolic pathways are reduction of the 4-en-3-one group in the A ring, various hydroxylations (at positions 2, 6 and 16) and conjugation to form both sulphate and glucuronide conjugates.[13] The 3α, 5β and 3β, 5β tetrahydro reduced metabolites are major metabolites present in urine as conjugates. Faecal excretion accounts for between 20 and 30% of an oral dose. Since absorption is complete this indicates enterohepatic circulation.

There is no presystemic metabolism of levonorgestrel and gut wall metabolism is minimal.[13] There are no known active metabolites.

Pharmaceutics

Table 1

Preparation	Manufacturer	LNG (µg)	NG (µg)	EE_2 (µg)
Levlen	Berlex (US)	150		30
Microgynon 30	Schering (UK)	150		30
Nordette	Wyeth (US)	150		30
Ovranette 30	Wyeth (UK)	150		30
Lo/Ovral	Wyeth (US)		300	30
Eugynon 30	Schering (UK)	250		30
Ovran 30	Wyeth (UK)	250		30
Eugynon 50	Schering (UK)		500	50
Ovral	Wyeth (US)		500	50
Ovran	Wyeth (UK)	250		50
Logynon	Schering (UK)	50	(6 tablets)	30
Trilevlen	Berlex (US)	75	(5 tablets)	40
Trinordiol	Wyeth (UK)	125	(10 tablets)	30
Triphasil	Wyeth (US)			
Microval	Wyeth (UK)	30		
Norgeston	Schering (UK)	30		
Neogest	Shering (UK)		75	
Ovrette	Wyeth (US)		75	

A variety of levonorgestrel-containing delivery systems (subdermal implants, intravaginal rings and steroid releasing IUDs) are at various stages of clinical trial worldwide.

Therapeutic use

Indications

1. Oral contraception
2. Control of menstrual disorders
3. Postcoital contraception
4. Hormone replacement therapy.

Contraindications[20]

1. Present or past circulatory system disease
a. Venous or arterial thrombosis
b. Stroke of any variety, including subarachnoid haemorrhage
c. Conditions which make thrombosis more probable or especially dangerous; e.g. planned operation
d. Coronary heart disease
e. Other heart disease, especially if associated with pulmonary hypertension or atrial fibrillation
f. Migraine if severe or focal
g. Sickle cell anaemia and some collagen diseases
2. Liver diseases
a. Impaired liver function
b. Congenital disorders of liver excretion and porphyrias
c. Liver tumours
3. Disturbance of lipid metabolism
4. Existing or treated carcinoma of breast or endometrium
5. Pregnancy
6. Hydatidiform mole (until HCG values negative for 3 months)
7. A history of serious condition deteriorating during pregnancy; e.g. otosclerosis, herpes gestationis or pruritus
8. Undiagnosed irregular genital tract bleeding.

Mode of use (contraception)

With combined oral contraceptive preparations 1 tablet is taken daily for 21 days starting on the first or fifth day of menstruation then followed by 7 tablet-free days. If the first course is started on the fifth day additional contraceptive precautions are necessary during the cycle.

With levonorgestrel-only preparations, 1 tablet is taken daily starting on the first day of menstruation. There is no interruption of tablet taking.

With the triphasic preparations, the first tablet (marked '1') is taken on the first day of menstruation, and then subsequently as marked to '21'. This is followed by 7 tablet-free days before the next course.

Indications

1. Oral contraception

Combined oral contraceptives (OCs) are the most effective reversible form of contraception known. In addition they have advantages not provided by other methods. Generally irregular periods are replaced by regular bleeding and heavy periods by lighter bleeding. Among the other beneficial effects that some women obtain from UC use are:[21]

Protection against pelvic inflammatory disease
Protection against ectopic pregnancy
Protection against endometrial cancer
Protection against ovarian cancer
Protection against benign breast disease

There are certain occasions when the benefits of OCs must be very carefully assessed against the risks. The use of any combined OC by women in the older age group (35+), especially those who smoke, is to be discouraged. Although hypertension is not an absolute contraindication in the younger patient, their use in the older hypertensive should be avoided if possible.

Progestogen-only preparations are suitable for women who do not want, or who for medical reasons are unable to take, combined pills.

2. Menstrual disorders

Some combined oestrogen–progestogen preparations are used for menstrual irregularities.

3. Postcoital contraception

As an occasional emergency measure 50 µg EE_2, 250 µg LNG tablet (×2) taken as soon as possible after unprotected intercourse and up to a maximum time of 72 hours. Two more tablets are taken 12 hours after the first dose. The mechanism may be a direct action of the drug on the endometrium or a consequence of the subtler change in the ovarian hormone milieu or both.[22]

4. Hormone replacement therapy

Some combined natural oestrogen (oestrogen conjugates)–progestogen preparations are used for HRT.

Adverse reactions (combined OC)

Potentially life-threatening effects

It is generally agreed that OC use increases the risk of three specific conditions: venous thromboembolism, ischaemic heart disease, and cerebrovascular disease or stroke.

However it is important to note that all the major Cohort studies have invariably provided information on brands of OCs containing 50 µg of oestrogen and higher doses of progestogens than now recommended. The low dose OCs now in use are likely to cause even less morbidity and mortality then the low rates which emerged from the original studies. Indeed, early results from new case-control studies suggest the possibility that the risk of myocardial infarction associated with OC use is now lower than indicated in the past although the observed small increase in risk of subarachnoid haemor-

Levonorgestrel

rhage appears to be unchanged. It should be noted that deaths in all the Cohort studies have been concentrated among older women who smoke[21]. Smoking is a very important risk factor for arterial disease.

Acute overdosage
There have been no reports of serious ill effects from overdosage, even when a considerable number of tablets have been taken by a small child. If overdosage is discovered within two to three hours and is large, then gastric lavage can be safely used.

Progestogen-only pills do not regulate the cycle as well as combined pills. There is a high incidence of abnormal bleeding.

Severe or irreversible adverse effects
There is some evidence that the incidence of hypertension in OC users is related to the progestogen. If hypertension is recognized during OC usage, then discontinuation is indicated.
OCs have no adverse effects on later childbearing. Return of fecundity is delayed for several months in some OC users but it does not seem to be permanently impaired.

The overall position with respect to breast cancer and OCs is equivocal. Most studies[23–26] have found no association between OC therapy and breast cancer, whereas one major study[27] claimed such an association. A causal link has not been proved.

Symptomatic adverse effects
These include nausea, vomiting, headaches, breast tension, changes in body weight, changes in libido and depressive moods. Some adverse effects with combined OCs are considered to result from the relative balance of oestrogenic and progestogenic effects.

Interference with clinical pathology tests
Combined oral contraceptives may cause technical interference with serum tests for adrenal corticosteroids, urine tests for 17-ketosteroids and 17-hydroxycorticosteroids and aldosterone, and the Thyopac method for measurement of T_3 levels.

High risk groups

Levonorgestrel is not used in neonates, children or pregnant women.

Drug interactions

A number of clinically significant drug interactions have been documented. Although most examples have related to combined oral contraceptives, caution should be exercised in relation to progestogen-only preparations and concurrent use of the drugs outlined below. Clinically significant interactions could be expected with the enzyme-inducing drugs phenobarbitone, phenytoin, primidone, carbamazepine and rifampicin, and in some patients with broad spectrum antibiotics.

Potentially hazardous interactions

Antiepileptic drugs. Phenobarbitone, phenytoin, primidone and carbamazepine are all recognized to be inducers of hepatic microsomal drug metabolizing enzymes in man.[28] Evidence, both from case reports and pharmacokinetic studies, have implicated these drugs in clinically important drug interactions with OCs.[29,31] Steroid plasma concentrations may be reduced below the therapeutic minimum concentration because of the increased rate of hepatic metabolism.

Rifampicin. Rifampicin is a lipophilic, enzyme-inducing drug which is a well-documented inducer of hepatic microsomal enzymes and has been shown to enhance the metabolism of OCs.[30,31]

Antibiotics. Well over 60 pregnancies have been reported to the Committee on Safety of Medicines in women on OCs who have taken an antibiotic concurrently. The most commonly implicated antibacterials have been ampicillin, the tetracyclines and co-trimoxazole.[32] The postulated mechanism is interference with the enterohepatic recirculation (EHC) mechanism of the oestrogenic component of OCs. It is thought that EHC may be important in some women for maintenance of adequate plasma concentrations of oestrogen for contraceptive purposes. Clinical studies have failed to show a consistent interaction between OCs and antibacterials[33–35] and it is clearly only a very few women who are at risk. As yet we have no procedure for detecting high risk patients.

Vitamin C. If Vitamin C (ascorbic acid) is administered at the same time as a combined OC then the plasma concentrations of ethinyloestradiol will increase due to competition for the sulphation mechanism.[34] Daily administration of 1 g of Vitamin C may then convert a low-dose preparation into a high-dose preparation.

Smoking. Smoking is a risk factor for cardiovascular disease in OC users. However plasma concentrations of OCs are apparently unaffected in smokers.[36]

Oral anticoagulants. Patients requiring anticoagulant therapy will almost certainly have an absolute contraindication to oestrogen-based hormonal contraception.

Antihypertensives. Concurrent prescription should not occur in clinical practice.

Other significant interactions
Impairment of oxidative drug metabolism by OCs is widespread[37] but probably of little clinical significance. One study demonstrating an increase in caffeine residence time in contraceptive users has postulated that adverse effects associated with OCs may be related to a reduction in the clearance of environmental toxins.[38]

Potentially useful interactions
No interactions of this kind have been reported.

Major outcome trials

Progestogen-only preparation

1. Rice-Wray E, Beristain I I, Cervantes A 1972 Clinical study of a continuous daily micro-dose progestogen contraceptive — d-Norgestrel. Contraception 5: 279–294

167 women used 30 µg d-norgestrel (levonorgestrel) for a total of 2019 cycles. Breakthrough bleeding was reported in 11.7% of cycles and 9 women discontinued the study for this reason. 45% of cycles were between 25 and 30 days. There were no pregnancies due to tablet failure; however there were four pregnancies due to tablet omissions.

2. Eckstein P, Whitby M, Fotherby K et al 1972 British Medical Journal 3: 195–200

Norgestrel was given in a dosage of 75 µg daily to 144 women for up to 30 months. The incidence of pregnancy was 2 per 100 women-years, or 1.3 if patient failure was excluded. Withdrawals from the trial totalled 94, 57 being connected with the method and 37 being unrelated to the method. Norgestrel caused a high proportion of irregular and generally short bleeding intervals. Norgestrel alone appeared to be a useful alternative to the combined pill for women unsuitable for or unable to tolerate oestrogen containing preparations.

Combined oral contraceptives

3. Apelo R, Veloso I 1975 Clinical experience with ethinyloestradiol and D-norgestrel as an oral contraceptive. Fertility and Sterility 26: 283–288

181 women received 30 µg ethinyloestradiol plus 150 µg levonorgestrel for a total of 1488 cycles. There were no pregnancies. Cycle control was excellent. Menstrual cycles lasted 25–32 days in 96.2% of treatment cycles. Breakthrough bleeding occurred in 2.0%, spotting in 0.1% and amenorrhoea in 0.8% of treatment cycles. See also:

4. Korba V D, Heil C G 1975 Eight years of fertility control with norgestrel-ethinyloestradiol (Ovral); an updated clinical review. Fertility and Sterility 26: 973–981

5. Lachnit-Fixson D 1980 Clinical investigation with a new triphasic oral contraceptive. In: Greenblat R B (ed) The development of a new triphasic oral contraceptive. MTP Press, Lancaster, pp 99–107

This study compared a triphasic regime with a daily fixed dose of 30 µg ethinyloestradiol plus 150 µg levonorgestrel. On the triphasic regimen, withdrawal bleeding occurred more reliably and during the first two cycles breakthrough bleeding and spotting were less common. There was no obvious loss of efficacy with the triphasic despite the reduction in total load of steroid and no pregnancies were reported in over 10 000 cycles of use.

Postcoital

6. Yuzpe A A, Smith R P, Rademaker A W 1982 A multicenter clinical investigation employing ethinyloestradiol combined with dl-norgestrel as a postcoital contraceptive

692 women were enrolled in a multi-centre clinical trial. For inclusion in the study unprotected intercourse had occurred within the previous 72 hours. The total dosage administered was 200 µg of ethinyloestradiol and 2 mg of dl-norgestrel, half at the initial visit (2 tablets of 50 µg EE_2 and 500 µg dlNG) and half 12 hours later. When compared with various formulas predicting the probability of pregnancy in this group, the number of pregnancies observed appeared to be reduced by 84%.

7. Van Stanten M R, Haspels A A 1985 Interception II; postcoital low-dose estrogens and norgestrel combinations in 633 women. Contraception 31: 275–293

A combination of ethinyloestradiol (200 µg) and either racemic norgestrel (2 mg) or levonorgestrel was used. A statistically significantly lower observed pregnancy rate was found compared to the expected number of pregnancies if no contraception was used.

Implants

8. Coutinho E 1978 Clinical experience with implant contraception. Contraception 18: 411–427

Subdermal implants of polysiloxane capsules containing a number of synthetic progestogens including levonorgestrel were studied in 4752 women over a period ranging from 6 months to 9 years. 67 087 women-months of use were recorded. 682 women had implants (1–12 capsules) containing levonorgestrel. The largest groups of patients had 6 capsules and were exposed for 6027 women-months; 47 pregnancies occurred. Abnormal bleeding patterns were a major disadvantage.

9. Robertson D N, Diaz S, Alvarez-Sanchez F et al 1985 Contraception with long-acting subdermal implants. A five year clinical trial with silastic covered rod implants containing levonorgestrel. Contraception 31: 351–359

A total of 189 women accepted subdermal implants for contraception. Each implant contained approximately 50 mg levonorgestrel. 78 women used 4 rods and 111 women 6 rods. In five years there were no pregnancies in either group. Termination of use because of menstrual problems were twice as frequent among the 4-rod users than among the users of 6 rods.

Intravaginal rings

10. Mishell D R, Moore D E, Roy S, Brenner P F, Page M A 1978 Clinical performance and endocrine profiles with contraceptive vaginal rings containing a combination of estradiol and d-norgestrel. American Journal of Obstetrics and Gynecology 130: 55–62

Contraceptive vaginal rings impregnated with levonorgestrel and estradiol were studied for up to 6 cycles in 10 subjects. Clinical acceptance was good. Ovulation was inhibited in all treatment cycles. Bleeding control was good.

Intrauterine device

11. Luukkainen T, Nilsson C G 1978 Sustained release of d-Norgestrel. Contraception 18: 451–454

Clinical experience with 72 first insertions of a levonorgestrel-releasing IUD is reported. No pregnancies occurred in 522 women-months of use. Removals were performed in six subjects for medical reasons and in seven subjects for other reasons. Plasma concentrations of levonorgestrel were highest during the first two weeks of use.

12. Sivin I, Alvarez F, Diaz J et al 1984 Intrauterine contraception with copper and with levonorgestrel: a randomized study of the TCu 380Ag and levonorgestrel 20 mcg/day devices

This was a randomized study of 1509 women. The levonorgestrel-releasing device was associated with significantly fewer bleeding days than the copper device. The cumulative gross pregnancy rate was 0.3 per 100 at one year.

Levonorgestrel

References

1. Diczfalusy E 1968 Mode of action of contraceptive drugs. American Journal of Obstetrics and Gynecology 100: 136–163
2. Moghissi K S, Marks C 1971 Effects of microdose norgestrel on endogenous gonadotrophic and steroid hormones, cervical mucus properties, vaginal cytology and endometrium. Fertility and Sterility 22: 424–434
3. Rice-Wray E, Beristain I I, Cervantes A 1972 Clinical study of a continuous daily micro-dose progestogen contraceptive -d-Norgestrel. Contraception 5: 279–294
4. Garmendia F, Kesseru E, Lierena L A 1973 Serum LH concentration in women under contraceptive treatment with estrogen-free progestogens. Hormones and Metabolic Research 5: 134–138
5. Spellacy W N, Buhti W C, Birk S A 1976 The effects of norgestrel on carbohydrate and lipid metabolism over one year. American Journal of Obstetrics and Gynecology 125: 984–986
6. Wynn V, Niththyananthan R 1982 The effect of progestins in combined oral contraceptives on serum lipids with special reference to high-density lipoproteins. American Journal of Obstetrics and Gynecology 142: 766–772
7. März W, Gross W, Gahn G, Romberg G, Taubert H-D, Kuhl H 1985 A randomized crossover comparison of two low-dose contraceptives: effects on serum lipids and lipoproteins. American Journal of Obstetrics and Gynecology 153: 287–293
8. Gaspard U J, Buret J, Gillian D, Romus M A, Lambotte R 1985 Serum lipid and lipoprotein changes induced by new oral contraceptives containing ethinyloestradiol plus levonorgestrel or desogestrel. Contraception 31: 395–408
9. Samsioe G 1982 Comparative effects of the oral contraceptive combinations 0.150 mg desogestrel and 0.030 mg ethinyloestradiol and 0.150 mg levonorgestrel and 0.030 mg ethinyloestradiol on lipid and lipoprotein metabolism in healthy female volunteers. Contraception 25: 487–504
10. Fotherby K 1984 Metabolic effects of low dose combined oral contraceptives. The British Journal of Family Planning 10: 15–19
11. Hümpel M, Wendt H, Pommerenke G, Weiss C, Speck U 1978 Investigations of pharmacokinetics of levonorgestrel to specific consideration of a possible first pass effect in women. Contraception 17: 207–220
12. Back D J, Bates M, Breckenridge A M et al 1981 The pharmacokinetics of levonorgestrel and ethinyloestradiol in women — studies with ovran and ovranette. Contraception 23: 229–240
13. Orme M L'E, Back D J, Breckenridge A M 1983 Clinical pharmacokinetics of oral contraceptive steroids. Clinical Pharmacokinetics 8: 95–136
14. Back D J, Orme M L'E 1984 Interindividual variability in oral contraceptive disposition. Trends in Pharmacological Sciences 5: 480–484
15. Victor A, Johansson E D B 1977 Effects of d-norgestrel-induced decreases in sex hormone binding globulin capacity on the d-norgestrel levels in plasma. Contraception 16: 115–123
16. Weiner E, Victor A, Johansson E 1977 New delivery systems for D-norgestrel. Acta Obstetrica et Gynecologica Scandinavica (suppl 54): 35–43
17. Croxatto H B, Diaz S, Brandels A, Pavez M, Johansson E D B 1985 Plasma levonorgestrel and progestogen levels in women treated with silastic covered rods containing levonorgestrel. Contraception 31: 643–654
18. Landgren B M, Johansson E, Xing S, Aedo A-R, Diczfalusy E 1985 A clinical pharmacological study of a new type of vaginal delivery system for levonorgestrel. Contraception 32: 581–601
19. Heikkila M, Haukkamaa M, Luukkainen T 1982 Levonorgestrel in milk and plasma of breast feeding women with a levonorgestrel-releasing IUD. Contraception 25: 41–49
20. Graham F M 1981 Problem patients and the 'pill'. Drugs 21: 152–156
21. Population Reports, Series A, No 6, 1982: A189–A224
22. Ling W Y, Wrixon W, Acorn T, Wilson E, Collins J 1983 Mode of action of dl-norgestrel and ethinyloestradiol combination in postcoital contraception III. Effect of preovulatory administration following the luteinizing hormone surge on ovarian steroidogenesis. Fertility and Sterility 40: 631–636
23. Centre for Disease Control and Steroid Hormone Study 1983 Long term oral contraceptive use and the risk of breast cancer. Journal of the American Medical Association 249: 1591–1595
24. Janerich D T, Polednak A P, Glebatis D M, Lawrence C E 1983 Breast cancer – and oral contraceptive use. A case control study. Journal of Chronic Diseases 36: 639–646
25. Stadel B V, Rubin G L, Webster L A, Schlesselman J J, Wingo P A 1985 Oral contraceptives and breast cancer in young women. Lancet 2: 970–973
26. Sattin R W, George L, Rubin M B et al 1986 The Centre for Disease Control Cancer and Steroid Hormone Study. Oral contraceptive use and the risk of breast cancer. New England Journal of Medicine 315: 405–411
27. Pike M C, Henderson B E, Krailo M D, Duke A, Roy S 1983 Breast cancer in young women and use of oral contraceptives; possible modifying effect of formulation and age at use. Lancet 2: 926–929
28. Park B K, Breckenridge A M 1981 Clinical implications of enzyme induction and enzyme inhibition. Clinical Pharmacokinetics 6: 1–24
29. Coulam C B, Annegers J F 1979 Do anticonvulsants reduce the efficacy of oral contraceptives? Epilepsia 20: 519–526
30. Back D J, Breckenridge A M, Crawford F E et al 1980 The effects of rifampicin on the pharmacokinetics of ethinyloestradiol in women. Contraception 21: 135–143
31. Orme M L'E, Back D J, Breckenridge A M 1984 Drug interactions with oral contraceptive steroids. British Journal of Family Planning 10: 19–23
32. Back D J, Grimmer S F M, Orme M L'E et al 1988 Evaluation of Committee on Safety of Medicines yellow card reports on oral contraceptive-drug interactions with anticonvulsants and antibiotics. British Journal of Clinical Pharmacology 25: 527–532
33. Friedman C I, Huneke A L, Kim M H, Powell J 1980 The effect of ampicillin or oral contraceptive effectiveness. Obstetrics and Gynecology 55: 33–37

L

34. Back D J, Breckenridge A M, Maciver M et al 1982 The effects of ampicillin on oral contraceptive steroids in women. British Journal of Clinical Pharmacology 14: 43–48
35. Grimmer S F M, Allen W L, Back D J, Breckenridge A M, Orme M L'E, Tjia A 1983 The effect of cotrimoxazole on oral contraceptive steroids in women. Contraception 28: 53–59
36. Beck D J, Breckenridge A M, Maciver M, Orme M L'E, Purba H, Rowe P H 1981 The interaction of ethinyloestradiol with ascorbic acid in man. British Medical Journal 282: 1516
37. Crawford F E, Back D J, Orme M L'E, Breckenridge A M 1981 Oral contraceptive steroid plasma concentrations in smokers and non-smokers. British Medical Journal 282: 1829–1830
38. Abernethy D R, Greenblatt D J, Ochs H R et al 1983 Lorazepam and Oxazepam kinetics in women on low dose oral contraceptives. Clinical Pharmacology and Therapeutics 33: 628–632
39. Rietvold E C, Broeitman M M, Houben J J G, Eskes T K A B, Van Rossum J M 1984 Rapid onset of an increase in caffeine residence time in young women due to oral contraceptive steroids. European Journal of Clinical Pharmacology 26: 371–373

Levorphanol (tartrate)

Levorphanol is a congener of the morphinan series of opioid analgesics.

Chemistry

Levorphanol tartrate
$C_{17}H_{23}NO.C_4H_2O_6.2H_2O$
3-Hydroxy-N-methylmorphinan tartrate dihydrate (alternatively 17-methyl-morphinan-3-ol tartrate dihydrate)

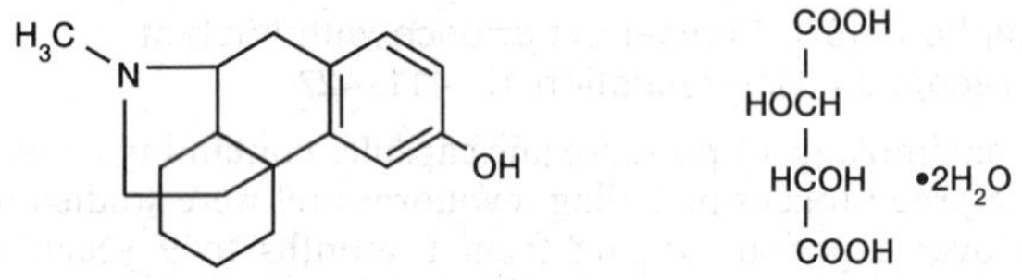

Molecular weight (base)	443.5 (257.4)
pKa	8.2
Solubility	
in alcohol	1 in 110
in water	1 in 40
Octanol/water partition coefficient	12.5

Levorphanol is a white, crystalline powder with a bitter taste. It lacks the oxygen bridge, the double bond and the 6-OH group of morphine. Chemical synthesis results in a racemic mixture of the (l)-enantiomer, levorphanol, and the (d)-enantiomer, the non-analgesic dextrorphan. This monograph refers to the (l)-enantiomer only.

Pharmacology

Levorphanol is a full agonist at μ opioid receptors to which it binds with high affinity.[1] Its binding to κ- and δ-receptors is not clear. Levorphanol is a potent analgesic with perhaps five times the potency of morphine (after subcutaneous injection) and with a similar duration of action (4–6 hours). It is said to be less sedative than morphine[2] and so may be more useful in the ambulatory patient with malignant disease causing pain. Most of the analgesic activity is retained when levorphanol is given orally. Levorphanol also causes more respiratory depression than morphine.

Toxicology

No information on toxicological studies in animals is available.

Clinical pharmacology

Levorphanol is a potent narcotic analgesic. A dose of 2 to 3 mg intravenously is equipotent[3] with morphine 10 mg, having a longer duration of action but with essentially similar effects. The longer period of pain relief is appreciated by both the patient and his attendants. Compared with morphine only half the number of intramuscular injections may be needed, and sufficient analgesia may be afforded after one evening dose to permit a full night's sleep. Oral potency is only 50% that of parenteral administration.[3] Levorphanol may also produce less nausea and vomiting than morphine. Otherwise its effects as a respiratory depressant and euphoric agent, and its effects on gastrointestinal motility, are similar to those of morphine.

Levorphanol (tartrate)

Pharmacokinetics

Analytical methods include HPLC with electrochemical detection,[4] a radioimmunoassay,[5] and gas chromatography with mass spectrometry.[6] The sensitivity of assay is 1 μg.l^{-1}. UV spectrophotometry lacks the sensitivity needed to measure therapeutic concentrations. The difficulties in assaying the drug have resulted in an incomplete picture of its pharmacokinetics in humans.

The drug is extensively distributed in the body[7,8] and its clearance is approximately 50% of hepatic blood flow, resulting in an elimination half life of 10 to 12 hours. It is easy to exceed the therapeutic concentration of 10 μg.l^{-1} after bolus intravenous injection.

Unlike morphine, levorphanol is well absorbed after oral administration. Analgesia is seen within 10 to 30 minutes, and lasts for 6 to 12 hours.[8] The 50% reduction in potency resulting from oral administration is due to presystemic metabolism. Levorphanol is well absorbed from an intramuscular injection site.

CSF concentrations are 60–70% of plasma concentrations, reflecting the plasma protein binding of 40%.[8] Some 15% exists as the free base at pH 7.0 and thus levorphanol and morphine have a similar ability to enter the central nervous system, and to cross the placenta.

The concentration–effect curve for levorphanol is quite steep so that any alteration in its kinetics is likely to require some adjustment of dosage. The elimination of the drug appears to be reduced in the elderly and it is very likely that hepatic and possibly renal impairment will result in reduced clearance of the drug and increased plasma concentrations.

Oral absorption	good
Presystemic metabolism	50%
Plasma half life	
range	10–12 h
Volume of distribution	10–13 l.kg^{-1}
Plasma protein binding	40%

Concentration–effect relationship

Concentrations exceeding 10 μg.l^{-1} produce analgesia in the non-tolerant surgical subject.[7]

Metabolism

Levorphanol is metabolized in the liver. The conjugate with glucuronic acid at the 3 position is the major metabolite, the levels of which reach 5 to 10 times the concentration of the parent drug in plasma. There is no information on the pharmacological activity of the 3-glucuronide in man. It has no activity on guinea-pig ileum,[9] but becomes active when injected intracerebrally because it is hydrolysed to levorphanol again. It is eliminated by the kidney. Little N-demethylation is thought to occur in humans. Levorphanol metabolism should be contrasted with that of morphine, where the additional OH group provides a starting place for another pathway of elimination, and the production of active metabolites.

Pharmaceutics

The manufacture of both oral and parenteral forms of this drug have been discontinued.

Therapeutic use

Indications

1. For the relief of moderate to severe pain
2. As an adjunct to general anaesthesia
3. As a premedicant.

Contraindications

Allergy to levorphanol is an absolute contraindication. As with other powerful opioids, levorphanol should be used with great care in the presence of the following:

1. Heart failure or hypovolaemia
2. Depression of consciousness induced by disease or other depressant drugs
3. Severe respiratory disease
4. Hepatic and renal impairment
5. There are no data relating to its safe use in pregnancy and paediatrics.

Mode of use

Oral dosing is commenced with 3–4.5 mg twice daily in the adult. The dose will require increasing for those tolerant to opioids. No paediatric prescribing information is available.

Parenteral administration is commenced at half the oral dosage. A slow intravenous injection of 0.5 to 3 mg can be titrated to effect or given intramuscularly. A similar dose is required to supplement general anaesthesia.

Elderly patients and those given other sedative drugs require a reduction in both the dose and the frequency of administration.

Indications

1. For the relief of moderate to severe pain

Levorphanol is an effective analgesic for the relief of severe postoperative pain.[2] It results in less depression of consciousness and less nausea than morphine or pethidine. It may have a particular value in patients suffering from the pain of terminal cancer who would appreciate its longer duration of action and reduced sedation.

2. As an adjunct to general anaesthesia[10]

Levorphanol has similar effects to morphine, but the duration of analgesia from an equipotent dose persists longer into the postoperative period.

3. As a premedicant[11,12]

Levorphanol has been compared with 10 other synthetic opioids and found to be the drug with the least side effects. However, the use of analgesics to produce sedation alone has been superseded by the more specific anxiolytic action of the benzodiazepines.

Contraindications

1. Heart failure or hypovolaemia

In common with other opioids, levorphanol produces peripheral vasodilation by a central action. Some of the fall in blood pressure seen with intravenous administration of morphine is due to direct release of histamine. There is no confirmation in the literature of the clinical impression that levorphanol has a lower tendency to release histamine.

2. Depression of consciousness induced by disease or other depressant drugs

Although levorphanol is only mildly sedative at analgesic concentrations, in common with other drugs of its class, it will potentiate the CNS depression produced by disease or other centrally acting drugs.

3. Severe respiratory disease

Levorphanol should be used with caution in patients sensitive to drug-induced respiratory depression, particularly as the effects can be expected to persist for several hours. Naloxone is an effective antagonist.

4. Hepatic and renal failure

Reduced elimination of levorphanol can be expected in the patient with hepatic or renal impairment, and the dose decreased accordingly.

5. Pregnancy

The usual precautions when prescribing drugs to pregnant and lactating mothers should be observed.

Adverse reactions

Potentially life-threatening effects

No allergic reactions have been reported. This may reflect a reduced potential to release histamine (cf. morphine) and the aqueous, preservative-free vehicle in the intravenous preparation. Fatalities have been attributed to respiratory arrest — an extension of the respiratory depressant action of opiates.

Acute overdosage

The clinical features of levorphanol overdose are typical of an opiate, with bradypnoea, hypoventilation and airway obstruction.

Levorphanol (tartrate)

L

Treatment consists of circulatory and respiratory support with tracheal intubation and mechanical ventilation if necessary, in conjunction with specific opiate antagonists. Levorphanol's long duration of action is likely to necessitate repeated doses of naloxone or an infusion. There is one report of a 30 mg oral dose leading to a fatality.

Severe or irreversible adverse effects
Depression of respiratory drive and the cough reflex, hypotension and urinary retention may occur.

Symptomatic adverse effects
Nausea and vomiting are not uncommon.

Interference with clinical pathology tests
None has been reported.

High risk groups

All of the observed actions of levorphanol are explicable in terms of opioid receptor binding, and contraindications and precautions are similar to those for morphine. Narcotic analgesics should always be prescribed according to patient response.

Neonates
There is insufficient information to recommend prescription to neonates.

Breast milk. There are no data in the literature on levels of the drug in breast milk, so it is probably best for patients who have received the drug to avoid breast-feeding.

Children
There are no references in the literature to paediatric prescribing. Infants are acknowledged to be sensitive to the action of narcotic analgesics.

Pregnant women
The safety of levorphanol in pregnancy has not been established. Extensive teratogenicity testing was not required at the time of its introduction.

The elderly
Altered pharmacokinetics are probably responsible for the observed sensitivity of the elderly to levorphanol.

Concurrent disease
Disease impairing drug elimination will affect dosing requirements. Increased sensitivity to narcotics is a feature of hypothyroidism, raised intracranial pressure and respiratory disease.

Drug interactions

Potentially hazardous interactions
Synergism can be anticipated with other central depressant drugs, such as benzodiazepines, phenothiazines, butyrophenones, tricyclic antidepressants, etc. The product data sheet suggests that combination with monoamine oxidase inhibitors should also be avoided.[3]

Other significant interactions
Decreased effect will be observed in those patients tolerant to the action of morphine, and may be seen in chronic alcoholism.

Potentially useful interactions
The therapeutic application of the interaction between levorphanol and naloxone has already been described.

Clinical trials

1. Morrison J D, Loan W B, Dundee J W 1969 Studies of drugs given before anaesthesia; the synthetic opiates. British Journal of Anaesthesia 41: 987–993
2. Dundee J W, Loan W B, Morrison J D 1970 Studies of drugs given before anaesthesia; the opiates. British Journal of Anaesthesia 42: 54–58
3. Morrison J D, Loan W B, Dundee J W 1971 Controlled comparison of the efficacy of 14 preparations in the relief of postoperative pain. British Medical Journal 3: 287–290

Levorphanol was compared with several analgesics for efficacy as a premedicant before surgery, and afterwards in the relief of postoperative pain. In a double-blind trial of pre-anaesthetic medication, involving over a thousand patients, levorphanol was compared with 10 other synthetic opioids for sedative properties and side effects. Levorphanol 2 mg produced the best sedation although this was at the expense of slightly more nausea and dizziness. Levorphanol was assessed as the most useful agent producing the least side effects.

General review articles

In addition to monographs in the larger pharmacology textbooks, a review article of levorphanol[3] is included in the reference list.

Clarke's Identification and isolation of drugs, 2nd edn. The Pharmaceutical Press, London, p 704

Remington's pharmaceutical sciences 1985 17th edn. Mark Publishing Company, Eaton, USA, pp 1104

The pharmaceutical codex 11th edn. The Pharmaceutical Press, London, p 924

Vickers M D, Wood-Smith F G, Stewart H C (eds) 1978 Drugs in anaesthetic practice 5th edn. Butterworths, London, p 185–186

References

1. Kuhar M, Pasternach G (eds) 1984 In: Analgesics — neurochemical, behavioral and clinical perspectives. Raven Press, New York
2. Morrison J D, Loan W B, Dundee J W 1971 Controlled comparison of the efficacy of 14 preparations in the relief of postoperative pain. British Medical Journal 3: 287–290
3. Eddy N B, Halbach H, Braeden O J 1957 Synthetic substances with morphine like effect; number 11. Morphinan derivatives. Bulletin of the World Health Organisation 17: 677–689
4. Lucek R, Dixon R 1985 Quantitation of levorphanol in plasma using high performance liquid chromatography with electrochemical detection. Journal of Chromatography 341: 239–243
5. Dixon R, Crewes T, Mohacsi E, Inturrusi C, Foley K 1981 Levorphanol: a simplified radio immunoassay for clinical use. Research Communications in Chemical Pathology and Pharmacology 31: 545–548
6. Min B H, Garland W A 1982 Determination of levorphanol in human plasma by gas chromatography negative ion mass spectrometry. Journal of Chromatography 231: 194–199
7. Dixon R, Crewes T, Inturrusi C, Foley K 1983 Levorphanol: pharmacokinetics and steady state plasma concentrations in patients with pain. Research Communications in Chemical Pathology and Pharmacology 42: 3–17
8. Dixon R 1986 Pharmacokinetics of levorphanol. In: Foley K M, Inturrusi C E (eds) Advances in pain research and therapy, vol 8. Raven Press, New York
9. Schulz R, Goldstein A 1972 Inactivity of narcotic glucuronides as analgesics and on guinea-pig ileum. Journal of Pharmacology and Experimental Therapeutics 183: 404–410
10. Dundee J W, Brown S S, Hamilton R C, McDowell S A 1969 Analgesic supplementation of light general anaesthesia. Anaesthesia 24: 52–61
11. Morrison J D, Loan W B, Dundee J W 1969 Studies of drugs given before anaesthesia; the synthetic opiates. British Journal of Anaesthesia 41: 987–993
12. Dundee J W, Loan W B, Morrison J D 1970 Studies of drugs given before anaesthesia; the opiates. British Journal of Anaesthesia 42: 54–58

Lignocaine (hydrochloride)

Lignocaine is a widely used local anaesthetic and cardiac antiarrhythmic. It is known officially as lidocaine in the USA.

Chemistry

Lignocaine hydrochloride (Xylocaine, Xylotox)
$C_{14}H_{12}N_2OHCl$
2-(Diethylamino)-N-(2,6-dimethylphenyl) acetamide

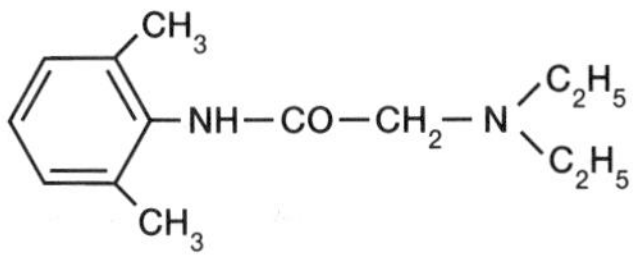

	Lignocaine	Hydrochloride
Molecular weight	234.33	288.8
pKa	7.86	—
Solubility		
in alcohol	1 in 1	1 in 1.5
in water	insoluble	1 in 0.7
Octanol/water partition coefficient	—	42

Lignocaine is the most widely used member of the amide group of local anaesthetic agents, which includes bupivacaine and prilocaine, as distinct from the ester group which includes cocaine and procaine. Lignocaine is a white or slightly yellow crystalline powder with a characteristic odour. It is prepared by chemical synthesis. Solutions are very stable and not decomposed by boiling.

It is also available in combination with prilocaine and other compounds.

Pharmacology

Lignocaine is primarily used for its local anaesthetic properties. Like other local anaesthetics lignocaine impairs the generation and conduction of the nerve impulses by slowing depolarization. This results from blocking of the large transient increase in permeability of the cell membrane to sodium ions that follows initial depolarization of the membrane. Lignocaine also reduces the permeability of the resting axon to potassium and to sodium ions. The site of action of lignocaine is on a specific receptor site in the sodium channel.

Lignocaine is more effective as a local anaesthetic on small non-myelinated nerve fibres, while myelinated A fibres are blocked before C fibres. The actions of lignocaine are prolonged by the use of a vasoconstrictor such as adrenaline.

Lignocaine has effects on the central nervous system to produce restlessness and tremor, and frank convulsions may occur. Central stimulation may be followed by depression and death due to respiratory failure. Lignocaine has weak neuromuscular blocking activity.

In the heart lignocaine's main activity is to reduce automaticity by decreasing the rate of diastolic (phase 4) depolarization. Lignocaine has little or no effect on conduction in the His–Purkinje system. The duration of the action potential is decreased due to blockade of the sodium channel and the effective refractory period is shortened.[1]

Toxicology

No teratogenic effects have been seen in dose levels up to 5 mg.kg^{-1} in the rat. There is no evidence of mutagenicity in the salmonella/rat liver microsomal assay system.

Clinical pharmacology

The local anaesthetic action is demonstrable in concentrations of 0.5 to 2.0% when the drug is injected close to the nerve and 4.0% when applied topically to mucous membranes. The recommended dose limit for infiltration anaesthesia is 3 mg.kg^{-1} without adrenaline and 7 mg.kg^{-1} with adrenaline. The addition of adrenaline 1:200 000 (5 μg.ml^{-1}) by its local vasoconstrictor action delays absorption of the lignocaine. More dilute solutions have a greater safety margin and the highest dose known to have been used is 14.6 mg.kg^{-1} of 0.26% solution with adrenaline, for infiltration anaesthesia.[2] The onset of action ranges from 5 minutes for infiltration anaesthesia to 20 minutes for regional anaesthesia. The duration of action is approximately one hour without adrenaline and one-and-a-half to two hours with adrenaline.

Lignocaine should not be used with adrenaline for anaesthesia of digits because of the risk of gangrene. Lignocaine stimulates the central nervous system and although this is unusual following local anaesthesia, both CNS stimulation followed by depression and cardiac depression have been recorded in this situation. These effects are more likely when lignocaine is used intravenously for the treatment of cardiac arrhythmias.

Lignocaine is usually administered intravenously when used to control arrhythmia, the effective dose being 1.0–1.5 mg.kg^{-1}, followed 5 minutes later by a second dose of half the first. These doses should be reduced for patients in heart failure. A therapeutic effect is best maintained by an intravenous infusion of 1–4 mg.min^{-1} to produce a plasma concentration of 1–5 mg.l^{-1}. Lignocaine can be given intramuscularly in emergencies in a dose of 4–5 mg.kg^{-1}.

Pharmacokinetics

Lignocaine can be assayed by high performance liquid chromatography or gas–liquid chromatography, the latter being sensitive down to 0.3 mg.l^{-1}.[3]

It is completely absorbed after oral administration but the presystemic metabolism is 65–70% so that this route is of little or no value clinically. It is, however, rapidly taken up from the oral mucous membranes and from the respiratory tract and dosage by topical spray must be monitored carefully. The uptake from the tissues into the blood is influenced by (1) site of injection and its vascularity, and (2) the associated use of a vasoconstrictor agent. Adrenaline constricts the cutaneous vascular bed but dilates muscle vessels so that it does not reduce uptake if injected into a muscle mass.

Following absorption of lignocaine there is a rapid distribution to all body tissues, the volume of distribution being approximately 100 l. Distribution takes place according to a two-compartment model involving first the highly vascular tissues and then those poorly perfused. Approximately 65% is bound to plasma protein, this figure being increased in cancer and uraemia in association with increased α_1-acid glycoprotein concentrations.[4] The drug crosses the blood–brain barrier freely and has a fetal/maternal plasma ratio of 0.5–0.7. Lignocaine has an elimination half life ($t_{\frac{1}{2}}\gamma$) of 1.6 hours.

Repetitive doses of local anaesthetics are used in continuous subarachnoid and extradural anaesthesia, and after a period of time the repeat dose produces a less effective and shorter-lasting blockade. This tachyphylaxis is due to accumulation of local acid hydrochloride, which favours the formation of ionized base and reduces penetration of the nerves. Systemic absorption of lignocaine from the extradural space is rapid, with a $t_{\frac{1}{2}}$ of approximately 1 hour, and repeated administration by this route can lead to toxic plasma levels.[5]

Oral absorption	>95%
Presystemic metabolism	65–70%
Plasma half life	1.6 h
Volume of distribution	1.3 l.kg^{-1}
Plasma protein binding	64%

Concentration–effect relationship

The antiarrhythmic effect is dose-related over the plasma range 2–5 μg.ml^{-1}, but toxic CNS effects may begin at 5–6 μg.ml^{-1} in unpremedicated patients. Anaesthesia has a protective effect and the safe concentration in anaesthetized patients rises to approximately twice the above.[6]

Metabolism

Lignocaine is metabolized in the liver to an extent of approximately 80%, only 3% being found unchanged in the urine (Fig. 1). None has been detected in the bile and there is no entero-hepatic circulation. There are three reactions involved:[7,8]

1. N-de-ethylation → monoethylglycinexylidide (MEGX) → glycinexylidide
2. Hydrolysis of glycinexylidide → 2.6 xylidine. The main excretion product in the urine (73%) is the 4-hydroxy derivative of this substance.
3. 5-hydroxylation of the benzene ring of both lignocaine and MEGX.

Both de-ethylation metabolites have antiarrhythmic activity, the monoethyl derivative being 33–83% as active as lignocaine and the glycinexylidide being 10–42% as active. Only the former has convulsive activity, having approximately 88% that of lignocaine.[9] Severe hepatic disease or reduced portal blood flow to the liver (as in congestive cardiac failure) decreases the rate of metabolism.[10]

Lignocaine (hydrochloride)

Pharmaceutics

Lignocaine hydrochloride is not available for oral medication. The solution (Xylocaine) is available as 0.5%, 1%, 1.5%, 2% plain (without adrenaline) and as 0.5%, 1% and 2% with adrenaline 1: 200 000. It is also available as a 2% solution with adrenaline 1: 80 000 for dental administration (Xylotox). Topical preparations include a 2% gel for urethral and vaginal anaesthesia, a 5% ointment for surface anaesthesia, a viscous 2% solution for anaesthesia of the upper digestive tract, 4% eye drops and a 4% topical solution for upper respiratory tract anaesthesia, and there are minor variations in these for special requirements. EMLA Local anaesthetic cream contains lignocaine 25 mg and priloiaine 25 mg.g^{-1}.

The multidose vials and topical applications contain hydroxybenzoate derivatives which may be allergenic.

Solutions containing adrenaline should be stored protected from light at a temperature of + 2 to + 15°C. The shelf-life of the various preparations is 2–5 years.

Fig. 1 The Metabolism of lignocaine

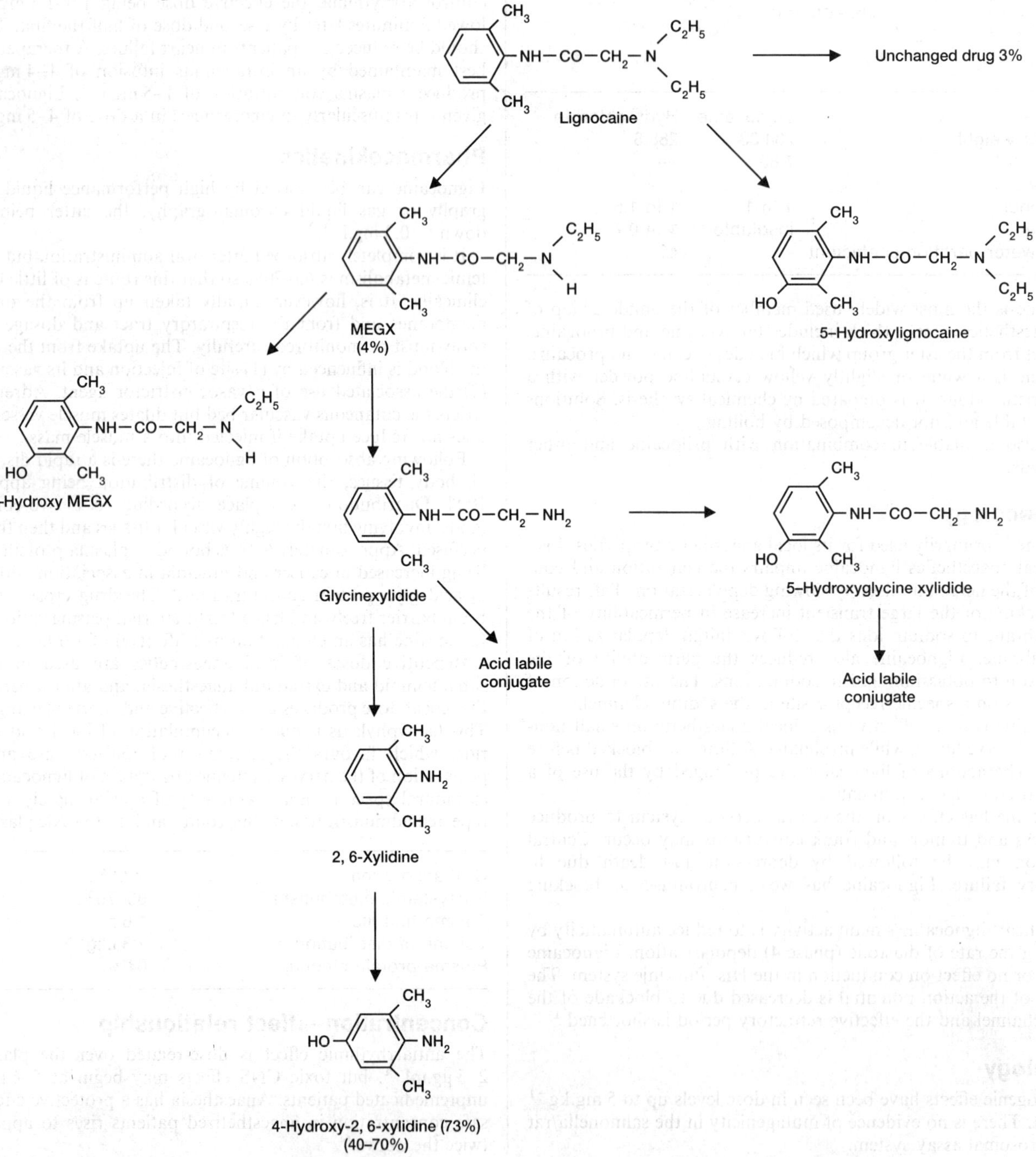

Lignocaine (hydrochloride)

Therapeutic use

Indications

Lignocaine has two main fields of use:

1. As a local anaesthetic for use in intrafiltration blockade and intravenous regional analgesia
2. For the prevention and treatment of ventricular tachyarrhythmias.

Contraindications

Contraindications include:

1. Hypersensitivity to local anaesthetics of the amide type, which is rare
2. Congestive cardiac failure, since it reduces clearance and volume of distribution, is an indication for reduction of the infused dosage by half.[16]

Mode of use

1. Local anaesthesia

The drug is introduced as close as possible to the nerves to be blocked in accordance with the relevant anatomy and clinical response.[11] The lowest concentration (usually 1% or 2%) and smallest dose to produce the required effect should be given. The maximum dose for healthy adults should not exceed 200 mg without adrenaline and 500 mg with adrenaline or 3 $mg.kg^{-1}$ and 7 $mg.kg^{-1}$, respectively, for children. Lignocaine can also be used for spinal, extradural and caudal block, adjusting the dose to the number of segments or area to be blocked. Hyperbaric 5% lignocaine is available for spinal anaesthesia. The 2% solution with 1:200 000 adrenaline has been used for extradural anaesthesia in obstetrics in preference to bupivacaine because of its rapid onset of action (20 min compared with 40 min).[12] In pregnancy the standard doses should be reduced by 30%.[13] In extradural blockade the dosage should also be reduced in the elderly because of the greater degree of spread of the drug.[14] Specific caudal doses for children have been recommended.[15]

2. Antiarrhythmic treatment

Lignocaine acts by preventing ventricular arrhythmias, particularly after myocardial infarction or cardiac surgery, and raising the threshold for ventricular fibrillation. It is of little value in suppressing supraventricular arrhythmias. An intravenous dose of 1 $mg.kg^{-1}$ may be given over 2 min and repeated after 5 min, but giving an infusion of 2–4 $mg.min^{-1}$ to produce a plasma level of 2–4 $mg.l^{-1}$ is a more satisfactory technique. To avoid a long delay in achieving a steady state, a loading dose of approximately 1 $mg.kg^{-1}$ is usually given intravenously over 2 min at the outset.

Adverse reactions

Potentially life-threatening effects

Central nervous system toxicity is usually due to accidental intravenous injection when carrying out local anaesthetic procedures. Early effects consist of dizziness, tinnitus, lightheadedness, nystagmus and fine twitching. These may progress to medullary depression and tonic and clonic convulsions. In general, the severity of the symptoms and signs is dependent on the speed of infusion or rapidity of absorption, rather than the plasma concentration.[17] Unconsciousness can occur at this stage but there is usually complete recovery without cardiac arrest if there is good general management. Convulsions may be treated with thiopentone or diazepam but respiratory and cardiovascular support will usually be necessary in addition. Oxygen should always be given by face mask before any sedative drugs. In over 36 000 regional block procedures Moore et al[18] found an incidence of CNS reactions of 1.5%.

Acute overdosage

An accidental overdose of 2 g to a patient has been successfully treated by cardiopulmonary bypass plus pacing until sinus rhythm and adequate cardiac output had returned.[19] Cardiovascular collapse commonly follows overdosage and results from depression of myocardial contraction, bradycardia and a fall in cardiac output. At the same time there is direct inhibition of the vascular smooth muscle, depression of the baroreceptor reflexes and of the vasomotor centre. Lignocaine is less toxic than bupivacaine and resuscitation after overdosage is more likely to be successful. The main consideration is to provide inotropic support.[20]

Severe or irreversible adverse effects

Allergic reactions are extremely rare, constituting only 2% of all toxic reactions.

Symptomatic adverse effects

Lignocaine infusions are well tolerated and the main CNS effects described above are an indication of excessive rapid infusion or overdosage. Many patients experience nausea, vomiting and abdominal discomfort after oral use but this route is not of practical importance.

Interference with clinical pathology tests

None is known.

High risk groups

Neonates

Neonates are more sensitive to lignocaine because the degree of protein binding is only 50% compared with the 64% in adults.

Breast milk. Not clinically important.

Children

Dosage should be reduced according to weight; 3 $mg.kg^{-1}$ without vasoconstrictors or 7 $mg.kg^{-1}$ with vasoconstrictors is appropriate.

Pregnant women

There are no specific contraindications during pregnancy.

The elderly

Healthy elderly patients do not appear to be abnormally sensitive to lignocaine.

Concurrent disease

Caution should be used in patients with severe liver disease since reduced metabolism may give rise to toxic blood levels. In epilepsy there is a possibility that the convulsive threshold may be lowered by lignocaine. Patients with impaired cardiac conduction and bradycardia are more sensitive to the cardiac depressant action of the drug.

Drug interactions

Potentially hazardous interactions

There appear to be few undesirable interactions with lignocaine itself. Concomitant administration of cimetidine (which inhibits hepatic metabolism) in patients receiving lignocaine may result in increased plasma concentrations of lignocaine and increased toxicity.[21] The maintenance dose of lignocaine may therefore need to be reduced in such patients. It was thought that ranitidine did not have this effect[22] but a 9% reduction in clearance has been shown following pretreatment with this drug also, presumably due to its effect in reducing hepatic blood flow.[23] Propranolol, however, reduces the systemic clearance of lignocaine in man by as much as 40% and in this case the effect is mainly due to direct inhibition of its hepatic metabolism.[24]

Other significant interactions

Lignocaine prolongs the duration of action of suxamethonium, due to both inhibition of acetylcholine release and postjunctional effects. Lignocaine also inhibits plasma cholinesterase activity but this probably has no clinical significance.[25]

Potentially useful interactions

A beneficial interaction, as indicated above, is that benzodiazepines and barbiturates raise the convulsive threshold to lignocaine.

General review articles

Covino B, Vassallo H 1976 Local anaesthetics: mechanisms of action and clinical use. Grune and Stratton, New York

Eriksson E 1979 Illustrated handbook of local anaesthesia. Astra, Copenhagen

Smith G, Scott D B (eds) 1986 Postgraduate educational issue: symposium on local anaesthesia. British Journal of Anaesthesia 58: 691–800

References

1. Liu P, Feldman H S, Covino B M, Giasi R, Covino B G 1982 Acute cardiovascular toxicity of intravenous amide local anesthetics in anesthetized ventilated dogs. Anesthesia and Analgesia 61: 317–322

2. Glauber D T, Buffington C W, Hornbein T F, Hamacher E N 1984 High dose lidocaine, ultradilute epinephrine and intravenous sedation for major plastic surgery. Anesthesia and Analgesia 63: 219
3. Abernethy D R, Greenblatt D J 1982 Lidocaine determination in human plasma with application to single low dose pharmacokinetic studies. Journal of Chromatography 232: 180–185
4. Jackson P R, Tucker G T, Woods H F 1982 Altered plasma drug binding in cancer: role of α_1-acid glycoprotein and albumin. Clinical Pharmacology and Therapeutics 32: 295–302
5. Tucker G T 1986 Pharmacokinetics of local anaesthetics. British Journal of Anaesthesia 58: 717–731
6. Gianelli R, Von der Groeben J O, Spicavk A P, Harrison D C 1967 Effect of lidocaine (xylocaine) on ventricular arrhythmias in patients with coronary heart disease. New England Journal of Medicine 277: 1215–1219
7. Keenaghan J B, Boyes R N 1972 The tissue distribution, metabolism and excretion of lidocaine in rats, guinea pigs, dogs and man. Journal of Pharmacology and Experimental Therapeutics 180: 454–463
8. Boyes R N 1975 A review of the metabolism of amide local anaesthetic agents. British Journal of Anaesthesia 47: 225–230
9. Burney R G, Difazio C A, Peach M J, Petrie K A, Silvester M J 1974 Antiarrhythmic effects of lidocaine metabolites. American Heart Journal 88: 765–769
10. Thomson P D, Melmon K L, Richardson J A et al 1973 Lidocaine pharmacokinetics in advanced heart failure, liver disease and renal failure in humans. Annals of Internal Medicine 78: 499–508
11. Eriksson E 1979 Illustrated handbook of local anaesthesia. Astra, Copenhagen, 1–152
12. Moir D D 1986 Local anaesthetic techniques in obstetrics. British Journal of Anaesthesia 58: 747–759
13. Fagraeus L, Urban B J, Bromage P R 1983 Spread of epidural anesthesia in early pregnancy. Anesthesiology 58: 184–186
14. Park W Y, Massengale M, Kim S I, Poon K C, MacNamara T E 1980 Age and the spread of local anesthetic solutions in the epidural space. Anesthesia and Analgesia 59: 768–771
15. Takasaki M, Dohi S, Kawabata Y, Takahashi T 1977 Dosage of lidocaine for caudal anesthesia in infants and children. Anesthesiology 47: 527–529
16. Benowitz N L, Meister W 1976 Pharmacokinetics in patients with cardiac failure. Clinical Pharmacokinetics 1: 389–405
17. Scott D B 1986 Toxic effects of local anaesthetic agents on the central nervous system. British Journal of Anaesthesia 58: 732–735
18. Moore D E, Bridenbaugh L D 1960 Oxygen: the antidote for systemic toxic reactions from local anesthetic drugs. Journal of the American Medical Association 174: 842–847
19. Noble J, Kennedy D J, Latimer R D et al 1984 Massive lignocaine overdose during cardiopulmonary bypass. Successful treatment with cardiac pacing. British Journal of Anaesthesia 56: 1439
20. Reiz S, Nath S 1986 Cardiotoxicity of local anaesthetic agents. British Journal of Anaesthesia 58: 736–746
21. Feely J, Wilkinson G R, McAllister C B, Wood A J J 1982 Increased toxicity and reduced clearance of lidocaine by cimetidine. Annals of Internal Medicine 96: 592–594
22. Feely J, Guy E 1983 Lack of effect of ranitidine on the disposition of lignocaine. British Journal of Clinical Pharmacology 15: 378–379
23. Robson R A, Wing L M H, Miners J O, Lillywhite K J, Birkett D J 1985 The effect of ranitidine on the disposition of lignocaine. British Journal of Clinical Pharmacology 20: 170–173
24. Bax N D S, Tucker G T, Lennard M S, Woods H F 1985 The impairment of lignocaine clearance of propranolol — major contribution from enzyme inhibition. British Journal of Clinical Pharmacology 19: 597–603
25. Viby-Morgensen J 1985 Interaction of other drugs with muscle relaxants. Seminars in Anesthesia 4: 52–64

Lincomycin hydrochloride

Lincomycin is an antibiotic used to treat serious infections with susceptible Gram-positive organisms.

Chemistry

Lincomycin hydrochloride (Lincocin, Albiotic, Mycivin, Frademicina, Lincocina, Sciroppo).
$C_{18}H_{34}N_2O_6S.HCl$[1]
Methyl-6,8-dideoxy-6-((2S,4R)-1-methyl-4-propyl-2-pyrrolidinecarboxamido)-1-thio-α-D-*erythro*-D-*galacto*-octopyranoside hydrochloride

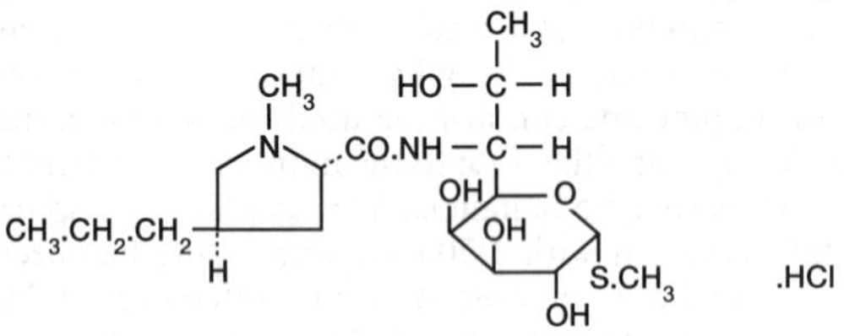

Molecular weight (free base)	443.5 (406.5)
pKa (amino group)	7.6
Solubility	
in alcohol	1 in 40
in water	1 in 1
Octanol/water partition coefficient	—

The hydrochloride is obtained as needle-like crystals by acetone precipitation from aqueous solution.[2] Lincomycin is produced by *Streptomyces lincolnensis* which is found in soil near Lincoln, Nebraska. Rotary optical dispersion measurements show it to be dextrorotatory.

Pharmacology

Lincomycin inhibits RNA-dependent protein synthesis by acting on the 50S subunit of the ribosomes of Gram-positive organisms.[3] Lincomycin can be displaced from the ribosomes by erythromycin,[3] temperature changes and by dilution. Studies with cell-free initiation systems have demonstrated the effects of lincomycin on the process of peptide chain initiation, especially at low magnesium concentrations.[4] Recent studies also suggest in vitro inhibition of enzyme synthesis in strains of *Staphylococcus aureus*. This inhibition seems to occur at lower concentrations than those causing growth inhibition.[5]

Toxicology

Lincomycin has low toxicity, and is usually well tolerated even when multiple large doses are given intravenously.[6] No carcinogenic effects have been described in association with the use of lincomycin.

Animal and human studies have not demonstrated teratogenicity.[7]

Clinical pharmacology[8,9]

Lincomycin is active against a wide range of organisms. At concentrations of less than 0.5 $mg.l^{-1}$ it inhibits the multiplication in vitro of *Streptococcus pyogenes*, *Strept. pneumoniae* and *Strept. viridans*. At concentrations of less than 2 $mg.l^{-1}$ the drug is active against *Corynebacterium diphtheriae*, *Clostridium tetani* and *Cl. perfringens*. Most strains of *Staphylococcus aureus* are also sensitive to this concentration of lincomycin although some strains will still grow in concentrations of 5 $mg.l^{-1}$. Lincomycin is also active against *Acti-*

Lincomycin hydrochloride

nomyces and *Bacteroides fragilis* and has some activity against *Haemophilus influenzae* and *Mycoplasma*. It is inactive against Gram-positive and most Gram-negative bacilli, enterococci and *Neisseria meningitidis*.

Pharmacokinetics

Gas–liquid chromatography has been used to determine the lincomycin content in bulk material; also to determine the amount of drug in capsules, syrups, ampoules and powders.[10] The microbiological assay was the official method used by the Food and Drug Administration in the certification of lincomycin and its dosage forms.[10] A modification of this assay with increased sensitivity is used in blood concentration determinations, using *Sarcina lutea* as an assay organism.[11]

Oral absorption	20–35%
Presystemic metabolism	—
Plasma half life	4.4 h
Volume of distribution	—
Plasma protein binding	72%

Serum concentrations

After a single oral dose of lincomycin, the peak serum concentration is achieved at 2–4 h and remains at significant levels for at least 12 h;[12] with multiple oral doses, the drug accumulates to steady state;[12,13] approximately 20–35% of an oral dose reaches the systemic circulation. Lower blood concentrations are obtained when lincomycin is taken orally with meals.[14] At oral dosages of 500 mg every 6 hours in adults, the antibiotic serum concentrations were maintained between 2.4–3.9 $mg.l^{-1}$.[9,12] After an intramuscular dose of 600 mg every 8 hours in adults, the peak and trough values were 12.2 and 6.4 $mg.l^{-1}$.[12] After an intravenous infusion of 600 mg (2 hour infusion period) every 6 hours in adults, the peak and trough concentrations were 17.5 and 8.2 $mg.l^{-1}$.[12] Ultrafiltration of serum, containing antibiotic in a concentration of 5 $mg.l^{-1}$, and tube dilution techniques have shown a high degree of serum protein binding of lincomycin; only 28% is found as free antibiotic.[15] Lincomycin is widely distributed to extracellular and intracellular fluids[9] penetrating well into peritoneal pleural spaces, joint fluid, soft tissue and bone. Subconjunctival injection of 75 mg results in therapeutic concentrations of lincomycin in ocular fluid for approximately 5 hours.[16]

Bone penetration

Studies in normal human bone have demonstrated that lincomycin penetrates readily in the bone marrow and its concentration is the same as that in the serum. Lower concentrations are found in spongy bone and compact bone, averaging 60% and 10% of serum values, respectively.[17]

Cerebrospinal fluid penetration

Lincomycin does not penetrate the blood–brain barrier of normal individuals in significant amounts.[18,19] In patients with active meningeal inflammation, concentrations of lincomycin of 7 $mg.l^{-1}$ in cerebrospinal fluid have been reported.[18] Intrathecal administration has been attempted in cases of meningitis without success.[20]

Pleural fluid, sputum and saliva penetration

The penetration of lincomycin into the pleural fluid after thoracotomy reaches 50% of serum concentration when given intramuscularly and 10–40% when given orally.[19,21] Sputum levels of $\frac{1}{10}$ of the serum have been found in cystic fibrosis patients after parenteral administration of lincomycin.[22] Saliva concentration after intramuscular administration attains a peak of approximately $\frac{1}{10}$ of the serum peak level.[23]

Peritoneal fluid

Peritoneal fluid concentrations are variable.[19]

Transplacental penetration

After a single intramuscular administration of lincomycin to mothers during labour, serum concentrations of 25% of maternal values are found in cord blood; clearance from the baby's serum follows the same linear regression as in the mother. The peak concentration of lincomycin in amniotic fluid approximates 25–50% of the maternal serum peak level.[19,24] Breast milk concentrations of 0.5 to 2.4 $mg.l^{-1}$ have been measured after conventional doses.

Bile penetration

Lincomycin concentrates into bile at levels 4 to 6 times those in serum,[25] immediately after a single intravenous dose.[19] After an oral dose, initial concentrations in bile are low, but slowly build up, prolonging the activity in serum. This is due in part to reabsorption from the intestinal tract after biliary excretion.[19]

Half life

Plasma half life of lincomycin after single intravenous administration in healthy adults is about 4.4 hours[26,9] with only small increases when repetitive oral doses are given. In patients with hepatic functional insufficiency, the calculated half life in serum is about 8.9 hours[27] with lower peak concentrations when compared with normal patients. In patients with severe azotaemia, the half life is about 12.6 hours; peak concentrations are also elevated three to fourfold when compared with patients with normal renal function.[28]

Renal excretion

Lincomycin is excreted mainly as unmetabolized drug. High serum concentrations seem to enhance renal excretion. The mean percentages of lincomycin recovered in the urine after 24 hours are 3–13% after oral dosing, 10–50% after a single intramuscular dose, and 13–73% after a single intravenous dose of 300 mg. Approximately 30–40% is excreted in faeces within 72 hours after oral administration and 5–15% after parenteral administration.[29] Lincomycin serum concentrations are not affected by peritoneal dialysis or haemodialysis.[28]

Concentration–effect relationship

The antimicrobial effect of lincomycin is related to the concentration of drug achieved in different body fluids.[14] Inhibition of extracellular virulence factors by lincomycin in some strains of *Staphylococcus aureus* occurs at subinhibitory concentrations.[5]

Metabolism

Lincomycin is partially metabolized in the liver[25] and excreted into bile. There is evidence of duodenal reabsorption of the drug. After parenteral administration, drug is present in stools up to 7 days after administration; susceptible intestinal flora are markedly decreased. Lincomycin is actively incorporated into macrophages and granulocytes.[30]

Pharmaceutics

Lincomycin, Lincocin (Upjohn UK/US) is available in 500 mg navy blue/light blue coloured capsules marked 'UPJOHN'. It is also available in 250 mg paediatric light blue coloured capsules (USA) or red raspberry flavoured syrup (UK) containing 250 mg lincomycin per 5 ml and 300 $mg.ml^{-1}$ of 2 ml and 10 ml vials. Benzyl alcohol is used as the preservative.

Aqueous solutions are stable for approximately 2 years. Dry crystalline lincomycin hydrochloride stored at 70°C showed no detectable degradation at 6 months.[2]

Therapeutic use

Lincomycin has been effective in the treatment of Gram-positive infections of the respiratory tract, genitourinary tract, soft tissue, bone and bloodstream.[20] Its main indications are for patients who cannot tolerate or are allergic to penicillins and cephalosporins or for infections due to bacteria resistant to penicillins and cephalosporins.[31] In general clindamycin is preferred to lincomycin.

Indications

These include:

1. Pneumococcal pneumonia[32]
2. Acute and chronic staphylococcal osteomyelitis[33]
3. Anaerobic infections following abdominal surgery[34]
4. Impetigo due to *Staphylococcus* or *Streptococcus*
5. Chronic middle ear infections in adults[35]
6. Group A streptococcal infections[36]
7. Infections caused by penicillin-resistant staphylococci[37]
8. Sensitive strains of *Corynebacterium diphtheriae*.[38]

Note: The sensitivity of above-named organisms to lincomycin must be determined for each patient, since several cases of resistance have

Lincomycin hydrochloride

L

been reported. These reports include: group A β-haemolytic *Streptococcus*,[39–42] *Staphylococcus aureus*,[43] *Streptococcus pneumoniae*,[44] *Neisseria gonorrhoeae*,[45] *Corynebacterium diphtheriae*[46] and *Streptococcus viridans*.[47]

Contraindications

Lincomycin is contraindicated in patients with known hypersensitivity to this drug or to clindamycin. Experimental challenge in CF 1 mice induced fatal anaphylaxis after sensitization to the drug.

Lincomycin has been given to newborns, but clinical experience is limited.

Mode of use

Oral dosage

In adults: 500 mg twice daily to 2 g daily. In children over 1 month of age: 30–60 mg.kg^{-1} daily, divided into three or four doses. Doses as high as 100 mg.kg^{-1} daily have been used in selected infections.

Lincomycin should be given on an empty stomach separated from meals by 1 to 2 hours.

Intravenous dosage

Adults: 600 mg to 1 g infused slowly every 8 to 12 hours. The rate of infusion should be no faster than 1 g per hour with a maximum dose of 8 g daily. Children older than 1 month: 10–20 mg.kg^{-1} daily in equally divided doses every 8 hours.

Intravenous infusions must be diluted in dextrose water, saline solution, or other compatible intravenous fluids in amounts of approximately 100 ml per gram of lincomycin.

Intramuscular dosage

Adults: 600 mg every 12 hours.

Children over 1 month of age: 10–20 mg.kg^{-1} per 24 h in equally divided doses every 12 hours.

Intravenous and intramuscular administration produces almost no local irritation or phlebitis.

Daily dosage in patients with severe impairment of renal function must be adjusted to 25–30% of the recommended dose for patients with normal renal function, or 200 mg intramuscularly every 8 to 12 hours for an average 70 kg individual.[28]

Adverse reactions

Potentially life-threatening effects

Syncope and hypotension may occur with poorly diluted and rapidly administered intravenous doses.[6,47] Anaphylaxis has occasionally occurred.

Cardiopulmonary arrest has occurred when the drug has been administered intravenously either rapidly and/or in high concentration.[48]

Pseudomembranous enterocolitis is most common after oral administration of lincomycin, but is also seen with other routes of administration. It occurs in 1–10% of cases; *Clostridium difficile* and/or its cytotoxin can be isolated in stools from these patients in approximately 90% of cases.[49,50] Treatment includes discontinuation of lincomycin, oral vancomycin or metronidazole and supportive intravenous fluids with potassium replacement. *Clostridium difficile* is a spore-forming organism and nosocomial contamination is possible; patients should be assigned enteric isolation precautions.[49]

Acute overdosage

No serious adverse effects or toxicities have been described after a large single dose of lincomycin, when given slowly and properly diluted. Very high serum concentrations have been achieved after repetitive intravenous administration of large doses in patients with severe azotaemia.

Severe or irreversible effects

Diarrhoea occurs in 10–50% of adult patients receiving large oral doses; it is less common in children.[49] Diarrhoea usually develops 7–10 days after the beginning of therapy with lincomycin, but can be seen as early as 24 hours or as late as 3 weeks.[51,52]

Intravenous administration of lincomycin can augment the neuromuscular-blocking effect of pancuronium.[53] This blockade can be effectively antagonized by neostigmine. Postoperative apnoea has also occurred after rapid intravenous administration.

Severe erythema multiforme and serum-sickness has occasionally been reported in association with the administration of lincomycin.

Granulocytopenia,[54] thrombocytopenia,[55] leukopenia and sideroblastic anaemia[56] have been reported occasionally. Prompt recovery usually occurs after cessation of therapy. Super-infections, including yeasts and resistant organisms, may occur. No evidence of hepatic or renal damage has been established but renal dysfunction as evidenced by azotaemia, oliguria, and/or proteinuria has been observed in rare instances.

Symptomatic adverse effects

Skin rashes, urticaria, fever, nausea, vomiting, stomatitis, tinnitus, vertigo, transient hepatic dysfunction, oesophagitis, and perianal, rectal and vaginal irritation.

High risk patient groups

Neonates

Lincomycin should not be given to neonates. The formulation contains benzyl alcohol which may cause apnoea in prematures.

Breast milk. Breast milk concentrations of lincomycin are similar to maternal serum concentrations.[19]

Children

The drug may be given to children in the doses mentioned earlier.

Pregnant women

Whether or not the drug is completely safe when given during pregnancy is not known.

The elderly

Therapy with lincomycin must be closely monitored in debilitated patients with severe renal impairment, liver disease, asthma and/or allergies, and a history of colitis, who might be more susceptible to dehydration secondary to diarrhoea.

Concurrent disease

Meningitis. Lincomycin should not be used to treat meningitis.

Renal failure. Dosage should be adjusted to 25–30% of the total daily dose, in patients with severe azotaemia.[28]

Hepatic failure. Lincomycin should be avoided in patients with liver disease.

Surgical operations. Lincomycin should be used cautiously in patients receiving neuromuscular blocking agents, since it may enhance the blockade produced by pancuronium,[57] d-tubocurarine, atracurium, besylate and gallamine triethiodide, affecting recovery of ventilation control after general anaesthesia.

Note. Periodic liver and renal function tests should be performed in several of the above categories and in patients treated for long durations.

Drug interactions

Some erythromycin-resistant strains of *Staphylococcus aureus* are resistant to lincomycin in the presence of erythromycin but fully sensitive in its absence. This interaction suggests antagonism between lincomycin and erythromycin due to the displacement of lincomycin from its ribosomal binding site.[3] Similar resistance is occasionally noted in *Streptococcus pneumoniae*,[44] group A β-haemolytic *Streptococcus*,[39–42] *Streptococcus viridans*,[47] and *Corynebacterium diphtheriae*.[46] Lincomycin resistance may occasionally develop in vivo; resistance seems to develop faster in *Staphylococcus aureus* resistant to erythromycin than in those that are susceptible. This pattern of resistance does not require previous exposure to either antibiotic.[43] In addition, cross-resistance with other antibiotics may also occur.[43] There is no evidence of rapid development of resistance to lincomycin.[58] Combinations of lincomycin and clindamycin demonstrate antagonism against *E. coli*[58] and indifference or equivalence against *Staphylococcus aureus*.[59] Lincomycin and erythromycin are synergistic against some strains of *Streptococcus* group A.[40]

Antidiarrhoeal agents should not be used in lincomycin-induced diarrhoea, since slowing of gastrointestinal motility increases the exposure time of the mucosa to the drug itself and to other potentially pathogenic agents and their toxins (e.g.*Clostridium difficile*); kaolin–pectin also prevents the absorption of lincomycin.[60]

Lincomycin hydrochloride

Major outcome trials

1. Donohoe R F, Swift J P 1967 Lincomycin therapy of pneumonia. Southern Medical Journal 60: 203–208[61]

Lincomycin was utilized in 50 patients with pneumonia secondary to Gram positives, especially *Streptococcus pneumoniae* with the following results:

Excellent clinical response: 15
Good clinical response: 24
Failures: 3
Unable to evaluate: 8
Total: 50

One death occurred in association with treatment failure. Two other deaths were not evaluable, and two were not associated with treatment failure. Most patients in this study had significant associated disease, belonged to a particular ethnic group, 80% were male and all were older than 28 years.

2. Novak E, Vitti T G, Panzer J D, Schlagel C, Hearron M S 1971 Antibiotic tolerance and serum levels after intravenous administration of multiple large doses of lincomycin. Clinical Pharmacology and Therapeutics 12 (5): 793–797

Double-blind study on males from a prison population ages 21 to 46 years. Large dosages of intravenous lincomycin (4.8–8 g daily) were infused into 32 healthy volunteers, 4 times a day for 7 days. No toxicity was detected, side effects were minor and few.

3. Leigh D A, Pease R, Henderson H, Simmons K, Russ R 1976 Prophylactic lincomycin in the prevention of wound infection following appendicectomy: a double blind study. British Journal of Surgery 63: 973–977

Double-blind study of the value of prophylactic use of a single dose of lincomycin in 100 patients undergoing appendectomy. Incidence of postoperative wound infection (most commonly due to *Bacteroides fragilis* and *E. coli*) was reduced from 17% to 6% when compared with similar control groups which consisted of patients who received sterile saline intramuscularly following closure of the wound.

References

1. Herr R R, Bergy M E 1962 Lincomycin, a new antibiotic. II. Isolation and characterization. Antimicrobial Agents and Chemotherapy 560–564
2. Mason D J, Dietz A, Deboer C 1962 Lincomycin, a new antibiotic. I. Discovery and biological properties. Antimicrobial Agents and Chemotherapy 554–559
3. Chang F N, Weisblum B 1967 The specificity of lincomycin binding to ribosomes. Biochemistry 6 (3): 836–843
4. Reusser F 1975 Effect of lincomycin and clindamycin on peptide chain initiation. Antimicrobial Agents and Chemotherapy 7 (1): 32–37
5. Shibl A M 1984 Selective inhibition of enzyme synthesis by lincomycin in *Staphylococcus aureus*. Journal of Antimicrobial Chemotherapy 13: 625–627

Novak E, Vitti T G, Panzer J D, Schlagel C, Hearron M S 1971 Antibiotic tolerance and serum levels after intravenous administration of multiple large doses of lincomycin. Clinical Pharmacology and Therapeutics 12 (5): 793–797

7. Mickal A, Panzer J D 1975 The safety of lincomycin in pregnancy. American Journal of Obstetrics and Gynecology 121 (8): 1071–1074
8. Holloway W J, Kahlbaugh R A, Scott E G 1963 Lincomycin: a clinical study. Antimicrobial Agents and Chemotherapy 200–203
9. Ma P, Lim M, Nodine J H 1963 Human pharmacological studies of lincomycin, a new antibiotic for gram positive organisms. Antimicrobial Agents and Chemotherapy 183–188
10. Margosis M 1968 Analysis of antibiotics by gas chromatography. I. Lincomycin. Journal of Chromatography 37: 46–54
11. Hanka L J, Mason D J, Burch M R, Treick R W 1962 Lincomycin, a new antibiotic. III. Microbiological assay. Antimicrobial Agents and Chemotherapy 565–569
12. Vavra J J, Sokolski W T, Lawson J B 1963 Absorption and excretion of lincomycin hydrochloride in human volunteers. Antimicrobial Agents and Chemotherapy 176–182
13. Wagner J G, Northam J I, Sokolski W T 1965 Biological half lives of the antibiotic lincomycin observed in repetitive experiments in the same subjects. Nature 207 (4993): 201–202
14. McGehee R F Jr, Smith C B, Wilcox C, Finland M 1968 Comparative studies of antibacterial activity in vitro, and absorption and excretion of lincomycin and clindamycin. The American Journal of the Medical Sciences 256: 279–292
15. Gordon R C, Regamey C, Kirby W M M 1973 Serum protein binding of erythromycin, lincomycin and clindamycin. Journal of Pharmaceutical Sciences 62 (7): 1074–1077
16. Becker E F 1969 The intraocular penetration of lincomycin. American Journal of Ophthalmology 67: 963
17. Nielsen M L, Hansen I, Nielsen J B 1976 The penetration of lincomycin into normal human bone. Acta Orthopedica Scandinavica 47: 267–270
18. Lerner P I 1969 Penetration of cephalothin and lincomycin into the cerebrospinal fluid. The American Journal of the Medical Sciences 257: 125–131
19. Medina A, Fiske N, Hjelt-Harvey I, Brown C, Prigot A 1963 Absorption, diffusion, and excretion of a new antibiotic, lincomycin. Antimicrobial Agents and Chemotherapy 189–196
20. Miyazaki Y 1973 Basic and chemical study of intrathecal administration of lincomycin. Arzneimittel-Forschung 27 (7): 940–945
21. Thomas P A, Jolly P C 1967 Lincomycin diffusion into pleural drainage fluid of post-thoracotomy patients. American Review of Respiratory Diseases 6 (5): 1044–1048
22. Saggers B A, Lawson D 1968 In vivo penetration of antibiotic into sputum in cystic fibrosis. Archives of Diseases of Children 43: 404–409
23. Smith R B, Lummis W L, Monovich R E, DeSante K A 1981 Lincomycin serum and saliva concentrations after intramuscular injection of high doses. Journal of Clinical Pharmacology 21: 411–417
24. Duignan N M, Andrews J, Williams J D 1973 Pharmacological studies with lincomycin in late pregnancy. British Medical Journal 14: 3 (871): 75–78
25. Nagar H, Berger S A 1984 The excretion of antibiotics by the biliary tract. Surgery, Gynecology and Obstetrics 158: 601–607
26. O'Connell C J, Plaut M E 1969 Intravenous lincomycin in high doses. Current Therapeutic Research 11 (7): 478–486
27. Bellamy H M Jr, Bates B B, Reinarz J A 1966 Lincomycin metabolism in patients with hepatic insufficiency: effect of liver disease on lincomycin serum concentrations. Antimicrobial Agents and Chemotherapy 36–41
28. Reinarz J A, McIntosh D A 1965 Lincomycin excretion in patients with normal renal function, severe azotemia, and with hemodialysis and peritoneal dialysis. Antimicrobial Agents and Chemotherapy 232–238
29. McCall C E, Steigbigel N H, Finland M 1967 Lincomycin: activity in vitro and absorption and excretion in normal young men. American Journal of the Medical Sciences 254: 144
30. Bartlett J G 1982 Anti-anaerobic antibacterial agents. The Lancet 2 (8296): 478–481
31. Sanders E 1969 Lincomycin versus erythromycin. A choice or an echo. Annals of Internal Medicine 70 (3): 585–590
32. Anderson R, Bauman M, Austrian R 1967 Lincomycin and penicillin G in the treatment of mild and moderately severe pneumococcal pneumonia. American Review of Respiratory Disease 97: 914–918
33. Hnatko S I 1967 The treatment of acute and chronic staphylococcal osteomyelitis and soft tissue infections with lincomycin. Canadian Medical Association Journal 97: 580–584
34. Leigh D A, Pease R, Henderson H, Simmons K, Russ R 1976 Prophylactic lincomycin in the prevention of wound infection following appendicectomy: a double blind study. British Journal of Surgery 63: 973–977
35. Trakas J C, Lind H E 1965 Lincomycin therapy in chronic middle ear infections. Antimicrobial Agents and Chemotherapy 717–720
36. Howie V M, Ploussard J H 1971 Treatment of group A streptococcal pharyngitis in children. American Journal of Diseases of Children 121: 477–480
37. Bentley J F R, Pollok D 1968 Lincomycin in the treatment of penicillin-resistant staphylococcal infections in children. Archives of Diseases of Children 43: 58–60
38. Harnecker J, Contreras J, Gilabert B, Ubilla V 1963 Bacteriological and clinical studies of lincomycin hydrochloride. Antimicrobial Agents and Chemotherapy 204–209
39. Sanders E, Foster M T, Scott D 1968 Group A, β-hemolytic streptococci resistant to erythromycin and lincomycin. The New England Journal of Medicine 278: 538–540
40. Annear D I 1977 Interaction between erythromycin and lincomycin in *streptococcus pyogenes*. Medical Microbiology 11: 193–196
41. Dixon J M S, Lipinski A E 1972 Resistance of group A β-hemolytic streptococci to lincomycin and erythromycin. Antimicrobial Agents and Chemotherapy 1 (4): 333–339
42. Hewitt J H, Fraser C A M 1968 Correspondence. Group A streptococci resistant to lincomycin. British Medical Journal March 1: 703
43. McGehee R F, Barrett F F, Finland M 1968 Resistance of *Staphylococcus aureus* to lincomycin, clindamycin and erythromycin. Antimicrobial Agents and Chemotherapy 392–397
44. Dixon J M S 1967 Pneumococcus resistant to erythromycin and lincomycin. Letters to the Editor. Lancet 1: 573
45. Kutscher E, Southern P M Jr, Sanford J P 1968 Clinical significance of lincomycin-resistant *Neisseria gonorrhoeae*. Antimicrobial Agents and Chemotherapy 331–334
46. Jellard C H, Lipinski A E 1973 *Corynebacterium diphtheriae* resistant to erythromycin and lincomycin. The Lancet, Jan 20, 1 (795): 156
47. Sprunt K, Leidy G, Redman W 1970 Cross resistance between lincomycin and erythromycin in viridans streptococci. Pediatrics 46 (1): 84–88
48. Waisbren B A 1968 Lincomycin in larger doses. Journal of the American Medical Association 206: 2118
49. O'Connor T W 1981 Pseudomembranous enterocolitis: a historical and clinical review. Diseases of Colon and Rectum 24 (6): 445–448
50. Berry D D, Brouhard B H, Box Q T 1981 Adverse reactions to parenteral lincomycin. Pediatrics 67 (3): 389–391
51. Borriello S P, Larson H E 1981 Antibiotic and pseudomembranous colitis. Journal of Antimicrobial Chemotherapy 7 (suppl A): 53–62
52. Gibson G E, Rowland R, Hecker R 1975 Diarrhoea and colitis associated with antibiotic treatment. Australian and New Zealand Journal of Medicine 5: 340–347
53. Navely S R, Hodges G R 1984 The neurotoxicity of antibacterial agents. Annals of Internal Medicine 101: 92–104
54. Martin J B Jr, Bleckley J E, Murray H L 1966 Probable side-effects of lincomycin. The Journal of the South Carolina Medical Association, July: 267–268
55. Raff M J 1973 Lincomycin: thrombocytopenia? Annals of Internal Medicine 78 (5): 779
56. Kokkini G, Tsianos E, Kappas A 1983 Sideroblastic anemia associated with lincomycin therapy. Postgraduate Medical Journal 59: 796–798

57. Boois L H D J, Miller R D, Crul J F 1978 Neostigmine and 4-aminopyridine antagonism of lincomycin–pancuronium neuromuscular blockade in man. Anesthesia and Analgesia 57: 316–321
58. Lewis C, Clapp H W, Grady J E 1962 In vitro and in vivo evaluation of lincomycin, a new antibiotic. Antimicrobial Agents and Chemotherapy 570–582
59. Heman-Ackah S M 1975 Microbial kinetics of drug action against Gram-positive and Gram-negative organisms. III: effect of lincomycin and clindamycin combinations on *Staphylococcus aureus* and *Escherichia coli*. Journal of Pharmaceutical Sciences 64 (10): 1621–1625
60. Nies A S 1974 Drug interactions. Medical Clinics of North America 58: 965–975
61. Donohoe R F, Swift J P 1967 Lincomycin therapy of pneumonia. Southern Medical Journal 60: 203–208

Lindane

It is a powerful parasiticide used against external parasites.

Chemistry

Lindane (Gamma benzene hexachloride, BHC, HCH, benzhexachlor; Lorexane; Lencid; Kwellada; Hexacid; Desantin; Aphtiria; Electol; Jacutin; Skabex; Atan; Gammene; Kwell, Quellada)
$C_6H_6Cl_6$
1α,2α,3β,4α,5α,6β-Hexachlorocyclohexane
The structural formula is approximately represented by the normal planar formula

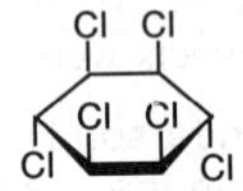

Molecular weight	290.8
pKa	not ionisable
Solubility	
in alcohol	1 in 19
in water	almost insoluble
Octanol/water partition coefficient	5000

Pure gamma BHC isomer is a white, crystalline chemical, with a slightly musty odour prepared by chemical synthesis. It is one of 8 isomers of BHC. It is an ingredient of Derbac soap with eresol.

Pharmacology

Lindane is a powerful parasiticide with a rapid action against the majority of external parasites, including *Pediculus humanus* var. *capitis*. Lindane is lipid soluble, is absorbed through the chitin of the insect's surface and is insecticidal by producing seizures. Lindane stimulates arachidonic acid release from macrophage phospholipids. It is also a powerful stimulator of leucotriene C_4 production.[1] The relevance of these facts to the actions of lindane as an insecticide is not clear.

Toxicology

Liver damage has been reported in dogs.[2] No significant teratogenic effect was produced by administration of oral doses of 5, 10 or 20 mg.kg^{-1} lindane on days 6–18 of gestation to the rabbit and days 6–15 gestation of the rat[3]

Daily doses of 0.5 mg.kg^{-1} lindane administered orally for 4 months to female rats produced disturbances of the oestrus cycle, inhibited capacity for conception and fertility, lowered the viability of embryos and delayed their physical development.[4] No effect was observed at 0.05 mg.kg^{-1} orally to female rats.[5] An increased incidence of stillborn pups was observed in litters of female beagle dogs administered 7.5 (30%) or 15 (18%) mg.kg^{-1} lindane orally from day 5 throughout gestation compared to control (2%).[6] Doses of 5 mg.kg^{-1} (equivalent to a dietary intake of 200 p.p.m.) produced toxic effects in non-pregnant beagle dogs during chronic oral administration.[7,8] These studies[5,6] have been interpreted as indicating that test animals do not reproduce normally at doses of lindane near maximal tolerated levels (US Environmental Protection Agency, 1980). Rasmussen[9] concludes that 'High doses of lindane may have a significant adverse effect on the pregnant test animal, and fetus. It dose not appear to be a teratogen however.'

Lindane was not mutagenic in the *Salmonella* assay[10] (metabolic activation not assessed), or host mediated assay.[11] No sex-linked recessive mutants were found in *Drosophila melanogaster* injected with lindane solution.[12] Unscheduled DNA synthesis was not induced in SVC40 transformed human fibroblasts by lindane.[13] Lindane caused a slight increase in the frequency of chromatic gaps and breaks in Chinese hamster fibroblasts in vitro[14] and a concentration related increase in chromatic breaks in human lymphocytes in vitro.[15] The US Environmental Protection Agency (1977) have stated that no presumption of mutagenicity is justified.

Reuber[2] found lindane to be highly carcinogenic in rats and mice. Wolff and others[16] concluded that the enhancement of susceptibility to neoplasia in experimental mice could be separated into two components. One of these is a direct sensitizing effect of the A^{vy} gene on cells which are already susceptible to neoplastic transformation due to their background genome. The other component is an indirect effect of the gene on promotion and progression of the transformed cells through its dysregulation of cellular metabolism resulting in increased lipogenesis and obesity.

Clinical pharmacology

Gamma benzene hexachloride is lipid soluble and this renders the drug easily absorbable through the skin after topical application. Although systemic effects are unusual in clinical practice, enough of the drug may be absorbed to have systemic effects, particularly in children. The drug may have affects on the central nervous system to produce irritability, insomnia, vertigo and even convulsions. A benzodiazepine is a suitable antagonist to these effects. Gamma benzene hexachloride may sensitize the myocardium to arrhythmias. The drug is also a potent enzyme inducer and this may occur with prolonged topical use. One application of gamma benzene hexachloride (1%) on to the skin remains effective for between 5–10 hours.[17]

Pharmacokinetics

There is little or no data available concerning the pharmacokinetics of lindane. The compound has been measured in plasma from factory workers exposes to the material. The method used was gas chromatography with electrochemical dection,[18] which has a sensitivity of $1 \mu g.l^{-1}$.

Lindane is readily absorbed after oral ingestion, inhalation and topical application. Topically applied lindane is absorbed through the skin in amounts varying from 9% to over 80% under occlusion. The dermal absorption rate is largest within 8 hours of dosing. Lindane is reported to have deleterious effects on the CNS in that it can cause brain damage and convulsions demonstrating that lindane crosses the blood–brain barrier. Rasmussen[8] refers to an earlier review by Solomon et al.[19] and examines more recent reports of toxicity.

Compounds such as lindane show a high affinity for body fat. The excretion of lindane in breast milk has been measured by Bakken and Seip.[20] The maximum allowed concentration of lindane in cow's milk approved by the WHO is 4 p.p.b.[21] The study quoted above stated that there was no positive evidence of harm to the babies although in some instances they were receiving higher doses than adults. It is likely that lindane crosses the placenta although data are not available. The half life of lindane based on urinary excretion data is approximately 2 l.h.

Concentration–effect relationship

Not relevant for a topically applied drug.

Metabolism

Lindane is eventually metabolized to much less toxic water-soluble products which are then excreted in the urine. More than 80 metabolites have been identified.[22,23] Mammalian biotransformation of lindane involves the formation of chlorophenols, which are excreted mainly in the urine in the free and conjugated forms.

Pharmaceutics

Shampoos

Lorexane Medicated Shampoo (ICI, UK) a shampoo containing 2% lindane in a detergent base.

Kwell (Reed and Carnrick, USA)/Quellada Application PC (Stafford-Miller, UK), Scabene (Stiefel, USA) contain 1% lindane in clear foaming shampoo bases.

Esoderm (Napp, UK) contains 1% lindane in a cream shampoo base.

Cream base, 1%

Lorexane Cream 1% (ICI, UK) contains 1% lindane in a white vanishing cream base.

Kwell (Reed and Carnrick, USA) includes lanolin.

Lotion 1%

Esoderm (Napp, UK) is a clear, colourless, alcohol based lotion

Kwell (Reed and Carnrick, USA)/Quellada (Stafford-Miller, UK)/Scabene (Stiefel, US) formulated in white, non-greasy, perfumed bases.

The Stiefel lotion contains parabens.

Formulations have a maximum shelf-life of two years when protected from the light.

Therapeutic use

Indications

1. Eradication of scabies
2. Treatment of pediculosis of the scalp, body and pubis.

Contraindications

1. For external use only. Isolated incidents of mild skin reactions have been reported; lindane preparations should not be applied to mucous membranes or broken skin.

Mode of use

In the treatment of pediculosis by shampoo, after thoroughly wetting the hair, rub in the shampoo and work well into the scalp. Rinse well with warm water, apply more shampoo and work up to a lather. Rinse thoroughly with warm water and then comb to remove any nits remaining. Dry the hair. Repeat the treatment one week later.

In the treatment of scabies of adults and children with the cream, the body should be washed liberally with soap and water and thoroughly dried before treatment. Lindane cream is then rubbed into the skin over the entire body surface, with the exception of the face and scalp, until completely absorbed.

In the treatment of pediculosis of adults and children, the affected area should be thoroughly washed with soap and water and dried. Lindane cream is then well rubbed into the involved skin and hair, and also adjacent areas. The hair may be combed with a dust comb after 24 hours to remove dead lice but, to ensure that any larvae which may subsequently develop from the nits are destroyed, the patient should be discouraged from washing the hair for a period of 7–10 days.

Contraindications

Lindane (Gamma benzene hexachloride) penetrates human skin and has been reported to cause signs of CNS irritation. This is more likely to occur in infants, children and pregnant women. Simultaneous applications of creams, ointments or oils may enhance the percutaneous absorption of lindane.

Welch et al[24] recorded a case of a child of 18 months who developed convulsions after the application of lindane. He had been given a hot bath before 2 consecutive applications. The authors concluded:

a. Lindane should not be used on pregnant women, small infants or those with grossly excoriated skin.
b. Lindane treatment, 2 applications one week apart, should not be repeated more than twice in a month.
c. Lindane should not be applied after a hot bath.
d. Application should be removed after six hours by bathing in water.
e. Infants should be prevented from licking the treated skin.

However, while washing the body within 6 hours of the application to the skin is thought to reduce the likelihood of toxic sequelae, there is no evidence that soap and water does remove the material.

Furthermore, the absorption of parathion and malathion from the skin has been shown to actually increase the absorption of these substances from the skin into the blood stream.[25]

Adverse reactions

Discussing the pros and cons of lindane, Rasmussen concluded that, considering the massive use of lindane in the USA, the number of adverse reactions is so small that lindane remains the treatment of choice for human clinical use, and that most adverse reactions are due to its misuse.[26] Shacter[27] held the view that lindane is the most effective treatment for scabies and pediculosis and that when used correctly it is the safest.

After decades of occupational exposure, 60 male workers in a Hamburg factory producing lindane were found to have no neurological defects on clinical examination or electromyographic studies.[28] Purves[29] commented that he had met several patients who had applied excessive amounts of lindane to the skin for long periods of time, but none had shown signs or symptoms of intoxication.

Potentially life-threatening effects

Aplastic anaemia. Fatal aplastic anaemia occurred following exposure to fumes of gamma benzene hexachloride from a vaporizer. An 8-year-old girl had been exposed to the fumes for about 2 hours daily for 2 years and a 52-year-old man for 8–15 hours weekly for about 3 months. Neither patient responded to blood transfusions or treatment with prednisone or methylestosterone.[30]

Another report on 6 patients has also been published.[31]

The lindane working group in Washington DC[32] have collected reports in the literature of aplastic anaemia, and also leukaemia, after normal exposure and accidental over exposure to lindane.

In 40 persons exposed in their work to gamma benzene hexachloride the concentration in blood was 0.0119 p.p.m. compared with 0.0001 p.p.m. in 40 persons not so exposed. In the exposed groups the creatinine concentration and the counts of erythrocytes were significantly higher; all other parameters were within normal limits. No evidence was found that gamma benzene hexachloride had any toxic effect on the bone marrow at these concentrations.[33]

Morgan et al[34] recorded a case of anaemia associated with lindane and reviewed 46 cases of haemotoxicity. 23 cases of fatal pancytopenia are included from studies in 9 countries.

Acute overdosage

Symptoms and signs of serious overdosage include vomiting, diarrhoea, restlessness, muscular spasm, loss of equilibrium, convulsions and collapse; and death may ensue.

A boy in a training centre for the mentally retarded was found unconscious with an empty 392 g bottle of 1% lindane shampoo beside him. Phenytoin sodium, diazepam and sodium phenobarbitone were all administered. Phenytoin was given to maintain a serum concentration of 10–20 $mg.l^{-1}$. Periodic administration of diazepam and curare was used to control seizures. In addition, cholestyramine 4 g was given every 8 hours to reduce the enterohepatic circulation of lindane. After five days of treatment with the above regime plus intravenous fluids and life-support facilities, the boy recovered.

7 ml of a bottle of 1% lindane was supplied for treatment of scabies in a 14-month-old infant. 2 ml was applied to the skin, and later that evening the child ingested the 5 ml which remained in the bottle. On examination that night the child was restless, but had recovered completely 12 hours later without specific treatment.[35]

In the event of ingestion gastric lavage should be performed and saline cathartics administered.

Oil laxatives, sympathomimetics, xanthines, anticholinergics, narcotic analgesics and tranquillizers should be avoided. If convulsions occur sedatives and 10% calcium gulconate (10 ml intravenously) should be given. Artificial respiration may be indicated to counteract pulmonary failure. The diet should be low fat, high protein and high carbohydrate. Milk or glucose should not be given.

Severe or irreversible adverse effects

Neurological symptoms. Chattopadhay et al[36] studied 45 male workers exposed to lindane during its manufacture, and compared them with 22 matched controls. Neurological symptoms reported were due to recent exposure to lindane, and were related to the intensity of exposure. Such symptoms were parasthesia of the face and extremities, headache, giddiness, vomiting, apprehension and loss of sleep.

These findings are at variance with those of Samuels and Milby,[37] who did not find any clinical or physical evidence of disease in workers exposed to HCH.

Lindane

Symptomatic adverse effects

Apart from those described above, there are none.

Interference with clinical pathology tests

No technical interferences of this kind have been reported.

High risk groups

Neonates

The use of lindane is contraindicated in neonates.

Breast milk. Lindane enters breast milk and its use is contraindicated in breast-feeding women.

Children

Lindane enhances hepatic microsomal enzyme activity. There has been some concern over the application of higher than normal concentrations of lindane to the skin in the treatment of scabies and pediculosis, children are considered to be particularly at risk.

Pregnant women

The use of the drug is contraindicated during pregnancy.

The elderly

The drug may be used in elderly patients.

Drug interactions

Potentially hazardous interactions

Aplastic anaemia and hypoplastic bone marrow. There are some reports of aplastic anaemia attributed to exposure to lindane and/or another possible haemotoxic agent. Albaharay et al.[38] described the case of a sanitation department employee who developed paramyelopthisis 9 days after exposure to DDT and lindane. Similarly, a teenage boy developed a fatal case of aplastic anaemia after being exposed to lindane and DDT for two months while working on a Calfornia farm.[39]

PERS Report 71-183[40] described a case of fatal aplastic anaemia in an Oregon farmer who was exposed to lindane and Toxaphene via the inhalation and dermal routes while spraying cattle in April 1969.

Other blood dyscrasias. Jedlicka et al.[41] described two 20-year-old cousins who lived and worked together and who, after simultaneous exposure to lindane and DDT, both developed paramyeloblastic leukaemia. The authors concluded that exposure to lindane caused the leukaemia in these cases. Hoshizzki et at.[42] also reported a case of leukaemia in a sanitation department employee who was regularly exposed to DDT and lindane.

Potentially useful interactions

No interactions of this type have been reported.

Clinical trials

Pediculosis and phthirus pubis

1. M M Cole et al 1960 Soap Chem. Spec. 36: 101
2. A B Ackerman 1968 New England Journal of Medicine 278: 950
3. L Wexler 1968 Clinical Medicine 75: 28
4. F A Ive 1973 British Medical Journal 4: 475
5. A J Singer 1977 British Medical Journal 2: 1608
6. Maunder J W 1981 Clinical Exp. Dermatology 6: 605

Clinical and laboratory trials employing Carbaryl against the human head louse. The results of extensive trials are recorded.

Scabies

1. E B Smith, T F Claypoole 1967 Journal of the American Medical Association 199: 59
2. J R Haydon, R M Caplan 1971 Archives of Dermatology 103: 168, per Clinical Medicine 1973, 80: 30
3. Further references: A B Cannon, M E McRae 1948 Journal of the American Medical Association 138: 557: B H E James (Letter) 1972. British Medical Journal 1: 178: R J G Rycroft, C D Calnan 1977 British Medical Journal 2: 303: Medical Letters, 1977, 19: 18

References

1. Meade C J, Harvey J, Boot J R, Turner G A, Bateman P E, Osborne D J 1984 Hexachlorocyclohexane stimulation of macrophage phospholipid hydrolysis and leukotriene production. Biochemical Pharmacology 33: 289
2. Reuber M D 1979 Carcinogenicity of lindane. Environment Research 19: 460

3. Palmer A K, Bottomley A M, Worden A M, Frohberg H, Bauer A 1978 Effect of lindane on pregnancy in the rabbit and rat. Toxicology 9: 239–247
4. Naishtein S U, Leibovich D L 1971 Effect of small doses of DDT and lindane and their mixture on sexual function and embryogenesis in rats. Hygiene and Sanitation 36: 190–195
5. Ahtenberg A I, Mametkuliev C 1976 The effect of gamma-isomer of hexachlorocyclohexane (HCCH) on the state of sexual glands in rats (Russ.) Voprosy Pitaniia 4: 62–67
6. Earl F L, Miller E, Van Loon E J 1973 Reproductive, teratogenic and neonatal effects of some pesticides and related compounds in beagle dogs and miniature swine. In: Deichmann, W B. (ed) Papers of the 18th Inter-American Conference on toxicology and Occupational Medicines, Pesticides and the Enviroment: Continuing Controversy, vol. 2. Stratton, New York, pp 253–266
7. Noel R B 1970 Lindane toxicity studies in beagle dogs. Dietary intake, 200 pm for thirty two weeks. Huntingdon Research Centre Report No. 3720/70/532
8. Petrescu S T, Dabre V, Leibovici M et al 1974 Studies of the effects of long term administration of organochlorate pesticides (lindane, DDT) on the white laboratory rat. Revista Medico-Chirurgicala Societatii Medici si Naturalisti Din Iasi 78: 831–842
9. Ramussen J E 1981 The problem of lindane. Journal of the American Academy of Dermatology 5: 507–516
10. Shiras Y, Moriya M, Kato K, Furutiashi A, Kada T 1976 Mutagenicity testing of pesticides in the microbial system. Mutation Research 40: 19–30
11. Buselnaier W, Rohrborn G, Propping P 1972 Mutagenicity investigations with pesticides in the host-mediated assay and the dominant lethal test in mice (Germ.) Biol. Zvl. 91: 311–325
12. Benes V, Sram R 1969 Mutagenic activity of some pesticides in Drosophila melanogaster. Indiana Medicine 38: 442–444
13. Amned F E, Hart R W, Lewis N J 1977 Pesticide-induced DNA damage and its repair in cultured human cells. Mutation Research 42: 161–174
14. Ishidate, M Jnr, Odashima S 1977 Chromosome tests with 134 compounds on Chinese hamster cells in vitro — a screening for chemical carcinogens. Mutation Research 48: 337–354
15. Tzoneva-Maneva M T, Kaloianova F, Georgieva V 1971 Influence of diazinon and lindane on the miotic activity and the caryotype of human lymphocytes, cultivated in vitro. In: Proceedings of the XII International Congress of the Society of Blood Transfusion, Moscow, 1969, Bibliotheca Haematologica No. 38, part 1, Basel, Karger, pp 344–347
16. Wolff G L, Roberts D W, Morrissey R L et al 1987 Tumorigenic response to lindane in mice. Potentiation by a dominant mutation. Carcinogenesis 8: 1889
17. Malhotra P R, Wal Y C, Petri S L 1972 Speed of toxic action of certain insecticides against body lice. Labdev Journal of Science and Technology 10B: 25
18. Radomski J et al 1970 Journal of Chromatographic Science 8: 108–114
19. Solomon L M et al 1977 A review: Gamma Benzene Hexachloride. Archives of Dermatology 113: 353–357
20. Bakken A F, Seip M 1976 Insecticides in human breast milk. Acta Paediatrica Scandinavica 65: 535–539
21. WHO Pesticide residue in food 19 679 Technical Report Series No. 417, Geneva
22. Menzie C V 1974 Metabolism of pesticides: an update. Special scientific report — wildlife No. 184. US Department of the Interior, Fish and Wildlife Service, Washington, DC
23. Macholz R M, Kujawa M 1985 Recent state of lindane metabolism part III. Residue Reviews 94: 119
24. Telch J, Jarvis D A 1982 Acute intoxication with lindane (gamma benzene hexachloride). Canadian Medical Association Journal 126: 662
25. Maibach H I 1974 Occupational exposure to pesticides. Federal Working Group on Pest Management, p 120
26. Rasmussen J E 1981 The problem of lindane. Journal of the American Academy of Dermatologists 5: 507
27. Shachter B 1981 The treatment of scabies and pediculosis with lindane preparations — an evaluation. Journal of the American Academy of Dermatologists 5: 517
28. Baumann K, Behling K, Brassow H L, Stapel K 1987 Occupational exposure to hexachlorocyclohexane. International Archives of Occupational and Environmental Health 48: 165
29. Purves J 1982 Letter. Journal of the American Academy of Dermatologists 7: 40
30. Loge J P 1965 Journal of the American Medical Association 193–110
31. West I 1967 Archives of Enviromental Health 15: 97
32. US Environemental Protection Agency 1977 Lindane. Position Document 1
33. Milby T H, Samuels A J 1971 Journal of Occupational Medicine 13: 256 per Abstr. Hyd. 1972, 47: 21
34. Morgan E P, Stockdale E M, Roberts R J, Walter A W 1980 Anaemia associated with exposure to lindane. Archives of Environmental Health 35: 307
35. Powell G M 1980 Letter. Central African Journal of Medicine 26: 170
36. Chattopadhyay P, Karnik A B, Thakore K N, Lakkad B C, Nigam S K, Kashyap S K 1988 Health effects among workers involved in manufacture of hexachlorocyclohexane. Journal Social and Occupational Medicine 38: 77–81
37. Samuels A J, Milby T H 1971 Journal of Occupational Medicine 13: 147
38. Albahary C, Dubrisay J, Guerin 1957 Obstinate aplastic anaemia caused by exposure to lindane. (Transl. from French.) Arch. Mal. Prof. 18: 687–691
39. Mendeloff A J, Smith D E (eds) 1955 Clinico-pathologic conference: exposure to insecticides, bone marrow failure, gastrointestinal bleeding, and uncontrollable infestions. American Journal of Medicine 19: 274–284
40. US Enviromental Protection Agency 1971 PERS report No. 71-183
41. Jedlicka V L, Hermanska S, Smida I, Kouba A 1958 Paramyeloblastic leukemia appearing simultaneously in two blood cousins after simultaneous contact with gammexane (hexachlorocyclonexane). Acta Medica Scandinavica 161: 447–451
42. Hoshizake H, Niki Y, Tahjinma B, Terada T, Kasahara A 1969 A case of leukemia following exposure to insecticide. Acta Heamatologica Japan 12: 672–677

Liothyronine sodium

Liothyronine is used in thyroid replacement therapy where a rapid onset and short duration of action are desired.

The abbreviation T3 is often used for liothyronine (tri-iodothyronine) in medical and biochemical reports.

Chemistry

l-Tri-iodothyronine sodium (liothyronine sodium, liothyroninum natricum, Tertroxin)

$C_{15}H_{11}I_3N\ NaO_4$

Sodium 4-O-(4-hydroxy-3-iodophenyl)-3,5-di-iodo-L-tyrosinate

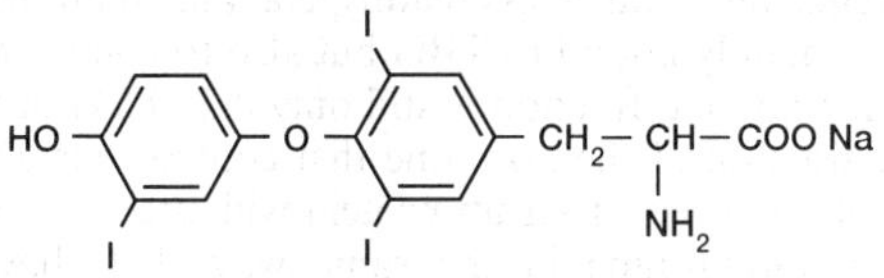

Molecular weight (free acid)	673.0 (651.0)
pKa	
(COOH)	2.2
(OH)	8.4
(NH_2)	10.1
Solubility	
in alcohol	1 in 500
in water	1 in 10 000
Octanol/water partition coefficient	—

Liothyronine is a white to buff-coloured odourless solid or crystalline powder which should be protected from light. It is prepared by chemical synthesis. Liothyronine is also available in combination with thyroxine in a ratio of 1:4 (Liatrix tablets, USP) but there is no advantage in this preparation.

Pharmacology

Tri-iodothyronine (T3) is a naturally occurring hormone produced in the thyroid gland and also by conversion from thyroxine (T4) in peripheral tissues.[1] It is qualitatively similar to thyroxine in its biological effects but it is much more potent on an equimolar basis. Many authorities now regard thyroxine as a pro-hormone which is converted into the metabolically active tri-iodothyronine (T3) or metabolically inactive reverse T3 (rT3). The thyroid hormones are required for normal growth and development, particularly of the nervous system. Tri-iodothyronine increases the resting or basal metabolic rate of the whole organism and has stimulatory effects on the heart, skeletal muscles, liver and kidney. Tri-iodothyronine enhances lipolysis and the utilization of carbohydrate. When used as a drug tri-iodothyronine is known as liothyronine.

Toxicology

Liothyronine sodium is not known to have either carcinogenic or teratogenic effects.

Clinical pharmacology

Liothyronine is more rapid in its effect and shorter in its duration of action than thyroxine, which remains the drug of choice for replacement therapy. Liothyronine nevertheless has a therapeutic role in those circumstances where either a rapid effect is required or a rapid

Liothyronine sodium

L

cessation of effect is required on removal of the drug. The dose required to maintain a patient in the euthyroid state is between 50 and 100 μg daily. Liothyronine sodium 25 μg is approximately equivalent to 90 μg of thyroxine sodium. The effect of liothyronine lasts for only a few hours so it has to be given in divided doses three or four times daily.

Correction of the hypothyroid state results in increased physical and mental well-being, weight reduction, improved tolerance of cold, relief of constipation, increased heart rate and peripheral vascular perfusion. The patient's metabolic rate is increased and there is a reduction of serum cholesterol and triglycerides with increased carbohydrate utilization.

Pharmacokinetics

The usual analytical method for measurement of tri-iodothyronine in serum or plasma is as for thyroxine, by radioimmunoassay, but other non-radioisotope methods are being developed which may shortly supersede radioimmunoassay. Limit of detection is 0.4 $nmol.l^{-1}$. The normal physiological range for total tri-iodothyronine is 1–3 $nmol.l^{-1}$ and for free (unbound) T3 it is between 5 and 10 $pmol.l^{-1}$.

Liothyronine is almost completely absorbed from the gastrointestinal tract and has a half life of approximately two days in subjects with normal thyroid function but this may be reduced in hyperthyroid states and prolonged in hypothyroid states due to altered rates of metabolism of the hormone. Like thyronine, tri-iodothyronine is largely bound to plasma proteins but is much less readily available than thyroxine. Like thyroxine it is mainly bound to TBG but also to a lesser extent to pre-albumin. The unbound fraction is still only 0.2–0.5% of the total, but it is the free fraction of the hormone that controls metabolic activity. Alterations of the levels of serum protein will affect the concentration of total tri-iodothyronine in the same way that they affect total thyroxine; thus pregnancy or oestrogens increase the binding of T3 and nephrotic syndrome and other protein-losing states will reduce total T3.[2] The liver is the major site of degradation of both thyroxine and tri-iodothyronine and both are conjugated with glucuronic and sulphuric acids and excreted in the bile. Iodothyronine and the inactive metabolite reverse T3 are both deiodinated to di-iodothyronines. Some free tri-iodothyronine is excreted in the urine together with deiodinated metabolites and conjugates.

Placental transfer of tri-iodothyronine is believed not to occur except possibly in the earliest few weeks of gestation before fetal production of thyroid hormones develops. The fetus produces very low amounts of tri-iodothyronine compared with thyroxine before birth. In the newborn infant there is a rapid surge in TSH within a few hours, followed in the next 24–48 hours by a rise in thyroxine and also in tri-iodothyronine levels. Tri-iodothyronine is excreted in breast milk, though there is no evidence that this is harmful to normal infants.

Oral absorption	almost complete
Presystemic metabolism	—
Plasma half life	
range	1–2 d
Volume of distribution	—
Plasma protein binding	99.5%

Concentration–effect relationship

Increasing concentrations of tri-iodothyronine beyond the normal physiological range (in the absence of any abnormality of binding proteins or other non-thyroid illness or interference by drugs) produce increasing symptoms and signs of hyperthyroidism. Lack of tri-iodothyronine results in symptoms and signs of hypothyroidism. Elevated serum tri-iodothyronine levels are the earliest biochemical feature of hyperthyroidism but are less helpful in the diagnosis of hypothyroidism as such patients may remain in a compensated state due to increased TSH drive with reduced thyroxine but normal tri-iodothyronine levels.[3]

Metabolism

Tri-iodothyronine is produced partly in the thyroid but largely by conversion from thyroxine in the peripheral tissues, mainly in the liver, kidney and anterior pituitary. Tri-iodothyronine is metabolized largely by conjugation with glucuronic acid or sulphate, by deiodination to di-iodo and mono-iodo-thyronines, and also by deamination and decarboxylation. Excretion is mainly in the bile and faeces, with enterohepatic re-circulation. The free compound, its metabolites and some iodide are also found in urine.

Metabolic clearance rate for T3 in normal humans has been estimated at between 20 litres per day and 26 litres per day, depending on the method used. Mean T3 production rate, derived from mean normal serum T3 concentrations and mean normal clearance rate, is estimated at approximately 26 μg per day. Estimates of the fraction of total T3 production from the thyroid vary widely from 10% to 38% and the true mean value is uncertain, but the estimates indicate that the generation of T3 from T4 peripherally accounts for most of T3 production in normal humans. The secretory product is derived from functionally heterogeneous pools which differ with respect to the rate at which their iodinated compounds turn over. The ratio of T3 to T4 in these pools may not be the same as the T3 to T4 ratios in extracts of the whole gland.

Pharmaceutics

1. Cytomel (SKF, USA): round white tablets containing 5 μg (coded 'D14'), 25 μg (scored and coded 'D16') and 50 μg (scored and coded 'D17') of liothyronine.
2. Tetroxin (Glaxo, UK): scored tablets containing 20 μg of tri-iodothyronine.
3. Tri-iodothyronine injection, a freeze-dried sterile white plug containing 20 μg of T3 with dextran. The drug is dissolved in water for preparation of an intravenous injection.

Therapeutic use

Indications

The indications for the use of liothyronine are the same as those for thyroxine[4,5] but thyroxine is usually preferred because of its longer half life. Indications for preferential use of liothyronine are:

Fig. 1

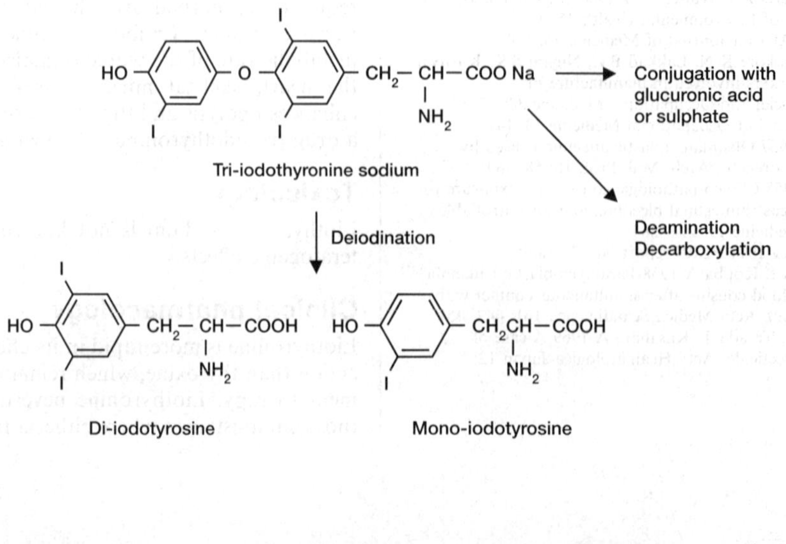

Liothyronine sodium

1. Myxoedema coma
2. Substitution therapy following thyroid ablation for differentiated thyroid cancer.

Contraindications

There are no absolute contraindications but greater care must be taken than with thyroxine in view of the increased potency and more rapid effects of liothyronine. This is particularly true in patients with angina or heart failure or adrenal failure and in the elderly.

Mode of use

In adults with hypothyroidism the initial daily dose should be 10 or 20 µg increasing every two weeks to 80 µg daily with reassessment of the patient's thyroid function on that dose. In myxoedema coma 10 to 25 µg of tri-iodothyronine can be given by intravenous injection and repeated at 12 hourly intervals until the patient is sufficiently improved to take oral replacement therapy. The dose can then be increased stepwise or replacement switched to thyroxine.[6]

In patients on maintenance thyroid hormone therapy after ablation for thyroid cancer, the dose of liothyronine used should be sufficient to suppress any TSH drive which might otherwise reactivate any residual TSH-sensitive tumour tissues.

Indications

1. Treatment of myxoedema coma

The treatment of myxoedema coma is empirical and treatment with either thyroxine or tri-iodothyronine has been advocated. The condition usually arises in a patient with long-standing neglected hypothyroidism and may be difficult to distinguish from hypothermia per se. Absorption of drugs by mouth is likely to be very slow as is the patient's whole metabolic rate. It therefore seems appropriate to advise intravenous therapy initially. Patients should be given steroid cover in view of the likelihood of relative adrenal insufficiency. Plasma cortisol should be taken for later assay and 100 µg of hydrocortisone given intravenously and repeated 6-hourly for the first 48 hours then gradually reduced towards a maintenance dose or tailed off if the initial plasma cortisol was raised. If the initial plasma cortisol was low or not significantly raised at the time of initial stress, hydrocortisone can be switched to an equivalent dose of dexamethasone (which does not interfere with cortisol assay) and a tetracosactrin test performed to determine that the adrenal response is adequate before discontinuing steroid replacement therapy.

General supportive measures to ensure adequate circulation and respiration and gradual rewarming are usually necessary. Thyroid hormone treatment is most rapidly effected by intravenous liothyronine 10 to 25 µg initially repeated at 12-hourly intervals. The dose can be increased gradually to a maximum of 100 µg daily as the patient shows improvement.[6]

Liothyronine can be given orally once the patient has an improved metabolic rate and can effectively absorb oral medication. Fortunately the condition is rare but it carries a high mortality rate.

2. Replacement therapy after thyroid ablation

Patients who have had total thyroidectomy followed by radioiodine in large doses to ablate any thyroid remnants, will need to be rechecked at intervals to determine that there has been no recurrence of tumour tissue. Whilst it is now common practice to measure thyroglobulin when patients are on long-term thyroxine replacement therapy as a measure of any residual activity, it may also be necessary to re-scan the patient. To do this thyroid hormone replacement therapy has to be stopped and a large dose of radioiodine given to try and detect any tissues that might take up the isotope. In view of the long half life of thyroxine it may be 3 weeks or so before the thyroxine is cleared sufficiently, during which time patients become hypothyroid. To minimize this source of discomfort and distress to the patient the thyroid hormone replacement therapy can be switched to liothyronine for a month prior to the anticipated scan date and discontinued only a week before scan. Therapy in the same dose as previously can be resumed promptly once the scan has been completed or any further radioisotope therapy given.

Adverse reactions

Potentially life-threatening effects

No reactions of this kind occur during treatment with conventional doses in patients who have no evidence of angina or ischaemic heart disease, but in patients with these conditions too rapid replacement can precipitate a myocardial infarction or dysrhythmias which can be fatal. T3 is best avoided in such patients, who are better treated with gradual low increments of T4, if necessary under cover with a β-adrenergic blocker such as propranolol.

Acute overdosage

Manifestations of toxicity due to liothyronine excess, like those of thyroxine excess, are those of thyrotoxicosis in varying degrees depending on the dose and the rapidity of ingestion. A massive acute overdosage is likely to produce thyrotoxicosis more rapidly than with thyroxine because of the more rapid action of liothyronine. Gastric lavage is indicated if the patient presents soon after ingestion of the acute overdose. Other treatment includes propranolol and supportive measures to maintain adequate circulation and prevent cardiovascular collapse.

Severe or irreversible adverse effects

Iatrogenic hyperthyroidism due to excessive liothyronine replacement or surreptitious ingestion of excess liothyronine may produce tachycardia or arrhythmias, diarrhoea, weight loss, heat intolerance, insomnia and agitation. Symptoms should disappear within a week of withdrawal of the drug.

Symptomatic adverse effects

Apart from those already described there are no adverse effects of this kind.

Interference with clinical pathology tests

Administration of liothyronine will suppress any endogenous thyroxine secretion, so measurement of thyroxine is not valid in this circumstance. Liothyronine will also suppress radioiodine uptake in normal individuals. Use has been made of this phenomenon to test for thyroid autonomy. Failure of suppression of a radioiodine uptake by 50% after T3 therapy (80 µg daily for 5 days) is taken to indicate thyroid autonomy. This so called T3 suppression test may be used in the assessment of patients treated for Graves' disease to determine whether or not the patient is in complete remission. It may have some predictive value in that patients who fail to suppress are more likely to relapse, but they do not invariably do so and the test is of limited practical value. Furthermore, it may be inadvisable to give T3 to anyone who is still toxic.

The factors which affect serum levels of thyroxine also affect serum levels of tri-iodothyronine and may give misleading results. Increased binding to TBG occurs during pregnancy and with oestrogen therapy and will result in elevated total, but not free, T3 levels. Protein loss due to nephrotic syndrome or liver disease will also lower total, but not free, T3 levels. Non-thyroidal illness may also result in low T3 levels and increased reverse T3 levels but these do not indicate hypothyroidism unless TSH is raised.

High risk groups

Neonates

Neonatal hypothyroidism is usually treated with thyroxine rather than liothyronine because the longer half life of the former makes it more suitable as a once-daily preparation.

Breast milk. Liothyronine is excreted in breast milk and may reach a higher concentration than expected physiologically but there is no evidence of harm to normal infants.

Children

Once-daily thyroxine replacement therapy is more suitable for children with hypothyroidism than liothyronine which has to be given two or three times a day to maintain equivalent therapeutic effect.

Pregnant women

Liothyronine is not the drug of choice in pregnant women who are on treatment for hypothyroidism. Such women are usually adequately maintained on thyroxine. Neither liothyronine nor thyroxine cross the placental barrier in any significant quantity. Should a patient be taking liothyronine then the serum total T3 levels are increased due to increased TBG binding in pregnancy as with thyroxine. Free T3 levels are maintained in the normal non-pregnant range.

The elderly

Thyroxine is preferred to liothyronine in the treatment of elderly patients. Compliance with thyroxine is likely to be greater because it only needs to be taken once a day. Caution is necessary with the use of either thyroid hormone for replacement therapy in patients with heart disease. Liothyronine is best avoided because it is more potent and more rapid in its effects and very gradual replacement is essential in anybody who has ischaemic heart disease or who is liable to an exacerbation of angina.

Concurrent disease

Severe non-thyroid illness may result in the conversion of thyroxine to reverse tri-iodothyronine rather than to the active tri-iodothyronine.[7] Reduction in serum proteins will also reduce the level of total tri-iodothyronine. Low levels of T3 in these circumstances do not indicate hypothyroidism unless accompanied by an increase in TSH. There is thus no indication for the introduction of liothyronine therapy in such circumstances.

Presence of arrhythmias, angina or heart failure necessitates very cautious use of thyroid hormone replacement therapy and in such circumstances liothyronine is best avoided.

Drug interactions

Potentially hazardous interactions

Thyroxine is known to potentiate the effect of warfarin and other dicoumarin anticoagulants, and it seems likely that liothyronine could do so, though no reports of such a reaction appear to have been published.

Other significant interactions

Drugs which interfere with the binding of thyroxine also interfere with the binding of tri-iodothyronine.

Phenylbutazone, carbamazepine and phenytoin and large doses of salicylates may cause false low total serum tri-iodothyronine levels but free T3 levels and TSH remain normal.[8]

Amiodarone, which is widely used in the treatment of cardiac arrhythmias, interferes with the conversion of T4 to T3. T4 levels are often elevated but T3 levels are usually normal as more thyroxine is converted to reverse tri-iodothyronine. Serum T3 and TSH levels may be used to monitor the patients thyroid status.[9,10]

Potentially useful interactions

No interactions of this kind appear to have been reported.

References

1. Chopra I J 1986 Nature, sources and relative biological significance of thyroid circulating hormones. In: Ingbar S H, Braverman L E (eds) Werner's The thyroid, 5th edn. J B Lippincott, ch 7, pp 136–153
2. Davies D M (ed) 1985 Endocrine disorders. In: Textbook of adverse drug reactions, 3rd edn. Oxford University Press, Oxford, pp 336–339
3. Gharib H 1974 Tri-iodothyronine: physiological and clinical significance. Journal of the American Medical Association 227: 302–304
4. Wise P H, Marion M, Pain R W 1973 Single-dose 'block-replace' drug therapy in hyperthyroidism. British Medical Journal 4: 143–145
5. Wilkin T J, Isles T E, Gunn A, Crooks J, Swanson-Beck J 1979 Short term tri-iodothyronine in prevention of temporary hypothyroidism after subtotal thyroidectomy for Graves' disease. Lancet 2: 63–66
6. Newmark S R, Himathongkam T, Shane J M 1974 Myxoedema coma. Journal of the American Medical Association 230: 884–885
7. Utiger R D 1980 Decreased extra thyroidal tri-iodothyronine production in non-thyroidal illness: benefit or harm? American Journal of Medicine 69: 807–810
8. Yeo P P B, Bates D, Howe J G et al 1978 Anticonvulsants and thyroid function. British Medical Journal 1: 1581–1583
9. Burger A, Dinichert D, Nicod P, Jenny M, Lemarchand-Beraud T, Valloton M B 1976 The effect of amidarone on serum T3, rT3, T4 and TSH: a drug influencing peripheral metabolism of thyroid hormones. Journal of Clinical Investigation 58: 255–259
10. Melmed S, Nademanee K, Allen K W, Henrickston J, Singh B N, Hershman J M 1981 Hyperthyroxinaemia with bradycardia and normal thyrotrophin secretion following chronic amidarone administration. Journal of Clinical Endocrinology and Metabolism 53: 997–1001

Lipid supplements

These are fat emulsions for parenteral feeding

Chemistry

The following fat emulsions for parenteral feeding are available in the UK, Europe and USA:
Intralipid, Lipofundin S.
The vast majority of published work relates to Intralipid.

Intralipid is an opaque white emulsion of fractionated soya bean oil in water produced using 1.2% fractionated egg yolk phospholipids. Glycerol is also present in a concentration of 2.25 g per 100 ml. The emulsion is available in 10% or 20% concentrations of the soya bean oil.

Lipofundin S is similar but contains 2.5 g glycerol per 100 ml. Lipofundin MCT/LCT 10% differs from Lipofundin S by the replacement of half the soya bean oil with medium-chain triglycerides.

Fat emulsion are almost insoluble in alcohol and are insoluble in water.

Pharmacology

These substances are a source of energy and essential fatty acids. They have no other important pharmacological effects.

Toxicology

Intralipid has not been observed to cause general toxicity or specific organ damage in animals given doses close to the equivalent doses used in man.[1]

Single infusions of as much as 15 g fat per kg have been given to rats and dogs without lethal effects and single doses of 0.6 g fat per kg over 2 minutes have been well tolerated in man. No teratogenicity, mutagenicity or carcinogenicity tests of this emulsion have been performed.

Clinical pharmacology

No pharmacological, as opposed to nutritional, effects have been noted in man.

Pharmacokinetics

The particles of Intralipid 20% have been compared electron microscopically with chylomicra collected from the thoracic ducts of rats fed corn oil and olive oil. Intralipid particles and corn oil chylomicra were strikingly similar and consisted of a pale core thought to be triglyceride surrounded by a 500–100 Å electron dense surface layer of phospholipid.[2] Particle size in Intralipid emulsions ranges between 0.1 and 0.5 µm. When infused, the average volume of distribution has been calculated to be 154% of plasma volume in critically ill patients, but in healthy volunteers and patients after elective surgery it is closer to the plasma volume.[3] The fat particle adsorbs apolipoprotein CII and CIII and circulates like chylomicrons.

The elimination of Intralipid has mainly been studied in terms of clearance of the triglyceride component. Above certain concentrations of the triglyceride, called the critical concentration (C), a maximal elimination rate (k_1) is observed (zero-order kinetics). Below C a fractional elimination rate (k_2) is seen (first-order kinetics). The relationship between these[4] is $k_1 = k_2 \times C$ expressed in mmol.l^{-1} or $\text{mmol.l}^{-1}.\text{min}^{-1}$.

The clearance is catalysed by lipoprotein lipase which has an apparent in vivo Michaelis–Menten constant of 521 ± 38 (SEM) $\mu\text{mol.l}^{-1}$ which is within the concentration range attained in therapeutic use. Average fractional clearance rates of 5 to 25% and

Lipid supplements

maximum rates of 91 to 157 $\mu mol.l^{-1}.min^{-1}$ have been reported in surgical patients.[5]

Heparin increases the elimination rate of both chylomicra and Intralipid particles more as a result of a change in distribution of lipoprotein lipase activity than of increasing enzyme activity.[4]

Elimination rates vary according to the clinical state of the patient. After surgery and starvation there is increased elimination from plasma.[6] Critically ill postoperative patients without sepsis may have relatively reduced maximal elimination capacity.[3]

The rate constants for the elimination of Intralipid from the blood permit estimations of the maximal 24-hour dose. After a 15-hour fast this is 3.8 ± 1.6 g (SD) fat per kg body weight per 24 hours.[1]

Concentration–effect relationship

Since no pharmacological effects are known there are no relevant data here.

Metabolism

That Intralipid is not only cleared from the blood but also metabolized can be inferred from many metabolic studies in various clinical situations. Infusion increases heat production, raises oxygen consumption and lowers the respiratory quotient. Studies of ^{14}C-labelled fat emulsions as early as 1948 showed that most of the label was excreted in expired air as carbon dioxide. However, clearance of Intralipid from the blood does not equate with its oxidation to carbon dioxide.[7]

Pharmaceutics

Intralipid 10% and 20% (Kabi Vitrum, Sweden) are white emulsions for intravenous use. They are available in bottles of 100 and 500 ml, which should be stored at below 25°C. They should not be frozen.

Lipofundin S is manufactured by B. Braun (W. Germany).

The maximum shelf-life is 18 months. Against a background of about 60 million patient doses administered there have been occasional single reports of hypersensitivity — see above. These reactions may be due to remaining traces of egg or soya bean proteins.

Therapeutic use

Indications

Soya bean fat emulsion is used in parenteral feeding

1. As a source of energy
2. As a source of essential fatty acids.

Contraindications

None.

Mode of use

With growing use of pharmacy-prepared mixtures of intravenous feeds there is increasing interest in the compatibility of Intralipid with other intravenous nutrients. Mixtures of fat emulsion with other nutrients have been administered for many years in Montpellier, France both in silicone rubber and, more recently, disposable plastic containers. Between 1972 and 1978 64 095 mixtures of this type were given to 2699 patients. Metabolic complications occurred in 1.4% of cases; none was serious and none could be directly attributed to the mixtures.

While amino acid mixtures may have a slight stabilizing effect on fat emulsions, dextrose and electrolyte solutions destabilize them. The destabilizing effect of dextrose may be related to its effect in lowering pH; the destabilizing effect of electrolytes increases markedly with valency.[8,9] Fat emulsions should only be added to mixtures of other nutrients in proportions previously shown to be stable and pharmacies not in a position to check emulsion stability are advised to mix fat emulsions and other electrolytes in the same containers only in these proportions.

Intralipid may leach out plasticizers used to soften the plastic of containers for parenteral nutrition mixtures.[9] However, bags without plasticizers have been developed for parenteral nutrition including fat emulsion. These bags are to be preferred.

The dosages recommended by the manufacturers are:

Intralipid 10%: 500–1550 ml per 24 h
Intralipid 20%: 500–1000 ml per 24 h
Lipofundin S 10%: 700–1400 ml per 24 h
Lipofundin S 20%: 350–700 ml per 24 h

Infusion rates of 10% emulsion should be at 20 drops per minute for the first 15 minutes, increasing to not more than 45 drops per minute. With the 20% emulsion the rate should be half of that recommended for the 10% formulation. Infusion rates in children or low body weight adults should be reduced accordingly.

Fat emulsions should not be mixed with electrolytes, drugs or any other additives in the infusion bottles.

Indications

1. As a source of energy

Throughout the first half of this century, studies of oral nutrients demonstrated that for optimal nitrogen preservation or restoration a small amount, approximately 100 g daily, of carbohydrate in the feed is desirable; after this has been supplied, a fat calorie seems to be closely equivalent to a carbohydrate calorie nutritionally. This seems to be broadly true in parenteral nutrition also and there is no convincing evidence that either carbohydrate or fat is superior to the other in energy terms or in its effects on nitrogen metabolism.

2. As a source of essential fatty acids

The essential fatty acid linoleic acid represents 54% of the fat content of Intralipid. Linolenic acid is also present. Daily dosages of between 10 and 20 g linoleic acid result in a normal or near normal ratio of oleic to linoleic acids in the plasma[10] (akin to the triene:diene ratio which is used as an indicator of essential fatty acid deficiency). Continued infusion of Intralipid sometimes results in an increase in cholesterol and phospholipid concentrations in the blood, present in the low density lipoprotein fraction, and in addition a lipoprotein identical with or similar to lipoprotein X which is seen in obstructive jaundice and congenital lecithin cholesterol acyl transferase (LCAT) deficiency. These changes are seen both in neonates[11] and in adults.[10,12] The abnormal lipoprotein clears within 2–4 days of cessation of Intralipid infusion.

Adverse reactions

Potentially life-threatening effects

No effects of this severity appear to have been reported.

Acute overdosage

No cases appear to have been studied.

Severe or irreversible adverse effects

The 'fat overload' syndrome of hyperlipidaemia, gastrointestinal disturbances, hepatosplenomegaly, impaired hepatic function, anaemia, thrombocytopenia, prolonged clotting and prothrombin times and spontaneous bleeding was a characteristic of cotton seed-oil-containing emulsions. In general this syndrome does not occur with Intralipid. However, occasional reports of similar syndromes associated with Intralipid are made.[13,14,15,16] It is not clear to what extent the common ability of 'acute phase' sera to agglutinate Intralipid in vitro[17] is relevant to this uncommon phenomenon in vivo, which appears to be more common in the neonate than the adult.

As with oral fat, Intralipid infusion results in decreased pulmonary membrane diffusion which is reversible with concomitant heparin infusion. This may be of clinical relevance to the patient with already diminished pulmonary diffusing capacity or tissue ischaemia.[18] However, in the patient with respiratory failure combined fat and glucose infusions result in a lower respiratory quotient than glucose infusions alone, and the resulting lower production of carbon dioxide by fat may be advantageous.[19]

Symptomatic adverse effects

Intralipid may produce 'chills' (1%), a sensation of warmth (8%), increased body temperature (2.7%). Mild eosinophilia is commonly seen during parenteral feeding which may occur also if Intralipid is not infused.[20]

Other effects

A rise in serum alkaline phosphatase and transaminases has been noted during parenteral nutrition and may occur whether or not

Intralipid is infused. Its relationship to Intralipid infusion is not clear.

Infusion of Intralipid results in a moderate reduction in platelet adhesiveness.[21]

Accumulation of Lipoprotein X has been linked with nephropathy in LCAT deficiency. Its relevance in parenteral feeding with Intralipid is not known.

Interference with clinical pathology tests
Intralipid may interfere with methods for measuring haemoglobin, bilirubin and protein in serum.

High risk groups

Neonates
Free fatty acids may displace drugs and other substances from plasma proteins. This displacement of bilirubin from albumin is potentially hazardous in newborns with hyperbilirubinaemia. Many centres start Intralipid administration only when the bilirubin concentration is below half the potential blood exchange level. A molar ratio of free fatty acids to plasma albumin below six is thought to decrease the risk of kernicterus. Measurements in the therapeutic situation gave figures below two in 90% of the observations.

Intralipid is cleared from the blood of pre-term 'light for dates' neonates more slowly than in normal neonates.[22–25] Such delayed clearance may be the basis of reported pulmonary fat accumulation in pre-term infants receiving Intralipid.[16]

Very-low-birth-weight or light-for-gestation-age neonates may not have fully developed the fat-metabolizing enzyme systems and the dosage should not exceed 2 g of fat per kg of body weight in 24 hours when serum triglycerides are not measured.

Breast milk. Patients being given Intralipid are unlikely to breast-feed their babies.

Children
There is no contraindication to the use of Intralipid in children.

Pregnant women
There are a number of reports of the use of parenteral nutrition during pregnancy. It has been suggested that the infusion of Intralipid may stimulate uterine contraction.[26] The triglyceride, but not the phospholipid, of Intralipid crosses the human placenta.[27]

The elderly
There are no special precautions necessary in older patients.

Concurrent disease
Hepatic disease. Relatively little information exists about Intralipid elimination and metabolism in liver disease and hepatic failure, and therefore in view of deranged fat metabolism caution must be exercised in these circumstances. However, in the normal subject little of an infused dose of Intralipid is cleared by the liver, and patients with very severe liver disease, though they have low circulating LDL triglyceride and cholesterol, exhibit normal clearance of Intralipid as judged by nephelometry.[28]

Renal disease. Intralipid is cleared from the blood more slowly in patients in renal failure whether they are undergoing haemodialysis or not.[29]

Drug interactions

A number of drugs interact with Intralipid when added to it, and no substance should be added unless specifically recommended by the manufacturers.

General review articles

Pelham L D 1981 Rational use of intravenous fat emulsions. American Journal of Hospital Pharmacy 38: 198–209

Munro H N 1951 Carbohydrate and fat as factors in protein utilization and metabolism. Physiological Reviews 31: 449–488

Rossner S 1974 Studies on an intravenous fat tolerance test. Methodological experimental and clinical experiments with Intralipid. Acta Medica Scandinavica 196 (suppl): 564

References

1. Hallberg D, Holm I, Obel A L, Schuberth O, Wretlind A 1967 Fat emulsions for complete intravenous nutrition. Postgraduate Medicine 42: A71–A152

Lipid supplements

2. Schoefl G I 1968 The ultrastructure of chylomicra and of the particles in an artificial fat emulsion. Proceedings of the Royal Society B 169: 147–152
3. Lindholm M, Rossner S 1982 Rate of elimination of the Intralipid fat emulsion from the circulation in ICU patients. Critical Care Medicine 10: 740–746
4. Boberg J, Hallberg D 1971 Studies on the elimination of exogenous lipids from the blood stream. Effect of heparin on the elimination. Acta Chirurgica Scandinavica 137: 749–755
5. Robin A P, Nordenstrom J, Askanazi J, Elwyn D H, Carpentier Y A, Kinney J M 1980 Plasma clearance of fat emulsion in trauma and sepsis use of a three stage lipid clearance test. Journal of Parenteral and Enteral Nutrition 4: 505–510
6. Hallberg D 1965 Studies on the elimination of exogenous lipids from the blood stream. The effect of fasting and surgical trauma in man on the elimination rate of a fat emulsion injected intravenously. Acta Physiologica Scandinavica 65: 153–163
7. Carpentier Y A, Nordenstrom J, Askanazi J, Elwyn D H, Gump F E, Kinney J M 1979 Relationship between rates of clearance and oxidation of 14c-intralipid in surgical patients. Surgical Forum 30: 72–74
8. Davis S S 1983 The stability of fat emulsions for intravenous administration. In: Johnson I D A (ed) Advances in clinical nutrition. MTP Press, Lancaster, pp 213–239
9. Hardy G, Cotter R, Dawe R 1983 The stability and comparative clearance of TPN mixtures with lipid. In: Johnson I D A (ed) Advances in Clinical Nutrition. MTP Press, Lancaster, pp 241–260
10. Jeejeebhoy K N, Marliss E B, Anderson G H, Greenberg G R, Kuksis A, Breckenridge C 1976 Lipid in parenteral nutrition: studies of clinic and metabolic features. In: Meng H C, Wilmore D W (eds) Fat emulsions in parenteral nutrition. American Medical Association, Chicago
11. Griffin E, Breckenridge W C, Kuksis A, Bryan M H, Angel A 1979 Appearance and characterization of lipoprotein X during continuous Intralipid infusions in the neonate. Journal of Clinical Investigation 64: 1703–1712
12. Miyahara T, Fujiwara H, Yae Y, Okano H, Okochi K, Torisu M 1979 Abnormal lipoprotein appearing in plasma of patients who received a ten per cent soybean oil emulsion infusion. Surgery 85: 566–574
13. Freund U, Krausz Y, Levij I S, Eliakim M 1975 Iatrogenic lipidosis following prolonged intravenous hyperalimentation. American Journal of Clinical Nutrition 28: 1156–1160
14. Belin R P, Bivins B A, Jona J Z, Young V L 1976 Fat overload with a 10% soybean oil emulsion. Archives of Surgery 111: 1391–1393
15. Hessov I, Melsen F, Haug A 1979 Postmortem findings in three patients treated with intravenous fat emulsions. Archives of Surgery 114: 66–68
16. Levene M I, Wigglesworth J S, Desai R 1980 Pulmonary fat accumulation after Intralipid infusion in the preterm infant. Lancet 2: 815–818
17. Hulman G, Fraser I, Pearson H J, Bell P R F 1982 Agglutination of Intralipid by sera of acutely ill patients. Lancet 2: 1426–1427
18. Greene H L, Hazlett D, Demaree R 1976 Relationship between Intralipid-induced hyperlipaemia and pulmonary function. American Journal of Clinical Nutrition 29: 127–135
19. Askanazi J, Nordenstrom J, Rosenbaum S H, Elwyn D H, Hyman A I, Carpentier Y A 1981 Nutrition for the patient with respiratory failure. Anesthesiology 54: 373–377
20. Kien C L, Chusid M J 1979 Eosinophilia in children receiving parenteral nutrition support. Journal of Parenteral and Enteral Nutrition 3: 468–469
21. Kapp J P, Duckert F, Hartmann G 1971 Platelet adhesiveness and serum lipids during and after Intralipid infusions. Nutrition and Metabolism 13: 92–99
22. Kerner J A, Cassani C, Hurwitz R, Berde C B 1981 Monitoring intravenous fat emulsions in neonates with the fatty acid/serum albumin molar ratio. Journal of Parenteral and Enteral Nutrition 5: 517–518
23. Andrew G, Chan G, Schiff D 1976 Lipid metabolism in the neonate. Journal of Pediatrics 88: 273–278
24. Shennan A T, Bryan M H, Angel A 1977 The effect of gestational age on Intralipid tolerance in newborn infants. Journal of Pediatrics 91: 134–137
25. Meurling S, Grotte G 1981 Complete parenteral nutrition in the surgery of the newborn infant. Acta Chirurgica Scandinavica 147: 465–473
26. Heller L 1972 Parenteral nutrition. Churchill Livingstone, London, p 180
27. Elphick M C, Filshie G M, Hull D 1978 The passage of fat emulsion across the human placenta. British Journal of Obstetrics and Gynaecology 85: 610–618
28. Rossner S, Johansson C, Walldius G, Aly A 1979 Intralipid clearance and lipoprotein pattern in men with advanced alcoholic liver cirrhosis. American Journal of Clinical Nutrition 32: 2022–2026
29. Russell G I, Davies T G, Walls J 1980 Evaluation of the intravenous fat tolerance test in chronic renal disease. Clinical nephrology 13: 282–286

Lisinopril

A potent, long-acting, oral converting enzyme inhibitor which is active without metabolism.

Chemistry

Lisinopril (Carace, Zestril)
$C_{21}H_{31}N_3O_5.2H_2O$
(S)-1-[N^2-(1-Carboxy-3-phenylpropyl)-L-lysyl]-L-proline dihydrate

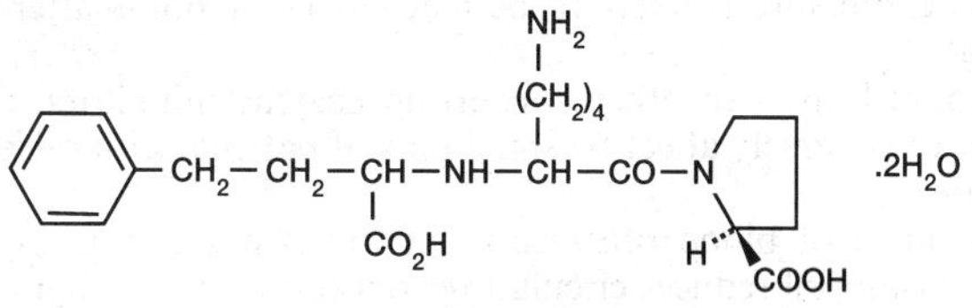

Molecular weight (anhydrous)	441.5 (405.5)
pKa	~2.5, 4.0, 6.7, 10.1
Solubility	
in alcohol	<1 in 10 000
in water	1 in 10
Octanol/water partition coefficient	10.2

Sparingly soluble in methanol. Lisinopril is prepared by chemical synthesis.[1,2]

Pharmacology

Lisinopril is a lysine derivative of enalaprilat (the active metabolite of enalapril) and does not require hydrolysis to become active.

Lisinopril is a competitive antagonist of angiotensin-converting enzyme (ACE). The enzyme renin cleaves the decapeptide angiotensin I from its substrate. The cleavage of the terminal two amino acids from angiotensin I by converting enzyme, which is widely distributed throughout the endothelium of blood vessels and within other tissues, produces the active octapeptide angiotensin II. Converting enzyme is a peptidyl peptide hydrolase identical with kininase II and also therefore breaks down the vasodilator bradykinin. Inhibition of this enzyme results in vasodilatation.

Lisinopril has a higher affinity for ACE than captopril as judged by the dissociation half lives of ACE–inhibitor complexes (105 min for lisinopril, 27 min for enalaprilat, 9 min for captopril).[3] Inhibition of ACE also appears to develop more slowly after lisinopril therapy than after captopril or enalapril treatment.[4]

Toxicology

Lisinopril has not been shown to have a mutagenic effect. No teratogenic effect has been found. Fetotoxicity can be induced in mice and rabbits and in large part seems to relate to the pharmacological effects of this class of drug on electrolyte status. Tests of carcinogenicity have not revealed untoward effects.

In common with other converting enzyme inhibitors, and therefore related to the mechanism of action of the drug, large doses will cause renal tubular degeneration. Administration of a low salt diet exacerbates the damage and saline administration or a high salt diet ameliorates the effect, which is thought to result from electrolyte depletion produced by the pharmacological action of this group of drugs.

Clinical pharmacology

Lisinopril is slowly absorbed after oral ingestion and peak concentrations in plasma are achieved 6–8 hours after a single dose. Plasma ACE activity falls progressively from 60 minutes after an oral dose of 10 mg, to reach its minimum value at 6 hours. The duration of the acute effects of lisinopril are dose-dependent up to a dose of 20 mg. Measurements of components of the renin–angiotensin system in the circulation in man show that a single oral dose of 10 mg of lisinopril, producing plasma concentrations of approximately 8–10 $\mu g.l^{-1}$ or more, can suppress converting enzyme activity to less than 20% of basal activity for 24 hours.[5] Circulating angiotensin II concentrations return towards pretreatment levels during 10–24 hours after a single dose but remain suppressed for longer during chronic dosing.[5,6] Tissue concentrations of ACE activity and angiotensin II may be more relevant to the drug's long-term effect.[7–9] Lower doses may provide 24 hours inhibition.

Lisinopril lowers blood pressure with maximum reductions occurring 6 hours after dosing and lasting for 24 hours.[10–12] This is accompanied by a fall in total peripheral vascular resistance.[13] Reflex tachycardia does not usually occur and cardiac output and ejection fraction do not alter in patients with hypertension.[14] In patients with congestive heart failure, lisinopril causes an increase in the cardiac index and a reduction in the peripheral vascular resistance as well as a fall in mean arterial pressure.[15] Renal blood flow is either unchanged or slightly increased.

Pharmacokinetics

The preferred analytical method for measuring lisinopril in plasma is radioimmunoassay by which method 0.4 $nmol.l^{-1}$ of plasma may be reliably measured.[16] but methods using separation by HPLC are also used.[17]

Lisinopril is slowly absorbed after oral ingestion and peak levels are reached 6–8 hours after a single dose.[5,6] Peak serum concentrations are achieved 6–8 hours after oral administration. Concomitant administration of food has no important effect on absorption or time to peak plasma concentration.[18] The bioavailability is 25–30% but this may be reduced in patients with heart failure.[15,19] Lisinopril is not metabolized and approximately 30% of an oral dose is found in urine and more than 60% in faeces (manufacturers data and Ref. 15).

Animal studies indicate that the drug may have differential effects on ACE inhibition in different tissues which may be relevant to its action.[19]

At pharmacologically effective concentrations 3–10% of plasma lisinopril binds to protein (manufacturers data). It is believed that this is binding to residual converting enzyme in the plasma.[20] Lisinopril is excreted largely through the kidney and the dose should be reduced in those with impaired renal function (see Mode of use).[21,22] With recommended doses the steady state is achieved in 2–3 days.

Lisinopril does cross the placental barrier and appears in cord blood. It is not known whether lisinopril is secreted in human milk.

Oral absorbtion	~25%
Presystemic metabolism	no significant quantity
Plasma half life[24]	12 h
Volume of distribution	31–36 l
Plasma protein binding	3–10%

Concentration–effect relationship

Absorption of lisinopril is slow, reaching a peak at 6–8 hours after a single dose, with low but detectable concentrations beyond 48 hours; serum ACE activity is closely associated with the concentration of lisinopril.[5] After a 10 mg dose, circulating concentrations of lisinopril reach 10 $\mu g.l^{-1}$ or more in 2–3 hours producing inhibition of plasma ACE activity. Circulating concentrations of renin and angiotensin I rise, and angiotensin II concentrations fall rapidly at this point. Larger doses will achieve this level of lisinopril in the circulation at an earlier point, inducing earlier changes in concentrations of renin and angiotensin; smaller doses will delay their onset. A dose of 10 mg or more will suppress circulating ACE activity to less than 20% of basal activity and angiotensin II levels for up to 24 hours.[5]

The initial fall in blood pressure in patients relates well to circulating angiotensin II concentrations and therefore substantial falls in pressure may occur usually 2 hours or more after dosing depending on the amount administered. Long-term pressure reduction does not relate well to the initial circulating concentrations of angiotensin II, to their reduction by treatment, or to plasma concentrations of lisinopril.

Metabolism

Careful study in man has revealed that there is no significant metabolism (<1%) of lisinopril. Of an orally administered dose 29±15% (mean±SD) is excreted unchanged in the urine and 69±23% recovered in the faeces. Enterohepatic circulation has not been documented and no metabolites identified in man (manufacturers' data).

Pharmaceutics

Lisinopril (Carace; Morson division of MSD/Zestril; ICI, UK) is available as 2.5, 5, 10 and 20 mg tablets for oral administration. A parenteral form containing 1 $mg.ml^{-1}$ and 5 $mg.ml^{-1}$ is available, but only for restricted use.

Carace tablets have the following colours: 2.5 mg blue, 5 mg white (scored), 10 mg yellow (scored) and 20 mg orange (scored). The corresponding colours for Zestril are white (2.5 mg), light pink (5 mg), pink (10 mg) and red (20 mg). The 5 mg strength is scored.

Lisinopril has a shelf-life of 36 months at room temperature protected from moisture (no dessicant is required).

Therapeutic use

Indications

1. Control of hypertension
2. Treatment of heart failure.

Contraindications

These are 'relative' and relate to the pharmacology of the drug and are relevant to all ACE inhibitors.

1. Bilateral renal artery stenosis and in some cases of unilateral renal artery stenosis when treatment may jeopardize the kidney with the stenosed vessel
2. Low blood pressure
3. High-dose diuretic therapy
4. Salt-deplete states
5. Renal impairment
6. Pregnancy
7. Potassium sparing diuretics
8. Angioneurotic oedema relating to previous treatment with an ACE inhibitor
9. Hypersensitivity to lisinopril.

Mode of use

This depends on the indication for treatment and renal function of the patient. A starting dose of 2.5–20 mg is used increasing to a usual effective dose of 5–20 mg with a maximum recommended dose of 40 mg daily in those with normal renal function; lower starting and maintenance doses are appropriate for patients with renal impairment. There seems little advantage in using the drug more than once daily. Withdrawal of the drug is not associated with untoward effects. Tolerance does not appear to be a problem. Dosage adjustment in liver impairment should not be required unless there is concurrent loss of kidney function.

Dosage adjustment in renal impairment[21–26]

The usual dose of lisinopril is recommended for patients with a creatinine clearance > 70 $ml.min^{-1}$. In hypertension, the dose would be 10–20 mg with the usual maintenance dose of 20 mg with a maximum of 40 mg daily. In patients with a creatinine clearance ⩽70 and >30 $ml.min^{-1}$ the initial dose should be 2.5–10 mg daily. In patients with a creatinine clearance ⩽30 and ⩾10 $ml.min^{-1}$ (serum creatinine > 165 $\mu mol.l^{-1}$) the initial dose is 2.5–5 mg lisinopril once daily. Maximum maintenance doses require similar reduction according to renal function. In patients with severe renal impairment (creatinine clearance < 10 $ml.min^{-1}$ and serum creatinine of 400–650 $\mu mol.l^{-1}$) the recommended initial dose is 2.5 mg lisinopril once a day and the maintenance dosage or frequency of administration should be reduced proportionately.

Patients with hypertension and proteinuria may show a decrease in protein excretion when treated with ACE inhibitors.[27] This has also been observed with lisinopril. The relation of this to pressure reduction or a specific drug effect is under evaluation.[28]

Indications

1. Hypertension

Converting enzyme inhibitors are effective antihypertensive agents with efficacy similar to other drugs currently available for reducing blood pressure.[29–32] In patients with contraindications to the use of β-antagonists or diuretics they make a sensible initial choice. Lisinopril is long acting and can be given once daily to produce 24-hour control. It combines particularly effectively with diuretics[29] (but see Contraindications) and the dihydropyridine calcium antagonists challenging the traditional 'step-care' approach with one, two or three drugs. Converting enzyme inhibitors when combined with β-antagonists reduce blood pressure further than either alone though some regard this as a less effective combination than with vasodilating antihypertensive drugs. Postural hypotension is not a problem unless patients are volume and/or 'salt-deplete' (see Contraindications). Apart from any immediate fall in pressure the optimal effect on blood pressure is likely to be reached 1–3 months after starting dosing.

Lisinopril, as with other converting enzyme inhibitors, does not appear to adversely affect plasma lipids of patients with raised blood pressure.

The mode of blood pressure reduction is not completely understood. Lisinopril reduces circulating concentrations of angiotensin II and aldosterone. Lowering tissue concentrations of angiotensin II may reduce noradrenaline release from adrenergic nerves. Antagonism of the intrarenal effects of angiotensin II causes a mild natriuresis. Inhibition of local angiotensin II formation within vessel walls may play a role. The drug also affects bradykinin degradation and probably indirectly prostaglandin formation but the importance of this effect in blood pressure control is far from clear. The outcome is reduction of peripheral resistance without compensatory increase in heart rate, and therefore reduction of blood pressure. Of patients considered to have essential hypertension 25% are usually classed as 'low renin' and probably respond equally as well to the drug in the long term as those with high circulating renin concentrations.

Renovascular hypertension In the presence of unilateral renal artery stenosis, the kidney distal to the obstruction becomes ischaemic and secretes renin. Converting enzyme inhibitors would be expected to be particularly effective in reducing pressure in this group. Lisinopril is no exception. Studies involving small groups of closely monitored patients have shown lisinopril monotherapy to control blood pressure without loss of renal function for up to 24 months providing care is taken to avoid dehydration, hypovolaemia and hyponatremia and to ensure dose reduction when appropriate.[33] Nevertheless, concern must exist over the fate of the kidney distal to the stenosis as the fall in pressure associated with removal of angiotensin II entering or being formed within the kidney may lead to a serious decline in function in this kidney. It has been suggested that renal artery occlusion may also be precipitated but the evidence that this is a drug-related problem is inconclusive. More seriously, if stenosis is bilateral, renal failure may develop particularly in those on concomitant diuretic therapy. This is reversible if recognized early enough. Concomitant diuretic therapy may exacerbate the renal impairment.

2. Heart failure

In common with other ACE inhibitors lisinopril has been found to be effective in treating patients with heart failure[34,35] whose symptoms are not adequately controlled by digoxin and diuretics (but see Contraindications). The drug is renally excreted and therefore its dosage should be reduced in patients with this condition as invariably they have some degree of renal impairment. Heart failure patients are particularly sensitive to these drugs due to activation of the renin–angiotensin system by concomitant diuretic therapy. Patients with less severe forms of heart failure may also benefit from the addition of lisinopril to diuretic therapy; a substantial part of the benefit may accrue from blocking the stimulating effects of diuresis on the renin–angiotensin–aldosterone system. Starting doses of 2.5 mg, with subsequent adjustment to the usual maintenance dose of 5–20 mg daily, are used depending on patient response.

Ischaemic heart disease

Although the majority of patients who have benefited from lisinopril therapy for heart failure have underlying ischaemic disease, the role of ACE inhibition in the setting of ongoing ischaemia manifesting as chest pain is unclear. Since these agents venodilate and reduce afterload and, at least when circulating angiotensin II levels are high, reduce coronary tone, they might be expected to benefit those with angina. Alternatively, they could impair perfusion across a critical stenosis by reducing blood pressure too far, though the simultaneous decrease of left ventricular pressure would be expected to compensate initially and allow adequate blood flow to the myocardium. Current evidence indicates that those with stable angina do not have worsening of symptoms or exercise capacity when taking lisinopril.

Contraindications

1. Renal artery stenosis

See renal vascular hypertension — above.

2–5. Hypotension, salt depletion and renal impairment

The initial fall in pressure on administration of an ACE inhibitor relates to the prevailing circulating concentration of angiotensin II. Patients who are volume or 'salt-deplete' through therapy with diuretics or illness, for example diarrhoea and vomiting, may have markedly elevated plasma angiotensin II levels. These individuals may therefore occasionally experience precipitous falls in blood pressure when angiotensin II concentrations are reduced after the first dose of an inhibitor. The slow absorption rate of lisinopril may delay the onset of hypotension for some hours. Interestingly, ACE inhibitors may 're-set' autoregulation of cerebral blood flow and marked pressure falls may be tolerated without symptoms. An appropriate reflex tachycardia often fails to occur in response to the fall in pressure induced by ACE inhibitors and thereby compounds the problem. Rarely, syncope with marked bradycardia may ensue.

Patients who have low initial blood pressure through a cardiovascular disorder, for example those in cardiac failure who are often also taking large doses of diuretics, may be particularly susceptible, though hypertensive patients on small doses of diuretics may also occasionally exhibit symptomatic hypotension with initial dosing.

Similarly, symptomatic hypotension may occur with long-term therapy in such patients, necessitating reduction of the diuretic therapy.

The combination of low blood pressure and removal of the renal actions of angiotensin II may lead to renal impairment and even renal failure. This appears to be reversible if recognized at an early stage.

6. Pregnancy

Insufficient data are available to allow use of this drug in patients of childbearing potential. Converting enzyme inhibitors have been used successfully in pregnant women with hypertension but their safety is not established and alternative agents should be used.

There is a potential risk of fetal hypotension, decreased birth weight and decreased renal perfusion or anuria in the fetus from in utero exposure to ACE inhibitors. Any neonate exposed to lisinopril in utero should be observed closely for adequate urine output and blood pressure. If required, appropriate medical measures should be initiated including administration of fluids and vasoconstricting agents, e.g. noradrenaline, angiotensin II or dialysis considered to remove lisinopril from the circulatory system though no satisfactory clinical experience is reported. Use of ACE inhibitors even during the later stage of pregnancy is, generally, not recommended.

7. Potassium-sparing diuretics

ACE inhibitors reduce the formation of angiotensin II and consequently also aldosterone. Combination with potassium-sparing diuretics or more rarely concurrent use of potassium supplement or potassium-containing salt substitutes may lead to dangerous hyperkalaemia especially if renal function is impaired, though the combination may occasionally be clinically useful with careful monitoring of renal function and serum potassium.

Adverse reactions

Potentially life-threatening effects

The major concerns are severe hypotension and renal failure. Administration of any ACE inhibitor may lead to renal failure especially in patients who have received high doses of loop diuretics. A reduction of diuretic dose or a 'diuretic holiday' before administration of lisinopril is wise, particularly in patients with severe heart failure.

Acute overdosage

A single report of lisinopril overdose resulted in full uneventful recovery of the patient[36]. Prolonged hypotension is the most likely immediate difficulty with renal impairment developing in certain situations. Restoration of pressure by increasing blood volume should suffice; this can be achieved by elevating the patient's legs and infusion of plasma volume expanders/saline. Converting enzyme inhibitors, possibly through removing angiotensin II, appear to 'switch off' sympathetic nerve activity and judicious infusion of noradrenaline (10 $\mu g.kg^{-1}.min^{-1}$ increasing according to pressure and ECG response) may restore the circulation through its inotropic and chronotropic effects as well as its α-agonist properties. In extreme cases infusion of angiotensin II can be undertaken, but this peptide is not readily available.

If restoration of blood volume and pressure with appropriate correction of any electrolyte abnormality fails to restore renal function then the management becomes that of acute renal failure.

Severe or irreversible adverse effects

Hypotension and renal failure may occur (see Contraindications). Severe angioedema leading to airway obstruction has been reported with ACE inhibitors.

Symptomatic adverse effects

In patients with hypertension and heart failure, headache, dizziness, diarrhoea, nausea, vomiting and rash have been reported but concomitant therapy and occurrence of similar effects in those receiving placebo obscure the exact relationship to lisinopril.[37] Palpitation, asthenia and impotence have also been reported. Cough and, extremely rarely, angioedema occur with ACE inhibitors.[38] In controlled trials of treatment of hypertension involving over 4000 patients the incidence of cough is reported to be between 0.4 to 1.6% of patients (manufacturers' data). Cough is reported more frequently in patients with heart failure, estimates of its incidence in patients taking part in clinical trials is 3% (manufacturers' data) and the time incidence may be higher still. Events indicative of angioedema are reported in only 13 hypertensive patients (0.3%) out of 4622 taking part in clinical trials and in 4 with heart failure (0.6%) out of 673 (manufacturers' data). Small increases in urea, creatinine and potassium may occur (see Contraindications).

Other effects

When converting enzyme inhibitors are administered renin concentrations rise markedly. Absolute concentrations of renin in the circulation are therefore difficult to interpret but renal vein sampling in patients with renal artery stenosis (but see Contraindications) may still be undertaken with the expectation of particularly high circulating levels for analysis.

Interference with clinical pathology tests

No technical interferences of this kind have been reported.

High risk groups

Neonates

The drug should not be used during pregnancy or the neonatal period.

Breast milk. Lisinopril should not be used during lactation.

Children

There is no experience of the use of the drug in children but there is no reason why it should not be used in children with hypertension, provided the dose is reduced pro rata to body weight and account taken of the relative contraindications.

Pregnant women

Insufficient data on the use of lisinopril during pregnancy and lactation in humans are available to permit assessment of the possible risk. ACE inhibitors cause intrauterine death of the fetus in some animal species. Pregnancy should be excluded before start of treatment with lisinopril and avoided during treatment.

The elderly

Renal function deteriorates with age and lower doses of ACE

inhibitors are appropriate. Cardiovascular reflexes may be more impaired and elderly patients therefore more at risk from hypotension than younger individuals.

Concurrent disease

Patients with collagen vascular disease. Agranulocytosis and bone marrow depression have been seen rarely in patients on angiotensin converting enzyme inhibitors. This is more frequent in patients with renal impairment, especially if they also have a collagen vascular disease. No cases of agranulocytosis have been reported to date with lisinopril. However, regular monitoring of white blood cell counts and protein levels in urine should be considered in patients with collagen vascular disease (e.g. lupus erythematosus and scleroderma), especially associated with impaired renal function and concomitant therapy of drugs particularly corticosteroids and antimetabolites.

Renal impairment. See Mode of use.

Drug interactions[39]

Potentially hazardous interactions

Diuretics and potassium-sparing diuretics. Concomitant administration may lead to serious hypotension with the former and, in addition, dangerous hyperkalaemia with the latter (see Contraindications). Some attempts have been made to exploit the increased antihypertensive efficacy of lisinopril when in combination with other antihypertensive agents such as diuretics (see Indications).

Lithium. Serum lithium concentrations may rise if patients are receiving an ACE inhibitor in addition to lithium.

Alcohol. When first administered the reduction in blood pressure may affect the ability to drive and operate machinery and this may be exacerbated by alcohol.

Other significant interactions

Non-steroidal anti-inflammatory agents like indomethacin may reduce the antihypertensive effects. In patients with stable renal impairment on an ACE inhibitor, administration of a cyclo-oxygenase inhibitor may cause a sharp reduction of renal function.

Potentially useful interactions

ACE inhibitors inhibit baroreflex-mediated tachycardia and can be used with vasodilator drugs.

General review articles

Armayor G M, Lopez L M 1988 Lisinopril: a new angiotensin-converting enzyme inhibitor. Drug Intelligence and Clinical Pharmacy 22: 365–372

Lancaster S G, Todd P A 1988 Lisinopril: a preliminary review of its pharmacodynamic and pharmacokinetic properties, and therapeutic use in hypertension and congestive heart failure. Drugs 35: 646–669

Noble T A, Murray K H 1988 Lisinopril: a non sulfhydryl angiotensin-converting enzyme inhibitor. Clinical Pharmacy 7: 659–669

1987 Current and future trends in hypertension. Journal of Cardiovascular Pharmacology 9 (suppl 3)

1989 ACE-inhibition — the next decade. Journal of Human Hypertension 3 (suppl 1)

References

1. Wu M T, Douglas A A W, Ondeyka D L et al 1985 Synthesis of N^2-[(S)-1-Carboxy-3-phenylpropyl]-L-lysyl-L-prolinen (Lisinopril). Journal of Pharmaceutical Sciences 74: 352–354
2. Blacklock T J, Butcher J W, Shuman R 1985 Large scale N-carboxyanhydride preparation of ALA-PRO and Ne-(TFA)-LYS-PRPO. In: Deber C M, Heuby V J, Kopplel K D (eds) Peptides: structure and function. Proceedings of the 9th American Peptide Symposium, Toronto, 23–28 June, pp 787–790
3. Bull H G, Thornberry N A, Cordes M H J, Patchell A A, Cordes E H 1985 Inhibition of rabbit lung angiotensin-converting enzyme by N-[(S)-1-carboxy-3-phenylpropyl]L-alanyl-L-proline and N-[(S)-1-carboxy-3-phenylpropyl] L-lysyl L-proline. Journal of Biological Chemistry 260: 2952–2962
4. Semple P F, Cumming A M M, Meredith P D, Morton J J 1987 Onset of action of captopril, enalapril, enalaprilic acid and lisinopril in normal man. Cardiovascular Drugs and Therapy 1: 45–50
5. Biollaz J, Schelling J L, Jacot des Combes B, Brunner D B, Desponds G, Brunner J R 1982 Enalapril maleate and a lysine analogue (MK-521) in normal volunteers; relationship between plasma drug levels and the renin angiotensin system. British Journal of Clinical Pharmacology 14: 363–368
6. Hodsman G P, Zabludowski J R, Zoccali C et al 1984 Enalapril (MK421) and its lysine analogue (MK 521): a comparison of acute and chronic effects on blood pressure, renin–angiotensin system and sodium excretion in normal man. British Journal of Clinical Pharmacology 17: 233–241
7. Jackson B, Cubela R, Sakaguchi K, Johnston C I 1987 Pharmacokinetics of angiotensin-converting enzyme inhibition in tissues following oral lisinopril: studies in the rat using quantitative radioinhibitor binding. Clinical and Experimental Pharmacology and Physiology 14: 343–347
8. Cushman D W, Wang F L, Fung W C et al 1989 Comparisons in vitro, ex vivo, and in vivo of the actions of seven structurally diverse inhibitors of angiotensin-converting enzyme (ACE). British Journal of Clinical Pharmacology 28 (suppl 2): 115S–131S
9. Johnson C I, Fabris B, Yamada H et al 1989 Comparative studies of tissue inhibition by angiotensin-converting enzyme inhibitors. Journal of Hypertension 7 (suppl 5): 511–516
10. Gomez H J, Cirillo V J, Sromovsky J A et al 1989 Lisinopril dose–response relationship in essential hypertension. British Journal of Clinical Pharmacology 28: 415–420
11. Herpin D, Conte D 1989 Assessment of the antihypertensive effect of lisinopril using 24 hour ambulatory monitoring. Journal of Human Hypertension 3 (suppl 1): 11–15
12. Graettinger W F, Lipson J L, Klein R C, Cheung D G, Weber M A 1989 Comparison of antihypertensive therapies by non-invasive techniques. Chest 96: 74–79
13. Millar J A, Derkx F H M, McLean K, Reid J L 1982 Pharmacodynamics of converting enzyme inhibition: the cardiovascular, endocrine and autonomic effects of MK421 (enalapril) and MK521. British Journal of Clinical Pharmacology 14: 347–355
14. Ajayi A A, Campbell B C, Howie C A, Reid J L 1985 Acute and chronic effects of the converting enzyme inhibitors enalapril and lisinopril on reflex control of heart rate in normotensive man. Journal of Hypertension 3: 47–53
15. Dickstein K 1987 Hemodynamic, hormonal, and pharmacokinetic aspects of treatment with lisinopril in congestive heart failure. Journal of Cardiovascular Pharmacology 9 (suppl 3): S73–S81
16. Worland P J, Jarrott B 1986 Radioimmunoassay for the quantitation of lisinopril and enalaprilat. Journal of Pharmaceutical Sciences 75: 512–516
17. Toco D J, de Luna F A, Duncan A E W, Vassil T C, Ulm E H 1982 The physiological disposition and metabolism of enalapril maleate (MK421) in laboratory animals. Drug Metabolism and Disposition 10: 15
18. Mojaverian P, Rocci M L, Vlasses P H, Hoholick C, Clementi R A, Ferguson R K 1986 Effect of food on the bioavailability of lisinopril, a nonsulfhydryl angiotensin-converting enzyme inhibitor. Journal of Pharmaceutical Sciences 74: 395–397
19. Ulm E H, Hichens M, Gomez H J et al 1982 Enalapril maleate and a lysine analogue (MK-521): disposition in man. British Journal of Clinical Pharmacology 14: 357–362
20. Gomez H J, Cirillo V J, Moncloa F 1987 The clinical pharmacology of lisinopril. Journal of Cardiovascular Pharmacology 9 (suppl 3): S27–S34
21. Begg E J, Bailey R R, Lynn K L, Robson R A, Frank G J, Olson S C 1989 The pharmacokinetics of angiotensin-converting enzyme inhibitors in patients with renal impairment. Journal of Hypertension 7 (suppl 5): S29–S32
22. Kelly J G, Doyle G D, Carmody M, Glover D R, Cooper W D 1988 Pharmacokinetics of lisinopril, enalapril and enalaprilat in renal failure: effects of haemodialysis. British Journal of Clinical Pharmacology 26: 781–786
23. Thomson A H, Kelly J G, Whiting B 1989 Lisinopril population pharmacokinetics in elderly and renal disease. British Journal of Clinical Pharmacology 27: 57–65
24. Beerman B, Junggren I, Cocchetto D et al 1985 Lisinopril steady state kinetics in healthy subjects. Journal of Clinical Pharmacology 25: 471
25. Kuntziger H E, Pouthier D, Bellucci A 1987 Treatment of hypertension with lisinopril in end-stage renal failure. Journal of Cardiovascular Pharmacology 10 (suppl 7): S157–S159
26. Van Schaik B A M, Geyskes G G, Boer P 1987 Lisinopril in hypertensive patients with and without renal failure. European Journal of Clinical Pharmacology 32: 11–16
27. Heeg J E, De Jong P E, Van Der Hem G K, De Zeeuw D 1987 Reduction of proteinuria by angiotensin-converting enzyme inhibition. Kidney International 32: 78–83
28. Keane W F, Anderson S, Aurell M, DeZeeuw D, Narins R G, Povar G 1989 Angiotensin-converting enzyme inhibitors and progressive renal insufficiency. Annals of Internal Medicine 3: 503–516
29. Pool J L, Gennari J, Goldstein R et al 1987 Controlled multicenter study of the antihypertensive effects of lisinopril, hydrochlorothiazide, and lisinopril plus hydrochlorothiazide in the treatment of 394 patients with mild to moderate essential hypertension. Journal of Cardiovascular Pharmacology 9 (suppl 3): S36–S42
30. Bolzano K, Arriaga J, Bernal R et al 1987 The antihypertensive effect of lisinopril compared to atenolol in patients with mild to moderate hypertension. Journal of Cardiovascular Pharmacology 9 (suppl 3): S43–S47
31. Morlin C, Baglivo H, Boeijinga J K et al 1987 Comparative trial of lisinopril and nifedipine in mild to severe essential hypertension. Journal of Cardiovascular Pharmacology 9 (suppl 3): S48–S52
32. Seedat Y K, Veriava Y, Cohen J D, Dateling F, Milne J F, Parag K B 1987 Evaluation of the antihypertensive effect of lisinopril compared to atenolol in black, mixed, and indian patients with mild-to-moderate essential hypertension. Current Therapeutic Research 41: 852–864
33. Fyhrquist F, Gronhagen Riska C, Tikkanen I, Junggren I-L 1987 Long-term monotherapy with lisinopril in renovascular hypertension. Journal of Cardiovascular Pharmacology 9 (suppl 3): S61–S65
34. Powers E W R, Chiaramida A, DeMaria A N et al 1987 A double-blind comparison of lisinopril with captopril in patients with symptomatic congestive heart failure. Journal of Cardiovascular Pharmacology 9 (suppl 3): S82–S88

35. Giles T D, Katz R, Facc M D 1989 Short and long-acting angiotensin-converting enzyme inhibitors: a randomised trial of lisinopril versus captopril in the treatment of congestive heart failure. Journal of the American College of Cardiology 13: 1240–1247
36. Dawson A H, Harvey D, Smith A J et al 1990 Lisinopril overdose. Lancet 335: 487–488
37. Rush J E, Merrill D D 1987 The safety and tolerability of lisinopril in clinical trials. Journal of Cardiovascular Pharmacology 9 (suppl 3): S99–S107
38. Cameron H A, Higgins T J 1989 Clinical experience with lisinopril. Observations on safety and tolerability. Journal of Human Hypertension 3: 177–186
39. Breckenridge A M 1989 Drug interactions with ACE-inhibitors. Journal of Human Hypertension 3: 133–138

Lisuride (hydrogen maleate)

A dopamine receptor agonist used to treat Parkinson's disease.

Chemistry

Lisuride hydrogen maleate, (lysuride hydrogen maleate, LHM, Dopergin, Revanil, Cuvalit)
$C_{20}H_{26}N_4O,C_4H_4O_4$
3-(9,10-Didehydro-6-methylergolin-8-α-yl)-1,1-diethylurea hydrogen maleate

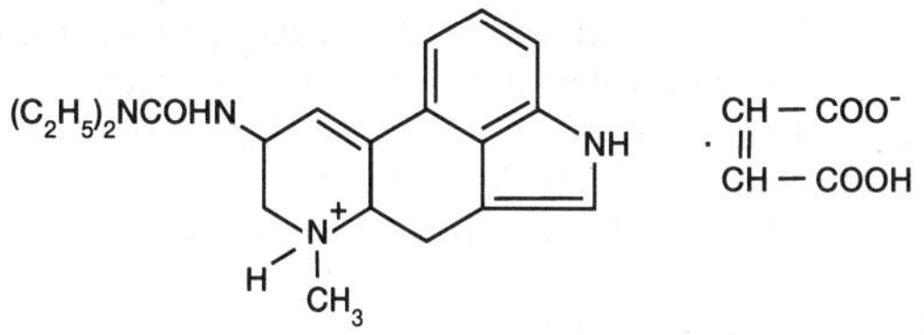

Molecular weight (free base)	454.5 (338.5)
pKa	7.0
Solubility	
in alcohol	—
in water	—
Octanol/water partition coefficient	26

Lisuride hydrogen maleate, LHM, is a semi-synthetic ergot derivative belonging to the 8-α-aminoergoline group. LHM is a white crystalline powder with a slightly bitter taste, sensitive to light (and, to a lesser degree, to heat and oxidants). It is not available in any combination preparations.

Pharmacology

Dopaminergic effects

LHM is a semi-synthetic ergot derivative which is a potent post synaptic D_2 dopaminergic receptor agonist. Studies of binding of tritium labelled lisuride to striatal membranes of rat brain, using 10^{-7}M (+) butaclamol as the displacing agent have shown high affinity binding with a K_D of 0.5 nmol and a Bmax of 490 fmol.mg^{-1} protein.[1] Although it has a high binding affinity, the intrinsic activity of lisuride is weaker and it can be regarded as a partial agonist.

As a consequence of the D_2 agonist activity lisuride induces stereotyped behaviour in naive as well as in reserpinized rodents, induces contralateral circling in rats with unilateral nigrostriatal lesions, reverses reserpine-induced immobility, rigidity and hypothermia, and causes hyperactivity, aggressiveness and mounting behaviour in rats maintained in groups. It also causes emesis in dogs and humans, and inhibits prolactin release. All these effects are competitively inhibited by haloperidol or specific D_2 receptor blockers, such as domperidone, although this antagonism is less marked than for bromocriptine.[2–5]

The effects of LHM are not inhibited or impaired by depletion of dopamine with reserpine or α-methyl-p-tyrosine, although this procedure reduces the activity of bromocriptine. Thus, the effect of LHM is due to direct activation of D_2 receptors and is independent of basal dopamine concentrations.

In competitive binding assays, LHM also has some affinity for D_1 sites, the clinical relevance of which is probably minimal.

Serotoninergic effects

LHM also activates 5-HT_1 and 5-HT_2 receptors. Depending on the neuronal system, preferential stimulation of the pre- or post-synaptic

L

5-HT receptors will result either in functional 5-HT antagonism or agonism. The action upon 5-HT receptors may probably account for the sedative action of the drug.

Adrenergic effects
High doses of LHM have antagonistic effects on α-adrenergic, and possibly also on β-adrenergic receptors but these actions are unlikely to be of significance at clinical doses.

Toxicology

Acute studies. Toxic symptoms of LHM in animals include hyperactivity, tremor, ataxic gait, apathy, prone posture, ptosis and convulsions. In rabbits and monkeys, respiratory abnormalities were noted. The LD_{50} for mice is $<30\ mg.kg^{-1}$ (intravenous), $550\ mg.kg^{-1}$ (subcutaneous) and $90–500\ mg.kg^{-1}$ (intragastric). Rats are much more sensitive ($1–4\ mg.kg^{-1}$ intravenous and subcutaneous, $10–60\ mg.kg^{-1}$ intragastric). Rabbits and monkeys have intragastric LD_{50} of <74 and above $200\ mg.kg^{-1}$ respectively.

Chronic studies. Chronic treatment in rhesus monkeys ($0.1–10\ mg.kg^{-1}$ daily intragastric for one year) produced only endocrinological changes (lowering of serum prolactin and diminution of prolactin cells, increased GH levels, hypoplasia of germinal epithelium in the testes and impaired spermatogenesis in the highest dosage). Carcinogenicity was not noted in mice, rats, monkeys and humans and in fact decreased incidence of pituitary and/or other tumours was noted in rodents. LHM was non-mutagenic in several in vitro tests and no teratogenic properties were observed.

Clinical pharmacology

The main interest in lisuride as a tool in clinical pharmacology and as a potential therapeutic agent has been its potency as a D_2 receptor agonist and its water solubility, which makes prolonged intravenous or subcutaneous infusion practical. The doses of lisuride used have ranged between 0.2 and 10 mg daily by mouth and up to 2.5 mg/24 hrs by sub-cutaneous infusion. Among the pharmacological effects that have been described in both normal volunteers and patients are nausea and emesis, dizziness, sedation, orthostatic hypotension and, with higher doses, dyskinesias, psychosis and hallucinations. These effects can be antagonised by sulpiride.[6] As there is extensive pre-systemic metabolism, parenteral doses are equivalent to substantially larger oral doses.

LHM has been investigated in various extrapyramidal disorders, particularly Parkinson's disease and related disorders, but also focal and generalized dystonia. In Parkinson's disease, LHM is usually used in combination with levodopa. There is evidence for some efficacy against the off stages of on–off symptoms. The average effective dose is 0.6–1.8 mg daily in 3–6 doses. Higher doses, up to 5.0 mg daily, are used uncommonly, especially when employed as monotherapy. The drug is also effective in reducing elevated prolactin levels.

A single dose of LHM (0.2 mg) was found to reduce ACTH levels in seven out of 14 patients with Cushing's disease.

Inconclusive suggestions were made for the efficacy of LHM in the prophylaxis of migraine. Relatively low doses are used for this indication, e.g. 0.025 mg tid.

Pharmacokinetics

The preferred analytical method for measuring LHM in body fluids is radioimmunoassay, which has high sensitivity and specificity.

Following intravenous injection, the plasma concentration of lisuride declines triphasically, with respective half lives of 5 min, 25 min and 120 min. The total plasma clearance is $800 \pm 250\ ml.min^{-1}$, similar to hepatic 'plasma flow'. The drug is widely distributed throughout the body, with a distribution volume of $2.3–2.4\ l.kg^{-1}$, indicating uptake by tissue.

Following oral administration, absorption is complete,[7,8] but there is extensive and variable pre-systemic metabolism.[8] The bioavailability of 100 µg oral LHM is $10 \pm 7\%$ and of 300 µg it is $22 \pm 7\%$. Peak plasma levels are reached 2–4 h after dosing. Lisuride is moderately bound to plasma proteins (70%).

Following the oral administration of radiolabelled drug to healthy volunteers (^{14}C-LHM), plasma levels (of total radioactivity) can be fitted by a two-compartment open model. Following absorption, the concentration of total radioactivity declines biphasically, with respective half lives of about one and eight h.

Independent of the route of administration, roughly equal proportions of the dose are eliminated via the renal and biliary route. The half life determined from urinary excretion data was 8–10 h for over 90% of the dose, and approximately 24 h for the remainder.

Whole-body autoradiography in the rat has shown that the highest concentrations are in the liver, gastrointestinal wall, lung and kidney. There does not appear to be any placental barrier in rabbits. In the brain, lisuride is concentrated in the pituitary gland. Lisuride is excreted in breast milk at concentrations about 10% of those in the blood.

Oral absorption	~100%
Presystemic metabolism	80–90%
Plasma half life	
mean	~8 h
Volume of distribution	$2.3–2.4\ l.kg^{-1}$
Plasma protein binding	70%

Concentration–effect relationship

There is no evidence of any correlation between the plasma concentration of lisuride and its therapeutic effects.

Metabolism

In man, five metabolites have been identified, the main one being the 2-keto-3-beta-hydroxy derivative. About one half of LHM undergoes N′-deethylation. None of the metabolites appear to contribute significantly to the effect of the drug.

Pharmaceutics

LHM is prescribed as white, round, convex, half-scored tablets of 0.025 (Cuvalit), 0.2 (Revanil) or 0.5 mg (Dopergin). They should be stored in a cool, dry condition and be protected from light.

Therapeutic use

The drug has been tried in a wide variety of conditions but the only licensed indication in the U.K. is for treatment of Parkinson's disease.

Indications

1. Parkinson's disease
2. Hyperprolactinaemia
3. The drug has also been studied in Cushing's syndrome and for migraine prophylaxis.

Contraindications

1. Pituitary tumour
2. Pregnancy.

Precautions

Great care should be taken in patients with severe peripheral vascular disease or coronary disease because of the possibility of inducing vasospasm.

Mode of use

1. Parkinson's disease
Oral lisuride has been used alone in the treatment of parkinsonism but it is usually combined with levodopa (and a decarboxylase inhibitor).[9] The starting dose is normally 0.2 mg which can be increased in increments of 0.2 mg. Most patients respond to doses between 1.5 and 4.5 mg daily. The manufacturers suggest a maximum dose of 5 mg daily although doses up to 10 mg daily have been given in trials. The daily dose should be fractionated because of the short half life. In some studies the drug has been given 2–3 times daily and in others as frequently as every 3 h.[10] Treatment for extended periods, up to 4 years, has shown sustained activity. McDonald and Horowski[11] reviewed approximately 375 patients from published (mainly open) clinical trials. Addition of lisuride to combination therapy with levodopa and a decarboxylase inhibitor resulted in a 20–50% improve-

Lisuride (hydrogen maleate)

ment in disability score and a 20–35% reduction in levodopa dosage. It has also been suggested that lisuride is more effective in controlling 'off' episodes and dyskinesias than levodopa.[9] Dystonia, particularly focal dystonia and dystonia with marked diurnal variations, is responsive to lisuride. On the other hand other parkinsonian syndromes, such as multiple system atrophies (progressive supranuclear palsy and Shy-Drager syndrome) are relatively resistant.

The side effect burden associated with use of lisuride is substantial and includes lightheadedness, drowsiness, vivid dreams and abdominal discomfort.[12] Most of the patients treated with lisuride have been refractory or advanced cases requiring high doses and the side effect profile should be interpreted with this in mind.

Since LHM is water-soluble, it can also be given by intravenous or subcutaneous infusion. In this way presystemic metabolism is circumvented and the daily dose can be reduced significantly. Infusion allows maintenance of constant blood levels which are thought to be helpful in the prevention of some side effects, e.g. peak dose dyskinesias, freezing and on–off fluctuations. For individual intravenous doses of 0.15 mg, the onset, peak effect and duration of action were at 5, 30 and 120 min respectively.

Long-term subcutaneous infusion of lisuride (2.5 mg/24 h) has been used to try and prevent motor fluctuations in Parkinson's disease. Domperidone, 10 mg 8 hourly, was used to control nausea and vomiting. Although treatment was initially successful in 3 patients with severe Parkinson's disease, chorea appeared in all the patients after 2–3 months.[13] In another study with an infusion pump, confusion, vivid dreams and memory disturbances occurred with dose increases.[14] Side effects appear to be too severe for this treatment to be generally applied in patients with on–off features. The doses used were large as the subcutaneous route avoids presystemic metabolism, which inactivates 75–90% of an oral dose.

2. Hyperprolactinaemia

LHM has been studied in the treatment of hyperprolactinaemic menstrual disorders, leading to reduction and normalization of prolactin levels, cessation of galactorrhoea and induction of menstruation and ovulation. The effective dose for lowering prolactin is 50–800 μg daily, usually given in two or three divided doses. Prolactinomas responded to LHM by a normalization of hormone release and reduction in size. Treatment of prolactinomas frequently required higher doses, up to 6 mg daily. However, an exact dose–response relationship has not yet been established and the manufacturers warn of the hazards associated with expansion of pituitary tumours during lisuride therapy. LHM is also effective for primary and secondary inhibition of lactation. In hyperprolactinaemic males, LHM similarly normalized prolactin and increased libido and sexual activity. Some acromegalics responded favourably to LHM. Bouloux et al concluded that the side effects of lisuride were more severe than with bromocriptine and that it could not be regarded as the first choice agent in hyperprolactinaemia. In their study two thirds of the patients stopped treatment because of side effects.

3. Other conditions

A single dose of LHM (0.2 mg) was found to reduce ACTH levels in seven of 14 patients with Cushing's disease.

For migraine prophylaxis, LHM was found to be superior to placebo, similar to methysergide in efficacy but with fewer side effects. The dose required was 75 μg daily in divided doses.[15]

Contraindications

1. Pituitary tumour

The manufacturers warn that extreme caution should be exercised in a patient who has, or has been treated for, a pituitary tumour. The tumour may enlarge, particularly during pregnancy, and visual field defects may develop.

2. Pregnancy

The drug has been taken during early pregnancy without apparent ill effect to mother or child but the numbers are small and the risk of teratogenicity has not been fully evaluated.

Adverse reactions

The adverse reactions so far reported for this drug all appear to be due to an excess of its known pharmacological actions, predominantly on the D_2 receptor.

Potentially life-threatening effects

None has been reported.

Acute overdosage

Deliberate overdose has not been reported but should be expected to induce ergotism as well as dopaminergic hyperstimulation. In two patients, bolus subcutaneous injection of about 3 mg resulted in deep sedation with a reduced level of consciousness but the patients recovered spontaneously within 24 h. In volunteer studies the dopamine antagonist, sulpiride, controlled most of the side effects of lisuride and this form of treatment might prove useful in case of overdose with features of excess dopaminergic stimulation.

Severe or irreversible adverse effects

CNS effects include drowsiness, memory disturbances and confusion, delirium and visual hallucinations, frequent and vivid dreams and, rarely, paranoid states. These are usually dose-related, the incidence is high and they can be severe. In some studies over half the patients have stopped treatment because of these adverse effects. Side effects sometimes appear after prolonged therapy without alteration of dosage. High doses often produce dyskinesias.

Autonomic effects related to dopaminergic activity include faintness and hypotension, particularly orthostatic hypotension. Patients who might be exposed to hazard if they became syncopal while standing should be warned. Other manifestations may be related to its ergot derivation, including cold extremities and digital vasospasm, burning of the skin and chest pain. These ergotism-like symptoms were reported, however, mainly in migraine sufferers who were also treated with other ergot-derived drugs.

Symptomatic adverse effects

Probably the most common adverse effects are nausea and vomiting which may occur early during therapy or after the dose is increased. Interestingly, this symptom is infrequent in women after childbirth (treated for suppression of lactation). The nausea can be prevented by pretreatment with a peripheral dopamine receptor blocker such as domperidone. Appetite changes in either direction have been noted. Weight gain following prolonged therapy has been reported.[9]

Other reported effects include headache, bradycardia, constipation, diarrhoea and xerostomia.

Interference with clinical pathology tests

No information is available.

High risk groups

Neonates

The drug is not used in neonates.

Breast milk. Lisuride is excreted in breast milk at concentrations about 10% of those in the blood so it would be inadvisable for a mother to breast-feed while taking the drug.

Children

The drug has been tried in the treatment of migraine in childhood but this is not an approved indication.

Pregnant women

The drug has been used successfully in the treatment of hyperprolactinaemia and infertility. Several women have ovulated and become pregnant before the drug has been stopped, sometimes months later. No ill effects on the mother or fetus have been reported thus far.

The elderly

Elderly subjects are more likely to develop confusion while taking lisuride, particularly against the background of dementia. Orthostatic hypotension is more likely to occur in very elderly patients and postural pressures should be checked.

Concurrent disease

Patients with peripheral vascular disease and coronary insufficiency may be susceptible to the ergot-like effects of LHM. Similarly a history of psychotic disease may predispose individuals to psychiatric side effects.

Drug interactions

The most obvious drug interaction is with other agents acting on dopamine receptors, whether as agonists (in which case synergism will occur) or as antagonists.

Lisuride (hydrogen maleate)

L

Lisuride has been combined with levodopa and dopa decarboxylase inhibitors in a number of studies. A moderate reduction of levodopa dose is often possible during treatment with the combination.

Centrally acting D_2 antagonists will block all the dopaminergic effects of LHM, while domperidone, which does not penetrate the brain readily, antagonizes primarily nausea, vomiting and orthostatic hypotension.

The effect of alcohol is not potentiated by LHM.

Clinical trials

Very few controlled studies of lisuride have been carried out and most of the available evidence of clinical efficacy is drawn from open studies.

1. LeWitt P A, Gopinathan G, Ward C D, Sanes J N, Dambrosia J M, Durso R, Calne D B 1982 Lisuride versus bromocriptine treatment in Parkinson's disease: a double-blind study. Neurology 32: 69–72

A double-blind crossover comparison of lisuride and bromocriptine was made in 28 patients with Parkinson's disease. The dose in each limb of the study was titrated for optimum effect. Each treatment period lasted 7–10 weeks. Other anti-parkinsonian medication, such as levodopa, was continued.

26 of the 28 patients completed the study. The mean daily dose of lisuride was 4.5 mg and of bromocriptine 56.5 mg. The only significant difference in efficacy was slightly better control of akinesia with bromocriptine. Many patients reported sedation but the incidence was similar with both drugs. Day-time hallucinations were more common on lisuride than bromocriptine (7 versus 1) but dry mouth was slightly less common on the former drug (9 versus 14).

2. Giovannini P, Scigliano G, Piccolo I, Soliveri P, Suchy I 1988 Lisuride in Parkinson's disease: a 4 year follow-up. Clinical Neuropharmacology 11: 201–211

This was an open study lasting 4 years in which parkinsonian patients were treated with lisuride alone in a dose of 3 mg daily or in combination with levodopa plus a dopa decarboxylase inhibitor. Half the 20 patients receiving lisuride alone withdrew because of lack of efficacy or side effects. Those who remained on monotherapy showed objective improvements. 14 of 36 patients on combination therapy withdrew, mainly because of side effects. In the patients maintained on combination therapy, resting tremor was improved at all time points but there was not a consistent improvement in akathisia or rigidity.

3. Bouloux P M G, Besser G M, Grossman A, Moult P G A 1987 Clinical evaluation of Lisuride in the management of hyperprolactinaemia. British Medical Journal 294: 1323–1324

42 patients with hyperprolactinaemia were treated with lisuride in incremental doses ranging from 0.1 mg daily to 1.2 mg daily. After a mean of 5.4 months, 8 patients had normal prolactin and in a further 15 the concentrations had been reduced. Five of 13 women with primary or secondary infertility became pregnant. The incidence of side effects was very high. Two thirds of patients stopped the drug because of side effects, the four most common being nausea, drowsiness, dizziness and depression.

General review articles

Calne D B, Horowski R, McDonald R J, Wuttke W 1983 Lisuride and other dopamine agonists. Raven Press, New York

Lieberman A N, Goldstein M, Gopinathan G, Neophytides A 1987 D-1 and D-2 agonists in Parkinson's disease. Canadian Journal of Neurological Sciences 14: 466–473

Lang A 1987 Update on dopamine agonists in Parkinson's disease: 'Beyond bromocriptine'. Canadian Journal of Neurological Sciences 14: 474–482

References

1. Fujita N, Saito K, Yonehara N, Watanabe Y, Yoshida H 1979 Binding of 3H-lisuride hydrogen maleate to striatal membranes of rat brain. Life Science 25: 969–974
2. Da Prada M, Bonetti E P, Keller H H 1977 Induction of mounting behaviour in female and male rats by lisuride. Neuroscience Letters 6: 349–353
3. Horowski R, Wachtel H 1976 Direct dopaminergic action of lisuride hydrogen maleate, an ergot derivative, in mice. European Journal of Pharmacology 36: 373–383
4. Kehr W 1977 Effect of lisuride and other ergot derivatives on monoaminergic mechanisms in rat brain. European Journal of Pharmacology 41: 261–273
5. Pieri L, Keller H H, Burkhard W, da Prada M 1978 Effect of lisuride and LSD on cerebral monoaminergic systems and hallucinosis. Nature 272:278–280
6. Horowski R, Dorow R, Loschmann P, Runge I, Wachtel H, Obeso J A 1989 Oral and parenteral use of lisuride in Parkinson's disease: Clinical pharmacology and implications for therapy. In: Calne D B et al (eds) Parkinsonisn and aging. Raven Press, New York, pp 269–285
7. Burn R S, Gopinatham G, Hümpel M, Dorow R, Calne D B 1984 Disposition of oral lisuride in Parkinson's disease. Clinical Pharmacology and Therapeutics 35: 548–556
8. Hümpel M 1983 Disposition of oral lisuride in Parkinson's disease. In: Calne D B et al (eds) Lisuride and other dopamine agonists. Raven Press, New York, pp 141–153
9. Rabey J M, Streifler M, Treves T A, Korczyn A D 1989 A long-term comparative study of lisuride and levodopa in Parkinson's disease. In: Calne D B et al (eds) Parkinsonism and aging. Raven Press, New York, pp 261–267
10. Lieberman A N, Leibowitz M, Gopinathan G, Walker R, Hiesinger E, Nelson J, Goldstein M 1985 Review: The use of pergolide and lisuride, two experimental dopamine agonists, in patients with advanced Parkinson's disease. American Journal of Medical Sciences 290: 102–106
11. McDonald R J, Horowski R 1983 Lisuride in treatment of Parkinsonism. European Neurology 22: 240–255
12. Ulm G 1983 Experiences with lisuride in the treatment of Parkinson's disease. In: Calne D B et al (eds) Lisuride and other dopamine agonists. Raven Press, New York, pp 463–472
13. Obeso J A, Luquin M R, Martinez-Lage J M 1986 Lisuride infusion pump: a device for treatment of motor fluctuations in Parkinson's disease. Lancet 1: 467–470
14. Castro-Caldos A, Costa C, Sampaio C 1986 Lisuride infusion pump for Parkinson's disease. Lancet 1: 1150–1151
15. Herrman WM, Horowski R, Dannehl K, Kramer U, Lurati K 1977 Clinical effectiveness of lisuride hydrogen maleate: a double-blind trial versus methysergide. Headache 17: 54–60

Lithium

Lithium was introduced into materia medica in about 1845[1,2] as a drug for treatment of diseases thought to be caused by gastric uric acid, i.e. 'the uric acid diathesis'. Lithium carbonate and lithium citrate were incorporated in the British Pharmacopoeia in 1864. In 1871, Hammond[3] recommended a high first-day dose of lithium followed by smaller maintenance doses for acute treatment of mania and depression, and in 1886 Lange[4] recommended prophylactic lithium for periodic depression. The rediscovery of the antimanic and prophylactic effects of lithium was made in 1949 by Cade[5] and in 1963 and 1964 by Hartigan[6] and Baastrup[7], respectively.

Chemistry

Lithium ion (Camcolit, Liskonum, Phasal, Priadel, Litarex) Li^+.
Lithium carbonate $Li_2\,CO_3$. Lithium citrate $C_6H_5Li_3\,O_7.\,4H_2O$.
Li is third in the periodic system and the lightest metallic element (specific gravity: 0.534). It is a member of the alkaline metals in group IA. Because of its large ionic radius in aqueous solution, it is close to calcium and magnesium of the neighbouring group IIA of the alkaline earths.

Molecular weight	
carbonate	73.9
citrate	282.0
pKa	—
Solubility	
in alcohol	insoluble
in water	
carbonate	1 in 100
citrate	1 in 2
Octanol/water partition coefficient	—

The pharmacological properties, therapeutic as well as prophylactic, of lithium salts are attached solely to the lithium ion, Li^+.

The tablet content of the active factor consequently varies with the type of salt used, depending on the chemical valency and molecular weight of the anion. Lithium doses should be stated as the molar weight of the Li^+, i.e. in practice in millimoles (mmol).

Pharmacology

Lithium is primarily used for its antimanic effect. However, its exact mode of action in the brain is uncertain, perhaps because the cause of the illness itself is unclear. Initially, lithium was thought to compete with Na^+, K^+ or other cations. However, lithium is not an adequate substitute for sodium in the 'sodium pump' and cannot maintain membrane potentials. In animal studies, lithium at therapeutic concentrations used in man (1 mM) has little effect on catecholamine-sensitive adenylate cyclase activity but does inhibit the calcium-dependent release of noradrenaline and dopamine. The release of 5HT may be slightly increased.[8]

Lithium, at a concentration of 1 mM, also inhibits the hydrolysis of myoinositol phosphate in brain,[1] and as a result lithium may reduce the cellular content of phosphatidylinositides. These substances act as second messengers in brain cells (particularly inositol trisphosphate) and depletion of phosphatidylinositides may reduce the sensitivity of neurones to endogenous neurotransmitters such as acetylcholine and noradrenaline.[9]

Toxicology

In 1876 Hesse[10] observed damage to the cerebrum and spinal cord or the heart (the latter possibly secondary to the cerebral effect) when lethal doses of lithium were administered to animals.

Animal studies at lower doses have shown that, depending on dosage size and treatment duration, lithium may induce varying degrees of histopathological, primarily distal, changes of the nephron.[11] Moderate enlargement of the thyroid may also occur. There is evidence that high lithium concentrations exert a teratogenic effect.[12]

Clinical pharmacology

Lithium is mainly used prophylactically in bipolar and unipolar manic–depressive illness for attenuation of both manic and depressive episodes[13] and, to a certain degree, therapeutically in mania.[14] In addition, it has been tried in treatment of endogenous depression and pathological aggression and prophylactically in attenuation of schizo-affective disorders.[15,16] The diuretic properties of lithium appear to be mediated via antagonism of the renal respone to ADH with a consequent reduction of the renal concentrating ability. The pathogenesis of lithium-induced nephrogenic diabetes insipidus which may persist for a time after the drug is stopped, is less certain.

Weight gain is common during lithium treatment. The most likely explanation may be that patients counteract the lithium-induced polyuria/polydipsia[17] by intake of calorie-rich drinks, but a direct action of lithium on thirst and appetite regulation cannot be excluded.

Lithium treatment often aggravates physiological hand tremor. The aetiology is unknown, but a possible explanation may be that lithium exerts a direct action on the spinal cord.

In most cases, lithium treatment affects depolarization of the heart, which is reflected in the ECG by low or inverted T waves and, infrequently, disturbances of the heart rhythm. In the brain lithium produces high voltage slow waves in the EEG.

Pharmacokinetics

Atomic emission or atomic absorption spectrophotometry are the only available methods for estimation of lithium, but alternatives, such as ion-selective electrodes, fluorometric, and conventional spectrophotometric determinations, are under development which may eventually fulfil the need for an easily available assay method. The atomic emission spectrophotometric method has a sensitivity for lithium in serum of $0.15\ mmol.l^{-1}$.

Lithium has simple pharmacokinetic properties; being a metallic ion it is not catabolized, neither is it protein-bound. Its distribution volume approximates to the body water volume but concentrations in white matter, thyroid, and bones are several-fold higher than the plasma concentration. Entry into the cerebrospinal fluid is relatively slow and the equilibrium concentration is about 40% of that in the plasma. Lithium is eliminated exclusively by the kidneys; it is filtered at the glomerulus and reabsorbed almost like sodium in the proximal tubules (i.e. to about 80%), but normally it is not reabsorbed in the distal parts of the nephron. Under sufficiently standardized circumstances the renal lithium clearance may be used as an approximate measure of the delivery of sodium from the proximal tubules.

The serum concentration curve of lithium taken orally (the only route of administration used in practice) shows rapid absorption, dependent upon the drug formulation. After intake of an aquous solution, the peak concentration occurs within about 30 min, after conventional tablets the absorption is variable starting at about 30 min with a maximum after 4–5 hours, and after slow-release tablets there is a broad maximum at about 5 hours. After the peak a biphasic fall occurs. The rapid α-phase lasts about 1.15 h and is followed by a slower β-phase with a half life ranging from 8 to 45 h with a mean of 24 h;[18] elimination can be simulated by a two-compartment model.[19]

Oral absorption	>97%
Presystemic metabolism	nil
Plasma half life	
range	8–45 h
Volume of distribution	$0.8\ l.kg^{-1}$
Plasma protein binding	<10%

Lithium

L

Concentration–effect relationship

The antimanic action of lithium was rediscovered on the basis of a treatment regimen using rather high maintenance doses.[5] Regardless of the reasons for this choice[3,20] it has largely determined the size of today's dosage regimens. Because the therapeutic ratio is narrow and both efficacy and toxicity are related to concentration, therapeutic monitoring of serum lithium concentrations is universal.[21]

The standardized (12 h post-dose serum lithium, abbreviated to 12 h-stSLi) is an indispensable tool in monitoring individual patients, but it should only be regarded as a very crude approximation concerning safety against poisoning on the one hand and failing efficacy on the other.[22] The concentration varies widely throughout the day, even with a twice daily regimen, the peak concentrations being about twice the trough values. Lithium concentrations in plasma correlate reasonably well with its antimanic effect. The therapeutic range[23] is usually stated to be from 0.75 to 1.25 $mmol.l^{-1}$ although a lower range of 0.5–0.8 $mmol.l^{-1}$ has also been proposed.[24] When plasma concentrations are used for treatment monitoring purposes, the time of dosing must be taken into account and trough concentrations, i.e. pre-dose values should be used.[25] The relationship between the desired effects and serum concentrations of lithium have not been fully validated and there is substantial interindividual variation[21,22,26,27] However, no better method of treatment monitoring for this toxic drug exists and variation within an individual is less than between individuals.

Metabolism

Being the ion of an element, lithium is not catabolized in the organism and is eliminated unchanged by the kidneys. Under normal circumstances lithium is only reabsorbed by the proximal renal tubules (about 80%), but unlike potassium, sodium, and water it is not reabsorbed by the distal parts of the nephron. The lithium concentration in the distal luminal fluid and in the bladder urine may therefore be 25–50 times a concentration which would be regarded as toxic for other tissues. However, even in long-term treatment this seems only exceptionally to entail serious sequelae.

Pharmaceutics

In the UK lithium is available in the formulations shown in Table 1.

Table 1

Proprietary name (Manufacturer)	Li (mmol)	Salt (mg)	Identification code (colour)
Camcolit-250 (Norgine)	6.8	carbonate (250)	'CAMCOLIT' (white)
Camcolit-400 (Norgine)*	10.8	carbonate (400)	'S' 'CAMCOLIT' (white)
Liskonum (SK&F)*	12.2	carbonate (450)	oblong (white)
Litarex (CP)*	6	citrate (564)	oval (white)
Phasal (Lagap)*	8.1	carbonate (300)	'P' in hexagon (white)
Priadel (Delandale)*	10.8	carbonate (400)	'PRIADEL' (white)
Priadel-200 (Delandale)*	5.4	carbonate (200)	'P 200' (white)
Priadel Liquid (Delandale)	5.4/5 ml	citrate (520)	pineapple/sugar free

*Sustained-release preparation.

In the USA lithium is available in the formulations shown in Table 2.

Table 2

Proprietary name (Manufacturer)	Li (mmol)	Salt (mg)	Identification code (colour)
Cibalith-S syrup (CIBA)	8.0/5 ml	citrate (752)	Raspberry/sugar-free
Eskalith capsules (SK&F)	8.1	carbonate (300)	'ESKALITH' (yellow/grey)
Eskalith tablets (SK&F)	8.1	carbonate (300)	'SKF' 'J09' (white)
Eskalith CR tablets (SK&F)*	12.2	carbonate (450)	'SKF' 'J10' (yellow)
Lithane (Miles)	8.1	carbonate (300)	'MILES' '951' (green)
Lithium carbonate capsules (Roxane)	4.05	carbonate (150)	'54 213' (white)
Lithium carbonate capsules (Roxane)	8.1	carbonate (300)	'54 463' (pink)
Lithium carbonate capsules (Roxane)	16.2	carbonate (600)	'54 702' (white/pink)
Lithium carbonate tablets (Roxane)	8.1	carbonate (300)	'54 452' (white)
Lithium citrate syrup (Roxane)	8.0/5 ml	citrate (752)	sugar-free
Lithium citrate syrup (Roxane)	10.0/10 ml	citrate (940)	sugar-free
Lithobid tablets (CIBA)*	8.1	carbonate (300)	'CIBA' '65' (pink)

*Sustained-release preparation.

Outside the UK and USA other lithium salts are in use as well such as sulphate, acetate, adipate, gluconate and glutamate.

When choosing between preparations their lithium content should be carefully considered. The dosage required by one patient with short(er) half life and high tolerance towards the toxicity of lithium is so high that it may be toxic to another patient with long(er) half life and low tolerance.

In addition the slow-release preparations Liskonum and Litarex with the suggested advantage of low maximum values may not be tolerated by certain patients because of loose stools or diarrhoea provoked by distal release of lithium in the intestines; in such cases conventional tablets or, better still, aqueous solutions with early high concentration peaks reflecting proximal absorption may be better tolerated.

Therapeutic use

Indications

1. Prophylaxis (prevention or attenuation) of recurrent mood disorders and schizo-affective psychosis
2. Acute treatment of mania
3. Acute treatment of depression
4. Use in other psychiatric conditions
5. Use in non-psychiatric conditions.

Contraindications

1. Kidney disorder
2. Heart disease
3. Disturbed electrolyte balance
4. Salt-poor diets
5. Major surgery
6. Pregnancy, delivery and lactation
7. Psoriasis
8. Acneiform eruptions.

Mode of use

Oral administration is used for lithium treatment.

A number of laboratory tests before and during treatment are considered mandatory.

Before starting treatment, body weight, blood pressure, ECG, haemoglobin, white blood cells, thyrotropin (TSH), serum creatinine, urine analysis for glucose, protein and casts and a pregnancy test should be carried out. During treatment, control serum lithium (SLi) (12 h-stSLi) and serum creatinine should be performed every 2–3 months, TSH every 6 months.

In spite of its shortcomings, the control SLi remains our only supplement to the difficult clinical evaluation of symptoms after start of treatment. During initiation of the treatment it is used as a guide in approximating individual maintenance dosage without risk of intoxication.

Treatment of acute mania should be started with a moderate dose, e.g. 30 mmol daily, and with daily measurement of 12 h-stSLi; the dosage should be adjusted taking account of accumulation.

During initiation of prophylactic treatment, time is available for a safer dose-titration procedure: a low dose, for example 3 or 4 mmol lithium, is given twice daily until a steady state is reached (about a week); the control SLi (12 h-stSLi) is checked daily for 3–4 consecutive days; the daily dose is then increased according to the mean of these check values (direct proportionality between dosage and the mean of 12 h-stSLi). During the next two months the control SLi should be checked weekly and the dosage adjusted accordingly; the reproducibility of the control SLi should also be observed during this phase. Thereafter, plasma concentrations should be monitored every 2–4 months, indefinitely.

A more rational, but less safe, starting procedure is to predict the maintenance dose by using a time-specified lithium concentration after a single pretest dose.[28–30]

Lithium treatment should not be stopped abruptly because of a risk of rebound of psychiatric symptoms.

Indications

1. Unipolar depression, bipolar depression, and schizo-affective psychosis

Strict diagnostic criteria should be applied before patients are regarded as candidates for prophylactic treatment with lithium. In general, they are unipolar patients who have experienced one episode within the last five years, bipolar patients with one episode within the last four years, and schizo-affective patients with one episode within the last three years.

The clinical trials so far published have differed in terms of diagnostic classification, treatment procedures, and rate of treatment compliance. This has made it difficult to estimate the response to be expected, but a realistic assessment may be that prevention of mood swings occurs in 30–60% of patients, attenuation of these episodes in 30–50% and non-response in 10–20% of patients with unipolar and bipolar depression.

Achieving the desired response depends on maintaining a consistent serum concentration over a prolonged time period.[18]

2. Mania

The onset of the antimanic effect of lithium takes place over a period of hours to some days. It is now common practice to start treatment of acute mania with a neuroleptic drug, often haloperidol, possibly in combination with lithium, and then gradually reduce the dose of neuroleptic. This custom may be the reason why the quick-acting neuroleptics are currently preferred in mania, so that lithium treatment is often neglected.

There have been surprisingly few clinical trials on the antimanic efficacy of lithium and those so far published are lacking in uniformity concerning exact diagnostic classification, disease severity, differentiation between statistical and clinical significance, and dosage and serum lithium concentrations. However, some conclusions have been drawn.

In violent patients, treatment with an antipsychotic drug is preferable to lithium treatment. In moderate manic excitement, a satisfactory response can be expected in about 75% of the patients treated with lithium. The response frequency apparently improves if the individual dosage (4–100 mmol daily) is increased somewhat during the first few weeks. In the middle of a manic episode such a high dose seems to be both required and well tolerated.

If after two weeks on this treatment, combined with a neuroleptic, the condition has not improved the patient should be considered a non-responder to lithium. In responsive patients, abrupt discontinuation of lithium usually results in relapse within a few days.

3. Depression

Hammond[3] and Garrod[31] both recommended lithium-containing salts for acute treatment of depression, and Lange used lithium carbonate alone against acute 'uric acid' depression.[32]

After Kraepelin's[33] union of mania and depression in the manic-depressive psychosis and Cade's[5] revival of lithium against mania, trials in acute depression[5,34] provided negative results only, lithium was deemed therapeutically ineffective in these patients. However, some acutely depressed patients do respond although lithium is not a treatment of first choice. It may be worth trying in patients who respond poorly or not at all to other antidepressive treatments, either alone or in combination with a tricyclic antidepressant.[35]

4. Other psychiatric conditions

Until recently, prophylactic lithium treatment has been regarded as 'specific' for conditions which are closely related to the manic-depressive disorders. Current investigations have suggested that prophylactic lithium may be useful in other periodic or recurrent psychiatric disorders. Only patients with unstable character disorders and episodic aggressiveness and assaultive behaviour, violent sociopaths, children, and mentally retarded persons are well-documented lithium responders. This use of lithium is limited by a general hesitation about administering drugs to children and to inmates of penal institutions[36].

5. Non-psychiatric indications

An inhibitory effect of lithium on the thyroid was discovered by Sedvall and co-workers[37] in a controlled animal study. The results are consistent with human studies assessing the usefulness of short-term lithium in similar doses in acute thyrotoxicosis. Lithium inhibits release of thyroxine (and thus of iodine) by the thyroid. A combination of lithium and radioactive iodine has been used in metabolizing thyroid cancer to prolong the radioactivity within the cancer cells.

Many lithium-treated patients develop impairment of the renal concentrating ability. Part of the explanation is that lithium inhibits the ADH-sensitive adenylate cyclase in the distal nephron. Reports on the effect of lithium treatment on the syndrome of inappropriate secretion of antidiuretic hormone have been somewhat contradictory and must be regarded as experimental.

Most lithium-treated patients have a moderate granulocytosis with increased granulocyte counts within the normal range; some patients show counts of up to 10 000–14 000 per mm^3, while counts above 20 000 are exceptional. In some cases this moderate leucocytosis is consistent, in others it is periodic. Its aetiology is probably increased colony-stimulating activity. There is no evidence whether this increase in neutrophil count can be used for therapeutic purposes in granulocytopenia.

Lithium also appears effective in the periodic type of cluster headache, especially in patients over 45 years of age. Lithium has mainly been tried in patients refractory to other treatments, and more conclusive controlled double-blind studies are needed.

An uncontrolled study has shown a statistically significant beneficial effect of lithium in Ménière's disease, but the results could not be replicated in a double-blind study by the same investigators and using almost the same patient material.

Contraindications

1. Kidney disorder

Stable renal function is a prerequisite for successful lithium treatment, which is therefore contraindicated in conditions with varying kidney function such as patients with active glomerulonephritis or pyelonephritis, or in uncontrolled heart failure. Once the condition has stabilized these are only relative contraindications.

The renal function usually decreases with advancing age. The lithium dosage may need a gradual reduction after the age of 60.

2. Heart disease

Apart from the possible influence of heart diseases on kidney function, lithium exerts a specific action on the electrocardiogram; the changes most often consist of lowering or inversion of T waves, but more serious disturbances of the conducting system occasionally appear. Lithium-treated patients should be taught to recognize an irregular pulse and if this occurs to contact a physician or cardiologist.

3. Disturbed electrolyte balance
Lithium clearance varies with sodium consumption, even with sodium intakes within the 'normal' range. If the sodium intake decreases below normal or there is non-renal loss of salt and water, and especially during hyponatraemia, the renal lithium clearance decreases. Close control of electrolyte status and 12 h-stSLi is particularly important during and after major surgery and other conditions with risk of disturbed salt and water balance. Temporary discontinuation of lithium may be necessary until rehydration has been established (but there is a risk of rapid relapse of mania).

4. Salt-poor diets
The first 'lithium scare' in 1949 was created by the death from lithium poisoning of several patients who had been put on a low sodium diet.[38] In this connection it should be remembered that many popular slimming diets are also salt-poor diets.[39].

5. Major surgery
Before planned major surgery the surgical team should take into account that lithium-induced polyuria often persists for weeks or months after withdrawal of long-term lithium. Very close attention should be paid to fluid balance during the postoperative period.

Lithium may potentiate the effect of muscular relaxants and should preferably be withdrawn at least three days before planned surgery involving use of muscle relaxants.

In order to avoid manic or depressive relapse lithium treatment should be resumed as soon as possible.

Adverse reactions

Potentially life-threatening effects
Death from lithium intoxication is well known.[39,40] Cade's very first patient died of lithium poisoning two years after the start of intermittent lithium therapy.[41]

For obvious reasons, our knowledge about lithium's toxicity stems from single case reports[39,42]. SLi has become more reliable for regulating treatment within one individual,[43] but substantial interindividual differences in the concentrations at which toxicity appears make caution essential. 12 h-SLi is often mistakenly regarded as being equal to the mean 24-hour SLi (MSLi), which may prove a pitfall in patients with shorter half life i.e. <20 hours. A concentration of no more than 0.8 $mmol.l^{-1}$ may indicate a dangerously high MSLi[22] and imply the start of a slowly progressing lithium poisoning[39,40] if the dosage has been adjusted by 12 h-stSLi.

Lithium poisoning should be assessed on the basis of symptoms, and if these are present treatment should be stopped immediately.[39,40]. Unfortunately, the clinical symptoms of intoxication often only manifest themselves after hours to days; even extremely high acute overdoses often produce only short-lasting gastrointestinal symptoms immediately after the dose. In this situation, 12 h-stSLi is a crude but useful guide.[22]

A 12 h-stSLi of >1.5 $mmol^{-1}$ usually indicates risk of an impending poisoning. It is, however, important to note that a SLi of 0.7–1.4 $mmol.l^{-1}$ may be toxic in persons with a shorter half life or in particularly susceptible patients.

A 12 h-stSLi of >2.5 $mmol.l^{-1}$ is most often accompanied by overt, but frequently mild, clinical features of poisoning.

A 12 h-stSLi of >3.5 $mmol.l^{-1}$ should always be regarded as potentially life-threatening.

Most lithium poisonings develop gradually over some days after start of treatment or an increase of dose. A vicious circle may also be initiated by temporarily reduced renal function due to kidney disorders, dehydration due to fever, vomiting, diarrhoea, salt-poor diets, and heavy sweating (residence in a hot climate, occupational, etc.).[44,45]

The clinical picture of lithium poisoning most often shows a period of latency followed by CNS symptoms of variable severity. Gastrointestinal symptoms are less frequent. Lithium intoxication has been classified into three grades of severity.[40,42,46]

The most severe grade (III) is characterized by a stupor-like state of semi-coma (manifest coma is seldom seen until just before death), complete muteness, convulsive muscular reactions to strong stimuli (often confined to the eyes), convulsions and acute renal failure.

Grade II is characterized by slightly impaired consciousness and mental concentration, slight muscular twitching, tremor, dysarthria, unsteady gait, increased tendon reflexes, and slightly increased serum creatinine.

Grade I (also called prodromal symptoms) resembles Grade II, but the symptoms are less severe. Fortunately, they are easily recognized by many patients because of their close resemblance to the transient 'initial side effects' occurring during the first weeks of treatment.

In severe intoxication haemodialysis, should be instituted and repeated until a sufficiently low lithium concentration has been achieved (SLi <1.0 $mmol.l^{-1}$ after rebound).[39,40]

Other countermeasures such as intravenous sodium loading[42] and forced diuresis have been suggested. However, sodium loading is not sufficiently effective against severe lithium poisoning and may involve a risk of dangerous hypernatraemia in patients with impaired renal concentrating ability.[40] Forced diuresis is also of dubious efficacy in more severe lithium poisoning; its only consequence may be that invaluable time is lost.

In mild poisoning (slight symptoms and moderately increased 12 h-stSLi) withdrawal of lithium and correction of water and electrolyte balance is usually all that is required.

It is important to be aware that serious toxicity may only become manifest when the lithium concentration has begun to fall. The most common permanent disabilities are characterized by cerebellar and extrapyramidal damage[42,47] and reduced renal function.[40] The acute renal toxicity of lithium may cause no symptoms at all; and a silent progressive impairment of renal function may take place.[40,42]

Acute overdosage
Intentional self-poisoning with lithium is uncommon. Even extremely high acute overdoses of lithium often cause only slight early signs of poisoning apart from abdominal distress or vomiting. After a latent period of several hours to a few days, however, many patients develop serious symptoms of poisoning, which may result in permanent disability or death. This may happen even when the progressively impaired but still functioning kidneys have reduced the lithium load to a 'normal' therapeutic level. The time for prompt haemodialysis, which might have been life-saving if it had been initiated earlier, has now been passed.[40,42]

Severe or irreversible adverse effects
Animal studies have shown severe renal adverse effects of lithium to occur with affection of the distal tubules of the nephron, resulting in histopathological changes, polyuria, and reduced concentrating ability during long-term administration.[11,38,48] In humans, however, severe histopathological changes in the kidney seem to be related to previous episodes of acute intoxication,[44] Some degree of increased diuresis, often deserving the designation polyuria, is almost universal during lithium treatment. A polyuria of more than 4 l daily may be very troublesome to the patient, but the problem can usually be reduced by lowering the MSLi, that is, the lithium dose, by 20–30%.

The reduction of the renal concentrating ability, with or without polyuria, may become irreversible and involve risk of a life-threatening dehydration.

Symptomatic adverse effects
Innumerable effects of this kind have been described, mainly based on single case reports,[49] but from a practical viewpoint only a few deserve mention.

Psoriasis. Lithium may occasionally cause exacerbation of psoriasis, and cases of lithium-provoked development of psoriasis have been published.[50]

Acneiform eruptions. Lithium-induced acneiform eruptions of unusual areas such as legs, forearms, and upper arms are not rare, in particular in younger persons; the face is less often affected.

Reduction of mental concentration. Although disturbing for the patient it seldom requires discontinuation of lithium.

Hand tremor. This problem may be reduced by lowering the lithium dose, but intermittent administration of β-blockers may be useful, for example, 10–20 mg of propranolol one hour before an important meeting.

Thyroid disorders. Lithium-induced hypothyroidism or goitre should be treated by moderate doses of levothyroxine until TSH has been normalized.[51]

Weight gain. This may, of course, be due to hypothyroidism but is more often the result of excessive intake of calorie-containing drinks.

Lithium

ECG changes. Flattened T waves in the ECG may be regarded as a harmless phenomenon.

Cardiac arrhythmias. Disturbances of the heart rhythm call for attention, and a cardiologist should be consulted.

High risk groups

Neonates

There is no indication for administration of lithium to neonates.

Breast milk. Lithium is excreted through the mother's milk and since the kidney function of neonates sets in only gradually, lactation may imply a potential risk of lithium accumulation and hence poisoning. In addition, neonates are more prone to dehydration which may result in a concurrent reduction of lithium elimination. However, some physicians regard the value of the intimate contact between child and mother during nursing to outweigh the limited potential risk of lithium exposure through the breast milk, since the child has already been exposed to the mother's lithium load during at least the last six months of pregnancy. However, a case of lithium intoxication in infancy has been published.[52]

Children

No special precautions are required when compared with lithium treatment of adults.

Pregnant women

Studies in experimental animals have shown lithium in high doses to exert some teratogenic action. The effect in humans during treatment with common therapeutic doses is under debate, but some relation between lithium treatment during the first trimester and the occurrence of serious heart defects in the infant cannot be excluded. Lithium-treated women in the fertile age-group should therefore use contraceptive measures, and lithium should be avoided during the first trimester of a planned pregnancy. If an unplanned pregnancy is discovered within the first three months, lithium treatment should be stopped.[12,53]

During pregnancy, the kidney function and hence the renal lithium clearance often show a gradual increase. If this is overlooked, 12 h-stSLi will decrease and treatment become less effective. If, on the other hand, the dosage is gradually increased in order to keep the SLi at a constant level there may be risk of lithium intoxication after delivery when kidney function returns to the prepregnancy level. After delivery, treatment should be resumed with very frequent control of 12 h-stSLi until the previous MSLi has been reached.

The elderly

No special precautions are required when the lithium dosage is adjusted by reference to the results of continual checks of the control SLi.

Concurrent disease

Heart disease. Relapse of manic excitement or agitated depression may be a more serious risk to such patients than lithium treatment, but careful control by physician and laboratory is needed.

Renal disease. The most serious problem is presented by patients with rapid and unpredictable variations of renal function. A more consistent and gradual reduction of renal function in chronic kidney disease requires close control. Even anuric patients being treated by haemodialysis can be treated with lithium by adding the correct amount of lithium to the dialysis fluid.

Drug interactions

Potentially hazardous interactions

Diuretics. Diuretics alter sodium and lithium excretion. Combined treatment with lithium and diuretics needs very careful consideration and the importance of strict compliance concerning both drugs should be stressed to the patient; the control SLi should be closely checked and the lithium dosage possibly readjusted.[54]

Non-steroidal anti-inflammatory drugs (NSAID). All NSAIDs, with the possible exception of acetylsalicylic acid (aspirin), seem to reduce lithium elimination and hence an increased MSLi on an unchanged lithium dosage. This is probably independent of any type of nephrotoxic adverse effects. MSLi may rise to the patient's point of acute renal toxicity and start progressive lithium poisoning.[39]

Neuromuscular-blocking agents. Although rare, the possibility of an unpredictable and prolonged synergistic effect of lithium and these drugs, especially pancuronium and suxamethonium, should be considered,[54] and lithium should cautiously be withdrawn at least three days before elective surgery.

Neuroleptics. Combined treatment with lithium and neuroleptic drugs is common and usually justifiable. The report by Cohen and Cohen[55] about serious sequelae in the form of encephalitis-like encephalopathy was based on only four patients and subsequent clinical investigations has shown this useful combination to be safe.[54]

Other significant interactions

Miscellaneous drugs. Questions pertaining to unusual combinations may be addressed in the USA, to The Lithium Information Center, Department of Psychiatry, University Hospital, 600 Highland Avenue, WI 53 792, USA. Telephone (608) 263-6171, or, in the UK, to the local Drug Information Service.

Food. Food in general has no significant effect on the metabolism of lithium in man. However, sodium-poor diets may cause a compensatory increase of the proximal renal sodium reabsorption and hence an increased reabsorption of lithium.

Alcohol. A suggested beneficial effect on chronic alcoholism is under discussion.

Potentially useful interactions

Antidepressants. Several case reports have shown lithium to augment antidepressants in cases of unsatisfactory response; an assessment was published in 1983.[35]

Monoamine oxidase inhibitors. When given in combination with lithium, these drugs may be useful in treatment of resistant depression, in break-through depression during prophylactic lithium treatment, and in rapid cyclers, i.e. patients with four or more cycles per year.

Carbamazepine and other anticonvulsant drugs. The anticonvulsant carbamazepine has been recommended in recent years as an alternative or adjunct to therapeutic and prophylactic lithium treatment as has a combination with some other anticonvulsants.

Classic descriptions

1. Hammond W A 1871 A treatise on diseases of the nervous system. D Appleton & Co, New York, Trubner & Co, London.

This book is a classical example of textbooks of the time. Chapter XV, section 5 describes in detail characteristic single cases of acute mania with exaltation and acute mania with depression and amplifies the text by showing a woodcut portrait of a 'characteristic' patient from each group.

2. Lange C 1896 Periodische Depressionszustände und Ihre Pathogenesis auf den Boden der harnsauren Diathese. Autorisierte deutsche Ausgabe nach der zweiten Auflage der Originals von Dr Hans Kurella. Verlag von Leopold Voss, Hamburg and Leipzig.

Major outcome trials

1. Noack C H, Trautner E M 1951 The lithium treatment of maniacal psychosis. Medical Journal of Australia 38: 219–222

The authors were inspired by Cade's[5] discovery of the antimanic effect of lithium carbonate and lithium citrate to try lithium in about 100 patients with psychotic excitement. The study design was open as was conventional at the time but the results still acceptable regarding this pronounced disease. Out of about 30 patients with the diagnosis of mania, 97% showed response. These authors also found it necessary to use near-toxic dosages: 'The dose varied greatly with each patient; some required amounts equal to those given in the acute phase whilst with others the dosage could be considerably reduced, or even stopped all together, to be recommenced at the first signs of recurring excitement. Patients whose maintenance dose was greater than 0.3 gramme of lithium carbonate (or 0.6 gramme of lithium citrate) three times per day were often allowed one lithium free day per week.'

2. Baastrup P C, Poulsen J, Schou M, Thomsen K, Amdisen A 1970 Prophylactic lithium: Double-blind discontinuation in manic-depressive and recurrent-depressive disorders. Lancet 2: 326–330

For methodological reasons Blackwell and Shepherd[56] questioned the results of the trial by Baastrup and Schou[57] on the prophylactic

Lithium

effects of lithium. These objections caused Baastrup et al. to initiate a discontinuation study on Baastrup's good responders: 50 manic-depressive patients and 34 patients with recurrent endogenous depression who had been in open lithium treatment for at least one year took part in double-blind discontinuation studies to compare lithium carbonate and placebo. Within each diagnostic groups matched pairs were randomly allocated to lithium carbonate or placebo. Relapses occurring first in the lithium partners constituted placebo preference and those occurring first in the placebo partners lithium preferences. Relapses were recorded when hospital admission or supervision with additional therapy at home was required. Serum lithium levels were monitored. The trials terminated in statistically significant preference for lithium in manic-depressive and in recurrent-depressive disorder; this happened when nine patients in each group had relapsed on placebo and none on lithium. During the whole trial, which lasted five months, 21 placebo patients relapsed and none of the lithium patients. Before the trials, the patients had been on lithium for up to 7 years; even after this long period there was still risk of relapse on withdrawal of the drug.

General review articles

Amdisen A, Hildebrandt J 1988 Use of lithium in the medically ill. Psychotherapy and Psychosomatics 49: 103–119

Johnson F N 1984 The history of lithium therapy. MacMillan, London, 198 pages

Johnson F N 1987 Depression and Mania. Modern lithium therapy. IRL Press, Oxford, 281 pages

Johnson F N 1987 Lithium combination treatment, lithium therapy monographs, vol 1. Karger, Basel, 273 pages

Muller-Oerlinghausen B, Greil W 1986 Die Lithiumtherapie. Nutzen, Risiken, Alternativen. Eine Einfuhrung für Ärzte aller Fachrichtungen. Springer, Berlin, 438 pages

References

1. Ure A 1843 Observations and researches upon a new solvent for stone in the bladder. Pharmaceutical Journal August: 71
2. Ure A 1844 Einführung des Lithions in die Materia medica. Repertorium fur die Pharmazie 84: 259–263
3. Hammond W A 1871 A treatise on diseases of the nervous system. D Appleton & Co, New York. Trubner & Co, London, pp 358–362
4. Lange C 1896 Periodische Depressionszustande und ihre Pathogenesis auf dem Boden der harnsauren Diathese. Autorisierte deutsche Ausgabe nach der zweiten Auflage des Originals von Dr Hans Kurella. Verlag von Leopold Voss, Hamburg and Leipzig
5. Cade J F J 1949 Lithium salts in the treatment of psychotic excitement. Medical Journal of Australia 36: 349–352
6. Hartigan G P 1963 The use of lithium salts in affective disorders. British Journal of Psychiatry 109: 810–814
7. Baastrup P C 1964 The use of lithium in manic-depressive psychosis. Comprehensive Psychiatry 5: 396–408
8. Treiser S L, Cascio C S, O'Donohue T L, Thoa N B, Jacobowitz D M, Kellar K J 1981 Lithium increases serotonin release and decreases serotonin receptors in the hippocampus. Science 213: 1529–1531
9. Berridge M J, Downes C P, Hanley M R 1982 Lithium amplifies agonist-dependent phosphatidylinositol responses in brain and salivary glands. Biochemistry Journal 206: 587–595
10. Hesse A 1876 Lithion. Inaugural-Dissertation zur Erlangung der Doctorwürde in der Medicin, Chirurgie and Geburtshülfe. W Fr Kaestner, Gottingen
11. Evan A P, Ollerich D A 1972 The effect of lithium carbonate on the structure of the rat kidney. American Journal of Anatomy 134: 97–106
12. Elia J, Katz I R, Simpson G M 1987 Teratogenicity of psychotherapeutic medications. Psychopharmacology Bulletin 23: 531
13. Johnson G F 1987 Lithium in depression: a review of the antidepressant prophylactic effects of lithium. Australian and New Zealand Journal of Psychiatry 21: 356–365
14. Tyrer S P 1985 Lithium in the treatment of mania. Journal of Affective Disorders 8: 251–257
15. Wickham E A, Reed J V 1987 Lithium for the control of aggressive and self-mutilating behaviour. International Clinical Psychopharmacology 2: 181–190
16. Tyrer S P 1988 Lithium in aggression. In: Birch N J (ed) Lithium: inorganic pharmacology and psychiatric use. IRL Press, Oxford, pp 39–42
17. King J R 1988 Review of significant side effects. In: Birch N J (ed) Lithium: inorganic pharmacology and psychiatric use. IRL Press, Oxford
18. Amdisen A, Carson S W 1986 Lithium. In: Evans W E, Schentag J J, Jusko W J (eds) Applied pharmacokinetcs. Principles of therapeutic drug monitoring. Applied Therapeutics, Spokane, pp 978–1008
19. Nielsen-Kudsk F, Amdisen A 1979 Analysis of the pharmacokinetics of lithium in man. European Journal of Clinical Pharmacology 16: 271–277
20. Culbreth D M R 1927 A manual of materia medica and pharmacology, 7th edn. Lea & Fibiger, Philadelphia, pp 743–745
21. Amdisen A, Nielsen-Kudsk F 1986 Relationship between standardized twelve-hour serum lithium, mean serum lithium of the 24-hour day, dose regimen, and therapeutic interval. An evaluation based on pharmacokinetic simulations. Pharmacopsychiatrica 19: 416–419
22. Amdisen A 1987 The 12-hour standardized serum lithium (12 h-stSLi). In: Johnson F N (ed) Depression and mania. Modern lithium therapy. IRL Press, Oxford, pp 88–91
23. Baldessarini R J 1985 Lithium salts and antimanic agents. In: Baldessarini R J (ed) Chemotherapy in psychiatry. Principles and practice. Harvard University Press, Cambridge, Massachusetts, pp 93–129
24. Vestergaard P, Thomsen K 1981 Renal side effects of lithium: the importance of the serum lithium level. Psychopharmacology 72: 203–204
25. Amdisen A, Nielsen-Kudsk F 1987 The coherence between daily maintenance dose and 12h-control concentrations of some psychotropic drugs in plasma. Nordisk Psykiatrisk Tidsskrift 41: 509–516
26. Müller-Oerlinghausen B 1981 Probleme der Langzeitprophylaxe. Bibliotheca Psychiatrica 161: 224–236
27. Amdisen A, Nielsen-Kudsk F 1986 Er 'det terapeutiske interval' og 12h-stSLi realiteten valide ved dosering pa basis af koncentrations-monitorering? Vurdering bl.a. ved hjaelp af en farmakokinetisk simulationsmodel. (Does any validity exist of a 'therapeutic interval' and 12 h-stSLi in dosing based on monitoring of 12 h serum lithium? — with an English summary). Nordisk Psykiatrisk Tidsskrift 40: 453–457
28. Cooper T B, Bergner P-E E, Simpson G M 1973 The 24-hour serum lithium level as a prognosticator of dosage requirements. American Journal of Psychiatry 130: 601–603
29. Tyrer S, Shaw D M 1983 Lithium carbonate. In: Tyrer S P (ed) Drugs in psychiatric practice. Butterworths, London, pp 280–312
30. Perry P J, Alexander B, Prince R A, Dunner F J 1986 The utility of a single-point dosing protocol for predicting steady-state lithium levels. British Journal of Psychiatry 148: 401–405
31. Garrod A B 1876 A treatise on gout and rheumatic gout, 3rd edn. Longmans, London, p 305
32. Lange Fr 1894 De vigtigste sindssygdomsgrupper i kort omrids. Gyldendalske Boghandels Forlag, Copenhagen
33. Kraepelin E 1913 Psychiatrie. Ein Lehrbuch für Studierende und Ärzte, 8th edn, vol 3, Klinische Psychiatrie. Verlag von Johann Ambrosius Barth, Leipzig
34. Schou M 1959 Lithium in psychiatric therapy. Stock-taking after ten years. Psychopharmacologia 1: 65–78
35. Heninger G R, Charney D S, Sternberg D E 1983 Lithium carbonate augmentation of antidepressant treatment. Archives of General Psychiatry 40: 1335–1342
36. Schou M 1987 Use in other psychiatric conditions. In: Johnson F N (ed) Depression & mania. Modern lithium therapy. IRL Press, Oxford, pp 44–46
37. Sedvall G, Jönsson B, Pettersson U, Levin K 1968 Effects of lithium salts on plasma protein bound iodine and uptake of ^{131}I in thyroid gland of man and rat. Life Sciences 7: 1257–1264
38. Radomski J L, Fuyat H N, Nelson A A, Smith P K 1950 The toxic effects, excretion and distribution of lithium chloride. Journal of Pharmacology and Experimental Therapeutics 100: 429–444
39. Amdisen A 1988 Clinical features and management of lithium poisoning. Medical Toxicology 3: 18–32
40. Hansen H E, Amdisen A 1978 Lithium intoxication (Report of 23 cases and review of 100 cases from the literature). Quarterly Journal of Medicine 47: 123–144
41. Davies B 1983 Historical note. The first patient to receive lithium. Australian and New Zealand Journal of Psychiatry 17: 366–368
42. El-Mallakh R S 1986 Acute lithium neurotoxicity. Psychiatric Developments 4: 3111–328
43. Amdisen A 1975 Monitoring of lithium treatment through determination of lithium concentration. Danish Medical Bulletin 22: 277–291
44. Hestbech J, Hansen H E, Amdisen A, Olsen S 1977 Chronic renal lesions following long-term treatment with lithium. Kidney International 12: 205–213
45. Olsen S 1976 Renal histopathology in various forms of acute anuria in man. Kidney International 10: S2–S8
46. Winchester J F 1983 Lithium. In: Haddad L M, Winchester J F (eds) Clinical management of poisoning and drug overdose. W B Saunders, Philadelphia, pp 372–379
47. Schou M 1984 Long-lasting neurological sequelae after lithium intoxication. Acta Psychiatrica Scandinavica 70: 594–602
48. Ottosen P D, Jacobsen N O, Christensen S 1988 Lithium-induced morphological changes in the rat kidney at different levels of urine flow. Pharmacology and Toxicology 63: 108–113
49. Reynolds J E F (ed) 1982 Martindale. The extra pharmacopoeia, 28th edn. The Pharmaceutical Press, London, pp 1535–1543
50. Skoven I, Thormann J 1979 Lithium compound treatment and psoriasis. Archives of Dermatology 115: 1185–1187
51. Amdisen A, Andersen C J 1982 Lithium treatment and thyroid function. A survey of 237 patients in long-term lithium treatment. Pharmacopsychiatrica 15: 149–155
52. Skausig O B, Schou M 1977 Diegivning under lithiumbehandling. (Breast-feeding during lithium treatment — with an English summary.) Ugeskrift for Laeger 139: 400–401
53. Weinstein M R 1980 Lithium treatment of women during pregnancy and in the post-delivery period. In: Johnson F N (ed) Handbook of lithium therapy. MTP Press, Lancaster, pp 421–429
54. Amdisen A 1982 Lithium and drug interactions. Drugs 24: 133–139
55. Cohen W J, Cohen N H 1974 Lithium carbonate, haloperidol and irreversible brain damage. Journal of the American Medical Association 230: 1283–1287
56. Blackwell B, Shepherd M 1968 Prophylactic lithium: another therapeutic myth? Lancet 1: 968–971
57. Baastrup P C, Schou M 1967 Lithium as a prophylactic agent. Its effect against recurrent depressions and manic-depressive psychosis. Archives of General Psychiatry 16: 162–172

Lofepramine (hydrochloride)

Lofepramine is a tricyclic antidepressant.

Chemistry

Lofepramine (hydrochloride) (Gamanil, Gamonil, Tymelyt, Emdalen, Deftan, Deprimil, Amplit)
$C_{26}H_{27}ClN_2O.HCl$
N-methyl-N-(3-clorophenacyl)-3-(10,11 dihydro-5H-dibenz[b,f]azepin-5-yl)-propylamine hydrochloride

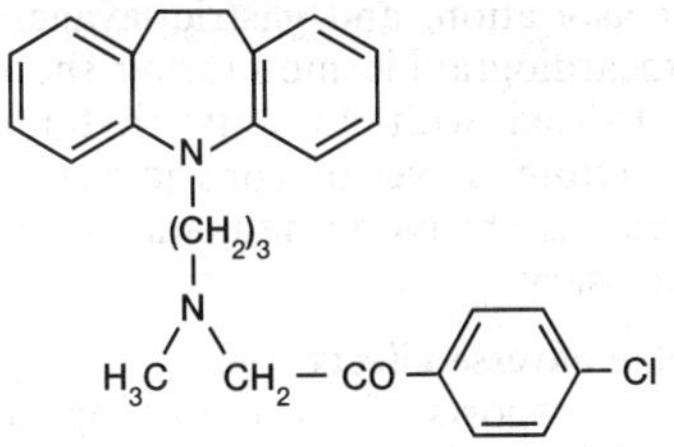

Molecular weight (freebase)	455.4 (419)
pKa (amino group)	7.5
Solubility	
in alcohol	freely
in water	sparingly
Octanol/water partition coefficient	–

It is a yellowish-white microcrystalline powder, freely soluble in methanol, ethanol, and chloroform, distribution between ether and water at pH3 > 95% in ether phase. It is sparingly soluble in water and is weakly basic. It is prepared by chemical synthesis and is not available in combination with other compounds.

Pharmacology

Lofepramine exhibits activity thought to be indicative of antidepressant activity in classical animal models. These include: the inhibition of the pressor response to tyramine in anaesthetized cats[1] and dogs;[2] potentiation of the noradrenaline pressor response in pithed rats (equivalent to that of imipramine); inhibition of the pressor responses to phenylephrine in anaesthetized rats (although less potently than imipramine);[3] antagonism of reserpine-induced ptosis, hypothermia and grooming behaviour in mice.[1]

In standard tests for peripheral and central anticholinergic potency lofepramine has been shown to have lower activity than imipramine.[1,3]

Toxicology

No teratogenic potential has been demonstrated in rats, rabbits or mice. No mutagenicity was observed in the Ames test, in human lymphocytes in vitro, or in the in vivo micronucleus test in developing mice erythrocytes. Tests for carcinogenicity have revealed no oncogenic potential for lofepramine.

The oral LD_{50} in rats[1] is 5580 mg.kg^{-1} and in mice[1] is greater than 2500 mg.kg^{-1}. These values are substantially higher than the corresponding values for other tricyclic antidepressants, consistent with the clinical evidence that lofepramine is less dangerous in overdose.

Clinical pharmacology

Lofepramine, in common with other tricyclic antidepressants, inhibits the re-uptake of monoamines in peripheral adrenergic nerves.[4] When compared with imipramine, lofepramine had significantly reduced anticholinergic side effects.[3] Whereas imipramine increases the intensity of delta, theta and beta frequencies of the EEG, lofepramine effects only the beta band.[5] Lofepramine produces a lesser increase in heart rate than that produced by amitriptyline when administered to normal individuals.[6]

Pharmacokinetics

The preferred analytical method is by gas chromatography[7] which has a sensitivity of 1 μg.l^{-1}. A high performance liquid chromatographic method has recently been developed[20] with a sensitivity of 0.5 μg.l^{-1}.

Lofepramine is rapidly absorbed with peak plasma concentrations being reached within 1 hour and having a plasma half life of 5 hours.[8] In common with imipramine, lofepramine appears to undergo significant presystemic metabolism. Plasma protein binding is approximately 99%. Volume of distribution has not yet been established, although according to animal data, this distribution is large, in common with other tricyclics such as imipramine. After oral administration higher concentrations of lofepramine and its metabolites can be found in blood, lungs, liver, kidney and brain.

Excretion in breast milk has not been established.

Oral absorption	rapid
Presystemic metabolism	extensive
Plasma half life	
mean	5 h
Volume of distribution	–
Plasma protein binding	99%

Concentration–effect relationship

A therapeutic window has not been established for lofepramine. In a double-blind comparison of lofepramine and imipramine, no correlation was found between plasma levels and therapeutic effect.[9]

Metabolism

Almost all of the drug is metabolized before excretion, which is mainly in urine and in faeces.[8] Lofepramine is metabolized by N-dealkylation, hydroxylation and glucuronidation. It is extensively metabolized to its principal metabolite, desmethylimipramine, on first pass through the liver. During chronic administration, the plasma level of desmethylimipramine is typically three times greater than that of lofepramine, except in the first few hours following administration of each dose, during which time the plasma level of the parent drug can exceed that of its metabolite.[10] Desmethylimi-

Fig. 1 The metabolism of Lofepramine

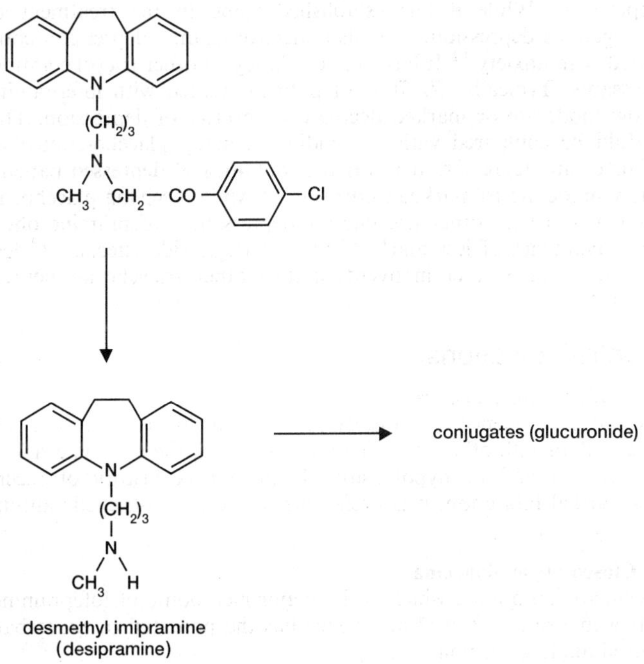

pramine, which is also known as desipramine, is itself an antidepressant.

Pharmaceutics

Lofepramine, Gamanil (E. Merck, UK) is available in oral dosage forms only. Tablets are round, lacquered, brownish-violet with a spindle-shaped scoring on one side. Each contains 70 mg of lofepramine as the hydrochloride.

This medication should be stored in its original container at room temperature and protected from light and moisture. Lofepramine has a 4 year shelf-life.

Therapeutic use

Indications

1. Treatment of the symptoms of depressive illness.

Contraindications

1. Cardiovascular diseases
2. Narrow angle glaucoma
3. Prostatic hypertrophy
4. Epilepsy
5. Hypersensitivity to dibenzazepines.

Mode of use

The initial dose is usually 70 mg twice daily, and an additional 70 mg is added to the evening dose if the balance between therapeutic effect and side effects indicates that an increase is appropriate. Although 210 mg is the upper limit of the usual daily dose, a daily total of 280 mg in divided doses is sometimes used, and use of a daily total as high as 490 mg has been reported. There is some evidence from controlled trials that the onset of the antidepressant effect is a little more rapid with lofepramine than with other tricyclic antidepressants. The majority of improvement occurs within two weeks and hence an increase of dose should be considered if there has not been an adequate response within this time. Because there is a high risk of relapse if antidepressant treatment is discontinued in the months following relief of symptoms, treatment should be continued for six months. Once symptoms have resolved, the dose should be reduced to the minimum necessary to sustain the improvement in mental state. It is advisable to avoid abrupt discontinuation because of the risk of rebound symptoms on abrupt discontinuation of tricyclic antidepressants.

Indications

1. Depression
Lofepramine is an effective treatment for moderate and severe depression. While it has established value in the treatment of endogenous depression, it is also effective against depression combined with anxiety.[11] It has similar efficacy to other tricyclic antidepressants. Typically, 60–70% of patients treated with lofepramine show moderate or marked decrease in severity of depression. This should be compared with the finding in many placebo-controlled trials of antidepressant drugs that about 40% of depressed patients show moderate to marked improvement while receiving placebo. In comparison with other tricyclic antidepressants, lofepramine offers the advantages of less marked anticholinergic side effects,[12,13] less sedation and is safer in overdose than other tricyclic antidepressants.[14,15]

Contraindications

1. Cardiovascular disease
Despite the evidence[16,17] suggesting a lower incidence of cardiac side effects than with other tricyclic antidepressants, there is some risk of arrhythmia and of hypotension. If there is a history of recent myocardial infarction, it is preferable to use a non-tricyclic antidepressant.

2. Closed angle glaucoma
Desmethylimipraine, which is the major metabolite of lofepramine, has a mydriatic effect,[18] and hence has the potential to exacerbate closed angle glaucoma.

3. Prostatic hypertrophy
The relatively mild anticholinergic effects might nonetheless be sufficient to cause retention of urine.

4. Epilepsy
Lofepramine should be used with caution in patients with epilepsy because tricyclic antidepressants lower the seizure threshold. However, the rarity of convulsions following overdose[14,15] suggests that the risk that lofepramine will precipitate seizures is low.

Adverse reactions

Potentially life-threatening effects
No potentially life-threatening effects have been clearly established.

Acute overdosage
In a study[14] of 13 patients who had overdoses ranging from 1100 mg to 4900 mg no patients suffered shock, convulsions or arrhythmias. A review[15] of 55 case reports of acute overdose of lofepramine, including cases in which several grams had been taken, found that hypotension was rare and no convulsions had been reported. There have been no reports of death due to lofepramine taken alone. Treatment of overdosage should include emptying of the stomach by induced emesis or aspiration, and gastric lavage. Haemodialysis is not useful. Electrocardiographic monitoring should be performed, and arrhythmias treated with an antiarrhythmic agent such as propanolol or phenytoin. Level of consciousness, respiration, and bowel sounds should also be monitored, and symptomatic treatment implemented if necessary.

Severe or irreversible adverse effects
There have been rare reports of thrombocytopenia, and reports of signs of hepatic toxicity such as jaundice and raised liver enzymes, but these signs have resolved on discontinuation of treatment.

Symptomatic adverse effects
Adverse effects, such as sedation, are similar to those observed with other tricyclics but tend to be mild and transient. Anticholinergic adverse effects occur less frequently.

Reported adverse effects have included dry mouth, constipation, blurring of vision, tachycardia, urinary retention, dizziness, drowsiness, hypotension, sweating and tremor. More rarely, reports of allergic skin reactions have occurred.

Interference with clinical pathology tests
Although not reported for lofepramine, drugs of this class have caused interference with thyroid function tests.

High risk groups

Neonates
The drug is not recommended for use in neonates.

Breast milk. Tricyclic antidepressants are excreted in breast milk. The risks to the infant are not well documented but it is likely that the metabolite, desmethylimipramine, is excreted in breast milk.

Children
Lofepramine is not recommended for use in this age group.

Pregnant women
The drug should not be used during pregnancy unless there are compelling medical reasons.

The elderly
The use in the elderly should be accompanied by routine monitoring in the initial stages of treatment. These patients may respond to initial doses below 140 mg.d^{-1}, and treatment may be commenced at 70 mg daily, increasing if necessary.

Concurrent disease
As with all tricyclic antidepressants, caution is advised in patients with liver, kidney and heart disease.

Drug interactions

Potentially hazardous interactions

Monoamine oxidase inhibitors. The concurrent administration of a tricyclic antidepressant and a monoamine oxidase inhibitor can result in a potentially fatal syndrome characterized by hyperpyrexia, convulsions and coma. The mechanism probably involves increased concentration of monoamines at postsynaptic receptors. Although rare, the severity of the interaction makes it advisable to avoid the combined use of lofepramine and a monoamine oxidase inhibitor. Because the effect of irreversible monoamine oxidase inhibitors is sustained for two weeks after cessation of treatment, treatment with lofepramine should not be started within two weeks of discontinuation of a monoamine oxidase inhibitor.

Sympathomimetic drugs. Desmethylimipramine, the major metabolite of lofepramine, potentiates the hypertensive effects of directly acting monoamines such as noradrenaline by virtue of inhibiting reuptake at the nerve terminal. It can antagonize the effects of indirectly acting sympathomimetic amines, such as tyramine, by preventing uptake of the drug into the nerve terminal.

Alcohol. Although lofepramine is usually less sedative than other tricyclic antidepressants such as amitriptyline, it can potentiate the sedative effects of alcohol and might impair the ability to drive a car or operate complex machinery.

Other significant interactions

Adrenergic neurone-blocking agents. The antihypertensive effect of the adrenergic neurone-blocking drugs such as guanethidine, bethanidine and debrisoquine is reduced by tricyclic antidepressants, making it advisable to review antihypertensive treatment with these agents during treatment with lofepramine.

Anaesthetic agents. While tricyclic antidepressants have been reported to increase the risk of arrhythmias during anaesthesia, the risk is not high enough to warrant discontinuation of the antidepressant prior to anaesthesia.[19] Nonetheless, the anaesthetist should be aware of the increased risk.

Barbiturates. Barbiturates are potent inducers of microsomal enzymes and hence increase the hepatic metabolism of tricyclic antidepressants. The influence of this interaction on the clinical effects of lofepramine is not clearly established.

Potentially useful interactions

None is known.

Clinical trials

1. Feighner J P, Meredith C H, Dutt J E, Hendrickson C G 1982 A double-blind comparison of lofepramine, imipramine and placebo in patients with primary depression. Acta Psychiatrica Scandinavica 66: 100–108

This was a multicentre trial in which 139 patients were assigned to receive lofepramine, imipramine or placebo. The entry criteria included having a score of at least 18 on the 21 item Hamilton Depression Scale. Dose was adjusted according to clinical estimate of need. In the majority of cases, the dose after 1 week was 210 mg in the group treated with lofepramine, and 130 mg in those treated with imipramine. At 6 weeks, the mean change in Hamilton Depression Scale score was 59% in the lofepramine group; 53% in the imipramine group; and 40% in the placebo group. If a reduction of at least 40% in the Hamilton Depression Scale score is taken as the criterion for response to treatment, 28 of the 46 patients in the lofepramine group; 25 of the 48 who received imipramine; and 21 of the 45 receiving placebo, were responders. Severe or moderate adverse effects were reported by 18 patients in the lofepramine group and 32 patients in the imipramine group. This difference in occurrence of adverse effects was statistically significant ($P < 0.001$). In particular, lofepramine produced fewer effects related to the autonomic nervous system. Dry mouth was the most common effect in both active treatment groups, occurring in 10 patients receiving lofepramine and 21 of those receiving imipramine. Therefore, the trial indicates that lofepramine is as effective as imipramine, but produces significantly fewer side effects.

2. Rickels K, Weise C C, Zal H M, Sanalosi I, Werblowsky J 1982 Lofepramine and imipramine in unipolar depressed outpatients. A placebo-controlled study. Acta Psychiatrica Scandinavica 66: 109–120

158 outpatients satisfying DSMIII criteria for major depressive disorder were assigned to receive lofepramine, imipramine or placebo in a double-blind manner. Significant therapeutic effect emerged in both active treatment groups after two weeks. On the basis of global improvement at end-point after 4–6 weeks treatment, there was moderate or marked improvement in 77% of those treated with lofepramine, 74% of those treated with imipramine and 44% of the placebo group. There was less sedation and fewer anticholinergic side effects in the lofepramine group than in the imipramine group

General review articles

Lancaster S G, Gonzalez J P 1989 Lofepramine. A review of its pharmacodynamic and pharmacokinetic properties, and therapeutic efficacy in depressive illness. Drugs 37: 123–140

References

1. Eriksoo E, Rohte D 1970 Chemistry and pharmacology of a new potential antidepressant. Arzneimittel Forschung 20: 1561–1569
2. Akashi A, Hashizume T, Tanaka M, Naka S, Suzuki I 1976 Pharmacological properties of lofepramine. Folia Pharmacologica Japan 72: 417–431
3. Sjogren C 1980 The pharmacological profile of lofepramine, a new antidepressant drug. Neuropharmacology 19: 1213–1214
4. Siwers B, Freyschuss U, Hamberger B, Tuck D, Malmfors T, Sjoqvist F 1970 A quantitative approach to the initial clinical trial of tricyclic antidepressants: a comparison of Leo 640 and nortriptyline. European Journal of Clinical Pharmacology 3: 12–17
5. Lehman E, Hopes H 1978 The effects of imipramine and lofepramine on EEG and their dependence on relative alpha-intensity. Pharmakopsychiate Neuropsychopharmakologic 11: 128–133
6. Stein H, Konetschny J, Hurman L, Sawe U, Belz G G 1985 Cardiovascular effects of single doses of the antidepressants amitriptyline and lofepramine in healthy subjects. Pharmacopsychiatry 18: 272–277
7. Lungren R, Olsson A, Plym Forshell G 1977 Gas chromatographic determination of lofepramine and desmethylimipramine in plasma. Acta Pharmaceutica Suecica 14: 18–94
8. Plym Forshell G 1975 Studies on the distribution and excretion of (^{3}H ^{14}C) labelled lofepramine in the rat. Xenobiotica 5: 73–82
9. Dutt J E 1982 On the clinical response/serum level relationship for antidepressants. II Lofepramine and imipramine. Psychopharmacological Bulletin 18: 17–27
10. Plym Forshell G, Siners B, Tuck J R 1976 Pharmacokinetics of lofepramine in man: relationship to inhibition of noradrenaline uptake. European Journal of Clinical Pharmacology 9: 291–298
11. Goncalves N, Wegener G 1979 Comparison of action of lofepramine and mianserin in depressive patients under double-blind conditions. International Pharmacopsychiatry 14: 310–318
12. Feighner J P, Meredith C H, Dutt J E, Hendrickson C G 1982 A double-blind comparison of lofepramine, imipramine and placebo in patients with primary depression. Acta Psychiatrica Scandinavica 66: 100–108
13. Rickels K, Weise C C, Zal H M, Sanalosi I, Werblowsky J 1982 Lofepramine and imipramine in unipolar depressed outpatients. A placebo-controlled study. Acta Psychiatrica Scandinavica 66: 109–120
14. Heath A, Hulten B-A 1983 Lofepramine toxicity in overdose. Proceedings of VI World Congress of Psychiatry, Vienna
15. Reid F, Henry J A 1990 Lofepramine overdosage. Pharmacopsychiatry 23 (suppl 1): 23–27
16. Seibel I 1978 Controlled double-blind study to compare lofepramine (leo 640) with imipramine in cyclothymic depression. MD Dissertation, University of Dusseldorf
17. Leonard B E 1987 A comparison of the pharmacological properties of the novel tricyclic antidepressant lofepramine with its major metabolite desipramine: a review. International Clinical Psychopharmacology 2: 281–291
18. Shur E, Checkley S 1982 Pupil studis in depressed patients: an investigation of the mechanism of action of desipramine. British Journal of Psychiatry 140: 181–184
19. Games G Y, Rees D I 1986 Electroconvulsive therapy and anaesthetic considerations. Anesthesia and Analgesia 65: 1345–1356
20. Virgili P, Henry J A 1989 Determination of lofepramine and desipramine using high performance liquid chromatography and electrochemical detection. Journal of Chromatography 496: 228–233

L

Loperamide (hydrochloride)

Loperamide is an antidiarrhoeal agent acting directly on the intestinal wall to inhibit peristalsis. It acts more rapidly and is longer acting than diphenoxylate or codeine.

Chemistry

Loperamide hydrochloride (Imodium, Arret, Suprasec, Imosec, Motilix, Enterol, Lopemin, Loperin, Fortasec, Seldiar)
$C_{29}H_{33}ClN_2O_2.HCl$
4-(4-p-Chlorophenyl-4-hydroxy-piperidino)-NN-dimethyl-2,2-diphenylbutyramide hydrochloride

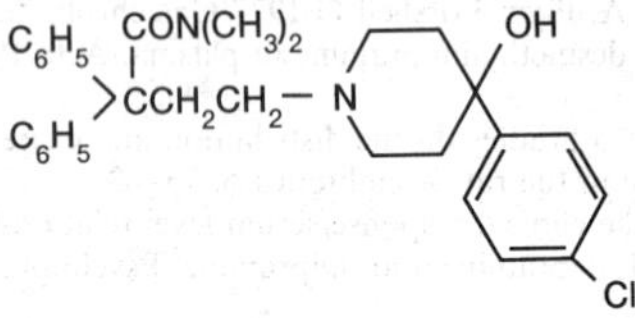

Molecular weight (free base)	513.5 (477.0)
pKa	8.7
Solubility	
in alcohol	>1 in 10
in water	1 in 50 000
Octanol/water partition coefficient	High

A white to slightly yellowish amorphous or microcrystalline powder, prepared by chemical synthesis.

Pharmacology

Loperamide inhibits the peristaltic activity of longitudinal and circular smooth muscle in the intestine by interacting with cholinergic and non-cholinergic neuronal mechanisms responsible for producing the peristaltic reflex. Loperamide binds to the opiate receptor in the gut wall, reducing propulsive peristalsis, and increasing intestinal transit time. Loperamide increases the tone of the anal sphincter.[1] Loperamide also inhibits electrolyte and fluid secretion in intestine.[2,3]

Loperamide acts as an anti-diarrhoeal agent by a combination of its actions on smooth muscle in the intestine and its effects on secretions.[4] It has no effect on the intestinal flora. Although loperamide binds to the opiate receptor it has virtually no analgesic activity.

Loperamide is an antidiarrhoeal agent with direct action on μ opiate receptors of the intestinal wall. In comparison to similarly acting agents such as diphenoxylate and codeine, the effects of loperamide are rapid, persist longer and are more selective for the intestine.[5–7]

The affinity of loperamide to μ opiate receptors is relatively high.[8] Intestinal receptors are reached following rapid absorption. Most of the absorbed drug does not leave the visceral organs, and the small fraction entering the systemic circulation does not cross a mature blood–brain barrier.[9]

Binding to μ opiate receptors of the intestine alters neuronal activity of the myenteric plexus. As a result, smooth muscle contractions induced by pressure, prostaglandins, fatty acid derivatives and other stimuli are inhibited. There is no direct antagonism of acetylcholine or VIP. Segmental contractions and anal sphincter tone increase. The short transit time, which is characteristic for diarrhoea, is lengthened.[5–7,10]

Hypersecretory responses to a variety of agents are reduced by loperamide. In healthy volunteers loperamide has antisecretory activity[11] or increases the absorptive capacity of the gut.[12]

Toxicology

No information of potential clinical relevance is available on toxicological tests in animals.

No embryotoxic or teratogenic effects at up to 10 mg.kg^{-1} were found in rats. Only 20% of animals at 40 mg.kg^{-1} were found to be pregnant. No embryotoxicity or teratogenicity at up to 40 mg.kg^{-1} was found in rabbits. Maternal toxicity occurred at 40 mg.kg^{-1}. In mutagenicity tests female dominant lethal test was negative. In an 18-month carcinogenicity study in rats, with doses up to 100 times the maximum dose no evidence of carcinogenesis was found.

Clinical pharmacology

Loperamide is an effective agent for the treatment of diarrhoea. Its action on smooth muscle and on intestinal secretions results in improvement in diarrhoeal symptoms within a few hours. Loperamide also increases the tone of the anal sphincter.

A dose–response relationship for single doses of loperamide has been demonstrated by Scheurmans et al.[13] In addition, these workers showed that loperamide was devoid of cardiovascular effects and side effects at doses at least 4 times higher than the constipating dose.

Loperamide is an effective and safe treatment for almost all forms of acute and chronic diarrhoea, for the reduction of ileostomy output and of incontinence. Loperamide compares very well with other agents in travellers' diarrhoea.

Loperamide is devoid of central opiate effects at therapeutic dosage,[13] partly because of its affinity for the opiate receptors in the gut wall and partly because of a high pre-systemic metabolism which results in low systemic plasma concentrations.

In adults loperamide is normally taken as two capsules initially (or 20 ml syrup) with 1 capsule (or 10 ml syrup) with each loose stool. In children (4–8 years) 5 ml syrup is given four times daily until the diarrhoea is controlled. In children over 8 years of age 10 ml of syrup is given four times daily until the diarrhoea is controlled.

Chronic diarrhoea. Adults: studies have shown that patients may need widely differing doses. The starting dosage should be between 2 and 4 capsules (or 20 and 40 ml syrup) per day in divided doses, depending on severity. If required this dose can be adjusted according to response.

Pharmacokinetics

The analytical method for drug in plasma is radioimmunoassay; this method can detect as little as 50 pg and can accurately assay 100 pg–10 ng loperamide in 0.5 ml plasma.[14]

The absorption is more than 65% by oral dosage. Absorption occurs at a modest rate, with peak serum levels of 2–3 μg.l^{-1} occurring at about 4 hours after oral administration.[15] Absorption of loperamide from the gut is at least 65%, since less than 35% is excreted unchanged in the faeces. The reason why systemic plasma levels are very low is that loperamide undergoes an extensive presystemic first-pass metabolism in the gut wall and in the liver. A recent study in dogs indicated that the absolute bioavailability of oral loperamide was 17.5%. Metabolism studies in rats demonstrated that part of loperamide was biliary excreted as its glucuronide, which could explain, at least partly, the presence of unchanged loperamide in the faeces (due to hydrolysis of loperamide glucuronide by the gut flora). Other metabolic pathways are: N-demethylation to mono- and didesmethylloperamide and oxidative N-dealkylation. The plasma half life is 10–12 hours,[16] and 96.5% is protein bound to plasma proteins.[17]

Loperamide does not act centrally because, due to its high affinity for the gut wall and its pre-systemic metabolism, very little reaches the systemic circulation. In rats the drug is distributed principally in the liver and kidney. Negligible amounts are found in the brain. In man, following intravenous administration, loperamide gradually concentrates in the small intestine.[18,19] Small amounts are excreted in human breast milk relative to the therapeutic dose. In hepatic disease, plasma levels of the drug may be elevated.

Loperamide (hydrochloride)

Oral absorption	>65%
Presystemic metabolism	some
Plasma half life	
range	10–12 hours
Volume of distribution	—
Plasma protein binding	96.5%

Concentration–effect relationship

There is no evidence of any correlation between the plasma concentration of loperamide and its antidiarrhoeal effect.

Metabolism

Loperamide is extensively metabolized in the liver.[20] The route of elimination is 0.63–1.4% in urine as unchanged drug; 58% is excreted in the bile (in the rat) and 15–23% appears in the faeces. There is enterohepatic recirculation with faecal excretion at 3 days after administration.[19,21]

Two primary pathways of metabolism have been described — demethylation and oxidative N-dealkylation in which the molecule is cleaved to yield 4(4-chlorophenyl)4-hydroxypiperidine (III).

The two desmethyl analogs (I) and (II) are potent antidiarrhoeal agents, but not as active as the parent compound.

Pharmaceutics

Three oral dosage forms are marketed by Janssen (UK/USA).

Imodium capsules (UK) are hard gelatin capsules with a dark green, opaque cap and a standard grey opaque body. Each capsule contains loperamide hydrochloride 2 mg.

Imodium in the USA is of a similar strength but the capsules have a dark green cap and a light green body. They are overprinted 'JANSSEN' and 'IMODIUM'.

Imodium syrup is a red raspberry and currant flavoured syrup containing loperamide hydrochloride 1 mg in 5 ml.

Arret capsules are packaged for over-the-counter sales in the UK. They are hard gelatin capsules with a brown, opaque cap and a turquoise opaque body. Each capsule contains loperamide hydrochloride 2 mg. All preparations have a shelf-life of 5 years. Capsules should be protected from light and moisture.

Potentially allergenic substances in the formulations

Imodium capsules: lactose, indigotine and erythrosin.

Imodium syrup: cochineal red and parabens.

Arret capsules: lactose and indigotine.

Therapeutic use

Indications

1. Acute diarrhoea
2. Chronic diarrhoea.

Contraindications

There are no specific contraindications but the drug is not recommended for use in pregnant women.

Mode of use

Acute diarrhoea

Adults: two capsules (or 20 ml syrup) initially followed by 1 capsule (or 10 ml syrup) after every loose stool. The usual dosage is 3–4 capsules a day; the maximum daily dose should not exceed 8 capsules.

Children 4–8 years: syrup 5 ml four times daily until diarrhoea is controlled. In children under 8 years further investigation may be necessary if diarrhoea has not responded to 3 days treatment.

Children 9–12 years: syrup 10 ml (or 1 capsule) four times daily until diarrhoea is controlled.

Chronic diarrhoea

Adults: studies have shown that patients may need widely differing amounts of the drug. The starting dosage should be between 2 and 4 capsules (or 20 and 40 ml syrup) per day in divided doses, depending on severity. If required this dose can be adjusted according to response.

Arret capsules

Adults and children over 12 years: two capsules initially followed by 1 capsule after every further loose bowel movement. The maximum daily dose should not exceed 8 capsules.

Indications

The drug should not be used for prolonged periods until the underlying cause of the diarrhoea has been investigated.

1. Acute diarrhoea

Loperamide provides rapid relief from acute diarrhoea in adults[13,22] and children.[23]

Loperamide is more potent than diphenoxylate and codeine phosphate[13] and has a considerably faster onset of action than kaolin and morphine.[22] Abdominal cramps associated with diarrhoea are also relieved.[22] The flexible dosage regimen means that the patient takes only that quantity of drug sufficient to control the symptoms.

2. Chronic diarrhoea

Loperamide has been shown to be superior to diphenoxylate in the symptomatic treatment of patients with chronic diarrhoea associated with irritable bowel, Crohn's disease, postgastric surgery, ulcerative colitis and diabetes.[24] The number of stools was reduced and the faecal consistency improved by loperamide treatment in patients with chronic diarrhoea due to intestinal resection,[25] irritable bowel[26] or irradiation/ radiotherapy of various tumours.[27] In one long-term study over 3–20 months, chronic diarrhoea during the day was controlled with a single dose of loperamide, while a second bedtime dose provided effective control in those patients with nocturnal or early morning diarrhoea.[28] A study in patients with ileostomy

Fig. 1 The metabolism of loperamide

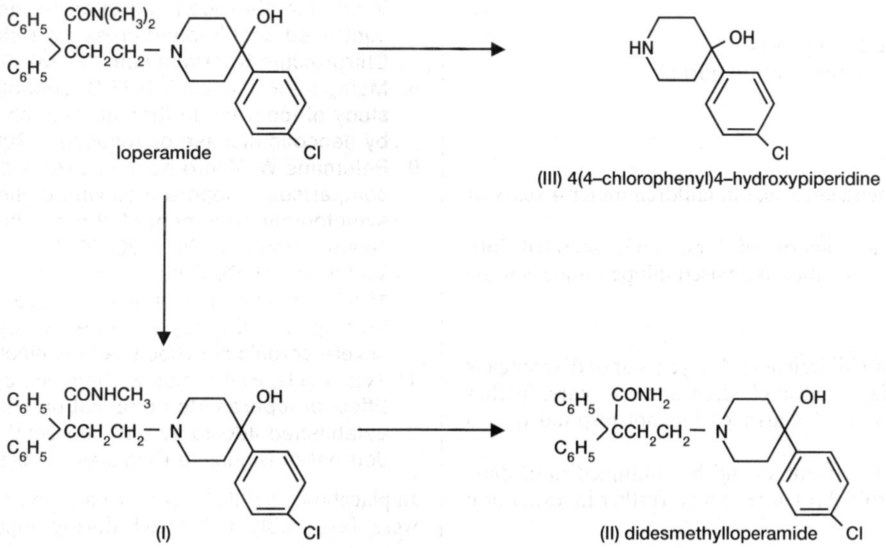

showed that total output and fluid content of diarrhoea were decreased by loperamide, compared with codeine phosphate,[29] while sodium and potassium loss were reduced.[30]

Contraindications

Diarrhoea is a common presentation of a number of serious gastrointestinal conditions. These must be investigated, particularly in patients over 40 years old. Loperamide should not be a substitute for proper investigations. Caution in the use of loperamide is necessary in patients with ulcerative colitis and Crohn's disease with extensive colonic disease, to avoid precipitating toxic dilatation of the colon. The drug is contraindicated in very severe disease. Loperamide must not be used when inhibition of peristalsis is to be avoided and in particular when ileus or constipation are present, or when abdominal distension develops particularly in severely dehydrated children or in patients with acute pseudomembranous colitis associated with broad spectrum antibiotics.[31–33]

Loperamide should not be used alone in acute dysentery, which is characterized by blood in the stool and elevated body temperature.

Loperamide must be used with caution when hepatic function, necessary for the drug's metabolism, is defective as in severe hepatic disturbances.

Adverse reactions

Potentially life-threatening effects
No effects of this kind have been reported.

Acute overdosage
Studies in animals suggest that overdosage in man may result in constipation, central nervous system depression, and gastrointestinal irritation. If spontaneous vomiting has occurred, 100 g of activated charcoal should be administered orally in a slurry as soon as fluids can be retained. If vomiting has not occurred, gastric lavage should be performed, followed by administration of 100 g of activated charcoal in a slurry. The patient should be monitored for signs of central nervous system depression for at least 24 hours which, if it occurs, may be responsive to naloxone administration. In view of the short duration of action of naloxone compared with loperamide, repeat doses may be required.

In clinical trials, an adult who took 60 mg (3 × 20 mg doses) within 24 hours was nauseated after 40 mg and vomited after 60 mg.

In case of overdosage the following effects may be observed: constipation, ileus and neurological symptoms (miosis, muscular hypertonia, somnolence and bradypnoea). Naloxone may be given as an antidote. Since the duration of action of loperamide is longer than that of naloxone, the patient should be kept under constant observation for at least 48 hours in order to detect any possible depression of the central nervous system.

Severe or irreversible adverse effects
No effects of this kind have been reported.

Symptomatic adverse effects
Abdominal cramps and skin reactions, including urticaria, have been reported.

Interference with clinical pathology tests
No interferences of this kind have been reported.

High risk groups

Neonates
Loperamide is not recommended for use in children under 4 years of age.

Breast milk. Whilst the fraction of loperamide secreted into human milk is extremely low, caution is advised if loperamide is to be given to a nursing mother.

Children
Loperamide can be used for children aged 4–8 years until diarrhoea is controlled or for up to 3 days, but in children under 8 years, further investigation may be necessary if diarrhoea has not responded to 3 days' treatment.

In children 9–12 years, treatment should be continued until diarrhoea is controlled for up to 5 days, after which further investigation is necessary.

Pregnant women
Safety in human pregnancy has not been established, though studies in animals have not demonstrated any teratogenic effects. It is not advisable to administer loperamide in pregnancy.

The elderly
No precautions are required and doses should be adjusted according to patient response.

Drug interactions

No interactions between loperamide and other drugs have been described.

Clinical trials

Controlled trials in acute diarrhoea

1. Amery W, Duyck F, Polak J, Van Den Bouwhuysen G 1975 A multicentre double-blind study in acute diarrhoea comparing loperamide (R 18 553) with two common antidiarrhoeal agents and a placebo. Current Therapeutic Research 17: 263–270
2. Rodriguez L 1975 The use of loperamide in acute non-specific diarrhoea. Gastroenterology 68: 974
   Zelvelder W G, Nelemans F A 1976 A double-blind placebo-controlled trial of loperamide in acute diarrhoea. Journal of Drug Research 2: 54
3. Dom J, Leyman R, Schuermans V, Brugmans J 1974 Loperamide (R 18 553), a novel type of antidiarrhoeal agent. Part 8: Clinical investigation. Use of a flexible dosage schedule in a double-blind comparison of loperamide with diphenoxylate in 614 patients suffering from acute diarrhoea. Arzneimittel-Forschung 24: 1660–1665
4. Cornett J W D, Aspeling R L, Mallegol D 1977 A double-blind comparative evaluation of loperamide versus diphenoxylate with atropine in acute diarrhoea. Current Therapeutic Research 21: 629

One single dose of loperamide (4 mg), compared to placebo significantly delays recurrence of diarrhoea (median of 24 hours for loperamide and only 2 hours for placebo) (Trial 1), and decreases the number of loose stools, as measured by the need for diphenoxylate as rescue medication (Trials 2).

In multidose studies (Trials 3 and 4) over 3 days, loperamide provided more rapid disappearance of diarrhoea (within 24 hours: 67, viz. 61% of patients) than diphenoxylate (58, viz. 40%), while the patient needed less frequent intake of loperamide.

Controlled trials in chronic diarrhoea

5. Demeulenaere L, Verbeke S, Muils M, Reyntjens A 1974 Loperamide: an open multicentre trial and a double-blind cross-over comparison with placebo in patients with chronic diarrhoea. Current Therapeutic Research 16: 32–39
6. Galambos J T, Hersh T, Spalding S, Wenger L 1976 Loperamide: a new antidiarrhoeal agent in the treatment of chronic diarrhoea. Gastroenterology 70: 1026–1029
7. Tytgat G N, Huibregtse K, Meuwissen S G M 1976 Loperamide in chronic diarrhoea and after ileostomy. A placebo-controlled double-blind cross-over study. Archivum Chirurgicum Neerlandicum 28: 13–20
8. Mainguet P, Fiasse R 1977 Double-blind placebo-controlled study of loperamide (Imodium) in chronic diarrhoea caused by ileocolic disease or resection. Gut 18: 575–579
9. Pelemans W, Vantrappen G 1976 A double-blind crossover comparison of loperamide with diphenoxylate in the symptomatic treatment of chronic diarrhoea. Gastroenterology 70: 1030–1034
10. Verhaegen H, De Cree J, Schuermans V 1974 Loperamide (R 18 553), a novel type of antidiarrhoeal agent. Part 7: clinical investigation. Efficacy and safety of loperamide in patients with severe chronic diarrhoea. Arzneimittel-Forschung 24: 1657–1660
11. Tytgat G N, Huibregtse K, Dagevos J, Van Den Ende A 1977 Effect of loperamide on faecal output and composition in well-established ileostomy and ileorectal anaastomosis. American Journal of Digestive Diseases 22: 669–676

In placebo-controlled studies frequency, consistency, weight of stools were favourably influenced during loperamide (Trials 5–7) and carmin red transit time significantly prolonged (Trial 8). In diphenoxylate controlled studies loperamide was also superior for onset of control of diarrhoea and reduction of stool frequency (Trials 9 and 10). In patients with ileostomy loperamide (8–12 mg per day) compared to placebo, significantly reduced the daily faecal weight and volume, the water content, sodium output, sodium potassium ratio and increased faecal viscosity and bulk density (Trial 11).

Major review articles

Heel R C, Brogden R N, Speight T M, Avery G S 1978 Loperamide: A review of its pharmacological properties and therapeutic efficacy in diarrhoea. Drugs 15: 33–52

Shriver R D; Rosenthale M, McKenzie B, Weintraub H, McGuire J 1981 In: Goldberg A (ed) Loperamide in pharmacological and biochemical properties of drug substances III. pp 461–476

Niemegeers C J E, Colpaert F C, Awouters F H L 1981 Pharmacology and antidiarrhoeal effect of loperamide. Drug Development Research 1: 1–20

Ooms L A A, Degryse A D, Janssen P A J 1984 Mechanisms of action of loperamide. Scandinavian Journal of Gastroenterology 19 (suppl 96): 145–155

References

1. Van Nueten J M, Sanssen P A J, Fontaine J 1974 Loperamide (R18 553) a novel type of antidiarrhoeal agent. Part 3: in vitro studies on the peristaltic reflex and other experiments on isolated issues. Arzneimittel Forschung 24: 1641–1645 (Abstract)
2. Sandhu B K, Milla P J, Hames J T 1983 Mechanisms of action in loperamide. Scandinavian Journal of Gastroenterology 18 (suppl 84) 85–92
3. Kachel G W, Ruppin H, Hagel J, Borina W, Meinhard M, Domschke W 1983 Effect of loperamide on jejunal fluid transport and propulsion in man. Gastroenterology 84(5): Part 2
4. Awouters F 1983 Loperamide: mechanisms of action. Annual Academy of Paediatrics meeting, San Francisco, October 27
5. Heel R C, Brogden R N, Speight T M, Avery G S 1978 Loperamide review. Its pharmacological properties and therapeutic efficacy in diarrhoea. Drugs 15: 33–52
6. Awouters F, Niemegeers C J E, Janssen P A J 1983 Pharmacology of antidiarrhoea drugs. Annual Review of Pharmacology and Toxicology 23: 279–301
7. Ruppin H 1987 Review: loperamide — a potent antidiarrhoeal drug with actions along the alimentary tract. Alimentary Pharmacology and Therapeutics 1: 179–190
8. Stahl K D, Van Bever W, Janssen P, Simon E J 1977 Receptor affinity and pharmacological potency of a series of narcotic analgesic, anti-diarrhoeal and neuroleptic drugs. European Journal of Pharmacology 46: 199–205
9. Niemegeers C J E, McGuire J L, Heykants J J P, Janssen P A J 1979 Dissociation between opiate-like and antidiarrhoea activities of antidiarrhoeal drugs. Journal of Pharmacology and Experimental Therapeutics 210(3): 327–333
10. Kachel G, Ruppin H, Hagel J, Barina W, Meinhardt M, Domschke W 1986 Human intestinal motor activity and transport: effects of a synthetic opiate. Gastroenterology 91(1): 85–93
11. Hughes S, Higgs N B, Turnberg L A 1984 Loperamide has anti-secretory activity in the human jejunum in vivo. Gut 23: 331–333
12. Schiller L R, Santa Ana C A, Morawski S G, Fordtran J S 1984 Mechanism of the antidiarrhoea effect of loperamide. Gastroenterology 86 (6)PB: 1475–1480
13. Scheurmans V, Van Lommel R, Dom J, Brugmans J 1974 Loperamide (R18 553) a novel type of antidiarrhoeal agent. Part 6: Clinical pharmacology. Placebo-controlled comparison of the constipating activity and safety of loperamide, diphenoxylate and codeine in normal volunteers. Arzneimittel Forschung 24: 1653–1657
14. Michiels M, Hendriks R, Heykants J 1977 Radioimmunoassay of antidiarrhoeal loperamide. Life Sciences 21: 451–460
15. Weintraub H S, Killinger J M, Fuller B L 1978 Human acute pharmacokinetics and comparative bio-availability of loperamide hydrochloride from capsule and syrup formulations. Gastroenterology 74: 1110 Abstract
16. Weintraub H S, Killinger J M, Heykants J, Kanzler M, Jaffe J H 1977 Studies on the elimination rate of loperamide in man after administration of increasing oral doses of Imodium. Current Therapeutic Research 21(6): 867–876
17. Hurkmans R, Meuldermans W, Heykants J 1977 The plasma protein binding and distribution of loperamide in human blood. Janssen preclinical research report no. 13 357 June (unpublished)
18. Wuester M, Hurz A 1978 Opiate agonist action of antidiarrhoeal agents in vitro and in vivo findings in support for selective action. Naunym Schmiedeberg's Archives of Pharmacology 301: 187–194
19. Heykants J, Michiels M, Knaeps A, Brugmans J 1974 Loperamide (R18 553) a novel type of antidiarrhoeal agent. Part 5: The pharmacokinetics of loperamide in rats and man. Arzneimittel Forschung 24: 1649–1653
20. Heykants J P, Mueldermans W E G, Knaeps A G, Michiels L J M 1977 The excretion and metabolism of the antidiarrhoeal loperamide in the Wistar rat. European Journal of Drug Metabolism and Pharmacology 2: 81–91
21. Michiels L M, Hendriks R, Heykants J, Scheijgrond H 1976 The absorption and excretion of loperamide in man after a single oral dose. Janssen clinical research report no 11 243, June 1976 (unpublished)
22. John G I 1977 Symptomatic treatment of acute self-limiting diarrhoea in adults. The Practitioner 219 (1311): 396–399
23. Anderson J 1984 Double-blind comparison of loperamide HCl and placebo in the treatment of acute diarrhoea in children. Advances in Therapy 1(1): 14–18
24. Palmer K R, Corbett C L, Holdsworth C D 1980 Double-blind cross-over study comparing loperamide codeine and diphenoxylate in the treatment of chronic diarrhoea. Gastroenterology 79(6): 1272–1275
25. Bergman L, Djarv L 1981 A comparative study of loperamide and diphenoxylate in the treatment of chronic diarrhoea caused by intestinal resection. Annals of Clinical Research 13: 402–405
26. Lishman A H, Sandle G I, Record C O 1982 The use of loperamide hydrochloride in the irritable bowel syndrome. Clinical Research Reviews 2(1): 45–49
27. Chapeaux J, Chapeaux P, Royer E 1978 Loperamide in patients with radiotherapy-induced diarrhoea. Arzneimittel Forschung/Drug Research 28(1)5: 864–866
28. Galambos J T 1978 Loperamide, a new antidiarrhoeal agent in the treatment of chronic diarrhoea. Schweizerische Medizinische Wochenschrift 108(28): 1080–1081
29. King R F G J, Norton T S, Hill C L 1979 Codeine or loperamide for ileostomy diarrhoea? A clinical trial. Gut 20(10): A906
30. King R F G J, Norton T, Hill G L 1982 A double-blind cross over study of the effect of loperamide hydrochloride and codeine phosphate on ileostomy output. Australian and New Zealand Journal of Surgery 52(2): A121–A124
31. Kirsner J B, Shorter R G 1988 In: Kirsner J B, Shorter R G (eds) Diseases of the colon, rectum and anal canal. Williams and Wilkins, Baltimore, p 280
32. Shearman D J C, Finlayson N D C 1982 In: Diseases of the gastrointestinal tract and liver. Churchill Livingstone, Edinburgh, p 890
33. Spiro H M 1970 Clinical gastroenterology, 2nd edn. Macmillan Publishing Co, p 742

L

Loratadine

Loratadine is a non-sedative H_1-histamine receptor antagonist with antiallergic properties, devoid of anticholinergic activity. It is rapidly effective and long-lasting, allowing once-a-day administration.

Chemistry

Loratadine (Loractin, Clarityn)
$C_{22}H_{23}N_2ClO_2$
Ethyl-4-(8-chloro-5,6-dihydro-11H-benzo-(5-6)-cyclohepta-(1,2-b)-pyridin-11-ylidine)piperidine-1 carboxylate

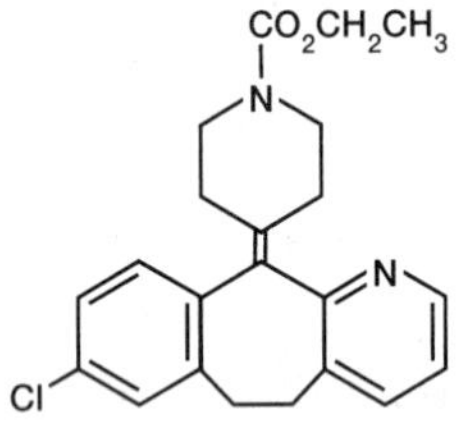

Molecular weight	382.88
pKa	5.0
Solubility	
in alcohol	1 in 10
in water	insoluble
Octanol/water partition coefficient	270

Loratadine is a white, odourless powder prepared by chemical synthesis. It is also available in an oral combination product with pseudoephedrine.

Pharmacology

Loratadine is derived from azatadine and is a potent and selective competitive antagonist at H_1-histamine receptors. It binds selectively to peripheral H_1-histamine receptors with a lower affinity to brain H_1-receptors.[1–4] It is therefore relatively free of CNS side effects, including sedation, as demonstrated by a relative lack of activity in assays of CNS function in animals. It also possesses antiallergic properties shown in vitro and in animal studies.[5] Loratadine has no anticholinergic properties at therapeutic doses.

Toxicology

Loratadine does not have mutagenic potential, and toxicological testing in animals at clinical doses have failed to demonstrate any results of potential clinical relevance. In a one-year study in rats, testicular atrophy and hypospermatogenesis were noted at doses equal to or greater than ten times the clinical dose. The results of teratogenicity tests showed no effect in rabbit at doses up to 480 times the clinical dose whereas in rats some effect was observed at 120 times the clinical dose.

Clinical pharmacology

Loratadine has been administered orally in safety and in tolerance studies at a maximal dose of 160 mg (single dose) or 40 mg twice daily for 28 days (multiple dose)[6–10] there was no evidence of toxicity.

Loratadine is a potent tricyclic H_1-receptor antagonist. It antagonizes the peripheral H_1-histamine receptors. Single or repeated oral doses of loratadine from 10 to 160 mg have shown that the drug decreases the wheal and flare reaction induced by histamine. The effect begins within 1–3 h, reaches a maximum at 8–12 h and lasts for more than 24 h.[11] The difference in activity between 10 mg once daily and 40 mg once daily was not great. Since studies of efficacy done in seasonal allergic rhinitis confirmed these clinical pharmacological studies, the dose of 10 mg once daily was chosen as the therapeutic dose.

Like other tricyclic compounds, loratadine also shows antiallergic activity, blocking the release of mediators by human chopped lung mast cells[12] and during nasal challenge with pollen grains[13] or by means of skin tests.[14] These data confirm previous animal studies.[5]

The effects of loratadine (10 mg once daily or 40 mg once daily) on CNS activity were tested and it was observed that it had little or no central effect.[15,16] In these experiments, diphenhydramine was found to increase daytime sleepiness and disrupt performance efficiency.

Pharmacokinetics

Radioimmunoassay is the preferred analytical method for loratadine, and HPLC is used for the active metabolite descarboethoxyloratadine. Both methods are highly specific and their sensitivity is under 1 $\mu g.l^{-1}$.

After oral administration, loratadine is rapidly and almost completely absorbed. It is rapidly metabolized to an active metabolite descarboethoxyloratadine. Plasma concentrations of loratadine reach a peak 1 h after its administration, and then decrease in two phases with mean half lives of 1 h and 10 h. Descarboethoxyloratadine appears rapidly in plasma, its maximal concentration is reached 2.4 h after the oral intake of loratadine. Plasma concentrations of the active metabolite decrease with a bi-exponential kinetic pattern with mean half lives of 2.3 h and 18 h.[17] These patterns explain the rapid onset of effect of the drug and its long-lasting activity. Loratadine, and to a lesser extent descarboethoxyloratadine, are highly bound to plasma proteins.

The distribution of loratadine in tissues has been studied in animals. The highest concentrations are found in lungs, liver and kidney.[18] On the other hand, there is very poor penetration into brain, and radioactivity in this tissue is not detectable by whole-body autoradiography. The volume of distribution has not been determined. Like other H_1-receptor antagonists, loratadine crosses the placental barrier. Loratadine is found in human breast milk, but only about 0.03% of the drug and active metabolite is excreted in milk in 48 h.[19]

Oral absorption	>90%
Presystemic metabolism	>90%
Plasma half life	
loratadine	
range	7–19 h
mean	12±4 h
descarboethoxyloratadine	
range	11–24 h
mean	18±4 h
Volume of distribution	—
Plasma protein binding	
loratadine	97–99%
descarboethoxyloratadine	73–76%

Loratadine has been administered to patients with renal or hepatic diseases and it was found that renal impairment has no significant effect on the bioavailability and disposition pharmacokinetics of loratadine and its active metabolite.[7] Haemodialysis does not clear loratadine and descarboethoxyloratadine so that it should not be used in cases of intoxication. In subjects with severe alcoholic liver disease the kinetics of loratadine (and to a lesser extent those of descarboethoxyloratadine) are altered but the differences do not appear to be clinically meaningful. Old age has been reported to have little effect on loratadine pharmacokinetics.[20]

Concentration–effect relationship

There is no evidence of a therapeutically useful correlation between the plasma concentration of loratadine or its active metabolite and the antihistaminic effects.

Metabolism

Loratadine is extensively and rapidly metabolized in the liver. It is excreted in urine (40% in 10 days) and faeces (42% in 10 days). There

Loratadine

is evidence of enterohepatic circulation in the rat. Three primary pathways of metabolism have been described.

hydrolysis of the carbamate moiety to form descarboethoxyloratadine
hydroxylation of descarboethoxyloratadine
glucuronidation.

Descarboethoxyloratadine has been found to be pharmacologically active, and has a half life compatible with the therapeutic effect of loratadine.

Pharmaceutics

Loratadine Clarityne (Schering Plough, Fr) Clarityn (Schering-Plough, UK) is available only in oral form. Clarityn are white to off-white tablets containing 10 mg micronized loratadine plus 90 mg of excipients including corn starch, lactose and magnesium stearate. There are no potentially allergenic substances in the excipients.

A syrup is also available for children at a concentration of 1 $mg.ml^{-1}$.

The maximal shelf-life is only given for the tablet formulation. Currently available data support a 48-month expiry date when the tablets are packaged in plastic bottles or blisters and stored between 2 and 30°C. This will probably be extended as longer-term data become available.

Therapeutic use

Indications

Loratadine has been submitted to licensing authorities in several countries and approved in a few others for the treatment of:

1. Seasonal allergic rhinitis
2. Perennial allergic rhinitis
3. Skin allergies including urticaria.

Contraindications

Loratadine is contraindicated in patients who have shown hypersensitivity or idiosyncrasy to its component.

Mode of use

All the clinical uses depend upon the antihistaminic and antiallergic activities of loratadine. The drug is given only by the oral route at doses of 10 mg once daily in adults and children over 30 kg of body weight and 5 mg once daily in children under 30 kg of body weight or under 5 years of age. A syrup is available for children.

Sudden withdrawal of loratadine is not hazardous but symptoms may reappear within 24–48 h.

Indications

Loratadine is indicated for relief of symptoms of seasonal and perennial allergic rhinitis[18,21–27] and skin allergic diseases.[28–31] The onset of relief of symptoms is rapid, improvement in allergy symptoms is observed within the first hour.[32] Owing to its lack of tachyphylaxis, loratadine can be administered over several weeks without any decreased activity.[33]

1. Seasonal allergic rhinitis
More than 4000 patients suffering from allergic rhinitis have been included in multi-centre double-blind, placebo/active controlled trials. The efficacy of loratadine in relieving symptoms of seasonal allergic rhinitis is similar to that of the classical or non-sedative antihistamines. In several studies it was found that the percentage improvement in mean total symptom scores (including nasal and ocular symptoms) was 49.6% in the loratadine-treated group vs. 48% in patients treated by clemastine (1 mg twice daily, 440 patients), 47.5% for mequitazine (5 mg twice daily, 68 patients), 46% for astemizole (10 mg once daily, 257 patients), 45% for terfenadine (60 mg twice daily, 232 patients) and 26% for the placebo group (841 patients).[18,21–26]

The clinical pharmacology wheal and flare studies showed that loratadine produced an effect within two hours of taking the first dose. Three clinical studies were specifically designed to determine the onset of allergy symptoms in patients with seasonal allergic rhinitis. In two studies patients estimated the time when relief of allergic symptoms first occurred in hours after the first dose. In both studies, the comparative antihistamine was astemizole 10 mg once daily and placebo. Loratadine demonstrated significantly earlier relief of symptoms than astemizole or placebo. Respectively, 28% and 73% of the patients of these two studies treated by loratadine experienced relief of symptoms within 4 h compared to 15% and 32% of the astemizole-treated patients. In the third study, the onset of relief was measured in minutes after the first dose. The mean onset of relief of allergy symptoms following the first dose was 27.1 min. Onset of relief began in as little as 10–20 min; by this time 30% of patients had experienced some relief of symptoms. By 40 min after the first dose, 100% of patients found relief from symptoms.[32]

2. Perennial rhinitis
More than 1300 patients suffering from perennial rhinitis have been included in multi-centre, double-blind, placebo/active controlled trials. In these studies, patients were treated for up to six months. Results confirmed the efficacy of loratadine, which improves symptoms of perennial rhinitis as much as the classical antihistamines used as a reference drug, such as clemastine and terfenadine.[27]

3. Chronic urticaria
Several multi-centre, double-blind, placebo/active controlled studies have shown that loratadine is effective in the treatment of chronic urticaria. Moreover, although many patients treated by placebo or terfenadine tend to drop out of the treatment very early, a higher percentage of patients treated by loratadine stayed on the treatment until the completion of the study (1 month).[28–31]

Adverse reactions

Potentially life-threatening effects
No effects of this kind have been encountered.

Acute overdosage
No cases of acute overdosage have been reported.

Severe or irreversible adverse effects
No effects of this degree of severity have been reported.

Symptomatic adverse effects
During double-blind, placebo-controlled trials in the treatment of allergic rhinitis, in which over 2000 patients were treated by loratadine, it was found to induce a very low rate of adverse effects, comparable to placebo, in particular for CNS effects (including sedation) and anticholinergic activity. The incidence of sedation was similar to that in the groups treated by the classical non-sedative antihistamines (astemizole and terfenadine) and was significantly lower than in the group of patients receiving clemastine. The lack of sedation by loratadine reported during clinical trials was confirmed by special psychomotor studies such as the driving performance test.[35–37] The most common effects reported were fatigue, dizziness, dry mouth, headache, sedation, nausea and pruritus.[18,21–34]

There is no information to indicate that abuse or dependency occurs with loratadine. No tachyphylaxis or tolerance has been observed during clinical trials.[18,21–34]

Interference with clinical pathology tests
No clinically significant changes in mean or median laboratory (standard battery of tests) values and no trends of changes were discernible for patients treated with loratadine, regardless of dose of loratadine or length of treatment.[18,21–33]

High risk groups

Neonates
The drug is not normally used in neonates.

Breast milk. Loratadine, as other H_1-receptor antagonists, is excreted in the breast milk so that nursing mothers are advised not to take the drug.

Children
There are no special precautions required in young children over 2 years. A recent study confirmed the efficacy of loratadine suspension in children[38].

Pregnant women
Although loratadine was not found to be teratogenic in animals, the safe use of loratadine during pregnancy has not been established and

Loratadine

L

therefore the compound should be used only if the potential benefit justifies the potential risk to fetus.

The elderly
No special precautions are required in the elderly.

Concurrent disease
Renal impairment has no clinically significant effects. Severe hepatic damage alters the pharmacokinetics of loratadine but has little clinical importance.

Drug interactions

Potentially hazardous interactions
To date, there are no reports of potentially hazardous interactions with other drugs. In contrast to many other H_1-receptor antagonists, loratadine has no potentiating effects when administered concomitantly with alcohol, as measured by psychomotor performance.

Potentially useful interactions
No interactions of this kind have been observed.

Clinical trials

1. Dockhorn R J, Bergner A, Connell J T et al 1987 Safety and efficacy of loratadine (SCH 29 851) a new non-sedating antihistamine in seasonal allergic rhinitis. Annals of Allergy 58: 407–411

330 patients with seasonal pollen-induced rhinitis were tested in a double-blind, parallel group, placebo-controlled study in which loratadine (10 mg once daily) was compared to clemastine 1 mg twice daily. Patients were randomly assigned to receive one of the three treatments for a period of 14 days. They were examined after 3, 7 and 14 days of treatment. Nasal and ocular symptoms due to pollen exposure were recorded.

This study shows that the incidence of sedation with loratadine is comparable to placebo and significantly lower than with clemastine. The incidence of anticholinergic side effects was low in the three groups of patients. The efficacy of loratadine is similar to that of clemastine and significantly superior to that of placebo.

Loratadine is as effective as clemastine, an efficacious conventional antihistamine, and induces less CNS depression.

2. Skassa-Brociek W, Bousquet J, Montes F et al 1988 Double-blind controlled study of loratadine, mequitazine and placebo in the symptomatic treatment of seasonal allergic rhinitis. Journal of Allergy and Clinical Immunology 81: 725–730

This is a double-blind, parallel group study examining the efficacy and safety of loratadine vs. placebo and a reference antihistamine (mequitazine) in the treatment of seasonal allergic rhinitis. 69 patients were evaluated over a period of two weeks using the same study design as Dockorn et al. Loratadine and mequitazine were found to be safe, inducing no more adverse reactions than placebo. Both drugs were significantly more effective than placebo in reducing nasal symptoms due to pollen allergy. Loratadine was significantly more effective than mequitazine after 3 days of treatment.

This study confirms the safety and efficacy of loratadine when compared to an H_1-receptor antagonist widely used in Europe. Moreover, the rapid onset of action of loratadine was confirmed in this study.

3. Saraceno E B, Falabella R, Dominguez L Comparative effects of loratadine and terfenadine in the treatment of chronic allergic disorders. Medicina Cutanea (in press)

The efficacy and safety of loratadine 10 mg once daily were compared with terfenadine 60 mg twice daily in controlling symptoms of allergic skin disorders. This study was a randomized, multi-centre, parallel group, double-blind design involving 101 patients divided into two groups receiving either loratadine or terfenadine for a period of 28 days. Patients had moderate to severe symptoms of urticaria before treatment. Both treatments significantly reduced symptoms compared to baseline. In particular, they were effective in relieving pruritus and itching. Sedation was nearly absent in each treatment group. No anticholinergic side effects were reported.

This study shows that loratadine is effective in chronic urticaria and elicits very few side effects.

Other trials

1. Bousquet J, Lebel B, Chanal I, Morel A, Michel F B 1988 Anti-allergic activity of loratadine and terfenadine assessed by nasal challenge. Journal of Allergy and Clinical Immunology 82: 881–887

This study examines the activity of loratadine 10 mg once daily, terfenadine 60 mg twice daily and placebo in nasal challenges with pollen grains in 15 patients highly allergic to grass pollens. The design is double-blind crossover. Nasal challenges were performed at 2-week intervals after a treatment course of 7 days. The positivity of the challenge was assessed by symptom scores.

It was found that both antihistamines had a significant and similar protective activity when compared to placebo. The release of histamine and PGD_2 in nasal secretions was examined. Loratadine blocked the release of histamine and delayed the release of PGD_2 whereas terfenadine had only a minor effect.

This study confirms by objective measurements that loratadine is effective in reducing nasal symptoms due to pollen exposure; its activity is similar to that of terfenadine. Loratadine possesses antiallergic activity.[39]

References

1. Barnett A, Iorio L C, Kreutner W, Tozzi S, Ahn H S, Gulbenkian A 1984 Evaluation of the CNS properties of SCH 29 851, a potential non-sedating antihistamine. Agents and Actions 14: 590–597
2. Ahn H S, Barnett A 1986 Selective displacement of ^{3}H-mepyramine from peripheral versus central nervous system receptors by loratadine, a non-sedating antihistamine. European Journal of Pharmacology 127: 153–155
3. Iorio L C, Cohen-Winston M, Barnett A 1986 Interaction studies in mice of Sch 29 851, a potential non-sedating anti-histamine, with commonly used therapeutic agents. Agents and Actions 18: 485–493
4. Villani F J, Magatti C V, Vashi D B, Wong J, Popper T L 1986 N-substituted 11-(4-piperidylene)-(5,6)-cyclohepta (1,2-b) pyridines; antihistamines with no sedating liability. Drug Research 36: 1311–1314
5. Kreutner W, Chapman R W, Gulbenkian A, Siegel M I 1987 Antiallergic activity of loratadine, a non-sedating antihistamine. Allergy 42: 57–63
6. Kassem N, Roman I, Gural R, Dyer G, Robillard N 1988 Effects of loratadine in suppression of histamine-induced skin wheals. Annals of Allergy 60: 505–507
7. Hilbert J M, Matzke G R, Radwanski E et al 1986 Loratadine pharmacokinetics in renal impairment. Journal of Allergy and Clinical Immunology 79: 206 (abstract)
8. Katelaris C H, 1986 A double-blind study of the effect of SCH 29851 in patients with seasonal allergic rhinitis. Asian Pacific Journal of Allergy and Immunology 4: 49
9. Batenhorst R L, Batenhorst A S, Graves D A et al 1986 Pharmacologic evaluation of loratadine, SCH 29 851, chlorpheniramine and placebo. European Journal of Clinical Pharmacology 31: 247–250
10. Radwanski E, Hilbert J, Symchowicz S, Zampaglione N 1987 Loratadine; multiple dose pharmacokinetics. Journal of Clinical Pharmacology 27: 530–533
11. Roman I J, Kassem N, Gural R P, Herron J 1986 Suppression of histamine-induced wheal response by loratadine (SCH 29 851) over 28 days in man. Annals of Allergy 57: 253–256
12. Temple D M, McCluskey M 1988 Loratadine, an antihistamine, blocks antigen- and ionophone-induced leukotriene release from human lung in vitro. Prostaglandins 35: 549–554
13. Bousquet J, Lebel B, Chanal I, Morel A, Godard P, Michel F B 1988 Anti-allergic activity of loratadine and terfenadine assessed by nasal challenge. Journal of Allergy and Clinical Immunology 82: 881–887
14. Skassa-Brociek W, O'Quigley J, Blizard R, Cougnard J, Michel F B, Bousquet J 1988 Differentiation between the anti-allergic and anti-histaminic effects of loratadine and astemizole. Journal of Allergy and Clinical Immunology 81: 175 (abstract)
15. Bradley C M, Nicholson A N 1987 Studies on the central effects of the H_1-antagonist, loratadine. European Journal of Clinical Pharmacology 32: 419–421
16. Roth T, Roehrs T, Koshorek G, Sicklesteel J, Zorrick F 1987 Sedative effects of antihistamines. Journal of Allergy and Clinical Immunology 80: 94–98
17. Katchen B, Cramer J, Chung M et al 1985 Disposition of ^{14}C-SCH 29 851 in humans. Annals of Allergy 55: 293 (abstract)
18. Friedman H M 1987 Loratadine, a potent, nonsedating, and long-acting H_1 antagonist. American Journal of Rhinology 1: 95–99
19. Hilbert J, Radwanski E, Affrime M B, Perentesis G, Symchowicz S, Zampaglione N 1988 Excretion of loratadine in human breast milk. Journal of Clinical Pharmacology 28: 234–239
20. Hilbert J, Moritzen V, Parks A et al 1988 Pharmacokinetics of loratadine in normal geriatric volunteers. Journal of International Medical Research 16: 50–60
21. Dockhorn R J, Bergner A, Connell J T et al 1987 Safety and efficacy of loratadine (SCH 29 851) a new non-sedating antihistamine in seasonal allergic rhinitis. Annals of Allergy 58: 407–411
22. Oei H D 1988 Double-blind comparison of loratadine (SCH 29 851), astemizole and placebo in hay fever with special regard to onset of action. Annals of Allergy 61: 436–439
23. Skassa-Brociek W, Bousquet J, Montes F et al 1988 Double-blind controlled study of loratadine, mequitazine and placebo in the symptomatic treatment of seasonal allergic rhinitis. Journal of Allergy and Clinical Immunology 81: 725–730

24. Kemp J P, Bahna S L, Chervinsky P et al 1987 A comparison of loratadine, a new nonsedating anti-histamine with clemastine and placebo in patients with fall seasonal allergic rhinitis. American Journal of Rhinology 1: 151–154
25. Gutowski A, Bedard P, Del Carpio J et al 1988 Comparison of the efficacy and safety of loratadine, terfenadine and placebo in the treatment of seasonal allergic rhinitis. Journal of Allergy and Clinical Immunology 81: 902–907
26. Horak F, Bruttmann G, Pedrali P et al 1988 A multicentric study of loratadine, terfenadine and placebo in patients with seasonal allergic rhinitis. Drug Research 38: 124–128
27. Bruttmann G, Charpin D, Germouty J, Horak F, Kunkel G, Wittman G 1989 Evaluation of the efficacy and safety of loratadine in perennial allergic rhinitis. Journal of Allergy and Clinical Immunology 83: 411–416
28. Saraceno E B, Falabella R, Dominguez L 1990 Comparative effects of loratadine and terfenadine in the treatment of chronic allergic disorders. Medicina Cutanea (in press)
29. Belaich S, Bruttman G, DeGreef H et al 1990 Comparative effects of loratadine and terfenadine in the treatment of chronic idiopathic urticaria. Annals of Allergy 64: 191–194
30. Monroe E W, Fox R W, Green A W et al 1988 Efficacy and safety of loratadine (10 mg OD) in the management of idiopathic chronic urticaria. Journal American Academy Dermatology 19: 138–139
31. Monroe E W 1989 Antihistamines in skin allergies. In: Kaliner M (ed) Management of allergy in the 1990's. Hans Huber Publishers, Toronto, pp 59–66
32. Soto Roman L Onset of action of loratadine in seasonal allergic rhinitis. British Journal of Clinical Pharmacology (in press)
33. Bousquet J, Chanal I, Skassa-Brociek W, Lemonier C, Michel F B 1990 Lack of subsensitivity to loratadine during long-term dosing over 12 weeks. Journal Allergy and Clinical Immunology 86: 248–252
34. Anonymous 1987 Loratadine. Drugs of the Future 12: 544–549
35. Betts T, Wild J, Ross K, Kenwood C, Yhirtle-Watts R 1989 A double-blind, single-dose study of the effects of loratadine on driving skills of normal volunteers. In: Kaliner M (ed) Management of allergy in the 1990's. Hans Huber Publishers, Toronto, pp 38–49
36. Riedel W J, Schoenmakers E A J M, O'Hanlon J F 1989 Sedation and performance impairment with anti-histamines. In: Kaliner M (ed) Management of allergy in the 1990's. Hans Huber Publishers, Toronto, pp 38–49
37. O'Hanlon J F 1988 Antihistamines and driving safety. Cutis 27: 10–13
38. Borier A L, Miglioranzi P, Richelli C, Marchesi E, Andreoli A 1989 Efficacy and safety of Loratadine suspension in the treatment of children with allergic rhinitis. Allergy 44: 437–441
39. Bousquet J, Chanez P, Michel F B 1989 Anti-allergic activity of antihistamines. In: Kaliner M (ed) Management of allergy in the 1990's. Hans Huber Publishers, Toronto, pp 21–37

Lorazepam

Lorazepam is a short-acting tranquillizer of the benzodiazepine group.

Chemistry

Lorazepam (Ativan)
$C_{15}H_{10}N_2O_2Cl_2$
7-Chloro-5-(2-chlorophenyl)-1,3-dihydro-3-hydroxy-2H-1,4-benzodiazepin-2-one

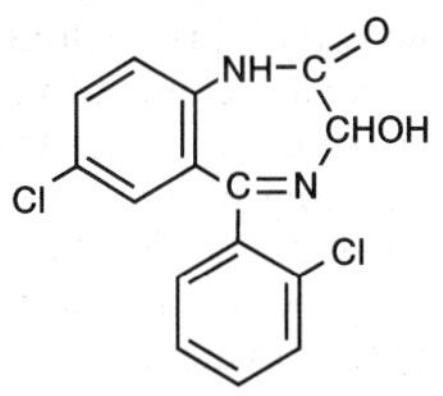

Molecular weight	321.2
pKa1	1.3
pKa2	11.5
Solubility	
in alcohol	1 in 71
in water	1 in 125 000
Octanol/water partition coefficient	73

Lorazepam is a white or almost white crystalline powder. It is prepared by chemical synthesis.

Pharmacology

Lorazepam is an agonist at benzodiazepine receptors in the CNS (central nervous system). It exerts a central depressant action on the (CNS) which may be mediated by potentiating the inhibitory actions of GABA in the CNS. This will result in diminution of the ascending activating systems, particularly the serotoninergic and noradrenergic pathway from brain stem or the mid-brain to the cerebral cortex. It is a highly potent benzodiazepine with a binding affinity to the benzodiazepine receptor in brain considerably greater than the binding affinity of nitrazepam or diazepam.[1]

Toxicology

Rats or dogs treated with doses in excess of 400 times those used therapeutically in humans have shown no toxic effects.

In male and female rabbits, tests indicated that lorazepam has no adverse effects on fertility, and no teratogenic action.

Clinical pharmacology

Lorazepam is an intermediate-acting benzodiazepine producing central depression of the CNS. Electrocardiographic recordings indicate that lorazepam begins to penetrate the CNS almost immediately following intravenous administration.

The CNS depression produced by lorazepam is dose-related. A 2 mg dose of lorazepam given intravenously produces perceptible sedation lasting 4 to 6 hours. An oral dose of 5 mg produces more obvious sedation. In addition, an oral dose of 5 mg produces anterograde amnesia. Doses greater than 7 mg produce initial stimulation with an EEG pattern consistent with stage I anaesthesia.[2] Sedation and anaesthesia are both dose-related.

In normal volunteers doses of 1 and 2 mg orally produce significant

Lorazepam

L

impairment of hand–eye coordination. There have been no other effects detected in peripheral visual tests.[3] Lorazepam produces dose-related impairment in other tests of psychomotor function, e.g. critical flicker fusion frequency and reaction time. Lorazepam, like all intermediate-acting benzodiazepines, may produce dependence but the dependence liability with lorazepam seems greater than with other benzodiazepines.

In comparison with other tranquillizers, 1 mg of lorazepam produces a similar degree of CNS depression to 5 mg of diazepam given orally.[4]

Lorazepam produces no significant change in blood pressure, pulse rate, ECG or cardiac output.[5]

In normal subjects lorazepam has mild if any effects on the respiratory system.[6] Parenteral doses of 2.5 mg or more may produce mild respiratory depression in patients with chronic obstructive lung disease.[6]

Pharmacokinetics

Lorazepam can be detected by electron-capture gas–liquid chromatography which has a limit of sensitivity of 1 μg.l^{-1}.

Following oral administration lorazepam is absorbed from the gastrointestinal tract. Peak plasma level is reached after approximately 2 hours. Oral bioavailability of lorazepam averages 90%.[8] The mean half life of lorazepam elimination in humans is 15 hours, with a usual range of 8 to 25 hours in healthy individuals.[8] The half life is not impaired by the aging process or renal disease but may be prolonged in the case of hepatic dysfunction.[9,10]

Lorazepam is extensively bound to plasma proteins with a free fraction of 8–12%.[11] There is evidence that it crosses the placenta.

Oral absorption	90%
Presystemic metabolism	—
Plasma half life	
range	8–25 h
mean	15 h
Volume of distribution	1–2 l.kg^{-1}
Plasma protein binding	88–92%

Concentration–effect relationship

Lorazepam has a longer duration of action than its half life would lead one to expect. The extent of its binding to benzodiazepine receptors in the brain correlates well with its duration of action.[12] However, in spite of its lack of active metabolites there is no evidence of a correlation between blood levels of lorazepam and its therapeutic effect.

Metabolism

The major metabolic pathway of lorazepam in humans involves conjugation at the 3 position with glucuronic acid in the liver. This yields a water-soluble metabolite which is pharmacologically inactive and is eliminated mainly by renal excretion.[13] Up to 75% of the dose is excreted as this metabolite within 5 days. A small amount of lorazepam is metabolized by other routes to hydroxylorazepam or to quinazolinine or quinazoline carboxylic acid derivatives. Unlike those of many other benzodiazepines, the metabolites are not responsible for the pharmacological effect to any significant degree.

Pharmaceutics

Lorazepam is available in oral and parenteral forms.

1. Lorazepam tablets contain lorazepam 1 or 2.5 mg.
2. Ativan tablets (Wyeth, UK) are capsule-shaped containing 1 mg or 2.5 mg lorazepam. They measure approximately 4 × 8 mm with a break bar on one side. The 2.5 mg tablets are yellow and marked with 'A2.5' and the 1 mg tablets are blue and marked with 'A1' on the other side. In the USA, Ativan tablets are white, five-sided and come in three strengths: 0.5 mg (coded '81'), 1 mg (coded '64') and 2 mg (coded '65').
3. Ativan injection (Wyeth, UK) is a clear, colourless solution containing lorazepam at a concentration of 4 mg.ml^{-1} supplied in 1 ml quantities in clear glass ampoules. A half-strength formulation is also available in the USA.

Tablets should be stored in a cool dry, place. Ativan injection should be stored in a refrigerator between 0°C and 4°C and should be protected from light. The shelf-life for tablets and injections is 2 years.

Therapeutic use

Indications

1. Treatment of anxiety states
2. Anxiety associated with phobic and obsessional states, psychosomatic, organic or psychotic illnesses
3. Insomnia associated with anxiety
4. As a premedicant before dental or general surgery or prior to investigative procedures where there may be discomfort
5. As an anticonvulsant.

Contraindications

Lorazepam should not be given to patients with a previous sensitivity to benzodiazepines.

Mode of use

Lorazepam tablets

In mild anxiety in adults 1–4 mg per day in divided doses can be given. In severe anxiety the dose can be increased to 8 mg per day. For insomnia, the dose is 1–4 mg before retiring. As a premedicant, 2–3 mg is given on the night before the operation with 2–4 mg 1 to 2 hours before the procedure.

In the elderly the dose required may be much lower than those referred to above and may be less than half the adult dose.

Lorazepam is not recommended for use in children.

Lorazepam injection

Ativan injection can be given intravenously or intramuscularly. Care should be taken to avoid injecting into small veins or arteries. Absorption from intramuscular injection may be no better than that achieved with oral administration of tablets.

Prior to injection the solution may be diluted 1:1 with normal saline or Water for Injections BP. This should always be done in the case of intramuscular administration.

Dosage. As a premedicant, the dosage is 0.05 mg.kg^{-1}. It should be administered 30 to 45 minutes before surgery when given intravenously, or 60 to 90 minutes before surgery when given intramuscularly.

In severe acute anxiety, 0.025–0.03 mg.kg^{-1} may be given repeated up to 6-hourly as necessary.

In status epilepticus, the dosage is 4 mg intravenously in adults; 2 mg intravenously in children.

The injection should be given slowly except in the case of status epilepticus where rapid injection is required.

Patients require observation following ativan injection and should not drive or operate machinery for at least 24 hours.

Fig. 1 Metabolism of lorazepam

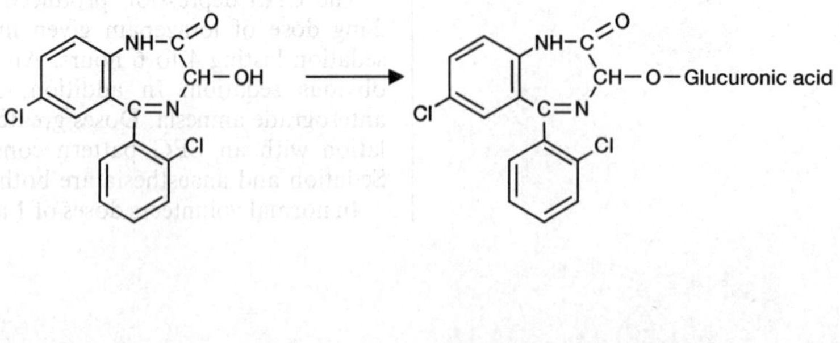

Indications

1, 2. Anxiety

Lorazepam is effective in alleviating the symptoms of pathological anxiety in anxiety states and in anxiety associated with other psychiatric disorders.[14] In general it should not be used in non-pathological anxiety where it may inhibit rather than enhance psychological adjustment. In the case of mixed depression and anxiety the therapeutic effect is on the anxiety symptoms only.[15,16]

Unless anxiety is severe and acute, initial dosage should be low and then increased slowly to achieve symptom control. Use of the lowest required dose reduces the incidence of unwanted side effects.

Comparisons with other benzodiazepines in terms of therapeutic effect in general show no great advantage of one component over the others.[17]

The length of the course of treatment should be kept to the minimum.[18] It is preferable that doses are taken at times when anxiety is more severe or when anxiety is anticipated rather than on a regular basis. In the case of severe, acute anxiety lorazepam injection may be used. When given intravenously, this is effective in five minutes.[19]

The usefulness of lorazepam in chronic anxiety with symptoms of longer duration than six weeks is, as is the case with other benzodiazepines, more doubtful. In such cases alternative methods of treatment, e.g. psychological therapies, should be considered.

With prolonged usage there is the risk of development of dependence with a resulting withdrawal syndrome when the medication is discontinued.[18] The longest safe course of treatment which avoids this risk is not known but it may be as short as six weeks.[20] There is some evidence that the withdrawal syndrome may occur earlier and be more severe in the case of shorter-acting drugs compared to those with longer half lives, e.g. diazepam.[21] Because of the problems of dependence it is advised that when a course of treatment is to be ended the dose should be reduced gradually to reduce the severity of the withdrawal syndrome.

3. Insomnia

In doses of 2 mg or more, lorazepam is more effective than placebo in promoting sleep.[22] It should be used for the shortest period of time and in conjunction with non-drug strategies. Administration when required is preferable to regular night-time use.

4. Premedicant

Parenteral injection of lorazepam is associated with sedation and relief of anxiety. Patients become calm and drowsy, though rousable to be able to cooperate with the procedure being undertaken. Most patients experience reduced recall or amnesia for the time of the procedure. Lorazepam has been used prior to gastroscopy, bronchoscopy and pneumoencephalography. Lorazepam tablets may be used as a premedicant, doses being given the night before the procedure and a second dose 1 to 2 hours before the procedure. The periods of amnesia associated with the use of lorazepam can be of advantage in the intensive care unit, e.g. during periods of assisted ventilation.

The amnesic effect varies but with doses of 4 mg amnesia occurs in 60–80% of cases within 15 minutes and persists for 4 hours.[23]

5. Status epilepticus

In status epilepticus intravenous lorazepam is rapidly effective. No adverse effects on cardiac or respiratory function have been reported. It has been reported that rapid injection is more effective than slow administration.[24]

Adverse reactions

Potentially life-threatening effects

No life-threatening adverse effects have been reported in humans. In 10 403 cases of acute overdose of lorazepam over eight years there was moderate central nervous system depression but no reported haemodynamic or respiratory problems.[25]

Acute overdosage

There is no specific treatment for acute overdosage. Management is symptomatic. If the patient is conscious an emetic may be given. A clear airway should be ensured at all times.

Severe or irreversible adverse effects

None has been reported.

Lorazepam

Symptomatic adverse effects

Reported side effects include daytime drowsiness, headache, dizziness, blurred vision, nausea and occasionally confusion. Drowsiness is common at the start of treatment. Ataxia when present often indicates excessive dosage.

The incidence of side effects in a pooled group of 3520 patients was:[26]

Sedation 15.9%
Dizziness 6.9%
Weakness 4.5%.

Most adverse effects occurred on the first day of treatment and could be managed without discontinuing treatment.

Other effects

In biochemical and haematological tests carried out on volunteers over a period of six months, taking up to 10 mg lorazepam per day, no drug-related abnormalities were found.[27]

Interference with clinical pathology tests

There is no known interference with the results of such tests.

High risk groups

Neonates

Lorazepam is not recommended in neonates.

Breast milk. Concentrations of most benzodiazepines in breast milk are very low but sedation may occur in the first 1–2 weeks of infant life perhaps due to slow metabolism of the drug by the infant.[28]

Children

Lorazepam is not recommended in anxiety states in children but may be used as a premedicant in a dose of 0.05 $mg.kg^{-1}$ in children aged 5–13 years.

Pregnant women

Lorazepam should not be administered during pregnancy or lactation unless in the judgement of the physician such administration is clinically justifiable. Special care should be taken in the first three months of pregnancy and also during labour.

The elderly

The elderly frequently require lower doses of lorazepam than the recommended adult dose. Care should be taken in the confused elderly patient, where tranquillizers including lorazepam may increase the degree of confusion. Similarly, lorazepam may reduce the level of consciousness and this should be borne in mind when an elderly person presents with drowsiness or confusion.

Concurrent disease

Lorazepam should be used with caution in patients with impairment of hepatic or renal function. Cirrhosis is associated with an increase in the elimination half life.[21]

Lorazepam should be used with caution in patients with acute or chronic pulmonary insufficiency.

Drug interactions

Potentially hazardous interactions

The most important drug interaction with lorazepam is the potentiation of the central depressant effect when combined with other drugs with central depressant action. Such drugs include alcohol, general anaesthetics, narcotic analgesics, tricyclic antidepressants and monoamine oxidase inhibitors. There were no interactions noted between lorazepam and the drugs used to treat hypertension or angina. No interaction was noted with anticoagulants, digitalis glycosides, anti-inflammatory agents, antimitotics, corticosteroids or intestinal antiseptics.

Potentially useful interactions

None has been reported.

Clinical trials

Richards D J 1978 Clinical profile of lorazepam, a new benzodiazepine tranquillizer. Journal of Clinical Psychiatry 39: 58–66

Richards pooled the results from 123 studies in which lorazepam had been used. These included 5966 patients of whom 3520 received lorazepam. Patients were rated by the clinician using a global rating scale and also the Hamilton Anxiety Rating Scale (HARS). Patients also completed self-rating assessments.

In those studies investigating anxiety neurosis, 12 used a twice daily regimen and 4 a three times daily regimen. Of the 2552 patients in this group 1446 received lorazepam. The dose range was generally 3–6 mg per day in divided doses. The pooled results of these trials indicated that lorazepam was more effective than placebo in reducing symptoms of anxiety up to four weeks. Similar results were found when comparing diazepam to placebo.

References

1. Speth R C, Wastek G J, Johnson P C, Yamamura H I 1978 Benzodiazepine binding in human brain: characterisation using [^{3}H]flunitrazepam. Life Sciences 22: 859–866
2. Comer W H, Elliot H W, Nomof N et al 1974 Pharmacology of parenterally administered lorazepam in man. Journal of International Medical Research 1: 216–225
3. Bell R W, Dickie D S, Stewart-Jones J, Turner P 1973 Lorazepam on visuo-motor coordination and visual function in man. (Letter) Journal of Pharmacy and Pharmacology 25: 87–88
4. Hedges A, Turner P, Harry T V A 1971 Preliminary studies on the central effects of lorazepam, a new benzodiazepine. Journal of Clinical Pharmacology 11: 423–427
5. Knapp R B, Fierro L 1974 Evaluation of the cardiopulmonary safety and effects of lorazepam as a premedicant. Anaesthesia and Analgesia Current Researches 53: 122–124
6. Dodson M E, Yousseff Y, Pleuvry B 1976 Respiratory effects of lorazepam. (Letter) British Journal of Anaesthesia 48: 611–612
7. Denault M, Yernault J C, DeCosta A 1975 A double-blind comparison of the respiratory effects of parenteral lorazepam and diazepam in patients with chronic obstructive lung disease. Current Medical Research and Opinion 2: 611–615
8. Greenblatt D J, Shader R I, Franke K et al 1979 Pharmacokinetics and bioavailability of intravenous, intramuscular and oral lorazepam in humans. Journal of Pharmaceutical Sciences 68: 57–63
9. Verbeeck R, Tjandramaga T B, Verberckmoes R, Schepper P J 1976 Biotransformation and excretion of lorazepam in patients with chronic renal failure. British Journal of Clinical Pharmacology 3: 1033–1039
10. Kraus J W, Desmond P V, Marshall J P, Johnson R F, Schenker S, Wilkinson G R 1978 Effects of aging and liver disease on the disposition of lorazepam. Clinical Pharmacology and Therapeutics 24: 411–419
11. Greenblatt D J 1981 Clinical pharmacokinetics of oxazepam and lorazepam. Clinical Pharmacokinetics 6: 89–105
12. Spirt N M, Bautz G, Zanko M, Horst W D, O'Brien R A 1981 Comparative receptor binding effects in brain after i.v. lorazepam and diazepam administration. Society of Neuroscience Abstracts 7: 865
13. Greenblatt D J, Schillings R T, Kyriakopoulos A A et al 1976 Clinical pharmacokinetics of lorazepam. I. Absorption and disposition of oral ^{14}C-lorazepam. Clinical Pharmacology and Therapeutics 20: 329–341
14. Haider I 1971 Evaluation of a new tranquillizer — WY 4036 — in the treatment of anxiety. British Journal of Psychiatry 119: 597–598
15. McCurdy L, Schatzberg A F 1978 Studies with oral lorazepam in anxiety neurosis associated with depressive symptomatology. Journal of Clinical Psychiatry 39 (No 10 Sect 2): 30–34
16. Benzodiazepines; dependence and withdrawal symptoms. Committee on Safety of Medicines, Current Problems No 21 Jan 1988
17. Ameer B, Greenblatt D 1981 Lorazepam, a review of its clinical pharmacological properties and therapeutic uses. Drugs 21: 161–200
18. Committee on the Review of Medicines 1980 Systematic review of the benzodiazepines. British Medical Journal 280: 910–921
19. Bacellar B B 1975 The treatment of acute anxiety states in neurotic patients with intravenous lorazepam. A placebo controlled study. Current Medical Research and Opinion 3: 16–21
20. Power K G, Jerrom R J, Simpson M 1985 Controlled study of withdrawal symptoms and rebound anxiety after six week course of diazepam for generalised anxiety. British Medical Journal 290: 1246–1248
21. Tyrer P, Rutherford D, Huggett T 1981 Benzodiazepine withdrawal symptoms and propranolol. Lancet 1: 520
22. Sechzer P H 1976 Demand method evaluation of hypnotics. Current Therapeutic Research 19: 637–644
23. Pandit S K, Heisterkamp D V, Cohen P J 1976 Further studies on the antirecall effect of lorazepam. A dose time–effect relationship. Anesthesiology 45: 495–500
24. Amand G, Evrard P 1978 Preliminary results on the use of injectable lorazepam in status epilepticus. Epilepsia
25. Garnier R, Riboulet-Delmas G, Gastot A, Efthymiou M L 1982 Acute lorazepam overdose a retrospective study at the Paris poison control centre. (January 1974–December 1981). Veterinary and Human Toxicology 24: 284
26. Richards D J 1978 Clinical profile of lorazepam a new benzodiazepine tranquillizer. Journal of Clinical Psychiatry 39: 58–66
27. Leube H, Hoffkes H 1971 Experience with the new tranquillizer WY 4036 (lorazepam) in the areas of psychiatric neurology and internal medicine. Arzneimittel-forschung 21: 1098
28. Whitelaw A G L et al 1981 The effect of maternal lorazepam on the neonate. British Medical Journal 1: 1106–1108

Lovastatin

Lovastatin is an inactive tricyclic lactone prodrug which is converted in vivo by esterases to the corresponding open hydroxyacid which is a potent inhibitor of endogenous cholesterol synthesis, and is a cholesterol-lowering agent. The lovastatin acid is a competitive inhibitor of 3-hydroxy, 3-methylglutaryl coenzyme A (HMG-CoA) reductase, the major rate-limiting step in cholesterol synthesis.

Chemistry

Lovastatin (Mevacor)
$C_{24}H_{36}O_5$
[1S,7S,8S,8aR]-1,2,3,7,8,8a-Hexahydro-3,7-dimethyl-8-[2-((2R,4R)tetrahydro-4-hydroxy-6-oxo-2H-pyran-2-yl)ethyl]-1-naphthyl-2-methylbutyrate

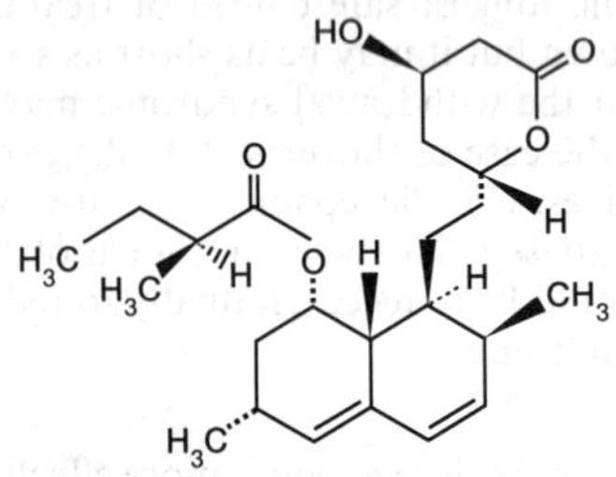

Molecular weight	404.6
pKa	
Solubility	
in alcohol	sparingly soluble
in water	insoluble
Octanol/water partition coefficient	—

Lovastatin is a white, odourless, non-hygroscopic crystalline powder. It is a metabolite derived from the fungus *Aspergillus terreus*.[1] The drug is not available in any combined preparations.

Pharmacology

After gastrointestinal absorption, lovastatin is readily hydrolyzed to the open hydroxyacid which is a competitive inhibitor of HMG-CoA reductase. This enzyme catalyzes the conversion of HMG-CoA to mevalonate, which is the major rate-limiting step in the cholesterol synthesis pathway. The Ki for the sodium salt of lovastatin to inhibit HMG-CoA reductase from rat liver microsomes[2] is 0.64 nmol.l^{-1}. Lovastatin causes a dose-dependent inhibition of reductase activity. The IC_{50} in rat liver microsomes (concentration causing 50% inhibition of HMG-CoA reductase activity)[3] was 2 mmol.l^{-1}.

In rats, inhibition of HMG-CoA reductase activity does not cause a fall in cholesterol in vivo. In vivo in the rat other products of the cholesterol synthetic pathway (e.g. oxysterols) inhibit cholesterol synthesis by feed back regulation and after lovastatin therapy this feedback inhibition is removed. The net result, in the rat, in vivo, is therefore a very large increase in HMG-CoA reductase activity (and its mRNA) without a fall in cholesterol.[2]

In other species (e.g. dogs) lovastatin produces a fall in plasma total cholesterol concentrations, with a marked fall in low density lipoprotein (LDL) cholesterol. The mechanism of the LDL lowering effect of lovastatin may involve reduction of the very low density lipoprotein (VLDL) cholesterol concentration. However, the main mechanism is that following HMG-CoA reductase inhibition, the LDL receptor density on the liver cells is increased (up-regulation)

Lovastatin

and this leads to increased removal of LDL cholesterol from the circulation. Inhibition of HMG-CoA reductase does not lead to a build up of intermediary metabolites, since this enzyme is involved early in the pathway of cholesterol synthesis and the precursor HMG-CoA is readily metabolized back to acetyl CoA which participates in many biosynthetic processes throughout the body's tissues. Despite the reduction in plasma lipids by lovastatin, cholesterol levels in brain, testis and lens are not reduced.

Toxicology

The oral LD_{50} of lovastatin in mice is approximately 20 $g.kg^{-1}$.

The active form of lovastatin, mevenolinic acid, is teratogenic in pregnant rats. This appears to be a mechanism-based effect because it can be prevented by administration of mevalonate, which circumvents the block on cholesterol synthesis.[4] In a 24 month study in rats receiving doses of up to 180 $mg.kg^{-1}$ daily (157 times the maximum recommended human dose (MRHD) assuming this to be 80 mg in a 70 kg person) no evidence of a tumourigenic effect was observed. In a 21 month carcinogenicity study in mice, a statistically significant ($P<0.05$) increase in the incidence of spontaneous hepatocellular carcinomas and adenomas was observed at doses of 500 $mg.kg^{-1}$ daily of lovastatin (approximately 437 times the MRHD). No similar changes were seen in the rat, and the changes were not seen in mice given doses of 20 and 100 $mg.kg^{-1}$ daily (18 and 90 times the MRHD).

In addition, an increase in the incidence of papilloma in the non-glandular mucosa of the stomach was observed in mice receiving 100 and 500 $mg.kg^{-1}$ daily (approximately 90 and 450 times the MRHD respectively); no increase was seen at a dosage of 20 $mg.kg^{-1}$ daily. The glandular mucosa was not affected. There is a strong association between this change and hyperplasia of the squamous epithelium (acanthosis) in this region. Acanthosis is a characteristic change observed in the non-glandular mucosa of rodents treated with HMG-CoA reductase inhibitors and is most probably a result of inhibition of reductase in this tissue. Similar squamous epithelium is found in the oesophagus and ano-rectal junction of the mouse and rat; however, no evidence of a similar hyperplastic response was observed in these tissues in studies of up to 21 months in the mouse given up to 500 $mg.kg^{-1}$ daily (450 times the MRHD), or in a study of 24 months in the rat given 180 $mg.kg^{-1}$ daily (157 times the MRHD).

A statistically significant increase ($P \leqslant 0.05$) in the spontaneous incidence of pulmonary adenomas was seen in female mice receiving 500 $mg.kg^{-1}$ daily. No similar changes were seen in males at any dose, or in females receiving 20 or 100 $mg.kg^{-1}$ daily. This incidence of pulmonary tumours was within the range seen in control groups in similar studies and the relationship of the change to treatment is therefore not known.

In a microbial mutagen test, using mutant strains of *Salmonella typhimurium* with or without rat or mouse liver metabolic activation, no evidence of mutagenicity was observed. In addition, no evidence of damage to genetic material was noted in an in vitro alkaline elution assay using rat or mouse hepatocytes, a V-79 mammalian cell forward mutation study, an in vitro chromosomal aberration assay in Chinese hamster ovary cells, or an in vivo chromosomal aberration assay in mouse bone marrow. These data indicate that the effects seen in the mouse study do not represent a primary carcinogenic effect of the drug.[5] In common with other HMG-CoA reductase inhibitors very high doses of lovastatin cause cataract formation in dogs exposed over long periods.[6]

Clinical pharmacology

Lovastatin has been shown to reduce both normal and elevated LDL cholesterol concentrations in plasma. The effect is dose-related over the range 5 to 40 mg twice daily. A twice daily regime is about 25% more effective than a once daily regime.[19] An effect is seen within one week and the maximum effect is seen within 4 weeks and is maintained during long term therapy. The mechanism is stimulation of expression of increased numbers of LDL receptors on hepatocytes with a resultant increase in LDL and apo B clearance.[7] As shown in Table 1 falls in total and LDL cholesterol of 20–40% can be expected. In addition there is usually a modest reduction of VLDL cholesterol and triglycerides with a slight rise in high density lipoprotein (HDL) cholesterol concentrations.[8] Concentrations of apolipoprotein B fall during lovastatin therapy by 20–40%. The reduction in apolipoprotein B concentration appears to be a result of the increased catabolism of LDL following up-regulation of the hepatic LDL receptor.

At therapeutic doses in man, HMG-CoA reductase activity is not completely inhibited and thus biologically necessary amounts of mevalonate are produced. Lovastatin has not been shown to have any effect on steroidogenesis, even though cholesterol is a precursor of steroid hormones. Response to ACTH in patients taking lovastatin is normal.[9,10] Lovastatin causes no increase in biliary lithogenicity and therefore would not be expected to increase the incidence of gall stones. Lovastatin competitively inhibits bile acid synthesis in man but the clinical significance of this is unclear at present.

A relatively selective effect of lovastatin upon the liver, the main target organ, depends upon kinetic factors. An oral dose must pass through the liver, which is the main site of formation of the active acid, probably by microsomal esterases. The acid is less diffusible that the lactone so enters other tissues less readily. Furthermore, a substantial fraction of the dose is excreted in bile and never reaches the systemic plasma.[11]

Pharmacokinetics

The preferred analytical method is reverse phase HPLC.[12] Lovastatin is an inactive lactone which is readily hydrolysed in vivo, presumably in the liver, to the corresponding β-hydroxyacid, a potent inhibitor of HMG-CoA reductase. Inhibition of HMG-CoA reductase is the basis of an assay for pharmacokinetic studies for the β-hydroxyacid metabolites (active inhibitors) and, following base hydrolysis, active plus latent inhibitors (total inhibitors) in plasma following administration of lovastatin.

Following an oral dose of ^{14}C-labelled lovastatin in man, 10% of the dose is excreted in urine and 83% in faeces. The latter represents absorbed drug equivalents excreted in bile as well as any unabsorbed drug.

Table 1 Effects on familial hypercholesterolaemic subjects: dose response to lovastatin

Dosage	Percentage change from baseline after 6 weeks					
	Total-C (mean)	LDL-C (mean)	HDL-C (mean)	LDL-C/ HDL-C (mean)	Total-C/ HDL-C (mean)	TG (median)
Placebo	−1	−2	+1	−1	0	+3
Lovastatin						
20 mg *	−18	−19	+10	−26	−24	−7
40 mg *	−24	−27	+10	−32	−29	−22
10 mg b.i.d.	−22	−25	+6	−28	−25	−11
20 mg b.i.d.	−27	−31	+12	−38	−34	−18
40 mg b.i.d.	−34	−39	+8	−43	−38	−12

C = cholesterol
TG = triglycerides
* = once daily in the evening

Absorption of lovastatin, estimated relative to an intravenous reference dose, in each of four animal species tested, averaged about 30% of an oral dose. Studies in the dog have indicated that the availability of the absorbed drug to the general circulation is limited by extensive first-pass extraction in the liver, its primary site of action, and that drug equivalents are subsequently excreted in the bile. A single dose study in four hypercholesterolaemic patients indicated that less than 5% of an oral dose of lovastatin reaches the general circulation as active inhibitors.

Peak plasma concentrations of both active and total inhibitors are attained within 2–4 h of drug administration.

Plasma concentrations of inhibitors increased linearly with doses up to 120 mg of lovastatin. With a once-daily dosing regimen, plasma concentrations of total inhibitors over a dosing interval achieve steady state between days 2 and 3 of therapy and are on average about 1.5 times those following a single dose. When the drug is given under fasting conditions, plasma concentrations of both active and total inhibitors are on average about two-thirds of those found when lovastatin is given immediately after a standard test meal.

Lovastatin and its β-hydroxyacid metabolite are both highly bound (>95%) to plasma proteins in man.

Animal studies demonstrated that lovastatin crosses the blood–brain and placental barriers. It is not known whether lovastatin is excreted in breast milk but it is likely that some such excretion occurs.

Oral absorption	incomplete
Presystemic metabolism	extensive
Plasma half life	
range	1.1–1.7 h
Volume of distribution	—
Plasma protein binding	>95%

As the excretion of lovastatin and its active metabolites in urine is insignificant, it is unlikely that renal impairment will cause any appreciable change in the elimination of the drug or its active products. In a study of patients with severe renal insufficiency (creatine clearance 10–30 $ml.min^{-1}$), the plasma concentrations of total inhibitors were approximately two fold higher than in healthy volunteers.

Concentration–effect relationship

There is insufficient data in man to establish concentration–effect relationships.

Metabolism

After oral ingestion in man lovastatin is extensively biotransformed, presumably in the liver (Fig. 1). 10% of the dose is excreted in the urine and 85% in the faeces as unchanged drug and metabolites.

The major active metabolites found in human plasma include the β-hydroxyacid of lovastatin, its 6′-hydroxymethyl and 6′-exomethylene derivatives, and two unidentified metabolites. In animal studies, at least five hepatic metabolites of lovastatin have been detected. The principal products are 6′-beta-hydroxy-lovastatin and the hydroxy acid form of lovastatin (a potent inhibitor of HMG-CoA), whereas hydroxylation at the ω-1 position of the side chain (3′-hydroxy-lovastatin) is a minor pathway.

Pharmaceutics

Lovastatin, Mevacor (MSD, US) is only available as 20 mg light blue, octagonal tablets.

Therapeutic use

Indications

1. Reduction of elevated total and LDL cholesterol levels in patients with primary hypercholesterolaemia, when the response to diet and other non-pharmacological measures has been inadequate.
2. Reduction of elevated cholesterol levels in patients with combined hypercholesterolaemia and hypertriglyceridaemia, when the hypercholesterolaemia is the abnormality of more concern.

Fig. 1 The metabolism of lovastatin

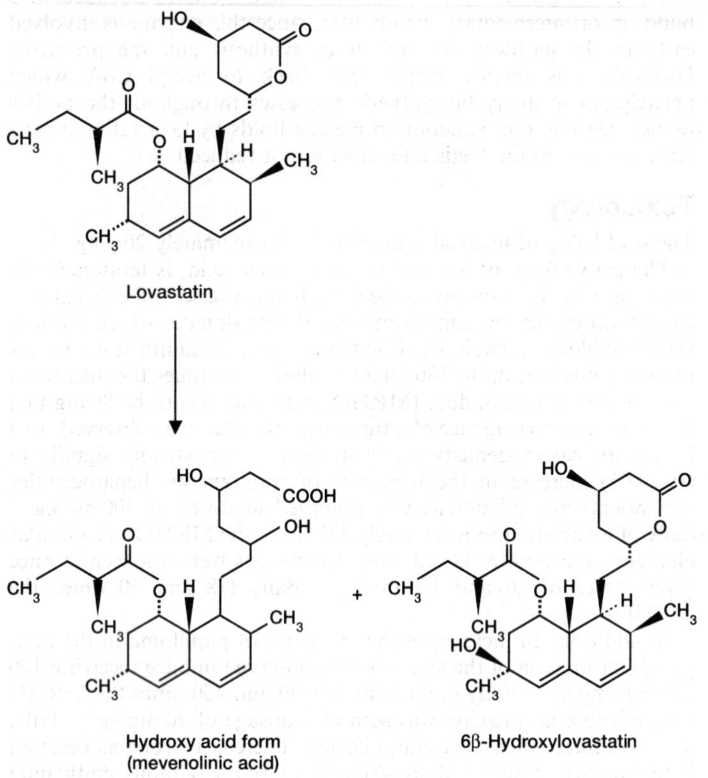

Contraindications

1. Hypersensitivity to any component of the preparation
2. Active liver disease or unexplained persistent elevations of serum transaminases
3. Pregnancy and nursing.

Mode of use

Lovastatin was the first HMG-CoA reductase inhibitor approved world-wide for marketing (in 1987).[16] Experience with this agent is much greater than with related newly marketed compounds such as simvastatin and pravastatin.

Prior to instituting therapy, attempts to control hypercholesterolaemia with appropriate diet, exercise and weight reduction in obese patients should be made[17] although the need for strict dietary restriction has been questioned.[18] A baseline physical examination, blood lipid profile, blood biochemistry including liver function tests and creatine phosphokinase, and urine microscopy should be performed. Lovastatin should be initially administered as 20 mg daily with the evening meal. The rationale for this is firstly that meals enhance the drugs absorption and secondly, since cholesterol synthesis is maximal in the early morning hours, administration of an evening dose optimizes its cholesterol-lowering effect.[19] One month following initiation of drug therapy, patients should be assessed and the baseline measurements repeated. In this way side effects and response to treatment may be evaluated. Thereafter patients should be reviewed and similar measurements undertaken at 2–3 monthly intervals. Drug therapy should be discontinued if there is a persistent increase greater than 3 times the upper limit of normal in serum transaminases or markedly elevated CPK levels (MM fraction) greater than 10 times the upper limit of normal.

Doses may be adjusted at intervals of 4 weeks (allowing time for optimal effects) increasing to a maximum of 80 mg daily orally in single or divided doses, except in patients receiving immunosuppressive therapy where 20 mg daily is the maximum recommended dose. There may be considerable variation in the magnitude of the individual patients response to the maximum 80 mg daily lovastatin dose, ranging from 20 to 50% reduction in LDL-cholesterol levels.[20]

In familial hypercholesterolaemia patients, lovastatin administered in doses of 20–80 mg daily is associated with a 23–33% reduction in total cholesterol, a 27–38% reduction in LDL-cholesterol, an 8–25% reduction in triglyceride and a 4–8% increase in

Lovastatin

HDL cholesterol.[21] Tendon xanthomas regress with treatment[22] Similar responses are noted when treating non-familial hypercholesterolaemic patients. Combination therapy is indicated in patients who, despite maximal doses (i.e. 80 mg daily) of lovastatin, fail to achieve desirable cholesterol levels as recommended by the European Atherosclerosis Society study group[23] or the National Cholesterol Education Program Expert Panel.[24] Combination of lovastatin 40–80 mg daily with colestipol 10–20 g daily leads to a further 13–17% reduction in total cholesterol and a 20–26% reduction in LDL cholesterol.[24] Using triple therapy i.e. colestipol 30 g daily, nicotinic acid 5.5 g daily and lovastatin 40–60 mg daily in familial hypercholesterolaemic patients, resulted in a 66% reduction in LDL-cholesterol. A recent 32 month duration study (see clinical trials) has demonstrated regression of atheroma with a therapeutic regime consisting of lovastatin 40 mg daily and colestipol 30 g daily.

Lovastatin has been used in comparative trials with a number of other lipid lowering agents such as cholestyramine, probucol and gemfibrozil.[25–29] Lipid reductions have generally been greater with lovastatin than with other agents with different types of action. Lovastatin has proved effective in a wide range of hyperlipidaemias both genetic and acquired including hyperlipidaemias in diabetes and after cardiac transplant.[30–32]

The combination of lovastatin with neomycin does not lead to any significant improvement in lipid profiles and this combination is therefore not recommended.[32]

Adverse reactions

Potentially life-threatening effects

In cardiac transplant patients who were receiving immunosuppressive drugs, including cyclosporin, there have been reports of severe rhabdomyolysis that precipitated acute renal failure.[33] Lovastatin therapy should be discontinued if marked elevation of creatine phosphokinase (CPK) levels occurs, and appropriate therapy should be instituted.

Consideration should be given to interrupting therapy with lovastatin in any patient with a risk factor predisposing to the development of renal failure (such as severe acute infection, hypotension, major surgery, trauma, severe metabolic, endocrine or electrolyte disorders and uncontrolled seizures) should rhabdomyolysis occur.

Patients should be advised to report promptly unexplained muscle pain, tenderness or weakness, particularly if accompanied by malaise or fever.

Acute overdosage

General measures should be adopted, and liver function should be monitored.

Five healthy human volunteers received up to 200 mg of lovastatin as a single dose without clinically significant adverse effects. A few cases of accidental overdosage have been reported; no patients had any specific symptoms, and all patients recovered without sequelae. The maximum dose taken was 5–6 g. The dialysability of lovastatin and its metabolites in man is not known at present.

Severe or irreversible adverse effects

A high incidence of lenticular abnormalities was observed in hypercholesterolaemic patients who were entering clinical trials of lovastatin. In the trials there were both increases and decreases in the reported prevalence of opacities. Of 431 patients examined with slit-lamp at base-line and during therapy with lovastatin, 34 had opacities at the final examination (5–15 months after starting therapy) which were not noticed at baseline. Conversely, 45 patients had opacities noted at baseline which were not noted at the final examination. These data may be more indicative of observer variation in the detection of minor lens opacities than an adverse effect of lovastatin on the human lens.

Symptomatic adverse effects

Myalgia occurs, although rarely, during treatment with lovastatin. Rhabdomyolysis has occurred, very rarely, and should be considered in any patient with diffuse myalgias, muscle tenderness and/or marked elevations of CPK (i.e. 10 times the upper limit of normal).

In controlled clinical studies, adverse effects (considered possibly, probably or definitely drug-related) occurring with a frequency of greater than 1% were flatulence, diarrhoea, constipation, nausea, dyspepsia, headache, dizziness, muscle cramps, myalgia, skin rashes and abdominal pain. Other adverse effects occurring in 0.5–1.0% of patients were: fatigue, pruritus, dry mouth, insomnia, sleep disorders and dysgeusia.[34]

Other effects

Transient mild elevations of CPK levels are commonly seen in patients treated with lovastatin. As such changes are readily provoked by minor muscle trauma or unusually heavy exercise, interpretation is often difficult. These changes have usually proved to be of no clinical significance but large elevation (> 10 times normal) without evident explanation must be taken more seriously. In a few patients taking part in clinical trials, increases in transaminases to more than three times the upper limit of normal occurred. These increases usually appeared 3–12 months after the start of therapy and were not accompanied by the development of jaundice or other clinical signs or symptoms. There was no evidence of hypersensitivity. A liver biopsy done in one of these patients showed mild focal hepatitis. In patients in whom the drug was interrupted or discontinued because of raised transaminases, including the one who underwent liver biopsy, the transaminase levels fell slowly to pre-treatment values.

It is, therefore, recommended that transaminase tests be performed before treatment begins, every 4–6 weeks during the first 12 months of therapy and periodically thereafter, particularly in patients who have abnormal liver function tests or who consume substantial quantities of alcohol. If serum transaminase levels show evidence of progression, particularly if they rise to more than three times the upper limits of normal and are persistent, the drug should be discontinued.

Marked and persistent increases of serum transaminases have been reported rarely, however, liver function test abnormalities have generally been mild and transient. Increases in serum (CPK) levels, attributable to the non-cardiac fraction of CPK, have been reported. These have usually been mild and transient; marked elevations have been reported rarely.

The drug should be used with caution in patients with a past history of liver disease.

Interference with clinical pathology tests

No information is available.

High risk groups

Neonates

Safety and effectiveness in neonates have not been established.

Breast milk. It is not known whether lovastatin is excreted in human milk, so mothers taking the drug should not breast-feed.

Children

Safety and effectiveness in children have not been established.

Pregnant women

Cholesterol and products of the cholesterol biosynthesis pathway are essential components for fetal development, including synthesis of steroids and cell membranes. Because of the ability of inhibitors of HMG-CoA reductase such as lovastatin to decrease the synthesis of cholesterol and possibly other products of the cholesterol biosynthesis pathway, lovastatin may cause fetal harm when administered to a pregnant woman. Therefore, lovastatin is contraindicated during pregnancy.

Lovastatin should be administered to women of childbearing age only when such patients are highly unlikely to conceive. If the patient becomes pregnant while taking the drug, lovastatin should be discontinued and the patient advised of the potential hazard to the fetus.

The elderly

In one controlled study in elderly patients over the age of 60, efficacy appeared similar to that in the population as a whole. There was no apparent increase in the frequency of clinical or laboratory adverse findings.

Concurrent disease

Renal insufficiency. As lovastatin does not undergo significant renal excretion, modification of the dosage should not be necessary in patients with renal insufficiency.

Homozygous familial hypercholesterolaemia. In patients with this condition lovastatin has been found to be less effective, probably because such individuals have no or few functional LDL receptors. In addition, lovastatin appears to be more likely to raise serum transaminases in these homozygous patients.[35,36]

Hypertriglyceridaemia. As lovastatin has only a moderate triglyceride-lowering effect, it is not indicated where hypertriglyceridaemia is the abnormality of most concern (i.e. hyperlipidaemia Types I, IV and V).

Drug interactions

Potentially hazardous interactions

Coumarin derivatives. When lovastatin and coumarin are administered concomitantly, prothrombin time may be increased in some patients. Because of this, in patients taking anticoagulants, prothrombin time should be determined prior to starting therapy with lovastatin and, thereafter, monitored at the intervals usually recommended for patients on coumarin anticoagulants.

Other significant interactions

Antipyrine. As lovastatin had no effect on the pharmacokinetics of antipyrine, interactions with drugs metabolized via the isoforms of cytochrome P-450 involved in antipyrine metabolism are not expected.

Propranolol. There was no clinically significant pharmacokinetic or pharmacodynamic interaction with concomitant administration of single doses of lovastatin and propranolol given to normal volunteers.

Digoxin. In patients with hypercholesterolaemia, concomitant administration of lovastatin and digoxin was without effect on digoxin plasma concentrations.

Other drugs. In various clinical studies lovastatin was used concomitantly with β-blockers, calcium entry blockers, diuretics, hypoglycaemic drugs (insulin, chloropropamide, glipizide, glyburide) and nonsteroidal anti-inflammatory agents without evidence of clinically significantly adverse interactions.

Potentially useful interactions

No interactions of this kind have been reported.

Clinical trials

Numerous short term and comparative studies have been reported but large scale outcome trials are not yet complete.

1. The Lovastatin Study Group III 1988 A multicenter comparison of lovastatin and cholestyramine therapy for severe primary hypercholesterolaemia. Journal of the American Medical Association 260 (3): 359–366

264 patients with severe primary hypercholesterolaemia were randomised to one of three regimens (i) cholestyramine 12 g twice daily, (ii) lovastatin 20 mg twice daily, (iii) lovastatin 40 mg twice daily for 12 weeks.

LDL cholesterol fell by 17% with cholestyramine, 27% with the lower lovastatin dose and 42% with the higher. Constipation and dyspepsia were the main side-effects and these were much more common with cholestyramine than with lovastatin.

2. Kannel W B, D'Agostino R B, Stephanians M, D'Agostino L C 1990 Efficacy and tolerability of lovastatin in a six-month study: analysis by gender, age and hypertensive status. American Journal of Cardiology 66 (Symp): 1–10

489 patients with hypercholesterolaemia were placed on a cholesterol reducing diet for 6 weeks followed by lovastatin 20–80 mg daily for 6 months.

61% attained a goal cholesterol of $<130\ \text{mg.dl}^{-1}$ with a mean lovastatin dose of 37.4 mg daily. Lovastatin was effective in both sexes, at all ages and in both hypertensives and normotensives. 17% of patients experienced adverse effects, mainly gastrointestinal or musculoskeletal symptoms. 21 withdrew because of adverse effects. One patient developed a slight subcapsular lens cataract.

3. Brown G, Albers J J, Fisher L D 1990 Regression of coronary artery disease as a result of intensive lipid-lowering therapy in men with high levels of apoliprotein B. New England Journal of Medicine 323: 1289–1298

146 men under 62 years old who had coronary disease and an apo B level of $\geqslant 125\ \text{mg.dl}^{-1}$ were randomly allocated to one of three treatment groups. One group received diet therapy plus placebo, the second lovastatin 20 mg twice daily and colestipol 10 g three times daily and the third nicotinic acid 1 g four times daily plus colestipol 10 g three times daily. 120 patients completed the 32 month study and has an entry and exit coronary arteriogram. Mean reductions of LDL in the three groups were 7%, 46% and 32% respectively. Progression of lessions occurred in 46%, 21 and 25% and regression in 11, 32 and 39%. Major cardiovascular events (death, acute MI, CABG) occurred in 10/52 of the diet/placebo groups, 3/46 of the lovastatin/colestipol groups and 2/48 of the nicotinic acid/colestipol group.

4. Bradford R H, Shear C L, Chremos A N, Dujovne C, Downton M et al 1991 Expanded clinical evaluation of lovastatin (EXCEL) Study Results. I. Efficacy in modifying plasma lipoproteins and adverse event profile in 8245 patients with moderate hypercholersterolaemia. Archives of International Medicine 151: 43–49

This was a double-blind diet and placebo-controlled trial in 8245 patients aged 18–70 years with primary hypercholersterolaemia (total cholesterol between 6.21 and 7.76 mmol/l). Patients were randomly assigned to placebo or lovastatin 20 mg once daily, 40 mg once daily, 20 mg twice daily or 40 mg twice daily for 48 weeks.

There was a dose-related reduction in LDL cholesterol with mean reductions of 24%, 30%, 34% and 40% in the four actively treated groups. Confirmed elevations of transaminase of greater than 3 times the upper limit of normal occurred in 0.9% of the 40 mg.d^{-1} group and 1.5% of the 80 mg.d^{-1} group. There was no case of a full myopathic syndrome. Five patients (1 on 40 mg.d^{-1}, 4 on 80 mg.d^{-1}) has plasma CPK levels greater than 10 times the upper limit of normal, although high risk groups were excluded from the trial (e.g. renal failure or treatment with gemfibrozil, cyclosporin or niacin).

General review articles

Henwood J M, Heel R C 1988 Lovastatin: a preliminary review of its pharmacodynamic properties and therapeutic use in hyperlipidaemia. Drugs 36: 429–454

Krukemyer J J, Talbert R L 1987 Lovastatin: a new cholesterol-lowering agent. Pharmacotherapy 7 (6): 198–210

O'Connor P, Feely J, Shepherd J 1990 Lipid-lowering drugs. British Medical Journal 300: 667–672

Loscalzo J 1990 Regression of coronary atherosclerosis. New England Journal of Medicine 323: 1337–1339

References

1. Alberts A W 1988 Discovery, biochemistry and biology of lovastatin. American Journal of Cardiology 62: 10–15J
2. Alberts A W, Chen J, Juron G et al 1980 Mevinolin: a highly potent competitive inhibitor of hydroxymethylglutaryl-coenzyme A reductase and a cholesterol-lowering agent. Proceedings of the National Academy of Science 77 (7): 3957–3961
3. Albers-Schonberg G, Joshua H, Lopez M B et al 1981 Dihydromevinolin, a potent hypocholesterolemic metabolite produced by Aspergillus terreus. Journal of Antibiotics 34 (5): 507–512
4. Minsker 1983 Mevalonate supplementation in pregnant rats suppresses the teratogenicity of mevinolinic acid an inhibitor of 3-hydroxy-3-methylglutaryl-coenzyme A reductase. Teratology 28: 449
5. MacDonald J S, Gerson R J, Kornburst D J et al 1988 Preclinical evaluations of lovastatin. American Journal of Cardiology 62: 16J–27J
6. Gerson R J, MacDonald J S, Alberts A W et al 1990 On the etiology of subcapsular lenticular opacities produced in dogs receiving HMG-CoA reductase inhibitors. Experimental Eye Research 50: 65–78
7. Brown M S, Goldstein J L 1983 Lipoprotein receptors in the liver control signals for plasma cholesterol traffic. Journal of Clinical Investigation 74: 743–747
8. The Lovastatin Study Group II 1986 Therapeutic response to lovastatin (Mevinolin) in non familial hypercholesterolaemia. A multicenter study. Journal of the American Medical Association 256 (20): 2829–2834
9. Thompson GR, Ford J, Jenkinson M, Trayner I 1986 Efficacy of Mevinolin as adjuvant therapy for refractory familial hypercholesterolaemia. Quarterly Journal of Medicine 232: 803–811
10. Illingworth D R, Corbin D 1985 The influence of Mevinolin on the adrenal cortical response to corticotrophin in heterozygous familial hypercholesterolaemia. Proceedings of the National Academy of Science USA 82: 6291–6294
11. Grundy S M, Bilheimer D W 1984 Inhibition of 3-hydroxy-3-methylglutanyl-6A reductase by Mevinolin in familial hypercholesterolaemia heterozygotes: effects on cholesterol balance. Proceedings of the National Academy of Science USA 81: 2538–2542
12. Stubbs R J, Schwartz M, Bayne W M 1986 Determination of mevinolin and mevinolinic acid in plasma and bile by reverse phase HPLC. Journal of Chromatography 383: 438–443

13. Vyas K P, Kari P H, Halpin R A et al 1990 Biotransformation of lovastatin. I. Structure elucidation of in vitro and in vivo metabolites in rat and mouse. Drug Metabolism and Disposition 18: 203–211
14. Duggan D E, Chen I W, Halpin R A et al 1989 The physiological disposition of lovastatin. Drug Metabolism and Disposition 17: 166–173
15. Chen I W, Vickers S, Duncan C A, Ellsworth R L, Duggan D E 1988 Tissue selectivities of three HMG-CoA reductase inhibitors. FASEB Journal 2: 1061
16. Henwood J M, Heel R C 1988 Lovastatin, a preliminary review of its pharmacodynamic properties and therapeutic use in hyperlipidaemia. Drugs 36: 429–454
17. Mevacor (Lovastatin, MSD) United States Food and Drug Administration package insert. West Point, Pa: Merck and Company
18. Miettinen T A, Tikkanen M J, Helve E, Ojala J P 1990 Inhibition of dietary cholesterol absorbtion by lovastatin (Mevinolin) treatment. Drug Investigation 2 (suppl 2): 29–35
19. Illingworth DR, 1986 Comparative efficacy of once versus twice daily Mevinolin in the therapy of familial hypercholesterolaemia. Clinical Pharmacology and Therapeutics 40: 338–343
20. Illingworth D R, Sextron G J 1984 Hypercholesterolaemic effects of Mevinolin in patients with heterozygous familial hypercholesterolaemia. Journal of Clinical Investigation 74: 1972–1978
21. Havel R J, Hunninglake D B, Illingworth D R 1987 Lovastatin (Mevinolin) in the treatment of heterozygous familial hypercholesterolaemia. Annals of Internal Medicine 107: 609–615
22. Illingworth D R, Cope R, Bacon S P 1990 Regression of tendon xanthomas in patients with familial hypercholesterolaemia treated with lovastatin. Southern Medical Journal 83: 1053–1057
23. European Artherosclerosis Society Study Group 1988 The recognition and management of hyperlipidaemia in adults: a policy statement of the European Atherosclerosis Society. European Heart Journal 9: 571–600
24. The Expert Panel. Report of the National Cholesterol Education Program Expert Panel on detection, evaluation and treatment of high blood cholesterol in adults. Archives of Internal Medicine 148: 36–69
25. Illingworth DR, 1984 Mevinolin plus colestipol in therapy for severe heterozygous familial hypercholesterolaemia. Annals of Internal Medicine 101: 598–604
26. Lovastatin Study Group III 1988 A multicenter comparison of lovastatin, a cholestyramine therapy for severe primary hypercholesterolaemia. Journal of the American Medical Association 260: 359–366
27. Helve E, Tikkanen M J 1988 Comparison of lovastatin and probucol in treatment of familial and non-familial hypercholesterolaemia: different effects on lipoprotein profiles. Atherosclerosis 72: 189–197
28. Lovastatin Study group IV 1990 A multicenter comparison of lovastatin and probucol for treatment of severe primary hypercholesterolaemia. American Journal of Cardiology 66 (Symp): 22–30
29. Tikkanen M J, Helve E, Jaattela A et al 1988 Comparison between lovastatin and gemfibrozil in the treatment of primary hypercholesterolaemia: the Finnish multi-centre study. American Journal of Cardiology 62: 35J–43J
30. Garg A, Grundy S M 1988 Treatment of dyslipidaemia in non-insulin dependent diabetes mellitus with lovastatin. American Journal of Cardiology 62: 44J–49J
31. Kuo P C, Kirshenbaum J M, Gordon J et al 1989 Lovastatin therapy for hypercholesterolaemia in cardiac transplant patients. American Journal of Cardiology 64: 631–635
32. Hoeg J M, Maher M B, Bailey K R, Brewer Jr H B 1986 The effects of Mevinolin and neomycin alone and in combination on plasma lipid and lipoprotein concentrations in type II hyperlipoproteinaemia. Atherosclerosis 60: 209–214
33. Norman D J, Illingworth D R, Murson J, Hosenpud J 1988 Myolysis and acute renal failure in a heart-transplant patient receiving lovastatin (Letter). New England Journal of Medicine 318: 46–47
34. Tobert J A 1988 Efficacy and long term adverse effect pattern of lovastatin. American Journal of Cardiology 62: 28J–34J
35. Illingworth D R, Bacon S P, Larsen K K 1988 Long term experience with HMGCoA reductase inhibitors in the therapy of hypercholesterolaemia. Atherosclerosis Review 18: 161–187
36. Vany R, Vega G L, Bilheimer D W 1987 Effect of lovastatin and LDL kinetics in homozygous familial hypercholesterolaemia (FH) Paediatric Research 24: 349A, Abstract

Lymecycline

Lymecycline is an antibiotic with a similar spectrum of activity to other tetracyclines. It is a very water-soluble derivative of tetracycline, the amino acid lysine and formaldehyde.[1] On absorption it is converted to tetracycline and lysine and thus should be considered as tetracycline in a more bioavailable form.

Chemistry

Lymecycline (tetracycline-L-methylene lysine, Tetralysal, Ciclolysal, Tancilina, Ciclisin, Lisinbiotic, Lisinciclina, Trasilin)
$C_{29}H_{38}N_4O_{10}$
(d)-N-(1-Amino-5-carboxypentylaminomethyl)-4-dimethylamino-1,4,4a,5,5a,6,11,12a-octahydro-3,6,10,12,12a-pentahydroxy-6-methyl-1,11-dioxonaphthacene-2-carboxamide

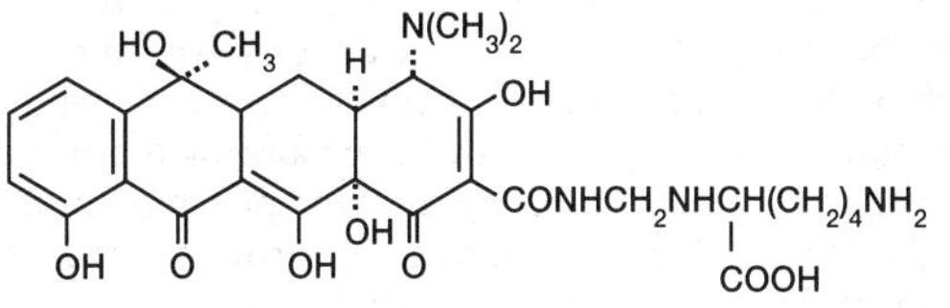

Molecular weight	603
pKa	9.7, 7.7
Solubility	
in alcohol	1 in 500
in water	>1 in 1
Octanol/water partition coefficient	low

A yellow very hygroscopic powder which darkens on exposure to light and air. Supplied with not more than 5% w/w of water. Prepared by chemical synthesis. Investigated mainly in the 1960s. The isomer used is dextrorotary.

Pharmacology

The pharmacology is essentially that of the tetracycline that is released in the body. Lymecycline has a wide spectrum of antibiotic activity with its main mechanism of action on protein synthesis. An energy-dependent active transport system pumps the drug through the inner cytoplasmic membrane. Once inside the bacterial cell, tetracycline inhibits protein synthesis by binding specifically to the 30S ribosomes. The drug appears to prevent access of aminoacyl tRNA to the acceptor site on the mRNA–ribosome complex. This prevents the addition of amino acids to the growing peptide chain. Tetracycline impairs protein synthesis in mammalian cells if used at very high concentrations. However, these cells lack the active transport system found in bacteria. There is also some evidence that tetracyclines may cause alterations in the cytoplasmic membrane thus allowing leakage of nucleotides from the cell. This would explain the rapid inhibition of DNA replication that ensues when cells are exposed to concentrations of tetracycline in excess of that required for inhibition of protein synthesis. Lymecycline appears not to chelate calcium or magnesium ions in the gut, unlike other tetracyclines.[1]

Toxicology

There is little published information available on the toxicology of lymecycline. There is only one report of possible fetal abnormality following clomocycline. In mice the intravenous LD_{50} is 253 $mg.kg^{-1}$ and given orally it is more than 2 $g.kg^{-1}$.

Clinical pharmacology

Lymecycline is primarily a bacteriostatic antibiotic and has a similar spectrum of activity to other tetracyclines. In the body it is broken down to lysine and tetracycline which produces the antibacterial activity. Tetracycline is active against most strains of *Haemophilus influenzae* and is particularly useful for infections with *H. ducreyi*, *Actinomyces*, *Brucella* and *Vibrio cholerae*. Tetracycline is also active against spirochaetes such as *Borrelia recurrentis*, *Treponema pallidum* and *T. pertenue*.

Tetracycline was initially useful for the treatment of Gram-positive infections but many strains are now resistant to the drug. The overall resistance in the UK of the pneumococcus is about 10%. Tetracycline possesses some activity against *Staphylococcus aureus*, particularly for community-acquired infections, but in hospitals the prevalence of resistance to staphylococci is high. Many Gram-negative organisms have acquired resistance to tetracycline and for *E. coli* more than 50% of strains may be resistant. Tetracycline has no activity against *Pseudomonas aeruginosa* while most strains of *Heliobacter* are sensitive. Tetracycline is also active against anaerobic species of bacteria and since concentrations of the drug are quite high in the gastrointestinal contents, the enteric flora are usually altered by the drug. Since lymecycline is better absorbed than tetracycline itself similar blood concentrations are produced by about half the oral dose of lymecycline compared to tetracycline. Lymecycline 204 mg is equivalent to 150 mg tetracycline in amount of tetracycline present.

Resistance to tetracyclines develops slowly and organisms that show resistance to one tetracycline frequently show resistance to others in the group (with some exceptions for minocycline and doxycycline). Most resistance is mediated by a plasmid and is an inducible trait, appearing only after exposure of the bacteria to the drug. Resistance seems to occur because the plasmid implants genetic material in the cell for a number of proteins and this affects penetration of the cell wall by tetracycline.

Pharmacokinetics

Lymecycline can be assayed either using *Staphylococcus aureus*[3] or HPLC,[4] the limits of sensitivity being about 50 μg.l^{-1} and about 500 μg.l^{-1} (depending on the bacterium used) respectively.

The drug is more completely absorbed from the gastrointestinal tract than tetracycline hydrochloride with peak plasma concentrations by 2 h. Plasma half life is 10 (7–14) h.[5] Lymecycline is broken down to tetracycline (the active molecule) and the amino acid lysine, possibly on passage through the gut wall. Although milk and other calcium-containing substances bind tetracycline in the gut this has not been demonstrated for lymecycline.[1] Divided doses of 600 mg per day provide blood levels of about 1–3 mg.l^{-1} regardless of whether the doses are taken on an empty stomach or not.[6] Lymecycline, following conversion to tetracycline, is distributed throughout the body with low concentrations in the CSF and 45% of that in the blood is bound to plasma proteins. Lymecycline, as active tetracycline, is known to enter skin,[5] maxillary sinus mucosa,[7] fallopian tube tissue[8] and the paranasal sinus mucosa. Sinus secretions contain similar levels to those found in blood.[9] Transfer of lymecycline (tetracycline) across the placenta occurs and it is excreted in breast milk. Approximately 30% is excreted via the urine.[10]

Oral absorption	>95%
Presystemic metabolism	—
Plasma half life	
range	7–14 h
Volume of distribution	–
Plasma protein binding	45%

Concentration–effect relationship

The therapeutic range will depend upon the minimum inhibitory concentration (MIC) of the antibiotic for the organism in question. Full susceptibility occurs when the MIC of tetracycline is less than 4.0 mg.l^{-1} and intermediate susceptibility is said to occur when the MIC is between 4.0 and 12.5 mg.l^{-1}. Concentrations of greater than 25 mg.l^{-1} are usually required to inhibit most strains of group B and group D streptococci and strains of *Staphylococcus aureus*. The MIC for *Streptococcus pyogenes* is usually about 1.0 mg.l^{-1} of tetracycline and for the pneumococcus it is often between 0.4 and 0.8 mg.l^{-1}.

Lymecycline

Metabolism

Lymecycline breaks down spontaneously to tetracycline. Therefore metabolism is as for tetracycline hydrochloride.

Pharmaceutics

Lymecycline (Tetralysal; Farmitalia, UK) is available in oral and intravenous forms. Hard gelatin white capsules are overprinted 'Farmitalia Carlo Erba' in black and contain either 150 or 300 mg. Their shelf-life is 18 months. The intravenous preparation is 135 mg of dry yellow powder supplied with 3 ml ampoules of solvent containing procaine hydrochloride (the shelf-life being 16 months). The powder should be stored below 25°C and stored in the dark. The dissolved drug should be used immediately after preparation.

Therapeutic use

Indications

1. Same as tetracycline.

Contraindications

1. Any individual with developing teeth (i.e. below 8 years and the latter half of pregnancy, due to placental transfer).

Mode of use

The use of lymecycline depends upon its bacteriostatic action which is of course identical to tetracycline. It interferes with bacterial protein synthesis. See Tetracycline hydrochloride monograph for further information.

Any effect in inappropriate ADH syndrome has not been demonstrated as it has for demeclocycline, another member of the tetracycline family.

Oral treatment is between 300 and 600 mg daily in divided doses. Used intravenously the dose is between 200 and 300 mg daily. Higher doses up to 1200 mg have been used. Up to 27 mg.kg^{-1} body weight per 24 hours have been used in children.

Adverse reactions

As for tetracycline hydrochloride. Gastrointestinal side effects are less than with tetracycline hydrochloride.[11,12]

High risk groups and drug interactions

As for tetracycline hydrochloride. It is important that no tetracycline is given in the last half of pregnancy and to children under 8 years due to reduced mineralization and discoloration of the teeth. Tetracyclines can further impair renal function and should not be given to patients with reduced renal function (doxycycline is least likely to do this).

Major outcome trials

The response of infections to lymecycline is the same as tetracycline hydrochloride. The main differences are that lymecycline is better absorbed (so lower doses are required) and fewer gastrointestinal side effects are observed. For example Pines et al.[11] compared 1.6 g of lymecycline (equivalent to 1.2 g of tetracycline) with 2 g of tetracycline hydrochloride in exacerbations of chronic bronchitis. The efficacy was similar but lymecycline was better tolerated. In a later study comparing chlortetracycline, methacycline and lymecycline (all given at a dose equivalent to 1.2 g of tetracycline) the same author[12] showed similar efficacy in exacerbations of chronic bronchitis, but less nausea, diarrhoea, vomiting and abdominal pain with lymecycline. Because of cost differences their recommendation was to start with chlortetracycline and to use lymecycline if gastrointestinal side effects were unacceptable. Essentially the same findings have obtained with infections in other systems.

General review articles

See Tetracycline hydrochloride monograph.

References

1. Ericson S, Gnarpe H 1979 Lymecycline and concurrent ingestion of milk. Journal of International Medical Research 7: 471–472
2. De-Carneri I, Coppi G, Lauria F, Lodgeman W 1961 A new soluble tetracycline: tetracycline-L methylene-lysine. Farmaco 16: 65–79
3. Lightbown J W, De Rossi P, Isaacson P 1972 International standards and international reference preparations. Bulletin of the World Health Organization 47: 343–356
4. Hermansson J, Andersson M 1982 Reversed-phase ion-pair chromatography of tetracycline, tetracycline analogues, and their potential impurities. Journal of Pharmaceutical Sciences 71: 222–229
5. Schreiner A, Digranes A 1985 Pharmacokinetics of lymecycline and doxycycline in serum and suction blister fluid. Chemotherapy 31: 261–265
6. Vitartali L, Pisani-Ceretti A 1968 Blood levels after lymecycline BD and QID. Lancet 1: 923–924
7. Ekedahl C, Holm S E, Bergholm A M 1978 Penetration of antibiotics into the normal and diseased maxillary sinus mucosa. Scandinavian Journal of Infectious Diseases (suppl) 14: 279–284
8. Bergholm A M, Holm S E, Wiklund D E 1982 Penetration of lymecycline (tetracycline) into the tissues of the fallopian tube. Acta Obstetrica et Gynecologica Scandinavica 61: 47–52
9. Lundin K, Brorson J E 1978 Secretory lymecycline concentrations in maxillary sinusitis. Journal of Antimicrobial Chemotherapy 4: 187
10. Whitby J L, Black H J 1964 Comparison of lymecycline with tetracycline hydrochloride. British Medical Journal 2: 1491–1495
11. Pines A, Plucinski K, Greenfield J S B, Mitchell R C 1964 Controlled comparison of lymecycline with tetracycline hydrochloride in exacerbations of chronic bronchitis. British Medical Journal 2: 1495–1498
12. Pines A, Raafat H, Pluczinski K 1968 Demethylchlortetracycline, lymecycline and methacycline compared in patients with purulent exacerbations of bronchitis. British Journal of Diseases of the Chest 62: 19–26

Lynoestrenol

Lynoestrenol is an orally active synthetic nortestosterone-derived progestogen which is primarily used as a component of a combined contraceptive preparation with the synthetic oestrogen ethinyloestradiol. It is also used in menstrual disorders. In some countries it is available alone for use as a progestogen-only contraceptive, or for other gynaecological therapeutic indications common to this group of drugs. In the latter case it is often combined with an oestrogen (e.g. for menstrual disorders). Its main application is as a component of combined oral contraceptives, containing also the synthetic oestrogen ethinyloestradiol.

Chemistry

Lynoestrenol (lynenol, lynestrenol, Exluton(a), Orgametril)
$C_{20}H_{28}O$
19-Nor-17α-pregn-4-en-20-yn-17β-ol

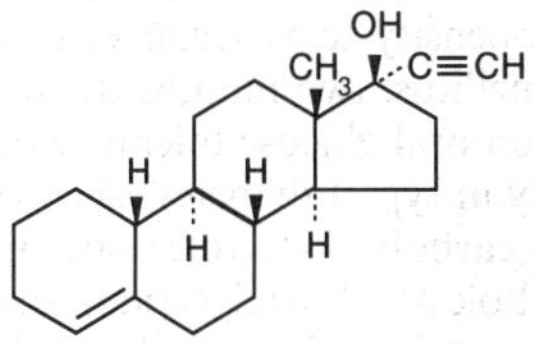

Molecular weight	284.4
pKa	not ionizable
Solubility	
in alcohol	1 in 15
in water	insoluble
Octanol/water partition coefficient	high

Lynoestrenol is a white, odourless, tasteless, crystalline powder, with melting point 158–160°C. It is prepard by chemical synthesis. It is present in combination with ethinyloestradiol in Minilyn.

Pharmacology

Lynoestrenol is a progestational pro-drug with weak intrinsic biological activity as judged by the Clauberg–McPhail test. Lynoestrenol is, however, converted quantitatively into the potent progestogen norethisterone,[1] through which it exerts its major biological effects. In practical terms, therefore, it shares the pharmacological properties of norethisterone. It is more potent than progesterone and has weak oestrogenic and androgenic properties as judged by standard biological tests.

Toxicology

Acute toxicity testing in a variety of animal species showed the LD_{50} to be greater than 1000 to 8000 $mg.kg^{-1}$. Chronic toxicity testing in rats, dogs and rhesus monkeys failed to reveal any results that were likely to be of clinical relevance.

The fetuses of rats treated from day 6 to day 19 of pregnancy showed no skeletal or visceral defects related to treatment and there was no increase in fetal loss.

Dominant lethal mutations were observed in female mice treated with combined mestranol 12.5 $\mu g.kg^{-1}$ and lynoestrenol 420 $\mu g.kg^{-1}$ for 3 days prior to mating. In 15 women who had discontinued combined treatment with lynoestrenol 2.5 mg and mestranol 75 µg daily within the period 0 to 12 months before conception, no increase in abnormal karyotypes was seen in spontaneous abortuses compared with controls.[2]

Lynoestrenol

Clinical pharmacology

Lynoestrenol is used alone as a progestogen-only contraceptive or in combination with either ethinyloestradiol or mestranol.

The mechanism of action of progestogen-only preparations is not clear; a number of different actions probably combine to produce antifertility effects. Probably the most important contraceptive, pharmacodynamic effect is a reduction in quantity and alteration in properties of cervical mucus, which acts as a barrier to sperm penetration. These changes have been studied in ovariectomized women.[3] Cervical mucus is reduced in volume and it becomes turbid. The spinnbarkeit (the degree to which cervical mucus may be lifted as a thread from a glass slide; maximal at the time of ovulation) is reduced and there is inhibition of ferning (the arborization of cervical mucus observed on microscopy). Vaginal cells show a reduced karyopyknotic index. Additionally, a number of other effects contribute to the antifertility properties of progestogens; these include the production of a semi-atrophic endometrium unsuitable for nidation, depression of the pituitary–ovarian axis leading to a 50% anovulatory cycle rate, and alteration in tubal and cervical transport function which impairs ovum motility.

Progestogen-only hormonal contraceptives do not appear to influence platelet function,[4] although this has not been specifically studied with lynoestrenol.

In combination with ethinyloestradiol 50 μg, higher doses of 1 and 2.5 mg lynoestrenol are employed to balance the oestrogenic effects of ethinyloestradiol and give good cycle control.

Because of the association between vascular disease and oral contraceptive steroids, attention has been paid to the changes in intermediary metabolism and haemostatic parameters which may be associated with a propensity to vascular disease. In 17 women with gestational diabetes mellitus, two months treatment with lynoestrenol 0.5 mg had no effect on oral glucose tolerance or total cholesterol and triglycerides.[5] A study in type I diabetes[6] showed lynoestrenol 0.5 mg to have no effect on carbohydrate tolerance or insulin requirements and to reduce total cholesterol, triglycerides and phospholipids, leaving high density lipoprotein (HDL) unchanged. The combination of ethinyloestradiol (50 μg) and lynoestrenol (2.5 mg) increased insulin requirements and triglycerides. Lynoestrenol in high doses (5–10 mg), as used in the treatment of endometriosis, increased low density lipoprotein (LDL) cholesterol and reduced HDL cholesterol.[7] These effects on carbohydrate and lipid metabolism are typical of those seen with other nortestosterone-derived progestogens.

As a result of its weak oestrogenic activity, lynoestrenol causes slight increases in cortisol binding globulin and caeruloplasmin and a reduction of sex hormone binding globulin.[8] These biochemical changes are reversed within one month of discontinuing therapy.[8]

Pharmacokinetics

As lynoestrenol is converted in vivo and in vitro to norethisterone, a specific radioimmunoassay for norethisterone derived from orally administered pro-drugs has been developed for pharmacokinetic studies.[9] This assay will detect 20 pg of norethisterone with a 95% confidence level and 35 pg with a confidence level of 99%. Additionally, a variety of adequate radioimmunoassays exists for the measurement of norethisterone itself.[10]

Lynoestrenol is almost completely absorbed from the gastrointestinal tract, with a time to maximum plasma concentrations following oral administration of tablets of about 2 hours.[11] Absorption is little affected by food. This study concluded that 5 mg lynoestrenol and 5 mg norethisterone gave similar peak plasma concentrations of about 23 $pmol.ml^{-1}$. The areas under the plasma concentration–time curves from 0–24 hours following 0.5 mg lynoestrenol and 0.3 mg norethisterone were identical.[11] A subsequent study[12] has shown that 1 mg lynoestrenol is equivalent to 0.7 mg norethisterone. With higher doses of lynoestrenol, peak norethisterone concentrations were higher but delayed and the elimination phase half life was longer, suggesting limitation of hepatic capacity for the conversion of lynoestrenol to norethisterone. In practice, lynoestrenol and norethisterone are virtually bioequivalent.

The half life of elimination for lynoestrenol is not available for the substance itself as it is rapidly converted in vivo to norethisterone. The half life of total radioactivity following administration of ^{14}C labelled drug was 2.5 ± 0.6 days but this is thought to reflect the persistence of polar metabolites retained in the plasma.[13] Norethisterone undergoes presystemic metabolism and has a bioavailability of 64%.[14] Since norethisterone concentrations after administration of lynoestrenol are of the same magnitude as those after an equivalent oral dose of norethisterone the systemic bioavailability of lynoestrenol is comparable to that of norethisterone.

The distribution half life of norethisterone following 1 mg lynoestrenol as a single dose is 2.5 ± 1.2 h[12] and 4.3 ± 1.6 h following a single dose of 5 mg lynoestrenol.[12] As Minilyn (lynoestrenol 2.5 mg and ethinyloestradiol 50 μg) the distribution half life is 3.7 ± 0.4 h.[13]

The volume of distribution of norethisterone following 5 mg lynoestrenol in combination with mestranol 75 μg is 35.7 l.[15]

The elimination half life of norethisterone may be dose dependant[12] but following a single oral dose of Minilyn was found to be 16.6 ± 0.7 h.[13]

For high-dose 5 mg lynoestrenol in combination with mestranol 150 μg, the plasma clearance is 0.61 $l.h^{-1}$.[15]

Lynoestrenol, like other progestogens, is highly protein bound (96%)[16] with high affinity and low capacity to sex hormone binding globulin (SHBG); binding to albumin is of high capacity low affinity type.

In practical terms the pharmacokinetics of lynoestrenol can be considered to be those of its major metabolite norethisterone. In lactating women orally treated with 4-14C-LYN/MEE 5000/150 μg daily 0.14% of the radioactivity administered with the LYN dose was excreted in breast milk.[15] Both lynoestrenol and its active metabolite norethisterone are likely to be transferred across the placenta.

Oral absorption	almost complete
Presystemic metabolism	rapid conversion to norethisterone (70% of administered dose); norethisterone bioavailability 64%
Plasma half life	
range (apparently dose-dependent)	2.5–16.6 h
Volume of distribution (norethisterone)	37.7 l
Plasma protein binding	96%

The conversion of lynoestrenol to norethisterone may be impaired in patients with hepatic dysfunction, although specific information is not available. The effects of renal disease on the kinetics of the drug are not known, but they are unlikely to be very marked.

Concentration–effect relationship

There is little information on the concentration–effect relationship for norethisterone as an hormonal contraceptive, although such evidence as there is does not suggest a strict correlation between the plasma concentration and the therapeutic effect.[17]

Metabolism

Lynoestrenol, a pro-drug of weak intrinsic activity, is rapidly and quantitatively metabolized, in the liver, possibly via 3α- and 3β-OH-

Fig. 1 The metabolism of lynoestrenol

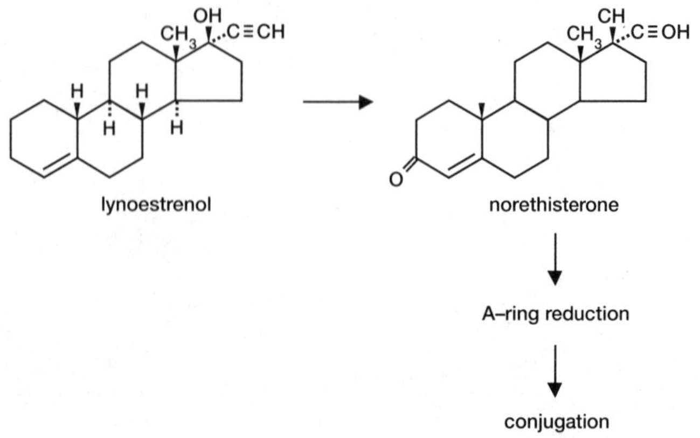

LYN[18] to norethisterone, the active metabolite, (Fig. 1) which subsequently undergoes saturation of the A-ring double bond and reduction of the 3-keto group, producing mainly $3\beta5\beta$-tetrahydro-norethisterone excreted as the sulphate and glucuronide conjugates which are inactive. Small amounts of $3\alpha5\beta$, $3\beta5\alpha$ and $3\alpha5\beta$-tetrahydro-norethisterone are also produced and excreted as inactive conjugates.

Pharmaceutics

Lynoestrenol is now marketed in the UK only as Minilyn (50 µg ethinyloestradiol and 2.5 mg lynoestrenol, Organon, UK). Minilyn is a white, round, flat tablet with a circle on one side and 'Organon' on the reverse. It is unavailable in the USA.

In other countries it is available under a variety of trade names in varying combinations with ethinyloestradiol and mestranol for hormonal contraception and alone for contraception and other gynaecological indications.

Therapeutic use

Indications

1. Hormonal contraception: this is the only marketed indication in the UK.

Other uses

Lynoestrenol alone may be used in the treatment of a variety of gynaecological disorders including:

2. Functional uterine bleeding
3. Endometriosis
4. Other occasional indications where drugs with a progestational activity are effective.

Contraindications

These are as for other progestogens when used alone or as for oestrogens if employed as part of a combined preparation.

Absolute contraindications to the use of combined preparations[19]

1. Vascular:
a. Venous thrombosis or arterial embolism
b. Cerebrovascular episodes, including subarachnoid haemorrhage
c. Elective surgery
d. Coronary heart disease
e. Valvular heart disease with pulmonary hypertension or atrial fibrillation
f. Focal migraine or symptomatic deterioration on introduction of the 'pill'
g. Sickle cell disease
h. Collagen vascular disease
i. Development of significant hypertension during therapy
2. Liver disease (since impairment of liver function may affect the metabolism of lynoestrenol):
a. Impaired liver function (cholestatic jaundice and hepatitis where liver function has failed to return to normal)
b. Congenital disorders of liver excretory function including the Rotor and Dubin–Johnson syndromes and the porphyrias
c. Hepatic tumours
3. Serious disorders of lipid metabolism, particularly familial hypercholesterolaemia
4. Existing or treated carcinoma of the breast or endometrium or other hormonally-dependent tumours
5. Pregnancy (undiagnosed amenorrhoea)
6. Hydatidiform mole (until HCG values negative for 3 months)
7. History of a serious condition deteriorating during pregnancy, e.g. otosclerosis, herpes gestationis or pruritis
8. Undiagnosed genital tract bleeding.

Relative contraindications to the use of combined oral contraceptive steroids:

1. Age over 35 years
2. Other factors associated with risk of accelerated atherogenesis:
a. Smoking
b. Obesity
c. Diabetes mellitus and prediabetes
3. Careful monitoring of patients with a depressive illness or history of such is necessary as depression may be exacerbated by sex steroids.

Lynoestrenol

Mode of use

1. Contraception

This is the major indication for lynoestrenol either in combination with an oestrogen or alone. In the UK, lynoestrenol is only available in combination with ethinyloestradiol as Minilyn. The first dose is given on the first day of menstruation and then for 22 consecutive days followed by a 6-day tablet-free interval. Treatment may also be started on the fifth day of the cycle and then as above, but in this case additional non-hormonal contraceptive precautions must be employed for the first 14 days of the contraceptive cycle.

2. Functional uterine bleeding

Appropriate investigations must be performed before initiating progestogen therapy. Doses of 2.5 to 5.0 mg may be employed.

3. Endometriosis

Lynoestrenol has been employed in the treatment of endometriosis but alternative pharmacological approaches and surgery are more appropriate.

Indications

1. Oral contraception

Combined oral contraceptive steroids are the most effective form of reversible fertility control known, with an intrinsic efficacy approaching 100%. They provide good cycle control with light, relatively painfree menstrual flow. It is now evident that they confer protection against a variety of diseases including tubal ectopic pregnancy,[20] pelvic inflammatory disease,[20] benign breast disease,[21] ovarian[22] and endometrial carcinoma,[23] and possibly rheumatoid disease.[26]

2. Functional uterine bleeding

Appropriate investigation must be performed before initiating progestogen therapy. The clinical circumstances will dictate the exact therapeutic approach, but often the disorder is self-limiting and a few cycles of treatment with a combined oestrogen preparation or lynoestrenol therapy alone will achieve cycle control, allowing spontaneous remission to occur.

3. Endometriosis

Lynoestrenol, like other progestogens, has been used to treat endometriosis, but alternative pharmacological approaches and surgery are more appropriate.

Contraindications to the use of lynoestrenol alone

These include hormonally dependent neoplasms, pregnancy and conditions deteriorating during pregnancy. With regard to vascular disease, progestogen-only preparations have not been implicated in venous or arterial thrombotic disease.[4] The oestrone progestogens, such as lynoestrenol, cause less upset of carbohydrate metabolism than the gonane progestogens,[24] and there is no evidence of increased blood pressure when these agents are used alone.[25]

The lower efficacy of progestogen-only preparations makes them less suitable than combined preparations when a high degree of contraceptive protection is required, particularly when compliance is in doubt and fertility is highest, in the young.

Adverse reactions

Potentially life-threatening effects

With combined preparations a very small increase in the incidence of fatal and non-fatal vascular episodes, including myocardial infarction, venous thromboemboli and cerebrovascular disease, has been observed. Such vascular events are more likely in smokers over the age of 35 years. Hormonal contraceptives have been implicated in breast neoplasia,[26] although the literature is conflicting and controversial,[27] and the role of the separate pharmacological moieties has not been discerned.

The use of lynoestrenol given alone is probably not a risk factor for accelerated vascular disease.

Acute overdosage

As with other contraceptive steroids, overdosage does not cause serious harm, even in children, although nausea, vomiting, transient breast swelling and mastalgia may occur. Withdrawal bleeding may occur in prepubertal girls. Treatment by emesis or gastric lavage may

Lynoestrenol

be considered if the overdose is discovered within about 3 hours of ingestion.

Severe or irreversible adverse effects

The effects of combined and progestogen-only preparations on carbohydrate and lipid metabolism have been discussed under Clinical pharmacology. The effect of these metabolic disturbances on premature atherogenesis is unclear. The biochemical effects are reversible on withdrawal of therapy.

Symptomatic adverse effects

Lynoestrenol alone or in combination with an oestrogen is well tolerated, but it may produce adverse effects common to all progestogens, including nausea, vomiting, weight gain, hyperphagia, changes in libido, breast tenderness, reduced vaginal secretion, irregular uterine bleeding, acne, greasy hair and alopecia. Progestogenic adverse effects are often balanced by the opposite effect of the oestrogen in the combined preparations.

Other effects

The effects of lynoestrenol on various metabolic parameters have been alluded to and are similar to those seen with norethisterone.

Interference with clinical pathology tests

Lynoestrenol does not interfere with analytical procedures per se. Many clinical pathology tests are very occasionally perturbed by lynoestrenol and other progestogens. Elevation of serum iron, copper and alkaline phosphatase may occur. Very occasional spurious elevations of the ESR and haematocrit may be seen. Indices of immunological function may be upset. Lynoestrenol amplifies the T-lymphocyte response to phytohaemagglutinin but the clinical relevance of this observation is obscure.[28] Antinuclear antigen positivity may be observed. These changes have been reviewed by Miale and Kent.[29]

High risk groups

Neonates

The drug is not indicated in neonates.

Breast milk. Norethisterone, the active metabolite, has a plasma to breast milk ratio of about 10:1.[30] Another study[31] in breast-fed infants of women using NET showed a norethisterone infant plasma concentration of 0.65 $nmol.l^{-1}$, which is unlikely to be of any pharmacodynamic significance.

Pregnant women

Lynoestrenol is contraindicated in pregnant women.

The elderly

There are no indications for the use of the drug in elderly patients.

Concurrent disease

Oral anticoagulant therapy. Any patient requiring oral anticoagulant therapy almost certainly has a contraindication to treatment with an oestrogen.

Hypertension. Combined preparations are relatively contraindicated. Progestogens alone such as lynoestrenol may be safe.[25]

Diabetes. Oral hypoglycaemic medication. Hormonal contraceptives cause minor deterioration in glycaemic control. Lynoestrenol appears to have minimal effect in this regard.

Drug interactions

Potentially hazardous interactions

No interactions of this type have been reported.

Other significant interactions

Contraceptive failure is the most serious result of drug interactions with contraceptive steroids. Most failures involve the co-prescription of combined contraceptive steroids with enzyme inducers or broad-spectrum antibiotics. The latter disrupt oestrogen enterohepatic circulation and would not be expected to interfere with progestogen efficacy except possibly by antibiotic-induced diarrhoea. Enzyme inducers may theoretically cause contraceptive failure with progestogen-only preparations in low dosage. The agents most frequently implicated in contraceptive failure with combined preparations include phenobarbitone, phenytoin, primidone, carbamazepine, dichloralphenazone and rifampicin. By the same mechanism, these drugs could impair the efficacy of lynoestrenol alone as a progestogen-only contraceptive agent, but no studies have been performed.

Inhibitors of steroid drug metabolism could theoretically increase the steroid load on the body, with toxicological consequences. Practical examples of this are not available.

As an enzyme inducer, alcohol may increase the metabolic breakdown of lynoestrenol but the effects are unlikely to be of clinical significance with social drinking.

Potentially useful interactions

Lynoestrenol is used with ethinyloestradiol in combined oral contraceptive preparations.

Major outcome trials

1. Ravn J 1972 Contraception with the lynoestrenol 'mini pill'. Arzneimittel-Forschung 22: 104–113

361 women (age range 19–40) were admitted to the trial. Patients were treated for a total of 3553 cycles (range 1–19 cycles) with 0.5 mg lynoestrenol at the same time each day.

There were no pregnancies and thus (confidence interval 0–1.1 pregnancies/100 women years). Irregular vaginal bleeding was frequent during the first two cycles of treatment, falling after 12 cycles to an incidence of 2.6%. During treatment there were no consistent changes in menstrual characteristics. Apart from the early occurrence of irregular bleeding, the regimen was well tolerated.

References

1. Shrinmanker K, Akpoviroro J, Fotherby K, Watson J 1980 Bioavailability of lynoestrenol. Arzneimittel-Forschung 30: 500–502
2. Lauritsen J G 1975 The significance of oral contraceptives in causing chromosome anomalies in spontaneous abortions. Acta Obstetrica Gynecologica Scandinavica 54: 261–264
3. Cullberg G, Eriksson O, Knutsson F, Steffensen K 1982 Desogestrel, a new progestational compound: a comparative study with lynoestrenol performed in ovariectomized women. Acta Obstetrica Gynecologica Scandinavica (suppl 111): 13–19
4. Poller L 1971 Oestrogen–progestogen oral contraception and blood clotting: a long-term follow up. British Medical Journal 4: 648–650
5. Pyorala T, Vahapassi J, Huntala M 1979 The effect of lynoestrenol and norethindrone on the carbohydrate and lipid metabolism in subjects with gestational diabetes. Annales Chirurgiae et Gynaecologiae 68 (2): 69–74
6. Radberg T, Gustafson A, Skryten A, Karlsson K 1982 Oral contraception in diabetic women. A cross-over study on serum and high density lipoprotein (HDL) lipids and diabetic control during progestogen and combined estrogen/progestogen contraception. Hormone and Metabolic Research 14 (2): 61–65
7. Malkonew M, Manninen V, Hirvonen E 1980 Effects of danazol and lynestrenol on serum lipoproteins in endometriosis. Clinical Pharmacology and Therapeutics 28: 602–604
8. Ruokonen A, Kaar K 1985 Effects of desogestrel, levonorgestrel and lynestrenol on serum sex hormone binding globulin, cortisol binding globulin, ceruloplasmin and HDL-cholesterol. European Journal of Obstetrics, Gynecology and Reproductive Biology 20: 3–18
9. Walls C, Vose C W, Horth C E, Palmer R F 1977 Radioimmunoassay of plasma norethisterone after ethynodiol diacetate administration. Journal of Steroid Biochemistry 8: 167–171
10. Orme M L'E, Back D J, Breckenridge A M 1983 Clinical pharmacokinetics of oral contraceptive steroids. Clinical Pharmacokinetics 8: 95–136
11. Odlind V, Weiner E, Victor A, Johansson E D B 1979 Plasma levels of norethindrone after single oral dose administration of norethindrone and lynestrenol. Clinical Endocrinology 10: 29–38
12. Kuhl H, Horst-Jurgen B, Hans-Dieter T 1982 Serum level and pharmacokinetics of norethisterone after ingestion of lynestrenol: its relation to dose and stage of menstrual cycle. Contraception 26: 303–315
13. Humpel M, Wendt H, Dogs G, Weib Chr, Rietz S, Speck U 1977 Intraindividual comparison of pharmacokinetic parameters of d-norgestrel, lynoestrenol and cyproterone acetate in 6 women. Contraception 16: 199–215
14. Back D J, Breckenridge A M, Crawford F E et al 1978 Pharmacokinetics of norethindrone in women. (2) Single dose pharmacokinetics. Clinical Pharmacology and Therapeutics 24: 448–453
15. Molen H J Van Der, Hart P G, Wijmenga H G 1969 Studies with 4-14C-lynestrenol in normal and lactating women. Acta Endocrinologica 61: 255–274
16. Hammond G L, Lahteenmaki P L A, Lahteenmaki P, Luukainen T 1982 Distribution and percentages of non-protein bound contraceptive steroids in human serum. Journal of Steroid Biochemistry 17: 375–380
17. Wynn V, Adams P W, Godsland et al 1979 Comparison of effects of different combined oral-contraceptive formulations on carbohydrate and lipid metabolism. Lancet 1: 1045–1049
18. Murata S 1968 Metabolism of 17α-ethynyl-19-nortestosterone and 17α-ethynylestradiol in vivo. Nippon Naibunpi Gakkai Zasshi 43: 1083–1096
19. Graham F M 1981 Problem patients and the 'pill'. Drugs 21: 152–156
20. Kay C R 1980 The happiness pill? Journal of the Royal College of General Practitioners 30: 8–19
21. The Centres for Disease Control, Cancer and Steroid Hormone Study 1983 Oral contraceptive use and the risk of ovarian cancer. Journal of the American Medical Association 249: 1596–1599

22. The Centres for Disease Control, Cancer and Steroid Hormone Study 1983 Oral contraceptive use and the risk of endometrial cancer. Journal of the American Medical Association 249: 1600–1604
23. Vandenbroucke J P, Valkenberg H A, Boersma J W et al 1982 Oral contraceptives and rheumatoid arthritis: further evidence for a preventive effect. Lancet 2: 839–842
24. Spellacy W N 1982 Carbohydrate metabolism during treatment with estrogen progestogen and low dose oral contraceptives. American Journal of Obstetrics and Gynecology 142: 732–734
25. Wilson E S B, Cruickshank J, Weir R J 1984 A prospective controlled study of the effect on blood pressure of contraceptive preparations containing different types and dosages of progestogens. British Journal of Obstetrics and Gynaecology 91: 1254–1260
26. Pike M C, Henderson B E, Krailo M D, Duke A, Roy S 1983 Breast cancer in young women and the use of oral contraceptives; possible modifying effects of formulation and age at use. Lancet 2: 926–929
27. McPherson K, Drife J O 1986 The pill and breast cancer: why the uncertainty? British Medical Journal 293: 709–710
28. Wybran J, Govaerts A, Dam D, Van Appelbroom T 1979 Stimulating properties of lynestrenol upon normal human blood T lymphocytes and leucocytes. International Journal of Immunopharmacology 1: 151–155
29. Miale J B, Kent J W 1974 The effect of oral contraceptives on the results of laboratory tests. American Journal of Obstetrics and Gynecology 120: 264–272
30. Toddywalla V S, Mehta S, Virkar K D, Saxena B M 1980 Release of 19-nortestosterone type of contraceptive steroids through different drug delivery systems into serum and breast milk or lactating women. Contraception 21: 217–223
31. Betrabet S S, Shikany Z K, Toddywalla V S, Toddywalla S P, Patel D, Saxena B N 1987 Transfer of norethisterone (NET) and levonorgestrel (LNG) from a single tablet into the infant's circulation through the mother's milk. Contraception 35: 517–522

Magnesium salts, oxides and hydroxide

Magnesium compounds are an essential part of many enzyme systems and are also widely used as antacids, as laxatives, as a central nervous depressant and in reducing cardiac muscle irritability.

Chemistry

Many magnesium compounds are available, including magnesium acetate, magnesium chloride, magnesium citrate, magnesium gluconate, magnesium sulphate, magnesium carbonate, magnesium hydroxide, magnesium oxide and magnesium trisilicate. The magnesium compounds are available in the pure forms listed above and are also widely used combined with aluminium compounds as antacids. The salts of magnesium compounds are white, odourless and usually tasteless powders. Except for the acetate, gluconate, sulphate and chloride, they are insoluble in water and alcohol but very soluble in dilute acids.[1]

Pharmacology

Magnesium is the second most plentiful cation in the intracellular fluids and is involved in a wide range of activities. It is essential for the activity of many enzymes and it is also important for the role that it plays in neurochemical transmission. The average individual (70 kg) contains about 2000 mEq of magnesium of which 50% is in bone. Magnesium compounds thus play a wide range of pharmacological roles. Magnesium salts are best known perhaps for their antacid properties[2,3] but they are also used as laxatives.[4] Magnesium sulphate (and other salts) acts as an osmotic laxative but in addition may stimulate the secretion of cholecystokinin thus increasing intestinal motility. Magnesium is also a depressant of both central nervous and neuromuscular function.[5] It decreases acetylcholine release by motor nerve impulses and reduces the sensitivity of the motor end plate to acetylcholine. Magnesium is also a depressant of cardiac muscle irritability and in these actions it is very similar to potassium and may act as a physiological calcium blocker.[6] Magnesium will block the transient inward current carried by calcium which is generated by cardiotonic drugs.[7] Because of this action magnesium will counteract ventricular irritability caused by excess digoxin. Magnesium overcomes the inhibition of the adenosine triphosphate system produced by digoxin, prolonging the refractory period and increasing the transmembrane potential.[8–10] These actions have the effect of electrically stabilizing the myocardium.[6]

Toxicology

Magnesium compounds have not been shown to have any mutagenic potential or carcinogenic activity.

Clinical pharmacology

Many of the pharmacological effects of magnesium salts are not widely used in therapeutics. Magnesium lengthens the PR and QRS intervals on the ECG and slows the rate of S-A nodal impulse formation. However, although it may abolish digitalis-induced premature ventricular contractions, it is rarely used for this purpose, except occasionally in the treatment of digitalis overdose. The effect of magnesium on the neuromuscular and central nervous systems is not relevant clinically except in magnesium poisoning. Hypermagnesaemia may occur if magnesium salts are given to patients with impairment of their renal function. Magnesium salts (sulphate, tartrate or phosphate) are used for their laxative effect. A full oral dose of compound (10–15 g) will produce a thorough semi-fluid evacuation in 3 hours or so, while lower doses (5 g) will have an effect 6–8 hours later. Magnesium sulphate (Epsom salts) has an intensely bitter taste that may induce nausea and is best given in citrus juice to mask the taste.

Magnesium containing antacid preparations are rarely used on their own because of the diarrhoea that they cause. Magnesium hydroxide is the most rapidly acting of the insoluble antacids. The solubility of $Mg(OH)_2$ is too low to be corrosive yet it quickly neutralizes acid to the end-point of pH 3.5. Magnesium carbonate is much slower acting as an antacid and magnesium trisilicate is too unreactive to be of much use as an antacid. The concurrent use of an aluminium- and magnesium-containing antacid provides both a fast-acting component and a more sustained effect. (See also Aluminium salts.) The delay in gastric emptying caused by aluminium is almost abolished in the presence of magnesium.

Pharmacokinetics

Except for the chlorides and sulphates, magnesium compounds are not absorbed, due to their intrinsic insolubility. However, the oxides, hydroxides and trisilicates are converted by acid gastric juice into soluble magnesium chloride which is absorbed. Magnesium compounds are widely distributed in nature, 50% being found in bones, 45% as an intracellular ion and 5% in extracellular fluid. About 30% of magnesium in a skeleton represents an exchangeable pool.[5,11]

The concentration of magnesium in intracellular fluid and plasma is about 15 and 0.75–1.1 $mmol.l^{-1}$ respectively. One-third is protein bound and the remainder is ionized.[12] It rapidly diffuses into all other tissues. Small and clinically irrelevant amounts are excreted in milk. The major excretory pathway of magnesium is renal and both oral and intravenous loads are rapidly eliminated.[13] In renal impairment there may be accumulation of magnesium.

Pharmaceutics

Magnesium salts are available in oral and parental forms, magnesium sulphate being the most commonly used parenteral form. When used as an antacid, the hydroxide or oxide and less commonly the trisilicate are used. Magnesium sulphate is used as a laxative but all magnesium compounds possess a laxative effect. Ideally, it should be stored in a cool environment in an airtight container.

Dried magnesium sulphate in glycerol is used as a paste for application to boils. It can only be used at the time the container is opened, since hydration renders it less effective.

A large number of preparations contain aluminium oxide and aluminium hydroxide gel in addition to magnesium salts. See aluminium hydroxide.

Therapeutic use

Indications

1. Antacids
2. Laxatives
3. In the treatment of hypomagnesaemia and in dialysis solutions
4. In the treatment of pre-eclampsia
5. In the treatment of massive digoxin overdose.

Other less common conditions where magnesium-containing medications have been used are listed by Mordes and Wacker.[13]

Contraindications

1. Long-term treatment of patients with renal failure[13]
2. Use as enema in patients with megacolon or intestinal obstruction.

Indications

1. Acid peptic disease

Magnesium oxide and hydroxide are combined with aluminium hydroxide gel in many antacid mixtures. This role is discussed in the monograph devoted to aluminium hydroxide (gel). In summary, magnesium antacids are combined in various preparations with aluminium hydroxide gel to maintain normal bowel function, the magnesium ion combating the constipating effect of the aluminium ion. Trials have shown that aluminium magnesium hydroxide gels accelerate the healing of both gastric ulcers and duodenal ulcers.[14–16] Aluminium magnesium hydroxide gels prevent acute stress ulcers.[17] Neither preparation should be used long-term, as long-term benefit has not been documented. The dosage used is limited by the ability of magnesium salts to produce diarrhoea. The preparation widely used in the treatment of acid peptic disease is the aluminium

Magnesium salts, oxides and hydroxide

M

hydroxide gel, Mylanta II, where the dose is 5–10 ml before and after the three main meals and before bed. This dose produces a healing effect equivalent to cimetidine or ranitidine in both gastric and duodenal ulcers but high-dose antacid therapy has a small role in management of acid pepsin-related diseases since the advent of potent anti-secretory drugs. They have a disadvantage of being costly, requiring frequent doses and being complicated by local side effects (constipation or diarrhoea) in about half the patients on therapeutically effective doses.

2. Cathartic
Magnesium sulphate is usually used and it acts to produce an osmotic diarrhoea. The recommended dose is 15 g but 5 g or less will produce a laxative effect when given in 200 ml of water in the fasting subject.[4] Each gram represents 4.1 mmol and 8.1 mEq of magnesium and sulphate.

3. Hypomagnesaemia and dialysis
Magnesium chloride is usually used in the treatment of magnesium depletion and as a source of magnesium ions in haemodialysis and peritoneal dialysis experiments. Each gram represents 4.9 mmol (4.8 mEq) of magnesium and 9.8 mmol (9.8 mEq) of chloride. The various preparations available include the sulphate, chloride, trisilicate, oxide, hydroxide and citrate.[12]

4. In the treatment of pre-eclampsia
An intravenous infusion of 4 g magnesium sulphate is given as a loading dose over 15 minutes, followed by a maintenance dose of 2 g per hour or more while the patellar reflexes, respiratory rate and urine output are maintained.[18]

5. Massive digitalis intoxication
Magnesium sulphate is given intravenously, 2–3 g initially followed by 2 g per hour for four to five hours.[19] However, the use of magnesium salts has probably been replaced by digoxin-specific FAB fragments.[20–22]

Adverse reactions

Potentially life-threatening effects
The only major adverse effects relate to the production of a hypermagnesaemic state consequent upon too rapid administration of the magnesium compounds parenterally or the prolonged administration of magnesium compounds to those with renal failure — see Acute overdosage.

Acute overdosage
Symptoms begin to appear when the serum magnesium concentration exceeds 2 $mmol.l^{-1}$ and include flushing, thirst, hypotension, weakness, drowsiness and loss of tendon reflexes. Respiratory depression, cardiac arrhythmias and ultimately cardiac arrest may result. The reaction was described in six patients in whom hypermagnesaemia was accidentally produced by the use of a dialysate solution containing 7.5 $mmol.l^{-1}$ (15 $mEq.l^{-1}$) instead of 0.75 $mmol.l^{-1}$ (1.5 $mEq.l^{-1}$). The patients complained of muscle weakness, blurred vision and ataxia, together with abnormal reflexes.[23] All recovered on using the correct dialysate solution. Other reactions due to excess administration of magnesium intravenously and occasionally after oral use are described above and in the review by Mordes and Wacker.[13]

Specific treatment of hypermagnesaemia. Intravenous injection of 10–20 ml of 10% calcium gluconate is required.[1] Dialysis may be needed in some patients. Any fluid deficit should be corrected.

Severe or irreversible adverse effects
Apart from those already mentioned there are none.

Symptomatic adverse effects
Diarrhoea results from orally administered magnesium compounds. The dose that produces diarrhoea is variable, but about 50% of those on a therapeutically effective dose will experience a disturbance of bowel function.

Interference with clinical pathology tests
An apparent increase in serum alkaline phosphatase levels can follow activation of the enzyme in vitro by magnesium salts or by interference in the Bessey procedure for estimating by bromsulphthalein. Magnesium may also interfere with methods for estimating serum and urinary calcium.

High risk groups

Neonates
There are no specific contraindications to the use of the drug in neonates, but adverse effects have occurred when magnesium sulphate enemas have been given to patients in this group.

Breast milk. Magnesium sulphate enters breast milk and may cause diarrhoea in the breast-fed infant.

Children
The drug may be given to children, if indicated.

Pregnant women
The drug may be used cautiously in pregnancy.

The elderly
Magnesium sulphate may be used in elderly patients provided that renal function is normal.

Concurrent disease
The drug should be avoided, if possible, in patients with renal or hepatic failure and in those with heart block and myocardial disease.

Unless used for the treatment of severe digoxin intoxication (see above), magnesium sulphate should be avoided by patients taking digitalis preparations.

Drug interactions

Potentially hazardous interactions
Magnesium sulphate use in pre-eclampsia potentiates the neuromuscular blockade produced by d-tubocurarine, and suxamethonium.

Other significant interactions
Antacids have been implicated in causing a reduced bioavailability or slower absorption of a number of drugs such as propranolol, isoniazid, prednisone, diflunisal and naproxen. This effect is predominantly due to the aluminium-based antacids. Magnesium-based antacids do not have this effect and will usually reverse the aluminium-based effect. Thus combined aluminium- and magnesium-based antacids will not affect the bioavailability of drugs except for tetracycline (due to the chelation of the cations by the antibiotic), and iron, whose bioavailability is decreased when the stomach contents are alkalinized.

Potentially useful interactions
The value of combining magnesium salts with aluminium-based antacids has been discussed above.

Major outcome trials

These relate to the healing of chronic duodenal and gastric ulcer. In all trials, magnesium antacids have been used in combination with aluminium hydroxide gel and the trials are described in relation to the latter drug.

General review articles

Mordes J P, Wacker W E C 1977 An extensive review of hypermagnesaemia and its effects. Pharmacological Review 29: 293

References

1. Reynolds J E F (ed) 1982 Martindale. The Extra Pharmacopoeia, 28th edn. The Pharmaceutical Press, London, pp. 81–84, 625–628
2. Piper D W, Fenton B H 1964 Antacid therapy of peptic ulcer. II Evaluation of antacids. Gut 5: 585–589
3. Fordtran J S, Marawski S G, Richardson C T 1973 In vivo and in vitro evaluation of liquid antacids. New England Journal of Medicine 288: 923–926
4. Fingl E 1980 Laxatives and cathartics. In: Gilman A G, Goodman L S, Gilman A (eds) The pharmacological basis of therapeutics, 6th edn. MacMillan, New York, pp 1002–1012
5. Mudge G H 1980 Agents affecting volume and composition of body fluids. In: Gilman A G, Goodman L S, Gilman A (eds) The pharmacological basis of therapeutics, 6th edn. MacMillan, New York, pp 848–884
6. Iseri L T, French J H 1984 Magnesium: nature's physiologic calcium blocker. American Heart Journal 108: 188–193
7. Kass R S, Lederer W J, Tsien R W et al 1978 Role of A calcium ions in transient inward currents and after contraction induced by strophanthidin in cardiac Purkinje fibres. Journal of Physiology (London) 281: 187–208

8. Seller R H, Cangiano J, Kim K E et al 1970 Digitalis toxicity and hypomagnesaemia. American Heart Journal 79: 57–68
9. Neff M S, Mendelssohn S, Kim K E et al 1972 Magnesium sulphate in digitalis toxicity. American Journal of Cardiology 29: 377–382
10. Parmintuan J C, Dreifus L S, Watanabe Y 1970 Comparative mechanisms of antiarrhythmic agents. American Journal of Cardiology 26: 512–519
11. Alfrey A C, Miller N L 1973 Bone magnesium pools in uraemia. Journal of Clinical Investigation 52: 3019–3027
12. Reynolds J E F (ed) Martindale. The Extra Pharmacopoeia, 28th edn. The Pharmaceutical Press, London, p 625
13. Mordes J P, Wacker W E C 1978 Excess magnesium. Pharmacological Review 29: 274–300
14. Peterson W L, Sturdevant R A L, Frankl H D et al 1977 Healing of duodenal ulcer with an antacid regimen. New England Journal of Medicine 297: 341–345
15. Ippoliti A F, Sturdevant R A L, Isenberg J I et al 1978 Cimetidine versus intensive antacid therapy for duodenal ulcer. Gastroenterology 74: 393–395
16. Lam S K 1988 Antacids: the past, the present and the future in peptic ulceration. Baillère's Clinics in Gastroenterology 2: 641–654
17. Robert A, Kauffman G L 1983 Stress ulcers. In: Sleisenger M H, Fordtran J S (eds) Gastrointestinal disease pathophysiology, diagnosis and management, 3rd edn. W B Saunders, Philadelphia, pp 612–624
18. Sibai B M, Graham J M, McCubbin J H 1984 A comparison of intravenous and intramuscular magnesium sulphate regimens in pre-eclampsia. American Journal of Obstetrics and Gynecology 150: 728–733
19. French J H, Thomas R G, Siskind A P 1984 Magnesium therapy in massive digoxin intoxication. Annals of Emergency Medicine 13: 562–566
20. Proudfoot A T 1986 A star treatment of digoxin overdose. British Medical Journal 293: 642–643
21. Jones M, Hawker F, Duggin G, Falk M 1987 Treatment of severe digoxin toxicity with digoxin-specific antibody fragments. Anaesthesia and Intensive Care 15: 234–236
22. Desantola J R, March Linski F E 1986 Response of digoxin toxic atrial tachycardia to digoxin specific Fab fragments. American Journal of Cardiology 58: 1109–1110
23. Govan J R, Porter C A, Cook J G H et al 1968 Acute magnesium poisoning as a complication of chronic intermittent haemodialysis. British Medical Journal 2: 278–279
24. Outerbridge E W, Papageorgiou A, Stern L 1973 Magnesium sulphate enema in a new born. Fatal systemic magnesium absorption. Journal of the American Medical Association 224: 1392–1393

Malathion

This substance is widely used as a topical insecticide and acaricide. It is also used in the control of mosquitoes.

Chemistry

Malathion, phosphothion
$C_{10}H_{19}O_6PS_2$
Diethyl 2-(dimethoxyphosphinothioylthio)succinate

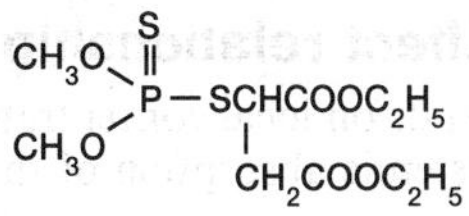

Molecular weight	330.4
pKa	–
Solubility	
in alcohol	miscible
in water	1 in 7000
Octanol/water partition coefficient	–

Malathion is a colourless to yellow liquid with a characteristic odour, rather like garlic. Its pKa is not known. Malathion is soluble in water at 145 ppm and in organic solvents. It is slightly soluble in mineral oils.

Pharmacology

Malathion is an anticholinesterase and will thus have all the pharmacological effects of compounds like neostigmine and pyridostigmine. Like other organophosphates it mainly interferes with cholinesterase in all tissues, causing parasympathetic over-activity and voluntary muscle paralysis. Despite lowered concentrations of cholinesterase in red blood cells, Goldin found no reduction in red cell survival time.[1] Malathion probably binds to the peripheral anionic site of the enzyme. Plasma carboxyl esterases cause rapid hydrolysis of the carboxyl ester linkage and thus in mammals malathion has a very short duration of action. If taken parenterally, e.g. by inhalation of insecticidal spray, malathion would be expected to cause symptoms such as salivation, miosis, gastrointestinal colic, bradycardia, fall in cardiac output, etc. When malathion was sprayed from three aircraft at a concentrations of 3 ounces per acre (212 g per hectare) to kill the mosquito vector during an epidemic of St Louis encephalitis in Corpus Christi, Texas, 119 volunteers were monitored. Six complained of symptoms but there was no correlation between plasma cholinesterase levels and symptoms, or exposure. It was concluded there was negligible risk to human health from such exposure.[2]

Malathion is rapidly pediculocidal and niticidal at concentrations as low as 0.06%. It is likely that insects are killed by the inhibition of acetylcholinesterases found at synaptic junctions in the insect's nervous system.[3]

Toxicology

The dermal LD_{50} in the female rat is 2500 mg.kg^{-1}. The dermal LD_{50} in the rabbit is 4100 mg.kg^{-1}.
Teratogenicity, mutagenicity and carcinogenicity tests have not been recorded. Kimborogh and Gains found congenital abnormalities in pregnant rats treated with malathion.[4] Only one case of congenital abnormalities in humans has been recorded.[5]

Malathion

Clinical pharmacology

Malathion is used clinically as a 0.5% solution or lotion for the treatment of head and pubic lice. It is applied topically and there is little evidence of transdermal absorption of the compound in the doses used. Since malathion is rapidly hydrolysed in man it is unlikely that any clinical pharmacological effects would be seen in normal use.

Pharmacokinetics

There is little direct information about malathion absorption through the skin, but as with other organophosphate compounds, it should be well absorbed through the skin, conjunctiva, gastrointestinal tract and lungs. Namba et al[6] showed that skin absorption of pesticide was rapid from palms, despite the thick keratin, very rapid from scalp, face and forearms where there are lots of hair follicles, and most rapid from the scrotum. Another study undertook extensive skin testing to estimate absorption through the skin of malathion and other pesticides.[7] The degree of poisoning could in many cases be correlated with the site of skin exposure and degree of skin exposure. Percutaneous absorption will increase in the presence of active eczema and in high ambient temperatures.[8]

Concentration–effect relationship

Therapeutic effect depends on local concentration and absorption by the parasite, not on systemic absorption of the drug.

Metabolism

Malathion is converted to the active malaoxon by cytochrome P450 mediated monooxygenases in the liver. The detoxication pathway involves hydrolysis of carboxylester linkages by tissue or plasma carboxylesterases (Fig. 1).

Fig. 1 Activation of malathion

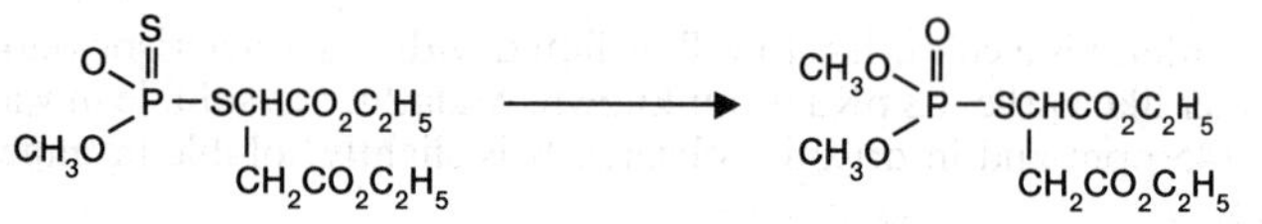

Malathion Malaoxon

Pharmaceutics

1. Derbac-M liquid (International Laboratories, UK): malathion 0.5% w/w aqueous liquid
2. Prioderm lotion (Napp, UK): malathion 0.5% w/v alcohol based lotion
3. Prioderm Shampoo (Napp, UK): malathion 1.0% w/w cream shampoo
4. Suleo-M lotion (International, UK): malathion 0.5% w/v alcohol based lotion

Therapeutic use

Indications

1. Eradication of head lice and pubic lice
2. Treatment of scabies.

Contraindications

There are no known contraindications.

Mode of use

1a. Head lice (adults and children)
Apply malathion liquid to the roots of the hair and scalp, paying special attention to the partings, back of the neck, fringes and around the ears. Leave the hair to dry naturally and wash in ordinary shampoo the next day. After shampoo, remove dead eggs (nits) with a metal nit comb while the hair is still wet.

1b. Pubic lice (adults and children)
Apply freely to all parts of the hair in the affected areas, paying special attention to the roots. Leave for at least one hour and then remove by washing with a bland shampoo or soap. If more convenient, malathion liquid can be left on overnight.

2. Scabies
The patient should take a fairly prolonged soap and water bath, rubbing the principal areas of involvement with a brush or wash cloth. Apply malathion liquid to the entire skin surface, excepting the head. This is best done by someone other than the patient to avoid missing some areas. Do not bathe for 24 hours. Put on fresh clothing. No special sterilization of clothing is necessary; ordinary laundering or dry cleaning and hot iron pressing are sufficient. The itching may not subside immediately; calamine lotion may be applied if necessary.

Malathion should not be used in children under the age of six months except under medical supervision.

Adverse reactions

Potentially life-threatening effects
A greenfly killer was blamed for the death of a man aged 65. He was found dead in his garage with a spilled container, and had inhaled malathion. He was found to have focal necrosis of the liver. He could have breathed in about 300 mg. This is much less than has been administered to volunteers without any toxic effect.[9] No other adverse effects of this severity have been reported.

Acute overdosage
Baker and others described an outbreak of epidemic poisoning among the mixers, spraymen and supervisors involved in spraying malathion for mosquito control.[10] Among the 7500 workers, 2800 cases occurred. Low red cell count cholinesterase was associated with signs and symptoms of organophosphate insecticide intoxication. Iso-malathion, a degradation product of malathion, was associated with the greatest toxicity seen in clinical cases. Poor work practices and excessive skin contact were blamed for the outbreak.

Extensive testing of malathion in malaria control programmes in Uganda, Nigeria and Central America yielded little evidence of human toxicity. Some workers allowed wet clothing smelling strongly of pesticides to remain in contact with the skin. Many of these had systemic symptoms, namely blurred vision, headache, nausea, sweating, vomiting and abdominal pain, and also had skin irritation and skin rashes. Two men died.

Gadoth and Fisher recorded late-onset neuromuscular block in organophosphorus poisoning.[11] In this case a 24-year-old pregnant girl took 150 ml of 50% malathion in xylene. After initial treatment following immediate resuscitation, she developed progressive muscular weakness and pulmonary oedema. The pulmonary oedema was thought to be due to xylene. Abortion was performed because of the danger of congenital abnormality.

Teitelbaum suggested that organophosphate insecticides should not be overlooked as a possible suicide weapon.[12] Three persons who took massive doses of malathion were revived by the use of pralidoxime and atropine.

Treatment consists of gastric lavage, assisted respiration, and, if necessary, administration of atropine and, possibly, pralidoxime or related compounds.[13,14]

Severe or irreversible adverse effects
No reactions of this kind have been described.

Symptomatic adverse effects
Apart from mild irritation at the site of application, no symptomatic adverse effects are to be expected.

Interference with clinical pathology tests
No technical interferences of this kind appear to have been reported.

High risk groups

Neonates
The drug should only be used in neonates under medical supervision.

Breast milk. There appears to be no contraindication to the use of the drug by lactating mothers.

Children
There is no contraindication to the use of the drug in children.

Pregnant women
While the general rule applies that no drug should be used during pregnancy unlesss absolutely necessary, there appears to be no absolute contraindication to the use of this drug during pregnancy.

The elderly
The drug may be used without special precautions in older patients.

Drug interactions

No interactions between locally applied malathion and other drugs used concurrently have been reported.

Clinical trials

1. Mathias R G, Huggins D R, Leroux S J et al. 1984 Comparative trial of treatment with Prioderm lotion and Kwellada shampoo in children with head lice. Canadian Medical Association Journal 130: 407–409

In this double-blind randomised study, 62 children with head lice were treated with 0.5% malathion lotion (Prioderm lotion) or 1% lindane shampoo (Kwellada shampoo). Malathion lotion proved to be safe and effective treatment for head lice. Ovicidal activity was incomplete in both drugs, and the authors recommended that both treatments should be used twice, with a one week gap, to achieve total eradication.

2. Taplin D, Castillero P M, Spiegal J et al 1982 Malathion treatment of Pediculus humanus var capitis infestations. Journal American Medical Association 247: 3103–3105

In this double-blind, randomised, controlled trial, 115 children with head lice were treated with either 0.5 malathion lotion or the alcoholic vehicle, to assess efficacy and safety of the drug. The results demonstrated that malathion 0.5% lotion was an effective pediculicide and ovicide and caused no side effects even when pre-existing scalp diseases were present.

3. Gomes-Urcuyo F, Zaias N 1986 Malathion lotion as an insecticide and ovicide in head lice infestations. International Journal Dermatology 25: 60–62

In this double-blind, parallel group study, 119 patients with head lice were treated with 0.5% malathion lotion or its vehicle. The malathion lotion proved to be an effective pediculicide and ovicide with no side effects.

General review articles

Pesticides for use in public health 1978 WHO Chronicle 32: 339–344

Hayes W J Jr, Mattson A M, Gordon Short J, Witter R F 1960 Safety of malathion dusting powder for louse control. Bulletin of the World Health Organization 22: 503–514

References

1. Goldin A, Rubenstein A H, Bradlow B A, Elliott G A 1964 Malathion poisoning with special reference to the effect of cholinesterase inhibition on erythrocyte survival. New England Journal of Medicine 1290–1293
2. Gardener A L, Inverson R E 1968 The effect of aerially applied malathion on an urban population. Archives of Environmental Health 16: 823–826
3. Metcalfe R L 1955 Organic insecticides, their chemistry and mode of action. Interscience Publishers Ltd
4. Kimborogh R D, Gains T B 1968 Effect of organic phosphorus compounds and alkylating agents on the rat fetus. Archives of Environmental Health 16: 805–808
5. Namba T, Nolte C T, Jackrel J, Grob D 1971 Poisoning due to organophosphate insecticide. American Journal of Medicine 50: 475
6. Namba T, Nolte C T, Nackrel J, Grob D 1971 Poisoning due to organophosphate insecticides, acute and chronic manifestations. American Journal of Medicine 50: 475
7. Maibach H I, Feldmann R J, Milby T H, Serat W F 1971 Regional variation in percutaneous penetration in man. Archives of Environmental Health 23: 208
8. Hamilton A, Hardy H L 1974 Industrial toxicology, 3rd edn. Publishing Sciences Group Inc, p 356).
9. Coroners Court Report — open verdict 1966 British Medical Journal 1: 304
10. Baker E L Jr, Warren M, Zack M et al 1978 Epidemic malathion poisoning in Pakistan malaria workers. Lancet 1: 31–34
11. Gadoth N, Fisher A 1978 Late onset of neuromuscular block in organophosphorus poisoning. Annals of Internal Medicine 88: 654–655
12. Teitelbaum D T 1971 Letter: organophosphate poisoning. Journal of the American Medical Association 217: 1704
13. Mathewson I, Hardy E A 1970 Treatment of malathion poisoning. Experience of two cases in Sarawak. Anaesthesia 25: 265
14. Crowley W J, Johns T R 1966 Accidental malathion poisoning. Archives of Neurology 14: 611–616

Mannitol

Mannitol is the most extensively employed of the osmotic diuretics.

Chemistry

Mannitol (Osmitrol, Manicol, Resectisol)
$C_6H_{14}O_6$
D-Mannitol

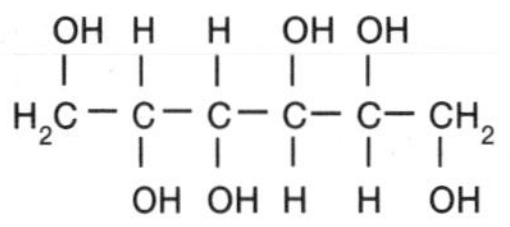

Molecular weight	182.2
pKa	—
Solubility	
in alcohol	1 in 83
in water	1 in 6
Octanol/water partition coefficient	low

Mannitol is white odourless crystalline powder or granules with a sweetish taste, prepared by chemical synthesis and it is practically insoluble in chloroform or ether. The D-enantiomer is used clinically. It is also available as a sterile solution with sodium chloride in water for injection [Mannitol and Sodium Chloride for Injection (USP)].

Pharmacology

Mannitol's structure makes it osmotically active. Its diuretic properties depend on its renal handling: complete glomerular filtration and minimal tubular reabsorption. The increased osmolality of tubular fluid impairs the proximal reabsorption of water and sodium; the resultant fluid and solute load overwhelms the reabsorptive capacity of distal segments of the nephron. Reduction of medullary hypertonicity with washout of the countercurrent osmotic gradient due to enhanced blood flow, and increased glomerular filtration rate also contribute to the extent of the diuresis.

Toxicology

No data are available.

Clinical pharmacology

After mannitol, urine flow and sodium excretion rise in proportion to the excreted osmotic load.[1] Changes in tubular free water and solute clearance in the hydropenic state and during maximal water diuresis support the importance of actions at distal tubular sites and on the renal medulla.[2] Mannitol increases glomerular filtration rate by increasing plasma flow as a result of plasma expansion and a direct vascular effect, and through acute reduction in systemic osmotic pressure.[3] The primary systemic effect of mannitol is a shift of fluid from the intracellular compartment to the extracellular space.[4] The movement of water is not accompanied by notable shifts of hydrogen or bicarbonate ions, and plasma pH falls. Plasma chloride and sodium concentrations typically fall acutely. Effects on plasma potassium are variable but acute increases are usual.[5]

Pharmacokinetics

The preferred analytical procedure is an enzymic method based on spectrophotometric measurement of the initial rate of NADH formation in the reaction between mannitol and NAD catalyzed by mannitol dehydrogenase.[6] There is a linear relationship between

Mannitol

M

plasma concentrations in the range 0.5–200 $mmol.l^{-1}$. This approach avoids the shortcomings of the more commonly applied but technically difficult and time consuming colorimetric method based on the measurement of formaldehyde formed by periodic acid oxidation of mannitol.[7] Only small amounts of mannitol are absorbed from the gastrointestinal tract.[8] Following intravenous administration, it is distributed uniformly in body water and concentration in serum is equivalent to that throughout the extracellular fluid volume.[9] Mannitol has a low volume of distribution (approximately 0.18 $l.kg^{-1}$) and a brief equilibrium time (less than one hour).[9,10] In patients with cardiac or renal impairment, volume of distribution is increased and equilibrium is delayed (three hours or more).[11] The elimination half life is around two hours but there is marked interindividual variability and elimination is greatly delayed in cardiac or renal failure (half life 6–36 hours).[12]

Oral absorption	negligible
Presystemic metabolism	negligible
Plasma half life	
range	2–36 h
mean	2.17 h
Volume of distribution	0.16–0.27 $l.kg^{-1}$
Plasma protein binding	—

No information is available on the excretion of mannitol in breast milk or on its passage across the placenta. It is unlikely that either would occur to any significant extent.

Concentration–effect relationship

No data are available.

Metabolism

After intravenous administration, over 80% of mannitol is excreted unchanged in urine within 24 hours.[10,11,13,14] Very little metabolism follows parenteral dosing[10,13–15] but unchanged mannitol is also lost in bile, particularly in renal failure.[14,16] Approximately 50% of an oral dose is excreted unchanged in urine and faeces, the remainder undergoing slow oxidation in the liver and, possibly, by bacteria in the gut.[13,17] There appears to be no difference in metabolism between cirrhotic subjects and those with normal hepatic function. As the oral dose increases, inducing diarrhoea, the proportion of mannitol in faeces increases.[13]

Pharmaceutics

Mannitol is available as 5%, 10%, 15% 20% and 25% sterile aqueous solutions in volumes of 50–1000 ml for intravenous injection or infusion. These are not suitable for subcutaneous or intramuscular injection. A 5.07% w/v solution in water is iso-osmotic with serum.

Mannitol is stable to heat and may be heated or autoclaved if crystals appear during storage. Plastic surfaces may act as nuclei for rapid crystallization when supersaturated (15% or greater) injections are used. Resolubilization by heating is of no benefit here as rapid recrystallization may occur. A filtration device should be used during administration of solutions containing 20% or more of mannitol. Mannitol should never be added to whole blood for transfusion or given through the same set by which blood is being infused because of the high risk of agglutination and irreversible crenation of erythrocytes.

Mannitol became permitted as a bulk sweetener in the UK in 1982. It is used as a tablet excipient in certain formulations.

Therapeutic use

Indications

1. Renal insufficiency
2. Raised intracranial pressure
3. Raised intraocular pressure
4. Management of poisoning
5. Oedematous states
6. Reperfusion injury
7. Termination of pregnancy
8. Bowel preparation
9. Bladder irrigation
10. Diluent and excipient.

Contraindications

1. Pulmonary oedema or congestive heart failure
2. Inadequate urine flow
3. Dehydration/acidosis
4. Intracranial bleeding.

Mode of use

The recommended range of doses in adults is 25–200 g by intravenous infusion over 24 hours although an adequate response is generally achieved with a dosage of 100 g. The rate of administration is adjusted to maintain a urine flow of at least 30–50 $ml.h^{-1}$. Careful monitoring of rate of administration is necessary to avoid fluid and electrolyte imbalance, and circulatory overloading. The infusion should be terminated if the patient develops signs of progressive renal dysfunction, heart failure or pulmonary congestion.

Indications

1. Renal insufficiency

Mannitol is useful in states of acute renal insufficiency, low renal perfusion or both; it is often used prophylactically where hypotension or sudden reduction in renal perfusion can be anticipated. Such circumstances include trauma, sepsis, haemolytic transfusion reactions, nephrotoxicity induced by radiocontrast media or amphotericin, surgery, or in the early stages of circulatory failure from other causes when underperfusion may progress to acute tubular necrosis.[18–22]

Since tubular permeability to mannitol is not greatly influenced by renal hypoperfusion of short duration and since the load of the agent filtered is not markedly altered in the presence of reduced glomerular filtration rate, mannitol often produces a diuresis in states refractory to other diuretics.

Mannitol may be used to treat oliguria provided a test dose of 200 $mg.kg^{-1}$ body weight (about 50 ml of a 25% solution in adults) given by intravenous infusion over 3–5 minutes produces a diuresis of at least 30-50 $ml.h^{-1}$ during the next 2–3 hours; a second test dose is permitted if the response to the first dose is inadequate. The usual dose is 50–100 g of a 15–25% solution over 24 hours. In states of shock, 200 g of mannitol over 24 hours may be required.

For prophylaxis of renal failure during major surgery, 500 ml of 5–10% mannitol solution is usually infused for 1–2 hours before the procedure and continued at a rate sufficient to ensure 1 ml $urine.min^{-1}$ for up to 48 hours afterwards (i.e. 50–100 g in total). Maintenance of an adequate flow of relatively dilute urine is probably the most important factor but hypertonic solutions increase extracellular osmolality which in turn may decrease the cellular swelling that accompanies renal ischaemia and hence improve renal blood flow.[3] In the absence of large prospective trials, however, there is little evidence that ultimate recovery of renal function occurs more quickly.

In cadaver kidney recipients, a regimen of mannitol (250 ml of 20% solution) and moderate rehydration reduces significantly the incidence of acute tubular necrosis and other problems following transplantation.[23] Mannitol may also prevent rapid osmolality changes in haemodialysis,[24] although this indication has not been explored extensively.

Mannitol is ineffective and hazardous in primary acute or chronic renal failure.

2. Raised intracranial pressure

By elevating plasma osmolality, mannitol enhances the diffusion of water from the cerebrospinal fluid. To provide a blood–brain osmotic gradient (10–30 mmol) sufficient to mobilize brain water rapidly, mannitol 1.0–1.5 $g.kg^{-1}$ administered as a 15–25% solution over 10 minutes is often necessary[25] but 0.5–2.0 $g.kg^{-1}$ infused for up to one hour may be effective. If mannitol is required more often than every three to four hours, serum osmolality rises above 320 m $osmol.l^{-1}$ and yet intracranial pressure remains elevated, administration of more mannitol is likely to lead to renal failure, metabolic acidosis and death.

Rapid administration may ameliorate cerebral oedema caused by tumour, ketoacidotic coma, Reye's syndrome or hypoxia after cardiac arrest and induces more substantial shift of water from brain cells during neurosurgery than does an osmotically equivalent dose of urea.[26] In severe head injury, mannitol is most likely to be of value in patients with focal damage, in those with very high intracranial pressure and in those in whom cerebral perfusion pressure is at or below the lower limit of autoregulation.[27]

3. Raised intraocular pressure
Since mannitol is confined to extraocular water with poor ocular penetration, it lowers intraocular pressure by creating an osmotic gradient between plasma and the ocular fluids. Dehydration of the vitreous gel leads to a shrunken vitreous and, on occasion, a soft eye is noted after treatment.

Mannitol is used for the short-term reduction of intraocular pressure in patients requiring ocular surgery, particularly for cataracts or for penetration keratoplasties. Given 30–60 minutes before surgery, 100 ml 20% mannitol effectively lowers intraocular pressure and increases anterior chamber depth. Larger volumes give almost identical responses although they act more rapidly and over a longer period.[28] A similar regimen is effective as adjuvant therapy in the prevention or treatment of acute glaucoma.

4. Management of poisoning
Mannitol has been applied to the management of acute drug intoxication with agents where a major route of elimination is through the kidney, such as certain barbiturates (phenobarbitone), salicylates, analgesics (pethidine) and psychotropic drugs (amphetamine). A 'forced diuresis' may be induced by employing mannitol alone or in combination with a potent natriuretic agent.

A 5% solution of mannitol is used, the aim being to produce a urine output of 150–500 $ml.h^{-1}$. Although it may be of value in paraquat poisoning, catharsis using an orally administered saturated solution of mannitol presents far too many hazards for routine application. The frequently associated loss of gut mobility favours increased absorption of the poison.

5. Oedematous states
Intravenous administration of mannitol to increase intravascular volume and thereby renal perfusion has been used to promote diuresis in patients with oedema refractory to conventional diuretics because of intravascualar hypovolaemia e.g. hepatic cirrhosis with ascites.[29] If there are no adverse effects following a test dose, 20% mannitol solution may be given at a rate of 25–50 $ml.h^{-1}$. Each 50 g mannitol obligates the intracellular to extracellular shift of one litre of water.

A similar beneficial effect may be obtained by oral administration of one to two litres of a 10–20% solution of mannitol over a period of one to four hours.[29,30] The mechanism is through fluid and sodium diffusion into the increased osmotic content of the gut. The results are massive diarrhoea and body loss of sodium, potassium and water.

The availability of loop diuretics, which are more effective and safer, has made the use of mannitol in oedematous states largely redundant.

6. Reperfusion injury
Hyperosmolar post ischaemic reflow with mannitol may be of some value in improving post ischaemic ventricular function, maintaining coronary blood flow during early reflow, and reducing myocardial oedema formation.[31] The beneficial action may be at least partly the result of hydroxyl radical elimination during reflow.

7. Termination of pregnancy
Mannitol (200 ml of a 25% solution) instilled into the amniotic cavity induces abortion in a high proportion of pregnancies.

8. Bowel preparation
Mannitol is effective in preparation of the bowel for barium enema or colonoscopy. Usually one litre of a 10% solution is consumed in less than 30 minutes early on the day of examination.

9. Bladder irrigation
A 2.5% solution of mannitol has been used for irrigating the bladder during transurethral resection of the prostate.

10. Diluent and excipient
Mannitol has been used as a diluent and excipient in pharmaceutical preparations.

Contraindications

1. Pulmonary oedema or congestive heart failure
In patients with diminished cardiac reserve and incipient failure, the sudden shift of water from cells to extracellular fluid which accompanies mannitol treatment may precipitate pulmonary oedema or fulminating congestive cardiac failure.

2. Inadequate urine flow
If urine flow is inadequate, as in acute tubular necrosis or obstructive uropathy, expansion of extracellular fluid may lead to acute water intoxication or pulmonary congestion, even in the absence of underlying heart disease.

3. Dehydration/acidosis
Because of its action on hydrogen and bicarbonate, use of mannitol may be hazardous in the presence of marked acidosis or dehydration.

4. Intracranial bleeding
Mannitol is contraindicated except during or immediately prior to craniotomy. Reduction in brain oedema may precipitate rebleeding.

Adverse reactions

Potentially life-threatening effects
Administration of hypertonic mannitol solutions in amounts sufficient to make a significant contribution to extracellular osmolality may be associated with severe fluid and electrolyte imbalance.[32] Pulmonary oedema, water intoxication, convulsions, and hypertension or hypotension may be provoked.

Oral mannitol may be associated with potentially explosive intracolonic hydrogen concentrations. Severe hypersensitivity (anaphylactic) reactions have also been reported. Over-rapid intravenous administration may lead to irreversible crenation of red blood cells.[33]

Acute overdosage
Overdosage with mannitol involves the central nervous system, leading to lethargy, confusion, stupor, coma and death.[35] These clinical findings are accompanied by fluid overloading, severe hyponatraemia and a large osmolality gap.

In such severe cases, the ideal treatment appears to be haemodialysis with rapid removal of mannitol and replacement with sodium. Peritoneal dialysis is a useful alternative. In less severe poisoning, treatment should be symptomatic, in particular directed to correction of fluid and electrolyte imbalance.

Severe or irreversible adverse effects
With long-term mannitol administration, dehydration and hypernatraemia may occasionally follow because of obligatory free water loss.[34] The risk of clinically significant hyperkalaemia and acidosis depends on dose, rate of infusion and presence of insulin response which regulates movements of potassium out of cells. When extracellular osmolality rises abruptly and induces water movement out of cells, a flux of potassium into the extracellular space occurs possibly by solvent drag. On the other hand, increased urine flow together with hyperaldosteronism due to extracellular fluid expansion promote urine potassium loss and severe hypokalaemia may ensue.

Hypersensitivity to intravenous mannitol may result in urticaria. Extravasation of the solution may cause oedema, inflammation, skin necrosis and thrombophlebitis.

Symptomatic adverse effects
Intravenous infusion of mannitol has been associated with thirst, headache, dizziness, chills, fever, tachycardia, chest pain, urinary retention and blurred vision. When given by mouth, mannitol invariably causes diarrhoea. Nausea and vomiting may follow administration by either route.

Interference with clinical pathology tests
Mannitol causes false positive estimations of ethylene glycol and interferes with some but not all methods for serum inorganic phosphate.[36]

High risk groups

Neonates
Very little information is available on the use of mannitol in neonates.

Breast milk. No information is available on the excretion of mannitol in breast milk.

Mannitol

M

Children

The usual test dose (200 mg.kg^{-1} by slow intravenous injection) is followed by 2 g.kg^{-1}. For cerebral and ocular oedema, a 15–20% solution is given over 30–60 minutes; for peripheral oedema and ascites, the same concentration is given over 2–6 hours.

Pregnant women

The safety of mannitol in pregnancy has not been established.

The elderly

No special precautions are necessary.

Drug interactions

Potentially hazardous interactions

Aminoglycosides. Mannitol potentiates their ototoxic effects.

Lithium. The renal excretion of lithium can be increased by administration of mannitol.

Neuromuscular-blocking drugs. Mannitol may enhance the effect of tubocurarine and other competitive or depolarizing neuromuscular-blocking drugs.

Oral anticoagulants. Mannitol may reduce the effect of oral anticoagulants by increasing the concentration of clotting factors secondary to dehydration.

Digoxin. If hypokalaemia follows mannitol treatment, there is increased risk of digoxin toxicity.

Other significant interactions

Potassium chloride, sodium chloride, other electrolytes or other drugs should not be added to 20 or 25% mannitol solutions because of the likelihood of salting-out (precipitating) mannitol.

Adrenocorticotrophic hormone, barbiturates, noradrenaline, metaraminol, suxamethonium, cisplatin or tetracycline should not be added to mannitol of any strength.

Potentially useful interactions

Mannitol reduces the renal toxicity of cisplatin.

Major outcome trials

Not available.

General review articles

1. Jacobson H R, Kokko J P 1976 Diuretics: sites and mechanisms of action. Annual Review of Pharmacology and Toxicology 16: 201–214
2. Gussin R Z 1977 Renal physiology and pharmacology. In: Antonaccio M (ed) Cardiovascular pharmacology. Raven Press, New York, pp 45–81
3. Warren S E, Blantz R C 1981 Mannitol. Archives of Internal Medicine 141: 493–497
4. Nissenson A R, Weston R E, Kleeman C R 1979 Mannitol. Western Journal of Medicine 131: 277–284
5. Gennari F J, Kassirer J P 1974 Osmotic diuresis. New England Journal of Medicine 291: 714–720
6. Goldberg M 1973 The renal physiology of diuretics. In: American Physiological Society (ed) Handbook of Physiology. American Physiological Society, Washington, pp 1003–1031

References

1. Goldberg M, McCurdy D K, Ramirez M A 1965 Differences between saline and mannitol diuresis in hydropenic man. Journal of Clinical Investigation 44: 182–192
2. Thurau K 1964 Renal haemodynamics. American Journal of Medicine 36: 698–719
3. Flores J, Di Bona D R, Beck C H, Leaf A 1972 The role of cell swelling in ischaemic renal damage and the protective effect of hypertonic solute. Journal of Clinical Investigation 51: 118–126
4. Lilieu O M, Jones S G, Mueller C B 1963 The mechanism of mannitol diuresis. Surgery, Gynaecology and Obstetrics 117: 221–228
5. Moreno M, Murphy C, Goldsmith C 1969 Increase in serum potassium resulting from the administration of hypertonic mannitol and other solutions. Journal of Laboratory and Clinical Medicine 73: 291–298
6. Blomquist C H, Snyder B D, Neihaus W G 1981 Improved enzymatic method for determining mannitol and its application to dog serum after mannitol infusion. Journal of Clinical Chemistry and Clinical Biochemistry 19: 139–143
7. Concoran A C, Page T H 1947 Determination of mannitol in plasma and urine. Journal of Biological Chemistry 170: 165–171
8. Hindle W, Code C F 1962 Some differences between duodenal and ileal sorption. American Journal of Physiology 203: 215–220
9. Elkinton J R 1947 The volume of distribution of mannitol as a measure of the volume of extracellular fluid with a study of the mannitol method. Journal of Clinical Investigation 26: 1088–1097
10. Dominguez R, Concoran A C, Page I H 1947 Mannitol: kinetics of distribution, excretion and utilization in human beings. Journal of Laboratory and Clinical Medicine 32: 1192–1202
11. Porter G A, Starr A, Kimsey J, Lenertz H 1947 Mannitol haemodilation-perfusion: the kinetics of mannitol distribution and excretion during cardiopulmonary bypass. Journal of Surgical Research 7: 447–456
12. Borges H F, Hocks J, Kjellstrand C M 1982 Mannitol intoxication in patients with renal failure. Archives of Internal Medicine 142: 63–66
13. Nasrallah S M, Iber F L 1969 Mannitol absorption and metabolism in man. American Journal of the Medical Sciences 258: 80–88
14. Schanker L S, Hogben A M 1961 Biliary excretion and insulin, sucrose and mannitol: analysis of bile formation. Journal of Physiology 200: 1087–1098
15. Clark J K, Barker H G 1948 Is mannitol metabolised? Proceedings of the Society for Experimental Biology and Medicine 69: 152–153
16. Young T K, Lees S C, Tai L N 1980 Mannitol absorption and excretion in uremic patients regularly treated with gastronintestinal perfusion. Nephron 25: 112–116
17. Wick A N, Morita T N, Joseph L 1954 The oxidation of mannitol. Proceedings of the Society for Experimental Biology and Medicine 85: 188–190
18. Byrne J J 1966 Shock. New England Journal of Medicine 275: 659–660
19. Dawson J L 1968 Acute post-operative renal failure in obstructive jaundice. Annals of the Royal College of Surgeons of England 42: 163–181
20. Forland M, Talley R C 1970 Treatment of renal abnormalities accompanying shock. Postgraduate Medicine 48: 128–133
21. Luck R J, Irvine W T 1965 Mannitol in the surgery of aortic aneurysm. Lancet 2: 409–411
22. Mazze R I, Barry K G 1967 Prevention of functional renal failure during anaesthesia and surgery by sustained hydration and mannitol infusion. Anaesthetics and Analgesia 40: 61–68
23. Figgeler R G W L, Berden J H M, Hoitsma A J, Koene R A P 1985 Prevention of acute tubular necrosis in cadaveric kidney transplantation by the combined use of mannitol and moderate hydration. Annals of Surgery 201: 246–251
24. Hagstram K E, Lindergard B, Tibbling G 1979 Mannitol infusion in regular haemodialysis treatment for chronic renal insufficiency. Scandinavian Journal of Urology and Nephrology 3: 257–263
25. Shapiro H M 1975 Intracranial hypertension: therapeutic and anaesthetic considerations. Anesthesiology 43: 445–471
26. Bucknell M 1964 Blood changes on intravenous administration of mannitol or urea for reduction of intracranial pressure in neurosurgical patients. Clinical Science 27: 223–227
27. Mendelow A D, Teasdale G M, Russell T, Flood J, Patterson J, Murray G D 1985 Effect of mannitol on cerebral blood flow and cerebral perfusion pressure in human head injury. Journal of Neurosurgery 63: 43–48
28. O'Keefe M, Nabil M 1983 The use of mannitol in intraocular surgery. Ophthalmic Surgery 14: 55–56
29. Shaldon S, McLaren J R, Sherlock S 1960 Resistant ascites treated by combined diuretic therapy (Spironolactone, mannitol and chlorothiazide). Lancet 1: 609–613
30. James J W, Evans R A 1970 The use of oral mannitol in the oedematous patients. British Medical Journal 1: 463–465
31. Magovern G J C, Bolling S F, Casale A S, Bulbley B H, Gardner T J 1984 The mechanism of mannitol in reducing ischemic injury: hyperosmolarity or hydroxyl scavanger. Circulation 70 (suppl 1): I91–I95
32. Feldman B H, Kjellstrand C M, Fraley E E 1971 Mannitol intoxication. Journal of Urology 106: 622–623
33. Roberts B E, Smith P H 1966 Hazards of mannitol infusion. Lancet 2: 421–422
34. Gunn D S, Wright H K, Newsome H H 1964 Prevention of sodium depletion during osmotic diuresis. Surgery, Gynaecology and Obstetrics 119: 265–268
35. Borges H F, Hocks J, Kjellstrand C M 1982 Mannitol intoxication in patients with renal failure. Archives of Internal Medicine 142: 63–66
36. Landerman P W, Lott J A, Zager R A 1982 Mannitol interferes with the Du Pont aca method for inorganic phosphorus. Clinical Chemistry 28: 1994–1995

Maprotiline hydrochloride

Maprotiline is an antidepressant marketed in the USA and the UK as Ludiomil.

Chemistry

Maprotiline hydrochloride (Ludiomil)
$C_{20}H_{23}N,HCl$
3-(9,10-Dihydro-9,10-ethanoanthracen-9-yl)-N-methylpropylamine

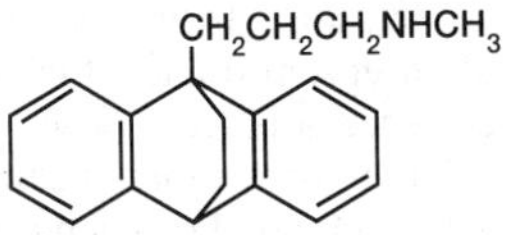

Molecular weight (free base)	313.9 (277.4)
pKa (amino)	10.5
Solubility	
in alcohol	soluble
in water	1 in 700
Octanol/water partition coefficient	—

Maprotiline is chemically distinct from the tricyclic antidepressants by the rigid flexure of its molecular skeleton and the presence of an ethylene-type bridge across the central ring. This bridge and its three-dimensional configuration define it as a tetracyclic. It is a white, odourless crystalline powder that is prepared by chemical synthesis.

Pharmacology

The mode of action of effective antidepressant drugs is unknown. Most are potent inhibitors of the uptake of noradrenaline and/or serotonin at presynaptic nerve terminals. These actions support the amine hypothesis of affective illness which, simply stated, is that in depression there is a functional deficiency of certain biogenic amines at synapses concerned with the regulation of mood. Maprotiline shares with effective antidepressant drugs some aspects of this common pharmacological profile. It is most potent in blocking uptake of noradrenaline but has little action on the uptake of serotonin. Although maprotiline was specifically developed as a novel antidepressant drug, it is less potent at noradrenaline uptake blockade than older drugs such as desipramine or nortriptyline, but more potent than imipramine or amitriptyline. Antidepressant drugs are also active at neurotransmitter receptor sites and these effects may be related to the amine hypothesis of depression. Maprotiline has many features in common with conventional tricyclic antidepressants in animal models of depression. Specifically, it exerts a dose-dependent protective effect against reserpine-induced ptosis and catalepsy in rats, being equipotent with imipramine in the latter setting and about eight times less active in the former. It also antagonizes in dose-dependent fashion the actions of tetrabenazine (which depletes catecholamine storage). Likewise, it reduces the rise in rat temperature produced by 4-α-dimethylmetatyramine.[1] In animals (chickens, rats and cats), maprotiline is a strong inhibitor of noradrenaline uptake in peripheral and central neurones. It also inhibits the depletion of endogenous noradrenaline by guanethidine. Antidepressant drugs (including monoamine oxidase inhibitors and many of the newer antidepressants such as maprotiline) cause decreased sensitivity of presynaptic α_2-adrenoceptors after chronic administration (down-regulation), while sensitivity to α_1-receptors is usually increased.

Additionally, knowledge of the actions of antidepressant drugs at neurotransmitter receptor sites may be of predictive value. Maprotiline is about 30-fold less active than amitriptyline at muscarinic cholinergic receptors and such data indicate that maprotiline is much less likely than amitriptyline to cause an antimuscarinic cholinergic side effect.

Maprotiline also differs from other antidepressants by its ability to decrease the number of benzodiazepine/β-carboline ester binding sites.

Toxicology

Maprotiline has fewer embryotoxic effects than imipramine, amitriptyline or mianserin when examined in chick embryos. It is without effect on organ development in mice, rats or rabbits in doses ranging from 1 to 30 $mg.kg^{-1}$ daily. It also appears to have fewer cardiotoxic actions than amitriptyline and imipramine and probably it has no or negligible effects on the cardiovascular system (see below).

Death following deliberate self-poisoning with maprotiline is extremely rare. The known maximum dose of maprotiline with full recovery is 5 g and acute animal studies have indicated LD_{50} values of 750 $mg.kg^{-1}$ in mice and 900 $mg.kg^{-1}$ in rats.

Clinical pharmacology

Maprotiline is an effective antidepressant drug in clinical practice. Like the tricyclic compounds, antidepressant activity may take 2–3 weeks to become fully effective, partly because of the time it takes for noradrenaline accumulation, and partly because, with its long half life, steady-state concentrations are not achieved until 7–10 days after starting therapy.

Unlike the tricyclic antidepressants, maprotiline has little influence on serotonin uptake and has few anticholinergic actions. In the platelet model of a presynaptic serotoninergic neurone, maprotiline does not alter serotonin uptake in human platelets when administered for four days in doses of 75 mg daily.[2] Turner and Ehsanullah[3] report only very weak inhibition and Muck-Seler[4] et al found maprotiline inhibited 5-HT uptake in the platelets of severely depressed patients. Long-term usage of maprotiline does not change the EEG of depressed patients. However, single oral doses in volunteers produce increased alpha activity, suggestive of increased relaxation. Maprotiline administration is associated with reduced time taken to fall asleep and increased total time spent in REM (or 'paradoxical') sleep and differs from imipramine in these respects.

Maprotiline has similar cardiovascular effects to the tricyclic antidepressants. Decrease in systolic blood pressure, prolongation of the QT interval on the ECG, and increase in heart rate may all occur and the drug may directly depress myocardial activity.

Pharmacokinetics

Maprotiline can be measured in blood by gas chromatography[5] with a sensitivity of 10 $\mu g.l^{-1}$.

Maprotiline is completely but slowly absorbed after oral administration. The half life is about 2 days and dose-dependent steady-state concentrations are attained in the second week of treatment. The mean plasma half life varies considerably between studies, however, and the range of 27 to 58 hours is probably a satisfactory clinical guide to the wide interindividual variations encountered in practice.

Like other lipophilic bases, maprotiline is widely distributed throughout the body following absorption and readily crosses body membranes. Peak plasma concentrations following a 50 mg oral dose are achieved between 9 and 16 h in healthy subjects. In man, about 30% of maprotiline is excreted in the faeces and about 70% in the urine. It is removed almost entirely as metabolites and only about 2% is unchanged maprotiline. Higher concentrations were noted in blood, lung, kidney, brain, adrenals and heart than in blood. The erythrocyte to plasma concentration ratio is 2.7. Binding to serum proteins is constant at about 88% and even at the high concentrations achieved during antidepressant therapy, saturation does not occur.

Maprotiline is also excreted in breast milk and during continuous therapy (150 mg daily for five days,[6]) the concentration ratio in milk to blood varies between 1.3 and 1.5.

Maprotiline hydrochloride

Oral absorption	>95%
Presystemic metabolism	—
Plasma half life	
range	27–58 h
mean	43 h
Volume of distribution	23–70 l.kg^{-1}
Plasma protein binding	~90%

Concentration–effect relationship

There is no established relationship between the blood concentrations of maprotiline (or any of its major metabolites) and its antidepressant action. High concentrations (above 300 μg.l^{-1}) are associated with increased frequency of unwanted side effects but are without any concomitant increase in antidepressant efficacy. Initially, a daily dose of 75–150 mg was recommended by the manufacturers and this yielded blood maprotiline concentrations between 50 and 550 μg.l^{-1}. Studies within this range did not indicate any relationship between blood concentration and outcome but did suggest that the best guide to dosage of maprotiline is provided by body weight. However, the manufacturers now recommend a much reduced starting dose of 25–75 mg daily before increasing to a maximum of 150 mg daily according to the response.

Metabolism

Maprotiline is eliminated almost entirely as its metabolites. In steady-state conditions, blood concentrations of its desmethyl derivative are highest and those of its phenolic derivatives are lowest. Other degradation products are detectable only in trace amounts. The major metabolite of maprotiline is, therefore, the desmethyl derivative and like the parent compound this is subject to further degradation into phenolic compounds. Numerous minor metabolites have been identified in urine. These are excreted in the urine as conjugated glucuronides and as aromatic methoxyethers. The inactivation of maprotiline follows first-order pharmacokinetics. The primary metabolic routes are N-demethylation, deamination, aromatic and aliphatic hydroxylations and the formation of aromatic methoxy derivatives (see Fig. 1).

Fig. 1 The metabolism of maprotiline

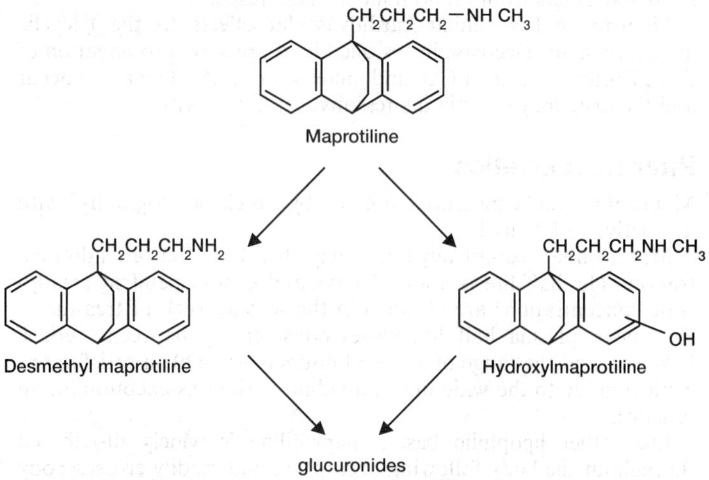

Pharmaceutics

Maprotiline, Ludiomil (CIBA, UK/USA), is available in oral form as tablets containing 10 mg, 25 mg, 50 mg and 75 mg maprotiline hydrochloride. The 10 mg tablets are pale yellow, circular, film-coated with 'CIBA' on one side and the code 'CO' on the reverse. The 25 mg tablets are greyish-red, circular, film-coated with 'CIBA' on one side and the code 'DP' on the reverse. The 50 mg tablets are light orange, circular, film-coated with 'CIBA' on one side and the code 'ER' on the reverse. The 75 mg tablets are brownish-orange, circular, film-coated with 'CIBA' on one side and the code 'FS' and a break line on the reverse. In the USA the codes are '110' (25 mg orange, ovoid tablet), '26' (50 mg orange round tablet) and '135' (75 mg white ovoid tablet).

Therapeutic use

Indications

1. Depressive illness.

Contraindications

1. Mania
2. Severe liver disease
3. Severe renal disease
4. Narrow-angle glaucoma
5. Urinary retention
6. Epilepsy
7. Recent myocardial infarction
8. Pregnancy.

Mode of use

The drug treatment of depression does not rely solely upon the administration of antidepressant drugs. Appropriate psychological and social support and intervention is often necessary and skilled nursing may be required when a patient poses a serious suicidal risk. Outpatient treatment with maprotiline usually starts with a daily dose between 25 and 75 mg. Divided doses have no advantage over a single dose. The daily dose may be increased up to a maximum of 150 mg, depending upon the clinical response. In early trials, doses of up to 225 mg daily were used, but these are no longer recommended. Severely depressed hospital inpatients may be started at a higher daily dose, between 100 and 150 mg. The daily dosage should never exceed 150 mg. Anticholinergic side effects increase in frequency with higher doses and there appears to be no antidepressant advantage associated with doses in excess of 150 mg daily. Discontinuation of maprotiline therapy should be gradual and not begun until remission of depressive illness has been maintained for at least three weeks.

Indications

1. Depressive illness

Maprotiline was initially marketed as a novel tetracyclic antidepressant with fewer side effects, lower toxicity in overdosage and a more rapid onset of antidepressant action than conventional tricyclic antidepressants. It continues to be used as a single agent in the treatment of depressive illness, in combination with electroconvulsive therapy (ECT) in the treatment of severe illnesses and with one of several types of sedative, hypnotic drugs in the treatment of depressive symptoms. The mode of action of maprotiline is not known but is usually related to the amine hypothesis of affective disorders (see Pharmacology).

Contraindications

1. Mania

As is the case with tricyclic antidepressants and ECT, maprotiline may precipitate hypomania or mania in susceptible depressed patients. In a double-blind comparison of amitriptyline and maprotiline three of four bipolar depressed patients receiving maprotiline developed hypomania while none of four bipolar patients receiving amitriptyline did so.[7]

2, 3. Liver/renal disease

Transient increases in alkaline phosphatase and hepatic transaminases with decreases in bilirubin are occasionally reported in patients receiving maprotiline. These are probably laboratory abnormalities that do not progress to liver disease. Nonetheless, maprotiline should be avoided in patients with hepatic or renal disease.

6. Epilepsy

Occasional seizures have been reported during maprotiline administration. Grand mal seizures are not uncommon during antidepressant treatment and their estimated incidence ranges between 0.1 and 4%. Most seizures that occur during maprotiline therapy have done so at doses equal to or greater than 150 mg per day. Bernard and Levine[8] report thirteen cases, in eleven of which the daily dose exceeded 150 mg. Most seizures appear to occur during long-term (more than six weeks) therapy and at doses greater than the manufacturer's revised guidelines. Dessain and others[9] have suggested that a long-acting maprotiline metabolite might be responsible for seizures.

7. Recent myocardial infarction
Maprotiline has been associated with increased heart rate and PR interval, flattening of T-waves, prolongation of the pre-ejection period, decrease in systolic blood pressure (erect) and lengthening of the QT interval. Cardiovascular effects of tricyclic antidepressants and maprotiline are probably similar and there are no advantages of maprotiline over conventional tricyclics with respect to clinical or ECG evidence of cardiotoxicity.[10]

Adverse reactions

Potentially life-threatening effects
Deaths caused by maprotiline are very unusual and all have been associated with self-poisoning. There are no idiosyncratic deaths reported.

Acute overdosage
Deliberate self-poisoning with maprotiline is not uncommon but very few deaths are recorded. In self-poisoning, patients have usually consumed more than one psychoactive substance, often in association with alcohol. Park and Proudfoot[11] observed six patients following acute poisoning with maprotiline. Seizures occurred in four patients and three were comatose (for 6–14 h) following doses between 750 and 3200 mg. The authors concluded that the acute toxic effects of maprotiline were based upon its anticholinergic effects. In a report of five children with maprotiline overdosage,[12] only two had toxic symptoms: one had repeated seizures following 525 mg of maprotiline.

Severe or irreversible adverse effects
Maprotiline is well tolerated and has few adverse effects. In general, it is similar to the tricyclic antidepressants. Severe idiosyncratic effects are agranulocytosis and cholestatic jaundice. Grand mal seizures have been reported in patients both with and without a history of epilepsy.

Symptomatic adverse effects
In the higher dose range (75–150 mg daily) there is little difference in the frequency of severity of adverse effects between maprotiline and the established tricyclic antidepressants. In the lower dose range (25–75 mg daily), adverse effects are less common with maprotiline than amitriptyline or imipramine.[13] Drowsiness and dry mouth are the most frequently reported adverse effects and others include headache, dizziness (which may be more common with maprotiline than other antidepressants), fainting, constipation, nausea, tremor, sweating, palpitations, hypotension and skin rash. Pinto et al[14] indicate that skin rashes are about twice as frequent with maprotiline as with amitriptyline or imipramine, falling within the range of 4–8% in various studies.[15] The rash resolves on cessation of therapy.

Maprotiline has a similar adverse effect profile in the cardiovascular system to that of the tricyclic antidepressants.[10] Most changes are mild and often disappear as treatment continues. Orthostatic hypotension and tachycardia are occasionally reported.[16]

Other effects
Laboratory investigations indicate that patients on maprotiline occasionally have short-lived increases in alkaline phosphatase and transaminases, and decreases in bilirubin. White blood cell counts may also increase and there are single case reports of granulocytopenia with a maculopapular rash induced by maprotiline that remitted on cessation of therapy.

Interference with clinical pathology tests
No technical interferences of this kind have been reported.

High risk groups

Neonates
The drug is not used in neonates. Abnormalities suggestive of maprotiline withdrawal have been observed in a neonate whose mother received maprotiline therapy.

Breast milk. Maprotiline is excreted in breast milk, and during continuous therapy (150 mg daily for five days) the concentration ratio in milk to blood varied between 1:3 and 1:5.

Maprotiline hydrochloride

Children
Maprotiline is not recommended for children.

Pregnant women
There is no evidence from animal studies or clinical reports that maprotiline is teratogenic, but its use during pregnancy is not recommended, especially during the first and last trimester.

The elderly
In common with tricyclic antidepressants, the elderly are more susceptible to adverse effects. These include postural hypotension, agitation, confusion and urinary hesitancy. Controlled trials with large numbers of elderly subjects indicate that there is nothing to distinguish maprotiline from amitriptyline or imipramine as far as adverse effects are concerned. Maprotiline should be introduced at low dose (10 mg daily) and gradually increased according to the patient's response and tolerability of any adverse effects that may occur.

Concurrent disease
Maprotiline should not be administered to patients with hepatic or renal impairment. In patients with cardiovascular disease, including recent myocardial infarction or cardiac arrhythmias, it should be introduced with caution. In one study[17], 126 patients who had recently suffered an acute myocardial infarction received either maprotiline 25 mg daily or diazepam 5 mg daily for an average of 2 weeks. There was no clinical or ECG evidence of cardiotoxicity associated with maprotiline. Maprotiline and imipramine have similar effects on cardiovascular function in depressed patients:[18] systolic blood pressure (erect) decreases, pulse rate (erect and supine) increases, and the QT interval lengthens. There are no clinically relevant differences in cardiovascular effects between maprotiline and the tricyclic antidepressants.

Drug interactions

Potentially hazardous interactions

Adrenaline. Maprotiline, like other antidepressants, may potentiate the cardiovascular effects of directly acting pressor amines.

Anaesthetic agents. Maprotiline may potentiate anaesthetic agents and anaesthetists should be advised accordingly.

Antihypertensive therapy. Some antihypertensive drugs may become ineffective when combined with maprotiline. Blood pressure control established by a previous antihypertensive therapy was lost on introduction of maprotiline, according to two reports.[19,20]

Alcohol. In common with other psychoactive drugs, especially the tricyclic antidepressants, maprotiline enhances the effects of alcohol and will reduce driving skills and increase sedation.

Potentially useful interactions
None is known.

Clinical trials

1. Jukes A M 1975 A comparison of maprotiline (Ludiomil) and placebo in the treatment of depression. Journal of International Medical Research 3: 84–88
2. Pinto O, Afeiche S P, Bartholini E 1972 International experience with Ludiomil. In: Kielholz P (ed) Depressive illness, diagnosis, assessment and treatment. Huber, Berne, pp 253–266

This is a meta-analysis of 13 double-blind studies, comparing maprotiline with tricyclic antidepressants.

General review articles

Diller N 1982 Worldwide clinical experience with Ludiomil. Activities Nervosa Superior (Praha) 24: 40–54
Grutr W, Pöldinger W 1982 Maprotiline. Modern problems of pharmacopsychiatry 18: 17–48
Kane J M, Lieberman J 1984 The efficacy of amoxapine, maprotiline and trazodone in comparison to imipramine and amitriptyline: a review of the literature. Psychopharmacology Bulletin 20: 240–249
Pinder R M, Brogden R N, Speight T M, Avery G S 1977 Maprotiline: a review of its pharmacological properties and therapeutic efficacy in mental depressive states. Drugs 13: 321–352

Richelson E 1984 The newer antidepressants: structures, pharmacokinetics, pharmacodynamics and proposed mechanisms of action. Psychopharmacology Bulletin 20: 213–223

Robinson D S 1984 Adverse reactions, toxicities and drug interactions of newer antidepressants: anticholinergic, sedative and other side effects. Psychopharmacology Bulletin 20: 280–290

References

1. Delini-Stula A 1972 The pharmacology of Ludiomil. In: Kielholz P (ed) Depressive illness. Diagnosis, assessment, treatment. Hans Huber, Berne, pp 113–124
2. Maitre L, Waldmeier P C, Greengrass P M, Jackel J, Sedlacek S, Delini-Stula A 1975 Maprotiline, its position as an antidepressant in the light of recent neuropharmacological and neurobiochemical findings. Journal of International Medical Research 3 (suppl 12): 2–15
3. Turner P, Ehsanullah R S B 1977 Clomipramine and maprotiline on human platelet uptake of 5-hydroxytryptamine and dopamine in vitro: relevance to their antidepressive and other central actions? Postgraduate Medical Journal 53 (suppl 4): 14–18
4. Muck-Seler D, Deanovic Z, Jamnicky B, Jakupcevic M, Mihovilovic M 1983 Maprotiline in the treatment of endogenous depression: comparison of therapeutic effect with serotonin level in blood platelets. Psychopharmacology (Berlin) 1979: 262–265
5. Alkalay D et al 1982 Measurement of mapotiline by gas chromatography. Analytical Letters (part B) 15: 1493–1503
6. Riess W 1976 The relevance of blood level determinations during the evaluation of maprotiline in man. In: Murphy J (ed) Research and clinical investigations in depression. Cambridge Medical Publications, Northampton, p 19
7. Amin M, Brahm E, Branheim L A et al 1973 A double-blind comparative clinical trial with Ludiomil (CIBA 34, 27b Ba) and amitriptyline in new admitted depressed patients. Current Therapy Research 15: 691–699
8. Bernard P G, Levine M S 1986 Maprotiline-induced seizures. Southern Medical Journal 79(9): 1179–1180
9. Dessain E C, Schatzberg A F, Woods B T, Cole J O 1986 Maprotiline treatment in depression. A perspective on seizures. Archives of General Psychiatry 43: 86–90
10. Glassman A H 1984 The newer antidepressive drugs and their cardiovascular effects. Psychopharmacological Bulletin 20: 272–279
11. Park J, Proudfoot A T 1977 Acute poisoning with maprotiline hydrochloride (letter). British Medical Journal 1: 1573
12. Crane P, Newman B 1977 Poisoning with maprotiline and mianserin (letter). British Medical Journal 2: 260
13. Wells B G, Gelenberg A J 1981 Chemistry, pharmacology, pharmacokinetics, adverse effects, and efficacy of the antidepressant maprotiline hydrochloride. Pharmacotherapy 1: 121–139
14. Pinto O de S, Afeiche S P, Bartholini E et al 1972 International experiences with Ludiomil. In: Kielholz P (ed) Depressive illness. Diagnosis, assessment, treatment. Hans Huber, Berne, pp 253–266
15. Warnock J K, Knesevich J W 1988 Adverse cutaneous reactions to antidepressants. American Journal of Psychiatry 145: 425–430
16. Edwards J G, Goldie A 1983 Mianserin, maprotiline and intracardiac conduction. British Journal of Clinical Pharmacology 15 (suppl 2): 249s–254s
17. Selvini A, Rossi C, Belli C et al 1976 Antidepressive treatment with maprotiline in the management of emotional disturbances in patients with acute myocardial infarction: a controlled study. Journal of International Medical Research 4: 42–49
18. Mielke D H, Koepke R P, Phillips J H 1979 A controlled evaluation of a tetracyclic (maprotiline) and a tricyclic (imipramine) antidepressant and their effects on the heart. Current Therapy Research 25: 738–742
19. Briant R H, George C F 1974 The assessment of potential drug interactions with a new tricyclic antidepressant drug. British Journal of Clinical Pharmacology 1: 113–118
20. Smith A J, Bant W P 1975 Interactions between post-ganglionic sympathetic blocking drugs and antidepressants. Journal of International Medical Research 3 (suppl 2): 55–60

Mebendazole

Mebendazole is a broad-spectrum antihelmintic developed in 1972.

Chemistry

Mebendazole (Vermox, Membutar, Nemasole, Pantelmin, Sirben, Vermirax)

$C_{16}H_{13}N_3$-O_3

Methyl 5-benzoyl-1H-benzimidazol-2-ylcarbamate

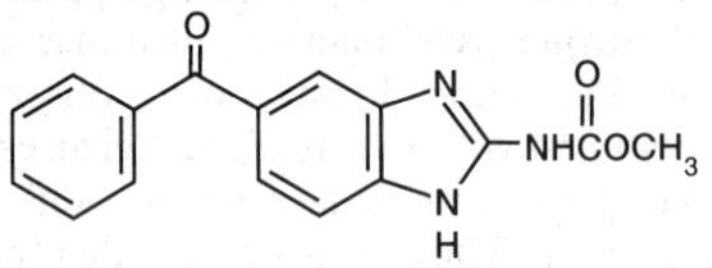

Molecular weight	295.3
pKa	—
Solubility	
in alcohol	insoluble
in water	insoluble
Octanol/phosphate buffer partition coefficient	191

Pharmacology

Initial in vitro and in vivo experiments have shown that mebendazole selectively and irreversibly blocks glucose uptake by adult intestinal dwelling nematodes and cestodes and their tissue dwelling larvae. Inhibition of glucose uptake appears to lead to depletion of parasite glycogen, decreased formation of ATP and ultimately, cell death.[1]

Toxicology

Toxicological studies in animals suggest that mebendazole has a high margin of safety and is generally well tolerated. Mebendazole is however teratogenic and embryotoxic in pregnant rats and for this reason should not be given to pregnant women. A dose of 40 $mg.kg^{-1}$ per day in rats was associated with mild alteration of spermatogenesis and with enlargement of the liver. All of these tests were conducted following oral administration. Since mebendazole is largely insoluble in aqueous solution and poorly absorbed from the gastrointestinal tract it is possible that systemic levels of the drug were insufficient for other toxic effects to be observed.

Clinical pharmacology

Mebendazole does not appear to affect blood glucose concentrations in the host. There are no reports of systemic effects of the drug in man due presumably to the poor absorption of the drug from the gastrointestinal tract.

Pharmacokinetics

Mebendazole has been measured by radioimmunoassay[2] and high performance liquid chromatography with ultraviolet[3–5] or electrochemical[6] detection. With uv detection, the limit of sensitivity of the HPLC assay is 10 $\mu g.l.^{-1}$ These are the only methods capable of providing the required degree of sensitivity and selectivity. Mebendazole is poorly absorbed after oral administration. Following the administration of a single 0.1 $mg.kg^{-1}$ body weight oral dose of ^{14}C-labelled mebendazole to three healthy adult volunteers only 5 to 10% was absorbed as assessed by the total recovery of urinary radioactivity. The peak level of radioactivity was reached in 2 to 4 hours. After administration of mebendazole tablets to three fasting volunteers

(1.5 g) plasma concentrations of mebendazole remained below 5 μg.$^{-1}$ in two volunteers and a maximal level of 5 μg.$^{-1}$ was observed in the third subject. When the same dose was given with a fatty breakfast within 2 to 4 hours plasma concentrations rose to 27, 33 and 42 μg. The terminal phase plasma half life was 1.4, 2.5 and 5.5 h. Administration of a similar dose of mebendazole to a patient with alveolar echinococcosis produced peak plasma concentrations 4 h after dosing of 112 μg and a terminal phase half life of 8 h.[8] When a further group of patients with cystic hydatid disease were studied following a 10 mg.kg^{-1} oral dose, plasma concentration–time profiles differed considerably between subjects. Terminal phase half lives ranged from 2.8 to 9.0 h, time to peak plasma concentration ranged from 1.5 to 7.25 h and peak concentrations from 17.5 to 500 μg.l^{-1}. Chronic administration of mebendazole emphasized these large inter-subject variations in plasma concentrations. There was no correlation between dosage and plasma concentrations which were subject to diurnal variation.[9]

Oral absorption	5–10%*
Presystemic metabolism	~80%
Plasma half life	
range	1.4–5.5 h
Volume of distribution	1.0–1.2 l.kg^{-1}
Plasma protein binding	95%

*From a tablet dose; absorption is limited by solubility. An oral solution is completely absorbed.[12]

That proportion of mebendazole which is absorbed from the gastrointestinal tract is extensively metabolized. Clearance of the two major metabolites of mebendazole, methyl 5-(6)(α-hydroxybenzyl)-benzimidazole carbamate and 2-amino-5-(6)[benzoyl] benzimidazole was less than that of the parent drug.[10] Conjugates of these and an additional metabolite of mebendazole have been found in bile together with a conjugate of the parent drug.[11] Impaired liver or biliary function results in higher plasma mebendazole levels in patients treated with the drug. Although no commercially available pharmaceutical formulation of mebendazole for intravenous use is available, a solution of radiolabelled mebendazole has been utilized to further define the pharmacokinetics of the drug in terms of bioavailability, half life and extent of first pass metabolism following oral administration of subtherapeutic doses (1.2 μg) in volunteers. Following intravenous administration, the mean distribution half life was 0.2 h (range 0.13–0.25 h), the mean plasma clearance was 1.06 l.min^{-1} (range 0.65–1.83) and the mean elimination half life was 1.12 h (range 0.83–1.36). The mean AUC was 22.7 pg.ml^{-1}.h (range 10–30). After oral administration of the same solution, the average time to peak plasma concentration was 0.42 h (range 0.28–0.50), the mean AUC was 4.63 pg.ml^{-1}.min (range 2.6–6.7) and the mean terminal elimination half life was 0.93 h (range 0.65–1.22). In addition, absorption is much more rapid from a tracer dose in solution than from the poorly soluble tablet formulations used in the treatment of systemic infections. Thus, the longer half life observed with higher doses of the tablet preparation probably reflects the rate of absorption rather than of elimination[12]. The apparent volume of distribution is 1.2 l.kg^{-1} (range 1.0–2.0). The mean bioavailability of mebendazole when given as a tracer dose in solution is 0.22 (range 0.12–0.35). Approximately 50% of the administered dose of radioactivity is excreted in the urine, with little unchanged compound, after both intravenous and oral administration. Thus, the low bioavailability reflects almost exclusively presystemic metabolism. At therapeutic doses of the tablet formulation the bioavailability is only 1–2%. The fraction of the dose subject to presystemic metabolism appears to be the same with tracer doses as with therapeutic doses. The difference in bioavailability of the latter is due to the very poor solubility of the therapeutic formulation of mebendazole, with only 5–10% of the dose being absorbed, the proportion decreasing with dose size. In healthy male volunteers, mebendazole was distributed with 63.3% in plasma and 36.7% in the cellular fraction. In plasma 95% was protein bound over the range 33 to 664 μg.l^{-1} and the blood/plasma concentration ratio (λ) was 0.79. Concentrations of mebendazole in liver tissue are considerably higher than those found in fatty tissue or parasitic material from patients with cystic hydatid disease. Analysis of cerebrospinal fluid from one patient receiving 200 mg.kg^{-1} daily gave a concentration of 8.6 μg.l^{-1}. (The maximum serum concentration was 93 μg.l^{-1}.[9])

Concentration–effect relationship

There is no correlation between the dose of mebendazole and plasma concentration due presumably to the poor solubility and the irregular and erratic absorption of the drug. Poor absorption is advantageous in the treatment of intestinal helminths but the successful therapy of systemic infections requires that a sufficient quantity of the administered dose is absorbed to achieve a therapeutic plasma concentration. In the treatment of echinococcosis this is estimated to be 100 μg.l^{-1} or 0.34 μmol.l^{-1}.[13,14]

Metabolism

The major proportion of an absorbed dose of mebendazole (I) is eliminated by metabolism in the liver. Its metabolites are present in the plasma, and appear in the urine and bile, principally as conjugates. The major plasma metabolites are the amide hydrolysis product 2-amino-5(6)benzoylbenzimidazole (II) and the product of ketone reduction, methyl-5(6)[α-hydroxybenzyl]benzimidazole carbamate (III) (Fig. 1). However, these are only minor urinary metabolites, accounting for only 12.4% of unconjugated material (0.17% of the dose) and 0.2% of unconjugated material (0.03% of the dose), respectively. The major unconjugated urinary metabolite is the product of both ketone reduction and hydrolysis, 2-amino-5(6)[α-hydroxybenzyl]benzimidazole (IV), which accounts for 87% of unconjugated material in urine (0.9% of the dose).[12] Low levels of this metabolite can be detected in plasma. Only 0.06% of the dose is excreted unchanged in the urine, and thus a total of 1.4% of the dose can be accounted for as unconjugated material in the urine. A large proportion of the absorbed dose is excreted in the urine as unidentified metabolites (approx. 4 times that accounted for by identified products), which does not liberate identifiable metabolites on enzymic hydrolysis.

Fig. 1 Metabolism of mebendazole

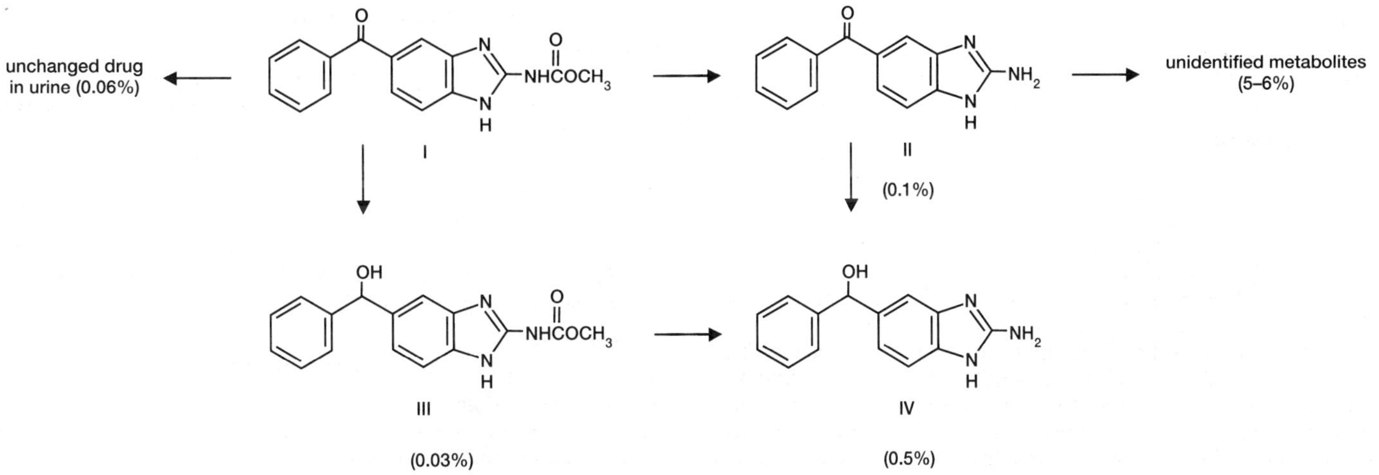

M

Mebendazole

M

Pharmaceutics

Mebendazole (Vermox Janssen, UK, US) is available in oral form only as a flavoured suspension containing 100 mg in each 5 ml, as pale pink, flat, scored chewable tablets containing 100 mg approximately 10 mm in diameter, and as Mebendazole 500, slightly beige circular scored tablets approximately 13 mm in diameter containing 500 mg Mebendazole. Vermox suspension has a shelf-life of three years under normal storage conditions.

Therapeutic use

Indications

1. *Capillaria* infection
2. Guinea worm
3. Hookworm (*Ancylostoma* and *Necator*)
4. Hydatid disease (*Echinococcus*)
5. Onchocerciasis
6. Roundworm (*Ascaris*)
7. Tapeworm (*Taenia*)
8. Threadworm (*Enterobius*)
9. *Trichinella*
10. Whipworm.

Contraindications

1. Pregnancy
2. Infants.

Mode of use

The poor intestinal absorption of mebendazole is obviously of therapeutic advantage in the treatment of intestinal helminthiases. For the treatment of tissue-dwelling organisms the drug must attain a therapeutic plasma concentration. Larger doses may therefore be desirable but these may be associated with a greater degree of side effect. Vermox suspension and tablets are for oral administration. The suspension is a banana-flavoured liquid formulation. Vermox tablets are orange-flavoured and may be chewed or swallowed whole. The same dosage applies to children aged two years and above. No special procedures such as purging, use of laxatives and/or dietary changes are required in the case of intestinal infection. However, it is recommended that patients treated for hydatid disease or other systemic infections take mebendazole with meals to enhance absorption.

Indications

1. *Capillaria*

Infection with *Capillaria philippinensis* is responsible for serious diarrhoea and malabsorption among the inhabitants of South East Asia. A 100% cure rate was reported in 33 new cases treated with 400 mg mebendazole daily for 20 days.[15]

2. Guinea worm

In 12 patients with guinea worm infection given mebendazole 200 mg four times daily for 6 days there was rapid relief from pain and inflammation and the worm was extracted.[16] A contrary report, however, indicated that mebendazole was without effect on the development of new worms.[17]

3. Hookworm

In cases of *Ancylostoma* 50 out of 53 patients receiving mebendazole 200 mg twice daily for four days were freed from infection without side effects. A similar regime is recommended for nectoriasis.[18,19]

4. Hydatid disease

Surgery was, until recently, the only therapy for hydatid (*Echinococcus granulosus*) and alveolar hydatid (*Echinococcus multilocularus*) disease. It is suggested that in cases of hydatid disease mebendazole therapy be considered in cases where surgery would be contraindicated, where cyst spillage may have occurred or preoperatively where there is a significant risk of spillage.[20] The optimum dose and duration of mebendazole therapy for hydatid disease are not clearly defined. Current recommendations vary depending upon the circumstances under which therapy is indicated. As an adjunct to surgery, chemotherapy should be started at least two weeks prior to the operation, ideally three months before, at 50 mg.kg^{-1} per day in two or three divided doses. Treatment should continue for at least three months after surgery especially if spillage has occurred. Where surgery is impossible, treatment should be as above with 50 mg.kg^{-1} per day for at least three months. Treatment may be necessary for two years or more to prevent the occurrence of a relapse. Short-term intensive therapy involves the administration of 50 mg.kg^{-1} daily for two weeks, then 200 mg.kg^{-1} daily for a further two weeks returning to 50 mg.kg^{-1} for at least another two weeks, preferably three months. Safety monitoring is essential, particularly at high doses where liver and renal function status should be assessed, together with full haematological screening and surveillance for adverse effects. Where mebendazole appears to eradicate *E. granulosus* it will only control or slow the growth of *E. multilocularis*. In alveolar hydatid disease, surgery is the therapy of choice with mebendazole being reserved for inoperable cases. It may be that albendazole will prove to be more effective.[21]

5. Onchocerciasis

There is some debate as to the efficacy of mebendazole in Onchocerciasis. One report suggests that mebendazole alone has only a very feeble microfilaricidal action against *O. volvulus*. It produces, however, severe temporary embryotoxic effects in the adult worm that last up to three months. In combination with levamisole, significant microfilarial destruction is produced with minimal side effects. Embryotoxic effects in the adult worm are of longer duration.[22] Another trial suggested that both mebendazole and the levamisole/mebendazole combination were equally effective, producing a slow but sustained fall in skin microfilarial counts which were maintained at 9 and 12 months. There was evidence of an embryotoxic effect in the adult worm on examination of the nodule.[23,24]

6. Roundworm

100 mg twice daily for three days produces high cure rates and almost complete egg eradication in cases of *Ascaris lumbricoides*.[25,26] There have been rare reports of abdominal pain and diarrhoea associated with mebendazole treatment of heavy roundworm infections.

7. Tapeworm

Mebendazole, in single (600 mg) or divided (200 mg twice daily) doses may be curative in *Taenia saginata* or *Taenia solium* infection.[27]

8. Threadworm

Cure rates using mebendazole for enterobiasis range from 91 to 100% after a single dose (100 mg).[7,26,28,29]

9. Whipworm

Mebendazole is the clear drug of choice in the treatment of *Trichuris trichiura* infection, being more effective than thiabendazole and with fewer side effects. High cure rates are achieved with prolonged therapy, with mean egg reductions of approximately 95%.[25,29–31]

10. *Trichinella*

Studies in mice indicate that intestinal adults and larvae as well as the developing and encysted muscle larvae of *Trichinella spiralis* may be susceptible to mebendazole.[32] Doses of 200–400 mg three times daily for three days then 400–500 mg three times daily for 10 days have been suggested.

Contraindications

1. Pregnancy

Mebendazole is teratogenic and embryotoxic in pregnant rats and for this reason is contraindicated in pregnancy.

2. Infants

In view of the limited experience with the use of the drug in children younger than two years of age, it is not currently recommended for this group.

Adverse reactions

Potentially life-threatening effects

One case of fatal leucopenia within the first two weeks of treatment in a patient with *Echinococcus multilocularis* has been reported.[33] This patient had severe pre-existing liver disease.

Acute overdosage

No case of overdose has so far been reported.

Severe or irreversible adverse effects

Alopecia, leucopenia and thrombocytopenia have been observed in patients treated for echinococcosis with mebendazole.[34,35]

Symptomatic adverse effects
Transient symptoms of diarrhoea and colic have occurred in heavily parasitized children during expulsion of *A. lumbricoides*.[36] Similar symptoms were also reported in two patients receiving mebendazole, 300 mg twice daily for taeniasis.[37] Slight headache and dizziness have been occasionally reported.[26] Pyrexia was reported in one patient receiving mebendazole 100 mg twice daily for three days.[38]

Interference with clinical pathology tests
No interference of this kind has been reported.

High risk groups

Neonates
Mebendazole should not be given to neonates.

Breast milk. No information on secretion into breast milk is available so mothers taking the drug should not breast feed.

Children
Mebendazole should not be given to children under two years of age.

Pregnant women
The drug should not be given during pregnancy.

The elderly
The drug may be used in the elderly in normal adult doses.

Concurrent disease
Mebendazole should not be given to pregnant women or children under two years. No dose reduction is warranted in patients with renal function impairment.[39] In patients with echinococcal infection, impairment of hepatic drug metabolizing capacity may produce elevated blood levels of mebendazole.[40]

Drug interactions

The absorption of mebendazole from the gastrointestinal tract is increased in the presence of fatty foods. The microfilaricidal effect of mebendazole in onchocerciasis is enhanced following treatment with levamisole but the mechanism is not understood.

Major outcome trials

1. Wilson J F, Davidson M, Rausch R L 1978 A clinical trial of mebendazole in the treatment of alveolar hydatid disease. American Review of Respiratory Disease 118: 747–757

This trial was initiated in 1974 in 4 patients with far advanced non-resectable lesions caused by *Echinococcus multilocularis*. A daily dose of 40 mg.kg^{-1} was administered to the patients for more than 3 years. No evidence of toxicity or adverse reactions has been observed. Detectable plasma mebendazole concentrations were achieved with high-dose mebendazole therapy. Although there was no evidence that the larval cestode was killed, the metastatic lesions were stabilized or diminished and overall clinical results were encouraging. Progressive enlarging thoracic metastases in two patients regressed during therapy and symptomatic improvement was observed in all patients.

2. Bekti A, Schaaps J-P, Capron M, Dessaint J-P, Santoro F, Capron A 1977 Treatment of hepatic hydatid disease with mebendazole. Preliminary results in four cases. British Medical Journal 2: 1047–1051

Mebendazole was given to four patients with hepatic hydatid disease. In three patients the disease had remained after surgery and in the fourth it could not be treated surgically. Mebendazole was given orally in maximum doses of 400–600 mg three times daily during courses lasting 21–30 days. Complete regression of the intrahepatic cysts was achieved in all four patients after 4–13 months. In three patients the course of treatment had to be repeated. Mebendazole also induced clinical improvement and a progressive lowering of specific IgE of *Echinococcus granulosus*.

3. (a) Rivas Alcala A R, Green B M, Taylor H R et al 1981 Chemotherapy of onchocerciasis: a controlled comparison of mebendazole, levamisole and diethylcarbamazine. Lancet 2: 484–490
   (b) Rivas Alcala A R, Green B M, Taylor H R et al 1981 Twelve month follow up of mebendazole therapy for onchocerciasis. Lancet 2: 1043

Mebendazole

This trial provides evidence that mebendazole may be a useful alternative to diethylcarbamazine in onchocerciasis. In a double blind study in 40 male patients with onchocerciasis the following 4 drug regimens were used: mebendazole 1 g twice daily for 28 days, levamisole 150 mg weekly for 5 weeks, the mebendazole and levamisole regimes together or diethylcarbamazine (DEC-C) citrate 100 mg twice daily for 28 days. DEC-C produced the more rapid fall in skin counts but on follow-up at six, nine and twelve months those receiving mebendazole alone or with levamisole showed similar or slightly greater reductions. Examination of adult worms in nodules excised at 2 months showed changes suggestive of an interruption of embryogenesis in those receiving the mebendazole-containing regimens only. Levamisole alone had no significant effect on microfilarial counts. In spite of corticosteroid administration during the initial stages of DEC-C therapy more systemic side effects occurred in the DEC-C group; ocular complications were also more common and more severe in those receiving DEC-C.

General review articles

Keystone J S, Murdock J K 1979 Mebendazole. Annals of Internal Medicine 91: 582–586

Van den Bossche H, Rochette F, Hörig C 1982 Mebendazole and related anthelmintics. Advances in Pharmacology and Chemotherapy 19: 67–128

References

1. Van den Bossche H 1972 Biochemical effects of the antihelmintic drug mebendazole. In: Van den Bossche H (ed) Comparative biochemistry of parasites. Academic Press, New York pp 1239–1257
2. Michiels M, Hendriks R, Thijssen J, Heykants J 1978 A sensitive radioimmunoassay for mebendazole (R17 635) and flubendazole (R17 889) Janssen research products information service. Preclinical Research Reports Nos R17 635/11 and R17 889/9
3. Allan R J, Goodman H T, Watson T R 1980 Two high-performance liquid chromatographic determinations for mebendazole and its metabolites in human plasma using a rapid Sep Pak C18 extraction. Journal of Chromatography, Biomedical Applications 183: 311–319
4. Alton K B, Patrick J E, McGuire J L 1979 High performance liquid chromatographic assay for the antihelmintic agent mebendazole in human plasma. Journal of Pharmaceutical Sciences 68: 880–882
5. Karlaganis G, Munst G J, Bircher J 1979 High pressure liquid chromatographic determination of the antihelmintic drug mebendazole in plasma. Journal of High Resolution Chromatography, Chromatography Communications 2: 141–144
6. Oosterhuis B, Wetsteyn J C F M, van Boxtel C J 1984 Liquid chromatography with electrochemical detection for monitoring mebendazole and hydroxymebendazole in echinococcosis patients. Therapeutic Drug Monitoring 6: 215–220
7. Brugmans J P, Thienpont D C, Van Wigngaarden I, Vanparijs O F, Scheurmans V L, Lauwers H L 1971 Mebendazole in enterobiasis; radiochemical and pilot clinical study in 1278 subjects. Journal of the American Medical Association 217: 313–316
8. Münst G J, Karlaganis G, Bircher J 1980 Plasma concentrations of mebendazole during treatment of enchinococcosus; preliminary results. European Journal of Clinical Pharmacology 17: 375–378
9. Witassek F, Burkhardt B, Eckert J, Bircher J 1981 Chemotherapy of alveolar echinococcosis: comparison of plasma mebendazole concentrations in animals and man. European Journal of Clinical Pharmacology 20: 427–433
10. Braithwaite P A, Roberts M S, Allan R J, Watson T R 1982 Clinical pharmacokinetics of high dose mebendazole in patients treated for cystic hydatid disease. European Journal of Clinical Pharmacology 22: 161–169
11. Witassek F, Allan R J, Watson T R, Woodtli W, Ammann R, Bircher J 1983 Preliminary observations on the biliary elimination of mebendazole and its metabolites in patients with echinococcosis. European Journal of Clinical Pharmacology 25: 81–84
12. Dawson M, Braithwaite P A, Roberts M A, Watson T R 1985 The pharmacokinetics and bioavailability of a tracer dose of [^{3}H]-mebendazole in man. British Journal of Clinical Pharmacology 19: 79–86
13. Bryceson A D M, Woestenborghs R, Michiels R, Van den Bossche H 1982 Bioavailability and tolerability of mebendazole in patients with inoperable hydatid disease. Transactions of the Royal Society of Tropical Medicine and Hygiene 76: 563–564
14. Woodtli W, Bircher J, Witassek F, Eckert J, Wuthrich B, Ammann R W 1985 Effect of plasma mebendazole concentrations in the treatment of human echinococcosis. American Journal of Tropical Medicine and Hygiene 34: 754–760
15. Singson C N, Banzon T C, Cross J H 1975 Mebendazole in the treatment of intestinal capillariasis. American Journal of Tropical Medicine and Hygiene 24: 932–934
16. Shafei A Z 1976 Preliminary Report on the therapeutic efficacy of mebendazole in guinea worm infection. Journal of Tropical Medicine and Hygiene 79: 197–200
17. Kale O O 1975 Mebendazole in the treatment of dracontiasis. American Journal of Tropical Medicine and Hygiene 24: 600–605
18. Banerjee D, Prakash O, Kaliyugaperunal V 1972 A clinical trial of mebendazole (R17 635) in cases of hookworm infection. Indian Journal of Medical Research 60: 562–566
19. Vakil B J, Dalal N J 1975 Comparative efficacy of new antihelminthics. Progress in Drug Research 19: 166–175

M

20. Beard T C, Rickard M D, Goodman H T Medical treatment for hydatids 1978. Medical Journal of Australia 1: 633–635
21. Morris D L, Dykes P W, Morrimer S et al 1985 Albenodazole — objective evidence of response in human hydatid disease. Journal of American Medical Association 253: 2053–2057
22. Awadzi K, Schulz-Key H, Howells R E, Haddock D R W, Gilles H M 1982 The chemotherapy of onchocerciasis VIII: levamisole and its combination with the benzimidazoles. Annals of Tropical Medicine and Parasitology 76: 459–473
23. Rivas Alcalá A R, Greene B M, Taylor H R et al 1981 Chemotherapy of Onchocerciasis; a controlled comparison of mebendazole levamisole and diethylcarbamazine. Lancet 2: 485–490
24. Rivas Alcalá A R, Greene G M, Taylor H R 1981 Twelve month follow up of mebendazole therapy for onchocerciasis. Lancet 2: 1043
25. Wolfe M S, Wershing J M 1974 Mebendazole: treatment of trichuriasis and ascariasis in Bahamian children. Journal of the American Medical Association 230: 1408–1411
26. Seah S K K 1976 Mebendazole in the treatment of helminthiasis. Canadian Medical Association Journal 115: 777–779
27. Chavarría A P, Villarejos V M, Zeledon R 1977 Mebendazole in the treatment of *Taenia solium* and *Taenia saginata*. American Journal of Tropical Medicine and Hygiene 26: 118–120
28. Goldsmid J M 1974 The use of mebendazole as a broad spectrum antihelminthic in Rhodesia (Zimbabwe). South African Medical Journal 48: 2265–2266
29. Miller M J, Krupp I M, Little M D, Santos C 1974 Mebendazole: an effective antihelmintic for trichuriasis and ascariasis. Journal of the American Medical Association 230: 1412–1414
30. Scragg J N, Proctor E M 1977 Mebendazole in the treatment of severe symptomatic trichuriasis in children. American Journal of Tropical Medicine and Hygiene 26: 198–203
31. Scragg J N, Proctor E M 1978 Further experience with mebendazole in the treatment of severe symptomatic trichuriasis in children. American Journal of Tropical Medicine and Hygiene 27: 255–257
32. Fernando S S E, Denham D A 1976 The effects of mebendazole on *Trichinella spiralis* in mice. Journal of Parasitology 62: 874–876
33. Wilson J F, Rausch R L 1980 Alveolar hydatid disease. A review of clinical features of 33 indigenous cases of *Echinococcus multilocularis* infection in Alaskan Eskimos. American Journal of Tropical Medicine and Hygiene 29: 1340–1355
34. Miskovitz P F, Javitt N B 1980 Leukopenia associated with mebendazole therapy of hydatid disease. American Journal of Tropical Medicine and Hygiene 29: 1356–1358
35. Kern P, Dietrich M, Volkmer K T 1979 Chemotherapy of echinococcosis with mebendazole: clinical observations in seven patients. Tropenmedizin und Parasitologie 30: 65–72
36. Pena Chavarria A, Swatzwelder J C, Villarejos V M, Zeledon M 1973 Mebendazole, an effective broad spectrum anthelmintic. American Journal of Tropical Medicine and Hygiene 22: 592–595
37. Vakil B, Dalal N J, Enjetti E 1975 Clinical trials with mebendazole, a new broad spectrum antihelminthic. Journal of Tropical Medicine and Hygiene 78: 154–158
38. Harris A 1979 Pyrexia and mebendazole. British Medical Journal 2: 1365
39. Allgayer H, Zahringer J, Back P and Bircher J 1985 Lack of effect of haemodialysis on mebendazole kinetics; studies in a patient with echinococcosis and renal failure. European Journal of Clinical Pharmacology 27: 243–245
40. Witassek F, Bircher J 1983 Chemotherapy of larval echinococcosis with mebendazole. Microsomal liver function and cholestasis as determinants of plasma drug level. European Journal of Clinical Pharmacology 25: 85–90

Mebeverine

Mebeverine is an antispasmodic agent used to treat bowel spasm. It was developed as a phenylethylamine derivative of reserpine specifically for its papaverine-like effects.

Chemistry

Mebeverine hydrochloride (Colofac, Duspatal, Duspatalin)
$C_{25}H_{35}NO_5.HCl$
Veratric acid 4-(ethyl(4-methoxy-α-methylphenethyl)amino)butyl ester hydrochloride

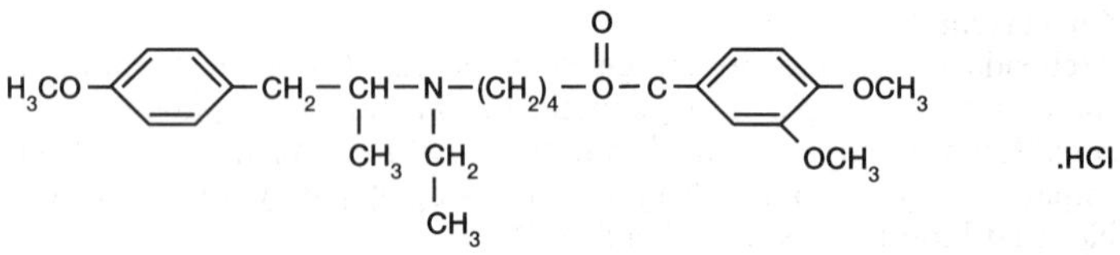

Molecular weight (free base)	466.0 (429.6)
pKa	8.1
Solubility	
in alcohol	>1 in 30
in water	>1 in 30
Octanol/water partition coefficient	—

A white crystalline powder with a very bitter taste. Mebeverine posesses a chiral centre. Mebeverine is also available as a combination product (Colven).

Pharmacology

Mebeverine has several pharmacological actions in vitro. It is an antagonist at muscarinic cholinergic receptors, being around 10–20 times less potent than atropine in vitro. Mebeverine also has an indirect antispasmodic effect on gastrointestinal smooth muscle and local anaesthetic effects.[1] In receptor–binding studies mebeverine was also found to bind to β_2 and uterine α-receptors; it also inhibits phosphodiesterase in preparations of rat brain and monkey artery.[2] It has been suggested that this latter action might also underlie the effect of mebeverine on the gut.[3]

Toxicology

In animal toxicological studies mebeverine appears free of teratogenic effects in rabbits and rats at doses of 100 $mg.kg^{-1}$ daily orally. There was also no effect on fertility in the rat. Behavioural and organ-specific toxicity was observed at 'very high doses'. No reports of mutagenicity tests are available.

Clinical pharmacology

Although there are no extensive dose–response studies, Prout[4] reported that increasing the dose from 400 to 800 mg daily did produce evidence of improvement in symptoms. This report was followed up in a controlled trial, the design of which was unfortunately suspect since the placebo phase was first for all patients, and the duration of treatment with mebeverine was twice as long as placebo. There was no significant difference between the two doses of mebeverine studied (405 and 810 mg) though not surprisingly, in view of the design, both the mebeverine treatment phases were significantly better than placebo.[5]

Mebeverine

Pharmacokinetics

There is no published data on the pharmacokinetics of mebeverine and no published analytical method.

Studies by the manufacturer using radiolabelled drug suggest that the label is well absorbed and has a half life of 2.5 h, though this may of course represent the half life of metabolites rather than the parent compound.

Protein binding to albumin of 75% is quoted by the manufacturers and radiolabelled tracer studies suggest a wide distribution, including the CNS. Small amounts of mebeverine are secreted in breast milk (approximately 10 µg after a 100 mg dose).

Oral absorption	well absorbed
Presystemic metabolism	—
Plasma half life	
mean	2.5 h
Volume of distribution	—
Plasma protein binding	75%

Concentration–effect relationship

No data are available.

Metabolism

Mebeverine is subject to hepatic metabolism and the metabolites are excreted into urine, and these include conjugates with glucuronide and products of the hydrolysis of the ester bond, to produce veratric acid and 4(2-(methoxyphenyl)-1 methyl-diethylamino)butanoic acid (see Fig. 1). The pharmacology of these compounds has not been reported.

Pharmaceutics

Available as white-sugar coated tablets 11 mm in diameter containing mebeverine hydrochloride 135 mg equivalent to 125 mg of base. Although not available in the UK 100 mg tablets and 200 mg capsules are also produced. Tablets have a shelf-life of 5 years if protected from light and stored at less than 20°C.

A banana flavoured liquid containing mebeverine 50 mg in 5 ml is also available. The undiluted product is stable for 3 years if stored in a similar manner to the tablets, but only for 14 days after dilution with water.

Therapeutic use

Indications

1. Irritable bowel syndrome
2. Gastrointestinal spasm.

Contraindications

Mebeverine has anticholinergic properties in vitro but since it is 10–20 fold less potent than atropine,[1] in clinical use anticholinergic adverse effects do not seem to occur.

Mode of use

Mebeverine is usually administered 135 mg three times a day, although higher doses have been used. Controlled studies in the irritable bowel syndrome suggest that mebeverine may be useful in addition to other therapy, including bulking agents and centrally acting drugs.[6]

Indications

1. Irritable bowel syndrome

Mebeverine has been shown in a number of short-term studies to be effective in the treatment of the irritable bowel syndrome.[5,7,8,9] The pharmacological mechanism of this effect is not established and may be a combination of direct effects of mebeverine on smooth muscle and its anticholinergic actions.

2. Gastrointestinal spasm

In view of the direct antispasmodic effect of mebeverine the drug has been evaluated in the reduction of spasm and pain during barium

Fig. 1 Metabolism of mebeverine

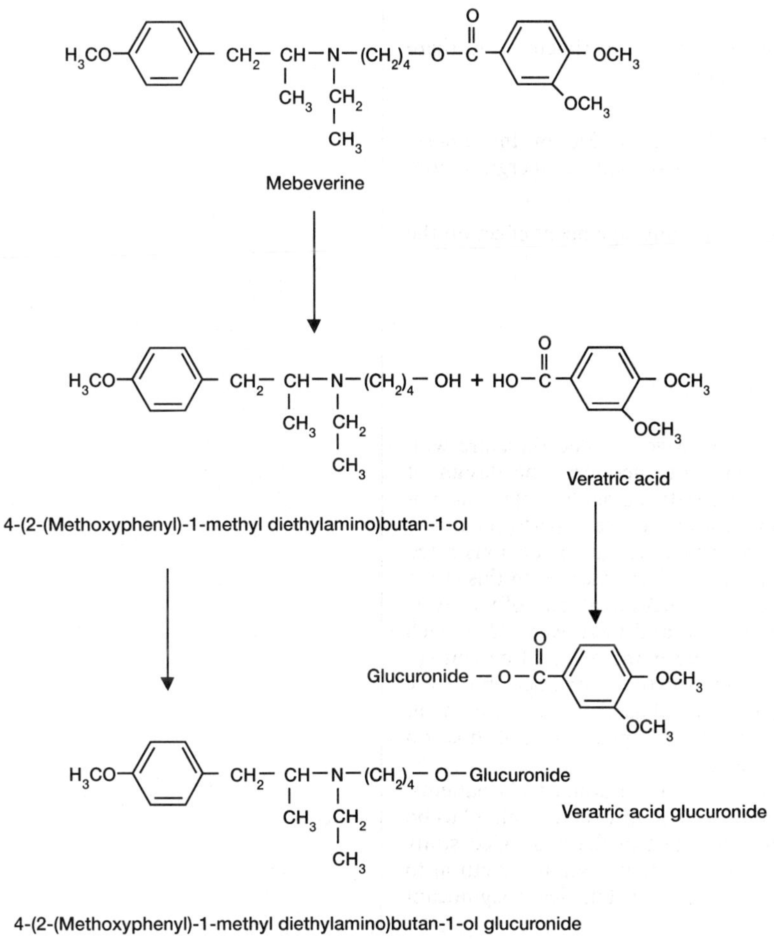

M

enema examination. In this study 270 mg was administered 2 h before the X-ray examination.[10] There was a significant reduction in spasm following mebeverine as judged fluoroscopically and by patient discomfort.

Adverse reactions

Potentially life-threatening effects
There are no known life-threatening toxic effects of mebeverine.

Acute overdosage
There are few reported cases of overdose with mebeverine. The manufacturers are aware of a fatality in which thioridazine was also taken and which was possibly associated with the inhalation of vomit rather than a specific effect of the overdose. Anticholinergic effects might be expected, but treatment should be symptomatic.

Severe or irreversible adverse effects
No effects of this kind have been reported.

Symptomatic adverse effects
These appear to be uncommon.

Other effects
In vitro inhibition of aspirin esterase has been reported.[11]

Interference with clinical pathology tests
None is known.

High risk groups

Neonates
Mebeverine is not recommended for neonates.

Breast milk. Small amounts of mebeverine are secreted in breast milk (approximately 10 µg after a 100 mg dose).

Children
Mebeverine is not recommended for children under 2 years. The tablet preparation is only recommended for patients over 10 years. There appear to be no specific toxicity problems in children over 10 years. If liquid doses are administered, a reduced dose is recommended for patients under 10 years.

Pregnant women
No teratogenicity has been shown in animal experiments, and there are no known teratogenic effects in man.

The elderly
There are no known problems with mebeverine in the elderly although they may be more susceptible to any anticholinergic action.

Concurrent disease
Concurrent disease is not known to have any significant effect on the actions of this drug.

Drug interactions

None is known.

Clinical trials

There are few controlled studies on mebeverine, and these are with relatively small numbers of patients. Furthermore, the design of many of these studies is generally unsatisfactory in that placebo-controlled cross-over studies have not usually been performed. The study by Connell[7] in 1965 was of sequential design and demonstrated significant advantage of active treatment over placebo. In this study patients were randomly allocated to 12 weeks treatment of mebeverine 100 mg four times daily or placebo, and there were 22 in each group, but 2 of active and placebo were withdrawn. 13 patients (6 active) were more compliant with the treatment regimen, but were still included in the analysis, and evaluated as at the time treatment was stopped. 5 patients had adverse effects (2 placebo), 2 of those on mebeverine complaining of depression.

A study published in the French literature[9] examined 111 patients. Although this did suggest symptomatic improvement all placebo responders were eliminated before the start of the controlled study leaving only 69 patients in the analysis. Analysis on an intention to treat basis seems unlikely to have produced a statistically significant result.

Mebeverine

References

1. Lindner A, Selzer H, Claasen V, Gans P, Offringa O R, Zwagemakers J M A 1963 Pharmacological properties of mebeverine, a smooth muscle relaxant. Archives Internationales de Pharmacodynamie et de Therapie 145: 370–395
2. Greenslade F C, Scott C K, Newquist K L, Krider K M, Chasin M 1980 Heterogenicity of biochemical actions among vasodilators. Journal of Pharmaceutical Sciences 71: 94–100
3. Saraya A 1981 Effect of mebeverine in smooth muscles. Mahidol University Journal of Pharmacological Science 7: 83–88
4. Prout B J 1975 Irritable bowel syndrome. Lancet 2: 1260
5. Prout B J 1983 The treatment of irritable bowel syndrome. Practitioner 227: 1607–1608
6. Ritchie J A, Truelove S C 1980 Comparison of various treatments for irritable bowel syndrome. British Medical Journal 231: 1317–1319
7. Connell A M 1965 Physiological and clinical assessment of the musculotropic agent mebeverine on the human colon. British Medical Journal 2: 848–851
8. Tasman-Jones C 1973 Mebeverine in patients with the irritable bowel syndrome: double blind study. New Zealand Medical Journal 77: 232–235
9. Berthelot J, Centoze M 1981 Controlled double blind trial of Duspatalin (mebeverine) against placebo, in the treatment of irritable colon. Gazette Medicale de France 83: 2341–2343
10. Messios N, Shaker M, Berry J M 1982 Oral mebeverine in barium enema preparation. Clinical Radiology 33: 271–272
11. Rylance H J, Wallace R C 1980 Drug inhibition of whole blood aspirin esterase. British Journal of Clinical Pharmacology 9: 520–521

Mebhydrolin

Mebhydrolin is an antihistamine which blocks H_1 receptors.

Chemistry

Mebhydrolin (Fabahistin tablets)
$C_{19}H_{20}N_2$
5-Benzyl-1,2,3,4-tetrahydro-2-methyl-γ-carboline

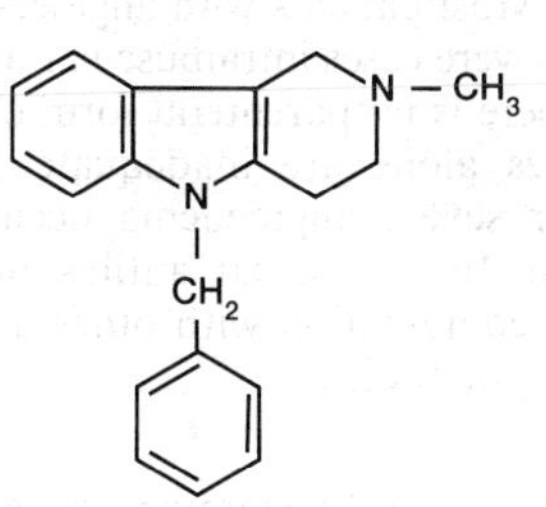

Molecular weight (napadisylate salt)	276.4 (841.1)
pKa	6.7
Solubility	
in alcohol (napadisylate salt)	~1 in 20 (~1 in 5000)
in water (napadisylate salt)	~1 in 10 000 (~1 in 5000)
Octanol/water partition coefficient	high

Mebhydrolin forms a salt with 1,5-naphthalene disulphonic acid (napadisylic acid) of the formula $(C_{19}H_{20}N_2)_2.C_{10}H_8O_6S_2$ (mebhydrolin naphthalene disulphonate, Fabahistin suspension, Incidal, Omeril). This compound is the active ingredient of most tablets (each of which contains 50 mg mebhydrolin equivalent to 76 mg of mebhydrolin napadisylate).

A white, tasteless, odourless powder. It is not present in any combination preparations.

Pharmacology

Mebhydrolin is an H_1 receptor blocking antihistamine. Very low concentrations of mebhydrolin (5×10^{-6} mol) markedly inhibit and a concentration of 1×10^{-6} mol completely abolishes a histamine-induced contraction of an isolated guinea-pig ileum strip.

Toxicology

There is no evidence of embryotoxicity or teratogenicity in rats and mice given either 50 mg.kg^{-1} or 150 mg.kg^{-1} mebhydrolin during pregnancy. The offspring developed normally in the postnatal period. There was no evidence of toxicity in rats given from 1 to 5 times the recommended maximum daily therapeutic dose over 13 weeks.

Clinical pharmacology

Antihistamine activity has been demonstrated in man by reduction in sneezing, nasal secretions and conjunctivitis in patients with allergic rhino-conjunctivitis and reduction in urticaria and pruritus.

Pretreatment with mebhydrolin reduces the size of the wheal and flare in response to histamine and itching is also relieved. The dose range in adults is 100–300 mg mebhydrolin daily.

Because sedation is a common side effect of many antihistamines, a number of controlled studies have been conducted to examine awareness and reactivity in patients taking mebhydrolin. There was no increase in reaction time,[1] reduction in reactivity in a simulator used for testing motorists,[2] or change in the electroencephalogram or level of vigilance during a 30-minute period after ingestion.[3] Nevertheless, sedation may be seen following the use of mebhydrolin and patients should be cautioned about driving cars or operating heavy machinery.

Pharmacokinetics

Following extraction mebhydrolin is detected by fluorescence with excitation and emission wavelengths of 290 or 350 nm. The limit of detection is 10 μg.l^{-1}.

Mebhydrolin is absorbed slowly but completely from the gastrointestinal tract, with a peak plasma concentration at 2 to 4 hours. The mean plasma half life is 5.5 hours. After 24 hours the plasma levels are at the lower limit of detection (11 μg.l^{-1}). No accumulation occurs after regular therapy. Fasting plasma levels recorded over a 10-day period at a daily dose of 50 mg three times a day were not higher than the peak values after a single dose of 50 mg. It is likely that the drug is excreted in breast milk and transferred across the placenta. Elimination may be reduced in renal impairment. Hepatic dysfunction is unlikely to alter the kinetics of the drug.

Oral absorption	~100%
Presystemic metabolism	nil
Plasma half life	5.5 h
Volume of distribution	—
Plasma protein binding	—

Concentration–effect relationship

There are no data on concentration–effect relationships.

Metabolism

There are very few data on metabolism. After a single dose, only 0.66% is excreted in the urine unchanged. About 50% of this is excreted in the first 8 hours, and about 80% in 24 hours.

Pharmaceutics

Mebhydrolin (Fabahistin; Bayer, UK) is available in oral form only. Tablets contain 50 mg of mebhydrolin as mebhydrolin napadisylate (naphthalene disulphonate) BPC. The tablets are orange, round, biconvex, and sugar-coated. Mebhydrolin suspension is orange and contains 50 mg per 5 ml. The shelf-life for tablets and suspension is about 5 years. Tragacanth mucilage is the recommended diluent for immediate use but methylcellulose suspending agent should be used if the storage time may be protracted. Both preparations contain the colouring agent Sunset yellow, CI 15 985. The tablets contain lactose and the suspension contains sucrose and sorbitol.

Therapeutic use

Indications

1. Hay fever
2. Rhinitis
3. Urticaria and angioedema
4. Eczema
5. Other allergic conditions.

Contraindications

1. Patients should be advised to exercise caution if they drive or use heavy machinery
2. Concomitant use of CNS depressants or alcohol
3. Mebhydrolin should not be readministered to a patient in whom it has previously been suspected to have caused agranulocytosis or neutropenia.

Mode of use

The usual dose in adults is 50–100 mg mebhydrolin three times a day. In children less than 10 years old 5–20 ml may be given daily in divided doses after meals. Although controlled studies suggest mebhydrolin has little sedative effect, sedation is seen in individual patients in clinical practice. Patients should be warned that drowsiness and impaired reactions may occur, and should be aware that it may be necessary to avoid operating machinery. Since alcohol can potentiate drowsiness, patients are advised to avoid alcohol during therapy.[4]

Mebhydrolin

M

Indications

Antihistamines are of value in the conditions discussed below. However, many antihistamines are of similar efficacy, and when selecting an antihistamine, mebhydrolin has the following disadvantages which need to be considered. It has the potential to cause sedation, and although this occurs in only a proportion of patients, this drawback is of more importance since the introduction of the non-sedative antihistamines. Furthermore, and of greatest importance, mebhydrolin may, although rarely, cause blood dyscrasias. It is therefore logical to select an alternative antihistamine unless it has been established that mebhydrolin offers a clear therapeutic advantage. This reservation applies to all of the potential indications considered below.

1. Hay fever

Mebhydrolin, like many other antihistamines, has been shown to be effective in the treatment of pollen-induced rhino-conjunctivitis, reducing sneezing, nasal secretions and eye symptoms, although usually with a lesser effect on nasal congestion or obstruction. In a placebo-controlled study, mebhydrolin 50 mg orally three times daily was effective in 19 of 28 patients with hay fever.[5] In another study, 47 of 52 students with hay fever improved on mebhydrolin.[6] Whilst many other antihistamines may have the same effect, it is not uncommon to find that in an individual patient one antihistamine is more effective or acceptable than another. This clinical observation has been confirmed in clinical trials, e.g. 12 of 19 cases successfully treated with mebhydrolin had failed to improve on other antihistamines.[5] It may therefore be necessary to try several antihistamines to determine the optimal effect.

In allergic rhino-conjunctivitis, antihistamines tend to be superior to topical therapy with corticosteroid or sodium cromoglycate nasal sprays and cromoglycate eye drops under the following circumstances:

a. if symptoms occur at several sites, e.g. nose, eyes, soft palate, pharynx and external auditory meatus;
b. in patients with nasal obstruction that limits the area of application and hence the efficacy of nasal sprays;
c. in patients with profuse rhinorrhoea where nasal sprays are rapidly washed out.

In patients with severe rhino-conjunctivitis, antihistamines are a useful adjunct to nasal sprays and eye drops.

2. Perennial allergic rhinitis

Antihistamines are often of value in perennial rhinitis. In allergic patients, particularly those with rhinitis, conjunctivitis and asthma, the use of a number of topical preparations several times each day throughout the year often leads to poor patient compliance. Under these circumstances, antihistamines can help to simplify therapy and improve compliance. They may also be a useful adjunct to other therapy in patients with more severe symptoms. In perennial rhinitis nasal obstruction is often a major feature, whereas sneezing and secretions tend to predominate in seasonal rhinitis. The topical preparations are less effective in the presence of nasal obstruction (see (1) above), and antihistamines may thus be of greater value in perennial rather than seasonal rhinitis.

3. Urticaria and angioedema

Antihistamines are the mainstay in the treatment of urticaria. In idiopathic urticaria either complete suppression or partial control of symptoms can be obtained with antihistamines in many patients. Mebhydrolin has been shown to be effective.[7,8] The same criteria for selection of a particular antihistamine, as discussed in (1) above, apply. Of the various disorders in which antihistamines are used, it is in urticaria that the greatest variation in efficacy of apparently similar antihistamines is observed. It is therefore important to try a number of H_1-receptor antihistamines, even if the first has had little or no effect, before concluding antihistamines are of no value.

Acute urticaria may be suppressed by a short course of oral antihistamines. In chronic urticaria, the duration and frequency of antihistamine therapy will depend on the nature and timing of the symptoms. Intermittent symptoms respond to intermittent therapy but it is best to start treatment immediately symptoms begin. In some patients urticaria responds to a single dose but in others several doses or a few days treatment are required. Chronic urticaria, with daily symptoms, is often more difficult to control. The most effective course of action is to obtain suppression of symptoms with regular antihistamine therapy (such as mebhydrolin 50–100 mg three times daily), titrating the dose according to response, then to continue with the same dose as maintenance therapy until the patient has remained symptom-free for 1 to 2 months. The dose can then be gradually reduced and the drug withdrawn over a period of 2–3 weeks, providing symptoms do not recur.

Many patients with urticaria complain of pruritus. Even in cases where the urticaria is relatively resistant to antihistamines, these drugs can be very helpful in reducing itching and discomfort.

Angioedema may also respond to antihistamines. Treatment is most effective if instituted early, for example at the onset of the prickling sensation at the corner of the mouth perceived by many patients with recurrent perioral oedema before the swelling is established. Periorbital, perioral and peripheral angioedema may all respond to oral antihistamines, but if the oedema is fully established by the time treatment begins less benefit is likely to be obtained. In such patients it is therefore worth determining whether the introduction of antihistamines speeds up resolution. If not, there may be little advantage in prescribing the drug. Most patients with angioedema do not complain of pruritus. In more severe cases intramuscular antihistamines may be required; however, there is no parenteral form of mebhydrolin.

Oral antihistamines alone are inadequate in the treatment of laryngeal oedema or severe angioedema occurring as part of an anaphylactic reaction. Intramuscular antihistamines are often indicated, but usually in combination with other drugs. In severe cases, adrenaline is the drug of choice.

4. Eczema

The main value of oral antihistamines in eczema is to reduce scratching. They are of particular value at night when a single oral dose may be adequate. Of 21 patients with eczema taking mebhydrolin 50 mg three times daily, all showed some improvement that was classified as excellent in 9, good in 6 and fair in 6.[8]

5. Other allergic conditions

Antihistamines are used in other disorders including drug reactions and pruritus.

Adverse reactions

Potentially life-threatening effects

No effects of this kind have been reported although serious but reversible blood dyscrasias have occurred.

Acute overdosage

There is little information on the effects of deliberate overdose, but one patient who took 140 tablets (7 g) is reported to have felt a little cold but had no other side effects and did not feel drowsy.[9]

Severe or irreversible adverse effects

Reversible agranulocytosis and neutropenia have been reported in patients taking mebhydrolin. Nine reports were submitted to the Committee on Safety of Medicines (CSM) in the UK in the 17 years up to 1981.[10] Up to November 1987, the CSM had received 13 reports of blood cell disorders: 6 cases of agranulocytosis, 4 of granulocytopenia, 1 of leucopenia, 1 of pancytopenia and 1 of thrombocytopenia. The Australian Adverse Drug Reactions Advisory Committee received 11 reports of agranulocytosis or neutropenia between 1973 and 1981.[11] In those reports, the blood dyscrasias occurred in middle-aged or older patients, and the majority of cases occurred after taking mebhydrolin for 4 to 49 days. Withdrawal of the drug was followed by recovery. In 1 patient who had a history of agranulocytosis 4 years previously when taking several drugs including mebhydrolin, inadvertent rechallenge with mebhydrolin was followed by agranulocytosis.

Symptomatic adverse effects

Drowsiness and sleepiness is the main symptomatic effect, although this probably occurs in only a small number of patients taking mebhydrolin. Overall, objective studies show little or no effect on reaction times or vigilance assessed in a number of ways.[1–3,5] One study showed impairment of mental processing time but not motor reaction time 2 hours after ingestion of 50 mg mebhydrolin, but this returned to normal at 4 hours.[2] In another study, although the mean motor reaction time was unaffected two subjects had increased reaction times.[5] In some studies mebhydrolin caused no more drowsiness than placebo,[2,5] whereas in another study drowsiness or sleepiness did occur (in 9 of 24 subjects taking mebhydrolin compared with 4 of 24 placebo-treated subjects) although more complicated indices of vigilance recorded simultaneously from electroencephalogram traces were unaffected.[3]

Other adverse effects are rare, but paradoxical excitement in children, anorexia, mild gastrointestinal disturbances, and dryness of the mouth have been reported.

Interference with clinical pathology tests
Mebhydrolin reduces the wheal and flare on skin prick testing, which is used in allergy diagnosis to detect specific IgE antibodies.[4] The drug should be stopped 24–48 hours before skin prick tests are performed.

High risk groups

Neonates
No special precautions are required in neonates, except for appropriate reduction of the adult dose.

Breast milk. No data on secretion in breast milk are available, but the manufacturers advise caution in the use of the drug during lactation.

Children
The drug may be given to children in appropriate doses.

Pregnant women
Between 1963 and 1987, the CSM received three reports of fetal malformations (leading to death in one case) where the mother had taken mebhydrolin during pregnancy. It is inadvisable to prescribe mebhydrolin during pregnancy, particularly in the first trimester.

The elderly
While agranulocytosis and neutropenia have occurred in older adults, this does not appear to be a special problem in the elderly.

Drug interactions

Potentially hazardous interactions
Mebhydrolin enhances ethanol-induced performance deficits, including visual and auditory reaction time, numerical reasoning and hand–arm coordination. Although neither alcohol nor mebhydrolin alone impairs finger dexterity, the combination does.[4]

Potentially useful interactions
No interactions of this kind appear to have been reported.

Clinical trials

1. Jones N 1960 Antihistamine treatment of hay fever with special reference to the effect upon reaction time. Practitioner 185: 334–339
2. Nini G 1974 Clinical results with a new antihistamine in various skin diseases. Giornale Italiano di Dermatologia Minerva Dermatologica 109: 276–278

References

1. Roberts C J 1972 Use of simple reaction time to determine the effects of an antihistamine on central nervous system function. A double-blind cross-over trial of mebhydrolin (Fabahistin). Clinical Trials Journal 9: 3–6
2. Muller-Limmroth W, Krueger H 1977 Study of effect of the daytime antihistamine mebhydrolin on motor reaction time and mental processing time. Clinical Therapeutics 1: 219–227
3. Kugler J, Thurmayr R, Rode C P 1972 The sedative action of several antihistamines. Electro-encephalographic and statistical studies. Arzneimittelforschung (Drug Research) 22: 1518–1522
4. Franks H M, Lawrie M, Schabinsky V V, Starmer G A, Teo R K C 1981 Interaction between ethanol and antihistamines: 3. Mebhydrolin. Medical Journal of Australia 2: 477–479
5. Jones N 1960 Antihistamine treatment of hay fever with special reference to the effect upon reaction time. Practitioner 185: 334–339
6. Schubert R, Fischer W 1954 Clinical experience with a new antihistamine. Deutsche Medizinische Wochenschrift 79: 809–811
7. Brett R 1954 Terapia dell'orticaria cronica. Medizinische 10: 336–337
8. Nini G 1974 Clinical results with a new antihistamine in various skin diseases. Giornale Italiano di Dermatologia Minerva Dermatologica 109: 276–278
9. Lidell K 1975 An unusual case of urticaria — cause and therapy. Current Medical Research and Opinion 3: 386–387
10. Committee on Safety of Medicines. Current problems (circular) 1981 Mebhydrolin (Fabahistin) and white cell disorders 7: 1
11. McEwan J, Strickland W J 1982 Mebhydrolin napadisylate: a possible cause of reversible agranulocytosis and neutropenia. Medical Journal of Australia 2: 523–525

Mecillinam

Mecillinam is a semisynthetic penicillin antibiotic developed by Leo Laboratories in Denmark and first described in 1972.[1] The US Adopted Name (USAN) is amdinocillin.

Chemistry

Mecillinam (Amdinocillin Selexidin, Selexid, Coactin, Selecidin)
$C_{15}H_{23}N_3O_3S$
6*β*-[(Hexahydro-1*H*-azepin-1-yl)-methyleneamino]penicillanic acid

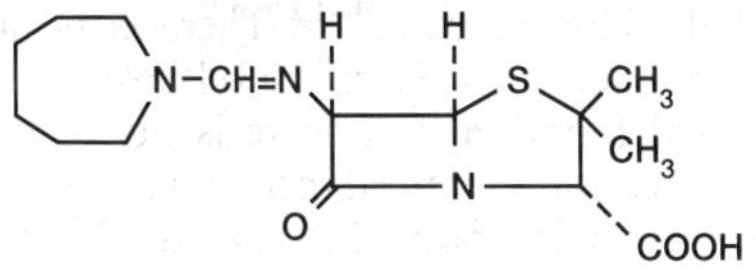

Molecular weight	325.4
pKa	3.4, 8.9
Solubility	
in alcohol	1 in 40
in water	1 in 1.7
Octanol/water partition coefficient	0.02

A white crystalline odourless powder with a bitter taste. It is a semisynthetic derivative of 6-aminopenicillanic acid. Unlike other penicillins, in which the side-chain is attached in an *N*-acyl linkage, mecillinam is an amidino derivative of 6-aminopenicillanic acid. It is not available in any combination preparations (but see pivmecillinam).

Pharmacology

Mecillinam is active primarily against Enterobacteriaceae.[2] Although it is a penicillin derivative its mechanism of action is different from that of most penicillins. The antibiotic acts in *Escherichia coli* by interfering with bacterial cell wall synthesis through inhibition of one of the high molecular weight penicillin-binding proteins (PBP-2) located in the bacterial cell membrane;[3] the mode of action in other susceptible organisms is probably the same. PBP-2 is involved in the maintenance of cell shape and susceptible Gram-negative bacilli exposed to mecillinam assume a spherical appearance and eventually succumb to lysis unless osmotic protection is given.[4,5] Bacterial growth is not prevented by mecillinam (in contrast to other *β*-lactam antibiotics) so that bacteria surviving osmotic lysis continue to grow in the presence of the antibiotic. In this way, phenotypically-resistant variants are readily selected from large bacterial populations.[4] Acquired resistance is otherwise usually due to *β*-lactamase production, but mecillinam is less susceptible to some of the common enterobacterial *β*-lactamases than is ampicillin, partly because of a low affinity for the enzymes.[6]

Toxicology

Toxicological studies in animals failed to reveal any adverse effects of potential clinical relevance. No teratological effects were observed in experiments with rats and mice (information supplied by manufacturers).

Clinical pharmacology

Mecillinam has poor activity against Gram-positive microorganisms. However it is highly active against Enterobacteriaceae. It is active against *E. coli*, *Klebsiella*, *Proteus*, *Enterobacter*, *Salmonella*,

Mecillinam

Shigella and *Yersinia*. Mecillinam has poor activity against *Pseudomonas aeruginosa*, and *Enterococcus faecalis* is for practical purposes resistant to mecillinam. Mecillinam has no other clinical pharmacological effects in man.

Pharmacokinetics

Mecillinam can be assayed by standard well-diffusion microbiological methods.[7] However, such tests are complicated by the natural instability of mecillinam, which deteriorates with a half life of approximately 5 h in serum.[8] For this reason, the preferred method of assay is high pressure liquid chromatography, with UV detection at 220 nm.[9] Serum samples must be first deproteinated with acetonitrile, but urine samples can be injected directly on to the chromatographic column. The limit of detection of the HPLC method is 0.25 $mg.l^{-1}$.

Mecillinam is poorly absorbed when given orally (but see pivmecillinam) and is administered by the intramuscular or intravenous routes.

Intravenous administration of 200 and 400 mg mecillinam to healthy volunteers results in mean peak plasma concentrations of about 12 and 25 $mg.l^{-1}$ respectively. Peak concentrations observed about 45 min after intramuscular injection of the same doses are approximately half these values.[10–12] There is no accumulation of the drug on multiple dosage.[13] Plasma levels are increased in patients with impaired renal function, but there is no accumulation of the drug,[14] probably because of natural instability of the compound. The volume of distribution is about 0.2–0.4 $l.kg^{-1}$ [12,13] and the compound is approximately 5–10% bound to plasma proteins. Mecillinam penetrates poorly into cerebrospinal fluid in the absence of meningeal inflammation[12] but limited evidence suggests that concentrations about one quarter of those observed in plasma may be achieved when the meninges are inflamed. Mecillinam is not detectable in breast milk, but the compound crosses the placenta.

Mecillinam is excreted into urine with a half life of about 1 h;[9,11] concentrations achieved in the urine on standard doses generally exceed 1000 $mg.l^{-1}$. About 60% of the total dose is recoverable from urine, mostly within 6 h.[11] A small proportion of the remainder finds its way into bile giving concentrations three times those in the serum, but most is lost by spontaneous hydrolysis into products that exhibit little or no antibacterial activity. Renal excretion is prolonged by the simultaneous administration of probenecid[11] suggesting that elimination is predominantly by tubular secretion. Mecillinam is slowly removed from circulation during haemodialysis, as would be expected of a compound with a small volume of distribution and low protein binding.[15]

Oral absorption	<10%
Presystemic metabolism	none
Plasma half life	
mean	~1 h
Volume of distribution	0.2–0.4 $l.kg^{-1}$
Plasma protein binding	5–10%

Mecillinam is eliminated largely unchanged in the urine, with virtually no metabolism. As a consequence, it is unlikely that hepatic disease would affect the pharmacokinetics of the drug. However, some adjustment of dose might be necessary in renal impairment. Old age does not appear to alter drug elimination, except where there is renal impairment.

Concentration–effect relationship

As with other antimicrobial agents, the efficacy of mecillinam depends on adequate concentrations being achieved at the site of infection. Bacteria that are inhibited in vitro by $\leqslant 1$ $mg.l^{-1}$ are generally regarded as fully susceptible; those inhibited by 1–8 $mg.l^{-1}$ as exhibiting reduced susceptibility; and those not inhibited by 8 $mg.l^{-1}$ as being resistant.

There is no difficulty in achieving concentrations of mecillinam in urine that are far in excess of those that are inhibitory to the common urinary pathogens.

Penicillins depend on active bacterial growth to achieve their effect and mecillinam is no exception. Since mecillinam is slowly bactericidal and displays a short plasma half life, the antibiotic may not be optimally suited to the treatment of systemic infection. Bacteria that are damaged, but not killed by mecillinam might be expected to exhibit enhanced susceptibility to host defences, such as serum bactericidal activity and phagocytosis, but attempts to demonstrate this have produced conflicting results.[16–18]

Metabolism

Mecillinam is not metabolized in the accepted sense and over 60% of a dose is eliminated unchanged in the urine. However, the compound is inherently unstable and the amidino side-chain and the β-lactam ring are both susceptible to aqueous hydrolysis. The products of hydrolysis are *N*-formyl-6-aminopenicillanic acid (which exhibits modest antibacterial activity) and the penicilloic acid derivatives of mecillinam and its *N*-formyl metabolite (which display no antibacterial activity).

Pharmaceutics

In the UK mecillinam (Selexidin; Leo, UK) is available as pure powder in vials containing 200 and 400 mg; in the USA the compound (Coactin; Roche, US) is dispensed in 500 mg and 1 g vials. For intravenous infusion, a 10% (w/v) solution is prepared in sterile water and infused slowly over 3–4 min; alternatively, the compound can be added to sodium chloride injection or to 5% dextrose solution and infused over 15–30 min.

Mecillinam is stable in the form of dry powder, but solutions are unstable and should be used immediately.

Although mecillinam may interact synergistically with some other β-lactam antibiotics, there are no pharmaceutical preparations in which it is combined with other agents (but see pivmecillinam).

Therapeutic use

Indications

1. Urinary tract infection
2. Enteric fever
3. Other serious infections caused by susceptible Gram-negative bacilli.

Contraindications

1. Hypersensitivity to penicillins or cephalosporins

Mode of use

Mecillinam is administered by intramuscular injection or by slow intravenous infusion in doses of 5–15 $mg.kg^{-1}$ given every 6-8 h. As much as 12 g daily has been administered intravenously without adverse effect, but such high dosage is not recommended.

Indications

1. Urinary tract infection

Since mecillinam is excreted by the renal route, high concentrations are achieved in the urine and urinary tract infection is the major indication for its use. However, it is usual to administer the drug in its oral prodrug form (see pivmecillinam) for this indication.

2. Enteric fever

Because of the impressive activity in vitro of mecillinam against salmonellae, considerable interest has been shown in the possibility of using the drug in the treatment of typhoid and paratyphoid fever. However, early optimism that mecillinam may be of value in enteric fever[19,20] has not been fully realized by subsequent experience[21,22] and the drug has not received acceptance as first-line therapy in this condition.

3. Other serious Gram-negative infections

Parenteral mecillinam has been used (generally in combination with another agent) in a wide variety of infections in adults, children and neonates.[23–26] Infections that have been successfully treated include septicaemia, pneumonia, bronchitis, meningitis and soft-tissue infections. The reasons for the use of mecillinam in combination with other agents are threefold: (a) avoidance of the risk of selection of variants that are resistant to mecillinam; such variants have been isolated from patients receiving the drug;[18,27] (b) the possibility of exploiting synergic interactions with other β-lactam agents;[28] (c) the need to reinforce the limited antibacterial spectrum in blind treatment situations.

Adverse reactions

Potentially life-threatening effects
Mecillinam shares with other β-lactam agents an excellent safety profile; apart from penicillin hypersensitivity, which may occur in 2–3% of patients treated with mecillinam, unwanted effects are uncommon. Anaphylactic reactions have not been reported, but since the compound is a penicillin, it is assumed that the risk of anaphylaxis exists.

Acute overdosage
Overdose has not been reported and is most unlikely with parenteral mecillinam. The drug can be removed by haemodialysis.

Severe or irreversible adverse effects
No serious reactions to this drug appear to have been reported.

Symptomatic adverse effects
These include thrombophlebitis, or pain at the injection site, nausea, diarrhoea, and vaginitis.

Other effects
A transient increase in alkaline phosphatase or transaminase levels may occur.

Interference with clinical pathology tests
No technical interferences of this kind appear to have been reported.

High risk groups

Neonates
Mecillinam appears to be safe in neonates.[25]

Breast milk. Mecillinam does not appear in breast milk.

Children
Young children tolerate the drug well.[26]

Pregnant women
Parenteral mecillinam has not been used extensively in pregnant women, but the oral prodrug form has been used in bacteriuria of pregnancy without untoward effect (see pivmecillinam). However, since mecillinam crosses the placenta, the manufacturers cautiously recommend that its use should be avoided in the first trimester of pregnancy.

The elderly
No special precautions are necessary when giving the drug to elderly patients.

Concurrent disease
In patients with impaired renal function a normal loading dose should be given, but subsequent doses should be reduced as follows:
Mild to moderate impairment (glomerular filtration rate 10–50 ml.min^{-1}): half the normal dose.
Severe impairment (glomerular filtration rate <10 ml.min^{-1}): one quarter the normal dose.
However, the dose should not be reduced below 200 mg 8 hourly in adults, or below 10 mg.kg^{-1} in children.

Drug interactions

Potentially hazardous interactions
Hazardous interactions between mecillinam and other drugs have not been reported.

Potentially useful interactions
Simultaneous administration of probenecid delays excretion of mecillinam by competition for renal tubular secretion.[11] Potentially useful synergy between mecillinam and ampicillin or other β-lactam antibiotics against some strains of enteric bacteria have been demonstrated in vitro[28,29] and in experimental animals.[30,31] The basis of the interaction probably rests on differential inhibition of the penicillin-binding proteins (PBPs) located in the bacterial cell membrane. Mecillinam binds exclusively to PBP-2 and bactericidal synergy is most evident when the compound is combined with β-lactam agents like cephalexin and cephradine, which preferentially inhibit PBP-3.[32]

Mecillinam

Major outcome trials

The results of most major clinical trials of parenteral mecillinam were presented in the course of a symposium sponsored by Hoffman-La Roche, who market mecillinam (amdinocillin) in the USA. The symposium proceedings were published as a supplement to the American Journal of Medicine (1983) 75 (2A). Most of the trial protocols specified the use of mecillinam in combination with another β-lactam antibiotic; a few of the studies were comparative and randomized. Among the wide variety of infections treated were: pneumonia and other pulmonary infections; septicaemia; urinary tract infection (simple and complicated); soft-tissue infections; neonatal and paediatric infections; and enteric fever.

Use of mecillinam in combination with another agent in the treatment of infections caused by susceptible microorganisms was generally found to be safe and effective, but no more so than alternative regimens. Reports of the use of mecillinam as monotherapy in serious infection do not support the view that the agent is reliable when used alone, except in urinary tract infection.

Other trials

1. Menday A P, Marsh B T 1979 Preliminary experience with parenteral mecillinam. Current Medical Research and Opinion 6: 221–228

This report is a collation by the Company's Medical Department of results obtained in various centres in an assortment of infections during the early clinical evaluation of mecillinam in the UK. The authors reviewed case reports of 26 patients treated with parenteral mecillinam, 23 of whom also received other antibiotics. Clinical improvement, or cure was observed in 17 of 25 patients who could be assessed; 3 of these 17 patients relapsed on cessation of treatment. Mecillinam was well tolerated.

2. Ekwall E, Scheja A, Cronberg S et al 1980 Mecillinam and ampicillin separately or combined in Gram-negative septicaemia. Infection 8: 37–40

24 patients with confirmed septicaemia received intravenous therapy with either: mecillinam alone (4 patients); ampicillin alone (11 patients); or a combination of mecillinam and ampicillin (9 patients). Patients were treated for 3 weeks and all were switched to oral therapy after 1–2 weeks of i.v. treatment. Two of the patients receiving mecillinam, three of those receiving ampicillin and one receiving the combination failed to respond to therapy. Therapy had to be discontinued in one patient receiving mecillinam alone because of the development of exanthema; otherwise, no serious side effects were noted.

General review articles

Geddes A M, Wise R (eds) 1977 Mecillinam. Journal of Antimicrobial Chemotherapy 3 (suppl B): 1–160
Moellering R C, Nelson J D, Neu H C (eds) 1983 An international review of amdinocillin: a new beta-lactam antibiotic. American Journal of Medicine 75 (2A): 1–138
Editorial 1976 Mecillinam. Lancet 2: 503–505

References

1. Lund F, Tybring L 1972 6β-amidinopenicillanic acids — a new group of antibiotics. Nature (New Biology) 236: 135–137
2. Reeves D S, Wise R, Bywater M J 1975 A laboratory evaluation of a novel β-lactam antibiotic mecillinam. Journal of Antimicrobial Chemotherapy 1: 337–344
3. Spratt B G 1977 The mechanism of action of mecillinam. Journal of Antimicrobial Chemotherapy 3 (suppl B): 13–19
4. Greenwood D, O'Grady F 1973 FL 1060: a new beta-lactam antibiotic with novel properties. Journal of Clinical Pathology 26: 1–6
5. Greenwood D 1976 Effect of osmolality on the response of *Escherichia coli* to mecillinam. Antimicrobial Agents and Chemotherapy 10: 824–826
6. Richmond M H 1977 In vitro studies with mecillinam on *Escherichia coli* and *Pseudomonas aeruginosa*. Journal of Antimicrobial Chemotherapy 3 (suppl B): 29–39
7. Andrews J M, Wise R 1978 Mecillinam. In: Reeves D S, Phillips I, Williams J D, Wise R (eds) Laboratory methods in antimicrobial chemotherapy. Churchill Livingstone, Edinburgh, pp 179–180
8. Menday A P, Tybring L 1978 Mecillinam. In: Reeves D S, Phillips I, Williams J D, Wise R (eds) Laboratory methods in antimicrobial chemotherapy. Churchill Livingstone, Edinburgh, pp 79–81
9. Lin E T, Gambertoglio J G, Barriere S L, Chen R R L, Conte J E, Benet L Z 1981 High pressure liquid chromatographic determination of mecillinam in human plasma and urine. Analytical Letters 14: 1433–1447

M

10. Williams J D, Andrews J, Mitchard M, Kendall M J 1976 Bacteriology and pharmacokinetics of the new amidino penicillin — mecillinam. Journal of Antimicrobial Chemotherapy 2: 61–69
11. Roholt K 1977 Pharmacokinetic studies with mecillinam and pivmecillinam. Journal of Antimicrobial Chemotherapy 3 (suppl B): 71–81
12. Garborg O 1981 Mecillinam in cerebrospinal fluid in children. Clinical Pharmacokinetics 6: 475–479
13. Barriere S L, Gambertoglio J G, Lin E T, Conte J E 1983 Multiple-dose pharmacokinetics of amdinocillin in healthy volunteers. Antimicrobial Agents and Chemotherapy 21: 54–57
14. Svarva P L, Wessel-Aas T, Maeland J A 1980 Mecillinam in the treatment of patients with severely impaired renal function. In: Nelson J D, Grassi C (eds) Current chemotherapy and infectious disease. American Society for Microbiology, Washington, pp 319–320
15. Bailey K, Cruickshank J G, Bisson P G, Radford B L 1980 Mecillinam in patients on haemodialysis. British Journal of Clinical Pharmacology 10: 177–179
16. Lorian V, Atkinson B A 1979 Effect of serum and blood on Enterobacteriaceae grown in the presence of subminimal inhibitory concentrations of ampicillin and mecillinam. Reviews of Infectious Diseases 1: 797–806
17. Taylor P W, Gaunt H, Unger F M 1981 Effect of subinhibitory concentrations of mecillinam on serum susceptibility of *Escherichia coli* strains. Antimicrobial Agents and Chemotherapy 19: 786–788
18. Verweij-van Vught A M J J, Namavar F, Smit A M, Sparrius M, MacLaren D M 1982 Virulence of mecillinam-resistant spherical mutants of *Klebsiella pneumoniae* and *Escherichia coli*. Journal of Antimicrobial Chemotherapy 9: 379–385
19. Clarke P D, Geddes A M, McGhie D, Wall J C 1976 Mecillinam: a new antibiotic for enteric fever. British Medical Journal 2: 14–15
20. Geddes A M, Clarke P D 1977 The treatment of enteric fever with mecillinam. Journal of Antimicrobial Chemotherapy 3 (suppl B): 101–102
21. Mandal B K, Ironside A K, Brennand J 1979 Mecillinam in enteric fever. British Medical Journal 1: 586–587
22. McKendrick M W, Geddes A M 1979 Mecillinam and amoxycillin in enteric fever. Journal of Antimicrobial Chemotherapy 5: 727–728
23. Menday A P, Marsh B T 1979 Preliminary experience with parenteral mecillinam. Current Medical Research and Opinion 6: 221–228
24. Demos C H, Green E 1983 Review of clinical experience with amdinocillin monotherapy and comparative studies. American Journal of Medicine 75 (2A): 72–81
25. de Louvois J, Mulhall A 1983 Efficacy, pharmacology and safety of amdinocillin in treatment of neonates. American Journal of Medicine 75 (2A): 119–124
26. Nelson J D, Kusmiesz H, Shelton S 1983 Randomized trial of cefamandole plus amdinocillin versus cefamandole in serious pediatric infections. American Journal of Medicine 75 (2A): 125–129
27. Barbour A G, Mayer L W 1980 Mecillinam resistance and small cell volume: the in vivo selection of an *Escherichia coli* mutant. In: Nelson J D, Grassi C (eds) Current chemotherapy and infectious disease. American Society for Microbiology, Washington, pp 715–716
28. Cleeland R, Squires E 1983 Enhanced activity of beta-lactam antibiotics with amdinocillin in vitro and in vivo. American Journal of Medicine 75 (2A): 21–29
29. Neu H C 1976 Synergy of mecillinam, a beta-amidino-penicillanic acid derivative combined with beta-lactam antibiotics. Antimicrobial Agents and Chemotherapy 10: 535–542
30. Grunberg E, Cleeland R, Beskid G, DeLorenzo W F 1976 In vivo synergy between 6β-amidinopenicillanic acid derivatives and other antibiotics. Antimicrobial Agents and Chemotherapy 9: 589–594
31. Gordin F M, Sande M A 1983 Amdinocillin therapy of experimental animal infections. American Journal of Medicine 75 (2A): 48–53
32. Greenwood D, O'Grady F 1973 The two sites of penicillin action in *Escherichia coli*. Journal of Infectious Diseases 128: 791–794

Medazepam

Medazepam is a benzodiazepine anxiolytic.

Chemistry

Medazepam (Ansilan, Diepin, Elbrus, Esmail, Medazepol, Mezepan, Megasedan, Nobrium, Pazital, Psiquium, Raporan, Resmit, Rudotel, Serenium, Siman)
$C_{16}H_{15}ClN_2$
7-Chloro-2,3-dihydro-1-methyl-5-phenyl-1H-1,4-benzodiazepine

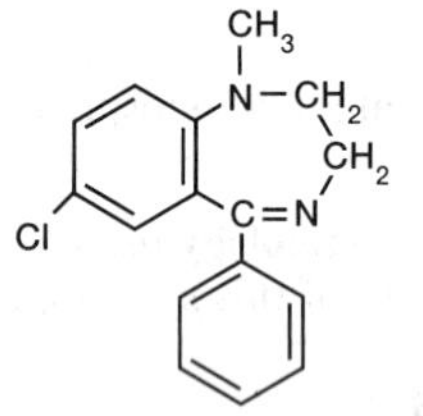

Molecular weight	270.8
pKa	6.2
Solubility	
in alcohol	1 in 8
in water	almost insoluble
Octanol/water partition coefficient	10 000

Medazepam appears as colourless prismatic crystals from ether + petroleum ether, melting point 95–97°C.

Medazepam hydrochloride ($C_{16}H_{15}ClN_2.HCl$) is an orange red crystalline powder, freely soluble in water and alcohol. It is prepared by chemical synthesis and the racemate is used clinically. Medazepam is also available in an oral combination product with amitriptyline (Nobritol).

Pharmacology

Medazepam has anxiolytic, sedative, muscle relaxant and anticonvulsant properties, like most benzodiazepines. However, its binding affinity to the benzodiazepine receptor is extremely low[1] whereas its metabolites, especially diazepam itself, show a high affinity to the benzodiazepine receptor. It is thus very likely that most, if not all, of the effects of medazepam are mediated via metabolites, notably diazepam and oxazepam (see these drugs for full details).

Toxicology

Medazepam has not been tested for mutagenicity and carcinogenicity. There is no evidence of teratogenicity or fetotoxicity in rats and rabbits.

Clinical pharmacology

Medazepam can be used as an anxiolytic or as a hypnotic. It has only mild suppressive effects on REM sleep, but increases total sleep time while suppressing the deeper phases (phases 3 and 4) of sleep. Via its metabolites it causes an increase in fast β activity on the EEG. Medazepam increases seizure threshold to some extent and could thus be used as an anticonvulsant. However, it is not in practice used for this indication and is not usually licensed in this area. Diazepam is likely to be of more use for the treatment of status epilepticus.

Medazepam in standard clinical doses causes a slight decrease in respiratory rate, blood pressure and in left ventricular stroke work.

On occasion an increase in heart rate and a decrease in stroke volume may occur. These effects are rarely of clinical significance.

Medazepam also has muscular relaxation effects, mainly through its effect on spinal reflexes.

Pharmacokinetics

The preferred analytical method is gas chromatography with electrochemical detection[2]. The limit of sensitivity is 40 μg.l^{-1}. Oral absorption of 10 mg of medazepam is 76.4%.[3] Plasma concentration peaks at 1–2 hours after oral administration of 10 to 50 mg of medazepam, with plasma level of 75 to 165 μg.l^{-1}. The mean plasma half life of unchanged medazepam is 2 to 5 hours. Then follows an irregular transitional phase lasting to the tenth hour after a single dose of 10 mg or up to 3 days after doses of 30 mg. It then enters the phase of approximate equilibrium. The half life of this latter phase is generally between 33 and 83 hours. However, extreme values of 20 and 360 hours can be observed.

Systemic bioavailability ranges between 49% and 76%.

Elimination half life of unchanged medazepam ranges from 1 to 7 hours but is 2 to 4 hours in most subjects.

Unchanged medazepam is almost completely bound to plasma proteins and does not penetrate blood cells. It enters the brain and other tissues as desmethyldiazepam.

The volume of distribution of desmethyldiazepam is 0.44 l.kg^{-1} (V_{ss}).

Placental transfer has been demonstrated for benzodiazepines. Desmethyldiazepam excretion in human breast milk has been documented.

Oral absorption	74.6%
Presystemic metabolism	<25%
Plasma half life	
range (desmethyldiazepam)	1–2 h, 40–100 h
Volume of distribution	0.44 l.kg^{-1}
Plasma protein binding	99.6%

Medazepam undergoes extensive hepatic biotransformation. Up to 75% of the dose is excreted in urine, with only 1% as unchanged drug. Approximately 20% of the dose is eliminated in the faeces.

Concentration–effect relationship

A concentration–effect relationship for medazepam has not been documented.

Metabolism

Medazepam is metabolized in the liver. Two primary pathways of metabolism have been described:[3]

1. 1-demethylation to desmethyldiazepam and oxazepam (active metabolites)
2. oxidation to 2-one hydroxymedazepam and diazepam (active metabolites).

Only 1% of unchanged medazepam is found in urine; other compounds are conjugated and non-conjugated metabolites, mainly conjugated oxazepam. 3-OH-diazepam, 4'-OH-diazepam and oxazepam are found in bile (15%) and in urine (48.9% of radioactivity).[4]

Pharmaceutics

Medazepam is available in oral form.

Nobrium capsules (Roche, UK) contain 5 mg (orange/ivory) and 10 mg (orange/black) medazepam. No special precautions for storage are required.

Medazepam carries the common risk of allergies to benzodiazepines.

Therapeutic use

Indications

1. Anxiety, tension, agitation, phobias, somatic manifestations of anxiety: cardiovascular reactions (tachycardia, pseudo angina), respiratory reactions (hyperventilation syndrome, sensations of pressure and tightness in chest), gastrointestinal reactions (nervous dyspepsia)

Medazepam

2. Insomnia, when associated with anxiety
3. Muscular contractures
4. Adjuvant to the treatment of: alcoholism, mild depression, organic illness associated with anxiety, behavioural disorders due to epilepsy and brain damage.

Contraindications

1. Allergy to benzodiazepines
2. Respiratory insufficiency and sleep apnoea syndrome
3. Myasthenia
4. Depression
5. Alcohol
6. Renal and hepatic insufficiency.

Mode of use

In most cases and in all elderly patients, the initial dosage is 5 mg, two or three times daily. Dosage may be gradually increased up to 40 mg a day, but usual doses range between 15 and 30 mg a day.

As for any benzodiazepines, especially short half life benzodiazepines (less than 24 hours), sudden withdrawal can provoke mild or severe symptoms: insomnia with nightmares, irritability, muscular pains, tremor, tension, abdominal pain, paraesthesias, sweating and exceptionally, confusion, isolated convulsions or myoclonic seizures. Withdrawal or reduction of doses should be performed slowly. Equivalent dosage of another benzodiazepine does not always prevent withdrawal syndrome.

Due to their potential addictive properties, benzodiazepines should not be used for prolonged periods of time.

Because of the sedative properties of medazepam, the patient should not drive for the first few days of treatment.[5] Alcohol should be avoided, due to reciprocal potentiation when taken concomitantly with medazepam.[6]

Indications

1. Anxiety[7–9]

Medazepam is effective in anxiety associated with neurosis. Its usefulness is less obvious in anxiety associated with psychosis. In cases of agitation or acute anxiety associated with phobia, medazepam should be used at higher doses (40 mg a day). It alleviates anxiety and agitation but not the phobias. In cases of somatizations of anxiety, medazepam, like other benzodiazepines does not necessarily alleviate the symptoms but it reduces the associated anxiety. Somatic manifestations of anxiety are more likely to be treated by β-blocking agents. It has also been used for the management of anxiety in children.[10]

2. Insomnia

Difficulty in getting to sleep or maintaining sleep during the first part of the night can be treated by medazepam taken at bedtime. If vesperal anxiety is important, medazepam can be given in the early evening (5 p.m.) in order to provide relaxation during the period preceding bedtime.

3. Muscular contractures

Like other benzodiazepines, medazepam has myo-relaxing properties and may be used at usual dosages as a relaxing agent when muscular pain is due to contractures.

4. Other uses

When anxiety is associated with alcoholism or alcohol withdrawal, a high dosage is recommended at the onset of treatment. In mild depression or organic illness, medazepam can be prescribed at normal doses. Like other benzodiazepines, medazepam has an anticonvulsant effect and may be used as an adjuvant agent to other antiepileptic treatments. It can be useful too for behavioural disorders associated with epilepsy and brain damage.

Contraindications

1. Allergy to benzodiazepines

Allergies to benzodiazepines are not frequently encountered.

2. Respiratory insufficiency

Respiratory insufficiency, when severe, represents a contraindication. Attention should be paid to the sleep apnoea syndrome which can be worsened by central depressants.

3. Myasthenia
Myasthenia can be worsened. Benzodiazepine prescription must be avoided in these cases. If not, special care should be taken.

4. Depression
In this condition, prescription of anxiolytics without antidepressants can be hazardous: with reduced anxiety, depressive symptoms can be increased and lead to suicide attempts.

5. Alcohol[6]
Due to possible reciprocal potentiation this association should be avoided.

Adverse reactions

Potentially life-threatening effects
There is no reported case of death directly linked to medazepam.

Acute overdosage
Cases (85) of deliberate overdoses (up to 500 mg and possibly 800 mg) have been reported. All subjects recovered, except one (male of 35 years who took 210 mg of medazepam with 115 g of alcohol, death was due to respiratory arrest).

Classic monitoring of coma is recommended.

Severe or irreversible adverse effects
Breakdown and elimination of medazepam and its metabolites may be delayed by liver or kidney insufficiency; doses should therefore be reduced or the interval between doses prolonged.

Addiction[11] to benzodiazepines have been described after long-term use.

Withdrawal symptoms[12] can be observed with high and normal doses of benzodiazepines but are usually more severe after long-term use. For this reason, medazepam should not be used for prolonged treatment without very careful consideration of risk and benefit.

Symptomatic adverse effects
Medazepam is usually well tolerated but sleepiness, fatigue, muscular hypotonia, drowsiness, paradoxical effects (irritability, aggressivity, excitation, oneiric confusional syndrome), anterograde amnesia, and skin eruptions with pruritus can be observed.

Interference with clinical pathology tests
None has been reported.

High risk groups

Neonates
There are no specific dosages for neonates.

Breast milk. As medazepam is excreted in the breast milk of nursing mothers, its use during this period is not recommended.

Children
Medazepam may be used,[10] but it must be remembered that longitudinal studies show that regular use of benzodiazepines during childhood can be correlated with drug addiction in adolescence.

Pregnant women
Though epidemiology does not suggest any teratogenic effect in animals, prescription of medazepam during the first three months of pregnancy is not recommended.

High doses should be avoided during the last three months of pregnancy because of the risk of hypotonia, hypothermia and respiratory insufficiency in the neonate.

The elderly
Because of the possible slowing of metabolism in elderly subjects, doses should be adjusted.

Concurrent disease
Renal and hepatic insufficiency. The dosage may need to be reduced in patients with renal and hepatic insufficiency.

Drug interactions

Potentially hazardous interactions
Centrally active drugs. Combination of medazepam with other centrally active drugs such as neuroleptics, tranquillizers, antidepressants, hypnotics, analgesics and anaesthetics can potentiate some of their effects such as hypotension, cardiovascular collapse and respiratory depression.

Alcohol. Despite a report of an experimental interaction study with medazepam and alcohol, without detrimental effect on driving ability,[9] the association alcohol–medazepam should be avoided, due to possible potentiation.

Potentially useful interactions
The mutual potentiation of centrally active drugs can be utilized therapeutically provided that the dose of each is kept low.

Major clinical trials

1. Kerry R J, McDermott C M 1971 Medazepam compared with amylobarbitone in treatment of anxiety. British Medical Journal 1: 151–152

This is a double-blind, crossover trial involving 29 patients suffering from neurotic anxiety. Each received a three weeks treatment period of the following: medazepam 30 mg daily, amylobarbitone 180 mg daily.

Subjective responses and relief of symptoms were assessed at the first visit and changes in the patients' condition were rated on subsequent visits.

The results show a superiority of medazepam over amylbarbitone: 24 out of 29 patients preferred the medazepam period when all the symptoms were rated as improved.

General review articles

McKenzie S 1983 Introduction to the pharmacokinetics and pharmacodynamics of benzodiazepines. Progress in Neuro-psychopharmacology and Biological Psychiatry 7: 623–627

Lader M H, Bond A J, James D C 1974 Clinical comparison of anxiolytic drug therapy. Psychological Medicine 4, 4: 381–387

References

1. Nakatsuka I, Shimizu H, Asami Y, Katoh T, Hirose A, Yoshitake A 1984 Benzodiazepines and their metabolites: relationship between binding affinity to the benzodiazepines receptor and pharmacological activity. Life Sciences 36: 113–119
2. de Silva J A F, Puglisi C V 1970 Determination of Medazepam (Nobrium), diazepam (Valium) and their major biotransformation products in blood and urine by electron capture gas–chromatography. Analytical Chemistry 42: 1725–1736
3. Randall L O 1970 Pharmacology of medazepam and its metabolites. Archives International of Pharmacology and Therapeutics 185: 135–148
4. Mahon W A, Inaba T, Umeda T, Tsutsumi E, Stone R 1976 Biliary elimination of diazepam in man. Clinical Pharmacology and Therapeutics 19 (4): 443–450
5. Moore N C 1977 Medazepam and the driving ability of anxious patients. Psychopharmacology 52: 103–106
6. Landauer A A, Pocock D A, Prott F W 1974 The effect of medazepam and alcohol on cognitive and motor skills used in car driving. Psychopharmacologia 37 (2): 159–168
7. Abrahams N 1971 General practitioner clinical trials, medazepam — a new tranquillizer. Practitioner 1235: 688–690
8. Daneman E A, Nutley N J, Gainsville F 1970 A comparative study of medazepam (Nobrium) in anxiety–depressive states. Psychosomatics 10 (6): 366–369
9. Committee on the review of medicines 1980 Systematic review of the benzodiazepines. Guidelines for data sheets on diazepam, chlordiazepoxide, medazepam, clorazepate, lorazepam, oxazepam, temazepam, triazolam, nitrazepam, and flurazepam. British Medical Journal 280: 910–912
10. Dahlström H, Fedor-Freybergh P, Käreland H, Vahlne L 1973 Benzoctamine and medazepam in treatment of anxiety of children and adolescents: a comparative study. Acta Psychiatrica Scandinavia 49: 735–743
11. Maletzky B M, Klotter J 1976 Addiction to diazepam. The International Journal of the Addictions 11: 95–115
12. Hallstrom C, Lader M 1981 Withdrawal phenomena in patients on high and normal doses of diazepam. International Pharmacology 16: 235–244

Medroxyprogesterone acetate

Medroxyprogesterone acetate has been available for over 20 years and has achieved wide therapeutic use as a progestational agent.

Chemistry

Medroxyprogesterone acetate (Provera, Clinovir, Farlutal, Depo-provera)
$C_{24}H_{34}O_4$
6α-Methyl-3,20-dioxopregn-4-en-17α-yl acetate

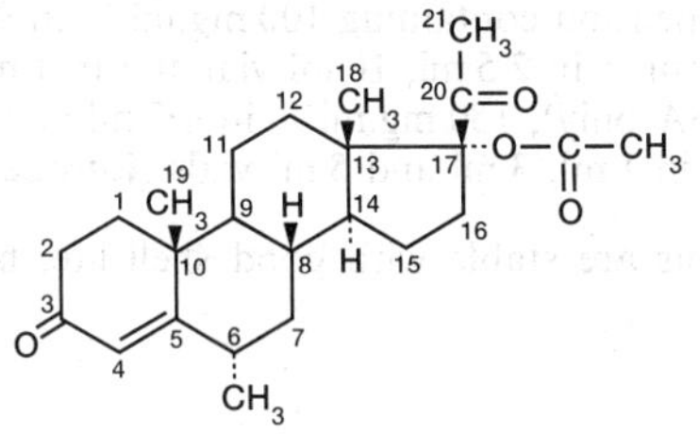

Molecular weight	386.5
pKa	—
Solubility	
in alcohol	1 in 800
in water	1 in 10 000
Octanol/water partition coefficient	1600[1]

Medroxyprogesterone acetate (MPA) is a white or almost white, odourless, crystalline powder, stable in air. It is prepared by chemical synthesis and is used clinically both in oral and injectable dose forms. The drug has been used in combination with ethinylestradiol (Provest) but is no longer available in any combination products.

Pharmacology

The methyl group at position 6 gives greater progestational activity than 17α-hydroxyprogesterone acetate.[2] Many effects of MPA are attributed to its ability to suppress pituitary gonadotrophins. In comparison with progesterone and other progestational agents, MPA has minimal androgenic activity and virtually no oestrogenic activity. At high doses, MPA has an anabolic effect. In animals MPA has a low adrenocortical effect. Following oral or intramuscular dosing MPA decreases cytoplasmic oestrogen receptors. Oral administration (100 mg MPA per day on cycle days 3 to 23) significantly reduced the number of cytosol progestin receptors in the endometrium of normal cycling pre-menopausal women, whereas nuclear concentrations of progestin and oestrogen receptors were not altered.[3]

Toxicology

Following extremely high doses of MPA, beagle bitches developed mammary nodules or breast malignancies but the relevance of these findings to clinical use is open to question. Because of the metabolism and sensitivity differences to progestogens between the human female and the beagle bitch, various regulatory agencies (including the World Health Organization and the Committee on Safety of Medicines) have concluded that the beagle bitch is an inappropriate species for long-term carcinogenicity testing of progestogens.

In long-term toxicology studies in the monkey,[3] in which very high intramuscular doses of MPA were given for 10 years, 2 out of 12 monkeys developed undifferentiated carcinoma of the uterus. At lower doses in the monkey no uterine malignancies were found. The relevance of the monkey data to humans is unknown. In humans, oestrogen stimulation is implicated in endometrial cancers but progestogens are considered protective. There is no evidence in women for an association between endometrial carcinoma and MPA therapy in over 10 million women-years of use.

Clinical pharmacology

MPA treatment decreases the levels of the hypophyseal gonadotrophins (LH and FSH), particularly in postmenopausal women and in men. In women inhibition of LH and FSH in turn limits ovarian production of oestrogens. In hormone-dependent neoplastic cells this may limit tumour growth and survival.[4] The effects of graded doses of OMPA (oral medroxyprogesterone acetate) on pituitary, ovarian and endometrial function have been studied in normal women. A dose of 2.5 mg a day on days 7–10 of the menstrual cycle did not affect the cycle, whereas a dose of 5 mg or 10 mg a day reduced the concentration in plasma of oestradiol, progesterone and LH.[5,6] It is, however, generally agreed that a clinical response in carcinoma of the breast cannot be achieved with a plasma concentration of less than 90 $\mu g.l^{-1}$. The response to MPA therapy in endometrial carcinoma appears to relate to the number of endometrial cytoplasmic progestin receptors.[7] MPA has an anti-oestrogenic effect, either direct or mediated. Early studies also showed that MPA inhibited RNA and DNA synthesis.[8]

Medroxyprogesterone acetate has no adrenocortical effect in women when used in standard contraceptive doses. However, when MPA is used in doses above 500 mg per day for the treatment of certain cancers, adrenocortical effects are seen.

Pharmacokinetics

None of the methods currently available in routine use is satisfactory for detailed kinetic studies. The vast majority of the data are derived from radioimmunoassay (RIA) which is non-specific and measures both MPA and its metabolites. Recently[9] HPLC data have become available which suggest that only 20%, or so, of the RIA-measured material in plasma following oral dosing is unchanged MPA. Because of the non-specificity of RIA and the lack of sensitivity of the HPLC techniques, formal pharmacokinetic studies have not been done. Instead MPA-like material, measured by RIA, has been used to describe qualitatively the pharmacokinetics of MPA. Unfortunately, many different RIA procedures have been used, which makes meaningful cross-comparisons of data impossible.

In general, MPA is absorbed from the gastrointestinal tract and food appears to enhance its absorption.[10] Following oral dosing, peak drug levels are seen within 2 to 6 hours. With daily oral dosing steady-state conditions are achieved within 2 to 3 weeks of dosing. Intramuscular (depot) injections of MPA result in lower C_{max} values but more persistent blood levels (apparent half life = 6 weeks) than with the equivalent oral dose. Examination from the RIA data indicates a biphasic disappearance of drug following oral dosing, with an overall elimination half life of 27 h. The terminal half life is estimated to be 60 h. Bioavailability of oral dose formulations is improved if rapid-dissolution, micronized drug is used.[11]

Unmetabolized MPA is about 94% bound to plasma proteins.[12] As would be expected from a lipophilic drug MPA is rapidly and widely distributed. The volume of distribution, which is probably an underestimate, is in excess of 20 l in women.[13] MPA crosses the blood–brain barrier[14] and accumulates in liver and kidneys. Orally administered MPA crosses the placental barrier in pregnant women[15] and enters breast milk in concentrations similar to those in the maternal plasma.[16]

MPA is extensively metabolized in the liver with less than 5% of the dose being excreted unchanged in the urine. Impaired renal or hepatic function does not appear to markedly affect the clearance of MPA.[17] Irrespective of the route of administration, MPA is eliminated mainly as conjugated metabolites in the faeces.[10] The average plasma clearance is estimated to be 1600–4000 l daily.
Bioavailability is reduced by smoking, due presumably to increased hepatic metabolism.

Medroxyprogesterone acetate

Oral absorption	<100%
Presystemic metabolism	—
Plasma half life	
mean (oral dosing)	~30 h
Volume of distribution	>20 l
Plasma protein binding	94%

Concentration–effect relationship

Concentrations of MPA in the low µg.l^{-1} range are effective for contraception.[18] In the oncology area there are conflicting views. Some investigators have related response rate, in responding patients, with serum MPA levels exceeding 90 µg.l^{-1}.[19] Other investigators have shown no correlation.[20] Reasons for this conflict probably relate to the marked differences in steady-state drug plasma levels between patients and between formulations.[21] Also, the oestrogen receptor status of responding individuals appears to be important.[22] Comparisons of drug concentrations between studies are made difficult by the plethora of RIA methods in use.

Metabolism

Metabolism of MPA is poorly documented by modern standards. The only comprehensive study of metabolites has been done by Sturm and Schulz.[23] These authors concluded that MPA metabolites are present in the plasma of high-dose-treated patients but that the clinical significance of these metabolites is not known, and that they could turn out to be therapeutically effective. The major MPA metabolite is a glucuronide thought to be conjugated to the 3-enol position of MPA.[24]

MPA is extensively metabolized in the liver by five primary pathways: hydroxylation at positions 6, 17 and 21; de-esterification and transesterification; demethylation; glucuronic acid conjugation and reduction. Only 5% of a dose is excreted unchanged in urine.

Over 26 metabolites have been identified but, where tested, these appear less active than MPA as progestins. The contribution of the metabolites as therapeutic agents in different disease states has not been studied.

Pharmaceutics

MPA is available in oral and parenteral forms.

1. Provera (Upjohn, UK/USA) is available as tablets containing medroxyprogesterone acetate 2.5, 5 and 10 mg in the USA, and 2.5, 5, 100, 200, 250, 400 and 500 mg in Europe. Farlutal (Farmitalia Carlo Erba, UK) is available at 250 and 500 mg.
2. Provera is also available as an oral suspension (400 mg MPA in 5 ml.
3. Depo-Provera (Upjohn, UK/USA) is supplied as a sterile aqueous suspension containing 100 mg.ml^{-1} in a 5 ml vial and 400 mg.ml^{-1} in 2.5 ml, 10 ml vial and in 1 ml disposable syringes (USA only), 150 mg.ml^{-1} in a 3 ml vial and 50 mg.ml^{-1} in 1 ml, 3 ml and 5 ml vials (Europe).

The preparations are stable with good shelf-life, but these factors

Fig. 1 Routes of medroxyprogesterone acetate metabolism

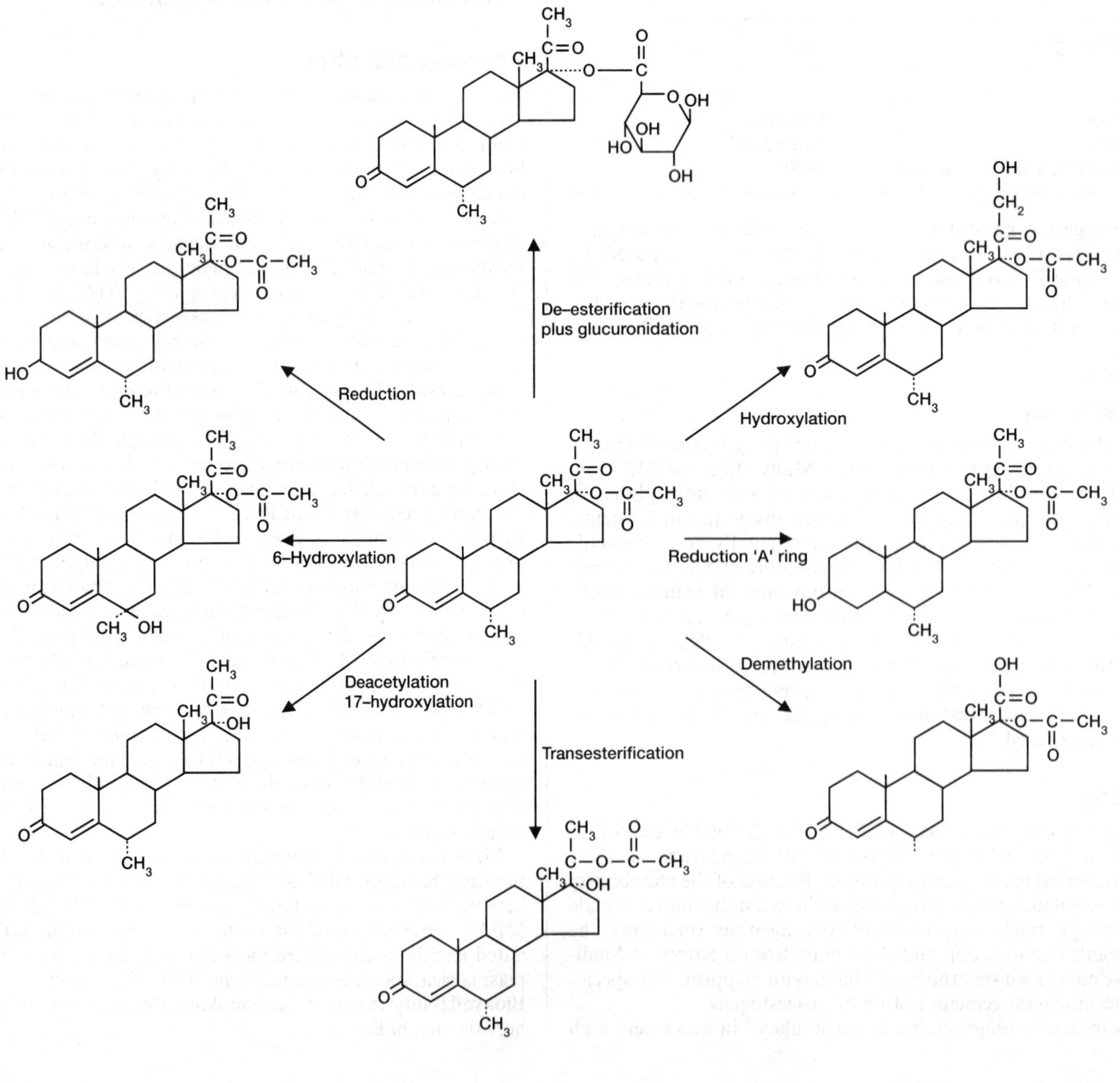

may vary between different generic preparations. The sterile aqueous suspension should be vigerously shaken before each use.

Therapeutic use

Indications

1. Contraception
2. The treatment of endometriosis
3. As adjunctive or palliative treatment of primary, recurrent or metastatic endometrial and renal carcinoma
4. The treatment of recurrent breast carcinoma
5. The regulation of dysfunctional uterine bleeding
6. The treatment of pelvic congestion.

Contraindications

There are few, because in general medroxyprogesterone acetate has been found to be an exceptionally safe drug with no serious side effects. Commonly accepted contraindications are:

1. Known sensitivity to medroxyprogesterone acetate
2. Undiagnosed abnormal uterine bleeding, haematuria and breast pathology before diagnosis
3. Pregnancy.

Conditions where special caution is required

4. History of phlebitis
5. Gross liver dysfunction.

Mode of use

MPA can be given orally (OMPA) or intramuscularly (DMPA). Both routes of administration achieve a similar concentration in the blood dose for dose. In general, OMPA is given for disorders requiring a short period of administration such as dysfunctional uterine bleeding, while DMPA is given for contraception. Although the intramuscular route has been widely used in the treatment of recurrent or metastatic carcinoma, it has no advantage over OMPA in terms of the blood concentration that can be achieved, and is obviously less acceptable to the patient.

Indications

1. Contraception

DMPA is used widely for contraception. Studies have shown that following a single injection of 150 mg of DMPA, the concentration of MPA remains above 1.0 $mg.l^{-1}$ for 2–3 months. Oritz et al[25] showed that at this concentration serum oestradiol levels remained low in the early to mid-follicular range, indicating suppression of normal follicular maturation. It appears that at this blood concentration the pattern of LH and FSH secretion is unaffected and it is only the midcycle surge of LH which is suppressed.[26] The recommended regimen of DMPA for contraception is 150 mg every three months. Salem and his co-workers[27] reported a randomized controlled trial comparing DMPA with Noristerat in 200 subjects. They found that DMPA at a dose 150 mg every 84–87 days was an effective contraceptive agent. Wilson[28] concluded that a dose of 200 mg every 105–112 days was a satisfactory contraceptive with continuation rates similar to those of the pill. These views are supported in a comprehensive review of injectable contraceptives by Fraser and Weisberg.[29]

Although there are no documented studies of MPA as an oral contraceptive agent, the study of Zelenyi et al[5] suggests that a dose above 10 mg a day would be effective for contraception.

2. Endometriosis

MPA is, in many ways, an ideal agent for the long-term treatment of endometriosis. It suppresses ovarian activity without inducing symptoms of severe oestrogen deficiency. It is also anti-androgenic.[30] Roland et al[31] treated 24 women using OMPA 30 mg a day for 90 days. Of these, 21 women became symptom free. Successful treatment appeared to be related to suppression of menses. The three women who were not cured continued to bleed intermittently vaginally.

3. Endometrial and renal carcinoma

Doses of 400 mg to 1000 mg of medroxyprogesterone acetate intramuscularly per week are recommended initially.[12] If improvement is noted within a few weeks or months and the disease appears stabilized, it may be possible to maintain improvement with as little as 400 mg per month. Medroxyprogesterone acetate is not recommended as primary therapy but as adjunctive and palliative treatment in advanced, inoperable cases and in recurrent or metastatic disease.

4. Breast cancer

The recommended dosage schedule is medroxyprogesterone acetate 400–600 mg daily orally or intramuscularly for 28 days.[12] The patient should then be placed on a maintenance schedule of up to 600 mg daily orally or 500 mg twice weekly intramuscularly as long as she is responding to treatment. Response to hormonal therapy for breast cancer may not be evident until after eight to ten weeks of therapy. Rapid progression of disease at any time during therapy should terminate treatment with medroxyprogesterone acetate.

5. Dysfunctional uterine bleeding

Systematic studies on the use of MPA for treating dysfunctional uterine bleeding are lacking, which is surprising in view of the central inhibitory effect of the drug on the release of gonadotrophins. Worstman et al[32] used a high dose of intramuscular MPA successfully to treat women with menstrual cycle irregularities and polycystic ovaries. Currently a dose of 2.5–10 mg daily in the last half of the cycle is recommended. Alternatively a low dose (2.5–5.0 mg a day) can be used continuously to treat women with irregular and/or heavy menses. OMPA 30–50 mg a day for 4 months has also been used successfully to treat women with cycle defects associated with cystic glandular hyperplasia or atypical hyperplasia of the endometrium. Unfortunately, good prospective studies of MPA in the treatment of menstrual cycle defects are lacking.

6. Pelvic congestion

Recent studies have shown that chronic lower abdominal pain in women is due to pelvic congestion.[33] OMPA has been used effectively to treat these women using doses of 30–50 mg a day for a minimum of 4 months.[34,35]

Adverse reactions

The anabolic and general side effects of MPA are extensively documented.[36] Unwanted side effects do not always follow a dose–response relationship. This is partly due to the many formulations of the drug. In general, MPA is well tolerated with easily controlled and infrequent side effects up to doses of 1000 mg a day.

Potentially life-threatening effects

Anaphylactic and anaphylactoid reactions have occasionally been reported in patients treated with Depo-Provera. Patients in whom signs and/or symptoms of thromboembolic disorders develop should be reevaluated before continuation of treatment.

Acute overdosage

High doses of MPA do not appear to be life-threatening.

Severe or irreversible adverse effects

In high dosage the drug may induce increased blood pressure, depression and thrombophlebitis.

Symptomatic adverse effects

Following repeated injections of MPA amenorrhoea and anovulation may persist for periods up to 18 months or longer in certain cases. At high doses (400 mg MPA daily or more) corticoid-like activity has been reported. This includes weight gain/fluid retention, Cushing's syndrome, slight tremors, muscular cramps, sweating, vaginal spotting, gluteal infiltration and hirsutism. When intramuscular injections are given, gluteal abscesses can occur. In most cases the symptoms clear if the dose is reduced or withdrawn. Other adverse effects include fatigue, insomnia, dizziness, headache, urticaria, rash, acne, hyperpylexia, depression, alopecia, nausea, breast tenderness, galactorrhoea, pain at injection site, and skin colour changes. A recent study[35] has shown that a dose of OMPA of 50 mg a day for 4 months is associated with a weight increase of 1.95 kg, which did not disappear up to 9 months after stopping treatment. Intermittent uterine bleeding ('spotting') can be troublesome at this dosage. No significant association with any other side effect was found.

Other effects

MPA, like other progestogens especially in the high doses used for cancer causes fluid retention and this may clinically influence other

Medroxyprogesterone acetate

conditions such as cardiac and renal dysfunction, epilepsy, migraine and asthma. MPA causes a decrease in glucose tolerance in some patients even at low dose but the reason for this is unknown. For this reason blood sugar in diabetic patients should be carefully monitored while on progestogen therapy.

Interference with clinical pathology tests
If endometrial or cervical tissue is submitted for examination the pathologist should be informed that the patient is on MPA. MPA can affect tests for liver function, gonadotrophin, progesterone, pregnanediol, testosterone, oestrogen, cortisol and glucose, and the metyrapone test. Hypercalcaemia can result during the management of breast cancer with MPA.

High risk groups

Neonates
No information is available on the use of MPA in neonates.

Breast milk. MPA is excreted into the breast milk of nursing mothers in concentrations similar to those in plasma. No special precautions are advised.

Children
Little information is available, but the drug has been used in the treatment of precocious puberty although this is not an approved use.

Pregnant women
The drug is contraindicated during pregnancy.

The elderly
No special precautions are needed other than those applicable to the younger age group.

Drug interactions

Potentially hazardous interactions
No interactions of this kind have been reported.

Other significant reactions

Food. Food appears to increase the bioavailability of MPA.

Alcohol. Alcohol appears to potentiate the effects of steroids which include MPA.

Smoking. Smoking reduces the bioavailability of steroids, presumably by enhancing liver metabolism.

Aminoglutethimide. When given uncomitantly, this drug significantly depresses the bioavailability of MPA.

Potentially useful interactions
In addition to the obvious interaction with oestrogens, MPA in high dose appears to make the use of other oncology agents more acceptable and more effective.[37] These include cyclophosphamide, methotrexate, tamoxifen, glutethimide, and 5-fluorouracil in breast cancer.

Major outcome trials

1. Wils J A, Bron H, Van Lange L et al 1985 A randomized comparative trial of combined versus alternating therapy with cytostatic drugs and high-dose medroxyprogesterone acetate in advanced breast cancer. Cancer 56: 1325

In a randomized, multi-centre trial, high-dose MPA was given either during or alternating with chemotherapy, to 155 patients with advanced breast cancer. The MPA dosage (intended to produce a high serum level within two weeks) was 600 mg orally on days 1 through 14, 500 mg intramuscularly on days 1 through 28, and twice weekly thereafter in the combination arm, vincristine. Adriamycin and cyclophosphamide were given intravenously on day 1 every four weeks in the alternating arm; the four-week cycles of the same chemotherapy were alternated with the above-mentioned MPA dose during eight weeks. Rates for complete plus partial response were 73% (26% CR) for the combination therapy groups and 76% (20% CR) for the alternating therapy group. Results in subsets of patients suggested that the alternating chemoendocrine approach may be better for ER-negative patients for those younger than 51 years, and for those with a disease-free interval of one year or less. No patient required dose reduction or postponement of therapy because of severe myelosuppression, and on day 14, patients receiving the combination therapy had leukocyte counts significantly higher ($p<0.005$) than the other group, suggesting a possible myeloprotective effect.

2. Izuo M, Yoshida M, Tominaga T et al 1985 A phase III trial of oral high-dose medroxyprogesterone acetate (MPA) versus mepitiostane in advanced postmenopausal breast cancer. Cancer 56: 2576

A double-blind controlled trial was performed to compare the therapeutic effects of oral high-dose MPA with those of mepitiostane (MS) in the treatment of women with postmenopausal breast cancer. MPA was given at a dosage of 1200 mg orally per day to 47 patients; 19 patients (40.4%) had an objective response; 14 (35.0%) of the 40 control patients given MS (20 mg orally per day) had an objective response. Among patients with bone metastases, 6 of 19 (31.6%) in the MPA group and 2 of 13 (15.4%) in the MS group had objective responses. Other benefits seen in the patients given MPA were improvement in performance status, increase in appetite, and myeloprotective effect.

Other studies

1. Silva A 1984 Medroxyprogesterone acetate versus tamoxifen in advanced breast cancer. Exhibit at 10th Congress of the European Society for Medical Oncology, Nice, France, 7–9 Dec 1984
2. Hortabagyi G, Buzdar A, Kau S et al 1985 Sequential combined hormonal therapy for metastatic breast cancer. Proceedings of ASCO vol 4, Mar 1985
3. Rendina G M, Donadio C, Fabri M et al 1984 Tamoxifen and medroxyprogesterone therapy for advanced endometrial cancer. European Journal of Obstetrics, Gynaecology and Reproductive Biology 17 (4): 285
4. Piver M S, Lele S B, Patsner B et al 1986 Melphalan, 5-fluorouracil, and medroxyprogesterone acetate in metastatic endometrial carcinoma. Obstetrics and Gynecology 67: 261

Other trials

The use of MPA as a contraceptive agent is well established. There are also many trials utilizing small numbers of patients in a variety of disease states, which should really be considered as pilot or hypothesis generating.

General review articles

Cavalli F, McGuire W L, Pannuti F, Pellegrini A, Robustelli Della Cuna G (eds) 1982 Proceedings of the International Symposium on MPA. Geneva, Switzerland, Feb 24-26, 1982. Excerpta Medica, IBSN 90 219 9560 3

Pellegrini A, Robustelli Della Cuna G, Pannuti F, Pouillart P, Jonat W (eds) 1984 Role of MPA in endocrine related tumours, vol 3. Raven Press, New York

Nash H 1975 Suppression of ovulation: a review. Contraception 12: 377

References

1. Biagi G L et al 1975 R-M values of steroids as an expression of their lipophilic character in structure H activity studies. Journal of Medicinal Chemistry 18: 873–883
2. Wied G R, Davis M E 1959 Obstetrics and Gynecology 14: 305
3. Kokko E, Jaenne O, Kauppila A et al 1982 Effects of tamoxifen, medroxyprogesterone acetate and their combination on human endometrial estrogen and progestin receptor concentrations, 17-beta hydroxy steroid dehydrogenase activity and serum hormone concentrations. American Journal of Obstetrics and Gynecology 143: 382
4. Izuo M 1982 Proceedings of the International Symposium on MPA, Geneva, Feb 1982, p 250
5. Zelenyi S, Aedo A R, Johanisson E, Landgren B M, Diczfalusy E 1986 Pituitary, ovarian and endometrial effects of graded doses of OMPA administered on cycle days 7–10. Contraception 33: 567–578
6. Stockdale A D, Rostom A Y 1989 Clinical significance of bioavailability of MPA preparations. Clinical Pharmacokinetics 16: 129–133
7. DiCarlo F, Pacillo G et al 1975 Tumori 61: 501
8. Nordqvist S 1972 Effect of progesterone on human endometrial carcinoma in different experimental systems. Acta Obstetrica Gynecologica Scandinavica 19: 25
9. Mould G P, Read J et al 1987 Comparison of HPLC and RIA measurements of MPA. Journal of Pharmaceutical and Biomedical Analysis (in press)
10. Information on file in Upjohn Limited

11. Johansson E D B et al 1986 Medroxyprogesterone acetate pharmacokinetics following oral high-dose administration in humans: a bioavailability evaluation of a new medroxyprogesterone acetate tablet formation. Acta Pharmacologica et Toxicologica 58: 311
12. Mathrubutham M, Fatherby K 1981 Medroxy progesterone acetate in human serum. Journal of Steroid Biochemistry 14: 783
13. Gupta C, Musto N A, Bullock L P et al 1977 The in vivo metabolism of progestins. Steroids 29: 669–677
14. Skatrud J B, Dempsey J A, Kaiser D G 1978 Ventilatory response to medroxyprogesterone acetate in normal subjects — time course and mechanism. Journal of Applied Physiology 44: 939
15. Besch P K, Vorys N, Ullery J C 1966 In-vivo metabolism of tritiated medroxyprogesterone acetate metab in pregnant and nonpregnant women and in the fetus. American Journal of Obstetrics and Gynecology 95: 288
16. Van Veelen H et al 1984 Adrenal suppression by oral high-dose medroxyprogesterone acetate breast cancer patients. Cancer Chemotherapy and Pharmacology 12: 83
17. Pannuti F et al 1982 Proceedings of the International Symposium on MPA, Geneva, Feb 1982, p 5
18. Fraser I S, Weisberg E 1981 A comprehensive review of injectable contraception with special emphasis on depot medroxyprogesterone acetate. Medical Journal of Australia special (suppl 1): 1
19. Tamassia V et al 1982 Pharmacokinetic approach to the selection of dose schedules for medroxyprogesterone acetate in clinical oncology. Cancer Chemotherapy and Pharmacology 8: 151
20. Hedley D W, Christie M, Whetherby R P et al 1987 Lack of correlations between plasma concentrations of MPA, hypothalamic–pituitary function and tumour response in patients with advanced breast cancer. Cancer Chemotherapy and Pharmacology (in press)
21. Stockdale A D et al 1987 Medroxyprogesterone acetate-variation in serum concentrations achieved with 3 commercially available preparations. Cancer Treatment Reports 71: 813
22. Ayoub J, Audet-Lapoint P, Methot Y et al 1984 Randomized trial of the addition of cyclical hormonal chemotherapy to conventional treatment for endometrial cancer. Proceedings ASCO 3: 167
23. Sturm G, Schulz K D 1984 MPA assays, measurement of plasma MPA levels in high dose MPA treated patients. In: Pellegrini A et al (eds) Role of medroxyprogesterone in endocrine related tumors, vol 3. Raven Press, New York, pp 23–42
24. Utaaker E, Lundgren S, Kvinnsland S, Aakvaag A 1988 Pharmacokinetics and metabolism of MPA in patients with advanced breast cancer. Journal of Steroid Biochemistry 31: 437–441
25. Oritz A, Hiroi M, Stanczyk F Z et al 1977 Serum medroxyprogesterone acetate concentrations and ovarian function following intramuscular injection of Depot MPA. Journal of Clinical Endocrinology and Metabolism 44: 32
26. Mishell D R, Kharma K M, Thorneycroft I M, Nakumura R H 1972 Estrogenic activity in women receiving an injectable progestogen for contraception. American Journal of Obstetrics and Gynecology 113: 372
27. Salem H T, Salah M, Aly M Y, Thabet A I, Shaaban M M, Fathalla M F 1988 Acceptability of injectable contraceptives in Assiut, Egypt. Contraception 38: 697–710
28. Wilson E 1976 Use of long acting DMPA in domiciliary family planning. British Medical Journal 2: 1435–1437
29. Fraser I S, Weisberg E 1981 A comprehensive reivew of injectable contraception with special emphasis on DMPA. Medical Journal of Australia 1 (suppl 1): 1–19
30. Nolten W E, Sholiton L J, Srivastava L S et al 1976 The effects of diethylstilbestrol and medroxyprogesterone acetate on kinetics and production rate of testosterone and dihydrotestosterone in patients with prostatic carcinoma. Journal of Clinical Endocrinology 22: 1018
31. Roland M, Leisten D, Kane R 1976 Endometriosis therapy with medroxyprogesterone acetate. Journal of Reproductive Medicine 17: 249–252
32. Worstman J, Singh K, Murray J 1981 Evidence for the hypothalamic origin of the polycystic ovary syndrome. Obstetrics and Gynaecology 58: 137–141
33. Beard R W, Highman J H, Pearce S, Reginald P W 1984 Diagnosis of pelvic varicosities in women with chronic pelvic pain. Lancet 2: 946–949
34. Reginald P W, Adams J, Franks S, Wadsworth J, Beard R W 1989 Medroxyprogesterone acetate in the treatment of pelvic pain due to venous congestion. British Journal of Obstetrics and Gynaecology 96: 1148–1152
35. Farquhar C M, Rogers V, Franks S, Pearce S, Wadsworth J, Beard R W 1989 A randomised controlled trial of medroxyprogesterone acetate and psychotherapy for the treatment of pelvic congestion. British Journal of Obstetrics and Gynaecology 96: 1153–1162
36. Hortobagyi G N, Buzdar A U, Frye D et al 1985 Oral MPA in the treatment of metastatic breast cancer. Breast Cancer Research and Treatment 5: 321–326
37. Ghilchik M W et al Cyclical sequential hormonotherapy in advanced breast cancer British Medical Journal 295: 1172

Mefenamic acid

This is a non-steroidal anti-inflammatory drug.

Chemistry

Mefenamic acid (Ponstan, Parkemed, Ponstel, Ponstyl)
N-(2,3-Xylyl) anthranilic acid
$C_{15}H_{15}NO_2$

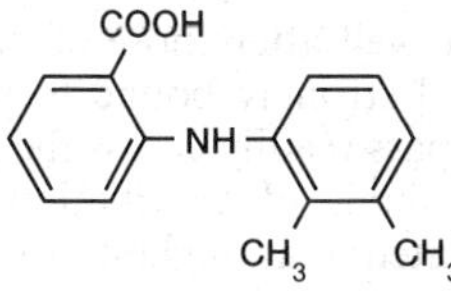

Molecular weight	241.3
pKa	4.2
Solubility	
in alcohol	1 in 185
in water	practically insoluble
Octanol/water partition coefficient	—

White or grey/white, odourless, tasteless, microcrystalline powder, soluble in alkali. Mefenamic acid is not available in combination preparations. It is prepared by chemical synthesis.

Pharmacology

Mefenamic acid inhibits the cyclooxygenase enzyme and thus exerts its anti-inflammatory activity by inhibition of prostaglandin synthesis. Mefenamic acid has antipyretic and analgesic properties acting by both central and peripheral mechanisms. This was originally demonstrated by studying the pain sensitivity of rats' paws when inflamed by brewer's yeast. A peripheral anti-inflammatory effect and an analgesic action in the sensory cortex was demonstrated by mefenamic acid in this model. In general its potency is about half that of phenylbutazone.[1] In addition to its actions as an inhibitor of prostaglandin synthesis, mefenamic acid antagonizes the $PGF_2\alpha$-induced contraction of isolated bronchial smooth muscle.[2]

Toxicology

Mefenamic acid does not have any known carcinogenic potential and is not teratogenic in mice or rats. Delayed parturition occurs in rats.

Clinical pharmacology

Mefenamic acid is an effective analgesic in doses up to 1.5 g daily. Its use as an analgesic may be because of its action on both central and peripheral pathways.[3] It has both anti-inflammatory and antipyretic effects. Mefenamic acid has no other significant effects in man.

Pharmacokinetics

The original analytical method involved fluorimetry. The current method of choice is high pressure liquid chromatography. A sensitivity in this assay method of 0.1 $mg.ml^{-1}$ can be expected.

Mefenamic acid is well absorbed after oral administration with peak plasma concentration occurring at 2–4 hours (see Fig. 1). A peak serum level of 10 $mg.l^{-1}$ occurs after a 1 g dose falling to low levels after 24 hours (0.1 $mg.l^{-1}$). The plasma half life is around 3 hours. There is no presystemic metabolism and peak levels of the two

Mefenamic acid

Fig. 1 Mean plasma levels of mefenamic acid and its metabolites in human subjects following single oral doses of 1 g (from: product information booklet Parke-Davis 1986).

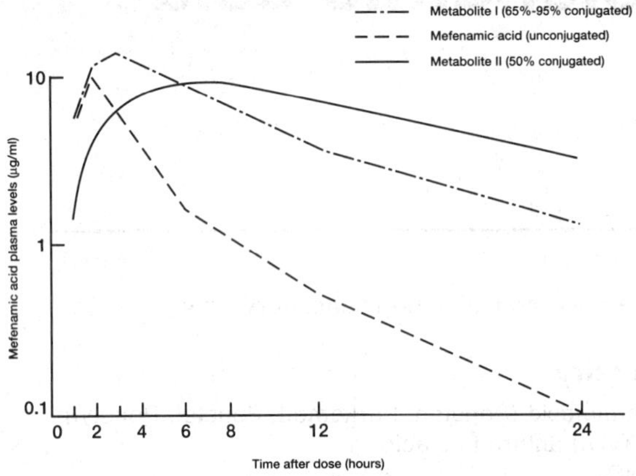

Fig. 2 Metabolism of mefenamic acid

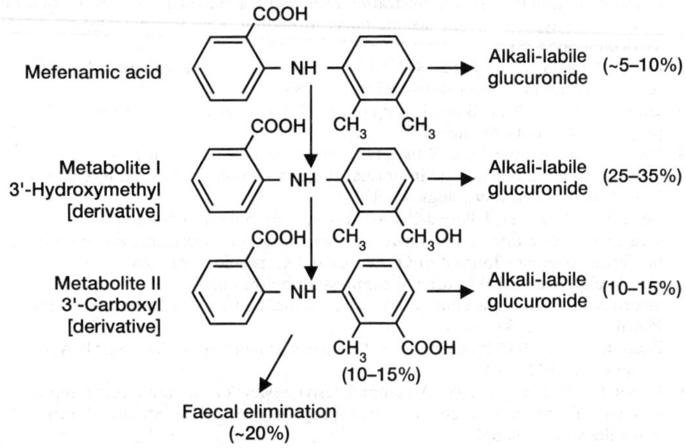

main metabolites occur well after those of mefenamic acid.[1] These three compounds are all strongly bound to plasma proteins (99%) though apparently can pass readily across the placental barrier in the rhesus monkey. The volume of distribution is 1.3 l.kg^{-1}. Animal studies have demonstrated that highest tissue levels occur in the kidney, liver and the gastrointestinal tract. A relatively small proportion passes into the brain. Very low levels appear in human breast milk. Mefenamic acid is apparently not dialysable.

Oral absorption	>90%
Presystemic metabolism	0
Plasma half life	
range	3–4 h
Volume of distribution	1.3 l.kg^{-1}
Plasma protein binding	99%

Concentration–effect relationship

There is no evidence of any correlation between the plasma concentration and the therapeutic effect of mefenamic acid.

Multiple-dose trials show that steady-state levels of drug in biological fluids is reached within 2–3 days, falling off promptly following termination of dosing.[4]

Metabolism

In man between 50 and 70% of a dose of mefenamic acid is excreted in the urine as conjugates of glucuronic acid almost, none excreted is unchanged drug. In urine, approximately half is the conjugated 3-hydroxymethyl derivative (metabolite I), and a little less than half is the 3-carboxyl derivative (metabolite II) and its conjugates. The remaining 10% is mostly conjugated mefenamic acid. 20% of the drug is recovered in the faeces mainly as unconjugated metabolite. Mefenamic acid is metabolized extensively in the liver into the two principal derivatives mentioned above and as shown in Fig. 2.

Metabolite I peaks somewhat later (see Fig. 1) than mefenamic acid and does not disappear as rapidly from the plasma; metabolite II peaks still later at 6–8 hours after an oral dose. Metabolite I is usually present in the form of an alkali-labile conjugate; approximately 50% of metabolite II is similarly conjugated. Neither derivative has significant pharmacological activity. Less than 5% of an oral dose is excreted in bile.

Pharmaceutics

Mefenamic acid is available only as an oral form. Yellow film-coated ovoid tablets containing 500 mg of mefenamic acid are inscribed 'Ponstan Forte' (Parke-Davis, UK) on one side. Ponstan (Parke-Davis, UK) capsules 250 mg contain an off-white powder in a No 1 hard gelatine shell with an ivory opaque body and aqua blue opaque cap and are radially printed 'Ponstan 250'. Ponstel (Parke-Davis, US) capsules are pale yellow with a tamper-proof blue seal. The cap is coded 'PD 540' and the proprietary name is printed on the base. Ponstan D tablets (Parke-Davis, UK) are flat, round, blue tablets containing 250 mg mefenamic acid. These dispersible tablets should be added to half a tumblerful of water before administration. They are marked 'Ponstan D' on one side.

A paediatric suspension contains mefenamic acid BP 50 mg in 5 ml. It is off-white with a banana-mint-chocolate flavour.

All preparations should be stored at below 30°C. The maximum shelf-life of available preparations is indicated by an expiry date.

Therapeutic use

Indications

1. As an anti-inflammatory analgesic for the symptomatic relief of rheumatoid arthritis (including juvenile chronic arthritis), osteoarthritis, and pain including muscular, traumatic and dental pain, headaches of most aetiology including migraine, postoperative and post partum pain
2. Analgesia and Pyrexia in children
3. Primary dysmenorrhoea
4. Menorrhagia due to dysfunctional causes and presence of an IUD when other pelvic pathology has been ruled out.

Contraindications

1. Inflammatory bowel disease
2. Peptic and/or intestinal ulceration
3. Renal and hepatic impairment
4. Asthma.

Indications

1. Analgesia

Mefenamic acid is an analgesic. A 500 mg dose should be given to adults and repeated up to three times (1.5 g total) per day. It may also be used in this dose for its anti-inflammatory properties in rheumatoid arthritis where it decreases joint tenderness, pain score duration and severity of morning stiffness. In osteoarthritis it improves stiffness, pain and function.

Mefenamic acid is also useful for controlling pain following extraction of teeth, endodontic therapy and dental surgery in general.[25]

Mefenamic acid has shown itself as effective as dextropropoxyphene/paracetamol in relief of low back pain[26] and equally effective in treatment of pain arising from soft tissue injuries and infections.

2. Children

Analgesia. Mefenamic acid may be used in the long-term treatment of juvenile chronic arthritis but it is otherwise not recommended for use longer than 7 days. The following dose regime is recommended using a paediatric suspension (50 mg per 5 ml).
Infants over six months: 25 mg.kg^{-1} of body weight daily in divided doses, i.e. six months to one year, one 5 ml spoonful.
2–4 years: 2 × 5 ml spoonfuls
5–8 years: 3 × 5 ml spoonfuls
9–12 years: 4 × 5 ml spoonfuls
These doses may be repeated as necessary up to three times daily.

Mefenamic acid

Pyrexia. Several studies suggest mefenamic acid provides an equally effective alternative to paracetamol and aspirin in the treatment of pyrexia in children. The usual dose is 4 $mg.kg^{-1}$ of body weight.[5]

3. Primary dysmenorrhoea
Mefenamic acid has been shown to be more effective than narcotic analgesics in the relief of symptoms in primary dysmenorrhoea when given at a dose of 500 mg three times daily for the duration of menstrual bleeding.[6] It has no effect on hormone levels. Primary spasmodic dysmenorrhoea results from incoordinate hyperactivity of the uterus resulting in uterine ischaemia and pain due to increased synthesis of endometrial prostaglandins. Mefenamic acid reduces uterine contractions by $>60\%$.[27]

4. Menorrhagia
Prostaglandins are involved in the process of myometrial contractions and endometrial shedding which accompanies menstruation. Haynes[20] found menorrhagic patients had higher levels of endometrial PGE_2 and $PGE_2\alpha$ in the premenstrual phase of the cycle compared to women with normal blood loss. Mefenamic acid significantly reduces blood loss. It should be given in standard dosage (500 mg three times daily for adults) starting on the first day of excessive bleeding and continued usually for five to seven days.

Contraindications

1. Inflammatory bowel disease
Diarrhoea is an occasional side effect of mefenamic acid therapy and may be associated with the development of proctocolitis in patients who continue to take the drug in the presence of persistent diarrhoea.

2. Peptic ulceration
All non-steroidal anti-inflammatory drugs (NSAIDs) have been associated with an increased risk of gastric and duodenal ulceration. Both bleeding[7] and perforation[8] may occur and all drugs in this class should be avoided in patients with active peptic ulceration and should only be given to patients with a previous history of gastric or duodenal ulcer, or to the elderly, after full consideration of other forms of treatment.

3. Renal and hepatic impairment
As a class, NSAIDs are known to affect hepatic and renal function in some patients and it is therefore inadvisable to administer them in the presence of pre-existing organ impairment. Very few case reports of hepatic injury due to mefenamic acid have been reported however. There have been abnormal enzyme tests but these have not permitted the identification or mechanism of injury.[29]

4. Asthma
Bronchospasm is precipitated in a minority of patients, in particular, those who are aspirin sensitive. This is also likely to occur in association with nasal polyps and late-onset asthma.[9,10]

Adverse reactions

Potentially life-threatening effects
Deaths caused by mefenamic acid are rare. NSAIDs as a class have principally been associated with deaths from haematological, gastrointestinal and hepatic adverse effects. Leucopenia, thrombocytopenia, agranulocytosis, pancytopenia, marrow hypoplasia and reversible autoimmune haemolysis have been associated with treatment with mefenamic acid.[11]

Acute overdosage
Deliberate overdose has been increasing though no deaths have yet been reported. Large doses produce excitement, incoordination, depression and convulsions in mice.[12] Grand mal convulsions appear to be the most regularly observed adverse effect in man.[13] These are commonly preceded by focal or generalized muscle twitching. If ingestion is recent, forced emesis or gastric lavage should be performed and activated charcoal then given (0.5 $g.kg^{-1}$) which may considerably reduce absorption.[4] Careful observation during the first few hours is recommended as convulsions are most likely to occur during this period. Very high serum levels may be associated with repeated convulsions which have been successfully suppressed with intravenous diazepam.[14]

Severe or irreversible adverse effects
Diarrhoea may occur early on or after several months. Prolonged use of the drug has been associated with proctocolitis and enteritis,[15] which may be complicated by steatorrhoea.[16,17] The drug should be withdrawn immediately and not given again should diarrhoea occur. Studies have compared incidence and severity of diarrhoea at dosages of 1 g, 2 g and 4 g daily. The number of subjects with diarrhoea increases, but not the severity. At 1 g daily 1 of 99 subjects have diarrhoea. At 4 g daily 8 of 25 patients have diarrhoea.[30] Continued use of mefenamic acid in patients with diarrhoea has been associated with proctocolitis. Large bowel perforation has been described.[22]

Renal impairment may occur via several mechanisms including renal hypoperfusion, interstitial nephritis[18] and non-oliguric renal failure, which is more likely in elderly dehydrated patients.[19,20] Acute tubular necrosis may supervene. Inhibition of important autoregulatory renal prostaglandins is thought responsible for some of these effects and for the relatively more frequent, mild, reversible elevation of blood urea seen in about 6% of patients taking mefenamic acid at a dose of 1 g per day.[21]

Dyspepsia and peptic ulceration which may be complicated by haemorrhage or perforation may occur. Mefenamic acid causes significantly less blood loss (1.7 ml per day) than aspirin (5 ml per day). The loss with ibuprofen is 2.6 ml per day and placebo 0.4 ml per day.[31]

Symptomatic adverse effects
Mefenamic acid is usually well tolerated though drowsiness and dizziness are well recognized. Skin rashes have been observed at all dose levels and therapy should be withdrawn should they occur.

Interference with clinical pathology tests
False positive tests for the presence of bile in the urine may occur due to the presence of the drug itself and its metabolites.

High risk groups

Neonates
Mefenamic acid is not recommended for use in neonates.

Breast milk. Very small amounts enter breast milk and may be transmitted to infants of nursing mothers.[23]

Children
In children from six months to twelve years, mefenamic acid is not recommended for use for longer than seven days, except in the treatment of juvenile chronic arthritis.

Pregnant women
The safety of mefenamic acid in pregnancy has not been established.

The elderly
Normal adult doses have been used in trials containing elderly subjects although no specific trials have been performed. Both renal and haematological adverse effects appear to be more prevalent in the elderly.[18,24] The minimum effective dose should be used and treatment stopped in the presence of diarrhoea or dehydration.

Drug interactions

Potentially hazardous interactions
Slight potentiation of oral anticoagulants is well documented,[21] but this is rarely significant.

Other significant interactions
The fenamates bind strongly to plasma proteins and therefore competition for non-specific binding sites on plasma albumin may occur.

Potentially useful interactions
No reactions of this kind have been reported.

Major outcome trials

Several clinical studies support the efficacy of mefenamic acid as an analgesic in inflammatory and non-inflammatory musculo-skeletal conditions.

1. Leslie D G 1977 Mefenamic acid compared with ibuprofen in the treatment of rheumatoid arthritis. Journal of International Medical Research 5: 161–163

A randomized double-blind within-patient study of mefenamic acid

M

compared with ibuprofen performed in 40 patients with rheumatoid arthritis concluding that analgesic, anti-inflammatory and side effects were similar.

2. Buchmann E 1966 Mefenamic acid compared with indomethacin and placebo in osteo-arthritis. Journal Phys Med 29: 119

A randomized double-blind study in 59 patients with osteoarthritis demonstrated similar symptomatic relief using mefenamic acid 500 mg and indomethacin 25 mg both given three times daily. Side effects were similar in each group.

3. Frazer I S, Pearse C, Shearman R P, Elliot T M, McIlveen J, Malcolm R 1981 Efficacy of mefenamic acid in patients with a complaint of menorrhagia. Obstetrics and Gynaecology 51: 543–551

A double-blind randomized placebo-controlled cross-over study of mefenamic acid performed in 69 patients who gave a history of menorrhagia was performed over 4 cycles. A definition of menorrhagia is given. A mean overall reduction in menstrual blood loss of 28.1% between placebo and mefenamic acid was seen. This varied with the underlying conditions and these are discussed.

References

1. Winder C V 1966 Pharmacology of the fenamates. Experimental observations of flufenamic, mefenamic and meclofenamic acids. I Pharmacology. Annals of Physical Medicine (suppl): 7–16
2. Collier H O J, Sweatman W J F 1968 Antagonism by fenamates of prostaglandin $F_{2\alpha}$ and of slow reacting substance on human bronchial muscle. Nature 219: 864–865
3. Winder C V 1959 Aspirin and algesimetry. Nature 184: 494–497
4. Glazko A J 1966 Pharmacology of the fenamates. Experimental observations on flufenamic, mefenamic and meclofenamic acids. III Metabolic disposition. Annals of Physical Medicine (suppl): 23–36
5. Simila S, Kouvalainen K, Keinanen S 1977 Oral antipyretic therapy: evaluation of mefenamic acid. Arzneimittelforschung 27: 687–688
6. Anderson A B M, Fraser L S, Haynes P J, Turnbull A C 1978 Trial of prostaglandin synthetase inhibitors in primary dysmenorrhoea. Lancet 1: 345–348
7. Somerville K, Faulkner G, Langman M 1986 Non-steroidal anti-inflammatory drugs and bleeding peptic ulcer. Lancet 1: 462–464
8. Walt R, Katschinski B, Logan R, Ashley J, Langman M 1986 Rising frequency of ulcer perforation in elderly people in the United Kingdom. Lancet 1: 489–492
9. Chafee F H, Settipane G A 1974 Aspirin intolerance I. Frequency in an allergic population. Journal of Allergy and Clinical Immunology 53: 193
10. Settipane G A, Chafee F H, Klein D E 1974 Aspirin intolerance II. A prospective study in an atopic and normal population. Journal of Allergy and Clinical Immunology 53: 200
11. Anon 1978 Around North America with mefenamic acid. Medical Letters and Drugs Therapeutics 20: 104
12. Kaump D H 1966 Pharmacology of the fenamates. Experimental observations on flufenamic, mefenamic and meclofenamic acids. II. Toxicology in animals. Annals of Physical Medicine (suppl): 16–23
13. Ballali-Mood M, Proudfoot A T, Critchley J A J H, Prescott L F 1981 Mefenamic acid overdosage. Lancet 1: 1354–1356
14. Shipton E A, Miller F O 1985 Severe mefenamic acid poisoning. South African Medical Journal 67: 823–824
15. Hall R I, Petty A H, Cobden I, Lendrum R 1983 Enteritis and colitis associated with mefenamic acid. British Medical Journal 287: 1182
16. Marks J S, Gleeson M H 1975 Steatorrhoea complicating therapy with mefenamic acid. British Medical Journal 4: 442
17. Chadwick R G, Hossenbocus A, Colin-James D G 1976 Steatorrhoea complicating therapy with mefenamic acid. British Medical Journal 1: 397
18. Adams D H, Michael J, Bacon P A, Howie A J, McConkey B, Adu D 1986 Non-steroidal anti-inflammatory drugs and renal failure. Lancet 1: 57–59
19. Taha A, Lenton R J, Murdoch P S, Peden N R 1985 Non-oliguric renal failure during treatment with mefenamic acid in elderly patients: a continuing problem. British Medical Journal 291: 661–662
20. Poultan S, Craft T, Severs M 1985 Non-oliguric renal failure during treatment with mefenamic acid in elderly patients. (Letter) British Medical Journal 291: 1048
21. Holmes E L 1966 Pharmacology of the fenamates. Experimental observations on flufenamic, mefenamic and meclofenamic acids. IV Toleration by normal human subjects. Annals of Physical Medicine (suppl): 36–49
22. Langman M J S, Morgan L, Worrall A 1985 Use of anti-inflammatory drugs by patients admitted with small or large bowel perforation and haemorrhage. British Medical Journal 290: 347–349
23. Buchanan R A, Eaton C J, Koeff S T, Kinkel A W 1968 The breast milk excretion of mefenamic acid. Current Therapeutic Research 10: 592–596
24. Burns A, Young R F 1984 Mefenamic acid induced leucopenia in the elderly. (Letter) Lancet 2: 46
25. Steinhauser E 1970 Application of Ponstan in painful and inflammatory conditions after dental surgery. Schweizerische Monatsschrift fur Zahnheileunde 80: 341–350
26. Evans D P, Burke M S, Newcombe R E 1980 Medicines of choice in low back pain. Current Medical Research and Opinion 6: 540–547
27. Smith R P, Powell J R 1982 Intrauterine pressure changes during dysmenorrhoea therapy. American Journal of Obstetrics and Gynecology 143: 286–292
28. Haynes P J et al 1980 Studies in menorrhagia. International Journal of Gynaecology and Obstetrics 17: 567–572
29. Lewis J H 1984 Hepatic toxicity of nonsteroidal anti-inflammatory drugs. Clinical Pharmacy 3: 128–137
30. Winder C V, Kaump D H, Glazko A J, Holmes E L 1966 Pharmacology of the fenamates. Annals of the Physical Medicine Symposium (suppl): 7–49
31. Bown R L, Martin B K 1983 Occult blood loss: a comparative study of mefanamic acid, ibuprofen and aspirin. Royal Society of Medicine International Congress Symposia Series 66: 15–21

Mefloquine (hydrochloride)

Mefloquine was the first synthetic quinolinemethanol compound to be introduced as an antimalarial drug.

Chemistry

Mefloquine hydrochloride (Lariam, Mephaquine)
$C_{17}H_{16}N_2OF_6.HCl$
(RS)-α-(2-Piperidyl)-2,8-bis(trifluoromethyl)-4-quinolinemethanol hydrochloride

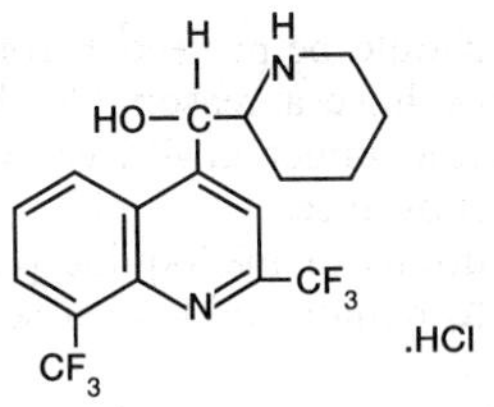

Molecular weight	
hydrochloride	414.8
(free base)	379.3
pKa (piperidyl group)	8.6
Solubility	
in alcohol	1 in 6
in water	1 in 250
Octanol/water partition coefficient	—

Mefloquine is a white odourless, amorphous powder with a brackish, slightly bitter taste. It is prepared by chemical synthesis and the racemate is used clinically. Mefloquine has also been produced as an oral combination with sulphadoxine and pyrimethamine (Fansimef).

Pharmacology

Mefloquine is believed to act against malaria parasites in a way similar to that of quinine to which it is structurally related. Its activity is directed against the parasite's protein metabolism during the intraerythrocytic trophozoite stage. Mefloquine is a potent and relatively fast-acting antimalarial drug. However, the lack of a formulation for parenteral administration restricts its use in the treatment of severe and complicated falciparum malaria. Mefloquine sensitivity is independent of resistance to 4-aminoquinolines and dihydrofolate reductase inhibitors.

Toxicology

Mefloquine showed no mutagenic potential in the standard test systems. Long-term studies in various animal species provided no evidence of carcinogenic or teratogenic activity. Animals given three times the human treatment dose daily for more than one month showed non-specific abnormalities of hepatic and renal function,[1] but at clinically relevant doses there were no toxic manifestations in rats, mice, dogs and monkeys.

Clinical pharmacology

Mefloquine is a blood schizontocidal drug with high affinity for erythrocyte membranes[2] where it preferentially binds with phospholipids.[3] It does not intercalate with DNA even at high concentrations.[4] Haemoglobin was found to bind mefloquine with low affinity, but exchange of the drug between haemoglobin and the erythrocyte membrane is rapid.[5] It has been proposed that uptake of mefloquine by infected erythrocytes is electrogenic, with both the proton gradient and the electrical potential contributing to the driving force.[6] The concentration of mefloquine in infected red blood cells is higher than that in non-infected erythrocytes. This is obviously due in part to the presence of phospholipids in the parasites, but also, more importantly, to binding with ferriprotoporphyrin IX (haematin) which is formed in the course of haemoglobin degradation by plasmodia. The mefloquine–ferriprotoporphyrin IX complex is toxic for the malaria parasite and believed to interfere with protease and peptidase activity in the acid environment of the parasite's food vacuoles. It is not known whether the mefloquine enantiomers have equal antimalarial activity.

Mefloquine is a non-competitive inhibitor of acetylcholinesterase and butyrylcholinesterase.[7] This may account for side effects involving the gastrointestinal system (e.g. nausea and vomiting) and central nervous system (e.g. hallucinations and disorientation) observed at relatively high drug concentrations. Since the inhibition of acetylcholinesterase is stereospecific, it is possible that the inhibitory effect of mefloquine may be greater with one of the enantiomers.[7]

At therapeutic concentrations mefloquine did not alter the proliferative responses of human lymphocytes to malaria antigens, pokeweed mitogen, concanavalin A and *Candida albicans*, but it significantly suppressed the response to phyto-haemagglutinin.[8]

Pharmacokinetics

Gas chromatographic methods for the determination of mefloquine use derivatization and electron capture or mass spectrographic detection. One such method has a detection limit of 13 $nmol.l^{-1}$.[9] An HPLC method using direct injection of plasma following precolumn enrichment and column switching techniques measures mefloquine and its main metabolite with a detection limit of 25 $nmol.l^{-1}$ for both substances.[10]

Following oral administration of mefloquine tablets (LARIAM), approximately 75–80% is absorbed, and peak plasma concentrations are observed after 2–12 hours. In fasting volunteers the apparent half life of absorption of mefloquine ranged from 0.36 to 2.0 hours.[11] In comatose malaria patients who had been given the drug by nasogastric tube, the mean values of absorption half life in two series were 1.8 and 1.5 hours.[12] Presystemic metabolism is negligible. The plasma half life is the longest so far observed in any antimalarial drug, with a range of 15–33 days and a mean of 21.4 days.[13] There is a significant difference in the elimination half life of mefloquine in healthy volunteers and patients with acute falciparum malaria.[14,15] Similarly, the whole blood and plasma mefloquine concentrations are higher in malaria patients as compared with healthy subjects.[15] Individual variation in plasma and whole blood concentration tends to be high.

Mefloquine, a highly lipid-soluble drug, is widely and rapidly distributed throughout the body, with an apparent volume of distribution of 16–25 $l.kg^{-1}$, indicative of drug accumulation in various tissues. There is a contraction of the volume of distribution of mefloquine in acute malaria, with mean values of 15.7 ± 4.9 $l.kg^{-1}$ in malaria patients, and 19.2 ± 7.0 in healthy subjects.[15] Mefloquine shows a high affinity for lung, liver and lymphoid tissue[16,17] and it has been suggested that apparent ethnic differences in the elimination half life of mefloquine are in fact to be ascribed to differences in the extent of body fat stores.[18] Mefloquine is highly bound (>98%) to plasma proteins.

Although lipid-soluble, mefloquine was not detectable in the CSF in samples from 17 patients all of whom had therapeutic mefloquine plasma concentrations.[12] Thus, mefloquine does not seem to cross the blood–brain barrier to any significant degree, which may be explained by the fact that the drug is highly protein bound. Mefloquine was detectable in the peritoneal dialysate of 3 patients with therapeutic mefloquine plasma concentrations.[12]

Mefloquine is excreted in breast milk. The milk-to-plasma ratio of mefloquine based on the area under the plasma and milk concentration curves was 0.13 and 0.16.[29] The amount of drug taken up by an infant through breast milk is far below the therapeutic or prophylactic level. Little is known about placental transfer of mefloquine in humans, but such transfer seems probable on account of its high lipid solubility.

Oral absorption	75–80%
Presystemic metabolism	negligible
Plasma half life	
range	15–33 days
mean	21.4 days
Volume of distribution	16–25 l.kg^{-1}
Plasma protein binding	>95%

A significant proportion of mefloquine undergoes hepatic transformation, mainly to 2,8-bis(trifluoromethyl)-4-quinoline carboxylic acid. Observations in steady state indicated that 9% of the drug is excreted unchanged in the urine. The carboxylic acid metabolite in urine accounted for 4% of the dose.[19] The bulk of mefloquine is eliminated through the bile in faeces. There is evidence of enterohepatic recirculation.

Studies of mefloquine pharmacokinetics in patients with renal and hepatic dysfunction have not yet been completed.

There are no published reports of the pharmacokinetics of mefloquine in children and pregnant women. Preliminary results in Thai children suffering from falciparum malaria indicate a relatively short elimination half life similar to that in malarious adults.[20]

A single therapeutic dose of 750 mg (base) produced peak plasma mefloquine concentrations of 1.69–6.60 μmol.l^{-1} in healthy Thai subjects and 2.25–7.97 μmol.l^{-1} in Thai malaria patients.[15]

With weekly prophylactic adult doses of 250 mg (base) steady state was reached within 8 weeks. The individual mean concentrations between the 8th and 22nd week varied between 1.49 and 3.30 μmol.l^{-1}, with a group mean of 1.98 μmol.l^{-1}.[21] Differences between trough and peak levels are relatively small as would be expected from the long half life of mefloquine.

The mefloquine concentrations in red blood cells are approximately twice those found in plasma.[11]

Concentration–effect relationship

As with the other blood schizontocidal drugs, mefloquine shows a distinct concentration–effect relationship against *Plasmodium falciparum*. This can be demonstrated in vitro. The response pattern for a natural *P. falciparium* population is log-dose normal.[22] Most of the *P. falciparum* isolates throughout the species' distribution are fully inhibited at a concentration of 1.6 μmol.l^{-1}. Schizont maturation at a concentration of 6.4 μmol.l blood can be considered as a sign of resistance.[22] Natural resistance of *P. falciparum* to mefloquine occurs sporadically throughout the species' distribution, but so far has not been a major practical problem. In areas where mefloquine is routinely used for treating the majority of *P. falciparum* infections, e.g. in Thailand, a problem may evolve when the MIC of mefloquine approaches the therapeutic concentrations of mefloquine.

Metabolism

A significant proportion of mefloquine, but probably less than half, is metabolized in the liver. Excretion is mainly through the bile into the faeces, but approximately 9% of a dose is eliminated unchanged in the urine.

Mefloquine is metabolized by hydrolytic loss of the piperidyl moiety and conversion to 2,8-bis(trifluoromethyl)-4-quinolinemethanol and the main metabolite, 2,8-bis(trifluoromethyl)-4-quinoline carboxylic acid (Fig. 1). Both metabolites are devoid of antimalarial activity. The main metabolite usually becomes detectable four hours after oral administration of mefloquine. The concentrations rise rapidly to levels higher than those of the parent drug, to reach a peak within two weeks.[21] It has only about 1/30 of the volume of distribution of mefloquine, but virtually the same half life. In rats and mice it has the same oral toxicity as mefloquine.

A multiple dose kinetic study with weekly doses of 250 mg (base) mefloquine provided no evidence of enzyme induction. In steady state the ratio of main metabolite to parent drug varied between 2.78 and 10.20, with a mean of 5.56.

Fig. 1 The metabolism of mefloquine

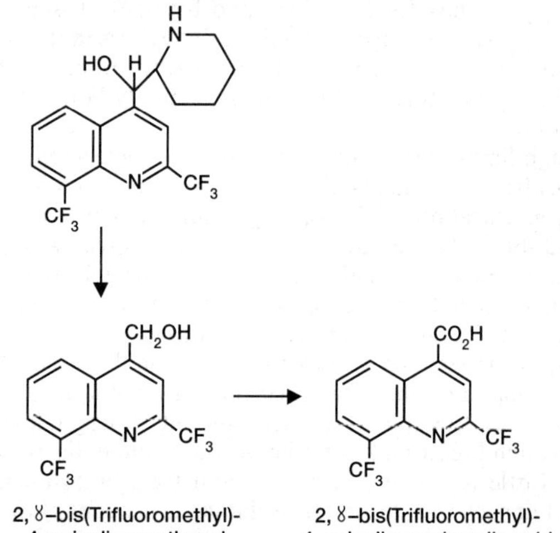

Pharmaceutics

Mefloquine, Lariam (Roche, UK) is available in an oral form only. Cross-scored white tablets containing mefloquine hydrochloride corresponding to 250 mg base content, packed in sealstrips or brown glass bottles.

Mefloquine tablets should be protected from light.

Properly stored, they have a reasonable shelf-life and, provided they have been produced under GMP, carry a minimal risk from potentially allergenic substances.

Sterile aqueous solutions of mefloquine prepared for laboratory purposes were found to remain stable over several years.[23]

Therapeutic use

Indications

1. Treatment of falciparum malaria
2. Malaria chemoprophylaxis in areas with chloroquine-resistant *P. falciparum*.

Contraindications

1. Treatment with quinine or quinidine during the preceding 24 hours
2. Treatment with cardioactive medicaments, such as β-blockers
3. Pregnancy
4. Use in infants
5. Prophylaxis in patients with renal insufficiency and severe impairment of hepatic function
6. Prophylaxis in occupational groups where fine co-ordination and spatial discrimination are essential.

Mode of use

Therapeutically, mefloquine is given by mouth in an adult dose of 15–25 mg base.kg^{-1} body weight. The dose for children is 25 mg.kg^{-1} body weight. Adults taking a low dose and children may be given a single dose, but for better tolerance adult doses over 750 mg (3 tablets) are divided, giving 3 tablets first, and the rest after 6–8 hours. Heavy patients requiring treatment with 6 tablets should receive 3 tablets first, 2 tablets 6–8 hours later, and 1 tablet after another interval of 6–8 hours.

For prophylaxis in adults, mefloquine is used in weekly doses of 250 mg (base). If prophylaxis with mefloquine is to be extended beyond 3 weeks, the weekly dose should be reduced to 125 mg in order to avoid excessive and potentially toxic drug levels. The corresponding doses for persons weighing less than 50 kg are 5 mg.kg^{-1} body weight weekly for the first three weeks, and 2.5 mg.kg^{-1} weekly as from the 4th week onward. Prophylaxis with mefloquine should be limited to 6 months.

Indications

1. Treatment of falciparium malaria

Mefloquine is an alternative drug for the treatment of falciparum malaria. Its use is indicated in *P. falciparum* infections which failed to respond adequately to chloroquine and/or sulfadoxine/pyrimethamine, or as a first line treatment of falciparum malaria if the infection was contracted in an area with a high prevalence of resistance to

Mefloquine (hydrochloride)

chloroquine and sulfadoxine/pyrimethamine. Hypersensitivity to chloroquine or sulfadoxine is also an indication for the use of mefloquine.

Infections with *P. vivax*, *P. ovale* and/or *P. malariae* do not require treatment with mefloquine since they respond to chloroquine which is both cheaper and better tolerated. However, where one or more of these species are associated with a *P. falciparum* infection that needs to be treated with mefloquine, no additional blood schizontocidal therapy is required since *P. vivax*, *P. ovale* and *P. malariae* respond adequately to mefloquine. Patients with *P. vivax* or *P. ovale* infections should also receive a course of primaquine for antirelapse treatment.

Infants below 1 year of age should not be given mefloquine. Children generally tolerate the drug better than adults. Mefloquine has not yet been cleared for use during pregnancy.

Vomiting is often associated with malaria. It may also be induced by mefloquine. This may lead to the loss of an undetermined quantity of the drug. Replacement dosing is contraindicated, as the absorbed amount of drug is unknown and the additional dose may cause toxic manifestations. In these cases clinical and parasitological response need to be monitored carefully.

Patients treated with mefloquine, especially with relatively high doses, may show deficiencies in spatial perception and fine co-ordination; these may last for up to four weeks.

2. Malaria chemoprophylaxis in areas with chloroquine-resistant *P. falciparum*

Mefloquine can be used for malaria prophylaxis against *P. falciparum*; its activity consists of a suppression of blood schizogony followed by suppressive cure if dose and duration of prophylaxis are adequate and the parasites sensitive. This does not exclude post-prophylaxis relapses of *P. vivax* or *P. ovale* since mefloquine lacks activity against hypnozoites.

Although experiences with mefloquine prophylaxis span up to two years, it is generally not recommended to extend the prophylactic use beyond 6 months. In view of the long half life of the drug and very marked individual differences in the pharmacokinetic parameters, including plasma concentration, there is a risk that toxic levels may be reached in some persons.

The most frequent prophylactic use of mefloquine is in short-term visits of non-immune travellers to areas with considerable malaria risk and where *P. falciparum* is resistant to chloroquine and/or sulfadoxine/pyrimethamine.

Pregnant women and children below 15 kg body weight should not be given mefloquine prophylaxis (for other exclusions see Contraindications).

Prophylaxis should start one week before exposure to malaria risk and continue until two weeks after last exposure. Dosages are as follows:

Adults (> 15kg) — 250 mg weekly (1 tablet)
Children 15–19 kg — 62.5 mg (1/4 tablet)
20–30 kg — 125 mg (1/2 tablet)
30–40 kg — 187.5 mg (3/4 tablet)

If the stay in the malarious area exceeds 3 weeks, the weekly dose should be halved as from the fourth week, or the dose interval extended to 2 weeks (maintaining the above mentioned dose level).

The medicament should be taken after a meal and with plenty of liquid (250 ml of a non-alcoholic beverage). It is advisable to take the prophylactic doses at the same time every week in order to establish a reliable routine. Mefloquine on an empty stomach may cause side effects, especially nausea and vomiting.

Women of child-bearing age engaging in sexual activity while under mefloquine prophylaxis should practice strict contraception.

Side effects under prophylaxis include dizziness, vertigo, nausea, vomiting (rarely), diarrhoea and, rarely, emotional disturbances.

Contraindications

1. Treatment with quinine or quinidine during the preceding 24 hours

Quinine, quinidine and mefloquine are similar in both chemical structure and their cardiovascular and neurological toxicity. If these drugs are used simultaneously or sequentially the risk is obviously increased. Since quinine and quinidine have relatively short half-lives, it will generally suffice to observe an interval of 24 hours between the last quinine or quinidine dose and the administration of mefloquine. The latter drug should, under these circumstances, be given in divided doses at 8-hour intervals. Monitoring for cardiovascular and neurological side effects is indicated.

2. Treatment with cardioactive medicaments such as β-blockers

Experience with drug interactions between cardioactive medicaments, e.g. β-blockers, and mefloquine is insufficient to rule out the potential occurrence of adverse reactions. The concurrent use of mefloquine and cardioactive agents should therefore be considered as contraindicated.

3. Pregnancy

Fetal damage was seen in mice and rats given 5–20 times the recommended human treatment dose daily during early pregnancy. There was no sign of fetal damage at normal treatment doses and/or normal dose intervals. Nevertheless, pending specific investigations, mefloquine should not be given to pregnant women. This applies to both treatment and prophylaxis. Women of child-bearing age engaging in sexual activity while exposed to malaria risk should practice strict contraception during prophylaxis with mefloquine, and for 2 months after the last dose of mefloquine.

4. Use in infants

There is little experience with mefloquine in infants below one year of age. In such infants mefloquine should only be used if there is a pressing medical reason, e.g. infection with multiresistant *P. falciparum* and hypersensitivity to quinine.

Although the risk is obviously small in view of the small drug quantities involved, it has been suggested that nursing mothers should not breast-feed their babies during treatment with mefloquine.[20]

5. Prophylaxis in patients with renal insufficiency and severe impairment of liver function

In the absence of adequate specific experiences with mefloquine in these patient groups, prophylaxis with mefloquine is contraindicated since it may lead to the accumulation of the parent drug and/or its metabolites, resulting in toxic concentrations.

6. Prophylaxis in occupational groups where fine coordination and spatial discrimination are essential

Dizziness and vertigo are relatively frequent side effects of mefloquine with both treatment and prophylaxis. This may interfere with spatial perception and fine co-ordination.[24] Persons whose tasks involve these faculties, e.g. air crews and surgeons, should not use mefloquine for prophylaxis. After treatment with mefloquine, an interval of 4 weeks should be observed before resuming work that requires full perception and co-ordination.

Adverse reactions

Potentially life-threatening effects

There has so far been no report of death due to an adverse reaction caused by mefloquine, although the number of treatments given either in the form of mefloquine or in association with sulfadoxine/pyrimethamine have now passed the 1 million mark.

Acute overdosage

There is so far no report of deliberate overdose of mefloquine. Where it is commercially available, the medicament is expensive; where it is used in malarious countries it is under strict control. This has probably kept the incidence of deliberate overdosing low. Cases of accidental overdose have occurred, with a maximum of 2 g (base). These patients showed the common adverse effects of mefloquine including neuropsychiatric disturbances, which were fully reversible.

Severe or irreversible adverse effects

Severe adverse effects of mefloquine are rare and relate to neuropsychiatric disturbances, especially behavioural disorders, hallucinations and convulsions. As these may occur at any time from shortly after drug administration until the fourth week after drug intake, the causative role of mefloquine has been unclear. However, evidence for an association between such adverse reactions and mefloquine has become stronger.[25–27] Although at times dramatic, the neuropsychiatric disturbances and convulsions respond to diazepam and all have so far resolved without residue.

Since the symptomatology resembles that produced by acetylcholinesterase (AChE) inhibitors, and as mefloquine is known to cause some inhibition of AChE,[7] it would be interesting to investigate

Mefloquine (hydrochloride)

possible alcohol drug or insecticide interactions or other predisposing factors in patients exhibiting neurological adverse effects.

Evidence for cardiotoxicity is remarkably scanty; however the occurrence of AV block, extrasystoles, sinus bradycardia and pulse irregularities suggests such toxic manifestations.

Symptomatic adverse effects

Among the symptomatic adverse effects associated with mefloquine treatment, dizziness and vertigo (19%) are the most frequent, followed by nausea (13%), vomiting (11%), diarrhoea (7%), headache (6%), sinus bradycardia (2%) and stomach pain (2%). Most of these ill effects are also part of the clinical picture of falciparum malaria. However, dizziness, vertigo, nausea, vomiting and diarrhoea are also seen in healthy subjects taking mefloquine for prophylaxis, though at lesser frequency. All these adverse effects spontaneously resolve after withdrawal of the drug.

Less frequent symptomatic adverse effects, mainly associated with curative doses, are pruritus, urticaria, anorexia, asthenia, pulse irregularities, constipation, insomnia, sialorrhoea, arthralgia and hearing disturbances.

Other effects

Mefloquine is a weak inhibitor of acetylcholinesterase (AChE), ranking in this respect behind the 4-aminoquinolines;[7] however, in view of the comparatively higher mefloquine plasma levels and a different specific tissue distribution, this inhibitory effect may be of some importance, especially in association with other agents or conditions conducive to reduced AChE levels.

At concentrations found in neutrophils, mefloquine stimulates the release of lysozyme, β-glucuronidase and myeloperoxide without loss of cell viability. It also inhibits the neutrophil iodination reaction.[28]

Interference with clinical pathology tests

Mefloquine interferes with the in vitro drug sensitivity tests in *P. falciparum*, where it may reduce schizont maturation in control and drug wells. This will result in erroneous readings due to the antiparasitic activity of mefloquine (the current in vitro drug sensitivity tests require blood free of antimalarial agents).

Mefloquine is not known to interfere with the usual clinical chemical or haematological tests used in the diagnosis and clinical management of malaria or other diseases.

High risk groups

Neonates

Because of the lack of specific experience in this group, mefloquine is contraindicated in the treatment of malaria in neonates (a very rare event).

Breast milk. Mefloquine is excreted in human milk. The milk/plasma ratio of mefloquine (based on the AUC) is 0.13–0.16.[29] Thus the total amount of mefloquine received by a fully breast-fed infant following the mother's treatment with normal therapeutic doses is less than 1 $mg.kg^{-1}$. Plasma clearance and V_d of mefloquine during lactation are approximately 50% less than those seen after the cessation of lactation.[29] It has been suggested that nursing mothers should not breast feed their babies during treatment with mefloquine.

Children

Infants below 12 months of age should not be treated with mefloquine. Children above 12 months of age and up to a body weight of 40 kg require a treatment dose of 25 $mg.kg^{-1}$ body weight. This can be given as a single dose, but dividing the dose (with a 6–8 hour interval) increases tolerance.

Children below 15 kg should not be given mefloquine for malaria prophylaxis. For children above 15 kg, the following weekly doses are indicated for short-term prophylaxis:

15–19 kg — 62.5 mg ($\frac{1}{4}$ tablet)
20–30 kg — 125 mg ($\frac{1}{2}$ tablet)
31–45 kg — 187.5 mg ($\frac{3}{4}$ tablet)
45 + kg — 250 mg (1 tablet)

The dose should be reduced to half the above mentioned doses, or the dose interval doubled after 3 weeks.

Pregnant women

Pending the results of specific continuing studies, mefloquine remains contraindicated during pregnancy, both for treatment and for prophylaxis.

The elderly

The presence of factors enhancing the occurrence of toxic manifestations, such as cardiovascular diseases, renal insufficiency and impaired liver function, calls for careful monitoring in these risk groups. Otherwise, healthy elderly persons tolerate mefloquine well.

Concurrent disease

Epileptic patients may be specially prone to develop neuropsychiatric adverse effects of mefloquine.[30] Such patients should not be given prophylaxis with mefloquine, and treated with the drug only under strict precautions when other suitable medication is not available.

Drug interactions

Potentially hazardous interactions

Quinine and quinidine. Quinine, quinidine and mefloquine are structurally related compounds and have similar cardiovascular and neurological toxicity. They should not be used simultaneously, and used sequentially only after an adequate safety interval.

Cardioactive agents. The cardiovascular adverse effects of mefloquine suggest the possibility of interactions with cardioactive agents, especially β-blockers. If mefloquine is used simultaneously with such drugs, this should be done with great caution.

Other drugs. Current experience does not suggest that mefloquine interacts with oral antidiabetic and anticoagulant drugs when given therapeutically. If such interactions occur at all, they are more likely to appear in persons under prophylaxis, since these constitute a sizeable part of the travelling population in contrast to the population residing in malarious areas. Unlike the structurally related quinine, mefloquine is not likely to interact specifically with antidiabetic drugs, since mefloquine does not cause hypoglycaemia.[31]

Other significant interactions

Acetylsalicylic acid. No interaction has been reported, although acetylsalicylic acid is extensively used in association with mefloquine in the management of malaria.

Paracetamol. This drug is often used in association with mefloquine in the management of severe malaria. No interactions have been reported.

Antipyrine. Mefloquine failed to show any significant effect on antipyrine metabolism.[32]

Potentially useful interactions

No interactions of this kind have been reported.

Major outcome trials

Mefloquine is one of the successful compounds originating from the development programme for antimalarial compounds conducted by the Walter Reed Army Institute of Research, Washington D.C.[33] The specific activity of mefloquine was recognized in 1971. Extensive toxicological, pharmacological and biological studies were subsequently carried out, and limited experience of its efficacy and safety was available by 1976, when further development of the drug was undertaken jointly by industry, the Walter Reed Army Institute of Research and the World Health Organisation (WHO). Since then, the majority of larger clinical and field trials has been conducted under the auspices of the UNDP/WHO/World Bank Special Programme for Research and Training in Tropical Diseases. A summary of the results of therapeutic and prophylactic trials can be found in reference 34. Some of the important Phase II and Phase III trials are summarized below.

1. Harinasuta T, Bunnag D, Wernsdorfer W H 1983 A phase II clinical trial of mefloquine in patients with chloroquine-resistant falciparum malaria in Thailand. Bulletin of the World Health Organisation 61: 299–306

This double blind, randomized, phase II dose-finding study of mefloquine included 147 adult male patients suffering from acute, uncomplicated falciparum malaria who were admitted to the Hospital for Tropical Diseases, Bangkok, Thailand. The treatment consisted of a single oral dose of 500 mg, 750 mg or 1000 mg mefloquine (base) in the form of the hydrochloride. In view of the long half life of mefloquine the patients were followed up for 63 days. The cure rates in the various groups were 95% for the 500 mg dose, 92.5% for the 750 mg dose and 100% for the 1000 mg dose. Clearance of parasitaemia and fever was fastest in the group receiving 1000 mg. Disease-

Mefloquine (hydrochloride)

associated pathological clinical and laboratory parameters tended to normalize quickly. There were no drug-associated changes of haematological and biochemical parameters. Side effects were generally mild, and included nausea, vomiting and diarrhoea. Reversible behavioural disorder (acute brain syndrome) was observed in one patient on day 21 (1000 mg group). Mefloquine was well tolerated by 10 patients with moderately severe malaria associated with jaundice, 13 patients with G6PD deficiency, one patient with thalassaemia and one with acute renal failure.

2. de Souza J M 1983 A phase II clinical trial of mefloquine in Brazilian male subjects. Bulletin of the World Health Organization 61: 815–820

This double blind, randomized trial included 97 patients with symptomatic falciparum malaria who were admitted to Barros Baretta Hospital, Belem, Brazil. One group of 49 patients received a single dose of 1000 mg mefloquine (base) as the hydrochloride. The other group of 48 patients was given a single dose of 1500 mg sulfadoxine and 75 mg pyrimethamine (3 tablets of Fansidar). The follow-up lasted for 63 days. All patients in the mefloquine group were cured. In the sulfadoxine/pyrimethamine group 73% were cured (S-response), 17% had R-I recrudescences, 6% R-II and 4% R-III responses. Clearance of parasitaemia and fever was faster under mefloquine as compared to sulfadoxine/pyrimethamine. Side effects with both medications were mild and transient. Neither drug caused pathological changes of haematological and biochemical parameters.

3. Ekue K J M, Ulrich A M, Rwabwogo-Atenyi J, Sheth U K 1983 A double-blind comparative clinical trial of mefloquine and chloroquine in symptomatic falciparum malaria. Bulletin of the World Health Organization 61: 713–718

In this double blind, randomized clinical trial 99 adult male Zambian patients with symptomatic falciparum malaria were treated either with 1000 mg mefloquine (base) as hydrochloride in a single dose or with a total dose of 1500 mg chloroquine (base) over 3 days. Chloroquine was at that time still effective in Zambia and all patients receiving the drug were cured. One patient in the mefloquine group (2%) showed a recrudescence during the post-treatment follow-up of 63 days. Both drugs were well-tolerated on the whole. Side effects, such as nausea, vomiting, dizziness, loose stools and pruritus, were mild and transient. Pruritus was significantly more common with chloroquine than with mefloquine.

Other trials

1. Harinasuta T, Bunnag D, Lasserre R, Leimer R, Vinijanond S 1985 Trials of mefloquine in vivax and of mefloquine plus 'Fansidar' in falciparum malaria. Lancet 1: 885–888
2. Chongsuphajaisiddhi T, Sabchareon A, Chantavanich P et al 1987 A phase-III clinical trial of mefloquine in children with chloroquine-resistant falciparum malaria in Thailand. Bulletin of the World Health Organization 65: 223–226
3. Harinasuta T, Kietinun S, Somlaw S B et al 1990 A clinical trial of mefloquine on multi-resistant falciparum malaria in pregnant women in Thailand. Bulletin de La Societé Française de Parsitologie 8 (Suppl. 1): 429
4. Anh T K, Kim N V, Arnold K et al 1990 Double-blind studies with mefloquine alone and in combination with sulfadoxine–pynmethamine in 120 adults and 120 children with falciparum malaria in Vietnam. Transactions of the Royal Society of Tropical Medicine and Hygiene 84: 50–53

References

1. Kim P 1985 Mefloquine hydrochloride. In: Florey K (ed) Analytical profiles of drug substances, vol 14. Academic Press, London, pp 157–180
2. Druilhe P, Danis M, Mazier D, Felix H, Gentilini M 1982 Biological activity of mefloquine and its serum metabolites on Plasmodium falciparum continuous cultures. Molecular and Biochemical Parasitology 1982 (suppl): 725–726
3. Chevli R, Fitch C D 1982 The antimalarial drug mefloquine binds to membrane phospholipids. Antimicrobial Agents and Chemotherapy 21: 581–586
4. Davidson M W, Griggs B G, Boykin D W, Wilson W D 1977 Molecular structural effects involved in the interaction of quinolinemethanolamines with DNA. Implications for antimalarial action. Journal of Medicinal Chemistry 20: 1117–1122
5. San George R C, Nagel D L, Fabry M E 1984 On the mechanism for the red-cell accumulation of mefloquine, an antimalarial drug. Biochimica et Biophysica Acta 803: 174–181
6. Vanderkool G, Prapunwattana P, Yuthavong Y 1988 Evidence for electrogenic accumulation of mefloquine by malarial parasites. Biochemical Pharmacology 37: 3623–3631
7. Lim L Y, Go M L 1985 The anticholinesterase activity of mefloquine. Clinical and Experimental Pharmacology and Physiology 12: 527–531
8. Bygbjerg I C, Theander T G, Andersen B J, Flachs H, Jepsen S, Larsen P B 1986 In vitro effect of chloroquine, mefloquine and quinine on human lymphocyte proliferative responses to malaria antigens and other antigens/mitogens. Tropical Medicine and Parasitology 37: 245–247
9. Heizmann P, Geschke R 1984 Determination of the antimalarial mefloquine in human plasma by gas chromatography with electron-capture detection. Journal of Chromatography 311: 411–417
10. Arnold P J, Stetten O V 1986 High-performance liquid chromatographic analysis of mefloquine and its main metabolite by direct plasma injection with pre-column enrichment and column switching techniques. Journal of Chromatography 353: 193–200
11. Schwartz D E, Eckert G, Hartmann D et al 1982 Single dose kinetics of mefloquine in man. Plasma levels of the unchanged drug and of one of its metabolites. Chemotherapy 28: 70–84
12. Chanthavanich P, Looareesuwan S, White N J et al 1985 Intragastric mefloquine is absorbed rapidly in patients with cerebral malaria. American Journal of Tropical Medicine and Hygiene 34: 1028–1036
13. World Health Organization 1984 Advances in malaria chemotherapy. WHO Technical Report Series no 711, World Health Organization, Geneva
14. Looareesuwan S, White N J, Warrell D A et al 1987 Studies of mefloquine bioavailability and kinetics using a stable isotope technique: a comparison of Thai patients with falciparum malaria and healthy Caucasian volunteers. British Journal of Clinical Pharmacology 24: 37–42
15. Karbwang J, Back D J, Bunnag D, Breckenridge A M 1987 Single dose mefloquine pharmacokinetics in healthy Thai subjects and Thai patients with falciparum malaria. In: Kager P A et al (eds) XIIth International Congress for Tropical Medicine and Malaria. Abstracts, no TUP-2-8, p 132. Excerpta Medica, Amsterdam
16. Mu J Y, Israili Z H, Dayton P G 1975 Studies of the disposition and metabolism of mefloquine HCl (WR 142 490), a quinolinemethanol antimalarial, in the rat. Limited studies with an analog, WR 30 090. Drug Metabolism and Disposition 3: 198–210
17. Rozman R S, Molek N A, Kobby R 1978 The absorption, distribution, and excretion in mice of the antimalarial mefloquine, erythro-2,8-bis(trifluoromethyl)-(2-piperidyl)-4-quinolinemethanol hydrochloride. Drug Metabolism and Disposition 6: 654–658
18. Schwartz D E, Warrell D A, Dubach U B, Ranalder N J, White N J, Looareesuwan S 1984 Pharmacokinetic parameters of mefloquine in adult male Thai patients and Swiss volunteers. In: XIIth International Congress of Tropical Medicine and Malaria. Abstracts. University of Calgary, Canada, p 136
19. Schwartz D E, Eckert G, Ekue J M 1987 Urinary excretion of mefloquine and some of its metabolites in African volunteers at steady state. Chemotherapy 33: 305–308
20. Hoffmann-La Roche & Co AG 1985 Lariam. Ref. 80. Hoffmann-La Roche, Basel, p 46
21. Schwartz D E, Jauch R 1982 Pharmacokinetics and metabolism of mefloquine. WHO document WHO/MAL/82.979
22. Wernsdorfer W H, Payne D 1988 Drug sensitivity tests in malaria parasites. In: Wernsdorfer W H, McGregor I A (eds) Malaria. Principles and practice of malariology. Churchill Livingstone, Edinburgh, pp 1765–1800
23. Reber-Liske R 1983 Note on the stability of mefloquine hydrochloride in aqueous solution. Bulletin of the World Health Organization 61: 525–527
24. Stockwell J R 1982 Aeromedical considerations of malaria prophylaxis with mefloquine hydrochloride. Aviation, Space and Environmental Medicine 53: 1011–1013
25. World Health Organization 1989 Prophylactic and therapeutic use of mefloquine. Weekly Epidemiological Record 64: 247–248
26. Bernard J, Le Camus J, Sarrouy J et al 1987 (Toxic encephalopathy caused by mefloquine?, Presse Medicale 16: 1654–1655
27. World Health Organization 1989 Central nervous system reactions related to the antimalarial drug, mefloquine. Unpublished WHO document WHO/MAL/89.1054 & WHO/MAL/89. 1054 Corr.1
28. Bates E J, Ferrante A 1988 Stimulation of human neutrophil degranulation by mefloquine. International Archive of Allergy and Applied Immunology 86: 446–452
29. Edstein M D, Veenendaal J R, Hyslop R 1988 Excretion of mefloquine in human breast milk. Chemotherapy 34: 165–169
30. Jallon P 1988 Use of mefloquine in epileptic patients. Journal of Neurology, Neurosurgery and Psychiatry 51: 732
31. Phillips R E, Looareesuwan S, White N J et al 1986 Hypoglycaemia and antimalarial drugs: quinidine and release of insulin. British Medical Journal 292: 1319–1321
32. Rivière J H, Back D J, Breckenridge A A, Howells R E 1985 The pharmacokinetics of mefloquine in man: lack of effect of mefloquine on antipyrine metabolism. British Journal of Clinical Pharmacology 20: 469–474
33. Rozman R S, Canfield C J 1979 New experimental antimalarial drugs. Advances of Pharmacology and Chemotherapy 16: 1–43
34. Fernex M, Leimer R 1986 (Pharmacology of antimalarials). Médecine et Hygiene 44: 2113–2114, 2117–2118, 2120–2122

M

Mefruside

Mefruside is a benzene disulphonamide derivative related to the benzothiadiazine or 'thiazide' diuretics. It was introduced into clinical use by Bayer Pharmaceuticals as Baycaron in 1971.

Chemistry

Mefruside (Baycaron, Mefrusal)
$C_{13}H_{19}ClN_2O_5S_2$
4-Chloro-N¹-methyl-N¹-(tetrahydro-2-methylfurfuryl)benzene-1,3-disulphonamide

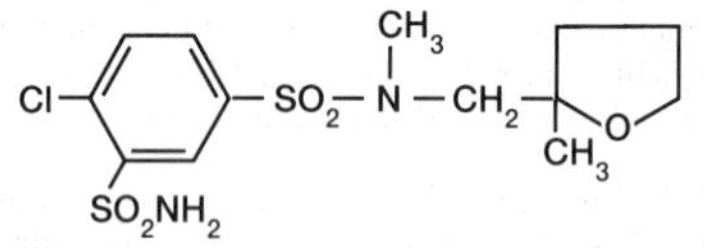

Molecular weight	382.9
pKa sulphonamide group	9.5
Solubility	
in alcohol	soluble
in water	practically insoluble
Ether/water (pH 7.4) partition coefficient	35

There are no commercially available drug combinations with mefruside in the UK. Mefruside is a 2-methyl, tetrahydrofurfuryl derivative of N-methyl, 4-chloro-1:3, disulphonamide and thus differs from the classical 'thiazides' in lacking a benzothiadiazine heterocycle. It shares, however, the chlorosulphamoyl benzene ring which is a common feature of all sulphonamide diuretics. Although the generic name mefruside suggests a close affinity in structure and function with frusemide, there are major differences between these two diuretics. Frusemide is a chlorosulphamoyl derivative of aminobenzoic acid, whereas mefruside has its chlorosulphamoyl benzene ring linked through a second sulphamoyl radical to the methylfurfuryl heterocycle. It is prepared by chemical synthesis as a white powder. Mefruside possesses an assymetric carbon atom.

Pharmacology

In doses over the range 0.02–5.0 mg.kg^{-1} orally, mefruside is saluretic in both rats and dogs. The saluretic action is independent of changes in urinary pH and is not accompanied by significant changes in glomerular filtration rate, though a slight rise in effective renal plasma flow has been noted in some studies.[1] Mefruside has weak carbonic anhydrase inhibitory activity of about $\frac{1}{30}$ that of acetazolamide; the comparative I_{50} values are 7.3×10^{-7}M for mefruside; 2.4×10^{-8}M for acetazolamide.[2,3] Micropuncture and clearance studies in the rat and stop–flow studies in the dog have localized the action of mefruside to the cortical diluting segment of the early distal nephron.[4]

In rats with experimentally-induced hypertension, mefruside showed a dose-dependent blood-pressure lowering effect over the oral dose range of 1.25–10.0 mg.kg^{-1} body weight.[4]

Toxicology

There are no published reports of toxicological results in animals given mefruside that have potential clinical relevance.

Long-term administration at oral doses of up to 500 mg.kg^{-1} in rats or of up to 240 mg.kg^{-1} in dogs did not cause any organ-specific damage attributable to the drug. No carcinogenic or teratogenic effects have been noted in the rat or rabbit, the two species tested.

Clinical pharmacology

Saluretic effects are seen in man after single oral doses of mefruside in the range 12.5–200 mg, with a peak attained at around the 100 mg dose level in healthy volunteers.[4] The maximal diuretic effect occurs between 6 and 12 hours after oral dosing, and some diuretic effects persist for up to 18–20 hours.[3,4] The diuretic effect of mefruside occurs later than that of frusemide (with which it is often confused) and it is a less potent diuretic than frusemide. Mefruside is essentially a thiazide-like diuretic. The actions of mefruside are partly due to its metabolites (5-oxo-mefruside and the carboxylic acid derivative see figure) both of which have similar but weaker diuretic actions than the parent drug. Overall, the drug causes insignificant changes in glomerular filtration rate as measured by inulin clearance of iodohippurate.[2,3] In acute studies, mefruside caused little change in potassium excretion. Significant increase in urinary magnesium has been noted, but serum calcium and magnesium remain unaltered.[15] Although uric acid clearance has not been noted to change, a dose-related increase in serum uric acid has been found with mefruside, reminiscent of that seen with other thiazide-like agents.[3]

Clearance studies in man have yielded similar results to those in animals, where the site of action of mefruside has been localized to the early part of the distal nephron.[3]

Acutely, the drug has no effect on glucose tolerance,[3] but in a group of 42 hospitalized diabetic patients treated chronically with 25 mg mefruside daily, glucose tolerance was found to be impaired in approximately 25% of cases.[5]

Pharmacokinetics

A gas chromatographic method, using extractive methylation and quantitation via a nitrogen detector, is able to selectively assay mefruside and its two major metabolites[10]. Sensitivity for unchanged mefruside is down to 5 µg.l^{-1}. Mefruside is rapidly absorbed from the gastrointestinal tract and peak plasma concentrations are encountered 2–3 h after oral dosing. The drug is widely distributed throughout the body, with an apparent volume of distribution of the order of 314–518 litres. Mefruside is about 64% bound to plasma protein. Following the absorption phase, plasma concentrations of the drug undergo a biphasic pattern of decline with a terminal half life for unchanged drug of approximately 2.9–12.5 h.[11] The elimination half life of the two major metabolites of mefruside, both of which possess intrinsic diuretic properties, is 10–14 h.[11]

Oral absorption	well absorbed
Presystemic metabolism	—
Plasma half life	
range	3–16 h
mean	7 h
Volume of distribution	310–520 l
Plasma protein binding	64%

Mefuside and its active metabolites are excreted in breast milk. There is evidence that mefruside can cross the placenta and enter the fetal circulation. The effects of hepatic disease on the kinetics of the drug are not known.

Concentration–effect relationship

There is no evidence of any correlation between the plasma concentration of mefruside and its therapeutic effects. The presence of an active metabolite will complicate any potential relationship.

Metabolism

Mefruside is metabolized by oxidative transformation into two main metabolites, a lactone formed by ketone formation at the 5-position of the tetrahydrofuran ring — 5-oxomefruside, (13% of the dose) an open hydroxycarboxylic acid derivative and its glucuronide conjugate (≤15%) of the dose (Figure 1). Both these metabolites are active as diuretics, but are distinctly less lipophilic than the parent molecule. Less than 1% of mefruside is excreted in unchanged form in the urine.[11] The main urinary metabolite is the open hydroxycarboxylic acid.[12] Approximately one-third of mefruside metabolites are ex-

Mefruside

Fig. 1 Metabolism of mefruside

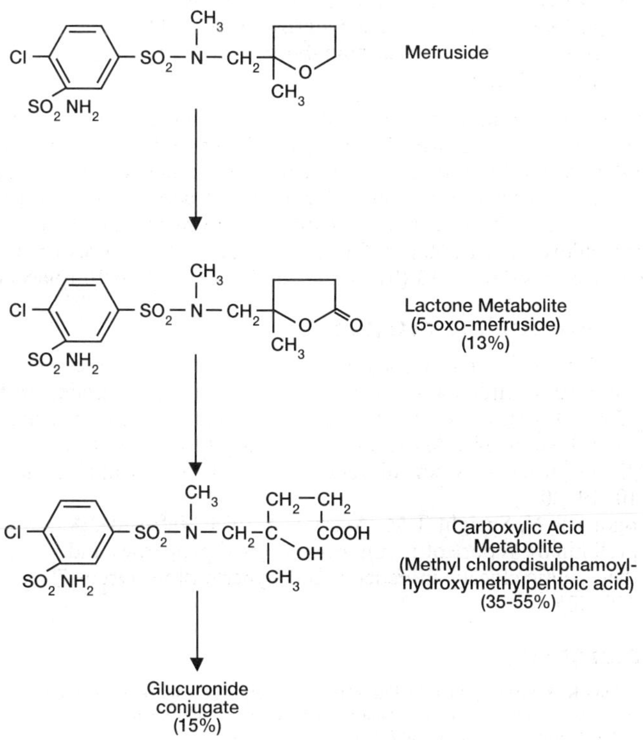

creted in bile via an enterohepatic circulation;[13] the remainder of the metabolites are excreted in the urine.[11]

Pharmaceutics

Mefruside is only available in the oral form.

Mefruside tablets Baycaron (Bayer, UK) 25 mg, white, round, one side scored L/1 with the reverse side marked with the Bayer cross.

Mefruside tablets require no special storage conditions and are stable in glass or PVC blister packs for 5 years.

Therapeutic use

Indications

1. Hypertension
2. Oedema.

Contraindications

1. Hypersensitivity to drugs of sulphonamide structure
2. Severe renal failure
3. Severe hepatic failure
4. Pregnancy
5. Addison's disease
6. Severe hypercalcaemia.

Mode of use

Mefruside should be taken after breakfast with some fluid.

Indications

1. Hypertension

Mefruside, 12.5–50 mg, taken as a single daily dose, may be used as monotherapy, or combined with any of the other first-line therapies for mild to moderate hypertension. In a double-blind, placebo-controlled trial, the antihypertensive effects of mefruside, 25 mg once daily, were compared with hydrochlorothiazide, 50 mg once daily, and a placebo, in 60 Caucasian and 60 Bantu patients with moderate to severe hypertension. Treatment continued for 12 weeks and the mean fall in BP was about the same with the two diuretics (mmHg): 21/12 with mefruside, 18/13, with hydrochorothiazide, as compared with 14/10 with placebo.[6] In open, uncontrolled studies, the mild hypotensive properties of mefruside have been demonstrated in variable dosages between 12.5 and 100 mg daily. Mean blood pressure fell from 181/110 to 161/97 mmHg in 15 patients treated with 25 mg once daily for 1 week;[7] whilst in a different study with variable doses, mean blood pressure fell from 210/115 to 177/103 mmHg in 11 patients treated for 10 weeks.[8] In a general practice study in the UK, mean blood pressure fell from 187/112 to 159/96 mmHg in a group of 840 patients treated for 2 months with an average daily dose of 35 mg mefruside.[9] In a dose of 25 mg daily, given over a period of 5 months in a group of eight hypertensive patients, there was no measurable change in intracellular potassium concentration when measured by needle biopsy of muscle.[14] In a different study in 52 hypertensive patients treated with 25 mg daily over 5 months, minimal hypokalaemia or hyperuricaemia was noted and usually little or no impairment of glucose tolerance or of disturbed lipid profiles.[15] As with most thiazide-like drugs, these metabolic sequelae of continued therapy are dose-related and may be minimized by employing the least effective antihypertensive dose of diuretic. It is important to note that the maximal blood pressure lowering effect may take 10–12 weeks to become manifest; the temptation to use higher doses in an attempt to produce more rapid blood pressure reduction should be resisted. In some patients, once satisfactory blood pressure control has been achieved, the dose frequency can be decreased to alternate days without loss of efficacy. There is no evidence of rebound hypertension on withdrawing drug therapy; it often takes 2–3 months before return to pre-treatment blood pressure levels.

2. Oedema

Mefruside is unsuitable for treating acute left ventricular failure or acute pulmonary oedema. In all other forms of oedema, the dosage is from 25 to 50 mg, taken as a single dose daily. In the presence of adequate renal function, further graded increase in dosage up to 100 mg daily may produce greater saluretic effects where these are required clinically. In the long-term management of mild to moderate cardiac failure, however, it is preferable to use the lower range of dosage, even on an intermittent basis. This avoids excessive stimulation of the renin–angiotensin–aldosterone (RAA) system with the attendant risks of increased renal wastage of potassium and other serious electrolyte disturbances such as hyponatraemia.

Contraindications

Use in pregnancy should be avoided. Hypovolaemia and increased plasma viscosity secondary to sustained saluretic effects may jeopardize placental function. Although no teratogenic effects have been noted with mefruside, occasional reports of fetal and neonatal jaundice or thrombocytopenia have been noted in instances where the drug has been used to treat toxaemia of pregnancy.

Adverse reactions

Potentially life-threatening effects

The principal metabolic abnormalities seen with long-term use of mefruside are those common to all thiazide-like drugs. Hypokalaemia is the most common, and is particularly likely to occur when doses in excess of 25 mg daily are used in the presence of impaired liver function, or in situations where dietary intake of potassium is poor as in the elderly, or where there is concurrent prescribing of potassium-wasting drug therapy such as with corticosteroids.[16]

Acute overdosage

There are no reported instances of deliberate overdosage with mefruside.

Severe or irreversible adverse effects

Hyperuricaemia is usually asymptomatic[15] but can be associated with acute gout in susceptible subjects. As with other sulphonamide diuretics, impaired glucose tolerance can occur and is not correlated with the intensity of the saluresis.[17]

Symptomatic adverse effects

Mefruside is a well-tolerated drug, which, because of its slow onset of action, is less likely to precipitate acute hypovolaemia or acute retention of urine where prostatic hypertrophy exists, as compared with loop diuretics. Occasional dyspepsia has been noted where higher doses of mefruside have been used. Nocturia can be a troublesome feature of continued therapy, as with other long-acting members of the thiazide and thiazide-like family of diuretics.

Other effects

The mechanisms that may be responsible for the above metabolic effects and on lipid metabolism are discussed in the monograph on Indapamide — effects on electrolyte, glucose and lipid metabolism.

Interference with clinical pathology tests

No technical interferences of this kind appear to have been reported.

High risk groups

Neonates

No information is available on the use of mefruside in neonates.

Breast milk. Since the drug and its metabolites pass into breast milk, mefruside should be avoided in lactating mothers.

Children

No information is available on the use of the drug in children.

Pregnant women

Mefruside is best avoided in the management of hypertension or oedema of pregnancy. No teratogenic effects have been reported with mefruside but a few instances of fetal and neonatal jaundice or thrombocytopenia have been observed when the drug has been used to treat toxaemia of pregnancy.

The elderly

Diuretics, in low dose, are effective and relatively safe in managing hypertension and oedema in the elderly. Doses of 12.5–25 mg mefruside daily should not be exceeded in this age group.

Drug interactions

Potentially hazardous interactions

Lithium. As with the use of other thiazide-like and loop diuretics, concurrent use with lithium salts will cause excessive systemic retention of lithium.

Non-steroidal anti-inflammatory drugs. The saluretic effects of thiazide-like drugs, including mefruside, are blunted by concurrent administration of non-steroidal anti-inflammatory agents; there may be acute deterioration of renal function when these two drug groups are given together.

Potentially useful interactions

In hypertension, mefruside may be used on its own as monotherapy, and provided sufficient time is allowed to elapse to judge attainment of full efficacy, the drug may, if necessary, be combined in low dosage with any one of the other first-line choices for managing essential hypertension, such as a β-blocker, ACE-inhibitor, calcium-channel blocker or selective α_1-blocker. Such combination therapy allows low doses of each partner drug to be employed with the minimizing of adverse reactions.

In the management of oedema, there is no logic in combining mefruside with another thiazide-like drug, since all these agents act in the same way and at the same locus in the nephron.[16] Additive effects may, however, be generated by the concurrent use of mefruside with a loop diuretic or with a potassium-sparing diuretic. Such combinations should only be used where clinical circumstances warrant the introduction of more potent saluresis than would be provoked by use of mefruside alone. Whenever such combination therapy is initiated, there must be knowledge of the state of renal function by concurrent administration of non-steroidal anti-inflammatory agents; there may be acute worsening of renal function when these two drug groups are given together.

Clinical trials

1. Auld W H R, Murdoch W R 1971 Clinical trial of mefruside, a new diuretic. British Medical Journal 2: 786–788

This is a controlled trial in three groups of subjects: 15 normal subjects, one day's treatment with oral mefruside, 50 mg or frusemide, 50 mg. One associated control day with matched urine collections before each diuretic challenge day.

15 oedematous patients: comparison of mefruside, 50 mg with frusemide, 50 mg (orally). Two doses of each diuretic according to a BAAB or ABBA pattern with a control day on either side of each diuretic challenge day. Result: greater diuretic effect per 24 h of mefruside, 50 mg as compared with frusemide, 50 mg.

15 hypertensive patients: open study of 7 days' treatment with mefruside, 50 mg (orally). Result: mefruside is a useful antihypertensive which was well tolerated with minimal side effects.

2. Dean G, Louw S, Hersch C, Kirsten H O, Brereton D N, Finnemore L, Dewar J 1971 A double-blind trial in hypertension comparing Baycaron (FBA 1500), hydrochlorothiazide and placebo. South African Medical Journal 45: 323

This report summarizes the results of a double-blind comparison of mefruside, 25 mg, hydrochlorothiazide, 50 mg and placebo, given in randomized fashion to 60 white and 60 Bantu patients with moderate to severe hypertension, over a period of 12 weeks. No significant difference was found between treatment with mefruside, 25 mg and hydrochlorothiazide, 50 mg. The average falls in blood pressure were 12/12 (mefruside); 18/13 (hydrochlorothiazide) and 14/10 (placebo).

General review articles

1967 Chemistry, pharmacodynamics and pharmacokinetics of 4-chloro-3-sulphonamido-benzolsulphonamide (mefruside, BAY 1500). A series of original articles in German, each with a short English summary. Arzneimittelforschung 17 (No. 6): 653–692

1972 Mefruside — a new diuretic. Drug and Therapeutics Bulletin 10: 19–20

Brogden R N, Speight T M, Avery G S 1974 Mefruside. A preliminary report of its pharmacological properties and therapeutic efficacy in oedema and hypertension. Drugs 7: 419–425

References

1. Meng K, Kroneberg G 1967 Pharmakologie von N-(4'-chloro-3'- sulfamoyl-benzol-sulfonyl)-N-methyl-2-aminomethyl-tetrahydrofuran), einer Arzneimittelforschung, 17: 659–671
2. Hesse L 1967 Die Wirkung von N-(4'-chloro-3'-sulfamoyl-benzolsulfonyl)-N-methyl-2-aminomethyl-2-methyl-tetrahydrofuran auf Elektrolytausscheidung, glomeruläre Filtrationsrate und Nierendurchblutung. Arzneimittelforschung 17: 691–692
3. Wilson C B, Kirkendall W M 1970 The acute effects of mefruside in man: a new diuretic compound. Journal of Pharmacology and Experimental Therapeutics 171: 288–299
4. Schwab M, Immich H 1967 Ergebnisse einer klinischpharmakologischen Gemeinschaftsuntersuchung mit einem neuen Saluretikum. In: Heilmeyer L, Holtmeier H J, Marongiu F, Mazzei E S (eds) Diureseforschung, Stuttgart, Thieme, pp 141–152
5. Mehnert H, Standl E, Stotter L et al 1967 Einfluss der BAY 1500 auf den Glucosestoffwechsel. In: Heilmeyer L, Holtmeier H J, Marongiu F, Mazzei E S (eds) Diureseforschung, Stuttgart, Thieme, p 196
6. Dean G, Louw S, Hersch C et al 1971 A double-blind trial in hypertension comparing Baycaron (FBA 1500), hydrochlorothiazide and placebo. South African Medical Journal 45: 323
7. Auld W H R, Murdoch W R 1971 Clinical trial of mefruside, a new diuretic. British Medical Journal 2: 786–788
8. Kühn K, Janocha C 1967 Über die Blutdruckwirkung eines neuen Diuretikums. In: Heilmeyer L, Holtmeier H J, Marongiu F, Mazzei E S (eds) Diureseforschung, Stuttgart, Thieme, pp 170–173
9. Allen H B, Lee D A 1973 A general practice assessment of mefruside ('Baycaron') in the treatment of oedema and hypertension. Current medical Research and Opinion 1: 547–553
10. Fleuren H L J, Verwey-van Wissen C P W, van Rossum J M 1980a Quantitative gas chromatographic determination of two oxidized metabolites of the diuretic mefruside in human urine, plasma and red blood cells. Journal of Chromatography 182: 179–190
11. Fleuren H L J, Verwey-van Wissen C P W, van Rossum H M 1980b Pharmacokinetics of mefruside and two active metabolites in man. European Journal of Clinical Pharmacology 17: 59–69
12. Schlossmann K, Pütter J 1973 Untersuchungen zur Enstehung der Lakton- und Säureform des Hauptmetaboliten des Mefrusid. Arzneimittelforschung 23: 255–262
13. Duhm B, Maul W, Medenwald H, Patzchke K, Wegner L A 1967 Untersuchungen mit ^{14}C-markiertem N-(4'-chloro-3'-sulfamoyl-benzol-sulfonyl)-N-methyl-2-aminomethyl-2-methyl-tetrahydrofuran. Stoffwechsel und Kinetik. Arzneimittelforschung 17: 672–687
14. Bergström J, Hultman E, Solheim S B 1973 The effect of mefruside on plasma and muscle electrolytes and blood pressure in7 normal subjects and in patients with essential hypertension. Acta Medica Scandinavica 194: 427–433
15. Henningsen N C, Bergengren B, Malmborg O et al 1980 Effects of mefruside treatment in hypertension. Acta Medica Scandinavica 208: 273–278
16. Lant A 1985 Diuretics: clinical pharmacology and therapeutic use. Drugs 29, Part I: 57–87; Part II: 162–188
17. Wales J K, Grant A, Wolff F W 1968 Studies on the hyperglycemic effects of nonthiazide diuretics. Journal of Pharmacology and Experimental Therapeutics 159: 229–235

Megestrol acetate

The use of the progestational agent megestrol acetate for the treatment of advanced breast cancer is now well established. It also has a role in the therapy of certain other hormone-dependent tumours.

There are two main groups of progestogens. These are progesterone and its analogues, and certain testosterone analogues. The naturally occurring progestogen progesterone, is the main hormone of the corpus luteum, the function of which was described so lucidly by Verheugen and Greenblatt.[1] Megestrol acetate is an orally active synthetic derivative of progesterone.

Chemistry

Megestrol acetate (Megace, Niagestin, Pallace)
$C_{24}H_{32}O_4$
6-Methyl-3,20-dioxopregna-4,6-dien-17α-yl acetate

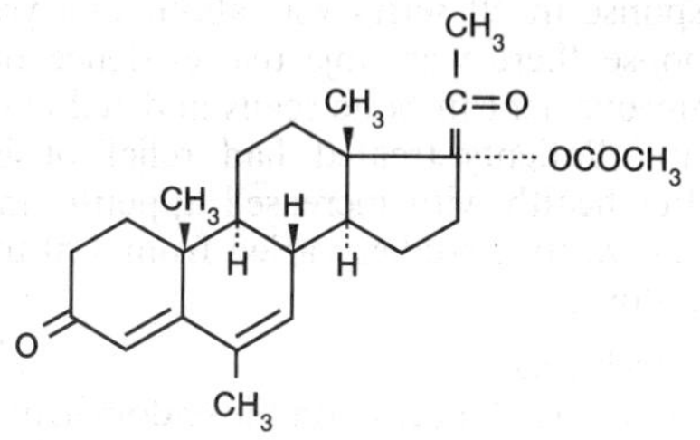

Molecular weight	384.5
pKa	not relevant
Solubility	
in alcohol	1 in 60
in water	<1 in 10 000
Octanol/water partition coefficient	high

It is a white to creamy-white crystalline powder that is prepared by chemical synthesis. A solution in chloroform is dextrorotatory. It is not available in any combination preparations.

Pharmacology

Megestrol acetate is a synthetic progestogen which modifies some of the effects of oestrogens, by acting on tissues sensitized to oestrogen. The pharmacological properties of megestrol are similar to those of natural progesterone. Megestrol changes the oestrogen-induced plentiful watery cervical secretions to a viscid scanty secretion. The oestrogen-induced maturation of the vaginal epithelium is modified by megestrol to a state more like the situation in pregnancy. The acini of the mammary glands proliferate under the influence of oestrogen and progestogen. Megestrol possesses significant antioestrogenic activity but has no androgenic effects. It has some antigonadotrophic effect and also has slight glucocorticoid and mineralocorticoid activity.[2]

The effect of chronic administration of megestrol acetate on the growth of the oestrogen-induced pituitary tumour '7315a' has been studied in the rat.[3] This transplantable tumour is prolactin- and adrenocorticotrophin (ACTH)-secreting. In the model used, megestrol acetate had some suppressive effect on tumour growth towards the end of the treatment period. There was also some suppressive effect on the ability to release prolactin, ACTH and luteinizing hormone of the pituitary gland of tumour-bearing rats. Megestrol probably acts by binding to the progesterone receptor, which in animal studies is a cytosolic receptor with a molecular weight of about 220 000. The amount of this receptor is increased following oestrogen therapy.

Toxicology

Animal toxicity studies on megestrol acetate have shown endometrial hyperplasia and depression of the adrenals, thymus, uterus, ovaries and the testes in the rat, on long-term administration of the agent. In a study by Weikel and Nelson,[4] megestrol acetate was administered continuously to female dogs for many years. They showed an increased incidence of both benign and malignant tumours of the breast in the dogs treated. Comparable studies in rats and monkeys, however, showed no increased incidence of such tumours.

Clinical pharmacology

Megestrol, although it has progestogenic effects in humans, is primarily used in the treatment of breast and other cancers. At the doses used it has progestogenic effects, as discussed under Pharmacology, and many patients gain weight. There are rarely any systemic clinical pharmacological effects although in some patients a rise in blood pressure may occur.

Pharmacokinetics

Megestrol acetate is readily absorbed following oral administration of 20, 40, 80 and 200 mg doses. Average peak serum concentrations for the four doses tested were 89, 190, 204 and 465 $\mu g.l^{-1}$, respectively. Most of the dose is excreted as metabolites in the urine, with 57–78% of a single oral dose being accounted for within 10 days. No unchanged drug is detected. Up to 30% is excreted via the faeces.[2] Tests have shown that a once-daily administration is suitable. A single daily administration of a 160 mg tablet delivers an equal amount of drug to the systemic plasma as does the administration of four 40 mg tablets daily. Mean peak serum concentrations are found 3 hours after single-dose administration. The serum concentration curve appears to be biphasic and the β-phase half life is 15 to 20 hours.[2] Megestrol acetate crosses the placenta and is excreted in breast milk.

Oral absorption	~100%
Presystemic metabolism	—
Plasma half life	
range	15–20 h
Volume of distribution	—
Plasma protein binding	—

Concentration–effect relationship

There is no clear evidence of any relationship between the plasma concentration of megestrol and its anticancer effects.

Metabolism

Three major metabolites have been identified as glucuronide conjugates in urine: 17α-acetoxy-2-α-hydroxy-6-methylpregna-4,6-diene-3,20-dione; 17α-acetoxy-2-α-hydroxy-6-hydromethylpregna-4,6-diene-3,20-dione; 17α-acetoxy-6-hydroxymethylpregna-4,6-diene-3,20-dione. No unchanged drug has been detected in urine, and there is no apparent A-ring aromatization to oestrogenic substances.

Pharmaceutics

Megace (Bristol-Myers, UK/US) is available as round, pale blue 20 mg and 40 mg tablets in the USA. In the UK 40 mg and 160 mg tablets are available. The 40 mg strength is a white circular tablet engraved '40' on one face and the 160 mg tablet is an off-white oval scored tablet engraved '160' on one face.

Therapeutic use

Indications

1. Breast carcinoma
2. Prostatic carcinoma
3. Endometrial carcinoma
4. It has also been used in the treatment of certain renal carcinomas and in cancer cachexia.

Megestrol acetate

M

Contraindications

1. The drug is contraindicated during pregnancy.

Indications

1. Breast carcinoma

The principle of megestrol acetate therapy in breast cancer is similar to that for all forms of endocrine treatment of the disease, that is, the alteration of the hormonal environment within which the cancer exists and thrives. This simplistic view tells us very little, but in reality there is no other explanation forthcoming. Certainly there is no factual evidence for any more specific effect.

Certainly, oestrogens have been shown to have a stimulating effect on malignant cell proliferation, mediated presumably through the oestrogen receptor. An oestrogen receptor is a macromolecule within a cell that selectively and actively takes up or binds oestrogen.[2] It is tempting to postulate, therefore, that the known antioestrogenic effect of megestrol is responsible for its 'anticancer' activity. The megestrol affects the oestrogen receptor cycle, possibly by interfering with the replenishment of cytoplasmic oestrogen receptors.[2] However, this acceptance of oestrogen as the essential culprit in breast cancer has its flaws. It hardly explains, for example, the often dramatic regression of advanced breast cancer that occurs in elderly women on stilboestrol therapy. Also, as long ago as 1962, Huggins and Yang,[5] using a dimethylbenzanthracene (DMBA)-induced rat mammary tumour, demonstrated that the administration of progesterone actually stimulated tumour growth.

If breast cancer hormonal responsiveness reflects a beneficial reaction to a change in the endocrine milieu, this presumably is mediated by altering the cell cycle. A temporary expansion of the 'resting-cell' fraction accords with the known clinical pattern of responsiveness. This entails a measurable shrinkage in the bulk of the responsive tumour, and may result in apparent disappearance of all active cancer. Ultimately and inevitably, however, tumour recrudescence occurs and there is active growth again.

Within this context, megestrol acetate has proved of value in the treatment of advanced incurable cancers of the breast and of metastatic disease. It has generally been used for progressive advanced disease, although there has been some use of the agent recently as adjuvant therapy where there is a strong likelihood of occult metastatic disease. Escher[6] is credited with first demonstrating the responsiveness of certain breast cancers to progestational therapy. Until recently, however, these agents have not been studied clinically with anything like the intensity of some of the other methods of endocrine therapy such as ovarian ablation, other antioestrogens and major endocrine ablation.

In man, to date, megestrol acetate has been used mainly as second-line therapy, subsequent to some other form of simple endocrine therapy. In such situations, either after relapse following beneficial response or after failure, megestrol acetate has a reasonably good record of success. In 1982, Ross and colleagues[7] showed a 64% beneficial response rate in 48 patients, with a median duration of response of 7 months. Subsequently, similar results have been published.[8,9]

As long ago as 1974, Ansfield et al.[10] recorded a 24% 'improvement rate' in 30 patients treated with megestrol acetate as the primary treatment for metastatic breast cancer. Recently there has been renewed interest in the use of the agent as first-line therapy. A number of studies[11–13] have reported beneficial response rates of around 60%. The median duration of response in these series varied according to whether there was complete objective response, partial objective response or stable disease, but was always worthwhile, being well beyond one year.

In all instances quoted above the dose schedule was 160 mg daily, usually given as 40 mg four times daily. More recently there has been a tendency to use a single dose of 160 mg given in the morning, as this results in plasma levels similar to the four times daily regime. There may be a place for the use of high-dose megestrol acetate for selected patients with metastatic disease which has been resistant to other simple endocrine therapy, including standard dose megestrol.[14] Doses of up to 1600 mg daily have been used and are well tolerated. In the above study, 7 of 9 patients who failed to respond to standard-dose megestrol had a beneficial response to high doses.

2. Prostatic carcinoma

Unfortunately a large proportion of prostatic cancers are only detected when they are no longer curable, usually due to the presence of skeletal metastases. Prolonged control of the disease is the best that can then be hoped for. In 1941, Huggins and Hodges[15] first showed the remarkable regressions that could be achieved with either castration or additive oestrogen therapy, through the mechanism of reduced circulating plasma testosterone. These treatments are not without side effects, however, and early relapses occur. Alternative methods have been sought over the years and in particular, progestational agents have been shown to be powerful androgen blockers.[16] More recently, the importance of dihydrotestosterone (DHT) as the final common pathway in prostatic cancer hormonal dependency has been recognized.

Megestrol acetate, at a dose of around 160 mg daily, has been shown to have appreciable androgen-blocking effects,[17] without major side effects. It has been postulated that the antiandrogenic effect is mediated by the pituitary or by direct action on the interstitial cells of the prostate.[18] It now has a regular place in the treatment of advanced prostatic cancer although there is still no clear consensus as to the optimum method of therapy. It remains uncertain whether the antiandrogenic effect is mediated by its action on the pituitary or by a direct effect on the prostate itself. Both probably apply, with the significant local action being its competition with DHT for the androgen receptors.

Subsequent clinical studies have confirmed the beneficial effect of megestrol acetate.[18–20] The reported response rates varied considerably, depending on the circumstances. Higher response rates were recorded when megestrol was used as first-line therapy. The median duration of response in all series was about one year. During the periods of response there was objective evidence of regression of disease, with improvement in bone scans and reduction of prostatic acid phosphatase. Patients treated had relief of bone pain and experienced better health with increased appetite and weight gain. Doses used in the various studies varied from 120 to 160 mg daily, given in divided doses.

3. Endometrial carcinoma

Progestogens have a direct effect upon the endometrium through their antioestrogen activity. Progestational agents have been used in the treatment of patients with advanced endometrial carcinoma, where their use in elderly patients is more feasible than cytotoxic drugs. They have been shown to control the disease successfully, for varying periods, in about 30% of patients treated. The response appears to be related to the extent of progestogen receptor activity within the tumour. This is usually greatest in well-differentiated carcinomas.[2]

Megestrol acetate now has an established place in the treatment of the advanced stages of endometrial carcinoma. The period of response varies considerably according to the circumstances and definitions used. With careful selection, improved response rates can be achieved. In a study reported by Wentz,[22] there appeared to be clear evidence that a good response to megestrol is associated with longer survival. The recommended dose of megestrol acetate for the treatment of advanced cancer of the endometrium is 80 mg four times daily. This total daily dose of 320 mg can be used safely with minimal side effects.

Cachexia often is a severe problem in the management of cancer. Megestrol therapy is valuable in the treatment by virtue of the increase in appetite and weight gain that occurs with its use. The evidence for this is anecdotal, however, and the exact mechanisms are not known.

Adverse reactions

Potentially life-threatening effects

The drug may predispose to thromboembolism, but there do not appear to be any confirmed reports.

Acute overdosage

No serious effects have resulted from ingestion of up to 800 mg daily.

Severe or irreversible adverse effects

Apart from thrombophlebitis, mentioned above, there appear to be no reactions of this kind.

Symptomatic adverse effects

The most constant symptomatic effect of the drug is gain in weight, associated not with fluid retention but with an increased appetite; this is not necessarily a disadvantage in the type of patient for whom the agent is prescribed.

Other symptomatic effects are nausea, which is usually transient, and urticaria.

A curious but rare complication of treatment is production of the carpel tunnel syndrome.

Interference with clinical pathology tests
No technical interferences of this kind appear to have been reported.

High risk groups

Neonates
The drug is not used in neonates.

Breast milk. The nature of the diseases for which the drug is used would usually contraindicate breast-feeding.

Children
Megestrol acetate is not used in children.

Pregnant women
The drug is contraindicated during pregnancy.

The elderly
No special precautions are necessary in older patients.

Concurrent disease
The drug should be avoided, if possible, in patients with a past history of thromboembolic disease.

Drug interactions

Potentially hazardous interactions
No interactions of this kind have been reported.

Potentially useful interactions
No therapeutically useful interactions are known.

References

1. Verheugen C, Greenblatt R B 1983 The use of progestational agents in clinical practice. Journal of New Developments in Clinical Medicine 1: 17–43
2. Bristol-Myers Oncology (undated) Megace-Megestrol acetate B.P. Product monograph. Bristol-Myers Company Limited
3. Lamberts S W J, Janssens E N W, Bons E G, Zuiderwisk J M, Utterlinden P, De Jong F H 1981 Effects of megestrol acetate on growth and secretion of a pituitary tumour. European Journal of Cancer and Clinical Oncology 17: 925–931
4. Weikel J H, Nelson L W 1977 Problems in evaluating chronic toxicity of contraceptive steroids in dogs. Journal of Toxicology and Environmental Health 3: 167–177
5. Huggins C, Yang N C 1962 Induction and extinction of mammary cancer. Science 137: 257–262
6. Escher G C 1951 In: White A (ed) Symposium on steroids in experimental and clinical practice. P Blukiston and Son Co, Philadelphia, p 402
7. Ross M B, Buzdar A U, Blumenschlein G R 1982 Treatment of advanced breast cancer with megestrol acetate after therapy with Tamoxifen. Cancer 49: 413–417
8. Carpenter J T, Peterson L 1985 Use of megestrol acetate in advanced breast cancer on a single daily dose schedule. Seminars in Oncology 12: 40–42
9. Benghiat A, Cassidy S A, Davidson H E, Mancero F S, Pickard J G, Tyrrell C J 1986 Megestrol acetate in the treatment of advanced post-menopausal breast cancer. European Journal of Surgical Oncology 12: 43–45
10. Ansfield F J, Davis H L, Ellerby R A, Ramirez G 1974 A clinical trial of megestrol acetate in advanced breast cancer. Cancer 33: 907–910
11. Gregory D, Cohen J C, Oines D W, Mims C H 1985 Megestrol acetate therapy for advanced breast cancer. Journal of Clinical Oncology 3: 155–160
12. Bonomi P, Johnson P, Anderson K et al 1985 Primary hormonal therapy of advanced breast cancer with megestrol acetate. Seminars in Oncology 12: 48–54
13. Morgan L R 1985 Megestrol acetate versus tamoxifen in advanced breast cancer in post menopausal patients. Seminars in Oncology 12: 43–47
14. Tehekmedyian N J, Tait N, Aisner J 1986 Phase I/II trial of high-dose (HD) megestrol acetate (MA) in breast cancer. Proceedings ASCO, p 281
15. Huggins C, Hodges C V 1941 Studies on prostatic cancer. The effect of castration of oestrogen and of androgens injection on serum phosphatases in metastatic carcinoma of the prostate. Cancer Research 1: 293–297
16. Geller J, Fruchtman B, Newman H, Roberts T, Silva R 1967 Effect of progestational agents on carcinoma of the prostate. Cancer Chemotherapy Reports 51: 41
17. Maltry E 1970 Use of megestrol acetate (a low progestational agent) in the treatment of carcinoma of the prostate. In: Proceedings of the Kimbrough urological seminar, 18th annual meeting, Norwich Eaton Laboratories, pp 135–137
18. Johnson D E, Kaesler K E, Ayala A G 1975 Megestrol acetate for treatment of advanced carcinoma of the prostate. Journal of Surgical Oncology 7: 9–15
19. Geller J, Albert J, Yen S S C 1978 Treatment of advanced cancer of prostate with megestrol acetate. Urology 12: 537–541
20. Bonomi P, Pressis D, Bunting N et al 1985 Megestrol acetate used as primary hormonal therapy in stage D prostatic cancer. Seminars in Oncology 12: 36–39
21. Wentz W B 1985 Progestin therapy in lesions of the endometrium. Seminars in Oncology 12: 23–27

Melarsoprol

Melarsoprol was introduced by Freidheim in 1949 for the treatment of human African trypanosomiasis,[1] and until recently was the only available therapy for meningoencephalitic trypanosomiasis due to *Trypanosoma brucei gambiense* and *T. b. rhodesiense*.

It is a condensation product of melarsen oxide, the trivalent equivalent of melarsen, and BAL (dimercaprol).

Chemistry

Melarsoprol (Mel B, Arsobal)
$C_{12}H_{15}AsN_6OS_2$
2-[4-(4,6-Diamino-1,3,5-triazin-2-yl)aminophenyl]-1,3,2-dithiarsolane-4-methanol

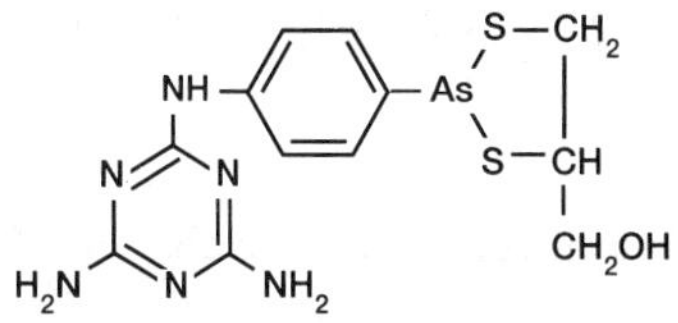

Molecular weight	398.3
pKa amino group	—
Solubility	
in alcohol	insoluble
in water	insoluble
Octanol/water partition coefficient	not determined

Melarsoprol is a slightly greyish/cream-coloured, almost odourless powder with a bitter taste containing 18.8% arsenic. It is prepared by chemical synthesis. It posesses a chiral centre.

Pharmacology

Melarsoprol is effective in the treatment of human African trypanosomiasis caused by *Trypanosoma brucei gambiense* and *T. b. rhodesiense*.

Trivalent arsenicals have a high affinity for sulphydryl groups and thus affect many enzymes, especially the glycolytic kinases. Trypanosomes are dependent upon glycolysis for energy generation. Pyruvate kinase in particular is inhibited in intact trypanosomes and is present in the cytoplasm of trypanosomes; hexokinase and phosphofructokinase are encapsulated within the glycosome. Trypanosome selectivity is thought to be related to three factors: selectivity of action in trypanosomes compared to mammalian cells; increased binding to trypanosomes; and trypanosome dependence on glycolysis for energy generation.

Toxicology

No information on toxicological activity, carcinogenicity or mutagenicity is available.

Clinical pharmacology

Melarsoprol is the treatment of choice for meningoencephalitic trypanosomiasis due to both *T. b. gambiense* and *T. b. rhodesiense*; it has also been used in the treatment of early *T. b. gambiense*. It is of particular value in the treatment of late-stage disease after the advent of meningoencephalitis, and is presently the treatment of choice in this situation. Melarsoprol crosses the blood–brain barrier and although only attaining levels 1% that of plasma this appears sufficient in exerting a trypanocidal effect in the central nervous

Melarsoprol

system. Injection of melarsoprol may cause transient abdominal and retrosternal pain, nausea and, rarely, vomiting. These effects may be reduced by slow intravenous administration. Both hypertension and hypotension have been described in association with melarsoprol and ECG changes suggestive of myocarditis. Meticulous attention to injection technique is essential with this very irritant substance. Extravascular leakage causes extensive tissue damage and destruction. Superficial thrombophlebitis is common even with good injection technique. Syringes and needles must be dry.

Pharmacokinetics

No pharmacokinetic studies have been carried out in man. It appears to be fairly well absorbed after oral administration but is not normally given by this route. Melarsoprol appears to be fairly rapidly excreted via bile and urine within days of administration. Concentrations of melarsoprol in the CSF are approximately 1% of plasma levels.[2] Hawking,[3,4] using a biological assay, found plasma levels immediately following intravenous administration of 10 $\mu g.l^{-1}$ falling rapidly to less than 1 μg within 6 hours.

Concentration–effect relationship

There are no data concerning this topic and there is a dearth of methods of analysis. Direct determination of arsenic in blood or CSF has been made by graphite furnace atomic absorption spectrometry. No standardized methods are available. There is a suggestion that there is a relationship between arsenic levels and toxicity but there are insufficient data.

Metabolism

No information is available on the metabolism of Melarsoprol.

Pharmaceutics

Sterile solutions of melarsoprol (Rhone Poulenc, France) in propylene glycol are sterilised by autoclaving, and contain a 3.6% (w/v) sterile solution in α-propylene glycol presented in 5 ml ampoules (36 $mg.ml^{-1}$). Ampoules should be stored at temperatures of less than 25°C and protected from light.

Therapeutic use

Indications

1. Meningo encephalitic trypanosomiasis due to a) *Trypanosoma brucei gambiense* b) *Trypanosoma brucei rhodesiense*.

Contraindications

In view of the uniformly fatal outcome in untreated trypanosomiasis and, until recently, the absence of alternative therapy there are no absolute contraindications to melarsoprol. Most authorities delay therapy in patients in poor physical condition or with intercurrent infections and short-term febrile episodes. Acute viral infections, especially influenza, have been associated with increased mortality during melarsoprol therapy. Other relative contraindications include impaired hepatic or renal function, G6PD deficiency and pregnancy. Under these circumstances a cautious approach to treatment regimes should be adopted.

Reintroduction of melarsoprol after reactive arsenical encephalopathy (RAE) has not been associated with a further episode.

The recent introduction of DFMO — difluoromethylornithine — in the treatment of *T. b. gambiense* infection suggests that this drug may replace melarsoprol, especially in the presence of relative contraindications to melarsoprol.

Mode of use

A variety of treatment regimes have been introduced in various geographical areas empirically and without access to pharmacokinetic information. These share the common principle of giving short courses of 3 or 4 days duration and separated by ‘rest periods’ of 7–10 days. Most regimes start with relatively low dosages which are increased over the early treatment period to a maximum daily dose of 5.0 ml for a 50 kg adult. Melarsoprol is usually reserved for late-stage disease, as alternative drugs are effective in treating the earlier haemolymphatic stages.

Prior to melarsoprol treatment, pretreatment with suramin (*T. b. rhodesiense* and *T. b. gambiense*) or pentamidine (*T. b. gambiense* only) is recommended both to reduce febrile Herxheimer-like reactions and to limit the potential of introducing parasites from the blood into the CSF during lumbar puncture, a necessary procedure to establish the presence of meningo encephalitis.

In Kenya, Uganda and Zambia schedules follow closely those developed by Apted,[4,5] in particular those utilizing low initial dosages. Most treatment regimes provide a total dosage of 35.0–37.5 ml of melarsoprol, with 9–12 doses over a period of 3–4 weeks. There are no comparative studies of the relative efficacy and toxicity of different treatment regimes, although workers, especially those in East Africa, have concluded that toxicity is reduced with regimes using a low initial dosage and modifying the initial three doses from daily to alternate days, especially in severely debilitated and advanced meningoencephalitic patients.[5,6] A widely used treatment schedule for late-stage *T. b. rhodesiense* (dosage for a 50 kg adult) is shown in Table 1.

In children the dosage of melarsoprol is usually based on body weight.

Table 1

Day		Vol.	$mg.kg^{-1}$
1	Suramin	2.5	5
3	Suramin	5.0	10
5	Suramin	10.0	20
7	Melarsoprol	0.5	0.36
8	Melarsoprol	1.0	0.72
9	Melarsoprol	1.5	1.1
16	Melarsoprol	2.0	1.4
17	Melarsoprol	2.5	1.8
18	Melarsoprol	3.0	2.2
25	Melarsoprol	3.0	2.2
26	Melarsoprol	4.0	2.9
27	Melarsoprol	5.0	3.6
34	Melarsoprol	5.0	3.6
35	Melarsoprol	5.0	3.6
36	Melarsoprol	5.0	3.6

A similar regime used in Tanzania and Uganda starts with a higher initial dose of melarsoprol and only three courses of injections, comprising: Course 1 — 2.5 ml, 3.0 ml, 3.5 ml; Course 2 — 3.5 ml, 4.0 ml, 4.5 ml; Course 3 — 5.0 ml, 5.0 ml, 5.0 ml. The complete treatment course, including pretreatment with suramin, can be completed within 25 days, but the more cautious regime is advised especially in those with advanced meningoencephalitic disease.

A proportion of patients relapse after treatment. This proportion varies from place to place, and is higher in patients that are inadequately or inappropriately treated. Relapse may occur up to three years following treatment.

Cure, relapse and death rates following melarsoprol appear to vary substantially from series to series reported and also geographically. Cure rates range from 50% to over 90%. Relapse rates of approximately 5–10% have been reported following effective melarsoprol therapy. Relapse patients may respond to further courses of the drug. Although resistance to melarsoprol occurs there is little information on the frequency in endemic areas. Mortality rates during treatment have ranged from 5% to almost 20%.

Although usually reserved for the treatment of meningoencephalitic stages of trypanosomiasis, melarsoprol has also been used for the treatment of early and late *T. b. gambiense* using a modified regime developed by Neujean.[7] This regime uses daily injections of 5.0 ml of melarsoprol for four days, and the number of series of injections is determined by the CSF cell count. Patients with less than 20 cells per μl receive one series of injections for four days; those with 21–100 cells per μl receive two series; and those with more than 100 cells per μl receive three series. Courses are separated by a one week ‘rest period’. Relapse is treated with four courses.

An alternative regime used in the Ivory Coast for late-stage *T. b. gambiense* provides three courses of injections, each series comprising 1.7 ml on day 1, 3.3 ml on day 2 and 5.0 ml on day 3. In both courses

2 and 3 a further 5.0 ml is given on day 4. Greenwood[9] recommends melarsoprol in the treatment of early *T. b. gambiense* giving 2.5 ml on day 1 and 3, and 5.0 ml on day 5 and 8.

Corticosteroids have been advocated for both the prevention and treatment of potentially fatal reactions, especially RAE, during melarsoprol therapy. Whilst earlier studies failed to demonstrate a reduced incidence of RAE, a recent randomized study in *T. b. gambiense* found that prednisolone 1 $mg.kg^{-1}$ up to a maximum of 40 mg daily during the first two courses of melarsoprol reduced the incidence of RAE from 11.1% to 4.1% ($p=0.002$).[10,11]

Melarsoprol must be given by slow intravenous injection. The propylene glycol component is extremely irritant and extravascular leakage causes severe local tissue damage and thrombophlebitis.

Adverse reactions

Potentially life-threatening effects

Reactive arsenical encephalopathy. The most serious adverse effect of melarsoprol is RAE. This is characterized by a rapid deterioration in conscious level, convulsions or a variety of neuropsychiatric features; it commonly occurs early in the course of treatment, especially between days 3 and 7. The frequency of RAE varies in different reported series from 2% to 10%, and has been observed in both early and late-stage disease, although more commonly in advanced, late-stage, meningo encephalitic disease. Mortality from RAE depends on the diagnostic criteria used but may reach 50–75%. Fulminant convulsive states have been associated with cerebral oedema and papilloedema. Pathologically, the condition is characterized by an acute vasculitis superimposed on the underlying trypanosomal damage.[12] A small proportion of patients developing coma whilst on melarsoprol have an acute, usually fatal haemorrhagic leucoencephalopathy, possibly related to relative or absolute overdosage as observed in the treatment of neurosyphilis.

Several workers have reported that RAE occurs more frequently when patients are febrile or in the presence of an intercurrent viral infection, and therefore advise delaying or suspending arsenical therapy under such circumstances.

Management of RAE has included temporary cessation of melarsoprol, administration of anticonvulsants and sedatives to control convulsions; the administration of ACTH and corticosteroids[10] and hypertonic solution such as Mannitol 25% 150 ml by rapid infusion followed by Mannitol 10% 500 ml by slow infusion as well as diuretics and subcutaneous adrenaline.[13]

Haemopoietic effects. Acute haemolysis may occur in patients with glucose-6-phosphate dehydrogenase (G6PD) deficiency. Infrequent instances of agranulocytosis, aplastic anaemia and thrombocytopenia have been reported.

Peripheral neuropathy. A peripheral neuropathy during melarsoprol therapy occurs in up to 10% of patients treated with melarsoprol.

Skin reactions. Vesicular or exfoliative dermatitis may occur; this may be fatal.

Gastrointestinal reactions. Severe dehydrating diarrhoea may occur (arsenical enteritis).

Acute overdosage

No cases of deliberate self-poisoning appear to have been reported.

Severe or irreversible adverse effects

Hepatotoxicity. Evidence of liver damage, including clinical jaundice, raised serum bilirubin and elevated liver enzymes, has been reported in patients on melarsoprol. In most instances hepatic toxicity has been reversible.

Renal effects. A small proportion of treated patients develop albuminuria and urinary casts; these abate in most instances.

Jarisch–Herxheimer-like reactions. Febrile reactions, associated with parasite destruction in either the blood or CSF, occur when melarsoprol is used in patients with a parasitaemia. These reactions are reduced by pretreatment with suramin or pentamidine.

Local reactions. Even with good injection technique, many patients develop thrombophlebitis. When injected extravascularly, severe tissue damage and extensive thrombophlebitis may develop.

Erythema nodosum leprosum. In one patient with concurrent leprosy, melarsoprol induced a severe ENL reaction.

Melarsoprol

Symptomatic adverse effects

Arthralgia and limb pains. Minor joint and limb pains commonly occur during melarsoprol therapy and may occasionally be severe.

Skin reactions. A wide variety of dermatological adverse effects may occur similar to those seen in the treatment of venereal syphilis with other arsenical preparations.[2,13]

Vesicular and exfoliative rashes have been mentioned above. Others include erythematous and urticarial reactions.

Gastrointestinal reactions. Abdominal pain, colic, nausea and vomiting are relatively common adverse effects of melarsoprol.

Other reactions. Other effects reported include angioneurotic and hypersensitivity reactions and hyperkeratosis of the soles of the feet.

Dimercaprol (BAL) in the treatment of toxicity

The value of dimercaprol in the treatment of RAE is uncertain. If there is evidence to indicate overdosage, either absolute or relative, then dimercaprol might prove beneficial, and by analogy with experience with other arsenical compounds, should also be used in the treatment of other severe, potentially fatal drug reactions.

High risk groups

Advanced late-stage disease

The mortality associated with treatment in advanced disease and in severely debilitated patients is substantially higher than in other stages of disease. Most authorities recommend that under these circumstances, especially in *T. b. rhodesiense*, dosage regimes should be reduced and spaced initially.

Neonates

The drug has been used in neonates and there is no evidence that they respond differently to adults with melarsoprol therapy when dosage is based on body weight.

Breast milk. Women receiving the drug should not breast-feed.

Children

As for neonates above.

Pregnant women

Despite the toxicity of melarsoprol, successful treatment during pregnancy has been reported.

The elderly

Melarsoprol has been used in the elderly. Given the severity of the disease, its rapid progression to a fatal outcome, and the absence of alternative drugs, any additional risk to this group has to be accepted.

Concurrent disease

Hepatic and renal disease. Caution is required in the presence of pre-existing hepatic or renal disease.

Intercurrent infection. Severe intercurrent infection should be treated prior to melarsoprol therapy. Treatment during outbreaks of viral infections, especially influenza, has been associated with an increased mortality on melarsoprol therapy, and under these circumstances treatment should be delayed.

Relapse and retreatment

There is no evidence that melarsoprol toxicity is increased during second or subsequent courses of treatment. Relapse usually responds to a second course of melarsoprol, but subsequent relapses are commonly associated with increasing resistance to the drug. There are no data on the longer term toxicity of melarsoprol.

Drug interactions

Potentially hazardous interactions

There are no well-documented hazardous interactions.

Potentially useful interactions

No interactions of this kind have been described.

References

1. Freidheim E A H 1949 Mel B in the treatment of human trypanosomiasis. American Journal of Tropical Medicine and Hygiene 29: 173–180
2. Crista B, Placidi M, Legait J P 1975 Etude de l'excrétion de l'arsenic chez le trypanosomé traité au mélarsoprol (Arsobal). Medicine Tropicale 35: 389–401
3. Hawking F 1963 Chemotherapy of trypanosomiasis. In: Schnitzer R J, Hawking F (eds) Experimental chemotherapy. Academic Press, New York, vol 1, pp 129–256

4. Hawking F 1962 The concentration of melarsoprol (Mel B) and Mel W in plasma and cerebrospinal fluid estimated by bioassay with trypanosomes in vitro. Transactions of the Royal Society of Tropical Medicine and Hygiene 56: 354–363
5. Apted F I C 1970 Treatment of human trypanosomiasis. In: The African trypanosomiases. Mulligan H W (ed) George Allen Unwin, London, pp 684–710
6. Robertson D H H 1963 The treatment of sleeping sickness (mainly due to *Trypanosoma rhodesiense*) with melarsoprol. Transactions of the Royal Society of Tropical Medicine and Hygiene 57 (2): 122–133
7. Neujean G 1959 Chimiothérapie et chimioprophylaxie de la maladie du sommeil à *T. b. gambiense*. Revue Médicale de Liege 14: 5–13
8. WHO 1986 Epidemiology and control of African trypanosomiasis. Technical Report Series 739. WHO, Geneva
9. Greenwood B M 1984 African trypanosomiasis. In: Weatherall D J, Ledingham J G G, Warrell D A (eds) Oxford Textbook of Medicine. Oxford University Press, vol 1, pp 5.406–5.410
10. Pepin J, Guern C, Ethier L, Lilord F, Mpia B, Mansinsa D 1989 Trial of prednisolone for prevention of melarsoprol-induced encephalopathy in gambiense sleeping sickness. Lancet i: 1246–1249
11. Foulkes J R 1974 An evaluation of prednisolone as a routine adjunct to the treatment of *T. rhodesiense*. Journal of Tropical Medicine and Hygiene 78: 72–74
12. Haller L, Adams H, Merouze F, Dago A 1986 Clinical and pathological aspects of human African trypanosomiasis (*T. b. gambiense*) with particular reference to reactive arsenical encephalopathy. American Journal of Tropical Medicine and Hygiene 35 (1): 94–99
13. Sina G C, Nicasio T, Bernard C, Suk B M 1979 L'adrénaline dans la prévention et le traitement des accidents de l'arsobalthérapie. A propos de 728 cas to trypanosomiase humaine africaine a *T. gambiense* traités dans les formations sanitaires de Fontem (RUC). Sixteenth meeting: International Scientific Council for Trypanosomiasis Research and Control. Yaounde (RUC) ed OAU/STRC, Scientific Publication Service, Nairobi
14. Rollo I 1980 Miscellaneous drugs used in the treatment of protozoal infections. In: Goodman A G, Goodman L S, Gilman A (eds) The pharmacological basis of therapeutics. Macmillan, New York, pp 1070–1079

Melphalan

Melphalan was one of the first rationally designed alkylating agents to be widely used in antitumour chemotherapy.

Chemistry

Melphalan (L-phenylalanine mustard, L-PAM, L-sarcolysin, sarcolorin, Alkeran, Compound CB 3025, NSC-8806)

$C_{13}H_{18}Cl_2\ N_2O_2$

4-bis(2-Chloroethyl)amino-L-phenylalanine

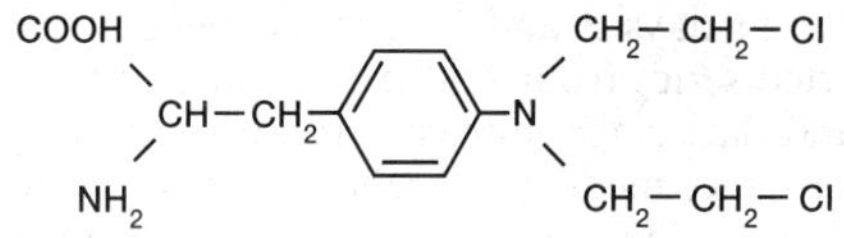

Molecular weight	305.2
pKa	2.1, 9.5
Solubility	
in alcohol	1 in 50
in water	—
Octanol/water partition coefficient	0.45

An odourless, white or buff powder, melphalan is available for oral use as a 2 or 5 mg tablet. For intravenous use, the drug is supplied as a kit comprising a vial of 100 mg (equivalent) melphalan, a 1.8 ml vial of acid–alcohol diluent and a 9 ml ampoule of final diluent. No drug combination product containing melphalan is available.

Pharmacology

Melphalan is a bifunctional alkylating agent used in the treatment of malignant disease.

The consequences of base alkylation include misreading and cross-linking of DNA, as well as both single- and double-strand breaks. This will consequentially interfere with synthesis of DNA, RNA and protein in rapidly dividing tissues. Alkylating agents such as melphalan that have two functional groups (the so-called 'bifunctional' agents) can cause cross-linkage of the two DNA strands, and the efficacy of these agents correlates closely with efficiency of cross-linkage.

Melphalan acts on cells at any stage in the cell cycle. However, the effects are usually seen when the cell enters the S phase and progress through the cell cycle is blocked at the G_2 (premitotic stage). The main target is cell DNA, and melphalan causes cross-linking of the DNA strands.[1] In low doses of the drug the number of cross-links is small and the DNA repair system is able to restore the DNA almost to normality. However, in larger doses the DNA cross-linking is extensive, DNA breakdown occurs and this results in cell death.

Toxicology

In a 30-day test, melphalan at a dose of 5 $mg.kg^{-1}$ daily proved fatal by 14 days in Wistar rats; 2.5 $mg.kg^{-1}$ daily produced severe damage in all tissues examined (including testis) and 0.5 $mg.kg^{-1}$ daily produced significant neutropenia by day 30.

In the same species, melphalan had no effects in teratogenicity tests at a dose of 33 $mg.kg^{-1}$ orally between days 6 and 16 of gestation; 1 $mg.kg^{-1}$ had no effect on the dams but reduced the number and body weight of the pups; 3 $mg.kg^{-1}$ resulted in maternal weight loss as well as reduction in number and weight of the pups. No dose was teratogenic.

In mutagenicity tests, melphalan has been shown to cause chromo-

Melphalan

somal damage and point mutations in bacteria[2] and is positive with all strains in the Ames test.[3] Melphalan (1 μg.ml^{-1}) causes transformation of C3H/10T cells in vitro and is clastogenic.[4]

Carcinogenicity studies have been extensively reviewed by IARC.[2] Of 33 female rats given melphalan 10 mg.kg^{-1} intraperitoneally, nine developed mammary fibroadenomas after 2–17 weeks. After administration of 0.9 or 1.8 mg.kg^{-1} intraperitoneally three times per week for six months, peritoneal sarcomas were seen by 12 months in both sexes.

Clinical pharmacology

Melphalan is a potent alkylating agent and this property determines all its known biological properties.

Melphalan has been primarily used in the treatment of multiple myeloma but beneficial effects have also been noted in the treatment of malignant melanoma and carcinoma of the breast and ovary. Toxic effects are primarily due to bone marrow suppression but nausea and vomiting are unusual and hair loss is only seen following intravenous therapy.

The dose administered has varied widely in different clinical studies, and references to specific applications should be consulted (see Indications). When given orally, the dose has usually been about 1 mg.kg^{-1} divided over five days, repeated every 3–4 weeks. 'Conventional' doses for intravenous use are also about 1 mg.kg^{-1}, but doses as high as 260 mg.m^{-2} have been safely administered in conjunction with autologous bone marrow rescue and cyclophosphamide 'priming' (see Concentration–effect relationship).[5]

Pharmacokinetics

The preferred analytical method is high performance liquid chromatography, which has a sensitivity of 5 ng.l^{-1} in plasma.[6]

Absorption of melphalan given orally is incomplete and highly variable. The time of first detection in plasma has been reported to vary between 15 min and 6 hours.[7]

Oral absorption	erratic
Presystemic metabolism	nil
Plasma half life	
oral administration	83±14 min
intravenous administration	92±27 min
Volume of distribution	0.62±0.21 l.kg^{-1}
Plasma protein binding	>80% at 4 h

Studies with tritiated melphalan have demonstrated ubiquitous distribution in tumour-bearing rats, with total tritium incorporation being greatest in the liver and kidney.[8] Melphalan is not thought to cross the blood–brain barrier in therapeutically useful concentrations.

There is no information available as to placental transfer or excretion in human breast milk. However, mothers receiving melphalan should not breast-feed.

Concentration–effect relationship

There is no information relating therapeutic effect or toxicity of melphalan to plasma concentration, but, as with other agents of this class, both effects are believed to be dose-related.[9] Against human malignant melanomas growing as xenografts in immune-deprived mice, melphalan shows a log-linear dose–response curve[10] over the range 5–25 mg.kg^{-1}. Clinical exploration of this relationship was encouraged by the observation that, while melphalan has only a 9% response rate in patients with malignant melanoma at conventional doses, the higher concentrations achievable by isolated limb perfusion are much more effective.[11] The observation that pretreatment ('priming') with a small dose of cyclophosphamide substantially reduced toxicity[12] has allowed doses as high as 260 mg.m^{-2} to be used in conjunction with autologous bone marrow rescue, with an increase in response rate to 43%.[5] The role of such high-dose therapy remains controversial.

Metabolism

In a study of the distribution and excretion of ^{14}C-labelled melphalan in man, up to 65% of the ^{14}C label was recovered in the urine by 7 days after intravenous administration. Following oral administration, 30% of the label was recovered in the urine by 9 days, and 20–25% in the faeces by 6 days.[13] There is no evidence of enterohepatic circulation.

No metabolites have been identified in man, but the compound hydrolyses spontaneously in vitro to form monohydroxy- and dihydroxy-melphalan (Fig. 1). Neither of the hydroxy compounds has been shown to have cytotoxic activity.[14] Dihydroxymelphalan is eliminated from the body more slowly than melphalan.[15] A recent study failed to demonstrate significant amounts of hydroxylated melphalan in plasma[16] and it is not known if the hydroxymelphalans have other pharmacological activities in man. By far the most important reaction products in man are alkylated DNA and protein.

Fig. 1 Metabolism of melphalan

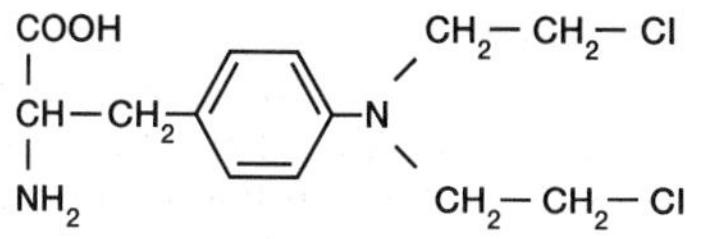

Melphalan

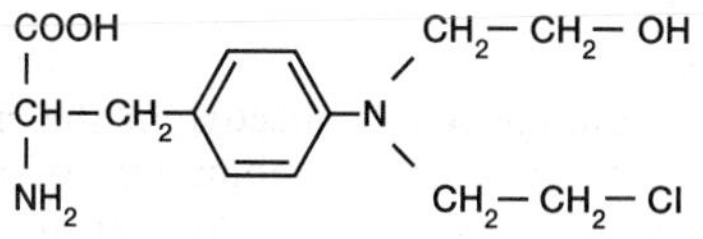

Monohydroxymelphalan

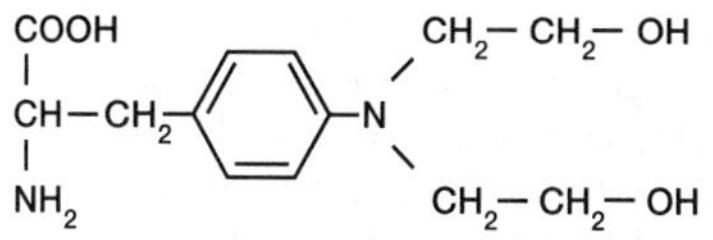

Dihydroxymelphalan

Pharmaceutics

Melphalan is available for oral and parenteral use (Alkeran; Burroughs Wellcome, USA/Calmic, UK). Tablets are available containing either 2 mg or 5 mg melphalan BP, and are white, round and biconvex with a pink core. Tablets containing 2 mg melphalan are coded 'Wellcome A2A', while those containing 5 mg are coded 'Wellcome B2A' (5 mg strength is not available in USA).

Melphalan for injection (Alkeran; Calmic, UK) is supplied as a tripack containing a 100 mg vial for sterile anhydrous melphalan BP, a 1.8 ml vial of acid–alcohol diluent containing 0.047 ml 37% hydrochloric acid made up to 1.8 ml with 96% ethanol, and a 9 ml ampoule of final diluent containing dipotassium phosphate 108 mg, propylene glycol 6 ml, and sterile water for injection to a final volume of 9 ml. Once reconstituted, the injection decomposes on storage, and should be used within 20 minutes of preparation.

Tablets should be stored in an airtight container in a dry area, and the parenteral preparation should be protected from light. Both should be stored at less than 25°C. However, storage of the parenteral pack in a refrigerator may cause precipitation when the drug is reconstituted, and storage at room temperature is recommended. If kept under these conditions, both preparations have a maximum shelf-life of three years.

Therapeutic use

Indications

1. Myelomatosis
2. Polycythaemia rubra vera
3. Carcinoma of breast
4. Carcinoma of ovary
5. Malignant melanoma
6. Soft-tissue sarcomas
7. Ewing's sarcoma
8. Neuroblastoma.

Contraindications

1. Myelosuppression, particularly neutropenia
2. Previous hypersensitivity
3. Impaired renal function.

Melphalan

M

Mode of use

The absorption of melphalan after oral administration is variable and, in some patients, dosage may need to be cautiously increased until myelosuppression is seen in order to achieve maximum therapeutic effect. Blood cell counts must be carefully monitored so that excessive myelosuppression (and the risk of irreversible bone marrow aplasia) is avoided.

Melphalan is usually given on an intermittent basis as the blood count may not reach its nadir for 3–4 weeks, full marrow recovery taking 4–6 weeks. Melphalan is unstable in infusion fluids, and should not be given in dextrose solutions. Infusions may be given in saline, but, at room temperature, the same solution must not be infused over longer than 2 hours. When given intravenously, melphalan must be given as a slow bolus injection, preferably into the tubing of a fast-running infusion in a large (or central) vein. The injection may be acutely painful at the injection site if administered too quickly. When given as an intravenous bolus, the injection should be prepared not more than 20–30 minutes prior to use.

Indications

1. Multiple myeloma

Melphalan is firmly established as effective in the chemotherapy of multiple myeloma,[17,18] and the combination of melphalan with prednisone has been shown in a controlled trial to be more effective than melphalan alone,[19] possibly as a result of non-specific benefit due to increased haemoglobin and control of hypercalcaemia. Early studies employed continuous low doses of melphalan, which have a theoretical advantage over intermittent use, but a typical dose regimen at present would be 0.15 $mg.kg^{-1}$ daily for four days together with 40 mg prednisolone for the same period, with intervals of six weeks between courses. If tolerated, the periods of treatment may be gradually extended to seven days.[20] However, many doses and schedules have been employed. Response rates of approximately 50% with median survival of 2–3 years may be expected.

Efforts to improve on these results have included the use of melphalan in high dose in conjunction with autologous bone marrow rescue (ABMR). A dose of 140 $mg.m^{-2}$ was evaluated in 58 patients aged < 63 years. Among previously untreated patients, 11/41 (27%) entered complete remission (no measurable myeloma protein and a normal bone marrow) and 21 (51%) entered a partial remission (> 50% reduction in myeloma protein and improvement in all other features).[21] Median duration of response was 19 months. The addition of high-dose methylprednisolone (1 $g.m^{-2}$ daily for 5 days) produced similar results (27% CR, 59% PR) but treatment mortality was substantially reduced. A prospective trial in which high-dose melphalan with and without steroids is compared with the best available conventional therapy is in progress (MRC VI Myelomatosis Trial).

2. Polycythaemia rubra vera

Melphalan has been regarded as one of the most effective treatments for the control of polycythaemia since the earliest reports of its use; 24 of 27 patients had responses described as good or excellent, with 14 patients free of disease after one year.[22] The usual dose for remission induction is 6–10 mg daily for 7–10 days followed by maintenance therapy according to a reducing dosage schedule.

3. Carcinoma of breast

Melphalan was originally reported to be active in patients with advanced breast cancer in 1966.[23] Of 40 evaluable patients (treated with 0.8–1.5 $mg.kg^{-1}$ over 4–6 days every 3–6 weeks depending on blood count recovery) 12 had objective responses with a median duration of 4 months. Melphalan alone has been compared with combination chemotherapy (cyclophosphamide, methotrexate and 5-fluorouracil) in previously untreated patients.[24] The combination was found to be superior (objective responses 53% versus 20%, median duration 25 weeks versus 13 weeks) but more toxic. Melphalan as adjuvant treatment in early breast cancer showed considerable promise in the National Surgical Adjuvant Breast Project trial comparing melphalan with placebo,[25] but this was not confirmed in subsequent studies.[26] Single agent adjuvant treatment has now given way to combinations of agents.

4. Carcinoma of ovary

Alkylating agents have been used more extensively in patients with advanced ovarian cancer than have any other class of chemotherapeutic agent. Melphalan is among the most active and widely used, with a response rate of 47% in pooled reports (complete response, 20%).[27] Although combination chemotherapy, incorporating newer agents such as cisplatin, is now more widely used, the lack of toxicity and oral route of administration make agents such as melphalan and chlorambucil attractive options in the therapy of older or more frail patients.

5. Malignant melanoma

Regional perfusion with melphalan (with or without hyperthermia) has been investigated in the treatment of patients with isolated peripheral recurrences[28] and as an adjuvant to surgical treatment of early disease,[29] the latter being the subject of a current multicentre prospective trial. In patients with advanced disease, conventional doses of melphalan (10 mg daily orally for 5 days every 4 weeks) have achieved response rates of only 9%.[30] A study employing melphalan in high dose (140–260 $mg.m^{-2}$ with ABMR) in 28 patients with life-threatening metastatic melanoma gave an overall response rate of 43%, with complete remission in 2 patients.[5] However, responses were short-lived and no patient survived more than 17 months from treatment.

6. Soft-tissue sarcomas

Regional perfusion with melphalan in combination with other cytotoxic agents (usually nitrogen mustard and/or actinomycin D with or without hyperthermia) has been used in the management of all stages of localized soft-tissue sarcomas, usually in conjunction with surgery. Reduced local recurrence rates and improved survival have been reported in patients with early disease, together with temporary remissions (with useful palliation of symptoms) in approximately 85% of patients with local recurrences.[31]

7. Ewing's sarcoma

High-dose melphalan (140–230 $mg.m^{-2}$ with ABMR) has been used in a small group of patients with Ewing's sarcoma refractory to conventional chemotherapy.[32] Of 5 patients reported 4 achieved a complete remission, with a median duration of response of 14 months.

8. Neuroblastoma

The European Neuroblastoma Study Group has investigated high-dose melphalan as late consolidation therapy in a randomized trial in children with advanced neuroblastoma who achieve complete remission after conventional induction therapy. In this trial 65 patients were randomized to high-dose melphalan (180 $mg.m^{-2}$ with marrow rescue) or no further therapy. Initial results have suggested an enhanced disease-free and overall survival for those receiving consolidation therapy.[33]

Contraindications

Melphalan should not be given to patients who have previously demonstrated an allergic reaction (see below). Melphalan should be given with extreme caution to patients who have recently received radiotherapy to bone-marrow-containing areas, or who have received other chemotherapy. Pre-existing myelosuppression from any cause is a contraindication to treatment with melphalan.

In patients with moderate to severe renal impairment, the initial intravenous dose should be reduced to 50% and subsequent doses determined according to extent of myelosuppression. Currently available pharmacokinetic data do not justify an absolute recommendation of reduction of oral dosage in such patients, but it would appear prudent to do so.[34] Patients with renal impairment should be monitored particularly carefully for myelosuppression; in myeloma patients with renal damage, temporary but significant increases in blood urea have been observed during melphalan therapy.[35]

Adverse reactions

Potentially life-threatening effects

In common with most alkylating agents, melphalan produces significant myelosuppression which may result in life-threatening anaemia, neutropenia and/or thrombocytopenia.[36] The risk is cumulative over time, and blood counts may continue to fall after treatment is stopped. Melphalan (particularly intravenous melphalan) should not be used by those inexperienced in the care of the neutropenic patient,

Melphalan

or in situations where vulnerable patients cannot be fully supported with blood products, etc. until marrow recovery.

Secondary acute leukaemia has been reported after prolonged treatment with melphalan for diseases such as amyloid,[37] melanoma[38] or ovarian cancer.[39]

Allergic reactions may occasionally be life-threatening. These are mentioned below.

Acute overdosage

Deliberate overdosage with melphalan has not been reported, but would be expected to produce severe myelosuppression and drug toxicity. There is no known antidote to melphalan poisoning, and full supportive measures (intravenous antibiotics, blood products, etc.) should be available until blood count recovery.

Severe or irreversible adverse effects

Severe immediate allergic reactions have been reported in 2.4% of patients treated with intravenous melphalan.[17] Whether the reaction is to melphalan itself or to the propylene glycol in the diluent is uncertain. There have also been case reports of pulmonary fibrosis[40] and haemolytic anaemia[41] after prolonged melphalan therapy; these have been considered to be allergic phenomena.

At the upper extreme of the dose range (<200 mg.m^{-2}), severe gastrointestinal disturbance, manifest as profuse diarrhoea with consequent electrolyte disturbance, may occur.[5]

Symptomatic adverse effects

Mild nausea and vomiting occur relatively infrequently after oral melphalan (30%),[42] but is universal after moderate or high-dose intravenous therapy. Prophylactic antiemetics should be prescribed routinely in these circumstances.

Hair loss is also infrequent after oral therapy but universal after higher dose intravenous treatment.[43] Regrowth is prompt.

Extravasation injuries have not been reported, but pain at the injection site is frequent if administration is too fast or into too small a vein.

Melphalan treatment of premenopausal patients with breast cancer can cause suppression of ovarian function resulting in failure of menstruation.[43] Recovery is more likely the younger the patient (i.e. the further from a normal menopause).

Maculopapular rashes and pruritis have occasionally been reported.[35]

Other effects

No clinically significant biochemical effects have been reported.

Interference with clinical pathology tests

Administration of melphalan may result in direct Coombs test positivity.[44]

High risk groups

Neonates

There is no clinical experience with melphalan in the neonatal age-group.

Breast milk. No information on excretion in human breast milk is available but mothers taking melphalan should not breast-feed.

Children

Experience with melphalan in the treatment of childhood malignancies has been limited and confined to investigation of consolidation treatment (e.g. in neuroblastoma[33]) or salvage therapy (e.g. Ewing's sarcoma[32]). The spectrum of adverse effects is similar to that in adults, and largely confined to myelosuppression at usual doses.

Pregnant women

Melphalan should not be used during pregnancy, particularly in the first trimester, unless the expected benefits to the mother are considered to outweigh the substantial risk to the fetus.

The elderly

Particular caution should be exercised in the use of melphalan in the elderly, as the toxicity (particularly myelosuppression) may be more marked.

Concurrent disease

The dose should be reduced by 50% in patients with impaired renal function (see above).

Drug interactions

Potentially hazardous interactions

Simultaneous administration of nalidixic acid with high-dose melphalan to children resulted in deaths due to severe gastrointestinal effects.[45] Simultaneous administration of cyclosporin and high-dose melphalan has been reported to exacerbate risks of renal damage due to cyclosporin alone.[46]

Other significant interactions

None has been reported.

Potentially useful interactions

Melphalan and prednisone together are a more effective treatment for multiple myeloma than is melphalan alone.[19] Pretreatment with cyclophosphamide (300 mg.m^{-2}) results in more rapid recovery of blood counts and reduced toxicity of high-dose melphalan (without loss of antitumour effect) in both experimental models[47] and patients.[5]

Clinical trials

1. Fisher B, Redmond C, Fisher E R and participating NSABP investigators 1980 The contribution of recent NSABP clinical trials of primary breast cancer therapy to an understanding of tumour biology—an overview of findings. Cancer 46: 1009–1025
2. Rubens R D, Hayward J L, Knight R K et al 1983 Controlled trial of adjuvant chemotherapy with melphalan for breast cancer. Lancet 1: 839–843
3. Pritchard J, Germond S, Jones D, de Kraker J, Love S 1986 Is high dose melphalan (HDM) of value in treatment of advanced neuroblastoma (AN)? Proceedings of the American Society of Clinical Oncology 5: 205

References

1. Alexander P, Swarcbort A, Stacey K A 1959 The reactivity of radiomimetic compounds — III. Crosslinking of nucleoprotein. Biochemical Pharmacology 2: 133–145
2. 1975 Melphalan, medphalan and merphalan. IARC monographs 9: 167–180
3. Benedict W F, Baker M S, Haroun L, Choi E, Ames B N 1977 Mutagenicity of cancer chemotherapeutic agents in the *Salmonella* microsome test. Cancer Research 37: 2209–2213
4. Benedict W F, Banerjee A, Gardner A, Jones P A 1977 Induction of morphological transformation in mouse C3H/10T½ clone 8 cells and chromosomal damage in hamster A(T_1)C1-3 cells by cancer chemotherapeutic agents. Cancer Research 37: 2202–2208
5. Cornbleet M A, McElwain T J, Kumar et al 1983 Treatment of advanced malignant melanoma with high-dose melphalan and autologous bone-marrow transplantation. British Journal of Cancer 48: 329–334
6. Bosanquet A G, Gilby E D 1982 Pharmacokinetics of melphalan following oral or intravenous administration in patients with malignant disease. Journal of Chromatography 232: 345–354
7. Alberts D S, Chang S Y, Chen H S et al 1979 Kinetics of intravenous melphalan. Clinical Pharmacology and Therapeutics 26: 73–80
8. Milner A N, Klatt O, Young S E, Stehlin J S 1965 The biochemical mechanism of activation of L-phenylalanine mustard: 1) Distribution of L-phenylalanine mustard-^{3}H in tumour bearing rats. Cancer Research 25: 259–264
9. Cornbleet M A, Leonard R C F, Smyth J F 1984 High-dose alkylating agent therapy: a review of clinical experience. Cancer Drug Delivery 1: 227–238
10. Selby P J, Courtenay V D, McElwain T J, Peckham M J, Steel G G 1980 Colony growth and clonogenic cell survival in human melanoma xenografts treated with chemotherapy. British Journal of Cancer 42(3); 438–447
11. Weaver P C, Wright J, Brander W L, Westbury G 1975 Salvage procedures for locally advanced malignant melanoma of the lower limb (with special reference to the role of isolated limb perfusion and radical lymphadenectomy). Clinical Oncology 1: 45–51
12. Hedley D W, Millar J L, McElwain T J, Gordon M Y 1978 Acceleration of bone-marrow recovery by pre-treatment with cyclophosphamide in patients receiving high-dose melphalan. Lancet 2: 966
13. Tattersall M H N, Jarman M, Newlands E S, Holyhead L, Milstead R A, Weinberg A 1978 Pharmacokinetics of melphalan following oral or intravenous administration in patients with malignant disease. European Journal of Cancer 14: 507–513
14. Ross W C J 1962 In: Biologic alkylating agents: fundamental chemistry and the design of compounds for selective toxicity. Butterworths, London
15. Ahmed A E, Hsu T F 1981 Quantitative analysis of melphalan and its major hydrolysate in patients and animals by reversed-phase high-performance liquid chromatography. Journal of Chromatography 222: 453–460
16. Osterheld H K, Musch E, von Unruh G E, Loos U, Rauschecker H, Muhlenbruch B J 1988 A sensitive high-performance liquid chromatographic assay for melphalan and its hydrolysis products in blood and plasma. Cancer Chemotherapy and Pharmacology 21: 156–162
17. Cornwell G G, Pajak T F, McIntyre O R 1979 Hypersensitivity reactions to intravenous melphalan during treatment of multiple myeloma; Cancer and Leukemia Group B experience. Cancer Treatment Reports 63: 399–403

18. Bergsagel D E, Griffiths K M, Haut A, Stuckey W J 1967 The treatment of plasma cell myeloma. Advances in Cancer Research 10: 311–359
19. Costa G, Engle R I, Schilling A et al 1973 Melphalan and prednisone: an effective combination for the treatment of multiple myeloma. American Journal of Medicine 54: 589–599
20. Malpas J S 1974 Blood and neoplastic diseases: myelomatosis. British Medical Journal 4: 520–522
21. Selby P J, McElwain T J, Nandi A C et al 1987 Multiple myeloma treated with high dose intravenous melphalan. British Journal of Haematology 66: 55–62
22. Logue G L, Gutterman J U, McGinn T G, Laszlo J, Rundles R W 1970 Melphalan therapy of polycythaemia vera. Blood 36: 70–86
23. Sears M E, Haut A, Eckles N 1966 Melphalan (NSC-8806) in advanced breast cancer. Cancer Chemotherapy Reports 50: 271–279
24. Canellos G P, Pocock S J, Taylor S G, Sears M E, Klaasen D J, Band P R 1976 Combination chemotherapy for metastatic breast carcinoma. Cancer 38: 1882–1886
25. Fisher B, Redmond C, Fisher E R and participating NSABP investigators 1980 The contribution of recent NSABP clinical trials of primary breast cancer therapy to an understanding of tumour biology — an overview of findings. Cancer 46: 1009–1025
26. Rubens R D, Hayward J L, Knight R K et al 1983 Controlled trial of adjuvant chemotherapy with melphalan for breast cancer. Lancet 1: 839–843
27. Young R C, Knapp R C, Fuks Z, DiSaia P J 1985 Cancer of the Ovary. In: DeVita V T, Hellman S, Rosenberg S A (eds) Cancer: Principles and practice of oncology. Lippincott, USA, pp 1083–1117
28. Rosin R D, Westbury G 1980 Isolated limb perfusion for malignant melanoma. Practitioner 224: 1031–1036
29. Sugarbaker E V, McBride C M 1976 Survival and regional disease control after isolation–perfusion for the invasive stage I melanoma of the extremities. Cancer 37: 188–198
30. Luce J K 1975 Chemotherapy of melanoma. Seminars in Oncology 2: 179–185
31. Krementz E T, Carter R D, Sutherland C M, Hutton I 1977 Chemotherapy of sarcomas of the limbs by regional perfusion. Annals of Surgery 185: 555–564
32. Cornbleet M A, Corringham R E T, Prentice G, Boesen E, McElwain T J 1981 High-dose melphalan in the treatment of Ewing's sarcoma. Cancer Treatment Reports 65: 241–244
33. Pritchard J, Germond S, Jones D, de Kraker J, Love S 1986 Is high-dose melphalan (HDM) of value in treatment of advanced neuroblastoma (AN)? Preliminary results of a randomized trial by the European Neuroblastoma Study Group (ENSG) (abstract). Proceedings of the American Society of Clinical Oncology 5: 205
34. Cornwell G G, Pajak T F, McIntyre O R, Kochwa S, Dosik H 1982 Influence of renal failure on myelosuppressive effects of melphalan: Cancer and Leukemia Group B experience. Cancer Treatment Reports 66: 475–481
35. Hoogstraten B, Sheehe P R, Cuttner J et al 1967 Melphalan in multiple myeloma. Blood 30: 74–83
36. Smith J P, Rutledge F N 1970 Chemotherapy in the treatment of cancer of the ovary. American Journal of Obstetrics and Gynecology 107: 691–703
37. Kyle R A, Pierre R V, Bayrd E D 1974 Primary amyloidosis and acute leukaemia associated with melphalan therapy. Blood 44: 333–337
38. Burton I E, Abbott C R, Roberts B E, Antonis A H 1976 Acute leukaemia after four years of melphalan treatment for melanoma. British Medical Journal 1: 20
39. Einhorn N 1978 Acute leukaemia after chemotherapy (melphalan). Cancer 41: 444–447
40. Codling B W, Chakera T M H 1972 Pulmonary fibrosis following therapy with melphalan for multiple myeloma. Journal of Clinical Pathology 25: 668–673
41. Eyster M E 1967 Melphalan (Alkeran) erythrocyte agglutinin and hemolytic anemia. Annals of Internal Medicine 66: 573–577
42. Fisher B, Carbone P, Economou S G et al 1975 L-phenylalanine mustard (L-PAM) in the management of primary breast cancer. New England Journal of Medicine 292: 117–122
43. Ahmann D L, Scanlon P W, Bisel H F et al 1978 Repeated adjuvant chemotherapy with phenylalanine mustard or 5-fluorouracil, cyclophosphamide and prednisone with or without radiation after mastectomy for breast cancer. Lancet 1: 893–896
44. Hansten P D 1971 Drugs in the production of direct Coombs' test positivity. American Journal of Hospital Pharmacy 28: 629–632
45. Voute P A, van der Nordaa J, Dobbelaar C D M 1982 Simultaneous administration of nalidixic acid (NA) and high-dose melphalan (HDM) in children causing death due to severe side-effects in the intestinal tract (abstract). European Journal of Cancer and Clinical Oncology 18: 1047
46. Morganstern G R, Powles R, Robinson B, McElwain T J 1982 Cyclosporin interaction with ketoconazole and melphalan (letter). Lancet 2: 1342
47. Millar J L, Hudspith B N, McElwain T J, Phelps T A 1978 Cyclophosphamide pretreatment reduces the toxic effect of high dose melphalan on intestinal epithelium in sheep. European Journal of Cancer 14: 1283–1285

Menotrophin

Menotrophin contains human menopausal gonadotrophin (HMG), which is used for induction of ovulation or superovulation in women and stimulation of spermatogenesis in men. Menotrophin is extracted from postmenopausal urine. Lunenfield began the therapeutic administration of menotrophin, culminating in the first pregnancy in 1962.[1]

Chemistry

Menotrophin (human menopausal gonadotrophin, HMG, Pergonal)
Menotrophin contains follicle stimulating hormone (FSH) and luteinizing hormone (LH) glycoproteins of pituitary origin, and is prepared from the urine of postmenopausal women. FSH and LH have two nonidentical and noncovalently linked peptide subunits, designated α and β subunits. The α subunit of each hormone is nearly identical. The biological specificity resides in the β subunit[2]

Molecular weight	~32 000
pKa	—
Solubility	
in alcohol	—
in water	soluble
Octanol/water partition coefficient	low

The carbohydrate content of menotrophin is greater than 30%. Analysis of the types of carbohydrate shows that sialic acid content is high — 8.5%.

Both FSH and LH are soluble in water but whereas FSH is soluble in acetate buffer (pH = 4.4, containing 20.5% sodium sulphate), LH is insoluble in this solution.

Each ampoule of menotrophin (Pergonal) contains 75 IU of FSH, 75 IU of LH and 10 mg of lactose, as a lyophilized (freeze-dried) powder. When subjected to chromatofocusing, HMG displays five immunoreactive FSH isohormones and nine luteinizing hormone (LH) isohormones.[3]

Pharmacology

Menotrophin contains approximately equal amounts of FSH and LH. The gonadotrophins bind to receptor sites within the gonads (ovaries and testes) and produce their effects via an adenosine 3,5-monophosphate (cAMP)-mediated second messenger mechanism. The main effects are as follows.

FSH binds to the granulosa cells to stimulate follicular growth and maturation. The role of LH in follicular development is questionable. Successful induction of follicular maturation and ovulation with FSH treatment in monkey[4] and human[5,6] studies during concomitant suppression of endogenous gonadotrophin secretion by gonadotrophin releasing hormone (GnRH) analogue has been reported. Also, pure FSH succeeded in the stimulation of follicular maturation in monkeys and gonadotrophin-deficient human females.[8] LH is not essential for ovarian steroidogenesis but, nonetheless, facilitates oestrogen biosynthesis.

LH stimulates thecal androgen production.[9]

FSH stimulates the induction of aromatase systems of the granulosa cells, enabling the aromatization of androgens, produced by theca cells, to oestrogen.

FSH induces LH receptor development on the granulosa cells of large antral follicles.[10]

FSH stimulates the synthesis of inhibin and plasminogen activator.

FSH and LH stimulate follicular steroidogenesis by activating adenylate cyclase. Cyclic AMP stimulates conversion of cholesterol to pregnenolone and sex steroid biosynthesis by mechanisms similar to those operative in the adrenal cortex.

LH induces luteinization of granulosa cells.[11]

Human menopausal gonadotrophin stimulates the change of undifferentiated spermatogonia type A to spermatogonia type A1 and then to spermatogonia type B.[12]

Toxicology

Menotrophin did not cause acute toxicity in mice at doses up to 150 000 IU.kg^{-1} body weight.

Clinical pharmacology

Menotrophin is used primarily to stimulate follicular development in infertile women. A course of menotrophin injections is usually followed by an injection of chorionic gonadotrophin (hCG) to induce ovulation.

Depending upon the dosages used, menotrophins are used to induce follicular development in women with hypothalamic hypogonadism (WHO group 1) or to stimulate multiple follicular development (superovulation) in women undergoing in vitro fertilization and other assisted conception techniques.

In men the drug can also be used to stimulate spermatogenesis in hypogonadotrophic hypogonadism, where 50% become fertile in response.

Menotrophin is also used in diagnostic tests of hypothalamic–pituitary–gonadal function.

Although menotrophin contains equal quantities of FSH and LH, the biological activity of FSH predominates as menotrophin is mainly used to stimulate follicular development or spermatogenesis. LH, however, is present as it plays a role in the production of oestrogens by the follicle.

Studies on cardiovascular and respiratory systems in animals have shown that menotrophin does not induce changes in heart rate, ECG pattern, arterial pressure or the breathing rate and pattern. No effects on the central nervous system have been noted.

Over a 14-day course of daily HMG administration of 1–4 ampoules, intended to mimic the follicular phase of the ovarian cycle in women with hypothalamic amenorrhoea, FSH levels gradually rise to twice their baseline level, and LH levels increase to 1.5 times the baseline.[13]

Marked individual differences were found in plasma FSH profiles, ovarian images and peripheral oestradiol levels after the administration of Humegon and Pergonal (150 IU daily for 8 days) and the approximate half life of FSH exceeded 40 h. There are marked individual differences in patient responsiveness, which are unrelated to the preparation administered.

Pharmacokinetics

The activities of FSH and LH in menotrophin are assessed by means of radioimmunoassay.[14,15] The potency of FSH and LH is defined in international units (IU) with respect to the first International Standard Preparation of human urinary FSH and LH. Menotrophin is well absorbed after intramuscular administration. Peak plasma concentrations of LH and FSH are seen at 4 and 6 h, respectively. Serum oestradiol increases by 88% in response to HMG, with the peak at 18 h.[14]

Following intravenous administration of 150 IU of FSH in the form of Pergonal and Metrodin, the maximum concentrations (C_{max}) were 24.1 and 26.5 IU.l^{-1} respectively which were reached after 15–16.9 min. The half lives were 2.3 and 2.0 h respectively (fast component) and 10 and 7.3 h, respectively (slow component).[16]

Oral absorption	poor
Presystemic metabolism	—
Plasma half life	
FSH	2 h
LH	20 min
Volume of distribution	—
Plasma protein binding	—

The half life of LH could only be estimated in a surgically hypophysectomized patient: the fast component was 1.3 h after the administration of Pergonal, and the slow component was 3.3 h.[16]

Menotrophin is eliminated via the kidneys.

No information is available on the excretion of menotrophin in breast milk. Similarly the effects of age and disease on the kinetics of this material are not known.

Concentration–effect relationship

Traditionally, patients who have undergone gonadotrophin induction of ovulation had been monitored by urinary or serum oestrogen levels and cervical mucus score. Despite monitoring, multiple gestation, ovarian hyperstimulation and poor response continued to occur. Recently, ultrasonographic monitoring has been advocated during gonadotrophin therapy[17] for improving the quality of ovulation and superovulation treatment cycles as well as reducing the incidence of multiple gestation, ovarian hyperstimulation and poor response. Some studies have advocated its use concurrently with serum oestradiol levels, and others have even suggested using ultrasonographic evaluation as the sole method for assessing follicular maturation. To conclude, ultrasound findings reflect growth, whereas serum oestradiol levels primarily detect functional activity of follicles.[4]

There is no evidence of any correlation between the plasma concentration of menotrophin and its various clinical effects.

Metabolism

Menotrophin is eliminated via the kidneys. The main pathway and structures of the metabolites are unknown.

Pharmaceutics

Menotrophin (Pergonal; Serono, UK/USA) is available in parenteral dosage only. Menotrophin contains human menopausal gonadotrophin (HMG) in a lyophilized (freeze-dried) powder form. An ampoule of menotrophin (Pergonal) contains 75 IU of FSH, 75 IU of LH and 10 mg of lactose. In the USA a double strength ampoule is also available. Each menotrophin ampoule is accompanied by a solvent ampoule containing 1 ml of 0.9% sodium chloride injection BP. Up to 5 ampoules may be dissolved in 1 ml of solvent. Menotrophin should be given by deep intramuscular injection.

One IU of human urinary FSH and one IU of human urinary LH are defined as the activities contained in 0.11 388 mg and 0.13 369 mg of the first international standard, respectively.

The maximum recommended shelf-life for menotrophin is three years, as the lyophilized ampoules of menotrophin have been found to be stable for 3 years when stored at 37°C, room temperature and deep frozen. It is recommended that menotrophin ampoules should be stored at temperatures preferably not exceeding 25°C. When reconstituted, menotrophin is stable for up to 14 days at 37°C and for up to 20 days at 25°C. Pergonal is tested and declared free from HBsAG and HIV.

Therapeutic use

Indications

In women

1. Follicular growth stimulation in anovulatory and amenorrhoeic patients
2. Follicular growth stimulation in hypothalamic amenorrhoea.
3. Follicular growth stimulation in combination with LHRH analogues particularly in Clomiphene citrate-resistant polycystic ovary (PCO)
4. Follicular growth stimulation for intrauterine insemination
5. Superovulation for IVF-ET and GIFT
   alone
   with clomiphene citrate either sequentially or concomitantly with GnRH analogues.

In men

6. With HCG in idiopathic male infertility
7. With HCG in hypogonadotrophic hypogonadism.

In children

8. In undescendent testes.

Contraindications

Women

1. Ovarian dysgenesis
2. Absent uterus
3. Premature menopause
4. Tubal disease (except in IVF).

Appropriate treatment should first be given for hypothyroidism, adrenocortical deficiency, hyperprolactinaemia or pituitary tumour.

Men

5. Primary testicular failure.

Elevated endogenous FSH levels are indicative of primary testicular failure. Such patients are usually unresponsive to menotrophin/chorionic gonadotrophins.

Mode of use

Dosage

The following are examples of dosage:

1. Follicular growth stimulation in anovulatory and amenorrhoeic patients: an initial dose of 2 ampoules is used.
2. Follicular growth stimulation in hypothalamic amenorrhoea. After pulsatile GnRH, when the dominant follicle reaches 7–8 mm, a low dose (such as 1.5–2 ampoules initially) menotrophin is given intramuscularly for three consecutive days. HCG produces presumptive evidence of ovulation.[18]
3. Follicular growth stimulation in combination with GnRH analogues particularly in clomiphene citrate-resistant polycystic ovary (PCO)[19]: a low dose such as 1–1.5 ampoules is recommended initially, but the dose should be adjusted every 5–7 days according to the responses of the ovary on serum oestradiol assays.
4. Follicular growth stimulation for intrauterine insemination:[20] a low dose such as 1.5–2 ampoules is recommended initially but the dose should be adjusted every 5–7 days according to the responses of the ovary on serum oestradiol assays.

1–4. Ovulation induction

The object is to develop a single mature Graffian follicle with individually tailored doses of menotrophin over several days and then give chorionic gonadotrophins to release the ovum. Follicular development is judged by the concentration of oestrogen, measured in blood or urine and/or by ultrasound measurement of follicular growth. The dose of menotrophin required to evoke the desired response is variable from patient to patient and in the same patient the ovarian response varies from cycle to cycle. Therefore, monitoring by hormone assay and/or ultrasound is essential (see Concentration–effect relationship).

There are only three essentially different types of therapy: fixed-dose regimens, individually adjusted schemes and combined therapy.

In the fixed-dose regimens, a certain amount of menotrophin is administered on predetermined cycle days followed by HCG. By using a fixed dose in each cycle, the patient's gonadotrophin requirements could be met only by successively increasing the dose in consecutive cycles.

The individually adjusted treatment scheme allows for successive increments of the gonadotrophin dose according to the patient's response during the same cycle. This tends to reduce the number of treatment cycles needed for successful ovulation induction and may reduce the incidence of ovarian hyperstimulation syndrome (OHSS).

Combined treatment in the form of clomiphene citrate and menotrophin has been widely used in most IVF programmes to stimulate a large enough crop of follicles. The claim is that this combination produces more uniform ovum maturation than does menotrophin alone.

Another form of combined treatment is to use GnRH analogues to suppress endogenous gonadotrophin to overcome the possible interference of untimely and/or unbalanced endogenous gonadotrophin secretion.

Menotrophin should be started within the first seven days of the menstrual cycle. Menotrophin could be administered daily or on alternate-day schedules and administration should continue till the mean diameter of the leading follicle is at least 17 mm with compatible oestrogen levels [>1100 pmol.l^{-1} (300 pg.ml^{-1}) for plasma oestradiol-17B or 180 nmol per 24 h (140 µg per 24 h) for total urinary oestrogens]. The optimal time for chorionic gonadotrophin administration is the day of the urinary oestrogen peak or the day after the plasma 17B-oestradiol peak. A single dose of up to 10 000 IU chorionic gonadotrophin is given.

The patient is recommended to have coitus on the day when chorionic gonadotrophin is given and on the following day.

5. Superovulation

The objective of superovulation for assisted conception techniques is to stimulate multiple follicular growth. Follicular development is judged by the assay of oestrogen in blood or urine, and/or by serial ultrasonography. Menotrophin could be administered within the first seven days of the menstrual cycle, in a dose of 2–3 ampoules daily, alone or following the administration of clomiphene citrate from days 2–6 in a dose of 50–150 mg (100 mg dose is commonly used) or after downregulation of the pituitary gland using GnRH analogues.[21,22]

Follicular development is judged by the assay of oestrogen in blood or urine, and/or by serial ultrasonography and the dose of menotrophin is adjusted accordingly.

A single dose of up to 10 000 IU chorionic gonadotrophin is administered when the mean diameter of at least three follicles are more than 17 mm with compatible oestrogen levels (>3500 pmol.l^{-1} (920 pg.ml^{-1}) for plasma oestradiol-17β or 630 nmol per 24 h (490 µg per 24 h) for total urinary oestrogens).

Egg collection is carried out using either ultrasound guided aspiration (vaginal, transabdominal or transurethral) or the laparoscope, about 34–36 h following the chorionic gonadotrophin injection.

To avoid OHSS, a small dose of menotrophin (2 ampoules daily) is recommended initially particularly for patients <36 years old. An even smaller dose (1–1.5 daily) is given initially to patients with polycystic ovarian disease or previous ovarian hyperstimulation syndrome. On the other hand, patients >36 years old or with a history of poor response to menotrophin are started on a higher dose (3 or 4 ampoules). The most predictive factor in identifying those patients who are at risk of OHSS is the level of oestradiol at the time of administering chorionic gonadotrophin.[23] If the oestradiol level of 13 000 pmol.l^{-1} is reached at or before the sonographic criteria of at least 3 follicles with a mean diameter of 17 mm, the administration of HCG is withheld, coitus avoided and the treatment cycle cancelled.

6, 7. Men

Treatment[24,25] should begin with chorionic gonadotrophin 2000 IU 2–3 times a week to produce a normal serum testosterone production and evidence of adequate masculinization. After six months of normal serum testosterone, menotrophin is added if necessary. The initial dose is 75 IU three times a week for four months, followed by 150 IU three times a week for a further four months.

8. Children with cryptorchidism

40 IU three intramuscular injections per week for eight weeks, plus HCG 500 IU one intramuscular injection weekly for four weeks. Testicular descent occurred in 50%.[26]

Adverse reactions

Potentially life-threatening effects

Ovarian hyperstimulation syndrome (OHSS). The ovarian hyperstimulation syndrome is the most serious of the complications affecting ovulation induction, and its severest manifestations take the form of massive ovarian enlargement, haemoconcentration and extravascular accumulation of fluid in the form of ascites, pleural and pericardial effusion. The full-blown clinical syndrome may be complicated by renal failure, oliguria, hypovolaemic shock, fever, arterial thromboembolism, adult respiratory distress syndrome, and even death.

The incidence of OHSS has been reported to vary from 8% to 23% in mild, <1% to 7% in moderate, and 1% to 1.8% in its severe form.[27] Young lean patients who after relatively few ampoules of menotrophin recruit more follicles with significantly more small follicles with high oestrogen levels in the early follicular phase are at risk of ovarian hyperstimulation.

Acute overdosage
No cases appear to have been reported.

Severe or irreversible adverse effects
Gynaecomastia occasionally occurs in men.

Symptomatic adverse effects
The drug may cause local reactions at the injection site. Fever, joint pains, headache, mood changes, tiredness and fluid retention have been reported rarely.

Other effects
Multiple births occur in 10–40% of the pregnant mothers following menotrophin/chorionic gonadotrophin therapy. However, the majority of multiple conceptions are twins.

Spontaneous abortion occurs in about 25% of those patients who conceive on a regimen of HMG with HCG.[28] This rate is higher than in a normal population but comparable with the rates in women with other fertility problems.[29]

The risks of congenital abnormalities are not increased by menotrophin.[30]

Interference with clinical pathology tests
No interference of this kind appears to have been reported.

High risk groups

Neonates
The drug is not used in neonates.

Breast milk. The drug is unlikely to be used in breast-feeding mothers.

Children
The drug is not used in children.

Pregnant women
Stimulation of multiple follicular development was induced concurrent with a viable early intrauterine pregnancy. The ovaries responded successfully to gonadotrophin stimulation. In addition, these recovered oocytes were successfully fertilized and two subsequently cleaved.[31]

The elderly
The drug is not used in this group of patients.

Drug interactions

No information is available.

Major outcome trials

For ovulation induction as a first-line therapy in amenorrhoeic patients with hypothalamo-pituitary failure

1. Hull M G R, Savage P E, Jacobs H S 1979 Investigations and treatment of amenorrhoea resulting in normal fertility. British Medical Journal 1: 1257–1261

This is a retrospective study of 59 patients with anovulatory amenorrhoea. The results are presented as cumulative rates of conception and delivery of a live baby. All ovulated and by the end of two years 55 (93%) had conceived, 42 (71%) had delivered at least one surviving child, while 5 others (8%) were pregnant and awaiting delivery.

2. Oelsner G, Seer D M, Mashiach S, Blankstein J, Snyder M, Lunenfeld B 1978 The study of induction of ovulation with menotrophins: analysis of results of 1897 treatment cycles. Fertility and Sterility 30 (5): 538–544

This is a retrospective analysis of 510 patients to whom 1897 treatment cycles with menotrophins were administered in a 15-year period. 708 treatment cycles were carried out to patients with hypogonadotrophic hypogonadism. 193 pregnancies occurred in 116 (60.4%) women.

3. Dor J, Itzkowic D, Mashiach S, Lunenfeld B 1980 Cumulative conception rates following gonadotrophin therapy. American Journal of Obstetrics and Gynaecology 136: 102–105

This is a retrospective analysis of 515 patients who were treated with HMG during the years 1963–1978. The cumulative pregnancy rate in 167 patients with absent endogenous oestrogen activity was 91.2% after six treatment cycles. In 77 patients, further treatment was given for a second pregnancy after the first gonadotrophin conception. In this group, the cumulative pregnancy rate was 93.6% after eight treatment cycles.

For ovulation induction as a second-line therapy in patients with hypothalamo-pituitary dysfunction who fail to conceive on anti-oestrogen agents

1. Oelsner G, Seer D M, Mashiach S, Blankstein J, Snyder M, Lunenfeld B 1978 The study of induction of ovulation with menotrophins: analysis of results of 1897 treatment cycles. Fertility and Sterility 30 (5): 538–544

This is a retrospective analysis of 510 patients to whom 1897 treatment cycles with menotrophins were administered in a 15-year period. 1189 treatment cycles were carried out to patients with normal endogenous gonadotrophin levels and distinct oestrogen activity. 85 pregnancies occurred in 68 (21.4%) of women.

2. Dor J, Itzkowic D, Mashiach S, Lunenfeld B 1980 Cumulative conception rates following gonadotrophin therapy. American Journal of Obstetrics and Gynecology 136: 102–105

This is a retrospective analysis of 515 patients who were treated with HMG during the years 1963–1978. The cumulative pregnancy rate in 348 patients with normal endogenous oestrogen activity was 50% after six treatment cycles.

3. Butler J K 1972 Clinical results with human gonadotrophins in anovulation, using two alternative dosage schemes. Postgraduate Medical Journal 48: 27–32

This is a retrospective analysis of 443 patients who were treated with HMG. 1280 treatment cycles were carried out to patients with normal endogenous gonadotrophin levels and distinct oestrogen activity. 126 pregnancies occurred.

For superovulation induction

1. Testart J, Belaisch-Allart J, Forman R et al 1989 Influence of different stimulation treatments on oocyte characteristics and in-vitro fertilizing ability. Human Reproduction 4 (2): 192–197
2. Rutherford A J, Subak-Sharpe R J, Dawson K J, Margara R A, Franks S, Winston R M L 1988 Improvement of in vitro fertilization after treatment with buserelin, an agonist of lutinising hormone releasing hormone. British Medical Journal 296: 1765–1768

Randomized controlled trials

1. Lavy G, Pellicer A, Diamond M, DeCherney A H 1988 Ovarian stimulation for in vitro fertilization and embryo transfer, human menopausal gonadotrophin versus pure human follicle stimulating hormone: a randomized prospective study. Fertility and Sterility 50 (1): 74–77

Other trials

1. Fleming R, Coutts J 1986 Induction of multiple follicular growth in normally menstruating women with endogenous gonadotrophin suppression. Fertility and Sterility 45: 226–230
2. Frydman R, Parneix I, Belaisch-Allart J, Forman R, Hazout A, Testar J 1988 LHRH agonists in IVF: different methods of utilization and comparison with previous ovulation stimulation treatments. Human Reproduction 3: 559–561
3. Porter R N, Smith W, Craft I L, Abdulwahid N A, Jacobs H S 1984 Induction of ovulation for in-vitro fertilization using Buserelin and gonadotrophins. Lancet 2: 1284–1285

General review articles

Hillier S G, Afnan A M M, Margara R A, Winston R M L 1985 Superovulation strategy before in vitro fertilisation. Clinics in Obstetrics and Gynaecology 12: 687–723
Insler V 1988 Gonadotrophin therapy: new trends and insights. International Journal of Fertility 33 (2): 85–97

References

1. Lunenfeld B, Sulimovizi S, Rabau E et al 1962 Compt Rendus Societé Français Gynecologie 35: 346
2. Pierce J G, Parsons T F 1981 Glycoprotein hormones: structure and function. Annual Review in Biochemistry 50: 465–495
3. Cook A S, Webster B W, Terranova P F, Keel B A 1988 Variation in the biologic and biochemical characteristics of human menopausal gonadotrophin. Fertility and Sterility 49 (4): 704–712
4. Kenigsberg D, Littman B A, Williams R F, Hodgen G D 1984 Medical hypophysectomy. I. Dose–response using a gonadotropin releasing hormone antagonist. Fertility and Sterility 42: 112–115
5. Venturoli S, Orsini L F, Paradisi R et al 1986 Human urinary follicle stimulating hormone and human menopausal gonadotropin in induction of multiple follicle growth and ovulation. Fertility and Sterility 45: 30
6. Martikainen H, Ronnberg L, Puistola U et al 1986 Comparison of the effects of follicle stimulating hormone and human menopausal gonadotropin on peripheral serum and follicular fluid hormones during ovarian stimulation. Fertility and Sterility 465: 317
7. Schenker R S, Williams R F, Hodgen G D 1984 Ovulation induction using pure follicle stimulating hormone in monkeys. Fertility and Sterility 41: 629
8. Couzinet B, Lestrat N, Brailly S, Forest M, Schaison G 1988 Stimulation of ovarian follicular maturation with pure follicle stimulating hormone in women with gonadotrophin deficiency. Journal of Clinical Endocrinology and Metabolism 66 (3): 552–556
9. Tsang B K, Armstrong D T, Whitfield J F 1980 Steroid biosynthesis by isolated human ovarian follicular cells in vitro. Journal of Clinical Endocrinology and Metabolism 51: 1407–1411
10. Zeleznik A J, Midgley A R, Reichart L E 1974 Granulosa cell maturation in the rat. Increased binding of human chorionic gonadotrophin following treatment with follicle stimulating hormone in vivo. Endocrinology 95: 818–825
11. Channing C P, Seymour J F 1970 Effects of dibutyryl cyclic 3′5′-AMP and other agents upon luteinization of porcine granulosa cells in culture. Endocrinology 87: 165–169
12. Kula K 1988 Induction of precocious maturation of spermatogenesis in infant rats by human menopausal gonadotropin and inhibition by simultaneous administration of gonadotropins and testosterone. Endocrinology 122 (1): 34–39
13. Anderson R E, Cragun J M, Chang R J, Stanczyk F Z, Lobo R A 1989 A pharmacodynamic comparison of human urinary follicle-stimulating hormone and human menopausal gonadotropin in normal women and polycystic ovary syndrome. Fertility and Sterility 52 (2): 216–220
14. Barttai G, Robertson D M, Diczfalusy E 1979 Biologically active luteinising hormone (LH) in plasma: IV. Comparison with immunologically active LH in plasma of men. Acta Endocrinological 90: 599–608
15. Marana R, Robertson D M, Suginami H, Diczfalusy E 1979 The assay of human follicle stimulating hormone preparations: the choice of a suitable standard. Acta Endocrinological 92: 599–614
16. Diczfalusy E, Harlin J 1988 Clinical–pharmacological studies on human menopausal gonadotrophin. Human Reproduction 3(1): 21–27
17. Hull M E, Moghissi K S, Magyar D M, Hayes M F, Zador I, Olson J M 1986 Correlation of serum estradiol level and ultrasound monitoring to assess follicular maturation. Fertility and Sterility 46 (1): 42–45
18. Corenblum B, Taylor P J 1987 Augmentation of gonadotropin-releasing hormone induced follicular growth with exogenous gonadotropins. Fertility and Sterility 48 (6): 954–957
19. Venturini P L, Remorgida V, Anserini P, De-Cecco L 1988 Use of combined exogenous gonadotropins and pulsatile gonadotropin-releasing hormone in patients with polycystic ovarian disease: a new approach to induction of ovulation. Gynecological Endocrinology 2 (3): 205–213
20. Kemmann E, Bohrer M, Shelden R, Fiasconaro G, Beardsley L 1987 Active ovulation management increases the monthly probability of pregnancy occurrence in ovulatory women who receive intrauterine insemination. Fertility and Sterility 48 (6): 916–920
21. Franks S, Sagle M, Mason H D, Kiddy D 1987 Use of LHRH agonists in the treatment of anovulation in women with polycystic ovary syndrome. Hormone Research 28 (2–4): 164–168
22. Awadalla S G, Friedman C I, Chin N W, Dodds W, Park J M, Kim M H 1987 Follicular stimulation for in vitro fertilization using pituitary suppression and human menopausal gonadotropins. Fertility and Sterility 48 (5): 811–815
23. Navot D, Relou A, Birkenfeld A, Rabinowitz R, Brezezinski A, Margalioth E J 1988 Risk factors and prognostic variables in the ovarian hyperstimulation syndrome. American Journal of Obstetrics and Gynaecology 159: 210–215
24. Namiki M, Nakamura M, Okuyama A et al 1988 Testicular follicle stimulating hormone receptors and effectiveness of human menopausal gonadotropin–human chorionic gonadotropin treatment in idiopathic male infertility. Hinyokika-Kiyo 34 (6): 957–961
25. Liu L, Banks S M, Barnes K M, Sherins R J 1988 Two-year comparison of testicular responses to pulsatile gonadotropin-releasing hormone and exogenous gonadotropins from the inception of therapy in men with isolated hypogonadotropic hypogonadism. Journal of Clinical Endocrinology and Metabolism 67 (6): 1140–1145
26. DeRosa G, Della-Casa S, Corsello S M et al 1987 Treatment of undescended testes with hMG and hMG plus hCG: clinical hormonal and sonographic evaluation. Annales d'Endocrinologie (Paris) 48 (6): 468–472
27. Schenker J G, Weinstein D 1978 Ovarian hyperstimulation syndrome: a current survey. Fertility and Sterility 30: 255
28. Bohrer M, Kemmann E 1987 Risk factors for spontaneous abortion in menotrophin treated women. Fertility and Sterility 48 (4): 571–575
29. Jansen R P 1982 Spontaneous abortion incidence in the treatment of infertility. American Journal of Obstetrics and Gynecology 143: 451
30. Caspi E, Ronen J, Scheyer P, Goldberg M D 1976 The outcome of pregnancy after gonadotropin therapy. British Journal of Obstetrics and Gynaecology 83: 967–973
31. Diamond M P, Tarlatzis B C, DeCherney A H 1987 Recruitment of multiple follicular development for in vitro fertilization in the presence of a viable intrauterine pregnancy. Obstetrics and Gynecology 70 (3 pt 2): 498–499

Meprobamate

Meprobamate was the most widely used of the propranediol carbamate anxiolytic sedatives. Since the advent of the benzodiazepines, use of meprobamate has declined. Its main use now is in combination with other agents.

Chemistry

Meprobamate (Equanil, Miltown, SK-Bamate, Meprate)
$C_9H_{18}N_2O_4$
2-Methyl-2-propyl-1,3-propanediol dicarbamate

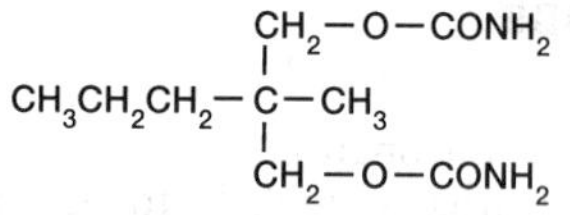

Molecular weight	218.3
pKa	14
Solubility	
in alcohol	1 in 7
in water	—
Octanol/water partition coefficient	—

Meprobamate occurs as odourless or almost odourless, colourless crystals or a white crystalline powder with a bitter taste.

Meprobamate is also available in oral combination products with aspirin (Equagesic, Heptogesic, Mepro Compound, Meprogesic), oestrogens (Milprem, PMB), bendrofluazide (Tenavoid), pentaerythritol tetranitrate (Miltrate), trihexethyl chloride (Milpath, Pathibamate), and benactyzine hydrochloride (Deprol).

Pharmacology

Meprobamate has a central nervous system depressant action similar to that of the barbiturates. The mechanism of action is not known. Meprobamate does not act on the benzodiazepine receptor or GABA system, nor is it related to the phenothiazine derivatives. It also has a relaxant effect on voluntary muscle.[1,2]

The effect of meprobamate on the EEG is similar to that caused by benzodiazepines and barbiturates resulting in an increase in the fast wave activity.[3]

Toxicology

Long-term studies in rats and dogs show no evidence of drug-related toxic effects. In humans no long-term toxic effects are known.[4]

Clinical pharmacology

Meprobamate has a generalized tranquillizing effect.[5] It also has muscle relaxant properties, although these may be secondary to the sedative actions.[6] In animals, anticonvulsant actions have been demonstrated, but these are not apparent in man. There is no effect on the autonomic nervous system. In toxic doses meprobamate depresses the respiratory and cardiovascular systems. Its actions make it suitable for combination with other drugs for the treatment of conditions in which a somatic and psychic component are present; for example with analgesics for the treatment of pain and with diuretics for the treatment of premenstrual tension.

Meprobamate use can result in psychological and physical dependence with a barbiturate-type withdrawal syndrome. The benzodiazepine tranquillizers have for the most part replaced meprobamate in clinical practice because of their greater safety and equal efficacy.

Meprobamate

Pharmacokinetics

Analytical methods for the determination of meprobamate in biological fluids include a colorimetric assay,[7] and gas chromatography with flame-ionization detection of the underivatized drug and of a silyl derivative of the hydrolysed drug.[8–10] The limit of detection is 5 mg.l^{-1}.

Meprobamate is readily absorbed from the gastrointestinal tract and peak concentrations in the plasma occur after 1 to 2 hours. The mean half life of meprobamate is about 10 hours. Half lives ranging from 6.4 to 16.6 hours have been shown after oral administration.[11,12] An oral dose of 400 mg meprobamate produces peak plasma concentrations of 5–30 mg.l^{-1}.

There is some evidence that meprobamate induces microsomal enzyme systems in the liver, resulting in accelerated metabolism, tolerance and interaction with the metabolism of other drugs such as warfarin.[13] Meprobamate is uniformly distributed through the body, with the exception of adipose tissue where time is taken for equilibration to occur.[14] It passes into the milk of lactating mothers and is found in concentrations up to four times that in the mother's plasma. It also crosses the placenta and is present in umbilical cord blood at a similar concentration to that in maternal blood.

Meprobamate is approximately 20% bound to plasma proteins.

Oral absorption	—
Presystemic metabolism	—
Plasma half life	
range	6–17 h
mean	10 h
Volume of distribution	—
Plasma protein binding	20%

Because meprobamate is partially excreted via the kidney, the dosage interval should be increased in patients with renal failure.[15]

Concentration–effect relationship

An oral dose of 400 mg meprobamate produces peak plasma concentrations of 5–30 mg.l^{-1}. In acute overdosage, blood concentrations between 100 and 200 mg.l^{-1} have been associated with deep coma. Concentrations above this may be fatal.[16]

Metabolism

Meprobamate is metabolized in the liver by microsomal enzymes: by oxidation of the propyl side-chain to hydroxymeprobamate, and to the N-glucuronide of the parent drug. About 10% of a single dose is excreted unchanged in the urine. Similarly, about 10% is excreted as hydroxymeprobamate and up to 65% is eliminated in the urine within 48 hours as the N-glucuronide. Less than 10% of the glucuronide appears in the faeces.[17]

Two pathways of metabolism have been described: side-chain oxidation and N-glucuronidation. Both metabolites are pharmacologically inactive (Fig. 1).

Pharmaceutics

Meprobamate is available in oral forms. Equanil tablets (Wyeth, UK) contain 200 mg and 400 mg. The 200 mg tablets are round, flat and white with bevelled edges. One face is plain, and the other has 'WYETH' impressed on it. The 400 mg tablets are similar, but have a scored face and the letter 'E' impressed on both halves. 600 mg tablets are oval in shape. Miltown tablets (Wallace, USA) contain 200 mg, 400 mg, and 600 mg. The 200 mg strength is a round, white, sugar-coated tablet marked '37' 'Wallace', '1101' in orange ink. Miltown 400 is a white, round, scored tablet debossed '37' 'Wallace', '1101'. The 600 mg strength is a white capsule-shaped tablet marked 'WALLACE' '37 1601'.

There are several combination preparations containing meprobamate available.

Meprobamate preparations are stable, with a shelf-life of up to 3 years. Tablets can be stored at room temperature.

Therapeutic use

Indications

1. Short-term treatment of anxiety states
2. Muscle tension
3. Somatic conditions where anxiety is present.

Contraindications

1. Known hypersensitivity to meprobamate or related compounds, carisoprodol or carbromal
2. Alcohol and drug dependence
3. Acute intermittent porphyria
4. Lactation.

Mode of use

The primary indication of meprobamate is as an anxiolytic/sedative drug. There is also a muscle relaxant action which is probably independent of the sedative action of the drug. The oral dose is usually 400 mg three to four times a day. The maximum daily dose is 2.4 g, although doses of up to 3200 mg have been used in clinical trials. Treatment should be limited to the short term and linked to other forms of help such as counselling, as appropriate in cases of anxiety, or physiotherapy in cases of muscle spasm. Caution should be exercised with longer-term use, as psychological and physical dependence can occur. Convulsions and severe anxiety may occur after sudden withdrawal.

Indications

1. Short-term treatment of anxiety states

Meprobamate is an effective anxiolytic agent.[18] It controls symptoms rapidly. Its effects are similar to those of the barbiturates. The dose should be adjusted to maximize the anxiolytic effect and to minimize the sedative action. A starting dose of 400 mg three times a day is usual, with an additional dose at bedtime. Since treatment is symptomatic it should only be continued for days, or at the most a few weeks, until the crisis resolves spontaneously. Failing this, medication should be linked to other therapeutic interventions such as psychological support and counselling.

In general, meprobamate has been superseded by the benzodiazepine tranquillizers. They are safer with regard to side effects and overdose, and are less likely to produce physical dependence.

2. Muscle tension

Meprobamate has been used in patients with a variety of musculoskeletal disorders associated with pain, muscle spasm, tension and

Fig. 1 Metabolism of meprobamate

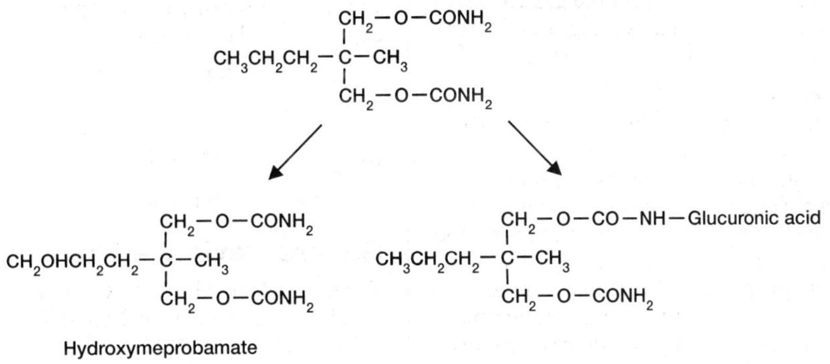

anxiety.[19,20] Most patients receive 400 mg meprobamate, three or four times a day, for periods of up to 3 to 4 weeks.

3. Somatic conditions where anxiety is present
Meprobamate is available in combination products. Meprobamate 200 mg combined with aspirin 325 mg is available as Equagesic. When given to patients with musculoskeletal disorders, Equanil produces significant improvements in a considerable proportion of patients. Pain, muscle spasm and emotional tension are reduced and mobility improved. Muscles are relaxed to enable patients requiring physiotherapy to exercise with less pain.[21] Meprobamate 200 mg in combination with oestrogens is available as a tablet for the treatment of premenstrual syndromes associated with anxiety. Meprobamate 200 mg with bendrofluazide 3 mg is available as Tenavoid, for use in premenstrual tension, in those cases where there is evidence of water retention as well as of emotional problems. The dose is one tablet three times a day beginning 5 to 7 days before the expected onset of the period.

Contraindications

1. Known hypersensitivity to meprobamate
Hypersensitivity is rare. The most frequent manifestations are skin reactions such as exanthematous reactions, eczematous dermatitis, urticaria, fixed eruptions and purpura.[22] These reactions appear to be more common in those with a history of skin diseases. Hypersensitivity reactions have been reported in about 2% of patients being treated with meprobamate. These reactions arise after one to four doses of the drug. A few cases of cross-reactions between meprobamate and carisoprodol or carbromal have been reported.[23]

2. Alcohol and drug dependence
Some degree of dependence may occur with meprobamate.[24,25] This is particularly likely in individuals with unstable personalities and the tendency to abuse alcohol and drugs. It should be prescribed cautiously and the patients supervised closely. Abrupt cessation is associated with a barbiturate-type withdrawal syndrome, characterized by anxiety, delirium and convulsions.

3. Acute intermittent porphyria
Meprobamate can precipitate attacks of acute intermittent porphyria in susceptible individuals. Such attacks are serious and potentially fatal. Meprobamate is contraindicated in patients at risk.[26]

4. Lactation
Meprobamate is found in the milk of lactating mothers at a concentration of up to four times the plasma concentration. Although the amounts of meprobamate ingested by the infant are likely to be small, women taking meprobamate should be advised not to breast-feed their infants.

Adverse reactions

Potentially life-threatening effects
Meprobamate is relatively free from adverse effects. It can, however, precipitate attacks of acute intermittent porphyria in susceptible individuals. Such attacks are serious and potentially fatal.

Acute overdosage
Acute poisoning with meprobamate produces coma, shock and vasomotor and respiratory collapse. Suicide attempts may prove successful. Documented fatal overdoses have ranged from 12 g to 47.6 g. The usual fatal dose is considered to be 40 g or more. Recovery has occurred after ingestion of similar large amounts (20–40 g).[27]

Gastric lavage is only effective within a short period of drug ingestion as meprobamate is rapidly absorbed from the gastrointestinal tract. Blood concentrations may be reduced by a regime of forced diuresis or haemodialysis. Assisted ventilation may be required.[16]

Severe or irreversible adverse effects
Meprobamate can cause allergic or hypersensitivity reactions, which are effects mediated through immunological mechanisms. They are not dose-related, occur in only a small minority of those who take the drug, and differ from the drug's usual pharmacological action.

Severe systemic reactions with shaking, chills and fever, nausea and vomiting, hypotension and collapse have occurred. Blood disorders, including non-thrombocytopenic purpura, and rarely, thrombocytopenia, have occurred. Rarely reported reactions, usually occurring as part of a generalized hypersensitivity reaction, include hyperpyrexia, angioneurotic oedema, bronchospasm and oliguria or anuria. Anaphylaxis, erythema multiforme, exfoliative dermatitis, stomatitis, proctitis, Stevens–Johnson syndrome and bullous dermatitis have also been reported.

Meprobamate may induce epileptic fits in susceptible individuals and may also cause fits on abrupt withdrawal. Its use in epileptic patients is not recommended.

Symptomatic adverse effects
Meprobamate generally acts as a central nervous system depressant. As such it causes sedation and psychomotor impairment. Caution has to be exercised in patients who drive motor cars or operate machinery. The most frequently reported adverse effects in 46 open or double-blind clinical trials of 4004 patients were drowsiness (12.6%), dizziness (1.6%), nausea (0.7%) and skin rashes (0.5%).

The incidence of other symptoms was low.

Interference with clinical pathology tests
Meprobamate has been reported to interfere with tests for:

1. Barbiturates causing a yellow spot with Frings' TLC procedure at 10 $mg.dl^{-1}$
2. Oestriol, by affecting the unmodified Brown–Kober procedure
3. 17-ketogenic steroids and 17-ketosteroids, by interference with the Zimmerman reaction
4. 17-hydroxy corticosteroids by its small effect on the modified Glenn–Nelson method and on the Porter-Silber reaction.

High risk groups

Neonates
Meprobamate is not recommended for use in neonates.

Breast milk. Meprobamate is found in the milk of lactating mothers at a concentration of up to four times the plasma concentration. As such it should not be given to mothers who are breast-feeding.

Children
It is not recommended for use in children.

Pregnant women
There are no human or animal studies which establish safety in pregnancy. Meprobamate should not be administered during pregnancy unless there are exceptional clinical circumstances. A higher incidence of birth defects has been suggested in women who took meprobamate in the first 42 days of pregnancy.[25] This has not been confirmed by other studies.[29] Special care should be exercised during the first trimester.

The elderly
The elderly have an increased sensitivity to sedative drugs and respond to lower doses. Half the normal adult dose or less may be sufficient.

Drug interactions

Potentially hazardous interactions
Alcohol potentiates the effects of meprobamate, causing greater sedation, incoordination and disinhibition. Their concurrent use is not recommended.

Other significant interactions
Meprobamate causes induction of liver enzymes and thus alters the metabolism of other drugs. The blood concentrations of drugs similarly metabolized will be reduced if meprobamate is given, or will increase if meprobamate is stopped. These drugs include: barbiturates and phenytoin, systemic steroids including oral contraceptives, warfarin, griseofulvin, rifampicin, phenothiazines and tricyclic antidepressants. The clinical importance of this effect is not established.

Potentially useful interactions
None is known.

Major outcome trials

None has been reported.

General review articles

Kaplan S, Jack M 1979 Minor tranquillizer pharmacokinetics. In: Schoolar J, Claghorn J (eds) The kinetics of psychiatric drugs. Brunner/Mazel, New York, ch 11, pp 191–214

Meprobamate

American Hospital Formulary Service–Drug Information Service 1985 Meprobamate. American Society of Hospital Pharmacists, Bethesda, pp 947–949

Harvey S 1980 Drugs and the treatment of psychiatric disorders. In: Goodman L, Gilman A (eds) The pharmacological basis of therapeutics 6th edn. Macmillan, New York, ch 17, pp 365–367

References

1. Ludwig B, Potterfield J 1971 The pharmacology of propanediol carbamates. Advances in Pharmacology and Chemotherapy 9: 173–240
2. Berger F 1956 Meprobamate. Its pharmacologic properties and clinical uses. International Record of Medicine and General Practice Clinics 169: 184–196
3. Fink M 1969 EEG and human psychopharmacology. American Review of Pharmacology 9: 241–258
4. Berger F 1954 The pharmacological properties of 2-Methyl-2-n-propyl-1,3-propanediol dicarbamate (Miltown), a new interneuronal blocking agent. Pharmacology and Experimental Therapeutics 112: 413–423
5. Domino E 1962 Human pharmacology of tranquillizing drugs. Clinical Pharmacology and Therapeutics 3: 599–664
6. Nyquist R, Bors E, Comart A 1958 A comparative study of antispasmodic drugs in patients with spinal cord injuries. Archives of Physical Medicine and Rehabilitation 39: 683–691
7. Hoffman A, Ludwig B 1959 An improved colorimetric method for the determination of meprobamate in biological fluids. Journal of the American Pharmaceutical Association 48: 740–742
8. Finkle B 1967 The identification, quantitative determination and distribution of meprobamate in biological materials. Journal of Forensic Science 12: 509–528
9. Douglas J, Kelley T F, Smith N B et al 1967 Gas chromatographic determination of meprobamate, 2-methyl-2-propyl-1,3-propanediol dicarbamate, in plasma and urine. Analytical Chemistry 39: 956–958
10. Martis L, Levy R 1974 GLC determination of meprobamate in water, plasma and urine. Journal of Pharmaceutical Science 63: 834–837
11. Meyer M, Melikian A, Straughn A 1978 Relative bioavailability of meprobamate tablets in humans. Journal of the American Pharmaceutical Association 67: 1290–1293
12. Hollister L, Levy G 1964 Kinetics of meprobamate elimination in humans. Chemotherapia 9: 20–24
13. Douglas J, Ludwig B, Smith N 1963 Studies on the metabolism of meprobamate. Proceedings of the Society of Experimental Biological Medicine 112: 436–438
14. Walkenstein S, Knebel C, Macmullen J, Seifter J 1958 The excretion and distribution of meprobamate and its metabolites. Journal of Experimental Therapeutics 123: 254–258
15. Bennett W, Singer I, Coggins C 1973 Guide to drug usage in adult patients with impaired renal failure. Journal of the American Medical Association 223: 991–997
16. Maddock R, Bloomer H 1967 Meprobamate overdosage. Journal of the American Medical Association 201: 999–1003
17. Baselt R 1982 Disposition of toxic drugs and chemicals in man. Biomedical Publications, 2nd edn, pp 470–479
18. Champlin F, Cotter C, Moskowitz M, Rossman M, Sheppard C, Merlis S 1968 A Comparison of chlormezanone, meprobamate and placebo. Clinical Pharmacology and Therapeutics 9: 11–15
19. Gillete H 1956 Relaxant effects of meprobamate in disabilities resulting from musculoskeletal and central nervous system disorders. International Record of Medicine and General Practice Clinics 169: 453–467
20. Smith R, Herman I, Kron K, Peak W 1957 Meprobamate (Miltown) in rheumatic diseases. Journal of the American Medical Association 163: 535–538
21. Winkelman N, Richards D 1975 Double blind evaluation of an analgesic tranquillizer combination for treating musculoskeletal pain associated with anxiety. Current Therapeutic Research 17: 352–360
22. Edwards J G 1981 Adverse effects of antianxiety drugs. Drugs 22: 495–514
23. Honeycutt W, Curtis A 1962 Fixed drug eruption to carisoprodol and cross reaction with meprobamate. Journal of the American Medical Association 180: 691–692
24. Bulla J, Ewing J, Buffaloe W 1959 Further controlled studies of meprobamate. American Practitioner and Digest of Treatment 10: 1961–1964
25. Haizlip T N, Ewing J A 1958 Meprobamate habituation: a controlled clinical study. New England Journal of Medicine 258: 1181–1186
26. Tschudy D P 1975 Acute intermittent porphyria: clinical and selected research aspects. American Int Med 83: 851–864
27. Felby S 1970 Concentrations of meprobamate in the blood and liver following fatal meprobamate poisoning. Acta Pharmacologica et Toxicologica 28: 334
28. Powell L W, Mann G T, Kaye S 1959 Acute meprobamate poisoning. New England Journal of Medicine 259: 716–718
29. Hartz S, Heinonen O, Shapiro S, Siskind V, Slone D 1975 Antenatal exposure to meprobamate and chlordiazepoxide in relation to malformation, mental development and childhood mortality. New England Journal of Medicine 292: 726–728

Meptazinol (hydrochloride)

Meptazinol is a centrally acting analgesic.

Chemistry

Meptazinol hydrochloride (Meptid)
$C_{15}H_{23}NO.HCl$
3-(3-Ethyl-1-methyl-hexahydro-1H-azepin-3-yl)-phenol hydrochloride

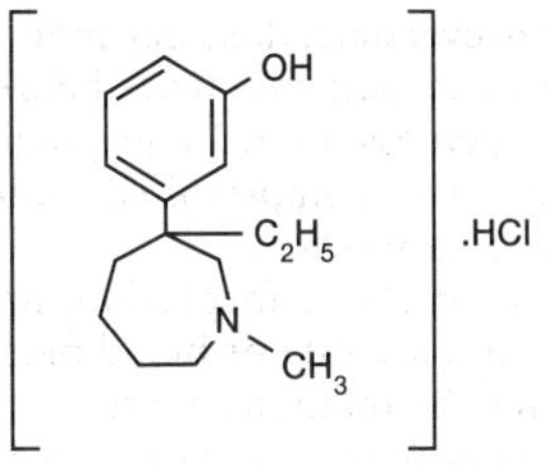

Molecular weight (free base)	269.8 (233.3)
pKa (phenol)	8.7
pKa (amino)	11.9
Solubility	
in alcohol	—
in water	—
Octanol/water partition coefficient	5.9

Meptazinol is a white or creamy white powder with a slight characteristic odour. The racemate is obtained from chemical synthesis and used in the marketed formulations.

Pharmacology

Meptazinol binds to the μ_1 opioid receptor,[1] but also has a central cholinergic activity which makes a significant contribution to the analgesic effect.[1] Although meptazinol behaves in vivo as a mixed agonist–antagonist, unlike classical opioids it is not active in the usual assay preparations such as guinea-pig ileum and both enantiomers are active in analgesic models.[3] In animals, meptazinol has no significant anti-inflammatory activity but has a weak local anaesthetic action.[4] As a separate and probably direct effect of prolonging the action potential duration of ventricular muscle, meptazinol reduces the incidence of experimentally-induced ventricular arrhythmias in animals.[5]

Toxicology

Toxicological testing in animals shows no effects of likely clinical relevance. Both carcinogenicity testing in rats, with dosing for up to two years, and mutagenicity tests were negative. Studies in rats and rabbits show no evidence of teratogenic effect.

Clinical pharmacology

Open studies of single intramuscular doses in the range 25–100 mg in patients with moderate to severe postoperative pain show a dose-related analgesic effect for doses exceeding 50 mg.[6,7] Controlled studies confirm the approximate analgesic equivalence of single intramuscular doses of 75–100 mg meptazinol to 100 mg pethidine,[8] 15 mg morphine, or 60 mg pentazocine.[9] The onset of analgesia is within 15–30 min, is maximal at 30–60 min, and lasts 3–4 h for the 100 mg dose. Multiple intermittent dosing studies in postoperative pain have generally shown analgesic consumption in agreement with

Meptazinol (hydrochloride)

M

that expected from the single-dose studies.[7] Patient-controlled analgesic techniques, involving self-administration of drug from a machine, appear to show higher consumption rates for parenteral meptazinol in the first 24 hours after surgery.[10,11] Parenteral administration has continued for up to 5 days in some studies.

Oral meptazinol 100 mg gave analgesia which was distinguished from placebo in a single-dose study.[12] Single oral doses up to 500 mg have been given without significant adverse effects. Daily oral doses of 800 mg show analgesia similar to that from standard oral analgesics including paracetamol,[13] pentazocine,[12] and a dextropropoxyphene/paracetamol combination.[14] Onset of effect is within 30–60 min, is maximal at 1.5–2 h and lasts 4–6 h. Oral administration has been reported for up to one year.[15]

Consistent with μ_1 opioid receptor selectivity, the ventilatory response to carbon dioxide and end-tidal carbon dioxide were significantly less affected by 100 mg meptazinol intramuscularly than morphine 10 mg intramuscularly in volunteer subjects:[16] some depressive effect was noted relative to placebo for some ventilatory parameters. Meptazinol has also been shown to have less ventilatory depressant effect than morphine in postoperative patients, although the magnitude of the difference was small and probably clinically irrelevant.[7] Naloxone-reversible, dose-dependent depression of ventilation has been shown in patients anaesthetized with halothane.[17] Reduced ventilatory depression with meptazinol may suggest its application to patients with compromised pulmonary function, but such use should still be cautious.

The haemodynamic effects of meptazinol appear to be minimal. No significant effect on pulse rate or blood pressure has been seen in analgesic studies,[7] and the pulmonary artery pressure is not raised. Antiarrhythmic effects in man have not been reported. Intravenous meptazinol and placebo had similar effects in opioid-dependent subjects on methadone maintenance.[18] This supports animal evidence,[4] suggesting that meptazinol has a low abuse potential. Meptazinol does not constrict the pupil, and its use is not associated with constipation.[4]

Pharmacokinetics

High performance liquid chromatography with fluorescence detection is the preferred analytical method for meptazinol.[19] The coefficient of variation of the method is less than 10% with a lower limit of detection of 3 µg.l^{-1}.

Oral absorption of meptazinol 50–200 mg is nearly complete, with peak plasma drug concentrations at 0.5–2 h after dosing. Systemic availability is low at 9% with a variability which can lead to ten-fold or greater plasma drug concentration differences between individuals at corresponding times after dosing. The mean half life in plasma, measured as 2 h in young volunteers, is significantly greater (3.4 h) in elderly (>70 years) patients. Other kinetic parameters are unaltered in the elderly and multiple dosing leads to similar plasma meptazinol concentrations in both groups.[4,20–22] Pathological or drug-induced changes in presystemic elimination have not been reported, but since meptazinol is mainly metabolized by hepatic glucuronidation any such alterations will probably be small. Animal studies suggest that more rapid absorption may reduce presystemic elimination,[23] possibly by saturating the conjugation mechanisms. Systemic plasma clearance after intravenous dosing is high[21] and close to estimated hepatic blood flow, consistent with a predominantly hepatic elimination. Terminal plasma half lives after parenteral and oral administration are similar. Absorption after intramuscular dosing is excellent with peak plasma concentrations 15–30 min after dosing: similar extensive and rapid absorption is seen after rectal administration.[4]

Meptazinol undergoes wide tissue distribution, as expected for a basic lipophilic molecule, and highly perfused tissues such as lung, liver, kidney and spleen show the highest concentrations of drug in animal studies. The apparent volume of distribution is about 3 l.kg^{-1} in man. Plasma protein binding of meptazinol is relatively low, being 27% in the young and somewhat higher (34%) in the elderly,[22] and is constant over the therapeutic plasma concentration range (25–250 µg.l^{-1}).

Meptazinol crosses the placenta to give a mean neonatal/maternal plasma concentration ratio of 0.57, and also passes freely into maternal milk. The plasma half life in the newborn is 3.4 h, implying that neonatal metabolism is comparatively well developed.

Oral absorption	~100%
Presystemic metabolism	92%
Plasma half life	
range	1.5–6 h
mean	1.9 h
Volume of distribution	3.1 l.kg^{-1}
Plasma protein binding	27%

Concentration–effect relationship

In rodents, good correlations were found between antinociceptive effect and plasma meptazinol concentration[24] over the approximate range 1000–2000 µg.l^{-1}. Such correlations have not been reported for pain relief in man. Although parenteral dosing can lead to similar plasma concentrations, acute or chronic oral dosing rarely leads to concentrations greater than 100 µg.l^{-1}.

Metabolism

Meptazinol is excreted primarily by the kidneys, with less than 10% of the administered dose appearing in the faeces in man. It is extensively metabolized, probably predominantly in the liver, so that less than 5% of the urinary recovery is unchanged drug. There are no long-lived pharmacologically active metabolites. The major metabolite is the inactive O-glucuronide. A minor inactive oxidative metabolite, accounting for about 7% of an administered dose, has been tentatively identified as the azepin-[2H]-2-one (Fig. 1). There is no evidence for N-demethylation.

Fig. 1 Metabolism of meptazinol

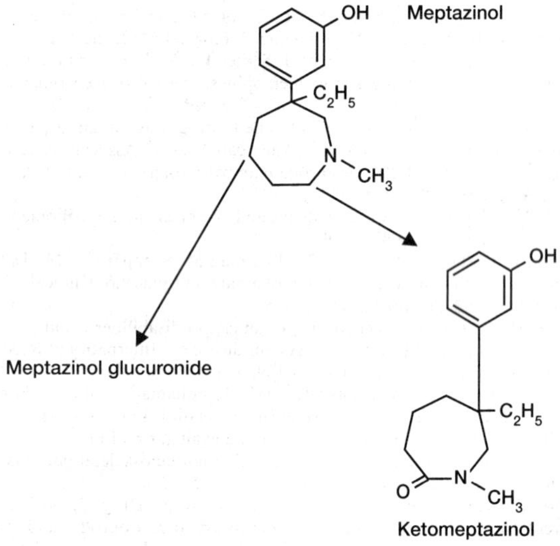

Pharmaceutics

Meptazinol is available in oral and parenteral forms.

1. Meptid tablets (Wyeth, UK) contain 200 mg meptazinol base as hydrochloride and are oval, orange, film-coated and impressed on one side with the name 'Wyeth'.
2. Meptazinol injection (Wyeth UK) for intravenous or intramuscular use contains 100 mg meptazinol base as hydrochloride per ml, and is supplied as a clear, preservative-free solution in 1 ml clear glass ampoules. (It is not suitable for administration by the epidural or intrathecal routes.)

The tablets require no special storage conditions. The injection should be stored in a cool place. Both formulations have a 3 year maximum shelf-life and contain no excipients with potential allergenic activity.

Meptazinol injection is compatible with all the usual intravenous crystalloid infusion solutions, but should not be mixed with other drugs in the same solution. Precipitation may occur with other injection solutions which are strongly alkaline (for example, sodium thiopentone).

Meptazinol (hydrochloride)

Therapeutic use

Indications

1. The treatment of acute or chronic pain of moderate intensity with the oral formulation (for example, acute or chronic backache, post-traumatic and musculoskeletal pain, and the pain associated with chronic rheumatoid or osteoarthritis, dysmenorrhoea, or the later stages of postoperative recovery).
2. The treatment of moderate to severe pain with the parenteral formulation (for example, pain associated with labour, renal colic, or the early stages of the postoperative course).

Contraindications

No specific contraindications are known.

Mode of use

With intermittent dosing, dose size and/or dosing interval should be adjusted within the recommended limits to achieve optimal control of pain as subjectively reported by the patient. 200 mg 3–6-hourly (usually 4-hourly) is used for oral treatment. Intramuscular dosage is generally 75–100 mg repeated up to every 2 hours as necessary, but in labour pain 100–150 mg (or approximately 2 $mg.kg^{-1}$) doses are recommended. 50–100 mg by slow injection may be used for intravenous bolus dosing, repeated up to every 2 hours as required.

In postoperative patients, meptazinol has also been given by continuous intravenous infusion at a rate of 0.45 $mg.h^{-1}.kg^{-1}$, and by patient-controlled analgesia, intravenous and intramuscular, where cumulative doses up to 1850 mg per 24 hours have been self-administered. Single doses by extradural or intrathecal administration give a relatively short duration of action and appear to have little advantage over parenteral routes.

Since meptazinol behaves clinically as a mixed agonist–antagonist, flattening of the dose–response relationship is expected at high (but presently undetermined) doses. The possibility of this effect, although not established as occurring within the clinical dose range, suggests that inadequate pain relief after full doses of meptazinol may require the addition or substitution of a complete agonist such as morphine. Clinical problems are not seen apparently when meptazinol and opioid agonists are administered concomitantly, even in opioid-dependent subjects.[18] However, such pharmacological complexity is preferably avoided, and meptazinol should be used with caution in opioid abusers.

Withdrawal effects have not been reported after stopping meptazinol, consistent with the absence of euphoric effects in man[18] and the lack of tolerance development in animals.[4]

Adverse reactions

Potentially life-threatening effects
No deaths attributable to meptazinol have been reported. Respiratory depression caused by meptazinol appears less than that caused by opioid agonists but is a potential source of patient danger, particularly if other central nervous system depressants are present.[17]

Acute overdosage
Overdosage with meptazinol has not been described. Large parenteral doses (up to seven times the recommended dose) have been used investigationally during anaesthesia without significant sequelae, and the oral route has a high first-pass effect.

In the event of overdose, appropriate measures would include general medical supportive therapy and the use of naloxone if ventilatory depression were present.

Severe or irreversible adverse effects
None is known.

Symptomatic adverse effects
Meptazinol is generally well tolerated with a frequency of adverse reactions comparable to that of opioid analgesics. In ambulant subjects treated with oral meptazinol, the most frequent adverse effect was nausea, which occurred in about 10% of patients.[25] Other ill effects with a frequency about 5% included dizziness, vomiting and gastrointestinal disturbances. Drowsiness occurred infrequently. Parenteral meptazinol generally has a similar adverse profile, except that vomiting displaces nausea as the most frequent disorder. Obstetric use leads to vomiting in as many as 25% of patients, but in part this probably reflects the clinical setting. In all situations, psychotomimetic effects have been rare (<0.5% with doses around 100 mg).

As with other opioids, nausea and vomiting from meptazinol is likely to involve a direct effect on the chemoreceptor trigger zone. Antiemetic drugs are effective in reducing the occurrence of these symptoms.

Other effects
An intramuscular dose of 100 mg meptazinol did not affect the postoperative rise of plasma glucose or cortisol. However, consistent with μ_1 opioid activity,[1] plasma prolactin levels were raised in comparison with morphine treatment.[26]

Interference with clinical pathology tests
No significant technical interferences of this kind have been reported.

High risk groups

Neonates
Neonatal use has not been directly investigated, but adverse effects in the newborn have not been seen after maternal use in labour.[27]

Breast milk. Meptazinol passes freely into breast milk, but its use in lactating women has not been evaluated.

Children
Not evaluated.

Pregnant women
Apart from its use in labour, no information is available about the safety of meptazinol during human pregnancy.

The elderly
Pharmacokinetic[22] and clinical[12] evidence suggests that dosing in young adults and the elderly will be comparable.

Concurrent disease
Hepatic or renal insufficiency. In the absence of kinetic or clinical studies in patients with hepatic or renal failure, the use of meptazinol in such subjects should be cautious.

Drug interactions

Potentially hazardous interactions
Pharmacokinetic. No pharmacokinetic interactions have yet been described in man.

Pharmacodynamic. Meptazinol and ethanol did not interact to affect psychomotor performance in volunteers. Caution is advisable with concomitant administration of central nervous system depressants.

Potentially useful interactions
None has been reported.

Clinical trials

1. Forrest W H 1985 Meptazinol and morphine in the treatment of postoperative pain (abstract). Clinical Pharmacology and Therapeutics 37: 196

Single intramuscular doses of 50, 100 or 200 mg meptazinol were compared with morphine in 151 patients with moderate to severe postoperative pain in this double-blind, parallel group study. 10 mg morphine was equivalent to 130 mg meptazinol based on peak effect, and to 190 mg meptazinol based on area-under-the-curve of analgesic effect over 6 hours. Duration of analgesia from meptazinol was about 4 hours, similar to that from morphine. The most frequent side effect with meptazinol was nausea, compared with sedation with morphine. Nausea and psychotomimetic effects (but not sedation) were dose-related with meptazinol. A 100 mg dose was concluded to be optimal.

2. Cohen D G, Major E, Jothilingham S, Clark G, Coutinho P 1983 Meptazinol in the treatment of severe post-operative pain: a comparison with morphine. Postgraduate Medical Journal 59 (suppl 1): 35–40

In this randomized, double-blind study, 63 patients with severe postoperative pain received parenteral doses of either 100 mg meptazinol or 15 mg morphine. After the first dose, pain relief was significantly faster in onset with meptazinol, with a similar duration

Meptazinol (hydrochloride)

M

of action. However, four patients in the meptazinol group required withdrawal for inadequate analgesia and morphine gave significantly better pain relief over a 24-hour period. Arterial PCO_2 was significantly higher in the morphine-treated patients. Symptomatic side effects were similar in both groups. The authors conclude that meptazinol gives satisfactory pain relief with apparently less ventilatory depression than morphine, but may not have adequate efficacy in some patients even on repeated dosing.

3. Nicholas A D G, Robson P J 1982 Double-blind comparison of meptazinol and pethidine in labour. British Journal of Obstetrics and Gynaecology 89: 318–322

Intramuscular doses of 75–150 mg of meptazinol or pethidine were compared in this randomized, double-blind trial in 358 patients in labour. Duration of action was similar at 1.5–3 hours, but meptazinol gave statistically better analgesia at around 1 hour after dosing. Maternal side effects were comparable in frequency and nature, with vomiting in about 20% of patients in both groups. Neonatal observations were similar in both groups, except that meptazinol gave a statistically greater number of high Apgar scores at 1 min. The authors conclude that meptazinol may have advantages over pethidine for the relief of labour pain.

Other trials

1. Teklu B, Habte-Michael A, Warrell D A, White N J, Wright D J M 1983 Meptazinol diminishes the Jarisch–Herxheimer reaction of relapsing fever. Lancet 1: 835–839

The effect of 300–500 mg meptazinol intravenously was compared with 30–40 mg naloxone in a double-blind, placebo-controlled trial in groups of eight Ethiopian patients experiencing the Jarisch–Herxheimer reaction following treatment of louse-borne relapsing fever with intravenous tetracycline. Meptazinol significantly reduced the clinical severity of the reaction relative to placebo. Naloxone was ineffective, as was high-dose corticosteroid treatment. The beneficial effect of meptazinol may or may not be related to its opioid antagonist properties, but is significant as the first effective therapy for this condition.

References

1. Spiegel K, Pasternak G W 1984 Meptazinol: a novel μ_1 selective opioid analgesic. Journal of Pharmacology and Experimental Therapeutics 228: 414–419
2. Bill D J, Hartley J E, Stevens R J, Thompson A M 1982 The antinociceptive activity of meptazinol depends on both opiate and cholinergic receptors. British Journal of Pharmacology 79: 191–199
3. Leading article 1983 Meptazinol. Lancet 2: 384–385
4. Stephens R J, Waterfall J F, Franklin R A 1978 A review of the biological properties and metabolic disposition of the new analgesic agent, meptazinol. General Pharmacology 9: 73–78
5. Fagbemi O, Kane K A, Lepran I, Parratt J R, Szekeres L 1983 Antiarrhythmic actions of meptazinol, a partial agonist at opiate receptors, in acute myocardial ischaemia. British Journal of Pharmacology 78: 455–460
6. Paymaster N J 1983 Clinical evaluation of meptazinol, a new analgesic, in postoperative pain. British Journal of Anaesthesia 48: 599–604
7. Robson P J 1983 Clinical review of parenteral meptazinol. Postgraduate Medical Journal 59 (suppl 1): 85–92
8. Hedges A, Turner P, Wadsworth J 1980 A double-blind comparison of meptazinol with pethidine in postoperative pain. British Journal of Anaesthesia 52: 295–298
9. Staquet M 1978 A double-blind comparison of meptazinol with pentazocine and placebo in cancer pain. Journal of Clinical Pharmacology 18: 76–79
10. Slattery P J, Harmer M, Rosen M, Vickers M D 1981 Comparison of meptazinol and pethidine given i.v. on demand in the management of post-operative pain. British Journal of Anaesthesia 53: 927–931
11. Harmer M, Slattery P J, Rosen M, Vickers M D 1983 Intramuscular on demand analgesia: double-blind controlled trial of pethidine, buprenorphine, morphine, and meptazinol. British Medical Journal 286: 680–682
12. Pearce V, Robson P J 1980 Double-blind crossover trial of oral meptazinol, pentazocine and placebo in the treatment of pain in the elderly. Postgraduate Medical Journal 56: 474–477
13. Wade A G, Ward P J 1982 A double-blind comparison of meptazinol versus paracetamol and placebo in acute and chronic painful conditions presenting to the general practitioner. Current Medical Research and Opinion 8: 191–196
14. Oro L 1984 A comparison between meptazinol and dextropropoxyphene plus paracetamol in elderly patients with musculoskeletal pains. Current Medical Research and Opinion 9: 240–245
15. Price R K J, Latham A N 1982 Long-term assessment of the efficacy and safcty of oral meptazinol (200 mg) in general practice. Current Therapeutic Research 31: 807–812
16. Jordon C, Lehane J R, Robson P J, Jones J G 1979 A comparison of the respiratory effects of meptazinol, pentazocine and morphine. British Journal of Anaesthesia 51: 497–502
17. Slattery P J, Harmer M, Rosen M, Vickers M D 1982 Naloxone reversal of meptazinol-induced respiratory depression. Anaesthesia 37: 1163–1166
18. Evans M, Robson P J, Chadd M A, Evans C M, Fry D M 1983 Administration of meptazinol to opiate-dependent patients. Postgraduate Medical Journal 59 (suppl 1): 78–84
19. Frost T 1981 Determination of meptazinol in plasma by high-performance liquid chromatography with fluorescence detection. Analyst 106: 999–1001
20. Franklin R A, Aldridge A, White C de B 1976 Studies on the metabolism of meptazinol, a new analgesic drug. British Journal of Clinical Pharmacology 3: 497–502
21. Norbury H M, Franklin R A, Graham D F 1983 Pharmacokinetics of the new analgesic, meptazinol, after oral and intravenous administration to volunteers. European Journal of Clinical Pharmacology 25: 77–80
22. Norbury H M, Franklin R A, Graham D F, Sinha B 1984 Pharmacokinetics of meptazinol after single and multiple oral administration to elderly patients. European Journal of Clinical Pharmacology 27: 223–226
23. Franklin R A 1977 The influence of gastric emptying on plasma concentrations of the analgesic, meptazinol. British Journal of Clinical Pharmacology 59: 565–569
24. Franklin R A, Pierce D M, Goode P G 1976 On the relation between the analgesic activity of meptazinol and its plasma concentration in rats, mice and monkeys. Journal of Pharmacy and Pharmacology 28: 852–853
25. Price R K J, Latham A N 1982 Meptazinol: a side-effect profile compared to placebo in general practice. Journal of International Medical Research 10: 219–224
26. Kay N H, Allen M C, Bullingham R E S et al 1985 Influence of meptazinol on metabolic and hormonal responses following major surgery. A comparison with morphine. Anaesthesia 40: 223–228
27. Jackson M B A, Robson P J 1983 Preliminary clinical and pharmacokinetic experiences in the newborn when meptazinol is compared with pethidine as an obstetric analgesic. Postgraduate Medical Journal 59 (suppl 1): 47–51

Mequitazine

A histamine receptor (H_1) antagonist used in the treatment of allergy.

Chemistry

Mequitazine (LM209, Metaplexan, Mircol, Primalan)
$C_{20}H_{22}N_2S$
10-(1-Aza bicyclo[2.2.2]oct-3-yl-methyl)-10H-phenothiazine

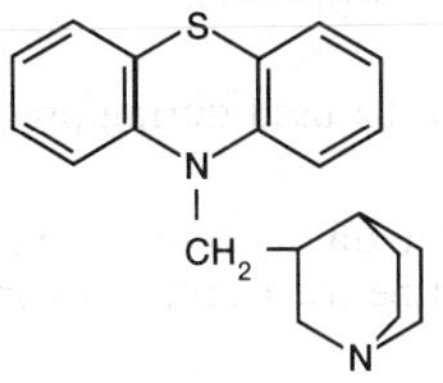

Molecular weight	322.5
pKa	8.66
Solubility	
in alcohol	soluble
in water	almost insoluble
Octanol/water partition coefficient	high

A white to creamy-white, odourless, amorphous powder with a bitter taste. It is prepared by chemical synthesis and posesses a chiral centre. Mequitazine is not available in any combination preparations.

Pharmacology

Mequitazine is a phenothiazine group histamine H_1-receptor antagonist active at both peripheral and central receptors in vitro,[1–6] and this accounts for its therapeutic effects in vivo. The affinity for peripheral receptors appears greater than for central H_1-receptors.[5–7] In the guinea-pig ileum and trachea preparations in vitro the drug is less active as an H_1-antagonist than clemastine or chlorpheniramine.[1] After oral dosing mequitazine has a long duration of action against histamine-induced acute death in mice.[1] The CNS sedation evoked by mequitazine is less marked than that produced by dexchlorpheniramine or brompheniramine.[8,9] Mequitazine also has some anticholinergic activity at higher doses[7] and this may account for the slight sedative properties of single 10 mg doses which have been used experimentally.[10–12] Other effects of the drug have been reported in in vitro studies e.g. mast cell stabilization and inhibition of cyclic nucleotide phosphodiesterase but these occur only at high drug concentrations.[13–15]

Toxicology

Subacute toxicity studies in dogs have revealed slight and reversible changes in liver, kidneys, mesenteric lymph nodes, palpebrail and conjunctival membranes after oral administration of 1–25 $mg.kg^{-1}$ daily for 14 weeks.[16] These observations suggest that mequitazine is not likely to have any serious toxicological problems at doses used clinically in man. Mequitazine has no mutagenic properties.[17] There are no published reports of carcinogenicity screening.

Clinical pharmacology

Mequitazine acts by antagonism of histamine H_1-receptors. The lesser affinity for central H_1-receptors is thought to explain the relative lack of sedation caused by mequitazine compared with brompheniramine or dexchlorpheniramine.[8,9] However, mequitazine can still cause sedation and patients should be warned not to drive shortly after taking the drug. Mequitazine will also enhance the sedative effects of alcohol. Its anticholinergic properties are not usually noted in low dosage but some patients will get dry mouth or blurred vision particularly in the early days of treatment.

Pharmacokinetics

The preferred method of analysis of mequitazine in plasma and urine is by capillary column gas chromatography/mass spectrometry.[18] The limit of detection in plasma is 0.5 $\mu g.l^{-1}$.

The drug is rapidly but incompletely (70%) absorbed following oral administration. Blood levels increase in proportion to the dose administered and peak plasma concentrations are attained 5–7 hours after administration in fasting subjects. The apparent elimination half life is approximately 40 hours, which is in agreement with the observation that more than 5 days treatment with two 5 mg doses of mequitazine per day is necessary to achieve steady-state plasma concentrations. This is probably due to extensive (90%) high affinity binding to blood and tissue proteins, and partially to enterohepatic shunting. The drug is widely distributed throughout the body with volumes of distribution in the range 3500–4000 l. After a single dose the drug concentrations in some tissues, particularly the liver and lung, are greater than the plasma concentration. There is no evidence of significant accumulation with further dosing, however.

The transport of mequitazine across the blood brain barrier is complex. Animal studies suggest the existence of a threshold of transfer from the circulating blood into the brain. Provided that this threshold is not exceeded little passage occurs and this may partly account for the reduced sedative effect of this drug compared with other antihistamines.

There is no information on the excretion of mequitazine in breast milk nor on its transfer across the placenta.

Mequitazine is excreted in both urine and faeces, the more prolonged faecal excretion representing the extensive enterohepatic shunting of the drug. In view of this, and the extensive protein binding of the drug, the pharmacokinetics of mequitazine may be altered in liver disease and acute illness. As with all phenothiazine-type drugs, patients with hepatic disease may be a risk group for mequitazine treatment. There is no information on the effects of old age on the kinetics of the drug.

Oral absorption	70%
Presystemic metabolism	—
Plasma half life	
mean	40 h
Volume of distribution	4000 l
Plasma protein binding	90%

Concentration–effect relationship

There is no clear evidence of a direct correlation between the plasma concentration of mequitazine and its therapeutic effect.

Metabolism

Mequitazine is extensively biotransformed by oxidation, presumably in the liver. Studies in animals have identified several metabolites, the structures of which indicate N-oxidation, S-oxidation or mono- or dihydroxylation. (See Fig. 1). With the exception of the sulphoxide metabolite, which is much less active at H_1-receptors,[19] no reports of the pharmacological activity of these metabolites have been published.

Less than 1% of the material excreted in the urine is unchanged mequitazine, although of the faecal metabolites identified the parent drug constitutes 83%. The pattern of metabolites in urine and faeces is as follows. Urine: parent, <1%; sulphoxide, 25%; sulphone, 4%; N-oxide, 2–5%; sulphoxide N-oxide, 3–7% (total, 35–42%). Faeces: parent, 83%; sulphoxide, 10%; N-oxide, 7% (total, 100%).

Pharmaceutics

Mequitazine (Rhone-Poulenc, UK) is available in an oral form as white biconvex tablets embossed 'Primalan' on one side. They are unmarked on the reverse side. Each tablet contains 5 mg mequitazine.

Preparations have a five year shelf-life when stored under normal pharmacy conditions.

M

M

Therapeutic use

Indications

1. Hayfever
2. Vasomotor and allergic rhinitis
3. Urticaria
4. Allergic pruritus
5. Allergic reactions to insect bites and stings.

Contraindications

1. Hepatic impairment.

Mode of use

All clinical uses depend upon the antagonism of histamine H_1-receptors. The normal dosage used is 5 mg given orally every 12 hours.

Indications

Mequitazine is used for symptomatic relief of many mild allergic conditions, especially where a non-sedative antihistamine is mandated.[20] These conditions include rhinitis,[8,9] urticaria, pruritus,[21,22] allergic conjunctivitis[9] and reactions to insect bites and stings. The usual dose employed is 5 mg every 12 hours. One study has suggested that mequitazine is more effective than terfenadine in allergy[23] and that this may be due to its broader spectrum of pharmacological activity.

Contraindications

The drug should be used cautiously in patients with hepatic dysfunction.

Adverse reactions

Potentially life-threatening effects
No information is available on such reactions.

Acute overdosage
No cases of this kind appear to have reported.

Severe or irreversible adverse effects
No reactions of this type have been reported.

Symptomatic adverse effects
Although less sedative than some H_1-receptor antagonists, some patients report mild drowsiness after taking mequitazine.

Although reported to be a non-sedative antihistamine, patients should be warned not to drive or operate machinery until it has been established that sedation does not occur.

Interference with clinical pathology tests
No technical interferences of this kind are known.

High risk groups

Neonates
The drug should not be used in neonates.

Breast milk. No information is available on whether the drug enters breast milk, so mothers taking it should not breast-feed.

Children
Mequitazine is not recommended for use in children under 12 years, although a clinical trial has reported its successful use in children with allergic disorders (mainly rhinitis), in whom the dosage ranged from one-half to two 5 mg tablets daily.[24]

Pregnant women
Mequitazine should not be used during pregnancy.

The elderly
No specific information on the use of the drug in the elderly is available, but it should be used cautiously in patients with compromised liver function.

Drug interactions

Potentially hazardous interactions
Mequitazine may potentiate the central effects of alcohol and other drugs with a CNS depressant effect.

Potentially useful interactions
No reactions of this kind are known.

Major outcome trials

1. Blamoutier J 1978 Comparative trial of two antihistamines, mequitazine and brompheniramine. Current Medical Research and Opinion 5: 366–370

Fig. 1

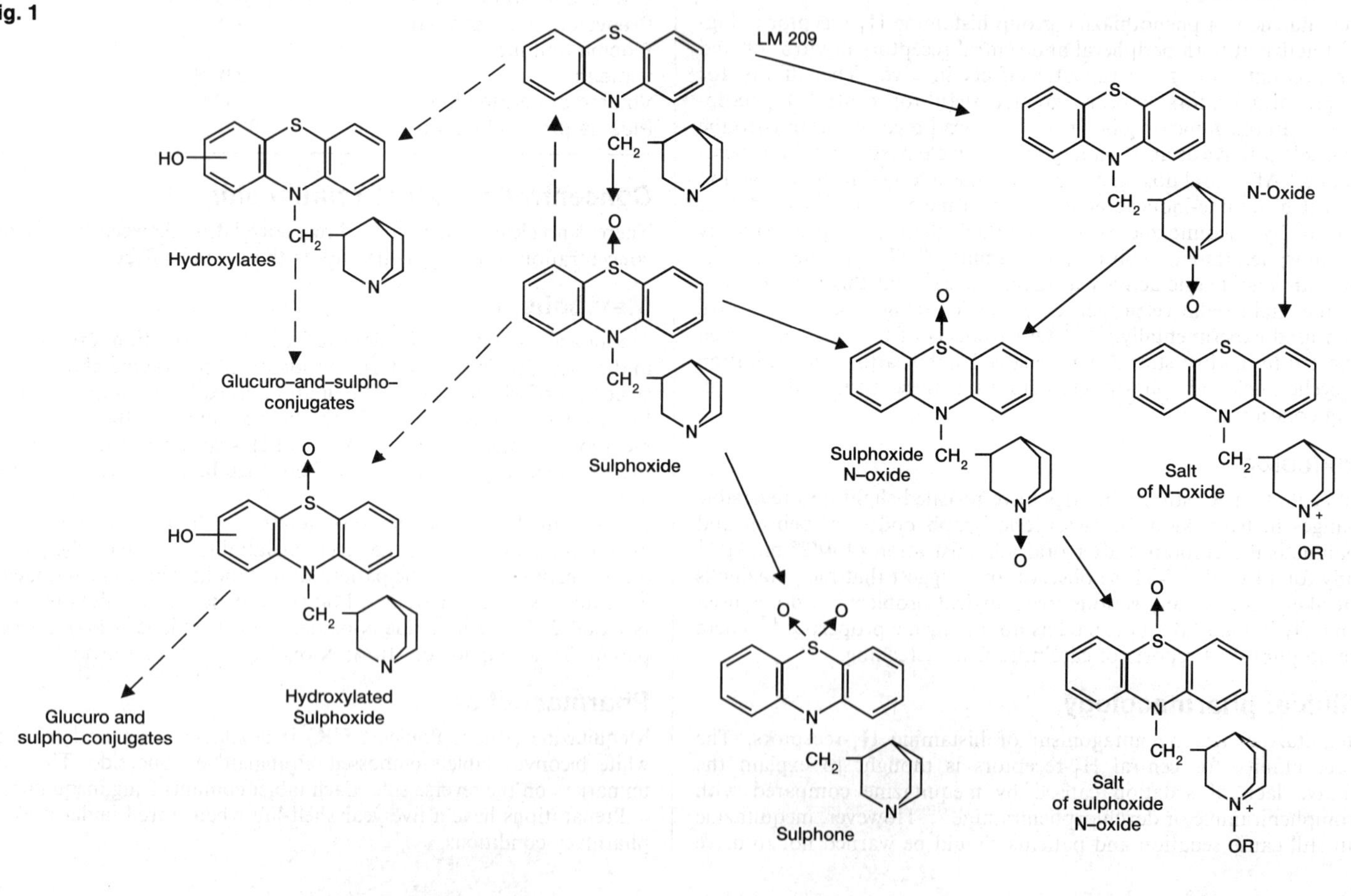

A double-blind evaluation in 48 patients with a variety of allergic disorders (pollenosis 8, ocular allergy 25, rhinitis 9, rhinopharyngitis 3, urticaria 1 and asthma 5). Mequitazine, 5 mg twice daily, was as effective over 14 days treatment as brompheniramine, 12 mg twice daily. However, mequitazine was subjectively assessed as causing significantly less drowsiness. There was no investigation of whether particular conditions responded more favourably than others to the therapeutic effect of mequitazine.

2. Muler H, Blum F 1978 Double-blind comparison of two antihistamines: mequitazine and dexchlorpheniramine. Current Medical Research and Opinion 5: 359–365

A double-blind 7 day evaluation of mequitazine (5 mg, twice daily) and dexchlorpheniramine (6 mg twice daily) in 49 patients with seasonal and perennial rhinitis and allergic sinusitis. One patient withdrew from each treatment group because of drug intolerance. There was no statistical difference between the effectiveness of the two drugs. After one week of treatment 9 out of 25 patients on mequitazine, and 4 out of those on dexchlorpheniramine showed marked improvement enabling treatment to be stopped. 11 patients in each group continued to receive the same dosage for a second week and improvement was maintained or increased in 8 patients on mequitazine and in 6 on dexchlorpheniramine. In 10 patients receiving reduced dosages during their second week of medication, only the 4 patients on mequitazine showed additional improvement.

3. Langier P, Orusco M 1978 Comparative trial of an antihistamine, mequitazine, and placebo. Current Medical Research and Opinion 5: 371–375

A double-blind randomized placebo-controlled study in which 40 patients suffering from dermatological conditions suitable for treatment with an antihistamine (urticaria and eczema) received mequitazine, 5 mg twice daily, or placebo over a 14 day period. Where justified, four patients taking mequitazine and seven taking placebo received topical support therapy with a hydrating cream or ichthyol paste. The overall response to treatment was significantly better in the mequitazine group. There was no significant difference between the levels of drowsiness experienced with mequitazine compared with placebo.

4. Leophonte P, Leophonte-Domairon S C, Carre J C, Goyeau E, Vayleux M 1984 Etude comparative de la mequitazine et de la terfenadine dans les rhinites allergiques. Allergie et Immunologie 16: 213–220

A double-blind study of the relative effectiveness and tolerance of mequitazine and terfenadine in 134 patients with allergic rhinitis. The treatment period was 7 days during which patients received either mequitazine (5 mg twice daily) or terfenadine (60 mg twice daily). Seven patients were ultimately excluded from study. Mequitazine was found to be significantly more effective than terfenadine, and it had a more rapid action. The incidence of somnolence was similar for both drugs ($<10\%$).

Other trials

Vialatte J, Paupe J 1977 La mequitazine dans le traitement des manifestations allergiques de l'enfant. Revue Internationale de Pediatre 74: 59–64

A study in 45 children aged between 13 months and 14½ years who were suffering from allergic rhinitis, eczema and rhinoconjunctivitis. Dosage and duration of treatment was very varied, depending upon the particular circumstances. In 71% of cases mequitazine produced marked improvement in or disappearance of the symptoms. In 9% no improvement was observed. Tolerance of mequitazine was found to be good, with few reports of drowsiness.

References

1. Fujimura H, Tsurumi K, Yanagihara M et al 1981 Pharmacological study of mequitazine (LM-209). I. Antagonistic actions of chemical mediators. Nippon Yakurigaku Zasshi 78: 279–289 (Japanese)
2. Fujimura H, Tsurumi K, Yanagihara M et al 1981 Pharmacological study of mequitazine (LM-209). II. Anti-allergic action. Nippon Yakurigaku Zasshi 78: 291–303 (Japanese)
3. Fujimura H, Tsurumi K, Yanagihara M et al 1981 Pharmacological study of mequitazine (LM-209). III. Action on the central nervous system. Nippon Yakurigaku Zasshi 78: 249–260 (Japanese)
4. Hojo M, Yoshida Y, Nagasaka Y, Katayama O, Serizawa I 1981 Pharmacological study of mequitazine (LM-209). IV. General pharmacological action. Nippon Yakurigaku Zasshi 78: 403–429 (Japanese)
5. Le Fur G, Malgouris C, Uzan A 1981 Effect of mequitazine, a non-sedative antihistamine, on brain H_1 receptors. Life Sciences 29: 547–552
6. Kanba S, Richelson E 1984 Histamine H_1 receptors in human brain labelled with [^{3}H]-doxepin. Brain Research 304: 1–7
7. Uzan A, Le Fur G 1979 Mequitazine et vigilance. Allergologica et Immunopathologia 11: 27–30
8. Muler H, Blum F 1978 Double-blind comparison of two antihistamines: mequitazine and dexchlorpheniramine. Current Medical Research and Opinion 5: 359–365
9. Blamoutier F 1978 Comparative trial of two antihistamines, mequitazine and brompheniramine. Current Medical Research and Opinion 5: 366–370
10. Nicholson A N, Stone B M 1983 The H_1-antagonist mequitazine: studies on performance and visual function. European Journal of Clinical Pharmacology 25: 563–566
11. Nicholson A N 1985 Central effects of H_1 and H_2 antihistamines. Aviation Space and Environmental Medicine 56: 293–298
12. Nicholson A N 1983 Antihistamines and sedation. Lancet 2: 211–212
13. Uzan A, Gueremy C, Le Fur G 1976 Absorption, distribution et excretion de la (quinuclidinyl-3-methyl)-10-phenothiazine (LM-209) un nouvel antiallergique. Xenobiotica 6: 633–648
14. Uzan A, Gueremy C, Le Fur G 1976 Biotransformation de la (quinuclidinyl-3-methyl)-10-phenothiazine (LM-209) un nouvel antiallergique et excretion des metabolites. Xenobiotica 6: 649–665
15. Uzan A, Le Fur G 1976 Inhibition de la phosphodiesterase de l'AMP-3',5' cyclique du poumon de cobaye par un nouvel antiallergique, la (quinuclidinyl-3-methyl)-10-phenothiazine (LM-209). Archives Internationale Pharmacodynamie et de Therapie 219: 160–168
16. Yano J, Igo H, Shiraiwa K, Miura M et al 1981 Subacute toxicity and recovery tests of mequitazine in beagle dogs. Journal of Toxicological Sciences 6: 129–157
17. Sono A, Kobayashi Y, Yamamoto H, Hayano K 1981 Mutagenicity tests on mequitazine. Journal of Toxicological Sciences 6: 123–128
18. Fourtillan J B, Girault J, Bouquet S, Lefebvre M A 1984 Determination of mequitazine in human plasma and urine by capillary column gas–liquid chromatography–mass spectrometry. Journal of Chromatography 309: 391–396
19. Hojo M, Nagasaka Y, Katayam O, Serizawa I 1981 Pharmacological study of mequitazine (LM-209). Pharmacological actions of a main metabolite of LM-209, mequitazine sulphoxide (LM-209 SO). Nippon Yakurigaku Zasshi 78: 431–438 (Japanese)
20. Brandon Ml 1985 Newer non-sedating antihistamines will they replace older agents? Drugs 30: 377–381
21. Langier P, Orusco M 1978 Comparative trial of an antihistamine, mequitazine and placebo. Current Medical Research and Opinion 5: 371–375
22. Gervais P, Gervais A, De Beule R, Van der Bijl W 1975 Comparative study of a new antihistamine, mequitazine and placebos. Acta Allergologica 30: 286–297
23. Leophonte P, Leophonte-Domairon S C, Carre J C, Goyeau E, Vayleux M 1984 Etude comparative de la mequitazine et de la terfenadine dans les rhinites allergiques. Allergie et Immunologie 16: 213–220
24. Vialatte J, Paupe J 1977 La mequitazine dans le traitement des manifestations allergiques de l'enfant. Revue Internationale de Paediatrie 74: 59–64

Mercaptopurine monohydrate

This is an anti-metabolite agent first tested against human tumours in 1951.

Chemistry

Mercaptopurine monohydrate (6-mercaptopurine monohydrate, 6MP, Puri-Nethol)

$C_5H_4N_4S.H_2O$

Purine-6-thiol monohydrate

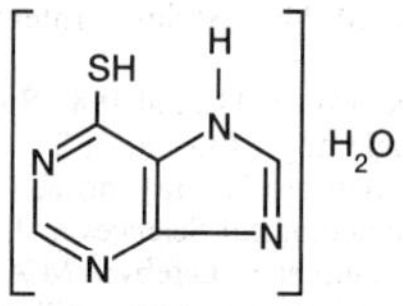

Molecular weight (anhydrous)	107.2 (152.2)
pKa 1	7.77
pKa 2	11.17
Solubility	
in alcohol	1 in 950
in water	very low <1 in 10 000
Octanol/water partition coefficient	—

Mercaptopurine is a yellow, practically odourless, crystalline powder that darkens on exposure to air and light. It is prepared by chemical synthesis. It is insoluble except in hot alcohol and solutions of alkali hydroxides. Dehydration occurs around 125°C.

Pharmacology

Mercaptopurine is converted to the ribonucleotide derivative which is the active form of the drug. This is capable of inhibiting several metabolic pathways. The identification of the primary mechanism whereby mercaptopurine has its cytotoxic effect is unknown.[1] Possible mechanisms are:

1. Incorporation into DNA. Several studies have correlated incorporation with cytotoxicity.[1] Against this possibility is the fact that drug-resistant cells incorporate more mercaptopurine derivatives than sensitive cells.[2]

Fig. 1

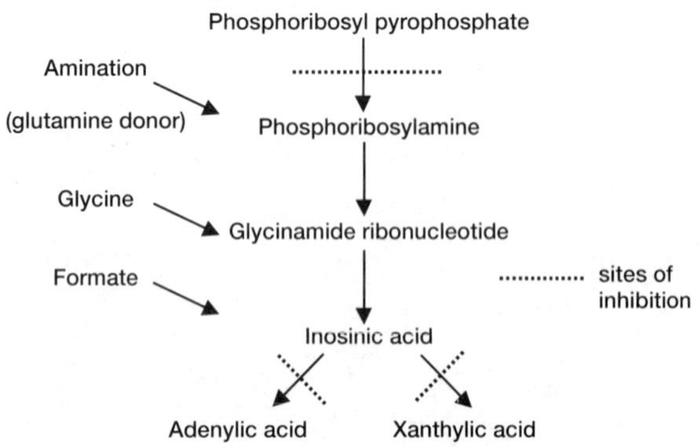

After McCormack & Jones 1982[2]

2. Inhibition of purine biosynthesis.[3] Figure 1 shows the three important sites where the synthesis of nucleic acid may be inhibited.
3. 6MP ribonucleotide inhibits the endonuclease repair activity of DNA polymerase.[4,5]

It is probable that mercaptopurine exerts its effect by a combination of all these mechanisms.[6]

Toxicology

Mercaptopurine showed three major manifestations of toxicity in animal studies. These are: myelosuppression giving rise to pancytopenia; damage to intestinal epithelium; and hepatocellular damage.

As mercaptopurine is a cytotoxic agent, teratogenicity is to be expected. In mice the drug is embryolethal or teratogenic at 3 $mg.kg^{-1}$ given intraperitoneally or by mouth. Similar findings occurred in the rat at higher doses of 60 $mg.kg^{-1}$. Teratogenicity was seen in the rabbit at only 1 $mg.kg^{-1}$ by mouth. These features have not been seen in man.

The drug is mutagenic in the Ames test. Carcinogenicity was not demonstrated in limited studies in animals.

Clinical pharmacology

Mercaptopurine in combination with cytotoxic drugs has an established place in the continuation or 'maintenance' phase of the management of acute lymphoblastic leukaemia in children and adults. It has been shown to be effective in inducing remission as well, but it is rarely used for this purpose now. Its chief use is in continuation therapy for acute lymphoblastic leukaemia; it has been replaced by thioguanine in the treatment of myeloblastic leukaemia.

It is unlikely to be used as a single agent now in the treatment of acute leukaemia. Estimates of activity of this drug when used as a single agent therefore come from much earlier work in the 1950s.[7] The range of drug dosage in childhood and adult acute lymphoblastic and myeloblastic leukaemia is given in Table 1.

The majority of the results in acute leukaemia shown in the table refer to the induction of complete remission, that is, the return of the patient to normal health with no symptoms or signs referable to leukaemia, a normal peripheral blood count, and a bone marrow showing less than 5% blasts with no obvious leukaemic blasts present. Short durations of remission were seen in a number of studies which were in the days before it was considered appropriate to give long-term continuation therapy.

A selection of studies in children and adults where modern treatment strategies have been employed have shown the value of mercaptopurine as a maintenance agent. A selection of these treatment programmes is shown in Table 2.

The highest dose of mercaptopurine used in combination chemotherapy is of the order of 800 $mg.m^{-2}$ weekly, but Esterhay et al (1978)[19] used 6-mercaptopurine alone in a study on solid tumours, giving it as a rapid intravenous infusion at a dose of 1000 $mg.m^{-2}$ daily for 5 days every 21 days. Mucositis, severe nausea and vomiting and diarrhoea, leucopenia and thrombocytopenia occurred, and there was one drug-related death. No response was seen in any of the patients treated. More recently the use of mercaptopurine in high doses is being studied in lymphoblastic leukaemias in children. The initial results are promising and details of these studies are awaited.

Conventional doses of mercaptopurine have ranged from 50 to 100 $mg.m^{-2}$ orally daily. It is very important that the drug is not administered except by physicians trained in its use. If the drug is given with allopurinol, the dose of 6-mercaptopurine must be reduced by 75%.

Pharmacokinetics

The preferred analytical method is by high pressure liquid chromatography. With this method mercaptopurine can be detected at levels of 5–10 $\mu g.l^{-1}$ in plasma.[20,21]

The drug is readily absorbed after oral administration, with peak plasma concentrations at 0.5–4 h (mean 2 h). Initial estimates of the bioavailability after oral dosing suggested that it was only 50%.[3,22] However, more recent studies, using improved analytical techniques, have shown that the bioavailability of oral mercaptopurine is very variable, with a mean of only 16%.[21] The low bioavailability is due to extensive presystemic metabolism in the liver. The drug is

Mercaptopurine monohydrate

rapidly eliminated from the body, with a plasma half life of only 0.9–1.5 h, and a clearance, following intravenous administration, of 700 ml.min^{-1}.m^{-2}. The extensive first-pass metabolism results in a much higher oral clearance, almost 5000 ml.min^{-1}.m^{-2}.

The drug is distributed rapidly throughout the body water, with an apparent volume of distribution of 0.9 l.kg^{-1}. Mercaptopurine is only weakly bound (20%) to plasma proteins.[22] The drug diffuses into CSF, but only poorly.[22]

Oral absorption	high
Presystemic metabolism	extensive
Plasma half life	
range	0.9–1.5 h
Volume of distribution	0.9±0.8 l.kg^{-1}
Plasma protein binding	20%

Mercaptopurine undergoes extensive hepatic metabolism, with only 8% of an oral dose being excreted in the urine as the unchanged drug over 24 h. Small amounts are also excreted in the faeces, but there is no evidence for enterohepatic circulation. Despite its short half life, small amounts of mercaptopurine can be detected in the urine for up to 17 days. In hepatic disease there is reduced elimination of mercaptopurine, and this may require a reduction in the dosage. The effects of old age on the pharmacokinetics of 6-mercaptopurine are not known. The drug crosses the placenta.

Metabolism

Mercaptopurine is extensively metabolized in the liver, with only small amounts of the drug being excreted unchanged. Excretion is largely in the urine (>50% over 24 h), with smaller amounts in the faeces. Only 8% of the dose is excreted unchanged in the urine in 24 h. The main metabolic reactions in man are oxidation to 6-thiouric acid, which is active, by xanthine oxidase[3] and methylation followed by oxidation, intracellular formation of 6-thioinosinic acid and methylmercaptopurine ribonucleotide[23–25] (see Fig. 2) which are biologically active. Mercaptopurine is a metabolite of azathioprine.

Pharmaceutics

1. Puri-Nethol (Wellcome, UK). Each tablet contains 50 mg of mercaptopurine BP, fawn coloured, scored and coded 'Wellcome 04A'. Product licence no. 0003/5227.
2. 10 mg tablets, white, unmarked, unlicenced, only directly from Wellcome.

Mercaptopurine should be stored below 25°C in a dry place protected from light, and under these conditions its maximum shelf-life is 5 years for the 50 mg tablet.

Injections have been prepared by dissolving 1 part in 99 parts of water and further diluting with dextrose injection or sodium chloride injection. This solution is stable for at least 7 days when stored refrigerated at 4°C.

Therapeutic use

Indications

1. Acute leukaemias

Mercaptopurine has been used in acute and chronic leukaemias and in non-Hodgkin lymphoma. Its major use now is in the continuation or 'maintenance' therapy of acute lymphoblastic leukaemia in children and adults (see Table 2). It has been used in a similar manner in combination therapy for high grade non- Hodgkin lymphoma.[26] Mercaptopurine has been used widely in lymphocytic leukaemia. When given in a comparative trial comparing methotrexate alone, methotrexate and mercaptopurine, methotrexate with mercaptopurine and cyclophosphamide, and then all three drugs together with cytosine arabinoside, in the continuation phase of therapy of childhood acute leukaemia, mercaptopurine and methotrexate was shown to be the safest combination, and was equally effective when com-

Table 1 Treatment of leukaemia with 6MP as a single induction agent

Dose	Type of leukaemia	No. of patients	% CR	Median duration (months)	Ref.
2.2 mg. kg.$^{-1}$ daily	Child AL	45	33		7
3.0 mg. kg.$^{-1}$ daily	Child ALL	43	27	147	8
2.5 mg. kg.$^{-1}$ daily	Child ALL	59	36	60	9
6.6 mg. kg.$^{-1}$ daily	Child ALL	64	34	50	
2.5 mg. kg.$^{-1}$ daily	Child AL	67	61		10
3.0 mg. kg.$^{-1}$ daily	Child AML	11	9		8
	Adult AML	31	10		
2.2 mg. kg.$^{-1}$ daily	Adult AML	14	14		7
2.5 mg. kg.$^{-1}$ daily	Adult AL	25	4	106	11
400 mg. m^{-2} twice weekly	Adult AL	25	0		12
800 mg. m^{-2} weekly	Adult AL	20	25		

CR = complete remission

Table 2

Induction	Dose of 6MP	Other maintenance agents	Type of leukaemia	No. of patients	Median duration of remission in months	Ref.
V+P or	50 mg. m^{-2}	MTX+C or	Adult ALL	—	23	13
V+P+Asp.		MTX, Asp.+c				
V+P+Daun.	—	MTX+V+P+Daun.	Adult ALL	—	13	14
V+P+Dox. +Asp. *or*	75 mg daily	MTX+C	Adult ALL	112	18	15
V+P+Dox.	+Asp.+C					
V+P	500 mg. m^{-2} daily ×5 by i.v. infusion	P+MTX *or* P	Childhood ALL	164	54 13	16
V+P±Daun ±Asp.	50 mg. m^{-2} daily per o.	MTX±Cyt.±C ±V+P		282	42	17
V+P+Asp.	50 mg. m^{-2} daily per o.	C+Dox.		58	24	18

Key: V = Vincristine; P = Prednisolone; C = Cyclophosphamide; MTX = Methotrexate; Asp. = Asparaginase; Daun. = Daunorubicin; Dox. = Doxorubicin; Cyt. = Cytosine

Mercaptopurine monohydrate

M

pared with the other three regimens.[17] This classic study established the role of mercaptopurine in continuation therapy. There are as yet no equally satisfactory studies on how long mercaptopurine should be given in combination. In a Medical Research Council Working Party study,[27] children who were in remission from acute lymphoblastic leukaemia at 18 or 24 months were randomized to a further 1 year of therapy including mercaptopurine, and showed no difference in relapse rate in girls. Boys, however, did less well if they received only 18 months of continuation therapy.

Contraindications

A considerable experience of its use has shown that there are no specific contraindications to the use of mercaptopurine.

Adverse reactions

Potentially life-threatening effects

Haematological reactions. Mercaptopurine is a moderately myelosuppressive drug; the nadir of suppression is seen 7 to 14 days after administration, and the duration is of between 14 and 21 days.[28] Haematological disturbance produced in man by mercaptopurine includes anaemia, leucopenia and thrombocytopenia. The severity is dose-related.

Severe or irreversible adverse effects

Severe or irreversible adverse reactions are unlikely to be seen with mercaptopurine administered as a single agent. The enhancement of myelotoxicity consequent upon administration with allopurinol has

Fig. 2 Metabolism of 6-mercaptopurine
After Chabner and Myers 1982[24]

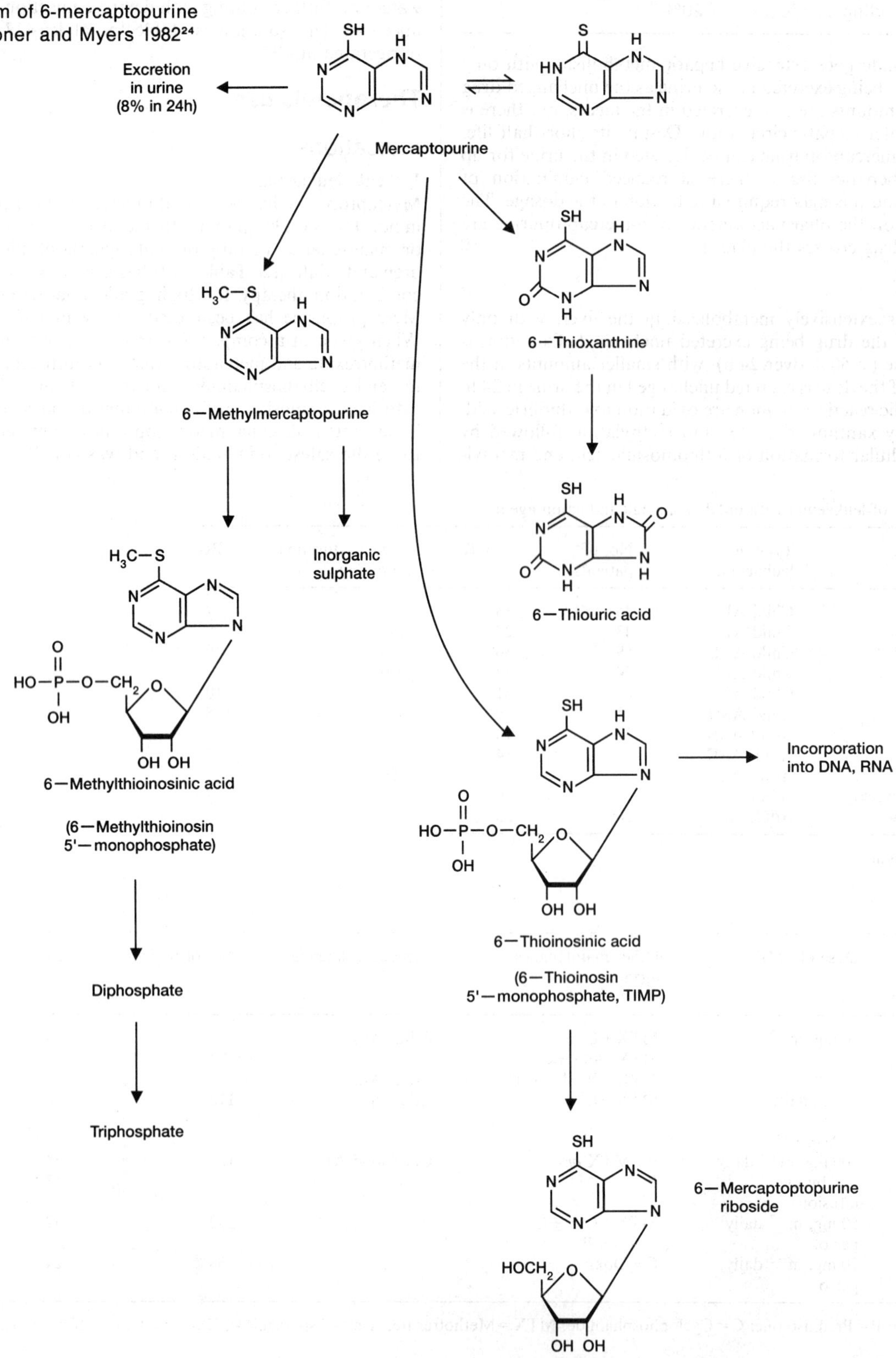

been mentioned earlier, and obviously if mercaptopurine is administered with another hepatotoxic agent, any propensity to liver damage will be increased. More recently, a marked enhancement of bioavailability of mercaptopurine has been noted when it is administered with methotrexate.[28] However, this interaction is not likely to be significant at standard low oral doses of mercaptopurine and methotrexate.

Carcinogenicity. No conclusions as to carcinogenicity in man are possible on existing evidence.

Gastrointestinal reactions. Stomatitis with gut ulceration giving rise to anorexia, nausea and vomiting are seen and are dose-dependent.

Liver damage. While the toxic effects on the haemopoietic system and gut are dose-related, liver dysfunction may occur in some patients treated with quite small doses of mercaptopurine. Usually this takes the form of a reversible cholestatic jaundice. In a few cases where this has not been recognized, and drug therapy prolonged, liver necrosis has occurred.

Mercaptopurine was first reported as a hepatotoxic agent by Farber (1954).[30] When the drug was stopped the jaundice cleared. Animal studies showed that it produced a mild hepatic necrosis. A number of case reports have been recorded subsequently.[31,32] Jaundice comes on about 30 days after the start of therapy, and is usually only seen if more than $2\,mg.kg^{-1}$ body weight per day is given. Mercaptopurine produces a mild hepatocellular or obstructive liver disease.[32]

Pulmonary reactions. Several cases of interstitial pneumonitis following therapy with 6-mercaptopurine have been described and are reviewed.[33] It is fortunately a very rare complication, and stopping the drug usually results in complete recovery.

Symptomatic adverse effects

Skin reactions. These are rare with mercaptopurine, but radiation recall reactions may occasionally occur.

Interference with clinical pathology tests

There is no evidence of interference with laboratory tests.

High risk groups

Neonates

There are no additional special risks attendant upon its use in neonates.

Breast milk. No information is available.

Children

There are no special additional risks when the drug is used in children.

Pregnant women

Mercaptopurine is very likely to be used in pregnancy when the mother has been diagnosed as having acute leukaemia, for which treatment will be required if she is to survive. Mercaptopurine is likely to be given with agents that are more toxic for the fetus, and it is almost impossible to distinguish the effect of mercaptopurine alone on the fetus from the reports in the literature. However, normal children have been born to mothers having mercaptopurine throughout pregnancy.[34]

Walden and Bagshawe (1976),[35] reporting on the reproductive performance of six women successfully treated for gestational trophoblastic tumours which included mercaptopurine, found that the number of abnormal pregnancies was increased when compared with a selected control group. It should be noted, however, that in this study mercaptopurine was never given alone. It was usually given in conjunction with methotrexate, which is certainly recorded as giving rise to fetal abnormality. After multidrug chemotherapy for acute leukaemia, fertility in the male is often impaired so that procreation is usually impossible. However, male patients have been recorded as fathering children, and one patient who had both mercaptopurine and methotrexate for 18 months fathered a child against medical advice. The baby was quite normal.[36]

The elderly

No special precautions are needed.

Concurrent disease

As the drug may be hepatotoxic, it should be avoided or carefully monitored in the presence of severe liver disease.

Mercaptopurine monohydrate

Drug interactions

Potentially hazardous interactions

Allopurinol. This drug affects the metabolism of mercaptopurine by inhibiting xanthine oxidase which converts active 6-thioinosinic acid to inactive 6-thiouric acid. Allopurinol therefore markedly increases the toxicity of mercaptopurine, and a reduction by 75% in the dose of mercaptopurine is advised if allopurinol is to be given concurrently.

Doxorubicin. Concurrent administration with other hepatotoxic agents such as doxorubicin must be avoided or carefully monitored.

Anticoagulants. The anticoagulant effect of warfarin has been reported to be inhibited by mercaptopurine, though this must be a rare occurrence.[37]

References

1. Bieber S, Dietrich L S, Elion G B, Hitchings G H, Martin D S 1961 The incorporation of 6-mercaptopurine-S35 into nucleic acids of sensitive and non sensitive transplantable month tumours. Cancer Research 21: 228–231
2. McCormack J J, Johns D G 1982 Purine antimetabolites. In: Chabner B (ed) Pharmacologic principles of cancer treatment. W B Saunders, Philadelphia, pp 213–228
3. Elion G B 1967 Biochemistry and pharmacology of purine analogues. Federation Proceedings 26: 898–903
4. Lee M Y W T, Byrnes J J, Downey K M, So A G 1980 Mechanisms of inhibition of deoxyribonucleic acid synthesis by 1β-D arabinofuranosyl adenosine triphosphate and its potentiation by 6-mercaptopurine ribonucleoside 5' monophosphate. Biochemistry 19: 215–219
5. Tidd D M, Patterson A R P 1974 A biochemical mechanism for the delayed cytotoxic action of 6-mercaptopurine. Cancer Research 34: 738–746
6. Calabresi P, Park R E 1980 Chemotherapy of neoplastic disease. In: Gilman A G, Goodman L S, Gilman A (eds) The pharmacological basis of therapeutics 6th edn. Macmillan, New York, pp 1282–1287
7. Burchenal J H, Murphy M L, Ellison R R et al 1953 Clinical evaluation of a new antimetabolite 6-mercaptopurine in the treatment of leukaemia and allied diseases. Blood 8: 965–999
8. Frei E III, Freireich E J, Gehan E et al 1961 Studies of sequential and combination antimetabolite therapy in acute leukaemia: 6-mercaptopurine and methotrexate from Acute Leukaemic Group B. Blood 18: 431–454
9. Sullivan M P, Bratti E C, Hyman C B, Murphy M L, Pierck M I, Severo N C 1962 A comparison of the effectiveness of standard dose 6-mercaptopurine, combination 6-mercaptopurine and DON, and high loading 6-mercaptopurine therapies in the treatment of acute leukaemia in children: results of a co-operative study. Cancer Chemotherapy Reports 16: 161–171
10. Heyn R M, Brubaker C A, Burchenal J H, Cramblett H G, Wolff J A 1960 The comparison of 6-mercaptopurine with the combination of 6-mercaptopurine and azaserine in the treatment of acute leukaemia in children: results of a co-operative study. Blood 15: 350–359
11. Ellison R R, Silver R T, Engel R L 1959 Comparative study of 6-chlorpurine and 6-mercaptopurine in acute leukaemia in adults. Annals of Internal Medicine 51: 322–338
12. Ellison R R, Hoogstraten B 1965 Intravenous 6-mercaptopurine and methotrexate in adults with acute leukaemia. Proceedings of American Association for Cancer Research 6: 17
13. Omura G A, Moffitt S, Voller W R, Salter M M 1980 Combination chemotherapy of adult lymphoblastic leukaemia with randomized central nervous system prophylaxis. Blood 55: 199–204
14. Willemze R, Haanen C, Dekker A et al 1982 Results of a multicentre study of the treatment of acute lymphoblastic leukaemia in adolescents and adults. Netherlands Journal of Medicine 25: 303–307
15. Barnett M J, Greaves M F, Amess J A L et al 1986 Treatment of acute lymphoblastic leukaemia in adults with OPAL and HEAV'D regimens. British Journal of Haematology 64 (3): 455–468
16. Berry D H, Fernback D J, Herson J, Pullen J, Sullivan M P, Vietti T J 1980 Comparison of prednisolone, vincristine, methotrexate and 6-mercaptopurine versus 6-mercaptopurine and prednisone maintenance therapy in childhood acute leukaemia. Cancer 46: 1098–1103
17. Aur R J A, Simone J V, Verzosa M S et al 1978 Childhood acute lymphocytic leukaemia (Study VIII). Cancer 42: 2123–2134
18. Camitta B M, Pinkel D, Thatcher L C, Caspar J, Kun L E, Lavers S 1980 Failure of early intensive chemotherapy to improve prognosis in childhood acute lymphocytic leukaemia. Medical and Pediatric Oncology 8: 383–389
19. Esterhay R J, Aisner J, Levi J A, Wiernik P H 1978 High-dose 6-mercaptopurine in advanced refractory cancer. Cancer Treatment Reports 62: 1229–1231
20. Varang P K, Yeager R L, Chatterji D C 1982 Quantitation of 6- mercaptopurine in biologic fluids using high performance liquid chromatography: a selective and novel procedure. Journal of Chromatography 230: 273–280
21. Zimm S, Collins J M, Riccardi R et al 1983 Variable bioavailability of oral mercaptopurine. Is maintenance chemotherapy in acute lymphoblastic leukaemia being optimally delivered. New England Journal of Medicine 308: 1005–1009
22. Loo T L, Luce J K, Sullivan M P, Frei E III 1967 Clinical pharmacologic observations on 6-mercaptopurine and 6-methylthiopurine ribonucleoside. Clinical Pharmacology and Therapeutics 9: 180–194
23. Zimmerman T P, Chu L C, Bugge C J L, Nelson D J, Lyon G M, Elion G B 1974 Identification of 6-methylmercaptopurine ribonucleoside-5'-diphosphate and 5'-triphosphate as metabolites of 6-mercaptopurine in man. Cancer Research 34: 221–224

24. Chabner B, Myers C E 1982 Clinical pharmacology of cancer chemotherapy. In: DeVita V T, Hellman S, Rosenberg S A (eds) Principles and practice of oncology. J B Lippincott, Philadelphia, pp 156–195
25. Tidd D M, Paterson R P 1974 Distinction between inhibition of purine nucleotide synthesis and the delayed cytotoxic reaction of 6-mercaptopurine. Cancer Research 34: 733–737
26. Lister T A, Cullen M H, Brearly R B et al 1978 Combination chemotherapy for advanced non-Hodgkin's lymphoma of unfavourable histology. Cancer Chemotherapy and Pharmacology 1: 107–112
27. Medical Research Council 1982 Duration of chemotherapy in childhood acute lymphoblastic leukaemia. Medical and Pediatric Oncology 10: 511–520
28. Hoagland H C 1982 Haematologic complications of cancer chemotherapy. Seminars in Oncology 5: 95–102
29. Balis F M, Holcenberg J S, Zimm S et al 1987 The effect of methotrexate on the bioavailability of oral 6-mercaptopurine. Clinical Pharmacology and Therapeutics 41: 384–387
30. Farber S 1954 Summary of experience with 6-mercaptopurine. Annals New York Academy of Sciences 60: 412–414
31. Clark P A, Hsia Y E, Huntsman R G 1960 Toxic complications of treatment with 6-mercaptopurine: two cases with hepatic necrosis and intestinal ulceration. British Medical Journal 1: 393–395
32. Einhorn M, Davidson I 1964 Hepatotoxicity of mercaptopurine. Journal of American Medical Association 188: 802–806
33. Ginsberg S T, Comis R L 1982 The pulmonary toxicity of antineoplastic agents. Seminars in Oncology 9: 34–51
34. Ravenna P, Stein P J 1963 Acute monocytic leukaemia in pregnancy. American Journal of Obstetrics and Gynaecology 85: 545–548
35. Walden P A M, Bagshawe K D 1976 Reproductive performance of women successfully treated for gestational trophoblastic tumours. American Journal of Obstetrics and Gynaecology 125: 1108–1114
36. Kroner T H, Tschumi A 1977 Conception of normal child during chemotherapy of acute lymphoblastic leukaemia in the father. British Medical Journal 1: 1322–1323
37. Spiers A S D, Mibashin R S 1974 Increased Warfarin requirement during mercaptopurine therapy: a new drug interaction. Lancet 2: 221–222

Mesalazine

Mesalazine is 5-aminosalicylic acid, the active moiety of sulphasalazine. Its major indication is to treat acute exacerbations of mild to moderate ulcerative colitis and maintain ulcerative colitis in remission, particularly in patients intolerant of sulphasalazine.

Chemistry

Mesalazine (5-aminosalicylic acid, Mesalamine, Asacol, Pentasa, Claversal, Salofalk, Nemasol, Parasol)
$C_7H_7NO_3$
5-Amino-2-hydroxybenzoic acid

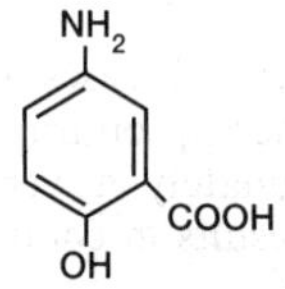

Molecular weight	153.1
pKa	2, 5.8, 12
Solubility	
in alcohol	1 in 20
in water	1 in 600
Octanol/water partition coefficient	log p = 0.87

An off-white powder or crystalline material, prepared by chemical synthesis.

Pharmacology

Mesalazine is 5-aminosalicylic acid. Sulphasalazine has long been used in the treatment of ulcerative colitis and this drug consists of 5-aminosalicylic acid joined to sulphapyridine by an azo bond which is split by intestinal bacteria to release the two components. It is now established that the active component in sulphasalazine as far as ulcerative colitis is concerned is 5-aminosalicylic acid.[1]

Mesalazine is a weak inhibitor of cyclo-oxygenase but this effect is model dependent. In the rabbit[2] mesalazine increases the synthesis of prostacyclin, $PGF_2\alpha$, PGE_2 and thromboxane B_2, while in human intestinal tissue PGE_1 metabolism was inhibited.[3] In human blood mononuclear cells prostaglandin production is also inhibited by mesalazine.[4]

Leucotrienes formed by the lipoxygenase pathway are also implicated in the pathogenesis of ulcerative colitis and mesalazine is an inhibitor of lipoxygenase.[5] Thus leucotriene release, particularly LTB_4, and the release of hydroxyeicosatetraenoic acids (HETE) are inhibited by mesalazine. Other actions of mesalazine are: 1) restricting the migration of macrophages into inflamed tissue; 2) acting as a free radical scavenger; 3) in the rat colon, suppressing the basal and deoxycholate-induced increases in reactive oxygen formation;[6] 4) inhibiting the synthesis of platelet activating factor; 5) suppressing mucosal fatty acid oxidation.

It is by no means clear which of these actions, if any, is responsible for the beneficial effect of mesalazine in ulcerative colitis; it is unlikely that it is cyclo-oxygenase inhibition because more potent inhibitors such as indomethacin are not effective agents for the treatment of colitis.

Toxicology

Mesalazine nephrotoxicity has been reported in rats given intravenous doses ten times greater per unit weight than the normal human oral dose.[7] Chronic toxicity studies in rats and rabbits given large oral doses have also provided evidence of nephrotoxicity, which is dose-dependent and reversible. The clinical relevance of these observations is unclear, but mesalazine preparations are consequently not recommended for patients with renal disease or impaired renal function. Toxicology studies in animals have otherwise been negative, and there is no evidence to suggest that mesalazine has teratogenic, mutagenic or carcinogenic properties.

Clinical pharmacology

Mesalazine is effective in the treatment of ulcerative colitis. There is good evidence that in patients with ulcerative colitis the generation of arachidonic acid metabolites is enhanced.[8] The prostaglandins (via the cyclo-oxygenase pathway) and the leucotrienes (via the lipoxygenase pathway) are increased and may act as highly potent inflammatory mediators, thus playing a major role in the pathogenesis of ulcerative colitis.[9] Mesalazine is a weak inhibitor of cyclo-oxygenase and drugs that are potent inhibitors of this pathway, such as indomethacin, do not improve ulcerative colitis and may make it worse.[10] It may be then that the clinical effects of mesalazine in improving ulcerative colitis are due to some of the other effects of mesalazine — notably its lipoxygenase inhibiting property. Mesalazine has been suggested to inhibit lymphocyte activation in man, to inhibit killer cell activity and to inhibit immunoglobulin synthesis by B lymphocytes. However, these actions have only been shown in vitro and no systemic effect in vivo has been consistently demonstrated other than its effect on arachidonic acid metabolism.

Pharmacokinetics

The preferred analytical method for mesalazine is high performance liquid chromatography. This technique can reliably distinguish mesalazine from closely related salicylates and has a sensitivity of 500 $\mu g.l^{-1}$. Orally ingested free mesalazine is efficiently absorbed by the small bowel and rapidly cleared from the circulation, with an elimination half life of about 1 hour. Therapeutic concentrations in the colon can only be achieved by oral ingestion of a delayed- or slow-release preparation, or by topical application in enema form. At steady state these preparations provide colonic luminal concentrations of the order of 1000-fold greater than plasma concentrations.[12,13]

The bioavailability in the colon of both delayed- and slow-release oral preparations is to some extent influenced by intestinal transit time and pH, and by the presence of small bowel disease, but this seems not to be of major clinical significance.[9,14] Delayed-release mesalazine (Asacol) is coated with Eudragit S, an acrylic-based resin which disintegrates above pH7 to release the active drug. In vivo, disintegration generally takes place in the terminal ileum or right colon,[15] and about 80% of the administered dose is available in the colonic lumen.[9]

Slow-release mesalazine (Pentasa) is prepared as microgranules coated with a thin layer of ethylcellulose. The rate of release of mesalazine increases above pH6 though, unlike Asacol, release is not critically pH dependent. Approximately 60% of the active drug is released in the small bowel and half of this is absorbed: the remaining 40% is released in the colon.[9] Thus, approximately 60% of the administered dose is available in the small bowel to exert a topical effect, and 70% in the colon.

10% of the mesalazine in Pentasa enema is in solution and so available for immediate activity. The remaining 90% dissolves slowly from suspension, with release of active drug continuing for about 6 hours after administration. The enema preparation is buffered to pH 4.8 to limit absorption of mesalazine.

The rapid clearance of mesalazine from the circulation is largely due to acetylation to form N-acetyl-5-aminosalicylic acid (Ac-5-ASA), which itself is swiftly cleared by glomerular filtration and active renal tubular secretion. Unlike Ac-5-ASA, very little mesalazine crosses the placenta or enters breast milk.[16] The systemic pharmacokinetic properties of mesalazine and Ac-5-ASA are as follows:[4,12–15]

Mesalazine

Oral absorption	high, depends on formulation
Presystemic metabolism	—
Plasma half life	
range	0.5–1 h
Volume of distribution	—
Plasma protein binding	50%

M

Concentration–effect relationship

Since the mechanism of therapeutic action has not been identified, no data are available.

Metabolism

The majority of an ingested dose of mesalazine is metabolized by N-acetylation in the intestinal epithelium and in the liver — polymorphism of the intestinal acetyl transferase has not been identified. The drug also undergoes conjugation with glycine. The major metabolites, N-acetyl-5-aminosalicylic acid, and 5-aminosalicyluric acid, appear to have no therapeutic activity or specific toxic effects (see Fig. 1).[9] For both Asacol and Pentasa tablets, total excretion of mesalazine (acetylated and unacetylated) is 20–40% of the ingested dose in the faeces and 30–50% of the ingested dose in the urine.[12–14,17,18]

Fig. 1 The metabolism of mesalazine

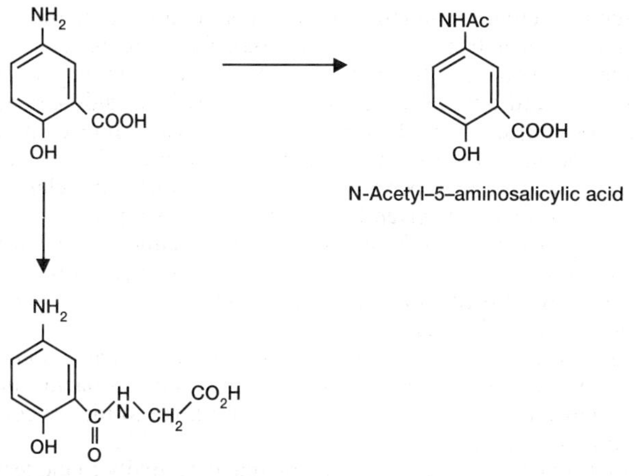

5–aminosalicyluric acid

Pharmaceutics

Mesalazine is available in delayed-release (Asacol) and slow-release form (Pentasa), which are designed to limit small bowel absorption and so enhance the delivery of active drug in the colon. Asacol is mesalazine coated with Eudragit S, an acrylic-based resin which disintegrates above pH 7 (also available as suppository). Pentasa consists of microgranules of mesalazine coated with a semipermeable layer of ethylcellulose.

Claversal and Salofalk are delayed-release mesalazine preparations not currently available in the UK.

Mesalazine is available in oral suppository and enema preparations:

Asacol tablets (SmithKline Beecham, UK) are red and oblong-shaped, containing 400 mg of mesalazine. Pentasa tablets (Ferring, UK) are round, scored on one side and coloured white flecked with grey. Each tablet contains 250 mg of mesalazine within slow-release microgranules. The shelf-life of both preparations is 2 years.

Pentasa enemas contain 1 g mesalazine in 100 ml. They are prepared under liquid nitrogen and individually foil-wrapped. The shelf-life of this preparation is 2 years. Asacol suppositories are opaque beige and contain 250 mg or 500 mg of mesalazine.

Therapeutic use

Indications

1. The treatment of mild to moderate acute exacerbations of ulcerative colitis

2. The maintenance of remission of ulcerative colitis including the maintenance of remission of ulcerative colitis in males hoping to induce conception in their partners
3. The induction of remission of mildly active ulcerative colitis in patients who cannot tolerate sulphasalazine.

Contraindications

1. Salicylate hypersensitivity
2. Renal disease/impaired renal function.

Mode of use

The recommended daily dose for adults, given in divided doses, is 1.2–2.4 g (Asacol) and 0.75–1.5 g (Pentasa), though higher doses have been used in some trials. For the maintenance of remission in proven ulcerative colitis, treatment should be continued indefinitely. Pentasa enemas may be given in the treatment of mild to moderately active colitis.

Indications

Sulphasalazine is the established drug of choice in the maintenance of remission of ulcerative colitis, but at least 10% of individuals are unable to tolerate sulphasalazine because of side-effects such as gastrointestinal disturbance, headache, cutaneous eruptions and haematological effects. These features are mostly attributable to the sulphapyridine moiety of sulphasalazine, which is not required for therapeutic activity in inflammatory bowel disease.[1] Preparations of mesalazine, the active moiety of sulphasalazine,[1] are just as effective as sulphasalazine in the maintenance of remission in ulcerative colitis[19–21] and are well tolerated by over 80% of sulphasalazine-intolerant subjects.[22–25] In one study, the relapse rate of patients given sulphasalazine was 38.6% compared with 37.5% in a group receiving Asacol over a period of 1 year.[20] Likewise, the relapse rate over 1 year in patients given Pentasa was 37% compared with 28% with sulphasalazine[37] Whether greater therapeutic efficacy will be obtained using higher doses of mesalazine is not yet known. As an alternative to oral therapy, daily mesalazine suppositories and enemas may reduce the relapse rate in distal colitis.[26]

Mesalazine does not cause the (reversible) oligospermia seen with sulphasalazine. It is therefore preferable to sulphasalazine in the maintenance treatment of male colitics who hope to induce conception in their partners.[27]

Mesalazine also has a role in the treatment of mildly to moderately active ulcerative colitis either by mouth[28,29] or in the case of distal disease by suppository or enema,[30–32,38,39] particularly in sulphasalazine-intolerant subjects.[22,24] There is some evidence that high dose mesalazine may be more effective orally than conventional doses of sulphasalazine,[28] and more effective topically than standard doses of corticosteroids.[30,31]

A role for mesalazine in the management of Crohn's disease remains to be proven. Unlike sulphasalazine and Asacol, Pentasa releases significant quantities of mesalazine in the small bowel, but a convincing therapeutic effect in small bowel Crohn's disease has not yet been demonstrated.[33]

Contraindications

1. Salicylate hypersensitivity
Mesalazine is a salicylate, and is therefore contraindicated in subjects with a history of salicylate hypersensitivity. Sulphasalazine hypersensitivity is not a contraindication, since most cases are due to the sulphapyridine moiety, but caution should be taken when introducing mesalazine in patients who have previously experienced a major hypersensitivity reaction to sulphasalazine.[23]

2. Renal disease/impaired renal function
On the basis of the structural resemblance of mesalazine to phenacetin and aspirin, and of animal toxicology studies (see above), the presence of renal disease or impairment of renal function is a contraindication to mesalazine therapy. There is currently no convincing evidence that therapeutic enteral doses of mesalazine are nephrotoxic in man, though long-term follow-up data is not yet available.

Mesalazine

Adverse reactions

Potentially life-threatening effects
There are no established adverse effects in this category.

Acute overdosage
The clinical features of mesalazine overdose in man are not documented. Gastric lavage and standard supportive measures are recommended following overdose.

Severe or irreversible adverse effects
Single cases of bronchospasm with pericarditis[22] and the nephrotic syndrome[34] have been reported, but a causal relationship is unproven.

Symptomatic adverse effects
A variety of symptomatic adverse effects have been reported, though all are infrequent, relatively minor and reversible. They include nausea, abdominal discomfort, diarrhoea, headache, rash, fever, unexplained chest pain, paraesthesia, relative leucopenia, hair loss and exacerbation of the underlying colitis.[20–25,28,29,31,33–35]

Other effects
Biochemical abnormalities are very uncommon. Minor elevations of serum creatinine[28] and liver enzyme levels[23] have occasionally been noted.

Interference with clinical pathology tests
Mesalazine may interfere with some assay methods for glucose, bilirubin, urobilinogen, phenylketones, VMA and urinary protein.[36] Interference with plasma salicylate assays is not a significant clinical problem.

High risk groups

Neonates
The drug is not recommended in neonates.

Breast milk. Mothers taking the drug should not breast-feed.

Children
The drug is not recommended in children.

Pregnant women
The drug should not be used during pregnancy unless considered essential.

The elderly
Mesalazine may be used in the elderly provided that renal function is normal.

Drug interactions

Potentially hazardous interactions
None is known.

Other significant interactions
Bacterial catabolism of lactulose and related agents generates organic acids which lower the luminal pH in the colon and so inhibit the disintegration of Eudragit S. They should therefore not be given with Asacol or other pH-dependent delayed release preparations.

Potentially useful interactions
None is known.

Major outcome trials

1. Riley S A, Mani V, Goodman M J, Herd M E, Dutt S, Turnberg L A 1988 Comparison of delayed-release 5-aminosalicylic acid (mesalazine) and sulphasalazine as maintenance treatment for patients with ulcerative colitis. Gastroenterology 94: 1383–1389

100 patients with inactive ulcerative colitis previously maintained on sulphasalazine were randomized in a double-dummy trial to receive Asacol (median dose 800 mg daily) or enteric-coated sulphasalazine (median dose 2 g daily). Cumulative clinical relapse at 48 weeks, confirmed by sigmoidoscopy, was 37.5% in the mesalazine group and 38.6% in the sulphasalazine group (NS). There was no significant difference in the mean time to relapse. The authors conclude that delayed-release mesalazine is as effective as sulphasalazine for the maintenance of remission in ulcerative colitis.

Mesalazine

2. Schroeder K W, Tremaine W J, Ilstrup D M 1987 Coated oral 5-aminosalicylic acid therapy for mild to moderately active ulcerative colitis. New England Journal of Medicine 317: 1625–1629

87 patients with mild to moderately active ulcerative colitis were randomized in a double-blind study to receive Asacol (4.8 g daily), Asacol (1.6 g daily) or placebo as the sole form of treatment. At six weeks, 18% in the placebo group were judged to have shown a partial or complete clinical response to therapy, compared to 27% in the low dose Asacol group (NS) and 74% in the high dose Asacol group ($P < 0.0001$). The authors conclude that high dose Asacol is effective therapy for mild to moderately active ulcerative colitis.

3. Danish 5-ASA Group 1987 Topical 5-aminosalicylic acid versus prednisolone in ulcerative proctosigmoiditis. Digestive Diseases and Sciences 32: 598–602

123 patients with mild to moderately active distal ulcerative colitis were randomized in a double-blind study to receive a daily enema containing 1 g Pentasa or 25 mg prednisolone. At four weeks, 77% in the Pentasa group were judged to have shown a partial or complete clinical response to therapy, compared to 72% in the prednisolone group (NS). The authors conclude that Pentasa enemas are as effective as topical prednisolone in the treatment of mild to moderately active distal ulcerative colitis.

General review articles

Martin F 1987 Oral 5-aminosalicylic acid preparations in the treatment of inflammatory bowel disease. Digestive Diseases and Sciences 32: 57s–73s

Arvind A S, Farthing M J G 1988 Review: new aminosalicylic acid derivatives for the treatment of inflammatory bowel disease. Alimentary Pharmacology and Therapeutics 2: 281–289

Peppercorn M A 1988 Update on the aminosalicylates: a promise fulfilled. Gastroenterology 95: 1677–1680

Ireland A, Jewell D P 1989 Sulphasalazine and the new salicylates. European of Journal of Gastroenterology and Hepatology 1: 43–50

References

1. Azad Khan A K, Piris J, Truelove S C 1977 An experiment to determine the active therapeutic moiety of sulphasalazine. Lancet 2: 892–895
2. Kolassa N, Becker R, Wiener H 1985 Influence of sulfasalazine, 5-aminosalicylic acid and sulphapyridine on prostanoid synthesis and metabolism in rabbit colonic mucosa. Prostaglandins 29: 133–142
3. Hiller K, Mason P, Smith C L 1981 Ulcerative colitis: prostaglandin metabolism and the effect of sulphasalazine, 5-aminosalicylic acid and indomethacin in human colonic mucosa. British Journal of Pharmacology 73: 217P
4. Keating I J, Maxwell W J, Hogan F P 1987 Effects of prednisolone, sulphasalazine, 5-aminosalicylic acid and indomethacin on prostaglandin E_2 and leucotriene B_4 production. Gut 28: A 1390
5. Nielsen O H, Bukhave K, Elmgreen J, Ahnfelt-Ronne I 1987 Inhibition of 5-lipoxygenase pathway of arachnidonic acid metabolism in human neutrophils by sulphasalazine and 5-aminosalicylic acid. Digestive Diseases and Sciences 32: 577–582
6. Craven P A, Pfanstiel J, Saito R, De Rubertis F R 1987 Actions of sulfasalazine and 5-aminosalicylic acid as reactive oxygen scavengers in the suppression of bile-acid induced increases in colonic epithelial cell loss and proliferative activity. Gastroenterology 92: 1998–2008
7. Calder J C, Funder C C, Green C R, Ham K N, Tange J D 1972 Nephrotoxic lesions from 5-aminosalicylic acid. British Medical Journal 1: 152–154
8. Donowitz M 1985 Arachidonic acid metabolites and their role in inflammatory bowel disease. Gastroenterology 88: 580–587
9. Bondesen S, Rasmussen S N, Rask-Madsen J et al 1987 5-aminosalicylic acid in the treatment of inflammatory bowel disease. Acta Medica Scandinavica 221: 227–242
10. Rampton D S, Hawkey C J 1984 Prostaglandins and ulcerative colitis. Gut 25: 1399–1413
11. Fischer C, Maier K, Klotz U 1981 Simplified high-performance liquid chromatographic method for 5-aminosalicylic acid in plasma and urine. Journal of Chromatography 225: 498–503
12. Al Mardini H, Lindsay D C, Deighton C M, Record C O 1987 Effect of polymer coating on faecal recovery of ingested 5-aminosalicylic acid in patients with ulcerative colitis. Gut 28: 1084–1089
13. Rijk M C M, Van Schaik A, Van Tongeren J H M 1988 Disposition of 5-aminosalicylic acid-delivering compounds. Scandinavian Journal of Gastroenterology 23: 107–112
14. Christensen L A, Slot O, Sanchez G et al 1987 Release of 5-aminosalicylic acid from Pentasa during normal and accelerated intestinal transit time. British Journal of Clinical Pharmacology 23: 365–369
15. Dew M J, Ryder R E J, Evans N, Evans B K, Rhodes J 1983 Colonic release of 5-aminosalicylic acid from an oral preparation in active ulcerative colitis. British Journal of Clinical Pharmacology 16: 185–187
16. Christensen L A, Rasmussen S N, Hansen S H, Bondesen S, Hvidberg E F 1987 Salazosulphapyridine and metabolites in fetal and maternal body fluids, with special reference to 5-aminosalicylic acid. Acta Obstetrica Gynaecologica Scandinavica 66: 433–435
17. Rasmussen S N, Bondesen S, Hvidberg E F et al 1982 5-aminosalicylic acid in a slow-release preparation: bioavailability, plasma level and excretion in humans. Gastroenterology 83: 1062–1070
18. Myers B, Evans D N W, Rhodes J et al 1987 Metabolism and urinary excretion of 5-aminosalicylic acid in healthy volunteers when given intravenously or released for absorption at different sites in the gastrointestinal tract. Gut 28: 196–200
19. Klotz U, Maier K E, Fischer C, Bauer K H 1985 A new slow-release form of 5-aminosalicylic acid for the oral treatment of inflammatory bowel disease. Arzneimittel-Forschung/Drug Research 35: 636–639
20. Riley S A, Mani V, Goodman M J, Herd M E, Dutt S, Turnberg L A 1988 Comparison of delayed-release 5-aminosalicylic acid (mesalazine) and sulphasalazine as maintenance treatment for patients with ulcerative colitis. Gastroenterology 94: 1383–1389
21. Dew M J, Hughes P, Harries A D, Williams G, Evans B K, Rhodes J 1982 Maintenance of remission in ulcerative colitis with an oral preparation of 5-aminosalicylic acid. British Medical Journal 285: 1012
22. Habal F M, Greenberg G R 1988 Treatment of ulcerative colitis with oral 5-aminosalicylic acid, including patients with adverse reactions to sulphasalazine. American Journal of Gastroenterology 83: 15–19
23. Turunen U, Elomaa I, Anttila V J, Seppala K 1987 Mesalazine tolerance in patients with inflammatory bowel disease and previous intolerance or allergy to sulphasalazine or sulphonamides. Scandinavian Journal of Gastroenterology 22: 798–802
24. Donald I P, Wilkinson S P 1985 The value of 5-aminosalicylic acid in inflammatory bowel disease for patients intolerant or allergic to sulphasalazine. Postgraduate Medical Journal 61: 1047–1048
25. Mulder C J J, Tytgat G N J, Dekker W, Terpstra I J 1988 Pentasa in lieu of sulphasalazine. Annals of Internal Medicine 61: 1047–1048
26. Biddle W L, Greenberger N J, Swan J T, McPhee M S, Miner P B 1988 5-aminosalicylic acid enemas: effective agent in maintaining remission in left-sided ulcerative colitis. Gastroenterology 94: 1075–1079
27. Riley S A, Lecarpentier J, Mani V, Goodman M J, Mandal B K, Turnberg L A 1987 Sulphasalazine induced seminal abnormalities in ulcerative colitis: results of mesalazine substitution. Gut 28: 1008–1012
28. Riley S A, Mani V, Goodman M J, Herd M E, Dutt S, Turnberg L A 1988 Comparison of delayed release 5-aminosalicylic acid (mesalazine) and sulphasalazine in the treatment of mild to moderate ulcerative colitis relapse. Gut 29: 669–674
29. Schroeder K W, Tremaine W J, Ilstrup D M 1987 Coated oral 5-aminosalicylic acid therapy for mild to moderately active ulcerative colitis. New England Journal of Medicine 317: 1625–1629
30. Campieri M, Bazzocchi G, Franzin G et al 1981 Treatment of ulcerative colitis with high-dose 5-aminosalicylic acid enemas. Lancet 2: 270–271
31. Danish 5-ASA Group 1987 Topical 5-aminosalicylic acid versus prednisolone in ulcerative proctosigmoiditis. Digestive Diseases and Sciences 32: 598–602
32. Willoughby C P, Campieri M, Lanfranchi G, Truelove S C, Jewell D P 1986 5-aminosalicylic acid (Pentasa) in enema form for the treatment of active ulcerative colitis. Italian Journal of Gastroenterology 18: 15–17
33. Rasmussen S N, Lauritsen K, Tage-Jensen U et al 1987 5-aminosalicylic acid in the treatment of Crohn's disease. Scandinavian Journal of Gastroenterology 22: 877–883
34. Novis B H, Korzets Z, Chen P, Bernheim J 1988 Nephrotic syndrome after treatment with 5-aminosalicylic acid. British Medical Journal 296: 1442
35. Kutty P K, Raman K R K, Hawken K, Barrowman J A 1982 Hair loss and 5-aminosalicylic acid enemas. Annals of Internal Medicine 97: 785–786
36. Tryding N, Roos K A (eds) 1986 Drug interferences and drug effects in clinical chemistry, 4th edn. Swedish Society for Clinical Chemistry
37. Mulder C J J, Tytgat G N J, Weterman I T et al 1988 Double-blind comparison of slow-release 5-aminosalicylate and sulfasalazine in remission maintenance of ulcerative colitis. Gastroenterology 65: 1449–1453
38. Campieri M, De Franchis R, Bianchi Porro G, Ranzi T, et al 1990 Mesalazine (5-aminosalicylic acid) suppositories in the treatment of ulcerative proctitis or distal proctosigmoiditis. Scandinavian Journal Gastroenterology 25: 663–668
39. Williams C N, Haber G, Aqvino J A 1987 Double-blind, placebo-controlled evaluation of 5-ASA suppositories in active distal proctitis and measurement of extent of spread using ^{99m}Tc-labeled 5-ASA suppositories. Digestive Diseases and Science 32(2): 71S–75S

M

Mesna

Mesna is a protective compound given in conjunction with ifosfamide or cyclophosphamide to prevent toxicity to the kidney and bladder from nucleophilic metabolites of these drugs. It also has mucolytic properties.

Chemistry

Mesna (mesnum, Uromitexan, Mistabron)
$C_2H_5O_3S_2Na$
Sodium 2-mercaptoethane sulphonate

$HS-CH_2-CH_2-SO_3^-Na^+$

Molecular weight	164.2
pKa	—
Solubility	
in alcohol	—
in water	>1 in 2.5
Octanol/water partition coefficient	—

Mesna is a white crystalline powder with a characteristic smell (rotten eggs). It is not present in any combination preparations.

Pharmacology

The oxazaphosphorines cyclophosphamide and ifosfamide are metabolized to a number of alkylating species. The presence of one of these — acrolein — in the urine is responsible for the toxicity to the bladder epithelium that is seen with both drugs and probably also the renal tubular toxicity resulting from ifosfamide therapy. Mesna contains a free sulphydryl moiety which reacts preferentially with the reactive nucleophiles, rendering them non-toxic.

The ability of mesna to provide uroprotection is a function of its disposition. Much of our knowledge of this comes from animal experiments. Orally administered mesna is readily absorbed in rats. It is rapidly oxidized in plasma to the inactive metabolite, dimesna, so that plasma concentrations of this greatly exceed those of mesna following both oral and intravenous administration.[1] Dimesna is not taken up into liver cells and neither this nor mesna appear in the bile.[1] Dimesna is filtered by renal glomeruli and much of it is reabsorbed into renal tubular cells. Here it undergoes reduction to mesna, which is secreted into the urine.[1,2] Glutathione and NADPH are cofactors in this reduction. Studies with ^{14}C mesna in rats have shown that at 20 minutes after intravenous injection 12% of the dose was present in the kidney — considerably more than could be accounted for by the presence of drug in urine. The amount in other organs corresponded closely with their blood content.[3] A consequence of this lack of entry of mesna into cells other than those of the kidney is that there is no blockade of the anti-tumour activity of synchronously administered alkylating agents.

Mesna produces mucolysis in vitro by disrupting the disulphide bonds of mucoprotein.

Toxicology

In mice, high doses of mesna gave slight excitation, and EEG changes were seen in the rabbit. Variable changes in heart rate and blood pressure have been seen in dogs and cats. Repeated intravenous injections produced nausea and vomiting in dogs. Solutions of $\geq 20\%$ mesna cause local irritation when injected intravenously.

Teratogenicity tests were negative in rats and rabbits.

Clinical pharmacology

In man mesna is absorbed after oral administration and 20% of the dose appears in the urine as mesna[4] or free thiols.[5] The drug is more commonly given intravenously, in which case 32% is excreted as mesna in the urine. Over 95% of the urinary mesna appears within four hours of intravenous administration. Oral dosing gives a delayed urinary peak.[4] Mesna should be given at the same time or shortly before giving ifosfamide. Because of its rapid elimination either repeated doses or continuous infusion should be used. It is probable that the dose required to protect the bladder and kidneys is similar to that of the coadministered oxazophosphorine. Because of the severity of the toxicity that may occur when mesna is omitted, very little work has been done to explore the minimum dose required. An early study gave doses of 50% by weight that of ifosfamide apparently with success.[1] Several subsequent ones have used a figure of 60% but incomplete protection has been noted on occasions.[6,7] As a result doses of 100–180% (by weight) that of the oxazophosphorine are now given.

Pharmacokinetics

Mesna in urine has been measured using Ellman's assay for free thiols.[8] Normally the quantity of naturally occurring free thiols in the urine is very low but during mesna therapy it is enhanced.[9] HPLC analysis of mesna has been described,[9,10] using either an electrochemical detector or, following post-column derivatization with Ellman's reagent, colorimetric detection. A method suitable for assay of mesna in plasma samples[10] involves the immediate mixing of the plasma with reagents to prevent metabolism by plasma components. Dimesna is measured using the assay for mesna following reduction with borohydride. The HPLC assay[10] allows detection of mesna in plasma and urine at concentrations as low as 6.2 $\mu mol.l^{-1}$.

Following intravenous administration, mesna concentrations in plasma are best fitted by a single-compartment, open pharmacokinetic model and decline with a mean half life of 22 minutes.[4] Dimesna concentrations, on the other hand, show an inflexion on a log concentration–time plot with a terminal half life of 1–2 hours.

Oral absorption	>76%
Presystemic metabolism	perhaps 25%
Plasma half life	
mean	22 min
Volume of distribution	0.65 $l.kg^{-1}$
Plasma protein binding	—

Following oral administration mesna is slowly and variably absorbed. Plasma levels of mesna are very variable and may be undetectable. Peak levels are reached in between one and four hours. Mean systemic bioavailability is 50%. Urinary bioavailability is more relevant to the action of mesna. It may be defined as the amount of mesna appearing in the urine following an oral dose compared to that after an intravenous dose. It is variable, with a mean of 53%.[4] Some indication of the extent of intestinal absorption of mesna may be gauged by measuring both mesna and its principal metabolite dimesna in the urine. Following an oral dose 49% of the drug is recovered in this way compared to 65% following an intravenous dose (suggesting that absorption is at least 76%).[4] Mesna has a volume of distribution of 0.65 $l.kg^{-1}$. The extent of placental transfer and excretion in breast milk, if any, are not known. The effects of hepatic and renal disease on the kinetics of mesna are not known.

Mesna is oxidized in the plasma and excreted in the urine, 16–32% as unchanged drug. Plasma protein binding is 10% in rats, but has not been ascertained in man.

Concentration–effect relationship

In this instance it is the urinary and not the plasma concentration that matters. The uroprotective effect of mesna in rats was tested following an intravenous injection of 65 $mg.kg^{-1}$ of ifosfamide. Some bladder toxicity was seen after a simultaneous intravenous dose of 7 $mg.kg^{-1}$ mesna but complete protection[11] occurred with 15 $mg.kg^{-1}$. This dose of mesna produces rather less than 90 $\mu mol.l^{-1}$ free thiols in the urine over a six-hour period.[12] As mesna detoxifies oxazaphosphorine metabolites by stoichiometric reaction, the required uroprotective concentration is a function of the toxin concentration. It has been suggested that 1.7 μmol.l^{-1} is a minimum effective concentration for urinary mesna following a therapeutic dose of ifosfamide.[13] A dose of 800 mg mesna intravenously produces peak urinary levels[4] of 10 μmol.l^{-1}. Following the same dose given by mouth, peak concentrations of 2.5 μmol.l^{-1} are seen either in the 0–4 hour or 4–8 hour urine.[4]

Metabolism

Mesna is rapidly oxidized in plasma, both in vivo and in vitro, to dimesna, which is inactive. Dimesna concentrations in plasma greatly exceed those of mesna following both oral and intravenous dosing. Neither mesna nor dimesna is excreted in bile. Dimesna is reduced in the kidney by glutathione reductase to mesna, which is excreted into the urine, where it is active. Following both oral and intravenous dosing with mesna, 33% of the drug appears in the urine as dimesna.[4] Following oral administration of dimesna, cysteine–mesna disulphide has also been found in the urine.[14] Up to 20% of an oral dose and 32% of an intravenous dose are excreted unchanged in the urine.

Fig. 1 Dimesna

$$NaO_3S - CH_2 - CH_2 - S - S - CH_2 - CH_2 - SO_3Na$$

Pharmaceutics

Uromitexan (Boehringer Ingelheim, UK) is a sterile clear solution containing mesna 100 mg.ml^{-1}, for intravenous or oral use. It is available in 400 mg and 1.0 g vials. When taken orally, the contents of the vial are mixed with fruit juice to disguise the taste.

Ampoules should be protected from light and stored below 30°C. The drug is stable in sodium chloride 0.9% solutions (with or without ifosfamide) for at least 24 hours.

Therapeutic use

Indications

1. Prevention of the urinary tract toxicity caused by therapy with ifosfamide and cyclophosphamide
2. As a mucolytic agent.

Contraindications

None.

Mode of use

1. Prevention of urinary tract toxicity

Ifosfamide is very toxic to the urinary tract and mesna should always be used with it. It is important to start the mesna at the same time as, or before, ifosfamide. As its half life is short, mesna, when given intravenously, is usually given by infusion. The duration of a mesna infusion should be equal to the duration of the ifosfamide infusion plus the time taken for the urinary concentration of toxic metabolites to fall to safe levels. Because of the comparatively long half life of ifosfamide this should be for 8–12 hours after the end of the ifosfamide administration.[15] Intermittent intravenous bolus mesna every 4 hours has been associated with a nephrotoxicity incidence as high as 17%.[6,7] It has been suggested that bladder protection is satisfactory on this schedule due to retention of urine in the bladder, whereas renal tubules experience wide fluctuations in mesna concentration. The dose of mesna administered on these occasions was only 60% by weight that of ifosfamide so it is not certain that the intermittent administration was the cause of the renal damage.

It is now customary to give mesna in a dose 100% by weight that of ifosfamide and by intravenous infusion. Ifosfamide and mesna may be mixed in the same infusion fluid without interaction.

Mesna may also be administered orally. Taken at 0, 4 and 8 hours after an ifosfamide injection it provided good urothelial protection in a total dose 112% that of ifosfamide.[16] In conjunction with oral ifosfamide which has a bioavailability of 100%, mesna given in four divided doses over 12 hours provided good protection when the total dose was 100% that of ifosfamide.[17] Given the urinary bioavailability of mesna (see above), twice the intravenous dose ought theoretically to be given. This has not been the practice, however, and until there are reports of adverse effects with the current oral dosage schedule clinicians will be unwilling to increase the dose; the taste of

Mesna

mesna is unpleasant and although it can be disguised in strongly flavoured drinks (cola or orange juice) this can be a problem in nauseated patients.

Cyclophosphamide is considerably less urotoxic than ifosfamide at conventional dosage and mesna is not routinely given. For high doses of cyclophosphamide, or when radiotherapy to the bladder is also contemplated, the administration of mesna becomes important and the mode of usage is as for ifosfamide.

Long-term oral cyclophosphamide is occasionally given for 'benign' conditions such as lupus nephritis and Wegener's granulomatosis. There is a small risk of developing bladder tumours in these patients. Concomitant oral mesna administration might obviate this risk, as has been described in rodents.[18] No clinical studies have yet been reported.

2. As a mucolytic agent

Inhaled via a nebulizer using a 20% solution, mesna caused chronic bronchitics to produce larger volumes of sputum than when 0.9% saline was used as the inhalant.[19] Pulmonary function tests were not improved. It is uncertain whether the effect on sputum production was due to true mucolysis or to bronchorrhoea.

Children with cystic fibrosis have also been treated with inhaled mesna. They showed significant improvement in lung function compared to the use of isosmolar saline.[20]

Adverse reactions

As mesna is nearly always given in conjunction with cytotoxic chemotherapy, adverse effects of the combined treatment are usually attributed to the cytotoxic drugs. There has only been one study investigating the toxicity of mesna and in fact this did produce adverse effects at doses only just above those used clinically.

Potentially life-threatening effects

None attributable to mesna has been observed.

Acute overdosage

A patient who was given 14 g of mesna inadvertently (a high dose to receive in one day) experienced only a transient mild headache. There are no reports of true overdosage.

Severe or irreversible adverse effects

None has been observed.

Symptomatic adverse effects

Six male volunteers were given 60–70 mg.kg^{-1} mesna intravenously for four consecutive days. They experienced exhaustion, diarrhoea, abdominal pains, headache and pains in the limbs and joints. Tachycardia and transient hypertension were seen shortly after each injection.[21] These limited data suggest that mesna can contribute to the subjective toxicity of chemotherapy.

Oral mesna has an unpleasant taste. Inhaled mesna can produce an irritative cough and bronchospasm, retrosternal burning and, with prolonged usage, yellowing of the teeth.

Interference with clinical pathology tests

Mesna therapy gives a false positive test for ketone bodies in the urine.[22]

High risk groups

Neonates

The drug is unlikely to be used in neonates.

Breast milk. The indications for the use of this drug make it highly unlikely that a woman receiving it would be able to breastfeed.

Children

The drug may be used in children in appropriate doses.

Pregnant women

The use of cytotoxic drugs and thus mesna is contraindicated during pregnancy.

The elderly

Mesna may be used in the elderly.

Concurrent disease

Mesna is unlikely to produce toxic effects in the presence of moderate hepatic or renal impairment.

M

Clinical trials

1. Burkert H, Schnitker H, Fichtner E 1979 Prevention of urinary tract toxicity of oxazaphosphorines by a uroprotector. Munchen Medizinische Wochenschrift 121: 760–762
2. Scheef W, Soemer G 1980 The treatment of solid malignant tumours with Holoxan and Uromitexan. Contributions to Oncology 5: 21–24

These two studies describe the outcome of chemotherapy in 581 patients treated with the oxazaphosphorines cyclophosphamide, ifosfamide and trofosfamide in combination with mesna. The majority of patients received ifosfamide. The incidence of gross haematuria was only 1.5% and 0.5%, respectively, whilst microscopic haematuria occurred in 5% and 3% of cases.

3. Varini M, Monfardini S 1981 Oral sodium 2-mercaptoethane sulfonate (Mesna, Uromitexan) in ifosfamide therapy: preliminary report. Contributions to Oncology 5: 47–51

Patients treated with ifosfamide received prophylaxis to the urothelium with either diuresis and urinary alkalinization (the first 17 patients) or with mesna (the subsequent 67). Microscopic and macroscopic haematuria were reduced from 24% and 18% to 7% and 3% respectively.

Other trials

1. Scheef W, Klein H O, Brock H et al 1979 Controlled clinical studies with an antidote against the urotoxicity of oxazaphosphorines: preliminary results. Cancer Treatment Reports 63: 501–505
2. Hows J M, Mehta A, Ward L et al 1984 Comparison of mesna with forced diuresis to prevent cyclophosphamide induced haemorrhagic cystitis in marrow transplantation: A prospective randomized study. British Journal of Cancer 50: 753–756

References

1. Ormstad K, Orrenius S, Lastbom T et al 1983 Pharmacokinetics and metabolism of sodium 2-mercaptoethane sulfonate in the rat. Cancer Research 43: 333–338
2. Ormstad K, Uehara N 1982 Renal transport and disposition of Na-2-mercaptoethane sulfonate disulfide (dimema) in the rat. FEBS Letters 150: 354–357
3. Shaw I C, Graham M I, Jones M S 1986 The fate of (14C)-Mesna in the rat. Arzneimittel-Forschung/Drug Research 36: 487–489
4. James C A, Mant T G K, Rogers H J 1987 Pharmacokinetics of intravenous and oral sodium 2-mercapto ethane sulphonate (mesna) in normal subjects. British Journal of Clinical Pharmacology 23: 561–568
5. Jones M S, Murrell R D, Shaw I C 1985 Excretion of sodium 2-mercaptoethanesulphonate (mesna) in the urine of volunteers after oral dosing. European Journal of Cancer and Clinical Oncology 21: 553–555
6. Stuart-Harris R, Harper P G, Kaye S B, Wiltshaw E 1983 High dose ifosfamide by infusion with mesna in advanced soft tissue sarcoma. Cancer Treatment Reviews 10 (suppl A): 163–164
7. Sangster G, Kaye S B, Calman K C, Dalton J F 1984 Failure of 2-mercaptoethane sulphonate sodium (mesna) to protect against ifosfamide nephrotoxicity. European Journal of Cancer and Clinical Oncology 20: 435–436
8. Ellman G L 1959 Tissue sulphydryl groups. Archives of Biochemistry and Biophysics 82: 70–77
9. Sidau B, Shaw I C 1984 Determination of sodium 2-mercaptoethane-sulphonate by high-performance liquid chromatography using post-column reaction colorimetry or electrochemical detection. Journal of Chromatography 311: 234–256
10. James C A, Rogers H J 1986 Estimation of mesna and dimesna in plasma and urine by high performance liquid chromatography with electrochemical detection. Journal of Chromatography 382: 394–398
11. Brock N, Pohl J, Stekar J 1981 Studies on the urotoxicity of oxazaphosphorine cystostatics and its prevention. 2. Comparative study on the uroprotective efficacy of thiols and other sulfur compounds. European Journal of Cancer and Clinical Oncology 17: 1155–1163
12. Brock N, Hilgard P, Pohl J, Ormstad K, Orrenius S 1984 Pharmacokinetics and mechanism of action of detoxifying low-molecular weight thiols. Journal of Cancer Research and Clinical Oncology 108: 87–97
13. Burkert H, Lucker P W, Wetzelsburger N, Bruel H P 1984 Bioavailability of orally administered mesna. Arzneimittel-Forschung 34: 1597–1600
14. Shaw I C, Weeks M S 1987 Excretion of disodium bis-2-mercaptoethanesulfonate (dimesna) in the urine of volunteers after oral dosing. European Journal of Cancer and Clinical Oncology 23: 933–935
15. Hilgard P, Burkert H 1984 Sodium-2-mercaptoethanesulfonate (Mesna) and ifosfamide nephrotoxicity. European Journal of Cancer and Clinical Oncology 20: 1451–1452
16. Araujo C E, Tessler J 1983 Treatment of ifosfamide induced urothelial toxicity by oral administration of sodium 2-mercaptoethane sulfonate (Mesna) to patients with inoperable lung cancer. European Journal of Cancer and Clinical Oncology 19: 195–201
17. Cerny T, Lind M, Thatcher N, Swindell R, Sout R 1989 A simple out-patient treatment with oral ifosfamide and oral etoposide for patients with small cell lung cancer. British Journal of Cancer 60: 258–261
18. Habs M R, Schmahl D 1983 Prevention of urinary bladder tumours in cyclophosphamide-treated rats by additional medication with the uroprotectors sodium 2-mercaptoethane sulfonate (Mesna) and disodium 2,2′-dithio-bis-ethane sulfonate (dimesna). Cancer 51: 606–609
19. Steen S N, Ziment I, Freeman D, Thomas J S 1974 Evaluation of a new mucolytic drug. Clinical Pharmacology and Therapeutics 16: 58–62
20. Weller P H, Ingram D, Preece M A, Matthew D J 1980 Controlled trial of intermittent aerosol therapy with sodium 2-mercaptoethane sulphonate in cystic fibrosis. Thorax 35: 42–46
21. Lucker P W, Facharztliches Goutackten zur Ermittlung der Toleranzschwelle von Na-2-mercepto-ethensulfonet (MESNA, ASTA D 7093). External research report No. 780 070
22. Matthiessen W, Wundrchack W, Have Z 1980 False positive test results for ketone bodies in the urine due to mesna (uromitexan). Joint Symposium of Study Group for Oncology of German Cancer Society and Asta-Werke A G Dusseldorf pp 63–67

Mestranol

Mestranol is a synthetic oestrogen, usually present in combined oral contraceptive steroid preparations. It achieves its oestrogenic effects largely through conversion to ethinyloestradiol by the process of demethylation. Mestranol is thus a pro-drug.

Chemistry

Mestranol (found only in combination products)
$C_{21}H_{26}O_2$
3-Methoxy-19-nor-17α-pregna-1,3,5(10)-trien-20-yn-17β-ol

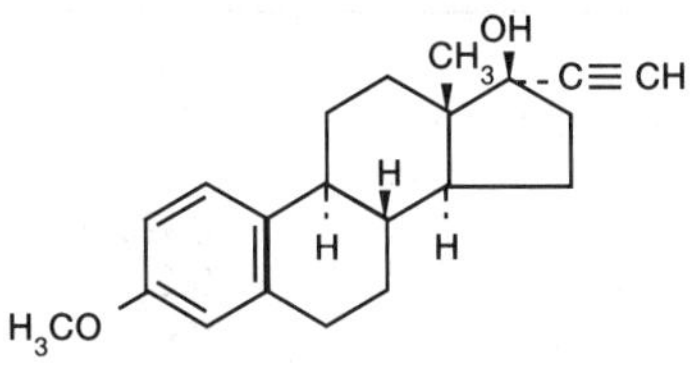

Molecular weight	310.4
pKa	—
Solubility	
in alcohol	1 in 44
in water	<1 in 40 000
Octanol/water partition coefficient	high

Mestranol is a white to creamy white, odourless crystalline powder. Its melting point is 146–154°C with a range of not more than 4°C. Mestranol is practically insoluble in water. It is soluble in 1 in 44 parts of ethyl alcohol, 1 in 23 parts of acetone and ether, and 1 in 12 parts of dioxan. Solutions should be protected from the light. Mestranol is chemically synthesized from oestrone.

Mestranol is found in a number of combination products together with a progestogen (Conovid, Enovid, Enavid, Menophase, Metrulen, Norinyl-1, Ortho-Novin 1/50, Orthonovum, Ovulen, Previson, C-Quens, Sequens).

Pharmacology

Mestranol is a potent synthetic oestrogen. However, it does not itself bind to the oestrogen receptor[1] and is demethylated in vivo to ethinyloestradiol which does bind to the oestrogen receptor. Mestranol is a weaker oestrogen than ethinyloestradiol. The methyl group on the 3 position renders the compound more lipid soluble than ethinyloestradiol.

Mestranol, through its active metabolite ethinyloestradiol, has oestrogenic effects on a variety of tissues, notably the reproductive tract, the breast, the liver and the brain. Mestranol produces proliferation of the vaginal mucosa followed by cornification and desquamation of the superficial layer. In the uterus it produces hyperaemia and oedema together with cell proliferation and hypertrophy of the endometrium. Mestranol also stimulates cervical secretion. In the breast, mestranol has a number of effects depending on the species.[2] In the rat or cat it produces mainly duct growth,[2] while in other species it also causes growth of the lobule-alveolar system. Oestrogens, by a feedback mechanism, suppress pituitary FSH secretion, probably via the hypothalamus. Mestranol, like other oestrogens, increases transcortin concentrations.[3] It increases glucose utilization and causes salt and water retention. Oestrogens affect lipid metabolism in most animal species. In general a rise in high density lipoprotein and a fall in low density lipoprotein is seen. Oestrogens induce specific proteins; in humans this particularly affects sex hormone binding globulin.

Toxicology

Long-term continuous administration of oestrogens to some animal species increases the frequency of carcinoma of the breast, cervix, vagina and liver, although the risk may be less for mestranol than for ethinyloestradiol. Administration of estrogens to mice produces a squamous cell carcinoma rather than an adenocarcinoma. In an 80-week study in mice, ethinyloestradiol slightly increased the incidence of malignant tumours of the uterine fundus and cervix, while mestranol caused no such change.[4] In beagle dogs, mestranol at a dosage of 0.05 $mg.kg^{-1}$ per day for 77 months caused no increase in mammary nodules compared with control dogs.[5] Mestranol given in a dose of 0.1 $mg.kg^{-1}$ daily to female rhesus monkeys in cyclical fashion produced a dose-dependent fall in haemoglobin and haematocrit but such changes have not been reported in other animal species or in humans.[5]

Clinical pharmacology

Mestranol reduces levels of gonadotrophin-releasing factors in the hypothalamus, and this reduces production of LH and FSH by the anterior pituitary gland, resulting in failure of ovarian follicle development, suppression of ovulation and reduction of endogenous ovarian steroid production. Daily doses of 50 µg or more inhibit ovulation. The synthetic oestrogen may stimulate prolactin secretion. There is no clear dose–response relationship for mestranol. There were originally two dose levels used, 80 µg and 50 µg per day, but nowadays the 80 µg preparation is rarely available because of increased toxicity compared to the 50 µg dose.

Oestrogens cause an increase in plasma volume, cardiac output and stroke volume, together with a decrease in peripheral resistance involving arteriolar dilation and increased venous distensibility. The resultant effect may be a slight rise in mean arterial blood pressure. Both systolic and diastolic blood pressure may rise and a change in blood pressure from 120/80 to 150/90 occurs in perhaps 1% of women on the combined oral contraceptive steroid. In rare cases a sustained rise in blood pressure to essential hypertension levels may occur. The rise in blood pressure recorded in women taking combined oral contraceptive steroids seems to be due to a combination of both steroids, rather than to either steroid on its own.[6] A significant rise in blood pressure is unusual with the standard doses of mestranol (50–80 µg daily).

There are considerable discrepancies in the literature on the effects of ethinyloestradiol on factors in the coagulation system. The amounts of the compound formerly available in combined oral contraceptives, 50–100 µg daily for weeks and months, may produce small increases in factors VII, VIII and IX and X, a small decrease in antithrombin III, increased noradrenaline-induced platelet aggregation and reduced fibrinolytic activity with an overall increase in tendency to thrombosis which may be manifested in a very few women.

Women taking mestranol 50–80 µg daily in assocation with a progestagen, tend to have higher plasma glucose and plasma insulin levels and a few, particularly gestational diabetics, develop abnormal glucose tolerance, which may not always revert to normal after the drugs have been taken for years.

Ethinyloestradiol tends to cause increased plasma triglyceride, free fatty acid and lipoprotein levels. Whether or not these effects are of any significance in healthy women taking low doses in oral contraceptives is doubtful. It is true that women over 40 who are obese, hypercholesterolaemic, have hypertension and smoke and who take oral contraceptives with 50–100 µg ethinyloestradiol a day have an increased risk of myocardial infarction[8] and stroke, but the exact cause of this is unclear. Oestrogens tend to raise the high density lipoprotein (HDL) and lower the low density lipoproteins (LDL). A rise of 5–10% in HDL and a fall of a similar magnitude in LDL cholesterol is quite common.[9]

Mestranol, via its metabolite, stimulates the hepatic synthesis of plasma sex hormone-binding globulin, cortisol-binding globulin, ceruloplasmin and some other proteins; it may inhibit haptoglobulin, orosomucoid and albumin synthesis. Ethinyloestradiol, 100 µg daily in oral contraceptives, causes increased bromsulphthalein retention in 10–15% of women. The changes are of no significance in healthy women, but the drug may have an adverse effect on hepatic function in women with impaired liver function. Exogenous oestrogen can, rarely, cause cholestatic jaundice in susceptible women, particularly those who have had this condition in pregnancy.

Oestrogens cause a degree of salt and water retention; they cause increases in circulating renin, plasma renin substrate, angiotensin and aldosterone excretion and this may be the mechanism for the oedema. Large doses of oestrogen cause a reduction in the ascorbic levels in plasma and blood vessels. Plasma folate may be decreased. Women taking oral contraceptives have an increased incidence of urinary tract infections but the mechanism is not clear.

Total plasma cortisol is slightly increased in patients taking ethinyloestradiol, 50 μg daily, and with 100 μg daily, plasma unbound cortisol is increased. Increases in the binding proteins, particularly thyroid-binding globulin, lead to raised plasma protein bound iodine levels and a decrease in red cell tri-iodothyronine uptake, but there is probably no change in plasma free thyroxine or in thyroid function.

Mestranol, in common with other oestrogens, will precipitate epiphyseal closure in the long bones in adolescents, and thereby limit stature. The drug will prevent osteoporosis in postmenopausal women.

Mestranol will relieve vasomotor symptoms, atrophic vaginitis and atrophic cystisis in postmenopausal women. On a longer-term basis it is claimed that it improves skin turgor and condition, relieves postmenopausal depression, improves libido and causes a sense of well-being in some women. It will cure kraurosis vulvae in older women.

Pharmacokinetics

There are no assays developed for mestranol as such. All available kinetic data have been based either on radioactive studies or on the radioimmunoassay of ethinyloestradiol (the major metabolite and active principle of mestranol) which has a sensitivity of 5 $ng.l^{-1}$. Anti-sera that have been developed against mestranol cross-react 100% with ethinyloestradiol.[10]

Mestranol is rapidly absorbed and extensively demethylated to ethinyloestradiol. Bolt and Bolt[11] have calculated that 54% of mestranol is converted to ethinyloestradiol while other authorities regard mestranol as being equipotent to ethinyloestradiol.[12] However, the general view is that mestranol is somewhat less potent as an oestrogen than ethinyloestradiol. After an oral dose of mestranol, plasma concentrations of ethinyloestradiol are very similar to those found after giving ethinyloestradiol itself, although the peak concentration (200–300 $ng.l^{-1}$) is slightly lower following mestranol.[13] The main compound circulating in plasma, as it is following ethinyloestradiol, is ethinyloestradiol 3-sulphate.[14] In a study of 89 women in various centres around the world given 50–100 μg doses of mestranol, the unchanged drug could just be detected in plasma 24 hours later but the ratio of mestranol to ethinyloestradiol was 0.24:1.[15] The ratio of mestranol to ethinyloestradiol sulphate was 1:3.4.[14] The absolute bioavailability of mestranol is unknown but that of ethinyloestradiol is on average 45% due to presystemic metabolism in the gut wall (largely sulphation).[16] Ethinyloestradiol in plasma is extensively bound to albumin with no variation in the binding due to the menstrual cycle. Free concentrations of unchanged ethinyloestradiol are 2.05 ± 0.02% of the total concentrations.[17]

The metabolic clearance rate of mestranol is between 1250[18] and 1750[14] litres per day. The plasma pharmacokinetics of ethinyloestradiol are best described by a two-compartment open model.[16] The half life of the α phase is 50–200 minutes and of the β phase is 6–20 hours. The plasma clearance of ethinyloestradiol is 375 ± 30 $ml.h^{-1}.kg^{-1}$ and the apparent volume of distribution is 3.8 ± 0.8 $l.kg^{-1}$.

Mestranol is excreted in breast milk only in very small amounts. After an oral dose of ^{14}C mestranol was given to four women only 0.0002–0.013% of the dose was excreted in the breast milk over a 4-day period. The authors calculated that a breast-fed infant would receive a daily dose equivalent to only 30–60 ng of mestranol.[19]

Ethinyloestradiol is excreted in the bile as conjugates and undergoes enterohepatic recirculation, though the importance of this to the overall kinetics is not clear.[16] Although mestranol is cleared from the body more rapidly than ethinyloestradiol, there is some evidence that the half life of the total metabolites of mestranol is longer, at 37–65 hours, than that of ethinyloestradiol itself,[20] no doubt due to conjugates such as ethinyloestradiol sulphate.

The rate of elimination of ethinyloestradiol is increased by enzyme-inducing agents such as rifampicin and anticonvulsants.

Ethinyloestradiol is extensively metabolized, largely in the gastrointestinal mucosa and to a lesser extent in the liver. Very little is excreted unchanged. The metabolites are excreted in both urine and bile.

Oral absorption	>90%
Presystemic metabolism	55%
Plasma half life	
range	6–20 h
Volume of distribution	3.8 ± 0.8 $l.kg^{-1}$
Plasma protein binding	98%

Concentration–effect relationship

Plasma concentrations of ethinyloestradiol at steady state vary from 6 to 190 $ng.l^{-1}$ after daily doses of 30–50 μg.[16] There are no similar data for mestranol but the values are unlikely to be very different. There is no evidence for a 'therapeutic range' of plasma concentration of ethinyloestradiol.[16]

Metabolism

Mestranol is initially metabolized by demethylation to ethinyloestradiol.[11] The site of demethylation is probably the liver. Mestranol is not extensively sulphated during first-pass metabolism in the gut wall (cf. ethinyloestradiol) because the methyl group on position 3 protects the molecule from sulphation. Once demethylation has taken place, sulphation on position 3 then occurs to give ethinyloestradiol sulphate. The main circulating metabolite is ethinyloestradiol sulphate[14] which is formed primarily by the gastrointestinal mucosa. Studies of the metabolism of mestranol using radiolabelled drug have shown that 9–36% of the drug is excreted in the urine over a 5-day period, almost entirely as conjugates.[19,21] If position 2 in the A ring is tritiated, between 14 and 45% of the radioactivity is released into body water, presumably due to hydroxylation of the 2 position.[22] If the 4 position is tritiated, less than 5% of the radioactivity is released into body water.[23] Once ethinyloestradiol or its sulphate conjugate is formed, the routes of metabolism are exactly as for ethinyloestradiol.

Fig. 1 Metabolism of mestranol

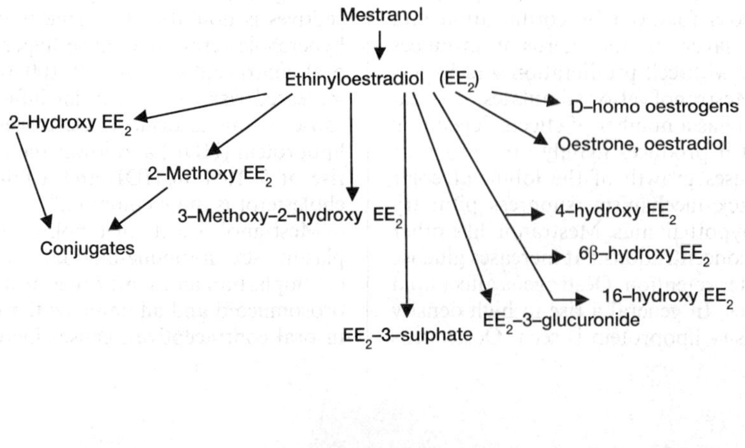

The main metabolite of ethinyloestradiol is 2-hydroxy-ethinyloestradiol, which can be directly conjugated or converted to the 2-methoxy form or the combined 2-hydroxy-3-methoxy metabolite. The catechol metabolite — 2-hydroxy-ethinyloestradiol — may also be converted in vitro to a quinone which is highly reactive and binds covalently to liver macromolecules.[24] Ethinyloestradiol is also hydroxylated at the 4, 6α and 16β positions and these are chiefly excreted as conjugates with glucuronic acid.[25] De-ethinylation of ethinyloestradiol may occur to form oestrone and oestradiol, suggesting minimal metabolism at the 4 position.[23] This is a minor pathway of metabolism in man and only 1–2% of a dose is metabolized in this way. The most unusual metabolic route for ethinyloestradiol is D-homo annulation. This step involves oxidation at the ethinyl triple bond, followed by rearrangement (ring D enlargement) and oxidative elimination of the ϕ-situated carbon atom. Ethinyloestradiol is itself conjugated directly with glucuronic acid and sulphate and these conjugates are excreted in bile. An enterohepatic circulation of ethinyloestradiol is formed when these conjugates are broken down by bacteria in the colon to liberate unchanged ethinyloestradiol which can then be reabsorbed.

Pharmaceutics

Mestranol is now only available in most countries combined with progestogen.

1. Norinyl-1 (Syntex, UK/USA) combines mestranol (50 µg) with 1 mg norethisterone in a white tablet marked with the manufacturer's name.
2. Orthonovin 1/50 (Ortho, UK) and Ortho Novum 1/50 (Ortho, USA) is an equivalent combination in a white tablet marked 'C/150' on both sides.
3. Ovulen-2 (Searle, USA) contains ethynodiol diacetate 1 mg and mestranol 0.1 mg.

For endometriosis, mestranol is available as a combination pack with variable doses of norethisterone as Menophase (Syntex, UK), and as Enovid (Searle, USA), a range of mestranol and norethynodiol combinations.

Therapeutic use

Indications

1. With progestagen for oral contraception
2. With progestagen for menopausal symptoms
3. With progestagen for disorders of menstruation.

Contraindications

1. Pregnancy
2. Undiagnosed abnormal bleeding from the genital tract
3. Untreated endometriosis
4. History of chloasma, cholestatic jaundice or herpes gestationis, in pregnancy or whilst on oestrogen treatment
5. Thrombophlebitis or thrombo-embolic disorders, past or current
6. Cerebrovascular or coronary artery disease
7. Suspected or known oestrogen-dependent malignant disease
8. Impaired liver function
9. Benign or malignant liver tumour
10. The known contraindications to oral contraceptives.

Relative contraindications

1. Sickle cell anaemia
2. Dubin Johnson/Rotor syndromes
3. Porphyria
4. Hypertension
5. Raynaud's disease
6. Migraine
7. Diabetes mellitus
8. Hyperlipidaemia
9. Gall stones
10. Epilepsy
11. Asthma
12. Chronic renal disease
13. Severe depression
14. Varicose veins
15. Cigarette smoking
16. Age over 30.

Mode of use

Mestranol is an orally effective oestrogen of high potency. To produce effects such as suppression of ovulation in women of reproductive age 50–80 µg are needed daily. Most formulations use 50 µg mestranol in combination with progestogen. For the relief of menopausal symptoms lower doses of mestranol are used, usually in combination with progestogen.

Indications

1. With progestagen for oral contraception

Mestranol is used in a dose of 50 µg to suppress ovulation, in combination with a progestogen to reinforce the contraceptive action and produce an endometrium that will shed when the course of pills is complete.

The combined preparations may be started on either day 5 or day 1 of the menstrual cycle and taken for 20 or 21 days, initiating the next cycle on the 5th day of withdrawal bleeding or 7 days after the last pill of the preceding cycle. Barrier contraception may be used during the first 14 days to reduce the small risk of failure in the first cycle. A day 1 start is now usual.

If, after regular menstrual withdrawal bleeding, menstruation fails to occur, barrier contraception may be used for that cycle to avoid any risk of an unsuspected pregnancy being exposed to exogenous hormones; and the contraceptive pill restarted after the next menstrual period. If a pill is forgotten it should be taken as soon as possible within 24 hours even if two taken together. If two tablets missed take a tablet as soon as possible to recommence medication and barrier contraception should be used in addition for the next 14 days. It is becoming clear that a missed pill is most likely to cause failure of contraception if it extends the 7-day-pill free period. Thus pills omitted on days 1 or 2 are the most likely to cause contraceptive failure.

When changing to another combined oral contraceptive, the first new pill should be started the day after the last of the previous pills, without any break.

2. With progestagen for menopausal symptoms

Oestrogen alone is no longer used for women in whom menstruation has not ceased. After the menopause, ethinyloestradiol, 10–30 µg daily, for three weeks out of four may be used for one or two cycles to relieve vasomotor symptoms and atrophic vaginitis or cystitis, but more prolonged use conveys a risk of causing endometrial hyperplasia and, rarely, endometrial carcinoma. The use of combined treatment of oestrogen with progestagen very much reduces this risk, and is preferable. The patient should be warned that she may have withdrawal bleeding but if she develops prolonged, heavy or intermenstrual bleeding, diagnostic endometrial sampling or formal curettage must be undertaken. Women who have had a hysterectomy may be treated safely with ethinyloestradiol, 10–30 µg daily, continuously for years if necessary. Oestrogen treatment for menopausal symptoms is known not to cause recurrence in women who have been treated successfully for intra-epithelial carcinoma of the cervix and is not known to be harmful in women who have had invasive carcinoma of the cervix fully treated. It is uncommon for oestrogen treatment to have any ill effect in women who have had endometriosis and are postmenopausal or have had a hysterectomy, even if the ovaries have been conserved.

Mestranol is available as a combination pack for the treatment of menopausal symptoms (Menophase).

3. With progestagen, for disorders of menstruation

A combination may be employed to suppress ovulation in the treatment of spasmodic dysmenorrhoea, or to regulate the menstrual cycle with dysfunctional uterine bleeding, when organic pathology has been excluded. Mestranol 50 µg daily, is given cyclically from days 5 to 25 of each cycle, and supplemented with a progestogen such as norethisterone throughout the cycle. The object of the oestrogen is to develop a proliferative endometrium and suppress ovulation, that of the progestogen is to develop a secretory change in the endometrium and, if given for 21 days, to assist in suppressing ovulation.

One of the combination contraceptive preparations containing mestranol may be used for this purpose.

Contraindications

1. Pregnancy
There are no indications for the use of mestranol during pregnancy. There are no known ill effects on the human fetus, but data are very limited.

2. Undiagnosed abnormal bleeding from the genital tract
There are risks that abnormal bleeding will be suppressed, diagnosis will be confused or endometrial hyperplasia or carcinoma exacerbated.

3. Untreated endometriosis
This is likely to be activated or exacerbated. The risk of this happening in postmenopausal women or those who have had a hysterectomy is small.

4. History of chloasma, cholestatic jaundice or herpes gestationis
Oestrogen treatment may precipitate recurrence.

5. Thrombophlebitis or thrombo-embolic disorders
With all oestrogens there is a slight hazard of increased tendency to coagulation. Mestranol has the same effect in this respect as equipotent doses of other oestrogens. It should be discontinued a month before major surgery. The cause of the clotting is probably the decrease in antithrombin III activity which may be quite marked in a few women.

6. Cerebrovascular or coronary artery disease
Similar remarks apply, particularly in women over 40.

7. Suspected or known oestrogen-dependent malignant disease
Although determination of the presence or absence of oestrogen receptors is being used in the attempt to ascertain sensitivity of tumours of the breast, uterus and ovaries to oestrogen, this can still only really be determined by exposing the patient to oestrogen, or by observing the response to ovarian ablation. Oestrogen risks of cerebrovascular and cardiovascular disease increase markedly[8] and it is best to use a non-oestrogen containing preparation.

Adverse reactions

Potentially life-threatening effects
Prolonged and particularly continuous use of synthetic oestrogens, without cyclical progestogens, may lead to endometrial hyperplasia and, rarely, to endometrial carcinoma.

Low incidences of the following conditions have been associated with the use of oral contraceptives containing ethinyloestradiol and a progestogen: venous thrombosis, pulmonary embolism, cerebral thrombosis, coronary thrombosis, hypertension, gall bladder disease, liver tumours, carcinoma of the breast and carcinoma of the cervix.

There has been much discussion about the potential carcinogenicity of the combined contraceptive steroid preparations. There is a small increased risk of developing carcinoma of the cervix with a risk ratio of about 1.6–2.0. However, this may be due to an indirect effect rather than a direct effect of the preparation. Induction of carcinoma of the breast is not proven at present and at least half of the long-term studies have shown no increased risk of developing breast carcinoma. To balance this, it should be remembered that women who take the combined contraceptive steroid preparations are relatively protected from developing a carcinoma of the ovary and uterine body.

Use of any drug is a balance of benefits against risk and this is especially true for the contraceptive steroids. Use of these preparations does convey benefits other than contraception and improvement of menstrual problems. Benign breast disease[6] is less common, as is pelvic inflammatory disease, peptic ulcer disease and hypothyroidism. In addition, women with rheumatoid arthritis generally have less severe disease while taking these steroid preparations.

Acute overdosage
No serious ill-effects have been reported. An overdose may cause nausea and vomiting, and subsequently withdrawal bleeding from the uterus in females.

Severe or irreversible adverse effects
It has been suggested that a predisposition to cerebrovascular, coronary artery and thromboembolic disorders, and breast cancer, may persist after cessation of treatment with oral contraceptives containing or producing ethinyloestradiol, but the evidence is not widely accepted. Chloasma developing in patients taking oral contraceptives may sometimes persist after they are discontinued; as may impairment of glucose tolerance.

Symptomatic adverse effects
Nausea and sometimes vomiting, and episodes of intermenstrual bleeding or spotting and other disturbances of the menstrual cycle, are common initially; they tend to resolve with continuing use. Sometimes fluid retention with oedema and breast discomfort occur. Weight gain may be due to fluid retention or to increased appetite. There may be changes in corneal curvature leading to intolerance of contact lenses. Cervical ectropion may develop or fail to resolve, and there may be an increased tendency to vaginal candidiasis. Pre-existing uterine fibromyomata may increase in size and become symptomatic. If mental depression occurs, it may sometimes be relieved with pyridoxine supplements. If the patient develops migraine, there may be an increased risk of the rare complication of cerebral thrombosis.

The following disorders are recorded as having occurred in patients taking ethinyloestradiol: erythema multiforme, erythema nodosum, haemorrhagic skin eruptions, loss of scalp hair, hirsuitism, sickle cell crises, exacerbation of symptoms of porphyria, dizziness, chorea, and increased or decreased libido.

Other effects
These have been detailed in the section on Clinical pharmacology. The most important clinically are the minor effects on the coagulation system, on liver function and on glucose tolerance, which may be of significance in patients with a predisposition to thrombosis or having a major surgical operation, patients with impaired liver function or those who are potential diabetics, respectively.

Interference with clinical pathology tests
Ethinyloestradiol stimulates hepatic protein synthesis, particularly the globulin carrier proteins, and thus increase the plasma level of a number of constituents — cortisol, thyroxine, vitamin A, iron, copper and cyanocobalamin. The previously described changes in glucose tolerance, bromsulphthalein retention, plasma lipids, coagulation factors and the renin–angiotensin system must be taken into account.

In the premenopausal woman ovulation is inhibited, with abolition of the midcycle peak and reduction in ovarian hormone secretion. Gonadotrophin levels and response to metapyrone are reduced; pregnanediol excretion is reduced.

Histopathologists need to be aware of mestranol treatment to permit interpretation of endometrial biopsies and uterine curettings.

High risk groups

Neonates
There is no indication for giving mestranol to neonates.

Breast milk. Ethinyloestradiol is no longer used to suppress lactation as the large doses required convey a small risk of thrombosis and pulmonary embolism. With the doses in oestrogen–progestogen oral contraceptives it is doubtful if lactation is affected, but with women to whom breast-feeding is important, alternative contraception is usually advised. The amounts of ethinyloestradiol reaching the baby in milk are minutely small in women taking mestranol-containing preparations.[19]

Children
The drug is not used in children.

Pregnant women
There is no indication for use; there is no evidence that mestranol affects the fetus adversely but data are sparse. There is a very low incidence, less than 1 in 1000, of congenital abnormalities, including limb reduction defects and vertebral, anal, cardiovascular, tracheal, oesophageal and renal anomalies, mainly affecting male fetuses, in the babies of women who continue to take oral contraceptives in the first trimester of pregnancy. The causative association is not proven.

The elderly
No special precautions are necessary other than those already detailed.

Drug interactions

Potentially hazardous interactions

Alcohol. Patients indulging in excess alcohol may forget to take their oral contraceptive pills.

Mestranol

Smoking. Women over 40 who smoke cigarettes heavily are at increased risk of myocardial infarction if they take preparations containing 50 μg mestranol a day.

Rifampicin. This drug induces the formation of hepatic microsomal enzymes that metabolize many drugs. Mestranol is metabolized in the liver and rifampicin undoubtedly increases the rate of disappearance of this drug from the plasma.[26] Unwanted pregnancies have occurred in women on oral contraceptives given rifampicin, and they should not rely on an oestrogen–progestagen oral contraceptive.

Anticonvulsants. Phenobarbitone, carbamazepine and phenytoin have all been shown to reduce plasma levels of ethinyloestradiol, and intermenstrual bleeding and unwanted pregnancies have resulted when epileptic women used oral contraceptives.[27] Such women should be advised of the risk, and in general control of contraception can be obtained by increasing the dose to overcome the enzyme-inducing effect of the anticonvulsant. Thus two tablets of a mestranol-containing preparation can be used daily, although more flexibility in dose can be obtained by using an ethinyloestradiol-containing preparation.

Antibiotics. Reports of intermenstrual bleeding and unwanted pregnancy in women taking oral contraceptives, during the administration of ampicillin, tetracycline, sulphonamides or chloramphenicol, have been recorded. The sparsity of such reports suggests that, at most, a very few women may be affected by an interaction. Formal trials have failed to demonstrate such an interaction in women taking contraceptive steroids.[28] Nevertheless, this interaction may occur occasionally in women who depend upon their enterohepatic circulation to maintain plasma concentrations of ethinyloestradiol. Thus alternative contraceptive precautions should be used if ampicillin or similar broad spectrum antibiotics are prescribed. The antibiotic co-trimoxazole does not reduce the efficacy of contraceptive steroids and may even enhance it.[29]

Vitamin C. Large doses of vitamin C compete for sulphate in the gut wall and thus enhance the bioavailability of ethinyloestradiol.[30] Whether this would be true for mestranol is not known but it would be wise to avoid taking large doses of ascorbic acid at the same time as the mestranol-containing preparation.

Other drugs. A number of other interactions are described between oestrogen-containing contraceptive preparations and other drugs.[31] Thus they may diminish the efficacy of oral anticoagulants such as warfarin but it would be rare for a patient to be taking both drugs. Patients taking oestrogen-containing preparations may be relatively resistant to the antidepressant effects of drugs such as imipramine. Because oestrogen-containing preparations may increase blood pressure they may impair the response to antihypertensive drugs, but it would again be rare for a patient to need both types of drug.

Potentially useful interactions

Mestranol is used in combination with a progestagen in oral contraceptive preparations.

Major outcome trials

There are no recent outcome trials concerning the pharmacodynamics or pharmacokinetics of mestranol-containing preparations. The reader is thus referred below to two recent books on the subject.

General review articles

Guillebaud J 1984 The pill. Oxford University Press, Oxford, 278 pp

Guillebaud J 1985 Contraception — your questions answered. Pitman Publishing Ltd, London, 310 pp

References

1. Korenman S G 1969 Comparative binding affinity of estrogens and its relation to estrogenic potency. Steroids 13: 163–177
2. Silver M 1953 Quantitative analysis of role of oestrogen in mammary development in rat. Journal of Endocrinology 10: 17–34
3. Doe R P, Mellinger G T, Swain W R, Seal U S 1967 Estrogen dosage effects on serum proteins: a longitudinal study. Journal of Clinical Endocrinology and Metabolism 27: 1081–1086
4. Committee on Safety of Medicines 1972 Carcinogenicity tests of oral contraceptives (a report). Her Majesty's Stationery Office. London
5. Geil R G, Lamar J K 1977 FDA studies of estrogen, progestogens and estrogen/progestogen combinations in the dog and monkey. Journal of Toxicology and Environmental Health 3: 179–193
6. Royal College of General Practitioners Oral Contraception Study 1977 Effect on hypertension and benign breast disease of progestagen component in combined oral contraceptives. Lancet 1: 624–628
7. Posner N A, Silverstone F A, Tobin E H 1975 Changes in carbohydrate tolerance during long term oral contraception. American Journal of Obstetrics and Gynecology 123: 119–126
8. Royal College of General Practitioners Oral Contraception Study 1981 Further analyses of mortality in oral contraceptive users. Lancet 1: 541–546
9. Demacker P N M, Schode R W B, Stalenhoef A F H, Stuyt P M J, Van't Laar A 1982 Influence of contraceptive pill and menstrual cycle on serum lipids and high density lipoprotein cholesterol concentrations. British Medical Journal 284: 1213–1216
10. Kundu N, Keenan S, Slaunwhite W R 1977 Production of anti sera against contraceptive steroids. Steroids 30: 85–98
11. Bolt H M, Bolt W H 1974 Pharmacokinetics of mestranol in man in relation to its oestrogenic activity. European Journal of Clinical Pharmacology 7: 295–305
12. Goldzieher J W, de la Pena A, Chenault C B, Wouterz T B 1975 Comparative studies of ethinylestrogens used in oral contraceptives. II Anti-ovulatory potency. American Journal of Obstetrics and Gynecology 122: 619–624
13. de la Pena A, Chenault C B, Goldzieher J 1975 Radioimmunoassay of unconjugated plasma ethynylestradiol in women given a single dose of ethynylestradiol or mestranol. Steroids 25: 773–780
14. Bird C E, Clark A F 1973 Metabolic clearance rates and metabolism of mestranol and ethynylestradiol in normal young women. Journal of Clinical Endocrinology and Metabolism 36: 296–302
15. Goldzieher J W, Dozier T S, de la Pena A et al 1980 Plasma levels and pharmacokinetics of ethynylestrogens in various populations II mestranol. Contraception 21: 17–27
16. Orme M, Back D, Breckenridge A 1983 Clinical pharmacokinetics of oral contraceptive steroids. Clinical Pharmacokinetics 8: 95–136
17. Orme M L'E 1982 Clinical pharmacology of oral contraceptive steroids. British Journal of Clinical Pharmacology 14: 31–42
18. Mills T M, Lin T J, Hernandez-Ayup S, Greenblatt R B, Ellegood Jo, Mahesh V B 1974 The metabolic clearance rate and urinary excretion of oral contraceptive drugs. II mestranol. American Journal of Obstetrics and Gynecology 120: 773–778
19. Wijmenga H G, Molen Van der H J 1969 Studies with 4-^{14}C mestranol in lactating women. Acta Endocrinologica 61: 665–667
20. Mills T M, Lin T J, Braselton W E, Ellegood J O, Mahesh V B 1976 Metabolism of oral contraceptive drugs. The formation and disappearance of metabolites of norethindrone and mestranol after intravenous and oral administration. American Journal of Obstetrics and Gynecology 126: 987–992
21. Kulkarni B D, Goldzieher J W 1970 Urinary excretion pattern and fractionation of radioactivity after injection of 4-^{14}C mestranol in women. Contraception 1: 131–136
22. Williams J G, Williams K I H 1975 Metabolism of 2-^{3}H- and 4-^{14}C-17α-ethynylestradiol-3-methyl ether (mestranol) by women. Steroids 26: 707–720
23. Williams J G, Longcope C, Williams K I H 1975 Metabolism of 4-^{3}H and 4-^{14}C-17α-ethynylestradiol-3-methyl ether (mestranol) by women. Steroids 25: 343–354
24. Purba H, Maggs J L, Orme M L'E, Back D J, Park B K 1987 The metabolism of 17α ethinyloestradiol by human liver microsomes in formation of catechol and chemically reactive metabolites. British Journal of Clinical Pharmacology 23: 447–453
25. Helton E D, Williams M C, Goldzieher J W 1976 Human urinary and liver conjugates of 17α ethinyloestradiol. Steroids 27: 851–867
26. Back D J, Breckenridge A M, Crawford F E et al 1980 The effect of rifampicin on the pharmacokinetics of ethinyloestradiol in women. Contraception 21: 135–143
27. Coulam C B, Annegers J F 1979 Do anticonvulsants reduce the efficacy of oral contraceptives. Epilepsia 20: 519–526
28. Back D J, Breckenridge A M, MacIver M et al 1982 The effects of ampicillin on oral contraceptive steroids in women. British Journal of Clinical Pharmacology 14: 43–48
29. Grimmer M, Allen W L, Back D J, Breckenridge A M, Orme M L'E, Tjia J 1983 The effect of cotrimoxazole on oral contraceptive steroids in women. Contraception 28: 53–59
30. Back D J, Breckenridge A M, MacIver M, Orme M L'E, Purba H, Rowe P H 1981 The interaction of ethinyloestradiol with ascorbic acid in man. British Medical Journal 282: 1516
31. Breckenridge A M, Back D J, Orme M 1979 Interactions between oral contraceptives and other drugs. Pharmacology and Therapeutics 7: 617–626

Metaraminol (bitartrate)

Metaraminol is a pressor drug used in certain hypotensive states.

Chemistry

Metaraminol bitartrate (Aramine, Araminium, Icoral B, Pressonex, Pressorol)
$C_9H_{13}NO_2.C_4H_6O_6$
(−)-2-Amino-1-(3-hydroxyphenyl)pronan-1-ol hydrogen (+)-tartrate

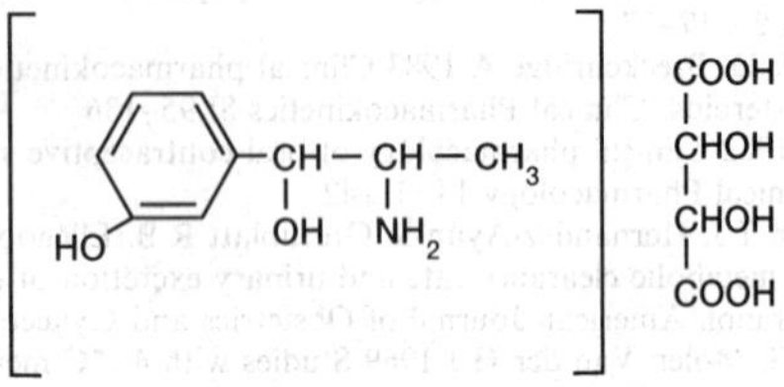

Molecular weight	317.2
pKa	
Solubility	—
in alcohol	slightly soluble
in water	freely soluble
Octanol/water partition coefficient	

Metaraminol bitartrate is a white, almost odourless crystalline powder with a bitter taste. The pH of a 1% aqueous solution is 3.5.

Pharmacology

Metaraminol is a potent sympathomimetic amine[1] which has agonist actions on both β- and α-adrenoceptors. Its chief effect, however, is agonist activity at α_1-receptors. This is achieved by direct action, as well as by indirect action through the release of noradrenaline. It is, in general, less potent than noradrenaline. Metaraminol produces a dose-dependent positive inotropic effect on the heart and has a marked peripheral vasoconstrictor effect.[2] It does not cause CNS stimulation.

Toxicology

Side effects and manifestations of toxicity are an exaggeration of the fundamental pharmacological properties of the drug. The acute toxicity (LD_{50}) of metaraminol administered intravenously in mice is obtained at a dose of about 39 $mg.kg^{-1}$. The oral LD_{50} in the rat and mouse is 240 $mg.kg^{-1}$ and 99 $mg.kg^{-1}$ respectively.

Clinical pharmacology

Due to its α and β stimulating properties, metaraminol exhibits a dose-related peripheral vasoconstrictor effect and an associated positive inotropic effect, both of which account for an elevation in blood pressure both systolic and diastolic. The pressor effect of metaraminol begins 1–2 minutes after intravenous injection, about 10 min after intramuscular administration, and 5–20 min after subcutaneous injection[3] and lasts about 20 min to 1 h.

The duration of the elevation in blood pressure varies from subject to subject. However, following subcutaneous and intramuscular injection a significant pressor effect persists for an average of 30 minutes. As regards the duration of action after a single dose injection, metaraminol exerts its effects two to three times longer than noradrenaline and phenylephrine.

Doses required to elevate blood pressure in adults range from 2 to 10 mg, administered either subcutaneously or intramuscularly, mainly depending on the condition of the patient.

Metaraminol usually causes a reflex bradycardia and thus in normotensive subjects cardiac output is unchanged. Cardiac output may be increased significantly in patients in shock and with hypotension, or whose reflex bradycardia is prevented by the use of atropine. Metaraminol decreases cerebral and renal blood flow. It causes an increase in pulmonary arterial pressure even when cardiac output is reduced.

Pharmacokinetics

Very few data exist on the pharmacokinetics and metabolism of metaraminol. From clinical studies it appears that the apparent half life of metaraminol is about two to three times longer than the half life of phenylephrine.

Monoamine oxidase has no effect on the metabolism of metaraminol.

Concentration–effect relationship

There are no data on this topic.

Metabolism

Nothing is known about the metabolism of metaraminol.

Pharmaceutics

Metaraminol bitartrate is available only in parenteral form. Metaraminol bitartrate injection (Aramine; MSD, UK/USA) is a sterile solution. Each 1 ml ampoule contains the equivalent of 10 mg of metaraminol. It is a clear isotonic solution containing the following preservatives: methylparaben, propylparaben and sodium bisulphite.

Therapeutic use

Metaraminol is now rarely used, even in anaesthesia and intensive care.

Indications

1. Prevention and treatment of acute hypotensive state occurring with spinal anaesthesia[4]
2. Adjunctive treatment of hypotension due to haemorrhage, reaction to medications, surgical complications, and shock associated with brain damage due to trauma or tumour.

Contraindications

1. The use of metaraminol with cyclopropane or halothane anaesthesia should be avoided
2. Hypersensitivity to any component of the injection solution
3. Children.

Mode of use

Metaraminol bitartrate may be given subcutaneously, intramuscularly or intravenously depending on the nature and the severity and the state of emergency of the patient's condition. In subcutaneous or intramuscular injections, the usual dose is 2–10 mg. In an intravenous infusion, the usual dose is 15–100 mg in 500 ml of sodium chloride injection, with a rate of infusion adjusted to maintain the blood pressure at an appropriate level. Direct intravenous injection of 0.5–5 mg (0.05–0.5 ml) followed by an infusion of 15–100 mg (1.5–10 ml) in 500 ml infusion liquid can be used in grave emergencies when immediate action is required to save life.

The blood pressure response to metaraminol may be poor in some patients, particularly in those with acidosis and coexistant shock. However, whatever the patient's condition, a 10 minute period of time should elapse before increasing the dose because the maximum effect is not immediately apparent.

In every case, an appropriate blood or fluid replacement must be performed prior to, or simultaneously with, the administration of metaraminol.

Indications

1. Acute hypotensive state occurring with anaesthesia
In this particular situation, the control of hypotension with metaraminol can be achieved, especially when hypotension is associated with aortic stenosis or achieved, especially when hypotension is associated with aortic stenosis or hypertrophic sub-aortic stenosis. In these specific situations, the direct cardiac stimulation induced by other vasopressor amines should be avoided.

Adverse reactions

Potentially life-threatening effects
Metaraminol, like other sympathomimetic amines, may cause sinus or ventricular tachycardia or arrhythmias, especially in patients with myocardial infarction.

Acute overdosage
Acute hypertension associated with pulmonary oedema especially in patients with heart failure may occur in cases of overdosage.[5]

Severe or irreversible adverse effects
Abscess formation or tissue necrosis or sloughing due to intense local vasoconstriction may follow the use of metaraminol.

If an adrenergic neuron blocking agent is being administered, the adrenergic receptors will be highly sensitive to metaraminol, leading to an overshoot in blood pressure just after the administration of this pressor drug. The pressor effect of metaraminol is decreased but not reversed by α-adrenergic blocking agents.

Symptomatic adverse effects
Apart from milder examples of the adverse effects already mentioned there is none.

Interference with clinical pathology tests
None is known.

High risk groups

Neonates
The drug is not used in this age-group.

Breast milk. No information is available.

Children
The drug is contraindicated in this age-group.

Pregnant women
The drug should be used with caution in pregnant women.

The elderly
As elderly patients may be sensitive to sympathomimetic drugs metaraminol should be used with caution in this group.

Concurrent disease

Hypovolaemic patients. Blood or plasma losses should be replaced prior to the administration of metaraminol when the principal reason for hypotension or shock is a decrease in circulating volume or is associated with such a decrease. If not corrected appropriately before using the vasopressor, metaraminol may aggravate the patient's situation and, in particular, precipitate renal failure. In case of prolonged use, the central venous pressure should be frequently monitored.

Asthmatics. Sodium bisulphite added to metaraminol injection as a preservative may cause severe allergic reactions in certain susceptible individuals.

Drug interactions

Potentially hazardous interactions

Anaesthetics. Of currently used general anaesthetic agents cyclopropane and halothane sensitive the myocardium to the effects of metaraminol and some other sympathominetic drugs, and serious cardiac arrhythmias may occur when metaraminol is used with these drugs.

Antidepressants. Since metaraminol has both direct and indirect effects on sympathetic nerve terminals, it may interact with both monoamine oxidase inhibitors and tricyclic antidepressants and cause severe hypertension.

Digitalis. Metaraminol in combination with digitalis and sympathomimetic amines is capable of causing ectopic arrhythmic activity.

Metaraminol (bitartrate)

References

1. Torchiana M L, Porter C C, Stone C A 1968 Relation between molecular configuration and certain biological actions of -methyldopamine and -methyl-meta-tyramine and their -hydroxylated products -methylnorepinephrine and metaraminol. Archives Internationales de Pharmacodynamie et de Therapie 174: 118–134
2. Harrison D C, Chidsey C A, Braunwald E 1963 Studies on the mechanism of action of metaraminol. Annals of Internal Medicine 59: 297–305
3. Weil M H 1955 Clinical studies on a vasopressor agent metaraminol (ARAMINE) 1. Observations in normotensive subjects. American Journal of the Medical Sciences 229: 661–669
4. Kajimoto Y, Nishimura N 1984 Metaraminol and dobutamine for the treatment of hypotension associated with epidural block. Resuscitation 12: 47–51
5. Laniado S, Kronson I, Mehta S S 1974 Pulmonary edema: a complication of metaraminol treatment of paroxysmal supraventricular tachycardia. Israel Journal of Medical Sciences 10: 504–508

Metformin (hydrochloride)

Metformin is the only antidiabetic biguanide available in most countries. Phenformin and buformin have been withdrawn because of their high risk of inducing lactic acidosis.

Chemistry

Metformin hydrochloride (Glucophage, Orabet)
$C_4H_{11}N_5.HCl$
N-1,1-Dimethylbiguanide hydrochloride

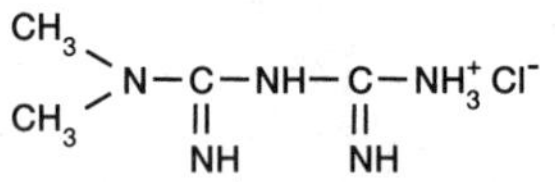

Molecular weight (free base)	165.6 (129.2)
pKa	11.5
Solubility	
in alcohol	1 in 100
in water	1 in 2
Octanol/water partition coefficient	very low

Metformin is a white, crystalline powder, which is almost odourless. It has a bitter taste, and is hygroscopic. It is prepared by chemical synthesis.

Metformin hydrochloride is also available in oral combination products: Glucosulpha in France (with tolbutamide) and Diabomet in Italy (with glibenclamide).

Pharmacology

Metformin reduces elevated blood glucose concentrations in patients with diabetes, but it does not increase insulin secretion. This is probably the reason why it does not cause hypoglycaemia. Accordingly, metformin should be labelled antihyperglycaemic rather than hypoglycaemic. Augmentation of muscular glucose uptake, reduction of increased gluconeogenesis and inhibition of intestinal glucose absorption explain the blood-glucose-lowering effect,[1–4] but the contribution of each process in different conditions is not known.

The mechanism of action involves binding of the apolar biguanide hydrocarbon side-chain to membrane phospholipids, evoking a change in the electrostatic surface potential.[3] Subsequently, various metabolic effects are elicited, depending on the target cell, tissue, organ, species[3,5] and metabolic regulation.[6] In healthy subjects counter-regulatory mechanisms mask the effect of the drug, and blood glucose remains unchanged. In diabetic subjects, on the other hand, the blood glucose elevation is reduced.

Metformin seems to potentiate insulin action by enhancing insulin binding to its receptors and/or postreceptor activity.[4,7] Apart from the glucose-lowering effect, metformin improves the blood lipoprotein profile not only in diabetics but also in non-diabetic subjects with hyperlipoproteinaemia.[1,8]

Toxicology

Administration of metformin for 12 months or more in dogs, rabbits and rats did not reveal any toxic effect on liver, kidneys, spleen, adrenals or bone marrow. Metformin does not pass through the placental barrier in mice. In rats no serious malformations were seen following 1000 mg.kg^{-1}. A 19% decrease in the average number of fetuses per litter was reported following 500 mg.kg^{-1}. There is no indication of a teratogenic effect in man. No tests on mutagenicity or carcinogenicity have been carried out.

Clinical pharmacology

There are no appropriate dose–response studies in man. Initially, daily doses of 0.5–1.0 g are used. No further effect on blood glucose seems to occur following doses above 3 g daily. However, higher doses (3.5 g daily) have been used successfully in hyperlipidaemic, non-diabetic subjects.[8]

In patients with diabetes metformin reduces the elevated fasting blood glucose concentration and improves both intravenous and oral glucose tolerance.[9,10] Metformin increases in vitro glucose uptake in human skeletal muscle.[11] Studies with the clamp technique[12–14] indicate a similar action in vivo. There is also evidence of improved insulin action by metformin from other studies,[10,15,16] and the drug can reduce insulin requirements in type 1 diabetes.[17,18] The presence of a small amount of circulating insulin seems necessary for the effect of metformin on blood glucose.

Metformin increases binding of insulin to its receptors both in vitro and in vivo.[4,19,20] Other studies indicate a postreceptor effect,[12,13,21,22] and this may be independent of the effect at the receptor level.[4] The increase in insulin binding is attributed mainly to an augmentation of low-affinity, high-capacity receptor sites.[19,20]

An increase of hepatic insulin sensitivity with reduced hepatic glucose output and without an increased glucose uptake in the periphery has been suggested recently.[23] Metformin seems to decrease gluconeogenesis from lactate (pyruvate) as well as from alanine.[24] Normally, serum lactate concentrations are not elevated during metformin therapy,[2,5] and metformin decreases lactate elimination to a lesser degree than phenformin at the same antihyperglycaemic level.[24,25]

An antilipolytic action of metformin has been suggested[26,27] and a lipid-lowering effect has been demonstrated, including reductions of plasma triglycerides and, to a lesser degree, of total cholesterol.[8,28–30] No deleterious effect on apolipoproteins has been observed in a long-term study.[30] Metformin seems to affect thrombohaemostatic mechanisms in a beneficial way, but this action has not been sufficiently elucidated. Metformin has been shown to improve peripheral vascular flow in patients with peripheral arterial disease.[31]

The suggested action of metformin on intestinal glucose absorption seems to play a minor role in the blood-glucose-lowering effect of the drug. Metformin may induce malabsorption of various substances, including vitamin B_{12} and possibly folic acid among the clinically most relevant ones. Other gastrointestinal effects include an action on some gastrointestinal hormones, and metformin may have an H_2-agonist capacity.[32]

Pharmacokinetics

Gas–liquid chromatography,[33] high pressure liquid chromatography[34] and mass fragmentography[35] have been employed for the determination of metformin concentrations in plasma and urine. These methods are highly specific and sensitive. The limit of detection is 50 µg.l^{-1}.

Metformin is incompletely absorbed, faecal recovery being about 30% of an oral dose.[33] The absorption is slower than the elimination.[36,37] Peak plasma concentrations of about 2 mg.l^{-1} are reached after 2 hours[33,36] or later.[37]

Oral bioavailability of usual doses is 50–60%.[33,35–37] The difference between absorbed and available drug may reflect minor presystemic clearance of the drug[33] or binding to the intestinal wall.[35] Higher doses are proportionally less available,[33,37] probably due to decreased absorption. Concomitant food intake may slightly impair metformin absorption.[38] Absorption is completed within 6 hours[33] and seems confined to the upper part of the intestine.[33]

The distribution of metformin is rapid,[36] but slow transfer to a deep compartment seems to occur.[37] Mean values for the apparent volume of distribution range from 63 to 276 litres in different pharmacokinetic studies.[33,35–37] Metformin accumulates in the walls of oesophagus, stomach and duodenum, and in salivary glands and kidneys.[1,3] Metformin is not bound to plasma proteins.[33,35,36] There is a slowly increasing binding to blood cells, indicated by an increasing blood:plasma drug concentration ratio with time.[33] Metformin is found in saliva, but in a lower concentration than in plasma.[36]

Metformin (hydrochloride)

The mean plasma elimination half life ranges from 1.5 to 4.5 hours.[33,35,36,37] It is prolonged in patients with renal impairment and is correlated to creatinine clearance.[35] Thus there may be some prolongation of the half life in the elderly due to deteriorating renal function. Urinary excretion data have revealed a quantitatively minor terminal elimination phase with a longer mean half life, ranging from 8.9 to 19 hours.[33,36,37] This suggests a small deep compartment with a slow elimination. Metformin is rapidly eliminated by renal excretion.[33,35–37] While metformin was completely excreted unchanged in one study,[36] only 80% of an intravenous dose was recovered as unchanged drug in the urine in two other studies.[33,35] Mean values (ml.min^{-1}) for renal/total clearance in these studies were 454/459,[36] 544/706[33] and 335/441.[35] The very high renal clearance considerably exceeds creatinine clearance, indicating that metformin is excreted by active tubular secretion. However, the renal clearance of metformin can be correlated with creatinine clearance.[33,35] Most of the drug is excreted within 8 hours after intravenous administration.[33] After oral administration of 0.5 g, 50% was recovered in the urine and 27% in the faeces.[33] No metformin seems to be exhaled by the lungs.[36] There are no data on excretion in breast milk or on placental transfer.

Under steady-state conditions plasma metformin concentrations were accurately predicted from single-dose data.[33] Once absorbed, metformin has linear pharmacokinetic properties; dose dependence has only been demonstrated for its absorption.[33,37]

Oral absorption	50–60%
Presystemic metabolism	negligible
Plasma half life	
range	1.5–4.5 h
Volume of distribution	63–276 l
Plasma protein binding	negligible

Although hepatic disease is unlikely to affect the kinetics of the drug, it is contraindicated in such patients for other reasons.

Concentration–effect relationship

There are no available data concerning the relation between plasma concentrations and therapeutic effect, but there is an association between high plasma metformin concentration and lactic acidosis.[39] Therapeutic plasma concentrations seem to be about 1–2 mg.l^{-1}, but level monitoring has little clinical value, except when lactic acidosis is suspected or present. However, there is no correlation between plasma lactate concentration and plasma metformin concentration at therapeutic drug levels.[35]

Metabolism

Metformin is excreted unmetabolized in the urine in laboratory animals.[3] This was also stated for humans on the basis of early pharmacokinetic studies[2] and confirmed in a study using a modern analytical method.[36] Although the same was concluded from another study,[35] the data showed only incomplete recovery in the urine after intravenous administration of the drug, in accordance with a further study,[33] in which 20% of the dose was not accounted for. Therefore, some metabolic transformation may occur. However, neither conjugates nor any other metabolites of metformin have been identified,[33] in contrast to the more lipophilic phenformin.

Pharmaceutics

Metformin hydrochloride is available as Glucophage (Lipha, UK) tablets of 500 mg and 850 mg. These are white, film-coated tablets, debossed circumferentially with the codes 'GL 500' and 'GL 850'. The maximum shelf-life is 5 years. A sustained-release preparation is also available.[40]

Therapeutic use

Indications

1. Type 2 diabetes (non-insulin-dependent diabetes, NIDDM)
2. Type 1 diabetes (insulin-dependent diabetes, IDDM) as adjuvant therapy in combination with insulin
3. Obesity and hyperinsulinaemia
4. Hyperlipoproteinaemia.

Contraindications

1. Ketosis-prone diabetes
2. Pregnancy
3. Acute complications (severe infections, major operations and trauma)
4. Diabetes with significant late complications (nephropathy, retinopathy)
5. Before intravenous urography or aortography
6. Impaired renal function
7. Liver damage
8. Alcoholism
9. Severe cardiovascular or respiratory disease
10. Deficiencies of vitamin B_{12}, folic acid and iron
11. General ill health (malnutrition, dehydration, etc.)
12. Old age.

Indications

1. Type 2 diabetes

The aim of using metformin is to reduce elevated blood glucose concentrations and to improve insulin sensitivity. Metformin may also promote weight reduction and influence associated hyperlipoproteinaemia.[2,3] It is possible that diabetic vascular complications can be reduced.

Metformin can be used as the only drug when the patient cannot be adequately controlled by diet alone. Metformin is used in this way mainly in type 2 diabetes associated with obesity. Adequate dietary treatment should be tried for at least 6–8 weeks before drug therapy is instituted. In non-obese patients metformin can also be used alone, but the most extensive use is in combination with a sulphonylurea,[2] whereby insulin can often be avoided.[41]

On average, metformin has a blood-glucose-lowering effect ranging from 25 to 30% or more of pretreatment values in 80% of the patients,[2,42] a figure comparable with that for sulphonylureas.[2,43,44] Metformin has a more favourable effect on body weight than chlorpropamide.[43,44] Combination therapy has been used mostly in patients with so-called sulphonylurea failure.[45–47] Even a small dose of metformin added to glibenclamide can improve metabolic control significantly.[48] Combination therapy is also possible by adding a sulphonylurea to patients already on metformin. Metformin reduces the circadian variation of glucose, insulin and FFA levels in diabetic patients,[49] and metabolic control deteriorates when metformin therapy is discontinued.[50] Glycosylated haemoglobin has been used only recently for evaluating the effect of the drug.

Treatment with metformin is usually initiated with 0.5–1.0 g daily, followed by a gradual increase if necessary. No further effect on blood glucose can be expected from doses above 3 g daily. When good control has been achieved, the dose may be gradually reduced. An adequate blood glucose control may not be apparent until after 1–2 weeks. In order to minimize gastrointestinal side effects, metformin should be taken together with meals. Metformin is usually given in two or three daily doses. There is little or no difference in metabolic control and side effects between a single and a divided dose schedule.[51]

2. Type 1 diabetes

The use of metformin as adjuvant therapy in combination with insulin has not been recommended generally because of the risk that these patients will develop keto- and lactic acidosis.[2] However, addition of metformin to insulin has been found to reduce insulin requirements[17,18] and glucose oscillations,[52] probably via improved insulin sensitivity.[14]

3. Obesity and hyperinsulinaemia

Metformin has been used occasionally in non-diabetic patients to support a weight-reducing regimen,[2,3] although the effect on body weight is less consistent in these patients than in diabetics with obesity. In a controlled study in borderline diabetics, metformin induced a significant weight reduction, as compared with both placebo and glibenclamide.[53] The weight-reducing effect is not correlated with the changes in blood glucose but may be related to the effect on insulin sensitivity. Anorexia cannot explain the weight loss.

4. Hyperlipoproteinaemia
The lipid-lowering effect of metformin has been utilized mainly in diabetic patients with associated hyperlipoproteinaemia,[2,3] but this effect has also been demonstrated in non-diabetic patients with hyperlipoproteinaemia, especially type IV and IIB.[8,28,29] An anti-atherosclerotic activity of metformin demonstrated in animal experiments[1] together with a rather extensive clinical experience[8] has been advocated as a basis for the use of metformin in lipid disorders.

Contraindications

The various contraindications are justified by the risk of lactic acidosis in these conditions. It is particularly important to avoid use of metformin in patients with impaired renal function, as the elimination of the drug is decreased.[35] A normal serum creatinine concentration is a prerequisite for treatment, and serum creatinine should be monitored regularly during therapy. Creatinine clearance can be estimated from nomograms.[39] Metformin should be stopped at least two days before intravenous urography and aortography, where a risk exists for temporary renal insufficiency. Metformin should also be stopped for a similar period before major operations. Discontinuation of the drug in these conditions and when acute complications are suspected or present must be followed by temporary insulin treatment until the condition of the patient is stable, and metformin can be reinstated. Apart from the renal function, liver function should also be monitored during metformin therapy, and serum B_{12} concentrations should be measured annually during long-term treatment.

Adverse reactions

Potentially life-threatening effects
Metformin has no direct toxic effects on bone marrow, liver or other organs, and tumour-inducing effects have not been encountered in man.

Metformin can provoke lactic acidosis. [2,3,5,6,39,54–58] A 1977–1982 review revealed 42 cases, of which 18 (43%) were fatal.[56–58] In 40 of these cases documented contraindications were present, and the remaining two patients had taken overdoses. Impaired renal function, mostly severe, was the predominant condition associated with the development of lactic acidosis, and this fits well with the fact that metformin is almost exclusively eliminated by renal excretion. Other predisposing conditions are hepatic dysfunction, cardiac failure and alcohol abuse.

Lactic acidosis may arise if lactate accumulates, due either to increased production (hypoxia) or to decreased elimination. Biguanides may provoke or augment lactic acidosis via both processes, particularly if the drug is present in high concentrations. Usually, the pathogenesis of lactic acidosis is complex, with several contributing factors.

Metformin carries a lower risk of lactic acidosis than do phenformin and buformin.[54] This may be due at least in part to differences in pharmacokinetic and membrane binding properties.[3] Phenformin is metabolized by ring hydroxylation, a process which is genetically impaired in 3–10% of European populations. Such subjects are hence particularly liable to accumulate phenformin.[5,38] Metformin, on the other hand, is mainly excreted by the kidneys without preceding metabolic transformation.

The true frequency of biguanide-associated lactic acidosis is not known, but for phenformin an estimate of 0.25–4 cases per 1000 patient years has been given,[2] that is approximately 1:500. The frequency for metformin appears to be about 20 times lower; hence, 1:10 000 will be the estimated frequency for metformin. From Sweden, 1.76 and 0.13 cases per million defined daily doses have been reported for phenformin and metformin.[55]

The risk of death from metformin-associated lactic acidosis has been estimated to be 0.0240 per 1000 patient-years,[56–58] a figure which is no higher than the risk of fatal glibenclamide-induced hypoglycaemia (0.0332). The incidence of metformin-associated lactic acidosis calculated in this study[56–58] was less than 1 per 10 000 patient-years. In Canada, clinical experience 1972–1983 has covered about 56 000 patient-years without a single documented case.[59]

Early symptoms of lactic acidosis are nausea, vomiting, diarrhoea and lower abdominal pain. Because these symptoms may mimic certain adverse effects of the drug, careful watch should be kept for their sudden onset or aggravation. The diagnosis of non-ketotic metabolic acidosis must give rise to suspicion, and the diagnosis of lactic acidosis should be confirmed by determination of plasma or blood lactate concentrations. Measurement of the so-called anion-gap may also be useful.[6,54] Treatment includes infusion of bicarbonate, glucose and insulin, but acute haemodialysis is often required as well.

Acute overdosage
In a recent review,[56–58] two cases of overdose have been reported. One patient took 7 g of metformin, and the other one was a suicidal case who took 20 g of metformin together with a barbiturate and an antidepressant agent. The clinical features of such deliberate overdose are those of lactic acidosis. Recovery from an overdose of 25 g metformin in an 83-year-old diabetic woman has been reported.[60]

Severe or irreversible adverse effects
During long-term treatment with metformin, malabsorption of vitamin B_{12} may occur.[2,3,5,61,62] In addition, folic acid absorption may be disturbed.[2,55] Two cases of megaloblastic anaemia due to B_{12} malabsorption associated with metformin treatment have been published.[63,64] B_{12} treatment was successful in these cases. Reversion of B_{12} absorption to normal has been observed when stopping metformin.[61] However, it has been suggested that metformin-induced B_{12} malabsorption can sometimes be permanent.[62] Disturbances in B_{12} absorption seems to occur in one-third of the patients on long-term therapy.[61,62] Therefore, serum B_{12} levels should be monitored annually in order to prevent B_{12} deficiency.

Symptomatic adverse effects
Gastrointestinal adverse effects have been reported in 5–20% of metformin-treated patients,[2,3] and seem to be dose-related. Discontinuation of treatment due to gastrointestinal effects may be necessary in less than 3%.[65] The symptoms are often seen initially and might be avoided by gradual dose increase.[2,65] The symptoms, which are metallic taste, abdominal distension, nausea, vomiting, diarrhoea and anorexia, may be attributed to the accumulation of the drug in the gastrointestinal mucosa.[3] Another contributing factor may be the proposed H_2-agonist capacity of metformin.[32]

The prevalence of diarrhoea is reported to be 20%, as compared to 6% in diabetic patients not on metformin.[66] The frequency was similar in patients on metformin alone and in patients on metformin plus sulphonylurea. Metformin-induced diarrhoea is often acute and disturbing but always disappears after cessation of therapy. It does not seem to be dose-related. The mechanism is not clear.

Very rarely, metformin has given rise to cutaneous hypersensitivity.[2,55]

Hypoglycaemia does not occur when metformin is given alone, but has been observed when the drug is given in combination with sulphonylureas and/or alcohol. [2,56–58]

Other effects
Various biochemical effects have been described under Clinical pharmacology. Effects exerted on lipid metabolism may be beneficial. The clinical relevance of minor elevations of intermediary metabolites is not known,[24] but elevations of lactate (pyruvate) and reductions of B_{12} and folate levels have clinical relevance under certain circumstances.

Interference with clinical pathology tests
No such interference is known.

High risk groups

Neonates
The drug is not used in this age group.

Breast milk. Metformin enters breast milk in small amounts and is best avoided in nursing mothers.

Children
Metformin is not recommended in children.

Pregnant women
The drug has been used in pregnant women[67] without any particular problems. Nevertheless, pregnancy is generally regarded as a contraindication, and insulin should be used in all pregnant diabetic women.

Metformin (hydrochloride)

M

The elderly
Caution is advised in elderly patients because of the reduced renal function with increasing age. Frequent monitoring of serum creatinine and dose reduction is recommended in this group.

Concurrent disease
The drug is contraindicated in renal, hepatic and cardiac failure.

Drug interactions

Potentially hazardous interactions
An increased elimination of phenprocoumon (Marcoumar) has been reported during metformin treatment.[68] This has been related to increased liver blood flow. No other drug interactions have been identified.

Alcohol potentiates the antihyperglycaemic and hyperlactataemic effect of metformin.[69] Hence, patients treated with metformin should preferably avoid alcohol, and alcoholism is a definite contraindication.

Potentially useful interactions
Metformin is extensively used in combination with a sulphonylurea, but it is not known whether there is an additive or potentiating effect between these drugs. A combination of metformin and clofibrate has been used,[2] and might have some advantages.

Major outcome trials

Clinical trials 1979–1980 have been reviewed earlier.[2,5] Some other efficacy trials published since then[42,47,48] have been commented on in this monograph. The major trials with metformin[43–45] have been reviewed separately.[65] Details from these trials are given below. A major randomized, comparative trial ('UK prospective diabetes study') is in progress.[70,71]

Three groups of patients were studied prospectively in Edinburgh:[65]

1. Obese type 2 diabetics uncontrolled by diet[43]
2. Non-obese type 2 diabetics uncontrolled by diet[44]
3. Non-obese type 2 diabetics uncontrolled by a sulphonylurea[45].

The overall aims were the evaluation of basic clinical responses in terms of success or failure of treatment and the blood glucose and body weight changes in those successfully controlled. Metformin (M) was used with a maximum daily dose of 3.0 g. Where possible, comparison was made with chlorpropamide (C) with a maximum daily dose of 375 mg.

1. Clarke B F, Duncan L J P 1968 Comparison of chlorpropamide and metformin treatment on weight and blood-glucose response of uncontrolled obese diabetics. Lancet 1: 123–126

This study included 139 patients with body weight greater than 120% of ideal body weight and postprandial blood glucose persistently > 14 mmol.l^{-1}. 124 patients completed one year's treatment with either M or C. Successful control was obtained in 94% (M) and 80% (C). There was a higher secondary failure rate with C. 77 successfully treated patients were studied by crossover, 1 year on each treatment. The blood glucose reduction (approximate values: 16 → 9 mmol.l^{-1}) was similar for both drugs, but body weight changes were different (−1.2 kg with M and +5.3 kg with C).

2. Clarke B F, Campbell I W 1977 Comparison of metformin and chlorpropamide in non-obese, maturity-onset diabetics uncontrolled by diet. British Medical Journal 2: 1576–1578

This study included 216 patients with blood glucose levels as in study 1. 189 patients completed 1 year's treatment with either M or C. Successful control was obtained in 82–83% (both groups). The number of failures was similar for both drugs. 58 successfully treated patients were studied by cross over, 1 year on each treatment. The blood glucose reduction (approximately values: 17 → 8 mmol.l^{-1}) was similar for both drugs, but body weight changes were different (−1.5 kg with M and +4.6 kg with C).

3. Clarke B F, Marshall R C, McGill A C, McCuish A C, Duncan L J P 1967 A 3-year evaluation of combined sulphonylurea-metformin treatment in 200 diabetic keto-acidosis resistant sulphonylurea-failures. In: Butterfield W J H, van Westering W (eds) Tolbutamide — after ten years. Excerpta Medica, New York, and Clarke B F, Duncan L J P 1965 Combined metformin-chlorpropamide therapy in 108 diabetic sulphonylurea-failures. Lancet 1: 1248–1251

This study included 200 patients with postprandial blood glucose persistently > 13.8 mmol.l^{-1} (patients over 60 years) and > 10 mmol.l^{-1} (patients under 60 years). 184 patients completed 3 years treatment on combined M and C. Successful control was obtained in approximately 50% of patients over 40 years (11, 47, 64% in the age groups 20–39, 40–59, 60–75). In 92 successfully controlled sulphonylurea failures treated by combined M and C the final blood glucose was 7–8 mmol.l^{-1} (initially 14–15 mmol.l^{-1}). Most patients were initially underweight and there was only a little weight gain (< 1 kg).

In these three studies 12 of 410 patients (2.9%) discontinued because of gastrointestinal side effects.

General review articles

In this monograph some review articles have been quoted.[2,3,6,38,54] While there are several reviews on biguanides (e.g.[3,6,54]) only one comprehensive review[2] deals specifically with metformin. Some updates have been published as proceedings of various symposia, and articles from these updates are quoted here.[1,4,5,7,8,37,56,57,65] All other references are original papers including clinical trials.[41,42,43,44,45,46–48,51,70,71]

References

1. Sterne J, Junien J L 1981 Metformin: pharmacological mechanisms of the antidiabetic and antilipidic effect and clinical consequences. In: van der Kuy A, Hulst S G T (eds) Biguanide therapy today, Royal Society of Medicine International Congress and Symposium Series, no. 48. Academic Press, Grune & Stratton, London, pp 3–13
2. Hermann L S 1979 Metformin: a review of its pharmacological properties and therapeutic use. Diabete et Metabolisme 5: 233–245
3. Schäfer G 1983 Biguanides: a review of history, pharmacodynamics and therapy. Diabete et Metabolisme 9: 148–163
4. Bailey C J 1985 The anti-hyperglycaemic action of metformin. In: Krans H M J (ed) Diabetes and metformin. A research and clinical update, Royal Society of Medicine International Congress and Symposium Series, no. 79. Royal Society of Medicine, London, pp 17–26
5. Hermann L S 1981 Metabolic effects of metformin in relation to clinical effects and side-effects. In: van der Kuy A, Hulst S G T (eds) Biguanide therapy today, Royal Society of Medicine International Congress and Symposium Series, no. 48. Academic Press, Grune & Stratton, London, pp 17–48
6. Hermann L S 1973 Biguanides and lactate metabolism: a review. Danish Medical Bulletin 20: 65–79
7. Schernthaner G 1985 Improvement of insulin action is an important part of the antidiabetic effect of metformin. Hormone and Metabolic Research Supplement Series 15: 116–120
8. Sirtori C R, Lovati M R, Franceschini G 1985 Management of lipid disorders and prevention of atherosclerosis with metformin. In: Krans H M J (ed) Royal Society of Medicine International Congress and Symposium Series, no. 79. Royal Society of Medicine, London, pp 33–44
9. Frayn K N, Adnitt P I, Turner P 1971 The hypoglycaemic action of metformin. Postgraduate Medical Journal 47: 777–780
10. Caporicci D, Mori A, Pepi R, Lapi E 1979 Effetti della dimetil-biguanide (metformina) sulla clearance periferica dell insulina e sulla biosintesi lipidica in pazienti obesi dislipidemici con e senza malattia diabetica. Clinica Terapeutica 88: 371–386
11. Frayn K N, Adnitt P I, Turner P 1973 The use of human skeletal muscle in-vitro for biochemical and pharmacological studies of glucose uptake. Clinical Science 44: 55–62
12. Tiengo A, Delprato S, Padovan D et al 1982 Improvement of postreceptor insulin defect in type 2 (non-insulin-dependent) diabetic patients by metformin. Diabetologia 23: 205 (abstract)
13. Prager R, Schernthaner G, Graf H 1984 Effect of metformin on peripheral insulin resistance in type 2 (non-insulin-dependent) diabetes mellitus. Diabetologia 27: 321A (abstract)
14. Gin H, Messerschmitt C, Brottier E, Aubertin J 1985 Metformin improved insulin resistance in type I, insulin-dependent, diabetic patients. Metabolism 34: 923–925
15. Hausmann L, Schubotz R 1975 Proinsulin- und Insulinsekretion bei übergewichtigen Frauen vor und nach Gabe von Metformin. Arzneimittel Forschung 25: 668–675
16. Von Lisch H-J, Sailer S, Braunsteiner H 1980 Die Wirkung von Biguaniden auf die Insulinempfindlichkeit von Altersdiabetikern. Wiener Klinische Wochenschrift 92: 266–269
17. Pagano G, Tagliaferro V, Carta Q et al 1983 Metformin reduces insulin requirement in type 1 (insulin-dependent) diabetes. Diabetologia 24: 351–354
18. Gin H, Slama G, Weissbrodt P et al 1982 Metformin reduces post-prandial insulin needs in type I (insulin-dependent) diabetic patients: assessment by the artificial pancreas. Diabetologia 23: 34–36
19. Holle A, Mangels W, Dreyer M, Kühnau J, Rüdiger W 1981 Biguanide treatment increases the number of insulin-receptor sites on human erythrocytes. New England Journal of Medicine 305: 563–566

20. Vigneri R, Gullo D, Pezzino V 1984 Metformin and insulin receptors. Diabetes Care 7 (suppl 1): 113–117
21. Prager R, Schernthaner G 1983 Insulin receptor binding to monocytes, insulin secretion, and glucose tolerance following metformin treatment. Diabetes 32: 1083–1086
22. Cigolini M, Bosello O, Zancanaro C, Orlandi P G, Fezzi O, Smith U 1984 Influence of metformin on metabolic effect of insulin in human adipose tissue in vitro. Diabete et Metabolisme 10: 311–315
23. Jackson R A 1986 Personal communication
24. Nattrass M, Todd P G, Hinks L, Lloyd B, Alberti K G M M 1977 Comparative effects of phenformin, metformin and glibenclamide on metabolic rhythms in maturity-onset diabetics. Diabetologia 13: 145–152
25. Björntorp P, Carlström S, Fagerberg S E et al 1978 Influence of phenformin and metformin on exercise induced lactataemia in patients with diabetes mellitus. Diabetologia 15: 95–98
26. Schönborn J, Heim K, Rabast U, Kasper H 1975 Oxidation rate of plasma free fatty acids in maturity-onset diabetics. Effect of metformin. Diabetologia 11: 375 (abstract)
27. Heim K 1979 Die Wirkung des Biguanides Metformin auf den Stoffwechsel der freien Plasmafettsäuren beim Altersdiabetiker. Inaugural – Dissertation. Julius-Maximilians-Universität Würzburg (ed), Schmitt & Meyer, Würzburg, pp 1–56
28. Gustafson A, Björntorp P, Fahlén M 1971 Metformin administration in hyperlipidaemic states. Acta Medica Scandinavica 190: 491–494
29. Descovich G, Montagutti U, Ceredi C, Cocuzza E, Sirtori C R 1978 Long-term treatment with metformin in a large cohort of hyperlipidaemic patients. Artery 4: 348–359
30. Taylor K G, John W G, Matthews K A, Wright A D 1982 A prospective study of the effect of 12 months treatment on serum lipids and apolipoproteins A-I and B in type 2 (non-insulin-dependent) diabetes. Diabetologia 23: 507–510
31. Sirtori C R, Franceschini G, Gianfranceschi G et al 1984 Metformin improves peripheral vascular flow in nonhyperlipidemic patients with arterial disease. Journal of Cardiovascular Pharmacology 6: 914–923
32. Molloy A M, Ardill J, Tomkin G H 1980 The effect of metformin treatment on gastric acid secretion and gastrointestinal hormone levels in normal subjects. Diabetologia 19: 93–96
33. Tucker G T, Casey C, Phillips P J, Connor H, Ward J D, Woods H F 1981 Metformin kinetics in healthy subjects and in patients with diabetes mellitus. British Journal of Clinical Pharmacology 12: 235–246
34. Charles B G, Jacobsen N W, Ravencroft P J 1981 Rapid liquid chromatographic determination of metformin in plasma and urine. Clinical Chemistry 27: 434–436
35. Sirtori C R, Franceschini G, Gallikienle M et al 1978 Disposition of metformin (N, N-dimethylbiguanide) in man. Clinical Pharmacology and Therapeutics 24: 683–693
36. Pentikäinen P J, Neuvonen P J, Penttilä A 1979 Pharmacokinetics of metformin after intravenous and oral administration to man. European Journal of Clinical Pharmacology 16: 195–202
37. Noel M 1979 Kinetic study of normal and sustained release dosage forms of metformin in normal subjects. In: Cudworth A G (ed) Metformin: current aspects and future developments. Research and Clinical Forms 1: 35–44
38. Melander A, Wåhlin-Boll E 1984 Clinical pharmacology or oral anti-diabetic agents. Acta Endocrinologica (suppl 262): 119–123
39. Hermann L S, Magnusson S, Möller B, Casey C, Tucker G T, Woods H F 1981 Lactic acidosis during metformin treatment in an elderly diabetic patient with impaired renal function. Acta Medica Scandinavica 209: 519–520
40. Karttunen P, Uusitupa M, Lamminsivu U 1983 The pharmacokinetics of metformin: a comparison of the properties of a rapid-release and a sustained-release preparation. International Journal of Clinical Pharmacology, Therapy and Toxicology 21: 31–36
41. Peacock I, Tattersall R B 1984 The difficult choice of treatment for poorly controlled maturity onset diabetes: tablets or insulin? British Medical Journal 288: 1956–1959
42. Wales J K 1980 Treatment of the obese diabetic patient. In: The proceedings of the 3rd international congress on obesity: recent advances in obesity research: III, Rome, ch 26, pp 184–189
43. Clarke B F, Duncan L J P 1968 Comparison of chlorpropamide and metformin treatment on weight and blood-glucose response of uncontrolled obese diabetics. Lancet 1: 123–126
44. Clarke B F, Campbell I W 1977 Comparison of metformin and chlorpropamide in non-obese, maturity-onset diabetics uncontrolled by diet. British Medical Journal 2: 1576–1578
45. Clarke B F, Marshall R C, McGill A C, McCuish A C, Duncan L J P 1967 A 3-year evaluation of combined sulphonylurea–metformin treatment in 200 diabetic keto-acidosis resistant sulphonylurea-failures. In: Butterfield W J H, van Westering W (eds) Tolbutamide — after ten years. Excerpta Medica, New York
46. Clarke B F, Duncan L J P 1965 Combined metformin–chlorpropamide therapy in 108 diabetic sulphonylurea-failures. Lancet 1: 1248–1251
47. Capretti L, Bonora E, Coscelli C, Butturini U 1982 Combined sulfonylurea–biguanide therapy for non-insulin dependent diabetics. Metabolic effects of glibenclamide and metformin or phenformin in newly diagnosed obese patients. Current Medical Research and Opinion 7: 677–683
48. Higginbotham L, Martin F I R 1979 Double-blind trial of metformin in the therapy of non-ketonic diabetics. Medical Journal of Australia 2: 154–156
49. Rigas A N, Bittles A H, Hadden D R, Montgomery D A D 1968 Circadian variation of glucose, insulin, and free fatty acids during long-term use of oral hypoglycaemic agents in diabetes mellitus. British Medical Journal 4: 25–28
50. Siitonen O, Huttunen J K, Järvinen R et al 1980 Effect of discontinuation of biguanide therapy on metabolic control in maturity-onset diabetics. Lancet 1: 217–220
51. Shenfield G M, Bhallia I P, Steel J M, Duncan L P J 1977 Metformin in the treatment of obese diabetics. Practitioner 219: 745–749
52. Coscelli C, Palmari V, Saccardi F, Alpi O, Bonora E 1984 Evidence that metformin addition to insulin induces an amelioration of glycaemic profile in type I (insulin-dependent) diabetes mellitus. Current Therapeutic Research 35: 1058–1064
53. Papoz L, Job D, Eschwege E et al 1978 Effect of oral hypoglycaemic drugs on glucose tolerance and insulin secretion in borderline diabetic patients. Diabetologia 15: 373–380
54. Luft D, Schmulling R M, Eggstein M 1978 Lactic acidosis in biguanide-treated diabetics. A review of 330 cases. Diabetologia 14: 75–87
55. Bergman U, Boman G, Wiholm B-E 1978 Epidemiology of adverse drug reactions to phenformin and metformin. British Medical Journal 2: 464–466
56. Campbell I W 1985 Metformin and sulphonylurea derivatives: the comparative risks. In: Krans H M J (ed) Diabetes and metformin. A research and clinical update, Royal Society of Medicine International Congress and symposium series, no. 79. Royal Society of Medicine, London, pp 45–50
57. Campbell I W 1984 Metformin and the sulphonylureas: the comparative risk. Hormone and Metabolic Research Supplement Series 15: 105–111
58. Campbell I W 1984 Metformin and glibenclamide: comparative risks. British Medical Journal 289: 289
59. Lucis O J 1983 Pharmacological update. The status of metformin in Canada. Canadian Medical Association Journal 128: 24–26
60. McLelland J 1985 Recovery from metformin overdose. Diabetic Medicine 2: 410–411
61. Tomkin G H, Hadden D R, Weaver J A, Montgomery D A D 1971 Vitamin B-12 status of patients on long-term metformin therapy. British Medical Journal 2: 685–687
62. Adams J F, Clark J S, Ireland J T, Kesson C M, Watson W S 1983 Malabsorption of vitamin B-12 and intrinsic factor secretion during biguanide therapy. Diabetologia 24: 16–18
63. Callaghan T S, Hadden D R, Tomkin G H 1980 Megaloblastic anaemia due to vitamin B-12 malabsorption associated with long-term metformin treatment. British Medical Journal 1: 1214–1215
64. Mourits-Andersen T, Ditzel J 1983 Megaloblastaer anaemi forårsaget af vitamin B12 malabsorption under langvarig metforminbehandling. Ugeskrift for Laeger 145: 25–26
65. Clarke B F, Duncan L J P 1979 Biguanide treatment in the management of insulin dependent (maturity-onset) diabetes: clinical experience with metformin. In: Cudworth A G (ed) Metformin: current aspects and future developments. Research and Clinical Forums 1: 53–63
66. Dandona P, Fonseca V, Mier A, Beckett A G 1983 Diarrhea and metformin in a diabetic clinic. Diabetes Care 6: 472–474
67. Coetzee E J, Jackson W P U 1979 Metformin in the management of pregnant insulin-dependent diabetics. Diabetologia 16: 241–245
68. Ohnhaus E E, Berger W, Duckert F, Oesch F 1983 The influence of dimethylbiguanide on phenprocoumon elimination and its mode of action. Klinische Wochenschrift 61: 851–858
69. Schaffalitzky de Muckadell O B, Mortensen H, Lyngsoe J 1979 Metabolic effects of glucocorticoid and ethanol administration in phenformin and metformin-treated obese diabetics. Acta Medica Scandinavica 206: 269–273
70. UK prospective study of therapies of maturity-onset diabetes 1983 I. Effect of diet, sulphonylurea, insulin or biguanide therapy on fasting plasma glucose and body weight over one year. Diabetologia 24: 404–411
71. UK prospective diabetes study 1985 II. Reduction in HbA_{1c} with basal insulin supplement sulphonylurea, or biguanide therapy in maturity-onset diabetes. Diabetes 34: 793–798

Methacycline (hydrochloride)

Methacycline hydrochloride is a semi-synthetic, tetracycline, broad-spectrum antibiotic. It is active against a wide range of Gram-negative and Gram-positive bacteria.

Chemistry

Methacycline hydrochloride (Rondomycin(e), Pluramycine, Apriclina)
$C_{22}H_{21}N_2O_8$.HCl
4-Dimethylamino-1,4,4α,5,5α,6,11,12α-octahydro-3,5,10,12,12α-pentahydroxy-6-methylene-1,11-dioxo-2-naphthacenecarboxamide

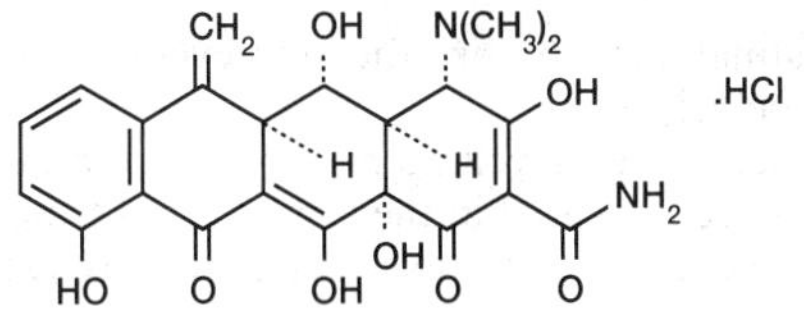

Molecular weight	478.9
pKa	3.1, 7.6, 9.5[1]
Solubility	
in alcohol	1 in 300
in water	1 in 100
Octanol/water partition coefficient	0.4[1]

A light yellow crystalline powder, methacycline is prepared by the exocyclic dehydration of 5-hydroxytetracycline.[2,3]

Pharmacology

Methacycline is a semisynthetic tetracycline antibiotic that became available for clinical use in 1961. Like other tetracyclines it has a wide spectrum of activity. In addition to its antibiotic activity it is also a chelating agent and will chelate Ca^{2+}, Mg^{2+} or Al^{3+} ions in the gut. Methacycline has its main mechanism of action on protein synthesis. Methacycline is relatively lipid-soluble and passes directly through the lipid bilayer of the bacterial cell wall. In addition, an energy-dependent active transport system pumps the drug, like all tetracyclines, through the inner cytoplasmic membrane. Once inside the bacterial cell, methacycline inhibits protein synthesis by binding specifically to 30S ribosomes. The drug appears to prevent access of aminoacyl-tRNA to the acceptor site on the mRNA ribosome complex.[4,5] This prevents the addition of amino acids to the growing peptide chain. Methacycline will impair protein synthesis in mammalian cells if used at very high concentrations. However, these cells lack the active transport system found in bacteria.

Toxicology

Results of animal studies indicate that tetracyclines cross the placenta, are found in fetal tissues and can have toxic effects on the developing fetus (often related to retardation of skeletal development). Evidence of embryotoxicity has also been noted in animals treated early in pregnancy.[6,7] Methacycline may cause teratogenic defects in mice.[8]

Photosensitivity manifested by an exaggerated sunburn reaction has been observed in some individuals taking tetracyclines. Patients apt to be exposed to direct sunlight or ultraviolet light should be advised that this reaction can occur with tetracycline drugs, and treatment should be discontinued at the first evidence of skin erythema.[6,9]

Acute toxicity studies[10] show that the LD_{50} of methacycline hydrochloride given intraperitoneally to rats was 252 mg.kg^{-1} of body weight.

Clinical pharmacology

Methacycline is primarily a bacteriostatic antibiotic and has a similar spectrum of activity to other tetracyclines.

Methacycline is active against most strains of *Haemophilus influenzae* and is particularly useful for infections with *H. ducreyi*, *Actinomyces*, *Brucella* and *Vibrio cholerae*. Methacycline is also active against *Nocardia*, *Chlamydia*, *Mycoplasma* and a wide range of *Rickettsia*. Methacycline is active against spirochaetes such as *Borrelia recurrentis*, *Treponema pallidum* and *T. pertenue*.

Methacycline was initially useful for the treatment of Gram-positive infections but many strains are now resistant to the drug. The overall resistance in the UK of the pneumococcus is about 10%. Methacycline possesses some activity against *Staphylococcus aureus*, particularly for community acquired infections, but in hospitals the prevalence of resistance to staphylococci is high. Many Gram-negative organisms have acquired resistance to methacycline and for *E. coli* more than 50% of strains may be resistant. Methacycline has no activity against *Pseudomonas aeruginosa* while most strains of *Campylobacter* are sensitive. Methacycline is also active against anaerobic species of bacteria and since concentrations of the drug are quite high in the gastrointestinal contents, the enteric flora are usually altered by the drug. Methacycline produces stable blood levels at a total daily dose of 600 mg given twice or four times daily.[11]

Resistance to tetracyclines develops slowly and organisms that show resistance to one tetracycline frequently show resistance to others in the group (with some exceptions for minocycline and doxycycline). Most resistance is mediated by a plasmid and is an inducible trait, appearing only after exposure of the bacteria to the drug. Resistance seems to occur because the plasmid implants genetic material in the cell for a number of proteins and this affects penetration of the cell wall by the tetracycline.

Pharmacokinetics

There are three useful analytical methods that can be used to determine tetracyclines in body tissues and fluids: microbiologic (the preferred method with a sensitivity of 0.1 μg.ml^{-1}), fluorometric and HPLC.[12–15]

In fasting adults, 60% of an oral dose of methacycline is absorbed from the gastrointestinal tract. After a single oral 150 mg dose of methacycline in fasting adults with normal renal function, a maximum serum concentration of 1.3–1.4 μg.ml^{-1} was attained in 2–3 h. Following a single 300 mg dose, a peak serum concentration of 2.4 μg.ml^{-1} was obtained.[16] The presence of food or milk can reduce the gastrointestinal absorption of methacycline by 50% or more. Since tetracyclines readily chelate divalent or trivalent cations including aluminium, calcium, iron and magnesium, concurrent oral administration of antacids and other drugs containing these cations may also decrease oral absorption of methacycline hydrochloride.

The serum half life of methacycline is 7–15 hours in adults with normal renal function and is reported to range up to 44 hours in patients with severe renal impairment. In one study in adults with normal renal function, the half life of methacycline was 7 hours following a single dose and 11 hours following multiple doses. In one study in patients with normal renal function, 30% of a single 150 mg oral dose of methacycline hydrochloride was excreted in urine and 13% in faeces within 48 hours as active drug.[16]

Oral absorption	60%
Presystemic metabolism	—
Plasma half life	
range	7–15 h
Volume of distribution	0.97 l.kg^{-1}
Plasma protein binding	79–90%

The long duration of action is in part due to greater binding by plasma and tissue proteins, which binding diminishes the effective plasma level of the drug and slows excretion in urine. Methacycline is 79 to 90% protein bound in plasma. The volume of distribution

M

is 0.97 l.kg^{-1}. The low rate of excretion results in a low urine concentration, so that it is less effective in urinary tract infections than the shorter-acting tetracyclines.[17]

Concentration–effect relationship

The therapeutic range will depend upon the minimum inhibitory concentration (MIC) of the antibiotic for the organism in question. Full susceptibility occurs when the MIC is less than 4.0 mg.l^{-1}, and intermediate susceptibility occurs when the MIC is between 4.0 and 12.5 mg.l^{-1}. Concentrations of greater than 25 mg.l^{-1} are usually required to inhibit most strains of group B and group D streptococci and strains of *Staphylococcus aureus*. The MIC for *Streptococcus pyogenes* is usually about 1.0 mg.l^{-1} while many strains of *Neisseria* have a similar MIC.

Metabolism

In one study in patients with normal renal function, 30% of a single 150 mg oral dose of methacycline hydrochloride was excreted in the urine and 13% was excreted in the faeces within 48 hours as methacycline.[16]

In another study,[18] the administration of methacycline hydrochloride 300 mg every 12 hours to 9 healthy subjects resulted in mean serum concentrations of about 0.9 μg.ml^{-1} after 2 hours, falling to 0.4 μg after 12 hours, rising and maintained between 1 and 2 μg after the first 24 hours of treatment. About 57 mg of the drug was recovered unchanged from the urine during the first 24 hours.

No metabolites of methacycline have been identified.

Pharmaceutics

Methacycline is available only in oral forms.[6]
Methacycline hydrochloride, Rondomycin (Wallace, US) is available for oral use as 300 mg in blue/white capsules marked 'Wallace 37-4101' on the white base and 150 mg in blue/white capsules marked 'Wallace 37-4001' on the white base. Methacycline hydrochloride capsules should be stored in a tight, light-resistant container at a temperature between 15–30°C.

Therapeutic use[6]

Indications

Methacycline hydrochloride is indicated in infections caused by the following microorganisms:

1. Rickettsiae (Rocky Mountain spotted fever, typhus fever and the typhus group, Q fever, rickettsialpox and tick fevers)
2. *Mycoplasma pneumoniae* (PPLO, Eaton Agent)
3. Agents of psittacosis and ornithosis
4. Agents of lymphogranuloma venereum and granuloma inguinale
5. The spirochaetal agent of relapsing fever (*Borrelia recurrentis*).

The following Gram-negative microorganisms:

1. *Haemophilus ducreyi* (Chancroid)
2. *Pasteurella pestis* and *Pasteurella tularensis*
3. *Bartonella bacilliformis*
4. *Bacteroides* species
5. *Vibrio comma* and *Vibrio fetus*
6. *Fusobacterium fusiforme* (Vincent's infection)
7. *Actinomyces* species
8. *Brucella* species (in conjunction with streptomycin).

Because many strains of the following microorganisms have been shown to be resistant to tetracyclines, culture and susceptibility testing are recommended.

Methacycline hydrochloride is indicated for treatment of infections caused by the following Gram-negative microorganisms, when bacteriologic testing indicates appropriate susceptibility to the drug:

1. *Escherichia coli*
2. *Enterobacter aerogenes* (formerly *Aerobacter aerogenes*)
3. *Shigella* species
4. *Mima* species and *Herellea* species
5. *Haemophilus influenzae* (respiratory infections)
6. *Klebsiella* species (respiratory and urinary infections).

Methacycline is indicated for treatment of infections caused by the following Gram-positive microorganisms when bacteriologic testing indicates appropriate susceptibility to the drug:

1. *Streptococcus* species: up to 44% of strains of *Streptococcus pyogens* and 74% of *Streptococcus faecalis* have been found to be resistant to tetracycline drugs. Therefore, tetracyclines should not be used for streptococcal disease unless the organism has been demonstrated to be sensitive. For upper respiratory infections due to group A β-haemolytic streptococci, penicillin is the usual drug of choice, including prophylaxis of rheumatic fever
2. *Diplococcus pneumoniae*
3. *Staphylococcus aureus*, skin and soft tissue infections. Tetracyclines are not the drugs of choice in the treatment of any type of staphylococcal infections.

When penicillin is contraindicated, tetracyclines are alternative drugs in the treatment of infection due to:

1. *Neisseria gonorrhoeae*
2. *Treponema pallidum* and *Treponema pertenue* (syphilis and yaws)
3. *Listeria monocytogenes*
4. *Clostridium* species
5. *Bacillus anthracis*
6. Fisobacterium fusiforme (Vincent's infection)
7. Actinomyces species.

In acute intestinal amoebiasis, the tetracyclines may be a useful adjunct to amoebicides.

In severe acne, the tetracyclines may be useful adjunctive therapy.

Tetracyclines are indicated in the treatment of trachoma, although the infectious agent is not always eliminated, as judged by immunofluorescence.

Inclusion conjunctivitis may be treated with oral tetracyclines or with a combination of oral and topical agents.

Contraindications

1. This drug is contraindicated in persons who have shown hypersensitivity to any of the tetracyclines
2. This drug should not be given to children or pregnant women since it may cause permanent discoloration of teeth
3. Photosensitivity may cause exaggerated sunburn reaction. Patients apt to be exposed to direct sunlight or ultraviolet light should be advised that this reaction can occur. Treatment should be discontinued at the first evidence of skin erythema
4. Methacycline should be used with caution in patients with renal impairment.

Mode of use[6]

The usual adult dosage of methacycline hydrochloride is 600 mg daily. This may be given in four divided doses of 150 mg each or two divided doses of 300 mg each. An initial dose of 300 mg may be followed by 150 mg every six hours or 300 mg every twelve hours may be used in the management of more severe infections. the recommended dosage schedule for children above eight years of age is 6.6–13.2 mg.kg^{-1} body weight per day divided into two or four equally spaced doses.

Indications

Some specific dosages along with information on mode of use as given by the manufacturer[6] are shown below:

1. Uncomplicated gonorrhoea
In uncomplicated gonorrhoea, when penicillin is contraindicated, methacycline hydrochloride may be used for treating both males and females in the following clinical dosage schedule: 900 mg initially, followed by 300 mg four times daily for a total of 5.4 g.

2. Syphilis
For treatment of syphilis, when penicillin is contraindicated, a total of 18–24 g of methacycline hydrochloride in equally divided doses over a period of 10–15 days should be given. Close follow-up including laboratory tests, is recommended.

3. Eaton Agent pneumonia
In Eaton Agent pneumonia, the usual adult dosage is 900 mg daily for six days.

Methacycline (hydrochloride)

Adverse reactions

Potentially life-threatening effects

Anaphylaxis may occur on rare occasions. If renal impairment exists, even usual oral or parenteral doses may lead to excessive systemic accumulation of the drug and possible liver toxicity. Under such conditions, lower than usual total doses are indicated, and, if therapy is prolonged, serum level determinations of the drug may be advisable.[6]

Acute overdosage

Apart from vomiting and diarrhoea, no effects are likely to result from a single overdose of the drug.

Severe or irreversible adverse effects

The antianabolic action of the tetracyclines may cause an increase in BUN. While this is not a problem in those with normal renal function, in patients with significantly impaired function, higher serum levels of tetracyclines may lead to azotaemia, hyperphosphataemia, and acidosis.[6]

Symptomatic adverse effects

The following adverse reactions have been reported:[6]

Gastrointestinal. Anorexia, nausea, vomiting, diarrhoea, glossitis, dysphagia, enterocolitis, and inflammatory lesions (with monilial overgrowth) in the anogenital region. These reactions have been caused by both the oral and parenteral administration of tetracyclines.

Skin. Maculopapular and erythematous rashes. Exfoliative dermatitis has been reported but is uncommon. Photosensitivity reactions may occur.

Hypersensitivity reactions. In addition to anaphylaxis, previously mentioned, urticaria, angioneurotic oedema, anaphylactoid purpura, pericarditis and exacerbation of systemic lupus erythematosus, can occur.

Intracranial hypertension. Bulging fontanelles in infants and benign intracranial hypertension in adults have been reported in individuals receiving full therapeutic dosages. These conditions disappeared rapidly when the drug was discontinued.

Superinfection. As with other broad-spectrum antibiotic preparations, use of this drug may result in overgrowth of non-susceptible organisms, including fungi. If superinfection occurs, the antibiotic should be discontinued and appropriate therapy instituted.

Other effects

Because tetracyclines have been shown to depress plasma prothrombin activity, patients who are on anticoagulant therapy may require downward adjustment of their anticoagulant dosage.[6]

Interference with clinical pathology tests

The tetracyclines, in general, may cause the following interference with some clinical pathology tests.[19]

In pregnant women, they may cause some elevation of serum amylase.

Tetracyclines may cause an increased fluorescence (false positive) in the Hingerty method for measuring urinary catecholamines.

With pre-existing renal impairment, tetracyclines may cause an increase in blood urea due to their antianabolic effect.

High risk groups

Neonates

Because of the risk of tooth staining, tetracyclines should not be given to neonates, unless absolutely essential.

Breast milk. There is probably negligible absorption of tetracyclines by breast-fed infants, because of chelation by the calcium in milk, but there is a remote possibility of tooth staining.

Children

What has been said above about neonates applies also to older children.

Pregnant women

The tetracyclines should be avoided in pregnant women, because of the risk of tooth staining and effect on bone growth in the fetus.

The elderly

Tetracyclines can be used in the elderly unless patients have renal or hepatic dysfunction.

Drug interactions

Potentially hazardous interactions

Antacids containing aluminium, calcium, or magnesium impair absorption and should not be given to patients taking oral tetracyclines.

Food and some dairy products also interfere with absorption. Oral forms of tetracycline should be given one hour before or two hours after meals. Paediatric oral dosage forms should be given at least one hour prior to feeding.

Jawetz[20] has reported an inhibition of the antimicrobial activity of penicillin when used in combination with a tetracycline.

Potentially useful interactions

No interactions of this kind have been reported.

General review articles

Achromycin — Tetracycline HCl 1975 Current concepts. Medical Advisory Department, Lederle Laboratories, Pearl River, New York

Conha B A, Comer J B 1982 The tetracyclines. Medical Clinics of North America 66: 294–302

Hlavka J J, Boothe J H (eds) 1985 The tetracyclines. In: Handbook of experimental pharmacology p 78. Springer-Verlag, Heidelberg, Germany

Mitcher L A 1978 The chemistry of the tetracycline antibiotics. Medicinal Research Service 9: 1–45

Ory E M 1980 The tetracyclines. Antimicrobial therapy, 3rd edn. ch 9, pp 117–126. W.B. Saunders Co., Phil., PA USA

References

1. Moffat A C (ed) 1986 Clarke's isolation and identification of drugs, 2nd edn. The Pharmaceutical Press, London, p 741
2. Blackwood R, Rennhard H, Beereboom J, Stephens C 1961 US Patent 2 984 686
3. Blackwood R 1962 U.S. Patent 3 026 354
4. Hlavka J J, Boothe J H (eds) 1985 The tetracyclines. In: Handbook of experimental pharmacology 78. Springer-Verlag, Heidelberg, p 331
5. Hogenawer G, Turnowsky F 1972 The effects of streptomycin and tetracycline on codon–anticodon interaction. FEBS Letters 26: 185–188
6. Rondomycin(e) (methacycline HCl), Brochure number IN-97A2-01. Wallace Laboratories, Division of Carter-Wallace Inc, Cranbury, New Jersey 08 512
7. Fillippi B, Mela V 1958 Congenital malformations and antibiotics. Archives Francoises de Pediatrie 15: 565–570
8. Rassoff I S 1974 Handbook of veterinary drugs. Springer, New York, pp 50–75
9. Hasan T, Kochevan I, McAuliffe D, Cooperman B, Abdulah D 1984 Mechanism of tetracycline phototoxicity. Journal of Investigative Dermatology 83: 179–183
10. Goldethal E I 1971 A compilation of LD_{50} values in new born and adult animals. Toxicology and Applied Pharmacology 18: 185–207
11. Bailey B 1980 Association of the British Pharmaceutical Industry data sheet compendium. Datapharm Publications Limited, England
12. Truant J P, Bolen J E, Mullins J 1965 Evaluation of susceptibility testing procedures with single and multiple antibiotic discs. In: Sylvester J C (ed) Antimicrobial agents and chemotherapy. American Society for Microbiology, Ann Arbor, pp 384–394
13. Koch M L 1955 An evaluation of the in vitro antibacterial activity of tetracyclines. Antibiotics and Chemotherapy June: 340–344
14. Saltzman A 1950 Fluorophotometric estimation of aureomycin in blood and urine. Journal of Laboratory and Clinical Medicine 35: 123–128
15. Mack G D, Ashworth R B 1978 A high performance liquid chromatographic system for the analysis of tetracycline drug standards, analogs, degradation products and other impurities. Journal of Chromatographic Science 16: 93–101
16. McEvoy G K, McQuarrie G M (eds) 1987 American hospital formulary service. American Society of Hospital Pharmacists, Bethesda
17. Gennaro A R 1980 Remington's pharmaceutical sciences. Mack Printing Co, Easton, PA, pp 1149–1150
18. Olon L P, Holvey D N 1968 Evaluation of tetracycline phosphate complex. Clinical Medicine 75: 33
19. Hansten P D 1971 Drug interactions. Lea and Febiger, Philadelphia, pp 1–100
20. Jawetz E 1968 The use of combination of antimicrobial drugs. Annual Review of Pharmacology 8: 15

Methadone (hydrochloride)

Methadone is an opioid analgesic similar to morphine, but with a longer duration of action. Though sometimes prescribed as an analgesic, it has been particularly used to substitute for other opioids in the management of dependence, and for the suppression of cough.

Chemistry

Methadone hydrochloride (Physeptone, Amidone, Dolophene, Eptadone, Heptanal, Ketalgin, Mephanon, Symoron, Tussol all use the dl-racemic mixture; L-Polamidon is the l-isomer)
$C_{21}H_{27}NO.HCl$
6-Dimethylamino-4,4-diphenyl-3-heptanone hydrochloride

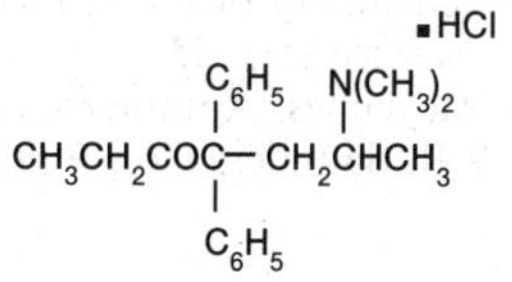

Molecular weight (free base)	345.9 (309.5)
pKa (amino group)	8.3
Solubility	
in alcohol	1 in 7
in water	1 in 12
Octanol/water partition coefficient	
l-isomer	57
d-isomer	28

A bitter-tasting white or colourless crystalline powder, it is prepared by chemical synthesis, and the racemate or l-isomer used clinically.

Pharmacology

Methadone is a strong opioid agonist with actions predominantly at the μ receptor. The analgesic activity of the racemate is almost entirely due to the l-isomer, which is at least 10 times more potent as an analgesic than the d-isomer.[1] The d-isomer lacks significant respiratory depressant activity but does have antitussive effects. Methadone also has some agonist actions at the κ and σ opiate receptors. These actions result in analgesia, depression of respiration, suppression of cough, nausea and vomiting (via an effect on the chemoreceptor trigger zone) and constipation. An effect on the nucleus of the oculomotor nerve, and perhaps on opioid receptors in the pupillary muscles, causes pupillary constriction. All these effects are reversible by naloxone with a pA_2 value similar to its antagonism of morphine. Like many basic drugs, methadone enters mast cells and releases histamine by a non-immunological mechanism. It causes a dependence syndrome of the morphine type.

Toxicology

The LD_{50} in rats is 95 mg.kg^{-1} and the intravenous LD_{50} in mice is 20 mg.kg^{-1} but little detailed information on toxicology has been published.

Clinical pharmacology

Methadone in an initial dose of 5–10 mg is an effective analgesic in man,[2] for most causes of pain; analgesia is accompanied by euphoria. Doses of up to 30 mg have been used, and doses up to 50 mg orally are useful in tolerant subjects. Doses less than 5 mg have little analgesic effect, but increasingly effective analgesia is produced by doses above that level throughout the therapeutic range. The effects of a single dose become apparent within 15 minutes of an intramuscular injection, and last for 3–5 hours. Epidural or intrathecal administration of an appropriate preparation also produces effective analgesia,[3] which is due to a local action on spinal cord neurones.[4] Low doses reduce mainly respiratory frequency while higher doses also diminish tidal volume; this respiratory depression can also be demonstrated in normal subjects as blunting of the increase in respiratory drive normally produced by inhalation of carbon dioxide. The related suppression of the cough reflex by even low doses of methadone is apparent in patients with respiratory disorder. Heart rate, systolic blood pressure and body temperature are all reduced.[5] A dose of 10–20 mg subcutaneously produces pupillary constriction for over 24 hours.[6] Methadone slows the α rhythm of the EEG but increases δ wave activity.[7]

With chronic administration, tolerance occurs to all effects other than pupillary constriction. There is cross-tolerance with other opioids, and so it suppresses the withdrawal symptoms due to morphine or heroin in physically dependent individuals. Physical dependence is established within a few days of long-term administration. Since, in chronic use, the plasma level of methadone is maintained by release of drug bound to tissues,[8] the effects of each dose become more prolonged and withdrawal symptoms may not occur until 1–2 days after the drug has been stopped, and are milder in degree than those following withdrawal of diamorphine, though they may persist for 3–6 weeks. A withdrawal syndrome also occurs in the neonates of dependent mothers.

Pharmacokinetics

The usual analytical method is gas chromatography with flame ionization detection[9] which can detect 5 μg.l^{-1}.

Methadone is one of the more lipid-soluble opioids, and is well absorbed from the gastrointestinal tract, but undergoes fairly extensive first-pass metabolism. It is bound to albumin and other plasma proteins[10] and to tissue proteins (probably lipoproteins), the concentrations in lung, liver and kidneys being much higher than in blood.[11] The pharmacokinetics of methadone are unusual, in that there is extensive binding to tissue proteins and fairly slow transfer between some parts of this tissue reservoir and the plasma. With an intramuscular dose of 10 mg, a peak plasma concentration of 75 μg.l^{-1} is reached in 1 hour. With regular oral doses of 100–120 mg daily, plasma concentrations rise from trough levels of approximately 500 μg.l^{-1} to a peak of about 900μg.l^{-1}in 4 hours.[12] Marked variations in plasma level occur in dependent persons on a stable dose of oral methadone, without any relationship to symptoms.[13] Methadone is secreted into sweat and found in saliva, and in high concentrations in gastric juice. The concentration in cord blood is about half the maternal level.[14]

Oral absorption	good
Presystemic metabolism	extensive
Plasma half life (single i.m. dose)	
range	6–8 h
mean	7.3 h
Volume of distribution	5 l.kg^{-1}
Plasma protein binding	60–90%

The half life of a single intramuscular dose is 6–8 (mean 7.3) hours and after a single oral dose is 12–18 (mean 15) hours, both figures partly reflecting distribution into tissue stores, as well as metabolic and renal clearance.[9,12] (An intramuscular dose is absorbed more rapidly, the half life is shorter, being more a matter of distribution than clearance. With regular doses, the tissue reservoir is already partly filled, and so the half life is extended to 13–47 (mean 25) hours[15] reflecting only clearance. In the first 96 h after administration, 15–60% can be recovered from the urine,[16] and as the dose is increased so a higher proportion of unchanged methadone is found there. Acidification of the urine can increase the renal clearance by a factor of at least three, and thus appreciably reduce the half time of elimination.

Concentration–effect relationship

There is a close relationship between the degree of pupillary constriction and the plasma concentration of methadone.[12] In this study peak concentrations of 70–80 μg.l^{-1} of methadone coincided with maximum pupillary constriction. In another study, plasma concentrations of methadone were seen to vary between 150 and 300 μg.l^{-1} and there was no correlation between these plasma levels and the change in symptoms.[13]

Metabolism

The chief metabolic pathways, which probably occur in the liver, are mono and di N-demethylation,[9,17] (Fig. 1) and studies with ^{14}C-labelled methadone[18] have identified additional, but minor, metabolic pathways. With a single dose, the urine contains an average of 20% excreted unchanged and 13% as demethylated product EDDP, these two accounting for one-third of the dose. Demethylation becomes more active with long-term treatment, so after 30 days EDDP made up 22% and unchanged compound 12%. In addition to these urinary values, 20–40% of the radioactive carbon appeared in the faeces, leaving a remaining one-third of the dose as minor metabolites in the urine. In rats, N-demethylation occurs more rapidly with the active l-isomer.[19] The metabolites are free from pharmacological effect. An N-oxide forms in the urine, but is not a true metabolite.[20]

Fig. 1 Metabolism of methadone

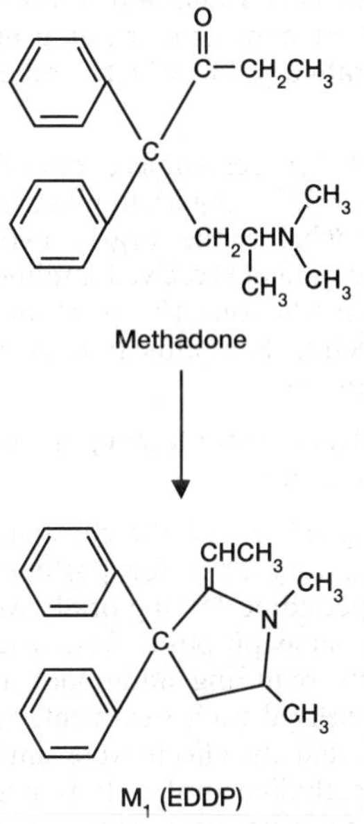

Pharmaceutics

Methadone is a Controlled Drug because of its potential for inducing dependence.

Methadone is available as tablets, an elixir and as a solution for injection. The white, biconvex, tablets of Physeptone contain 5 mg methadone hydrochloride in a lactose base, and are marked 'Wellcome L4A'. Both 5 mg and 10 mg tablets are available in the USA (Dolophine, Lilly and Roxane). A 40 mg dispersible tablet (Lilly, USA) is round, peach coloured and cross-scored. The pale brown elixir contains 2 mg per 5 ml methadone hydrochloride in a syrup base. The solution for injection is in ampoules of 1 ml, containing 10 mg methadone hydrochloride; it is somewhat irritant, and the intramuscular route is preferable to subcutaneous administration, especially for repeated doses. Preparations may be sterilised by autoclaving. Methadone is physically incompatible with alkalis, amaranth, chlorocresol, oxidising agents, iodides, mercury salts and saccharin, sodium. None of the preparations contains any potentially allergenic excipient.

Methadone mixture 1 mg per ml is used orally for the management of opioid dependence. A viscous syrup, coloured bright green, has been used for supply to addicts to discourage intravenous use of the oral preparation.

The injection and linctus require to be protected from light and all preparations have a shelf-life of 5 years at 25°C.

Methadone (hydrochloride)

Therapeutic use

Indications

1. The control of severe pain
2. Suppression of cough
3. Management of opioid dependence.

Contraindications

1. Respiratory depression or respiratory failure, e.g. due to airways obstruction
2. Monoamine oxidase inhibitor drugs given concurrently, or within two weeks before methadone
3. Obstetric use.

Mode of use

As with any opioid that carries a substantial danger of producing dependence, methadone is used only if less dangerous drugs have failed to be effective, or are unlikely to be effective, or when — as in patients with advanced malignancy — dependence will not be a problem.

Indications

1. The control of severe pain

Methadone is an alternative to morphine or diamorphine in the control of severe pain, such as visceral pain or the pain of advanced malignancy. An initial dose of 5–10 mg six to eight hourly is usual, but should soon be followed by observation of the patient to check that this is sufficient. A higher initial dose may be selected if the patient is being transferred to methadone from treatment with another opioid, according to the dose of the other drug (which the patient is likely to have become tolerant to). In chronic pain (e.g. due to advanced malignant disease), the dose is then gradually increased, with no limit on the dose that may be used, until pain is relieved, or adverse effects occur that prevent further increase in dose. Treating nausea due to methadone with an antiemetic, or constipation with a stimulant laxative, may allow a higher dose of methadone to be used.

In long-term use, the tissue reservoir of methadone allows less frequent administration than for morphine. But, given regularly for more than two or three days, substantial accumulation of methadone can occur unless the dose is reduced as the tissue stores are saturated, and the half life gets longer because distribution is no longer contributing to it. In particular, careful observation of respiration is required in the first two weeks of treatment, in case the dose should be reduced.

2. Suppression of cough

Methadone can be used as an alternative to diamorphine linctus to relieve severe and distressing cough, when codeine linctus has proved ineffective.

3. Management of opioid dependence

There is some reason to believe that to give an opioid-dependent patient a single daily dose of methadone designed for oral use is less damaging to the addict, and to society, than leaving the individual to seek diamorphine (heroin) for intravenous use. The intentions are that the methadone occupies opioid receptors, so reducing craving for other opioids, and the effect of any taken; the slower onset of effect of an oral preparation reduces the reward and consequent reinforcement of dependence; and the slower offset reduces the intensity of withdrawal symptoms. There is a risk of methadone being diverted into abuse by persons other than the person for whom it was prescribed. There may be a substantial benefit if abuse of injectable opioids (with the risks of infection, including with HIV and hepatitis B) is suppressed, but methadone maintenance is a cure only if it is the first step towards complete opioid withdrawal by progressive reduction of the methadone dose. Not many addicts achieve this, and of those who do, many relapse later.

Contraindications

1. Respiratory depression or respiratory failure e.g. due to airways obstruction

The respiratory depression caused by methadone can summate with respiratory depression from any other cause to result in serious, or even fatal, respiratory failure. When methadone is used as an analgesic, the stimulation of respiration by pain makes this only a relative contraindication, which emphasizes the special danger of an overdose in any patient with pre-existing respiratory depression. However, it would seldom be safe to use methadone to suppress cough in such a patient.

2. Monoamine oxidase inhibitor drugs given concurrently, or within two weeks before methadone
The manufacturer warns against this, but see Drug Interactions.

3. Obstetric use
The long duration of action is inappropriate for this purpose.

Adverse reactions

Potentially life-threatening effects
The only really serious adverse effect of methadone is respiratory depression. Accumulation of methadone can result in this lasting for several days, especially in children and the elderly.

Acute overdosage
Self-poisoning with methadone is common among dependent individuals with access to it, and iatrogenic overdose is not unknown. Almost always, the main danger to life is from depression of respiration or pulmonary oedema. Antagonism of the methadone by naloxone is usually sufficient, using an infusion of naloxone after the initial dose because the antagonist has a much shorter half life than methadone; naltrexone is a longer-acting alternative to naloxone, and so preferable as an antagonist to methadone. Acidification of the urine will increase the clearance of methadone, if measures other than giving an antagonist are necessary.

Severe or irreversible adverse effects
The use of methadone, like that of may other opioids, is constrained by its potential for producing physical and psychological dependence. Hypotension and the exacerbation of existing asthma may occur due to histamine release.

Symptomatic adverse effects
In common with other opioids, methadone can produce nausea, vomiting and constipation. Sedation and dizziness are common. Euphoria occurs, but may be regarded as beneficial, except in so far as it promotes dependence.

Interference with clinical pathology tests
Methadone may interfere with Frings TLC procedure for measuring urinary alkaloids, and with some pregnancy tests on urine.

High risk groups

Neonates
Particular care is needed to avoid respiratory depression in neonates.

Breast milk. No data are available on passage of methadone into breast milk, but general considerations suggest that the quantity received by the infant by this route would be negligible.

Children
Particular care is needed to avoid respiratory depression in young children.

Pregnant women
Respiratory depression of the neonate precludes the use of methadone near the time of delivery.

The elderly
The reduced renal and hepatic function of the elderly affect both routes of elimination of methadone, but the observed special risk of respiratory failure is not necessarily entirely a pharmacokinetic effect.

Concurrent disease
Liver disease. In common with other opioids, methadone would be expected to precipitate porto-systemic encephalopathy in patients with liver disease.

Drug interactions

Potentially hazardous interactions
Cerebral depressants may have an effect additive to the sedation due to methadone, and this would be expected with alcohol.

Other significant interactions
Pharmacokinetic interactions may pass unnoticed when methadone is used for pain relief, but have been reported as causing overdose or withdrawal in dependent patients stabilized on oral methadone. A decrease in methadone effect is to be expected if the urine is made acid with ammonium chloride, and an increase with sodium bicarbonate or acetazolamide. The acceleration of metabolism by enzyme-inducing drugs (e.g. phenytoin[21] or rifampicin[22]) can diminish the effect of methadone, though other mechanisms may also be at work. A single, but by no means clear-cut, case of increased methadone effect due to enzyme inhibition by cimetidine[23] has been reported.

A serious interaction between monoamine oxidase inhibitors and pethidine does occur in some patients exposed to this drug combination, but despite warnings of this interaction with other opioids, including methadone, there is no evidence that it occurs with opioids other than pethidine.

Potentially useful interactions
The use of antiemetics such as cyclizine[24] to reduce nausea and vomiting, and stimulant laxatives to antagonize constipation, has been referred to, as has the antagonism of methadone overdose by naloxone.

Clinical trials

1. Morrison J D, Loan W B, Dundee J W 1971 Controlled comparison of the efficacy of fourteen preparations in the relief of post-operative pain. British Medical Journal 2: 287–290

This is a double-blind, between-subject trial of different opioids for postoperative analgesia following abdominal surgery, patients being stratified according to whether the surgery involved the upper or the lower abdomen. Some patients received a saline control, and among the opioids used was methadone 10 mg intramuscularly, which was significantly more effective than saline in respect of both the patients' and the observer's estimates.

2. Stetson J B 1974 The clinical testing of weak oral analgesics. Anaesthesia 29: 349–365

A trial primarily designed to test the effectiveness of an oral non-steroidal anti-inflammatory drug for postoperative analgesia was adapted to compare pethidine 150 mg orally with methadone 10 mg orally, given for the same purpose. Response was judged by the proportion of patients requiring additional analgesia within four hours. Ten patients received each treatment, and a between-patient comparison indicated that the effects were similar, and greater than the effect of 75 mg pethidine orally. It is unclear how effectively patients and observers were kept blind, and the nature of the operation varied, but the trial is of interest as an evaluation of oral methadone for postoperative pain.

3. Beaver W T, Wallenstein S L, Houde R W, Rogers A 1967 A clinical comparison of the analgesic effects of methadone and morphine administered intramuscularly, and of orally and parenterally administered methadone. Clinical Pharmacology and Therapeutics 8: 415–426

These double-blind within-patient trials were conducted using brief periods of treatment with each preparation in patients with pain due to malignant disease. Methadone and morphine were compared by giving two doses of each drug intramuscularly, and four such trials using different dose levels were carried out in groups of from 15 to 32 patients. The duration of effect and side effects of morphine and methadone were similar, but methadone was slightly more potent.

In a separate trial, oral and intramuscular methadone were compared in 21 such patients, using a double-dummy technique. The oral preparation of methadone had the expected lower but more prolonged time/effect curve than the same intramuscular dose, so that the oral route was about one-sixth as potent in peak effect, but about one-half as potent in total effect over the time of observation.

General review articles

Eddy N B, Halbach H, Braendon O J 1957 Synthetic substances with morphine like effect. Bulletin of the World Health Organization 17: 619–643

Martin W R 1976 Pharmacology of opioids. Pharmacological Reviews 35: 283–324
Säwe J 1986 High-dose morphine and methadone in cancer patients; clinical pharmacokinetic considerations of oral treatment. Clinical Pharmacokinetics 11: 87–106

References

1. Scott C C, Robbins E B, Chen K K 1948 Pharmacologic comparison of the optical isomers of methadone. Journal of Pharmacology and Experimental Therapeutics 93: 282–286
2. Scott C C, Chen K K 1946 The action of 1,1-diphenyl-1-(dimethylaminoisopropyl)-butanone-2, a potent analgesic agent. Journal of Pharmacology and Experimental Therapeutics 87: 63–71
3. Beeby D, MacIntosh K C, Bailey M et al 1984 Postoperative analgesia for caesarian section using epidural methadone. Anaesthesia 39: 61–63
4. Shir Y 1989 Intrathecal opioids, potency and lipophilicity. Pain 38: 235
5. Isbell H, Eisenmann A J, Wikler A, Frank K 1948 The effects of single doses of 6-dimethylamino-4-4-diphenyl-3-3heptanone (Amidone, Methadon or '10 820') on human subjects. Journal of Pharmacology and Experimental Therapeutics 92: 83–89
6. Martin W R, Jasinski D R, Haertzen C A et al 1973 Methadone — a reevaluation. Archives of General Psychiatry 28: 286–295
7. Martin W R, Kay D C 1977 Effects of Opioid Analgesics and Antagonists on the EEG. In: Longo V G (ed) Handbook of electroencephalography and clinical neurophysiology. Elsevier/North Holland, Amsterdam, vol 7 part C, pp 7C-97–7C-132
8. Dole V P, Kreek M J 1973 Methadone plasma levels sustained by a reservoir of drug in tissue. Proceedings of the National Academy of Sciences USA 70: 10
9. Inturrussi C E, Verebely K 1972 A gas–liquid chromatographic method for the quantitative determination of methadone in human plasma and urine. Journal of Chromatography 65: 361–369
10. Olsen G D 1973 Methadone binding to human plasma proteins. Clinical Pharmacology and Therapeutics 14: 338–343
11. Robinson A E, Williams F M 1971 The distribution of methadone in man. Journal of Pharmacy and Pharmacology 23: 353–358
12. Inturrussi C E, Verebely K 1972 Disposition of methadone in man after a single oral dose. Clinical Pharmacology and Therapeutics 13: 923–930
13. Horns W H, Rado M, Goldstein A 1975 Plasma levels and symptom complaints in patients maintained on daily dosage of methadone hydrochloride. Clinical Pharmacology and Therapeutics 17: 636–649
14. Rosen T S, Pippenger C E 1976 Pharmacologic observations on the neonatal withdrawal syndrome. Journal of Pediatrics 88: 1044–1048
15. Inturrussi C E, Verebely K 1972 The levels of methadone in the plasma in methadone maintenance. Clinical Pharmacology and Therapeutics 13: 633–637
16. Baselt R C, Caserett L J 1972 Urinary excretion of methadone in man. Clinical Pharmacology and Therapeutics 13: 64–70
17. Pohland A Boaz H E, Sullivan H R 1971 Synthesis and identification of metabolites resulting from the biotransformation of d,l-methadone in man and in the rat. Journal of Medicinal Chemistry 14: 194–197
18. Anggard E, Gunne L-M, Holmstand J, McMahon R E, Sandberg C-G, Sullivan H R 1975 Disposition of methadone in methadone maintenance. Clinical Pharmacology and Therapeutics 17: 258–266
19. Misra A L, Mulé S J 1972 Stereospecificity and differential metabolism in vivo of dextro and laevo-methadone-1-^{3}H. Nature 241: 281–283
20. Sullivan H R, Due S L, McMahon R E 1973 Methadone N-oxide in the urine of methadone maintenance subjects — an artifact? Journal of Pharmacy and Pharmacology 25: 1009–1010
21. Finelli P F 1976 Phenytoin and methadone tolerance. New England Journal of Medicine 294: 227
22. Kreek M J, Garfield J N, Gutjahr C L, Giusti L M 1976 Rifampicin-induced methadone withdrawal. New England Journal of Medicine 294: 1104–1106
23. Sorkin E M, Ogawa C S 1983 Cimetidine potentiation of narcotic action. Drug Intelligence and Clinical Pharmacy 17: 60–61
24. Dundee J W, Jones P O 1968 The prevention of analgesic-induced nausea and vomiting by cyclizine. British Journal of Clinical Practice 22: 379–382

Methimazole

Methimazole is the active metabolite of carbimazole and is widely used in the treatment of hyperthyroidism. Apart from that which follows, all details are contained in the section on Carbimazole.

Chemistry

Methimazole (Tapazole)
$C_4H_6N_2S$
1-Methylimidazole-2-thiol

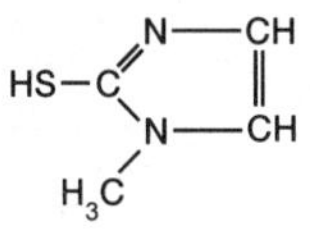

Molecular weight	114.2
pKa	—
Solubility	
in alcohol	1 in 5
in water	1 in 5
Octanol/water partition coefficient	—

Methimazole is a white to pale buff crystalline powder with a faint characteristic odour and slightly bitter taste.

Pharmacokinetics

Methimazole is rapidly and virtually completely absorbed from the gastrointestinal tract. Following a single oral dose of 60 mg given to 11 subjects, peak serum levels of 0.5–2.5 $mg.ml^{-1}$ (mean 1.3) were attained in about 1–3 hours.[1] The plasma half life of methimazole is approximately 3–5 hours, and is prolonged in hepatic and renal disease. Although the plasma half life is relatively short, the biological effects of the drug are much longer lasting.

Methimazole is weakly bound to plasma proteins (approximately 40%) and has a volume of distribution of about 40 l. The drug readily crosses the placenta and is excreted in breast milk (plasma:milk concentration ratio approximately 1).

Methimazole is excreted in the urine, about 12% of the administered dose being eliminated by this route within 24 hours.

Oral absorption	90–100%
Presystemic metabolism	—
Plasma half life	
range	3–5 h
Volume of distribution	0.5 $l.kg^{-1}$
Plasma protein binding	40%

Pharmaceutics

Methimazole USP is available as 5 and 10 mg tablets. It can be formulated for rectal administration for patients unable to take oral medication, producing plasma levels similar to those obtained after oral dosage.[2] Although no preparation exists for intravenous use, methimazole is freely soluble in neutral aqueous solutions and could be prepared for use in severely ill patients with thyrotoxic crisis.

The dosage schedule is similar to that recommended for carbimazole.

M

References

1. Melander A et al 1980 Comparative in vitro effects and in vivo kinetics of antithyroid drugs. European Journal of Clinical Pharmacology 17: 295–299
2. Nabil N, Miner D J, Amatruda J M 1982 Methimazole: an alternative route of administration. Journal of Clinical Endocrinology and Metabolism 54: 180–181

Methionine

Methionine is an essential amino acid.

Chemistry

L-, or DL-Methionine (race methionine)
$C_5H_{11}NSO_2$
Amino-4-(methylthio)butyric acid

$CH_3S{-}CH_2{-}CH_2{-}CHNH_2COOH$

Molecular weight	149.2
pKa (carboxyl)	2.28
pKa (amino)	9.21
Solubility	
in alcohol	very slight
in water	1 in 55
Octanol/water partition coefficient	low

White crystalline flakes or powder with a characteristic rather unpleasant odour. Both the L- and DL-isomers have been used clinically.

The racemic mixture is available in combination with paracetamol (Pameton) it is also an ingredient of Amino-Cerv.

Pharmacology

Methionine plays an essential role in intermediary metabolism. It must first be activated by conversion to S-adenosylmethionine and, as the primary biological methyl donor, is involved in the transmethylation of nucleic acids, proteins, lipids and other metabolites, and in the synthesis of compounds such as choline. Methionine is also converted in the liver to cysteine, which is an important precursor of glutathione. It is demethylated to homocysteine and this condenses with serine to form cystathione which on cleavage yields cysteine. Methionine is claimed to have a so-called lipotrophic action in preventing the development of fatty liver, and it stimulates the release of insulin from the pancreas.

Toxicology

Systematic toxicity studies have not been carried out with methionine. Growth was inhibited in rats fed 2.5 and 4% methionine in their diet for 30 days. Other findings included microcytic hypochromic anaemia, bone marrow hyperplasia and histological changes in the pancreas, gastrointestinal tract, salivary glands, kidney, spleen, thymus, thyroid and adrenals resembling those produced by ethionine.[1,2] In guinea pigs 1.5 g methionine daily produced fatty liver, hypoglycaemia and aminoacidaemia followed by hypothermia, profound hypoglycaemia and death.[3] Methionine depletes hepatic adenosine triphosphate (ATP), and in large doses it causes metabolic acidosis through conversion to inorganic sulphate.

Metabolism

Methionine is converted to homocysteine via S-adenosylmethionine, and about 80% is then sequentially metabolized to cystathione, cysteine, taurine and inorganic sulphate. Cysteine serves as a precursor for the synthesis of glutathione. The D-isomer is converted to the L-form in vivo.

Pharmaceutics

Tablets contain DL-methionine, 250 mg. Pameton (Sterling-Winthrop, UK) contains paracetamol 500 mg with DL-methionine

250 mg. L-Methionine is also one of the amino acids present in solutions for parenteral nutrition. Amino-Cerv cervical cream for use post-cauterization contains urea 8.34% together with selected amino acids including DL-methionine 0.83%.

Therapeutic use

Indications

1. The treatment of severe paracetamol poisoning particularly if N-acetylcysteine is not available, and in patients who are unable to tolerate N-acetylcysteine
Liver damage following overdosage of paracetamol is caused by its metabolic activation and the formation of a reactive arylating intermediate (N-acetyl-p-benzoquinineimine) which is normally conjugated with glutathione.[4] Liver damage does not occur unless glutathione is depleted and methionine is thought to act by facilitating glutathione synthesis via conversion to S-adenosylmethionine, homocysteine, cystathione and cysteine. Methionine added to paracetamol prevented liver injury and death in rats pretreated with phenobarbitone.[5]

Methionine is given orally in a dose of 2.5 g (10 tablets) every four hours to a total dose of 10 g in adults. It must be given within 8 to 10 hours after ingestion of the paracetamol: after this time its protective action falls off rapidly and it is ineffective after 12 to 15 hours. Methionine cannot be considered the treatment of choice for severe paracetamol poisoning since the associated nausea and vomiting may make absorption unreliable and oral administration impracticable. It has been suggested that late treatment with methionine might precipitate or aggravate hepatic encephalopathy, but there is no good evidence for this.

2. In parenteral nutrition as a component of amino-acid mixtures
As an essential amino-acid, methionine is included in the mixture of amino-acids used in solutions for parenteral nutrition.

In the past, oral methionine has been used as an adjunct in the treatment of acute and chronic liver disease. There is no evidence of clinical efficacy for this indication.

Contraindications

1. Advanced chronic liver disease, hepatic failure
Methionine may cause neurological deterioration and encephalopathy in patients with hepatic cirrhosis and portal hypertension.

2. Schizophrenia
Methionine has been reported to precipitate acute reactions in schizophrenic patients.

3. Severe acidosis
In large doses, methionine may aggravate metabolic acidosis.

Adverse reactions

Potentially life-threatening effects
In daily doses of 6 to 20 g, methionine can cause neurological changes and precipitate encephalopathy in patients with hepatic cirrhosis, particularly in the presence of portal hypertension.[6]

Severe or irreversible adverse effects
Doses of 10 to 20 g daily may provoke an acute exacerbation of symptoms in schizophrenic patients.[7]

Symptomatic adverse effects
Nausea, vomiting, drowsiness and irritability may occur.[3]

Major outcome trials

1. Vale J A, Meredith T J, Goulding R 1981 Treatment of acetaminophen poisoning. The use of oral methionine. Archives of Internal Medicine 141: 394–396

132 patients with severe paracetamol poisoning were treated with oral methionine. Of 96 patients given methionine within 10 hours of ingestion of the paracetamol, 7 suffered severe liver damage in comparison with 33 of 57 similarly poisoned patients studied elsewhere before effective treatment became available. Severe liver damage occurred in 17 of the 36 patients given methionine 10 to 24 hours after taking the paracetamol, and 2 died.

Methionine

2. Prescott L F, Park J, Sutherland G R, Smith L J, Proudfoot A T 1976 Cysteamine, methionine and penicillamine in the treatment of paracetamol poisoning. Lancet 2: 109–113

20 patients with severe paracetamol poisoning were given a total dose of 20 g of methionine intravenously over 20 hours within 12 hours of ingestion of the paracetamol. Three developed severe liver damage compared with 28 of 54 patients receiving supportive therapy only.

References

1. Klavins J V, Kinney T D, Kaufman N 1963 Body iron levels and hematologic findings during excess methionine feeding. Journal of Nutrition 79: 101–104
2. Klavins J V, Kinney T D, Kaufman N 1963 Histologic changes in methionine excess. Archives of Pathology 75: 661–673
3. Hardwick D F, Applegarth D A, Cockcroft D M, Ross P M, Calder R J 1970 Pathogenesis of methionine-induced toxicity. Metabolism 19: 381–391
4. Mitchell J R, Thorgiersson S S, Potter W Z, Jollow D J, Keiser H 1974 Acetaminophen-induced hepatic injury: role of glutathione in man and rationale for therapy. Clinical Pharmacology and Therapeutics 16: 676–684
5. McLean A E M, Day P A 1974 The effect of diet on the toxicity of paracetamol and the safety of paracetamol–methionine mixtures. Biochemical Pharmacology 24: 37–42
6. Phear E A, Ruebner B, Sherlock S, Summerskill W H J 1965 Methionine toxicity in liver disease and its prevention by chlortetracycline. Clinical Science 15: 93–117
7. Bowman W C, Rand M J 1980 Textbook of Pharmacology, 2nd edn. Blackwell Scientific Publications, Edinburgh, pp 15–30

M

Methohexitone (sodium)

Methohexitone, a methylated oxybarbiturate, is the only drug of this group which offers any competition to thiopentone as an induction agent. Its use is normally limited to circumstances where its more rapid recovery offers advantages over the older drug.

Chemistry

Methohexitone sodium (Methohexital sodium, Brietal Sodium, Brevital Sodium)
$C_{14}H_{17}N_2NaO_3$
Sodium α-dl-1-methyl-5-allyl-5-(1-methyl-2-pentynyl) barbiturate; 1-methyl-5-(1-methyl-2-pentynyl)-5-(2-pentenyl)-2,4,6(1H,3H,5H)-pyrimidinetrione monosodium salt

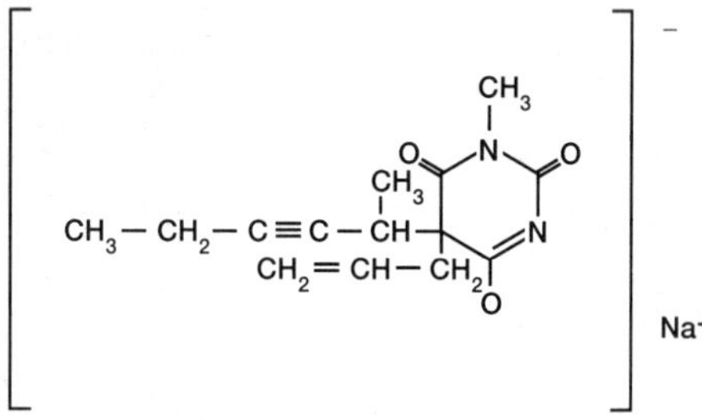

Molecular weight (free acid)	284.3 (262.3)
pKa	8.3
Solubility	
in alcohol	—
in water	>1 in 30
Octanol/water partition coefficient	100

The molecule contains two asymmetric carbon atoms, thus two dl pairs of enantiomers exist. The most desirable configuration is α-dl which is used clinically. The drug is prepared by chemical synthesis, as minute white crystals.

It is not present in any compound preparations.

Pharmacology

Methohexitone reversibly depresses the activity of all excitable tissues. The central nervous system (CNS) is particularly sensitive to its action and single anaesthetic induction doses have remarkably little effect on cardiac or smooth muscle, but induction doses are frequently accompanied by mild excitatory effects (extraneous muscle movement or hypotonus). In healthy subjects it is only with large doses and/or prolonged administration that one encounters serious cardiovascular or respiratory depression and deleterious effects on other systems.

The exact mode of action of the barbiturates is not known, but a likely mechanism is a direct effect on the specialized portions of the neural membrane, modifying synaptic transmission. The ability of a number of agents to depress sodium-dependent excitatory synaptic transmission can be correlated with hydrophobicity which, in turn, is strongly correlated with anaesthetic potency in vivo. Available evidence suggests that excitatory synaptic transmission is mainly depressed by barbiturates while inhibitory synaptic transmission is usually unaffected or enhanced. The site of action appears to be at a component of the GABA-modulated chloride channel rather than on the associated receptor.

The effects of barbiturates on the various pathways and subsystems of the CNS represent the total effect of these complex and diverse actions of the drugs on many millions of individual neurones. For obvious reasons, pathways subserving the maintenance of consciousness and centripetal transfer of sensory information have been the main objects of study in investigations of barbiturate action. The spinal cord dorsal horn has an important modulatory role in the onward transfer of sensory information. Monosynaptic spinal reflexes are depressed by barbiturates, as are spontaneous and evoked activity in dorsal horn cells. Thus, action at spinal cord level contributes to the overall picture of barbiturate anaesthesia. In contrast, the classical sensory pathways of the spinal cord and brain stem, which contain only two or three synapses, appear to be relatively resistant to the effects of barbiturates.

However, information also travels cortically in the multisynaptic reticular formation. The demonstration[1] that stimulation of the reticular formation causes electroencephalographic (EEG) and behavioural arousal suggests that the formation might have a role in the production of the anaesthetic state. Pentobarbitone blocks sensory and auditory cortical evoked responses by a direct action on the reticular formation,[2] while EEG arousal in response to direct reticular stimulation is also blocked by barbiturates.[3] Analysis of the effects of thiopentone on the human sensory evoked response shows that the late component of the response, which is believed to be due to reticular stimulation, is blocked by anaesthetic doses of the drug, while the early, specific component remains intact.[4] These results suggest that reticular formation blockade is an essential component of the mechanism of barbiturate action on the brain. Depression by barbiturates of transmission through the ventrobasal thalamus, has also been attributed to an effect on reticular tone.[5]

Functional denervation of the cortex, through increased inhibitory and decreased facilitatory reticular stimulation of the ventrobasal thalamus, might be a general mechanism of anaesthesia. However, there is no simple relationship between the concentration of a drug which produces anaesthesia and that which blocks cortical evoked responses.[6] Furthermore, the complex effects of barbiturates and other anaesthetics on synaptic transmission in isolated slices of cortex provide evidence of the probable importance of direct cortical effects, as well as effects on ascending systems, in the mechanism of barbiturate anaesthesia.

Toxicology

In a subacute intravenous toxicity study in dogs, there were no effects on haematopoietic, hepatic or renal systems. No drug-induced changes were seen at necropsy and no microscopic changes were seen where the tissues were examined.

Teratogenicity studies in rats and rabbits show no fetal defects related to treatment. No study to determine the mutagenic potential has been performed.

Clinical pharmacology

Adequate doses of methohexitone will induce anaesthesia in one arm–brain circulation time and maximum depression of vital centres occurs within one minute of administration. The plasma concentration necessary for anaesthesia is 10–12 mg.l^{-1} in fit adults.[7,8] The loss of consciousness is accompanied by slight spontaneous muscle movement or tremor of the upper limbs or by hypotension and by hiccough in about 25% of unpremedicated subjects. Methohexitone, like thiopentone, is predictable in its anaesthetic action, but resistance can occur in patients who have developed tolerance to alcohol or other cerebral depressants.

Methohexitone has no analgesic action and small doses may increase sensitivity to somatic pain. This hyperalgesia (antanalgesic) action limits its use as sole anaesthetic, and it has also been demonstrated in the postoperative period following large doses.

The EEG changes with methohexitone have not been studied in the same detail as with thiopentone, but they follow the general pattern of the barbiturates. Likewise its effect on cerebral blood flow has not been studied.

Induction of anaesthesia is accompanied by a fall of around 10% in arterial pressure and a compensatory rise in heart rate of 10–20 beats per minute. The decrease in arterial pressure is due to a decrease in systemic vascular resistance. Cardiac output may fall slightly.

Methohexitone (sodium)

Maintenance of anaesthesia with an infusion of methohexitone is associated with a fall in arterial pressure of 13–33%, a fall in cardiac output of 26–38% and a decrease of 13% in systemic vascular resistance.[9] The incidence of respiratory depression is dose-related and results in some hypoventilation. Apnoea is not uncommon, but is transient (< 30 s). Respiratory upsets such as cough or hiccup have been shown to occur in 20–50% of patients on induction.

Pharmacokinetics

The preferred method of analysis is gas chromatography with nitrogen-selective detection, which has a limit of detection[10] of 50 μg.l^{-1}. Other authors give a sensitivity of 30 μg.l^{-1} for gas chromatography and 20 μg.l^{-1} for HPLC.[11,12]

Methohexitone is not administered by the oral route, being given by intravenous infusion. It is very lipid-soluble and will be largely unionized at the pH of plasma. Hence, it distributes rapidly and extensively throughout the body, rapidly crossing the blood–brain barrier. Drug continues to accumulate in the brain for 30–60 s, and then there is redistribution so that it is localized in body fat, though to a lesser extent than thiopentone. This quickly leads to a decline in the brain levels of the drug.

Methohexitone is quite extensively bound (about 73%) to plasma proteins, presumably mainly albumin. The volume of distribution is approximately 1 l.kg^{-1}. The drug is rapidly eliminated, with a half life of only 1–2 h. The elimination of methohexitone is described by an initial rapid phase, due to distribution to highly perfused tissues, including the brain. This is followed by redistribution to lean tissues, with some contribution from body fat stores. The terminal phase reflects metabolism of the drug and redistribution to poorly perfused fat stores.

Methohexitone is very extensively metabolized in the liver, with less than 1% of the dose being excreted unchanged in the urine in 24 h.[13]

Oral absorption	—
Presystemic metabolism	—
Plasma half life	
range	1–2 h
Volume of distribution	1 l.kg^{-1}
Plasma protein binding	~73%

There is no information on the excretion of methohexitone in breast milk. However, although it is likely that this does occur, its short half life means that refraining from nursing for a relatively short interval (about 12 h) should avoid any potential problems in the infant. It is likely that the drug crosses the placenta.

The effects of age, renal disease and age on the pharmacokinetics of methohexitone are not known.

Metabolism

Methohexitone is extensively metabolized in the liver, the products being excreted in the urine. Less than 1% of the dose is recovered unchanged in the urine in 24 h. The principal route of metabolism is oxidation of the pentynyl side chain, to give 4′-hydroxymethohexitone, which possesses hypnotic activity.[14]

Pharmaceutics

Methohexitone is formulated for parenteral use as Brietal Sodium (Lilly, UK), in vials containing 100 mg, 500 mg and 2.5 g of methohexitone sodium powder. Brevital sodium (Lilly, USA): 500 mg, 2.5 g and 5 g. Anhydrous sodium carbonate is included in the formulation.

Methohexitone is usually prepared freshly before use. A 1% aqueous solution is recommended, although some prefer a 2% solution, because a smaller volume needs to be injected. Solutions are incompatible with silicone or acid solutions. Cloudy solutions should be discarded.

Therapeutic use

Indications

1. For induction of anaesthesia, particularly for short procedures
2. For induction followed by other agents for more prolonged anaesthesia.

Fig. 1 Metabolism of methohexitone

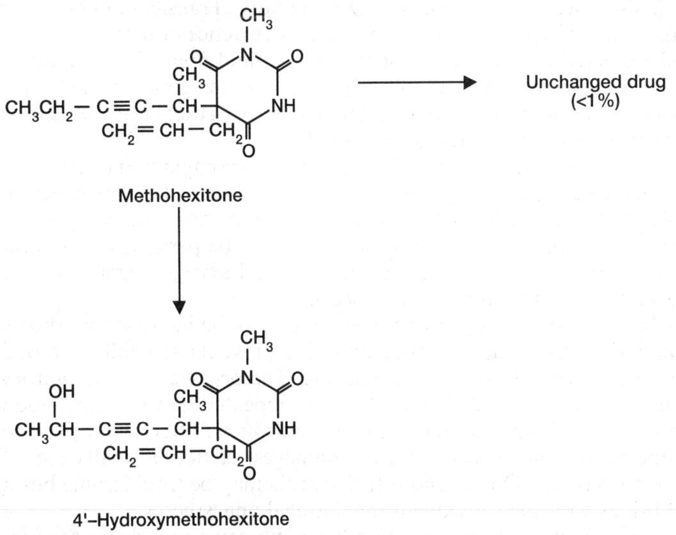

Other uses

3. The use of dilute solutions for maintenance of anaesthesia is being investigated.[8]

Contraindications

1. Hypersensitivity to barbiturates
2. Contraindication to general anaesthesia
3. Patients with a history of porphyria should not receive barbiturates
4. The drug is best avoided in patients taking coumarin-type anticoagulants (see Drug interactions below)
5. A history of epilepsy.

There are, however, some absolute and relative contraindications to intravenous anaesthesia which should be observed. The general contraindications are:

1. Known or suspected full stomach
2. Unavailability of means of resuscitation
3. Inadequate access to patient and airway
4. Lack of facilities for recovery or attendants to take home day-cases.

The following poor risk patients require extra caution in its use:

5. Marked hypovolaemia including blood loss
6. Uraemia
7. History of severe asthma
8. Severe cardiac disease.

Mode of use

Methohexitone is the barbiturate of choice for outpatient anaesthesia.

The drug is given intravenously in doses of 1–1.5 mg.kg^{-1} or 1 or 2% solution, over 30–60 seconds.

The induction dose varies with:

1. Age of the patient
2. Fitness of the patient
3. Premedication
4. Pretreatment with opioids immediately prior to induction.

The normal dose of 1–1.5 mg.kg^{-1} can be as high as 2 mg.kg^{-1} in children and as low as 0.3 mg.kg^{-1} in the elderly.

Subjects with an acquired tolerance to sedatives, hypnotics, opioids or even alcohol, have increased requirements of methohexitone and this may occur in patients with a degree of cardiovascular or other disease which would engender sensitivity to the toxic effects of such doses. This situation is best dealt with by prior administration of a suitable dose of fentanyl or alfentanil.

Indications

1, 2. Induction of anaesthesia

The injection of methohexitone is followed by spontaneous muscle movement and some degree of hypertonus of the upper limbs in about 25% of unpremedicated subjects. The incidence and severity is highest when a large dose is injected rapidly. Transient apnoea may also occur if injection is too rapid. The occurrence of these excitatory effects is reduced to acceptable limits by opioid premedication, but is increased to an unacceptable degree by antanalgesic premedicants such as promethazine and hyoscine. Excitatory effects rapidly subside when inhalational anaesthesia is used.

Hiccough and occasionally coughing accompany induction of anaesthesia in about 25% of unpremedicated subjects. Slow injection of small doses reduces the incidence, as does atropine or hyoscine premedication. On occasions, hiccough may be persistent and upset the course of the subsequent anaesthesia. Laryngospasm is a rare adverse effect in atropinized subjects.

In contrast to thiopentone, heart rate may be increased markedly on induction of anaesthesia, and this prevents the fall in blood pressure seen with the thiobarbiturate. The occurrence of excitatory effects often makes it difficult to make repeated non-invasive blood pressure readings after induction, as patients will frequently react to superficial stimuli because of the antanalgesic action of small doses of the barbiturate. On occasions tachycardia may be troublesome but it subsides with the subsequent inhalational anaesthesia.

Like other barbiturates, methohexitone causes marked vasodilation, with blood shunted from the central pool to the periphery. However, even on repeat administration or prolonged infusion, systolic blood pressure is well maintained because of the compensatory tachycardia. The response to methohexitone varies with the condition of the patient, particularly with regard to blood volume, acid–base balance and cardiovascular disease and hypertension: these relate mainly to the ability to compensate for the effects of peripheral vasodilation. Concurrent or previous administration of drugs which themselves cause vasodilation or reduce compensatory tachycardia will also enhance the hypotensive effect of methohexitone. It abolishes the compensatory vasoconstriction produced by an increase in intrathoracic pressure and persistent hypotension can accompany hyperventilation. In the absence of hypercarbia, arrhythmias are uncommon after methohexitone.

In clinical doses methohexitone causes a greater degree of respiratory depression, but this is of shorter duration than with thiopentone. It is not a problem in fit patients except after 'heavy' opiate premedication. As with most anaesthetics, the sensitivity of the respiratory centre to carbon dioxide is depressed proportionately to the depth of anaesthesia. In deep anaesthesia the action of hypoxia on the carotid sinus plays an important part in the maintenance of respiration but the shift of control of respiration from carbon dioxide retention may be particularly difficult to detect since the thiopentone may also obtund the usual rise in pressure which it causes.

In common with other anaesthetics, oliguria occurs during methohexitone anaesthesia — partly as the result of reduction in renal blood flow and partly from an increase in circulating antidiuretic hormone. This is of no clinical importance. Therapeutic doses have no effect on the tone of the gravid uterus, but tone is reduced in deep anaesthesia.

Theoretically methohexitone can induce an acute attack in patients with latent porphyria. This is brought about by stimulation of ALA synthetase, the enzyme which catalyses the rate-limiting reaction for haem production. The outcome is so serious that any suspicion of porphyria should be an absolute contraindication to the use of methohexitone.

Other uses

3. Maintenance of anaesthesia

Methohexitone has been used to maintain anaesthesia by incremental bolus dosing and by infusion. Incremental bolus dosing has been used during bronchoscopy, tonsillectomy and dental surgery.[15,16] Methohexitone has also been used as an infusion at rates[9,17] of 60–120 $\mu g.kg^{-1}.min^{-1}$. However, cumulation has been noted after a total dose of 600 mg and an upper limit of 2 h for infusion has been recommended.[18] Methohexitone has been administered rectally as 1, 2 and 10% solutions to induce anaesthesia in children.[19]

Adverse reactions

Potentially life-threatening effects

Hypersensitivity reactions. These are rare with methohexitone, occurring in about 1 in 30 000 patients.[20] It is often difficult to distinguish between relative overdose ('normal' dose given to an unfit patient) and true hypersensitivity to methohexitone. The latter resembles the effects of histamine liberation and might involve this as an intermediary. The clinical picture is one of sudden onset of pallor, cardiovascular collapse (tachycardia and hypotension) and bronchospasm. The latter is most difficult to treat, but the hypotension, due to sudden expansion of the cardiovascular tree, usually responds rapidly to rapid colloid infusion and vasopressors. There is also usually a slight delay in onset of action of the anaesthetic.

Acute overdosage

The main effects of mild or moderate overdosage are respiratory depression and hypotension, which should be managed by assisted ventilation and cautious plasma volume expansion. Intentional self-poisoning with massive doses by the intravenous route is unlikely, but should be managed by respiratory and cardiovascular support. Forced diuresis will be ineffective. No data are available on the use of haemodialysis or haemoperfusion.

Severe or irreversible adverse effects

Accidental intra-arterial injection may be followed by the production of platelet aggregates and thrombosis, starting in arteriole distal to the site of injection. The resulting necrosis may lead to gangrene, which may require amputation.

Symptomatic adverse effects

Local effects. Pain on injection will be noted by the patient in 20–30% of cases, especially where small veins on the back of the hand are used. This is a transient experience and patients should be warned in advance of its possibility. Methohexitone given subcutaneously will cause less tissue damage than thiopentone, and the drug has been given intramuscularly to children. Sequelae after intra-arterial injection are less severe than after thiopentone.

High risk groups

Neonates

The drug may be used in neonates if indicated, in appropriate doses.

Breast milk. No data are available, but it seems likely that a mother receiving the drug could resume breast-feeding within a few days.

Children

Methohexitone may be used in children in appropriate doses.

Pregnant women

The safety of methohexitone in pregnancy has not been established.

The elderly

The drug may be used in elderly patients, but special care should be exercised in the presence of circulatory, respiratory, endocrine, hepatic or renal disease.

Concurrent disease

The drug is contraindicated in patients suffering from porphyria.

Methohexitone is not recommended for use in patients with a history of epilepsy as psychomotor seizure may be provoked.

Drug interactions

The effects of various premedicants on the incidence of excitatory upset and respiratory complications during induction have already been discussed. All barbiturates are inducers of hepatic microsomal drug-metabolizing enzymes, but the significance of this in anaesthetic practice has not been studied. If it behaves like thiopentone[21] this will be of no significance.

Clinical trials

The clinical use of methohexitone has been compared with that of thiopentone, etomidate and propofol.

Thiopentone

Dundee J W, Moore J 1961 Thiopentone and methohexitone. A comparison as main anaesthetic agents for a standard operation. Anaesthesia 16: 50

Induction time is similar. There is a lower incidence of hypotension with methohexitone and more rapid recovery. There is a higher incidence of excitatory phenomena with methohexitone.

Etomidate and propofol

Wells J K G 1985 Comparison of ICI 35 868, etomidate and methohexitone for day-case anaesthesia. British Journal of Anaesthesia 59: 732

Induction time is similar with all three drugs. There is a greater fall in arterial pressure with propofol than with methohexitone or etomidate. The increase in heart rate is greater with methohexitone. Excitatory phenomena were noted with all agents: propofol 12%, methohexitone 55%, etomidate 64%.

References

1. Moruzzi G, Magoun H W 1949 Brain stem reticular formation and activation of the EEG. Electroencephalography and Clinical Neurophysiology 1: 455–473
2. French J D, Verzeano M, Magoun H W 1953 An extralemniscal sensory system in the brain. Archives of Neurology and Psychiatry 69: 505–518
3. Arduini A, Arduini M G 1954 Effect of drugs and metabolic alterations on brain stem arousal mechanism. Journal of Pharmacology and Experimental Therapeutics 110: 76–85
4. Abrahamian H A, Allison T, Goff W R, Rosner B S 1963 Effects of thiopental human cerebral evoked responses. Anaesthesiology 24: 650–657
5. King E E, Naquet R, Magoun H W 1957 Alterations in somatic afferent transmission through thalamus by central mechanisms and barbiturates. Journal of Pharmacology and Experimental Therapeutics 119: 48–63
6. Clarke D L, Rosner B S 1973 Neurophysiologic effects of general anaesthetics. I: The electroencephalogram and sensory evoked responses in man. Anaesthesiology 38: 564–582
7. Dundee J W, McMurray T J 1984 Clinical aspects of total intravenous anaesthesia. Journal of the Royal Society of Medicine 77: 669–672
8. McMurray T J, Robinson F P, Dundee J W, Riddell J G, McClean E 1986 A method for producing constant plasma concentrations of drugs. British Journal of Anaesthesia 58: 1085–1090
9. Prys-Robert C, Sear J W, Low J M, Phillips K C, Dagnino J 1983 Hemodynamic and hepatic effects of methohexital infusion during nitrous oxide anaesthesia in humans. Anesthesia and Analgesia 62: 317
10. Heusler H et al 1981 Journal of Chromatography 226. Biomedical Applications 15: 403–412
11. Brand L, Mark L C, Snell M M Vrindten P, Dayton P G 1963 Physiological disposition of methohexital in man. Anesthesiology 24: 331
12. Breimer D D 1976 Pharmacokinetics of methohexitone following intravenous infusion in man. British Journal of Anaesthesia 48: 643
13. Murphy P J 1974 Biotransformation of Methohexital. Internation Anesthesiology Clinics 12: 139
14. Welles J S, McMahon R E, Doran W J 1963 The metabolism and excretion of methohexital in the rat and dog. Journal of Pharmacology and Experimental Therapeutics 139: 166–171
15. Hargrove R L, Pearce D J 1964 An anaesthetic technique for bronchoscopy. Anaesthesia 19: 226
16. Mann P E, Hatts S D, Dixon R A, Griffin K D, Perks E R, Thornton J A 1971 A minimal increment methohexitone technique in conservative dentistry. Anaesthesia 26: 3
17. Jessop E, Grounds R M, Morgan M, Lumley J 1985 Comparison of infusions of propofol and methohexitone to provide light general anaesthesia under regional blockade. British Journal of Anaesthesia 57: 1173
18. Sear J W 1983 General kinetic and dynamic principles and their application to continuous infusion anaesthesia. Anaesthesia 38: 10
19. Forbes R B, Murray D J, Dillman J B, Dull D L 1989 Pharmacokinetics of 2% rectal methohexitone in children. Canadian Journal of Anaesthesia 36: 160
20. Clarke R S J 1981 Adverse effects of intravenously administered drugs used in anaesthetic practice. Drugs 22: 26–41
21. Fee J P H, Dundee J W 1986 Antipyrine elimination is not increased by a single induction dose of thiopentone. British Journal of Clinical Pharmacology 22: 224P

Methotrexate

Methotrexate is an antimetabolite that is an analogue of folic acid. It is widely used in cancer chemotherapy and immunosuppresion.

Chemistry

Methotrexate, amethopterin

$C_{20}H_{22}N_8O_5$

L-(d)-N-[4-([2,4-Diamino-6-pteridinylmethyl]methylamino) benzoyl glutamic acid

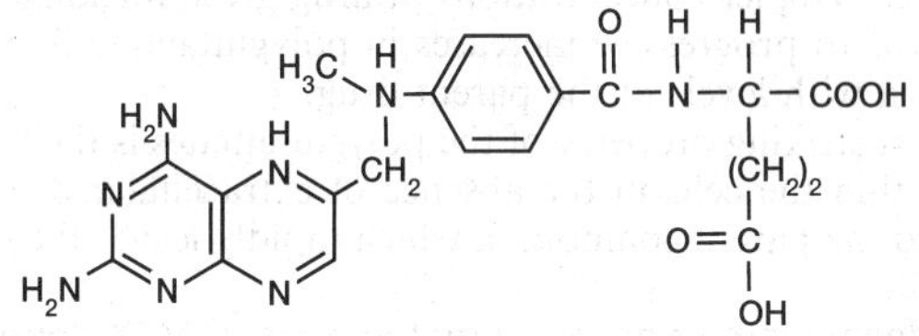

Molecular weight	454.5
pKa (of designated functional group)	4.8, 5.5
Solubility	
in alcohol	practcally insoluble
in water	practcally insoluble
Octanol/water partition coefficient	—

It is a yellow to orange-brown crystalline powder. Methotrexate is also prepared for use as the sodium salt (Maxtrex).

Pharmacology

Methotrexate (MTX), the most widely used antimetabolite, is a folic acid antagonist. It has an essential role in the treatment of acute lymphocytic leukaemia, choriocarcinoma, non-Hodgkin's lymphoma, osteosarcoma, head and neck cancer, and breast cancer.[1,2] It is a therapeutic alternative in the treatment of severe psoriasis,[3] suppression of graft-versus-host disease after bone marrow transplantation[4] and various rheumatic diseases.[5]

MTX is the 4-NH_2, N^{10}-methyl analogue of folic acid. Current concepts of the drug's mechanism of action are illustrated in Fig. 1. MTX enters cells through the active transport system used by the physiologic circulating folate N^5-methyltetrahydrofolate (5m-FH_4) and by N^5-formyl-F_4 (leucovorin or folinic acid), which is used as a rescue agent after high-dose therapy.[6–8] There is a second, albeit less efficient, drug entry mechanism that comes into play at high concentrations of MTX (in excess of 20–50 μM).[9–11] Because this second mechanism accounts for the major fraction of drug that enters the cell at high concentrations, this carrier-independent uptake provides a rationale for the clinical use of high-dose methotrexate. After entering the cells, MTX quickly binds to and inactivates dihydrofolate reductase (DHFR). This enzyme plays a crucial role in maintaining intracellular reduced folate (FH_4) pools by reducing dihydrofolic acid (FH_2),which is produced during thymidylate synthesis. Since the latter is the only reaction that converts the reduced folate to the inactive oxidized FH^2, the underlying rate of thymidylate synthesis is an important determinant of cytotoxicity.[12–15]

The critical result produced by inhibition of DHFR is depletion of intracellular pools of reduced folate (FH^4). In the presence of active thymidylate synthesis, this inhibition leads to accumulation of FH^2. High FH_2concentrations then compete with MTX for binding to

M

DHFR. Because of this competition, an excess of unbound, or 'free', MTX, above the amount required for simple titration of DHFR binding sites, is required in the cytosol to block FH_2 reduction to FH_4.[16–18]

Thymidylate synthetase is the enzyme most sensitive to the depletion of FH_4, or actually N^{5-10}-methylene-FH_4. The synthesis of thymidylate ceases at concentrations of 1×10^{-8} M MTX. 19 N10-formyl-FH_4, the folate involved in both folate-dependent steps of purine synthesis,[20] is also depleted by blockade of DHFR. The cessation of purine synthesis occurs at MTX concentrations of 1×10^{-7} M.[21] The lack of either thymidylate or purines blocks synthesis of DNA.

Like the physiological folates, MTX is extensively metabolized intracellularly to polyglutamate derivatives (Fig. 1). Although first observed in red cells,[22] polyglutamates of methotrexate have been found in livers[23] and other tissues[24–26] of patients who had received MTX.[23] MTX polyglutamate synthesis increases with drug concentration and duration of exposure to the drug. In human breast cancer cells, notable formation of MTX polyglutamates occurs only after 6 hours of incubation at a concentration of 2 μM MTX, a concentration–time profile easily achieved with high-dose MTX therapy but not with small 'conventional' doses[26,27] of 15–50 $mg.m^{-2}$ of body surface area. Higher concentrations of drug given for longer periods of time lead to progressive increases in polyglutamate formation in comparison with levels of the parent drug.

The most striking property of the polyglutamates is their ability to remain within the cells in the absence of extracellular drug,[26,27] in contrast to the parent compound, which rapidly leaves the cells after the extracellular drug disappears. Retention is clearly influenced by chain length: the derivatives that contain three or four additional glutamates are retained for up to 24 hours in the absence of external drug,[26] whereas the compounds with a shorter chain length have proportionally shorter retention times. Longer retention is associated with prolonged inhibition of DHFR and extended cytotoxicity.[27]

In addition to inhibiting DHFR, the MTX polyglutamates inhibit other folate-requiring enzymes not affected directly by MTX. It is well established that physiologic folate polyglutamates have a much greater affinity for folate-requiring enzymes than do the corresponding monoglutamated derivatives.[28] The addition of one additional glutamyl residue to MTX transforms the drug into a potent direct inhibitor of both thymidylate synthetase[29] and aminoimidazole carboxamide ribonucleotide transformylase;[30] the latter is one of the enzymes involved in de novo purine synthesis.

From studies of experimental MTX resistance, it is clear that resistant cells may display any one or more of the following changes.

Decreased membrane transport. Tumour cells exposed to MTX in vitro may become drug resistant because of impairment of the active uptake system[10,31] through a decrease in the affinity of the carrier for MTX.

Decreased affinity of DHFR for MTX. Experimental tumour cells resistant to MTX may have an altered DHFR that may differ in molecular weight[32] from the wild-type enzyme, may have a binding affinity for MTX that is decreased from 2.5- to 270-fold,[33–35] or may retain its affinity for antifolates other than MTX.[36]

Increased levels of DHFR. Experimental tumour cells and human tumours have both been found to express increased amounts of

Fig. 1 Mechanism of action of methotextrate. MTX denotes methotrexate, DHFR dihydrofolate reductase, TS thymidylate synthase, FH_4 tetrahydrofolate, FH_2 dihydrofolate, Glu glutamyl, dTMP thymidylate, and dUMP dioxyuridylate. Broken lines indicate enzyme inhibition

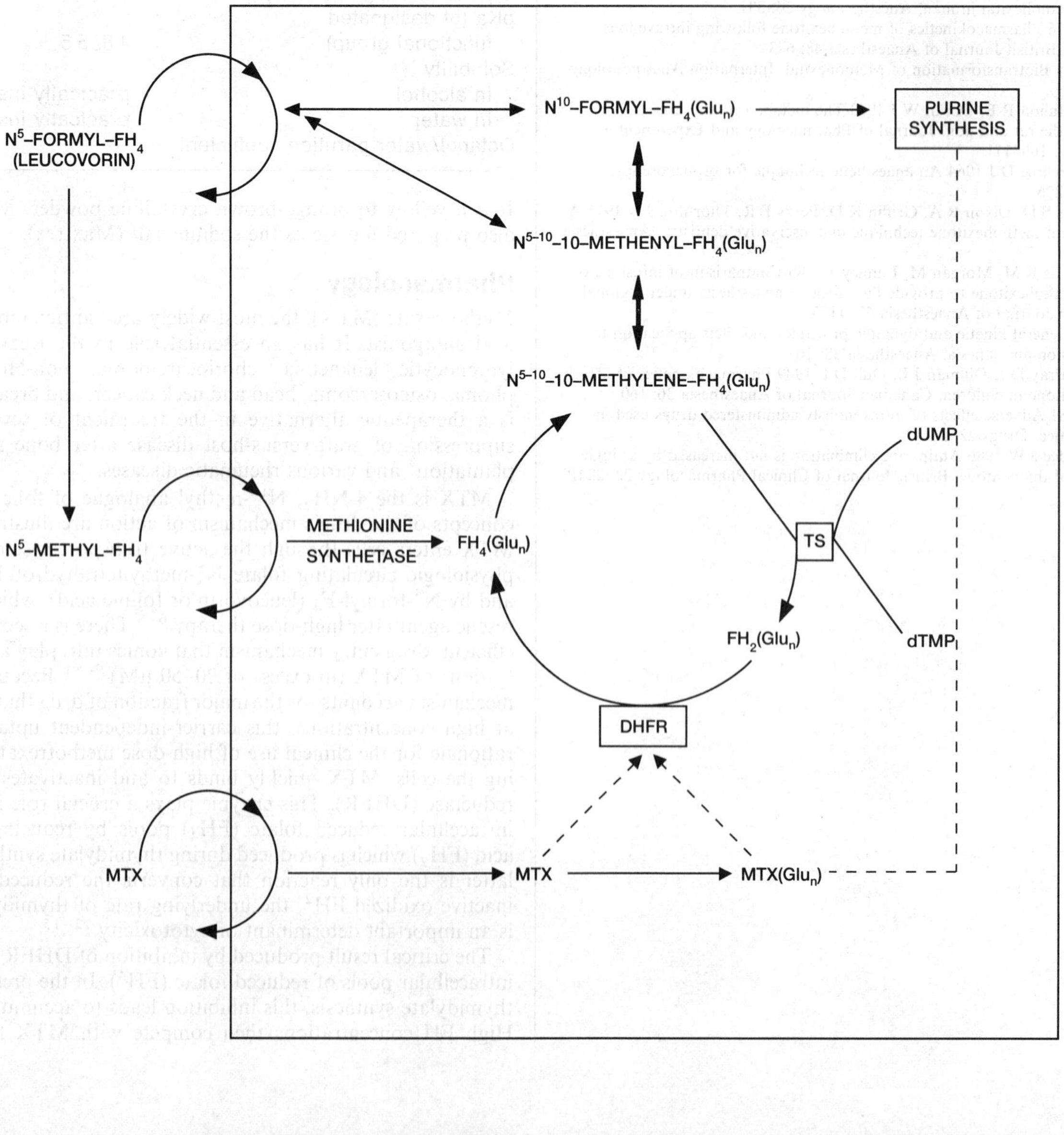

DHFR due to increased numbers of genes coding for the enzyme. This process is known as gene amplification. It can be expressed as an expanded homogeneously staining region (HSR) on elongated chromosomes[32,37,38] or as small bodies of extrachromosomal DNA, termed 'double minutes'.[39,40] The latter has been reported from human tumour cell lines isolated from patients who have received MTX.[40]

The type of cytogenetic abnormality present in drug-resistant cells determines the stability of resistance. Since double minutes lack centromeres, they segregate unequally into daughter cells during mitosis. In the absence of selective pressure, such as that from the cytotoxic drug, the daughter cells containing double minutes do not have a growth advantage and the tumour population may revert to sensitivity if the drug is withdrawn.

Decreased polyglutamation. Although it is clear that polyglutamation allows enhanced accumulation of free drug, extends drug action, and promotes inhibition of additional enzymes, evidence that the absence of polyglutamation may be responsible for resistance is still preliminary. A resistant human breast cancer cell line in which decreased polyglutamate formation played a part in drug resistance has been described.[41] The biochemical defect in this resistant cell line has not been extensively characterized. Studies of three cell lines from patients with small-cell carcinoma indicated that drug sensitivity in these cells was correlated with the ability to form long-chain polyglutamates.

Thymidylate synthetase activity. As noted above, many investigators have found that the underlying rate of thymidylate synthesis is an important determinant of MTX cytotoxicity. Lower rates of thymidylate synthesis make cells less susceptible to MTX.[12–15] Further studies of human tumours will be required to determine the role of this pathway in clinical MTX resistance.

Toxicology

MTX seriously interferes with embryogenesis.

Clinical pharmacology

The critical determinants of MTX cytotoxicity are drug concentration and duration of cell exposure. Cells in cycle are sensitive to methotrexate, with the epithelial cells of the mouth and gastrointestinal tract more sensitive than those of the bone marrow. Myelosuppression and mucositis reach their maximum in 5–14 days after a bolus dose or short-term infusion, and recovery is usually rapid thereafter. The threshold for the sensitivity of human tumour cells to MTX has not been established, but it is clear that drug concentrations much higher than 1×10^{-8}M may be required to inhibit DNA synthesis in resistant cells. Cells with greatly increased DHFR levels may be resistant to drug concentrations above achievable plasma levels (>1 mM).[42,43] Under experimental conditions, there is evidence of a dose–response relationship. High doses are able to overcome drug resistance due to a transport defect[9] and will penetrate sanctuary sites more effectively. Although pharmacologically very logical, there remains some doubt about the clinical effectiveness of high dose methotrexate and convincing evidence from randomized clinical trials is lacking and further studies are needed. Since in vitro experiments have established that cell kill increases with increasing drug concentration,[44] support for regimens that achieve drug concentrations above 1×10^{-6}M is justified. Additionally, since duration of exposure is important, brief periods of exposure (under 6 hours) are less effective than longer periods in producing cell kill.[44,45] The duration of action of methotrexate is difficult to quantify but clearly dependant on both serum and cellular concentrations. Methotrexate is usually administered intravenously every one to three weeks, the time between treatments allowing recovery of normal cells.

Pharmacokinetics

A necessary element in a rational treatment design is a method for monitoring drug concentrations in plasma. The methods include competitive protein binding,[46] radioimmunoassay,[47] and the enzyme-linked immunoassay.[48] They provide extremely sensitive measurements at drug concentrations of 10^{-8}M or less in biological fluids as well as being rapid and fairly specific.[1]

MTX is well absorbed from the gastrointestinal tract by the active transport system, which is also used by physiologic folates[49,50] at doses below 30 mg.m^{-2}. With optimal absorption, doses of 20 mg.m^{-2} produce peak blood levels of approximately 1×10^{-6}M. The peak occurs between one and five hours after drug administration, and drug levels remain at above 1×10^{-7}M for approximately six hours.[51] At higher doses there is strong evidence for reduced MTX bioavailability. The bioavailability of 50 mg.m^{-2} is only 20–50%, as determined by pharmacokinetic comparison of plasma drug concentration after oral versus intravenous administration.[52] With still larger doses (200 mg.m^{-2}) absorption decreases to approximately 25%.

It should be remembered that drug absorbed in the intestine enters the portal circulation and thus must pass through the liver, where hepatocellular uptake, polyglutamation, and storage all occur. Orally administered drug is further subject to degradation by intestinal flora to DAMPA (2,4-diamino-N^{10}-methyl pteroic acid), a metabolite that is inactive pharmacologically[53] but which cross-reacts in the commonly used radioimmunoassay system for MTX. Drugs taken orally are also subject to the variability of intestinal absorption created by drug-induced epithelial denudation, motility changes, and alterations in flora. Other factors such as food,[54] presence of other drugs such as metoclopramide, and dosage form of MTX, liquid versus tablet,[55] can all affect the bioavailability of MTX.

The volume of distribution of MTX is approximately that of total body water. The drug is loosely bound to serum albumin, with approximately 60% binding at or above 1×10^{-6}M concentration in plasma.[56] It can be displaced from this binding by weak organic acids such as aspirin,[57] but this displacement has no proven clinical significance. As a weak organic acid, MTX is negatively charged at neutral pH, has limited lipid solubility, and therefore diffuses slowly across physiologic membranes. At steady state, drug levels in the cerebrospinal fluid (CSF) are 3% of those in plasma during a constant intravenous drug infusion.[58] This slow rate of diffusion that inhibits influx into a compartment may become an advantage in slowing egress from the same site, and has become the basis for direct intracavitary therapy such as into the abdominal, pleural, or lumbar or cranial cavities.[59]

Intrathecally injected drug distributes in a total volume of approximately 120 ml for persons over 3 years of age. Thus a maximal total dose of 12 mg is advised for all persons over 3 years. For those patients younger than 3, the following dosages have been advised: 6 mg for age 1 and younger, 8 mg for ages 1 to 2, and 10 mg for ages 2 to 3.[60] MTX administered into the lumbar space distributes poorly over the cerebral convexities and into the ventricular space,[58] a problem that can be corrected by direct intraventricular injection via an Ommaya reservoir.[61] Distribution is further impaired if the patient is allowed to assume an upright position immediately after the lumbar puncture.[62]

Intravenous infusions of extremely large doses (15–30 g.m^{-2}) of MTX are required to achieve CSF drug levels that approximate those achieved by intrathecal therapy with 12 mg. Regimens employing lower doses of MTX (500 mg.m^{-2}) have not been effective in preventing meningeal leukaemic relapse,[63] probably in part because of substantial interpatient variability in the level achieved in the CSF.[64] The relative efficacy and toxicity of systemic versus intrathecal MTX regimens are now being evaluated in ongoing trials with patients who have childhood leukaemia.

Conventional doses of 25–100 mg.m^{-2} produce peak plasma concentrations of $1–10 \times 10^{-6}$M, while high-dose infusion regimens using 1.5 g.m^{-2} or greater yield peak levels of $1–10 \times 10^{-4}$M.[65] Following the initial distribution phase, which lasts a few minutes, at least two phases of drug disappearance from plasma are observed. The first has a half life of 2–3 hours, is unrelated to dose, and is largely determined by renal excretion of MTX.[66] The final phase of drug disappearance has a considerably longer half life of 8–10 hours, is affected by dose, and may further lengthen in patients with renal dysfunction or third-space fluid.[65,67] Following conventional doses of 25–100 mg.m^{-2}, this terminal phase begins at drug concentration above the threshold for toxicity to bone marrow (1×10^{-8}M) and gastrointestinal epithelium (5×10^{-9}M).[19] Prolongation of the terminal half life is likely to be associated with significant and unexpected toxicity, and this can occur because of third-space retention of drug. In patients with ascites or pleural fluid, there is a slow re-entry of sequestered drug into the bloodstream.[67] Additional intrathecally injected MTX will also provide a slow-release reservoir of MTX into the bloodstream. No strict guidelines for dose and adjustment have been provided by the few studies of MTX pharmacokinetics in patients with third-space accumulations; however, it is advisable to evacuate this fluid before treatment, to monitor plasma drug concentration, and to reduce dosage in proportion to the terminal half life of the drug.

Intrathecal MTX in a dose of 12 mg gives a peak CSF concentration of 1×10^{-4}M. The lumbar CSF concentration declines in a biphasic pattern with half lives of 1.7 and 6.6 hours.[68] MTX exits from the CSF by two mechanisms: as a passive passenger in the reabsorption of CSF (bulk flow) and by an active transport process. The terminal phase of elimination may be prolonged in patients with active meningeal disease, increased intracranial pressure,[68] in those of older age,[69] or in the presence of probenecid.[68]

The use of MTX by constant infusion offers the advantage of providing predictable blood and CSF concentrations for a specific period. The following formulae have been used for achieving a desired plasma concentration in a patient with normal renal function:[60]

1. Priming dose ($mg.m^{-2}$) = (1.5×10^7).[MTX]plasma
2. Infusion dose ($mg.m^{-2}.h^{-1}$) = (3×10^6).[MTX]plasma.

An approximate correction for renal function may be made by reducing the infusion doses in proportion to the reduction in creatinine clearance, based on a normal creatinine clearance of 60 $ml.min^{-1}.m^{-2}$.

The bulk of drug is excreted in the urine in the first 12 hours after administration. Estimates of the percentage of renal excretion vary from 44% to virtually 100% of the administered dose,[65,70–72] and the higher figure is likely to be correct in patients with normal renal function. MTX clearance by the kidney has been found to exceed creatinine clearance in most studies.[73,74]

The renal excretion mechanism of MTX has not been elucidated in man, but in the dog and monkey active secretion of MTX takes place in the proximal renal tubule, with reabsorption in the distal tubule.[75] The high clearance values in excess of creatinine clearance suggest active tubular secretion occurs in the human kidney.

MTX secretion is inhibited by the weak organic acid, aspirin,[57] and by probenecid, an inhibitor of organic acid secretion.[76] Simultaneous folinic acid (leucovorin) administration blocks MTX reabsorption, suggesting the folinic acid might accelerate MTX excretion in high-dose rescue regimens.

During high-dose infusions, rapid drug excretion may lead to MTX concentrations approaching 1×10^{-2}M that exceed the solubility of the drug below pH 7.0 and are believed to be responsible for intrarenal precipitation of drug leading to renal failure. Thus, in high-dose regimens, hydration ($1.5\ l.m^{-2}$ 12 hours prior to treatment and continuing for 24 hours after treatment) and alkalinization (100 mEq bicarbonate per litre hydration fluid) of the urine are recommended in order to avoid renal toxicity. Intensive hydration does not affect the clearance of MTX or the plasma pharmacokinetics, aside from its effects that are related to prevention of renal damage.[77,78] A study has looked at the effect of vitamin C (1–3 g daily) on low-dose MTX excretion and found no change in excretion.[79] However, caution should be observed in administering vitamin C, an inhibitor of organic acid tubular secretion, to patients receiving high-dose MTX, as levels of 4–8 g per day of vitamin C could possibly cause urine acidification.

Oral absorption (dose-dependent)	25–50%
Presystemic metabolism	—
Plasma half life	
range	8–10 h
Volume of distribution	1 $l.kg^{-1}$
Plasma protein binding	60%

Concentration–effect relationship

As with most cytotoxic drugs there is no clear relationship between the plasma concentration of methotrexate and its therapeutic effect. However, plasma levels of less than 1×10^{-8}M are unlikely to achieve antineoplastic effects.[19] Some cells may require much higher concentrations.[42,43] Duration of exposure to the drug seems to be as important as the actual concentration.

Plasma concentrations of methotrexate are important in predicting toxicity (see Table 3). Therefore monitoring of methotrexate concentrations is usually recommended at 24 or 28 hours after dose initiation.

Concentrations of more than 5×10^{-6}M at 24 hours or more than 1×10^{-7}M at 48 hours usually need high-dose leucovorin to prevent toxicity to the bone marrow and gastrointestinal epilethium.[98]

Metabolism

MTX undergoes uptake, storage, and metabolism in the liver. It is transported into hepatocytes by an active uptake system that has a high-affinity, low-capacity carrier[80] and by a low-affinity, high-capacity mechanism.[81] The low-affinity system appears to be distinct from that used by the naturally occurring reduced folates. In the hepatocyte, MTX is converted to polyglutamate forms that can persist for several months after drug administration.[23] The parent drug also undergoes excretion into the biliary tract and is reabsorbed into the systemic circulation from the small intestines. Hepatic uptake and biliary excretion of MTX is affected by other chemotherapeutic agents.[82] Vincristine and cyclophosphamide inhibit both hepatic uptake and biliary excretion, but the net effect of these actions is to produce a fall in intrahepatic drug concentration. Actinomycin D strongly inhibits biliary secretion of MTX, with little effect on hepatic uptake, and causes a marked increase in intrahepatic levels of the drug. The pharmacokinetic effects of these drug interactions have not been examined in detail in man; the possibility exists that the combination of MTX and actinomycin D may increase MTX levels in liver and enhance its hepatic toxicity.

There are widely divergent estimates of the quantitative importance of biliary excretion of MTX in man.[72,83,84] Recent studies indicate that probably a high percentage enters the biliary system but is reabsorbed by the intestines.[72,85] Less than 10% of an intravenous dose of MTX is eliminated in the faeces. An undefined fraction is, however, metabolized to the inactive derivative DAMPA.[86] The intraluminal metabolism of MTX by intestinal flora can be reduced by non-absorbable antibiotics such as kanamycin.[84]

Fig. 2 Metabolism of methotrexate

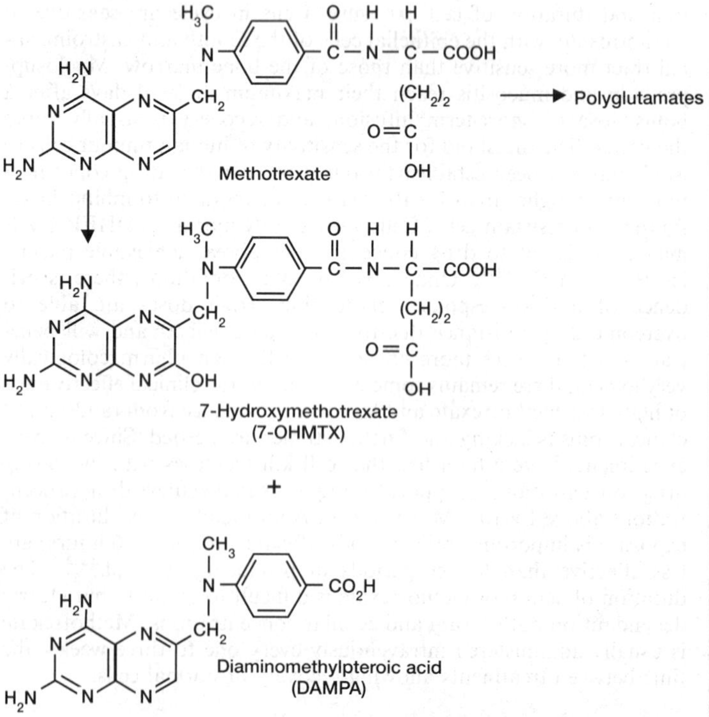

MTX is metabolized to 7-hydroxy methotrexate (7-OH-MTX) and 2,4-diamino-N^{10}- methyl pteroic acid (DAMPA) (Fig. 2). 7-OH-MTX constitutes 20–46% of material excreted in the urine in the time interval between 12 and 24 hours after the start of the infusion. The fraction of drug in the form of metabolite was estimated to be as high as 86% in the time period from 24 to 48 hours.[87] DAMPA becomes an important fraction of drug-derived material at later time points, comprising a mean of 25% of material excreted in the time interval

Methotrexate

from 24 to 48 hours.[53] Neither of these metabolites contributes a majority fraction of total material excreted in the urine, but both are known to accumulate in plasma in increasingly high percentages at later time points, at 24 to 48 hours after high-dose MTX administration. They account for most of the MTX-derived material found in plasma. In fact, 7-OH-MTX has been found to reach equivalent plasma levels with MTX 10 hours after bolus administration. At 24 hours, the ratio of 7-OH to MTX was between 1:1 and 30:1 in eight patients studied.[88]

The sites of MTX metabolism have not been definitively identified. The 7-OH metabolite is probably formed by aldehyde oxidase in the liver. This reaction has been clearly demonstrated in rabbits but not in man. Dosage adjustment does not appear to be necessary for patients with hepatic dysfunction or a history of previous methotrexate treatment. The pteroic acid metabolite, DAMPA, is probably formed by the action of bacterial carboxypeptidases in the gastrointestinal tract; enzymes specific for glutamate terminal peptide bonds have been characterized from bacterial sources,[89] but not from mammalian tissues.

The role of these metabolites in producing MTX toxicity or therapeutic activity is uncertain. Both 7-OH-MTX and DAMPA have lesser solubility than the parent drug. More than 50% of precipitated intrarenal material was 7-OH-MTX in MTX-induced renal failure in monkeys,[87] but the role of either metabolite in the clinical syndrome of renal toxicity secondary to MTX is unproved.

Neither metabolite retains significant ability to inhibit DHFR. The 7-OH metabolite has one-tenth the activity of MTX, and DAMPA has less than one-hundredth the inhibitory activity. Transport of 7-OH-MTX into cells is mediated by the MTX-tetrahydrofolate cofactor carrier, having a K_m twice that of MTX. It also causes efflux of MTX from cells. Thus, in high-dose regimens the presence of high concentrations of 7-OH-MTX in the plasma may cause reduced cellular uptake and/or increased efflux of MTX from cells.[90,91]

As mentioned previously, MTX may also be converted to polyglutamate forms in the liver and probably other tissues as well, but as yet there is no evidence that this conversion significantly affects the plasma pharmacokinetics of MTX.

Pharmaceutics

Methotrexate is available as 2.5 mg (Lederle, USA/UK) and 10 mg (Lederle, UK) tablets for oral use. For parenteral administration it comes as a dry white powder in 2.5 mg, 20 mg or 25 mg vials or in a 2 ml solution of sodium chloride as 2.5 mg.ml^{-1} or 25 mg.ml^{-1}. (Lederle, USA) and in solution as Folex (Adria, USA) 50 mg, 100 mg and 200 mg vials. Ready-for-use high-dose oncology formulations include 500 mg, 1 g and 5 g vials. All liquid formulations are preservative free and adjusted to pH 8.5 (DBL, Australia/Lederle, UK/Nordic, UK)

Therapeutic use

Methotrexate has antitumour activity against a wide variety of tumours. However, the drug is used most often in combination chemotherapy regimens. It is also used in severe disabling psoriasis and occasionally in other severe immunologically mediated disease states.

Indications

1. Acute lymphocytic leukaemia
2. Acute non-lymphocyctic leukaemia
3. Diffuse histiocyctic lymphoma
4. Mycosis fungoides
5. Breast carcinoma
6. Ovarian cancer
7. Choriocarcinoma
8. Osteosarcoma
9. Head and neck carcinoma
10. Small-cell lung carcinoma
11. Medulloblastoma
12. Severe psoriasis
13. Prevention of graft-versus-host disease in bone marrow transplantation.

Other possible indications include:

14. Hydatidiform mole
15. Chorioadenoma destruens
16. Dermatomyositis
17. Rheumatoid arthritis
18. Wegener's granulomatosis
19. Pityriasis rubra pilaris.

Contraindications

Caution should be used in administering the drug to patients with renal or haematological failure.

Mode of use

Methotrexate is most commonly used in combination chemotherapy protocols and, in fact, is only occasionally used as a single agent in maintenance therapy of leukaemia and in the treatment of head and neck carcinomas, choriocarcinomas, and psoriasis. However, single-agent MTX is gaining in popularity with the use of high-dose regimens employing folinic acid (leucovorin) rescue. The dose of MTX varies widely, usually based on the protocol being employed for a certain disease. It is a drug that should be used only by physicians experienced in the use of antineoplastic agents.

In leukaemia, MTX has been used in a daily oral dose of 2.5–10 mg. Since it induces remission slowly, it has been supplanted by vincristine, prednisone, and daunorubicin for the induction cycle in the treatment of leukaemia. It is frequently used in the maintenance of remission either orally, intramuscularly, or intravenously in various schedules.[92,93]

It is also used intrathecally in a dosage of 12 mg (see above) either to prevent leukaemic or choriocarcinoma involvement/relapse or in situations of carcinomatous meningitis caused by a variety of neoplasms. In the systemic therapy of leukaemia, the blood–brain barrier prevents the chemotherapeutic drugs from entering the brain, creating a 'sanctuary' site for the leukaemic cells; intrathecal MTX or cytarabine (ara-C) have been employed as effective antileukaemic agents in this site.

There is a high remission rate with the use of MTX with or without dactinomycin in the treatment of choriocarcinoma and related trophoblastic tumours of women.[94] In addition, there appears to be great utility for MTX with the non-metastatic, but probably premalignant, trophoblastic diseases, hydatidiform mole, and chorioadenoma destruens.[95]

Although many tumours are treated at conventional dosages of MTX, it is more frequently being used in high doses (1–30 g.m^{-2}) followed by leucovorin rescue. The use of high-dose MTX leading to high plasma levels (10^{-4} to 10^{-5}M) for prolonged periods (12 to 36 hours) has several appealing features based on the drug's biochemical pharmacology: (i) at high plasma levels, passive entry of MTX into tumour cells can potentially overcome drug resistance due to defective active transport; (ii) the increased free intracellular MTX levels achieved can overcome drug resistance secondary to increased DHFR or altered enzyme binding; (iii) the high and prolonged plasma drug levels can promote increased MTX polyglutamate formation, resulting in more prolonged drug action and accessory sites of action; and (iv) prolonged drug administration can expose more cells to MTX during DNA synthesis. Furthermore, high – dose therapy may prevent or delay MTX resistance,[96] since in experimental systems drug resistance emerges most readily when cells are exposed to concentrations that are barely cytotoxic. Leucovorin rescue is an important feature of the high – dose regimen and there is evidence that this rescue is selective for normal cells but not tumour cells.[97] In contradiction to this are experiments in mice that have shown that excessive leucovorin can decrease the response to subsequent doses of MTX.[104] This may result from the inhibition of MTX polyglutamate formation by leucovorin,[105] thus preventing the accumulation of derivatives that may play an important part in prolonging the drug's antitumour effect.

High – dose MTX with leucovorin rescue has been administered in a wide variety of dosage schedules, and typical regimens are shown in Table 1. Some basic precautions are necessary to prevent undue toxicity. They are (i) establishment of alkaline diuresis to prevent nephrotoxicity, and (ii) monitoring of plasma MTX levels during therapy to identify patients at high risk for toxicity and who will require higher doses of leucovorin. An example of dose escalation of leucovorin is shown in Table 2. Prediction of toxicity from plasma MTX levels can be accomplished in several ways, as seen in Table 3.

Table 1 High-dose methotrexate (MTX) therapy

Prehydration
In 12 hours before treatment, establish diuresis with 1.5 $l.m^{-2}$ containing 100 mmol of bicarbonate and 20 meq of potassium chloride per litre. Test urine pH to ensure neutrality (pH 7.0 or higher) at time of drug infusion.

Drug infusion
Jaffe regimen: 50–250 $mg.kg^{-1}$ MTX over 6-hour infusion. Continue hydration for 24 hours. Begin leucovorin 2 hours after end of infusion: 15 $mg.m^{-2}$ intramuscularly every 6 hours for 7 doses. Alternate regimen. Bolus administration of 50 $mg.m^{-2}$ of MTX intravenously, followed by infusion of MTX over 36-hour period at dose of 1.5 $g.m^{-2}$. At 36 hours, begin leucovorin infusion, 200 $mg.m^{-2}$ for 12 hours. At 48 hours, give leucovorin as follows: 25 $mg.m^{-2}$ intramuscularly every 6 hours for 6 doses.

Monitor points For Jaffe regimen and for 36-hour infusion, drug levels above 5×10^{-7} M at 48 hours require additional leucovorin rescue.

Table 2 Folinic acid dose required for methotrexate rescue

methotrexate drug level (M)	Folinic acid dose ($mg.m^{-2}$)
$>5 \times 10^{-5}$	1000 every 6 h i.v.
5×10^{-5} to 5×10^{-6}	100 every 3 h i.v.
5×10^{-6} to 5×10^{-7}	30 every 6 h; 10 every 3 h } i.v. i.m. or oral
$<5 \times 10^{-7}$	10 every 6 h orally until plasma MTX $<5 \times 10^{-8}$ M

Drug levels should be measured every 24–48 hours and leucovorin dose adjusted until drug concentration is less than 5×10^{-8} M.[121,122]

Table 3 Methotrexate (MTX) levels indicating a high risk of toxicity

Dosage regimen	MTX level (M)	Reference
50–250 $mg.kg^{-1}$ over 6 h	$>9 \times 10^{-7}$ 48 h after start of infusion	98
8 $g.m^{-2}$ over 4 h	$>10^{-5}$ at 24 h $>10^{-6}$ at 48 h $>10^{-7}$ at 72 h	70
50–200 $mg.kg^{-1}$ over 4 h	$>10^{-5}$ at 24 h $>5 \times 10^{-7}$ at 48 h	21
1–15 $g.m^{-2}$ by bolus	$>5 \times 10^{-7}$ at 48 h	99
725–15 000 $mg.m^{-2}$ over 6 h	$>5 \times 10^{-6}$ at 24 h	100

Although trials of high – dose MTX have shown it is effective, it has often not dramatically improved the therapeutic results obtained with lower doses. Several factors may contribute to a diminished response to high – dose MTX. MTX exposure leads to acute increases in the intracellular levels of DHFR by rapid (3–6 hour) increases in protein synthesis.[101] A similar acute increase in DHFR occurs in cells with genetically amplified levels of the enzyme.[102,103] This rapid increase could result in a failure to saturate and inhibit DHFR.[103] However, since the intracellular levels of MTX are more than 6-fold greater, this would seem to be an important argument for high – dose MTX. None the less, given our current state of knowledge concerning drug resistance, high – dose MTX regimens have a compelling pharmacological logic and are receiving extensive controlled testing to prove or disprove their value.

Adverse reactions

Potentially life threatening effects

Myelosuppression and gastrointestinal mucositis are the primary toxic effects of folate antagonists. The intestinal and oral epithelium is somewhat more sensitive than granulocyte and platelet precursors, in that schedules that produce intense mucositis (particularly those with prolonged low drug concentrations) may cause little marrow suppression. The threshold plasma concentration of MTX required to inhibit DNA synthesis in bone marrow has been estimated to be 1×10^{-8}M, whereas gastrointestinal epithelium is inhibited at 5×10^{-9}M plasma concentration.[19] This greater sensitivity of gastrointestinal epithelium is believed to result from greater accumulation and persistence of MTX in intestinal epithelium, as opposed to bone marrow.[106] Mucositis usually appears 3–7 days after drug administration, and precedes the onset of a fall in leucocyte and platelet count by several days. The duration and intensity of these acute toxicities are generally determined by drug dose and individual pharmacokinetics. Doses as small as 25 mg in patients with renal failure may provide cytotoxic blood levels for 3–5 days and may result in serious bone marrow toxicity. Myelosuppression and mucositis usually resolve within 2 weeks, unless drug excretion mechanisms are severely impaired.

The introduction of high-dose MTX regimens,[107] with leucovorin rescue, has led to the appreciation of a new spectrum of clinical toxicities and has required a more careful monitoring of drug pharmacokinetics in individual patients. Besides causing severe myelosuppression and mucositis, high-dose MTX has been associated with nephrotoxicity, especially when alkaline diuresis has not been optimal.

True anaphylactic reactions of MTX are rare, and in the two cases described, both patients were also receiving BCG.[116]

Acute overdosage

Although accidental overdoses of MTX do occur, the more common situation is persistence of high concentrations of MTX in plasma during standard or high-dose therapy. The most effective rescue is with oral or intravenous leucovorin every 6 hours until the MTX concentration is measured to be 5×10^{-8}M or less. Table 3 gives examples of various plasma concentrations of MTX that are considered potentially toxic for a given dose. In general, a time point well into the final phase of drug disappearance, such as 24–48 hours after the start of infusion, should be chosen. Doses of leucovorin needed to accomplish rescue from methotrexate are given in Table 2.

Early detection of elevated concentrations of MTX allows institution of specific clinical measures. Continuous medical surveillance is warranted until the severity and duration of myelosuppression can be determined. Patients with plasma MTX concentrations above 1×10^{-5}M may not be rescued by folinic acid; in these patients, supportive care (including antibiotics, platelet transfusion, and hydration) must be relied on to carry them through the prolonged period of myelosuppression. Both haemodialysis and peritoneal dialysis are ineffective in removing significant quantities of MTX. Clearance by the former was estimated to be 40 $ml.min^{-1}$, but only 5 $ml.min^{-1}$ by the latter[73]. Although haemodialysis produces a substantial decrease in plasma concentration of MTX, a rapid rebound to predialysis levels is observed upon cessation of the procedure. This rebound results from re-entry of drug into the plasma space from deeper compartments. Charcoal haemoperfusion columns are capable of removing MTX and other antineoplastic drugs from whole blood, but again this encounters the problem of re-entry from deeper compartments;[118] in addition, platelets adhere to these columns, leading to thrombocytopenia.

Accidental overdose of intrathecal MTX can be reversed, if discovered within the first few hours, by exchange removal of CSF.[119]

Severe or irreversible adverse effects

Hepatotoxicity. Acute elevations of liver enzymes (AST, ALT, LDH) are commonly found and usually return to normal within 10 days. Liver biopsy in such patients has revealed fatty infiltration, but no evidence of hepatocellular necrosis or periportal fibrosis. The late occurrence of cirrhosis in patients treated with high-dose MTX in the adjuvant situation has not been reported. However, chronic low-dose MTX therapy, as used in the treatment of psoriasis, has been associated with portal fibrosis and occasionally cirrhosis. The incidence of frank cirrhosis has been estimated to be 10% in MTX-treated psoriatic patients, but reaches 25% in those treated for 5 or more years.[109] In these cases cirrhosis does not always progress with continued antifolate treatment. Of 11 psoriatic patients with cirrhotic changes on liver biopsy who received continued treatment, only 3 showed progression on subsequent biopsy, and 3 had no pathologic findings on subsequent biopsy.[109]

Neurotoxicity. Three types of neurotoxic reactions to intrathecal MTX have been observed.[60] The most common is an acute chemical arachnoiditis (severe headache, nuchal rigidity, vomiting, fever, and inflammatory cell pleocytosis of the spinal fluid). This constellation of symptoms may be a function of frequency and/or dose of drug administered and may be ameliorated by dosage reduction or a change in therapy to intrathecal cytosine arabinoside. The second type of neurotoxicity is subacute and appears during the second or third week of treatment in approximately 10% of adult patients. It is manifested as motor paralysis of the extremities, cranial nerve palsy, seizures, or coma. Because of the associated abnormal drug pharmacokinetics found in these toxic patients, it is suspected that this toxicity may be the result of high drug concentrations present for an extended time period.[69] Finally, a more chronic demyelinating encephalopathy has been observed in children months or years after intrathecal MTX. The primary symptoms are dementia, limb spasticity, and, in more advanced cases, coma. Computerized axial tomography has revealed ventricular enlargement, cortical thinning, and diffuse intracerebral calcifications. Most affected children had also received cranial irradiation (greater than 2000 rads) and all had received systemic chemotherapy. A few treated only with repeated courses of high-dose intravenous MTX therapy also developed encephalopathy;[117] in these patients, dementia and paretic symptoms developed in the second or third month after treatment was begun. There is no evidence that leucovorin can ameliorate either acute or chronic neurotoxic symptoms. The aetiology of the CNS toxicity of MTX is unknown.

Symptomatic adverse effects

Nausea and vomiting have been seen in approximately 20% of patients.[108] More unusual adverse effects include ocular irritation,[110] erythema and desquamation,[111] pleuritis,[112] vasculitis,[113] and a poorly characterized, self-limiting pneumonitis with fever, cough, and an interstitial pulmonary infiltrate.[114,115]

Interference with clinical pathology tests

The drug may cause falsely high readings in tests for measuring protein in cerebrospinal fluid.

High risk groups

Neonates

The drug is unlikely to be used in neonates.

Breast milk. Very small amounts enter breast milk, breast-feeding is contraindicated.

Children

The drug may be used in children in appropriate doses.

Pregnant women

Teratogenicity. MTX seriously interferes with embryogenesis. The drug affects embryonic mesenchyme but not decidual and placental tissues.

Methotrexate is a potent teratogen which may cause defective oogenesis and spermatogenesis. Although fertility may be impaired, successful pregnancies after methotrexate treatment for choriocarcinoma are frequent.[123]

Young embryos are more susceptible than older ones. Patients should be cautioned to avoid pregnancy during administration of this drug because of the great hazard to the fetus.

Carcinogenicity. There is no evidence that methotrexate is carcinogenic. A follow-up study of 457 women with choriocarcinoma receiving methotrexate has been reported.[124] After a mean of 7.8 years only 2 had developed a second malignancy, less than the statistically expected 3.5 cases.

The elderly

The drug may be used in elderly patients who have normal renal function.

Drug interactions

In experimental tumour systems, MTX has significant synergistic or antagonistic interactions with other antineoplastic drugs. These are briefly summarized in Table 4. Most of these interactions are highly dependent on the specific sequence and timing of administration of MTX and the second agent. The reader is referred to the comprehensive review of Warren and Bender[120] for further discussion of MTX-related drug interactions. It should be remembered that these inter-

Table 4 Interactions of methotrexate with other neoplastic agents*

Agent	Drug 1	Drug 2	Time (h)	Interaction	Effect	Reference
Fluoropyrimidines	MTX	FU	3–24	MTX enhances FU	Synergism	71
	FU	MTX	0–24	MTX effect negated by prior inhibition of thymidylate synthase	Antagonism	60
Asparaginase	MTX Asp	Asp MTX	24 ?	MTX cytotoxicity attenuated by block in protein synthesis	Decreased MTX toxicity, permitting administration of higher MTX doses	72, 73
Cytarabine	MTX	Ara-C	1–72	Increased ara-C nucleotide formation; mechanism unknown	Synergism	74
Vincristine	VCR	MTX	0–1	MTX efflux blocked (only at high VCR concentrations)	None in vivo	77
Thiopurines	MTX	6-TG or 6-MP	–	Increased TG or MP nucleotide formation; MTX selectively toxic to TG- or MP-resistant cells	Synergism	75, 76

*MTX, methotrexate; FU, fluorouracil; Asp, asparaginase; Ara-C, cytarabine; VCR, vincristine; TG, thioguanine; MP, mercaptopurine.

Methotrexate

actions have no proven importance in the clinical use of MTX, although in the absence of evidence to the contrary, they should logically be taken into consideration in the design of clinical protocols.

Clinical trials

Shiner R J, Nunn A J, Chung A F, Geddes D M. 1990 Randomised, double-blind, placebo-controlled trial of methotrexate in steroid dependent asthma. Lancet 336: 137–140.

69 patients with steroid-dependent asthma took part in a randomised study taking methotrexate 15 mg daily for 24 weeks or placebo. The patients were seen every 4 weeks by a physician who reduced the prednisolone dose in accordance with diary card responses and lung function test results.

After 24 weeks the prednisolone dose had been reduced by 50% in the methotrexate group and only by 14% in the placebo group ($p<0.005$). Six patients were weaned off all steroids. Abnormalities of liver function tests occurred in 12 of 38 patients given methotrexate and three of them were withdrawn because the aminotransferase concentrations were more than 4 times the baseline value. In two others, who continued, aminotransferase results were still deteriorating at 24 weeks. Gastrointestinal symptoms (heartburn, nausea, bloating, diarrhoea) were common and two patients were withdrawn because of them. The authors comment that many questions still remain about steroid therapy in asthma.

General review articles

Because methotrexate is rarely used as a single agent there are no obvious phase III controlled clinical trials to summarise the place of methotrexate in cancer chemotherapy. The reader is recommended to refer to the relevant clinical sections of a standard text such as:

De Vita V T, Hellman S, Rosenberg S A (eds) 1989 Cancer principles and practice of oncology, 3rd edn. J B Lippincott, Philadelphia

References

1. Chabner B A 1982 Methotrexate. In: Chabner B A (ed) Pharmacologic principles of cancer treatment. W B Saunders Co, Philadelphia, pp 229–255
2. Jolivet J, Cowan K H, Curt G A, Clendeninn N J, Chabner B A 1983 The pharmacology and clinical use of methotrexate. New England Journal of Medicine 309: 1094–1104
3. Weinstein G D 1977 Methotrexate. Annals of Internal Medicine 86: 199–204
4. Blume R G, Beutler E, Briss J et al 198 Bone-marrow ablation and allogeneic marrow transplantation in acute leukaemia. New England Journal of Medicine 302: 1041–1046
5. Willkens R F, Watson M A 1982 Methotrexate: a perspective of its use in the treatment of rheumatic diseases. Journal of Laboratory and Clinical Medicine 100: 314–321
6. Goldman I D, Lichtenstein N S, Oliverio V T 1978 Carrier-mediated transport of the folic acid analogue methotrexate in the L1210 leukaemia cell. Journal of Biological Chemistry 243: 5007–5017
7. Bender R A 1975 Membrane transport of methotrexate in human neoplastic cells. Cancer Chemotherapy Reports 6: 73–82
8. Schilisky R L, Bailey B D, Chabner B A 1981 Characteristics of membrane transport of methotrexate by cultured human breast cancer cells. Biochemical Pharmacology 30: 1537–1542
9. Warren R D, Nichols A P, Bender R A 1978 Membrane transport in human lymphoblastoid cells. Cancer Research 38: 668–671
10. Hill B T, Bailey B D, White J C, Goldman I D 1979 Characteristics of transport of 4-amino antifolates and folate compounds by two lines of L5178Y lymphoblasts, one with impaired transport of methotrexate. Cancer Research 39: 2440–2446
11. Henderson G B, Zevely E M 1984 Transport routes utilized by L1210 cells for the influx and efflux of methotrexate. Journal of Biological Chemistry 254: 1526–1531
12. Moran R G, Mulkins M, Heidelberger C 1979 Role of thymidylate synthetase activity in development of methotrexate cytotoxicity. Proceedings of the National Academy of Sciences USA 76: 5924–5928
13. White J C, Goldman I D 1981 Methotrexate resistance in an L1210 cell line resulting from increased DHFR, decreased thymidylate synthetase activity and normal membrane transport: computer simulations based on network thermodynamics. Journal of Biological Chemistry 256: 5122–5127
14. Aynsawa D, Koyama N, Seno T 1981 Resistance to metotrexate in thymidylate synthetase-deficient mutants of cultured mouse mammary tumour FM3A cells. Cancer Research 41: 1497–1501
15. Washtien W L 1982 Thymidylate synthetase levels as a factor in 5-fluorodeoxyuridine and methotrexate cytotoxicity in gastrointestinal tumour cells. Molecular Pharmacology 21: 723–728
16. Cohen M, Bender R A, Donehower R C, Myers C E, Chabner B A 1978 Reversibility of high-affinity binding of methotrexate in L1210 murine leukaemia cells. Cancer Research 38: 866–870
17. White J C, Loftfield S, Goldman I D 1975 The mechanism of action of methotrexate. III. Requirement of free intracellular methotrexate for maximal suppression of [^{14}C] formate incorporation into nucleic acids and proteins. Molecular Pharmacology 11: 287–297
18. White J C 1979 Reversal of methotrexate binding to DHFR by dihydrofolate studies with pure enzyme and computer modelling using network thermodynamics. Journal of Biological Chemistry 254: 10 889–10 895
19. Chabner B A, Young R C 1973 Threshold methotrexate concentrations for in vivo inhibition of DNA synthesis in normal and tumorous target tissues. Journal of Clinical Investigation 52: 1804–1811
20. Smith G K, Benkovic D A, Benkovic S J 1981 L(-)-10-formyl-tetrahydrofolate is the cofactor for glycinamide ribonucleotide transformylase from chicken liver. Biochemistry 20: 4034–4036
21. Zaharko D S, Fung W P, Yang K H 1977 Relative biochemical aspects of low and high doses of methotrexate in mice. Cancer Research 37: 1602–1607
22. Baugh C M, Kdrumdieck C L, Nau M G 1973 Polygammaglutamyl metabolites of methotrexate. Biochemical and Biophysical Research Communications 52: 27–39
23. Jacobs S A, Derr C J, Johns D G 1977 Accumulation of methotrexate diglutamate in human liver during methotrexate therapy. Biochemical Pharmacology 26: 2310–2313
24. Rosenblatt D S, Whitehead V M, Dupont M M, Vuchich M J, Vera N 1978 Synthesis of methotrexate polyglutamates in cultured human cells. Molecular Pharmacology 14: 210–214
25. Krakower G R, Nylen P A, Kamen B A 1982 Separation and identification of sub-picomole amounts of methotrexate polyglutamates in animal and human biopsy material. Analytical Biochemistry 122: 412–416
26. Jolivet J, Chabner B A 1983 Intracellular pharmacokinetics of methotrexate polyglutamates in human breast cancer cells: selective retention and less dissociable binding of 4-NH_2-10-CH_3PteGlu$_4$ and Glu$_5$ to dihydrofolate reductase. Journal of Clinical Investigation 72: 773–775
27. Jolivet J, Schilsky R L, Bailey B D, Drake J C, Chabner B A 1982 Synthesis, retention, and biological activity of methotrexate polyglutamates in cultured human breast cancer cells. Journal of Clinical Investigation 70: 351–360
28. McGuire J J, Hsieh P, Coward J K, Bertino J R 1980 Enzymatic synthesis of folylpolyglutamates: characterization of the reaction and its products. Journal of Biological Chemistry 255: 5776–5788
29. Allegra C J, Chabner B A, Drake J C, Lutz R, Rodbard D, Jolivet J Enhanced inhibition of thymidylate synthetase by methotrexate polyglutamates. Journal of Biological Chemistry, in press
30. Baggott J E 1983 Inhibition of purified avial liver aminoimidazolecarboxamide ribotide transformylase by polyglutamates of methotrexate and oxidized folates (Abstract). Federation Proceedings 42: 667
31. Sirotnak F M, Moccio D M, Kelleher L E, Goutas L J 1981 Relative frequency and kinetic properties of transport-defective phenotypes among methotrexate-resistant L1210 clonal cell lines derived in vivo. Cancer Research 41: 4447–4452
32. Malera P W, Lewis J A, Biedler J L, Hession C 1980 Antifolate-resistant Chinese hamster cells: evidence for DHFR gene amplication among independently-derived sublines overproducing different DHFRs. Journal of Biological Chemistry 255: 7024–7028
33. Flintoff W F, Essani K 1980 Methotrexate-resistant Chinese hamster ovary cells contain a DHFR with an altered affinity for methotrexate. Biochemistry 19: 4321–4327
34. Haber D A, Beverley S M, Kiely M L, Schimke R T 1981 Properties of an altered DHFR encoded by amplified genes in cultured mouse fibroblasts. Journal of Biological Chemistry 256: 9501–9510
35. Jackson R C, Niethammer D 1977 Acquired methotrexate resistance in lymphoblasts resulting from altered kinetic properties of DHFR. European Journal of Cancer 13: 567–575
36. Dedhar S, Freisheim J H, Hynes J B, Goldie J H 1983 Inhibition of a methotrexate-sensitive DHFR from L5178Y cells by substituted triazines and quinazolines. Biochemical Pharmacology 32: 922–924
37. Biedler J L, Spengler B A 1976 Metaphase chromosome anomaly: association with drug resistance and cell-specific products. Science 191: 185–187
38. Cowan K H, Goldsmith M E, Levine R M et al 1982 DHFR gene amplification and possible rearrangement in estrogen-responsive methotrexate-resistant human breast cancer cells. Journal of Biological Chemistry 257: 15 079–15 086
39. Kaufman R J, Brown P C, Schimke R T 1979 Amplified DHFR in unstable methotrexate-resistant cells is associated with double minute chromosomes. Proceedings of the National Academy of Sciences USA 76: 5669–5673
40. Curt G A, Carney D N, Cowan K H et al 1982 Unstable methotrexate resistance in human small cell carcinoma associated with double-minute chromosomes. New England Journal of Medicine 308: 199–202
41. Cowan K H, Jolivet J 1983 A novel mechanism of resistance of methotrexate in human breast cancer cells: lack of methotrexate polyglutamate formation. Clinical Research 31: 508
42. Bostock C J, Clark E M, Harding N G et al 1979 The development of resistance to methotrexate in a mouse melanoma cell line. I. Characterization of DHFRs and chromosomes in sensitive and resistant cells. Chromosoma 74: 153–177
43. Alt F W, Kellems R E, Schimke R T 1976 Synthesis and degradation of folate reductase in sensitive and methotrexate-resistant lines of S-180 cells. Journal of Biological Chemistry 251: 3063–3074
44. Pinedo H M, Zaharko D S, Bull J, Chabner B A 1977 The relative contribution of drug concentration and duration of exposure to mouse bone marrow toxicity during continuous methotrexate infusion. Cancer Research 37: 445–450
45. Eichholtz H, Trott K R 1980 Effect of methotrexate concentration and exposure time on mammalian cell survival in vitro. British Journal of Cancer 41: 277–284
46. Myers C E, Lippman M E, Eliot H M, Chabner B A 1975 Competitive protein binding assay for methotrexate. Proceedings of the National Academy of Sciences 72: 3683–3686

Methotrexate

47. Bertino J R, Isacoff W H 1978 Methods of measuring methotrexate in body fluids. In: Pinedo H M (ed) Clinical pharmacology of antineoplastic drugs. Elsevier/North Holland, Amsterdam, pp 3–11
48. Oellerich M, Engelhardt P, Schaadt M, Diehl V 1980 Determination of methotrexate in serum by a rapid, fully mechanized enzyme immunoassay (EMIT). Journal of Clinical Chemistry and Clinical Biochemistry 18: 169–174
49. Chungi V S, Bourne D W A, Dittert L W 1978 Drug absorption. VIII. Kinetics of gastrointestinal absorption of methotrexate. Journal of Pharmaceutical Sciences 67: 560–561
50. Henderson E S, Adamson R M, Oliverio V T 1965 The metabolic fate of tritiated methotrexate. II. Absorption and excretion in man. Cancer Research 25: 1018–1024
51. Canfell C, Sadee W 1980 Methotrexate and 7-hydroxymethotrexate: serum level monitoring by high-performance liquid chromatography. Cancer Treatment Reports 64: 165–169
52. Smith D K, Omura G A, Ostroy F 1980 Clinical pharmacology of intermediate-dose oral methotrexate. Cancer Chemotherapy and Pharmacology 4: 117–120
53. Donehower R C, Hande K R, Drake J C, Chabner B A 1979 Presence of 2,4-diamino-N^{10}-methyl pteroic acid after high-dose methotrexate. Clinical Pharmacology and Therapeutics 26: 63–72
54. Pinkerton C R, Glasgow J F T, Welshman S G, Bridges J M 1980 Can food influence the absorption of methotrexate in children with acute lymphoblastic leukemia. Lancet 2: 944–945
55. Mahoney M J, Murphy M S, Wadsworth J, Mott M G 1984 Modification of oral methotrexate absorption in children with leukemia. Cancer Chemotherapy and Pharmacology 12: 131–133
56. Steele W H, Lawrence J R, Stuart J B, Mitchel C R The protein binding of methotrexate in the serum of normal subjects. European Journal of Clinical Pharmacology 150: 363–366
57. Liegler D G, Henderson E S, Hahn M A, Oliverio V T 1969 The effect of organic acids on renal clearance of methotrexate in man. Clinical Pharmacology and Therapeutics 10: 849–857
58. Shapiro W R, Young D R, Mehta B M 1975 Distribution in cerebrospinal fluid after intravenous ventricular and lumbar injections. New England Journal of Medicine 293: 161–166
59. Jones R B, Collins J M, Myers C E et al 1981 High-volume intraperitoneal chemotherapy with methotrexate in patients with cancer. Cancer Research 41: 55–59
60. Bleyer W A 1978 The clinical pharmacology of methotrexate. Cancer 41: 36–51
61. Bleyer W A, Poplack D G, Simon R M 1978 'Concentration × time' methotrexate via a subcutaneous reservoir: a less toxic regimen for intraventricular chemotherapy of central nervous system neoplasms. Blood 51: 835–842
62. Echelberger C K, Riccardi R, Bleyer A, Levine A S, Poplack D G 1981 Influence of body position on ventricular cerebrospinal fluid methotrexate concentration following intralumbar administration (Abstract). Proceedings of the American Association of Cancer Research/American Society for Clinical Oncology 22: 365
63. Freeman I, Weinberg V, Brecher M L 1983 Comparison of intermediate-dose methotrexate with cranial irradiation for the post-incubation treatment of acute lymphocytic leukemia in children. New England Journal of Medicine 308: 477–484
64. Evans W E, Hutson P R, Stewart C F 1983 Methotrexate CSF and serum concentrations after intermediate-dose methotrexate infusion. Clinical Pharmacology and Therapeutics 33: 301–307
65. Stoller R G, Jacobs S A, Drake J C, Lutz R J, Chabner B A 1975 Pharmacokinetics of high-dose methotrexate. Cancer Chemotherapy Reports 6: 19–24
66. Kristenson L, Weisman K, Hutters L 1975 Renal function and the rate of disappearance of methotrexate from serum. European Journal of Clinical Pharmacology 8: 439–444
67. Chabner B A, Stoller R G, Hande K R, Jacobs S, Young R C 1978 Methotrexate disposition in humans: case studies in ovarian cancer and following high-dose infusion. Drug Metabolism Reviews 8: 107–117
68. Bode U, Magrath I T, Bleyer W A, Poplack D G, Glaubiger D L 1980 Active transport of methotrexate from cerebrospinal fluid in humans. Cancer Research 40: 2184–1287
69. Bleyer W A, Drake J C, Chabner B A 1973 Neurotoxicity and elevated cerebrospinal fluid methotrexate concentration in meningeal leukemia. New England Journal of Medicine 298: 770–773
70. Nirenberg A, Mosende T, Mehta B, Gisolfi A L, Rosen G 1977 High-dose methotrexate with citrovorum factor rescue: predictive value of serum methotrexate concentrations and corrective measures to avert toxicity. Cancer Treatment Reports 61: 779–783
71. Isacoff W H, Morrison P F, Aroesty J, Willis J L, Block J B, Lincoln T L 1977 Pharmacokinetics of high-dose methotrexate with citrovorum factor rescue. Cancer Treatment Reports 61: 1665–1674
72. Calvert A H, Bondy P K, Harap K R 1977 Some observations on the human pharmacology of methotrexate. Cancer Treatment Reports 61:
73. Hande K R, Drake J C, Balow A, Rosenberg S A, Chabner B A 1977 Clearance of methotrexate by peritoneal dialysis and hemodialysis. Annals of Internal Medicine 87: 495
74. Monjanel S, Rigault J P, Cano J P, Carcassone Y, Fame R 1979 High-dose methotrexate: preliminary evaluation of a pharmacokinetic approach. Cancer Chemotherapy and Pharmacology 3: 189–196
75. Huang K C, Wenczak B A, Liu Y K 1979 Renal tubular transport of methotrexate in the rhesus monkey and dog. Cancer Research 39: 4843–4848
76. Aherne G W, Piall E, Marks V, Meald A, White W F 1978 Prolongation and enhancement of serum methotrexate concentrations by probenecid. British Medical Journal 1: 1097–1099
77. Romolo J L, Goldberg N H, Hande K R, Rosenberg S A 1977 The effects of hydration on plasma methotrexate levels. Cancer Treatment Reports 61: 1393–1395
78. Sasaki K, Tanaka J, Fujimoto T 1984 Theoretically required urinary flow during high-dose methotrexate infusion. Cancer Chemotherapy and Pharmacology 13: 9–13
79. Sketnis I S, Farmer P S, Fraser A 1984 Effect of vitamin C on the excretion of methotrexate. Cancer Treatment Reports 68: 446–447
80. Gewirtz D A, White J C, Goldman I D 1979 Transport, binding and polyglutamation of methotrexate in freshly isolated hepatocytes. Proceedings of the American Asociation of Cancer Research 24: 147
81. Strum W B, Liem H H 1977 Hepatic uptake, intracellular protein binding and biliary excretion of amethopterin. Biochemical Pharmacology 26: 1235–1240
82. Strum W B, Liem H H, Muller-Eberhard U 1978 Effect of chemotherapeutic agents on the uptake and excretion of amethopterin by the isolated perfused rat liver. Cancer Research 38: 4734–4736
83. Leme P R, Creaven P J, Allen L M, Berman M 1975 A kinetic model for the disposition and metabolism of moderate and high-dose methotrexate in man. Cancer Chemotherapy Reports 59: 811–817
84. Shen D D, Azarnoff D L 1978 Clinical pharmacokinetics of methotrexate. Clinical Pharmacokinetics 3: 1–13
85. Valerino D M, Johns D G, Zaharko D S 1972 Studies of the metabolism of methotrexate by intestinal flora. Biochemical Pharmacology 21: 821–831
86. Hendel J, Brodthagen H 1984 Enterohepatic cycling of methotrexate estimated by use of the D-isomer as a reference marker. European Journal of Clinical Pharmacology 26: 103–107
87. Jacobs S A, Stoller R G, Chabner B A, Johns D G 1976 7-Hydroxy-methotrexate as a urinary metabolite in human subjects and rhesus monkeys receiving high-dose methotrexate. Journal of Clinical Investigation 57: 534–538
88. Lankelma J, van der Klein E 1980 The role of 7-hydroxy-methotrexate during methotrexate anticancer chemotherapy. Cancer Letters 9: 133–142
89. McCullough J L, Chabner B A, Bertino J R 1971 Purification and properties of carboxypeptidase G1. Journal of Biological Chemistry 246: 7203–7213
90. Fabre G, Matherly L J, Fabre I, Cano J P, Goldman I D 1984 Interactions between 7-hydroxymethotrexate and methotrexate at the cellular level in the Ehrlich ascites tumor in vitro. Cancer Research 44: 970–975
91. Gaukroger J M, Wilson L 1984 Protection of cells from methotrexate toxicity by 7-hydroxymethotrexate. British Journal of Cancer 50: 327–333
92. Jacobs A D, Gale R P 1984 Recent advances in the biology and treatment of acute lymphoblastic leukemia in adults. New England Journal of Medicine 311: 1219–1231
93. Lister T A, Rohatinen A Z S 1982 The treatment of acute myelogenous leukemia in adults. Seminars in Hematology 19: 172–192
94. Hertz R, Lewis J, Lipsett M B 1962 Five-year experience with the chemotherapy of metastatic trophoblastic diseases in women. Medical Annals of Obstetrics 31: 663–668
95. Hertz R, Ross G T, Lipsett M B 1963 Primary chemotherapy of title nonmetastatic trophoblastic disease in woman. American Journal of Obstetrics and Gynecology 86: 808–814
96. Schrecker A W, Mead J A R, Greenberg W H, Goldin A 1971 Dihydro-folate reductase activity of leukemia L1210 during development of methotrexate resistance. Biochemical Pharmacology 20: 716–718
97. Frei E III, Jaffe N, Tattersall M H N, Pitman S, Parker L 1975 New approaches to cancer chemotherapy with methotrexate. New England Journal of Medicine 292: 846–851
98. Stoller R G, Hande K R, Jacobs S A, Rosenberg S A, Chabner B A 1977 Use of plasma pharmacokinetics to predict and prevent methotrexate toxicity. New England Journal of Medicine 297: 630–634
99. Tattersall M H N, Parker L M, Pitman S W, Frei E 1975 Clinical pharmacology of high-dose methotrexate. Cancer Treatment Reports 6: 25–29
100. Evans W E, Pratt C B, Taylor R H, Barker L F, Crom W R 1979 Pharmacokinetic monitoring of high-dose methotrexate: early recognition of high-risk patients. Cancer Chemotherapy and Pharmacology 3: 161–166
101. Bertino J R, Cashmore A, Fink M, Calabresi P, Lefkowitz E 1965 The 'induction' of leukocyte and erythrocyte dihydrofolate reductase by methotrexate. II. Clinical and pharmacologic studies. Clinical Pharmacology and Therapeutics 6: 763–770
102. Domin B A, Grill S P, Bastow K F, Cheng Y C 1982 Effect of methotrexate on dihydrofolate reductase activity in methotrexate-resistant human KB cells. Molecular Pharmacology 21: 478–482
103. Jolivet J, Levine R M, Cowan K H 1983 The regulation of DHFR in gene-amplified methotrexate-resistant human breast cancer cells. Clinical Research 31: 509A
104. Sirotnak F M, Moccio D M, Dorick D M 1978 Optimization of high-dose methotrexate with leucovorin rescue therapy in the L1210 leukemia and sarcoma 180 murine tumor models. Cancer Research 38: 345–353
105. Galivan J, Nimec Z 1983 Effects of folinic acid on hepatoma cells containing methotrexate polyglutamates. Cancer Research 43: 551–555
106. Sirotnak F, Moccio D M 1980 Pharmacokinetic basis for differences in methotrexate sensitivity of normal proliferative tissues in the mouse. Cancer Research 40: 1230–1234
107. Jaffe N 1972 Recent advances in the chemotherapy of metastatic osteogenic sarcoma. Cancer 30: 1627–1631
108. Frei E III, Blum R H, Pitman S W et al 1980 High-dose methotrexate with leucovorin rescue: rationale and spectrum of antitumor activity. American Journal of Medicine 68: 370–376
109. Zachariae H, Kragball K, Sogaard H 1980 Methotrexate-induced cirrhosis. British Journal of Dermatology 102: 407–412
110. Doroshow J H, Locker G Y, Gaasterland D E, Hubbard S P, Young R C, Myers C E 1981 Ocular irritation from high-dose methotrexate therapy: pharmacokinetics of drug in the tear film. Cancer 48: 2158–2162
111. Doyle L A, Berg C, Bottino G, Chabner B A 1983 Erythema and desquamation after high-dose methotrexate. Annals of Internal Medicine 98: 611–612
112. Urban C, Nirenberg A, Caparros B, Anac S, Cacavio A, Rosen G 1983 Chemical pleuritis as the cause of acute chest pain following high-dose methotrexate treatment. Cancer 51: 34–37

M

113. Marks C R, Willkens R F, Wilsne K R, Brown P B 1984 Small-vessel vasculitis and methotrexate. Annals of Internal Medicine 100: 916
114. Clarysse A M, Catney W J, Cartwright G E et al 1969 Pulmonary disease complicating intermittent therapy with methotrexate. Journal of the American Medical Association 204: 1861–1864
115. Sostman H D, Matthay R A, Putman C et al 1976 Methotrexate-induced pneumonitis. Medicine 55: 371–388
116. Goldberg N H, Romolo J L, Austin E H et al 1978 Anaphylactoid type reactions in two patients receiving high-dose intravenous methotrexate. Cancer 41: 52–55
117. Shapiro R, Allen J C, Horten B C 1980 Chronic methotrexate toxicity to the central nervous system. Clinical Bulletin, Memorial Sloan-Kettering 10: 49–52
118. Djerassi I, Ciesielda W, Kim J S 1977 Removal of methotrexate by filtration–adsorption using charcoal filters or by hemodialysis. Cancer Treatment Reports 61: 751–752
119. Addiego J E, Ridgway D, Bleyer W A 1977 The acute management of intrathecal methotrexate overdose: pharmacologic rationale and guidelines. Journal of Pediatrics 98: 825–828
120. Warren R D, Bender R A 1977 Drug interactions with antineoplastic drugs. Cancer Treatment Reports 61: 1231–1241
121. Bleyer W A 1978 The clinical pharmacology of methotrexate. Cancer 41: 36–51
122. Bleyer W A 1981 Therapeutic drug monitoring of methotrexate and other antineoplastic drugs. In: Baer D M, Sito W R (eds) Interpretations in therapeutic drug monitoring. American Society of Clinical Pathology, Chicago, pp 169–186
123. Rustin G J S, Booth M, Dent J et al 1984 Pregnancy after cytotoxic chemotherapy for gestational trophoblastic tumours. British Medical Journal 288: 103–106
124. Rustin G J S, Rustin F, Dent J, Booth M, Salt S, Bagshawe K D 1983 No increase in second tumors after cytotoxic chemotherapy for gestational trophoblastic tumors. New England Journal of Medicine 308: 473

Methotrimeprazine (hydrochloride and maleate)

Methotrimeprazine is a sedative antipsychotic phenothiazine with analgesic properties, especially useful in terminal care.

Chemistry

Methotrimeprazine maleate (Nozinan), Methotrimeprazine hydrochloride
$C_{19}H_{24}N_2OS.C_4H_4O_4$ or .HCl
2-Methoxy-10-(2-methyl-3-dimethylaminopropyl)phenothiazine maleate or hydrochloride

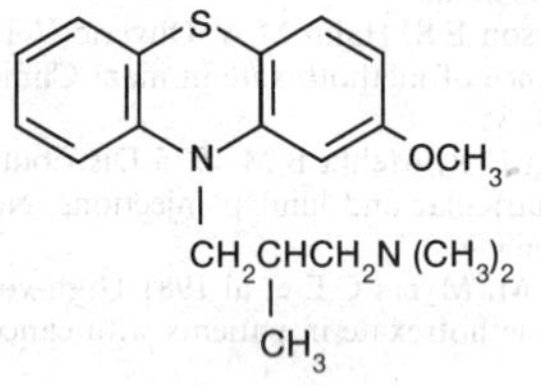

Molecular weight maleate (free compound)	444.5 (328.5)
pKa (dimethylaminopropyl group)	9.15
Solubility	
in alcohol	slightly soluble
in water	slightly soluble
Octanol/water partition coefficient	high

The maleate is a fine, crystalline, virtually odourless, white powder, prepared by chemical synthesis. The hydrochloride is a yellowish white slightly hygroscopic powder which deteriorates on exposure to air and light. The hydrochloride injection is prepared from the base and hydrochloric acid.

Pharmacology

Methotrimeprazine has antidopaminergic, antiadrenergic, antiserotoninergic, antihistaminic and anticholinergic actions. Its action on the central nervous system in animals produces analgesic, sedative, antiemetic, cataleptic, and hypothermic effects.[1,2] It also has hypotensive and antishock effects.

Methotrimeprazine binds to dopamine D_2 adrenoceptors with an affinity approximately equal to that of chlorpromazine. In the rat striatum, the binding constant K_1 for binding to D_2 receptors in the rat striatum is 27 (SD 7), while that for chlorpromazine is 23 (SD 6).[3] Like chlorpromazine, it has a strong affinity for α_1-adrenoceptors ($K_1=2.6$, SD 1.4)[3] but only a weak affinity for α_2-receptors ($K_1=1060$, SD 192).[3] Long-term administration results in increased sensitivity of serotoninergic 5-HT_2 receptors, resembling the effect of chronic administration of antidepressants such as clomipramine.[4]

Toxicology

Methotrimeprazine is not teratogenic when administered subcutaneously to rats at daily doses of 15–50 $mg.kg^{-1}$, but does reduce fertility when fed to male and female rats at high doses equivalent to 50 $mg.kg^{-1}$ daily. No studies of mutagenicity or carcinogenicity have been reported.

Clinical pharmacology

In man, methotrimeprazine 15 mg intramuscularly or subcutaneously has an analgesic effect equivalent to morphine sulphate 10 mg intramuscularly[5,6] or pethidine 75 mg intramuscularly.[7,8] Uncontrolled clinical studies suggest that methotrimeprazine has stronger analgesic effects than other phenothiazine drugs, but it is difficult to exclude the possibility that the analgesic effects are due at least in part to sedation. In contrast to the situation in rats, where methotrimeprazine potentiates the analgesic effects of morphine at a dose below the threshold for producing detectable sedation, Petts and Pleuvry[10] found that in healthy human volunteers, 7.5 mg methotrimeprazine intramuscularly was sufficient to produce detectable sedation, but did not potentiate the analgesic effect of 5 mg morphine intramuscularly.

In a study of the effects of methotrimeprazine on respiration in healthy volunteers, Pearson and Dekornfeld[11] found that a dose of 15 mg intramuscularly produced significant sedation, but did not exacerbate the decreased ventilatory response to carbon dioxide produced by 10 mg of morphine. At 0.15 $mg.kg^{-1}$ intramuscularly it does produce some exacerbation of respiratory depression induced by pethidine.[12] In a study of former opiate addicts, it was demonstrated that methotrimeprazine does not cause opiate-like addictiveness.[13]

Oral methotrimeprazine has an antipsychotic effect approximately equivalent to an equal dose of chlorpromazine, and there is some evidence of a therapeutic effect in schizophrenic patients previously resistant to treatment with other antipsychotic agents.[14–16]

Methotrimeprazine has a hypotensive effect in middle-aged and elderly patients[7] and in particular may cause postural hypotension. It also has an antiemetic effect.[17] The anticholinergic effect may cause dry mouth and difficulty in micturition in men. The antagonist action at 5-hydroxytryptamine receptors may lead to weight gain.

Pharmacokinetics

The preferred analytical method is high performance liquid chromatography using electrochemical detection.[18] The limit of detection is 100 pg, at a concentration of 500 $\mu g.l^{-1}$.

Approximately 50% of an oral dose reaches the systemic circulation. A substantial proportion is metabolized to methotrimeprazine sulphoxide, apparently presystemically.[19] Peak plasma concentration is achieved in 1–3 hours.[19] The plasma half life is in the range 15–30 hours[19] and the volume of distribution is 23–42 $l.kg^{-1}$, indicating that the drug accumulates in tissues.

Oral absorption	well absorbed
Presystemic metabolism	~50%
Plasma half life	
range	15–30 h
Volume of distribution	23–42 $l.kg^{-1}$
Plasma protein binding	—

Concentration–effect relationship

There are no reports indicating that the therapeutic effects of methotrimeprazine occur within a defined range of plasma concentrations.

Metabolism

Virtually all of the drug is metabolized before excretion. Excretion is mainly in urine and faeces. The major metabolic pathways are sulphoxidation,[20] N-demethylation (Fig. 1)[20] and also hydroxylation at the 3 and 7 positions.[21] The sulphoxide is found only after oral administration. The steady-state serum concentration of the sulphoxide is generally 1.5 to 3 times as high as the concentration of methotrimeprazine.[19] Being more polar than the parent compound, it is likely that the sulphoxide has a smaller volume of distribution in the body and, therefore, a higher serum concentration does not necessarily indicate that there is more sulphoxide than parent compound in the body. In urine, the concentration of the sulphoxide is approximately 10 times greater, and the concentration of monodesmethylmethotrimeprazine is approximately 5 times greater than the concentration of unmetabolized methotrimeprazine, 5 hours after ingestion during steady-state treatment.[20]

The pharmacological effects of the metabolites are not well established. The sulphoxide has cardiodepressive effects when applied to isolated rat atria.[22] The sulphoxide produces a greater increase in refractory period, but a lesser reduction in contractile force than methotrimeprazine itself. The pattern of antagonism of the effects of apomorphine in the mouse suggests that 3-hydroxymethotrimeprazine might have antipsychotic effects, while N-desmethylmethotrimeprazine might be sedative.[23]

Fig. 1 Metabolism of methotrimeprazine

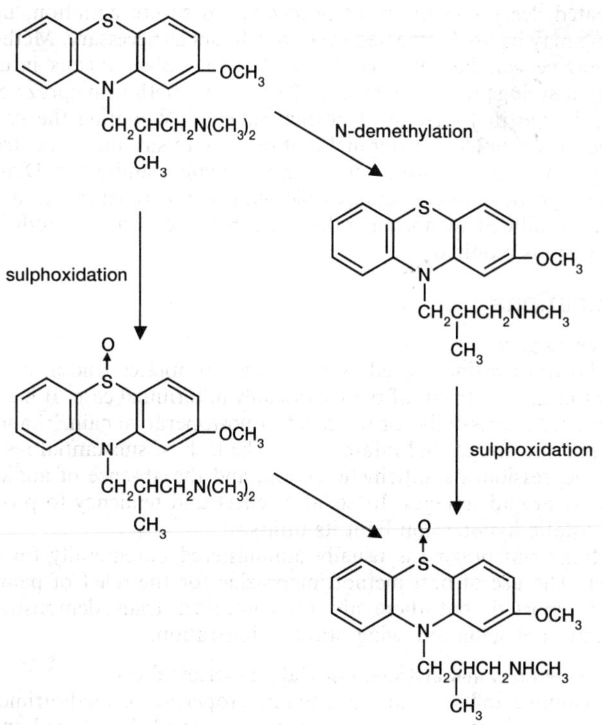

Pharmaceutics

Methotrimeprazine is available in oral and parenteral forms.

Nozinan (Rhone Poulenc, UK) contains 25 mg of methotrimeprazine maleate. The tablets are white, varnished, round and impressed with the legend ‘NOZINAN 25’ (formerly ‘VERACTIL 25’) on one face and scored with a break line on the obverse. There is no slow-release formulation.

Methotrimeprazine is available as a clear solution containing methotrimeprazine hydrochloride 25 $mg.ml^{-1}$ for intramuscular injection, or for intravenous injection after dilution with an equal volume of 0.9% sodium chloride injection immediately before use.

All preparations should be protected from light. Both the tablet and injectable formulations have a maximum shelf-life of 5 years, and carry a minimal risk from potentially allergenic substances.

Therapeutic use

Indications

1. Severe pain
2. Restlessness and distress, especially in terminal care
3. Schizophrenia and related psychoses.

Contraindications

1. Coma caused by CNS depressants
2. Bone-marrow depression
3. Closed-angle glaucoma
4. Liver disease
5. Cardiac disease.

Mode of use

The initial dose for oral treatment of ambulant patients should not exceed 25–50 mg per day, delivered in divided doses. A larger portion of the dosage may be taken at bed time to minimize day time sedation. The dose is then increased according to the individual response of the patient to provide the most effective level coupled with minimal side effects, such as sedation and hypotension. For patients in bed, the initial dose may be 100–200 mg, usually divided into three doses. The dose may be increased to a total of 1 g daily if necessary. When the patient is stable, the dose should be gradually reduced to an adequate maintenance level.

The usual dose for intramuscular injection is 12.5 to 25 mg, repeated every 6–8 hours as necessary. In severe agitation, up to 50 mg may be used, repeated every 6–8 hours as necessary. Methotrimeprazine can be delivered by continuous subcutaneous infusion using a syringe driver, delivering 25–200 mg methotrimeprazine per day, diluted in 10–20 ml of normal saline.[24] Mounting the syringe driver in a shoulder holster makes it possible to sustain the control of symptoms while allowing the patient to remain ambulant. Diamorphine hydrochloride is compatible with methotrimeprazine hydrochloride diluted in normal saline and may be added if additional analgesia is required.

Indications

1. Severe pain

Methotrimeprazine is used as an adjunct to opiates, and as a single agent in the treatment of pain, especially in terminal care. It has also been used successfully for the relief of postoperative pain,[5,7] and for the pain of myocardial infarction.[25] The lack of substantial respiratory depression, its antiemetic action, and the absence of addiction liability are advantages. Its sedative effect and tendency to produce orthostatic hypotension limit its utility.

Methotrimeprazine is usually administered parenterally for pain relief. The use of oral methotrimeprazine for the relief of pain has been reported, but there are no controlled trials demonstrating effective analgesia following oral administration.

2. Restlessness and distress, especially in terminal care

The calming influence and antiemetic properties of methotrimeprazine, coupled with its analgesic properties, have led to its widespread use in terminal care.[26] For this purpose, it can be administered either parenterally or orally.

3. Schizophrenia and related psychoses

Like other phenothiazine neuroleptics with an aliphatic chain at the 10-position, methotrimeprazine is an antipsychotic drug with relatively strong sedative effects. There is evidence that methotrimeprazine can be of benefit in cases previously unimproved by treatment with other antipsychotics.[14–16] Sedation is potentially a major problem when long-term treatment is required. By starting at an oral dose of 25 mg morning and evening and increasing the evening dose by steps of 25 mg, the patients are enabled to continue their daily activities.[16]

Contraindications

1. Coma caused by CNS depressants

Although Pearson and Dekornfeld[11] found that methotrimeprazine did not exacerbate the decreased ventilatory response to carbon dioxide induced by morphine, it can produce a degree of respiratory depression in some circumstances. In particular, at a dose of $0.15\ mg.kg^{-1}$ it has been reported to exacerbate the respiratory depression produced by pethidine.[12] Therefore it is contraindicated in coma produced by CNS depressants.

2. Bone-marrow depression

Methotrimeprazine can suppress bone-marrow function, and produce agranulocytosis.[27] It should generally be avoided if there is a history of bone-marrow suppression, but previous use of cytotoxic agents with marrow depressant activity would not be an absolute contraindication in terminal care.

3. Closed-angle glaucoma

The anticholinergic effects of methotrimeprazine are liable to exacerbate closed-angle glaucoma.

4. Liver disease

Liver disease is a relative contraindication. Phenothiazines have a propensity to be hepatotoxic and can precipitate coma.

5. Cardiac disease

Cardiac disease is a relative contraindication. Methotrimeprazine has pharmacological effects on the heart. Motomura et al[28] found a decrease in the coefficient of variation in the RR interval which they consider might indicate interference with vagal regulation of the heart. Furthermore, the hypotensive effects of methotrimeprazine indicate the need for caution when cardiac function is impaired. Nonetheless, methotrimeprazine has been used for the treatment of the pain of myocardial infarction. In a double-blind comparison of methotrimeprazine with pethidine, the mortality was significantly less at both 4 weeks and one year in those treated with methotrimeprazine.[25]

Adverse reactions

Potentially life-threatening effects

Agranulocytosis[27] is potentially fatal. It usually occurs within the first three months of treatment, but in one of the three cases reported by Anath et al,[27] agranulocytosis developed after 22 months of treatment with methotrimeprazine. The neuroleptic malignant syndrome has occurred in patients taking methotrimeprazine.[29]

Acute overdosage

Fatal cases in which several drugs, including methotrimeprazine, were taken have been reported.[30] Treatment of overdosage should include adoption of a supine or head down position to counter hypotension; avoiding the use of adrenaline because phenothiazines can reverse the effect of adrenaline, exacerbating hypotension. If necessary, the plasma volume should be expanded with intravenous fluids (warmed to avoid aggravation of hypothermia). Positive inotropic agents such as dopamine may be used if other intravenous fluids are insufficient to correct for the circulatory collapse. Haemodialysis is ineffective.[31] Body temperature should be allowed to recover naturally unless it falls below 29.4°C, at which level cardiac arrhythmias may develop. The patient should be observed for evidence of intestinal or urinary bladder distention.

Severe or irreversible adverse effects

Tardive dyskinesia can occur after prolonged administration, even when the dose is relatively small.[32] Intrahepatic cholestasis[33] can arise as a result of hypersensitivity. Lens opacities[34] and maculopathy[35] occur occasionally. Methotrimeprazine can lower the seizure threshold, leading to seizures, especially in the elderly.[36] Paralytic ileus can be severe.[37]

Symptomatic adverse effects

On account of its multiple pharmacological actions, methotrimeprazine, like other phenothiazines, can produce a wide range of adverse effects. Sedation, asthenia, hypotension, parkinsonism, and weight gain are common. Patients should not drive vehicles for at least several days at the start of treatment, until any sedation or hypotensive effects have subsided. Dermatological effects include erythematous rashes, photosensitivity and contact dermatitis.[38] The anticholinergic effect can lead to dry mouth. Impaired temperature regulation predisposes to heat stroke. Priapism occurs rarely.[39]

Other effects

The ESR is elevated rarely. Despite the potential for interference with liver function, Linnet et al[40] found no effect on measurements of alkaline phosphatase, aspartate aminotransferase or bile acids in patients receiving long-term treatment with methotrimeprazine. Methotrimeprazine does increase the rate of clearance of bromosulphthalein,[41] implying that it induces liver enzymes.

Interference with clinical pathology tests

Methotrimeprazine can interfere with serum and urinary cortisol estimations.[42]

High risk groups

Neonates

Methotrimeprazine is not recommended for use in the neonate because phenothiazines are liable to produce extrapyramidal effects and irritability.

Breast milk. Methotrimeprazine is not recommended for use by lactating women because phenothiazines are secreted in breast milk, and can cause extrapyramidal effects and irritability in the neonate.

Children

Children are especially sensitive to the hypotensive and sedative effects of methotrimeprazine. The total daily oral dose for a child should not exceed 40 mg.

Pregnant women

Because its safety in pregnancy has not been established, methotrimeprazine should be avoided in pregnancy. Phenothiazines are prone

Methotrimeprazine (hydrochloride and maleate)

to cause extrapyramidal signs and irritability in the neonate. Nonetheless, methotrimeprazine has been used to treat labour pain at or near term, and in a double-blind comparison with pethidine was found to be safe and as effective as pethidine alone but less effective than pethidine plus scopolamine.[43]

The elderly
The hypotensive effects of methotrimeprazine are enhanced in the elderly, making it necessary to exercise great caution in prescribing for ambulant patients over age 50.

Concurrent disease
Methotrimeprazine should be avoided in liver disease because of the risk of precipitating coma. It should be used with caution in cardiac disease because of the risk of arrhythmias and hypotensive effects. In renal disease there is a risk of increased cerebral sensitivity to phenothiazines, and treatment should be initiated with a reduced dose.

Drug interactions

Potentially hazardous interactions

Adrenaline. Phenothiazines can reverse the pressor effect of adrenaline because of their α-adrenergic receptor blocking action.

Monoamine oxidase inhibitors. Unexplained fatalities have occurred in patients receiving methotrimeprazine coadministered with pargyline and with tranylcypromine.[44]

Other significant interactions

Hypotensive agents. Because of its α-adrenergic receptor blocking action, methotrimeprazine may enhance the effects of hypotensive drugs.

Anticholinergics. Extrapyramidal symptoms have been reported in patients premedicated with scopolamine and methotrimeprazine, implying that anticholinergics should be administered with caution in patients receiving methotrimeprazine.[45] Discontinuation of anticholinergic medication produces an increase in the plasma level of methotrimeprazine.[46]

CNS depressants. Methotrimeprazine is liable to enhance the effects of other CNS depressants. Dosage reduction may be necessary. Patients should be warned of the potential enhancement of the CNS depressant effects of alcohol.

Potentially useful interactions

Analgesics. On account of its analgesic effect and lack of substantial potentiation of the respiratory depression produced by opiates, methotrimeprazine can be a useful adjunct to opiate analgesics.

Clinical trials

1. Baker A A, Thorpe J G 1958 Assessing a new phenothiazine. Journal of Mental Science 104: 855–859

This was a randomized double-blind comparison of methotrimeprazine and chlorpromazine performed in a group of 28 chronic schizophrenic patients who had previously relapsed on withdrawal of chlorpromazine. Dose was adjusted according to clinical requirement. At eight weeks, the patients in both treatment groups had improved significantly in both the schizophrenic withdrawal score and restlessness score of the Baker and Thorpe Psychotic Behaviour Scale. The improvement in the group treated with methotrimeprazine did not differ significantly from that in the chlorpromazine group. At eight weeks, the methotrimeprazine group was receiving a mean daily dose of 261 mg, and the chlorpromazine group a mean daily dose of 348 mg. By 20 weeks, there had been further improvement in the schizophrenic withdrawal score in both treatment groups.

2. Quinn P J G, Johnson J, Latner G, Kiloh L G 1960 A comparative controlled trial of methotrimeprazine in chronic schizophrenia. Journal of Mental Science 106: 160–170

This was a randomized double-blind comparison of methotrimeprazine, chlorpromazine and placebo in 146 chronic schizophrenic patients, many of whom had severe persistent symptoms. For both active treatments, the initial dose was 25 mg daily and this was increased in 25 mg steps over a period of seven weeks to a total daily dose of 300 mg. The outcome measure was the change in clinical state over the first nine weeks of treatment. Both drugs were significantly superior to placebo, but there was no significant difference between the two active treatment groups. 20 of 48 cases treated with methotrimeprazine, and 15 of 48 cases treated with chlorpromazine had improved. Weight gain, drowsiness and parkinsonism were the most common side effects in the group treated with methotrimeprazine.

M

3. Minuck M 1972 Post-operative analgesia — comparison of methotrimeprazine (nozinan) and meperidine (demerol) as post-operative analgesia agents. Canadian Anaesthetists Society Journal 19: 87–96

In this double-blind study, 197 patients with postoperative pain were randomly allocated to receive either 10 $mg.ml^{-1}$ methotrimeprazine intramuscularly, 50 $mg.ml^{-1}$ pethidine intramuscularly or normal saline. Pain relief was rated on a scale from 1 (excellent) to 4 (unsatisfactory) at 20–30 minutes after injection. The mean ratings of efficacy in pain relief were 2.83 for methotrimeprazine, 2.91 for pethidine and 3.22 for saline. The difference between methotrimeprazine and pethidine was not statistically significant, but both active drugs were significantly superior to the saline placebo. Methotrimeprazine produced a greater fall in systolic blood pressure, but less nausea and vomiting than pethidine. 11 of the 66 patients in the methotrimeprazine group were drowsy, compared with 2 of the 65 in the group treated with pethidine.

Other trials

1. Davidson O, Lindeneg O, Walsh M 1979 Analgesic treatment with levomepromazine in acute myocardial infarction. Acta Medica Scandinavica 205: 191–194

A double-blind comparison of methotrimeprazine and pethidine for the alleviation of pain in 328 consecutive cases of myocardial infarction was performed. Efficacy in pain control was equal, but there was significantly lower mortality at 4 weeks and 1 year in the group treated with methotrimeprazine.

General review articles

Council on Drugs 1968 A non-narcotic analgesic agent. Journal of the American Medical Association 204: 159–160

Caprietti G 1962 The value of methotrimeprazine in the treatment of cancer pain. Minerva Medica 53: 3300–3306

References

1. Courvoisier S, Ducrot R, Fournel J, Julou L 1957 Proprietes pharmacodynamiques generales de la levomepromazine. Comptes Rendus de la Societe de Biologie (Paris) 151: 1378–1382
2. Courvoisier S, Leau O 1959 Activite analgesique experimental de la levomepromazine. Comptes Rendus de l'Academie des Sciences 248: 3227–3228
3. Hals P A, Hall W, Dahl S G 1986 Phenothiazine drug metabolites: dopamine D_2 receptor α_1 and α_2 adrenoreceptor binding. European Journal of Pharmacology 125: 373–381
4. Ankiewicz M L 1986 The influence of chronic treatment with antidepressant neuroleptics on the central serotonin system. Polish Journal of Pharmacology and Pharmacy 38: 359–370
5. Lasagna J, Dekornfeld T J 1961 Methotrimeprazine, a new phenothiazine derivative with analgesic properties. Journal of the American Medical Association 178: 887–890
6. Bloomfield S, Simard-Savoie S, Bernier J, Tetrault L 1964 Comparative analgesic activity of levopromazine and morphine in patients with chronic pain. Canadian Medical Association Journal 90: 1156–1159
7. Minuck M 1972 Post-operative analgesia — comparison of methotrimeprazine (Nozinan) and meperidine (demerol) as post-operative analgesia agents. Canadian Anaesthetists Society Journal 19: 87–96
8. DeKornfeld T J, Pearson J W, Lasagna L 1964 The use of methotrimeprazine for the treatment of labour pain. New England Journal of Medicine 270: 391–394
9. Sigwald J, Boultier D 1959 Analgesic action of phenothiazines. I. Treatment of severe or intractable pain by levomepromazine. Therapie 14: 978–984
10. Petts H V, Pleuvry B J 1983 Interactions of morphine and methotrimeprazine in mouse and man with respect to analgesia, respiration and sedation. British Journal of Anaesthesia 55: 437–441
11. Pearson J W, Dekornfeld T J 1963 Effects of methotrimeprazine on respiration. Anesthesiology 24: 38–40
12. Zsigmund E K, Flynn K 1988 The effect of methotrimeprazine on arterial blood gases in human volunteers. Journal of Clinical Pharmacology 28: 1033–1037
13. Fraser H F, Rosenberg D E 1963 Observations on the human pharmacology and addictiveness of methotrimeprazine. Clinical Pharmacology and Therapeutics 4: 596–601
14. Quinn P J G, Johnson J, Latner G, Kiloh L G 1960 A comparative controlled trial of methotrimeprazine in chronic schizophrenia. Journal of Mental Science 106: 160–170
15. Payne P, Verinder D 1960 Levomepromazine in the treatment of neuroleptic resistant psychotics. Journal of Mental Science 106: 1429–1431

16. Teulie G, DeVerbizier J, Poyart E 1958 Essais therapeutiques par la levomepromezine des psychoses ayant resiste aux traitements anterieurement utilises. Annales Medico-Psychologiques 116: 159
17. Higi M, Niederle N, Bierbaum W, Schmidt G G, Seeber S 1980 Pronounced antiemetic activity of the antipsychotic drug levomepromazine in patients receiving cancer therapy. Journal of Cancer Research and Clinical Oncology 97: 81–86
18. Murakami K, Murakami K, Ueno T, Hijikata J, Shirasana K, Muto T 1982 Simultaneous determination of chlorpromazine and levomepromazine in human plasma and urine by high performance liquid chromatography using electrochemical detection. Journal of Chromatography 227: 103–112
19. Dahl S G 1976 Pharmacokinetics of methotrimeprazine after single and multiple doses. Clinical Pharmacology and Therapeutics 19: 435–442
20. Dahl S G, Garle M 1977 Identification of non-polar methotrimeprazine metabolites in plasma and urine by GLC-Mass Spectrometry. Journal of Pharmaceutical Science 66: 190–193
21. Dahl S G, Kaufmann E, Mompon B, Purcell T 1987 Nuclear Magnetic Resonance analysis of methotrimeprazine hydroxylation in humans. Journal of Pharmaceutical Science 76: 541–544
22. Dahl S G, Refsum H 1976 Effects of levomepromazine, chlorpromazine and their sulfoxides on isolated rat atria. European Journal of Pharmacology 37: 241
23. Morel E, Lloyd K G, Dahl S G 1987 Anti-apomorphine effects of phenothiazine drug metabolites. Psychopharmacology — Berlin 92: 68–72
24. Oliver D J 1985 The use of the syringe driver in terminal care. British Journal of Clinical Pharmacology 20: 515–516
25. Davidson O, Lindeneg O, Walsh M 1979 Analgesic treatment with levomepromazine in acute myocardial infarction. Acta Medica Scandinavica 205: 191–194
26. Oliver D J 1985 The use of methotrimeprazine in terminal care. British Journal of Clinical Practice 39: 339–340
27. Anath J V, Lehmann H E, Ban T A 1970 Agranulocytosis associated with methotrimeprazine (Nozinan). Canadian Medical Association Journal 102: 1286–1287
28. Motomura N, Ashaba H, Sakai T 1989 R-R interval during neuroleptic treatment. Biological Psychiatry 26: 219–220
29. Padgett R, Lipman E 1989 Use of neuroleptics after an episode of neuroleptic malignant syndrome. Canadian Journal of Psychiatry 34: 323–325
30. Klys M, Brandys J 1988 Gas chromatography in multidrug overdose fatalities. Forensic Science International 38: 185–192
31. Andersson S B, Forskell G P, Schulman A, Wellerberg L, Ashaba W 1983 Levomepromazine elimination in patients during active and sham haemodialysis. Artificial Organs 7: 340–343
32. Basset A, Renwick R A, Blasberg B 1986 Tardive dyskinesia: an unrecognized cause of orofacial pain. Oral Medicine, Oral Surgery and Oral Pathology 61: 570–572
33. Pierson H, Priess H A, Perrin F, Cuny G 1987 Hepatite cholestastique chez une patiente prenant de la levomepromazine. Annales de Gastroenterologie et d'Hepatologie — Paris 23: 101
34. Kassman J, Wetterberg L 1987 Lens opacities and porphorobilinogen-like substance in urine associated with levomepromazine. Acta Psychiatrica Scandinavica 43: 163–168
35. Deodati F, Bec P, Labro J B, Arne J L, Chambon P 1973 Maculopathie et levomepromazine. Bulletins et Memoires de la Societe Francaise d'Ophtalmologie 86: 191–197
36. Van Sweden B 1985 Toxic 'ictal' confusion in middle age: treatment with benzodiazepines. Journal of Neurology, Neurosurgery and Psychiatry 48: 472–476
37. Warnes H, Lehmann H E, Ban T A 1967 Adynamic ileus during psychoactive medication: a report of three fatal and five severe cases. Canadian Medical Association Journal 96: 1112–1113
38. Johansson G 1988 Contact urticaria form levomepromazine. Contact Dermatitis 19: 304
39. Bourgeouis M 1972 Priapismus sous neuroleptiques (trois cas). Nouvelle Presse Medicale 1: 1161
40. Linnet K, Anderson J R, Morup L 1983 Acta Psychiatrica Scandinavica 67: 315–318
41. Denis P, LeLeannec A M, Benhamou J P 1973 Augmentation de la clearance de la brome-sulfone-pthaleine par les phenothiazines. Nouvelle Presse Medicale 2: 2881–2883
42. Rado J P, Simon T, Johos E, Tako J, Nagy O 1974 Interference of psychotropic drugs with cortisol determination. Hormone and Metabolic Research 6: 530–531
43. Cullaghan P E, Zelenik J S 1966 Methotrimeprazine for obstetric analgesia. American Journal of Obstetrics and Gynaecology 95: 636–639
44. Sjoqvist F 1965 Psychotropic drugs (2): Interaction between MAO inhibitors and other substances. Proceedings of the Royal Society of Medicine 58: 967–978
45. Stockley I 1981 Drug interactions. Blackwell, Oxford
46. Gautier J, Jus M, Villeneuve A, Jus K, Pres P, Villaneuve R 1977 Influence of the anti-parkinsonism drugs on the plasma level of neuroleptics. Biological Psychiatry 12: 389–399

Methyclothiazide

Methyclothiazide is a thiazide diuretic.

Chemistry

Methyclothiazide (Enduron, Aquatensen)
$C_9H_{11}Cl_2N_3O_4S_2$
6-Chloro-3-(chloromethyl)-3,4 dihydro-2-methyl-2H-1,2,4-benzothiadiazine-7-sulphonamide-1,1-dioxide

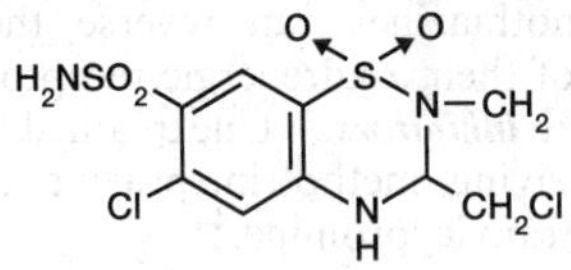

Molecular weight	360.25
pKa (sulphonamide)	9.4
Solubility	
in alcohol	soluble
in water	almost insoluble
Octanol/water partition coefficient	—

Methyclothiazide is an off-white to colourless powder prepared by chemical synthesis.

It is available in a number of combination formulations (Enduronyl, Enduronyl Forte, Diutensen, Diutensen-R).

Pharmacology

The actions of methyclothiazide are similar to those of other benzothiadiazine (thiazide) diuretics. These drugs cause their natriuretic effect by decreasing sodium and chloride reabsorption to a minor degree at the proximal tubule with their major effect at the cortical segment of the thick ascending limb of the loop of Henle (also referred to as the diluting segment).[1] Because of this latter effect, these agents decrease the ability to dilute the urine and thereby impair the ability of patients to respond to a water load.[2–5] This can result in hyponatraemia.

The increased sodium excretion caused by these agents is also associated with increased potassium excretion because of an increased tubular fluid flow rate and increased sodium delivery to the distal tubule and collecting duct.[2–4] Both effects independently increase potassium secretion at distal nephron sites, causing a kaliuresis.

The mild volume depletion caused by thiazide diuretics results in increased proximal tubular reabsorption of cations such as lithium and calcium and also of uric acid. Hence, decreased lithium excretion occurs which mandates a decrease in the maintenance dose of lithium.[6,7] Similarly, decreased calcium excretion occurs which can be therapeutic in patients with nephrolithiasis[8–10] or undesirable if it causes hypercalcaemia[11] (particularly in patients with overt or occult hyperparathyroidism). Lastly, the increased uric acid can be asymptomatic or, rarely, can precipitate gout.[12–15]

By unknown mechanisms thiazide diuretics decrease peripheral vascular resistance during chronic therapy, which accounts for their efficacy as antihypertensive agents.[16]

Toxicology

Much larger doses than those used in man have been well tolerated in mice, rats, dogs and monkeys with both acute and chronic administration. Effects observed were those of the known pharmacology of

Methyclothiazide

the drug. The vast majority of toxic effects of thiazides observed in clinical use in man are also extensions of the pharmacology of the drug. The remainder are accounted for by unexpected hypersensitivity reactions including rashes, and rarely bone marrow depression, and vasculitiis.[17] Neither mutagenicity nor carcinogenicity data are available.

Clinical pharmacology

The clinical pharmacology of methyclothiazide is identical to that of other thiazide diuretics.[18–34] These properties can be conveniently divided into renal as opposed to extra-renal effects:

a. Renal effects of methyclothiazide

It is presumed that methyclothiazide must gain entry into the urine to cause its renal effects. All thiazides and the chemically similar loop diuretics which have been studied block tubular solute reabsorption from the lumen (urine) side of the tubule as opposed to the peritubular (blood) side.[35] In turn, all similar agents are highly bound to serum albumin and cannot enter the urine by filtration at the glomerulus. Instead, they are actively secreted via the organic acid transport pump of the proximal tubule.[36] Whether methyclothiazide behaves similarly can only be assumed, since specific studies have not been performed with this drug.

Upon entering the luminal contents, thiazides have a minor effect to block sodium chloride reabsorption in the proximal tubule with a dominant effect at the cortical segment of the thick ascending limb of the loop of Henle (diluting segment).[1] The proximal effect is sufficiently small that solute rejected from this site is reclaimed at the medullary segment of the thick ascending limb of the loop of Henle. Hence, the overall natriuretic effect is the result of the thiazide's effect at the diluting segment less the sodium reabsorbed at more distal sites in exchange for potassium and/or hydrogen.[1] Thiazides have recently been shown to inhibit an electroneutral NaCl reabsorption pathway in the distal nephron.[37,38]

Because of their natriuretic and diuretic effects, thiazides are used to treat oedematous states and for hypertension. With the latter, an additional extra-renal effect of these drugs is also important (see below). However, in addition to their obvious use to cause losses of sodium chloride, these agents have other effects on renal function that can be used therapeutically.

The mild volume depletion caused by the thiazide diuretics results in increased proximal tubular reabsorption of sodium, other solutes and water. This can be advantageous in patients with nephrolithiasis from hypercalciuria[8–10] and in patients with nephrogenic diabetes insipidus.[39] Increased proximal tubular reabsorption of calcium parallels that of sodium, such that chronic thiazide therapy results in decreased urinary calcium excretion which is often sufficient to curtail stone formation.[8–10] Importantly, this effect requires chronic thiazide administration and mild volume depletion.[9] Acute administration of a thiazide diuretic causes increased calcium excretion by blocking calcium reabsorption at distal nephron sites; the decreased calcium excretion does not occur until increased proximal reabsorption of solute supervenes with chronic therapy.

A similar pharmacology occurs in patients with nephrogenic diabetes insipidus. The indirect effect of increasing proximal tubular reabsorption of water coupled with the direct effect more distally of decreasing the maximal ability to dilute the urine culminates in a diminished urine volume which may be sufficient to improve these patients' quality of life.[39]

The beneficial clinical pharmacology described above is also coupled with predictable potential side effects of thiazide diuretics. Increased distal tubular lumen flow rates enhance potassium secretion.[2–5] Similarly, reabsorption of sodium in exchange for potassium and/or hydrogen at this same nephron segment also increases potassium secretion.[2–5] Hence, patients receiving these drugs are subject to potassium and hydrogen ion loss culminating in a hypokalaemic metabolic alkalosis.

Epidemiologically, it would appear that this condition develops only infrequently,[40] probably because dietary intake of potassium is sufficient to match urinary potassium losses in the majority of patients.

The decreased excretion of calcium can result in hypercalcaemia, particularly in patients with hyperparathyroidism.[11] In fact, the development of hypercalcaemia on institution of therapy with thiazide diuretics may be the first clue that occult hyperparathyroidism is present.

Lastly, the diminished ability to dilute the urine maximally renders patients unable to excrete a hypotonic fluid load. If free water intake exceeds the capacity to excrete it, hyponatraemia will ensue. Thiazide diuretics are one of the most common causes of hyponatraemia and its development may preclude their use in some patients.

b. Extra-renal effects of methyclothiazide

Thiazide diuretics including methyclothiazide are extensively used as single agents or as adjunctive therapy for hypertension.[16,18] Early in the course of therapy with thiazides, the blood pressure lowering effect most likely occurs via the natriuretic-induced volume depletion. However, with chronic therapy with these agents, homeostatic mechanisms restore blood volume to or toward normal while the antihypertensive effect persists. It appears that the blood pressure lowering with chronic treatment with thiazides occurs by a decrease in peripheral vascular resistance, the mechanism of which is unknown.[16] This effect is also associated with a diminished response to vasoconstrictors such as catecholamines, and angiotensin, but how it occurs is not understood.

Pharmacokinetics

No formal studies of the pharmacokinetics of methyclothiazide are available, most likely because the drug was developed before the utility of such data was perceived and before sensitive and specific analytical methods were available. Subsequent investigators have demonstrated thin layer chromatography,[41] gas chromatography,[42] and high performance liquid chromatography[43,44] to be sensitive and specific measurement techniques. The last is the most efficient method of assay. However, these techniques have not been applied to defining methyclothiazide's pharmacokinetics. If this drug is similar to other thiazides, it is highly protein bound with a volume of distribution approximating intravascular volume, with little or no metabolic degradation and with excretion of most of a dose into the urine as unchanged drug.[45]

Clinical pharmacology studies have shown the effective dose of methyclothiazide to be 2.5 to 10.0 mg.[18–34] Since the drug seems to have a long duration of action (approximately 24 h), it can be administered once a day. Like all other thiazide diuretics, the dose–response curve is shallow, with little difference between the minimally effective and the maximally effective dose. In addition, the maximal effect is the same as occurs with all other thiazides.[17] Consequently, methyclothiazide is interchangeable with other thiazides with the only differentiating features among them being duration of action and cost.

Concentration–effect relationship

No studies have evaluated the relationship between concentrations of methyclothiazide and effect. If this drug is similar to other thiazide diuretics on which studies have been conducted, urinary amounts, rather than serum concentrations, of the drug will be the best correlate of response, for the drug probably must reach the urine to be effective.[35,36]

Metabolism

It appears that methyclothiazide is not metabolized and is excreted unchanged in the urine in its entirety.

Pharmaceutics

1. Enduron (Abbott, UK/USA): Monogrammed, grooved, square-shaped tablets; the 2.5 mg strength is orange coloured; the 5.0 mg strength is salmon coloured.
2. Aquatensen (Wallace, USA): also contains 5 mg methyclothiazide.
3. Enduronyl and Enduronyl Forte (Abbott, USA): also contain deserpidine.
4. Diutensen (Wallace, USA): contains methyclothiazide and cryptenamine (vevatrum alkaloid).
5. Diutensen R (Wallace, USA): contains methyclothiazide and reserpine.

No special storage conditions are needed and the shelf-life is 36 months.

Dyes include AZO and Ponceau 4R.

M

Therapeutic use

Indications

Therapeutic indications for the use of methyclothiazide include:

Renal actions

1. Oedematous disorders
2. Hypercalciuric nephrolithiasis
3. Diabetes insipidus
4. Hypertension.

Non-renal actions

5. Hypertension.

Contraindications

There are few absolute contraindications to thiazide diuretics, which are drugs of low toxicity, but there are several circumstances where they are best avoided.

1. Maturity onset diabetes
2. Gout
3. Hyponatraemia
4. Previous hypersensitivity reactions to thiazides
5. Pregnancy, in which fetal exposure can cause jaundice, thrombocytopenia, haemolytic anaemia and electrolyte abnormalities.

Mode of use

1. Oedematous disorders

Methyclothiazide, like all thiazides, is a mild diuretic that can be used in all of the oedematous disorders. Therapy should commence with a 2.5 mg dose and if insufficient be increased to 5.0 and then 10.0 mg once a day. If the maximum dose is not effective, the thiazide should be abandoned and a more potent diuretic used. In addition, in patients with diminished renal function (creatinine clearance < 50 ml.min^{-1}) thiazides are usually not effective diuretics as single agents and more potent drugs should be used instead.[2–4] The mechanism of this lack of effect is probably an inability of the diuretic to gain access to its urinary site of action when renal function is impaired.[36] Rarely, patients are encountered who are refractory to large doses of loop diuretics. In such patients, the addition of a thiazide diuretic, including methyclothiazide, can sometimes be effective.[46–48] If used in this fashion, it is probably reasonable to start with the maximum dose.

2. Hypercalciuric nephrolithiasis

As discussed previously, the mild volume depletion associated with chronic thiazide (and presumably methyclothiazide) therapy causes decreased urinary calcium excretion which can ameliorate stone formation in patients with hypercalciuric nephrolithiasis.[8–10] This therapeutic effect can usually be obtained with a low dose. The patient's urinary calcium excretion can be followed to judge the need for higher doses. This effect is probably best assessed after several weeks of therapy.

3. Nephrogenic diabetes insipidus

Thiazide diuretics can also be effective in patients with nephrogenic diabetes insipidus.[39] A beneficial effect can usually be obtained with a low dose, with further dose escalation based on the easily monitored urinary output of the patient.

4. Hypertension

Probably the most prevalent indication for use of thiazide diuretics, including methyclothiazide, is for hypertension.[16] In this setting, they are useful as single agents in mild hypertension and in combination with other drugs (e.g. β-adrenergic antagonists, central acting α-adrenergic stimulants, peripheral α-adrenergic antagonists, directly acting vasodilators, etc.) in more severe hypertension.[27–34] Therapy should begin with a low dose and increase as described for oedematous disorders. Importantly, it may take several weeks for the effect to become maximal, so escalation of doses should occur at approximately monthly intervals. In general, dose increases are not beneficial in the treatment of hypertension and response is usually best at low dosages. An increase in the dose may only enhance the chance of side effects occurring.

Methyclothiazide

Adverse reactions

Potentially life-threatening effects

As discussed under Pharmacology and Clinical pharmacology, hyponatraemia and hypokalaemia can occur with use of any thiazide, including methyclothiazide. The former occurs because of the effect of these drugs in impairing the ability to dilute the urine maximally. If free water intake is sufficient to exceed excretion, hyponatraemia can develop. Usually, this is asymptomatic and of mild degree; however, profound, life-threatening hyponatraemia can occur.

Though most patients receiving thiazide diuretics do not become potassium depleted or develop hypokalaemia, approximately 5% do.[40] This can occasionally be life-threatening, particularly in patients with cardiac disease and especially if they are being treated with digitalis glycosides.

A variety of allergic reactions have been reported with thiazide diuretics.[17] These usually manifest as minor skin rashes but rarely more serious conditions such as anaphylaxis, Stevens–Johnson syndrome or necrotizing vasculitis may occur and can be life-threatening.

Blood dyscrasias, including aplastic anaemia, agranulocytosis, and thrombocytopaenia have been attributed to treatment with thiazide diuretics.

Acute pancreatitis has been reported as an adverse reaction to methyclothiazide and to related oral diuretics.

Acute overdosage

Overdose of thiazides can result in depression of central nervous system function, but most commonly results in the predictable pharmacological effects of these drugs.[17] Treatment is supportive.

Severe or irreversible adverse effects

Loss of libido and impotence are recognized as complications of thiazide therapy.

Cholestatic jaundice has been associated with the administration of drugs of the thiazide group.

Symptomatic adverse effects

All thiazide diuretics can cause hyperuricaemia by two mechanisms: (1) mild volume depletion causes increased proximal tubular reabsorption of uric acid and (2) the thiazide itself inhibits renal secretion of uric acid.[49] This side effect is usually asymptomatic but can occasionally result in gout. Moreover, the asymptomatic hyperuricaemia does not adversely affect renal function.[12–15] Consequently, unless gout occurs, the hyperuricaemia does not need to be treated.

By the same mechanisms that cause urinary calcium to decrease, serum calcium concentration may concomitantly increase.[11] The degree of elevation is usually minor and asymptomatic. Its importance is only to raise the question of co-existent occult hyperparathyroidism.

All thiazide diuretics can decrease glucose tolerance by mechanisms that are unclear.[50] In most patients this effect is not sufficient to cause overt, symptomatic diabetes mellitus. However, in non-insulin-dependent diabetics, the requirement for oral hypoglycaemics may be increased or a need to change to therapy with insulin may occur.

Recent evidence has indicated that thiazide therapy can cause 10–15% increases in VLDL and LDL cholesterol by unknown mechanisms.[50] The effect, however, appears to occur by biochemical mechanisms rather than by volume depletion. Some investigators feel the effect is linked to glucose intolerance which in turn is linked to potassium depletion. The majority of data argues against this mechanism, implying that the effect cannot be prevented by potassium supplementation. Whether the increase in LDL cholesterol could adversely affect cardiac risk is unclear, but the potential is unsettling and has resulted in more cautious use of thiazides in the treatment of hypertension.

Interference with clinical pathology tests

No technical interferences of this kind have been reported.

High risk groups

Neonates

The drug is not used in patients of this age group.

Breast milk. All thiazides tested appear in breast milk and presumably this would also be the case for methyclothiazide.[17] The amount received by a breast-fed infant is very small and breast-feeding is not contra-indicated.

Children

The drug may be used in children in appropriate doses.

Pregnant women

Thiazides, and presumably methyclothiazide, cross the placenta and the drug is best avoided in pregnancy. Fetal exposure can cause jaundice, thrombocytopenia, haemolytic anaemia and electrolyte abnormalities.

The elderly

The elderly have mildly diminished renal function which makes them less responsive to the renal effects of thiazide diuretics. Presumably, this phenomenon relates to decreased access of these diuretics to their urinary site of action.[36] Hence, elderly patients may require larger doses or more potent diuretics. A corollary of the diminished renal excretion of thiazides in the elderly would be the prediction that overall clearance would be less and thereby serum concentrations would be increased. This might result in an increased antihypertensive effect though this possibility has not been studied. However, overall the elderly might need lower doses of methyclothiazide as an antihypertensive and a higher dose as a diuretic.

Concurrent disease

In general, patients with renal insufficiency and creatinine clearances $< 50\ ml.min^{-1}$ do not respond to thiazides as diuretics. The mechanisms and implications are the same as discussed above for the elderly.

Patients with cardiac disease are most likely at greater risk of complications from potassium depletion caused by methyclothiazide, particularly if they are receiving digitalis glycosides.

Patients with cirrhosis are sensitive to diuretic-induced changes in volume and electrolyte status. Hence, volume depletion, potassium depletion and/or hyponatraemia can precipitate hepatic encephalopathy in such patients.

Drug interactions

Potentially hazardous interactions

Methyclothiazide presumably has the same capacity as other thiazide diuretics to decrease the renal elimination of lithium.[6,7] If maintenance doses of the latter are not decreased by approximately 25 to 50%, toxicity may ensue. Lithium is reabsorbed in the proximal tubule. The mild volume depletion of chronic thiazide therapy causes increased proximal tubular reabsorption of lithium, thereby diminishing its renal clearance.[6,7]

Patients treated with digitalis glycosides are more sensitive to toxicity from these compounds when they are potassium or magnesium depleted as can occur with methyclothiazide.

Potassium depletion of any cause can also potentiate the effect of neuromuscular blocking agents.

The volume depletion that occurs with methyclothiazide can cause postural hypotension which can be accentuated by other conditions causing volume depletion or other drugs which decrease venous tone such as some α-adrenergic antagonists, nitrates, tricyclic antidepressants, ethanol and barbiturates.

Potentially useful interactions

All thiazide diuretics have additive antihypertensive effects when combined with other blood pressure lowering medications.[27–34] The classical example of this phenomenon is use of these drugs to prevent the fluid retention associated with potent vasodilators.

Similarly, combining thiazide diuretics with diuretic agents affecting different nephron sites (e.g. loop diuretics, or potassium-retaining diuretics) results in an additive or even supra-additive effect.[46–48]

Nonsteroidal anti-inflammatory drugs may reduce the antihypertensive effect (but not apparently the diuretic effect) of thiazide diuretics.[51]

Major outcome trials

None.

References

1. Kunau R T, Weller D R, Webb H L 1975 Clarification of the site of action of chlorothiazide in the rat nephron. Journal of Clinical Investigation 56: 401–407

2. Frazier H S, Yager H 1973 The clinical use of diuretics: renal regulation of salt and water balances. New England Journal of Medicine 288: 246–249, 455–457
3. Jacobson H R, Kokko J P 1976 Diuretics: sites and mechanisms of action. Annual Review of Pharmacology and Toxicology 16: 201–214
4. Seely J F, Dirks J H 1977 Site of action of diuretic drugs. Kidney International 11: 1–8
5. Seldin D W, Eknoyan G, Suki W N, Rector F C 1966 Localization of diuretic action from the pattern of water and electrolyte excretion. Annals of the New York Academy of Science 139: 328–343
6. Amdisen A 1977 Serum level monitoring and clinical pharmacokinetics of lithium. Clinical Pharmacokinetics 2: 73–92
7. Thomsen K, Schou M 1968 Renal lithium excretion in man. American Journal of Physiology 215: 823–827
8. Brickman A S, Massry S G, Coburn J W 1972 Changes in serum and urinary calcium during treatment with hydrochlorothiazide: studies on mechanisms. Journal of Clinical Investigation 51: 945–954
9. Breslau N, Moses A M, Weiner I M 1976 The role of volume contraction in the hypocalciuric action of chlorothiazide. Kidney International 10: 164–170
10. Coe F L 1977 Treated and untreated recurrent calcium nephrolithiasis in patients with idiopathic hypercalciuria, hyperuricosuria, or no metabolic disorder. Annals of Internal Medicine 87: 404–410
11. Duarte C G, Winnacker J L, Becker K L, Pace A 1971 Thiazide-induced hypercalcemia. New England Journal of Medicine 284: 828–830
12. Berger L, Yu T-F 1975 Renal function in gout. IV. An analysis of 524 gouty subjects including long-term follow-up studies. American Journal of Medicine 59: 605–613
13. Yu T-F, Berger L, Dorph D J, Smith H 1979 Renal function in gout. V. Factors influencing the renal hemodynamics. American Journal of Medicine 67: 766–771
14. Fessel W J 1979 Renal outcomes of gout and hyperuricemia. American Journal of Medicine 67: 74–82
15. Johnson M W, Mitch W E 1981 The risks of asymptomatic hyperuricaemia and the use of uricosuric diuretics. Drugs 21: 220–225
16. Shah S, Khatri I, Freis E D 1978 Mechanism of antihypertensive effect of thiazide diuretics. American Heart Journal 95: 611–618
17. Gilman A G, Goodman L S, Rall T W, Murad F 1985 Goodman and Gilman's The pharmacological basis of therapeutics, 7th edn. Macmillan, New York, pp 892–896
18. Seller R H 1962 The clinical pharmacology of methyclothiazide. Geriatrics 17: 577–582
19. Wilson S A 1963 Clinical and laboratory observations on methyclothiazide, an oral diuretic. Current Therapeutic Research 5: 63–69
20. Ford R V, Bush J 1960 Clinical-pharmacologic investigation of methyclothiazide, a new oral diuretic. Current Therapeutic Research 2: 422–429
21. Ford R V, Bush J 1960 Comparative clinical effects of hydrochlorothiazide and methyclothiazide. Current Therapeutic Research 2: 430–441
22. Patel N, Mock D C Jr 1963 A comparative study of diuretic agents, methyclothiazide and dihydrochlorothiazide. Current Therapeutic Research 5: 127–134
23. Stern F H 1962 The use of methyclothiazide (Enduron) in geriatric patients. Journal of the American Geriatric Society 10: 256–263
24. Soghikian K, Bartenbach D E 1977 Influence of dosage and duration of therapy on the rate of response to methyclothiazide in essential hypertension. Southern Medical Journal 70: 1397–1404
25. Bushnell L F 1965 Methyclothiazide in the management of premenstrual tension. Western Medicine 6: 168–169
26. Walker J L Methyclothiazide in excessive weight gain and edema of pregnancy. Obstetrics and Gynecology 27: 247–251
27. Kravitz B J, Hutchinson J C 1968 The hypoglycemic effect of pargyline hydrochloride on the fasting blood sugar of patients receiving methyclothiazide. Current Therapeutic Research 10: 18–23
28. Sutnick A I, Frankl W S, Fewell J W, Esbenshade J H Jr, Bello C T 1966 Antihypertensive effect of pargyline and methyclothiazide in combination. Vascular Diseases 3: 145–155
29. Fletcher F W 1968 A unique antihypertensive combination — pargyline hydrochloride and methyclothiazide: a controlled study of twenty-five patients over a nine-month period. Current Therapeutic Research 10: 394–398
30. Waldmann E B, Nickas G 1967 Pargyline hydrochloride combined with methyclothiazide in the treatment of hypertension. Arizona Medicine 24: 343–346
31. Kimmerling H W 1967 Methyclothiazide and deserpidine in the treatment of the elderly hypertensive. Current Therapeutic Research 9: 75–78
32. Hamm H J 1966 Pargyline hydrochloride combined with methyclothiazide in the treatment of essential hypertension. Current Therapeutic Research 8: 378–383
33. Shafer N 1966 Combined therapy for the treatment of hypertension: pargyline hydrochloride and methyclothiazide. Vascular Diseases 3: 59–66
34. Breall W S 1966 Treatment of hypertension with a combination of pargyline hydrochloride and methyclothiazide. Journal of the American Geriatric Society 14: 85–87
35. Odlind B 1979 Relation between renal tubular secretion and effects of five loop diuretics. Journal of Pharmacology and Experimental Therapeutics 211: 238–244
36. Brater D C 1983 Pharmacodynamic considerations in the use of diuretics. Annual Review of Pharmacology and Toxicology 23: 45–62
37. Shimizu T, Yoshitomi K, Namkamura M, Imai M 1988 Site and mechanism of action of trichlormethiazide in rabbit distal nephron segments perfused in vitro. Journal of Clinical Investigation 82: 721–730
38. Stokes J B 1984 Sodium chloride absorption by the urinary bladder of the winter flounder. A thiazide-sensitive electrically neutral transport system. Journal of Clinical Investigation 74: 7–16
39. Crawford J D, Kennedy G C 1959 Animal physiology: chlorothiazide in diabetes mellitus. Nature 183: 891–892
40. Lawson D H 1974 Adverse reactions to potassium chloride. Quarterly Journal of Medicine 43: 433–440
41. Osborne B G 1972 A thin-layer chromatography screening technique for thiazide diuretics in urine. Journal of Chromatography 70: 190–193

42. Fagerlund C, Hartvig P, Lindstrom B 1979 Extractive alkylation of sulphonamide diuretics and their determination by electron-capture gas chromatography. Journal of Chromatography 168: 107–116
43. Moskalyk R E, Locock R A, Chatten L G, Veltman A M, Bielech M F 1975 Determination of polythiazide in pharmaceutical dosage forms by high-pressure liquid chromatography. Journal of Pharmaceutical Sciences 64: 1406–1408
44. Hartman C A, Kucharozyk N, Sofia R D, Perhach J L Jr 1981 Determination of methyclothiazide in human plasma by high-performance liquid chromatography. Journal of Chromatography 226: 510–513
45. Beermann B, Groschinsky-Grind M 1980 Clinical pharmacokinetics of diuretics. Clinical Pharmacokinetics 5: 221–245
46. Sigurd B, Olesen K H, Wennevold A 1975 The supra-additive natriuretic effect of addition of bendroflumethiazide and bumetanide in congestive heart failure. American Heart Journal 89: 163–170
47. Wollam G L, Tarazi R C, Bravo E L, Dustan H P 1982 Diuretic potency of combined hydrochlorothiazide and furosemide therapy in patients with azotemia. American Journal of Medicine 72: 929–938
48. Oster J R, Epstein M, Smoller S 1983 Combined therapy with thiazide-type and loop diuretic agents for resistant sodium retention. Annals of Internal Medicine 99: 405–406 (editorial)
49. Manuel M A, Steele T H 1974 Changes in renal urate handling after prolonged thiazide treatment. American Journal of Medicine 57: 741–746
50. Ames R P 1983 Metabolic disturbances increasing the risk of coronary heart disease during diuretic-based antihypertensive therapy: lipid alterations and glucose intolerance. American Heart Journal 106: 1207–1214
51. Faure L, Glasson P L, Riondel A, Valloton M B 1983 Interaction of diuretics and nonsteroidal anti-inflammatory drugs in man. Clinical Science 64: 407–415

Methylcellulose

Methylcellulose is a semi-synthetic carbohydrate laxative.

Chemistry

Methylcellulose BPC (Cologel, Celevac, Cellucon, Methocell, Syncelose, Bagolax, Cellylose, Cethytin, Cellumeth, Hydrolose, Nicel, Tearisol, Tylose)

Methylcellulose is a white or creamy white powder or granules, odourless, and somewhat hygroscopic. It is prepared from wood pulp or chemical cotton by treatment with alkali and methylation of the alkali cellulose with methyl chloride. It is present in the compound preparation Nilstim.

Pharmacology

Methylcellulose acts by increasing stool moisture uptake in the colon. In addition it delays gastric emptying, accelerates small intestinal transit and changes faecal bile acids and colonic bacteria.

Toxicology

It is not known if methylcellulose has mutagenic potential. There is no evidence of toxic effects in animals or man. Carcinogenicity testing in rats has failed to show any carcinogenic properties.[1]

Clinical pharmacology

Methylcellulose produces a laxative effect partly by increasing small bowel transit time by absorbing fluid, thus increasing the intestinal contents.[2] Methylcellulose is itself non-absorbable and so remains in the gastrointestinal tract. There is also a complex interaction that increases colonic bacteria and is likely to result in an increase in faecal bile acids, short-chain fatty acid production and gas formation. These factors are thought to cause an increase in faecal bulk and water output.[3,4]

Doses of 1–10 g per day produce a variable increase in stool volume and frequency. Doses up to 25 $mg.kg^{-1}$ have been used safely.

Pharmacokinetics

Analytical analysis of the compound in vitro or in vivo has not been performed. Methylcellulose is excreted into the faeces. There is no systemic absorption.[5]

Concentration–effect relationship

There are no data on this subject and methylcellulose is not absorbed.

Pharmaceutics

Methylcellulose is only available as oral forms.

1. Cellucon (Medo, UK): tablets containing 500 mg of methylcellulose '2500' BP. The tablets are chocolate coloured and flavoured, uncoated.
2. Celevac (Boehringer Ingelheim, UK): plain pink coloured, uncoated tablets, containing 500 mg methylcellulose '450'.
3. Cologel (Lilly, UK) is an aromatized solution with 900 mg methylcellulose per 10 ml in a lemon flavoured vehicle with 5% alcohol.
4. Methylcellulose mixture, 900 mg of methylcellulose '450' per 10 ml, is a suspending agent for crushed tablet or liquid preparations. It may be sterilized by autoclaving. The life of the diluted mixture is 14 days. If stock solutions cannot be autoclaved they should include a preservative such as phenylmercuric nitrate 0.001%.

Methylcellulose is compatible with most hydroxybenzoates. All methylcellulose preparations are stable with a long shelf-life. Preparations should be protected from moisture and high temperatures to prevent gel formation. The liquids should not be frozen. The Cologel preparation contains 0.4 mg per 100 ml of tartrazine.

Therapeutic use

Indications

1. Idiopathic constipation
2. Diverticular disease
3. Irritable bowel syndrome
4. Control of chronic diarrhoea
5. To reduce food intake in the treatment of obesity.

Contraindications

1. Intestinal obstruction
2. Dehydration.

Mode of use

The clinical use of methylcellulose depends on the interaction with intestinal fluid, resulting in a bulking effect, and a varied effect on intestinal bacteria resulting in an increased production of fatty acids, bile acids and intestinal gas. It is likely that these latter effects are predominantly involved in the laxative action. Treatment begins at a dose of 500 mg daily and can be increased at 500 mg to 1g intervals until the desired effect is obtained. Doses up to 15g have been used from time to time, but it is unusual to use more than 6 g per day. Doses as low as 1 g daily have proved effective.[6] Where a laxative action is required, it is important to maintain an adequate fluid intake. However, where it is used to thicken faeces, extra fluid should be avoided.

Indications

1. Constipation
Methylcellulose may be helpful in simple constipation as an alternative to increasing dietary fibre intake.[7] Should the daily fibre intake be less than 30 g despite encouragement, methylcellulose may be of value. It is important to ensure an adequate fluid intake. A dose of 500 mg–1 g after each meal and at bedtime is adequate to promote the passage of formed soft stools within 3–4 days.[8] Should a more rapid or a more potent effect be required, an alternative type of agent should be tried.

2. Diverticular disease
In those patients with diverticular disease and constipation who are intolerant of a high fibre diet, methylcellulose may help. Care is required to avoid faecal impaction through a strictured area.

3. Irritable bowel syndrome
In the type of irritable bowel syndrome in which bowel performance is either alternating diarrhoea and constipation, or predominantly constipation, then a high fibre diet or a bulk-laxative like methylcellulose may provide symptomatic improvement. These agents usually do not improve the painless diarrhoea variant of the condition.

4. Control of chronic diarrhoea
The hygroscopic qualities of methylcellulose are of value in mild ileostomy or colostomy diarrhoea, in an attempt to thicken the ileostomy effluent. It is important that the patient ingests as little fluid as possible with their tablets or mixture. This makes the preparation less palatable. There is little evidence to justify the claims that it is of value in other forms of chronic diarrhoea.

Contraindications

1. Intestinal obstruction
Any patient with intestinal obstruction or severe narrowing of the intestinal lumen due to a stricture should avoid all bulk type laxatives.

2. Dehydration
Any patients, particularly children, who are dehydrated may have their condition worsened by the ingestion of methylcellulose by virtue of its hygroscopic properties.

Adverse reactions

Potentially life-threatening effects
No effects of this kind have been described.

Acute overdosage
No cases have been described, but overdose is unlikely to be harmful provided an adequate fluid intake is maintained.

Severe or irreversible adverse effects
No effects of this kind have been described.

Symptomatic adverse effects
Symptomatic adverse effects are rare, but have included nausea, bloating distension, fluid retention and diarrhoea. In all cases symptoms resolve on either dosage reduction or drug withdrawal.

Interference with clinical pathology tests
No interferences of this kind have been reported.

High risk groups

Neonates
The drug is not used in neonates.

Breast milk. As the drug is unabsorbed, it should be safe to use during lactation.

Children
Dosage reduction is necessary according to body size.

Pregnant women
As the drug is unabsorbed, it is considered safe for use during pregnancy.

The elderly
There are no known problems in elderly patients.

Drug interactions

There are no known clinically relevant interactions.

General review articles

Gullikson G W, Bass P 1984 Mechanism of action of laxative TZ drugs. In: Csaky T Z (ed) Pharmacology of intestinal permeation II. Springer-Verlag, Berlin ch 28: 419–461

Tainter M L, Buchanan O H 1954 Quantitative comparisons of colloidal laxatives. Annals of the New York Academy of Science: 438–452

WHO 1974 Microcystalline cellulose in thickening agents. A Celluloses. World Health Organisation, Geneva 14 H 5 297–315

References

1. Shelanksi H A, Clark A M 1942 Sodium carboxymethylcellulose; its physiological action on laboratory animals and humans. Food Research 13: 29
2. Malagelada J R, Carter S G, Brown M G, Carlson G L 1980 Radiolabelled fibre and physiological marker for gastric emptying and intestinal transit of solids. Digestive Diseases and Sciences 25: 81–87
3. Spiller G A, Chernoff M C, Hill R A, Gates S E, Nassar J J, Shipley E A 1980 Effect of purified cellulose, pectin and a low residue diet on faecal volatile fatty acids, transit time and faecal weight in humans. American Journal of Clinical Nutrition 33: 754–759
4. Tainter M L 1943 Methylcellulose as a colloid laxative. Proceedings of the Society for Experimental Biology and Medicine 54: 77–79
5. Mackle W, Heyroth F F, Witherup S 1944 The fate of methylcellulose in the human digestive tract. Journal of Biological Chemistry 153: 551–559
6. Hamilton J W, Wagner J, Burdick B B, Buss P 1988 Clinical evaluation of methylcellulose as a bulk laxative. Digestive Diseases and Sciences 33: 993–998
7. Schweig K 1948 The use of methylcellulose as a bulk laxative. New York State Journal of Medicine 48: 1822–1823
8. Bangen J A 1949 A method of improving function of the bowel, the use of methylcellulose. Gastroenterology 13: 275–279

M Methyldopa

Methyldopa is a widely used antihypertensive agent. It was first shown to have hypotensive properties by Oates.[1]

Chemistry

Methyldopa (alpha-methyldopa, Aldomet, Aldometil, Alphamex, Baypresol, Co-Caps Methyldopa, Dopamet, Dimal, Dopegyt, Grospisk, Hy-po-tone, Medimet-250, Medomet, Medopal, Medopren, Novomedopa, Presinol, Sembrina, Hyperpax (racemic), Hyperpaxa (racemic), Mulfasin (racemic))
$C_{10}H_{13}NO_4.1\frac{1}{2}H_2O$
α-Methyl-3,4-dihydroxy-L-phenylalanine sesquihydrate

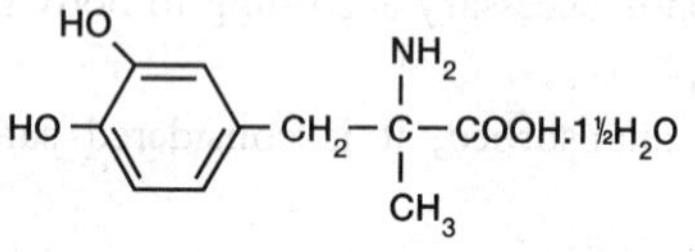

Molecular weight (anhydrous)	238.2 (211.21)
pKa(–COOH,–OH–NH_2,–OH)	2.2, 9.2, 10.6, 12
Solubility	
in alcohol	1 in 400
in water	1 in 100
Octanol/water partition coefficient	0.22 (calc.)[2]

Methyldopa is a colourless or almost colourless crystalline solid or a white to yellowish-white odourless, almost tasteless, fine powder which may contain friable lumps. It is prepared by chemical synthesis. Methyldopate hydrochloride is a more soluble ethyl ester, available for intravenous use.

Methyldopa is also available in an oral combination product with hydrochlorothiazide (Hydromet, Aldoril).

The (l)-isomer is used in most preparations, though a few contain the racemate.

Pharmacology

Hypotheses about the mechanisms of action of methyldopa have undergone several changes since the hypotensive effect was first reported in 1960. Early studies proposed a peripheral site of action for methyldopa by which stores of noradrenaline in sympathetic nerve endings were decreased, either by inhibition of l-aromatic amino acid decarboxylase, or by replacing noradrenaline with a metabolite of methyldopa, α-methylnoradrenaline, which would act as a 'false transmitter'.

Current evidence indicates the main site of action for methyldopa is within the central nervous system, although some contribution by peripheral mechanisms cannot be ruled out.[3] In central noradrenergic neurones methyldopa is metabolized to α-methylnoradrenaline, which is stored in synaptic vesicles and released by nerve stimulation. α-Methylnoradrenaline is a relatively specific agonist for α_2-receptors, suggesting that its effect is mediated by stimulation of α_2-receptors within the central nervous system. There is a resulting decrease in efferent sympathetic tone and a fall in arterial pressure. There is also evidence suggesting that central serotonergic pathways may be involved in the action of methyldopa.

Toxicology

Acute and chronic toxicity studies have established that methyldopa possesses a low order of toxicity. LD_{50} for intravenous methyldopa is in the range 700–1900 $mg.kg^{-1}$ in animals.[4] The minimum toxic or lethal dose for man has not been established. One adult female died following acute ingestion of 25 g of methyldopa.

Doses of methyldopa (6–12 mg subcutaneously) completely inhibit ovulation in mice,[5] but smaller doses are without effect. Methyldopa given throughout rat pregnancy showed no teratogenic effects at subcutaneous doses of 75 $mg.kg^{-1}$ daily.[6]

No teratogenic effects have been observed in man,[7] although male children of women who commenced treatment with methyldopa at 16–20 weeks of gestation had smaller head circumferences than sons of untreated women, but no difference in mean intelligence quotient.[7]

Methyldopa is non-mutagenic by the Ames test. Mutation studies in the hamster indicate an effect on lung somatic cells at a concentration[8] of 37 $mg.l^{-1}$. Tumour-inducing effects in man have not been described.

Clinical pharmacology

Oral administration of methyldopa in single doses of 250–1000 mg to patients with essential hypertension significantly reduces systolic and diastolic blood pressure, with an effect maximal at 4–6 hours and persisting for 10–12 hours with some residual effect at 24 hours after dosing.[9] The response to intravenous administration of the same dose of the ester, methyldopate, the commercially available parenteral form, is more variable or absent due to a slow hydrolysis to the active form in vivo in man and a much larger volume of distribution.

Methyldopa reduces total peripheral resistance without altering cardiac output or heart rate.[10,11] There is an increased total blood volume, which is not reflected in changes in cardiopulmonary blood volume due to the venodilation which results from reduced sympathetic outflow.[10,11]

The blood pressure and heart rate response to standing or feet-down tilt are attenuated by methyldopa as there is a modest fall in systolic pressure and only a small increase in heart rate.[12] The orthostatic effects of methyldopa on the blood pressure are of clinical significance, as approximately 15% of patients receiving the drug complain of postural light-headedness.[13] In most patients the blood pressure and heart rate responses to dynamic and static exercise are unchanged by treatment with methyldopa. The results of studies of the action of methyldopa on autonomic reflexes are not entirely consistent. With acute dosing the pressor response to the Valsalva manoeuvre is abolished or attenuated,[14] but the pressor response to cold stress is not affected.[11] There is an increase in responsiveness to intravenous noradrenaline and the indirect-acting sympathomimetic, tyramine,[14] suggesting enhanced sensitivity or number of peripheral α-adrenoceptors and increased storage and release of amines from nerve terminals.[15]

The hypotensive effect of methyldopa is accompanied by increases in renal blood and plasma flow[16,17] and decreases in renal vascular resistance with no change in glomerular filtration rate.[17] There is a moderate reduction in plasma renin activity, but this is unlikely to be sufficient to have a major hypotensive effect. Methyldopa given acutely causes an increase in urine volume.[17] On chronic administration most individuals have a tendency to fluid retention associated with an increased plasma volume.[18]

Methyldopa increases plasma prolactin concentration which may be associated with decreased libido, impotence and galactorrhoea.[19] There is no long-term impairment of glucose metabolism, or ACTH, thyrotropin or growth hormone release in man.[15]

In addition to the centrally mediated hypotensive effect, methyldopa produces other effects within the central nervous system. It has little or no effect on motor performance but in some patients extrapyramidal symptoms of rigidity and hypokinesia may be provoked, or a parkinsonian syndrome worsened.[20] Drowsiness and sedation occur frequently on initiation of therapy, possibly due to α receptor stimulation in other areas of the brain. Some tolerance to this sedative effect occurs with long-term treatment.

Methyldopa can increase the proportion of rapid eye movement (REM) sleep.[1]

Pharmacokinetics

For detection of methyldopa and its principal metabolites in plasma, urine and tissues, the preferred analytical method is by high performance liquid chromatography with electrochemical detection, which is specific and extremely sensitive.[21]

The absorption of orally administered methyldopa is incomplete and variable. It appears to be absorbed, at least in part, by the active transport process used by dietary l-aromatic amino acids. Oral bioavailability is approximately 25% (range 8–62%),[22] reflecting first-pass metabolism in the liver and also the gut wall. Food, in particular protein-rich meals, reduces both the rate and extent of bioavailability.[23]

During the absorption phase after oral dosing acid-labile conjugates, mainly methyldopa-O-sulphate, are found in plasma. As they are found in very small amounts after intravenous dosing, but account for approximately 40% of a dose after oral administration, they are probably formed in intestinal mucosal cells.[24,25]

The apparent volume of distribution in the central compartment is 0.23 $l.kg^{-1}$ (range 0.19–0.32 $l.kg^{-1}$) and the total apparent volume of distribution (V_d area) in healthy males is calculated to be 0.60 $l.kg^{-1}$ (range 0.41–0.72).[23] The commercially available parenteral dose form, methyldopate, has a much larger volume of distribution in man (estimated to be approximately 2 $l.kg^{-1}$)[24]. Animal studies with ^{14}C-methyldopa show a wide tissue distribution with the highest concentrations in the kidneys, heart and brain.[23]

Plasma protein binding of methyldopa is 10–15%. The acid-labile metabolites are about 50–60% protein bound.[23]

Methyldopa is excreted in breast milk in significant amounts as free (0–0.2 $\mu g.ml^{-1}$) and conjugated (0.1–0.9 $\mu g.ml^{-1}$) methyldopa .[26] Since most of the drug is conjugated it is most unlikely to affect the infant adversely. In infants delivered to mothers treated with methyldopa in pregnancy, the concentration of unconjugated methyldopa in umbilical cord plasma and maternal plasma at time of delivery are similar, indicating relatively complete distribution through the placenta.[27] These concentrations persist for some days after birth, with the potential to exert pharmacological effects.

Total drug clearance is 207 $ml.min^{-1}.m^{-2}$ (range 174–266). Renal clearance is 95 $ml.min^{-1}.m^{-2}$ (range 75–120), accounting for about 50% of drug elimination.[23]

The plasma elimination is biphasic with an α (distribution) phase half life of 0.21 h (range 0.16–0.26) and a β (elimination) phase of 1.38 h (range 1.0–1.7 h).[23] These figures may be an underestimate because of lack of sensitivity of available assays, as urinary data strongly suggest plasma elimination is not complete until 24–48 h after administration.

Oral absorption	incomplete
Presystemic metabolism	40–90%
Plasma half life	
range	1–2 h
mean	1.4 h
Volume of distribution	0.4–0.7 $l.kg^{-1}$
Plasma protein binding	10–15%

Methyldopa is metabolized in both the liver and the small intestine (after oral administration), with relatively large amounts eliminated in the faeces. After intravenous dosing 52–82% of the dose is excreted in the urine in 36 h.

Concentration–effect relationship

There is no correlation between plasma concentrations and antihypertensive effects of methyldopa.[24] Hypotensive effects of single doses may last up to 24 hours[9] with maximum effect on blood pressure at approximately 6–10 hours,[24,28] although the time of maximum plasma concentration varies between 1 and 6 hours after oral dosing and elimination half life is approximately 2 hours. Failure to demonstrate a relationship between plasma concentration of the drug and pharmacological activity is consistent with the drug's action through an active metabolite. Therapeutic plasma concentration monitoring is thus of no value, but the readily measurable end-point, blood pressure, is a good guide to the therapeutic dose.

In patients with renal impairment, an increased responsiveness to the hypotensive effect of methyldopa has been noted. Hypotensive effects are observed with lower plasma concentrations than in patients with normal renal function. One possible explanation is that excess accumulation of methyldopa-O-sulphate, or other metabolites, contributes to the hypotensive effect in renal failure patients, although a direct correlation between hypotensive response and plasma levels of the conjugate has not been shown. Recent work suggests the enhanced response may be due in part to α-methyldopamine found in elevated plasma concentrations in children with renal insufficiency.[29] The drug and the possibly active metabolites are removed by dialysis and harmful or prolonged hypotension may be effectively treated with dialysis. At present, there is no evidence that accumulation of methyldopa metabolites is harmful in renal failure, and dose requirements should be determined by blood pressure responses and presence or absence of side effects. In one study of methyldopa in patients with renal impairment methyldopa doses ranged from 250 to 1000 mg twice daily.[30]

Metabolism

Metabolism, largely in the liver and small intestine, accounts for approximately 50% of the total clearance of methyldopa. From a pharmacological viewpoint the most important metabolic steps are those which occur within adrenergic nerve endings in the brain and periphery where methyldopa is converted to its active metabolites, methyldopamine and methylnoradrenaline. Quantitatively the production of these active metabolites accounts for only a small proportion of the dose.

After an oral dose, the major metabolite is methyldopa-O-sulphate (30–60% of the dose), which is generally thought to be inactive in man but has been shown to have a hypotensive effect in animals.[23] Only small amounts of this metabolite are found after intravenous dosing, suggesting that it is predominantly formed during the first pass through the intestinal wall.

Other metabolites which have been identified in human urine in significant amounts include the O-methylated compound 3-methoxymethyldopa and its analogue 3-methoxy-methyldopamine and their sulphate conjugates (see Fig. 1). These result from the action of catechol-O-methyltransferase, a widely distributed enzyme.

Small amounts of the deaminated metabolites, including 3,4-

Fig. 1 The metabolism of methyldopa

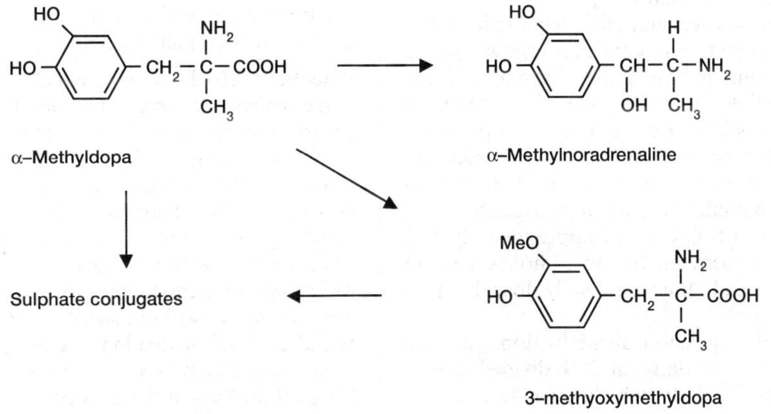

M

M

dihydroxyphenylacetone, may be found, although the main metabolites of methyldopa are not extensively metabolized by monoamine oxidase. Methyldopa and methylnoradrenaline are not good substances for phenylethanolamine-N-methyltransferase.[15]

Pharmaceutics

Methyldopa is available as Aldomet (MSD, UK/USA) in oral form and parenteral forms.

1. Tablets contain 125 mg, 250 mg or 500 mg of methyldopa BP. The tablets are yellow, film-coated, round, biconvex and are impressed with the legend 'Aldomet' on one face and the code 'MSD135', 'MSD401', 'MSD516' on the 125, 250 and 500 mg strengths respectively.
2. The oral creamy suspension contains methyldopa 250 mg/5 ml in an orange/pineapple flavoured vehicle.
3. A combination tablet containing methyldopa 250 mg and hydrochlorothiazide 15 mg is available in some countries.

Methyldopate hydrochloride

4. Methyldopate hydrochloride Methyldopa is available for intravenous use as a colourless solution containing the more soluble ethyl ester, methyldopate hydrochloride, 50 mg.ml^{-1} in 5 ml vials. However, de-esterification in the systemic circulation is so slow that peak effect may not be seen for 12 hours.

Tablets and injection should be stored in a cool place, protected from light. The injection should be protected from freezing. Under correct storage methyldopa tablets and methyldopate injection have a shelf-life of 5 years, and methyldopa suspension 2 years.

Most formulations do not include potentially allergenic substances such as tartrazine, although this may vary with different generic preparations.

Therapeutic use

Indications

1. Control of blood pressure in primary hypertension
2. Renal hypertension
3. Hypertension in pregnancy
4. Postmenopausal flushing (this is not a licensed indication in the UK).

Contraindications

1. Patients with known hypersensitivity to the drug
2. Pre-existing postural hypotension
3. Active hepatic disease.

Indications

1. Essential hypertension

Methyldopa as monotherapy has been shown to reduce blood pressure by an average of 20/13 mmHg in mild hypertension (mean maximum daily dose 2 g) and by 38/22 mmHg in moderate to severe hypertension (mean maximum dose 3.8 g daily) producing satisfactory blood pressure control in up to 75% of patients.

Oral treatment is usually begun with 250 mg twice daily, for at least two days, and then the dose is adjusted by 250–500 mg daily at intervals of not less than two days, depending on the therapeutic response. The maximum daily dose is usually 3 g.

Since the use of β-adrenoceptor blockers and thiazide diuretics in the treatment of uncomplicated hypertension have been shown to be equally efficacious to methyldopa and to have a lower incidence of side effects, methyldopa is now mainly used in patients in whom a contraindication to the use of β-blockers or thiazides exists. For severe hypertension methyldopa may be a valuable addition to diuretics and β-blockers although other alternatives such as peripheral vasodilators and angiotensin-converting enzyme inhibitors are now available.

Although methyldopa has a short half life of approximately 1–2 hours, its hypotensive effect varies between 10 and 24 hours. Not all patients will be adequately controlled on a single daily dose, hence a twice daily dose is recommended.[29]

In paediatric patients the oral suspension of methyldopa may be used. The initial dose is 10 mg.kg^{-1} daily in 2–4 divided doses. Maximum dose is 65 mg.kg^{-1} or 3 g daily, whichever is less.

2. Renal hypertension

As methyldopa has the ability to lower blood pressure without reducing renal function, it has been the treatment of choice for hypertension in association with renal impairment, often in combination with a loop diuretic such as frusemide.

A dose of 0.5–2.0 g daily of methyldopa has been shown to produce satisfactory blood pressure control in 90% of patients with renal impairment, from a pretreatment mean of 199/129 mmHg to 137/88 mmHg.[31]

3. Hypertension in pregnancy

Drugs used to treat hypertension in pregnancy must not reduce uterine blood flow, nor adversely affect the fetus. Methyldopa appears to be safe to use for the treatment of hypertension in pregnancy under close medical supervision.

242 women completed a controlled trial of methyldopa for moderate hypertension in pregnancy.[32,33] The hypotensive effect of methyldopa was similar to its action in non-pregnant individuals and greatly reduced the frequency of severe hypertension occurring antenatally and in labour.[33] Active treatment was associated with a significantly improved fetal outcome.[32] (See under Major outcome trials.) In a further study of these children up to the age of 7 years there was no evidence of any deleterious effect on cardiovascular or psychomotor indices in children of the methyldopa-treated group.[7]

Other uses

4. Postmenopausal flushing

Methyldopa 250 mg three times daily has been shown to reduce hot flushes in postmenopausal women,[34] but side effects preclude its routine use. In a further double-blind crossover study methyldopate 100 mg intravenously significantly decreased the number of subjective flushes.[35] These studies indicate that α-adrenergic mechanisms (central and/or peripheral) play a role in the pathophysiology of menopausal flushing.

Contraindications

1. Known hypersensitivity to the drug

A number of immune-mediated adverse reactions may occur associated with the use of methyldopa, such as fever, skin rashes, hepatotoxicity, Coombs'-positive haemolytic anaemia and systemic lupus erythematosus (see section on Adverse reactions for details). Although rare, these reactions are potentially serious and thus for any patient who has manifested such a reaction on previous exposure to methyldopa, further exposure to the drug is contraindicated.

2. Pre-existing postural hypotension

Patients with pre-existing symptoms due to orthostatic fall in blood pressure associated with an autonomic neuropathy or impaired baroreceptor reflex mechanism (e.g. the elderly) may show a worsening of their symptoms if treated with methyldopa.

3. Active hepatic disease

As methyldopa may unpredictably cause hepatic damage it is relatively contraindicated in patients with known hepatic disease.

Adverse reactions

A wide range of adverse effects has been reported following methyldopa administration. Many of the side effects are related to the action of methyldopa on the central and peripheral autonomic nervous system. In addition, a number of immunologically mediated adverse reactions occur which, although rare, are the most serious reactions associated with methyldopa.

Potentially life-threatening effects

Haemolytic anaemia. The development of a positive Coombs' test occurs in about 20% of patients taking methyldopa, usually after 6–12 months of therapy.[36] The incidence rises with increasing dosage and tends to reverse within a few weeks or months of ceasing therapy. The presence of the abnormal antibody may lead to problems in cross-matching blood for transfusion. Only 0.1–0.2% of patients with a positive Coombs' test will develop haemolytic anaemia, necessitating the withdrawal of methyldopa. Although deaths have occurred, haemolysis usually resolves without specific treatment when the drug is stopped.[37] Withdrawal of methyldopa or administration of steroids seem to be equally effective in producing rapid improvement in clinical and haematological findings in the majority of patients.[37]

Methyldopa

Hepatitis. Disturbances in liver function tests have been noted in 5 to 35% of patients.[38] The mechanism of liver damage may be direct toxicity or an immune-mediated reaction. Patients developing symptoms of hepatitis may be divided into two groups based on length of exposure to methyldopa. Patients with an exposure of less than six months have a clinical course similar to viral hepatitis and on liver biopsy may show marked parenchymatous changes with focal, confluent or massive necrosis and associated inflammation. Death from hepatic failure has occurred. The mechanism is probably a hypersensitivity-type reaction. The second group of patients develop symptoms, which are usually milder in degree, after a delay of several years. On liver biopsy, cellular changes consisting of fatty accumulation and increased fibrous trabeculae occur. Several mechanisms may be involved after chronic exposure, one of which may be an excess of reactive metabolites reducing hepatic protective mechanisms by reducing glutathione reserve.[39] Chronic active hepatitis has also been reported. Generally complete recovery occurs following withdrawal of methyldopa. Care should be taken to avoid a second exposure to methyldopa in patients who develop hepatitis associated with this drug.

Myocarditis. This is an unexpected reaction which has been reported following methyldopa therapy. Five cases of myocarditis circumstantially associated with methyldopa were reported in one study.[40] In all instances death occurred and the inflammatory changes in the hearts were consistent with a hypersensitivity reaction. In addition four of the patients had a severe hepatitis.

Acute overdosage

Acute overdosage of methyldopa may result in severe hypothermia, dry mouth, hypotension, dizziness, weakness, coma and bradycardia.[41] There are insufficient data in the literature to assess accurately the minimum toxic or lethal dose. One adult female died following acute ingestion of methyldopa 25 g. A 19-year-old who ingested methyldopa 2.5 g and became sedated and hypotensive had a 10-hour serum concentration of 19.2 $\mu g.ml^{-1}$, compared to peak concentrations of approximately 1 $\mu g.ml^{-1}$ which follow ingestion of 250–750 mg daily. This patient made a full recovery by three days after ingestion of the overdose.[42]

Severe or irreversible adverse effects

Lightheadedness or dizziness related to postural hypotension has been reported in about 15% of patients and sometimes necessitates cessation of therapy.[11]

Fever is reported to occur in 3% of patients, often associated with elevations of hepatic transaminase activities in blood, skin rashes, eosinophilia and gastrointestinal intolerance, and is likely to be an immune-mediated reaction.[43]

Pancreatitis, with increased serum and urinary amylase activity accompanied by fever, has occurred two or three weeks after commencement of therapy with methyldopa. The pancreatitis was reversible and recurred on re-challenge with the drug.[44]

Acute colitis, reversible on cessation of methyldopa, may occur and has been associated with the development of a haemolytic anaemia, due to an immune reaction. A possible case of retroperitoneal fibrosis has also been reported.[45] Methyldopa has been associated with the development of antinuclear antibodies, and rare cases of a lupus-like syndrome induced by methyldopa have been reported.[46] There have been rare reports of immune thrombocytopenia and granulocytopenia.[47]

Adverse effects attributable to the central adrenergic action of methyldopa include precipitation or exacerbation of parkinsonism by interference with dopaminergic activity in the stratium,[48] and depression which may be severe.

Symptomatic adverse effects

Treatment with methyldopa produces a relatively high incidence of symptomatic effects which are most evident either during the initial period of therapy or following dosage increments. These effects are probably related to the pharmacological effects of the drug.

Sedation is a frequent dose-related adverse effect and nightmares and sleep disturbances also occur, although less frequently. Other relatively common adverse effects are dry mouth, probably also a central effect, nasal congestion secondary to decreased sympathetic tone, and loss of libido, impotence and failure of ejaculation, which are reported with varying degrees of frequency. Diarrhoea occurs in about 5% of patients; the mechanism is uncertain although increased peristalsis due to reduced sympathetic tone may contribute. Galactorrhoea secondary to increase in prolactin secretion has been reported rarely. Headache occurs with a reported incidence of 9% and nausea 3%.[47] A variety of skin rashes has been reported.

Some changes in the blood lipid profile have been demonstrated in hypertensive patients treated with methyldopa.[49] There was no significant change in total cholesterol and triglyceride levels but there was a significant 10% decrease in HDL cholesterol and an increase in total cholesterol to HDL cholesterol ratio. The mechanism of the change in lipid profile and the significance of these findings remains to be elucidated.

Withdrawal symptoms from methyldopa have been reported in a number of studies. Symptoms of increased activity of the sympathetic nervous system include insomnia, agitation, nausea and headache, and a reported 13% incidence of blood pressure rebound.[50] The rise in blood pressure was less common and less severe than that reported with clonidine.

Interference with clinical pathology tests

1. A positive Coombs' test interferes with cross-matching of blood.
2. Methyldopa gives false positive results in the Watson–Schwartz method of testing for porphobilinogen.
3. Creatinine determination by the alkaline picrate method may be inaccurate in patients taking methyldopa.
4. Serum aspartate aminotransferase measurement with colorimetric methods may be altered in patients on methyldopa therapy.
5. As methyldopa fluoresces in urine samples at the same wavelengths as catecholamines, falsely high values for urinary catecholamines may be reported if a fluorimetric method is used. In addition, there is similar interference with the fluorimetric method for measurement of vanillylmandelic acid (VMA) in urine, although not with the gas chromatographic method. Falsely high values for VMA or catecholamines in urine in the presence of methyldopa may inappropriately suggest the diagnosis of phaeochromocytoma.
6. After ingestion of high doses of methyldopa a false positive test for glucose may occur using Clinitest tablets (cupric sulphate, sodium hydroxide, sodium carbonate and sodium citrate).
7. Measurement of urinary 5-hydroxyindoleacetic acid may be falsely low.
8. Urine colour changes from red to brown/black have been noted.[51]

High risk groups

Neonates

The disposition of methyldopa has been studied in babies from mothers treated with methyldopa for hypertension in pregnancy. Plasma levels at birth were similar in mothers and babies. The rate of elimination of methyldopa in the newborn is three to four times longer than in the adult. The newborn appears readily able to metabolize methyldopa to methyldopa-O-sulphate. Methyldopa tends to be conjugated to a greater extent in the newborn than in adults. It is postulated that elimination in the neonate is mainly controlled by the rate of renal excretion.[52]

Breast milk. Concentrations of methyldopa measured in milk samples are very low. Most of the drug in milk is conjugated. The concentration in milk is unlikely to be sufficient to affect the nursing infant.[26]

Children

Methyldopa may be used as indicated under Therapeutic use. No particular problems have been reported.

Pregnant women

Results of a major study indicate that methyldopa appears to be safe to use in pregnancy.[32] It also appears that when the drug is used from early pregnancy there may be a reduction in fetal loss, resulting largely from fewer mid-trimester abortions. In a follow-up study at age 7 years of children born to hypertensive women, there was no evidence of any deleterious effect on cardiovascular or psychomotor indices in children of the methyldopa-treated group.[7]

The elderly

Provided that special care is taken to avoid postural hypotension, the elderly appear to tolerate methyldopa at least as well as younger

M

patients,[13] although sedation and confusion may occur and in practice limit the usefulness of methyldopa in this group.

Concurrent disease

Renal failure. Methyldopa is 50% excreted by the kidney and lower doses may be required in patients with renal impairment. As indicated under Concentration–effect relationship, patients with renal impairment have an increased responsiveness to the hypotensive effect of methyldopa.

Hepatic failure. Use of methyldopa is relatively contraindicated in patients with known hepatic disease (see Therapeutic use).

Drug interactions

Potentially hazardous interactions

General anaesthetic agents. These may enhance the effect of methyldopa, causing hypotension and bradycardia.

Tricyclic antidepressants. Antagonism of the hypotensive effect of methyldopa by tricyclics has been reported in animals[53] but only a single case report describes such an interaction in man. Methyldopa may induce depression and so may not be appropriate for depressed patients requiring antihypertensive treatment.

Haloperidol. A reversible form of dementia has been reported when haloperidol was used in three patients treated with methyldopa.[54,55] The mechanism is not understood and should not preclude concurrent use.

Levodopa. Although methyldopa occasionally causes parkinsonian-like symptoms, it can enhance the actions of levodopa, and permit a reduction in dosage in some patients.[52] However, the adverse effects of levodopa are sometimes made worse. A small enhancement of the effects of methyldopa can also occur.

Salbutamol. Severe hypotension attributed to the use of salbutamol infusion has been reported during premature labour in women receiving methyldopa.[52] It has been suggested that this reaction is caused by peripheral vasodilation due to β_2-receptor stimulation.

Phenothiazines. Reduction of blood pressure by methyldopa may be potentiated by concurrent use of some phenothiazines (e.g. chlorpromazine).

Lithium. Lithium toxicity has been reported, apparently induced by concurrent administration of methyldopa.[56] The mechanism is not understood but the potential seriousness of this interaction suggests that careful monitoring of clinical state and lithium serum concentrations is necessary if these two drugs are given together.

Direct-acting sympathomimetics. The pressor effects of noradrenaline are increased and prolonged by concurrent treatment with methyldopa. It is not certain whether other direct-acting sympathomimetics interact similarly but the mydriasis due to phenylephrine appears not to be affected.

Monoamine oxidase inhibitors. Increased stimulation of the central nervous system and variable effects on blood pressure have occurred with concurrent use of methyldopa and monoamine oxidase inhibitors.

Potentially useful interactions

Thiazide diuretics. A clinically useful additive effect may occur when methyldopa is combined with a thiazide diuretic. The increase in plasma renin activity and reduction in glomerular filtration rate attributable to the thiazide can be prevented by methyldopa and the tendency to develop fluid retention with methyldopa can be prevented by the thiazide.

Levodopa. See above.

Major outcome trials

Methyldopa as a single agent

1. Bayliss R I S, Harvey-Smith, E A 1962 Methyldopa in the treatment of hypertension. Lancet 1: 763–768

In 20 patients with severe or moderately severe hypertension, methyldopa in a dosage range of 750–2250 mg daily produced a satisfactory reduction of diastolic blood pressure from a mean of 125 ± 2 (SE) mmHg to 95 ± 3 mmHg. One patient failed to respond and six initial responders showed evidence of tolerance. Side effects were limited to drowsiness, fluid retention and dry mouth.

2. Dollery C T, Harrington M 1962 Methyldopa in hypertension — clinical and pharmacological studies. Lancet 1: 759–763

This study reported the use of methyldopa in 59 patients with moderate to severe hypertension (most with blood pressure greater than 220–120 mmHg) when treatment was begun. Satisfactory control of blood pressure was achieved in 32 patients. In one-third of patients the drug in a maximum dosage of up to 4 g daily failed to control blood pressure adequately or produced intolerable side effects. The onset of hypotensive effect began 4–5 hours after oral or intravenous dosing. Five patients received a thiazide diuretic which potentiated the hypotensive effect. Blood pressure control was less successful in patients with the severest grades of hypertension.

3. Gillespie L, Oates J A, Grant J R, Sjoerdsma A 1962 Clinical and chemical studies with α-methyldopa in patients with hypertension. Circulation 25: 281–291

In this study a comparison was made of the d- and l-isomers of methyldopa and the pharmacological effect was shown to reside in the l-isomer. 20 hypertensive patients with diastolic pressures greater than 110 mmHg were given l-α-methyldopa with or without chlorothiazide to evaluate the antihypertensive effect and side effects on a chronic basis. Effective reduction in blood pressure occurred in 18 patients without development of tolerance to the drug. Side effects recorded included excessive sedation, sexual impotence, psychic depression, and febrile reactions.

4. Connolly M E, Briant R H, George C F, Dollery C T 1972 A crossover comparison of clonidine and methyldopa in hypertension. European Journal of Clinical Pharmacology 4: 222–227

The results of a titrated dose crossover comparison of clonidine with methyldopa are reported. Only one-third of those entering the trial completed it. The blood-pressure-lowering effect of the two drugs was seen to be similar. The mean daily dose of methyldopa used was 4.5 g and of clonidine 1.33 mg. At these dosages the incidence of moderate or severe side effects was high. These doses are higher than those normally used in clinical practice where a diuretic would be introduced to the regimen rather than increasing the dose of methyldopa to this level.

Methyldopa in combination with a diuretic

5. Prichard B N C, Boakes A J, Graham B R 1976 A within-patient comparison of bethanidine, methyldopa and propranolol in the treatment of hypertension. Clinical Science and Molecular Medicine 51: 567s–570s

17 patients (16 with essential and 1 with renal hypertension) completed a within-patient comparison. In 10 patients there was a significant reduction in blood pressure compared with placebo on the addition of Moduretic (hydrochlorothiazide plus amiloride) to a constant dose of methyldopa. All three antihypertensives produced similar effects on resting blood pressure and on the blood pressure effects of posture and exercise. Unlike bethanidine, propranolol did not produce postural and exercise hypotension. Methyldopa was intermediate in effect. Overall side effects were of a similar incidence with each drug although there were differences in the patterns of particular side effects.

6. Webster J, Jeffers T A, Galloway D B, Petrie J C, Barker N P 1977 Atenolol, methyldopa, and chlorthalidone in moderate hypertension. British Medical Journal 1: 76–78

14 patients with moderate hypertension on continuous treatment with chlorthalidone were treated additionally with either atenolol or methyldopa, or low doses of atenolol and methyldopa in combination. All doses of methyldopa and atenolol used were effective in reducing blood pressure. Doubling the dose of methyldopa from 750 mg daily to 1500 mg daily did not increase the hypotensive effect significantly. More side effects, including dreaming, increased sleeping and tiredness, were reported during treatment with methyldopa than with atenolol or chlorthalidine.

Methyldopa in renal insufficiency

7. Mohammed S, Hanenson I B, Magenheim H G, Gaffney T E 1968 The effects of α-methyldopa on renal function in hypertensive patients. American Heart Journal 76: 21–27

In eight patients with hypertension and renal insufficiency, treatment with methyldopa for 7 to 13 days decreased arterial pressure without changing glomerular filtration rate. Renal plasma flow and urine volume increased in supine and tilted positions. The results of this study provide a rational basis for the use of methyldopa in the treatment of ambulatory hypertensive patients with impaired renal function.

8. Stenbaek O, Myhre E, Brodwall E K, Hansen T 1971 Hypotensive effect of methyldopa in renal failure associated with hypertension. Acta Medica Scandinavica 191: 333–337

The reduction in supine blood pressure following methyldopate 200 mg intravenously was significantly greater in patients with hypertension due to advanced renal disease than in patients with little or no renal impairment. A similar response was observed following oral dosing. The increased sensitivity to the hypotensive action of methyldopa was not associated with increased methyldopa serum concentration.

Dosage regimens for methyldopa

9. Wright J M, Orozco-Gonzalez M, Polak G, Dollery C T 1982 British Journal of Clinical Pharmacology 13: 847–854

Ten patients were studied in a double-blind crossover study designed to determine the duration of antihypertensive effect of methyldopa by comparing hourly supine and standing blood pressures throughout the day, during placebo, single morning, and single evening dose therapy. The antihypertensive effect of methyldopa peaked 6–9 hours after a dose and declined thereafter with an approximate pharmacological half life of 10 hours. Little antihypertensive effect remained at 24 hours post-dose. The results suggest a twice-daily dosing regime is appropriate for most patients.

Methyldopa in the elderly

10. Mortality and morbidity results from the European Working Party on High Blood Pressure in the Elderly (EWPHE) 1985 Lancet 1: 1349–1354

In this double-blind, randomized, placebo-controlled trial of antihypertensive treatment in patients over the age of 60, 840 patients were randomized either to active treatment (hydrochlorothiazide 25 mg plus triameterene 50 mg daily) or to matching placebo. If the blood pressure remained above 160/90, methyldopa was added to the active regimen and matching placebo added in the placebo group. 145/416 patients in the actively treated group required methyldopa 250–2000 mg daily.

The blood pressure was significantly lower in the actively treated patients than in those on placebo. An overall intention-to-treat analysis revealed that the actively treated group had a non-significant 27% reduction in cardiovascular mortality due to a significant 38% reduction in cardiac mortality and a non-significant 32% decrease in cerebrovascular mortality. Study-terminating morbid cardiovascular events were reduced significantly by 60% by active treatment. The authors conclude that hypertensive patients in this age group benefited from antihypertensive therapy.

Methyldopa in pregnancy

11a. Redman C W G, Beilin L J, Bonnar J, Ounstead M K 1976 Fetal outcome in trial of antihypertensive treatment in pregnancy. Lancet 2: 753–756

11b. Redman C W G, Beilin L J, Bonnar J 1977 Treatment of hypertension in pregnancy with methyldopa: blood pressure control and side effects. British Journal of Obstetrics and Gynaecology 84: 419–426

In this randomized controlled trial of treatment of moderate hypertension in pregnancy (reported in two separate papers), treatment with methyldopa (0.5–4.0 g daily) significantly improved fetal survival. There was one fetal loss in 117 treated patients compared to nine losses, including four mid-pregnancy abortions, in 125 untreated patients. The occurrence of the pre-eclamptic complications of proteinuria and hyperuricaemia was not affected by treatment. The birthweight and maturity of viable infants were similar in treated and control groups.

The hypotensive effect of methyldopa was similar to its action in non-pregnant individuals and greatly reduced the frequency of severe hypertension occurring antenatally and in labour. As pregnancy advanced, an increasing daily dose of methyldopa was needed and there was a greater use of additional hypotensive therapy. 17 women stopped methyldopa because of side effects (none serious); 14 then received alternative treatment.

Methyldopa

M

The authors concluded that methyldopa is safe to use for the treatment of hypertension in pregnancy in the context of close medical and obstetric supervision.

Use of methyldopa in menopausal flushing

12. Nesheim B-1, Saetre T 1981 Reduction of menopausal hot flushes by methyldopa. European Journal of Clinical Pharmacology 20: 413–416

In a double-blind, placebo-controlled study of 28 women suffering from menopausal hot flushes, methyldopa (in doses of 250–1000 g daily) was shown to be significantly more effective than placebo in reducing the number of hot flushes. The magnitude of the reduction was essentially the same as that reported for oestrogens and clonidine. The results of this study suggest a role of α_2-adrenoceptors, possibly within the central nervous system, in the physiology of menopausal hot flushes.

Quality of life

13. Croog S H, Levine S, Testa M A, Brown B, Bulpitt C J, Jenkins C J, Klerman G L, Williams G H, 1986 The effects of antihypertensive therapy on the quality of life. New England Journal of Medicine 314: 1657–1664

626 men with mild to moderate hypertension participated in a multicentre randomized double-blind clinical trial to determine the effects of methyldopa, propranolol and captopril on their quality of life. Hydrochlorothiazide was added as needed to 'control' blood pressure. After 24 weeks, all three groups had similar blood pressure control, with approximately 30% of the methyldopa- and captopril-treated patients and 20% of the propranolol group requiring additional diuretic therapy.

39(20%) of the methyldopa group withdrew from the study due to adverse reactions, the most frequent being fatigue and lethargy, whereas 27(13%) withdrew from the propranolol group and 17(8%) from the captopril group. More subjects receiving captopril had improvements in their quality-of-life scores for general well-being, physical symptoms and sexual dysfunction than in the methyldopa and propranolol groups, whereas more of those in the latter groups showed worsening in these scores compared to the captopril group. The addition of a diuretic was associated with deterioration in quality-of-life measures in all three treatment groups, although the relative advantage of captopril was maintained.

The authors concluded that the effects of antihypertensive agents on quality of life depend on the pharmacological class of the agent. The agents interfering with sympathetic nervous function (methyldopa, propranolol) had more adverse effects on quality of life than did the angiotensin-converting enzyme inhibitor, captopril.

General review articles

Zanchetti A (ed) 1978 Methyldopa in hypertension: a review of long-term clinical experience with methyldopa. Merck Sharp & Dohme International, Rahway, New Jersey

Maxwell M H (ed) 1978 Current update: Aldomet (methyldopa, MSD) in the management of hypertension. Merck Sharp & Dohme, West Point, Pennsylvania

Connolly M E, Oates J A 1977 The clinical pharmacology of antihypertensive drugs: III Methyldopa. In: Gross F (ed) Handbook of Experimental Pharmacology XXXIX: Antihypertensive agents, Springer-Verlag, Heidelberg, New York, ch 13, p 577–583

McMahon F G 1978 Management of essential hypertension, Futura Publishing Company Inc., Mount Kisco, New York, ch IX, p 251–276

Frohlich E D 1980 Methyldopa: mechanisms and treatment 25 years later. Archives of Internal Medicine 140: 954–959

Reid J L, Elliot H L 1984 Methyldopa In: Doyle A E (ed) Handbook of hypertension. 5: Clinical pharmacology of antihypertensive drugs. Elsevier, Amsterdam, ch 4, pp 92–112

References

1. Oates J A, Gillespie L, Udenfriend S, Sjoerdsma A 1960 Decarboxylase inhibition and blood pressure reduction by alpha-methyl,4-dihydroxy-DL-phenylalanine. Science 131: 1890–1891
2. Leo A, Jow P Y C, Sillipo C, Hansch C 1975 Calculation of hydrophilic constant (log P) from pi and f constants. Journal of Medicinal Chemistry 18: 865–868

M

3. Van Zwieten P A, Timmermans P B M W M, Van Brummelen P 1984 The role of α-adrenoceptors in hypertension and in antihypertensive drug treatment. American Journal of Medicine 77: 17–25
4. Usdin E, Efron D H (eds) 1972 Psychotropic drugs and related compounds, 2nd edn, Washington DC
5. Brown P S 1966 The effect of reserpine, 5-hydroxytryptamine and other drugs on induced ovulation in immature mice. Journal of Endocrinology 35: 161–168
6. West G B 1962 Drugs and rat pregnancy. Journal of Pharmacy and Pharmacology 828–830
7. Cockburn J, Moar V A, Ounstead M, Redman C W G 1982 Final report of study on hypertension during pregnancy: the effects of specific treatment on the growth and development of children. Lancet 1: 647–649
8. Ishidate M I, Sofuni T, Yoshikawa K 1981 Chromosomal aberration tests in vitro as a primary screening tool for environmental mutagens and/or carcinogens. GANN Monograph on Cancer Research 27: 95–108
9. Dollery C T, Harrington M 1962 Methyldopa in hypertension: clinical and pharmacological studies. Lancet 1: 759–763
10. Safar M E, London G M, Levenson J A 1979 The effect of α methyldopa on cardiac output in hypertension. Clinical Pharmacology and Therapeutics 25: 266–272
11. Mancia G, Ferrari A, Gregorini L et al 1980 Methyldopa and neural control of circulation in essential hypertension. American Journal of Cardiology 45: 1237–1243
12. Kersting F, Reid J L, Dollery C T 1977 Clinical and cardiovascular effects of α-methyldopa in combination with decarboxylase inhibitors in man. Clinical Pharmacology and Therapeutics 21: 547–555
13. Lawson D H, Gloss D, Jick H 1978 Adverse reactions to methyldopa with particular reference to hypotension. American Heart Journal 96: 572–579
14. Dollery C T, Harrington M, Hodge J V 1963 Haemodynamic studies with methyldopa: effect on cardiac output and response to pressor amines. British Heart Journal 25: 670–676
15. Reid J L, Elliott H L 1984 Methyldopa. In: Doyle A E (ed) Handbook of hypertension. 5: Clinical pharmacology of antihypertensive drugs. Elsevier, Amsterdam, ch 4, pp 92–112
16. Alcocer L, Aspe J 1978 Haemodynamic, metabolic and ventricular function effects of methyldopa in the treatment of hypertension. In: Zanchetti A (ed) Methyldopa in hypertension. Merck, Sharp & Dohme International, New Jersey, pp 33–49
17. Mohammed S, Hanenson I B, Magenheim H G, Gaffney T E 1968 The effects of alpha-methyldopa on renal function in hypertensive patients. American Heart Journal 76: 21–27
18. Hansen J 1968 Alpha-methyldopa (Aldomet) in the treatment of hypertension. Acta Medica Scandinavica 183: 323–327
19. Alexander W D, Evans I 1975 Side effects of methyldopa. British Medical Journal 2: 501
20. Rosenblum A M, Montgomery E B 1980 Exacerbation of parkinsonism by methyldopa. Journal of the American Medical Association 224: 2727–2728
21. Ong H, Sved S, Beaudoin N 1982 Assay and stability of alpha-methyldopa in man using high-performance liquid chromatography with electrochemical detection. Journal of Chromatography 229: 433–438
22. Kwan K C, Foltz E L, Breault G O, Baer J E, Totaro J A 1976 Pharmacokinetics of methyldopa in man. Journal of Pharmacology and Experimental Therapeutics 198: 264–277
23. Myhre E, Rugstad H E, Hansen T 1982 Clinical pharmacokinetics of methyldopa. Clinical Pharmacokinetics 7: 221–233
24. Saavedra J A, Reid J L, Jordan W, Rawlins M D, Dollery C T 1975 Plasma concentration of α-methyldopa and sulphate conjugate after oral administrationof methyldopa and intravenous administration of methyldopa and methyldopa hydrochloride ethyl ester. European Journal of Clinical Pharmacology 8: 381–386
25. Stenbaek O, Myhre E, Rugstad H E, Arnold E, Hansen T 1977 Pharmacokinetics of methyldopa in healthy man. European Journal of Clinical Pharmacology 12: 117–123
26. Jones H M R, Cummings A J 1978 A study of the transfer of alpha-methyldopa to the human fetus and newborn infant. British Journal of Clinical Pharmacology 6: 432–434
27. Jones H M R, Cummings A J, Setchell K D R, Lawson A M 1979 A study of the disposition of α-methyldopa in newborn infants following its administration to the mother for the treatment of hypertension during pregnancy. British Journal of Clinical Pharmacology 8: 433–440
28. Wright J M, Orozco-Gonzalez M, Polak G, Dollery C T 1982 Duration of effect of single daily dose of methyldopa therapy. British Journal of Clinical Pharmacology 13: 847–384
29. Verbeeck R K, Branch R A, Wilkinson G R 1981 Drug metabolites in renal failure: Pharmacokinetics and clinical implications. Clinical Pharmacokinetics 6: 329–345
30. Lowenstein I, Alterman L, Zelen R, Bank D E, Bank N 1984 Comparison of long-term renal haemodynamic effects of methyldopa and propranolol in patients with hypertension and renal insufficiency. Journal of Clinical Pharmacology 24: 436–445
31. Luke R G, Kennedy A C 1964 Methyldopa in treatment of hypertension due to chronic renal failure. British Medical Journal 1: 27–30
32. Redman C W G, Beilin L J, Bonnar J, Ounstead M K 1976 Fetal outcome in trial of antihypertensive treatment in pregnancy. Lancet 2: 753–756
33. Redman C W G, Beilin L J, Bonnar J 1977 Treatment of hypertension in pregnancy with methyldopa: blood pressure control and side effects. British Journal of Obstetrics and Gynaecology 84: 419–426
34. Hammond M G, Hatley L, Talbert L M 1984 A double-blind study to evaluate the effect of methyldopa in post menopausal vasomotor flushes. Journal of Clinical Endocrinology and Metabolism 58: 1158–1161
35. Tulandi T, Kinch R A, Guyda H, Mazella L, Lal S 1984 Effect of methyldopa on menopausal flushes, skin temperature and luteinizing hormone secretion. American Journal of Obstetrics and Gynecology 150: 709–712
36. Carstairs K C, Breckenridge A, Dollery C T, Worlledge S M 1966 Incidence of a positive direct Coombs' test in patients on alpha-methyldopa. Lancet 2: 133–135
37. Worlledge S M, Carstairs K G, Dacie J V 1966 Autoimmune haemolytic anaemia associated with α-methyldopa therapy. Lancet 2: 135–139
38. Toghill P J, Smith P G, Benton P, Brown R C, Matthews H L 1974 Methyldopa liver damage. British Medical Journal 3: 545–548
39. Arranto A J, Sotaniemi E A 1981 Morphologic alterations in patients with alpha-methyldopa-induced liver damage after short-and long-term exposure. Scandinavian Journal of Gastroenterology 16: 853–863
40. Mullick F G, McAllister H A 1977 Myocarditis associated with methyldopa therapy. Journal of the American Medical Association 237: 1699–1701
41. Poisindex (R) Australian edition, Micromedisc Inc. 1974–1985
42. Shnaps Y, Almog S, Halkin H, Tirosh M 1982 Methyldopa poisoning. Journal of Toxicology. Clinical Toxicology 19: 501–503
43. Steiner J A 1984 Antihypertensive drugs In: Dukes M N G (ed) Meyler's side effects of drugs, 10th edn. Elsevier, Amsterdam, ch 21, pp 358–360
44. Van der Heide H, ten Haaft M A 1981 Pancreatitis caused by methyldopa. British Medical Journal 282: 1930–1931
45. Ahmed S 1983 Methyldopa and retroperitoneal fibrosis. American Heart Journal 105: 1037–1038
46. Dupont A, Six R 1982 Lupus-like syndrome induced by methyldopa. British Medical Journal 285: 693–694
47. McMahon F G 1978 Management of essential hypertension. Futura Publishing, New York, ch IX, p 265
48. Rosenblum A M, Montgomery E B 1980 Exacerbation of parkinsonism by methyldopa. Journal of the American Medical Association 244: 2727–2728
49. Leon A S, Agre J, McNally C et al 1984 Blood lipid effects of antihypertensive therapy: a double-blind comparison of the effects of methyldopa and propranolol. Journal of Clinical Pharmacology 24: 209–217
50. Whitsett T I 1983 Abrupt cessation of treatment with centrally acting antihypertensive agents. Chest 83 (suppl): 400–402
51. Cardwell J B 1969 Red urine associated with methyldopa treatment. Lancet 2: 326
52. Cummings A J, Whitelaw A G L 1981 A study of conjugation and drug elimination in the human neonate. British Journal of Clinical Pharmacology 12: 511–515
53. Stockley I 1981 Drug interactions: a source book of adverse reactions, their mechanisms, clinical importance and management. Blackwell Scientific Publications, Oxford, p 238
54. Thornton W E 1976 Dementia induced by methyldopa with haloperidol. New England Journal of Medicine 243: 1222
55. Nadel I, Wallach M 1979 Drug interaction between haloperidol and methyldopa. British Journal of Psychiatry 135: 484
56. Byrd G J 1975 Methyldopa and lithium carbonate: suspected interaction. Journal of the American Medical Association 233: 320

Methylene blue

Methylene blue is used in the treatment of drug-induced and some forms of genetic methaemoglobinaemia. It is also used medically as a dye to delineate body cavities or fistulae, and is an important histological stain.

Chemistry

Methylene blue is methylthionine hydrochloride (Methylene Blue, Methylene Blue Injection)
$C_{16}H_{11}N_3SCl.3H_2O$
3,7-Bisdimethylamino-phenazathionium chloride trihydrate

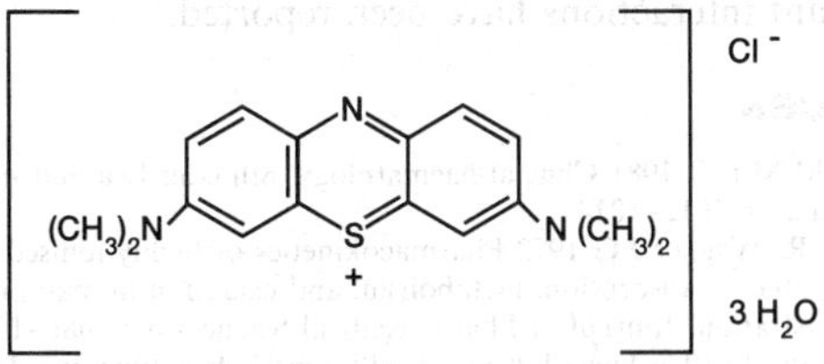

Molecular weight	373.9
pKa	0–1
Solubility	
in alcohol	1 in 65
in water	1 in 25
Octanol/water partition coefficient	—

Methylene blue exists as dark green crystals, or crystalline powder, with a bronze lustre, but is dark blue in solution. It is almost odourless. Commercial methylene blue contains zinc chloride and is not suitable for medical use.

Pharmacology

Methylene blue at low concentrations accepts electrons from NADPH-dependent methaemoglobin reductase and is thus reduced to leuco methylene blue, which in turn rapidly reduces methaemoglobin to haemoglobin. However, at high concentrations the drug oxidizes ferrous ions in haemoglobin to ferric ions, hence forming methaemoglobin.[1]

Toxicology

Animal studies have been of limited value as the pharmacokinetics of methylene blue may be different to the situation in man. In the dog, methylene blue was poorly absorbed after oral administration, only 2.4% of the 15 mg.kg^{-1} dose being recovered in catheter collection of urine in the first 10 hours.[2] In contrast, the mean urinary recovery of methylene blue in humans[2] following an oral dose of 10 mg.kg^{-1} was 74%. The dog is therefore not a suitable animal model to study toxic effects of methylene blue.

There is no evidence in the literature of carcinogenic or teratogenic effects. Toxicity in humans will be discussed later.

Clinical pharmacology

Methaemoglobin is reduced to haemoglobin via the Embden–Myerhof pathway. Two enzymes are involved in this reduction, NADPH-dependent methaemoglobin reductase and diaphorase (NADH-methaemoglobin reductase). Methylene blue is an effective electron acceptor from NADPH-dependent methaemoglobin reductase and is converted to leucomethylene blue. This rapidly and non-enzymatically reduces methaemoglobin to haemoglobin. Methylene blue is therefore an effective treatment for drug-induced methaemoglobinaemias and for genetic methaemoglobinaemias due to enzyme deficiency. Methaemoglobinaemia due to structural abnormality of haemoglobin will not respond to methylene blue.

The usual dose range is 1–2 mg.kg^{-1} by slow intravenous bolus injection of 1% solution, or 3–6 mg.kg^{-1} per 24 h orally in divided doses for non-urgent treatment. Higher doses increase the risk of toxic effects. Of particular importance is the oxidation of ferrous ions to ferric ions by high dose methylene blue, therefore converting haemoglobin to methaemoglobin. Symptomatic haemolysis may occur after high doses. A four-year-old boy (weighing 12.5 kg) given 1000 mg of intravenous methylene blue during surgery developed tachycardia and hypotension and remained intensely blue for several days.[3] Two infants developed haemolytic anaemia during treatment of methaemoglobinaemia with methylene blue — the higher dose used was 75 mg in an infant weighing just over 2 kg.[4] Haemolytic jaundice has been reported in a neonate following the intra-amniotic injection of 7 ml of 1% solution of methylene blue as a diagnostic test for premature rupture of the membranes.[5]

Pharmacokinetics

Methylene blue and its pharmacologically active metabolite leucomethylene blue can both be measured in blood, urine, or tissue by an extraction spectrophotometric assay[6] with sensitivity for methylene blue of 0.02 mg.l^{-1}.

Oral absorption	53–97%
Presystemic metabolism	negligible
Plasma half life	—
Volume of distribution	—
Plasma protein binding	—

Methylene blue is well absorbed from the gastrointestinal tract in man, around 75% of an oral dose being recovered from the urine as methylene blue or a metabolite. It is distributed fairly evenly between erythrocytes and plasma[6,7] and has been shown in rats to be rapidly taken up by lungs, liver, kidney and heart after intravenous administration.[8] Almost 80% of methylene blue excreted in the urine is in the form of leucomethylene blue[2] which is colourless. Plasma concentration of the drug are raised in patients with reduced renal function.

Concentration–effect relationship

The concentration produced by intravenous administration of 1–4 mg.kg^{-1} body weight is effective in the treatment of methaemoglobinaemia.[1,7,9] Higher doses may cause methaemoglobinaemia and haemolysis.

Metabolism

After a dose of 10 mg in human volunteers, urinary excretion was 53–97% of the oral dose (mean 74%) of which 65–85% (mean 78%) was in the reduced form, leucomethylene blue.[2]

Pharmaceutics

Methylene blue is available as Methylene blue injection USP (Elkins Sinn, US), a sterile solution of methylene blue in water for injection. This contains 9.5–10.5 mg of methylene blue trihydrate in each millilitre (i.e. approximately 1% solution). It should be stored in airtight containers as it is readily oxidized to other dyes (azure A, B and C; methylene violet). This solution is usually diluted further for use as a tracer dye. Solutions are sterilized by autoclaving.

Therapeutic use

Indications

1. Treatment of drug–induced methaemoglobinaemia.
2. Treatment of genetic methaemoglobinaemia (not due to structural abnormality of haemoglobin) — often used in conjunction with ascorbic acid.
3. Used as a trace dye to demonstrate fistulae (particularly in female genitourinary tract), gastric reflux, leakage during

peritoneal dialysis, premature rupture of membranes, and to delineate structures during surgical operations.[7,9–12]

Contraindications

1. Methylene blue should be used with caution in severe renal impairment.
2. In glucose-6-phosphate dehydrogenase deficiency methylene blue may cause haemolytic anaemia.[13]
3. It should not be given subcutaneously or intrathecally.

Mode of use

The emergency treatment of drug-induced methaemoglobinaemia consists of the intravenous injection of 1–4 mg methylene blue per kg body weight (usually 1–2 $mg.kg^{-1}$) of a 1% solution over 5 minutes, repeated if necessary after 1 hour.[1,8,9] Emergency treatment is indicated if methaemoglobinaemia is in excess of about 40–50% of haemoglobin, symptoms of acute anaemia generally being present at levels of 50–60%. Untreated, progressively increasing methaemoglobinaemia may lead to circulatory collapse, coma and death. Methylene blue treatment is appropriate for methaemoglobinaemia due to any drug or chemical causing oxidation of haemoglobin, and may therefore be used for treatment of poisoning with ferricyanide, bivalent copper, chromates, chlorate, quinones, nitrates, nitrites, dyes with high redox potential (such as aniline dyes) and drugs (phenacetin, primaquine, and sulphonamides).

Oral therapy of genetic methaemoglobinaemias is with methylene blue 3–6 $mg.kg^{-1}$ (generally 300 mg daily in adults in divided doses) with ascorbic acid 500 mg daily. Although congenital deficiency of NADPH-dependent methaemoglobin reductase is not associated with methaemoglobinaemia, significant methaemoglobinaemia may result from deficiency of several of the variants of diaphorase which is a major cause of hereditary methaemoglobinaemia in many populations.[1]

Contraindications

Use of the dye should be avoided in patients with renal insufficiency or those suffering from glucose-6-phosphate deficiency.

Adverse reactions

Potentially life-threatening effects

Intravenous injection of methylene blue has occasionally caused hypotension and cardiac arrhythmias, and such disorders might prove fatal on rare occasions.

Severe or irreversible adverse effects

Low grade haemolytic anaemia has been reported in patients with glucose-6-phosphate dehydrogenase deficiency after oral administration of 390 mg of methylene blue daily,[13] and a more acute haemolysis has occurred in a neonate after intra-amniotic injection.

Necrotic ulcers have been reported at the site of subcutaneous injection of methylene blue.[14] Spinal cord necrosis causing paraplegia occurred in a patient in whom methylene blue was administered intrathecally.[15] Haemolytic anaemia, hyperbilirubin and methaemoglobinaemia have been reported in neonates following intra-amniotic injection of methylene blue for diagnosis of premature rupture of the membranes.[5,12] The authors suggest that its use for this purpose should be discontinued.

Symptomatic adverse effects

In addition to the severe toxic effects discussed above, the following may occur.[1,9,16] Nausea, vomiting, diarrhoea and dysuria have been reported in patients treated with oral methylene blue. Intravenous administration may also cause abdominal pain, headache, dizziness, tremors, apprehension, confusion, chest pain, dyspnoea, tachycardia and sweating. However, several of these are also symptoms of methaemoglobinaemia.

Blue colouration of urine, faeces and saliva occurs. Topical use will stain skin blue but the colour may be removed with a hypochloride solution.

Interference with Clinical Pathology tests

No interference with currently used tests have been reported.

High risk groups

Neonates

There appears to be a high risk of haemolytic anaemia after intra-amniotic use of methylene blue.

Breast milk. Use of the dye is best avoided in mothers who are breast feeding.

Children

In general, doses should be determined by body weight. For emergency treatment, symptomatic infants should be treated with 2 $mg.kg^{-1}$ initially.[1]

Pregnant women

If the drug is given to pregnant women there is a risk of neonatal haemolytic anaemia.

The elderly

No specific toxic effects have been reported on the elderly with reasonable renal function but reduce dose in renal impairment.

Concurrent disease

In the presence of severe renal impairment toxic blood concentrations may occur with conventional doses.

Drug interactions

No significant interactions have been reported.

References

1. Wintrobe M M (ed) 1981 Clincial haematology, 8th edn. Lea and Febinger, Philadelphia, pp 1012–1014
2. DiSanta A R, Wagner J G 1972 Pharmacokinetics of highly ionised drugs. II: Methylene blue — absorption, metabolism, and excretion in man and dog after oral administration. Journal of Pharmaceutical Sciences 61: 1086–1090
3. Blass N, Fung D 1976 Dyed but not dead — methylene blue overdose. Anesthesiology 45: 458–459
4. Goluboff N, Wheaton R 1961 Methylene blue induced cyanosis and acute haemolytic anaemia complicating the treatment of methaemoglobinaemia. Journal of Pediatrics 58: 86–89
5. Crooks J 1982 Haemolytic jaundice in a neonate after intra-amniotic injection of methylene blue. Archives of Disease in Childhood 57: 872–873
6. DiSanto A R, Wagner J G 1972 Pharmacokinetics of highly ionised drugs. I: Methylene blue — whole blood, urine, and tissue assays. Journal of Pharmaceutical Sciences 61: 598–602
7. The Pharmaceutical Codex, 11th edn. 1979. The Pharmaceutical Press, London
8. DiSanto A R, Wagner J G 1972 Pharmacokinetics of highly ionised drugs. III: Methylene blue — blood levels in the dog and tissue levels in the rat following intravenous administration. Journal of Pharmaceutical Science 61: 1090–1094
9. Reynolds J E F 1982 Martindale. The Extra Pharmacopoiea, 28th edn. The Pharmaceutical Press, London
10. Dudley N E 1971 Methylene blue for rapid identification of the parathyroids. British Medical Journal 3: 680–681
11. Giradi G, Fritas E, Vial L et al 1978 Diagnosis of gastro-oesophageal reflux in infants and children by methylene-blue test. Lancet 1: 1236
12. McEnerney J K, McEnerney L N 1983 Unfavourable neonatal outcome after intraamniotic injection of methylene blue. Obstetrics and Gynaecology 61: 35s–37s
13. Beutler E 1969 Drug induced haemolytic anaemia. Pharmacological Reviews 21: 73–103
14. Perry P M, Meinhard E 1974 Necrotic subcutaneous abscesses following injection of methylene blue. British Journal of Clinical Practice 28: 289–291
15. Sharr M M, Weller R O, Brice J G 1978 Spinal cord necrosis after intrathecal injection of methylene blue. Journal of Neurology, Neurosurgery and Psychiatry 41: 384–386
16. Nadler J E, Green H, Rosenbaum A 1934 Intravenous injection of methylene blue in man with reference to its toxic symptoms and effects on the electrocardiogram. American Journal of the Medical Sciences 188: 15–21

Methylergometrine (maleate)

Methylergometrine is an ergot alkaloid used as an oxytocic agent, due to its potent α-adrenoceptor stimulating properties. It is very similar in properties to ergometrine maleate.

Chemistry

Methylergometrine maleate (methylergonovine maleate, Methergine)
$C_{20}H_{25}N_3O_2.C_4H_4O_4$
9,10-Didehydro-N-[(S)-1(hydroxymethyl)-propyl]-6-methylergoline-8β-carboxamide maleate

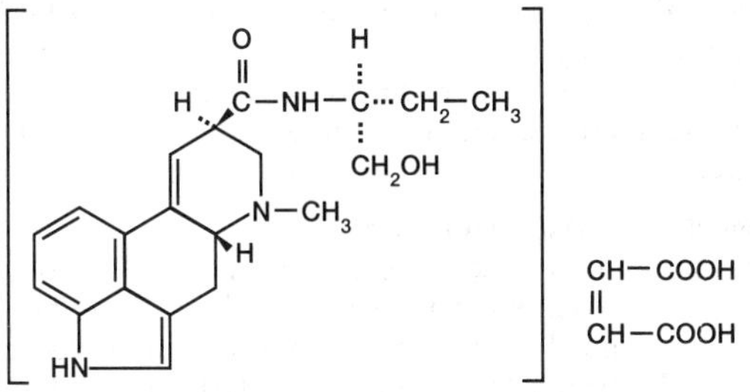

Molecular weight of maleate (free base)	455.5 (339.4)
pKa (amino)	6.65[1,2]
Solubility	
in alcohol	1 in 140
in water	1 in 200
Octanol/water partition coefficient	—

Methylergometrine maleate is a white to pinkish-tan microcrystalline powder, with a bitter taste. It darkens with age and on exposure to light. Injectable preparations of the drug are clear colourless solutions with a pH of 2.7–3.5. Commercially it is produced by chemical synthesis.

Pharmacology

Methylergometrine is an oxytocic amine alkaloid which causes contraction of uterine smooth muscle with an increase in contraction frequency and amplitude at low doses and an elevation of uterine basal tone at higher doses. At higher doses, contractions become much more forceful with a marked increase in resting tones. The mechanism of action involves direct uterine smooth muscle stimulation through α-adrenergic receptors.[2,3] The drug produces vasoconstriction, mainly of capacitance vessels, however the effects on vascular smooth muscle are much less than that of ergotamine.

Toxicology

In teratological experiments in animals, ergometrine, the parent compound of methylergometrine, inhibited embryonic implantation,[4] but was a relatively non-potent agent as compared to other ergot derivatives. Methylergometrine can cause fetal death but at moderately high doses.[5]

Clinical pharmacology

Through α-adrenergic receptor stimulation, which can be blocked by α-adrenergic blocking drugs such as phentolamine and dihydroergotamine,[2,3] the main pharmacological action of ergometrine and methylergometrine is uterine smooth muscle contraction. Studying the postpartum human uterus in situ, dose–response curves of methylergometrine and ergometrine were compared and found to be parallel, with ergometrine about 1.5 times as active as methylergometrine.[6] A small dose of methylergometrine can cause intense uterine smooth muscle contractions followed by periods of relaxation. High doses of the drug cause sustained uterine contraction with elevation of basal tone. Blood flow through the spiral arteries is decreased by the contraction of the myometrium, and not as an effect of the drug on the uterine vasculature.[7]

Methylergometrine also causes constriction of vascular smooth muscle, affecting mainly capacitance vessels. This may result in an elevation in central venous pressure and in an elevated blood pressure. In initial studies methylergometrine seemed to cause less elevation of blood pressure than ergometrine,[8,9] but in randomized trials this has not been confirmed.[10,11]

In lactating puerperal women, methylergometrine has been shown not to cause any change in prolactin levels or milk secretion.[12]

Prolonged use of the drug can produce signs of ergotism.

Pharmacokinetics

Since the total daily dose of methylergometrine is usually less than 1 mg, the concentrations found in biological fluids are very low. Therefore, the assay of choice is usually radioimmunoassay. The antiserum is prepared against lysergic acid and is thus not specific for methylergometrine, but also reacts with ergometrine, lysergic acid, ergotamine, dihydroergotamine, and dihydro-ergotoxine.[13] Although the antiserum apparently measures the unmetabolized drug, some cross-reactivity with metabolites is possible. The lower limit of detection of the assay is 0.5–1.0 $\mu g.l^{-1}$. A high pressure liquid chromatographic assay, which utilizes fluorescence detection, has also been developed.[14] This has a lower limit of detection of 100 $ng.l^{-1}$.

Methylergometrine is rapidly and almost completely absorbed after oral dosing or intramuscular injection. The bioavailability is approximately 60% after oral dosing.[15] Peak plasma concentrations of the drug after an oral dose occur at 30 min. The uterine contractile effect starts 5–15 min after oral administration, and 2–5 min after intramuscular administration. When given intravenously, the uterine contractile effect is virtually instantaneous.[16,17] Uterine contractions can last for 3 or more hours after an oral or intramuscular dose and can last for up to 2 hours after intravenous administration.

Methylergometrine is rapidly distributed, with an apparent volume of distribution of 0.33–0.67 $l.kg^{-1}$, corresponding to total body water. When given intravenously, the distribution half life is 1–3 min.[15,18] The drug is extensively metabolized, with only 2–3% of the unchanged drug being excreted in the urine in 24 h. As a consequence, elimination is rapid, the elimination half life reported as 32.1 ± 9.6 min in postpartum females[18] and approximately 115 min in male volunteers.[15]

In studies on the oral administration of methylergometrine it was shown that a dose of 0.125 mg three times a day produced plasma levels of 0.5 $\mu g.l^{-1}$ in male volunteers and in postpartum patients.[19] However, peak levels of the drug did not occur until 3 hours after dosing in the postpartum patients, compared with 30 min in the male volunteers, the delay attributed to decreased gastrointestinal motility in pregnancy.[19] However, these studies may have been confounded by the cross-reactivity of the antiserum used in the radioimmunoassay with metabolites of the drug. Methylergometrine is bound to plasma proteins only weakly (35%).

The milk:plasma ratio of methylergometrine is 0.3. However, the amount of drug present in breast milk is insufficient to affect the infant. On an oral dose of 0.125 mg of the drug three times per day, the calculated daily amount in maternal milk is only 1.3 μg.[20]

Oral absorption	almost complete
Presystemic metabolism	30–40%
Plasma half life	
range	0.5–2.0 h
Volume of distribution	0.33–0.67 $l.kg^{-1}$
Plasma protein binding	35%

The drug is not used in the elderly, so it is not known whether old age has any effect on its pharmacokinetics. There is no information on

Methylergometrine (maleate)

M

the effect of renal or hepatic disease on the elimination of the compound. Hepatic dysfunction is likely to reduce the elimination of methylergometrine.

Concentration–effect relationship

The contractile effect that these drugs exert on the uterus is dose-dependent with a steep dose–response curve.[6] However, plasma levels do not seem to correlate with uterine effect since the elimination phase half life is 0.5 h in puerperal women but the uterine effect has been shown to last for 3 or more hours.[17]

Metabolism

Ergot alkaloids are eliminated primarily by hepatic metabolism and excretion in the faeces.[21,22] (Fig. 1)

Fig. 1

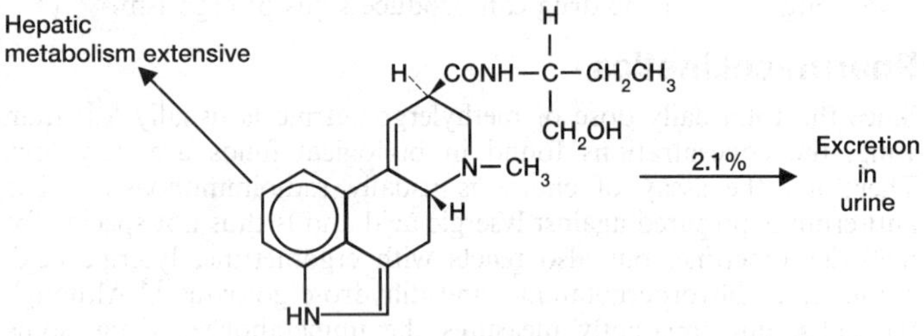

Methylergometrine is extensively metabolized in the liver, with only approximately 3% of the orally administered drug appearing in urine. The specific routes of metabolism of methylergometrine have not been well studied, but they are likely to be similar to those of ergometrine. These include hydroxylation and glucuronidation, and possibly also N- demethylation. In the rat, the drug (ergometrine) undergoes hydroxylation of the benzene ring and subsequent glucuronic acid conjugation. There is also glucuronidation of the terminal hydroxyl group of the side chain.[23]

Pharmaceutics

Methylergometrine maleate is available in sugar coated pinkish-red tablets containing 0.2 mg and marked with the black numbers '78–54'. The injectable form is available as a clear solution with a concentration of $0.2\ mg.ml^{-1}$, which should be stored at temperatures below 8°C and should be protected from light.

Therapeutic use

Indications

1. Prevention and treatment of postpartum and postabortal haemorrhage due to uterine atony
2. Treatment of uterine subinvolution
3. Under careful obstetric supervision to shorten the third stage of labour by administration after the delivery of the anterior shoulder of the fetus.

Contraindications

1. Use before delivery of a living fetus for induction or augmentation of labour
2. Pregnancy-induced hypertension (pre-eclampsia, eclampsia)
3. The presence or prior history of arterial-venous shunts
4. Heart disease
5. Peripheral obliterative vascular disease
6. Threatened spontaneous abortion.

Mode of use

Methylergometrine produces sustained tetanic contraction of the postpartum and postabortal uterus, and appears to be as effective as its parent compound, ergometrine, for this purpose.[10] Methylergometrine is preferred by many clinicians because in initial reports it appeared to produce hypertension less frequently than ergometrine.[8,9] However, in two randomized clinical trials, no difference was found between the two drugs in their ability to cause hypertension.[10,11]

Indications

1. Prevention and treatment of postpartum and postabortal haemorrhage due to uterine atony
In the prevention and treatment of postpartum and postabortal haemorrhage due to uterine atony ergometrine and methylergometrine are preferred by many clinicians over oxytocin for sustained tonic uterine contractions. Initial treatment is administration of 0.2 mg of methylergometrine intramuscularly which usually produces a firm contraction of the uterus within 3 to 5 minutes. However, in obstetrical emergencies where a quicker response is needed and where shock may delay absorption from intramuscular sites, methylergometrine may be administered intravenously over no less than 60 seconds with careful monitoring of blood pressure and pulse. The intramuscular dose can be repeated in 2 to 4 hours; however, refractoriness to a second dose of methylergometrine has been observed in the first few hours after delivery[24] and in the advanced puerperium.[16] If calcium deficient patients fail to respond to therapy, response may be restored by intravenous administration of calcium salts. Once the haemorrhage has subsided, therapy may be continued orally in a dosage of 0.2 mg of methylergometrine three to four times per day for 2 to 7 days to reduce postpartum bleeding, puerperal uterine atony and subinvolution. Uterine cramping can be reduced by decreasing dosage.

Mild postpartum haemorrhage occurring later in the puerperium may be treated by methylergometrine orally in a dose of 0.2 mg three to four times per day.

In all treatment of postabortal or postpartum haemorrhage the possibility that there are retained products of conception in the uterus must be kept in mind.

2. Treatment of uterine subinvolution
Methylergometrine is used in postabortal[25] and in postpartum[26] uterine subinvolution, clinically evidenced by a large, boggy, tender uterus and continued heavy and irregular uterine bleeding. Initial therapy may be begun either intramuscularly or orally, depending upon the clinical situation, and continued orally for 2 to 7 days.

3. Under careful obstetric supervision to shorten the third stage of labour by administration after the delivery of the anterior shoulder of the fetus
Because postpartum haemorrhage is a leading cause of maternal morbidity and mortality there has been active interest in pharmacologic management of the third stage of labour. The goals have been to reduce the time to placental expulsion, reduce the incidence of postpartum haemorrhage, and reduce the incidence of placental retention. Whether or not this drug actually is effective in achieving these goals and should be used in this manner is controversial. When employed the clinician must be certain that there is not a multiple gestation and must be willing to accept the possibility of occasionally trapping the placenta. If used, 0.2 mg of methylergometrine is administered intramuscularly after the delivery of the anterior shoulder of the infant. Alternatively 10 IU of oxytocin can be given intramuscularly at the birth of the anterior shoulder followed by 0.2 mg methylergometrine intramuscularly after the delivery of the placenta.[27]

Contraindications

1. Use before delivery of a living fetus for induction or augmentation of labour
The pregnant uterus is very sensitive to methylergometrine and even a small dose can produce sustained tetanic contraction of the uterus which may interfere with uteroplacental circulation and fetal respiratory function. Since contractions produced by this agent are irregular, unpredictable, and not readily reversible, it is not used prior to delivery.

2. Pregnancy-induced hypertension (pre-eclampsia, eclampsia)
Methylergometrine can acutely produce severe and sustained hypertension particularly in patients with pregnancy-induced hypertension.[28] However, patients with only a history of hypertension without signs of pregnancy induced hypertension do not seem to be at increased risk for acutely developing hypertension. The drug should not be used in any patient with pregnancy-induced hypertension.

3. The presence or prior history of arterial-venous shunts
Patients in whom a cerebral arterial-venous malformation has been diagnosed or who have had corrective surgery should not receive this

drug, since acute elevation of blood pressure could induce a cerebral haemhorrage.

4. Heart disease
Use of methylergometrine may cause spasm of the coronary arteries and is particularly contraindicated in patients with a history of angina or prior myocardial infarction.

In patients with other forms of heart disease consideration must be given as to whether or not an acute hypertensive episode could be tolerated without severe sequelae.

5. Peripheral obliterative vascular disease
Since methylergometrine causes vasoconstriction, use of this agent in patients with peripheral obliterative vascular disease could produce circulatory compromise of a limb with possible gangrene.

Adverse reactions

Potentially life-threatening effects
Severe reaction to methylergometrine is manifested by nausea, vomiting, diarrhoea, severe thirst, cold extremities, confusion, coma, hypotension or hypertension, and seizures. One death is reported from use of the parent compound, ergometrine, given to a neonate inadvertently.

Acute overdosage
Principal manifestations of severe methylergometrine overdosage are gangrene and seizures. Other effects are nausea, vomiting, diarrhoea, dizziness, hypertension, angina, palpitations, dyspnoea, confusion, loss of consciousness and intense vasoconstriction of the extremities.

Treatment is first directed toward withdrawal of the drug. In oral ingestions, particularly in children, emesis or gastric lavage followed by administration of activated charcoal is indicated.[29] Other therapeutic measures are supportive and directed at symptoms present. Seizures should be treated with anticonvulsants. Hypertension should be treated with hydralazine or nitroprusside. The drug of choice for treatment of severe vasospasm is nitroprusside due to its direct action on smooth muscle and its rapid onset and cessation of action.[30] Venous thrombosis caused by stasis and endothelial damage should be treated with heparin or low molecular weight dextran.

Severe or irreversible adverse effects
Chronic toxicity produces vascular complications presenting most commonly in the legs with a cold, pale, pulseless extremity and in severe cases with ischaemia and gangrene. Withdrawal of the drug will effect a reversal of toxicity in the majority of cases. However, treatment of vasospasm and prevention of thrombosis may be indicated.

Symptomatic adverse effects
Adverse effects do not appear as frequently during treatment with methylergometrine as they do when other ergot alkaloids are used. The major adverse effects reported are nausea and vomiting. This is important to remember since this drug is used in an obstetrical setting with anaesthesia, and its use may increase the risk of aspiration of stomach contents. Other adverse effects include headache, vertigo, tinnitus, abdominal pain, palpitations, angina and shortness of breath.

Interference with clinical pathology tests
No significant interference of this kind has been reported.

High risk groups

Neonates
The drugs are not used in this patient group but inadvertent administration to neonates reportedly has caused peripheral cyanosis, apnoea, myoclonic movements, purpura, mild jaundice, and one death.

Breast milk. Methylergometrine, as compared to ergometrine, does not appear to affect prolactin levels or milk production.[12] Methylergometrine has been detected in breast milk; however, the daily amount excreted should not affect the infant.[20]

Children
The drug is not used in this patient group.

Pregnant women
Methylergometrine is particularly contraindicated before delivery.

Methylergometrine (maleate)

The elderly
The drug is not used in this patient group.

Concurrent disease
The drug is contraindicated in patients with pregnancy-induced hypertension, arterial-venous shunts, ischaemic heart disease or peripheral obliterative vascular disease.

Drug interactions

Potentially hazardous interactions
The vasoconstrictive effects of methylergometrine are enhanced by sympathomimetic drugs.

Potentially useful interactions
When methylergometrine is used with oxytocin, postpartum haemorrhage due to uterine atony is controlled by two different mechanisms, oxytocin producing an immediate response and methylergometrine producing a sustained response.

Major outcome trials

Sorbe B 1978 Active pharmacologic management of the third stage of labor. Obstetrics and Gynecology 52: 694–697

A randomized clinical trial of intravenous use of either 10 IU oxytocin or 0.2 mg methylergometrine given to 1049 parturients with the birth of the anterior shoulder. The study examines duration of the third stage of labour, immediate postpartum blood loss, and the incidence of retained placenta. A large historical control group given 0.2 mg methylergometrine after delivery provides an additional comparative group.

The mean duration of the third stage of labour was not significantly different in any group. Blood loss and the incidence of postpartum haemorrhage was significantly less in the groups treated with methylergometrine or oxytocin at the birth of the anterior shoulder as compared with the control group treated only after delivery of the placenta. Postpartum haemorrhage was significantly less in patients treated with oxytocin. Methylergometrine significantly increased the incidence of retained placenta, and for this reason blood loss was slightly greater in the methylergometrine group as compared to the oxytocin group.

Groeber W R, Bishop E H 1960 Methergine and ergonovine in the third stage of labor. Obstetrics and Gynecology 15: 85–88

This is a block-randomized, double-blind study of 2887 parturients, comparing methylergometrine and ergometrine given intravenously after the delivery of the anterior shoulder of the infant. The study examines blood loss, the incidence of haemorrhage, and the incidence of hypertension.

No difference could be found between the two drugs.

Friedman E A 1957 Comparative clinical evaluation of postpartum oxytocics. American Journal of Obstetrics and Gynecology 73: 1306–1313

This study compares methylergometrine, ergometrine, oxytocin and dihydroergotamine administered randomly to parturients in the third stage of labour. Blood loss, the incidence of hypertension, and the incidence of haemorrhage were found to be equivalent for methylergometrine and ergometrine. However, oxytocin caused less blood loss, less postpartum haemorrhage, and no incidents of hypertension.

General review articles

Mantyla R, Kanto J 1981 Clinical pharmacokinetics of methylergometrine (methylergonovine). International Journal of Clinical Pharmacology, Therapeutics and Toxicology 19: 386–391

References

1. Maulding H V, Zoglio M A 1970 Physical chemistry of ergot alkaloids and derivatives I: ionization constants of several medicinally active bases. Journal of Pharmaceutical Science 59: 700–701
2. Rothlin E, Bircher R 1952 Allergy, the autonomic nervous system and ergot alkaloids. Progress in Allergy 3: 434
3. Konzett H 1960 Specific antagonism of dibenamine to ergometrine. In: Wolstenholme G E W, O'Connor M (eds) Ciba Foundation Symposium on Adrenergic Mechanisms. Churchill, London, pp 463–465

4. Grauwiler J, Schon H 1973 Teratological experiments with ergotamine in mice, rats, and rabbits. Teratology 7: 227–235
5. Griffith R W, Grauwiler J, Hochel C H, Leist K H, Matter B 1978 Toxicologic considerations in ergot alkaloids and related compounds. In: Berde B, Schild H O (eds) Handbook of experimental pharmacology, Vol 49. Springer-Verlag, p 828
6. Myerscough P R, Schild H O 1958 Quantitative assays of oxytocic drugs on the human postpartum uterus. British Journal of Pharmacology 13: 207–212
7. Kofler E 1972 Ueber die mikrozirkulation an der portio vaginalis uteri. Wiener Klinische Wochenschrift 84 (suppl 3): 3–16
8. Schade F F 1951 Methergine: a study of its vasomotor properties. American Journal of Obstetrics and Gynecology 61: 188–192
9. Fitzgerald W J 1956 Methergine: a study of its effect on blood pressure. Obstetrics and Gynecology 8: 167–169
10. Groeber W R, Bishop E H 1960 Methergine and ergonovine in the third stage of labor. Obstetrics and Gynecology 15: 85–88
11. Friedman E A 1957 Comparative clinical evaluation of postpartum oxytocics. American Journal of Obstetrics and Gynecology 73: 1306–1313
12. del Pozo E, Brun del Re E, Hinselmann M 1975 Lack of effect of methyl-ergonovine on postpartum lactation. American Journal of Obstetrics and Gynecology 123: 845–846
13. Kleimola T 1978 Quantitative determination of ergot alkaloids in biological fluids by radioimmunoassay. British Journal of Clinical Pharmacology 6: 255
14. Edland P O 1981 Journal of Chromatography 226 Biomedical Applications 15: 107
15. Mantyla R, Kleimola T, Kanto J 1978 Methylergometrine (methylergonovine) concentrations in the human plasma and urine. International Journal of Clinical Pharmacology 16: 254
16. Gill R C 1947 The effect of methyl-ergometrine on the human puerperal uterus. Journal of Obstetrics and Gynecology of the British Empire 54: 482–488
17. Roth-Brandel U, Bygdeman M, Wizvist N 1970 A comparative study on the influence of prostaglandin E_1, oxytocin and ergometrine on the pregnant human uterus. Acta Obstetrica Gynecologica Scandinavica 49 (suppl 5): 1–7
18. Mantyla R, Kleimola T, Kanto J 1977 Pharmacokinetics of methylergometrine (methylergonovine) in the rabbit and man. Acta Pharmacolica et Toxicologica 40: 561–569
19. Allonen H, Juvakoski J, Kanto J, Laitinen S, Mantyla R, Kleimola T 1978 Methylergometrine: comparison of plasma concentrations and clinical response. International Journal of Clinical Pharmacology 16: 340
20. Erkkola R, Kanto J, Allonen H, Kleimola T, Mantyla R 1978 Excretion of methylergometrine (methylergonovine) into the human breast milk. International Journal of Clinical Pharmacology 16: 579
21. Aellig Wh, Nuesch F 1977 Comparative pharmacokinetic investigations with tritium labelled ergot alkaloids after oral and after intravenous administration in man. International Journal of Clinical Pharmacology 15: 106
22. Nimmerfall F, Rosenthaler J 1976 Ergot alkaloids: hepatic distribution and estimation of absorption by measurement of total radioactivity in bile and urine. Journal of Pharmacokinetics and Biopharmaceutics 4: 57
23. Slaytor M B, Wright S E 1962 The metabolites of ergometrine and lysergic acid diethylamide in rat bile. Journal of Medicinal and Pharmaceutical Chemistry 5: 483–491
24. Muller H A, Stroker W 1959 Studien uber die Uterusmotilitat. Die spontane Motilitat in der Postplacentarperiode und Metherginwirkung. Arch Gynak. 191: 369–376
25. Hern W M 1984 Management of complications. In: Abortion Practice. J B Lippincott, New York, ch 7, p 185
26. Pritchard J A, MacDonald P C, Gant N F 1985 Other disorders of the puerperium. In: Williams Obstetrics 17th edn. Appleton-Century-Crofts, Norwalk, Connecticut, ch 36, p 737
27. Pauerstein C J 1973 Use and abuse of oxytocic agents. Clinics in Obstetrics and Gynecology 16: 262–277
28. Baillie T W 1963 Vasopressor activity of ergometrine. British Medical Journal 1: 585–588
29. Kunkel D B, Jallo D S 1983 Ergot. In: Haddad L M, Winchester J F (eds) Clinical management of poisoning and drug overdose. W B Saunders, Philadelphia, ch 94, pp 876–881
30. Husted J W, Ring E J, Hirsh L F 1978 Intra-arterial nitroprusside treatment for ergotism. American Journal of Roentgenology 131: 1090–1092

Methylphenidate

Methylphenidate is a centrally active sympathomimetic agent used clinically in the management of attention deficit disorders and narcolepsy.

Chemistry

Methylphenidate hydrochloride (Ritalin)
$C_{14}H_{19}NO_2.HCl$
Methyl-phenyl-2-piperidineacetate hydrochloride

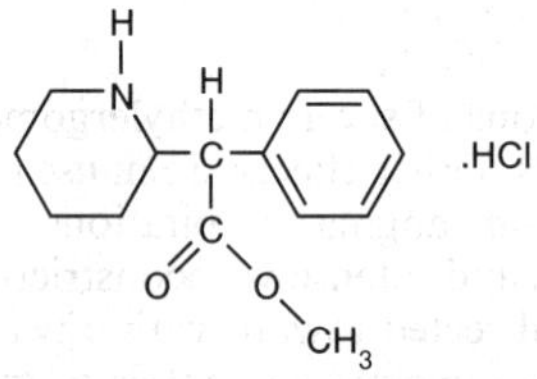

Molecular weight hydrochloride (free base)	269.3 (233.3)
pKa (amino group)	8.5
Solubility	
in alcohol	freely soluble
in water	freely soluble
Octanol/water partition coefficient	—

A white odourless, fine crystalline powder prepared by chemical synthesis. Although there are two asymmetric carbon atoms in the molecule, only one racemate with the *threo* configuration is used therapeutically, (d)-*threo* methylphenidate. The stability of this compound in acid environments, such as the stomach, is presumed to be due to its complete protonation and intramolecular hydrogen bonding, which is only possible for the *threo* form.

Pharmacology

Methylphenidate is a sympathomimetic agent with its main actions in the central nervous system (CNS). It blocks the uptake of noradrenaline (NA) into peripheral adrenergic nerves, and the uptake of both dopamine (DA) and NA into synaptosomes from several brain areas. Methylphenidate differentially releases DA from striatal synaptosomes, in contrast to (S)-(d)-amphetamine, which releases similar amounts of DA and NA. *Threo* methylphenidate has weak activity as an inhibitor of monoamine oxidase activity in liver, kidney and brain, but this is not thought to be responsible for its pharmacological actions.

The overall pharmacological profile of methylphenidate resembles that of amphetamine and other phenyl isopropylamines, with the exception that its anorexic effects and actions on the peripheral circulation are less marked. Locomotor stimulation is only seen with the *threo* diastereoisomer, which is about one-seventh as active as (S)-(d)-amphetamine. Stereotypic behaviour induced by methylphenidate at higher doses are blocked by antipsychotic agents, suggesting that DA is involved.

The mechanisms of the locomotor stimulation induced by methylphenidate and by amphetamine are different. Reserpine pretreatment antagonizes the effects of methylphenidate, whilst α-methyltyrosine has no effect. The opposite situation is found with amphetamine. These observations, together with other biochemical studies, suggest that the action of methylphenidate is on reserpine-sensitive amine pools, with increased release of both DA and NA, together with increased accumulation of their O-methylated derivatives, 3-methoxytyramine and normetanephrine. Amphetamine acts on reserpine-resistant pools of DA, and in this case, it is only the increased normetanephrine that is blocked by pretreatment with reserpine.

Toxicology

No published information relating to carcinogenicity or teratological effects is available.

Clinical pharmacology

At clinically effective doses, methylphenidate is a CNS stimulant in normal individuals, and frequently causes insomnia and some anorexia. The clinical pharmacology of methylphenidate is similar to that of amphetamine, although the peripheral sympathomimetic actions are less evident. Doses of methylphenidate in the range of 0.2 $mg.kg^{-1}$ daily to 2.0 $mg.kg^{-1}$ daily given in two or three divided doses are required for therapeutic effect in hyperactive children with attention deficit disorder (ADD). Treatment is started at low doses with weekly dose adjustments made empirically until a clinical response is obtained or until toxicity becomes a problem. Variable tolerance is produced and doses in the order of 60–100 mg daily are not unusual. Confusion, and occasionally, frank hallucinations, may be produced in some individuals in this dose range. Methylphenidate may cause significant increases in diastolic blood pressure in adolescents.[1]

In children with ADD, the drug decreases hyperactivity, allows more purposeful activity, and improves learning capacity. In this age group, long-term use of methylphenidate in doses greater than 20 mg daily may be associated with impairment of growth and development, which is reversible on withdrawal of the drug.[2]

Recently the use of positron emission tomography (PET) has demonstrated that children with ADD have decreased blood flow (low striatal neuronal activity) in the white matter of the prefrontal cortex and striatal regions. The investigators claim that the strial hypoperfusion, which was partially reversible by treatment with the CNS stimulant, methylphenidate, may be an essential feature of ADD.[3]

Pharmacokinetics

The bioavailability of orally administered methylphenidate is low and very variable (10.5–52.5%), although this does not appear to be influenced by food.[4,5] Peak concentrations in the plasma are seen about two hours after an oral dose, but the drug is absorbed more slowly from extended-release tablets which are available in some countries. Its half life of elimination from plasma is in the order of 1–2 hours. Concentrations in the brain exceed those in plasma.

Oral absorption	80%
Presystemic metabolism	50–90%
Plasma half life range	1–2 h
Volume of distribution	—
Plasma protein binding	15%

Concentration–effect relationship

Whilst there have been suggestions that the relationship between dose and response may be non-linear and there are reports of relationships between drug concentration and neuroendocrine responses, a number of studies in adults and hyperactive children have failed to establish any useful relationships between drug concentrations in the blood and behavioural or laboratory measures of response.[6]

Metabolism

Methylphenidate is rapidly metabolized in man. After oral administration, little parent drug can be identified in plasma with doses less than 20 mg. This extensive presystemic metabolism probably explains the low and variable oral bioavailability. Parenterally administered methylphenidate tagged with ^{14}C is largely recovered as metabolites in the urine within 30 hours. Three metabolites have been identified in the urine by radiochromatography techniques. The main urinary metabolite is retalinic acid, a de-esterified product which accounts for 80% of the dose. Most of the remaining drug is oxidized by the hepatic mixed function oxidase to oxomethylphenidate and p-hydroxymethylphenidate (Fig. 1). These oxidized products may be further hydrolysed by esterases to oxoretalinic acid and p-hydroxyretalinic acids, respectively. The p-hydroxy metabolites may have significant pharmacological activity, but this has not yet been clarified.

Fig. 1 The metabolism of methylphenidate

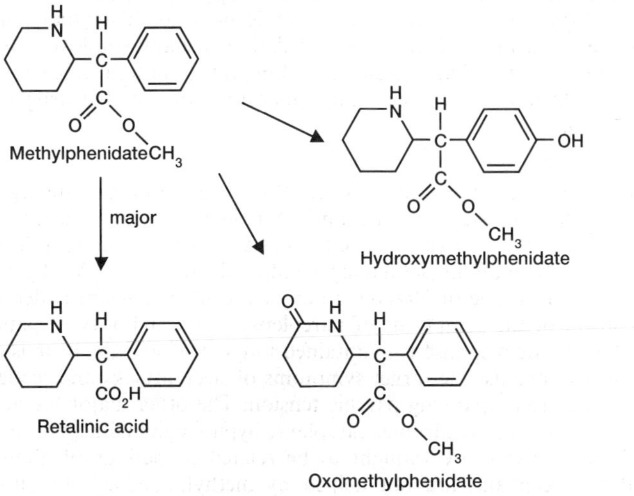

One hour after an oral dose, ritalinic acid is also the major circulating form of the drug. With long-term administration of the drug, there may be significant accumulation of this compound and other polar metabolites, which have longer elimination half lives than the parent drug.

Pharmaceutics

Methylphenidate is available in the form of tablets in the USA containing 5 mg, 10 mg, 20 mg of methylphenidate hydrochloride (Ritalin, CIBA white and scored tablet marked AB, CIBA on the reverse) and as a sterile injection (Ritalin, CIBA) containing 20 mg of methylphenidate hydrochloride in a single use ampoule. Dosage forms vary in different countries.

Therapeutic use

Indications

1. Attention deficit disorder
2. Narcolepsy
3. Other clinical uses.

A number of clinical uses for methylphenidate have been suggested but, at the present time, its utility has not been confirmed or established. Amongst the claimed indications are: chronic fatigue, stuttering in children, drug-induced lethargy, psychoneuroses, apathetic or withdrawn senile behaviour, and as a provocative test of the need for antipsychotic therapy in controlled schizophrenia.

Contraindications

1. Alcoholics
2. Emotionally unstable patients
3. Drug abusers
4. Marked anxiety
5. Tension and agitation
6. Glaucoma
7. Motor tics or family history of Gilles de Tourettes syndrome
8. Hypertension
9. Cardiac arrhythmias
10. Psychoses
11. Epilepsy.

Indications

1. Attention deficit disorder

Methylphenidate has an established place in the management of hyperactive children who meet the diagnostic criteria for attention deficit disorder (ADD). There is not general agreement about its role

M

in the management of adolescents and adults with the disorder, but recent studies suggest the drug is useful, especially in those with a history extending from childhood. About 80% of children with hyperactivity associated with ADD show a worthwhile, and sometimes dramatic, response to the drug. Treatment is usually started with a dose of 5 mg in the morning and at midday taken with, or before, meals to avoid gastrointestinal side effects. Dosage is usually increased in 5 mg increments until a therapeutic response, or toxicity, develops. Most patients benefit with doses of 20–40 mg daily and an upper limit in the order of 80 mg daily is usually employed. Whilst there is good evidence of short- and intermediate-term efficacy, long-term efficacy is less clear. The mode of action of the drug is not known.

2. Narcolepsy
It is now over 50 years since Prinzmetal and Bloomberg first suggested the use of amphetamine for the treatment of narcolepsy,[7] and more than 30 years since the initial reports of the usefulness of methylphenidate in the management of the disorder.[8] Methylphenidate in a dosage of 20–60 mg daily as divided doses provides good control of the symptoms of narcolepsy in the majority of patients. Therapeutic response is maintained long-term[9] and the drug is most effective against the target symptoms of sleep attacks and tendency, and the accompanying psychic tension. The other major features of the narcoleptic syndrome, cataplexy, hypnogogic hallucinations and sleep paralysis, are thought to be related to periods of abnormal REM sleep and are not helped by methylphenidate, but usually respond to tricyclic antidepressants, which are thought to work by suppressing REM sleep. It is important to keep the dosage of methylphenidate as low as possible to minimize the risk of side effects and to reduce the risk of paradoxical sleepiness which is seen in about 14% of narcoleptic patients treated with the drug. If the narcoleptic symptoms are only mild, it may be possible to administer the methylphenidate only before driving or other important events.

Contraindications

1–3. Alcoholism, drug abuse and emotional instability
Because of the risks of tolerance and the development of psychological dependence on the drug, methylphenidate should be avoided in these high risk patients.

4, 5. Anxiety states
Like other sympathomimetic agents, methylphenidate may cause or exacerbate anxiety. The drug is best avoided in patients with agitation or anxiety from any cause.

6. Glaucoma
Methylphenidate is contraindicated in patients with narrow-angle glaucoma as the drug causes mydriasis and may elevate intraocular pressure.

8, 9. Hypertension and cardiac disease
Significant increases in systemic blood pressure may be seen following the administration of methylphenidate. The risk is high in patients also treated with tricyclic antidepressants and hypertension and tachycardia are more likely after parenteral administration. Cardiac arrhythmias are also well documented after both oral and parenteral administration. As with other sympathomimetic agents, the drugs are best avoided in patients with hypertension or with cardiac disease.

10. Schizophrenia
Methylphenidate may induce or exacerbate psychotic symptoms when given to patients with schizophrenia who are acutely ill or who are in partial remission. This property of the drug has been used as a test to determine the necessity for continuing antipsychotic therapy,[10] although the test is not in general use.

11. Epilepsy
In large doses, methylphenidate may cause convulsions and the drug is best avoided if there is a history of epilepsy.

Adverse reactions

Potentially life-threatening effects
Cardiac arrhythmias and convulsions are the main threats to life with overdosage.

Acute overdosage
The minimal lethal dose in man is not known as there are insufficient reports available. Both children and adults have survived large overdoses with the drug. Thus, there are records of a 37-year-old woman surviving the ingestion of 500 mg over a 12-hour period; a 14-year-old girl surviving the ingestion of 300 mg in association with primidone; and a record of the survival of an 18-month-old boy who ingested 40 mg of methylphenidate.

The main features of overdosage with methylphenidate are due to overstimulation of the CNS and excessive sympathomimetic effects peripherally. The patients may be pale or flushed. Sweating can be profuse, although mucous membranes remain dry. Vomiting is common and the pupils are dilated. Stimulation of respiratory centres produces hyperventilation, although with severe poisoning Cheyne-Stokes respiration and respiratory depression may follow. Tachycardia, with the risk of cardiac arrhythmias, is to be expected and the blood pressure is usually elevated. More severe poisoning may be associated with depression of the heart and circulation, with a low blood pressure and cardiac insufficiency. Stimulation of the CNS produces euphoria and may lead to hallucinations, confusion, delusions and impairment of consciousness, up to and including coma. Hyperreflexia, tremor and muscle twitching are common features and may be followed by convulsions.

The management of overdosage with methylphenidate is directed at limiting oral absorption and control of the specific features of the poisoning. Gastric lavage followed by the instillation of activated charcoal and manitol is indicated to limit absorption unless the patient is severely agitated, in which case initial sedation may be indicated. Supportive measures may be indicated to maintain the circulation and respiration, and to lower the core temperature if hyperpyrexia supervenes. Convulsions should be controlled along standard lines using intravenous diazepam or phenytoin.

There is no established role for peritoneal dialysis or extracorporeal haemoperfusion.

Severe or irreversible adverse effects
Psychotic reactions may be seen especially with parenteral abuse of the drug and, on withdrawal of the drug after high-dose use, severe depression with agitation and hyperactivity can be precipitated. There are reports of the precipitation of angina, tachycardias and tachyarrhythmias of various types.

Symptomatic adverse effects
The common adverse reactions are those shared with other sympathomimetics, namely, nervousness, restlessness and insomnia. Anorexia is common especially with short-term use and palpitations, nausea, dizziness and headache are not uncommon. Weight loss, abdominal pain and tachycardia are all reported to be more commonly seen with long-term treatment in children rather than adults.

Interference with clinical pathology tests
Methylphenidate may interfere with some tests for the measurement of alkaloids and amphetamine in urine.

Chemical dependency and abuse
Chronic abuse of methylphenidate can lead to marked tolerance and psychic dependence. Psychotic episodes may occur, particularly after parenteral use. Careful supervision is required during drug withdrawal as severe depression can be unmasked.

The intravenous injection of dissolved methylphenidate tablets containing the fillers talc and corn starch has resulted in pulmonary granuloma (2 patients), tricuspid valve granuloma (1 patient) and cutaneous reactions in 16 patients. The death of a drug abuser from pulmonary hypertension due to widespread obstruction of the pulmonary vascular bed by talc granulomas has also been described. Talc retinopathy has recently been described in some 17 drug addicts who had injected methylphenidate solution prepared from methylphenidate tablets.[11] Similarly, injection of tablet-derived material into or adjacent to the brachial artery may cause severe ischaemic lesions in the hand, including gangrene and severe intractable ischaemic neuritis.[12]

High risk groups

Neonates
There are no indications for the use of methylphenidate in neonates.

Methylphenidate

Breast milk. The safe use of methylphenidate during lactation has not been established.

Children
Methylphenidate is not recommended for children under 6 years of age as safety and efficacy in this age group have not been established. Three children have been reported to have developed gross behavioural changes with hallucinations following treatment with methylphenidate. In two, the reactions occurred after short-term administration of modest doses and in the third, an adolescent, an excessive amount of medication was taken after long-term drug use.

Pregnant women
The safe use of methylphenidate in pregnant women has not been established.

The elderly
As with other sympathomimetic agents, methylphenidate should be administered with special care in the elderly because of the risk of the precipitation of arrhythmias.

Drug interactions

Potentially hazardous drug interactions
The elimination of phenytoin is slowed by methylphenidate due to inhibition of p-hydroxylation. A similar mechanism underlies the slowed elimination of ethyl biscoumacetate and phenylbutazone caused by methylphenidate.

Methylphenidate should be used with great caution in patients treated with MAO inhibitors, because of the risks of hypertensive reactions.

Other significant interactions
Pressor agents. Methylphenidate should be used with caution in patients taking other pressor agents.

Coumarin anticoagulants. Methylphenidate may increase anticoagulant action by slowing the rate of p-hydroxylation of ethyl biscoumacetate.

Tricyclic antidepressants. Methylphenidate increases serum concentrations of imipramine and desipramine because of its inhibition of aromatic hydroxylation and demethylation. This interaction is well documented and may result in increased antidepressant action. There are several reports of hypertensive episodes occurring in adults after taking methylphenidate together with tricyclic antidepressants. The combination is best avoided.

Other drugs. Methylphenidate is a moderately potent general (type 1) inhibitor of hepatic microsomal drug metabolism, although aromatic hydroxylation appears to be more sensitive to inhibition than other pathways. Clinically significant interactions have been recorded with phenytoin, imipramine, chlorpromazine, ethyl biscoumacetate, thiopentone and phenylbutazone.

Phenytoin plasma concentrations increase after the administration of methylphenidate due to inhibition of the p-hydroxylation of phenytoin to p-hydroxy-phenylhydantoin, and the dosage of phenytoin should be adjusted by frequent plasma concentration monitoring.

Potentially useful interactions
Although methylphenidate and imipramine interact as indicated above, the combination is most useful in the management of narcolepsy where only small doses of tricyclic antidepressants are needed.

Major outcome trials

Attention deficit disorder

1. McBride M C 1988 An individual double-blind crossover trial for assessing methylphenidate response in children with attention deficit disorder. Journal of Pediatrics 113 (1 pt 1): 137–145

To obtain more objective data on response to therapy and to overcome parents', teachers', psychologists' and physicians' concerns about potential overuse, I instituted individual double-blind crossover trials of methylphenidate for children with attention deficit disorder (ADD). Each child is given 0.3 $mg.kg^{-1}$ dose twice daily for 2 weeks and placebo for 2 weeks in random order and in double-blind fashion. Parents and teachers record observations of behaviour and academic performance. Analysis of 70 trials and follow-up clinical data demonstrated that (1) 51 children showed improvement in one of the 2-week periods and that period corresponded with methylphenidate therapy in 48 (69%); (2) 6 of the 22 who did not respond to methylphenidate experienced worsening of function while taking the drug; (3) history and physical findings were not helpful in predicting methylphenidate response; (4) there were no serious side effects during the trial; and (5) all but three of the responders took methylphenidate for at least 1 year with sustained improvement in behavioural function, academic function, or both. Individual double-blind crossover trials can be used in an office setting to identify objectively which children with ADD respond to treatment with methylphenidate. Because the trial demonstrates to parents, teachers, psychologists, and physicians that methylphenidate is or is not beneficial to a particular child, this clinical tool is associated with a high level of confidence that the drug is being appropriately prescribed.

2. Tannock R, Schachar R J, Carr R P, Logan G D 1989 Dose–response effects of methylphenidate on academic performance and overt behaviour in hyperactive children. Pediatrics 84 (4): 648–657

In this study, the effects of 0.3 $mg.kg^{-1}$ and 1.0 $mg.kg^{-1}$ of methylphenidate on the overt behaviour and academic functioning of 12 children with an established diagnosis of attention deficit disorder with hyperactivity were evaluated. A double-blind, placebo-control, within-subject (crossover) design was used, in which each child was tested four times in each drug condition. Drug conditions were alternated on a bi-daily basis and each child received two different drug conditions each day. The academic tasks were designed for evaluation of the relationship between task complexity and dose. Whereas overt behaviour improved with increasing dose, academic functioning was improved with methylphenidate at both doses.

3. Wender P H, Reimherr F W, Wood D, Ward M 1985 A controlled study of methylphenidate in the treatment of attention deficit disorder, residual type, in adults. American Journal of Psychiatry 142: 547–552

4. Sebrechts M M, Shaywitz S E, Shaywitz B A, Jatlow P, Anderson G M, Cohen D J 1986 Components of attention, methylphenidate dosage, and blood levels in children with attention deficit disorder. Paediatrics 77: 222–228

Other trials

Attention deficit disorder

1. Kutcher S P 1986 Assessing and treating attention deficit disorder in adolescents. The clinical application of a single case-study research design. British Journal of Psychiatry 149: 710–715
2. Eichlseder W 1985 Ten years experience with 1000 hyperactive children in a private practice. Paediatrics 76: 176–184

Narcolepsy
There are no randomized controlled trials in this indication.

1. Yoss R E, Daly D D 1959 Treatment of narcolepsy with Ritalin. Neurology 9: 171–173
2. Akimoto H, Honda Y, Takahashi Y 1960 Pharmacotherapy in narcolepsy. Diseases of the Nervous System 21: 704–706
3. Guilleminault C, Carskadon M, Dement W C 1974 On the treatment of rapid eye movement narcolepsy. Archives of Neurology 30: 90–93
4. Honda Y, Hishikawa Y, Takahashi Y 1979 Long-term treatment of narcolepsy with methylphenidate (Ritalin). Current Therapeutic Research 25: 288–298

General review articles

Taylor E A 1986 Childhood hyperactivity. British Journal of Psychiatry 149: 562–573
Varley C K 1985 A review of studies of drug treatment efficacy for attention deficit disorder with hyperactivity in adolescents. Psychopharmacology Bulletin 21: 216–221

M

References

1. Brown R T, Sexson S B 1989 Effects of methylphenidate on cardiovascular responses in attention deficit hyperactivity disordered adolescents. Journal of Adolescent Health Care 10 (3): 179–183
2. Safer S, Allen R, Barr E 1972 Depression of growth in hyperactive children on stimulant drugs. New England Journal of Medicine 287: 217–220
3. Lou H C, Henriksen L, Bruhn P, Borner H, Nielsen J B 1989 Striatal dysfunction in attention deficit and hyperkinetic disorder. Archives of Neurology 48: 48–52
4. Chan Y-P M, Swanson J M, Soldin S S, Thiessen J J, Macleod S M, Logan W 1983 Methylphenidate hydrochloride given with or before breakfast. II. Effects on plasma concentration of methylphenidate and ritalinic acid. Paediatrics 72: 56–59
5. Swanson J M, Sandman C A, Deutsch C, Baren M 1983 Methylphenidate hydrochloride given with or before breakfast: 1. Behavioural, cognitive, and electrophysiologic effects. Paediatrics 72: 49–55
6. Gualtieri C T, Hicks R E, Kennerly P, Shroeder S R, Breese G R 1984 Clinical correlates of methylphenidate blood levels. Therapeutic Drug Monitoring 6: 379–392
7. Prinzmetal M, Bloomberg W 1935 The use of benzedrine for the treatment of narcolepsy. Journal of the American Medical Association 105: 2051–2054
8. Daly D D, Yoss R E 1956 Treatment of narcolepsy with methylphenidate. Proceedings of the staff meeting of the Mayo Clinic 31: 620
9. Honda Y, Hishikawa Y, Takahashi Y 1979 Long-term treatment of narcolepsy with methylphenidate (Ritalin). Current Therapeutic Research 25: 288–298
10. Liberman J A, Kane J M, Gadaleta D, Benner R, Lesser M S, Kinon B 1984 Methylphenidate challenge as a predictor of relapse in schizophrenia. American Journal of Psychiatry 145: 633–638
11. Tse D T, Ober R R 1980 Talc Retinopathy. American Journal of Ophthalmology 90: 624–640
12. Begg E J, McGrath M A, Wade D N 1980 Inadvertant intra-arterial injection — A problem of drug abuse. Medical Journal of Australia 2: 561–563

Methylprednisolone (sodium succinate)

Methylprednisolone (sodium succinate) is a soluble glucocorticoid suitable for oral, intravenous or intramuscular administration. It has been widely used in high dose 'pulse' therapy.

Chemistry

Methylprednisolone (Medrone, Depo-Medrone, Solu-Medrone, Solu-Medrol)

$C_{26}H_{33}NaO_8$

11β,17α-21-Trihydroxy-6α-methyl pregna-1,4-diene-3,20-dione-21-succinate sodium salt

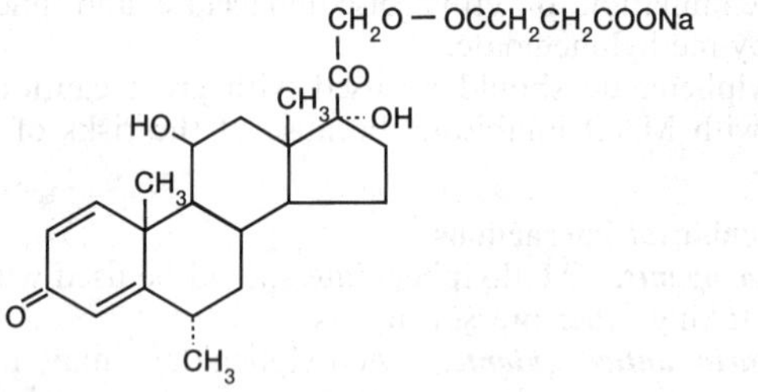

Molecular weight	496.5
pKa	
Solubility	
in alcohol	1 in 12
in water	1 in 1.5
Octanol/water partition coefficient	66

It is a white, or nearly white, odourless, hygroscopic amorphous solid. Chemically related compounds are methylprednisolone acetate, and methylprednisolone hemisuccinate. Methylprednisolone sodium succinate 53 mg is approximately equivalent to 40 mg of methylprednisolone. It is also available in combination with lignocaine.

Pharmacology

Methylprednisolone has 4 to 5 times the glucocorticoid activity per unit weight of cortisol. In common with other glucocorticoids, methylprednisolone binds to an intracytoplasmic receptor. This receptor is a 95kD protein, which is present in most cells of the body and which has been cloned.[1] The steroid-receptor complex is translocated to the nucleus where it binds to DNA and alters the transcription of the genes for a large number of proteins. The rate of synthesis of some proteins, such as lipomodulin, is increased while that of many others, such as collagen, is decreased. In consequence, glucocortocoids have very widespread actions which affect the function of many different cells and tissues and many of which are still not understood in detail.[2] Among the more important of these are:

i. Inhibition of phospholipase A2 by increased production of lipomodulin. This action reduces the supply of free arachidonic acid and thereby diminished the production of prostaglandins and leukotrienes.
ii. Reduction of production of soluble mediators such as IL-1.
iii. Membrane effects, e.g. reducing the likelihood that mast cells will degranulate.
iv. Complex effects on the lymphoid system. These include an acute reduction of circulating lymphocytes which is caused by sequestration rather than lysis. Prolonged administration decreases the mass of lymphoid tissue. The lymphocytopenia is

mainly due to decreased circulating numbers of T cells. At lower doses T-helper cells are reduced and at higher doses cytotoxic T-cell numbers also fall.

v. Inhibition of chemotactic responses in macrophages (but not in neutrophils).

vi. Reduction of synthesis of collagen and other structural proteins. This leads to thin skin, weak bones, myopathy etc.

vii. Endocrine effects. These include suppression of ACTH secretion with inhibition of endogenous cortisol production and, during prolonged administration, partial atrophy of the adrenal cortex. Glucose tolerance is reduced and blood sugar increases.

viii. Mineralocorticoid effects. Methylprednisolone has less than half the minealocorticoid effect of cortisol but in some species (e.g. rat) high doses cause fluid retention and hypertension although others species (e.g. dog and sheep) do not show this response.

The net effect of these diverse actions upon inflammatory and immune responses is not always easy to predict. For example, the glomerulonephritis caused by anti-GBM antibody in rabbits was little affected by methylprednisolone 2 $mg.kg^{-1}$ in 12 h. However, when sub-threshold doses of anti-GBM antibody were preceded by rabbit anti-sheep IgG, the nephritic response which occurred in control animals was almost completely inhibited by the same dose of the steroid.[3]

In mice the lung injury caused by butylated hydroxytoluene (BHT) was exacerbated by treatment with methylprednisolone 30 $mg.kg^{-1}$ twice daily.[4] However, rabbits were partially protected from the hypotension and they increased prostacyclin production (a marker of endothelial injury) caused by endotoxin when given methylprednisolone 40 $mg.kg^{-1}$ intravenously 10 min beforehand.[5]

Toxicology

No data specific to methylprednisolone is available.

Clinical pharmacology

Methylprednisolone is a moderately potent glucocorticoid which has only slight mineralocorticoid activity. When used in oral treatment with doses in the range 16–96 mg daily it has the expected anti-inflammatory and immunomodulatory effects, such as are seen with a somewhat lower dose of prednisolone. It has been shown to be effective in a wide range of conditions such as asthma, systemic lupus, rheumatoid arthritis, renal transplant rejection, as a component of cancer chemotherapy regimes and in certain skin (Stevens–Johnson syndrome) and eye inflammatory disorders. It has been shown to be ineffective and/or hazardous in septic shock, and adult respiratory distress syndrome. The main interest of the compound lies in its potential for use in very high parenteral doses. Very high dosage regimens have been tried in a variety of acute medical conditions in which morbidity/mortality is high and standard treatment relatively ineffective.

The systemic bioavailability of methylpredisolone is high following oral doses, so the main justification of high parenteral doses would be for patients who are unable to take the drug by mouth, or to achieve a more rapid onset of action. The onset of action of glucocorticoids takes hours rather than minutes because it depends upon alterations in the rate of protein synthesis. Therefore, the difference in onset between an oral and a parenteral dose is unlikely to be more than one and three-quarter hours (the time to peak plasma concentration after an oral dose) in several hours, unless very high 'pulse' doses recruit different pharmacological effects. It is not clear whether very high doses (e.g. 1–2 grams daily) are supramaximal in terms of receptor occupancy but it seems quite possible that they are.

Construction of dose–response curves to a glucocorticoid in man presents considerable difficulties and the data available are limited. In a small study, 18 renal transplant patients with acute rejection were randomized to receive either 250 mg or 1 g of methylprednisolone (MP) daily for 4 days. There was no significant difference in the response of the two groups in the early or one year responses.[5] A randomised controlled trial in 100 renal transpant patients compared a regimen of MP 160 mg daily intravenously for 3 days followed by oral 0.8 $mg.kg^{-1}$ daily which was tapered by 4 mg per week to a maintenance dose of 16 mg with a regimen involving half those doses. There was no significant difference between them.[6] A double-blind randomised controlled trial of MP in 333 patients with acute spinal cord injury compared 1,000 mg by bolus daily for 10 days with 100 mg by bolus daily for 10 days. There was no significant difference, and little evidence of response in either group.[7] A double-blind controlled trial in 29 patients with rheumatoid arthritis compared 1000 mg intravenously with 320 mg either intravenously or intramuscularly. Clinical benefit was noted in all groups but there was no significant difference between them.[8,9] A double-blind controlled trial in 21 patients with severe systemic lupus compared 100 mg with 1000 mg of MP daily for 3 days. There was no significant difference between the clinical states after the 2 doses.[10] None of these studies

Fig. 1 The metabolism of Methylprednisolone

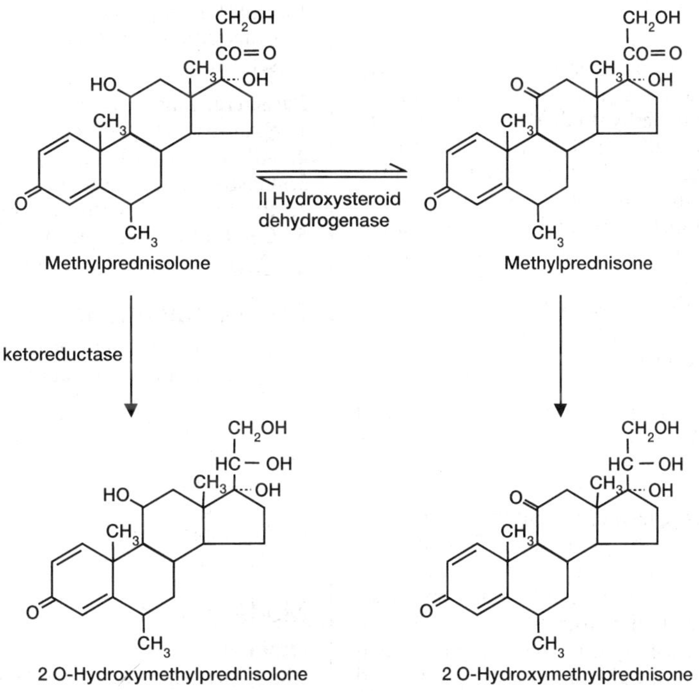

Methylprednisolone (sodium succinate)

provides clear evidence that very high doses convey any advantage compared with somewhat lower ones but most were not large enough to settle the issue.

Pharmacokinetics

Methylprednisolone plasma concentrations may be measured using thin layer chromatography, high pressure liquid chromatography (HPLC), or a radioimmune assay (RIA). The preferred method is HPLC[11] which has a sensitivity of 1 $\mu g.l^{-1}$. Methylprednisolone sodium succinate is a pro-drug which is rapidly hydrolysed in vivo to methylprednisolone with a half life of about 1.4 minutes. Studies with doses of about 1 $mg.kg^{-1}$ have shown elimination half lives of 1.1–3.1 h, although most estimates have been about 2.5 h, and a volume of distribution of 1.0–1.5 $l.kg^{-1}$. Higher doses of 10 $mg.kg^{-1}$ have been reported to show a longer elimination half life of 3.6 h, but the evidence of dose-dependent kinetics is not very convincing.[12] Following an intravenous dose the peak plasma concentration is seen immediately but after an intramuscular dose it is delayed for about 2 hours. The time-to-peak plasma concentration following an oral dose averaged 1–2 h in different studies. The systemic bioavailability of oral doses is high, with estimates ranging from 80% to 99%.[13,14] Plasma clearance averages 6.5 $ml.min^{-1}.kg^{-1}$ and is independent of dose over the range 10 to 3000 mg.[15–19].

Animal studies using radiolabelled drug showed that MP is widely distributed and enters nearly every organ in as little as 15 min after administration, although concentrations in the brain are lower than in other tissues such as liver and kidney.[16] Plasma protein binding is 77%, but little is bound to the corticosteroid-binding protein, transcortin.[17] Methylprednisolone is haemodialysable with an average dialysance of 18.4 ± 6.1 $ml.min^{-1}$. There is no accumulation with renal impairment. Kinetics are little changed by disease, apart from severe liver disease, and dosing requires no adjustment.[21,22]

Oral absorption	high
Presystemic metabolism	—
Plasma half life	
range	1.1-3.1 h
mean	2.5
Volume of distribution	1–1.5 $l.kg^{-1}$
Plasma protein binding	77%

Concentration–effect relationship

There is no data concerning any correlation between the plasma concentration of methylprednisolone and its immunomodulating effects.

Metabolism

Methylprednisolone sodium succinate is a pro-drug which is very slowly hydrolysed in vitro (>7days) but which is very rapidly hydrolysed in vivo (4.5 mins) to free methylprednisolone. When high intravenous doses are given, up to 10% of the unhydrolysed drug may be excreted in the urine.[19] When given by other routes, very little of the hemisuccinate appears in the urine but 2–5% of the dose appears in urine as unmetabolized methylprednisolone. When radiolabelled doses were given to cancer patients 20% of the label was excreted in the bile.[20] Methylprednisolone differs from prednisolone only in the presence of the 6-α methyl group on the A ring. Delta-1 saturation and the 6-α methyl group prevent hydroxylation at the 2 and 6 positions but otherwise the metabolic routes are similar to those of prednisolone.

The compound undergoes reduction of the C-20 keto function and oxidation of C-11. The 20-β-hydroxysteroid dehydrogenase enzyme is present in the liver and kidney[23] yielding 20α-hydroxy-6α-methylprednisolone which is subsequently conjugated. The action of the 11,β-hydroxy steroid dehydrogenase enzyme, present in liver, kidney, lung, muscle and placenta[24], yields methylprednisone. This action is reversible (Fig. 1) although the plasma concentrations of methylprednisone are only about one tenth that of the parent methyl prednisolone in man. The main plasma metabolites formed in man are 20β-hydroxy-6α-methylprednisone and 20β-hydroxy-6α-methylprednisolone, both of which are inactive. In urine glucuronides, sulphates and free compounds are present. 6,7 dehydro analogues of the 11-keto and 20-hydroxy metabolites have been detected. Both 20-α and 20-β isomers are formed during metabolism of MP.

Pharmaceutics

The tablet preparations of methylprednisolone (Medrone; Upjohn, UK) include oval double scored pink 2 mg tablets, and similar white 4 mg tablets. There are also oval double scored white 16 mg tablets marked 'Upjohn 73'. The intramuscular preparation (Depo-Medrone) contains methylprednisolone acetate in a white sterile aqueous suspension of 40 $mg.ml^{-1}$. Methylprednisolone sodium succinate (Solu-Medrone) is supplied in vials of 40 mg, 125 mg, 500 mg, 1 g and 2 g. After reconstitution with the diluent provided the volume for injection measures respectively 1 ml, 2 ml, 8 ml, 16 ml, and 30.6 ml. The pHs of the reconstituted solutions range from 7 to 8, and their tonicities from 0.40–0.50 osmolar. The introduction by Upjohn of a two-compartment vial Mix-o-Vial has simplified the mixing procedure. In the USA certain strengths of Solu-Medrol are supplied in vials, vials with diluent or in ACT-O-VIALs. The reconstituted methylprednisolone can be administered intravenously by first adding it to a small bag of 50 ml of dextrose 5% in water or normal saline. Mixtures in dextrose 5% in water, normal saline, dextrose 5% in 0.45% or 0.9% sodium chloride are stable for 48 h (L 1). Because of possible incompatibilities with other drugs it is recommended that concomitant administration through the same infusion system should be avoided. In particular precipitation is likely to occur if mixed with aminophylline, calcium gluconate, cephalothin, cytarabine, insulin, nafcillin, penicillin G and tetracycline.

Therapeutic use

Methyl predisolone has been used in a very wide range of clinical conditions as a glucorticoid, particularly as one whose formulation permits very high parenteral doses. As a result of clinical trials the approved indications are more restricted, although still very wide.

Indications

Oral route

1. Collagen diseases
2. Some allergic and autoimmune dieases
3. Certain dermatological diseases
4. Acute and chronic ocular inflammatory diseases
5. As a component of treatment regimens for some leukaemias and lymphomas
6. Ulcerative colitis and Crohn's disease
7. Nephrotic syndrome
8. Transplant rejection
9. Endocrine disorders requiring treatment with a glucorticoid
10. Other uses: glucorticoids have been used in a wide variety of other conditions such as traumatic injury to the CNS, multiple sclerosis etc.

Parenteral route

1. Skin disease e.g severe erythema multiforme
2. Allergy e.g. asthma, angioneurotic oedema, anaphylaxis
3. Gastrointestinal disease e.g. ulcerative colitis or Crohn's disease
4. Respiratory disease e.g. inhalation of gastric contents
5. Cerebral oedema secondary to cerebral tumour
6. Organ transplant rejection.

Contraindications

1. Tuberculosis, latent or active
2. Systemic fungus infections
3. Vaccinia and varicella
4. Herpes simplex keratitis
5. Cerebral oedema due to malaria
6. Peptic ulcer
7. Cushing's syndrome
8. Acute psychosis
9. Hypersensitivity to the drug.

Mode of use

Oral route

Methylprednisolone is available in 2, 4 and 16 mg tablets. The initial

Methylprednisolone (sodium succinate)

dose depends upon the severity of the condition and clinical judgement of the amount likely to be required to suppress inflammation. In adults the doses commonly used range from 16 to 96 mg daily. These should be taken in four divided doses with meals. As soon as a satisfactory response has been elicited the dose should be reduced. A reduction of 2 mg every 7 days is suggested by the manufacturers, with the maintenance dose (if needed) at the lowest possible level.

In children lower doses are recommended. In the adrenogenital syndrome 4–12 mg daily, in generalized infantile eczema 8–12 mg daily and in acute rheumatic fever 1.1 mg.kg^{-1} daily until the ESR is normal for a week.

Parenteral route

Methylprednisolone sodium succinate is usually employed parenterally to provide high dose glucocorticoid treatment for a relatively short time. As oral doses have almost complete systemic bioavailability the need for intravenous or intramuscular doses in many conditions has been questioned.

A daily dose of 0.5 to 2 g is commonly administered for three days. In life-threatening conditions, doses of 30 mg.kg^{-1} repeated every four to six hours for 48 h have been used. The reconstituted drug, if administered intravenously, should be given slowly over a period of 15–30 minutes, to minimize adverse circulatory effects (see below). Dosage may be reduced appropriately for infants and children. Concomitant administration of antacid therapy is advisable when treatment is likely to be prolonged.

Indications

1. Collagen diseases

Methylprednisolone is effective in acute exacerbations of systemic lupus erythematosus, systemic dermatomyocytis (polymyositis) and acute rheumatic carditis. Intravenous methylprednisolone has been used in systemic lupus erythematosus when there is thrombocytopenia, haemolytic anaemia, nephritis or CNS disturbances[25] but lupus patients are particularly susceptible to the complications of steroid treatment, and high dose methylprednisolone should be used with great caution.[26,27] Methylprednisolone has also been used successfully in rheumatoid arthritis but use of steroids in this condition is now very restricted[28]

2. Allergic disease

Methylprednisolone is effective in the treatment of asthma if systemic treatment is required. Intravenous high dose therapy has been used in the initial treatment of severe asthma in the emergency room but the added benefits are small and probably do not justify the risks.[29–32] Other allergic states including contact dermatitis, atopic dermatitis, serum sickness, drug hypersensitivity reactions, urticarial transfusion reactions and autoimmune haemolytic anaemia are among those which may respond to the drug.

3. Dermatological diseases

Methylprednisolone is useful in dermatological diseases with severe systemic features. These include pemphigus, severe erythema multiforme (Stevens–Johnson syndrome), exfoliative dermatitis and bullous dermatitis herpetiformis.

4. Ophthalmic disease

Methylprednisolone has been used in a variety of severe, acute and chronic allergic and inflammatory processes that involve the eye. These include iritis, irido-cyclitis, posterior uveitis, and allergic conjunctivitis. Great care is needed to exclude an infective cause before using the drug.

5. Leukaemia and lymphoma

In chronic lymphocytic leukaemia, steroid therapy, usually in conjunction with an alkalating agent, will produce a rapid reduction in the size of the liver, spleen and lymph nodes. High doses are required in patients where chronic lymphatic leukaemia is associated with auto-immune features such as haemolytic anaemia and thrombocytopenia.[33] Steroids are also employed in the treatment of other lymphoid malignancies such as acute lymphoblastic leukaemia, multiple myeloma, Hodgkin's disease, and non-Hodgkin's lymphoma. Methylprednisolone is a component of some of the standard chemotherapy regimes such as MOCCA (vincristine, methylprednisolone and three alkylating agents) and MOPP.

6. Gastrointestinal disease

A short course of steroids will often control an acute exacerbation of ulcerative colitis, regional ileitis or Crohn's disease. For severe attacks, when treatment cannot be taken by mouth, intravenous methylprednisolone may be indicated. Conditions associated with Crohn's disease can also improve with such treatment. These include sacro-ileitis, iritis, hepatitis and skin rashes.

7. Renal disease

Steroids have been used for many years to treat nephrotic syndrome. Methylprednisolone has been found to be effective when given in high doses to patients with minimal change disease. Its place in the management of other glomerulopathies is less certain.[34]

8. Transplant rejection

It has been known since the 1960s that high doses of steroids will frequently reverse rejection in an organ transplant. High doses of oral prednisone were used initially but were replaced by intravenous methylprednisolone following reports of success with its use.[35] A controlled clinical trial, however, has not shown methylprednisolone to have clear advantages over the former treatment.[36–37] In bone marrow transplantation the host response is manifested as graft versus host disease. This acute illness usually responds rapidly to high dose infusions of methylprednisolone.[38,39]

9. Endocrine disorders

Methylprednisolone may be used in acute cases of adrenocortical insufficiency, although mineralocorticoid supplementation may be necessary and hydrocortisone or cortisone is preferable for long term maintenance. High dose methylprednisolone was once used in septic shock, on the hypothesis that relative adrenal insufficiency played a part in the pathogenesis, but two large randomised controlled trials showed no benefit and an increased risk of secondary infection. The drug should not be used in septic shock unless there is independent evidence of adrenal insufficiency (see clinical trials).

10. Other uses

Methylprednisolone has been tried in traumatic injury of the spinal cord but the benefits are uncertain. Multiple sclerosis is a disease that is known to show some response to steroids.[40] In a controlled clinical trial five daily treatments of 0.5 g methylprednisolone improved symptoms in 77% of patients (controls 25%).[41] While relapses of the disease may show a short-term response, methylprednisolone is not indicated in the long term management of multiple sclerosis.

Like dexamethazone, methylprednisolone will reduce, acutely, the intracerebral pressure in patients with cerebral tumours.

Parenteral route

The main indication for use of the parenteral route is in a patient who cannot take oral medication or where initiation of treatment is extremely urgent. In the latter case only the first dose need be given parenterally. The indications are the same as those for the oral route. While there is good evidence of efficacy for high dose parenteral therapy there is relatively little to show that it conveys any advantage over oral therapy when that route is available.

Adverse reactions

Potentially life-threatening effects

Anaphylactic reactions, which may be life-threatening occur, rarely, after intravenous adminitration. Cardiovascular collapse with hypotension, bronchospasm, cardiac arrest or cardiac arrhythmias have been reported.[42–43] Most cases have been described in patients with renal disease or following renal transplantation. Reactions often followed rapid infusion of methylprednisolone and hypotensive episodes have been observed under similar conditions in animals. For these reasons slow infusion of the drug is necessary and special care should be taken in any patient with a history of drug allergy.

Acute overdosage

There is no clinical syndrome of acute overdosage with methylprednisolone doses up to several g in 24 h, although rises in blood sugar and blood urea have been reported. Following chronic overdosage the possibility of adrenal suppression should be guarded against by gradual diminution of dose levels over a period of time.

Severe or irreversible adverse effects

As with other corticosteroids, methylprednisolone, particularly when given for a prolonged period in high doses, can induce a number of serious adverse events. Causation or exacerbation of peptic ulceration is a common complication. High doses increase the risk of haemorrhage or perforation of a peptic ulcer. The latter may pose diagnostic problems because of the anti-inflammatory action of the drug. Loss of mineral and matrix from bone may lead to vertebral compression fractures and other pathological fractures. Urinary calcium excretion is increased and nitrogen balance is negative. Patients may develop aseptic necrosis of femoral or humeral heads. Other effects include suppression of growth in children.

Patients are at increased risk of bacterial, viral and fungal infections. Resistance to infection is decreased so that patients become vulnerable to opportunistic infections, latent infections (e.g. tuberculosis) may be activated and the clinical signs may be masked.

Sodium and fluid retention may provoke or exacerbate congestive heart failure or hypertension. Potassium loss may lead to a hypokalaemic alkalosis. Carbohydrate intolerance may develop and in diabetic patients there may be increased requirements for insulin or oral hypoglycaemic agents.

Insomnia, personality changes, mood swings and even acute psychosis may occur and special care is needed in patients with a history of major psychological illnesses. Increased intracranial pressure and pseudotumour cerebri are rare, but serious, complications. Epileptic attacks may be precipitated in susceptible individuals and great care is needed if high dose steroids are required in a patient with a history of seizures. Ocular changes from prolonged treatment include glaucoma and its complications, subcapsular cataracts and an increased risk of fungal or viral infections.

Intramuscular injections may cause subcutaneous or cutaneous atrophy and sterile abcesses.

All of these effects emphasise the importance of using the lowest effective dose for the shortest possible time and not using high-dose daily systemic corticosteroids when other forms of therapy are available. Restriction of sodium intake and administration of potassium supplements may be helpful, particularly in cardiac patients.

Symptomatic adverse effects

Patients on prolonged high doses develop a cushingoid appearance with round face, buffalo hump, thin wasted limbs etc. Skin changes include facial erythema, increased sweating, hypo- or hyperpigmentation, ecchymoses and thin fragile skin which is slow to heal. Large parenteral doses may provoke nausea and vomiting. Headaches, vertigo, weakness, proximal myopathy, wasting and menstrual abnormalities may occur.

Other effects

Prolonged suppression of the pituitary–adrenal axis may lead to secondary failure of adrenocortical response to accidental trauma or surgery. Increased doses of a rapidly acting steroid are often required to cover the period of acute trauma.

Interference with clinical pathology tests

ACTH secretion and endogenous cortisol production are suppressed by high doses.

Antigen skin test responses may be suppressed.

High risk groups

Neonates

The use of Solu-Medrol sterile powder is contraindicated in premature infants because the 40 mg, 125 mg and 1 g ACT-O-VIALs and the accompanying diluent for the 500 mg, 1 g and 2 g vials contain benzyl alcohol which has been reported to cause a fatal 'Gasping Syndrome'.

Breast milk. Methylprednisolone is excreted in the breast milk and mothers taking the drug should not breast feed.

Children

Because corticosteroids cause growth retardation in infancy and childhood, treatment should be limited to the minimum dosage for the shortest possible time. Alternate day dosing causes less suppression of the hypothalamo–pituitary–adrenal axis, and yet may confer adequate immunosuppression in some children with organ transplants.

Pregnant women

The drug crosses the placenta and and methylprednisolone has been detected in cord plasma of mothers give intravenous methylprednisolone hemisuccinate during labour.[46] It should be used in early pregnancy only if there is an overriding clinical need. There may be a very small risk of cleft palate and intra-uterine growth retardation in the fetus. Neonates of mothers who receive therapy during pregnancy should be observed for signs of hypoadrenalism.

The elderly

Methylprednisolone can be used in elderly patients but the reduced rate of tissue repair enjoins special care over the use of high doses or prolonged therapy because of the increased risks of peptic ulcer, vertebral collapse, skin ulceration etc.

Concurrent disease

Patients harbouring latent infections may experience a recrudescence of the infections. Slowing of wound healing puts patients with recent intestinal anastomoses at particular risk. Perforation may also occur in severe ulcerative colitis or diverticulitis. Patients with ocular herpes simplex infection may proceed to corneal perforation. Patients with existing emotional instability or psychotic tendencies may be aggravated by corticosteroids.

The effect of methyprenisolone may be enhanced in patients with hypothyroidism or severe liver disease because its metabolism is retarded.

Drug interactions

Potentially hazardous interactions

Aspirin and NSAIDs. The ulcerogenic effects of non-steroidal anti-inflammatory drugs and aspirin may be potentiated.

Patients should not be vaccinated against smallpox while on steroids.

Immunization. Immunization procedures should not be undertaken because the response may be inhibited and the risk of neurological complications increased.

Rifampicin, carbamazepine, phenytoin and barbiturates. These drugs (and other enzyme inducers) may diminish the corticosteroid effect by as much as 50% by increasing its rate of metabolism.

Cyclosporin. Convulsions have been reported in patients treated with methylprednisolone and cyclopsorin, probably due to mutual inhibition of metabolism.

Amphotericin and thiazide diuretics. These drugs (and frusemide and other potassium–depleting diuretics) may further increase potassium loss in the urine.

Hypoglycaemic drugs. Steroid hyperglycaemia may partially antagonize the effect of hypoglycaemic drugs.

Cyclophosphamide. The efficacy of cyclophosphamide may be reduced because its metabolic activation is decreased.

Oestrogens. Oestrogens may enhance the effect by slowing metabolism of methylprednisolone.

Potentially useful interactions

Glucorticoids and β-receptor agonists may have a synergistic effect in asthma.

Methylprednisolone reduces cisplatin-induced vomiting.

Troleandomycin,a macrolide antibiotic, inhibits steroid metabolism and thereby enhances the effect of methylprednisolone. This combination has been used clinically in the treatment of asthma and hypereosinophilic syndrome and a synergistic effect has been claimed[47–48] Erythromycin appears to have a similar but smaller effect.

Major outcome trials

The efficacy of methylprednisolone as a glucorticoid is not in doubt. Major outcome trials have mainly addressed the effectiveness of high 'pulse' doses in septic shock, adult respiratory distress syndrome, transplant rejection etc.

1. The Veterans Administration Systemic Sepsis Cooperative Study Group 1987 Effect of high-dose glucocorticoid therapy on mortality in patients with clinical signs of systemic sepsis. New England Journal of Medicine 317: 659–665

This was a multicentre, randomized, double-blind, placebo-controlled trial of high-dose methylprednisolone sodium succinate in 223 patients with clinical signs of systemic sepsis. Patients received antibiotics and intravenous fluids and, in addition, 112 received methylprednisolone (30 $mg.kg^{-1}$ intravenously over 15 min) and 111 received placebo.

Methylprednisolone (sodium succinate)

The main end point was mortality at 14 days, which was almost identical in the placebo (22%) and glucocorticoid (21%) groups. Resolution of secondary infection within 14 days was significantly higher in patients receiving placebo (12 of 23) than in those receiving glucocorticoid (3 of 16) ($P=0.03$).

2. Bone R C, Fisher C J Jr, Clemmer T P, Slotman G J, Metz C A, Balk R A A 1987 Controlled clinical trial of high-dose methylprednisolone in the treatment of severe sepsis and septic shock. New England Journal of Medicine 317: 653–658

This was a randomized, double-blind, placebo-controlled trial of high-dose methylprednisolone sodium succinate in 383 patients with septic shock given either methylprednisolone sodium succinate (30 mg.kg^{-1}) or placebo. No significant differences were found in the prevention or reversal of shock, or overall mortality. Among actively treated patients, significantly more deaths were related to secondary infection.

3. Bernard G R, Luce J M, Sprung C L et al 1985 High-dose corticosteroids in patients with the adult respiratory distress syndrome. New England Journal of Medicine 317: 1565–1570

This was a randomized, double-blind, placebo-controlled trial of methylprednisolone therapy in 99 patients with ARDS defined as refractory hypoxemia, diffuse bilateral infiltrates on chest radiography and absence of congestive heart failure documented by pulmonary artery catheterization. Fifty patients received methylprednisolone (30 mg.kg^{-1} every six hours for 24 hours), and 49 received placebo at the same times.

There was no significant differences between groups at entry, five days and forty-five days after entry. There were no difference in mortality which was 60% and 63% respectively.

4. De Vecchi A, Rivolta E, Tarantino A et al 1985 Controlled trial of two different methylprednisolone doses in cadaveric renal transplantation. Nephron. 41: 262–266

This was a controlled trial the effects of two different methylprednisolone dosage schedules in 100 adult cadaver kidney recipients. Half were given 160 mg daily intravenously for 3 days, then oral methylprednisolone (0.8 mg.kg^{-1} daily), which was tapered by 4 mg each week to a maintenance dose of 16 mg daily up to the 6th month. The other half were given 80 mg daily intravenously for 3 days followed by 0.4 mg.kg^{-1} daily; the dose was reduced by 2 mg each week to 16 mg daily. In both groups, the dose was further reduced bimonthly to a final dose of 8 mg daily. There were no significant differences between the two groups in patients and kidney survival or in the incidence of complications. The number of patients with at least one rejection episode was significantly higher in the lower dose group.

5. Ponticelli C, Zucchelli P, Imbasciati E et al 1984 Controlled trial of methylprednisolone and chlorambucil in idiopathic membranous nephropathy. New England Journal of Medicine 310: 946–950

67 adults with idiopathic membranous nephropathy and the nephrotic syndrome were randomly allocated to symptomatic treatment or methylprednisolone alternating with cholambucil, every other month. After a mean of 31 to 37 months follow-up, 12 of the treated and 2 of the control patients were in complete remission. In the treated group there no change in serum creatinine but there was a significant deterioration in the control group.

General review articles

Kirby B 1989 A review of the rational use of corticosteroids. Journal of International Medical Research 17: 493–505

Rebuck A S 1986 Asthma: non-responsiveness to conventional therapy. European Journal of Respiratory Diseases 69 (suppl 147) 105–109

Hughes R A C, 1986 Immunological treatment of multiple sclerosis II Journal of Neurology 233: 566–68

Cameron J S 1989 Treatment of primary glomerulonephritis using immunosuppressive agents. American Journal of Nephrology 9 (suppl 1): 33–40

Davis G F 1986 Adverse effects of corticosteroids: II systemic. Clinics in Dermatology 4: 161–169

References

1. Disterhorst C W 1989 Recent insight into the structure and function of the glucocorticoid receptor. Journal of Laboratory Clinical Medicine 113: 404–412
2. Rugstad H E 1988 Antiinflammatory and immunoregulatory effects of glucocorticoids: mode of action. Scandinavian Journal of Rheumatology (suppl) 76: 257–264
3. Bult H, Herman A G, Rampart M 1985 Modification of endotoxin-induced haemodynamic and haematological changes in the rabbit by methylprednisolone, F(ab')2 fragments and rosmarinic acid. British Journal of Pharmacology 84: 317–327
4. Kehrer J P, Klein-Szanto A J, Sorensen E M, Pearlman R, Rosner M H 1984 Enhanced lung damage following corticosteroid treatment. American Review of Respiratory Diseases 130: 256–261
5. Park G D, Bartucci M, Smith M C 1984 High- versus low-dose methylprednisolone for acute rejection episodes in renal transplantation. Nephron 36: 80–83
6. De-Vecchi A, Rivolta E, Tarantino A et al 1985 Controlled trial of two different methylprednisolone doses in cadaveric renal transplantation. Nephron 41: 262–266
7. Bracken M B, Collins W F, Freeman D F et al 1984 Efficacy of methylprednisolone in acute spinal cord injury. Journal of the American Medical Association 251: 45–52
8. Vischer T L, Sinniger M, Ott H, Gerster J C 1986 A randomised, double-blind trial comparing a pulse of 1000 mg with 250 mg methylprednisolone in rheumatoid arthritis. Clinical Rheumatology 5: 325–326
9. Radia M, Furst D E 1988 Comparison of three pulse methylprednisolone regimens in the treatment of rheumatoid arthritis. Journal of Rheumatology 15: 242–246
10. Edwards J C, Snaith M L, Isenberg D A 1987 A double-blind controlled trial of methylprednisolone infusions in systemic lupus erythematosus using individualised outcome assessment. Annals of Rheumatic Diseases 46: 773–776
11. Ebling W F, Szefler S J, Jusko W J 1985 Methylprednisolone disposition in rabbits. Analysis, pro-drug conversion, reversible metabolism, and comaparison with man. Drug Metabolism and Disposition 13: 296–304
12. Szefler S J, Ebling W F, Georgitis J W et al 1986 Methylprednisolone versus prednisolone pharmacokinetics in relation to dose in adults. European Journal of Clinical Pharmacology 30: 323–329
13. Derendorf H, Mollman H, Rohdewald P 1987 Pharmacokinetics and pharmacodynamics of high dose glucocorticoid esters. Clinical Pharmacology and Therapeutics 41: 198
14. Derendorf H, Mollman H, Rohdewald P 1988 Pharmacokinetics and pharmacodynamics of methylprednisolone phosphate and hemisuccinate. Clinical Pharmacology and Therapeutics 43: 176
15. Weber D J, Vanderlugt J T, Olanoff L S, Shah J A 1988 Comparative pharmacokinetics of methylprednisolone (MP) and its prodrugs following intravenous doses of methylprednisolone sodium succinate (MPSS) and methylprednisolone suleptanate (MPSP) in humans. Clinical Pharmacology and Therapeutics 43: 189 (abstract)
16. Kitagawa H, Esumi Y, Ohtsuki T et al 1977 Metabolic fate of 6-alphamethylprednisolone sodium succinate: 1. Absorbtion, distribution and excretion in rats. Pharmacometrics 13: 235–247
17. Ebling W F, Milsap R L, Szefler S J et al 1986 6-alpha-methylprednisolone and 6-alpha-methylprednisone plasma protein binding in humans and rabbits. Journal of Pharmeutical Science 75: 76–763
18. Szefler S J, Rose J Q, Ellis E F, Spector S L, Green A W, Jusko W J 1980 The effect of troleandomycin on methylprednisolone elimination. Journal of Allergy and Clinical Immunology 66: 447–451
19. Al-Habet S M H, Rogers H J 1989 Methylprednisolone pharmacokinetics after intravenous and oral administration. British Journal Clinical Pharmacology 27: 285–290
20. Slaunwhite W R, Sandberg A A 1961 Disposition of radioactive 17-alpha-hydroxyprogesterone, 6-alpha-methyl-17-alpha-acetoxyprogesterone and 6-alpha-methylprednisolone in human subjects. Journal of Endocrinological Metabolism 21: 753–764
21. Tornatore K M, Morse G D, Jusko W J, Wawhe J J 1989 Methylprednisolone disposition in renal transplant recipients receiving triple-drug immunosuppression. Transplantation 48: 962–965
22. Kung A N, Jungbluth G L, Pasko M T, Beam T R, Jusko W J 1990 Pharmacokinetics of methylprednisolone sodium succinate and methylprednisolone in patients undergoing cardiopulmonary bypass. Pharmacotherapy 10: 29–34
23. Recknagel R O 1957 Adrenocortical steroid C-20 keto reductase. Journal of Biological Chemistry 227: 273–284
24. Bush I E, Hunter S A, Meigs R A 1968 Metabolism of 11-oxygenated steroids. Biochemical Journal 107: 239–258
25. Kimberley R P 1988 Systemic lupus erythematosus: Treatment. Corticoids and anti-inflammatory drugs. Rheumatic Disease Clinics of North America 14: 203–217
26. Wofsy D 1987 New approach to treating systemic lupus erythematosus. Western Journal of Medicine 147: 181–186
27. Mackworth Young C G, David J, Morgan S H, Hughes G R 1958 A double-blind, placebo controlled trial of intravenous methylprednisolone in systemic lupus erythematosus. Annals of the Rheumatic Diseases 47: 496–502
28. Smith M D, Ahern M J, Roberts Thomson P J 1988 Pulse steroid therapy in rheumatoid arthritis: can equivalent doses of oral prednisolone give similar clinical results to intravenous methylprednisolone? Annals of the Rheumatic Diseases 47: 28–33
29. Garrity E R, Gross N J 1987 Prompt management for status asthmaticus. Journal of Respiratory Diseases 8: 21–32
30. Haskell R J, Wong B M, Hansen J E 1983 A double-blind randomized clinical trial of methylprednisolone in status asthmaticus. Archives of Internal Medicine 143: 1324–1327
31. Littenberg B, Gluck E H 1986 A controlled trial of methylprednisolone in the emergency treatment of acute asthma. New England Journal of Medicine 314: 150–152

M

32. Younger R E, Gerber P S, Herrod H G, Cohen R M, Crawford L V 1987 Intravenous methylprednisolone efficacy in status asthmaticus of childhood. Pediatrics 80: 225–230
33. Shaw J, Bochner F, Brooks P M, Moulds R F W, Ravenscroft P J, Smith A J 1986 Corticosteroid drugs: their role in oncological practice. Medical Journal of Australia 144: 81–84
34. Ponticelli C, Fogazzi G B 1989 Methylprednisolone pulse therapy for primary glomerulonephritis. American Journal of Nephrology 9 (suppl 1): 41–46
35. Clarke A G, Salaman J R 1974 Methylprednisolone as the treatment of renal transplant rejection. Clinical Nephrology 2: 230–234
36. Gray D, Shepherd H, Daar A, Oliver D O, Morris P J 1978 Oral versus high-dose steroid treatment of renal allograft rejection. Lancet 1: 117–118
37. Kaufman H M, Sampson D, Fox P J, Stanicki B S 1977 High dose (bolus) intravenous methylprednisolone at the time of kidney transplantation. Annals of Surgery 186: 631–634
38. Kendra J, Barrett A J, Lucus C et al 1981 Response of graft versus host disease to high doses of methylprednisolone. Clinical Laboratory Haematology 3: 19–26
39. Kennedy M S, Deeg H J, Storb R et al 1985 Treatment of acute graft-versus-host disease after allogeneic marrow transplantation. Randomized study comparing corticosteroids and cyclosporine. American Journal of Medicine 78: 978–983
40. Compston D A S 1989 The management of multiple sclerosis. Quarterly Journal of Medicine. New Series 70: 93–101
41. Milligan N M, Newcombe R, Compston D A S 1987 A double-blind controlled trial of high doses methylprednisolone in patients with multiple sclerosis. 1. Clinical effects. Journal of Neurology, Neurosurgery and Psychiatry 50: 511–516
42. Erstad B L 1989 Severe cardiovascular adverse effects in association with acute, highdose corticosteroid administration. DICP, Annals of Pharmacotherapy 23: 1019–1023
43. Ditzian-Kadanoff R, Ellman M H 1987 How safe is it? High-dose intravenous methylprednisolone. Illinois Medical Journal 172: 432–434
44. Pryse-Phillips W E, Chandra R K, Rose B 1984 Anaphylactoid reaction to methylprednisolone pulsed therapy for multiple sclerosis. Neurology 34: 1119–1121
45. Ueda N, Yoshikawa T, Chihara M, Kawaguchi S, Niinomi Y, Yasaki T 1981 Atrial fibrillation following methyprednisolone pulse therapy. Pediatric Nephrology 2: 29–31
46. Anderson G G, Rothchell Y, Kaiser D G 1981 Placental transfer of methylprednisolone following maternal intravenous administration. American Journal of Obstetrics and Gynecology 140: 699–701
47. Jungnickel P W, Cave J A 1988 Troleandomycin–methylprednisolone therapy in asthma. Drug Intelligence Clin Pharm 22: 611–613
48. Edwards D A, Wald J A, Dobozin B S et al 1987 Troleandomycin and methylprednisolone in the treatment of the hypereosinophilic syndrome. New England Journal of Medicine 317: 573–574

Methyprylone

Methyprylone is a non-barbiturate sedative hypnotic agent used in the short-term treatment of insomnia.

Chemistry

Methyprylone (Methyprylon, Noludar)
$C_{10}H_{17}NO_2$
3,3-Diethyl-5-methylpiperidine-2,4-dione

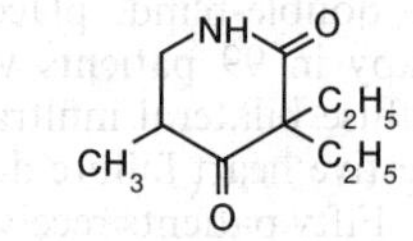

Molecular weight	183.2
pKa (>NH)	12.0
Solubility	
in alcohol	1 in 0.7
in water	1 in 14
Octanol/water partition coefficient	—

A white crystalline powder with a slight characteristic odour, a burning taste and bitter after-taste. It is prepared by chemical synthesis.[1]

Pharmacology

Methyprylone is a non-barbiturate hypnotic that produces sedation similar to that seen with barbiturates. The exact mechanism of action is unknown, though in animal studies methyprylone increases the threshold of arousal centres in the brain.

Toxicology

No information is available.

Clinical pharmacology

Methyprylone acts as both a sedative and as a hypnotic. In a dose of 200–400 mg it is a hypnotic. A 300 mg dose of methyprylone is very similar in hypnotic effects to 200 mg secobarbitone.[2] In hypnotic doses, methyprylone suppresses the REM stage of sleep in a similar way to barbiturates.[3] In spite of its short half life, methyprylone may produce a hangover effect next morning. Habituation, dependence and tolerance may occur, similar to that seen with barbiturates. Tolerance does develop to the suppression of REM sleep and the rebound sleeplessness when methyprylone is stopped may be due to REM rebound. Methyprylone is a potent inducer in animals of hepatic microsomal drug metabolizing enzymes as well as of δ-amino levulinic acid synthetase. However, the relevance of this to man is not clear. Methyprylone has no analgesic activity.

Pharmacokinetics

Research into the pharmacokinetics of methyprylone has been hampered until fairly recently by the lack of a specific assay for the parent drug in the presence of its metabolites.[4,5] Initially, the preferred analytical method was colorimetry.[6,7] This has been superseded by gas chromatography with flame ionization,[8,9] which has a limit of sensitivity of 1 mg.l^{-1}, and by a more recently developed high performance liquid chromatographical technique, which distinguishes between the drug and its known metabolites.[4,10]

Methyprylone is rapidly absorbed after oral administration and peak plasma levels are seen within 1–2 hours in fasting subjects.[6] The plasma half life has been reported to be 3–6 hours[11] although recent work suggests a range of 9–11 hours.[5,12] However, elimination may be concentration-dependent and the biological half life may approach 50 hours as was observed in a girl of 14 years admitted 24 hours after taking a large overdose.[13]

Methyprylone is highly lipid soluble with a volume of distribution[5] of 0.97 $l.kg^{-1}$. Though little other information is available, tissue distribution in four fatal cases was nearly uniform.[14] In plasma, approximately 60% is protein bound. It is not known whether methyprylone crosses the placenta or is excreted in milk.

Oral absorption	—
Presystemic metabolism	—
Plasma half life	
range	probably 9–11 h
Volume of distribution	0.97 $l.kg^{-1}$
Plasma protein binding	60%

Methyprylone is extensively biotransformed in the liver. Only 3% is excreted unchanged in the urine while another 3% is excreted as the active metabolite 5-methylpyrithyldione.[14] Approximately 60% of a dose of methyprylone is excreted in urine as other metabolites or their glucuronide conjugates.

Concentration–effect relationship

Therapeutic effects are produced by plasma concentrations of 10 $mg.l^{-1}$. Although toxic plasma concentrations have not been clearly defined, concentrations in excess of 30 $mg.l^{-1}$ are associated with stupor[7] or coma[12] and concentrations over 100 $mg.l^{-1}$ are potentially lethal.

Metabolism

Methyprylone is extensively metabolized in the liver and only 3% is excreted unchanged in urine.

There are two important metabolic pathways:[6,14] dehydrogenation to 5-methylpyrithyldione with subsequent oxidation to the alcohol and corresponding acid; and oxidation to 6-oxomethyprylone.

The metabolite 5-methylpyrithyldione is believed to be an active hypnotic and it is likely that 6-oxomethyprylone also exhibits hypnotic activity.

Fig. 1 Metabolism of methyprylone

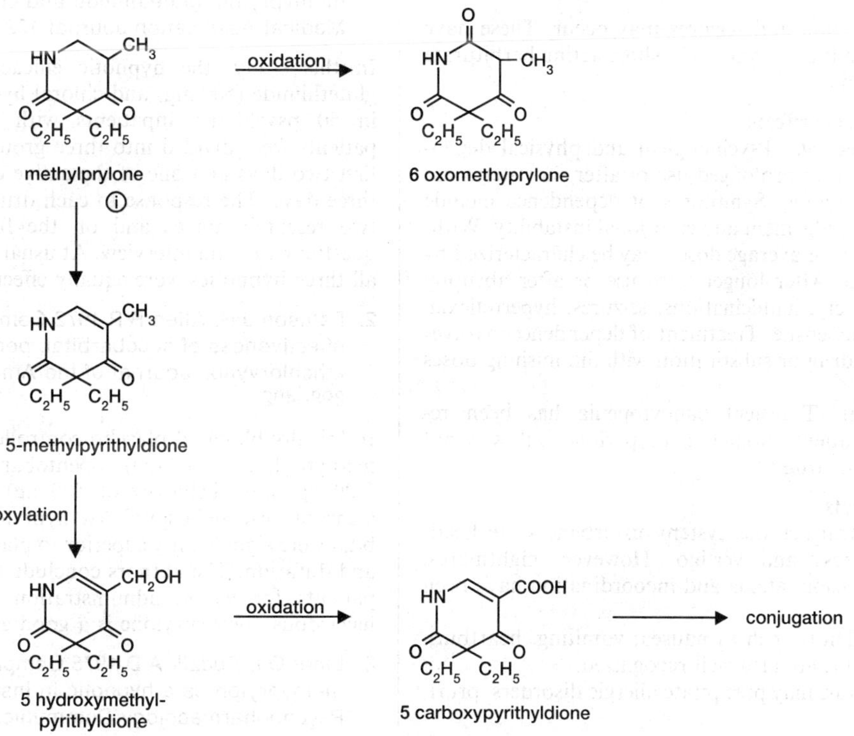

Methyprylone

Pharmaceutics

Methyprylone is administered orally.

Tablets contain 200 mg methyprylone (Noludar; Roche, UK/USA) in the form of white, round, flat discs with 'Noludar' imprinted across one face and two break bars across the other and coded '17'. In the USA, Noludar is also available as a 50 mg white, round, flat, scored tablet, marked 'ROCHE 16' on one side.

Capsules containing 300 mg methyprylone USP are available in a spheroid formation, the cap being amethyst pink and the base white. Each half is marked 'ROCHE'.

Methyprylone preparations should be protected from light except in the case of sugar-coated tablets.

Therapeutic use

Indications

1. Insomnia and sedation.

Contraindications

1. Depression
2. History of alcohol or drug abuse
3. Acute intermittent porphyria
4. Sleep apnoea.

Mode of use

The clinical uses depend upon the production of central nervous system depression. The precise mechanism of this is not known. Methyprylone may be the drug of choice in patients who do not respond to or are unable to tolerate other drugs, but otherwise offers no particular advantage over barbiturates or other hypnotic agents.

Indications

1. Insomnia and sedation

The usual dose for sedation in adults is 150–400 mg of methyprylone daily in three or four divided doses. Children have received 150–200 mg daily in divided doses.

The hypnotic dose in adults is 200–400 mg. Larger doses do not significantly increase the hypnotic effect. Children older than 12 years of age have been given 50 mg at bedtime though this may be increased to 200 mg if necessary. Sleep follows a hypnotic dose within 15–60 minutes and lasts for 5–8 hours.

Contraindications

1. Depression or suicidal tendencies
Although methyprylone is considered relatively safe, its use in suicidal attempts has been reported[7,15–17] and it has been implicated in at least one fatal poisoning.

2. History of alcohol or drug abuse
Methyprylone has high potential for addiction of the barbiturate–alcohol type. Either prolonged administration or short-term use of high doses may lead to tolerance and subsequently to physical and psychological dependence.

3. Acute intermittent porphyria
Patients with this condition should not be administered methyprylone.

4. Sleep apnoea
Methyprylone causes respiratory depression and should not be given to these patients.

Adverse reactions

Potentially life-threatening effects
Doses of more than 6 g methyprylone usually produce prolonged coma frequently accompanied by haemodynamic, respiratory and hepatic dysfunction. Although a similar dose has been fatal in one patient,[17] others have recovered after ingestion of up to 30 g.[7] Death may result from hypotension, respiratory depression or complications such as pulmonary oedema.

Acute overdosage
Deliberate overdosage with methyprylone has been reported[7,12,15] and in one patient has been fatal.[17] Clinical features include hypothermia or hyperpyrexia, hypotension, respiratory depression, nystagmus, pupillary abnormalities, dysarthria, drowsiness, confusion and coma. ST segment and T-wave changes on ECG have been ascribed to methyprylone overdose in a 45-year-old man, although it is noteworthy that he had also developed a tachycardia of 120 per minute.[15]

Treatment consists of gastric lavage and general supportive measures. In the presence of severe hypotension, noradrenaline and metaraminol have been administered to maintain blood pressure.[7,16] In severe acute poisoning, peritoneal dialysis may be useful[18] though haemodialysis probably effects an earlier response.[7,13] Charcoal haemoperfusion has also been employed with good results.[19]

During recovery, excitation and seizures may occur. These have been treated by cautious administration of a short-acting barbiturate such as thiopental sodium.

Severe or irreversible adverse effects
Dependence and withdrawal. Psychological and physical dependence occur, particularly after prolonged use or after short-term use of high doses of methyprylone. Symptoms of dependence include confusion, impairment of judgement and emotional instability. Withdrawal after short-term use of average doses may be characterized by nightmares and insomnia. After longer term use or after abruptly stopping high doses, anxiety, hallucinations, seizures, hyperreflexia, sweating and polyuria may ensue. Treatment of dependence involves gradual reduction of the drug or substitution with diminishing doses of a barbiturate.

Haematological effects. Transient pancytopenia has been reported in two related patients taking methyprylone but was not definitely attributed to the drug.[20]

Symptomatic adverse effects
Frequently reported central nervous system disturbances are headache, dizziness, drowsiness and vertigo. However, nightmares, anxiety, excitation, depression, ataxia and incoordination have been described.

Gastrointestinal complaints such as nausea, vomiting, heartburn and changes in bowel habit are also well recognized.

In addition, methyprylone may precipitate allergic disorders, pruritus and skin eruptions.

Interference with clinical pathology tests
Methyprylone may interfere with in vitro determination of 17-ketosteroids using the Holtorff–Koch modification of the Zimmerman reaction.[21]

High risk groups

Neonates
There is no information on the safety or efficacy of methyprylone in children under the age of 12 years.

Breast milk. It is not known whether methyprylone is excreted in breast milk, so it is best avoided during breast-feeding.

Children
Children older than 12 years have been given 50 mg of methyprylone at night as a hypnotic dose and 150–200 mg daily in divided doses for sedation.

Pregnant women
Methyprylone should not be used in this group. There is no evidence of safety in human pregnancy although a $3\frac{1}{2}$-month pregnant woman is reported to have taken an 800 mg overdose without ill effect.[15]

The elderly
Doses in elderly and debilitated patients should not exceed half those normally recommended.

Concurrent disease
Methyprylone should be used with caution in patients with renal or hepatic insufficiency.

Drug interactions

Potentially hazardous interactions
Barbiturates. Barbiturates and other central nervous system depressant drugs increase the sedative effect of methyprylone when administered together.

Alcohol. Concurrent use of alcohol with methyprylone may have an additive effect depending on individual susceptibility.

Other significant interactions
There is little information on concurrent use of methyprylone and oral contraceptives or anticoagulants but caution is advised.

Potentially useful interactions
No interactions of this type have been reported.

Clinical trials

1. Brown W T 1970 A comparative study of three hypnotics: methyprylon, glutethimide and chloral hydrate. Canadian Medical Association Journal 102: 510–511

In this study, the hypnotic efficacy of methyprylone (300 mg), glutethimide (500 mg) and chloral hydrate (1000 mg) was compared in 50 psychiatric inpatients with long-standing insomnia. The patients were divided into three groups and given a placebo on the first two days and one of the active drugs on each of the following three days. The response to each drug was assessed during sleep by two research nurses and on the following day by means of a questionnaire and interview. At usual levels of statistical significance, all three hypnotics were equally effective.

2. Pattison J H, Allen R P 1972 Comparison of the hypnotic effectiveness of secobarbital, pentobarbital, methyprylon and ethchlorvynol. Journal of the American Geriatrics Society 20: 398–402

In this double-blind placebo-controlled study, the hypnotic effect of methyprylone (300 mg), pentobarbital (100 mg), secobarbital (100 mg) and ethchlorvynol (500 mg) was compared in 50 patients in a chronic disease hospital. Methyprylone, pentobarbital and secobarbital were significantly superior to placebo with respect to sleep onset and duration. The authors conclude that in elderly or chronically ill patients for whom administration of barbiturates is considered hazardous, methyprylone is a good alternative hypnotic.

3. Linet O I, Rudzik A D 1975 Comparison of triazolam and methyprylon as a hypnotic in insomniacs. Psychopharmacology Communications 1: 473–480

In this more recent double-blind study, a preference technique was used to compare the efficacy of methyprylone with that of the benzodiazepine triazolam. One of these drugs was administered on the first night and the alternate medication was given on the following night. 28 insomniacs were involved on an outpatient basis. Of these 21 preferred triazolam, 5 preferred methyprylone and 2 had no preference (P = 0.001).

References

1. Rudy B C, Senkowski B Z 1973 Methyprylon. An analytical profile. In: Florey K (ed) Analytical profiles of drug substances. Academic Press, New York, vol 2, pp 363–382
2. Rickels K, Bass H 1963 A comparative controlled clinical trial of seven hypnotic agents in medical and psychiatric inpatients. American Journal of the Medical Sciences 245: 142–152
3. Kales A, Preston T A, Tjiauw-Ling T, Allen C 1970 Hypnotics and altered sleep dream patterns. I. All night EEG studies of glutethimide, methyprylon and pentobarbital. Archives of General Psychiatry 23: 211–218
4. Pankaskie M C 1983 Determination of methyprylon and its dehydro metabolite, 5 methylpyrithyldione, in plasma by high performance liquid chromatography. Journal of Chromatography 278: 458–463
5. Gwilt P R, Pankaskie M C, Thornburg J E, Zustiak R, Shoenthal D R 1985 Pharmacokinetics of methyprylon following a single oral dose. Journal of Pharmaceutical Sciences 74: 1001–1003
6. Randall L O, Iliev V, Brandman O 1956 Metabolism of methyprylon. Archives Internationales de Pharmacodynamie et de Therapie 56: 388–394
7. Xanthaky G, Freireich A W, Matusiak W, Lukash L 1966 Hemodialysis in methyprylon poisoning. Journal of the American Medical Association 198: 1212–1213
8. Dickson S J 1974 The determination of methyprylon and its metabolites in biological fluids by gas chromatography. Forensic Science 4: 177–182
9. Werner M, Mohrbacher R J, Riendeau C J 1979 Gas–liquid chromatography of underivatized drugs after chromatographic extraction from blood. Clinical Chemistry 12: 2020–2025
10. Van Veldhuizen J E, Hartmann A E 1981 Hypnotic–sedative screen by high performance liquid chromatography. Journal of Liquid Chromatography 4: 501–514
11. Hoffman-La Roche Inc. Personal communication
12. Bailey D N, Shaw R F 1983 Interpretation of blood glutethimide, meprobamate and methyprylon concentrations in non-fatal and fatal intoxications involving a single drug. Journal of Toxicology and Clinical Toxicology 20: 133–145
13. Pancorbo A S, Palagi P A, Piecoro J J, Wilson H D 1977 Hemodialysis in methyprylon overdose. Some pharmacokinetic considerations. Journal of the American Medical Association 237: 470–471
14. Baselt R C 1978 Disposition of toxic drugs and chemicals in man. Biomedical publications, Canton, Connecticut, pp 299–301
15. Pellegrino E D, Henderson R R 1957 Clinical toxicity of methyprylon (Noludar). Case report and review of twenty three cases. Journal of the Medical Society of New Jersey 54: 515–518
16. Burnstein N, Strauss H K 1965 Attempted suicide with methyprylon. Journal of the American Medical Association 194: 1139–1140
17. Reidt W U 1956 Fatal poisoning with methyprylon (Noludar), a nonbarbiturate sedative. New England Journal of Medicine 255: 231–232
18. Polin R A, Henry D, Pippinger C E 1977 Peritoneal dialysis for severe methyprylon intoxication. Journal of Pediatrics 90: 831–833
19. Koffler A, Bernstein M, La Sette A, Massry S G 1978 Fixed-bed charcoal hemoperfusion. Treatment of drug overdose. Archives of Internal Medicine 138: 1691–1694
20. McLaren G D, Doukas M A, Muir A 1978 Methyprylon-induced bone marrow suppression in siblings. An inherited defect? Journal of the American Medical Association 240: 1744–1745
21. Borushek S, Gold J J 1964 Commonly used medications that interfere with routine endocrine laboratory procedures. Clinical Chemistry 10: 41–52

Methysergide (hydrogen maleate)

Methysergide is a potent and specific serotonin antagonist, which must be used with care.

Chemistry

Methysergide hydrogen maleate (Deseril, Desernil, Deserril, Sansert)
$C_{21}H_{27}N_3O_2, C_4H_4O_4$
(+)-9,10-Didehydro-N-(1-hydroxy-2-butyl)-1,6- dimethylergoline-8 β-carboxamide hydrogen maleate

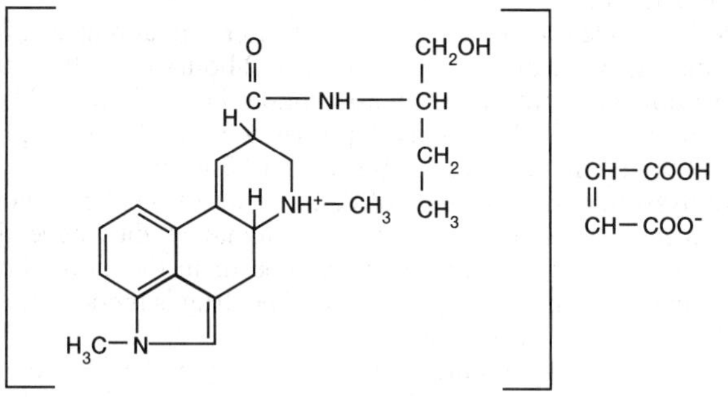

Molecular weight (free compound)	469.5 (353.45)
pKa	—
Solubility	
in alcohol	1 in 165
in water	—
Octanol/water partition coefficient	—

Methysergide, a white or off-white crystalline powder, odourless or with only a slight odour. It is a semisynthetic ergot alkaloid formed by the methylation of the indole nitrogen of lysergic acid hydroxybutylamide (methylergonovine). Methysergide hydrogen maleate is not available in combination with other drugs.

Pharmacology

Methysergide is one of the most potent and specific serotonin antagonists available, acting as a reversible competitive antagonist and, at low doses, as a partial agonist. It has only slight oxytocic and direct vasoconstrictor effects. Bradley and others (1986)[1] have proposed a classification for the nomenclature of functional receptors for 5-hydroxytryptamine. They classify them into three groups: $5HT_1$, $5HT_2$, and $5HT_3$. Methysergide has its main action on the $5HT_2$ receptors but is also a partial agonist at $5HT_1$.

Toxicology

Methysergide does not have mutagenic potential and toxicological testing in animals of 3 to 156 weeks in six species (rat, guinea pig, dog, minipig, rhesus monkey, rabbit) does not show any organ-specific damage. Teratogenicity tests in the rat and rabbit show no adverse effects on organogenesis. Carcinogenicity tests have not been done.

Clinical pharmacology

No published studies have been specifically designed to evaluate human tolerance. Efficacy and dose ranging in the prophylaxis of migraine and related headaches[2] and the symptomatic treatment for carcinoid syndrome[3,4] have been well established since 1959–1961.

For the prophylactic treatment of headaches, doses of 2–6 mg daily have been recommended and for the treatment of carcinoid syndrome 12–20 mg daily have been successfully tolerated.

The major pharmacological actions of methysergide in man are outlined below.

5-HT antagonism is demonstrated in various experimental models including: inhibition of 5-HT induced constriction of isolated human temporal[5] and intracranial arteries;[6] saphenous vein; [7] hand veins in situ[8]; umbilical vessels;[9] jejunum;[10] ileum;[7,11] inhibition of 5-HT-induced blood platelet aggregation.[12,13]

Methysergide acts as agonist at low doses (while antagonism occurs at higher doses) as observed in the potentiation of the constrictor effect of 5-HT on hand veins[14] and on isolated extra- and intracranial arteries.[15]

Methysergide potentiates the constrictor effect of noradrenaline on extracranial vessels[5,16] and acts as a weak vasoconstrictor on isolated human temporal and intracranial arteries and on hand veins.[17]

Pharmacokinetics

There is no specific analytical method for the measurement of methysergide; analysis has been done using ^{14}C labelled drug[18] in which total radioactivity is measured (i.e. unchanged drug together with metabolites).

Methysergide is completely absorbed after oral administration and peak plasma levels are expected within 1–2 hours in healthy subjects. Absorption is rapid with an absorption half life of 0.38 hours. Elimination takes place in two phases with a shorter α-phase of 1.0–1.7 hours and a longer β- phase of 10.0 hours.

Methysergide has a volume of distribution of 50 $l.kg^{-1}$ indicating drug accumulation in some tissues. Animal studies have demonstrated that the highest concentrations occur in the kidneys and the lowest in the brain and adipose tissue. The drug is moderately bound (66%) to proteins in plasma.

Animal studies show concentrations of drug in the CSF to be seven times less than in plasma with a CSF/plasma ratio of 0.14. Information concerning excretion in human breast milk is not available but studies in lactating rats have shown that concentrations in the milk are twice as high as plasma concentrations. As the drug is lipid soluble, placental transfer is expected and has been demonstrated in animals but not in man.

Information on presystemic metabolism is not available. It has been found that the greater part of the dose is excreted via the kidneys in the urine. Thus, after a 2 mg oral dose the total radio-activity excreted was found to be 56.4%.

When migraine patients who had developed retroperitoneal fibrosis as a result of chronic treatment with methysergide and normal volunteers were given radioactively labelled methysergide, they showed no difference in the amount of radioactivity excreted in the urine nor in the quantity of $^{14}CO_2$ in expired air. Also the time course of the elimination of radioactivity in urine and expired air were no different. Thus, there was no alteration in the kinetics due to disease.[19]

Oral absorption	100%
Presystemic metabolism	—
Plasma half life	
range	1–2.7 h
mean	1.85
Volume of distribution	50 $l.kg^{-1}$
Plasma protein binding	66%

Concentration–effect relationship

Daily oral medication with a therapeutic dose of 2 mg three times daily produces from the second day on, blood levels fluctuating between 17 and 60 $\mu g.l^{-1}$ with ^{14}C-methysergide.[18]

Metabolism

Much work still needs to be done on the metabolism of methysergide and other ergot alkaloids in many respects; including the elucidation of structure of respective metabolites in body tissues and the relationship between structure and metabolic degradation.

The main route of elimination of the drug is via the kidneys in the urine — 56.4% (unchanged drug and metabolite) of a 2 mg oral dose of methysergide is excreted in the urine.[18]

Information concerning entero-hepatic circulation is not available. The main metabolic reaction in man is N-demethylation; the main metabolite being methylergonovine which has uterotonic properties.

Pharmaceutics

Methysergide is available in oral dosage forms only (parenteral dosage forms in ampoules are no longer available).

Tablets contain 1 mg methysergide maleate. The tablets are either whitish or yellow (depending on the country), sugar coated, circular biconvex. The Deseril (Sandoz, UK) white tablets are coded 'DSL'on one side. Deseril is white in the UK but similary coded. The Sansert (Sandoz USA) tablets are yellow and bear the code number '78-58'. They contain tartrazine which is potentially allergenic. The tablets have good stability with a maximum shelf-life of 5 years in both temperate and hot climates.

Therapeutic use

Indications

1. Prophylactic treatment of migraine, in patients who, despite other attempts at control, experience attacks of such severity or regularity that their social or economic life is seriously disrupted
2. Cluster headache (Horton's syndrome)
3. To control profuse diarrhoea associated with carcinoid disease.

Contraindications

1. Pregnancy
2. Breast-feeding
3. Cardiac and peripheral vascular diseases —
   Phlebitis or cellulitis of lower limbs
   Clinical arteriosclerosis
   Coronary artery disease
   Valvular heart disease
   Severe hypertension
4. Collagen diseases
5. Impaired kidney or liver function
6. States of cachexia or sepsis.

Mode of use

In the prophylaxis of migraine headaches 1 mg by mouth taken two or three times a day with meals is recommended. The initial 1 mg is preferably given at bedtime and dosage is increased gradually to effective levels over a period of approximately two weeks so that the minimal effective dose is employed which will prevent 75% of attacks (rather than increase the dose to a high level in an effort to prevent all headaches). It should be explained at the outset to patients that regular clinical supervision and periodic interruptions in treatment are imperative in order to recognise and minimize any side effects.

In the treatment of diarrhoea in carcinoid disease, high oral doses are usually necessary. Doses recorded range between 12 and 20 mg daily.

Methysergide should be withdrawn for 3–4 weeks at least after 6 months of treatment; the dose should be reduced gradually over 2–3 weeks in order to avoid rebound headache.

Indications

1, 2. Prophylaxis of migraine attacks

Methysergide is one of the most effective drugs in the prophylactic treatment of migraine but has many serious side effects. While not efficient in aborting acute attacks, it is of use in preventing cluster headache but is less effective in chronic cluster headaches.

In view of its side effects, methysergide is restricted to those patients who do not respond to any other form of treatment. In order to avoid fibrotic complications, withdrawal of the drug is recommended at the first signs of impaired peripheral circulation.

3. Carcinoid syndrome

In carcinoid syndrome, the risk of untoward side effects due to the higher dose of the drug must be weighed against the therapeutic benefit.

Contraindications

1. Pregnancy
Methysergide should not be given in pregnancy due to the uterotonic property of the main metabolite — methyergonovine.

2. Breast-feeding
Animal data indicates that the drug passes into breast nilk; therefore mothers should not breast-feed.

3. Cardiac and peripheral vascular disorders
In cases of cardiac and peripheral vascular diseases the drug is contraindicated due to the possibility of vasoconstrictor reactions.

4. Collagen diseases
The drug should not be administered to those suffering from collagen diseases as fibrotic reactions are a possibility.

5. Impaired kidney or liver functions
In patients suffering from kidney or liver impairments methysergide should not be given as there is the risk of accumulation due to reduced excretion.

6. States of cachexia or sepsis
Certain conditions may aggravate toxic effects of ergot drugs (such as methysergide); these include febrile states, hepatic and renal diseases, sepsis and malnutrition, the latter two commonly occurring in cachexia. The drug is therefore contraindicated in states of cachexia and sepsis.

Adverse reactions

Potentially life-threatening effects
The most serious potentially lethal toxic effect associated with long-term treatment with methysergide is the development of fibrotic disorders, mainly retroperitoneal fibrosis resembling the idiopathic form, producing a compression of the urinary tract with presenting symptoms such as girdle or flank pain, dysuria, increased blood nitrogen and vascular insufficiency of the lower limbs. More exceptional are pleuro-pulmonary fibrosis with chest pain, dyspnoea, pleural friction rub or pleural effusion and fibrosis with cardiac murmurs and vascular bruits. These disorders are usually reversible with the withdrawal of the drug but in some cases surgical treatment is necessary. The incidence of fibrotic disease has been estimated at 1 case in 5000 patients treated continuously with the drug for 6 months. According to the manufacturers fibrosis can usually be avoided if drug therapy is limited to a maximum of 6 months with at least a 3–4 week interval before recommencing medication.

Acute overdosage
In patients taking a single dose of up to 200 mg, headache, mydriasis, tachycardia and agitation are reported. No deaths due to acute overdosage have been reported. Treatment of overdosed patients is not specific. In case of peripheral vasospasm, vasodilators such as nitroprusside sodium or calcium antagonists should be used.

Severe or irreversible adverse effects
Severe adverse effects of methysergide occur if the drug is given in certain disease states such as cardiac and peripheral vascular disease where vasoconstrictor reactions may occur; in collagen diseases in which there is a possibility of fibrotic reactions and in cases of impaired liver and kidney function, in which the drug may accumulate and cause further complications due to reduced excretion.

Symptomatic adverse effects
Nausea and vomiting may occur but these can often be minimized by taking the drug with food. Insomnia, vertigo, transient slight mental changes, skin reactions, oedema and vasoconstriction, affecting both large and small arteries, are observed. Depending on the vessel involved, this complication may present as chest pain, abdominal pain or cold, numb, painful extremities with or without paraesthesia and diminished or absent pulses.
Fibrotic complications, mainly retroperitoneal, may occur if the drug is not carefully regulated.

Interference with clinical pathology tests
There have been no reported interferences with clinical pathology tests during treatment with methysergide.

Methysergide (hydrogen maleate)

High risk groups

Neonates
Methysergide is contraindicated in neonates.

Breast milk. The drug should not be used by nursing mothers. Animal data shows that methysergide is excreted in breast milk, and its inherent toxicity is such that it cannot be recommended for nursing mothers.

Children
Methysergide is not recommended for use in children.

Pregnant women
Methysergide is contraindicated in pregnant women as the main metabolite, methyergonovine, has uterotonic properties.

The elderly
No extra-special precautions are required in the elderly as doses are adjusted according to patient response.

Concurrent disease
The drug should be avoided in the presence of renal or hepatic disease or in patients suffering from ischaemic heart disease, peripheral vascular disease, collagen disorders or cachectic or septic disorders.

Drug interactions

Potentially hazardous interactions
No potentially hazardous reactions are known, but in patients undergoing methysergide therapy, the dose of ergotamine required to control acute attacks of migraine may have to be reduced.

Potentially useful interactions
No therapeutically useful interactions have been recorded.

Major outcome trials

1. Southwell N, Williams J D, Mackenzie J 1964 Methysergide in the prophylaxis of migraine. Lancet 1: 523–524

This was a double-blind trial of methysergide versus placebo lasting 12 weeks. 53 patients of mean age 38.8 years suffering from at least 1 migraine per fortnight participated. The initial dose of 6 mg of methysergide daily had to be reduced to 3 mg per day in some patients due to side effects. 34 patients completed the study; 17 withdrew due to side effects and 2 were excluded due to incomplete data. Results showed that patients had fewer headaches whilst on the drug than on placebo. The difference between the two groups was most significant ($p = 0.01$) in the second week of the trial. The authors suggest that methysergide may therefore continue to be effective after medication has ceased and conclude that the drug is a useful prophylactic agent for those suffering from frequent and severe migraine headaches and that the side effects may be controlled be a change of dose.

2. Whewell J 1966 Methysergide in prophylaxis of migraine: a clinical trial in general practice. British Medical Journal 2: 394–395

This was a double-blind cross-over trial of methysergide versus placebo lasting 6 months. 50 migraine patients of average age 42 years completed the trial. The dose of methysergide was 4 mg daily in divided doses, side effects at this dose were not troublesome. The duration of severe headaches in patients on methysergide was reduced significantly ($p < 0.05$) when compared to placebo. The number of headaches was also reduced with severe headaches being reduced to a greater extent than moderate or mild ones. The drug was most effective when given after placebo. Patients suffering with oedema and subsequent diuresis benefited most.

3. Friedman A P, Elkind A H 1963 Treatment of vascular headaches of migraine type. Journal of the American Medical Association 184: 125–128

This comprises both a double-blind and an open study with 421 patients suffering from migraine — common, classical and cluster headaches — lasting for up to 29 months in cases. Patients received methysergide or placebo, or methysergide alone, respectively. The dose of methysergide ranged from 6 to 16 mg daily in divided doses.

Results showed that methysergide reduced the frequency of headaches by at least 50% in 83% of patients treated for more than 2 months: a result significantly better than placebo. In all patients who had taken the drug a 64% improvement in migraine frequency was obtained. The authors conclude that methysergide is a useful prophylactic drug for use in all forms of migraine and that the frequent side effects may be controlled by an adjustment of the dose.

Other trials

Melmon K L, Sjoerdsma A, Oates J A, Laster L 1965 Treatment of malabsorption and diarrhoea of the carcinoid syndrome with methysergide. Gastroenterology 48: 18–24

Methysergide was shown to be more effective than placebo in controlling malabsorption, diarrhoea and resulting weight loss in 2 patients with carcinoid syndrome. The drug was administered in maximum doses of 4 mg every 6 hours initially to one patient. Prolonged administration of methysergide (6 to 12 mg daily) over 6 to 7 months resulted in weight gain and control of diarrhoea in both patients. Also in 4 or 5 other patients with only diarrhoea, methysergide in a maximal dose of 8 to 12 mg per day over 7 to 28 days greatly improved gastrointestinal symptoms.

General review articles

Graham J R 1967 Methysergide. Practitioner 198: 302–311
Graham J R, Suby H I, Le Compte P R, Sadowski N L 1966 Fibrotic disorders associated with methysergide therapy for headache. New England Journal of Medicine 274: 359–368
Griffith R W, Grauwiler J, Hodel Ch, Leist K H Matter B 1978 Toxicologic considerations In: Berde B Schild H O (eds) Ergot alkaloids and related compounds. Handbook of Experimental Pharmacology. Springer, Berlin, 49: 805–851

References

1. Bradley P B, Engel G, Feniuk W et al 1986 Proposals for the classification and nomenclature of functional receptors for 5-hydroxytryptamine. Neuropharmacology 25: 563–576
2. Graham J R 1964 Methysergide for prevention of headache: experience in five hundred patients over three years. New England Journal of Medicine 270: 67–72
3. Peart W S, Robertson J I S 1961 The effect of a serotonin antagonist (UML 491) in carcinoid disease. Lancet 2: 1172–1174
4. Dubach U C, Gsell O R 1962 Carcinoid syndrome: alleviation of diarrhoea and blushing with Deseril and RO 5-1025. British Medical Journal 1: 1390–1391
5. Carroll P R, Ebeling P W, Glover W E 1974 The responses of the human temporal and rabbit ear artery to 5-hydroxytryptamine and some of its antagonists. Australian Journal of Experimental Biology and Medical Science 52: 813–823
6. Müller-Schweinitzer E 1983 Vascular effects of ergot alkaloids: a study on human basilar arteries. General Pharmacology 14: 95–102
7. Metcalfe H L, Turner P 1969 Pharmacological studies of cinanserin in human isolated smooth muscle. British Journal of Pharmacology 37: 519
8. Collier J N, Nachev C, Robinson B F 1972 Effect of catecholamines and other vasoactive substances on superficial hand veins in man. Clinical Science 43: 455–467
9. Astrom A, Samelius U 1957 The action of 5-hydroxytryptamine and some of its antagonists on the umbilical vessels of the human placenta. British Journal of Pharmacology 12: 410–414
10. Fishlock D J, Parks A G, Dewell J V 1965 Action of 5-hydroxytryptamine on the human stomach, duodenum and jejunum in vitro. Gut 6: 338–342
11. Fishlock D J 1964 The action of 5-hydroxytryptamine on the circular muscle of human ileum and colon in vitro. Journal of Physiology (London) 170: 11–12
12. Hilton B P, Cumings J N 1971 An assessment of platelet aggregation induced by 5-hydroxytryptamine. Journal of Clinical Pathology 24: 250–258
13. Michal F, Motamed M 1975 Time-dependent potentiation and inhibition by 5-hydroxytryptamine of platelet aggregation induced by ADP. British Journal of Pharmacology 54: 221–222
14. Fanciullacci M, Granchi G, Sicuteri F 1976 Ergotamine and methysergide as serotonin partial agonists in migraine. Headache 16: 226–231
15. Hardebo J E, Edvinason L, Owman C H, Svendgaard N Aa 1978 Potentiation and antagonism of serotonin effects on intracranial and extracranial vessels. Possible implications in migraine. Neurology 28: 64–70
16. Dalessio D J 1963 Recent experimental studies on headache. Neurology (Minneap.) 13: 7–10
17. Aellig W H 1976 Influence of ergot compounds on compliance of superficial hand veins in man. Postgraduate Medical Journal 52 (suppl 1): 21–23
18. Meier J, Schreier E 1976 Human plasma levels of some antimigraine drugs. Headache 16: 96–104
19. Bianchine J R, Friedman A P 1970 Metabolism of methysergide and retroperitoneal fibrosis. Archives of Internal Medicine 126: 252–254

Metoclopramide (hydrochloride)

Metoclopramide was developed in France as a derivative of orthoprocainamide in the early 1960s.[1] It was introduced into clinical use in the UK in 1967. It was the first of the benzamides with motor effects on the gut. Metoclopramide also has actions within the central nervous system.

Chemistry

Metoclopramide (Maxolon, Primperan)
$C_{14}H_{23}Cl_2N_3O_2$
4-Amino-5-chloro-2-methoxy-N-[(2-diethylamino)ethyl]benzamide
or 4-amino-5-chloro-N-(2-diethylaminoethyl)-2-methoxybenzamide

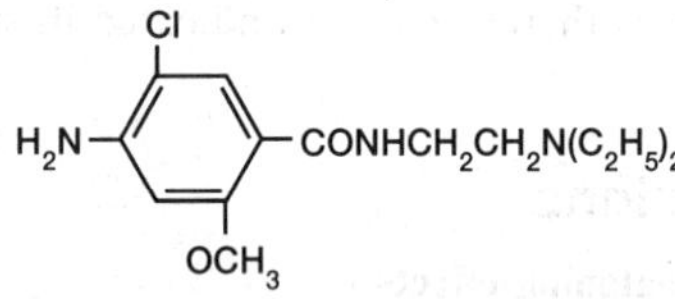

The pharmacological preparation is either the mono- or dihydrochloride monohydrate

Molecular weight (free base)	354.3 (299.8)
pKa	4.45, 9.2
Solubility	
in alcohol	1 in 3
in water	1 in 0.7
Octanol/water partition coefficient	high

Metoclopramide is a white or off-white powder.
It is also available orally in combination with paracetamol (Paramax) and aspirin (Migravess).

Pharmacology

Metoclopramide has at least two pharmacological actions at clinical doses. It is an antagonist at D_2 dopamine receptors.[2] It also has actions on muscarinic cholinergic systems within the gut increasing the release of acetylcholine.[3] The precise mechanism of this effect is still unclear, and may result from presynaptic anticholinergic activity,[4] or an action on 5HT receptors at presynaptic muscarinic neurones.[5] This effect does not appear to be dependent on dopamine receptor antagonism.[6]

Toxicology

Metoclopramide increases prolactin release in animals and man, and may therefore be expected to produce mammary tumours in experimental animals. There is no suggestion that metoclopramide is teratogenic, though the manufacturers in the UK do not recommend use of metoclopramide in pregnancy unless there are compelling reasons and it is not advised during the first trimester.

Clinical pharmacology

Metoclopramide has effects on the upper gastrointestinal tract of man, increasing lower oesophageal sphincter pressure, increasing gastric emptying rate and gastroduodenal coordination.[7–9] Metoclopramide's effects on the gut may result from a local action on acetylcholine release or be in part related to its actions within the central nervous system which are mediated primarily via an action on dopamine receptors in the chemoreceptor trigger zone. Antagonism at dopamine receptors in the basal ganglia results in adverse effects

Metoclopramide (hydrochloride)

including in particular acute dystonia, akathisia, parkinsonism and tardive dyskinesia. Actions on dopamine receptors in the pituitary result in an increase in prolactin secretion occasionally with galactorrhoea as an adverse effect. Metoclopramide has been used to investigate prolactin release.

Nausea and vomiting in patients receiving cytotoxics may be controlled by administering large doses of metoclopramide (up to 10 mg.kg^{-1} body weight over a day in divided doses).[10] The pharmacological properties that result in effective antiemesis at those doses are unclear, since the maximal effect on the dopamine receptors involved in controlling prolactin release has been observed with intravenous doses of 10 mg or less. Some of the effects of 'high-dose' metoclopramide are mediated by antagonism of $5HT_3$ receptors.

Pharmacokinetics

The first analytical method reported involves GCMS with a stable isotope internal standard.[11] More recently a number of HPLC and GC techniques have been published.[12] The limit of sensitivity of these methods is 5–10 μg.l^{-1}.

Metoclopramide is almost completely absorbed following oral dosing, and peak plasma concentrations are seen within 0.5–2 hours in fasted healthy volunteers. Metoclopramide undergoes first-pass metabolism with bioavailability of between 32 to 98%.[13] There have been no studies of the effects of other drugs or environmental factors on the bioavailability of metoclopramide.

Metoclopramide has a volume of distribution of 2.2 to 3.4 l.kg^{-1} after intravenous administration. It is rapidly distributed following intravenous administration ($t_{\frac{1}{2}}\alpha$ 5 to 21 min). Protein binding of metoclopramide is around 40% and protein binding interactions are therefore unlikely. The clearance of metoclopramide is principally by hepatic metabolism; only 20% is excreted in urine unchanged, and the total plasma clearance is between 4 and 7 l.kg^{-1}.h^{-1}.

The half life of metoclopramide after oral and intravenous administration is between 2.5 to 5 hours, the mean being around 4.5 hours.

Metoclopramide is excreted into breast milk at concentrations above those in plasma; nevertheless, the amount being absorbed by a breast-fed infant is likely to be extremely low.[14]

The clearance and volume of distribution of metoclopramide in children is similar to that in adults. The elderly handle high-dose metoclopramide in a similar manner to younger adults.

The only disease state known to alter metoclopramide kinetics is renal failure.[15] In renal failure patients the clearance of metoclopramide is approximately one half that found in normals, with a terminal half life in the region of 14 hours. The precise mechanisms underlying these changes in kinetics have not been elucidated, but may, in part, be due to enterohepatic recirculation of metoclopramide conjugates.

Metoclopramide exhibits linear kinetics at 'high-dose' levels and kinetic parameters in cancer patients without severe hepatic and renal impairment appear similar to those in healthy volunteers.

Oral absorption	>90%
Presystemic metabolism	0–68%
Plasma half life	
range	2.6–5.4 h (normal dose)
mean	4.5 h (normal dose) 5.5 h (high dose)
Volume of distribution	2.2–3.4 l.kg^{-1}
Plasma protein binding	40%

Since there is no clear therapeutic drug concentration, changes in pharmacokinetics are probably of little practical importance, except in determining the frequency of adverse events, particularly extrapyramidal syndromes in patients with renal impairment.

Concentration–effect relationship

There have been few studies on concentration–effect relationships for metoclopramide. Akathisia occurs in young adult volunteers at plasma concentrations around 100 μg.l^{-1}.[16] Gastric emptying increased with 10 mg intravenous metoclopramide, though the effect was not seen with the same dose orally. This suggests that the plasma concentration may be relevant to the effects of the drug on the gut and concentrations above 40 μg.l^{-1} appear necessary for an effect on gastric emptying. In the treatment of cytotoxic drug-induced nausea, high doses of metoclopramide are more efficacious than standard doses and this suggests a dose–response relationship.

Metabolism

Metoclopromide is extensively metabolised. The major route of excretion is in the urine (≤80%). The principal identified route of metabolism of metoclopramide in man is by N-4-sulphate formation (≤50%). In addition a small amount of metoclopramide N-glucuronide has been identified.[12] The site of metabolism has not been positively identified. A small amount is excreted as 2-(4-amino-5-chloro-2-methoxybenzamido)acetic acid.

Pharmaceutics

Potency is expressed as the equivalent amount of anhydrous monohydrochloride.

Metoclopramide hydrochloride is available in oral and parenteral form:

1. Tablets containing metoclopramide hydrochloride 10 mg, as small white, scored tablets engraved 'Maxolon' or 'Primperan'. Primperan is prepared with the monohydrochloride monohydrate in the UK, but in some countries it is prepared with the dihydrochloride monohydrate.
2. Syrup containing metoclopramide hydrochloride 5 mg in 5 ml in a clear yellow lemon/lime solution.
3. Solution for injection, a clear colourless solution containing 10 mg in 2 ml ampoules, pH 3–5, sterilized by autoclaving. It is prepared using water for injection free of dissolved air and stabilizing and buffering agents are necessary.

A 'high-dose' preparation for injection is available containing 100 mg in 20 ml of solution. The syrup and ampoules for injection should be stored away from light. If exposed to light the ampoules for injection may discolour, and should be discarded. Once dispensed the paediatric syrup should be stored for not more than 14 days. Metoclopramide is also marketed in two combination preparations, metoclopramide hydrochloride 5 mg with paracetamol 500 mg (Paramax) as white scored tablets or sachets and metoclopramide hydrochloride 5 mg with aspirin 450 mg, sodium bicarbonate PhEur 1230 mg and citric acid PhEur 850 mg (Migravess) a white tablet, effervescent in water. These preparations are specifically marketed for use in migraine.

Therapeutic use

Indications

1. Treatment of motility disorder of upper GI tract, particularly delayed gastric emptying
2. Gastro-oesophageal reflux
3. Nausea and vomiting from causes other than motion sickness
4. Migraine, particularly to increase the absorption of analgesics
5. Diagnostic radiology, to speed the passage of contrast media into the small bowel
6. In the treatment of non-specific upper gastrointestinal symptoms, including 'gastritis', flatulence and 'heartburn'
7. Diagnostic investigation of pituitary function, particularly prolactin release
8. Specifically in high doses for treatment of cytotoxic-induced nausea
9. Defective lactation
10. Tardive dyskinesia
11. Antipsychotic activity
12. Postural hypotension.

Contraindications

1. Parkinsonism
2. Phaeochromocytoma (risk of hypertensive crisis)
3. Previous history of dystonia with dopamine receptor antagonists
4. Pyloric stenosis.

Mode of use

Metoclopramide is usually administered orally 10 mg three times daily for the treatment of short duration disturbance of upper gastrointestinal motility and nausea and vomiting. It may also be used parenterally, the latter route being obviously more appropriate in a vomiting patient.

In the prophylaxis of cytotoxic-induced vomiting metoclopramide may be given in a loading dose before chemotherapy (around 3 $mg.kg^{-1}$ body weight) and can then be given by continuous infusion. Alternatively, intermittent injections can be given, but appear less logical (see below). It is probably useful to add antiemetics such as dexamethasone and a benzodiazepine in patients at particular risk (e.g. those receiving cisplatin). Doses of up to 10 mg/kg/24 hours may be given to patients under these circumstances. Unwanted adverse effects with high doses of metoclopramide are predominantly sedation, increased bowel frequency and acute dystonia. The latter is more common in young adults.

Long-term therapy with metoclopramide is associated with the risk of tardive dyskinesia; this appears to be a particular problem in the elderly.[18]

Indications

1. Motility disorders of upper GI tract — gastrokinetic action

Delayed gastric emptying is associated with diabetic autonomic neuropathy and may occur post vagotomy. In these situations metoclopramide has been shown in several studies[7,19,20] to increase gastric emptying when given in doses of between 30 and 60 mg per day. Metoclopramide is also of use in two other situations where an increase in the rate of gastric emptying is desirable. First for patients in labour who have received opiate analgesics and require emergency surgery. Second, for delayed gastric emptying as a feature of migraine,[21] since this may result in delay in the absorption of co-administered analgesics. This action of metoclopramide on the gut can be inhibited by anticholinergic drugs and, similarly, metoclopramide will reverse the effects of anticholinergics on gastric emptying.

There is still extensive debate as to whether these actions of metoclopramide on the stomach involve an action on dopamine receptors, or are due to its alternative action on postsynaptic cholinergic muscarinic nerves via 5HT receptors.

2. Gastro-oesophageal reflux

Metoclopramide increases oesophageal motility and increases the lower oesophageal sphincter pressure.[22] These effects are more easy to demonstrate in volunteers than patients with gastro-oesophageal reflux. It has therefore been suggested that the therapeutic benefit of metoclopramide results from a combination of actions on the oesophagus and stomach, and that increased gastric emptying is an important factor in the therapeutic effect.[23] The effect of metoclopramide on the lower oesophageal sphinter may, in part, be due to dopamine receptor antagonism at dopamine receptors within the oesophagus.[24] This is a contentious point since dopamine receptors have not been demonstrated in the lower oesophagus in man.

3. Nausea and vomiting

Metoclopramide has been shown to be effective in the treatment of nausea and vomiting in postoperative patients in a number of trials when the drug is given pre- or peri-operatively. This is by no means a universal finding however, though several double blind studies do suggest that in high risk patients metoclopramide 10 mg is more effective than placebo.[9]

Metoclopramide is not effective in motion sickness, though it may alleviate symptoms of nausea in patients with vertigo.[7,25] Although it is extensively used in general practice for the treatment of acute episodes of nausea and vomiting, there is little controlled evidence to suggest that metoclopramide is effective in this situation.

Metoclopramide has been shown to be effective in the treatment of nausea and vomiting in pregnancy. There is no evidence that metoclopramide is teratogenic, but this drug is not recommended by the manufacturers for use in pregnancy unless there are compelling reasons.

Metoclopramide may also be effective in radiation sickness. Where nausea and vomiting are associated with drugs, particularly opioid analgesics, there is good evidence that metoclopramide is an effective therapy.

The therapeutic benefit of metoclopramide in the above conditions is probably due to a combination of its effects on the chemoreceptor trigger zone and on the upper gastrointestinal tract. The manufacturers recommend the dose of metoclopramide be adjusted according to age. This is with the aim of reducing acute dystonia which appears to be a particular problem in children and young adults. Total daily dosage of metoclopramide, especially for children and young adults, should not normally exceed 0.5 μg/kg/day. The dose recommendations are complex and do not have a clear scientific basis. Long-term treatment in the elderly carries with it a substantial risk of induction of tardive dyskinesia, and is best avoided.

Dose recommendations

Up to 1 year, 1 mg twice daily
1–3 years, 1 mg 2–3 times daily
3–5 years, 2 mg 2–3 times daily
5–9 years, 2.5 mg 3 times daily
9–14 years, 5 mg 3 times daily
14–20 years, 5–10 mg 3 times daily
over 20 years, 10 mg 3 times daily

Akathisia was almost universal in normal volunteers given metoclopramide 10 mg intravenously, and occurs more frequently than most physicians appreciate with this and other dopamine receptor antagonists.

4. Migraine

As mentioned above gastric emptying is delayed in migraine. There is good evidence that parenteral metoclopramide will increase the rate of absorption of analgesics in patients suffering a migraine attack.[21] The efficacy of oral metoclopramide has not been so convincingly demonstrated, although the absorption of aspirin is increased.[26] Two combination preparations are available in the UK, Paramax (metoclopramide and paracetamol) and Migravess (metoclopramide and aspirin). Although these preparations appear logical at first sight, there is little controlled evidence to support their use. Furthermore, since to be effective metoclopramide first requires absorption from the small bowel, the patients with established migraine may not benefit from these combination tablets because of gastric stasis.

5. Diagnostic radiology

Metoclopramide 10 mg intravenously (reduced doses in children: under 3 years 1 mg; 3–5 years 2 mg; 6–12 years 2.5–5 mg) will increase the emptying of barium from the stomach, and has therefore been used to speed the passage of contrast in small bowel meals.

6. Non-specific upper gastrointestinal symptoms

Metoclopramide was initially studied in the management of many non-specific symptoms attributed to the upper GI tract. These trials were generally uncontrolled, and although widely used for this indication there is still no large well-conducted study to support this indication. Metoclopramide should not be used on a chronic basis for this type of indication in view of potential adverse effects, particularly tardive dyskinesia.[18] In one study on 40 patients metoclopramide was significantly better than placebo in treating flatulent dyspepsia.[27]

7. Diagnostic tests of pituitary function

Metoclopramide causes release of prolactin, due to its antagonistic effects on D_2 receptors in the pituitary. Intravenous metoclopramide has been used in the diagnostic investigation of the dynamics of prolactin release. The high incidence of akathisia makes it less suitable for this purpose than domperidone which has superseded it.

8. Prophylaxis of chemotherapy-induced vomiting

High doses of metoclopramide have been shown to be efficacious in the prophylaxis of vomiting associated with cancer chemotherapy.[10] The initial regimens were pharmacokinetically illogical,[12] since they advocated equal 2-hourly doses of the drug over 8 hours. Metoclopramide can be given by a loading dose, followed by infusion to obtain a steady state concentration.[17] The optimum level is unknown but should probably be at least 1 $mg.l^{-1}$. This can be achieved by a loading dose of 3.1 $mg.kg^{-1}$ followed by an infusion of 0.4 $mg.kg^{-1}.h^{-1}$, providing the patient has normal renal and hepatic function. High oral doses of metoclopramide also appear efficacious,[30] though the optimum regimen should probably also include steroids and a benzodiazepine. Adverse effects include drowsiness, diarrhoea and dystonia, particularly in younger patients. Dystonia can be treated with a parenteral anticholinergic or a benzodiazepine.

Metoclopramide (hydrochloride)

9. Defective lactation
Since metoclopramide raises serum prolactin a number of workers have investigated its use orally as a means of improving lactation. There is some evidence that this does indeed occur, though the place of metoclopramide for this indication is conjectural, and the drug is not marketed for this purpose. Breast-fed babies of mothers receiving metoclopramide had higher prolactin than controls suggesting a biological effect in the baby.[28]

10. Tardive dyskinesia
Metoclopramide has been shown to reduce signs of tardive dyskinesia both acutely and chronically.[29,30] The treatment of tardive dyskinesia is difficult, but in view of the occurrence of this effect during long-term therapy with metoclopramide, this does not appear to be an appropriate therapy.

11. Antipsychotic effects
Since the dose required to produce effects on the gut did not produce symptomatic improvement in psychotics, metoclopramide was thought to lack antipsychotic activity. Recent evidence suggests this is not the case and that metoclopramide may be an effective antipsychotic at high doses.[31]

12. Postural hypotension
Metoclopramide reversed postural hypotension in a case report,[32] and in low doses had a small effect in patients with orthostatic hypotension related to Parkinson's disease.[33] It seems that small doses of metoclopramide (30 mg per day) might be worth a trial in patients in whom more conventional therapy has failed.

Adverse reactions

Potentially life-threatening effects
Death associated with metoclopramide is very rare though it has occurred in association with dystonia. A rise in blood pressure was observed in a patient with a phaeochromocytoma given metoclopramide intravenously, and it should therefore not be given to patients with this condition.[34] Acute porphyria is said to have been precipitated by metoclopramide given intramuscularly.[35]

Acute overdosage
Metoclopramide is relatively safe in overdose.[36] Doses well above the recommended therapeutic ranges are given without ill effect for vomiting induced by cancer chemotherapy.

Treatment of a large overdose should include monitoring blood pressure and pulse, but symptomatic treatment is all that is required. Dystonia may be more likely to occur with overdose in children, and will usually respond to an intravenous injection of diazepam or an anticholinergic drug.

Severe or irreversible adverse effects
The most common adverse effects of metoclopramide are due to its action as a dopamine antagonist in the basal ganglia. Metoclopramide produces both acute adverse effects, including akathisia, dystonia and acute dyskinesia occasionally severe enough to produce fever,[37] and effects after chronic ingestion (parkinsonism and tardive dyskinesia).

Acute dystonias appear more frequently in children[38] and young adults. Acute dystonias can be treated with a parenterally administered anticholinergic or benzodiazepine and will usually resolve within 24 hours. Parkinsonism will usually respond to withdrawal of the drug but, in common with drug-induced parkinsonism from dopamine antagonists, may take several months to resolve. Tardive dyskinesia is a particularly difficult adverse effect to manage since it may become symptomatically worse when the offending drug is stopped.[18] Consequently, if at all possible, metoclopramide should therefore not be given long-term and particular care is required in the elderly.

Symptomatic adverse effects
Drowsiness, diarrhoea and hyperprolactinaemia with galactorrhoea may all be caused by metoclopramide.

A small fall in arterial blood pressure and increase in heart rate was observed in the first 5 minutes following acute intravenous administration of metoclopramide to normal volunteers,[39] and hypotension has been reported in patients given metoclopramide after surgery.[40] No change had been observed in earlier studies when cardiac output was monitored. There is one report of multifocal supraventricular extrasystoles after metoclopramide given intramuscularly[41] and bradycardia has also been reported in one patient. In general, metoclopramide is relatively free of adverse effects outside the central nervous system.

Interference with clinical pathology tests
None is known.

High risk groups

Neonates
Metoclopramide can be used in appropriate reduced doses.

Breast milk. Only small amounts are excreted in breast milk.

Children
Acute dystonia is more common in children and young adults. Dosage should be adjusted accordingly, though this adverse effect is not clearly dose related.

Pregnant women
Metoclopramide does not appear to be teratogenic.

The elderly
The elderly are at greater risk of parkinsonism and tardive dyskinesia. The elimination of metoclopramide is prolonged in renal failure, with clearance being reduced by around 50% of values in normal volunteers. The dose should be appropriately reduced. Theoretically, liver disease might delay elimination, though there is no data published on this point.

Concurrent disease
There is evidence that metoclopramide causes a higher incidence of extrapyramidal reactions in patients with renal impairment, and this may be related to changes in the pharmacokinetics of the drug in this group.[15] Metoclopramide may cause acute hypertension in patients with phaeochromocytoma and should therefore not be used in this group; similarly, there is some suggestion that acute porphyria may be precipitated.[34,35]

Drug interactions

Metoclopramide increases the rate of gastric emptying and decreases small bowel transit; it will therefore increase the rate of absorption, but not usually the degree of absorption of drugs given concurrently. When given with drugs that have a poor bioavailability metoclopramide may make this worse, but this does not seem to be a problem that is often encountered in practice. Metoclopramide will reverse the impairment of gastrointestinal motility caused by opiates and anticholinergics.

Major outcome trials

Clinical trials with metoclopramide have all been of short duration. Important short-duration studies have been mentioned in the monograph under the appropriate sections. Probably the most common reason for prescribing metoclopramide in general practice is for nausea and vomiting associated with a concurrent illness, usually viral, or with 'gastroenteritis'. There are no controlled studies of metoclopramide efficacy in this situation and these would be extremely difficult to mount.

1. Johnson A G 1971 Controlled trial of metoclopramide in the treatment of flatulent dyspepsia. British Medical Journal 2: 25–26

This study examined the effect of metoclopramide 10 mg three times daily before meals for 2 weeks in a double-blind study against placebo in 47 patients with flatulent dyspepsia, essentially epigastric discomfort after meals with distention relieved by eructation. The patients who benefited most were those whose symptoms came on within one hour of the meal. Six patients complained of drowsiness on active drug, and 4 withdrew because of this; 2 had drowsiness on placebo, 1 withdrawing from the study; 42 completed the study.

2. McCallum R W, Fink S M, Winnan G R, Avella J, Callachan C 1984 Metoclopramide in gastrooesophageal reflux disease: rationale for its use and results of a double-blind trial. American Journal of Gastroenterology 79: 165–172

Metoclopramide (hydrochloride)

M

This study examined the effect of metoclopramide 10 mg 4 times daily in 19 patients with reflux oesophagitis in a 4 week treatment period double-blind cross-over study. The improvement in symptoms (60%) was better than that with placebo (32%), but this advantage appeared principally in the daytime. In this study gastric emptying and lower oesophageal sphincter pressures were measured. Metoclopramide significantly increased both gastric emptying rate and lowered oesophageal sphinder pressure. The authors suggest both these actions are important in the efficacy of metoclopramide in reflux oesophagitis. The dose used in this study is higher than that recommended by the manufacturer in the UK.

3. Gralla R J, Itri L M, Pisco S E et al 1981 Antiemetic efficacy of high-dose metoclopramide: randomised trials with placebo and prochlorperazine in patients with chemotherapy-induced nausea and vomiting. New England Journal of Medicine 305: 905–909

The efficacy of metoclopramide in high doses for cytotoxic vomiting was first shown by Gralla and colleagues who studied 41 patients receiving cisplatin, and compared in two groups of patients, metoclopramide 2 mg.kg^{-1} body weight for 5 hours over 8.5 hours to standard doses of prochlorperazine or placebo. 60% of patients had less than two vomits on metoclopramide, and this was significantly better than either control group. The principal adverse effect was sedation.

General review articles

Pinder R M, Brogden R N, Sawyer P R, Speight T M, Avery G S 1976 Metoclopramide: a review of its pharmacological properties and clinical use. Drugs 12: 81–131

Schulze-Delrieu K 1981 Metoclopramide. New England Journal of Medicine 305: 28–33

Harrington R A, Hamilton C W, Brogden R W, Linkewich J A, Romankiewicz J A, Heel R C 1983 Metoclopramide — an updated review of its pharmacological properties and clinical use. Drugs 25: 451–494

Bateman D N 1983 Clinical pharmacokinetics of metoclopramide. Clinical Pharmacokinetics 8: 523–529

References

1. Justin-Besancon J-L, Laville C, Thominet M 1964 Le metoclopramide et ses homologues: introduction a lur etude biologique. Compte Rendue d'Acadamie Sciences (Paris) 258: 4384–4386
2. Jenner P, Marsden C D 1979 The substituted benzamides — a novel class of dopamine antagonists. Life Sciences 25: 479–485
3. Hay A M 1977 Pharmacological analysis of the effects of metoclopramide on the guinea-pig isolated stomach. Gastroenterology 72: 864–869
4. Fosbraey P, Hird M F, Johnson E S 1980 The effects of some dopamine antagonists of cholinergic mechanisms in the guinea-pig ileum. Journal of Autonomic Pharmacology 1: 17–25
5. Kilbinger H, Kruel R, Pfeuffer-Friederich J, Wessler I 1982 The effects of metoclopramide on acetylcholine release and on smooth-muscle response in the isolated guinea pig ileum. Naungn-Schmiedeberg's Archives of Pharmacology 319: 231–238
6. Zar M A, Ebong O O, Bateman D N 1982 Effects of metoclopramide in guinea-pig ileum longitudinal muscle: evidence against dopamine mediation. Gut 23: 66–70
7. Pinder R M, Brogden R N, Sawyer P R, Speight T M, Avery G S 1976 Metoclopramide: a review of its pharmacological properties and clinical use. Drugs 12: 81–131
8. Schulze-Delrieu K 1981 Metoclopramide. New England Journal of Medicine 305: 28–33
9. Harrington R A, Hamilton C W, Brogden R W, Linkewich J A, Romankiewicz J A, Heel R C 1983 Metoclopramide — an updated review of its pharmacological properties and clinical use. Drugs 25: 451–494
10. Gralla R J, Itri L M, Pisco S E et al 1981 Antiemetic efficacy of high-dose metoclopramide: randomised trials with placebo and prochlorperazine in patients with chemotherapy-induced nausea and vomiting. New England Journal of Medicine 305: 905–909
11. Bateman D N, Kahn C, Mashiter K, Davies D S 1978 Pharmacokinetic and concentration effect studies with intravenous metoclopramide. British Journal of Clinical Pharmacology 6: 401–407
12. Bateman D N 1983 Clinical pharmacokinetics of metoclopramide. Clinical Pharmacokinetics 8: 523–529
13. Bateman D N, Kahn C, Davies D S 1980 The pharmacokinetics of metoclopramide in man with observations in the dog. British Journal of Clinical Pharmacology 9: 371–377
14. Lewis P J, Devenish C, Kahn C 1980 Controlled trial of metoclopramide in the institution of breast feeding. British Journal of Clinical Pharmacology 9: 217–219
15. Bateman D N, Gokal P, Dodd T R P, Blain P G 1981 The pharmacokinetics of single doses of metoclopramide in renal failure. European Journal of Clinical Pharmacology 19: 437–441
16. Bateman D N, Kahn C, Davies D S 1979 Concentration effect studies with oral metoclopramide. British Journal of Clinical Pharmacology 8: 179–182
17. Taylor W B, Proctor S J, Bateman D N 1984 Pharmacokinetics and efficacy of high-dose metoclopramide given by continuous infusion for the control of cytotoxic drug-induced vomiting. British Journal of Clinical Pharmacology 18: 679–684
18. Wiholm B E, Mortimer O, Boethius G, Haggstrom J E 1984 Tardive dyskinesia associated with metoclopramide. British Medical Journal 288: 545–547
19. Longstreth G F, Malagelada J-R, Kelly K A 1977 Metoclopramide stimulation of gastric motility and emptying in diabetic gastroparesis. Annals of Internal Medicine 86: 195–196
20. Malagelada J R, Rees W D W, Mazzotta L J, Gov L W 1980 Gastric motor abnormalities in diabetic and postvagotomy gastroparesis: effects of metoclopramide and bethanechol. Gastroenterology 78: 286–293
21. Volans G N 1975 The effects of metoclopramide on the absorption of effervescent aspirin in migraine. British Journal of Clinical Pharmacology 2: 57–63
22. McCallum R W, Kline M M, Curry N, Sturdevert R A L 1975 Comparative effects of metoclopramide and bethanechol on lower oesophageal sphincter pressure in reflex patients. Gastroenterology 68: 1114
23. McCallum R W, Fink S M, Lerner E, Berkowitz D M 1983 Effects of metoclopramide and bethanecol on delayed gastric emptying present in gastrooesophageal reflex patients. Gastroenterology 84: 1573–1577
24. DeCarle D J, Christensen J 1976 A dopamine receptor in oesophageal smooth muscle of the opossum. Gastroenterology 70: 216–219
25. Marshall N W 1970 A double-blind trial of metoclopramide and prochlorperazine in general practice. British Journal of Clinical Practice 24: 25–28
26. Ross-Lee L, Heazlewood V, Tyrer J H, Eadie M J 1982 Aspirin treatment of migraine attacks. Plasma drug lunch data. Cephalgia 2: 9
27. Johnson A G 1971 Controlled trial of metoclopramide in the treatment of flatulent dyspepsia. British Medical Journal 2: 25–26
28. Arvela P, Jouppila R, Kauppila A, Pakarinen A, Pelkinen O, Tuimala R 1983 Placental transfer and hormonal effects of metoclopramide. European Journal of Clinical Pharmacology 24: 345–348
29. Bateman D N, Dutta D K, McClellant H A, Rawlins M D 1979 Metoclopramide and haloperidol in tardive dyskinesia. British Journal of Psychiatry 135: 505–508
30. Karp I M, Penkel M S, Hersh T, McKinney A S 1981 Metoclopramide treatment of tardive dyskinesia. Journal of the American Medical Association 246: 1934–1935
31. Stanley M, Lautin A, Rotrosen J, Gershun S, Kleinberg D 1980 Metoclopramide: antipsychotic efficacy of a drug lacking potency in receptor models. Psychopharmacology 71: 219–225
32. Kuchel O, Buu N T, Gutkowska J, Genest J 1980 Treatment of some orthostatis hypotension by metoclopramide. Annals of Internal Medicine 93: 841–843
33. Bateman D N, Kahn C, Legg N J, Reid J L 1978 Metoclopramide in Parkinson's Disease. Clinical Pharmacology and Therapeutics 24: 459–464
34. Abe M, Orita Y, Nakashima Y, Nakamura M 1984 Hypertensive crisis induced by metoclopramide in patient with phaeochromocytoma. Angiology 35: 122–128
35. Doss M, Becker U, Peter N-J, Kaffarnik H 1981 Drug safety in prophyria: risks of valproate and metoclopramide. Lancet 2: 91
36. Bar J 1966 Attempted suicide with metoclopramide without serious consequences. Therapie 21: 349–353
37. Wandlass I, Evans J G, Jackson M 1980 Fever associated with metoclopramide-induced dystonia. Lancet 1: 1255–1256
38. Castaels van Dael M, Jaeken J, Van Der Schueren P, Zimmerman A T, Van Den Bon P 1970 Dystonic reactions in children caused by metoclopramide. Archives of Diseases of Childhood 45: 130–133
39. Park G R 1981 Hypotension following the intravenous injection of metoclopramide. Anaesthesia 36: 75–76
40. Pegg M S 1980 Hypotension following metoclopramide injection. Anaesthesia 35: 615
41. Shaklai M, Pinkhaj J, De Uries A 1974 Metoclopramide and cardiac arrhythmia. British Medical Journal 2: 385
42. McCallum R W, Fink S M, Winnan G R, Avella J, Callachan C 1984 Metoclopramide in gastroesophageal reflux disease: rationale for its use and results of a double-blind trial. American Journal of Gastroenterology 79: 165–172

Metolazone

Metolazone is a thiazide-related diuretic.

Chemistry

Metolazone (Metenix 5, Zaroxolyn)
$C_{16}H_{16}ClN_3O_3S$
7-Chloro-1,2,3,4-tetrahydro-2-methyl-4-oxo-3-o-tolyl-6-quinazoline-6-sulphonamide

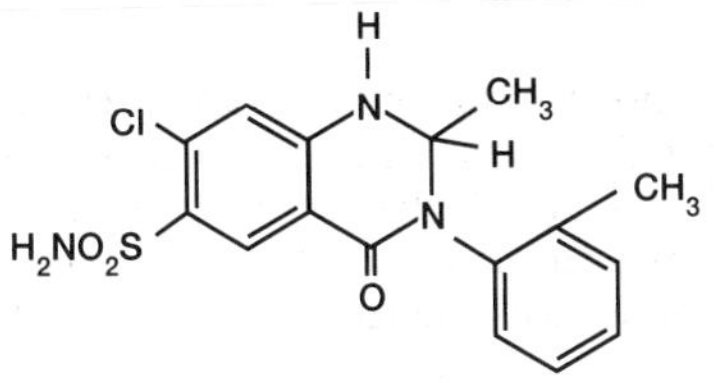

Molecular weight	365.8
pKa	9.72
Solubility	
in alcohol	high
in water	>1 in 100
Octanol/water partition coefficient (37°C)	42

Colourless crystals, to be protected from light. A quinazolinone derivative prepared by chemical synthesis.

Metolazone is optically active and is used clinically as the racemate.

Pharmacology

Metolazone is a diuretic having about twice the potency on a weight basis compared to hydrochlorothiazide. Metolazone acts directly on the cortical segment of the distal convoluted tubule. It inhibits sodium, chloride, and water reabsorption but the exact mechanism of action is unclear. The maximal rate of sodium excretion that metolazone can achieve is modest compared to loop diuretics. Metolazone has some effects on the proximal convoluted tubule due to its active secretion into the tubule but the effects on sodium reabsorption here are minor in importance compared to the distal tubule. Metolazone has weak carbonic anhydrase activity being 1000 times weaker in this regard than acetazolamide. Metolazone also increases the urinary excretion of potassium, phosphate, calcium and magnesium.

Toxicology

Metolazone has low acute toxicity in mice, rats and dogs, with LD_{50} (p.o. or i.p.) higher than 0.5 $g.kg^{-1}$. One month's treatment in dogs caused some hypokalaemia and a rise in blood urea nitrogen. No toxic effects of potential clinical significance were shown by rats, dogs and monkeys chronically treated with metolazone. The drug had no teratological effects in mice, rats and rabbits.

Clinical pharmacology

Metolazone has a dose-related natriuretic effect, evident within 2 hours of oral administration and lasting 12–24 hours. Chloride excretion rises in parallel with the natriuresis.[1] Potassium excretion is increased by metolazone, as with most thiazide-like diuretics; the drug-induced enhancement of urine flow is a stimulus to potassium excretion. Initial reports with metolazone suggested a lesser potassium loss in the urine compared to other thiazide-like diuretics but this has not been confirmed in clinical practice.[2,3] Hypokalaemia is quite common in metolazone treated patients. Unlike other thiazide-related diuretics, metolazone is an effective diuretic in patients with severe impairment of renal function.[1,2] This has led to a view that metolazone is intermediate in potency between loop diuretics and thiazides. Metolazone has been shown to be effective in cases of oedema resistant to frusemide (see ref. 16) and can produce profound hyponatraemia.

Metolazone increases the concentration of urate in the plasma by inhibiting the tubular secretion of urate in the distal tubule as well as by enhancing the absorption of urate from the proximal tubule. Metolazone may increase the blood glucose and can produce diabetes after prolonged usage. Metolazone lowers blood pressure in prolonged therapy by its effects on sodium excretion as well as by a vasodilatory effect on resistance blood vessels.

Pharmacokinetics

Only two assays of metolazone have been published; they use high-performance liquid chromatography. One is suitable only for urine,[4] the other, coupled with fluorimetric detection, for plasma.[5] However, to our knowledge no pharmacokinetic studies have been published using these assays. All pharmacokinetic data have been obtained using ^{14}C-labelled drug.[6] Metolazone is partially absorbed (64%) after oral administration; its systemic bioavailability after oral administration is around 60% and there is no noteworthy presystemic metabolism. A lower proportion of the oral dose (40%) is absorbed in patients with congestive heart failure.[6]

Metolazone is widely distributed in the body and its volume of distribution is larger than 1 $l.kg^{-1}$. Studies in the rat have shown that the drug distributes homogeneously throughout the body, with low concentrations in the central nervous system.

Oral absorption	64%
Presystemic metabolism	very low
Plasma half life	
range	4–5 h
Volume of distribution (steady state)	113 l*
Plasma protein binding	95%

* subject's body weight was not reported.

Metolazone is excreted 80% unchanged in urine, and 10% as metabolites; about 10% is excreted in the bile as unchanged drug and metabolites. Elimination seems to be prolonged in renal failure. In four patients with chronic renal failure, clearance from the central compartment was about five times less than in normal patients. Metolazone crosses the placental barrier and is excreted in milk. Metolazone plasma concentrations are not reduced by haemodialysis.[7,8]

The very small number of subjects and patients studied make the pharmacokinetic characterization of the drug largely incomplete. Consequently a therapeutic range has not been established.

Concentration–effect relationship

There are no data available relating the plasma concentration of metolazone and its diuretic effect.

Metabolism

Only 5–10% of an intravenous dose of metolazone is excreted as metabolites in urine; these are mainly produced by hydroxylation and oxidation. About 10% of the dose is excreted through non-renal routes. Thus there should be no active metabolites reaching noteworthy concentrations in plasma.

Pharmaceutics

Metolazone is available in oral forms:
Metenix 5 (Hoechst, UK) tablets containing 5 mg of metolazone, blue, flat, uncoated, round, 6 mm in diameter, marked with a figure '5' on one side and the Hoechst insignia on the other. Metolazone preparations should be stored in a cool dark place.

Zaroxolyn (Pennwalt, USA)/Diulo (Searle, USA) tablets containing 2.5, 5, 10 mg of metolazone are round, biconvex and uncoated. The colours are pink (2.5 mg), blue (5 mg) and yellow (10 mg). Diulo tablets are coded '501', '511' and '521' respectively. (no longer available in the UK)

Therapeutic use

Indications

1. The control of mild to moderate hypertension (essential and renal)
2. The management of renal failure
3. The management of congestive heart failure
4. The management of oedema in hepatic disorders.

Contraindications

1. Diabetes (relative)
2. Patients with frequent ventricular arrhythmias in presence of heart disease.

Mode of use

The duration of action of metolazone allows a once-a-day dosage schedule, starting with 2.5–5 mg in essential hypertension and raising the dose, in case of non-response, usually up to 10 mg. In refractory cases of fluid retention in severe renal or hepatic failure, daily doses as high as 150 mg have been used with success.

Indications

1. Hypertension
Metolazone can be used alone, but is most often employed in combination with β-adrenergic blocking drugs and/or vasodilators, to control mild to moderate hypertension. It lowers systolic and diastolic blood pressure in standing and supine positions. Full therapeutic response develops 1 to 4 weeks after the beginning of treatment when both systolic and diastolic blood pressure drop about 20% in patients who respond (50 to 90% of the patients studied). As stated above, in view of its long duration of action (12 to 24 hours) the drug is usually given once a day at doses from 1 to 10 mg, most commonly 2.5 and 5 mg. The hypotensive response appears to be sustained for several years.[9,10] In two comparative studies, metolazone showed similar therapeutic efficacy to hydrochlorothiazide in 21 patients with primary hypertension[11] and as chlorthalidone in 57 non-oedematous, hypertensive patients.[2]

2. Renal failure
Metolazone increases urine volume, sodium and potassium urinary output and lowers blood pressure in patients with renal disease. A sustained decrease over 3 months in blood pressure, body weight and oedema were obtained in more than half the patients treated with up to 25 mg daily of metolazone, with creatinine clearance ranging from 4 to 50 $ml.min^{-1}$ (mean 37.4 $ml.min^{-1}$).[12] A single oral dose of metolazone, 20–150 mg, induced a diuretic and natriuretic effect in patients, with average creatinine clearance of 4 $ml.min^{-1}$.[13] However, in similar patients, a daily dose of only 5 mg did not have any effect on blood pressure.[8] Increased diuresis, control of oedema and decreased blood pressure may be observed within the first week and can be maintained over months to years.[14]

Metolazone's diuretic and natriuretic effects, in patients with reduced filtration rates, seem to be intermediate between the less effective thiazides and the loop diuretics, frusemide and ethacrynic acid. It has been found effective to associate metolazone with loop diuretics, especially frusemide, to reduce oedema. Synergism of action has been reported, attributed to the prevention of compensatory sodium reabsorption at the distal convoluted tubule.[24] This observation has been made by several authors, also in cases of oedema from other causes, like congestive heart failure and liver failure.[15,16] Though doses as high as 150 mg of metolazone have been used with success in this indication,[3,13] the usual effective maintenance doses are between 2 and 25 mg daily. Metolazone has been reported to be effective in cases of oedema resistant to 320 mg daily of frusemide.[17]

3. Congestive heart failure
Metolazone has been shown to reduce oedema in congestive heart failure, in combination with other non-diuretic drugs. Daily doses from 1.25 to 20 mg have been used. A synergism with frusemide in diuretic effect and oedema reduction has been reported.[17] Metolazone, added to conventional treatments including frusemide, potassium sparing agents, nitrates and ACE inhibitors, caused a decrease in NYHA class from IV to II or III in 12 out of 17 previously unresponsive patients with severe congestive heart failure.[25] However, it is not known whether survival was increased.

4. Hepatic disorders
Metolazone can increase diuresis and reduce ascites in liver disease, such as cirrhosis, alone or in combination with frusemide. Doses from 1 to 150 mg daily have been used. The drug did not offer advantages over traditional diuretics, except for a low incidence of azotaemia, suggesting that it might be helpful when renal function is greatly reduced.[3]

Contraindications

In view of the scarcity of ad hoc studies, the same precautions suggested for chlorothiazide, a better-studied drug, should be applied. Two cases specifically discussed in the literature for metolazone are reported here.

1. Diabetes
Metolazone can raise fasting blood glucose levels in non-diabetic patients; in some diabetics the drug has to be withdrawn because of excessive increases in blood glucose, and in one case it has been reported to cause hyperosmolar non-ketotic diabetes mellitus.[19] This adverse effect is shared with thiazide diuretics.[2,9,11]

2. Ventricular arrhythmias with heart disease
Patients with frequent cardiac arrhythmias in the presence of heart disease (enlargement or ECG abnormalities) are more prone to suffer worsening of their baseline arrhythmia as a consequence of diuretic-induced hypokalaemia.

Adverse reactions

Potentially life-threatening effects
No deaths caused by metolazone have been reported.

Acute overdosage
No cases of this kind appear to have been reported.

Severe or irreversible adverse effects
Metolazone increases urinary excretion of potassium, like thiazide and loop diuretics, and can thus cause hypokalaemia. Preliminary claims that metolazone did not increase urinary potassium loss, based on studies performed in animals and healthy volunteers,[1] have not been borne out by further clinical work.[2,3,9–11] Potassium supplements have to be given in many cases, particularly when metolazone is associated with frusemide. Metolazone has been reported to raise serum creatinine and uric acid, leading in rare cases to clinical gout.[9,14,18]

A case has been reported of the induction of renal failure by the association of captopril with metolazone.[20]

As already stated, metolazone can worsen diabetic control, raising blood sugar levels.

Symptomatic adverse effects
Several subjective side effects have been reported, but never validated against placebo. Rashes, nocturia, constipation, vertigo, headache and muscle cramps have been seen in groups of patients, but their attribution to drug treatment was mostly presumptive. In general, the profile of side effects and toxicity of metolazone seems to be very similar to that of thiazides.

Interference with clinical pathology tests
No technical interferences of this type have been reported.

High risk groups

Neonates
The drug is not recommended in neonates.

Breast milk. The drug enters breast milk, so nursing mothers should not breast-feed their infants while taking the drug.

Children
The drug is not recommended in children.

Pregnant women

There is little evidence of safety during pregnancy. Metolazone crosses the placenta but animal studies have shown no ill effects.

The elderly

There are no specific contraindications to the use of the drug in elderly patients, but, as with all diuretics, dosage and tolerance should be carefully monitored.

Concurrent disease

Little is known in this area for metolazone. Metolazone always increases potassium loss, and this side effect may be more pronounced and dangerous in oedematous patients, patients with congestive heart failure or liver cirrhosis. Serum potassium levels should be regularly monitored and potassium supplements should be given when needed.

Signs of overdosage of the drug arising from pharmacokinetic alterations due to organ failure have not been described, and even in patients with creatinine clearance < 50 $ml.min^{-1}$ no clinical evidence was found of accumulation of the drug or its metabolites.[12] However, the scarcity of kinetic studies, mainly because of the lack of a sensitive assay of drug concentrations in biological fluids, limits our knowledge. Using radiolabelled metolazone it was shown that its renal clearance was reduced in patients with renal failure, in parallel with creatinine clearance.

Drug interactions

Potentially hazardous interactions

Captopril. A case has been reported of the induction of renal failure by the association of captopril with metolazone.[20]

Potentially useful interactions

The synergistic effect of metolazone added to a maximal dose regimen of frusemide in refractory oedema has been reported by several studies reviewed by Oster et al.[21] The mechanism for this infection has still to be fully clarified[22] and seems to be shared by other thiazide-like diuretics. A pharmacokinetic interaction with frusemide has been ruled out.[23] The synergistic action with frusemide, though clinically useful, may cause severe potassium losses. Serum potassium should be carefully monitored during concomitant treatment with digitalis because of the increased risk of cardiac toxicity in presence of hypokalaemia.

References

1. Suki W N, Dawoud F, Eknoyan G, Martinez-Maldonado M 1972 Effects of metolazone on renal function in normal man. Journal of Pharmacology and Experimental Therapeutics 180: 6–12
2. Fotiu S, Mroczek W J, Davidov M, Finnerty F A Jr 1974 Antihypertensive efficacy of metolazone. Clinical Pharmacology and Therapeutics 16: 318–321
3. Hillenbrand P, Sherlock S 1971 Use of metolazone in the treatment of ascites due to liver disease. British Medical Journal 4: 266–270
4. Vose C W, Muirhead D C, Evans G L, Stevens P M, Burford S R 1981 Quantitation of metolazone in plasma and urine by high-performance liquid chromatography with fluorescence detection. Journal of Chromatography 222: 311–315
5. Hinsvark O N, Zazulak W, Cohen A I 1972 Liquid chromatography: its use in the biological characterization and study of metolazone. A new diuretic. Journal of Chromatographic Science 10: 379–383
6. Tilstone W J, Dargie H, Dargie E N, Morgan H G, Kennedy A C 1974 Pharmacokinetics of metolazone in normal subjects and in patients with cardiac or renal failure. Clinical Pharmacology and Therapeutics 16: 322–329
7. Bennett W M, Muther R S, Parker R A, Feig P, Morrison G, Golper T A, Singer I 1980 Drug therapy in renal failure: dosing guidelines for adults. II. Sedatives, hypnotics, and tranquilizers; cardiovascular, antihypertensive, and diuretic agents; miscellaneous agents. Annals of Internal Medicine 93: 286–325
8. Bennett W M, McDonald W J, Kuehnel E, Hartnett M N, Porter G A 1977 Do diuretics have antihypertensive properties independent of natriuresis? Clinical Pharmacology and Therapeutics 22: 499–504
9. Dornfeld L, Kane R E 1975 Metolazone in essential hypertension: the long-term clinical efficacy of a new diuretic. Current Therapeutic Research 18: 527–533
10. Cangiano J L 1976 Effects of prolonged administration of metolazone in the treatment of essential hypertension. Current Therapeutic Research 20: 745–750
11. Pilewski R M, Scheib E T, Misage J R, Kessler E, Krifcher E, Shapiro A P 1971 Technique of controlled drug assay in hypertension. V. Comparison of hydrochlorothiazide with a new quinethazone diuretic, metolazone. Clinical Pharmacology and Therapeutics 12: 843–848
12. Bennett W M, Porter G A 1973 Efficacy and safety of metolazone in renal failure and the nephrotic syndrome. Journal of Clinical Pharmacology 13: 357–364
13. Dargie H J, Allison M E M, Kennedy A C, Gray M J B 1972 High dosage metolazone in chronic renal failure. British Medical Journal 4: 196–198
14. Paton R R, Kane R E 1977 Long-term diuretic therapy with metolazone of renal failure and the nephrotic syndrome. Journal of Clinical Pharmacology 17: 243–251
15. Ram C V S, Reichgott M J 1977 Treatment of loop-diuretic resistant oedema by the addition of metolazone. Current Therapeutic Research 22: 686–691
16. Ghose R R, Gupta S K 1981 Synergistic action of metolazone with 'loop' diuretics. British Medical Journal 282: 1432–1433
17. Epstein M, Lepp B A, Hoffman D S, Levinson R 1977 Potentiation of furosemide by metolazone in refractory edema. Current Therapeutic Research 21: 656–667
18. Levey B A, Palmer R F 1975 Biochemical and clinical effects of metolazone in congestive heart failure. Current Therapeutic Research 18: 641–651
19. Rowe P A, Mather H G 1985 Hyperosmolar non-ketotic diabetes mellitus associated with metolazone. British Medical Journal 291: 25–26
20. Hogg K J, Hillis W S 1986 Captopril/metolazone induced renal failure. Lancet 1: 501–502
21. Oster J R, Epstein M, Smoller S 1983 Combined therapy with thiazide-type and loop diuretic agents for resistant sodium retention. Annals of Internal Medicine 99: 405–406
22. Brater D C, Pressley R H, Anderson S A 1985 Mechanisms of the synergistic combination of metolazone and bumetanide. Journal of Pharmacology and Experimental Therapeutics 233: 70–74
23. Marone C, Muggli F, Lahn W, Frey F J 1985 Pharmacokinetic and pharmacodynamic interaction between furosemide and metolazone in man. European Journal of Clinical Investigation 15: 253–257
24. Puschett J B 1986 Clinical pharmacologic implications in diuretic selection. American Journal of Cardiology 57: 6A–13A
25. Kiyingi A, Field M J, Pawsey C C, Yiannikas J, Lawrence J R, Arter W J 1990 Metolazone in treatment of severe refractory congestive cardiac failure. Lancet 335: 29–31

Metolazone

M Metoprolol (tartrate)

Metoprolol is a β_1-selective adrenoceptor blocking drug which has achieved wide therapeutic use.

Chemistry

Metoprolol tartrate (Betaloc, Betaloc-SA, Seloken, Lopresor, Lopresor SR)
$(C_{15}H_{25}NO_3)_2.C_4H_6O_6$
(dl)-1-Isopropylamino-3-[4-(2-methoxyethyl) phenoxy]propan-2-ol L-(d)-tartrate

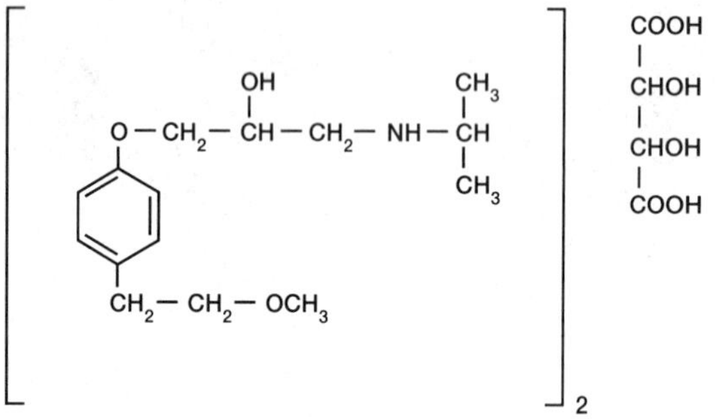

Molecular weight (free base)	684.8 (267.4)
pKa (amino group)	9.5
Solubility	
in alcohol	soluble
in water	very high
Octanol/water partition coefficient	0.5

A white, almost odourless powder with a bitter taste, it is prepared by chemical synthesis and the racemate is used clinically. The n-octanol/water partition coefficient is 0.98 at pH 7.4. Metoprolol tartrate is also available in an oral combination product with hydrochlorothiazide (Co-Betaloc, Co-Betaloc SA).

Pharmacology

Metoprolol is a competitive β_1-selective antagonist. Metoprolol is an effective antagonist of the inotropic and chronotropic responses to isoprenaline, with potency similar to propranolol. However to inhibit the vasodilator response to isoprenaline (mediated via β_2-adrenoceptors) the dose of metoprolol must be some 50 times greater than propranolol. Metoprolol reduces the plasma renin activity in both normal subjects and patients and inhibits the rise in renin activity induced by standing. Metoprolol has no direct agonist activity and its membrane stabilizing activity is only seen at doses much higher than those used clinically.[1–4]

Toxicology

Toxicology studies have not revealed any toxic effect other than the acute effects observed after administration of single high doses.[5] In teratological tests in rats (up to 200 mg.kg^{-1} daily) and rabbits (up to 25 mg.kg^{-1} daily) there were no effects on parent animals, as assessed by clinical signs, mortality, and body weight; offspring, as assessed by litter size, fetal loss, litter, and mean pup weight; and embryonic and fetal development, as assessed by incidence of abnormalities. The *salmonella*/mammalian microsome mutagenicity test revealed no mutagenic effect of metoprolol. Carcinogenicity tests on mice and rats revealed no carcinogenic effect.

Clinical pharmacology

Blockade of β_1-receptors resulting in a reduction of heart rate and blood pressure has been demonstrated in dose–response studies (25, 50 and 100 mg) in healthy subjects[6–8] and in disease.[9,10] The effect on heart rate lasts longer than expected from plasma half life and a significant antihypertensive effect persists for 24 h.[11–17] Metoprolol has been shown to reduce cardiac output[18,19] and inhibit renin release.[20–24]

Metoprolol has electrophysiological effects in that it slows the conduction velocity in sinus node and AV node.[25–27]

Metoprolol is a β_1-selective (cardioselective) β-blocker and since there is less blockade of β_2-receptors than that produced by non-cardioselective β-blockers there is less potential for bronchoconstriction and less inhibition of β_2-stimulant bronchodilators in both asthmatics[28,29] and bronchitics.[30] Metoprolol has similar cardioselectivity to atenolol.[31–34]

In comparison with non-cardioselective β-blockers metoprolol produces a smaller reduction in peripheral blood flow,[35] and a smaller increase in peripheral resistance and diastolic blood pressure in the presence of adrenaline or isoprenaline in both normals[36,37] and hypertensives.[38] Furthermore, during hypoglycaemia metoprolol, in comparison with non-cardioselective β-blockers, causes less inhibition of tachycardia, less increase of blood pressure and less delay in blood glucose recovery in normals[39] and diabetics.[40] In maturity onset diabetics metoprolol causes less interference with glucose tolerance.[41,42]

Metoprolol, in comparison with non-selective agents, causes less interference with the release of free fatty acids, glucose and insulin[43] and less effect on exercise capacity and metabolism during exercise.[44,45]

Pharmacokinetics

The most widely used analytical method has been gas–liquid chromatography of a fluorinated derivative with electron capture detection. The limit of sensitivity is approximately 5 µg.l^{-1}. However, liquid chromatography is now the preferred method in most laboratories.[46]

The drug is a racemic mixture and the pharmacologically active (S) enantiomer has slightly different pharmacokinetic properties from the less active (R) enantiomer.

Metoprolol is almost completely absorbed after oral administration, though the systemic bioavailability varies widely owing to extensive presystemic metabolism. Bioavailability may be increased by food.[47] Peak plasma concentrations are achieved after 2–3 h. The plasma half life is about 4 h (range 2.5–9.5 h in healthy subjects) and the liver is the main metabolizing organ. For any given dose there is a 10–20-fold variation in total plasma concentration between individuals as a consequence of presystemic metabolism, which ranges from $<5\%$ to 50% or more.[48] Metabolism of metoprolol by hydroxylation is subject to genetic polymorphism and poor metabolizers of debrisoquine/sparteine are also poor metabolizers of metoprolol. Poor metabolizers, who constitute about 8% of a Caucasian population, may develop very high plasma concentrations when given standard doses of metoprolol, largely because of much-reduced presystemic metabolism. (See reviews by Lennard, McDevitt and Smith.)

Metoprolol is rapidly and widely distributed throughout the body, with a high volume of distribution of 3–6 l.kg^{-1}. The drug crosses the blood–brain barrier and is found in brain tissue in concentrations 6–7 times those in plasma and is also found in cerebrospinal fluid in concentrations slightly lower than in plasma.[49] Metoprolol is found in the lung, liver and kidney in concentrations significantly higher than that in plasma. High concentrations of the drug are present in bile but very little is eliminated in the faeces, due presumably to reabsorption. Metoprolol is not bound to plasma proteins to any appreciable extent (12%). The pharmacokinetics of metoprolol have been reviewed by Regardh.[50]

Metoprolol is excreted in breast milk in concentrations 3.5 times higher than those in plasma. However, the amount of the drug ingested by a breast-feeding infant would be less than 0.1 mg.kg^{-1} daily and so it is unlikely to induce adverse reactions in the infant unless its liver function was severely under-developed. Metoprolol readily crosses the placenta into the fetus.[51,52]

Oral absorption	>95%
Presystemic metabolism	40–60%
Plasma half life	
range	3–5 h
mean	3 h
Volume of distribution	3–6 l.kg^{-1}
Plasma protein binding	12%

Metoprolol is extensively biotransformed in the liver, with only 10% of the drug eliminated unchanged, by excretion in the urine. In severe liver disease the elimination of metoprolol is impaired, with significant elevation of peak plasma concentrations and a prolonged half life in some patients.[53]

There is no evidence for any effect of renal disease on the pharmacokinetics of metoprolol.[54] Old age has no significant effect on the pharmacokinetics of the drug.[55] Thyrotoxicosis may result in an increase in the metabolism of metoprolol, with decreased plasma concentrations.

Concentration-effect relationship

Measurement of plasma concentration is not generally of value as a guide to dosage, although it may be of value in patients who suffer severe side effects at normal doses and lead to detection of poor metabolizers. Reduction of exercise-induced tachycardia is proportional to the logarithm of the plasma concentration over the range 20–100 μg.l^{-1} and effects are detected[52] at 5–10 μg.l^{-1}. There is no defined relationship between plasma levels of metoprolol and antihypertensive activity[9,56] although there may be some correlation.[57] In angina pectoris no correlation has been established between the plasma concentration and the antianginal effects.[58]

Metabolism

Metoprolol is extensively metabolized by the liver, with very little of the drug excreted unchanged. Excretion is almost entirely (>90%) in the urine, with less than 5% in the faeces. There is no evidence of entero-hepatic circulation.

Three primary pathways of metabolism have been described (see Fig. 1).

O-demethylation to O-desmethylmetoprolol (1%) and subsequent rapid oxidation to the corresponding acid, 4-(2-hydroxy-3-isopropylaminopropoxy)phenylacetic acid (65%); oxidative deamination to 2-hydroxy-3-[4-(2-methoxyethyl)phenoxy]propionic acid (10%); aliphatic hydroxylation to α-hydroxymetoprolol (10%).

Two of these metabolites, O-desmethylmetoprolol and α-hydroxymetoprolol, are β_1-blocking agents, but they are substantially less potent than the parent drug, and do not contribute to the β-blocking activity of metoprolol. The plasma half life of α-hydroxymetoprolol is 4 to 12 h (mean 6 h). The oxidation of metoprolol is polymorphic, sharing the same genetic regulation as the 4-hydroxylation of debrisoquine, due to the involvement of the same form of cytochrome P-450 in the two activities. Plasma concentrations of metoprolol are 3–4 times higher in poor metabolizers than in extensive metabolizers.[59] The pathways of metoprolol oxidation that are impaired in poor metabolizers include aliphatic oxidation and O-demethylation. The clinical implications of this are not clear, although a small number of cases of excessive pharmacological effect have been reported in poor metabolizers.[59,60]

Pharmaceutics

Metoprolol is available in oral and parenteral forms:

White Betaloc tablets (Astra, UK) contain 50 mg and 100 mg of metoprolol tartrate BP and are coded A/BB and A/ME respectively. Pale red, scored 'Lopresor' 100 mg tablets (Geigy Pharmaceuticals,

Fig. 1 Metabolism of metoprolol

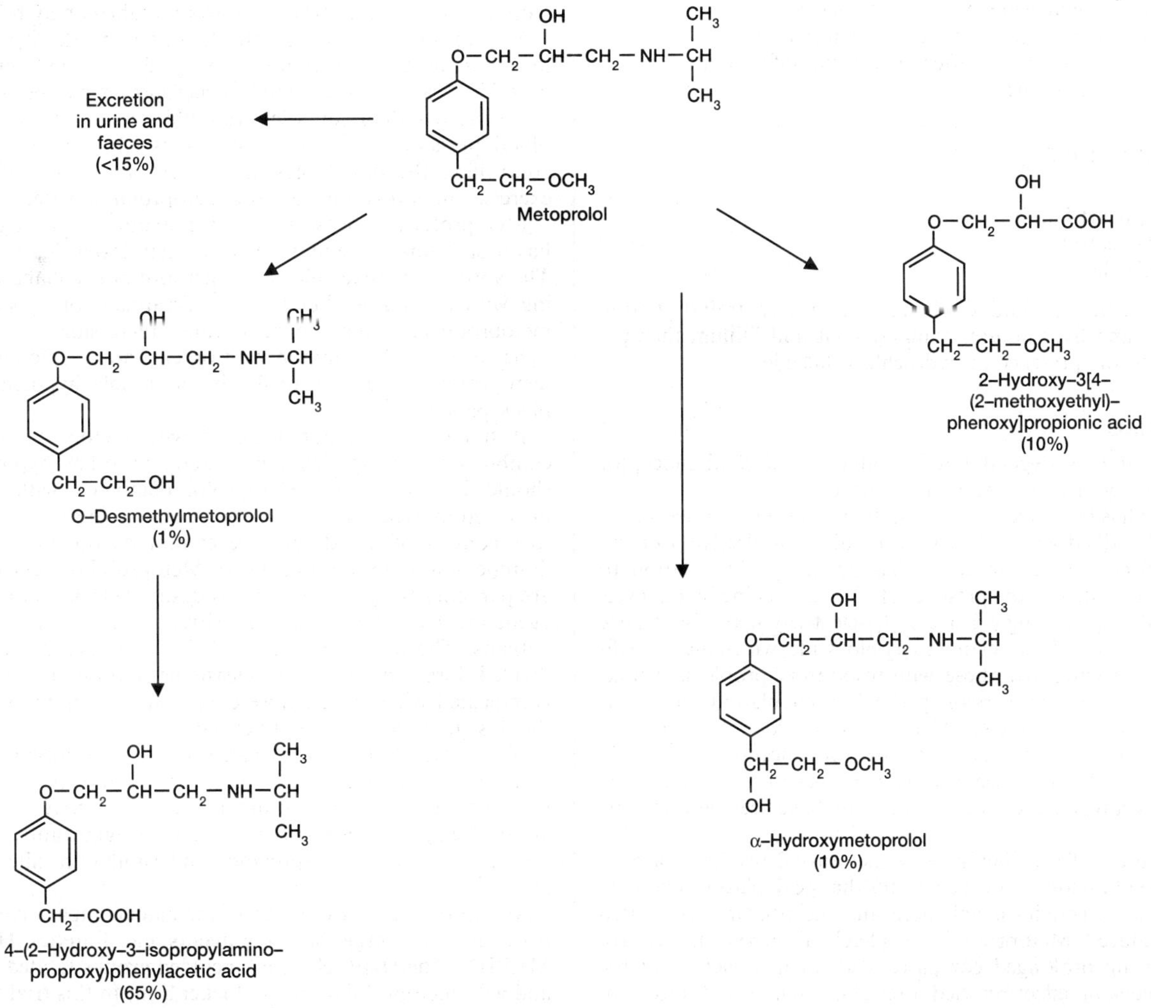

UK/USA) contain 50 mg metoprolol tartrate BP engraved Geigy on one side. Light blue scored tablets (Geigy UK) contain 100 mg metoprolol tartrate BP and are labelled Geigy on one side.

In addition white scored 'Co-Betaloc' tablets coded A/MH contain 100 mg metoprolol tartrate BP and 12.5 mg hydrochlorothiazide BP. 'Lopresoretic' are off-white scored on one side, impressed GEIGY on the other side and contain 100 mg metoprolol tartrate BP and 12.5 mg chlorthalidone BP.

Sustained-release tablets containing 200 mg metoprolol tartrate in a formulation based on the Durule principle which is an inert plastic matrix. These white tablets are coded A/MD and are called 'Betaloc SA'. A combination formulation, 'Co-Betaloc SA', consists of a yellow biconvex film-coated tablet engraved A/MC and comprises 200 mg metoprolol tartrate BP in a white layer which is a sustained-release formulation based on the Durule principle, and a yellow layer containing 25 mg hydrochlorothiazide BP which is rapidly released. 'Lopresor SR' (Geigy UK) are pale yellow tablets containing 200 mg metoprolol tartrate with Geigy imprinted on one side and CDC on the other. These are sustained-release tablets using the wax matrix principle.

Metoprolol is available for intravenous use as a solution containing metoprolol tartrate 1 mg per ml in 5 ml ampoules (Betaloc, Astra; Lopresor, Geigy UK). It is a clear solution which should be protected from the light. Metoprolol preparations are stable with a shelf-life of 3 years, and carry a minimal risk from potentially allergenic substances. All preparations should be stored in a cool dry place and protected from light, heat and moisture.

Therapeutic use

Indications

1. The management of hypertension
2. The management of angina pectoris
3. The control of cardiac arrhythmias, especially supraventricular tachyarrhythmias
4. The adjunctive management of thyrotoxicosis
5. Early intervention in acute myocardial infarction
6. The reduction of mortality after myocardial infarction
7. Prophylaxis of migraine.

Contraindications

1. AV block
2. Refractory heart failure
3. Severe bradycardia
4. Cardiogenic shock.

In addition 'Co-Betaloc' and 'Co-Betaloc SA' are contraindicated in severe kidney and liver failure, manifest gout and lithium therapy, which relate to the presence of hydrochlorothiazide.

Mode of use

All the clinical uses depend upon production of β-adrenoceptor blockade, usually of β_1-receptors in the heart.

Metoprolol has been found to be effective and well tolerated in the indications described above. In contrast with non-selective β-blockers, its β_1-selective blocking action has advantages in relation to blood pressure control in the presence of high adrenaline blood levels as in physical or physiological stress. β_1-selectivity may also reduce the incidence of side effects related to β_2-blockade, which may benefit many patients, particularly those with respiratory problems, smokers, diabetics, those with poor peripheral circulation, or those carrying out physical exercise. Metoprolol should not be used in patients with known asthma as higher doses or concentrations (e.g. in poor metabolizers) may cause appreciable blockade of β_2-mediated responses. The advantages of cardioselectivity have been described by Kendall.[61]

Administration of sustained-release metoprolol results in a controlled release of metoprolol which means that peak plasma levels are reduced and so selectivity is enhanced and the risk of dose-related side effects reduced. Metoprolol is completely absorbed, the absorption phase being prolonged compared with plain tablets, and the maximal β-blocking effect reached after about 4 h. The duration of effect is extended and so sustained-release metoprolol is effective in hypertension and angina when taken once daily which may aid patient compliance.

The sustained-release formulation of metoprolol ('Lopresor SR') has been compared with 'Betaloc SA'.[62] Only 'Betaloc SA' was associated with significantly higher plasma metoprolol concentrations at the end of a dosing interval. The mean reduction in exercise tachycardia at the end of a dosing interval was significantly greater with 'Betaloc SA' than with 'Lopresor SR' and conventional metoprolol.

The dose of metoprolol must always be adjusted to the individual requirements of the patient and the dosage guidelines depend on the indication.

Sudden withdrawal of metoprolol can be hazardous for patients who have ischaemic heart disease. When discontinuing treatment with metoprolol, therefore, the drug should usually be withdrawn gradually, i.e. over 7–10 days. Currently it is thought that metoprolol administration should be continued up to and including surgery for patients undergoing anaesthesia. If withdrawal of therapy or reduction of dosage is considered necessary, this should be done gradually in hospital.

Indications

1. Hypertension

Metoprolol has been found to be effective in the treatment of hypertension[63,64] and can lower the blood pressure to normotensive levels in about 50–75% of patients with mild to moderate hypertension when used as monotherapy in plain tablets. Higher response rates have been reported with sustained-release metoprolol and with metoprolol in combination formulations with a diuretic.

In hypertension the starting dose of metoprolol is 100 mg daily. This may be increased by 100 mg daily at weekly intervals until the total daily dose is in the range 100–400 mg, usually divided into a twice-daily dose.

Sustained-release metoprolol dosage is usually one tablet, once daily in the morning. In rare cases two tablets may be indicated.

Metoprolol is at least as effective as non selective β-blockers in lowering the blood pressure when given in equipotent β-blocking doses[65–67] and in some studies metoprolol has been found to be more effective than non-selective β-blockers in lowering the diastolic blood pressure.[68–71] Metoprolol is as effective as methyldopa in controlling the blood pressure at rest and more effective during exercise and stress: furthermore metoprolol is better tolerated.[72,75]

Metoprolol is at least as effective as diuretics in high dose[74] and has been found to be more effective than lower doses of diuretics.[75] The antihypertensive efficacy of metoprolol is enhanced by combining with a thiazide diuretic.[76,77] Treatment of hypertension with metoprolol has been shown to cause regression of left ventricular hypertrophy.[78] In common with other β-adrenergic blocking drugs, metoprolol is relatively ineffective as a sole hypotensive agent in black patients.[79]

If full control is not achieved with metoprolol monotherapy, combination therapy with a diuretic or other hypotensive agent should be considered. Metoprolol combined with a diuretic is indicated in hypertension and may be suitable for use when satisfactory control of blood pressure cannot be obtained with either a diuretic or a β-blocker used alone. Metoprolol/diuretic combinations are particularly suitable when it is desirable to keep the dose of each agent low as in particularly sensitive patients, for example elderly patients. The dosage is usually 1–3 tablets per day as a single or divided dose. The sustained-release metoprolol/diuretic formulation is indicated when higher dose combination therapy is required and the dosage is usually one tablet daily.

Metoprolol/diuretic combinations have been found to be effective and well tolerated in elderly patients[80,81] and the sustained-release preparations have been found to be an effective antihypertensive agent when given once daily,[82,73] and are significantly more effective over 24 h than slow oxprenolol and similar in efficacy to atenolol.[84–87]

Metoprolol was used in two of the main comparative clinical trials between β-adrenergic blocking agents and diuretics, HAPPHY and MAPHY. The HAPPHY trial included groups treated with atenolol and with metoprolol in the β-blocker arm. In this trial there were no significant differences between the outcome on the two regimes. The MAPHY trial was a continuation of the metoprolol group from the HAPPHY trial. This trial showed a greater reduction in cardiovascular events in the metoprolol-treated group than in the diuretic-treated patients. Unlike the MRC trial, which used propranolol, benefit was seen in both smokers and non-smokers. There has been a great deal of debate about the statistical validity of continuing the MAPHY study in a 'sub-group' of the HAPPHY trial. See Major Outcome trials and reviews by Furberg, Moser and Berglund.

2. Angina pectoris

In patients with angina pectoris metoprolol reduces the attack rate and increases the physical working capacity in both young and elderly patients.[88–90] Metoprolol tablets are usually given 50–100 mg twice or three times daily and sustained-release metoprolol as one tablet once daily. It is at least as effective as propranolol in the treatment of angina pectoris.[7,91,92] A decrease in ST-segment depression during exercise after long-term treatment with metoprolol has been observed suggesting a gradual improvement in myocardial ischaemia.[93]

Sustained-release metoprolol has been shown to be effective and well tolerated in elderly patients[90] and to be effective in angina when given once daily.[94,95]

3. Cardiac arrhythmias

Metoprolol controls heart rate in supraventricular tachycardia. Its use often re-establishes sinus rhythm or reduces ventricular rate in patients with paroxysmal atrial tachycardia. In patients with atrial fibrillation or flutter metoprolol can reduce ventricular rate and may also restore sinus rhythm. Metoprolol also reduces the number of ventricular extrasystoles. As a result of the diappointing results of the CAST trial with the type-1 antiarrhythmics, encainide and flecainide, there is renewed interest in the use of β-blockers in ventricular arrhythmias. Hypotension has been reported when metoprolol injection has been given to patients with congestive heart failure, idiopathic hypotension or acute myocardial infarction, but the incidence of hypotension after metoprolol injection in patients without risk factors is low.[96–103] It is very important to remember that parenteral dosing bypasses presystemic metabolism in the liver so the dose given intravenously may be equivalent to twice to twenty times the same dose given by mouth.

Initially up to 5 mg of metoprolol by injection, at a rate of 1–2 mg.min^{-1}, is given. The injection can be repeated at 5-minute intervals until a satisfactory response has been obtained. Because of the risk of a pronounced drop of blood pressure the intravenous administration of metoprolol to patients with a systolic blood pressure below 100 mgHg should only be given with special care. Following the treatment of an acute arrhythmia with injections, continuation therapy with oral metoprolol should be initiated 4–6 h later with an initial oral dose not exceeding 50 mg three times daily. Metoprolol tablets 50 mg twice daily or three times daily should usually control the condition. If necessary the dose can be increased up to 300 mg per day in divided doses.

The use of metoprolol premedication in patients undergoing elective surgery may protect the heart against the effects of excessive sympathetic stimulation including arrhythmias or acute coronary insufficiency.[104–108] Metoprolol, 2–4 mg injected slowly intravenously at induction is usually sufficient to prevent the development of arrhythmias during anaesthesia, or to control arrhythmias developing after anaesthesia. Further injections of 2 mg may be given as required to a maximum dose of 10 mg.

4. Thyrotoxicosis

Metoprolol is effective in reducing the clinical manifestations of hyperthyroidism. It gives rapid symptomatic relief and may be used concomitantly with all antithyroid treatment. Metoprolol bridges the time lag until antithyroid treatment is effective.[109–113] The usual dose of metoprolol is 50 mg four times daily.

5. Myocardial infarction

Early intervention with metoprolol in acute myocardial infarction reduces infarct size[114] and the incidence of ventricular fibrillation.[115] Pain relief has been demonstrated[116] and this may decrease the need for opiate analgesics. Metoprolol has been shown to reduce mortality at 3 months when administered orally to patients with acute myocardial infarction[117] for 3 months. In addition the safety of metoprolol[118] and its ability to reduce heart failure[119] have been demonstrated. More recently treatment with intravenous metoprolol within 24 h of the onset of symptoms followed by oral metoprolol treatment for 15 days demonstrated a 13% difference in mortality compared with placebo (NS). A retrospective analysis of a high risk group category, however, demonstrated a 29% reduction in mortality compared with placebo.[120]

In early intervention optimal benefits from intravenous metoprolol are obtained if patients are presented within 12 h of the onset of chest pain. Therapy should commence with 5 mg intravenously every two minutes to a maximum of 15 mg total as determined by blood pressure and heart rate. Oral therapy should commence 15 minutes after the injection with 50 mg every 6 h for 48 h. Patients who fail to tolerate the full intravenous dose should be given half the suggested oral dose. The usual maintenance dose is 200 mg daily.

Metoprolol has been used in several large secondary prevention trials in myocardial infarction such as MIAMI, TIMI, Lopressor Intervention Trial etc. The results have been mixed, with the large MIAMI and Lopressor Intervention Trials showing no significant benefit but the metoprolol group in some of the other trials showing reduced mortality and reinfarction in line with experience from other β-blocker trials in patients who have suffered a myocardial infarction. See Major outcome trials.

Contraindications

1. AV block

Since metoprolol prolongs the conduction velocity at the AV node and slows the idioventricular rate, it is contraindicated in second and third degree heart block.[25,26]

2. Refractory heart failure

Because of the negative inotropic effects of metoprolol due to β_1-receptor blockade metoprolol is contraindicated in digitalis or diuretic refractory or uncompensated heart failure.

3. Severe bradycardia

Metoprolol is contraindicated in marked bradycardia because of the negative chronotropic effects of the drug due to β_1-receptor blockade. Physically fit hypertensive patients with slow heart rates due to athletic training do not appear to suffer any adverse effects from further moderate bradycardia induced by metoprolol, provided their ECG shows normal conduction.

4. Cardiogenic shock

Metoprolol has negative chronotropic effects due to β_1-receptor blockade and for this reason it is contraindicated in cardiogenic shock and in patients with a low cardiac output who may not yet be in shock.

Adverse reactions

Potentially life-threatening effects

The myocardial depressant effects of β-blockers may occasionally have fatal results.

Acute overdosage

Cases of deliberate overdose have occurred and deaths have been recorded. One patient who took a fatal overdose had a plasma concentration[121] of 19.8 mg.l^{-1}. The main clinical features of massive overdose include symptoms of cardiodepression particularly hypotension and bradycardia. Metoprolol has not been found to be conclusively the cause of death, as salicylate and traces of barbiturate have also been found.[122] A fatal case occurred following ingestion of 75 × 100 mg tablets,[123] but non-fatal cases occurred following the ingestion of 25 × 100 mg tablets and 200 × 50 mg tablets.[124,125]

The marked bradycardia may be treated by intravenous atropine sulphate (0.5–3.0 mg) and in severe cases by slow intravenous infusion of about 5 µg.l^{-1}.min^{-1} of isoprenaline. Alternatively, prenalterol 2–5 mg intravenously at 2–5-minute intervals until the desired effect is achieved may be tried. Glucagon may be useful and is more generally available.

Severe or irreversible adverse effects

Severe bradycardia and/or myocardial depression may occur.

Symptomatic adverse effects

Metoprolol is generally well tolerated and adverse effects are mild and have been infrequently reported. The commonest appear to be lassitude, cold peripheries, gastrointestinal disturbances, and disturb-

Metoprolol (tartrate)

ances of sleep pattern. If patients suffer these side effects severely at normal doses the possibility that they are poor metabolizers who have very high plasma concentrations should be considered. In many cases these effects have been transient and have disappeared after a reduction in dosage. There has been a small reported incidence of skin rashes and/or dry eyes. In most cases the symptoms have cleared when treatment was withdrawn. Discontinuation of the drug should be considered if any such reaction is not otherwise explicable. In large-scale, long-term studies, when data on adverse effects has been included with a questionnaire, the incidence of such effects was low and similar to that in patients on placebo in both hypertension[126] and angina.[127] The incidence of CNS adverse effects is low[128] but greater than those observed with hydrophilic β_1-blockers.[129,130]

Other effects

Alterations in serum lipid levels have been reported in patients taking metoprolol. These comprise significant increases in total triglyceride and very low density lipoproteins (VLDL) triglyceride, and reduction in high density lipoprotein (HDL) cholesterol and ratio of HDL and LDL cholesterol.[131]

Interference with clinical pathology tests

There are no significant effects of metoprolol on common laboratory tests.[132]

High risk groups

Neonates

Metoprolol is not recommended for therapeutic use in neonates. However pharmacologically significant blood levels of metoprolol occur in neonates of mothers treated with metoprolol but no adverse effects have been observed.[133]

Breast milk. The concentrations of metoprolol in breast milk are unlikely to cause harm to the breast-fed infant unless its liver function is grossly underdeveloped.

Children

Metoprolol is not recommended for children, as the safety and efficacy have not been established.

Pregnant women

Metoprolol is not recommended during pregnancy. However, metoprolol has been found to be an effective and well tolerated antihypertensive agent in pregnancy. The drug crosses the placenta and slows the fetal heart rate.[134]

The elderly

There is no significant difference in the volume of distribution, elimination half life, total body clearance, or bioavailability of metoprolol in healthy elderly patients.[55] There is no evidence of an increased risk of metoprolol therapy provided standard contraindications are observed.

Concurrent disease

Heart disease. Digitalization with or without diuretics should be considered in patients with a history of heart failure or with poor cardiac reserve. In patients with renal failure no dose adjustment of metoprolol is needed since this disease has no important effect on either the pharmacokinetics or the β-blocking effect of metoprolol.[54] In severe liver disease peak blood levels of metoprolol are significantly increased and the half life is significantly prolonged in a few. Hence it is advisable to reduce the dosage initially in patients with portacaval shunts or signs of advanced liver disease.[53]

Lung disease. In chronic obstructive lung disease caution in administering metoprolol is advised despite its relative cardioselectivity. Formgren recommended that the total daily dose of metoprolol should not exceed 100 mg.[135] In patients with mild seasonal asthma, additional therapy with a β_2-stimulant (eg. terbutaline) may be advisable.[135,136]

Diabetes. In labile and insulin-dependent diabetes it may be necessary to adjust the hypoglycaemic therapy.[121]

Thyrotoxicosis. In thyrotoxicosis the metoprolol blood levels are decreased and therefore it may be necessary to increase the dose.

Drug interactions

Potentially hazardous interactions

Verapamil. Although oral verapamil can be coprescribed with a β-blocker with relative safety, great care should be taken in the presence of AV nodal and left ventricular dysfunction. The concurrent treatment of metoprolol and verapamil may result in bradycardia, hypotension and asystole particularly after intravenous administration.

Hypoglycaemic agents. Hypoglycaemic symptoms are uncommon in patients taking β-blockers and most insulin-requiring diabetics may be given β-blockers. There is evidence that non-selective, compared to selective, β-blockers caused a fall in blood glucose during and after submaximal exercise. Hypoglycaemia is undoubtedly a rare but important adverse effect with non-selective β-blockade. The concurrent administration of metoprolol and hypoglycaemic agents may alter the response to hypoglycaemia but it presents only a minor clinical problem.

Propafenone. Combined use of metoprolol and propafenone increases the plasma concentration of the former agent by approximately a factor of two.[137]

Cimetidine. Maximum plasma concentrations of the (R) enantiomer of metoprolol were increased by 40% and of the active (S) enantiomer by 20% when cimetidine was added to treatment[138].

General anaesthesia. The concurrent administration of metoprolol and anaesthetic agents may give rise to additive negative inotropic effects and therefore anaesthetics with minimum negative inotropic effects are preferred. The anaesthetist must be informed if the patient is taking metoprolol. It appears that cyclopropane, diethylether, fluroxene, trichlorethylene, methoxyflurane, and, possibly, enflurane should not be used in β-blocked patients. By comparison, provided that carbon dioxide retention is avoided, halothane, isoflurane, nitrous oxide, the available intravenous induction agents, muscle relaxants, narcotic analgesics, and local anaesthetics are all compatible with β-blockade.

Other significant interactions

The bioavailability of metoprolol may be enhanced by food.[47]

Potentially useful interactions

Nifedipine. Combining metoprolol and nifedipine leads to an enhancement of antianginal efficacy.[139–141]

Verapamil. As with other β-blockers the oral combination of metoprolol and verapamil may be advantageous in anginal patients in whom response to either drug alone is inadequate.

Nitrates. Combining metoprolol and nitrates leads to an enhancement of antianginal efficacy.

Diuretics and vasodilators. The antihypertensive efficacy of metoprolol is enhanced by combining it with diuretics and vasodilators (e.g. hydralazine and nifedipine).[142]

Class I antiarrhythmic agents. Metoprolol can safely be combined with Class I antiarrhythmic agents such as tocainide.[143,144]

Digitalis. In patients with congestive cardiomyopathy metoprolol has been combined with digitalis (or diuretics) to good effect.[145] The combination with digitalis is also useful in supraventricular arrhythmias, notably atrial fibrillation.

β_2-stimulants. Metoprolol given in a normal therapeutic dose does not block the bronchodilating action of a β_2-stimulant but might do so in a poor metabolizer with a high plasma concentration.

Major outcome trials

Ischaemic heart disease

1. Hjalmarson A, Elmfeldt D, Herlitz J, Holmberg S, Malek I et al 1981 Effect on mortality of metoprolol in acute myocardial infarction. A double-blind randomised trial. Lancet 2: 823–827

The effect of metoprolol on mortality was compared with that of placebo in a double-blind randomized trial in patients with definite or suspected acute myocardial infarction. Treatment with metoprolol or placebo started on average 11.1 h after the onset of chest pain and was continued for 90 days. Metoprolol was given as a 15 mg intravenous dose followed by oral administration of 100 mg twice daily. 1395 patients (697 on placebo and 698 on metoprolol) were included in the trial. Definite acute myocardial infarction developed in 809 and probable infarction in 162. Patients were allocated to various risk groups and within each group patients were randomly assigned to treatment with metoprolol or placebo. There were 62 deaths in the placebo group (8.9%) and 40 deaths in the metoprolol group (5.7%), a reduction of 36% ($p < 0.03$) at 3 months. There was

Metoprolol (tartrate)

no reduction in mortality during the first week of treatment so that benefit from early intervention could not be established.

2. The MIAMI Trial Research Group 1985 Metoprolol in acute myocardial infarction (MIAMI). A randomized placebo-controlled international trial. European Heart Journal 6: 199–226

The effect of metoprolol on mortality and morbidity after 15 days was compared with that of placebo in a double-blind randomized international trial in patients with definite or suspected acute myocardial infarction. Treatment with intravenous metoprolol (15 mg) or placebo was started shortly after the patient's arrival in hospital within 24 h of the onset of symptoms, and then oral treatment (200 mg daily) was continued for the study period (15 days). Of the 5778 patients included, 2901 were allocated to placebo and 2877 to metoprolol. There were 142 deaths in the placebo group (4.9%) and 123 deaths in the metoprolol group (4.3%) a non-significant difference of 13%.

Previously recorded risk indicators of mortality were analysed in retrospect. In this higher risk category the mortality rate in the metoprolol-treated group was 29% less than in the placebo group.

There was no significant effect on ventricular fibrillation but the number of episodes tended to be lower in the metoprolol-treated patients during the later phase (6–15 days). The incidence of supraventricular tachyarrhythmias, the use of cardiac glycosides and other antiarrhythmics, and the need for pain-relieving treatment were significantly diminished by metoprolol amongst all randomized patients. Adverse effects associated with metoprolol were infrequent, expected and relatively mild.

3. Olsson G, Rehnqvist N, Sjogren A, Erhardt L, Lundman T 1985 Long-term treatment with metoprolol after myocardial infarction: effect on 3 year mortality and morbidity. Journal of the American College of Cardiology 5(6): 1428–1437

This was a study on 301 patients with acute myocardial infarction who represented 66% of a total of 556 patients under 70 years of age admitted to two hospital coronary care units within 48 h of onset of symptoms and living in a circumscribed catchment area. The excluded patients were 37 from outside the catchment area, 157 who did not meet the inclusion criteria and 61 who died in the coronary care unit.

The patients were randomized to treatment with metoprolol 100 mg or placebo and they were followed up for 36 months. The major findings were non-significant reduction in death rates overall; 31 out of 147 in the placebo group and 25 out of 154 in the metoprolol group. However, there was a significant reduction in mortality in the sub-group of patients with large infarcts, a significant reduction in sudden deaths in the metoprolol group and a significant reduction in non-fatal infarcts in the metoprolol group. The beneficial effect of long-term metoprolol treatment was continuous over the three years of the study.

4. Lopressor Intervention Trial Research Group 1987 The Lopressor intervention trial: multicentre study of metoprolol in survivors of acute myocardial infarction. European Heart Journal 8: 1056–1064

2395 patients with acute myocardial infarction were treated with metoprolol 200 mg daily or placebo for up to 1 year. There was no significant difference in mortality at 12 and 18 months of follow-up.

5. Herlitz J, Kjalmarson A, Swedberg K, Ryden K, Waagstein F 1988 Effects on mortality during five years early intervention with metoprolol in suspected acute myocardial infarction. Acta Medica Scandinavica 223: 227–231

In a randomized double-blind study 1395 patients with chest pain of >30 minutes duration and ECG/enzyme evidence of myocardial infarction received metoprolol 15 mg intravenously followed by 200 mg daily by mouth, or placebo, for 3 months. At 3 months the mortality was 5.7% in the metoprolol group and 8.9% on placebo ($p = 0.02$). At 2 years the mortality was 13.2% and 17.2% respectively ($p = 0.04$) and at 5 years 24.2% and 25.7% (NS).

6. The TIMI Study Group 1989 Comparison of invasive and conservative strategies after treatment with intravenous tissue plasminogen activator in acute myocardial infarction. Results of the Thrombolysis in Myocardial Infarction (TIMI) phase II trial. New England Journal of Medicine 320: 618–627

This was primarily a trial of conservative therapy (alteplase) versus invasive therapy (alteplase plus early PTCA) in patients with acute myocardial infarction. Within the trial, 1390 patients were randomized to immediate intravenous metoprolol or deferred treatment with oral metoprolol beginning at 6 days. Immediate β-blocker therapy was associated with fewer deaths and recurrent infarctions.

Hypertension

7. Wilhelmsen L, Berglund G, Elmfeldt D et al 1987 Beta blockers versus diuretics in hypertensive men. Main results from the HAPPHY trial. Journal of Hypertension 5: 561–72

The HAPPHY trial included 6568 patients. It was constructed by bringing together two studies both of which involved a β-blocker diuretic comparison, in one case atenolol and the other metoprolol. The β-blocker groups were not separated in the presentation of the results. There were a total of 96 deaths in the β-blocker group and 101 in the diuretic-treated patients. There were 50 cardiovascular deaths on diuretics and 54 on β-blockers. None of these differences was statistically significant.

8. Wikstrand J, Warnold I, Olsson G, Tuomilheto J, Elmfeldt D, Berglung G 1988 Primary results with metoprolol in patients with hypertension. Mortality results from the MAPHY study. Journal of the American Medical Association 259: 1976–1982

The study included 3234 patients, 1609 randomized to metoprolol and 1625 to the diuretic. The study was drawn from 66 of the 70 investigators using metoprolol in the HAPPHY trial. Patients were followed for at least 842 days, although the median follow-up was 4.2 years. At 842 days there were 15 deaths in the metoprolol group and 27 on diuretics. The cumulative death rate was low in non-smokers ($n = 2097$) and not significantly different on the two regimes. The death rate was nearly 4 times higher in smokers ($n = 1059$) and was significantly less in those treated with metoprolol ($p = 0.013$)

General review articles

Brogden R N, Heel R C, Speight T M Avery G S 1977 Metoprolol: a review of its pharmacological properties and therapeutic efficacy in hypertension and angina pectoris. Drugs 14: 321–348

Koch-Weser J 1979 Metoprolol. New England Journal of Medicine 301: 698–703

Regardh C-G, Johnsson G 1980 Clinical pharmacokinetics of metoprolol. Clinical Pharmacokinetics 5: 557–569

Kendall M J 1981 Are selective β-adrenoceptor blocking drugs an advantage? Journal of the Royal College of Physicians, London 15: 33–40

Ablad B 1979 In: Goldberg F (ed) Pharmacological and biochemical properties of drug substances, Volume II, pp 188–228

Ablad B 1980 In: Scriabine E (ed) Pharmacology of antihypertensive drugs. Raven Press, New York, pp 247–262

Ablad B, Bork K O, Carlsson E, Johnsson G, Malmfors T, Regardh C-G 1975 Animal and human pharmacological studies on metoprolol — a new selective adrenergic β-receptor antagonist. Acta Pharmacologica et Toxicologica 36 (suppl V)

Lennard MS, Tucker GT, Silas JH, Woods HF 1986 Debrisquine polymorphism and the metabolism and action of metoprolol, timolol, propranolol and atenolol. Xenobiotica 16: 435–37

McDevitt DG 1987 Comparison of pharmacokinetic properties of beta adrenoceptor blocking drugs. European Heart Journal 8 (suppl M): 9–14

Smith RL 1985 Polymorphic metabolism of beta-adrenoceptor blocking drugs and its clinical relevance. European Journal of Clinical Pharmacology 28 (suppl): 77–84

Berglund G 1989 Beta blockers and diuretics. The HAPPHY and MAPHY studies. Clinical and Experimental Hypertension 11: 1137–48

Moser M, Sheps S 1989 Confusing messages from the newest of the beta-blocker/diuretic hypertension trials. The Metoprolol Atherosclerosis Prevention in Hypertension Trial. Archives of Internal Medicine 149: 2174–2175

Furberg CD, Cutler JA 1989 Diuretic agents versus beta blockers. Comparison of effects on mortality, stroke and cardiovascular events. Hypertension 13: 157–161

References

1. Ablad B, Carlsson E, Ek L 1973 Pharmacological studies of two new cardioselective adrenergic β-receptor antagonists. Life Sciences 12, Part 1: 107–119
2. Lundgren B, Carlsson E, Herrmann I 1979 β-adrenoceptor blockade by atenolol, metoprolol and propranolol in the anaesthetized cat. European Journal of Pharmacology 55: 263–268
3. Ablad B, Borg K O, Carlsson E, Ek L, Johnsson G, Malmfors T, Regardh C-G 1975 A survey of the pharmacological properties of metoprolol in animals and man. Acta Pharmacologica et Toxicologica 36 (suppl V): 7–23
4. Ablad B, Carlsson B, Carlsson E 1974 Cardiac effects of β-adrenergic receptor antagonists. Advances in Cardiology 12: 290–302
5. Bodin N-O, Flodh H, Magnusson G, Malmfors T, Nyberg J-A 1975 Toxicological studies on metoprolol. Acta Pharmacologica et Toxicologica 36 (suppl) V: 96–103
6. Johnsson G, Regardh C-G, Solvell L 1975 Combined pharmacokinetic and pharmacodynamic studies in man of the adrenergic β-1-receptor antagonist metoprolol. Acta Pharmacologica et Toxicologica 36 (suppl V): 31–44
7. Regardh C-G, Johnsson G, Jordo L, Lungborg P, Persson B-A, Ronn O 1980 Plasma concentrations and β-blocking effects in normal volunteers after intravenous doses of metoprolol and propranolol. Journal of Cardiovascular Pharmacology 2: 715–723
8. Gugler R, Krist R, Raczinski H, Hoffgen K, Bodem G 1980 Comparative pharmacodynamics and plasma levels of β-adrenoceptor blocking drugs. British Journal of Clinical Pharmacology 10: 337–343
9. Myers M G, Thiessen J J 1980 Metoprolol kinetics and dose response in hypertensive patients. Clinical Pharmacology and Therapeutics 27: 756–762
10. Uusitalo A, Keyrilainen O, Johnsson G 1981 A dose-response study on metoprolol in angina pectoris. Annals of Clinical Research 13: 54–57
11. Regardh C-G, Johnsson G, Jordo L, Solvell L 1975 Comparative bioavailability and effect studies on metoprolol administered as ordinary and slow-release tablets in single and multiple doses. Acta Pharmacologica et Toxicologica 36 (suppl V): 45–58
12. Carlsson E, Ablad B 1978 Receptorfarmakologin: β-adrenoceptor blockerarnas verkan vid kardiovaskulaera sjukdomar. Lakartidningen 75: 4028–4033
13. Reybrouck T, Amery A, Fagard R, Jousten P, Lijnen P, Meulepas E 1978 β-blockers: once or three times a day. British Medical Journal 1: 1386–1388
14. Johnsson G, Jordo L, Lundborg P, Regardh C-G, Ronn O 1980 Plasma levels and pharmacological effects of metoprolol administered as controlled release (Durules) and ordinary tablets in healthy volunteers. International Journal of Clinical Pharmacology, Therapy and Toxicology 18: 292–297
15. Harron D W G, Shanks R G 1981 Comparison of the duration of effect of metoprolol and a sustained release formulation of metoprolol ('Betaloc SA'). British Journal of Clinical Pharmacology 11: 518–520
16. Van den Bergh J H, Van Herwaarden C L 1981 Ventilatory effects of ordinary and slow-release tablets of metoprolol in asthmatic patients. European Journal of Respiratory Disease 62: 168–172
17. Ravid M, Lang R, Jutrin I 1985 The relative antihypertensive potency of propranolol, oxprenolol, atenolol, and metoprolol given once daily. A double-blind, crossover, placebo-controlled study in ambulatory patients. Archives of Internal Medicine 145: 1321–1323
18. Stenberg J, Wasir H, Amergy A, Sannerstedt R, Werko L 1975 Comparative hemodynamic studies in man of adrenergic β-1-receptor agents without (H93/26 = metoprolol) or with (H87/07) intrinsic sympathicomimetic activity. Acta Pharmacologica et Toxicologica 36 (suppl V): 76–84
19. Sannerstedt R, Wasir H 1977 Acute haemodynamic effects of metoprolol in hypertensive patients. British Journal of Clinical Pharmacology 4: 23–26
20. Attman P O, Aurell M, Johnsson G 1975 Effects of metoprolol and propranolol on furosemide-stimulated renin release in healthy subjects. European Journal of Clinical Pharmacology 8: 201–204
21. Isbary J, Greding H, Nechwatal W, KIoenig E 1978 Haemodynamische veraenderungen bei hypertonikern nach β-sympathikolyse mit propranolol und metoprolol. Zeitschrift fur Kardiologie 67: 857–862
22. Lund-Johansen P, Ohm O-J 1977 Haemodynamic long-term effects of metoprolol at rest and during exercise in essential hypertension. British Journal of Clinical Pharmacology 4: 147–151
23. Hansson B-G, Dymling J-F, Hedeland H, Hulthen U L 1977 Long term treatment of moderate hypertension with the β-1-receptor blocking agent metoprolol. European Journal of Clinical Pharmacology 11: 239–245
24. Spence J D, Paterson N A M 1979 Long-term oral metoprolol versus propranolol in essential hypertension. Exercise studies of blood velocity, cardiac output, systolic time intervals and expiratory flow rates. Current Therapeutic Research 26: 941–950
25. Rizzon P, Di Biase M, Chiddo A, Mastrangelo D, Sorgente L 1978 Electrophysiological properties of intravenous metoprolol in man. British Heart Journal 40: 650–655
26. Hillis S 1979 In: MacFarlane P W (Ed) Progress in electrocardiology, Pitman Med Ltd London, pp 441–443
27. Edvardsson N, Olsson S B 1981 Effects of acute and chronic β-receptor blockade on ventricular repolarization in man. British Heart Journal 45: 628–636
28. Thiringer G, Svedmyr N 1976 Interaction of orally administered metoprolol, practolol and propranolol with isoprenaline in asthmatics. European Journal of Clinical Pharmacology 10: 163–170
29. Formgren H 1976 The effect of metoprolol and practolol on lung function and blood pressure in hypertensive asthmatics. British Journal of Clinical Pharmacology 3: 1007–1014
30. Sinclair D J M 1979 Comparison of effects of propranolol and metoprolol on airways obstruction in chronic bronchitis. British Medical Journal 1: 168
31. Lofdahl C-G, Svedmyr N 1981 Cardioselectivity of atenolol and metoprolol. European Journal of Respiratory Disease 62: 396–404
32. Harms H 1977 In: Cardioselective β-adrenoceptor blocking agents. Human and animal studies in vitro and in vivo. Enroprint B V, Rijswijk
33. Lawrence DS S, Sahay J N, Chatterjee S S, Cruickshank J M 1982 Asthma and β-blockers. European Journal of Clinical Pharmacology 22: 501–509

Metoprolol (tartrate)

34. Decalmer P B S, Chatterjee S S, Cruickshank J M, Benson M K, Sterling G M 1978 β-blockers and asthma. British Heart Journal 40: 184–189
35. McSorley P D, Warren D J 1978 Effects of propranolol and metoprolol on the peripheral circulation. British Medical Journal 2: 1598–1600
36. Johnsson G 1975 Influence of metoprolol and propranolol on hemodynamic effects induced by adrenaline and physical work. Acta Pharmacologica et Toxicologica 36 (suppl V): 59–68
37. Johnsson G, Nyberg G, Solvell L 1975 Influence of metoprolol and propranolol on hemodynamic effects induced by physical work and isoprenaline. Acta Pharmacologica et Toxicologica 36 (suppl V): 69–75
38. Van Herwaarden C L A, Binkhorst R A, Fennis J F M, Laar A 1977 Effects of adrenaline during treatment with propranolol and metoprolol. British Medical Journal 1: 1029
39. Davidson N McD, Corrall R J, Shaw T R, French E B 1977 Observations in man of hypoglycaemia during selective and non-selective β-blockade. Scottish Medical Journal 22: 69–72
40. Lager I, Blohme G, Smith U 1979 Effect of cardioselective and non-selective β-blockade on the hypoglycaemic response in insulin-dependent diabetics. Lancet 1: 458–462
41. Waal-Manning H J 1976 Metabolic effects of β-adrenoreceptor blockers. Drugs 11 (suppl 12): 121–126
42. Groop L, Totterman K-J, Harno K, Grodin A 1982 Influence of β-blocking drugs on glucose metabolism in patients with non-insulin dependent diabetes mellitus. Acta Medica Scandinavica 211: 7–12
43. William-Olsson T, Fellenius E, Bjorntorp P, Smith U 1979 Differences in metabolic responses to β-adrenergic stimulation after propranolol or metoprolol administration. Acta Medica Scandinavica 205: 201–206
44. Lundborg P, Astrom H, Bengtsson C, Fellenius E, Von Schenck H, Svensson L, Smith U 1981 Effect of β-adrenoceptor blockade on exercise performance and metabolism. Clinical Science 61: 299–305
45. Franz I W, Lohmann F W 1979 Der Einfluss einer chronischen sog kardioselektiven und nichtkardioselektiven β-rezeptoren-blockade auf den Blutdruck, die O_2-aufnahme und den Kohlenhydratstoffwechsel, ergometrische Untersuchungen beim hochdruckkranken. Zeitschrift fur Kardiologie 68: 503–509
46. Devi KP, Rao KV, Baveja SK, Leeman T, Dayer P 1988 Determination of alprenolol and metoprolol in plasma by column liquid chromatography. Journal of Chromatography 434: 265–270
47. Melander A, Danielson K, Schertsen B, Wahlin E 1977 Enhancement of the bioavailability of propranolol and metoprolol by food. Clinical Pharmacology and Therapeutics 22: 108–112
48. Cruickshank J M 1980 The clinical importance of cardioselectivity and lipophilicity in β-blockers. American Heart Journal 100: 160–178
49. Neil-Dwyer G, Bartlett J, McAinsh J, Cruickshank J M 1981 β-adrenoceptor blockers and the blood-brain barrier. British Journal of Clinical Pharmacology 11: 549–553
50. Regardh C-G, Johnsson G 1980 Clinical pharmacokinetics of metoprolol. Clinical Pharmacokinetics 5: 557–569
51. Sandstrom B, Regardh C-G 1980 Metoprolol excretion into breast milk. British Journal of Clinical Pharmacology 9: 518–519
52. Lindeberg S, Lundborg P, Regardh CL, Sandstrom B 1987 Disposition of the adrenergic blocker metoprolol and its metabolite OH-metoprolol in maternal plasma, amniotic fluid and capillary blood of the neonate. European Journal of Clinical Pharmacology 33: 363-368
53. Regardh C-G, Jordo L, Errik M, Lundborg P, Olsson R, Rönn O 1981 Pharmacokinetics of metoprolol in patients with hepatic cirrhosis. Clinical Pharmacokinetics 6: 375–388
54. Jordo L, Attman P O, Aurell M, Johansson L, Johnsson G, Regardh C-G 1980 Pharmacokinetic and pharmacodynamic properties of metoprolol in patients with impaired renal function. Clinical Pharmacokinetics 5: 169–180
55. Regardh C-G, Landahl S, Larsson M, Lundborg P, Steen B, Hoffmann K-J, Lagerstrom P-O 1983 Pharmacokinetics of metoprolol and its metabolite OH metoprolol in healthy, non-smoking, elderly individuals. European Journal of Clinical Pharmacology 24: 221–226
56. Von Bahr C, Collste P, Frisk-Holmberg M, Haglund K, Jorfelt L, Orme M, Ostman J, Sjoqvist F 1976 Plasma levels and effects of metoprolol on blood pressure, adrenergic β-receptor blockade, and plasma renin activity in essential hypertension. Clinical Pharmacology and Therapeutics 20: 130–137
57. Edvardsson N, Fritz H, Haellen J, Larsson R, Norlander S, Kasmussen P A 1978 Effekt och koncentration i plasma av metoprolol efter dosering morgon och kvaell vid essentiell hypertoni. Lakartidningen 75: 1069–1072
58. Uusitalo A, Keyrilaeinen O, Johnsson G 1981 A dose-response study on metoprolol in angina pectoris. Annals of Clinical Research 13: 54–57
59. Lennard M S, Silas J H, Freestone S, Ramsey L E, Tucker G T, Woods H G 1982 Oxidation phenotype — a major determinant of metoprolol metabolism and response. New England Journal of Medicine 307: 1558–1560
60. Alvan G, Von Bahr C, Seideman P, Sjoqvist F 1982 High plasma concentrations of β-receptor blocking drugs and deficient debrisoquine hydroxylation. Lancet 1: 333
61. Kendall M J 1981 Are selective β-adrenoceptor blocking drugs an advantage? Journal of the Royal College of Physicians London 15: 33–40
62. Freestone S, Silas J H, Lennard M S, Ramsey L E 1982 Comparison of two long-acting preparations of metoprolol with conventional metoprolol and atenolol in healthy men during chronic dosing. British Journal of Clinical Pharmacology 14: 713–718
63. Andreassen P H, Drivenes A 1977 Ny selektiv β-1-receptorantagonist, En sammenligning av metoprolol ('Seloken') med placebo ved mild til moderat hypertsjon. Tidsskr Nor Laegeforen 97: 1081–1083
64. Bengtsson C 1981 Seven years on a selective β-blocker — metoprolol. A long-term study of women with arterial hypertension. Annals of Clinical Research 13: 7–15
65. Bengtsson C 1976 Comparison between metoprolol and propranolol as antihypertensive agents. A double-blind cross-over study. Acta Medica Scandinavica 199: 71–74

Metoprolol (tartrate)

66. Clausen N, Damsgaard T, Mellemgaard K 1979 Antihypertensive effect of a non-selective (propranolol) and a cardioselective (metoprolol) β-adrenoceptor blocking agent at rest and during exercise. British Journal of Clinical Pharmacology 7: 379–383
67. Davidson C, Thadani U, Singleton W, Taylor S H 1976 Comparison of antihypertensive activity of β-blocking drugs during chronic treatment. British Medical Journal 2: 7–9
68. Sjoberg K H 1981 Metoprolol and propranolol in the treatment of essential hypertension — a long-term comparative study. Annals of Clinical Research 13: 23–29
69. Bosman A R, Goldberg B, McKechnie J K, Offermeier J, Oosthuizen O J 1977 South African multicentre study of metoprolol and propranolol in essential hypertension. South African Medical Journal 51: 57–61
70. Tuomilehto J, Nissinen A 1979 Double-blind comparison of metoprolol, alprenolol and oxprenolol in hypertension. European Journal of Clinical Pharmacology 16: 369–374
71. Tuomilehto J, Pohjola M 1978 A comparison between metoprolol and pindolol in the treatment of essential hypertension. Annals of Clinical Research 10: 24–29
72. Lorimer A R, Barbour M, Hillis W S, Lawrie T D, Stoker J B, Steeharan N, Leanage R U, Linden R J 1980 Long-term comparison of metoprolol and methyldopa in the treatment of hypertension. Clinical Cardiology 3: 36–41
73. Bergstrand R H, Vedin J A, Wilhelmsson C E, Berglund G 1976 Comparative study of metoprolol and α-methyldopa in untreated essential hypertension. European Journal of Clinical Pharmacology 10: 375–379
74. Lederballe Pedersen O 1976 Comparison of metoprolol and hydrochlorothiazide as antihypertensive agents. European Journal of Clinical Pharmacology 10: 381–385
75. Stokkeland O M, Sangvik K, Lindseth Ditlefsen E-M 1975 A comparative study of metoprolol and trichloromethiazide in hypertension. Current Therapeutic Research 18: 755–768
76. Asplund J 1981 A fixed-ratio combination of metoprolol and hydrochlorothiazide ('Co-Betaloc') in essential hypertension: A comparison between the individual drugs. Current Therapeutic Research 29: 387–394
77. Bengtsson C 1979 Metoprolol and hydrochlorothiazide in fixed combination in the treatment of arterial hypertension. Current Therapeutic Research 26: 394–401
78. White WB, Schulman P, Karimeddini MK, Smith VE. 1989 Regression of left ventricular mass is accompanied by improvement in rapid left ventricular filling following anti-hypertensive therapy with metoprolol. American Heart Journal 117: 145–150.
79. Cruickshank JK, Anderson NM, Wadsworth J, Young SM, Jepson E 1988 Treating hypertension in black compared with white non-insulin dependent diabetics: a double blind trial of verapamil and metoprolol British Medical Journal 297:1155–1159.
80. Goodfellow R M, Westberg B 1981 The treatment of high blood pressure in the elderly: a multicentre evaluation of a fixed combination of metoprolol and hydrochlorothiazide ('Co-Betaloc') in general practice. Current Medical Research Opinion 7: 536–542
81. Penman W A, Smith R G 1982 Pilot study of antihypertensive treatment in the elderly. Practitioner 226: 1180–1182
82. Oro L 1979 Once-daily administration of metoprolol Durules in hypertension: A comparison with ordinary tablets administered twice daily. Current Therapeutic Research 25: 778–785
83. Asplund J, Ohman P 1981 Metoprolol administered once daily in the treatment of hypertension. A double-blind crossover comparison between conventional tablets and metoprolol Durules. Annals of Clinical Research 13: 30–36
84. Wilcox R G, Hampton J R 1981 Comparative study of atenolol, metoprolol, metoprolol Durules, and slow-release oxprenolol in essential hypertension. British Heart Journal 46: 498–502
85. Comerford M B, Besterman E M 1982 A comparison of the effects of the slow release formulations of metoprolol and oxprenolol in hypertension. Annals of Clinical Research 14: 27–31
86. Morley C A, Cavalcanti C, Perrins E J, Sutton R 1983 A comparison of once daily atenolol and metoprolol and oxprenolol in hypertension. British Journal of Clinical Pharmacology 15: 715–717
87. Scott A K, Rigby J W, Webster J, Hawksworth G M, Petrie J C, Lovell H G 1982 Atenolol and metoprolol once daily in hypertension. British Medical Journal 284: 1514–1516
88. Keyrilaeinen O, Uustialo A 1975 Effects of the cardioselective β-blocker metoprolol in angina pectoris. A subacute study with exercise tests. Annals of Clinical Research 7: 433–441
89. Ekelund L-G, Olsson A G, Oro L, Rossner S 1976 Effects of the cardioselective β-adrenergic receptor blocking agent metoprolol in angina pectoris. Subacute study with exercise tests. British Heart Journal 38: 155–161
90. Howe A 1982 Once-daily treatment of stable angina pectoris. Practitioner 226: 1621–1624
91. Borer J S, Comerford M B, Sowton E 1976 Assessment of metoprolol, a cardioselective β-blocking agent, during chronic therapy in patients with angina pectoris. Journal of International Medical Research 4: 15–22
92. Frick M H, Luurila O 1976 Double-blind titrated-dose comparison of metoprolol and propranolol in the treatment of angina pectoris. Annals of Clinical Research 8: 385–392
93. Comerford M B, Besterman E M M 1976 An eighteen months' study of the clinical response to metoprolol, a selective β-1-receptor blocking agent, in patients with angina pectoris. Postgraduate Medical Journal 52: 481–486
94. Uusitalo A J, Keyrilaeinin O 1979 Slow-release metoprolol in angina pectoris. A comparative study of a cardioselective β-blocking drug, metoprolol, in ordinary and slow-release tablets (Durules) in the treatment of angina pectoris. Annals of Clinical Research 11: 199–204
95. Comerford M B, Besterman E M 1982 A clinical evaluation of sustained release metoprolol Durules in the treatment of angina pectoris. Clinical Cardiology 5: 131–135
96. Wasir H S, Mahapatra R K, Bhatia M L, Roy S B, Sannerstedt R 1977 Metoprolol — a new cardioselective β adrenoceptor blocking agent for treatment of tachyarrhythmias. British Heart Journal 39: 834–838
97. Stroobandt R, Kesteloot H 1981 Intravenous metoprolol for the treatment of acute supraventricular tachyarrhythmias. A multicentre study. Acta Cardiologica 36: 155–165
98. Rehnqvist N 1981 Clinical experience with intravenous metoprolol in supraventricular tachyarrhythmias. A multicentre study. Annals of Clinical Research 13: 68–72
99. Quan S F, Fenster P E, Hanson C D, Coaker L A, Basista M P 1983 Suppression of atrial ectopy with intravenous metoprolol in chronic obstructive pulmonary disease patients. Journal of Clinical Pharmacology 23: 341–347
100. Fenster P E, Quan S F, Hanson C D, Coaker L A 1984 Suppression of ventricular ectopy with intravenous metoprolol in patients with chronic obstructive pulmonary disease. Critical Care Medicine 12: 29–32
101. Khalsa A, Advardsson N, Olsson S B 1978 Effects of metoprolol on heart rate in patients with digitalis treated chronic atrial fibrillation. Clinical Cardiology 1: 91–95
102. Pratt C M, Yepsen S C, Bloom M G K, Taylor A A, Young J B, Quinones M A 1983 Evaluation of metoprolol in suppressing complex ventricular arrhythmias. American Journal of Cardiology 52: 73–78
103. Olsson G, Rehnqvist N 1984 Ventricular arrhythmias during the first year after acute myocardial infarction: influence of long-term treatment with metoprolol. Circulation 69: 1129–1134
104. Whitehead M H, Whitmarsh V B, Horton J N 1980 Metoprolol in anaesthesia for oral surgery. The effect of pretreatment on the incidence of cardiac dysrhythmias. Anaesthesia 35: 779–782
105. Rollason W N, Russell J G 1980 Intravenous metoprolol and cardiac dysrhythmias. An evaluation in the management of dysrhythmias in outpatient dental anaesthesia. Anaesthesia 35: 783–789
106. Coleman A J, Jordan C 1980 Cardiovascular responses to anaesthesia. Influence of β-adrenoreceptor blockade with metoprolol. Anaesthesia 35: 972–978
107. Ward-Booth P, Rubin P, Macfarlane P, Hillis S 1983 Metoprolol in the prevention of dysrhythmias during minor dental surgery. American Heart Journal 105: 689–690
108. Hanna M H, Heap D G, Kimberley P S 1983 Cardiac dysrhythmia associated with general anaesthesia for oral surgery. Its prevention by the prophylactic use of an oral β-adrenergic blocker. Anaesthesia 38: 1192–1194
109. Murchison L E, How J, Bewsher P D 1979 Comparison of propranolol and metoprolol in the management of hyperthyroidism. British Journal of Clinical Pharmacology 8: 581–587
110. Nilsson O R, Melander A, Tegler L 1980 Effects and plasma levels of propranolol and metoprolol in hyperthyroid patients. European Journal of Clinical Pharmacology 18: 315–320
111. Nilsson O R, Karlberg B E, Soderberg A 1980 Plasma catecholamines and cardiovascular responses to hypoglycaemia in hyperthyroidism before and during treatment with metoprolol or propranolol. Journal of Clinical Endocrinology and Metabolism 50: 906–911
112. Nilsson O R, Kagedal B, Tegler L 1980 Insulin release and carbohydrate tolerance in hyperthyroid patients during non-selective or selective β-1-adrenoceptor blockade. Acta Endocrinologica 93: 179–185
113. Nilsson O R, Anderberg B, Karlberg B E, Kagedal B 1980 Cortisol, growth hormone and prolactin response to insulin-induced hypoglycaemia in hyperthyroid patients before and during β-adrenoceptor blockade. Clinical Endocrinology 12: 581–588
114. Herlitz J, Elmfeldt D, Hjalmarson A et al 1983 Effect of metoprolol on indirect signs of the size and severity of acute myocardial infarction. American Journal of Cardiology 51: 1282–1288
115. Ryden L, Ariniego R, Arnman K et al 1983 A double-blind trial of metoprolol in acute myocardial infarction. New England Journal of Medicine 308: 614–618
116. Herlitz J, Hjalmarson A, Holmberg S et al 1984 Effect of metoprolol on chest pain in acute myocardial infarction. British Heart Journal 51: 438–444
117. Hjalmarson A, Elmfeldt D, Herlitz J et al 1981 Effect on mortality of metoprolol in acute myocardial infarction. Lancet 2: 823–827
118. Ronnevik PK, Gundersen T, Abrahamsen AM, Knutsen H, Woie L 1989 Effect of metoprolol on early exercise-induced ST segment changes and ventricular arrhythmia in patients with suspected acute myocardial infarction. International Journal of Cardiology 22: 31–57
119. Herlitz J, Hjalmarson A, Holmberg S et al 1984 Development of congestive heart failure after treatment with metoprolol in acute myocardial infarction. British Heart Journal 51: 539–544
120. The Miami Trial Research Group 1985 Metoprolol in acute myocardial infarction (MIAMI). A randomized placebo-controlled international trial. European Heart Journal 6: 199–226
121. Rohrig TP, Rundle DA, Leifer WN 1987 Fatality resulting from metoprolol overdose. Journal of Analytical Toxicology 11: 231–232.
122. Holzbecher M, Perry R A, Ellenberger H A 1982 Report of a metoprolol-associated death. Journal of Forensic Science 27: 715–717
123. Shore E T, Cepin D, Davidson M J 1981 Metoprolol overdose. Annals of Emergency Medicine 10: 524–527
124. Moller B H J 1976 Massive intoxication with metoprolol. British Medical Journal 1: 222
125. Sire S 1976 Metoprolol intoxication. Lancet 2: 1137
126. Rosengard S 1977 Antihypertensive effect and tolerability of metoprolol during long-term treatment: a multicentre study. Journal of International Medical Research 5: 199–206
127. Keyrilainen O, Uusitalo A 1976 Effects of metoprolol in angina pectoris. A subacute study with exercise tests and a long-term tolerability study. Acta Medica Scandinavica 199: 491–497
128. Lyngstam O, Ryden L 1981 Metoprolol and atenolol administered once daily in primary hypertension. A clinical comparison of the efficacy of two selective β-adrenoceptor blocking agents. Acta Medica Scandinavica 209: 261–266

M

129. Betts T A, Alford C 1983 β-blocking drugs and sleep. A controlled trial. Drugs 25: 268–272
130. Westerlund A 1983 A comparison of the central nervous system side-effects caused by lipophilic and hydrophilic β-blockers. Drugs 25: 280–281
131. Day J L, Metcalfe J, Simpson C N 1982 Adrenergic mechanisms in control of plasma lipid concentrations. British Medical Journal 284: 1145–1148
132. Wright L W, Foster M G 1980 Effect of some commonly prescribed drugs on certain chemistry tests. Clinical Biochemistry 13: 249–252
133. Lundborg P, Agren G, Ervik M, Lindeberg S, Sandstrom B 1981 Disposition of metoprolol in the new born. British Journal of Clinical Pharmacology 12: 598–600
134. Sandstrom B 1978 Antihypertensive treatment with the adrenergic β-receptor blocker metoprolol during pregnancy. Gynecologic and Obstetric Investigation 9: 195–204
135. Formgren H 1976 The effect of metoprolol and practolol on lung function and blood pressure in hypertensive asthmatics. British Journal of Clinical Pharmacology 3: 1007–1014
136. Johnsson G, Svedmyr N, Thiringer G 1975 Effect of intravenous propranolol and metoprolol and their interaction with isoprenaline on pulmonary function, heart rate and blood pressure in asthmatics. European Journal of Clinical Pharmacology 8: 175–180
137. Wagner F, Kaluschke D, Trenk D, Jaehnchen E, Roskamm H 1987 Drug interaction between propafenone and metoprolol. British Journal of Clinical Pharmacology 24: 213–220
138. Toon S, Davidson EM, Garstang FM, Batra H, Bowes RJ et al 1988 The racemic metoprolol H2-antagonist interaction. Clinical Pharmacy and Therapeutics 43: 283–289
139. Ekelund L G, Oroe L 1979 Antianginal efficiency of nifedipine with and without a β-blocker, studied with exercise test. A double-blind, randomized subacute study. Clinical Cardiology 2: 203–211
140. Schmidt J F, Baadsgaard O 1981 Kombinationsbehandling af angina pectoris med nifedipin og metoprolol. Ugeskr Laeger 143: 2580–2581
141. Jenkins R M, Nagle R E 1982 The symptomatic and objective effects of nifedipine in combination with β-blocker therapy in severe angina pectoris. Postgraduate Medical Journal 58: 697–700
142. Tuomilehto J, Pakarinin P 1977 Effects of metoprolol as monotherapy and in combination with hydralazine in hypertensive patients previously considered to be treatment failures. Current Therapeutic Research 21: 257–264
143. Ikram H 1980 Hemodynamic and electrophysiologic interactions between antiarrhythmic drugs and β-blockers, with special reference to tocainide. American Heart Journal 100: 1076–1080
144. Renard M B, Bernard R M, Ewalenko M B, Englert M 1983 Hemodynamic effects of concurrent administration of metoprolol and tocainide in acute myocardial infarction. Journal of Cardiovascular Pharmacology 5: 116–120
145. Waagstein F, Swedberg K, Wallentin I, Baandrup U, Hjalmarson A 1981 The role of β-adrenoceptor blockade in congestive cardiomyopathy. In: Delius W (ed) Catecholamines heart international symposium, Munich May 28–30th

Metriphonate

Metriphonate is an organophorus compound used in the treatment of *Schistosoma haematobium* infections.

Chemistry

A simple description of the pharmaceutical product metriphonate is complicated by the confusing number of names used in the literature to delineate three compounds, trichlorfon,[1] metriphonate and dichlorvos. The demonstration of the transformation of both trichlorfon and metriphonate in man to produce the direct-acting acetylcholinesterase inhibitor dichlorvos (DDVP; 2,2-dichlorovinyl dimethylphosphate)[2] clarified the fact that trichlorfon and metriphonate are different formulations of the same substance and both act as prodrugs to the active form dichlorvos.

Unlike the vast majority of drugs, the organophosphorus ester metriphonate was introduced originally as a commercial chemical in 1952 and was used as an agricultural insecticide for the control of insects on crops and animals, as a forest insecticide, and as a veterinary anthelmintic, under the name trichlorfon.[1]

Dichlorvos itself is used as an insecticide, as an anthelmintic for swine and dogs, in flea collars for pet animals, in the control of external parasites on livestock, in the control of insects either in buildings or on certain greenhouse crops (e.g. mushrooms, tomatoes) and also for mosquito and fly control.[3]

Metriphonate

Metriphonate (metrifonate, metrifonate, trichlorfon, trichlorphon, Chlorophos, Bilarcil, Dipterex, Dylox)
$C_4H_8Cl_3O_4P$
O,O-Dimethyl-2,2,2-trichloro-1-hydroxyethylphosphonate;
phosphoric acid 2,2,2-trichloro-1-hydroxyethyl dimethyl ester

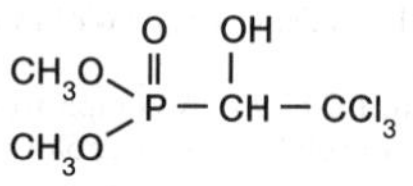

Molecular weight	257.5
pKa	—
Solubility	
in alcohol	soluble
in water	1 in 7
Octanol/water partition coefficient	—

At least 20 synonyms and 70 trade names have been used,[1] among the commonest of the latter being Dipterex and Dylox.

The pure substance occurs as colourless crystals, with a melting point of 83–84°C.

It is soluble in water, benzene, ethanol and most chlorinated hydrocarbons; it is poorly soluble in carbon tetrachloride and diethyl ether and insoluble in petroleum oils.[1]

It is stable at room temperature; decomposes at higher temperatures in water and at pH < 5.5 to form dichlorvos.

Dichlorvos

Dichlorvos (dichlorophos, DDVP, dichlorovos, Vapona)
$C_4H_7Cl_2O_4P$
2,2-Dichloroethenyldimethylphosphate;

2,2-dichlorovinyldimethylphosphate

$$Cl_2C{=}CH-O-\overset{\displaystyle O}{\overset{\|}{P}}(OCH_3)_2$$

Molecular weight	221.0
pKa	—
Solubility	
in alcohol	—
in water	1 in 100
Octanol/water partition coefficient	high

Dichlorvos[3] is a colourless-to-amber liquid with a boiling point of 140°C at 20 mm; 84°C at 1 mm; density $d^{25}{}_4$ 1.1415; refractive index of $n^{25}{}_D$ 1.4523.

It is miscible with aromatic and chlorinated hydrocarbon solvents. It is moderately volatile (the vapour pressure is 1.2×10^{-2} mm at 20°C) and practically nonflammable. A saturated aqueous solution is hydrolysed at the rate of 3% per day.

Dichlorvos hydrolyses rapidly in alkali. It is corrosive to iron and mild steel but noncorrosive to stainless steel, aluminium, nickel, Hastelloy 13 and Teflon.

Pharmacology

Like other organophosphorus compounds, trichlorfon (metriphonate) produces, in various species at different doses, inhibition of plasma, erythrocyte and brain acetylcholinesterases. After many years of usage as an insecticide and veterinary anthelmintic, empirically conducted trials of trichlorfon pointed to its utility as an antiparasitic compound.[4–6] The pharmaceutically purified form is known as metriphonate when used as an antischistosomal drug.

The mode of action of metriphonate on the parasite in man is not known. The two basic theories on the mode of action of metriphonate may be termed the chemical and the mechanical.[7] Acetylcholinesterase (AChE) activity in *S. mansoni* adults was demonstrated in 1952.[8] It was thus logical to expect that an organophosphorus compound (e.g. Dipterex, trichlorfon, metriphonate) would have an inhibitory effect on worm cholinesterases. In 1966, it was postulated that acetylcholine (ACh) functioned as an inhibitory neurotransmitter in *S. mansoni* adults since it was shown that the cholinergic receptors in *S. mansoni* were not identical to those in man and that cholinesterase inhibition in the worms was confirmed.[9–13] This theory, however, does not explain all the known facts.

A 'mechanical' theory of the mode of action[14,15,16] was advanced that the adult schistosomes, under the paralysing influence of the drug, drifted from their original locations in the perivesical plexus, via the inferior vena caval system to the small arterioles of the lung where they became trapped, encased by leucocytes and died. The reason advanced for the failure of metriphonate in *S. mansoni* or *S. japonicum* infections was that since adult schistosomes of these species live within the draining areas of the portal venous system, they are able, on recovery from the action of metriphonate and/or its metabolites, to retrace a migratory path down the portal system and return to their preferred sites of anatomical location to resume egg laying.

Progress is slow in the elucidation of the mode of action of metriphonate and to date[17–23], no really satisfactory explanation has been advanced. One suggestion of the differential species susceptibility to metriphonate is that genetic differences in cholinesterase may occur.[24]

Toxicology

Metriphonate

Acute toxicity

As metriphonate is potentially a toxic compound and has been used in population-based chemotherapeutic control of urinary schistosomiasis, its safety is of major importance. Whereas metriphonate, the pharmaceutical preparation, is given nowadays solely by mouth, trichlorfon, the pesticide, can be absorbed by inhalation or through the skin.[25]

After single doses, the LD_{50} of metriphonate in male rats was 630 mg.kg^{-1} and in female rats 560 mg.kg^{-1}. On dermal application the LD_{50} in rats of either sex was >2800 mg.kg^{-1} and in rabbits 5000 mg.kg^{-1}.

Extended and long-term studies

Such studies in several species have revealed no effects in animals of clinical relevance in man (but see Neurotoxicity – below).[26]

Carcinogenicity studies

Studies in several species have shown no evidence of carcinogenicity.[26]

Mutagenicity

Metriphonate induced a low degree of gene mutation in direct *Salmonella* tests with different strains,[27] with an *E. coli* strain, but no mutagenic effect was seen in the *Drosophila melanogaster* assay.[24]

In tests for chromosomal effects (dominant lethal studies in male mice), whether given the drug intraperitoneally or by mouth, in a dose corresponding to one-third of the LD_{50}, no induction of dominant lethals was observed.[24] In the micronucleus test in mice given doses of 2×125 mg and 2×250 mg.kg^{-1} metriphonate by mouth no mutagenic effects were observed.[24]

In later cytogenetic investigations of test systems based on bone marrow and testis in mice given metriphonate 100 mg.kg^{-1} intraperitoneally, no clastogenic effects were seen or, alternatively, when metriphonate was given chronically at 0.5 ppm five days a week for seven weeks. In a dominant lethal test, metriphonate did not produce any effect. These data were derived by comparison with those obtained with trimethylphosphate and methyl methane sulphonate used as positive controls.[28]

Teratogenicity

No teratogenic effects have been observed in animals (but see High risk groups — Pregnant women).

Reproductive studies

A two-generation, two-year feeding study of trichlorfon at concentrations of 100, 300 and 1000 ppm, fed as an additive in diet, was performed in pathogen-free, CD, Long-Evans rats. Ingestion of trichlorfon by the F_o generation parents did not affect reproductive performance. This generation and their progeny, the F_1 generation, were observed for approximately 105 weeks.[29] In a study in 1970 in dogs, a reduced testicular weight was found at 800 ppm but histology revealed no inhibition of spermatogenesis despite earlier suggestions of adverse effects on the gonads [26,30–32]

Dichlorvos

Dichlorvos is formed nonenzymatically from metriphonate after ingestion.

Dichlorvos itself is a volatile organophosphorus insecticide, directly active without having to be metabolized first. It is of a high toxicity but its rapid metabolism renders it safe under correct conditions of use.[33]

It is absorbed by the intact skin, by inhalation and from the gastrointestinal tract. Its mode of action is by cholinesterase inhibition and it is rapidly metabolized in mammals. Hydrolytic metabolism occurs in all species and leads presumably to dichloroacetaldehyde which is further metabolized by (i) reduction to dichloroethanol and excretion in the urine as the glucuronide and (ii) dechlorination followed by incorporation of the carbon atoms into endogenous biosynthesis and excretion as carbon dioxide and hippuric acid in the urine.

Acute toxicity

In single dose toxicity studies, the rat was the most susceptible species; the oral LD_{50} was 56–80 mg.kg^{-1}. The mouse appeared more susceptible than the rat to inhalation.

Repeated dosage was conducted through dietary studies. A dietary concentration of only 50 mg.kg^{-1} soon produced detectable inhibition of plasma and erythrocyte cholinesterase in rats but a dietary level of 1000 mg.kg^{-1} (about 50 mg.kg^{-1} daily) was tolerated for 90 days without diminution of growth or sign of intoxication. In a 2-year study in rats there was slight plasma and erythrocyte cholinesterase inhibition at about 50 mg.kg^{-1} (2.5 mg.kg^{-1} daily) but not at about 5 mg.kg^{-1} (0.25 mg.kg^{-1} daily). Some hepatocellular changes were however seen at about 50 mg.kg^{-1} (2.5 mg.kg^{-1} daily) and above.[33]

Mutagenicity and related short-term tests
No significant effect of dichlorvos was found in any in vivo mammalian study.[34,35]

Carcinogenicity studies
Neither in mice nor rats receiving various dietary doses for 78 and 80 weeks respectively were there significant trends in tumour incidences and control and treated animals showed broadly similar patterns of tumour yields.[3]

Areas of particular toxicological importance in relation to trichlorfon and dichlorvos

Alkylation
Possible alkylating effects of organophosphates have been discussed widely in recent years. The difficulties of interpretation of much of the data in this field arise because the purity of the compound used has not always been clearly defined by authors. Thus, doubts exist as to whether an effect can be attributed to the compound itself or to some impurity as additive.[36]

Any genetic risk to patients treated with metriphonate for urinary schistosomiasis would be due to the methylating capacity of metriphonate and dichlorvos (DDVP) and to the mutagenic activity of dichloroacetaldehyde.[37,38] which appear to be quite small.

Neurotoxicity
Compounds such as Mipafox (N,N^1-di-isopropyl phosphordiamidofluorate) and TOCP (triorthocresyl phosphate) are known to produce polyneuritis with flaccid paralyses of distal muscles in arms and legs in man.[39–43]

No signs of neurotoxicity were found in chickens or hens in a variety of experiments when metriphonate or dichlorvos were given by different routes in both short-term and long-term studies.[36]

Metriphonate has been used as a drug with a very high margin of safety. In contrast, many cases of trichlorfon intoxication have been reported from the USSR and Eastern Europe. Mostly involving suicidal attempts, delayed polyneuropathy occurred in various samples with a highest incidence of 23.7%.[36] The polyneuropathy thus caused could have been due to a very large dose of trichlorfon, or some unknown contaminant. No convincing explanation has yet been adduced.

Contamination of agricultural trichlorfon with the ethyl analogue would greatly increase the neurotoxic hazard but analysis of a few samples has not revealed such impurities. Simultaneous ingestion of alcohol does not appear to increase neuropathic hazard.

Clinical pharmacology

In man, evidence on the absorption and effect of metriphonate in schistosome-infected children was gathered by monitoring acetylcholinesterase activities in red cells, whole blood and plasma during and after treatment.[44] Acetylcholinesterase activity was determined by a sensitive spectrophotometric technique.[45–47]

A few hours after each dose of a three-dose regime of 7.5, 10.0 or 12.5 mg.kg^{-1} of metriphonate given once every 14 days, plasma cholinesterase was almost completely inhibited, regardless of the amount given in this dose range, but erythrocyte cholinesterase was inhibited, in a dose-dependent fashion, down to some 40–60% of the individual patient's pre-treatment activity. Inhibited plasma cholinesterase returned to normal activity fairly rapidly. After 14 days, plasma cholinesterase activities, having been completely inhibited within 24 hours of each dose, were some 75% of the 'normal' activity for each individual patient. At 4 weeks after the last dose of a three-dose regime, activities were 'normal'. However, erythrocyte cholinesterase activities, considered the closest parallel monitoring measurement of brain cholinesterase, although inhibited to a lesser extent and at a slower rate than plasma cholinesterases, were also slower to recover. Activities were not regained within 14 days of a dose of metriphonate and the subsequent dose depressed red cell cholinesterase activity further to 35–50% of the level existing at the time of dosing. After the last dose of a three-dose treatment, erythrocyte cholinesterase activities did not return to 'normal' for times varying between 8 and 15 weeks. The main problem of using red cell measurements is that these are non-nucleated cells and cannot synthesize acetylcholinesterase. The long duration of action measured in red cells may simply reflect the red cell life.

Despite these inhibitions of erythrocyte and plasma cholinesterases, no correlation could be established between the degree of cholinesterase inhibition and any symptom after treatment. Thus, enzyme inhibition occurring after metriphonate treatment in man should be regarded as indicative of satisfactory absorption and biotransformation of the compound into dichlorvos the actual inhibitory substance, rather than evidence of drug toxicity.

Initial empirical experimental trials of Dipterex (trichlorfon) in humans suggested evidence of therapeutic activity in schistosomiasis,[14,15,48–50] hookworm, creeping eruption, ascariasis, trichiuriasis,[6] and onchocerciasis.[51] Further studies with metriphonate confirmed a partial microfilaricidal effect in infections due to *Onchocerca volvulus*[52–54] but no macrofilaricidal action, and no macrofilaricidal or microfilaricidal effect against *Wuchereria bancrofti*.[53]

Both cerebral[55,56] and cutaneous[57] cysticercosis due to infection with the larval stages of *Taenia solium*, the pork tapeworm, have been treated by metriphonate with claims of high success.

Since the efficacy of metriphonate is inconstant in the majority of the parasitic infections noted, the sole indications for its use are in the treatment of infections due to *S. haematobium* or, rarely, as an alternative treatment to praziquantel or albendazole in cysticercosis due to *T. solium*. Trials using quantitative techniques of parasitological assessment, the methodologies of the randomized control trial (RCT) and the pharmaceutically pure form of metriphonate (trichlorfon) showed that the optimum individual dose for schistosomiasis was 7.5–10 mg.kg^{-1} and a widely adopted schedule of 7.5 mg.kg^{-1}, given in three oral doses, at an interval of 14 days, became the 'standard' treatment regime.[44,58] In fact, all investigations have shown that doses of 5 mg.kg^{-1} are too low and that some strains of *S. haematobium* in Egypt, Sudan and various areas in Africa seem to respond best to three doses each of 10 mg.kg^{-1}.[7,59] Whether each individual dose is given at intervals of two or four weeks is immaterial.[58]

Pharmacokinetics

Methods for the study of the action of metriphonate and dichlorvos have traditionally been indirect, e.g. direct polarographic measurements of reaction rates at 25 and 37°C at pH 7.4, or indirect calculation of acetylcholinesterase and cholinesterase from different enzyme sources in metriphonate solutions at 25 and 37°C and pH 7.4.[60]

A major advance occurred when specific techniques for the determination of both metriphonate and dichlorvos became available.[61] This necessitated the use of mass fragmentography and several compounds labelled with stable isotopes:

1. ^{1}H-metriphonate for injection and standard curve;
2. ^{1}H-dichlorvos for injection and standard curve;
3. $^2H_6$-metriphonate as internal standard for determination of metriphonate;
4. $^2H_4$-dichlorvos as internal standard for determination of dichlorvos;
5. $^2H_6$-dichlorvos used in standard curve to calculate amount of $^2H_6$-dichlorvos from $^2H_6$-metriphonate during the work-up procedure.

When these isotopic variants were used in the determination of metriphonate, dichlorvos or acetylcholinesterase activity in mice after the administration of metriphonate, dichlorvos was found in the brains and the in vivo identity was established by comparing the retention time with the retention time of a reference substance, the mass spectrum of which was recorded.[2]

From kinetic calculations using the results obtained with the multiple stable isotopes, the total amount of ^{1}H-dichlorvos measured and the amount of ^{1}H-dichlorvos formed in vivo can be estimated.[2] It was concluded that non-enzymatic formation of dichlorvos, which is known to occur in solutions, in all probability occurs in the body and metriphonate in this way acts as a slow-release formulation for the direct acting cholinesterase inhibitor dichlorvos.

Following these animal studies, the methods of mass fragmentography and the use of internal standards labelled with stable isotopes, being both highly specific and sensitive, were used to quantify metriphonate and dichlorvos in human blood in patients with schistosomiasis undergoing metriphonate treatment.[62] The amount of dichlorvos formed in plasma was approximately 1% of the metriphonate levels. Peak levels of both organophosphates occurred at 1 hour and 1.5 hours in the two patients studied, which coincided with the time at which the erythrocyte cholinesterase reached its lowest level, and showed considerable reductions eight hours after dosage. The plasma levels of the organophosphate compounds did not correlate with the curves of cholinesterase inhibition in erythrocytes, whole blood or plasma in which it is known that action is prolonged for days or weeks.[44] On analysis of the Bilarcil (metriphonate) tablets, no dichlorvos was detected.

Thus, overwhelming evidence exists for the formation of dichlorvos in body fluids. There is no reason to believe that the dichlorvos formed in man during treatment with metriphonate is anything but the result of a chemical transformation unrelated to enzymatic metabolism.[2] Metriphonate in man acts as a slow-release formulation for dichlorvos; the latter is known to be a directly acting cholinesterase inhibitor, giving rise to a dimethylphosphorylated enzyme. This mechanism of inhibition is less prone to the phenomenon of 'ageing', although it does occur, and may well be the explanation for the well-known prolonged enzyme inhibition observed after metriphonate treatment.

Concentration–effect relationship

There appears to be little correlation between plasma concentrations of DDVP and anticholinesterase inhibition in erythrocytes.[44]

Metabolism

Studies using ^{32}P-, ^{36}Cl-, [vinyl-^{14}C]- and [methyl-^{14}C]-dichlorvos in pigs, rats and mice,[63] have shown that dichlorvos is degraded rapidly, whether it is administered orally or by inhalation. After oral administration of [vinyl-1-^{14}C]-dichlorvos to male rats, 42% of the radioactivity was recovered as metabolites during the first 24 hours. After 4 days, 39% of the radioactivity was recovered as $^{14}CO_2$. 13% was excreted in the urine and 3.4% in the faeces, and 16% was found in the carcass. At least nine metabolites were detected in the urine: ^{14}C-labelled metabolites were dichloroethyl β-D-glucopyranosiduronic acid, desmethyldichlorvos, hippuric acid, N-benzoyl glycine and urea. Four days after dosing, 5% of the radioactivity of the administered dose was associated with liver, largely in the protein fraction as ^{14}-glycine and ^{14}C-serine. Similar results were obtained in rats exposed by inhalation to ^{14}C-dichlorvos.

Exposure of rats to 10 mg.m^{-3} (1.1 ppm) for 4 h was required before dichlorvos could be detected reliably, and then only in kidneys; the half-life of dichlorvos in kidneys of animals exposed to 50 mg.m^{-3} (5.5 ppm) for 4 h was 13.5 min. With 90 mg.m^{-3} (10 ppm), which is equivalent to 60% of full air saturation, dichlorvos could be detected in most tissues. In mice similarly exposed, dichlorvos was found in most tissues, but at one-tenth of the levels found in rats.

Dichlorvos is metabolized via two major pathways, hydrolysis and O-demethylation (see Fig. 1). The primary products of the esterase-catalysed hydrolysis of the P–O (vinyl) bond are dimethylphosphate, which is excreted in the urine, and dichloroacetaldehyde, which is rapidly degraded to dichloroethanol. This may be glucuronidated and excreted in the urine or dehalogenated to a 2-carbon fragment, which may then enter pathways of intermediary metabolism. O-Demethylation of dichlorvos can proceed via oxidative demethylation catalysed by microsomal monooxygenases, with formation of formaldehyde and desmethyldichlorvos, or S-methyltransferase-catalysed monomethylation, to yield S-methyl-glutathione and desmethyldichlorvos. Of the two major metabolic routes, esterase-catalysed hydrolysis is quantitatively more important and occurs in a wide range of tissues. The tissue distribution of methyltransferases is less well defined, but such activities have been demonstrated in liver and kidney.

There is no information available on protein or tissue binding of metriphonate. The major pathways of metabolism of dichlorvos found in the rat have been shown to operate in pigs, mice, hamsters, and man.[36]

Fig. 1 Metabolism of metriphonate

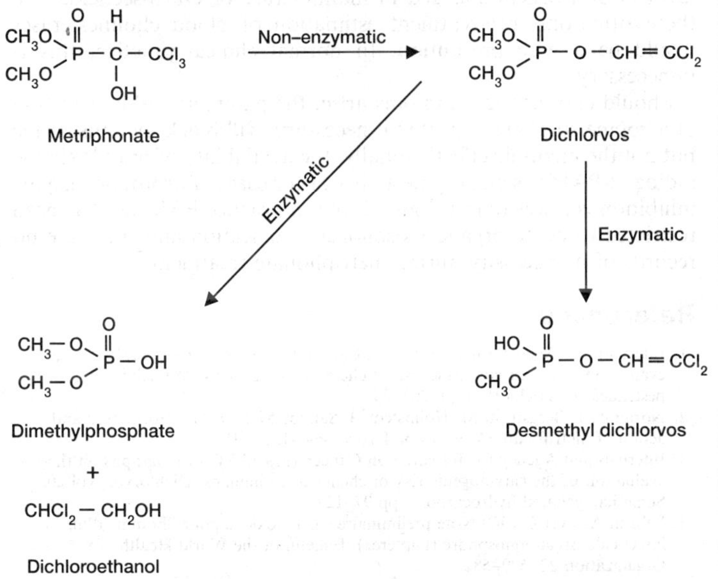

Pharmaceutics

Metriphonate (Bilarcil) is available as a white scored tablet containing 100 mg of active substance and is usually supplied in tins containing 1000 tablets. Tablets of metriphonate are estimated to have a shelf-life of two years in warm climates, i.e. storage temperature 25°C, and of four years in moderate climates, i.e. storage temperature of approximately 20°C. In general, metriphonate tablets must be moisture-proof packed, stored in a cool place, preferably in a refrigerator at 4°C, and the contents of opened tins should be used as soon as possible. Storage at high temperatures may cause discoloration of the tablets, which are then no longer suitable for treatment.[7]

Therapeutic use

Indications

1. Schistosomiasis due to infection with *S. haematobium*
2. Other uses.

Contraindications

1. Occupational exposure to anticholinesterase agents.

Indications

1. Schistosomiasis

For the treatment of patients with urinary schistosomiasis (*S. haematobium*) the standard dose is 7.5–10.0 mg.kg^{-1} body weight, given in three oral doses at an interval of 14 days. Whether an individual dose of 7.5 or 10 mg.kg^{-1} is used depends on the therapeutic results gained from local experience. On these regimes, cure rates, which are inversely proportional to pretreatment urinary egg outputs when measured quantitatively, vary between 60 and 90% in different population samples. Variable proportions of low density infections are cured after one or two doses and relapses are rare.

Although a fixed dose schedule of three doses is commonly used, there is no reason, patient tolerance permitting, why four or more doses should not be given at appropriate intervals.[7] In Zimbabwe, multiple monthly doses given to uninfected, yet constantly exposed, children appeared to possess a prophylactic effect against the acquisition of *S. haematobium* infection.[64]

Population-based chemotherapy with metriphonate

Following the first major use of metriphonate as a spearhead in the control of epidemic urinary schistosomiasis on Lake Volta, Ghana,[65] in which repetitive, annual, population-based chemotherapy with metriphonate at a total dosage of 7.5 mg.kg^{-1} body weight once every two weeks for three doses was given for 5 years to minimize morbidity and assist in the control of transmission in this hyperendemic area, much experience has been accrued.

In Egypt, where the population at risk of infection is about 33

M

million persons, large control programmes using metriphonate at $10\,mg.kg^{-1}$ for three doses at 2-weekly intervals have been implemented since 1974; in middle Egypt, the population of 4.5 million is screened annually and those found infected are treated (selective population chemotherapy); in upper Egypt, the population of 5.1 million is dealt with similarly. Naturally, many millions of infected people have been treated with metriphonate, many repeatedly.[66]

In Morocco, metriphonate is the basis for the national control programme in which infected people are treated on a population basis, annually if necessary. The population at risk is 650 000.[66]

In many other countries in Africa, smaller schemes of population-based chemotherapy of urinary schistosomiasis are underway. Many millions of individuals of different ethnic origins have been treated, frequently repeatedly, and this experience of mass drug administration in urinary schistosomiasis is a unique phenomenon.

Because, in many developing countries, patients are unable or unwilling to return to centres for administration of a second and third dose of metriphonate, a 'delivery system' must be devised to optimize the known good therapeutic results of the three-dose regime. In parallel, many attempts have been made to shorten the time of treatment by using either single-dose treatments[67–71] of $10\,mg.kg^{-1}$ on a large scale or by giving metriphonate combined with other antischistosomal agents.[68] Results have been disappointing with either variant and the three-dose regime retains its popularity despite the cost of the delivery system.

In summary, it can be said that where an efficient health delivery system exists, the three-dose metriphonate regime will give good results in population-based chemotherapy programmes for control of urinary schistosomiasis. Where an efficient system does not exist, consideration must be given to the use of praziquantel in a single oral dose regime. The costs of delivery are area-specific and must be carefully calculated before embarking on large morbidity control programmes with chemotherapy.

When metriphonate is used in large community treatment projects — as it frequently is — in areas where highly endemic hookworm infection is co-existent with *S. haematobium*, then a useful peripheral 'spin-off' is seen in its modest therapeutic effect on hookworms although, with clearance rates of only 40–50%, it is not recommended as a primary drug for either *Ancylostoma duodenale* or *Necator americanus* infections.

Other uses

Metriphonate possesses some activity against *S. mansoni* and *S. japonicum*[72] but insufficient to recommend its use against these species.

Initial empirical studies in man in the 1950s provided evidence of therapeutic activity not only in schistosomiasis, but also in hookworm infection, creeping eruption, ascariasis,[73,74] trichuriasis[6] and onchocerciasis;[51–54] yet in another filarial infection due to *Wucheraria bancrofti* no macro- or microfilaricidal effects were found.[53]

Claims of success in the treatment of both cerebral[55,56] and cutaneous cysticercosis[57] due to infection with the larval stages of the pork tapeworm *Taenia solium* have been advanced.

These studies were not conducted in accordance with the principles of the randomized clinical trial and the consensus of current opinion is that since the antiparasitic efficacy of metriphonate is inconstant in the majority of the infections noted above, the sole indication for its routine use is in the treatment of infections due to *S. haematobium*.

Adverse reactions

Potentially life-threatening effects

No effects of this kind are to be expected from therapeutic doses.

Acute overdosage

Even in the rare recorded examples of therapeutic errors, where patients received single doses ranging from $30\,mg.kg^{-1}$ to $72\,mg.kg^{-1}$, recovery from cholinergic symptoms, usually with the help of atropine, occurred in 24–48 hours. Monitoring of hepatic, renal and haematological function has not revealed any changes of clinical significance. In short, metriphonate is a safe and effective drug for *S. haematobium* infections.[7]

Severe or irreversible adverse effects

No effects of this kind appear to have been reported in patients given therapeutic doses.

Symptomatic adverse effects

The enormous accumulated experiences of very large-scale chemotherapy campaigns have made it abundantly clear that, at levels of $7.5–10\,mg.kg^{-1}$ per individual dose, patient tolerance has been extremely good. Since metriphonate, like other organophosphorus compounds, inactivates the enzyme destroying acetylcholine, thus allowing the chemical transmitter to persist, cholinergic symptoms would be anticipated during treatment. These symptoms include fatigue, muscular weakness, muscle tremor, sweating, fainting, abdominal colic, diarrhoea, nausea or vomiting and bronchospasm, all reflecting stimulation of cholinergic synapses in the autonomic nervous system, ganglionic and postganglionic sites in both parasympathetic and sympathetic divisions, the neuromuscular junction and several sites in the cardiovascular system. However, metriphonate provides an excellent example of the dictum that each anticholinesterase drug does not necessarily produce every theoretical effect, nor are such effects necessarily seen at a therapeutic dose.[7]

The frequency of cholinergic side effects is extremely low, their severity is mild and they disappear spontaneously in a few hours. One constant accompaniment of metriphonate treatment is depression of acetylcholinesterases in both plasma and erythrocytes but, as noted, this appears to be an inseparable pharmacological adjuvant rather than an adverse effect.

High risk groups

Neonates

The drug is unlikely to be used in this age group.

Breast milk. No information is available on the secretion of the drug in breast milk, so it is probably best for mothers taking the drug not to breast-feed.

Children

The drug is used in children in the vast majority of endemic areas of *S. haematobium* infection, in the recommended doses, with excellent tolerance and safety.

Pregnant women

Although there is no evidence of teratogenicity in animals, a case has been described in which a mother who took the drug during the second month of pregnancy gave birth to an infant with massive hydrocephalus and a large meningomyelocoele.[75] The authors of the report conclude that while there is no firm evidence of a causal relationship, caution is necessary when prescribing the drug for pregnant women.

The elderly

No special precautions are necessary in older patients.

Occupational exposure

Since potentiation of the effects of one organophosphorus (OP) compound by another may occur, and since seasonal use of OP compounds in agriculture is not uncommon, special care must be taken with occupational groups such as spraymen, unsupervised farmers or workers engaged in manufacture of OP insecticides. In these situations, pretreatment estimation of blood cholinesterases would be a wise precaution. In normal clinical practice, this is unnecessary.

Should cholinergic symptoms arise, the parenteral administration of atropine sulphate, repeated if necessary, will block the muscarinic but not the nicotinic effects. Finally, the availability of pralidoximine iodide (2-PAM) as an enzyme activator for cases of profound enzyme inhibition is a welcome safeguard, but in practice PAM use has been restricted to acute organophosphorus intoxication and there are no records of its necessity during metriphonate treatment.[7]

References

1. International Agency for Research on Cancer 1983 IARC Monographs on the evaluation of the carcinogenic risk of chemicals to humans. Miscellaneous pesticides 30, Trichlorfon, pp 207–231
2. Nordgren I, Bergström M, Holmstedt B, Sandoz M 1978 Transformation and action of metrifonate. Archives of Toxicology 41: 31–41
3. International Agency for Research on Cancer 1979 IARC Monographs on the evaluation of the carcinogenic risk of chemicals to humans. Dichlorvos, vol 20, Some halogenated hydrocarbons, pp 97–127
4. Lebrun A, Cerf C 1960 Note préliminaire sur la toxicité pour l'homme d'un insecticide organophosphoré (Dipterex). Bulletin of the World Health Organization 22: 579–582

5. Beheyt P, Lebrun A, Cerf J, Dierickx J, Degroote V 1961 Etude de la toxicité pour l'homme d'un insecticide organophosphoré. Bulletin of the World Health Organization 24: 465–472
6. Cerf J, Lebrun A, Dierickx J 1962 A new approach to helminthiasis control: the use of an organophosphorous compound. American Journal of Tropical Medicine and Hygiene 11: 514–517
7. Davis A 1982 Management of the patient with schistosomiasis. In: Jordan P, Webbe G (eds) Schistosomiasis. Epidemiology, treatment and control. William Heinemann Medical Books, London, pp 184–226
8. Bueding E 1952 Acetylcholinesterase activity of *Schistosoma mansoni*. British Journal of Pharmacology 7: 563–566
9. Barker L R, Bueding E, Timms A R 1966 The possible role of acetylcholine in *S. mansoni*. British Journal of Pharmacology 26: 656–665
10. Bueding E, Liu C L, Rogers S H 1972 Inhibition by metriphonate and dichlorvos of cholinesterases in schistosomes. British Journal of Pharmacology 46: 480–487
11. Gear N R, Fripp P J 1974 Comparison of the characteristics of acetylcholinesterase present in four species of *Schistosoma*. Comparative Biochemistry and Physiology 47: 743–752
12. Gear N R 1976 The effect of inhibitors on the hydrolysis of acetylcholine by four species of *Schistosoma*. Comparative Biochemistry and Physiology 55: 5–10
13. Fripp P J 1967 Histochemical localisation of esterase activity in schistosomes. Experimental Parasitology 21: 380–390
14. Forsyth D M, Rashid C 1967 Treatment of urinary schistosomiasis. Practice and theory. Lancet 1: 130–133
15. Forsyth D M, Rashid C 1967 Treatment of urinary schistosomiasis with trichlorphone. Lancet 2: 909–912
16. Forsyth D M 1965 Treatment of urinary schistosomiasis — practice and theory. Lancet 2: 354–358
17. James C, Webbe G 1974 The susceptibility of *Schistosoma japonicum* in hamsters to metrifonate. Annals of Tropical Medicine and Parasitology 68: 487
18. James C, Webbe G, Preston J M 1972 A comparison of the susceptibility to metrifonate of *Schistosoma haematobium*, *S. matthei* and *S. mansoni* in hamsters. Annals of Tropical Medicine and Parasitology 66: 467–474
19. James C, Webbe G 1974 Treatment of *Schistosoma haematobium* in the baboon with metriphonate. Transactions of the Royal Society of Tropical Medicine and Hygiene 68: 413
20. Bloom A 1981 Studies of the mode of action of metrifonate and DDVP in schistosomes — cholinesterase activity and the hepatic shift. Acta Pharmacologica et Toxicologica 49: 109–113
21. Omer A H S, Teesdale C H 1978 Metriphonate trial in the treatment of various presentations of *Schistosoma haematobium* and *S. mansoni* in the Sudan. Annals of Tropical Medicine and Parasitology 72: 145–150
22. Doehring E, Poggensee U, Feldmeier H 1986 The effect of metrifonate in mixed *Schistosoma haematobium* and *Schistosoma mansoni* in humans. American Journal of Tropical Medicine and Hygiene 35: 323–329
23. Taylor M G, Nelson G S 1971 A comparison of the susceptibility to niridazole of two geographical strains of *S. mansoni* in mice with a note on the susceptibility of *S. matthei*. Transactions of the Royal Society of Tropical Medicine and Hygiene 65: 169–174
24. Frohberg H, Schulze Schencking M 1981 Toxicological profile of praziquantel, a new drug against cestode and schistosome infections, as compared to some other schistosomicides. Arzneimittel Forschung 31: 555–565
25. World Health Organization/Food and Agriculture Organization 1977 Data sheets on pesticides No. 27, Trichlorfon. VBC/DS/77.27. Unpublished document
26. Machemer L 1981 Chronic toxicity of metrifonate. Acta Pharmacologica et Toxicologica 49 (suppl V): 15–28
27. Batzinger R P, Bueding E 1977 Mutagenic activities in vitro and in vivo of five antischistosomal compounds. Journal of Pharmacology and Experimental Therapeutics 200: 1–9
28. Dahmen-Moutschen J, Damen-Moutschen M, Degraeve N 1981 Metrifonate and dichlorvos: cytogenetic investigations. Acta Pharmacologica et Toxicologica 49 (suppl V): 29–39
29. Bayer A G 1984 Manufacturer's information supplied to WHO
30. Doull J D, Vesselinovitch M, Root J, Conan J, Meskausas M, Fitch J 1962 Chronic oral toxicity of Dylox to male and female rats. Unpublished report by Department of Pharmacology, University of Chicago. Cited in WHO Pesticide Residues Series No 1 1971 Evaluations of some pesticide residues in food, WHO, Geneva, 1972, p 183 ff
31. Doull J D, Vesselinovitch M, Fitch J, Meskausas M, Root J, Cowan J 1965 Chronic oral toxicity of Dylox to male and female rats. Unpublished report by Department of Pharmacology, University of Chicago. Cited in WHO Pesticide Residues Series No 1 1971 Evaluations of some pesticide residues in food, WHO, Geneva, 1972, p 183 ff
32. Doull J D, Root D, Vesselinovitch J, Meskausas M, Fitch J 1962 Chronic oral toxicity of Dylox to male and female dogs. Unpublished report by Department of Pharmacology, University of Chicago. Cited in WHO Pesticide Residues Series No 1 1971 Evaluations of some pesticide residues in food, WHO, Geneva, 1972, p 183 ff
33. World Health Organization/Food and Agriculture Organization 1975 Data sheets on pesticides No 2, Rev. 1, Dichlorvos. VBC/DS/75.2(Rev. 1). Unpublished document
34. Fischer G W, Schneider P, Scheufler H 1977 Mutagenicity of dichloroacetaldehyde and 2,2-dichloro-1,1-dihydroxy-ethane-phosphoric acid methyl esters, possible metabolites of the organophosphorus pesticide trichlorphon (in German). Chemico-Biological Interactions 19: 205–213
35. Epstein S S, Arnold E, Andrea J, Bass W, Bishop Y 1972 Detection of chemical mutagens by the dominant lethal assay in the mouse. Toxicology and Applied Pharmacology 23: 288–325
36. Holmstedt B, Nordgren I, Sandox M, Sundwall A 1978 Metrifonate. Summary of toxicological and pharmacological information available. Archives of Toxicology 41: 3–29
37. Segerbäck D, Ehrenberg L 1981 Alkylating properties of dichlorvos (DDVP). Acta Pharmacologica et Toxicologica 49 (suppl V): 56–66
38. Löfroth G 1978 The mutagenicity of dichloroacetaldehyde. Zeitschrift fur Naturforschung 33C: 783–785
39. Johnson M K 1975 Review articles: organophosphorus esters causing delayed neurotoxic effects. Mechanism of action and structure–activity studies. Archives of Toxicology 34: 259–288
40. Johnson M K 1975b The delayed neuropathy caused by some organophosphorus esters: mechanism and challenge. Critical Reviews in Toxicology 3: 289–316
41. Kimmerle G, Lorke D 1968 Toxicology of insecticidal organophosphorates. Pflanzenschutz-Nachrichten, Bayer 21: 111–142
42. Johnson M K 1981 Delayed neurotoxicity — do trichlorfon and/or dichlorvos cause delayed neuropathy in man or in test animals. Acta Pharmacologica et Toxicologica 49 (suppl V): 87–98
43. Slott V, Ecobichon D J 1984 An acute and subacute neurotoxicity assessment of trichlorfon. Canadian Journal of Physiology and Pharmacology 62: 513–518
44. Plestina R, Davis A, Bailey D R 1972 Effect of metrifonate on blood cholinesterases in children during the treatment of schistosomiasis. Bulletin of the World Health Organization 46: 747–759
45. Ellman G L, Courtney K D, Andres V, Featherstone R M 1961 A new and rapid colorimetric determination of acetylcholinesterase activity. Biochemical Pharmacology 7: 88–95
46. Vandekar M, Hedayat S, Plestina R, Ahmandy G 1968 A study of the safety of O-isopropoxyphenylmethylcarbamate in an operational field trial in Iran. Bulletin of the World Health Organization 38: 609–623
47. Wilhelm K 1968 Determination of human plasma cholinesterase activity by adapted Ellman's method. Arhiv za Higijenu Rada 19: 199–207
48. Abdallah A, Saif M, Taha A et al 1965 Evaluation of an organophosphorus compound, Dipterex, in the treatment of bilharziasis. Journal of the Egyptian Medical Association 48: 262–273
49. Hanna S, Basmy K, Selim O, Shoeb S M, Awny A Y 1966 The effects of administration of an organophosphorus compound as an antibilharzial agent, with special reference to plasma cholinesterase. British Medical Journal 1: 1390–1392
50. Katz N, Pellegrino J, Pereira J P 1968 Experimental chemotherapy of schistosomiasis. III. Laboratory and clinical trials with trichlorphone, an organophosphorus compound. Revista Societa Brasil Medicina Tropicale II, 5: 237–245
51. Salazar-Mallen M, González-Barranco D, Mitrani-Levy D 1968 Tratamiento experimental de la oncocercosis con trichlorfon. Revista de Investigacion en Salud Publica de Mexico 28: 231–246
52. Fuglsang H, Anderson J 1977 Effects of a single dose of metrifonate on the forest strain of *Onchocerca volvulus* in Cameroon. World Health Organization, WHO/ONCHO/77.139 WHO/FIL/77.147. Unpublished document
53. Abaru D E, McMahon J E 1977 Metrifonate in onchocerciasis and lymphatic filariasis. World Health Organization, WHO/ONCHO/77.135 WHO/FIL/77.147. Unpublished document
54. Kale O O 1982 Further trials of mebendazole and metrifonate in the treatment of onchocerciasis. Bulletin of the World Health Organization 60: 109–113
55. Trujillo-Valder V M, González-Barranco D, Sandoval-Islas M E, Villanueva-Diaz G, Orozco-Bohne R Chemotherapy of human cysticercosis using metrifonate. Bayer de Mexico, SA de CV, Depto. Veterinario, M. Cervantes Saavedra 259, Mexico
56. Trujillo-Valdez V M, González-Barranco D, Orozco-Bohne R, Villanueva-Diaz G, Sandoval-Islas M E 1981 Experimental treatment of cysticercosis with metrifonate. Archives of Investigative Medicine (Mexico) 12: 15–28
57. Tschen E H, Tschen E A, Smith E B 1981 Cutaneous cysticercosis treated with metrifonate. Archives of Dermatology 117: 507–509
58. Davis A, Bailey D R 1969 Metrifonate in urinary schistosomiasis. Bulletin of the World Health Organization 41: 209–224
59. Davis A 1986 Recent advances in schistosomiasis. Quarterly Journal of Medicine [illegible] 110
60. Reiner E, Krauthacker B, Simeon B, Ŝkrinjaric-Ŝpoljar M 1975 Mechanism of inhibition in vitro of mammalian acetylcholinesterase and cholinesterase in solutions of 0,0-dimethyl 2,2,2-trichloro-1-hydroxyethyl phosphonate (Trichlorfon). Biochemical Pharmacology 24: 717–722
61. Holmstedt B, Palmer L 1973 Mass fragmentography: principles, advantages and future possibilities. In: Costa E, Holmstedt B (eds) Advances in biochemical psychopharmacology, 7. Raven Press, New York, pp 1–14
62. Nordgren I, Holmstedt B, Bengtsson E, Finkel Y 1980 Plasma levels of metrifonate and dichlorvos during the treatment of schistosomiasis with Bilarcil. American Journal of Tropical Medicine and Hygiene 29: 426–430
63. Miyata T, Saito T 1973 Metabolism of NS 2662 in the mouse (in Japanese). Botyu-Kagaku 38: 81–86
64. Jewsbury J M, Cooke M J 1977 Field trial of metrifonate in the treatment and prevention of schistosomiasis infection in man. Annals of Tropical Medicine and Parasitology 71: 67–83
65. World Health Organization 1979 Research on the epidemiology and methodology of schistosomiasis control in man-made lakes. (RAF/71/217). Project findings and recommendations. Report prepared for the United Nations Development Programme and the Governments of Ghana and Egypt. PDP/79.2, unpublished document
66. World Health Organization 1985 The control of schistosomiasis. WHO Technical Report Series No. 728, pp 73, 77
67. Wilkins H A, Moore P J 1980 Single dose of metriphonate. Transactions of the Royal Society of Tropical Medicine and Hygiene 74: 692
68. Pugh R N, Teesdale C H 1983 Single dose oral treatment in urinary schistosomiasis: a double blind trial. British Medical Journal 286: 429–432
69. Pugh R N, Teesdale C H 1984 Long term efficacy of single-dose oral treatment in schistosomiasis haematobium. Transactions of the Royal Society of Tropical Medicine and Hygiene 78: 55–59
70. Rey J L, Nouhou H, Sellin B 1984 Comparaison de trois posologies de metriphonate en chimiothérapie de masse contre *Schistosoma haematobium*. Médecine Tropicale (Marseilles) 44: 57–60

71. El-Kholy A, Boutros S, Tamara F, Warren K S, Mahmoud A A 1984 The effect of a single dose of metrifonate on *Schistosoma haematobium* infection in Egyptian school-children. American Journal of Tropical Medicine and Hygiene 33: 1170–1172
72. World Health Organization 1981 Abstracts of recent Chinese publications on schistosomiasis. WHO/SCHISTO/81.56 Nos 49,50. Unpublished document
73. Cervoni W A, Oliver-González J, Kaye S, Slomka M B 1969 Dichlorvos as a single-dose intestinal anthelmintic therapy for man. American Journal of Tropical Medicine and Hygiene 18: 912–919
74. Peña-Chavarria A, Swartzwelder J C, Villarejos V M, Kotcher E, Argvedas J 1969 Dichlorvos, an effective broad-spectrum anthelmintic. American Journal of Tropical Medicine and Hygiene 18: 907–911
75. Monson M H, Alexander K 1984 Metriphonate in pregnancy Transactions of the Royal Society of Tropical Medicine and Hygeine 78:565.

Metronidazole

Metronidazole was the first clinically effective 5-nitroimidazole drug that received widespread therapeutic use in the treatment of various infections. It was synthesized in 1957 following investigations with azomycin, a structurally related naturally occurring antibiotic isolated from a *Streptomyces* species which had shown activity against *Trichomonas vaginalis*.[1,2] Other nitroimidazoles include tinidazole, ornidazole and nimorazole.

Chemistry

Metronidazole (Flagyl, Elyzol, Metrolyl, Zadstat)
$C_6H_9O_3N_3$
1-(2-Hydroxyethyl)-2-methyl-5-nitroimidazole

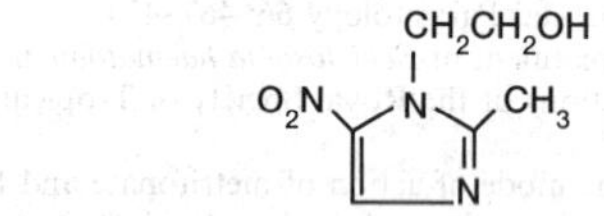

Molecular weight	171.15
pKa	2.62[3,4]
Solubility	
in alcohol	1 in 200
in water	1 in 100
Octanol/water partition coefficient	1.18[5]

Metronidazole is a white to cream crystalline solid or powder, with a slight odour and a bitter taste. It is obtained by chemical synthesis. Metronidazole is also available in combination with nystatin as a vaginal suppository (Flagystatin).

Pharmacology

Metronidazole is an antimicrobial drug that is primarily active against obligate anaerobic microorganisms, both bacteria and protozoa. The 5-nitro group undergoes reductive transformation to an active intermediate which then exerts an inhibitory or lethal effect against DNA.[6,7] Not only is DNA synthesis inhibited but the reduced metabolite also causes a loss of the helical structure of DNA with subsequent DNA strand breakage. The structure of the intermediate has not been determined. Other reduction–oxidation processes within anaerobic organisms may also be inhibited (for example, the phosphoroclastic reaction in clostridia),[8] which also contribute to cell death. In vitro, metronidazole demonstrates a consistently rapid bactericidal effect with the minimal bactericidal concentration approximating very closely to the minimal inhibitory concentration.[9,10]

Toxicology

Metronidazole and some of its metabolites have been shown to be mutagenic in certain bacterial test systems (Ames test).[11,12] The basis for the mutagenic effect (and antimicrobial effect) appears to be dependent upon the reduction of the 5-nitro group which normally would not occur to any significant degree in normal mammalian cells.[13] It could possibly occur in very hypoxic or necrotic tissue. The tumourgenicity of metronidazole has been demonstrated in certain laboratory animals,[14] but not in others or in humans.[15,16] Moreover, there is no firm evidence for teratogenicity or embryotoxicity with metronidazole in animals or in humans.[17] At dose levels approximately 5–10 times those used in humans, metronidazole caused microscopic changes in the liver in monkeys and central nervous system effects (ataxia, tremors, prostration) in dogs.[13] Evidence that

Metronidazole

caused concern regarding cytogenic effects has not been corroborated.[15]

Clinical pharmacology

Metronidazole is very active against the clinically important protozoa *Trichomonas vaginalis*, *Giardia lamblia* and *Entamoeba histolytica* with minimal inhibition concentrations[18–20] of approximately 1 mg.l^{-1}. Of various anaerobic bacteria, metronidazole is especially active against strains of *Bacteroides fragilis* and related species, *Fusobacterium*, *Clostridium*, *Peptococcus*, and *Peptostreptococcus* species.[21–23] Most obligate anaerobes are inhibited by concentrations of 6 mg.l^{-1} or less. It is also moderately active against the facultative anaerobes, *Gardnerella vaginalis*[24] and *Campylobacter fetus*.[25] The hydroxy metabolite of metronidazole is less active against obligate anaerobes but more active against *Gardnerella vaginalis*[26] than the parent compound.

Metronidazole does not inhibit DNA synthesis in normal human cells because oxygen prevents the reduction of the 5-nitro group. However, it does act as a chemical radiosensitizer for hypoxic malignant cells because of its high affinity for electrons.[27] In addition, it can produce a disulfuram-like effect (nausea, vomiting, flushing, headache) with concurrent ethyl alcohol ingestion.[28]

Pharmacokinetics

HPLC methods are the preferred analytical assays for the measurement of metronidazole and its individual metabolites.[29–31] The limit of detection in one assay was approximately 10 μg.l^{-1} and the limit of accurate quantification[30] 20–50 mg.l^{-1}. Microbiological assays, developed first and usually employing *Clostridium* species,[32] can also be used but measure both the parent compound and the microbiologically active metabolites.

The bioavailability of oral metronidazole approaches 90–100%.[33] Peak serum levels of metronidazole after a single 500 mg oral dose range between 9 and 13 mg.l^{-1} and occur 0.33 to 3 hours after the dose.[34] With multiple oral doses, there is some drug accumulation, with minimum serum levels averaging 17 mg.l^{-1} on day 3 on a dose of 500 mg 6-hourly with no evidence of further accumulation by day 7. On a multiple dose regimen of 250 mg 8-hourly, minimum serum levels[35] were approximately 4 mg.l^{-1}. Serum levels are directly proportional to the dose over a broad therapeutic range.[36]

Pharmacokinetic parameters have been derived from several studies in which serum concentration/time data from intravenous infusions of metronidazole were analysed. There is considerable variation in these parameters among individual patients or volunteers.

Oral absorption	90–100%
Presystemic metabolism	negligible
Plasma half life	
range	7.9–9.8 h[36,39]
Volume of distribution	0.76–1.02 l.kg^{-1} [36,37,38]
Plasma protein binding	0–20%

When metronidazole is given as a rectal or vaginal suppository, the bioavailability is approximately 50–70% and 25%, respectively.[33,39] Peak serum levels after rectal administration are usually delayed up to 4 hours after the dose and reach only 50% of those of an equivalent oral dose. After an intra-vaginal dose, the serum levels are only 15% of an equivalent oral dose.

Metronidazole is widely and rapidly distributed throughout the body. This is reflected in its large volume of distribution. Therapeutic levels of metronidazole are found in various tissues, including bile, breast milk, synovial fluid and saliva, in which serum and tissue levels are approximately the same.[37,40–42] Levels in the CSF vary between 60 and 100% of the serum level concentration.[33] In the aqueous humour, levels are approximately 40% of that of the serum[43] and in bone the levels of metronidazole are approximately 75% those of serum.[44] Metronidazole penetrates amoebic and pyogenic abscesses very well, including cerebral abscesses.[45]

The major route of elimination of metronidazole and its metabolites is through the urine. Approximately 60–80% of the total administered dose is recovered as (a) the parent drug (10–20%) and (b) its major metabolites (the hydroxy (30–40%) and acid metabolites (10–20%)) over 48 hours as determined by HPLC.[46]

Concentration–effect relationship

Metronidazole exerts a very rapid bactericidal effect in anaerobic microorganisms at concentrations slightly above those producing an inhibitory effect. The radiosensitizing property of metronidazole requires approximately 5–10 times the usual dose given for its antimicrobial effect.[36]

Metabolism

Metronidazole is metabolized primarily in the liver to various oxidative metabolites which are excreted partially conjugated as glucuronides in the urine. The major metabolites of metronidazole are 1-(2-hydroxyethyl)-2-hydroxymethyl-5-nitroimidazole, the hydroxy metabolite, and 1-acetic acid-2-methyl-5-nitroimidazole, the acid metabolite.[47] A very small percentage may be reduced in the gut to acetamide.[48]

Approximately 14% of the administered dose of metronidazole is detected in the faeces as determined by ^{14}C tracer studies.[49]

After a single intravenous dose of metronidazole, peak levels of the hydroxy metabolite are measured in the serum at concentrations 10–20% those of unchanged drug at approximately 8 hours.[29] The acid metabolite, in contrast, is usually not measurable after a single dose in the serum. After multiple doses, there is accumulation of the metabolites in the serum (hydroxy metabolite 30% of unchanged drug and acid metabolite 3%). In patients on oral therapy, the concentrations of the hydroxy metabolite became quite constant and averaged 7.50 and 3.20 mg.l^{-1} on doses of 1000 and 400 mg daily, respectively.[50] The half life of the hydroxy metabolite was shown to be approximately 11 hours in one study.[46]

Fig. 1 Metabolism of metronizadole

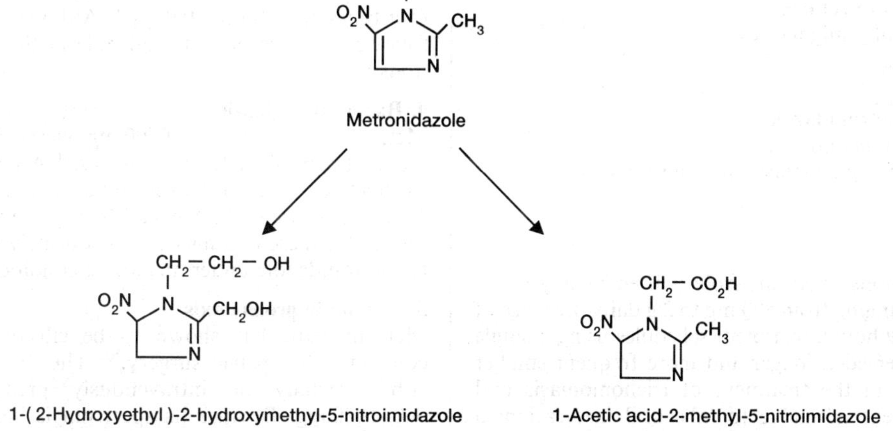

M

Pharmaceutics

Metronidazole is available in oral and parenteral formulations, as vaginal/rectal suppositories, and as a topical cream. UK and USA formulations are listed in Table 1.

Table 1 Metronidazole formulations (UK/USA)

Tablets 200 mg	250 mg	400 mg	500 mg
Flagyl (M&B, UK) cream, round	Flagyl (Searle, USA) blue, round	Flagyl (M&B, UK) cream, round	Flagyl (Searle, USA) blue, oblong
Metrolyl (Lagap, UK)	Metric 21 (Fielding, USA)	Metrolyl Lagap, UK)	Metryl (Lemmon, USA)
Nidazol (Steinhard, UK)	Metryl (Lemmon, USA)	Vaginyl (DDSA, UK)	Protostat (Ortho, USA)
Vaginyl (DDSA, UK)	Protostat (Ortho, USA)		Satric (Savage, USA)
Zadstat (Lederle, UK)	Satric (Savage, USA)		

IV infusion 500 mg/100 ml	Suppositories 500 mg	Suspension 200 mg/5 ml
Flagyl (M&B, UK/Searle, USA)	Elyzol (CP, UK)	Flagyl S (M&B, UK)
Metrolyl (Lagap, UK)	Flagyl (M&B, UK)	
Zadstat (Lederle, UK)	Metrolyl (Lagap, UK)	
	Zadstat (Lederle, UK)	

Metronidazole Flagyl is available for injection as 500 mg in 100 ml infusate (containing sodium chloride, sodium phosphate, and citric acid). It is recommended that this preparation be stored away from direct light and at temperatures lower than 30°C.

Vaginal/rectal inserts contain 500–1000 mg of metronidazole. Flagystatin vaginal inserts contain 500 mg metronidazole and 100 000 units of nystatin and are available in some countries. Vaginal cream contains 10% metronidazole in a cream base.

In the UK Flagyl compak contains 200 mg tablets of oral metronidazole and vaginal tablets containing 100 000 units of nystatin.

Therapeutic use

Indications

1. The treatment of trichomoniasis, giardiasis, and amoebiasis
2. The treatment of serious anaerobic bacterial infections.

Other uses

3. The treatment of *Clostridium difficile* colitis
4. The treatment of bacterial vaginosis
5. The prophylaxis of colorectal and pelvic surgery
6. The treatment of Crohn's disease
7. The treatment of dental infections
8. The radiosensitization of malignancies.

Contraindications

1. Known sensitivity to metronidazole
2. Concurrent use of ethyl alcohol
3. History of serious neurologic disease, including seizures
4. Severe hepatic failure.

Mode of use

In the treatment of infections, metronidazole is used mainly as an oral medication in doses ranging from 500 mg to 2 g daily. Because of its long half life of about 9 hours, treatment schedules using a single large daily dose have superseded longer and more frequent smaller dose regimens, especially in the treatment of trichomoniasis and giardiasis. When the patient is unable to take oral medication, a rectal suppository may be used, although the bioavailability is reduced and absorption is delayed.

The intravenous form of metronidazole is used in seriously ill patients and in patients in whom therapeutic levels are required immediately. It is very expensive compared to the oral or rectal forms of the drug and substituting these preparations as soon as possible is strongly recommended.

The topical formulation as the suppository or cream is used for vaginal trichomoniasis when the oral form is contraindicated or not tolerated. Although metronidazole is absorbed systemically from the vaginal suppository, its bioavailability is only 25% compared to the oral form. It is generally less convenient to use than the oral medication.

Very large doses of metronidazole are used (6 g.m^{-2} body surface area) when it is used as a chemical radiosensitizer.

Indications

1. Protozoal infections

Metronidazole is the drug of choice for the treatment of trichomoniasis. A single 2 g dose is as effective as the original, longer regimen consisting of 250 mg two to three times daily for 7–10 days. Male partners can also be treated with the single dose. Topical therapy as the vaginal suppository or cream is rarely used as an alternative because of the inconvenience and long duration of treatment (1 insert or 1 application of cream nightly for 10–20 days). For cases that persist after oral treatment and where 'resistant' trichomonads are suspected,[51] a combination of oral and topical therapy may be effective. In clinical circumstances where low systemic levels would be desirable, for example in pregnancy, topical treatment might be indicated.

In giardiasis, 2 g daily for 3 days is as effective as a longer course of 250 mg two to three times daily for 5–10 days.[52] In children, the usual dose is 25–35 mg.kg^{-1} daily in two divided doses.

Metronidazole is effective in symptomatic amoebic intestinal disease and amoebic abscess at a dose of 750 mg three times daily for 5–10 days. It is less effective in asymptomatic intestinal infection.[53] In children, the dose is 35–50 mg.kg^{-1} daily in three divided doses.

2. Anaerobic bacterial infections

For serious anaerobic bacterial infections, metronidazole is usually given at a dose of 500 mg three times daily. Although it is effective against most clinically important anaerobes, its marked activity against lower gut anaerobes, including *Bacteroides fragilis* (and related strains), *Fusobacterium* and *Clostridium* species make it very useful in the treatment of intra-abdominal and pelvic sepsis in which these organisms are implicated. The excellent distribution into most body tissues and its consistently bactericidal effect make it also the drug of choice for many serious infections, including meningitis, cerebral abscess, and endocarditis.

Because many infections in which anaerobes are present are mixed and include aerobic bacteria, treatment with metronidazole is usually combined with an antibiotic effective against aerobes (a penicillin, cephalosporin or aminoglycoside).

Other uses

3. *Clostridium difficile* colitis

Oral metronidazole is an alternative and less expensive agent than vancomycin in antibiotic-associated colitis. The usual dose is 250 mg four times daily for 5–10 days.[54] Although rare, *C. difficile* colitis has followed the use of metronidazole in the treatment of other infections.[55]

4. Bacterial vaginosis

Metronidazole at a dose of 500 mg twice daily for 7 days is effective in the treatment of bacterial vaginosis.[56] A single 2 g dose appears to be as effective.[57] The organisms implicated in this clinical entity include *Gardnerella vaginalis*, *Mobiluncus* spp., and various anaerobic organisms. All these organisms are exquisitely or moderately susceptible to metronidazole under anaerobic conditions.

5. Antibiotic prophylaxis

Metronidazole has shown to be effective in the prophylaxis of colorectal and pelvic surgery.[58] The drug is usually administered either rectally or intravenously preoperatively at doses of 500–1000 mg. Because its spectrum is limited to anaerobes, other drugs effective against aerobic organisms are often also administered concurrently.

6. Treatment of Crohn's disease
In a large multi-centre trial, metronidazole at a dose of 400 mg twice daily orally for four months was shown to be slightly more effective than sulfasalazine in active Crohn's disease.[59] Failure to respond to sulfasalazine may warrant a trial of metronidazole.

7. Dental infections
Anaerobic bacteria play a major role in various dental infections, including pericoronitis, acute ulcerative gingivitis, periapical infections, and osteitis (including dry socket). Metronidazole is used at a dose of 200 mg three times daily for 3–7 days.[60]

8. Radiosensitization of malignancies
Metronidazole given as a radioenhancer was shown to delay tumour regrowth in patients with glioblastoma multiforme.[61] However, in patients with metastatic epidural spinal cord compression treated with metronidazole prior to radiotherapy, no significant beneficial long-term effect was noted.[62] This application of metronidazole therefore may be limited.

Contraindications

1. Hypersensitivity to metronidazole
This is very rare and usually is manifested as a maculo-papular rash on the trunk and neck. A fixed drug eruption due to metronidazole has also been reported. Acute neurological deterioration within hours of ingestion of metronidazole can also occur.

2. Concurrent use of alcohol
Metronidazole produces a disulfuram-like effect with hypotension and flushing when used concurrently with ethyl alcohol. Patients should abstain from alcoholic beverages for at least 48 hours following discontinuation of therapy with metronidazole.

3. Patients with neurological disease
Because of its potential neurotoxicity, metronidazole may aggravate pre-existing neurological disease, including patients with a convulsive disorder. This is a relative contraindication, since metronidazole is very effective in the treatment of cerebral abscesses and meningitis caused by susceptible anaerobes.

4. Severe hepatic failure
Metronidazole is primarily metabolized by the liver and therefore toxic accumulation of the parent compound could occur in patients with severe hepatic failure.

Adverse reactions

Potentially life-threatening effects
Although the potential tumourgenicity of metronidazole has been intensively reviewed following the report of increased tumours in animals, there is no evidence to date to substantiate an increase of cancer in humans.[16,63]

Acute overdosage
One case report of a voluntary overdose of 4200 mg in a 16-year-old pregnant woman reported that the patient developed disorientation which resolved without specific treatment.[64] Larger doses than this reported overdose have been given to patients as a radiosensitizer without severe toxicity.

Severe or irreversible adverse effects
Patients who have received unusually large doses of metronidazole have developed various central neurological effects, including seizures, ataxia, headaches and encephalopathy.[65–67] Seizures have also been reported in patients without known neurological disease who have received usual therapeutic doses. EEG changes have also been noted in patients on metronidazole and it is postulated that the drug may have a specific effect on the limbic structures in the brain.[68]

A sensory peripheral neuropathy has been caused by metronidazole in patients who have received high doses for radiosensitization or prolonged treatment regimens, as in patients with Crohn's disease.[69,70] Doses of metronidazole larger than 30 g have usually been given in these cases. The peripheral neuropathy is often asymptomatic and is reversible in the majority of patients over a period of weeks to months, although in a minority complete reversal has not occurred after two years.[71]

Metronidazole

A reversible neutropenia is also seen in approximately 2% of patients who have received prolonged high doses of metronidazole.[72]

Symptomatic adverse effects
Gastrointestinal upset, including anorexia, nausea, vomiting, and epigastric pain, is the most common adverse effect but is usually very mild. These symptoms are more pronounced and occur quite commonly after the massive doses of metronidazole that are given for radiosensitization purposes. After single large doses for the treatment of trichomoniasis, giardiasis and bacterial vaginitis, the incidence of reported gastrointestinal upset is usually less than 5%.[57] A metallic taste and mouth dryness, probably due to the presence of high concentrations of metronidazole in the saliva, and furring of the tongue are also reported.

Dermatological reactions are very rare and include a maculopapular rash resembling pityriasis rosaceae, usually on the trunk and neck, pruritus and fixed drug eruptions.[73] Palpitations and chest pain have also been reported. Darkening of the urine with a reddish-brown discoloration is often reported and is probably due to an azo-group-containing metabolite.

There is a low incidence of phlebitis associated with the intravenous injection of metronidazole.

Microbiologically, administration of metronidazole appears to predispose to vaginal candidiasis through the alteration of the vaginal microflora.

Single case reports have implicated metronidazole in producing gynaecomastia[74] and acute pancreatitis.[75]

Other effects
Metronidazole was shown to reduce serum levels of cholesterol and triglycerides up to 40% in patients taking 750 mg three times daily.[76]

Interference with clinical pathology tests
Metronidazole interferes with the assay of aspartate aminotransferase by simulating the presence of reduced nicotinamide adenine dinucleotide (NADH).[77]

High risk groups

Neonates
Metronidazole has been administered to full-term and premature infants without deleterious effect. The half life of metronidazole was prolonged to 75 hours in patients less than 32 weeks gestation, 35 hours from 32–35 weeks gestation, and 25 hours in infants 36–40 weeks gestation. The total body clearance is proportionately decreased.[78] In a 6-week-old infant, the half life and total body clearance was similar to that seen in adults.[37] It is recommended that term infants receive a loading dose of 15 $mg.kg^{-1}$ and then 7.5 $mg.kg^{-1}$ every 24 hours. Pre-term infants, after a similar loading dose, should receive 7.5 $mg.kg^{-1}$ every 48 hours.

Breast milk. Metronidazole penetrates well into breast milk.[41] If exposure of the neonate to metronidazole is to be avoided, breast-feeding should be delayed until 48 hours after discontinuing metronidazole in the mother.

Children
Children should receive a dose of 7.5 $mg.kg^{-1}$ of metronidazole every 8 hours for serious infections.

Pregnant women
When metronidazole has been administered during pregnancy, no adverse effects have been noted in the mother or fetus.[77] However, it is recommended that metronidazole not be given during the first trimester of pregnancy and avoided during the latter trimesters if possible. If use is deemed necessary, short high-dose regimens are not recommended. The efficacy of metronidazole in serious anaerobic infections has to be weighed against potential, but unproved, mutagenic and teratogenic effects. From limited data, metronidazole appears to cross the placenta, as would be expected from its lipid solubility.[79]

The elderly
No dosage change is usually necessary. Metronidazole should be used with caution in patients with known neurological disease.

Concurrent disease

Renal failure
Renal failure does not change the half life of metronidazole. How-

ever, since the major metabolites of metronidazole, the acid and hydroxy metabolites, are primarily excreted in the urine, these accumulate in renal failure.[38] The half life of the hydroxy metabolite in one study was 34 hours and for the acid metabolite 138 hours.[80] Adverse reactions to the metabolites, which accumulate in renal failure, could occur, and reducing the dose by approximately one-third of the normal dose per day may be desirable.

The type of dialysis required in renal failure patients will affect the elimination of metronidazole and its metabolites. Haemodialysis reduces the half life of metronidazole from 9 hours to approximately 3 hours.[81] The half lives of the metabolites of metronidazole are also reduced, with the half life of the hydroxy metabolite decreasing from 34 hours to 8 hours and the acid metabolite from 138 to 7.9 hours.[81] The type of dialyser membrane appears to affect the clearances of metronidazole and the hydroxy metabolite.[82] Full doses of metronidazole therefore can be given if the patient is on haemodialysis but it is recommended that they be given after dialysis to ensure adequate levels.

Peritoneal dialysis does not appear to affect the elimination of metronidazole or its metabolites, and therefore the recommendations for patients in severe renal failure would pertain.[83]

Hepatic disease

Since metronidazole is metabolized in the liver by oxidative mechanisms, it would be expected that its pharmacokinetics would be affected in patients with impaired liver function. In one study involving 10 patients with severe liver disease,[84] after a single intravenous dose, the total body clearance of metronidazole was reduced by approximately 66% and the terminal serum half life (β phase) was increased to 19.9 hours from 7.9 hours in normal patients. The production of the hydroxy metabolite was delayed, with peak serum levels occurring at 22 hours in liver failure patients, in contrast to 8 hours in normal patients. The total urinary excretion of the hydroxy and acid metabolites was markedly reduced over 48 hours. The excretion of unchanged metronidazole, in contrast, was not significantly different in normal patients and patients with liver failure. The degree of conjugation of the metabolites did not appear affected in patients with liver failure. No studies examining the fate of metronidazole or its metabolites in patients with severe liver failure on multiple dose regimens have been reported, but a reduction in the daily dose by 50% may be prudent with measurement of serum levels.

Drug interactions

Potentially hazardous interactions

Metronidazole interacts with racemic and S(−) warfarin and increases the blood levels of warfarin and causes a hypothrombinaemic effect. It is postulated that metronidazole inhibits ring oxidation of S(−) warfarin and therefore impairs total body clearance of warfarin.[85]

Other significant interactions

Premedication with metronidazole did not affect the metabolic disposition of phenytoin, diazepam or antipyrine, whose metabolism depends upon oxidative drug metabolism (a cytochrome P-450 system).[86] Theophylline pharmacokinetics were also not affected, although theophylline is metabolized by dealkylation and hydroxylation in the liver.[87] Cimetidine, in contrast, prolongs the half life of metronidazole through reduction of its total plasma clearance.[88]

Metronidazole and disulfiram when given concurrently have caused an acute psychosis.[89]

Potentially useful interactions

Metronidazole can be combined with other antimicrobials for an additive or synergistic effect.[90] There is no evidence to suggest that metronidazole antagonizes the activity of other antimicrobials.

Major outcome trials

1. Canadian metronidazole–clindamycin study group 1983 Prospective, randomized comparison of metronidazole and clindamycin, each with gentamicin, for the treatment of serious intra-abdominal infection. Surgery 93: 221–229

141 patients were evaluated in this study, 72 receiving gentamicin and metronidazole, and 69 clindamycin and gentamicin. Appendicitis and diverticulitis were the most common infections. Patients were categorized as cured, improved or treatment failures, and results were similar in both groups with cure rates of approximately 85%. Side effects of rash, diarrhoea and superinfection were the same in both groups.

2. Marti M C, Aukenthaler R 1983 Antibiotic prophylaxis in large bowel surgery. Results of a controlled clinical trial. Surgery 93: 190–196

Gentamicin and metronidazole were compared with gentamicin and clindamycin given three times daily prior to and for 48 hours after surgery. 52 patients were evaluated after receiving gentamicin and clindamycin, and 57 after gentamicin and metronidazole. The post-operative infection rate was 8.4% and was similar in both groups and aerobic organisms were the major pathogens. Side effects were minimal in both groups.

3. Swedberg J, Steilner J F, Deiss F, Steiner S, Driggers D A 1985 Comparison of single-dose vs. one week course of metronidazole for symptomatic bacterial vaginosis. Journal of the American Medical Association 254: 1046–1049

In a prospective, single-blind study of 82 women with symptomatic bacterial vaginosis, 46 were treated with a single 2 g dose of metronidazole and 36 with 500 mg twice daily for 7 days. The cure rates at 7–10 days after treatment were 86% and 97% for the single and 7-day regimen, respectively. However, at 21 days post treatment, only 46% were cured after the single 2 g dose compared to 86% for the longer dose regimen.

4. Austin T W, Smith E A, Darwish R, Ralph E D, Pattison F L M 1982 Metronidazole in a single dose for the treatment of trichomoniasis. Failure of a single 1-g dose. British Journal of Venereal Disease 58: 121–123

In this prospective single-blind study, a single 2 g dose of metronidazole in 86 patients was more effective (84% cure rate) than a single 1 g dose in 77 patients (55% cure rate). Patients in either treatment group who failed to respond initially were treated with a single 2 g dose. 86% in the failed 1 g dose group were cured and 70% in the failed 2 g dose group.

5. Teasley D G, Gerding D, Olson M M et al 1983 Prospective randomized trial of metronidazole versus vancomycin for Clostridium-difficile-associated diarrhoea and colitis. Lancet 2: 1043–1046

94 patients with diarrhoea from whom *C. difficile* was either cultured or the cytotoxin detected were treated with oral metronidazole (250 mg four times daily) or vancomycin (500 mg four times daily) for 10 days. Of 42 patients receiving metronidazole, there were 2 treatment failures and 2 relapses. For 52 patients treated with vancomycin, there were no failures but 6 relapses. The cost of metronidazole was approximately forty times less.

General review articles

Brogden R N, Heel R C, Speight T M, Avery G S 1978 Metronidazole in anaerobic infections: a review of its activity, pharmacokinetics and therapeutic use. Drugs 16: 387–417

Molavi A, LeFrock J L, Prince R A 1982 Metronidazole. Medical Clinics of North America 66: 121–133

Brook I 1983 Treatment of anaerobic infections in children with metronidazole. Developmental Pharmacology and Therapeutics 6: 187–198

Anderson K E 1981 Pharmacokinetics of nitroimidazoles. Spectrum of adverse reactions. Scandinavian Journal of Infectious Diseases (suppl) 26: 60–67

Finegold S M 1980 Metronidazole. Annals of Internal Medicine 93: 585–587

References

1. Jolles G E 1977 Original and anti-infective activities of metronidazole. In: Finegold S M (ed) McFadzean J A, Roe F J C (assoc eds) Metronidazole. Proceedings of the International Metronidazole Conference, Montreal, Quebec, Canada, May 26–28 1976. Excerpta Medica, Princeton, New Jersey, pp 3–11
2. Maeda K, Osata T, Umezawa H 1953 A new antibiotic azomycin. Journal of Antibiotics 6A: 182
3. Raymond G G, Born J L 1986 An updated pKa listing of medicinal compounds. Drug Intelligence and Clinical Pharmacy 10: 683–686

4. Cho M, Kwtz R, Lewis C et al 1982 Metronidazole phosphate — a water-soluble pro-drug for parenteral solutions of metronidazole. Journal of Pharmaceutical Sciences 71: 410–414
5. May & Baker Ltd. Unpublished data
6. Muller M 1981 Action of clinically utilized 5-nitroimidazoles on microorganisms. Scandinavian Journal of Infectious Diseases (suppl) 26: 31–41
7. Sigeti J S, Guiney D G, Davis C E 1983 Mechanism of action of metronidazole on *Bacteroides fragilis*. Journal of Infectious Diseases 148: 1083–1089
8. Lockerby D L, Rabin H R, Laishley E J 1985 Role of the phosphoroclastic reaction of *Clostridium pasteurianum* in the reduction of the metronidazole. Antimicrobial Agents and Chemotherapy 27: 863–867
9. Ralph E D, Kirby W M M 1975 Unique bactericidal action of metronidazole against *Bacteroides fragilis* and *Clostridium perfringens*. Antimicrobial Agents and Chemotherapy 8: 409–414
10. Tally F P, Sutter V L, Finegold S M 1972 Metronidazole versus anaerobes. California Medicine 117: 22–26
11. Voogd C E, Van Der Stel J J, Jacobs J J J A A 1974 The mutagenic action of nitroimidazoles, metronidazole, nimorazole, dimetridazole, and ornidazole. Mutation Research 26: 483–490
12. Conner T H, Stoeckel M, Evrard J, Legator M S 1977 The contribution of metronidazole and two metabolites to the mutagenic activity detected in urine of treated humans and mice. Cancer Research 37: 629–633
13. Bost R G 1977 Metronidazole: mammalian mutagenicity. In: Finegold S M (ed) McFadzean J A, Roe F J C (assoc eds) Metronidazole. Proceedings of the International Metronidazole Conference, Montreal, Quebec, Canada, May 26–28 1976. Excerpta Medica, Princeton, New Jersey, pp 126–131
14. Rustia M, Shubik P 1972 Induction of lung tumors and malignant lymphomas in mice by metronidazole. Journal of National Cancer Institute 48: 721–726
15. Roe F J C 1979 A critical appraisal of the toxicity of metronidazole. In: Phillips I, Collier J (eds) Metronidazole. Proceedings of the 2nd International Symposium on Anaerobic Infections, Geneva, April 25–27. The Royal Society of Medicine, London Academic Press, London; Grune and Stratton, New York, pp 215–222
16. Beard C, Noller K L, O'Fallon M, Karland L T, Dockerty M B 1979 Lack of evidence for cancer due to use of metronidazole. New England Journal of Medicine 301: 519–522
17. Morgan I 1978 Metronidazole treatment in pregnancy. International Journal of Gynecology and Obstetrics 15: 501–502
18. Ralph E D, Darwish R, Austin T W, Smith E A, Pattison F L M 1983 Susceptibility of *Trichomonas vaginalis* strains to metronidazole: response to treatment. Sexually Transmitted Diseases 10: 119–122
19. Cederno J R, Krogstad D T 1983 Susceptibility testing of *Entamoeba histolytica*. Journal of Infectious Diseases 148: 1090–1095
20. Jokipii L, Jokipii A M M 1980 In vitro susceptibility of *Giardia lamblia* trophozoites to metronidazole and tinidazole. The Journal of Infectious Diseases 1412: 317–325
21. Chow A W, Bednorz D, Guze L B 1977 Susceptibility of obligate anaerobes to metronidazole: an extended study of 1054 clinical isolates. In: Finegold S M (ed) McFadzean J A, Roe F J C (assoc eds) Metronidazole. Proceedings of the International Metronidazole Conference, Montreal Quebec, Canada, May 26–28 1976. Excerpta Medica, Princeton, New Jersey, pp 286–292
22. Wust J 1977 Susceptibility of anaerobic bacteria to metronidazole, ornidazole, and tinidazole and routine susceptibility testing by standardized methods. Antimicrobial Agents and Chemotherapy 11: 631–637
23. Dubrevil L, Devos J, Neut C, Romond C 1984 Susceptibility of anaerobic bacteria from several French hospitals to three major antibiotics. Antimicrobial Agents and Chemotherapy 25: 764–766
24. Ralph E D, Austin T W, Pattison F L M, Schieven B 1979 Inhibition of *Haemophilus vaginalis* (*Corynebacterium vaginale*) by metronidazole, tetracycline, and ampicillin. Sexually Transmitted Diseases 6: 199–202
25. Hof H, Sticht-Groh V, Muller K M 1982 Comparative in vitro activities of niridazole and metronidazole against anaerobic and microaerophilic bacteria. Antimicrobial Agents and Chemotherapy 22: 332–333
26. Ralph E D, Amatnieks Y E 1980 Relative susceptibilities of *Gardnerella vaginalis* (*Haemophilus vaginalis*), *Neisseria gonorrhoeae*, and *Bacteroides fragilis* to metronidazole and its two major metabolites. Sexually Transmitted Diseases 7: 157–160
27. Foster J L, Willson R L 1973 Radiosensitization of anoxic cells by metronidazole. British Journal of Radiology 46: 234–235
28. Taylor J A T 1964 Metronidazole, a new agent for combined somatic and psychic therapy of alcoholism. A case study and preliminary report. Bulletin of Los Angeles Neurological Society 29: 158–162
29. Wheeler L A, DeMeo M, Halula M, George L, Hesseltine P 1978 Use of high pressure liquid chromatography to determine plasma levels of metronidazole and metabolites after intravenous administration. Antimicrobial Agents and Chemotherapy 13: 205–209
30. Gulaid A, Houghton G W, Lewellen O R W, Smith J, Thorne P S 1978 Determination of metronidazole and its two major metabolites in biological fluids by high pressure liquid chromatography. British Journal of Clinical Pharmacology 6: 430–432
31. Hackett L P, Dusci L J 1979 Determination of metronidazole and tinidazole in human plasma using high performance liquid chromatography. Journal of Chromatography 175: 347–349
32. Ralph E D, Kirby W M M 1975 Bioassay of metronidazole with either anaerobic or aerobic incubation. Journal of Infectious Diseases 132: 587–591
33. Ralph E D 1983 Clinical pharmacokinetics of metronidazole. Clinical Pharmacokinetics 8: 43–62
34. Houghton G W, Thorne P S, Smith J, Templeton R, Collier J 1979 Comparison of the pharmacokinetics of metronidazole in healthy female volunteers following either a single oral or intravenous dose. British Journal of Clinical Pharmacology 8: 337–381
35. Ralph E D, Clarke J T, Libke R D, Luthy R P, Kirby W M M 1974 Pharmacokinetics of metronidazole as determined by bioassay. Antimicrobial Agents and Chemotherapy 6: 691–696
36. Rabin H R, Urtasun R C, Partington J, Koziol D, Sharon M, Walker K 1980 High dose metronidazole: pharmacokinetics and bioavailability using an iv preparation and application of its use as a radiosensitizer. Cancer Treatment Reports 63: 1087–1095
37. Amon I, Amon K, Sharp H, Franke G, Nagel F 1983 Disposition kinetics of metronidazole in children. European Journal of Clinical Pharmacology 24: 113–119
38. Kreeft J H, Olgivie R I, Dufresne L R 1983 Metronidazole kinetics in dialysis patients. Surgery 93 (Part 2): 149–153
39. Mattila J, Mannisto P T, Mantyla R, Nykanen S, Lamminsivu U 1983 Comparative pharmacokinetics of metronidazole and tinidazole as influenced by administration route. Antimicrobial Agents and Chemotherapy 23: 721–725
40. Nielsen M L, Justeben T 1977 Excretion of metronidazole in human bile. Investigations of hepatic bile, common duct bile, and gall bladder bile. Scandinavian Journal of Gastroenterology 12: 1003–1008
41. Erickson S H, Oppenheim G L, Smith G H 1981 Metronidazole in breast milk. Obstetrics and Gynaecology 57: 48–50
42. Sattar M A, Sankey M G, Cawley M I D, Kaye C M, Holt J E 1982 The penetration of metronidazole into the synovial fluid. Postgraduate Medical Journal 58: 20–24
43. Mattila J, Nerdrum K, Rouhianen H, Mannisto P, Tuovinen E, Lamminsivu U 1983 Penetration of metronidazole and tinidazole into the aqueous humor in man. Chemotherapy 29: 188–191
44. Rood J P, Collier J 1979 Metronidazole levels in alveolar bone. In: Phillips I, Collier J (eds) Metronidazole. Proceedings of the 2nd International Symposium on Anaerobic Infections, Geneva, April 25–27. The Royal Society of Medicine, London Academic Press, London; Grune and Stratton, New York, pp 45–47
45. George R H, Bint A J 1976 Treatment of a brain abscess due to *Bacteroides fragilis* with metronidazole. Journal of Antimicrobial Chemotherapy 2: 101–106
46. Jenson J C, Gugler R 1983 Single and multiple-dose metronidazole kinetics. Clinical Pharmacology and Therapeutics 34: 481–487
47. Stambaugh J E, Feo L G, Manthei R W 1968 The isolation and identification of the urinary oxidative metabolites of metronidazole in man. Journal of Pharmacology and Experimental Therapeutics 161: 373–381
48. Koch R L, Krystal E J T, Beaulieu B B Jr, Goldman P 1979 Acetamide — a metabolite of metronidazole formed by the intestinal flora. Biochemical Pharmacology 28: 3611–3615
49. Schwartz D E, Jeunet F 1976 Comparative pharmacokinetic studies of ornidazole and metronidazole in man. Chemotherapy 22: 19–29
50. Schneider M U, Reimann J F, Laudage G 1984 Serum concentrations of metronidazole and its main metabolite in patients with active Crohn's disease: correlation with disease activity and therapeutic efficacy. Chemotherapy 30: 345–352
51. Meingassner J G, Thurner J 1977 Strain of *Trichomonas vaginalis* resistant to metronidazole and other 5-nitroimidazoles. Antimicrobial Agents and Chemotherapy 15: 254–257
52. Wright S G, Tomkins A M, Ridley D S 1977 Giardiasis: clinical and therapeutic aspects. Gut 18: 343–350
53. Adams E B, MacLeod I N 1977 Invasive amoebiasis. I. Amebic dysentery and its complications. II. Amebic liver abscess and its complications. Medicine, Baltimore 56: 315–334
54. Pashby N L, Bolton R P, Sherriff R J 1979 Oral metronidazole in *Clostridium difficile* colitis. British Medical Journal 1: 1605–1606
55. Thomson G, Clark A H, Hare K, Spilg W G 1981 Pseudomembranous colitis after treatment with metronidazole. British Medical Journal 282: 864–865
56. Pheifer T A, Forsyth P S, Durfee M A, Pollock H M, Holmes K K 1978 Nonspecific vaginitis. Role of *Haemophilus vaginalis* and treatment with metronidazole. New England Journal of Medicine 298: 1429–1434
57. Minkowski W L, Baker C J, Alleyne D, Baghai M, Friedlander L, Schultz B 1983 Single oral dose metronidazole therapy for *Gardnerella vaginalis* vaginitis in adolescent females. Journal of Adolescent Health Care 4: 113–116
58. Willis A T, Fiddian R V 1983 Metronidazole in the prevention of anaerobic infection. Surgery 93: 174–179
59. Blichfeldt P, Blomhoff J P, Myhre E, Gjone E 1978 Metronidazole in Crohn's disease. A double blind cross-over clinical trial. Scandinavian Journal of Gastroenterology 13: 123–127
60. Mitchell D A 1984 Metronidazole: its use in clinical dentistry. Journal of Clinical Peridontology 11: 145–158
61. Urtasun R C, Band P R, Chapman J D, Feldstein M L, Mielke B, Fryer C 1976 Radiation and high dose metronidazole in supratentorial glioblastomas. New England Journal of Medicine 294: 1364–1367
62. Obbens E A M T, Kim J H, Thaler H, Deck M D F, Posner J B 1984 Metronidazole as a radiation enhancer in the treatment of metastatic epidural spinal cord compression. Journal of Neuro-oncology 2: 99–104
63. Friedman G D 1980 Cancer after metronidazole. New England Journal of Medicine 302: 519
64. Fluker J L 1961 Two unusual cases. British Journal of Venereal Diseases 36: 280–281
65. Frytak S, Moertal C G, Childs D S, Albers J W 1978 Neurologic toxicity associated with high dose metronidazole. Annals of Internal Medicine 88: 361–362
66. Kusumi R K, Plouffe J F, Wyatt R H, Fass R J 1980 Central nervous system toxicity associated with metronidazole therapy. Annals of Internal Medicine 93: 59–60
67. Bailes J, Willis J, Priebe C, Strub R 1983 Encephalopathy with metronidazole in a child. American Journal of Diseases in Children 137: 290–291
68. Placidi G F, Masuoka D, Alcaraz A et al 1970 Distribution and metabolism of ^{14}C-metronidazole in mice. Archives of International Pharmacodynamic Therapy 188: 168–179

69. Coxon A, Pallis C A 1976 Metronidazole neuropathy. Journal of Neurology, Neurosurgery and Psychiatry 39: 403–405
70. Bradley W G, Karlson I J, Rassol C G 1977 Metronidazole neuropathy. British Medical Journal 3: 610–611
71. Duffy L F, Daum F, Fisher S E et al 1985 Peripheral neuropathy in Crohn's disease patients treated with metronidazole. Gastroenterology 8: 681–684
72. Smith J A 1980 Neutropenia associated with metronidazole therapy. Canadian Medical Association Journal 123: 202
73. Naik R P C, Singh G 1977 Fixed drug reaction due to metronidazole. Dermatologica 155: 59–60
74. Fagan T C, Johnson D G, Grosso D S 1985 Metronidazole-induced gynecomastia. Journal of the American Medical Association 254: 3217
75. Plotkin B H, Cohen I, Tsang T, Cullinane T 1985 Metronidazole-induced pancreatitis. Annals of Internal Medicine 103: 891–892
76. Davis J L, Schultz T A, Mosley C A 1983 Metronidazole lowers serum lipids. Annals of Internal Medicine 99: 43–44
77. Rissing J P, Newman C, Moore W L 1978 Artifactual depression of serum glutamine oxaloacetic transaminase by metronidazole. Antimicrobial Agents and Chemotherapy 14: 636–638
78. Jager-Roman E, Doyle P E, Baird-Lambert J, Cvejic M, Buchanan N 1982 Pharmacokinetics and tissue distribution of metronidazole in the newborn infant. Journal of Paediatrics 100: 651–654
79. Amon K, Amon I, Huller H 1972 Maternal–fetal passage of metronidazole. Proceedings of the 7th International Congress of Chemotherapy 1: 113–115
80. Gabriel R, Page C M, Weller I V D et al 1979 The pharmacokinetics of metronidazole in patients with chronic renal failure. In: Phillips I, Collier J (eds) Metronidazole. Proceedings of the 2nd International Symposium on Anaerobic Infections, Geneva, April 25–27. The Royal Society of Medicine, London Academic Press, London; Grune and Stratton, New York, pp 50–54
81. Roux A F, Moirot E, Delhotal B, Leroy J A, Bonmarhand G P, Humbert G, Flouvat B 1984 Metronidazole kinetics in patients with acute renal failure on dialysis: a cumulative study. Clinical Pharmacology and Therapeutics 36: 363–368
82. Lau A H, Chang C W, Sabatini S 1986 Hemodialysis clearance of metronidazole and its metabolites 29: 235–238
83. Guay D R, Meatherall R C, Baxter H, Jacyk W R, Penner B 1984 Pharmacokinetics of metronidazole in patients undergoing continuous ambulatory peritoneal dialysis. Antimicrobial Agents and Chemotherapy 25: 306–310
84. Farrel G, Baird-Lambert J, Cuejic M, Buchanan N 1984 Disposition and metabolism of metronidazole in patients with liver failure. Hepatology 4: 722–726
85. O'Reilly R A 1976 The stereoselective interaction of warfarin and metronidazole in man. New England Journal of Medicine 295: 354–357
86. Jensen J C, Gugler R 1985 Interaction between metronidazole and drugs eliminated by oxidative metabolism. Clinical Pharmacology and Therapeutics 37: 407–410
87. Reitberg D P, Klarnet J P, Carlson J K, Schentag J J 1983 Effect of metronidazole on theophylline pharmacokinetics. Clinical Pharmacology 2: 441–444
88. Gugler R, Jensen J C 1983 Interaction between cimetidine and metronidazole. New England Journal of Medicine 309: 1518–1519
89. Rothstein E, Clancy D D 1969 Toxicity of disulfiram combined with metronidazole. New England Journal of Medicine 280: 1006
90. Ralph E D, Amatnieks Y 1980 Potentially synergistic antimicrobial combinations with metronidazole against *Bacteroides fragilis*. Antimicrobial Agents and Chemotherapy 17: 379–382

Metyrapone

Metyrapone (Metopirone) is an inhibitor of 11β-hydroxylase, an important cytochrome P450 enzyme involved in the biosynthesis of cortisol and aldosterone. It also inhibits most microsomal cytochromes P450 induced by phenobarbitone treatment.

Chemistry

Metyrapone (Methopyrapone, Metopiron(e))
$C_{14}H_{14}N_2O$
2-Methyl-1,2-di-(3′-pyridyl)propan-1-one

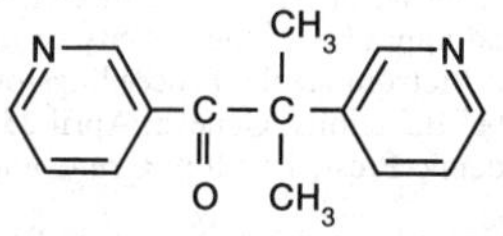

Molecular weight	226.3
pKa	
Solubility	
in alcohol	1 in 3
in water	1 in 100
Octanol/water partition coefficient	high

Metyrapone is a white to light amber crystalline powder, which darkens on exposure to light. It is not available in any combination preparations.

Pharmacology

Metyrapone is an inhibitor of two classes of cytochrome P450 enzymes: adrenal 11β-hydroxylase and most phenobarbitone-inducible forms of cytochrome P450. These enzymes are important in the oxidation of a variety of lipophilic compounds including corticosteroids, drugs and polycyclic aromatic hydrocarbons.

Toxicology

Studies in mice indicated that there was a marked circadian variation in susceptibility to metyrapone toxicity. The peak occurred at 1600 h when lights were on from 0600 to 1800 h.[1] This coincided with an elevated level of plasma corticosterone. The lethal doses of metyrapone (300–400 $mg.kg^{-1}$) are much greater than those required to inhibit corticosteroid biosynthesis. Doses of metyrapone from 100 to 200 $mg.kg^{-1}$ produced signs of central nervous system depression in the mice with ataxia and drowsiness. Further increase in dose led to general anaesthesia (250–400 $mg.kg^{-1}$). It has also been suggested that there might be a negative inotropic effect.[2] Little is known about the teratological or carcinogenic properties of this drug. Because of the risk that the drug could impair the biosynthesis of fetoplacental steroids it would seem unwise to administer it during pregnancy.

Clinical pharmacology

Inhibition of 11β-hydroxylase in the inner zones of the adrenal in man has been shown by demonstrating a reduction of plasma cortisol associated with elevation of plasma 11-deoxycortisol consequent on the increase in adrenocorticotrophin (ACTH) secretion. The 11β-hydroxylase enzyme in the zona glomerulosa is also inhibited as evidenced by the fall in plasma aldosterone and the rise in plasma deoxycorticosterone levels. In the absence of ACTH the effect of metyrapone on the cleavage of 20,22-dihydroxycholesterol to form pregnenolone becomes a significant effect of the drug.[3]

The 11β-hydroxylase and 18-hydroxylase are the same enzyme and thus it is not surprising that metyrapone also blocks 18-hydroxylation in man (e.g. formation of 18-OH-deoxycorticosterone).

Levin and colleagues[4] studied the extra-adrenal effects of metyrapone in man using ^{14}C-cortisol. Metyrapone caused an increase in the volume of distribution of cortisol (34%) and in the metabolic clearance rate (75%). The half life of cortisol fell by 25%. Previous investigations had shown this and it had been thought to be due to an effect demonstrated in vitro of metyrapone decreasing the binding of cortisol to albumin.[5] However, the changes in cortisol metabolism as indicated by the urinary steroid metabolites suggest an alternative explanation. There appears to be a block in the conversion of cortisone to cortisol. This prevents the recycling of cortisol by cortisol–cortisone shuttle and thus shortens the half life. It would be anticipated that urinary tetrahydrocortisone levels would increase but the reverse is the case. This seems to be the result of stimulation of the 20-oxosteroid reductase, which converts tetrahydrocortisone to β-cortolone.

Pharmacokinetics

The pharmacokinetics and metabolism of metyrapone have not been extensively investigated. The usual analytical method is by fluorometry;[6] an alternative is HPLC with ultraviolet detection at 254 nm.[7]

The absorption of metyrapone has been investigated by Sprunt and colleagues.[8] Following a light breakfast subjects were given three 250 mg capsules between 0900 and 0930 h together with some milk. The assay used was a bioassay based on the ability of plasma to inhibit the hydroxylation of deoxycorticosterone by rat adrenal homogenate. The results are thus difficult to compare with those from other methods. Absorption was extremely variable. The majority of individuals showed a peak plasma level at 1 hour (mean 3.7 mg.l^{-1}). In one subject the peak was at 2 hours and in another extremely low levels (<0.3 mg.l^{-1}) were found during the 4 hours of the study. The plasma half life following 600 mg metyrapone ditartrate intravenously ranged from 20 to 26 min. Much lower plasma levels of metyrapone have been reported.[9]

Plasma levels of metyrapone were maintained above 0.3 mg.l^{-1} throughout the dosing interval when the drug was administered at a dose of 750 mg every 4 h, but fell rapidly after stopping treatment.[9] After intravenous administration of metyrapone higher blood levels were achieved than with the oral route. Plasma levels were greater than 0.3 mg.l^{-1} until 4 hours after the infusion. The plasma half life was 30 minutes.

No information is available on plasma metyrapone levels in patients with renal or hepatic dysfunction.

Metyrapone is extensively metabolized in the liver. The main route of excretion is via the kidneys. Less than 1% of the dose is excreted unchanged. No formal studies on protein binding have been reported. However, addition of metyrapone to normal plasma samples resulted in an increased free, non-protein-bound cortisol.[5] The authors suggested that the drug decreased the binding of cortisol to albumin but not to transcortin.

Oral absorption	variable
Presystemic metabolism	—
Plasma half life	30 min
Volume of distribution	—
Plasma protein binding	—

Concentration–effect relationship

Plasma metyrapone levels above 0.3 mg.l^{-1} over a 24 h period are associated with marked inhibition of cortisol biosynthesis and progressive elevation of plasma 11-deoxycortisol levels, indicative of satisfactory 11β-hydroxylase inhibition.[9] The effect of the drug is dependent on the time of day when it is administered. A four-hour intravenous infusion starting at 0800 h lowered plasma cortisol to nearly undetectable levels by the end of the infusion. In comparison an infusion starting at midnight when plasma cortisol levels are low had little immediate effect. However, the levels rose significantly at four hours after the infusion and at 14 h were above normal. The magnitude of the ACTH response was greater with the midnight than with the morning infusion. However, the plasma 11-deoxycortisol levels were not significantly different.

Metyrapone

Metabolism

Metyrapone is extensively metabolized in the liver. Reported metabolites include the keto reduction product metyrapol (MPOL) (see Fig. 1), two isomeric metyrapone mono-N-oxides and an α-pyridone.[10–12] In the rat, MPOL levels increase rapidly after administration of metyrapone and exceed those of metyrapone within 30 min, the half life of the metabolite exceeding that of the parent drug. There is minimal conversion of MPOL to metyrapone. It has been suggested that as MPOL is also active as an inhibitor of cytochrome P450, even though it is less potent than metyrapone, its high blood concentration and long half life may result in it contributing a large proportion of the active principle in vivo.

Fig. 1 Metabolism of metyrapone

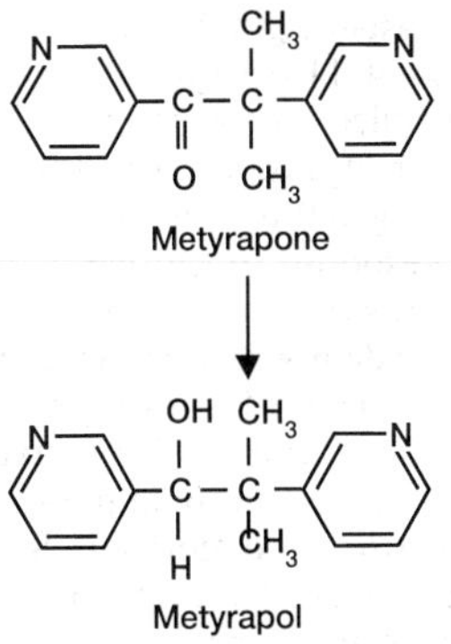

About 50% of a dose is excreted in urine over 72 h, 5.3% as metyrapone (9.2% free form; 90.8% conjugated with glucuronic acid) and 38.5% as MPOL (8.1% free; 91.9% conjugated with glucuronic acid).

Pharmaceutics

Metyrapone is available in 250 mg capsules and tablets. The capsules (Metopirone; CIBA, UK) are opaque, cylindrical, soft gelatine coloured, white and coded 'CIBA LN'. They should be protected from heat and moisture. Metopirone tablets (CIBA, USA) are round, biconcave, off-white debossed on one side 'CIBA' and on the other with the recognition code '130'.

Therapeutic use

Indications

1. Investigation of anterior pituitary function in patients with suspected hypopituitarism
2. The differential diagnosis and management of patients with Cushing's syndrome
3. In conjunction with glucocorticoids in the treatment of resistant oedema associated with secondary hyperaldosteronism.

Contraindications

1. Severe adrenocortical insufficiency
2. Hypersensitivity to metyrapone
3. Pregnancy: since the drug can impair the biosynthesis of steroids by the fetoplacental unit it should not be given during pregnancy. It is unknown whether the drug is passed into breast milk and thus it should not be used in mothers who are breast-feeding.

Mode of use

This is entirely dependent on the indication for which the drug is being used. In the case of testing the responsiveness of the hypothalamic–pituitary–adrenal axis the aim is to lower plasma cortisol to subnormal levels and thus activate negative feedback control of corticotrophin releasing factor (CRF) and ACTH. The response to the drug can then be assessed by measuring either ACTH, the steroid immediately prior to 11β-hydroxylation block (11-deoxycortisol) or its urinary metabolites (17-oxogenic steroids).

In the control of Cushing's syndrome the aim is to lower plasma cortisol levels to normal (levels of approximately 300–400 nmol.l^{-1}

throughout the 24 hours). This usually requires a lower dose than that which is used diagnostically.

Much less information is available on the treatment of secondary hyperaldosteronism.

Indications

1. Investigation of anterior pituitary function in patients with suspected hypopituitarism

A variety of different tests have been proposed based on either the oral or intravenous administration of metyrapone. The methods used to assess the response have changed considerably with the advent of specific assays for the measurement of plasma ACTH and plasma 11-deoxycortisol.

Oral metyrapone test. The standard test was introduced by Liddle and colleagues.[13] This was originally based on the measurement of the urinary metabolites of 11-deoxycortiocosteroids as 17-hydroxy-corticosteroids. Urine collections were made for the day before, the day of and the day after metyrapone. The drug was given orally in six doses with 750 mg being given four hourly starting at 0800 h. Liddle considered a positive response to be one in which the urinary 17-hydroxycorticosteroids rose above control values either by a two-fold factor or 10 mg daily. He demonstrated that in patients with pituitary disease this was a useful means of assessing the pituitary reserve with regard to ACTH secretion. Many others have confirmed this. The test has, however, been subsequently improved by the measurement of plasma 11-deoxycortisol and cortisol. Strott and colleagues[14] showed that by measuring 11-deoxycortisol after metyrapone it was easy to distinguish between normal subjects and those with diminished ACTH reserve. This test was further improved by the simultaneous measurement of plasma cortisol. This gives a direct indication of the degree of inhibition of 11β-hydroxylation produced by metyrapone.[15] Obviously, if an effective block is not achieved then negative feedback control will not be activated and hence there will be no rise in ACTH or 11-deoxycortisol. It is important to recognize that the marked rise in plasma 11-deoxycortisol may produce levels which interfere in several cortisol radioimmunoassays.

In an attempt to simplify the oral test several authors have looked at the effect of giving single oral doses. Staub and colleagues[16] showed that this can produce an ACTH response equivalent to the standard insulin hypoglycaemia test. In a similar test proposed by Jubiz and others[17] Dolman and colleagues[18] measured both ACTH and 11-deoxycortisol and found the single-dose test to be useful in distinguishing primary from secondary adrenal insufficiency. The single-dose test was further evaluated by Feek and colleagues.[19] They gave 2 g metyrapone with a snack at 2300 h and measured plasma ACTH at 0800 h the next morning. Plasma ACTH concentrations following metyrapone were significantly lower in patients with pituitary disease with no evidence of anterior pituitary deficiency (as judged by a normal response to insulin-induced hypoglycaemia) than in normal subjects. The levels in these patients were significantly greater than in those with definite anterior pituitary insufficiency. It remains to be determined whether those who have an impaired response to metyrapone but a normal response to insulin-induced hypoglycaemia have a clinically significant deficit in cortisol production. These results, however, suggest that this is a sensitive method for assessing minor abnormalities of the hypothalamic–pituitary–adrenal axis. The authors stress the importance of the time when ACTH blood samples are taken and suggest that sampling before 0800 h might improve the discrimination of the test.

Leisti reported a 3-hour morning test which appeared satisfactory in children.[20] Others have looked at this in adults and have suggested that it is not a valuable test and was associated with a high incidence of unpleasant side effects.[21]

Intravenous metyrapone test. This was introduced by Gold and colleagues.[22] They gave 30 mg.kg^{-1} of metyrapone tartrate dissolved in 1 litre of 0.9% saline over 4 hours. Urine was collected for the measurement of 17-oxogenic steroids. Urine collections were made on a control day and for 24 hours after starting the infusion. The test appeared to be useful. Their results differed from those of Liddle and colleagues[13] in that there was a subnormal response in both hypo- and hyperthyroidism. It was suggested that there might be more rapid metabolism of metyrapone in hyperthyroidism as judged by the fact that doubling the dose of metyrapone improved the 17-oxogenic steroid responses in these patients. It has also been suggested that the response may be subnormal in patients with cirrhosis or on phenothiazines.

Cushman[23] produced an 8-hour intravenous metyrapone test, which he claimed enhanced precision and utility. However, the difficulty with all these studies is that there is no 'gold standard' with which to compare the test.

Arguelles and colleagues[24] compared intravenous and oral metyrapone tests performed on the same subjects using the Gold protocol and a variation of that of Liddle (500 mg metyrapone orally for 8 doses every 2–3 hours). The mean increase in 17-oxogenic steroids in the intravenous test was 47% above control as compared to 132% in the oral test ($P<0.01$). This striking difference would suggest that oral administration over a 24-hour period was a more potent stimulus to ACTH production than a 4-hour infusion.

2. Differential diagnosis and management of patients with Cushing's syndrome

Patients with pituitary-dependent Cushing's syndrome (Cushing's disease) show an exaggerated rise in plasma 11-deoxycortisol in response to metyrapone (usually above 1000 nmol.l^{-1} at 24 hours after 750 mg metyrapone 4 hourly for 6 doses). This distinguishes them from nearly all patients with the ectopic ACTH syndrome in whom a much smaller rise is usually seen. The measurement of plasma 11-deoxycortisol during the metyrapone test provides better discrimination than that using plasma ACTH. Liddle and others[13] studied 7 patients with Cushing's disease and showed that the urinary 17-hydroxycorticosteroid levels following metyrapone were higher than those in normal subjects. Similar results were found using the intravenous metyrapone test.[22]

In patients with Cushing's syndrome secondary to functioning adrenal adenomas or carcinomas, ACTH levels are usually undetectable and would not be expected to rise with metyrapone. Under these circumstances one might imagine that the drug would simply effect an equimolar substitution of 11-deoxycortisol for cortisol. However, in many patients the levels of 11-deoxycortisol actually fall because of the inhibiting effect of metyrapone on the side-chain cleavage enzyme. This effect is readily overcome by ACTH but this is suppressed in these patients.

There have been few comparisons of the metyrapone test with other methods for establishing the differential diagnosis of Cushing's syndrome. Sindler and colleagues[25] investigated 25 unselected patients with Cushing's syndrome (14 Cushing's disease, 2 adrenal adenoma, 8 adrenal carcinoma, 1 ectopic ACTH syndrome). They compared high-dose dexamethasone (8 mg daily) with metyrapone and concluded that the metyrapone test was more accurate in differentiating Cushing's disease from adrenocortical neoplasm (100% v. 81%). In practice, however, this distinction can usually be made on a basal plasma ACTH level. The real difficulty lies in distinguishing some cases of the ectopic ACTH syndrome from those with Cushing's disease.

Metyrapone has been extensively used in the treatment of Cushing's syndrome. In many cases this has been to improve the condition of the patient prior to definitive therapy with surgery or irradiation. In others the drug has been used whilst awaiting the beneficial effects of radiotherapy. Jeffcoate and colleagues[26] used metyrapone in the long-term management of 13 patients with pituitary-dependent bilateral adrenal hyperplasia. Eight of the patients had received radiotherapy and one transfrontal surgery. The aim of metyrapone therapy was to reduce the mean plasma fluorogenic corticosteroid concentration to 300–400 nmol.l^{-1} (mean of 4–7 samples over 24 h). The dose of metyrapone required to do this ranged from 250 mg twice daily to 1.0 g four times daily. Despite the rise in plasma ACTH the drug was able to maintain the block in cortisol biosynthesis. On metyrapone the clinical features of the disease rapidly improved and this improvement was maintained. The only side effect of note was mild hirsutism in 4 of the 7 women who had received the drug for more than 6 months. Plasma testosterone should be monitored.

Some authors have elected to use higher doses of metyrapone to block cortisol biosynthesis virtually completely and to replace glucocorticoid in these patients. Such blockade can be very difficult in Cushing's disease. Child and colleagues[27] used a combination of metyrapone 2 g daily, aminoglutethimide 500–750 mg daily, dexa-

Metyrapone

M

methasone 0.5 mg twice daily and fludrocortisone 0.1 mg daily in 4 patients with Cushing's disease and successfully controlled the condition for up to one year. Metyrapone has also been used with benefit in patients with the ectopic ACTH syndrome[27–29] and in those with cortisol-secreting adrenal tumours.[27,30]

3. Treatment of resistant oedema
Early studies showed that patients with resistant oedema might benefit from a combination of metyrapone together with a thiazide diuretic.[31] Further diuresis ensued when spironolactone was added. Prednisone was also given to suppress the compensatory ACTH response and hence the rise in deoxycorticosterone (DOC). In the absence of any steroid measurements it is difficult to assess these studies and to determine the mechanism of action of metyrapone. In patients with chronic liver disease and ascites treated by Holub and Jailer[32] a variable response to metyrapone was seen. In one patient with intractable ascites metyrapone produced a natriuresis but in two others this was not the case. They demonstrated in both of these a marked rise in tetrahydrodeoxycorticosterone, the metabolite of DOC. They then looked at metyrapone together with prednisone and showed that this produced an effective natriuresis. A number of other papers in the 1960s confirmed these results. However, no studies appear to have been performed comparing metyrapone and prednisolone with more recent therapies for secondary hyperaldosteronism. One advantage that this treatment with metyrapone might have over angiotensin converting enzyme (ACE) inhibition therapy is that it would not produce the hypotensive effect observed in many of these patients when an ACE inhibitor is given.

Adverse reactions

Potentially life-threatening effects
No effects of this kind directly due to the drug have been described. This is surprising in view of the inhibition of cortisol biosynthesis. There would appear to be two reasons why severe adrenocortical insufficiency is rare. The first is the compensatory rise in ACTH, which thus overcomes the enzyme blockade. The second is the increase in deoxycorticosterone, which offsets the reduction in aldosterone. This is similar to the situation when low doses of the intravenous anaesthetic agent etomidate are given.[33]

Acute overdosage
There is surprisingly little information on this. In one child aged 6, with a craniopharyngioma, 2000 mg daily was given for 2 days. On the first evening she lost consciousness, had stereotyped movements of tongue and extensor spasm of the fingers: she subsequently had a convulsion and eventually respiratory followed by cardiac arrest. At autopsy in addition to the craniopharyngioma there was marked cerebral oedema. Apart from this there are no specific reports. It would be anticipated that an overdose would produce glucocorticoid insufficiency. The mineralocorticoid status would be more difficult to anticipate as the initial elevation in deoxycorticosterone would offset the reduction in aldosterone. Intravenous hydrocortisone and saline would be appropriate emergency therapy with induction of vomiting and/or gastric aspiration with lavage if the drug had only recently been swallowed.

Severe or irreversible adverse effects
None has been reported.

Symptomatic adverse effects
It is sometimes difficult to distinguish the adverse effects of metyrapone from those of adrenal insufficiency that may result from its use. Thus nausea, vomiting, dizziness, headache and hypotension have been reported as adverse effects but may occur with adrenal insufficiency alone. It is normally recommended that the drug should be taken with milk or after food to reduce nausea and vomiting.

Interference with clinical pathology tests
No technical interferences of this kind have been reported.

High risk groups

Neonates
The drug is unlikely to be used in neonates.

Breast milk. The drug should not be given to lactating mothers.

Children
Metyrapone has been widely used as a diagnostic test in children. A variety of protocols have been performed. These have included the short test (oral metyrapone in a single dose 30 $mg.kg^{-1}$ body weight at midnight with a snack, with measurement of plasma 11-deoxycortisol and cortisol at 0800 h) and the prolonged test (3 $g.m^{-2}$ body surface area given in 6 doses every 4 hours from 0800 h to 0400 h with blood sampling at 0800 h after the last dose). Comparison of the two tests showed that there was a positive correlation between them but 2 out of 27 with a subnormal short test responded normally to the prolonged test.[34] The data sheet recommends 6 four-hourly doses of 15 $mg.kg^{-1}$ with a minimum dose of 250 mg every 4 hours.

Pregnant women
For reasons given earlier, the drug should not be given to pregnant women.

The elderly
Several authors have used metyrapone to assess hypothalamic–pituitary–adrenal function in the elderly. It is possible that there may be an age-related difference in response. Jensen and Blichert-Toft[35] showed that a group of elderly subjects had a similar cortisol response to surgery as a younger group. However, in response to metyrapone the elderly patients showed a significantly higher 11-deoxycortisol response.

Concurrent disease

Obese patients. Measurement of corticosteroid metabolites (17-hydroxycorticosteroids, 17-oxogenic steroids) and of cortisol secretion rate have shown that these may be elevated in obesity. Simkin and Arce[36] looked at the response of obese patients to metyrapone and showed that those who had normal baseline 17-oxogenic steroid excretion had a normal rise in 17-oxogenic steroids with metyrapone ($208 \pm 39.5\%$). However, those whose baseline values were elevated had a minimal further rise with metyrapone ($11 \pm 14.7\%$). The reason for this difference is unclear but it helps to distinguish such patients from those with Cushing's disease who would have an exaggerated rise in 17-oxogenic steroids but not from other causes of Cushing's disease.

Drug interactions

Potentially hazardous interactions
No interactions of this type have been reported.

Other significant interactions
Patients on enzyme-inducing drugs (e.g. phenytoin and barbiturates), antidepressants and neuroleptics should be carefully reviewed before considering metyrapone administration as the usual doses may be inappropriate. Corticosteroid therapy may not only affect the result of metyrapone tests by suppressing the hypothalamic–pituitary–adrenal axis but may also invalidate the plasma and urinary steroid assays.

Potentially useful interactions
No interactions of this kind have been described.

References

1. Ortel R J, Halberg F, Ungar F 1964 Circadian system phase-dependent toxicity and other effects of methopyrapone (SU-4885) in the mouse. Journal of Pharmacology and Experimental Therapeutics 146: 395–399
2. Lefer A M, Nadzam G R 1964 Cardiovascular effects of SU-4885 (mepyrapone), an inhibitor of corticosteroid biosynthesis. Proceedings of the Society for Experimental Biology and Medicine 115: 356–359
3. Carballeira A, Fishman L M, Jacobi J D 1976 Dual sites of inhibition by metyrapone of human adrenal steroidogenesis: correlation of in vivo and in vitro studies. Journal of Clinical Endocrinology and Metabolism 42: 687
4. Levin J, Zumoff B, Fukushima D K 1978 Extraadrenal effects of metyrapone in man. Journal of Clinical Endocrinology and Metabolism 47: 845–849
5. Kehlet H, Binder C 1976 Effect of metyrapone on cortisol binding capacity in plasma. Acta Endocrinologica 81: 787–792
6. Meikle A W, Jubiz W, West C D et al 1969 A simple fluorometric method for assay of plasma metyrapone. Journal of Laboratory and Clinical Medicine 74: 515–520
7. Usansky J I, Damani L A, Houston J B 1984 The pharmacokinetics of metyrapone and metyrapol in the rat. Journal of Pharmacy and Pharmacology 36 (suppl): 28P
8. Sprunt J G, Browning M C K, Hannah D M 1968 Some aspects of the pharmacology of metyrapone. Memoirs of the Society of Endocrinology 17: 193–203

9. Jubiz W, Matsukura S, Meikle A W, Harada G, West C D, Tyler F H 1970 Plasma metyrapone, adrenocorticotropic hormone and deoxycortisol levels: sequential changes during oral and intravenous metyrapone administration. Archives of Internal Medicine 125: 468–471
10. Damani L A, Crooks P A, Cowan D A 1981 Metabolism of metyrapone. 2 — Chromatographic and mass spectral properties of the N-oxides of metyrapone and metyrapol. Biomedical Mass Spectrometry 8: 270–277
11. Damani L A, Crooks P A, Cowan D A 1981 Metabolism of metyrapone. III. Formation of an alpha-pyridone metabolite by rat hepatic soluble enzymes. Drug Metabolism and Disposition: The Biological Fate of Chemicals 9: 270–273
12. Usansky J I, Damani L A 1983 Oxidation of metyrapone to an α-pyridone metabolite by a mammalian molybdenum hydroxylase. Journal of Pharmacy and Pharmacology 35 (suppl): 72P
13. Liddle G W, Estep H L, Kendall J W, Carter Williams W, Townes A W 1959 Clinical application of a new test of pituitary reserve. Journal of Clinical Endocrinology and Metabolism 19: 875–894
14. Strott C A, West C D, Nakasawa K et al 1969 Plasma 11-deoxycorticosteroid and ACTH responses to metyrapone (plasma metyrapone test). Journal of Clinical Endocrinology and Metabolism 29: 6–11
15. Spark R F 1971 Simplified assessment of pituitary–adrenal reserve. Annals of Internal Medicine 75: 717–723
16. Staub J J, Noelpp B, Girard J, Banmann J B, Graf S, Ratcliffe J G 1979 The short metyrapone test: comparison of the plasma ACTH response to metyrapone and insulin-induced hypoglycaemia. Clinical Endocrinology 10: 595–601
17. Jubiz W, Meikle A W, West C D et al 1970 Single-dose metyrapone test. Archives of Internal Medicine 125: 472–474
18. Dolman L I, Nolan G, Jubiz W 1979 Metyrapone test with adrenocorticotrophic levels. Journal of the American Medical Association 241: 1251–1253
19. Feek C M, Bevan J S, Ratcliffe J G, Gray C E, Blundell G 1981 The short metyrapone test: comparison of the plasma ACTH response to metyrapone with the cortisol response to insulin-induced hypoglycaemia in patients with pituitary disease. Clinical Endocrinology 15: 75–80
20. Leisti S 1977 Evaluation of 3 hour metyrapone test in children and adolescents. Clinical Endocrinology 6: 305–320
21. Best J D, Alford F P, Donald R A 1980 Evaluation of the three hour metyrapone test in adults. Clinical Endocrinology 13: 69–76
22. Gold E M, Kent J R, Forsham P H 1961 Clinical use of a new diagnostic agent, methopyrapone (SU-4885), in pituitary and adrenocortical disorders. Annals of Internal Medicine 54: 175–188
23. Cushman P 1968 Hypothalamic–pituitary–adrenal function in thyroid disorders; effects of methopyrapone infusions on plasma corticosteroids. Metabolism 17: 263–270
24. Arguelles A E, Martin H, Chekherdemian M, Moloeznik I 1967 Comparison of intravenous and oral metyrapone tests performed on the same subjects. Journal of Endocrinology 37: 471–472
25. Sindler B H, Griffing G T, Melby J C 1983 The superiority of the metyrapone test versus the high dose dexamethasone test in the differential diagnosis of Cushing's syndrome. American Journal of Medicine 74: 657–662
26. Jeffcoate W J, Rees L H, Tomlin S, Jones A E, Edwards C R W, Besser G M 1977 Metyrapone in long-term management of Cushing's disease. British Medical Journal 2: 215–217
27. Child D F, Burke C W, Burley D M, Rees L H, Russell Fraser T 1976 Drug control of Cushing's syndrome. Acta Endocrinologica 82: 330–341
28. Liddle G W, Nicholson W F, Island D P, Orth D N, Abe K, Lowder S C 1969 Clinical and laboratory studies of ectopic humoral syndromes. Recent Progress in Hormone Research 25: 283–314
29. Sugawara M, Hagen G A 1977 Ectopic ACTH syndrome due to salivary gland adenoid cystic carcinoma: response to metyrapone. Archives of Internal Medicine 137: 102–105
30. Daniels H, Amstel W J Van, Schopman W et al 1963 Effect of metopirone in a patient with adrenal cortical carcinoma. Acta Endocrinologica 44: 346–354
31. Shaldon S, McLaren J R 1960 An 11β-hydroxylase inhibitor in the treatment of resistant ascites. Lancet 2: 1330–1332
32. Holub D A, Jailer J W 1960 Sodium and water diuresis in cirrhotic patients with intractable ascites following chemical inhibition of aldosterone synthesis. Annals of Internal Medicine 53: 425–444
33. Sear J W, Edwards C R W, Atherden S M 1988 Dual effect of etomidate on mineralocorticoid biosynthesis. Acta Anaesthetica Belgica 39: 87–94
34. Limal J M, Basmaciogullari A, Rappaport R 1976 Evaluation of single oral dose metyrapone tests in children with hypopituitarism. Acta Paediatrica Scandinavica 65: 177–183
35. Jensen H K, Blichert-Toft M 1971 Investigation of pituitary–adrenocortical function in the elderly during standardized operations and postoperative metyrapone test assessed by plasma cortisol, plasma compound S and eosinophil cell determinations. Acta Endocrinologica 67: 495–507
36. Simkin B, Arce R 1962 Response of obese patients to an 11β-hydroxylase inhibitor, Methopyrapone (SU-4885). Proceedings of the Society for Experimental Biology and Medicine 111: 780–783

Mexiletine (hydrochloride)

Mexiletine is an antiarrhythmic drug, active chiefly against ventricular arrhythmias.

Chemistry

Mexiletine hydrochloride (Mexitil)
$C_{11}H_{16}NO.HCl$
1-(2′,6′-Dimethylphenoxy)-2-aminopropane hydrochloride

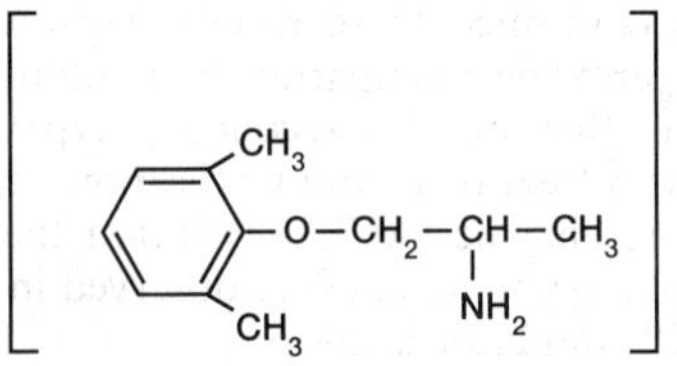

Molecular weight (free base)	215.7 (179.3)
pKa (−NH_2)	8.4
Solubility	
in alcohol	1 in 3
in water	1 in 2
Octanol/water partition coefficient	1.46

Mexiletine hydrochloride is a white, odourless, crystalline substance which is not available in any drug combinations. It is prepared by chemical synthesis. It posseses an assymetric carbon.

Pharmacology

The main pharmacological actions are as follows.[1–6]

1. It is a Class IB antiarrhythmic agent, producing fast sodium channel inhibition with decrease of the maximal upstroke rate (phase 0) of the action potential and shortening of the action potential duration without alteration of resting membrane potential
2. Mexiletine also has some inhibitory effect on nodal tissue and shortens the refractory period of atrial tissue; therefore it has mild quinidine-like antiarrhythmic activity
3. Mexiletine has a local anaesthetic effect
4. It inhibits ventricular and supraventricular arrhythmias.

Toxicology

Ataxia and tonic–clonic spasms appear in Rhesus monkeys at doses of 12 $mg.kg^{-1}$ or more. The results of teratogenicity tests in mice, rats and rabbits were negative. Two Ames tests for mutagenicity were negative. Carcinogenicity tests were negative over 18 months in mice and over 24 months in rats.

Clinical pharmacology

Mexiletine has been extensively used in patients with ventricular arrhythmias.[7–9] The usual oral dose is 200–400 mg three times daily[10] or 10–14 $mg.kg^{-1}$ per day in divided doses.[11] The following pharmacological features have been demonstrated in man:

1. Inhibition of ventricular premature systoles[12] and ventricular tachycardia[13]
2. A variable effect on sinus node recovery time;[3] prolonged ventricular conduction time;[14] prolonged AV (atrioventricular) nodal conduction time and HV (his-ventricular) interval;[15] inhibition of conduction times along the bypass tract in patients with Wolff–Parkinson–White syndrome

3. There are no marked haemodynamic effects[16,17] except in the presence of prior myocardial depression.[3]

Pharmacokinetics

The preferred analytical method for the drug in plasma is gas–liquid chromatography[18] with a sensitivity of 30–50 μg.l^{-1}; high performance liquid chromatography[19] has a sensitivity of 10 μg.l^{-1}. Absorption from the gastrointestinal tract is virtually complete within 2–4 h[7] but delayed in acute myocardial infarction. Peak plasma levels are normally reached in 2–4 h. There is presystemic hepatic metabolism by oxidative–reductive processes so that 90% of the orally absorbed mexiletine is broken down in the liver to inactive metabolites.

In patients, the plasma half life is 10–17 h, mean 12.6 h,[20] and the volume of distribution[7,21] 5.5–9.0 l.kg^{-1}. In normal volunteers the mean half life is 9.3 h.[8] 60–70% is reversibly bound to plasma proteins.

Mexiletine is lipophilic and enters the brain. There is considerable tissue penetration (high volume of distribution). Mexiletine is excreted in human breast milk at concentrations slightly higher than those in the maternal plasma and crosses the placenta.

Oral absorption	>95%
Presystemic metabolism	80–90%
Plasma half life	
range	10–17 h
mean	12.6 h
Volume of distribution	5.5–9.0 l.kg^{-1}
Plasma protein binding	60–70%

The kinetics of mexiletine are likely to be altered in patients with hepatic or severe renal disease such that some adjustment of dosage might be necessary.

Concentration–effect relationship

As the dose is increased, there is a greater antiarrhythmic effect as judged by suppression of ventricular premature systoles.[22] There is evidence that the therapeutic effect occurs within a well-defined plasma concentration range[21,23] which is 1–2 mg.l^{-1}. However, there is no clear correlation between the plasma concentration and the therapeutic effect in individual patients.

Metabolism

The main routes of elimination from the human body are: urine 75–90%, mostly after hepatic metabolism, but 5–20% as unchanged mexiletine. There is an increase in excretion of unchanged drug when the pH of the urine is acidic; 10% is eliminated through the bile. There is no evidence of any enterohepatic circulation.

The main metabolic reactions are:

1. 4′-hydroxylation to 4′-hydroxymexiletine
2. 2′-hydroxymethylation to 2′-hydroxymethylmexiletine.

Both metabolites may be deaminated to the corresponding alcohols. None of the metabolites is thought to be pharmacologically active.

Pharmaceutics

Mexiletine is available in oral and parenteral forms as the hydrochloride from Boehringer Ingelheim.

1. Mexitil capsules (UK, USA): 200 mg, red/red. In the UK, marked with strength and company symbol. In the USA, coded ‘B167’
2. Mexitil capsules (USA): 150 mg, red/orange, coded ‘BI66’
3. Mexitil low-dose capsules (UK): 50 mg, red/purple, marked with the strength and company symbol
4. Mexitil sustained-release capsules (USA): 250 mg, red/aqua green, coded ‘BI68’
5. Mexitil ampoules (UK/USA): 250 mg in 10 ml
6. Sustained-release capsules (Perlongets) (UK) contain 360 mg, turquoise/scarlet, marked ‘Mexitil PL’.

None of the preparations includes potentially allergenic substances. There are no special conditions required for any of the formulations and the maximum shelf-life of each formulation is 3 years.

Therapeutic use

Indications

In the USA, oral mexiletine is licensed for suppression of symptomatic ventricular arrhythmias including premature ventricular contractions, couplets and ventricular tachycardia. The following are reported uses of the drug:

1. Ventricular arrhythmias and ectopic beats especially in and after acute myocardial infarction[24]
2. Lignocaine-resistant arrhythmias and other refractory ventricular arrhythmias[13,25]
3. Post-infarction arrhythmias[26]
4. Symptomatic and/or serious ventricular tachycardia[27]
5. Wolff–Parkinson–White arrhythmias[28]
6. Supraventricular tachycardia[29,30]
7. Digitalis-related arrhythmias.

Contraindications

Intravenous use

1. Serious conduction system defects (second-or third-degree heart block without pacemaker)
2. Cardiogenic shock.

Relative contraindications

Conduction system defects, sick sinus syndrome, bradycardia, hypotension and cardiac, hepatic or renal failure (although pharmacokinetics are not markedly altered in heart or renal failure).[31]

Mode of use

A therapeutic blood level (1–2 μg.ml^{-1}) is aimed at by the following dose schedules:

Fig. 1 Metabolism of mexiletine

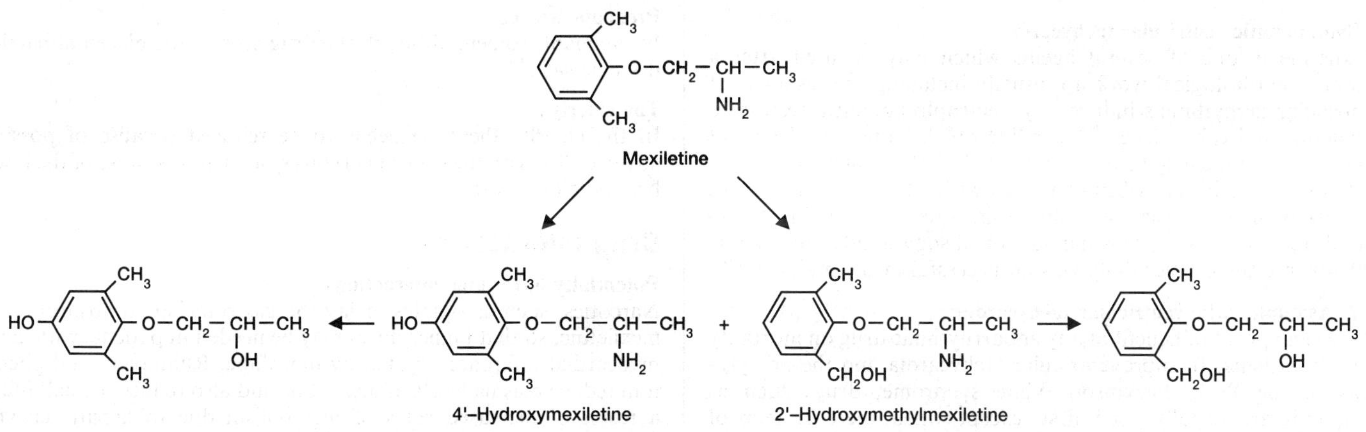

1. Intravenous loading dose followed by infusion
The intravenous dose (not licensed for USA) currently recommended in the package insert in Germany is 100–250 mg (2.5 $mg.kg^{-1}$) at 12.5 $mg.min^{-1}$, then 2.0 $mg.kg^{-1}.h^{-1}$ for 3.5 h, then 0.5 $mg.kg^{-1}.h^{-1}$ as long as indicated. A commonly used intravenous dosage[3] is an initial loading dose of 150–250 mg over 5 min followed by an infusion to a maximum dose of 750 mg over 3 h, then 0.5–1.0 $min.mg^{-1}$.

2. Oral loading dose followed by chronic oral dosage
The oral loading dose is 400 mg if high initial blood levels are required, followed by 300–1200 mg in three divided daily doses starting 2–6 h after the loading dose. In patients with acute myocardial infarction, absorption may be delayed, particularly after opiates; the oral loading dose is 600 mg followed by 200 mg 2 h later (omit the latter if arrhythmia is controlled or side effects occur).

A dose of 200–300 mg mexiletine 8-hourly produces therapeutic steady-state levels (1–2 $\mu g.ml^{-1}$) in about two-thirds of patients.[7] The usual daily dose for sustained-release capsules is 360 mg twice daily with a loading dose of 720 mg.

The dose needs individual adjustment according to tolerance and effects.

3. Intravenous loading dose followed by oral dosage
In 2. above, replace oral by intravenous loading dose.

Depending on the urgency, the oral or intravenous route is chosen and the dose built up to the therapeutic blood level which should ideally be measured. Otherwise, the dose is increased until the desired effect is obtained or side effects such as tremor, dizziness or nystagmus appear, whereupon the dose is cut back. When the drug is abruptly stopped after prolonged oral therapy, any of the arrhythmias suppressed by the drug may recur and require re-introduction of the drug or of another antiarrhythmic agent.

Indications

Critical to the possible benefit of mexiletine as an antiarrhythmic agent is whether it is used as a first-line agent when it is much more likely to work, or whether it is used after other agents such as lignocaine (lidocaine). Once several other agents have failed to work, mexiletine is less likely to be beneficial. The drug has a narrow therapeutic range and this, and unpredictable variations in the plasma concentration, make it a difficult drug to use in chronic treatment.

1, 2. Acute myocardial infarction
Life-threatening or symptomatic ventricular tachyarrhythmias requiring urgent treatment are usually first treated by lignocaine (lidocaine); thereafter mexiletine is one of several agents that may be used. However, as both mexiletine and lidocaine belong to the same group of agents (IB), it would be more logical to switch from lidocaine to another category of agent, e.g. procainamide or flecainide. Nonetheless, mexiletine has some electrophysiological properties that differ from lignocaine and can be clinically effective when lignocaine is not.[32]

3. Post-infarct arrhythmias
Oral mexiletine is frequently given as post-infarct therapy if the patient has responded to lignocaine in the acute phase. Proof of benefit on mortality or morbidity of this procedure is lacking.

4. Symptomatic ventricular tachycardia
Mexiletine is one of several agents which may be used after a complete cardiological work-up, usually including the response of ventricular arrhythmias induced by electrophysiological testing to mexiletine and other drugs. Depending on the category of patient chosen, mexiletine may be of benefit in only 20% of such patients,[22] with up to 35% benefit when combined with a Class IA agent.[33] In patients with drug-resistant tachycardia, previously failing to respond to quinidine, procainamide or disopyramide, mexiletine 200–400 mg three times daily was unsuccessful in the majority.[20]

5–7. Asymptomatic ventricular tachycardia
There is no proof of benefit of any antiarrhythmic drug on mortality in such patients. In supraventricular tachycardia and the arrhythmias of the Wolff–Parkinson–White syndrome, drugs such as verapamil are usually used first, except when there is fear of antegrade conduction down the bypass tract. Then mexiletine becomes one of a number of other agents of choice.

Adverse reactions

Potentially life-threatening effects
In about 5% of patients, bradycardia and hypotension may occur[10] if the drug is given intravenously.

Acute overdosage
In a patient with overdosage and blood levels of 34–37 $\mu g.ml^{-1}$ (normal value 1–2 $\mu g.ml^{-1}$) there were convulsions, complete heart block and ventricular asystole.[43]

Decreasing the urinary pH will block tubular reabsorption of mexiletine to enhance urinary excretion. Diazepam reduces central nervous effects, according to animal studies.

To prevent toxicity, the dose of mexiletine should be reduced in renal disease (creatinine clearance below 10 $mg.min^{-1}$), hepatic disease,[35] or heart failure.

Severe or irreversible adverse effects
Jaundice has complicated mexiletine treatment in rare instances. Convulsions may occur with higher doses and are unpredictable.

Symptomatic adverse effects
A serious problem is the narrow therapeutic–toxic margin of mexiletine[36] with more adverse effects as the dose is increased, so that a mean total daily dose of 950 mg (150 mg more than the dose recommended by the manufacturers) caused significant adverse effects in 17 of 21 patients before there was arrhythmia suppression.[37] Symptomatic adverse effects are dizziness and mild disorientation with single oral doses of 400 mg.[8] During the therapy of ventricular arrhythmias the adverse effects include tremor/nystagmus in 40%, indigestion in 10%, and toxic confusional states in less than 10%.[10,12] These effects depend on the blood concentration and are present in the majority of patients with blood levels[10] exceeding 1.5 $\mu g.ml^{-1}$. Blood concentrations vary greatly even when patients are on the same dose[32] so that the degree of toxicity for any given dose cannot be predicted. Dizziness and vomiting can be decreased by giving 12.5 mg prochlorperazine intravenously 5 minutes before the mexiletine injection.[33]

A major advantage of mexiletine is that, like lignocaine, there is little haemodynamic depression with its use,[10,38] even when mild left ventricular failure is present.[27]

Other effects
Mexiletine does not cause any modification of blood biochemistry.

Interference with clinical pathology tests
Mexiletine does not interfere with clinical pathology tests.

High risk groups

Neonates
The drug is unlikely to be used in neonates.

Breast milk. The drug enters breast milk and mothers taking it should not breast-feed.

Children
In children the dose should be titrated according to the blood levels.[38]

Pregnant women
In pregnant women, although the drug crosses the placental barrier, it seems safe.[39]

The elderly
In the elderly, the dose needs to be reduced because of possible adverse effects on the central nervous system and because of the lower hepatic blood flow.

Drug interactions

Potentially hazardous interactions
Narcotics, such as opiates, delay the gastrointestinal absorption of mexiletine, so that higher doses may be needed in patients with acute myocardial infarction treated by morphine. Rifampicin and phenytoin reduce plasma levels of mexiletine and also reduce the half life as a result of increased rates of metabolism due to hepatic enzyme

induction. Disopyramide predisposes to a negative inotropic effect.[40] Urinary alkalinization delays the tubular clearance of mexiletine in the urine.

Potentially useful interactions
These include interactions with Type 1A antiarrhythmic agents such as quinidine[36] or procainamide.[41] Mexiletine has also been used in combination with β-adrenoceptor blocker therapy[41] and with amiodarone.[42] Mexiletine does not interact with digoxin.

Major outcome trials

1. Impact Research Group 1984 International mexiletine and placebo antiarrhythmic coronary trial: I. Report on arrhythmia and other findings. Journal of the American College of Cardiology 4: 1148–1163

The major clinical trial in which mexiletine has been used in a double-blind prolonged comparison with placebo is for post-infarct arrhythmias. 630 patients with recent myocardial infarction were subject to Holter monitoring for 24 h within 3–25 days of admission to hospital and followed for up to 1 year. Frequent or complex ventricular arrhythmias were reduced by mexiletine at the first and fourth months, but were unchanged after 12 months. There was no improvement in mortality over 1 year in patients treated by mexiletine; in fact there were more deaths in the mexiletine than in the placebo group (7.6 vs 4.8%, p = NS). However, therapeutic blood levels were not reached in the majority of patients, possibly because the dose of the slow-release preparation was too low (Mexitil-Perlongets, 360 mg twice daily).

2. Campbell N P S, Pantridge J F, Adgey A A J 1978 Long-term oral antiarrhythmic therapy with mexiletine. British Heart Journal 40: 796–801

In a non-blinded study, oral mexiletine 200–300 mg 8-hourly for a mean period of 3 months had no benefit on major ventricular arrhythmias in 48 patients with ischaemic heart disease, despite therapeutic plasma concentrations at the time of the arrhythmia. At the same time side effects were frequent.

3. Bell J A, Thomas J M, Isaacson J R, Snell N J C, Holt D W 1982 A trial of prophylactic mexiletine in home coronary care. British Heart Journal 48: 285–290

Mexiletine has also been given to 157 patients with acute myocardial infarction when first seen at home by a general practitioner. Over a period of 6 weeks, mexiletine reduced the incidence of ventricular tachycardia when compared with placebo but mortality was unchanged. However, the dose of mexiletine used (200 mg three times daily) was likely to give blood concentrations at the lower end of the therapeutic range[9] with probably only modest antiarrhythmic effects.[22]

Objective evidence of the benefit of mexiletine in drug-resistant ventricular tachycardia measured by electrophysiological induction techniques shows only a modest success at most.[8,27]

Major comparative trials

4. Nademanee K, Feld G, Hendrickson J et al 1985 Mexiletine: double-blind comparison with procainamide in PVC suppression and open-label sequential comparison with amiodarone in life-threatening ventricular arrythmias. American Heart Journal 110: 923–931
   Campbell R W F, Dolder M A, Prescott L F, Talbot R G, Murray A, Julian D G 1975 Comparison of procainamide and mexiletine in prevention of ventricular arrhythmias after acute myocardial infarction. Lancet 1: 1257–1260

In the chronic oral prophylaxis of ischaemic ventricular arrhythmias after myocardial infarction, mexiletine 300 mg 8-hourly is about as effective as procainamide although much less effective than amiodarone.

5. Campbell N P S, Pantridge J F, Adgey A A J 1977 Mexiletine in the management of ventricular dysrhythmias. European Journal of Cardiology 6/4: 245–258

In patients with recurrent ventricular tachycardia mexiletine is about as effective as quinidine in approximately equal mean doses (1000 mg daily) although with a different side effect profile; the combination of the two agents with mean doses of each of about 800 mg daily produced a better antiarrhythmic response.

6. Frank M J, Russell S L, Watkins L O, Abdulla A M 1985 Relative efficacy of mexiletine and quinidine in consecutive trials. Circulation 72 (suppl 3): 111–164

In a prolonged study with repetitive trials on 114 patients, mexiletine had to be discontinued for side effects less frequently than quinidine and arrhythmia aggravation occurred less frequently; during a 14-month follow-up period mexiletine was as effective as quinidine in arrhythmia control.

General review articles

Chew C Y C, Collett J, Singh B H 1979 Mexiletine: a review of its pharmacological properties and therapeutic efficacy in arrhythmias. Drugs 17: 161–181
Danilo P 1979 Mexiletine. American Heart Journal 97: 399–403
1977 Postgraduate Medical Journal 53 (suppl 1): 10–171

References

1. Weld F M, Bigger J T, Swistel D, Bordiuk J 1977 Effects of mexiletine (Ko 1173) on electrophysiological properties of sheep cardiac Purkinje fibers. American Journal of Cardiology 39: 292
2. Hering S, Bodewei R, Wollenberger A 1983 Sodium current in freshly isolated and in cultured single rat myocardial cells: frequency and voltage-dependent block by mexiletine. Journal of Molecular and Cellular Cardiology 15: 431–444
3. Chew C Y C, Collett J, Singh B H 1979 Mexiletine: a review of its pharmacological properties and therapeutic efficacy in arrhythmias. Drugs 17: 161–181
4. Singh B N, Vaughan Williams E M 1972 Investigation of the mode of action of a new antidysrhythmic drug, Ko 1173. British Journal of Pharmacology 44: 1–9
5. Allen J D, James R G G, Kelly J G, Shanks R G, Zaidi S A 1977 Comparison of the effects of lignocaine and mexiletine on experimental ventricular arrhythmias. Postgraduate Medical Journal 53 (suppl 1): 35–45
6. Okuma K, Sugiyama S, Wada M et al 1976 Experimental studies on the antiarrhythmic action of a lidocaine analogue. Cardiology 61: 289–297
7. Pottage A 1977 Oral dosage schedules for mexiletine. Postgraduate Medical Journal 53 (suppl 1): 155–157
8. Prescott L F, Pottage A, Clements J A 1977 Absorption, distribution and elimination of mexiletine. Postgraduate Medical Journal 53 (suppl 1): 50–55
9. Campbell N P S, Pantridge J F, Adgey A A J 1978 Long-term oral antiarrhythmic therapy with mexiletine. British Heart Journal 40: 796–801
10. Podrid P J, Lowin B 1981 Mexiletine for ventricular arrhythmias. American Journal of Cardiology 47: 895–902
11. Campbell N P S, Pantridge J F, Adgey A A J 1977 Mexiletine in the management of ventricular dysrhythmias. European Journal of Cardiology 6: 245–258
12. Mehta J, Conti C R 1982 Mexiletine, a new antiarrhythmic agent, for treatment of premature ventricular complexes. American Journal of Cardiology 49: 455–460
13. Dimarco J P, Garan H, Ruskin J N 1981 Mexiletine for refractory ventricular arrhythmias. Results using serial electrophysiological testing. American Journal of Cardiology 47: 131–138
14. Harper R W, Olsson S B 1979 Effect of mexiletine on conduction of premature ventricular beats in man: a study using monophasic action potential recordings from the right ventricle. Cardiovascular Research 13: 311–319
15. Roos J C, Paalman A C A, Dunning A J 1976 Electrophysiological effects of mexiletine in man. British Heart Journal 38: 1262–1271
16. Campbell N P S, Zaidi S A, Adgey A A J, Patterson G C, Pantridge J F 1979 Observations on haemodynamic effects of mexiletine. British Heart Journal 41: 182–186
17. Stein J, Podrid P, Lown B 1984 Effects of oral mexiletine on left and right ventricular function. American Journal of Cardiology 54: 575–578
18. Kelly J G, Nimmo J, Rae R, Shanks R G, Prescott L F 1973 Spectrophotofluorimetric and gas-liquid chromatographic methods for the estimation of mexiletine (Ko 1173) in plasma and urine. Journal of Pharmacology and Pharmacotherapy 25: 550–553
19. Breithaupt H, Wilfling M 1982 Determination of mexiletine in biological fluids by high-performance liquid chromatography. Journal of Chromatography 230: 97–105
20. Heger J J, Nattel S, Rinkenberger R L, Zipes D P 1980 Mexiletine therapy in 15 patients with drug-resistant ventricular tachycardia. American Journal of Cardiology 45: 627–632
21. Campbell N P S, Kelly J G, Adgey A A J, Shanks R G 1978 The clinical pharmacology of mexiletine. British Journal of Clinical Pharmacology 6: 103–108
22. Nademanee K, Feld G, Hendrickson J et al 1985 Mexiletine: double-blind comparison with procainamide in PVC suppression and open-label sequential comparison with amiodarone in life-threatening ventricular arrythmias. American Heart Journal 110: 923–931
23. Rutledge J C, Harris F, Amsterdam E A 1985 Clinical evaluation of oral mexiletine therapy in the treatment of ventricular arrhythmias. Journal of the American College of Cardiology 6: 780–784
24. Campbell R W F, Dolder M A, Prescott L F, Talbot R G, Murray A, Julian D G 1975 Comparison of procainamide and mexiletine in prevention of ventricular arrhythmias after acute myocardial infarction. Lancet 1: 1257–1260
25. Manz M, Steinbeck G, Nitsch J, Luderitz B 1983 Treatment of recurrent sustained ventricular tachycardia with mexiletine and disopyramide. Control by programmed ventricular stimulation. British Heart Journal 49: 222–228

26. Impact Research Group 1984 International mexiletine and placebo antiarrhythmic coronary trial: I. Report on arrhythmia and other findings. Journal of the American College of Cardiology 4: 1148–1163
27. Waspe L E, Waxman H L, Buxton A E, Josephson M E 1983 Mexiletine for control of drug-resistant ventricular tachycardia: clinical and electrophysiologic results in 44 patients. American Journal of Cardiology 51: 1175–1181
28. Touboul P, Gressard A, Kirrorian G, Atallah G 1981 Effects of mexiletine in Wolff–Parkinson–White syndrome. Archives des Maladies du Coeur et des Vaisseaux 74: 1315–1323
29. Neumann G, Simon H, Aulepp H, Otten H, Grube E, Schaede A 1978 Untersuchungen ober die Wirksamkelt von oral verabreichtem Mexiletin (Ko 1173) in der Behandlung unterschiedicher Herzrhythmusstorungen. Herz/Kreislauf 10: 34–40
30. Salem H H 1977 Persistent supraventricular tachycardia treated with mexiletine. Lancet 2: 94
31. Nitsch J, Steinbeck G, Luderitz B 1983 Increase of mexiletine plasma levels due to delayed hepatic metabolism in patients with chronic liver disease. European Heart Journal 4: 810–814
32. Santinelli V, Chiariello M, Stanislao M, Condorelli M 1983 Intravenous mexiletine in management of lidocaine-resistant ventricular tachycardia. American Heart Journal 105: 680–685
33. Greenspan A M, Spielman S R, Webb C R, Sokoloff N M, Rae A P, Horowitz L N 1985 Efficacy of combination therapy with mexiletine and a type IA agent for inducible ventricular tachyarrhythmias secondary to coronary artery disease. American Journal of Cardiology 56: 277–284
34. Jequier P, Jones R, Mackintosh A 1976 Fatal mexiletine overdose. Lancet 1: 429
35. Palileo E V, Welch W, Hoff J et al 1982 Lack of effectiveness of oral mexiletine in patients with drug-refractory paroxysmal sustained ventricular tachycardia. American Journal of Cardiology 50: 1075–1081
36. Duff H J, Roden D, Primm R K, Oates J A, Woosley R L 1983 Mexiletine in the treatment of resistant ventricular arrhythmias: enhancement of efficacy and reduction of dose-related side-effects by combination with quinidine. Circulation 67: 1124–1128
37. Campbell N P S, Pantridge J F, Adgey A A J 1977 Mexiletine in the management of ventricular dysrhythmias. European Journal of Cardiology 6/4: 245–258
38. Holt D W, Walsh A C, Curry P V, Tynan M 1979 Paediatric use of mexiletine and disopyramide. British Medical Journal 2: 1476–1477
39. Timmis A D, Jackson G, Holt D W 1980 Mexiletine for control of ventricular dysrhythmias in pregnancy. Lancet 2: 647–648
40. Breithardt G, Selpel L, Abendroth R R 1980 Comparative cross-over study of the effects of disopyramide and mexiletine on stimulus-induced ventricular tachycardia. Circulation 62 (suppl III): 153
41. Leahey E B, Heissenbuttel R H, Giardina E G V, Bigger J T 1980 Combined mexiletine and propranolol treatment of refractory ventricular tachycardia. British Medical Journal 2: 357–358
42. Waleffe A, Mary-Rabine L, Legrand V, Demoulin J C, Kulbertus H E 1980 Combined mexiletine and amiodarone treatment of refractory recurrent ventricular tachycardia. American Heart Journal 100: 788–793

Mezlocillin

Chemistry

Mezlocillin sodium monohydrate (Baypen)
$C_{21}H_{24}N_5O_8S_2NaH_2O$
The sodium monohydrate salt of 6-{(R)-2-[3-methylsulphonyl-2-oxo-1-imidazolidinecarboxamido]-2-phenylacetamido}-penicillanic acid

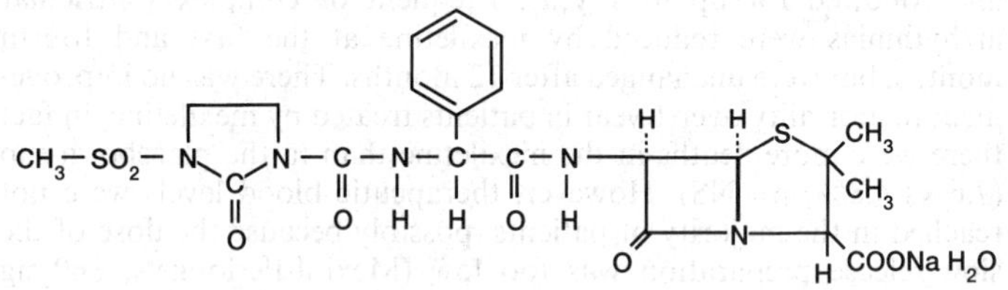

Molecular weight	579.6
pKa	2.7
Solubility	
in alcohol	—
in water	1 in 3
Octanol/water partition coefficient	low

A semi-synthetic acylureidopenicillin derived from ampicillin by substitution at the 6-carbon position of one of the hydrogen atoms at the amino group for a 2-oxo-imidazolidin-1-carboxamido substituent with a terminal methyl sulphonyl group. The latter group is the only difference between mezlocillin and azlocillin. The D-isomer is used clinically. Supplied as the sodium monohydrate salt, it is a white to slightly yellow crystalline substance which is almost odourless and is readily soluble in water (about 30% w/v). Each gram contains about 1.85 mmol sodium.

Pharmacology

Mezlocillin binds to penicillin sensitive enzymes (penicillin binding proteins, PBP) in the bacterial cell wall and thereby inhibits the final stages of peptidoglycan synthesis. It has a particularly high affinity for PBP 3 which is responsible for septum formation and thus induces filament formation of the bacterial cell.[1] These filaments are non-viable. Although the stability of mezlocillin to many β-lactamases is relatively weak, this is compensated by its high affinity for PBP 3 and ability to penetrate rapidly the outer membrane of Gram-negative bacteria, thus ensuring a high degree of activity against most isolates.

Toxicology

Animal studies have shown no evidence of acute or chronic toxicity in various animal species, except for reversible histological damage to veins in dogs which is dose dependent. Mezlocillin has no demonstrable mutagenic potential or carcinogenic effects. Tests in rats and mice show no impairment of fertility or reproduction, or any teratogenic effects in their offspring.

Clinical pharmacology

Mezlocillin has a range of activity similar to but wider than that of carbenicillin and ticarcillin, with greater potency against certain sensitive strains. It is relatively unstable to many of the commonly occurring β-lactamases found in Gram-positive and Gram-negative bacteria, but still retains excellent activity against many such isolates.

Most of the clinically relevant Enterobacteriaceae are susceptible to achievable serum concentrations of mezlocillin, with activity generally being greater than carbenicillin, ticarcillin and azlocillin. The majority of *E. coli* are inhibited by 4–8 mg.l^{-1} or less, although β-lactamase producing strains will be more resistant.[2,3] Activity against *Klebsiella* is considerably greater than that of carbenicillin or ticarcillin, with the number of sensitive strains varying depending on the prevalence of β-lactamase-producing strains.[2,3] Mezlocillin is also active against a proportion of *E. coli* and klebsiellae resistant to carbenicillin and ticarcillin.[3] *Proteus mirabilis* is highly susceptible; 95% of isolates are inhibited[3] by 2 mg.l^{-1}. Indole-positive *Proteus* are less sensitive with MICs of 8–32 mg.l^{-1}. Mezlocillin is more active than the earlier penicillins against *Serratia* and *Enterobacter* (about 70% of strains having MICs[2–4] of 4–8 mg.l^{-1}), and substantially more active against *Citrobacter*.[4]

Activity against *Pseudomonas aeruginosa* is comparable with ticarcillin, though less than azlocillin and piperacillin, with most strains inhibited[3–6] by 8–32 mg.l^{-1}. Mezlocillin may also be active against some ticarcillin and carbenicillin resistant strains, although the MIC tends to be higher.[3]

Non-β-lactamase-producing *Neisseria gonorrhoeae* and *Haemophilus influenzae* are highly susceptible to mezlocillin (MIC 0.01 mg.l^{-1} and 0.25 mg.l^{-1} or less respectively), more so than to ampicillin or penicillin.[3,7] However, β-lactamase-producing strains are more resistant, although mezlocillin still retains good activity against such strains of gonococci, with the MIC often only increasing ten-fold.[7] The meningococcus is also highly susceptible.

Mezlocillin possesses greater activity against Gram-positive cocci than either carbenicillin or ticarcillin.[4,8] Penicillin sensitive staphylococci are moderately sensitive, with 90% inhibited by 2 mg.l^{-1} or less.[8] However, most strains of *Staphylococcus aureus* produce a β-lactamase which inactivates mezlocillin and such strains should be considered resistant. The activity of mezlocillin against pneumococci is similar to that of ampicillin but less than penicillin (MIC 0.1 mg.l^{-1} or less).[8] It is also highly active against β-haemolytic streptococci and non-enterococcal streptococci (MIC 0.1–1.0), being almost as active as penicillin.[7] Mezlocillin has good activity against enterococci and is comparable to ampicillin; MIC 1 mg.l^{-1} or less.[4]

The activity of mezlocillin against anaerobic bacteria is similar to that of penicillin, with most being highly susceptible. However, the majority of *Bacteroides fragilis* produce a β-lactamase and are therefore less susceptible: 50% of strains inhibited by 8 mg.l^{-1} and 90% by 32 mg.l^{-1}.[10] Other *Bacteroides*, anaerobic cocci, *Fusobacteria* and *Clostridia* are inhibited by much lower concentrations, although mezlocillin offers no advantage over penicillin against these isolates.[2,4,10]

Pharmacokinetics

The preferred assay method is high performance liquid chromatography, which has a sensitivity[11] of 1.5 mg.l^{-1}.

Mezlocillin is poorly absorbed from the gastrointestinal tract and must therefore be administered parenterally. Intramuscular administration results in peak serum levels being reached in 60–90 min; a single 1 g dose giving mean levels of about 40 mg.l^{-1} which decline to about 1 mg.l^{-1} after 6 h.[12] Serum levels after intravenous use depend on the mode of administration. A bolus injection of 2 g produces peak levels[12] at 30 min of 110–140 mg.l^{-1} while five minute infusions of 2 g and 4 g give peak levels within 15 min of 105–118 mg.l^{-1} and 155–410 mg.l^{-1} respectively.[13–15] A 5 g infusion over 15 min gives a mean serum concentration at 1 h of 164–220 mg.l^{-1}, falling to 12–21 mg.l^{-1} after 6 h.[6]

Mezlocillin, like other acylureidopenicillins, exhibits dose-dependent pharmacokinetic characteristics. Therefore with increasing doses, serum levels are higher than expected, serum half life is longer and clearances are lower.[13] Serum bactericidal activity is also prolonged; consequently longer administration intervals may be as therapeutically effective when using higher dosages.[16] The protein binding is relatively low and diminishes as serum concentration increases, being 42, 35 and 27% at 2, 20 and 200 mg.l^{-1} respectively.[17] Similarly, the volume of distribution varies according to the amount of drug administered; 0.55 l.kg^{-1} after 1 g falling to 0.38 l.kg^{-1} after 5 g.

Elimination of mezlocillin from the body is primarily via the kidneys by glomerular filtration and active tubular secretion. Probenecid reduces renal clearance by about one third, producing higher

Mezlocillin

and more prolonged serum levels. Approximately 7 dose of mezlocillin is excreted in the urine, the unchanged active drug.[14] Urinary levels are the peak levels being approximately 2000 and 8000 mg.l 4 g dose respectively, [15] although renal impairment will values. The serum half life in normal subjects is about although variations have been reported particularly after differ doses, ranging from 0.9 h after a 1 g dose to 1.2 h after a 5 g dose. [1-] Impaired renal function causes an increase in half life giving higher, more prolonged serum levels, and reduces renal clearances.[15] Anuric patients have a serum half life of 2–5 h.[18,19]

A variable amount of mezlocillin is excreted via the biliary tract; up to 30% of the total administered dose.[20] A lower proportion is excreted when hepatobiliary function is reduced (approximately 0.2–6.2% of a given dose).[20,21] Biliary concentrations can be in excess of 8000 mg.l^{-1} in normal subjects but are much lower in patients with hyperbilirubinaemia.[12,21] Biliary clearance is also markedly reduced in the presence of jaundice,[21] falling from around 90 ml.min^{-1} in normal subjects to 0.2–7.8 ml.min^{-1}. However, levels in excess of 10 mg.l^{-1} are consistently attained[23] which exceeds the MIC of most pathogens.

Mezlocillin is distributed widely throughout the body with levels in various organs reaching 25–50% of corresponding serum levels. Wound fluid (skin window) levels range from 10 to 64 mg.l^{-1} after a 2 g dose and have a longer half life than corresponding serum levels.[22] Concentrations in bronchial mucosa after only 1 g intramuscularly[23] range from 0.7 to 10.0 mg.l^{-1}; corresponding levels in bronchial aspirates are much lower, as are sputum levels, and are not a reliable guide to tissue concentrations. Penetration into bone is poor although concentrations of 57 mg.l^{-1} after a 2 g dose have been measured in spongy bone with cortical bone levels somewhat lower[22] at 35 mg.l^{-1}. CSF levels tend to be low, with CSF/serum ratios ranging from 0 to 10%,[12,24] although therapeutic levels may be more reliably attained in the presence of inflammation. Mezlocillin readily passes into the fetus with levels in amniotic fluid and cord blood approximating to those in maternal serum. Very little crosses into breast milk.

Oral absorption	negligible
Presystemic metabolism	not relevant
Plasma half life	
range	0.9–1.2 h
mean	1.0 h
Volume of distribution	0.38–0.55 l.kg^{-1}
Plasma protein binding	27–42%

Concentration–effect relationship

There is no evidence to suggest any further therapeutic benefit once the MIC of the infecting organism has been surpassed. Larger doses are employed for less sensitive bacteria or when penetration of the antibiotic to the site of infection is likely to be limited. Due to dose-dependent pharmacokinetics, serum bactericidal activity is prolonged when using higher dosages.[16]

Metabolism

The majority of a dose of mezlocillin is excreted in the urine (~70%) largely as the unchanged drug. Most of the remainder is excreted unchanged via the biliary tract.

Mezlocillin is converted in the liver to the corresponding penicilloate and penilloate derivatives (Fig. 1). Approximately 10–15% of the total dose is accounted for by these metabolites, which are then excreted predominantly in the urine. They possess no significant antibacterial activity.

Pharmaceutics

Mezlocillin (Baypen Bayer, UK) is normally given by the parenteral route but may be given intramuscularly if required. Baypen is available as vials containing 0.5 g, 1 g and 2 g of the sodium monohydrate salt, or as infusion packs containing 5 g. Vials containing 3 g and 4 g are also available in the USA and Germany. Mezlin (Miles, US) vials contain mezlocillin sodium equivalent to 1 g, 2 g, 3 g

Fig. 1 Metabolites of mezlocillin. R = side chain

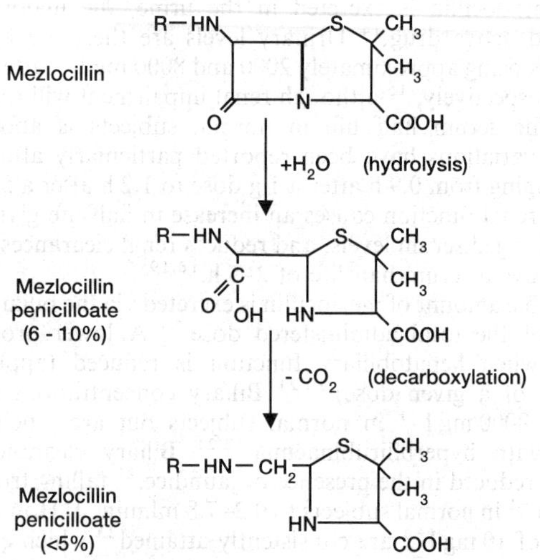

and 4 g. Mezlin infusion bottles contain 2 g, 3 g or 4 g. Each gram contains about 1.85 mEq of sodium. When reconstituted as a 10% aqueous solution, it is isotonic.

Mezlocillin should be stored in temperatures not exceeding 25°C and will then have a shelf-life of 5 years. (The powder may darken slightly but potency is not affected.) It should be freshly prepared prior to administration; water for injection BP is the preferred diluent for reconstitution. Mezlocillin is also compatible with dextrose 5 and 10%, laevulose 5%, Ringers solution and physiological saline. It should be administered separately from other intravenous preparations and must not be mixed together with an aminoglycoside due to possible inactivation of the latter due to physical incompatibility. Injectable tetracyclin derivatives, ciprofloxacin and metronadizole, have also proved to be incompatible with mezlocillin and must therefore be administered separately. Compatibility with rarely used solutions must be ascertained prior to administration; possible incompatibility is indicated by precipitation, cloudiness or discolouration.[25]

Therapeutic use

Indications

1. The treatment of serious infections of the respiratory, urogenital and biliary tracts, soft tissues, bone and joints, and for septicaemia, peritonitis and meningitis when due to susceptible bacteria.
2. The treatment of proven or suspected infections in the immunocompromised.
3. The prophylaxis of postoperative sepsis following abdominal (including biliary) surgery and vaginal hysterectomy.

Contraindications

1. Hypersensitivity to penicillin-class antibiotics.
2. Mezlocillin, as with all new drugs, should not be used during the first three months of pregnancy unless the potential benefits clearly outweigh the risk, although studies have shown no evidence of teratogenic or embryotoxic effects of mezlocillin.

Mode of use

The recommended dosage for most therapeutic indications is 2 g every 6–8 h. However, for severe infections and those due to less susceptible bacteria such as *Ps. aeruginosa*, this can be increased up to a maximum of 5 g every 6–8 h. At such dosages the longer administration interval could be used due to the dose-dependent pharmacokinetic characteristics of mezlocillin.[16] Acute gonorrhoea may be treated by a single intramuscular injection of 1 g. For prophylactic use, 5 g given intravenously immediately preoperatively as a single dose should suffice, although an alternative regimen of 2 g immediately preoperatively followed by two further 2 g injections at 8 hourly intervals is also recommended.

Intravenous administration can be achieved by firstly dissolving the powder in water for injection to make a 10% solution. This is then administered either by bolus injection over 2–4 min for dosages up to 2 g, or by an infusion over 15–20 min when a 3–5 g dose is given. Mezlocillin can also be given by deep intramuscular injection into the buttocks, up to a maximum dose of 2 g. Each gram should be dissolved in 3.5 ml water to achieve solution.

Indications

Mezlocillin has been used to treat a wide variety of infections with overall success rates of 80–90%.[10,12,26,27] It has also been used extensively in many centres for prophylaxis in certain surgical procedures.

1. Treatment of serious infections in the normal host

Urinary tract infection. Mezlocillin's activity against most of the common urinary pathogens, including *Ps. aeruginosa* and enterococci, has proved successful in many complicated urinary tract infections. Clinical responses range from 66% in complicated infection to 87% in cystitis.[26,28] Comparative studies with ticarcillin show an improved, though not clinically significant, cure rate.[29]

Respiratory tract infection. A good clinical response has been demonstrated in about 90% of adults and children with pneumonia.[30,31] These high cure rates include a large percentage of Gram-positive aerobic pathogens and *Ps. aeruginosa* although the latter often persists after treatment. If staphylococcal pneumonia is suspected, mezlocillin should not be used even though occasional successes have been reported.[10]

Biliary tract infections. Mezlocillin's spectrum of activity encompasses the important biliary pathogens and it is also excreted in high levels in bile. Reduced amounts are found in patients with jaundice, but therapeutic levels are still attained.[21] (See also Major outcome trials.)

Septicaemia. Mezlocillin has been used alone as empirical therapy for suspected septicaemia both in adults[12,26] and the newborn.[32] High cure rates have been recorded when the causative organism is sensitive, including *Ps. aeruginosa* and *B. fragilis*. Poor activity against β-lactamase producing *S. aureus* suggests that mezlocillin may not be the best single agent for empirical therapy in all cases. For infections due to *Pseudomonas*, combination therapy with an aminoglycoside is recommended.

Other infections. Mezlocillin has been used successfully to treat a wide variety of infections: meningitis in both adults and neonates,[32] osteomyelitis,[10] soft tissue infections[10,26] and pelvic infections[33] due to a variety of aerobic and anaerobic bacteria. Successful use for the treatment of acute gonorrhoea has also been reported.[27] Other more appropriate agents are now available and it is unlikely that mezlocillin would be considered as first line therapy in any of these infections unless laboratory investigations suggest otherwise.

2. Empirical therapy in the immunocompromised host

Like other anti-pseudomonal penicillins, mezlocillin has been used for empirical therapy in this group of patients. When used alone, response rates of only about 50% were obtained.[34,35] Particularly poor responses were recorded for proven bacteraemia, especially when due to *S. aureus* or *Ps. aeruginosa*. Better results are achieved when combined with an aminoglycoside.[36]

3. Prophylaxis

Mezlocillin has been used extensively as single agent prophylaxis for operations where postoperative infection due to aerobic and anaerobic bacteria may occur. In appendicectomy, a single 5 g preoperative dose of mezlocillin was comparable to metronidazole, giving infection rates of 6% and 8% respectively.[37] For colorectal procedures the same regimen was as effective as three doses of cefuroxime and metronidazole.[38] The high biliary levels achieved by mezlocillin, even in the presence of stasis, is reflected in its successful use in biliary tract surgery. A single 5 g dose reduces wound infection rate from 10% (placebo) to 4% in one prospective double blind trial.[39] Other applications are in vaginal hysterectomy and following transurethral prostatectomy.[40]

Adverse reactions

Potentially life-threatening effects

Acute anaphylaxis may occur in penicillin allergic patients receiving mezlocillin and its use is therefore contraindicated in such patients.

Acute overdosage

Overdosage should be treated by standard monitoring and supportive measures. Serum levels of mezlocillin may be reduced by dialysis.

Severe or irreversible adverse effects

Hepatotoxicity has been occasionally reported although in most instances this has been a reversible rise in AST (SGOT) and ALT (SGPT) only. Similarly hyperbilirubinaemia has also been noted but its relationship to mezlocillin administration is doubtful.[34]

Acute interstitial nephritis has been recorded in two patients each infected with *Ps. aeruginosa* and each receiving other antibiotics. The diagnosis was confirmed by renal biopsy and mezlocillin administration considered the most likely cause.[41]

Leucopenia is a well described complication of penicillin therapy although its incidence following mezlocillin use is probably less than with many other penicillin derivatives. Mezlocillin, like carbenicillin, causes platelet dysfunction and a prolonged bleeding time, but the risk of its producing a bleeding disorder is much less.[43,26] Neurological effects reported after high-dose penicillin therapy have not been reported after mezlocillin use.

Symptomatic adverse effects

The commonest adverse reactions are those at the site of administration of mezlocillin such as thrombophlebitis, erythema or cellulitis. The overall incidence is 3% with thrombophlebitis accounting for the majority. Most reactions tend to occur after several days of therapy.[10,26,42] Allergic cutaneous reactions are unusual (<2%), the commonest being a nondescript maculopapular or urticarial rash. These reactions may occur at any stage of mezlocillin therapy.

Gastrointestinal disturbances are unusual, occurring in about 1% of patients and tending to be mild and reversible on discontinuing therapy.

Other effects

Eosinophilia has been found in about 2% of patients receiving mezlocillin, especially when therapy continues for over a week.[42] Other haematological effects such as thrombocytopenia, thrombocytosis and a positive Coombs test have been reported in individual patients but appear to be extremely unusual.

Hypokalaemia may occur due to a non-reabsorbable anion effect in the renal tubule and is related to the dose given.[34,42] Its overall incidence (0.7%) is less than for carbenicillin or ticarcillin as would be expected from its lower sodium content, and is easily reversed with potassium supplements.

Interference with clinical pathology tests

A positive test for proteinuria may occur if the sulphosalicylic acid precipitation test is used.

High risk groups

Neonates

The recommended dosage for neonates and premature babies is 75 $mg.kg^{-1}$ every 12 h as a prolonged intravenous infusion. Using this regimen the maximum serum concentration in neonates tends to be similar to that in adults although the half life is 2–4 times as long. This is related more to age rather than weight or maturity at birth.[44]

Breast milk. Very little mezlocillin crosses into breast milk and so use during lactation should present no problems. However, the risk of sensitization of the infant to penicillins should be borne in mind, and alternative methods of feeding considered.

Children

The recommended dosage for children is 75 $mg.kg^{-1}$ every 8 h given as a bolus injection or a short intravenous infusion. Pharmacokinetic parameters in children are comparable to those in adults.

Pregnant women

Although there is no evidence to suggest teratogenic effects, mezlocillin is best avoided in the first trimester unless considered absolutely necessary.

The elderly

Provided renal function is not impaired, no special precautions are required.

Concurrent disease

Renal failure. Because the route of elimination is mainly renal, dosage adjustments are only required when renal function is markedly impaired. When creatinine clearance is b 30 $ml.min^{-1}$ the normal adult dose should be red especially if higher doses are being used. For s (creatinine clearance < 10 $ml.min^{-1}$) reduce the dos In each case the same dosage interval can be used. Alterna the half life is not appreciably increased except in severe renal another suggested schedule is to give the normal adult dose but 12 h intervals when the creatinine clearance is 10–15 $ml.min^{-1}$ or less.[15,18]

Haemodialysis removes approximately 25% of an administered dose and reduces the half life in anuric patients by about 50% to almost normal.[18,19] During dialysis the dosage interval should be doubled. Peritoneal dialysis does not remove significant amounts of mezlocillin from the body (<5% of a given dose), and therefore no extra adjustment needs to be made other than that required for the level of renal impairment.[18]

Hepatic failure. Small increases in half life and serum levels can be measured in severe hepatobiliary dysfunction. Alterations in dosage are only required if there is concomitant severe renal failure, when monitoring of serum levels might then be advisable.

Drug interactions

Potentially hazardous interactions

Several β-lactams, particularly cefoxitin, have been shown to be antagonistic to mezlocillin in vitro against certain bacteria such as *Ps. aeruginosa*, *Enterobacter* and *Serratia*.[45] These agents act as β-lactamase inducers causing these bacteria to produce large amounts of this enzyme which inhibits the access of the antibiotic to target proteins.

Mezlocillin can inactivate aminoglycosides due to physical incompatibility when mixed together in the same infusion bottle. The extent of inactivation is greater with increasing mezlocillin concentration, contact time and temperature.[25] Similar effects may be seen in vivo in patients with renal failure and high serum levels of mezlocillin.

Patients being treated with mezlocillin and concomitant heparin or other anticoagulants need more frequent control of coagulation parameters.

Potentially useful interactions

Synergy can be demonstrated between aminoglycosides and mezlocillin against a variable number of strains of Enterobacteriaceae including some gentamicin resistant species, and against *Ps. aeruginosa*. Synergy against enterococci can also be demonstrated.

Major outcome trials

Gerecht W B, Henry N K, Hoffman W W, Muller S M, La Russo N F, Rosenblatt J E, Wilson W R (1989) Prospective randomised comparison of mezlocillin therapy alone or with combined ampicillin and gentamicin therapy for patients with cholangitis. Archives of Internal Medicine 149: 1279–1284

This was a randomized trial comparing mezlocillin with a combination of ampicillin and gentamicin in 46 patients with cholangitis. The mezlocillin group had a cure rate of 83% (compared to 41%) and showed fewer toxic or adverse reactions. Biliary concentrations of mezlocillin were 112 and 778 times higher than those of ampicillin and gentamicin respectively.

General review articles

Bergan T 1981 Overview of acylureidopenicillin pharmacokinetics. Scandinavian Journal of Infectious Diseases 29 (suppl): 33–48

Eliopoulos G M, Moellering R C 1982 Azlocillin, mezlocillin and piperacillin: new broad-spectrum penicillins. Annals of Internal Medicine 97: 755–760

Neu H C, Wise R (eds) 1982 Mezlocillin. Journal of Antimicrobial Chemotherapy 9 (suppl A)

Neu H C, Reeves D S, Leigh D A (eds) 1983 Mezlocillin — a broad spectrum penicillin: an update. Journal of Antimicrobial Chemotherapy 11 (suppl C)

References

1. Curtis N A C, Orr D, Ross G W, Boulton M G 1979 Affinities of penicillins and cephalosporins for the penicillin-binding proteins of *Escherichia coli* K-12 and their antibacterial activity. Antimicrobial Agents and Chemotherapy 16: 533–539

2. Thadepalli H, Roy I, Bach V T, Webb D 1979 In vitro activity of mezlocillin and its related compounds against aerobic and anaerobic bacteria. Antimicrobial Agents and Chemotherapy 15: 487–490
3. Wise R, Gillett A P, Andrews J M, Bedford K A 1978 Activity of azlocillin and mezlocillin against Gram-negative organisms: comparison with other penicillins. Antimicrobial Agents and Chemotherapy 13: 559–565
4. Fass R J 1980 In vitro activities of β-lactam and aminoglycoside antibiotics. A comparative study of 20 parenterally administered drugs. Archives of Internal Medicine 140: 763–768
5. Harris R L, Smith N J, Dietrich J E et al 1984 In vitro bactericidal effect of azlocillin, mezlocillin, piperacillin and ticarcillin against Gram-negative bacilli. Current Therapeutic Research 35: 633–642
6. Coppens L, Klastersky J 1979 Comparative study of anti-*Pseudomonas* activity of azlocillin, mezlocillin and ticarcillin. Antimicrobial Agents and Chemotherapy 15: 396–399
7. Baker C N, Thornsberry C, Jones R N 1980 In vitro antimicrobial activity of cefoperazone, cefotaxime, moxalactam (LY 127 935), azlocillin, mezlocillin, and other β-lactam antibiotics against *Neisseria gonorrhoeae* and *Haemophilus influenzae*, including β-lactamase producing strains. Antimicrobial Agents and Chemotherapy 17: 757–761
8. Sanders C C 1981 Comparative activity of mezlocillin, penicillin, ampicillin, carbenicillin and ticarcillin against Gram-positive bacteria and *Haemophilus influenzae*. Antimicrobial Agents and Chemotherapy 20: 843–846
9. Aldridge K E, Sanders C V, Janney A, Faro S, Marier R L 1984 Comparison of the activities of penicillin G and new β-lactam antibiotics against clinical isolates of *Bacteroides* species. Antimicrobial Agents and Chemotherapy 26: 410–413
10. Thadepalli H, Rao B, Dhawan V K, Bach V T 1982 Evaluation of mezlocillin in aerobic and anaerobic infections. Journal of Antimicrobial Chemotherapy 9 (suppl A): 115–119
11. Hildebrandt R, Gundert-Remy U 1982 Improved procedure for the determination of the ureidopenicillins azlocillin and mezlocillin in plasma by high-performance liquid chromatography. Journal of Chromatography 228: 409–412
12. Ellis C J, Geddes A M, Davey P G 1979 Mezlocillin and azlocillin: an evaluation of two new β-lactam antibiotics. Journal of Antimicrobial Chemotherapy 5: 517–525
13. Bergan T 1978 Pharmacokinetics of mezlocillin in healthy volunteers. Antimicrobial Agents and Chemotherapy 14: 801–806
14. Pancoast S J, Neu H C 1978 Kinetics of mezlocillin and carbenicillin. Clinical Pharmacology and Therapeutics 24: 108–116
15. Frimodt-Moller N, Maigaard S, Toothaker R D et al 1980 Mezlocillin pharmacokinetics after single intravenous doses to patients with varying degrees of renal function. Antimicrobial Agents and Chemotherapy 17: 599–607
16. Flaherty J F, Barriere S L, Mordenti J, Garbertoglio J G 1987 Effect of dose on pharmacokinetics and serum bactericidal activity of mezlocillin. Antimicrobial Agents and Chemotherapy 31: 895–898
17. Rosenkrantz H, Forster D 1979 Comparative study of the binding of acylureidopenicillins and carbenicillin to human serum proteins. Infection 7: 102–108
18. Kampf D, Schurig R, Weihermuller K, Forster D 1980 Effects of impaired renal function, haemodialysis and peritoneal dialysis on the pharmacokinetics of mezlocillin. Antimicrobial Agents and Chemotherapy 18: 81–87
19. Janicke D M, Mangione A, Schulz R W, Jusco W J 1982 Mezlocillin disposition in chronic haemodialysis patients. Antimicrobial Agents and Chemotherapy 20: 590–594
20. Brogard J M, Kopferschmitt J, Arnaud J P, Dorner M, La Villaureix J 1980 Biliary elimination of mezlocillin: an experimental and clinical study. Antimicrobial Agents and Chemotherapy 18: 69–76
21. Dooley J S, Gooding A, Hamilton-Miller J M T, Brumfitt W, Sherlock S 1983 The biliary excretion and pharmacokinetics of mezlocillin in jaundiced patients with external bile drainage. Liver 3: 201–206
22. Wittman D H, Schassan H H, Schreiner P 1980 Pharmacokinetic investigations into the penetration of azlocillin and mezlocillin into bone and wound tissue fluid. In: Siegenthaler (ed) International Symposium Acylureidopenicillins, Vienna 1979. Excerpta Medica, Amsterdam, pp 85–86
23. Pirali F, Santus G, Spedini C, Turano A 1987 Antibiotic levels in bronchopulmonary tissue. Lancet 1: 505
24. Modai J, Pierre J, Bergogne-Berezin E, Vril M F 1979 Cerebrospinal fluid penetration of mezlocillin. Arzneimittelforschung 29: 1967–1969
25. Henderson J L, Polk R E, Kline B J 1981 In vitro inactivation of gentamicin, tobramycin and netilmicin by carbenicillin, azlocillin or mezlocillin. American Journal of Hospital Pharmacy 38: 67–70
26. Pancoast S J, Jahre J A, Neu H C 1979 Mezlocillin in the therapy of serious infections. American Journal of Medicine 67: 747–752
27. Lassus A, Renkonen O V 1979 Mezlocillin in the treatment of gonorrhoea. British Journal of Venereal Disease 55: 191–193
28. Cox C E 1982 Multi-institutional study of mezlocillin therapy of urinary tract infections. Journal of Antimicrobial Chemotherapy 9 (suppl A): 173–177
29. Madsen P O, Nielsen O S 1982 Treatment of complicated urinary tract infections with mezlocillin and ticarcillin, a comparative study. Journal of Antimicrobial Chemotherapy 9 (suppl A): 179–181
30. McCloskey R V, Killebrew D, Tutlane V, Bentley J 1982 A randomized double blinded comparison of mezlocillin and ticarcillin for the treatment of respiratory infections. Journal of Antimicrobial Chemotherapy 9 (suppl A): 209–213
31. Nishimura T 1980 Clinical comparative double blind study with mezlocillin and ampicillin in the treatment of bacterial pneumonia in children. In: Siegenthaler (ed) International Symposium on Acylureidopenicillins, Vienna 1979. Excerpta Medica, Amsterdam, pp 123–126
32. Chiu T, Garrison R D, Fakhreddine F, Ayoub E M 1982 Mezlocillin in neonatal infections: evaluation of efficacy and toxicity. Journal of Antimicrobial Chemotherapy 9 (suppl A): 251–255
33. Marshall J R, Chow A W, Sorrell T C 1982 Effectiveness of mezlocillin in female genital tract infections. Journal of Antimicrobial Chemotherapy 9 (suppl): 149–158
34. Wade J C, Schimpff S C, Newman K A et al 1980 Potential of mezlocillin as empiric single-agent therapy in febrile granulocytopenic cancer patients. Antimicrobial Agents and Chemotherapy 18: 299–306
35. Issel B F, Bodey G P 1980 Mezlocillin for treatment of infections in cancer patients. Antimicrobial Agents and Chemotherapy 17: 1008–1013
36. Melikian V, Wise R, Allum W H, Wells W D 1981 Mezlocillin and gentamicin in the treatment of infections in seriously ill and immunosuppressed patients. Journal of Antimicrobial Chemotherapy 7: 657–663
37. McIntosh G S, Jacob G, Townell N H, Noone P 1984 Prevention of post-appendicectomy sepsis by mezlocillin and metronidazole: a prospective, randomised, double-blind trial. Journal of Antimicrobial Chemotherapy 14: 537–542
38. Stubbs R S, Griggs N J, Kelleher J P, Dickinson I K, Moat N, Rimmer D M D 1987 Single dose mezlocillin versus three dose cefuroxime plus metronidazole for the prophylaxis of wound infection after large bowel surgery. Journal of Hospital Infection 9: 285–290
39. Elke R, Widmer M, Gerber H, Trippel M, Gruber U F 1983 Mezlocillin single-dose prophylaxis in biliary tract surgery. European Surgical Research 15: 297–301
40. Allan W R, Kumar A 1985 Prophylactic mezlocillin for transurethral prostatectomy. British Journal of Urology 57: 46–49
41. Cushner H M, Copley J B, Bauman J, Hill S C 1985 Acute interstitial nephritis associated with mezlocillin, nafcillin and gentamicin treatment for *Pseudomonas* infection. Archives of Internal Medicine 145: 1204–1207
42. Parry M F, Neu H C 1982 The safety and tolerance of mezlocillin. Journal of Antimicrobial Chemotherapy 9 (suppl A): 273–280
43. Copelan E A, Kusumi R K, Miller L, Fass R J 1983 A comparison of the effects of mezlocillin and carbenicillin on haemostasis in volunteers. Journal of Antimicrobial Chemotherapy 11 (suppl C): 43–49
44. Rubio T, Wirth F, Karotkin E 1982 Pharmacokinetic studies of mezlocillin in newborn infants. Journal of Antimicrobial Chemotherapy 9 (suppl A): 241–244
45. Sanders C C, Sanders W E, Goering R V 1982 In vitro antagonism of beta-lactam antibiotics by cefoxitin. Antimicrobial Agents and Chemotherapy 21: 968–975

Mianserin

Mianserin was introduced in 1976 as an antidepressant with a novel tetracyclic structure and a pharmacological action which differed from previous antidepressant drugs.

Chemistry

Mianserin hydrochloride (Bolvidon, Norval, Tolvon)
$C_{18}H_{20}N_2.HCl$
1,2,3,4,10,14b-Hexahydro-2-methyldibenzo [c,f] pyrazino [1,2,-a]azepine hydrochloride

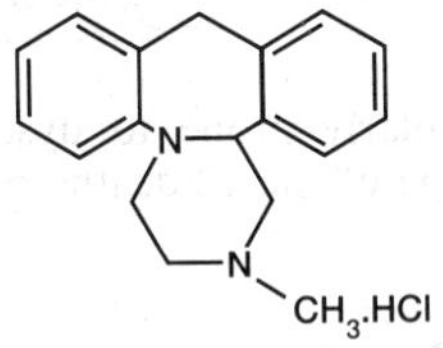

Molecular weight (free base)	300.8 (264.4)
pKa	7.05
Solubility	
in alcohol	1 in 100
in water	1 in 50
Octanol/water partition coefficient	>1000

White to almost white crystals or crystalline powder; bitter taste; odourless. Mianserin is not present in any combination products.

Pharmacology

Although mianserin inhibits noradrenaline uptake in vitro, it does not do so in vivo possibly because it does not bind to the desipramine receptor which is coupled to the noradrenaline transporter.[1] Rather its effects upon noradrenaline can be attributed to its ability to antagonize α_2 and α_1-adrenoceptors.[2,3] In acute experiments mianserin reduces brain concentrations of MHPG and prevents the α_2-adrenoreceptor-mediated suppression of MHPG by clonidine.[4] In acute experiments therefore mianserin increases noradrenaline release by inhibiting the α_2 mediated inhibition of noradrenaline release.

During chronic treatment, brain concentrations of MHPG remain elevated but clonidine is able to suppress MHPG concentrations.[4] The mechanisms by which chronic mianserin treatment apparently increases noradrenaline turnover is therefore not understood. Chronic treatment with mianserin also results in reduced activity of the brain noradrenaline sensitive adenylate cyclase without change in the number of β adrenoceptors.[5]

Mianserin does not inhibit the uptake of 5-hydroxytryptamine (5HT) or dopamine[2] but it is an antagonist at $5HT_2$ and $5HT_{1c}$ receptors.[6] Mianserin is also a potent antihistamine which binds to histamine H_1 receptors:[7] it also inhibits H_2 mediated adenylate cyclase in rat brain.[8]

Compared to tricyclic antidepressants mianserin is a very weak muscarinic antagonist.[9]

Toxicology

Acute and chronic experiments have failed to detect abnormalities in routine toxicology. Body weight loss in parent animals and fetuses were the only abnormalities noted in mice and rabbits given at least 10 times the therapeutic dose. There is no evidence for carcinogenicity or teratogenicity.

Clinical pharmacology

Mianserin is an effective antidepressant in patients suffering from mild depression. Like most members of its class the full antidepressant effects take two to three weeks to be evident. It is relatively free of anticholinergic side effects and thus does not reduce salivary flow.[10] Mianserin equally does not inhibit the miotic effects of pilocarpine eye drops.[11] Anticholinergic side effects are unusual. Although mianserin has α_1 adrenoceptor antagonist activity it has relatively few cardiovascular effects. The drug has no effects on the ECG and His bundle cardiography studies show no untoward effects.[12] Mianserin does not prolong the pre-ejection period[13] and changes in heart rate or blood pressure are unusual. Mianserin does reduce the spontaneous and pentagastrin-evoked secretion of gastric acid,[14] possibly by its actions at the H_2 receptor complex.

Pharmacokinetics

Mianserin can be measured by gas chromatography with nitrogen detection,[15] the limit of detection being 1 μg.l^{-1} or by liquid chromatography with electrochemical detection,[16] the limit of detection being 5 μg.l^{-1}.

Mianserin is rapidly absorbed after oral administration and peak plasma concentrations are achieved within 3 hours of administration of a 60 mg dose.[17] As a result of high presystemic metabolism the systemic bioavailability of mianserin is only 20–30%.[19] In different studies the mean elimination half life in normal volunteers has varied between 10 and 20 hours[17–20] and in elderly subjects the half life is 40 hours.[19] During chronic treatment steady-state levels are achieved by the sixth day of treatment and because the volume of distribution is large there is little day-to-day variation in plasma drug concentrations.

Oral absorption	>70%
Presystemic metabolism	~60–80%
Plasma half life	
range	10–20 h
mean	16 h
Volume of distribution	13 l.kg^{-1}
Plasma protein binding	96.4±0.2%

Mianserin is extensively metabolized in the liver, with only 5% of the dose excreted unchanged in the urine. About 70% of the dose can be recovered in the urine as unchanged drug and metabolites. Little drug is excreted in breast milk.

Concentration–effect relationship

In depressed patients no relationship has been found between plasma concentrations of mianserin and antidepressant response.

Metabolism

In man mianserin is extensively metabolized in the liver by hydroxylation to 8-hydroxymianserin and 8-hydroxydesmethylmianserin, by demethylation to 2-desmethylmianserin, and by 2(N) oxidation to mianserin-N-oxide,[21] which are excreted largely as their conjugates (see Fig. 1). The desmethyl metabolite is a major plasma metabolite. Of an oral dose of mianserin, 5% is excreted unchanged in the urine. The total urinary excretion of mianserin and its metabolites is 64–74% of the total dose. Both 8-hydroxymianserin and desmethylmianserin are pharmacologically active as relatively weak α_2 antagonists.[22]

Pharmaceutics

Film-coated tablets for oral use are made by Organon, Holland (parent company AKZO); Bolvidan tablets contain 10 mg, 20 mg or 30 mg of mianserin. The tablets are white, round, bi-convex, coded CT 4 (for the 10 mg tablet), CT 6 (20 mg) and CT 7 (30 mg) on one side and marked 'ORGANON' on the other side. The tablets which are stable for 5 years should be stored protected from light and moisture.

Therapeutic use

Indications

Mianserin is an effective antidepressant in mildly depressed outpatients.[23–26] It is free of anticholinergic side effects and is safer in overdose than are tricyclic antidepressants.[27] It does not interact with hypotensive drugs[1,28] and it has no unwanted cardiovascular effects.[13,14] Consequently, it is an appropriate treatment for mildly depressed outpatients particularly if they are sensitive to the anticholinergic side effects of other antidepressants, or if they have cardiovascular disease, hypotension, prostration or glaucoma.

In view of its relative safety in overdose it is also an appropriate antidepressant in moderately depressed patients with impulsive and self destructive behaviour.

Contraindications

1. Mania.

Mode of use

Mianserin treatment is started with 30 mg daily administered either as a single dose at night or in divided doses. Thereafter the dose is adjusted according to the clinical response. An effective dose usually ranges from 30–90 mg (mostly 60 mg) daily. Higher doses (up to 150 mg daily) may be necessary in some cases. In elderly patients, a lower than normal maintenance dose may be sufficient for a satisfactory clinical response. A dosage scheme for children cannot be given as there is not sufficient clinical experience. As with other antidepressants, the full antidepressant effect of mianserin may not be apparent for 2–3 weeks.

Patients should be warned about drowsiness which is usually greatest in the first 1–2 weeks. They should avoid driving or using complex machinery and they should be warned of the interaction with alcohol.

Haematological screening should be performed before treatment and at monthly intervals for the first three months of treatment. Treatment should be discontinued if patients develop fever, rash, arthropathy, jaundice, convulsions or blood dyscrasias and screening of haematology and liver function should be performed.

Adverse reactions

Potentially life-threatening effects
The UK Committee on Safety of Medicines estimated that between 1976 and 1982 there were 200 reported adverse reactions for every million prescriptions of mianserin.[29] Of these blood dyscrasias were the most serious and accounted for 12 deaths. Aplastic anaemia, and agranulocytosis have been reported particularly after 4–6 weeks of treatment.[30] Treatment should be discontinued if patients develop fever, sore throat, stomatitis or other signs of infection and a full blood count should be obtained. Monthly blood counts are recommended for the first 3 months of treatment.

Acute overdosage
Drowsiness is the main feature of overdoses with mianserin[27] but the serious cardiovascular effects of overdoses caused by tricyclic antidepressants or monoamine oxidase inhibitors are virtually never seen with mianserin. Occasional fatalities have been reported but much less frequently than with other antidepressant drugs.[27]

Severe or irreversible adverse effects
Hepatic reactions have been reported particularly in the elderly with jaundice and hepatocellular damage[30] but deaths due to this cause have not been reported. Cases of fever with rash and polyarthropathy have also been described.

Symptomatic adverse effects
Drowsiness is a common adverse effect. Less frequently reported side effects include increased appetite, weight gain and giddiness. Clinical trials in which mianserin has been compared with tricyclic antidepressants have shown a lower incidence of adverse effects in the patients receiving mianserin. The absence of dry mouth is particularly notable in patients receiving mianserin.

Fig. 1 Metabolites of mianserin

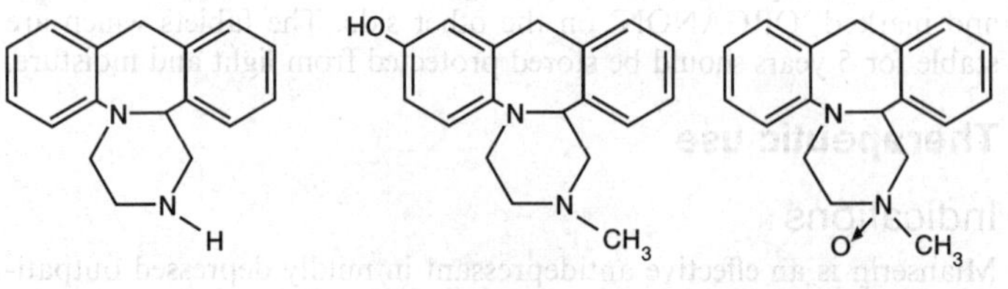

desmethylmianserin 8-hydroxymianserin mianserin-N-oxide

Interference with clinical pathology tests
None has been reported.

High risk groups

Neonates
The drug is not used in neonates.

Breast milk. Little mianserin is excreted in breast milk in animals, but human studies have not been reported and in view of the incidence of blood dyscrasias in adults mianserin should probably not be prescribed for nursing mothers.

Children
Small groups of children have been treated for depression, with a low incidence of adverse reactions.

Pregnant women
Transfer across the placenta has not been measured, but fetal abnormalities have not been reported in man or animals following the administration of mianserin. In view of the reports of blood dyscrasias in adults, the prescription of mianserin during pregnancy is not advisable.

The elderly
The elderly are particularly prone to dyscrasias associated with mianserin. The mean age of the 12 deaths reported to the CSM by 1982 was 75.[29]

Drug interactions

Potentially hazardous interactions
As a sedative drug mianserin enhances the CNS depressant action of other sedative drugs particularly alcohol.

Other significant interactions
In contrast to tricyclic antidepressants mianserin does not antagonize the hypotensive action of clonidine, methyldopa, bethanidine, and guanethidine.[28]

It is not known whether mianserin interacts with monoamine oxidase inhibitors.

Potentially useful interactions
No interactions of this type have been reported.

Clinical trials

Placebo controlled evidence for the antidepressant efficacy of mianserin is limited to studies of mildly depressed outpatients.[23–26,28]

1. Perry G F, Fitzsimmons B, Shapiro L, Irwin P 1978 Clinical study of mianserin, imipramine and placebo in depression: blood level and MHPG correlation. British Journal of Clinical Pharmacology 5 (suppl): 35–41
2. Smith A H W, Naylor G S, Moody J P 1978 Placebo-controlled double-blind trial of mianserin hydrochloride. British Journal of Clinical Pharmacology 5 (suppl): 67–70
3. Edwards J G, Goldie A 1983 Placebo controlled trial of mianserin and maprotiline in primary depressive illness: a preliminary report. British Journal of Clinical Pharmacology 15: 239–248

Of the two inpatient studies, Smith et al reported a superiority of mianserin to placebo but the treatments lasted for only two weeks and the mianserin dose was only 30 mg daily; in the other study by Perry et al patients were exposed to intensive psychotherapy and this might explain the finding that neither imipramine nor mianserin were better than placebo. The study of the most severely depressed outpatients also yielded negative results (Edwards et al).

4. Russell G F M, Niaz U, Wakeling A et al 1978 Comparative double-blind trial of mianserin hydrochloride (Org GB94) and diazepam in patients with depressive illness. British Journal of Clinical Pharmacology 5 (suppl): 57–66

As mianserin has mild sedative properties it has been compared with that of a minor tranquillizer, diazepam, in the depressive illness.[34] Mianserin was superior to diazepam, suggesting that the antidepressant effect of mianserin could not be attributed to its sedative properties.

General review articles

Pinder R M, Fink M 1982 Mianserin. Modern Problems of Pharmacopsychiatry 18: 70–101

References

1. Pinder R M, Fink M 1982 Mianserin. Modern Problems of Pharmacopsychiatry 18: 70–101
2. Baumann P A, Maitre L 1977 Blockade of presynaptic alpha receptors and of amino uptake in the rat brain by the antidepressant mianserin. Naunyn Schmiedeberg's Archives of Pharmacology 300: 31–37
3. Doggrell S A 1980 Effect of mianserin on noradrenergic transmission in the rat anococcygeus muscle. British Journal of Clinical Pharmacology 68: 241–250
4. Sugrue M F 1980 The inability of chronic mianserin to block central alpha adrenoceptors. European Journal of Pharmacology 68: 377–380
5. Mishra R, Janowsky A, Sulser F 1980 Action of mianserin and zimelidine on the norepinephrine receptor coupled adenylate cyclase system in brain: subsensitivity without reduction in beta adrenergic receptor coupling. Neuropharmacology 19: 983–987
6. Pazos A, Hoyer D, Palacios J M 1984 The binding of serotonergic ligands to the porcine choroid plexus: characterization of a new type of serotonin recognition site. European Journal of Pharmacology 106: 539–546
7. Nickolson V J, Wiering J A, Van Delft A M L 1982 Comparative pharmacology of mianserin its main metabolites and 6-azamianserin. Naunyn Schmiedeberg's Archives of Pharmacology 19: 48–55
8. Kanoff P D, Greengard L 1978 Brain histamine receptors as targets for antidepressant drugs. Nature 272: 329–333
9. Brogden R M, Heel R C, Speight T M et al 1978 Mianserin: a review of its pharmacological properties and therapeutic efficacy in depressive illness. Drugs 16: 273–301
10. Ghose K, Coppen A, Turner P 1976 Autonomic actions and interactions of mianserin hydrochloride and amitriptyline in patients with depressive illness. Psychopharmacology 49: 201–204
11. Shur E, Checkley S A, Delgado I 1983 Acta Psychiatrica Scandinavica 67: 50–55
12. Burrows G D, Davies B, Hamer H et al 1979 Effect of mianserin on cardiac conduction. The Medical Journal of Australia 2: 97–98
13. Burgess C D, Wadsworth J, Montgomery S, Turner P 1979 Cardiovascular effects of amitriptyline, mianserin, zimeledine and nomifensine in depressed patients. Postgraduate Medical Journal 55: 704–708
14. Wilson J A, Read J R M, Boyd E J S, Wormsley K G 1983 Inhibition of pentagastrin-stimulated and overnight gastric acid secretion by mianserin. British Journal of Clinical Pharmacology 15 (suppl 2): 329–333
15. Vink J, Van Hal H H M 1980 Simplified method for determination of the tetracyclic antidepressant mianserin in human plasma using gas chromatography with nitrogen detection. Journal of Chromatography 181: 25–31
16. Suckow R F, Cooper Th B, Quirkin F M et al 1982 Determination of mianserin and metabolites in plasma by liquid chromatography with electrochemical detection. Journal of Pharmaceutical Science 71: 889–892
17. Maguire K P, Norman T R, Burrows G D 1982 A pharmacokinetic study of mianserin. European Journal of Clinical Pharmacology 21: 517–520
18. Hodina P D, Lapierre Y D, McIntosh B et al 1983 Mianserin kinetics in depressed patients. Clinical Pharmacology and Therapeutics 33: 747–762
19. Shani N, Elliott H L, Kelman A, Whiting B 1983 The pharmacokinetics of mianserin. British Journal of Clinical Pharmacology 15 (suppl 2): 313–322
20. Timmer C J, Pourbaix S, Desager M et al 1985 Absolute bioavailability of mianserin tablets and solution in healthy volunteers. European Journal of Drug Metabolism and Pharmacokinetics 10: 315–323
21. Jongh G, Dide van den Wildenberg H M, Nieuwenhuyse H et al 1981 The metabolism of mianserin in women, rabbits and rats. Identification of the major metabolites. Drug Metabolism and Disposition 9: 48–53
22. Marshall R J 1983 The pharmacology of mianserin — an update. British Journal of Clinical Pharmacology 15 (suppl 2): 263–268
23. Murphy J E, Donald J F, Molla A L 1976 Mianserin in the treatment of depression in general practice. Practitioner 217: 135–138
24. Magnus R V 1979 Mianserin — a study of different dosage regimens. British Journal of Clinical Practice 33: 251–258
25. Branconnier R J, Cole J D, Ghazvinian S 1981 The therapeutic profile of mianserin in mild elderly depressives. Psychopharmacology Bulletin 17: 129–131
26. McGrath P J, Rabkin J G, Stewart J W et al 1985 Placebo controlled study of mianserin in depressed outpatients. Neuropsychobiology 14: 128–132
27. Cassidy S, Henry J 1987 Fatal toxicity of antidepressant drugs in overdose. British Medical Journal 295: 1021–1024
28. Elliott H L, Whiting B, Reid J L 1983 Assessment of the interaction between mianserin and centrally acting hypotensive drugs. British Journal of Clinical Pharmacology 15 (suppl 2): 323–328
29. Committee on Safety of Medicines 1985 Adverse reactions to antidepressants. British Medical Journal 291: 1638
30. Mashford M H 1984 Mianserin: an example of benefits and risks in therapy. Medical Journal of Australia 141: 308–310

Miconazole (nitrate)

Miconazole was one of the first azole antifungal drugs to achieve wide therapeutic use.

Chemistry

Miconazole (Daktarin, Monistat)
$C_{18}H_{14}Cl_4\text{-}N_2O$
Miconazole nitrate (Daktarin, Dermonistat, Gyno-Daktarin, Monistat, Monistat 7, Micatin)
$C_{18}H_{14}Cl_4\text{-}N_2O\ HNO_3$
1[[2(2,4-dichlorophenyl)-2-[(2,4-dichlorophenyl)methoxy]ethyl]-1H-imidazole (nitrate)

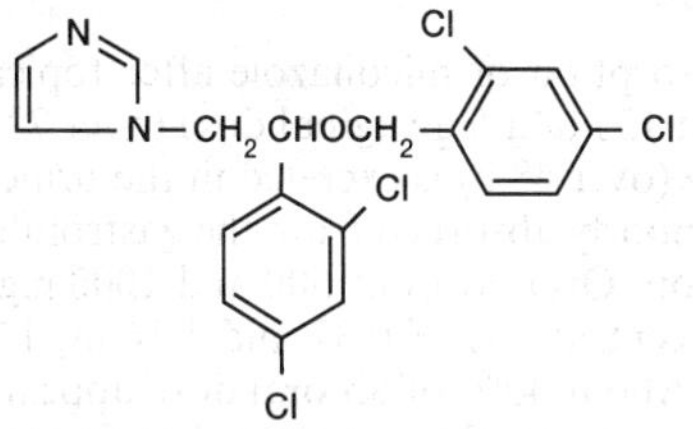

Molecular weight (base)	416.1
(nitrate)	479.1
pKa	6.65
Solubility	
in alcohol (nitrate)	1 in 140
in water	—
Octanol/water partition coefficient	—

A white or almost white, odourless or almost odourless, crystalline or microcrystalline powder. It is prepared by chemical synthesis and the base and nitrate are used clinically. Miconazole nitrate is also available in a cream combination product with hydrocortisone (Daktacort).

Pharmacology

Miconazole is an imidazole antifungal agent. At low concentrations, it interacts with fungal cytochrome P450 which results in inhibition of a demethylation step in the biosynthesis of ergosterol. The depletion of ergosterol and concomitant accumulation of lanosterol leads to alterations in a number of membrane-associated functions.[1] At high concentrations, miconazole interacts with membrane lipids causing direct membrane damage which results in leakage of fungus cell constituents.[1] It appears that fungistatic effects result from the inhibition of membrane sterol synthesis and fungicidal effects from impairment of the barrier function of the membrane.

Toxicology

Toxicological testing in animals produced few results of potential clinical relevance. Intravenous injection of miconazole base (10, 20 or 40 mg.kg^{-1} for 4 weeks) in dogs produced a number of gross pathological and histopathological effects in both dosed and control (1 mg.kg^{-1} Cremophor EL) animals. These effects were attributed to the histamine-releasing effects of the Cremaphor EL carrier solution. Oral administration of miconazole was well tolerated for periods of up to 18 months in the rat and 12 months in the dog. Pathological findings in both the rat and the dog indicated that the liver is a target organ for miconazole. Increased liver weight with slight histological

Miconazole (nitrate)

effects occurred at doses around 40 mg.kg^{-1} in the dog and above 80 mg.kg^{-1} in the rat.

No teratological effects have been found in rats or rabbits.

Clinical pharmacology

Miconazole is an imidazole antifungal agent. It is effective against a broad spectrum of fungal pathogens including: *Trichophyton, Microsporum* and *Epidermophyton* spp.; *Candida albicans* and related species; *Cryptococcus neoformans; Coccidioides immitis*; and *Paracoccidioides brasiliensis*.

Pharmacokinetics

Miconazole concentrations in serum and other biological fluids can be determined by a microbiological method,[2] by gas–liquid chromatography,[3] or by high pressure liquid chromatography.[4] The sensitivity of the HPLC assay is about 0.1 mg.l^{-1}.

Oral absorption	20%
Presystemic metabolism	—
Plasma half life	
mean	24.1 h
Volume of distribution	20 l.kg^{-1}
Plasma protein binding	91–93%

There is little absorption of miconazole after topical application of 2% cream. About 1% of a 5 g vaginal dose (over 72 h) and 0.35% of a 1 g topical dose (over 48 h) is excreted in the urine as metabolites.[5]

Miconazole is poorly absorbed from the gastrointestinal tract after oral administration. Oral doses of 500 and 1000 mg produced mean peak plasma concentrations of 0.37 and 1.16 mg.l^{-1}, 2 to 4 h after administration.[6] About 40% of an oral dose appears in the faeces in unchanged form; another 40% is excreted in faeces as metabolites.[5] About 20% of an oral dose is excreted in the urine, but less than 1% of this is in unchanged form.[5]

In a formal analysis of drug kinetics,[7] 12 subjects were given 522 mg of miconazole as a single infusion over 15 min. Four were normal subjects, four had mild renal impairment, and four were undergoing haemodialysis. Mean peak plasma concentrations 15 min after the infusion were 6.18 mg.l^{-1} (range 2.0–9.1), 21.85 mg.l^{-1} (range 3.3–33.0) and 13.98 mg.l^{-1} (range 2.4–31.8). Mean concentrations 1 h after the infusion were 1.90, 6.76 and 4.55 mg.l^{-1}; after 4 h the mean concentrations were 0.44, 0.90 and 0.77 mg.l^{-1} in the three groups.

Information on plasma levels in patients with fungal infection is limited. In 10 patients mean peak plasma concentrations of 1.8, 2.3, 7.5 and 7.5 mg.l^{-1} were noted 15 min after infusion of 400, 600, 800 and 1000 mg of miconazole.[9] Information on levels in children is also limited.[10]

The pharmacokinetics of miconazole in man fit a three-compartment open model with half life values of 0.4, 2.1 and 24.1 h.[7] Apparent volumes of distribution show a significant difference between normal subjects and patients with renal impairment not undergoing haemodialysis.[7] The mean apparent volume of distribution is about 1400 l in normal subjects. In patients with renal impairment, the volume can fall to 800 l without a change in the rate of elimination, resulting in a tripling of the usual plasma levels.[7] Plasma levels in patients undergoing haemodialysis are not altered, since the drug is not dialysable.[7]

Miconazole appears to be widely distributed in man, although certain sites do not achieve therapeutic concentrations. Penetration into the CSF is poor. Concentrations ranging from less than 3% to 48% of the simultaneous plasma level have been detected in the CSF of patients with meningitis;[11] in half of the CSF specimens, the peak levels[11] were less than 0.1 mg.l^{-1}.

Intrathecal administration of 20 mg miconazole produced cisternal CSF concentrations of 6.2, 2.4, 0.7 and 0.24 mg.l^{-1} at 12, 24, 48 and 72 h.[9] This method of administration achieves higher concentrations which are maintained longer than those following intravenous administration.

Miconazole penetrates well into infected joints: peak concentrations in synovial fluid in three patients with coccidioidomycosis ranged from 0.5 to 1.35 mg.l^{-1} following intravenous doses of 200, 600 and 1200 mg.[12]

Miconazole appears to penetrate the vitreous humour. In one patient with fungal endophthalmitis given an intravenous infusion of 1000 mg over 1 h, the drug concentration in the vitreous humour was 0.6 mg.l^{-1}, 2 h after a peak plasma level of 0.8 mg.l^{-1} had been reached.[13]

In one patient with peritonitis, a level of 1.2 mg.l^{-1} was detected in the peritoneal fluid 2 h after a 600 mg intravenous dose.[14]

Miconazole is 91–93% bound to plasma protein, in particular albumin.[15] This in part explains the poor penetration of the drug into CSF and other fluids such as sputum.

Concentration–effect relationship

There is no established relationship between plasma concentration and therapeutic effect in patients with deep fungal infection. Nor has it been established whether treatment failure is related to low plasma concentrations. Thus, the need for therapeutic drug monitoring has not been defined.

Metabolism

Miconazole is metabolized in the liver and is eliminated in the urine and faeces as inactive metabolites. About 20% of an oral dose appears in the urine as metabolites, but 40% is eliminated in faeces as unchanged drug.[5] About 14 to 22% of an intravenous dose is excreted in the urine; however, only 1% of this is present as unchanged miconazole.[5]

Two major pathways of metabolism are believed to exist:[5] oxidative O-dealkylation and oxidative N-dealkylation. The major metabolite is α-(2,4-dichlorophenyl)-1H-imidazole ethanol, derived by O-dealkylation (Fig. 1).

Miconazole metabolism is not altered by repeated administration.[5]

Fig. 1

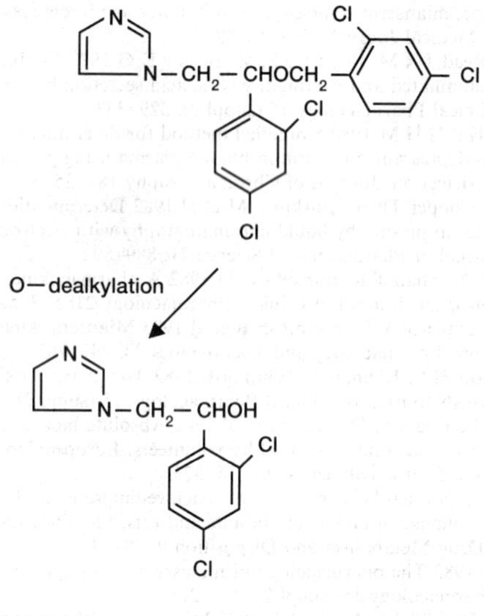

Pharmaceutics

Miconazole base is available in oral and parenteral forms; miconazole nitrate is supplied in several forms for topical application.

Miconazole base is supplied for intravenous or intrathecal administration as a sterile solution in 20 ml amounts with 10% Cremophor EL included as solvent; 1 ml of this solution contains 10 mg of miconazole base (Daktarin intravenous solution).

The tablets contain 250 mg of miconazole base. They are white, round and marked with the legend 'Janssen' and 'M250' (Daktarin oral tablets).

The sugar-free orange-flavoured oral gel contains miconazole base 2% (25 mg.ml^{-1}). This is supplied in 40 g tubes (Daktarin oral gel).

None of the above formulations are marketed in the USA.

The cream contains miconazole nitrate 2%. The cream is white, non-staining and water miscible. It is supplied in 78 g tubes with disposable applicators for intravaginal use (Gyno-Daktarin cream; Monistat cream). For topical application it is supplied in 30 g tubes (Daktarin cream; Janssen, UK Monistat-Derm; Ortho, USA).

Pessaries contain 100 mg of miconazole nitrate. They are white and non-staining (Gyno-Daktarin pessaries; Monistat 3, vaginal suppositories).

Ovules contain 1200 mg of miconazole nitrate (Gyno-Daktarin).

The tampons are coated with 100 mg of miconazole nitrate (Gyno-Daktarin tampons).

A cream containing miconazole nitrate 2% and hydrocortisone 1% is available. The cream is white, non-staining and water miscible and is supplied in 30 g tubes (Daktacort cream).

Cream preparations and pessaries should be stored in a cool place.

The intravenous solution should be stored at room temperature and should be mixed with the recommended diluents (sodium chloride injection BP or 5% dextrose injection BP) before use.

Therapeutic use

Indications

1. Topical treatment of fungal infection of the skin and nails
2. Topical treatment of vulvo-vaginal candidosis and fungal balanitis
3. Oral treatment of oral and oesophageal candidosis
4. Oral treatment for eradication of fungal colonization of the mouth and gastrointestinal tract
5. Parenteral treatment of deep fungal infection.

Contraindications

1. Hypersensitivity

Indications

1. Treatment of fungal infection of the skin and nails

Miconazole nitrate cream should be applied to skin lesions in the mornings and in the evenings. Treatment should be continued for two weeks after the lesions have cleared. Cream containing miconazole nitrate and a steroid is sometimes useful in reducing initial inflammation. This formulation should not be used unless a definite diagnosis has been obtained and should be discontinued once the inflammation has subsided.

Miconazole nitrate cream should be applied to infected nails once daily and the nail should be covered with an occlusive dressing. Nails should be clipped short at regular intervals and treatment continued uninterrupted until the growth of the new nail is established.

2. Treatment of vulvo-vaginal candidosis and balanitis

One applicator (about 5 g) of miconazole nitrate cream or one pessary should be inserted high into the vagina each night for 14 nights. 10 g of cream or two pessaries can be used for 7 nights. Patients should be instructed not to discontinue treatment upon relief of symptoms, but to complete the prescribed course. Tampons coated with miconazole are also available. These should be inserted morning and evening for one week. Treatment should be continued even if menstruation occurs. A single 1200 mg ovule should be inserted high into the vagina as a single dose at night.

To prevent reinfection, the male partner can be treated with an antifungal cream at the same time. This should be applied to the penis in the morning and in the evening.

Vaginal applications can be supplemented with cream for vulvitis and other superficial sites of infection.

Balanitis in men can be treated with local applications of miconazole nitrate cream. This should be applied in the morning and evening for one week.

3. Treatment of oral and oesophageal candidosis

Oral and oesophageal lesions can be treated with miconazole oral gel. For best results, the gel should be retained in the mouth for as long as possible. Miconazole oral tablets can also be used: these should be allowed to dissolve in the mouth before swallowing. The usual adult dose is one tablet (250 mg) or 5 to 10 ml oral gel (125–250 mg miconazole base) at 6 h intervals. In children aged over 6, the recommended dose of oral gel is 5 ml at 6 h intervals; in children aged 2 to 6, 5 ml at 12 h intervals; and in children under 2, 2.5 ml at 12 h intervals.

Treatment should be continued for 48 h after symptoms have cleared or until mycological tests prove negative.

4. Eradication of fungal colonization of the gastrointestinal tract

Eradication of oral and intestinal reservoirs of infection is sometimes indicated in patients with recurrent vaginal candidosis or in immunocompromised patients at risk of developing serious fungal infection. This can be attempted with oral miconazole treatment. The usual adult dose is one tablet (250 mg) at 6 h intervals.

5. Treatment of deep fungal infection

Miconazole intravenous solution is supplied in 20 ml amounts (containing 200 mg miconazole base) and must be diluted with either sodium chloride injection BP or 5% dextrose injection BP. The intravenous infusion must be given over a period of at least 30 min.

Optimal dosage regimens for specific deep fungal infections or particular sites of infection have not been developed. The adult dose can range from 200 to 1200 mg per infusion diluted in 200 to 500 ml of fluid. The usual adult dose is 600 mg given at 8 h intervals.

In children older than 12 months, the recommended dose is 20–40 $mg.kg^{-1}$ per 24 h. A dose of 15 $mg.kg^{-1}$ per infusion should not be exceeded.

Treatment should be continued until tests indicate that active fungal infection is no longer present. Inadequate periods of treatment often lead to a poor response. The dosage, dosing interval, site(s) and duration of treatment will differ from patient to patient and depend upon the nature and extent of the infection.

Local treatment with miconazole intravenous solution is sometimes useful as an adjunct to intravenous treatment. In patients with fungal meningitis, intrathecal administration of 1.5–2 ml of undiluted injectable solution (15–20 mg miconazole base) may be indicated. Injections can be given at 12 or 24 h intervals and alternated between lumbar and cisternal sites.

Miconazole has been used to irrigate bone, joints, the bladder, infected wounds, the ear and other sites;[16] 100 mg of miconazole (undiluted) can be instilled into the bladder at 12 h intervals. If discomfort is experienced with undiluted drug, the dose can be given as a 12-hourly continuous irrigation in 500 ml of sterile sodium chloride solution.

Miconazole has been used to treat coccidioidomycosis and paracoccidioidomycosis.[16] However, relapse and failure rates have been high. Its role in candidosis and cryptococcosis remains unclear and it cannot now be recommended for the treatment of these infections.[17]

Contraindications

1. Hypersensitivity

In animal tests, Cremophor EL has been shown to produce adverse effects associated with histamine release. Similar anaphylactoid reactions have been reported in occasional patients receiving miconazole intravenous solution.[18]

Adverse reactions

Potentially life-threatening effects

Major adverse effects have been reported in patients with haematological neoplasia who were given intravenous miconazole diluted in less than 200 ml of fluid.[18] These effects included cardiac arrest and anaphylactic reactions after the drug was administered. The patients all recovered.

Acute overdosage

No cases of deliberate overdosage have been reported.

Severe or irreversible adverse effects

Cardiac arrhythmias. Rapid injection of miconazole can produce transient tachycardia or cardiac arrhythmia. These effects, if not transient, respond to lignocaine.[9] Infusions over periods of 30 min or more are well tolerated by most patients with pre-existing cardiovascular disorders or with cardiovascular reactions to other antifungal drugs.

Phlebitis. Phlebitis has been reported to occur in about 30% of patients receiving miconazole through a peripheral vein.[11,16,19] The manufacturer recommends using a subclavian catheter or changing the infusion site at 48–72 h intervals if phlebitis is a problem.

Pruritus. Pruritus has been reported in 25% of patients receiving miconazole infusions.[16] Severe pruritus has necessitated discontinuation of treatment in some patients.

Arachnoiditis. Arachnoiditis has been reported in several patients following intrathecal administration of miconazole.[11]

Symptomatic adverse effects

Adverse side effects reported during the use of miconazole intravenous solution have included nausea and vomiting, febrile reactions, rash, drowsiness, diarrhoea, anorexia and flushes. Nausea and vomiting can be mitigated with antihistaminic or antiemetic drugs given prior to an infusion or by reducing the dose, decreasing the rate of infusion or avoiding administration at meal times.

Topical or intravaginal treatment with miconazole cream can cause local irritation. Local sensitization, necessitating discontinuation of treatment, has also been reported.

Mild gastrointestinal upsets have been reported on occasion following the use of miconazole oral tablets or oral gel. However, an oral dose of 1 g given at 8 h intervals caused diarrhoea in five of six patients.[20] In four cases, this was controlled with antiemetics or antacids and an intestinal absorbent, but treatment had to be discontinued in the fifth patient.

Other effects
Intravenous infusion of miconazole in large amounts of fluid has been reported to cause transient decreases in haemoglobin, haematocrit and serum sodium levels. Haematological and biochemical tests performed during and after treatment have demonstrated no adverse effects on renal or hepatic function.

Patients receiving intravenous miconazole sometimes develop increased serum lipid levels. Erythrocyte aggregation can also occur. These effects have been attributed to the carrier solution, Cremophor EL, but are transient, abating on cessation of treatment. It is unusual for these effects to warrant discontinuation of treatment.

Interference with clinical pathology tests
No cases of interference with clinical pathology tests have been reported.

High risk groups

Neonates
Doses of miconazole nitrate cream for topical application are as recommended for adults, but there is little information available.

Doses of miconazole oral gel for treatment of oral lesions have not been established, but should not exceed 5 ml per 24 h.

Doses of miconazole intravenous solution have ranged from 10 to 30 $mg.kg^{-1}$ per 24 h.[21-23] However, as in adult patients, miconazole is best regarded as a drug of second choice for infants with deep fungal infection and should be reserved for those instances where treatment with amphotericin B and flucytosine has been unsuccessful.

Breast milk. There is no information on whether miconazole or its metabolites are excreted in breast milk, nor whether it has a harmful effect on the newborn.

Children
Doses of miconazole nitrate cream for topical application are as recommended for adults.

Doses of miconazole oral gel and miconazole oral tablets should be determined according to the age or weight of the child.

Doses of miconazole intravenous solution should be determined according to the weight of the child. The manufacturer recommends a dose of 40 $mg.kg^{-1}$ per 24 h in children older than 12 months, but a dose of 15 $mg.kg^{-1}$ per infusion should not be exceeded.

Pregnant women
Miconazole nitrate pessaries are effective in the treatment of vaginal candidosis in pregnant women. However, safety of the drug in pregnancy has not been established and it should not be used unless the expected benefit outweighs any potential risk. If there is a strong need for the use of miconazole nitrate vaginal cream or pessaries during pregnancy, in particular during the first trimester, the patients should be advised to exercise caution in the insertion of a vaginal applicator.

There is no information concerning the safety of miconazole oral gel, oral tablets or intravenous solution during pregnancy and their use in pregnant women should be avoided if possible.

The elderly
No special precautions are required in this age group.

Drug interactions

Potentially hazardous interactions
Anticoagulants. Miconazole intravenous solution has been reported to enhance the anticoagulant effect of warfarin and other coumarin drugs.[11,24] The mechanism of this interaction is probably inhibition of drug metabolism, since many imidazole compounds are known to be inhibitors of hepatic microsomal enzymes. In cases of simultaneous treatment, the anticoagulant effect should be carefully titrated and reduction of the anticoagulant dose will usually be needed.

Hypoglycaemic agents. Miconazole intravenous solution may potentiate the effect of hypoglycaemic drugs, the dosage of which may require adjustment.

General review articles

Craven P C, Graybill J R 1983 Antifungal agents used in systemic mycoses. Activity and therapeutic use. Drugs 25: 41–62

Daneshmend T K, Warnock D W 1983 Clinical pharmacokinetics of systemic antifungal drugs. Clinical Pharmacokinetics 8: 17–42

Fromtling R A 1988 Overview of medically important antifungal azole derivations. Clinical Microbiology Reviews 1: 187–217

Heel R C, Brogden R N, Pakes G E, Speight T M, Avery G S 1980 Miconazole: a preliminary review of its therapeutic efficacy in systemic fungal infections. Drugs 19: 7–30

Sawyer P R, Brogden R N, Pinder R M, Speight T M, Avery G S 1975 Miconazole: a review of its antifungal activity and therapeutic efficacy. Drugs 9: 406–423

Stevens D A 1983 Miconazole in the treatment of coccidioidomycosis. Drugs 26: 347–354

Stranz M H 1980 Miconazole. Drug Intelligence and Clinical Pharmacy 14: 86–95

Walsh T J, Pizzo A 1988 Treatment of systemic fungal infections; recent progress and current problems. European Journal of Clinical Microbiology and Infectious Diseases 7: 460–475

References

1. Van den Bossche H 1985 Biochemical targets for antifungal azole derivatives: hypothesis on the mode of action. In: McGinnis M R (ed) Current Topics in Medical Mycology 1. Springer Verlag, New York, pp 313–351
2. Espinel-Ingroff A, Shadomy S, Fisher J F 1977 Bioassay for miconazole. Antimicrobial Agents and Chemotherapy 11: 365–368
3. Mannisto P T, Mantyla R, Nykanen S, Lamminsivu U, Ottoila P 1982 Impairing effect of food on ketoconazole absorption. Antimicrobial Agents and Chemotherapy 21: 730–733
4. Brodie R R, Chasseaud L F, Walmsley L M 1978 High-pressure liquid chromatographic determination of the antimycotic agent, econazole in plasma. Journal of Chromatography 155: 209–213
5. Brugmans J, Van Cutsem J, Heykants J, Schuermans V, Thienpont D 1972 Systemic antifungal potential, safety, biotransport and transformation of miconazole nitrate. European Journal of Clinical Pharmacology 51: 93–99
6. Boelaert J, Daneels R, Van Landuyt H, Symoens J 1976 Miconazole plasma levels in healthy subjects and in patients with impaired renal function. Chemotherapy 6: 165–169
7. Lewi P J, Boelaert J, Daneels R et al 1976 Pharmacokinetic profile of intravenous miconazole in man: comparison of normal subjects and patients with renal insufficiency. European Journal of Clinical Pharmacology 10: 49–54
8. Hoeprich P D, Lawrence R M, Goldstein E 1980 Treatment of coccidioidomycosis with miconazole. Journal of the American Medical Association 243: 1923–1926
9. Sung J P, Grendahl J G, Levine H B 1977 Intravenous and intrathecal miconazole therapy for systemic mycoses. Western Journal of Medicine 126: 5–13
10. Sung J P, Rajani K, Chopra D R, Grendahl J G, Haws E B 1979 Miconazole therapy for systemic candidiasis in a conjoined twin and a premature newborn. American Journal of Surgery 138: 688–691
11. Deresinski S C, Lilly R B, Levine H B, Galgiani J N, Stevens D A 1977 Treatment of fungal meningitis with miconazole. Archives of Internal Medicine 137: 1180–1185
12. Deresinski S C, Stevens, D A 1979 Bone and joint coccidioidomycosis treated with miconazole. American Review of Respiratory Disease 120: 1101–1107
13. Lutwick L I, Galgiani J N, Johnson R H, Stevens D A 1976 Visceral fungal infections due to *Petriellidium boydii* (*Allescheria boydii*). In vitro drug sensitivity studies. American Journal of Medicine 61: 632–640
14. Deresinski S C, Galgiani J N, Stevens D A 1977 Miconazole treatment of human coccidioidomycosis: status report. In: Ajello L (ed) Coccidioidomycosis: current clinical and diagnostic status. Symposium Specialists, Miami, pp 267–292
15. Stevens D A, Levine H B, Deresinski S C 1976 Miconazole in coccidioidomycosis. II. Therapeutic and pharmacologic studies in man. American Journal of Medicine 60: 191–202
16. Stevens D A 1977 Miconazole in the treatment of systemic fungal infections. American Review of Respiratory Disease 116: 801–806
17. Bennett J E, Remington J S 1981 Miconazole in cryptococcosis and systemic candidiasis: a word of caution. Annals of Internal Medicine 94: 708–709
18. Fainstein V, Bodey G P 1980 Cardiorespiratory toxicity due to miconazole. Annals of Internal Medicine 93: 432–433
19. Negroni R, Rubinstein P, Herrmann A, Gimenez A 1977 Results of miconazole therapy in twenty-eight patients with paracoccidioidomycosis (South American blastomycosis). Proceedings of the Royal Society of Medicine 70 (suppl 1): 24–28
20. Lima N S, Teixeira G, Miranda J, do Valle ACF 1977 Treatment of South American blastomycosis (paracoccidioidomycosis) with miconazole by the oral route: an on-going study. Proceedings of the Royal Society of Medicine 70 (suppl 1): 35–39

21. Clarke M, Davies D P, Odds F, Mitchell C 1980 Neonatal systemic candidiasis treated with miconazole. British Medical Journal 281: 354
22. Tettenborn M, Gould J D M, Tayler P 1982 Problems of treating systemic fungal infections in the neonate: role of IV miconazole. Clinical Research Reviews 2: 51–55
23. McDougall P N, Fleming P J, Speller D C E, Daish P, Spiedel B D 1982 Neonatal systemic candidiasis: a failure to respond to intravenous miconazole in two neonates. Archives of Disease in Childhood 57: 884–886
24. Watson P G, Lochan R G, Redding V J 1982 Drug interaction with coumarin derivative anticoagulants. British Medical Journal 285: 1045–1046

Midazolam (hydrochloride)

Midazolam is a water-soluble imidazo benzodiazepine derivative which may be given orally or intramuscularly as a sedative, or intravenously as a sedative or as an induction agent prior to general anaesthesia.

Chemistry

Midazolam (Hypnovel, Dormicum)
$C_{18}H_{13}ClFN_3$
8-Chloro-6-(2-fluorophenyl)-1-methyl-4H-imidazo (1,5-a)(1,4)] benzodiazepine

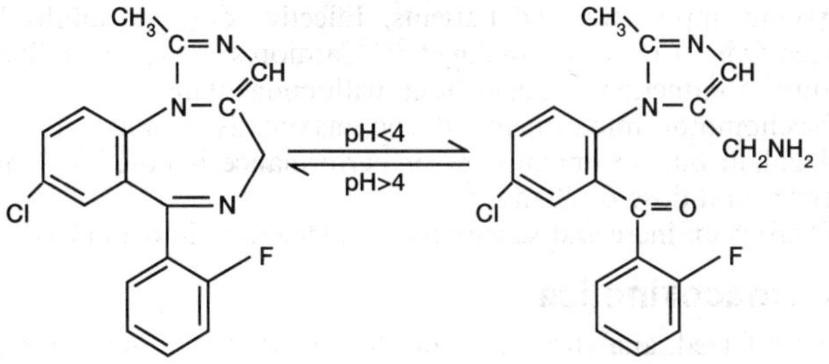

Molecular weight of hydrochloride (free base)	392.3 (325.8)
pKa	6.2
Solubility	
in alcohol	—
in water	soluble
Octanol/water partition coefficient	—

A colourless solution, supplied as the hydrochloride, with a pH of less than 4.0 and available in concentrations of 0.2 and 0.5%. At the physiological pH, the ring structure closes and the drug becomes lipid-soluble and rapidly penetrates the blood–brain barrier. It is prepared by chemical synthesis.

Pharmacology

Midazolam is an imidazo benzodiazepine with properties very similar to those of other benzodiazepines. Thus it binds to benzodiazepine receptors in various regions of the brain such as the spinal cord, brain stem, cerebellum, limbic system and the cerebral cortex. Benzodiazepines like midazolam block EEG arousal from stimulation of the brain stem reticular formation. Midazolam acts as a CNS depressant on CNS reflexes via the brain stem reticular formation. Midazolam is an anxiolytic in animal test systems such as the fear of electroshock in rats or monkeys. It is sedative as judged by reduction of fighting in mice or monkeys. The hypnotic effects of midazolam which are demonstrable in man are difficult to show in animals even in very high doses. Midazolam produces anterograde amnesia similar to that produced by diazepam but neither benzodiazepine produces retrograde amnesia. Midazolam has a more rapid onset of action and shorter duration of effect than diazepam in most animal test systems.

Toxicology

In vitro and in vivo microbial and mammalian test systems have revealed no evidence of mutagenicity. No evidence of carcinogenic potential was seen in rats or mice given oral midazolam maleate in doses up to 9 mg.kg^{-1} daily for 2 years (about 25 times the recommended human dose).

Reproductive studies in rabbits and rats using parenteral midazolam maleate in doses of 350 μg.kg^{-1} have not revealed evidence of fetal malformation. The intravenous and oral LD_{50} in mice are reported to be 86 and 760 mg.kg^{-1} respectively. The lethal oral dose in rats is 1600 mg.kg^{-1}.

Clinical pharmacology

Midazolam is a water-soluble benzodiazepine drug producing sedation, anxiolysis and hypnosis. Doses of 3–6 mg intramuscularly produce a similar degree of sedation and anxiolysis to papaveretum and hyoscine when used for premedication, but with significantly more anterograde amnesia.[1] It is commonly used intravenously to produce conscious sedation before unpleasant procedures such as dentistry, upper gastrointestinal endoscopy and bronchoscopy. There is a wide variation in response and it should not be used in doses greater than 0.1 mg.kg^{-1} for the latter procedures.[2] Satisfactory sedation can be achieved in the majority of patients with a dose of 0.07 mg.kg^{-1},[3] although excessive sedation may still occur, albeit rarely. At these doses, most patients do not recall passage of the endoscope. A dose of 0.08 mg.kg^{-1} administered slowly intravenously produced excellent sedation during surgery performed under regional anaesthesia.[4]

For induction of anaesthesia, midazolam is less reliable than thiopentone, but preferable to diazepam. Sleep does not occur in one arm–brain circulation time and the delay in onset is more prolonged in young unpremedicated patients. Effective doses in adults have ranged from 0.15 to 0.5 mg.kg^{-1}.[5,6] Cardiorespiratory stability is a feature of induction of anaesthesia with midazolam.

Psychomotor impairment is seen maximally 1 hour after oral midazolam but no impairment of performance is noted 7–9 hours after an oral dose of 30 mg.[15]

There is an increased sensitivity to midazolam in the elderly.

Pharmacokinetics

The preferred analytical method for detection of midazolam in plasma involves extraction with benzene and estimation by gas chromatography with Ni^{63} electron capture detection which has a sensitivity of 500 ng.l^{-1}.[7]

Following oral administration of 10, 20 and 40 mg in volunteers, peak plasma levels occur within 30 minutes with a linear relationship between plasma levels and dosage.[8] Bioavailability is between 31% and 72% due to high liver extraction. Absorption is almost complete following intramuscular injection, peak plasma levels being attained within 45 minutes. After rapid injection of midazolam 0.15 mg.kg^{-1} intravenously, plasma levels at 5 minutes varied from 291 to 425 µg.l^{-1} and due to its rapid distribution had fallen to approximately 10% of these values within 2 hours.[8]

At physiological pH, midazolam is highly lipophilic, but this decreases with decreasing pH. Following intravenous administration, it is rapidly and widely distributed, with a steady-state volume of distribution of 39–68 l (0.8–1.7 l.kg^{-1}).[8] The kinetics are adequately described by a two-compartment model with an elimination half life of 2–3 hours; this is prolonged in the elderly[9] and half lives of over 10 hours have been reported.[10] The $t_{\frac{1}{2}}\beta$ is short compared with other benzodiazepines. Total body clearance is 6.4–11.1 ml.min^{-1}.kg^{-1} (plasma clearance 268–630 ml.min^{-1}). There is no evidence of any significant enterohepatic circulation.

Midazolam is extensively bound to plasma proteins (94–98%) and small changes in protein binding will produce large changes in the amount of available free drug, which has important consequences in clinical practice.[11] The free fraction is higher in patients with chronic renal failure.[12]

Less than 1% of midazolam is excreted unchanged in the kidneys[13] and the drug is cleared virtually entirely by liver metabolism. The effects of liver disease on elimination of midazolam have not been studied, but theoretically it should be delayed. Prolonged sedation has resulted from use of the drug in severely ill patients with reduced hepatic blood flow.[14]

Oral absorption	100%
Presystemic metabolism	30–70%
Plasma half life	
range	2–3 h
Volume of distribution	0.8–1.7 l.kg^{-1}
Plasma protein binding	94–98%

Midazolam is oxidized by a member of the P450 IIIA sub-family and thus concentrations of the drug may be reduced in patients receiving inducers of these microenzymes, such as macrolide antibiotics (eg rifampicin) and anticonvulsants (eg phenytoin).

Concentration–effect relationship

Clinical sedation, assessed objectively and subjectively parallels plasma concentrations after intravenous and oral administration.[15–17] Sleep occurs with plasma concentrations greater than 100 µg.l^{-1}.[15] Objective tests of sedation did not differ from baseline when plasma midazolam concentrations were between 20 and 80 µg.l^{-1}.[15,16] The minimum effective concentration is from 30 to 100 µg.l^{-1}. At identical plasma concentrations, the oral dose produces more marked effects than the intravenous due to the activity of the α-hydroxy metabolite.[16] The correlation between effect and drug concentration is closer when the midazolam and α-hydroxymidazolam concentrations are considered together. Following infusions of midazolam to maintain sedation in the intensive care unit, patients with normal metabolism awake at plasma midazolam concentrations of 100 µg.l^{-1} and α-hydroxymidazolam levels about 30 µg.l^{-1}.

Metabolism

Midazolam is extensively metabolized by the P450 dependent mixed-function oxidase system in the liver (Fig. 1).[18] The principal metabolite is α-hydroxymidazolam, which is rapidly conjugated with glucuronic acid, although a small proportion is further hydroxylated to α,4-dihydroxymidazolam. The other metabolite is 4-hydroxymidazolam. The α-hydroxymidazolam is biologically active, but has a shorter half life than midazolam (less than one hour).[16] It may contribute to the pharmacological activity of the drug after oral administration. The discovery of metabolites following injection of 10 mg midazolam during the an-hepatic period of liver transplantation indicates extrahepatic sites of metabolism of the drug.[19]

Pharmaceutics

Blue scored tablets of 15 mg midazolam are available only in Switzerland. For injection, midazolam is supplied as a colourless aqueous solution containing midazolam hydrochloride.

Fig. 1 Metabolism of midazolam

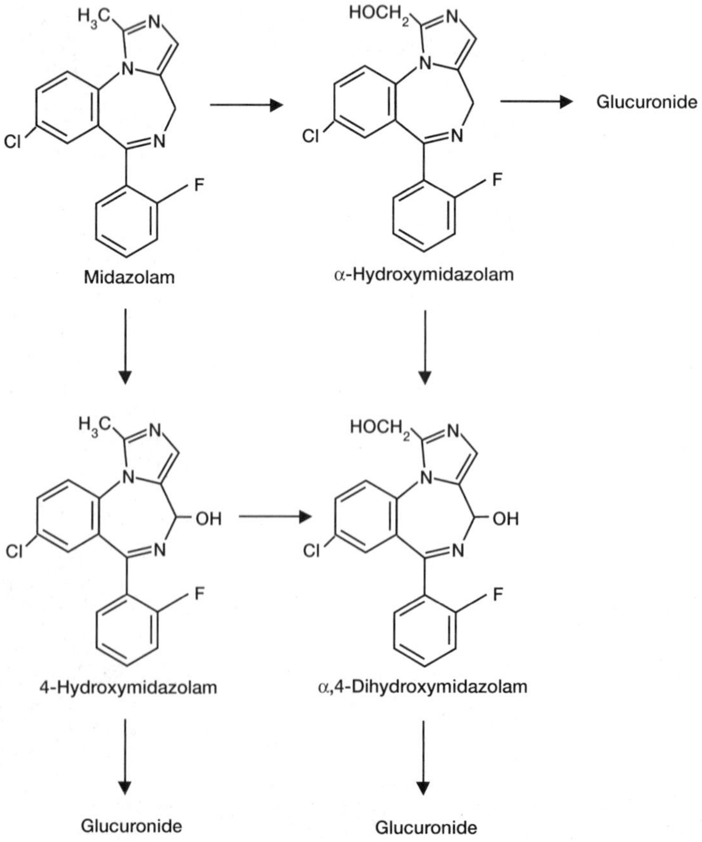

Hypnovel (Roche, UK) injections contain the equivalent of 2 mg or 5 mg.ml^{-1}. Versed (Roche, USA) injections contain the equivalent of 1 mg or 5 mg.ml^{-1}. The pH is adjusted to 3 and benzyl alcohol is used as the preservative for Versed, whilst sodium benzoate is used in the Hypnovel formulation.

Therapeutic use

Indications

1. As a hypnotic
2. Preoperative medication
3. As a sedative/hypnotic for procedures such as dentistry, upper gastrointestinal endoscopy, bronchoscopy and surgery performed under regional anaesthesia
4. To produce long-term sedation in patients requiring artificial ventilation of the lungs in the intensive care unit
5. Induction of general anaesthesia.

Contraindications

1. Known benzodiazepine sensitivity
2. General precautions for all intravenous anaesthetic agents
3. Respiratory insufficiency.

Mode of use

By intramuscular injection as a hypnotic or as a sedative/anxiolytic for premedication. Intravenously it should be given slowly in a diluted form and titrated until the desired effect is obtained. Elderly patients tend to be particularly sensitive. Monitoring of vital signs is mandatory, particularly so when an anaesthetist is not present. Great care must be taken during endoscopies, where sedation is usually carried out by the endoscopist and which is usually performed in a darkened room.

Indications

1. Hypnotic

Midazolam 15 mg orally at night is an effective hypnotic, increasing the total duration of sleep and decreasing the number of awakenings. There is no carryover of sedation to the morning and it is most useful as a hypnotic in patients in whom absence of daytime sedation is important.

2. Preoperative medication

Intramuscular midazolam is an effective sedative and anxiolytic when given preoperatively and in a dose of 0.07 and 0.08 mg.kg^{-1} produced greater sedation and antianxiety effects than hydroxyzine.[20] It also produced greater anterograde amnesia for up to 60 minutes than hydroxyzine with and without hyoscine.[20] In doses of 3–6 mg, midazolam proved to be a satisfactory agent for premedication compared with papaveretum 10–20 mg and hyoscine 0.2–0.4 mg, producing a similar degree of sedation and anxiolysis, but causing significantly more amnesia.[1]

3. Sedative hypnotic ('conscious sedation')

Midazolam is used in this field because of its ability to allay apprehension and produce amnesia in sub-hypnotic doses, but allowing a relatively rapid recovery. The short-term anterograde amnesia allows an injection of local anaesthetic to be carried out without recall, which is particularly important in dental practice.

Endoscopy. Fibreoptic endoscopy of the upper gastrointestinal tract and of the lungs is an unpleasant experience and requires some form of sedation. Midazolam administered intravenously provides good operating conditions with lack of coughing, gagging, laryngospasm and retching. Early studies[2] found that 0.15 mg.kg^{-1} produced unacceptably deep levels of sedation during gastroscopy and even 0.1 mg.kg^{-1} produced excessive sedation in 10% of patients. A dose of 0.07 mg.kg^{-1} produced satisfactory conditions in the majority of patients, with 64% failing to recollect passage of the endoscope.[3] The same dose of midazolam was found to produce satisfactory conditions when used by the endoscopist.[21]

Dentistry. The initial sedation following intravenous midazolam can be great and there might therefore be problems in assessing the adequacy of the local anaesthetic block. The drug should thus be titrated against the desired end-point, which in these circumstances is taken as a noticeable reduction in the patient's anxiety and apprehension, some slurring of speech and half-ptosis of the eyelids.[22] The dose of midazolam should not exceed 0.1 mg.kg^{-1}, and preferably less, and should be given over at least one minute. The undue sensitivity of the elderly to midazolam and their slower circulation times should be remembered in titrating their dose requirements.

Whenever midazolam is being used as a sedative by an operator/anaesthetist it is essential that verbal contact be maintained with the patient.

Regional anaesthesia. Midazolam in an initial dose of 0.08 mg.kg^{-1} with supplementary doses of 0.04 mg.kg^{-1} when indicated produced excellent sedation in patients undergoing surgery with the aid of regional anaesthesia.[4] Comparable effects were produced by an emulsion formulation of diazepam with respective doses of 0.15 and 0.075 mg.kg^{-1}. There were no detectable differences in the rate of recovery between the two drugs, although some patients given diazepam tended to drift back to sleep, which was not seen with midazolam. A highly significantly greater degree of anterograde amnesia followed the use of midazolam. Similar results have been found by others using midazolam 0.1 mg.kg^{-1} with incremental doses of 0.05 mg.kg^{-1} for the same purpose, and who also noted no significant cardiorespiratory changes.[23]

4. Long-term sedation

Sedation is a necessary part of the management of patients in the intensive care unit, particularly those requiring artificial ventilation of the lungs. This is most commonly met by a combination of a benzodiazepine and an opioid and midazolam has generally replaced diazepam in this respect.[24] Grounds and others[25] found that midazolam in incremental doses of 2.5 mg intravenously provided excellent sedation in patients whose lungs were being artificially ventilated after open-heart surgery, analgesia being provided by papaveretum in doses of 2.5 mg intravenously. The mean dose of midazolam used was 1.125 mg.h^{-1}, but this will be considerably influenced by other drugs that the patient has received.

Because of its relatively short elimination half life and high plasma clearance, midazolam has been used as continuous infusion in a strength of 1 mg.ml^{-1} in seriously ill patients in the intensive care unit, the infusion rate being adjusted to maintain the desired level of sedation.[26] In critically ill patients, prolonged sedation may follow the use of midazolam infusions due to delayed elimination.[14,27] Suggestions that prolonged sedation following infusions of midazolam might be due to a pharmacogenetic abnormality have been discounted.[28] Although the effects of midazolam are readily reversed by the specific antagonist flumazenil, great care must be taken because of the discrepancies in the half lives of the two drugs[29] and the antagonist may have to be given over prolonged periods.[26]

5. Induction of general anaesthesia

Midazolam may be used intravenously to induce general anaesthesia, but the main difference with thiopentone is the delay in onset of anaesthesia, the latter in adequate doses always producing its effect in one arm–brain circulation time. Effective adult doses of midazolam range from 0.1 to 0.5 mg.kg^{-1}.[5,6] There is a considerable variation in response to midazolam, which is reduced by opioid premedication.[6] Slow induction times are particularly seen in young, unpremedicated patients, in some of whom anaesthesia is not induced in 3 minutes with the recommended dose of 0.3 mg.kg^{-1}.[30]

The changes in heart rate and arterial blood pressure in healthy patients following induction of anaesthesia with midazolam are less pronounced than after thiopentone.[31] It has proved a satisfactory induction agent in patients with coronary artery disease.[2,32] It also lessens the haemodynamic response to tracheal intubation to a greater extent than thiopentone in such patients.[33]

In healthy patients the respiratory depressant effects of midazolam induction are less than those of thiopentone, but in patients with chronic obstructive airways disease, the respiratory depressant effect is greater than in normal subjects.[34]

Overall, induction of anaesthesia with midazolam is very smooth, but slower and less reliable than with thiopentone, and with minimal cardiorespiratory depression.

M

Contraindications

1. Known benzodiazepine sensitivity
Cross-sensitivity occurs with other benzodiazepines.

2. General precautions for all intravenous anaesthetic agents
Midazolam is a potent sedative agent and there is a wide variation in susceptibility to its effects. Deaths have been reported to the UK Committee on Safety of Medicines associated with respiratory and cardiovascular depression. It is therefore essential that the drug is only used intravenously by those skilled in resuscitation and tracheal intubation and that full resuscitative apparatus and a means of ventilating the lungs must always be available when midazolam is given intravenously.

3. Respiratory insufficiency
Patients with chronic respiratory disease may be particularly sensitive to the respiratory depressant effects of intravenous midazolam and exhibit a more marked and prolonged depression than healthy subjects.

Adverse reactions

Potentially life-threatening effects
Midazolam can cause respiratory[35] and cardiovascular depression,[36] ventricular irritability[37] and a change in the baroreflex control of heart rate.[38] There is a wide variation in susceptibility to its effects, the elderly being particularly sensitive. Respiratory depression, respiratory arrest, hypotension and even death have been reported following its use, usually during conscious sedation.[29] Respiratory obstruction can easily occur if sedation is too deep, and may not be noticed by the endoscopist, who has usually provided sedation as well. Desaturation of haemoglobin occurs to an average of less than 90% in a significant proportion of patients and to less than 80% in some.[39] Supplemental oxygen will readily compensate for the decreased saturation.[40] It is mandatory that proper monitoring of these patients be carried out during midazolam sedation and that full resuscitation apparatus and appropriately trained staff are present.

Acute overdosage
There is little information available on overdose of midazolam, but the results would likely be an extension of the usual pharmacological effects of the benzodiazepines with sedation, somnolence, confusion, impaired coordination, diminished reflexes, and coma. The effects would be rapidly reversed with flumazenil, although central depression may return after use of the latter,[41] because of its shorter duration of action.

Severe or irreversible adverse effects
Apart from dose-related central nervous system depression, no irreversible effects have been reported.

Symptomatic adverse effects
Systemic. These are an extension of the normal pharmacological actions of the drug. Adverse effects following intravenous midazolam include agitation, involuntary movements, confusion, slurred speech, blurred vision, lethargy, and dizziness and occur in less than 1% of patients receiving midazolam parenterally. Nausea and vomiting occur in 2–3% of patients following intravenous use.

Local. Pain on injection is rare following intravenous midazolam, while thrombophlebitis and thrombosis occur in less than 1% of cases and is less common than with diazepam with organic solvents.[42] Following intramuscular midazolam, local erythema, induration, and muscle stiffness occurs in less than 1% of patients, while pain at the site of injection occurs in about 4% of cases.

Other effects
Midazolam is not known to cause any modification of body biochemistry per se, although like other anaesthetics it is known to depress renal blood flow and renal function[43] and also liver blood flow in experimental animals.

Interference with clinical pathology tests
Midazolam is not known to interfere with any clinical pathological measurements.

High risk groups

Neonates
The newborn, particularly if premature, are very susceptible to the central depressant effects of benzodiazepines and they also have a reduced capacity for the elimination of these drugs and their metabolites. The use of diazepam in late pregnancy may result in infants who have apnoeic spells, fail to breathe or suckle normally, and may remain hypotonic and hypothermic for several days. There is no reason to suppose that midazolam would behave any differently in this respect.

Breast milk. It is not known whether midazolam enters breast milk, but this is likely as it is known to occur with other benzodiazepines.

Children
Little information is available on its use in children. Midazolam 0.2 $mg.kg^{-1}$ intramuscularly has been shown to produce effective sedation and anxiolysis when used as premedication in a limited number of children aged 2–10 years, who were also significantly more awake in the early postoperative period than those who received papaveretum and hyoscine.[44] Oral midazolam 7.5–15.0 mg was found to be an effective anxiolytic when given preoperatively in children aged 6–15 years.[45]

Pregnant women
Specific information on the effects of midazolam in pregnancy is not available, and although an increased risk of congenital malformations associated with the use of benzodiazepines has been suggested by retrospective studies, the association is tenuous. Midazolam does cross the placenta in humans. It should only be used in pregnancy where its benefits are thought to outweigh the possible risks.

The elderly
The elderly are particularly sensitive to midazolam. The dose should be reduced and the drug given slowly intravenously in a diluted form until the desired response is achieved.

Drug interactions

Potentially hazardous interactions
Alcohol. Midazolam will potentiate the central nervous depressant effects of alcohol. Its amnesic effects are potentiated following the co-administration of alcohol.[46]

Opioids, barbiturates, sedatives and anaesthetics. Midazolam will also potentiate the central depressant effects of opioids, barbiturates, and other sedatives and anaesthetics, and profound and prolonged respiratory depression might result. Severe hypotension has occurred when midazolam was used concomitantly with high dose fentanyl.

Other significant interactions
Plasma midazolam concentrations were increased by about 30% following oral administration of cimetidine, while levels following oral midazolam 15 mg were consistently increased after pretreatment for 24 hours with ranitidine, resulting in subjects being more sleepy than when they did not receive the H_2 receptor antagonists.[47]

Potentially useful interactions
Midazolam will attenuate the increase in heart rate and arterial blood pressure produced by anaesthetic doses of ketamine[48] and will also reduce the psychotic sequelae following ketamine anaesthesia.[49]

Clinical trials

1. Bell G D, Spickett G P, Reeve P A, Morden A, Logan R F A 1987 Intravenous midazolam for upper gastrointestinal endoscopy: a study of 800 consecutive cases relating dose to age and sex of patient. British Journal of Clinical Pharmacology 23: 241–243

Midazolam was given, in an initial dose of 2.5 mg, intravenously to 800 patients until they were dysarthric and drowsy but still cooperative. If this state was not achieved in 2 minutes, further increments were given until the appropriate conscious level was reached. The dose of midazolam decreased markedly with age in both male and female patients and there was a highly significant correlation in both sexes between age and dose of midazolam. There was only a small difference in dose between men and women. In patients over 70 years

Midazolam (hydrochloride)

the dose of midazolam necessary for endoscopy was often so small that an overdose could easily be given.

2. Bell G D, Reeve P A, Moshiri M et al 1987 Intravenous midazolam: a study of the degree of oxygen desaturation occurring during upper gastrointestinal endoscopy. British Journal of Clinical Pharmacology 23: 703–708

A fall in oxygen saturation was noted in 100 patients given a mean of 6.3 mg midazolam intravenously for upper gastrointestinal endoscopy. In 7% it fell to below 80% during procedure. Age, sex, dose of midazolam and pre-endoscopy respiratory function tests failed to identify those patients at risk of hypoxia during the endoscopy.

General review article

Dundee J W, Halliday N J, Harper K W, Brogden R N 1984 Midazolam. A review of its pharmacological properties and therapeutic use. Drugs 28: 519–543

References

1. McAteer E J, Dixon J, Whitwam J G 1984 Intramuscular midazolam. A comparison with papaveretum and hyoscine for intramuscular premedication. Anaesthesia 39: 1177–1182
2. Al-Khudairi D, Whitwam J G, McCloy R F 1982 Midazolam and diazepam for gastroscopy. Anaesthesia 37: 1002–1006
3. Whitwam J G, Al-Khudairi D, McCloy R F 1983 Comparison of midazolam and diazepam in doses of comparable potency during gastroscopy. British Journal of Anaesthesia 55: 773–777
4. Dixon J, Power S J, Grundy E M, Lumley J, Morgan M 1984 Sedation for local anaesthesia. Comparison of intravenous midazolam and diazepam. Anaesthesia 39: 372–376
5. Fragen R J, Gahl F, Caldwell N 1978 A water soluble benzodiazpine, R0 21-3981 for induction of anaesthesia. Anesthesiology 49: 41–43
6. Gamble J A S, Kawar P, Dundee J W, Moore J, Briggs L P 1981 Evaluation of midazolam as an intravenous induction agent. Anaesthesia 36: 868–873
7. Howard P J, McLean E, Dundee J W 1985 The estimation of midazolam, a water-soluble benzodiazepine by gas liquid chromatography. Anaesthesia 40: 664–668
8. Heizmann P, Eckert M, Ziegler G 1983 Pharmacokinetics and bioavailability of midazolam in man. British Journal of Clinical Pharmacology 16: 43S–49S
9. Collier P, Kawar P, Gamble J A S, Dundee J W 1982 Influence of age on pharmacokinetics of midazolam. British Journal of Clinical Pharmacology 13: 602P
10. Harper K W, Collier P S, Dundee J W, Elliott P, Halliday N J, Lowry K G 1985 Age and nature of operation influence the pharmacokinetics of midazolam. British Journal of Anaesthesia 57: 866–871
11. Dundee J W, Halliday N J, Loughran P G 1984 Variation in response to midazolam. British Journal of Clinical Pharmacology 17: 645P–646P
12. Vinik H R, Reves J G, Greenblatt D J, Abernethy D R 1983 Pharmacokinetics of midazolam in chronic renal failure patients. Anesthesiology 59: 390–394
13. Smith M T, Eadie M J, Brophy T O'R 1981 The pharmacokinetics of midazolam in man. European Journal of Clinical Pharmacology 19: 271–278
14. Shelly M P, Mendel I, Park G R 1987 Failure of critically ill patients to metabolise midazolam. Anaesthesia 42: 619–626
15. Allonen H, Ziegler G, Klotz U 1981 Midazolam kinetics. Clinical Pharmacology and Therapeutics 30: 653–661
16. Crevoisier Ch, Ziegler W H, Eckert M, Heizmann P 1983 Relationship between plasma concentration and effect of midazolam after oral and intravenous administration. British Journal of Clinical Pharmacology 16: 51S–61S
17. Kanto J, Aaltonen L, Erkkola R, Aarimaa L 1984 Pharmacokinetic and sedative effect of midazolam in connection with Caesarean section performed under epidural analgesia. Acta Anaesthesiologica Scandinavica 28: 116–118
18. Gerecke M 1983 Chemical structure and properties of midazolam compared with other benzodiazepines. British Journal of Clinical Pharmacology 16: 11S–16S
19. Park G R, Manara A, Dawling S 1989 Extra-hepatic metabolism of midazolam. British Journal of Clinical Pharmacology 27: 634–637
20. Fragen R J, Funk D I, Avram M J, Costello C, De Bruine K 1983 Midazolam versus hydroxyzine as intramuscular premedication. Canadian Anaesthetists Society Journal 30: 136–141
21. Kawar P, Porter K G, Hunter E K, McLaughlin J, Dundee J W 1984 Midazolam for upper gastrointestinal endoscopy. Annals of the Royal College of Surgeons of England 66: 283–285
22. O'Neil R, Verrill P J 1969 Intravenous diazepam in minor oral surgery. British Journal of Oral Surgery 7: 12–14
23. McLure J H, Brown D T, Wildsmith J A W 1983 Comparison of the i.v. administration of midazolam and diazepam as sedation during spinal anaesthesia. British Journal of Anaesthesia 55: 1089–1093
24. Gast P H, Fisher A, Sear J W 1984 Intensive care sedation now. Lancet 2: 863–864
25. Grounds R M, Lalor J, Lumley J, Royston D, Morgan M 1987 Propofol sedation for sedation in the intensive care unit: preliminary report. British Medical Journal 294: 397–400
26. Bodenham A, Brownlie G, Dixon J S, Park G R 1988 Reversal of sedation by prolonged infusion of flumazenil (Anexate, R0 15-1788). Anaesthesia 43: 376–378
27. Byatt C M, Lewis L D, Dawling S, Cochrane G M 1984 Accumulation of midazolam after repeated dosage in patients receiving mechanical ventilation in an intensive care unit. British Medical Journal 289: 799–800
28. Kassai A, Toth G, Eichelbaum M, Klotz U 1988 No evidence of genetic polymorphism in the oxidative metabolism of midazolam. Clinical Pharmacokinetics 15: 319–325
29. Editorial 1988 Midazolam — is antagonism justified. Lancet 1: 140–142
30. Dundee J W, Halliday N J, Loughran P G, Harper K W 1985 The influence of age on the onset of anaesthesia with midazolam. Anaesthesia 40: 441–443
31. Lebowitz P W, Cote M E, Daniels A L et al 1982 Comparative cardiovascular effects of midazolam and thiopental in healthy patients. Anesthesia and Analgesia 61: 771–775
32. Reves J G, Paul N, Samuelson P N, Lewis S 1979 Midazolam maleate induction in patients with ischaemic heart disease. Haemodynamic observations. Canadian Anaesthetists Society Journal 26: 402–409
33. Boralessa H, Senior D F, Whitwam J G 1983 Cardiovascular response to intubation. A comparative study of thiopentone and midazolam. Anaesthesia 38: 623–627
34. Gross J B, Zebrowski M E, Carel W D, Gardner S, Smith T C 1983 Time course of ventilatory depression after thiopental and midazolam in normal subjects and in patients with chronic obstructive pulmonary disease. Anesthesiology 58: 540–544
35. Forster A, Gardaz J-P, Suter P M, Gemperle M 1980 Respiratory depression by midazolam and diazepam. Anesthesiology 53: 494–497
36. Massant J, D'Hollander A, Barvais L, Dubois-Primo J 1983 Haemodynamic effects of midazolam in the anaesthetised patient with coronary artery disease. Acta Anaesthesiologica Scandinavica 27: 299–302
37. Arcos G J 1987 Midazolam-induced ventricular irritability. Anesthesiology 67: 612
38. Marty J, Ganzit R, Lefevre P et al 1986 Effects of diazepam and midazolam on baroreflex control of heart rate and on sympathetic activity in humans. Anesthesia and Analgesia 65: 113–119
39. Bell G D, Spickett G P, Reeve P A, Morden A, Logan R F A 1987 Intravenous midazolam for upper gastrointestinal endoscopy: a study of 800 consecutive cases relating dose to age and sex of patients. British Journal of Clinical Pharmacology 23: 241–243
40. Bell G D, Reeve P A, Moshiri M et al 1987 Intravenous midazolam: a study of the degree of oxygen desaturation occurring during upper-gastrointestinal endoscopy. British Journal of Clinical Pharmacology 23: 703–708
41. Knudsen L, Lonka L, Sorensen B H, Kirkegaard L, Jensen O V, Jensen S 1988 Benzodiazepine intoxication treated with flumazenil (Anexate, R015-1788). Anaesthesia 43: 275–276
42. Kawar P, Dundee J W 1982 Frequency of pain on injection and venous sequelae following the i.v. administration of certain anaesthetics and sedatives. British Journal of Anaesthesia 54: 935–939
43. Lebowitz P W, Cote M E, Daniels A L, Bonventre J 1982 Comparative renal effects of midazolam and thiopental. Anesthesiology 57: A35
44. Taylor M B, Vine P R, Hatch D J 1986 Intramuscular midazolam premedication in small children. A comparison with papaveretum and hyoscine. Anaesthesia 41: 21–26
45. Sjovall S, Kanto J, Iisalo E, Himberg J-J, Kangao L 1984 Midazolam versus atropine plus pethidine as premedication in children. Anaesthesia 39: 224–228
46. Subhan Z, Hindmarch I 1983 The effects of midazolam in conjunction with alcohol on iconic memory and free recall. Neuropsychobiology 9: 220–234
47. Elwood R J, Hildebrand P J, Dundee J W, Collier P S 1983 Ranitidine influences the uptake of oral midazolam. British Journal of Clinical Pharmacology 15: 743–745
48. White P F 1982 Comparative evaluation of intravenous agents for rapid sequence induction — thiopental, ketamine and midazolam. Anesthesiology 57: 279–284
49. Cartwright P O, Pingel S M 1984 Midazolam and diazepam in ketamine anaesthesia. Anaesthesia 39: 439–442

M Mifepristone

Mifepristone (Mifegyne) is a synthetic antiprogesterone that can be used as an abortifacient.

Chemistry

Mifepristone (Mifegyne)
$C_{29}H_{35}NO_2$
17-β-Hydroxy-11β-(4-dimethyl-aminophenyl)-17α-1-propynyl)-oestra-4.9-diene-3-one

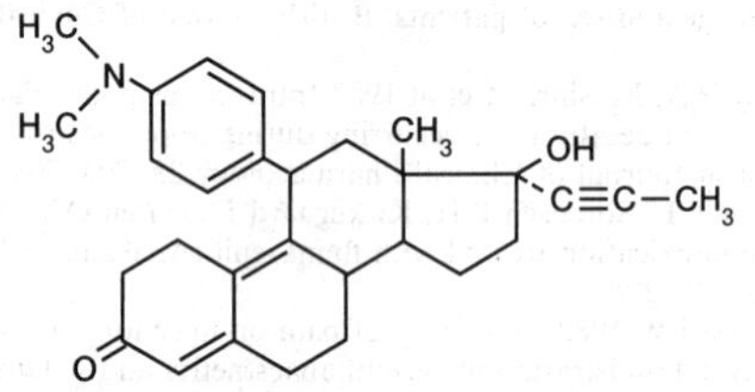

Molecular weight	429.6
pKa	3.7
Solubility	
in alcohol	1 in 20
in water	—
Octanol/water partition coefficient	—

Mifepristone is prepared by chemical synthesis.[1]

Pharmacology

Mifepristone is a synthetic 19-norsteroid related to norethisterone. It binds to the intracellular progesterone receptor where it competitively inhibits progesterone attachment and this is thought to be how it antagonizes the effects of endogenous progesterone.[2] In animal studies it binds to progesterone receptors with an affinity five times that of progesterone itself. Mifepristone does not inhibit progesterone synthesis by ovarian cells.[3] In early pregnancy the most important site of action of mifepristone seems to be on the endometrium. In late pregnancy it is suggested that mifepristone acts on the myometrium to increase contractility by interfering with the effects of progesterone.[4] Mifepristone binds to androgen receptors but inhibition of the action of androgens is minimal.

Mifepristone has an antiglucocorticoid action with an affinity for the glucocorticoid receptor three times greater than that of dexamethasone. Antagonism of dexamethasone has been demonstrated in vivo with abolition of the inhibition of ACTH secretion by dexamethasone in rats and also prevention of the thymolytic actions of dexamethasone.[5] There is no antimineralocorticoid activity.

Toxicology

Mifepristone had no mutagenic effect in vitro or in vivo. Toxicological studies do not show any effects other than the endocrine consequences of competitive antagonism of progesterone receptors.[5,6] Smaller doses than those required to induce abortion were not teratogenic in either rats or mice. Cranial malformations in rabbits were not dose-related and also occurred in controls. Antiglucocorticoid activity in long term animal use is compensated for by increased ACTH release.

Clinical pharmacology

Mifepristone antagonizes progesterone at receptors in the decidualized endometrium. Decidual necrosis follows and there is increased local prostaglandin production. Prostaglandins E_2, $F_2\alpha$ and 6-keto $F_1\alpha$ seem to be the most important.[7] During the earliest luteal phase normal corpus luteum formation is prevented, but from the mid luteal phase onwards decidual necrosis can be caused by a dose of mifepristone that does not cause the corpus luteum to break down.[8]

In the human endometrium, in the absence of endogenous progesterone, there may be some partial agonist activity and mifepristone can induce secretory change in the endometrium of postmenopausal women stimulated by oestrogen.[9]

The relatively weak antagonist action of mifepristone at glucocorticoid receptors in humans results in an increase in endogenous steroid production which compensates for this effect.[10]

Pharmacokinetics

The preferred analytical method for mifepristone is radioimmunoassay with a sensitivity of 10 pg per assay tube and ultraviolet spectrometry after separation by high pressure liquid chromatography[11] with a detection limit of $0.01\ mg.l^{-1}$.

Mifepristone is well absorbed after oral administration with over 90% of an oral dose entering the body.[12] Peak plasma levels are reached after 1.5 hours. The plasma concentration remains stable over 12 hours and then declines.[13] The half life of mifepristone is approximately 24 hours.[14,15] Approximately 98% of mifepristone in plasma is protein bound, to both albumin and α-1 acid glycoprotein.

The pharmacokinetic data for mifepristone do not conform to standard open compartment models for distribution and elimination. The discrepancy between quoted half lives has been thought to be the result of an enterohepatic circulation[13] as the main route for excretion of the drug is in bile.[12]

Oral absorption	90.6
Presystemic metabolism	—
Plasma half life	
range	12–72 h
Volume of distribution	$1.22–1.72\ l.kg^{-1}$
Plasma protein binding	98%

Concentration–effect relationship

There is inadequate information from which to derive any conclusions about concentration–effect relationships for free and bound drug: at doses of $1\ mg.kg^{-1}$ mifepristone antagonizes the action of progesterone on the endometrium and myometrium. With doses of $5\ mg.kg^{-1}$ there is partial or complete luteolytic activity. These effects occur after single doses or very short term use. The relative efficacies of various regimens have been discussed;[12] twelve hours after administration of mifepristone there was no difference in plasma concentration of the drug between those women who aborted and those who did not.

Metabolism

Mifepristone is metabolized in the liver to N-didesmethyl and N-monodesmethyl compounds which have similar but reduced bioactivity.[16] Tritiated mifepristone and its metabolites are excreted in bile. The main route of elimination of mifepristone is faecal. There is no information available as to the amount of mifepristone that is excreted unchanged or the proportions of the metabolites that are excreted.

Pharmaceutics

Mifepristone 'RU486' (Roussel) is presented as tablets (not yet commonly available) containing 200 mg of mifepristone itself with: colloidal silica 3 mg; maize starch 102 mg; polyvidone excipient 12 mg; microcrystalline cellulose 30 mg; magnesium stearate 350 mg.

Therapeutic use

Indications

1. Menstrual regulation
2. Postcoital contraception
3. Missed abortion and intrauterine death
4. Induction of abortion (with prostoglandins)
5. Induction of labour

Other proposed indications
6. Ectopic pregnancy.

Contraindications

1. Desired pregnancy.

Mode of use

Mifepristone is given as a single oral dose of 600 mg for the induction of menstruation or to cause early abortion. Repeated doses may be needed to induce labour after intra uterine death.

Indications

1. Induction of menstruation
The monthly use of mifepristone as a once-a-month birth control pill to ensure menstruation in sexually active women is under study. It is taken regularly, or administered within days of the expected date of an overdue menstrual period, early in the fifth week of amenorrhoea. A failure rate of 20% has been reported.[17]

2. Postcoital contraception
Mifepristone has been used for postcoital contraception after occasional exposure to the risk of pregnancy with mixed results.[18]

3. Missed abortion and intrauterine death
Mifepristone is effective in evacuating the uterus with second trimester missed abortion. It is also effective in inducing labour with intrauterine death of the fetus.[20] It is well tolerated. The recommended dose is 600 mg orally, which may have to be repeated.

4. Induction of abortion
Mifepristone has been used to induce abortion from 10 days after the expected date of the missed period. 85% of patients aborted completely after 400–800 mg orally as a single dose. The remaining 15% threatened to abort and suction evacuation of the uterine contents was facilitated by the treatment with mifepristone.[16] The recommended dose is 600 mg by mouth. Because of the risk of failed or incomplete abortion and prolonged uterine bleeding close medical

Fig. 1 Metabolism of mifepristone

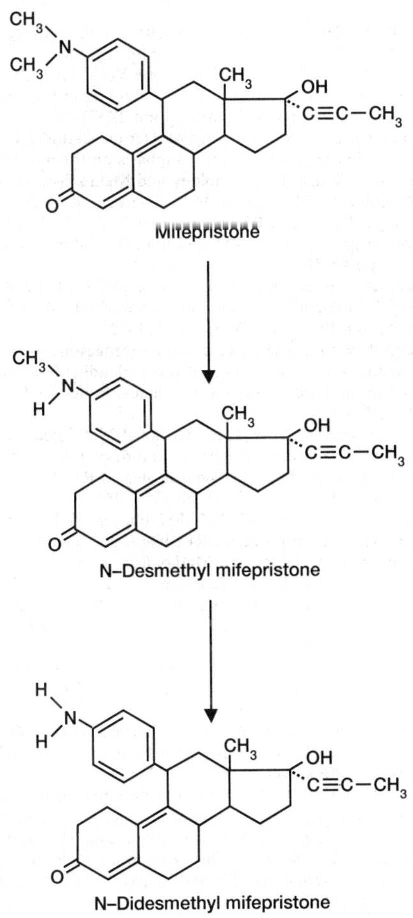

supervision is needed. The addition of a vaginal pessary containing 1 mg of the prostaglandin E_1 analogue, gemeprost, increases the proportion of patients aborting.[14,21] With pregnancies with 7 weeks amenorrhoea or less abortion is usually complete, between 7 and 10 weeks 7% are likely to need surgical evacuation of the uterus to complete abortion. Severe bleeding requiring hospital admission occurs in approximately 1% of cases. Ectopic pregnancy should be excluded before this level of dosage is used.

5. Induction of labour
In late pregnancy mifepristone is thought to act by increasing myometrial contractility. The use of 100–400 mg oral mifepristone for up to 4 days has been suggested[20] as an alternative to prostaglandin or artificial rupture of the amniotic membranes for induction of labour. Although it has been used successfully to induce labour after intrauterine death and with abnormal fetuses the safety of mifepristone for the fetus has not yet been established.

6. Ectopic pregnancy
Pre-operative oral mifepristone, 200 mg orally for 4 days, has been suggested as an adjunct to conservative surgery of the fallopian tube to facilitate embryo extraction in ectopic pregnancy.[19]

Contraindications

1. Desired pregnancy
Mifepristone is an effective abortifacient.

Adverse reactions

Potentially life-threatening effects
No effects of this kind have been reported.

Acute overdosage
There is no information on the effects of overdose in humans.

Severe or irreversible adverse effects
None of the problems that might have been anticipated because of antiglucocorticoid activity have materialized in short-term use.

Symptomatic adverse effects
No significant symptomatic adverse effect has been recorded. Vomiting and diarrhoea have been recorded but were thought to be due to either pregnancy or to prostaglandin used as an adjunct to mifepristone.

Rarely heavy bleeding requiring blood transfusion has followed pregnancy termination.

Other effects
Mifepristone in the dose range used to terminate pregnancy, has been reported to cause a significant increase in plasma cortisol levels but without interfering with diurnal patterns of either ACTH or cortisol secretion. It appears that mifepristone has some antagonist action at glucocorticoid receptors but that this is easily countered by an increase in ACTH and cortisol secretion. To obtain effective blockade of glucocorticoid receptors much higher doses than those used to block progesterone are needed.[10] The use of mifepristone in Cushing's disease has been advocated.[22] There is an elevation in serum prolactin 12 hours after ingestion of mifepristone which returns to normal after 24 hours.

Interference with clinical pathology tests
Both plasma adrenocorticotrophic hormone (ACTH) and plasma cortisol levels may be elevated by mifepristone.

High risk groups

Neonates
There is no indication for the use of mifepristone in the neonate.

Breast milk. There is no information as to the excretion of mifepristone in breast milk, nor is there any information on any possible effects on the suckling infant.

Children
There is no indication for the use of mifepristone in children.

Pregnant women
Mifepristone is an effective abortifacient in pregnancy and has been shown to be effective in inducing abortion or labour in all three trimesters. Insufficient evidence is available to comment definitively on the effects of mifepristone in women on a pregnancy which

continued after mifepristone was given. A very small number of such pregnancies have produced apparently normal babies. Normal pregnancies have been reported after conception which occurred as little as one month following a mifepristone-induced abortion.[23]

The elderly
There is no indication for the use of mifepristone in the elderly.

Drug interactions

Potentially hazardous interactions
No potentially hazardous interactions have as yet been reported.

Potentially useful interactions
Complete abortion of early pregnancy occurred in 95% of women given a vaginal pessary of the prostaglandin E_1 analogue, gemeprost, 48 hours after a single oral dose of mifepristone.[21]

Clinical trials

1. Couzinet B, LeStrat N, Ulman A, Baulieu E E, Schaison G 1986 Termination of early pregnancy by the progesterone antagonist RU 486 (mifepristone). New England Journal of Medicine 315: 1565–1570

This study involved 100 women recruited early in unwanted pregnancy, within 10 days of the expected onset of the missed period. Dates were confirmed both clinically and by ultrasound. Three regimens were used for mifepristone: 50 mg twice daily for 4 days; 50 mg thrice daily for 4 days, and 400 mg daily for 2 days. Plasma B-HCG, oestriol, progesterone and mifepristone were measured. Completeness of abortion was assessed clinically and by ultrasound.

The overall abortion rate was 85% with no apparent differences between the mifepristone regimens. 15 women bled vaginally but did not abort completely with medical treatment alone. Surgical evacuation of the uterus was thought to be facilitated by mifepristone with softening of the uterine cervix. The women who aborted bled for 6–17 days compared with 2–5 days for those women who did not abort. Mifepristone was well tolerated. Vaginal bleeding was equivalent to a heavy period except for 18 subjects in whom the bleeding was felt to be excessive. None required blood transfusion. In comparison with the painful uterine contractions and gastrointestinal disturbance that would have been expected from an equipotent prostaglandin analogue regimen; mifepristone was better tolerated. A normal period occurred within 8 weeks. The authors could find no apparent difference between treatment groups to explain the failure of mifepristone to secure complete abortion in 15 subjects.

2. Rodger Mary W, Baird D T 1987 Induction of therapeutic abortion in early pregnancy with mifepristone in combination with prostaglandin pessary. Lancet 2: 1415–1418

100 women in early pregnancy (56 days amenorrhoea or less) were given either 150 mg of mifepristone orally for 4 days or single doses of 400 mg, 500 mg or 600 mg of mifepristone. After 48 hours, a single 0.5 mg gemeprost pessary was inserted into the vagina, with a further 0.5 mg if abortion did not occur. Duration of pregnancy had been confirmed by the menstrual history, clinical examination and ultrasound. Haemoglobin, cortisol, HCG, oestradiol and progesterone were measured before and after treatment. Vaginal blood loss was measured in 72 women. Abortion was considered complete if vaginal bleeding had ceased within 4 weeks, the cervix was closed and a pregnancy test was negative.

The effectiveness of the 4 treatment regimens used was similar. Only 14% required a second 0.5 mg gemeprost pessary. 95 women were thought to have aborted completely, 3 were found at curettage to have aborted completely after all and only 2 had significant retained products of conception. There were no continuing viable pregnancies in any of the treatment groups. The median measured blood loss was 72.5 ml. No significant change in haemoglobin concentration was found between groups and no individual required blood transfusion. Bleeding lasted longer than would be expected after vacuum aspiration of pregnancy. 94 women complained of pain; 44 requiring oral analgesia and 9 an intramuscular opiate. Almost one third of the women vomited during the study although half of these had vomited before treatment began. Diarrhoea, more clearly likely to be due to treatment than to pregnancy, affected 10% and was attributed to the prostaglandin analogue rather than to mifepristone.

This study confirmed the effectiveness of a single dose of mifepristone and showed that the addition of gemeprost, a prostaglandin E_1 analogue, resulted in a 95% rate of medically-induced complete abortion. There was an acceptable low rate of severe pain and gastrointestinal side effects. Because of the possibility of incomplete abortion, follow up was recommended.

3. Silvestre L, Dubois C, Renault M, Rezvani Y, Baulieu E-E, Ulmann A 1990 Voluntary interruption of pregnancy with mifepristone (RU 486) and a prostaglandin analogue: a large scale French experience. New England Journal of Medicine 322: 645–648

The authors studied 2115 women seeking termination of pregnancy after 49 days or less of amenorrhoea. A single 600 mg dose of mifepristone was given followed 36–48 hours later by either gemeprost (vaginal suppository) or sulprostone (intramuscular injection at 3 different dose levels).

The overall efficacy was 96.0%. Failures included persisting pregnancy (1%), incomplete expulsion (2.1%) and need for haemostatic procedures (0.9%). The mean time to expulsion was shortest (4.5 hours) with mifepristone and the highest dose of sulprostone (0.5 mg intramuscularly).

Other trial

1. Grimes D A, Mishell D R, Sharpe D, Lacora M 1968 Early abortion with a single dose of the antiprogestin RU 486. American Journal of Obstetrics and Gynecology 158: 1307–1312

General review articles

Cousinet B, Schaison B 1988 Mifegyne (mifepristone) A new antiprogestagen with potential therapeutic use in human fertility control. Drugs 35: 187–191

References

1. Teutsch G 1985 Analogues of RU 486 for the mapping of the progestin receptor: synthetic and structural aspects. In: Baulieu E E, Segal S J (eds) The antiprogestin steroid RU 486 and human fertility control, ch 2. Plenum Press, New York, pp 27–47
2. Baulieu E E 1985 RU 486: an antiprogestin steroid with contragestive activity in women. In: Baulieu E E, Segal S J (eds) The antiprogestin steroid RU 486 and human fertility control, ch 1. Plenum Press, New York, pp 1–25
3. Schrieber J R, Hsueh A J W, Baulieu E E 1983 Binding of the antiprogestin RU 486 to rat ovary steroid receptors. Contraception 28: 77–85
4. Garfield R E, Baulieu E E 1987 The antiprogesterone steroid RU 486: a short pharmacological and clinical review, with emphasis on the interruption of pregnancy. Balliere's Clinical Endocrinology and Metabolism 1: 207–221
5. Philibert D, Mogiulewsky M, Lecaque M D, Tournemine C, Secchi J, Deraedt R 1985 Pharmacological profile of RU 486 in animals. In: Baulieu E E, Segal S J (eds) The antiprogestin steroid RU 486 and human fertility control, ch 3. Plenum Press, New York, pp 49–68
6. Deraedt R, Vannier B, Fournex R 1985 Toxicological study on RU 486. In: Baulieu E E, Segal S J (eds) The antiprogestin steroid RU 486 and human fertility control, ch 10. Plenum Press, New York, pp 123–126
7. Smith S K, Kelly R W 1987 The effect of the antiprogestins RU486 and ZK 98 734 on the synthesis and metabolism of prostaglandins $F_{2\alpha}$ and E_2 in separated cells from early human decidua. Journal of Clinical Endocrinology and Metabolism 65: 527–534
8. Hermann W L, Schindler A M, Wyss R, Bischof P 1985 Effects of the antiprogesterone RU 486 in early pregnancy and during the menstrual cycle. In: Baulieu E E, Segal S J (eds) The antiprogestin steroid RU 486 and human fertility control, ch 16. Plenum Press, New York pp 179–198
9. Gravanis A, Schaison C, George M et al 1985 Endometrial and pituitary responses to the steroidal antiprogestin RU 486 in post menopausal women. Journal of Clinical Endocrinology and Metabolism 60: 156–163
10. Gaillard R C, Riandel A, Muller F, Hermann W, Baulieu E E 1985 RU 486: Studies of its antiglucocorticoid activity in man. In: Baulieu E E, Segal S J (eds) The antiprogestin steroid RU 486 and human fertility control, ch 31. Plenum Press, New York, pp 331–337
11. Salmon J, Mouren M 1985 Radioimmunoassy of RU 486 In: Baulieu E E, Segal S J (eds) The antiprogestin steroid RU 486 and human fertility control, ch 8. Plenum Press, New York, pp 99–101
12. Deraedt R, Bannat C, Busigny M et al 1985 Pharmacokinetics of RU 486. In: Baulieu E E, Segal S J (eds) The antiprogestin steroid RU 486 and human fertility control, ch 9. Plenum Press, New York, pp 103–122
13. Liu J H, Garzo V G, Jen S S C 1988 Pharmacodynamics of the antiprogesterone RU 486 in women after oral administration. Fertility and Sterility 50: 245–249
14. Swahn M L, Cekan S, Wang, Lundstrom V, Bygdeman M 1985 Pharmacokinetics and clinical studies of RU 486 for fertility regulation. In: Baulieu E E, Segal S J (eds) The antiprogestin steroid RU 486 and human fertility control, ch 22. Plenum Press, New York, pp 242–258

15. Kawai S, Nieman L K, Brandon D D et al 1987 Pharmacokinetic properties of the antiprogesterone steroid RU 486 in man. Journal of Pharmacology and Experimental Therapeutics 241: 401–406
16. Couzinet B, LeStrot N, Ulman A, Baulieu E E, Schaison G 1986 Termination of early pregnancy by the progesterone antagonist RU 486 (mifepristone) New England Journal of Medicine 315: 1565–1570
17. Dubois C, Silvestre L, Ulmann A 1989 Utilisation de la mifépristone dans l'interuption volontaire de grossesse. Expérience française. la Presse Medical 18: 757–760
18. van Santen, Haspels 1987 Interception III: postcoital luteal contragestion by an antiprogestin (mifepristone RU 486) in 62 women. Contraception 35: 433–431
19. Paris F X, Henry-Suchet J, Tesquier L 1984 Le traitment medical des grossesses extro-utérines par le RU 486. La Presse Medical B 1219
20. Cabrol D, Bouvier d'Ivoire M, Mermot E, Cedard L, Sureau C, Baulieu E E 1985 Induction of labour with mifepristone after intrauterine fetal death. Lancet 2: 1019
21. Rodger M W, Baird D T 1987 Induction of therapeutic abortion in early pregnancy with mifepristone in combination with prostaglandin pessary. Lancet 2: 1415–1418
22. Nieman L K, Chrousos G P, Kellner C et al 1985 In: Baulieu E E, Segal S J (eds) The antiprogestin steroid RU 486 and human fertility control, ch 32. Plenum Press, New York, pp 339–346
23. Hermann W, Wyss R, Riondel A et al 1982 Effet d'un steroid anti progesterone chez la femme: interruption de la cycle menstrual at de la grossesse au debut. Comptes-Rendus de Seances de l'Academie des Sciences 294: 933–938

Minocycline (hydrochloride)

This drug was developed in the 1960s and is produced from deep tank fermentation followed by chemical transformation. It is a broad-spectrum antibiotic used for the treatment of infections caused by tetracycline-sensitive organisms. It is also effective against some tetracycline-resistant strains of staphylococci.

Chemistry

Minocycline (Minocin)[1]
$C_{23}H_{27}N_3O_7.HCl$
7-Dimethylamino-6-demethyl-6-deoxytetracycline hydrochloride

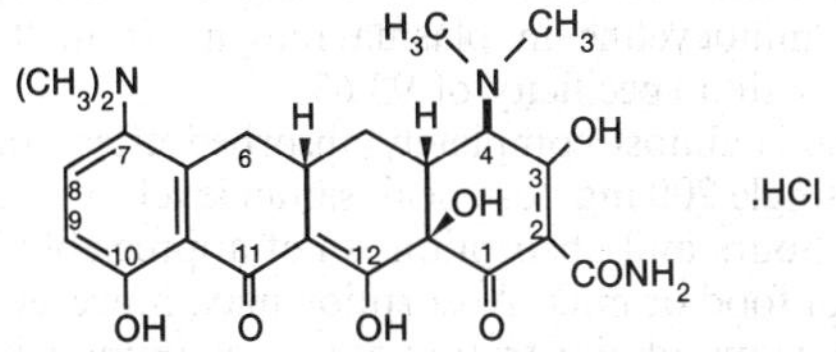

Molecular weight (free base)	493.9 (457.5)
pKa	2.8, 5.0, 7.8, 9.3
Solubility	
in alcohol	>1:100
in water	>1:30
Octanol/water partition coefficient	1.48

(The presence of various ionizable groups in the minocycline molecule leads to different degrees of dissociation (pKa) in each group when the compound is in solution.)

The pharmaceutical powder is yellow, odourless and crystalline with a bitter taste. It is slightly hygroscopic and is sensitive to light. The compound used clinically is laevorotary.

It is not available in combination with other products.

Pharmacology

Minocycline is a semi-synthetic tetracycline antibiotic that first became available in 1972. Like other tetracyclines it has a wide spectrum of activity. In addition to its antibiotic activity it is also a chelating agent and will chelate Ca^{2+}, Mg^{2+} or Al^{3+} ions in the gut. It has its main mechanism of action on protein synthesis. Minocycline is more lipophilic than other tetracyclines and passes directly through the lipid bilayer of the bacterial cell wall. In addition, an energy-dependent active transport system pumps the drug, like all tetracyclines, through the inner cytoplasmic membrane. Once inside the bacterial cell, minocycline inhibits protein synthesis by binding specifically to the 30S ribosomes. The drug appears to prevent access of aminoacyl tRNA to the acceptor site on the mRNA–ribosome complex.[3] This prevents the addition of amino acids to the growing peptide chain. Minocycline will impair protein synthesis in mammalian cells if used at very high concentrations.[4] However, these cells lack the active transport system found in bacteria.

Toxicology

Toxicological testing in animals failed to demonstrate any results of potential clinical relevance. There are no data available for long-term carcinogenicity and mutagenicity studies in animals. Teratogenic effects have been shown to occur in rats and rabbits (not dog or monkey).[1,5]

M

Clinical pharmacology

50–100 mg twice daily (see Mode of use) is the most commonly used dose but up to 400 mg has been given.[6]

Minocycline is primarily a bacteriostatic antibiotic. It has a similar spectrum of activity to other tetracyclines but in particular is more active against *Staphylococcus aureus* and *Nocardia*. The drug is often active against penicillin-resistant strains of *Staph. aureus* and against strains of those organisms that are resistant to other tetracyclines.[7]

Apart from chlortetracycline, minocycline is also more active than other tetracyclines against β-haemolytic streptococci.[8]

Certain Gram-negative strains of *E. coli*, *Proteus mirabilis* and *Klebsiella* which are often resistant to tetracyclines may be sensitive to minocycline.[9]

Minocycline is active against most strains of *Haemophilus influenzae* and is particularly useful for infections with *H. ducreyi*, actinomycetes, *Brucella* and *Vibrio cholerae*. It is also active against *Nocardia*, *Chlamydia*, mycoplasmas, and a wide range of rickettsiae. Minocycline is active against spirochaetes such as *Borrelia recurrentis*, *Treponema pallidum* and *T. pertenue*. Like all tetracyclines, minocycline will alter the enteric flora.

Pharmacokinetics

The preferred analytical method is by liquid chromatography.[11] It will measure minocycline in plasma ranging from 0.5 $\mu g.ml^{-1}$ to 2.55 $\mu g.ml^{-1}$ with a specificity of 93.6%.

Minocycline is almost completely absorbed after oral administration. After a single 200 mg dose peak serum levels of 2–3 $\mu g.ml^{-1}$ are attained in 2 hours and absorption is not appreciably influenced by the presence of food or milk. Absorption may, however, be decreased by the simultaneous administration of iron-containing haematinics or antacids (containing calcium, magnesium and iron).[12,13]

Presystemic metabolism does not occur. Plasma half life is 12–16 hours, in patients with normal renal or hepatic functions.[14] In severe renal impairment the plasma half life increases to approximately 32 hours.[15,16]

Minocycline is widely distributed in human body tissue and fluids (no published data for volume of distribution). It has better penetration into most tissues as compared with oxytetracycline and in most instances tissue levels exceed serum levels with highest concentrations in bile, thyroid, lung, and liver but also good penetration into breast, skin and sinuses, for example.[16] Minocycline penetrates CSF better than other tetracyclines but levels are still low. It also has better penetration into tears and saliva. Minocycline is excreted in breast milk and crosses the placenta.

This tetracycline also becomes bound to teeth and bones (whilst growing), causing yellow fluorescence.[17]

Minocycline is more highly protein bound than oxytetracycline (76% vs c. 30%).[16]

Oral absorption	100%
Presystemic metabolism	<5%
Plasma half life range	12–16 h
Volume of distribution	78.6±10.8 l
Plasma protein binding	76%

Concentration–effect relationship

The therapeutic range will depend upon the minimum inhibiting concentration (MIC) of the antibiotic for the organism in question. Full susceptibility occurs when the MIC is less than 4.0 $mg.l^{-1}$, and intermediate susceptibility occurs when the MIC is between 4.0 and 12.5 $mg.l^{-1}$. Concentrations of greater than 25 $mg.l^{-1}$ are usually required to inhibit most strains of group B and group D streptococci and strains of *Staph. aureus*. The MIC for *Streptococcus pyogenes* is usually about 1.0 $mg.l^{-1}$ while many strains of *Neisseria* have a similar MIC.

Metabolism

Minocycline is partially degraded to microbiologically inactive metabolites by chemical conversion in the body.[13] The identification of these substances is still under investigation. Animal studies have shown conversion to 4-epiminocycline.[18]

Minocycline is more slowly excreted in urine than oxytetracycline: 5% in the first 24 hours. Urinary recovery of minocycline increases as duration of therapy continues[1,19] and persists for some time after the dosage is stopped. Minocycline is extremely soluble in fat, and also has a high serum protein binding; it will thus be released slowly into the bloodstream whence it is excreted.

32% of minocycline is recovered as an active drug; about 12% in urine and 20% in faeces. High concentrations have also been found in the bile.[13]

Pharmaceutics

Minocycline is available under the proprietary name Minocin.

1. Orange, film-coated tablet containing 100 mg minocycline marked 'LL' and 'M/100' (Lederle, UK) or 'LL' with 'M/5' (Lederle, US). A red and orange and purple capsule is available in the US marked 'Lederle M4'.
2. Film-coated tablets containing 50 mg minocycline are beige and marked 'LL' and 'M/50' (Lederle, UK) or are orange and marked 'LL' with 'M/3' (Lederle, US). An orange capsule is available in the US marked 'Lederle M2'.

The UK Minocin 100 mg tablet no longer contains a potentially allergenic substance, tartrazine. The 50 mg tablet and the US formulations do not contain this or any other potentially allergenic substance.

The shelf-life of both tablets is 3 years. They should be stored between 10°C and 30°C in the original pack or in containers which prevent access of moisture.

In the USA 'custard-flavoured' suspension is available containing 50 mg per 5 ml. It is preserved with parabens and 5% alcohol. A 100 mg vial for intravenous injection is available on a named patient basis.

Therapeutic use

Indications

1. Respiratory infection
2. Cholera
3. Gonorrhoea
4. Chlamydial infections
5. Chancroid and granuloma inguinale
6. Syphilis
7. Chemoprophylaxis of meningococcal infections
8. Nocardiosis
9. Staphylcoccal infections
10. Acne.

Contraindications

1. Hypersensitivity to tetracyclines
2. Women who are or may become pregnant
3. Patients less than 12 years of age
4. Patients who have systemic lupus erythematosus.

Mode of use

The causative organism should be isolated for minocycline susceptibility testing. Minocycline should be administered as follows: 200 mg initially, followed by 200 mg daily in divided doses, unless specifically indicated — see treatment of gonorrhoea, prophylaxis of meningococcal carriers, and treatment of acne.

Indications

1. Respiratory infections
Minocycline can be used to treat respiratory infections. It has the advantage of requiring twice-daily dosage, and may be active against some organisms which are resistant to the older tetracyclines.

2. Cholera
Minocycline is as effective as tetracyclines for the treatment of cholera but does not clear the faeces of vibrios as rapidly as tetracyclines.[20]

3. Gonorrhoea
A single dose of 300 mg of minocycline is only 50% effective, so longer courses are necessary. An older tetracycline or doxycycline is usually used.[21]

4. Chlamydial infections
Lymphogranuloma venereum. Minocycline has been used to treat this disease, and is effective in courses lasting 15–21 days.[22]
Non-specific urethritis. Minocycline has been used to eradicate *Chlamydia* from the male and female genital tract, and can also be used to treat ureaplasma infection.[23]
Psittacosis and trachoma. Older tetracyclines are usually used.

5. Chancroid and granuloma inguinale
Minocycline is effective if given for 2 weeks in treating these infections.[22]

6. Syphilis
Minocycline in a dose of 100 mg twice daily for 15 days appears to be satisfactory for primary and secondary syphilis.[22]

7. Chemoprophylaxis of meningococcal infections
Minocycline at the dose of 200 mg initially, then 100 mg 12-hourly for five days is moderately effective for the elimination of sulphonamide-resistant meningococci from nasopharyngeal carriers.[24] It is, however, no longer advocated for use because of its propensity to cause vestibular problems, and rifampicin is used instead.

8. *Nocardiosis*
Minocycline is quite active against this organism with most *N. asteroides* strains being inhibited by 1.6–3.1 $\mu g.ml^{-1}$. Other tetracyclines are less active against this species.[25]

9. Staphylococcal infection
Minocycline is effective in staphylococcal skin tissue infections including those caused by tetracycline-resistant but minocycline-sensitive organisms.[26]

10. Acne
A low dose of minocycline (50 mg twice daily) is effective in the treatment of this skin condition. Treatment should be continued for a minimum of 6 weeks. A low dosage (250 mg four times daily) of the older tetracyclines can be used if vestibular side effects occur with minocycline.[27]

Use of other tetracyclines
Older tetracyclines are usually used for the following conditions:

Mycoplasma pneumonia
Brucellosis
Rickettsial infections
Q fever
Relapsing fever, tulaeraema and plague
Actinomycin, gas gangrene and anthrax
Meliodosis
Malaria
Urinary tract infections

Contraindications

1. Hypersensitivity to tetracyclines
This is uncommon and may take the form of urticaria, asthma or facial oedema (review article A).

2. Women who are or may become pregnant
After the first trimester tetracyclines may cause staining of the deciduous teeth.[17]

3. Patients under 12 years
Tetracyclines have been found to cause permanent tooth discoloration, enamel hypoplasia and depressed bone growth in children under 12 years.[17]

4. Systemic lupus erythematosus
Tetracyclines are thought to exacerbate this condition.[28]

Adverse reactions

Potentially life-threatening effects
No effects of this kind appear to have been reported.

Minocycline (hydrochloride)

Acute overdosage
A woman in her 20s took 50 minocycline tablets but after gastric lavage recovered in two days (anecdotal report). There have been no published reports of acute overdosage with Minocin.

Severe or irreversible adverse effects
Minocycline can usually be used safely in patients with renal failure, but in severe cases it should be used with caution.[29]

Symptomatic adverse effects
Gut. Gastrointestinal disturbances including nausea and vomiting have been reported. Their frequency is probably directly related to higher doses, with few problems at the 50 mg twice-daily dosage.[30]
Skin. Dermatological reactions are rare. However, erythema multiforme, Stevens–Johnson syndrome, exfoliate dermatitis and photosensitivity have been reported.
Vestibular disturbance. Minocycline (but not other tetracyclines) can cause reversible dizziness, vertigo, ataxia, nausea and tinnitus.[32] Earlier studies showed that vestibular dysfunction occurred in 4.5–7.2% of patients.[31] Further trials in volunteers, however, showed that the disturbances occurred in 50–90% of patients and more frequently in women. These disturbances are reversible within 3–48 hours of discontinuing therapy[27,28] and are less when a low dose (50 mg twice daily) is given.

Other effects
Tetracyclines have been reported to exert an antianabolic action which may lead to increased blood urea concentrations.[33]
They also cause decreased plasma prothrombin activity due to inhibition of vitamin-K-producing flora in the gut.

Interference with clinical pathology tests
Tetracyclines may produce an interference fluorescence in the Hungarty methods for measuring urinary catecholamines.[34] They also may reduce bacteria converters of bilirubin to urobilinogen in the gut. This may affect urinary urobilinogen excretion methods.[35]

High risk groups

Neonates
The drug is contraindicated because of tooth staining, enamel hypoplasia and depressed bone growth.[39]
Breast milk. Tetracyclines should not be given, as the antibiotics pass to the child in the milk.

Children
Minocycline is contraindicated in children under 12 for the same reasons as for neonates above. For children over 12 years 50 mg of minocycline every 12 hours is recommended.

Pregnant women
Minocycline is contraindicated during pregnancy because of tooth staining in the fetus.

The elderly
Care needs to be taken only in patients with severe renal or liver dysfunction.

Drug interactions

Potentially hazardous interactions
Tetracyclines may enhance methoxyflurane-induced nephrotoxicity.[36] Sodium bicarbonate may inhibit dissolution of tetracyclines in the gastrointestinal tract by increasing the pH.[37]
Minocycline may decrease plasma prothrombin activity due to inhibition of vitamin-K-producing flora in the gut. Great care should be taken if a broad-spectrum antibiotic is given to patients taking coumarin anticoagulants.
Antacids containing divalent or trivalent cations chelate tetracyclines, impairing oral absorption. These cations are contained in foods, particularly dairy products, and iron preparations have the same effect.[38]
The bacteriostatic action of the tetracyclines may interfere with the bactericidal action of penicillin.

Potentially useful interactions
There are no interactions of this kind.

Minocycline (hydrochloride)

General review articles

A. Kucers A, Bennett N Mck 1979 Tetracyclines. In: The use of antibiotics. Heinemann, London, pp 592–645

B. Garrod L P, Lambert H P, O'Grady F 1981 In: Antibiotics and chemotherapy, 5th edn. Churchill Livingstone, Edinburgh, ch 7, pp 169–182

References

1. MINOCIN White Book, Medical Advisory Dept, Lederle Laboratories, Pearl River, NY 10 965
2. Colaizzi J L, Klink P R 1969 pH partition behaviour of tetracyclines. Journal of Pharmaceutical Sciences 58 (10): 1184–1189
3. Green R, Brown J R, Calvert R T 1976 The disposition of four tetracyclines in normal subjects. European Journal of Clinical Pharmacology 10: 245–250
4. Pato M L 1977 Tetracycline inhibits propagation of deoxyribonucleic acid replication and alters membrane properties. Antimicrobial Agents and Chemotherapy 11: 318–323
5. Jackson B A 1975 Effect of maternally administered minocycline on embryonic and foetal development in the rhesus monkey. Toxicology and Applied Pharmacology 33 (1): 156
6. Thatcher R W, Paxin G, Domescik G 1970 Gonorrhoeal urethritis in males treated with a single oral dose of minocycline. Public Health Report 85: 160–162
7. Mitchell A A B 1974 Comparative activity of minocycline and tetracyclines. British Medical Journal 1: 576
8. Finland M, Garner C, Wilcox C, Sabath C D 1976 Susceptibility of beta-haemolytic streptococci to 65 antibacterial agents. Antimicrobial Agents and Chemotherapy 9: 11
9. Candanoza C, Ellner P D 1975 Differences in susceptibilities of entero bacteriaceae and penicillin resistant *Staphylococcus aureus* to tetracycline and minocycline. Antimicrobial Agents and Chemotherapy 7: 27
10. Del Bene V E, Rogers M 1975 Comparison of tetracycline and minocycline transport in *Escherichia coli*. Antimicrobial Agents and Chemotherapy 7: 801–806
11. Leenheer A P, De Nelis H J 1979 Liquid chromatographic determination of minocycline in human serum. Journal of Pharmaceutical Sciences 68 (12): 1527–1530
12. Smith C, Woods G C, Wood M J 1984 Absorption of minocycline. Journal of Antimicrobial Chemotherapy 13: 93
13. MacDonald H, Kelly R G, Allen E S, Noble J F, Kanegis L A 1973 Observations on the pharmacokinetic properties of a new tetracycline antibiotic — minocycline. Clinical Pharmacology and Therapeutics 14: 852
14. Carney S, Butler R A, Dawborn J K, Pattison G 1974 Minocycline excretion distribution in relation to renal function in man. Clinical and Experimental Pharmacology and Physiology 1: 299
15. Devulder B, Cuvelier D, Tacquer A 1974 Pharmacokinetic studies of minocycline in subjects with chronic renal insufficiency receiving or not receiving treatment by haemodialysis. Lille Medicale 19: 287
16. Kunin C M 1967 A guide to use of antibiotics in patients with renal disease. Annals of Internal Medicine 67: 151
17. Cohlan S Q 1977 Tetracycline staining of teeth. Teratology 15: 127–131
18. Kelly R G, Kaneyis L A 1967 Metabolism and tissue distribution of radioisotopically labelled minocycline. Toxicology and Applied Pharmacology 11: 171
19. Jonas M, Cunha B A 1982 Minocycline. Therapeutic Drug Monitoring 4: 137–145
20. Mazumder D N G, Sikar B K, De S P 1974 Minocycline in the treatment of cholera. A comparison with tetracycline. Indian Journal of Medical Research 62: 712–718
21. Baytch H 1974 Minocycline in single dose therapy in the treatment of gonococcal urethritis in male patients. Medical Journal of Australia 1: 831–832
22. Velasco J E, Miller A E, Zaius N 1972 Minocycline in the treatment of venereal disease. Journal of the American Medical Association 220: 1323
23. Prentice M J, Taylor-Robinson D, Csonka G M 1976 Non specific urethritis, a placebo controlled trial of minocycline in conjunction with laboratory investigations. British Journal of Venereal Disease 52 (2): 69
24. Devine L F, Johnson D P, Hagerman C R, Pierce W E, Rhode S L, Peckinpaugh R O 1970 The effect of minocycline on meningococcal nasopharyngeal carrier state in navy personnel. American Journal of Epidemiology 93: 337–345
25. Bach M C, Sabath L D, Finland M 1973 Susceptibility of *Nocardia asteroides* to 45 antimicrobial agents in vitro. Antimicrobial Agents and Chemotherapy 3: 1
26. Candanoza C, Ellner P D 1975 Differences in susceptibilities of *Enterobacteriaceae* and penicillin resistant *Staphylococcus aureus* to tetracyclines and minocycline. Antimicrobial Agents and Chemotherapy 7: 227
27. Cullen S I 1978 Low dose minocycline therapy in tetracycline recalcitrant acne vulgaris. Cutis 101–105
28. Doniz C A 1969 Tetracycline provocation in lupus erythematosus. Annals of Internal Medicine 50 (5): 1217–1225
29. Welling P G, Shaw K W R, Kuman S W, Tse F L S, Craig W A 1975 Pharmacokinetics of minocycline in renal failure. Antimicrobial Agents and Chemotherapy 8: 532–537
30. Fanning W L, Crump D W, Sofferman R A 1977 Side effects of minocycline. A double blind study. Antimicrobial Agents and Chemotherapy 11: 712
31. Allen J C 1976 Minocycline. Annals of Internal Medicine 8: 482
32. Kucers A, Bennett N McK 1979 Tetracyclines. In: The use of antibiotics. Heinemann, London, pp 592–645
33. Shils M E 1973 Renal disease and the metabolic effects of tetracycline. Annals of Internal Medicine 58: 389
34. Klotz M O, Richter H, Meuffels M et al 1964 Interference by formaldehyde forming drugs in the determination of urinary catecholamines. Clinical Chemistry 10: 372–374
35. Levinson S A, MacFate R P 1969 Clinical laboratory diagnosis, 7th edn. Lea and Febiger, Philadelphia, pp 646–647
36. Kuzneu E Y 1970 Methoxyflurane, tetracyclines and renal failure. Journal of the American Medical Association 221 (1): 62
37. Barr W H, Adir J, Garrettson L 1971 Decrease of tetracycline absorption in man by sodium bicarbonate. Clinical Pharmacology and Therapeutics 12 (5): 779–784
38. Neuvonen P J 1976 Interactions with the absorption of tetracyclines. Drug 11: 45
39. Cohlan S Q 1977 Tetracycline staining of teeth. Teratology 15: 127–130

Minoxidil

Minoxidil is a potent resistance vessel dilator used in the treatment of severe hypertension.

Chemistry

Minoxidil (Loniten)
$C_9H_{15}N_5O$
2,6-Diamino-4-piperidinopyrimidine 1-oxide

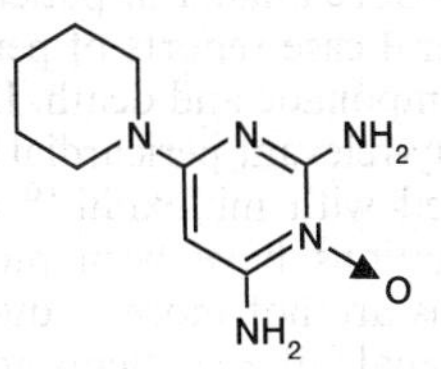

Molecular weight	209.3
pKa	4.6
Solubility	
in alcohol	1 in 25
in water	1 in 500
Octanol/water partition coefficient log p	1.24

Minoxidil is a white or off-white crystalline solid. It is prepared by chemical synthesis.

Pharmacology

Minoxidil is a directly acting vascular smooth muscle relaxant. The mechanism of action is unknown but is believed to involve a reduction in cytosolic calcium possibly through an action upon transmembrane calcium flux.

Toxicology

Administration of minoxidil to dogs, rats and mice has shown no evidence of carcinogenicity. Mutagenicity testing of minoxidil and two of its metabolites was negative. Administration of doses several times those employed clinically to pregnant rats and rabbits has not had a teratogenic effect. When minoxidil was administered to dogs, haemorrhagic necrosis of the right atrium occurred with doses of 20 $mg.kg^{-1}$ body weight and less frequently with lower doses.[1] These were not seen with low doses or in other species. Myocardial focal necrosis has also been described in the papillary muscles of the left ventricle of dogs or rats. No right atrial lesions of this type were observed in 242 autopsies performed on patients who had received minoxidil.[2] When minoxidil was administered in therapeutic doses to dogs with experimental myocardial infarction, blood flow to the ischaemic area was reduced and ischaemic damage increased.[3] Since blood flow to the normal myocardium was increased, this seems to be a manifestation of a 'steal' phenomenon.

Clinical pharmacology

Minoxidil lowers elevated systolic and diastolic blood pressure by decreasing peripheral resistance: there is a compensatory tachycardia with increased cardiac output and elevated plasma renin.[4] The fall in blood pressure is dose-related. Thus progressive increments in serial doses from 2.5 mg to 20 mg are associated with progressively greater falls in blood pressure in hypertensive subjects. The drug has little action on the blood pressure of normotensive subjects.[5] Sodium and water retention occur, probably as an indirect result of widespread vasodilation and concomitant diuretic therapy is nearly always needed. Hypertrichosis is not associated with a disturbance of sex hormones and is probably the result of increased skin blood flow.

Pharmacokinetics

Minoxidil can be measured spectrophotometrically at 272 nm following methylene dichloride extraction[6] or by high pressure liquid chromatography. The preferred method, however, is now radioimmunoassay; the limit of detection is 3 $\mu g.l^{-1}$. At least 90% of minoxidil is absorbed from the gastrointestinal tract. It appears in the blood within half an hour and peak plasma concentrations are reached after approximately one hour. The elimination half life is 2.8–4.2 hours. Neither this value nor the area under the plasma concentration–time curve is affected by chronic administration of the drug.[5] Minoxidil has a large volume of distribution, variably estimated at between 200 and 526 litres.[8] This suggests extravascular binding. Minoxidil is preferentially bound by vascular smooth muscle but not by cardiac or skeletal muscle.[6] It is not protein bound to any significant degree.

Minoxidil is predominantly metabolized by the liver: only 12% of the drug is excreted unchanged in the urine. The drug and its metabolites are filtered at the glomerulus with no evidence for tubular secretion or reabsorption. 3% or slightly more of the administered dose is excreted in the faeces.[8]

Renal excretion of the drug and its metabolites is reduced in renal failure whilst faecal excretion increases.[9] The glucuronide metabolite accumulates. Since this has antihypertensive activity (although this is less than the parent compound), it has been suggested that dosage regimens may have to be slightly reduced in renal failure patients. Minoxidil and its metabolites can be removed by haemodialysis,[5] although insufficient amounts are removed to affect half lives appreciably.

Oral absorption	100%
Presystemic metabolism	—
Plasma half life	
range	2.8–4.2 h
Volume of distribution	200–526 l
Plasma protein binding	negligible

Concentration–effect relationship

There is no relationship between plasma levels of minoxidil and the hypotensive effect, which reveals a peak much later than the peak plasma level and persists beyond the time at which significant drug can be detected in the plasma. This has been attributed both to vascular binding of the drug and also to possible active metabolites of minoxidil.[6,10]

Metabolism

Four pathways of hepatic metabolism have been proposed:

1. Conjugation with glucuronic acid at the N-oxide position in the pyrimidine ring to form minoxidil-O-glucuronide (67%)
2. Hydroxylation to 3'-minoxidil and 4'-minoxidil (2.5%)
3. Conversion to an uncharacterized polar compound
4. Sulphation by liver sulphotransferases.

The glucuronide, which is the major circulatory metabolite has reduced pharmacological activity.

Pharmaceutics

Minoxidil is available in oral form for the treatment of severe hypertension. It has, however, also been marketed as Regaine (Upjohn, UK), a 1% lotion for the treatment of alopecia.[11] Loniten (Upjohn, UK) are round, white, biconvex tablets with the dosage strength imprinted on one side and scored on the other with a 'U' on either side of the score. Each tablet contains 2.5 mg, 5 mg, 10 mg or 25 mg minoxidil.

In the USA two strengths are available (Upjohn, USA): 2.5 mg and 10 mg. In addition to the above markings, they are imprinted under the 'U' symbol with the code '121' on the 2.5 mg tablets.

The tablets are stable and have a shelf-life of 5 years at controlled room temperature. They should be protected from light.

Minoxidil

M

Therapeutic use

Indications

1. Minoxidil is used in the treatment of severe hypertension.
2. It is used in topical form in the treatment of male pattern baldness.

Contraindications

1. Phaeochromocytoma.
2. Hypersensitivity to any of the components of the preparation.

Mode of use

Minoxidil is usually only employed after more conventional antihypertensive drugs have failed to control blood pressure. The initial adult daily dose is usually 5 mg. This may be given as a single or divided dosage. The dose may first be increased to 10 mg daily and subsequent increases should be by increments of 10 mg in the daily dose. Dosage adjustments should be made at intervals of not less than three days, until optimum control of blood pressure is achieved. It is seldom necessary to exceed 50 mg per day although in exceptional circumstances doses up to 100 mg per day have been used. Once or twice-daily dosage is satisfactory. Where diastolic pressure reduction of less than 30 mg Hg is required, once-daily dosing has been reported as effective. Usually the patient will already be receiving antihypertensive therapy. If this includes a β-blocker or diuretic these should be maintained. If β-blockade is not contraindicated it is preferable to combine treatment with a β-blocker (equivalent of 80–160 mg propranolol daily) to limit reflex cardiovascular sympathetic activity. There is some evidence that sympathetic activation and therefore the need for β-blockade become less important with the passage of time.[12] Sodium retention requires simultaneous diuretic treatment in almost all cases. The dose and potency of diuretic regime varies greatly, but in general more potent diuretics are necessary in patients with renal failure. Milder sodium retention can be treated with hydrochlorothiazide 50–100 mg daily (or other thiazides), whilst more severe sodium retention in renal failure patients may require a loop diuretic (e.g. frusemide 40–500 mg daily).

In the treatment of alopecia 1.0 ml of minoxidil lotion or 0.5 g of minoxidil ointment are applied to affected areas twice daily (total daily dose should not exceed 2 ml).[11]

Indications

1. Severe hypertension

Minoxidil is particularly useful in hypertension that is symptomatic or associated with target organ damage. It is used in the treatment of hypertension not controlled adequately by a combination of a diuretic and β-blocker or by maximum therapeutic doses of a diuretic plus two other hypertensive drugs.

2. Male pattern baldness

Evidence of hair growth was seen after 4 months of treatment and continued through one year of treatment. As systemic absorption of the topically-applied drug may occur, the contraindications for minoxidil should still apply.

Contraindications

The clinical manifestations of phaeochromocytoma may be precipitated by minoxidil.

Adverse reactions

Potentially life-threatening effects

Electrocardiographic changes are often observed shortly after beginning minoxidil therapy (within two weeks). These take the form of ST depression and T-wave inversion. They are particularly apparent in left ventricular leads.[13,14] These changes have been observed in as many as 90% of patients.[15] They may revert after 3–6 months or may persist. They are not associated with elevation of cardiac enzymes or other evidence of cardiac damage. Reflex tachycardia, uncontrolled by β-blockade may produce angina in patients with ischaemic heart disease. There are several case reports of pericardial effusion, sometimes progressing to tamponade and death. In a retrospective review, 91 instances of clinically-relevant pericardial effusions were identified in 1869 patients treated with minoxidil.[16] In 21 cases tamponade occurred. Two explanations have been put forward. It has been suggested that effusions are not more frequent in minoxidil-treated patients than in other renal failure patients not taking this drug.[16] On the other hand, rechallenge with minoxidil has resulted in reappearance of the effusion.[8] It seems more likely therefore that pericardial effusion is a manifestation of the same changes as cause fluid accumulation in other tissues, that is, redistribution of Starling forces in the pericardial and superficial myocardial capillaries.

Patients have been described in whom pulmonary hypertension occurred when minoxidil was used as part of a combination regime.[17] This has been attributed to an increase in cardiac output and pulmonary blood flow with a lesser decrease in pulmonary vascular resistance. The effect is probably not of great clinical importance as most patients will also be receiving β-adrenoceptor blockers which will limit the rise in cardiac output.

Rebound hypertension has been reported,[18] although this is not recorded elsewhere and may simply reflect loss of blood pressure control in patients with severe hypertension.

Acute overdosage

A two-year-old boy who took approximately 20 tablets of minoxidil suffered no symptoms other than tachycardia.[19] Excessive hypotension as a result of minoxidil should be treated by administration of volume expanders and if absolutely necessary vasoconstrictor agents other than adrenaline or noradrenaline.

Fig. 1 Metabolism of minoxidil

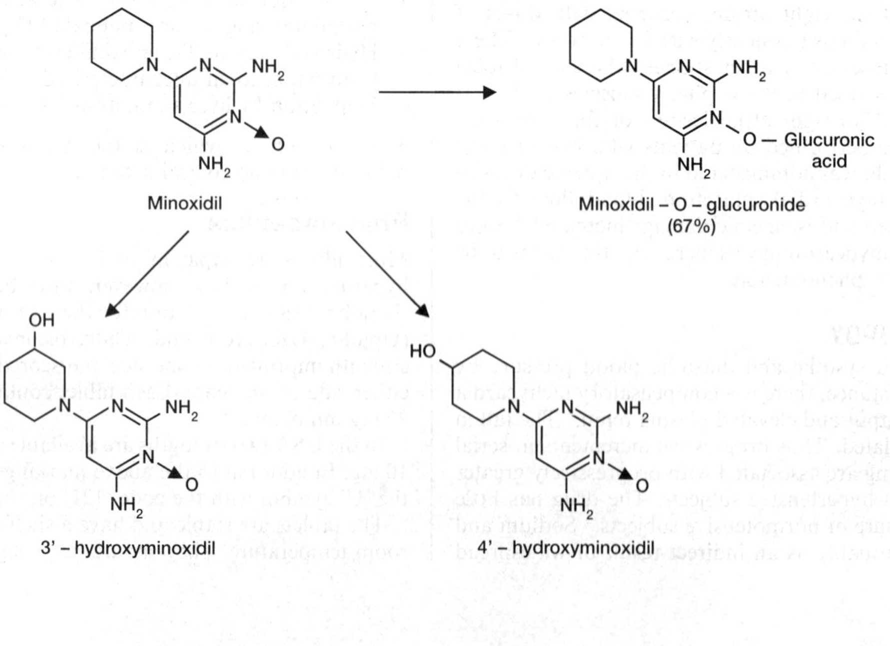

Minoxidil

Severe or irreversible adverse effects

Fluid retention manifested by oedema and ascites is probably due to a local action of minoxidil increasing the capillary hydrostatic pressure and therefore encouraging the formation of interstitial fluid. Renal retention of sodium and water is probably secondary to this. It is noteworthy that fluid retention can also be demonstrated in anuric patients on dialysis.[20]

Symptomatic adverse effects

Hypertrichosis of some degree occurs in nearly all patients. Increased growth, thickening and enhanced pigmentation of lanugo hair involves particularly the temples, forehead, face, pinnae of the ear, eyebrows, forearm and finally all the hair-bearing surfaces. It is particularly apparent in dark-haired individuals and is often intolerable in women. It disappears within 1–6 months of discontinuing the drug. Depilatories and shaving are the only effective treatment. Mild nausea and breast tenderness occasionally occur.

Adverse effects common to other vasodilators, for example flushing, palpitations and headache, are often seen in patients not simultaneously under treatment with β-blockers. Hypersensitive skin rashes have occasionally been reported and rarely Stephens-Johnson Syndrome. Redness of the conjunctivae, menstrual disturbances and thrombocytopenia have been described but the relationship to minoxidil treatment is uncertain.

Other effects

Glucose intolerance has been described,[21] but this has not been observed in other series.

Interference with clinical pathology tests

Stimulation of catecholamine release may cause a false positive when catecholamine measurements are used for diagnosing phaeochromocytoma.

High risk groups

Neonates

There is no clinical experience with minoxidil in this group.

Breast milk. Minoxidil is excreted into breast milk: slightly higher plasma concentrations than those found in milk are observed in the first hour. Thereafter similar concentrations occur in milk and plasma. Breast-feeding should not, as a general rule, be carried out by women on minoxidil.

Children

Minoxidil has been used successfully in treating hypertension in children.[22] For patients of 12 years of age or under, the initial dose should be 0.2 $mg.kg^{-1}$ given as a single or divided daily dose. Incremental increases of 0.1–0.2 $mg.kg^{-1}$ in the daily dose are recommended at intervals of not less than three days until optimum blood pressure control has been achieved. Effective dosage range is usually 0.25–1.0 $mg.kg^{-1}$ daily with a maximum daily dosage of 50 mg.

Pregnant women

Although no teratologenic effects have been observed in pregnant rats and rabbits treated with doses several times that employed in man, the safety of minoxidil in pregnancy has not been established and it should only be used where it is considered to be essential.

The elderly

The elderly may be more sensitive to the hypotensive action of minoxidil and a lower starting dose (e.g. 2.5 mg) may be necessary. There have been no pharmacokinetic studies of minoxidil in the elderly.

Drug interactions

Potentially hazardous interactions

There is a report of an enhanced hypotensive effect when minoxidil was given with neuroleptics.[23] Topical minoxidil absorption may be increased by topical corticosteroids, retinoids, petrolatum or other agents which enhance cutaneous drug absorption.

Potentially useful interactions

β-blockers inhibit the baroreceptor-mediated tachycardia, whilst diuretics oppose sodium retention produced by minoxidil therapy. There is probably a synergistic effect when converting enzyme inhibitors are combined with minoxidil; this may be therapeutically useful, although there is a risk of excessive blood pressure lowering. Clonidine and methyldopa may also have an additive effect by central inhibition of sympathetic outflow.

Major outcome trials

1. Devine B L, Fife R, Trust P M 1977 Minoxidil for severe hypertension after failure of other hypotensive drugs. British Medical Journal 2: 667–669

44 patients were studied in an open uncontrolled investigation who could either not tolerate other antihypertensive medication or whose blood pressure was not controlled. Treatment with minoxidil was combined routinely with β-blockade and diuretics. Outpatient blood pressure fell from 221/134 mmHg to 162/98 mmHg. 11 patients required additional or alternative antihypertensive therapy. Hirsuites was observed in all patients and was unacceptable to three women.

2. Mehta P K, Mamdani B, Shansky R M, Mahurkar S D, Dunea G 1975 Severe hypertension: treatment with minoxidil. Journal of the American Medical Association 233: 249–252

17 patients who were partially or totally refractory to maximal doses of conventional antihypertensive agents were treated with minoxidil in combination with propranolol and diuretics. Control was excellent in 16 but blood pressure was resistant to doses of minoxidil up to 60 mg daily in the seventeenth. Blood pressure rose again in three patients and guanethidine was required to control it. The major side effects of minoxidil were fluid retention, hypertrichosis and coarsening of facial features.

3. Swales J D, Bing R F, Heagerty A M, Pohl J E F, Russell G I, Thurston H 1982 Treatment of refractory hypertension. Lancet 1: 894–896

126 patients are reported in whom blood pressure was unacceptably high despite maximal doses of agents in a conventional, stepped care regime. One of four regimes was used: oral diazoxide, captopril, quadruple therapy (diuretic, β-blocker, hydralazine and prazosin) and minoxidil. Minoxidil was the most frequently used therapy (70 patients) in doses up to 60 mg daily. Oedema was a particular problem requiring up to 1 g frusemide per day to control it. 49 patients remained on minoxidil long-term with good blood pressure control; four patients were taken on to a dialysis programme; two patients were taken off minoxidil because of side effects (rash and recurrent arrhythmias). In two patients blood pressure could not be controlled and other therapy was used. Minoxidil treatment was unacceptable in one woman who defaulted from the clinic. Seven patients died and the remainder showed a sustained fall in blood pressure following myocardial infarction and no longer required minoxidil.

Controlled trials

1. Dargie H J, Daniel J, Dollery C T 1978 Minoxidil in resistant hypertension. Lancet 2: 515–518

In this trial, 30 patients were included in whom diastolic blood pressure was more than 110 mmHg despite large doses of three or more standard drugs. They were then randomly allocated to a minoxidil group or a control group. Drugs in the control group patients were adjusted to gain optimal control of blood pressure. Patients in the minoxidil group were admitted to hospital and all drugs except for propranolol and a diuretic withdrawn. Minoxidil was then started in doses up to 40 mg daily. Blood pressure was followed for 6 months. Blood pressure reduction in the minoxidil group was significantly better than in the control group (supine BP from 191/115 to 153/93 in the minoxidil group and 189/114 to 176/106 in the control group). The main problem in the minoxidil group was fluid retention. Patients felt better on minoxidil with less sleepiness, postural dizziness or dryness of the mouth, although hypertrichosis was observed in all patients.

General review articles

Editorial: Minoxidil for severe hypertension. Drugs and Therapeutics Bulletin 19: 5–7

Pettinger W A 1980 Minoxidil and the treatment of severe hypertension. New England Journal of Medicine 303: 922–926

M

References

1. Gilmore E, Weil J, Chidsey C 1970 Treatment of essential hypertension with a new vasodilator in combination with beta adrenergic blockade. New England Journal of Medicine 282: 521–527
2. Sobota J T 1989 Review of cardiovascular findings in humans treated with minoxidil. Toxicological Pathology 17: 193–202
3. Radvany P, Davis M A, Muller J A, Maroko P R 1978 Effects of minoxidil on coronary collateral flow and acute myocardial injury following experimental coronary artery occlusion. Cardiovascular Research 12: 120–126
4. O'Malley K, Velasco M, Wells J, McNay J L 1975 Control plasma renin activity and changes in sympathetic tone as determinants of minoxidil induced increased in plasma renin activity. Journal of Clinical Investigation 55: 230–235
5. Lowenthal D T, Affrime M B 1980 Pharmacology and pharmacokinetics of minoxidil. Journal of Cardiovascular Pharmacology 2 (suppl 2): S93–S106
6. Pluss R G, Orcutt J, Chidsey C A 1972 Tissue distribution and hypotensive effects of minoxidil in normotensive rats. Journal of Laboratory Clinical Medicine 79: 639–647
7. Royer M E, Ko H, Golbertson T J, McCall J M, Johnston K T, Stryd R 1977 Radioimmunoassay of minoxidil in human serum. Journal of Pharmaceutical Science 66: 1266–1269
8. Campese V M 1981 Minoxidil: a review of its pharmacological properties and therapeutic use. Drugs 22: 257–278
9. Bennett W M, Golper T A, Muther R S, McCarron D A 1980 Efficacy of minoxidil in the treatment of severe hypertension in systemic disorders. Journal of Cardiology Pharmacology 2 (suppl 2): S142–S148
10. Gottlieb T B, Thomas R C, Chidsey C A 1972 Pharmacokinetic studies of minoxidil. Clinical Pharmacology Therapeutics 13: 436–441
11. Fenton D A, Wilkinson J D 1983 Topical minoxidil in the treatment of alopecia areata. British Medical Journal 287: 1015–1017
12. Brunner Hr, Jaeger P, Ferguson R K, Jequier E, Turini G, Gavras H 1978 Need for beta-blockade in hypertension reduced with long-term minoxidil. British Medical Journal 2: 385–388
13. Ryan J R, Jain A K, McMahon R G 1975 Minoxidil treatment of severe hypertension. Current Therapeutic Research 17: 55–66
14. Bryan R K, Hoobler S W, Rosenzweig J, Weller J M, Purdy J M 1977 Effect of minoxidil on blood pressure and hemodynamics in severe hypertension. American Journal of Cardiology 39: 796–801
15. Hall D, Froer K L, Rudolph W 1980 Serial electrocardiographic changes during long-term treatment of severe hypertension with minoxidil. Journal of Cardiological Pharmacology 2 (suppl 2): S200–S205
16. Martin W B, Spodick D H, Zins G R 1980 Pericardial disorders occurring during open study of 1869 severely hypertensive patients treated with minoxidil. Journal of Cardiological Pharmacology 2 (suppl 2): S217–S227
17. Hall D, Froer K L, Loracher L 1976 Treatment of severe hypertension with minoxidil and its effect on systemic and pulmonary haemodynamics. Clinical Science and Molecular Medicine 51 (suppl 1): 587s–589s
18. Makker S P, Morthy B 1980 Rebound hypertension following minoxidil withdrawal. Journal of Paediatrics 96: 762
19. Isles C, Mackay A, Barton P J M, Mitchell I 1981 Accidental overdose of minoxidil in a child. Lancet 1: 97
20. Keusch G W, Weidmann P, Campese V, Lee D B N, Uphan A, Massry S G 1978 Minoxidil therapy in refractory hypertension: analysis of 155 patients. Nephron 21: 4–15
21. Oka M, Makela M 1978 Minoxidil in severe hypertension. Acta Medica Scandinavica 203: 43–47
22. Pennisi A J, Takahashi M, Berstein B H et al 1977 Minoxidil therapy in children with severe hypertension. Journal of Pediatrics 90: 813–819
23. Sakman C, Hoffman S A 1983 Clinical interaction between psychotropic and other drugs. Hospital Community Psychiatry 34: 397–402

Misoprostol

Misoprostol is a prostaglandin E_1 analogue developed for the treatment of peptic ulcers and which is used in the treatment and prevention of non-steroidal anti-inflammatory drug-induced gastro-intestinal damage.

Chemistry

Misoprostol (Cytotec)
$C_{22}H_{38}O_5$
DL-Methyl-11α-16-dihydroxy-16-methyl-9-oxoprost-13E-en-1-oate
Misoprostol is a synthetic prostaglandin E_1 methyl ester analogue and exists in a 1:1 mixture of two diastereoisomers. The structure of the parent prostaglandin E_1 is also shown for comparison

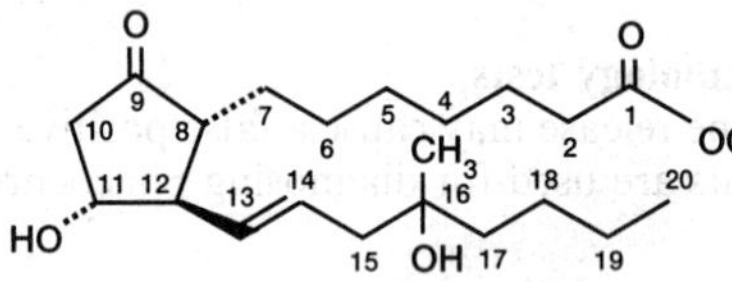

Misoprostol

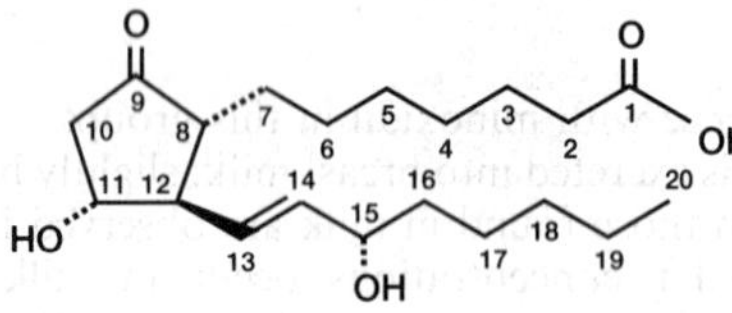

Prostaglandin E_1

Molecular weight	382.5
pKa	not relevant
Solubility	
in alcohol	1 in 100
in water	1 in 2500
Octanol/water partition coefficient	—

Pure misoprostol is a viscous, clear, yellowish oil with a musty odour. Misoprostol (Cytotec) tablets contain the following excipients: hydroxypropyl methylcellulose 2910, microcrystalline cellulose, sodium starch glycolate and hydrogenated castor oil.

Pharmacology

Misoprostol has gastric antisecretory[1–4] and mucosal 'cytoprotective'[5,6] effects in man as well as in various animal models. The antisecretory activity of misoprostol is thought to be mediated through a class of high affinity E-type prostaglandin receptors on the gastric parietal cell surface (approx. 8000 receptors per cell).[7] In preparations of enriched canine gastric parietal cells misoprostol, as well as its major acid metabolite (SC-30 695), binds to these receptors saturably, reversibly, and stereospecifically. This receptor-binding activity correlates well with the ability of misoprostol, and of its acid metabolite, to inhibit histamine-stimulated acid production by the parietal cells. The mechanisms underlying the mucosal cytoprotective effects of misoprostol are less clear, and will be discussed later (see Clinical pharmacology).

Toxicology

The oral LD_{50} values in mice, rats and dogs are approximately 27–138 $mg.kg^{-1}$, 81–100 $mg.kg^{-1}$ and 9 $mg.kg^{-1}$ respectively (these are single oral doses). Dogs given overdoses of misoprostol develop tremors, mydriasis and diarrhoea.

Misoprostol has no mutagenic potential. Over a 2-year testing period in rats, no evidence of carcinogenicity appeared. Large doses of misoprostol (e.g. 300 μg.kg^{-1}) result in gastric mucosal hyperplasia in animals. This is a characteristic response to prostaglandins of the E series, and the mucosa reverts to normal on discontinuation of the compound. No such changes have been noted in humans after treatment with misoprostol for up to one year.

Although there is no evidence of embryotoxicity, very large doses (above 1600 μg.kg^{-1}) have reduced the number of implantations in rat fertility studies.

Clinical pharmacology

In man, misoprostol has clinically significant antisecretory activity mediated by direct action on gastric parietal cells, as well as mucosal cytoprotective properties in the stomach and duodenum.

In the recommended therapeutic doses, the drug achieves significant reductions in unstimulated nocturnal gastric acid secretion, as well as in basal, food-, histamine-, pentagastrin-, betazole- and coffee-stimulated gastric acid secretion.[1–4,6,8,9] Thus, in a healthy adult, a single 200 μg oral dose reduces nocturnal acid output by over 50% in the 2–4 hour post-dose period. Doses of 100 μg or less do not significantly reduce nocturnal acid, but 100 μg given orally will significantly inhibit histamine- and food-stimulated acid production. Studies of the duration of antisecretory effects of misoprostol have shown that the peak inhibitory effect of misoprostol is reached 30–90 minutes after administration, and that acid output is reduced by 58% over a period of 7 hours.[9] The proteolytic activity of gastric juice is concomitantly reduced.

The mechanisms underlying the mucosal cytoprotective effects of misoprostol and other prostaglandins and their derivatives have been much debated,[10–12] and are less clearly understood than the mechanisms behind its antisecretory activity. Cytoprotection may be defined as the ability to protect the gastrointestinal mucosa against damage by injurious agents through mechanism(s) independent of acid inhibition. Cytoprotection is believed to result from an enhancement of physiological mucosal defence mechanisms that are normally achieved by endogenous mucosal prostaglandins. These activities include:

1. Stimulation of gastric mucus secretion
2. Stimulation of duodenal bicarbonate secretion
3. Stimulation of gastric mucosal blood flow
4. Other activities, including the strengthening of intercellular tight junctions.

Misoprostol achieves each of the first three foregoing functions in human volunteers. Thus, it increases gastric mucus[8] and duodenal bicarbonate[13] secretion dose dependently. The mucus–bicarbonate barrier protects against mechanical abrasion of the gastric epithelium, and the damaging effects of hydrogen ions. In addition, endoscopic organ reflectance spectrophotometry shows a 10–25% increase in mucosal blood volume measured at 20 different gastric locations after a 200 μg dose.[14]

Cytoprotection has been confirmed against a range of injurious agents, including alcohol, hypertonic solutions and thermal injury.[5,6] Most notably, however, cytoprotection appears to be conferred against damage by the non-steroidal anti-inflammatory drugs (NSAIDs), which are widely prescribed for arthritis, and are associated with gastroduodenal bleeding and ulceration. As cyclo-oxygenase inhibitors, NSAIDs inhibit the production of mucosal prostaglandins. Exogenous prostanoids, such as misoprostol, may therefore be a logical choice in the protection against such damage and, indeed, studies using aspirin and a range of non-aspirin NSAIDs confirm the ability of misoprostol to prevent as well as heal gastric and duodenal damage in healthy subjects[15–21] as well as in patients with arthritis.[22–24]

Misoprostol reduces small bowel transit time, and increases stool water and electrolyte losses, in volunteers given 400 μg four times daily orally. This effect is greater than that seen at the recommended therapeutic dose (200 μg four times daily for ulcer healing), and is also significantly less marked when the tablets are taken after meals. No significant effects are noted on the rate of gastric emptying. No significant effects on blood pressure or cardiac function have been noted during misoprostol therapy.

Pharmacokinetics

Misoprostol, and its major active metabolite misoprostol acid, are estimated by sensitive radioimmunoassays, with a detection limit of 23 ng.l^{-1} for the latter.

In man misoprostol is rapidly absorbed, extensively metabolized and rapidly excreted. It is estimated that 88% of an oral dose of misoprostol is absorbed in man. Absorption of misoprostol and its active de-esterified derivative misoprostol acid is extremely rapid. However, almost no unchanged misoprostol is detectable in plasma 5 minutes after dosing.[25] This is because misoprostol is rapidly metabolized by fatty acid oxidizing systems present in organs throughout the body. The major active metabolite, misoprostol acid, peaks 15–30 minutes after an oral dose, and disappears with an elimination half life of approximately 21 minutes.[25] Steady-state plasma concentrations of misoprostol acid on twice daily misoprostol dosing are achieved by day 2.[25] Following the first dose of misoprostol the C_{max}, AUC and half life values were 634 ± 113 ng.l^{-1}, 353 ± 82 ng.h.l^{-1} and 26.9 ± 12.1 min, respectively. At steady state on day 4 these values were 688 ± 268 ng.l^{-1}, 294 ± 87 ng.h^{-1}.l^{-1} and 17.6 ± 7.1 min, respectively. There were no statistically significant differences between the day 1 and 4 values for these parameters.[25] No plasma accumulation of misoprostol or misoprostol acid occurs after repeated dosing of 400 μg twice daily. Serum protein binding of misoprostol acid is approximately 81–89%, and is age independent.

Given with a high-fat meal, the absorption of misoprostol is markedly slowed, although there is no substantial decrease in the net absorption. Administration with large doses of antacids does, however, reduce the bioavailability of misoprostol. NSAIDs do not affect misoprostol absorption.

Elderly subjects show no significant differences in peak plasma concentrations (C_{max}) after an oral dose, nor in elimination half life but they do show a somewhat higher AUC. This may be due to a reduced volume of distribution in the elderly. This finding is not considered clinically relevant as clinical trials show no differences in the efficacy or side effect profiles between young and elderly patients.

Oral absorption	88%
Presystemic metabolism	extensive
Plasma half life	
misoprostol acid	21 min
Volume of distribution	858 l
Plasma protein binding	
misoprostol acid	81–89%

Concentration–effect relationship

No studies have investigated the relationship between plasma levels of misoprostol (or misoprostol acid) and antisecretory activity. Considering the short plasma half life of misoprostol such correlations would be unlikely.

Metabolism

Misoprostol is metabolized by fatty acid oxidizing systems (β and ω oxidation) present throughout the body.

The metabolism of misoprostol in man has been studied with the 17,18-tritium labelled compound. Healthy subjects ingesting this compound show no plasma radioactivity associated with unchanged misoprostol after 5 minutes. This reflects rapid metabolism of misoprostol during and/or prior to gastrointestinal absorption. Several metabolites are formed, and < 1% unchanged drug is detected in the plasma or urine.[25] One of the major metabolites in the plasma is the active de-esterified compound, misoprostol acid, and others are the more polar inactive dinor and tetranor acid metabolites.

In similar studies, 73 ± 11% of the radioactivity of an oral dose of 17,18-^{3}H-misoprostol appears in the urine during a 7-day period, mostly in the first 24 hours. Less than 1% of the dose, however, is as unchanged misoprostol or misoprostol acid. Excretion of radioactivity in the faeces amounts to 15 ± 8% of the dose, and this is attributed to biliary excretion.

Renal excretion of misoprostol or its active acid metabolite is not the major pathway of elimination of active drug. Thus, while C_{max}, AUC and elimination half life are all greater in subjects with renal impairment, the figures overlap with those for normal volunteers, and a change in dosing schedule in renal impairment is not considered necessary. Likewise, as the misoprostol oxidizing enzymes are present in several organs, its metabolism and plasma levels are unlikely to be affected significantly in patients with hepatic impairment.

Pharmaceutics

For routine clinical use, misoprostol (Cytotec; Searle, UK/USA) is available only as an oral tablet preparation. Cytotec tablets (Searle, UK) are white/off-white and hexagonal. They are scored on both sides, and engraved 'Searle 1461' on one side. Each tablet contains 200 µg of misoprostol.

Therapeutic use

Indications

1. Prophylaxis of gastric and duodenal ulceration in NSAID users
2. Healing of established NSAID-induced gastric and duodenal damage
3. Healing of gastric and duodenal ulcers in the absence of NSAID therapy
4. Miscellaneous uses, some requiring further evaluation.

Contraindications

1. Pregnant women
2. Women of childbearing age (relative contraindication, see below)
3. Allergy to prostaglandins.

Mode of use

All treatment regimes employ doses of misoprostol that achieve gastric antisecretory activity as well as mucosal cytoprotection.

For the healing of gastric and duodenal ulcers the recommended daily dose is 800 µg daily in four divided doses. It is recommended the tablets be taken after breakfast, after each main meal and at bedtime. The initial treatment period is 6 weeks, whether or not symptomatic relief has been achieved sooner. Treatment should be continued until ulcer healing has occurred; this may be confirmed by a second endoscopy. During the early phase of ulcer healing symptomatic relief of ulcer pain is best achieved with antacids in modest quantities, noting that large quantities of antacids can reduce the bioavailability of misoprostol. Whilst it has been demonstrated that misoprostol has the ability to accelerate the healing of peptic ulcers despite continued NSAID use, the decision as to whether to continue the NSAID during the phase of ulcer healing should, in the author's opinion, be based on the symptoms and clinical condition of the patient, as well as on the size and appearance of the ulcer. Appearances suggesting active or recent bleeding, for example, warrant discontinuation of the NSAID until ulcer healing has been demonstrated.

For the prophylaxis of NSAID-associated inflammation and ulceration, 200 µg given two or three times a day after meals, if possible with the NSAID, is recommended. It is suggested that the clinical condition of the patient and the dose of NSAID he/she is receiving may be used as guidelines in the choice of dose frequency.

No change of dosage is required in the elderly or in patients with mild or moderate renal or hepatic impairment (see High risk groups).

Indications

1. Prophylaxis of gastric and duodenal ulceration in NSAID users
A multicentre clinical trial has established the efficacy of misoprostol in the prevention of NSAID-associated gastric ulcers in patients with osteoarthritis.[24] The patients studied were all taking an NSAID (either ibuprofen, naproxen or piroxicam) and were expected to require it for at least a further 3 months. After an 'entry' endoscopy, patients without ulcers were admitted to the prevention phase of the study in which they received misoprostol or placebo in addition to the respective NSAID. The incidence of gastric ulcers at the end of the 3 months was 21.7% in the placebo group, 5.6% in the 100 µg four times daily misoprostol group and 1.4% in the 200 µg four times daily misoprostol group. Both misoprostol doses were superior to placebo in gastric ulcer prevention ($p<0.001$), but not significantly different from each other ($p=0.103$).

A more recent study in 130 healthy volunteers demonstrated that misoprostol in cytoprotective (50 µg four times daily) as well as full antisecretory (200 µg four times daily) doses reduces acute aspirin-induced gastric erosions and duodenal ulceration, determined endoscopically.[26]

2. Treatment of established NSAID-induced gastric damage
Misoprostol has been shown to reduce established aspirin-induced gastrointestinal blood loss in patients with arthritis.[23] However, in another study of patients on indomethacin, misoprostol failed to reduce daily blood loss.[27]

Using direct endoscopic assessment of gastric damage, misoprostol reverses established aspirin-induced gastric lesions, including gastric and duodenal ulcers, in patients with rheumatoid arthritis. Thus, after 8 weeks of treatment misoprostol (200 µg four times daily) was found to be superior to placebo in healing the gastric mucosal lesions (70% versus 25%, $p=0.0001$).[22]

3. Healing of gastric and duodenal ulcers in the absence of NSAID therapy
In the absence of NSAID therapy, misoprostol is effective in accelerating the healing of duodenal[28,29] as well as gastric ulcers;[30,31] 800 µg daily in two or four divided doses are required to achieve satisfactory healing rates.

4. Miscellaneous uses, some requiring further evaluation
A role for misoprostol in the maintenance of duodenal ulcer remission is being investigated.

Misoprostol (200 µg 4-hourly) is as effective as high-dose antacid in the prevention of stress ulceration and bleeding in postsurgical ICU patients.[32]

Although initial studies suggested that misoprostol may reduce lesion size and transfusion requirement in patients with upper gastrointestinal bleeding, other studies have failed to confirm this, and the patient numbers are small.

Concurrent administration of misoprostol with NSAIDs reduces the increase in small intestinal permeability due to NSAIDs. This permeability change may be the prerequisite of NSAID-induced small intestinal inflammation (I Bjarnason, personal communication).

Finally, a possible role for misoprostol in the prevention of renal transplant rejection is currently being investigated.

Contraindications

1. Pregnancy
Misoprostol should not be used in pregnancy as it has been noted to increase uterine tone and contractions. This may induce a miscarriage.

2. Women of childbearing age
Misoprostol should be avoided in women of childbearing age unless the patient requires NSAID therapy and is considered to be at high risk of complications from NSAID-induced ulceration. In such patients misoprostol may be used only if the patient uses effective contraceptive measures, and has been advised of the risks of taking misoprostol if pregnant.

The efficacy and safety of misoprostol in pregnancy has not yet been fully evaluated.

It should be noted that the efficacy and safety of misoprostol in children has not yet been fully evaluated.

3. Allergy to prostaglandins
This is a rare contraindication to misoprostol therapy.

Adverse reactions

Potentially life-threatening effects
Life-threatening complications of misoprostol therapy in man have not been described.

Acute overdosage
The toxic dose of misoprostol in humans, and its effects in overdosage, have not been described. Divided daily doses of 1600 µg have been tolerated, except for gastrointestinal discomfort. In animals, the acute toxic effects include central nervous system and smooth muscle effects with resulting sedation, convulsions, diarrhoea and hypotension.

It is not known whether misoprostol acid is dialysable. However, because misoprostol is metabolized quickly to fatty acids, it is

Misoprostol

unlikely that dialysis would be of benefit in overdosage. No specific antidote is available.

Severe or irreversible adverse effects
In pregnancy, the adverse effects of misoprostol can be serious. In studies of women undergoing elective termination of pregnancy during the first trimester, misoprostol caused partial or complete expulsion of the products of conception in 11% of the patients, and increased uterine bleeding in 41%. Therefore, misoprostol should not be used in pregnancy.

Symptomatic adverse effects
The most frequent symptomatic adverse effects of misoprostol are gastrointestinal, and include dose-dependent diarrhoea, abdominal pain, and flatulence. The incidence of diarrhoea in clinical studies was about 11%, usually being mild and disappearing within one week despite continuation of misoprostol therapy. This has required discontinuation of misoprostol therapy in approximately 2% of cases. Nausea and headache have also been noted. Misoprostol-associated diarrhoea, resulting from an increase in gut motility, may be minimized by taking the drug after meals, temporarily reducing the dose, and by avoiding magnesium-containing antacids which can themselves cause diarrhoea.

Gynaecological adverse effects include spotting, cramps, dysmenorrhoea and hypermenorrhoea, but these are rare.

Other effects
Using the Fogarty International Commission guidelines[33] to determine any potential hepatotoxicity of misoprostol, small numbers of patients were found to have developed abnormal liver function tests whilst on misoprostol, but these were generally considered to be unrelated to the study medication.

Interference with clinical pathology tests
No technical interferences of this kind have been described.

High risk groups

Neonates
The use of misoprostol in neonates has not been studied.

Breast milk. It is not known whether misoprostol's active metabolite, misoprostol acid, is excreted in human milk. Use in this group of women is also contraindicated.

Children
Use of misoprostol in children should await formal studies of efficacy and safety.

Pregnant women
Misoprostol can cause uterine bleeding and miscarriage and must not be used in pregnancy.

Pre-menopausal women
The use of misoprostol in pre-menopausal women is discussed under Contraindications.

The elderly
Despite minor pharmacokinetic differences the safety and efficacy profile of misoprostol is the same in the elderly population as it is in young adults. Therefore, no additional precautions in the elderly are required.

Concurrent disease
In renal impairment no change of dosage is needed. This is because misoprostol and its active metabolite are inactivated by fatty acid oxidizing systems and renal excretion is not the mode of active drug elimination.

Drug interactions

Potentially hazardous interactions
None is known.

Other significant interactions
There is no evidence of clinically significant interactions between misoprostol and cardiac, pulmonary or central nervous system drugs, or with NSAIDs. Misoprostol has no significant effects on the cytochrome P450 enzyme system.

Food. High fat foods slow down the absorption of misoprostol, but do not affect its bioavailability. This is a potentially useful interaction, for administration of misoprostol after food may ameliorate the symptomatic gastrointestinal adverse effects.

Antacids. Antacids in high doses can significantly reduce the bioavailability of misoprostol.[34] 'As required' usage, however, for example during ulcer healing studies for symptomatic relief, has no effect on the efficacy of misoprostol.

Potentially useful interactions
The only potentially useful interaction is that with food mentioned above.

Major outcome trials

1. Roth S, Agrawal N, Mahowald M et al 1989 Misoprostol heals gastroduodenal injury in patients with rheumatoid arthritis receiving aspirin. Archives of Internal Medicine 149: 775–779

This study was designed to test the efficacy of misoprostol in reversing established aspirin-induced damage in patients with rheumatoid arthritis. 238 patients were endoscoped and then randomly assigned to receive either misoprostol 200 µg four times daily or placebo. Each subject received aspirin (650–1300 mg four times daily) concurrently. Initially, all subjects had significant mucosal lesions (a score greater than 3 on a 7 point rating scale). Endoscopic assessments were repeated after 4 and 8 weeks of treatment. After 8 weeks, misoprostol was found to be superior to placebo in the healing of gastric mucosal lesions (70% versus 25%, $p=0.0001$) as well as duodenal mucosal lesions (86% versus 53%, $p=0.0014$).

2. Ryan J R, Vargas R, Clay G A, McMahon F G 1987 Role of misoprostol in reducing aspirin-induced gastrointestinal blood loss in arthritic patients. American Journal of Medicine 83 (1A): 41–44

This study assessed the ability of misoprostol to reduce aspirin-induced gastrointestinal blood loss in patients with rheumatoid or osteoarthritis. 41 patients completed the study. Each patient received 3.6 g of aspirin daily for 4 weeks. After 2 weeks of aspirin, patients underwent a 7-day ^{51}Cr faecal blood loss estimation. Those who had a mean daily blood loss in excess of 1.5 ml entered the fourth week of the study during which they received 200 µg misoprostol four times daily or placebo. Stools were collected again for assessment of blood loss. 11 of 19 patients who received misoprostol (57%), and only 1 of 22 patients who received placebo (4.5%), showed reductions in faecal blood loss of 50% or more ($p=0.0003$).

3. Graham D Y, Agrawal N M, Roth S H 1988 Prevention of NSAID-induced gastric ulcer with misoprostol: multicentre, double-blind, placebo-controlled trial. Lancet 2: 1277–1280

This was a multicentre placebo controlled clinical trial of the efficacy of misoprostol in preventing the development of NSAID-associated gastric ulcers in patients with osteoarthritis. The 420 patients studied were all receiving either ibuprofen, naproxen or piroxicam, and were expected to require their respective NSAID for at least a further 3 months. The mean age was 58.9 years (range 22–90 years). Approximately 15% of patients were smokers. Patients had an 'entry' endoscopy and were admitted to the study only if an ulcer was not present. They then entered the prophylaxis phase and received, in addition to the NSAID, either placebo, 100 µg misoprostol four times daily, or 200 µg misoprostol four times daily. This medication was continued for 3 months, during which, at 4-weekly intervals, patients were re-endoscoped. The incidence of gastric ulcers at the end of 3 months was 21.7% ($n=138$) in the placebo group, 5.6% ($n=143$) in the 100 µg misoprostol group, and 1.4% ($n=139$) in the 200 µg misoprostol group. Both misoprostol doses were superior to placebo in gastric ulcer prevention ($p=0.001$), but there was no statistically significant difference between the two misoprostol dose regimes ($p=0.103$).

4. Moran M, Mozes M F, Maddux M S et al 1990 Prevention of acute graft rejection by the prostaglandin E_1 analogue misoprostol in renal-transplant recipients treated with cyclosporine and prednisone. New England Journal of Medicine 322: 1183–1188

A randomized double-blind placebo-controlled trial was carried out in 77 renal allograft recipients. The actively treated patients received

M

misoprostol 200 μg four times daily for 12 weeks after transplant and were observed for a further 4 weeks after its cessation.

10 of 38 patients who received misoprostol developed acute rejection episodes against 20 of 39 on placebo (p = 0.03). Blood levels of cyclosporine, and nephrotoxicity due to it, were higher in the misoprostol group but infectious complications were fewer.

General review articles

Bauer R F 1985 Misoprostol preclinical pharmacology. Digestive Diseases and Sciences 30: 118S–125S

Herting R L, Clay G A 1985 Overview and clinical safety with misoprostol. Digestive Diseases and Sciences 30: 185S–193S

Konturek S J, Pawlik W 1986 Physiology and pharmacology of prostaglandins. Digestive Diseases and Sciences 31: 6S–19S

Roth S H, Bennett R E 1987 Non-steroidal anti-inflammatory drug gastropathy: recognition and response. Archives of Internal Medicine 147: 2093–2100

References

1. Bauer R F 1985 Misoprostol preclinical pharmacology. Digestive Diseases and Sciences 30: 118S–125S
2. Makamura T, Niwa H, Muto H 1986 Misoprostol inhibits basal gastric secretion in humans (abstract). Gastroenterology 90: 1562
3. Akdamar K, Agrawal N, Ertan A 1982 Inhibition of nocturnal gastric secretion in normal human volunteers by misoprostol: a synthetic prostaglandin E_1 methyl ester analog. American Journal of Gastroenterology 77: 902–904
4. Davis G R, Fortran J S, Dajani E Z 1988 Dose response, meal-stimulated gastric antisecretory study of prostaglandin E_1 analog, misoprostol, in man. Digestive Diseases and Sciences 30: 298–302
5. Dajani E Z, Nissen C H 1985 Gastrointestinal cytoprotective effects of misoprostol. Digestive Diseases and Sciences 30: 194S–200S
6. Wilson D E 1987 Antisecretory and mucosal protective actions of misoprostol: potential role in the treatment of peptic ulcer disease. American Journal of Medicine 83 (suppl 1A): 3–8
7. Tsai B S, Kessler L K, Bauer R F 1986 Correlation of ^{3}H-misoprostol free acid binding and anti-secretory activity in enriched canine parietal cells. Gastroenterology 90: 1671
8. Wilson D E, Quadros E, Rajapaksa T, Adams A, Noar M 1986 Effects of misoprostol on gastric acid and mucus secretion in man. Digestive Diseases and Sciences 31: 126S–129S
9. Mutoh H, Niwa H, Nakamura T, Yanaka A 1988 Misoprostol inhibits nocturnal gastric secretion in humans. Digestive Diseases and Sciences 31: 200S
10. Konturek S J, Pawlik W 1986 Physiology and pharmacology of prostaglandins. Digestive Diseases and Sciences 31: 6S–19S
11. Jacobson E D 1986 Direct and adaptive cytoprotection. Digestive Diseases and Sciences 31: 28S–31S
12. Robert A 1976 Antisecretory, antiulcer, cytoprotective and diarrheogenic properties of prostaglandins. In: Samuelsson B, Paoletti R (eds) Advances in prostaglandin and thromboxane research, vol 2. Raven Press, New York
13. Selling J A, Hogan D L, Koss M A, Isenberg J I 1985 Prostaglandin E_1 (misoprostol) stimulates human duodenal mucosal bicarbonate secretion (Abstract). Gastroenterology 85: 1580
14. Sato N, Kawano S, Fukada M, Tsuji S, Kamada T 1987 Misoprostol-induced changes in gastric mucosal hemodynamics. American Journal of Medicine 83 (suppl 1A): 15–21
15. Cohen M M, Clark L, Armstrong L, D'Souza J 1985 Reduction of aspirin-induced fecal blood loss with low-dose misoprostol tablets in man. Digestive Diseases and Sciences 30: 605–611
16. Silverstein F E 1986 Gastric protection by misoprostol against 1300 mg of aspirin: an endoscopic study. Digestive Diseases and Sciences 31: 137S–141S
17. Silverstein F E, Kimmey M B, Jiranek R A, Wilson R A, Saunders D R 1988 Misoprostol protects the normal gastroduodenum against 7 days of aspirin (abstract). Gastroenterology 94: A428
18. Lanza F, Peace K E, Gustitus L, Rack M F, Dickson B 1988 A blinded endoscopic comparative study of misoprostol versus sucralfate and placebo in the prevention of aspirin-induced gastric and duodenal ulceration. American Journal of Gastroenterology 83: 143–146
19. Aadland E, Fausa O, Vatn M, Cohen H, Quinlan D 1987 Protection by misoprostol against naproxen-induced gastric mucosal damage. American Journal of Medicine 83 (suppl 1A): 37–40
20. Lanza F L 1986 Prophylactic effect of misoprostol on lesions of the gastric mucosa induced by oral administration of tolmetin in healthy subjects. Digestive Disorders and Sciences 31: 131S–136S
21. Lanza F L, Aspinall R, Swabb E, Davies R, Rack M, Rubin A 1988 Double-blind, placebo-controlled endoscopic comparison of the mucosal protective effects of misoprostol versus cimetidine on tolmetin-induced mucosal injury to the stomach and duodenum. Gastroenterology 95: 289–294
22. Roth S, Agrawal N, Mahowald M et al 1989 Misoprostol heals gastroduodenal injury in patients with rheumatoid arthritis receiving aspirin. Archives of Internal Medicine 149: 775–779
23. Ryan J R, Vargas R, Clay G A, McMahon F G 1987 Role of misoprostol in reducing aspirin-induced gastrointestinal blood loss in arthritic patients. American Journal of Medicine 83 (suppl 1A): 41–44
24. Graham D Y, Agrawal N M, Roth R H 1988 Prevention of NSAID-induced gastric ulcer with misoprostol: multicenter, double-blind placebo-controlled trial. Lancet 2: 1277–1280
25. Karim A 1986 Antiulcer prostaglandin misoprostol: single and multiple dose pharmacokinetic profile. Prostaglandins 33 (suppl): 40–50
26. Jiranek G C, Kimmey M B, Saunders D R, Willson R A, Shanahan W, Silverstein F E 1989 Misoprostol reduces gastroduodenal injury from one week of aspirin: an endoscopic study. Gastroenterology 96: 656–661
27. Jallad N S, Garg D C, Heal A V, Weidler D J 1986 Effects of misoprostol on previously established and continuing fecal blood loss in arthritic patients receiving indomethacin (abstract). Journal of Clinical Pharmacology 26: 559
28. Sontag S J, Mazure P A, Pontes J F, Beker S G, Dajani E Z 1985 Misoprostol in the treatment of duodenal ulcer: a multicenter double-blind placebo-controlled study. Digestive Diseases and Sciences 30: 159S–163S
29. Brand D L, Roufail W M, Thomson A B R Tapper E J 1985 Misoprostol synthetic PGE_1 analog, in the treatment of duodenal ulcers: a multicenter double-blind study. Digestive Diseases and Sciences 30: 147S–158S
30. Agrawal N M, Saffouri B, Kruss D M, Callison D A, Dajani E Z 1985 Healing of benign gastric ulcer: a placebo-controlled comparison of two dosage regimens of misoprostol. Digestive Diseases and Sciences 30: 164S–170S
31. Rachmilewitz D, Chapman J W, Nicholson P A 1986 A multicenter international controlled comparison of two dosage regimens of misoprostol with cimetidine in treatment of gastric ulcer in outpatients. Digestive Diseases and Sciences 31: 75S–80S
32. Zinner M J, Rypins E B, Martin L R et al 1990 Misoprostol: Another agent to prevent stress gastritis. Gastroenterology 99: 566–567
33. Davidson C D, Levey C M, Chamberlayne E D (eds) 1979 Guidelines for detection of hepatotoxicity due to drugs and chemicals. US Department of Health, Education and Welfare, NIH publication no 79-313, ch 7
34. Karim A, Rozek L F, Smith M E et al 1989 Effects of food and antacid on oral absorption of misoprostol, a synthetic prostaglandin E_1 analog. Journal of Clinical Pharmacology 29: 439–443

Mitomycin C

Mitomycin C is an antitumour antibiotic produced by the actinomycete *Streptomyces caespitosus*; it has a wide spectrum of activity.

Chemistry

Mitomycin C (Mitomycin X, Mitomycin C Kyowa, Mutamycin, NSC 26 980)

$C_{15}H_{18}N_4O_5$

6-Amino-8a-methoxy-5-tethylazirino [2',3':3,4]pyrrolo [1,2-a] indole-4,7-dione carbamate

The structure consists of a quinone ring linked to an indole group, and two side groups, the first a methoxyformamide side-chain and the second an aziridine ring

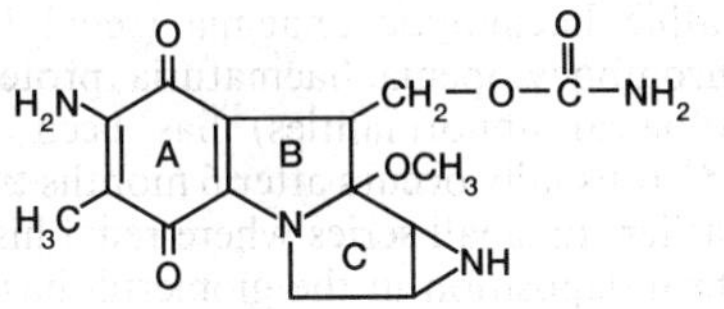

Molecular weight	334.3
pKa	—
Solubility	
in alcohol	high
in water	high
Octanol/water partition coefficient	low

A blue-violet crystalline powder supplied in a vial for dilution and parenteral administration. It is produced by *Streptomyces caespitosus*. Mitomycin C is not available in any combined preparations.

Pharmacology

Mitomycin is thought to act via a metabolite produced following a bioreductive alkylation reaction. Mitomycin loses the methoxy group and the quinone group is reduced followed by activation of the resulting metabolites. It inhibits DNA synthesis and cross-links DNA to an extent that is proportional to its content of guanine and cytosine.[1] Both the carbamate side chain and aziridine C_1 carbone are highly reactive. Mitomycin may also act through the generation of superoxide and hydroxyl radicals, and as a result may be selectively toxic to hypoxic cells.[2] Mitomycin C via its metabolites causes alkylation at the O-6 residue of guanine and this results in single strand breaks in DNA.[3] Its action is most marked in the late G_1 and early S phases of the cell cycle. Mitomycin C also inhibits RNA and protein synthesis.

Toxicology

The major toxic effect is myelosuppression, predominantly severe depression of the leucocytes and platelets. Tissue concentrations in mice show relatively high levels in lung, kidney, muscle and skin, and absence of detectable drug in the brain, and in this species the LD_{50} is 7.5 mg.kg^{-1}. There is little evidence of nephrotoxicity in animals, but the drug is both teratogenic and carcinogenic.

Clinical pharmacology

Mitomycin C is cytotoxic to tumour cells and normal body tissues, and in common with other antineoplastic agents has a low therapeutic ratio. Bone marrow suppression can be a major side effect, particularly if used in conjunction with an alkylating agent. Nephrotoxicity has also limited the use of higher doses in combination, and over the last 10 years there has been a significant reduction in the dose employed based on empirical criteria rather than as a result of randomized trials comparing efficacy or toxicity. The gastrointestinal tract is also frequently affected by toxicity. The cytotoxic effects of mitomycin C are not phase-specific, and the activity should therefore be related to length of drug exposure, but clinical studies have suggested an intermittent schedule to be more efficacious than a low dose continuous one.[5] Toxicity to normal tissues may, however, be reduced by leaving 4–8 weeks between courses in some cases to allow delayed myelosuppression to recover. The relevance of the putative mechanisms of action derived from in vitro observations to the clinical use of mitomycin is not clear, but it may be used either alone or in combination with antimetabolites (e.g. methotrexate, fluorouracil), anthracyclines or vinca alkaloids at doses of 8–10 mg.m^{-2} every 3–4 weeks. Up to 90 mg.m^{-2} has been given followed by autologous bone marrow transplantation. There is also some evidence for lymphocyte inactivation.[4]

Pharmacokinetics

High performance liquid chromatography is the most widely used technique for assay of the drug and has a sensitivity of 1 μg.l^{-1}.[6] After bolus intravenous administration, mitomycin C shows dose-dependent pharmacokinetics with rapid distribution into the intracellular compartment.[6] Early studies showed the plasma disappearance curve to be prolonged at higher doses, such as those more than 20 mg.m^{-2}. This was presumed to be due to saturation of drug metabolism, but recent studies have shown linearity at doses up to 60 mg.m^{-2}.[7] There is considerable variation in the elimination half life and total body clearance (1–46 l.h^{-1}.m^{-2}) of mitomycin C, but liver function, renal function and age would not appear to be important in determining its duration of action.[7] Renal excretion of the unchanged drug is in the range 2–15%.[6] In patients with liver damage the blood concentrations are maintained longer compared with patients with normal liver function. Intra-arterial infusion gives a 3-fold greater regional exposure, but the small proportion of hepatic extraction makes this route not so useful.[8] The drug has also been given by the intravesical route, but data are not available on its fate in man, although in the beagle dog absorption from the bladder was minimal.[9] Oral absorption is erratic and toxicity does not correlate with dose.[5]

Mitomycin C crosses the placenta and is teratogenic in animals.

Oral absorption	variable
Presystemic metabolism	—
Plasma half life α	5 min (2.9–12.4 min)
β	54 min (26–89 min)
Volume of distribution	25 l.m^{-2}
Plasma protein binding	—

Concentration–effect relationship

There is no evidence of a correlation between the plasma concentration of mitomycin C and its therapeutic effect.

Metabolism

Mitomycin C requires activation by chemical or enzymatic reduction of the parent compound to the hydroquinone or semiquinone. There is a close relationship between the mechanism of action of mitomycin C and its metabolism, which leads to unstable, highly reactive species, which involve free radical intermediates with short half lives. If these reactions take place adjacent to DNA, or possibly other critical macromolecules, cytotoxicity, or at least cellular damage will occur as a result of formation of irreversible cross-links. Inactivation occurs predominantly in the liver, and to a lesser extent in the kidney, heart and brain, and is promoted by compounds such as nicotinamide, vitamin B_6 and glutathione. Quantitation of these routes of elimination or the compounds formed have not been fully evaluated. In the mouse, metabolism is impaired following carbon-tetrachloride induced hepatic damage. In the dog, recovery in the urine rises from 7% after 0.5 mg.kg^{-1} mitomycin C, to 30% after 2 mg.kg^{-1}.

Pharmaceutics

Mitomycin C is only available in parenteral form: Vials (Mutamycin: Bristol-Myers, US) contain 2 mg with 48 mg sodium chloride, 10 mg with 240 mg sodium chloride and 20 mg with 480 mg sodium chloride for dissolving in water. The reconstituted solution at 1 $mg.ml^{-1}$ is stable with refrigeration for 7 days. Administration should be into a running saline or dextrose infusion, taking care to avoid extravasation. For intravesical instillation, 10–40 mg should be dissolved in 20–40 ml of water and instilled via a catheter.

Therapeutic use

Mitomycin C has been available for many years and has activity against a wide range of tumours, but proved too toxic for general use at the doses originally used (around 20 $mg.m^{-2}$). With administration at lower doses, it has found a role as a useful second-line agent often in combination with other cytotoxic drugs.

Indications

1. Stomach cancer
2. Breast cancer
3. Bladder cancer
4. Lung cancer
5. Cervical cancer
6. Miscellaneous tumours, including pancreas, colon, soft tissue sarcomas and carcinomas of unknown origin have also been shown to respond to mitomycin C.

Contraindications

1. Cumulative myelosuppression with thrombocytopenia and leucopenia is the major toxicity, and patients pretreated with radiotherapy or chemotherapy should be monitored carefully
2. Severe renal toxicity may supervene rapidly and renal function should be carefully monitored.

Mode of use

The usual dose is 10 $mg.m^{-2}$ given as a single dose into a running saline infusion every 4–6 weeks. The dose may be divided into 2 $mg.m^{-2}$ daily for 5 days. The cycles are repeated once the bone marrow nadir has passed. In some experimental regimes, doses up to 20 $mg.m^{-2}$ are employed, but bone marrow and renal toxicity can be major limiting factors. For intravesical instillation the dose employed is between 10 and 40 mg.

Indications

1. Gastric cancer
This tumour is moderately responsive to chemotherapy, but the duration of response has been short and the survival benefit modest. Mitomycin C has been an important component of most regimes, and has been used in combination with 5-fluorouracil, adriamycin and CCNU, in regimes which achieve an overall response rate of the order of 35%.[10,11] However, these results show insufficient evidence of activity to translate into a survival benefit when similar regimes are used in the adjuvant setting.[12]

2. Breast cancer
Mitomycin C is one of a number of agents in breast cancer which achieve a satisfactory response rate of the order of 30%.[12] The myelosuppression associated with this drug has led to difficulty in incorporating it into first-line combinations with an alkylating agent, but it has found a useful place as a second-line agent often in conjunction with a vinca alkaloid.[14–16]

3. Bladder cancer
Mitomycin C achieves a response rate of about 70% in patients with superficial tumours.[17] These lesions have a long and poorly defined natural history which makes interpretation of the overall benefit of such treatment difficult, but studies have also been carried out where the instillations are given prophylactically.[18] The optimum duration of treatment has not been established.

4. Lung cancer
In contrast to small cell lung cancer, few agents exert significant anticancer activity against non-small cell lung cancer, but along with vindesine, ifosfamide and cisplatin, mitomycin C is one of the most active drugs.[19] The overall response rate is low and of short duration even when used in combination chemotherapy, but a small proportion of the squamous cell tumours are particularly responsive.

5. Cervical cancer
Combination chemotherapy can now achieve moderate response rates of the order of 40–60% in this disease. However, patients with prior radiation therapy and compromised renal function respond less well. The duration of response is usually less than 6 months. Mitomycin C has been used in combination with bleomycin, cisplatinum and vincristine.[20,21]

6. Miscellaneous tumours
Colorectal carcinomas and pancreatic carcinoma respond poorly to conventional chemotherapy, but responses are seen in some patients treated with combinations developed for gastric carcinoma.[22,23] These remain experimental and the benefits questionable at present.[25] Squamous cell carcinoma of the head and neck has also been shown to respond to mitomycin C.[24,26] In the treatment of hepatocellular carcinoma intra-arterial mitomycin C has been used. Arterial embolization with microencapsulated drug has been used in experimental studies.[27]

Adverse reactions

Potentially life-threatening effects
A microangiopathic haemolytic anaemia (renal failure syndrome with anaemia, thrombocytopenia, haematuria, proteinuria, hypertension and neurological abnormalities) has been reported and is frequently fatal.[31] It usually occurs after 6 months treatment, but has been reported earlier. In small series where renal histopathology has been studied, fibrin deposition in the glomeruli has been noted, but the precise mechanism is not known. Hepatic veno-occlusive disease has been reported in one high-dose study.

Acute overdosage
Following acute overdose, cardiac monitoring should be performed for 24–36 hours, but the principal risk would be from later severe myelosuppression.

Severe or irreversible adverse effects
The dose-limiting toxicity is myelosuppression, which may be delayed with a nadir at 4–8 weeks. The effect is cumulative,[28] and affects both leucocytes and platelets. Diffuse pulmonary infiltration has also been recorded,[29] and exposure to oxygen in high concentration may be contributory. This side effect is thought to be related to generation of free radicals following activation of the drug.

Symptomatic adverse effects
Nausea and vomiting of moderate severity are seen in about 25% of patients and alopecia, stomatitis and diarrhoea are also observed. Local tissue necrosis is observed if the solution is extravasated from a vein or artery.

Interference with clinical pathology tests
No technical interferences of this kind appear to have been reported.

High risk groups

Neonates
The drug is not used in neonates.

Breast milk. As the metabolic pathways involved in degradation are not clear, and the drug is known to be both mutagenic and teratogenic, its use should be avoided during lactation.

Children
Mitomycin C is rarely used in children.

Pregnant women
The drug should be avoided during pregnancy.

The elderly
As bone marrow reserve may be impaired in the elderly, mitomycin C should be used with care.

Concurrent disease
Renal failure is a relative contraindication to the use of this drug.

Drug interactions

Potentially hazardous interactions

As free radical generation is noted with this drug, there may be some synergistic cardiotoxicity with adriamycin.[30] The possible enhancement of lung damage by nitrosoureas and doxorubicin has been reported.

Microsomal enzyme inducers such as barbiturates or liver enzyme inhibitors such as cimetidine may alter activity by an effect on host and tumour metabolism.

Potentially useful interactions

Mitomycin C may show synergy with 5-fluorouracil.[32]

Mitomycin C may enhance cell kill induced by radiation therapy, particularly under hypoxic conditions.

Major outcome trials

1. The Gastrointestinal Tumour Study Group 1984 Randomised study of combination chemotherapy in unresectable gastric cancer. Cancer 53: 13–17
2. Fielding J W L, Fagg S L, Jones B G 1983 An interim report of a prospective randomised controlled study of adjuvant chemotherapy in operable gastric cancer: British Stomach Cancer Group. World Journal of Surgery 7: 390–399

The Gastrointestinal Tumour Study Group reported on a randomized three-arm study in unresectable gastric cancer and found no difference between 5-fluorouracil and doxorubicin alone or with the addition of mitomycin C. The British Stomach Cancer Group reported on a large randomized trial in which patients received adjuvant 5-fluorouracil and mitomycin or no treatment. There was no survival difference between the groups, but 8.5% of the 281 patients given mitomycin C developed a haemolytic uraemic syndrome.

3. Niijima T, Koiso K, Akasa H and the Japanese Urological Cancer Research Group 1983 Randomised trial on chemoprophylaxis of recurrence in cases of superficial bladder cancer. Cancer Chemotherapy and Pharmacology 11 (suppl): 79

This was on a randomized trial on 707 Ta and T_1 cases of resected bladder cancer, given either doxorubicin, mitomycin C or no treatment. The recurrence rate was 48% for doxorubicin, 57% for mitomycin C and 62% for the control group, a result significant at $P<0.05$.

In non-small cell lung cancer there have been no randomized trials on which to base a measure of activity against other treatment options.

Other trials

1. Godfrey T E 1979 Mitomycin C in breast cancer. In: Carter S K, Crooke S T (eds) Mitomycin C: current status and new developments. Academic Press, New York, ch 10, pp 91–99

This study reviews the results of treating 129 patients with breast cancer and shows a response rate up to 33% with a range of duration of response 1½–10 months.

General review articles

Den Hartigh J, Pinedo H M 1984 Mitomycin C. In: Pinedo H M, Chabner B A (eds) Cancer chemotherapy 7. Elsevier, Amsterdam, pp 83–90

Doll D C, Weiss R B 1983 Chemotherapeutic agents and the erythron. Cancer Treatment Reviews 10: 185–200

Doll D C, Weiss R D, Issell B 1985 Mitomycin: ten years after approval for marketing. Journal of Clinical Oncology 3: 276–286

Lawn J W 1979 The molecular mechanism of antitumour action of the mitomycins. In: Carter S K, Crooke S T (eds) Mitomycin C: current status and new developments. Academic Press, New York, ch 2, pp 5–26

Shingleton H M, Orr J W 1983 Recurrent cervical cancer. In: Cancer of the cervix: diagnosis and treatment. Churchill Livingstone, Edinburgh, ch 7, pp 145–192

Straus M J, Selawry O S, Wallach R A 1983 Chemotherapy in lung cancer. In: Straus M J (ed) Lung cancer: clinical diagnosis and treatment. Grune and Stratton, New York, ch 16, pp 261–283

References

1. Iyer V N, Szybaloki W 1964 Mitomycin and porfiromycin: chemical mechanism of activation and cross-linking of DNA. Science 145: 55
2. Lawn J W, Sim S K, Chen H H 1978 Hydroxyl radical production by free and DNA-bound aminoquinone antibiotics and its role in DNA degradation. Electron spin resonance detection of hydroxyl radicals by spin trapping. Canadian Journal of Biochemistry 56: 1042
3. Lawn J W, Begleiter A, Johnson D 1976 Studies relating to antitumour antibodies. Part V. Reactions of mitomycin C with DNA examined by ethidium fluorescence assay. Canadian Journal of Biochemistry 54: 110
4. Etheridge E E, Shono A R, Hohenthanes K L 1973 Mitomycin C inactivation of leukocytes in the mixed leucocyte culture. Transplantation 15: 331
5. Reich S D 1979 Clinical pharmacology of mitomycin C. In: Carter S K, Crooke S T (eds) Mitomycin C: current status and new developments. Academic Press, New York, 243–250
6. Den Hartigh J, McVie J G, Van Dort W J, Pinedo H M 1983 Pharmacokinetics of mitomycin C in humans. Cancer Research 43: 805
7. Schilcher R B, Young R D, Ratanatharathom V et al 1984 Clinical pharmacokinetics of high dose mitomycin C. Cancer Chemotherapy and Pharmacology 13: 186
8. Hu E, Howell S B 1983 Pharmacokinetics of intraarterial mitomycin C in humans. Cancer Research 43: 4474
9. Schmidbauer C P, Porpaczy P, Georgopoulos A, Rameis H 1984 Absorption of doxorubicin-hydrochloride and mitomycin C after instillation into non-infected and infected bladders of dogs. Journal of Urology 131: 818
10. Panattiere F J, Haas C, McDonald B et al 1984 Drug combinations in the treatment of gastric adenocarcinoma: a randomized South West Oncology Group Study. Journal of Clinical Oncology 2: 420
11. Macdonald J S, Schein P S, Woolley P V et al 1980 5 Fluorouracil, doxorubicin and mitomycin (FAM) combination chemotherapy for advanced gastric cancer. Annals of Internal Medicine 93: 533–536
12. Ogawa M, Taguchi T 1985 Upper gastrointestinal tumours. In: Pinedo H M, Chabner B A (eds) Cancer chemotherapy 7. Elsevier, Amsterdam, pp 322–331
13. Buzdar A U, Tashima C K, Blumenschein G R et al 1978 Mitomycin C and megestrol acetate in treatment of breast cancer refractory to hormone and combination chemotherapy. Cancer 41: 392–395
14. Perez D J, Powles T J, Gazet J C, Ford H T, Coombes R C 1984 Mitomycin C, melphalan and methotrexate combination chemotherapy for palliation of disseminated breast cancer. Cancer Chemotherapy and Pharmacology 13: 36–38
15. Howell A, Morrison J M, Bramwell V H C, Harland R N L, Monneypenny I J 1984 Dibromudolcitol, mitomycin C and vinblastine (DMV) chemotherapy in advanced breast cancer. European Journal of Clinical Oncology 20: 873–876
16. Luikart S D, Witman G B, Portlock C S 1984 Adriamycin, vinblastine and mitomycin C combination chemotherapy in refractory breast carcinoma. Cancer 54: 1252–1255
17. Soloway M S 1983 Treatment of superficial bladder cancer with intravesical mitomycin C: analysis of immediate and long term response in 70 patients. Journal of Urology 134: 1107–1109
18. Jauhiainen K, Alfthan O 1987 Instillation of mitomycin C and doxorubicin in the prevention of recurrent superficial (Ta–T1) bladder cancer. British Journal of Urology 601: 54–59
19. Bakowski M T, Crouch J C 1983 Chemotherapy of non-small cell lung cancer: a reappraisal and a look to the future. Cancer Treatment Reports 10: 159–172
20. Baker L H, Opipari M I, Wilson H, Bottomley R, Coltman C A 1978 Mitomycin C, vincristine and bleomycin therapy for advanced cervical cancer. Obstetrics and Gynecology 52: 146–150
21. Trope C, Johnson J, Simonsen E et al 1983 Bleomycin, mitomycin C in advanced squamous cell carcinoma of the cervix: a third book. Cancer 51: 591–593
22. Bonomi P D, Chambra G, Rossat A H, Klaasen D 1980 Mitomycin C, methyl CCNU and 5-fluorouracil in the treatment of metastatic colorectal carcinoma. Cancer Chemotherapy and Pharmacology 5: 39–42
23. Smith F P, Hoth D F, Levin B et al 1980 5-fluorouracil, adriamycin and mitomycin C (FAM) chemotherapy for advanced adenocarcinoma of the pancreas. Cancer 46: 2014–2018
24. O'Connell M J 1985 Colorectal carcinoma, pancreatic carcinoma and malignant hepatomas. In: Pinedo H M (ed) Cancer Chemotherapy 5. Elsevier, Amsterdam, pp 335–348
25. Misra N C, Jaiswal M S D, Singh R V, Das B 1977 Intrahepatic arterial infusion of combination of mitomycin C and 5-fluorouracil in treatment of primary and metastatic liver carcinoma. Cancer 39: 1425–1429
26. Wheeler R H, Baker S R, Liepman M K, Ensminger W D 1983 Intensive sequential chemotherapy with bleomycin, oncovin, mitomycin C and methotrexate followed by adriamycin, cisplatin and cyclophosphamide in squamous cell cancer of the head and neck. Medical and Paediatric Oncology 11: 12–19
27. Kato T, Nemoto R, Mori H et al 1981 Arterial chemoembolisation with microencapsulated anticancer drug. An approach to selective cancer chemotherapy with sustained effects. Journal of the American Medical Association 245: 1123–1127
28. Glaubiger D, Ramu A 1982 Antitumour antibiotics. In: Chabner B A (ed) Pharmacologic principles of cancer treatment. W B Saunders, Philadelphia, ch 19, pp 407–410
29. Arwoll E S, Kressling P J, Patterson J R 1978 Interstitial pneumonia from mitomycin. Annals of Internal Medicine 89: 352
30. Buzdar A U, Legha S S, Tashima C K et al 1978 Adriamycin and mitomycin C: possible synergistic cardiotoxicity. Cancer Treatment Reports 62: 1005–1008
31. Pavy M D, Wiley E L, Abeloff M D 1982 Haemolytic uraemic syndrome associated with mitomycin therapy. Cancer Treatment Reports 66: 457–461
32. Kowal C, Diven W, Kozikowski A 1983 Mitomycin–nucleotide interactions: formation of a covalently linked mitomycin C (MMC) fluorodeoxyuridylate (FdUMP) molecule and kinetics of aziridine ring opening. Proceedings of the Second European Conference on Clinical Oncology 18

Mitozantrone (hydrochloride)

Mitozantrone (originally named mitoxantrone: the chemical name has since been altered to mitozantrone in the UK) is an anthracenedione antineoplastic agent which has structural similarities to the anthracycline antibiotics doxorubicin and daunorubicin. It has been in use since 1979.

Chemistry

Mitozantrone hydrochloride (Mitoxantrone, Novantrone)
$C_{22}H_{28}N_4O_6.2HCl$
1,4-Dihydroxy-5,8-bis [2-(2-hydroxyethyl amino)-ethylamino]-9,10-anthracenedione dihydrochloride

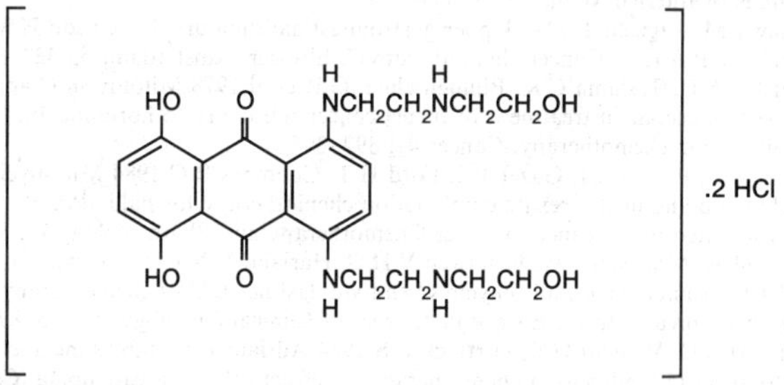

Molecular weight (free base)	517.4 (444.1)
pKa	5.99, 8.13
Solubility	
in alcohol	slight
in water	sparing
Octanol/water partition coefficient	—

Mitozantrone hydrochloride is a blue-black, crystalline solid prepared by chemical synthesis. The octanol/water partition coefficient has not been measured, but it would be expected that very little would be extracted into the octanol phase. Mitozantrone is not available in any combination product.

Pharmacology

Mitozantrone is a potent inhibitor of RNA and DNA synthesis. It intercalates DNA, causing inter- and intra-strand cross-linking with preference for G–C base pairs. Mitozantrone is a non-cell-cycle specific agent, although proliferating cells are more sensitive to inhibition than stationary ones with the most sensitive phase being in the S phase of the cell cycle. The cytotoxicity to the DNA appears to be greatly increased by a small increase in temperature from 37°C to 42.4°C.

Mitozantrone reacts with microsomal cytochrome P-450 reductase in the presence of NADPH to form semiquinone radicals which can themselves produce superoxide anions after reaction with oxygen. These and hydroxyl radicals are highly toxic to cells. Mitozantrone reacts with cell membranes and may alter the functions of these membranes.

Toxicology

The carcinogenic potential of mitozantrone is unknown in man but it is known to be mutagenic in vitro and in vivo in the rat. It has also been implicated in the development of malignant neoplasia in the rat. In microbial mutagenicity tests, mitozantrone caused frame-shift mutations consistent with its proposed mechanism of action, that is, intercalation in the DNA molecule. In teratology studies, pregnant rats and rabbits were given mitozantrone but no gross foetal malformations were observed in either species. The effects of mitozantrone on human fertility or pregnancy have not been established but patients and their partners should avoid conception during treatment and for six months after.

Clinical pharmacology

Mitozantrone is an effective antitumour drug used primarily in the treatment of advanced breast carcinoma and acute non-lymphocytic leukaemia, in combination with other drugs. Mitozantrone may interact with cell membranes thus altering their function. This action seems to be responsible for the cardiac toxicity of mitozantrone which directly damages the cardiac muscle myofibrils. Mitozantrone is immunosuppressive and use of live vaccines may produce systemic disease. Mitozantrone is generally used at maximal tolerated doses in line with previous experience with other cytotoxic agents. Alberts et al[1] showed a direct relationship between the degree of mitozantrone uptake into tumour and cytotoxic effect, according to mitozantrone tissue deposition data, and it may be therefore that clinical response may depend more upon adequate drug uptake into tumour tissue than plasma levels of drug.

Pharmacokinetics

Mitozantrone is poorly absorbed after oral administration but has been administered by the intravenous,[1–4] intra-arterial,[5] intrathecal[6] (NB: this route is not recommended by the manufacturers) and intraperitoneal[7] routes. It is most commonly administered intravenously, which is the manufacturers' recommended route. The pharmacokinetics of the drug have been studied using high performance liquid chromatography (HPLC) techniques, with limits of detection to 1 $\mu g.l^{-1}$, and radiolabelled methods. It has been shown that the plasma disappearance of mitozantrone is best described by a three-compartment model.

All studies of plasma mitozantrone disappearance indicate an initial rapid α phase representing a rapid distribution of the drug into the red blood cells, white blood cells and platelets. This is then followed by a second β distribution phase which is associated with a redistribution from blood cells into the tissues (autopsy studies and animal pharmacokinetic studies have shown extensive dose-related distribution into most tissues, but little penetration into the central nervous system).

However, although it is clear that the α and β half lives are relatively short (α 0.1–0.14 h, β 0.38–3.12 h) (see Table 1 for summary of published pharmacokinetic studies), the terminal γ half life of mitozantrone has not yet been adequately defined and measured; values have ranged from 1 to 215 hours.[1–4] A prolonged terminal half life is consistent with data from autopsy studies[3] where > 15% of the administered dose of mitozantrone appeared in autopsy tissues 35 days after dosing (the liver contained the highest amount, followed by the heart, lungs, spleen, kidney and thyroid gland in that order). A prolonged elimination half life suggests that mitozantrone distributes into a deep tissue compartment from which it is slowly released and this is consistent with the extremely large volume of distribution which has been reported for the drug (see Table 1). Mitozantrone has been reported to bind to albumin (76%) and α_1-acid glycoprotein (66%) in in vitro studies.[8]

Elimination of mitozantrone is slow and occurs via the hepatobiliary and renal systems. Work by Alberts et al.[3] showed that only a mean of 10.1% of the total administered dose of mitozantrone was recovered in the urine over the first 5 days after dosing (with 6.5% as unchanged drug) and of this the majority (62%) of urinary recovery was within the first four hours. Total drug-related material recovered in the faeces over 5 days averaged 18.3% of the dose administered, therefore the most important route of mitozantrone elimination appears to be faecal.

Limited salivary secretion data obtained by Alberts et al.[3] show prolonged but low salivary concentrations of mitozantrone up to 120 hours after drug administration but because of the very low amounts of drug detected this route is unlikely to be of importance in the evaluation of mitozantrone pharmacokinetics. There is no information available with regard to excretion of mitozantrone in breast milk. However, the manufacturers recommend that mitozantrone should not normally be administered to breast-feeding mothers.

As administration of mitozantrone to patients with hepatic dysfunction is thought to be associated with a more prolonged body clearance, caution in the use of this drug in patients with impaired hepatic function should be advised. However, it is likely that the pharmacokinetics of mitozantrone are only significantly influenced by severe hepatic dysfunction and that mild or moderate impairment will have little effect. It is unlikely, however, that dosage adjustments of mitozantrone are required for patients with renal impairment because of the small amount of drug that is cleared by the renal route.

Mitozantrone has several features which make it a suitable drug for administration into the peritoneal space (e.g. for the treatment of advanced ovarian cancer). They include a high molecular weight and hydrophilic properties which should lower peritoneal absorption rates, and also its fairly high hepatic metabolism following portal circulation distribution which should limit its systemic availability. Thus higher doses than those routinely administered intravenously can be given without an increased risk of side effects, e.g. bone marrow depression. Only limited pharmacokinetic data are available for mitozantrone following intraperitoneal administration. Alberts et al.[7] administered mitozantrone intraperitoneally to 17 patients in a dose of 12–23 $mg.m^{-2}$ in 2 l of dialysate which was left in situ for 1–4 hours. The resulting areas under the curve (AUC) reflected a wide interpatient variation and much more work appears to be required before evaluation of its efficacy as an intraperitoneal agent can be made.

Oral absorption	low
Presystemic metabolism	—
Plasma half life	
range	3.87–214.8 h
Volume of distribution	212.9–2248 $l.m^{-2}$
Plasma protein binding	~76%

Concentration–effect relationship

There is no evidence of any relationship between the plasma concentration of mitozantrone and its therapeutic effect.

Metabolism

Evidence exists to show that mitozantrone is most probably metabolized in the liver. Studies by Ehninger et al[4] demonstrated that four metabolites of mitozantrone could be isolated from urine and it was probable that the two major metabolites were the mono and dicarboxylic acid derivatives which result from oxidation of the terminal hydroxy groups of the side-chain(s) of mitozantrone (Fig. 1).

So far metabolites III and IV have not been identified but metabolite III was detected only during the first hours after mitozantrone administration. Metabolite IV appears in the urine only after a few days post-dosing although it is still observed 4 weeks later. Metabolites I, II and III were blue coloured, indicating the presence of the anthracenedione ring system, whereas metabolite IV was reddish-brown, pointing to a change of substituents in the anthracenedione ring (therefore the metabolic pathway leading to metabolite IV may be different from that of I and II). Within 48 hours of drug administration a mean value of 4.4% of the administered dose was excreted in the urine as mitozantrone, 0.5% as metabolite I and 0.3% as metabolite II. However, the excretion of mitozantrone and the two major metabolites showed interpatient variability and it was suggested

Fig. 1 Monocarboxylic (I) and dicarboxlic (II) acid derivatives of mitozantrone

I

II

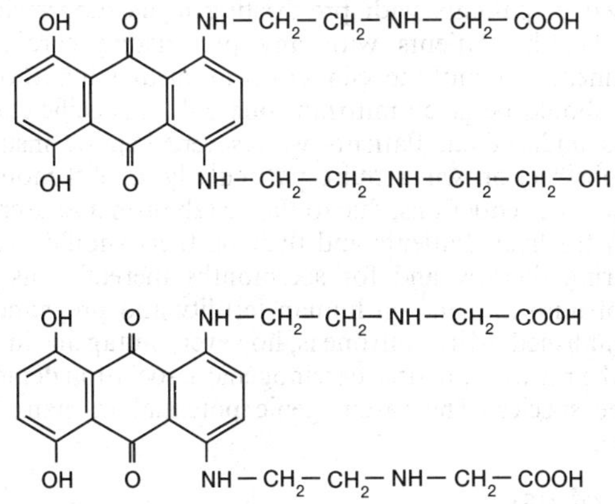

that this may be related to the general condition of the patients, concurrent drug therapy and the capacities of the excretory organs.

Synthetic samples of metabolites I and II were both inactive when tested against P388 leukaemia in mice (against which mitozantrone exhibits high activity) and are therefore regarded as biologically inactive metabolic detoxification products.

Pharmaceutics

Novantrone injection (2 $mg.ml^{-1}$) (Lederle, UK/USA) is a sterile, dark-blue, aqueous isotonic solution of mitozantrone hydrochloride equivalent to 20 mg, 25 mg and 30 mg mitozantrone, together with sodium chloride and a buffer of sodium acetate and acetic acid to approximately pH3.

Novantrone injection should be stored at room temperature (refrigerated storage may cause precipitation), and has a shelf-life of 2 years. The drug suffers no detrimental effects from light. It can be diluted in sodium chloride 0.9% or dextrose 5%, but the injection does not contain an antimicrobial preservative, so dilutions should be discarded within 24 hours. Lack of specific data on compatibility necessitates that Novantrone should not be mixed with other drugs in the same infusion. Care should be taken to avoid contact of the drug with the skin, mucous membrane or eyes. It can cause staining and skin accidentally exposed should be rinsed copiously with warm water. A green discoloration of urine is common for up to 24 hours following drug administration due to metabolism and excretion of the drug. Postmortem examination often reveals blue discoloration of organs.

Therapeutic use

Indications

1. Advanced breast carcinoma
2. Leukaemias
3. Lymphomas
4. Other tumour types.

Contraindications

Demonstrated hypersensitivity to the drug.

Precautions

Mitozantrone is an antiproliferative drug which should be used where there are facilities for careful monitoring of clinical and haematologi-

Table 1 Pharmacokinetics of mitozantrone

Study	No. of patients	1 h dose /$mg.m^2$	Mean half lives (hours) α	β	γ	Mean volume of distribution /$l.m^{-2}$
Smyth et al.[1]	11	14	0.156	1.6	23	1565
Miser et al.[2]	17	12–20	0.057	0.378	3.87	212.9
Alberts et al.[3]	5	12	0.1	1.1	42.6	1875
Ehninger et al.[4]	7	14	0.14	3.12	214.8	2248

M

Mitozantrone (hydrochloride)

M

cal parameters during treatment and subsequently. Dose adjustments may be required on the basis of the haematological findings. Caution is advised in patients with pre-existing myelosuppression or poor general health. Patients with any pre-existing cardiac problem, pretreatment with anthracyclines or prior mediastinal/thoracic radiotherapy should be given mitozantrone only if specific cardiac monitoring is undertaken. Patients with severe hepatic insufficiency or biliary obstruction will require particularly careful monitoring and probable dose reductions, due to the metabolism and excretion of the drug via the liver. Patients and their partners should avoid conception during therapy and for six months thereafter as the overall effects of mitozantrone on human fertility and pregnancy have not been established. Mitozantrone is, however, mutagenic in vitro and in vivo in the rat with possible carcinogenic association demonstrated in the same species. The carcinogenic potential in man, however, is unknown.

Mode of use

Mitozantrone is a cytotoxic drug for use in malignant disorders. The drug is administered intravenously only, as safety for intrathecal use has not been established. Mitozantrone should be made up to the required volume of at least 50 ml of sodium chloride 0.9%, glucose 5% or sodium chloride 0.18% and glucose 4%. It is recommended that the resulting solution be administered in the tubing of a freely running intravenous infusion of the above fluids over not less than 3 minutes. The drug should not be mixed with other drugs in the same infusion. If extravasation occurs then it is recommended that the drip be discontinued and resited. Severe local reaction following extravasation is very unlikely. The appropriate dose and schedule is discussed under the following disease indications.

Indications

1. Advanced breast carcinoma

There is now considerable experience in the use of mitozantrone in the treatment of advanced breast carcinoma and it has established a role due to its relatively good therapeutic index. There is evidence of activity at all metastatic sites with the exception of brain and there is evidence for lack of cross-resistance with anthracyclines. It will normally be indicated for advanced breast cancer refractory to hormonal therapy or in advanced disease where chemotherapy is indicated as initial therapy. There is evidence of non-cross, resistance with doxorubicin.[10]

Single-agent dosage. The recommended dosage of mitozantrone as a single agent is 14 $mg.m^{-2}$ (body surface area) and given as a single intravenous dose this may be repeated at 21-day intervals. If, however, patients have had prior chemotherapy or are in poor general condition then a dose of 12 $mg.m^{-2}$ or less may be considered. Alteration of dose and subsequent dosing interval may be required depending on the degree and duration of myelosuppression on the basis of clinical judgement. In untreated patients a response rate (i.e. tumour reduction by 50% or more of measurable disease) may be expected in between 30 and 40% of patients, with a response being maintained for a median of 8–9 months. The total duration of treatment is dependent on clinical judgement and a knowledge of the recommended maximum dosage.

Combination therapy. Mitozantrone has been given as part of combination cytotoxic chemotherapy in the treatment of advanced breast carcinoma but at present such usage remains in the province of clinical research and dosage and combination recommendations cannot be given.

2. Leukaemias

Mitozantrone has been used in the treatment of acute non-lymphocytic leukaemia (ANLL) in second or subsequent relapse or in leukaemia refractory to conventional therapy. Only limited data are available on the treatment of relapsed acute lymphocytic leukaemia and on chronic myeloid leukaemia in blast crisis. The use of mitozantrone in paediatric leukaemia is limited and as yet dosage recommendations cannot be given. There is evidence of non-cross-resistance with doxorubicin and daunorubicin in the treatment of leukaemia.

Single agent therapy. Approximately ⅓ of patients with relapse or refractory ANLL are likely to respond to single-agent mitozantrone therapy with a complete remission rate of the order of 15%.[11] The duration of complete response is usually short, with a median of just over 3 months, but several patients have had remissions lasting over 1 year. The recommended dose for remission induction is 12 $mg.m^{-2}$ of body surface area given daily for 5 consecutive days as a single intravenous dose (total 60 $mg.m^{-2}$).

Combination therapy. Mitozantrone has been combined with cytosine arabinoside with a 54–56% complete response rate.[12,13] Response duration was again quite short but several sustained remissions were seen and mitozantrone may well be incorporated into front-line chemotherapy in the future. At present, however, dosage recommendations for combination therapy cannot be advised until further studies of its use in combination have been done.

3. Lymphoma

Mitozantrone has activity against all types of intermediate and high grade lymphoma. Phase II trials demonstrated that approximately ⅓ of patients with previously treated lymphoma respond to mitozantrone as a single agent, with a median response duration extending over 6 months.[14] The recommended single-agent dose is 14 $mg.m^{-2}$ of body surface area given as a single intravenous dose and repeated at 21-day intervals. Depending on the degree and duration of myelosuppression the subsequent dose and timing may require alteration based on clinical judgement.

Combination therapy. Although mitozantrone has been used in combination in phase II and phase III regimens the data are still too premature to give clear guidelines on combination of drug and dose.

4. Other tumour types

Mitozantrone is not at present licensed for use in other solid tumours but there is evidence of activity against epithelial ovarian carcinoma and this may prove to be a future use for the drug.[15] In addition, activity has been demonstrated against hepatocellular carcinoma.[16] A summary of activity in other tumour types can be found in the article by Smyth, 1984.[17]

Adverse reactions

Potentially life-threatening effects

The major dose-limiting toxicity of mitozantrone is myelosuppression. Patients at risk of developing profound myelosuppression are those who have had heavy pretreatment with chemotherapy and/or radiotherapy which has compromised marrow reserves and patients who have extensive bone marrow involvement by tumour. Dose prescription and dosing interval require sound clinical judgement if the risk of profound neutropenia and thrombocytopenia is to be avoided. Caution should be exercised in patients who have pre-existing cardiac disease which compromises ventricular function and also if patients have received prior mediastinal radiotherapy or anthracycline therapy. Such patients are at risk of developing further cardiotoxicity which may precipitate cardiac failure (see Severe or irreversible adverse effects).

Acute overdosage

There is no specific antidote for mitozantrone. In the event of error in dosing then supportive measures will have to be undertaken for the expected haemopoietic toxicity with the need for monitoring of the blood count over the succeeding few weeks of myelosuppression. Gastrointestinal toxicity may also be seen with acute nausea and vomiting, acute diarrhoea and subsequent mucositis. Occasional hepatic or renal toxicity may be experienced depending on the pre-existing condition of these organs. Close haematological and biochemical monitoring is mandatory throughout this period with resort to antibiotics, antifungal agents, antiviral agents and blood products as appropriate.

Severe or irreversible adverse effects

Prolonged therapy with mitozantrone, particularly in the presence of a compromised bone marrow, may lead to marrow hypoplasia. There is a mild risk of cardiotoxicity following the use of mitozantrone. A total dose of 160 $mg.m^{-2}$ can be administered to the patient before there is a significant increase in the incidence of cardiac toxicity. The risk of developing any significant cardiotoxicity below this level is low but is increased in the presence of pre-existing poor ventricular function, previous treatment with anthracyclines and prior mediastinal irradiation.[18] Patients with pre-existing risk factors should have

Mitozantrone (hydrochloride)

left ventricular ejection fraction measured by radionucleotide scanning, or echocardiogram, together with frequent electrocardiographs. Microscopic evidence of endomyocardial damage has been demonstrated, with damage to sarcotubular elements and myofibril damage and loss. These findings are usually minor, haemodynamically insignificant and are seldom clinically significant.[19]

Symptomatic adverse effects
The most commonly encountered adverse effects are nausea and vomiting which occur in approximately 40% of courses administered but are generally mild and transient. The concomitant administration of an effective antiemetic can usually abolish this adverse effect. Approximately 5% of patients will develop complete reversible alopecia. A further 10% will experience patchy alopecia and others may experience mild hair thinning. Allergic reactions are very infrequent but female patients should be counselled concerning the possibility of developing amenorrhoea. Other reported adverse effects are anorexia, constipation, diarrhoea, stomatitis, fever, weakness, fatigue, gastrointestinal bleeding, dyspnoea, and non-specific neurological side effects. Extravasation of the drug outwith the vein should be avoided although serious necrosis following extravasation is extremely rare. Side effects in patients with leukaemia are likely to be more severe due to the higher dose given and more severe stomatitis, mucositis and myelosuppression may be expected.

Other effects
Infrequent elevated serum creatinine and blood urea nitrogen levels have been demonstrated and, although occasional reports of severe impairment of hepatic function in patients with leukaemia have been made, liver enzyme elevation is infrequent.

With a single dose every 21 days, suppression of white blood count will reach its nadir at 10 days after dosing with recovery usually occurring by day 21. Suppression of white blood count below 1000 mm^{-3} is uncommon; less frequently thrombocytopenia can occur and following repeated administration anaemia is possible. Table 2 suggests modification of dose depending on the white blood count nadir after the preceding dose.[20]

Interference with clinical pathology tests
Mitozantrone may cause blue-green discoloration of the urine for 24 hours after administration.

High risk groups

Neonates
The drug is not used in neonates.

Breast milk. Nursing mothers receiving mitozantrone should be counselled to discontinue breast-feeding.

Children
Mitozantrone has been used in the treatment of paediatric leukaemias but experience with the drug here remains limited and its use should be restricted to experienced clinicians. The monitoring of cardiac function is important for this age group.

Pregnant women
Mitozantrone should not be used during pregnancy and patients and their partners should be counselled against conception during treatment with mitozantrone and for six months after treatment.

The elderly
As with other cytotoxic drugs mitozantrone should be used with great caution in the elderly due to diminishing marrow tolerability.

Drug interactions

Potentially hazardous interactions
No major hazardous drug interactions have been reported to date. Mitozantrone has been used as part of combination chemotherapy with a variety of other cytotoxic drugs but further evaluation of such combinations is required before they can be recommended for widespread use.

Potentially useful interactions
Mitozantrone appears to have synergistic activity with 5-fluorouracil, vincristine and dacarbazine against transplantable mouse tumours[21] and with methotrexate in murine LI20 leukaemia.[22]

Major outcome trials

1. Cornbleet M A, Stewart-Harris R C, Smith I E et al 1984 Mitozantrone for the treatment of advanced breast cancer: single agent therapy in previously untreated patients. European Journal Cancer and Clinical Oncology 20: 1141–1146

In 99 evaluable patients, an overall response rate of 35% was demonstrated although only 6 patients achieved complete response. The median time to treatment failure was in excess of 46 weeks. Mitozantrone was well tolerated, with myelosuppression being the dose-limiting toxicity. In this study, 4 patients developed clinically significant cardiotoxicity after cumulative mitozantrone doses of 174–256 $mg.m^{-2}$. Responses were seen in all metastatic sites (brain excluded). The study concluded that mitozantrone had comparable efficacy but less acute toxicity compared with other cytotoxic agents used as single agents in advanced breast cancer.

2. Prentice H G, Robbins G, Ma D D F, Ho A D 1984 Mitozantrone in relapsed and refractory acute leukaemia. Seminars in Oncology 11 (suppl 1): 32–35

Two separate studies were performed, one using a slow infusion of mitozantrone at an initial dose of 20 $mg.m^{-2}$ which proved ineffective in the treatment of refractory or relapsed acute myeloid leukaemia, acute lymphoblastic leukaemia and chronic myeloid leukaemia in blast crisis. The second study, however, using a 5-day treatment regimen at a dose of 10 $mg.m^{-2}$ per day for 5 days, demonstrated a 59% response in 17 evaluable patients with 5/17 achieving complete remission. These patients had acute myeloid leukaemia either refractory to previous treatment or in first relapse, acute lymphoblastic leukaemia refractory or in relapse, and (3 patients) with blast crisis of chronic myeloid leukaemia. Four patients were non-evaluable due to early death. Non-haematological toxicities were not considered severe in this study. In the study mitozantrone was established as an active single agent in refractory leukaemia.

3. Gamms R A, Steinberg J, Posner L 1984 Mitozantrone in malignant lymphoma. Seminars in Oncology 11 (suppl 1): 47–49

This study demonstrated useful activity of mitozantrone against all histological types of malignant lymphoma. Two separate schedules were evaluated with the dose of 14 $mg.m^{-2}$ given every 3 weeks providing a better response rate and less toxicity than a weekly schedule of 5 $mg.m^{-2}$. There was an overall response rate of 53% in 28 evaluable patients, with 2 patients achieving a complete response.

Other trials

Breast

1. Leonard R C F, Cornbleet M A, Kaye S B et al 1987 Mitozantrone versus doxorubicin in combination chemotherapy for advanced carcinoma of the breast. Journal of Clinical Oncology 5: 1056–1063
2. Powels T J, Ashley S E, Forgeson G V et al 1987 Treatment of advanced breast cancer with mitomycin C, mitozantrone and methotrexate (3M) compared with vincristine, an anthracycline and cyclophosphamide. In: Bonadonna G (ed) Clinical progress with mitozantrone. Royal Society of Medicine Services International Congress and Symposium Series No 110. Royal Society of Medicine Services Ltd, pp 1–7

Leukaemia

3. Hiddemann W, Kreutzmann H, Straif K et al 1987 High-dose cytosine arabinoside in combination with mitoxantrone for the treatment of refractory acute myeloid and lymphoblastic leukaemia. Seminars in Oncology 14 (2 suppl 1): 73–77
4. Brito-Babapulle F, Catovsky D, Newland A C, Goldman J M, Galton D A 1987 Treatment of acute myeloid leukaemia with intermediate-dose cytosine arabinoside and mitoxantrone. Seminars in Oncology 14 (suppl 1): 51–52

References

1. Smyth J F, Macpherson J S, Warrington P S, Leonard R C F, Wolf C R 1986 The clinical pharmacology of mitozantrone. Cancer Chemotherapy and Pharmacology 17: 149–152

2. Miser J S, Malspa S L, Staubus A E et al 1963 Plasma pharmacokinetics in paediatric patients. Proceedings of the American Association for Cancer Research 24: 132
3. Alberts D S, Peng Y M, Leigh S, Davis T P, Woodward D L 1985 Disposition of mitozantrone in cancer patients. Cancer Research 45: 879–884
4. Ehringer G, Proksch B, Heinzel G, Schiller E, Woodward D L 1986 Clinical pharmacology of mitozantrone. Cancer Treatment Reports 70: 1373–1378
5. Van Belle S J P, De Planque M M, Smith I E 1986 Pharmacokinetics of mitozantrone in humans following single agent infusion of intra-arterial injection therapy of combined agent infusion therapy. Cancer Chemotherapy and Pharmacology 18: 27–32
6. La Porte J P, Godefray W, Verny A et al 1985 Intrathecal mitozantrone. Lancet 2: 1391
7. Alberts D S, Peng K M, Bowden G T, Dalton W S, Mackel C 1985 Pharmacology of mitozantrone: mode of action. Investigational New Drugs 3: 101–107
8. Lederle Laboratories 1985 Brochure for clinical investigations. Pearl River, NY, October
9. Alberts D S, Peng Y M, Bowden G T, Mackel C, Dalton W S 1985 Mechanisms of action and pharmacokinetics of Novantrone in intravenous and intraperitoneal therapy. Proceedings of Symposium on the Current Status of Mitozantrone, pp 15–21
10. Yap H Y, Blumenschein G R, Schell F C, Budzar A U, Valdivieso M, Bodey G P 1981 Dihydroxyanthracenedione: a promising new drug in the treatment of metastatic breast cancer. Annals of Internal Medicine 95: 694–697
11. Prentice H G, Robbins G, Ma D D F, Ho A D 1983 Sequential studies on the role of mitoxantrone in the treatment of acute leukaemia. Cancer Treatment Reviews 10 (suppl B): 57–63
12. Hiddemann W, Kreutzmann H, Straif K et al 1987 High dose cytosine arabinoside in combination with mitoxantrone for the treatment of refractory acute myeloid and lymphoblastic leukaemia. Seminars in Oncology 14 (2 suppl 1): 73–77
13. Brito-Babapulle F, Catovsky D, Newland A C, Goldman J M, Galton D A 1987 Treatment of acute myeloid leukaemia with intermediate dose cytosine arabinoside and mitozantrone. Seminars in Oncology 14 (2 suppl 1): 51–52
14. Gams R A 1984 Mitoxantrone therapy in malignant lymphomas. In: Smyth J F (ed) A comprehensive guide to the therapeutic use of Novantrone. Pharmalibra Publishers, Chicago, pp 107–117
15. Lawton F, Blackledge G, Mould J, Latief T, Watson R, Chetiyaw A D 1987 Phase II study of mitoxantrone in epithelial ovarian cancer. Cancer Treatment Reports 71: 627–629
16. Falkson G, Coetzer B J, Terblanche A P S 1984 Phase II trial of mitoxantrone in patients with primary liver cancer. Cancer Treatment Reports 68: 1311–1312
17. Smyth J F 1984 Other tumours: Phase II review. In: Smyth J F (ed) A comprehensive guide to the therapeutic use of Novantrone. Pharmalibra Publishers, Chicago, pp 119–125
18. Dukart G 1984 Cardiac events in patients receiving mitoxantrone. In: Smyth J F (ed) A comprehensive guide to the therapeutic use of Novantrone. Pharmalibra Publishers, Chicago, pp 65–74
19. Billingham M E 1984 Mitoxantrone cardiotoxicity in humans: an endomyocardial biopsy assessment. In: Smyth J F (ed) A comprehensive guide to the therapeutic use of Novantrone. Pharmalibra Publishers, Chicago, pp 51–64
20. Novantrone (mitozantrone) Product Information Booklet. Lederle Laboratories, Gosport, Hants
21. Corbett T H, Roberts B J, Trader M W, Laster W R, Griswold D P, Schabel F M 1982 Response of transplantable tumours of mice to anthracenedione derivatives alone and in combination with clinically useful agents. Cancer Treatment Reports 66: 1187–1200
22. Schabel F M, Corbett T H, Griswold D P, Laster W R, Trader M W 1983 Therapeutic activity of mitoxantrone and ametantrone against murine tumours. Cancer Treatment Reviews 10 (suppl B): 13–21

Molsidomine

Molsidomine is a vasodilator used in the treatment and prophylaxis of angina pectoris.

Chemistry

Molsidomine (Corangor, Corvasal, Corvaton, Duracoron, Mobidain, Mobidolat, Morial)
$C_9H_{14}N_4O_4$
N-(Ethoxycarbonyl)-3-(4-morpholinyl)sydnon imine ethyl ester

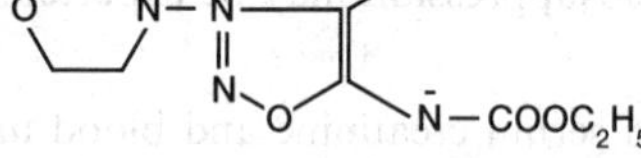

Molecular weight	242.2
pKa	3.0
Solubility	
in alcohol	soluble
in water	sparingly soluble
Octanol/water partition coefficient	—

Colourless crystals or a white crystal powder, practically tasteless and odourless. It is prepared by chemical synthesis. It is not available in combination with other drugs.

Pharmacology

Molsidomine is a non-benzene, heterocyclic compound used mainly for its vasodilator properties. Molsidomine is primarily active through its metabolites. Metabolism in the liver produces 3-morpholino-sydnonimine (SIN-1), which is converted non-enzymatically in the blood to N-morpholino-N-nitrosoaminoacetonitril (SIN-1A) which is the active metabolite.[1–4] The free nitroso group in SIN-1A activates soluble guanylate cyclase in vascular smooth muscle and induces vascular relaxation. In the dog, dilatation of peripheral veins occurs and this decreases preload on the heart. There is some increase in the diameter of large coronary arteries.[5] Molsidomine, in addition to its dose-dependent effects in reducing preload, also prevents coronary thrombotic occlusion and reduces the wet weight of thrombus.[6] This effect is independent of venous dilatation since it is not possessed by nitrate. This effect appears to be related to the reduction of thromboxane levels in coronary blood. Tolerance to molsidomine occurs in vitro and is associated with cysteine deficiency.

Molsidomine also increases cyclic GMP in platelets and this inhibits platelet aggregation.

Toxicology

No information on teratogenicity or carcinogenicity in man is available.

Clinical pharmacology

Molsidomine causes a marked reduction in left ventricular loading conditions, resulting in reduced diastolic filling and improved systolic emptying.[1] These effects are due to a direct effect on the veins that results in peripheral venous pooling of blood and, to a lesser extent, dilatation of systemic arteriolar beds.[1,7,8] The effects on preload predominate at rest since stroke volume and cardiac output are reduced.[1,7,8] These effects are similar to those of nitroglycerin except that the actions of molsidomine are more prolonged.[1,2] During exercise the effects are compounded by direct arteriolar dilatation, which lowers systemic vascular resistance and consequently impedance to left ventricular ejection.[1] Molsidomine also has some platelet-inhibiting effect but the importance of this in clinical practice is not clear.

Doses of 2 mg three times daily have been shown to be effective in treating exercise-induced angina pectoris.[1] A clinical effect of the drug is present for at least 6 hours after one oral dose of 2 mg.[1] The heart rate and blood pressure response of the patient to exercise are similar to nitroglycerin.[1,2] However, unlike nitroglycerin, tolerance does not seem to develop during chronic therapy.[9–11]

Pharmacokinetics

The preferred analytical method for molsidomine is by liquid column chromatography.[12,13] Molsidomine is completely absorbed from the gastrointestinal tract and peak plasma levels are reached 0.5 to 1.0 hours after an oral dose.[12] Systemic bioavailability is approximately 44%.[12] The mean plasma half life[12,14] is between 1.6 and 2.1 h. The volume of distribution is 98 ± 48 litres and the drug is not plasma protein bound. Less than 2% of the drug appears unchanged in the urine;[12] 90–95% of the metabolized drug is excreted in the urine.[12] Faecal excretion is around 3 to 4%.[12]

Oral absorption	complete
Presystemic metabolism	56%
Plasma half life	1–9 h
Volume of distribution	98 ± 48 l
Plasma protein binding	nil

Concentration–effect relationship

There are no satisfactory data supporting a correlation between levels of molsidomine or its metabolites and its antianginal efficacy. However, correlations between plasma levels of molsidomine and SIN-1, and arterial effects in man have been shown.[14] These authors showed that the maximal arterial effects of molsidomine after a single oral dose of 4 mg correlated with its peak plasma concentration of 76.1 ± 33.7 μg.l^{-1}. Thereafter the plasma concentration of molsidomine fell and the arterial effects declined with a similar slope as the corresponding molsidomine concentration. A similar relationship between arterial effects and concentration of SIN-1 has also been shown.[14] The 50% effective concentration of molsidomine was 32.5 ± 20.9 μg.l^{-1} whereas that for SIN-1 was substantially smaller[14], 4.4 ± 2.6 μg.l^{-1}. The clinical value of plasma concentration monitoring has yet to be shown.

Metabolism

Molsidomine is extensively metabolized in the liver by enzyme hydrolysis and decarboxylation to SIN-1 (Fig. 1)[3] In a subsequent nonenzymatic and pH dependent step, the oxazolidine ring is opened and a labile intermediate compound, SIN-1A, is formed.[3] SIN-1A carries the pharmacologically active NNO-group.[3] SIN-1A is rapidly

Fig. 1 Metabolism of molsidomine

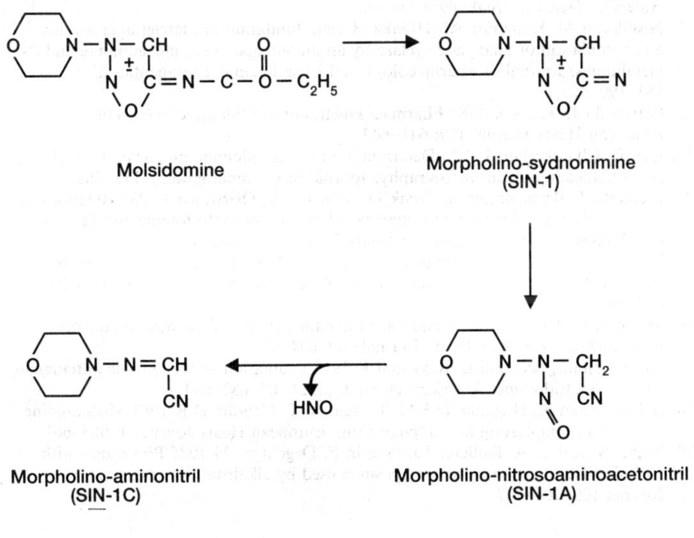

Molsidomine

denitrosylated to the inactive metabolite SIN-1C.[3] Following a single oral dose of molsidomine (8 mg) SIN-1 is measurable in the plasma almost immediately and reaches a maximal value before the peak level of molsidomine, SIN-1 and SIN-1C decline with the same slopes.[14] It is likely that the formation of SIN-1 is the rate-limiting step in the metabolic sequence. Excretion of the metabolites is almost entirely in the urine (95%) with very little in the faeces.

Pharmaceutics

Molsidomine is not available for clinical use in the UK or USA. It is available elsewhere in 2 and 4 mg tablets and as a slow-release preparation containing 8 mg molsidomine.[14] It is also available as an intravenous preparation.

Therapeutic use

Indications

1. Treatment of angina pectoris
2. Chronic cardiac failure.

Contraindications

There are no specific contraindications to treatment with molsidomine. Care should be taken, as with all vasodilator drugs in patients with low systolic blood pressures and cardiac failure.

Indications

1. Treatment of angina pectoris

Molsidomine produces a reduction in cardiac preload with consequent reduced diastolic filling and reduced cardiac output due to dilatation of the venous system.[1,7,8] This causes a reduction in cardiac work. A small degree of arteriolar dilatation occurs, reducing peripheral vascular resistance but this effect is only apparent on exercise.[1] It has been shown to be more effective than placebo[1,2,15–17] and is as effective as propranolol[18] in doses of up to 2 mg three times daily in the treatment of angina pectoris, improving symptoms and the duration of exercise to ST segment depression on exercise testing. Preliminary data suggest that it may prevent coronary spasm.[19]

Treatment with molsidomine is usually begun with 2 mg three times daily and this may be increased to 4 mg four times daily according to clinical response.[1,15,17,18,20]

2. Treatment of chronic heart failure

Molsidomine has been used for the treatment of both chronic and acute heart failure but there are no satisfactory controlled trials.

Larbig and colleagues[21] showed that in patients with chronic heart failure molsidomine (4 mg four times daily) decreased pulmonary artery, pulmonary capillary wedge and right atrial pressures whilst cardiac output and systemic blood pressure were unchanged. These effects persisted for at least 3 weeks. A symptomatic improvement in patients with chronic heart failure treated with molsidomine in addition to their usual treatment of diuretic and digoxin was reported by Acar and colleagues.[22] No exercise tolerance was reported however.[22]

In patients with acute left ventricular failure due to myocardial infarction molsidomine has been shown to have beneficial haemodynamic effects, with a lowering of pulmonary artery diastolic pressure and minimal change in systemic blood pressure compared to controls.[23] There was, however, no improvement in cardiac output.

The effects of molsidomine in patients with both acute and chronic heart failure are consistent with predominantly a reduction in preload due to venodilatation[21–23] and are therefore similar to nitroglycerin.

Adverse reactions

Potentially life-threatening effects

None has been reported.

Acute overdosage

No cases of self-poisoning have been reported. It is expected that hypotension would occur and this should be treated by appropriate cardiovascular support.

Severe or irreversible adverse effects

None has been reported.

Symptomatic adverse effects
Molsidomine frequently causes headache.[1] Other adverse effects are much less frequent and include loss of appetite, nausea, vomiting, diarrhoea, facial flushing and orthostatic hypotension.

Other effects
Molsidomine does not cause any clinically significant biochemical abnormalities.[1]

Interference with clinical pathology tests
No technical interferences of this kind have been reported.

High risk groups

Neonates
The drug is not indicated for use in neonates.

Breast milk. No data are available on the excretion of molsidomine into human breast milk. Molsidomine should therefore not be given to breast-feeding women.

Children
The drug is not used in children.

Pregnant women
There are no data supporting safety of molsidomine in pregnant women and it should therefore not be administered.

The elderly
Though no special precautions are necessary, as doses of molsidomine are adjusted according to the patient response, it must be remembered that elderly patients are more susceptible to the hypotensive effects of all vasodilating agents, and so the starting dose of molsidomine should be reduced.

Drug interactions

Potentially hazardous interactions
No potentially dangerous drug interactions have been reported.

Potentially useful interactions
Molsidomine may be usefully combined with a β-adrenoceptor blocking drug in the treatment of angina pectoris,[24] since both drugs have different though complimentary modes of action.

Clinical trials

1. Majid P A, DeFeyter P J F, Van der Wall E E, Wardeh R, Roos J P 1980 Molsidomine in the treatment of patients with angina pectoris. Acute hemodynamic effects and clinical efficacy. New England Journal of Medicine 302: 1–6

This is a placebo-controlled study comparing molsidomine 2 mg three times daily with placebo in 14 patients with stable exertional angina pectoris. Patients were assessed by symptoms, nitroglycerin consumption and treadmill exercise testing. Molsidomine reduced the frequency of angina pectoris attacks and the consumption of nitroglycerin tablets compared to placebo. On exercise testing, though exercise capacity was not improved by molsidomine, the magnitude of ST segment depression was significantly reduced and this effect lasted for up to 6 hours.

2. Takeshita A, Nakamura M, Tajimi T et al 1977 Long-lasting effect of molsidomine on exercise performance. A new antianginal agent. Circulation 55: 401–407

In this study molsidomine was compared with placebo in a randomized crossover study of 8 patients with chronic stable angina pectoris. Exercise testing was performed 2 hours after oral administration of either molsidomine, 2 mg, or placebo. Molsidomine increased exercise capacity in all 8 patients and increased the duration of exercise before the onset of ST segment depression compared with placebo. These data indicate that molsidomine offers prophylaxis for angina pectoris that lasts for at least 2 hours after oral administration.

3. Messin R 1985 Exercise tolerance in coronary patients: randomized trial of two-week treatment with molsidomine versus placebo. American Heart Journal 109: 667–669

Molsidomine was compared with placebo in a randomized, double-blind, crossover study in 25 patients with coronary artery disease. Molsidomine increased exercise capacity and reduced the magnitude of ST segment depression compared to placebo. Symptomatic changes were not reported.

Other trials

1. Balakumaran K, Hugenholtz P G, Tijssen J G P, Chadha D R 1983 Molsidomine, an effective long-lasting anti-anginal drug. European Heart Journal 4: 655–661

Molsidomine was compared with propranolol in a double-blind, crossover study in 39 patients with stable angina pectoris on effort. The frequency of angina pectoris was similar with both drugs though propranolol was more effective in reducing nitroglycerin consumption. Exercise tolerance was increased by both drugs to a comparable extent. The rate–pressure product was lower with propranolol compared with molsidomine, indicating that these drugs achieve their anti-anginal effect via different mechanisms.

2. Van Mantgem J P, Lie K I, Matroos A W 1985 Combination of metoprolol with molsidomine in the treatment of angina pectoris. European Journal of Clinical Pharmacology 28: 109–111

This was a randomized, parallel, double-blind study in which 31 patients, who were being unsuccessfully treated with metoprolol, 100 mg two times daily, for severe angina pectoris were given either molsidomine, 2 mg three times daily, or placebo. There was a small and significant improvement in exercise capacity in the molsidomine-treated group. Exercise heart rate and blood pressure response were similar in the two groups. There was no difference between the two groups in terms of frequency of angina attacks and nitroglycerin consumption was similar in the two groups.

References

1. Majid P A, DeFeyter P J F, Van der Wall E E, Wardeh R, Roos J P 1980 Molsidomine in the treatment of patients with angina pectoris. Acute haemodynamic effects and clinical efficacy New England Journal of Medicine 302: 1–6
2. Takeshita A, Nakamura M, Tajimi T et al 1977 Long-lasting effect of oral molsidomine on exercise performance. A new antianginal agent. Circulation 55: 401–407
3. Bassenge E, Kukovetz 1984 Molsidomine. In: Scriabine A (ed) New drugs annual: cardiovascular drugs, vol 2. Raven Press, New York, pp 177–191
4. Tanayama S, Fujita T, Shirakawa Y, Suzvoki Z 1970 Metabolic fate of 5-ethoxycarbonyl-3-morpholinosydnonimine (SIN10). Absorbtion, excretion and tissue distribution in rats and mice. Japanese Journal of Pharmacology 20: 413–423
5. Bassenage E, Pohl U 1985 Effect of molsidomine on cardiac preload, coronary artery diameter and coronary resistance. American Heart Journal 109: 627–630
6. Nitz R E, Martorana P A 1985 The activity of molsidomine in experimental models of ischemic cardiac disease. American Heart Journal 109: 631–636
7. Karsch K R, Rentrop K P, Blanke H, Kreuzer A 1978 Haemodynamic effects of molsidomin. European Journal of Clinical Pharmacology 13: 241–245
8. Kikichi K, Hirato M, Nagaoka A 1970 Hypotensive action of N-ethoxycarbonyl-3-morpholinosydnonimine, SIN-10. Japanese Journal of Pharmacology 20: 102–115
9. Luscher T F 1989 Endothelium-derived relaxing contracting factors: potential role in coronary artery disease. European Heart Journal 10: 847–857
10. Kukovetz W R, Holzman S 1985 Mechanisms of vasodilation by molsidomine. American Heart Journal 109: 637–640
11. Nishikawa M, Kanamori M, Hidaka H 1982 Inhibition of platelet aggregation and stimulation of guanylate cyclase by an antianginal agent molsidomine and its metabolites. Journal of Pharmacology and Experimental Therapeutics 220: 183–190
12. Ostrowski J, Resag K 1985 Pharmacokinetics of molsidomine in humans. American Heart Journal 109: 641–643
13. Dell D, Chamberlain J 1978 Determination of molsidomine in plasma by high performance liquid chromatography. Journal of Chromatography 146: 465
14. Meinertz T, Brandstatter A, Trenk D, Jahnchen E, Ostrowski J 1985 Relationship between pharmacokinetics and pharmacodynamics of molsidomine and its metabolites in humans. American Heart Journal 109: 644–648
15. Messin R 1985 Exercise tolerance in coronary patients: randomised trial of two week treatment with molsidomine versus placebo. American Heart Journal 109: 667–669
16. Malcolm A D 1985 Clinical and haemodynamic effects of the new dilator drug molsidomine. American Heart Journal 109: 674–677
17. Dalla-Volta S, Scorzelli L, Razzolini R 1985 Evaluation of the chronic antianginal effect of molsidomine. American Heart Journal 109: 682–684
18. Balakumaran K, Hugenholtz P G, Tijssen J G P, Chadha D R 1983 Molsidomine, an effective long-lasting anti-anginal drug. European Heart Journal 4: 655–661
19. Weber S, Kahan A, Pailleret J J, Guerin F, Degeorges M 1985 Prevention with molsidomine of coronary artery spasm caused by alkalosis. American Heart Journal 109: 704–707

20. Rudolph W, Dirschinger J 1985 Effectiveness of molsidomine in the long-term treatment of exertional angina pectoris and chronic heart failure. American Heart Journal 109: 670–674
21. Larbig D T, Milstrey H R, Nasse H, Kahle T 1985 The influence of molsidomine on the hemodynamics of patients with chronic heart failure at rest and during exercise. American Heart Journal 109: 688–690
22. Acar J, Kulas A, Escudier B 1985 Long-term clinical and hemodynamic results of molsidomine treatment in patients with refractory heart failure. American Heart Journal 109: 685–687
23. Reifart N, Neidl K, Kaltenbach M, Bussman W D 1985 Hemodynamic effects of molsidomine in patients with acute myocardial infarction. American Heart Journal 109: 708–712
24. De Backer G G, Derese A 1985 Double-blind randomized, placebo-controlled study of molsidomine in patients with stable effort angina receiving β-blocker therapy with atenolol. American Heart Journal 109: 678–681

Morphine

Morphine was isolated from an opium extract in 1803 by Serturner,[1] but the chemical structure was not elucidated until 1925[2] and chemical synthesis was not achieved until 1952.[3] Nevertheless, morphine is still the opiate drug with which all new drugs with suspected opioid activity are compared and it is frequently considered by many doctors to be the 'drug of choice' for the treatment of severe acute pain (e.g. postoperative and trauma) and pain related to cancer.

Chemistry

Morphine (Duromorph, MST Continus, Oramorph)
$C_{17}H_{17}NO_3.H_2O$
7,8-Didehydro-4,5-epoxy-3,6-dihydroxy-n-methylmorphinan

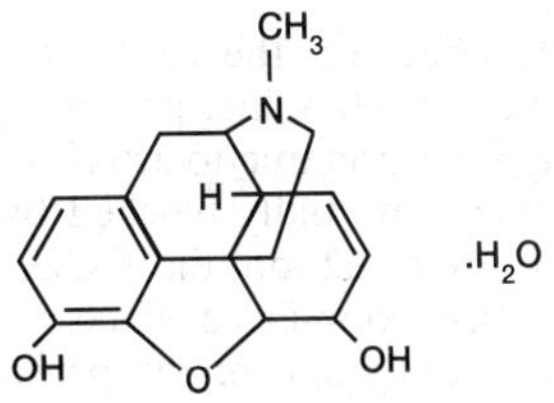

Molecular weight (anhydrous)	303.4 (285.3)
pKa (tertiary amine, phenolic hydrogen)	7.93, 9.63
Solubility	
in alcohol	1 in 250
in water	1 in 5000
Octanol/water partition coefficient	6.03

Morphine occurs as a colourless white crystalline powder with a bitter taste. It is prepared from opium, the dried sap obtained by lancing the unripe seed pods of the opium poppy (*Papaver somniferum*), or by solvent extraction of poppy straw (the dried seed pods and stalk of the poppy). The preparation used clinically is laevorotary. Morphine and salts of morphine are available as tablets (sometimes in combination with aspirin or other pharmacological agents), a variety of mixtures (also in combination with other drugs) and parenteral formulations (alone or in combination with other drugs).

Pharmacology

Morphine is a potent analgesic with competitive agonist actions at the μ receptor which is thought to mediate many of its other actions of respiratory depression, euphoria, inhibition of gut motility and physical dependence. It is possible that analgesia, euphoria and dependence may be due to the effects of morphine on a μ-1 receptor subtype, while respiratory depression and inhibition of gut motility may be due to actions on a μ-2 receptor subtype. Morphine is also a competitive agonist at the κ receptor which mediates spinal analgesia, miosis and sedation. Morphine has no significant actions at the other two major opioid receptors, the δ and the σ receptors.

Morphine directly suppresses cough by an effect on the cough centre in the medulla. Morphine also produces nausea and vomiting by directly stimulating the chemoreceptor trigger zone in the area postrema of the medulla. Morphine provokes the release of histamine.

Toxicology

Morphine, like the majority of other opioids, has been shown experimentally to induce nervous system defects in the offspring

Morphine

following administration to pregnant hamsters and mice,[4] which may be related to hypoxaemia and subsequent hypoglycaemia. However, the evidence for these effects in man is far from conclusive.

Clinical pharmacology

The occupancy of the μ receptor by morphine results in pain relief, a feeling of calmness and respiratory depression. The dose of morphine required for pain relief does vary from individual to individual, depending on the cause of the pain amongst other reasons and thus doses need to be individually adjusted. Morphine also induces drowsiness and this effect is paramount when the drug is given to normal pain-free individuals. Elsewhere in the central nervous system morphine suppresses cough and may cause nausea and vomiting due to stimulation of the chemoreceptor trigger zone. Respiratory depression may occur within 7 minutes of an intravenous injection of morphine and is manifest by a reduced responsiveness of the brain stem respiratory centre to increasing concentrations of inhaled carbon dioxide.

Morphine has effects on the hypothalamus and pituitary–adrenal axis resulting in an increased secretion of antidiuretic hormone, thyroid stimulating hormone and prolactin. Cortisol production is diminished[5,6] due to decreased secretion of corticotrophin releasing factor (CRF) while decreased secretion of gonadotrophin releasing hormone (GnRH) leads to a reduction in the secretion of FSH and LH. Morphine induces a shift in the EEG toward lower frequencies and increased voltage.

Morphine has little effect on the cardiovascular system in the supine patient. However, on standing, patients given morphine may experience postural hypotension due to arteriolar and venous dilatation. This vasodilatation is partially blocked by the histamine (H_1) antagonists. There is no effect on the ECG or on the cerebral circulation. Morphine has pronounced effects on the gastrointestinal tract which results in a reduction in the peristaltic activity of the intestines leading to constipation.[7] Morphine causes some decrease in gastric acid secretion, as well as in biliary and pancreatic secretions. The rate of gastric emptying is markedly reduced.[8,9] Morphine causes an increase in the pressure in the biliary tract and this may explain why the pain of biliary colic is not always helped by morphine.[10]

Morphine has effects on smooth muscle elsewhere resulting in occasional urgency of micturition and prolongation of labour. Tolerance and physical dependence with repeated use of morphine are common.

Pharmacokinetics

There are many analytical methods reported for the quantitation of morphine including gas–liquid chromatography[11] usually following derivatization and radioimmunoassay.[12,13] The radioimmunoassay (RIA) procedure is subject to interference by the glucuronide metabolites of morphine to a variable extent.[14–16] However, the preferred method is by high pressure liquid chromatography (HPLC) with electrochemical detection which is both a sensitive (with a lower limit of 1 μg.l^{-1}) and selective assay procedure.[17–20] The analytical method used to quantitate morphine concentrations in blood or plasma (for example, HPLC or RIA) will affect the derived pharmacokinetic parameters because of the significant cross-reactivity of the glucuronide metabolites with the antibody to morphine in RIA procedures.

Morphine is rapidly, but variably, absorbed from the gastrointestinal tract following oral administration with peak blood concentrations occurring 30–120 min following the dose.[21,22] However, the mean oral bioavailability is approximately 30% within the range of 10–50%.[21,23] These data indicate that the mean oral/parenteral ratio for an equivalent pain relieving effect is 3 but the extremes in this ratio are 2–10. The reason for the poor oral bioavailability is the extensive hepatic presystemic metabolism of morphine which results in a marked 'first-pass effect' following oral doses. In addition, animal studies[24,25] have shown that morphine is metabolized by the intestinal mucosa prior to absorption and intestinal metabolism accounts for 50–66% of the first-pass effect. It is probable that a similar situation occurs in man but the actual percentage contribution of intestinal metabolism may be different from the data obtained in animals.

The mean elimination half life for morphine in blood[21] and plasma[26] is 2.7 h (range 1.2–4.9 h) and 2.95 h (range 1.8–5 h) respectively. The mean blood[21] and plasma[26] clearance is 1.16 l.min^{-1} (range 0.32–1.7 l.min^{-1}) and 1.09 l.min^{-1} (range 0.77–1.1 l.min^{-1}), respectively. There are, however, other studies[27,28] which report lower estimates of morphine clearance, but these measurements were made under the influence of anaesthesia in surgical patients which could alter the results obtained. This high clearance value is approximately 75% of hepatic blood flow (HBF) and suggests that HBF rather than the capacity of the liver enzymes to metabolize morphine is the major determinant of morphine clearance. Therefore, drugs and environmental agents which induce drug metabolism will have only a minor effect on morphine clearance and half life, although they may alter bioavailability of oral doses.

Both single[29] and multiple[30] dose pretreatment of volunteers with cimetidine had no significant effect on morphine half life, clearance and volume of distribution at steady state. In addition, morphine-induced miosis, the extent of which is correlated with morphine plasma concentration,[31] was similar in placebo and cimetidine-pretreated volunteers.[30] However, the situation is clouded by the finding of a statistically significant but clinically insignificant shift in the carbon dioxide response curves in volunteers treated with cimetidine plus morphine compared with that obtained with morphine alone.[29] Cimetidine alone had minimal effects on the carbon dioxide response curves suggesting an elevation in morphine blood concentration as a result of the inhibition of morphine metabolism by cimetidine.

Morphine is relatively hydrophilic and therefore has a lower volume of distribution than the majority of the other commonly used opioid drugs. The apparent volume of distribution at steady state is usually 2–3 l.kg^{-1} [21,23,32] but a mean value of 1.02 l.kg^{-1} was reported for cardiac surgery patients.[27] The blood or plasma concentration–time data are usually best fitted by a two or three term polyexponential equation suggesting slow but extensive distribution throughout the body. Animal studies have shown that the highest levels of morphine occur in liver, kidney, lung, heart, cerebellum, spleen, thymus, adrenals, and thyroid.[33] In humans undergoing autopsy, the highest concentrations of morphine were found in blood, bile, lung and liver.[34] A similar profile was obtained in neonates from heroin-dependent mothers who died 3–5 days after birth where high morphine concentrations were found in brain stem, thymus, spleen, lungs, liver and cerebellum.[33] The authors suggest that the low morphine concentrations in the CNS combined with the pronounced central nervous system effects of morphine indicate that the nervous system of neonates is immature and sensitive to morphine.

Animal studies have indicated that there is a significant 'blood–brain barrier' controlling the entry of morphine into the CNS. For example, morphine is significantly more potent (approximately 900 times) when administered intraventricularly when compared with systemic administration.[35] Further, there is a longer time delay to maximal effects (e.g. the use in anaesthesia to suppress noxious stimuli and pain relief) with morphine than with other more lipophilic opioids such as pethidine, fentanyl and methadone.

A recent study[36] has revealed that the concentration of morphine in CSF samples collected following a 10 mg intramuscular dose was between 1 and 30 μg.l^{-1}. Further, an apparent equilibrium between CSF and blood occurred after 3 h providing a mean CSF/plasma ratio of 0.89 (S.D. 0.14). A similar study[37] undertaken in cancer patients indicated a mean CSF/plasma concentration ratio of 0.3 for morphine, but the ratio for morphine-3-glucuronide was only 0.07.

There was a linear relationship between the morphine dose and morphine concentrations in both plasma and CSF at steady state following the epidural administration of morphine to treat pain in cancer patients.[38] The mean CSF/plasma concentration ratio was 132 at steady state.

Morphine is bound to plasma proteins only to the extent of 25–35% and therefore factors that change the extent of protein binding will have only a minor impact on its pharmacodynamic effects.[39,40]

Morphine is excreted in human breast milk but the amount is generally considered to be less than 1% of any dose.[41] It should be noted that the withdrawal signs observed in newborn infants probably occur as a result of exposure to opioids in utero as the severity of these effects can be correlated to the length of maternal dependence and time since the last opioid dose.[42]

Oral absorption	25–50%
Presystemic metabolism	50–66%
Plasma half life	
range	1–5 h
mean	3 h
Volume of distribution	1.5–4.0 l.kg^{-1}
Plasma protein binding	25–35%

Liver disease does not appear to have a marked effect on morphine pharmacokinetics as the terminal half life, plasma clearance and volume of distribution were similar in cirrhotic patients and normal volunteers.[37,43] Therefore, the morphine doses required to provide an equivalent extent of pain relief in patients with liver disease should be similar to those used in patients with normal hepatic function. Nevertheless, animal studies have shown that there is a significant prolongation of morphine effects in hepatectomized dogs confirming the central role of the liver in the elimination of morphine.[44] Although renal excretion is a minor route of elimination for unchanged morphine, it constitutes the major mechanism of elimination of conjugated metabolites of morphine.[45,46] The renal clearances of morphine, morphine-3-glucuronide and morphine-6-glucuronide were 99 ± 41, 79 ± 32 and 103 ± 47 ml.min^{-1} respectively.[46] There have been reports of prolonged narcosis lasting 3-5 days following normal doses of morphine in patients with renal failure.[47] The specific opioid antagonist, naloxone, reversed these effects suggesting that morphine or one of its metabolites was responsible. Morphine-6-glucuronide, a minor metabolite (approximately 5% of a dose),[45] has been shown to be approximately 40 times as active as morphine[48] in suppressing nociceptive stimuli (hot plate test in rats) following intracerebral administration and therefore could be responsible for the prolonged narcosis. Alternatively, the biliary excretion of morphine glucuronides and the enterohepatic recycling of morphine resulting from the hydrolysis of the glucuronides in the gastrointestinal tract could also explain this effect. There is considerable debate regarding the extent to which the kidney contributes to the overall metabolism of morphine[49] and therefore the influence of renal disease on morphine pharmacokinetics. Aitkenhead et al.[32] have shown that morphine clearance and terminal half life are similar in patients with chronic renal failure compared with normal patients. This finding has recently been confirmed by Sawe and Odar-Cederlof.[50] However, the mean (±S.D.) terminal half life of morphine-3-glucuronide was increased from 4 ± 1.5 hours (range 2.4–6.7 hours) in patients with normal renal function to 49.6 ± 36.9 hours (range 14.5–118.8 hours) in patients with renal failure and there was a significant correlation (r = 0.91) between the elimination half life of morphine-3-glucuronide and serum urea. The half life of the active metabolite, morphine-6-glucuronide was similar to that found for morphine-3-glucuronide in the patients with renal failure.[50] Nevertheless, care must be exercised in the choice of the morphine dose and dosing interval in patients with renal disease.

Age has been shown to be an important factor in determining an effective dose of morphine, with older patients exhibiting an apparently greater sensitivity to a standard dose of morphine. The older patients did not differ from younger patients in peak intensity of pain relief, but the older patients had a longer duration of pain relief for an equivalent dose. However, morphine pharmacokinetic studies suggest that older patients have a lower morphine clearance and a reduced volume of distribution compared with younger patients, which would result in higher morphine concentrations for a given dose.[51]

Concentration–effect relationship

A relationship between blood (or plasma) concentration of morphine and effect has been proposed for postoperative pain,[52,53] cancer pain[21,37] and the suppression of intraoperative surgical stimuli.[54] The minimum effective concentration (MEC) for morphine varies from 10 to 50 µg.l^{-1} for the provision of postoperative pain control while concentrations of 40–70 µg.l^{-1} were required to suppress surgical stimuli. The MEC for morphine in patients with cancer varies from 10 to 45 µg.l^{-1} when estimated soon after the commence ment of morphine therapy.[21] The MEC value would be expected to increase in cancer patients due to the possible combination of effects of a more painful stimulus resulting from progression of the disease and the development of tolerance to morphine. There is also a correlation between the extent of miosis and the plasma morphine concentration.[31]

Metabolism

Morphine is extensively metabolized by hepatic biotransformation and animal studies suggest a significant degree of metabolism in the intestine prior to absorption.[24,25] The kidney has been shown to have the capacity to form morphine glucuronides and only a small percentage of a dose is excreted unchanged in the urine (5–10% of the dose). Morphine-3-glucuronide is the major metabolite (approximately 45% of a dose) while morphine-6-glucuronide is a quantitatively minor (5% of a dose) but active metabolite (see Fig. 1). Other minor metabolites include normorphine (1–5% of the dose) and normorphine-3-glucuronide (3% of the dose), morphine-3,6-diglucuronide, morphine ethereal sulphate and normorphine glucuronides.[45] There has been a report of the conversion of morphine to codeine by O-methylation.[55] Further, biliary excretion of morphine metabolites could occur resulting in the enterohepatic circulation of morphine and ultimately, faecal excretion of both morphine and its metabolites (5–10% of the dose). While the relative contribution of the different routes of metabolism varies between oral and parenteral doses, there are no routes of metabolism specific to a particular mode of administration. Morphine is the active metabolite of diamorphine and is also an active metabolite of codeine.

Fig. 1 Metabolism of morphine

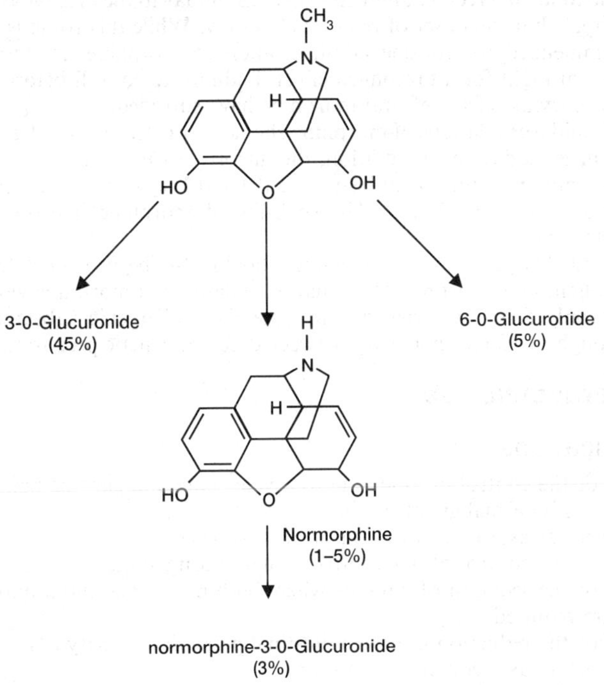

Pharmaceutics

Morphine is available in oral (in both tablet and liquid preparations) and parenteral formulations.

It must be remembered that morphine has been used to provide pain relief for centuries and therefore morphine formulations are not usually patented. Consequently, many manufacturers provide similar formulations containing a particular morphine dose, which precludes a detailed list in this monograph. However, the following is a compendium of generally available strengths and formulations of morphine, which is usually present as the acid salt (either hydrochloride, sulphate or tartrate).

Tablets. Morphine strength of either 10, 15 or 30 mg. Some formulations include either aspirin, atropine or tacrine (tetrahydroaminacrine, which is suggested to be a CNS stimulant which reduces the extent of respiratory depression of morphine therapy allowing larger doses to be administered. However, there is no acceptable experimental evidence to support this claim).

Sustained release tablets. A sustained release formulation (MST; Napp, UK/MS Contin; Purdue-Frederick, US) is available in some countries with morphine strengths of 10, 30, 60 and 100 mg. Although the recommended dosage interval is 12 hourly for the sustained release formulation, clinical experience suggests a more realistic estimate of the dosage interval is 8 hourly.

Oral solutions. The usual strengths of oral morphine mixtures are 5 $mg.ml^{-1}$ or 10 $mg.ml^{-1}$ (MSIR; Purdue-Frederick, US/Oramorph; Boehringer, UK), and these are used mainly in the treatment of cancer pain. Additional pharmacological agents such as cocaine, alcohol, gin, or brandy have been added in various amounts to the morphine mixture to produce a variety of formulations collectively known as 'Brompton's mixture'. However, morphine solution alone has been shown to be as effective in providing pain relief as the equivalent morphine dose in Brompton's mixture.[56]

Injections. The usual strengths of morphine injections are 10 $mg.ml^{-1}$ or 15 $mg.ml^{-1}$. More concentrated injections are available in some countries for use in patients requiring terminal care and these can be as strong as 80 $mg.ml^{-1}$ (for example, morphine tartrate injection). There are formulations containing morphine (10 $mg.ml^{-1}$) and either atropine (0.6 $mg.ml^{-1}$) or hyoscine (0.4 $mg.ml^{-1}$) for use as premedication prior to anaesthesia and surgery.

Suppositories. Morphine has been incorporated into various types of suppository base at a usual concentration of 15 mg per suppository, for patients who cannot take morphine by mouth. The strength of morphine in the suppository can be varied depending on patient requirements. The efficacy of rectal administration of opioids including morphine depends on the type of formulations used (e.g. suppository versus rectal solution).[57] However, the bioavailability of morphine following rectal administration was similar to the oral bioavailability,[58] but the onset of pain relief is slow. While this route is not recommended for routine administration of morphine, it may be useful at night for a prolonged effect if administered well before the pain-relieving effects of oral morphine have subsided.

All liquid formulations of morphine should be protected from light to minimize oxidation. In addition, the majority of injectable formulations contain sodium metabisulphite (0.05–0.1%) to prevent discoloration due to oxidation. The shelf-life of morphine injections is greater than two years.

Solid dosage forms of morphine should also be protected from both light and moisture. The usual formulations of morphine would pose only a minimal risk due to potentially allergenic substances, although this factor may vary between different generic preparations.

Therapeutic use

Indications

1. For the control of moderate to severe acute and chronic pain (mostly of malignant origin)
2. For use as a premedication prior to surgery
3. For the control of nociceptive stimuli during surgery
4. For the sedation of patients where both pain relief and sedation are required
5. For the reduction in gastrointestinal peristaltic activity
6. For use as a cough suppressant
7. For the relief of severe dyspnoea in terminal lung cancer or other terminal respiratory disease.

Contraindications

1. In patients with significant pre-existing respiratory disease
2. In patients with head injuries where there is a potential for raised intracranial pressure
3. In patients with biliary colic
4. In patients with poor coronary perfusion.

Mode of use

The clinical uses of morphine depend on the interaction of morphine with opioid receptors in the brain, spinal cord and gut. The morphine dose for pain relief and the dosing interval must be titrated against the patient's report of pain provided that the clinical condition of the patient does not preclude additional doses. The *major* factor to ensure effective pain control with morphine or any other opioid in both acute and chronic pain is to constantly review the efficacy of the dosage regimen and to be prepared to make appropriate adjustments to the dose, dosage interval or both. The correct dose is the dose that provides good pain relief with minimal or no side effects. However, extreme caution should be exercised in the long-term use of morphine in patients with non-terminal conditions.

Prolonged use of morphine in any patient will result in physical dependence; sudden withdrawal of morphine, or the administration of a specific antagonist (for example, naloxone), will result in an abstinence syndrome.

Indications

1. Acute and chronic pain

Acute pain. Morphine is still considered by many practitioners to be the 'drug of choice' for the control of acute pain. Various routes of administration have been used including intravenous bolus, continuous intravenous infusion, intramuscular, intrathecal, epidural and 'patient-controlled analgesia'.[59] As indicated previously, the dose and dosing interval must be titrated against the patients' report of pain and frequent adjustments may be necessary to achieve optimal pain control.

Recommended starting dosage regimens for a fit adult of 70 kg for the various routes of administration are as follows:

Intravenous boli: 2.5 mg every 5 minutes until analgesia is achieved. Monitor the duration of pain relief and adjust the dose and dosing interval accordingly.
Continuous intravenous infusion: a loading dose of 5–15 mg over 30 minutes, then 2.5–5 mg every hour.
Intramuscular: 5–15 mg every 2–4 hours.
Epidural: 2–15 mg every 12–24 hours.[60] It should be noted that latent and severe respiratory depression has been reported in opioid-naive patients with a suggested incidence of approximately 1 in 1100 cases.[61] Therefore, care should be exercised in the epidural administration of morphine in this group of patients. Epidural pethidine (50–100 mg) is recommended in opioid-naive patients as the epidemiological evidence suggests a very low incidence of delayed respiratory depression with pethidine.
Intrathecal: 0.25–1 mg every 12–24 hours.[62]
Rectal: 15 mg every 2–4 hours.

At the present time, sustained-release morphine preparations are contraindicated for postoperative pain control because of possible delayed gastric emptying, which could result in respiratory depression as a consequence of several doses reaching the duodenum simultaneously.

Chronic pain. Morphine is a valuable drug in the treatment of chronic pain particularly in patients with terminal disease. There is a wide variability in the morphine dose required by these patients, due to both the progressive nature of the terminal disease, which is frequently associated with an increasing pain stimulus, and also a degree of receptor tolerance. Titration of the dose and dosing interval to the patients' requirements will enhance the degree of pain relief. Nevertheless, recommended initial dosage regimens are as follows:

Oral: 10–200 mg every 2–4 hours.[62]
Intravenous: 10–100 mg every 2–4 hours.
Continuous intravenous infusion:[63] 5–200 mg hourly. Similar infusion rates have been administered subcutaneously in the treatment of cancer pain.
Intramuscular: similar to the intravenous regimen.
Epidural: 5–100 mg every 8–24 hours.[60,64]
Subarachnoid: 0.5–5 mg every 8–24 hours.[60]
Subarachnoid infusion: 0.5–30 mg per day.[60,65]
Intraventricular: 0.25–1 mg every 12–24 hours.[66]
Rectal/vaginal: 10–30 mg every 2–4 hours.

It should be noted that the delayed respiratory depression that can occur following epidural or subarachnoid morphine in opioid-naive patients does not occur in patients who have been exposed to opioids for a period of one week or more. There is considerable debate regarding the use of epidural versus intrathecal routes for the spinal administration of morphine.[66,67] It should also be noted that the inappropriate administration of morphine by any route may result in respiratory depression, even in cancer pain patients on long-term opioid therapy.

2. Premedication prior to surgery
Morphine and omnopon are still widely used as a premedication prior to surgery.[68] The usual morphine dose varies between 5 and 15 mg while the equivalent omnopon dose varies from 10 to 30 mg. Frequently, atropine or hyoscine are co-administered with morphine for this indication. The sedative and calming properties of morphine are the main reasons for its frequent use as premedication for surgery. This is often offset by nausea so that benzodiazepines may be a better choice unless sedation and pain relief are required. The usual route of administration is by intramuscular injection at least one hour prior to induction of anaesthesia. If anaesthesia is to be induced in less than one hour, the anaesthetist may elect to administer a lower dose (5–10 mg) by intravenous injection.

3. The suppression of nociceptive stimuli during surgery
Morphine is very effective in the suppression of response to intra-operative surgical stimuli. The dose of morphine varies widely depending on the type of surgery, the duration of surgery and the nature and concomitant use of other anaesthetic agents. For example, the morphine dose could be as low as 2 mg for minor surgical procedures, but as high as 4 $mg.kg^{-1}$ body weight for the induction and maintenance of cardiac surgery patients.[69] These higher intravenous morphine doses can be associated with profound hypotension. In recent times, the synthetic opioid fentanyl has replaced morphine in cardiac surgery because of greater haemodynamic stability. The preferred route of administration is by repeated intravenous bolus doses or continuous intravenous infusion.

4. Sedation where sedation and pain relief are indicated
It should be noted that morphine is *not* indicated as a sedative drug for long-term use. Rather, the use of morphine *is* indicated where the requirement for pain relief and sedation co-exist such as in patients admitted to intensive care units and other high-dependency areas.[70] The patients who satisfy this indication frequently have painful injuries and require ventilation and therefore sedation. The preferred route of administration is by continuous intravenous infusion or repeated intravenous boli with a hourly morphine dose usually varying from 1.25 to 10 mg. The morphine dose should be titrated to provide pain relief and an appropriate level of sedation. Frequently, other pharmacological agents (e.g. benzodiazepines) are added to this regimen to increase the level of sedation.

5. For the reduction of gastrointestinal peristaltic activity
In addition to the interaction of morphine with the receptors in the brain and spinal cord to provide pain relief, morphine also interacts with receptors in the gastrointestinal tract resulting in a reduction in peristaltic activity.[7] While the end result of this interaction is the troublesome side effect of constipation in the majority of patients administered morphine on a long-term basis, it can be used to treat diarrhoea in some patients. For diarrhoea of short duration, the short-term administration of morphine, usually with adsorbants such as kaolin is recommended. However, the long-term administration of morphine in the treatment of chronic diarrhoea should be restricted for patients with diarrhoea associated with a terminal disease in whom a clearcut diagnosis has been made. The effects of morphine on the gut occurs at lower doses and an initial starting oral dose between 2 and 10 mg six-hourly is recommended.

6. For the suppression of cough
Morphine has been used as a cough suppressant although this indication is currently not recommended for routine use. An effective oral dose varies between 5 and 10 mg every four to six hours for coughs of the irritative type usually associated with terminal cancer. Other opioid drugs such as codeine, dihydrocodeine and dextromethorphan have now largely replaced morphine for this indication. Morphine has the potential to increase the incidence of postoperative chest complications by the suppression of a productive cough.

7. For the relief of severe dyspnoea in terminal cancer
Morphine is the drug of choice for the relief of ‘air hunger’ associated with terminal respiratory failure, for example, associated with disseminated cancer of the lungs. The morphine dose is titrated to provide maximal relief of suffering. Morphine is only used for this indication after other means, such as supplemental oxygen, have failed.

Contraindications

1. Significant pre-existing respiratory disease
Extreme caution should be exercised in the use of morphine to provide pain relief in patients with significant pre-existing respiratory insufficiency; for example, patients with bronchial asthma, emphysema, significant bronchial or pulmonary infection, clinically significant arterial oxygen desaturation and respiratory obstruction. Such patients may have a reduced respiratory reserve and therefore the superimposition of the respiratory depressant effects of morphine (or any other opioid agonist) and associated retention of bronchial secretions could result in a life-threatening situation. If possible, non-opioid methods of providing pain relief (for example, regional block techniques) should be employed in these patients, unless adequate respiratory support is available at short notice.

2. Head injuries and raised intracranial pressure
The respiratory depression associated with morphine may increase intracranial pressure as a result of cerebral vasodilatation due to carbon dioxide retention. These effects may be markedly exaggerated in the presence of head injuries, intracranial space occupying lesions or a pre-existing increase in intracranial pressure. Morphine should only be administered under such circumstances when considered essential and then with extreme caution.

3. Biliary colic
Morphine has been shown to induce spasm of the sphincter of Oddi.[10] Therefore, morphine is contraindicated in the treatment of biliary colic. Pethidine has, for a considerable period of time, been proposed as the only opioid agonist not to induce spasm of the sphincter of Oddi.

4. Patients with poor coronary perfusion
Morphine induces variable histamine release resulting in peripheral vasodilatation and a decrease in end-diastolic pressure. This could be an advantage in patients with congestive heart failure following recent myocardial infarction, but a disadvantage in patients with aortic valve disease and significant coronary artery disease. This effect, when combined with concomitant respiratory disease, may constitute a contraindication to the use of morphine in favour of more cardiac-stable opioids such as the fentanyl derivatives. It remains common practice to administer morphine in patients with acute left ventricular failure to reduce ventricular preload as a result of histamine-induced vasodilatation. However, this can be achieved by the use of more specific vasodilators.

Adverse reactions

Potentially life-threatening effects
Although deaths are relatively rare from the medical use of morphine, they are a frequent occurrence following the illicit use of this drug. Following overdoses of morphine, there is significant respiratory depression resulting in cyanosis, hypotension (which sometimes can be profound), and then shock and coma. Death occurs as a result of respiratory failure. The abrupt withdrawal of morphine from patients or recreational users who have been administering the drug on a long-term basis and are therefore dependent upon it will result in an abstinence syndrome characterized by sweating, tachycardia, nausea and vomiting, piloerection, cramps, muscle tremor, yawning, lacrimation, sneezing, headache, insomnia, anxiety, diarrhoea, dehydration, a rise in body temperature and vasomotor disturbances. However uncomfortable these effects are, they are most unlikely to result in death. These effects may be modified by the intravenous, oral or transdermal administration of clonidine.

Anaphylactic shock is a rare adverse reaction to morphine.

Acute overdosage
The main clinical features of massive overdose include respiratory depression leading to respiratory failure, coma, and hypotension. In mild overdose, symptoms include nausea and vomiting, tremor, miosis, dysphoria, hypothermia, hypotension, confusion, and sedation.

The medical management of overdose involves the prompt institution of respiratory support, and the intravenous administration of naloxone. The initial intravenous naloxone dose (0.4 mg) should be

M

repeated at 1–2 minute intervals to a maximum dose of 1.2–1.6 mg. Following the initial response, repeated doses at 1–2 hourly intervals or a naloxone infusion may be required for optimal management. If the patient has not responded to the initial doses of 0.4–1.6 mg, it is most likely that some other CNS depressant has been administered possibly in combination with morphine. Both respiratory and cardiovascular support is given; the latter consists of intravenous fluids and inotropic agents if hypotension is a serious problem.

Severe or irreversible adverse effects

Psychological and physical dependence is discussed elsewhere.

Symptomatic adverse effects

The symptomatic adverse effects of morphine are mediated by occupancy of receptors in the CNS and periphery, notably the gastrointestinal tract. The CNS effects include itching, nausea and vomiting, sedation, respiratory depression, mental clouding, hallucinations and dreams, dizziness, and alterations to mood. The latter changes in mood need not necessarily be considered undesirable as the ability of morphine to induce a sensation of calmness to the point of euphoria can be advantageous when morphine is used as a premedicant prior to surgery and in the treatment of cancer pain. Other highly undesirable CNS effects include psychological dependence, physical dependence (not a problem in acute and cancer pain), orthostatic hypotension, miosis, bradycardia, dry mouth, sweating, facial flushing, and hypothermia. Morphine has endocrine and metabolic effects. For example, morphine increases the secretion of pituitary hormones with the exception of ACTH which is decreased. Thyroid secretion is decreased by morphine but adrenaline secretion from the adrenals is increased.

Other adverse effects associated with actions of morphine in the periphery include constipation, spasm of the sphincter of Oddi resulting in biliary colic, and spasm of the sphincter of the urinary bladder which can result in urinary retention. Further, morphine can induce histamine release which may be partly responsible for asthma, pruritis, and urticaria. Morphine has a depressant effect on gonadal hormone secretion which can result in a reduction of testosterone secretion leading to regression of secondary sexual characteristics in men on long-term therapy. A disruption in ovulation and amenorrhoea can occur in women. While morphine can significantly suppress lactation, only small amounts of morphine are secreted in breast milk.

Other effects

Morphine has been reported[71] to increase the blood, plasma or serum levels of the following enzymes: amylase, hydroxybutyric acid dehydrogenase, lipase, the transaminases (alanine aminotransferase [ALT, SGPT] and aspartate aminotransferase [AST, SGOT]), alkaline phosphatase, leucine aminopeptidase, and lactate dehydrogenase, due to spasm of the sphincter of Oddi. Increased bilirubin levels together with bromosulphthalein retention time and decreased indocyanine green clearance have been reported for the same reason. The liver enzymes can remain elevated for longer than 24 hours, which may complicate the diagnosis of acute abdominal pain.

Morphine has been reported to decrease the basal metabolic rate and decrease gastric acidity by reducing the secretion of acid. There can be increased levels of creatinine kinase as a response to frequent intramuscular injections of morphine. Morphine has the metabolic effect of increasing adrenaline while decreasing noradrenaline concentrations in plasma; the rise in adrenaline is probably mediated by a central action on the brain. Plasma histamine concentrations can be increased following intravenous morphine administration.

Morphine can cause hypercapnia by reducing ventilation which needs to be considered in the interpretation of blood gas results. Urinary volume may be decreased as morphine stimulates antidiuretic hormone release. Plasma and urinary 17-ketosteroids and 17-hydroxycorticosteroids can be reduced as morphine inhibits ACTH and pituitary gonadotrophin release.

Interference with clinical pathology tests

Morphine can react with the Folin–Ciocalteau reagent in the Lowry method of protein estimation.[71] Morphine can also interfere with the determination of urinary 17-ketosteroids due to chemical structure effects in the Zimmerman procedure.

High risk groups

Clinical observation and experimental data indicate that premature, term neonates, infants, and children differ from one another in response to opioid drugs. Further, the altered response to morphine is probably greater than that observed for the new opioids such as fentanyl.

Neonates

The administration of morphine (or any other opioid) to neonates requires very careful control of dosage and conditions of continuous surveillance, because of the immaturity of their nervous systems and altered pharmacokinetics. The terminal half life was 13.9 ± 6.4 hours (range 5.2–28 hours) in neonates with a gestational age varying from 35 to 41 weeks[72] and studied with a mean postnatal age of 9.5 ($\pm$S.D. 4.3) days when a morphine infusion was used for postoperative pain relief. The morphine clearance, estimated from the steady-state blood morphine concentrations, varied from 1.7 to 39 $ml.kg^{-1}.min^{-1}$ with a mean ($\pm$S.E.) value of 7.8 ± 1.9 $ml.kg^{-1}.min^{-1}$. There was a tendency for the steady-state blood morphine concentration to decrease with time during a constant rate intravenous infusion suggesting an improvement in the morphine clearance rate.[72] There was significant correlation ($p < 0.02$) between steady-state blood morphine concentration and the infusion rate, but the blood concentration at 20 hours varied from 15 to 100 $\mu g.l^{-1}$ in patients receiving a morphine infusion at the rate of 20 $\mu g.kg^{-1}.h^{-1}$. Two infants had grand mal seizures 3–5 hours after the initiation of infusion rates of 32 and 40 $\mu g.kg^{-1}.h^{-1}$ which resulted in morphine concentrations of 61 and 90 $\mu g.l^{-1}$ at the time of the seizure.[73] Morphine concentrations of this magnitude have been associated with the suppression of surgical stimuli in children[54] and the control of both postoperative[52,53] and cancer pain[21,37] in adults, suggesting an immature nervous system in neonates. Koren et al.[72] recommended that the preferred infusion rate should be less than 15 $\mu g.kg^{-1}.h^{-1}$ to minimize the possibility of seizures. The only exception to this recommendation should be the administration of morphine (preferably by anaesthetists) to control nociceptive stimuli as a result of surgery. There is now evidence that preterm[74] and term neonates have a stress response to surgical stimulation[75] and that outcome is improved by the administration of opioid drugs.[74] When opioids are given in such situations, fentanyl, or its analogues[75] may be better choices than morphine because of their higher therapeutic index.

Infants

Studies of greater respiratory depression due to morphine in neonates compared with adults[76] have been extrapolated by stating that infants as well as neonates are 'sensitive' to the respiratory depressant effects of opioids. However, studies with fentanyl report that infants older than 3 months were not more sensitive and may even be more resistant than adults to respiratory depressant effects.[77] Some of the adverse respiratory effects of opioids in infants may have resulted from inappropriately high-dose regimens. Opioid drugs are required to treat pain in infants and it is unacceptable to attempt to imply that pain is 'not perceived' at this age.[74] Until more data are available for morphine, it may be wise to use fentanyl because of its documented respiratory effects and greater cardiovascular stability.

Breast milk. While morphine can suppress lactation, the quantity that may reach the neonate via breast milk is probably insufficient to cause major problems of dependence or adverse effects.[41]

Children

Morphine is used in children to treat pain associated with operations and trauma, as premedication prior to surgery, and in anaesthesia to suppress nociceptive stimuli. Van den Berghe et al.[78] studied morphine pharmacokinetics during morphine infusions in children aged from 3 months to 5 years. The mean ($\pm$S.D.) morphine clearance was estimated to be 20.5 ± 2.8 $ml.kg^{-1}.min^{-1}$ (range 15.1–23.7 $ml.kg^{-1}.min^{-1}$) during infusions of 60–120 $\mu g.kg^{-1}.h^{-1}$ which resulted in apparent steady-state morphine concentrations ranging from 31.7 to 98.7 $\mu g.l^{-1}$. However, Dahlstrom et al.[54] reported clearance values of approximately 6–7 $ml.kg^{-1}.min^{-1}$ in children aged from 1 to 15 years following intravenous doses administered perioperatively. Lynn et al.[79] provided postoperative pain relief with a morphine infusion at a rate varying from 10 to 30 $\mu g.kg^{-1}.h^{-1}$ following cardiac surgery in patients aged from 14 months to 17 years (mean age was 6.5 years). There was a non-linear relationship between the mean serum morphine concentration at 24 hours

(10 μg.l^{-1}, 17 μg.l^{-1} and 21 μg.l^{-1}) and the morphine infusion rate (10, 20 and 30 μg.kg^{-1}.h^{-1}, respectively). Serum morphine concentrations of less than 30 μg.l^{-1} did not affect baseline respiratory control values as shown by blood gas analysis.

Postoperative pain relief has been achieved by both epidural[80] and intrathecal[81] administration of morphine in children with a mean age of approximately 7 years. The epidural dose varied from 0.5 to 2 mg and provided pain relief lasting from 8 to 25 hours. The intrathecal morphine dose varied from 0.02 to 0.03 mg.kg^{-1}, and respiratory depression occurred in 16% of the patients usually from 3.5 to 4.5 hours after the administration of intrathecal morphine. In all of these indications, the dose of morphine should be titrated to achieve the desired effect.

Pregnant women

Morphine has been extensively used in the past for obstetric analgesia. Morphine undoubtedly causes respiratory depression in the neonate as shown by a shift to the right in the CO_2 response curve.[76] In addition, morphine has clinically significant effects on fetal heart rate[82] and on fetal heart rate variability.[83] Factors influencing the severity of these effects include the magnitude of the morphine dose and the time latency between delivery and the last morphine dose. With respect to the latter effect, more pronounced neonatal effects are observed if delivery occurs between 1 and 6 hours from the last morphine dose. Therefore, parenteral administration of morphine is now rarely used for pain relief in labour when safer alternative techniques are available such as inhalational analgesia (nitrous oxide) or epidural local anaesthetic or opioid.

There is a significantly increased incidence of complications in neonates delivered of opioid-dependent mothers. These include tremor, irritability, hypertonus, respiratory distress, fever, diarrhoea, convulsions, and vomiting, which are associated with opioid abstinence. However, the incidence of congenital malformations is no greater than that observed in the general population.[42] The higher incidence of complications in neonates may be associated with the lower socio-economic status and hence poorer nutritional status of the mother. In addition, there is a greater incidence of infection and disease as a result of using communal needles for injecting opioids during pregnancy.[42]

The elderly

Age has been shown to be highly correlated with the effects of pain relief in that older patients report greater pain relief from a standard 10 mg dose of intramuscular morphine for the control of postoperative pain.[84] Age has been shown to have an influence on morphine elimination. A review of pharmacokinetic studies[51,85] has suggested that morphine clearance decreases and half life increases in older patients. Therefore, morphine doses should be reduced in elderly patients and titrated to provide optimal pain relief with minimal side effects.

Concurrent disease

Severe respiratory disease and general debility

Clinical observation indicates that patients with severe respiratory disease, and also those severely debilitated from any advanced systemic disease, are more sensitive to the respiratory depressant effects of opioids. Unfortunately, precise experimental data are lacking, so that morphine should be administered in such patients with great care in small incremental intravenous doses. Epidemiological evidence also suggests that such patients are more sensitive to the respiratory depressant effects of epidural and intrathecal opioids.[61]

While the requirement to scale the morphine dose according to the age and size of the patient is essential for all patients ranging from neonates to the elderly, no useful relationship has been shown between body weight and blood morphine concentration. Therefore, doses or infusion rates which are normalized for body weight must only be taken as a guide and the dose and dosing interval optimized for that particular patient.

Renal disease. Care should be exercised in the use of morphine in patients with renal failure because such patients can show signs of morphine overdose even following conservative dosage regimens. The hypothesis proposed to explain this observation is the accumulation of the minor metabolite, morphine-6-glucuronide as a result of decreased renal function.[47] There may also be an increased response to standard doses of morphine in severe renal disease, although precise data are lacking. While the administration of naloxone will reverse the overdose effects of morphine in this situation, care and increased observation of such patients to ensure adequate pain relief and to minimize any adverse effects is recommended.

Liver disease. The use of morphine in patients with liver disease does not appear to be a major clinical problem[37,43] in that conventional dosage regimens are required to provide adequate pain relief. However, animal studies have indicated that there is a marked increase in terminal half life and the pharmacodynamic effects of morphine in the absence of liver function.[44] These results support the hypothesis that the liver is the primary site of morphine biotransformation.

Drug interactions

Potentially hazardous interactions

Monoamine oxidase inhibitors. Such drugs intensify the effects of morphine and other opioid drugs which can cause anxiety, confusion and significant depression of respiration, sometimes leading to coma.

Phenothiazines. These drugs potentiate the depressant effects of morphine on the CNS, particularly with respect to respiration. The simultaneous administration of morphine and phenothiazines can also result in significant hypotension.

Hypnotics and neuroleptics. The depressant effects of morphine on respiration is significantly greater if the patient is simultaneously taking hypnotics or neuroleptics.

Alcohol. The respiratory depressant effects of morphine are significantly increased by all CNS depressant drugs, including alcohol. The use of morphine in patients who are intoxicated with alcohol is especially dangerous, and low doses can be fatal when there is a high concentration of alcohol in the blood. One of the commonest drug interactions in hospitals is severe sedation and respiratory depression due to the administration of inappropriate combinations of opioids and other drugs with CNS depressant effects.

Muscle relaxants. Patients recovering from relaxant anaesthesia are especially vulnerable to the respiratory depressant effects of morphine. A respiratory acidosis, secondary to acute hypercapnia, can result in reactivation of the long-acting relaxant reversed at the completion of anaesthesia, resulting in further depression of respiration. The combination of the above with the interference of morphine on efferent motor innervation of respiratory muscles could result in a rapidly progressive respiratory crisis.[86]

Other significant interactions

Cimetidine. There is a report[87] of confusion and severe respiratory depression when a haemodialysis patient was given morphine and cimetidine.

Diuretics. Morphine reduces the efficacy of diuretics by inducing the release of antidiuretic hormone. Morphine may also lead to acute retention of urine by causing spasm of the sphincter of the bladder, particularly in men with early prostatism.

Food. Recent studies[88] have indicated that there was a 34% increase in the area-under-curve of blood morphine concentration versus time curve when morphine (50 mg as a solution) was administered immediately after a high fat breakfast compared with an equivalent dose in the fasting state. However, there was no significant difference between the fed and fasted states with respect to the maximum blood morphine concentration or the time to maximum concentration. Further, the shape of the blood morphine concentration–time profile was consistently altered in the fed compared with the fasting state, in that the blood morphine concentrations were maintained at a higher level from 240 to 600 min when the morphine was administered with food. There appears to be some similarity with respect to the influence of food on the pharmacokinetics of both morphine and propranolol and it is significant to note that the glucuronidation pathway is a major route of metabolism for both drugs.

Smoking. There are no data concerning the influence of smoking on morphine pharmacokinetics. However, there was no influence of smoking on the pharmacokinetics of codeine where both morphine and codeine concentrations were quantified following oral and intramuscular injections.[89]

Potentially useful interactions

Hydroxyzine. The simultaneous administration of morphine and hydroxyzine potentiates the pain-relieving effects of morphine.[90]

Morphine

Dexamphetamine. There was a dose-dependent increase in the extent of pain relief when either 5 or 10 mg doses of dexamphetamine were administered with morphine in the treatment of postoperative pain.[91] However, there was also a greater frequency of adverse effects such as nausea, dizziness, and increased sweating in these patients given both morphine and dexamphetamine.

Tricyclic antidepressants. Tricyclic antidepressants have been shown to have pain-relieving properties in a wide variety of chronic pain states.[92] Further, when these drugs are combined with morphine there is improved pain relief in the treatment of cancer pain.[93]

Other analgesic adjuvants. The simultaneous administration of morphine with aspirin or other NSAIDs in patients with bone metastases may increase analgesia and decrease the dose of morphine required. Anticonvulsant drugs such as carbamazepine may add to the pain-relieving (and sedative) effects of morphine in patients with pain involving a neuralgic component. In pure neuralgic pain, morphine may be ineffective, and drugs such as carbamazepine and tricyclic antidepressants may be required instead of morphine. In pain states such as the thalamic syndrome and spinal cord damage, morphine may also be ineffective. In such situations, anticonvulsant, antidepressant, or long-acting phenothiazines are used instead of morphine.

General review articles

Bonica J J (ed) Advances in pain research and therapy, vols 5, 7, 8 and 9. Raven Press, New York

Lipton S, Miles J 1983 Persistent pain: modern methods of treatment. Grune and Stratton, London

Stimmel B 1983 Pain, analgesia, and addiction: the pharmacologic treatment of pain. Raven Press, New York

Twycross R, Lack S 1984 Oral morphine in advanced cancer. Beaconsfield Publishers Ltd, Beaconsfield, England

References

1. Casey A F, Parfitt R T 1986 Opioid analgesics. Chemistry and receptors. Plenum Press, New York, pp 9–10
2. Gulland J M, Robinson R 1925 The constitution of codeine and thebaine. Memoirs and proceedings of the Manchester Literary and Philosophical Society 69: 79–86
3. Gates M, Tschudi G 1952 The synthesis of morphine. Journal of the American Chemical Society 74: 1109–1110
4. Ciociola A A, Gautieri R F 1983 Evaluation of the teratogenicity of morphine sulphate administered via a miniature implantable pump. Journal of Pharmaceutical Sciences 72: 742–745
5. Zis A P, Haskett R F, Albala A A, Carroll B J 1984 Morphine inhibits cortisol and stimulates prolactin secretion in man. Psychoneuroendocrinology 9: 422–427
6. Delitala G, Grossman A, Besser M 1983 Differential effects of opiate peptides and alkaloids on anterior pituitary hormone secretion. Neuroendocrinology 37: 275–279
7. Ruskis A F 1982 Effects of narcotics on the gastrointestinal tract, liver and kidneys. In: Kitahata L M, Collins J G (eds) Narcotic analgesics in anesthesiology. Williams & Wilkins, Baltimore, pp 143–156
8. Nimmo W S 1982 Gastrointestinal function following surgery. Regional Anesthesia 7: S105–S109
9. Crone R S, Ardran G M 1957 The effect of morphine sulphate on gastric motility: some radiological observations in man. Gastroenterology 32: 88–95
10. Radnay P A, Brodman E, Mankikar D et al 1980 The effect of equi-analgesic doses of fentanyl, morphine, meperidine and pentazocine on common bile duct pressure. Anaesthesist 29: 26–29
11. Dahlstrom B, Paalzow L 1975 Quantitative determination of morphine in biological samples by gas–liquid chromatography and electron capture detection. Journal of Pharmacy and Pharmacology 27: 172–176
12. Catlin D H 1977 Pharmacokinetics of morphine by radioimmunoassay: the influence of immunochemical factors. Journal of Pharmacology and Experimental Therapeutics 200: 224–235
13. Moore R A, Baldwin D, Allen M C et al 1984 Sensitive and specific morphine radioimmunoassay with iodine label: pharmacokinetics of morphine in man after intravenous administration. Annals of Clinical Biochemistry 21: 318–325
14. Aherne G W 1983 The specificity of morphine radioimmunoassays. Royal Society of Medicine (International Congress and Symposium Series) 58: 21–28
15. Walsh T D 1983 Measurement of morphine: clinical pharmacokinetic considerations during chronic administration. Royal Society of Medicine (International Congress and Symposium Series) 58: 3–8
16. Grabinski P Y, Kaiko R F, Walsh T D et al 1983 Morphine radioimmunoassay specificity before and after extraction of plasma and cerebrospinal fluid. Journal of Pharmaceutical Science 72: 27–30
17. White M W 1979 Determination of morphine and its major metabolite, morphine-3-glucuronide, in blood by high-performance liquid chromatography with electrochemical detection. Journal of Chromatography 178: 229–240
18. Wallace J E, Harris S C, Peek M W 1980 Determination of morphine by liquid chromatography with electrochemical detection. Analytical Chemistry 52: 1328–1330
19. Svensson J O, Rane A, Sawe J, Sjoquist F 1982 Determination of morphine, morphine-3-glucuronide and (tentatively) morphine-6-glucuronide in plasma and urine using ion-pair high performance liquid chromatography. Journal of Chromatography 230: 427–432
20. Gourlay G K, McLean C F, Murphy G A, Badcock N R 1985 A rapid method for the determination of blood morphine concentration suitable for use in studies involving acute and chronic pain. Journal of Pharmacological Methods 13: 317–324
21. Gourlay G K, Cherry D A, Cousins M J 1986 A comparative study of the efficacy and pharmacokinetics of oral methadone and morphine in the treatment of severe pain in patients with cancer. Pain 25: 297–312
22. Welsh J, Stuart T, Habeshaw R et al 1983 A comparative pharmacokinetic study of morphine sulphate solution and MST CONTINUS 30 mg tablets in conditions expected to allow steady-state drug levels. Royal Society of Medicine (International Congress and Symposium Series) 58: 9–12
23. Sawe J, Dahlstrom B, Paalzow L, Rane A 1981 Morphine kinetics in cancer patients. Clinical Pharmacology and Therapeutics 30: 629–635
24. Dahlstrom B, Paalzow L 1978 Pharmacokinetic interpretation of the enterohepatic recirculation and first pass metabolism of morphine in the rat. Journal of Pharmacokinetics and Biopharmaceutics 6: 505–519
25. Iwamoto K, Klaassen C D 1977 First pass effect of morphine in rats. Journal of Pharmacology and Experimental Therapeutics 200: 236–244
26. Stanski D R, Greenblatt D J, Lowenstein E 1978 Kinetics of intravenous and intramuscular morphine. Clinical Pharmacology and Therapeutics 24: 52–59
27. Stanski D R, Greenblatt D G, Lappas J et al 1976 Kinetics of high-dose intravenous morphine in cardiac surgery patients. Clinical Pharmacology and Therapeutics 19: 752–756
28. Bennett M R D, House A C, Pearce R M et al 1983 Morphine kinetics during anaesthesia: IV bolus and infusions. British Journal of Anaesthesia 55: 906P
29. Lam A M, Clement J L 1984 Effect of cimetidine premedication on morphine-induced ventilatory depression. Canadian Anaesthetists Society Journal 31: 36–43
30. Mojaverian P, Fedder I L, Vlasses P M et al 1982 Cimetidine does not alter morphine disposition in man. British Journal of Clinical Pharmacology 14: 809–813
31. Fedder I L, Vlasses P M, Mojaverian P et al 1984 Relationship of morphine-induced miosis to plasma concentration in normal subjects. Journal of Pharmaceutical Sciences 73: 1496–1497
32. Aitkenhead A R, Vater M, Achola K et al 1984 Pharmacokinetics of single dose IV morphine in normal volunteers and patients with end-stage renal failure. British Journal of Anaesthesia 56: 813–819
33. Ostrea E M, Lynn S M, Wayne R N, Stryker J C 1980 Tissue distribution of morphine in the newborns of addicted monkeys and humans. Developmental Pharmacology and Therapeutics 1: 163–170
34. Cravey R H, Reed D 1977 The distribution of morphine in man following chronic intravenous administration. Journal of Analytical Toxicology 1: 166–167
35. Herz A, Teschemacher H J 1971 Activities and sites of antinociceptive action of morphine-like analgesics and kinetics of distribution following intravenous, intracerebral and intraventricular application. In: Harper N J, Simmonds A B (eds) Advances in drug research, vol 6. Academic Press, New York, pp 79–119
36. Nordberg G, Borg L, Hedner T, Mellstrand T 1985 CSF and plasma pharmacokinetics of intramuscular morphine. European Journal of Clinical Pharmacology 27: 677–681
37. Sawe J 1986 High dose morphine and methadone in cancer patients: clinical pharmacokinetic considerations of oral treatment. Clinical Pharmacokinetics 11: 87–106
38. Samuelsson H, Nordberg G, Hedner T, Lindqvist J 1987 CSF and plasma morphine concentrations in cancer patients during chronic epidural morphine therapy and its relationship to pain relief. Pain 30: 303–310
39. Hollt V, Teschemacher H J 1975 Hydrophobic interactions responsible for unspecific binding of morphine like drugs. Naunyn-Schmiedeberg's Archives of Pharmacology 288: 163–177
40. Olsen G D 1975 Morphine binding to human plasma proteins. Clinical Pharmacology and Therapeutics 17: 31–35
41. Wilson J T, Brown R D, Cherek D R et al 1980 Drug excretion in human breast milk: principles, pharmacokinetics and projected consequences. Clinical Pharmacokinetics 5: 1–66
42. Tuchmann-DuPlessis K 1975 Drug effects on the fetus. Adis Press, New York, pp 163–164
43. Patwardhan R V, Johnson R F, Hoyumpa A et al 1981 Normal metabolism of morphine in cirrhosis. Gastroenterology 81: 1006–1011
44. Greene N M, Hug C C 1982 Pharmacokinetics. In: Kitahata L M, Collins J G (eds) Narcotic analgesics in anesthesiology. Williams and Wilkins, Baltimore, pp 1–41
45. Yeh S Y, Gorodetzky C W, Krebs H A 1977 Isolation and identification of morphine 3- and 6-glucuronides, morphine-3,6-diglucuronide, morphine-3-ethereal sulphate, normorphine, and normorphine-6-glucuronide as morphine metabolites in humans. Journal of Pharmaceutical Sciences 66: 1288–1293
46. Sawe J 1986 Morphine and its 3- and 6-glucuronides in plasma and urine during chronic oral administration in cancer patients. In: Foley K M, Inturrisi C E (eds) Advances in pain research and therapy, vol 8. Raven Press, New York, pp 45–55
47. Osborne R J, Joel S P, Slevin M L 1986 Morphine intoxication in renal failure: the role of morphine-6-glucuronide. British Medical Journal 292: 1548–1549
48. Shimomura K, Kamata O, Ueki S et al 1971 Analgesic effect of morphine glucuronides. Tohoku Journal of Experimental Medicine 105: 45–52
49. Moore R A, Sear J W, Bullingham R E S, McQuay H J 1986 Morphine kinetics in renal failue. In: Foley K M, Inturrisi C E (eds) Advances in pain research and therapy, vol 8. Raven Press, New York, pp 65–72
50. Sawe J, Odar-Cederlof I 1987 Kinetics of morphine in patients with renal failure. European Journal of Clinical Pharmacology 32: 377–382
51. Kaiko R F, Wallenstein S L, Rogers A G et al 1982 Narcotics in the elderly. Medical Clinics of North America 66: 1079–1089

Morphine

52. Dahlstrom B, Tamsen A, Paalzow L, Hartvig P 1982 Patient controlled analgesic therapy, part IV: pharmacokinetics and analgesic plasma concentrations of morphine. Clinical Pharmacokinetics 7: 266–279
53. Gourlay G K, Willis R J, Lamberty J 1986 A double blind comparison of the efficacy of methadone and morphine in post operative pain control. Anesthesiology 64: 322–327
54. Dahlstrom B, Bolme P, Flychting H et al 1979 Morphine kinetics in children. Clinical Pharmacology and Therapeutics 26: 354–365
55. Boerner U, Abbott S 1973 New observations in the metabolism of morphine. The formation of codeine from morphine in man. Experientia 29: 180–181
56. Melzack R, Mount B M, Gordon J M 1979 The brompton mixture versus morphine solution given orally: effects on pain. Canadian Medical Association Journal 120: 435–438
57. deBoer A G, Moolenaar F, deLeede L G, Breimer D D 1982 Rectal drug administration: clinical pharmacokinetic considerations. Clinical Pharmacokinetics 7: 285–311
58. Westerling D, Lindahl S, Andersson K E, Anderson A 1982 Absorption and bioavailability of rectally administered morphine in women. European Journal of Clinical Pharmacology 23: 59–64
59. Tamsen A 1985 Comparison of patient controlled analgesia with constant infusion and intermittent intramuscular regimens. In: Harmer M, Rosen M, Vickers MD (eds) Patient-controlled analgesia. Blackwell Scientific Publications, Oxford, pp 111–125
60. Cousins M J, Cherry D A, Gourlay G K 1988 Acute and chronic pain: use of spinal opioids. In: Cousins M J, Bridenbaugh P O (eds) Neural blockade in clinical anesthesia and management of pain, 2nd edn. J B Lippincott, Philadelphia, pp 955–1029
61. Rawal N, Arner S, Gustafsson L L, Allvin R 1987 Present state of extradural and intrathecal opioid analgesia in Sweden: a nationwide followup study. British Journal of Anaesthesia 59: 791–799
62. Twycross R G 1983 Narcotic analgesics in clinical practice. In: Bonica J J, Lindblom U, Iggo A (eds) Advances in pain research and therapy, vol 5. Raven Press, New York, pp 435–459
63. Portenoy R K, Moulin D E, Rogers A G et al 1986 Intravenous infusion of opioids in cancer-related pain: review of cases and guidelines for use. In: Foley K M, Inturrisi C E (eds) Advances in pain research and therapy, vol 8. Opioid analgesics in the management of clinical pain. Raven Press, New York, pp 413–426
64. Cherry D A 1987 Drug delivery systems for epidural administration of opioids. Acta Anaesthesiologica Scandinavica 31 (suppl 85): 54–59
65. Ventafridda V, DeConno I, Tamburini M, Pappalettera M 1986 Clinical evaluation of chronic infusion of intrathecal morphine in cancer pain. In: Foley K M, Inturrisi C E (eds) Advances in pain research and therapy, vol 8. Opioid analgesics in the management of clinical pain. Raven Press, New York, pp 391–397
66. Lobato R D, Madrid J L, Fatela L V et al 1985 Analgesia elicited by low dose intraventricular morphine in terminal cancer patients. In: Field H L, Dubner R, Cevero F (eds) Advances in pain research and therapy, vol 9. Raven Press, New York, pp 673–681
67. Cherry D A, Gourlay G K 1987 The spinal administration of opioids in the treatment of acute and chronic pain: bolus doses, continuous infusion, intraventricular administration and implanted drug delivery systems. Palliative Medicine 1: 89–106
68. Smith G, Aitkenhead A R 1985 Preoperative assessment and premedication. In: Textbook of anaesthesia. Churchill Livingstone, Edinburgh, pp 216–222
69. Smith G, Aitkenhead A R 1985 Anaesthesia for cardiac surgery. In: Textbook of anaesthesia. Churchill Livingstone, Edinburgh, pp 379–393
70. Mather L E, Phillips G D 1986 Opioids and adjuvants: principles of use. In: Cousins M J, Phillips G D (eds) Acute pain management. Churchill Livingstone, New York, pp 77–103
71. Young D S, Pestaner L C, Gibberman V 1975 Effect of drugs on clinical laboratory tests. Clinical Chemistry 21: 1D–432D
72. Koren G, Butt W, Chinyanga H et al 1985 Postoperative morphine infusion in newborn infants: assessment of disposition characteristics and safety. Journal of Pediatrics 107: 963–967
73. Koren G, Butt W, Pape K, Chinyanga H 1985 Morphine induced seizures in newborn infants. Veterinary and Human Toxicology 27: 519–520
74. Anand K J S, Sipell W G, Aynsley-Green A 1987 Randomized trial of fentanyl anesthesia in preterm babies undergoing surgery: effects on the stress response. Lancet 1: 243–248
75. Anand K J S, Hickey P R 1987 Randomized trial of high dose sufentanil anesthesia in neonates undergoing cardiac surgery: effects on the metabolic stress response. Anesthesiology 67: A502
76. Way W L, Costley E C, Way E L 1965 Respiratory sensitivity of the newborn infant to meperidine and morphine. Clinical Pharmacology and Therapeutics 6: 454–461
77. Hertzka R E, Fisher D M, Gauntlett I S, Spellman M 1987 Are infants sensitive to respiratory depression from fentanyl. Anesthesiology 67: A512
78. Van Den Berghe H, MacLeod S, Chinyanga H et al 1983 Pharmacokinetics of intravenous morphine in balanced anaesthesia: studies in children. Drug Metabolism Reviews 14: 887–903
79. Lynn A M, Opheim K E, Tyler D C 1984 Morphine infusion after pediatric cardiac surgery. Critical Care Medicine 12: 863–866
80. Shapiro L A, Ledeikin R J, Shalen D, Hoffman S 1984 Epidural morphine analgesia in children. Anesthesiology 61: 210–212
81. Jones S E F, Beasley J M, MacFarlane D W R 1984 Intrathecal morphine for postoperative pain relief in children. British Journal of Anaesthesia 56: 137–140
82. Grimwade J, Walker D, Wood C 1971 Morphine and the fetal heart rate. British Medical Journal 3: 373
83. Petrie R H, Yeh S Y, Murata Y 1978 The effect of drugs on fetal heart rate variability. American Journal of Obstetrics and Gynecology 130: 294–299
84. Bellville J W, Forrest W H, Miller E, Brown B W 1971 Influence of age on pain relief from analgesics. Journal of the American Medical Association 217: 1835–1841
85. Kaiko R F, Wallenstein S I, Rogers A G et al 1986 Clinical analgesic studies and sources of variation in analgesic responses to morphine. In: Foley K M, Inturrisi C E (eds) Advances in pain research and therapy, vol 8. Opioid analgesics in the management of clinical pain. Raven Press, New York, pp 13–23
86. Bellville J W, Cohen E N, Hamilton J 1964 The interaction of morphine and D-tubocurarine on respiration and grip strength in man. Clinical Pharmacology and Therapeutics 5: 35–43
87. Fine A, Churchill D N 1981 Potentially lethal interaction of cimetidine and morphine. Canadian Medical Association Journal 124: 1434–1436
88. Gourlay G K, Plummer J L, Cherry D A, Foate J A, Cousins M J 1989 Influence of a high fat meal on the absorption of morphine from oral solutions. Clinical Pharmacology and Therapeutics 46: 463–468
89. Hull J H, Findlay J W A, Rogers J F et al 1982 An evaluation of the effects of smoking on codeine pharmacokinetics and bioavailability in normal human volunteers. Drug Intelligence and Clinical Pharmacy 16: 849–854
90. Stimmel B 1983 Pain, analgesia and addiction: the pharmacologic treatment of pain. Raven Press, New York, pp 170–201
91. Forrest W H, Bronn B W, Cherek D R et al 1977 Dextroamphetamine with morphine for the treatment of post operative pain. New England Journal of Medicine 296: 712–715
92. Monks R, Merskey H 1984 Psychotropic drugs. In: Wall P D, Melzack R (eds) Textbook of pain. Churchill Livingstone, Edinburgh, pp 526–537
93. Walsh T D 1987 Management of cancer pain by the oncologist. In: Burrows G D, Elton D, Stanley G V (eds) Handbook of chronic pain management. Elsevier, Amsterdam, pp 347–369

Mupirocin

Mupirocin is a recently introduced topical antibiotic with a novel chemical structure and mode of action.

Chemistry

Mupirocin previously known as pseudomonic acid A (Bactroban)
$C_{26}H_{44}O_9$
9-[(2E)-4[(2S,3R,4R,5S)-5[(2S,3S,4S,5S)-2,3-Epoxy-5-hydroxy-4-methylhexyl] tetrahydro-3,4-dihydroxy-pyran-2-yl]-3-methylbut-2-enoyloxyl] nonanoic acid

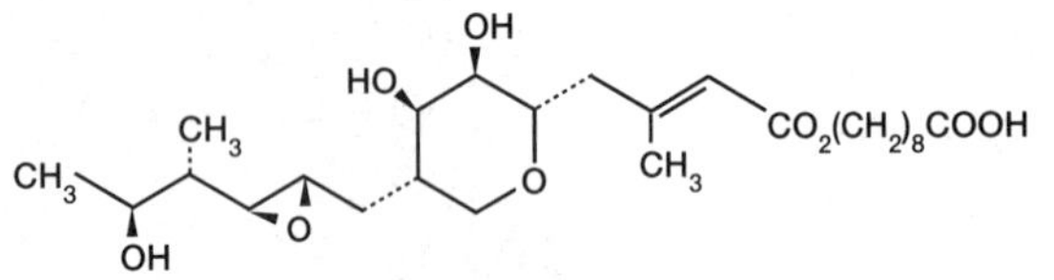

Molecular weight	500.6
pKa	5.0
Solubility	
in alcohol	—
in water	1g in 1 l
Octanol/water partition coefficient	—

Mupirocin is prepared by solvent extraction of the fermentation broth from a mutant of a strain of *Pseudomonas fluorescens*. The crude antibiotic mixture is a family of structurally related substances termed the 'pseudomonic acids' of which mupirocin comprises 90–95%. Mupirocin is available as a 2% ointment in polyethylene glycol for use on the skin, and in soft paraffin for use in the nose.

Pharmacology

Mupirocin acts by formation of a stable complex with isoleucyl transfer RNA synthetase. This in turn causes depletion of isoleucyl transfer RNA in the cell and the arrest of protein synthesis. The antibiotic has an 8000-fold greater inhibitory effect on the enzyme of *Escherichia coli* B than on that of rat liver.[1] Only one other antibiotic, furanomycin, which is not clinically useful, acts in this way.

Toxicology

In vitro testing did not demonstrate any mutagenic potential for mupirocin itself. Both parenteral and topical toxicity studies in animals showed no results of clinical relevance. There was no evidence of teratogenicity or embryotoxicity in doses of up to 160 $mg.kg^{-1}$ daily although radiolabelled sodium pseudomonate was shown to cross the placental barrier.[2]

Clinical pharmacology

Mupirocin has several features which make it especially suitable for topical use.[3] The drug is most active against the common skin pathogens, that is *Staphylococcus aureus* and *Streptococcus pyogenes* and less so against the commensal flora of the skin. Mupirocin is not itself a valuable systemic antibiotic nor does it show cross-resistance with other antibiotics; thus any resistance developing would not alter the treatment choices for systemic infections.

Over 1000 clinical isolates of *Staph. aureus* in two studies[3,4] were all very susceptible (minimum inhibitory concentration, MIC, of 0.5 $mg.l^{-1}$ or less) as were selected strains resistant to several antibiotics including methicillin. However, the minimum bactericidal concentration of mupirocin for 40 of these isolates was up to 16 $mg.l^{-1}$ indicating a degree of tolerance. Some reports have detailed an increasing incidence of low level (MIC of 8–64 $mg.l^{-1}$) resistance in vivo,[5] and high level resistance (MIC > 700 $mg.l^{-1}$) has also been reported.[6]

The commensal flora of the skin, which may have a protective role, is less sensitive to mupirocin. Strains of corynebacteria, micrococci and *Propionibacterium acnes* were all relatively resistant (MIC 32–128 $mg.l^{-1}$) although *Staph. epidermidis* is usually sensitive.

The majority of anaerobic and Gram-negative bacteria so far examined have reduced sensitivity (MIC in the range of 64–128 $mg.l^{-1}$). However, since mupirocin is applied in such high concentration it is possible that activity will be demonstrated against many of these organisms. Some notable exceptions are the gonococcus, *Haemophilus influenzae* and *Pasteurella* sp., strains of which were very sensitive, and *Pseudomonas aeruginosa* which was highly resistant (MIC > 1000 $mg.l^{-1}$).

The resistance of strains of *Staph. aureus* trained in vitro is slow to develop and of a low order.[3,4] There is no evidence of cross-resistance with other systemically useful antibiotics in either direction, i.e. the mutants are sensitive to other antibiotics and strains of *Staph. aureus* resistant to several other antibiotics, including methicillin, remain sensitive to mupirocin.

The activity of mupirocin against *Chlamydia* and fungi is poor.

When applied to the skin the activity of a single application of mupirocin persists for at least 24 hours under occlusion. Some activity remains for at least 24 hours after the last application of antibiotic.

Pharmacokinetics

Mupirocin and its metabolites are assayed in body fluids and tissue homogenates by high pressure liquid chromatography. The sensitivity of the assay is normally set at 2.5 $mg.l^{-1}$, but may be increased to 1 $mg.l^{-1}$.[6] Sensitivity tests of bacterial isolates for mupirocin in agar or broth are little affected by the medium or inoculum used. Mupirocin is more active in an acid environment but is 95% bound to the protein in human serum. MIC are 10–25 times higher in the presence of 50% serum.[3,4]

The sodium salt of mupirocin has been injected intravenously in healthy volunteers at four dose levels of 31.3, 61.2, 125 and 252 mg of pure free acid (pfa).[7] At the two lower doses more than 90% of the monic acid moiety in the dose of mupirocin sodium was recovered in the urine as monic acid. No mupirocin was recovered in the urine. At the higher doses sufficient reached the plasma to allow calculation of pharmocokinetic data. The mean peak plasma concentration was 7.12 mg $pfa.l^{-1}$ following an infusion of 125 mg over 25 min, and fell to undetectable levels after 3 h. The plasma concentration time curve fitted a two compartment model, with a β phase half life of 16.9 and 20.9 min respectively in two subjects. Most of the dose was eliminated as monic acid, with 71.1% and 73.6% appearing in the urine of the two subjects within 12 h. However, mupirocin itself was detected in the urine at levels of less than 1% of the initial dose.

Monic acid levels in the plasma peaked at a mean of 2.6 mg $pfa.l^{-1}$ one hour after the beginning of the infusion. The half life of monic acid elimination was 75.2 and 77.9 min respectively in each of the two subjects.

After a dose of 252 mg mupirocin the peak level was 14.1 mg $pfa.l^{-1}$, with a β phase half life of 35.5 min. More mupirocin appeared in the urine, 4.59% of the dose, but recovery of monic acid fell to 57.7%. The elimination phase half life of monic acid was 73.1 min in two subjects and 32.3 min in a third.

When 2% mupirocin ointment is applied to normal human skin less than 0.3% of the applied dose is absorbed; 24 hours following application 1–4% is present in the stratum corneum. There is no data on absorption from damaged skin, although this might be expected to be greater[5] the levels absorbed are still small.

Concentration–effect relationship

Since this drug is used topically and transcutaneous absorption is very low plasma concentrations are irrelevant to the actions of mupirocin. Minimum inhibitory concentrations (MICs) are given in the clinical pharmacology section.

Metabolism

The skin itself is capable of some metabolism; 2.7% of an applied dose is metabolized to monic acid over 48 hours. There is little data on the metabolism of mupirocin given systemically. Although it would not normally be administered in this way, absorption might occur when large amounts are applied to damaged skin. In human volunteers at doses under 125 mg, over 90% of the injected dose can be detected in the urine as monic acid. At higher doses the proportion of the injected dose appearing in the urine as monic acid drops, and a very small percentage, less than 1%, appears as unchanged mupirocin. When 252 mg is given nearly 40% of the initial dose is unaccounted for by urinary excretion after 12 h. At the higher doses another route of elimination may be appearing, or metabolic conversion may be saturated. Biliary excretion in humans has not been studied,[7] but in the rat 36% of an injected dose is excreted as monic acid in the bile; this has been suggested as a route of excretion at higher doses in humans (see Fig. 1).[5] 252 mg is equivalent to the instantaneous absorption of 12 g of mupirocin ointment. No ill effects were observed.[7]

Mupirocin is stable in whole human blood, with a half life of 9 days.[7]

Pharmaceutics

Mupirocin is available as a 2% w/w formulation in a polyethylene glycol base Bactroban (SmithKline Beecham, UK). It is a sterile, white, translucent water-soluble ointment. Polyethylene glycols may be minor irritants and produce some sensitization in 0.3% of people exposed.[8] If absorbed through damaged skin polyethylene glycol may also cause reversible exacerbation of pre-existing renal damage.

This preparation is not suitable for intranasal or ophthalmic application. Recently a 2% preparation in a white soft paraffin base has been marketed for use in the nose alone. This contains a glycerin ester to improve spreading properties. Nasal mupirocin has been shown to be effective in eliminating carriage of methicillin-resistant *Staphylococcus aureus* from the nose.[9]

Mupirocin may be stored at room temperature below 25°C. Tubes once opened should be discarded at the end of a course of treatment.

Therapeutic use

Indications

1. Acute primary skin infections
2. Secondary infection of skin lesions
3. Elimination of nasal staphylococcal carriage, particularly strains of *Staph. aureus* resistant to several other antibiotics including MRSA.

Fig. 1 Metabolism of mupirocin after intravenous injection

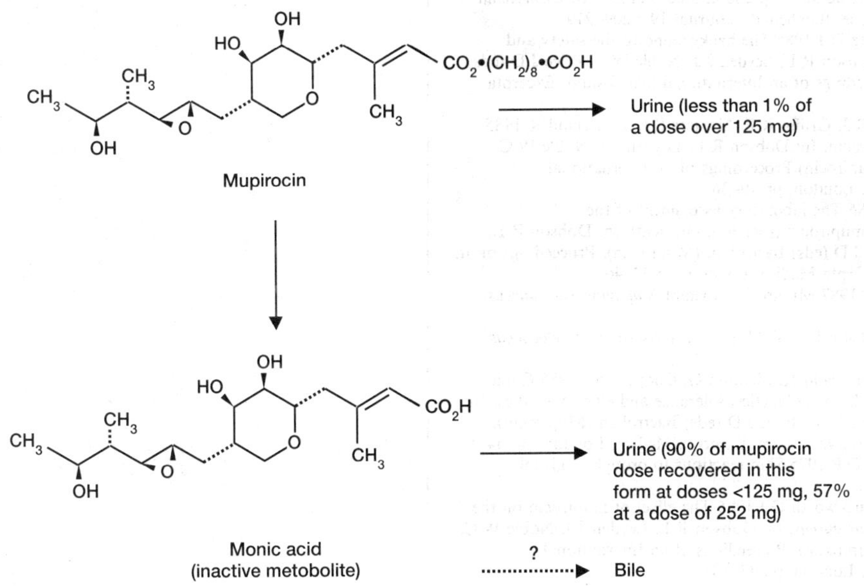

Contraindications

1. Hypersensitivity to mupirocin or constituents of the ointment base
2. Use in the eye.

Mode of use

In trials, applications have been made to affected areas 2–4 times daily. Periods of treatment have varied from 5–14 days, the majority being 7–10 days. No clear differences in cure rates or side effects have so far emerged with varying frequencies or duration of treatment. A dressing or occlusion may be used if required.

Indications

1. Acute primary skin infections

Some patients with folliculitis, furunculosis, impetigo or other primary skin infections have been treated apparently successfully with mupirocin. However, the published studies so far including controls have had very small numbers of patients making meaningful analysis difficult. In the treatment of impetigo caused by *Staph. aureus* or *Strep. pyogenes* mupirocin is clearly superior to the vehicle and at least as effective as fucidin,[10] neomycin[11] or other topical antibiotics frequently prescribed for this condition.

2. Secondary skin infections

Mupirocin has been used for the infected dermatoses, principally eczema, and a variety of traumatic lesions such as burns, minor abrasions, surgical wounds and chronic ulcers. The antibiotic is certainly effective in clearing superficial lesions of *Staph. aureus* and *Strep. pyogenes*[12,13] and possibly some Gram-negative species, but not *Pseudomonas*. This may or may not contribute to cure of the underlying lesion. Mupirocin may be particularly useful for lesions colonized with MRSA.[14,15] Few studies including patients with infected surgical wounds give details of the type of wound treated but mupirocin may have a role in the elimination of bacteria from chronically infected surgical wounds where it appears to be superior to Eusol dressings.[13]

3. Elimination of nasal staphylococcal carriage

Mupirocin may be the agent of choice for the elimination of nasal carriage of *Staph. aureus* and particularly MRSA. Although mupirocin in polyethylene glycol base has been used for this purpose it is not recommended and may result in local discomfort.[17] A five day course of 2% mupirocin in a white soft paraffin and softisan base applied four times daily to the anterior nares was successful where 1% chlorhexidine obstetric cream had failed. It is possible that even shorter courses may be equally effective.[9] It might be expected that mupirocin would also be effective in eliminating *Staph. aureus* from sites of skin carriage.[17]

M

M

Adverse reactions

Potentially life-threatening effects
No reactions of this kind have been described.

Acute overdosage
No cases of overdosage have been described.

Severe or irreversible adverse effects
No effects of this kind are known.

Symptomatic adverse effects
Pain or stinging on application, itching and rashes have been reported. The incidence of such reaction is similar when either the polyethylene vehicle alone or with mupirocin is used, suggesting that the antibiotic itself causes few adverse reactions.

Interference with clinical pathology tests
None has been described.

High risk groups

Neonates
The drug has been used to control an outbreak of MRSA in a special care baby unit.[21]

Breast milk. No information is available on the appearance of the drug in breast milk but it seems unlikely that any harm would come to a breast-fed infant of a mother using the drug in the recommended way.

Children
Mupirocin has been used safely in children.[18,19]

Pregnant women
Animal studies do not show any evidence of teratogenicity. There are no published data of the use of mupirocin during pregnancy in humans.

The elderly
Mupirocin has been used safely in the elderly without special precautions.[13,20]

Drug interactions

There are no available data on this subject.

General review articles

Dobson R L, Leyden J J, Noble W C, Price J D (eds) 1985 Bactroban (Mupirocin). Proceedings of an International Symposium. Excerpta Medica, London

Wilkinson D S, Price J D (eds) 1984 Mupirocin — a novel topical antibiotic for the treatment of skin infection. Royal Society of Medicine International Congress and Symposium Series No 80

References

So far very little work independent of the manufacturers has been published.

1. Hughes J, Mellows G 1980 Interaction of pseudomonic acid A with *Escherichia coli* B isoleucyl-tRNA synthetase. Biochemical Journal 191: 209–219
2. Cockburn A, Jackson D, White D J 1985 The background to the safety and tolerance of mupirocin. In: Dobson R L, Leyden J J, Noble W C, Price J D (eds). Bactroban (Mupirocin). Proceedings of an International Symposium. Excerpta Medica, London, pp 11–18
3. White A R, Beale A S, Boon R J, Griffin K E, Masters P J, Sutherland R 1985 Antibacterial activity of mupirocin. In: Dobson R L, Leyden J J, Noble W C, Price J D (eds) Bactroban (Mupirocin) Proceedings of an International Symposium. Excerpta Medica, London, pp 19–36
4. Casewell M W, Hill R L R 1985 The laboratory assessment of the antistaphylococcal activity of mupirocin (pseudomonic acid). In: Dobson R L, Leyden J J, Noble W C, Price J D (eds) Bactroban (Mupirocin). Proceedings of an International Symposium. Excerpta Medica, London, pp 37–46
5. Kavi J, Andrews J M, Wise R 1987 Mupirocin-resistant *Staphylococcus aureus*. Lancet 2: 1472
6. Rahman M, Noble W C, Cookson B 1987 Mupirocin-resistant *Staphylococcus aureus*. Lancet 2: 387
7. Jackson D, Tasker T C G, Sutherland R, Mellows G, Cooper D L 1985 Clinical pharmacology of Bactroban; pharmacokinetics, tolerance and efficacy studies. In: Dobson R L, Leyden J J, Noble W C, Price J D (eds) Bactroban (Mupirocin). Proceedings of an International Symposium. Excerpta Medica, London, pp 54–67
8. Hannuksela M, Pirila V, Salo O P 1975 Skin reactions to propylene glycol. Contact Dermatitis 1: 112–116
9. Casewell M W, Hill R L R, Duckworth G J 1985 The effect of mupirocin on the nasal carriage of *Staphylococcus aureus*. In: Dobson R L, Leyden J J, Noble W C, Price J D (eds) Bactroban (Mupirocin). Proceedings of an International Symposium. Excerpta Medica, London, pp 47–53
10. Lewis-Jones S, Hart C A, Vickers C F H 1985 Bactroban ointment versus fucidic acid in acute primary skin infections in children. In: Dobson R L, Leyden J J, Noble W C, Price J D (eds) Bactroban (Mupirocin). Proceedings of an International Symposium. Excerpta Medica, London, pp 103–108
11. Kennedy C T C, Watts J A, Speller D C E 1985 Bactroban ointment in the treatment of impetigo; a controlled trial against neomycin. In: Dobson R L, Leyden J J, Noble W C, Price J D (eds) Bactroban (Mupirocin). Proceedings of an International Symposium. Excerpta Medica, London, pp 11–18
12. Wilkinson J D, Lever L R, Leigh D A 1985 Infected eczema and Bactroban. In: Dobson R L, Leyden J J, Noble W C, Price J D (eds) Bactroban (Mupirocin). Proceedings of an International Symposium. Excerpta Medica, London, pp 177–182
13. Leyden J J 1985 Double-blind vehicle-controlled studies of Bactroban ointment in secondary infections. In: Dobson R L, Leyden J J, Noble W C, Price J D (eds) Bactroban (Mupirocin). Proceedings of an International Symposium. Excerpta Medica, London, pp 183–189
14. Rode H, Hanslo D, Davies M R Q, Cywes S, Swanepoel C 1985 The efficacy of Bactroban ointment in the treatment of multiple antibiotic-resistant *Staphylococcus aureus* burn wound infections in children. In: Dobson R L, Leyden J J, Noble W C, Price J D (eds) Bactroban (Mupirocin). Proceedings of an International Symposium. Excerpta Medica, London, pp 235–240
15. Duckworth G J, Lothian J L E, Williams J D 1988 Methicillin-resistant *Staphylococcus aureus*: report of an outbreak in a London teaching hospital. Journal of Hospital Infection 11: 1–15
16. Huizinga W K J, Robbs J V, Kritzingga N A et al 1985 Chronic wound infections; eradication of pathogens by topical application of Bactroban ointment. In: Dobson R L, Leyden J J, Noble W C, Price J D (eds) Bactroban (Mupirocin). Proceedings of an International Symposium. Excerpta Medica, London, pp 216–223
17. Dacre J E, Emmerson A M, Jenner E A 1983 Nasal carriage of gentamicin and methicillin-resistant *Staphylococcus aureus* treated with topical pseudomonic acid. Lancet 2: 1036
18. McLinn S E 1985 The use of Bactroban ointment in common skin infections in children. In: Dobson R L, Leyden J J, Noble W C, Price J D (eds) Bactroban (Mupirocin). Proceedings of an International Symposium. Excerpta Medica, London, pp 216–223
19. Eaglstein W H 1985 The efficacy and safety of Bactroban ointment and its vehicle in the treatment of secondarily infected skin lesions in children. In: Dobson R L, Leyden J J, Noble W C, Price J D (eds) Bactroban (Mupirocin). Proceedings of an International Symposium. Excerpta Medica, London, pp 120–123
20. Levenstein J H, Penman J and Partners, Kritzings N A, Tattersal M 1985 The efficacy of Bactroban ointment in the treatment of common skin infections encountered in general practice. In: Dobson R L, Leyden J J, Noble W C, Price J D (eds) Bactroban (Mupirocin). Proceedings of an International Symposium. Excerpta Medica, London, pp 216–223
21. Davies E A, Emmerson A M, Hogg G M, Patterson M F, Shields M D 1987 An outbreak of infection with a methicillin resistant staphylococcus aureus in a special care baby unit: value of topical mypirocin and of traditional methods of infection control. Journal of Hospital Infection 10: 120–128

Nabumetone

Nabumetone is a recently introduced non-steroidal anti-inflammatory drug.

Chemistry

Nabumetone (Relifex)
$C_{15}H_{16}O_2$
4-(6-methoxy-2-naphthyl)-butan-2-one

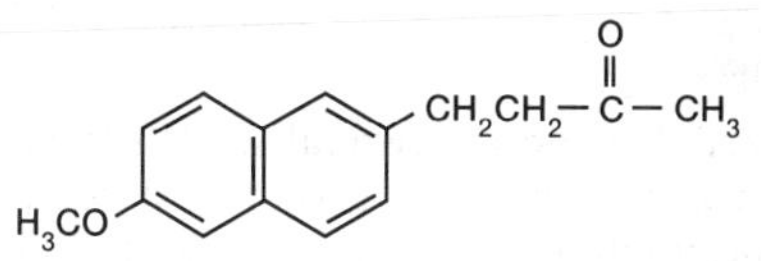

Molecular weight	228.3
pKa	not relevant
Solubility	
in alcohol	sparingly soluble
in water	1 in 17 000
Octanol/water partition coefficient	high

A white non-hygroscopic powder prepared by chemical synthesis. Nabumetone is not present in any combination preparations.

Pharmacology

Nabumetone is a non-steroidal anti-inflammatory agent that is a prodrug and exerts its pharmacological effects via the metabolite 6-methoxy-2-naphthylacetic acid (6-MNA). Nabumetone itself is non-acidic and only a weak inhibitor of prostaglandin synthesis. Following absorption, it undergoes extensive first-pass metabolism and the main circulating metabolite (6-MNA) is a much more potent inhibitor of cyclooxygenase than the parent compound. Via 6-MNA, nambumetone, is a potent inhibitor of prostanglandin synthesis and also reduces the influx of neutrophils into inflamed tissues.[2] It has analgesic and anti-inflammatory activity and inhibits the formation of carrageenin-induced oedema in the rat in a dose-dependent manner.[1] Nabumetone is less potent than indomethacin or naproxen in this regard. Nabumetone also inhibits the development of ultraviolet-induced erythema. Nabumetone has long-term anti-inflammatory activity as shown by the inhibition of adjuvant-induced arthritis and cotton pellet-induced granuloma in the rat.[1] Nabumetone, via its metabolite, is a potent inhibitor of prostaglandin synthesis and also reduces the influx of polymorphonuclear leucocytes into inflamed tissues.[2] Nabumetone also has analgesic and antipyretic activities.

Toxicology

Compared with other non-steroidal anti-inflammatory compounds, nabumetone has less nephrotoxicity and gastrointestinal irritancy. Unlike most NSAIDs, nabumetone is not acidic and thus unlikely to cause direct gastric mucosal injury. However, systemic inhibition of prostaglandin production does predispose to gastro-intestinal ulceration so this difference is relative rather than absolute. Animal studies have shown that the drug is well tolerated at doses which have systemic anti-infiammatory activity. No adverse effects on the liver or haemopoietic system have been observed in long-term animal toxicity studies[3] and the drug has no mutagenic or carcinogenic activity.[4] There is no teratogenic potential in experimental animals.

Clinical pharmacology

Nabumetone, like other non-steroidal anti-inflammatory drugs has been shown to be effective in reducing pain and inflammation in patients with osteoarthritis; and pain, inflammation and stiffness in patients with rheumatoid arthritis. The pharmacological benefit in animal models is therefore confirmed by clinical studies in man. Nabumetone has not been shown to alter the progression of the disease process.

Nabumetone has weak effects on the platelet through the inhibition of thromboxane A_2 production by the platelet. Nabumetone renders the platelets less sticky but the effect is much less than that of naproxen and the bleeding time is not prolonged.[1,5] The drug may cause salt and water retention and patients with moderate or severe renal impairment may suffer a reduction in GFR. Although nabumetone itself is not a gastric irritant the systemic effects of 6-MNA may cause dyspepsia and nausea.

Three dosage regimens have been studied in healthy volunteers. These were 500 mg twice daily, 1000 mg at night and 1000 mg twice daily. Steady state for each regimen was reached on day three with a mean morning steady-state concentration of 17.4–20.6 $mg.l^{-1}$; 27.0–42.0 $mg.l^{-1}$; and 34.6–41.7 $mg.l^{-1}$ respectively. On the basis of these values, a single nocturnal daily dose of 1.0 g nabumetone was judged the preferred regimen, though this has not formally been compared to other regimens in groups of patients, often elderly, suffering from arthritis. In those patients for whom the dose of 1.0 g at night is judged effective, the drug appears equally efficacious in the reduction of different aspects of inflammation such as pain, stiffness and swelling.

Pharmacokinetics

The preferred analytical method is HPLC which has been adapted for the measurement of both the parent compound nabumetone and its active metabolite 6-methoxy-2-naphthylacetic acid (6-MNA)[6] Nabumetone is readily absorbed, largely intact, from the gastrointestinal tract. However, it is almost completely metabolized presystemically in the liver to produce a range of metabolites amongst which the major one is also the active principle, 6-methoxy-2-naphthylacetic acid. This compound is the result of oxidative cleavage of the side chain on the parent molecule, accounting for 70–90% of the plasma radioactivity in radiotracer studies. Additional metabolites are produced by demethylation and reduction of the ketone moiety to an alcohol. The metabolite 6-MNA is itself metabolized to desmethyl-6-MNA, though this and the other metabolites of nabumetone appear to have minimal pharmacological action compared to 6-MNA. Thus, nabumetone can be considered a non-acidic prodrug. Absorption of the drug is not affected by antacids. The bioavailability of 6-MNA is not affected by food but it is increased when nabumetone is ingested with milk.

Plasma concentrations of unchanged nabumetone are below the limit of detection in most subjects after oral administration.[7] The mean absolute bioavailability of 6-MNA, the active metabolite, in six healthy young subjects, after oral administration of nabumetone, is 38%. Healthy subjects receiving nabumetone, either 500 mg twice daily or 1000 mg each evening for 10 days, achieve steady-state plasma concentrations after three days. Morning pre-dose steady-state plasma concentrations with twice daily administration are 17–21 $mg.l^{-1}$ while morning pre-dose steady-state plasma concentrations are 27–42 $mg.l^{-1}$ with the once daily regimen. Increasing the dosage to 1000 mg twice daily does not increase the morning steady-state plasma concentration (35–42 $mg.l^{-1}$) above that found with 1000 mg administered once daily in the evening.[8]

After the oral administration of a single dose of 1.0 g nabumetone to patients with rheumatoid arthritis or osteoarthritis, peak synovial fluid concentrations of the active metabolite are about 10–12 $mg.l^{-1}$ and are generally attained between 4–12 hours after administration.[9] The active metabolite is extensively bound to human plasma protein (>99%) which may result in transient increases in the free concentrations of other highly bound drugs such as warfarin, phenytoin and sulphonylurea hypoglycaemics. It has a volume of distribution of 7.5 $l.kg^{-1}$. 6-MNA distributes into breast milk and crosses the placenta of rats. Nabumetone is extensively metabolized in the liver as is its principal active metabolite, 6-MNA. Essentially no nabumetone and < 1% of the major active metabolite are excreted unchanged in the

Nabumetone

urine. The main route of excretion is the urine, in which 80% of the dose can be recovered, with a further 10% eliminated in the faeces.

Excretion maybe delayed in patients with hepatic impairment.[10] In elderly patients there is considerable variation between subjects such that the plasma concentrations of the active metabolites are higher than in younger subjects.[11] Alcohol does not appear to alter the kinetics of the drug.

Oral absorption	~80%
Presystemic metabolism (to 6-MNA)	~100%
Plasma half life of active metabolite (6-MNA)	
range	16–27 h
mean	22 h
Volume of distribution of 6-MNA	$7.5\ l.kg^{-1}$
Plasma protein binding of 6-MNA	~99%

Concentration–effect relationship

There is no data concerning any correlation between the clinical effects of nabumetone and plasma concentrations of its metabolite 6-MNA.

Metabolism

Nabumetone is absorbed largely intact from the gastrointestinal tract and undergoes extensive presystemic hepatic metabolism in animals and humans producing a range of metabolites. The minor metabolites have been found mainly as conjugates and several others have been detected in the urine, largely as conjugates. Three interrelated metabolic pathways appear to be operating: O-demethylation; reduction of the ketone to an alcohol; and oxidative cleavage of the side chain to yield acetic acid derivatives (Fig. 1).[3,12]

Both free and conjugated 6-MNA, the active form of the drug, and its O-demethylated metabolite are found in the urine accounting for 32% of urinary recovery (24% of the dose). Less than 1% of the nabumetone reaches the urine as a major active metabolite.[13] Two non-acidic metabolites account for another 23% of urinary recovery (16% of the dose) and the remaining 45% is made up of numerous minor metabolites resulting from further metabolism. Overall, 80% of the administered dose of nabumetone is excreted in the urine and about 10% in the faeces.

Pharmaceutics

Nabumetone (Relifex; Bencard division of SmithKline, Beecham, UK) is only available in oral form. Tablets containing 500 mg nabumetone are red, film-coated and marked 'Relifex' on one side and '500' on the other.

Therapeutic use

Indications

1. Osteoarthritis
2. Rheumatoid arthritis.

Other uses

3. Ankylosing spondylitis
4. Soft tissue rheumatism.

Contraindications

1. Active peptic ulceration
2. Severe hepatic impairment (e.g. cirrhosis)
3. Hypersensitivity to the drug.

Mode of use

The recommended daily dose is two tablets (1.0 g) nabumetone taken as a single dose at bedtime. For severe or persistent symptoms or during acute exacerbations, an additional dose of one or two tablets (500 mg to 1 g) may be given as a morning dose. The dose should be reduced in elderly patients when often 500 mg daily may give satisfactory relief.

There is inadequate clinical data to recommend the use of nabumetone in children.

Indications

1. Osteoarthritis

Some 15 clinical trials have been described. Most are of short duration but in four treatment was for periods of up to one year or longer. Two of these are comparisons with placebo. In both studies[14,15] nabumetone 1 g once and twice daily, respectively, were superior to placebo both statistically and clinically. The treatments were similarly well tolerated though nabumetone caused more 'moderate' side effects than placebo in one of the studies. The majority of studies against other non-steroidal anti-inflammatory drugs show nabumetone to be as effective as aspirin, diclofenac, indomethacin

Fig. 1 Pathways of biotransformation of nambumetone

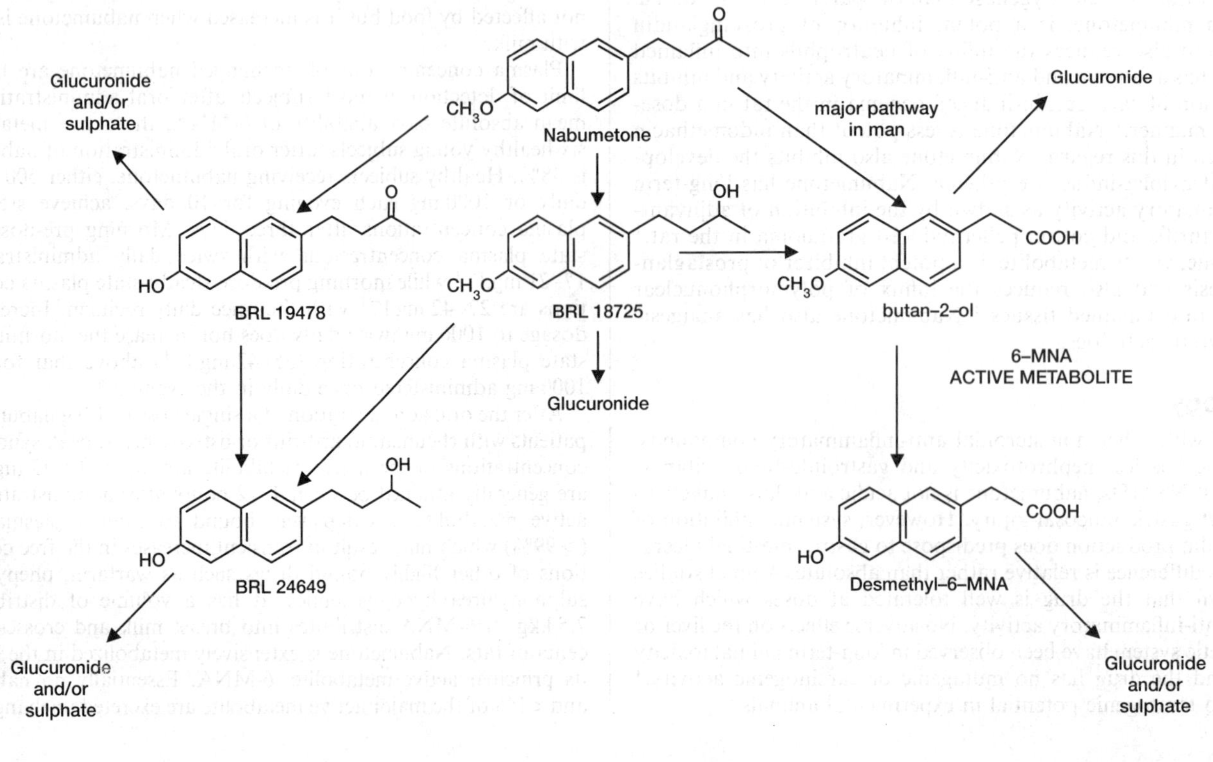

Nabumetone

and naproxen in standard doses. Two well designed studies of adequate duration including a run-in period on placebo and adequate numbers of patients perhaps suggest that some patients withdraw because of unsatisfactory efficacy at the recommended dose of 1 g daily.[16,17] The optimum therapeutic dose range might therefore lie between 1.0 and 2.0 g a day.

The use of non-steroidal anti-inflammatory drugs in osteoarthritis remains controversial. Although some patients undoubtedly have an element of inflammatory synovitis, the main pathology is felt to be degenerative and the use of non-steroidal anti-inflammatory drugs in the elderly group of patients who are susceptible to the condition is associated with a high risk of side effects, particularly gastrointestinal. Simple analgesic therapy may be preferred and no studies have to date compared nabumetone with paracetamol or co-proxamol (dextropropoxyphene and paracetamol) in osteoarthritis.

2. Rheumatoid arthritis

There have been 17 studies of nabumetone in rheumatoid arthritis. In some the numbers of patients are small and in others the duration of treatment is relatively short (2–4 weeks). In four studies, the duration of treatment was 3–6 months. The use of non-steroidal anti-inflammatory agents for this inflammatory condition is without controversy.

No formal dose-ranging studies have been published for nabumetone in rheumatoid arthritis though 1.0 g once daily in the evening is the dosage most frequently used. The evening dose may be more effective than a dose administered at other times of the day.[18] An impression derived from several trials is that 1.5–2.0 g daily in divided doses may be more effective than 1.0 g daily as a single dose.

The short-term analgesic and anti-inflammatory effect of nabumetone 1.0 g daily and evening has been confirmed, relative to that of placebo.[19,20] In comparative studies with other non-steroidal anti-inflammatory drugs, nabumetone appears to have been better tolerated than most other non-steroidal anti-inflammatory drugs with the exception of sulindac. In some trials the doses selected for the comparator drugs have been lower than those in conventional use and new trials using higher doses are now being carried out. Aspirin (not frequently used in British rheumatological practice) certainly produced more gastrointestinal and central nervous sysstem complaints[21] and indomethacin[22,23] produced more gastrointestinal side effects than nabumetone. An open extension to one of the studies,[24] in which patients were allowed to continue on nabumetone titrated to achieve an optimum therapeutic response, also confirmed that the current recommended dose may be too low. After three years, only seven patients were taking 1.0 g daily while 24 had increased to 1.5 g daily and 30 were receiving 2.0 g daily.

An endoscopic study showed gastroduodenal lesions in 19 out of 25 patients treated with naproxen 500 mg twice daily compared with only 1 out of 20 treated with nabumetone 1.0 g daily.[25] This may reflect the value of a prodrug on the gastric mucosa though endoscopic appearances do not always correlate with the symptoms experienced by patients with arthritis. In a further 12 week double-blind study involving 37 patients, nabumetone 1.0 g daily was significantly less damaging to the gastrointestinal tract than naproxen 250 mg twice a day. Arguably, the doses of both drugs used in this study were suboptimal.

3. Ankylosing spondylitis

One single double-blind parallel trial in 29 patients suggested that nabumetone in a dose of 1.5 g daily was slightly less effective than indomethacin up to 175 mg daily in ankylosing spondylitis.[26]

4. Soft tissue rheumatism

A group of five studies in soft tissue rheumatism have suggested that the drug is effective and well tolerated compared to aspirin, ibuprofen and naproxen.

Adverse reactions

In comparative clinical trials, the overall incidence of adverse effects, resulting from the use of nabumetone appears similar to the incidence with diclofenac, ibuprofen, naproxen and sulindac. Gastrointestinal adverse effects are less frequently seen with nabumetone than with indomethacin, and both gastrointestinal and central nervous system complaints are significantly less frequently seen with nabumetone than with aspirin.

In British trials 26% of patients have reported one or more unwanted effects. Dyspepsia occurred in 7%, nausea or vomiting in 5%, diarrhoea in 2% and a rash in 1%. A total of seven peptic ulcers have been reported during clinical studies, six occurring in the USA and one in Europe although these were not necessarily drug related.

Potentially life-threatening effects

Deaths attributed entirely to nabumetone are extremely rare. Hypersensitivity to the drug in patients who display hypersensitivity to aspirin and other acidic non-steroidal anti-inflammatory drugs represents the main risk. The increased incidence of serious morbidity (perforation or haemorrhage) in elderly patients with peptic ulceration receiving non-steroidal anti-inflammatory drugs should be borne in mind. There is insufficient long-term epidemiological evidence to compare the risk of treatment with nabumetone in unselected elderly patients with other widely used NSAIDs although withdrawals from clinical trials due to side-effects have been similar in patients above and below 65 or 70 years.

Acute overdosage

There is no specific antidote and little information is available. Treatment with activated charcoal, using up to 60 g orally in divided doses with appropriate supportive therapy, might be helpful.

Severe or irreversible adverse effects

Complications of gastrointestinal ulceration, particularly in the elderly, are the main risk.

One case of cholestatic jaundice has been described[27] but the rare severe side effects, such as renal failure, anaphylaxis, photosensitivity reactions and blood dyscrasias that are sometimes seen with other non-steroidal anti-inflammatory drugs, have not to date been reported in the literature on nabumetone. It is claimed that this is a reflection of its 'prodrug' activity, though may alternatively reflect limited experience with its use since marketing began.

Symptomatic adverse effects

Reviews of adverse effects in 6000 patients receiving nabumetone in clinical trials are available from the USA.[28,29] In addition 40 000 patients have paticipated in past nabumetone surveillance studies. In common with other non-steroidal anti-inflammatory drugs, gastrointestinal adverse effects (e.g. abdominal pain, dyspepsia, diarrhoea, nausea and flatulence) were the most common. These were followed less frequently by central nervous system complaints (headache, tinnitus, dizziness) and dermatological effects (e.g. rash, pruritus).

Interference with clinical pathology tests

No interferences of this kind have been reported.

High risk groups

Neonates

Breast milk. Animal studies have shown 6MNA is excreted in breast milk, so used during lactating is not recommended. Safety of the drug during lactation has also not been established so use is not recommended.

Children

The use of the drug is not recommended for children.

Pregnant women

Safety in human pregnancy has not been established. At present, the use of nabumetone is not recommended in pregnancy.

The elderly

A reduction in dose may be necessary (see above).

Drug interactions

Potentially hazardous interactions

Anticoagulants. Since the drug is highly protein bound, patients receiving concurrent treatment with oral anticoagulants might suffer transient loss of anticoagulant control. However, use of a drug of this type in a patient on anticoagulants is unwise because of the risk of gastrointestinal haemorrhage.

Other significant interactions

Antacids. The co-administration of antacids has been shown to decrease the bioavailability of some non-steroidal anti-inflammatory drugs but not nabumetone.

Antihypertensive drugs. Although interactions have been reported

N

N

between some non-steroidal anti-inflammatory drugs and antihypertensive drugs, these have not been reported with nabumetone.

Diuretics. Although diuretics may interact with non-steroidal anti-inflammatory drugs, no significant increases in weight during treatment with nabumetone have been seen, suggesting lack of antagonism of diuretic effect.

Food. The bioavailability of 6-MNA is unaffected by food but is increased following the co-administration of nabumetone with milk.

Clinical trials

1. Gillgrass J, Grahame R 1984 Nabumetone: a double-blind study in osteoarthrosis. Pharmatherapeutica 3: 592–594

An outpatient double-blind crossover study of nabumetone 1 g twice daily versus placebo in 18 patients with osteoarthritis (mean age 51.2 years). A statistically significant drug-related beneficial effect was shown both for patient preference and clinical response. No drug-related adverse events were noted.

2. Lanier B G, Turner R A, Collins R L, Serter R G Jnr 1987 Evaluation of nabumetone in the treatment of active adult rheumatoid arthritis. American Journal of Medicine 83: 40–43

An outpatient double-blind parallel group study of nabumetone 1.0 g at night against placebo in 139 patients with rheumatoid arthritis (mean age 48 years). Patients treated with nabumetone had a greater degree of improvement of modest statistical significance. More patients withdrew from the placebo group because of lack of efficacy. The profiles of adverse experiences were similar for both groups.

3. Brobyn R D 1986 Proceedings of the conference on new NSAIDs: criteria of therapeutics selection, San Diego Abstract 16

An outpatient double-blind parallel group study over six months in 100 patients with rheumatoid arthritis (mean age 54 years) randomized to either nabumetone 1.0 g at night or naproxen 250 mg twice daily (a relatively low dose). There was no statistically significant difference between the two drugs in terms of efficacy or adverse experiences.

4. Pease C T, Storr J, Earle J, Barnardo D E 1985 Royal Society of Medicine International Congress Symposium Series, vol 69, pp 105–112

A double-blind outpatient crossover study of four weeks duration comparing nabumetone 1.0 g at night versus naproxen 500 mg twice daily in 28 patients with osteoarthritis (range 45–84 years). There was no statistical difference between the two treatments for any of the clinical parameters measured and some trends suggested that endoscopically, nabumetone was better tolerated by the gastric mucosa though these trends did not reach statistical significance in favour of nabumetone superiority.

General review articles

Friedel H A, Todd P A 1988 Nabumetone: a preliminary review of its pharmacodynamic and pharmacokinetic properties and therapeutic efficacy in rheumatic disease. Drugs 35: 504–524

Mangan F R, Flack J D, Jackson D 1987 Pre-clinical overview of nabumetone: pharmacology, bioavailability, metabolism and toxicology. American Journal of Medicine 83: 6–10

References

1. Boyle E A, Freeman P C, Mangan F R, Thomson M J 1982 Nabumetone (BRL 14 777, 4-(6-methoxy-2-naphthyl) butane-2-one a new anti-inflammatory agent. Journal of Pharmacy and Pharmacology 34: 562–569
2. Freeman A M, Undre N A, Thawley A R, Golding D N 1985 Plasma and synovial fluid concentrations of nabumetone and BRL 10 720 in patients given nabumetone. Royal Society of Medicine International Congress and Symposium Series, vol 69, pp 37–42
3. Jackson D, Hardy T L, Langley P F, Von Schrader H W 1985 Pharmacokinetic, toxicological, and metabolic studies with nabumetone. Royal Society of Medicine International Congress and Symposium Series, vol 69, pp 15–27
4. Mangan F R 1986 Proceedings of the Conference on new NSAIDs: criteria for therapeutic selection. San Diego, Abstract 7
5. Nunn B, Chamberlain P D 1982 Effect of nabumetone (BRL 14 777), a new anti-inflammatory drug, on human platelet reactivity ex vivo: comparison with naproxen. Journal of Pharmacy and Pharmacology 34: 576–579
6. Ray J E, Day R O 1984 High-performance liquid chromatographic determination of a new anti-inflammatory agent, nabumetone, and its major metabolite in plasma using fluorimetric detection. Journal of Chromatography 336: 234–238
7. Von Schrader H W, Thawley A R, Buscher G, Undre N A 1984 Metabolism and pharmacokinetics of nabumetone (BRL 14 777) in healthy volunteers. Abstract presented at the 2nd European Congress of Biopharmaceutics and Pharmacokinetics, Salamanca, Spain
8. Von Schrader H W, Buscher G, Dierdorf D, Mugge H, Wolfe D 1984 Nabumetone — a novel anti-inflammatory drug: bioavailability after different dosage regimens. International Journal of Clinical Pharmacology, Therapy and Toxicology 22: 672–676
9. Bourke B, Under N A, Thawley A R 1985 An investigation into the penetration of nabumetone and its metabolites into synovial fluid in patients with rheumatoid arthritis. Royal Society of Medicine International Congress and Symposium Series, vol 69, pp 31–35
10. Clarke A K, Hawkins S, Henderson R C, Undre N A, Thawley A R 1984 Pharmacokinetics of nabumetone (BRL 14 777) and its safety at steady state in patients with moderately impaired renal function. Abstract presented to the 2nd European Congress of Biopharmaceutics and Pharmacokinetics, Salamanca, Spain
11. Hamdy R C, Price J D, Undre N A, Thawley A R, Rotman H 1985 The pharmacokinetics of nabumetone in elderly patients. Royal Society of Medicine International Congress and Symposium Series, vol 69, pp 173–183
12. Mangan F R 1985 A review of the pharmacology of nabumetone. Royal Society of Medicine International Congress and Symposium Series, vol 69, pp 5–14
13. Haddock R E, Jeffery D J, Lloyd J A, Thawley A R 1984 Metabolism of nabumetone (BRL 14 777) by various species including man. Xenobiotica 14: 327–337
14. Blechman W J 1987 Nabumetone therapy of osteoarthritis. American Journal of Medicine 83: 70–73
15. Gillgrass J, Grahame R 1984 Nabumetone: a double-blind study in osteoarthrosis. Pharmatherapeutica 3: 592–594
16. Appelrouth D J, Baim S, Chang R W et al 1987 Comparison of the safety and efficacy of nabumetone and aspirin in the treatment of osteoarthritis in adults. American Journal of Medicine 83: 78–81
17. Pisco E J, Bockow B I, Box P, Brodsky A L, Burch F X 1987 Six month multicenter study comparing nabumetone and naproxen in the treatment of osteoarthritis. American Journal of Medicine 83: 86–91
18. Pownall R, Knapp M S, Kowanko I C, Rudge S, Swannell A J 1985 The therapeutic effectiveness of nabumetone given at different times of day including domiciliary self-measurement of circadian variations in the signs and symptoms of rheumatoid arthritis. Royal Society of Medicine International Congress and Symposium Series, vol 69, pp 113–123
19. Lanier B G, Turner Jr R A, Collins R L, Serter Jr R G 1987 Evaluation of nabumetone in the treatment of active adult rheumatoid arthritis. American Journal of Medicine 83: 40–43
20. Turner R A, Brindley D A, Mitchell F M 1987 Nabumetone: a single center three-week comparison with placebo in the treatment of rheumatoid arthritis. American Journal of Medicine 83: 36–39
21. Bernhard G C, Appelrouth D J, Bankhurst A D et al 1987 Long-term treatment of rheumatoid arthritis comparing nabumetone with aspirin. American Journal of Medicine 83: 44–49
22. Wojtulewski J A 1985 A double-blind study of nabumetone in rheumatoid arthritis. Royal Society of Medicine International Congress and Symposium Series, vol 69, pp 79–88
23. Zoma A, Capell H 1985 Double-blind study to compare the effectiveness and tolerance of nabumetone with indomethacin in patients with rheumatoid arthritis attending a hospital outpatient clinic. Royal Society of Medicine International Congress and Symposium Series, vol 69, pp 73–78
24. Brobyn R D 1987 Nabumetone in the treatment of active adult rheumatoid arthritis. American Journal of Medicine 83: 50–54
25. Bianchi Porro G, Caruso I, Petrillo M, Montrone F, Price J D 1985 Endoscopic evaluation of the effect of naproxen and nabumetone on gastric and duodenal mucosa. Royal Society of Medicine International Congress and Symposium Series, vol 69, pp 97–101
26. Short D J, Brierley J, Hajiroussou V, Webley M 1985 Comparison of nabumetone with indomethacin in the treatment of ankylosing spondylitis. Royal Society of Medicine International Congress and Symposium Series, vol 69, pp 125–130
27. Shadforth M F, Crook P R 1985 A study comparing nabumetone and ibuprofen in osteoarthritis of the knee. Royal Society of Medicine International Congress and Symposium Series, vol 69, pp 133–138
28. Jackson R E, Mitchell F N, Brindley D A 1987 Safety evaluation of nabumetone in United States clinical trials. American Journal of Medicine 83: 115–120
29. Jenner P N, Johnson E S 1987 Review of the experience with nabumetone in clinical trials outside the United States. American Journal of Medicine 83: 110–114

Nadolol

Nadolol is a hydrophilic non-selective β-adrenoceptor blocking drug with a long half life, which is devoid of partial agonist activity (intrinsic sympathomimetic activity) and membrane activity.

Chemistry

Nadolol (Corgard, Solgol)
$C_{17}H_{27}NO_4$
(2R,3S)-5-(3-tert-Butylamino-2-hydroxypropoxy)-1,2,3,4-tetrahydronaphthalene-2-3-diol

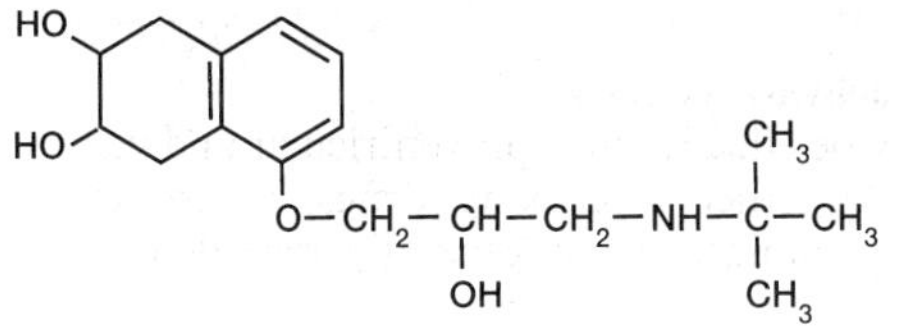

Molecular weight	309.4
pKa	9.67
Solubility	
in alcohol	freely soluble
in water	soluble
Octanol/water partition coefficient	0.066, at pH 7.4, 37°C

Nadolol is a white crystalline powder prepared by chemical synthesis. It is also available with bendrofluazide in the compound formulation Corgaretic.

Pharmacology

Nadolol is a competitive antagonist at both the β_1 and β_2 adrenoceptor, it is therefore a non-selective β-blocking drug. In anaesthetized dogs, a 7.5 μg.kg^{-1} intravenous dose of nadolol gave over 50% inhibition of the heart rate response to isoprenaline (1 μg.kg^{-1} intravenously), whereas a 60 μg.kg^{-1} intravenous dose of propanolol gave about 40% inhibition. The fall of diastolic blood pressure caused by 1 μg.kg^{-1} isoprenaline was inhibited by about 70% by 7.5 μg.kg^{-1} of nadolol. A similar inhibition was obtained with propanolol 15 μg.kg^{-1}.[1] Nadolol does not possess any agonist activity or membrane stabilizing activity. It is hydrophilic and has a very long half life.[1,2] It does not readily cross the blood–brain barrier because of its hydrophilicity.

Toxicology

Nadolol has low toxicity and tests have not shown evidence of damage that is relevant to its use in man. No teratogenicity was found in tests in mice, rats, hamsters, rabbits and dogs. No evidence of carcinogenicity has been found in mice or rats at doses of 500 and 1000 mg.kg^{-1} respectively. Mutagenicity tests have not been done.[3]

Clinical pharmacology

Nadolol inhibits the effect of isoprenaline on the heart in man. The haemodynamic effects of nadolol are overall similar to those of propranolol, reducing exercise tachycardia and exercise systolic blood pressure and lowering cardiac output at rest and on exercise.[4,5] In a study in normal volunteers it was found that 80 mg of nadolol gave a 42% reduction in exercise double product (systolic blood pressure × heart rate) compared to a 32% inhibition from the same dose of propranolol, while 160 mg of nadolol gave the same effect as 80 mg. Higher doses of propranolol were not studied.[4] Nadolol has a long duration of action with a 'pharmacodynamic half life' of 39 h compared to 11 h for propranolol.[4]
Nadolol decreases maximal exercise tolerance in normal individuals but in patients with angina, exercise tolerance is increased, due to a reduction in total myocardial oxygen consumption. Nadolol lowers blood pressure in both the lying and standing position although the exact mechanism of this effect is in doubt. Nadolol increases peripheral resistance, reducing peripheral blood flow and thus causing cold hands and feet. The reduction in cardiac output may lead to the precipitation of heart failure in susceptible individuals. Although there has been some suggestion that nadolol has a special dilator action on renal blood vessels (i.e. with blood pressure falling and glomerular filtration rate maintained)[6] this has not been fully confirmed.[7] Nadolol has no effect on cerebral blood flow.[8]

In addition to reducing the heart rate, particularly on exercise, nadolol slows conduction in the atria and in the A-V node and decreases the spontaneous rate of depolarization of ectopic pacemakers. These effects all contribute to the antiarrhythmic effects of nadolol. The drug blocks the action of adrenaline on β-receptors in other tissues. In particular, airways resistance is increased by nadolol and this may be dangerous in patients with obstructive airways disease. Nadolol probably shares the various endocrine and metabolic effects of propranolol, although relatively few studies have been done. Thus it is likely to alleviate the somatic manifestations of hyperthyroidism, and to improve essential tremor. Nadolol has been reported to lower plasma renin levels and inhibits catecholamine-induced lipolysis. It reduces the HDL lipoprotein fraction, increasing VLDL.[7]

Pharmacokinetics

The preferred analytical method is by HPLC.[9–11] The detection limit is 0.5 μg.l^{-1} for plasma, 0.1 mg.l^{-1} for urine.[11]

Nadolol is poorly absorbed after oral administration; on average it is about 30% bioavailable. Absorption is variable, so individual dosage adjustment is advisable.[10] There is no presystemic, or other, metabolism so that the bioavailability of about 30% is a reflection of the level of absorption of unchanged drug. Peak concentration occurs 1–4 h after oral administration. Nadolol is excreted unchanged by the kidneys and has a long plasma half life, 17–24 h.[5]

Nadolol is widely distributed, with a relatively high volume of distribution of 2 l.kg^{-1}. However, dog studies indicated poor brain penetration, with levels about 25% of that in blood, which is a reflection of its low lipid solubility. No studies on brain penetration have been done in man. It is about 30% protein bound. Animal experiments indicated that nadolol crosses the placenta; data in man are not available. It is concentrated about three to five times in breast milk.[5,12]

Nadolol is excreted unchanged by the kidney and in the bile; 23% of an intravenous dose has been recovered from the faeces (73% in the urine). Predictably, half life is progressively prolonged with increasing renal insufficiency. With a creatinine clearance at an average of 10.7 ± 2.3 ml.min^{-1}, for instance, the half life averaged 38.6 ± 4.4 h with a range 29.7–58.2 h.[13]

Data are not available for the very young and the elderly, but in the latter, as renal function declines with age, a moderately prolonged half life would be expected. Dosage of nadolol should be reduced in patients with renal failure.

Oral absorption	30%
Presystemic metabolism	—
Plasma half life	
range	17–24
Volume of distribution	2 l.kg^{-1}
Plasma protein binding	30%

Concentration–effect relationship

Concentrations of nadolol measured 6 h after the oral administration of dosages between 20 and 80 mg were found to be linearly related to exercise-induced changes in the rate–pressure product.[14] However, there is no evidence of a correlation between the plasma concentration of nadolol and its antihypertensive effect.

N

Metabolism

Nadolol is not metabolized, it is excreted unchanged.[5,7]

Pharmaceutics

Nadolol is available only in oral form from Squibb/Princeton (UK/USA).

1. Corgard 40 mg: pale blue, round biconvex tablets, unscored, with 'Squibb 207' engraved on one side.
2. Corgard 80 mg: pale blue, round, biconvex tablets, scored on one side and engraved 'Squibb 241'.
3. Corgard (Squibb/Princeton, USA) is available as 20, 40, 80, 120 and 160 mg tablets in the United States.

It is also available in combination with the diuretic bendrofluazide:

5. Corgaretic 40/Corzide 40/5 (Squibb/Princeton, UK/USA): white, blue-speckled, round biconvex tablets containing 40 mg nadolol and 5 mg bendrofluazide. Engraved 'Squibb' and '283' on one side with a bisect bar on the other.
6. Corgaretic 80/Corzide 80/5 (Squibb/Princeton, UK/USA): white, blue-speckled, round biconvex tablets containing 80 mg nadolol and 5 mg bendrofluazide. Engraved 'Squibb' and '284' on one side with a bisect bar on the other.

A shelf-life of 4 years is quoted for nadolol. It can be stored at room temperature but should be protected from excessive heat and moisture. Corgard is not thought to contain any allergenic substances.

Therapeutic use

This would be expected to be the same as for propranolol, but as evaluation has not been so wide the approved indications are fewer.

Indications

1. Long-term management of hypertension
2. Long-term management of angina pectoris
3. Cardiac tachyarrhythmias
4. Relief of hyperthyroid symptoms and pre-operative preparation for thyroidectomy
5. Prophylaxis of migraine.

Contraindications

1. Obstructive airways disease
2. Cardiac insufficiency and cardiogenic shock
3. Heart block
4. Hypoglycaemia.

Mode of use

Clinical use is dependent on β-blockade, most particularly of receptors in the heart. Although both β_1 and β_2 receptors are present in the heart, receptors mediate nerve impulses and thus β_1 block is more important.

Oral treatment is usually commenced with 40 mg once daily. Dosage may be increased up to 160 or 240 mg; occasionally, higher doses have been used in hypertension. The long half life allows once daily dosage.

Exacerbations of ischaemia in patients at risk, increased angina and myocardial infarction have been reported after abrupt withdrawal of β-adrenoceptor blocking drugs. Nadolol, like other similar drugs, should not be abruptly stopped before anaesthesia. Although there is no evidence for nadolol it is likely that, as has been reported with other non-agonist β_1-blocking drugs, there is an up-regulation of β-receptors during drug administration. Evidence from other β-blocking drugs suggests that no post β-blockade hypersensitivity occurs, provided a very small dose (possibly 10 mg a day of nadolol) is continued for two weeks.[15]

Indications

1. Hypertension

Nadolol may be used as a first choice drug for the treatment of hypertension. It is similar in efficacy to propranolol or hydrochlorothiazide.[5] When necessary, nadolol may be given in combination with a diuretic or other treatment, e.g. methyldopa[16] or nifedipine.[17]

The usual initial dose for hypertension is 80 mg once daily, increasing to 240 mg daily if required. Occasionally larger doses are used, but it is usually more useful to add a second drug, or try alternative treatment if no response has been obtained. In most studies supine diastolic blood pressure has been lowered by about 10%, systolic by 6 to 20%,[5] a mean fall in arterial pressure of 10–25 mmHg.[10] How nadolol and other β-adrenoceptor blocking drugs lower the blood pressure is not clear, although reduction of cardiac output without a full compensatory rise in peripheral resistance seems to be the main haemodynamic change.[7]

2. Angina pectoris

Nadolol is an effective prophylactic in angina pectoris.[5,18] Nadolol 40–240 mg reduced angina attacks by 59% compared to baseline and increased acute exercise tolerance by 38%.[19] It is similar in efficacy to propranolol. Nadolol has been used in combination with isosorbide which gave a further reduction in angina attacks, while nifedipine reduced exercise ST segment changes.[18,20]

Dosage in angina is usually commenced at 40 mg a day and increased as required up to 160 or 240 mg a day. The value of still higher doses has not been demonstrated. The optimum dose of a β-adrenoceptor blocking drug in angina, provided it is tolerated, generally is the dose which gives maximum inhibition of exercising heart rate.

3. Cardiac tachyarrhythmias

Nadolol may be effective in supraventricular and ventricular arrhythmias, but like other β-blocking drugs, except in catecholamine-induced arrhythmias, is not generally regarded as a drug of first choice.[10,20,21]

The starting dose is 40 mg a day which can be increased to 160 mg a day if required.

4. Thyrotoxicosis

Nadolol is similar to propranolol in its ability to suppress the signs and symptoms of thyrotoxicosis.[21–23] The dosage range is 80–160 mg once daily. Most patients require 160 mg once daily. Conventional antithyroid treatment may be used concomitantly. For the preparation of patients for partial thyroidectomy, nadolol should be administered with potassium iodide for 10 days prior to operation. It should also be administered on the morning of operation. Nadolol dosage should be slowly reduced postoperatively and withdrawn when clinical stability is attained.

5. Migraine

The starting dose is 40 mg a day which may be increased to obtain optimal prophylaxis, the usual maintenance dose being 80–160 mg a day. Treatment should be discontinued after 4 to 6 weeks if a satisfactory response has not been obtained, withdrawing treatment gradually over two weeks.[24]

Contraindications

These apply to all non-selective β-adrenoceptor blocking drugs.[7]

1. Obstructive airways disease

Nadolol should not be given to patients with asthma, as a severe attack may be precipitated[25] due to the blocking action of nadolol on the β_2-dilator action of adrenaline. There is a possibility that some patients with allergic rhinitis may experience bronchospasm, and patients with chronic obstructive airways disease may also be worsened. Patients who have received nadolol will be unresponsive to usual doses of β_2-stimulant drugs.

2. Cardiac insufficiency and cardiogenic shock

A major compensatory mechanism in myocardial insufficiency, either left or right sided, is sympathetic stimulation leading to an increase in heart rate. β-blockade, with nadolol for instance, will interfere with this compensatory mechanism and worsen the failure.

3. Heart block

Nadolol should be avoided in second or third degree heart block and in patients with an already slow heart rate, 45–55 beats.min^{-1}. A slow heart rate in an asymptomatic patient who is otherwise well in sinus rhythm need not necessarily be a cause for concern.

4. Hypoglycaemia

Muscle glycogenolysis is β_2-receptor mediated, and hepatic glycogenolysis is also β-mediated, although here α-receptors also play a part. As might be expected, therefore, nadolol has been shown to prolong insulin-induced hypoglycaemia. Additionally, the cardiovascular responses to hypoglycaemia would be expected to be modified, the β-mediated vasodilator action of liberated adrenaline being inhibited leaving the α-vasoconstrictor action unopposed, and consequently there is an increased rise of blood pressure.

Adverse reactions

Potentially life-threatening effects
No specific toxicity has been reported. Dangerous reactions reported are consequent on β-blockade. A severe asthma attack has been reported in a young hypertensive who had hitherto only experienced mild episodes, leading to unconsciousness for 4 days.[25]

Nadolol should not be withdrawn suddenly in patients with ischaemic heart disease such as those with myocardial infarction or angina pectoris in whom symptoms may be worsened.

Acute overdosage
Overdosage with nadolol has not been reported. Haemodialysis might be useful in severe cases as it would reduce the serum concentration.

Management of overdosage would be similar to that for other β-blocking drugs.[26] Excessive bradycardia may be treated with intravenous atropine.

Isoprenaline, if given, should be administered as an infusion in graded doses increased rapidly (e.g. minute intervals) until heart rate increases to an adequate level. Impracticable dosage levels may be required, hospital supplies being inadequate. Glucagon may be a useful cardiac stimulant as the adenyl cyclase system is stimulated independently of the β-receptor. Digitalization and diuretics may be employed. Bronchospasm may be treated with aminophylline, or again, extremely large doses of isoprenaline or salbutamol (arrived at by a graded approach).

Severe or irreversible adverse effects
Severe adverse effects from nadolol are most likely to be associated with poor patient selection and to occur at the beginning of treatment. It is in this situation that the long half life of nadolol is a disadvantage.

Asthma is likely to be dramatically worsened in an asthmatic. Heart failure may be worsened or precipitated in patients in or on the verge of heart failure.

Symptomatic adverse effects
Symptomatic adverse effects are similar to those of other β-blocking drugs and seldom require withdrawal of treatment. Sometimes dosage reduction will relieve adverse effects without loss of therapeutic efficacy. Those reported infrequently include gastrointestinal effects, alopecia, bradycardia, fatigue, light-headedness, cold extremities, insomnia, paraesthesia and dryness of the mouth. Cardiac insufficiency, hypotension and A-V block have occurred on rare occasions.

In a multi-centre study using 14 870 hypertensive patients, the incidence of adverse effects was 6.2%, which compares favourably with other β-blockers under similar conditions.[27]

Other effects
Nadolol would be expected to produce biochemical changes similar to those induced by non-selective agents. There is a modest increase in serum potassium and urate but creatinine and urea have been reported as unchanged.[28] Insulin hypoglycaemia can be prolonged.[29] Nadolol, like propranolol, reduces HDL and increases VLDL.[30] It is not clear whether these changes are clinically important.

Interference with clinical pathology tests
There are no known interferences of this kind.

High risk groups

Neonates
There are no data on the use of nadolol in neonates.

Breast milk. Caution is required in nursing women as concentrations in breast milk are 3–5 times higher than steady-state blood concentrations.[31]

Children
There are no data on the use of nadolol in children.

Pregnant women
The safety of nadolol in pregnancy has not been established.

The elderly
In both angina pectoris and hypertension, dosage with nadolol should be titrated gradually, say at one week intervals, so that no problem should arise. However, it should be remembered that the decline in renal function associated with ageing will prolong the half life of renally excreted nadolol, leading to greater accumulation and thus a lower dosage than otherwise would be expected in the elderly for all indications.

Drug interactions

As nadolol is not metabolized in the liver a major possible source of drug interactions is removed.

Potentially hazardous interactions

Adrenaline. As with other non-selective β-blockers, marked increases in blood pressure and bradycardia would be expected from the administration of adrenaline in the presence of nadolol, isoprenaline or verapamil.

Anaesthetic agents. Heart rate and cardiac output may fall in anaesthesia to a greater degree in patients taking β-blockers. This can be counteracted by atropine 1–2 mg intravenously. Nadolol should not be abruptly stopped before anaesthesia as potentiation of the effects of any liberated catecholamines would be expected. Myocardial depressants such as lignocaine and procanamide may potentiate the hypotensive action of nadolol.

Clonidine. Rebound hypertension following abrupt withdrawal of clonidine may be potentiated by a β-blocker such as nadolol. Clonidine should not be discontinued until several days after nadolol withdrawal.

Insulin. Care should be taken in giving nadolol to insulin-dependent diabetics. The signs of hypoglycaemia will be masked and the rise of blood pressure associated with hypoglycaemia will be enhanced.

Other significant interactions

Indomethacin. It is possible that the hypotensive action of nadolol may be reduced by indomethacin.

Food. Food does not appear to significantly affect absorption of nadolol.[5]

Alcohol. There are no data, but hydrophilic nadolol would not be expected to influence the CNS effects of alcohol.

Smoking. In view of its β_2-blocking action on the vasodilator component of the actions of adrenaline, nadolol might be expected to enhance the rise of blood pressure that has been reported with smoking, particularly in combination with caffeine, although no data are available.

Potentially useful interactions
Nadolol inhibits the tachycardia associated with some vasodilators such as minoxidil.

References

1. Lee R J, Evans D B, Baky S H, Laffan R J 1975 Pharmacology of nadolol (SQ 11 725), a β-adrenergic antagonist lacking direct myocardial depression. European Journal of Pharmacology 33: 371–382
2. Evans D B, Peschka M T, Lee R J, Laffan R J 1976 Anti-arrhythmic action of nadolol a β-adrenergic receptor blocking agent. European Journal of Pharmacology 35: 17–27
3. Sibley P L, Keim G R, Kulesza J S et al 1978 Preclinical toxicologic evaluation of nadolol, a new β-adrenergic antagonist. Toxicology and Applied Pharmacology 44: 379–389
4. Vukovich R A, Foley J E, Brown B et al 1979 Effect of β-blockers on exercise double product (systolic blood pressure × heart rate). British Journal of Clinical Pharmacology 7 (suppl 2): 167S–172S
5. Heel R C, Brogden R N, Pakes G, Speight T M, Avery G S 1980 Nadolol: a review of its pharmacological properties and therapeutic efficacy in hypertension and angina pectoris. Drugs 20: 1–23
6. Textor S C, Fouad F M, Bravo E L, Tarazi R C, Vidt D G, Gifford R W Jr 1982 Redistribution of cardiac output to the kidneys during oral nadolol administration. New England Journal of Medicine 307: 601–605
7. Cruickshank J M, Prichard B N C 1988 β-Blockers in Clinical Practice. Churchill Livingstone, Edinburgh, p 1003
8. Steiner J A, Hughes R J D, James I M 1981 The effect of nadolol on cerebral blood flow. In: Gross F (ed) International experience with nadolol. The Royal Society of Medicine International Congress Symposium Series No. 37. Academic Press/Royal Society of Medicine, London, pp 99–102

N

9. Funke P T, Malley M F, Ivashkiv E, Cohen A I 1978 Determination of serum nadolol levels by GLC-selected ion monitoring mass spectrometry: comparison with a spectrofluorimetric method. Journal of Pharmaceutical Sciences 67: 653–656
10. Frishman W H 1981 Nadolol: a new β-adrenoceptor antagonist. New England Journal of Medicine 305: 678–682
11. Liu L K, Robinson M L 1985 The determination of nadolol in biological samples using high-performance liquid chromatography. Journal of Pharmaceutical and Biomedical Analysis 3: 351–358
12. Delvin R G, Duchin K L, Fleiss P M 1981 Nadolol in human serum and breast milk. British Journal of Clinical Pharmacology 12: 393–396
13. Herrera J, Vukovich R A, Griffith D L 1979 Elimination of nadolol by patients with renal impairment. British Journal of Clinical Pharmacology 7 (suppl 2): 227S–231S
14. Duchin K L, Vukovich R A, Dennick L G, Groel J T, Willard D A 1980 Effects of nadolol β-blockade on blood pressure in hypertension. Clinical Pharmacology and Therapeutics 27: 58–63
15. Prichard B N C, Walden R J, Tomlinson B, Liu J-B 1988 The cardiovascular effect of withdrawal of β-adrenoceptor blocking drugs. Current Opinions in Cardiology vol. 3 (suppl 2): S19–S29
16. Jenkins A C, Rosenthal J, Stumpe K O 1981 Mediation of blood pressure by nadolol and α methyldopa. Practitioner 225 (1353): 405–409
17. Myers M A, Leenen F H, Burns R, Frankel D 1986 Nifedipine tablets vs. hydralazine in patients with persisting hypertension who receive combined diuretic and β-blocker therapy. Clinical Pharmacology and Therapeutics 39: 409–413
18. Shapiro W, Park J, DiBianco R, Singh S N, Katz R J, Fletcher R 1981 Comparison of nadolol, a new long-acting β-receptor blocking agent, and placebo in the treatment of stable angina pectoris. Chest 80: 425–430
19. Ling A S C, Groel T T 1979 Improved physical performance as a therapeutic objective in patients with angina. British Journal of Clinical Pharmacology 7 (suppl 2): 161S–166S
20. Mir M A, Tirlapur V G 1982 Circadian rhythm of ventricular arrhythmias and antiarrhythmic efficacy of the long-acting β-adrenoceptor blocker. In: Hollenberg N (ed) The haemodynamics of nadolol, second international symposium. Royal Society of Medicine International Congress Symposium Series No. 51. Academic Press/Royal Society of Medicine, London, pp 101–107
21. Coumel P, Leclercq J-F, Attuel P 1980 Nadolol in arrhythmia. In: Gross F (ed) International experience with nadolol. The Royal Society of Medicine International Congress Symposium Series No. 37. Academic Press/Royal Society of Medicine, London, pp 103–130
22. Peden N R, Isles T E, Stevenson I H, Crooks J 1982 Nadolol in thyrotoxicosis. British Journal of Clinical Pharmacology 13: 835–840
23. Wilkinson R, Burr W 1981 The effect of nadolol on thyroid function. In: Gross F (ed) International experience with nadolol, a long-acting β-blocking agent. The Royal Society of Medicine International Congress Symposium Series No. 37. Academic Press/Royal Society of Medicine, London, pp 51–56
24. Ryan R E Sr, Ryan R E Jr 1984 A comparison study of nadolol and propranolol. Headache 24: 165–166
25. Raine J M, Palazzo M G,Kerr J H, Sleight P 1981 Near-fatal bronchospasm after oral nadolol in a young asthmatic and response to ventilation with halothane. British Medical Journal 282: 548–549
26. Prichard B N C, Battersby L A, Cruickshank J M 1984 Overdosage with β-adrenergic blocking agents. Adv. Drug React. Ac. Pois. Rev. 3: 91–111
27. Schimert G, Buschbeck K 1981 Multicentre study with nadolol in hypertension. In: Gross F (ed) International experience with nadolol, a long-acting β-blocking agent. The Royal Society of Medicine International Congress Symposium Series No. 37. Academic Press/Royal Society of Medicine, Lonodn, pp 197–205
28. Waal-Manning H J, Hobson C H 1980 Renal function in patients with essential hypertension receiving nadolol. British Medical Journal 9 Aug. 423–424
29. Blanford M F 1980 New drug evaluations. Nadolol. Drug Intelligence and Clinical Pharmacy 14: 825–830
30. Peden N R, Dow R J, Isles T E, Martin B T 1984 β-adrenoceptor blockade and responses of serum lipids to a meal and to exercise. British Medical Journal 288: 1788–1790
31. McKinstry D N, Dreyfuss J 1981 Pharmokinetics of nadolol. In: Gross F (ed) International experience with nadolol, a long-acting β-blocking agent. The Royal Society of Medicine International Congress Symposium Series No. 37. Academic Press/Royal Society of Medicine, London, pp 31–38

Naftidrofuryl oxalate

Naftidrofuryl oxalate is a vasodilator.

Chemistry

Naftidrofuryl oxalate (Nafronyl oxalate, Praxilene, Dusodril, Iridus, Iridux)
$C_{26}H_{37}NO_7$
2-Diethylaminoethyl 3-(1-naphthyl)-2-tetrahydrofurfurylpropionate; hydrogen oxalate

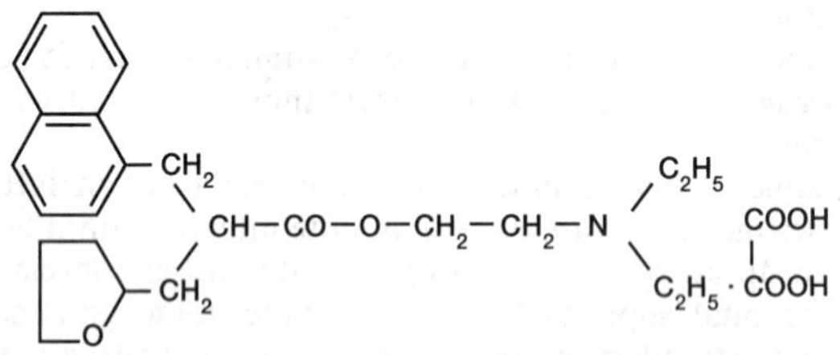

Molecular weight (free base)	473.6 (383.5)
pKa	8.7
Solubility	
in alcohol	—
in water	readily soluble
Octanol/buffer pH 6.8 coefficient	57

It is a white microcrystalline powder (melting point 108°C) of sharp odour and bitter taste prepared by chemical synthesis, producing very marked anaesthesia of the tongue. Naftidofuryl posesses a chiral centre.

Pharmacology[1,2]

Naftidrofuryl is a powerful vasodilator agent with an antagonist effect on 5-HT_2 receptors of the smooth muscle cells. The vasodilator effect, which occurs in both the cerebral and peripheral circulation, is probably the main action. Actions demonstrated include release of endothelial-derived relaxing factor (EDRF), prejunctional inhibition of noradrenergic transmission and non-selective relaxation of smooth muscle.[3] The relative importance of these actions is not clear. However, the drug has also been shown to activate intracellular aerobic metabolism as demonstrated by a reduction of lactic acid level and an increased level of ATP. It is claimed that this action protects cells against the metabolic effects of ischaemia.

Toxicology

Orally the safety margin is wide. When given intravenously at rates of infusion approximately six times that given to man, studies in the anaesthetized dog have demonstrated a slowing in intracardiac conduction and an increase in the refractory period of the contractile atrial tissue.

Clinical pharmacology

The data available is confined to single doses. A dose-dependent improvement in finger blood flow, measured by plethysmography, has been demonstrated in normal volunteer subjects following contralateral hand cooling, using doses between 100 and 1200 mg. Naftidrofuryl caused a significant reduction in lactate/pyruvate ratios in exercising healthy volunteers and a significant reduction of lactate levels and increase in ATP levels in patients with severe peripheral vascular disease.[4,5]

Naftidrofuryl has been shown to cause significant increases in transcutaneous pH and oxygen in patients with severe peripheral vascular disease.

The recommended dose range is between 300 and 600 mg orally daily and 200–400 mg by infusion. The highest oral dose known to have been used is 1600 mg daily and the highest intravenous dose is 2000 mg daily by continuous infusion over 24 hours.

Pharmacokinetics

The preferred analytical method is HPLC. The limit of detection is 5 µg.l^{-1}. Peak plasma levels are attained at 0.5–0.75 h after an oral dose. Some 24% of drug (range 17–32%) is absorbed from the gastrointestinal tract. There is some pre-systemic metabolism. The plasma half life is approximately 1 hour (range 0.8–1.6 hours). Following intravenous administration the volume of distribution is 61.5 l (range 52.7–69.4). The drug penetrates brain and other tissues. It is, however, 80% bound to albumin.

Oral absorption	17–32%
Presystemic metabolism	some
Plasma half life	
range	0.8–1.6 h
mean	1 h
Volume of distribution	61.5 l (53–70 l)
Plasma protein binding	80%

Concentration–effect relationship

Few studies have been performed but there is evidence that objective improvement in the skin flow in patients with Raynaud's disease occurs at levels of 100 µg.l^{-1}.

Metabolism

Studies have been conducted in man with labelled compound. 80% of the orally administered dose was recovered in the urine during 5 days and about 15% in the faeces. Naftidrofuryl undergoes enterohepatic circulation. Six metabolites have been isolated in urine; none is pharmacologically active.

Pharmaceutics

Naftidrofuryl (Praxilene; Lipha, UK) is available in oral and parenteral forms:

Tablets containing 200 mg of naftidrofuryl oxalate are white and round.

Capsules containing 100 mg of naftidrofuryl oxalate are pink.

There are no slow-release formulations.

There are two parenteral dosage forms. Praxilene, the standard injection 40 mg per 5 ml, and the 'forte' injection (Praxilene Forte), 200 mg per 10 ml. All formulations should be stored in a cool place away from light.

The maximum shelf-life for capsules and the 200 mg injection is 3 years in temperate climates.

Therapeutic use

Indications

1. Intermittent claudication due to peripheral vascular disease
2. Raynaud's syndrome.

Other proposed uses

3. Alzheimer's disease
4. Multi-infarct dementia
5. Acute stroke.

Contraindications

1. Hypersensitivity to the drug
2. Patients with atrioventricular block (for parenteral form only).

Mode of use

The manufacturer recommends a fixed dosage schedule. For cerebrovascular lesions treatment is given at a dosage of 300 mg orally daily. If no improvement is noted within 2 months treatment should be discontinued.

For peripheral vascular disease treatment is given at a dosage of 600 mg daily by mouth for at least 3 months. If no improvement occurs treatment should be discontinued.

Indications

Judging the clinical response in conditions such as multi-infarct dementia and peripheral vascular disease is difficult and the value of vasodilators in treatment is not fully established. It is also difficult to reconcile the short half life of this drug with a sustained therapeutic effect.

Data are still insufficient to allow critical evaluation of the benefits of naftidofuryl. In intermittent claudication the drug can increase pain-free walking distance, but probably to not more than 200 metres.[6] The drug cannot be recommended in patients with dementia until further evidence emerges.[6]

Contraindications

Atrioventricular block contraindicates the use of the parenteral form. This is based on animal experiments. Dogs given six times the recommended human dose had slowing of intracardiac conduction and sustained an increase in refractory period of the contractile atrial tissue.

Adverse reactions

Potentially life-threatening effects

There are no reports of life-threatening effects at normal clinical doses.

Acute overdosage[8]

Three patients have died from self-poisoning. In two it is known that a total dose of between 8 and 10 g was swallowed. In all cases other drugs and/or alcohol were also taken. Symptoms reported in these cases and others where accidental overdosage (too rapid infusion) was involved include loss or impairment of consciousness, convulsions, and hypotension.

Severe or irreversible adverse effects

There are no known reactions of this kind to normal doses.

Symptomatic adverse effects

The most common side effects are nausea and epigastric pain occurring in some 5% of patients. These are usually of minor severity, rarely warranting discontinuation of treatment.

Other effects

The drug alters lactate/pyruvate ratios as a part of its therapeutic effect (see above).

Interference with clinical pathology test methods

None has been reported.

High risk groups

Neonates

Naftidrofuryl is not indicated for use in neonates.

Breast milk. No information is available on the secretion of this drug in breast milk.

Children

No special precautions are necessary in children.

Pregnant women

No special precautions are necessary during pregnancy.

The elderly

No special precautions are necessary in the elderly.

Concurrent disease

There is no evidence of any toxic effects occurring in patients with renal or hepatic disease.

Drug interactions

Intravenous naftidrofuryl should be given with caution, if at all, if the patient is already on an antiarrhythmic or β-adrenoceptor blocking drug.

Controlled clinical trials

1. Admani A K 1978 New approach to treatment of recent stroke. British Medical Journal 2: 1661–1732

91 patients with acute stroke were studied in a double-blind, placebo-controlled trial of naftidrofuryl. Treatment was allocated at random and given over 12 weeks. Neurological and neurophysical scores were obtained before treatment and at weeks 2, 4, 8 and 12. Improvement occurred in both groups over the 12 week period but the naftidrofuryl-treated patients made greater neurological progress. Of patients discharged, those given naftidrofuryl spent only half as long in hospital as the controls. Deaths attributable to stroke were significantly fewer in the active treatment group, but the death rate in the whole series was only 24%.

2. Adhoute et al 1986 Naftidrofuryl in chronic arterial disease. Results of a 6 month controlled multicentre study using naftidrofuryl tablets 200 mg. Angiology 37: 160–167

This study was carried out on 118 patients with intermittent claudication who received naftidrofuryl 600 mg per day or a placebo for 6 months. The pain-free walking distance (measured on a treadmill) increased by 94% with naftidrofuryl compared to 46% with placebo ($p<0.02$).

3. Steiner T J 1986 Towards a model stroke trial. The single-centre naftidrofuryl study. Neuroepidemiology 5: 121–147

In this randomized double-blind study, naftidrofuryl 300 mg per day for 9 months was compared with placebo in 89 patients hospitalized for acute stroke. The mean duration of hospitalization was significantly reduced by the naftidrofuryl compared to the placebo group (about 50%). The recovery from hemiplegia was also better in the naftidrofuryl-treated group.

Other trials

Cox J R, Shaw A M 1981 Controlled trial of naftidrofuryl in dementia in old age. Journal of Clinical and Experimental Gerontology 3 (4): 339–343

A controlled trial of naftidrofuryl in 32 carefully selected hospital patients with mild to moderate dementia was performed. The author claimed to have shown improvement in behavioural rating scores after one and two months treatment.

General review articles

Coffman J D 1975 Vasodilator drugs in peripheral vascular disease. American Journal of Hospital Pharmacy 32: 1276–1281

Cook P, James I 1981 Cerebral vasodilators I+II. New England Journal of Medicine 305: 1508–1513, 1560–1564

Sandercock P 1987 Important new treatment for acute ischaemic stroke. British Medical Journal 295: 1224–1225

References

1. Meynaud A, Grand M, Fontaine L 1973 Effect of naftidrofuryl upon energy metabolism of the brain. Arzneimittel Forschung 23: 1431–1436
2. Meynaud A, Grand M, Belleville M, Fontaine L 1975 Effect du naftidrofuryl sur le metabolisme energetique cerebral chez la souris. Deuxieme partie. Therapie 30: 777–888
3. Zander J F, Aarhus L L, Katusic Z S, Rubanyi G M, Vanhoutte P M 1986 Journal of Pharmacology and Experimental Therapeutics 239: 760–767
4. Shaw S W J, Johnson R H 1975 The effect of naftidrofuryl on the metabolic response to exercise in man. Acta Neurologica Scandinavica 52: 231–237
5. Elert C, Niebel W, Karuse E, Satter P 1976 The effect of naftidrofuryl on energy metabolism in the musculature of limbs with impaired blood flow. Therapiewoche 23: 3947–3950
6. Naftidofuryl (Praxiline). Drug and Therapeutics Bulletin 26 No 7: 25–27
7. Meehan S E, Preece P E, Walker W F 1982 The usefulness of naftidrofuryl in severe peripheral ischaemia — a symptomatic assessment using linear analogue scales. Angiology 33 (10): 625–634
8. Rey J L, Quiret J C, Gamain J, Errasti M 1976 Etat de mal convulsif et troubles transitoires de la conduction intracardiaques provoques par une perfusion intraveineuse trop rapide de naftidrofuryl. Nouvelle Presse Medicale 7: 1864

Nalbuphine (hydrochloride)

Nalbuphine is an opioid agonist/antagonist analgesic of the nalorphine type.

Chemistry

Nalbuphine hydrochloride (Nubain)
$C_{21}H_{27}NO_4.HCl$
(l)-(−)-(5R,6S,14S)-9a-(Cyclobutylmethyl)-4,5-epoxymorphinan-3,6α,14-triol hydrochloride

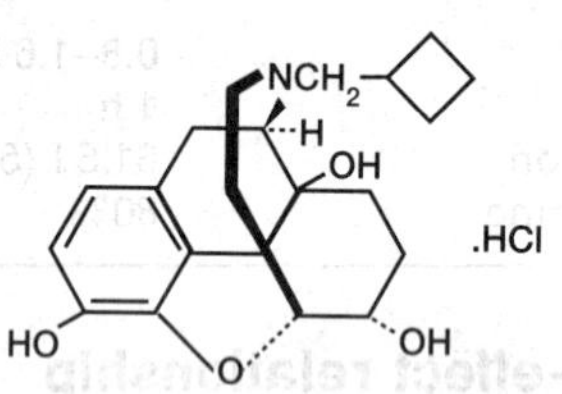

Molecular weight (free base)	393.9 (357.4)
pKa	8.71, 9.96
Solubility	
in alcohol	soluble
in water	soluble
Octanol/water partition coefficient	—

It is a white to off-white powder that is prepared by chemical synthesis. Nalbuphine is not present in any combination preparations.

Pharmacology

Nalbuphine is chemically closely related to naloxone, the specific opioid antagonist and to oxymorphone a strong opioid agonist. Nalbuphine is an agonist and antagonist at different opioid receptors with a spectrum of effects that resemble those of pentazocine. Nalbuphine is an agonist at kappa (κ) opioid receptors and an antagonist at mu (μ) receptors.[1,2] It is without significant effects on delta (δ) opioid receptors. Nalbuphine produces typical opioid effects in the central nervous system, such as analgesia and depression of respiration but may also act as an opioid antagonist.

Toxicology

Testing in animals has shown no signs of acute toxicity of potential clinical relevance. Multiple dose studies (2 weeks; 6 months) of subcutaneously or intravenously administered nalbuphine in rats and dogs resulted in reversible hair loss in both species. No such effects have been reported in humans. No evidence of impaired fertility has been found in rats, or of teratogenicity in rats or rabbits.

Nalbuphine does not substitute for morphine in morphine-dependent monkeys[3] and studies in rodents indicate a much lower abuse potential for nalbuphine compared to morphine.

Clinical pharmacology

Given by intramuscular injection nalbuphine is a powerful analgesic almost equipotent with morphine,[4] and 3 to 4 times as potent as pentazocine.[5] When given by mouth the analgesic action of nalbuphine is much weaker. Oral nalbuphine is $\frac{1}{4}$ to $\frac{1}{5}$ as potent as intramuscular nalbuphine in terms of intensity and duration of analgesia, and only $\frac{1}{10}$ as potent in terms of peak effects.[6] Nalbuphine 30 mg by mouth has a similar effect to 90 mg codeine or 650 mg of paracetamol.[7,8] No oral formulation is available for clinical use at present.

The usual parenteral dose is 10–20 mg by subcutaneous, intramuscular or intravenous injection. The onset of action is similar to that of morphine (2–3 minutes after intravenous injection and 15 minutes after intramuscular or subcutaneous administration) as is the duration of action of 3–6 hours.

At usual therapeutic doses nalbuphine has a respiratory depressant effect equivalent to that of morphine.[9] Unlike morphine, there appears to be a ceiling to both the respiratory depression[10] and the analgesic action[11,12] of nalbuphine at single doses of 20–30 mg. Animal studies also indicate a ceiling to the anaesthetic sparing effect of nalbuphine.[13] The respiratory depression may be reversed by naloxone.

Other opioid effects may occur including miosis and sedation, and less commonly nausea, vomiting, constipation, and psychotomimetic effects. Nalbuphine has minimal haemodynamic effects and in particular does not produce the adverse haemodynamic disturbances associated with pentazocine.[14–16]

Opioid antagonist activity has been demonstrated in both animals and man. In morphine-dependent human subjects, nalbuphine precipitated a typical nalorphine-like abstinence syndrome and was $\frac{1}{4}$ as potent as nalorphine.[17] Nalbuphine has also been used to reverse the respiratory depression caused by intraoperative opioids without affecting analgesia.[18,19]

Pharmacokinetics

Several assay methods for nalbuphine have been developed, most of which involve high performance liquid chromatography (HPLC) with electrochemical detection. Limits of sensitivity[20,21] range from 0.1 μg.l^{-1} to 1 μg.l^{-1}.

There are only limited data on the pharmacokinetics of nalbuphine in man. Nalbuphine is readily absorbed after oral administration but is subject to extensive presystemic metabolism. As a consequence oral bioavailability is about 10–20%.[22] After intravenous administration the elimination half life is 2–4 hours[21,23] and total body clearance[20,21] is 1.42–1.50 l.min^{-1}. Peak plasma concentrations after intramuscular injection are achieved after 15–30 minutes.[24] Peak plasma concentrations after oral administration are achieved at $\frac{3}{4}$ to 1 hour, and the mean elimination half-life is about 5 hours.[21,24] Nalbuphine is distributed throughout the body, with a volume of distribution of 160-500 l. The drug crosses the placenta and enters the fetal circulation producing concentrations comparable to those in maternal blood.[25]

Oral absorption	~100%
Presystemic metabolism	90%
Plasma half life	
range (i.v.)	2–4 h
(oral)	2.8–8 h
Volume of distribution	160–500 l
Plasma protein binding	minimal

There is no information of the excretion of nalbuphine in breast milk. Nalbuphine is extensively metabolized in the liver. The drug and its metabolites are excreted largely in the urine (70%) though some excretion into bile also occurs.

It is likely that liver disease will delay the elimination of nalbuphine. The effects of renal disease and old age on the kinetics of the drug are not known.

Concentration–effect relationship

There are no reliable data on the relationship between analgesic activity and plasma concentrations of nalbuphine.

Metabolism

There is little published information on the metabolism of nalbuphine,[24,26] although it appears that the drug undergoes extensive biotransformation in the liver. Unchanged nalbuphine and its glucuronide and sulphate conjugates are the major excretion products (see Fig. 1). The major metabolite is the nalbuphine glucuronide, which is inactive. Oxidation to 6-oxonalbuphine and N-dealkylation to 7,γ-dihydro-14-hydroxy-normorphine also occurs. Conjugates are also secreted in the bile and eliminated in the faeces.

Nalbuphine (hydrochloride)

Fig. 1 Urinary metabolites of nalbuphine

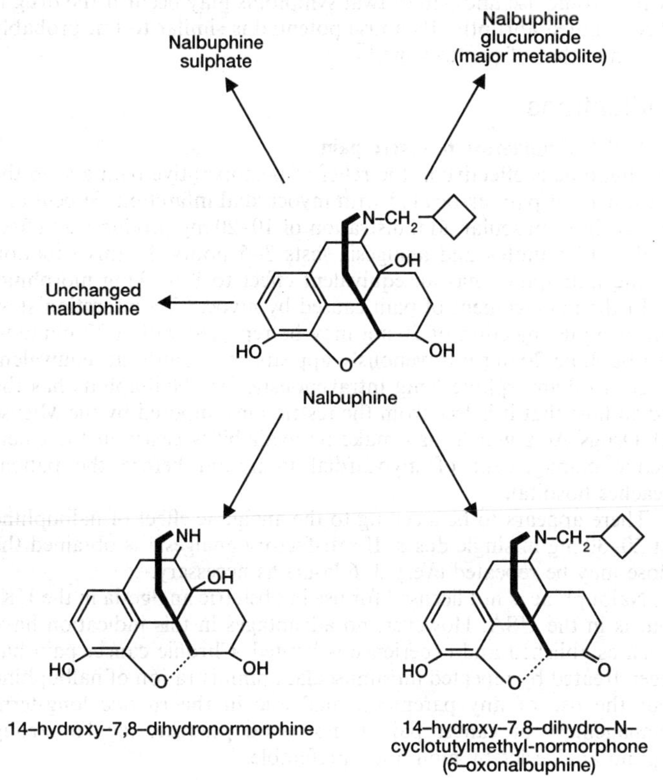

Pharmaceutics

Nalbuphine (Nubain; Dupont UK/USA) is only available for intravenous, intramuscular or subcutaneous use. Ampoules of 1 and 2 ml containing nalbuphine hydrochloride 10 mg.ml^{-1} as a clear colourless aqueous solution are available in the UK. In the USA also available are 10 ml vials containing 10 mg.ml^{-1}; 1 ml ampoules containing 20 mg.ml^{-1}; 1 ml disposable pre-filled syringes containing 20 mg.ml^{-1}; and 10 ml vials containing 20 mg.ml^{-1}.

Ampoules should be stored at controlled room temperature (15–30°C) and protected from light.

Nalbuphine is not subject to any restrictions under the Misuse of Drugs Act in the UK or the Federal Controlled Substance Act in the USA.

Therapeutic use

Indications

1. Relief of moderate to severe pain
2. Premedication, and as a supplement to surgical anaesthesia.

Contraindications

The only absolute contraindication to the use of nalbuphine is known sensitivity to the drug. Caution is required in the following circumstances:

1. Established respiratory depression
2. Individuals physically dependent on opioid analgesics
3. Conditions where clouding of consciousness is undesirable
4. Raised intracranial pressure.

Mode of use

Nalbuphine is only available for parenteral use. The usual recommended dose is 10–20 mg for a 70 kg individual by subcutaneous, intramuscular or intravenous injection, repeated every 3–6 hours as necessary. The maximum recommended single dose in non-tolerant patients is 20 mg, and maximum daily dose 160 mg.

In children an initial dose of 0.3 mg.kg^{-1} should be given (intramuscularly, intravenously, or subcutaneously) and may be repeated once or twice as necessary.

Although nalbuphine has low abuse potential compared with

N

N

morphine and other strong opioid agonists, dependence may develop with chronic use and withdrawal symptoms may occur if the drug is discontinued abruptly. Its abuse potential is similar to but probably less than that of pentazocine.[17]

Indications

1. Relief of moderate to severe pain

Nalbuphine is effective in the relief of postoperative pain and in the treatment of pain associated with myocardial infarction. Subcutaneous or intramuscular administration of 10–20 mg produces an effect within 15 minutes and analgesia lasts 3–5 hours. In this situation 10 mg nalbuphine has an equivalent effect to 8 or 9 mg morphine.

In the management of pain caused by myocardial infarction slow intravenous injection of 20 mg may be repeated within 30 minutes. Nalbuphine 20 mg intravenously appears to produce an equivalent effect to diamorphine 5 mg intravenously.[16,27] Nalbuphine has the advantage that it is free from the restrictions imposed by the Misuse of Drugs Acts which may make its availability easier in the emergency management of myocardial infarction before the patient reaches hospital.

There appears to be a ceiling to the analgesic effect of nalbuphine at 20–30 mg in single doses. If satisfactory analgesia is obtained the dose may be repeated every 3–6 hours as necessary.

Nalbuphine is not licensed for use in obstetric analgesia in the UK, but is in the USA. However, no advantages in this indication have been established and experience is limited. Chronic cancer pain has been treated by repeated intramuscular administration of nalbuphine but the use of any parenteral analgesic in the *routine* long-term management of cancer pain is not good practice: regular strong opioid analgesics by mouth are preferable.

2. Premedication, and as a supplement to surgical anaesthesia

Like other potent analgesics nalbuphine has been used as a premedicant before general anaesthesia and as a supplement to surgical anaesthesia.[28] However, the published data on such use are limited and no particular advantages of nalbuphine in these indications have been established.

The manufacturers' dosage recommendations are: premedication: 0.1–0.2 mg.kg^{-1}; anaesthesia induction: 0.3–1.0 mg.kg^{-1} intravenously over 10–15 minutes; maintenance: 0.25–0.5 mg.kg^{-1} at 30 minute intervals

Precautions

1. Established respiratory depression

In common with all drugs having opioid agonist activity nalbuphine has a respiratory depressant effect, and at usual therapeutic doses this is similar to that of morphine. Care is required in patients with impaired respiratory drive.

2. Individuals physically dependent on opioid analgesics

Withdrawal effects may occur following administration of nalbuphine to patients who are physically dependent on opioids because of its opioid antagonist action. Its use in such patients should therefore be avoided.

3. Conditions where clouding of consciousness is undesirable

Following head injury and in certain other acute conditions the patient's level of consciousness is an important clinical sign. Where analgesia is required sedative drugs, including nalbuphine, should be avoided. Nalbuphine also causes pupillary constriction[17] which, though less marked than with other opioid agonists, may further obscure signs of raised intracranial pressure.

4. Raised intracranial pressure

In patients with brain damage or where intracranial pressure is already raised due to a space-occupying lesion an increase in intracranial and spinal fluid pressure may occur with opioid analgesics. These changes are not seen in normal patients, nor in patients with brain damage who are mechanically ventilated, suggesting that mild respiratory depression with an associated intracranial vasodilatation secondary to a rise in P_aCO_2 may be the underlying cause. This problem has not been reported specifically in relation to nalbuphine, but it is unlikely that nalbuphine will differ in this respect from pentazocine and other opioids which do cause a rise in intracranial pressure.

Adverse reactions

Potentially life-threatening effects

No such effects have been reported.

Acute overdosage

No cases of nalbuphine overdose have been documented. The management of overdosage should be with the specific opioid antagonist naloxone and supportive measures, as for other strong opioid analgesics.

Severe or irreversible adverse effects

The abuse potential of nalbuphine is similar to but probably less than that of pentazocine. There are, however, only isolated reports of misuse or abuse of nalbuphine.

Symptomatic adverse effects

The commonest adverse effect reported in clinical studies is sedation. This does not appear to be any more of a problem than with other strong opioid analgesics. The incidence of nausea and vomiting seems to be less than that associated with morphine. Psychotomimetic reactions are much less frequent than with pentazocine (estimated to be in the region of 1% overall compared with the 10–20% reported with pentazocine).

Other nonspecific effects (dizziness, sweating, dry mouth and headache) have been reported but in general nalbuphine is well tolerated in usual therapeutic doses. There have been one or two reports of transient pain at the injection site following intramuscular[29] or intravenous administration.

Interference with clinical pathology tests

No significant interference with clinical laboratory tests has been reported.

High risk groups

Neonates

The drug is not recommended for use in neonates.

Breast milk. There is no information on nalbuphine and lactation but the use of the drug during lactation should be avoided.

Children

There are some published reports on the use of nalbuphine in children and the drug is licensed for such use. An initial dose of 0.3 mg.kg^{-1} should be given (intramuscularly, intravenously or subcutaneously) and may be repeated once or twice as necessary.

Pregnant women

Nalbuthine is licensed for use in obstetric analgesia in the USA. However no advantages in this indication have been established and experience is limited. Nalbuphine may produce respiratory depression in the neonate if used during labour and pregnancy.

The elderly

No specific problems are seen in the elderly following nalbuphine. However, certain conditions which may be more common in the elderly, in particular impairment of hepatic or renal function, may adversely affect the metabolism and excretion of the drug. This may predispose to increased toxicity and care is required in these situations.

Drug interactions

Potentially hazardous drug interactions

No specific hazardous interactions have been identified, though excessive sedation may be produced by interaction with CNS depressants, including alcohol.

Other significant reactions

Opioid analgesics. Withdrawal symptoms may be precipitated by nalbuphine if it is given to patients who are physically dependent on opioid analgesics.

CNS depressants. When nalbuphine is administered with any CNS depressant increased sedation may occur.

Alcohol. As with other opioid analgesics, increased sedative effects are likely if alcohol is taken together with nalbuphine.

Potentially useful interactions

Naloxone. The opioid agonist effects of nalbuphine can be reversed by the specific competitive antagonist naloxone.

Fentanyl. The respiratory depression caused by fentanyl and other intraoperative opioids may be reversed by nalbuphine with no deleterious effect on pain control.[18,19,30] However, there is a report of acute pulmonary oedema resulting from this procedure[31] which is a recognized hazard of the use of naloxone in this way.

Clinical trials

1. Beaver W T, Feise G A 1978 A comparison of the analgesic effect of intramuscular nalbuphine and morphine in patients with postoperative pain. Journal of Pharmacology and Experimental Therapeutics 204: 487–496

The relative analgesic potency of intramuscular nalbuphine and morphine was determined in 56 postoperative patients who had undergone a variety of surgical procedures. Assessments were based on patients' subjective reports of pain and pain relief and the study used a double-blind, twin crossover design to compare single doses of 4 and 8 mg morphine with 3 and 6 mg nalbuphine, or 6 and 12 mg nalbuphine.

Nalbuphine was 0.8–0.9 times as potent as morphine in terms of intensity and duration of analgesia, and 0.7–0.8 times as potent as morphine in terms of peak analgesic effect. Nalbuphine appeared to have a slightly longer duration of action. Morphine-like side-effects were similar with both drugs. No psychotomimetic effects were observed with nalbuphine.

2. Hew E, Foster K, Gordon R, Hew-Sang E 1987 A comparison of nalbuphine and meperidine in treatment of post-operative pain. Canadian Journal of Anaesthesia 34: 462–465

The analgesic effect and side-effects of nalbuphine 20 and 40 mg intravenously and meperidine (pethidine) 75 mg intramuscularly were evaluated in postoperative patients who experienced moderate or severe pain following abdominal or orthopaedic surgery. A group comparative design was used and 150 patients (50/group) were included.

There was no significant difference between the three treatments for any of the efficacy measures. The lower dose of nalbuphine was associated with significantly less nausea and vomiting than pethidine.

The lack of difference in analgesic efficacy between 20 and 40 mg nalbuphine intravenously may reflect a ceiling to the analgesic effect of the drug.

3. Beaver W T, Feise G A, Robb D 1981 Analgesic effect of intramuscular and oral nalbuphine in postoperative pain. Clinical Pharmacology and Therapeutics 29: 174–180

The relative analgesic potency of oral and intramuscular nalbuphine was evaluated in a double-blind crossover comparison of single doses of 3 and 9 mg intramuscular nalbuphine with 15 and 45 mg oral nalbuphine in 104 postoperative patients. Nalbuphine by mouth was $\frac{1}{4}$ to $\frac{1}{5}$ as potent as intramuscular nalbuphine in terms of intensity and duration of analgesia, but only $\frac{1}{10}$ as potent in terms of peak effect. No psychotomimetic reactions were observed.

Other trials

Randomized controlled trials

1. Lee G, Low R I, Amsterdam E A, DeMaria A N, Huber P W, Mason D T 1981 Hemodynamic effects of morphine and nalbuphine in acute myocardial infarction. Clinical Pharmacology and Therapeutics 29: 576–581
2. Greenbaum R A, Kaye G, Mason P D 1987 Experience with nalbuphine, a new opioid analgesic, in acute myocardial infarction. Journal of the Royal Society of Medicine 80: 418–421

General review articles

Errick J K, Heel R C 1983 Nalbuphine: a preliminary review of its pharmacological properties and therapeutic efficacy. Drugs 26: 191–211

Miller R R 1980 Evaluation of nalbuphine hydrochloride. American Journal of Hospital Pharmacy 37: 942–949

Wilkinson D J 1987 Opioid agonist/antagonists in general anaesthesia. British Journal of Hospital Medicine 38: 130–133

Nalbuphine (hydrochloride)

N

References

1. Schmidt W K, Tam S W, Shotzberger G S, Smith D H, Clark R, Vernier V G 1985 Nalbuphine. Drug and Alcohol Dependence 14: 339–362
2. De Souza E B, Schmidt W K, Kuhar M J 1988 Nalbuphine: an autoradiographic opioid receptor-binding profile in the central nervous system of an agonist/antagonist analgesic. Journal of Pharmacology and Experimental Therapeutics 244: 391–402
3. Villareal J E, Karbowski M G 1974 The actions of narcotic antagonists in morphine-dependent Rhesus monkeys. In: Braude M C, Harris L S, May E L et al (eds) Narcotic antagonists. Raven Press, New York, pp 273–289
4. Beaver W T, Feise G A 1978 A comparison of the analgesic effect of intramuscular nalbuphine and morphine in patients with postoperative pain. Journal of Pharmacology and Experimental Therapeutics 204: 487–496
5. Houde R W, Wallenstein S L, Rogers A, Kaiko R F 1976 Annual report of the analgesic studies section of the Memorial Sloan-Kettering Cancer Center. In: Report of the 38th Annual Scientific Meeting of the Committee on Problems of Drug Dependence. Richmond: 149–168
6. Beaver W T, Feise G A, Robb D 1981 Analgesic effect of intramuscular and oral nalbuphine in postoperative pain. Clinical Pharmacology and Therapeutics 29: 174–180
7. Okun R 1982 Analgesic effects of oral nalbuphine and codeine in patients with postoperative pain. Clinical Pharmacology and Therapeutics 32: 517–524
8. Forbes J A, Kolodny A L, Chachich B M, Beaver W T 1984 Nalbuphine, acetaminophen, and their combination in postoperative pain. Clinical Pharmacology and Therapeutics 35: 843–851
9. Klepper I D, Rosen M, Vickers M D, Mapleson W W 1986 Respiratory function following nalbuphine and morphine in anaesthetized man. British Journal of Anaesthesia 58: 625–629
10. Romagnoli A, Keats A S 1980 Ceiling effect for respiratory depression by nalbuphine. Clinical Pharmacology and Therapeutics 27: 478–485
11. Gal T J, DiFazio C A, Moscicki J 1982 Analgesic and respiratory depressant activity of nalbuphine: a comparison with morphine. Anesthesiology 57: 367–374
12. Hew E, Foster K, Gordon R, Hew-Sang E 1987 A comparison of nalbuphine and meperidine in treatment of post-operative pain. Canadian Journal of Anaesthesia 34: 462–465
13. Murphy M R, Hug C C 1982 The enflurane-sparing effect of morphine, butorphanol, and nalbuphine. Anesthesiology 57: 489–492
14. Lee G, Low R I, Amsterdam E A, DeMaria A N, Huber P W, Mason D T 1981 Hemodynamic effects of morphine and nalbuphine in acute myocardial infarction. Clinical Pharmacology and Therapeutics 29: 576–581
15. Lake C L, Duckworth E N, DiFazio C A, Durbin C G, Magruder M R 1982 Cardiovascular effects of nalbuphine in patients with coronary or valvular heart disease. Anesthesiology 57: 498–503
16. Greenbaum R A, Kaye G, Mason P D 1987 Experience with nalbuphine, a new opioid analgesic, in acute myocardial infarction. Journal of the Royal Society of Medicine 80: 418–421
17. Jasinski D R 1979 Human pharmacology of narcotic antagonists. British Journal of Clinical Pharmacology 7: 287S–290S
18. Magruder M R, Delaney R D, DiFazio C A 1977 Reversal of narcotic-induced respiratory depression with nalbuphine hydrochloride. Anesthesiology Review 9: 34–37
19. Moldenhauer C C, Roach G W, Finlayson D C et al 1985 Nalbuphine antagonism of ventilatory depression following high-dose fentanyl anaesthesia. Anesthesiology 62: 647–650
20. Lo M-W, Juergens G P, Whitney C C 1984 Determination of nalbuphine in human plasma by automated high-performance liquid chromatography with electrochemical detection. Research Communications in Chemical Pathology and Pharmacology 43: 159–168
21. Aitkenhead A R, Lin E S, Achola K J 1988 The pharmacokinetics of oral and intravenous nalbuphine in healthy volunteers. British Journal of Clinical Pharmacology 25: 264–268
22. Lo M-W, Schary W L, Whitney C C 1987 The disposition and bioavailability of intravenous and oral nalbuphine in healthy volunteers. Journal of Clinical Pharmacology 27: 866–873
23. Sear J W, Keegan M, Kay B 1987 Disposition of nalbuphine in patients undergoing general anaesthesia. British Journal of Anaesthesia 59: 572–575
24. Bullingham R E S 1984 The pharmacokinetics of nalbuphine. In: Nimmo W S, Smith G (eds) Opioid agonist/antagonist drugs in clinical practice. Excerpta Medica, Amsterdam, pp 115–122
25. Wilson S J, Errick J K, Balkon J 1986 Pharmacokinetics of nalbuphine during parturition. American Journal of Obstetrics and Gynaecology 155: 340–344
26. Lake C L, DiFazio C A, Duckworth E N, Moscicki J C, Engle J S, Durbin C G 1982 High performance liquid chromatographic analysis of plasma levels of nalbuphine in cardiac surgical patients. Journal of Chromatography 233: 410–416
27. Jamidar H A, Crooks S W, Adgey A A J 1987 Nalbuphine versus diamorphine early in the course of suspected myocardial infarction. European Heart Journal 8: 597–602
28. Zsigmond E K, Winnie A P, Raza S M A, Wang X Y, Barabas E 1987 Nalbuphine as an analgesic component in balanced anesthesia for cardiac surgery. Anesthesia and Analgesia 66: 1155–1164
29. Chestnutt W N, Clarke R S J, Dundee J W 1987 Comparison of nalbuphine, pethidine and placebo as premedication for minor gynaecological surgery. British Journal of Anaesthesia 59: 576–580
30. Zsigmond E K, Durrani Z, Barabas E, Wang X Y, Tran L 1987 Endocrine and hemodynamic effects of antagonism of fentanyl-induced respiratory depression by nalbuphine. Anesthesia and Analgesia 66: 421–426
31. DesMarteau J K, Cassot A L 1986 Acute pulmonary edema resulting from nalbuphine reversal of fentanyl-induced respiratory depression. Anesthesiology 65: 237

N Nalidixic acid

Nalidixic acid is a bactericidal antimicrobial agent used mainly in the treatment and prophylaxis of urinary tract infections.

Chemistry

Nalidixic acid (Negram, Uriben)
$C_{12}H_{12}N_2O_3$
1-Ethyl-1,4-dihydro-7-methyl-4-oxo-1,8-naphthyridine-3-carboxylic acid

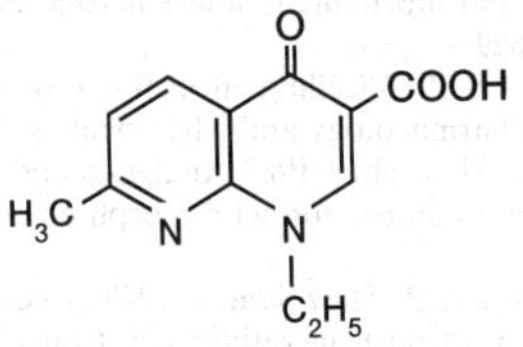

Molecular weight	232.2
pKa	6.7
Solubility	
in alcohol	<1 in 910
in water	<1 in 10 000
Octanol/water partition coefficient	—

Nalidixic acid is a colourless or pale yellow crystalline powder prepared by chemical synthesis. It is soluble in solutions of alkali. It is available as a combination product with sodium citrate BP, anhydrous citric acid BP and sodium bicarbonate BP (Mictral) which, when added to water, disperses with slight effervescence.

Pharmacology

Nalidixic acid exerts its antibacterial activity by inhibiting DNA replication in the bacterial cell by inhibition of the enzyme DNA gyrase.[1,2] Although acquired resistance to nalidixic acid occurs, this is not R-factor determined and consequently not transferable. It is effective in vitro against most Gram-negative bacilli with the notable exception of *Pseudomonas* species.

Toxicology

Animal studies have shown that nalidixic acid causes cleft palate and skeletal defects in rats but not in rabbits or primates.[3] In a few animals nalidixic acid has produced some disorganization of the epiphyseal plates.[4] A study of small numbers of paediatric patients suggested no difference in the occurrence of arthralgia between those patients receiving nalidixic acid and those not receiving the drug, and no skeletal growth abnormalities were seen.[5] A phototoxic reaction has been demonstrated in mice and this is a recognized adverse effect in man.[6,7]

Clinical pharmacology

In dose-ranging studies, normal human volunteers showed excellent tolerance to regular doses of nalidixic acid for up to 180 days. The maximum sustained dose was 8 g daily for 56 days and most individuals tolerated an initial dose of 4 g. No significant alterations were observed in blood pressure, heart rate, haemoglobin, haematocrit, blood cell picture, urine analysis or alkaline phosphatase during this study (Sterling-Winthrop Research Institute, unpublished data).

The recommended normal dosage is 1 g four times daily for a minimum of seven days. For Mictral it is one sachet three times daily for three days.

Pharmacokinetics

The preferred analytical method is reverse phase high pressure liquid chromatography. The sensitivity[8] of this method is 0.5 $\mu g.l^{-1}$.

The absorption of nalidixic acid is >90% after oral administration.[9] Peak plasma concentrations occur within 2 hours of oral dosing.[10] The plasma elimination half life ranges from 1.5 to 2 hours. Nalidixic acid is 93% protein bound. It does not normally cross the blood–brain barrier.

Nalidixic acid is excreted mainly in the urine, and only about 4% of a single oral dose is excreted in faeces. About 12% of the administered dosage is excreted in an extractable (i.e. biologically available) form and the remainder in the conjugated form and as the dicarboxylic acid derivative. The elimination rate of nalidixic acid is pH dependent, clearance increasing as the urine becomes more alkaline. The concurrent administration of sodium bicarbonate or citrate to make the urine alkaline increases the proportion of active antibacterial metabolites excreted in the urine from about 12% to 30% by reducing the glucuronides in the urine without altering the ratio of free nalidixic acid to free hydroxynalidixic acid.[10]

Nalidixic acid has been detected in human breast milk at a measured concentration of 3.9 $\mu g.l^{-1}$ one hour after an oral dose.[11] Another study suggested that 0.05% of an oral dose was excreted in the milk in 24 hours.[12] Haemolytic anaemia in a newborn child due to nalidixic acid transmitted via breast milk has been described.

The drug is extensively transformed, mainly in the liver. Most of the dose is excreted in the urine, with only 2–3% as the unchanged drug.

Oral absorption	>90%
Presystemic metabolism	minimal
Plasma half life	~90 min
Volume of distribution	0.4 $l.kg^{-1}$
Plasma protein binding	93%

Concentration–effect relationship

The usual plasma concentration in therapeutic dosage[13] is 20–50 $mg.l^{-1}$. Most strains of bacteria are sensitive to concentrations <16 $mg.l^{-1}$.

Metabolism

Nalidixic acid is metabolized in the liver to free 7-hydroxynalidixic acid, 7-carboxynalidixic acid, and the glucuronide conjugates of the parent substance and the hydroxy metabolite, NA glucuronide and HNA glucuronide respectively (Fig. 1). Both the parent substance and the free 7-hydroxy metabolite have antibacterial properties but the glucuronide conjugates and the 7-carboxynalidixic acid are devoid of activity against pathogenic organisms. Approximately 85% of the drug in the urine is in an inactive form, the remainder being free 7-hydroxynalidixic acid and unchanged nalidixic acid (both active). The ratio of free HNA to free NA in the urine is about 7:1 and this is not markedly changed with bicarbonate supplementation.

Pharmaceutics

Nalidixic acid is available in tablet and suspension form:

1. Negram tablets (Sterling-Winthrop, UK) contain 500 mg nalidixic acid BP. They are beige, bi-convex, marked 'Negram' on one side and with the company trade mark on the other.
2. NeGram Caplets (Winthrop, US) are available as three scored beige tablets: 250 mg, oblong; 500 mg, oblong and 1 g, ovoid.
3. NeGram suspension (Winthrop, US) contains 250 mg nalidixic acid per 5 ml. It is raspberry-flavoured, sugar-free and preserved with parabens.
4. Negram suspension (Sterling Winthrop, UK) is deep pink and viscous with a raspberry odour and taste, containing 300 mg nalidixic acid BP/5 ml.

The suspension remains stable for 2–3 weeks when diluted with syrup BP.

Nalidixic acid

Tablet preparations are stable with a reasonable shelf-life.

3. Mictral (Winthrop, UK) is formulated as granules, each 7 g containing
   nalidixic acid BP 660 mg
   sodium citrate BP 3.750 g
   anhydrous citric acid BP 250 mg
   sodium bicarbonate BP 250 mg.
   When reconstituted with water it forms a citrus-flavoured suspension.

Therapeutic use

Indications

1. Treatment of urinary tract infections with sensitive Gram-negative organisms
2. Treatment of intestinal infections due to *Salmonella* or *Shigella*.

Contraindications

1. Patients with a history of convulsive disorders.

Mode of use

In adults the usual dose of tablet or suspension is 1 g four times daily for at least seven days, reducing to 0.5 g four times daily for chronic infections. The granular formulation is prescribed as 1 sachet (660 mg nalidixic acid three times daily) for three days.

Indications

1. Urinary tract infections
Nalidixic acid can be used in the treatment of patients with Gram-negative urinary tract infections, particularly those caused by *E. coli*, *Aerobacter*, *Proteus* and *Klebsiella*. It can be administered before the initial laboratory reports are received because of its wide activity against Gram-negative organisms commonly encountered in urinary tract infections. It is not usually used in urinary tract infections with systemic manifestations because it is not effective outside the urinary tract.

2. Gastrointestinal infections
Nalidixic acid is effective against gastrointestinal *Salmonella* and *Shigella* infections, although if antibiotic therapy is to be used other drugs are usually preferred.

Contraindications

Convulsions have been reported both following overdosage and during therapy in patients with pre-existing brain disorders including epilepsy, atherosclerosis and Parkinson's disease.[14] Since there are many other alternative antibiotics there is rarely a need to give nalidixic acid in this group.

The manufacturers recommend caution with patients whose creatinine clearance is less than 20 ml.min^{-1}.

Adverse reactions

Potentially life-threatening effects
There has been one report of anaphylaxis in a diabetic patient one hour after 660 mg of citrated nalidixic acid.[15] Fatal immune haemolytic anaemia has been described in a patient with previous episodes of haemolytic anaemia.[16]

Acute overdosage
Symptoms of overdose include nausea, drowsiness, lightheadedness, hallucinations, teichopsia, ataxia, disorientation, hyperpnoea, sometimes glycosuria and possibly hyperglycaemia.[17] Severe metabolic acidosis has been reported following ingestion of 28 g of nalidixic acid. The patient recovered after the intravenous administration of 844 mmol sodium bicarbonate over 60 hours.[18] If more than 10 tablets have been taken a stomach wash-out is recommended with maintenance of fluid balance and control of electrolytes. The fatal dose is probably over 30–50 tablets.

Severe or irreversible adverse effects
These include photosensitivity, haemolytic reaction (in patients with glucose 6-phosphate dehydrogenase deficiency),[19] cholestatic jaundice, raised intracranial pressure in infants and young children,[20,21] thrombocytopenia,[22] leucopenia,[23] pancytopenia,[24] and eosinophilia.[18,22,25] Severe arthralgia has been reported in a 22-year-old woman who received 2 g of nalidixic acid.[26]

Symptomatic adverse effects
Nausea, vomiting and other gastrointestinal disturbances may occur. Dizziness, drowsiness and weakness are sometimes encountered, as are pruritus, urticaria and other rashes, and subjective visual disturbances.

Interference with clinical pathology tests
When testing for glycosuria in patients receiving nalidixic acid, a glucose-specific method should be used, as glucuronic acid liberated from the metabolites of nalidixic acid can produce false positive results with glucose estimations based on copper reduction.[14]

Nalidixic acid in therapeutic doses can interfere with the estimation of 17-ketosteroids[27] and may cause high results in the Pisano assay of urinary estimation of vanillylmandelic acid.[28]

High risk groups

Neonates
The drug is not suitable for infants under 3 months due to immaturity of liver enzymes, impaired elimination and risk of haemolysis of

Fig. 1 Metabolism of nalidixic acid

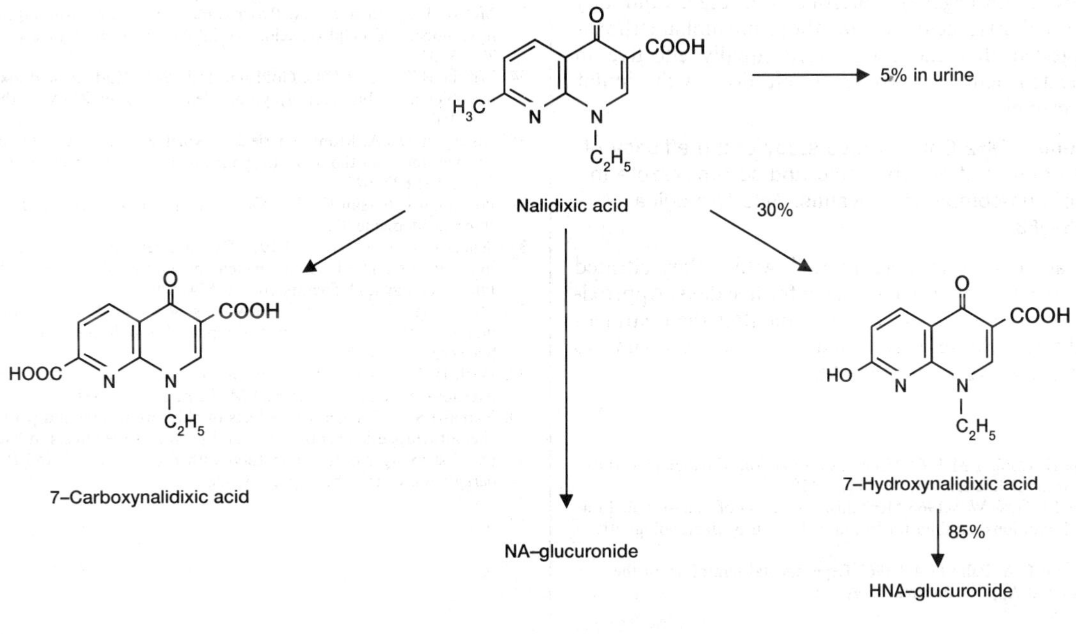

Nalidixic acid

N

neonatal erythrocytes. Coma following a single therapeutic dose of 100 mg of nalidixic acid has been reported in a 17-month-old patient with normal renal function.[29] Convulsions, intracranial hypertension, metabolic acidosis and hyperglycaemia were found 24 hours after beginning treatment in a 45-day-old infant.[30]

Breast milk. Nalidixic acid is excreted in breast milk and there is a report of haemolytic anaemia in a breast-fed child of an azotaemic mother.

Children

The maximum recommended dose is 50 $mg.kg^{-1}$ body weight per 24 hours in divided doses. However, concern over the potential for cartilage damage, although not yet reported in humans,[31] lead the authors to recommend that nalidixic acid should not be used in patients whose skeletal growth is incomplete or in pregnant women, particularly where alternative therapies exist.

Pregnant women

There were no congenital abnormalities in the offspring of 63 women treated with nalidixic acid during pregnancy.[32] However, nalidixic acid as a DNA-gyrase inhibitor is capable of causing DNA damage.[33,34]

The elderly

If creatinine clearance is <20 $ml.min^{-1}$ half dosage is recommended.

Drug interactions

Potentially hazardous interactions

There is some evidence that nalidixic acid prolongs the prothrombin time in patients on oral anticoagulants. The dose may have to be reduced.[35–37]

Following concomitant use of nalidixic acid with nelphalan there have been reports of serious gastrointestinal toxicity.

Other significant interactions

Food may delay the absorption of the drug from the gastrointestinal tract.[38]

Tests in healthy volunteers suggest that probenecid can prolong the serum half life of nalidixic acid so use of the two together may result in raised serum levels of nalidixic acid.[39]

Potentially useful interactions

Chlorpromazine and perphenazine have been shown to potentiate the antibacterial effect of nalidixic acid in vitro.[40]

Clinical trials

1. Iravani A, Richard G A, Baer H, Fennell R 1981 Comparative efficacy and safety of nalidixic acid versus trimethoprim/sulphamethoxazole in treatment of acute urinary tract infections in college-age women. Antimicrobial Agents and Chemotherapy 19: 598–604

This was a study of 135 college-age women with acute urinary tract infection caused by Gram-negative Enterobacteriaeceae, randomly allocated to either nalidixic acid or trimethoprim/sulphamethoxazole. Results suggested that the drugs were equally effective in treating uncomplicated acute urinary tract infection, with similar resistance and adverse effects.

2. Van Erps P, Denis I 1982 Comparative study of the efficacy of a new formula of citrated nalidixic acid and cotrimoxazole in the treatment of non-complicated cystitis. Acta Urologica Belgica 50: 376–383

92 patients with acute cystitis were treated with either citrated nalidixic acid for three days or co-trimoxazole for five days. Approximately 85% of each group were free of infection after the treatment period. No significant relapse was found on follow-up and no significant adverse effects were encountered.

References

1. Goss W A, Deitz W H, Cook T M 1964 Mechanism of action of nalidixic acid on *Escherichia coli*. Journal of Bacteriology 88: 1112–1118
2. Deitz W H, Cook T M, Goss W A 1966 Mechanism of action of nalidixic acid on *Escherichia coli*. 3. Conditions required for lethality. Journal of Bacteriology 91: 768–773
3. Courtney K D, Valerio D A, Pallotta A J 1967 Experimental teratology in the monkey. Toxicology and Applied Pharmacology 10: 378
4. Ingham B, Brentnall D W, Dall E A, McFadzean J A 1977 Arthropathy induced by antibacterial fused n-alkyl-4-pyridone-3-carboxylic acids. Toxicology Letters 1: 21–26
5. Schaad V B, Wedgwood-Krucko J 1987 Nalidixic acid in children: retrospective matched controlled study for cartilage toxicity. Infection 15: 165–168
6. Ljunggren B, Moller H 1978 Drug phototoxicity in mice. Acta Dermato-venereologica 58: 125–130
7. Kaidbey K H, Kligman A M 1978 Identification of systemic phototoxic drugs by human intradermal assay. Journal of Investigative Dermatology 70: 272–274
8. Cuisinaud G, Ferry N, Seccia M, Bernard N, Sassard J 1980 Determination of nalidixic acid and its two major metabolites in human plasma and urine by reverse phased high performance liquid chromatography. Journal of Chromatography 181: 399–406
9. Harrison L H, Cox C E 1970 Bacteriologic and pharmacodynamic aspects of nalidixic acid. Journal of Urology 104: 908–913
10. McChesney E W, Froelich E J, Lesher G Y, Crain A V R, Rosi D 1964 Absorption, excretion and metabolism of a new antibacterial agent nalidixic acid. Toxicology and Applied Pharmacology 6: 292–309
11. Richer C, Giudicelli J F 1976 Excretion des medicaments dans le lait maternelle. Revue Medicale 17: 1149–1157
12. Belton E M, Vaughan-Jones R 1965 Haemolytic anaemia due to nalidixic acid. Lancet 2: 691
13. Stamey T A, Nemoy N J, Higgins M 1969 The clinical use of nalidixic acid: a review and some observations. Investigative Urology 6: 582–592
14. Ronald A R, Turck M, Petersdorf R G 1966 A critical evaluation of nalidixic acid in urinary-tract infections. New England Journal of Medicine 275: 1081–1089
15. Beeley L 1984 Personal communication to the editor. Quoted in Dukes M N G Side-effects of drugs Annual 8, Amsterdam, Oxford Excerpta Medica p 283
16. Tafani O, Mazzoli M, Landini G, Alterini B 1982 Fatal acute immune haemolytic anaemia caused by nalidixic acid. British Medical Journal 285: 936–937
17. Fraser A G, Harrower A D B 1977 Convulsions and hyperglycaemia associated with nalidixic acid. British Medical Journal 2: 1518
18. Nogue S, Bertran A, Mas A, Nadal P, Anguita A, Milla J 1979 Metabolic acidosis and coma due to an overdose of nalidixic acid. Intensive Care Medicine 5: 141–142
19. Mandal B K, Stevenson J 1970 Haemolytic crisis produced by nalidixic acid. Lancet 1: 614
20. Gedroyc W, Shorvon S D 1982 Acute intracranial hypertension and nalidixic acid therapy. Neurology 32: 212–215
21. Deonna T, Guignard J P 1974 Acute intracranial hypertension after nalidixic acid administration. Archives of Diseases in Childhood 49: 743
22. Meyboom R H B 1984 Thrombocytopenia induced by nalidixic acid. British Medical Journal 289: 962
23. Swinney J 1964 Nalidixic acid. Practitioner 192: 701–706
24. Swanson M, Cook R 1977 Drugs, chemicals and blood dyscrasias. Drug Intelligence Publication, Hamilton 11: 667–669
25. Westerholm B 1974 Adverse reactions from chemotherapeutic agents as seen in a national monitoring centre. International Journal of Clinical Pharmacology, Therapy and Toxicity 9: 276–282
26. Bailey R R, Natale R, Linton A L 1972 Nalidixic acid arthralgia. Canadian Medical Association Journal 107: 604–605
27. Llerena O, Pearson O H 1968 Interference of nalidixic acid in urinary 17-ketosteroid determinations. New England Journal of Medicine 279: 983–984
28. Anonymous 1972 Interference of drugs with chemical diagnostic tests. Drug and Therapeutics Bulletin 10: 69–72
29. Corsini C, Tanghetti B, Valenti F 1982 Observation about a case of coma following the administration of nalidixic acid. Anesthesie, Analgesie Reanimation 23: 31–34
30. Ulivelli A, Minelli F 1984 Intossicazione acuta da acido nalidixico in un lattante. Minerva Paediatrica 36: 55–59
31. Ball P 1986 Ciprofloxacin: an overview of adverse experiences. Journal of Antimicrobial Chemotherapy 18 (suppl D): 187–193
32. Murray E D S 1981 Nalidixic acid in pregnancy. British Medical Journal 282: 224
33. McCoy E C, Petrullo L A, Rosenkranz H S 1980 Non-mutagenic genotoxicants: novobiocin and nalidixic acid, two inhibitors of DNA-gyrase. Mutation Research 79: 33–34
34. Wright H T, Nurse K C, Goldstein D J 1981 Nalidixic acid, oxolinic acid and novobiocin inhibit yeast glycyl- and leucyl-transfer RNA synthetases. Science 213: 455–456
35. Gallagher D J A, Montgomerie J Z, North J D K 1965 Acute infections of the urinary tract and the urethral syndrome in general practice. British Medical Journal 1: 622–626
36. Potasman I, Bassan H 1980 Nicoumalone and nalidixic acid interaction. Annals of Internal Medicine 92: 571
37. Sellers E M, Koch-Weser J 1970 Displacement of warfarin from human albumin by diazoxide and ethacrynic, mefenamic and nalidixic acids. Clinical Pharmacology and Therapeutics 2: 524–529
38. McChesney E W, Portmann G A, Koss R F 1967 Pharmacokinetic model for nalidixic acid in man 3. Effect of repeated oral dosage. Journal of Pharmaceutical Sciences 56: 594–599
39. Dash H, Mills J 1976 Severe metabolic acidosis associated with nalidixic acid overdosage. Annals of Internal Medicine 84: 570–571
40. Yamabe S 1978 Synergistic effects of chlorpromazine and perphenazine on several chemotherapeutic agents. I. General profile of the effects measured by the filter paper strip–agar diffusion method with *Escherichia coli* and *Pseudomonas aeruginosa*. Chemotherapy 24: 81–86

Naloxone (hydrochloride)

Naloxone was the first opioid antagonist developed which is devoid of agonist activity.

Chemistry

Naloxone hydrochloride (Narcan, Narcan Neonatal)
$C_{19}H_{21}NO_4$.HCl
(I) 17-Allyl-6-deoxy-7,8-dihydro-14-hydroxy-6-oxo-17-normorphine hydrochloride

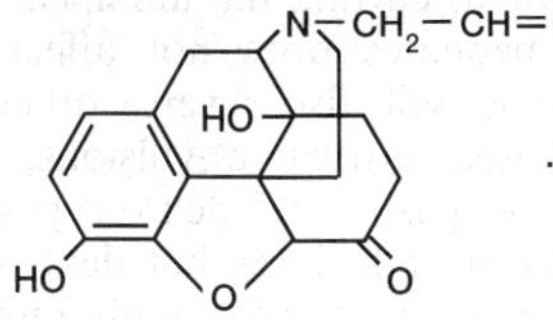

Molecular weight (free base)	363.8 (327.4)
pKa	7.9
Solubility	
in alcohol	<1 in 100
in water	>in 30
Octanol/water partition coefficient	34

A white or slightly off-white powder, being a semisynthetic derivative of thebaine. It is not present in any combination preparation.

Pharmacology

Naloxone is a competitive antagonist at μ-, κ-, and σ- opiate receptors with lesser effects at δ- and ε-receptors. The competitive nature of the opioid antagonism has been demonstrated by parallel right shift of the dose–response curves of opiate agonists in isolated animal preparations.[1] Naloxone is more potent as an antagonist at μ-receptors than at other receptors. From various animal preparations the dissociation constant (K_e) for naloxone at μ receptors has been estimated at 2–3 nM while at κ- and δ-receptors it is 20–30 nM.[2] It has no intrinsic agonist properties and appears devoid of other pharmacological actions.

Toxicology

Animal toxicity and reproductive studies have not revealed any mutagenic, carcinogenic, teratogenic or embryotoxic effects.

Clinical pharmacology

All the observed effects of naloxone are related to antagonism of endogenous or exogenous opioids. It produces no effects when administered in clinical doses to normal human volunteers. In larger doses (up to 4 mg.kg^{-1}) behavioural disturbances are seen including reluctance to move, sweating, yawning, anxiety, anger, depression, confusion and decreased cognitive function. These effects may persist for two or more days following a single dose, and are thought to suggest the involvement of opioid systems in the tonic regulation of mood, behaviour and cognition.[3] A rise in systolic arterial blood pressure is also seen in normal individuals given high doses (0.3 mg.kg^{-1}) of naloxone.

When administered to humans in pain who have not received exogenous opioids, some studies have demonstrated a biphasic response dependent on the dose used, low doses producing analgesia and higher doses hyperalgesia.[4,5] A similar biphasic effect has been observed in animals.

Naloxone will reverse all the effects of exogenous opioids, i.e. analgesia, respiratory depression, pupillary constriction, delayed gastric emptying, dysphoria, coma and convulsions. It will also reverse the analgesia produced by stress, transcutaneous electrical nerve stimulation, acupuncture, electro-acupuncture and placebo response.

Pharmacokinetics

Naloxone has been estimated in plasma by gas chromatography, radioimmunoassay and more recently by high performance liquid chromatography with electrochemical detection (limit of sensitivity 2–5 μg.l^{-1})[6] which is the method of choice.

It is rapidly absorbed following oral administration but high presystemic metabolism makes this route unreliable. The oral parenteral potency ratio has been estimated as 1:50. Effects are seen within 1–2 minutes of an intravenous dose and 2–5 minutes of a subcutaneous dose.

Naloxone is highly lipid soluble and is thus rapidly distributed throughout the body, with a volume of distribution[7] of approximately 5 l.kg^{-1}. High concentrations occur in brain, kidney, lung, heart and skeletal muscle.[8] The brain/serum ratio has been estimated to be 1.5–4.6, approximately 15 times that of morphine. High central nervous system levels are short-lived as rapid redistribution takes place and this might account for the relatively short duration of action seen clinically.[8,9] Approximately 50% of the drug is bound to plasma proteins, principally albumin.[10] The plasma half life is 1–2 h.

Naloxone crosses the placenta easily but it is unknown to what extent it is excreted in breast milk. Naloxone undergoes extensive biotransformation in the liver, and almost none of the drug is excreted unchanged. The metabolites are excreted largely in the urine, with 70% of the dose recoverable over 72 h. The elimination half life in the neonate is prolonged, presumably as a result of reduced hepatic metabolism.[11] The effects of renal and hepatic failure on the metabolism and disposition of naloxone in man have not been studied.

Oral absorption	95%
Bioavailability	very low
Elimination half life	
adults	60–90 min
neonates	180 min
Volume of distribution	5 l.kg^{-1}
Plasma protein binding	50%

Concentration–effect relationship

Although a dose–response relationship may be seen in the naloxone-induced reversal of opioid effects, there is no evidence of any correlation between the plasma concentration of naloxone and those biological effects.

Metabolism

Extensive hepatic metabolism takes place with approximately 70% of an administered dose appearing in the urine within 72 hours. Metabolism is by conjugation, mainly with glucuronic acid, N-dealkylation and 6-keto reduction (Fig. 1). The principal metabolite, naloxone-3-glucuronide, is inactive but 6-β-naloxol is also produced and this may have opioid antagonist activity.[12]

Pharmaceutics

Naloxone is available in parenteral form as the hydrochloride in a clear solution in 1 ml ampoules containing 400 μg (Narcan, Dupont UK/USA) or 2 ml ampoules containing 20 μg per ml (Narcan Neonatal). Pre-filled disposable syringes are available containing 400 μg in 1 ml and 800 μg in 2 ml. Preparations include methylparaben and propylparaben as preservatives and should be protected from light. The injection may be given intramuscularly, intravenously or subcutaneously. When given by continuous intravenous infusion it is diluted with glucose 5% or sodium chloride 0.9% to a concentration of 4 μg.ml^{-1}.

Naloxone has been incorporated into a pentazocine tablet (Talwin Nx; Winthrop Breon, USA) as a deterrent to illicit injectable use of crushed pentazocine tablets. The tablets contain pentazocine 50 mg and naloxone 0.5 mg (both as their hydrochloride salt).

Therapeutic use

Indications

1. Reversal of effects of opioid drugs
2. Diagnosis and treatment of opioid addiction.

There are also a number of further potential uses under investigation.

3. Reversal of central nervous system depressant effects of non-opioid drugs
4. Management of spinal injury and cerebral ischaemia
5. Treatment of mental illness
6. Treatment of endotoxic and hypovolaemic shock
7. Treatment of acute and chronic pain
8. Treatment of pain insensitivity.

Contraindications

1. Known hypersensitivity.

Mode of use

Naloxone may be administered by intravenous, intramuscular or subcutaneous routes.

In opioid overdose, 5–10 μg.kg^{-1} is the usual initial intravenous dose and may be repeated at 2–3 minute intervals until the desired response is seen. At least 2 mg should be used to constitute an adequate trial in overdose of unknown cause. If no response is seen after approximately 150 μg.kg^{-1} then the diagnosis of opioid overdose must be questioned. The duration of action of long-acting opioids may outlast that of an intravenous dose of naloxone so patients should be carefully monitored for signs of returning opioid depression. Intravenous infusions have been employed to avoid this problem commencing at 2.5 μg.kg^{-1} hourly and adjusted according to response. Absorption is good from intramuscular and subcutaneous sites but rate of onset is slower than the intravenous route. While some workers have used oral naloxone for control of opioid addiction, there is no oral preparation available in this country and newer orally active opioid antagonists are being introduced.

Naloxone (hydrochloride)

Indications

1. Reversal of effects of opioid drugs

The treatment of the life-threatening consequences of known or suspected opioid overdose is the prime indication for naloxone and the only licensed use in the UK. Administration in cases of opioid overdosage in adults is as above. In children the initial dose range is 5–10 μg.kg^{-1}. Treatment may need to be continued for 2 to 3 days in cases of overdose involving long-acting opioids, e.g. methadone; this may be achieved either by intermittent doses or by continuous infusion. In cases of overdose following therapeutic use of opioids e.g. postoperatively, a smaller initial dose is used in an attempt to reverse respiratory depression without loss of the opioid analgesia. In such cases 0.1 mg doses may be administered at 2–3 minute intervals until the required effect is achieved. Careful observation is again required to detect recurrence of opioid effects.

In neonates 0.01 mg.kg^{-1} can be administered intravenously, subcutaneously or intramuscularly to reverse the effects of analgesics given to the mother prior to delivery. Larger doses, 0.2 mg, given intramuscularly to infants whose mothers had received pethidine in labour produced significant changes in alveolar ventilation for 48 hours after birth.[13] Naloxone is also effective if administered to the mother 15 minutes prior to cutting the umbilical cord. Administration of naloxone to neonates does not affect their subsequent development.[14] Naloxone will also reverse other effects of opioid agents and it has been used to treat convulsions, dysphoria, itching, urinary retention, biliary spasm, and delayed gastric emptying. All opioids are convulsants in high doses but dextropopoxyphene and pethidine are the two agents most commonly implicated. Naloxone can be administered by slow intravenous injection until the fit stops, and usually no further doses are required. Due to the lower affinity of naloxone for the σ-receptor the treatment of psychotogenic and dysphoric effects of σ-agonists may require higher than usual doses of naloxone.[15]

2. Diagnosis and treatment of opioid addiction

The precipitation of a withdrawal reaction by naloxone has been used as a diagnostic test in cases of suspected opioid dependence, though care must be taken to avoid a severe withdrawal reaction.[16,17]

Naloxone may be used as a screening test prior to administration

Fig. 1 Metabolism of naloxone

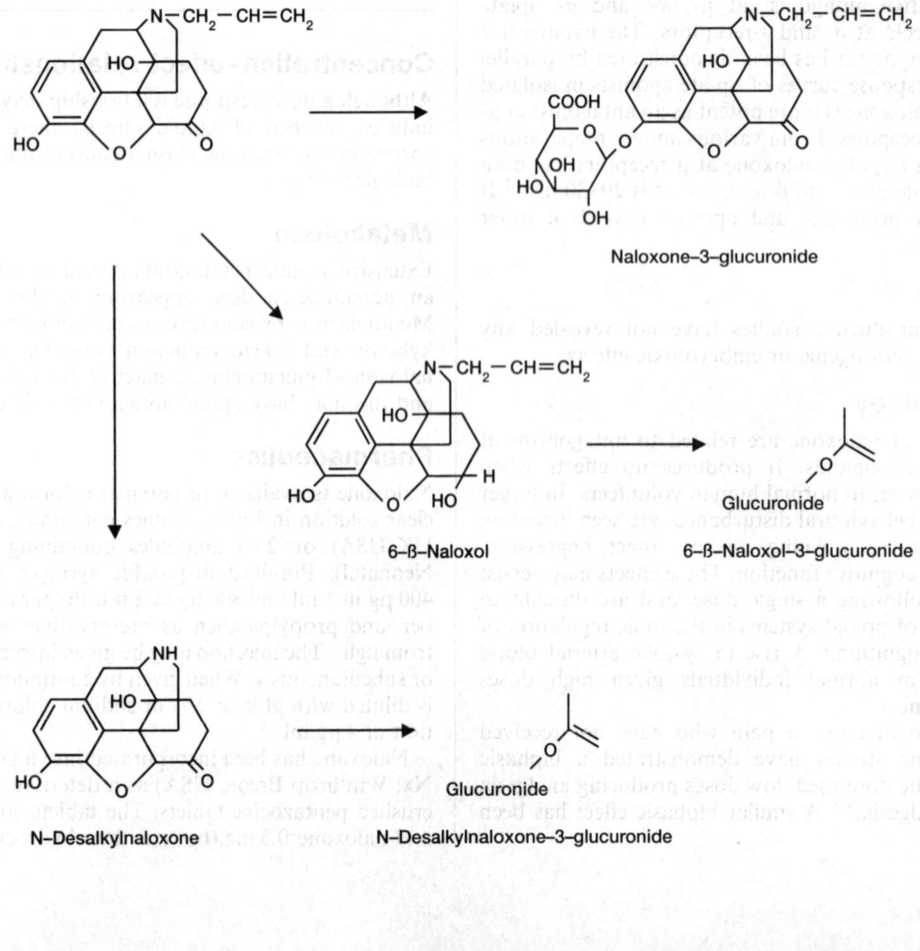

Naloxone (hydrochloride)

of naltrexone in a detoxification programme, so as to avoid a prolonged withdrawal reaction being precipitated by the longer-acting drug.[18] It has also been used as a method of rapidly weaning from opioid dependence to naltrexone maintenance without precipitation of the abstinence syndrome.[19] Because of its low oral activity, the incorporation of naloxone into tablets with methadone does not reduce the activity of the methadone component; however, if the tablets are dissolved for intravenous use (abuse) then the naloxone is active and will precipitate a withdrawal reaction in an addict.[20]

Other uses

Naloxone is under investigation for a number of non-approved uses.

3. Reversal of central nervous system depressant effects of non-opioid drugs

Naloxone has been reported to reverse some of the effects of non-opioid drugs. Respiratory depression caused by diazepam may be reversed by naloxone but changes in the level of consciousness less so.[21–24] Studies of naloxone reversal of alcohol intoxication have yielded conflicting results.[25,26] It has been suggested that nitrous oxide is an opioid agonist[27] and naloxone seems to be partially effective in reversing nitrous oxide analgesia, though paradoxical increases in analgesia have been observed.[28–30] Naloxone does not reverse the non-analgesic effects of nitrous oxide[31,32] nor does it have any effect on anaesthesia produced by thiopentone or halothane.[33–35] Naloxone has been used to treat coma and respiratory depression following clonidine overdose, but precipitation of hypertension severe enough to warrant treatment has been reported and therefore its routine use in this situation cannot be advised.[36]

4. Management of spinal injury and cerebral ischaemia

In many animal models of spinal cord and cerebral ischaemia naloxone administered after the ischaemic insult has been shown to limit the degree of neurological impairment.[37–39] There is some evidence that this may also be the case in humans though further study is required.[40,41] It has been demonstrated that the improvement is not due to changes in systemic cardiovascular dynamics and it may be that endogenous opioids are involved in the pathogenesis of central nervous system ischaemia.[42] In the dog, however, naloxone has been shown to produce relaxation of vascular smooth muscle in the cerebral circulation.[43]

5. Treatment of mental illness

Naloxone has been shown to decrease symptoms in manic patients and to alter hallucinations but not disordered thought in schizophrenics. The therapeutic role for opioid antagonist agents has yet to be established in these conditions.

6. Treatment of endotoxic and hypovolaemic shock

Animal experiments indicate that endogenous opioids may be important in the pathogenesis of a variety of shock states primarily by central inhibition of sympathomedullary activity, possibly by action on δ-receptors. Naloxone produces haemodynamic improvement in many animal models of shock though survival is not uniformly improved and in some studies may be worsened.[44] In humans, encouraging early uncontrolled and anecdotal reports of the use of naloxone in shock have given way to disappointing results in later controlled studies.[45,46] Also, the high doses used in the treatment of shock have led to a high incidence of reported side effects including arrhythmias, pulmonary oedema, hypertension and convulsions. The role of naloxone in the treatment of shock states has still to be fully established.

7. Treatment of acute and chronic pain

No therapeutic use has been found for the analgesia produced by low doses of naloxone, but a synergistic effect with partial opioid agonists has been demonstrated and used clinically.[47] Patients suffering chronic pain as a result of the thalamic syndrome may experience long-lasting relief after large doses of naloxone. The mechanism of the effect is unknown.

8. Treatment of pain insensitivity

Naloxone reduces the nociceptive threshold in patients suffering from congenital pain insensitivity though further studies are necessary to establish the role of opioid antagonists in this condition.

Adverse reactions

Potentially life-threatening effects

Deaths attributed to naloxone are extremely rare and all follow reversal of opioid effects. Two deaths have occurred in previously fit young women,[48] the remainder occurring in patients with known myocardial disease. All were non-addicts given naloxone to reverse the effects of perioperatively administered opiates. Ventricular tachycardia and fibrillation and acute pulmonary oedema have also been reported in patients following naloxone reversal of opioids and occur most frequently in those with existing cardiovascular disease.[49]

Acute overdosage

There have been no reported cases of deliberate or accidental overdose with naloxone.

Severe or irreversible adverse effects

Extreme hypertension may follow naloxone administration both in opioid addicts and after large therapeutic doses of opioids for pain relief. This may be a manifestation of the withdrawal syndrome or a result of sudden reversal of analgesia in the postoperative patient; however, other mechanisms have been postulated. Naloxone has little or no effect on the arterial blood pressure of normal individuals or hypertensives who have not previously received opioid agents. Naloxone appears not to affect the tonic control of blood pressure in awake volunteers;[50] however, it does prevent the fall in blood pressure seen during sleep.[51] The mechanism for this is assumed to be inhibition of endogenous opioid substances.

Symptomatic adverse effects

Nausea and vomiting have been reported following reversal by naloxone of opioid respiratory depression postoperatively. In addicts a typical acute withdrawal syndrome will be seen which even large doses of agonist agents will not alleviate.

Other effects

Naloxone produces no significant biochemical effects.

Interference with clinical pathology tests

Naloxone is not known to interfere with any clinical pathology tests.

High risk groups

Neonates

Naloxone is safe for use in neonates to reverse the effects of opioids given to mothers during labour.

Breast milk. It is unknown to what extent naloxone is excreted in breast milk but transfer by this route is unlikely to be of clinical significance.

Children

There are no special problems related to the use of naloxone in children.

Pregnant women

There are no special restrictions on the use of naloxone in pregnancy.

The elderly

There are no special problems related to the use of naloxone in the elderly.

Drug interactions

Potentially hazardous interactions

Clonidine. Severe hypertension has been reported following naloxone reversal of coma due to clonidine overdose.

Other significant interactions

Alcohol. Naloxone has been reported to reverse alcohol-induced intoxication, though the evidence for this is inconclusive.

Potentially useful interactions

Buprenorphine. Administration of naloxone to postoperative patients in pain who have received buprenorphine as a perioperative analgesic may result in the restoration of full analgesia. This effect is thought to be a consequence of the bell-shaped dose–response curve seen with buprenorphine, with diminishing analgesia at high doses.[46]

General review articles

Budd K 1987 Naloxone. In: Clinical anesthesiology — update in opioids. Ballierre Press

Naloxone (hydrochloride)

N

McNicholas L F, Martin W R 1984 New and experimental therapeutic roles for naloxone and related opioid antagonists. Drugs 27: 81–93
Martin W R 1976 Naloxone. Annals of Internal Medicine 85: 765–768

References

1. Kosterlitz H W, Watt A J 1968 Kinetic parameters of narcotic agonists and antagonists, with particular reference to N-allylnoroxymorphone (naloxone). British Journal of Pharmacology and Chemotherapy 33: 266–276
2. Leslie F M 1987 Methods used for the study of opioid receptors. Pharmacological Reviews 39: 197–249
3. Cohen M R, Cohen R M, Picker D, Weingartner H, Murphy D L, Bunney W E 1981 Behavioral effects after high dose naloxone administration to normal volunteers. Lancet 2: 1110
4. Levine J D, Gordon N C, Fields H L 1979 Naloxone dose dependently produces analgesia and hyperalgesia in postoperative pain. Nature 278: 740–741
5. Lasagna L 1965 Drug interactions in the field of analgesic drugs. Proceedings of the Royal Society of Medicine 58: 978–983
6. Derendorf H, El-Din A, El-Koussi A, Garrett E R 1984 Electrochemical chromatographic determinations of morphine antagonists in biological fluids with applications. Journal of Pharmaceutical Sciences 73: 621–624
7. Aitkenhead A R, Derbyshire D R, Pinnock C A, Achola K, Smith G 1984 Pharmacokinetics of naloxone in healthy volunteers. Anesthesiology 61: A381
8. Berkowitz B A, Ngai S H, Hempstead J, Spector S 1975 Disposition of naloxone: use of a new radioimmunoassay. Journal of Pharmacology and Experimental Therapeutics 195: 499–504
9. Ngai S H, Berkowitz B A, Yang J C, Hempstead J, Spector S 1976 Pharmacokinetics of naloxone in rats and in man. Anesthesiology 44: 398–401
10. Asali L A, Brown K F 1984 Naloxone protein binding in adult and foetal plasma. European Journal of Clinical Pharmacology 27: 459–463
11. Moreland T A, Brice J E H, Walker C H M, Parija A C 1980 Naloxone pharmacokinetics in the newborn. British Journal of Clinical Pharmacology 9: 609–612
12. Weinstein S H, Pfeffer M, Schor J M, Indindoli L, Mintz M 1971 Metabolites of naloxone in human urine. Journal of Pharmaceutical Sciences 60: 1567–1568
13. Wiener P C, Hogg M I J, Rosen M 1977 Effects of naloxone on pethidine induced neonatal depression. British Medical Journal 2: 228–231
14. Weiner P C, Wallace S 1980 Effects of naloxone on pethidine induced neonatal depression. British Medical Journal 280: 252
15. Martin W R 1976 Naloxone. Annals of Internal Medicine 85: 765–768
16. Blachly P H 1973 Naloxone for diagnosis in methadone programs. Journal of the American Medical Association 224: 334–335
17. Wang R I H, Weisen R L, Lamid S, Roh B L 1974 Rating the presence and severity of opiate dependence. Clinical Pharmacology and Therapeutics 16: 653–658
18. Judson B A, Himmelberger D U, Goldstein A 1980 The naloxone test for opiate dependence. Clinical Pharmacology and Therapeutics 27: 492–501
19. Resnick R B, Kestenbaum R S, Washton A, Poole D 1977 Naloxone precipitated withdrawal: a method for rapid induction onto naltrexone. Clinical Pharmacology and Therapeutics 27: 409–413
20. Nutt J G, Jasinski D R 1974 Methadone–naloxone mixtures for use in methadone maintenance programs. Clinical Pharmacology and Therapeutics 15: 156–166
21. Bell E F 1975 The use of naloxone in the treatment of diazepam poisoning. Journal of Pediatrics 87: 803–804
22. Bell E F 1980 Naloxone reversal of diazepam effects. Anesthesiology 53: 264
23. Christensen K, Huttel M 1979 Naloxone does not antagonise diazepam induced sedation. Anesthesiology 51: 187
24. Jordan C, Tech B, Lehane J R, Jones J G 1980 Respiratory depression following diazepam: reversal with high dose naloxone. Anesthesiology 53: 293–298
25. Guerdin J M, Freidberg G 1982 Naloxone and ethanol intoxication. Annals of Internal Medicine 97: 932
26. Mattila M J, Nuotto E, Seppala T 1981 Naloxone is not an effective antagonist of ethanol. Lancet 1: 775–776
27. Daras C, Cantrill R C, Gillman M A 1983 [^{3}H] Naloxone displacement: evidence for nitrous oxide as opioid receptor agonist. European Journal of Pharmacology 89: 177–178
28. Berkowitz B A, Finck D, Ngai S H 1977 Nitrous oxide analgesia: reversal by naloxone and development of tolerance. Journal of Pharmacology and Experimental Therapeutics 203: 539–547
29. Yang J C, Crawford Clark W, Ngai S H 1980 Antagonism of nitrous oxide analgesia by naloxone in man. Anesthesiology 52: 414–417
30. Gillman M A, Kok L, Lichtigfeld F J 1980 Paradoxical effect of naloxone on nitrous oxide analgesia in man. European Journal of Pharmacology 61: 175–177
31. Smith R A, Wilson B S, Miller K W 1978 Naloxone has no effect on nitrous oxide anesthesia. Anesthesiology 49: 6–8
32. Willer J-C, Bergeret S, Gaudy J-H, Dauthier C 1985 Failure of naloxone to reverse the nitrous oxide induced depression of a brain stem reflex: an electrophysiologic and double blind study in humans. Anesthesiology 63: 467–472
33. Harper M H, Winter P M, Brynte M D, Johnson H, Eger E I 1978 Naloxone does not antagonise general anesthesia in the rat. Anesthesiology 49: 3–5
34. Bennett P B 1978 Naloxone fails to antagonise the righting response in rats anesthetised with halothane. Anesthesiology 49: 9–11
35. Duncalf D, Nagashima H, Duncalf R M 1978 Naloxone fails to antagonise thiopental anesthesia. Anesthesia and Analgesia 57: 558–562
36. Gremse D A, Artman M, Boerth R C 1986 Hypertension associated with naloxone treatment for clonidine poisoning. Journal of Pediatrics 776–778
37. Faden A I, Jacobs T P, Holaday J W 1981 Opiate antagonist improves neurologic recovery after spinal injury. Science 211: 493–494
38. Young W, Flamm E S, Demopoulos H G, Tomasula J H, DeCrescito V 1981 Effect of naloxone on post traumatic ischaemia in experimental spinal contusion. Journal of Neurosurgery 55: 209–219
39. Hosobuchi Y, Baskin D S, Woo S K 1982 Reversal of induced ischaemic neurologic deficit in gerbils by the opiate antagonist naloxone. Science 215: 65–71
40. Baskin D S, Hosobuchi Y 1981 Naloxone reversal of ischaemic neurologic deficits in man. Lancet 2: 272–275
41. Iselin H U, Weiss P, Gonzalez-Miranda F, Gillman M A, Lichfield F J 1981 Naloxone reversal of ischaemic neurologic deficits. Lancet 2: 642
42. Baskin D S, Kieck C F, Hosobuchi Y 1982 Naloxone reversal of ischaemic neurologic deficit in baboons is not mediated by systemic effects. Life Sciences 31: 2201–2204
43. Mayer F B, Sundt T M, Yanagihara T, Anderson R E 1987 Focal cerebral ischaemia: pathophysiologic mechanisms and rationale for future avenues of treatment. Mayo Clinic Proceedings 62: 35–55
44. Hinds C J, Donaldson M D J 1988 Endogenous opioids in shock. In: Ledingham I (ed) Recent advances in critical care medicine 3. Churchill Livingstone, Edinburgh, ch 11, pp 175–194
45. Hughes G S 1984 Naloxone and methylprednisolone sodium succinate enhance sympathomedullary discharge in patients with septic shock. Life Sciences 35: 2319–2326
46. DeMaria A, Craven D E, Hefferman J J, McIntosh T K, Grindlinger G A, McCabe W R 1985 Naloxone versus placebo in treatment of septic shock. Lancet 1: 1363–1365
47. Pedersen J E, Chraemmer-Jorgensen B, Schmidt J F, Risbo A 1985 Naloxone, a strong analgesic in combination with buprenorphine. British Journal of Anaesthesia 57: 1045–1046
48. Andree R A 1980 Sudden death following naloxone administration. Anesthesia and Analgesia 59: 782–784
49. Pallasch T J, Gill C J 1981 Naloxone associated morbidity and mortality. Oral Surgery 52: 603–603
50. Fuenmayor N, Cubeddu L 1986 Cardiovascular and endocrine effects of naloxone compared in normotensive and hypertensive patients. European Journal of Pharmacology 126: 189–197
51. Rubin P, Blaschke T F, Guilleminault C 1981 Effect of naloxone, a specific opioid inhibitor, on blood pressure fall during sleep. Circulation 63: 117–121

Naltrexone

Naltrexone is an opioid antagonist, first synthesized by Blumberg et al in 1965.

Chemistry

Naltrexone hydrochloride (Nalorex)
$C_{20}H_{23}NO_4HCl$
17-(Cyclopropylmethyl)-4,5α-epoxy-3,14-dihydroxymorphinan-6-one hydrochloride

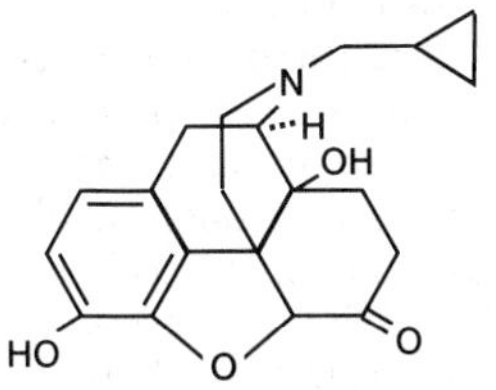

Molecular weight	377.9
pKa	8.13 at 37°C
Solubility	
in alcohol	—
in water	—
Octanol/water partition coefficient (pH7)	2.95

Naltrexone is an analogue of naloxone, where the nitrogen atom of oxymorphone is substituted by a cyclopropylmethyl group. Naltrexone hydrochloride is a white crystalline solid with a bitter taste.

Pharmacology

Naltrexone is a long acting opioid antagonist, modifying responses at the μ, κ and δ opiate receptors in isolated smooth muscle experiments.[1] In binding studies using guinea pig brain membrane, naltrexone's affinity for μ sites is almost 10 times that for κ sites.[2] Following long term naltrexone administration in animal studies, the number of μ, κ and δ brain opioid receptors increased, but not that of the sigma subclass.[3] It has weak agonist actions of its own, which are clinically insignificant.

Toxicology

Animal studies at doses of at least 20 mg.kg^{-1}, which is 20 times greater than the recommended clinical dose, showed no toxicity[4] and no evidence of carcinogenicity has been found.[5] Naltrexone had no effects on fertility and reproduction in rats, and was not teratogenic in rats or rabbits.[4,6]

Clinical pharmacology

As an opioid antagonist, naltrexone is twice as potent as naloxone.[7] It causes a parallel rightward shift of the dose–response curve of opiate agonist, indicating competitive blockade.[8] Opioids differ in their relative sensitivity to naltrexone as an antagonist. In a study of the effects of opioids on the performance of a fixed-rate discrimination test in rats, naltrexone 0.1 mg.kg^{-1} shifted the morphine dose curve to the right by 0.75 log units, whereas the κ agonist ketocyclazocine dose curve was shifted to the right by less than 0.5 log units. Naltrexone failed to antagonize the effects of the σ agonist phencyclidine.[9] Duration of action is dose-related and much longer than that of naloxone, and a single dose can be effective for up to three days.[10] The euphoric effects of intravenous diamorphine 25 mg are antagonized in a dose-related manner; 50 mg of naltrexone blocked the euphoric effects for nearly all subjects. The duration of effect produced by naltrexone 200 mg was 72 hours.[11] The drug has been given to ex-addicts in doses up to 800 mg per day with no related side effects.[4] The analgesia, respiratory depression and miosis produced by opioids are also blocked by naltrexone and it will precipitate an acute withdrawal reaction in subjects who are physically dependent on opiates.

Naltrexone can affect neuro-endocrine functions, possibly due to its effect on endogenous opioids. In former opioid addicts who received naltrexone 350 mg per week for an average of 5 months, 47% had elevated levels of β-endorphins with loss of its diurnal variations. The mean morning β-endorphin level of 19.5 ng.l^{-1} was significantly above those of normal controls (12.1 ng.l^{-1}).[12] Similar changes have also been seen with cortisol levels. Naltrexone was associated with a 50% increase in plasma luteinizing hormone levels in normal subjects, but only a 23–35% increase in opioid-dependent men.[13] The effects of naltrexone on adrenocorticotrophic hormone, prolactin and follicular-stimulating hormones are inconclusive.[14]

Naltrexone or its metabolites may also have weak agonist activity resulting in a lowered respiratory rate and oral temperature, dysphoria and, on chronic dosing, pupillary miosis. These effects are probably clinically insignificant.[15]

Pharmacokinetics

Gas–liquid chromatography is the preferred method of analysis in plasma and, using electron capture detection of halogenated derivatives of naltrexone, the sensitivity of this method[16–18] is 0.25 μg.l^{-1}. However, these methods are expensive and time-consuming, and thus not practical for routine clinical analysis. A simpler method for monitoring the compliance with naltrexone therapy is the qualitative detection of its major metabolite, 6β-naltrexol in urine using thin layer chromatography. The lower limit of sensitivity of this technique for naltrexone and 6β-naltrexol is 0.5 μg, and it should be able to detect the excretion of 6β-naltrexol for up to 72 hours after a therapeutic dose of naltrexone.[19]

After oral administration, naltrexone is rapidly absorbed, reaching peak plasma concentration at one hour. It undergoes extensive presystemic metabolism in the liver; only 5% of the unchanged drug reaches the systemic circulation.[20] The plasma concentration declines in a bi-exponential manner for up to 24 hours. The elimination half life has been quoted as 1.1–10.3 hours; the discrepancies may be due to enterohepatic recycling and intersubject variation.

There are no data on the tissue distribution of naltrexone in humans. In animal studies, tritiated naltrexone given intravenously was rapidly distributed from plasma to the tissues, with less than 4% of the drug present in plasma at one minute after the injection. At 1–5 minutes post injection, the drug was distributed in rough proportion to the tissue wet weight, but after 15 minutes was concentrated in the organs of elimination — the kidney, liver and gastrointestinal tract. The amount of radioactivity in the brain reached a maximum at 5 minutes.[21] The volume of distribution at steady state after oral administration of 100 mg averaged 16.1 l.kg^{-1}, and 14.2 l.kg^{-1} with long-term dosing.[22] Intracellular as well as extracellular distribution of the drug may account for these large values. The plasma protein binding is 20%, and is consistent with the large apparent volume of distribution.

Oral absorption	100%
Presystemic metabolism	95%
Plasma half life (elimination)	
range	1.1–10.3 h
Volume of distribution	14–16 l.kg^{-1}
Plasma protein binding	~20%

Concentration–effect relationship

The minimum effective plasma concentration of naltrexone[25] for opioid antagonism is 0.2 μg.l^{-1}.

Metabolism

Naltrexone is rapidly and extensively reduced to 6β-hydroxynaltrexone (6β-naltrexol), which is its main metabolite. Peak plasma levels of

Naltrexone

this metabolite are achieved in 2–4 hours and its elimination half life is 12.7 hours.[10] 6β-naltrexol is a weaker opioid antagonist than naltrexone, having only $\frac{1}{25}$–$\frac{1}{50}$ the antagonist potency.[23] However, 6β-natrexol's antagonism may be clinically significant as it persists in plasma in larger amounts than naltrexone. Other minor metabolites include 2-hydroxy-3-methoxy-6β-naltrexol and 2-hydroxy-3-0-methyl naltrexone.[24]

Naltrexone and its metabolites undergo extensive glucoronide conjugation in the liver. Most of the drug is present in the conjugated form in a ratio of 3:1. The main route of elimination of naltrexone and its metabolites is by urinary excretion, 40–70% of the drug being recovered from the urine. Multiple dosing increased urinary recovery, possibly due to tissue binding sites becoming saturated, and more of the drug being available for excretion. Less than 5% of orally administered naltrexone is eliminated in the faeces.[10]

Fig. 1 Metabolism of naltrexone

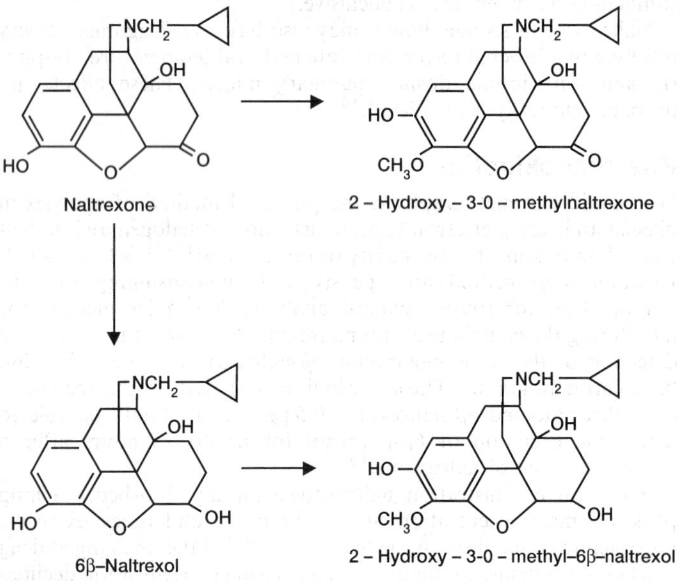

Pharmaceutics

Naltrexone is marketed as Trexan (Dupont UK/USA) in tablet form for oral administration only. Each tablet contains 50 mg of naltrexone hydrochloride. The tablets are a pale orange mottled colour, round, flat faced, bevelled-edged, and scored on one side. The tablets should be stored at room temperature and protected from light.

Therapeutic use

Indications

1. Management of opioid addiction
2. Induction of ovulation in hypothalamic amenorrhoea.

Other uses

1. Mental illness
2. Appetite suppression
3. Chronic pulmonary disease.

Contraindications

1. Patients currently dependant on opioids
2. Patients using opioid-containing medicines
3. Hypersensitivity to naltrexone
4. Acute hepatitis or liver failure.

Mode of use

Naltrexone is available commercially only in tablet form. Its main use is to help detoxified opiate addicts to remain abstinent. Treatment should be initiated in a drug addiction centre. The patient should be completely detoxified and opiate-free before starting naltrexone, to avoid precipitating acute withdrawal. The opiate-free period should be 7 days for short-acting opiates such as heroin, morphine or pethidine, and at least 10 days for longer-acting ones such as methadone. To make sure that a patient is opiate free, the urine should be screened for opiates. As urine toxicology may yield false negatives, a naloxone challenge should also be performed, as the longer-acting naltrexone can cause a very protracted withdrawal reaction which may last up to 48 hours. If no signs of opiate withdrawal are elicited, oral naltrexone treatment can be started with a single dose of 25 mg. The patient is observed for 1 hour, and if no withdrawal signs are seen the rest of the daily dose may be given.

Daily dosage is 50 mg but a more flexible dosage regimen may be adopted to improve patient compliance e.g. 100 mg three times per week. A sustained-release preparation in the form of subcutaneous beads results in adequate absorption, but also causes local tissue irritation, and has only been used on study patients.[26] Liver function should be monitored monthly for the first 6 months during the use of naltrexone.

Indications

1. Management of opiate addiction
Naltrexone has been developed for its treatment of opiate addiction and has been tested in the USA under the guidance of the National Institute of Drug Abuse. In the UK, it is only licensed as an adjunctive prophylactic therapy in the maintenance of detoxified, formerly opiate-dependent patients.

Naltrexone is not a cure for opiate dependence, but is used in conjunction with other therapy in an overall rehabilitation programme. Its main role is to prevent the detoxified patient from relapsing into opiate addiction through its blockade of the effects of subsequent opiate abuse. Patients receiving naltrexone were less likely to continue illicit opiate drug-taking than were those on placebo,[27] as detected by urine toxicology. Even so, there is a high drop-out rate in most trials of naltrexone treatment because of poor patient compliance. Withdrawal symptoms do not result from abrupt cessation of naltrexone treatment.

The three areas where naltrexone are of particular use are: firstly, in patients who can't resist the temptation of opiates where it can be used as a maintenance medication throughout a treatment programme; secondly for short term only to provide protection during the early transition from opiates to abstinence; and thirdly for short term during periods of crises where the patient may relapse to opiate-use or have an irresistible craving for opiates.

2. Induction of ovulation in hypothalamic amenorrhoea
Hypothalamic amenorrhoea is characterized by low levels of circulating gonadotrophins, and endogenous opiates can decrease hypothalamic gonadotrophin-releasing hormone secretion. Naltrexone at a daily dose of 50 mg for 8 days induced ovulatory menstrual cycles in 3 women suffering from secondary hypothalamic amenorrhoea.[28]

Other uses
Naltrexone has been tried in a number of other conditions in which endogenous opioids may play a part. These include mental illness, appetite suppression and chronic pulmonary disease. These uses are speculative and not approved.

1. Mental illness. In controlled and open trials, naltrexone 50–800 mg daily given to schizophrenic patients showed a spectrum from worsening of the psychosis to some improvement.[29] The drug has also been tried in Alzheimer's disease. The results from various trials have been inconclusive[30,31]

2. Appetite suppression. The endogenous opiate system is thought to be associated with the regulation of food intake and body weight. Animal studies suggest that the acute administration of naltrexone may reduce food intake, and that chronic administration may inhibit weight gain in animals on palatable diets that could induce obesity. This has not been reproduced in human studies.[32] Naltrexone failed to regulate appetite in children with Prader Willi syndrome.[33]

3. Chronic pulmonary disease. Raised level of β-endorphins have also been reported in pulmonary disease. There is an anecdotal report of the benefit of naltrexone 100–200 mg daily in patients with hypercapnic, hypoxic chronic obstructive pulmonary disease.[34] Conclusive trials have not been performed.

Contraindications

1. Patients currently dependent on opioids
Naltrexone causes severe and protracted withdrawal symptoms in patients still taking opioids.

2. Patients using opioid-containing medicine
Naltrexone will render the opioid ineffective.

3. Hypersensitivity to naltrexone

4. Acute hepatitis or liver failure
Naltrexone is extensively metabolized in the liver and should not be used in patients with severe liver disease. Its use in patients with marginal evidence of hepatocellular dysfunction must be considered on an individual basis. There is also the possibility that naltrexone itself can cause liver toxicity.

Adverse reactions

Potentially life-threatening effects
Naltrexone is still a relatively new drug, and few side effects have been reported. There have been no lethal or irreversible toxic effects reported in humans.

Acute overdosage
There is no clinical experience of overdosage with naltrexone.

Severe or irreversible adverse effects
There has been one case of reversible idiopathic thrombocytopenic purpura and several of skin rashes, suggesting that naltrexone can cause immune reactions.[35]

There is evidence that naltrexone can cause dose-related hepatocellular damage. In studies where naltrexone has been given in doses of 100–300 mg to obese patients, significant elevation of liver enzymes has been found (serum glutamate-pyruvate transaminase). Following cessation of treatment, the transaminase activity returned to normal levels over a period of a few weeks to months.[32,36]

In drug addicts treated with 350 mg naltrexone weekly, those whose pretreatment hepatic enzymes were above normal range, actually experienced falls in LDH and SGOT to within normal levels. However, for those whose pretreatment levels were normal, there were increases to above the base-line enzyme levels although they remained within normal limits.[37] There are no available data on liver histological changes with naltrexone. Thus, it is inconclusive as to whether naltrexone causes significant liver toxicity.

Symptomatic adverse effects
In opiate addicts, a protracted withdrawal syndrome can be precipitated by naltrexone. Overlap of a mild withdrawal syndrome with concurrent use of naltrexone makes evaluation of the incidence of side effects difficult. Gastrointestinal irritation is common in these patients.

Naltrexone has not been well studied in non-addicts, and it may have adverse effects unrelated to its opiate antagonist properties. Fatigue, nausea, decreased food intake, mental depression and irritability have been reported in a series of normal volunteers.[38]

Other effects
As a result of its effects on the neuroendocrine system, naltrexone can cause changes in hormone levels. Those which have been consistently reproduced include elevation of β-endorphins, cortisol and luteinizing hormone.[12,13]

Interference with clinical pathology tests
Naltrexone is not known to cause any interference with such tests.

High risk groups

Neonates
There are no published reports on naltrexone's safety or use in neonates.

Breast milk. There is little information on the use of naltrexone in lactating women, so the drug should only be given to these patients when the benefits outweigh possible risks to the infant.

Children
Safe use in children has not been established.

Pregnant women
As naltrexone is a new drug, there is little data on its use in pregnant women. Naltrexone should not be used during the first three months of pregnancy.

The elderly
Liver function test abnormalities have been reported in elderly patients taking naltrexone who have had no history of drug abuse.

Concurrent disease
As naltrexone is extensively metabolized by the liver and excreted mainly in the urine, care should be taken when giving the drug to patients with impaired hepatic or renal function. It is not uncommon for opiate drug abusers for whom naltrexone is specifically indicated to have impaired liver function tests and these patients should be screened and monitored.

Drug interactions

Potentially hazardous interactions

Concomitant opiate use. Patients should be warned that attempts to overcome the opiate blockade by naltrexone may cause acute opioid overdose which may be life-threatening. In an emergency requiring opiate analgesia, much larger amounts of opiates need to be given, and the resulting respiratory depression may be more profound and prolonged. In such circumstances, a rapidly-acting analgesic that minimizes respiratory depression is recommended, and the dose titrated to the needs of the patient. In addition, the large doses of opiates needed may cause significant histamine release; this is not countered by the opiate blockade of naltrexone, so that facial swelling, itching and generalized erythema result. Patients needing reversal of naltrexone blockade should be closely monitored for evidence of respiratory depression and other adverse effects by appropriately trained personnel in hospital.

Opiate-containing drug products. Naltrexone will also interfere with the action of opiate-containing drug products. Patients receiving naltrexone may not benefit from opiate-containing medicines, such as cough and cold preparations and antidiarrhoeal preparations. A non-opiate alternative should be used instead if one is available. Special cards are available from drug addiction centres which warn medical personnel that the patient is on naltrexone should they require other medical treatment. The card also warns the patient of the danger of trying to overcome the opiate blockade themselves with large doses of illicit opioids.

Potentially useful interactions
No useful interactions between naltrexone and other drugs have been publicized.

Major outcome trials

1. Brahan L S, Capone T, Wiechart V, Desiderio D 1977
Naltrexone and cyclazocine — a controlled treatment study.
Archives of General Psychiatry 34: 1181–1184

40 male detoxified addicts were randomly assigned to one of four groups. 10 patients received cyclazocine, achieving 4 mg on the 10th day by daily 0.4 mg incremental doses; 10 received placebo for 10 days initially and were then started on the induction treatment of cyclazocine, again building up to a dose of 4 mg over a 10-day period; a further 10 started naltrexone at 10 mg which was increased daily to 50 mg by the fifth day, and were then continued on 50 mg daily for the following 5 days; five patients received placebo for 5 days and then converted to naltrexone induction therapy; and 5 patients were given placebo for 10 days before starting on naltrexone induction. The drugs were given on a double-blind basis, and a drug effect questionnaire was filled in by the patient, nurse or medical officer. The study showed that naltrexone produced fewer induction side effects than cyclazocine; these ranged from tiredness to headaches. In addition, the minor effects of naltrexone induction can be eliminated by preceding placebo treatment.

2. Report of the National Research Council Committee on Clinical Evaluation of Narcotic Antagonists 1978 Clinical evaluation of naltrexone treatment of opiate-dependent individuals. Archives of General Psychiatry 35: 335–341

This was a multicentre controlled trial of naltrexone in recently detoxified addicts, methadone-controlled addicts and former addicts who were drug free at the time of study. The subjects were randomly allocated to a placebo group (98 patients) or naltrexone group (94 patients), and treatment was carried out in a double-blind manner. In the naltrexone group, graduated doses of naltrexone were given on a daily basis starting with 50 mg daily from Monday to Friday and 100 mg on Saturday and increasing to 100 mg on Monday and Wednesday, and 150 mg on Friday. The five criteria used to assess the efficacy of naltrexone were: urinalysis to detect continued opioid usage; compliance with treatment; social and psychological data; post study assessment by clinic staff and patient; and patient assessment of their craving for heroin.

Of the patients who had an initial positive urinalysis for opioid substances, those in the naltrexone group had a better outcome on subsequent testing; 26% were still found to be positive in the naltrexone group and so were presumably still taking opioids, compared with 38% positive urinalysis for the placebo group. There was a high drop-out rate from the programme; 140 patients completed the 2 weeks, but only 13 patients remained for the full 9 months. The naltrexone group reported less craving towards the end of their evaluation time. The conclusion was that, although differences between the naltrexone and placebo patient groups were slight, both retention in treatment and opioid-free urine testing favoured the naltrexone group.

3. Mello N K, Mendelson J H, Kuehnle J C, Sellars M S 1980 Operant analysis of human heroin self-administration and the effects of naltrexone. Journal of Pharmacology and Experimental Therapeutics 216: 45–54

12 male heroin addict volunteers lived in a clinical research ward for 34 days. After a 9-day, drug-free period, naltrexone or placebo were given and the subjects were allowed to earn heroin (up to 40 mg per day) or money, according to their performance on a specific behavioural task, for a period of 10 days. The 3 subjects in the naltrexone group, taking 50 mg daily chose to use only 2.5–7.5% of the available heroin, while the 9 subjects in the placebo group used 57.5–100% of the available heroin. Thus naltrexone suppressed heroin self-administration.

General review articles

Budd K 1987 Naltrexone. Clinical use of optical antagonists. Clinical Anaesthesiology 1: 993–1011

Crabtree B L 1984 Review of naltrexone: a long-acting opiate antagonist. Clinical Pharmacy 3: 273–280

Gonzalez J P, Brogden R N 1988 Naltrexone. A review of its pharmacodynamic and pharmacokinetic properties and therapeutic efficacy in the management of opioid dependence. Drugs 35: 192–213

Pinkert T M, Ginzburg H M 1983 Naltrexone clinics. In: Anaesthesiology — opiate analgesia. vol 1, no 1: 168–179

References

1. Takemori A E, Portoghesee P S 1984 Comparative antagonism by naltrexone and naloxone of μ; κ; δ agonists. European Journal of Pharmacology 104: 101–104
2. Schwyzer R 1988 Estimated membrane structure and receptor subtype selection of an opioid allocated peptide hybrid. International Journal of Peptide Protein Research 32: 476–483
3. Tempel A, Zukin R S, Gardner E L 1982 Supersensitivity of brain opiate receptor subtypes after chronic naltrexone treatment. Life Sciences 31: 1401–1404
4. Braude M C, Morrison J M 1976 Preclinical toxicity studies of naltrexone. National Institute of Drug Abuse Research Monograph Series 9: 16–26
5. Rosenkrantz H 1984 Physiologic and morphologic changes in mice and rats fed naltrexone HCI for 24 months. Journal of Clinical Psychiatry 45: 11–14
6. Christian M S 1984 Reproductive toxicity and teratology evaluations of naltrexone. Journal of Clinical Psychiatry 45: 7–10
7. Martin W R, Jasinski D R, Mansky P A 1973 Naltrexone, an antagonist for the treatment of heroin dependence. Archives of General Psychiatry 28: 784–791
8. Howell L L, Bergman J, Morse W H 1988 Effect of levorphanol and several κ-selective opioids on respiration and behaviour in rhesus monkeys. Journal of Pharmacology and Experimental Therapeutics 245: 364–356
9. Moerschbaecher J M, Devia C, Brocklehurst C 1987 Differential antagonism by naltrexone of the effects of opioids on a field-atio discrimination in rats. Journal of Pharmacology and Experimental Therapeutics 244: 237–244
10. Verebey K, Volavka J, Mule S J, Resnick R B 1976 Naltrexone: Disposition, metabolism and effects after acute and chronic dosing. Clinical Pharmacology and Therapeutics 20: 315–328
11. Resnick R B, Volavka J, Freedman A M, Thomas M 1974 Studies of EN-1639A (Naltrexone): a new narcotic antagonist. American Journal of Psychiatry 131: 646–650
12. Kosten T R, Kreek M J, Ragunath J, Kleber H D 1986 A preliminary study of betaendorphin during chronic naltrexone maintenance treatment in ex-opiate addicts. Life Sciences 39: 55–59
13. Mendelson J H, Ellingboe J, Kuehnle J C, Mello N K 1980 Heroin and naltrexone effects on pituitary-gonadol hormones in man: interaction of steroid feedback effects, tolerance and supersensitivity. Journal of Pharmacology and Experimental Therapeutics 214: 503–506
14. Volavka J, Mallya A, Bauman J, Pevnick J, Cho D, et al 1979 Hormonal and other effects of naltrexone in normal men. Advances in Experimental Medicine and Biology 116: 291–305
15. Gritz E R, Shifman S M, Jarvik M E, Schlesinger J, Charuvastra V C 1976 Naltrexone: physiological and pharmacological effects of single doses. Clinical Pharmacology and Therapeutics 19: 773–776
16. Reuning R H Ashcraft S B, Morrison B E 1980 An electron-capture gas chromatographic assay for naltrexone in biological fluids. National Institute on Drug Abuse Research Monograph Series 28: 25–35
17. Verebey K 1980 Quantitative determination of naltrexone, 6β-naltrexol and 2-hydroxy-3-methoxy-6β-naltrexol (HMN) in human plasma, red blood cells, saliva and urine by gas liquid chromatography. National Institute on Drug Abuse Research Monograph Series 28: 37–39
18. Wall M E, Brine D R 1980 Analytical methods for quantitative and qualitative analysis of naltresone in biological fluids. National Institute on Drug Abuse Research Monograph Series 28
19. Verebey K, Alarazi J, Lehrer M, Mule S J 1986 Determination of 6-naltrexol and naltrexone by bonded-phase absorption thin-layer chromatography. Journal of Chromatography 378: 261–266
20. Meyer M C, Straughn A B, Lo M W, Schary W L, Whitney C C 1984 Bioequivalence, dose-proportionality and pharmacokinetics of naltrexone after oral administration. Journal of Clinical Psychiatry 45: 15–19
21. Ludden T M, Malspeis L, Baggot J D, Sokolski T D, Frank S F et al 1976 Tritiated naltrexone binding in plasma from several species and tissue distribution in mice. Journal of Pharmaceutical Sciences 65: 712–716
22. Kogan M J, Verebey K, Mule S J 1977 Estimation of the systemic availability and other pharmacokinetic parameters of naltrexone in man after acute and chronic oral administration. Research Communications in Chemical Pathology and Pharmacology 18: 29–34
23. Misra A 1980 Current status of preclinical research on disposition, pharmacokinetics and metabolism of naltrexone. National Institute on Drug Abuse Research Monograph 28: 133–146
24. Wall M E, Brine D R, Perez-Reyes M 1981 Metabolism of naltrexone in man after oral and intravenous administration. Drug Metabolism and Disposition 9: 369–375
25. Verebey K 1980 The clinical pharmacology of naltrexone: pharmacology and pharmacodynamics. National Institute on Drug Abuse Research Monograph Series 28: 147–158
26. Chiang C N, Hollister L E, Kishimoto A, Barnett G 1984 Kinetics of a naltrexone sustained release preparation. Clinical Pharmacology and Therapeutics 35: 704–708
27. Report of the National Research Council Committee on Clinical Evaluation of Narcotic Antagonists 1978 Clinical evaluation of naltrexone treatment of opiate-dependent individuals. Archives of General Psychiatry 35: 335–340
28. Wildt L, Leyendecker G 1987 Induction of ovulation by the chronic administration of naltrexone in hypothalamic amenorrhea. Journal of Clinical Endocrinology and Metabolism 64: 1334–1335
29. Volavka J, Anderson B, Koz G 1982 Naloxone and naltrexone in mental illness and tardive dyskinesia. Annals New York Academy of Sciences 398: 97–102
30. Tennant F S Jr 1987 Preliminary observations of naltrexone for treatment of Alzheimer's type demential (letter). Journal of the American Geriatrics Society 35: 369–370
31. Hyman B T, Eslinger P J, Damasio A R 1985 Effect of naltrexone on senile dementia of the Alzheimer type. Journal of Neurology Neurosurgery and Psychiatry 48: 1169–1171
32. Atkinson R L, Berke L K, Drake C R, Bibbs M L, Williams F L, Kaiser D L et al 1985 Effects of long-term therapy with naltrexone on body weight in obesity. Clinical Pharmacology and Therapeutics 38: 419–422
33. Zlotkin S H, Fettes I V, Stallings V 1986 The effects of naltrexone on oral β-endorphin antagonist in children with Prader-Willi Syndrome. Journal of Clinical Endocrinology and Metabolism 63: 1229–1232
34. Reents S B, Beck C A 1988 Naloxone and naltrexone-application in COPD Chest 92: 217–219
35. O'Brien C P, Greenstein R A, Mintz J, Woody G E 1975 Clinical experience with naltrexone. American Journal of Drug and Alcohol Abuse 2: 365–377
36. Mitchell J E 1986 Naltrexone and hepatotoxicity. Lancet 1: 1215
37. Brahen L S 1988 Naltrexone: lack of effects on hepatic enzymes. Journal of Clinical Pharmacology 28: 64–70
38. Hollister L E, Johnson K, Boukhabza D, Gillespie H K 1981 Aversive effects of naltrexone in subjects not dependent on opiates. Drug and Alcohol Dependence 8: 37–41

Nandrolone decanoate

Nandrolone decanoate is the most widely used injectable anabolic steroid.

Chemistry

Nandrolone decanoate (nortestosterone decylate, Deca-Durabolin, Anabolin LA-100, Androlone D, Hybolin Decanoate)
$C_{28}H_{44}O_3$
3-Oxoestr-4-en-17β-yl-decanoate

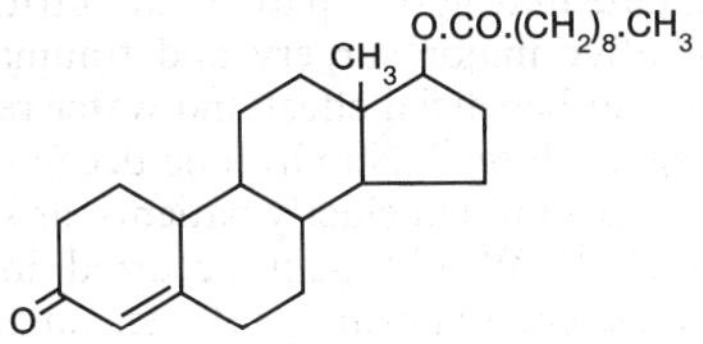

Molecular weight	428.7
pKa	—
Solubility	
in alcohol	1 in 1
in water	almost insoluble
Octanol/water partition coefficient	—

Nandrolone decanoate is a white to creamy-white crystalline powder with a faint characteristic odour, which is prepared by chemical synthesis.

Pharmacology

Nandrolone decanoate has anabolic, androgenic, progestagenic and erythropoietic activity. The steroid maintains the anabolic (myotrophic) activity of testosterone but the androgenic action is markedly diminished. The dissociation of these activities is not due to differences in the selectivity of receptors in different target tissues but to the virtual absence of 5α reductase activity from muscle tissue and its high concentration in tissues with a characteristic androgenic response.[1] The 5α reduced metabolite of testosterone has a higher affinity for the androgen receptor than testosterone itself. The 5α reduced metabolite of nandrolone, by contrast, has a much lower affinity for the androgen receptor than nandrolone. The activity of nandrolone in tissues with a high concentration of 5α-reductase activity is therefore reduced.[2] The dissociation of the anabolic/androgenic activities has been quantitated by treating young castrated male rats with subcutaneous injections of nandrolone decanoate. The anabolic activity is represented by the increase in weight of the levator ani muscle while the androgenicity is assessed by the increase in weight of the ventral prostate. The anabolic/androgenic quotient after 2 weeks treatment was 12 times that obtained with testosterone decanoate.[3] The use of the levator ani muscle has been criticized because it is not a typical skeletal muscle.[4] It is certainly much more responsive to male hormone than other skeletal muscles but this appears to be due to a higher concentration of androgen receptors rather than to differences in 5α-reductase concentration.[1]

In rats nandrolone decanoate produces a dose-related reduction in gonadal weights.[5] In female rats treated with a high dosage of nandrolone there was inhibition of pituitary function.[6]

Toxicology

No evidence of acute or chronic toxic effects of nandrolone decanoate have been demonstrated in studies on rats and dogs lasting for up to 6 months, apart from the expected androgenic and gonad inhibiting effects. Studies of carcinogenicity were not carried out before the drug was introduced but extensive use in the last 25 years has not indicated a carcinogenic potential. Since the androgenic properties preclude use during pregnancy, teratogenic studies are not relevant.

Clinical pharmacology

Nandrolone is primarily anabolic and its androgenic effect is very weak. Nevertheless, in long-term use in females, virilization may occur with acne, hirsutism, deeper voice and coarse skin. Its anabolic effects may lead to premature closure of the epiphysis in children. Nandrolone stimulates erythropoetic activity by a direct effect on erythropoetin production and this has been used in the treatment of chronic renal failure. Nandrolone may cause fluid retention and oedema due to sodium retention by the kidney.

Pharmacokinetics

Several methods are available for quantifying the urinary excretion of either unchanged nandrolone by radioimmunoassay[7] or the major metabolites by isotope dilution–mass spectrometry.[8] The preferred analytical method for measuring concentrations in blood uses isolation of nandrolone by high performance liquid chromatography and quantitation by radioimmunoassay.[9] Although the nandrolone antiserum cross-reacts 8% with testosterone and 14% with dihydrotestosterone, specificity is ensured by the HPLC. The sensitivity of the assay is 0.09 $mmol.l^{-1}$.

The pharmacokinetics of the drug have been studied only after intramuscular injection of depot preparations. In one study[9] injection of nandrolone decanoate (50 mg) into six normal men resulted in peak nandrolone concentrations of 4.6 ± 3.2 (range 2.8–9.7) $nmol.l^{-1}$ after 24 h. The mean plasma half life was 8 ± 5 days (range 5–17 days). In a second study[10] it was found that the mean half life for release of the ester from the depot into the general circulation was 6 days, whereas the mean half life for the combined processes of hydrolysis of nandrolone decanoate and elimination of free nandrolone was only 4.3 h. In vitro studies revealed that nandrolone decanoate undergoes rapid hydrolysis in serum with a half life < 1 h.

Oral absorption	—
Presystemic metabolism	—
Plasma half life	
range	8 ± 5 d
mean	5–17 d
Volume of distribution	—
Plasma protein binding	—

Concentration–effect relationship

The concentrations of testosterone and dihydrotestosterone in six normal men injected with 50 mg nandrolone decanoate were reduced from day 1 to day 15 during which time the mean concentration of nandrolone in the plasma declined from 4.6 to 1.0 $nmol.l^{-1}$. The suppression was not statistically significant.[9]

Metabolism

The prolonged action of nandrolone decanoate (I) is due to its slow absorption from the oily solution at the site of injection and subsequent rapid hydrolysis to nandrolone (II), the active form of the preparation. There is no excretion of the ester. Subsequent metabolism (Fig. 1) is similar to that of testosterone and presumably takes place mainly in the liver with the formation of the tetrahydro metabolites 19-norandrosterone (III), 19-norepiandrosterone (IV), and 19-noraetiocholanolone (V)[11] These reduced metabolites are conjugated to glucuronic and sulphuric acids and excreted in the urine. The proportion of drug excreted in the form of the 5α, 3β-hydroxy metabolite, 19-norepiandrosterone, is much greater than in the case of testosterone and thus is conjugated mainly with sulphuric acid.[12]

Pharmaceutics

Nandrolone decanoate is available as Deca-Durabolin (Organon, UK/USA) in oily solutions at concentrations of 50 and 100 $mg.ml^{-1}$

and at concentrations of 25 mg.ml⁻¹ (UK only) and 200 mg.ml⁻¹ (USA only). Administration is by deep intramuscular injection. In the USA injections are supplied in pre-filled syringes.

Therapeutic use

Indications

1. Established osteoporosis
2. Disseminated breast cancer in women
3. Protein deficiency states occurring after major surgery or trauma
4. Anaemia
a. due to chronic renal failure
b. aplastic anaemia
c. due to cytotoxic chemotherapy.

Other possible uses

5. Chronic debilitating disease in the elderly
6. Postsurgical and post traumatic catabolism
7. During glucocorticosteroid therapy.

Contraindications

1. Prostatic carcinoma
2. Male breast carcinoma
3. Pregnancy.

Indications

1. Established osteoporosis
During the Joint WHO/EOPF/NIAMS(NIH) Consultation on Osteoporosis in 1988 it was concluded that anabolic steroids do increase bone mass in women with established osteoporosis but some concerns remain about their side-effects, particularly following oral administration.[12] The recent discovery of the existence of androgen receptors in human bone[13] supports the concept that their action is in part a direct effect on the skeleton. Clinical trials using modern methods of assessment of bone mass have demonstrated a significant increase in bone mineral content in the axial and peripheral skeleton in postmenopausal women with established osteoporosis during treatment with nandrolone decanoate for one year.[15–21] The effect on forearm bone mass appears to level off during the second year of treatment but was still significant after two years' treatment in one study.[15] Patients may experience rapid relief of bone pain,[17] but effects on fracture rate are not yet known. Doses of 50 mg every three weeks are appropriate.

2. Disseminated breast cancer in women (palliative therapy)
The 20% regression rate in unselected human breast cancers achieved with injections of testosterone esters led to a search for less virilizing agents. Nandrolone decanoate used in doses of 50 mg every 3 weeks gave similar rates of remission (10%) or arrest (24%) in patients with intact pituitaries.[22] The duration of the favourable effect was 3–24 months and most patients experienced subjective improvement (increased appetite and well-being). Slight virilization is seen in less than 10% of patients at this dose level.

3. Protein deficiency states occurring after major surgery or trauma
The administration of an anabolic agent would appear to be a rational therapy to speed recovery from protein deficiency conditions when dietary intake is adequate. However, although a large number of studies have been carried out over the past 30 years using a variety of natural and synthetic anabolic steroid preparations, the overall result has been disappointing.[23,24] The accurate evaluation of the benefits of treatment are complicated by the difficulty of adequate control of the many variables and the undesirable effects and side effects of the treatment. In respect of the undesirable consequences, nandrolone decanoate is better than most anabolic steroids because of its low toxicity to the liver. Also, because of the inactivating effect of the 5α-reductase enzyme on this particular steroid, it suffers less from the normal virilizing action of the male hormone.

There are a number of reports of controlled studies suggesting that nandrolone decanoate may add to parenteral nutrition in minimizing the nitrogen loss after major surgery and trauma.[22–28] However, other studies show no beneficial effect and water retention may be a problem at the higher dose.[29] Nandrolone decanoate may promote body weight gain in debilitated elderly patients, as shown in placebo-controlled studies.[30,31] Weight gain occurred in the absence of oedema and did not decrease abruptly after termination of treatment, suggesting that it is not due to water retention.[32,33] Although there is no proof of the efficacy of nandrolone decanoate in catabolic and chronic debilitating states or of any improvement in the underlying disease processes, several reports suggest an improvement in appetite and general well-being.[32,34] Treatment regimens given are 50 mg every 2–3 weeks, a single 100 mg injection, and 100 mg every 4 weeks for up to 12 weeks.

4. Anaemia

a. Anaemia due to chronic renal failure
The anaemia found in these patients is mainly due to suppressed erythropoiesis. This condition is probably the one in which the benefit conferred by treatment with anabolic steroids is most firmly established but, even here, the advantage is limited.[35] Nandrolone decanoate stimulates erythropoiesis. Its mode of action appears to be twofold: it stimulates erythropoietin production and it also appears to stimulate stem cells in the bone marrow directly. Doses are high, in the range 50–200 mg per week and some female patients may suffer from virilization. The availability of pure erythropoietin has largely superseded this use.

Fig. 1 Metabolism of nandrolone decanoate

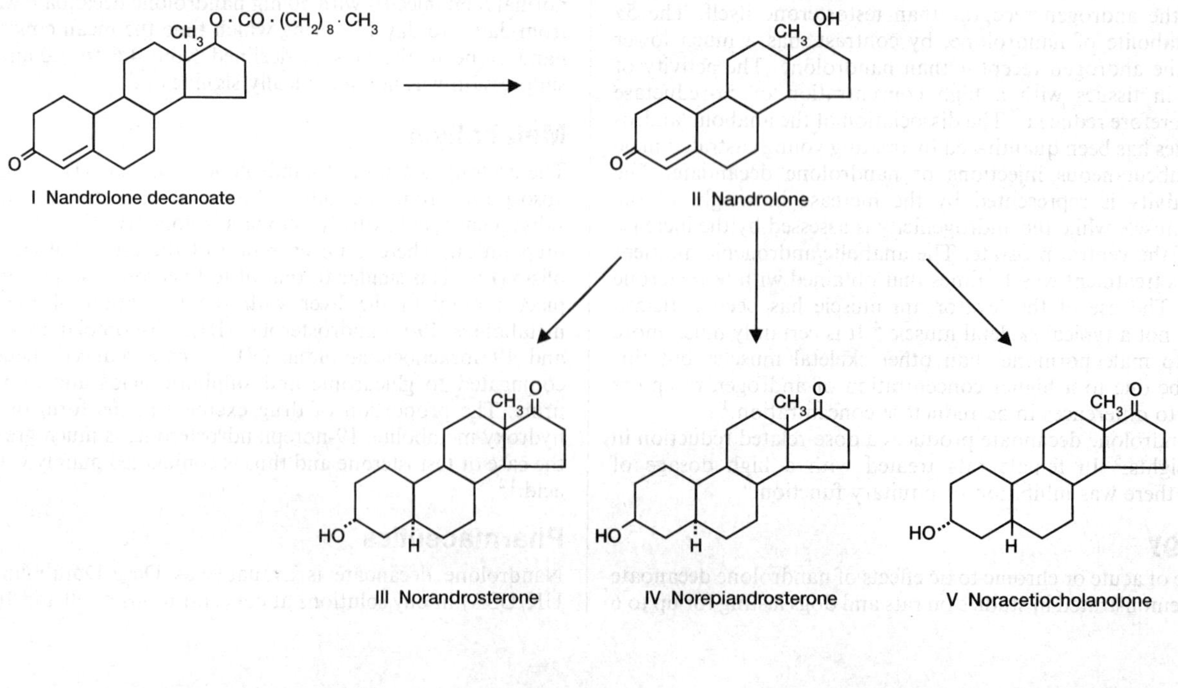

Nandrolone decanoate

b. Aplastic anaemia
Severe cases are best treated with bone marrow transplantation, but in milder cases and where this treatment cannot be used, anabolic steroids may be effective. Controlled studies in this condition are few and success rates vary widely, probably because of the heterogeneity of the patients studied in the different reports. The degree of hypoplasia is obviously important here and the nature of the damage to the haematopoietic cells and their responsiveness to treatment may depend on the aetiologic agents responsible for the aplastic anaemia. Patients with acquired aplastic anaemia in general respond better than those in whom the disease is constitutional and children respond better than adults. Doses of 50–150 mg nandrolone decanoate per week often in conjunction with glucocorticosteroid therapy, are used. Haematomas at the site of injection are sometimes reported, due to the low initial platelet count in these patients.

c. Anaemia due to cytotoxic therapy
In cancer patients, adjuvant treatment with nandrolone decanoate can reduce the suppressive effects of chemotherapy on bone marrow. Doses of 200 mg per week are most often used. However, the introduction of granulocyte colony stimulating factor (GCSF, GMCSF) is likely to offer a more effective alternative.

Other uses

5. Chronic debilitating disease in the elderly
Nandrolone decanoate has been used in elderly subjects with degenerative and debilitating changes to improve their general physical and mental condition. Treatment regimes vary from a single 100 mg injection to 100 mg every 4 weeks for up to 12 weeks.

6. Postsurgical and post-traumatic catabolism
Major surgery is usually followed by a catabolic phase lasting 3–5 days and this is succeeded by an anabolic phase of 5–10 days. The precise duration and intensity of these phases depends on a number of factors including the preoperative condition, the anaesthesia, the extent of the surgical trauma and of blood loss and the postoperative care.

Nandrolone decanoate has been found to be of benefit in some studies in minimizing the early nitrogen loss.[26] However, not all studies show a beneficial effect and water retention may be a problem.[29]

7. During glucocorticosteroid therapy
Among the undesirable effects of treatment with corticosteroids in pharmacological doses are negative balances of nitrogen and potassium and loss of bone minerals. Animal experiments indicated that these effects could be prevented by administration of anabolic steroids but with human subjects the effects on protein catabolism seemed to be only transient. Nevertheless there may be occasions during long-term glucocorticosteroid therapy when intermittent use of nandrolone decanoate may be of value.[36]

Contraindications

1. Prostatic carcinoma
Because androgens are growth promoters in carcinoma of the prostate, nandrolone decanoate should not be used in this condition.

2. Male breast carcinoma
Androgens are also growth promoters in carcinoma of the male breast and should be avoided in this condition.

3. Pregnancy
Because of the danger of masculinization of the female fetus nandrolone decanoate should not be used during pregnancy.

The non-therapeutic use of nandrolone esters in sport

Of the six classes of drugs whose use is banned by the International Olympic Committee, anabolic steroids are quantitatively by far the most important. In 1988 more than half of all positives found by IOC accredited testing laboratories were anabolic steroids and the single most common steroid found was nandrolone. The incidence of abuse varies between types of athletic ability although there is probably no activity that can claim to be free of the use of steroids. The frequency of abuse and the largest doses are probably to be found in events most dependent on muscular power, e.g. weight-lifting, throwing (discus, shot, etc.) and sprinting.

Scientific evidence for a direct anabolic effect of these steroids in adult men is conflicting. There may, however, be an indirect effect brought about by the action of the steroid on the CNS, causing an increase in aggression and competitiveness. Stimulation of erythropoiesis may be a factor in the use of these steroids in endurance events.

Adverse reactions

Potentially life-threatening effects
There are no acute lethal toxic effects of nandrolone decanoate. Male and female athletes taking anabolic steroids, including nandrolone decanoate, have been found to have high serum total cholesterol, low HDL2-C, low HDL-C to total cholesterol ratio and low apo A-1 levels.[37] This lipoprotein profile may increase the risk of atheroma deposition.

Acute overdosage
The only circumstance in which overdose of nandrolone decanoate is likely to occur is in its use to improve performance in sport. In this application, use of doses of up to 200 mg daily have been reported for men. No adverse effects have been recorded although azoospermia is probable at this dose level.

Severe or irreversible adverse effects
Although nandrolone decanoate has a diminished androgenicity relative to testosterone, when administered in higher doses its effects can be troublesome in women. The only irreversible effects are deepening of the voice in some women and stunting of growth in children by premature fusion of the epiphyses.

Symptomatic adverse effects
These include disturbances of the menstrual cycle, acne, male pattern growth of the hair on face and body, temporal recession of scalp hair, water retention, increase of libido, and, rarely, cliteromegaly.

Other effects
Slight changes in the serum HDL cholesterol may occur, but serum triglycerides remain unaffected.[38,39] Unlike the C-17 alkylated anabolic steroids, nandrolone decanoate is almost free of adverse effects on the liver even when administered in high dosage. Exceptionally, abnormalities of liver function (increased serum transaminases or cholestasis[40,41] and, on long-term treatment, liver tumours and peliosis hepatis[42] have been recorded but the causal relationship with drug treatment is not clear. The hypercalcaemia which is often present in patients with disseminated breast cancer may be transiently exacerbated at the start of nandrolone therapy.[44]

Interference with clinical pathology tests
None is known.

High risk groups

Neonates
Not appropriate.

Breast milk. The drug should not be given to lactating women.

Children
If treatment with nandrolone decanoate is necessary, skeletal maturation must be monitored.

Pregnant women
Not appropriate.

The elderly
No special precautions are needed.

Concurrent disease
Patients with nephritis, nephrosis or cardiac decompensation should be carefully monitored during treatment with nandrolone decanoate because of possible excessive retention of sodium, calcium and water.

Drug interactions

Potentially hazardous interactions

Anticoagulants
Nandrolone decanoate may potentiate anticoagulants such as phenindione and warfarin and may therefore enhance a bleeding tendency.

Cyclophosphamide
A much reduced response to combination treatment with cyclophosphamide and nandrolone decanoate compared with cyclophosphamide on its own was found in patients with advanced breast cancer.[45] It was suggested that nandrolone may interfere with the activation of cyclophosphamide in the liver.

Potentially useful interactions
No interactions of this kind have been described.

Clinical trials

Osteoporosis

1. Geusens P, Dequeker J 1986 Long-term effect of nandrolone decanoate, 1α-hydroxy vitamin D_3 or intermittent calcium infusion therapy on bone mineral content, bone remodelling and fracture rate in symptomatic osteoporosis: a double-blind controlled study. Bone and Mineral 1: 347–357

In this double-blind controlled study of 60 patients having at least one vertebral crush fracture, an injection of 50 mg of nandrolone decanoate every 3 weeks was compared with 1 α-hydroxy vitamin D_3 or intermittent calcium infusion therapies. Nandrolone decanoate statistically significantly increased the bone mineral content at the radius, reduced the endosteal bone loss at the metacarpals and statistically significantly reduced urinary calcium and hydroxyproline excretion.

2. Hassager C, Riis B J, Podenphant J, Christiansen C 1989 Nandrolone decanoate treatment of post-menopausal osteoporosis for 2 years and effects of withdrawal. Maturitas 11: 305–317

In this double-blind, placebo-controlled study, the effects of two-year treatment with nandrolone decanoate on forearm and lumbar spine bone mineral content are reported. The nandrolone-treated groups (14 patients) showed statistically significant increases in forearm bone mineral content (+3.5% and 2.7% with two dose regimens) during the first year. This effect partly levelled off during the second year of treatment (also observed by the Dequeker group). The lumbar spine bone mineral density increased by 0.8% during the first year and by 4.6% during a subsequent year of nandrolone therapy, but the difference with the placebo group (1.9% increase) was not statistically significant.

3. Need A G, Horowitz M, Bridges A, Morris H A, Nordin B E C 1989 Effects of nandrolone decanoate and antiresorptive therapy on vertebral density in osteoporotic postmenopausal women. Archives Internal Medicine; 149: 57–60

In this comparative study, using quantitative computed tomography as assessment method, vertebral (lumbar spine) mineral density (VMD) was measured in 71 postmenopausal osteoporotic women before and after treatment with either nandrolone decanoate (23 women) or antiresorptive therapy (calcium with or without calcitriol, with or without ovarian hormones, given to 48 women). After a mean treatment period of 14 months, there was a mean increase of 20% ($p<0.01$) in VMD in the former group, and no significant change in the latter group. There was no significant change in VMD in the reference group on anti-resorptive therapy for 15 months.

4. Need A G, Horowitz M, Walker C J, Chatterton B E, Chapman I C, Nordin B E C 1989 Cross-over study of fat-corrected forearm mineral content during nandrolone decanoate therapy for osteoporosis. Bone; 10: 3–6

In this cross-over study, using single photon absorptiometry as assessment method, the effects of nandrolone decanoate (50 mg every 2 or 3 weeks for 6–7 months) on fat-corrected forearm bone mineral content (BMC) were studied in 70 postmenopausal women with established osteoporosis. There was a statistically significant rise in the mean forearm fat-corrected BMC on nandrolone decanoate and a non-significant fall in mean fat-corrected BMC off the drug. The authors concluded that nandrolone decanoate produced a significant gain in forearm mineral content even after allowing for changes in forearm fat content during therapy.

Nandrolone decanoate

Other controlled trials

Osteoporosis

1. Need A G, Chatterton B E, Walker C J, Steurer T A, Horowitz M, Nordin B E C 1986 Comparison of calcium, calcitriol, ovarian hormones and nandrolone in the treatment of osteoporosis. Maturitas 8: 275–280

In this study there was a highly significant increase in the forearm mineral density of 42 patients given nandrolone decanoate (50 mg) every 2 weeks and in 38 patients in whom it was administered every 3 weeks ($p<0.001$). The 3-weekly regime is advocated because of the much lower incidence of side effects, with hoarseness of voice in only 5% instead of 48% on the 2 weekly regime. It is suggested that nandrolone decanoate stimulates bone formation as well as inhibiting bone reabsorption.

Anaemias

2. Hendler E D, Goffinet J A, Ross S, Longnecker R E, Bakovic V 1974 Controlled study of androgen therapy in anaemia of patients on maintenance haemodialysis. New England Journal of Medicine 291: 1046–1051

This is a double-blind cross-over trial involving 14 patients in the centre and 8 at home. During the 5-month period of androgen administration the mean red cell mass rose from 946 to 1173 ml ($p<0.001$) and mean haematocrit from 23 to 27% ($p<0.005$). There was no improvement in the red cell mass or haematocrit when placebo was given. Blood transfusion requirements fell from 0.35 to 0.16 units/patient/month ($p<0.05$) during the use of androgen. All the patients were men and no adverse effects were noted on the dose of 100 mg per week.

Other trials

1. Neff M S, Goldberg J, Slifkin R F, et al 1985 Anaemia in chronic renal failure. Acta Endocrinolgica 110: (suppl) 271: 80–86
2. Spiers A S D, De Vita S F, Allar M J, Richards S, Sedransk N 1981 Beneficial effects of an anabolic steroid during cytotoxic chemotherapy for metastatic cancer. Journal of Medicine 12: 433–445
3. Daiber A, Herve L, Con I, Donoso A 1970 Treatment of aplastic anaemia with nandrolone decanoate. Blood 36: 748–753

General review of all aspects of anabolic steroids

Kochakian C D (ed) 1976 Anabolic–androgenic steroids. Springer-Verlag, Berlin

Review articles

Turner R 1985 Deca Durabolin R and cytotoxic drugs. Acta Endocrinologica 110: (suppl 271): 70–79

References

1. Krieg M, Voigt K 1977 Biochemical substrate of androgenic actions at a cellular level in prostate, bulbocavernous/levator ani and in skeletal muscle. Acta Endocrinologica (suppl 214): 43–89
2. Toth M, Zakar T 1982 Relative binding affinities of testosterone, 19-nortestosterone and their 5α-reduced derivatives to the androgen receptor and to other androgen-binding proteins: a suggested role of 5α-reductive steroid metabolism in the dissociation of 'myotropic' and 'androgenic' activities of 19-nortestosterone. Journal of Steroid Biochemistry 17: 653–660
3. Overbeek G A, de Visser J 1961 A comparison of the myotropic and androgenic activities of the phenyl propionates and decanoates of testosterone and nandrolone. Acta Endocrinologica 38: 285–292
4. Hayes K J 1965 The so-called 'Levator Ani' of the rat. Acta Endocrinologica 48: 337–347
5. de Visser J, Overbeek G A 1960 Pharmacological properties of nandrolone decanoate. Acta Endocrinologica 35: 405–412
6. Vanha-Perttula T, Lehto J 1963 The effect of anabolic hormones on the reproductive system of intact mature female rats. Anales Medicinae Experimentalis et Biologiae Fennicae 41: 297–304
7. Brooks R V, Jeremiah G, Webb W A, Wheeler M 1979 Detection of anabolic steroid administration to athletes. Journal of Steroid Biochemistry 11: 913–917
8. Bjorkhem J, Ek H 1982 Detection and quantitation of 19-norandrosterone in urine by isotope dilution–mass spectrometry. Journal of Steroid Biochemistry 17: 447–451

Nandrolone decanoate

9. Belkien L, Schurmeyer T, Hano R, Gunnarsson P O, Nieschlag E 1985 Pharmacokinetics of 19-nortestosterone esters in normal men. Journal of Steroid Biochemistry 22: 623–629
10. Wijnand H P, Bosch A M G, Donker C W 1985 Pharmacokinetics parameters of nandrolone (19-nortestosterone) after intramuscular administration of nandrolone decanoate (Deca Durabolin R) to healthy volunteers. Acta Endocrinologica 110 (suppl 271): 19–30
11. Masse R, Laliberte C, Tremblay L, Dugal R 1985 Gas chromatographic/mass spectrometric analysis of 19-nortestosterone urinary metabolites in man. Biomedical Mass Spectrometry 12: 115–121
12. Kicman A, Brooks R V 1988 A radioimmunoassay for the metabolites of the anabolic steroid nandrolone. Journal of Pharmaceutical and Biomedical Analysis 6: 473–483
13. World Health Organization 1988 Report of the Joint WHO/EOPF/NIAMS(NIH) Consultation on Osteoporosis. Geneva, 13–15 July 34 (1–43)
14. Colvard D S, Eriksen E F, Keeting Ph E et al 1989 Identification of androgen receptors in normal human osteoblast-like cells. Proceedings of the National Academy of Science, USA 86: 854–857
15. Geusens P, Dequecker J 1986 Long-term effect of nandrolone decanoate, 1-alpha hydroxyvitamin D_3 or intermittent calcium infusion therapy on bone mineral content, bone remodelling and fracture rate in symptomatic osteoporosis. A double-blind controlled study. Bone and Mineral 1: 347–357
16. Geusens P, Dequecker J, Verstraeten A, Nijs J, van Holsbeeck M 1986 Bone mineral content, cortical thickness and fracture rate in osteoporotic women after withdrawal of treatment with nandrolone decanoate, 1-alpha hydroxyvitamin D_3, or intermittent calcium infusions. Maturitas 8: 281–289
17. Gennari C, Agnus Dei D, Gonnelli S, Nardi P 1989 Effects of nandrolone decanoate therapy on bone mass and calcium metabolism in women with established osteoporosis: a double-blind placebo-controlled study. Maturitas 11: 187–197
18. Hassagar C, Riis B J, Podenphant J, Christiansen C 1989 Nandrolone decanoate treatment of post-menopausal osteoporosis for 2 years and effects of withdrawal. Maturitas 11: 305–317
19. Need A, Chatterton B E, Walker C J, Steurar T A, Horowitz M, Nordin B E C 1986 Comparison of calcium, calcitriol, ovarian hormones and nandrolone in the treatment of osteoporosis. Maturitas 8: 275–281
20. Need A G, Horowitz M, Bridges A, Morris H A, Nordin B E C 1989 Effects of nandrolone decanoate and antiresorptive therapy on vertebral density in osteoporotic postmenopausal women. Archives of Internal Medicine 149: 57–60
21. Need A G, Horowitz M, Walker C J, Chatterton B E, Chapman I C, Nordin B E C 1989 Cross-over study of fat-corrected forearm mineral content during nandrolone decanoate therapy for osteoporosis. Bone 10: 3–6
22. Hortling H, Malmio K 1967 Treatment of metastasising mammary carcinoma with anabolic steroids. Nordisk Medicin 77: 275–279
23. Wynn V 1968. The anabolic steroids. The Practitioner 200: 509–518
24. Wilson J D, Griffin J E 1980 The use and misuse of androgens. Metabolism 29: 1278–1295
25. Tweedle D, Walton C, Johnston I D A 1973 The effect of an anabolic steroid on postoperative nitrogen balance. British Journal of Clinical Practice 27: 130–132
26. Michelson C B, Askenazi J, Kinney J M, Gump F E, Elwyn D H 1982. Effect of an anabolic steroid on nitrogen balance and amino acid patterns after total hip replacement. Journal of Trauma 22: 410–413
27. Moseback K O, Hausmann D, Caspari R, Stoeckel H 1985 Deca Durabolin R and parenteral nutrition in post traumatic patients. Acta Endocrinologica 110 (suppl 271): 60–69
28. Martin M F, Brabant G V, Forse R A, Shizgal H M 1985 Efficacy of anabolic steroids in patients receiving total parenteral nutrition. Surgical Forum 36: 42–45
29. Yule A G, Macfie J, Hill FL 1981. The effect of anabolic steroid on body composition in patients receiving intravenous nutrition. Australian and New Zealand Journal of Surgery 51: 280–284
30. Kalliomäki J L, Markkanen T K, Pirilä A M, Ruikka I Norandrostenolone decanoate — a new anabolic steroid with prolonged effect. Annals Medicine Internal Fennicae 50: 177–84
31. Page C W 1962 The treatment of debility: a controlled experience. Paper presented at the Symposium on Anabolic Therapy held by the Michigan and Wayne County Academies of General Practise, Detroit, Michigan March 21 pp 71–83
32. Martins J K 1965 Clinical; evaluation of an anabolic agent, nandrolone decanoate. Clinical Medicine 72: 844–850
33. Johnson Jr J P C 1962 Weight gain in geriatric patients. Paper presented at the Symposium on Anabolic Therapy held by the Michigan and Wayne County Academies of General Practise, Detroit Michigan March 21 pp 85–95
34. Berkowitz D 1962 Anabolic agents in gastroenterology. Paper presented at the Symposium on Anabolic Therapy held by the Michigan and Wayne County Academies of General Practise, Detroit, Michigan March 21 pp 105–114
35. Editorial 1977 Androgens in the anaemia of chronic renal failure. British Medical Journal 2: 417–418
36. Lindholm B 1967 Body cell mass during long-term treatment with cortisone and anabolic steroids in asthmatic subjects. Acta Endocrinologica 55: 222–239
37. Cohen J C, Faber W M, Bernade A J S, Noakes T D 1986 Altered serum lipoprotein profiles in male and female power lifters ingesting anabolic steroids. Physician and Sports Medicine 14: 131–136
38. Bertolini S, Maglio M L, Seriolo B et al 1985 Interferences of three slow-release anabolic steroids in lipoprotein metabolism. Paper presented at the fourth European Symposium on Metabolism held at Padua, Italy May 27–29
39. Hassager C, Podenphant J, Riis B J, Johansen J S, Jensen J, Christiansen C 1989 Changes in soft tissue body composition and plasma lipid metabolism during nandrolone decanoate therapy in postmenopausal osteoporotic women. Metabolism 38: 238–242
40. Naik R B, Gibbons A R, Gyde O H B, Harris B R 1978 Androgen trial in renal anaemia. Proceedings of the European Dialysis and Transplant Association 15: 136–143
41. Teruel J L, Quereda C, Martin E, Orofino L, Liano F, Ortuno J 1983 Androgen therapy in nonferropenic patients on hemodialysis. Kidney International 24: 269
42. Carrasco D, Prieto M, Pallardo L et al 1985 Multiple hepatic adenomas after long-term therapy with testosterone enanthate. Journal of Hepatology 1: 573–578
43. Turani H, Levi J, Zevin D, Kessler E 1983 Hepatic lesions in patients on anabolic androgenic therapy. Israel Journal of Medical Sciences 19: 332–337
44. Gordon G S 1976 Cancer in Man. In: Kochakian C D (ed) Anabolic–androgenic steroids. Springer-Verlag, Berlin, ch VII D, pp 499–513
45. Cole M P, Todd I D, Wilkinson P M 1973 Cyclophosphamide and nandrolone decanoate in the treatment of advanced carcinoma of the breast: results of a comparative controlled trial of the agents used singly and in combination. British Journal of Cancer 27: 396–399

N Naproxen

Naproxen is a derivative of propionic acid which inhibits the cyclo-oxygenase enzyme and is widely used to treat patients with rheumatic diseases. In controlled clinical trials naproxen was found to be of comparable potency to aspirin and to other non-steroidal anti-inflammatory drugs, including ibuprofen, indomethacin, fenoprofen, ketoprofen and diclofenac.

Chemistry

Naproxen (Naprosyn); Naproxen sodium (Anaprox)
$C_{14}H_{14}O_3$
(d)-6-Methoxy-α-methyl-2-naphthalene acetic acid

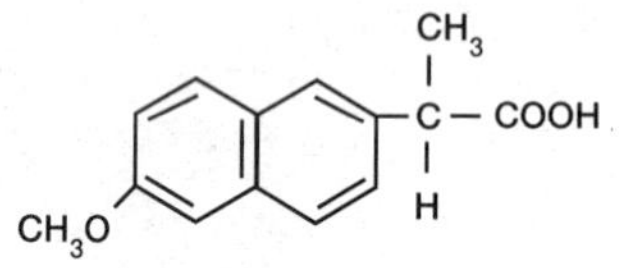

Molecular weight (sodium salt)	230.25 (252.2)
pKa (COOH)	4.39
Solubility	
in alcohol	1 in 25 (>1 in 100)
in water	<1 in 10 000 (>1 in 30)
Octanol/water partition coefficient	1514

Naproxen is a white or off-white odourless crystalline powder with a bitter taste. It is prepared by chemical synthesis and only the dextrorotatory isomer is pharmacologically active and used clinically.

Pharmacology

Naproxen reduces the synthesis of prostaglandins primarily by inhibiting the enzyme cyclo-oxygenase. Naproxen is approximately 20 times as potent in this regard as aspirin. Naproxen has been shown to have anti-inflammatory activity in a number of experimental models. It is anti-inflammatory in the carrageenin-induced paw oedema model, in cotton pellet granuloma formation in rats and adjuvant-induced arthritis in rats. Naproxen inhibits prostaglandin E_2 synthesis in vitro by human rheumatoid synovial microsomes. It also inhibits prostaglandin E_2 production by phytohaemagglutin-stimulated peripheral blood mononuclear cells. At 10^{-4} M (23 mg.l^{-1}) naproxen inhibits neutral protease activity derived from human polymorphonuclear leucocytes. Naproxen also inhibits in vitro the activity of cathepsin-β and other hydrolytic enzymes derived from lysosomes.[1] Naproxen is a potent inhibitor of leucocyte migration and produces effects comparable to those of colchicine.

Toxicology

Naproxen does not have mutagenic potential. It causes gastric erosions when given orally or subcutaneously to fasting rats. There is no evidence of carcinogenicity in tests lasting up to two years in rats, and no evidence of teratogenicity in mice, rats or rabbits.

Clinical pharmacology

Naproxen has useful anti-inflammatory, analgesic and antipyretic activity in man. At a dose of 7.5 mg.kg^{-1} in children, it has similar antipyretic activity to 15 mg.kg^{-1} of aspirin. Naproxen inhibits collagen-induced platelet aggregation and thus the bleeding time may be prolonged. It causes salt and water retention by the kidney through the reduced intrarenal synthesis of prostaglandin E_2 which has local vasodilatory activity. The same mechanism may lead to a deterioration in renal function in patients whose kidney function is dependent on local prostaglandin E_2. The effect on leucocyte migration may have some clinical importance since this effect is seen at concentrations of naproxen readily achievable with standard dosage.

Pharmacokinetics

Naproxen can be analysed by high pressure liquid chromatography which has a sensitivity of 2 μg.l^{-1} in plasma and 50 μg.l^{-1} in urine.[2]

Naproxen is completely absorbed from the gut after oral administration, with no presystemic metabolism, and peak plasma concentrations are seen at about 2 hours in fasted subjects.[3] It is also well absorbed after rectal administration. The rate of absorption is diminished by the concomitant administration of food or antacids; however, the overall area under the plasma level time curve remains similar. The plasma half life is between 12 and 15 hours. Plasma levels rise proportionately with dosage after oral administration of up to 500 mg, but thereafter the increase is less than linear. This is due to a disproportionate increase in excretion rates following saturation of plasma protein binding. Concomitant administration of probenecid results in a 50% increase in steady-state naproxen concentration and a 5.3 hour increase in half life. These changes are accompanied by a significant (66%) decrease in the urinary excretion of unmetabolized naproxen and naproxen conjugates and an increase in excretion of the inactive metabolite 6-O-desmethylnaproxen.

The half life of naproxen in the plasma of children aged more than 1 year is similar to that in adults; no data are available for children of less than one year. The unbound plasma fraction of naproxen is increased in the elderly, although total plasma concentrations of the drug are unchanged. In renal failure, free naproxen levels remain largely unchanged; free naproxen excretion by the kidneys falls but this is counterbalanced by increased metabolism of naproxen to its inactive metabolite 6-O-desmethylnaproxen. This metabolite of naproxen is dialysed although the parent drug is not.

The drug is highly bound to albumin (>99%), resulting in a volume of distribution of only 0.9 l.kg^{-1}. Binding to albumin is reduced in cirrhosis and in the elderly. Synovial fluid concentrations of naproxen increase from 50% of serum levels at three to four hours, to 74% at 15 hours. It crosses the placenta within 20 to 30 minutes of oral administration, and appears in the milk of lactating women at approximately 1% of maternal plasma concentrations.

Oral absorption	100%
Presystemic metabolism	<5%
Plasma half life	
range	12–15 h
Volume of distribution	0.9 l.kg^{-1}
Plasma protein binding	>99%

Concentration–effect relationship

Naproxen shows increased therapeutic activity as the dose is increased up to 1500 mg daily. However, it is difficult to show any clear correlation between the plasma concentration of naproxen and its therapeutic effects. There is a clear correlation between the plasma concentration of naproxen and the decrease in prostaglandin $F_{2\alpha}$ production by platelets.[4] In patients with rheumatoid arthritis, those who have higher levels of naproxen in the plasma have a better therapeutic response than those patients who have lower levels of the drug. However, the variability of the response is so great that this information is of little help in clinical practice.

Metabolism

Naproxen is extensively metabolised in the liver. Excretion is almost entirely via the kidneys (97.5%–99%) with only a very small percentage excreted in the faeces. Less than 10% of the dose is excreted unchanged. Two primary pathways of metabolism have been described, demethylation at the 6-methoxy position and glucuronic acid conjugation.

Naproxen is eliminated in the urine primarily as the conjugated glucuronide of naproxen (60%) or as the unchanged drug (10%).

30% of naproxen undergoes hepatic demethylation at the 6-methoxy position and is excreted as 6-O-desmethylnaproxen or its conjugates. The metabolic products of naproxen appear to be pharmacologically inactive.

Pharmaceutics

Naproxen (Naprosyn Syntex, UK/USA) is available as tablets, suppositories, suspension or granules.

1. A round, scored, buff-coloured, low excipient tablet containing 250 mg of naproxen, inscribed 'Naproxen 250' on one side and 'Syntex' on the other
2. An oval, scored, pink, low excipient tablet containing 375 mg of naproxen, inscribed 'Naprosyn 375' on one side and 'Syntex' on the other
3. An oblong, scored, buff-coloured, low excipient tablet containing 500 mg of naproxen, inscribed 'Naprosyn 500' on one side and 'Syntex' on the other
4. A more rapidly absorbed sodium salt is available as Anaprox (Syntex, USA). The ovoid, pale-blue tablets contain 275 mg naproxen sodium, equivalent to 250 mg naproxen. They are inscribed '274' and 'Syntex'. In the UK, naproxen sodium is available as Synflex (Syntex, UK), an opaque, orange, film-coated oval tablet marked 'Syntex' on one face, containing naproxen sodium 275 mg (equivalent to naproxen 250 mg)
5. Suppositories each containing 500 mg naproxen
6. A flavoured orange suspension containing 25 $mg.ml^{-1}$ naproxen
7. A dry powder formulation containing 500 mg naproxen to be dispersed in water to form a flavoured suspension.

Therapeutic use

Indications

1. Rheumatic diseases — for anti-inflammatory and analgesic action in rheumatoid arthritis, juvenile chronic arthritis, osteoarthritis, ankylosing spondylitis, gout
2. Periarticular and musculoskeletal indications — for analgesia in bursitis, tendinitis, synovitis, tenosynovitis, lumbago
3. Prophylaxis and treatment of migraine headache
4. Surgical and traumatic uses — for analgesic action for sports injuries, orthopaedic manipulations, dental extractions, surgery
5. Infectious diseases — for analgesic, anti-inflammatory and anti-pyretic purposes
6. Gynaecological uses — in dysmenorrhoea, following IUCD insertion and for uterine relaxation and analgesia in the post-partum non-nursing mother.

Contraindications

1. Patients with a history of asthma, rhinitis or urticaria induced by aspirin or other non-steroidal anti-inflammatory drugs
2. Peptic ulceration
3. Hypersensitivity to naproxen or naproxen sodium.

N

Mode of use

Oral treatment is usually begun with 250–500 mg of naproxen given orally twice daily. A total dose of 1500 mg daily has been given in a number of studies but there is no evidence for increasing therapeutic benefit above this dose. For most indications the maximum benefit of the drug is seen within a few days; however, a trial of two weeks is probably justified in inflammatory rheumatic diseases. The drug may be stopped suddenly or substituted with an equivalent dose of an alternative non-steroidal anti-inflammatory drug without adverse effects.

Indications

1. Rheumatic diseases

Rheumatoid arthritis. Several controlled studies[5] have shown naproxen to have comparable anti-inflammatory and analgesic properties to 4 g daily of aspirin or to 150 mg daily of indomethacin.[5] Naproxen is usually administered twice daily in a dose titrated between 375 mg and 1000 mg daily according to the clinical response. Doses of 1500 mg daily have been administered without adverse effects.[7,8] A nocturnal dose may alleviate nocturnal pain and reduce morning stiffness. A two-week trial is sufficient to establish any benefit from the drug. No study has conclusively shown which is the non-steroidal anti-inflammatory drug of choice in rheumatoid arthritis. Variability in response seems idiosyncratic and is not related to measurable pharmacological parameters. There is no clear evidence for additional benefit from concurrent medication with naproxen and other non-steroidal anti-inflammatory drugs such as non-acetylated salicylate.[8]

Juvenile chronic arthritis. Trials have suggested that naproxen is as effective as soluble aspirin.[9] A dose of 10 $mg.kg^{-1}$ daily in two divided doses is usual, although 15 $mg.kg^{-1}$ daily has been used.

Ankylosing spondylitis. Naproxen is of similar potency to indomethacin and phenylbutazone in the treatment of ankylosing spondylitis.

Osteoarthritis. Naproxen was shown to have greater activity than placebo and comparable activity to aspirin[10] and indomethacin[11] in the management of pain associated with osteoarthritis.

Acute gout. A dose-ranging study in acute gout showed that a loading dose of 750 mg followed by 250 mg every eight hours was associated with rapid resolution of pain and tenderness.[12,13] Various other regimes have been used with initial doses varying between 375 mg and 1 g followed by 250 mg every eight hours. In one study, patients who had experienced many previous attacks of gout generally responded less than those who had had few attacks.

2. Periarticular and musculoskeletal indications

Naproxen has similar activities to other non-steroidal drugs in the management of bursitis, tendonitis, synovitis, tenosynovitis and lumbago. In a non-placebo-controlled study, diclofenac and naproxen had similar activities in alleviating the effects of soft tissue rheumatic complaints apart from lesions around the shoulder where diclofenac 75 mg was more effective than naproxen 500 mg.[14]

Fig. 1 The metabolism of naproxen

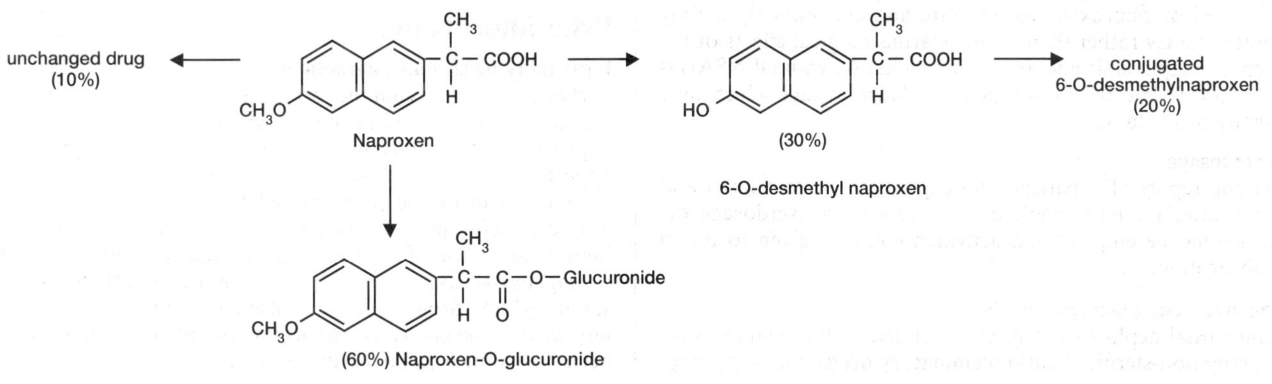

3. Prophylaxis and treatment of migraine headache
Several studies have shown the effectiveness of naproxen and other non-steroidal anti-inflammatory drugs as prophylactic agents in the prevention of migraine headaches. One double-blind, placebo-controlled study observed the effect of naproxen sodium, given at a dose of 550 mg twice daily, in the prophylaxis of migrainous headaches in 34 patients with frequent headaches.[15] There was a significant reduction in headache severity, duration and concomitant medication during the active phase of treatment.

4. Surgical and traumatic uses
Naproxen has been used in studies of the relief of postoperative pain after dental, orthopaedic and general surgical procedures. Naproxen 400 mg was more effective than acetylsalicylic acid 325 mg plus codeine 30 mg after dental surgery[16] and equivalent to meperidine 75 mg after a variety of other surgical procedures. In this study remedication was frequently required after the administration of naproxen, suggesting that it was only acting as a moderately potent analgesic.[17] Pain arising from sporting injuries may be relieved by naproxen 750 mg daily.

5. Antipyretic uses
In a study of fever due to a variety of causes (mainly upper respiratory tract infections) in children aged between 3 and 12, naproxen 7.5 $mg.kg^{-1}$ given as a single dose had a similar antipyretic effect[18] to aspirin 15 $mg.kg^{-1}$. Naproxen had a greater antipyretic effect in patients with pyrexia due to Hodgkin's disease than in patients with pyrexias due to Hodgkin's disease with superadded infection.[19]

6. Gynaecological uses
Controlled studies have been published showing that naproxen provides symptomatic relief in primary and secondary dysmenorrhoea,[20] and pain associated with IUCD insertion, suction curettage and postpartum uterine pain.[21] The activity of naproxen for these indications is comparable with that of other non-steroidal anti-inflammatory drugs including diflunisal, indomethacin and ibuprofen.

Contraindications

1. Bronchospasm
Patients with rhinitis, nasal polyps and asthma associated with aspirin may show cross-sensitivity with other non-steroidal anti-inflammatory drugs including naproxen.

2. Peptic ulceration
Naproxen causes a slight increase in faecal occult blood loss but is relatively infrequently associated with peptic ulceration. It should, nevertheless, be used with great caution in patients with a history of peptic ulceration and should not be used in patients with active peptic ulceration.

3. Severe renal impairment
The fall in glomerular blood flow induced by naproxen and other non-steroidal anti-inflammatory drugs may precipitate irreversible renal failure in patients with pre-existing severe impairment of renal function.

Adverse reactions

Potentially life-threatening effects
Deaths caused by naproxen are very rare and are probably mainly due to idiosyncrasy rather than to the pharmacological effects of the drug such as anaphylaxis and aplastic anaemia. As with all NSAIDs there is a risk of intestinal ulceration and haemorrhage which may occasionally prove fatal.

Acute overdosage
There is one report of a patient who experienced mild nausea and indigestion after taking a single dose of 25 g.[21] In overdosage the stomach should be emptied and activated charcoal given to try to reduce absorption.

Severe or irreversible adverse effects
Acute interstitial nephritis has been associated with the administration of many non-steroidal anti-inflammatory drugs, including naproxen.[23] This may be accompanied by sufficient proteinuria to cause the nephrotic syndrome.[24] Patients with renal impairment, cardiac failure or hepatic cirrhosis may show a reversible decline in renal function due to a reduction in glomerular blood flow secondary to a reduction in intrarenal vasodilatory prostaglandin synthesis.[25,26] Rare adverse effects associated with the administration of naproxen include anaphylactic reactions, hepatitis, haemolytic anaemia, aplastic anaemia, granulocytopenia, and pseudoporphyria.[27]

Symptomatic adverse effects
Central nervous system. Naproxen is generally well tolerated compared with other non-steroidal anti-inflammatory drugs. Headache, dizziness, drowsiness and tinnitus are the most commonly reported effects. Less frequent are light-headedness, vertigo, and hearing and visual disturbances. Cognitive dysfunction, depression, malaise and dream abnormalities are rare. All of these effects are more common in patients taking higher doses of naproxen.
Gastrointestinal. Gastrointestinal disturbance is common,[28] but occurs less frequently than in patients taking 3.6–4.0 g of aspirin or 150 mg of indomethacin. Heartburn, abdominal pain, nausea and constipation are most frequently reported, with dyspepsia, stomatitis and diarrhoea occurring less frequently. In the United Kingdom 332.8 serious gastrointestinal reactions per million prescriptions were reported to the Committee on Safety of Medicines, a rate comparable with the majority of non-steroidal anti-inflammatory drugs.[29]

Other effects
Non-steroidal anti-inflammatory drugs have been associated with a fall in creatinine clearance. This is discussed above under Severe or irreversible adverse effects.

Interference with clinical pathology tests
Naproxen administration may lead to artefactual elevation in the measured urinary concentrations of 17-ketogenic steroids and of 5-hydroxyindoleacetic acid using certain assays. This may be obviated by stopping naproxen for 48 hours before the collection of urine for measurement of these metabolites.

High risk groups

Neonates
There is very little information on treatment of this group of subjects and naproxen is not recommended.
Breast milk. Naproxen is excreted in the breast milk of nursing mothers and should be avoided in lactating women, although the amounts in breast milk are small.

Children
The drug is not recommended for use in children, other than those over 5 years of age with juvenile rheumatoid arthritis.

Pregnant women
Most non-steroidal anti-inflammatory drugs may have an adverse effect on the fetus through their pharmacological properties. Naproxen causes a delay in parturition in animals and has been associated with premature closure of the ductus arteriosus and severe pulmonary hypertension in infants born to mothers taking naproxen.[30]

The elderly
The unbound fraction of naproxen is increased in elderly subjects and naproxen should be used at reduced dosage.[31] Naproxen should be avoided in elderly subjects with cardiac, renal or hepatic failure.

Drug interactions

Potentially hazardous interactions
Warfarin. Although the serum free fraction of warfarin in vitro is increased after the concomitant administration of warfarin and naproxen,[32] the effect may not be important. Naproxen has no apparent effect on the steady-state serum concentrations of free or total warfarin or the prothrombin time. However, since naproxen interferes with platelet function,[33] and may cause peptic ulcers. Simultaneous use of the two drugs should be monitored closely.
Sulphonylureas. Although there is a theoretical risk of displacing sulphonylurea drugs from their protein binding sites, the effect does not seem to be clinically important. No pharmacological effect has been shown in patients taking tolbutamide.

Naproxen

Phenytoin. Plasma phenytoin levels may be increased in patients receiving naproxen and should be closely monitored.

Beta-blockers. Naproxen may reduce the antihypertensive effect of β-blockers and diuretics.

Lithium. Increases in plasma lithium concentration have been reported because of an inhibition of renal lithium excretion.

Other significant interactions

Antacids. Antacids which increase the aqueous solubility of naproxen enhance its absorption rate. In contrast, the concomitant administration of naproxen with magnesium oxide or with aluminium hydroxide significantly reduces the absorption of naproxen.[34] Commercial magnesium/aluminium hydroxide gel reduces the time taken to reach peak naproxen plasma levels.

Probenecid. Probenecid induces marked alterations in the metabolism and excretion of naproxen.[35] The net effect is of a marked decrease in urinary excretion of native naproxen and an increase inurinary 6-O-desmethylnaproxen. The half life of naproxen increased from 14 to 37 hours following a single dose of 500 mg of naproxen given to subjects receiving regular probenecid.

Methotrexate. Fatal toxicity has been reported in patients receiving high-dose methotrexate in conjunction with a number of non-steroidal anti-inflammatory drugs including naproxen.[34] A patient who mistakenly took 23.5 mg of methotrexate whilst taking naproxen died. The mode of action of non-steroidal anti-inflammatory drugs in causing this effect is not certain, but may be via inhibition of the tubular secretion of methotrexate.

Frusemide. Like other non-steroidal anti-inflammatory drugs, naproxen slightly inhibits the sodium diuresis induced by frusemide.

Potentially useful interactions

No interactions of this kind have been reported.

Clinical Trials

1. Henzl M R, Buttram V, Segre E J, Bessler S 1977 The treatment of dysmenorrhoea with naproxen sodium. A report of two independent double-blind trials. American Journal of Obstetrics and Gynecology 127: 818

2. Bowers D E, Dyer H R, Fosdick W M et al 1975 A controlled trial of naproxen in rheumatoid arthritis. Annals of Internal Medicine 83, 4: 470

3. Furst D E, Block A K, Cassell S et al 1987 A controlled study of concurrent therapy with a nonacetylated salicylate and naproxen in rheumatoid arthritis. Arthritis and Rheumatism 30: 146–154

4. Barnes C G, Goodman H V, Eade A W 1975 A double-blind comparison of naproxen with indomethacin in osteoarthritis. Journal of Clinical Pharmacology 15: 347–354

General review articles

Brogden R N, Heel R C, Speight T M, Avery G S 1979 Naproxen up to date: a review of its pharmacological properties and therapeutic efficacy and use in rheumatic diseases and pain states. Drugs 18: 241–277

Dumas K (ed) 1973 Naproxen. Scandinavian Journal of Rheumatology (suppl 2)

Segre E J 1979 Naproxen. Clinics in Rheumatic Diseases 5: 411–426

References

1. Kruze D, Fehr K, Menninger H, Boni A 1976 Effect of anti-rheumatic drugs on neutral protease from human leucocyte granules. Zeitschrift fur Rheumatologie 35: 337
2. Upton R A, Buskin J N, Guentert T W, Williams R L, Riegelman S 1980 Convenient and sensitive high-performance liquid chromatography assay for ketoprofen, naproxen and other allied drugs in plasma and urine. Journal of Chromatography 190: 119–128
3. Runkel R, Chaplin M, Boost G, Segre E, Forchielli E 1972 Absorption, distribution, metabolism and excretion of naproxen in various laboratory animals and human subjects. Journal of Pharmaceutical Sciences 61: 703–708
4. Tomson G, Lunell N-O, Oliw E, Rane A 1981 Relation of naproxen kinetics to effect on platelet prostaglandin release in man and dysmenorrhoea in women. Clinical Pharmacology and Therapeutics 29: 168–173
5. Bowers D E, Dyer H R, Fosdick W M et al 1975 A controlled trial of naproxen in rheumatoid arthritis. Annals of Internal Medicine 83, 4: 470
6. Castles J J, Moore T J, Vaughan J H et al 1978 Multicenter comparison of naproxen and indomethacin in rheumatoid arthritis. Archives of Internal Medicine 138: 362
7. Day R O, Furst D E, Dromgoole S H, Damm B, Roe R, Paulus H E 1982 Relationship of serum naproxen concentration to efficacy in rheumatoid arthritis. Clinical Pharmacology and Therapeutics 31: 733–740
8. Furst D E, Block A K, Cassell S et al 1987 A controlled study of concurrent therapy with a nonacetylated salicylate and naproxen in rheumatoid arthritis. Arthritis and Rheumatism 30: 146–154
9. Moran H, Hanna D B, Ansell B M, Hall M, Engler C 1979 Naproxen in juvenile chronic polyarthritis. Annals of Rheumatic Diseases 38: 152
10. Melton J W, Lussier A, Ward J R, Neustadt D, Multz C 1978 Naproxen vs aspirin in osteoarthritis of the hip and knee. Journal of Rheumatology 5: 338–346
11. Barnes C G, Goodman H V, Eade A W 1975 A double-blind comparison of naproxen with indomethacin in osteoarthritis. Journal of Clinical Pharmacology 15: 347–354
12. Wilkens R F, Case J B, Huix F J 1975 The treatment of acute gout with naproxen. Journal of Clinical Pharmacology 15: 363–366
13. Sturge R A, Scott J T, Hamilton E B D et al 1977 Multicentre trial of naproxen and phenylbutazone in acute gout. Annals of the Rheumatic Diseases 36: 80–82
14. Valtonen E J 1978 A comparative short-term trial with voltaren (diclofenac sodium) and naproxen in soft-tissue rheumatism. Scandinavian Journal of Rheumatology (suppl 22): 69
15. Ziegler D K, Ellis D J 1985 Naproxen in prophylaxis of migraine. Archives of Neurology 42: 582–584
16. Ruedy J 1973 A comparison of the analgesic efficacy of naproxen and acetylsalicylic acid–codeine in patients with pain after dental surgery. Scandinavian Journal of Rheumatology (suppl 2): 60–63
17. Stetson J B, Robinson K, Wardell W, Lasagna L 1973 Analgesic activity of oral naproxen in patients with postoperative pain. Scandinavian Journal of Rheumatology (suppl 2): 50–55
18. Cashman T M, Starns R J, Johnson J, Oren J 1979 Comparable effects of naproxen and aspirin on fever in children. Journal of Pediatrics 95: 626–629
19. Geisler C, Gotzche P C, Schadehansen S, Juul K, Plesner A M, Nissen N I 1985 Naproxen has greater antipyretic effect on Hodgkin's disease-related fever than on other tumours or infection. Scandinavian Journal of Haematology 35: 325–328
20. Henzl M R, Buttram V, Segre E J, Bessler S 1977 The treatment of dysmenorrhoea with naproxen sodium. A report of two independent double-blind trials. American Journal of Obstetrics and Gynecology 127: 818
21. Edgren R A, Morton C J 1986 Naproxen sodium for ob/gyn use, with special reference to pain states: a review. International Journal of Fertility 31 (2): 135–142
22. Fredell E W, Strand L J 1977 Naproxen overdose. Journal of the American Medical Association 238: 938
23. Clive D N, Stoff J S 1984 Renal syndrome associated with nonsteroidal anti-inflammatory drugs. New England Journal of Medicine 310: 563–572
24. Brezin J H, Katz S M, Schwartz A B, Chinitz J L 1979 Reversible renal failure and nephrotic syndrome associated with nonsteroidal anti-inflammatory drugs. New England Journal of Medicine 301: 1271–1273
25. Kimberly R P, Bowden R E, Keiser H R, Plotz P H 1978 Reduction of renal function by newer non-steroidal anti-inflammatory drugs. American Journal of Medicine 64: 804–807
26. Brater D C, Anderson S, Baird B, Campbell W B 1983 Effects of ibuprofen, naproxen and sulindac on prostaglandins in men. Kidney International 27: 66–73
27. Judd L E, Henderson D W, Hill D C 1986 Naproxen-induced pseudoporphyria. Archives of Dermatology 122: 451–454
28. Pemberton R E, Strand L J 1979 A review of upper gastrointestinal effects of the new nonsteroidal anti-inflammatory agents. American Journal of Digestive Diseases 24: 53–64
29. Anon 1986 CSM update: non-steroidal anti-inflammatory drugs and serious gastrointestinal adverse reactions — 2. British Medical Journal 292: 1190–1191
30. Wilkinson A R, Aynsley-Green A, Mitchell M D 1979 Persistence of pulmonary hypertension and abnormal prostaglandin levels in preterm infants after maternal treatment with naproxen. Archives of Disease in Childhood 54: 942–945
31. Upton R A, Williams R L, Kelly J, Jones R M 1984 Naproxen pharmacokinetics in the elderly. British Journal of Clinical Pharmacology 18: 207–214
32. Jain A, McMahon F G, Slattery J T, Levy G 1979 Effect of naproxen on the steady-state serum concentration and anti-coagulant activity of warfarin. Clinical Pharmacology and Therapeutics 25: 61
33. Nadell J, Bruno J, Varady J, Segre E J 1974 Effect of naprosyn and aspirin on bleeding time and platelet aggregation. Journal of Clinical Pharmacology 14: 176
34. Singh R R, Malaviya A N, Pandey J N, Guleria J S 1986 Fatal interaction between methotrexate and naproxen. Lancet 1: 1390
35. Segre E J, Sevelius H, Varady J 1974 Effects of antacids on naproxen absorption. New England Journal of Medicine 291: 582
36. Runkel R, Mroszczak E, Chaplin M, Sevelius H, Segre E 1978 Naproxen–probenecid interaction. Clinical Pharmacology and Therapeutics 24: 706–713

Nedocromil sodium

Nedocromil sodium inhibits the release of inflammatory mediators from a range of cells found in the bronchi under certain pathological conditions.[1] Although preliminary research indicates that nedocromil sodium may also affect nerves,[2–4] the precise mechanism of action of this compound is not known. Nedocromil sodium is used for the regular prophylactic treatment, as opposed to symptomatic relief, of reversible obstructive airways diseases exemplified by asthma.

Chemistry

Nedocromil sodium (Tilade)
$C_{19}H_{15}N\ Na_2O_7$
Disodium 9-ethyl-6,9-dihydro-4,6-dioxo-10-propyl-4H-pyrano(3,2-g) quinoline-2,8-dicarboxylate

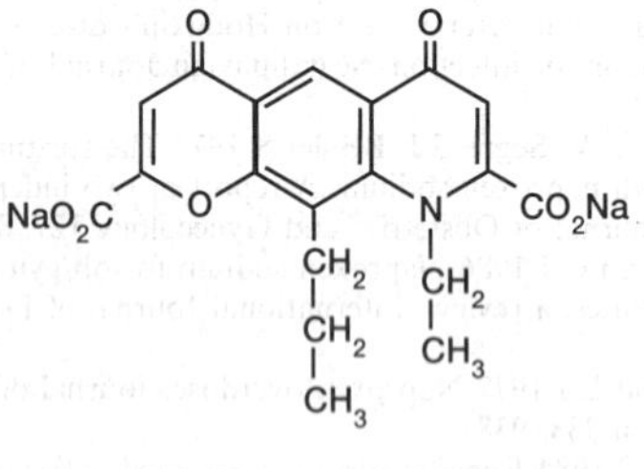

Molecular weight	415.3
pKa_1, pKa_2	0.95, 1.99
Solubility	
in alcohol	1 in 410
in water	1 in 40
Octanol/water partition coefficient	log $D_{7.4}$ 9.1

Nedocromil was identified from a series of chemically synthesized 4,6-dioxopyranoquinolines[5] and the disodium salt, a pale yellow powder, is used clinically.

Pharmacology

In vitro, nedocromil sodium inhibits the activation of (IC_{50} 5×10^{-9} M)[6] and release of mediators from eosinophils (10^{-4} M)[7] and neutrophils (10^{-5} M).[8] The release of preformed and newly synthesized mediators from mast cells lavaged from the macaque model is inhibited by nedocromil sodium (IC_{30} antigen challenge: histamine 2.1×10^{-6} M, LTC_4 2.3×10^{-6} M and PGD_2 1.9×10^{-6} M).[9] Similar results have been found with rodent[10] and human lung mast cells.[11] Nedocromil sodium also inhibits the IgE-mediated activation of mononuclear phagocytes and platelets from rat[12] and man.[13]

In the subhuman primate model of bronchoconstriction (the macaque model), nebulized nedocromil sodium (approximately 4 mg) inhibits the antigen-induced changes in airway resistance and lung compliance.[14] Nedocromil sodium (20 mg) inhibits both the early and late response to antigen in the allergic sheep model[15] and blocked the associated increase in airway responsiveness.[16] In vivo, 2% nedocromil sodium inhibits citric acid-induced cough in conscious dogs[2] and the increase in bronchial reactivity in dogs exposed to sulphur dioxide.[17] The reduction in bronchial reactivity is associated with a reduction in the accumulation of neutrophils in the lavage fluid.[18] Nedocromil sodium (0.2–2.0 $mM.kg^{-1}$) inhibits the increase in lung resistance induced by adenosine in the rat.[4] In a sensitized guinea-pig model, nedocromil sodium (100 $\mu g.kg^{-1}$ intravenously) reduced the increase in pulmonary vascular permeability induced by ovalbumin challenge.[19] Nedocromil sodium is also effective in classical models of antiallergic activity (passive cutaneous anaphylaxis and passive lung anaphylaxis in the rat; ID_{50} 2.2 $mg.kg^{-1}$ and 0.9 $mg.kg^{-1}$, respectively).[20]

Toxicology

Extensive toxicological testing in animals using inhaled and systemic routes of administration has failed to demonstrate any results of potential clinical relevance.[21]

Clinical pharmacology

Nedocromil sodium has no significant bronchodilator action. Nedocromil sodium is effective in patients with antigen[22,25–27] and exercise-induced bronchoconstriction.[23,24,28–30] Doses of nedocromil sodium of 0.5, 1.0 or 2 mg significantly reduced the immediate fall in pulmonary function following antigen challenge, attenuating the fall in FEV_1[25–27] and FVC[25] by 50% and 63%, respectively. Administration of nedocromil sodium 2–3 hours before challenge[25–27] suggested that clinically significant protection may last several hours.

After exercise challenge 4 or 8 mg doses of nedocromil sodium have been shown to be significantly more effective than 1.0 mg, the higher doses reducing the mean maximum percentage fall in PEFR to 15% and 22%, respectively.[28] Pretreatment with 2 mg nedocromil sodium led to a mean maximum percentage fall in FEV_1 of 10% compared with a greater than 30% fall in placebo-treated patients.[30] This protective effect of nedocromil sodium is seen in children[23] and teenagers[29] as well as in adult patients.[30] In comparative exercise challenge studies with sodium cromoglycate, nedocromil sodium shows similar efficacy, although there are minor differences owing to the doses used.[24,31,32]

Using metabisulphite or sulphur dioxide to induce a fall in airway conductance, nedocromil sodium is significantly more effective than oxitropium bromide[33] or sodium cromoglycate.[33,34] Nedocromil sodium completely inhibited the induced bronchoconstriction after the maximum dose (120 μmol) of metabisulphite (PD_{35} 49.9 μmol and 27 μmol for sodium cromoglycate and oxitropium bromide, respectively). Nedocromil sodium also protects against the bronchoconstriction produced by fog,[35] hyperventilation of cold air[36] and inhaled adenosine.[37,38] These studies have shown nedocromil sodium to be more potent and more effective than sodium cromoglycate in extrinsic and intrinsic asthma patients.

Pharmacokinetics

A large proportion of the dose of a drug administered by inhalation is deposited in the oropharyngeal region and swallowed.[39,40] Hence the study of the pharmacokinetics of a drug administered by inhalation involves the measurement of plasma and urine concentrations after both oral dosing and inhalation. A comparison with data obtained from intravenous dosing allows the determination of the extent of absorption from the lungs and the fate of the drug once absorbed.[41]

Plasma and urinary concentrations of nedocromil sodium, measured using a sensitive radioimmunoassay[42] (limit of detection, 0.25 $\mu g.l^{-1}$), have been determined after separate oral, inhaled and intravenous administration to healthy volunteers.[41] Dosing schedules were 1 $mg.kg^{-1}$ orally, single (2×2 mg) and multiple dose (2×2 mg four times daily for seven days) by inhalation and slow intravenous infusion of 0.2 $\mu g.kg^{-1}.min^{-1}$ for 30 minutes.

A peak plasma concentration of 13.7 ± 1.3 $\mu g.l^{-1}$ occurred at the end of the intravenous infusion. Plasma levels then fell biphasically, and, following an initial rapid fall ($t_{\frac{1}{2}\alpha}$ 5 min) β nedocromil sodium was not detectable at 6 hours ($t_{\frac{1}{2}\beta}$ 54 min).[43] Clearance (10.2 ± 1.3 $ml.min^{-1}.kg^{-1}$) from the plasma was high owing largely to rapid elimination; 88% of the total urinary excretion (81% of the dose) occurred within 2 hours of the start of the infusion. Urinary excretion half life was subsequently 13.8 h.

Following inhalation of a single dose, the plasma concentration rose rapidly (15 min) to around 3 $\mu g.l^{-1}$, remained at this level for an hour and then declined. The half life (2.3 h) for this phase being longer than the β-phase after intravenous infusion. The results from the inhalation studies require a model with two absorption components, with the lower component being rate-limiting.

After multiple dosing by inhalation no accumulation was observed.[41]

Nedocromil sodium

Following oral administration, a peak plasma concentration of 5.8 μg.l^{-1} was reached one hour after dosing. There followed an initial rapid fall, then a much slower decline ($t_{\frac{1}{2}}$ 21 h). Oral absorption was low (bioavailability 2–3% of the dose) and had little influence on the plasma profile after administration by inhalation (bioavailability 7–9% of the dose).

Inhalation absorption	7–9%
Oral absorption	2–3%
Presystemic metabolism	nil
Plasma half life	
oral	21.1±2.4 h
inhalation	2.3±0.3 h
Volume of distribution	0.8 l.kg^{-1}
Plasma protein binding	80%

Concentration–effect relationship

There is no direct correlation between the plasma concentration of nedocromil sodium and its therapeutic effects. The effects are the result of local administration.

Metabolism

Studies in man used ^{14}C-labelled drug have shown no detectable metabolism of nedocromil sodium[41]. Nedocromil sodium is thus excreted unchanged in the urine; 80.7±3.0% after intravenous administration, 1.7±0.3% after oral administration and 5.6±1.0% after administration via inhalation.[41]

Pharmaceutics

Nedocromil sodium is available in the UK as TILADE (Fisons), a metered dose aerosol for administration by inhalation.

Each aerosol contains 112 inhalations of 2 mg nedocromil sodium per actuation. Nedocromil sodium is a pale yellow powder. The aerosol device is yellow in colour with a brown cover. The aerosol container is pressurized and must not be punctured or burnt even when empty.

In addition to the UK, TILADE is available in several other countries (France, The Netherlands, Italy, etc).

Therapeutic use

Indications

1. Management of reversible obstructive airways disease
2. Bronchial hyperresponsiveness.

Contraindications

There are no specific contraindications for the use of nedocromil sodium.

Mode of use

Nedocromil sodium is used in reversible obstructive airways disease including bronchial asthma, whether extrinsic or intrinsic; asthmatic bronchitis; late onset asthma; exercise-induced asthma and bronchospasm provoked by a variety of stimuli such as cold air, inhaled allergens, atmospheric pollutants and other irritants.

The drug improves pulmonary function, reduces the frequency and severity of attacks and reduces bronchospasm, cough and bronchial hyperreactivity. The clinical use of nedocromil sodium is governed by its preventive mode of action. Thus it does not provide immediate symptomatic relief in the same manner as a bronchodilator but is taken regularly to reduce the frequency and severity of respiratory symptoms and when taken prior to a challenge situation, for example exercise, to prevent attacks occurring. Nedocromil sodium is a preventive therapy; it will not relieve symptoms during an acute attack.

The recommended dose of nedocromil sodium is 4 mg (2×2 mg actuations) twice daily, increased to four times daily if necessary. At present nedocromil sodium is recommended only for adults and children over 12 years of age.

In common with any drug formulated as an aerosol for inhalation, the correct method of administration is crucial to the effectiveness of the therapy.[44] The patient should be taught to synchronize a slow deep inhalation through the mouth with the actuation of the aerosol. Head position (tilted slightly back), breath holding (for 10 seconds after the inhalation) and pausing prior to the second inhalation of drug will aid the correct deposition of the drug.

Nedocromil sodium has been given to patients also receiving other therapeutic agents used in the treatment of the reversible airways obstruction; inhaled and oral corticosteroids[45,46] and inhaled and oral bronchodilators, both β_2-agonists and methylxanthines.[47–49] No evidence of drug–drug interaction or a decrease in efficacy of the steroid or bronchodilator has been observed. The addition of nedocromil sodium to existing regimens frequently provides additional therapeutic benefit and can result in a reduction in concomitant therapy.[45,47]

N

Indications

1. Bronchial asthma

The clinical evaluation of an agent intended to exert long-term protective effects in the management of patients with chronic reversible airways obstruction, such as adult patients with chronic asthma, is complicated by the fact that virtually all such patients are maintained on regular bronchodilator therapy or on regular inhaled corticosteroid therapy plus inhaled bronchodilators 'as required' to relieve acute symptoms. When asthma is adequately controlled by such maintenance therapy it is difficult to demonstrate therapeutic benefit from the addition of a new preventive agent which does not exert short-term effects. The majority of efficacy studies have been of double-blind, placebo-controlled, group-comparative design where nedocromil sodium has been administered in conjunction with, and as a potential substitute for, existing regimens. Response to test treatments has been assessed by analysis of patient-generated data recorded on daily diary cards, by lung function tests and physician's examination at clinic visits.

Addition of nedocromil sodium to the therapy of patients maintained solely on inhaled or oral bronchodilators has resulted in significant improvements in day and night-time asthma and the symptoms of morning tightness and cough.[47,49,50] Although the patients assessed their symptoms on entry to the study as predominantly mild, night-time asthma and cough were reduced to half the baseline level of severity, concurrent with a 25% reduction in inhaled bronchodilator use.[47] Nedocromil sodium appeared to substitute completely for sustained-release theophylline preparations, with either a return to baseline levels[50] or a continued improvement[49] in symptom severity following their withdrawal.

A similar level of symptom control has been observed when nedocromil sodium has been added to inhaled corticosteroid therapy,[51] or when inhaled corticosteroids have been reduced prior to treatment;[52,53] with nedocromil sodium substituting largely for 330 μg daily inhaled corticosteroid.[52] Nedocromil sodium has compared favourably with inhaled corticosteroids (400 μg daily) for control of asthma symptoms under the scrutiny of direct comparative studies.[54,55] Experience has shown that nedocromil sodium can be used to reduce the total dose of steroid in inhaled corticosteroid-dependent patients[53,56] but any reduction in their use should be carried out gradually to avoid rebound deterioration.[57–59]

Significant improvements in twice or three times daily measurements of peak expiratory flow have occurred with nedocromil sodium. Treatment with nedocromil sodium resulted in increases of 23–70 l.min^{-1} after a reduction in inhaled corticosteroid[52,53,60] or bronchodilator therapy[48] and increases of approximately 25 l.min^{-1} when nedocromil sodium was added to maintenance therapy.[47,51]

Cosinor analysis[61] of morning, afternoon and evening peak expiratory flow measurements of patients treated with nedocromil sodium in addition to either bronchodilators[47] or a combination of inhaled corticosteroids and bronchodilators[62] has demonstrated an increase in the mean daily peak flow and a significant decrease in the diurnal (daily) variation.

Trends for or significant improvements in physician assessment of asthma severity have been monitored at clinic visits or by the end of several studies, irrespective of whether nedocromil sodium was added to existing therapy,[47,51,62] compared directly with inhaled corticosteroids[54] or existing maintenance therapies were reduced[45,48,49,53,60,63] The improvement in severity has been up to one point[49,51,54,60] on a five-point scale of severity.

2. Bronchial hyperresponsiveness

Nedocromil sodium, (4 mg) twice daily, significantly reduced the seasonal increase in responsiveness to histamine (PC_{10} FEV_1 and PC_{40} Vp_{30}) in grass pollen sensitive asthmatics[64] and at a dose of 4 mg four times daily in atopic grass pollen rhinitic patients.[65]

Chronic treatment with nedocromil sodium reduced the responsiveness of the airways to methacholine ($PD_{20}FEV_1$,[66–68] $PD_{15}FEV_1$[69]) to a similar extent to inhaled corticosteroids[66] but to a greater extent than sodium cromoglycate.[68] During the first phase of a crossover study comparing inhaled corticosteroids and nedocromil sodium both treatments reduced histamine responsiveness significantly[59]. Beclomethasone dipropionate alone reduced responsiveness after the crossover, emphasizing the need for a gradual reduction in steroid dose,[59] and was significantly different compared with nedocromil sodium for both phases.

Further evidence of a decrease in bronchial responsiveness as a result of treatment with nedocromil sodium comes from the reduction in peak flow diurnal variation.[47,62] A wide diurnal variation indicates poorly controlled asthma[60] and is correlated with increased bronchial responsiveness.[70]

Adverse reactions

Potentially life-threatening effects

None has occurred in any of the clinical trials or bronchial challenge studies with nedocromil sodium.

Acute overdosage

No cases of this kind have yet been reported.

Severe or irreversible adverse effects

No effects of this kind are known.

Symptomatic adverse effects

Analysis of reports of side effects has revealed that these effects have been relatively infrequent, mild and transient and insufficient in nearly all cases (3% nedocromil sodium, 1.7% placebo)[39] to cause withdrawal. The most frequently reported side effects are headache (4.8%) and nausea (4%).

A distinctive taste of nedocromil sodium has been reported by 13.6% of patients; in only a very few cases did this lead to withdrawal from therapy.[39] A flavoured version of Tilade is now available in Germany.

In the period of general use to date, there have been no published cases of possible adverse reactions to nedocromil sodium. Spontaneous reports have not so far suggested any change in the adverse reactions profile.

Interference with clinical pathology tests

No technical interferences of this kind have been reported.

High risk groups

Neonates

There is no experience at present of the use of nedocromil sodium in neonates.

Breast milk. Small amounts of nedocromil sodium are excreted in breast milk in the rat. There is no information on breast milk excretion in women.

Children

Experience with nedocromil sodium in children is extremely limited,[71,72] and paediatric use is currently not approved.

Pregnant women

Studies in pregnant animals have shown no adverse fetal or maternal effects. As with all recently introduced drugs, nedocromil sodium should be used with caution during pregnancy, particularly in the first trimester.

The elderly

Clinical experience to date has been predominantly in middle-aged and elderly patients with reversible obstructive airways disease. There has been no indication that in the elderly there is any difference in pharmacokinetics or therapeutic effect.

Drug interactions

No drug interactions with nedocromil sodium have been reported to date.

Clinical trials

Two long-term open assessment studies have examined the safety and efficacy of nedocromil sodium in a total of 130 adult asthmatic patients. Each study employed a four-week baseline followed by a 12-month open assessment period during which nedocromil sodium 4 mg four times daily was added to existing routine maintenance therapy.

1. Lal S, Malhotra S, Gribben D, Hodder D 1986 An open assessment study of the acceptability, tolerance and safety of nedocromil sodium in long-term clinical use in patients with perennial asthma. European Journal of Respiratory Disease 69 (suppl 147): 136–142

51 adult moderate asthmatic patients (age range 22–60, mean 41.2 years) entered this year-long study. The majority (44) were diagnosed as extrinsic asthmatics. Two were intrinsics and five were of mixed aetiology. Seven patients, one of whom died, withdrew for reasons unconnected with the trial treatment.

The patients were encouraged to reduce their use of inhaled steroids after one month of add-on therapy with nedocromil sodium. By the end of the study 28 patients (out of 48) had stopped using inhaled steroids and 10 had significantly reduced the mean daily dosage. 10 patients (out of 16) had ceased using sodium cromoglycate and three had reduced the dose. Inhaled bronchodilator use fell significantly in the first three months, when the dose of inhaled steroid was still relatively high, but returned to baseline with the reduction in inhaled steroid usage. Significant improvements in wheeze and dyspnoea were observed particularly in the early months of the study. The authors conclude that the addition of nedocromil sodium to current therapy can provide significant benefit and, in some patients, replace or allow a reduction in the use of an existing drug.

2. Carrasco E, Sepulveda R 1988 The acceptability, safety and efficacy of nedocromil sodium in long-term clinical use in patients with perennial asthma. Journal of International Medical Research 16: 394–401

79 moderate to severe adult asthmatic patients (age range 15–64, mean 37 years) of mainly extrinsic aetiology (n=72) participated in this one year study of add-on nedocromil sodium therapy. 19 patients withdrew during the course of the study for various reasons (pregnancy, removal outside the area, uncontrolled asthma and non-cooperation), including two who withdrew owing to severe sore throats and one who withdrew after 49.5 weeks of treatment owing to a severe cough.

Whilst expressing caution in the interpretation of open assessment efficacy data, the authors reported a significant reduction in the use of oral bronchodilator therapy and a definite and highly significant improvement in both morning and evening PEF ($>30\,l.min^{-1}$). Symptom scores improved from the third month — an improvement which continued throughout the study.

No clinically significant treatment-related changes were observed in the results from routine laboratory tests carried out in these two studies. No serious adverse effects were reported and nedocromil sodium was well tolerated in routine clinical use.

3. Cherniack R M, Wasserman S I, Ramsdell J W, Selner J C, Koepke J W, Rogers R M, Owens G R, Rubin E M, Wanner A (North American Tilade Study Group) 1990 A double-blind multicenter group comparative study of the efficacy and safety of nedocromil sodium in the management of asthma. Chest 97: 1299–1306.

121 adult, chronic bronchial asthma patients (age range 12–70, mean 35.2 years), treated solely with bronchodilator drugs (sustained release theophyllines and inhaled and oral β_2-bronchodilators) were randomised to receive 4 mg nedocromil sodium four times daily or placebo for 14 weeks. Sustained release theophyllines were withdrawn after 2 weeks and oral β_2-bronchodilators were withdrawn after 6 weeks on study treatments. Immediate release theophyllines could be used if inhaled β_2 bronchodilators did not provide relief.

Nedocromil sodium

The use of nedocromil sodium produced a rapid (three days), significant ($P<0.05$) improvement in asthma symptoms. This improvement was sustained over the following two weeks despite a spontaneous reduction in bronchodilator use. When sustained release theophyllines were removed, the improvements gained during the first two weeks of concurrent therapy with nedocromil sodium were maintained (with the exception of night-time asthma). After the withdrawal of oral β_2-bronchodilators (used by 16 patients), the majority of the diary card and clinic variables remained at the previous level of improvement and night-time asthma severity returned to pre-theophylline withdrawal levels. Theophylline use decreased to 36% of baseline usage during the final 8 weeks of the study in the nedocromil sodium-treated group. All clinic assessments (lung function, asthma severity and evaluation of treatment efficacy) significantly ($P\leq0.01$) favoured nedocromil sodium. Nedocromil sodium, which was well tolerated, improved the patients' asthma despite a reduction in bronchodilator therapy.

General review articles

Auty R M 1986 The clinical development of a new agent for the treatment of airway inflammation, nedocromil sodium (Tilade). European Journal of Respiratory Disease 69 (suppl 147): 120–131

Eady R P 1986 The pharmacology of nedocromil sodium. European Journal of Respiratory Disease 69 (suppl 147): 112–119

Gonzalez J P, Brogden R N 1987 Nedocromil sodium. A preliminary review of its pharmacodynamic and pharmacokinetic properties, and therapeutic efficacy in the treatment of reversible obstructive airways disease. Drugs 34: 560–577

1986 Nedocromil sodium. Drugs of the Future 11: 756–758

References

1. Chu S S 1987 Nedocromil sodium. Drugs of Today 23: 136–143
2. Jackson D M 1988 The effect of nedocromil sodium, sodium cromoglycate and codeine phosphate on citric acid-induced cough in dogs. British Journal of Pharmacology 93: 609–612
3. Dixon C M S, Barnes P J 1989 Bradykinin-induced bronchoconstriction: inhibition by nedocromil sodium and sodium cromoglycate. British Journal of Clinical Pharmacology 27: 831–836
4. Pauwels R A, Van Der Straeten M E 1987 An animal model for adenosine-induced bronchoconstriction. American Review of Respiratory Disease 136: 374–378
5. Cairns H, Cox D, Gould K J, Ingall A H, Suschitzky J L 1985 New antiallergic pyrano[3,2-g]quinoline-2,8-dicarboxylic acids with potential for the topical treatment of asthma. Journal of Medicinal Chemistry 28: 1832–1842
6. Moqbel R, Cromwell O, Walsh G M, Wardlaw A J, Kurlak L, Kay A B 1986 Effects of nedocromil sodium (Tilade) on the activation of human eosinophils and neutrophils and release of histamine from mast cells. Allergy 43: 268–276
7. Spry C J F, Kumaraswami V, Tai P C 1986 The effect of nedocromil sodium on secretion from human eosinophils. European Journal of Respiratory Disease 69 (suppl 147): 241–243
8. Bradford P G, Rubin R P 1986 The differential effects of nedocromil sodium and sodium cromoglycate on the secretory response of rabbit peritoneal neutrophils. European Journal of Respiratory Disease 69 (suppl 147): 238–240
9. Wells E, Jackson C G, Harper S T, Mann J, Eady R P 1986 Characterization of primate bronchoalveolar mast cells. II. Inhibition of histamine, LTC_4 and PGD_2 release from primate bronchoalveolar mast cells and a comparison with rat peritoneal mast cells. Journal of Immunology 137: 3941–3945
10. Broide D, Marquardt D, Wasserman S 1986 Effect of nedocromil sodium and sodium cromoglycate on connective tissue and bone marrow derived mast cells: acute and chronic studies. European Journal of Respiratory Disease 69 (suppl 147): 196–198
11. Leung K B P, Flint K C, Brostoff J et al 1988 Effects of sodium cromoglycate and nedocromil sodium on histamine secretion from human lung mast cells. Thorax 43: 756–761
12. Thorel T, Joseph M, Vorng H, Capron A 1988 The regulation of IgE-dependent anti-parasite functions of rat macrophages and platelets by nedocromil sodium. International Archives of Allergy and Applied Immunology 85: 227–231
13. Thorel T, Joseph M, Tsciopoulos A, Tonnel A B, Capron A 1988 Inhibition by nedocromil sodium of IgE-mediated activation of human mononuclear phagocytes and platelets in allergy. International Archives of Allergy and Applied Immunology 85: 232–237
14. Eady R P, Greenwood B, Jackson D M, Orr T S C, Wells E 1985 The effect of nedocromil sodium and sodium cromoglycate on antigen-induced bronchoconstriction in the *Ascaris*-sensitive monkey. British Journal of Pharmacology 85: 323–325
15. Abraham W M, Stevenson J S, Chapman G A, Tallent M W, Jackowski J 1987 The effect of nedocromil sodium and cromolyn sodium on antigen-induced responses in allergic sheep in vivo and in vitro. Chest 92: 913–917
16. Abraham W M, Stevenson J S, Eldridge M, Garrido R, Nieves L 1988 Nedocromil sodium in allergen-induced bronchial responses and airway hyperresponsiveness in allergic sheep. Journal of Applied Physiology 65: 1062–1068
17. Jackson D M, Eady R P, Farmer J B 1986 The effect of nedocromil sodium on non-specific bronchial hyperreactivity in the dog. European Journal of Respiratory Disease 69 (suppl 147): 217–219
18. Jackson D M, Eady R P 1988 Acute transient SO_2-induced airway hyperreactivity: effects of nedocromil sodium. Journal of Applied Physiology 65: 1119–1124
19. Evans T W, Rogers D F, Aursudkij B, Chung K F, Barnes P J 1988 Inflammatory mediators involved in antigen-induced airway microvascular leakage in guinea-pigs. American Review of Respiratory Disease 138: 395–399
20. Riley P A, Mather M E, Keogh R W, Eady R P 1987 Activity of nedocromil sodium in mast-cell-dependent reactions in the rat. International Archives of Allergy and Applied Immunology 82: 108–110
21. Clark B, Clarke A J, Bamford D G, Greenwood B 1986 Safety evaluation studies: a preliminary report. European Journal of Respiratory Disease 69 (suppl 147): 248–251
22. Svendsen U G, Nielsen N H, Frolund L, Madsen F, Weeke B 1986 Effects of nedocromil sodium and placebo delivered by pressurized aerosol in bronchial antigen challenge. Allergy 41: 468–470
23. Chudry N, Correa F, Silverman M 1987 Nedocromil sodium and exercise-induced asthma. Archives of Disease in Childhood 62: 412–414
24. Konig P, Hordvik N L, Kreutz C 1987 The preventive effect and duration of action of nedocromil sodium and cromolyn sodium on exercise-induced asthma in adults. Journal of Allergy and Clinical Immunology 79: 64–68
25. Youngchaiyud P, Lee T B 1986 Effect of nedocromil sodium on the immediate response to antigen challenge in asthmatic patients. Clinical Allergy 16: 129–134
26. Bonifazi F, Antonicelli L, Pieretti C et al 1987 Double-blind crossover trial to compare the activity of nedocromil sodium and placebo in antigen challenge. Allergologia et Immunopathologia 15: 151–153
27. Robuschi M, Simone P, Fasano W, Bianco S 1986 The efficacy and duration of action of nedocromil sodium compared with placebo in bronchial antigen challenge. European Journal of Respiratory Disease 69 (suppl 147): 289–291
28. Vilsvik J, Schaanning J 1988 A comparative study of the effect of three doses of nedocromil sodium and placebo given by pressurized aerosol to asthmatics with exercise-induced bronchoconstriction. Annals of Allergy 61: 367–370
29. Debelic M 1986 Nedocromil-sodium in effort-induced asthma in teenagers. Atemwegs und Lungenkrankheiten 12: S110–S113
30. Shaw R J, Kay A B 1985 Nedocromil, a mucosal and connective tissue mast cell stabilizer, inhibits exercise-induced asthma. British Journal of Diseases of the Chest 79: 385–389
31. Patel K R, Albazzaz M K 1987 Protective effect of cromolyn sodium and nedocromil sodium in exercise-induced asthma. Journal of Allergy and Clinical Immunology 79: 187
32. Magnussen H 1986 The protective effect of sodium cromoglycate (SCG) and nedocromil sodium on effort-induced bronchial asthma. Atemwegs und Lungenkrankheiten 12: S107–109
33. Dixon C M S, Ind P W 1989 Metabisulphite-induced bronchoconstriction: mechanisms. American Review of Respiratory Disease 137: 238
34. Altounyan R E C, Cole M, Lee T B 1986 Inhibition of sulphur dioxide-induced bronchoconstriction by nedocromil sodium and sodium cromoglycate in non-asthmatic atopic subjects. European Journal of Respiratory Disease 69 (suppl 147): 274–276
35. Del Bufalo C, Fasano L, Patalano F, Gunella G 1989 Inhibition of fog-induced bronchospasm by nedocromil sodium and sodium cromoglycate in intrinsic asthma: a double-blind, placebo-controlled study. Respiration 55: 181–185
36. Juniper E F, Kline P A, Morris M M, Hargreave F E 1987 Airway constriction by isocapnic hyperventilation of cold, dry air: comparison of magnitude and duration of protection by nedocromil sodium and sodium cromoglycate. Clinical Allergy 17: 523–528
37. Crimi E, Palermo F, Oliveri R et al 1988 Comparative study of the effects of nedocromil sodium (4 mg) and sodium cromoglycate (10 mg) on adenosine-induced bronchoconstriction in asthmatic subjects. Clinical Allergy 18: 367–374
38. Phillips GD, Scott VL, Richards R, Holgate ST 1989 Effect of nedocromil and sodium cromoglycate against bronchoconstriction induced by inhaled adenosine 5'-monophosphate. European Respiratory Journal 2: 210–217
39. Gonzalez J P, Brogden R N 1987 Nedocromil sodium. A preliminary review of its pharmacodynamic and pharmacokinetic properties, and therapeutic efficacy in the treatment of reversible obstructive airways disease. Drugs 34: 560–577
40. Newman S P, Moren F, Pavia D, Moren F, Sheahan N F, Clark S W 1981 Deposition of pressurized aerosols in the human respiratory tract. Thorax 36 (1): 52–55
41. Neale M G, Brown K, Foulds R A, Lal S, Morris D A, Thomas D 1987 The pharmacokinetics of nedocromil sodium, a new drug for the treatment of reversible obstructive airways disease, in human volunteers and patients with reversible obstructive airways disease. British Journal of Clinical Pharmacology 24: 493–501
42. Gardner J J, Preston J R, Gilbert C M, Wilkinson D J, Lockley W J S, Brown K 1988 A radioimmunoassay method for the determination of nedocromil sodium in plasma and urine. Journal of Pharmaceutical and Biomedical Analysis 6: 285–297
43. Auty R M, Clarke A J 1986 Kinetics and disposition of nedocromil sodium in man: a preliminary report. European Journal of Respiratory Disease 69 (suppl 147): 246–247
44. Newman S P 1983 The correct use of inhalers. In: Clark T J H Steroids in asthma: a reappraisal in the light of inhalation therapy. ADIS Press, New Zealand, pp 210–226
45. Fyans P G, Chatterjee P C, Chatterjee S S 1986 A trial comparing nedocromil sodium (Tilade) and placebo in the management of bronchial asthma. Clinical Allergy 16: 505–511
46. Bianco S, Del Bono L, Grassi V, Orefice U 1989 Effectiveness of nedocromil sodium versus placebo as additions to routine asthma maintenance therapy: a multicentre, double-blind group comparative trial. Respiration 56: 204–211
47. Fairfax A J, Allbeson M 1988 A double-blind comparative trial of nedocromil sodium and placebo in the management of bronchial asthma. Journal of International Medical Research 16: 216–224

48. Cua-Lim F, Agbayani B F, Lachica D 1985 A double-blind comparative trial of nedocromil sodium and placebo in the management of bronchial asthma. Philippine Journal of Internal Medicine 23: 181–190
49. Van As A, Chick T W, Bodman S F et al 1986 A group comparative study of the safety and efficacy of nedocromil sodium (Tilade) in reversible airways disease: a preliminary report. European Journal of Respiratory Disease 69 (suppl 147): 143–148
50. Callaghan B, Teo N C, Clancy L 1989 The use of Tilade in theophylline treated asthmatics. American Review of Respiratory Disease 139: A65
51. Fyans P G, Chatterjee P C, Chatterjee S S 1989 Effects of adding nedocromil sodium (Tilade) to the routine therapy of patients with bronchial asthma. Clinical and Experimental Allergy 19: 521–528
52. Bone M F, Kubik M M, Keaney N P et al 1989 Nedocromil sodium in adults with asthma dependent on inhaled corticosteroids: a double-blind, placebo controlled study. Thorax 44: 654–659
53. Dorow P 1986 A double-blind group comparative trial of nedocromil sodium and placebo in the management of bronchial asthma in steroid-dependent patients. European Journal of Respiratory Disease 69 (suppl 147): 317–319
54. Bergmann K-Ch, Bauer C P, Overlack A 1989 A placebo-controlled, blind comparison of nedocromil sodium and beclomethasone dipropionate in bronchial asthma. Current Medical Research and Opinion 11: 533–542
55. Harper G D, Neill P, Vathenen A S, Cookson J B, Ebden P 1989 A comparison of inhaled beclomethasone dipropionate and nedocromil sodium as additional therapy in asthma. American Review of Respiratory Disease 139: A432
56. Ruffin R, Alpers J, Rubinfeld A, Pain M, Bowes G, Czarny D 1986 A 4-week Australian multicentre study of nedocromil sodium in asthmatic patients. European Journal of Respiratory Disease 69 (suppl 147): 336–339
57. Chadwick G, Lane D J 1986 A double-blind comparative trial of nedocromil sodium versus placebo as replacement therapy for inhaled corticosteroids in patients with bronchial asthma. European Journal of Respiratory Disease 69 (suppl 147): 327–329
58. Paananen M, Karakorpi T, Kreus K E 1986 Withdrawal of inhaled corticosteroid under cover of nedocromil sodium. European Journal of Respiratory Disease 69 (suppl 147): 330–335
59. Svendsen U G, Frolund L, Madsen F, Nielsen N H 1989 A comparison of the effects of nedocromil sodium and beclomethasone dipropionate on pulmonary function, symptoms, and bronchial responsiveness in patients with asthma. Journal of Allergy and Clinical Immunology 84: 224–231
60. Greif J, Fink G, Smorzik Y, Topilsky M, Bruderman I, Spitzer S A 1989 Nedocromil sodium and placebo in the treatment of bronchial asthma. Chest 96: 583–588
61. Hetzel M R, Clark T J H 1980 Comparison of normal and asthmatic circadian rhythms in peak expiratory flow rate. Thorax 35: 732–738
62. Williams A J, Stableforth D 1986 The addition of nedocromil sodium to maintenance therapy in the management of patients with bronchial asthma. European Journal of Respiratory Disease 69 (suppl 147): 340–343
63. Greco D B, Brum Negreiros E, Chaieb J A, Ferreira-Lima P, Croce J 1986 A multicentre double-blind group comparative trial of two dose levels of nedocromil sodium and placebo in the management of perennial extrinsic asthma. European Journal of Respiratory Disease 69 (suppl 147): 323–326
64. Dorward A J, Roberts J A, Thomson N C 1986 Effect of nedocromil sodium on histamine airway responsiveness in grass-pollen sensitive asthmatics during the pollen season. Clinical Allergy 16: 309–315
65. Altounyan R E C, Cole M, Lee T B 1985 Effects of nedocromil sodium on changes in bronchial hyperreactivity in non-asthmatic atopic rhinitic subjects during the grass pollen season. Progress Respiratory Research 19: 397–400
66. Bel E H, Timmers M C, Hermans J, Dijkman J H, Sterk P J 1990 The long-term effects of nedocromil sodium and beclomethasone dipropionate on bronchial responsiveness to methacholine in nonatopic asthmatic subjects. American Review of Respiratory Disease 141: 21–28
67. Di Maria G U, Bellofiore S, Ciancio N, Ruggieri F, Mistretta A 1989 Nedocromil sodium prevents the increase in airway responsiveness to methacholine induced by platelet activating factor. American Review of Respiratory Disease 139: A109
68. Orefice U, Struzzo P L, Pitzalis G 1989 Non specific bronchial hyperresponsiveness study in asthmatic subjects before and after medium-term treatment with nedocromil sodium and sodium cromoglycate. American Review of Respiratory Disease 139: A509
69. Orefice U, Ferrazzano P L, Patalano F, Ruggieri F 1987 Changes in bronchial reactivity to methacholine induced by nedocromil sodium. In: Stam J et al (eds) The lung and the environment. CIP — Gegevens Koninklijke Bibliotheek, The Haag, p 49
70. Ryan G, Latimer K M, Dolovich J, Hargreave F E 1982 Bronchial responsiveness to histamine: relationship to diurnal variation of peak flow rate, improvement after bronchodilator, and airway calibre. Thorax 37: 423–429
71. Strinati R 1987 Nedocromil sodium. Medico Bambino 10: 794–796
72. Kerstjens J M, Griffioen R W, Van Aalderen W M C 1989 Tolerability and efficacy of nebulized nedocromil sodium in asthmatic children. European Respiratory Journal 2 (suppl 8): 836S

Nefopam (hydrochloride)

Nefopam is an analgesic drug for the treatment of moderate to moderately severe pain. It is chemically and pharmacologically distinct from any other class of analgesics.

Chemistry

Nefopam hydrochloride (Acupan, Ajan, Sinalgico)
$C_{17}H_{19}NO.HCl$
3,4,5,6-Tetrahydro-5-methyl-1-phenyl-1H-2,5-benzoxazocine hydrochloride

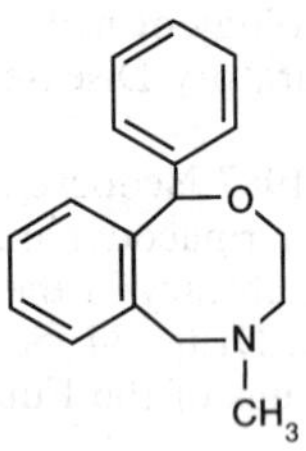

Molecular weight (free base)	289.8 (253.3)
pKa	9.2
Solubility	
in alcohol	1 in 312
in water	1 in 43
Heptane/water partition coefficient	5.8

A white to off-white crystalline powder with negligible odour and a bitter, numbing taste, which is produced by chemical synthesis. It has a unique heterocyclic structure produced by cyclization of diphenhydramine to produce a topomeric analogue.[1]

Pharmacology

Nefopam is a potent inhibitor of synaptosomal uptake of dopamine, noradrenaline and serotonin.[2,3] Its analgesic properties can be blocked by reserpine[3] suggesting mediation, at least in part, by an enhancement of monoaminergic function. Detailed studies have suggested that descending serotonergic pathways are involved in nefopam-induced antinociception.[4] Analgesia is not mediated by prostaglandin inhibition or opiate receptors and is not reversed by naloxone.[2,5] At higher concentrations nefopam also has anticholinergic, mild antihistaminic and local anaesthetic activity.[1,2] Evidence of an antidepressant effect has been seen in animals.[6,7]

Toxicology

Acute toxicological studies in rats, mice and dogs[8] showed oral LD_{50} values of 80–178 $mg.kg^{-1}$, intramuscular LD_{50} values of 30–75 $mg.kg^{-1}$ and intravenous LD_{50} values of 20–45 $mg.kg^{-1}$. Longer term toxicological studies[9] showed dose-dependent weight loss and fatty liver changes in rats and convulsions in some dogs. At a daily dose of 24 $mg.kg^{-1}$ nefopam potentiated the hepatotoxicity of paracetamol overdose. These effects were only seen at doses very much higher than those used in clinical practice. There was no evidence of teratogenicity, dependence or tolerance[5] or carcinogenicity (unpublished data, 3M Health Care).

Clinical pharmacology

Analgesia has been demonstrated in acute and chronic pain states after administration by oral or parenteral routes.[10–25] Nefopam is more potent than aspirin but less potent than morphine. The potency ratio with respect to aspirin is 1:8.4–10.4[20,25] and with respect to morphine, 1:0.18–0.56.[18,23] Long-term use of nefopam does not appear to result in the development of tolerance or dependence.[26]

Clinical studies demonstrating an enhancement of spinal stretch reflexes[16] contrast with early animal studies which showed a potent central muscle relaxant effect.[1]

Nefopam has a chronotropic and slight positive inotropic effect due to potentiation of endogenous catecholamines. After a dose of 0.3 mg.kg^{-1} intravenously, mean arterial pressure rose by 13% and cardiac output by 10%.[27]

Significantly less respiratory depression was seen after intramuscular administration of nefopam 20 mg or 40 mg than after morphine 5 mg or 10 mg[28] but these results may reflect hyperventilation resulting from the sensation of nausea associated with the former group. A significant reduction in the slope of the ventilatory response curve to carbon dioxide was shown after oral administration.[29]

Nefopam is neither anti-inflammatory nor antipyretic but has a hypothermic effect, significantly depressing core temperature for six hours after an oral dose of 60 mg. This may be a reflection of the increased sweating that occurs.[30]

Gastrointestinal blood loss is not increased by nefopam;[30] it does not cause constipation but gastric emptying is delayed.[31]

Pharmacokinetics

The preferred analytical method is by gas–liquid chromatography using a nitrogen selective detector.[32] The limit of sensitivity is 5 μg.l^{-1}

Virtually complete absorption occurs from the gastrointestinal tract following oral dosing but there is extensive presystemic metabolism. Peak plasma levels ranging from 29 to 67 μg.l^{-1} occur 1–3 h after an oral dose of 60 mg. Peak plasma levels of 32–49 μg.l^{-1} were reported 90 min after 20 mg intramuscularly. The mean plasma half life is 4 h with a range of 3–8 h and there is no change after regular administration for seven days.

Steady-state concentrations in the cerebrospinal fluid of five patients taking nefopam 60 mg 8 hourly were 25% of the corresponding plasma concentration,[33] reflecting the 71–76% plasma protein binding and free penetration of the blood–brain barrier. The volume of distribution of nefopam is not quoted nor are levels in other tissues. It is known to be excreted in breast milk and would be expected to cross the placenta, though direct evidence for this is not available.

Oral absorption	95–100%
Presystemic metabolism	extensive
Plasma half life	
range	3–11 h
mean	4 h
Volume of distribution	~10 kg.l^{-1}
Plasma protein binding	71–76%

Hepatic and renal insufficiency may impair the metabolism and excretion of nefopam. This is unlikely to be of clinical significance except perhaps in end-stage organ failure.

Concentration–effect relationship

A linear dose–response relationship has been shown in many clinical studies,[17–19,23,25] though there are reports suggesting a ceiling effect at higher doses. Plasma nefopam levels correlate well with the dose administered[17] but a concentration–effect profile has not been established.[20] The duration of analgesia increases with dose, with 3–4 h following low dose (7.5–10 mg intramuscularly) and 5–6 h following a higher dose (30 mg intramuscularly).[10,18]

Metabolism

Nefopam is extensively metabolized with less than 5% being excreted unchanged. After a 20 mg intravenous dose of labelled drug, 87% of the activity was recovered in the urine and 8% in the faeces over the subsequent five days.

Seven metabolites have been identified of which five have been shown to be devoid of analgesic activity with the other two accounting for less than 2% of the nefopam dose. Urinary excretion half lives of these metabolites range from 2.2 to 9.2 h.

Nefopam (hydrochloride)

Fig. 1 Metabolism of nefopam

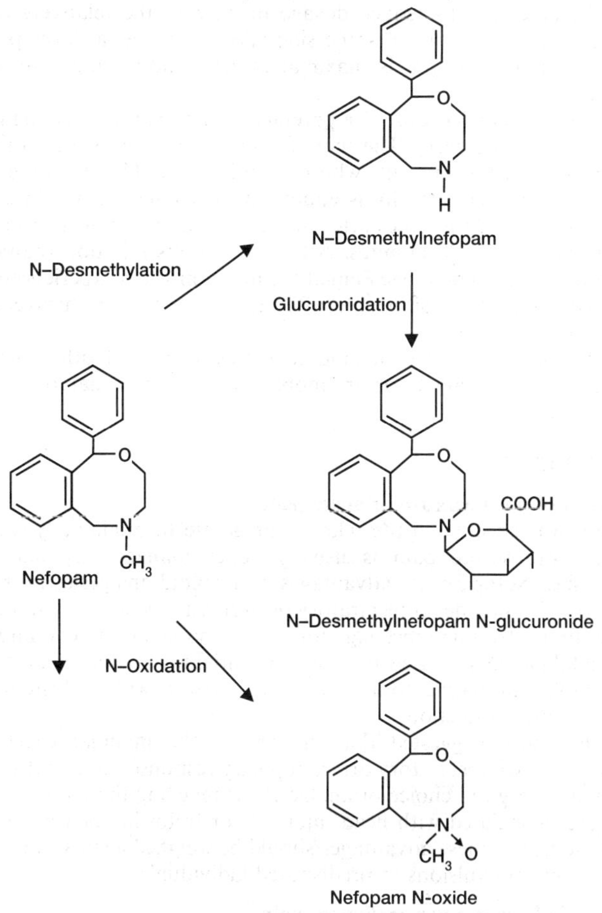

The three principal metabolic pathways are: N-desmethylation, glucuronidation of the latter, and N-oxidation (Fig. 1)

Pharmaceutics

Nefopam (Acupan; 3M Health Care, UK) is available in oral and parenteral forms.

Tablets are white, film-coated, biconvex and round, measuring 7 mm in diameter and marked 'APN' on one side. Each tablet contains 30 mg of nefopam hydrochloride. There are no other tablet strengths and no combination preparations.

The injectable preparation is a clear, colourless solution containing 20 mg of nefopam hydrochloride in 1 ml of solution, presented in clear glass ampoules.

Both preparations should be stored in a cool dry place. Tablets have a shelf-life of five years, and the parenteral preparation three years.

Neither formulation contains any recognized allergens.

Therapeutic use

Indications

1. Relief of postoperative or acute pain
2. Relief of chronic non-malignant pain
3. Relief of cancer pain
4. Intraoperative use.

Contraindications

1. History of convulsive disorder
2. Concurrent or recent use of monoamine oxidase inhibitors
3. Recent myocardial infarction
4. Glaucoma
5. Prostatic hypertrophy or urinary retention.

Mode of use

Oral therapy should usually commence at a dose of 30 mg 8 hourly increasing to 60 mg or 90 mg 8 hourly if the response is inadequate.

The maximum dosage level reported has been 360 mg per 24 hours. It may be necessary to reduce dosage in view of the relatively high incidence of minor but irksome side effects. Analgesia develops 30 minutes after ingestion, is maximal at 1.5–2 hours and lasts 4–6 hours.

The recommended dose for parenteral administration is 20 mg 6 hourly intramuscularly. The manufacturers recommend that this is given to recumbent patients who remain lying for 15–20 minutes. A dose of 20 mg parenterally is equivalent to 60 mg orally. Onset of analgesia is 15–20 minutes after intramuscular injection with maximum effect at 60–90 minutes. After intravenous injection the peak effect is seen at 15 minutes. Pain at the injection site is experienced by approximately 20% of people after intramuscular or intravenous injection.

Nefopam is indicated in mild to moderate pain if other simple analgesics have failed, or in more severe pain if narcotics are contraindicated.

Indications

1. Relief of postoperative or acute pain

Nefopam is effective in the relief of moderate to moderately severe pain. More severe pain is usually better managed by narcotic analgesics. Nefopam has advantages over opioid analgesics in those patients with significant respiratory problems and where constipation tends to be troublesome, e.g. following anorectal surgery and in postnatal patients. In view of its low potential for abuse, it represents a suitable alternative to narcotics in patients with a history of previous drug addiction.

It has been suggested that in view of the minimal effect on conscious level, respiratory drive, pupillary responses and vital signs, nefopam is a good choice of analgesic for relieving the pain of limb fractures associated with head injuries[34] or following neurosurgical operations, but these advantages should be weighed against the risks of inducing convulsions in predisposed individuals.

2. Relief of chronic non-malignant pain

Although it is in this population that nefopam shows greatest promise, there have been few studies reporting on its use in chronic pain. At a dose of 60 mg three times daily it is an effective supplement to anti-inflammatory drugs in rheumatoid arthritis, with improvement of function as well as pain relief.[14] In a study on severe chronic back pain with a mean duration of 8 years, only a small proportion of patients obtained significant relief but this was sustained over a period of years and, considering the repeated failure of other therapeutic endeavours in this population, suggests a useful role for nefopam.[17]

If side effects are not seen when treatment is initiated, they are unlikely to limit long-term use. Nefopam does not increase gastrointestinal blood loss or cause constipation, it is not sedative and present evidence suggests a low dependence liability. These properties suggest that nefopam may prove useful for long-term administration but further studies are required to determine this role.

3. Relief of cancer pain

Nefopam may be effective in the relief of cancer pain either by oral or parenteral routes.[11]

4. Intraoperative use

The intraoperative use of nefopam has been described and advantages claimed with respect to papaveretum for spontaneously breathing patients and specifically for paediatric ear, nose and throat operations.[15] In a similar population, however, the use of nefopam as an oral premedicant resulted in a very high incidence of vomiting during emergence from anaesthesia.[35]

Contraindications

1. History of convulsive disorders

This is an absolute contraindication to the use of nefopam following the occurrence of seizures in three patients with a history of previous convulsions and in a fourth after a cerebrovascular accident. Convulsions occurred 10–21 days after starting oral treatment with a dose of 30–60 mg three times daily.

2. Monoamine oxidase inhibitors

Nefopam is absolutely contraindicated in patients taking monoamine oxidase inhibitors (MAOIs) and within three weeks of cessation of such therapy. Nefopam reduces synaptosomal reuptake of monoamines and if the alternative pathway of elimination by oxidation is inhibited, catastrophic hypertension may ensue.

3. Recent myocardial infarction

The tachycardia and elevation of mean arterial pressure seen especially after parenteral use of nefopam will increase myocardial oxygen consumption and decrease coronary perfusion, representing a risk to critically ischaemic cardiac muscle.

In patients with ischaemic heart disease or arterial hypertension it is recommended that the intravenous dose of 20 mg be given over a period of not less than 10 minutes.[27]

4. Glaucoma

Because of the anticholinergic properties of nefopam, it should be used with caution, if at all, in patients with glaucoma.

5. Prostatic hypertrophy or urinary retention

The anticholinergic properties of nefopam may precipitate or exacerbate urinary retention in predisposed individuals.

Adverse reactions

Potentially life-threatening effects

No life-threatening side effects have been reported in therapeutic dosage.

Acute overdosage

Ten cases of overdosage with nefopam have been described, including one fatality.[36] Non-fatal overdosage was characterized by convulsions, agitation, hallucinations, and tachycardia. The fatal case described developed generalized convulsions and a subsequent respiratory arrest. She had a temperature of 41.9°C and a tachycardia of 150 beats per minute with right bundle branch block and first-degree heart block progressing to alternate nodal and ventricular tachycardia with subsequent cardiac arrest. She had gross haematuria and developed a coagulopathy. Unresponsive anuria ensued. Necropsy revealed cerebral oedema and signs of coning. The lungs, liver, and kidneys were congested and the gastric mucosa showed patchy necrosis. A plasma level of 11.9 $mg.l^{-1}$ was measured compared with observed therapeutic peak plasma levels of approx. 0.1 $mg.l^{-1}$, representing massive ingestion. One further death has occurred subsequent to this report.

Management of overdosage is supportive with gastric lavage, administration of diazepam for agitation and convulsions, and possibly β-adrenoceptor blockade for tachyarrhythmias.

Severe or irreversible adverse effects

Convulsions in four predisposed individuals constitute the only reported adverse effects of nefopam. This may represent an increase in monoaminergic neurotransmitters or possibly a central anticholinergic phenomenon.

Symptomatic adverse effects

In contrast to its relative lack of severe adverse effects, the use of nefopam is associated with a high incidence of minor ill effects, especially after parenteral use. The most frequently reported are sweating, nausea, headache, and dry mouth. Others include sleep disturbances, dizziness, light-headedness, loss of appetite, and difficulty in swallowing.

Nausea appears to be dose-related and occurs in 10–30% but is generally of brief duration, and the incidence of vomiting is low. This may be a direct dopaminergic effect on the chemoreceptor trigger zone.

There are conflicting reports of the sedative effect of nefopam, a number of studies reporting drowsiness as a common adverse effect.[12,16] Comparative studies, however, agree that nefopam is less sedative than the opiates,[10,11,21,23,24] and some recipients have reported a stimulant effect,[13,17] while others have expressed anxiety, restlessness, or a sense of panic.[30] Insomnia has been a problem in longer term usage.[17,26] Both euphoric and dysphoric effects have been reported.

Sweating, sometimes profuse,[23] is seen in 10–30% of people. This generally occurs within 30 minutes of a parenteral dose and seldom lasts more than 10 minutes.

Sweating, headache, tachycardia, insomnia, anxiety, and loss of appetite reflect the sympathomimetic properties of the drug, while dry mouth, drowsiness, and blurred vision are anticholinergic effects.

Nefopam (hydrochloride)

Other effects

No changes were observed in full blood count, blood urea nitrogen, alkaline phosphatase, bilirubin, transaminases, or urinalysis in 25 subjects receiving nefopam 60 mg three times daily for 12 weeks.[26] A minor elevation of alkaline phosphatase was reported in 2 patients after taking nefopam for four weeks.[14] No studies have reported an analysis of blood glucose levels.

Interference with clinical pathology tests

Nefopam has similar retention times to codeine, diazepam, and pentazocine in some chromatographic analyses and may interfere with assays.[37]

High risk groups

Neonates

Nefopam is not recommended for use in neonates.

Breast milk. Nefopam is excreted in breast milk, but the effects on children of nursing mothers are unknown.

Children

Nefopam is not recommended for children under 12 years of age.

Pregnant women

The safety of nefopam in pregnancy has not been established and at present its use cannot be recommended. Although use of nefopam in labour is unlikely to cause neonatal respiratory depression, no studies have been reported.

The elderly

It is advisable to start treatment with a lower dose in elderly patients.

Drug interactions

Potentially hazardous interactions

Monoamine oxidase inhibitors. See Contraindications.

Tricyclic antidepressants. The manufacturers recommend caution with the concurrent use of tricyclic antidepressants and nefopam, based on theoretical considerations rather than on reports of adverse reactions.

Anaesthetics. Intraoperative use of nefopam in conjunction with halothane may produce an increased incidence of dysrhythmias.

Other significant interactions

An assessment of possible interactions between nefopam and eight different drugs (aspirin 650 mg, diazepam 5 mg, phenobarbitone 60 mg, propoxyphene 65 mg, codeine 60 mg, pentazocine 50 mg, indomethacin 25 mg, and hydroxyzine pamoate 50 mg) showed no alterations in the bioavailability of nefopam but an overall increase in the incidence and severity of adverse effects when given in combination with codeine, pentazocine, or propoxyphene.[37]

Reserpine has been shown to block the analgesic action of nefopam.[3]

Potentially useful interactions

The combination of nefopam 20 mg intravenously and diazepam 10 mg intravenously has been described as an alternative to general anaesthesia for the manipulation of closed fractures and the reduction of dislocated joints in emergency situations. The combination is reported to provide muscle relaxation and analgesia with preservation of consciousness but retrograde amnesia. The adverse effects are reported to be mutually antagonistic.[38]

Major outcome trials

1. Emery P, Gibson T 1986 A double blind study of the simple analgesic nefopam in rheumatoid arthritis. British Journal of Rheumatology 25: 72–76

This is a double-blind, crossover study, balanced for order effects, in 27 patients with rheumatoid arthritis of 4–30 years duration who were suffering pain despite maximal anti-inflammatory therapy. The study compared nefopam 60 mg 8 hourly for 4 weeks with an identical placebo regime. Pain, morning stiffness, joint tenderness, joint swelling and grip strength were assessed by a single observer before and 2 and 4 weeks after starting each treatment.

A significant improvement in pain, stiffness and joint tenderness was seen with nefopam. Grip strength improved but this difference did not achieve statistical significance.

2. Stamp J, Rhind V, Haslock I 1989 A comparison of nefopam and flurbiprofen in the treatment of osteoarthrosis. British Journal of Clinical Practice 43:
3. McLintock T T C, Kenny G N C, Howie J C, McArdle C S, Lawrie S, Aitken H 1988 Assessment of the analgesic efficacy of nefopam hydrochloride after upper abdominal surgery: a study using patient controlled analgesia. British Journal of Surgery 75: 779–781.

General review articles

Heel R C, Brogden R N, Pakes G E, Speight T M, Avery G S 1980 Nefopam: a review of its pharmacological properties and therapeutic efficacy. Drugs 19: 249–267

Nefopam — a new analgesic 1979 Drug and Therapeutics Bulletin 17: 59–60

References

1. Klohs M W, Draper M D, Petracek F J, Ginzel K H, Re O N 1972 Benzoxacines: a new chemical class of centrally acting skeletal muscle relaxants. Arzneimittelforschung 22: 132–133
2. Tresnak-Rustad N J, Wood M E 1981 In vitro biochemical effects of nefopam hydrochloride, a new analgesic agent. Biochemical Pharmacology 30: 2847–2850
3. Vonvoigtlander P F, Lewis R A, Neff G L, Triezenberg H J 1983 Involvement of biogenic amines with the mechanisms of novel analgesics. Progress in Neuro-Psychopharmacology and Biological Psychiatry 7: 651–656
4. Hunskaar S, Fasmer O B, Broch O J, Hole K 1987 Involvement of central serotonergic pathways in nefopam-induced antinociception. European Journal of Pharmacology 138: 77–82
5. Conway A C, Mitchell C L 1977 Analgesic studies with nefopam hydrochloride. Archives Internationale de Pharmacodynamie et de Therapie 226: 156–171
6. Bassett J R, Cairncross K D, Hacket N B, Story M 1969 Studies on the peripheral pharmacology of fenazoxine, a potential antidepressant drug. British Journal of Pharmacology 37: 69–78
7. Hammerbeck D M, Conway A C, Mitchell C L 1974 Pharmacologic evaluation of nefopam hydrochloride (Acupan). Pharmacologist 16: 247–254
8. Case M A, Smith J K, Nelson R A 1975 Reproductive, acute and subacute toxicity studies with nefopam in laboratory animals. Toxicology and Applied Pharmacology 33: 46–51
9. Case M A, Smith J K, Nelson R A 1976 Chronic oral toxicity studies of nefopam hydrochloride in rats and dogs. Toxicology and Applied Pharmacology 36: 301–306
10. Beaver W T, Feise G A 1977 A comparison of the analgesic effect of intramuscular nefopam and morphine in patients with postoperative pain. Journal of Clinical Pharmacology 17: 579–591
11. de Thibault de Boesinghe L, Van Daele M J, Van Severen G 1976 Open study of the analgesic effects of nefopam hydrochloride (Acupan) on cancer patients with pain. Current Therapeutic Research 20: 59–61
12. Campos V M, Solis E L 1980 The analgesic and hypothermic effects of nefopam, morphine, aspirin, diphenhydramine and placebo. Journal of Clinical Pharmacology 20: 42–49
13. Cohen A, Hernandez C M 1976 Nefopam hydrochloride: a new analgesic. Journal of International Medical Research 4: 138–143
14. Emery P, Gibson T 1986 A double blind study of the simple analgesic nefopam in rheumatoid arthritis. British Journal of Rheumatology 25: 72–76
15. Hannington-Kiff J G 1985 The need for analgesic cover after ENT surgery — comparison of nefopam and papaveretum. Anaesthesia 40: 76–78
16. Gassel M M, Daimantopoulos E, Petropoulos V, Hughes A C R, Fernandez Ballesteros M L, Re O N 1976 Controlled clinical trial of oral and parenteral nefopam hydrochloride. A novel and potent analgesic drug. Journal of Clinical Pharmacology 16: 34–42
17. McQuay H J, Moore R A, Poppleton P, Bullingham R E S, Lloyd J W 1986 Nefopam in chronic back pain: analgesic efficacy and plasma concentrations after single and multiple dose use. The Pain Clinic 1: 15–22
18. Sunshine A, Laska E 1975 Nefopam and morphine in man. Clinical Pharmacology and Therapeutics 18: 530–534
19. Sunshine A, Laska E, Slafta J 1978 Oral nefopam and aspirin. Clinical Pharmacology and Therapeutics 24: 555–559
20. Tigerstedt I, Tammisto T, Leander P 1979 Comparison of the analgesic dose–effect relationships of nefopam and oxycodone in postoperative pain. Acta Anaesthesiologica Scandinavica 23: 555–560
21. Tigerstedt I, Sipponen J, Tammisto T, Turunen M 1977 Comparison of nefopam and pethidine in postoperative pain. British Journal of Anaesthesia 49: 1133–1138
22. Trop D, Kenny L, Grad B R 1979 Comparison of nefopam hydrochloride and propoxyphene hydrochloride in the treatment of postoperative pain. Canadian Anaesthetic Society Journal 26: 296–304
23. Wallenstein S L, Kaiko R F, Rogers A, Houde R W 1978 A clinical assay of nefopam and morphine. Clinical Pharmacology and Therapeutics 23: 134
24. Conway M, Lipton S 1982 A comparison of a new analgesic, nefopam hydrochloride, with morphine sulphate, pentazocine and pethidine hydrochloride in postoperative pain. Current Medical Research and Opinion 7: 580–597
25. Workmon F C, Winter L Jr 1974 A clinical evaluation of nefopam hydrochloride (Acupan): a new analgesic. Current Therapeutic Research 16: 609–616
26. Klotz A L 1974 Long-term safety of nefopam hydrochloride (Acupan), a new analgesic formulation. Current Therapeutic Research 16: 602–608
27. Hagemann K, Platte G, Meyer J, Effert S 1978 Hamodynamische wirkung von nefopam (Haemodynamic effect of nefopam). Deutsche Medizinische Wochenschrift 103: 1040–1043

28. Gasser J C, Bellville J W 1975 Respiratory effects of nefopam. Clinical Pharmacology and Therapeutics 18: 175–179
29. Bhatt A M, Pleuvry B J, Maddison S E 1981 Respiratory and metabolic effects of oral nefopam in human volunteers. British Journal of Clinical Pharmacology 11: 209–211
30. Baltes B J 1977 Gastrointestinal blood loss study with a new analgesic compound: nefopam hydrochloride. Journal of Clinical Pharmacology 17: 120–124
31. Todd J G, Nimmo W S 1983 Effect of premedication on drug absorption and gastric emptying. British Journal of Anaesthesia 55: 1189–1193
32. Chang S F, Hansen C S, Fox J M, Ober R E 1981 Quantitative determination of nefopam in human plasma, saliva and cerebrospinal fluid by gas–liquid chromatography using a nitrogen-selective detector. Journal of Chromatography 226: 79–89
33. Hesla P E 1982 Influence of plasma concentrations of nefopam hydrochloride on enkephalin concentrations in cerebrospinal fluid of patients being treated for chronic pain. Acta Neurologica Scandinavica 65 (suppl 90): 62–63
34. Subhedar V Y, Hashemi K 1983 Use of nefopam for pain relief in patients with head injury. (Abstract) VIth International Congress of Emergency Surgery, Dubrovnik, Yugoslavia, June 6–10
35. Wilkinson P A 1984 A double-blind comparison of nefopam and placebo used as a premedication in children. Anaesthesia 39: 815–819
36. Piercy D M, Cumming J A, Dawling S, Henry J A 1981 Death due to overdose of nefopam. British Medical Journal 283: 1508–1509
37. Lasseter K C, Cohen A, Back E L 1976 Nefopam hydrochloride interaction study with eight other drugs. Journal of International Medical Research 4: 195–201
38. Bauer J 1982 Hypalgesia with an Ajan–Valium combination. Wehrmedizin 2: 84–88

Neomycin (sulphate)

This aminoglycoside antibiotic was found in cultures of *Streptomyces fradiae* in 1949, only five years after the discovery of streptomycin. Although more widely used initially it is now restricted to topical and oral (non-systemic) use.

Chemistry

Neomycin base (Nivemycin)
$C_{23}H_{46}N_6O_{13}$
2-Deoxy-4-O-(2,6-diamino-2,6-dideoxy-α-D-glucopyranosyl)-5-O-[3-O-(2,6-diamino-2,6 dideoxy-β-L-idopyranosyl)-β-D-ribofuranosyl]-D-streptamine
It is a mixture of neomycin B (indistinguishable from framycetin; 70–90%) neomycin C (10–30%) and less than 5% of the inactive, degradation product neamine. Neomycins B and C are isomers with very similar biological properties.[1]

At the core of the neomycin B structure is the 6-membered aminocyclitol-2-deoxystreptamine, which is common to all the aminoglycosides with the exception of streptomycin. To this are linked 2,6-diamino-substituted d glucose and, indirectly through a molecule of d-ribose, another 2,6-diamino-substituted l-hexose. There is, therefore, a chain of four ring structures united by glycosidic links; most aminoglycosides contain only three rings

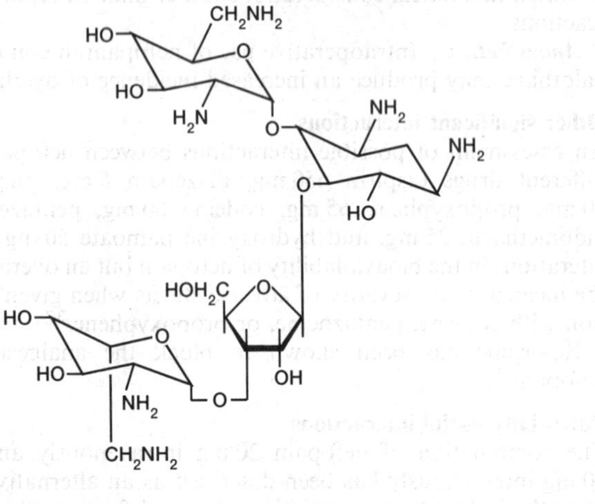

Molecular weight (free base)	711.7 (614.6)
pKa	—
Solubility (sulphate)	
in alcohol	very slightly soluble
in water	slowly soluble 1 in 1
Octanol/water partition coefficient	—

Multiple OH groupings make the molecule very polar; it is highly soluble in water (1:1) and virtually insoluble in hexane. The amino groups make the molecule very basic; it is usually handled in the form of the sulphate salt. The dried powder is white or yellow-white; 1 g neomycin sulphate should contain not less than 600 mg neomycin base.

Pharmacology

Neomycin shares all the main features of the aminoglycoside antibiotics. It is rapidly bactericidal and diffuses readily through the aqueous channels formed by porin proteins in the outer membrane of Gram-negative bacteria. Transport of neomycin across the inner

Neomycin (sulphate)

cytoplasmic membrane is an energy-dependent process and can be blocked by calcium ions or reduced pH. Neomycin binds to polysomes and thus inhibits protein synthesis. It binds to the 30S ribosomal subunit and also, unlike streptomycin, to the 50S ribosomal subunit. Neomycin disrupts the normal cycle of ribosomal function by interfering at least in part with the first step of protein synthesis. Neomycin also causes a misreading of the genetic code of the mRNA template and this causes incorrect amino acids to be incorporated into the growing polypeptide chain, producing nonsense proteins.

Toxicology

Damage to hearing was recognized very soon after the introduction of neomycin into therapeutic use. Animal studies have often used proportionately much greater doses than those used in man. In these circumstances degenerative changes can be demonstrated in the auditory nerve and its projections in the brain stem.

Skeletal muscle paralysis, kidney failure and impairment of intestinal absorption have all been demonstrated in animal and human studies.

Clinical pharmacology

Neomycin is active against a wide range of Gram-negative bacteria including *Escherischia coli*, *Haemophilus influenzae*, *Enterobacter aerogenes*, *Klebsiella* spp., *Proteus* spp., *Salmonella* spp. and *Shigella* spp. It is effective against *Staphylococcus aureus*, *Streptococcus faecalis*, and has some activity against *Mycobacterium tuberculosis*. It is ineffective against *Pseudomonas aeruginosa*.

The aerobic bacteria of the colon include a wide range of coliform bacilli and other species which live symbiotically with the predominantly anaerobic population in a complex and relatively stable ecological system. Neomycin is bactericidal to many of the coliforms but not directly toxic to the anaerobes. The overall effect of oral neomycin on the large bowel flora has been demonstrated in healthy volunteers by the measurement of ammonia production by fresh stool samples.[2] After a large loading dose of neomycin, ammonia production fell gradually to about 20% of the baseline rate by 3 days. Thereafter a smaller daily dose maintained a low production rate indefinitely, except in individuals with neomycin-resistant flora. After neomycin was stopped, some subjects took several weeks to regain the baseline rate.

Neomycin has other effects on the gastrointestinal tract. Neomycin produces crypt cell necrosis in the intestine and this may account for the lowered synthesis of cholesterol which occurs with neomycin. The drug also precipitates bile salts within the lumen of the intestine. By inhibiting pancreatic lipase activity, neomycin inhibits intraluminal hydrolysis of long-chain triglycerides. There is also an increase in faecal bile acid excretion. These changes cause a moderate degree of malabsorption of fat, protein, cholesterol, lactose, calcium, vitamin B_{12} and iron. They occur with 3–4 g neomycin daily but were more marked when higher doses were used.

The fall in serum cholesterol that is seen is more than can be accounted for by the malabsorption. Neomycin disrupts the micellar structure, leading to reduced absorption of cholesterol. The multicharged neomycin cation interacts with fatty acids and bile salts, causing precipitation.[4]

Pharmacokinetics

Most published work relating to serum concentration/time patterns is based on the classical plate diffusion assay. *Bacillus subtilis* is a commonly used test organism.[5] Sensitivity seldom extends below 0.5 mg.l^{-1} and the expected coefficient of variation is about 10%. Other antibiotics interfere but more specific methods, enzyme based assay for example,[6] and high performance liquid chromatography,[7] have been applied to other aminoglycosides and could be adapted for the assay of neomycin.

It is important to remember that a neomycin sulphate standard is only partly neomycin base and that the base itself is a mixture of two active isomers (see Chemistry).

The introduction of less toxic aminoglycosides has made the systemic use of neomycin obsolete. Recent pharmacokinetic studies are therefore based on the handling of oral doses. All the aminoglycosides which are given by injection appear to have similar pharmacokinetic properties, however,[8] and there is no reason to believe that neomycin is an exception.

Urinary recovery of neomycin after oral administration of tablets or elixir indicates that seldom is more than 3% absorbed. The remainder is excreted unchanged in the faeces. Absorption may be increased in children with enteritis,[9] but apparently not in cases of active ulcerative colitis treated by neomycin given by enema.[10] 5% of a dose of 2–4 g per 24 h is not negligible, however, in a patient with substantial renal impairment.[11] When a solution of neomycin sulphate (10 g.l^{-1}) was used to irrigate the surgical area during hip replacement systemic absorption was clearly shown.[12]

The volume of distribution probably corresponds with the general value for other aminoglycosides,[8] namely 0.25 l.kg^{-1}, which is slightly larger than the extracellular water.

The mean serum concentration half time in the healthy adult is 2 h but varies according to renal function. It is prolonged in the infant (3–4 h), in the newborn (mean 5.6 h) and particularly in the premature newborn (4–10 h).[13] Similarly, in end-stage renal disease the half time is very substantially prolonged (12–24 h).[14]

Oral absorption	<5%
Presystemic metabolism	—
Plasma half life	
mean	2 h
Volume of distribution	0.25 l.kg^{-1}
Plasma protein binding (aminoglycosides)	20%

Plasma protein binding of aminoglycosides in general is not quantitatively important. Estimates seldom exceed 20%. Clearance of aminoglycosides from plasma is by glomerular filtration. There is a close parallel between kanamycin clearance and inulin clearance, for example,[15] but there is no comparable data for neomycin.

Concentration–effect relationship

When used as a systemic antibiotic, plasma concentrations of 5–10 mg.l^{-1} were considered therapeutic. Deafness has occurred, however, in patients whose measured concentrations did not exceed this (0.4–1.2 cg.l^{-1}).[16] Duration of exposure has a major influence on the severity of both oto- and nephro-toxicity. Systematic studies of concentration–effect relationships are lacking, but clearly the therapeutic index is low. Susceptible microorganisms are usually inhibited by concentrations of neomycin ranging from 0.5 to 10 mg.l^{-1}.

Metabolism

No products of in vivo metabolism have been identified. It is likely that most of the dose systemically absorbed is excreted unchanged, chiefly in the urine but also in the bile.

Pharmaceutics

Numerous topical formulations of neomycin sulphate are available from several manufacturers. Skin formulations include creams, ointments, dusting powders, and sprays and suspensions. Eye formulations include single-use sterile solutions and ointments. Ear formulations include drops, ointments and sprays. Nasal creams, drops and sprays are also available. Dental formulations are pastes for application to the root canal.

These formulations generally contain neomycin sulphate at a concentration of 0.25 to 0.5 g.dl^{-1}. This is often combined with other 'non-systemic' antibiotics (bacitracin, polymyxin B) or corticosteroids (betamethasone, hydrocortisone, prednisolone).

Neomycin is cationic and incompatible with some anionic substances such as sodium lauryl sulphate. Preparations for oral use include 500 mg tablets of neomycin sulphate (Nivemycin; Boots, UK) and generic preparations (Lederle/Roxane, USA)). Nivemycin elixir contains 100 mg in 5 ml. There is a recommended ceiling to the total dose used[17] (4 g daily, see Acute overdosage).

Solid dosage forms are stable almost indefinitely. Concentrated solutions should be protected from direct light.

Neomycin sulphate is also available in combination with bacitracin and polymyxin B as Polybactrin Soluble G.U. (Calmic). This is a sterile powder intended for the preparation of an antibacterial solution to be instilled into the urinary bladder. A preparation of

Neomycin (sulphate)

neomycin sulphate alone intended for the same purpose has been withdrawn; this removes the risk of the solution being administered in error by parenteral injection. Dilute solutions intended for use in the bladder should be discarded within a few hours if not used.

Skin or eye contact can give rise to a neomycin allergy of the delayed hypersensitivity type in patients or other handlers of the formulations.

Therapeutic use

Indications

1. Superficial bacterial infections
2. Bladder infection
3. Hepatic encephalopathy
4. Prophylaxis of sepsis associated with colonic surgery.

Former indications

5. Hypercholesterolaemia
6. Acute bacterial enteritis
7. Management of wounds.

Contraindications

To topical use

1. Allergy to an aminoglycoside
2. Perforation of the ear drum.

To uses with significant systemic absorption

3. Pregnancy
4. Renal impairment
5. Myasthenia gravis.

To oral use

6. Intestinal obstruction
7. Inflammatory or ulcerative gastrointestinal disease.

Indications

1. Superficial bacterial infections

The large number of topical formulations demonstrates the popularity of neomycin for the treatment of bacterial infections of skin, eye, ear and nose. Evaluation of efficacy is complicated by the use of antibiotic mixtures.

Neomycin is effective against staphylococcal impetigo, although penetration of crusts may be poor and systemic penicillin or erythromycin is often preferred. The combination with corticosteroids in formulations for eczema is justified by the presence of secondary bacterial infection. There is a significant risk of allergy to neomycin, however, and prolonged use is discouraged. Allergy to some deodorants may be attributable to neomycin.

Neomycin-containing drops or ointment are used in bacterial conjunctivitis. Penetration of the cornea/conjunctiva is poor although subconjunctival injection has been used to treat infections of the anterior chamber.

Nasal creams have been used to treat carriers of *Staphylococcus aureus* but the emergence of resistance has reduced efficacy.

Neomycin sulphate is included in some antibacterial pastes for application to the dental root canal; the Eastman Dental Hospital endodontic compound contains 10 g in 36.6 g polyethylene glycol together with bacitracin, nystatin and polymyxin B. Although sensitive coliforms are sometimes isolated from apical infections, the main isolates are strict anaerobes including Bacteroides, which are all neomycin-resistant. Neomycin is therefore now seen as a minor component of such pastes. Since the pastes can physically interfere with the bonding of the root filling to the dentine, greater reliance is placed on thorough debridement and irrigation with dilute antiseptic solutions.

The prevalence of aminoglycoside-resistant bacteria is commonly linked to the local use of topical formulations. Although neomycin is not used for systemic treatment, cross-resistance to other aminoglycosides does occur and may reduce the effectiveness of gentamicin, for example.

2. Bladder infections

Instillation into the urinary bladder of dilute solutions of neomycin sulphate (for example, 100 mg.l^{-1}) can be used to kill bacteria introduced by urethral catheterization or instrumentation.

This route may also be used to treat established infection in the presence of gross abnormality of the urinary tract. When kidney function is impaired, the systemic administration of aminoglycoside antibiotics carries an increased risk of toxicity; dosage must accordingly be reduced and the resulting urinary concentrations are lowered. Direct instillation allows higher urinary concentrations to be achieved with a small total dose. Absorption of the antibiotic from the bladder is very slow so long as the mucosal lining is intact.

3. Hepatic encephalopathy

Early studies showed improved tolerance to dietary protein and reduction of neuro-psychiatric symptoms in patients with chronic portal-systemic encephalopathy.[18,19] Improvement was usually associated with lowering of arterial blood ammonia concentrations but the relationship was not simple. Some cases failed to relapse despite a rise of ammonia to pretreatment levels.[18] Placebo-treated controls were not studied, although in some individual cases it was shown that purgation alone could not maintain remission after neomycin withdrawal.

Patients with acute encephalopathy also improved with neomycin treatment,[18] although other measures were taken including protein-free diet, blood transfusion and enemas. An alternative approach to the treatment of encephalopathy involves the use of lactulose by mouth or enema. Osmotic purgation occurs and bacterial ammonia production is discouraged by the provision of an alternative energy source. Fermentation produces organic acids which lower the colon pH, thus trapping ammonia within the lumen as ammonium ion. Recent studies have compared the efficacy of neomycin with lactulose/lactose. A randomized comparison of oral lactulose with oral neomycin was carried out in 173 patients with biopsy-proven cirrhosis and evidence of encephalopathy. Approximately one-third of the patients improved in each treatment group (see Major outcome trials). Similar results were obtained in a double-blind trial of neomycin against a lactose enema.[20] Blindness was preserved by the use of placebo tablets and a starch enema.

The comparable efficacy of neomycin and lactulose must lead to a preference for lactulose in patients with impairment of renal function or a history of vertigo or deafness. The two agents are often used together. This practice has been questioned.[21] Nevertheless, lactulose still lowers the stool pH when the colonic flora has been reduced by neomycin and there is no evidence of antagonism (see Drug interactions).

4. Prophylaxis of sepsis associated with colonic surgery

From 1960 to 1980 there were many trials of poorly absorbed antibiotics in preparing the large bowel for surgery. Oral neomycin reduced the aerobic bacteria in rectal washings and the frequency of postoperative infections,[22–24] but the best drug and dosage schedule remained uncertain. Metronidazole was added when the importance of anaerobes was appreciated but in 1979 (see Major outcome trials) it was shown that systemic administration was more effective than oral. Instead of pre-treating for several days by mouth, two antibacterial drugs were given by injection immediately before and after surgery. This result was confirmed several years later when single-dose systemic metronidazole and ceftriaxone proved more effective in preventing postoperative wound infection than oral neomycin and erythromycin.[25] Some workers have found that a single systemic anti-anaerobic agent is sufficient[26] but more typically it has been found that a combination which includes an anti-aerobic agent is necessary.[27]

Oral pre-treatment with antibiotics including neomycin is still practised but to a reduced extent. Increasingly the systemic route is used peri-operatively after preliminary cleansing of the large bowel by the oral administration of large volumes of electrolyte solutions.

Former indications

5. Hypercholesterolaemia

In 1959 neomycin was shown to lower the serum cholesterol concentration. It has since been used to treat severe hypercholesterolaemia which has not responded adequately to other measures. This use has declined with the advent of safer drugs and the greater awareness of neomycin toxicity.

At modest dosage (500 mg three times in 24 h) neomycin produced a 20% reduction in serum cholesterol in patients with familial hypercholesterolaemia. This was accompanied by a similar increase

Neomycin (sulphate)

in the excretion of cholesterol in the faeces but there was no malabsorption of bile salts.[28] Neomycin was more efficient than cholestyramine, which produced a similar lowering of serum cholesterol at a much greater dose (32 g per 24 h) and at the cost of a 2–3 fold increase in faecal cholesterol excretion in the form of bile salts.[28] The hepatocyte appears to respond to cholesterol depletion partly by increased cholesterol biosynthesis but also by increased clearance of low density lipoprotein (LDL) cholesterol from the plasma. This results in a selective lowering of LDL cholesterol concentration.[28] HDL cholesterol and triglyceride concentrations are virtually unchanged.[29]

6. Acute bacterial enteritis

In the absence of systemic spread of infection, antibacterial drugs now play no part in the treatment of bacterial enteritis. There is much evidence that oral neomycin treatment does not shorten the illness and many even prolong carrier states in infections with salmonellae, shigellae and enteropathic *E. coli* in infants.

A recent controlled study in adults showed a better response in patients who received a freeze-dried lactic acid-producing enterococcus than in those who received a bacitracin and neomycin preparation.[30]

7. Management of wounds

Solutions of neomycin were used to irrigate surgical wounds and body cavities with the intention of reducing postoperative sepsis. There was no barrier to absorption,[12] however, and there were many reports of toxicity.[31,32] The evidence of therapeutic effectiveness which might justify this hazard was lacking[33] and the practice has ceased.

The incidence of bacterial infection of surgical prostheses, for example artificial joints, is low but the secondary consequences are very serious. Accordingly, several methods of prophylaxis have been used including incorporation of antibiotics, for example neomycin, into bone cement. This practice is contrary to experience in other areas of prophylaxis against bacterial infection; a high plasma concentration at the time of possible introduction of infection has proved more effective than sustained low concentrations of antibiotics. The danger of hypersensitivity also militates against the implantation of a slowly absorbed depot of neomycin.

Adverse reactions

Potentially life-threatening effects

Superinfection. Reduction of colonic flora by oral neomycin clearly carries the risk of secondary infection with opportunistic organisms. This is probably the basis of the mild diarrhoea which is a common adverse effect in patients on long-term oral treatment for hypercholesterolaemia.[28] In more severe cases staphylococcal enterocolitis or pseudomembranous colitis[34] associated with infection by *Clostridium difficile* can be life-threatening.

Renal failure. The aminoglycosides are selectively concentrated in tubular cells; even a single, systemic therapeutic dose will impair tubular function as measured by the reabsorption of β_2 microglobulin. This may represent competition for a common transport system. The risk of renal damage with oral neomycin is probably small when the dose is no more than 4 g per 24 h and renal function is not impaired. Higher doses gave potentially toxic plasma concentrations, however, in patients with hepatic cirrhosis and a raised blood urea.[11] Most cases of acute renal failure have been caused by the overenthusiastic use of irrigating solutions, poor aspiration technique or even unintended intramuscular injection. All aspects of renal function are affected, glomerular filtration rate (GFR) falls and severe oliguria or anuria can result. A substantial degree of recovery is usual with adequate haemodialysis treatment in the interim.[14,32]

Skeletal muscle paralysis. Potentially fatal respiratory arrest has been reported, usually after the application of neomycin to wounds or cavities.[31,32] Transmission at the neuromuscular junction is impaired either by reduction of acetylcholine release or by antagonism at cholinoceptors. This property is common to the aminoglycosides; patients with myasthenia gravis and patients who have received tubocurarine or related drugs are particularly at risk[35] as are patients with severe renal impairment.

Acute overdosage

Deliberate overdosage is rare; reported cases are usually therapeutic accidents in which excessive amounts or inappropriate routes were employed. The number of deaths and cases of permanent deafness demonstrates the need for clear guidelines.

Neomycin should never be used as a systemic antibiotic; there is no place for intramuscular, intravenous or subcutaneous injection.

Powders, sprays or solutions containing neomycin should not be applied to body cavities or closed wounds.

The irrigation of open surgical wounds has questionable efficacy but undoubted risk. It is no longer recommended procedure. When neomycin-containing solution is instilled into the bladder of a patient with normal renal function, the total daily dose used should not exceed 1 g and the period of use should not exceed seven days. Neomycin is absorbed from body surfaces after local irrigation and toxicity has been reported following this procedure.

Oral dosage should not exceed 4 g per 24 h in the adult; in many cases of hepatic encephalopathy 1 g twice daily will be sufficient and less is needed in hypercholesterolaemia. Monitoring by pure tone audiometry and serum neomycin assay is good practice, particularly in cases requiring long-term treatment or repeated courses.

Topical formulations of neomycin should not be used on large areas of skin made permeable by abrasion, burns or eczema. This applies particularly when the surface is then to be occluded.

Apart from topical use on a small area, neomycin should not be used at all in patients with substantial renal impairment. Renal failure commonly plays a part in overdosage, either as a predisposing factor or as a secondary result. Haemodialysis gives effective clearance of neomycin.[14] Prolonged assisted ventilation may also be required.[31,32]

Severe or irreversible adverse effects

Ototoxicity. Reports of ototoxicity attributed to neomycin are numerous.[16] All routes of administration are implicated, even oral, but the risk is greatest with injection or irrigation of wounds. Documentation is often poor; baseline audiometry and serum neomycin concentration profiles are seldom available. Nevertheless, it is clear that prolonged treatment, large doses and renal impairment all predispose. The effects of repeated courses or systemic doses of other aminoglycosides are cumulative and progressive. The risk is great when serum concentrations exceed 10 $mg.l^{-1}$ for long periods but deafness has occurred at lower levels.[16]

Acuity for high-pitched sounds is lost first. Conversational frequencies are relatively preserved, and therefore detection is often delayed. Even if dosage is stopped at the first suspicion there is seldom improvement. More commonly, hearing continues to deteriorate for weeks or even months. Vestibular function is usually relatively spared.

Temporal bone studies show that hair cells of the cochlea are destroyed;[36] there is no capacity for regeneration. Kinetic studies in animals suggest very slow equilibration of aminoglycoside concentrations between plasma and inner ear fluids. Once a high concentration is established in these fluids it is slow to decline.

Perforation of the drum allows passage of topical neomycin preparations into the middle ear. Despite slow diffusion characteristics, the steepness of the concentration gradient then allows direct penetration of toxic amounts into the inner ear.

Allergy. Severe systemic manifestations (anaphylactic shock, angioneurotic oedema, blood dyscrasias) occur rarely, as with the other aminoglycosides; indeed there may be a cross-sensitivity.

Symptomatic adverse effects

Skin rashes. Milder manifestations are primarily skin rashes which affect 6–8% of patients using topical preparations. Rashes may be erythematous, morbilliform, maculopapular or urticarial.

Diarrhoea. Withdrawals from clinical trials of oral neomycin in hypercholesterolaemia were most commonly due to the passage of frequent or unformed stools.[28] This is attributed chiefly to changes in the colonic flora.

Steatorrhoea. Oral doses of 500 mg three times in 24 h cause increased excretion of cholesterol in faeces. It is only at higher doses that there is substantial excretion of fatty acid or triglyceride.[28] Disruption of micelle function[4] and toxic effects on the jejunal mucosa are probably both involved. The effects of neomycin are usually reversible on stopping the drug.

Changes in the jejunal mucosa have been shown in before-and-after biopsy studies in healthy volunteers who received treatment for only 6 days.[37] Shortening and clubbing of villi were seen in some cases and reduced levels of Mg^{2+}-activated ATP-ase, 5'-nucleotidase and alkaline phosphatase were found.

Absorption of D-xylose was reduced. Other studies have shown impaired absorption of nutrients and drugs including fat, nitrogen, carotene, glucose, lactose, sodium, calcium, iron and cyanocobalamin (see Drug interactions).

Interference with clinical pathology tests

Neomycin can interfere with amino acid analysis in urine. A ninhydrin-positive spot was produced on paper chromatography and high voltage electrophoresis.[38]

High risk groups

Neonates

The plasma concentration half time can be markedly prolonged, particularly in the premature infant.[13] Without a measurement of GFR, however, there is no way of predicting handling in the individual case.

Breast milk. Aminoglycosides enter breast milk and in some circumstances neomycin given to the mother might appear in breast milk. There is little risk of ototoxicity to the infant, but abnormal development of gut flora in the infant might occur.

Children

Hearing loss at high frequency was detected in some infants given oral neomycin for acute enteritis.[9] In the absence of renal disease the GFR is higher relative to surface area than in later life; there is, therefore, no special predisposition to neomycin toxicity.

Pregnant women

Systemic aminoglycosides are avoided in pregnancy because of the risk to the developing cochlea and vestibule. This must also apply to the irrigation of burns or wounds with neomycin solutions, nor can the oral use of neomycin be justified, since for most indications there are less hazardous treatments.

The application of small amounts of cream, drops or ointment to intact mucosa or skin is unlikely to harm the fetus or the breast-fed baby.

The elderly

This group is particularly vulnerable; hearing is already impaired, vestibular function is critical, and the GFR may be reduced two or three-fold without any tell-tale rise in serum creatinine concentration.

Concurrent disease

There is no justification for the exposure of patients with renal impairment to the risk of neomycin absorption. This effectively restricts usage to topical application to intact mucosa or skin in all patients with a reduced GFR — the newborn, the elderly and patients with systemic or renal disease leading to renal impairment.

Drug interactions

Potentially hazardous interactions

Neomycin augments the nephrotoxic effects of other aminoglycosides, the neuromuscular blocking action of tubocurarine, pancuronium and related drugs[31,35] and the ototoxic effects of loop diuretics.[39]

The enhancement of the action of warfarin[40] is attributed to interference with the absorption of vitamin K. This in turn may be caused by inhibition of bacterial synthesis or by impairment of lipid absorption. However, the interaction is usually of minor clinical significance.

Interference with drug absorption has been reported for digoxin,[41] phenoxymethylpenicillin[42], vitamin B_{12}, methotrexate, 5-flurouracil and spironolactone.[43] In the last, the rate was reduced but extent was unchanged. Most of these studies were conducted on healthy volunteers who received a few doses of neomycin and a single oral dose of the test drug. The magnitude of the effect on steady-state concentrations of the test drug during multiple dosage is not generally known.

Potentially useful interactions

The cholesterol-lowering effect of neomycin is enhanced by combination with cholestyramine,[28] clofibrate[44] and d-thyroxine.[29] The evidence does not suggest a greater than additive effect. Similarly, the combination of neomycin with lactulose in patients with hepatic cirrhosis has an additive effect in reducing gut ammonia production.[45]

Neomycin (sulphate)

Major outcome trials

1. Orlandi F, Freddara U, Candelaresi M T et al 1981. Comparison between neomycin and lactulose in 173 patients with hepatic encephalopathy: a randomized clinical study. Digestive Diseases and Sciences 26: 498–506

The authors reviewed 10 controlled clinical studies encompassing 127 patients and giving equivocal results about the relative efficacy of neomycin and lactulose. They believed theirs was the first large-scale study on hepatic encephalopathy.

The study occupied 4 years and 6 clinical units. Patients with biopsy-proven cirrhosis and clinical, biochemical and EEG evidence of encephalopathy were admitted. Severity was graded 1 to 3. Patients with uraemia and hypokalaemia were excluded because of the unacceptable risks associated with neomycin and purgation respectively.

Treatments were allocated randomly within centres and the two groups were balanced with respect to clinical grade and other factors known to influence outcome. Assessors were not aware of the treatment allocated. 24 patients were excluded before randomization and 17 before analysis. 82 patients received neomycin 1–2 g four times in 24 h (depending on grade) and magnesium sulphate 30–60 g per 24 h. 91 patients received 50% lactulose syrup 10–35 ml three times in 24 h; dosage was adjusted to give not less than two bowel motions in 24 h. The treatment and observation period was 14 days.

There were no significant differences between the two treatment groups in the number of deaths (12 on neomycin; 11 on lactulose) nor in the number of patients who attained a less severe grade of encephalopathy (34 on neomycin; 28 on lactulose). It was concluded that neomycin had no clear advantage over lactulose and that the latter should therefore be preferred because of its lower toxicity.

2. Keighly M R B, Alexander-Williams J, Arabi Y, Youngs D, Burdon D W 1979 Comparison between systemic and oral antimicrobial prophylaxis in colorectal surgery. Lancet 1: 894–897

The results of this trial have played an important part in the decline of oral neomycin in preoperative bowel preparation. The experimental design demanded an aminoglycoside which could be given both orally and by injection. Accordingly kanamycin was substituted for neomycin.

93 patients undergoing elective colorectal surgery for carcinoma were allocated randomly to the two treatment groups. 47 patients received 3 days treatment with kanamycin (3 g in 24 h) and 2 days treatment with metronidazole (1.2 g in 24 h) all by mouth. 46 patients received 3 doses of 1 g kanamycin and 0.5 g metronidazole both by intravenous or intramuscular routes; the first dose was given immediately before surgery and the last about 24 h later.

Sepsis was substantially less frequent in the group receiving antibiotics by injection (3 cases) than in the group receiving oral pretreatment (17 cases). There was also a lower incidence of pseudomembranous colitis in the injection-treated group (1 case to 6).

The authors conclude that 'systematic preoperative anti-microbial prophylaxis is safer and more effective'.

General review articles

Bailey R R 1981 The aminoglycosides. Drugs 22: 321–327

Bint A J, Burtt I 1980 Adverse antibiotic drug interactions. Drugs 20: 57–68

Mawer G E 1979 Aminoglycoside pharmacology. In: Reeves D, Geddes A (eds) Recent advances in infection, No.1. Churchill Livingstone, Edinburgh, ch 8, pp 121–135

Phillips I 1982 Aminoglyocosides. Lancet 2: 311–315

Waksman S A 1953 Neomycin: nature, formation, isolation and practical application. Rutgers University Press, New Brunswick

References

1. Hewitt W 1977 Assay of mixtures of antibiotics. In: Microbiological assay. Academic Press, New York, ch 5, pp 136–137
2. Reynolds A V, Smith J T 1979 Enzymes which modify aminoglycoside antibiotics. In: Reeves D, Geddes A (eds) Recent advances in infection, No 1. Churchill Livingstone, Edinburgh, ch 11, pp 165–181
3. Byungse S, Stephens J L, Kunin C M 1979 Oral neomycin dosage schedules for suppression of ammonia production by bowel flora. Antimicrobial Agents and Chemotherapy 16: 519–522

4. Thompson G R, Barrowman J, Gutierrez L, Dowling R H 1971 Action of neomycin on the intraluminal phase of lipid absorption. Journal of Clinical Investigation 50: 319–323
5. Sabath L D, Casey J I, Ruch P A, Stumpf L L, Finland M 1971 Rapid microassay of gentamicin, kanamycin, neomycin, streptomycin and vancomycin in serum or plasma. Journal of Laboratory and Clinical Medicine 78: 457–463
6. Broughall J M, Reeves D S 1975 The acetyltransferase enzyme method for the assay of serum aminoglycoside concentrations and a comparison with other methods. Journal of Clinical Pathology 28: 140–145
7. Crugers Dagneaux P G L C, Klein Elhorst J T 1981 HPLC estimation of tobramycin in serum. Pharmaceutisch Weekblad 3: 582–586
8. Bochner F, Carruthers G, Kampmann J, Steiner J 1983 Aminoglycosides. In: Handbook of clinical pharmacology. Little, Brown, Boston, pp 106–108
9. Zelenka J, Tomes D, Zilkova B 1966 Possibilités d'effets ototoxiques de la neomycine administrée per os dans la dyspepsies du nourrisson. Etude experimentale et audiometrique. Pediatrie 21: 573–583
10. Breen K J, Bryant R E, Levinson J D, Schenker S 1972 Neomycin absorption in man; studies of oral and enema administration and effect of intestinal ulceration. Annals of Internal Medicine 76: 211–218
11. Kunin C M, Chalmers T C, Leevy C M, Sebastyen S C, Lieber C S, Finland M 1960 Absorption of orally administered neomycin and kanamycin with special reference to patients with severe hepatic and renal disease. New England Journal of Medicine 262: 380–385
12. Weinstein A J, McHenry M C, Gavan T L 1977 Systemic absorption of neomycin irrigating solution. Journal of the American Medical Association 238: 152–153
13. Axline S G, Yaffe S J, Simon H J 1967 Clinical pharmacology of antimicrobials in premature infants. II ampicillin, methicillin, oxacillin, neomycin and colistin. Pediatrics 39: 97–107
14. Krumlovsky F A, Emmerman J, Parker R H, Wisgerhof M, Del Greco F 1972 Dialysis in treatment of neomycin overdose. Annals of Internal Medicine 76: 443–446
15. Orme B M, Cutler R E 1969 The relationship between kanamycin pharmacokinetics: distribution and renal function. Clinical Pharmacology and Therapeutics 10: 543–550
16. Kavanagh K T, McCabe B F 1983 Ototoxicity of oral neomycin and vancomycin. Laryngoscope 93: 649–653
17. Fitzgerald R H 1976 Invited editorial comment. Archives of Surgery 111: 825
18. Dawson A M, McLaren J, Sherlock S 1957 Neomycin in the treatment of hepatic coma. Lancet 2: 1263–1268
19. Fisher C J, Faloon W W 1957 Blood ammonia levels in hepatic cirrhosis. New England Journal of Medicine 256: 1030–1035
20. Uribe M, Berthier J M, Lewis H et al 1981 Lactose enemas plus placebo tablets vs neomycin tablets plus starch enemas in acute portal systemic encephalopathy. A double-blind randomised controlled study. Gastroenterology 81: 101–106
21. Martin A J 1981 Portal systemic encephalopathy — should lactulose and neomycin be used together. British Journal of Clinical Practice 35: 323–324
22. Montori A, Viceconte G W, Pietropaulo V, Viceconte G, Bosliolo G 1980 Neomycin and the combination of neomycin and bacitracin in the prevention of bacterial infection in surgery of the colon and/or rectum. Chemotherapy 26: 72–79
23. Sellwood R A, Burn J I, Waterworth P M, Welbourn R B 1969 A second clinical trial to compare two methods for pre-operative preparation of the large bowel. British Journal of Surgery 56: 610–612
24. Clarke J S, Condor R E, Bartlett J G 1977 Preoperative oral antibiotics reduce septic complications of colon operations: results of a prospective randomised double-blind clinical study. Annals of Surgery 186: 251–259
25. Weaver M, Burdon D W, Youngs D J, Keighly M R 1986 Oral neomycin and erythromycin compared with single-dose systemic metronidazole and ceftriaxone prophylaxis in elective colorectal surgery. American Journal of Surgery 151: 437–442
26. Mitchell N J, Evans D S, Pollock D 1983 Single dose metronidazole with and without cefuroxime in elective colorectal surgery. British Journal of Surgery 70: 668–669
27. Bergman L, Solhaug J H 1987 Single-dose chemoprophylaxis in elective colorectal surgery: comparison between doxycycline plus metronidazole and doxycycline. Annals of Surgery 205: 77–81
28. Miettinen T A 1979 Effects of neomycin alone and in combination with cholestyramine on serum cholesterol and fecal steroids in hypercholesterolaemic subjects. Journal of Clinical Investigation 64: 1485–1493
29. Vogelberg K H, Koschinsky T, Hein H, Gries F A 1982 Effect of neomycin sulphate alone and in combination with D-thyroxine on serum lipoproteins in hypercholesterolaemic subjects. European Journal of Clinical Pharmacology 22: 33–38
30. Cammari E, Belvisi A, Guidoni G, Marini G, Frigerio G 1981 A double-blind comparison of two different treatments for acute enteritis in adults. Chemotherapy 27: 466–470
31. Pridgeon J E 1956 Respiratory arrest thought to be due to intraperitoneal neomycin. Surgery 40: 571–574
32. Davia J E, Siemsen A W, Anderson R W 1970 Uraemia, deafness and paralysis due to irrigating antibiotic solution. Archives of Internal Medicine 125: 135–139
33. Nachamie B W, Siffert R S, Bryer M S 1968 A study of neomycin instillation into orthopedic surgical wounds. Journal of the American Medical Association 204: 687–689
34. Weidma W F, Von Myenfeldt M F, Soeters P B, Wesdorp R I C, Greep J M 1980 Pseudomembranous colitis after whole gut irrigation with neomycin and erythromycin base. British Journal of Surgery 67: 895–896
35. Giala M, Sareyiannis C, Cortsaris N, Paradelis A, Lappas D G 1982 Possible interaction of pancuronium and tubocurarine with oral neomycin. Anaesthesia 37: 776
36. Lowry L D, May M, Pastore P 1973 Acute histopathologic inner ear changes in deafness due to neomycin in a human. Laryngoscope 70: 382–392
37. Gonciarz Z, Lelek E, Kaminiski M, Kaminiska O 1982 Enzyme alteration in human jejunal mucosa associated with neomycin induced malabsorption. Scandinavian Journal of Gastroenterology 17 (suppl): 279

Neomycin (sulphate)

38. Potter J L 1974 Further observations on ninhydrin reacting compounds in urine. Journal of Paediatrics 84: 250–251
39. Mathog R H, Klein W J 1969 Ototoxicity of ethacrynic acid and aminoglycoside antibiotics in uraemia. New England Journal of Medicine 280: 1223–1224
40. Udall J A 1970 Drug interference with warfarin therapy. Clinical Medicine 77: 20–25
41. Lindenbaum J, Maulitz R M, Saha J R, Shea N, Butler V P 1972 Impairment of digoxin absorption by neomycin. Clinical Research 20: 410
42. Cheng S H, White A 1962 Effect of orally administered neomycin on the absorption of penicillin V. New England Journal of Medicine 267: 1296–1297
43. Bartle W R, Coates P E, Fisher M M, Louman F J 1979 Effect of neomycin on the bioavailability of spironolactone: a single dose study. American Journal of Hospital Pharmacy 36: 1701–1703
44. Samuel P, Holtzman C M, Meilman E, Sekowski I 1970 Reduction of serum cholesterol and triglyceride levels by the combined administration of neomycin and clofibrate. Circulation 41: 109–114
45. Weber F L Jr, Fresard K M, Lally B R 1982 Effects of lactulose and neomycin on urea metabolism in cirrhotic subjects. Gastroenterology 82: 213–217

N

Neostigmine (bromide and methylsulphate)

The drug is a potent reversible inhibitor of acetylcholinesterase whose main use is in the treatment of myasthenia gravis.

Chemistry

Neostigmine bromide
Neostigmine bromide (Prostigmin, Juvastigmin, Prostigmina, Prostigmine, Injectable Neostigmine)
$C_{12}H_{19}BrN_2O_2$
3-(Dimethylcarbamoyloxy)-NNN-trimethylanilinium bromide

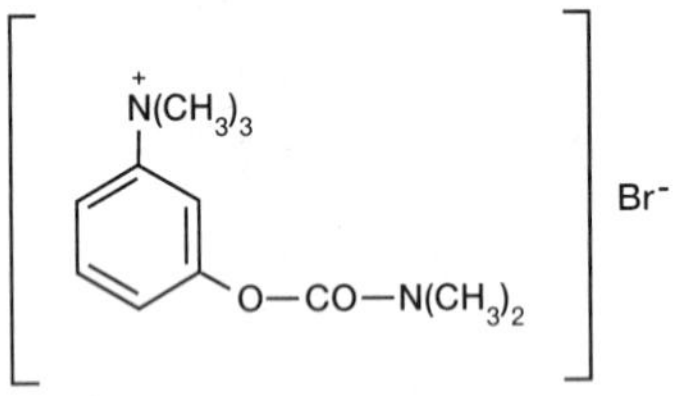

Molecular weight	303.2
pKa	12.0
Solubility	
in alcohol	1 in 8
in water	1 in 0.5
Octanol/water partition coefficient	low

Neostigmine bromide is a quaternary ammonium compound prepared by chemical synthesis as colourless crystals or a white, crystalline, slightly hygroscopic powder with a bitter taste. It is not available in any combined preparations.

Neostigmine methylsulphate
Neostigmine methylsulphate (Neostigmine Injection, Neostigmine Methylsulphate Injection, Prostigmin, Intrastigmina, Juvastigmin, Prostigmina)
$C_{13}H_{22}N_2O_6S$
3-(Dimethylcarbamylocy)-NNN-trimethylanilinium methylsulphate

Molecular weight	334.4
pKa	12.0
Solubility	
in alcohol	1 in 6
in water	1 in 0.5
Octanol/water partition coefficient	low

Neostigmine methylsulphate is a quaternary ammonium compound prepared by chemical synthesis as odourless, colourless crystals or a white crystalline powder with a bitter taste. It is available in a compound preparation for injection with glycopurronium bromide as Robinul-Neostigmine.

Pharmacology

Neostigmine is a reversible antagonist to acetylcholinesterase, the enzyme that destroys acetylcholine. Acetylcholinesterase exists in two molecular forms: a simple oligomer of 70 000 dalton subunits and a complex elongated structure with a molecular weight of 10^6. The active centre of the enzyme consists of a negative subsite and an esteratic subsite where nucleophilic attack occurs on the acyl carbon of acetylcholine. Neostigmine has a carbamyl ester linkage that is hydrolysed by acetylcholinesterase[1] but much more slowly than is acetylcholine itself. The enzyme is thus carbamylated at the active centre and the duration of inhibition of acetylcholinesterase by the carbamylating agents is about 4 hours.

Neostigmine potentiates both the nicotinic and muscarinic effects of naturally occurring acetylcholine. In addition, it probably also has direct effects on acetylcholine receptors in skeletal muscle. In many species neostigmine inhibits the muscle relaxant effects of curare-like drugs.

Toxicology

Neostigmine has not been reported to have mutagenic or carcinogenic potential. In rats, acute and chronic exposure causes changes in the fine structure at the end-plate region of muscle.[2] The files of the Committee on Safety on Medicines from 1969 to date do not hold any reports of suspected carcinogenicity resulting from neostigmine.

Clinical pharmacology

Neostigmine is used mainly for its effects on skeletal muscle in myasthenia gravis[3] and in anaesthesia for termination of the effects of competitive neuromuscular blocking drugs. It is also used for its effect on smooth muscle in treating atony of the gut and bladder in paralytic ileus and primary and secondary glaucoma. Adverse effects include salivation, anorexia, nausea and vomiting, abdominal cramps and diarrhoea. Paradoxical effects can occur because of an interaction between the nicotinic and muscarinic actions of neostigmine.

Neostigmine is an effective cholinesterase inhibitor with an onset of action after an oral dose of 30–60 min and a duration of action of 2–4 h. Neostigmine produces miosis and although the pupil is small, it usually reacts further to light. Accommodation is usually blocked temporarily and intraocular pressure is reduced, although a transient rise in intraocular pressure may be seen initially.

Neostigmine acts on the gastrointestinal tract to increase gastric and intestinal contractions which may cause abdominal colic. It also affects skeletal muscle by increasing contraction, both directly and by inhibiting cholinesterase activity. In standard doses, this is primarily due to the effects of acetylcholine in initiating a propagated muscle action potential. However, in higher doses or after prolonged use, depolarization of the motor end plate may follow, leading to decreased muscle activity and paralysis.

Neostigmine will reverse the effects of competitive neuromuscular blocking drugs such as tubocurarine and is usually given by the intramuscular route for this purpose. Neostigmine causes increased secretion by secretory glands innervated by postganglionic cholinergic fibres. This results in increased salivation, increased intestinal secretions which may lead to diarrhoea, and increased bronchial secretions. The predominant effect of neostigmine on the cardiovascular system is bradycardia due to the peripheral accumulation of acetylcholine. Blood pressure is not usually affected, although the cardiac output may fall. In the central nervous system neostigmine may initially cause stimulation followed by depression, and this may lead to depression of respiration and anoxia, especially with larger than standard doses. The usual oral dose of neostigmine is in the range of 15–90 mg daily given in divided doses every 4–6 h. The optimal dose in myasthenia gravis can be determined by giving an oral dose of 7.5 mg and measuring muscle strength and vital capacity. When the observations have returned to pretreatment values, a larger dose of neostigmine ($1\frac{1}{2}$ times as great as previously) is given and the tests are repeated. This sequence is continued until an optimal response is obtained.

Pharmacokinetics

The assay of cholinesterase inhibitors presents technical problems because of the very low concentrations present in plasma and the tendency of these compounds to undergo spontaneous in vitro hydrolysis in blood, plasma and buffer solutions. This hydrolysis can be inhibited by the addition of dyflos.[4] The analytical techniques currently employed include gas chromatography with electron-capture, nitrogen or mass spectrometric detection, or liquid chromatographic techniques.[5] The limit of sensitivity with nitrogen detection is 1 $\mu g.l^{-1}$ and with mass spectrometric detection it is 1 $\mu g.l^{-1}$.

Neostigmine, a quaternary ammonium drug, is poorly absorbed from the gastrointestinal tract.[25] The actual absorption mechanism for neostigmine has not been determined but animal studies suggest that it is absorbed intact and that no hydrolysis takes place in the intestinal wall.[6] Bioavailability has been estimated at between 1% and 2%.[7] Peak plasma concentrations occur at between one and two hours after ingestion in fasting patients. Plasma concentrations after a 30 mg oral dose of neostigmine vary from 1 to 5 µg.l^{-1}. The time to peak concentration is delayed by about 90 min by the ingestion of food, although the area under the plasma concentration–time curve (AUC) is unaffected. The mean plasma half life of neostigmine bromide is very short, between 0.06 and 0.09 h for the α phase[8,9] and between 0.40 and 1.32 h for the β phase.[10,11] The elimination half life in infants and children is lower than that in adults.

Neostigmine is extensively hydrolysed in the body by plasma cholinesterases, although there may be some metabolic conversion by the liver and enterohepatic recirculation. For a given dose, there is a large variation in total plasma concentration between individuals.[5] The apparent volume of distribution of neostigmine bromide varies between 0.1 and 1.08 l.kg^{-1}. Similar values have been reported for infants, children and adults.

The mean values for the plasma half life of neostigmine methylsulphate given by the intravenous route are 0.015–0.14 h (α phase) and 0.38–1.74 h (β phase). The apparent volume of distribution of neostigmine methylsulphate when given by the intravenous route ranges from 0.53 to 1.56 l.kg^{-1}. The kinetics of neostigmine methylsulphate are otherwise the same as for the bromide.

Neostigmine and its metabolites are not bound to plasma proteins or to red blood cells. Following oral administration, 20% of the dose is excreted in urine, with 5% dose as unchanged drug. About half of the dose is excreted in the faeces. Following intramuscular administration, 80% of the dose is excreted in urine with 50% as unchanged drug. Thus neostigmine is eliminated by both extrarenal and renal mechanisms. The plasma clearance of neostigmine, normally 11 ml.min^{-1}.kg^{-1}, is substantially reduced in anephric patients and the mean elimination half life is prolonged from 113 to 379 min. Liver disease is unlikely to affect the kinetics of the drug. Neither the presence of myasthenia gravis nor its surgical treatment by thymectomy appear to affect the pharmacokinetics of neostigmine.

	Bromide	Methylsulphate
Oral absorption	<40%	<40%
Presystemic metabolism	—	—
Plasma half life		
range	0.4–1.3 h	—
mean	~1 h	0.38 h
Volume of distribution	0.1–1.1 l.kg^{-1}	0.53–1.56 l.kg^{-1}
Plasma protein binding	negligible	negligible

Neostigmine is unlikely to be excreted in breast milk in significant amounts, given its hydrophilicity. Neostigmine can cross the placenta.

Concentration–effect relationship

In the management of patients with previously untreated myasthenia gravis, there is a linear correlation between the log plasma concentration and the effect on muscle response decrement in the range 1–10 µg.l^{-1} after oral and intravenous administration of neostigmine.

No clear relationship has been established between the plasma concentration of neostigmine and its effect as an antagonist of non-depolarizing neuromuscular blockade in anaesthetized patients. This results from the fact that the effects of neostigmine are superimposed on a complex interaction of changing depth and spontaneous recovery from anaesthesia.

Metabolism

Neostigmine is extensively hydrolysed at the ester linkage by cholinesterases in the blood. The main metabolite is 3-hydroxyphenyltrimethyl ammonium which possesses some biological activity. This compound and other, as yet unidentified, metabolites account for 30% of urinary excretion in the first 24 h after oral administration. Large amounts of the drug, about 50%, are excreted in the faeces.

Neostigmine (bromide and methylsulphate)

Fig. 1 Metabolism of neostigmine

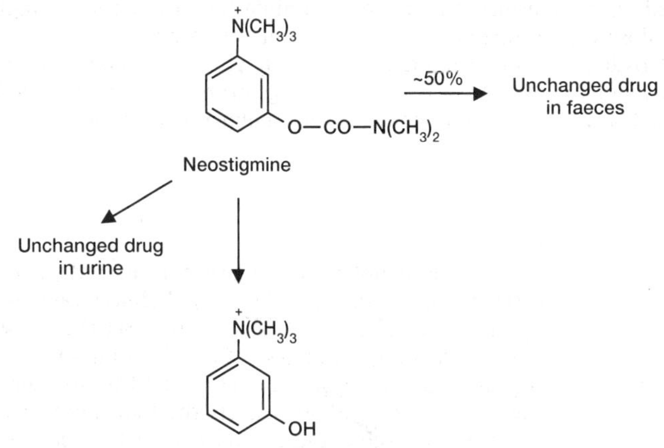

3–Hydroxyphenyl–trimethylammonium

Only 20% of the dose is recovered in urine after oral administration. This increases to 80% after intramuscular administration, 15% as 3-hydroxyphenyl-trimethyl ammonium (Fig. 1).

Pharmaceutics

1. Prostigmin tablets (Roche, UK/USA): white, round, scored tablets containing 15 mg neostigmine bromide, marked 'Prostigmin'.
2. Prostigmin injection (Roche, UK/USA): neostigmine methylsulphate is available in ampoules containing 0.5 mg and 2.5 mg of the drug in 1 ml Water for Injections as a colourless to pale yellow solution. In the USA multidose vials are available containing either 0.5 mg.ml^{-1} or 1 mg.ml^{-1}. The recommended maximum storage temperature for the solution is 25°C and it should be protected from light. The ampoule solution may be further diluted with Water for Injections but the stability of the resulting solution cannot be guaranteed.

Therapeutic use

Indications

1. Myasthenia gravis
2. Non-depolarizing neuromuscular block induced by the muscle relaxants used in anaesthesia
3. To combat the neuromuscular block induced by aminoglycoside antibiotics and antiarrhythmic agents.

Other uses

4. Management of paralytic ileus
5. Retention of urine.

Contraindications

1. Intestinal obstruction
2. Urinary obstruction
3. Hypersensitivity.

Mode of use

In the treatment of myasthenia gravis, tablets of neostigmine bromide are taken at intervals throughout the day when maximal strength is needed. In a typical regime, the tablets are taken on rising and before meals. The usual duration of action of an oral dose is between 2 and 4 h. The optimal dose can be determined by giving 7.5 mg and measuring changes in muscle strength and vital capacity. When these observations have returned to pretreatment values, then a dose 1½ times as great is administered and the observations repeated. This sequence is repeated until the optimal response is obtained. The normal adult dose is between 15 and 90 mg daily given in divided doses every 4–6 h. Alternatively, dosage can be optimized by recording the variables above and following the effects of successive small (0.125 mg) intravenous increments of neostigmine methylsulphate given at intervals of a few minutes. Atropine (0.6 mg) should be given intravenously before injecting neostigmine to prevent muscarinic side effects. When the optimal total intravenous dose has been established, and confirmed by the edrophonium test, the optimal single oral dose can be calculated as 30 times that amount.

Neostigmine methylsulphate is normally given very slowly by the intravenous route. A syringe containing atropine sulphate should always be available to counteract severe cholinergic reactions, should they occur.

Indications

1. Myasthenia gravis

The primary action of anticholinesterase drugs is to reduce the hydrolysis of acetylcholine by the enzyme acetylcholinesterase. Although these drugs have no effect on the underlying disease process, which is the loss of acetylcholine receptors as the result of immunological damage, they do allow the acetylcholine released by the nerve ending to act over a longer time. This permits the total number of interactions between acetylcholine and its receptor to be increased. The dosage must be determined empirically. Patients with myasthenia gravis require widely differing doses of anticholinesterase drugs, and although it was originally presumed that variability in absorption and metabolism were responsible,[12] the blood levels in fact vary greatly among both well and poorly controlled patients.[13] It is important to establish the dose of anticholinesterase which gives the maximum therapeutic response. This often does not restore muscle strength to normal and many patients have to live with some degree of disability. If the dose is increased above the maximum response level in an attempt to improve physical activity, the opposite effect will be produced and progressive muscular weakness may end in cholinergic crisis. The short-acting anticholinesterase, edrophonium (Tensilon), may be used to decide whether a patient is under- or overdosed. A 2 mg dose is injected intravenously initially and if there is no deterioration in muscle strength a further 3–8 mg may then be injected. An increase in muscle strength suggests that the patient requires an increase in medication of anticholinesterase drugs, whereas a deterioration in muscle strength suggests that the patient is overdosed. Facilities for artificial ventilation should be readily available in case a cholinergic crisis is precipitated.

Anticholinesterase drugs have no effect on the underlying disease process. Thymectomy is the only certain way to induce permanent remission and improvement can be anticipated in 80% of patients without thymoma, although 3 to 5 years may elapse before the benefits of the operation become apparent. Both corticosteroids and immunosuppressants, such as azathioprine, frequently induce remission, although there is a significant relapse rate when these drugs are discontinued.

Profound weakness may accompany the early stages of treatment with corticosteroids in patients already receiving anticholinesterase drugs. The weakness does not occur in patients not on anticholinergic preparations.[14] Increasing the dose of anticholinesterase aggravates the weakness and it has been found that reducing the dose of anticholinesterase drugs in patients starting corticosteroids avoids this initial deterioration. It seems probable that steroids render the patient more sensitive to anticholinergic drugs and thus produce in effect a cholinergic crisis.

2, 3. Neuromuscular block

Neostigmine 40–50 $\mu g.kg^{-1}$ with atropine 20 $\mu g.kg^{-1}$ is the treatment of choice to reverse the block induced by muscle relaxants used in anaesthesia and to combat the neuromuscular block induced by aminoglycoside antibiotics and antiarrhythmic agents. There are in fact more than 30 drugs in current clinical use that may interfere with neuromuscular transmission,[15] but the aminoglycoside antibiotics which have both a presynaptic and postsynaptic action and the antiarrhythmic drugs such as quinidine, procainamide and disopyramide are the most important. Cholinesterase inhibitors have a place in the treatment of anticholinergic drug overdosage[16] and tricyclic antidepressant overdosage[17] but penetration of the blood–brain barrier in this situation is of obvious importance and therefore physostigmine is the drug of choice.

A number of neurotransmitter deficiencies have been identified in the brain and replacement therapy on the lines of levodopa in Parkinson's disease holds out some hope for the future. The importance of a cholinergic defect in Alzheimer's disease is now established.[18] Theoretically, there are several ways of augmenting cholinergic transmission, such as administration of the precursors choline and lecithin, but the most widely studied drugs are the cholinesterase inhibitors and especially the drug physostigmine which penetrates the blood–brain barrier. Cholinesterase inhibitors may have a theoretical place in the management of dementia caused by a defect in the cholinergic neurotransmitter, such as occurs in Alzheimer's disease, but this is unproven. Penetration of the blood–brain barrier is of obvious importance so that pyridostigmine and neostigmine would have no place in the management of this disorder. Instances of improvement in cognitive function have been reported with physostigmine[19,20] and also following the administration of tetrahydroaminoacridine.[21] This latter, partly double-blind, trial of oral tetrahydroaminoacridine in the long-term treatment of Alzheimer's dementia suggested that this drug improved the condition of patients. However, a fully double-blind study[22] did not confirm any benefit.

4, 5. Other uses

The other therapeutic application of cholinesterase inhibitors is in the management of paralytic ileus and retention of urine.

Adverse reactions

Potentially life-threatening effects

Excessive doses may impair neuromuscular transmission by causing a depolarizing block. This may precipitate a state of profound weakness described as a cholinergic crisis. Clinically this may be difficult to distinguish from a myasthenic crisis. Usually, however, in a cholinergic crisis there is evidence of muscarinic signs of parasympathomimetic action, such as sweating, abdominal pain, diarrhoea, hypersalivation and bradycardia. The Tensilon test (see Indications) helps to differentiate myasthenic from cholinergic weakness.

Acute overdosage

Signs of overdosage include those due to muscarinic effects, such as abdominal cramps, increased peristalsis, diarrhoea, nausea and vomiting, increased bronchial secretion, salivation, sweating and miosis. Nicotinic effects may include muscular cramps, fasciculation and general weakness. Bradycardia and hypotension may also occur. Artificial ventilation should be instituted if respiratory depression is severe. Atropine sulphate 1–2 mg can be given intravenously to counteract the muscarinic effects.

Severe or irreversible adverse effects

There is a rare syncopal reaction in which the patient feels dizzy after the injection of an anticholinergic drug. There may be transient loss of consciousness but recovery without treatment is the rule.

Central toxic effects occur with anticholinesterase preparations that cross the blood–brain barrier, such as physostigmine. These include anxiety, disorientation, hallucination and epilepsy.

Symptomatic adverse effects

Muscarinic adverse effects are not uncommon in patients with myasthenia gravis receiving treatment with anticholinergic drugs. These usually take the form of abdominal pain and diarrhoea. Hypersalivation is not uncommon and occasionally patients complain of sweating.

High risk groups

Neonates

No special problems occur in neonates. Neonatal myasthenia occurs in the offspring of 20% of myasthenic mothers. The delay in onset of the weakness in the baby has been attributed to the passage of the mother's anticholinesterase drugs across the placenta.[23] The half life of this is much shorter than that of the acetylcholine receptor antibody so that children of myasthenic mothers tend to develop muscular weakness at 12 h after birth and the transient myasthenia persists for 4 to 6 weeks.

Breast milk. Only negligible amounts of neostigmine are excreted in breast milk, but due regard should be paid to possible effects on the breast-fed infant.

Children

No special problems occur in children.

Pregnant women

The use of neostigmine in pregnant patients with myasthenia gravis has revealed no untoward effect of the drug on the course of pregnancy.

Neostigmine (bromide and methylsulphate)

The elderly
There is no particular problem with this group.

Concurrent disease
Bronchial asthma. Neostigmine should be given to patients with bronchial asthma with great caution.

Drug interactions

Potentially hazardous interactions
Quarternary ammonium ions are poorly absorbed and their absorption may be completely inhibited by bulk laxatives such as methylcellulose.[11] Drugs that interfere with neuromuscular transmission will antagonize the effects of anticholinesterase preparations and this is particularly important in patients with myasthenia gravis where a serious relapse may occur when such preparations are used. The aminoglycoside antibiotics inhibit the release of acetylcholine. These include neomycin, streptomycin, kanamycin and gentamicin. The polypeptide antibiotics polymixin and colistin may have effects similar to those of the aminoglycosides. Oxytetracycline has also been reported to aggravate myasthenia gravis, and both lincomycin and clindamycin as a result of their curare-like action, may also aggravate myasthenia.

Antiarrhythmic drugs such as quinidine and procainamide and even propranolol block the acetylcholine receptor and may aggravate myasthenia gravis. Indeed, quinidine was once used as a provocative diagnostic test for myasthenia gravis. A myasthenic syndrome may develop in patients on long-term treatment with penicillamine. It tends to occur in those patients receiving penicillamine for rheumatoid arthritis and is rarely encountered in patients receiving penicillamine for Wilson's disease. The patients also develop acetylcholine receptor antibodies and the myasthenia usually remits when the penicillamine is withdrawn. Lithium and chlorpromazone also interfere with neuromuscular conduction and there are reports of the development of myasthenia gravis as a result.[24]

Major outcome trials

The immediate effects of anticholinesterase drugs are so dramatic that there is no need for a controlled trial to be convinced of their benefit. This is the reason that there are no published controlled trials of cholinesterase inhibitors in myasthenia gravis. Indeed, most physicians would regard the therapeutic response as part of the definition of the disease. Nor have there been comparative trials to compare the relative effects of pyridostigmine and neostigmine. Most patients tend to choose pyridostigmine as there are fewer muscarinic side effects. Otherwise there is no convincing evidence that one drug is better than the other, or that one drug can be effective when the other has failed.

References

1. Nowell P T, Scott C A, Wilson A 1962 Hydrolysis of neostigmine by plasma cholinesterase. British Journal of Pharmacology and Chemotherapy 19: 498–502
2. Hudson C S, Rash J E, Tiedt T N, Alberquerque E X 1978 Neostigmine-induced alterations at the mammalian neuromuscular junction II. Ultrastructure. Journal of Pharmacology and Experimental Therapeutics 205: 340–356
3. Aquilonius S M, Eckernas S A, Hartvig P, Linstrom B, Osterman P O 1983 Clinical pharmacology of neostigmine and pyridostigmine in patients with myasthenia gravis. Journal of Neurology, Neuro-surgery and Psychiatry 46: 929–935
4. Nowell P T, Scott C A, Wilson A 1962 Determination of neostigmine and pyridostigmine in the urine of patients with myasthenia gravis. British Journal of Pharmacology 18: 617
5. Aquilonius S M, Hartvig P 1986 Clinical pharmacokinetics of cholinesterase inhibitors. Clinical Pharmacokinetics 11: 236–249
6. Kunze H, Blime K, Vogt W 1981 Intestinal absorption of a monoquaternary drug ^{14}C-neostigmine. Nauyn Schmeideberg's Archives of Pharmacology 270: 161–168
7. Aquilonius S M, Eckernas S A, Hartvig P, Lindstrom B, Osterman P O 1980 Pharmacokinetics and oral bioavailability of pyridostigmine in man. European Journal of Clinical Pharmacology 48: 423–428
8. Morris R B, Cronnelly R, Miller R D, Stanski D, Fahey M R 1981 Pharmacokinetics of edrophonium and neostigmine when antagonising d-tubocurarine neuromuscular blockade in man. Anesthesiology 54: 399–402
9. Calvey T N, Waring M, Williams N E, Chan K 1978 Pharmacokinetics and pharmacological effects of neostigmine in man. British Journal of Clinical Pharmacology 7: 149–155
10. Williams N E, Calvey T N, Chan K 1978 Clearance of neostigmine from the circulation during antagonism of neuromuscular block. British Journal of Anaesthesia 50: 1065–1067
11. Cronnelly R, Stansky D R, Miller R D 1980 Pyridostigmine kinetics with and without renal failure. Clinical Pharmacology and Therapeutics 28: 78–81
12. Calvey T N, Chan K 1977 Plasma pyridostigmine levels in patients with myasthenia gravis. Clinical Pharmacology and Therapeutics 21: 187–193
13. White M C, de Silva P, Havard C W H 1981 Plasma pyridostigmine levels in myasthenia gravis. Neurology 31: 145–150
14. Warmolts J R, Engel W K 1972 Benefit from alternate day prednisolone in myasthenia gravis. New England Journal of Medicine 286: 17–20
15. Argov Z, Mastalgia F L 1979 Disorders of neuromuscular transmission caused by drugs. New English Journal of Medicine: 409–413
16. Duvoisin R C, Katz R 1968 Reversal of anticholinergic syndrome in man by physostigmine. Journal of the American Medical Association 206: 5
17. Petit J M, Biggs J T 1977 Tricyclic antidepressants overdose in adolescent patients. Paediatrics 52: 449–451
18. Coyle J T, Price D T, DeLong M R 1983 Alzheimer's disease: a disorder of cortical cholinergic innervation. Science 219: 1184–1190
19. Thal L J, Fuld P A, Masur D M, Sharpless N S 1983 Oral physostigmine and lecithin improve memory in Alzheimer's disease. Annals of Neurology 13: 491–496
20. Mohs R C, Davis B M, Johns C A et al 1985 Oral physostigmine treatment of patients with Alzheimer's disease. American Journal of Psychiatry 142: 28–33
21. Summers W K, Majovski L V, Marsh F M, Tachiki K, Kling A 1986 Oral tetrahydroaminoacridine in long-term treatment of senile dementia, Alzheimer-type. New England Journal of Medicine 315: 1241–1245
22. Chatelier G, Lacomblez L 1990 Tacrine (tetrahydroaminoacridine; THA) and lecithin in senile dementia of the Alzheimer type: a multicentre trial. British Medical Journal 300: 495–499
23. Buckley G A, Roberts D V, Roberts J B, Thomas B H, Wilson A 1986 Drug induced neonatal myasthenia. British Journal of Pharmacology 34: 203–204
24. Granacher R P 1977 Neuromuscular problems associated with lithium. American Journal of Psychiatry 134: 702
25. Chan K, Davison S C, Dehghan A, Hyman N 1981 The effect of neostigmine and pyridostigmine bioavailability in myasthenic patients after oral administration. Methods and Findings in Experimental Clinical Pharmacology 3: 291–296

N

Netilmicin (sulphate)

Netilmicin sulphate is an aminoglycoside antibiotic.

Chemistry

Netilmicin sulphate (Netillin, Netromycin, Nettacin, Netrocin, Netilyn, Certomycin, Vectacin, Netromicine, Netromycine)
$(C_{21}H_{41}N_5O_7)_2 5H_2SO_4$
4-O-[(2S,3S)-3-Amino-y-(aminomethyl)-3,4-dihydro-2H-pyran-2-yl]2-deoxy-6-O-[3-deoxy-4-C-methyl(3-methylamino-β-L-arabinopyranosyl]-N¹-ethyl-D-streptamine sulphate

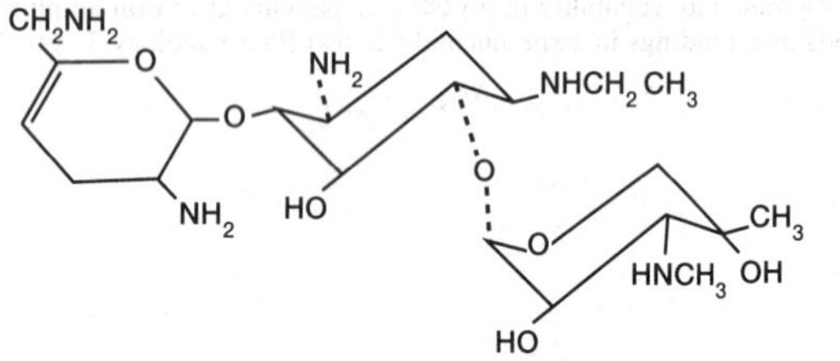

Molecular weight (free base)	1441.6 (475)
pKa	8.1
Solubility	
in alcohol	—
in water	soluble
Octanol/water partition coefficient	>0.001

Netilmicin sulphate is an odourless, white to buff powder, free from foreign matter. It is a semi-synthetic derivative of sisomicin, derived chemically by ethylation of the 1-N position of the deoxystreptamine ring of sisomicin. Netilmicin is not present in any combined preparations.

Pharmacology

Netilmicin is active against a wide range of aerobic Gram-negative bacilli. The mode of action of netilmicin is almost certain to be the same as its more extensively investigated predecessor aminoglycosides[1] which are first actively transported across the bacterial cell membrane by an oxygen-dependent system. Factors determining the rate of intracellular accumulation include the concentration of divalent cations (Mg^{2+} and Ca^{2+}), environmental pH and oxygen tension. Aminoglycosides are inactive under anaerobic conditions.

Aminoglycosides bind irreversibly to the 30S subunit of the bacterial ribosome, blocking protein synthesis by inhibiting the movement of peptidyl-tRNA associated with translocation, as well as increasing the frequency of misreading of the genetic code due to incorrect codon–anticodon interaction. The effect is bactericidal.

Toxicology

Toxicological studies in animals show that netilmicin is substantially less toxic to the kidneys and demonstrates less ototoxicity than other aminoglycosides.[2,3] Lifetime carcinogenicity tests have been undertaken in the mouse and rat and no drug-related tumours were observed. Mutagenicity tests with netilmicin have also proved negative. Teratogenicity tests have shown no adverse effects in rabbits and only an increased incidence of wavy ribs in rats. Moreover, no impairment in fertility has been observed in the rat.[4]

Clinical pharmacology

Netilmicin is poorly absorbed from the gastrointestinal tract and is therefore administered intravenously or intramuscularly. Peak serum concentrations occur between 30 and 40 minutes after intramuscular administration, and follow a biphasic curve after a 'slow bolus' given intravenously.[5] It has no important pharmacological effects apart from the action upon bacteria.

Netilmicin is a broad-spectrum aminoglycoside antibiotic active against a wide range of Gram-negative organisms and against some Gram-positive organisms. All Enterobacteriaceae such as *E. coli*, *Klebsiella*, *Enterobacter*, *Serratia* spp., *Proteus*, *Yersinia* and *Neisseria* spp. are sensitive to netilmicin.[6,7] Netilmicin is inactive against *B. fragilis* and other anaerobic Gram-negative bacteria. It is particularly useful for its activity against *Pseudomonas aeruginosa* and the Enterobacteriaceae that acquire resistance to gentamicin.[8]

Netilmicin is active against *Staphylococcus aureus* and *Staphylococcus epidermis*. However, an increasing number of methicillin-resistant strains of these organisms are also resistant to all aminoglycosides. *Streptococcus pyogenes* and *Streptococcus faecalis* are both relatively netilmicin resistant.[7] *Nocardia asteroides* and some other *Nocardia* species are netilmicin sensitive.[9] All Gram-positive anaerobic bacteria are resistant to netilmicin.

Pharmacokinetics

As for other aminoglycosides, a variety of techniques is available for the assay of netilmicin in blood, urine and other tissues. These include microbiological bioassays, high pressure liquid chromatography, radioimmunoassays and enzyme immunoassays. Commercial kits are available, including enzyme modified radioimmunoassay, radioimmunoassay and fluorescence polarization immunoassay.[10] Using fluorescence polarization immunoassay, the sensitivity of the system for netilmicin detection is 0.09 $mg.l^{-1}$.

Netilmicin, like other aminoglycosides, is poorly absorbed after oral administration, and must therefore be given parenterally. Following intramuscular administration peak serum concentrations are achieved at 30–40 min. After a 'slow bolus' given intravenously, serum concentrations follow a biphasic curve.[5]

The mean plasma half life is 2.5 hours after both intravenous and intramuscular administration. The half life increases as the dose increases, and decreases in severely burnt, anaemic and febrile patients. Like other aminoglycosides, netilmicin is excreted via the kidney tubules by glomerular filtration and reabsorbed in the tubules to a limited extent. The unchanged drug appears in the urine in high concentrations, with >80% of the dose excreted by this route within 24 h.[11]

Haemodialysis will remove varying amounts of netilmicin from the blood (for example, an eight-hour haemodialysis may remove 63% of a dose of netilmicin).[12] The recommended dose at the end of each dialysis period is 2 $mg.kg^{-1}$ (2.0–2.5 $mg.kg^{-1}$ in children). Dosage should then be adjusted according to netilmicin serum levels.

The volume of distribution is approximately 270 $ml.kg^{-1}$ body weight (i.e. 20% body weight) and netilmicin exhibits low plasma protein binding. Following parenteral administration, netilmicin is rapidly distributed into tissues and can be detected in serum, tissue, sputum and in pericardial, pleural, synovial and peritoneal fluids. As with gentamicin, netilmicin accumulates in the body with multiple dosage, probably predominantly in renal cortical cells.[13] Since aminoglycosides diffuse poorly into the subarachnoid space after parenteral administration, netilmicin concentrations in CSF are often low and dependent upon dose and degree of meningeal inflammation. Small amounts of the drug may be excreted in the breast milk of lactating women. It is not known to what extent the drug crosses the placenta.

Oral absorption	poor
Presystemic metabolism	nil
Plasma half life	
range	2.5 h
mean	
Volume of distribution	270 $ml.kg^{-1}$
Plasma protein binding	low

Netilmicin (sulphate)

The elimination of netilmicin is reduced in renal disease and in the elderly as renal function declines. Appropriate adjustment of dosage is necessary. A urine concentration about 150 mg.l^{-1} is often achieved after a dose[14,15] of 2 mg.kg^{-1}. After several days of treatment, the amount of netilmicin excreted in the urine approaches the daily dose administered. Minute quantities of aminoglycosides can be detected in the urine for weeks after discontinuation of drug administration.[16] Concentrations in bile are relatively low, suggesting minimal biliary excretion. There is no evidence of enterohepatic circulation.

Concentration–effect relationship

With the administration of netilmicin injection in two or three daily doses, the peak serum concentration should be 4–12 mg.l^{-1}. Prolonged levels above 16 mg.l^{-1} and trough concentrations less than 4 mg.l^{-1} should be avoided.[13]

For an individual patient, serum concentrations appear to be highly predictable after a given dose of netilmicin injection.[14,17]

Metabolism

There is no evidence that netilmicin sulphate is subject to metabolic transformation and hence it has no active metabolites.[15,18]

Pharmaceutics

Netilmicin sulphate, Netillin (Schering-Plough Ltd, UK)/Netromycin (Schering, USA), is only available for parenteral form as an aqueous solution. Each millilitre contains 10 mg, 25 mg, 50 mg or 100 mg of netilmicin base and is available in ampoules and multiple doses of 150 mg vials. Netilmicin injection ranges in colour from water white to pale yellow. Dark yellow solutions should not be used.

The required dose may be administered intramuscularly or injected directly into a vein or intravenous tubing slowly over a period of 3–5 minutes. For adults, a single dose may be diluted in 50–100 ml of normal saline, 5% or 10% dextrose in water. Netilmicin injection contains sodium metabisulphate and sodium sulphite. Netilmicin is stable chemically and physically for 60 months when packaged in ampoules and stored between 2° and 30°C.

Therapeutic use

Netilmicin is a highly effective aminoglycoside with a low potential for oto- and nephrotoxicity. Because of these characteristics, netilmicin is not only suitable for all standard aminoglycoside indications, but may be preferred for the treatment of patients where side effects are of major concern, e.g. patients who have pre-existing renal disease or cochlear-vestibular damage or patients requiring prolonged or repeated courses of aminoglycoside therapy. It should also be considered as the aminoglycoside of choice in elderly patients with decreased hearing, and especially in blind patients, for whom any hearing loss could be disastrous.

Indications

1. Septicaemia and other severe infections due to aerobic Gram-negative bacilli
2. Severe Gram-negative sepsis in children
3. Urinary tract infections
4. Prophylaxis in open heart surgery
5. Some other infections (see below).

Contraindications

1. Hypersensitivity.

Mode of use

The recommended dosage for adults with normal renal function and weighing 50–90 kg is 150 mg every 12 hours or 100 mg every 8 hours. For adults smaller or larger than the above range, dosage should be calculated in mg.kg^{-1} of lean body weight, i.e. 4.0–6.0 mg.kg^{-1} daily given in three equal doses every 8 hours, or two equal doses every 12 hours or once daily. No difference in efficacy has been found between single versus multiple daily dosage in the use of netilmicin for Gram-negative bacteraemia.[19] The duration of therapy is usually seven to fourteen days. In general, the lower dosage is used for urinary tract infections and the higher dosage for systemic infections. The upper limit of dosage may be increased to 7.5 mg.kg^{-1} daily in life-threatening infections, but reduced again as soon as clinically indicated, usually within 48 hours.

The dosage for paediatric patients is as follows:

Premature or full-term neonates, one week of age or less: 6 mg.kg^{-1} daily in two divided doses.

Neonates over one week of age and infants: 7.5–9.0 mg.kg^{-1} daily in three divided doses.

Children: 6.0–7.5 mg.kg^{-1} daily in three divided doses.

The dosage of netilmicin must be individualized in patients with impaired renal function. In such patients, following a loading dose, subsequent dosage must be adjusted either with reduced doses administered at 8-hour intervals or with normal doses given at prolonged intervals.[12] Serum netilmicin levels should be monitored during therapy. The initial or loading dose is the same as that recommended for a patient with normal renal function. In anephric patients undergoing chronic haemodialysis, a dose of 2 mg.kg^{-1} at the end of each dialysis session is usually sufficient.[12] Nomograms are available to calculate dosage in patients with renal impairment but these should be regarded as rough guidelines only and dosage monitoring must be performed.

Indications

1. Septicaemia and other infections

Netilmicin is a useful drug for treatment of septicaemias due to sensitive organisms, although it is not as extensively used as gentamicin. Netilmicin has a wider therapeutic ratio than all other clinically available aminoglycosides except amikacin, and the low incidence of nephrotoxicity and eighth cranial nerve dysfunction resulting from netilmicin administration confirm the excellent safety profile observed in animal studies.[1]

It may be used preferentially in the treatment of gentamicin-resistant infections, e.g. *Pseudomonas* bacteraemic illnesses.[20] Like other aminoglycosides, netilmicin is only recommended in combination with a β-lactam antibiotic for the treatment of septicaemia in neutropenic patients.[21]

Netilmicin may be combined with β-lactams, clindamycin or metronidazole in intra-abdominal or female genital tract infections. Netilmicin has been used successfully in combination with antipseudomonal β-lactam antibiotics for life-threatening infections caused by *Pseudomonas aeruginosa*.

2. Severe Gram-negative sepsis in children

Netilmicin is considered a safe and effective aminoglycoside with low toxicity in children and neonates. In neonates, it has been used successfully as a single agent in bacteraemic illness[22] and has been found to be as effective as other aminoglycosides in the treatment of severe pneumonias.[23]

3. Urinary tract infections

Netilmicin has been used successfully in the treatment of complicated urinary tract infections caused by a variety of organisms including *Klebsiella*, *E. coli*, *Proteus* spp. and *Pseudomonas aeruginosa*.[24–26] Like other aminoglycosides, it is not indicated for most uncomplicated urinary tract infections which usually respond to safer oral agents.

4. Prophylaxis in open heart surgery

Netilmicin combined with an isoxazolyl penicillin has been found to provide good antistaphylococcal cover in open heart surgery.[27]

5. Other uses

Various types of subcutaneous, postoperative and traumatic wound infections have been successfully treated with netilmicin, as have bone and joint infections.[28]

Contraindications

Contraindications to the use of netilmicin include hypersensitivity reactions to the agent, which are rare. Cross-hypersensitivity with other aminoglycosides exists. A relative contraindication to its use is the presence of impaired renal function in which the dosage must be adjusted and regular blood level monitoring performed as described earlier.

Adverse reactions

Potentially life-threatening effects
Anaphylaxis has rarely been reported.

Nephrotoxicity. See section on Severe and irreversible adverse effects below.

Neuromuscular blockade. As with other aminoglycosides, the possibility that prolonged or secondary apnoea may occur should be considered if netilmicin is administered to anaesthetized patients who are also receiving neuromuscular blocking agents. This effect may be reversed by the administration of calcium salts. Netilmicin should be administered with caution in patients with myasthenia gravis or parkinsonism because of its potential curare-like effect on neuromuscular junctions.

Acute overdosage
In the event of overdose or toxic reaction with netilmicin, haemodialysis will reduce serum levels. Peritoneal dialysis also helps, but is less effective.

No deliberate overdoses have been reported. As toxic levels will increase the likelihood of severe renal toxicity or ototoxicity, serum levels and renal function should be monitored carefully.

Severe or irreversible adverse effects

Nephrotoxicity. In a review of results of 150 clinical studies, Lane et al reported a 6.9% incidence of nephrotoxicity probably or possibly related to netilmicin.[29] This is less than that reported with other aminoglycosides, and is generally mild, demonstrated by the presence of casts, cells or protein in the urine or by rising levels of blood urea and serum creatinine. Nephrotoxicity is more likely to occur in patients receiving high doses for a long period, those with a history of renal impairment or concomitant use of other nephrotoxic drugs, and the elderly. Nephrotoxicity is usually reversible after treatment. Kahlmeter and Dahlager surveyed aminoglycoside-induced nephrotoxicity in some 10 000 patients described in clinical trials published between 1975 and 1982. Average frequencies of nephrotoxicity for gentamicin, tobramycin, amikacin and netilmicin were 14%, 12.9%, 9.4% and 8.7% respectively.[30]

Ototoxicity. Unlike other aminoglycosides, the incidence of vestibular and cochlear toxicity with netilmicin injection is very low, possibly 1% or less.[29] Impairment of vestibular function may be transient due to compensatory mechanisms. The rarely reported cochlear impairment is usually irreversible. Factors which increase the risk of ototoxicity include previous renal impairment coupled with high doses of netilmicin, dehydration, concomitant administration of ethacrynic acid or frusemide, or previous exposure to other ototoxic drugs. Kahlmeter and Dahlager surveyed aminoglycoside ototoxicity in approximately 10 000 patients described in clinical trials published between 1975 and 1982. The average frequency of cochlear toxicity was 13.9% for amikacin, 8.3% for gentamicin, 6.1% for tobramycin and 2.4% for netilmicin.[30]

Symptomatic adverse effects

Local reactions. Local reactions such as pain at the site of injection, phlebitis and skin reactions may occur with parenteral netilmicin.

Hypersensitivity reactions. Urticaria and maculopapular rashes have been reported in association with its use.

Other effects
Transient elevations in liver enzymes, nausea, vomiting and headache have all been occasionally reported.[31] These reactions are generally of a mild or moderate severity, do not usually require discontinuation of netilmicin and occur in less than 1% of patients treated with netilmicin.

Interference with clinical pathology tests
None has been reported.

High risk groups

Neonates
Infants and neonates over one week of age should receive 7.5–9.0 mg.kg^{-1} daily in three divided doses. Premature or full-term neonates one week of age or less should receive 6 mg.kg^{-1} daily in two divided doses. The incidence of adverse effects is low, but patients treated for longer than 14 days should be carefully monitored for changes in renal, auditory and vestibular function.

Breast milk. Small amounts of the drug may enter breast milk, but apart from the possibility of sensitization of the infant or mild gastrointestinal upset no serious harm is likely.

Children
The dosage is 6.0–7.5 mg.kg^{-1} daily in three divided doses.

Pregnant women
Aminoglycoside antibiotics cross the placenta. Serious adverse effects have so far only been reported with streptomycin (irreversible bilateral congenital deafness in children born to mothers who received the drug). It is not known whether netilmicin can cause fetal harm or affect reproductive capacity. However, studies in animals have shown no such problems.

The elderly
The risk of nephrotoxicity is greater in elderly patients. One should reduce the dose if renal function is impaired.

Concurrent disease
The most important of these is impaired renal function in which, as has been mentioned before, dosage modification must be made.

Drug interactions

Potentially hazardous interactions
Aminoglycosides should not be given concurrently with potent diuretics such as ethacrynic acid and frusemide, since these enhance their toxicity. Concurrent or sequential use of other neurotoxic or nephrotoxic drugs such as other aminoglycosides, cephaloridine, polymixin B, cisplatinin and vancomycin should be avoided. The aminoglycosides potentiate the effect of neuromuscular blocking agents.

Other significant interactions

Physical incompatibility. In vitro mixing of an aminoglycoside with β-lactam antibiotics may result in significant mutual inactivation.

Potentially useful interactions
In serious infections where the causative microorganisms are unknown, netilmicin may be used in combination with a penicillin or cephalosporin. In vitro netilmicin frequently demonstrates synergy with a variety of β-lactam antibiotics and patients treated with such combinations often exhibit a high bactericidal activity in their serum. It has been used successfully in combination with ticarcillin and other antipseudomonal β-lactams for the treatment of life-threatening infections caused by *Ps. aeruginosa*.[20,32]

Major outcome trials

1. 1979 Clinical evaluation of netilmicin therapy in serious infections. American Journal of Medicine 66: 67–73

Netilmicin was evaluated in the therapy of 33 episodes of infections in 30 patients. 18 patients had documented bacteraemia. Infection sites included pulmonary, urinary tract and soft tissue. A complete bacteriological and clinical cure rate was achieved in 85% of all cases: there were no treatment failures in the bacteraemic group. Netilmicin was the sole antibiotic in all but two cases, when concomitant penicillin was given. Despite uniform dosage, a wide range of netilmicin serum levels was obtained.

2. 1981 Multicentre comparative evaluation of netilmicin and gentamicin in adult patients. Arzneimittel-Forschung/Drug Research 31 (1) 2: 366–370

Netilmicin and gentamicin were compared in a multi-centre clinical trial in 12 worldwide locations. The two aminoglycosides were randomly assigned to hospitalized adult patients with systemic infections (4–6 mg.kg^{-1} daily of netilmicin, or 3–5 mg.kg^{-1} daily of gentamicin). Lower doses were given in the presence of renal impairment. In some cases, patients received other antibiotics as well. Efficacy was evaluated when the aminoglycoside given was the only antimicrobial used that was active against the isolated organism. Organisms in the evaluable group included *Escherichia coli* (40%), *Klebsiella–Enterobacter–Serratia* group (24%), *Proteus* spp. (14%) and *Pseudomonas aeruginosa* (13%).

Netilmicin was favoured over gentamicin for both clinical and

Netilmicin (sulphate)

bacteriological responses by a small margin ($p=0.085$ and $p=0.012$ respectively). Both drugs appeared relatively safe. The toxicity noted was generally mild and reversible.

General review articles

1984 Netilmicin. Symposium proceedings. Journal of Antimicrobial Chemotherapy 3 (suppl A)

Schwarz A J, Lorber R 1982 Netilmicin. A clinical review. Royal Society of Medicine International Congress Symposium 50: 127–135

1984 Aminoglycoside toxicity, a review of clinical studies published between 1975 and 1982. Antimicrobial Agents and Chemotherapy 13 (suppl A): 9–22

References

1. Kabins S A, Nathan C, Cohen S 1976 In vitro comparison of netilmicin, a semi-synthetic derivative of sisomicin, and four other aminoglycoside antibiotics. Antimicrobial Agents and Chemotherapy 10: 139–145
2. Luft F C, Block R, Sloan R S et al 1978 Comparative nephrotoxicity of aminoglycoside antibiotics in rats. Journal of Infectious Disease 138: 541–545
3. Luft F C 1978 Netilmicin: a review of toxicity in laboratory animals. Journal of International Medical Research 6: 286–299
4. Schering Corporation: data on file Pathology and Toxicology Department
5. Riff L J, Moreschi G 1977 Netilmicin and gentamicin: comparative pharmacology in humans. Antimicrobial Agents and Chemotherapy 11 (4): 609–614
6. Briedis D J, Robson H G 1976 Comparative activity of netilmicin, gentamicin, amikacin and tobramycin against *Pseudomonas aeruginosa* and *Enterobacteriaceae*. Antimicrobial Agents and Chemotherapy 10 (4): 592–597
7. Eickhoff T C, Ehret J M 1977 In vitro activity of netilmicin compared with gentamicin, tobramycin, amikacin and kanamycin. Antimicrobial Agents and Chemotherapy 11 (5): 791–796
8. Digranes A, Dibb W L, Ostervold B 1980 The in vitro activity of netilmicin against 357 clinical isolates of *Enterobacteriaceae*, *Ps aeruginosa* and *Staphylococcus aureus*. Scandinavian Journal of Infectious Diseases (suppl 123): 30
9. Martin-Luengo F, Valero Guillen P L 1983 In vitro activity of netilmicin against nocardia. Journal of Antimicrobial Chemotherapy 12: 413
10. Van Remmerden C, Brouwers J R, Berk J A, Boskma R J 1984 Evaluation of five immunological methods for the assay of serum netilmicin. Pharmaceutisch Weekblad Scientific Edition 6: 68–74
11. Chiu P J S, Miller G H, Brown A D et al 1977 Renal pharmacology of netilmicin. Antimicrobial Agents and Chemotherapy 11: 821–825
12. Luft F C, Brannon D R, Stropes L L et al 1978 Pharmacokinetics of netilmicin in patients with renal impairment and patients on dialysis. Antimicrobial Agents and Chemotherapy 14: 403–407
13. Edwards D J, Mangione A, Cumbo T J et al 1981 Predicted tissue accumulation of netilmicin in patients. Antimicrobial Agents and Chemotherapy 20 (6): 714–717
14. Hensely M J 1977 A crossover study comparing the pharmacokinetics of netilmicin and gentamicin administered intramuscularly. Clinical Pharmacology and Therapeutics 21: 116–117
15. Phillips I, Smith A, Shannon K 1977 Antibacterial activity of netilmicin, a new aminoglycoside antibiotic, compared with that of gentamicin. Antimicrobial Agents and Chemotherapy 11 (3): 402–406
16. Madsen P O 1978 Dose range of study of the tolerance and efficacy of netilmicin in patients with complicated urinary tract infections. Clinical Therapeutics 1: 224–250
17. Yap B, Stewart D, Bodey G P 1977 Clinical pharmacology of netilmicin. Antimicrobial Agents and Chemotherapy 12: 717–720
18. Miller G H, Arcieri G, Weinstein M J et al 1976 Biological activity of netilmicin. A broad-spectrum semi-synthetic aminoglycoside antibiotic. Antimicrobial Agents and Chemotherapy 10 (5): 827–836
19. Sturm A W 1989 Netilmicin in the treatment of Gram-negative bacteraemia single daily versus multiple daily dosage. Journal of Infectious Diseases 159 (5): 931–937
20. Lorber R R, Linzmayer M I 1985 Netilmicin in the treatment of psuedomonal bacteraemia. Clinical Therapeutics 7 (3): 338–346
21. Noone P 1984 Netilmicin in the treatment of immuno-compromised patients. Antimicrobial Agents and Chemotherapy 13 (suppl A): 51–58
22. Henriksson P, Svenningsen N, Juhlin I, Haeher K 1978 Netilmicin in moderate to severe infections in neonates and infants: a study of efficacy, tolerance and pharmacokinetics. Current Therapeutic Research 24 (3)
23. Brook I 1989 Tolerance and efficacy of netilmicin in paediatric patients with Gram-negative pneumonia. Chemotherapy 26: 452–460
24. Madsen P O, Baumiecller A, Frimodt-Møller N et al 1980 Netilmicin treatment of complicated urinary tract infections. Scandinavian Journal of Infectious Diseases (suppl 23): 128–131
25. Alfthan O, Renkonen O V, Haeger K 1978 Netilmicin therapy in patients with complicating Gram negative urinary tract infections. Clinical Trials Journal 15 (2): 55–61
26. Cox C E 1979 Comparison of multiple-dose regimens of netilmicin in patients with urinary tract infections. Journal of International Medical Research 7: 370–374
27. Stanbridge T N, Greenall D J B 1984 Netilmicin prophylaxis in open-heart surgery. Journal of Antimicrobial Chemotherapy 13 (suppl A): 59–66
28. Schwarz A J, Lorber R 1982 Netilmicin. A clinical review. Royal Society of Medicine International Congress Symposium 50: 127–135
29. Lane A Z 1984 Clinical experience with netilmicin. Journal of Antimicrobial Chemotherapy 13 (suppl A): 67–72
30. Kahlmeter G, Dahlager J I 1984 Aminoglycoside toxicity — a review of clinical studies published between 1975 and 1982. Journal of Antimicrobial Chemotherapy 13 (suppl A): 9–22
31. Young L S 1978 Comparison, efficacy on tolerance of netilmicin and amikacin in the treatment of patients with serious systemic infections. Current Chemotherapy 2: 908–910
32. Jackson G G 1978 Tolerance and efficacy of netilmicin in patients with serious systemic infections. Antimicrobial Agents in Chemotherapy 13: 170–176

N

Nicardipine

Nicardipine is a calcium entry blocking drug.

Chemistry

Nicardipine (Cardene, Perdipine, Vasonase, Rycardene, Ridene)
$C_{26}H_{29}N_3O_6$.HCl
1,4-Dihydro-2,6-dimethyl-4-(3-nitrophenyl)-3,5-pyridinedicarboxylic acid, methyl-2-[methyl(phenylmethyl)amino]-ethyl ester monohydrochloride

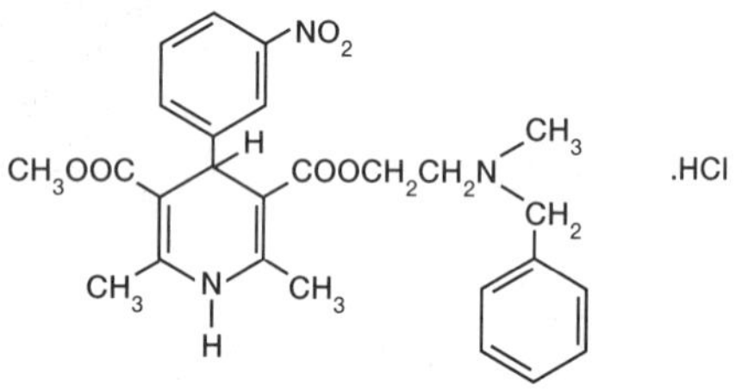

Molecular weight (free base)	515.99 (479.5)
pKa	7.2±0.4
Solubility	
in alcohol	—
in water	—
Octanol/water partition coefficient	—

Nicardipine is a greenish yellow, odourless, crystalline powder, prepared by chemical synthesis.

Pharmacology

Nicardipine is an inhibitor of calcium ion influx (slow calcium channel blocker or calcium entry blocker) and inhibits the transmembrane influx of calcium ions into cardiac muscle and vascular smooth muscle without changing serum calcium concentrations. The vascular smooth muscle is more sensitive to this effect than cardiac muscle,[1–4] because depolarization of vascular smooth muscle is dependent on calcium ion influx whereas cardiac muscle depolarization involves both sodium and calcium ion influx. In addition, nicardipine shows voltage dependant block; the resting potential of cardiac muscle (at −90 mV) is about 50 mV greater than that in vascular smooth muscle (at −40 mV), and nicardipine is much more effective as a calcium channel blocker when the resting potential is less negative. Although nicardipine does interfere with the binding of calcium ions to calmodulin inside the cell, higher concentrations of the drug are needed to achieve this compared to those which inhibit calcium ion influx.

Toxicology

Nicardipine does not have mutagenic potential. Carcinogenicity studies in mice and long-term studies in dogs have shown no evidence of neoplasia of any tissue. No adverse effects on mating, fertility or reproductive indices were found in male or female rats. At high doses, dystocia occurred in rats and weight gains of pups were suppressed. Nicardipine was not teratogenic in rat or rabbit.

Rats treated with high doses of nicardipine for two years showed a dose-dependent increase in thyroid hyperplasia and neoplasia. Studies in the rat have indicated these results are linked to a combination of pharmacological effects on the thyroid and liver leading to a reduction in plasma T4. This results in a chronic elevation of TSH, causing hyperstimulation of the thyroid. In animal safety studies these effects occurred only in the rat. In man, nicardipine does not have an analogous combination of effects on the liver and thyroid. Results of tests in rats showed thyroid changes consistent with excessive TSH stimulation. These changes were further investigated and the results showed that the administration of nicardipine had two effects on rat thyroid hormones:

1. it primarily induced the liver enzymes associated with metabolism of the thyroid hormones, and
2. it partially inhibited the release of thyroid hormones.

Both of these effects resulted in a prolonged decrease in free thyroxine and thus an elevation of thyroid-stimulating hormone. It is generally accepted that substances with this mechanism of action do not represent a significant human risk, provided that the therapeutic dose does not alter thyroid function and thyroxine blood concentrations in man. There was no evidence of thyroid change in mice or in dogs. Laboratory tests conducted during the clinical development programme showed no consistent changes in thyroid function. Furthermore, nicardipine does not induce liver enzymes in man.

Clinical pharmacology

In man nicardipine produces a significant decrease in systemic vascular resistance. The degree of vasodilation and the resultant hypotensive effects are more prominent in hypertensive patients.[5] In hypertensive patients, nicardipine reduces the blood pressure at rest and during isometric and dynamic exercise.[6] In normotensive patients, a small decrease in systolic and diastolic blood pressure may accompany this fall in peripheral resistance. An increase in heart rate occurs as a baroreflex response to the vasodilation and decrease in blood pressure. Haemodynamic studies in patients with coronary artery disease and normal left ventricular function have shown significant increases in cardiac output and coronary blood flow, with no significant change or a small decrease in left ventricular end-diastolic pressure (LVEDP).[7] The ejection fraction is often significantly increased by nicardipine. In a study of patients with coronary artery disease, intracoronary administration of nicardipine caused no direct myocardial depression.[8] Nicardipine improves both rest and exercise cardiac performance in patients with congestive heart failure.[9–11] However, nicardipine does have a negative inotropic effect in some patients with severe left venricular dysfunction.

In patients with chronic stable angina, nicardipine increases exercise tolerance and reduces nitroglycerin consumption. The frequency of anginal attacks decreases, and some patients remain symptom-free without additional medication. The onset of exercise-induced angina and ST segment depression is delayed, and the ST segment depression is less at a given exercise load. Nicardipine may afford more metabolic protection than propranolol to the myocardium under circumstances of pacing-induced tachycardia.[12] Nicardipine protects ischaemic tissue in animal models and may therefore reduce cell damage or loss.[13] Short-term controlled studies on the efficacy and safety of the concomitant use of nicardipine and β-blockers showed additive effects and the drugs were well tolerated. Nicardipine decreases the frequency of spontaneous pain episodes in patients with coronary artery spasm (Prinzmetal's variant angina).

Nicardipine increases the heart rate when given intravenously during acute electrophysiological studies and prolongs the corrected QT interval to a minor degree. The minor QTc prolongation does not lead to any significant clinical findings. More importantly, the PA, AH, and HV intervals and the functional and effective refractory periods of the His–Purkinje system are not prolonged by nicardipine.

Nicardipine is a potent cerebral artery dilator. As such it can increase the cerebral blood flow and oxygen supply to the brain and decrease cerebral vascular resistance.[14] Nicardipine has little effect as a venodilator in man.

Nicardipine has not been shown to exert any consistent effect on hepatic function. It does not impair renal function and, in hypertensive subjects, may increase renal blood flow and the rate of glomerular filtration.[15–17] There is a transitory increase in renal clearance and elimination of electrolytes, including sodium, even when urine flow is unchanged.[18] Nicardipine dose not cause fluid retention.

Nicardipine

Pharmacokinetics

Nicardipine and its M5 metabolite (Fig.1) are extracted from the plasma, purified by extraction and analysed by chromatography on a fused silica capillary column. The assay is sensitive to 1 μg.l^{-1} of nicardipine or the M5 metabolite.

Nicardipine is rapidly ($t_{max}=1$ h) and almost completely absorbed.[19] Nicardipine undergoes extensive presystemic (first-pass) metabolism. Bioavailability increases from 5–10% to 30–45% as the oral dose is increased from 10 to 40 mg. The elimination half life ranges from 0.5 to 12 hours, but steady state is reached within 2–3 days of dosing three times a day.

Nicardipine disposition is not significantly affected by age, but AUC is significantly higher in patients with renal impairment and is even higher in patients with hepatic cirrhosis. The volume of distribution is 1.7 l.kg^{-1}. Nicardipine is highly protein bound (>95%) over a wide concentration range. There is very low penetration into the brain and CSF. Significant concentrations of nicardipine appear in maternal milk following oral administration.

Oral absorption	>95%
Presystemic metabolism	55–95%
Plasma half life	
range	0.5–12 h
mean	8.6 h
Volume of distribution	1.7 l.kg^{-1}
Plasma protein binding	>95%

Concentration–effect relationship

Oral dosing with nicardipine in doses of 30 mg every 8 hours produces both higher plasma concentrations and a greater reduction in systemic vascular resistance than does 20 mg every 8 hours.[20] However, there is no clear correlation between the plasma concentration of nicardipine and its therapeutic effects.

Metabolism

Nicardipine is completely metabolized prior to excretion. The metabolites are excreted into urine (59%) and faeces (35%) to account for 94% of the oral dose.[21] There is no apparent enterohepatic circulation of the parent drug. There are three major pathways of metabolism (Fig. 1):

1. Oxidation of the dihydropyridine ring to M5 (5% of plasma ^{14}C).
2. Cleavage of side-chain at position 3 as follows: N-debenzylation followed by N-demethylation followed by oxidative deamination to S16 (15%).
3. Further oxidation of side-chain and dihydropyridine ring to form M9 (15%) and hydrolysis to M6 (20%).

The major plasma metabolites are formed by reaction 3. None of the metabolites possesses significant biological activity.

Pharmaceutics

Nicardipine (Cardene, Syntex, UK) is available in oral form. Capsules with opaque blue cap and opaque white body, marked 'Syntex 20', contain 20 mg nicardipine hydrochloride. Capsules with opaque blue cap and opaque pale blue body, marked 'Syntex 30', contain 30 mg nicardipine hydrochloride.

In the USA a 20 mg capsule is available; an opaque white hard gelatin capsule with a bright blue band and printed 'Cardene 20' on the cap.

An intravenous formulation is currently under development for the indications of postoperative hypertension, hypertensive emergencies

Fig. 1 Metabolism of nicardipine

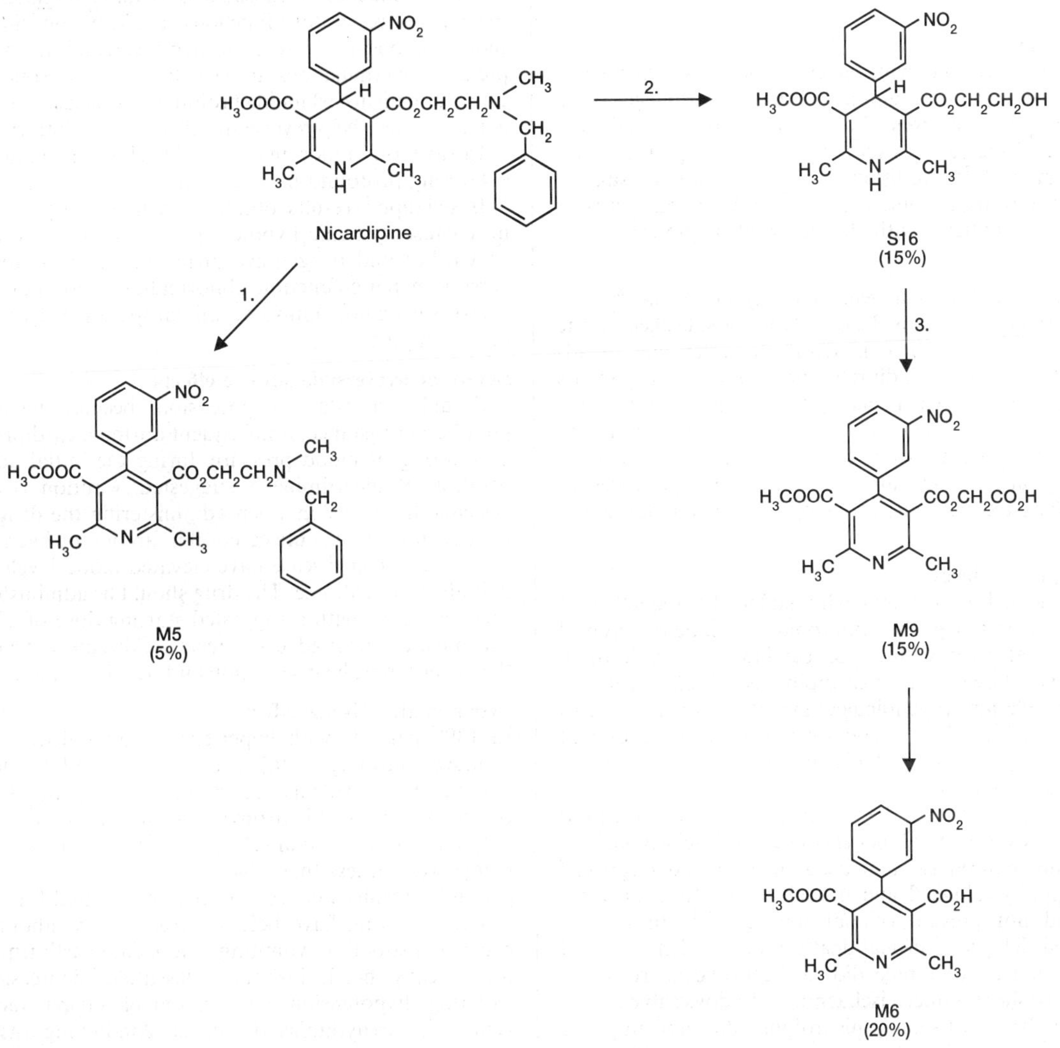

N

and subarachnoid haemorrhage. Controlled-release and sustained-release formulations are currently in development.

All preparations should be protected from light. The maximum shelf-life is 3 years.

No formulations include potentially allergenic substances.

Therapeutic use

Indications

1. Treatment of vasospastic angina
2. Treatment of chronic stable angina
3. Treatment of hypertension
4. Treatment of cerebrovascular insufficiency.

Contraindications

1. Hypersensitivity to nicardipine hydrochloride
2. Advanced aortic stenosis.

Mode of use

The usual effective dose is 30 mg three times a day, with a range of 60–120 mg per day. A starting dose of 20 mg three times a day is recommended, titrating rapidly upwards as necessary. The dose ranges are:
Hypertension: 60–120 mg daily
Angina: 60–120 mg daily
Cerebrovascular insufficiency: 60 mg daily.

Indications

1. Vasospastic angina
Nicardipine is indicated for the management of angina due to coronary artery spasm (vasospastic, Prinzmetal's or variant angina). Nicardipine effectively treats the coronary artery spasm associated with either fixed obstructive coronary disease or non-obstructed coronary arteries.[22,23]

2. Chronic stable angina
Nicardipine is indicated for the management of patients with chronic stable angina (effort-associated angina).[24,25] In controlled trials of up to 52 weeks duration, nicardipine has been effective in reducing angina frequency and increasing exercise tolerance in patients with chronic stable angina.[26–28] Additional controlled studies suggest that concomitant use of nicardipine with either β-blocking agents or nitrates is beneficial in patients with chronic stable angina.[29]

3. Hypertension
Nicardipine is indicated for management of hypertension.[18,30–33] It has been shown to be effective as the initial and/or sole agent in the treatment of patients with mild to moderate hypertension. In addition, the use of nicardipine with diuretics or with β-blocking agents is effective and well tolerated when concomitant therapy is needed for proper patient response. Parenteral nicardipine, currently under investigation, lowers blood pressure promptly. The addition of a single dose of oral captopril to parenteral nicardipine produces an additive hypotensive effect without producing additional reflex tachycardia.[34]

4. Cerebrovascular insufficiency
Nicardipine is indicated in patients who suffer the sequellae of cerebrovascular ischaemia (e.g. the symptomatic residue of cerebral infarction, of cerebral haemorrhage, or cerebral arteriosclerosis). Clinical trials have shown that nicardipine is effective for the treatment of subjective and psychological symptoms (e.g. enhances cognitive and interpersonal skills, mood, or interest in self-care), and some neurological symptoms due to the disturbance of cerebral blood flow in these chronic conditions.

Nicardipine has been shown to be useful in maintaining cerebral blood flow in several experimental models of cerebral ischaemia.[35,36] In rats, nicardipine reduced calcium accumulation and improved behavioural, electrophysiological and mitochondrial function after ischaemia, but did not prevent cellular damage.[37,38] In gerbils, nicardipine reduced delayed neuronal death after transient cerebral ischaemia.[39] In rabbits, nicardipine did not improve neurological outcome after microsphere-induced ischaemia.[40] In dogs subjected to 10 minutes of cerebral ischaemia, nicardipine did not improve neurological outcome in comparison to controls, despite preserving cerebral blood flow.[36]

Nicardipine has also been studied in subarachnoid haemorrhage. At a dose of 0.15 $mg.kg^{-1}.h^{-1}$, nicardipine prevented vasospasm and cerebral ischaemia.[41] In another study, nicardipine, 6 $mg.m^{-2}$, in combination with aminocaproic acid, appeared to reduce the incidence of ischaemic complications in 27 patients with subarachnoid haemorrhage.[42]

Larger controlled trials are needed to determine the role of nicardipine in managing patients with cerebral ischaemia or subarachnoid haemorrhage.

Contraindications

1. Hypersensitivity to nicardipine

2. Advanced aortic stenosis
Reduction of diastolic blood pressure in patients with severe aortic stenosis may worsen myocardial oxygen balance.

Adverse reactions

Potentially life-threatening effects
Atrial fibrillation, increased angina, myocardial infarction, pericarditis, exertional hypotension, syncope and ventricular tachycardia have been observed during nicardipine therapy. It is difficult to distinguish such events from the natural history of the disease process being treated.

Acute overdosage
Several overdosages with nicardipine have been reported. One adult patient allegedly ingested 600 mg of nicardipine (standard capsules), and another patient, 2 160 mg of the sustained release formulation of nicardipine. Symptoms included marked hypotension, bradycardia, palpitations, flushing, drowsiness, confusion and slurred speech. All symptoms resolved without sequelae.

For treatment of overdose standard measures including monitoring of cardiac and respiratory functions should be implemented. The patient should be positioned so as to avoid cerebral anoxia. Frequent blood pressure determinations are essential. Vasopressors are clinically indicated for patients exhibiting profound hypotension. Intravenous calcium gluconate may help reverse the effects of calcium entry blockade.

Intravenous fluids may also be clinically indicated for patients exhibiting profound hypotension.

Based upon results obtained in laboratory animals, overdosage may cause systemic hypotension, bradycardia (following initial tachycardia) and progressive atrioventricular conduction block. Reversible hepatic function abnormalities and sporadic focal hepatic necrosis were noted in some animal species receiving very large doses of nicardipine.

Severe or irreversible adverse effects
Although orthostatic hypotension, because nicardipine decreases peripheral resistance, is infrequent during nicardipine therapy careful monitoring of blood pressure during the initial administration and titration of nicardipine is suggested. Caution is advised to avoid systemic hypotension when administering the drug to patients who have sustained an acute cerebral infarction or haemorrhage. Patients with severe liver disease have elevated blood levels and a prolonged half life of nicardipine. The drug should be administered cautiously in those patients, with a suggested starting dose of 20 mg twice a day. The most frequent adverse effects are dizziness, headache, oedema of the lower limbs, heat sensation and flushing, palpitations and nausea.

Symptomatic adverse effects
In 1390 patients with hypertension, administration of nicardipine produced flushing in 9.7% of patients and headache in 8.2% of patients. Pedal oedema occurred in 8% of patients. These effects are common to most dihydropyridine calcium antagonists. In addition, palpitations occurred in 4.1% of patients, and dizziness, asthenia and tachycardia in less than 4%.

Similar results were seen in patients treated for angina.

The following have been reported rarely: abdominal pain, diarrhoea, constipation, vomiting, anorexia, heartburn, tinnitus, drowsiness, heavy head, insomnia, lassitude, depression, nervousness, sweating, hypotension, aggravation of angina, tachycardia, supraventricular arrhythmias, dyspnoea, skin itching, rash, salivation, dry mouth, backache, myalgia, paraesthesia, frequent micturition, and renal and hepatic impairment. Some of these effects may occasionally come into the serious or irreversible category, discussed above.

Interference with clinical pathology tests
Nicardipine has no significant effect on clinical pathology tests.

High risk groups

Neonates
Safety and efficacy in neonates has not been established.

Breast milk. Nicardipine should not be given to women who intend to breast-feed.

Children
Safety and efficacy in patients under the age of 18 have not been established.

Pregnant women
Use of nicardipine has not been studied in pregnant women. It is recommended that this drug be taken by pregnant women only if clearly indicated and if the potential benefits outweigh the unknown potential hazards to the fetus.

The elderly
Although clinical and pharmacokinetic studies in the elderly generally showed no significant differences from the younger adult population, nevertheless careful titration of the dose in elderly patients, starting with 20 mg three times a day, is advised.[43]

Drug interactions

Potentially hazardous interactions
There is a possibility that serum digoxin levels may be increased when concomitant therapy with nicardipine is initiated and therefore careful monitoring of patients is advised.[44] Cimetidine can increase nicardipine plasma levels. Patients receiving the two drugs concomitantly should be carefully monitored.

Coadministration of cyclosporin resulted in a $110 \pm 92\%$ increase in cyclosporin levels. Close monitoring of cyclosporin dosing is needed when nicardipine is introduced.[45]

A multiple interaction has been reported in patients receiving a β-blocker, a calcium blocker and fentanyl anaesthesia. Increased volume of circulation fluids may be required to compensate for potentially severe hypotension if it should occur.

Other significant interactions

Food. Food consumption reduces the bioavailability of nicardipine. Plasma levels of nicardipine 30–60 min after a dose are 40–60% lower when the drug is given with food than if it is given separately from a meal. However, levels 90 min to 8 h after a dose are no different with or without meals.[46]

Potentially useful interactions
Clinical studies have shown that nicardipine may be used concomitantly with nitrates, β-blockers or diuretics where appropriate. Coadministration of nicardipine and angiotensin converting enzyme inhibitor may be therapeutically useful in some circumstances.[34,47]

References

1. Wagner J G et al Single intravenous dose and steady-state oral pharmacokinetics of nicardipine in healthy subjects. Biopharmaceutics and Drug Disposition (in press)
2. Bongrani S, Razzetti R, Schiantarelli P 1985 Cardiovascular effects of nicardipine in anesthetized open-chest dogs in the absence and presence of beta-adrenergic receptor blockade: a comparison with nifedipine and verapamil. Journal of Cardiovascular Pharmacology 7: 899–905
3. Nakayama K, Kurihara J, Miyajima Y, Ishii K, Kato H 1985 Calcium antagonistic properties of nicardipine, a dihydropyridine derivative assessed in isolated cerebral arteries and cardiac muscle. Arzneimittel-Forschung 35: 687–693
4. Lambert C R, Hill J A, Nichols W W, Feldman R L, Pepine C J 1985 Coronary and systemic hemodynamic effects of nicardipine. American Journal of Cardiology 55: 652–656
5. Hulth'en U L, Bolli P, Bühler F R 1985 Vasodilatory effect of nicardipine and verapamil in the forearm of hypertensive as compared with normotensive man. British Journal of Clinical Pharmacology 20 (suppl 1): 62S–66S
6. Littler W A, Young M A 1985 The effect of nicardipine on blood pressure, its variability and reflex cardiac control. British Journal of Clinical Pharmacology 20 (suppl 1): 115S–119S
7. Lambert C R, Hill J A, Feldman R L, Pepine C J 1986 Effects of nicardipine on left ventricular function and energetics in man. International Journal of Cardiology 10: 237–250
8. Rousseau M F, Vincent M F, Cheron P, van den Berghe G, Charlier A A, Pouleur H 1985 Effects of nicardipine on coronary blood flow, left ventricular inotropic state and myocardial metabolism in patients with angina pectoris. British Journal of Clinical Pharmacology 20 (suppl 1): 147S–157S
9. Ryman K S, Kuba S H, Lystash J, Stone G, Cody R J 1986 Effect of nicardipine on rest and exercise hemodynamics in chronic congestive heart failure. American Journal of Cardiology 58: 583–588
10. Greenbaum R A, Wan S, Evans T R 1986 The acute hemodynamic effects of nicardipine in patients with chronic left ventricular failure. European Journal of Clinical Pharmacology 30: 383–386
11. Lahiri A, Robinson C W, Kohli R S, Caruana M P, Raftery E B 1986 Acute and chronic effects of nicardipine on systolic and diastolic left ventricular performance in patients with heart failure: a pilot study. Clinical Cardiology 9: 257–261
12. Rousseau M F, Hanet C, Pardonge-Lavenne E, Van den Berghe G, Van Hoof F, Pouleau H 1986 Changes in myocardial metabolism during therapy in patients with chronic stable angina: a comparison of long-term dosing with propranolol and nicardipine. Circulation 73: 1270–1280
13. Endo T, Nejima J, Fujita S, Kiuchi K, Iida N, Kikuchi K, Hayakawa H, Okumura H 1986 Comparative effects of nicardipine, a new calcium antagonist, on size of myocardial infarction after coronary artery occlusion in dogs. Circulation 74: 420–430
14. Montero J L, Grau M, Balasch J 1986 Nicardipine: protection against brain hypoxia. Drugs under Experimental and Clinical Research 12: 377–380
15. Chaignon M, Bellet M, Lucsko M, Rapoud C, Guedon J 1986 Acute and chronic effects of a new calcium inhibitor, nicardipine, on renal hemodynamics in hypertension. Journal of Cardiovascular Pharmacology 8: 892–897
16. Baba T, Ishizaki T, Ido Y, Aoyagi K, Murabayashi S, Takebe K 1986 Renal effects of nicardipine, a calcium entry blocker, in hypertensive type II diabetic patients with nephropathy. Diabetes 35: 1206–1214
17. Baba T, Boku A, Ishizaki T, Sone K, Takebe K 1986 Renal effects of nicardipine in patients with mild-to-moderate essential hypertension. American Heart Journal 111: 552–557
18. Fagan T C, Brown R, Schnaper H, Smolens P, Montijo M, Michelson E, O'Neill W, Conrad K A, Lessem J, Freedman D 1989 Nicardipine and hydrochlorothiazide in essential hypertension. Clinical Pharmacology and Therapeutics 45: 429–438
19. Higuchi S, Sasaki H, Seki T 1980 Pharmacokinetic studies on nicardipine hydrochloride, a new vasodilator, after repeated administration to rats, dogs, and humans. Xenobiotica 10: 897–903
20. McCredie R M, McKenzie W B, McGill D A 1985 The acute haemodynamic effects of oral nicardipine. British Journal of Clinical Pharmacology 20 (suppl 1): 163S–168S
21. Rush W R, Alexander O, Hall D J, Cairncross L, Dow R J, Graham D J 1986 The metabolism of nicardipine hydrochloride in healthy male volunteers. Xenobiotica 16: 341–349
22. Pepine C J, Gelman J S 1985 Prevention of vasospastic angina with nicardipine. British Journal of Clinical Pharmacology 20 (suppl 1): 187S–194S
23. Gelman J S, Feldman R L, Scott E, Pepine C J 1985 Nicardipine for angina pectoris at rest and coronary arterial spasm. American Journal of Cardiology 56: 232–236
24. Bowles M J, Khurmi N S, O'Hara M J, Raftery EB 1986 Randomized double-blind placebo-controlled comparison of nicardipine and nifedipine in patients with chronic stable angina pectoris. Chest 89: 260–265
25. McGill D, McKenzie W, McCredie M 1986 Comparison of nicardipine and propranolol for chronic stable angina pectoris. American Journal of Cardiology 57: 39–43
26. Scheidt S, LeWinter M M, Hermanovich J, Venkataraman K, Freedman D 1986 Efficacy and safety of nicardipine for chronic, stable angina pectoris: a multicenter randomized trial. American Journal of Cardiology 58: 715–721
27. Gheorghiade M, St Clair C, St Clair J, Freedman D, Schwemer G 1985 Short- and long-term treatment of stable effort angina with nicardipine, a new calcium channel blocker: a double-blind, placebo-controlled, randomised, repeated cross-over study. British Journal of Clinical Pharmacology 20 (suppl 1): 195S–205S
28. Scheidt S, LeWinter M M, Hermanovich J, Venkataraman K, Freedman D 1985 Nicardipine for stable angina pectoris. British Journal of Clinical Pharmacology 20 (suppl 1): 178S–186S
29. Silke B, Verma S P, Frais M A, Reynolds G, Jackson N, Taylor S H 1985 Haemodynamic analysis of the effects of nicardipine and metoprolol alone and in combination in coronary artery disease. European Heart Journal 6: 930–938
30. Bellet M, Loria Y, Lallemand A 1985 First-step treatment of mild to moderate uncomplicated essential hypertension by a new calcium antagonist: nicardipine. Journal of Cardiovascular Pharmacology 7: 1149–1153
31. Coruzzi P, Biggi A, Musiari L, Ravanetti C, Novarini A 1985 Cardiovascular, baroreflex and humoral responses in hypertensive patients during nicardipine therapy. European Journal of Clinical Pharmacology 29: 371–374
32. Taylor S H, Frais M A, Lee P et al 1985 A study of the long-term efficacy and tolerability of oral nicardipine in hypertensive patients. British Journal of Clinical Pharmacology 20 (suppl 1): 130S–134S
33. Asplund J 1985 Nicardipine hydrochloride in essential hypertension — a controlled study. British Journal of Clinical Pharmacology 20 (suppl 1): 120S–124S
34. Conrad K A, Fagan T C, Mayshar P, McAllister E 1987 Pharmacodynamics of nicardipine alone and in combination with captopril in essential hypertension. Clinical Pharmacology and Therapeutics 42: 113–118
35. Iwatsuki N, Ono K, Koga Y, Amaha K 1987 Prevention of postischemic hypoperfusion after canine cardiac arrest by nicardipine. Critical Care Medicine 15: 313–317
36. Sakabe T, Nagai T, Ishikawa T et al 1986 Nicardipine increases cerebral blood flow but does not improve neurologic recovery in a canine model of complete cerebral ischaemia. Journal of Cerebral Blood Flow and Metabolism 6: 684–690
37. Hadani M, Young W, Flamm S 1988 Nicardipine reduces calcium accumulation and electrolyte derangements in regional cerebral ischaemia in rats. Stroke 19: 1125–1132

38. Grotts J, Pettigrew L, Rosenbaum D, Reid C, Rhoades H, McCandless D 1988 Efficacy and mechanism of action of a calcium channel blocker after global cerebral ischaemia in rats. Stroke 19: 447–454
39. Alps B, Calder C, Hass W, Wilson A 1988 Comparative protective effects of nicardipine, flunarizine, lidoflazine and nimodipine against ischaemic injury in the hippocampus of the Mongolian gerbil. British Journal of Pharmacology 93: 877–883
40. Lyden P, Zivin J, Kochhar A, Mazzarella V 1988 Effects of calcium channel blockers on neurologic outcome after focal ischemia in rabbits. Stroke 19: 1020–1026
41. Flamm E, Adams H, Beck D et al 1988 Dose–escalation study of intravenous nicardipine in patients with aneurysmal subarachnoid hemorrhage. Journal of Neurosurgery 68: 393–400
42. Beck D, Adams H, Flamm E, Godersky J, Loftus C 1988 Combination of aminocaproic acid and nicardipine in treatment of aneurysmal subarachnoid hemorrhage. Stroke 19: 63–67
43. Forette F, Bellet M, Henry J F et al 1985 Effect of nicardipine in elderly hypertensive patients. British Journal of Clinical Pharmacology 20 (suppl 1): 125S–129S
44. Lessem J, Bellinetto A 1983 Interaction between digoxin and the calcium antagonists nicardipine and tiapamil. Clinical Therapeutics 5: 595
45. Graham D J M, Dow R J, Freedman D, Mroszczak E, Ling T 1984 Pharmacokinetics of nicardipine following oral and intravenous administration in man. Postgraduate Medical Journal 60 (suppl 4): 7–10
46. Graham D J, Dow R J, Hall D J, Alexander O F, Mroszcsak E J, Freedman T 1985 The metabolism and pharmacokinetics of nicardipine hydrochloride in man. British Journal of Clinical Pharmacology 20 (suppl 1): 23S–28S
47. Bourbigot B, Guiserix J, Airiau J, Bressollette L, Morin J F, Cledes J 1986 Nicardipine increases cyclosporin blood levels. Lancet 1: 1447

Niclosamide

Niclosamide is an effective and safe taeniacide, used since the late 1960s. It expels the worm from the gut, and is therefore not effective to treat cysticercosis in extraintestinal tissue.

Chemistry

Niclosamide (Yomesan, Nicloxide)
$C_{13}H_8Cl_2N_2O_4$
2′,5′-Dichloro-4′-nitrosalicylanilide

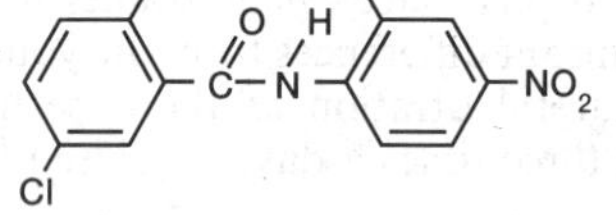

Molecular weight	327.1
pKa	—
Solubility	
in alcohol	1 in 150
in water	<1 in 10 000
Octanol/water partition coefficient	high

A cream-coloured, odourless, tasteless powder, soluble in fat solvents and practically insoluble in water.

Pharmacology

Niclosamide has potent activity against most of the cestodes that infect man. At low concentrations the drug stimulates oxygen uptake by the worm but at higher concentrations respiration is inhibited. It appears to inhibit anaerobic phosphorylation of adenosine diphosphate by the mitochondria of the cestode.[1] As a result the worm dies and, aided by the proteolytic enzymes in the gut, the scolex and segments of the cestode are digested. The scolex may not be identifiable in the stools. The ova of the tapeworm which are present in the segments of the worm are not affected.

Toxicology

Very small amounts of niclosamide are absorbed from the gut, and the single oral lethal dose in the rat[2] is around 5000 $mg.kg^{-1}$.

Toxicity is mainly due to its ability to uncouple oxidative phosphorylation. Mammalian toxicity is much lower compared with pentachlorophenol, a chemical having the same mode of action as niclosamide, and the small concentrations after oral absorption seem to indicate a safe therapeutic index.

Clinical pharmacology

Niclosamide appears to have little clinical pharmacological effect in man. Very little of the drug is absorbed into the body and there is no evidence of a direct irritant action on the gut of man. No changes of hepatic or renal function have been observed.[3] Niclosamide also has some action against *Enterobius (Oxyuris) vermicularis*.

Pharmacokinetics

About 15–20% of the drug is absorbed from the oral route and this is transformed into the amino derivative. Very little is known about its further fate in the human body.

Concentration–effect relationship

Because of the local effect on the tapeworm in the gut, and the relatively bad absorption of the drug, no studies on concentration of niclosamide in the blood that relates to its effectiveness seem relevant.

Metabolism

Apart from transformation into its amino derivative (Fig. 1), little is known of the metabolism of niclosamide.

Fig. 1 Metabolism of niclosamide

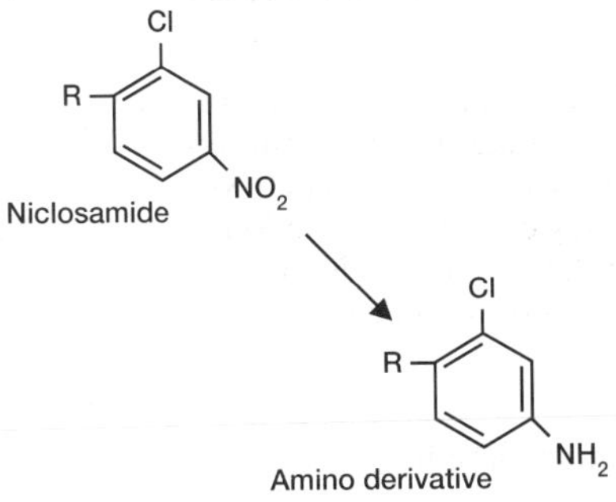

Pharmaceutics

Niclosamide is available as round, light-yellow, chewable tablets, vanilla-flavoured, containing 500 mg niclosamide BP. In most countries it is marketed by Bayer under the proprietary name Yomesan and is marked on one side of the tablet with 'FE', and on the other side with the Bayer cross. In the USA it is marketed by Miles as Niclocide chewable tablets 500 mg. These are yellow, round, scored tablets marked 'Miles-721'.

Therapeutic use

Indications

1. For most tapeworm infestations in the gut, like: *Taenia saginata* (beef tapeworm), *Taenia solium* (pork tapeworm), *Diphyllobothrium latum* (fish tapeworm), and *Hymenolepsis nana* (dwarf tapeworm).

It has no effect on cysticercosis and echinococcosis due to tapeworm larvae infesting the extraintestinal tissue and organs.

Contraindications

There are no known contraindications of niclosamide as a taeniacide. Although no known teratogenicity has been recorded in man, it may be convenient to postpone treatment of pregnant women in the first trimester until delivery.

The consumption of alcohol during treatment must be avoided to minimize absorption. No special diet or fasting is needed.

Mode of use

The following dosage for *Taenia saginata* (beef tapeworm), *Taenia solium* (pork tapeworm), and *Diphyllobothrium latum* (fish tapeworm) are recommended:
adults and children over 6 years, 4 tablets;
children from 2 to 6 years, 2 tablets;
children under 2 years, 1 tablet.
The tablets should be chewed thoroughly or pulverized when given to small children to allow appropriate contact with the worm.

In infestation with *Taenia solium* the tablets are taken as a single dose after a light breakfast, but in the case of *Taenia saginata* and *Diphyllobothrium latum* the dose may be divided in two, the first taken after breakfast and the second one hour later.

A mild laxative may be given two hours afterwards, but a drastic purge (magnesium sulphate or sodium sulphate) is needed for *Taenia solium* to eliminate possible viable ova liberated from the dead segments, which may lead to cysticercosis. In *Taenia saginata* infection there is no danger of cysticercosis, and purging is not necessary. *Hymenolepsis nana* (dwarf tapeworm) infestation should be treated for 7 days as follows:
First day: dose as above (as single dose);
Subsequent 6 days: half the dose as above (as single dose).
Sour fruit juice may dislodge intestinal mucus and promote contact of the drug with the worms.

Adverse reactions

Potentially life-threatening effects
None has been reported.

Acute overdosage
No cases of overdosage have been documented. Its property of uncoupling oxidative phosphorylation may result in fever and increased metabolism when toxic amounts are ingested.

In the event of overdose a fast-acting laxative and enema may be given. Vomiting should not be induced.

Severe or irreversible adverse effects
None has been reported.

Symptomatic adverse effects
Such effects may occur occasionally and include gastrointestinal irritation, light-headedness, and pruritus.

High risk groups

Neonates
The drug is not used in this patient group.

Breast milk. Since the drug is not absorbed from the gut in significant amounts, it seems unlikely that any would appear in breast milk.

Children
See Mode of use for appropriate dosage in children.

Pregnant women
Experience with this drug in the first trimester of pregnancy is limited[1] to a few cases. The mothers delivered healthy children when treated with niclosamide at 8–10 weeks of pregnancy. If possible, treatment should be postponed until after delivery.

The elderly
There are no known special risks in the elderly or debilitated patient.[4]

Drug interactions

No information is available other than that alcohol may enhance absorption of the drug.

Major outcome trials

Jones W E 1979 Niclosamide as a treatment for *Hymenolepsis diminuta* and *Dipylidium caninum* infection in man. American Journal of Tropical Medicine and Hygiene 28 (No 2): 300–302

86 patients were treated with niclosamide (Yomesan, Bayer) chewable tablets between 1973 and 1977. The drug was given to physicians who requested it for the treatment of human infections with *Hymenolepsis diminuta* (43 patients) and *Dipylidium caninum* (43 patients). Diagnosis was confirmed in each case by identification of eggs or proglottids in stools. For *Dipylidium caninum* 2 g niclosamide was given as a single dose for adults and 1.5 or 1 g for children weighing > 34 kg or 11–34 kg respectively. For *Hymenolepsis diminuta* 5–7 days treatment was used.

Only 13 *Dipylidium caninum* cases were adequately followed up with complete cure in all; two were previously unsuccessfully treated with quinacrine.

19 cases of *Hymenolepsis diminuta* were followed up, and 17 were cured with the first course of treatment. The two who had positive stool findings after therapy were given a second course, which resulted in cure.

Adverse effects were nausea (3 patients), abdominal cramps and sweat (1 patient).

Other trials

1. Prashara K G 1966 Treatment of taeniasis with Yomesan. East African Medical Journal 65:
2. Abdallah A, Saif M 1961 The efficacy of N-2′-chloro-4′-nitrophenyl-5-chlorosalicylamide in the treatment of taeniasis. Journal of the Egyptian Medical Association 44: 379–381

N

General review articles

Brown H W 1968 Anthelmintics, new and old. Clinical Pharmacology and Therapeutics 10: 5–21

Keeling J E D 1968 The chemotherapy of cestode infections. Advanced Chemotherapy 3: 109–152

References

1. Scheibel L W, Saz H J, Bueding E 1968 The anaerobic incorporation of ^{32}P into adenosinetriphosphate by *Hymenolepsis diminuta*. Journal of Biological Chemistry 243: 2229–2235
2. World Health Organization Technical Report Series 1973 No 513 Safe use of pesticides, pp 35–36
3. Abdallah A, Saif M 1961 The efficacy of N-2′-chloro-4′-nitrophenyl-5-chlorosalicylamide in the treatment of taeniasis. Journal of the Egyptian Medical Association 44: 379–381
4. Gönnert R, Schraufstätter E 1960 Experimentelle untersuchungen mit N-(2′-chlor-4′-nitrophenyl)-5-chlor-salicylamid, einen neuen bandwurmmitel. Arzneimittel Forschung 10: 881–884
5. Ruttenber A J, Weniger B G, Sorvillo F, Murray R A, Ford S L 1984 Diphyllobotriasis associated with salmon consumption in Pacific Coast States. American Journal of Tropical Medicine and Hygiene 33: 455–459
6. Vermund S H, MacLeod S, Goldstein R G 1986 Taeniasis unresponsive to single dose of niclosamide: case report of persistent infection with *Taenia saginata* and a review of therapy. Reviews of Infectious Diseases 8: 423–426

Nicotinamide

The water-soluble vitamin nicotinamide is incorporated into the coenzymes nicotinamide adenine dinucleotide (NAD) and nicotinamide adenine dinucleotide phosphate (NADP), which serve as cofactors for numerous oxidation/reduction reactions of cell respiration, glycolysis, and fat synthesis. NAD serves as a donor for ADP-ribosylation of macromolecules.

Chemistry

Nicotinamide, niacinamide
$C_6H_6N_2O$
3-Pyridinecarboxylic acid amide

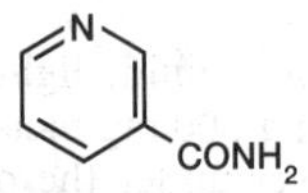

Molecular weight	122.1
pKa (acidic)	
Solubility	
in alcohol	1 in 1.5
in water (sodium salt)	1 in 1
Octanol/water partition coefficient	—

Nicotinamide is an odourless, white crystalline solid with a bitter taste.

It is available in many combination preparations.

Pharmacology

Nicotinamide is an essential nutrient. The term 'niacin' is often used to refer to both nicotinamide and nicotinic acid; some use niacin as a synonym for nicotinic acid, which can also be converted to the coenzyme forms. The significant hypolipidaemic and vasodilatory effects of nicotinic acid are not shared by nicotinamide.[1,2]

Chronic dietary deficiency of niacin results in the disorder pellagra, which is characterized by dermatitis, diarrhoea, dementia, and ultimately death. Administration of the antimetabolite, 6-aminonicotinamide, to mice produced pathologic lesions of the skin, intestine, and central nervous system that were characteristic of those described in human pellagra.[3] Nicotinamide is needed for the coenzymes NAD and NADP that catalyse tissue oxidation–reduction reactions.

Recommended dietary allowances for adults range from 13 to 18 mg daily. Some dietary tryptophan is converted to nicotinamide by a vitamin B^6-dependent pathway. For estimating dietary requirements, 60 mg of tryptophan is considered equivalent to 1 mg of niacin, although the efficacy of conversion varies among individuals. Dietary requirements for niacin are usually estimated on the basis of energy expenditure,[1] e.g. for adults, $6.6\ mg.1000\ kcal.^{-1}$

Toxicology

In acute toxicity testing, the estimated LD_{50} for subcutaneous administration was $1.7\ g.kg^{-1}$ in rats.[4] In rats fed a choline-deficient diet, large doses of nicotinamide resulted in growth inhibition, decreased food intake and weight gain per food intake, liver and kidney hypertrophy, and fatty liver. These effects were attributed to methyl deficiency induced by methylation of nicotinamide to N^1-methylnicotinamide, the major excretory product.[5] Nicotinamide toxicity may also impair RNA and DNA synthesis due to ATP and 5-phosphoribosyl-1-pyrophosphate depletion.[6]

Nicotinamide

In patients taking 3 g daily of nicotinamide for 3--36 months, side effects included heartburn, nausea, headaches, hives, fatigue, sore throat, dry hair, tautness of the face, and inability to focus the eyes.[2] Hepatotoxicity resulting in jaundice, cholestatic hepatitis, and portal fibrosis has been reported with large doses of up to 9 g daily of nicotinamide.[7] However, the incidence of adverse reactions to doses of 6 g daily or less appears to be low.[8,9]

Clinical pharmacology

Nicotinamide is predominantly utilized for the prevention and treatment of niacin deficiency. High doses of nicotinamide (300–2500 mg. daily have been of use in the treatment of various inflammatory skin lesions, including acne, dermatitis herpetiformis, erythema elevatum diutinum, generalized granuloma annulare, bullous pemphigoid, polymorphous light eruption and others.[10–13] Inhibitory effects of nicotinamide on lymphocyte proliferation and transformation, histamine release from mast cells and neutrophil function may be responsible for the therapeutic response. Unconfirmed reports of the effectiveness of nicotinamide in the treatment of schizophrenia have not been substantiated by controlled trials.[14] Neither the significant hypolipidaemic effect nor the vasodilating effect of nicotinic acid, which are unrelated to its role as a nutrient, is shared by nicotinamide.

Pharmacokinetics

The usual clinical assay method is microbiological assay with *Lactobacillus plantarum*[15] although a radiometric–microbiologic approach with *Klockera brevis*[16] and several high performance liquid chromatographic methods applicable to biological samples have been reported, which have a sensitivity of.[17–19]

In the diet, niacin is present mainly as the coenzyme forms NAD(H) and NADP(H).[20] The bioavailability of food forms of niacin varies significantly, and bound forms in wheat and corn may be largely unavailable. NAD has been demonstrated to undergo extensive digestion prior to intestinal absorption. In the rat, Gross and Henderson demonstrated that NAD was first converted to nicotinamide ribonucleotide by a pyrophosphatase, with subsequent rapid hydrolysis of the nicotinamide ribonucleotide to nicotinamide riboside, which accumulated in the intestinal lumen.[21] The rate-limiting step was conversion of nicotinamide riboside to nicotinamide. Baum and colleagues, et al who studied NAD hydrolysis by rat small intestinal brush border membranes, demonstrated two independent pathways of hydrolysis: one formed nicotinamide through hydrolysis of the ribosyl-pyridinium bond, and the other formed nicotinamide mononucleotide through hydrolysis of the pyrophosphate bond with subsequent dephosphorylation to nicotinamide riboside.[19] Nicotinamide appears to be the major form absorbed by the intestine, although some nicotinamide riboside may also be absorbed. In addition, some nicotinamide may be converted to nicotinic acid by gut bacteria.

The mechanism of intestinal absorption of nicotinamide remains controversial. Many animal studies suggest passive diffusion, whereas others support carrier-mediated facilitated diffusion.[19, 22–24] Conversion of nicotinamide to coenzyme forms in the intestine complicates interpretation of transport data. Perfusion studies in the rat indicated that nicotinamide was readily absorbed, more rapidly than nicotinic acid.[24]

Nicotinamide is the major circulating form of the vitamin. It is readily taken up into tissues and utilized for synthesis of the coenzyme forms. The liver plays a major role in regulating nicotinamide metabolism. Newly ingested nicotinamide appears to enter a hepatic storage pool of NAD. Glycohydrolases release nicotinamide from NAD to supply the nicotinamide for peripheral tissues.[5] Nicotinamide is taken up by most tissues by simple diffusion with metabolic trapping as nucleotides and dinucleotides, although specific transport systems are involved in red blood cells and kidney. Nicotinamide readily enters the cerebrospinal fluid, choroid plexus, and brain.[25] Nicotinamide and its coenzyme forms are present in all tissues that have been examined; however, concentrations are variable. It is particularly abundant in liver, heart, kidney, muscle, and brain. The principal bound forms are NAD and NADH, and NADP and NADPH.

Urinary excretion of nicotinamide is dose-related. At physiologic doses, N^1-methyl-2-pyridone-5-carboxamide and N^1-methylnicotinamide are the major metabolites. At larger doses, free nicotinamide is also excreted.[26] The normal range for urinary N^1-methylnicotinamide excretion is above 1.6 mg.g^{-1} creatinine for adults, with values less than 0.5 mg.g^{-1} creatinine the usual criterion for deficiency. The normal range for the circulating total niacin concentration in whole blood is 3.5–7.0 mg.l^{-1} using microbiological assay. Values below 2.3 mg.l^{-1} are considered deficient.

Concentration–effect relationship

No data are available.

Metabolism

Nicotinamide is converted to NAD and NADP enzymatically via the Dietrich pathway. Nicotinamide ribonucleotide (NMN) is an intermediate in the pathway and 5-phosphoribosyl-1-pyrophosphate and ATP are cosubstrates. Nicotinamide is degraded in liver and other organs to a number of products that are excreted in the urine, including N^1-methylnicotinamide, N^1-methyl-2-pyridone-5-carboxamide, N^1-methyl-4-pyridone-5-carboxamide and nicotinamide-N^1-oxide (see Fig. 1).[4,25] At doses of less than 1000 mg, the 2-pyridone is the major excretory product, whereas at a dose of 3000 mg daily N^1-methylnicotinamide predominates and some free nicotinamide appears in urine.

Pharmaceutics

Nicotinamide is available in oral and parenteral forms. Oral nicotinamide is available in 50, 100, 500 and 1000 mg tablets. Injectable nicotinamide is available in 30 ml vials, containing 100 mg.ml^{-1}. Nicotinamide is present in most oral multivitamin preparations and in multivitamin formulations for intravenous use, providing 20–40 mg daily. Topically administered nicotinamide was successful in reversing both cutaneous and systemic manifestations of pellagra.[27]

Therapeutic use

Indications

1. Niacin deficiency

Fig. 1 Metabolism of nicotinamide

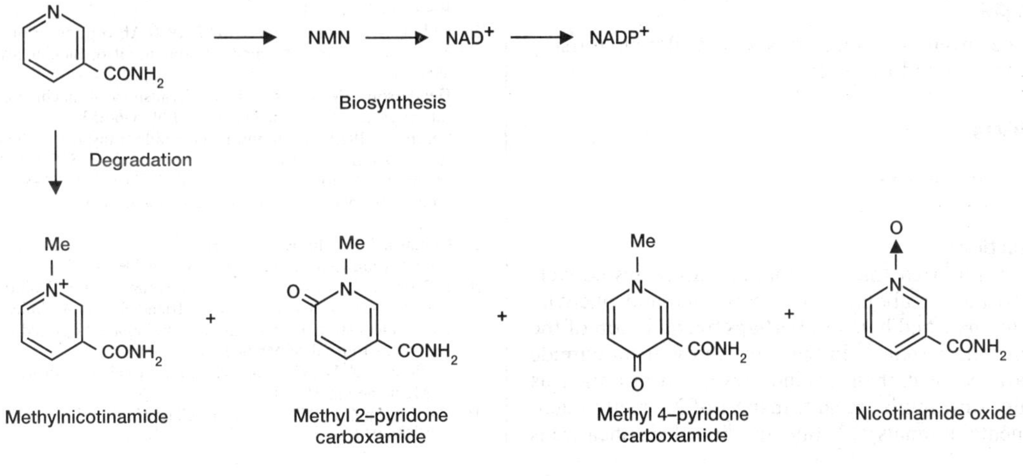

2. Hartnup disease
3. Inflammatory skin disease.

Contradictions

There are none.

Indications

1. Niacin deficiency
The major therapeutic use of nicotinamide is for the prevention or treatment of niacin deficiency. For patients with severe acute niacin deficiency, high doses are recommended, 500–1000 mg orally or 100–250 mg parenterally daily. Patients at risk of nicotinamide deficiency include those with a history of alcoholism, energy/protein malnutrition, malabsorption, and small bowel disease. Patients with malignant carcinoid tumours may develop niacin deficiency attributable to conversion of tryptophan to 5-hydroxytryptamine and other compounds rather than niacin synthesis.[29] Patients on isoniazid therapy for tuberculosis occasionally develop pellagra-like skin lesions that respond to niacin treatment.[30,31] In one young patient, pellagra was the presenting manifestation of Crohn's disease.[32]

2. Hartnup disease
Patients with Hartnup disease, a rare metabolic disorder of renal and intestinal transport of tryptophan and other monoamino/monocarboxylic acids, develop clinical and biochemical niacin deficiency,[28] which can be reversed by oral therapeutic doses of nicotinamide or nicotinic acid (50 mg, given 3 to 10 times daily).

3. Inflammatory skin diseases
High doses of nicotinamide (300–2500 mg daily) may be useful in treating inflammatory skin diseases such as dermatitis herpetiformis, erythema elevatum diutinum, generalized granuloma annulae, and bullous pemphigoid.

Adverse reactions

Potentially life-threatening effects
Large doses of nicotinamide (3–9 g daily) can result in hepatotoxicity with cholestasis and portal fibrosis.[7]

Acute overdose
A single large overdose of nicotinamide is unlikely to have serious ill effects, though transient abnormalities of liver function might occur.

Severe or irreversible adverse effects
Apart from the liver damage described above, none appears to have been described.

Symptomatic adverse effects
Doses of about 3 g daily can cause heartburn, nausea, headaches, hives, fatigue, sore throat, dry hair, tautness of the face and inability to focus the eyes.[2]

Nicotinamide does not produce the flushing, itching, burning, or tingling associated with nicotinic acid and is, therefore, preferable in treating deficiency states.

Interference with clinical pathology tests
No clinical interferences of this kind have been reported.

High risk groups

Nicoinamide may be given in normal doses to children, nursing mothers, pregnant women and the elderly.

Drug interactions

Potentially hazardous interactions
No interactions of this kind have been reported.

Other significant reactions
Bourgeois and others reported that nicotinamide decreases conversion of primidone to the metabolites phenobarbitone and phenylethylmalonamide in animals and humans, perhaps by inhibition of the cytochrome P450 enzyme system.[33] In the same study, nicotinamide also decreased clearance of carbamazepine. Several drugs such as cisplatin and cephaloridine inhibit renal transport of N^1-methylnicotinamide in experimental animals,[34,35] but the clinical significance is uncertain. Nicotinamide treatment reduced acute paraquat toxicity in rats.[36]

Potentially useful interactions
None has been described.

Clinical trials

No data are available except in schizophrenia where nicotinamide has not been proven efficacious.[14]

References

1. Committee on Dietary Allowances, Food and Nutrition Board 1980 Recommended dietary allowances, 9th edn. National Academy of Sciences, Washington, DC, pp 92–96
2. Hankes L V 1984 Nicotinic acid and nicotinamide. In: Machlin L J (ed) Handbook of vitamins. Nutritional, biochemical, and clinical aspects. Dekker, New York, ch 8, pp 329–377
3. Aikawa H, Suzuki K 1986 Lesions in the skin, intestine, and central nervous system induced by an antimetabolite of niacin. American Journal of Pathology 122: 335–342
4. Brazda F G, Coulson R A 1946 Toxicity of nicotinic acid and some of its derivatives. Proceedings of the Society for Experimental Biology and Medicine 62: 19–20
5. Kang-Lee Y A E, McKee R W, Wright S M, Swendseid M E, Jenden D J, Jope R S 1983 Metabolic effects of nicatinamide administration in rats. Journal of Nutrition 113: 215–221
6. Bernofsky C 1980 Physiologic aspects of pyridine nucleotide regulation in mammals. Molecular and Cellular Biochemistry 33: 135–143
7. Winter S L, Boyer J L 1973 Hepatic toxicity from large doses of vitamin B_3 (nicotinamide). New England Journal of Medicine 239: 1180–1182
8. Hawkins D R 1968 Treatment of schizophrenia based on the medical model. Journal of Schizophrenia 2: 3--10
9. Hoffer A 1969 Safety, side effects and relative lack of toxicity of nicotinic acid and nicotinamide. Schizophrenia 1: 78–87
10. Ma A, Medenica M 1983 Response of generalized granuloma annulare to high-dose niacinamide. Archives of Dermatology 119: 836–839
11. Kohler I K, Lorincz A L 1980 Erythema elevatum diutinum treated with niacinamide and tetracycline. Archives of Dermatology 116: 693–695
12. Berck M A, Lorincz A L 1986 The treatment of bullous pemphigold with tetracycline and niacinamide. Archives of Dermatology 122: 670–674
13. Neumann R, Rappold E, Pohl-Markl H 1986 Treatment of polymorphous light eruption with nicotinamide: a pilot study. British Journal of Dermatology 115: 77–80
14. Lipton M A, Mailman R B, Nemeroff C B 1979 Vitamins, megavitamin therapy, and the nervous system. In: Wurtman R J, Wurtman J J (eds) Nutrition and the brain, vol 3. Raven, New York, pp 183–264
15. The United States Pharmacopeia, 21st edn. 1984 U.S. Pharmacopeial Convention, Rockville, Maryland, pp 1204–1206
16. Guilarte T R, Pravlik K 1983 Radiometric-microbiologic assay of niacin using *Klockera brevis*: analysis of human blood and food. Journal of Nutrition 113: 2587-2594
17. Kalhorn T F, Thummel K E, Nelson S D, Slattery J T 1985 Analysis of oxidized and reduced pyridine dinucleotides in rat liver by high-performance liquid chromatography. Analytical Biochemistry 151: 343-347
18. Schuette S A, Rose R C 1983 Nicotinamide uptake and metabolism by chick intestine. American Journal of Physiology 245: G531-G538
19. Baum C L, Selhub J, Rosenberg I H 1982 The hydrolysis of nicotinamide adenine dinucleotide by brush border membranes of rat intestine. Biochemical Journal 204: 203-207
20. Robinson J, Levitas N, Rosen F, Perlzweig W A 1947 Fluorescent condensation product of n^1-methyl nicotinamide and acetone; rapid method for determination of pyridine nucleotides in animal tissues; coenzyme content of rat tissues. Journal of Biological Chemistry 170: 653-659
21. Gross C J, Henderson L M 1983 Digestion and absorption of NAD by the small intestine of the rat. Journal of Nutrition 113: 412-420
22. Elbert J, Daniel H, Rehner G 1986 Intestinal uptake of nicotinic acid as a function of microclimate-pH. International Journal of Vitaminology and Nutrition Research 56: 85-93
23. Sadoogh-Abasian F, Evered D F 1980 Absorption of nicotinic acid and nicotinamide from rat small intestine in vitro. Biochimica Biophysica Acta 598: 385-391
24. Henderson L M, Gross C J 1979 Transport of niacin and niacinamide in perfused rat intestine. Journal of Nutrition 109: 646-653
25. Spector R 1979 Niacin and niacinamide transport in the central nervous system. In vivo studies. Journal of Neurochemistry 33: 895-904
26. Mrochek J E, Jolley R L, Young D S, Turner W J 1986 Metabolic response of humans to ingestion of nicotinic acid and nicotinamide. Clinical Chemistry 22: 1821-1827
27. Comaish J S, Felix R H, McGrath H 1976 Topically applied nicotinamide in isoniazid-induced pellagra. Archives of Dermatology 112: 70-72
28. Halvorsen K, Halvorsen S 1963 Hartnup disease. Pediatrics 31: 29-38
29. Sjoerdsma A, Weissbach H, Udenfriend S 1956 A clinical, physiologic and biochemical study of patients with malignant carcinoid (argentaffinoma). American Journal of Medicine 20: 520-532
30. Griffiths W A D 1976 Isoniazid induced pellagra. Proceedings of the Royal Society of Medicine 69: 313-314
31. Harrington C I 1977 A case of pellagra induced by isoniazid therapy. Practitioner 218: 716-717

32. Pollack S, Enat R, Haim S, Zinder O, Barzilai D 1982 Pellagra as the presenting manifestation of Crohn's disease. Gastroenterology 82: 948-952
33. Bourgeois B F D, Dodson W E, Ferrendelli J A 1982 Interactions between primidone, carbamazepine, and nicotinamide. Neurology 32: 1122-1126
34. Williams P D, Hottendorf G H 1985 Effect of cisplain on organic ion transport in membrane vesicles from rat kidney cortex. Cancer Treatment Reports 69: 875-880
35. Williams P D, Hitchcock M J M, Hottendorf G H 1985 Effect of cephalosporins on organic ion transport in renal membrane vesicles from rat and rabbit kidney cortex. Research Communications in Chemical Pathology and Pharmacology 47: 357-371
36. Brown O R, Heitkamp M, Song C-S 1981 Niacin reduces paraquat toxicity in rats. Science 212: 1510-1512

Nicotine

Nicotine is one of the few natural liquid alkaloids. Its primary action is at the nicotinic receptors for acetylcholine where an initial agonist effect is followed by a more prolonged blocking effect.

As the main and most potent alkaloid of tobacco, *Nicotiana tabacum*, the major interest of nicotine is concerned more with its widespread use as a recreational and addictive drug than with its therapeutic use in medical practice. It has been used in the past for the treatment of many ailments, but its return to the modern pharmacopoeia has been as an aid to giving up smoking. It is also widely used as an insecticide.

Chemistry

Nicotine
$C_{10}H_{14}N_2$
(S)-3-(1-Methyl-2-pyrolidinyl)pyridine

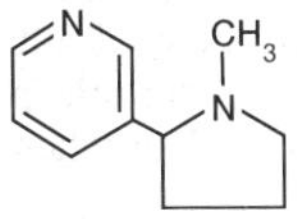

Molecular weight	162.2
pKa (−N=, −N<)	3.2, 8.0
Solubility	
in alcohol	>1 in 30
in water	>1 in 30
Octanol/water partition coefficient	—

A volatile strongly alkaline liquid, it is colourless when pure but undergoes auto-oxidation and turns yellow to brown on exposure to air or light and gives off the pungent, characteristic smell of tobacco. It has an acid, peppery taste. It is highly soluble in water and forms water-soluble salts and double salts with many metals and acids. Under atmospheric pressure, it boils at 246°C. It is volatilized in the cone of burning tobacco, 800–900°C, and the free base is present in the minute (0.3–1.0 μm) semi-liquid droplets of the so-called particulate phase of the smoke. Natural nicotine is mainly laevorotatory, and l-nicotine (S-isomer) is much more potent than d-nicotine.

Nicotine is a natural product in tobacco plants (*Nicotiana tabacum* and *N. rustica*), from which it is obtained.

A nicotine resin complex (Nicotine Polacrilex) is manufactured using nicotine from natural sources. It is a white to faintly yellow fine powder. The nicotine resin complex has been incorporated into a chewing gum (Nicorette) which is available for clinical use.

Pharmacology

The acute action of nicotine is as a nicotinic cholinergic agonist causing depolarization and hence stimulation at the nicotinic receptors of acetylcholine. But the action is biphasic in that the depolarization is prolonged and further excitation of the receptor is blocked for as long as it remains occupied by nicotine. Thus the overall effect of large doses is to produce a depressant or blocking effect after initial stimulation, whereas repeated small doses have a stimulant effect until acute tolerance develops when sufficient receptors are occupied. Nicotinic cholinergic receptors in the CNS appear to resemble those in autonomic ganglia more closely than those at neuromuscular junctions where larger doses of nicotine are necessary to produce blockade.

Nicotine also stimulates the release of many neurotransmitters including acetylcholine, noradrenaline, dopamine, serotonin and β-endorphin. Some of these effects appear to be due to a direct action at presynaptic receptors on nerve terminals,[1] whereas others occur indirectly via its action at postsynaptic nicotinic cholinergic receptors, for example in autonomic ganglia. Evidence for the presence of functional nicotinic receptors at noncholinergic sites within the CNS is controversial.

In moderate doses the stimulant effect of nicotine on sympathetic ganglia and the release of adrenaline and noradrenaline from the adrenal medulla cause an increase in heart rate and blood pressure together with peripheral vasoconstriction, whereas larger toxic doses cause a drop in blood pressure due to ganglionic blockade and may in extreme cases lead to circulatory collapse. If the intake of nicotine is rapid (e.g. intravenous injection), excessive doses may cause vasovagal attacks due to the stimulant effect on parasympathetic ganglia and vasomotor centres.

The central and peripheral actions of nicotine are blocked by mecamylamine which appears to act as a noncompetitive antagonist at nicotinic cholinergic receptors.

Toxicology

Nicotine is a highly toxic drug and is used as an insecticide. However, the margin is wide between those doses required to produce mild toxic effects and the more serious and life-threatening toxic doses. The acute LD_{50} and LDL_0 values of nicotine vary widely across different species and for different routes of administration. Animals appear to tolerate far higher doses than is the case with humans. In rats the LD_{50} dose for a subcutaneous injection is 35–50 $mg.kg^{-1}$ whereas only 0.4 $mg.kg^{-1}$ is required to produce plasma nicotine concentrations equivalent to those of human smokers.[2] Mecamylamine pretreatment affords considerable protection against the toxic effects of nicotine but has no effect when administered after nicotine dosage.[3]

Apart from local irritancy nicotine has no other acute effects of a non-pharmacological nature. There is no clear evidence that nicotine has a role in the toxicity of tobacco smoke to cilia.

Clinical pharmacology

Within the smoking range there is a dose-related increase in heart rate and blood pressure during the early stages of administration but, due to the development of acute tolerance within 30–60 minutes, the changes after repeated or more prolonged administration are relatively small.[4–6] The peripheral vasoconstrictor effect, in contrast, does not appear to be subject to acute tolerance and a clear dose–effect relationship persists throughout the day.[5] Due probably to lack of tolerance to central effects, non-smokers frequently develop nausea at blood nicotine levels in the range of 10–20 $\mu g.l^{-1}$. This may be accompanied by pallor, faintness and a drop in blood pressure, but it is not clear how much these effects are due to reflexes associated with the development of nausea or to ganglionic blockade emerging at lower doses than is the case with smokers.

The central effects of smoking doses of nicotine are numerous but are less dramatic and obvious than is the case with many other psychoactive and dependence-producing drugs. Although nicotine can act as a primary reinforcer in many species of animal[7] and although regular tobacco users find their habit pleasurable, the source of the pleasurable effects remains elusive. Nicotine taken in rapidly via infusion, injection or nasal drops has no subjectively striking euphoriant, stimulant or sedative effect apart from a vague and transient 'heady' or 'dizzy' feeling which smokers find pleasant but which nonsmokers dislike.[8–12] Furthermore, this effect is subject to acute tolerance[11,12] and regular smokers tend to experience it only during the first cigarette of the day or after a few hours of abstinence.

Nicotine has both stimulant and sedative effects over the smoking range of dosage.[13–17] Like a sedative it promotes relaxation and reduces anxiety and tension. Like other stimulants it allays fatigue and increases the subjective sense of arousal and ability to concentrate. On objective tests it enhances performance on a number of psychomotor and mental tasks, improves memory and increases tolerance to pain. It also reduces hunger. Although EEG studies in animals have shown a dose-related biphasic response with small doses producing the patterns of arousal and larger doses having a sedative effect,[18] the EEG effects in humans of nicotine dosage within the smoking range are predominantly stimulant and closely reflect the patterns of natural arousal.[19–21] Nicotine has also been shown to decrease the P300 latency, a putative measure of stimulus evaluation time.[22] In contrast to these purely stimulant effects, a biphasic response to smoking and intravenous nicotine has been demonstrated in humans using another electrocortical measure of attention and arousal, the expectancy wave or CNV.[23] Lower doses of nicotine increase the magnitude of the CNV similarly to stimulant drugs, while higher doses decrease the magnitude as with sedative drugs.

Other actions of nicotine may also contribute to the calming and relaxing effects reported by smokers. For example, nicotine increases the rate of habituation to irrelevant stimuli such as a repeated loud noise.[24] Nicotine has a stimulant effect on inhibitory interneurones (Renshaw cells) in the spinal cord with consequent depression of tendon reflexes which may contribute to subjective feelings of relaxation and reduced muscle tension.[25] These effects, however, may be undermined by another effect of higher doses, which induce tremor.[26] Nicotine also reduces aggression.[27]

The widespread metabolic and endocrine effects of smoking doses of nicotine are discussed under Adverse reactions. One of the first to have been clearly documented is the antidiuretic effect mediated by the release of arginine-vasopressin.

Pharmacokinetics

The preferred analytical method is gas–liquid chromatography with nitrogen detection,[28–30] sensitivity 0.1 to 0.5 $\mu g.l^{-1}$.

Cigarette smokers absorb about 90% of the nicotine content of the smoke which they inhale, the amount depending on the depth of inhalation.[31] The bioavailability of nicotine retained in human lungs is not known. However, in the isolated perfused dog lung about 30% of the nicotine absorbed from smoke is metabolized within the lung to cotinine and nicotine-N-oxide before entering the pulmonary venous system, although nicotine introduced via the pulmonary artery undergoes first-pass metabolism to a very small extent, about 7%.[32] Nicotine is completely absorbed after oral administration but its bioavailability by this route has not been studied adequately. Data obtained in two subjects suggest a value of about 30%.[33] Although buccal absorption of nicotine avoids first-pass metabolism by the liver, the bioavailability from the use of nicotine gum may be as low as 30–40%.[34] This is due to a number of factors including expectoration, excessive salivation and swallowing of saliva, and incomplete extraction of nicotine from the gum due to inadequate chewing.

Absorption of nicotine through the lungs is rapid and concentrations of nicotine in venous blood peak within one minute after the last puff of a cigarette. The decline of nicotine in plasma is biexponential. The half life of the initial phase ranges from 7 to 10 minutes (mean 9 minutes) and that of the terminal phase ranges from 1 to 4 hours (mean 2 hours).[5,35] Nicotine is a high clearance drug with a total clearance averaging 18 $ml.min^{-1}.kg^{-1}$ (range 9–27) of which 85% to 95% is accounted for by metabolic clearance. The renal clearance depends on urinary pH and averages about 10% of total clearance under natural conditions. The high value of metabolic clearance approaches that of the hepatic circulation suggesting that presystemic metabolism by the liver may be greater, and the oral bioavailability lower, than indicated by the values cited above.

Blood nicotine concentrations vary widely between different smokers, as do smoking habits, and depend more on the way that cigarettes are puffed and inhaled than on the nicotine yield or number smoked per day.[31,36] Peak levels, sampled two minutes after smoking during the afternoon of a typical smoking day, range from below 5 to just short of 100 $\mu g.l^{-1}$, but the levels of individual smokers tend to be fairly constant from one day to the next. The peak levels of regular smokers of 15 or more cigarettes per day average about 35 $\mu g.l^{-1}$ (SD 13) and trough levels just before smoking average about 10 $\mu g.l^{-1}$ less.[36–38] Similar levels are found in regular users of 'wet' and 'dry' snuff[37,39] and in former cigarette smokers who have switched to a pipe or cigars.[40,41] Data from more than 2000 human subjects show no values in excess of 100 $\mu g.l^{-1}$ resulting from the recreational use of tobacco.[36,38,42]

The dose of systemically available nicotine absorbed by regular smokers averages about 1 mg per cigarette.[35,42,43] However, there is great variation between smokers. By intensive puffing and inhalation it is possible to obtain 3 mg nicotine or more from a cigarette having

Nicotine

a standard machine-smoked yield of only 1 mg nicotine. Also, smokers tend to take in a little more nicotine from the first cigarette of the day, about 1.5 mg on average.[44] The daily nicotine intake of smokers averages about 25 mg (around 0.4 mg.kg^{-1} daily), but ranges from negligible amounts in non-inhalers up to 50 mg or more.[35,38,42–45] Since the blood nicotine concentrations are similar in men and women, less nicotine is required to produce these levels in women due to their lower body weight.

Nicotine is widely and rapidly distributed throughout the body as would be expected with a highly lipid soluble drug, with an apparent volume of distribution averaging 2.6 l.kg^{-1} (range 1.3 to 3.8) indicating drug accumulation in some tissues. Animal studies have demonstrated that within one minute after intravenous administration the highest levels of nicotine occur in the kidney, brain and liver reflecting blood flow to these tissues.[46] The levels decline rapidly within the first hour but the brain to blood nicotine concentration ratio remains at about 5:1 throughout this period.[47] Nicotine also accumulates in some sites such as the stomach, kidney, bladder and salivary glands due to pH partitioning.[46] The binding of nicotine to plasma proteins is low (5%) and is not affected by nicotine concentration.[5] Consistent with its high lipid solubility nicotine crosses the placenta readily. It is also found in many body fluids including saliva, breast milk and cervical mucus in concentrations which reflect the balance between blood levels and the pH of the fluid in question. It can also be measured in human hair. Nicotine is extensively biotransformed, largely in the liver but also in the lung and kidney. Only 10% of the dose is excreted unchanged in the urine.

Oral absorption	100%
Presystemic metabolism	>70%
Plasma half life	
range	1–4 h
mean	2 h
Volume of distribution	2.6 l.kg^{-1}
Plasma protein binding	5%

Concentration–effect relationship

The relationship between the plasma concentration of nicotine and its effects is complex due to the rapid development of tolerance.

Pharmacological effects of smoking appear at relatively low blood nicotine concentrations in the 10–15 μg.l^{-1} range. Cardiovascular and central effects become detectable at these low levels and many of the unpleasant symptoms of tobacco withdrawal are alleviated.[48] Although mild acute toxic effects may be experienced by novices at these levels, tobacco users regulate their nicotine intake with great precision and seldom experience unpleasant toxic effects. However, the upper limit tolerated by regular tobacco users varies considerably from about 30 to 100 μg.l^{-1} so that some users may experience mild toxic effects such as nausea, vomiting, pallor and tremor at levels that others require for full satisfaction. Serious acute toxic effects discussed in the section on toxicology do not occur with tobacco use and have been reported only in the context of accidental or deliberate poisoning by nicotine-containing insecticides. Blood nicotine concentrations of 300–400 μg.l^{-1} have been recorded in such cases, followed by gradual recovery over 12 h.[49]

Hiccups and mild dyspeptic symptoms are well-known side effects of nicotine gum (see below). The fact that they occur at low blood nicotine concentrations and are much less common during smoking suggests that local actions are involved.

Metabolism

Nicotine is extensively metabolized, mainly in the liver but also in the lungs and kidneys though not in the brain.[32,46,50] Four primary pathways have been identified: alpha-carbon oxidation of the pyrrolidine ring, N-oxidation of the pyrrolidine ring, N-methylation of the pyridine ring and N-demethylation of the pyrrolidine ring.

Alpha-carbon oxidation to cotinine is the major metabolic pathway in most species including man. It is a complex process, mediated by cytochrome P-450 and involving at least two intermediates.[51] One of these, an iminium ion, is not pharmacologically active and may be an antagonist at nicotinic receptors. Cotinine has a relatively long half life (about 20 hours on average)[52] so that concentrations in the blood of regular smokers build up to steady-state levels almost ten times higher than those of the parent compound and average[38] about 300 μg.l^{-1}. Cotinine concentrations in blood, saliva or urine are widely used as biochemical measures of nicotine intake from active or passive smoking.[53] Cotinine is metabolized to 3-hydroxycotinine, which is the main urinary metabolite of nicotine.[54]

N-oxidation to nicotine l'-N-oxide is another important route of metabolism and concentrations of this N-oxide in urine average about one third of those of cotinine. This N-oxide is not metabolized further but is reduced back to nicotine by bowel flora and small amounts of nicotine are subject to enterohepatic recycling in this way.[55] The nicotine isomethonium ion formed by N-methylation of the pyridine ring is not metabolized further.[50] Nornicotine arises by N-demethylation of nicotine. Nornicotine and cotinine are both degraded through many stages to form 3-pyridylacetic acid which appears to be the end-product of nicotine metabolism in humans. None of the numerous metabolites of nicotine have been shown to have significant pharmacological effects in the concentrations found after nicotine administration. However, it has been suggested that certain carcinogenic nitrosamines may be formed endogenously from one or more metabolites of nicotine.[56]

Pharmaceutics

Nicotine is available as a resin complex (USA approved name Nicotine Polacrilex) incorporated into a chewing gum, Nicorette (Lakeside, USA/Lundbeck, UK). The chewing gums, containing 2 mg or 4 mg nicotine, are square pieces 14 × 14 × 4.5 mm weighing 1 g. The 2 mg gum has a beige colour; the 4 mg gum is yellowish.

The nicotine gum is a slow-release preparation, the rate of release of nicotine depending on the rate of chewing. It takes 20–30 minutes of vigorous chewing to release 95% of the nicotine content of the gum. Without chewing or if the gum is accidentally swallowed negligible amounts of nicotine are released.

The nicotine gum is a fairly stable preparation with a shelf-life of about 2 years. It should be stored at no more than 25°C and protected from light. The 4 mg preparation contains quinoline yellow, but the gum is otherwise free of potential allergens.

Preliminary tests have been done to explore the therapeutic potential of a nasal nicotine spray and smoke-free cigarettes delivering nicotine vapour,[57,58] and a transdermal nicotine patch is available in some countries.[59]

Therapeutic use

Indications

1. Treatment of tobacco withdrawal symptoms.

Contraindications

1. Non-users of tobacco
2. Gastritis or active peptic ulcer disease.

Precautions

1. Pregnancy
2. Angina and coronary disease
3. Severe hypertension
4. Peripheral vascular disease.

Mode of use

Nicotine gum is usually taken ad libitum, starting on the day that smoking or other forms of tobacco use are abandoned. One piece of 2 mg gum is taken as necessary whenever there is a strong urge to smoke and should be chewed for about 30 minutes. The stronger 4 mg gum may be used after a few days if 10 or more 2 mg gums per day are not sufficiently effective. Like the smoking habits and blood nicotine levels of smokers, ad libitum use of nicotine gum varies widely. Some are helped sufficiently to give up smoking on only 2–3 pieces of 2 mg gum per day while a few may need the maximum dose of 15 pieces of 4 mg gum per day (mean about 8 × 2 mg per day).

To achieve good results it is important that it is chewed correctly and that its effects and limitations are understood. Its main effect is to reduce withdrawal symptoms after smoking has ceased. Due to the slower rate of nicotine absorption through the buccal mucosa it does not produce the same pleasurable effects as smoking. In fact it usually

N

tastes slightly unpleasant at first and may be irritating to the mouth and throat over the first 2–3 days until the subject has got used to it. Ideally, it should not be chewed continuously. After every 10–20 chews, it should be parked in the side of the mouth for 1–2 minutes before chewing again. The bioavailability of nicotine absorbed through the buccal mucosa is greater than that absorbed after swallowing. Excessive chewing increases the rate of release of nicotine from the gum and also increases salivation and swallowing of nicotine.

If complete abstinence from smoking has not been achieved after 2–3 weeks of nicotine gum use the treatment should probably be abandoned until a further attempt is made in the future. Those who achieve long-term success tend to stop smoking in the early stages of treatment. The optimal duration of gum treatment for those who do stop smoking is contentious. Most successful ex-smokers are able to reduce and discontinue gum use within two months. Since the risk of relapse is high in the first 3–4 months after stopping smoking, it seems unwise to forcibly restrict gum use during this period so that it is usual practice to permit the gum to be used ad libitum for at least 3–4 months provided that abstinence from smoking is maintained. After this point weaning from the gum should be encouraged, but if forced too hard, relapse to smoking is more likely. A proportion of smokers transfer their dependence to the gum. Of those who initially receive nicotine gum about 7% continue to use it for a year or more if prescriptions are maintained. Abrupt withdrawal in these cases gives rise to effects similar to those of tobacco withdrawal. However, many of these cases are able to give up the gum after using it for a year or more without relapsing to smoking.

Indications

Although many people give up smoking without any formal help or treatment, there are as many who are dependent and continue smoking despite numerous unsuccessful attempts to stop. Nicotine gum is not a panacea which makes it easy to stop smoking, but acts rather as an aid which makes the task a little less difficult. It follows therefore that it is suitable only for smokers who are well motivated to stop and who are sufficiently committed to maintain their efforts and determination through a withdrawal period that may present difficulties for several weeks or even months. Although nicotine gum appears to be more helpful to highly dependent smokers who smoke heavily, it can also be helpful to lighter smokers. In summary, its use is indicated in any smoker (or smokeless tobacco user) who is well motivated to stop and who has tried unsuccessfully in the past or has little confidence in succeeding without some help. Its use is also indicated in light smokers who meet these criteria.

Contraindications

Nicotine gum is contraindicated in non-smokers. Having less tolerance to nicotine they would be more sensitive to toxic effects and could risk developing dependence.

Due to the possibility of adverse local effects of nicotine in the stomach, nicotine gum is contraindicated in people with gastritis or active peptic ulcer disease and should be used with caution in those with a past history of such disorders.

Precautions

Nicotine may have adverse effects on the fetus and in people with coronary disease, hypertension and peripheral vascular disease (see above). However, blood nicotine concentrations during ad libitum clinical use of nicotine gum average about one third of those produced by cigarette smoking and are, furthermore, free of the sharp peaks and post-inhalation high-nicotine boli which are characteristic of inhaled cigarette smoking. Nicotine gum is therefore likely to be far less hazardous than continued smoking to people with these disorders and has the additional advantage of being free of carbon monoxide and other harmful substances present in tobacco smoke. Its cautious use, therefore, is probably justified in pregnant women and smokers with these disorders who smoke heavily and who have been unable to stop smoking despite repeated warnings. Indeed, it could be argued that the indication to prescribe nicotine gum is stronger in such cases than in those for whom stopping smoking is less urgent. However, gum dosage should probably be kept lower and discontinued earlier in the absence of success.

Adverse reactions

Potentially life-threatening effects

In high risk groups such as those with coronary disease there may be a risk of inducing cardiac arrhythmia but the risks are likely to be less than those of continued smoking.

Acute overdosage

Severe and even fatal acute toxic effects can occur as a result of nicotine overdosage through cutaneous absorption of nicotine from exposure to nicotine insecticides or as a result of accidental or deliberate ingestion of insecticide, cigarettes or other tobacco products. Such extreme overdose is characterized by circulatory collapse with pallor, sweating and tachycardia, tremor, hyperpnoea, abdominal pains, vomiting and diarrhoea, muscular spasms and, occasionally, epileptic fits. Death may occur as a result of circulatory failure or by respiratory arrest as the hyperpnoea is superseded by the development of muscular paralysis. Death can occur within a few minutes of ingestion, but recovery is rapid after peak absorption and is usual if survival exceeds 2–3 hours. The textbook figure of 30–60 mg for the lethal dose of oral nicotine in humans is traceable to the German literature of the 1920s and 1930s and may be an underestimate.[4] The toxic threshold is obviously considerably less for parenteral dosage, and intravenous doses as low as 25 μg.kg^{-1} require considerable caution if the rate of administration is rapid.[35]

No incidents of overdose with nicotine chewing gum have been reported. Several pieces at a time would have to be chewed vigorously for 15 minutes or more to produce significant acute intoxication and since nausea and vomiting would occur before more serious effects it is unlikely that the gum could be used to threaten life. Similarly overdose by ingestion is not a risk. The gums are more awkward to swallow than pills or capsules, bioavailability of swallowed nicotine is extremely low and the resin complex of which the gum is made releases little of its nicotine during transit through the gastrointestinal tract.

Severe or irreversible adverse effects

A major problem with nicotine is that it is so highly addictive. At least nine out of ten smokers are to some extent dependent on nicotine. Some 75% are moderately to strongly dependent and continue smoking despite wanting and trying to stop. Nicotine fulfils all the criteria of an addictive drug. It is psychoactive, it affects mood, it can act as a primary reinforcer, it induces tolerance, and physical as well as psychological changes occur on withdrawal. Chronic exposure to nicotine induces upregulation of nicotinic cholinergic receptors in many parts of the brain, and post-mortem studies show higher densities of nicotinic receptors in the brains of smokers.[60] Evidence of the addictive properties of nicotine is fully documented in the 1988 US Surgeon General's Report,[61] and nicotine dependence and nicotine withdrawal are now recognized as forms of mental disorder in ICD9 and DSM-III-R[62] alongside dependence on other drugs such as heroin and cocaine.

There is no direct evidence from which an assessment can be made of the chronic human toxicity of nicotine as opposed to tobacco products. The effects of tobacco use are confounded by many other factors, not least by the near 4000 other toxic, irritant and carcinogenic chemical compounds that have been identified in tobacco smoke.[63] Numerous effects of chronic exposure to nicotine in experimental animals have been documented.[64–69] However, in many cases, the dosage was far in excess of exposures resulting from tobacco use, and their value for extrapolation to humans is limited. Epidemiological studies have identified a number of diseases which are associated with smoking and other forms of tobacco use but there is no clear evidence that nicotine has a causal role in any of the smoking-related diseases. However, it may be a contributory factor in certain cases and its role in the major smoking-related diseases is considered below.

Cancer. There is no evidence that nicotine is teratogenic or carcinogenic. It is not mutagenic, neither does it act as a tumour initiator, promoter or cocarcinogen. Tobacco, and especially tobacco smoke, contains several potent carcinogens which are present in sufficient quantities to account for the raised incidence of lung cancer and other cancers in smokers and other forms of tobacco user. None of the major metabolites of nicotine is carcinogenic but concern has been raised about the possibility that certain tobacco-specific nitrosamines which are highly carcinogenic may be formed endogenously

Nicotine

from a metabolite of nicotine.[56,70] This has not been clearly established, however, in either animals or humans.

Bronchitis and chronic obstructive lung disease. There is no evidence that nicotine contributes significantly to the toxic effects of tobacco smoke on the cilia or epithelium of the respiratory tract, the effects on immune mechanisms, the balance of elastase production and inhibition, or other processes which may be involved in the harmful effects of tobacco smoke on the lungs of smokers.

Cardiovascular disease. The cardiovascular risks of smoking are closely linked to the degree of inhalation and are minimal in smokers who do not inhale.[71] Absorption and retention of most smoke components also depends on the degree of inhalation. In some cases, carbon monoxide (CO) for example, absorption is negligible in non-inhalers. Nicotine, in contrast, is absorbed through the buccal mucosa especially if the pH is high. Thus pharmacologically effective doses can be absorbed from non-inhaled pipe and cigar smoking and also from snuff and chewing tobacco, whereas the absorption from cigarettes is negligible without inhalation. The fact that the cardiovascular risks are high in inhaling cigarette smokers who absorb nicotine, CO and tar but low in non-inhaling pipe and cigar smokers who absorb nicotine but little CO has lead some epidemiologists to suggest that CO or a tar component, but not nicotine, is responsible for smoking-related cardiovascular disease.[40] Another possibility, however, is that nicotine may be an important factor but that its adverse effects depend on the rate of absorption, buccal absorption being far slower than through the lung alveoli.

Nicotine could affect atherogenesis and thrombogenesis in many ways, predominantly by activation of peripheral adrenergic systems. Nicotine has been shown to cause damage to vascular endothelium,[72,73] to impair the synthesis of prostacyclin (PGI_2) in vitro[74,75] and to increase platelet activity in vitro, but the relevance of these observations is uncertain.[63] Nicotine probably is responsible for the increase in platelet adhesiveness,[76] enhanced ADP-induced platelet aggregation[77,78] and decreased platelet survival[79] which occur on smoking a single cigarette. Chronic cigarette smokers have increased excretion of thromboxane metabolites in their urine which suggests platelet activation. Regular smokers also have raised plasma fibrinogen levels, raised blood viscosity, reduced fibrinolytic activity and a shortened coagulation time,[78,80] but it is not yet clear whether these effects are attributable to nicotine.

Nicotine administration, like smoking, causes an increase in plasma free fatty acids, LDL and triglycerides, mediated by catecholamine release.[81–83] The effect on free fatty acids appears to be more pronounced in patients who have suffered a myocardial infarction.[84] Rapid development of tolerance means that these effects are less prominent in chronic smoking.

Through sympathetic stimulation and the release of noradrenaline, nicotine might lower the ventricular fibrillation threshold during an episode of myocardial ischaemia.[69,85] By increasing heart rate, blood pressure, stroke volume and cardiac output[85–89] and thereby increasing the load and oxygen demand of the myocardium, nicotine could trigger or exacerbate angina in patients with established coronary artery disease. The deleterious effects of smoking on mortality following a first heart attack are largely abolished by propranolol indicating that adrenergic mechanisms are involved. This strongly implicates nicotine which is the only smoke component with effects on adrenergic systems.[90] Lastly, nicotine-induced peripheral vasoconstriction[86,91,92] and consequent reduction in blood flow to the distal parts of the limbs[93] might exacerbate the effect of peripheral vascular disease.

Peptic ulcers. A dose-related association between smoking and peptic ulcers is well-established by epidemiological studies.[69] However, it is not clear whether smoking causes peptic ulcers although both gastric and duodenal ulcers tend to heal more slowly in smokers and, once healed, are more likely to recur.[69,94]

Chronic nicotine administration does not produce ulcers in animals, but potentiates and increases the number of duodenal ulcers induced by pentagastrin and other stimulants of gastric secretion.[95,96] Studies of the effects of nicotine or smoking on gastric acid secretion have had conflicting results.[69] Larger doses appear to reduce secretion but this may be due to the inhibitory effect of nausea induced by nicotine or the investigation procedures. Intravenous infusion of 2 mg nicotine had no effect on pentagastrin-stimulated acid and pepsin secretion in one study of human subjects.[97]

In animal studies, nicotine has a dose-related inhibitory effect on pancreatic bicarbonate secretion and on the flow and bicarbonate content of bile.[98] These effects are mediated by nicotine-induced noradrenaline release and are prevented by α-blockers.[99] Similar effects occur during smoking in human subjects, the magnitude being related to plasma nicotine levels. However, smoking does not affect plasma gastrin or secretin concentrations.[100]

Smoking has been shown to delay gastric emptying time,[101] impair pyloric competence[102] and increase duodenogastric reflux[103] in human subjects, but no studies have examined the capacity of nicotine to reproduce these effects.

Prostaglandins increase the resistance of the gastric mucosa to injury[119] and smoking impairs prostaglandin synthesis in both fundal and central human gastric mucosa.[120] This action is probably mediated by nicotine which has been shown to impair in vitro synthesis of prostaglandins in other tissues.[74,75]

Endocrine and metabolic effects. Apart from increasing plasma adrenaline, noradrenaline and vasopressin concentrations,[85] nicotine increases blood levels of ACTH, cortisol and growth hormone.[104–107] Although the blood levels of prolactin are increased in acute studies,[106,107] the chronic effects of nicotine are probably responsible for the lower levels of serum prolactin in smokers.[108] A distinction between short-term and longer term effects has been found in rats in studies which show that the inhibition of the secretion of prolactin and luteinizing hormone produced by cigarette smoke and nicotine is mediated by dopaminergic and noradrenergic systems in the hypothalamus.[109,110] Women who smoke have lower levels of luteal phase urinary oestrogens[111] due probably to enhanced hepatic metabolism to less active metabolites.[112] C-2 hydroxylation of oestradiol, for example, is mediated by cytochrome P-450 enzymes which are powerfully induced by benzpyrene and other PAH compounds in tobacco smoke.[113] These antioestrogenic effects may be implicated in the early menopause of women who smoke and the attendant risks of cardiovascular disease and osteoporosis.[114,115]

Nicotine may also affect thyroid function. Heavy smokers have reduced serum levels of thyroxine (T_4) and triiodothyronine (T_3).[116] These effects appear to be mediated by nicotine or its N-oxide metabolite, chronic administration of which produces in rats a thyroid function profile similar to that of the 'low $T3_3$ syndrome' seen clinically in humans.[117,118]

Through its effects on the release of catecholamines and glucocorticoids nicotine has multiple effects on carbohydrate, fat and protein metabolism. These include stimulation of lipolysis leading to increases in serum FFAs and triglycerides,[121] increases in blood glucose and lactate[122] in acute studies, and decreases in blood insulin levels during chronic administration of nicotine.[123] However, it is not known to what extent these metabolic effects may lead to adverse consequences. Nicotine is responsible for the weight reducing effects of smoking.[124] Smokers as a group weigh about 5 kg less than non-smokers of equivalent age and sex, and the tendency for them to put on weight after giving up smoking is reduced by nicotine chewing gum.[125,126] Studies in animals and humans have shown that nicotine decreases the consumption of sweet-tasting foods and carbohydrates.[124] In addition, nicotine reduces body weight even when food consumption is unchanged[124] suggesting that it affects energy expenditure as well as intake. The rise in metabolic rate and body oxygen consumption induced by smoking and nicotine injections appears to be mediated through increased mobilization and consumption of FFAs, for the effect can be abolished if lipolysis is inhibited with β-piridylcarbinol.[127]

Symptomatic adverse effects

Smokers and other forms of tobacco user learn to regulate their nicotine intake with great skill and precision and seldom experience acute toxic effects. They are also partially protected by the development of tolerance to nicotine. Mild toxic effects such as pallor, faintness, sweating, palpitations, tremor, parasthesiae, coolness of the extremities, nausea, vomiting and headache occur commonly in novice tobacco users. Such effects have also been reported as a result of cutaneous absorption of nicotine in tobacco croppers (Green tobacco sickness).[128]

The nicotine gum is a slow-release product. In view of the slow rate of absorption and low bioavailability of nicotine from the gum (30–40%) its potential to produce toxic nicotine effects is substanti-

N

ally less than that of cigarette smoking. Although the 4 mg nicotine gum can in time build up blood nicotine concentrations similar to or above those of normal smoking, its free ad libitum use by heavy smokers seldom results in blood nicotine concentrations amounting to half the smoking levels so that serious toxic effects do not occur in clinical use in normal smokers. The gum is generally well tolerated although minor adverse effects are common in the first few days of treatment. They usually arise from excessive chewing and can be prevented or diminished by adequate instructions and guidance on how to chew the gum correctly. The adverse effects include: irritation to the mouth and throat, sticking of the gum to dentures and dislodgement of loose fillings, tired and aching jaws, borborygmi due to air swallowing, indigestion, hiccups, nausea and, rarely, vomiting. Occasional reports of mouth ulcers are no more common than after stopping smoking without the gum. A slightly more serious adverse effect is palpitations (incidence about 5/1000).[129]

Interference with clinical pathology tests
Nicotine may interfere with the Frings thin-layer chromatographic method for measuring urinary alkaloids.

High risk groups

Neonates
The drug is not used in neonates.

Breast milk. Nicotine enters breast milk in small amounts that do not appear to have any acute effects on the neonate. However, the long-term effects on the child are unknown, and breast-feeding mothers should be strongly advised against the use of nicotine-containing substances.

Children
The drug should not be taken by children.

Pregnant women
While carbon monoxide may contribute to the effect of maternal smoking on reducing the size, and hence increasing the vulnerability, of the fetus in utero and during the perinatal period, it has been shown that administration of nicotine chewing gum to pregnant women affects the breathing movements and heart rate of the fetus whereas carbon monoxide via nicotine-free herbal cigarettes has no effect.[130,131] This acute effect is probably mediated through the vasoconstrictor action of nicotine, although nicotine and smoking have also been shown to cause pathological changes in the umbilical arteries.[73]

The elderly
In theory, the elderly are more likely than the young to have coronary artery disease and so be more susceptible to the risks of nicotine-induced cardiac arrhythmias.

Drug interactions

Potentially hazardous interactions
The risks of vascular disease induced by the contraceptive pill appear to be increased by smoking tobacco. Due to induction of liver enzymes cigarette smoking reduces the bioavailability and increases clearance rates of many drugs. This effect is not thought to be due to nicotine but to other components of tobacco smoke, particularly polycyclic hydrocarbons.

Potentially useful interactions
None has been reported.

Clinical trials

1. Jarvis M J, Raw M, Russell M A H, Feyerabend C 1982 Randomised controlled trial of nicotine chewing-gum. British Medical Journal 285: 537–540

This was a double-blind trial with biochemical validation of self-reported smoking status and categorization of drop-outs and non-respondents as failures. Cigarette smokers attending a smokers clinic were randomly assigned to treatment with 2 mg nicotine gum ($n=58$) or placebo gum ($n=58$). The placebo gum contained 1 mg nicotine to reproduce the nicotine taste, but was unbuffered to lower its bioavailability. Abstinence rates at one year were 47% and 21% respectively ($P<0.025$) and the rates using a stringent criterion of lapse-free abstinence throughout the year were 31% and 14% respectively ($P<0.05$).

Subjects receiving active gum experienced less severe withdrawal symptoms and rated their gum as more helpful than did the placebo group. Minor side effects were common but only hiccups and indigestion were more frequent with the active gum. The number of gums used daily correlated significantly with pretreatment blood nicotine concentrations in the active treatment group but not in the placebo group. Active gum was also used for longer than the placebo but most subjects stopped using it within six months. Four subjects (7%) developed longer-term dependence on active gum, but there were no such cases in the placebo group.

2. Hjalmarson A I M 1984 Effect of nicotine chewing gum in smoking cessation: a randomized, placebo-controlled, double-blind study. Journal of the American Medical Association 252: 2835–2838

This double-blind study among smokers attending a smoking cessation clinic compared 2 mg nicotine chewing gum with a placebo gum flavoured with capsaicin to imitate the sharp taste of nicotine. After one year, 29% of the 106 subjects treated with nicotine gum had remained abstinent throughout the year compared with 16% of 99 subjects treated with placebo ($P<0.05$). The results were confirmed by measurement of expired air carbon monoxide. More subjects in the nicotine group reported that the gum reduced the craving to smoke. Side effects were few and not serious. Hiccups and flatulence were more frequent in those treated with nicotine gum. In the nicotine group, 3% were still using the gum after two years, but no subjects used placebo gum beyond six months.

Other trials

1. Fagerstrom K O 1984 Effects of nicotine chewing gum and follow-up in physician-based smoking cessation. Preventive Medicine 13: 517–527

This study examined the effect of supportive advice and counselling, with and without nicotine gum, and of two levels of support, short and long, using a 2×2 factorial design. 16 family physicians (GPs) randomly assigned a total of 145 patients who wanted to stop smoking to one of the four treatment conditions. At one year follow-up the abstinence rate in those who received nicotine gum and were supported longer was 27%, compared with 22% for those who received nicotine gum and brief support, 15% in those who had longer support but no gum and 3% of those on brief support without gum. Nicotine gum had the major effect ($P<0.05$) but the effect of the level of support was not statistically significant.

Effect on withdrawal symptoms

1. West R J 1984 Psychology and pharmacology in cigarette withdrawal. Journal of Psychosomatic Research 28: 379–386

This report presents and discusses data from three double-blind placebo-controlled studies, each of which showed that 2 mg nicotine chewing gum alleviates many of the unpleasant symptoms of cigarette withdrawal.

General review articles

Russell M A H 1976 Tobacco smoking and nicotine dependence. In: Gibbens R J, Israel Y, Kalant H, Popham R E, Schmidt W, Smart R J (eds) Research advances in alcohol and drug problems, vol 3. Wiley & Sons, New York, pp 1–47

Cohen A J, Roe F J C 1981 Monograph on the pharmacology and toxicology of nicotine. Tobacco Advisory Council Occasional Paper 4. Sinclair Pride, London

Benowitz N L 1988 Pharmacologic aspects of cigarette smoking and nicotine addiction. New England Journal of Medicine 319: 1318–1330

Wonnacott S, Russell M A H, Stolerman I P (eds) 1990 Nicotine psychopharmacology: molecular, cellular and behavioural aspects. Oxford University Press, Oxford

References

1. Balfour D J K 1982 The effects of nicotine on brain neurotransmitter systems. Pharmacology and Therapeutics 16: 269–282
2. Pratt J A, Stolerman I P, Garcha H S, Giardini V, Feyerabend C 1983 Discriminative stimulus properties of nicotine: further evidence for mediation at a cholinergic receptor. Psychopharmacology 81: 54–60

3. Stolerman I P, Pratt J A, Garcha H S, Giardini V, Kumar R 1983 Nicotine cue in rats analyzed with drugs acting on cholinergic and 5-hydroxytryptamine mechanisms. Neuropharmacology 22: 1029–1037
4. Russell M A H, Feyerabend C 1978 Cigarette smoking: a dependence on high-nicotine boli. Drug Metabolism Reviews 8: 29–57
5. Benowitz N L, Jacob P, Jones R T, Rosenberg J 1982 Interindividual variability in the metabolism and cardiovascular effects of nicotine in man. Journal of Pharmacology and Experimental Therapeutics 221: 368–372
6. Russell M A H, Jarvis M J, Jones G, Feyerabend C 1990 Nonsmokers show acute tolerance to subcutaneous nicotine. Psychopharmacology 102: 56–58
7. Spealman R D, Goldberg S R 1982 Maintenance of schedule-controlled behavior by intravenous injections of nicotine in squirrel monkeys. Journal of Pharmacology and Experimental Therapeutics 223: 402–408
8. Johnston L M 1942 Tobacco smoking and nicotine. Lancet 2: 742
9. Henningfield J E, Miyasato K, Jasinski D R 1983 Cigarette smokers self-administer intravenous nicotine. Pharmacology, Biochemistry and Behaviour 19: 887–890
10. Russell M A H, Jarvis M J, Feyerabend C, Ferno O 1983 Nasal nicotine solution: a potential aid to giving up smoking? British Medical Journal 286: 683–684
11. Jones R T, Farrell T R, Herning R I 1978 Tobacco smoking and nicotine tolerance. In: Krasnegor N A (ed) Self-administration of abused substances: methods for study. NIDA Research Monograph. 20. Department of Health, Education and Welfare, Washington, DC, pp 202–208
12. West R J, Russell M A H 1987 Cardiovascular and subjective effects of smoking before and after 24 hr of abstinence from cigarettes. Psychopharmacology 91: 118–121
13. Wesnes K, Warburton D M 1983 Smoking, nicotine and human performance. Pharmacology and Therapeutics 21: 189–208
14. Ashton H, Stepney R 1982 Smoking: psychology and pharmacology. Tavistock Publications Ltd, London
15. Russell M A H 1976 Tobacco smoking and nicotine dependence. In: Gibbins R J et al (eds) Research advances in alcohol and drug problems, vol 3. Wiley and Sons, New York, pp 1–47
16. West R J, Russell M A H 1985 Nicotine pharmacology and smoking dependence. In: Iversen S D (ed) Psychopharmacology: recent advances and future prospects. Oxford University Press, Oxford, pp 303–314
17. Jaffe J H 1985 Nicotine and tobacco. In: Gilman A G, Goodman L S, Rall T W, Murad F (eds) The pharmacological basis of therapeutics, 7th edn. MacMillan Publishing Co, New York, pp 554–558
18. Armitage A K, Hall G H, Sellers C M 1969 Effects of nicotine on electrocortical activity and acetylcholine release from the cat cerebral cortex. British Journal of Pharmacology 35: 152–160
19. Ulett J A, Itil T M 1969 Quantitative electroencephalogram in smoking and smoking deprivation. Science 164: 969–970
20. Herning R I, Jones R T, Bachman J 1983 EEG changes during tobacco withdrawal. Psychophysiology 20: 507–512
21. Knott V J, Venables P H 1977 EEG alpha correlates of nonsmokers, smokers, smoking and smoking deprivation. Psychophysiology 14: 150–156
22. Herning R I, Pickworth W B 1985 Nicotine gum improved stimulus processing during tobacco withdrawal. Psychophysiology 22: 594
23. Ashton H, Marsh V R, Millman J E, Rawlins M D, Telford R, Thompson J W 1978 The use of event-related slow potentials of the brain as a means to analyse the effects of cigarette smoking and nicotine in humans. In: Thornton R (ed) Smoking behaviour: physiological and psychological influences. Churchill Livingstone, Edinburgh, pp 54–68
24. Friedman J T, Horvath T, Meares R 1974 Tobacco smoking and a 'stimulus barrier'. Nature 248: 455–456
25. Domino E F, von Baumgarten A M 1969 Tobacco, cigarette smoking and patella reflex depression. Clinical Pharmacology and Therapeutics 10: 72–79
26. Frankenhauser M, Myrsten A L, Post B 1970 Psychophysiological reactions to cigarette smoking. Scandinavian Journal of Psychology 11: 237–245
27. Schechter M D, Rand M J 1974 Effect of acute deprivation of smoking on aggression and hostility. Psychopharmacologia 35: 19–28
28. Feyerabend C, Russell M A H 1980 Assay of nicotine in biological materials: sources of contamination and their elimination. Journal of Pharmacy and Pharmacology 32: 178–181
29. Jacob P, Wilson M, Benowitz N L 1981 Improved gas chromatographic method for the determination of nicotine and cotinine in biologic fluids. Journal of Chromatography and Biomedical Applications 222: 61–70
30. Feyeraband C, Russell M A H 1990 A rapid gas–liquid chromatographic method for the determination of cotinine and nicotine in biological fluids. Journal of Pharmacy and Pharmacology 42: 450–452
31. Armitage A K, Dollery C T, George C F, Houseman T H, Lewis P J, Turner D M 1975 Absorption and metabolism of nicotine from cigarettes. British Medical Journal 4: 313–316
32. Turner D M, Armitage A K, Briant R H, Dollery C T 1975 Metabolism of nicotine by the isolated perfused dog lung. Xenobiotica 5: 539–551
33. Beckett A H, Gorrod J W, Jenner P 1971 The analysis of nicotine 1'-N-oxide in urine in the presence of nicotine and cotinine and its application to the study of in vivo nicotine metabolism in man. Journal of Pharmacy and Pharmacology 23: 55–61S
34. Benowitz N L, Jacob P, Savanapridi C 1987 Determinants of nicotine intake while chewing nicotine polacrilex gum. Clinical Pharmacology and Therapeutics 4: 467–473
35. Feyerabend C, Ings R M J, Russell M A H 1985 Nicotine pharmacokinetics and its application to intake from smoking. British Journal of Clinical Pharmacology 19: 239–247
36. Russell M A H, Jarvis M J, Iyer R, Feyerabend C 1980 Relation of nicotine yield of cigarettes to blood nicotine concentrations in smokers. British Medical Journal 280: 972–975
37. Russell M A H, Jarvis M J, Devitt G, Feyerabend C 1981 Nicotine intake by snuff users. British Medical Journal 283: 814–817
38. Russell M A H, Jarvis M J, Feyerabend C, Saloojee Y 1986 Reduction of tar, nicotine and carbon monoxide intake in low tar smokers. Journal of Epidemiology and Community Health 40: 80–85
39. Gritz E R, Baier-Weiss V, Benowitz N L, Van Vunakis H, Jarvik M E 1981 Plasma nicotine and cotinine concentrations in habitual smokeless tobacco users. Clinical Pharmacology and Therapeutics 30: 201–209
40. Wald N J, Idle M, Boreham J, Bailey A, Van Vunakis H 1981 Serum cotinine levels in pipe smokers: evidence against nicotine as a cause of coronary heart disease. Lancet 2: 775–777
41. Wald N J, Idle M, Boreham J, Bailey A, Van Vunakis H 1984 Urinary nicotine concentrations in cigarette and pipe smokers. Thorax 39: 365–368
42. Gori G B, Lynch C J 1985 Analytical cigarette yields as predictors of smoke bioavailability. Regulatory Toxicology and Pharmacology 5: 314–326
43. Benowitz N L, Jacob P 1984 Daily intake of nicotine from cigarette smoking. Clinical Pharmacology and Therapeutics 35: 499–504
44. Russell M A H, West R J, Jarvis M J 1985 Intravenous nicotine simulation of passive smoking to estimate dosage to exposed non-smokers. British Journal of Addiction 80: 201–206
45. Galeazzi R L, Daenens P, Gugger M 1985 Steady-state concentration of cotinine as a measure of nicotine intake by smokers. European Journal of Clinical Pharmacology 28: 301–304
46. Schmiterlow C G, Hansson E, Andersson G, Applegren L E, Hoffman P C 1967 Distribution of nicotine in central nervous system. Annals of the New York Academy of Science 142: 2–14
47. Stalhandske T 1970 Effects of increased liver metabolism of nicotine on its uptake, elimination and toxicity in mice. Acta Physiologica Scandinavica 80: 222–234
48. Russell M A H 1988 Nicotine replacement: the role of blood nicotine levels, their rate of change and nicotine tolerance. In: Pomerleau O F, Pomerleau C S (eds) Nicotine replacement: a critical evaluation. Alan R Liss Inc, Nwe York, pp 63–94
49. Benowitz N L, Lake T, Keller K H, Lee B L 1987 Prolonged absorption with development of tolerance to toxic effects after cutaneous exposure to nicotine. Clinical Pharmacology and Therapeutics 42: 119–120
50. Gorrod J W, Jenner P 1975 The metabolism of tobacco alkaloids. In: Essays in Toxicology 6: 35–78
51. Peterson L A, Trevor A, Castagnoli N 1987 Stereochemical studies on the cytochrome P-450 catalyzed oxidation of (S)-nicotine to the (S)-nicotine δ1'(5')-iminium species. Journal of Medicinal Chemistry 30: 249–254
52. Benowitz N L, Kuyt F, Jacob P, Jones R T, Osman A L 1983 Cotinine disposition and effects. Clinical Pharmacology and Therapeutics 34: 604–611
53. Curvall M, Vala E K, Enzell C R, Wahren J 1990 Simulation and evaluation of nicotine intake during passive smoking: cotinine measurements in body fluids of nonsmokers given intravenous infusions of nicotine. Clinical Pharmacology and Therapeutics 47: 42–49
54. Neurath G B, Dunger M, Orth D, Pein F G 1987 Trans-3'-hydroxycotinine as a main metabolite in urine of smokers. International Archives of Occupational and Environmental Health 59: 199–201
55. Jenner P, Gorrod J W, Beckett A H 1973 The absorption of nicotine-1'N-oxide and its reduction in the gastro-intestinal tract in man. Xenobiotica 3: 341–349
56. Hoffmann D 1989 Nicotine, a tobacco-specific precursor for carcinogens. In: Wald N, Froggatt P (eds) Nicotine, smoking and the Low Tar Programme. Oxford University Press, Oxford, pp 24–40
57. Jarvis M J, Hajek P, Russell M A H, West R J, Feyerabend C 1987 Nasal nicotine solution as an aid to cigarette withdrawal: a pilot clinical trial. British Journal of Addiction 82: 983–988
58. Russell M A H, Jarvis M J, Sutherland G, Feyerabend C 1987 Nicotine replacement in smoking cessation: absorption of nicotine vapor from smoke-free cigarettes. Journal of the American Medical Association 257: 3262–3265
59. Abelin T, Muller P, Buehler A, Vesanen K, Imhof P R 1989 Controlled trial of transdermal nicotine patch in tobacco withdrawal. Lancet 1: 7–10
60. Benwell M E M, Balfour D J K, Anderson J M 1988 Evidence that tobacco smoking increases the density of nicotine binding sites in human brain. Journal of Neurochemistry 50: 1243–1247
61. US Public Health Service 1988 The health consequences of smoking: nicotine addiction. A report of the Surgeon General: 1988: US Government Printing Office, Washington, DC
62. Diagnostic and statistical manual of mental disorders (DSM-III-R), 3rd edn, revised. American Psychiatric Association, Washington, DC
63. US Public Health Service 1983 The health consequences of smoking: cardiovascular disease. A report of the Surgeon General: 1983. US Department of Health, Education and Welfare, Public Health Service, DHHS Pub. No. (PHS) 84-50 204
64. Larson P S, Haag H B, Silvette H 1961 Tobacco: experimental and clinical studies. A comprehensive account of the world literature. Williams & Wilkins Co, Baltimore
65. Larson P S, Silvette H 1968 Tobacco: experimental and clinical studies. A comprehensive account of the world literature, suppl I. Williams & Wilkins Co, Baltimore
66. Larson P S, Silvette H 1971 Tobacco: experimental and clinical studies. A comprehensive account of the world literature, suppl II. Williams & Wilkins Co, Baltimore
67. Larson P S, Silvette H 1975 Tobacco: experimental and clinical studies. A comprehensive account of the world literature, suppl III. Williams & Wilkins Co, Baltimore
68. Cohen A J, Roe F J C 1981 Monograph on the pharmacology and toxicology of nicotine. Tobacco Advisory Council Occasional Paper 4. Sinclair Pride Ltd, London
69. US Public Health Service 1979 Smoking and health: a report of the Surgeon General: 1979. US Department of Health, Education and Welfare, Public Health Service, DHSS Pub. No. (PHS) 79-50 066
70. Hoffmann D, Lavoie E J, Hecht S S 1985 Nicotine: a precursor for carcinogens. Cancer Letters 26: 67–75
71. Wald N J, Howard S, Smith P G, Kjeldsen K 1973 Association between atherosclerotic diseases and carboxyhaemoglobin levels in tobacco smokers. British Medical Journal 1: 761–765

Nicotine

72. Booyse F M, Osikowicz G, Quarfoot A J 1981 Effects of oral consumption of nicotine on the rabbit aortic endothelium. American Journal of Pathology 102: 229–238
73. Asmussen I, Kjeldsen K 1975 Intimal structure of human umbilical arteries from newborn children of smoking and non-smoking mothers. Circulation Research 36: 579–589
74. Wennmalm A 1978 Effects of nicotine on cardiac prostaglandin and platelet thromboxane synthesis. British Journal of Pharmacology 64: 559–563
75. Adler B, Gimbrone M A, Schafer A I, Handin R I 1981 Prostacyclin and beta-adrenergic catecholamines inhibit arachidonate release and PGI_2 synthesis by vascular endothelium. Blood 58: 514–517
76. Ashby P, Dalby A M, Miller J H D 1965 Smoking and platelet stickiness. Lancet 2: 158–159
77. Levine P H 1973 An acute effect of cigarette smoking on platelet function. A possible link between smoking and arterial thrombosis. Circulation 48: 619–623
78. Hawkins R I 1972 Smoking, platelets and thrombosis. Nature 236: 450–452
79. Mustard J F, Murphy E A 1963 Effect of smoking on blood coagulation and platelet survival in man. British Medical Journal 1: 846–849
80. Meade T W, Chakrabarti R, Haines A P, North W R S, Stirling Y 1979 Characteristics affecting fibrinolytic activity and plasma fibrinogen concentrations. British Medical Journal 1: 153–156
81. Kershbaum A, Bellet S, Khorsandian R 1965 Elevation of serum cholesterol after administration of nicotine. American Heart Journal 69: 206–210
82. Kershbaum A, Jimenez J, Bellett S, Zanuttini D 1966 Modification of nicotine-induced hyperlipidaemia by antiadrenergic agents. Journal of Athersclerosis Research 6: 524–530
83. Bizzi A, Tacconi M T, Medea A, Garattini S 1972 Some aspects of the effect of nicotine on plasma FFA and tissue triglycerides. Pharmacology 7: 216–224
84. Kershbaum A, Bellet S, Dickstein E R, Fineberg L T 1961 Effect of cigarette smoking and nicotine on serum free fatty acids: based on a study in the human subject and the experimental animal. Circulation Research 9: 631–638
85. Cryer P E, Haymond M W, Sartiago J V, Shah S D 1976 Norepinephrine and epinephrine release and adrenergic mediation of smoking-associated hemodynamic and metabolic events. New England Journal of Medicine 295: 573–577
86. Roth G M, McDonald J B, Sheard C 1944 The effect of smoking cigarettes. Journal of the American Medical Association 125: 761–767
87. Herxheimer A, Griffiths R L, Hamilton B, Wakefield M 1967 Circulatory effects of nicotine aerosol inhalations and cigarette smoking in man. Lancet 2: 754–755
88. Lucchesi B R, Schuster C R, Emley G S 1967 The role of nicotine as a determinant of cigarette smoking frequency in man with observations of certain cardiovascular effects associated with the tobacco alkaloid. Clinical Pharmacology and Therapeutics 8: 789–796
89. Pentecost B, Shillingford J 1964 The acute effects of smoking on myocardial performance in patients with coronary arterial disease. British Heart Journal 26: 422–429
90. Jafri S M, Tilley B C, Peters R, Schultz L R, Goldstein S 1990 Effects of cigarette smoking and propranolol in survivors of acute myocardial infarction. American Journal of Cardiology 65: 271–276
91. Gershon-Cohen J, Borden A G B, Hermel M B 1969 Thermography of extremities after cigarette smoking. British Journal of Radiology 42: 189–191
92. Burn J H, Rand M J 1958 Noradrenaline in artery walls and its dispersal by reserpine. British Medical Journal 1: 903–908
93. Sarin C L 1974 Effects on smoking on digital blood-flow velocity. Journal of the American Medical Association 229: 1327–1328
94. Sontag S, Graham D Y, Belsito A et al 1984 Cimetidine, cigarette smoking, and recurrence of duodenal ulcer. New England Journal of Medicine 311: 689–693
95. Robert A, Stowe D F, Nezamis J E 1971 Possible relationship between smoking and peptic ulcer. Nature 233: 497–498
96. Konturek S J, Radecki T, Thor P, Dembinski A, Jacobson E D 1971 Effects of nicotine on gastric secretion and ulcer formation in cats. Proceedings of the Society for Experimental Biology and Medicine 138: 674–677
97. Debas H T, Cohen M M 1972 Effect of smoking on gastric secretion stimulated by pentagastrin. Lancet 1: 43–44
98. Konturek S J, Solomon T E, McCreight W G, Johnson L R, Jacobson E D 1971 Effects of nicotine on gastrointestinal secretions. Gastroenterology 60: 1098–1105
99. Solomon T E, Solomon N, Shanbour L L, Jacobson E D 1974 Direct and indirect effects of nicotine on rabbit pancreatic secretion. Gastroenterology 67: 276–283
100. Murthy S N S, Dinoso V P, Clearfield H R, Chey W Y 1977 Simultaneous measurement of basal pancreatic, gastric acid secretion, plasma gastrin, and secretin during smoking. Gastroenterology 73: 758–761
101. Schnedorf J G, Ivy A C 1939 The effect of tobacco smoking on the alimentary canal. Journal of the American Medical Association 112: 898–903
102. Valenzuela J E, Defilippi C, Csendes A 1976 Manometric studies on the human pyloric sphincter: effect of cigarette smoking, metoclopramide, and atropine. Gastroenterology 70: 481–483
103. Read N W, Grech P 1973 Effect of cigarette smoking on competence of the pylorus: preliminary study. British Medical Journal 3: 313–316
104. Kershbaum A, Pappajohn D J, Bellet S, Hirabayashi M, Shafiiha H 1968 Effect of smoking and nicotine on adrenocortical secretion. Journal of the American Medical Association 203: 275–278
105. Pomerleau O F, Fertig J B, Seyler L E, Jaffe J 1983 Neuroendocrine reactivity to nicotine in smokers. Psychopharmacology 81: 61–67
106. Seyler L E, Pomerleau O F, Fertig J B, Hunt D, Parker K 1986 Pituitary hormone response to cigarette smoking. Pharmacology, Biochemistry and Behaviour 24: 159–162
107. Wilkins J N, Carlson H E, Van Vunakis H, Nill M A, Gritz E, Jarvik M E 1982 Nicotine from cigarette smoking increases circulating levels of cortisol, growth hormone and prolactin in male chronic smokers. Psychopharmacology 78: 305–308
108. Baron J A, Bulbrook R D, Wang D Y, Kwa H G 1986 Cigarette smoking and prolactin in women. British Medical Journal 293: 482–483
109. Andersson K, Fuxe K, Eneroth P, Mascagni F, Agnati L F 1985 Effects of acute intermittent exposure to cigarette smoke on catecholamine levels and turnover in various types of hypothalamic DA and NA nerve terminal systems as well as on the secretion of adenohypophyseal hormones and corticosterone. Acta Physiologica Scandinavica 124: 277–285
110. Andersson K, Eneroth P, Agnati L F 1981 Nicotine-induced nerve increases in noradrenaline turnover in discrete noradrenaline nerve terminal systems of the hypothalamus and the median eminence of the rat and their relationship to changes in the secretion of adenohypophyseal hormones. Acta Physiologica Scandinavica 113: 227–231
111. MacMahon B, Trichopoulos D, Cole P, Brown J 1982 Cigarette smoking and urinary oestrogens. New England Journal of Medicine 307: 1062–1065
112. Michnovicz J J, Hershcopf R J, Naganuma H, Bradlow H L, Fishman J 1986 Increased 2-hydroxylation of oestradiol as a possible mechanism for the anti-estrogenic effect of cigarette smoking. New England Journal of Medicine 315: 1305–1309
113. Welch R M, Harrison Y E, Gommi B W, Poppers P J, Finster M, Conney A H 1969 Stimulatory effect of cigarette smoking on the hydroxylation of 3,4-benzpyrene and the N-demethylation of 3-methyl-4-monoethylaminoazobenzene by enzymes in the human placenta. Clinical Pharmacology and Therapeutics 10: 100–109
114. Baron J A, La Vecchia C, Levi F 1990 The antiestrogenic effect of cigarette smoking in women. American Journal of Obstetrics and Gynaecology 162: 502–514
115. Jick H, Porter J, Morrison A S 1977 Relation between smoking and age of natural menopause. Lancet 1: 1354–1355
116. Sepkovic D W, Haley N J, Wynder E L 1984 Thyroid activity in cigarette smokers. Archives of Internal Medicine 144: 501–503
117. Sepkovic D W, Haley N J, Axelrad C M, Lavoie E J 1984 Thyroid hormone concentrations in rats after chronic nicotine metabolite administration. Proceedings of the Society for Experimental Biology and Medicine 177: 412–416
118. Cavalieri R R, Rapaport B 1977 Impaired peripheral conversion of thyroxine to triiodothyronine. Annual Review of Medicine 28: 57–65
119. Miller T A 1983 Protective effects of prostaglandins against gastric mucosal damage: current knowledge and proposed mechanisms. American Journal of Physiology 245: 601–623
120. Quimby G F, Bonnice C A, Burstein S H, Eastwood G L 1986 Active smoking depresses prostaglandin synthesis in human gastric mucosa. Annals of Internal Medicine 104: 616–619
121. Kershbaum A, Bellet S 1968 Cigarette, cigar and pipe smoking: some differences in biochemical effects. Geriatrics 23: 126–134
122. Spohr U, Hofmann K, Steck W et al 1979 Evaluation of smoking-induced effects on sympathetic, hemodynamic and metabolic variables with respect to plasma nicotine and COHb levels. Athersclerosis 33: 271–283
123. Grunberg N E, Popp K A, Bowen D J, Nespor S M, Winders S E, Eury S E 1986 Biochemical effects of nicotine: relevance to nicotine/body weight relationship. Paper presented at the Annual Meeting of the American Psychological Association, Washington, DC
124. Grunberg N E 1985 Nicotine, cigarette smoking and body weight. British Journal of Addiction 80: 369–377
125. Russell M A H, Raw M, Jarvis M J 1980 Clinical use of nicotine chewing gum. British Medical Journal 280: 1599–1602
126. Fagerstrom K O 1987 Reducing the weight gain after stopping smoking. Addictive Behaviours 12: 91–93
127. Ilebekk A, Miller N E, Mjos O D 1975 Effects of nicotine and inhalation of cigarette smoke on total body oxygen consumption in dogs. Scandinavian Journal of Clinical and Laboratory Investigation 35: 67–72
128. Gehlbach S H, Williams W A, Perry L D et al 1975 Nicotine absorption by workers harvesting green tobacco. Lancet 1: 478–480
129. Hughes J R, Miller S A 1984 Nicotine gum to help stop smoking. Journal of the American Medical Association 252: 2855–2858
130. Manning F, Walker D, Feyerabend C 1978 The effect of nicotine on fetal breathing movements in conscious pregnant ewes. British Journal of Obstetrics and Gynaecology 52: 563–568
131. Manning F, Feyerabend C 1976 Cigarette smoking and fetal breathing movements. British Journal of Obstetrics and Gynaecology 83: 262–270

Nicotinic acid

Nicotinic acid (niacin) is an essential water-soluble vitamin. However, when given in pharmacological doses it lowers plasma lipids by a mechanism unrelated to its role as a vitamin.

Chemistry

Nicotinic acid (niacin)
$C_6H_5NO_2$
Pyridine-3-carboxylic acid

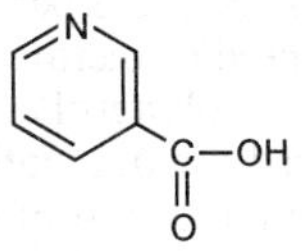

Molecular weight	123.1
pKa (−N<, COOH)	2.0, 4.8
Solubility	
in alcohol	1 in 100
in water	1 in 60
Octanol/water partition coefficient	low

Nicotinic acid is an odourless, white, crystalline powder with a slight acid taste. It is synthesized by oxidation of nitric acid.

Nicotinamide is the amide derivative of nicotinic acid. It is available in compound vitamin preparations such as Vitamins B and C Injection and Parentrovite. Nicofuranose (Bradilan) is tetranicotinoyl fructofuranose; it is metabolized to nicotinic acid. Acipimox (Olbetam) is 5-methylpyrazine carboxylic acid 4-oxide.

Pharmacology

Nicotinic acid is converted in the body to nicotinamide adenine dinucleotide (NAD) and nicotinamide adenine dinucleotide phosphate (NADP), two cofactors essential for a variety of oxidation–reduction reactions that comprise tissue respiration. Deficiency of nicotinic acid leads to the clinical condition known as pellagra. This is characterized by symptoms and signs referable to the skin (dermatitis), gastrointestinal tract (glossitis and enteritis) and central nervous system (headache, depression, delusions and dementia).

In large doses nicotinic acid has a number of pharmacological effects which are not shared by nicotinamide and are therefore unrelated to its role as a vitamin. Principal among these are its effects on lipid metabolism.[1] Nicotinic acid reduces production of VLDL[2] which in turn results in decreased production of IDL and LDL. The mechanism by which it lowers VLDL synthesis is uncertain but is thought to be due to a combination of inhibition of lipolysis in adipose tissue, decreased esterification of triglycerides in the liver, increased activity of lipoprotein lipase and a possible direct effect on hepatic production of apolipoprotein B.

Nicotinic acid also has a vasodilating action,[3] probably related to its ability to stimulate prostacyclin synthesis. An inhibitory effect on platelet aggregation and a transient fibrinolytic action have also been reported.[4,5]

Toxicology

Data are limited, but no evidence of fetal toxicity has been found with doses up to 2 $g.kg^{-1}$ administered during pregnancy.[6]

Clinical pharmacology

The normal daily requirement of nicotinic acid is 10–20 mg and can be met by either nicotinic acid or nicotinamide. The action of nicotinic acid on serum lipids is dose-related and significant effects are seen with doses of 1 g or more per day. Studies in healthy subjects and patients with hyperlipidaemia have shown that 1 g three times daily lowers serum triglycerides by 25–30% and serum cholesterol by 10–15%; the major reduction is in VLDL and LDL, while a mild to moderate increase in HDL-cholesterol may be produced.[7,8]

The effect of large doses of nicotinic acid on serum triglycerides can be seen within 1–4 days of starting treatment and a fall in LDL-cholesterol is apparent within 5–7 days. However, the rapid introduction of pharmacological doses of nicotinic acid is invariably accompanied by unpleasant cutaneous vasodilation. This occurs within minutes of oral ingestion and is most marked over the upper part of the body. The flushing diminishes with continued treatment but can be avoided or reduced in severity by introducing the drug gradually, building to a maintenance dose over 1–3 weeks. Aspirin (325 mg) taken 30 minutes before nicotinic acid prevents flushing.[4] Nicotinic acid has been shown to increase forearm blood flow[3] but it is of dubious value as a vasodilating agent for vascular disease.

Pharmacokinetics

The preferred analytical method for nicotinic acid is HPLC, which has a limit of detection[9] of 100 $\mu g.l^{-1}$. Bioassays (microbiological)[10] and biochemical assays[11–13] for nicotinic acid have also been described. The bioassays are less specific for nicotinic acid, and also measure precursors and metabolites that can substitute for nicotinic acid as growth factors. The method described by Carlson[12] is specific for nicotinic acid and plasma levels in healthy subjects[12,14] range from 0 to 0.8 $mg.l^{-1}$.

Nicotinic acid is rapidly and completely absorbed from the upper gastrointestinal tract. Following a large (e.g. 1 g) oral dose the peak plasma concentration reaches about 25 $mg.l^{-1}$ within 30–60 min (average 45 min).[14] Nicotinic acid diffuses freely across lipid membranes. Studies in animals show that 5 min after a single intravenous injection of labelled compound most of the material is found in adipose tissue and kidney, but after 15 min, it has redistributed in such a way that the liver is the predominantly labelled organ.[15] Protein binding is approximately 15–30%.[13] The volume of distribution of nicotinic acid in man is not known.

The half life of nicotinic acid is short, approximately 45 min. The major route of clearance from the circulation is by hepatic metabolism. Animal studies suggest that at low doses there is extensive presystemic metabolism although precise figures for man are not available. However, it is clear that the metabolic pathways are saturable, as at higher doses increasing amounts of the unchanged compound appear in the urine.[16] Nicotinic acid and its metabolites are excreted in the urine. Following therapeutic doses of the compound, up to 34% of the dose is excreted in the urine in 6 h.

Oral absorption	>90%
Presystemic metabolism	Saturable
Plasma half life	
range	15–50 min
mean	45 min
Volume of distribution	—
Plasma protein binding	15–30%

Concentration–effect relationship

The effect of nicotinic acid on serum lipids is dose-related. It has been estimated that a plasma nicotinic acid concentration of 1–2 $mg.l^{-1}$ is necessary to reduce circulating free fatty acid levels.[14] Moderate increases in plasma nicotinic acid levels of 0.1–0.3 $mg.l^{-1}$ increase blood flow through skin and muscle.[3] Further elevation of the plasma level to 2–4 $mg.l^{-1}$ leads to a further rise in blood flow through muscle but not skin. There is no threshold concentration at which flushing is produced; rather it is related to a rising plasma level of nicotinic acid and abates when plasma levels are stable.[3]

Nicotinic acid

N

Metabolism

Nicotinic acid is extensively metabolized in the liver, with up to 34% of a therapeutic dose excreted unchanged in the urine over 6 h. The major pathways of metabolism of nicotinic acid are shown in Fig. 1. The urinary metabolite profile varies with the dose of the drug, indicating that some of the pathways are saturable. The principal route of metabolism of endogenous nicotinic acid is to nicotinamide and subsequently to N-methylnicotinamide, which is further converted to N-methyl-2-pyridone-5-carboxamide and N-methyl-4-pyridone-3-carboxamide. The glycine conjugate of nicotinic acid is present in urine only in trace amounts and no free nicotinic acid is found. However, following oral administration of 3 g per day, an appreciable amount of the drug is excreted as nicotinuric acid (about one-fourth) or unchanged (one-sixth) with increased amounts of N-methylnicotinamide and 2-pyridone derivatives but not 4-pyridone.[16] Only nicotinamide is an active metabolite, but it has no lipid-lowering activity.

Pharmaceutics

A number of generic preparations of nicotinic acid are marketed. It is available as tablets in the following strengths: 25, 50, 100, 250 and 500 mg. In some countries extended-release preparations are also available, as tablets 150 mg (Span niacin, Scrip) and capsules 125, 250, 300, 400 and 500 mg (Rorer).

Therapeutic use

Indications

1. Prophylaxis and treatment of pellagra
2. Treatment of hyperlipidaemia.

Contraindications

1. Hepatic disease
2. Peptic ulcer
3. Gout
4. Diabetes mellitus.

Mode of use

Nicotinic acid is usually given orally in divided doses but may be given intravenously in severe pellagra when oral medication is difficult. It is given with or after meals to reduce gastric irritation. Relatively low doses (50–500 mg daily) are required for the prophylaxis and treatment of pellagra.

In the treatment of hyperlipidaemia, nicotinic acid is used in conjunction with dietary measures and higher doses (1–8 g daily) are necessary, although the dose is often limited by side effects, particularly cutaneous vasodilation. This is maximal during the first weeks of therapy but thereafter a degree of tolerance develops. It is recommended that treatment is initiated with low doses (100–250 mg three times a day) and gradually increased over 1–3 weeks to a maximum tolerated dose. Aspirin (325 mg) given 30 min beforehand helps minimize nicotinic acid-induced flushing.[4] Nicotinic acid may be usefully combined with a bile acid binding resin to achieve effective reduction of plasma lipids with more conservative doses of each agent.

Indications

1. Prophylaxis and treatment of pellagra

Pellagra may occur due to dietary deficiency or in the course of two metabolic diseases, Hartnup's disease or carcinoid syndrome. In the former, there is defective intestinal and renal transport of tryptophan, a nicotinic acid precursor, while in carcinoid syndrome large amounts of tryptophan may be utilized by the tumour for serotonin production. Treatment can be given as nicotinic acid or nicotinamide 50–500 mg daily, the dose depending on the severity of the condition. When oral administration is difficult, intravenous administration of nicotinamide 25 mg (slowly) two or three times daily is recommended. The symptoms and signs of established pellagra (cutaneous, gastrointestinal and cerebral) improve rapidly with effective treatment. Attention should also be given to the possibility of co-existing nutritional deficiencies, e.g. thiamine, riboflavin and pyridoxine.

2. Hyperlipidaemia

Nicotinic acid is particularly useful in hyperlipidaemia types IIb, IV and V. All three types have in common hypertriglyceridaemia due to excess VLDL; hypertriglyceridaemia is most marked in type V where excess VLDL is accompanied by chylomicroaemia. Nicotinic acid would be more commonly employed if it were not for its side effects. The usual maintenance dose is 1–3 g per day although higher doses (up to 8 g per day) may be used if tolerated. Used alone, 3 g daily has been shown to reduce serum cholesterol and triglycerides by 10% and 28% respectively.[8] Prolonged use of nicotinic acid and colestipol has been shown to result in the regression of xanthomas[17] and to arrest the progression of angiographically defined lesions in the coronary arteries.[18] Nicotinic acid has been shown to potentiate a neomycin-induced decrease in lipoprotein Lp(a) levels while offsetting the decrease in HDL-cholesterol induced by neomycin.[19]

Contraindications

1. Hepatic disease

Disturbance of liver function is common, particularly with doses of nicotinic acid in excess of 3 g daily, but the degree of elevation of circulating liver enzymes is generally not marked and usually transient. Nonetheless, severe hepatotoxicity has been reported in association with use of the drug for treating hyperlipidaemia.[20–22] Therefore, nicotinic acid is contraindicated in patients with active hepatic disease.

2. Peptic ulcer

Gastric ulceration is common, particularly with high doses of nicotinic acid. Its use in patients with a history of peptic ulceration is generally not recommended, although there is no evidence that nicotinic acid increases the risk of activating peptic ulcer disease.

3. Gout

Nicotinic acid increases plasma uric acid levels and appears to increase the incidence of acute gouty arthritis.[6] It should therefore be used with caution in patients with a history of gout.

4. Diabetes mellitus

Nicotinic acid has been shown to increase plasma glucose and impair glucose tolerance.[6] In most patients without diabetes the changes in blood glucose are small and remain within the normal range. Patients

Fig. 1 Metabolism of nicotinic acid

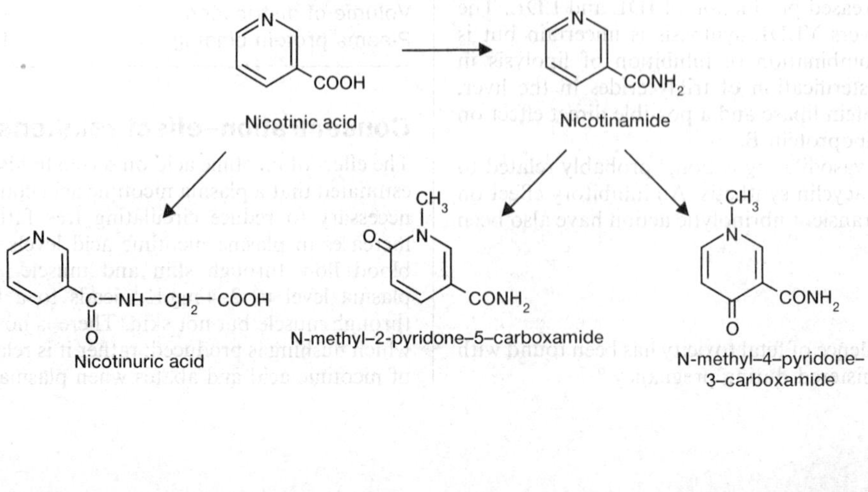

with diabetes mellitus should be closely monitored for worsening of plasma glucose control, and their medication titrated accordingly.

Adverse reactions

Potentially life-threatening effects

An uncommon adverse effect of nicotinic acid is severe hepatotoxicity. Hepatitis,[20] fulminant hepatic failure[21] requiring liver transplantation, and hepatic fibrosis[22] have been associated with nicotinic acid treatment. In all but one report the patients were receiving 3 g or more per day of the drug, which would suggest a dose-related direct mechanism of toxicity rather than hypersensitivity. Severe hepatotoxicity has been reported within weeks of reaching a maintenance dose for hyperlipidaemia but may also occur during the course of long-term treatment. Regular (3–6-monthly) liver function tests are therefore advised.

Acute overdosage

Experience with acute nicotinic acid overdose is limited. The clinical features reflect the vascular and gastrointestinal effects of the drug and comprise flushing, pruritus, headache, nausea, abdominal pain, diarrhoea, hypotension and tachycardia. Treatment consists of supportive measures.

Severe or irreversible adverse effects

Long-term treatment produces a brown pigmentation in up to 25% of patients. An increased incidence of urticaria, ichthyosis, acanthosis nigrans and loss of hair has also been reported.

Occasionally, ophthalmological effects have also been noted, in particular toxic amblyopia and blurred vision due to cystoid macular oedema. These are reversible on discontinuation of treatment but recur when nicotinic acid is reintroduced.

A myopathy comprising myalgia, cramps and elevated serum concentrations of aspartate transaminase and creatine kinase has also been described.[23] Atrial dysrhythmias have also been attributed to nicotinic acid therapy.

Symptomatic adverse effects

The commonest adverse effect of nicotinic acid treatment is flushing, experienced by 92% of patients (versus 4.3% in the placebo group) in one large study and often associated with pruritus. A degree of tolerance develops with time and the problem is less severe if treatment is initiated with low doses. Gastric irritation is also common, sometimes associated with nausea, bloating and diarrhoea; this is alleviated by taking the drug with food.

Other effects

The potentially important biochemical effects of nicotinic acid treatment comprise elevated liver function enzymes, hyperuricaemia and hyperglycaemia. The disturbance of liver function is more common with doses in excess of 3 g daily and is usually mild and transient. If liver enzymes become more markedly elevated (for example more than twice the upper normal range) a dose reduction is recommended.

Interference with clinical pathology tests

Nicotinic acid may produce fluorescent substances which cause false elevations in some fluorimetric determinations of urinary catecholamines. It may also produce false positive reactions with copper (II) sulphate solution (Benedict's reagent) used for urinary glucose determination.

High risk groups

Neonates

There is no indication for the use of high doses of nicotinic acid in neonates and no information is available regarding the safety of the drug.

Breast milk. Nicotinic acid is excreted into breast milk and should be avoided in nursing mothers unless the benefits of treatment outweigh the potential harm to the baby.

Children

The toxic effects of nicotinic acid suggest that it should be used with particular care in the treatment of hyperlipidaemia in children. It is recommended that it should be avoided until after puberty.

Nicotinic acid

Pregnant women

Nicotinic acid crosses the placenta to the fetus and should be avoided in pregnancy unless absolutely essential to prevent life-threatening pancreatitis due to hypertriglyceridaemia.

The elderly

No special precautions are required for the older patient.

Concurrent disease

Patients with Gilbert's syndrome are more sensitive to the hepatic effects (see Other effects above) of nicotinic acid, and more marked elevations of unconjugated bilirubin are seen in this group.

Nicotinic acid may precipitate attacks of gout in predisposed individuals and worsen plasma glucose control in diabetics. These patients should be closely monitored and their medication titrated accordingly.

Drug interactions

Potentially hazardous interactions

Nicotinic acid has been reported to enhance the hypotensive effects of ganglion-blocking agents. It is conceivable that it could also enhance the effects of vasodilating hypotensive agents, but formal studies have not been done.

Other significant interactions

Ingestion with food has not been shown to impair absorption and is recommended to reduce gastric irritation. Hot drinks and alcohol may magnify flushing and pruritus with nicotinic acid and should be avoided at the time of ingestion of the drug.

Potentially useful interactions

Nicotinic acid may be combined with a bile acid binding resin or an HMG-CoA reductase inhibitor to treat mixed hyperlipidaemias or to achieve a synergistic effect in refractory cases of severe hyperlipidaemia.

Major outcome trials

1. (a) The Coronary Drug Project Research Group 1975 Clofibrate and niacin in coronary heart disease. Journal of the American Medical Association 231: 360–381
(b) Canner P L, Berge K G, Wenger N K et al for the Coronary Drug Project Research Group 1986 Fifteen year mortality in Coronary Drug Project patients: long-term benefit with niacin. Journal of the American College of Cardiologists 8: 1245–1255

The Coronary Drug Project was a secondary prevention study conducted between 1966 and 1975, and enrolled 8341 men aged 30 to 64 years with electrocardiographic evidence of previous myocardial infarction. The men were randomly allocated to one of six groups: placebo, two different doses of oestrogen, α-thyroxine, clofibrate and nicotinic acid. The trial for the groups taking oestrogen and α-thyroxine was terminated early because of adverse effects. After a mean period of 6.2 years no therapeutic benefit could be attributed to clofibrate with respect to prevention of myocardial infarction. Treatment with nicotinic acid (3 g per day) produced significant reductions in cholesterol (9%) and triglyceride (27%) and was associated with a lower incidence of non-fatal myocardial infarction compared with the placebo group.

The subjects were followed for a further 9 years off treatment, giving a total follow-up period of 15 years. Total mortality in each drug group was similar to that of the placebo group with the exception of the group that had received nicotinic acid. In this group there was a 12% reduction in fatal myocardial infarction and an 11% lower total mortality rate.

2. Carlson L A, Rosenhamer G 1988 Reduction of mortality in the Stockholm Ischaemic Heart Disease Secondary Prevention Study by combined treatment with clofibrate and nicotinic acid. Acta Medica Scandinavica 223: 405–418

555 survivors of myocardial infarction under 70 years of age received dietary and anti-smoking advice and were randomly assigned (non-blind) to a control or treatment group. The latter comprised clofibrate 2 g and nicotinic acid 3 g daily for 5 years. During this period, serum cholesterol and triglyceride were 13% and 19% lower respec-

tively in the treatment group compared to the controls. This was associated with a 36% reduction in mortality from coronary heart disease and a 26% reduction in total mortality.

Other trials

1. Blankenhorn D H, Nessim S A, Johnson R L, Sanmarco M E, Azen S P, Cashin-Hemphill J 1987 Beneficial effects of combined colestipol–niacin therapy on coronary atherosclerosis and coronary venous bypass grafts. Journal of the American Medical Association 257: 3233–3240

162 non-smoking men aged 40–59 years with previous coronary bypass surgery were randomly assigned to placebo or treatment with colestipol (30 g daily) plus nicotinic acid (3–12 g daily). After 2 years, the actively treated group showed a 26% reduction in total colestipol with a 37% elevation of HDL-cholesterol. Repeat angiography showed that these changes were associated with a significant reduction in the average number of lesions that progressed in native coronary arteries. The percentage number of subjects with new lesions in native or coronary bypass grafts was also significantly reduced. Atherosclerosis regression, as judged by an improvement in overall coronary status, occurred in 16.2% of colestipol–nicotinic acid-treated subjects compared with 2.4% in the placebo group.

General review articles

Gey K F, Carlson L A (eds) 1971 Metabolic effects of nicotinic acid and its derivatives. Hans Huber, Bern

References

1. Altschul R, Hoeffer A, Stephen J D 1955 Influence of nicotinic acid on serum cholesterol in man. Archives of Biochemistry and Biophysics 54: 558–559
2. Grundy S M, Mok H Y I, Zack L, Berman M 1981 The influence of nicotinic acid on metabolism of cholesterol and triglycerides in man. Journal of Lipid Research 22: 24–36
3. Svedmyr N, Harthon L, Lundholm L 1969 The relationship between plasma concentration of free nicotinic acid and some of its pharmacologic effects in man. Clinical Pharmacology and Therapeutics 10: 559–570
4. Olsson A G, Carlson L A, Anggard E, Ciabattioni G 1983 Prostaglandin production augmented in the short-term by nicotinic acid. Lancet 2: 565–567
5. Weiner M, Devinis K, Redisch W, Steele J 1959 Circulation 19: 845
6. Knodel L C, Talbert R L 1987 Adverse effects of hypolipidaemic drugs. Medical Toxicology 2: 10–32
7. Shepperd J, Packard C J, Patsch J R, Grotto A M Jr, Taunton O D 1979 The effects of nicotinic acid therapy on plasma high density lipoprotein subfraction distribution and composition and on apolipoprotein A metabolism. Journal of Clinical Investigation 63: 858–867
8. The Coronary Drug Project Research Group 1975 Clofibrate and niacin in coronary heart disease. Journal of the American Medical Association 231: 360–381
9. Takikawa K, Miyazaki K, Takaichi A 1982 High performances liquid chromatographic determination of nicotinic acid and its metabolites, nicotinuric acid and nicotinamide in plasma Journal of Chromatography 233: Biomedical Applications 22: 343–348
10. Baker H, Sobotke H 1962 Microbiological assay methods for vitamins Advances in Clinical Chemistry 5: 173–235
11. Friedemann T E, Frazier E I 1950 The determination of nicotic acid Archives of Biochemistry and Biophysics 26: 361–376
12. Carlson L A 1966 Determination of free nicotinic acid in blood plasma. Clinica Chimica Acta 13: 349–351
13. Robinson W T, Cosyns L, Kraml M 1978 An automated method for the analysis of nicotinic acid in serum Clinical Biochemistry 11: 46–49
14. Carlson L A, Oro L, Ostmann J 1968 Effect of a single dose of nicotinic acid on plasma lipids in patients with hyperlipoproteinaemia. Acta Medica Scandinavica 183: 457–465
15. Carlson L A, Hanngren A 1964 Initial distribution in mice of ^3H labelled nicotinic acid. Life Sciences 3: 867–871
16. Mrochek J E, Jolly R L, Young D S, Turner W J 1976 Metabolic response of humans to ingestion of nicotinic acid and nicotinamide. Clinical Chemistry 22: 1821–1827
17. Kane J P, Malloy M J, Tun P et al 1981 Normalization of low density lipoprotein levels in heterozygous familial hypercholesterolemia with a combined drug regimen. New England Journal of Medicine 304: 251–258
18. Blankenhorn D H, Nessim S A, Johnson R L, Sanmarco M E, Azen S P, Cashin-Hemphill J 1987 Beneficial effects of combined colestipol–niacin therapy on coronary atherosclerosis and coronary venous bypass grafts. Journal of the American Medical Association 257: 3233–3240
19. Gurakar A, Hoeg J M, Kostner G, Papadopoulos N M, Brewer H B 1985 Levels of lipoprotein Lp(a) decline with neomycin and niacin treatment. Atherosclerosis 57: 293–301
20. Patterson D J, Dew E W, Gyorkey F, Graham D Y 1983 Niacin hepatitis. Southern Medical Journal 76: 239–241
21. Mullin G E, Greenson J K, Mitchell M C 1989 Fulminant hepatic failure after ingestion of sustained-release nicotinic acid. Annals of Internal Medicine 11: 253–255

Nicotinic acid

22. Kohn R M, Montes M 1969 Hepatic fibrosis following long acting nicotinic acid therapy. American Journal of the Medical Sciences 258: 94–99
23. Litin S C, Anderson C F 1989 Nicotinic acid associated myopathy: a report of three cases. American Journal of Medicine 86: 481–483

Nicoumalone

Nicoumalone, a derivative of 4-hydroxycoumarin, is an oral anticoagulant agent.

Chemistry

Nicoumalone (acenocoumarol, acenoc(o)umarin, Sinthrome)
$C_{19}H_{15}NO_6$
3-(α-*p*-Nitrophenyl-β-acetylethyl)-4-hydroxycoumarin

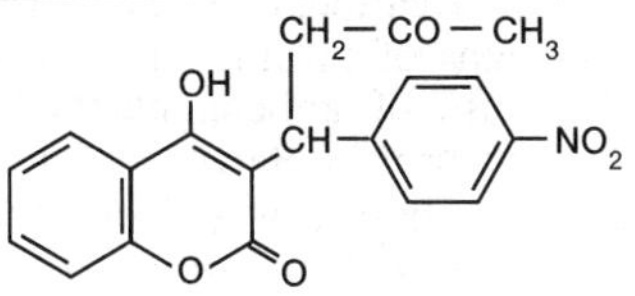

Molecular weight	353.3
pKa	—
Solubility	
in alcohol	1 in 400
in water	virtually nil
Octanol/water partition coefficient	—

Nicoumalone is an almost white to buff, odourless powder with a slightly sweet taste becoming bitter.

Pharmacology

Nicoumalone is an oral anticoagulant drug that affects the synthesis of the vitamin K-dependent clotting factors (factors II, VII, IX, X and protein C). Nicoumalone blocks the action of a microsomal epoxide reductase that is responsible for conversion of vitamin K epoxide back to vitamin K. Vitamin K is responsible for the γ-carboxylation of the coagulation factors II, VII, IX and X. Factor VII, like prothrombin, has 10 glutamic acid residues that undergo γ-carboxylation, whereas factors IX and X have 12 such residues. The presence of the γ-carboxyglutamic acid residues enables the coagulation factors to bind calcium ions and phospholipid. Vitamin K is also required for the formation of the anticoagulant proteins C and S. Protein C also has a direct fibrinolytic role. Proteins C and S seem less important when nicoumalone is given than the effect on factors II, VII, IX and X.

Toxicology

The administration of 0.5–5 $mg.kg^{-1}$ of nicoumalone to rabbits prolonged the prothrombin times to a potentially therapeutic range for a number of months without evidence of toxic liver damage or internal bleeding. There were no abnormalities seen of clinical chemistry or routine haematological parameters. However, rats and mice receiving daily doses of up to 50 $mg.kg^{-1}$ for 12 days developed excessive bleeding with marked disturbances of coagulation and a significant mortality. This drug was introduced into clinical use at a time before drug regulations demanded the recent more stringent toxicological studies, so data are limited. There is evidence that nicoumalone is probably teratogenic.[1]

Clinical pharmacology

Nicoumalone is well absorbed in man with a half life of about 8 h. It is extensively bound to albumin in the plasma. Nicoumalone inhibits clotting factor synthesis and this is reflected in an increased prothrombin time, usually expressed as a ratio compared to a standardized control sample. After a dose of nicoumalone the prothrombin time reaches a maximum after 36–48 h. Nicoumalone has two enantiomers, R and S, and the commercial product is a 50–50 mixture of the two enantiomers. The anticoagulant potency of R-nicoumalone is greater than that of S-nicoumalone, in contrast to the situation with warfarin.[2]

Pharmacokinetics

Nicoumalone may be quantified by gas chromatography with electron capture detection, with a limit of detection[3] of 0.5 $\mu g.l^{-1}$.

Nicoumalone is well absorbed from the upper gastrointestinal tract. Peak plasma concentrations in healthy volunteers are achieved after 3 h. The decay of plasma nicoumalone does not follow first-order kinetics. For the main elimination phase, between 6 and 24 hours after administration, the half life in two healthy volunteers was 8.7 h and 8.2 h. A figure of 24 h has also been obtained. Nicoumalone is highly (98%) bound to protein in plasma. Animal data have demonstrated drug accumulation in liver, kidney, muscle, brain, heart and spleen. It has a volume of distribution of approximately 0.3 $l.kg^{-1}$.

Nicoumalone can cross the placenta and is excreted in very small quantities into breast milk.

Oral absorption	extensive
Presystemic metabolism	—
Plasma half life	
mean	8 h
Volume of distribution	0.3 $l.kg^{-1}$
Plasma protein binding	98%

Concentration–effect relationship

There is no direct relationship between the plasma concentration of nicoumalone and its therapeutic effect. The effect of nicoumalone is delayed, as measured by the prothrombin time (or thrombotest), by some 24–36 h after taking the dose of the drug. Since it is easy to measure the therapeutic effect it is rarely necessary to measure the plasma concentration. If necessary, the rate of synthesis of the clotting factors can be calculated and there is a direct negative correlation between the plasma concentration of nicoumalone and the rate of synthesis.

Metabolism

The drug is extensively metabolized in the liver, resulting in both reduction and oxidation of the molecule. Amino, acetoamido and alcohol metabolites are found in plasma. This extensive metabolism may account for the lack of a relationship between the plasma concentration of nicoumalone and the degree of prolongation of clotting times. Approximately 60% of the orally administered dose appears in the urine, most being in the form of metabolites, with only 1% of the dose present as the unchanged drug. Approximately 30% of the dose is eliminated in the faeces.

Pharmaceutics

Nicoumalone (Sinthrome; Geigy, UK) is available only in an oral form as white, compressed, scored tablets, approximately 7 mm in diameter, with the legend 'GEIGY' impressed on one side, containing 4 mg in each tablet. Pink compressed tablets, approximately 5 mm diameter, contain 1 mg per tablet.

Nicoumalone has been shown to be light-sensitive and should be stored in a metal or dark glass container. The shelf-life is 5 years.

Therapeutic use

This is identical to that of warfarin sodium which is the most commonly used and preferred oral anticoagulant in the UK and North America.

Indications

1. Prevention of deep venous thrombosis after surgery in high risk groups

2. Management of deep venous thrombosis and pulmonary embolism
3. Prevention of embolism associated with artificial cardiac valves
4. Prevention of embolism associated with rheumatic heart disease.

Other uses

5. Possible role in postmyocardial infarction
6. Possible role in cerebrovascular disease.

Mode of use

Providing the prothrombin time is normal before treatment with nicoumalone is commenced, a dose of 8–12 mg should be given on the first day, followed by 4–8 mg the next day. Nicoumalone should be administered as a single daily dose. Thereafter the dose should be adjusted according to the prothrombin time. When an oral anticoagulant is being introduced to a patient on heparin the two drugs should be overlapped for 3 days before the heparin is stopped, to ensure that the full antithrombotic effect of the oral agent is established.

In the UK a standardized thromboplastin (produced in Manchester) is used by most laboratories. The results are commonly expressed as a British Ratio (BR) which is the ratio of results obtained from patient and control plasmas using this standard thromboplastin. Efforts are now being made to ensure that results from thromboplastins produced by different manufacturers are expressed with reference to an international thromboplastin standard. The relationship between the reference thromboplastin and the commercial thromboplastin allows an International Normalized Ratio (INR) to be calculated. The BR is almost identical to the INR over the range 2.0–4.0. The current recommended intensities of anticoagulation[4] depend on the indication for therapy and are given in Table 1.

Table 1 Recommended intensity of anticoagulant therapy

BR (INR)	Indication
2.0–2.5	Prophylaxis of deep venous thrombosis
2.0–3.0	Treatment of deep venous thrombosis and/or pulmonary embolism; prophylaxis for hip surgery
3.0–4.5	Recurrent deep venous thrombosis and/or pulmonary embolism; prosthetic valves and grafts

It is important that all patients on anticoagulant therapy are educated prior to commencing treatment regarding the potential hazards of therapy. Control should be assessed regularly and the patient interviewed to determine if any complications are being encountered.

Patients with a long-term risk of thrombosis, such as those with rheumatic heart disease or certain artificial heart valves, require long-term anticoagulation. Important members of this group are patients who have familial deficiency of the naturally occurring anticoagulants antithrombin III or Protein C which predispose to recurrent thromboembolism.

In patients who have had a single episode of deep venous thrombosis or pulmonary embolism, there is no definite evidence that treatment for longer than 6 weeks is beneficial.[5] Although there have been reports of 'rebound' thrombosis if an oral anticoagulant is stopped abruptly, others have not documented such a risk.

Indications

Most studies have involved the use of warfarin but it is reasonable to expect the same results with nicoumalone if it is given in doses resulting in an equivalent intensity of anticoagulation.

1. Prevention of deep venous thrombosis

Controlled studies have demonstrated the effectiveness of oral anticoagulants in the prophylaxis of deep venous thrombosis in patients undergoing surgery.[6,7] The efficacy of oral anticoagulants in such high risk situations has to be balanced against the risk of bleeding. However, conventional low-dose heparin is relatively ineffective in these situations and if the intensity of treatment is in the range BR 2–3 the benefit would appear to outweigh the risk.[8]

2. Acute deep venous thrombosis and/or pulmonary embolism

Prior to consideration of treatment the diagnosis should be made objectively, as clinical signs of thromboembolic disease are notoriously unreliable.[9] The use of anticoagulants became established following the randomized trial of Barritt and Jordan,[10] in which a higher rate of recurrent embolism was documented in the placebo group, compared to the treatment group. The trial in fact was stopped before its completion and has been further criticized for its method of randomization, small number of patients, and lack of reliable objective assessments. However, recent studies comparing follow-up patients with deep venous thrombosis, treated initially with heparin and then randomized to either warfarin or heparin, appear to confirm the value of oral anticoagulants.[11,12]

3. Prosthetic heart valves

No randomized controlled trials have conclusively demonstrated the role of oral anticoagulants in patients with prosthetic valves. Clinical experience, however, suggests a higher embolism rate in unprotected patients.[13] The combination of an oral anticoagulant agent and an antiplatelet drug may be a more effective form of therapy.[14] Tissue values are less thrombogenic and there is no need for life-long anticoagulation.

4. Rheumatic heart disease

Again, no randomized controlled trials have been performed. However, early trials indicated less embolism in treated patients compared to patients off treatment.[15]

Controversial indications

5. Myocardial infarction

Trials conducted in the 1950s and 1960s reported conflicting results regarding the role of oral anticoagulants after myocardial infarction. These studies failed to fulfil the criteria necessary for good trial design, but Douglas and McNicol,[16] reviewing 12 reports, considered that a small benefit did accrue from treatment. This view was supported by a

Fig. 1 Metabolism of nicoumalone

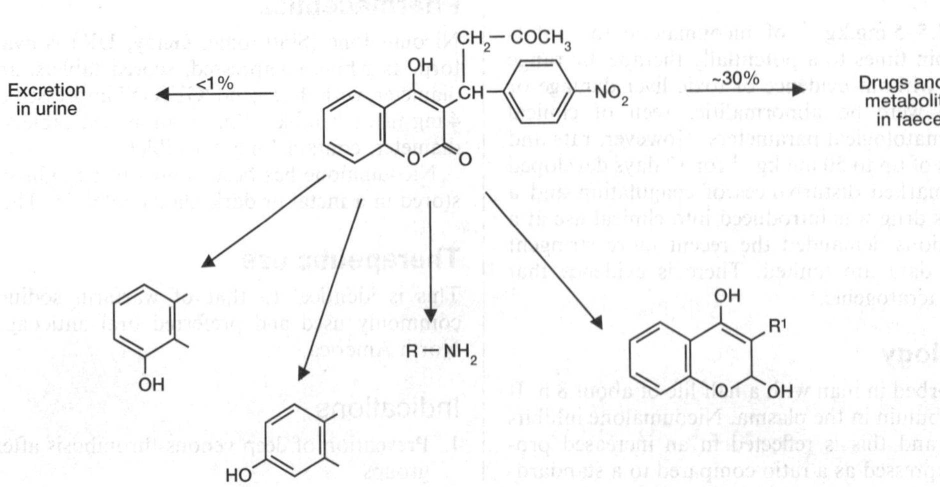

'Collaborative analysis of long-term anticoagulant administration after myocardial infarction'.[17] In this, nine soundly designed trials were re-evaluated by going back to the authors and collecting in a uniform way the simple essential data. The numbers when pooled were 2205 men and 282 women. In men under 55 years of age the results were: at the end of two years 91% of the anticoagulant group were alive compared to 85% of the comparative group. This difference was significant at $P<0.01$. In men over 55 years of age at the end of three years 75% of the anticoagulant group were alive compared to 69% of the comparative group. This difference was significant at $P<0.05$. Overall there was a reduction of death by about 20%, not too dissimilar to that being reported by the use of β-blockers. In the anticoagulant study when patients with no previous history of coronary heart disease were excluded, the benefit was found to be limited almost entirely to those with previous angina or a previous event of myocardial infarction. Peripheral thrombotic and embolic events did seem to be prevented.[18,19] The debate has been renewed following the results of a trial conducted in the Netherlands.[20] Patients on anticoagulants (nicoumalone was one of the drugs) following infarction were randomized to stop treatment or to continue. Increased reinfarction and mortality was demonstrated in the placebo group over the study period of two years. Further studies are still required to definitely define the role of anticoagulants after myocardial infarction but the balance of evidence indicated a degree of benefit from their use.

6. Cerebrovascular disease

Completed stroke. Development of new scanning techniques has helped considerably in the differentiation between a stroke caused by cerebral haemorrhage and that related to thrombosis or embolism. Anticoagulation would be contraindicated in the former situation but theoretically might be beneficial in the latter problems. However, trial data do not support the use of anticoagulants in thrombotic cerebral infarction, although there is some evidence of benefit in the presence of embolism.[21]

Transient ischaemic attacks. Trials have again led to conflicting results and many studies have been criticized on methodological grounds.[21] Not only has there been a failure to demonstrate a definite reduction in strokes and mortality, but the use of anticoagulants has been associated with a significant risk of intracranial haemorrhage. However, it must be said that the exact role of anticoagulants in transient ischaemic attacks remains to be delineated by well designed trials.

Adverse reactions

Potentially life-threatening effects

The incidence of haemorrhage varies, depending on the age of the patient, intensity of treatment, and indication for using an anticoagulant. Figures are very variable and are reviewed by Mackie and Douglas.[22] In general, a 20% incidence might be expected although half of these episodes at least will be minor. More serious haemorrhage (10%) might be expected after hip surgery and with the treatment of transient ischaemic attacks. Haematuria, bruising and gastrointestinal bleeding are the commonest signs of bleeding in general medical patients. An underlying lesion is often present. Bleeding might be expected in certain sites in particular patient populations, for example wound haematoma postsurgery. The most common site of fatal haemorrhage is intracranial.

Acute overdosage

Vitamin K is the antidote to oral anticoagulants. If excessive prolongation of the prothrombin time occurs but the patient is not bleeding then the anticoagulant should merely be withheld and the prothrombin time rechecked daily. A small oral dose of vitamin K_1 (2.5–5 mg) can also be used to hasten the return of the prothrombin time towards normal. If bleeding is present or there is very marked prolongation of the time (ratio > 5) then vitamin K_1 should be given. Intravenous vitamin K_1 (10 mg) should be given slowly and this will significantly shorten the prothrombin time in 6–10 h. The patient may well be relatively refractory to reinstitution of anticoagulant therapy after vitamin K_1. If more rapid correction is required, as in the presence of major haemorrhage, fresh frozen plasma should be given in addition. 'Prothrombin' concentrate (contains all vitamin K-dependent factors) should only be used with extreme caution because of reports of thromboembolic complications.

Severe or irreversible adverse effects

Skin necrosis is a rare early complication of treatment with oral anticoagulants of the coumarin family.[23] It usually occurs between the first and tenth days and affects predominantly females. Histologically there is thrombosis in venules and capillaries, and areas of the body with abundant fat (e.g. breast, buttocks) are principally involved. The lesions may resolve spontaneously but skin grafting may be required. Intravenous heparin therapy has also been reported as beneficial. Patients with this complication should not be given further oral anticoagulant therapy, as repeat episodes have occurred. There is recent suggestive evidence that this complication occurs in patients with inherited protein C deficiency given oral anticoagulants.

High risk groups

Neonates

The drug is not recommended for use in neonates.

Breast milk. Although nicoumalone may appear in the breast milk it is thought that the amounts excreted are unlikely to result in a clinical problem in the neonate. If there is no alternative (e.g. heparin) then it would be prudent to check the infant's prothrombin time.

Children

The drug is not recommended for use in children.

Pregnant women

Nicoumalone should be avoided in the first and third trimesters, but may be used with caution at other times.

The elderly

Elderly patients may be more susceptible to the effects of oral anticoagulants and thus require a lower dosage. This is probably related to pharmacodynamic changes.

Concurrent disease

Any severe illness may increase the sensitivity to oral anticoagulants and special care is required in the presence of alcoholism, cardiac failure, liver disease, renal failure, diarrhoea and thyrotoxicosis.

The major complication of nicoumalone is haemorrhage. The use of this drug in patients considered at special risk of bleeding or in whom bleeding would be particularly catastrophic, should always be considered in comparison with the risk of thromboembolism. If anticoagulation is felt to be mandatory, measures should obviously be taken to correct, if possible, any of the following situations: presence of a congenital or acquired disorder with coagulation factor deficiency or disorders; those with abnormal renal or hepatic function; postsurgical patients; patients with a history of recent peptic ulceration; patients with severe uncontrolled hypertension; patients on other drugs which alter haemostasis.

Drug interactions

The anticoagulant action of nicoumalone may be potentiated or inhibited by drugs.[24] The latter is usually caused by stimulation of liver microsomal enzymes by the offending drug, whereas the former may be related to inhibition of metabolism.

Particular care is required when any alterations are made to the drug regimen given to a patient on nicoumalone. No list of interacting drugs is complete and the lists shown below need to be continuously updated.

Potentially hazardous interactions

Drugs causing gastric erosions or ulceration. Drugs causing damage to the gastric wall (e.g. aspirin) may precipitate haemorrhage in patients taking nicoumalone.

Other drugs affecting haemostasis. Antiplatelet drugs (e.g. aspirin) will have an additive effect with nicoumalone on haemostasis. High doses of aspirin decrease prothrombin synthesis and therefore may potentiate the effect of nicoumalone.

Non-steroidal anti-inflammatory drugs and analgesics. A number of these drugs enhance the effect of nicoumalone by inhibiting its metabolism; the best documented example is phenylbutazone.

Sulphinapyrazone. This may enhance the effect of nicoumalone, probably by inhibiting its metabolism.

H_2-antagonists. Cimetidine is likely to enhance the nicoumalone effect by inhibiting its metabolism.

Antibiotics. Co-trimoxazole and metronidazole probably interfere with the metabolism of nicoumalone, thus potentiating its effect.

N

Some of the newer cephalosporins may lead to a prolongation of the prothrombin time and thus could potentiate the nicoumalone effect. Broad-spectrum antibiotics in general can cause suppression of vitamin K-producing bowel flora and thus, particularly in patients with reduced dietary intake of vitamin K, potentiate the effect of nicoumalone.

Hepatic microsomal enzyme induction. Drugs such as phenobarbitone and carbamazepine induce enzymes to increase the metabolism of nicoumalone and thus reduce its anticoagulant effect.

Vitamin K. A high vitamin K intake will tend to reduce the effect of nicoumalone. This may be a problem in patients receiving parenteral nutrition, using fluids with high vitamin K additions.

Diuretics. The treatment of cardiac failure by diuretics may result in higher availability of vitamin K and therefore a reduction in the nicoumalone effect.

Potentially useful interactions

None is known.

References

1. Pettifor J M, Benson R 1975 Congenital malformations associated with the administration of oral anticoagulants during pregnancy. Journal of Paediatrics 86: 459–462
2. Meinertz T, Kasper W, Karl C, Jähnchen E 1978 Anticoagulant activity of the enantiomers of acenocoumarol. British Journal of Clinical Pharmacology 5: 187–188
3. Bianchetti G, Latini R, Morselli P L 1976 Gas chromatographic determination of acenocoumarin in human plasma. Journal of Chromatography 124: 331–335
4. Poller L 1985 Therapeutic ranges in anticoagulant administration. British Medical Journal 290: 1683–1686
5. Sullivan E F 1972 Duration of anticoagulant therapy in venous thromboembolism. Medical Journal of Australia 2: 1104–1107
6. Sevitt S, Gallagher N G 1959 Prevention of venous thrombosis and pulmonary embolism in injured patients. Trial of anticoagulant prophylaxis with phenindione in middle-aged and elderly patients with fractured necks of femur. Lancet 2: 981–989
7. Taberner D A, Poller L, Burslem R W, Jones J B 1978 Oral anticoagulants controlled by British comparative thromboplastin versus low dose heparin prophylaxis of deep vein thrombosis. British Medical Journal 1: 272–274
8. Morris G K, Mitchell J R 1976 Warfarin sodium in prevention of deep venous thrombosis and pulmonary embolism in patients with fractured neck of femur. Lancet 2: 869
9. Gallus A S, Hirsh J 1976 Diagnosis of venous thromboembolism. Seminars in Thrombosis and Hemostasis 2: 203–231
10. Barritt D W, Jordan S C 1960 Anticoagulant drugs in the treatment of thromboembolism. A controlled trial. Lancet 1: 1309–1312
11. Hull R, Delmore T, Genton E 1979 Warfarin sodium versus low dose heparin in long term treatment of venous thrombosis. New England Journal of Medicine 301: 855–858
12. Hull R, Delmore T, Carter C 1982 Adjusted subcutaneous heparin versus warfarin sodium in the long-term treatment of venous thrombosis. New England Journal of Medicine 306: 189–194
13. Gadboys H L, Litwak R S, Neimetz J, Wisch N 1967 Role of anticoagulants in preventing embolisation from prosthetic heart valves. Journal of the American Medical Association 202: 282–280
14. Sullivan J M, Harken D E, Gorlin R 1968 Pharmacologic control of thromboembolic complications of cardiac valve replacement. A preliminary report. New England Journal of Medicine 279: 576–580
15. Coulshed N, Epstein E J, McKendrick C S, Galloway R W, Walker E 1970 Systemic embolism in mitral valve disease. British Heart Journal 32: 26–34
16. Douglas A S, McNicol G P 1970 In: Biggs R (ed) Human blood coagulation, haemostasis, and thrombosis, 2nd edn. Blackwell Scientific Publications, Oxford, pp 585–586
17. International Anticoagulant Review Group 1970 Collaborative analysis of long term anticoagulant administration after acute myocardial infarction. Lancet 1: 203–209
18. Report of the Working Party on anticoagulant therapy in coronary thrombosis to the Medical Research Council 1969 Assessment of short-term anticoagulant administration after cardiac infarction. British Medical Journal 1: 335–342
19. Co-operative Clinical Trial 1973 Anticoagulants in acute myocardial infarction. Journal of the American Medical Association 225: 724–729
20. Sixty Plus Reinfarction Group 1980 A double blind trial to assess long term oral anticoagulant therapy in elderly patients after myocardial infarction. Lancet 2: 989–994
21. Mackie M J, Douglas A S 1978 Oral anticoagulants in arterial disease. British Medical Bulletin 34: 177–183
22. Mackie M J, Douglas A S 1991 Drug-induced disorders of coagulation. In: Ratnoff O D, Forbes C D (eds) Disorders of haemostasis. W B Saunders Co., Philadelphia, ch 17, pp 493–518
23. Nalbandian R M, Mader I J, Barret J L, Pearce J F, Rupp E C 1965 Petichial, euhymosis, and necrosis of skin. Induced by coumarin congeners. Journal of the American Medical Association 192: 603–608
24. Standing Advisory Committee for Haematology of the Royal College of Pathologists 1982 Drug interaction with coumarin derivative anticoagulants. British Medical Journal 285: 274–275

Nifedipine

Nifedipine is a calcium antagonist, which inhibits the entry of calcium ions through the slow channel in the cell membrane of cardiac and smooth muscle cells.

Chemistry

Nifedipine (Adalat, Procardia)

$C_{17}H_{18}N_2O_6$

Dimethyl-1,4-dihydro-2,6-dimethyl-4-(2-nitrophenyl)pyridine-3,5-dicarboxylate

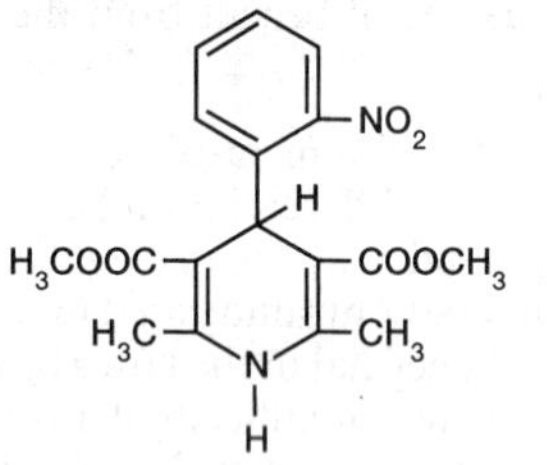

Molecular weight	346.3
pKa	—
Solubility	
in alcohol	sparingly soluble
in water	practically insoluble
Octanol/water partition coefficient	—

Nifedipine is a yellow crystalline powder prepared by chemical synthesis. Nifedipine is also available as an oral combination product with atenolol (Tenif or Beta-Adalat).

Nifedipine should be protected from strong light, which degrades it.

Pharmacology

Nifedipine is an inhibitor of calcium ion influx (slow calcium channel blocker or calcium entry blocker) and blocks the transmembrane influx of calcium ions into muscle cells. Nifedipine also binds to intracellular calcium binding proteins. Normally, calcium is released intracellularly from the sarcoplasmic reticulum and this, combined with the influx of extracellular calcium, results in enhanced binding of calcium to calmodulin. Calcium channel blockers such as nifedipine act as arteriolar dilators by inhibiting this calcium entry into the channel. The effects are seen more on vascular smooth muscle because depolarization of cardiac muscle cells is dependent on sodium ion influx as well as on calcium ion influx. In addition, nifedipine has little effect on cardiac muscle cells because although calcium ion influx is reduced, the drug has little effect on the rate of recovery of the slow calcium channel (unlike verapamil). Nifedipine, unlike verapamil, has no effect on atrioventricular conduction and does not depress the sinus node pacemaker. Separate high affinity binding sites on the ion channel have been identified for dihydropyridine (nifedipine-like) and aralkylamine (verapamil-like) type calcium entry blocking drugs.[1,2]

The major source of 'activating' cytosolic calcium ions for excitation–contraction coupling in cardiac and smooth muscle is still controversial.[3,4] Dihydropyridine calcium antagonists appear to bind to sarcolemmal membranes rather than the sarcoplasmic reticulum, suggesting that the former is the major site of action.[5] However, some contribution from the sarcoplasmic reticulum is possible,[6] while

Nifedipine

other investigators have suggested that the T-tubules are the major source of dihydropyridine calcium antagonist binding sites.

Toxicology

No teratogenic effect of nifedipine has been recorded during use in human pregnancy. Carcinogenicity is unrecorded.

The acute toxicity of nifedipine has been tested in the mouse, rat, rabbit and cat. The ratio between pharmacologically effective and lethal doses in animals ranges from 1:100 to 1:1000. Acute intoxication leads to convulsions, breathlessness, and death with necropsy demonstrating pulmonary oedema.

Dogs have tolerated one year of treatment with doses up to 100 $mg.kg^{-1}.day^{-1}$ without any toxic damage. In rats, daily doses up to 7 $mg.kg^{-1}$ body weight did not lead to any toxic effect. Dosing up to 200 $mg.kg^{-1}$ body weight per day over two years led to a reduction in weight increments.

Doses up to 10 $mg.kg^{-1}.day^{-1}$ have been given to pregnant mice, rats and rabbits. This caused no teratogenic effect. Higher doses (30–100 $mg.kg^{-1}.day^{-1}$) caused malformations in mice and rat fetuses.

Rat fertility was unimpaired by doses up to 100 $mg.kg^{-1}.day^{-1}$. However, this led to a prolongation of the gestation period resulting in fetal death, the consequence of uterine relaxation. At doses of 30 $mg.kg^{-1}.day^{-1}$ animals that were born showed a disturbed postnatal development presumably due to the prolongation of gestation.

Clinical pharmacology

Nifedipine is given for the treatment of angina pectoris and hypertension in doses from 15 to 80 mg per day in divided doses. Nifedipine is usually given by mouth but it can be given intravenously (0.5–1 mg by slow injection over 3 minutes) or into the coronary arteries (0.1 mg by slow injection which can be repeated up to 1.2 mg in any 3-hour period).

Nifedipine has a selective effect as a dilator of arterial vessels. This causes dilation of pulmonary, coronary and peripheral arteries. As a result blood pressure falls and this elicits a sympathetic reflex response causing tachycardia and an increase in cardiac output. Pulmonary arterial pressure also falls. Nifedipine has direct negative inotropic effects on cardiac muscle but these effects are seen at higher doses than cause arterial vasodilation. As a result the usual response is an improvement in left ventricular performance but heart failure can be precipitated in some patients. There is no change in venous tone with nifedipine. Nifedipine also has weak effects as an inhibitor of platelet aggregation, and it causes oesophageal relaxation. Nifedipine also causes a diuresis. The mechanism of the diuresis is uncertain but is possibly mediated by direct effects on the renal tubule or perhaps cardiac output.[7]

Pharmacokinetics

Numerous assays have been developed for the measurement of plasma nifedipine. The preferred methods are gas–liquid chromatography with electron capture (sensitivity 1–5 $\mu g.l^{-1}$) or high performance liquid chromatography (sensitivity 2–10 $\mu g.l^{-1}$).[8,9] However, as nifedipine is not heat-stable, non-reproducible amounts of the pyridine derivative may be formed during assay with gas–liquid chromatography.

Although the absorption of nifedipine appears to be over 90%,[10] the measured mean systemic bioavailability is between 45 and 70%.[10,11] Substantial presystemic metabolism may take place, though no evidence of saturation is observed with doses between 5 and 60 mg. With sublingual dosing nifedipine appears in the plasma within 10 minutes. Absorption may be even more rapid if the capsule is bitten and swallowed.[12] Two distinct patterns of absorption have been observed after oral capsules, one with peak levels between 30 and 60 minutes and the other between 120 and 240 minutes.[13] The absorption of tablets (as opposed to capsules) is delayed with peak plasma levels occurring between 120 and 240 minutes, but bioavailability does not appear to be reduced. Food delays the time to peak plasma concentration, but probably does not substantially reduce nifedipine's bioavailability.[14]

Nifedipine is widely distributed in the tissues. The steady-state volume of distribution[10,15,16] is between 0.3 and 1.2 $l.kg^{-1}$. It is highly bound to plasma proteins, particularly albumin.[17] In patients with renal failure and liver cirrhosis, protein binding of nifedipine is reduced, which may enhance the drug effect in those conditions.

Nifedipine appears to undergo hepatic oxidation to three inactive metabolites, which are excreted in the urine (80%) and faeces (20%).

Fig. 1 Metabolism of nifedipine

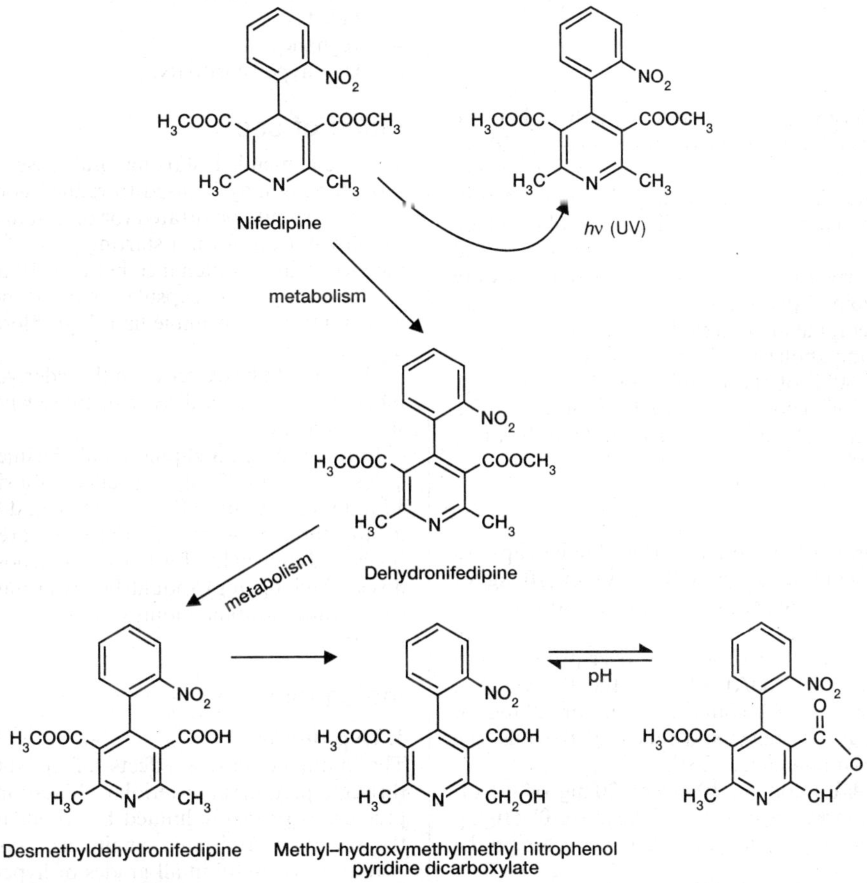

Metabolism involves enzyme systems other than cytochrome P450. Only small amounts of unchanged nifedipine are excreted in the urine. There is evidence of slow and fast 'metabolizers' of nifedipine with the latter in the majority. The latter produce more of the hydroxy carboxylic derivatives.[18]

The elimination half life of an intravenous dose is 80–120 minutes. The elimination half life of orally administered nifedipine capsules is 4–8 hours,[10,16] while after tablets it is apparently prolonged by 2–3 hours. The discrepancy between oral and intravenous metabolism reflects delay in absorption. The mean systemic plasma clearance is high at 27 $l.h^{-1}$.

Oral absorption	>90%
Presystemic metabolism	substantial
Plasma half life	
range	2–6 h
Volume of distribution	0.3–1.2 $l.kg^{-1}$
Plasma protein binding	>90%

Renal failure, haemodialysis or peritoneal dialysis appear to have little effect on plasma concentrations.[19,20]

Concentration–effect relationship

The minimal effective plasma concentration to produce cardiovascular effects[10] is about 15 $\mu g.l^{-1}$. A 1 mg parenteral dose will produce a peak plasma concentration of about 40 $\mu g.l^{-1}$ and a 10 mg oral dose about 160 $\mu g.l^{-1}$. Chronically administered nifedipine tablets at a dose of 20 mg twice daily will produce[21] trough concentrations of 11 ± 4 $\mu g.l^{-1}$ and peak concentrations of 37 ± 14 $\mu g.l^{-1}$. There appears to be wide interindividual variation in the plasma concentration and clinical effect of a given dose of nifedipine. However, several investigators have found a good relationship between plasma concentration and hypotensive effect both in normal subjects and in patients with hypertension. The plasma level required to produce 50% of the maximal effect[22,23] was between 25 and 35 $\mu g.l^{-1}$. Similarly, a relationship between plasma concentration and oesophageal relaxation has been noted.[24] However, the relationship between antianginal efficacy and plasma concentration appears to be poor though plasma concentrations between 30 and 90 $\mu g.l^{-1}$ have been suggested as effective.[25,26] Monitoring of plasma levels is not thought to be of great clinical use.

Metabolism

Nifedipine appears to undergo hepatic oxidation to three inactive metabolites, which are excreted in the urine (80%) and faeces (20%). Metabolism involves enzyme system such as cytochrome P450, but the drug is light-sensitive and photo oxidation may also occur. About 70% of nifedipine is rapidly oxidized to a pyridine metabolite, which is then further hydrolysed; 3–5% is further oxidized to hydroxy and methoxy carboxylic acid derivatives (Fig. 1). These metabolites are thought to be relatively devoid of pharmacological effects. Only small amounts of unchanged nifedipine are excreted in the urine. There is evidence of slow and fast metabolizers of nifedipine with the latter comprising approximately 80% of the population. Those subjects exhibiting a reduced rate of oxidative metabolism of nifedipine excreted less than 25% of the carboxylic acid metabolite in the urine over an eight-hour period.[18]

Pharmaceutics

Nifedipine is available in oral and parenteral forms. Adalat capsules (Bayer, UK/Miles, USA) contain 5 mg (UK only) or 10 mg of nifedipine. The capsules are orange, ovoid and of soft gelatin containing a bitter-tasting, viscous, yellow fluid; in the UK they are flavoured with peppermint oil. The capsule is over-printed with 'ADALAT 5' (5 mg capsule) or 'ADALAT' and the Bayer cross.

Procardia capsules (Pfizer, USA) contain 10 mg or 20 mg of nifedipine. The 10 mg strength is orange and coded '260', whilst the 20 mg strength is light brown and coded '261'.

'Adalat' tablets (Bayer, UK) contain 10 mg or 20 mg of nifedipine. The tablets are pink–grey lacquered and bear 'A10' (10 mg tablet) or '1U' (20 mg tablet) on one side and the Bayer cross on the other.

An intracoronary injection contains nifedipine 0.1 mg per ml. This is marketed in yellow, semi-opaque, pre-filled syringes containing 2 ml of solution.

Beta-Adalat and Tenif are combination products with atenolol. The former is presented as a reddish-brown capsule with the name 'Beta-Adalat' and the Bayer cross or 'Tenif' and the Stuart logo. Both contain atenolol 50 mg and nifedipine 20 mg in tablet form.

All preparations should be protected from strong light.

Therapeutic use

Indications

1. Hypertension
a. Essential hypertension
b. Accelerated hypertension
c. Hypertension in pregnancy
d. Hypertension during coronary bypass surgery
e. Renal hypertension
2. Ischaemic heart disease
a. Stable exertional angina pectoris
b. Variant angina
c. Unstable angina
d. Myocardial infarction
e. Postinfarction prophylaxis
f. Prevention of atherosclerosis
g. Silent ischaemia
3. Miscellaneous
a. Raynaud's phenomenon
b. Heart failure
c. Pulmonary hypertension
d. Hypertrophic cardiomyopathy
e. Asthma
f. Renal and genitourinary effects
g. Gastrointestinal effects
h. Endocrine effects
i. Effects on platelets.

Contraindications

1. Hypotension
2. Poor left ventricular function
3. Diabetes
4. Pregnancy
5. Drug hypersensitivity.

Mode of use

The recommended starting oral dose is 10 mg three times daily, though 5 mg may be used to reduce side effects in selected patients. The dose should be titrated for optimum effect up to 60 mg daily. For the slow-release form a starting dose of 10 mg twice daily is recommended, with maintenance between 10 and 40 mg twice daily.

The soft gelatin capsules may be bitten to achieve sublingual absorption and an immediate high blood level during an attack of angina pectoris.

Care should be exercised in the elderly, those who have a low initial blood pressure, liver disease or those who are on other antihypertensive medication.

Intracoronary nifedipine should be injected slowly over 90–120 s at a dose of 0.2 mg (2 ml). The effect of a single application lasts about 15 minutes. No more than 1.2 mg (six doses) should be administered in any three-hour period. Extreme care should be exercised at all times and especially if a left main stenosis is present, when reduced doses (0.05–0.1 mg) should be given initially. Arterial pressure and electrocardiographic monitoring should be available during intracoronary use.

Indications

1. Hypertension

The antihypertensive effects of nifedipine are largely mediated through peripheral arteriolar dilatation. The reduction in blood pressure is probably limited by secondary activation of the sympathetic nervous and renin–angiotensin systems.

It appears useful in all grades of hypertension as monotherapy or in combination with other hypotensive agents including diuretics, methyldopa, β-blockers and ACE inhibitors.

However, it should be kept in mind that there is as yet no firm evidence that any of the calcium antagonists can reduce the increased morbidity or mortality associated with hypertension.

a. Essential hypertension

Nifedipine has generally been shown to be as effective in the treatment of mild to moderate hypertension as other calcium antagonists,[27] β-blockers,[28] ACE inhibitors[29] thiazide diuretics[30] and α-blockers.[31] Continued efficacy has been demonstrated up to four years,[32] while brief interruptions of therapy lead to a rise in pressure, confirming a continuing hypotensive effect. Long-term therapy in conjunction with methyldopa has been reported to reduce ECG evidence of left ventricular strain, reduce heart size and cause regression of hypertensive changes in the optic fundus.[32] In combination with a β-blocker, nifedipine reduces blood pressure during exercise, though it is not clear if nifedipine monotherapy is effective.[33] In patients with hypertension despite treatment with β-blockers, diuretic and/or another vasodilator, the addition of nifedipine appears to control pressure in about 60% of cases.[34]

Some studies have indicated a relatively high incidence of side effects, such as flushing, headache and ankle swelling.

b. Accelerated hypertension

Nifedipine has been administered in doses of 5 mg orally or sublingually to patients with hypertensive emergencies. The onset of effect has generally been within 10 minutes and the maximal fall in systolic blood pressure between 40 and 80 mmHg and diastolic pressure between 10 and 60 mmHg. Rarely, an excessive hypotensive effect may occur and it is wise to start with a 5 mg dose, which can be repeated and increased if the initial response is inadequate. In patients with heart failure a beneficial haemodynamic response is generally observed with relief of pulmonary oedema.[35] In those with disturbed consciousness improvement has also been observed, which may be related to cerebral vasodilatation as the blood pressure falls.[36]

c. Hypertension during pregnancy

Nifedipine has been used for hypertensive emergencies during pregnancy and the puerperium without any adverse effects on the fetus.[37] Blood pressure was lowered by about 26/20 mmHg within 20 minutes. Side effects included headache and facial flushing.

In pre-eclampsia unresponsive to atenolol, nifedipine has also been effective, and although laboratory indices of the pre-eclamptic process were not improved,[38] fetal outcome seems favourable. The product license of nifedipine in the UK states that nifedipine should not be used in women capable of child bearing and this includes women who are already pregnant (see Toxicology).

d. Hypertension during coronary bypass surgery

One-third of patients will develop intraoperative hypertension during coronary bypass surgery, which predisposes to myocardial ischaemia and increases perioperative morbidity. Nifedipine given intravenously in doses of 0.7–5 $\mu g.kg^{-1}.min^{-1}$ effectively reduces pressure without compromising ventricular function.[39,40] Nifedipine has also been added (0.2 $\mu g.kg^{-1}$) to cardioplegic solution in an attempt to reduce cellular calcium overload during relative myocardial ischaemia.[41] This led to a more rapid recovery of myocardial function on coming off bypass with reduced requirements for balloon pumping. Therapy can be continued postoperatively by sublingual or nasogastric administration.

e. Renal hypertension

Nifedipine is effective in patients with renal failure.

2. Ischaemic heart disease

a. Stable exertional angina pectoris

Several placebo-controlled studies have demonstrated the superiority of nifedipine over placebo[42–44] for exercise-induced and pacing-induced angina. Nifedipine reduces blood pressure, but increases tachycardia during exercise. Consequently, the rate–pressure product, an index of myocardial oxygen consumption, is not markedly altered. This suggests that the predominant effects of nifedipine are mediated through afterload reduction and/or coronary vasodilatation. Comparative studies suggest that β-blockers, diltiazem and verapamil, have superior antianginal efficacy, probably by limiting the increase in heart rate during exercise.[45–50] Only one double-blind study has suggested that nifedipine is as effective as propranolol[51] for exercise-induced angina, although another study has suggested that nifedipine may be superior during exercise in the cold.[52]

The combination of nifedipine with a β-blocker appears superior to a β-blocker alone in most but not all studies.[50,53] Though cases have been reported of this combination causing ventricular depression and heart failure, the vasodilator effect of nifedipine generally reduces β-blocker-induced myocardial depression. Chronic oral nitrate therapy is of questionable value in stable angina, and though good trial data are lacking, the addition of nifedipine to β-blocker therapy is to be preferred. There are few data on the effects of combining nifedipine with other calcium antagonists.

Careful titration of the dose of nifedipine seems to be necessary to optimize the therapeutic effect and minimize adverse effects. Paradoxical worsening of angina has been noted, and may be more common in older subjects. A fall in arterial perfusion pressure in the presence of a fixed severe coronary stenosis which cannot dilate to maintain coronary blood flow and reflex tachycardia are possible mechanisms which could induce ischaemia. Nifedipine may also be ineffective in patients who have angina due to an occluded coronary artery supplied by collaterals.[54]

Smoking attenuates the antianginal efficacy of nifedipine[55] and other antianginal agents.[56] In contrast to β-blockers, nifedipine is safe in patients with chronic obstructive airways disease.[57]

There is no evidence that nifedipine reduces the morbidity or mortality associated with chronic stable angina.

b. Variant angina

Compared to placebo, nifedipine is highly effective in the treatment of patients with variant angina,[58,59] though nifedipine does not appear to be clearly superior to long-acting nitrates.[60,61] The various calcium antagonists appear to be of equal efficacy in this situation. Calcium antagonists may have a favourable effect on survival.[62] Intracoronary administration of nifedipine is highly effective in relieving spasm at the time of coronary angiography. Sudden withdrawal of nifedipine may precipitate instability and even infarction in some patients.

c. Unstable angina

Nifedipine may be superior to placebo in patients with unstable angina, especially if there is evidence of a vasospastic component,[63] while it may also be usefully combined with a β-blocker.[64] A comparative trial with propranolol suggested that both drugs were equally effective.[65] The HINT study compared nifedipine with metoprolol and that combination. Nifedipine monotherapy was considerably less effective than metoprolol, though the combination tended to be most efficacious.[66] Nifedipine may also be usefully combined with aspirin, nitrates or heparin for the management of patients with unstable angina.

d. Myocardial infarction

Animal studies have suggested that nifedipine may reduce calcium overload in ischaemic cardiomyocytes and may also improve coronary collateral flow.

However, there is no evidence that nifedipine can abort a developing infarct or reduce infarct size in man.[67–69] One small study suggested an increase in early postinfarct mortality with nifedipine though no difference was seen at six months.[67]

e. Postinfarction prophylaxis

Nifedipine may be useful in the management of recurrent chest pain in the postinfarction period. Large studies have confirmed that nifedipine does not reduce postinfarction mortality.[70,71]

f. Prevention of atherosclerosis

Calcium antagonists can prevent the increase in arterial wall calcium associated with aging.[72,73]

Nifedipine has also been shown to prevent atheroma formation in rabbits fed a cholesterol-rich diet.[74] It is not clear if this effect is specific or merely related to blood pressure reduction. However, initial reports from the INTACT Study[75] suggesting that nifedipine prevents the progression of mild coronary atheroma in man are not convincing. Nifedipine therapy was associated with excess total mortality.

g. Silent myocardial ischaemia
Although nifedipine is effective in reducing electrocardiographic evidence of 'silent' myocardial ischaemia, it is not at all clear that this condition requires treatment.

3. Miscellaneous

a. Raynaud's phenomenon
Nifedipine in doses of 30–80 mg daily is probably the drug of choice for the management of Raynaud's[76,77] and is superior to prazosin.[78] It may also reduce the frequency of associated migraine. There is some evidence that it is more efficacious in the idiopathic form of the disease. Poor results have been reported in systemic sclerosis,[79] though healing of cutaneous ulceration has been reported.

b. Heart failure
The product licence in the UK cautions against using this drug in patients with poor ventricular function.

The potent vasodilator properties of nifedipine offset much of its direct myocardial suppression. However, compared with a pure vasodilator the negative inotropic effects of nifedipine become apparent.[80]

Controlled studies have suggested that nifedipine has beneficial haemodynamic effects that are maintained over a period of two weeks.[81] However, this does not appear to be translated into clinical benefit.[82] Controlled studies also show that nifedipine is inferior to captopril.[83]

c. Pulmonary hypertension
Many case reports exist on the treatment of pulmonary hypertension with nifedipine, but carefully documented series are few.[84,85] Acute administration of nifedipine can lead to a reduction in pulmonary vascular resistance, but this is usually associated with a rise in cardiac output and therefore pulmonary artery pressure changes little. Acute haemodynamic effects may be predictive of long-term haemodynamic benefit, which is seen in about 50% of patients with doses up to 120 mg daily.

In some cases systemic vasodilatation may occur without a concomitant fall in pulmonary vascular resistance. The resultant fall in arterial pressure can be fatal.[86]

d. Hypertrophic cardiomyopathy
Nifedipine may reduce left ventricular hypertrophy in this condition,[87] but this awaits confirmation. Due to its pronounced vasodilator action nifedipine may exacerbate symptoms. Nonetheless, some encouraging observations have been made.[88] In general, verapamil or a β-blocker are preferred.

e. Asthma
Nifedipine has a protective effect on exercise-induced asthma. It is not clear if this is a direct effect on bronchial muscle or by stabilizing mast cells.[89] Nifedipine may actually increase FEV_1 in patients with chronic bronchitis and angina.[90] A bronchodilator effect in other situations is more controversial.

f. Renal and genitourinary effects
Nifedipine inhibits the contractile activity of the uterus in pregnancy and in dysmenorrhoea. Nifedipine has been reported to reverse the onset of premature labour. Nifedipine increases bladder capacity and reduces uninhibited detrusor contractions in women with urge incontinence. Diuretic, natriuretic, kaliuretic and uricosuric effects of nifedipine have also been reported. These appear most prominent at low doses and disappear at higher doses, presumably as blood pressure falls and neuroendocrine systems are activated.[91]

g. Gastrointestinal effects
Nifedipine can relax the lower oesophageal sphincter, and diminish the size and duration of peristaltic waves. It may also reduce diffuse oesophageal spasm.

h. Endocrine effects
Acute administration of nifedipine increases sympathetic activity and activates the renin–angiotensin system. Aldosterone does not seem to rise, which may represent an effect of nifedipine on the adrenal cortex. During chronic administration neuroendocrine activation is not consistently seen. Animal studies suggest that nifedipine reduces glucose-induced insulin release. Despite case reports, short-term and long-term studies have failed to demonstrate a worsening of glucose tolerance in diabetics and non-diabetics.[92]

Nifedipine

i. Effects on platelets
Nifedipine inhibits platelet aggregation in vitro at clinically toxic levels. Collagen-induced platelet aggregation appears to be inhibited after therapeutic doses of nifedipine in man.[93]

Contraindications

These are relative apart from known previous allergic reaction to the drug, which is rare.

1. Hypotension
In patients with angina or myocardial infarction excessive lowering of arterial pressure is unwise.

2. Poor left ventricular function
Nifedipine has mild negative inotropic effects, which may be exacerbated by β-blockade or treatment with cardiodepressant antiarrhythmic agents. Fortunately afterload reduction compensates for this in most cases.

3. Diabetes
This appears to be more of theoretical than practical concern.

4. Pregnancy
Nifedipine has ben used successfully in pregnancy without harm to mother or fetus. Nonetheless, it is not officially recommended in pregnancy.

5. Drug hypersensitivity
This is rare, but isolated reports of allergic hepatitis, rash, immune complex glomerulonephritis and acute psychosis exist.

Adverse reactions

Potentially life-threatening effects
Deaths caused by nifedipine are rare. In severe pulmonary hypertension nifedipine can cause cardiovascular collapse if the pulmonary vascular resistance does not fall, as this prevents the necessary rise in cardiac output to maintain blood pressure during systemic vasodilatation. Patients with low arterial pressure (e.g. cardiogenic shock) may not tolerate a further reduction in pressure. Life-threatening allergic reactions are rare. In general, studies in patients with hypertension or ischaemic heart syndromes have shown no difference in mortality comparing placebo and nifedipine (though individual studies reporting in both directions exist).

Acute overdosage
Reports are few. Hypotension and bradycardia have been observed with loss of consciousness. Intravenous calcium gluconate or calcium chloride are effective specific antagonists in the majority of cases. Calcium gluconate may be given as 10–20 ml of calcium gluconate 10% given over 5–10 minutes by infusion or 10–20 ml of calcium chloride 10%, diluted in 50–100 ml dextrose 5% and infused over 10–20 minutes.

Atropine may be added if bradycardia persists, while metaraminol has been used experimentally. Gastric lavage and charcoal instillation may be of use if the patient is seen early after overdose.

Severe or irreversible adverse effects
Flushing, dizziness, palpitation and headache may be severe and disconcerting to the patient when they occur with the first dose. Withdrawal of nifedipine in patients with variant angina may precipitate a severe relapse. Occasionally, nifedipine may exacerbate angina.

Allergic reactions (see above) are rare.

Symptomatic adverse effects
About 20–30% of patients will develop symptomatic adverse effects.[94,95] These may respond to a reduction in dose or the addition of a β-blocker. Most of these effects are related to its vasodilator action. Headache, flushing, paraesthesia, palpitation, dizziness, ankle swelling and gastrointestinal upset are all common (5–12%). As with all antihypertensive drugs, hypotension exacerbated by upright posture may occur. Reversible gingival hyperplasia is an uncommon effect of long-term therapy. At higher doses patients may complain of dizziness.

Other effects
Potential diabetogenic effects[96] have not been confirmed.

Nifedipine

Interference with clinical pathology tests
There is one report of nifedipine interfering with an assay for urinary catecholamine metabolites.

High risk groups

Neonates
Little information exists, but no adverse outcome has been reported in babies born to mothers treated with nifedipine.

Breast milk. Some nifedipine is excreted in breast milk,[97,98] and so breast feeding is not recommended.

Children
Nifedipine has been used to treat hypertensive emergencies in children with renal disease at reduced doses (0.25–0.5 $mg.kg^{-1}$).

Pregnant women
While nifedipine is not officially recommended in pregnancy, it has been used for maternal hypertension with good effect.

The elderly
Elderly patients may be more prone to such adverse effects as postural hypotension. Most reports of exacerbation of angina have come from the elderly population.

Concurrent disease
Caution is advised in those with severe liver disease, severe pulmonary hypertension, hypertrophic cardiomyopathy and aortic stenosis.

Drug interactions

Potentially hazardous interactions

Digoxin. Initial reports that nifedipine reduced renal digoxin clearance are unsupported.

β-Blockers. Nifedipine and β-blockers may have synergistic effects in angina and hypertension. Reports of a serious depression of ventricular function and hypotension are uncommon. In fact nifedipine may reverse the depression of cardiac function caused by β-blockers by its vasodilatory action.

Quinidine. Plasma levels may be reduced by nifedipine.

Theophylline and phenytoin. Plasma levels may be increased by nifedipine.

Other significant interactions

Cimetidine. Cimetidine but not ranitidine appears to increase the bioavailability of nifedipine and may potentiate the latter's hypotensive action.

Potentially useful interactions
As mentioned above, nifedipine and β-blockers may have synergistic effects in angina and hypertension and serious depression of ventricular function and hypotension are uncommon.

Major outcome trials

Few large studies of nifedipine in hypertension or angina have been published, while no large placebo-controlled studies exist.

1. Report of the Holland Interuniversity Nifedipine/Metoprolol Trial (HINT) Research Group 1986 Early treatment of unstable angina in the coronary care unit: a randomised double blind, placebo controlled comparison of recurrent ischaemia in patients treated with nifedipine or metoprolol or both. British Heart Journal 56: 400–413

A multicentre, double-blind, placebo-controlled, randomized trial of nifedipine, metoprolol and the combination in 515 patients with unstable angina. The end-points were recurrent ischaemia or myocardial infarction over the subsequent 48 hours. Nifedipine monotherapy led to increased risk relative to placebo, though this was not significant.

Metoprolol alone or in combination with nifedipine led to a reduction in events though again no statistically significant differences were observed. In contrast, in 177 patients who had nifidepine added to pre-existing, long-term β-blockade, there was a significant reduction in new events.

2. Wilcox R G, Hampton J R, Banks D C et al 1986 Trial of early nifedipine in acute myocardial infarction: the TRENT Study. British Medical Journal 293: 1204–1208

A randomized double-blind study on 9292 patients with suspected acute myocardial infarction, comparing placebo and nifedipine (10 mg four times daily). 4491 fulfilled the entry criteria, the others being rejected largely due to age, duration of pain greater than 24 hours, prior treatment with a calcium antagonist and protocol violations. Only 64% of patients randomized actually had a confirmed infarct. Patients were given the first capsule of nifedipine sublingually to achieve a more rapid effect. The one-month mortality was 9.3% for placebo and 10.2% for nifedipine (not significant) in those with a confirmed infarct. Despite the large number of patients considered for study only 2874 were strictly appropriate. Furthermore, 572 patients were withdrawn from placebo, largely for persisting angina, while 608 withdrew from nifedipine largely because of side effects. However, the number of patients is probably still large enough to exclude a clinically important effect of nifedipine in either direction.

3. The Israeli Sprint Study Group 1988 Secondary prevention reinfarction Israeli nifedipine trial (SPRINT). A randomized intervention trial of nifedipine in patients with acute myocardial infarction. European Heart Journal 9: 354–364

A randomized double-blind study of 2276 survivors of acute myocardial infarction comparing placebo and nifedipine (10 mg three times daily). 4545 patients were screened and inability or refusal to cooperate was the major cause of dropouts at this stage. 334 dropped out during the study because of need for further therapy, side effects or refusal to continue. Medication was started 7–21 days after infarction. Comparing placebo and nifedipine, mortality (5.7% vs 5.8%) and non-fatal reinfarction (4.8% vs 4.4%) were virtually identical at 10 months. It seems unlikely that nifedipine exerts a clinically significant effect in either direction.

4. Hugenholtz P G, Rafflenbeul W, Hecker H, Jost S, Deckers J W on behalf of the INTACT Group Investigators 1990 Retardation of angiographic progression of coronary artery disease by nifedipine (results of the International Nifedipine Trial on Anti-atherosclerotic therapy [INTACT]). Lancet 335: 1109–1113

This was a randomized double-blind placebo-controlled multicentre study comparing the effects of nifedipine and placebo in a group of patients defined as having mild coronary artery disease. The eligible group were under the age of 65, had been referred for a diagnostic coronary angiogram, but were not scheduled to undergo invasive therapeutic procedures. A majority of their coronary segments had to be angiographically normal. The majority of patients were equally divided between one, two and three vessel disease.

425 patients were enrolled into this study. A second coronary angiogram was carried out in 175 patients who received placebo and 173 patients who received nifedipine. On average, patients had been treated for around three years.

Nifedipine did not effect progression or regression of existing lesions over the study period. Nifedipine also failed to reduce the number of patients developing a new coronary lesion, although it did reduce the number of new lesions developing per patient (by 28%). However, there were 8 cardiac deaths in those treated with nifedipine versus only 2 in those treated with placebo. If these had been taken into account by the analysis, it is unlikely that any influence of nifedipine would have been seen on the progression of coronary disease. In addition to the cardiac deaths reported in the paper, there were 3 deaths from cancer in those treated with nifedipine and 1 death as a result of surgery for resection of abdominal aortic aneurysm. Thus, overall there were 12 deaths in the nifedipine-treated group versus 2 in the placebo group.

References

1. Holck M, Thorens S, Haeusler G et al 1982 Characterisation of [3H] nifedipine binding sites in rabbit myocardium. European Journal of Pharmacology 85: 305–315
2. Godfraind T, Morel N 1977 An upper limit to the number of calcium channels in smooth muscle as estimated with cinnarizine. European Journal of Pharmacology 41: 245–246
3. Lullman H, Ziegler Z 1987 Calcium, cell membrane, and excitation–contraction coupling. Journal of Cardiovascular Pharmacology 10: S2–S8
4. Somlyo A P 1985 Excitation–contraction coupling and the ultra-structure of smooth muscle. Circulation Research 57: 497–507

Nifedipine

5. Sarmiento J G, Janis R A, Colvin R A, Triggle D J, Katz A M 1983 Journal of Molecular and Cellular Cardiology 15: 135–138
6. Williams L T, Jones L R 1983 Journal of Biological Chemistry 258: 5344–5347
7. Zanchetti A, Leonetti G 1985 Natriuretic effect of calcium antagonists. Journal of Cardiovascular Pharmacology 7: S33–S37
8. Bach P R 1983 Determination of nifedipine in serum or plasma by reversed phase liquid chromatography. Clinical Chemistry 29: 1344–1348
9. Hamann S R, McAllister R G 1983 Measurements of nifedipine in plasma by gas–liquid chromatography and electron-capture detection. Clinical Chemistry 29: 158–160
10. Kleinbloesem C G, van Harten J, de Leede L G J, van Brummelen P, Breimer D D 1984 Nifedipine kinetics and dynamics during rectal infusion to steady state with an osmotic system. Clinical Pharmacology and Therapeutics 36: 396–401
11. Jaiprakash S S, Chatterjee S S, Sahay J N, MacDonald G 1980 Efficacy of nifedipine in the treatment of angina pectoris and chronic airways obstruction. Postgraduate Medical Journal 56: 624–628
12. Love S J, Yeh K, Kann J, Levitt M J, Reitberg D P 1985 Effect of mode of administration on nifedipine pharmacokinetics (Abstract). Clinical Pharmacology and Therapeutics 37: 209
13. Nakashima T, Inoki M, Nakanishi Y 1984 Nifedipine serum concentration: Effects upon blood pressure and heart rate in normotensive volunteers. European Journal of Drug Metabolism and Pharmacokinetics 9: 73–78
14. Hirsawa K, Shen W F, Kelly D T, Roubin G, Tateda K, Shibtat J 1985 Effect of food ingestion on nifedipine absorption and haemodynamic response. Journal of Clinical Pharmacology 28: 105–107
15. Raemsch K D, Sommer J 1983 Pharmacokinetics and metabolism of nifedipine. Hypertension 5: II-18–II-24
16. Foster T S, Hamann S R, Richards V R, Bryant P J, Graves D A, McAllister Jr R G 1983 Nifedipine kinetics and bioavailability after single intravenous and oral doses in normal subjects. Journal of Clinical Pharmacology 23: 161–170
17. Otto J, Lesko J 1986 Protein binding of nifedipine. Journal of Pharmacy and Pharmacology 38: 399–400
18. Kleinbloesem C H, van Brummelen P, Faber H, Danhof M, Vermeulen N P E, Breimer D D 1984 Variability in nifedipine pharmacokinetics and dynamics: a new oxidation polymorphism in man. Biochemical Pharmacology 33: 3721–3724
19. Bogaert M G, Rosseel M T, Joos R, Boelaert J 1984 Plasma concentrations of nifedipine in patients with renal failure. Arzneimittel-Forschung 34: 307–308
20. Kleinbloesem C H, van Brummelen P, van Harten J, Danhof M, Breimer D D 1985 Nifedipine: influence of renal function on pharmacokinetic/haemodynamic relationship. Clinical Pharmacology and Therapeutics 37: 563–574
21. Kleinbloesem C H, van Brummelen P, Faber H, Breimer D D 1987 Pharmacokinetics and haemodynamic effects of long term nifedipine treatment in hypertensive patients. Journal of Cardiovascular Pharmacology 9: 202–208
22. Traube M, Hongo M, McAllister R G, McCallum R W 1985 Correlation of plasma levels of nifedipine and cardiovascular effects after sublingual dosing in normal subjects. Journal of Clinical Pharmacology 25: 125–129
23. Aoki K, Sato K, Kawaguchi Y, Yamamoto M 1982 Acute and long-term hypotensive effects and plasma concentrations of nifedipine in patients with essential hypertension. European Journal of Clinical Pharmacology 23: 197–201
24. Hongo M, Traube M, McAllister Jr R G, McCallum R W 1984 Effects of nifedipine on esophageal motor function in humans: correlation with plasma nifedipine concentration. Gastroenterology 86: 8–12
25. Chaitman B R, Wagniart P, Pasternac A et al 1984 Improved exercise tolerance after propranolol, diltiazem or nifedipine in angina pectoris: comparison at 1, 3 and 8 hours and correlation with plasma drug concentration. American Journal of Cardiology 53: 1–9
26. Silke B, Verma S P, Nelson G I C et al 1984 The effects on left ventricular performance of nifedipine and verapamil in exercise-induced angina-pectoris. British Journal of Clinical Pharmacology 17: 735–742
27. Schulte K L, Meyer-Sabellek W A, Distler A, Gotzen R 1984 Long-term treatment with diltiazem and nifedipine in essential hypertension. Journal of Hypertension 2: 93
28. De Divitiis O, Petitto M, Di Somma S et al 1984 Acebutolol and nifedipine in the treatment of arterial hypertension: efficacy and acceptability. Arzneimittel-Forschung 34: 710–715
29. MacGregor G A, Markandu N D, Smith S J, Sagnella G A 1985 Captopril: contrasting effects of adding hydrochlorothiazide, propranolol or nifedipine. Journal of Cardiovascular Pharmacology 7 (suppl 1): S82–S87
30. Hallin L, Andren L, Hansson L 1983 Controlled trial of nifedipine and bendroflumethiazide in hypertension. Journal of Cardiovascular Pharmacology 5: 1083–1085
31. Corea L, Bentivoglio M, Cosmi F, Alunni G, Carnovali M 1981 Nifedipine versus prazosin in essential hypertension: A double-blind study. Current Therapeutic Research 30: 708–717
32. Guazzi M D, Polese A, Diorentini C, Bartorelli A, Moruzzi P 1983 Treatment of hypertension with calcium antagonists: review. Hypertension 5 (suppl II): 85–90
33. Lejeune Ph, Gunselmann W, Hennies L et al 1985 Effects of BAY 15 240, a fixed combination of low dose nifedipine and acebutolol on hypertension: comparison with standard dose nifedipine. European Journal of Clinical Pharmacology 28: 17–21
34. Sloane P J M, Beevers D G 1983 Nifedipine in combination therapy for resistant hypertension. Pharmatherapeutica 3: 349–353
35. Polese A, Fiorentini C, Olivari M I, Guazzi M D 1979 Clinical use of a calcium antagonist (nifedipine) in acute pulmonary oedema. American Journal of Medicine 66: 825–830
36. Kuwajima I, Ueda K, Kamata C et al 1978 A study on the effects of nifedipine in hypertensive crises and severe hypertension. Japanese Heart Journal 19: 455–467
37. Walters B N J, Redman C W G 1984 Treatment of severe pregnancy-associated hypertension with the calcium antagonist nifedipine. British Journal of Obstetrics and Gynaecology 91: 330–336
38. Rubin P C, McCabe R, Low R A L 1984 Calcium channel blockade with nifedipine combined with atenolol in the management of severe pre-eclampsia. Clinical and Experimental Hypertension B3: 379
39. Hess W, Schulte-Sasse U, Tarnow J 1984 Nifedipine versus nitroprusside for controlling hypertensive episodes during coronary artery bypass surgery. European Heart Journal 5: 140–145
40. Bovill J G, Wezel H V, Schuller J, Hoeneveld M 1984 Comparison of nitroglycerine, verapamil and nifedipine in coronary artery surgery. British Journal of Anaesthesiology 56: 804P
41. Clark R E et al 1981 Laboratory and initial clinical studies of nifedipine, a calcium antagonist for improved myocardial prevention. Annals of Surgery 193: 719–732
42. Mueller H S, Chahine R A 1981 Interim report of multicenter double-blind, placebo-controlled studies of nifedipine in chronic stable angina. American Journal of Medicine 71: 645–657
43. Sherman L G, Liang C S 1983 Nifedipine in chronic stable angina: A double-blind placebo-controlled crossover trial. American Journal of Cardiology 51: 706–711
44. Van der Wall E E, De Jong J P, Eenige Van M J, Scholtalbers A G, Roos J P 1983 Long-acting effects of nifedipine on exercise tolerance in patients with stable angina pectoris. Current Therapeutic Research 34: 574–580
45. Dargie H J, Lynch P F, Krikler D M, Harris L, Krikler S 1981 Nifedipine and propranolol: a beneficial drug interaction. American Journal of Medicine 71: 676–682
46. Findlay I N, MacLeod K, Ford M, Gillen G, Elliott A T, Dargie H I 1983 Treatment of angina pectoris with nifedipine and atenolol: efficacy and effect on cardiac function. British Heart Journal 55: 240–245
47. Bala Subramanian V, Bowles M J, Khurmi N S, Davies A B, Raftery E B 1982 Randomized double-blind comparison of verapamil and nifedipine in chronic stable angina. American Journal of Cardiology 50: 696–707
48. Schurtz C I, Lesbre J P, Kalisa A, Jarry G, Fardelonne P 1983 Interet des inhibiteurs calciques dans l'angor d'effort stable. Diltiazem versus nifedipine. Annales de Cardiologie et d'Angeiologie 32: 337–341
49. Kenmure A C F, Scruton J H 1979 A double-blind controlled trial of the anti-anginal efficacy of nifedipine compared with propranolol. British Journal of Clinical Practice 33: 49–51
50. Keyrilainen O, Bae E, Rytkonen U, Mathiesen M S, Wendelin H 1984 Metoprolol, nifedipine and the combination in effort angina pectoris (Abstract). European Heart Journal 5: 293
51. Higginbotham M B, Morris K G, Coleman R E, Cobb F R 1986 Comparison of nifedipine alone with propranolol alone for stable angina pectoris including hemodynamics at rest and during exercise. American Journal of Cardiology 57: 1022–1028
52. Peart I, Bullock R E, Albers C, Hall R J 1989 Cold intolerance in patients with angina pectoris: effect of nifedipine and propranolol. British Heart Journal 61: 521–28
53. Katz R I, Weintraub W S, Bodenheimer M M, Agarwal J B, Banka V S, Helfant R H 1982 Failure of low dose nifedipine to improve exercise tolerance in stable angina (Abstract). American Journal of Cardiology 49: 895
54. Schultz W, Jost S, Kober G, Kaltenbach M 1985 Relation of antianginal efficacy of nifedipine to degree of coronary arterial narrowing and to presence of coronary collateral vessels. American Journal of Cardiology 55: 26–32
55. Fox K M, Deanfield J, Selwyn A, Krikler S, Wright C 1982 Treatment of chronic stable angina pectoris with nifedipine. 5th International Adalat Symposium, pp 197–208
56. Deanfield J, Wright C, Krikler S, Ribeiro P, Fox K 1984 Cigarette smoking and the treatment of angina with propranolol, atenolol and nifedipine. New England Journal of Medicine 310: 941–954
57. Jaiprakash S S, Chatterjee S S, Sahay J N, MacDonald G 1980 Efficacy of nifedipine in the treatment of angina pectoris and chronic airways obstruction. Postgraduate Medical Journal 56: 624–628
58. Schick E C, Liang C S, Heupler F A et al 1982 Randomized withdrawal from nifedipine: Placebo-controlled study in patients with coronary artery spasm. American Heart Journal 104: 690–697
59. Antman E, Muller J, Goldberg S et al 1980 Nifedipine therapy for coronary artery spasm. New England Journal of Medicine 302: 1269–1273
60. Ginsburg R, Lamb J H, Schroeder J S, Hu M, Harrison D C 1982 Randomized double-blind comparison of nifedipine and isosorbide dinitrate therapy in variant angina pectoris due to coronary artery spasm. American Heart Journal 103: 44–48
61. Hill J A, Conti C R 1983 Coronary spasm: uses of nifedipine and isosorbide dinitrate. Primary Cardiology 9: 104–113
62. Walters D D, Miller D D, Szlachcic J et al 1983 Factors influencing the long-term prognosis of treated patients with variant angina. Circulation 68: 258–265
63. Gerstenblith G, Ouyang P, Achuff S C et al 1982 Nifedipine in unstable angina. A double-blind randomized trial. New England Journal of Medicine 306: 885–889
64. Muller J E, Turi Z G, Pearle D L et al 1984 Nifedipine and conventional therapy for unstable angina pectoris: a randomized, double-blind comparison. Circulation 69: 728–739
65. Moll M G, Dominguez J M, Obrador D, Oter R, Tomas L 1984 Nifedipine (N) vs. propranolol (P) in unstable angina (A): a prospective randomized study. European Heart Journal 5: 238
66. Report of the Holland Interuniversity Nifedipine/Metoprolol Trial (HINT) Research Group 1986 Early treatment of unstable angina in the coronary care unit: a randomised, double blind, placebo controlled comparison of recurrent ischaemia in patients treated with nifedipine or metoprolol or both. British Heart Journal 56: 400–413
67. Muller J E, Morrison J, Stone P H et al 1984 Nifedipine therapy for patients with threatened and acute myocardial infarction: a randomized double-blind, placebo-controlled comparison. Circulation 69: 740–747
68. Sirnes P A, Overskeid K, Pedersen T R et al 1984 Evolution of infarct size during the early use of nifedipine in patients with acute myocardial infarction: the Norwegian nifedipine multicentre trial. Circulation 70: 638–644

69. Walker L J E, MacKenzie G, Adgey A A J 1988 Effect of nifedipine on enzymatically estimated infarct size in the early phase of acute myocardial infarction. British Heart Journal 59: 403–410
70. Wilcox R G, Hampton J R, Banks D C et al 1986 Trial of early nifedipine in acute myocardial infarction: the Trent Study. British Medical Journal 293: 1204–1205
71. The Israeli Sprint Study Group 1988 Secondary prevention reinfarction Israeli nifedipine trial (SPRINT). A randomized intervention trial of nifedipine in patients with acute myocardial infarction. European Heart Journal 9: 354–364
72. Buhler F R, Hulthen L 1982 Calcium channel blockers: a pathophysiologically based antihypertensive treatment concept for the future? European Journal of Clinical Investigation 12: 1–3
73. Frey M, von Witzleben H, Keidel J, Fleckenstein A 1980 Restriction of calcium overload of the arterial walls of spontaneously hypertensive rats by calcium antagonists. Naunyn Schmiedebergs Archives of Pharmacology 313: 48
74. Henry P D, Bentley K I 1981 Suppression of atherosclerosis in cholesterol-fed rabbits treated with nifedipine. Journal of Clinical Investigation 68: 1366–1369
75. Lichtlen P R, Hugenholtz P G, Rafflenbeul W, Hecker H, Jost S, Deckers J W on behalf of the INTACT Group Investigators 1990 Retardation of angiographic progression of coronary artery disease by nifedipine (results of the International Nifedipine Trial on Anti-atherosclerotic therapy (INTACT)). Lancet 335: 1109–1113
76. Sarkozi J, Bookman A A H, Mahon W, Ramsay C, Yetsky A S, Keyston E C 1986 Nifedipine in the treatment of idiopathic Raynaud's syndrome. Journal of Rheumatology 13: 331–336
77. Hawkins C M A, Fletcher A W, Bulpitt C J, Pike L A 1988 The effects of verapamil and propranolol on quality of life in hypertension. British Journal of Clinical Pharmacology 25: 98P–99P
78. Kahan A, Foult J, Weber S, Amor B, Menkes C J, Degeorges M 1985 Nifedipine and alpha-adrenergic blockade in Raynaud's phenomenon (Abstract). European Heart Journal 61: 702–705
79. Lindsey G, McCullough R G, Seaman J, Hawkins R, Weil J, Steigerwald J 1985 Nifedipine may be harmful in the treatment of Raynaud's phenomenon secondary to systemic sclerosis (Abstract). Arthritis and Rheumatism 28 (suppl): S18
80. Fifer M A, Colucci W S, Lorell B H, Jaski B E, Barry W H 1985 Inotropic, vascular and neuroendocrine effects of nifedipine in heart failure: comparison with nitroprusside. Journal of the American College of Cardiology 5: 731–737
81. Corea L, Bentivoglio M, Verdecchia P 1983 Captopril compared with nifedipine in the treatment of heart failure: A randomized study. Drugs Under Experimental and Clinical Research 9: 901–910
82. Camerini F, Alberti E, Benussi B, Fioretti P, Klugmann S, Salvi A 1983 Nifedipine as an afterload reducing agent; 5th International Adalat Symposium 64–80
83. Agostoni P G, De Cesare N, Doria E, Polese A, Tamborini G, Guazzi M D 1986 Afterload reduction: a comparison of captopril and nifedipine in dilated cardiomyopathy. British Heart Journal 55: 391–399
84. McKenzie W B, Lee C L, Wilcken D E L 1983: Acute and long-term effects of nifedipine in patients with primary and secondary pulmonary hypertension. Australian and New Zealand Journal of Medicine 13: 423
85. Rubin L J, Nicod P, Hillis L D, Firth B G 1983 Treatment of primary pulmonary hypertension with nifedipine. A hemodynamic and scintigraphic evaluation. Annals of Internal Medicine 99: 433–438
86. Dalat J J, Griffiths B E, Henderson A H 1981 Primary pulmonary hypertension: Effects of nifedipine. British Heart Journal 46: 230–231
87. Strauer B E, Atef Mahmoud M, Bayer F, Bohn I, Motz U 1984 Reversal of left ventricular hypertrophy and improvement of cardiac function in man by nifedipine. European Heart Journal 5 (suppl F): 53–60
88. Ruddy T D, Koilpillai C, Liu P P et al 1982 Evaluation of chronic nifedipine therapy in non-obstructive hypertrophic cardiomyopathy (Abstract). Circulation 66 (suppl 11): 11–24
89. Nair N, Townley R G, Againdra B, Nair C K 1984 Safety of nifedipine in subjects with bronchial asthma and COPD Chest 86: 515–518
90. Barnes P J, Wilson N M, Brown M J 1981 A calcium antagonist, nifedipine, modifies exercise-induced asthma. Thorax 36: 726–730
91. Ene M D, Williamson P J, Roberts C J C, Waddell G 1985 The natriuresis following oral administration of the calcium antagonists — nifedipine and nitrendipine. British Journal of Clinical Pharmacology 19: 423–427
92. Trost B N, Weidmann P 1987 Effects of calcium antagonists on glucose homeostasis and serum lipids in non-diabetic and diabetic subjects: a review. Journal of Hypertension 5: S81–S104
93. Dale J, Landmark K H, Myhre E 1983 The effects of nifedipine, a calcium antagonist, on platelet function. American Heart Journal 105: 103–105
94. Lewis J G 1983 Adverse reactions to calcium antagonists. Drugs 25: 196–222
95. Terry R W 1982 Nifedipine therapy in angina pectoris: Evaluation of safety and side effects. American Heart Journal 104: 681–689
96. Bhatnagar S K, Amin M M A, Al-Yusuf A R 1984 Diabetogenic effects of nifedipine. British Medical Journal 289: 19
97. Ehrenkranz R A, Ackerman B A, Hulse J D 1989 Nifedipine transfer into human milk. The Journal of Pediatrics 114: 478–480
98. Penny W J, Lewis M J 1989 Nifedipine is excreted in human milk. European Journal of Clinical Pharmacology 36: 427–428

Nifurtimox

Nifurtimox is the first compound that proved effective in human therapy of the South American trypanosomiasis caused by *Trypanosoma cruzi.*

Chemistry

Nifurtmox (Lampit)
$C_{10}H_{13}N_3O_5S$
4-[(5-Nitrofurfurylidene)amino]-3-methylthiomorphiline-1,1-dioxide

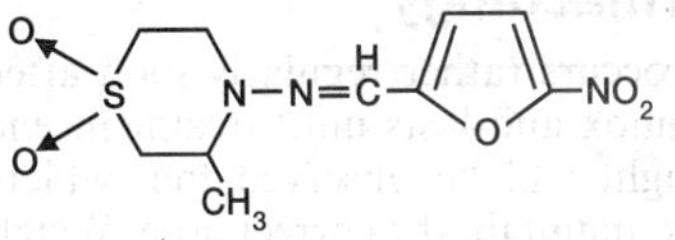

Molecular weight	287.3
pKa	—
Solubility	
in alcohol	—
in water	1 in 20
Octanol/water partition coefficient	—

The active substance is hygroscopic. This nitrofurfurylidene derivate is an intense yellow tasteless and odourless crystalline powder. It is manufactured by chemical synthesis[1] and is stable under normal conditions.

Pharmacology

Nifurtimox is trypanocidal against both the amastigote and the trypanomastigote form of *Trypanosoma cruzi*, and is effective in the acute as well as in the chronic phase of infection.[2,3] Concentrations of 1 μM have been shown to affect intracellular amastigotes in vitro and to inhibit their development. Ultrastructural observations showed severe alterations within the parasite, particularly the appearance of dense masses in the mitochondrial matrix.[4] The trypanomastigotes are less sensitive, and concentrations of 10 μM are needed to inhibit penetration of vertebrate cells by the parasite. Nifurtimox increases the intracellular generation of superoxide anions and hydrogen peroxide, both of which are very toxic to the parasite. The parasite seems to lack catalase and glutathione peroxidase so that detoxification of these toxic substances is not possible for the parasite.[5,6] Nifurtimox has not been shown to have any other pharmacological effects. In particular, even at high dosage, it has no effect on blood pressure, diuresis and blood clotting, or on acetylcholine, histamine and nicotine receptors in the guinea-pig ileum.

Toxicology

Individual members of the nitrofurane group of chemicals differ in their toxicity. The LD_{50} of nifurtimox is high: 3720 mg.kg^{-1} (3130–4420) in the mouse, 4050 mg.kg^{-1} (3490–4690) in the rat, and approximately 2000 mg.kg^{-1} in the rabbit. Symptoms of toxicity, particularly in rats, include paralysis, convulsions and respiratory distress. The same symptoms appeared after a few weeks during studies of subacute and subchronic toxicity at doses of 100 mg.kg^{-1}. Atrophy of testes and inhibition of spermatogenesis were also observed. Higher doses produced histopathological changes in midbrain, cerebellum and medulla oblongata, resulting finally in death. Doses of 25 mg.kg^{-1} were, however, well tolerated by male and female animals.[7] In tests of subchronic neurotoxicity in chickens, all animals receiving 250 mg.kg^{-1} died. Those receiving 100 mg.kg^{-1} did not develop the degenerative changes in neurones or axons, or loss of myelin in the central nervous system and the sciatic nerve, which were seen at the higher dose.[96] In chronic toxicity studies dogs tolerated 120 $mg.kg^{-1}$ for 52 weeks; a dose of 30 $mg.kg^{-1}$ was regarded as the no-effect dose. Impairment of spermatogenesis led to studies in the mouse. Immediately after treatment with 120 and 224 $mg.kg^{-1}$, no mature sperm cells were found. Their production was inhibited completely in the higher, and partially in the lower, dose-group. Inhibition of spermatogenesis, however, was reversed entirely nine weeks after treatment. From results of studies of embryotoxicity and teratogenicity it was concluded that nifurtimox was not teratogenic or embryotoxic in rats and mice. No malformation was ever seen even after doses of 125 $mg.kg^{-1}$. Fertility was impaired in males only as long as inhibition of spermatogenesis lasted.

Nifurtimox is clearly mutagenic[9,10,11] particularly in the TA 100 strain. Since the only other antichagassic compound, benznidazole, appears to be even more mutagenic these findings should be considered carefully when the need for treatment of this rather dangerous infection has to be decided. No oncogenic activity was observed in SPF wistar rats.[12]

Clinical pharmacology

Loss of appetite occurs rather regularly soon after beginning treatment with nifurtimox and lasts until treatment ends. Consequently, loss of body weight will be observed too, which requires regular control in order to maintain the correct dose. Weight will be regained with return of appetite soon after termination of treatment. Concomitant gastrointestinal troubles such as nausea and pain are often relieved by aluminium hydroxide preparations. Also during treatment, occasional disturbances in sexual functions may be recorded. Rarely there are psychic alterations such as excitement, sleeplessness, and periods of depression which — very exceptionally — may develop into a suicidal tendency. However, previously abnormal EEGs will return to normal with nifurtimox treatment.[16] Fevers occurring early in acute infection will usually subside in a few days after onset of treatment.

Pharmacokinetics

The serum concentration is measured by extracting the compound with a suitable organic solvent followed by chromatographic separation and estimation with a spectrophotometer.[22] Only limited information is available on the kinetics of nifurtimox. It is well absorbed after oral administration. Levels of the drug reach a maximum concentration 1–3 hours after medication; they then decrease rapidly and are no longer discernible at 24 hours after drug intake. Only 0.5–1.0% of the dose is excreted in urine as unchanged nifurtimox; the rest is metabolized. There were slightly raised concentrations in the kidneys, liver, lungs, aorta wall, adrenals, thyroid and Cowper's gland. Nifurtimox passes the placental barrier as well as the blood–brain barrier.[23] The extent to which nifurtimox is excreted in breast milk is not known.

Concentration–effect relationship

No data are available on this topic.

Metabolism

Nifurtimox is metabolized almost completely; only 1% of unchanged drug is excreted in the urine of man, dog and rat.[22] By using high voltage electrophoresis, more than 10 radioactive products were detected in the 24-hour urine of rats after an oral dose of 25 $mg.kg^{-1}$. Basic, acidic and neutral metabolites were present.[23] The enzyme nitroreductase present in *E. coli* of human intestines forms the nitro anion radical ($R{-}NO_2^{-}$). This radical was also detected within intact *T. cruzi* cells exposed to nifurtimox. Formation of superoxide and hydrogen peroxide was stimulated and this contributed substantially to the antiparasitic activity of nifurtimox.[24–30]

Pharmaceutics

For human therapy the compound is available in tablets only. There are two formulations; one contains 120 mg of active substance for administration to adults, the other contains 30 mg for treatment of children. The tablets are of an intense yellow colour and have one score thus providing segments of 60 and 15 mg respectively; this enables dosages to be adjusted exactly to the patient's body weight.

The tablets must be protected against light. A minimum three years expiry pertains when stored at room temperature in subtropical climates.

No known allergens are used in the formulation of the tablets.

Because Chagas' infection only occurs in Latin America there is no production of nifurtimox in Bayer AG's factories in the USA or Europe. The drug is produced by Bayer subsidiary companies in Buenos Aires, Argentina, and São Paulo, Brazil.

Therapeutic use

Indications

1a. South American trypanosomiasis due to *T. cruzi*
b. South American trypanosomiasis due to *T. rangeli*
2a. Infections by *Trypanosoma* species outside Latin America
b. African trypanosomiasis due to *T. gambiense*
3. (Muco-) cutaneous leishmaniasis
4. Onchocerciasis
5. Others.

Contraindications

The seriousness of this infection is such that no absolute contraindication exists. However, some precautions should be strictly observed whenever one or more of the following conditions are present or recorded in history:

1. Convulsions and cerebral impairment such as epilepsy, psychosis, behavioural disorder
2. Allergies, especially of the skin
3. Disorders of renal excretion
4. Chronic abuse of alcohol and/or drugs.

Mode of use

Initially treatment with nifurtimox was based on experience with other nitrofurane compounds such as nitrofurazone.[13,14,90] Therefore the starting daily dose of treatment was 30 $mg.kg^{-1}$ but a high incidence of myalgia, vomiting, polyneuritis and CNS stimulation led to dose-limiting trials in order to reduce untoward side effects. A scheme was then tested that started with a rather low daily dose (5 $mg.kg^{-1}$), which was then increased stepwise up to the amount regarded necessary to destroy all forms of *T. cruzi.* Although promising at first, this scheme was given up for two reasons:

1. The type and frequency of side effects could not be reduced significantly.
2. It could not be excluded that using less than trypanosmocidal doses over weeks would provoke resistance to the drug.

Administration is always by the oral route; injectable formulations did not prove stable. In some regions of developing countries in Latin America where Chagas' infection is frequent, the local nutritional status may be poor. In the case of a poorly nourished individual the dose should be based more on body weight than on age. Patients who are overweight should be given a dose based on normal weight corresponding to their height. Experience has shown that nitrofurane compounds are better tolerated by children than by adults.

In general, doses should be fixed according to age and body weight:

1. Babies with congenital infection 15 $mg.kg^{-1}$ daily $= 3 \times \frac{1}{2}$ tablet of 30.0 mg
2. Children up to 10 years of age or weighing up to 26.0 kg — 15–20 mg daily $= 3 \times \frac{1}{2}$–4 tablets of 30.0 mg or 3×1 tablet of 120 mg
   weighing up to 32.0 kg— $= 3 \times 1\frac{1}{4}$ tablets of 120 mg daily
3. Adolescents from 11–16 years of age or weighing up to 60.0 kg — 12.5–15 mg daily $= 3 \times 1\frac{1}{4}$–3×2 tablets of 120 mg
4. Adults from 17 years onwards or weighing 45–100.0 kg 8.0–10.0 mg daily $= 3 \times 1$–$3 \times 2\frac{1}{4}$ tablets of 120 mg

Tablets should be taken after meals. When newborn or small children are to be treated, tablets should be crushed, mixed with some pulpy food and given at the beginning of a meal.

As regards duration of therapy it is recommended that acute infection in children and adolescents is treated for 90 consecutive days, and in adults for 120 days. For the treatment of chronic disease administration for 120 days is required irrespective of age. In a case where untoward side effects make continuous medication difficult interruption of treatment for 3–4 weeks after the first 60 days has been practised by some Brazilian physicians, usually with success.

Occasionally adverse drug reactions may require additional treatment to alleviate complaints such as gastralgia, insomnia or excitation. No incompatibility with other drugs has been reported so far. Corticosteroids should be avoided because they may provoke an exacerbation of the infection.[110]

Indications

1a. South American trypanosomiasis (Chagas' infection) due to *Trypanosoma cruzi*

Causal treatment of this hazardous infection has become possible for the first time with the advent of nifurtimox. A number of earlier drugs eliminated the blood-borne forms of the parasite, but they did not prevent recrudescence of new trypamastigote forms from pseudocysts in muscular tissue. The walls of those cysts were impermeable to those drugs. Thus, every 4–5 days a new parasite generation appeared in the bloodstream able to invade new host cells. Nifurtimox penetrates the cyst walls and destroys the amastigote stage as well as the trypamastigote blood forms.[31–41] However, experience with the drug has revealed some new problems which cannot yet be entirely explained:

1. Knowledge of the infection in man has depended largely upon individual case reports. Regional differences in the clinical picture have been described, but it is not clear that these are due to differences in substrains of the parasite.
2. Laboratory methods of diagnosis have varied. Xenodiagnosis with too few organisms has been prone to observer error. The complement fixation reaction (CFR) of Machado-Guerreiro has also proved unreliable. Agreement has now been reached to use the immunofluorescence test (IFT) and the indirect haemagglutination test (IHT) in addition to CFR, and to use at least 20 triatomes for each xenodiagnosis in order to obtain reproducible results.[42,60,69–72]
3. Clinical criteria for judging therapeutic response have also posed problems. Parasites seemed to disappear from the bloodstream coincidently with a decrease of the symptoms of acute infection. But after an asymptomatic interval, sometimes many years, serious impairments of health can appear abruptly, even causing sudden death. Thus, a distinction between acute and chronic infection has been made. During a chronic infection new generations of parasites with unchanged antigenic properties appear approximately every five days. Koeberle's statement that 'the fate of the patient with Chagas' disease is decided by the acute infection',[61,62] led to the conclusion that drug treatment of the chronic infection was useless. However, studies stimulated by the availability of effective treatment revealed that parasites persisted (in low numbers) in damaged organs, such as the heart muscle, and could provoke autoimmune responses.[63–65] It has been suggested that the complete elimination of the antigenic parasite is necessary in order to halt or, at least, to slow down further disease progression. Thus treatment of the chronic stage of disease is now regarded as fully justified by many physicians although there is still some controversy.

Efficacy in acute infection, the stage which mainly occurs in children, has now been determined. Acute infection is regarded as present if an early diagnosis can be made by demonstrating *T. cruzi* in blood smears. Around day 14 after parasite invasion the IFT turns to positive. In untreated patients the two other tests will follow inevitably until about the end of the third month, CFR being the last. Their positivity marks the end of the acute phase and the beginning of the subacute to early chronic phase.

Curative drug efficacy can be judged from:

1. Return to negative of all 3 serological tests.[43,47,48,50,54,57–59]

Nifurtimox

2. A negative xenodiagnosis in a previously positive case using 20 organisms each time and repeating both tests at 1–3-month interval for a minimum of one year.[14,45,52,55]
3. Marked clinical improvement in a shorter time than can be observed in untreated or placebo-treated patients[18,21,66–73,111] (see Table 1).

Table 1 Patients treated n = 298 placebo treated n = 38

Symptoms after	Already regressed (%)		In days of observation
	Nifurtimox	Placebo	
Chagoma (Romanas Sign)	87.4	34.2	<30
Temperature	78.4	11.1	<90
Tachycardia	47.3	16.7	<90
Oedema generalized	72.1	0	<90
Hepatomegaly	55.1	7.1	<90
Splenomegaly	76.2	6.3	<90
Lympharmoplasma generalized	21.2	5.3	<90

According to figures reported from 232 Argentine patients treated and followed up carefully for 24 months post-treatment[91] 81% were regarded as cured parasitologically, 8.6% had the disease suppressed temporarily, 4.3% did not respond to therapy, and 6.1% became positive again, probably due to reinfection.

Assessment of efficacy in the chronic stage of disease presents the following difficulties.[14,16,56,75,80,89]

1. Positive serological tests may not revert to negative, e.g. as in acute infection.[50,54,63,89]
2. Parasitaemia can be very low due to increased immunological defence of the host; demonstration of the parasite's presence or absence can be almost impossible.[46,74,77,81,86]
3. The parasite may have caused irreversible damage, e.g. in the myocardium; in this case, the clinical response to treatment is not a useful criterion.[14,76]

Establishing reliable parameters to prove parasitological cure in chronic infections has been attempted. Most investigators reported decreased titres of the three serological tests.[49,60,81,82,86,88,91] Attempts have also been made to increase the sensitivity of xenodiagnosis by using 70–80 bugs, but this is impractical for routine purposes. In agreement with findings in experimental therapy[3] good results have been reported in adult patients from Argentina,[53,88,91] Chile,[44,51,78,85] Southern Brazil,[82] Venezuela[60] and Uruguay.[87] Less favourable results have been obtained in parts of Brazil but the explanation is disputed. A lower susceptibility to chemotherapy of local *T. cruzi* strains has been suggested,[34,37,41,93] and primary resistance has been reported.[92,79,83,84] Some clinical observations point to unusual properties of the local *T. cruzi* strains since they cause deformation of hollow organs more frequently than is observed elsewhere. Doubts have also been expressed about compliance, because of lack of close surveillance of drug intake and the many untoward side effects which these patients experienced.

Nifurtimox has been tested for its potential to cause resistance in comparison with nitrofurazone, in the laboratory. The parasite used experimentally was *T. cruzi Tulahuen*. With nitrofurazone a completely resistant strain had been developed after 20 passages within 8½ months; however, a strain fully resistant to nifurtimox was still not detected after 45 passages in over two years.

1b. South American trypanosomiasis due to *Trypanosoma rangeli*

This parasite is not pathogenic to man. Human infections occur occasionally, for example in Colombia, but being morphologically rather similar, distinction between the species can be difficult. Mixed infections have been observed. However, it has been established that *T. rangeli* is fully susceptible to nifurtimox.[94,95]

2a. Infections by *Trypanosoma* species outside Latin America

The following parasites have been studied for response to nifurtimox both in experimental animals and in vitro: *Trypanosoma brucei*, *T. congolense*, *T. equinum*, *T. equiperdum*, *T. evansi*, *T. lewisi*, *T. gambiense*, *T. rhodesiense* and *T. vivax*. The drug was active against all of them but considerable differences were observed both in sensitivity of species and subspecies, and in the effective dosage schedules.[30,97]

2b. African trypanosomiasis due to *Trypanosoma gambiense*

Nifurtimox proved lifesaving when given as a last resort to desperately ill patients with advanced sleeping sickness due to *T. gambiense*. Four patients received suramine as premedication over 1–5 days. Both these four and a further eight patients had been completely refractory to repeated treatments with arsenical preparations. An additional seven patients in the same poor clinical condition were treated without arsenicals. The dosage was the same as for Chagas' infection, and duration of therapy was 60 days in most cases. After follow-up of about 30 months, 14 of these 19 patients were cured and two others improved.[98,99] Favourable results have been documented in a further 99 patients but are not yet published in detail.[100–102,112] Tolerability was acceptable to good in all cases. Haemolytic reactions have not been observed but G6PD deficiency has not been investigated satisfactorily.

Nifurtimox appears very promising, but further studies are needed to establish its place in relation to arsenicals.[112]

3. (Muco-) cutaneous leishmaniasis

Morphological resemblance between trypanosomes and leishmania suggested that nifurtimox might be useful. Results obtained have not been consistent. Favourable results were achieved in 17 Columbian[103,104] and 16 Peruvian[105] patients with 17 and 10 cures respectively; however, these results have not been reproduced in Brazil,[106,107] where only eight out of 26 patients were regarded as cured. The drug has been given in doses of approximately 10.0 $mg.kg^{-1}$ body weight to adults, and 15 $mg.kg^{-1}$ to children over a period of about 30 days. Marsden[106] considers varying susceptibility to nifurtimox by the *L. mexicana* group and the *L. brasiliensis* group to be a possible reason for this discrepancy. Assessment of response has been rendered difficult because of spontaneous healing of some lesions, and because reinfection could not be excluded in non-responders.

4. Onchocerciasis

Based on the experience that trypanocidal compounds may be effective against filarial infections,[108] nifurtimox was tested against *O. volvulus*. There was no microfilaricidal effect, but hints of macrofilaricidal activity with higher doses have been suggested. In a few human infections with *O. volvulus* and *W. bancrofti* nifurtimox had been given after premedication with a reliable microfilaricidal drug. Results have been unsatisfactory, however, and never published.

5. Other indications

The influence of nifurtimox on intra- and extracellular development stages of *Toxoplasma gondii* has been studied experimentally. No effect has been observed by nifurtimox, either alone or in combination with other drugs, as regards cysts or trophozytes of *Toxoplasma gondii*.[109]

Adverse reactions

Potentially life-threatening effects

A very few cases of intermittent leucopenia have been reported during clinical investigation, where very high doses had been used initially.

Acute overdosage

Only one case of overdose has been reported, and this caused no additional impairment of health. Treatment was interrupted for 10 days.

Severe or irreversible adverse effects

There have been no irreversible adverse effects. Adverse reactions disappeared shortly after terminating treatment.

Cerebral reactions, including convulsions, vertigo, excitation, disturbance of equilibrium, disorientation, psychosis, depression, insomnia, and centrally induced vomiting, have occurred. However, during treatment a previously abnormal EEG will usually return to normal.[16]

Symptomatic adverse effects

Symptoms of infection[8] and untoward side effects of nifurtimox are often alike. Thus a symptom or sign can either be due to one of them alone or to both simultaneously, and so the cause can be difficult to distinguish.

Reactions affecting the peripheral nervous system have included paraesthesia, neuralgia and myalgia.

Skin manifestations include urticaria and morbiliforme exanthema. The slightly higher frequency of skin manifestations during treatment has been explained by allergic reactions towards foreign protein set free by parasites killed abruptly by nifurtimox.

Anorexia is the main adverse reaction to nifurtimox, leading to loss of weight of up to a maximum of 9.0 kg within 90 days. Weight gain begins immediately after termination of therapy. Closely connected are nausea/vomiting and gastralgia, with an incidence of 15% and 12% respectively.

Interference with clinical pathology tests

No observations have been reported in this respect.

High risk groups

Neonates

Newborns infected in utero with *T. cruzi* (Chagas' congenital infection) have been successfully treated. No impairment of physical and psychological development, and no adverse influence on vital functions and organs, has been reported.[18–21]

Breast milk. No adverse experience has been reported.

Children

Mortality due to acute infection in children is high, and children of all ages have been successfully treated.[1,14,17,18,66–72]

Pregnant women

In animal experiments no impairment of pregnancy has been observed, except moderate loss of weight.[8] Although the manufacturer does not recommend the drug for treatment of pregnant women, nifurtimox has been used in order to prevent miscarriage, which is observed not infrequently in pregnant patients. No harm due to such treatment has been reported.[19,20]

The elderly

No special precautions are required, except that dosage must be carefully adjusted to body weight.

Drug interactions

Potentially hazardous interactions

No such interaction has been observed.

Other significant reactions

Considering the great number of patients treated and the length of treatment (90–120) days the drug has been well tolerated.

Alcohol. Evidence suggests that nifurtimox may reduce patient tolerance of a high alcohol intake.

Potentially useful interactions

Lack of appetite and consequent loss of body weight has occasionally been considered an advantage in the treatment of overweight patients. However, the manufacturer has not recommended this indication or supported its further investigation.

Major outcome trials

1. Lugones H 1972 Tratamiento de la enfermedad de Chagas aguda. In: Cervisola J A, Lugones H, Rabinovich L B Tratamiento de la enfermedad de Chagas, Sección II: 31–47, 6º Premio Cientifico 'F. Antonio Rizzuto', Asociación de Caballeros Argentinos de la Soberana Orden Militar de Malta, Buenos Aires

This is the fundamental trial concerning treatment of acute infection with *T. cruzi*. It was carried out in the highly endemic region of Santiago del Estero over 36 months. Out of an initial 713 patients, 601 completed treatment and were followed up for 24 months after medication. Treatment had to be discontinued in 15 patients due to side effects; another 97 patients either did not receive drug regularly or did not return for follow-up examinations. Of those who completed treatment, 36.5% were under one year of age, 48% were between 2 and 10 years, 12.4% were adolescents of 11–19 years and only 3.2% were over 20 years. In cases where the exact date of parasite invasion could be determined, parasitological diagnosis was made within 10 days in 39.9%, between 11 and 15 days in 29%, between 16 and 20 days in 19%, and from day 21 onwards in 12.2%.

Nifurtimox

Forty patients received nifurtimox at a dose of 15 $mg.kg^{-1}.d^{-1}$ for 90 days and 510 patients were given 25 $mg.kg^{-1}.d^{-1}$ for the first 15 days, followed by 15 $mg.kg^{-1}.d^{-1}$ for a further 75 days in order to complete treatment of 90 days. 51 patients received placebo. Follow-up tests were carried out every 15–30 days during the first six months and monthly thereafter up to two years. Each inspection consisted of:

1. Parasitological examinations of a blood smear
2. Serological tests:
   — Complement fixating reaction (CFR) of Machado-Guerreiro
   — Indirect haemagglutination test (IHT)
   — Immunofluorescence test (IFT).

In actively treated patients, parasites disappeared permanently from the blood and could not be demonstrated even with highly sensitive concentration methods.

In placebo-treated patients, parasites remained demonstrable first directly and later for up to two years by means of xenodiagnosis using 80 bugs each time.

Among actively treated patients 34.9% had positive CFR at the start of therapy. After 4 months this had fallen to 10.7% and was still 13.0% after 24 months. In patients receiving placebo, the percentage of positive CFR had risen to 100% after 6 months and was 92.9% after 24 months.

Argentina

2. Rabinovich L B 1972 Tratamiento de la infección chagásica crónnica con el Bay 2502 (Lampit). Simpósio Internacionál sobre Enfermedad de Chagas. Sociedad Argentina de Parasitología, Buenos Aires: 277–285

After consent by an ethical board 50 out of 187 male inmates of a neuropsychiatric hospital were chosen for this study. Each one had had all three serological tests simultaneously positive, as well as repeated positive xenodiagnoses using 8 bugs in each of 10 boxes.

30 patients were treated with nifurtimox 8–10 $mg.kg^{-1}.d^{-1}$ for 120 days. They were between 27 and 71 years of age (average 45.3 years). 20 patients received placebo. Serological examinations using CFR, IHT and IFT were repeated monthly. None became negative although a slight decrease in titres was observed in the CFR of some of the treated patients.

In both groups 2–4 pretherapeutic xenodiagnoses (XD) had been positive in every patient. During therapy four xenodiagnoses were performed for every patient. 1–4 were positive in the placebo group, while each was negative in the treated group. In the follow-up period, 8–30 (average 13) XDs were performed in each patient of the placebo group and 1–32 (average 20) in the treated group. Placebo cases showed an average of 5.8 positive XDs, but no XD was positive in a treated patient.

Southern Brazil

3. Neves da Silva N, Kuhn I, Cardoso dos Santos J F, Eye G von, Braga Chaher J A 1972 Avaliação da eficácia e tolerância de um derivado nitrofurfurilidénico (Bay 2502) na fase crônica da doença de Chagas. Simpósio Internacionál sobre Enfermedad de Chagas. Sociedad Argentina de Parasitología, Buenos Aires: 293–302

25 male inmates of the psychiatric hospital 'San Pedro', Porto Alegre were chosen and — after clearance by an ethical board — included in a therapeutic trial under strictest conditions. They were between 23 and 52 years of age and had spent over four years in hospital where reinfection could be excluded. Criteria for their participation had been simultaneously positive CFR, IHT and IFT as well as repeatedly positive XD. Follow-up examinations were carried out monthly for 13 months after terminating treatment. Of the serological tests, none turned to negative although some titres in treated patients were lower than those of the placebo cases. The investigators concluded that, in chronic Chagas' disease, a serological situation exists similar to that found in syphilis, yaws and other chronic diseases where, in spite of curative treatment, serological tests remain positive.

The parasitological response was based on four pretreatment XDs, all of which were highly positive in each patient. Of four intratreatment XDs, at least two and usually all four were positive in the placebo cases, but all were negative in virtually all patients receiving nifurtimox. Of 13 post-treatment XDs most were highly positive (10.8 times in 13 months) in the placebo patients, but all were negative in the treated patients.

Venezuela

4. Maekelt G A 1972 Tratamiento de la infección Chagásica crónica. Experiencia en Venezuela. Simpósio Internacionál sobre Enfermedad de Chagas. Sociedad Argentina de Parasitología, Buenos Aires: 303–311

Forty-six male patients of the out-patient department of the Institute of Tropical Medicine, University, Caracas, were included in this study. 10 received placebo and served as a control group. Only five patients were hospitalized; the other 31 were treated as out-patients. Follow-up was for an average period of 10 months in 18 drug-treated patients, and 20 months for the placebo group.

Comparison of positive findings in pretreatment XDs with those observed in intra- and post-treatment XDs showed a statistically significant improvement in the actively treated group.

Every case showed the well-known persistence of seropositivity during treatment and follow-up. However, on comparing the titres in drug-treated patients with those observed in placebo cases, a highly significant reduction was observed.

General review articles

Cerisola J A 1977 Chemotherapy of Chagas' disease in man. Pan American Health Organization Scientific Publication No 347: 35–47

Cerisola J A, Lugones H, Rabinovich L B 1972 Tratamiento de la Enfermedad de Chagas. 6º Premio Cientifico 'F. Antonio Rizzuto' 1972 Fundación Rizzuto para la Asociación de Caballeros Argentinos de la Soberana Orden Militar de Malta, Buenos Aires

Gutteridge W E 1976 Chemotherapy of Chagas' Disease. The present situation. Tropical Diseases Bulletin 73 (9): 699–705

Haberkorn A 1979 The effect of nifurtimox on experimental infection with Trypasomatidae other than *Trypamosoma cruzi*. Zentralblatt für Bakteriologie und Hygiene, I. Abteilung, Originalien A 244: 331–338

Wegner D H G 1975 La infección de Chagas y su tratamiento con lampit. Revista de Información Médico-Terapéutica, Año L 5-6: 67–73

Wegner D H G, Rohwedder R W 1972 The effect of nifurtimox in acute Chagas' infection. Arzneimittelforschung/Drug Research 22 (9a): 1624–1635

Wegner D H G, Rohwedder R W 1972 Experience with nifurtimox in chronic Chagas' infection. Arzneimittelforschung/Drug Research 22 (9a): 1635–1641

References

1. Bock M, Haberkorn A, Herlinger H, Mayer K H, Petersen S 1972 The structure–activity relationship of a 4-(5'-nitrofurfurylidene-amino)-tetrahydro-4H-1,4-thiazine-1,1-dioxides active against *Trypanosoma cruzi*. Arzneimittelforschung/Drug Research 22 (9a): 1564–1569
2. Gönnert R 1972 Nifurtimox: causal treatment of Chagas' disease. Arzneimittelforschung/Drug Research 22 (9a): 1563
3. Haberkorn A, Gönnert R 1972 Animal experimental investigation into the activity of nifurtimox against *Trypanosoma cruzi*. Arzneimittelforschung/Drug Research 22 (9a): 1570–1582
4. Villatta F, de Souza W, Leon W 1979 The effect of Lampit on *Trypanosoma cruzi* in mice organs and in the bloodstream. Zeitschrift für Parasitenkunde 61 (1): 21–27
5. Docampo R, Moreno S N J 1984 Free radical metabolites in the mode of action of chemotherapeutic agents and phagocytic cells on *Trypanosoma cruzi*. Reviews of Infectious Diseases 6 (2): 223–229
6. Goijman S, Frasch A A C, Moreno S N J, Docampo R, Stoppani A O M 1982 Cleavage of *Trypanosoma cruzi* DNA by nifurtimox metabolites. Journal of Protozoology 29 (2): 332–333
7. Hofmann K 1972 Toxicological investigations on the tolerability of nifurtimox. Arzneimittelforschung/Drug Research 22 (9a) 1550–1603
8. Lorke D 1972 Embryotoxicity studies of nifurtimox in rats and mice and study of fertility and general reproductive performance. Arzneimittelforschung/Drug Research 22 (9a): 1603–1607
9. Onishi T, Ohashi Y, Nozu K, Inoki S 1980 Mutagenicity of nifurtimox in *Escheria coli*. Mutation Research 77: 241–244
10. Nagel R, Nepomaschy I 1983 Mutagenicity of two antichagassic drugs and their metabolic deactivation. Mutation Research 117 (3–4): 237–242
11. Ferreira R C C, Ferreira L C S 1986 Mutagenicity of nifurtimox and benznidazole in the Salmonella-microsome assay. Brazilian Journal of Medical Biology Research 19: 19–25

12. Steinhoff D, Grundmann E 1972 Test for carcinogenicity of nifurtimox on oral and subcutaneous administration to rats. Arzneimittelforschung/Drug Research 22(9a): 1607–1612
13. Marra U D 1969 Comparación de la tolerancia medicamentosa de la nitrofurazona, levofuraltadona y el preparado Bay 2502. Boletín Chileno de Parasitología 24 (1–2): 38–42
14. Bustos A G, Sosa E V, Constanco S, Wybert L A, DeLucía A, Carrizo F A 1969 Evolución clínico-parasitológica y de laboratorio en niños y adolescentes con infección chagásica crónica tratados con Bay 2502 y con placebo. Boletín Chileno de Parasitología 24 (1–2): 63–65
15. Jörg M E, Orlando A S 1967 Encefalopatía en la tripanosomiasis cruzi crónica. Prensa Médica Argentina 54: 1665–1681
16. Girardelli M A 1972 Electroencefalografia y enfermedad de Chagas crónica. Boletín Chileno de Parasitología 24 (1–2): 32–35
17. Girardelli M A 1972 Evolución electroencefalográfica en niños y adultos jóvenes con infección chagásica crónica tratados con Bay 2502. Boletín Chileno de Parasitología 24 (1–2): 35–38
18. Rubio M, Donoso F 1972 Enfermedad de Chagas en niños y tratamiento con Bay 2502. Boletín Chileno de Parasitología 24 (1–2): 43–48
19. Bittencourt A L, Sadigursky M, Barbosa H S 1975 Doença de Chagas congenita. Estudo de 29 casos. Revista do Instituto de Medicina Tropical, Saõ Paulo 17: 146–159
20. Bittencourt A L 1976 Congenital Chagas' Disease. American Journal of Diseases in Childhood 130: 97–103
21. Gonzalez O 1972 Chagas congenito. In: Cerisola J A, Segura E L (eds) Simpósio Internacionál sobre Enfermedad de Chagas. Sociedad Argentina de Parasitologiá, Buenos Aires, pp 101–108
22. Medenwald H, Brandau K, Schlossmann K 1972 Quantitative determination of nifurtimox in body fluids of rat, dog and man. Arzneimittelforschung/Drug Research 22 (9a): 1613–1617
23. Duhm B, Maul W, Medenwald H, Patzschke K, Wegner L A 1972 Investigations on the pharmacokinetics of nifurtimox-^{35}S in the rat and dog. Boletín Chileno de Parasitología 24 (1–2): 1617–1624
24. Andrews P, Haberkorn A, Thomas H 1987 Antiparasitic drugs. Mechanism of action, pharmacokinetics, and in vitro and in vivo assays of drug activity. In: Lorian V (ed) Antibiotics in laboratory medicine, 2nd edn. Williams and Wilkins, Baltimore, pp 282–309
25. Docampo R, Moreno S N 1984 Free radical intermediates in the antiparasitic action of drugs and phagocytic cells. In: Pryor W A (ed) Free radicals in biology, vol VI. Academic Press, New York, pp 264–266
26. McLane K E, Fisher J, Ramakrishnan K 1983 Reductive drug metabolism. Drug Metabolism Review 14 (4): 763–778
27. Docampo R 1981 Mechanism of nifurtimox toxicity in different forms of *Trypanosoma cruzi*. Biochemistry in Pharmacology 30 (14): 1947–1951
28. Docampo R, Stoppani A O M 1980 Sobre el mecanismo de la acción tripanocida del nifurtimox y otros nitro-derivados en *Trypanosoma cruzi*. Medicina (Buenos Aires) 40 (suppl 1): 10–16
29. Masana M, Toranzo E G de, Castro J A 1984 Studies on nifurtimox nitroreductase activity in liver and other rat tissues. Archives of Internal Pharmacodynamic Therapy 270 (1): 4–10
30. Groijman S G, Stoppani A O M 1985 Effects of nitroheterocyclic drugs on macromolecule synthesis and degradation in *Trypanosoma cruzi*. Biochemical Pharmacology 34 (8): 1331–1336
31. Gönnert R, Bock M 1972 The effect of nifurtimox on *Trypanosoma cruzi* in tissue cultures. Arzneimittelforschung 22 (9a): 1582–1586
32. Voigt W-H, Bock M, Gönnert R 1972 Ultrastructural observations on the activity of nifurtimox on the causative organism of Chagas' disease. Arzneimittelforschung/Drug Research 22 (9a): 1586–1589
33. Voigt W-H, Haberkorn A, Gönnert R 1973 Licht-und elektronenmikroskopische Untersuchungen mastigoter und amastigoter Formen von *Trypanosoma cruzi* unter dem Einfluss von Lampit. Zeitschrift für Parasiten-Kunde 41: 255–267
34. Andrade S G, Figueira R M, Carvalho M L, Grozini D F 1975 Influêcenca da cepa do *Trypanosoma cruzi* na resposta à terapêutica experimental pelo Bay 2502. Revista do Instituto de Medicina Tropical Saõ Paulo 17 (6): 380–385
35. Andrade S G, Andrade Z A 1976 Aspectos anatomo-patológicos e resposta terapêutica na infeccão chagásica crônica experimental. Revista do Instituto de Medicina Tropical Saõ Paulo 18 (4): 268–274
36. Rimoldo M T, Cardoni R L, Manni J A 1976 Efecto in vivo e in vitro del nifurtimox sobre las formas infectivas de *T. cruzi*. Medicina 36 (6): 616
37. Brener Z, Costa C A, Chiari C 1976 Differences in the susceptibility of *Trypanosoma cruzi* strains to active chemotherapeutic agents. Revista do Instituto de Medicina Tropical Saõ Paulo 18 (6): 450–455
38. Morrow D T, Wescott R B, Davis W C 1977 Effect of length of treatment with Bayer 2502 on isolation of *Trypanosoma cruzi* and resistance to challenge in the mouse. American Journal of Tropical Medicine and Hygiene 26 (3): 382–386
39. Villalta F, De Souza W, Leon W 1979 The effect of Lampit on *Trypanosoma cruzi* in mice organs and the bloodstream. Zeitschrift für Parasiten-Kunde 61: 21–27
40. Cabeza Meckert P, Gelpi R, Chambo G, Laguens R 1984 *T. cruzi* reinfection in Chagasic mice treated with nifurtimox. Journal of Protozoology 31 (4): 39
41. Andrade S G, Magalhaes J B, Pontes A L 1985 Evaluation of chemotherapy with benznidazole and nifurtimox in mice infected with *Trypanosoma cruzi* strains of different type. Bulletin of the World Health Organization 63 (4): 721–726
42. Alvarez M, Cerisola J A, Rohwedder R W 1968 Test de immunofluorescencia para el diagnóstico de la enfermedad de Chagas. Boletín Chileno de Parasitología 23 (1–2): 4–9
43. Cerisola J A, Rohwedder R W, Di Corleto C 1968 Estimación de la especifidad de reacciones serológicas para enfermedad de Chagas. Boletín Chileno de Parasitología 23 (1–2): 2–3
44. Schenone H, Alfaro E, Reyes H, Taucher E 1968 Valór del xenodiagnostico en la infección chagásica crónica. Boletín Chileno de Parasitología 23 (3–4): 149–154
45. Schenone H, Alfaro E, Reyes H, Taucher E 1969 Rendimento del xenodiagnóstico en las formas aguda y congénita de la enfermedad de Chagas. Boletín Chileno de Parasitología 24 (1–2): 105–106
46. Abreu Salgado A de 1969 Consideraciones sobre metodologia y sensibilidad del xenodiagnóstico. Boletín Chileno de Parasitología 24 (1–2): 9–13
47. Cerisola J A, Alvarez M, Lugones H, Rebosolán J B 1969 Sensibilidad de las reacciones serológicas para el diagnóstico de la enfermedad de Chagas. Boletín Chileno de Parasitología 24 (1–2): 2–8
48. Cerisola J A 1969 Evolución serológica de pacientes con enfermedad de Chagas aguda tratados con Bay 2502. Boletín Chileno de Parasitología 24 (1–2): 54–59
49. Maekelt G A 1969 Evolución clínica y serológica de la droga Bay 2502 en pacientes con infección chagásica crónica. Boletín Chileno de Parasitología 24 (1–2): 95–96
50. Cerisola J A, Alvarez M, De Rissio A M 1970 Imunodiagnôstico da doença de Chagas. Revista do Instituto de Medicina Tropical. Saõ Paulo 12 (6): 403–411
51. Schenone H, Concha L, Aranda R et al 1970 Valor do xenodiagnôstico na avaliaçaõ do tratamento de infecçaõ crônica pelo *Trypanosoma cruzi*. Revista de Goîana Medical 16: 19–181
52. Cerisola J A, Russo M C, Del Prado C E, Jozami L B de, Rohwedder R W 1972 Estudio comparativo de diversos métodos parasitológicos en la enfermedad de Chagas aguda. Proceedings: Simpósio Internacionál sobre Enfermedad de Chagas, Sociedad Argentina de Parasitología, Buenos Aires: 97–100
53. Cerisola J A, Rohwedder R W, Del Prado C E 1972 Sensibilidad del xenodiagnóstico en infección chagasica crónica. Proceedings: VIII Congresso Sociedade Brasileira de Medicina Tropical, Belo Horizonte
54. Cerisola J A 1972 Valor del inmunodiagnóstico en la infección chagásica. Proceedings: Simpósio Internacionál sobre Enfermedad de Chagas, Sociedad Argentina de Parasitología, Buenos Aires: 115–121
55. Schenone H, Alfaro E, Rojas A 1972 Bases y rendimiento del xenodiagnóstico en la infección chagásica. Proceedings: Simpósio Internacionál sobre Enfermedad de Chagas, Sociedad Argentina de Parasitología, Buenos Aires: 111–114
56. Almeida J O, Cerisola J, Cedillos R, Maekelt G A 1972 Sôro de referência internacional para moléstia de Chagas. Proceedings: Simpósio Internacionál sobre Enfermedad de Chagas, Sociedad Argentina de Parasitología, Buenos Aires: 125–133
57. Knierim F, Sandoval J, Alfaro E, Sandoval L, Muñoz E, Eskuche G 1972 Reacción de hemaglutinación indirecta o passiva en enfermedad de Chagas. Proceedings: Simpósio Internacionál sobre Enfermedad de Chagas, Sociedad Argentina de Parasitología, Buenos Aires: 135–139
58. Camargo M E, Hoshino S 1972 Reaçaõ de hemaglutinaçaõ passiva con hemácias preservadas para o diagnôstico da tryposomiase americana. Proceedings: Simpósio Internacionál sobre Enfermedad de Chagas, Sociedad Argentina de Parasitología, Buenos Aires: 142–147
59. Alvarez M 1972 Test de inmmunofluorescéncia para el diagnóstico de la enfermedad de Chagas. Proceedings: Simpósio Internacionál sobre Enfermedad de Chagas, Sociedad Argentina de Parasitología, Buenos Aires: 149–154
60. Maekelt G A 1972 Tratamiento de la infección chagásica crónica, experiéncia en Venezuela. Proceedings: Simpósio Internacionál sobre Enfermedad de Chagas, Sociedad Argentina de Parasitología, Buenos Aires: 303–311
61. Köberle I 1957 Patogenía da moléstia de Chagas. Revista de Goiana Medical 3: 155–180
62. Köberle F 1970 The causation and importance of nervous lesions in American trypanosomiasis. Bulletin of the World Health Organization 42: 739–743
63. Marsden P D 1984 74.3 American trypanosomiasis. In: Strickland G Th (ed) Hunter's tropical medicine, 6th edn. Protozoal infections. W B Saunders, Philadelphia, pp 565–571
64. Kierszenbaum F 1985 Is there autoimmunity in Chagas' disease? Parasitology Today 1 (1): 4–6
65. Hudson L 1985 Autoimmune phenomena in chronic chagasic cardiopathy. Parasitology Today 1 (1): 6–9
66. Bocca Tourres G L 1969 La enfermedad de Chagas en período agudo y su tratamiento con Bay 2502. Boletín Chileno de Parasitología 24 (1–2): 24–27
67. Fernandez J J, Cedillos R A, Godoy G A 1969 Reporte preliminar sobre el ensayo de una nueva droga de la seria de los nitrofuranos — el Bayer 2502 – en el tratamiento de la enfermedad de Chagas aguda. Archives Collegio de Medicina El Salvador 22 (1): 46–66
68. Lugones H, Peralta F, Canal-Feijôo D, De Marteleur A E A 1969 Evolución de la Sintomatología clínica y la función hepática en la enfermedad de Chagas aguda tratada con Bay 2502. Boletín Chileno de Parasitología 24 (1–2): 19–24
69. Oliveira Ferreira H de 1967 Tratamento da doença de Chagas (fasa aguda) com Bayer 2502. Revista do Instituto de Medicina Tropical Saõ Paulo 9 (5): 343–345
70. Wegner D H G 1970 Über de Behandlung der akuten Chagas-Krankheit mit Lampit. Proceedings V International Congress of Infectious Diseases, Wien, vol IV: 153–156
71. Lugones H S 1972 Tratamiento de la enfermedad aguda. Experiencia en Santiago del Estero. Proceedings: Simpósio Internacionál sobre Enfermedad de Chagas, Sociedad Argentina de Parasitología, Buenos Aires: 255–259
72. Oliveira Ferreira H de, Anis Rassi A 1972 Tratamiento da fasa aguda de doença de Chagas. Proceedings: Simpósio Internacionál sobre Enfermedad de Chagas, Sociedad Argentina de Parasitología, Buenos Aires: 261–269
73. Western K A, Schultz M G, Farrar W E, Kagan I G 1969 Laboratory acquired Chagas' disease treated with Bay 2502. Boletín Chileno de Parasitología 24 (1–2): 94
74. Cichero J A, Segura E, Quatrochi J C 1969 Evolución clínico-parasitológica chagásica crónica tratada con Bay 2502. Boletín Chileno de Parasitología 24 (1–2): 59–62
75. Ejden J 1969 Efecto del Bay 2502 in adultos asintomaticos con infección chagásica crónica. Boletín Chileno de Parasitología 24 (1–2): 99–100
76. Valecillos-V R I 1969 Investigación terapéutica del Bay 2502 en pacientes con miocardiopatía chagásica crónica. Observaciones sobre tolerância clínica y de los parenquimas. Boletín Chileno de Parasitología 24 (1–2): 96–97
77. Schenone H, Concha L, Aranda R, Rojas A, Alfaro E 1969 Experiencia terapéutica con el Bay 2502 en la infección chagásica crónica del adulto. Importancia del uso adecuado del xenodiagnóstico. Boletín Chileno de Parasitología 24 (1–2): 66–69

Nifurtimox

78. Schenone H, Concha L, Aranda R, Rojas A, Knierim F, Rojo M 1972 Tratamiento de la infección chagásica crónica humana: experiencia en Chile. Proceedings: Simpósio Internacionál sobre Enfermedad de Chagas, Sociedad Argentina de Parasitología, Buenos Aires: 287–291
79. Cançado J R, Marra U D, Lopes M et al 1969 Toxiciadad y valór terapéutico en tres esquemas posológicos. Boletín Chileno de Parasitología 24 (1–2): 28–32
80. Romero G 1969 Investigación terapéutica del Bay 2502 en adultos jovenes con infección chagásica crónica. Boletín Chileno de Parasitología 24 (1–2): 97–99
81. Wagner Pinto L, Fourniol D, Di Santo L 1969 Experiencia terapéutica con el Bay 2502 en un grupo homogénico de pacientes adultos con infección chagásica crónica. Boletín Chileno de Parasitología 24 (1–2): 103–104
82. Neves da Silva N, Kuhn G, Cardoso dos Santos J F, von Eye G, Braga Chaher J A 1972 Avaliazão da eficácia e tolerância de um derivado nitrofurfurolidenico (Bay 2502) na fasa crônica da doença de Chagas. Proceedings: Simpósio Internacionál sobre Enfermedad de Chagas, Sociedad Argentina de Parasitología, Buenos Aires: 293–302
83. Cançado J R 1972 Experiencia clínica com o tratamento específico. Proceedings VIII Congresso Sociedade Brasileira da Medicina Tropical, Belo Horizonte
84. Prata A 1972 Experiencia clínica com o tratamento específico. Proceedings VIII Congresso Sociedade Brasileira da Medicina Tropical, Belo Horizonte
85. Schenone H 1972 Tratamiento de la infección chagásica crónica con Lampit. Proceedings VIII Congresso Sociedade Brasileira da Medicina Tropical, Belo Horizonte
86. Rabinovich L B 1972 Evaluación de la actividad del Bay 2502 (Lampit) en el tratamiento de la infección chagásica crónica. Proceedings VIII Congresso Sociedade Brasileira da Medicina Tropical, Belo Horizonte
87. Lopez-Fernandez J R, Franca-Rodriguez M E, Pignataro de Vinas F, Zanela de Alves E 1969 Primeros estudios en el Uruguay sobre tratamiento de la enfermedad de Chagas con un derivado nitrofurfuridinico (Bayer 2502). Revista Uruguyana de Patología Clínica 1969: 66–73
88. Rabinovich L B 1972 El tratamiento de la infección chagásica crónica con el Bayer 2502 (Lampit). Proceedings: Simpósio Internacionál sobre Enfermedad de Chagas, Sociedad Argentina de Parasitología, Buenos Aires: 277–285
89. Cerisola J A, Rohwedder R 1972 Comportamiento de la parasitémia y el inmunodiagnóstico de la infección chagásica crónica. Proceedings: Simpósio Internacionál sobre Enfermedad de Chagas, Sociedad Argentina de Parasitología, Buenos Aires: 271–275
90. Oliveira Ferreira H de 1969 Comparación de la tolerancia medicamentosa de la nitrofurazona, la levafuraltadona (NF602) y el Bay 2502. Boletín Chileno de Parasitología 24 (1–2): 101–103
91. Cerisola J A 1971 Studies on the efficacy of Lampit, a useful model for the evaluation of antichagasic drugs. Proceedings V Tagung der Deutschen Tropenmedizischen Gesellschaft, Tübingen: 45–57
92. Andrade S G, Andrade Z A, Figueira R M 1977 Estudo experimental sobre a resistência de uma cepa do *Trypanosoma cruzi* ao Bay 2502. Revista do Instituto de Medicina Tropical, São Paulo 19 (2): 124–129
93. Wegner D H G 1973 Clinical studies with the anti-Chagasic drug Lampit. Proceedings: IX International Congress for Tropical Medicine and Malaria, Athens. Abstracts II/83: 56
94. Marinkelle C J 1982 The effect of Lampit on *Trypanosoma rangeli* in experimentally infected mice. Tropenmedicine and Parasitology 33 (3): 151–152
95. Marinkelle C J, Vallejo G A, Guhl F, Sánchez N de 1985 Diferenciación entre *Trypanosoma cruzi* y *Trypanosoma rangeli* en el intestino del vector Rhodnius prolixus en base al comportamiento de estos flagelados frente a la actividad litica del complemento. Revista Latinamericana de Microbiología 27 (1): 21–25
96. Dieckmann W, Sawada S, Hobik H P 1972 Histopathological changes in the CNS of the rat after peroral administration of high doses of nifurtimox (German). Verhandlungen der Deutschen Gesellschaft für Pathologie 56: 417–419
97. Kaddu I B, Njogu A R 1980 The action of Lampit and a new compound on *Trypanosoma rhodesiense*. 1. Annual Medical Science Conference of the Kenya Medical Research Institute Nairobi: 166–172
98. Janssens P G, De Muynck 1977 Clinical trials with nifurtimox in African trypanosomiasis. Annales de la Societé Belge de Médicine Tropicale 57 (4–5): 475–480
99. Moens F, De Wilde M, Kola Ngato 1984 Essai de traitement au Nifurtimox de la trypanosomiase humaine africaine. Annales de la Societé Belge de Médicine Tropicale 64: 37–43
100. Van Nieuvenhove S 1985 Alternative treatment in African human sleeping sickness. World Health Organization Expert Committee on the Epidemiology and Control of African Trypanosomiasis. TRY/EC/WP 85.24: 3–4
101. Van Nieuvenhove S, Declercq J 1981 Nifurtimox (Lampit) treatment in late stage of gambiense sleeping sickness. International Scientific Council for Trypanosomiasis Research and Control, 17th Meeting, Arusha, Tanzania, Publication No 112: 206–208
102. De Raadt P, Van Nieuvenhove S 1987 Session on human trypanosomiasis. International Scientific Council for Trypanosomiasis Research and Control, Lome, Togo, MS. Alternative Drugs: 3–4
103. Restrepo M, Velasquez J P 1973 Treatment of leishmaniasis with a nitrofurfurylidene derivative (Bayer 2502). Transactions of the Royal Society of Tropical Medicine and Hygiene 67: 616
104. Restrepo M, Restrepo F 1976 Tratamiento de pacientes con leishmaniasis. Tribuna Medica 54 (4): 36–38
105. Lumbreras H 1975 Sobre el tratamiento de 16 patientes con leishmaniasis mediante el uso oral de Lampit un derivado nitrofuranico. Resumenes de la II. Jornada Peruviana de Microbiolgía y Parasitología, Trujillo, Perú III: 4
106. Marsden P D, Cuba C C, Barreto A C, Sampaio R N, Rocha R A A 1979 Nifurtimox in the treatment of South American leishmaniasis. Transactions of the Royal Society of Tropical Medicine and Hygiene 73 (4): 391–394
107. Sampaio R N, Sampaio J H, Marsden P D 1985 Pentavalent antimonial treatment in mucosal leishmaniasis. Lancet 1 (8437): 1097
108. Duke B O L 1977 The effects of some drugs: — Pentamidine, Stilbocaptate, Hoechst 33 258, F151, compound 'E' and nifurtimox — on *Onchocerca volvulus* in chimpanzees. Tropenmedizin und Parasitologie 28 (4): 447–455
109. Werner H, Gönnert R 1974 Der Einfluss von Nifurtimox auf intra- und extrazelluläre Entwicklungsstadien von *Toxoplasma gondii*. Arzneimittelforschung/Drug Research 24 (5): 700–793
110. Andrade S G, Macêdo V 1973 Tratamento combinado da doença de Chagas con Bayer 2502 e corticóide (Estudo experimental e clinico). Revista do Instituto de Medizina Tropical, São Paulo 15 (6): 421–430
111. Hofflin S M, Sadler P H, Araujo F G, Page W E, Remington J S 1987 Laboratory-acquired Chagas' disease. Transactions of the Royal Society of Tropical Medicine and Hygiene 81 (3): 437–440
112. Pepin J, Milord F, Mpia B et al 1989 An open clinical trial of nifurtimox for arseno-resistant *Trypanosoma brucei gambiense* sleeping sickness in central Zaire. Transactions of the Royal Society of Tropical Medicine and Hygiene 83: 514–517

N

Nimodipine

Nimodipine is a calcium slow channel antagonist of the dihydropyridine class.[1]

Chemistry

Nimodipine (Nimotop)
$C_{21}H_{26}N_2O_7$
1,4-Dihydro-2,6-dimethyl-4-(3-nitrophenyl)-3,5-pyridinedicarboxylic acid 2-methoxyethyl-1-methylethyl ester

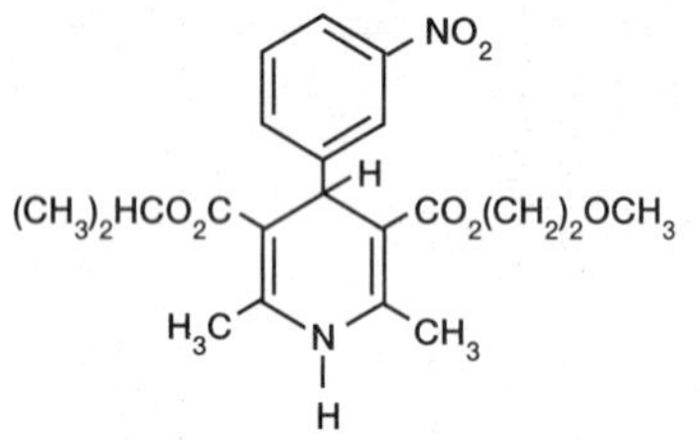

Molecular weight	418.5
pKa	—
Solubility	
in alcohol	soluble
in water	insoluble
Octanol/water partition coefficient	—

Nimodipine is heat-stable, non-hygroscopic and is sensitive to light. In pure form it is a yellow, finely crystalline compound prepared by chemical synthesis.

Pharmacology

Nimodipine is a calcium channel antagonist with its major site of action at the sarcolemma.[2] The major mechanism of action is stabilization of calcium channels in the inactive mode, thereby producing blockade of calcium entry. Nimodipine is most effective on arterioles with a diameter $< 100\ \mu m$.[3,4]

The drug is relatively selective for cerebral vessels. There have been a number of in vitro studies using various agonist-contracted isolated arterial preparations which have indicated relative selectivity of nimodipine for vessels of cerebral origin. Selectivity has been demonstrated in the rabbit where potassium, 5HT, CTXA2 and blood have been used as agonists.[5–8] In the cat, nimodipine was selective in its antagonism of potassium-induced vasoconstriction.[9] In the dog, nimodipine was selective in its antagonism of vasoconstriction induced by the 5HT.[10] In these various animal studies, the selectivity of nimodipine for cerebral vessels was approximately three- to ten-fold in comparison to various peripheral vessels. In the human, nimodipine was selective in antagonizing potassium-induced vasoconstriction in the pial vessel as compared to mesenteric vessels. Selectivity was approximately three-fold.[11]

The cellular basis of cerebral selectivity is unknown, but may in part be due to greater dependence of cerebral blood vessels on exogenous calcium for maintenance of the contractile state. The high lipid solubility of nimodipine may result in higher drug concentrations at the site of action in the cerebral vessels. Nimodipine increases cerebral blood flow in animal models of cerebral ischaemia. As little as $1\ \mu g.kg^{-1}$ given intravenously increases cerebral blood flow in dogs. Doses of $10\ \mu g.kg^{-1}$ increase cerebral blood flow by more than 50%.[1] The drug reduces infarct size in rats with middle cerebral artery occlusion. Administration of nimodipine prior to cerebral ischaemia in dogs reduced postischaemic hypoperfusion and improved neurological outcome. Treatment of monkeys after a 17 minute period of ischaemia also improved neurological outcome.[12]

Intravenous administration of $10–100\ \mu g.kg^{-1}$ nimodipine to dogs lowers systemic arterial pressure. Much lower doses of $0.3\ \mu g.kg^{-1}$ increase cardiac output.[13]

Toxicology

The intravenous LD_{50} ranges from $2.5\ mg.kg^{-1}$ in rabbits to $33\ mg.kg^{-1}$ in mice. The oral LD_{50} is at least 40 times larger. Chronic toxicity is low; doses of $10\ mg.kg^{-1}$ daily to dogs slowed the rate of weight gain, reduced appetite and produced sedation and salivation. There is no evidence of mutagenic activity. Teratogenic studies are complicated by the fact that the solvent (PEG 400) produced diarrhoea leading to reduced weight in pregnant animals. Occasional malformations and an increase in mortality among offspring occurred in initial studies but later studies showed no teratogenic or embryotoxic effects.

Clinical pharmacology

Single doses of 1–30 µg intravenous nimodipine had no consistent effects upon blood pressure or heart rate in normal volunteers. Intravenous infusions of $15–45\ \mu g.kg^{-1}$ over a period of three hours produced falls of 16.5% in the systolic blood pressure in hypertensive patients.

Single sublingual doses of $0.05–0.2\ mg.kg^{-1}$ nimodipine produced no effect on blood pressure or heart rate. Sublingual doses of $0.3\ mg.kg^{-1}$ produced drops of more than 10 mmHg systolic in 10/35 measurements and a similar change in diastolic blood pressure.

Single oral doses of 120 mg nimodipine to healthy volunteers produced falls of 8 mmHg in systolic blood pressure. Diastolic blood pressure fell by 20 mmHg. The heart rate rose 15 beats per minute. Nimodipine 20–40 mg three times daily lowered mean supine systolic blood pressure by 14–18 mmHg in hypertensive patients. Diastolic blood pressure was reduced in both the supine and standing positions.

Nimodipine has the potential for lowering blood pressure in a dose-dependent fashion. Changes of blood pressure are more likely to occur in patients who had initially elevated blood pressure, as would be expected with a calcium antagonist.[14]

Nimodipine produces variable effects on cerebral blood flow in patients with stroke. Patients with cerebrovascular insufficiency generally show slight increases in cerebral blood flow. There has been no evidence of intracerebral steal in any of these studies. A single dose of 40 mg nimodipine inhibited ADP-induced platelet aggregation in five healthy volunteers.

Pharmacokinetics

Measurement of nimodipine in humans is by gas chromatography or HPLC. The detection limit for gas chromatography is $0.5–1.0\ \mu g.l^{-1}$, although some groups[15,16] have been able to lower this to $0.1–0.2\ \mu g.l^{-1}$.

The pharmacokinetics of intravenous nimodipine $30\ \mu g.kg^{-1}$ were studied in six volunteers.[17] The plasma concentration–time curve showed an initial distribution phase with a half life of about 10 minutes and a slower log-linear decay. The elimination half life averaged 1.1 ± 0.2 h, but sampling was concluded at 5 hours after dosing, thereby possibly missing a longer elimination phase. Clearance was $14.0 \pm 4\ ml.min^{-1}.kg^{-1}$ and the volume of distribution at steady state $0.9 \pm 0.4\ l.kg^{-1}$. Oral administration of three 20 mg nimodipine tablets showed that bioavailability was 5–10%. The elimination half life in this study was 1.7 ± 1.1 h, but sampling was limited to 8 hours post dose. The maximal plasma concentration was $20.6 \pm 11.8\ \mu g.l^{-1}$ at 0.8 ± 0.3 hours after drug administration.

After administration of 20 mg ^{14}C-labelled nimodipine, 53% of the radioactivity was recovered in the urine. Over 30% of the dose was recovered in the faeces. It appears that nimodipine is subject to an extensive presystemic hepatic metabolism. Nimodipine kinetics are linear in the dose range 10–90 mg. Less than 1% of the drug appears in the urine as unchanged drug. About 30–40% of an orally administered dose appears in the urine in the form of nine acidic inactive metabolites.

Oral clearance of nimodipine was reduced in six patients with cirrhosis. Oral clearance was 187 ± 163 l.h^{-1} in cirrhotics compared to 469 ± 198 l.h^{-1} in normals.[15] The elimination half life after oral administration was 7.9 ± 1.9 hours in patients with liver disease and 5.7 ± 1.0 hours in age-matched normals.

Autoradiographic and distribution studies have been carried out in rats using ^{14}C-labelled nimodipine. It has been shown that following intravenous injection, radioactive material was distributed rapidly throughout all tissues and organs. After about one hour there were relatively greater levels of radioactive material in the gastrointestinal tract, fat deposits around the kidneys, adrenal glands and liver. Single-dose studies using pregnant animals showed the placental transfer of nimodipine was limited; radioactivity levels were 8 to 15 times lower in the fetus than in the dam.[18] It appears that nimodipine does cross the blood–CSF barrier. Ramsch et al.[17] measured the concentration of nimodipine in cerebrospinal fluid samples taken from 15 patients with subarachnoid haemorrhage. These patients had received a constant intravenous infusion of nimodipine 2 mg.h^{-1} for up to 14 days. The mean CSF concentration during the intravenous infusion was 0.3 ± 0.2 μg.l^{-1} the mean plasma concentration was 76.9 ± 34 μg.l^{-1}. It is not known whether nimodipine enters into breast milk.

Fig. 1 The metabolism of nimodipine[23]

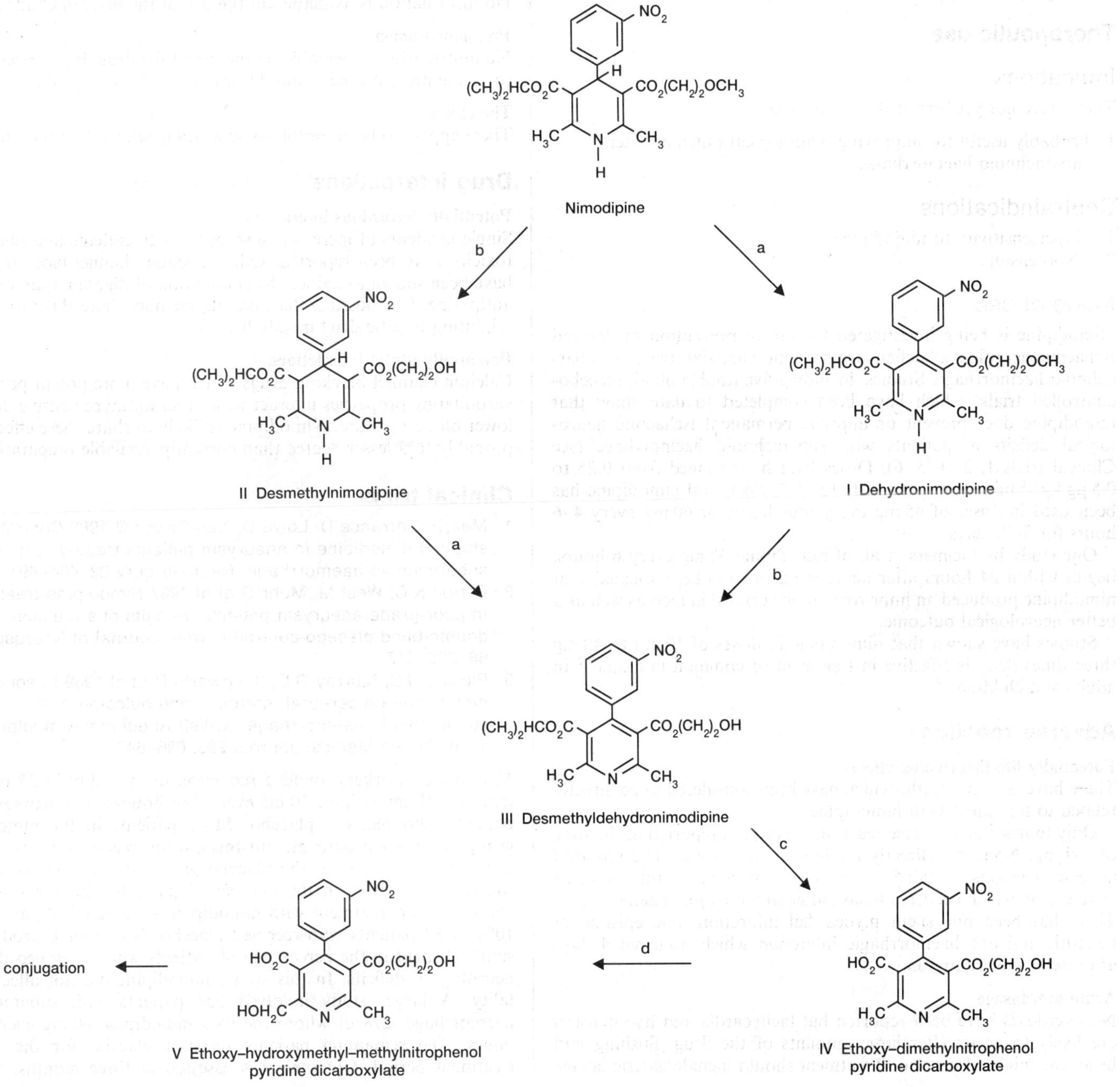

Oral absorption	53%
Presystemic metabolism	80%
Plasma half life	
range	1.1–5.7 h[15,17]
mean	8–9 h[19]
Volume of distribution	0.9–2.3 l.kg^{-1}
Plasma protein binding	95%

Concentration–effect relationship

There is no evidence of any relationship between the plasma concentration of nimodipine and its therapeutic effects.

Metabolism

The major routes of nimodipine metabolism are demethylation of the ethoxymethoxy ether, dehydrogenation to the pyridine analogue III, cleavage of the ester groups by hydrolysis to carboxylic acids and hydroxylation of the methyl groups with subsequent glucuronide conjugation[19] (Fig. 1). Only the demethylated dihydropyridine analogue metabolite was active, but its activity was 20 times lower than that of nimodipine.[20,21]

N

Administration of nimodipine 60 mg orally produces a peak plasma concentration of approximately 20 $\mu g.l^{-1}$ at approximately 30 minutes after drug administration. In contrast, metabolite III has a peak plasma concentration of nearly 100 $\mu g.l^{-1}$ at approximately 45 minutes after drug administration. The peak plasma concentration of metabolite II is approximately 50 $\mu g.l^{-1}$ whereas that of metabolite I is approximately 20 $\mu g.l^{-1}$. Therefore, the area under the plasma concentration–time curve is greatest for metabolite III which is still measurable at approximately 5 $\mu g.l^{-1}$ 8 hours after drug administration. Measurable concentrations of metabolite II are present 5 hours after administration, but not at 8 hours, and metabolite I is gone within 3 hours after drug administration.[17]

Pharmaceutics

1. Nimodipine is available in the USA as 30 mg capsules (Nimotop; Miles, USA).
   In the UK the 30 mg strength is available as a yellow, film-coated tablet (Nimotop; Bayer, UK).
2. Nimodipine (Nimotop; Bayer, UK) is also available in a solution (10 mg per 50 ml) for intravenous use. The formulation of the intravenous solution includes 15–17% polyethylene glycol (macrogol) 400 and 20% ethanol. It should be administered via an infusion pump through a Y-piece into a central catheter. It is incompatible with PVC giving sets. Polyethylene or polypropylene apparatus should therefore be used.

Therapeutic use

Indications

These have not yet been firmly established.

1. Probably useful for improving neurological outcome after subarachnoid haemorrhage.

Contraindications

1. Hypersensitivity to nimodipine
2. Hypotension.

Mode of use

Nimodipine is being investigated for use in prevention of delayed ischaemic neurological deficits from cerebral arterial spasm in subarachnoid haemorrhage. Studies, including five double-blind, placebo-controlled trials, which have been completed to date show that nimodipine does prevent or improve permanent ischaemic neurological deficits in patients with subarachnoid haemorrhage (see Clinical trials 1, 2, 4, 5, 6). Doses used have ranged from 0.25 to 0.5 $\mu g.kg^{-1}.min^{-1}$ intravenously for 5–7 days; oral nimodipine has been used in doses of 45 mg every four hours or 60 mg every 4–6 hours for 3–21 days.

One study by Gelmers et al. of nimodipine 30 mg every 6 hours, begun within 24 hours after acute ischaemic stroke, indicated that nimodipine produced an improvement in survival in men as well as a better neurological outcome.

Studies have shown that nimodipine in doses of 10 mg to 40 mg three times daily is effective in treatment of common migraine[22] in adults and children.[24]

Adverse reactions

Potentially life-threatening effects

There have been no deaths which have been considered to be directly related to treatment with nimodipine.

Only four serious adverse reactions have been reported at the time of writing. None has directly implicated nimodipine. The reported adverse reactions included one case of disseminated intravascular coagulation which occurred 8 days after subarachnoid haemorrhage. There has been one silent myocardial infarction, one episode of hepatitis and one haemorrhagic infarction which occurred 4 days after ischaemic infarction.

Acute overdosage

No overdoses have been reported but tachycardia and hypotension are likely to occur after large amounts of the drug; flushing and headache might also occur. Treatment should include gastric lavage with charcoal. Hypotension can be managed with pressor agents in addition to other supportive measures such as proper positioning and fluid infusion.

Severe or irreversible adverse effects

There have been no severe or irreversible effects other than those described above.

Symptomatic adverse effects

Adverse experiences have been reported in 32.3% of one series of patients. The most frequent complaints have been headache (5%), muscle pain (4%), dizziness (4%), nausea (4%), gastrointestinal symptoms (4%), fatigue (3%), joint pain (2%), flushing (2%), decreased blood pressure (2%), rash (2%) and constipation (2%).

Interference with clinical pathology tests

No interferences of this kind appear to have been reported.

High risk groups

Neonates

No information is available on the use of the drug in neonates.

Breast milk. No information is available on the secretion of nimodipine in breast milk, so women taking the drug should not breast-feed.

Children

No information is available on the use of the drug in children.

Pregnant women

No information is available on the use of the drug during pregnancy, so at the present time it should not be given to pregnant women.

The elderly

There appear to be no problems specifically related to elderly patients.

Drug interactions

Potentially hazardous interactions

Single incidents of increased susceptibility to caffeine and phenytoin toxicity have been reported. Other calcium channel-blocking drugs have been shown to reduce the elimination of digoxin, quinidine and antipyrine. It is possible that nimodipine may share this property of inhibiting hepatic drug metabolism.

Potentially useful interactions

Calcium channel blocking drugs which have more potent peripheral vasodilating properties interact with other antihypertensive drugs to lower blood pressure. Nimodipine is likely to share these effects, but probably to a lesser degree than currently available preparations.

Clinical trials

1. Mee E, Dorrance D, Lowe D, Neil-Dwyer G 1988 Controlled study of nimodipine in aneurysm patients treated early after subarachnoid haemorrhage. Neurosurgery 22: 484–491
2. Petruc K C, West M, Mohr G et al 1987 Nimodipine treatment in poor-grade aneurysm patients. Results of a multicenter double-blind placebo-controlled trial. Journal of Neurosurgery 68: 505–517
3. Pickard J D, Murray G D, Illingworth R et al 1989 Effect of oral nimodipine on cerebral infarction and outcome after subarachnoid haemorrhage: British Aneurysm Nimodipine Trial. British Medical Journal 298: 636–642

Mee and co-workers found a reduction in mortality in 25 patients treated with nimodipine 60 mg every four hours in comparison to 25 patients who received placebo. More patients in the nimodipine group had a good outcome but this did not reach statistical significance in comparison to the placebo group. Petruc and co-workers showed an increase in the number of patients who made a good recovery after treatment with nimodipine — 29% of 72 patients vs. 10% of 82 patients who received placebo. Nimodipine produced a similar benefit in the percentage of patients who developed delayed neurological deficits. In this study, nimodipine did not affect mortality. A larger study involved 554 patients with subarachnoid haemorrhage, 278 of whom received nimodipine 60 mg every four hours. The remaining patients received placebo for the 21-day treatment period. Outcome was assessed at three months. In this study, the number of patients who were judged to have had a poor outcome was again significantly reduced by nimodipine — 55 compared to 91 patients. Additionally, nimodipine reduced the incidence of cerebral infarction from 92 patients in the placebo group to 61 patients in the nimodipine group.

4. Tettenborn D, Porto L, Ryman T, Strugo V, Taquoi G, Battye R 1987 Survey of clinical experience with nimodipine in patients with subarachnoid haemorrhage. Neuorsurgery Review 10: 77–84
5. Neil-Dwyer G, Mee E, Dorrance D, Lowe D 1987 Early intervention with nimodipine in subarachnoid haemorrhage. European Heart Journal 8 (suppl K): 41–47
6. Phillipon J, Grob R, Dagreou F, Guggiari M, Rivierez M, Viars P 1986 Prevention of vasospasm in subarachnoid haemorrhage. A controlled study with nimodipine. Acta Neurochirurgia 82: 110–114
7. Gelmers H J, Gorter K, de Weerdt C J, Wiezer H J 1988 A controlled trial of nimodpipine in acute ischemic stroke. New England Journal of Medicine 318: 203–207
8. Trust study group 1990 Randomised double-blind, placebo controlled trial of nimodipine in acute stroke. Lancet 336: 1205–1209

Oral nimodipine, 120 mg daily was compared with placebo in 1215 patients who had suffered an acute stroke within the past 48 h. At 6 months 55% of the nimodipine group and 58% of the placebo group were living independently. The nimodipine group had a slightly higher mortality than the placebo group (29% dead at 24 weeks versus 25%).

The results do not support any beneficial effect of nimodipine in acute stroke.

References

1. Scriabine A, Battye R, Hoffmeister F et al 1985 Nimodipine. New Drugs Annual: Cardiovascular Drugs 3: 197–218
2. Towart R, Kazda S 1979 The cellular mechanism of action of nimodipine (BAY e 9736), a new calcium antagonist. British Journal of Pharmacology 67: 409–410
3. Schmidt J, Santillan G G, Saeed M, Dalmieri D, Bing P J 1985 The effect of nimodipine, a calcium antagonist on intracortical arterioles in the cat brain. Current Therapeutic Research 38: 94–103
4. Tanaka K, Gotoh F, Muramatsu F et al 1980 Effects of nimodipine (BAYe9736) on cerebral circulation in cats. Arzneimittel-Forschung 30: 1494–1497
5. Towart R, Kazda S 1985 Effects of calcium antagonist nimodipine on isolated cerebral vessels. In: Betz et al (eds) Nimodipine: pharmacological and clinical properties. Schattauer Verlag, Stuttgart, pp 147–161
6. Towart R 1981 The selective inhibition of serotonin-induced contractions of rabbit cerebral vascular smooth muscle by calcium antagonistic dihydropyridines. Circulation Research 48: 650–657
7. Towart R, Perzborn E 1981 Nimodipine inhibits carbocyclic-induced contractions of cerebral arteries. European Journal of Pharmacology 69: 213–215
8. Towart R 1981 Predilective relaxation by the calcium antagonist nimodipine (BAY e9736) of cerebral blood vessels, contracted with autologous blood. British Journal of Pharmacology 74: 268–269
9. Andersson K E, Edvinsson L, MacKenzie E T, Skarby T, Young A R 1983 Influence of extra-cellular calcium and calcium agonists on contractions induced by potassium and prostaglandin $F_2\alpha$ in isolated cerebral and mesenteric arteries of the cat. British Journal of Pharmacology 79: 135–140
10. Muller-Schweinitzer E, Neumann P 1983 In vitro effects of calcium antagonists PN200-110, nifedipine, and nimodipine on human and canine cerebral arteries. Journal of Cerebral Blood Flow and Metabolism 3: 354–361
11. Brandt L, Andersson K E, Edvinsson L, Ljunggren B 1981 Effects of extracellular calcium and of calcium antagonists on the contractile responses of isolated human pial and mesenteric arteries. Journal of Cerebral Blood Flow and Metabolism 1: 339–347
12. Newberg L A, Steen P A, Milde J H, Gisvold S E, Lanier W L 1984 Effects of nimodipine on cerebral blood flow and neurologic function following complete global ischemia in dogs and primates. In: First International Nimotop Symposium. Schattauer Verlag, Stuttgart
13. Kazda S, Garthoff B, Krause H P, Schlossmann K 1982 Cerebrovascular effects of the calcium antagonistic dihydropyridine derivative nimodipine in animal experiments. Arzneimittel Forschung 32: 331–338
14. Tettenborn D, Dycka J, Volberg E, Dudden P 1985 Blood pressure and heart rate during treatment with nimodipine in patients with subarachnoid hemorrhage. Neurochirurgia 28: 84–86
15. Gengo F M, Fagan S C, Krol G, Bernhard H 1987 Nimodipine disposition and haemodynamic effects in patients with cirrhosis and age-matched controls. British Journal of Clinical Pharmacology 23: 47–53
16. Ramsch K D, Ahr G, Tettenborn D, Auer L M 1985 Overview on pharmacokinetics of nimodipine in healthy volunteers and in patients with subarachnoid hemorrhage. Neurochirurgia 28: 74–78
17. Ramsch K, Graefe K H, Scherling D, Sommer J, Ziegler R 1986 Pharmacokinetics and metabolism of calcium-blocking agents nifedipine, nitrendipine and nimodipine. American Journal of Nephrology 6 (suppl 1): 73–80

Nimodipine

18. Suwelack D, Weber H 1985 Assessment of enterohepatic circulation of radioactivity following a single dose of ^{14}C nimodipine in the rat. European Journal of Drug Metabolism and Pharmacokinetics 10: 231–239
19. Data on File, Miles Pharmaceuticals, West Haven, Ct
20. Ramsch K D, Graefe K H, Scherling D, Sommer J, Ziegler R 1986 Pharmacokinetics and metabolism of calcium blocking agents nifedipine, nitrendipine and nimodipine. American Journal of Nephrology 6: 73–89
21. Meyer H, Wehinger E, Bosserk F, Scherling D 1983 Nimodipine: synthesis and metabolic pathway. Arzneimittel-Forschung 33(1): 106–112
22. Jonsdottir M, Meyer J S, Rogers R L 1987 Efficacy, side effects and tolerance compared during headache treatment with three different calcium blockers. Headache 27: 364–369
23. Langley M S, Sorkin F M 1989 Nimodipine: a review of its pharmacodynamic and pharmacokinetic properties and therapeutic potential in cerebrovascular disease. Drugs 37: 669–699
24. Battistella P A, Ruffill R, Moro R, Fabiani M, Bertok S, Antolini A, Zacchello F 1990 A placebo-controlled crossover trial of nimodipine in paediatric migraine. Headache 30: 264–268

N

Nitrazepam

Nitrazepam was the first benzodiazepine hypnotic to be widely used in Europe. It was never introduced to the USA.

Chemistry

Nitrazepam (Mogadon, Nitrados, Noctesed, Somnite, Remnos, Surem, Unisomnia). Generic equivalents available.
$C_{15}H_{11}N_3O_3$
1,3-Dihydro-7-nitro-5-phenyl-2H-1,4-benzodiazepin-2-one

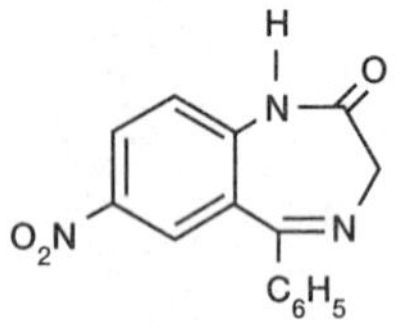

Molecular weight	281.3
pKa	3.2, 10.8
Solubility	
in alcohol	1 in 120
in water	<1 in 10 000
Octanol/water partition coefficient	125

A yellow, odourless, tasteless crystalline powder. It is not available in combination preparations.

Pharmacology

Nitrazepam is a typical benzodiazepine. It binds to benzodiazepine receptors in the brain, thereby potentiating the inhibitory actions of gamma aminobutyric acid (GABA) in the spinal cord, brain stem, cerebellum, limbic system and cerebral cortex. The potentiation of GABA inhibition diminishes the activity in ascending activating systems, particularly noradrenergic and serotonergic pathways from brain stem and mid-brain to the cerebral cortex. Sedation and muscle relaxant actions are typical of benzodiazepines and nitrazepam has also powerful anticonvulsant effects.

Toxicology

As with other benzodiazepines, the toxicology of nitrazepam is low. The LD_{50} in animal species is far beyond the psychoactive doses giving an extremely high therapeutic index. There is no evidence of carcinogenicity or teratogenicity.

Clinical pharmacology

Nitrazepam has useful sedative properties, allaying anxiety and inducing sleep. At moderate doses nitrazepam probably promotes sleep by a tranquillizing effect, lessening sensory input and emotional arousal. At higher doses, a direct depressant effect supervenes lessening the activity of the arousal centres of the brain.

Doses of 5–10 mg by mouth induce sleep within 15–30 minutes. Nitrazepam delays the first appearance of REM sleep during the night, reduces whole-night duration of REM sleep, shortens the delay of sleep onset, reduces the time spent in stage 1 (drowsiness) during the night, reduces restless movements at night, and lessens time spent in the deep stages of sleep (3 and 4; slow-wave sleep).[1–3] Thus, most of the night is spent in stage 2 sleep. The effects of nitrazepam on sleep architecture are dose-related.

Nitrazepam lessens the 'bizarreness' of dreams during its administration, followed by increased bizarreness during withdrawal.

Because of the relatively long elimination half life, residual effects are detectable the next day.[4] These residual effects comprise impairment of psychomotor ability, cognitive functions and memory and a subjective feeling of drowsiness and lightheadedness. The effects generally wane during the day.

'Rebound' occurs when nitrazepam is discontinued. For example, withdrawal after two weeks of drug administration each night caused abnormalities of longer paradoxical (REM) sleep and its earlier onset during the night.[5] It took 4 weeks for the rebound phenomena to disappear.

Nitrazepam's anticonvulsant properties are important in the treatment of some forms of childhood epilepsy.

Pharmacokinetics

The usual method of analysis is by gas–liquid chromatography, with electron capture detection.[6,7] The limit of detection is 1 μg.l^{-1}.

Nitrazepam is readily absorbed from the gastrointestinal tract with a rapid entry to the brain. The α-redistribution phase is fairly short, the decline in plasma concentrations being biphasic.[8] The time to peak concentration is 0.5–4 h. Bioavailability is high.

The half life of elimination after intravenous injection is 22.9–30.8 h (mean 26.6 h)[9] and after oral administration is 20–48 h (mean 30.7 h).[10] Maximum plasma concentrations after oral administration,[8] reached after 81 (45–240) min, are 37 (28–45) μg.l^{-1}.

Steady-state concentrations are reached after 4 days. Nitrazepam does not induce its own metabolism.

The plasma half life of nitrazepam averaged 24 hours in 25 healthy subjects aged 21 to 38 years who took nitrazepam 5 mg daily for 14 days and 40 hours in 12 hospitalized patients aged 66–89 years who took this dosage for 2 months. Peak plasma concentrations were 40 and 22 μg.l^{-1} in young and old, respectively and volumes of distribution were 2.4 and 4.8 l.kg^{-1}, respectively.[11] Penetration to and elimination from CSF is relatively slow.

Traces are found in breast milk and nitrazepam crosses the placenta quite readily reaching fetal concentrations similar to those in the maternal plasma, in late pregnancy.

The drug is extensively metabolized in the liver, with <4% of the dose excreted unchanged. Metabolites are excreted in the urine and about 20% of an oral dose is found in the faeces.

Oral absorption	95%
Presystemic metabolism	6–47%
Plasma half life	
range	20–48 h
mean	25 h
Volume of distribution	1.8–4.7 l.kg^{-1}
Plasma protein binding	87%

It is to be expected that the half life will be prolonged in liver disease, and adjustment of dose may be necessary. It has been shown that clearance of unbound nitrazepam is reduced in cirrhosis. Renal dysfunction alone is unlikely to affect the pharmacokinetics of nitrazepam.

Concentration–effect relationship

No 'therapeutic range' has been established.

Metabolism

Metabolism is mainly by reduction of the nitro group to the corresponding amine, which is psychotropically inactive. Further metabolism by acetylation leads to the major metabolite, the 7-acetamido derivative. This reaction has been reported to be polymorphic. Hydroxylation in the 3 position also occurs, yielding both the hydroxylated amide and acetamido compounds, both minor metabolites (Fig. 1). Cleavage of the benzodiazepine ring also occurs (Fig. 2), to form after hydroxylation, 2-amino-3-hydroxy-5-nitrobenzophenone. Only the parent nitrazepam is active.[12]

Pharmaceutics

Nitrazepam is available as Mogadon (Roche, UK) as round white tablets with Roche and two semicircles imprinted on one side and a single score line on the other. Each tablet contains 5 mg of nitrazepam. Many generic equivalents are available in Europe.

Mogadon capsules (5 mg) are black/purple with 'Roche' printed in red/brown.

Nitrazepam suspension Somnite (Norgine, UK) contains 2.5 mg per 5 ml. Diluted with syrup it has a shelf-life of 14 days. Suspensions of crushed tablets turn black on exposure to light, unless specially formulated.

Nitrazepam is not available in the USA.

Therapeutic use

Indications

1. Insomnia where daytime sedation is acceptable
2. Some forms of epilepsy.

Contraindications

Sensitivity to benzodiazepines.

Mode of use

Treatment of insomnia is usually initiated with a dose of 5 mg at night although 2.5 mg is more appropriate in the elderly. The dose may be increased to 10 mg at night if insomnia is severe. Further dosage increases suggest that tolerance is supervening and should be avoided. Intermittent use for a few nights at a time may help avoid tolerance. Another strategem is to hold off from taking the hypnotic until it seems evident that a sleepless night is in the offing.

The dosage for the treatment of the following forms of epilepsy must be more flexible and often higher than that for insomnia.

1. Myoclonic seizures
2. Lennox syndrome
3. Infantile spasms (West syndrome)
4. Grand mal during sleep.

Children should be treated with half-doses.

Fig. 1 Metabolism of nitrazepam

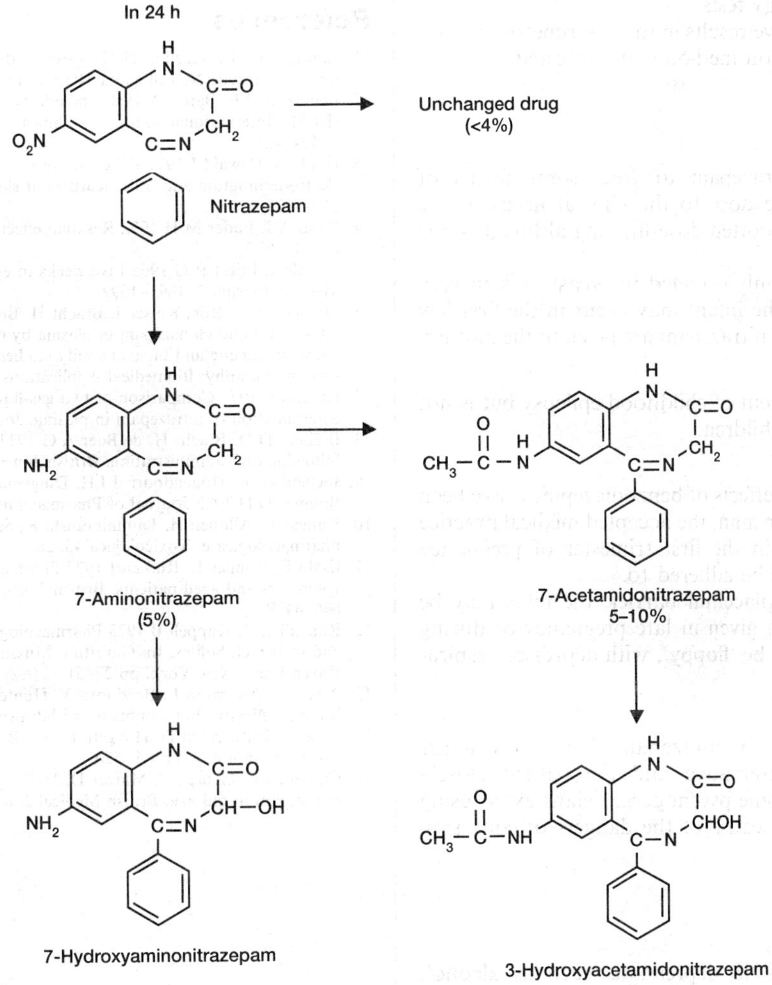

Nitrazepam

Fig. 2 Products of cleavage of benzodiazepine ring

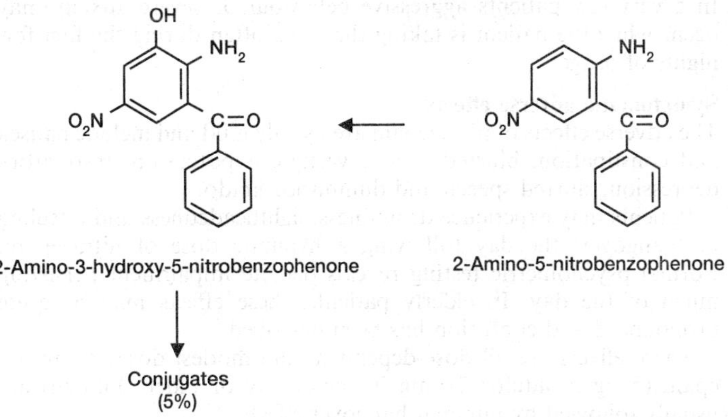

Adverse reactions

Potentially life-threatening effects
Apart from acute anaphylactic reactions in some patients with sensitivity to benzodiazepines serious adverse effects are almost unknown.

Acute overdosage
As with other benzodiazepines, it is unusual for overdoses to be fatal. The patient typically sleeps for 24–48 hours but is usually rousable. Less severe cases present with dysarthria, ataxia and drowsiness. Treatment of overdose is symptomatic and supportive.

Severe or irreversible adverse effects
In a very few patients aggressive behaviour or severe anxiety may occur while the patient is taking the drug, often during the first few nights of usage.

Symptomatic adverse effects
The adverse effects of nitrazepam are usually mild and include nausea and constipation, blurred vision, vertigo, hypotension, respiratory depression, slurred speech and diminished libido.

Patients may experience drowsiness, lightheadedness and a feeling of 'hangover' the day following a hypnotic dose of nitrazepam. Formal psychometric testing reveals definite impairment persisting much of the day. In elderly patients, these effects may be quite pronounced and confusion has been described.

These effects are all dose-dependent and modest doses of nitrazepam (5 mg in adults; 2.5 mg in the elderly or older children) are usually followed by minimal hangover effects.

Other effects

Rebound and withdrawal. As with most other benzodiazepine hypnotics, regular nightly use is followed by rebound insomnia on withdrawal.[13] Rebound with nitrazepam usually occurs 3–5 nights after discontinuation with a prolongation of time to fall asleep, disturbed sleep, and reduced total sleep time.

Longer periods of use may be attended by a withdrawal syndrome on cessation of the nitrazepam. Withdrawal symptoms may be seen after as little as six weeks therapy.[14] As well as rebound insomnia, anxiety and tension, the patient may experience perceptual phenomena such as photophobia and hyperacusis. The management of such problems is similar to that of other benzodiazepines such as diazepam. Gradual tapering of the dose with adequate psychological support is essential. It is better, however, to prevent the onset of dependence by avoiding the use of nitrazepam as much as possible and reserving its use for the intermittent relief of severe insomnia. Indeed, in view of the 'hangover' effects, accumulation especially in the elderly,[15] and the risk of rebound and withdrawal syndromes, it is doubtful if nitrazepam has any place in modern therapeutics.

Interference with clinical pathology tests
Nitrazepam may give false positive results in the colorimetric method of Baer,[16] although the Broughton method is not affected.[17]

High risk groups

Neonates
Paediatric neurologists use nitrazepam to treat some forms of infantile epilepsy and adjust the dose to the clinical needs of the patient. Nevertheless, sedation is often dose-limiting although some tolerance does occur.

Breast milk. Nitrazepam is only excreted in breast milk in very small amounts but sedation of the infant may occur in the first few days post partum if high doses of nitrazepam are given to the mother.

Children
Nitrazepam is used in the treatment of childhood epilepsy but is not recommended as a hypnotic in children.

Pregnant women
Although no definite teratogenic effects of benzodiazepines have been demonstrated either in animals or man, the accepted medical practice of only prescribing medication in the first trimester of pregnancy when absolutely essential should be adhered to.

As benzodiazepines pass the placental barrier, the fetus may be adversely affected by nitrazepam given in late pregnancy or during labour. The new-born baby may be 'floppy', with depressed respiration and failure to feed actively.

The elderly
The elderly are more sensitive to nitrazepam than are younger adults.[15] Dosage must be conservative and the patient closely observed for signs of toxicity. Some psychogeriatricians avoid using benzodiazepines in the elderly because of the dangers of confusion and ataxia.

Drug interactions

Potentially hazardous interactions
Nitrazepam potentiates other CNS depressants such as alcohol, barbiturates, sedative antidepressants and antihistamines, and antipsychotic drugs.

Other significant interactions
Antacids may delay the absorption of benzodiazepines. Metabolic interactions, for example with cimetidine, do not seem to be of clinical significance.

Major outcome trial

Oswald I, French C, Adam K, Gilham J 1982 Benzodiazepine hypnotics remain effective for 24 weeks. British Medical Journal 284: 860–863

97 poor sleepers aged 40–68 years took medication nightly for 32 weeks and filled out rating scales of quality of sleep, time to fall asleep, hangover effects and daytime anxiety. Nitrazepam 5 mg appeared to be still improving sleep after 24 weeks of intake when compared with continuous placebo intake. There was even some tendency for the ratings of quality of sleep to gradually improve on nitrazepam 5 mg but to remain unchanged on placebo. After withdrawal, rebound occurred so that for 2 or 3 weeks quality of sleep and sleep latency were significantly worse than baseline values. The impairment was most marked on the fourth night after withdrawal of nitrazepam.

Other trial

Hindmarch I 1977 A repeated dose comparison of three benzodiazepine derivatives (nitrazepam, flurazepam and flunitrazepam) on subjective appraisals of sleep and measures of psychomotor performance the morning following night-time medication. Acta Psychiatrica Scandinavica 56: 373–381

Repeated doses of 5 mg nitrazepam improved subjective perceptions of quality of sleep in 30 healthy volunteers. However, subjects also perceived difficulty in awakening from sleep the morning after medication. Some mental tests such as serial sevens were affected but psychomotor performance seemed unimpaired.

References

1. Lob I, Papy J J, Gastaut H 1966 Action du Ro 4-5360 (Mogadon) sur le sommeil nocturne. Revue Neurologique (Paris) 115: 545–546
2. Lehmann H E, Ban T A 1968 The effects of hypnotics on rapid eye movement (REM). International Journal of Clinical Pharmacology Therapy and Toxicology 5: 424–427
3. Haider I, Oswald I 1971 Effects of amylobarbitone and nitrazepam on the electrodermogram and other features of sleep. British Journal of Psychiatry 118: 519–522
4. Bond A J, Lader M H 1972 Residual effects of hypnotics. Psychopharmacologia 25: 117–132
5. Oswald I, Priest R G 1965 Five weeks to escape the sleeping-pill habit. British Medical Journal 2: 1093–1099
6. De Boer A G, Röst-Kaiser J, Bracht H, Breimer D D 1978 Assay of underivatized nitrazepam and clonazepam in plasma by capillary gas chromatography applied to pharmacokinetic and bioavailability studies in humans. Journal of Chromatography: Biomedical Applications 245: 105–114
7. Kangas L 1977 Comparison of two gas-liquid chromatographic methods for the determination of nitrazepam in plasma. Journal of Chromatography 136: 259
8. Breimer D D, Bracht H, de Boer A G 1977 Plasma level profile of nitrazepam following oral administration. British Journal of Clinical Pharmacology 4: 709
9. Jochemsen R, Hogendoorn J J H, Dingemans J, Hermans J, Boeijinga J K, Breimer D D 1982 Journal of Pharmacokinetics and Biopharmaceutics 10: 231
10. Kangas L, Allonen H, Lammintausta R, Salonen M, Pekkarinen A 1979 Acta Pharmacologica et Toxicologica 45: 20
11. Iisalo E, Kangas L, Ruikka I 1977 Pharmacokinetics of nitrazepam in young volunteers and aged patients. British Journal of Clinical Pharmacology 4: 646–647P
12. Randall L O, Kappell B 1973 Pharmacological activity of some benzodiazepines and their metabolites. In: Garattini, Mussini, Randall (eds) The Benzodiazepines. Raven Press, New York, pp 27–51
13. Adam K, Adamson L, Brezinova V, Hunter W M, Oswald I 1976 Nitrazepam: lastingly effective but trouble on withdrawal. British Medical Journal 1: 1558–1560
14. Tyrer P, Rutherford D, Huggett T 1981 Benzodiazepine withdrawal symptoms and propranolol. Lancet 1: 520
15. Castleden C, George C, Marcer D, Hallett C 1977 Increased sensitivity to nitrazepam in old age. British Medical Journal 1: 10–12

Nitrofurantoin

A semisynthetic antibacterial agent. One of many 5-nitrofurans, effective for the treatment and prophylaxis of urinary infections.

Chemistry

Nitrofurantoin microcrystals (Furadantin, Furadantine, Furadan)
Nitrofurantoin macrocrystals (Macrodantin, Furadantin macrocrystals, Furadantine macrocrystals, Furadantin retard, Furadan macrocrystals, Furadantina macrocrystals)
Nitrofurantoin sodium (Ivadantin)
$C_8H_6N_4O_5$
1-[(5-Nitro-2-furfurylidine)amino]hydantoin

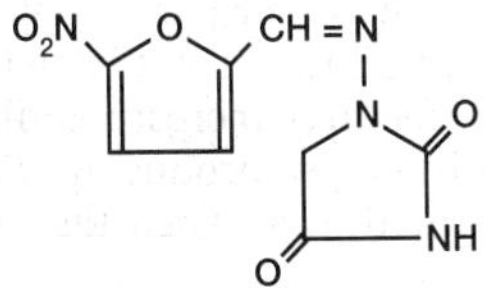

Molecular weight	238.2
pKa (acidic)	7.0
Solubility	
in alcohol	1 in 1960
in water (sodium salt)	1 in 440 (1 in 20)
Octanol/water partition coefficient	—

Yellow, odourless crystals or powder with a bitter taste, discoloured by exposure to light,[1] synthesized from furfural derived from pentosans obtained from bran, oat husks and corncobs.

The macrocrystals are absorbed and excreted more slowly and are less bioavailable than the micro-form, but urinary levels are sufficient and treatment is effective. They may be tolerated by those who suffer from gastrointestinal symptoms resulting from treatment with the microcrystals.[2]

Nitrofurantoin is more soluble in urine than in water due to the presence of urea and creatinine in the former. As a consequence, crystalluria is not a problem, despite high urine levels of the drug.[3]

Pharmacology

Nitrofurantoin is active against most common causes of urinary tract infection, especially *E. coli* but also Gram-positive cocci, including *Strep. faecalis* and *Staph. saprophyticus*. *Salmonella*, *Shigella* and anaerobes, including *Bacteroides fragilis*, are also sensitive. Bacteria naturally resistant include all *Pseudomonas* and some strains of *Klebsiella–Aerobacter*. The minimal inhibitory concentration (MIC) of fully sensitive species is 0.4–10.0 $mg.l^{-1}$. *Klebsiella–Aerobacter* are less sensitive, with an MIC of 50 $mg.l^{-1}$, but treatment of acute infection usually succeeds. *Proteus* species are more resistant, with MIC values of about 100 $mg.l^{-1}$ and the urease which they produce makes the urine highly alkaline, reducing antibacterial activity. Thus nitrofurantoin is not suitable for the treatment of acute *Proteus* infection.[4]

The antibacterial action is normally inhibitory at concentrations near the MIC and bactericidal at concentrations little higher than this, especially in acid solution.

There is no cross-resistance with other important antibacterial agents.

Resistance is chromosomal and is much less common than resistance to antibacterial agents acquired by R-factor transduction. This is a distinct advantage, especially in the treatment of hospital patients. The mode of antibacterial action is still poorly understood. Reduction of nitrofurantoin to unstable metabolites within the bacterial cell leads to fracture of DNA strands.[5] *E. coli* contains three distinct nitrofuran reductases and loss of one of these will confer resistance on some strains.[6]

Toxicology

Because of their effect on DNA, nitrofurans are radiometic, mutagenic and can both induce and inhibit experimental oncogenesis.[7] Nitrofurantoin is toxic for hamster ovarian cells.[8] In doses near those used in man, however, tests, including long-term studies of carcinogenicity, have not revealed toxicity in animals. Moreover, after more than 30 years of use in the treatment of urinary tract infection, no data have been presented to associate nitrofurantoin with human cancer.

Clinical pharmacology

The beneficial action of nitrofurantoin is its inhibitory and killing power on bacteria in urine. Because of low serum levels tissue concentrations were believed to be too low to kill most sensitive bacteria in the kidney. However, tissue levels bactericidal for urinary pathogens have now been found in normal human kidneys.[9] Nitrofurantoin is undoubtedly an effective urinary antiseptic; its role in pyelonephritis is, at present, unproven.

Pharmacokinetics

Until recently, the preferred analytical method for the determination of nitrofurantoin in body fluids was the nitromethane–hyamine method.[10] However, it is by no means certain that all drug estimated in this way is biologically active. Methods employing bacteria have also been used.[11] More recently, a method utilizing high pressure liquid chromatography with UV detection, providing a limit of detection of 20 $\mu g.l^{-1}$, has been reported.[12]

Following oral administration, nitrofurantoin is rapidly and almost completely absorbed, achieving peak plasma concentrations after about 1–4 h in fasting subjects. The systemic bioavailability is almost 100%, with no first-pass metabolism. Elimination is rapid, with a mean half life of only 0.3–1 h.

Nitrofurantoin is rapidly distributed throughout the body, with an apparent volume of distribution of only 0.6 $l.kg^{-1}$. Binding of the drug to plasma proteins is moderately high (60–77%). Plasma levels of the drug do not exceed 2.0 $mg.l^{-1}$ on normal doses.

Oral absorption	95%
Presystemic metabolism	negligible
Plasma half life	
range	0.3–1 h
mean	0.75 h
Volume of distribution	0.6 $l.kg^{-1}$
Plasma protein binding	60–77%

Nitrofurantoin is rapidly and extensively excreted in urine,[1] both by filtration and by tubular secretion with 40% of the unchanged drug eliminated in 24 h. Urine levels are 15–46 $mg.l^{-1}$, and a concentration above the MIC for most sensitive organisms can be detected for about 6 h.[4]

Following conventional oral doses insignificant concentrations of nitrofurantoin are found in breast milk,[13] as might be expected from its poor lipid solubility. Penetration into amniotic fluid is negligible and concentrations in cord blood are lower than in maternal blood.[14]

The excretion of nitrofurantoin in urine is linearly related to creatinine clearance, so that in patients with impaired glomerular function the concentration of the drug in the glomerular filtrate may fall below a suitable therapeutic level, yet the plasma concentration may increase to levels at which systemic toxicity occurs. The renal tubular excretion of nitrofurantoin is inhibited by uricosuric drugs such as probenicid and sulphinpyrazone, due to competition for the acid secretory system, increasing the plasma concentration of the drug. The effect of old age on the pharmacokinetics of nitrofurantoin have not been reported, but it is likely that its elimination will decrease with decreasing renal function in such subjects.

N

Concentration–effect relationship

The therapeutic effect of nitrofurantoin is independent of its concentrations in blood, which are clinically insignificant.

Metabolism

Considerable amounts of nitrofurantoin are excreted unchanged in the urine (⩽40% of the dose). There is also substantial excretion in the bile, although the unchanged drug is only occasionally found in faeces.

Some nitrofurantoin is reduced to aminofurantoin in several tissues including liver and by the intestinal microflora. The amount of this metabolite excreted in the urine is approx. 17% of the dose (Fig. 1).

Fig. 1 Metabolism of nitrofurantoin

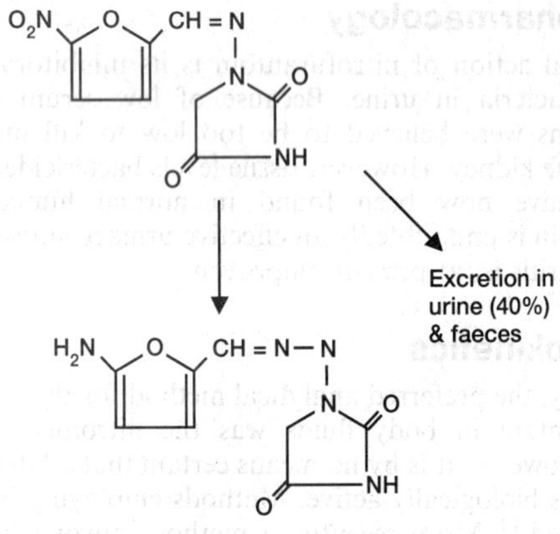

Pharmaceutics

Nitrofurantoin is available in oral form.

1. Furadantin (Norwich Eaton, UK, USA) tablets: contain 50 mg or 100 mg. They are yellow, slightly convex, pentagonal, bearing a 50 or 100 monogram on one face and a single break-line on the other. They contain the microcrystal form of the drug and cornstarch. A number of generic equivalents are available.
2. Macrodantin (Norwich Eaton, UK, USA) capsules: are yellow/white and contain either 50 or 100 mg of the macrocrystal form. They are labelled 'Macro 50' or 'Macro 100' on one half and 'Dantin 50' or 'Dantin 100' on the other. They also contain cornstarch and lactose.
3. Furadantin suspension: yellow, flavoured carboxymethylcellulos suspension contains 5 mg.ml^{-1}, using nitrofurantoin microcrystal form. It contains parabens but is sugar-free.

The tablets and capsules should be stored in light-proof containers.
The suspension should also be protected from light.
The maximum shelf-life for all three preparations is 3 years.

Therapeutic use

Indications

1. Infection
2. Prophylaxis.

Contraindications

1. Neonates
2. Anuria, oliguria and renal failure.

Indications

1. Infection
Urinary tract infection caused by bacteria sensitive to nitrofurantoin: cystitis, pyelitis, pyelonephritis, postoperative infection.

2. Prophylaxis
Prophylaxis during catheterization or instrumentation of the urinary tract. Prevention in those liable to recurrent urinary tract infection.

Contraindications

1. Neonates
Infants less than 1 month old should not receive nitrofurantoin since haemolytic anaemia is more likely to develop in patients with immature glucose-6-phospate dehydrogenase activity.[15]

2. Anuria, oliguria and renal failure
Patients suffering from anuria or marked oliguria or those suspected of renal failure (creatinine clearance less than 60 ml.min^{-1} and/or increased serum creatinine) should not receive nitrofurantoin because urinary concentration sufficient for cure is uncertain and there is a danger of polyneuropathy.[15]

Mode of use

Acute infection
Nitrofurantoin is not regarded as a drug of choice in the absence of laboratory sensitivity tests. It is, however, a drug of first choice for testing. When other treatment has failed and Gram-positive cocci are a likely cause of infection it should be given. A course of treatment, 50–100 mg by mouth four times daily for 7–10 d, is indicated. The dose should be given with food or immediately after meals to avoid gastric intolerance, the last dose just before bedtime, in order to maintain a high level of drug in the urine which will prevent bacterial growth in the bladder during the night. The patient should drink copiously to maintain a brisk urinary flow. Fluid intake is very unlikely to be sufficient to dilute the antibacterial effect significantly.

Acidification of the urine may increase antibacterial activity. This will be impossible with urease-producing *Proteus* infection, and treatment is contraindicated even when the organism is apparently sensitive in the laboratory.

In acute pyelonephritis lack of high tissue concentration does not necessarily prevent cure but drugs which give higher levels in kidney tissue may be preferred.[4]

Prophylaxis
Nitrofurantoin is a particularly suitable prophylactic agent against urinary infection because it is active against most urinary pathogens yet it fails to penetrate sufficiently to other sites to interfere with the patient's resident bacteria. Moreover, acquired resistance during treatment is rare. It is unfortunate that some patients cannot tolerate it because of side effects.

Nitrofurantoin has been very successfully used for the prevention of urinary infection during surgical manipulation. It should be given at the time of urinary tract surgery and continued only as long as there is continuing surgical intervention. There may be superinfection with naturally resistant bacteria, such as *Pseudomonas*, but the spread of nitrofurantoin-resistant bacteria as a result of treatment in surgical wards is not a problem.[17] Long-term therapy for patients, including children, often succeeds in preventing recurrent infection. A small dose, 50 mg or the equivalent in children, is all that is required and even a single nightly dose may be sufficient when treatment is established.

Recurrent cystitis related to coitus is often caused by Gram-positive cocci. A single dose of nitrofurantoin taken after coitus is often effective.[18]

The possibility of serious side effects with insidious onset must be borne in mind when patients have to receive nitrofurantoin for long periods.

Pregnancy
This is considered to be a contraindication in the USA, but not in Britain. When treatment of urinary tract infection in pregnancy is essential and the bacteria are sensitive, nitrofurantoin may be the drug of choice because penetration to the fetus in significant amounts is very unlikely.[13,15]

Adverse reactions

Potentially life-threatening effects
Serious reactions are rare. Pulmonary disease is the most common to be cited as a contributory cause of death. Hepatitis is very rare and no deaths were reported from long-term therapy until 1980[19] despite widespread use of nitrofurantoin for about 30 years. Haemolytic anaemia may contribute to or cause death in those with G-6-PD deficiency.

Nitrofurantoin

Pulmonary disease. Nitrofurantoin is one of the commoner causes of drug-induced pulmonary disease.[20,21] It has occasionally been reported as a contributory cause of death. It takes three forms: the acute pneumonitis syndrome consists of chills, fever, dyspnoea, cough and cyanosis, with rapid resolution of the acute pulmonary infiltrates after withdrawal of the drug. It is an allergic reaction. The subacute form is most often found in elderly women on prolonged therapy. Symptoms include dyspnoea, orthopnoea and cough. Pulmonary infiltrates are found and pleural effusion may be present.[22]

Chronic interstitial fibrosis is also seen in patients undergoing treatment for 6 months or more. Provided the condition is recognized and the drug is discontinued the prognosis is good. The presenting symptoms are usually dyspnoea and non-productive cough. Women are more often affected than men.[23]

The most important aspect of the treatment of any lung reaction to nitrofurantoin is to stop giving that patient the drug. In many instances, this is all the treatment necessary.

Steroids have been most commonly employed in the treatment of the chronic lung reactions. Since it is impossible to conduct clinical studies on the treatment of nitrofurantoin lung reactions, the efficacy of steroid administration is not known. Anecdotal information indicates that steroids are helpful in hastening recovery or alleviating symptoms of the more severe reactions. They seem to be of value in those cases in which the nitrofurantoin was given continuously, long after the first clinical symptoms appeared.

The true incidence of pulmonary reaction is hard to assess. Between 1959 and 1969 237 cases were reported[24] but between 1969 and 1980 there are only about 200 cases in the English language literature.

Hepatitis. Acute hepatocellular and cholestatic injury due to nitrofurantoin was reported in 1974.[25] Chronic active hepatitis occurs rarely, its onset may be insidious and patients receiving long-term therapy should be monitored for changes in liver function. When abnormalities are found the drug must be withdrawn immediately. Fatalities have been reported.[26]

Jaundice caused by nitrofurantoin can be due to two different mechanisms. The first is haemolytic anaemia, as in patients with G-6-PD deficiency. The jaundice here is due to the rapid destruction of red blood cells and the overloading of the bilirubin elimination system. The second is liver injury, in which the jaundice is due to damage of part of the bilirubin elimination system.

Haemolytic anaemia. Haematological changes are rarely caused by nitrofurantoin. Haemolytic anaemia, granulocytopenia, agranulocytosis, leukopenia, thrombocytopenia, eosinophilia and megaloblastic anaemia have all been reported. Aplastic anaemia is very rare.[27]

Nitrofurantoin in concentrations obtained after conventional oral doses inhibits ADP-induced platelet aggregation.[27] Patients with G-6-PD deficiency are likely to suffer haemolytic episodes during nitrofurantoin therapy.[28]

Acute overdosage

Incidents of acute overdosage have not resulted in reports of any specific symptoms other than vomiting. In case vomiting does not occur soon after an acute ingestion, and if the amount ingested is considered dangerous or excessive, vomiting should be induced unless the patient is convulsing, is comatose or has lost the gag reflex, in which case gastric lavage should be performed, using a large-bore tube. If indicated, this should be followed with activated charcoal and a saline cathartic. There is no specific antidote and treatment is symptomatic and supportive. A high fluid intake should be maintained to promote urinary excretion of the drug.

Severe or irreversible adverse effects

Neuropathy. Peripheral neuropathy has been reported in patients on long-term therapy particularly associated with renal failure, not necessarily severe enough to raise the blood urea.[28] Symptoms are usually paraesthesiae beginning in the extremities and ascending bilaterally and symmetrically followed by paralysis of varying degree. Occasionally motor symptoms only are seen. Complete recovery usually occurs within weeks or months and this depends on the severity of the symptoms rather than the quantity of drug given, the dose, or failure to recognize the cause of symptoms and withdraw the drug promptly.[30] In most patients symptoms occur within the first 45 d of treatment. They should be warned to report parasthaesiae immediately. The mode of action of the drug on the peripheral nerves is unknown but in normal people given the recommended dosage symptomless decrease in conduction velocities of peripheral nerves has been noted.[31]

Symptomatic adverse effects

Gastrointestinal. Anorexia, nausea and vomiting are common. Diarrhoea, abdominal pain and gastrointestinal bleeding are also encountered, especially in women. The symptoms are dose-related. They were found in 1.6% of patients receiving less than 4 $mg.kg^{-1}$ (the average recommended dose) but in 23.6% of those receiving more than 7 $mg.kg^{-1}$ body weight.[31] Nausea and vomiting have also resulted from intravenous therapy.[32] Reduction of the dose may be all that is needed to relieve symptoms, or the macrocrystalline form of the drug may be better tolerated.

Allergy. Hypersensitivity is less frequent than gastrointestinal symptoms.[34] Drug fever is the commonest manifestation but serum sickness and vasculitis have been reported. Acute pulmonary infiltration, hepatic injury and polyneuritis (all described above) may also be hypersensitivity reactions.

Skin reactions. These range from mild pruritus to severe eczematous eruptions and angioedema. The overall incidence is difficult to assess, but has been reported as 2% in hospitalized patients.

Interference with clinical pathology tests[35–37]

Nitrofurantoin therapy may interfere with the following:

Clinitest (Ames): false positive result — trace to 1+

Benedict's test: false positive (urine glucose tests depending on glucose oxidase — e.g. Clinistix — are not affected)

Urinary alkaline phosphatase: produces a decreased value

Urinary lactic dehydrogenase: produces a decreased value

Specific gravity of urine: depends on concentration of drug

Urine colour: deepens the normal yellow colour of urine

Urine pH: decreased

Bilirubin and icteric index: false positive or enhanced effect

High risk groups

Neonates

The drug is contraindicated in this age group.

Breast milk. Trace amounts are found in human milk.

Children

Nitrofurantoin has proved very successful as a prophylactic agent in those with recurrent infection. No reasons for special precautions for this age group are known.

Pregnant women

When treatment is essential, nitrofurantoin may be the drug of choice for urinary infection because of its wide antibacterial spectrum and low penetration to maternal plasma, fetus and amniotic fluid.[15]

The elderly

Patients on long-term therapy are liable to pulmonary reactions and other adverse effects. Supervision and monitoring of liver function is desirable.[32]

Drug interactions

Potentially hazardous interactions

Magnesium trisilicate reduces the rate and extent of nitrofurantoin absorption.

Uricosuric drugs: probenecid and sulphinpyrazone inhibition of renal tubular excretion of nitrofurantoin is likely to result in lower urinary concentration, i.e. reduced efficiency and high serum concentration leading to increased toxicity.

Nalidixic acid and related drugs are antagonized by nitrofurantoin in vitro and the combination is therefore contraindicated.

Potentially useful interactions

Increased (possibly doubled) urinary excretion if pyridoxine is given concomitantly. Antibacterial action may be increased by combination with drugs which acidify the urine.

Major outcome trials

1. Richards W A, Riss E, Kass E H, Finland M 1955 Nitrofurantoin: clinical and laboratory studies in urinary tract infections. Archives of Internal Medicine 96: 437–450

This is a study of 39 hospitalized patients aged 14–93 years. They received 100–200 mg nitrofurantoin orally 6-hourly for 2–13 d (average 7 d). Ten had acute pyelonephritis, 9 had mixed infections. There were 17 *E. coli*, 13 *Aerobacter aerogenes*, 11 *Proteus*, 8 Gram-positive cocci and 3 *Ps. aeruginosa* infections. *E. coli* was eliminated from the urine of all patients. There was superinfection in nine patients, five due to *Ps. aeruginosa*, 2 *Proteus*, 1 *Klebsiella* and 1*Enterobacter*. Two patients had to stop treatment because of nausea and vomiting on the second day. Nine suffered less severe nausea and vomiting; four of these failed to finish the course, the remaining five continued on a lower dose.

The investigators conclude that nitrofurantoin is useful in uncomplicated infections of the urinary tract.

2. Williams D K, Garrod L P, Waterworth P M 1962 Prevention of urinary infection after vaginal surgery with nitrofurantoin. Journal of Obstetrics and Gynaecology of the British Commonwealth 69: 403–405

This is a controlled study of 82 patients undergoing vaginal repair with bladder drainage for 1 week. They received either 100 mg nitrofurantoin 4 times daily until the catheter was removed at the end of a week or no prophylactic treatment. There were 54 treated patients aged 38–88 years and 55 control patients aged 33–70 years. Frequency of infection was reduced from 86% in the untreated to 10% in the treated patients. There were no significant side effects. Four of the treated patients became infected with *Ps. aeruginosa*. The infections in the untreated patients were mainly caused by *E. coli* but there were some *Proteus* and *Strep. faecalis* infections.

Routine prophylaxis with nitrofurantoin for such patients was adopted as a result of this trial.

3. Smellie J M, Katz G, Gruneberg R N 1978 Controlled trial of prophylactic treatment in childhood urinary tract infection. Lancet 2: 175–178

This study included 45 children aged 2–12 years suffering from repeated urinary infections without X-ray abnormality of the urinary tract. After initial successful treatment with co-trimoxazole, 13 children were maintained on a low dose of co-trimoxazole, 12 received nitrofurantoin 1–2 mg.kg^{-1} in either twice-daily dose or a single evening dose. 22 children received no prophylaxis.

None of the treated children developed infection during the year of treatment and no resistance to nitrofurantoin in faecal organisms developed. Half of the 22 controls without treatment had a further infection during this time. On follow-up, 8 of the treated patients had an infection within the first year after completion of the trial compared with 13 infections in the untreated group.

Other trials

Jawetz E, Hopper J, Smith D R 1957 Nitrofurantoin in chronic urinary tract infection. Archives of Internal Medicine 100: 549–557

Davis A, Patterson D K, Winn W R, Hertzer J, Finegold S M 1966 Additional studies comparing in vitro drug susceptibility with clinical bacteriological response. In: Hobby G L (ed) Symposium 6 of the American Society for Microbiology. Antimicrobial Agents and Chemotherapy

Hobby G L (ed) American Society for Microbiology, Ann Arbor, Michigan

Bailey R R, Gower P E, Roberts A P, de Wardener H E 1971 Prevention of urinary tract infection with low dose nitrofurantoin. Lancet 2: 1112–1114

Morgan D, Kraft W, Bender M, Pearson A 1988 Nitrofurans in the treatment of gastritis associated with *Campylobacter pylori*. Gastroenterology 95: 1178–1184

General review articles

Gleckman R, Alvarez S, Joubert D W 1979 Drug therapy reviews: nitrofurantoin. American Journal of Hospital Pharmacy 36: 342–351

D'Arcy P F 1985 Nitrofurantoin. Drug Intelligence and Clinical Pharmacology 19: 540–547

D'Arcy P F 1985 The comparative safety of therapies for urinary tract infection, with special reference to nitrofurantoin. In: Recent advances in the treatment of urinary tract infections. Proceedings of the Royal Society of Medicine Services, Amsterdam, pp 45–49

References

1. Conklin J D 1978 The pharmacokinetics of nitrofurantoin and its related bioavailability. Antibiotics and Chemotherapy 25: 233–252
2. Kalowski S, Radford N, Kincaid-Smith P 1974 Crystalline and macrocrystalline nitrofurantoin in the treatment of urinary tract infection. New England Journal of Medicine 290: 385–387
3. Chen L, Cadwallader D E, Jun H W 1976 Nitrofurantoin solubility in aqueous urea and creatinine solutions. Journal of Pharmaceutical Science 65: 868–872
4. Garrod L P, Lambert H P, O'Grady F 1981 In: Antibiotic and chemotherapy, 5th edn. Churchill Livingstone, Edinburgh
5. McCalla D R 1977 Biological effects of nitrofurans. Journal of Antimicrobial Chemotherapy 3: 517–520
6. McCalla D R, Olive P, Tu Y, Fan M L 1975 Nitrofurazone-reducing enzymes in *E. coli* and their role in drug activation in vivo. Canadian Journal of Microbiology 21: 1484–1491
7. Ebinger L, Jurasek A, Konicek J, Konikova M, Lahitova N, Trubacik S 1976 Mutagenic action of nitrofurans on *Euglena gracilis* and *Mycobacterium phlei.* Antimicrobial Agents and Chemotherapy 9: 682–689
8. Mohinra J K, Rauth A M 1976 Increased cell killing by metronidazole and nitrofurazone of hypoxic compared to aerobic mammalian cells. Cancer Research 36: 930–936
9. Boileau M A, Corriere J H Jr, Liss R H et al 1983 Visualisation of bactericidal concentrations of nitrofurantoin macrocrystals in primate and human urinary tract tissue. Journal of Urology 130: 1010–1012
10. Cadwallader D E 1975 Nitrofurantoin. Journal of the American Pharmaceutical Association 15: 409–412
11. Hamilton-Miller J M T, Kerry D W, Reynolds A V, Brumfitt W 1977 Two new bioassay techniques for nitrofurans. Chemotherapy 23: 236
12. Kree T B, Hekster Y A, Baars A M, Damsma J E, Van Der Kleijn E 1979 Determination of nitrofurantoin (Furadantine) and hydroxymethylnitrofurantoin (Urfadyn) in plasma and urine of man by means of high-performance liquid chromatography. Journal of Chromatography 162 (Biomedical Applications 4): 110–116
13. O'Brien T E 1974 Excretion of drugs in human milk. American Journal of Hospital Pharmacy 31: 844–854
14. Perry J E, LeBlanc A L 1967 Transfer of nitrofurantoin across the human placenta. Texas Reports on Biology and Medicine 25: 265–269
15. Brumfitt W, Hamilton-Miller J M T 1980 Nitrofurans. In: Kagan B M (ed) Antimicrobial chemotherapy, 3rd edn. W B Saunders, Philadelphia
16. Sachs J, Geer T, Noel P, Kunin C M 1968 Effect of renal function on urinary recovery of orally administered nitrofurantoin. New England Journal of Medicine 278: 1032–1035
17. Williams D K, Garrod L P, Waterworth P M 1962 Prevention of urinary infections after vaginal surgery with nitrofurantoin. Journal of Obstetrics and Gynaecology of the British Commonwealth 69: 403–405
18. Vosti K L 1975 Recurrent urinary tract infections: prevention by prophylactic antibiotics after sexual intercourse. Journal of the American Medical Association 231: 934–940
19. Rosenow E C III 1972 The spectrum of drug-induced pulmonary disease. Annals of Internal Medicine 77: 977–991
20. Prakash U B S 1980 Pulmonary reaction to nitrofurantoin. Seminars in Respiratory Medicine 2: 70–75
21. Fisk A A 1957 Anaphylactoid reaction to nitrofurantoin. New England Journal of Medicine 256: 1054
22. Sollacio P A, Ribando C A, Grace W J 1966 Subacute pulmonary infiltration due to nitrofurantoin. Annals of Internal Medicine 65: 1284–1286
23. Robinson B W S 1983 Nitrofurantoin-induced interstitial pulmonary fibrosis. Medical Journal of Australia 1: 72–76
24. Hailey F J, Grascock W W Jr, Hewitt W F 1969 Pleuropneumoniac reactions to nitrofurantoin. New England Journal of Medicine 281: 1087–1090
25. Goldstein L I, Ishak K G, Burns W 1974 Hepatic injury associated with nitrofurantoin therapy. American Journal of Digestive Diseases 19: 987–995
26. Sharp J R, Ishak K G, Zimmerman H J 1980 Chronic active hepatitis and severe hepatic necrosis associated with nitrofurantoin. Annals of Internal Medicine 92: 14–19
27. Rossi E C, Mieyal J J, Strone J M 1975 The molecular components of nitrofurantoin critical to its inhibitory effect on platelet aggregation. Molecular Pharmacology 11: 751–758
28. Hoigne R, Lubbers P, Gautschi M 1980 Nitrofurantoin. In: Dukes M N G (ed) Meyler's side effects of drugs, 9th edn. Excerpta Medica, Amsterdam
29. Craven R S 1971 Furadantin neuropathy. Australian and New Zealand Journal of Medicine 1: 246–249
30. Morris S J 1966 Nitrofurantoin and peripheral neuropathy with megaloblastic anaemia. Journal of Neurology, Neurosurgery and Psychiatry 27: 224–228
31. Toole J F, Gergen J A, Hayes D M 1968 Neural effects of nitrofurantoin. Archives of Neurology 18: 680–687
32. Delaney R A, Douglas A M, Gerbino P P 1977 Adverse effects resulting from nitrofurantoin administration. American Journal of Pharmacy 149: 26–29
33. Halliday A, Jawetz E 1962 Sodium nitrofurantoin administered intravenously: a limited study to define its clinical implications. New England Journal of Medicine 266: 427–432
34. Koch-Weser J, Sidal V W, Dexter M, Parish C, Finer D C, Kanarek P 1971 Adverse reactions to sulphisoxazole, sulphamethoxazole and nitrofurantoin. Archives of Internal Medicine 128: 399–404

35. Elking M P, Kabat H F 1968 Drug induced modifications of laboratory test values. American Journal of Hospital Pharmacy 25: 485
36. Nosal T, Kiser W S, Robitaille M L, King J W 1966 Urinary alkaline phosphatase and lactic dehydrogenase activity in the diagnosis of urologic neoplasm. Clinical Chemistry 12: 542
37. Smellie J M, Katz G, Gruneberg R N 1978 Controlled trial of prophylactic treatment in childhood urinary tract infection. Lancet 2: 175–178

Nitrous oxide

This gas was first used as an anaesthetic in 1844 in the UK by Horace Wells for dental extraction, but it did not attain widespread popularity until the 1860s. It has remained in continuous use since then, and is still a very important anaesthetic drug.

Chemistry

Nitrous oxide
N_2O

Molecular weight	440
Boiling point	−88.5°C at 1 atmosphere
Critical temperature	36.4°C
Minimum alveolar concentration (age 20–30 y)	105%
Partition coefficients at 37°C:	
Blood/gas	0.47
Oil/gas	1.4
Tissue/blood (heart, lung, brain, liver, muscle) approx.	1.0
Fat/blood (assuming fat consists of 65% oil and 35% blood)	2.3

Nitrous oxide is a colourless, odourless gas which is very stable and relatively inert chemically at room temperature. It is a good oxidizing agent with a latent tendency to decompose into nitrogen and oxygen. It is, however, inert to halogens and alkali metals. It supports combustion.

It is manufactured by heating solid or liquid ammonium nitrate at a carefully controlled temperature. Nitric acid and ammonia are also produced, together with higher oxides of nitrogen. The gas is very carefully purified before being dried, compressed and liquefied by cooling. It is denser than air.

It is available in combination with oxygen (Eatonox).

Pharmacology

Nitrous oxide depresses the activity of the central nervous system. In low concentrations, analgesia is the main feature; at higher concentrations, it is an anaesthetic in some individuals, but it is only an anaesthetic in all individuals at hyperbaric pressure.[1] There is some evidence that its analgesic effect is mediated via encephalinergic nerve endings in the spinal cord, perhaps by activation of a supraspinal descending pain-inhibiting system which increases the activity of encephalinergic nerve endings in the substantia gelatinosa.[2]

Toxicology

A most important toxic effect of nitrous oxide is its ability to oxidize vitamin B_{12} and thus reduce the activity of the enzyme methionine synthetase. Inactivation of this enzyme decreases the formation of thymidine which is an essential part of DNA. This interference with DNA synthesis is the mechanism whereby nitrous oxide causes megaloblastic anaemia and neuropathy, and raises the possibility that N_2O could be teratogenic. N_2O is lethal to chick embryos when these are exposed to a high concentration for a prolonged period of time, but no increase in fetal abnormalities was seen. Pregnant rats exposed to much lower concentrations of 500 or 1000 p.p.m. for 24 hours had a higher incidence of both fetal deaths and abnormalities, but reducing the exposure to 12 hours was followed by little evidence of fetotoxicity.[3] The results of human epidemiological studies suggest that there is an increased abortion rate in females exposed occupationally to N_2O, but the evidence for an increase in fetal abnormalities after such exposure is less conclusive.[3,4]

Neither human nor animal studies have produced evidence that N_2O is mutagenic or carcinogenic.

The effects of occupational exposure to N_2O have been studied in dentists and their assistants.[4] In addition to the increased incidence of abortions mentioned earlier, higher incidences of liver, kidney and neurological disease were observed. A more recent study demonstrated abnormal vitamin B_{12} metabolism in 3 of 22 dentists examined.[5] It is considered that reducing exposure to levels of less than 200 p.p.m. N_2O would prevent these problems and that scavenging systems should be installed to prevent occupational exposure to higher concentrations. However, lower safe levels than 200 p.p.m have been suggested.[6]

Clinical pharmacology

N_2O is always an anaesthetic if it is administered at a pressure of 1.1 atmospheres. At a higher pressure of 1.5 atmospheres, unconsciousness in volunteers not subjected to surgery was accompanied by excessive muscle tone, tachypnoea and signs of increased sympathetic activity such as sweating and dilated pupils.

At normal pressures, the effects of increasing concentrations of N_2O have been summarized as:[7]

6–25% Moderate analgesia; slight sedation and sensory impairment.
26–45% Dissociation analgesia; dreaming; a sense of detachment; paraesthesiae; dizziness; light sedation; slight amnesia.
46–65% Analgesic anaesthesia; response to command retained; marked amnesia and somnolence; dreaming.
66–85% Light anaesthesia; contact with patient lost; amnesia; involuntary movements.

However, even at the higher concentrations compatible with adequate oxygenation, some subjects will be aware and not have any amnesia.

Effects on the autonomic nervous system

Nitrous oxide causes signs of sympathoadrenal stimulation such as sweating, pupillary dilation and increases in blood pressure and cardiac output. These changes occur in the absence of surgical stimulation. However, tolerance appears to develop and these effects disappear on continued administration. It is postulated that this stimulation is centrally mediated as N_2O acts as a depressant to the sympathetic nervous system when given to decerebrate animals.[8] There is no consistent effect of N_2O on adrenaline or noradrenaline blood levels,[9] though noradrenaline levels rose in most patients when N_2O was added to halothane/oxygen anaesthesia.[10] Any increase in noradrenaline levels may be mediated by inhibition of uptake of noradrenaline by the lung.[11]

Effects on the cardiovascular system

N_2O has some direct depressant effects on the isolated heart.

In volunteers, inhalation of N_2O 60% caused an initial increase in heart rate, stroke volume, cardiac output, blood pressure and systemic vascular resistance, but after about 15–60 minutes of continued inhalation, the values all returned to the pre-N_2O levels.[12] In contrast, inhalation of a lower concentration of N_2O, 40%, was accompanied by a decrease in heart rate, cardiac output and arterial pressure, possibly related to the sedation produced by this concentration.[9] Even this lower concentration caused vasoconstriction and a decrease in forearm blood flow, largely due to an effect on cutaneous capillaries. N_2O causes an increase in venous tone.[9]

Renal blood flow and urine output changes follow the changes in systemic vascular resistance. Splanchnic blood flow decreased with an increase in systemic vascular resistance in volunteers given thiopentone, d-tubocurarine and nitrous oxide.[13] N_2O may increase cerebral blood flow.[14]

Effects on the respiratory system

Slight rises in $PaCO_2$ can occur during the administration of N_2O, but these are never large, as an increase in respiratory rate compensates for the decrease in tidal volume.[1,12]

No consistent effects of N_2O on the ventilatory response to CO_2 are seen, but the ventilatory response to hypoxia is obtunded.[15,16]

Like all other inhaled anaesthetic agents, N_2O decreases functional residual capacity. There was a greater incidence of postoperative atelectasis in patients who were given nitrous oxide as part of their anaesthetic compared with those in whom nitrogen replaced the N_2O.[17]

Effects on intracranial pressure

N_2O causes a small increase in intracranial pressure (i.c.p.) in patients without intracranial lesions, but this increase is smaller than that caused by other inhalation anaesthetic agents.[18] An increase in i.c.p. was also caused by N_2O in patients with intracranial lesions, and the pressure was restored to normal by hyperventilation.[19]

Pharmacokinetics

Analysis of N_2O in discrete blood and gas samples can be carried out using gas chromatography, with a katharometer detector for analgesic levels of the drug. A microionization cross-section detector has been used to measure trace levels of N_2O in blood[20] over the range 0.03 to 0.78 $mg.l^{-1}$.

N_2O enters the alveoli and diffuses across the alveolar membrane to reach the bloodstream. It is then carried to all the tissues of the body. A brief discussion of the rate of rise of the alveolar partial pressure of inhaled gases and vapours is given under Ether. Because of the low blood/gas solubility of N_2O, the alveolar partial pressure rises rapidly, and within 5 minutes of starting to inhale a constant inspired concentration of the gas, the alveolar concentration will have reached about 80% of the inspired concentration. Thus induction of a state of analgesia or anaesthesia with N_2O is very rapid, despite its low potency as expressed by MAC. In contrast to more soluble anaesthetic gases or vapours, changes in cardiac output and ventilation have very little effect on the rate of rise of alveolar concentration of N_2O.

The uptake of large volumes of N_2O, when administration of this gas is first started, has two effects called the 'concentration effect' and the 'second gas effect'. These are of relatively little clinical importance. After the administration of N_2O is stopped, the partial pressure of the gas in the alveoli falls, creating a pressure difference across the alveolar membrane. Immediately, N_2O starts to diffuse out of the bloodstream to equalize this pressure difference. Because N_2O is not a very soluble gas, and has been given in a high concentration, a large volume of gas will enter the alveoli in a short period of time. Thus if after stopping the N_2O the patient is allowed to breathe air, the air which enters the alveoli will be 'diluted' by the N_2O which is leaving the blood, with the result that the alveoli will contain less than 21% oxygen. This period of 'diffusion hypoxia' usually lasts only a few minutes, and can be completely prevented by the administration of 100% oxygen instead of air after discontinuing the administration of N_2O.

N_2O moves readily through tissues and cell membranes and also across the skin and mucous membranes. It can thus enter closed body spaces.[21] If these contain air, the pressure within them can rise as N_2O enters more rapidly than nitrogen leaves. The resultant rise in pressure and volume may be of clinical importance in (i) intestinal obstruction, when abdominal closure at the end of surgery is impeded; (ii) closed pneumothorax or a pulmonary cyst; (iii) air embolus; (iv) surgical emphysema. Postoperative deafness in patients with blocked eustachian tubes can be caused by the use of N_2O. Early after the anaesthetic, this is caused by an increase in the pressure in the middle ear as N_2O diffuses into it. Later, the deafness is due to a decrease in the pressure in the middle ear, N_2O diffusing more rapidly out than nitrogen diffuses in. N_2O can also diffuse into the cuffs of endotracheal tubes and cause a considerable increase in the pressure exerted by the cuff on the tracheal wall. Endotracheal tubes with low pressure cuffs are available to minimize this effect.

Concentration–effect relationship

The relationship between inspired concentrations of N_2O and effect is described in the section on Clinical pharmacology.

In a study of the arterial concentration of N_2O when a mixture of the gas with 50% oxygen was administered for labour pains, the mean concentration 5 seconds after the start of inhalation was 26.7 $mg.l^{-1}$ and at the end of the contraction, when inhalation stopped, it was 201.5 $mg.l^{-1}$. The concentration had dropped to 40 $mg.l^{-1}$ by 60 seconds after stopping inhalation.[22]

The blood levels of N_2O in anaesthetists exposed to approximately 2000 p.p.m. were up to 2.2 mg.l^{-1}. After scavenging, the blood levels were reduced[23] to less than 0.4 mg.l^{-1}.

Metabolism

N_2O is not metabolized by rat liver homogenates. It is metabolized by anaerobic intestinal bacteria in humans with the formation of free radicals, but it is not known whether this is important clinically.

Pharmaceutics

N_2O is supplied compressed as a liquid in cylinders which in the UK are coloured blue. Various sizes of cylinder are available. The smaller ones can be attached directly to anaesthetic machines; the larger are usually used in banks which supply several outlets at the same time. The cylinder pressure is 13 470 kPa, but only about 90% of the volume of the cylinder is filled with liquid N_2O. The cylinders are filled by weight.

The purity of the gas is 98% (BP) or 99% (USP), the rest being largely air, with some carbon dioxide (30 p.p.m.) and water vapour (less than 200 p.p.m.). Very strict limits (less than 1 p.p.m.) are laid down for the presence of the toxic higher oxides of nitrogen.

N_2O is also available in cylinders as a concentration of 50% with oxygen (Entonox). These cylinders are blue with a blue and white quartered shoulder, and the gas inside is at a pressure of 13 470 kPa. At low temperatures, the N_2O separates out as a liquid. Regulations have been formulated for the storage and use of cylinders of Entonox to ensure that all the N_2O is in gaseous form before use.[24]

Therapeutic use

Indications

1. Surgical anaesthesia
2. Dental anaesthesia
3. Dental analgesia
4. Obstetric analgesia
5. Other analgesia.

Contraindications

1. Intracranial air, e.g. pneumoencephalogram
2. Tension pneumothorax
3. The presence of an air embolus: some would consider that N_2O is contraindicated in patients in whom there is a risk of this complication
4. Prolonged use, especially in the critically ill, for example, on the Intensive Care Unit (see Toxicology)
5. Specific contraindications to its use in general dental practice.[25]

Indications

1. Surgical anaesthesia
Concentrations of 50–75% are given with oxygen. This provides some degree of analgesia, but unconsciousness cannot be assured and muscle relaxation will not occur. Thus N_2O is usually used as part of a balanced anaesthetic technique in which other agents are used to induce anaesthesia, to ensure unconsciousness and to produce muscle relaxation. The effect of N_2O is potentiated by all other hypnotic, sedative and analgesic drugs which are commonly used in anaesthesia. It is administered via anaesthetic machines which reduce the pressure in the cylinder and provide a means of measuring the flow of gas. There is always the danger of hypoxia due to failure of oxygen supply when separate flows of N_2O and O_2 are used.

2. Dental anaesthesia
This can sometimes be achieved in children using only N_2O and O_2 when the procedure is very short. More often, however, N_2O alone would not provide anaesthesia of sufficient depth or duration, and intravenous induction agents and/or a more potent inhalation agent are also used.

3. Dental analgesia
Concentrations of 15–50% N_2O in oxygen can be used to provide analgesia, sedation, euphoria or relaxation for dental procedures. Contact with the patient is maintained throughout the procedure as the aim is never to produce anaesthesia. Local anaesthetic drugs are often also used.

4. Obstetric analgesia
This can be provided by self-administration of Entonox, especially during the pains of late first-stage or second-stage labour. Inhalation of the drug should start when the contraction starts and before it is actually felt as pain.

5. Other analgesia
Entonox can be self-administered for analgesia during painful procedures such as dressing burns, wound dressing or probing, removal of drains, or physiotherapy after abdominal or thoracic surgery. If unconsciousness should supervene during self-administration, N_2O intake automatically stops as the patient releases the mask. Entonox is also provided in ambulances in the UK for use by casualties at the site of an accident or during transport to hospital.

Adverse reactions

Potentially life-threatening effects
1After prolonged exposure to N_2O to treat tetanus, granulocytopenia and aplastic anaemia were observed.[26] Although these changes were reversible after even prolonged exposure, in most cases returning to normal in about 4 days, a few deaths occurred due to sepsis or haemorrhage. In normal patients given nitrous oxide for anaesthesia, mobilization of stored mature leucocytes prevents leukopenia. However, stores are inadequate for replacement if N_2O administration is continued for 24 hours. Patients given N_2O for 6 hours after cardiac surgery had mild megaloblastic bone marrow depression.[27] The toxicity of this gas to the bone marrow is greater in more severely ill patients, abnormalities of vitamin B_{12} metabolism being seen in some patients who had only been given N_2O for anaesthesia lasting 2–6 h.[28]

N_2O may be able to precipitate malignant hyperpyrexia,[29] but it is used for anaesthesia for muscle biopsy in the diagnosis of this syndrome.

Acute overdosage
Potentially life-threatening hypoxia can occur if no oxygen is administered with the N_2O. This can occur accidentally and warning devices are now incorporated in most anaesthetic machines to indicate failure of the oxygen supply.

Severe or irreversible adverse effects
Peripheral neuropathy develops after prolonged use by those abusing this drug. This is due to vitamin B_{12} deficiency and resembles the subacute combined degeneration that occurs in pernicious anaemia. There is also some evidence of neuropathy in oral surgeons experiencing heavy occupational exposure.[30,31] Numbness, paraesthesiae, ataxia and clumsiness appear first, with impotence and loss of sphincter control after more prolonged exposure.

Symptomatic adverse effects
Nausea and vomiting occurred in all volunteers exposed to hyperbaric N_2O,[1] and N_2O may contribute to postoperative vomiting in patients undergoing laparoscopy.[32]

Impairment of driving skills can be detected for up to 30 minutes after the administration of 50% or 70% N_2O in oxygen.[33]

Interference with clinical pathology tests
No technical interferences of this kind are known.

High risk groups

Neonates
Nitrous oxide is safely used.

Breast milk. There is no evidence that nitrous oxide is transmitted to the infant in breast milk.

Children
Nitrous oxide is safely used.

Pregnant women
Prolonged occupational exposure to low concentrations of nitrous oxide should be avoided in early pregnancy because of the small risk of abortion. There is no evidence that nitrous oxide given during the course of an anaesthetic during early pregnancy will increase the risk of abortion. Nitrous oxide given during delivery does not cause depression of the baby, nor does it relax the uterus.

The elderly
Nitrous oxide is safely used, but see below.

Concurrent disease
There are no absolute contraindications to nitrous oxide, but care should be taken in the following situations:

Lung bullae. Nitrous oxide can enter these and cause them to expand.

Intestinal obstruction. The gut may distend further with the passage of nitrous oxide into the bowel lumen.

Blocked eustachian tubes. Nitrous oxide will increase middle ear pressure and can rupture the tympanic membrane.

The critically ill. These patients should not be given nitrous oxide for periods of more than 2 hours, and a shorter period of exposure may be preferable if adverse effects on haemopoiesis are to be avoided.

Severe coronary disease. The cardiac depressant effects of nitrous oxide may be of clinical importance in patients with severe coronary disease.

Drug interactions

Important drug interactions occur between nitrous oxide and other drugs used in anaesthesia. These drugs vary in the degree of seriousness in any individual patient. In some patients, they may be life-threatening; in others they are of no clinical importance, or may even be beneficial.

Inhalation agents
The combination of nitrous oxide with halothane 0.8% or 1.0% may be less depressant to the cardiovascular system (CVS) than halothane alone, or may even produce cardiovascular stimulation with increased systemic vascular resistance and blood pressure.[34–36] A similar stimulant effect may also be seen with enflurane[37] and isoflurane.[36,38] However, in patients with cardiovascular disease, the addition of N_2O to a volatile agent may have only a depressant effect on the CVS[39,40]

Nitrous oxide reduces the threshold for adrenaline-induced arrhythmias in dogs given halothane.[41]

Opioids
A decrease in cardiac index occurs when N_2O is administered to patients who have been given morphine.[42] The degree of myocardial depression is related to the concentration of N_2O over the range of 10–50%.[43] A similar decrease is seen when N_2O is given to patients who have received a large dose of fentanyl (25 $\mu g.kg^{-1}$).[44] The CVS depressant effect of N_2O and opioids may be more marked in patients with coronary or other cardiac disease, and in some studies a decrease in both systemic and pulmonary vascular resistance was seen. A possible mechanism of these effects is attenuation of the α- and β-stimulating effects of N_2O by opioids. Pancuronium can reverse the CVS depression caused by N_2O and pethidine, but systemic vascular resistance, blood pressure and heart rate can rise to levels higher than those present before induction of anaesthesia.[48]

N_2O administered to patients receiving an infusion of fentanyl or alfentanil depressed minute volume, respiratory frequency and the ventilatory response to carbon dioxide.[49]

Muscle rigidity can occur when N_2O is given to patients who have received large doses of some opioids, e.g. morphine[50,51] 2 $mg.kg^{-1}$.

General review articles

Eger E I II (ed) 1985 Nitrous oxide. Edward Arnold, London

References

1. Hornbein T F, Eger E I II, Winter P M, Smith G, Wetstone D, Smith K H 1982 The minimum alveolar concentration of nitrous oxide in man. Anesthesia and Analgesia 61: 553–556
2. Finck A D 1985 Nitrous oxide analgesia. In: Eger E I II (ed) Nitrous oxide. Edward Arnold, London, ch 3, pp 41–55
3. Baden J M 1985 Mutagenicity, carcinogenicity, and teratogenicity of nitrous oxide. In: Eger E I II (ed) Nitrous oxide. Edward Arnold, London, ch 14, pp 235–247
4. Cohen E N, Brown B W, Wu M L et al 1980 Occupational disease in dentistry and chronic exposure to trace anaesthetic gases. Journal of the American Dental Association 101: 21–31
5. Bingham R M, Sweeney B, Cole P V 1985 Bone marrow changes after inhalation of atmospheric nitrous oxide. British Journal of Anaesthesia 57: 342P
6. Nunn J F, Chanarin I 1985 Nitrous oxide inactivates methionine synthetase. In: Eger E I II (ed) Nitrous oxide. Edward Arnold, London, ch 13, pp 211–233
7. Parbrook G D 1967 The levels of nitrous oxide analgesia. British Journal of Anaesthesia 39: 974–982
8. Fukunaga A F, Epstein R M 1973 Sympathetic excitation during nitrous oxide–halothane anesthesia in the cat. Anesthesiology 39: 23–36
9. Eisele J H, Smith N T 1972 Cardiovascular effects of 40 percent nitrous oxide in man. Anesthesia and Analgesia 51: 956–963
10. Smith N T, Eger E I II, Stoelting R K, Whayne T F, Cullen D, Kadis L B 1970 The cardiovascular and sympathomimetic responses to the addition of nitrous oxide to halothane in man. Anesthesiology 32: 410–421
11. Naito H, Gillies C N 1973 Effects of halothane and nitrous oxide on removal of norepinephrine from the pulmonary circulation. Anesthesiology 39: 575–580
12. Kawamura R, Stanley T H, English J B, Hill G E, Liu W-S, Webster C R 1980 Cardiovascular responses to nitrous oxide exposure for two hours in man. Anesthesia and Analgesia 59: 93–99
13. Cooperman L H, Warden J C, Price H L 1968 Splanchnic circulation during nitrous oxide anesthesia and hypocarbia in normal man. Anesthesiology 29: 254–258
14. Frost E A M 1985 Central nervous system effects of nitrous oxide. In: Eger E I II (ed) Nitrous oxide. Edward Arnold, London, ch 9, pp 157–176
15. Knill R L, Clement J L 1982 Variable effects of anaesthetics on the ventilatory response to hypoxaemia in man. Canadian Anaesthetists' Society Journal 29: 93–99
16. Yacoub O, Doell D, Kryger M H, Anthonisen N R 1976 Depression of hypoxic ventilatory response by nitrous oxide. Anesthesiology 54: 385–389
17. Browne D R G, Rochford J, O'Connell U, Jones J G 1970 The incidence of postoperative atelectasis in the dependent lung following thoracotomy: the value of added nitrogen. British Journal of Anaesthesia 42: 340–346
18. McDowell D G, Barker J, Jennett W B 1966 Cerebrospinal fluid pressure measurements during anaesthesia. Anaesthesia 21: 189–201
19. Henriksen H T, Jorgensen P B 1973 The effect of nitrous oxide on intracranial pressure in patients with intracranial disorders. British Journal of Anaesthesia 45: 486–492
20. Saloojee Y, Cole P V 1978 Estimation of nitrous oxide in blood. Anaesthesia 33: 779–783
21. Munson E S 1974 Transfer of nitrous oxide into body air cavities. British Journal of Anaesthesia 46: 202–209
22. Latto I P, Molloy M J, Rosen M 1973 Arterial concentrations of nitrous oxide during intermittent patient-controlled inhalation of 50% nitrous oxide in oxygen (Entonox) during the first stage of labour. British Journal of Anaesthesia 45: 1029–1034
23. Krapez J R, Saloojee Y, Hinds C J, Hackett G H, Cole P V 1980 Blood concentrations of nitrous oxide in theatre personnel. British Journal of Anaesthesia 52: 1143–1148
24. Cole P V, Crawford J S, Doughty A G et al 1970 Specifications and recommendations for nitrous oxide/oxygen apparatus to be used in obstetric analgesia. Anaesthesia 25: 317–327
25. Smith R A, Beirne O R 1985 The use of nitrous oxide by dentists. In: Eger E I II (ed) Nitrous oxide. Edward Arnold, London, ch 17, pp 281–304
26. Lassen H C A, Henriksen E, Neukirch F, Kristensen H S 1956 Treatment of tetanus. Severe bone marrow depression after prolonged nitrous oxide anaesthesia. Lancet 1: 527–530
27. Amess J A L, Burman J F, Rees G M, Nancekievill D G, Mollin D L 1978 Megaloblastic haemopoiesis in patients receiving nitrous oxide. Lancet 2: 339–342
28. Amos R J, Amess J A L, Hinds C J, Mollin D L 1982 Incidence and pathogenesis of acute megaloblastic bone marrow change in patients receiving intensive care. Lancet 2: 835–839
29. Ellis F R, Clarke I M C, Appleyard T N, Dinsdale R C W 1974 Malignant hyperpyrexia induced by nitrous oxide and treated with dexamethasone. British Medical Journal 4: 270–271
30. Brodsky J B, Cohen E N, Brown B W, Wu M L, Whitcher C E 1981 Exposure to nitrous oxide and neurological disease among dental professionals. Anesthesia and Analgesia 60: 297–301
31. Brodsky J B 1985 Toxicity of nitrous oxide. In: Eger E I II (ed) Nitrous oxide. Edward Arnold, London, ch 16, pp 259–279
32. Lonie D A, Harper N J N 1986 Nitrous oxide anaesthesia and vomiting. Anaesthesia 41: 703–707
33. Moyes D G, Cleaton-Jones P, Lelliott T 1979 Driving after anaesthetics. British Medical Journal 1: 1425
34. Hornbein T F, Martin W E, Bonica J J, Freund F G, Parmentier P 1969 Nitrous oxide effects on the circulatory and ventilatory responses to halothane. Anesthesiology 31: 250–260
35. Bahlman S H, Eger E I II, Smith N T et al 1971 The cardiovascular effects of nitrous oxide–halothane in man. Anesthesiology 35: 274–285
36. Eisele J H 1985 Cardiovascular effects of nitrous oxide. In: Eger E I II (ed) Nitrous oxide. Edward Arnold, London, ch 8, pp 125–156
37. Smith N T, Calverley R K, Prys-Roberts C, Eger E I II 1978 Impact of nitrous oxide on the circulation during enflurane anesthesia in man. Anesthesiology 48: 345–349
38. Dolan W W, Stevens W C, Eger E I II et al 1974 The cardiovascular and respiratory effects of isoflurane–nitrous oxide anaesthesia. Canadian Anaesthetists' Society Journal 21: 557–568
39. Moffitt E A, Sethna D H, Gary R J, Raymond M J, Matloff J M, Bussell J A 1983 Nitrous oxide added to halothane reduces coronary flow and myocardial oxygen consumption in patients with coronary disease. Canadian Anaesthetists' Society Journal 30: 5–9
40. Ramsay J G, Arvieux C C, Foëx P, Ryder W A, Jones L A, Jeavons P 1985 Myocardial function when nitrous oxide is added to halothane in the presence of critical coronary artery constriction. British Journal of Anaesthesia 57: 817P
41. Liu W, Wong K C, Port J D, Andriano K P 1982 Epinephrine-induced arrhythmias during halothane anesthesia with the addition of nitrous oxide, nitrogen or helium in dogs. Anesthesia and Analgesia 61: 414–417

42. Wong K C, Martin W E, Hornbein T F, Freund F C, Everett J 1973 The cardiovascular effects of morphine sulphate with oxygen and with nitrous oxide in man. Anesthesiology 38: 542–549
43. McDermott R W, Stanley T H 1974 The cardiovascular effects of low concentrations of nitrous oxide during morphine anesthesia. Anesthesiology 41: 89–91
44. Lunn J K, Stanley T H, Eisele J, Webster L, Woodward A 1979 High dose fentanyl anesthesia for coronary artery surgery: plasma fentanyl concentrations and influence of nitrous oxide on cardiovascular responses. Anesthesia and Analgesia 58: 390–395
45. Lappas D G, Buckley M J, Laver M B, Daggett W M, Lowenstein E 1975 Left ventricular performance and pulmonary circulation following addition of nitrous oxide to morphine during coronary artery surgery. Anesthesiology 43: 61–69
46. Stoelting R K, Gibbs P S 1973 Hemodynamic effects of morphine and morphine–nitrous oxide in valvular heart disease and coronary artery disease. Anesthesiology 38: 45–52
47. Philbin D M, Foëx P, Lowenstein E, Ryder W A, Jones L A 1983 Nitrous oxide causes myocardial dysfunction. Anesthesiology 59: A80
48. Stanley T H, Lui W 1977 Cardiovascular effects of meperidine–N_2O anesthesia before and after pancuronium. Anesthesia and Analgesia 56: 669–673
49. Andrews C J H, Sinclair M, Dye A, Dye J, Harvey J, Prys-Roberts C 1982 The additive effects of nitrous oxide on respiratory depression in patients having fentanyl or alfentanil infusions. British Journal of Anaesthesia 54: 1129
50. Sokoll M D, Hoyt J L, Gergis S D 1972 Studies in muscle rigidity, nitrous oxide and narcotic analgesic agents. Anesthesia and Analgesia 51: 16–26
51. Freund F G, Martin W E, Wong K C, Hornbein T F 1973 Abdominal-muscle rigidity induced by morphine and nitrous oxide. Anesthesiology 38: 358–362

Nizatidine

Nizatidine is a histamine H_2-receptor antagonist for use in the treatment of peptic ulcer disease.

Chemistry

Nizatidine (Axid)
$C_{12}H_{21}N_5O_2S_2$
N-[2-[[[-2[(Dimethylamino)methyl]-4-thiazolyl]-methyl]thiol]-ethyl]-N-methyl-2-nitro-1,1-ethenediamine

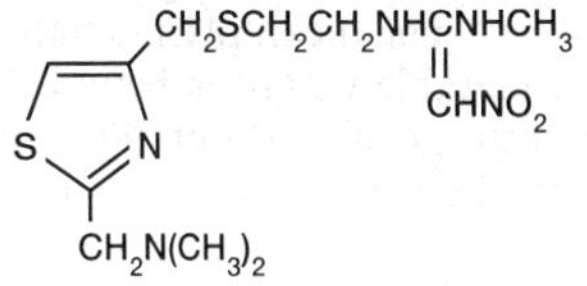

Molecular weight	331.5
pKa	—
Solubility	
in alcohol	soluble
in water	soluble
Octanol/water partition coefficient	0.3

An off-white to buff crystalline solid with a bitter taste, prepared by chemical synthesis.

Pharmacology

Nizatidine is a potent competitive antagonist at the histamine H_2-receptor, and on a weight-for-weight basis is about 10 times as potent as cimetidine.[4] High concentrations of nizatidine (10 μmol.l^{-1}), about 100 to 1000 times higher than those found in plasma during therapy, stimulated contractions in an in vitro preparation of guinea-pig duodenum. This effect of nizatidine was inhibited by atropine, and by the histamine H_1-receptor antagonist pyrilamine. Both agents produced non parallel shifts of the dose–response curves with depression of the maximum. There have been no further studies and it is not clear whether the apparent stimulatory effects of nizatidine on muscarinic and histamine H_1-receptors are direct or indirect.[2] Nizatidine has no H_1-antagonist activity and therefore selectively inhibits the stimulatory effect of histamine on gastric parietal and chief cells. Nizatidine has no adrenergic or serotoninergic agonist properties.[1] Nizatidine, unlike cimetidine, does not possess antiandrogenic activity.

Toxicology

Nizatidine is not mutagenic and had no carcinogenic effect in mice and rats, when given for up to 2 years. Nizatidine is not teratogenic in rats or rabbits and reproduction is not affected in the rat. High doses given to rabbits produced maternal weight loss and underweight offspring. Rats given high doses of nizatidine for 2 years showed dose-dependent increases in the gastric mucosal enterochromaffin-like (ECL) cell density consistent with suppression of gastric acid secretion leading to hypergastrinaemia. Although the density of ECL cells was increased, there was no histological evidence of gastric tumours, gastrin carcinoids or dysplastic changes which might be considered to be precancerous.[1]

Clinical pharmacology

Suppression of gastric acid secretion is considered to be the main mechanism by which histamine H_2-receptor antagonists promote relief of symptoms and healing of peptic ulceration.

Nizatidine

N

Nizatidine, like other H_2-antagonists, inhibits gastric acid secretion in the basal state,[3–5] and during stimulation by histamine itself,[1] pentagastrins,[6,7] meals,[4,6] sham feeding[6] or caffeine.[8] The duration of action of nizatidine is 8–10 hours. Typically, evening doses of 30 mg and 300 mg inhibited overnight acid secretion by 57% and 90% respectively, but had no effect on meal-stimulated secretion on the following morning.[4] Nizatidine diminished aspirin-induced gastric mucosal damage to human stomach.[9]

Nizatidine treatment in normal subjects does not affect plasma concentrations of testosterone, oestrogen, growth hormone, follicle stimulating hormone, androstenedione, luteinizing hormone, thyroid stimulating hormone, prolactin,[10] antidiuretic hormone or urinary cortisol.[6] Plasma gastrin concentrations were not altered.[4] Nizatidine does not influence the metabolism of drugs by the mixed function oxidase system in the liver.

Pharmacokinetics

Nizatidine is measured in body fluids by high performance liquid chromatography (HPLC). The limit of sensitivity[11] is about 10 μg.l^{-1}.

Nizatidine is almost totally absorbed after oral administration and peak plasma concentrations occur at 1–2 h. Concurrent administration of food,[6] antacids or anticholinergic agents[12] does not affect absorption of nizatidine.[6] The mean plasma half life is about 1.5 h,[13] but there may be considerable variation between individuals.[7] Elimination is predominantly renal. About 90% of an oral dose of nizatidine appeared in the urine, mostly unchanged, within 16 h of administration.[11]

Nizatidine is widely distributed in the bodies of experimental animals.[13] The volume of distribution in man is 1 l.kg^{-1}. In human blood about 30% is bound to plasma proteins, mainly α_1-acid glycoprotein, and another 30% is associated with blood cells.[11]

Nizatidine crosses the human placenta[14] and has been found to appear in human breast milk.[15]

Oral absorption	>70%
Presystemic metabolism	<7%
Plasma half life	
range	1.5–1.6 h
Volume of distribution	1 l.kg^{-1}
Plasma protein binding	30%

Hepatic dysfunction did not affect the disposition of nizatidine,[6] consistent with predominant excretion of unchanged drug in the urine. Renal impairment significantly delays elimination and prolongs the plasma half life of nizatidine.[6,16] The plasma half life was prolonged from 1.5 h in normal subjects to 1.9 h in elderly patients with mild renal dysfunction and to 3.5–11 h in anephric subjects. It is therefore recommended that the dose be reduced to 150 mg daily if creatinine clearance is 20–50 ml.min^{-1} and 150 mg on alternate days if the creatinine clearance is <20 ml.min^{-1}. Age does not appear to affect the pharmacokinetics of nizatidine, but elimination may be affected by the associated diminution of renal function in old age.

In practice, since the therapeutic range of nizatidine is not narrow, the clinical significance of mild to moderate alterations in pharmacokinetics may be slight.

Concentration–effect relationship

Oral doses of nizatidine from 30 to 300 mg,[4] and intravenous bolus doses from 25 to 250 mg progressively inhibited gastric acid secretion.[4] The mean plasma concentration of nizatidine which produced 50% inhibition of pentagastrin-stimulated secretion[7] was 154 μg.l^{-1}. However, there is considerable individual variation among the concentration–effect curves and there is little clinical benefit in measuring the plasma concentration of nizatidine.

Metabolism

Metabolites account for only about 35% of nizatidine excreted in urine, the remainder being intact drug.[11]

The metabolites of nizatidine that have been identified in urine are N-2-monodesmethyl nizatidine, nizatidine N-2-oxide and nizatidine sulphoxide (see Fig. 1). These accounted for 8%, 6% and 6% of an administered dose respectively. N-2-Monodesmethyl nizatidine has H_2-receptor antagonist activity and was 60% as active as nizatidine in inhibiting gastric secretion in dogs. Nizatidine N-2-oxide had no H_2-receptor antagonist activity and nizatidine sulphoxide was not tested.[11] High concentrations of N-2-monodesmethyl nizatidine were present in the plasma of anephric patients after administration of nizatidine; apparently the result of increased formation, as well as increased elimination of this metabolite.[6,16] Nizatidine does not appear to inhibit P450 dependant oxidation reactions.

Pharmaceutics

Nizatidine (Axid; Lilly, UK) is only available for oral use: capsules containing 150 mg are pale yellow/dark yellow and coded '3144'; capsules containing 300 mg are pale yellow/brown and coded '3145'.

Nizatidine preparations are believed to be stable but their shelf-life is unknown. Allergy to nizatidine is very rare.

Therapeutic use

Indications

1. Therapy of duodenal ulceration
2. Therapy of benign gastric ulcer
3. Prevention of relapse of duodenal ulceration.

Contraindications

1. Known hypersensitivity to nizatidine or other H_2-receptor antagonists.

Fig. 1 Metabolism of nizatidine

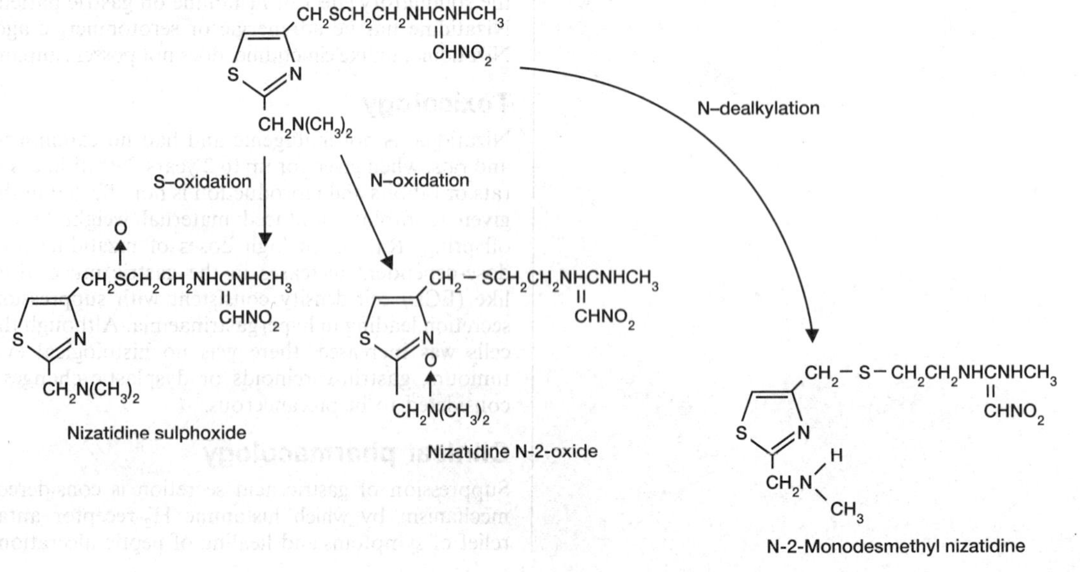

Mode of use

Clinical use depends on histamine H_2-receptor blockade suppressing the secretion of acid and pepsin. The recommended daily dose for treatment of duodenal and gastric ulcers is 300 mg, taken in the evening. Similar results are obtained if nizatidine 150 mg is taken twice daily, but once-daily administration is more convenient and has the theoretical advantage of not affecting daytime acid secretion or gastrin release.[4] Four weeks' treatment will heal most ulcers but therapy may be continued for a further four weeks if necessary. For the prevention of relapse of duodenal ulcers nizatidine 150 mg may be taken each evening for up to one year.

Indications

1. Therapy of duodenal ulceration
Treatment of duodenal ulcer disease with nizatidine 300 mg in the evening or with 150 mg twice daily produced healing of duodenal ulcers in about 70 and 90% of patients at 4 and 8 weeks respectively. Healing of duodenal ulcers on nizatidine is significantly faster than healing on placebo which is about 30% and 50% at 4 and 8 weeks respectively.[13,17,18]

Treatment with nizatidine also significantly decreased abdominal pain and the consumption of concomitant antacids.[17]

2. Therapy of benign gastric ulcer
The effect of nizatidine on the healing of gastric ulcers has been studied in a European multicentre study. After 8 weeks' therapy, 66% healed on nizatidine 150 mg twice daily and 65% healed on nizatidine 300 mg at night. There was no placebo group but ranitidine, which has been shown to promote healing of gastric ulcers,[19] also healed 66% of gastric ulcers in the same trial.[20]

3. Prevention of relapse of duodenal ulceration
Maintenance therapy with nizatidine 150 mg at night reduces recurrence of duodenal ulcers during a one-year period from 64% to 34%.[21] The protective effect of nizatidine 150 mg nightly is not significantly different from that produced by ranitidine 150 mg nightly.[13]

Contraindications

1. Hypersensitivity to nizatidine or other histamine H_2-receptor antagonists
Hypersensitivity to this group of drugs is rare and at the time of writing there have been no reports of cross-sensitivity between nizatidine and other H_2-receptor antagonists.

Adverse reactions

Potentially life-threatening effects
No lethal, or potentially life threatening adverse effects have been reported during treatment with nizatidine.

Acute overdosage
There is no experience of overdose in humans. Very high doses are relatively non-toxic in experimental animals. Such studies suggest that overdose in man might cause cholinergic-type effects such as lacrimation, salivation, emesis, miosis and diarrhoea.[1]

General supportive measures should be taken. Activated charcoal may reduce nizatidine absorption[12] and haemodialysis may remove absorbed nizatidine.

Severe or irreversible adverse effects
No adverse effects of this kind have been reported.

Symptomatic adverse effects[22]
Nizatidine is remarkably well tolerated and the incidence of adverse effects is close to that experienced on placebo. Urticaria, sweating and somnolence occurred more frequently with nizatidine, but several non-gastrointestinal disorders such as acne, eczema, palpitation and eye disorder have occurred more frequently on placebo.[13]

Other effects
Nizatidine has been reported to cause a slight elevation in serum cholesterol and uric acid.[13,22] Ranitidine has a similar effect on uric acid levels. These effects are probably not of great clinical significance.

Mildly abnormal liver function tests occur quite frequently during treatment with nizatidine but may be mainly due to coincidental causes because abnormalities also occurred in the placebo group. In one study, mildly abnormal alkaline phosphatase levels occurred in 11% and 7% of patients on nizatidine and placebo respectively.

There have been rare instances of markedly increased transaminases (>500 $IU.l^{-1}$), sometimes associated with jaundice, during treatment with nizatidine but causality has not been established. The abnormality reversed when the drug was discontinued.

Interference with clinical pathology tests
None is known.

High risk groups

Neonates
Nizatidine is not recommended for neonates and children because safety and efficacy have not been tested.

Breast milk. Nizatidine is excreted into human breast milk so nizatidine should be used in nursing mothers only if absolutely necessary.[15]

Children
What has been said about neonates also applies to older children.

Pregnant women
It has not been established that nizatidine is safe in human pregnancy but there was no evidence of impaired fertility or of teratogenicity in experimental animals. Nizatidine should not be used in women who are pregnant, or likely to become so, unless absolutely necessary.

The elderly
Age does not alter the efficacy or safety of nizatidine but, in the presence of renal impairment, the dose should be reduced.

Concurrent disease
Renal impairment. Nizatidine is excreted mainly via the kidneys. If the creatinine clearance rate is reduced to 20–50 $ml.min^{-1}$, the dose of nizatidine used to heal ulcers should be reduced to 150 mg daily. If the creatine clearance rate is <20 $ml.min^{-1}$, the dose should be 150 mg on alternate days. The dose used to maintain remission in duodenal ulcer disease should be reduced to 150 mg on alternate days if the creatinine clearance rate is reduced to 20–50 $ml.min^{-1}$. For patients with creatinine clearance rates <20 $ml.min^{-1}$ the maintenance dose should be 150 mg every three days.

Drug interactions

Potentially hazardous interactions
No interactions of this type have been observed.

Other significant interactions
Enzyme induction. Unlike cimetidine, nizatidine has little or no effect on the cytochrome P450-linked mixed function oxygenase system of the liver. Nizatidine does not impair the metabolism or potentiate the activity of warfarin, phenobarbitone, propantheline, diazepam,[23,24] propranolol,[11] chlordiazepoxide, theophylline, aminophylline, lorazepam,[25] ibuprofen,[13] lignocaine, metoprolol, antipyrine or amidopyrine.[13]

Food. Food does not significantly affect the absorption of nizatidine.[6]

Alcohol. Alcohol does not appear to alter the absorption, excretion or action of nizatidine (information from Lilly).

Smoking. Smoking delays the healing of duodenal ulcers during treatment with H_2-antagonists,[18] but there is currently no information to suggest that cigarette smoking affects the absorption or excretion of nizatidine, or the inhibitory effect of nizatidine on gastric secretion.

Potentially useful interactions
No interactions of this type have been observed.

Major outcome trials

1. Cloud M L, Offen W W, Matsumoto C 1987 Efficacy and safety of nizatidine 150 mg twice daily in the treatment of duodenal ulcer disease. Gastroenterology 92: 1348

In this endoscopically controlled, double-blind, multi-centre trial 555 patients with duodenal ulcers were randomized to receive nizatidine

Nizatidine

N

150 mg twice daily or placebo. On the respective regimes 76% and 39% patients healed at 4 weeks. Patients who failed to heal at 4 weeks were then reallocated nizatidine 150 mg twice daily or placebo. On the respective regimes 53% and 26% of these patients healed after a further 4 weeks. Adverse events on nizatidine were no more frequent than on placebo.

2. Dyck W P, Cloud M L, Offen W W, Matsumoto C 1987 Treatment of duodenal ulceration in the United States. Scandinavian Journal of Gastroenterology 22 (suppl 136): 47–55

In this multi-centre, endoscopically controlled, double-blind study 418 patients were randomized to receive either nizatidine 300 mg at bedtime, nizatidine 150 mg twice daily, nizatidine 25 mg twice daily or placebo. After 4 weeks' therapy 67%, 68%, 50% and 29% of ulcers had healed on the four regimes respectively. Patients whose ulcers had not healed at 4 weeks were randomly allocated to receive either nizatidine 150 mg twice daily or placebo for a further 4 weeks. Of these patients, about 50% healed on nizatidine and about 20% healed on placebo, irrespective of therapy during the first 4 weeks. Ulcer healing was associated with relief of symptoms and adverse events on nizatidine were not more frequent than on placebo.

3. Cloud M L, Matsumoto C, Offen W W 1986 Two night time doses of nizatidine compared in the treatment of acute duodenal ulcer. American Journal of Gastroenterology 81: 899

In this multi-centre, endoscopically controlled, double-blind study 284 patients with duodenal ulcers were randomized to receive either nizatidine 300 mg at night, nizatidine 100 mg at night or placebo. On the respective regimes 61%, 54% and 33% healed at 4 weeks and 82%, 77% and 49% healed at 8 weeks. Nizatidine 300 mg at night produced significantly greater symptom relief and ulcer healing than nizatidine 100 mg at night. Adverse events on nizatidine were no more frequent than on placebo.

Other randomized trials

1. Simon B, Cremer M, Dammann H G et al and members of the European Duodenal Ulcer Study Group 1987 300 mg nizatidine at night versus 300 mg ranitidine at night in patients with duodenal ulcer. Scandinavian Journal of Gastroenterology 22 (suppl 136): 61–70
2. Cheyner J A, Cloud M L, Offen W W et al 1989 Comparison of nizatidine and cimetidine as once-nightly treatment of acute duodenal ulcer. American Journal of Gastroenterology 84: 769–774
3. Naccaratto R, Cremer M, Dammann H G et al 1987 Nizatidine versus ranitidine in gastric ulcer disease. Scandinavian Journal of Gastroenterology 22 (suppl 136): 71–78
4. Cerulli M A, Cloud M L, Offen W W, Chernish S M, Matsumoto C 1987 Nizatidine as maintenance therapy of duodenal ulcer disease in remission. Scandinavian Journal of Gastroenterology 22 (suppl 136): 79–83
5. Hentschel E, Schutze K, Reichel W et al 1987 Nizatidine versus ranitidine in the prevention of duodenal ulcer relapse: six month interim results of a European multicentre study. Scandinavian Journal of Gastroenterology 22 (suppl 136): 84–88 The results at one year are described in reference 11.

References

1. Morton D M 1987 Pharmacology and toxicology of nizatidine. Scandinavian Journal of Gastroenterology 22 (suppl 136): 1–8
2. Lin T M, Evans D C, Warrick M W, Pioch R P 1986 Actions of nizatidine, a selective histamine H_2 receptor antagonist, on gastric acid secretion in dogs, rats and frogs. Journal of Pharmacology and Experimental Therapeutics 239: 406–410
3. Dammann H G, Gottlieb W R, Walter T A, Muller P, Simon B, Keohane P 1978 The 24-hour acid suppression profile of Nizatidine. Scandinavian Journal of Gastroenterology 22 (suppl 136): 56–60
4. Kovacs T O G, Van Deventer G M, Maxwell V, Sytnik B, Walsh J H 1987 The effect of an oral evening dose of nizatidine on nocturnal and peptine-stimulated gastric acid and gastrin secretion. Scandinavian Journal of Gastroenterology 22 (suppl 136): 41–46
5. Cunningham M, Male P J, Griessen M, Striberni R, Loizeau E 1985 24-hour H^+ activity, nocturnal acid and pepsin output on a new H_2-receptor antagonist, nizatidine. American Journal of Gastroenterology 80: 839
6. Callaghan J T, Bergstrom R F, Rubin A et al 1987 A pharmacokinetic profile of nizatidine in man. Scandinavian Journal of Gastroenterology 22 (suppl 136): 9–17
7. Welage L S, Grasela T H, Thomas R W, Wing P E, Mueller L S 1987 The concentration effect relationship of nizatidine on stimulated gastric acid secretion. Clinical Pharmacology and Therapeutics 41: 225
8. Linscheer W G, Raheja K L, Hirose N 1985 A double-blind controlled study proves nizatidine to be much more potent than cimetidine. Gastroenterology 88: 1478
9. Callaghan J T, Ridolfo A S, Crabtree R E, Obermeyer B D, Offen W W, De Sante K A 1987 Nizatidine: effect on aspirin-induced gastro-intestinal red blood cell loss. Gastroenterology 92: 1336
10. Van Thiel D H, Gavaler J S, Heyl A, Susen B 1987 An evaluation of the antiandrogen effects associated with H_2-antagonist therapy. Scandinavian Journal of Gastroenterology 22 (suppl 136): 24–28
11. Knadler M P, Bergstrom R F, Callaghan J T, Rubin A 1986 Nizatidine, an H_2-blocker; its metabolism and disposition in man. Drug Metabolism Disposition 14: 175–182
12. Knadler M P, Rubin A, Bergstrom R F, Callaghan J T 1984 Effects of gelusil, charcoal and propantheline on the bioavailability of the H_2-blocker nizatidine. The Pharmacologist 26: 236
13. 1988 AXID nizatidine. Eli Lilly Company Limited, Basingstoke, Hampshire
14. Schenker S, Johnson R, Mor L, Henderson G, Dicke J 1986 Human placental transport of cimetidine (C), ranitidine (R) and nizatidine (N). Clinical Research 34: 445A
15. Obermeyer B D, Bergstrom R F, Callaghan J T, Golichowsky A, Knadler M P, Rubin A 1988 Secretion of nizatidine into human breast milk. Pharmacologist 30: A13
16. Aronoff G R, Sloan R S, Bopp R J, Walters J B, Bergstrom R F, Callaghan J T 1986 Nizatidine kinetics in patients with renal insufficiency. Clinical Pharmacology and Therapeutics 39: 178
17. Dyck W P, Cloud M L, Offen W W, Matsumoto C, Chernish S M 1987 Treatment of duodenal ulceration in the United States. Scandinavian Journal of Gastroenterology 22 (suppl 136): 47–55
18. Simon B, Cremer M, Dammann H G et al 1987 300 mg nizatidine at night versus 300 mg ranitidine at night in patients with duodenal ulcer. A multicentre trial in Europe. Scandinavian Journal of Gastroenterology 22 (suppl 136): 61–70
19. Ryan F P 1982 A comparison of ranitidine and placebo in the acute treatment of gastric ulcer. In: Misiewicz J J, Wormsley K G (ed) The clinical uses of ranitidine: proceedings of the second international symposium on ranitidine. Medicine Publishing Foundation, Oxford, pp 201–206
20. Nacarratto R, Cremer M, Dammann H G et al 1987 Nizatidine versus ranitidine in gastric ulcer disease. A European multicentre trial. Scandinavian Journal of Gastroenterology 22 (suppl 136): 71–78
21. Cerulli M A, Cloud M L, Offen W W, Chernish S M, Matsumoto C 1987 Nizatidine as maintenance therapy of duodenal ulcer. Scandinavian Journal of Gastroenterology 22 (suppl 136): 79–83
22. Cloud M L 1987 Safety of nizatidine in clinical trials conducted in the USA and Europe. Scandinavian Journal of Gastroenterology 22 (suppl 136): 29–36
23. Klotz U 1987 Lack of effect of nizatidine on drug metabolism. Scandinavian Journal of Gastroenterology 22 (suppl 136): 18–23
24. Pasanen M, Arvela P, Pelkonen O, Sotaniemi E, Klotz U 1986 Effect of five structurally diverse H_2-receptor antagonists on drug metabolism. Biochemical Pharmacology 35: 4457–4461
25. Secor J W, Speeg K V, Meredith G G, Johnson R F, Snowdy P, Schenker S 1985 Lack of effect of nizatidine on hepatic drug metabolism in man. British Journal of Clinical Pharmacology 20: 710–713
26. Price A H, Brogden R N 1988 Nizatidine: a preliminary review of its pharmacodynamic and pharmacokinetic properties, and its therapeutic use in peptic ulcer disease. ADIS Press, Auckland, pp 522–539

Noradrenaline (acid tartrate)

Noradrenaline (norepinephrine) is an endogenous catecholamine released from sympathetic nerve endings.

Chemistry

Noradrenaline acid tartrate (norepinephrine bitartrate, Levophed)
$C_8H_{11}NO_3.C_4H_6O_6.H_2O$
(R)-β,3,4-Trihydroxyphenethylammonium hydrogen tartrate

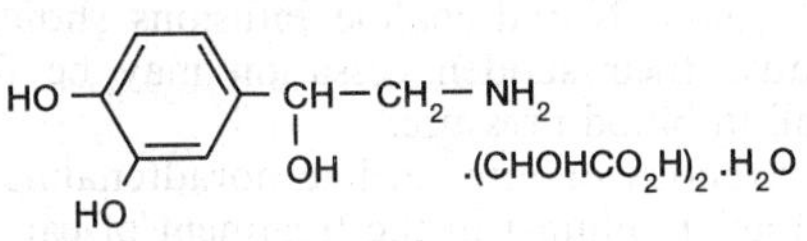

Molecular weight (free base)	337.3 (169.2)
pKa	8.6, 9.8, 12
Solubility	
in alcohol	1 in 300
in water	1 in 2.5
Octanol/water partition coefficient	—

Noradrenaline acid tartrate is an odourless, white or faintly grey, crystalline powder with a bitter taste. It slowly darkens on exposure to air and light, and turns brown in alkaline or neutral solutions. Noradrenaline occurs naturally and can be prepared by chemical synthesis. The (l)-enantiomer is used clinically. Noradrenaline is available in combination with lignocaine (Lignostab-N).

Pharmacology

Noradrenaline is a potent agonist at the α-adrenergic receptor and, when injected intravenously, shows predominantly α-mediated effects. It also possesses β-stimulating properties which can be best demonstrated after α-receptor blockade. It is equipotent to adrenaline at β_1-receptors but has little action on β_2-receptors.

Toxicology

Chronic administration of hypertensive or even sub-hypertensive doses of noradrenaline to dogs results in significant cardiac hypertrophy.[1,2] Intra-amniotic injections of noradrenaline to pregnant mice produce haemorrhagic lesions of the fetal extremities.[3]

Clinical pharmacology

Infusion of noradrenaline into man produces α-adrenergic receptor mediated vasoconstriction with an increase in total peripheral resistance and elevation of both diastolic and systolic blood pressure.[4,5] This is accompanied by a vagal mediated reflex fall in heart rate. Cardiac output is unchanged or reduced. Peripheral vascular resistance increases in most vascular beds and the blood flow through the kidney, liver and skeletal muscle is decreased.

Infusion of noradrenaline at incremental rates (10–75 $ng.kg^{-1}.min^{-1}$) produces dose-dependent increases in systolic and diastolic blood pressure and depression of heart rate. The changes induced in plasma noradrenaline, blood pressure and heart rate are near maximal by the tenth minute of a constant-rate continuous infusion. The pressor response can be maintained throughout a ten hour infusion but depression of heart rate may be variable over the infusion period. Blood pressure and heart rate return to basal levels within several minutes of stopping an infusion.[6]

Non-cardiovascular responses to noradrenaline in man are not as prominent as those observed with adrenaline. Infusion of noradrenaline in normal subjects increases circulating glycerol, acetoacetate, β-hydroxybutyrate and glucose levels. Circulating levels of insulin, lactate, pyruvate and alanine are decreased but plasma glucagon, cortisol and growth hormone levels remain unchanged.[5] Based on the plasma catecholamine thresholds required to produce various haemodynamic and metabolic effects, noradrenaline has been estimated to be ten times less potent than adrenaline.[7]

Pharmacokinetics

The preferred analytical techniques are high performance liquid chromatography (HPLC) or radioenzymatic assay (REA).[7–10] The sensitivity of both the HPLC and REA assays is 20 $ng.l^{-1}$.

Noradrenaline is rapidly and extensively metabolized in the gut and liver and consequently ineffective after oral administration. It is poorly absorbed from subcutaneous injection sites due to local vasoconstriction. Animal studies show that noradrenaline is rapidly but unequally distributed in tissues. Heart, spleen and glandular tissues show the highest uptake and skeletal muscle the lowest. Noradrenaline is extensively metabolized in man and only small amounts are excreted unchanged in the urine. It is rapidly cleared, at 20–100 $ml.kg^{-1}.min^{-1}$. This, together with a small volume of distribution, 0.09–0.40 $l.kg^{-1}$, results in a very short half life, which ranges from 0.6 to 2.9 min.

Oral absorption	good
Presystemic metabolism	>95%
Plasma half life	
range	0.6–2.9 min
Volume of distribution	0.09–0.40 $l.kg^{-1}$
Plasma protein binding	~50%

Noradrenaline is not excreted in breast milk to any appreciable extent. Any of the compound ingested by an infant by this route will be degraded before reaching the systemic circulation. Although noradrenaline does not cross the placenta in significant amounts it can affect the placenta itself.

Noradrenaline is extensively metabolized in the liver and a variety of other tissues. Most of a dose is excreted in the urine, up to 16% as the unchanged compound following intravenous administration. Virtually no free noradrenaline is excreted from endogenous sources in normal subjects. The kinetics of noradrenaline are not significantly affected by renal or hepatic disease. Although noradrenaline is metabolized by the liver, it is most significantly cleared by uptake into nerve endings and extraneuronal tissues. The excretion of noradrenaline is significantly increased in patients with phaeochromocytoma who may excrete as much as 15 mg per day. None of the metabolites of noradrenaline is active.

Concentration–effect relationship

Intravenous infusion of noradrenaline at increasing rates leads to concentration-dependent increases in diastolic and systolic blood pressure and decrease in heart rate.[6] Infusions which produced mean steady-state plasma concentrations between 0.275 and 2.15 $pg.l^{-1}$ showed that levels in excess of 1.8 $pg.l^{-1}$ are required to produce haemodynamic and metabolic effects. Highly significant parabolic concentration–effect relationships have been found for blood pressure and circulating glycerol, acetoacetate, β-hydroxybutyrate and glucose (increased) and heart rate and circulating insulin, lactate, pyruvate and alanine (decreased).[5]

Metabolism

Noradrenaline is extensively metabolized in the liver and other tissues. Both the parent compound and its metabolites are excreted largely in the urine.

Noradrenaline undergoes O-methylation catalysed by catechol O-methyltransferase (COMT) to form normetanephrine. Normetanephrine is deaminated (a reaction catalysed by monoamine oxidase [MAO]) to form a short-lived product, 3-methoxy-4-hydroxymandelic aldehyde, which undergoes further oxidation or reduction to 3-methoxy-4-hydroxymandelic acid or 3-methoxy-4-hydroxyphenylethyleneglycol, respectively. The reaction sequence also occurs in

Noradrenaline (acid tartrate)

N

reverse with the action of monoamine oxidase producing 3,4-dihydroxymandelic acid which is then methylated to 3-methoxy-4-hydroxymandelic acid; the metabolites are conjugated with glucuronic acid or sulphate or further metabolized. The paths by which noradrenaline is metabolized vary with the route of administration, and in particular there is a greater proportion of deaminated metabolites when noradrenaline is released from sympathetic nerve endings than when it is infused into the bloodstream.[11,12] Up to 16% of an intravenous dose is excreted unchanged in the urine, whereas negligible amounts of endogenous noradrenaline are excreted unchanged in normal subjects.

Pharmaceutics

Noradrenaline acid tartrate is available in two formulations for intravenous administration:

1. Noradrenaline acid tartrate 2 $mg.ml^{-1}$ injection, Levophed (Winthrop, UK/Winthrop-Breon, USA) in 2 and 4 ml ampoules.
2. Noradrenaline acid tartrate 200 $\mu g.ml^{-1}$ special injection, Levophed Special (Winthrop, UK) in a 2 ml ampoule, for intravenous or intracardiac injection.

Noradrenaline acid tartrate solution should be protected from light. It must not be used if brown in colour. (See also Mode of use).

Therapeutic use

Indications

1. The treatment of acute hypotension
2. Adjunctive use in local anaesthesia.

Contraindications

1. Hypertension
2. Hyperthyroidism
3. Ischaemic heart disease
4. Myocardial infarction.

Fig. 1 Metabolism of noradrenaline

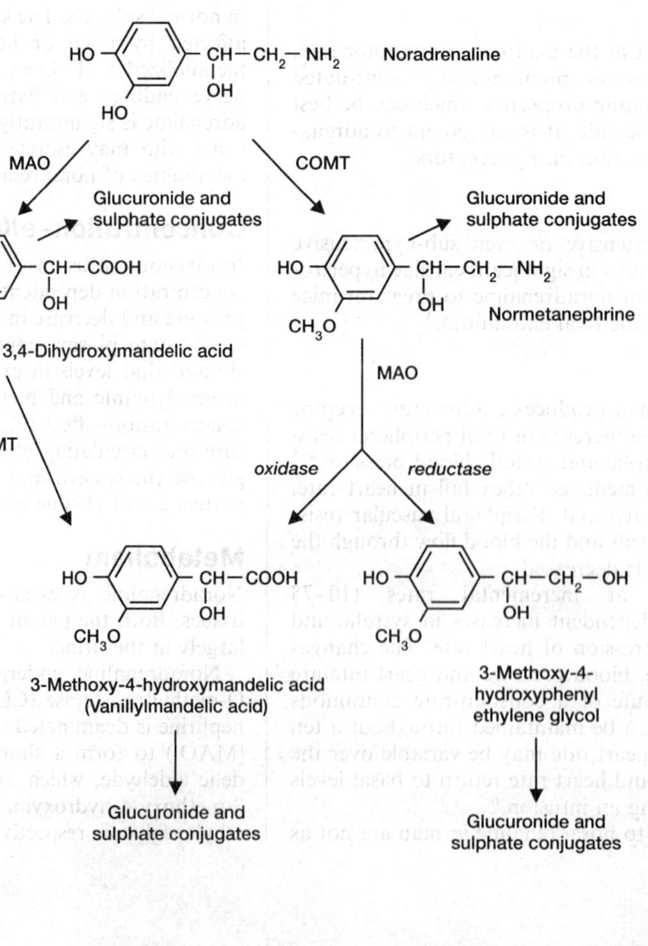

Mode of use

Noradrenaline must be diluted and given as an intravenous infusion. An infusion is prepared by diluting to 250 times its volume (8 $mg.l^{-1}$ acid tartrate; 4 $mg.l^{-1}$ base) with glucose 5% or sodium chloride and glucose infusion. Sodium chloride 0.9% should not be used for dilution as the pH of the infusion must be below 6 for maximum stability.

(See Adverse reactions for treatment if extravasation occurs.)

The response to noradrenaline is dependent on the rate of infusion, which must be adjusted accordingly with close monitoring of blood pressure and the electrocardiogram. Blood pressure must be taken at 5 minute intervals and more frequently at the beginning of the infusion.

It has been suggested that the cardiovascular response to a test dose of 0.1–0.2 $\mu g.kg^{-1}$ of noradrenaline base be observed carefully before adjustment of the infusion rate to obtain the desired pressor response. The usual dose range is 2–4 μg of base per minute (1 $ml.min^{-1}$). Blood pressure should not be raised to more than normotensive levels.

In order to minimize the risk of tissue necrosis due to impaired circulation and extravasation, the infusion site should be changed at least every 12 hours. Noradrenaline infusions should be stopped gradually because their sudden cessation may be followed by a catastrophic fall in blood pressure.

A rapid intravenous or intracardiac noradrenaline injection has been suggested as an adjunct in the treatment of cardiac arrest but there is little evidence of its value and it is best avoided.

Indications

1. Acute hypotension

Noradrenaline has limited therapeutic value in the treatment of acute hypotension. Volume expansion is almost always a more appropriate measure. It should be emphasized that hypotension per se is not an indication for the use of noradrenaline. The main danger of noradrenaline administration is reduced perfusion through the kidney, liver, skin and skeletal muscle with tissue ischaemia. Coronary blood flow, however, is usually increased.[13,14]

Noradrenaline should be considered in the treatment of shock only if there is evidence that hypotension is the cause of inadequate perfusion of vital organs. It should be noted that, except in neurogenic shock and shock associated with spinal anaesthesia, peripheral resistance is probably already high due to reflex vasoconstriction mediated by the sympathetic nervous system. Noradrenaline may further compromise blood flow to vital organs.

The haemodynamic response to noradrenaline may vary depending on the circulatory status of the patient on initiation of treatment.[15] Noradrenaline may be used in an emergency to raise the blood pressure and sustain the coronary and cerebral circulation until measures can be taken to restore an adequate circulating blood volume. It may also be of value where volume expansion has been ineffective or is unacceptable. In general, however, the risks and difficulties of administering noradrenaline far outweigh the potential benefits to the patient.

2. Adjunctive use in local anaesthesia

Noradrenaline is used in concentrations of 1 in 80 000 or less to reduce and delay the absorption of local anaesthetics. The effects of local anaesthetics are thus localized and prolonged.

Contraindications

1. Hypertension

Hypertensive patients may be more sensitive to the pressor effects of noradrenaline.

2. Hyperthyroidism

Patients suffering from hyperthyroidism are hypersensitive to the effects of noradrenaline and toxicity may occur in low doses.

3. Ischaemic heart disease

Coronary blood flow is generally increased by noradrenaline but patients with Prinzmetal's variant angina are hypersensitive to the α-adrenergic vasoconstrictor effects of noradrenaline. In such patients, coronary blood flow may be reduced to such an extent and duration as to cause myocardial infarction.

4. Myocardial infarction

Unequivocal diagnosis of hypotension and shock is required for the use of noradrenaline in patients with myocardial infarction since animal studies suggest that infarct size may be extended in normotensive subjects.[16]

Adverse reactions

Potentially life-threatening effects

The potentially life-threatening effects of noradrenaline stem from its dose-related hypertensive action. Acute hypertension with cerebral haemorrhage and pulmonary oedema may occur.

Acute overdosage

Overdoses or conventional doses in hypertensive individuals lead to severe hypertension with violent headache, photophobia, stabbing retrosternal pain, pallor, intense sweating and vomiting. An overdose may be treated with an intravenous dose of the α-adrenergic blocker phentolamine.

Severe or irreversible adverse effects

Extravasation of noradrenaline during an intravenous infusion leads to sloughing and necrosis around the infusion site. Gangrene of the extremities may follow prolonged infusions. Impaired circulation at infusion sites, with or without extravasation, may be relieved by hot packs and infiltration of the area with phentolamine (5 mg diluted to 10 ml with normal saline).

Symptomatic adverse effects

Anxiety, palpitations, bradycardia and transient headache are common adverse effects.

Other effects

Noradrenaline has been shown to increase circulating levels of glycerol, acetoacetate, β-hydroxybutyrate and glucose. Plasma insulin, lactate, pyruvate and alanine levels are decreased by noradrenaline.

Interference with clinical pathology tests

There are no well documented reports of the effect of exogenous noradrenaline on commonly used clinical laboratory tests.

Noradrenaline (acid tartrate)

High risk groups

Neonates

The particular effects of noradrenaline in neonates are not well documented.

Breast milk. Since noradrenaline does not achieve pharmacologically active levels after oral administration, breast-feeding should not present any hazard to the infant.

Children

Similar care must be exercised in giving noradrenaline to children as in adults. An initial dose of $0.05\ \mu g.kg^{-1}.min^{-1}$ of noradrenaline base may be infused with blood pressure monitoring and adjusted up to $0.5\ \mu g.kg^{-1}.min^{-1}$ base.

Pregnant women

Noradrenaline should be avoided in pregnancy, as placental perfusion may be reduced, and fetal bradycardia has been reported.[17] The contractile action of noradrenaline on the pregnant uterus may lead to fetal asphyxia in late pregnancy.

The elderly

The elderly are particularly susceptible to the effects of sympathomimetic agents and noradrenaline must be used cautiously.

Drug interactions

Potentially hazardous interactions

Tricyclic antidepressants. Intravenous infusion of noradrenaline in healthy subjects or patients receiving tricyclic antidepressants produces several fold increases in the pressor response to noradrenaline.[18,19] Noradrenaline should be avoided or given with great caution in patients on tricyclic antidepressant therapy.

Halogenated anaesthetic agents. Noradrenaline is less likely to induce arrhythmias than adrenaline but must be used with great caution in patients receiving halothane and other halogenated anaesthetics.

Other significant interactions

Adrenergic-neurone blocking agents. The pressor effect of noradrenaline may be enhanced in patients receiving guanethidine and the risk of cardiac arrhythmias may be increased.[20]

Methyldopa. Only a slight increase in the pressor response to noradrenaline has been observed in patients receiving methyldopa but the duration of the pressor response is considerably prolonged.[21]

Digoxin. Digoxin and other drugs which sensitize the myocardium may increase the risk of arrhythmias in patients receiving noradrenaline.

Potentially useful interactions

Noradrenaline is sometimes combined with local anaesthetic agents to localize and prolong the action of the anaesthetic drugs.

General review articles

Axelrod J 1963 The formation, metabolism, uptake and release of noradrenaline and adrenaline. In: Varley H, Gowenlock A H (eds) The clinical chemistry of monoamines. Elsevier, Amsterdam

Weiner N 1985 Norepinephrine, epinephrine and the sympathomimetic amines. In: Goodman L S, Gilman A G (eds) The pharmacological basis of therapeutics, 7th edn. Macmillan, New York, pp 145–180

Tarazi R C 1974 Sympathomimetic agents in the treatment of shock. Annals of Internal Medicine 81: 364–371

References

1. Gans J H, Cater M R 1970 Norepinephrine-induced cardiac hypertrophy in dogs. Life Sciences 9: 731–736
2. Laks M M, Morady F, Swan H J C 1973 Myocardial hypertrophy produced by chronic infusion of sub-hypertensive doses of norepinephrine in the dog. Chest 64: 75
3. Davies J, Robson J M 1970 The effects of vasopressin, adrenaline and noradrenaline on the mouse fetus. British Journal of Pharmacology 38: 446P
4. Allwood M J, Cobbold A F, Ginsburg J 1963 Peripheral vascular effects of noradrenaline, isopropylnoradrenaline and dopamine. British Medical Bulletin 19: 132–136
5. Silverberg A B, Shah S D, Haymond M W, Cryer P E 1978 Norepinephrine: hormone and neurotransmitter in man. American Journal of Physiology 234: E252–E256

N

6. Fitzgerald G A, Hossmann V, Hamilton C A, Reid J L, Davies D S, Dollery C T 1979 Interindividual variation in kinetics of infused norepinephrine. Clinical Pharmacology and Therapeutics 26: 669–675
7. Clutter W E, Brier D M, Shah S D, Cryer P E 1980 Epinephrine plasma metabolic clearance rates and physiologic thresholds for metabolic and haemodynamic actions in man. Journal of Clinical Investigation 66: 94–101
8. Causon R C 1985 High performance liquid chromatographic separation and determination of catecholamines. In: Marks N, Rodnight R (eds) Research methods in neurochemistry, vol 6. Plenum Publishing Corporation, New York pp 211–241
9. Brown M J, Jenner D A 1981 Novel double isotope technique for the enzymatic assay of catecholamines, permitting high precision, sensitivity and plasma sample capacity. Clinical Science 61: 591–598
10. Causon R C, Brown M J, Boulou P M, Perret D 1983 Analytical differences in measurement of plasma catecholamines. Clinical Chemistry 29: 735–736
11. Nagatsu T 1973 Biochemistry of catecholamines: the biochemical method. University Park Press, Baltimore, pp 94–101
12. Brown M J 1984 Simultaneous assay of noradrenaline and its deaminated metabolite, dihydroxyphenylglycol, in plasma: a simplified approach to the exclusion of phaeochromocytoma in patients with borderline elevation of plasma noradrenaline concentration. European Journal of Clinical Investigation 14: 67–72
13. Mueller H, Ayres M, Giannelli S, Conklin E F, Mazzara J T, Grace W J 1972 Effect of isoproterenol, 1-norepinephrine and intraaortic counterpulsation on haemodynamics and myocardial metabolism in shock following acute myocardial infarction. Circulation 45: 335–351
14. Mueller H, Ayres S M, Gregory J J, Giannelli S, Grace W J 1970 Haemodynamics, coronary blood flow and myocardial metabolism in coronary shock: response to 1-norepinephrine and isoproterenol. Journal of Clinical Investigation 49: 1885–1902
15. Cohn J N, Luria M H 1965 Studies in clinical shock and hypotension. II. Haemodynamic effects of norepinephrine and angiotensin. Journal of Clinical Investigation 44: 1494–1504
16. Lesch M 1976 Inotropic agents and infarct size: theoretical and practical considerations. American Journal of Cardiology 37: 508–513
17. Beard R W 1962 Response of human foetal heart and maternal circulation to adrenaline and noradrenaline. British Medical Journal 1: 443–446
18. Boakes A J, Laurence D R, Teoh P C, Barar F S K, Benedikter L T, Prichard B N C 1973 Interactions between sympathomimetic amines and antidepressant agents in man. British Medical Journal 1: 311–315
19. Mitchell J R, Cavanaugh J H, Arias L, Oates J A 1970 Guanethidine and related agents. III. Antagonism by drugs which inhibit the norepinephrine pump in man. Journal of Clinical Investigation 49: 1596–1604
20. Muelheims G H, Estrup R W, Paiewonsky D, Mierzwiak D S 1965 Increased sensitivity of the heart to catecholamine-induced arrhythmias following guanethidine. Clinical Pharmacology and Therapeutics 6: 757–762
21. Dollery C T, Harington M, Hodge J V 1963 Haemodynamic studies with methyldopa: effect on cardiac output and response to pressor amines. British Heart Journal 25: 670–676

Norethisterone, (acetate, heptanoate)

Norethisterone was the first highly active oral progestational agent to be synthesized and to achieve widespread use. It was patented in 1951.

Chemistry

Norethisterone (norethindrone)
$C_{20}H_{26}O_2$
17α-Ethinyl-19-nortestosterone, 17β-hydroxy-19-nor-17α-pregn-4-en-20-yn-3-one, 17α-ethinyl-17β-hydroxy-19-nor-androst-4-en-3-one

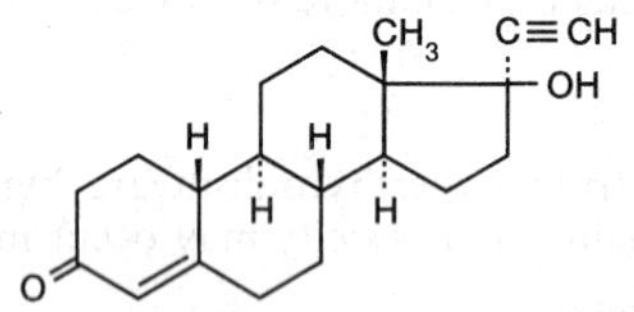

Molecular weight	298.4
pKa	—
Solubility	
in alcohol	1 in 150
in water	1 in 10 000
Octanol/water partition coefficient	—

Norethisterone is a white or creamy white, odourless, crystalline powder with a slightly bitter taste. It is practically insoluble in fixed oils, soluble in dioxane and most alcohols and slightly soluble in ether. It is prepared by chemical synthesis, usually from precursors obtained from the Mexican yam (*Dioscorea*). Both the 17β-acetate and the 17β-heptanoate (oenanthate) are used clinically and are rapidly converted to norethisterone in vivo. Some other orally active synthetic progestogens, including ethynodiol diacetate, lynoestrenol and norethynodrel, are metabolized to norethisterone in vivo.

Two ester forms are used. The acetate is rapidly hydrolysed after oral administration. The heptanoate is only used by intramuscular injection. It is probably fairly rapidly hydrolysed once taken up from the injection site; long duration of action depends on delayed absorption from the injection site.

Trade names of the compound and its esters used in Great Britain include Micronor, Noriday, Noristerat, Primolut N, SH420, Utovlan. Names used abroad include Aygestin, Conludag, Gesta Plan, Micronovum, Milligynon, Mini-Pe, Mini-Pill, Norfar, Norgestin, Norlutate, Norluten, Norlutin, Nor-QD, Nur-Isterate (the heptanoate) and Prolutеasi. Some oral preparations contain norethisterone acetate but this is rapidly hydrolysed to norethisterone and the two can be considered as equivalent. Norethisterone is also available with ethinyloestradiol in Anovlar 21, BiNovum, Brevinor, Gynovlar 21, Loestrin 20 and 30, Minovlar, Minovlar ED, Neocon 1/35, Norimin, Norlestrin, Orlest 21, Ovysmen, Synphase and TriNovum, principally used as oral contraceptives; and Controvlar, used to control menstrual symptoms. Norethisterone is combined with mestranol in the oral contraceptives Norinyl-1 and Ortho-Novin 1/50 and in Menophase and Estrapak, used in menopausal symptoms. Trisequens is a combination of norethisterone, oestradiol and oestriol, used for menopausal symptoms.

Pharmacology

Like progesterone, norethisterone will produce secretory changes in the oestrogen-primed endometrium and affect the activity of many

Norethisterone (acetate, heptanoate)

enzymes. Stimulation of carbonic anhydrase in rabbit uterus has been used for bioassay. Enzymes related to liver function including transaminases such as γ-glutamyl transpeptidase, liver monoamine oxidase, and the enzymes of the glycolytic pathways can be inhibited by norethisterone, and some of the metabolic effects of the drug are enzyme mediated.

Norethisterone exerts its biological activity mainly by interaction with receptors which exist in many tissues, principally those of the reproductive tract, breast, liver and brain. In some tissues, particularly endometrium, the progesterone receptor to which norethisterone binds is oestrogen induced. The binding affinity for norethisterone to the receptors in the endometrium is similar to that of progesterone itself.

Norethisterone will not support pregnancy in animals from which the corpus luteum has been removed but in rats it will delay parturition.

In experimental animals other endocrinological effects include an androgenic and anabolic action, with a potency of approximately 2% and 10% respectively of that of testosterone propionate; it will also bind to rat prostate androgen receptors. There is little oestrogenic activity in acute assays but norethisterone has about 0.3% of the oestrogenic potency of ethinyloestradiol on long-term administration to rats. This activity may result from in vivo conversion to oestrogen in this species, though norethisterone has been found to bind to a small degree to oestrogen receptors in both rats and rabbits. In mice, norethisterone will antagonize oestrogen-stimulated uterine growth and vaginal changes. In progestogenic tests such as stimulation of decidual reaction and pregnancy maintenance, and in receptor binding, norethisterone can act as a competitive antagonist of progesterone itself. In addition, norethisterone will inhibit androgen-induced comb growth in chicks.

Like other progestogens, norethisterone has a thermogenic effect, resembling that of progesterone, seen in the second half of the menstrual cycle. In addition to receptor mechanisms, the drug may act directly on membrane excitability and affect hypothalamic and cerebral functions. Behavioural changes such as those occurring in oestrus and in mating can be influenced in animals, but similar effects are less obvious in humans.

Toxicology

The toxicity of norethisterone is very low, given either alone or with oestrogen. Large doses of the progestogen can be given without causing death. In subacute and chronic studies only minimal differences between treated and control animals are observed. Loss of fertility occurs in treated animals as a result of pituitary inhibition but fertility is rapidly restored at the end of the treatment period. Reports of teratogenic effects in animals are uncommon, but masculinization of fetuses, estimated by changes in the anogenital distance, has been reported at doses greater than 5 mg daily in rats. In the mouse, with 1–10 mg daily from days 8 to 15 of pregnancy there was no virilization but some fetuses had cleft palate. No carcinogenic effects have been found even in long-term studies.

Clinical pharmacology

Hypothalamus and anterior pituitary gland

Norethisterone depresses the production of LH but has less effect on FSH secretion. Since simultaneous administration of LH-releasing factor can restore LH levels it seems likely that the effect is mediated by reduction of endogenous production of LH-releasing factor in the hypothalamus. Small doses of norethisterone (350 µg daily) used as an oral contraceptive only suppress ovulation in less than half the patients so treated. Intermediate doses (5–10 mg daily) do suppress ovulation. Large doses of norethisterone hexanoate, given in intramuscular depot injections, inhibit ovulation. These injections can produce blood levels as high as 8000 ng.l^{-1} two weeks later, falling to low levels only 10 to 12 weeks later. Repeated doses at 8-week intervals can produce prolonged inhibition of pituitary gonadotrophin production.

Ovary

Large doses of norethisterone heptanoate reduce ovarian steroidogenesis so that circulating oestradiol levels are in the low follicular phase range. In women taking small doses of norethisterone the structure of the corpus luteum seems normal, but function as estimated by pregnanediol production is impaired. In this respect norethisterone differs from 17α-hydroxyprogesterone derivatives, which do not affect luteal function.

Endometrium

Norethisterone will produce secretory transformation of the oestrogen-primed endometrium, with development of subnuclear vacuoles, but it alters the development of the endometrial stroma and glands. The stroma is excessively vascularized, is oedematous and has the appearance of decidua, contrasting with the glands, which are atrophic, with absent mucus secretion. This can deter implantation of blastocysts. Norethisterone postpones menstruation when administered before and during the time when menstrual bleeding is due. The effect is enhanced by concurrent administration of oestrogen. Prolonged exposure to progestogens can cause dilated endometrial sinusoids. In three-quarters of women who take 5 mg of norethisterone daily for 5 years proliferation of the endometrium is absent. Norethisterone heptanoate, 200 mg intramuscularly, causes atrophy of the endometrial glands, reduced mucus secretion and oedema and increased vascularity of the endometrial stroma. In some cases normal cyclical changes resume during the second month after injection, in others atrophic change is more prolonged. Larger doses of norethisterone of the order of 20–50 mg daily can cause not only atrophy of uterine endometrium, but also atrophy and necrosis in ectopic endometriotic deposits.

Myometrium

In women with proliferative phase oestrogen levels, or given small oestrogen supplements, norethisterone 5–20 mg daily induces over several days a myometrial contraction pattern with high amplitude, long duration and low frequency of contractions, resembling that seen physiologically in the late secretory phase of the cycle.

Fallopian tube

Progestogens such as norethisterone tend to reduce numbers and height of cilia on the cells lining the tube. In addition, they cause increase in frequency but decrease in amplitude of smooth muscle contractions in the tube. Both these effects could delay tubal transport of ova.

Cervical mucus

Norethisterone administration increases the protein and sialic acid content of cervical mucus. This enhances the binding between the glycofibrils of the mucus, increasing viscosity and reducing elasticity and inhibiting the liquefaction normally produced by increased endogenous oestrogen at the mid-cycle. This tends to prevent penetration of the mucus by spermatozoa. The effect of norethisterone on cervical mucus is antagonized by concurrent administration of oestrogen. It has been suggested that progestogens can induce biochemical changes in cervical mucus which reduce the respiration and motility of spermatozoa and prevent capacitation.

Androgen activity

This is not seen in humans unless the drug is administered in very large doses.

Systemic effects

Norethisterone has little significant action on the cardiovascular system or on coagulation mechanisms. Prolonged administration of small doses (350 µg daily) have been reported to be associated with slight reductions in blood pressure. When given in combination with synthetic oestrogens in oral contraceptives, a small incidence of hypertension related to dose of norethisterone results. Norethisterone alone (350 µg daily) does not affect plasma coagulation factors VII, IX or X, or antithrombin III, or cause thrombosis or embolism, but when given in larger doses (1 mg daily) with ethinyloestradiol, the combination causes a minor elevation of prothrombin and plasma factors VII, VIII, IX and X, which is not reproduced by a combination of norgestrel and ethinyloestradiol. With norethisterone heptanoate (200 mg intramuscularly), a minor reduction of recalcification and thromboplastin times and an increase in haemoglobin level have been observed, but there have been no observations of thrombosis or embolism. Combination with synthetic oestrogens leads to changes in coagulation factors which are associated with thromboembolic disease, particularly in women over 40 who are hyperlipidaemic, obese, hypertensive smokers.

Norethisterone (acetate, heptanoate)

Low doses (350 μg daily) of norethisterone given alone have little or no effect on plasma cortisol or on thyroid function. Larger doses (norethisterone heptanoate, 200 mg intramuscularly) do not affect basal cortisol but may reduce dexamethasone suppression. When norethisterone is given with oestrogen, increase in plasma binding proteins leads to elevated total plasma levels of cortisol. Serum protein-bound iodine may be increased and tri-iodothyroxine uptake diminished. Free thyroxine is unaltered.

Progestogens in general have a mood-stabilizing, mildly sedative effect in large doses and electroencephalographically have a profile similar to that of a minor tranquillizer. They may block the impairment of performance caused by lysergic acid diethylamide, they may protect against stress reactions and they relieve premenstrual and perimenopausal irritability.

Norethisterone has no consistent effect on body weight. Norethisterone heptanoate, 200 mg intramuscularly, may cause subjective symptoms of bloating but marked increases of weight are rare.

Metabolic effects

With doses used clinically, the incidence of serious metabolic effects is low. Small doses have no effect on carbohydrate metabolism, plasma triglyceride levels, or liver function. Large doses decrease high density lipoprotein cholesterol, and there may be some increase in the low density fraction; other blood lipids such as triglycerides and phospholipids may increase. Combination with oestrogen results in inhibition of ovulation in association with reduced levels of pituitary gonadotrophins and oestrogen and progesterone in the plasma and, on prolonged administration, a small increase in plasma androgens. Liver function changes, with increase in bromsulphthalein retention, are slight and of no consequence in normal individuals, though they may be significant if liver function is chronically impaired. Fasting blood sugar is unchanged but glucose tolerance may be impaired and plasma insulin raised. There is an increase in amino acid utilization with a corresponding fall in plasma amino acid levels. Total plasma protein and albumin fall, but globulins, including the binding fraction, rise.

Serum folate may be reduced.

Pharmacokinetics

The most widely used method for estimation of norethisterone in blood is radioimmunoassay, which has a sensitivity of 20 $ng.l^{-1}$. The drug is rapidly and completely absorbed after oral administration, peak plasma concentrations occurring in the majority of subjects between 1 and 3 hours. Due to a 'first-pass' presystemic metabolism in the intestinal wall and liver, blood levels after oral administration are only 60% of those after intravenous administration. Norethisterone is rapidly and widely distributed throughout the body tissues, with the highest levels accumulating and being metabolized in liver, kidney, intestine and bile. There is no enterohepatic circulation. Less than 5% exists in plasma in the unbound state, with about 60% bound to albumin and 35% to sex hormone binding globulin. Most tissues can metabolize norethisterone. The half life of elimination varies from 5 to 12 hours, with a mean of 7.6 hours. With single daily doses a steady-state concentration is reached in 5 to 10 days.

Small amounts of norethisterone pass into breast milk, the concentration being 10 to 20% of that in plasma.

Oral absorption	100%
Presystemic metabolism	~40%
Plasma half life	
range	5–12 h
mean	7.6 h
Volume of distribution	—
Plasma protein binding	95%

Concentration–effect relationship

Norethisterone heptanoate, 200 mg intramuscularly, gives plasma levels of about 10 000 $ng.l^{-1}$ in the first week, falling to about 500 $ng.l^{-1}$ at 60 days. This is effective for contraception. The levels are undetectable after 74 days.

With use in combination with oestrogen, a single daily oral dose (norethisterone 1 mg, ethinyloestradiol 50 μg) produces a peak plasma level of norethisterone of about 5000 $ng.l^{-1}$ in 1 to 2 hours, falling to about 100 $ng.l^{-1}$ in 24 hours. The combination is effective as an oral contraceptive.

Metabolism

Norethisterone is metabolized mainly in the liver. A little, probably less than 1%, is excreted unchanged. The major pathway is reduction of the α,β-unsaturated oxo group in ring A with the production of tetrahydronorethisterone, the $5\beta,3\alpha$-hydroxy configuration predominating. This is then conjugated with glucuronic acid and excreted in the urine (Fig. 1). Both sulphate conjugation and hydroxylation of norethisterone occur as minor metabolic pathways. The ethinyl group does not appear to undergo metabolism. The formation of 'active' metabolites such as the 4,5-epoxide has been claimed. Of the dose of norethisterone about 60% is excreted as metabolites in urine and faeces.

Fig. 1 Metabolism of norethisterone

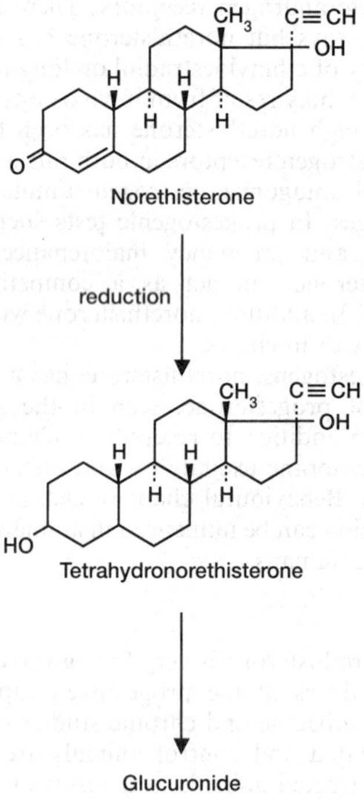

Enzyme systems are present in the body which will convert androstane steroids to oestranes, but their substrate specificity is such that they show little or no activity with respect to progestogens.

Norethisterone heptanoate, injected intramuscularly, undergoes partial hydrolysis to norethisterone. Release is from the primary depot site and possibly from a secondary depot in fat.

Pharmaceutics

Norethisterone is available as tablets containing 350 μg intended for use as a continuous low-dose progestogen oral contraceptive:

1. Micronor (Cilag, UK): white tablets marked 'Ortho 0.35';
2. Noriday (Syntex, UK): yellow tablets marked 'Noriday' on one side, 'Syntex' on the other.

For treatment of disorders of menstruation, 5 mg tablets are used:

3. Primolut N (Schering, UK): white tablets marked 'AN' in a hexagon
4. Utovlan (Syntex, UK): white scored tablets.
5. Aygestin (Wyeth-Ayerst, USA) oval, white tablets debossed '5'.
6. Norlutate (Parke-Davis, USA) round, pink tablets debossed 'P-D 918'.
7. SH 420 (Schering, UK): for treatment of breast cancer 10 mg tablets of norethisterone acetate, white, quarter-scored and marked with 'AR' in a hexagon.

8. Noristerat (Schering, UK): Norethisterone heptanoate (oenanthate) 200 mg.ml^{-1} as a solution in castor oil and benzyl benzoate (6/4, v/v) in ampoules, for intramuscular use as a depot contraceptive.

For combination oral contraceptives see Ethiryloestradiol and Mestranol.

It is said that tablets should be protected from light under cool dry conditions, with a shelf-life of 5 years, and norethisterone hexanoate should be stored away from strong sunlight, again with a shelf-life of 5 years.

Therapeutic use

Indications

1. Control of menorrhagia and menstrual irregularity in the absence of organic pathology, alone or with an oestrogen
2. For premenstrual tension
3. For spasmodic dysmenorrhoea
4. Management of endometriosis
5. Management of perimenopausal symptoms
6. As a continuous low-dose progestogen oral contraceptive
7. As an intramuscular depot long-acting contraceptive
8. In depot contraceptive devices
9. For the treatment of inoperable cancer of the breast
10. In combination with an oestrogen, as an oral contraceptive.

Contraindications

1. Pregnancy
2. History of herpes gestationis
3. History of cholestatic or idiopathic jaundice or pruritus in pregnancy
4. Severe disturbance of liver function, Dubin-Johnson and Rotor syndromes
5. Undiagnosed abnormal vaginal bleeding
6. Amenorrhoea due to pituitary gonadotrophic failure
7. Hirsutism
8. Desire for pregnancy during continuous treatment
9. In conjunction with oestrogen, the known contraindications to combined oral contraceptives.

Indications

1. Control of menstruation

It is possible to defer normal menstruation with norethisterone, 15 mg daily in divided doses, starting 3 days before the expected onset of menstrual bleeding. Usually menstruation occurs 2 to 3 days after discontinuing treatment. The manoeuvre, sometimes adopted for social reasons, is considered to be inadvisable by some as subsequent menstrual cycles may be disturbed. If withdrawal bleeding does not follow withdrawal of norethisterone, early pregnancy should be suspected. Prolonged suppression of menstruation may be achieved using this or larger doses of oral norethisterone if these are needed, or norethisterone heptanoate, 100 or 400 mg intramuscularly every 4 to 6 weeks. This is sometimes attempted for medical reasons, such as patients with menorrhagia and a bleeding diathesis or women having chemotherapy for leukaemia. Again, this may be undesirable, as prolonged pituitary suppression and an atrophic endometrium can result, and occasionally heavy breakthrough bleeding from a hypertrophied lax uterus can result. A cyclical regimen in combination with oestrogen or the use of danazol are preferable.

Teenage menstrual abnormalities such as polymenorrhoea or menorrhagia are commonly associated with anovulation and hence with failure of progesterone withdrawal. If endocrine abnormality has been excluded by physical examination and the pelvic organs are normal, with ovarian cysts excluded by ultrasound examination, it is reasonable and logical to proceed to treatment with cyclical norethisterone, 2.5 to 10 mg daily from days 16 to 26, for several months. It is not reasonable to treat infrequent or scanty menstruation per se with cyclical hormones as there is no medical indication and the onset of a natural cycle may be delayed.

With mature teenagers and adults it is usual to require a diagnostic curettage to eliminate pelvic pathology such as retained products of conception, inflammatory conditions or malignant disease before treating menorrhagia with hormones.

Norethisterone in doses as high as 30 mg daily in divided doses may be necessary for 1 to 3 days to arrest heavy menstruation on the second or third day of bleeding, even after a curettage. The dose is then reduced to 15 mg daily in divided doses, continued until day 26. If there is breakthrough bleeding, oestrogen is added to the regimen. In subsequent cycles control is best achieved with a high-progestogen oral contraceptive preparation containing oestrogen, unless there is a real contraindication to the use of the latter.

Less severe menstrual disturbances are often associated with anovular cycles, the best characterized form being metropathia haemorrhagica, and may often be treated successfully with norethisterone, 2.5 to 15 mg daily, either from days 3 to 26 or from days 16 to 26, for three to six cycles in the first place. Others will respond better to norethisterone with an oestrogen from days 5 to 25, in a combined preparation designed for oral contraception.

Menorrhagia or polymenorrhoea without pelvic abnormality occurring in ovular cycles is best treated with a cyclical norethisterone–oestrogen combination which will suppress ovulation.

A short course of norethisterone (10–15 mg daily for 3 days) may be used to induce withdrawal bleeding in women with amenorrhoea, as a preliminary to a cycle of ovulation stimulant treatment of infertility. If withdrawal bleeding fails to occur from an anatomically normal uterus, this suggests ovarian failure with abnormally low oestrogen levels.

2. Premenstrual tension

A proportion of patients in whom pyridoxine has failed to give relief of the premenstrual syndrome respond to norethisterone, 5–15 mg daily from days 19 to 26, for two to three cycles at a time.

3. Spasmodic dysmenorrhoea

Dysmenorrhoea in the absence of pelvic pathology is treated by suppression of ovulation, provided there is no immediate desire for pregnancy. This is best achieved with a norethisterone and oestrogen combination. If there is a reason for avoiding oestrogen, the same result may usually be obtained with norethisterone, 15 mg daily from days 5 to 26 of the cycle, but anovulation and contraception cannot be guaranteed with the same degree of confidence.

4. Endometriosis

When norethisterone was introduced for the management of endometriosis it was considered necessary always to give very large doses to suppress menstruation completely. It is now generally believed that it is the hormone causing atrophy and necrosis in the ectopic deposits of endometrium that is the major factor.

Minor degrees of endometriosis can often be treated successfully with 6–12 months of cyclical norethisterone 10–20 mg daily, from days 5 to 25 or even with a cyclical preparation containing 2–4 mg norethisterone daily and added oestrogen.

With more severe endometriosis endometriotic masses may require surgical removal before treatment is initiated. Norethisterone is then given continuously, starting with 10 mg daily, and increasing until symptomatic relief is obtained; the dose taken may be up to 35 mg daily but should be limited by the occurrence of side effects such as nausea, even if menstrual spotting still occurs. If menstruation is completely suppressed it may be possible to reduce the dose again with continuing therapeutic effect. Norethisterone has been widely used in this way in conjunction with ethinyloestradiol, but it is not clear if the oestrogen component of the regimen is helpful, and it may contribute to side effects. Treatment should be for a minimum of 6 months and may be continued up to 18 months if reappraisal by laparoscopy and symptomatology indicates continuing improvements.

5. Management of perimenopausal symptoms

Cyclical norethisterone 2.5–10 mg daily from days 5 to 26 in premenopausal women or for 3 weeks out of 4 in postmenopausal women is sometimes effective in relieving climacteric symptoms when the use of oestrogen is contraindicated. Postmenopausal osteoporosis can also be prevented with norethisterone, 10 mg daily, and treated with 1α-hydroxycholecalciferol combined with norethisterone.

More commonly, norethisterone combined with oestrogen is used for this purpose. The norethisterone, given cyclically, is intended to

Norethisterone (acetate, heptanoate)

protect the uterus from unopposed exogenous oestrogen, which can give rise to endometrial hyperplasia and even endometrial carcinoma. A preparation (Menophase) containing mestranol 12.5 μg for 5 days, mestranol 25 μg for 8 days, mestranol 25 μg with norethisterone 1 mg for 3 days, mestranol 30 μg with norethisterone 1.5 mg for 6 days and mestranol 20 μg with norethisterone 0.75 mg for 4 days is intended to be taken continuously for 6 to 12 months. It is intended to simulate the hormone changes of a normal menstrual cycle, but will in fact tend to suppress residual endogenous steroidogenesis. Other approaches to the relief of menopausal symptoms include the use of cyclical combined norethisterone–oestrogen contraceptives containing minimal doses of hormones, and the use of transdermal oestrogen or oestrogen implants, together with courses of oral norethisterone, 0.35 to 1.05 mg daily for 12 days each month, to produce regular withdrawal bleeding and prevent endometrial hyperplasia.

6. Progestogen oral contraception

Norethisterone, 0.35 mg, is taken daily. The failure (pregnancy) rate is somewhat higher than with combined oestrogen and progestogen oral contraceptives, as ovulation is not always inhibited, the contraceptive effect being attributed only to rendering the cervical mucus less easily penetrated by spermatozoa and the endometrium hostile to implantation. For these reasons 'progestogen only' oral contraceptives are less effective in preventing ectopic pregnancy than they are in preventing intrauterine pregnancy. In the attempt to reduce failures, it is usually advised that (a) treatment is started on the first day of a menstrual period, (b) the tablet is taken at the same time each day, preferably between 4 and 20 hours of when intercourse may be anticipated, (c) barrier contraception be used in addition for the first 14 days of treatment, (d) if a tablet is missed it should be taken as soon as possible and barrier contraception employed in addition until the next menstrual period, and (e) if any gastrointestinal disturbance occurs barrier contraception should be used in addition until the next menstrual period.

To enhance the protection against conception given by norethisterone alone, barrier contraception can be used in addition at the mid-cycle.

7. Long-acting intramuscular contraception

Norethisterone heptanoate, 200 mg in oily solution, is given intramuscularly each 8 weeks or each 60 days. An alternative is to give the second dose after 60 days, and thereafter use an 84-day interval. Ideally the first dose should be given in the first five days of a normal menstrual cycle, but there is no established risk to an early conception. With the 8-week interval the proportion of failures (pregnancies) is low but the incidence of complete amenorrhoea is high; with longer intervals failure rates increase but fewer women develop amenorrhoea. Irregular bleeding is common and unacceptable in a proportion of women.

Norethisterone heptanoate, 50 mg, with an oestradiol ester, for example oestradiol valerate 5 mg, has been used as a monthly contraceptive injection, but this procedure must be regarded as experimental.

8. Depot contraceptive devices

The subcutaneous implantation of biodegradable pellets containing 30 mg norethisterone as a depot contraceptive is currently under study. Two, three or four pellets are implanted subcutaneously in the forearm, and maintain plasma levels of norethisterone which have a contraceptive action for at least 6 months.

Vaginal rings made of silicone rubber containing norethisterone, released at a rate of about 250 μg daily, are also being studied as low-dose progestogen contraceptives. Trials of intrauterine contraceptive devices releasing norethisterone are in progress.

9. Disseminated carcinoma of the breast

Norethisterone may be used in inoperable primary or recurrent carcinoma of the breast, or as an adjunct to surgery or radiotherapy. If it is effective, the mechanism of action may be by pituitary inhibition or by an anti-oestrogen or direct effect on the tumour deposits. Norethisterone or its acetate, 30–40 mg daily in divided doses, is given. If no subjective or objective response occurs within 6 weeks, the dose is increased to 60 mg daily and may be continued indefinitely. If no remission is obtained within 9 weeks of starting treatment, none is to be expected.

Norethisterone has been used in a similar way in other supposedly hormone-dependent cancers, particularly carcinoma of the endometrium, and also as an adjunct to operative treatment. There is no good evidence of its efficacy in this context.

10. Combined norethisterone–oestrogen oral contraceptives

These contain ethinyloestradiol, 20 to 50 μg, or mestranol, 50 μg, to suppress ovulation, in combination with 0.5 to 4.0 mg of norethisterone or its acetate to reinforce the contraceptive action and produce an endometrium which will shed when the course of pills is complete.

Patients should start treatment on the first day of a menstrual period and take one pill daily for 21 days. Subsequent courses are started after a 7 day break. Others suggest that if, after previously regular withdrawal bleeding, menstruation fails to occur, barrier contraception should be employed for that cycle and the contraceptive pill restarted on the first day of the next menstrual period. This is to avoid the very small risk (probably less than 1 in 1000) of a drug-associated congenital abnormality if the contraceptive pill continues to be taken in the early months of an unsuspected pregnancy.

Missed pills. If the pill is forgotten for less than 12 hours it should be taken as soon as it is remembered, and the next one at its normal time. If a pill is forgotten for more than 12 hours additional contraceptive precautions should be taken for the next 7 days concurrently with restarting one pill per day, i.e. if a tablet is missed from the last 7 of a pack, the next pack must be started without a break. Some authors feel that unless pills have been missed on consecutive days at the start of the cycle, the risk of pregnancy is very small.

Intestinal hurry. Diarrhoea may interfere with absorption of contraceptive steroids. With a short-term episode, additional (barrier) contraceptive precautions should be taken for the rest of the cycle. Patients with chronic gastrointestinal disorders need a higher dose pill and should be advised that there is a small risk of failure (pregnancy).

Changing combined oral contraceptives. The first new pill should be started the day after the last of the previous pills has been taken, with no break, and continued daily for 21 days.

Contraindications

1. Pregnancy

There is no established risk from either norethisterone or oral contraceptives containing this drug taken before conception or during the month in which conception takes place. On the other hand, there is somewhat equivocal evidence of a very small risk, probably less than 1 in 1000, of a range of drug-associated congenital anomalies, if combined oral contraceptives, and possibly norethisterone alone, are ingested in the early months of pregnancy. Some reports suggest that male fetuses are at greater risk.

If norethisterone is given in the early months of pregnancy there is a small chance of 'masculinization' of a female fetus. In most of the cases reported, this consists merely of enlargement of the clitoris, which resolves during the first year or two of life, but a few cases where there was fusion of the labio-scrotal fold were reported.

The balance of evidence suggests that norethisterone supplements tend to diminish rather than enhance the chance of a successful pregnancy in women with habitual abortion.

2, 3. Herpes gestationis, cholestatic jaundice, pruritus in pregnancy

There is a chance of recurrence if women with a history of these conditions are given norethisterone.

4. Defective liver function, Dubin–Johnson and Rotor syndromes

Norethisterone may exacerbate defects of liver function. This is not usually considered to contraindicate use of oral contraceptives containing modest doses of the drug in women with moderate degrees of quiescent liver disease, but liver function should be closely monitored and the drug discontinued if there is deterioration.

5. Abnormal vaginal bleeding

This should not be treated symptomatically with norethisterone until a firm diagnosis has been made; otherwise there is a serious risk of failing to treat endocrine problems, infection, early pregnancy complications, or major pelvic pathology, including malignant disease. Normally, in women over 25, pelvic examination, a cervical smear, examination under anaesthesia and dilatation and curettage are required to make a diagnosis of dysfunctional uterine bleeding, for which treatment with norethisterone may be appropriate.

Norethisterone (acetate, heptanoate)

6. Amenorrhoea due to pituitary gonadotrophic failure
Use of cyclical hormones to produce regular withdrawal bleeding in this condition may delay the spontaneous return of normal menstrual cycles, and consequently impair future fertility.

7. Hirsutism
Use of cyclical hormone treatment in undiagnosed hirsutism may obscure diagnosis. In idiopathic or constitutional hirsutism, large doses of norethisterone may occasionally appear to exacerbate the symptom. This is unlikely with doses used for contraception.

8. Desire for pregnancy during treatment
Norethisterone given throughout the menstrual cycle will tend to prevent pregnancy by preventing ovulation in a proportion of women, according to dose, and by acting as a progestogen-only contraceptive. Norethisterone given only in the second half of the menstrual cycle to enhance progesterone effects is of little if any value and may inhibit endogenous progesterone production.

9. With oestrogen in combined oral contraceptives
The principal contraindications include existing thrombophlebitis, thromboembolic disorders, cerebrovascular disease, myocardial infarction, or a past history of these disorders; markedly impaired liver function, Dubin–Johnson and Rotor syndromes, congenital or existing disorders of lipid metabolism, known or suspected oestrogen-dependent neoplasia, including carcinoma of the breast; history of cholestatic jaundice or of idiopathic jaundice, herpes gestationis or gestational diabetes; undiagnosed abnormal genital tract bleeding; and suspected or known pregnancy.

Other conditions provide relative contraindications which need a balanced clinical decision in individual cases and close monitoring of the patient. These include varicose veins; history of thrombosis or pulmonary embolism; hypertension; migraine; liver disease of any sort; gall bladder disease; diabetes mellitus; renal disease in women over 35 in association with obesity, hyperlipidaemia, hypertension or cigarette smoking; age over 40, without or with these conditions; fluid retention; depression; wearing of contact lenses; uterine fibromyomata.

There is no substantiation of contentions that combined oral contraceptives might be contraindicated in sickle cell disease, porphyria, otosclerosis or multiple sclerosis.

Adverse reactions

Adverse effects are unusual with doses of norethisterone up to 15 mg daily, apart from the placebo effects of any oral medication.

Potentially life-threatening effects
Norethisterone alone (350 µg daily) used for continuous low-dose progestogen oral contraception has been found not to have adverse cardiovascular effects but there is no good evidence on this point with larger doses. The heptanoate (200 mg intramuscularly) has been used in women with previous venous thrombosis, without ill effects, but larger doses do reduce high density lipoprotein cholesterol levels.

Norethisterone is combined with oestrogen in some oral contraceptives, and an increased risk of the following disorders has been associated with the use of such preparations: thromboembolism, pulmonary embolism, coronary thrombosis, cerebral thrombosis, cerebral haemorrhage, hypertension, gall bladder disease, liver tumours and congenital anomalies.

There is limited evidence of an association with mesenteric thrombosis, but the association cannot be regarded as having been confirmed. These risks are increased by obesity and hyperlipidaemia, cigarette smoking, increasing age and the presence of pre-existing vascular disease, including hypertension.

Acute overdosage
Treatment is usually unnecessary or symptomatic. Gastric lavage, if felt to be indicated, can be used with safety. Nausea and withdrawal bleeding may occur.

Severe or irreversible adverse effects
With extremely high doses there may be cholestatic liver changes which resolve on withdrawing the drug. An increase in the size of uterine myomata has been reported.

Mental depression, retinal thrombosis, optic neuritis, reduced carbohydrate tolerance, cataract, loss of scalp hair, cholestatic jaundice, gall bladder disease, erythema multiforme, porphyria, chorea, impaired renal function, and the haemolytic uraemic syndrome have been reported, but not all have been confirmed.

Symptomatic adverse effects
Exacerbation of epilepsy or migraine and allergic rashes, with or without pruritus, have been reported.

Irregular ingestion, inconsistent with the menstrual cycle, may cause irregular uterine bleeding. In particular, stopping a regular dose often causes withdrawal bleeding.

Doses above 15 mg daily, used to treat endometriosis or malignant disease, are usually tolerated but sometimes give rise to nausea, other gastrointestinal disturbances, and fluid retention.

Women having 200 mg injections of norethisterone heptanoate every 8 weeks for contraception have reported bloating, breast discomfort, dizziness, and transient nausea and vomiting. Weight increases attributable to the drug are uncommon. Menstrual irregularity, intermenstrual spotting and delayed menstruation are common and do not require treatment. Persistent intermenstrual bleeding calls for diagnostic procedures to exclude disease; a cycle of a combined oestrogen–progestogen oral contraceptive may restore a normal menstrual cycle. Amenorrhoea is fairly common, a situation which can cause anxiety — if it persists, a pregnancy test should be performed before the next dose is given.

Other effects
Effects which may be drug-associated include abdominal cramps; dysmenorrhoea; infertility after discontinuation; oedema; chloasma or melasma; breast tenderness, enlargement and secretion; decrease in weight; change in cervical erosions or secretion; diminution in lactation; migraine; allergic rashes; vaginal candidiasis; steepening of corneal curvature; and intolerance of contact lenses.

Symptomatic effects which have been reported but not confirmed are premenstrual syndrome, changes in libido, changes in appetite, symptoms of cystitis, headaches, nervousness, dizziness, hirsutism, erythema nodosum, haemorrhagic eruptions, and vaginitis.

Regular cyclical treatment with norethisterone may mask the onset of the climacteric.

Interference with clinical pathology tests
Norethisterone can affect tests for gonadotrophin, progesterone, pregnanediol, testosterone, oestrogen, cortisol, and glucose, and interfere with the metyrapone test.

High risk groups

Neonates
The drug is not used in neonates.

Breast milk. Daily oral doses of 350 µg for contraception were reported in one study to reduce milk volume somewhat but do not usually affect volume or composition. Intramuscular injections of 200 mg each 8 weeks do not interfere with lactation. The plasma/milk ratio of the heptanoate is about 10 and only 0.1% of the dose, estimated as a maximum of 1.5 µg daily, reaches the baby. This is unlikely to affect the baby and is undetectable in the baby's plasma at the time of the peak maternal plasma level. There is a theoretical risk of all steroids interfering with bilirubin conjugation, and maternal use of norethisterone should probably be avoided whilst a baby has neonatal jaundice.

Oral contraceptives containing norethisterone with an oestrogen have been thought to affect milk volume and persistence of lactation adversely in some women, and are best avoided in breast-feeding mothers, whose risk of conception is relatively small.

Children
The drug is not used in children.

Pregnant women
The use of norethisterone in pregnancy is contraindicated, as there is a small risk of androgenic effects on a female fetus, resulting in enlargement of the clitoris and, very rarely, other minor deformities of the genitalia. There is believed to be a very small risk of other congenital deformities, including limb reduction defects and heart defects, associated with taking synthetic female sex hormones, including oral contraceptives, during the first three months of pregnancy. There are reports that the effects occur mainly in male fetuses. If the association is real, it affects less than 1 in 1000 exposed fetuses.

The elderly
The use of the drug in postmenopausal women and in disseminated carcinoma of the breast has been discussed earlier.

Concurrent disease
The risks of using the drug in the presence of liver disease have been discussed earlier.

Drug interactions

Potentially hazardous interactions
Interactions occur between oral contraceptives and a number of other drugs and may lead to loss of efficacy of progestogen and particularly oestrogen components. The interactions may not necessarily be of such an extent that significant changes in the biological activity of the drugs occur, and present evidence suggests that it is only a small number of women taking contraceptive steroids who are affected. Interactions impairing steroid efficacy might be expected to be more common with the low-dose contraceptive preparations now widely used but evidence for this seems not to be available. A decrease in bioavailability of the steroids would be demonstrated mainly by intermenstrual spotting or bleeding, though in some instances the reduction in activity may be of sufficient magnitude to lead to pregnancy.

Drugs which induce hepatic microsomal drug metabolism. The antituberculosis drug rifampicin, the antifungal drug griseofulvin and anticonvulsant drugs such as phenobarbitone and phenytoin are enzyme inducers which may impair the efficacy of the contraceptive steroids, including norethisterone, by increasing their rate of metabolic degradation.

Drugs influencing intestinal flora. Antibiotics may change the bacterial flora in the intestine with reduction in hydrolysis of some steroid conjugates excreted with bile into the intestine. This does not occur with norethisterone, which is inactivated before conjugation in the liver and has no such enterohepatic circulation, but it may reduce plasma oestrogen levels in patients taking combined oral contraceptives.

Effect on activity of other drugs. Some evidence suggests that the activity of a wide range of drugs, including anticoagulants, antihypertensives, oral antidiabetic drugs and antidepressants, may be reduced by concurrent administration of contraceptive steroids, including norethisterone. The interaction appears to be minimal.

Potentially useful interactions
No interactions of this kind have been reported.

Major outcome trials

1. Pincus G, Rock J, Garcia C R 1958 Effects of certain 19-nor steroids upon reproductive processes. Annals of the New York Academy of Sciences 71: 676–690

This was the first study in women of the effects of pure norethisterone, containing no oestrogen contaminant. The authors demonstrated in 21 cycles that norethisterone, 10 to 20 mg daily from days 5 to 25 of the cycle, prevented ovulation as judged by basal temperatures, endometrial biopsy, vaginal smears and pregnanediol excretion, compared with 56 control cycles, and that 'breakthrough' bleeding was uncommon. The endometrial changes indicated an initial progestational effect followed by partial glandular regression and stromal stimulation, with shedding in a normal menstrual period following withdrawal of the norethisterone.

This work provided the basis for the use of norethisterone in control of menstrual disorders, including dysmenorrhoea.

2. Toppozada H K et al 1983 Multinational comparative trial of long-acting injectable contraceptives; norethisterone enanthate given in two dosage schedules and depo-medroxyprogesterone acetate. Final report. Contraception 28: 1–20

Norethisterone heptanoate, 200 mg intramuscularly, was given to 789 women at 60-day intervals (10 361 woman-months) and at 796 women at 84-day intervals (10 331 woman-months). The respective failure (pregnancy) rates at 24 months were 0.4% and 1.4%. Discontinuation rates were 33 to 86% after 1 year, 56 to 100% after 2 years. The commonest reason was disturbance of menstruation. Blood pressures tended to fall a little.

Other trials

1. Dalton K 1959 Comparative trials of new oral progestogenic compounds in treatment of premenstrual syndrome. British Medical Journal 2: 1307–1309
2. Ylöstalo P, Kauppila A, Puolakka J, Rönnberg L, Jänne O 1982 Bromocriptine and norethisterone in the treatment of premenstrual syndrome. Obstetrics and Gynecology 59: 292–298
3. Kistner R W 1960 The use of steroidal substances in endometriosis. Clinical Pharmacology and Therapeutics 1: 525–537
4. Grant A 1961 The non-surgical treatment of endometriosis by progestogens. Medical Journal of Australia 2: 936–938
5. Abdalla H I, Hart D M, Lindsay R, Leggate I, Hooke A 1985 Prevention of bone mineral loss in postmenopausal women by norethisterone. Obstetrics and Gynecology 66: 789–792
6. Nordin B E C, Jones M M, Crilly R G, Marshall D H, Brooke R 1980 A placebo-controlled trial of ethinyl oestradiol and norethisterone in climacteric women. Maturitas 2: 247–251
7. Howard G, Blair M, Fotherby K, Elder M G, Bye P 1985 Seven years clinical experience of the injectable contraceptive, norethisterone oenanthate. British Journal of Family Planning 11: 9–16
8. Program for Applied Research on Fertility Regulation 1985 Phase II clinical study of implanted norethindrone pellets for longterm contraception in women. Advances in Contraception 1: 295–304
9. Curwen S 1970 Treatment of carcinoma of the breast with SH 420. Clinical Radiology 21: 219–221
10. Edelstyn G A 1973 Norethisterone acetate (SH_{420}) in advanced breast cancer. Cancer 32: 1317–1320
11. Earl H M, Rubens R D, Knight R K, Hayward J L 1984 Norethisterone acetate in the treatment of advanced breast cancer. Clinical Oncology 10: 103–109

General review articles

Back D J, Breckenridge A M, Orme M, Rowe P H 1980 Clinical pharmacology of oral contraceptive steroids: drug interactions. Journal of Obstetrics and Gynaecology 1: 126–138

Dorflinger L 1985 Relative potency of progestins used in oral contraceptives. Contraception 31: 557–571

Elder M G 1984 Injectable contraception. Clinics in Obstetrics and Gynaecology 11: 723–741

Filshie M, Guillebaud J (eds) 1989 Contraception, science and practice. Butterworths, London

Fotherby K 1981 Factors affecting the duration of action of the injectable contraceptive norethisterone oenanthate. Contraceptive Delivery Systems 2: 249–257

Fotherby K 1984 A new look at progestogens. Clinics in Obstetrics and Gynaecology 11: 701–722

Fotherby K 1985 Oral contraceptives, lipids and cardiovascular disease. Contraception 31: 367–394

Fotherby K 1986 Pharmacokinetics of progestational compounds. Maturitas 8: 123–132

Gregoire A T, Blye R T (eds) 1986 Contraceptive steroids, pharmacology and safety. Plenum Press, New York

Hawkins D F, Elder M G 1979 Human fertility control. Theory and Practice. Butterworths, London, pp 28–38, 49–130

Hümpel M 1982 Pharmacokinetics and biotransformation of norethisterone in animals. A review. Contraception 26: 83–95

International Symposium on Contraception 1987 American Journal of Obstetrics and Gynecology 157: 1019–1092

Liskin L, Blackburn R, Ghani R 1987 Hormonal contraception: new long-acting methods. Population Reports, series K, number 3, K58–K87

Masson G M, Klopper A 1981 Medical management of menstrual disorders; sex hormones and related drugs in gynaecology. In: Hawkins D F (ed) Gynaecological therapeutics. Baillière-Tindall, London, pp 37–63

Orme M L L, Back D J, Breckenridge A M 1983 Clinical pharmacokinetics of oral contraceptive steroids. Clinical Pharmacokinetics 8: 95–136

Realini J P, Goldzieher I W 1985 Oral contraceptives and cardiovascular disease. American Journal of Obstetrics and Gynecology 152: 729–798
Whitelock O V S, Furness F N, Stahl F S, Rakoff A E (eds) 1958 New steroid compounds with progestational activity. Annals of the New York Academy of Sciences 71: 479–806
Population Reports, Series A, No 1, 1974, pp A1–A26; No 2, 1975, pp A29–A52; No 4, 1977, pp A105–A132; No 5, 1979, pp A136–A186; No 6, 1982, pp A189–A222
These reports provide extensive reviews of clinical trials with combined oestrogen–progestogen oral contraceptives containing norethisterone.

Norfloxacin

Norfloxacin is an antimicrobial drug of the fluoroquinolone class.

Chemistry

Norfloxacin (Noroxin, Utinor)
$C_{16}H_{18}FN_3O_3$
1-Ethyl-6-fluoro-1,4-dihydro-4-oxo-7-(1-piperazinyl)-3-quinoline carboxylic acid

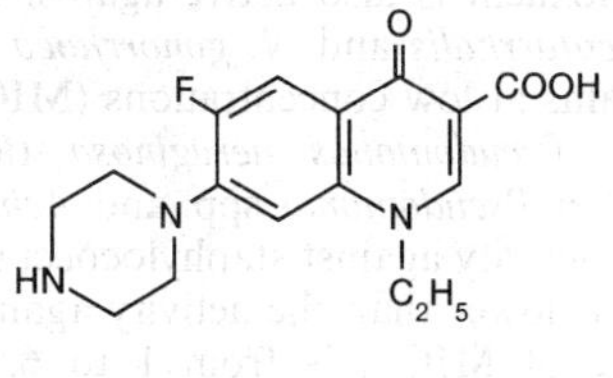

Molecular weight	319.3
pKa (carboxylic acid, amino group)	6.2–6.4, 8.7–8.9
Solubility	
in alcohol	1 in 500
in water	1 in 500–1 in 100
Octanol/water partition coefficient	0.46

Norfloxacin is prepared by chemical synthesis. The compound is a white to pale yellow crystalline powder that is odourless and has a bitter taste.

Pharmacology

Norfloxacin, like other quinolones, appears to inhibit DNA synthesis and/or conformation by inhibiting the activity of DNA gyrase (topoisomerase II), an enzyme responsible for ATP-dependent negative supercoiling of bacterial DNA.[1–4] Some investigators believe that the drug acts directly on DNA producing a covalent attachment of DNA gyrase to DNA, which forms a complex that is inaccessible to the action of DNA polymerase.[5] The bactericidal effect of norfloxacin is antagonized by rifampicin and chloramphenicol and seems to involve interruption of protein synthesis. The mechanism responsible for the lethal effect of norfloxacin on bacteria has not been completely elucidated.[6]

Toxicology

Irreversible erosions of articular cartilage and clinical signs of lameness on 3–5-month-old dogs have been observed following chronic administration of norfloxacin in doses of 60 $mg.kg^{-1}$ daily. Crystalluria (crystals consisting of the dihydrate and magnesium salt of norfloxacin) can cause urinary obstruction in rats and dogs on moderate or high doses when the urine pH is 6.0 or above.

There is no evidence that norfloxacin has any teratogenic effect in small animals or monkeys. All in vivo and in vitro mutagenicity studies have been negative except weakly positive impairment in an assay of DNA repair. No carcinogenic effect has been detected in a 19-month study of chronic administration of norfloxacin to rats.

The inhibition of DNA synthesis in bacteria and the weak impairment of DNA repair detected in an assay in rat cells caused concern about the potential fetotoxicity of norfloxacin, in the preclinical and early clinical phases of use. No substantial data have borne this out other than a suggestion from studies in pregnant rabbits. The latter effects cannot be related directly to drug toxicity and are most likely species-specific effects caused by alterations of the fecal flora resulting from the antimicrobial action of the drug. Such alterations can produce severe reactions in rabbits and guinea-pigs. Restraint in the use of norfloxacin during pregnancy is recommended as a matter of principle, rather than because of demonstrated fetotoxicity.

Clinical pharmacology

Norfloxacin is absorbed after oral administration with the production of serum and tissue levels that enable the effective treatment of local infections caused by susceptible bacteria.

Norfloxacin in general is more active, with a broader spectrum of inhibition, than earlier quinolones; it is less active with a narrower spectrum than ciprofloxacin. The antimicrobial activity in vitro is diminished by acidic pH, high concentrations of Mg^{2+} ions in the medium and an inoculum size of $>10^7$ CFU.ml^{-1}. More than 90% of strains (MIC_{90}) among the species of Enterobacteriaceae are inhibited at concentrations lower than 2 mg.l^{-1}. The exceptions are *Serratia marcescens* and *Providencia stuartii*, which are more resistant with an MIC_{90} of 3.1 mg.l^{-1}. Pathogenic enteric bacteria, including *Salmonella* spp., *Shigella* spp., *Yersinia enterocolitica*, *Aeromonas hydrophila*, *Plesiomonas shigelloides*, *Vibrio parahaemolyticus*, *Vibrio cholera* and *Campylobacter jejunii* are very susceptible with an MIC_{90} of <1 mg.l^{-1}. Norfloxacin is also active against *Neisseria meningitidis*, *Branhamella catarrhalis* and *N. gonorrhoea* including β-lactamase-producing strains at low concentrations ($MIC_{90}<0.06$ mg.l^{-1}).

The MIC_{90} for *Pseudomonas aeruginosa* ranges from 1 to 3.1 mg.l^{-1} while other *Pseudomonas* spp. and *Acinetobacter* spp. are more resistant. The activity against staphylococci including methicillin-resistant strains is lower than the activity against Gram-negative bacteria. The range of MIC_{90} is from 1 to 6.1 mg.l^{-1}. Activity against streptococci is even less and more variable than against staphylococci[2,7–11] with an MIC_{90} of 0.5–32 mg.l^{-1}. Norfloxacin is generally inactive against most clinically important anaerobic bacteria, mycobacteria, *Mycoplasma*, *Chlamydia* and *Ureaplasma*. Synergy between norfloxacin and amphotericin B has been reported for *Candida* spp. and *Cryptococcus* spp.

No plasmid-mediated norfloxacin resistance has been reported.[12] In contrast, there is evidence that the quinolone group of drugs inhibits conjugal transfer of plasmids and also eliminates some plasmids from bacteria.[13] Isolates resistant to norfloxacin both in vitro and in vivo have been reported. Cross-resistance among quinolones and infrequently with other classes of drugs has been described.[14,15] Species vary in their ability to engender resistant variants, the frequency being higher with non-fermenting organisms than with Enterobacteriaceae.[16]

Pharmacokinetics

The concentrations of norfloxacin in body fluids can be determined satisfactorily by either microbiological or high pressure liquid chromatography (HPLC). HPLC with fluorescence detection is recommended since it is simple, rapid, sensitive and specific. Metabolites can be detected only by HPLC. Limitations on the sensitivity of identification of the parent compound and metabolites are variable according to method and equipment. HPLC can be expected to detect 0.05–0.1 mg.l^{-1}; the sensitivity of the bioassay is in the same range.

After an oral dose of 200 or 400 mg mean peak serum concentrations of 0.8 ± 0.3 and 1.5 ± 0.6 mg.l^{-1} respectively are achieved within 60–90 minutes. Absorption is slightly impaired when norfloxacin is administered with food as evidenced by a reduction of approximately 30% in the peak serum concentration. Administration of 400 mg orally every 12 hours produces slight accumulation with minimal changes in the serum concentration.

Studies in animals show that the distribution volume of norfloxacin is very large, about 50% of the body weight, and the bioavailability 50–80%. The same is probably true for humans, but an intravenous preparation has not been available for studies in man to accurately determine the bioavailability and the volume of distribution. Approximately 15% of the drug in serum is bound to plasma proteins.

There is little information on the penetration of norfloxacin into different tissues. The penetration into a mild inflammatory exudate induced by a cantharides-impregnated plaster showed a peak blister fluid level of about 1 mg.l^{-1} after a 400 mg dose, approximately 67% of the peak serum level. Following oral administration of 200 mg the concentration in tonsillar tissue, maxillary sinus mucosa, vaginal tissue, cervical tissue, salpinges, ovaries, renal cortex and the gallbladder wall were only slightly lower than the serum concentrations. Bile, liver and renal medulla had drug concentrations higher than serum. Concentrations in sputum were relatively low. Norfloxacin has not been found in human milk after a single oral dose of 200 mg. Following ingestion of 400 mg of norfloxacin, the peak urine and faecal concentrations are >300 mg.l^{-1} or Gm respectively, which is several hundred times higher than the MIC of the majority of pathogenic bacteria causing urinary and enteric infections.

Norfloxacin is cleared from the body through the kidneys, biliary excretion and metabolism. The elimination half life is 3 h (2.6–4.5 h). Within 24 hours of drug administration, 26–32% of the administered dose is recovered in the urine as norfloxacin and an additional 5–8% as metabolites. Faecal recovery accounts for 30% of the administered dose, 2–3% is excreted in the bile.

Renal excretion of norfloxacin occurs by both glomerular filtration and tubular secretion. Renal clearance is 275 ± 71 ml.min^{-1}. Probenecid reduces urinary recovery of the drug by 50%.[17–21]

Oral absorption	50–80%
Presystemic metabolism	—
Plasma half life	
range	2.6–4.5 h
mean	3 h
Volume of distribution	2.5–3.1 l.kg^{-1}
Plasma protein binding	15%

Concentration–effect relationship

The drug is bactericidal at 1–4 times the MIC against most susceptible strains of bacteria. Paradoxical effect of decreased killing at higher drug concentrations has been observed in *E. coli*.[6] The effect of sub-inhibitory concentrations of norfloxacin on ultrastructure of bacteria and their virulence factors has not been studied. Examples of MIC values for some bacteria are shown in the Clinical pharmacology section.

Metabolism

Quinolones may be conjugated with glucuronic acid at the 3-position, but this is a minor metabolite of norfloxacin. The major metabolites are derived from chemical substitutions on the piperazine ring. These occur by modification of the amino nitrogen with formation of formyl and acetyl derivatives; or by oxidation of a carbon atom in the piperazine ring to a keto group designated as the oxo derivative. Open ring metabolites are developed by hydroxylation or carboxylation of the piperazine ring, yielding acetylaminoethyl, desethyl and amino compounds from progressive metabolism of the ring structure (see Fig. 1).

More than 70% of the amount of norfloxacin recovered in the urine is in the parent form and somewhat less than 30% as the collective metabolites. The oxo-piperazine metabolite is the most common derivative of norfloxacin accounting for about 5% of the dose. Acetyl and formyl piperazine derivatives of norfloxacin make up only about 0.5% of the dose excreted in the urine. Among the open ring metabolites, desethyl accounts for more than twice as much as the acetylamino and amino metabolites combined. Overall one-half of the dose of norfloxacin is recovered in the urine, as parent compound and metabolites; the other half is excreted by extrarenal routes. Metabolites excreted by extrarenal routes are inadequately quantitated, but the available information suggests that the proportion of drug metabolites is higher than observed in the urine.

Pharmaceutics

Norfloxacin Noroxin (MSD, USA) is supplied in 400 mg tablets dark pink in colour, oval shaped, film-coated, coded 'MSD 705' on one side and 'NOROXIN' on the other (US) and white oval, marked Utinor in the UK. The tablets should be stored in a tightly-closed container protected from light and the storage temperature should not exceed 40°C. Norfloxacin is not available for parenteral administration.

Norfloxacin

Therapeutic use

Norfloxacin has been effective, but not necessarily the drug of first choice, in the treatment of the following infections.

Indications

1. Urinary tract infections
2. *Neisseria gonorrhoea* urethritis and/or cervicitis
3. Bacterial enteric infections
4. Prophylaxis in granulocytopenic patients.

Contraindications

1. Norfloxacin should not be given to patients with known hypersensitivity to norfloxacin or other quinolones
2. As with other drugs of this class, norfloxacin should not be used in patients with a history of convulsions unless there is an overwhelming clinical need.

Mode of use

The dosage of norfloxacin that has been used for the treatment of various infections ranges from 800 mg as a single dose to 1200 mg daily. In the treatment of urinary tract infection, the usual adult dosage is 400 mg twice a day for 7–10 days. Women with uncomplicated acute cystitis can be treated for 3 days, whereas patients with chronic relapsing urinary tract infection need therapy for a longer period of time (400 mg twice daily for up to 12 weeks).

In acute bacterial gastroenteritis, the recommended regimen is 400 mg twice daily for 5 days.

In acute gonococcal urethritis and/or cervicitis the dose is 800 mg given as a single dose.

In the prophylaxis of sepsis in granulocytopenic patients, the recommended dosage is 400 mg three times daily for the duration of neutropenia (neutrophil count $< 100.mm^{-3}$).

Indications

1. Urinary tract infections

The antimicrobial spectrum of norfloxacin encompasses the majority of pathogenic bacteria causing urinary tract infections (UTI) including *Ps. aeruginosa* and other Gram-negative bacilli with multiple drug resistance. The drug is well absorbed orally, achieves good tissue penetration and high levels in the urine, which provides an inexpensive regimen for inpatient treatment and permits effective treatment of outpatients. A by-product of treatment of potential advantage in the cure and prevention of urinary tract infections is the ability of the drug to eradicate pathogenic aerobic bacteria from the periurethral and faecal flora.[22] This property might be important in the prophylaxis of recurrent urinary tract infections.

The efficacy of norfloxacin in the treatment of urinary tract infection has been assessed with promising results in several studies, the majority of which were open-label trials. When comparison of norfloxacin with nalidixic acid, amoxycillin and co-trimoxazole was made in randomized, non-blinded studies in patients with an anatomically normal urinary tract, higher or equivalent rates of cure were demonstrated with norfloxacin.[22–26] In several studies, including patients with an abnormal urinary tract or catheterized patients, norfloxacin was shown to be superior or at least equally effective in comparison with pipedimic acid, amoxycillin, ciprofloxacin or co-trimoxazole.[27–31] The dose used in most studies was 400 mg by mouth twice daily for 3–10 days. Although more experience is needed with larger controlled trials in the treatment of complicated UTI, it is expected that norfloxacin will be a useful and effective drug with an increasing role in the treatment of UTI in the future. The efficacy of norfloxacin in the treatment of UTI caused by *Ps. aeruginosa* or Gram-positive cocci has been studied in a limited number of patients. It appears, however, to be similar to that of infections caused by Gram-negative bacilli.

Development of bacterial resistance during norfloxacin treatment has been infrequent; therapeutic failures have been associated with

Fig. 1 Major metabolites of norfloxacin

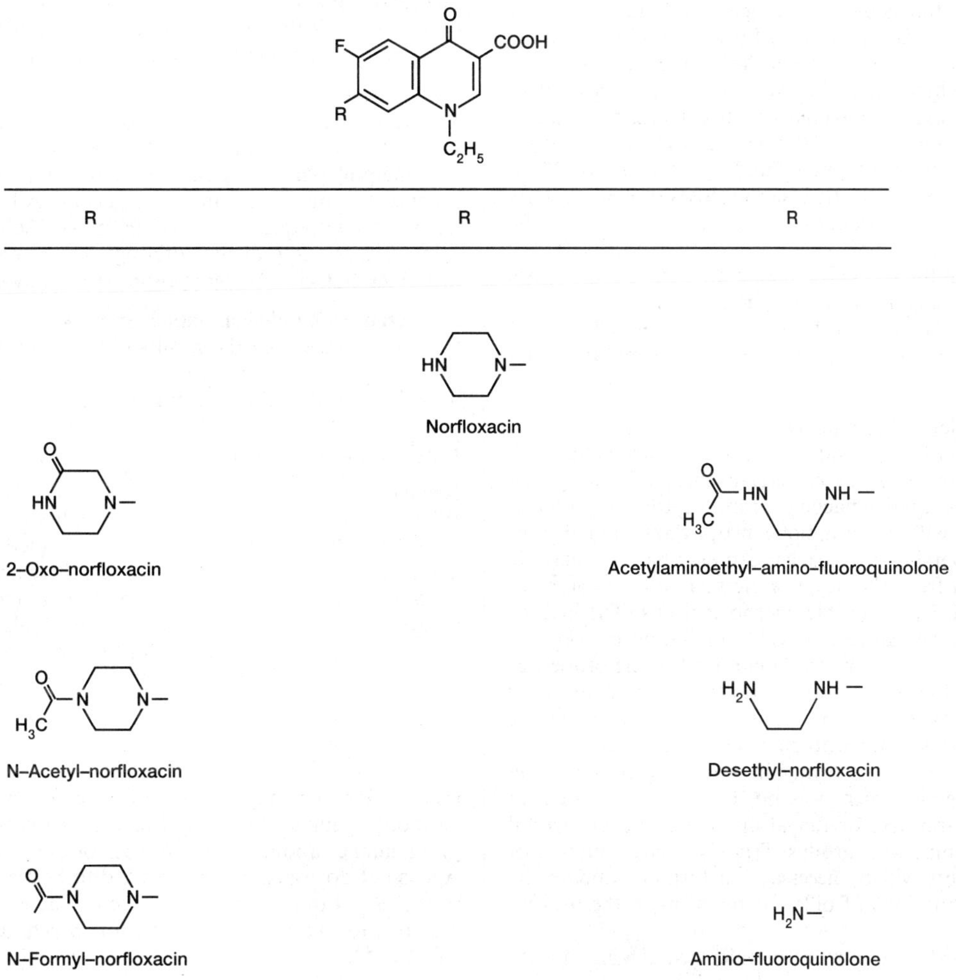

N

bacterial resistaince in 1.0% of the cases. A subgroup of patients with functional or structural abnormalities of the urinary tract appears to be in high risk to acquire resistant organisms during or shortly following treatment.

It remains to be determined whether or not single dose therapy and long-term prophylaxis in selected groups of patients will be effective.

2. *Neisseria gonorrhoea* urethritis and/or cervicitis

In vitro studies have shown that norfloxacin is a highly active agent against both β-lactamase positive and β-lactamase negative strains of *N. gonorrhoea* and several clinical trials have shown its efficacy in the treatment of gonococcal urethritis and/or cervicitis. Two doses of norfloxacin (600 mg orally) given 4 hours apart or a single dose of 800 mg were equally effective as a single dose of spectinomycin (2 g intramuscularly) or as the combination of ampicillin (3.5 g orally) plus probenecid (1.0 g orally) in men and women with gonococcal urethritis and/or cervicitis. It is noteworthy to mention that norfloxacin eliminated concurrent infection in the rectum or pharynx, sites at which the ampicillin–probenecid combination is known to fail.[32–34]

The efficacy of this new quinolone for the treatment of gonococcal salpingitis or disseminated gonococcal infection remains to be determined.

Few studies to date have addressed the effectiveness of norfloxacin in the treatment of chancroid[46].

Norfloxacin demonstrates limited in vitro activity against *Chlamydia trachomatis*. The marginal activity and limited clinical experience make it appear unlikely that norfloxacin will be useful treatment for urethritis, pelvic inflammatory disease, and other infections caused by chlamydiae.[35]

3. Gastrointestinal infections

The high concentrations of norfloxacin produced in the stools and the high level of activity against the majority of pathogenic enteric bacteria make the potential for effective treatment and prophylaxis of the most common bacterial gastrointestinal infections extremely promising. Clinical efficacy has been assessed by different investigators and in different countries.[36–38] Norfloxacin (400 mg twice or three times daily for five days) was as effective as co-trimoxazole or nalidixic acid in the treatment of bacterial gastroenteritis caused by enterotoxigenic *E. coli* or *Shigella* species. Further studies are desirable to confirm the effectiveness of oral norfloxacin as treatment for typhoid fever (400 mg three times daily for 14 days). In a double-blind, controlled clinical trial of patients with cholera, norfloxacin was superior to co-trimoxazole and placebo in reducing stool output, duration of diarrhoea, fluid requirement, and vibrio excretion.[39]

Norfloxacin used as a prophylactic agent in doses of 400 mg daily for two weeks among US students arriving in Mexico was 93% effective in preventing diarrhoea while 36 of 59 students (61%) experienced diarrhoea in the placebo group.[40] Its indiscriminate use, however, for this purpose is not recommended. In a limited number of chronic carriers of *Salmonella typhi* the apparent efficacy of norfloxacin in eradicating the organism from the intestinal tract and tissues is promising.

4. Prophylaxis in granulocytopenic patients

Oral non-absorbable antibiotics and co-trimoxazole are commonly used to reduce the level of faecal bacteria as prophylaxis against bacteraemia with Gram-negative bacilli in granulocytopenic patients. Their effect compared with no antibiotic prophylaxis and barrier isolation is still controversial. Norfloxacin can eliminate the aerobic Gram-negative bacteria from the bowel while maintaining colonization resistance provided by anaerobic microorganisms. The lack of plasmid-mediated resistance and the possible inhibition of conjugal plasmid transfer by norfloxacin are additional favourable properties of this new quinolone that make it an alternative consideration for prophylaxis against bacterial infections in granulocytopenic patients.[41] Norfloxacin was shown to be as effective as co-trimoxazole and superior to vancomycin–polymyxin or placebo in preventing Gram-negative bacteraemia. There was no difference, however, on the frequency of Gram-positive or fungal infections and on overall survival between the comparable groups. Trials in a large number of granulocytopenic patients will be necessary to further evaluate the relative efficacy and limitations of different regimens in the prevention of infection.

A recent report regarding treatment of falciparum malaria with norfloxacin justifies further investigation, as this agent might prove important in dealing with the present problems in malaria chemotherapy.[42]

Adverse reactions

Potentially life-threatening effects

No adverse effects of a lethal or potentially life-threatening nature have been observed in clinical experience or presumed on the basis of experimental and theoretical knowledge of norfloxacin.

Acute overdosage

Involuntary overdosing is rare and has a large margin of safety owing to the size and number of tablets required. Single overdoses are unlikely to produce serious acute toxicity other than gastrointestinal signs and symptoms. No cases of voluntary overdose with intent to produce drug toxicity from norfloxacin have been reported; therefore, neither the signs and symptoms nor their duration or reversibility are known. In the event of acute overdosage, the stomach should be emptied by inducing vomiting or by gastric lavage. Adequate hydration without administration of alkali will avoid the possible development of crystalluria.

Severe or irreversible adverse effects

Severe or irreversible adverse effects caused by norfloxacin have not been reported.

Symptomatic adverse effects

Norfloxacin is well tolerated, with few adverse reactions involving less than 10% of patients in most studies. In comparative studies, the incidence of adverse effects reported with norfloxacin was similar to, or significantly less frequent than, those reported with the comparison drugs, which included co-trimoxazole, amoxycillin and nalidixic acid.

The most common adverse experiences were either gastrointestinal (nausea, vomiting, heartburn, constipation, diarrhoea), or neurological (headache, dizziness, depression, insomnia, seizures). Additional reactions that have been attributed to norfloxacin are rash, dry mouth, fever, arthralgias, tendonitis, and crystalluria. There has been one report of acute renal failure during therapy with norfloxacin and desipramine. With the exception of crystalluria, the symptoms and signs are non-specific and their mechanisms unknown.

Other effects

Abnormal laboratory values observed in clinical trials include elevated blood concentrations of AST (SGOT) and ALT (SGPT), LDH, alkaline phosphatase, urea, creatinine; and eosinophilia, granulocytopenia, thrombocytopenia and anaemia. All of these manifestations have been infrequent enough to make their separation from the primary diseases difficult, although pharmacogenetic differences in drug metabolism or drug idiosyncrasies may exist.

Interference with clinical pathology tests

No interference with the results obtained in routine clinical laboratory tests has been observed. The antibacterial activity of the drugs must be considered in any biologic assays.

High risk groups

Neonates

What is said below about children applies to neonates.

Breast milk. Norfloxacin was not detected in human milk following a single dose of 200 mg. However, there are few if any conditions in which the use of norfloxacin in a nursing mother would be indicated until more information is available about its secretion in breast milk and the potential risk to the baby.

Children

Erosions or toxicity of joint cartilage observed in beagle puppies has not been reported in humans. The effect is believed to be unique to the species and age of the dogs. Children treated with fluoroquinolones, often for long periods of time for cystic fibrosis, have not developed joint complaints. Further experience is accumulating to give guidance about the relative risk of use of quinolones in children. Age is not documented or perceived to be a serious contraindication to the use of quinolones, but current practice is to limit their use in children to specific indications for which other treatment is not effective.[43]

Occasional reports of arthritis or tendonitis among patients receiving norfloxacin are probably not related to the articular erosions observed in young animals. It is an infrequent side effect, not age related, is benign and the pathogenic mechanism is unknown.

Pregnant women
The safety of norfloxacin for the fetus from exposure resulting from treatment of the mother during pregnancy has not been established.

The elderly
In elderly patients with normal renal function for their age (GFR > 30 ml.min^{-1}) no alterations in dosage are recommended.

Concurrent disease
In renal failure the serum half life of norfloxacin increases only slightly with moderate impairment of creatinine clearance (< 20–30 ml.min^{-1}) compared with normal volunteers. With greater degrees of renal failure there is an increase in serum half life. When the creatinine clearance falls below 10 ml.min^{-1} the half life approximately doubles, from 3 to 7.7 hours. Opinions differ as to whether dosage modifications are necessary in patients with impaired renal function. There is general agreement, however, on doubling the interval or halving the dose when the creatinine clearance is < 10 ml.min^{-1}. Some authorities claim that modifications are necessary when the creatinine clearance is < 30 ml.min^{-1}. Haemodialysis does not appear to influence the elimination of drug and substitution after dialysis is not indicated.[44,45]

In moderately severe renal failure the concentration of norfloxacin in the urine is decreased, but the levels attained are several times above the MIC for the majority of bacteria causing urinary tract infections. However, the efficacy of treatment of urinary tract infections, specifically in patients with advanced renal failure, remains to be determined.

Drug interactions

Potentially hazardous interactions

Antacids. Co-administration with antacids decreases the absorption of norfloxacin from the gastrointestinal tract, which might be hazardous during the treatment of a serious infection.

Theophylline. Simultaneous administration of other quinolones with theophylline interferes with theophylline disposition resulting in high theophylline levels. Close monitoring of theophylline levels is recommended when theophylline and norfloxacin are co-administered.

Cyclosporins. Elevated serum levels of cyclosporin have been reported with concomitant use of norfloxacin.

Warfarin. The effects of warfarin may be enhanced by quinolones through its displacement from serum albumin-binding sites.

Probenecid. Probenecid reduces the urinary excretion of norfloxacin.

Potentially useful interactions
No interactions of this kind have been reported.

Clinical trials

1. Urinary Tract Infection Study Group 1987 Co-ordinated, multicentre study of norfloxacin versus trimethoprim–sulphamethoxazole treatment of symptomatic urinary tract infections. Journal of Infectious Diseases 155: 170–177

This study was a double-blind multicentre trial designed to compare the safety and efficacy of 400 or 200 mg of norfloxacin with TMP-SMX for the treatment of urinary tract infections. 886 patients were randomized to receive 200 mg of norfloxacin (333 patients), 400 mg of norfloxacin (335 patients), or 160/800 mg of TMP-SMX (218 patients) twice daily for seven days. In patients with complicated infections and in men, the efficacy for the group receiving 200 mg of norfloxacin was lower than that for the other two groups. In patients with recurrent infections, bacterial elimination was greater for those receiving TMP-SMX. Significantly fewer adverse reactions occurred in patients receiving norfloxacin than in those treated with TMP-SMX. The 200 mg dosage of norfloxacin seemed to cause fewer side effects than the 400 mg dosage.

Norfloxacin

2. Crider S R, Colby S D, Miller L K, Harrison W O, Kerbs S B, Berg S W 1984 Treatment of penicillin-resistant *Neisseria gonorrhoea* with oral norfloxacin. New England Journal of Medicine 311: 137–140

In this comparative study, norfloxacin given by mouth to 59 men as two doses of 600 mg proved as effective as a single dose of 2 g of spectinomycin in 33 men. Approximately half of the strains of *N. gonorrhoea* in that investigation produced β-lactamase. Two patients with gonococcal pharyngitis were included in the norfloxacin group. All patients in both groups were cured.

3. Karp J E, Merz W G, Hendricksen C et al 1987 Oral norfloxacin for prevention of Gram-negative bacterial infections in patients with acute leukemia and granulocytopenia. Annals of Internal Medicine 106: 1–7

This prospective, randomized, double-blind, placebo-controlled trial was conducted to evaluate the efficacy of norfloxacin in reduction of bacterial infections in adult patients with acute leukaemia who had chemotherapy-induced prolonged granulocytopenia. Gram-negative infections were documented in 13 of the 33 patients receiving placebo, but only in 4 of the 35 patients receiving norfloxacin. Patients receiving norfloxacin developed first infectious fevers later than did those receiving placebo, had more rapid resolution of that fever after systemic antibiotic treatment, and spent less time febrile. No difference was shown, however, on the frequency of Gram-positive or fungal infections and on the overall survival of two groups.

General review articles

Acar J F, Norrby R (eds) 1983 Norfloxacin: microbiology-pharmacology—clinical evaluation. European Journal of Clinical Microbiology

Daikos G K, Acar J F (eds) 1983 Proceedings of a symposium: norfloxacin, a new oral anti-bacterial in the treatment of urinary tract infections. European Journal of Chemotherapy and Antibiotics 3:(1)

Fass R J 1985 The quinolones (editorial) Annals of Internal Medicine 102: 400–402

Holmes B, Brogden R N, Richards D M 1985 Norfloxacin, a review of its antibacterial activity, pharmacokinetic properties and therapeutic uses. Drugs 30: 482–513

Hooper D C, Wolfson J S 1989 Treatment of genitourinary tract infections with fluoroquinolones. Antimicrobial Agents and Chemotherapy 33: 1662–1667

Leigh D A, Wise R (eds) 1984 Norfloxacin: a new quinolone for urinary infections. Journal of Antimicrobial Chemotherapy 13 (suppl B)

Moellering R C (ed) 1987 Norfloxacin, the first of a new generation of quinolone antibiotics. American Journal of Medicine 82 (suppl 6B): 1–92

Norby S R 1986 Norfloxacin: targeted antibiotic therapy. Scandinavian Journal of Infectious Diseases 48 (suppl): 1–91

Norfloxacin (Noroxin) 1987 Medical Letter on Drugs and Therapeutics 29: 27

Rubenstein E, Adam D, Moellering R, Waldvogel F 1988 International symposium on new quinolones. Reviews of Infectious Diseases 10 (suppl 1): S1–S271

Rubenstein E, Adam D, Moellering R, Waldvogel F 1989 Second international symposium on new quinolones. Reviews of Infectious Diseases 11 (suppl 5): S897–S1431

Wolfson J S, Hooper D C 1988 Norfloxacin: A new targeted fluoroquinolone antimicrobial agent. Annals of Internal Medicine 108: 238–251

References

1. Cozzarelli N R 1980 DNA gyrase and the supercoiling of DNA. Science 207: 953–960
2. Wolfson J S, Hooper D C 1985 The fluoroquinolones: structures, mechanisms of action and resistance, and spectra of activity in vitro. Antimicrobial Agents and Chemotherapy 28: 581–586
3. Benbrook D M, Miller R V 1986 Effects of norfloxacin on DNA metabolism in *Ps. aeruginosa*. Antimicrobial Agents and Chemotherapy 29: 1–6
4. Hooper D C, Wolfson J S 1989 Mode of action of the quinolone antimicrobial agents. Review of recent information. Reviews of Infectious Diseases 11: S902–S911

Norfloxacin

N

5. Engle E C, Manes S H, Drlica K 1983 Differential effects of antibiotics inhibiting gyrase. Journal of Bacteriology 149: 92–98
6. Crumplin G C, Kenwright M, Hirst T 1984 Investigations into the mechanism of action of the antibacterial agent norfloxacin. Journal of Antimicrobial Chemotherapy 13 (suppl B): 9–23
7. Ito A, Hirai K, Inone M et al 1980 In vitro antibacterial activity of AM-715, a new nalidixic acid analog. Antimicrobial Agents and Chemotherapy 17: 103–108
8. King A, Warren C, Shannon K, Phillips J 1982 In vitro antibacterial activity of norfloxacin. Antimicrobial Agents and Chemotherapy 21: 604–607
9. Norrby S R, Jonsson M 1983 Antibacterial activity of norfloxacin. Antimicrobial Agents and Chemotherapy 23: 15–18
10. Neu H C, Labthavikul P 1982 In vitro activity of norfloxacin, a quinolone carboxylic acid, compared with that of β-lactams, aminoglycosides and trimethoprim. Antimicrobial Agents and Chemotherapy 22: 23–27
11. Mitsuhashi S 1988 Comparative antibacterial activity of new-quinolone carboxylic acid derivatives. Reviews of Infectious Diseases 10 (suppl 1): S27–S31
12. Courvalin P 1990 Plasmid mediated 4-quinolone resistance: a real or apparent absence? Antimicrobial Agents and Chemotherapy 34: 681–684
13. Hooper D C, Wolfson J S, McHugh G L, Swartz M D, Tung C, Swartz M N 1984 Elimination of plasmid pMG110 from E. coli by novobiocin and other inhibitors of DNA gyrase. Antimicrobial Agents and Chemotherapy 25: 586–590
14. Barry A L, Jones R N 1984 Cross resistance among cinoxacin, ciprofloxacin, DJ-6783, enoxacin, nalidixic acid, norfloxacin and oxolinic acid after in vitro selection of resistant populations. Antimicrobial Agents and Chemotherapy 25: 775–777
15. Sanders C C, Sanders W E, Goering R V, Werner V 1984 Selection of multiple antibiotic resistance by quinolones, β-lactams and amino-glycosides with special reference to cross- resistance between unrelated drug classes. Antimicrobial Agents and Chemotherapy 26: 797–801
16. Duckworth G J, Williams J D 1984 Frequency of appearance of resistant variants to norfloxacin and nalidixic acid. Journal of Antimicrobial Chemotherapy 13 (suppl B): 33–38
17. Norrby S R 1983 Pharmacokinetics of norfloxacin: clinical implications. European Journal of Chemotherapy and Antibiotics 3: 19–25
18. Wise R 1984 Norfloxacin — a review of pharmacology and tissue penetration. Journal of Antimicrobial Chemotherapy 13 (suppl B): 59–64
19. Bergeron M G, Thabet M, Roy R, Lessard C, Foucault P 1985 Norfloxacin penetration into human renal and prostatic tissues. Antimicrobial Agents and Chemotherapy 28: 349–350
20. Cofsky R D, DuBonchet L, Lendesman S H 1984 Recovery of norfloxacin in feces after administration of a single oral dose to human volunteers. Antimicrobial Agents and Chemotherapy 26: 110–111
21. Swanson B N, Boppana V K, Vlasses P H, Rotmensch H H, Ferguson R K 1983 Norfloxacin disposition after sequentially increasing oral doses. Antimicrobial Agents and Chemotherapy 23: 284–288
22. Haase D A, Harding G K M, Thomson M Y, Kennedy J K, Urias B A, Ronald A R 1984 Comparative trial of norfloxacin and trimethoprim–sulfamethoxazole in the treatment of women with localized acute, symptomatic urinary tract infections and antimicrobial effect on periurethral and faecal microflora. Antimicrobial Agents and Chemotherapy 26: 481–484
23. Sabbaj J, Hoagland V L, Shih W J 1985 Multi-clinic comparative study of norfloxacin and trimethoprim–sulfamethoxazole for treatment of urinary tract infections. Antimicrobial Agents and Chemotherapy 27: 297–301
24. Gimarelou H, Tsagarakis J, Petrikkos G, Daikos G K 1983 Norfloxacin vs. cotrimoxazole in the treatment of lower urinary tract infections. European Journal of Clinical Microbiology 2: 266–269
25. Reeves D S, Lacey R W, Mummery R V, Mahendran M, Biut A J, Newsom S W B 1984 Treatment of acute urinary infection by norfloxacin or nalidixic acid/citrate: a multi-center comparative study. Journal of Antimicrobial Chemotherapy 13 (suppl B): 99–105
26. Hooper D C, Wolfson J S 1985 The fluoroquinolones: pharmacology, clinical uses and toxicities in humans. Antimicrobial Agents and Chemotherapy 28: 716–721
27. Kumamoto Y, Ishigami J 1983 Clinical experience with norfloxacin in urinary tract infections. European Journal of Chemotherapy and Antibiotics 3: 31–39
28. Leigh D A, Emmanuel F X S, Petch V J 1986 Treatment of complicated urinary tract infections due to *Pseudomonas aeruginosa* with ciprofloxacin and norfloxacin. ICAAC Abstract 404
29. Leigh D A, Smith E L, Marriner J 1984 Comparative study using norfloxacin and amoxicillin in the treatment of complicated urinary tract infections in geriatric patients. Journal of Antimicrobial Chemotherapy 13 (suppl B): 79–83
30. Cherubin C, Stilwell S 1986 Norfloxacin versus parenteral therapy in the treatment of complicated urinary tract infections and resistant organisms. Scandinavian Journal of Infectious Diseases 48 (suppl): 32–37
31. Sabba J, Hoagland V L, Cook T 1986 Norfloxacin versus cotrimoxazole in the treatment of recurring urinary tract infections in men. Scandinavian Journal of Infectious Diseases 48 (suppl) 48–53
32. Crider S R, Colby S D, Miller L K, Harrison W O, Kerbs S B J, Berg W 1984 Treatment of penicillin-resistant *Neisseria gonorrhoea* with oral norfloxacin. New England Journal of Medicine 311: 137–140
33. Romanowski B, Wood H, Draker J, Tsianco M C 1986 Norfloxacin in the therapy of uncomplicated gonorrhea. Antimicrobial Agents and Chemotherapy 30: 514–515
34. Kaplowitz L G, Vishniavsky N, Evans T et al 1987 Norfloxacin in the therapy of uncomplicated gonococcal infections. American Journal of Medicine 82 (suppl 6B): 35–39
35. Bowie W R, Willetts V, Sibau L 1986 Failure of norfloxacin to eradicate *Chlamydia trachomatis* in nongonococcal urethritis. Antimicrobial Agents and Chemotherapy 30: 594–597
36. Dupont H L, Corrado M L, Sabbaj J 1987 The use of norfloxacin in the treatment of acute diarrheal disease. American Journal of Medicine 82 (suppl 6B): 79–83
37. Ruiz-Palacios G M 1986 Norfloxacin in the treatment of bacterial enteric infections. Scandinavian Journal of Infectious Diseases 48 (suppl): 55–63
38. Rogerie F, Ott D, Vandepitte J, Verbist L, Lemmens P, Habiyaremye I 1986 Comparison of norfloxacin and nalidixic acid for treatment of dysentery caused by *Shigella dysenteriae* type 1 in adults. Antimicrobial Agents and Chemotherapy 29: 883–886
39. Battacharya S K, Battacharya M K, Dutta P et al 1990 Double-blind, randomized, controlled clinical trial of norfloxacin for cholera. Antimicrobial Agents and Chemotherapy 34: 939–940
40. Johnson P C, Ericsson C D, Morgan D R, Dupont H L, Cabada F J 1986 Lack of emergence of resistant fecal flora during successful prophylaxis of traveler's diarrhoea with norfloxacin. Antimicrobial Agents and Chemotherapy 30: 671–674
41. Winston D J, Ho W G, Nakao S L, Gale R P, Champlin R E 1986 Norfloxacin versus vancomycin/polymyxin for prevention of infections in granulocytopenic patients. American Journal of Medicine 80: 884–890
42. Sarma P S 1989 Norfloxacin: a new drug in the treatment of falciparum malaria. Annals of Internal medicine 111: 336–337
43. Douidar S M, Snodgrass W R 1989 Potential role for fluroquinolones in pediatric infections. Reviews of Infectious Diseases 11 (suppl 5): S878–S889
44. Eandi M, Viano I, DiNola F, Leone L, Genazzani E 1983 Pharmacokinetics of norfloxacin in healthy volunteers and patients with renal and hepatic damage. European Journal of Clinical Microbiology 2: 253–259
45. Hughes P J, Webb D B, Asscher A W 1984 Pharmacokinetics of norfloxacin (MK 366) in patients with impaired kidney function — some preliminary results. Journal of Antimicrobial Chemotherapy 13 (suppl B): 55–57
46. Ariyarit C, Mokamukkul B, Chitwarakorn A et al 1988 Clinical and microbiological efficacy of a single dose of norfloxacin in the treatment of chancroid. Scandinavian Journal Infections Diseases Suppl. 56: 55–68

Nortriptyline (hydrochloride)

Nortriptyline is used in the treatment of depression. It is a secondary amine and is the first metabolite of amitriptyline.

Chemistry

Nortriptyline hydrochloride (Allegron, Aventyl, Altilev, Noritren, Nortab, Nortrilen, Pamelor, Psychostyl, Sensival, Vividyl)

$C_{19}H_{21}N.HCl$

3-(10,11-Dihydro-5H-dibenzo[a,d]cyclohepten-5-ylidene)-N-methylpropylamine hydrochloride

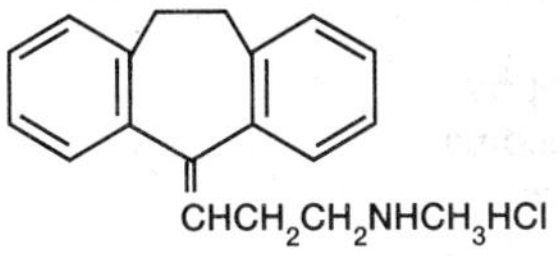

Molecular weight (free base)	299.8 (263.4)
pKa (amino)	9.7
Solubility	
in alcohol	1 in 10
in water	1 in 50
Octanol/water partition coefficient	50.1

Nortriptyline hydrochloride is a white or off-white powder with a slight characteristic odour and a burning, bitter taste followed by a sensation of numbness. It is prepared by chemical synthesis.

Pharmacology

Nortriptyline inhibits the uptake of noradrenaline and serotonin at nerve terminals. In contrast to its parent compound amitriptyline, which is equally potent in inhibiting the uptake of noradrenaline and serotonin, nortriptyline has a greater effect on noradrenaline reuptake than on serotonin reuptake.[1,2] It does not affect reuptake of dopamine. The inhibition of reuptake of noradrenaline and serotonin is an immediate effect, whereas in clinical practice the antidepressant effect is not usually observed until after two weeks of treatment, suggesting that changes in receptor sensitivity might be required for the therapeutic effect. Chronic administration of nortriptyline results in decreased sensitivity of presynaptic α_2-adrenoceptors. However, it is not known if this change plays a part in the therapeutic effect.

Nortriptyline is a potent antagonist at muscarinic acetylcholine receptors and has weak antagonist effects at histamine (H_1) receptors and at α_1-adrenoceptors. The antimuscarinic effects are likely to be partially responsible for the cardiac effects, such as tachycardia and arrhythmias, experienced in clinical practice. In rabbit atrial tissue, nortriptyline exhibits an antimuscarinic effect approximately equal to that of imipramine, but less than that of amitriptyline.[3] In mice, nortriptyline hydrochloride administered subcutaneously at doses in the range 0.125–0.50 mg.kg^{-1} potentiates the pressor responses to noradrenaline given either subcutaneously or into the lateral cerebral ventricles.[4] Paradoxically, nortriptyline and other tricyclic antidepressants antagonize the hypothermic effects of intracerebral injection of noradrenaline.[5] However, subcutaneous administration of noradrenaline has a hyperthermic effect which is potentiated by nortriptyline,[4] suggesting that the paradoxical antagonism of the hypothermic effect of intraventricular noradrenaline arises through potentiation of the hyperthermic effect of noradrenaline that has leaked to the periphery, rather than direct antagonism of the central effects of noradrenaline.

Toxicology

In tests of acute toxicity of nortriptyline hydrochloride,[6] the LD_{50} in mice is 327 mg.kg^{-1} for oral administration and 145 mg.kg^{-1} for subcutaneous administration. In rats, the LD_{50} is 502 mg.kg^{-1} for oral administration and 666 mg.kg^{-1} for subcutaneous administration. In tests of toxicity during chronic administration,[6] rats tolerated daily subcutaneous administration of 20 mg.kg^{-1} for 246 days without suffering drug-induced changes, except for ulceration at the site of injection. There were no detectable effects on either reproduction or development of the offspring of rats fed nortriptyline hydrochloride at levels as high as 0.03% in the diet. Dogs survived daily doses of 20 mg.kg^{-1} for one year without deleterious effects, but succumbed within a few days to daily doses of 40 mg.kg^{-1}. Thus there is a wide margin between the pharmacologically active dose of nortriptyline and the toxic dose in animals.

Clinical pharmacology

Nortriptyline is an effective antidepressant drug in clinical practice. While blockade of amine uptake is established quickly following oral administration, full antidepressant activity is not apparent clinically for 2–3 weeks, steady-state concentrations in plasma are achieved after about 10 days therapy. Nortryptiline is less sedative than amitryptiline because of its lesser blockade of serotonin reuptake, but is more sedative than imipramine. Nortryptiline helps depressed patients to sleep, although it is not primarily hypnotic. It decreases the number of awakenings and decreases the time spent in rapid eye movement (REM) sleep. There are few long-term effects on the EEG but in the short term there is an increase in alpha activity.

Nortryptiline causes postural hypotension by virtue of its actions primarily on α_1-receptors. In addition, tachycardia may occur (also due to anticholinergic action) and the effects on the ECG include inversion of the T-wave and prolonged conduction. Direct myocardial depression may occur. Cardiac arrhythmias may ensue in overdosage. Nortryptiline may have anticholinergic effects, including dry mouth, blurred vision, constipation and retention of urine.

Pharmacokinetics

The preferred analytical method for the drug in plasma is gas chromatography, the lower limit of detection[7] being 20 μg.l^{-1}.

Nortriptyline is readily and completely absorbed from the gastrointestinal tract. Presystemic metabolism has been estimated to be in the order of 40–50%,[8] so that approximately 60% of an oral dose will reach the systemic circulation.

Oral absorption	100%
Presystemic metabolism	40–50%
Plasma half life	
range	18–60 h
mean	36
Volume of distribution	14–40 l.kg^{-1}
Plasma protein binding	90–95%

Nortriptyline is bound to plasma proteins to a variable extent.[9] Twin studies have shown that although plasma protein binding is partly under genetic control, environmental factors also play a role.[10] Plasma steady-state levels for nortriptyline are reached in 1–2 weeks.[11]

A positive correlation between age and steady-state plasma levels has been shown to exist for nortriptyline. In general, the therapeutic doses for the elderly are lower than those recommended for adult dosage.[12,13]

Approximately 62% of the initial dose of nortriptyline is excreted as its metabolites in the urine, most within the first 24 hours.[14,15]

It has been demonstrated that nortriptyline can be used safely in renal failure, and that its concentration is unaffected by haemodialysis or peritoneal dialysis.[16]

Concentration–effect relationship

Asberg et al 1971[17] found that clinical improvement was greatest in patients with plasma levels of nortriptyline in the range of

Nortriptyline (hydrochloride)

50–139 $\mu g.l^{-1}$, and that patients with a lower or higher plasma level did less well.

Further studies have demonstrated a poor clinical response when the plasma levels of nortriptyline were high, above[18] 170 $\mu g.l^{-1}$ and above[19] 150 $\mu g.l^{-1}$. Ziegler[20] showed that there was a significantly better response when the plasma level was lower than 140 $\mu g.l^{-1}$; however, he was not able to identify any lower limit to the therapeutic range. In contrast, Burrows[21] failed to find any relationship between plasma levels and clinical improvement after 4–6 weeks of treatment. However, in a second trial,[22] when larger numbers of patients were considered, he identified a sub-group of patients who showed a positive correlation between plasma levels of drug and therapeutic response.

The balance of evidence confirms a curvilinear relationship between plasma level and clinical response, and the recommended plasma levels for nortriptyline are 50–150 $\mu g.l^{-1}$. However, it is unclear to what extent the curvilinear relationship reflects a decrease in the specific antidepressant effect at higher plasma levels. It is possible that a decrease in clinical benefit at higher doses might at least in part reflect distress associated with side effects. The relationship between plasma concentration and subjective side effects is difficult to establish. There is evidence that in cases of overdose with the parent compound, amitriptyline, the cardiotoxic effects are correlated with the plasma levels of both amitriptyline and nortriptyline.[23]

Metabolism

Nortriptyline is metabolized by 10-hydroxylation, demethylation and conjugation with glucuronic acid (Fig. 1). During chronic administration, the plasma concentration of 10-hydroxynortriptyline usually exceeds that of nortriptyline, but there is pronounced variation between individuals in the plasma concentrations of the parent drug and of the metabolite.[24] Genetic effects influence the E-10-hydroxylation of nortriptyline in a manner parallel to the polymorphic 4-hydroxylation of debrisoquine.[25] The rate of plasma clearance of nortriptyline is slower in individuals who are slow hydroxylators of debrisoquine. The nortriptyline clearance rate ranges from 0.30 $l.h^{-1}.kg^{-1}$ to 0.89 $l.h^{-1}.kg^{-1}$.

10-Hydroxynortriptyline has half the potency of nortriptyline for blocking reuptake of noradrenaline,[26,27] but less than 6% of its antimuscarinic activity.[28] The major proportion of 10-hydroxynortriptyline is conjugated, while a small proportion is oxidized.

Pharmaceutics

Nortriptyline is available only in oral formulations.

1. Allegron (Dista, UK): tablets, 10 mg (white, round, marked 'Dista') and 25 mg (orange, scored, round, marked 'Dista').
2. Aventyl (Lilly, UK): capsules are 10 mg (white/yellow, coded 'H17') and 25 mg (white/yellow, coded 'H19').
3. Pamelor (Sandoz, USA): capsules, 10 mg (orange/white, coded '78-86'), 25 mg (orange/white, coded '78-87'), 50 mg (white, coded '78-78') and 75 mg (orange, coded '78-79'). They are also overprinted with 'Pamelor', 'Sandoz' and the capsule strength.
4. A colourless syrup was also available (Lilly, UK) and this contains 10 mg of nortriptyline hydrochloride per 5 ml.

The 25 mg Allegron tablet contains sunset yellow as a colorant, which is a potentially allergenic substance.

Fig. 1 The metabolism of nortriptyline

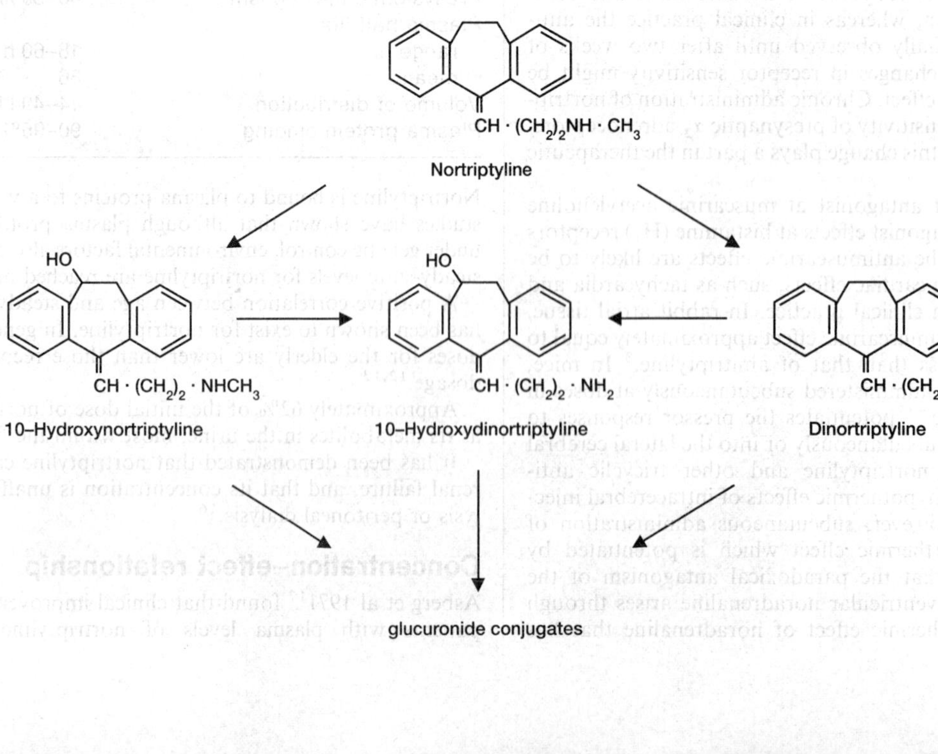

Therapeutic use

Indications

1. Treatment of depression
2. Treatment of enuresis
3. Treatment of nausea and vomiting during chemotherapy
4. Panic disorders
5. Urticaria.

Contraindications

1. Mania
2. Hypersensitivity to nortriptyline
3. Recent myocardial infarction or in heart block
4. Epilepsy
5. Prostatic hypertrophy
6. Closed-angle glaucoma
7. Severe liver disease.

Indications

1. Depression

The antidepressant effects of nortriptyline have been recognized since the 1960s.[29] As with the other tricyclic antidepressants, it is more effective in the treatment of endogenous depression than reactive depression. There is some evidence that nortriptyline may have a more rapid onset of action than the other tricyclic antidepressants,[30] but that after 4 weeks of treatment this effect is no longer evident.

There is a substantial relief of depression in about 60% of depressed patients treated with nortriptyline. However, the outcome of depression in the absence of specific treatment is often quite good, and in addition the benefits of psychological support can be substantial. In placebo-controlled treatment trials, it is usual to find moderate or marked improvement in about 40% of the cases treated with placebo. The evidence suggests that nortriptyline treatment is responsible for an increase of 20% in the number of cases obtaining relief from depression within a period ranging from 2 weeks to 2 months after the beginning of treatment.

Nortriptyline (hydrochloride)

The initial recommended dosage is 10 mg three times daily, gradually increasing to a maximum of 100 mg daily. The usual maintenance dose is 30–75 mg daily. Since nortriptyline has a long half life this can be given as a once-daily dosage.[31]

2. Enuresis
The antienuretic effect of nortriptyline is similar to that reported with imipramine; its effects are immediate, in contrast to the delay in onset of its antidepressant actions. Its presumed mode of action in enuresis is via the noradrenergic receptors in the bladder. The dose should be administered 30 min before bedtime. Recommended doses are, for a child of 7, 10 mg, children aged 7–11, 10–20 mg, and children over the age of 11, 25–35 mg. The maximum period of treatment should not exceed 3 months, including the time required to gradually taper off the treatment.[32,33]

3. Nausea and vomiting
In patients receiving chemotherapy for carcinoma of the breast, nortriptyline 30 mg daily has been shown to have an antiemetic effect when combined with fluphenazine 1.5 mg daily.[34]

4. Panic disorders
Nortriptyline has been demonstrated to be effective in treating patients with panic disorder or agoraphobia with panic attacks. 67% of patients treated completely lost their attacks while only 10% showed no improvement.[35]

5. Urticaria
Nortriptyline has been used successfully to treat urticarial wheals or dermographism; however, maintenance dosage was required for continued control of the urticaria.[36] The presumed mode of action is nortriptyline's antihistaminic properties.

Contraindications

1. Mania
Care should be taken when treating patients with a history of bipolar illness, since mania may be precipitated.

2. Hypersensitivity to nortriptyline
Nortriptyline should not be used when there is a history of previous hypersensitivity to the drug.

3. Recent myocardial infarction
Nortriptyline is contraindicated during the acute recovery period after a myocardial infarction, since it is sympathomimetic and has anticholinergic properties, thus causing increased frequency of discharge and encouraging ectopic impulse formation. For these reasons it is also contraindicated where there is any degree of heart block or other cardiac arrhythmia.

4. Epilepsy
Nortriptyline, in common with other tricyclic antidepressants, lowers the seizure threshold.

5. Prostatic hypertrophy
Nortriptyline should be used with caution in patients with a history suggestive of prostatism, since acute retention can be precipitated.

6. Closed-angle glaucoma
In principle the anticholinergic effects of nortriptyline might exacerbate closed-angle glaucoma by causing mydriasis. However, the autonomic effects of nortriptyline reflect a complex interplay between effects on the cholinergic and adrenergic systems, and there is some evidence that moderate doses of nortriptyline do not produce mydriasis.[37]

Adverse reactions

Potentially life-threatening effects
Agranulocytosis is a rare but potentially fatal adverse effect of all the tricyclic antidepressants. It is thought to be immunological in nature, occurs in the second month of treatment and is more common in women and in the elderly.[38]

Acute overdosage
Deliberate overdosage using antidepressants is well recognized. Doses of up to 1250 mg of nortriptyline have been taken with subsequent full recovery. The major cardiac signs are sinus tachycardia and arrhythmias. Hypotension can occur, but is less common than with imipramine, possibly because nortriptyline has less antagonistic activity at α_1-adrenoceptors. The CNS signs include hyperreflexia, convulsions and coma. A period of excitement might occur, but can precede the development of coma in severe cases. There can be respiratory complications leading to hypoxia and acid–base disturbances. Common anticholinergic effects are dry mouth, blurred vision, constipation and urinary retention. Temperature regulation can be disturbed.

In treating acute overdosage, the stomach should be emptied by emesis or aspiration. Oral administration of activated charcoal might reduce absorption of nortriptyline from the gastrointestinal tract. Haemodialysis is not useful, possibly on account of the large volume of distribution. The use of physostigmine, an anticholinesterase agent that crosses the blood–brain barrier, to counter atrial tachycardia, gut immotility and somnolence remains controversial, because of the risk that physostigmine itself might induce respiratory difficulties or cardiac arrhythmias.

It is essential to perform cardiac monitoring. Cardiac arrhythmias can be treated with propanolol or phenytoin, but quinidine and procainamide should be avoided because they could exacerbate slowed conduction and rhythm disturbances due to the nortriptyline. Serum electrolytes should be monitored and imbalances corrected. Metabolic acidosis should be corrected with bicarbonate.[39] Convulsions can be treated with diazepam.

Severe or irreversible adverse effects
Cardiovascular. Nortriptyline causes an increase in the heart rate,[40] in the region of 3–16 beats per minute. However, this is thought to be of clinical significance only when there is co-existing coronary artery disease.

Cardiac conduction is slowed, and a prolongation of the P-R interval on the electrocardiograph occurs at levels above the therapeutic window. The effects of nortriptyline on the heart's conduction system was further studied,[41] and the finding that none of 11 patients with first degree heart block went on to develop complete heart block, in comparison to 3 of 24 patients with bundle branch block who did so, confirms the evidence that the tricyclic antidepressants seem to exert their major effect on the distal conduction system.

Nortriptyline appears less likely than imipramine to cause significant postural hypotension in patients when plasma levels within the 'recommended' range are achieved.[42]

Neurological. Nortriptyline may lower the seizure threshold, which may cause fits in susceptible individuals. Peripheral neuropathy has been reported as a rare adverse effect in patients taking nortriptyline.

Hepatic. Nortriptyline has rarely been associated with the development of cholestatic jaundice.

Symptomatic adverse effects
As with the other members of the group, nortriptyline may cause anticholinergic effects, which may lead to dry mouth, constipation, urinary hesitancy, confusional states and blurred vision.

Interference with clinical pathology tests
Nortriptyline may interfere with the nitrobenzo-oxo-diazole chloride reaction used to measure urinary amphetamines.

High risk groups

Neonates
The drug is not recommended for use in neonates.

Breast milk. Nortriptyline is not recommended in nursing mothers. Like the other tricyclic antidepressants, it is excreted in breast milk.

Children
Nortriptyline is not recommended in children under the age of 6. Above this age it can be used as a treatment of depression or, in the short term, for the treatment of enuresis.

The pharmacokinetics of nortriptyline in children have been studied,[43] and as with adults a logarithmically linear rate of elimination and a wide interindividual rate of metabolism were found. Children under 12 were shown to have a significantly shorter half life of nortriptyline, and a significantly greater mean apparent oral clearance than those over the age of 12, suggesting that a twice-daily dosage regime may be necessary in treating children with depression.

Pregnant women
The safety of nortriptyline during pregnancy has not been established.

The elderly
Nortriptyline has been demonstrated to be an effective antidepressant in the elderly,[44] but it may take up to four weeks before symptom relief is seen.[45] Pharmacokinetic studies of nortriptyline in the elderly have confirmed that the half life, plasma clearance and volume of distribution are similar to those obtained in studies of younger adults.[46]

Drug interactions

Potentially hazardous interactions

Monoamine oxidase inhibitors. Nortriptyline should not be used in conjunction with a monoamine oxidase inhibitor, or within 14 days of stopping one, since severe hyperpyretic reactions can occur.

Sympathomimetic amines. The pressor effects of directly acting sympathomimetic amines are potentiated by nortriptyline, which may result in severe headache or even death.

Antihypertensive drugs. Nortriptyline, in common with other tricyclic antidepressants, antagonizes the hypotensive effects of drugs such as guanethidine, bethanidine and debrisoquine. Nortriptyline may also antagonize the effects of centrally acting hypotensive drugs such as clonidine.

Major tranquillizers. Phenothiazines can inhibit the metabolism of tricyclics,[47] the probable mechanism being blocking of hydroxylation which, in turn, leads to high levels of excretion of unchanged drug.

Anticoagulants. Nortriptyline increases the half life of coumarin anticoagulants.[48]

Other drugs. Interactions have also been reported with cimetidine, reserpine, fluoxetine, barbiturates and excessive alcohol.

Potentially useful interactions
None has been described.

Major outcome trials

1. White K, Razani J, Cadow B, Gelfand, Palmer R, Simpson G, Sloane R 1985 Tranylcypromine vs nortriptyline vs placebo in depressed outpatients: a controlled trial. Psychopharmacology 82: 258–262

122 depressed outpatients, including both endogenous and non-endogenous cases, were assigned to receive tranylcypromine, nortriptyline or placebo under double-blind conditions. Dose was adjusted according to clinical estimate of need. The mean daily dose of tranylcypromine was 44.4 mg and that of nortriptyline was 104.4 mg. Depression was assessed according to several scales and, in addition, overall clinical improvement was rated according to the Clinical Global Improvement scale. At 4 weeks, there was moderate or marked improvement in 25 of 37 cases receiving tranylcypromine (68%); 25 of 40 cases receiving nortriptyline (62%) and 19 of 45 cases receiving placebo (42%). The number of cases with moderate or marked improvement in both groups receiving active treatment was significantly greater than that in the group receiving placebo. The small difference between the nortriptyline group and the tranylcypromine group was not statistically significant.

2. Mendells J 1968 Comparative trial of nortriptyline and amitriptyline in 100 depressed out-patients. American Journal of Psychiatry 124 (suppl): 59–62

This was a double-blind comparison of nortriptyline with amitriptyline in 100 consecutive inpatient and outpatient cases suffering from primary depressive illness. Severity of depression was assessed using the Hamilton Depression Scale administered at 0, 2, 3, 4, 6 and 8 weeks. Dose was adjusted according to clinical estimate of need. In the group receiving nortriptyline, mean Hamilton Depression Scale scores were 26.2 at week 0; 11.74 at week 3; and 5.3 at week 8. In the group receiving amitriptyline, the mean scores were 25.9 at week 0; 14.89 at week 3; and 7.08 at week 8. The small differences at week 0 and at week 8 were not statistically significant, but the mean score for the nortriptyline group was significantly lower than that for the amitriptyline group at week 3 ($P < 0.001$). Thus both groups achieved similar levels of relief of depression, but the therapeutic effect had a more rapid onset in the group treated with nortriptyline.

Nortriptyline (hydrochloride)

References

1. Waldmeier P C, Greengrass P M, Baumann P, Maitre L 1976 Effects of clomipramine and other tricyclic antidepressants on the biogenic amine uptake and turnover. Postgraduate Medical Journal 52 (suppl 3): 33
2. Horn A S 1980 The mode of actions of the tricyclic antidepressants: a brief review of recent progress. Postgraduate Medical Journal 56 (suppl 1): 9–12
3. Somogyi G J, Perel J M 1989 Antagonism by tricyclic antidepressants of the muscarinic receptors located in the adrenergic nerve endings in rabbit heart atrium. Journal of Pharmacology and Experimental Therapeutics 251: 922–928
4. Cowell P, Davey M J 1968 The reversal of the central effects of noradrenaline by antidepressant drugs in mice. British Journal of Pharmacology 34: 159–168
5. Brittain R J 1966 The intracerebral effects of noradrenaline and its modification by drugs in the mouse. Journal of Pharmacy and Pharmacology 18: 621–623
6. Meyers D B, Small R M, Anderson R C 1966 Toxicology of nortriptyline hydrochloride. Toxicology and Applied Pharmacology 9: 152–159
7. Braithwaite R A, Widdop B 1971 A specific gas-chromatographic method for the measurement of 'steady state' plasma levels of amitriptyline and nortriptyline in patients. Clinica Chemica Acta 35: 461–472
8. Alexanderson B, Borga O, Alvan G 1973 The availability of orally administered nortriptyline. European Journal of Clinical Pharmacology 5: 181–183
9. Borga O, Hamberger B, Malmfors T, Sjoqvist 1970 The role of plasma protein in binding in the inhibitory effect of nortriptyline on the neuronal uptake of norepinephrine. Clinical Pharmacology and Therapeutics 11: 581–588
10. Alexanderson B, Borga O 1973 Prediction of steady state plasma levels of nortriptyline from single dose kinetics: a study in twins. European Journal of Clinical Pharmacology 6: 44–53
11. Alexanderson B 1972 Pharmacokinetics of nortriptyline in man after single and multiple oral doses. The predictability of steady state plasma concentrations from single-dose plasma level data. European Journal of Clinical Pharmacology 4: 82–91
12. Nies A, Robinson D S, Friedman M J et al 1977 Relationship between age and tricyclic antidepressant levels. American Journal of Psychiatry 134: 790–793
13. Dawling S, Crome P, Braithwaite R 1980 Pharmacokinetics of single oral doses of nortriptyline in depressed elderly hospital patients and young healthy volunteers. Clinical Pharmacokinetics 5: 394–401
14. Alexanderson B, Borga O 1973 Urinary excretion of nortriptyline and five of its metabolites in man after single and multiple oral doses. European Journal of Clinical Pharmacology 5: 174–177
15. Amundsen M E, Manthey J A 1966 Excretion of nortriptyline in man. Detection and determination of urinary nortriptyline. Journal of Pharmacological Science 55: 277–280
16. Bennett W M 1977 Guidelines for drug therapy in renal failure. Annals of Internal Medicine 86: 754
17. Asberg M, Cronholm B, Sjoqvist F, Tuck D 1971 Relationship between plasma level and the therapeutic effect of nortriptyline. British Medical Journal 3: 331–334
18. Kragh-Sorenson P, Asberg M, Eggert-Hansen C 1973 Plasma nortriptyline levels in endogenous depression. Lancet 1: 113–115
19. Montgomery S A, Braithwaite R A, Crammer J L 1977 Routine nortriptyline levels in the treatment of depression. British Medical Journal 2: 166–167
20. Ziegler V E, Clayton P J, Taylor J R, Co B T, Biggs J T 1976 Nortriptyline plasma levels and therapeutic response. Clinical Pharmacology and Therapeutics 20: 458–463
21. Burrows G D, Davies B, Scoggins B A 1972 Plasma concentrations of nortriptyline and clinical response in depressive illness. Lancet 2: 619–623
22. Burrows G D, Scoggins B A, Turecek L R, Davies B 1974 Plasma nortriptyline and clinical response. Clinical Pharmacology and Therapeutics 16: 639–644
23. Petit J M, Spiker D G, Ruwitch J F, Zeigler V E, Weiss A N, Biggs J T 1977 Tricyclic antidepressant plasma levels and adverse effect after overdose. Clinical Pharmacology and Therapeutics 21: 47–51
24. Nordin C, Bertilsson L, Siwers B 1985 CSF and plasma levels of nortriptyline and its 10-hydroxy metabolite. British Journal of Clinical Pharmacology 20: 411–413
25. Melstrom B, Bertilsson L, Sawe J, Schulz H-U, Sjoqvist F S 1981 E- and Z-10-hydroxylation of nortriptyline: relationship to polymorphic debrisoquine hydroxylation. Clinical Pharmacology and Therapeutics 30: 189–193
26. Bertilsson L, Melstrom B, Sjoqvist F 1979 Pronounced inhibition of noradrenaline uptake by 10-hydroxymetabolites of nortriptyline. Life Sciences 25: 1285–1292
27. Nordin C, Bertisson L, Siwers B 1987 Clinical and biochemical effects during treatment of depression with nortriptyline, the role of 10 hydroxy nortriptyline. Clinical Pharmacology and Therapeutics 42: 10–19
28. Wagner A, Ekqvist B, Bertilsson L, Sjoqvist F 1984 Weak binding of 10-hydroxymetabolites of nortriptyline to rat brain muscarinic acetylcholine receptors. Life Sciences 35: 1379–1383
29. Maclean R, Rees L 1966 Clinical Trials Journal 3: 567
30. Mendels J 1968 Comparative trial of nortriptyline and amitriptyline in 100 depressed patients. American Journal of Psychiatry 124: 59–62
31. Ziegler V E, Clayton P J, Biggs J T 1977 A comparative study of amitriptyline and nortriptyline with plasma levels. Archives of General Psychiatry 34: 607–612
32. Lake B 1968 Controlled trial of nortriptyline in childhood enuresis. Medical Journal of Australia 5, 2 (suppl 14): 582–585
33. Forsythe W I, Merrett J D 1969 A controlled trial of imipramine and nortriptyline in the treatment of enuresis. British Journal of Clinical Practice 23: 210–215
34. Morran C, Smith D C, Anderson D A, McCardle C S 1979 Incidence of nausea and vomiting with cytotoxic chemotherapy; a prospective randomized trial of anti-emetics. British Medical Journal 1: 1323–1324
35. Munjack D J, Usigli R, Zulueta A, et al 1988 Nortriptyline in the treatment of panic disorder and agoraphobia with panic attacks. Journal of Clinical Psychopharmacology 8: 204
36. Morley W N 1969 Nortriptyline in the treatment of chronic urticaria. British Journal of Clinical Practice 23: 305–306

37. Bye C E, Clubley M, Henson T, Peck A W, Smith S A, Smith S E 1979 Changes in the human light reflex as a measure of the anticholinergic effects of drugs. A comparison with other measures. European Journal of Clinical Pharmacology 15: 21–25
38. Mielke D H 1975 Psychiatry Annual 5: 473–483
39. Brackenridge R G, Peter T J, Watson J M 1968 Myocardial damage in amitriptyline and nortriptyline poisoning. Scottish Medical Journal 13: 208–210
40. Glassman A, Bigger J C 1981 Vascular effects of therapeutic doses of tricyclic antidepressants. Archives of General Psychiatry 38: 815–820
41. Roose S P, Glassman A J, Giardinia E G V, Walsh B T, Woodring S, Bigger J T 1987 Tricyclic antidepressants in patients with cardiac conduction disease. Archives of General Psychiatry 44: 272–275
42. Smith R C, Chajnacki M, Hu R et al 1980 Cardiovascular effects of therapeutic doses of tricyclic antidepressants: the importance of blood level monitoring. Journal of Clinical Psychiatry 41: 12 Sec 2: 57–63
43. Geller B, Cooper T B, Schluchter M D, Warham J E, Carr L G 1987 Child and adolescent nortriptyline single dose pharmacokinetic parameters: final report. Journal of Clinical Pharmacology 7: 321–323
44. Georgotas A, McCue R E, Kim O M, Friedman E, Hapworth W, Welkowitz J, Cooper T B 1986 Comparative efficacy and safety of monoamine oxidase inhibitors vs tricyclic antidepressants in the treatment of depressed elderly. Biological Psychiatry 21: 1155–1166
45. Georgotas A, McCue R E, Friedman E, Cooper T B 1987 Response of depressive symptoms to nortriptyline, phenelzine and placebo. British Journal of Psychiatry 151: 102–106
46. Dawling S, Crome P, Braithwaite R A, Lewis R R 1980 Nortriptyline therapy in elderly patients. Dosage prediction after single dose pharmacokinetic study. European Journal of Clinical Pharmacology 18: 147–150
47. Gram L F, Overo K F 1972 Drug interaction; inhibitory effect of neuroleptics on the metabolism of tricyclic antidepressants in man. British Medical Journal 1: 463–465
48. Stockley I H 1973 Interaction with oral anticoagulants. Pharmacology Journal 210: 339–342

Noxythiolin

A broad spectrum antiseptic acting mainly via its breakdown product formaldehyde.

Chemistry

Noxythiolin, Noxytiolin (Noxyflex S R)
$C_3H_8N_2OS$
1-Hydroxymethyl-3-methyl-2 thiourea

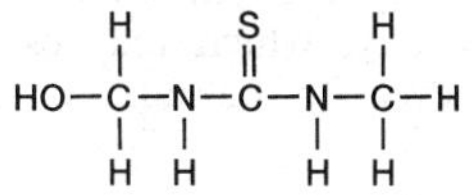

Molecular weight	120.2
pKa	not relevant
Solubility	
in alcohol	1 in 25
in water	1 in 10
Octanol/water partition coefficient (apparent)	0.189

Noxythiolin is a white crystalline powder prepared by chemical synthesis. Noxythiolin decomposes to formaldehyde upon heating to 90°C. When 1% solutions in an aqueous buffer (pH 4,7 and 10) were stored at 37°C for 18 h, most of the theoretical content of formaldehyde was released. However, in urine at pH 5.5 only 15% of the maximum was released.[1] This release occurred gradually. The stability characteristics have been studied by Irwin.[2] Noxythiolin is assayed by HPLC.[2,3] Fluorimetric and 14C–labelled techniques do not differentiate between noxythiolin and N-methylthiourea.

Pharmacology

Weak solutions of noxythiolin slowly release formaldehyde to give an antimicrobical effect. The contact time required for maximum bacteriostatic effect is 1–2 h.[4] Nuclear magnetic resonance spectroscopy has shown[5] that the antibacterial effect resides mainly in the free formaldehyde. N-methylthiourea does not exert any detectable antibacterial effect at the concentrations which develop in clinical use. A third metabolite has not yet been identified. The low levels of formaldehyde detected have led some workers[6] to deduce that the concentration is too low for a bactericidal effect. These workers recommend that formaldehyde assays are performed by a non–destructive pulse polarographic technique rather than a destructive assay (eg. Hantzsch reaction) which may result in estimations of formaldehyde levels which are too high.

Toxicology

Noxythiolin's cytotoxic effect is weak compared with other common antiseptic agents[7,8] but one writer claims that unlike chlorhexidine it is selectively cytotoxic against some established neoplastic cell lines but not against normal control (non–neoplastic) cells.[9] This is at variance with the work of Umpleby[8] who found only 80% of colorectal tumour cells were rendered non–viable by noxythiolin. Similarly Garett[7] did not find an increased survival rate in 242 patients treated for bladder carcinoma.

Tissue distribution studies with ^{14}C labelled noxythiolin have shown that radioactivity is selectively associated with the thyroid gland and may have anti-T4 activity, since it lowers T4 levels in rat serum.[10] No serious effects have been seen in rat models. The LD_{50} orally in mice exceeds 3 $g.kg^{-1}$. The lethal intraperitoneal dose in mice is 1650 $mg.kg^{-1}$.[11] This is over forty times the highest equivalent clinical dose.

In addition to the possible toxic effects of low concentrations of formaldehyde (op. cit.), a number of adverse effects include the sensation of burning pain. This is the most frequently observed problem, which led to an alternative formulation containing 0.01% amethocaine hydrochloride, a local anaesthetic. This was in use until the late 1980s, when a specification for a product with a less acidic pH was adopted by the manufacturer.

Clinical pharmacology

Noxythiolin solutions are bactericidal in vitro. In vivo evidence is limited but irrigation of the upper and lower urinary tract with noxythiolin has been shown to reduce bacteriuria. Most bacteria are susceptible to noxythiolin, but resistance is not uncommon.[12] Disc perfusion sensitivity tests should, therefore, be performed. *Chlamydia* spp. are susceptible[13] but the effect on viruses is inferior to glutaraldehyde or povidone-iodine.[14] Noxythiolin is known to have an effect, when used intraperitoneally, which reduces bacterial adhesion.[15] This effect is not believed to be due to free formaldehyde or N-methylthiourea.[16,17]

Pharmacokinetics

The assay of noxythiolin, as described by Irwin[2] involved using a HPLC with a UV detector operating at 250nm with a sensitivity of 0.32 AUFS. The stainless steel column was packed with a reversed-phase stationary phase. The final concentrations of noxythiolin injected were in the region of 0.0025% and 0.001% thiourea was used as the internal standard. Calibration was performed using standards containing varied proportions of noxythiolin and N-methylthiourea.

Metabolism

The stability of noxythiolin is both concentration and pH-dependent. The pH of the 1% or 2.5% aqueous solutions currently in use are in the range of 6.3–7.0. Significant spontaneous degradation occurs at a pH below 4 and above 7 (see Fig. 1).

Fig. 1 The metabolism of noxythiolin

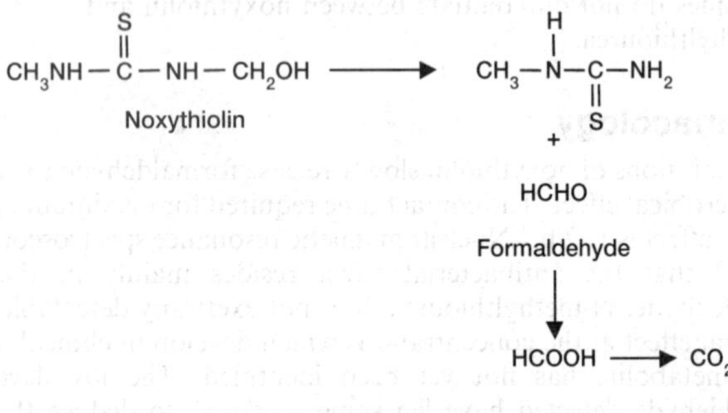

It has been estimated[2] that a 2.5% noxythiolin solution would degrade in the pH of fluid in a body cavity by about 1.8% in a minimum contact time of 30 minutes. This would yield a concentration of formaldehyde of 100 $ng.l^{-1}$. This is substantially in excess of the bacteriostatic concentration of 20 $ng.ml^{-1}$ required for formaldehyde activity. However, formaldehyde is rapidly inactivated in contact with organic macromolecules so it is unlikely that this figure is attained in vivo.

Although water is essential for decomposition, the degradation pathway in vivo is by a base-catalyzed elimination reaction to N-methylthiourea. The reaction is, however, reversible, and in an excess of formaldehyde it would be theoretically possible for a dihydroxymethyl polymer of noxythiolin to be produced. In practice, the N-methylthiourea is excreted via the kidney. At least 50% of an intraperitoneal dose of noxythiolin is excreted unchanged.[10] The breakdown product, formaldehyde is not excreted either in the urine or in the expired air, but is metabolized via formate to carbon dioxide.

Pharmaceutics

Noxythiolin, Noxyflex S (Geistlich UK/Switz) is a white powder supplied as (a) 2.5g in a 20 ml vial or (b) 2.5g in a 100 ml vial for aseptic reconstituion with water for injection or sodium chloride 0.9% infusion. Noxythiolin should not be used intravenously. Reconstituted solutions may be stored in a refrigerator for using up to seven days after admixture. Dissolution of noxythiolin is only achieved with vigorous shaking. For bladder instillation a formulation containing amethocaine was available; Noxyflex (Geistlich UK/Switz). The manufacturer claims that the current specification for a pH range of 6.3–7.0 has decreased the need for a product containing amethocaine. Noxythiolin solutions may be stored in polypropylene containers without adsorption occurring.[18]

Therapeutic use

Indications

Noxythiolin has been used as an antiseptic in the following circumstances:

1. Peritoneal eg. per and post-operative treatment
2. Bladder, for which the preparation containing amethocaine is preferred
3. Abscess cavities
4. Wounds, fistulae and burns.

The drug is bactericidal in vitro to most pathogens and resistance does not arise quickly. The use of antiseptic washes and irrigations is at best a backup to effective antibacterial chemotherapy.

Contraindications

Noxythiolin should not be administered concurrently with other pharmaceutical preparations. 10g is regarded as the maximum daily dose.

Mode of use

Whenever possible noxythiolin solutions should be warmed to body heat before use, 30–60 minutes of contact time is necessary.

Indications

1. Peritoneal infections

Noxythiolin has been used in infra-mesocolic peritonitis.[19] and in empyema.[20] In comparison to povidone iodine, it is less toxic and believed to be superior in *E. Coli* infections.[21,22] In peritonitis secondary to perforated appendix all antibiotic/antiseptic lavage was judged to be of benefit by Stewart.[23] Most experts believe that the systemic antibiotics administered concurrently are the mainstay of treatment and added benefits of antiseptic lavage have not yet been demonstrated in well controlled outcome trials.[24]

Chlorhexidine is a more potent antiseptic in Gram positive infections[14] and chlorhexidine-cetrimide preparations are more effective as cytotoxic agents in contact with neoplastic cell-lines.[8] Rosenfeldt recommends use of the drug by irrigation but this results in more nausea due to the systemic effect of noxythiolin, absorbed from the peritoneal cavity.[11,25] The most common intraperitoneal use is the instillation of 100 ml of a 25% solution prior to closure. The manufacturer also recommends repeated instillation of 200 ml of a 2.5% solution. Contact time should be for a minimum of two hours. Repeated instillation using an umbilical catheter may be repeated twice daily for five days. A post-operative irrigation of a 1% solution is occasionally used. 500 ml is dripped in over each twelve hour period for one to three days. Use of noxythiolin to treat peritonitis associated with chronic ambulatory peritoneal dialysis (CAPD) is not recommended.

2. Bladder infections

Controlled trials have demonstrated a reduction of bacteriuria after irrigation of the upper or lower urinary tract with 2.5% or 1% noxythiolin (see Clinical trials). However, the number of complications was not altered and some authors have expressed concern about possible damage to the uroepithelial cells which might predispose to reinfection. Initial use in the purulent infected bladder is often accompanied by an intense reaction including the passage of large

Noxythiolin

clumps of fibrin. 100 ml of a 2.5% solution is instilled slowly via a catheter into the bladder. The manufacturers recommend that the solution is retained in the bladder for 60 minutes.[6] For particularly heavy infections, two consecutive instillations are recommended. Treatment should continue once or twice daily for five days and the condition reviewed with microbiological advice. If infection is known to be caused by *Pseudomonas* spp a microbiological sensitivity test should be undertaken before therapy with noxythiolin is initiated.[13] For the treatment of trichomonal infections, chlorhexidine or picloxidine are more effective than noxythiolin and povidone-iodine.[27]

3, 4. Other infections

Abscess cavities are irrigated with a 2.5% solution via a polythene tube, twice daily. Noxythiolin has been used as a dental root application[28] between treatments, either as a 5 mg impregnated cotton pellet or by application of the formerly marketed methylcellulose gel containing 2.5% noxythiolin (Gynaflex).

For infected wounds and fistulae a 1% or 2.5% solution has been used twice daily for five days. Noxythiolin is now only rarely used for infected burns. It is applied as a dressing moistened with a 2.5% solution twice daily.

Adverse reactions

Potentially life-threatening effects

No effects of this kind have been reported.

Burning pain on contact with the bladder epithelium and mucous surfaces remains the most significant side effect. This problem, it is claimed, is reduced in the most recent formulation with a higher pH.

Acute overdosage

No case of deliberate self-poisoning with noxythiolin appears to have been reported.

Severe or irreversible adverse effects

Bleeding due to the drugs anticoagulant effect, with the release of fibrin clots from the bladder wall, are common on the first instillation.

The formation of adhesions in peritoneal cavities has been ascribed to noxythiolin, but some workers have used noxythiolin under the impression that it lowers the incidence of adhesions.

Symptomatic adverse effects

Foetid breath is a reaction common to thiol-containing compounds. Nausea, appetite loss and malaise are all associated with noxythiolin use. Levels of the drug reach a peak in the circulation approximately one hour after initial contact. Some of these effects may be due to its breakdown product formaldehyde.

Interference with clinical pathology tests

Blood levels are likely to be too low to interfere with any biochemical tests.

High risk groups

Noxythiolin has been used in all age groups. However, it would be prudent to use solutions of 1%, or less, in neonates and infants.

Concurrent disease

Intraperitoneal use of noxythiolin during surgery in patients with grossly impaired renal function should be avoided.

Drug interactions

Potentially hazardous interactions

No such interactions have been reported. Experience with the drug is only using sodium chloride 0.9% or water for injection as the vehicle. It is not recommended that other agents are instilled in the same solution as noxythiolin formulations. Noxythiolin is physically incompatible with hypochlorite, iodine, lactic acid and organo-mercurial compounds.

Potentially useful interactions

None has been described.

Clinical trials

1. Buck A C 1988 The use of noxythiolin (Noxyflex 'S') as an antiseptic irrigant in upper urinary tract drainage following percutaneous nephrolithotomy. British Journal of Urology 62: 306–10

A double-blind, placebo controlled study was carried out in 20 patients undergoing a single-stage percutaneous nephrolithotomy to evaluate the use of a 2.5% solution of noxythiolin as an upper urinary tract antiseptic. In the treated patients significant bacterial infection was eliminated from the nephrostomy urine and colonisation of the catheter tip was markedly reduced. The authors concluded that irrigation of the upper urinary tract with noxythiolin solution is safe and may be a useful adjunct to reduce the risk of sepsis in patients undergoing percutaneous drainage procedures.

2. Jones M A, Hasan A 1988 Controlled trial of intravesical noxythiolin in the prevention of infection following outflow tract surgery. British Journal of Urology 62: 379–404

Ths was randomised control trial in 100 consecutive patients undergoing endoscopic surgery for bladder outflow tract obstruction. 1% noxythiolin or sterile water was instilled at the time of catheter removal. The incidence of bacteriuria in the treated group (7/50) was significantly lower than in the control group (19/50). There was no difference in the complication rate despite a reduction of infection in the treated group.

3. Querleu D, Vankeerberghen-Deffense F, Boutteville C 1989 Adjuvant treatment of tubal surgery. Randomized prospective study of systemically administered corticoids and noxythiolin. Journal de Gynecologie, Obstetrique et Biologie de la Reproduction 18: 935–40

This was a randomized study of the effect of dexamethasone and/or noxythiolin versus no treatment in 126 patients having been operated upon by tubal microsurgery. Adhesions were assessed by a score derived from the American Fertility Society endometriosis classification, before operation and by laparoscopy 3 to 6 months later. The mean improvement on adhesion score was 23.2 in the corticosteroid treated group, 19.3 in the noxythiolin group, 15.7 in the noxythiolin and corticosteroid group, 10.2 in the control group. The authors conclude that their results support the use of corticosteroids to reduce adhesions in infertility surgery.

4. Elliott T S, Reid L, Rao G G, Rigby R C, Woodhouse K 1989 Bladder irrigation or irritation? British Journal of Urology 64: 391–4

The authors studied exfoliation rates of urothelial cells following bladder irrigation in patients with long-term indwelling catheters and chronic urinary tract infections. Irrigations were associated with an increased shedding and disruption of urothelial cells. The authors suggest that use of bladder irrigation should be reviewed as damage to the uroepithelium might predispose to reinfection.

Other studies

Gilmore O J A, Springell R G 1983 Local management of surgical sepsis. British Journal of Hospital Medicine 29: 440

Noxythiolin was assessed as being ineffective in three studies of appendicectomies and two studies on general surgical wounds.

References

1. Kingston D 1965 Release of formaldehyde from polynoxylin and noxythiolin. Journal of Clinical Pathology 18: 666–667
2. Irwin W J, Li-Wan-Po A, Stephens J S 1984 Noxythiolin — high performance liquid chromatography and assay. Journal of Clinical Hospital Pharmacy 9: 41–51
3. Debruyne D, Moulin M A, Bricard H, Bigot M C 1985 Liquid chromatographic determination of noxythiolin and 1-methyl-2-thiourea in serum: application to pharmacokinetic. Journal of Pharmaceutical Science 74: 224–226
4. Stickler D J, Plant S, Bunni N H, Chawla J C 1981 Some observations on the activity of three antiseptics used as bladder irrigants in the treatment of urinary tract infection in patients with indwelling catheters. Paraplegia 19: 325–333
5. Gidley M J, Sanders J K 1983 Mechanisms of antibacterial formaldehyde delivery from noxythiolin adn other 'masked-formaldehyde' compounds. Journal of Pharmacy and Pharmacology 35: 712–717
6. Woolfson A D, McCafferty D F, Gorman S P, Anderson L 1985 Differential pulse polarographic determination of formaldehyde in stored noxythiolin solutions. Journal of Clinical Hospital Pharmacy 10: 177–183
7. Garett M J, Arthur W 1981 A study of the efficacy of noxythiolin instillation as adjunctive to radiotherapy in carcinoma of the bladder; a clinical trial. Clinical Radiology 32: 237–239
8. Umpleby H C, Williamson R C 1984 The efficacy of agents employed to prevent anastomotic recurrence in colorectal carcinoma. American Journal of the College of Surgeons Eng. 66: 192–194
9. Blenkharn J I 1987 The differential cytotoxicity of antiseptic agents. Journal of Pharmacy and Pharmacology 39: 477–479

10. Jones A R, Mashford P M 1983 The fate of N-methyl-N' (hydroxymethyl) thiourea in the rat Xenobiotica 13: 73–79
11. Rosenfeldt F L, Glover J R, Marossy D 1981 Systemic absorption of noxythiolin from the pleural cavity in man and in the rabbit. Thorax 36: 278–281
12. Chattopadhyay B 1977 Noxythiolin — resistant organisms in a district general hospital. British Medical Journal 2: 1121–1122
13. Platt J, Bucknall R A 1984 An experimental evaluation of antiseptic wound irrigation. Journal of Hospital Infections 5: 181–188
14. Boudouma M, Enjalbert L, Didier J 1984 A simple method for the evaluation of antiseptic and disinfectant virucidal activity. Journal of Virological Methods 9: 271–276
15. Gilmore O J, Reid C 1976 Noxythiolin and peritoneal adhesion formation. British Journal of Surgery 63: 978–980
16. Gilmore O J, Reid C 1979 Prevention of intraperitoneal adhesions; a comparison of noxythiolin and a new providone iodine/PVP solution. British Journal of Surgery 66: 197–199
17. Carbasse D, Regnier C, Berthat J, Watrelot A, Racinet C 1981 Prevention of peritoneal adhesions: An experimental study using noxythiolin. Journal of Gynaecologie Obstetrique et Biologie de la Reproduction 10: 425–429
18. McCafferty D F, Furness K, Anderson L 1984 Stability of noxythiolin solutions stored in plastic and glass containers. Journal of Clinical Hospital Pharmacy 9: 241–247
19. Migliori G, Codinach F, Marsan A, Inglesakis J A 1978 Resultats de l'utilization de la noxythioline au cours des peritonites aigues. Annals of Anesthesiology of France 19: 903–907
20. Migueres J, Jover A, Krempf M 1981 La noxythioline dans le traitement local des epanchements pleuraux purulents. Nouvelle Presse Medicale 10: 3379–3381
21. Browne M K, Leslie G B, Pfirrman R W 1978 A comparison of noxythiolin and povidone-iodine in experimentally induced peritoneal infection in mice. British Journal of Surgery 65: 601–602
22. Platt J, Jones R A, Bucknall R A 1984 Intra-peritoneal antiseptics in experimental bacterial peritonitis. British Journal of Surgery 71: 626–628
23. Stewart D J, Matheson N A 1978 Peritoneal lavage in appendicular peritonitis. British Journal of Surgery 65: 54–56
24. McAvinchey D J, McCollum P T, Lynch G 1984 Towards a rational approach to the treatment of peritonitis: an experimental study in rats. British Journal of Surgery 71: 715–717
25. Rosenfeldt F L, McGibney D, Braimbridge M V, Watson D A 1981 Comparison between irrigation and conventional treatment for empyema and pneumonectomy space infection. Thorax 36: 272–277
26. Elliott T S, Reid L, Rao G G, Rigby R C, Woodhouse K 1989 Bladder irrigation or irritation? British Journal of Urology 46: 391–394
27. Thomas D, Osfila F, Bissac E 1984 Action de differents antiseptiques sur chalmydia trachomitis. Pathologie Biologie 32 (5, part 2): 544–546
28. Kennedy G D C, Stevenson A G, MacFarlane T W, Mason W N 1977 Root treatment of pulpless anterior teeth. British Dental Journal 143: 77–82

Nystatin

Nystatin was one of the first polyene antibiotics discovered and used clinically, although it is employed exclusively for mycoses involving epidermal and mucosal surfaces.

Chemistry

Nystatin (Mycostatin, Mystadin, Nystan)
$C_{44}H_{75}NO_{17}$
Nystatin A_1 is 19-(3-Amino-3,6-dideoxy-β-D-mannopyranosyloxy)-16-carboxy-3,5,7,10,11,15,17,35-octahydroxy-34,36-dimethyl-13-oxo-octatriaconta-20,22,24,26,30,32-hexaen-37-olide

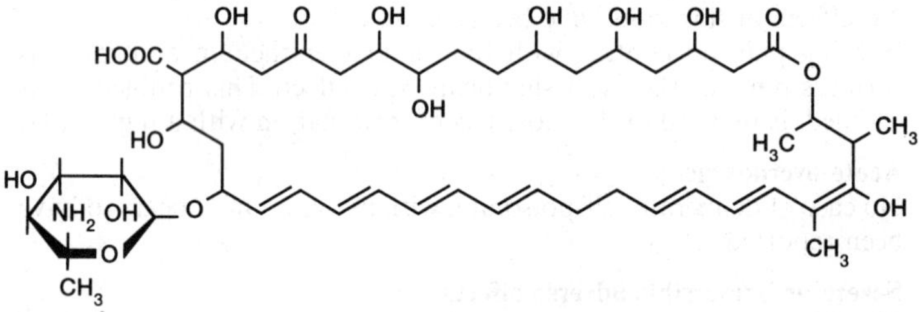

Molecular weight	926
pKa	4.5, 8.64
Solubility	
in alcohol	—
in water	very low
Octanol/water partition coefficient	—

Nystatin is a yellow to light brown hygroscopic powder with an odour suggestive of cereal. It is a product of *Streptomyces noursei.*[1] Nystatin is a mixture of four different tetranes, primarily nystatin A1, along with two other tetranes, most commonly nystatin A2 or A3 and polyfungin B.

Pharmacology

Nystatin exerts its effect by interaction with cell walls and cell membranes. Early work demonstrated that interaction with polyene antibiotics and cell walls resulted in leakage of ions, amino acids, sugars, and other metabolites.[2,3] Sterols, present in the cell membrane, were necessary for this effect to occur.[4–6] Amphotericin B has demonstrated irreversible binding to sterols, which results in disruption of the cell wall and membranes. This allows the passage of ions and disrupts active transport mechanisms, leading to complete equilibration of all constituents between the extracellular environment and the cell. This results in cell death. The molecular events and sterol chemical alterations that occur when nystatin interacts with the cell membrane have yet to be elucidated. The nature of the interaction of nystatin has been pursued using a variety of model membrane systems.[7–11] These experiments demonstrated that cholesterol/ergosterol are required to permit polyenes to disrupt membranes (i.e. to alter membrane rigidity, permeability characteristics, membrane fluidity).[12,13] Elegant experiments by Beezer[14–16] have demonstrated that the interaction is a two-phase phenomenon (the first which occurs within 5 minutes — fast phase — and a second phase which requires up to one hour for equilibration). The initial phase is not energy dependent whereas the latter requires transport from cell wall to cell membrane and is energy and temperature dependent. Other authors have demonstrated that this initial uptake is in part dictated by the fatty acid/fatty acid ester composition of the cell wall.[9,10]

Nystatin

Inhibition of chitin synthetase by polyenes has also been demonstrated in in vitro preparations.[17]

Toxicology

Mutagenic potential and teratological effects of nystatin have not been reported.

Clinical pharmacology

Nystatin is one representative of the group of polyene antibiotics that are known to affect the membrane characteristics of cells containing sterols in their wall. It has both fungistatic and fungicidal effects. The drug is effective against *Candida*, *Cryptococcus*, *Histoplasma* and *Blastomyces* although its prime use is for *Candida* infections. Nystatin is less affected by changes in pH than other antifungal drugs and it has no effect on protozoa, bacteria or viruses. Resistance to nystatin rarely develops in clinical practice, although it can be produced in vitro, particularly with species of *Candida* other than *Candida albicans* (e.g. *C. tropicalis* or *C. krusei*). Nystatin has no other pharmacological effects in man.

Pharmacokinetics

No data on systemic kinetics are available, as most of the use is topical. Little or no data have been collected about the persistence of the polyenes on mucosal surfaces or about gastrointestinal availability. No data on detection of the antibiotic in stool have been published.

Concentration–effect relationship

Concentrations that inhibit the growth of organisms have been shown to be in the range 3 to 6 $mg.l^{-1}$. Full inhibition of membrane motility (maximal at pH 3.5–4.5) requires a concentration[5] of 10 $mg.l^{-1}$.

Metabolism

Nystatin is not metabolized in vitro or in vivo.

Pharmaceutics

Nystatin is available in powder, tablet, pastille, cream, ointment, dusting powder, gel, pessary and suspension forms.

1. Sterile powder: vials of 500 000 U
2. Non-sterile powder: bottles of 3 MU
3. Tablets: brown, round, sugar-coated, containing 500 000 IU, coded '480' in the USA
4. Pastilles: yellow–brown, aniseed flavoured, containing 100 000 IU. The preparation contains sugar and cinnamon
5. Cream: containing 100 000 $U.g^{-1}$ in a vanishing cream base
6. Ointment: containing 100 000 $U.g^{-1}$ in a yellow plasticized hydrocarbon gel (polyethylene and mineral oil)
7. Gel: opaque amber-coloured base containing 100 000 $U.g^{-1}$
8. Dusting powder: containing 100 000 $U.g^{-1}$ in a white sterilized talc base
9. Pessary: pale yellow, diamond-shaped vaginal tablet containing 100 000 IU and marked 'Squibb 457' (Squibb, UK/USA) or 'N6' (Lederle, USA). Also pale yellow, diamond-shaped pessary containing 100 000 U in an effervescent matrix, and marked 'Squibb' (Nystavescent, Squibb, UK)
10. Oral suspension Nystatin-Dome (Bayer, UK): yellow, cherry-mint flavoured ready to use suspension containing 100 000 $IU.ml^{-1}$. The preparation contains sugar;
    OR sugar-free granules for reconstitution with 22 ml of purified water, to give a similar user concentration (100 000 $U.ml^{-1}$).

The commonest proprietary names are Mycostatin (Squibb, US), Nilstat (Lederle, US) and Nystan (Squibb, UK).

Therapeutic use

Indications

Candidiasis

1. In the mouth and palate
2. In the intertriginous regions and other areas of skin
3. In the nails
4. In the gastrointestinal tract
5. In the vagina.

Contraindications

Prior history of allergic reaction on exposure to the drug.

Mode of use

Nystatin has been used as a cream, ointment or solution when applied to the skin or mucosal surfaces with the average dose being 100 000 to 400 000 units per application. Pessaries have been used for vaginal infections and tablets for attempts at eradicating *Candida* from the gastrointestinal tract.

The dose requirement varies with site and severity of infection, ranging from 100 000 units two to three times daily to 400 000 units every four hours. A few studies have used higher doses. The recommended dosage of the oral suspension and tablets for infants is 200 000 units four times daily with no dose adjustment for children or adults.

Indications

1. Oral candidiasis

Neonates

The incidence of oral candidiasis in the newborn is approximately 5%. Studies with nystatin in established candidal infection have demonstrated cure rates varying from 75% to 100%. However there was a relapse rate that varied from 0% to 25%.[18–20] Depending on the demographics of the population studied, Harris[20] has demonstrated that the use of prophylactic nystatin can reduce the incidence of thrush in neonates from 4% to zero. The utility of routine prophylaxis must be weighed against the low incidence and the self-limiting nature of the illness. When *Candida* has an adverse effect on the nutrition of the infant this can be minimized by rapid clearing of the infection with nystatin.

Nystatin appears to be superior to gentian violet and placebo therapy but less effective than miconazole gel.[21] The latter has the disadvantage of a higher incidence of gastrointestinal side effects.

Adults

Nystatin has been used to treat oral candidiasis in the elderly. The results have been variable, with a good response seen in the majority of patients but a considerable incidence of relapse.[22–25] Those individuals with 'denture sore mouth' with isolation of yeast but no evidence of oral plaques appeared to do well; however, this was an uncontrolled study.[27]

2. Candidiasis of the skin

Infants. Infants with diaper rash due to *Candida albicans* demonstrate a complete response to nystatin applied locally.[27–32] There is no advantage in adding oral nystatin therapy.[29] Comparative trials with other agents have not been performed. Relapse rates are low.

Adults. The use of topical therapy in other situations of localized infection have demonstrated excellent results with localized nystatin creams.[33] Some studies have suggested that a combination of steroid and nystatin may be superior in the rate and extent of resolution of cutaneous candidiasis.[34]

3. Onychomycosis

Good responses have been claimed for the local application of nystatin to Candidal onchomycosis. However there are no controlled data to define the optimal route or duration of therapy. The use of nystatin creams for protracted time periods has been suggested but the numbers of patients so treated has been very limited.

4. Gastrointestinal candidiasis

Treatment of infants with presumed candidal diarrhoea with nystatin has been successful, with the eradication of the organism.[35]

Nystatin has been used to eradicate oesophageal candidiasis in adults with no underlying malignant process,[36,37] but the duration of therapy was protracted. No relapse rates were given and no follow-up of the patients was reported.

Elimination of *Candida* from the stool in adults is difficult and the reported results are very variable.[36,37] Recent studies have failed to demonstrate a useful effect.[38–40] This is particularly true of prophy lactic use of nystatin in patients with haematological malignancies where the results have been disappointing in the majority of studies.[38–44]

Nystatin was also ineffective in oesophageal candidiasis in leukaemic patients.[36,44–47]

5. Vulvovaginal candidiasis[51–58]
Nystatin creams and pessaries have high response rates;[49] however, relapse rates may also be high (up to 50%)[56] and some patient populations have lower response rates (50–76%) than that reported with localized therapy with the newer imidazoles (85–100%).[48,50,58] Combined oral therapy does not augment the response rates and the overall response rate does not increase with successive courses of therapy.[57]

Adverse reactions

Potentially life-threatening effects

One case of unexplained death has occurred, after the second dose in a child.[18] Further details with regard to this child are not available.

Acute overdosage

Because of lack of absorption by conventional routes, this is highly unlikely to occur. However, if topical preparations of nystatin are applied extensively over denuded or burned surfaces or as part of a solution for wound irrigation, systemic absorption can occur. Nephrotoxicity may result. It should be emphasized that use of nystatin in this manner is never indicated under any circumstance.

Severe or irreversible adverse effects

None has been reported.

Symptomatic adverse effects

Contact dermatitis is seen rarely and occurs primarily with the cream preparations and is not associated with any specific patient characteristics. This type of rash has not been reported with the oral preparation. A fixed drug eruption has been reported after oral administration.

Tablets which are allowed to dissolve in the mouth leave an unpleasant aftertaste. This does not occur with the nystatin suspension. Gastrointestinal disturbances including nausea, vomiting, and diarrhoea have been reported after oral dosing.

Interference with clinical pathology tests

None has been described although the absorption in the ultraviolet spectrum of this drug may interfere with drug assays using UV spectrophotometric measurements of mucosal secretions (e.g. saliva, gastrointestinal or vaginal secretions).

High risk groups

Neonates

No alterations of dosage are required.

Breast milk. The drug can be used during lactation.

Children

No alteration of dosage is required.

Pregnant women

No precautions or adverse effects have been noted in the studies in which nystatin was used in pregnant women.

The elderly

No dosage adjustment is required in elderly patients.

Drug interactions

No interactions have been described.

References

1. Hazen E L, Brown R 1950 Two antifungal agents produced by a soil *Actinomycete*. Science 12: 423
2. Kinsky S E 1961 The effect of polyene antibiotics on the permeability in *Neurospora crassa*. Biochemical and Biophysical Research Communications 4: 353–357
3. Schlosser E, Shaw P D, Gottleib D 1969 Sterols in species of *Pythium*. Archives of Microbiology 66: 147–153
4. Bulder C J E A 1971 Anaerobic growth, ergosterol content and sensitivity to a polyene antibiotic of the yeast *Schizosaccharomyces japonicus*. Antonie van Leewenhoek 37: 353–358
5. Medoff G, Kobayashi G A 1980 The polyenes. In: Spiller D C E (ed) Antifungal chemotherapy. J Wiley and Sons, Chichester, pp 1–33
6. Rast D M, Bartnicki-Garcia S 1981 Effects of Amphotericin B, nystatin and other polyene antibiotics. Proceedings of the National Academy of Sciences of the United States of America 78 (2): 1233–1236
7. Kotler-Brajtburg J, Medoff G et al 1979 Classification of polyene antibiotics according to chemical structure and biological effects. Antimicrobial Agents and Chemotherapy 15: 716–722
8. Kitajima Y, Sekiya T, Nozawa Y 1976 Freeze-fracture ultrastructural alterations induced by filipin, pimaricin, nystatin, and amphotericin B in the plasma membranes of *Epidermophyton*, *Saccharomyces*, and red complex-induced membrane lesions. Biochemica Biophysica Acta 455 (2): 452–465
9. Karst F, Jund R 1976 Sterol replacement in *Saccharomyces cerevisiae*. Biochemical and Biophysical Research Communications 71 (2): 535–543
10. Johnson B, White R J, Williamson G M 1978 Factors influencing the susceptibility of *Candida albicans* to the polyene antibiotics, nystatin and amphotericin B. Journal of General Microbiology 104 (2): 325–333
11. Russell J M, Eaton D C, Brodwick M S 1977 Effects of nystatin on membrane conductance and internal ion activities in *Aplysia* neurons. Journal of Membrane Biology 37: 137–156
12. Sunger M A 1975 Interaction of amphotericin B and nystatin with the phospholipid bilayer membrane: effect of cholesterol. Canadian Journal of Physiology and Pharmacology 53 (6): 1072–1079
13. Mark A, Finkelstein A 1975 Pores formed in a lipid bilayer membrane by nystatin. Differences in its one sided and two sided action. Journal of General Physiology 65 (4): 515–526
14. Beezer A E, Chowdhry B Z 1980 Flow microcalorimetric study of the effects of pH, metal ions and sterols on the interaction of polyene antibiotics with *Saccharomyces cerevisiae NCYC239*. Microbios 28: 107–121
15. Beezer A E, Sharma P B 1981 On the uptake of nystatin by *Saccharomyces cerevisiae*. Microbios 30: 139–151
16. Beezer A E, Sharma P B 1981 On the uptake of nystatin by *Saccharomyces cerevisiae*. 2. Effects of pH, ionic strength, sterol concentration, and protecting ions. Microbios 31: 7–16
17. Rast D M, Bartnicki-Garcia S 1981 Effects of amphotericin B, nystatin and other polyene antibiotics on chitin synthetase. Proceedings of the National Academy of Sciences of the United States of America 78: 1233–1236
18. Dioxiadis S A 1959 Oral thrush in infancy treated with nystatin. Lancet 2: 916
19. Graham R D 1959 Oral thrush in infancy treated with nystatin. Lancet 2: 600–601
20. Harris L J 1960 Further observations on a simple procedure to eliminate thrush from hospital nurseries. American Journal of Obstetrics and Gynecology 80: 30–31
21. Schaad U B, Bachman D 1983 Prospective therapeutic trial of miconazole gel and nystatin suspension in oral candidiasis. Schweizerische Medizinische Wochenschrift 113: 1356–1362
22. Wright B M, Fenwick F 1981 Candidiasis and atrophic tongue lesions. Oral Surgery 51 (1): 55–61
23. Epstein J B, Pearsall N N, Truelove E L 1981 Oral candidiasis: effects of antifungal therapy upon clinical signs and symptoms, salivary antibodies, and mucosal adherence of *Candida albicans*. Oral Surgery 51 (1): 32–36
24. Stritzler C 1966 Cutaneous candidiasis treated with topical amphotericin B. Archives of Dermatology 93: 101–105
25. Bergenal T, Isacssin G 1980 Effect of nystatin in the treatment of denture stomatitis. Scandinavian Journal of Dental Research 88: 446–454
26. Cawson R A 1963 Denture sore mouth and angular cheilitis. Oral candidiasis in the adult. British Dental Journal 115: 411–449
27. Munz D, Powell K R, Pai C H 1982 Treatment of candidal diaper dermatitis. A double blind placebo controlled comparison of topical nystatin with topical plus oral nystatin. Journal of Pediatrics 101 (6): 1022–1027
28. Rudolph N, Tariq A A, Peale M R, Goldberg P K, Koznin P J 1977 Congenital cutaneous candidiasis. Archives of Dermatology 113: 1101–1103
29. Taschdjian C L, Koznin P J 1957 Laboratory and clinical studies in candidiasis in the newborn infant. Journal of Pediatrics 50: 426–433
30. Kam L A, Giacoia G P 1975 Congenital cutaneous candidiasis. American Journal of Diseases of Children 129: 1215–1218
31. Leyden J J, Klignin A M 1978 The role of micro-organisms in diaper dermatitis. Archives of Dermatology 114: 57–59
32. Weston W L, Lane A T, Weston A M 1980 The role of micro-organisms in diaper dermatitis. Pediatrics 66: 532–536
33. MacMillan B G, Law E J, Holdor I A 1972 Experience with candidal infections in burn patients. Archives of Surgery 104: 509–514
34. Beveridge G W, Fairburn E, Finn O A, Scott O L S, Stewart T W, Summerly R 1977 A comparison of nystatin cream with nystatin/triamcinolone acetonide combination cream in the treatment of candidal inflammation of the flexures. Current Medical Research and Opinion 4: 584–587
35. Koznin P J, Taschdjian C L 1962 Enteric candidiasis. Diagnosis and clinical considerations. Pediatrics; 71–85
36. Holt J M 1968 Candidal infection of the esophagus. Gut 9: 227–231
37. Kodsi B E, Wickremesinghe P C, Koznin P J, Iswara K, Goldberg P K 1976 Candida esophagitis. Gastroenterology 71 (5): 715–719
38. Degregorio M W, Lee W F, Ries C A 1982 Candida infections in patients with acute leukemia: ineffectiveness of nystatin prophylaxis and relationship of nystatin prophylaxis between oral and systemic candidiasis. Cancer 50 (12): 2780–2784
39. Jones P G, Kauffman C A, McAuliffe L S, Leipman M K, Bergman A G 1984 Efficacy of ketoconazole versus nystatin in prevention of fungal infection in neutropenic patients. Archives of Internal Medicine 144: 549–557
40. Carpentiere U, Haggard M E, Lockhart L H, Gustavson L P, Box Q T, West E F 1978 Clinical experience in the prevention of candidiasis by nystatin in children with acute lymphoblastic leukemia. Journal of Pediatrics 92: 593–595
41. Shepp D H, Klosterman A, Siegel M S, Meyers J D 1985 Comparative trial of ketoconazole and nystatin for prevention of fungal infection in neutropenic patients treated in a protective environment. Journal of Infectious Diseases 152: 1257–1263

42. Hann I M, Prentice H G, Corrangle R et al 1982 Ketoconazole versus nystatin plus amphotericin B for fungal prophylaxis in immuno-compromised patients. Lancet 1: 826–829
43. Meunier-Carpentier F, Cruciani M, Klastersky J 1983 Oral prophylaxis with miconazole or ketoconazole of invasive fungal disease in neutropenic cancer patients. European Journal of Cancer and Clinical Oncology 19: 43–48
44. Tusham A, Conners J M 1987 Ketoconazole vs nystatin as prophylaxis against fungal infections for lymphoma patients receiving chemotherapy. American Journal of Clinical Oncology 10 (4): 355–359
45. Gonazalez-Crussi F, Iung O S 1965 Esophageal moniliasis as a cause of death. American Journal of Surgery 109: 634–638
46. Bjorn-Jensen K, Stenderup A, Brown-Thomsen J, Bichel J 1964 Oesophageal moniliasis in malignant neoplastic disease. Acta Medica Scandinavica 175 (4): 455–459
47. Eras P, Goldstein M J, Sherlock P 1972 Candidal infection of the gastrointestinal tract. Medicine 51: 367–379
48. Bentley S, Bourne M S, Powell A 1978 A comparative study of miconazole nitrate pessaries and nystatin vaginal tablets in the treatment of vaginal candidiasis. British Journal of Clinical Practice 32: 258–259
49. McNellis D, McLeod M, Lawsen J, Pasquale S A 1977 Treatment of vulvo-vaginal candidiasis in pregnancy. A comparative study. Obstetrics and Gynecology 50: 674–678
50. Wallenburg H C, Wladimiroff J W 1976 Recurrence of vulvo-vaginal candidiasis during pregnancy. Comparison of miconazole versus nystatin treatment. Obstetrics and Gynecology 48: 491–494
51. Higton B K 1974 A trial of clotrimazole and nystatin in vaginal candidiasis. Postgraduate Medical Journal 50 (suppl 1): 95–98
52. Marks H J 1974 A double blind comparison of clotrimazole and nystatin vaginal tablets in Candida vaginitis. Postgraduate Medical Journal 50 (suppl 1): 105–108
53. Tan C G, Good C S, Milne L J, Loudon J D 1974 A comparative trial of six day therapy of clotrimazole and nystatin in pregnant patients with vaginal candidiasis. Postgraduate Medical Journal 50 (suppl 1): 102–105
54. Binghan J S, Steele C E 1981 Treatment of vaginal candidosis with econazole nitrate and nystatin. A comparative trial. British Journal of Venereal Diseases 57: 204–207
55. Dennerstein G J, Langley R 1982 Vulvovaginal candidiasis. Treatment and recurrences. Australian and New Zealand Journal of Obstetrics and Gynecology 22: 231–233
56. Milne J D, Warnoch D W 1979 Effect of simultaneous oral and vaginal treatment on the rate of cure and relapse in vaginal candidiasis. British Journal of Venereal Diseases 55: 362–365
57. Eliot B W, Howat R C L, Mack A E 1979 A comparison between the effects of nystatin, clotrimazole, and miconazole on vaginal candidiasis. British Journal of Obstetrics and Gynaecology 86: 572–577
58. Davies J E, Frudenfeld J A, Goddard J L 1974 Comparative evaluation of monistat and mycostatin in the treatment of vulvo-vaginal candidiasis. Obstetrics and Gynecology 44: 403–406

Octreotide (acetate)

Octreotide is a long-acting octapeptide analogue of somatostatin, the first to be commercially available, which inhibits the secretion of peptides from the gastroenteropancreatic system and of growth hormone from the pituitary gland. It is used to relieve symptoms associated with gastroenteropancreatic endocrine tumours, carcinoid tumours and acromegaly.

Chemistry

Octreotide acetate (Sandostatin, SMS 201-995)

H_2N— D-Phe — Cys — Phe — D-Trp — Lys — Thr — Cys — Thr — OH

Molecular weight	1019.3
pKa (α amino group, ε amino group)	6.8, 9.7
Solubility	
in alcohol	—
in water	>1 in 100
Octanol/buffer (pH 6.8) partition coefficient	0.12

It is a synthetic peptide that is prepared by the use of conventional fragment condensation techniques.[1]

Pharmacology

Octreotide is a synthetic 8 amino acid peptide (octapeptide) that shares some amino acid homology with somatostatin (SMS) Fig. 1. It binds specifically and with high affinity to SMS receptors in various systems. It exhibits pharmacological effects similar to somatostatin but it has a much longer duration of action than the parent compound due to its protection against degradation by a D-phenylalanine residue at the N terminus and by an amino alcohol terminal at the C terminus. Inhibition of growth hormone in preclinical studies (rat, 15 min after intramuscular injection) was 70 times that of somatostatin, that of glucagon 23 times and that of insulin 3 times.[1] Unlike the parent compound there is no rebound hypersecretion of these hormones following cessation of its action.

Toxicology

In animal toxicity studies octreotide treatment caused minor growth retardation of offspring in high-dose regimes (>1 mg.kg^{-1} daily) probably because of the specific endocrine profiles of the species tested. There is no evidence of fetotoxicity, or teratogenic or other reproductive effect.

Clinical pharmacology

Following subcutaneous or intravenous administration, octreotide by stimulating somatostatin receptors has been shown in man to inhibit exercise-stimulated growth hormone secretion, sleep-induced growth hormone release and growth hormone secretion during insulin-induced hypoglycaemia.[2,3] These studies used between 50 and 250 μg octreotide. Single dose subcutaneous octreotide (50 or 100 μg) has also been shown significantly to inhibit thyrotrophin releasing hormone (TRH)-induced thyroid stimulating hormone (TSH) secretion.[2] In normal subjects it does not have any effects on other anterior pituitary secretions.

Octreotide, like native somatostatin, exerts a potent inhibitory effect on the release of peptides of the gastroenteropancreatic endocrine system, and subcutaneous administration of 50 μg suppresses both basal and postprandial plasma concentrations of insulin, glucagon, pancreatic polypeptide, gastric inhibitory peptide, secretin and gastrin.[4,5] One of these studies also demonstrated transient inhibition of insulin release in a dose-dependent manner following subcutaneous administration of octreotide in doses of 25, 50 and 100 μg.[4] There is a mild transient elevation of plasma glucose postprandially due to suppression of insulin but this is an effect that wears off with continued administration of octreotide.

Besides gastroenteropancreatic hormones, octreotide, like somatostatin, has other effects on the gastrointestinal tract. It markedly inhibits pentagastrin-stimulated gastric acid secretion and is a strong inhibitor of pancreatic enzyme secretion stimulated by secretin and cholecystokinin (CCK).[6,7] This effect decreases with time.

It also inhibits gall bladder contraction and may accelerate gastric emptying while prolonging intestinal transit time.[8] It increases fluid and electrolyte absorption from the gut and reduces intestinal blood flow.[9,10]

Pharmacokinetics

The preferred analytical method is by radioimmunoassay using ^{125}I-labelled 203-422 (the tyrosine analogue of SMS 201-995) as tracer. The radioimmunoassay has a sensitivity of 0.01–0.02 μg.l^{-1}. The drug is poorly absorbed orally. Following subcutaneous and intravenous administration, octreotide is rapidly and completely absorbed with peak levels occurring 30–60 minutes after subcutaneous administration and 4 minutes after intravenous administration.[2,11] There are linear dose-dependent increases in peak plasma concentration and the area under the plasma concentration time curve after both intravenous and subcutaneous administration of octreotide.[11]

The elimination half life after intravenous administration ranges between 72 and 98 minutes[11] and that following subcutaneous administration from 88 to 113 minutes.[2,11]

Preliminary reports suggest that hepatic metabolism of octreotide is extensive with up to 30–40% hepatic extraction ratio in healthy volunteers.[11] It has also been reported that approximately 11% and less than 2% of an administered dose are excreted unchanged in the urine and faeces, respectively.[12] The total body clearance of octreotide in healthy volunteers is slow[11] being approximately 11.4 l.h^{-1}.

Using the equation for a two-compartment model,[11] the volume of distribution of the central compartment of octreotide following intravenous administration is calculated to be in the range of 18–30 l. Plasma protein binding is calculated to be 65%.

There are no published data on levels of octreotide in the CSF and breast milk. Transplacental passage has not been studied although because of its molecular size it is unlikely to cross the placental barrier.

There are no published studies investigating the extent of octreotide tissue distribution in man. No studies are available of its use in patients with liver disease but in view of the importance of this metabolic pathway it should clearly be used cautiously in such patients. Patients with reduced renal function have been shown to have a reduced clearance of the drug (75 ml.min^{-1} vs 175 ml.min^{-1}).[13] There is no evidence of reduced tolerability or altered dose requirements in the elderly.

Fig. 1 Native somatostatin 14

H_2N— Ala — Gly — Cys — Lys — Asn — Phe — Phe — Trp — Lys — Thr — Phe — Thr — Ser — Cys — COOH

Oral absorption	not absorbed
Presystemic metabolism	—
Plasma half life	
intravenous	72–98 min
subcutaneous	88–113 min
Volume of distribution	0.27 l.kg^{-1} (18–30 l)
Plasma protein binding	65%

Concentration–effect relationship

In 15 patients with acromegaly being treated with continuous subcutaneous infusion of octreotide in increasing doses from 200 to 1600 μg per 24 hours by 200 μg increments each week, optimum suppression of growth hormone occurred at a dosage of 600 μg per 24 hours.[14] However the manufacturers report that 100 μg three times daily leads to optimum growth hormone suppression.

Metabolism

Data not available.

Pharmaceutics

Octreotide (Sandostatin; Sandoz, UK) is available for parenteral use only.

Ampoules contain 1 ml of clear colourless solution of octreotide acetate. Three strengths are available: 50 μg.ml^{-1}, 100 μg.ml^{-1}, 500 μg.ml^{-1} diluted in glacial acetic acid, sodium acetate, sodium chloride and water. Ampoules should be stored between 2 and 8°C and may be stored at room temperature for up to 2 weeks.

Therapeutic use

Indications

1. Carcinoid tumours
2. Vipoma
3. Glucagonoma
4. Acromegaly.

Contraindications

Pregnant women and breast-feeding mothers should not be given octreotide to avoid effects on the fetus or baby.

Mode of use

For patients with gastroenteropancreatic tumours, a subcutaneous dose of 50 μg once or twice daily is usual for the initiation of treatment. The dose may be increased and there is no clearly defined maximum but up to 500 μg 8 hourly may safely be administered.

In acromegaly it is usual to start off with 100 μg twice daily or 8 hourly and similarly to increase the dose, if suppression of growth hormone is considered to be insufficient, to up to 500 μg 8 hourly.

The local discomfort observed after injecting the compound may be reduced by allowing the solution to reach room temperature before administration.

Octreotide may increase the depth and duration of hypoglycaemia in patients with insulinoma because of the more potent inhibition of growth hormone and glucagon than that of insulin.[15] When used in patients with insulinoma, patients on this compound should be carefully observed and blood glucose regularly monitored. Octreotide may reduce insulin and oral hypoglycaemic requirements in patients with diabetes mellitus.

It is wise to monitor thyroid function tests because of the suppression of TSH. Hypothyroidism has not been observed in clinical practice except in a carcinoid tumour patient treated with 150 μg daily.

Indications

Octreotide is used for the relief of symptoms in patients with gastroenteropancreatic endocrine tumours, carcinoid tumours and acromegaly. It does not have an antitumour effect and thus only improves symptoms but not the ultimate prognosis.

1. Carcinoid tumours[16]
Octreotide improves symptoms in patients with carcinoid tumours. In the majority, flushing is reduced and diarrhoea may improve although this is more variable. Treatment has been given for up to 48 months and this may be associated with a recurrence of symptoms despite continued treatment. Doses in the range of 50–500 μg three times daily have been used subcutaneously. Associated with this is a fall in serotonin and a reduction in 5-hydroxyindole acetic acid excretion. However, levels of the latter do not always become normal.

Intravenous octreotide has been used successfully in the treatment of carcinoid crisis.

Prospective trials are underway to further evaluate the effect of octreotide in patients with malignant carcinoid tumours. These have not hitherto been possible due to the rarity of such tumours.

2. Vipoma[17,18]
Octreotide relieves the severe secretory diarrhoea in patients with vipoma. This effect is seen in most patients with pancreatic tumours secreting VIP. After doses of between 50 and 100 μg twice daily the secretory diarrhoea is usually considerably alleviated after between 12 and 48 hours. Furthermore electrolyte imbalances, particularly hypokalaemia and hypercalcaemia, are improved. On octreotide, patients no longer require glucocorticoid medication.

Doses of up to 1500 μg per day have been used. VIP levels often fall in the normal range. With continued treatment relapse of diarrhoea may occur thus necessitating an increase in dose.

3. Glucagonoma[17,19]
Octreotide improves the necrolytic migratory rash characteristic of glucagonoma. In non-comparative trials of doses between 50 and 400 μg per day, the rash takes between 1 to 4 weeks to disappear. This is associated with a decrease in glucagon but in some patients despite continued treatment levels rise again. Glucagon levels rarely become normal on treatment. Despite continued treatment the rash may recur requiring an increase in dose.

Data regarding the effect of octreotide on weight loss, abdominal pain and diarrhoea are sparse but it appears on preliminary evidence that there is little effect on either these or diabetes mellitus.

4. Acromegaly[20,21,22]
Octreotide causes suppression of abnormal growth hormone secretion for 6–8 hours after a single dose of 50–200 μg of subcutaneous octreotide. In non-comparative trials using daily doses of between 75 and 1500 μg for up to 27 months the majority of acromegalic patients show clinical improvement with suppression of insulin-like growth factor 1 (IGF1) and growth hormone secretion in around 80%. IGF1 levels become normal in 60%. If the same dose of octreotide is continued, a gradual fall in growth hormone occurs over a 24-month period. Desensitization to octreotide has not been observed. Responses can be predicted by the test administration of 50 μg octreotide subcutaneously.

In a proportion of patients pituitary tumour size decreases.

Comparisons with growth hormone reduction obtained by the dopamine agonist bromocriptine suggest that octreotide is often more effective than bromocriptine — patients are more often responsive to octreotide and it more frequently suppresses growth hormone to normal.

Ocreotide may be used preoperatively or after hypophysectomy in patients with persistent acromegaly and in patients awaiting the full effects of external pituitary irradiation.

Adverse reactions

Potentially life-threatening effects
None have been reported.

Acute overdosage
One patient has been reported who was given 250 μg per hour intravenously instead of 25 μg per hour. This was continued for 48 hours. No side effects were noted.

In general, management of overdosage is symptomatic. No antagonists exist.

Severe or irreversible adverse effects
No effects of this kind have been reported.

Octreotide (acetate)

Symptomatic adverse effects
In general the drug is well tolerated, but octreotide causes both local and gastrointestinal adverse effects.

Local pain and stinging or tingling at the site of injection can occur with occasional redness and swelling which usually settles within 15 minutes of the injection. This side effect is due to the acidic solvent and may be reduced by allowing the injection to warm up to room temperature.

Gastrointestinal effects, which occur in about 30% of patients, include anorexia, nausea, vomiting, abdominal pain, bloating, flatulence, loose stools and steatorrhoea. The faecal fat excretion may rise transiently but there is no evidence of nutritional deficiency developing due to malabsorption during long-term treatment. All these effects usually wear off with continued administration of the compound. Gastrointestinal adverse effects are sometimes avoided by timing the injection between meals. Rarely, abdominal distension with epigastric pain, tenderness and guarding has been described. An increased incidence of gallstones has been reported due to the effects of octreotide in suppressing CCK secretion and thereby decreasing gall bladder motility.[23]

Other effects
There are no long-term effects on haematological or biochemical parameters.

Octreotide may impair postprandial glucose tolerance because of the suppression of insulin secretion, but this usually wears off in patients on long-term treatment and no rise in HbA_{1C} is observed. Hepatic dysfunction has been observed occasionally with a hepatitic picture associated with cholestasis or the slow development of hyperbilirubinaemia in association with elevated transaminase, alkaline phosphatase and gamma-glutamyl transpeptidase (γ-GT).

Interference with clinical pathology tests
No technical interferences of this kind have been observed.

High risk groups

Neonates
No information is available on the use of the drug in neonates.

Breast milk. No data are available, so women taking the drug should not breast-feed their infants.

Children
No data are available on the use of the drug in children.

Pregnant women
There are no data available. If a pregnant women developed one of these tumours the risks of treatment would have to be balanced against the potential benefit.

The elderly
There is no evidence of reduced tolerability or altered dose requirement.

Concurrent disease
There are no useful data on the administration of octreotide in patients with hepatic and cardiac disease. In patients with renal disease clearance is significantly reduced.

Drug interactions

Potentially hazardous interactions
None is known.

Other significant interactions
Octreotide reduces the intestinal absorption of cyclosporin and delays the absorption of cimetidine.

Potentially useful interactions
None is known.

Major outcome trials

None have been reported.

Other trials

1. Kvols L K, Moertel C G, O'Connell M J, Schutt A J, Rubin J, Hahn R G 1986 Treatment of the malignant carcinoid syndrome: evaluation of a long-acting somatostatin analogue. New England Journal of Medicine 315: 663–666

In this uncontrolled study 25 patients were evaluated having previously had chemotherapy with one or more cytotoxic drugs, on 450 µg per day subcutaneously (150 µg three times daily) of octreotide given for between 1 and 18 months. 22 out of 25 had improvement in flushing and/or diarrhoea and in 18 out of 25 there was a decrease in 5-hydroxyindole acetic acid excretion of 50% or more.

2. Anderson J V, Bloom S R 1986 Neuroendocrine tumours of the gut: long term therapy with the somatostatin analogue SMS 201-995. Scandinavian Journal of Gastroenterology 21 (suppl 119): 115–128

This uncontrolled trial assessed four patients who had previously had a combination of surgery, chemotherapy, hepatic artery embolism and fluid and electrolyte replacement therapy. These were given between 100 and 600 µg daily of subcutaneous octreotide for up to 18 months. There was a reduction in 24-hour stool volume in 3 out of 4 and a reduction in plasma VIP in 2 out of 4. No patient showed any evidence of tumour shrinkage.

3. Lamberts S W J, Uitterlinden P, Del Pozo E 1987 SMS 201-995 induces a continuous decline in circulating growth hormone and somatomedin-C levels during therapy of acromegalic patients for over two years. Journal of Endocrinology and Metabolism 65: 703–710

This uncontrolled study of 10 patients with acromegaly previously treated with pituitary surgery and/or radiotherapy used 200–300 µg daily of subcutaneous octreotide and studied the effect over a period of 4–24 months. In 5 out of 10 patients IGF1 levels returned to normal and pituitary tumour shrinkage was seen in 3 out of 6.

General review articles

Battershill P E, Clissold S P 1989 Octreotide. A preliminary review. Drugs 38: 658–702

Gorden P 1989 Somatostatin and somatostatin analogue (SMS 201-995) in treatment of hormone-secreting tumors of the pituitary and gastrointestinal tract and non-neoplastic diseases of the gut. Annals of Internal Medicine 110: 35–50

Lamberts S W J 1988 The role of somatostatin in the regulation of anterior pituitary hormone secretion and the use of its analogs in the treatment of human pituitary tumours. Endocrine Reviews 9: 417–436

Leading article 1989 Octreotide. Lancet 2: 541–542

Rosenberg J M 1988 Octreotide: a synthetic analog of somatostatin. Drug Intelligence and Clinical Pharmacy 22: 748–754

Van Thiel D H, Dindzans V J, Schade R R 1988 Somatostatin: its uses in gastroenterology. Drugs Today 24: 743–753

References

1. Bauer W, Briner U, Doepfner W et al 1982 SMS 201-995: a very potent and selective octapeptide analogue of somatostatin with prolonged action. Life Sciences 31: 1133–1140
2. Del Pozo E, Neufeld M, Schlüter K et al 1986 Endocrine profile of a long-acting somatostatin derivative SMS 201-995: study in normal volunteers following subcutaneous administration. Acta Endocrinologica 111: 433–439
3. Lightman S L, Fox P, Dunne M J 1986 The effect of SMS 201-995, a long-acting somatostatin analogue, on anterior pituitary function in healthy male volunteers. Scandinavian Journal of Gastroenterology 21 (suppl 119): 84–95
4. Fuessl H S, Burrin J M, Williams G, Adrian T E, Bloom S R 1987 The effect of a long-acting somatostatin analogue (SMS 201-995) on intermediary metabolism and gut hormones after a test meal in normal subjects. Alimentary Pharmacology and Therapeutics 1: 321–330
5. Kraenzlin M E, Wood S M, Neufeld M, Adrian T E, Bloom S R 1985 Effect of long-acting somatostatin-analogue, SMS 201-995, on gut hormone secretion in normal subjects. Experientia 15; 41: 738–740.
6. Olsen J A, Loud F B, Christiansen J 1987 Inhibition of meal stimulated gastric acid secretion by an octapeptide somatostatin analogue SMS 201-995. Gut 28: 464–467
7. Jenkins S A, Baxter J N, Leinster S J et al 1986 Effects of subcutaneous SMS 201-995 on exocrine pancreatic secretion and function in man. British Journal of Surgery 73: 1029–1030
8. Füessl H S, Carolan G, Williams G, Bloom S R 1985 Accelerated gastric emptying but prolonged mouth-to-caecum transit by a long-acting somatostatin analogue. Regulatory Peptides 13: 101
9. Primi M P, Bueno L 1987 Influence of centrally administered somatostatin and two related peptides on intestinal absorption of water and electrolytes in conscious dogs. Peptides 8: 619–623
10. Christiansen J, Yotis A 1986 The role of somatostatin and a long-acting analogue, SMS 201-995, in acute bleeding due to peptic ulceration. Scandinavian Journal of Gastroenterology 21 (suppl 119): 109–114

O

11. Kutz K, Nüesch E, Rosenthaler J 1986 Pharmacokinetics of SMS 201-995 in healthy subjects. Scandinavian Journal of Gastroenterology 21 (suppl 119): 65–72
12. Longnecker S M 1988 Somatostatin and octreotide: literature review and description of therapeutic activity in pancreatic neoplasia. Drug Intelligence and Clinical Pharmacy 22: 99–106
13. Kallivretakis N, Yotis A, Del Pozo E et al 1985 Pharmacokinetics of SMS 201-995 in normal subjects and in patients with severe renal failure. Neuroendocrinology Letters. 7: 92
14. James R A, Chatterjee S, White M C, Hall K, Moller N, Kendall-Taylor P 1989 Continuous infusion of octreotide in acromegaly. Lancet 2: 1083–1087
15. Stehouwer C D A, Lems W F, Fischer H R A, Hackeng W H L, Naafs M A B 1989 Aggravation of hypoglycaemia in insulinoma patients by the long-acting somatostatin analogue octreotide (Sandostatin). Acta Endocrinologica 121: 34–40
16. Kvols L K, Moertel C, O'Connell M J et al 1986 Treatment of the malignant carcinoid syndrome. New England Journal of Medicine 315: 663–666
17. Anderson J V, Bloom S R 1986 Neuroendocrine tumours of the gut: long term therapy with the somatostatin analogue SMS 201-995. Scandinavian Journal of Gastroenterology 21 (suppl 119): 115–128
18. Eriksson B, Oberg K, Andersson T et al 1988 Treatment of malignant endocrine pancreatic tumors with a new long-acting somatostatin analogue, SMS 201-995. Scandinavian Journal of Gastroenterology 23: 508–512
19. Kvols L K, Buck K, Moertel C G et al 1987 Treatment of metastatic islet cell carcinoma with a somatostatin analogue (SMS 201-995). Annals of Internal Medicine 107: 162–168
20. Lamberts S W J, Uitterlinden P, Del Pozo E 1987 SMS 201-995 Induces a continuous decline in circulating growth hormone and somatomedin-C levels during therapy of acromegalic patients for over two years. Journal of Clinical Endocrinology and Metabolism 65: 703–710
21. Tolis G 1988 Long-term management of acromegaly with sandostatin. Hormone Research 29: 112–114
22. Lamberts S W J, Uitterlinden P, Schuijff P C, Klijn J G M 1988 Therapy of acromegaly with Sandostatin: the predictive value of an acute test, the value of serum somatomedin-C measurements in dose adjustment and the definition of a biochemical 'cure'. Clinical Endocrinology 29: 411–420
23. Wass J A H, Anderson J V, Besser G M, Dowling R H 1989 Gall stones and treatment with octreotide for acromegaly. British Medical Journal 299: 1162–1163

Oestradiol

Oestradiol-17β is the most important oestrogen secreted by the ovary.

Chemistry

Oestradiol-17β (estradiol)
$C_{18}H_{24}O_2$
1,3,5-(10)-Oestratriene-3,17β-diol

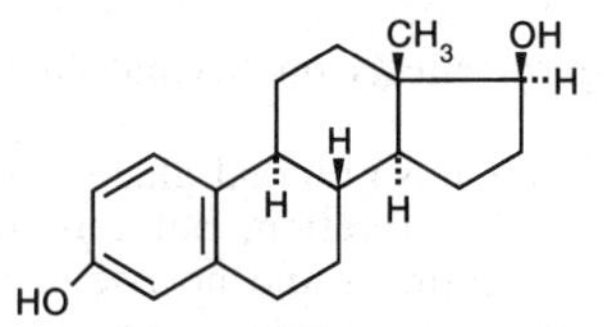

Molecular weight	272.4
pKa	—
Solubility	
in alcohol	1 in 28
in water	1 in 10 000
Octanol/water partition coefficient	high

Oestradiol is a creamy-white odourless and tasteless crystalline powder prepared by reduction of oestrone. It is also available in esterified form, e.g. oestradiol benzoate, oestradiol valerate, or oestradiol phenylpropionate and in combination with oestrone in Hormonin.

Pharmacology

Oestradiol is the most potent of the naturally occurring oestrogens. It promotes the growth and maintenance of the female reproductive tract and secondary sexual characteristics.

Toxicology

In many experimental species, oestradiol promotes the development of a range of tumours, including tumours of the mammary glands, uterus and cervix. There are no studies of the carcinogenicity of oestradiol alone in humans, but long-term administration of oestrogens appears to be associated with an increased incidence of endometrial carcinoma.[1] The role of oestradiol in the aetiology of breast cancer in women is controversial.

Animal studies indicate that oestradiol has teratogenic effects on the genital tract, and that offspring exposed to oestradiol in utero may have impaired fertility. Evidence for a teratogenic effect in humans is limited.[1]

The action, toxicity and uses of the oestradiol esters are those of oestradiol.

Clinical pharmacology

The pharmacological effects of oestradiol are exerted via specific oestrogen receptors in target tissues.[2] The steroid–receptor complex binds to the cell's DNA and stimulates the synthesis of specific proteins.

Oestradiol promotes growth of the endometrium, and its withdrawal leads to vaginal bleeding; hyperplasia of the endometrium during oestrogen treatment can be reduced by concurrent administration of a synthetic progestogen.[3] Oestrogens suppress gonadotrophin secretion by the pituitary, and implants of oestradiol have been used for contraception,[4] but oestradiol is not normally used for this purpose.

Oestradiol

The decline in ovarian oestrogen production at the menopause leads to vaginal atrophy and, in many women, vasomotor symptoms ('hot flushes'). These postmenopausal symptoms can be reversed by treatment with oestrogens such as oestradiol. Postmenopausal osteoporosis is also prevented by oestradiol, which promotes calcium absorption from the intestine, while reducing urinary calcium excretion and bone resorption. Oestradiol also has widespread metabolic effects, including a reduction in low-density lipoproteins (LDL) and increases in high-density lipoproteins (HDL) and triglycerides.

Pharmacokinetics

Plasma oestradiol concentrations are usually measured by radioimmunoassay. The method is extremely sensitive, typical sensitivities being less than 10 $ng.l^{-1}$ and usually highly specific, although some form of chromatographic separation may be necessary to remove cross-reacting oestrone or oestriol. Gas–liquid chromatography with mass spectrometry has been used as a reference method for oestrogen determinations.[5]

After oral administration, oestradiol is absorbed from the gastrointestinal tract, but undergoes extensive metabolism in the gut wall and liver. The bioavailability of oral oestradiol is therefore low, and the oral dose is 5–10 times that required by intramuscular injection. Micronized preparations of oestradiol have however been found to be well absorbed and effective when given orally.[6,7] Doses of 2–4 mg daily produce plasma oestradiol concentrations of between 300 and 800 $pmol.l^{-1}$, with maximum concentrations occurring within 0.5–5 h. Concentrations then decline over a period of 24–30 h.[7,8,9] Similar concentrations have been reported after administration of 600 µg oestradiol in a compound preparation with 1.4 mg oestrone and 270 µg oestriol.[10] These concentrations are similar to those seen during the follicular phase of the menstrual cycle.

Since oestradiol is extensively converted to oestrone in the gut and liver, oral administration leads to high circulating oestrone concentrations,[7,10,11] and high oestrone:oestradiol ratios; in this respect, oestradiol does not restore the premenopausal condition, in which the oestrone:oestradiol ratio is normally less than unity. This is sometimes cited as a disadvantage of oral preparations, but it should be noted that the significance of the oestrone:oestradiol ratio is unknown.

Oestradiol has also been administered by subcutaneous implants or percutaneously; sublingual, intranasal and vaginal administration have also been used, although less frequently. Subcutaneous implants of 50 or 100 mg oestradiol lead to circulating levels similar to those seen after oral administration,[12] which are maintained for several months. In contrast to the situation after oral administration, the corresponding increases in oestrone concentrations are less than those of oestradiol, leading to oestrone:oestradiol ratios resembling those in premenopausal women. Percutaneous administration also leads to follicular phase concentrations of oestradiol, and low oestrone:oestradiol ratios.[8,13] Both percutaneous and subcutaneous administration of oestradiol cause slower and more prolonged increases in oestradiol concentrations than oral administration.

After intravenous administration, oestradiol has an initial half life of approximately 20 minutes, followed by a second half life of approximately 70 minutes.[14] Its metabolic clearance rate (MCR), defined as the volume of blood irreversibly cleared of oestradiol per unit time, is 600–800 l per 24 $h.m^{-2}$ in premenopausal women and about 500–600 l per 24 $h.m^{-2}$ in postmenopausal women. (For references, see review by Reed and Murray.)

Being highly lipid-soluble, oestradiol is distributed throughout the body but the apparent volume of distribution is only 9–15 l because of extensive protein binding. Circulating oestradiol is almost completely bound to plasma proteins; about 60% is bound to albumin, 38% to sex hormone binding globulin (SHBG), and 2–3% is unbound. Binding to SHBG is increased in some clinical conditions, such as hyperthyroidism, cirrhosis, pregnancy and during oestrogen treatment.

Oral absorption	good
Presystemic metabolism	extensive
Plasma half life	
1.	approx. 20 min
2.	approx. 70 min
Volume of distribution	9–15 l
Plasma protein binding	97–99%

Oestradiol undergoes extensive biotransformation, and is excreted primarily in the urine as glucuronide or sulphate conjugates; some double conjugates are also formed. Between 40 and 100% (average 80%) of a dose of oestradiol is excreted in the urine within 96–120 h.[14] About 40% of oestradiol metabolites are excreted into the bile, but of these about 80% are reabsorbed into the enterohepatic circulation; only a small proportion (about 7%) of a dose of oestradiol is excreted in the faeces.[14]

Although oestradiol is excreted in breast milk, the concentrations achieved are unlikely to pose any threat to the nursing infant.

Oestradiol can cross the placenta and should be avoided in pregnancy.

Concentration–effect relationship

The plasma oestradiol concentrations produced by either oral or parenteral administration (300–800 $pmol.l^{-1}$) are sufficient to relieve menopausal symptoms such as hot flushes, and to reduce elevated postmenopausal gonadotrophin concentrations.[6,9,12,15] Menopausal symptoms have been reported to return when plasma oestradiol concentrations[16] fall below 100–120 $pmol.l^{-1}$.

There is some evidence that the degree of efficacy depends on the plasma concentration. Dickerson et al[17] reported that following vaginal administration of oestradiol cream, the greatest improvement in menopausal symptoms was shown by women with very high oestradiol concentrations (about 300–500 $pmol.l^{-1}$), and the least by women with relatively low concentrations (about 150–200 $pmol.l^{-1}$). It has also been reported that after transdermal administration of oestradiol, the degree of suppression of gonadotrophins is related to the delivery rate.[13]

Metabolism

Oestradiol is converted to oestrone by a 17β-hydroxysteroid dehydrogenase and it is oestrone which is the substrate for further metabolism.

A major route of oestrogen metabolism involves hydroxylation of the aromatic A-ring at position C-2. Hydroxylation can also occur at C-16 on the D-ring to form 16α-hydroxyoestrone, which is then reduced to oestriol. Hydroxylation reactions at C-2 and C-16 are competitive. Hydroxylation can also occur at positions C-4, 6, 7, 11, 14, 15, 16 and 18.

Catechol oestrogens formed by A-ring hydroxylation can undergo methylation of the hydroxyl groups. In addition, catechol oestrogens may form covalent bonds with sulphydryl groups of liver proteins, probably via a semiquinone intermediate.

Oestrone, oestradiol and their metabolites are conjugated in the liver to yield glucuronides and sulphates. Notable among these is oestrone-3-sulphate. This is the major circulating oestrogen metabolite, and its concentration in plasma greatly exceeds that of oestradiol.[18] It is readily deconjugated to free oestrone, which is reduced to oestradiol; oestrone sulphate may therefore have a storage function, providing a readily available pool of free oestradiol.

Pharmaceutics

Oestradiol is available in oral and parenteral and transdermal formulations.

Oral preparations

1. Cyclo-Progynova 1 mg (Schering, UK) is a biphasic preparation. Each pack contains a total of 21 tablets; 11 beige tablets contain 1 mg oestradiol valerate and 10 brown tablets contain 1 mg oestradiol valerate and 0.25 mg (levonorgestrel. Cyclo-Progynova 2 mg is also available. Each pack contains 11 white tablets (2 mg oestradiol valerate) and 10 brown tablets (2 mg oestradiol and 0.5 mg norgestrel).
2. A triphasic preparation Trisequens (Novo, UK) is available, consisting of 28 tablets supplied in a calendar date-pack. All tablets are round and biconvex, with a diameter of 6 mm: (a) 12 blue tablets marked 'NOVO 270' on one face, containing 2 mg oestradiol and 1 mg oestriol; (b) 10 white tablets marked 'NOVO 271' on one face, containing 2 mg oestradiol, 1 mg oestriol and 1 mg norethisterone acetate BP; (c) 6 red tablets, marked 'NOVO 272' on one face, containing 1 mg oestradiol and 0.5 mg oestriol.

3. Progynova (Schering, UK) contains oestradiol valerate (1 mg, beige tablets; 2 mg, blue tablets).
4. Estrace (Mead Johnson, USA) tablets contain 1 mg oestradiol in a lavender-coloured scored tablet. A 2 mg Estrace tablet is turquoise coloured.
5. Hormonix (Carnrick, UK) tablets contain 600 μg oestradiol with 270 μg oestriol and 1.4 mg oestrone. They are pink, scored tablets.

Parenteral preparations

1. Oestradiol implants (Organon, UK) are sterilized pellets containing 25, 50 or 100 mg. They are supplied individually in glass tubes. A vaginal cream containing 0.01% oestradiol is marketed under the name Estrace by Mead Johnson, USA. It contains parabens.
2. Estraderm TTS (CIBA, UK/US) is a self-adhesive, transdermal formulation patch which releases oestradiol at a constant rate over 4 days. Three strengths are available designated by their release rates: 25, 50 and 100 μg for 24 hours (total oestradiol contents being 2, 4 and 8 mg respectively).

Oestradiol preparations should be protected from light and kept in a cool place. Under these conditions, oestradiol has a shelf-life of approximately 5 years. Oestradiol preparations contain no allergenic materials with the exception of Estrace vaginal cream.

Oestradiol esters are insoluble in water and are injected in oily (e.g. ethyl oleate) solution to provide a depot from which oestradiol is slowly released.

Therapeutic use

Indications

1. Hormone replacement in cases of oestrogen deficiency, e.g. after the menopause or ovariectomy
2. The treatment of prostatic carcinoma.

Contraindications

1. Known or suspected pregnancy
2. Cardiovascular or cerebrovascular disorders such as thrombophlebitis, or a history of such conditions
3. Acute or chronic liver disease (oestradiol is not contraindicated, however, if liver function is normal after previous liver disease)
4. Oestrogen-dependent tumours
5. Hypertension
6. Endometrial hyperplasia
7. Undiagnosed vaginal bleeding
8. Haemoglobinopathies such as sickle-cell anaemia
9. Porphyria
10. Hyperlipoproteinaemia
11. History during pregnancy of general pruritus, pemphygoid gestationis, or a deterioration of otosclerosis.

Mode of use

Oestradiol is widely used for postmenopausal hormone replacement, but synthetic oestrogens — chiefly ethinyloestradiol — are preferred for oral contraception. Since oestrogens given alone are associated with an increased risk of endometrial cancer, oestradiol is normally given with a short concurrent course of a synthetic progestogen in order to induce withdrawal bleeding and prevent endometrial hyperplasia. The use of oestrogen alone is not recommended except in hysterectomized women. Oestrogen replacement is not routinely indicated in postmenopausal women, but may be appropriate if symptoms are severe. The duration of treatment depends on the severity and persistence of symptoms, and it may be necessary to withdraw oestradiol gradually over 1–2 years.

Oestradiol may also be used in high doses in the treatment of androgen-dependent prostatic carcinoma.

Indications

1. Treatment of menopausal symptoms

Oestradiol is normally given orally, but subcutaneous implants and transdermal preparations are increasingly being used. An oral dose of 1–2 mg daily is recommended, and treatment is normally given in 21-day cycles to avoid excessive endometrial stimulation. An appropriate progestogen, such as norethisterone 5 mg daily, should be given for at least 10 days during the second half of the treatment cycle to induce withdrawal bleeding and to protect against the development of endometrial carcinoma. Oestrogen replacement after ovariectomy should be continued at least until the expected time of menopause.

Parenteral administration of oestradiol by implant avoids gastrointestinal metabolism, and produces a low oestrone:oestradiol ratio, but the dosage is necessarily less precise. Oestradiol implants

Fig. 1 Major routes of oestradiol metabolism

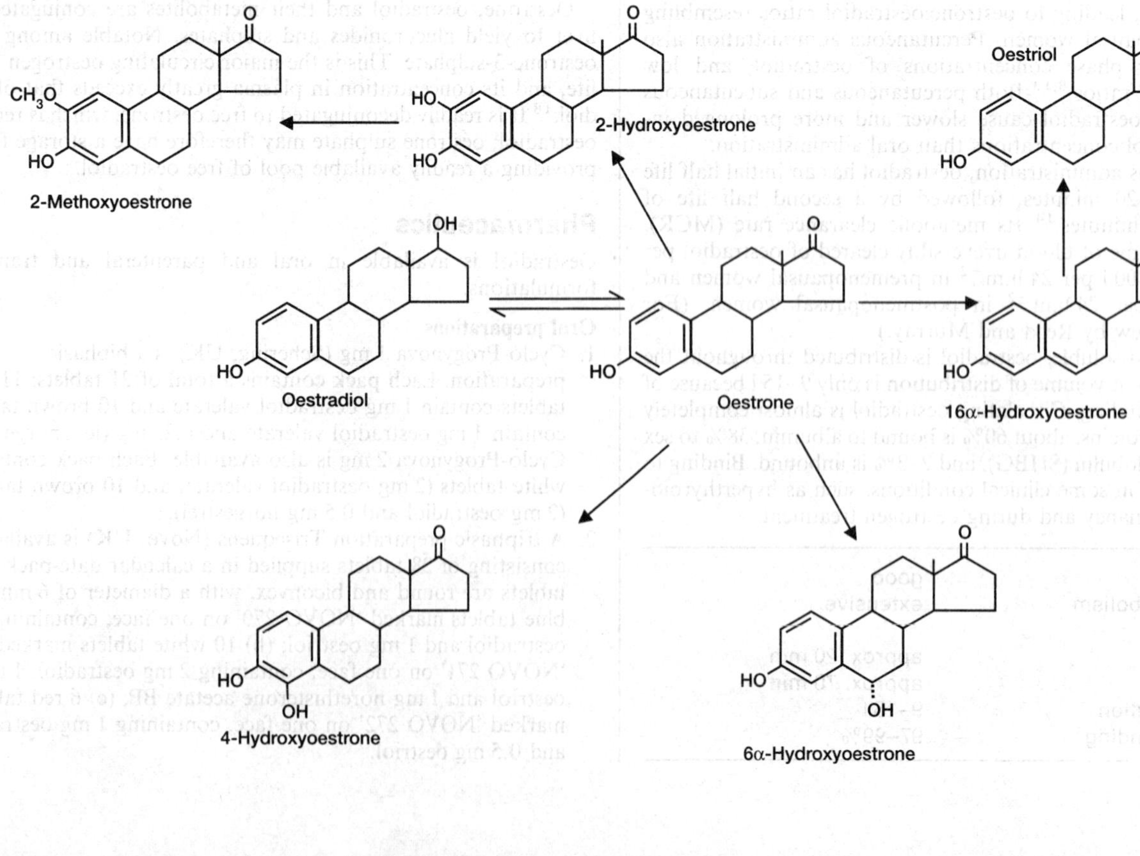

Oestradiol

(25–50 mg) are inserted, usually by trocar and cannula, into the subcutaneous fat of the lower abdomen or buttock. The rate of release of oestradiol from such implants varies, and may initially produce excessive oestrogen levels, leading to endometrial hypertrophy. Implants must therefore be placed superficially, in case they have to be removed. Implants remain active for up to 4–6 months.

Oestradiol replacement causes significant improvement of vasomotor symptoms, genitourinary atrophy, and osteoporosis. Oestradiol appears to reduce vasomotor symptoms via some hypothalamic mechanism; one possibility is that oestradiol is metabolized in the hypothalamus to catechol oestrogens which interact with monoaminergic synapses.[19] Vasomotor symptoms may return on cessation of treatment, and thus it is sometimes necessary to withdraw oestrogens gradually over a period of 1–2 years, during which time the severity of symptoms usually diminishes.

The effects of oestradiol on genitourinary atrophy are due to local actions on the vaginal epithelium and mucosa, accompanied by an oestrogen-dependent stimulation of the local circulation.

The protective effect of oestradiol against osteoporosis is well established, but the mechanism is unclear; stimulation of parathyroid hormone may be involved. Oestradiol treatment of osteoporosis should be started as soon as possible after the menopause and continued indefinitely. Cessation of treatment may be associated with an increased risk of fractures, since bone loss accelerates if oestradiol is withdrawn.[20]

2. Treatment of prostatic cancer
Oestrogen-responsive prostatic carcinoma can be treated by deep intramuscular injection of Estradurin (polyoestradiol phosphate), a water-soluble polymer in which oestradiol molecules alternate with phosphate groups. The polymer is slowly broken down by phosphatases, and so behaves as a long-acting oestradiol preparation. The initial dosage is 80–160 mg every four weeks for 2–3 months, which can then be reduced as appropriate to 40–80 mg every four weeks. Oestrogenic side effects such as gynaecomastia are claimed to be less severe with this preparation than with stilboestrol. The mode of action of oestradiol involves suppression of pituitary gonadotrophin secretion, thereby reducing androgen production, and inhibition of androgen action in the tumour cells.

Contraindications

1. Pregnancy
Although evidence for a teratogenic effect of oestradiol is limited, other oestrogens, notably stilboestrol, have been shown to be teratogenic.[1] For this reason, oestradiol should not be administered during pregnancy.

2. Cardiovascular or cerebrovascular disease
Oestrogen therapy may increase the risk of thrombosis, but natural oestrogens appear not to be thrombogenic per se, although they may predispose susceptible individuals to a thromboembolic state. Therapy should if possible be stopped approximately six weeks before elective surgery.

3. Liver disease
Oestrogens have widespread metabolic effects in the liver[21] and their use is therefore contraindicated if liver function is impaired.

4. Oestrogen-dependent carcinomas
Oestrogens stimulate the growth of some tumours of the breast and endometrium.[1]

5. Hypertension
Some oestrogen preparations increase plasma renin activity and are associated with an increased incidence of hypertension.[22]

6. Endometrial hyperplasia
Endometrial hyperplasia is believed to be a potentially premalignant condition since a proportion of cases progress to endometrial carcinoma. Since oestradiol will further stimulate the hyperplastic endometrium, its use is contraindicated in this condition.

7. Undiagnosed vaginal bleeding
Oestradiol is contraindicated in cases of undiagnosed vaginal bleeding since this may be a symptom of endometrial hyperplasia or carcinoma.

8. Haemoglobinopathies
There may be an increased risk of thromboembolism in conditions such as sickle-cell anaemia.

9. Porphyria
Oestrogens stimulate hepatic porphyrin synthesis[21] and have been reported to induce porphyria when used in replacement therapy.[23]

10. Hyperlipoproteinaemia
Oestradiol alters lipoprotein synthesis, causing in particular an increase in the high-density lipoprotein (HDL) fraction.[21]

11. Pruritis, etc.
General pruritis or pemphigoid gestationis may occur during pregnancy as a result of high oestrogen concentrations. Similarly, otosclerosis may be exacerbated by oestrogens.

Adverse reactions

Potentially life-threatening effects
Unopposed oestradiol replacement in postmenopausal women is associated with an increased risk of endometrial cancer, the magnitude of the risk depending on the dosage and duration of treatment (see general review articles by Hammond and Maxson, and Nicholls et al). This increased risk results from excessive stimulation of the endometrium. Oestrogen therapy has also been reported to increase the risk of breast cancer, but the evidence for this is controversial.

Acute overdosage
There appear to be no reports of ill-effects from acute overdosage. Treatment is symptomatic. Subcutaneous implants can be removed if necessary.

Severe or irreversible adverse effects
Abnormal uterine bleeding may occur during oestradiol treatment, which may necessitate endometrial biopsy to rule out the possibility of carcinoma. Gynaecomastia may occur in men receiving oestradiol treatment for prostatic carcinoma.

Symptomatic adverse effects
A number of minor but undesirable side effects can occur during oestradiol therapy. These include dose-related nausea and vomiting, painful or tender breasts, weight gain, fluid retention, headaches and depression.

Other effects
Oestradiol has widespread metabolic effects, including increases in high-density lipoproteins and hepatic protein and in haem and porphyrin synthesis.[21] Glucose tolerance may be slightly reduced, although overt diabetes mellitus is unlikely.[24] Hypercalcaemia and sodium and fluid retention may also occur.

Interference with clinical pathology tests
Oestradiol may influence thyroid function tests, plasma cortisol and urinary 17-oxogenic steroid determinations by increasing concentrations of specific binding proteins.[25]

High risk groups

Neonates
There are no indications for the use of oestradiol in neonates.

Breast milk. There are few indications for the use of oestradiol in nursing mothers. Oestradiol is excreted into breast milk, but the amounts appearing in the milk are very small — probably less than 0.02% of the maternal dose per day.[26] Thus women taking oestradiol may breast-feed their infants.

Children
Oestradiol has occasionally been used to inhibit growth in tall girls.[27] Adverse effects include nausea, weight gain and menorrhagia, and the benefits of treatment are uncertain.[28]

Pregnant women
Synthetic oestrogens such as stilboestrol increase the risk of vaginal and cervical adenocarcinoma in daughters exposed in utero. Although there are no adequate data on the carcinogenicity of oestradiol in humans, it is prudent to avoid oestradiol administration during pregnancy.[1]

The elderly
Some patients may receive oestradiol replacement for postmenopau-

sal osteoporosis into the sixth or seventh decades, with the attendant risk of endometrial hyperplasia and carcinoma. Furthermore, bone loss increases on cessation of oestrogen treatment,[20] so there may be an increased risk of fractures. The benefit of long-term oestrogen therapy for osteoporosis seems to be debatable.[20]

Drug interactions

Potentially hazardous interactions

Cigarette smoking has not been shown to affect the efficacy of oestradiol, but increases the risk of thromboembolism in women receiving oestrogen therapy.

Other significant interactions

Hepatic enzyme-inducing drugs such as rifampicin, barbiturates and phenytoin have been reported to increase the rate of metabolism of oestrogens. Most published reports have concerned oral contraceptive steroids, and there are few data on oestradiol itself. It seems likely, however, that the efficacy of oestradiol should also be reduced by such drugs; an interaction between a conjugated oestrogen preparation and phenytoin has been reported.[29]

Oestrogens may also enhance the activity of phenytoin by inhibiting its metabolism.[30]

Potentially useful interactions

There appear to be no such interactions.

Major outcome trials

1. Callantine M R, Martin P L, Bolding O T, Warner P O, Greaney M O 1975 Micronized 17β-estradiol for oral estrogen therapy in menopausal women. Obstetrics and Gynecology 46: 37–41

This is a multi-centre study of 319 patients with menopausal symptoms. Micronized oestradiol was given daily for 21 days with a 7-day interval; the mean duration of treatment was approximately 6 months. The starting dose was 1–2 mg daily, which was adjusted as required to a maximum of 4 mg daily. In total, 96% of patients obtained adequate or complete relief of symptoms (flushes, genitourinary atrophy, etc.) and of these, symptoms disappeared completely in about 80%. In general, oestradiol was well tolerated, with only about 6% of patients withdrawing because of side effects. Endometrial hyperplasia occurred in 7 patients, all of whom had previously received oestrogen for 1–3 years. The authors conclude that oral oestradiol is a highly effective treatment for menopausal symptoms related to oestrogen deficiency.

Other trials

1. Staland B 1981 Continuous treatment with natural oestrogens and progestogens. A method to avoid endometrial stimulation. Maturitas 3: 145–146

This is an uncontrolled study of 265 patients treated for up to 52 months with a compound preparation containing 2 mg oestradiol, 1 mg oestriol and 1 mg norethisterone acetate. If necessary, the daily dose was increased by ½–1 tablet. All except one patient reported relief from vasomotor symptoms and few side effects except for uterine bleeding during the first few months of treatment. In most cases, the endometrium became atrophic during therapy, even when it was initially hyperplastic. It is suggested that this implies a lower risk of endometrial cancer, and that this form of oestrogen replacement may be useful in cases of endometrial atypia.

2. Brincat M, Magos A, Studd J W W et al 1984 Subcutaneous hormone implants for the control of climacteric symptoms. Lancet 1: 16–18

This is a prospective randomized study of 55 postmenopausal women who received either oestradiol (50 mg) and testosterone (100 mg) implants or placebo for 8 months. Patients with a uterus were also given norethisterone 5 mg daily for 7 days every four weeks. Oestradiol brought about significant improvement in menopausal symptoms (flushes, headaches, urethral syndrome, etc.) which lasted for up to six months. Some symptoms, notably urethral syndrome, deteriorated after 4 months, and symptoms returned when treatment was stopped. There was no significant effect with placebo. The authors conclude that the return of climacteric symptoms is associated with a fall in oestrogen concentrations rather than low concentrations per se.

Oestradiol

General review articles

Anonymous 1969 Oestrogens. British Medical Journal 3: 285–287

Bolt H M 1979 Metabolism of estrogens — natural and synthetic. Pharmacology and Therapeutics 4: 155–181

Furuhjelm M 1976 Estrogenic hormones — general considerations. Acta Obstetrica et Gynecologica Scandinavica (suppl) 54: 29–34

Gower D B 1979 Steroid hormones. Croome Helm, London

Hammond C B, Maxson W S 1982 Current status of estrogen therapy for the menopause. Fertility and Sterility 37: 5–25

Nichols K C, Schenkel L, Benson H 1984 17β-estradiol for postmenopausal estrogen replacement therapy. Obstetrical and Gynecological Survey 39: 230–245

Reed M H, Murray M A F 1979 The oestrogens. In: Gray C H, James V H T (eds) Hormones in blood, 3rd edn. Academic Press, London, vol 3, ch 6, pp 263–353

References

1. World Health Organisation 1979 International Agency for Research on Cancer monographs on the evaluation of the carcinogenic risk of chemicals to humans. Vol 21, Sex hormones (11). IRAC, Lyon
2. Jenson E V, DeSombre E R 1971 Estrogen–receptor interactions. Science 182: 126–134
3. Fink B J 1984 Endometrial changes after long-term use of continuous oestrogen and cyclic progestogen. Maturitas 5: 277–280
4. Greenblatt R B, Asch R H, Mahesh V B, Bryner J R 1977 Implantation of pure crystalline pellets of estradiol for conception control. American Journal of Obstetrics and Gynecology 127: 520–524
5. Wilson D W, John B M, Groom G V, Pierrepoint C G, Griffiths K 1977 Evaluation of an oestradiol radioimmunoassay by high-resolution mass fragmentography. Journal of Endocrinology 74: 503–504
6. Martin P L, Burnier A M, Greaney M O 1972 Oral menopausal therapy using 17β-micronized estradiol. Obstetrics and Gynecology 39: 771–774
7. Englund D E, Johansson E D B 1981 Oral versus vaginal absorption in (sic) oestradiol in postmenopausal women. Effects of different particle sizes. Upsala Journal of Medical Science 86: 297–307
8. Lyrenas S, Carlstrom K, Backstrom T, von Schoultz B 1981 A comparison of serum oestrogen levels after percutaneous and oral administration of oestradiol-17β. British Journal of Obstetrics and Gynaecology 88: 181–187
9. Yen S S C, Martin P L, Burnier A M, Czekala N M, Greaney M O, Callantine M R 1975 Circulating estradiol, estrone and gonadotrophin levels following the administration of orally active 17β-estradiol in postmenopausal women. Journal of Clinical Endocrinology and Metabolism 40: 518–521
10. Townsend P T, Dyer G I, Young O, Whitehead M I, Collins W P 1981 The absorption and metabolism of oral oestradiol, oestrone and oestriol. British Journal of Obstetrics and Gynaecology 88: 846–852
11. Schindler A E, Bolt H M, Zwirner M, Hochlehnert G, Goser R 1982 Comparative pharmacokinetics of oestradiol, oestrone, oestrone sulfate and 'conjugated oestrogens' after oral administration. Arzneimittel-forschung — Drug Research 32: 787–791
12. Thom T H, Collins W P, Studd J W W 1981 Hormonal profiles in postmenopausal women after therapy with subcutaneous implants. British Journal of Obstetrics and Gynaecology 88: 426–433
13. Powers M S, Schenkel L, Darley P E, Good W R, Balestra J C, Place V A 1985 Pharmacokinetics and pharmacodynamics of transdermal dosage forms of 17β-estradiol: comparison with conventional oral estrogens used for hormone replacement. American Journal of Obstetrics and Gynecology 152: 1099–1106
14. Sandberg A, Slaunwhite W R 1957 Studies on phenolic steroids in human subjects. 11 The metabolic fate and hepato-biliary-enteric circulation of C^{14}-estrone and C^{14}-estradiol in women. Journal of Clinical Investigation 36: 1266–1278
15. Padwick M L, Endacott J, Whitehead M I 1985 Efficacy, acceptability, and metabolic effects of transdermal estradiol in the management of postmenopausal women. American Journal of Obstetrics and Gynecology 152: 1085–1091
16. Staland B 1978 Treatment of menopausal oestrogen deficiency symptoms in hysterectomized women by means of 17β-oestradiol pellet implants. Acta Obstetrica et Gynecologica Scandinavica 57: 281–285
17. Dickerson J, Bressler R, Christian C D, Hermann H W 1979 Efficacy of estradiol vaginal cream in postmenopausal women. Clinical Pharmacology and Therapeutics 26: 502–507
18. Hawkins R A, Oakey R E 1974 Estimation of oestrone sulphate, oestradiol-17β and oestrone in peripheral plasma: concentrations during the menstrual cycle and in men. Journal of Endocrinology 60: 3–17
19. Gosden R G 1985 Somatic, metabolic and behavioural consequences of menopause. In: Biology of menopause. Academic Press, London.
20. Anonymous 1980 Oestrogen-replacement in old age. British Medical Journal 281: 572–573
21. Song C S, Rifkind A B, Gillette P N, Kappas P 1969 Hormones and the liver. American Journal of Obstetrics and Gynecology 105: 813–847
22. Pfeffer R I 1978 Estrogen use, hypertension and stroke in postmenopausal women. Journal of Chronic Diseases 31: 389–398
23. Stein K M, Raque C J, Zeigerman J H, Shrager J D 1971 Porphyria cutanea tarda induced by natural estrogens. Obstetrics and Gynecology 38: 755–760
24. Thom M, Chakravarti S, Oram D H, Studd J W W 1977 Effect of hormone replacement therapy on glucose tolerance in postmenopausal women. British Journal of Obstetrics and Gynaecology 84: 776–784
25. Anonymous 1972 Interference of drugs with chemical diagnostic tests. Drug and Therapeutics Bulletin 10: 69–72

26. Nilsson S, Nygren K G, Johansson E D 1978 Transfer of oestradiol to human milk. American Journal of Obstetrics and Gynecology 13: 653–659
27. Colle M L, Alperin H, Greenblatt R B 1977 The tall girl. Archives of Diseases in Childhood 52: 118–120
28. Anonymous 1975 Excessive height. British Medical Journal 2: 648–649
29. Notelovitz M, Tjapkes J, Ware M 1981 Interaction between estrogen and Dilantin in a menopausal woman. New England Journal of Medicine 304: 788–789
30. Kutt H, McDowell F 1968 Management of epilepsy with diphenylhydantoin sodium. Journal of the American Medical Association 203: 969–972

Ofloxacin

Ofloxacin is a quinolone antibiotic.

Chemistry

Ofloxacin (Tarivid, Oflocet, Tabrin, Visiren)
$C_{18}H_{20}FN_3O_4$
9-Fluoro-2,3-dihydro-3-methyl-10-(4-methyl1-1-piperazinyl)-7-oxo-7H-pyrido-[1,2,3-de] [1,4] benzoxazine-6-carboxylic acid

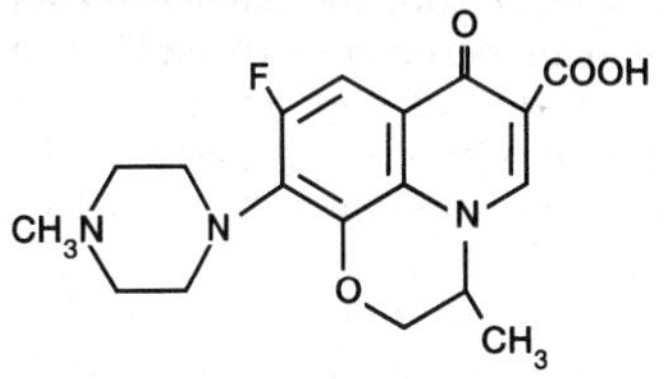

Molecular weight	361.37
pKa	7.9
Solubility	
in alcohol	poorly soluble
in water	poorly soluble
Octanol/water partition coefficient	0.278

Ofloxacin possesses an oxazine ring. The methyl group attached to this ring can exist in either the D or L configuration. The L-isomer is two-fold more active than the D-isomer.[1]

A mixture of the two isomers is used clinically. Ofloxacin is a synthetic, fluorinated 4-quinolone derivative and is structurally related to nalidixic acid. It is a yellow, opalescent, odourless powder with a bitter taste.

Pharmacology

A primary bacterial target of ofloxacin, like other quinolones is the enzyme DNA gyrase. DNA gyrase contains four subunits; two 'A' and two 'B' subunits. Genetic and biochemical studies have identified the A subunit of DNA gyrase (type II topoisomerase) as the target of quinolones.[2,3] Quinolones inhibit all the enzymatic activities of DNA gyrase, including inhibition of negative supercoiling, the joining and separation of interlocked DNA circles.[4]

In addition ofloxacin has a second mechanism of action, independent of its effect on RNA synthesis. Rifampicin, which inhibits RNA synthesis, prevents the bactericidal action of quinolones such as nalidixic acid but has much less effect on the action of ofloxacin.

Ofloxacin has bactericidal activity against sensitive bacteria, in general the minimal bactericidal concentration (MBC) is the same as, or no more than, one-fold concentration higher than the minimal inhibitory concentration (MIC).[5]

Toxicology

Acute toxicity was evaluated following oral administration of ofloxacin to rats, mice, dogs and monkeys, subcutaneous administration to mice and rats and intravenous administration to rats, mice and dogs.[6] Overt signs included ptosis, hypoactivity, sedation, prostration, hypopnoea, dyspnoea and convulsions. At necropsy, pulmonary congestion was a common finding. These studies suggested that acute toxicity of ofloxacin was minimal, within the safety margin of 13 to 67 times the proposed human dose.

An arthropathic effect of ofloxacin was shown in four-week-old rats and immature beagle dogs. Ofloxacin caused erosions, blister formation on cartilage and increased synovia in these animals.[6–8]

Toxicology studies in animals revealed that there was no impairment of fertility and no adverse effects on late fetal development, labour, delivery, lactation, neonatal viability or growth of offspring. Target organ studies showed no evidence of ocular, nephrotoxicity or ototoxicity. In rats, there was evidence of maternal and embryotoxicity, but no teratogenicity was observed.[6]

Clinical pharmacology

Ofloxacin is essentially 100% absorbed following oral administration. Very high concentrations of the drug are achieved in serum and most body fluids and tissues. These levels are sufficient to inhibit most bacteria at the site of infection.

Ofloxacin is very active against both nalidixic acid-susceptible and resistant strains of the *Enterobacteriaceae*.[9–12] MIC_{90} values for *E. coli, Klebsiella* spp, *Enterobacter* spp, *Citrobacter* spp, and *Proteus* spp are $\leq$0.25 mg.l^{-1}. The MIC_{90} for *Serratia* spp is $\leq$2 mg.l^{-1}. Like other quinolones, ofloxacin is highly active against enteric pathogens, such as *Shigella* spp, *Salmonella* spp, *Vibrio cholera, Campylobacter jejuni*, and *Yersinia enterocolitica*, including multi-resistant strains of *Shigella* spp, and *Salmonella* spp.[13] Higher MIC_{90} values for *Pseudomonas aeruginosa* (4 mg.l^{-1}), other *Pseudomonas* spp (4–8 mg.l^{-1}), *Acinetobacter* spp (1 mg.l^{-1}), and *Providencia* spp (1 mg.l^{-1}) are reported. Ofloxacin is highly active against *Neisseria gonorrhoea, Neisseria meningitidis, Haemophilus influenzae, Morexella catarrhalis*, and *Legionella species* (MIC_{90} $\leq$0.25 mg.l^{-1}). Ofloxacin is also active against *Brucella melitensis*.[14]

The MIC_{90} value for methicillin-sensitive and resistant *Staphylococcus aureus* is 0.5 mg.l^{-1}. For other Gram-positive cocci the values are as follows: *Staphylococcus epidermidis* 0.5 mg.l^{-1}, group A *Streptococcus* 2 mg.l^{-1}, group B *Streptococcus* 2 mg.l^{-1}, *Enterococcus* 4 mg.l^{-1} and *Streptococcus pneumoniae* 2 mg.l^{-1}.

Ofloxacin shows in-vitro activity against *Chlamydia trachomatis, Mycoplasma hominis, Mycoplasma pneumoniae*, and *Ureaplasma urealyticum*.[15–17] The drug also has a high activity against *Mycobacterium*.[18]

Human topisomerases are sufficiently different from those in bacteria for there to be no inhibition of them by quinolone antibiotics. Ofloxacin has no other pharmacological effects in man but occasional central nervous system disturbances have been reported in clinical trials. These include tremor, restlessness, agitation, confusion, visual disturbances and psychotic reactions. The mechanism behind these effects is not clear but it is recommended that ofloxacin is not used in patients with a history of epilepsy.

Resistance

Spontaneous resistant mutants can be selected by all of the quinolones, including ofloxacin. The frequency of resistant mutants is much less for the new fluoroquinolones than for nalidixic acid. The ofloxacin-resistance mutation rates[19] for *E. coli* and *S. aureus* were 1×10^{-8}. The quinolone resistance in clinical settings is likely to be due to an altered DNA gyrase and decreased drug permeation.[20–22] Plasmid mediated resistance to new quinolones has not been noted.[23]

Pharmacokinetics

The concentration of ofloxacin in plasma and other fluids can be determined by high pressure liquid chromatography or by bioassay.[24,25]

Ofloxacin is rapidly and uniformly absorbed after oral administration. There is negligible presystemic metabolism. Maximum serum concentrations (Tmax) are usually achieved in under two hours (0.5–1.6 h).[24–27] Following an oral dose of 100 mg ofloxacin, the peak serum concentration (Cmax) is 1.3 mg.l^{-1}, which increase to 3.8 mg.l^{-1} with 300 mg, 5.5 mg.l^{-1} with 400 mg, and 7–10 mg.l^{-1} with 600 mg, respectively. The plasma elimination half life ($t_{\frac{1}{2}}$) is about 6–7 hours. The apparent volume of distribution is 1–2.5 l.kg^{-1}. More than 70% of the drug is recovered unchanged in the urine in 24 h, and 80% in 48 h. Renal clearance is 180–190 ml.min^{-1}. Less than 10% of the dose is recovered as metabolites. Ofloxacin exhibits low plasma protein binding (20–25%).

When the pharmacokinetics of ofloxacin are compared with those of other quinolones, the following conclusion can be reached:[26,28] Ofloxacin is more rapidly absorbed; serum concentrations are highest with ofloxacin and its elimination half life is longer than that of most.

Oral absorption	100%
Presystemic metabolism	
Plasma half life	
range	4.9–6.9 h
Volume of distribution	1–2.5 l.kg^{-1}
Plasma protein binding	20–25%

Because ofloxacin is eliminated almost entirely via the kidneys, some adjustment of dose is necessary in patients with renal failure. In patients with mild renal failure (creatinine clearance > 50 ml.min – 1) there is little change in the pharmacokinetics of ofloxacin. In patients with moderate to severe renal failure C_{max} does not change, but T_{max} and $t_{\frac{1}{2}}$ increase significantly.[24,29,30] In patients with renal failure the following dosage recommendations are made: for patients with a creatinine clearance between 20–50 ml.min^{-1} 100 mg every 24 h, for patients with a creatinine clearance less than 20 ml.min^{-1} 50 mg every 24 h. An initial loading dose of 200 mg should be given to all patients irrespective of renal function.[29] Ofloxacin and its metabolites are only slightly removed by haemodialysis.[30,31]

Peak serum levels of ofloxacin are higher in elderly persons.[28,32] However, if renal function is normal, there is no need for dose adjustment in this group. Liver disease does not affect the kinetics of ofloxacin.

The pharmacokinetics of ofloxacin after parenteral infusion are very similar to those observed after oral administration.[24,33–35] After intravenous infusion of 200 mg ofloxacin C_{max} is 2.3 ± 0.6 mg.l^{-1}, and with 400 mg dose it is 4.5 ± 0.8 mg.l^{-1}. The elimination half life is 4–5 h. Urinary recovery is 73–82% of the administered dose, and renal clearance is 190 ml.min^{-1}.

Ofloxacin penetrates well into many body fluids. Very high concentrations of the drug are found in saliva, nasal secretions, tears, blister fluid, bronchial secretions, and sputum.[25,26,37] Ofloxacin penetration into sputum and bronchial secretions is 70–115%. Bronchial secretion penetration studies suggest that ofloxacin, at a 400 mg oral dose, is likely to achieve therapeutic activity against most respiratory pathogens.[38] After oral administration of ofloxacin 200 mg, 42–71% penetration is found in the cerebrospinal fluid.[39,40]

Ofloxacin penetration into lung tissue is quite high (with tissue/serum levels of 17.7/8.7 mg.l^{-1}, to give a ratio of 2).[41] Ofloxacin penetration into bone has also been studied.[42] The ratio of bone to serum levels was 0.61%. Penetration of up to 112% into prostatic tissue were reported.[43]

Like other quinolones, ofloxacin penetrates into human cells (polymorphonuclear leukocytes) in very high concentrations. In one study, the ratio of intracellular to extracellular concentration was 8.15.[44] The extent to which ofloxacin crosses the placenta or enters breast milk is not known.

Concentration–effect relationship

There is no indication to measure ofloxacin concentrations in everyday clinical practice. The aim should be to obtain plasma concentrations in excess of the MIC_{90} value (see Clinical pharmacology).

Metabolism

Ofloxacin is extensively excreted by the kidneys as the unchanged drug with up to 80% of an oral dose eliminated in the urine as the parent compound within 48 h.

Metabolism plays a very limited role in the elimination of ofloxacin. Three metabolites of ofloxacin have been found: ofloxacin-glucuronide, desmethyl-ofloxacin, and ofloxacin-N-oxide (see Fig. 1). Urinary recovery of desmethyl and N-oxide ofloxacin accounts for less than 5% of an administered oral dose.[45,46]

Pharmaceutics

Ofloxacin is supplied in 100 mg and 200 mg tablets. Its parenteral form is for intravenous infusion, a vial contains 100 mg ofloxacin in 50 ml of infusion fluid, or 200 mg in 100 ml. 200 mg tablets, Tarivid

Ofloxacin

(Hoechst, Roussel, UK) are yellowish-white, biconvex, oblong and scored on one side.

Therapeutic use

Indications

Clinically, ofloxacin has been shown to be effective in various bacterial infections. Available data suggest that the drug can be used with the following indications:

1. Urinary tract infections
2. Sexually transmitted diseases
3. Gastrointestinal infections
4. Pulmonary infections
5. Other infections (osteomyelitis, skin and soft tissue infections, use in immunocompromised host).

In all these clinical situations, ofloxacin was clinically effective and in comparative studies it was found to be as effective as or better than the comparative agent.

Contraindications

Ofloxacin should not be used in patients with known allergy to older or new quinolones. Its use in children with incomplete skeletal growth, pregnant women, and nursing mothers is not recommended.

Indications

1. Urinary tract infections

Ofloxacin, like other quinolones, covers the spectrum of organisms that cause urinary tract infections, including nosocomial ones. The drug is well absorbed after oral administration and is excreted as the parent, active form, in urine. Renal tissue concentration is very high. Ofloxacin achieves high levels in prostatic tissue. Because of these favourable pharmacokinetics, ofloxacin is used in the treatment of urinary tract infections.

Clinical studies have demonstrated efficacy of ofloxacin in uncomplicated acute cystitis in women, complicated lower urinary tract infections, and upper urinary tract infections.[16,47–50] Single dose ofloxacin (100, 200 and 400 mg) was found to be as effective as a 3-day course of therapy in acute cystitis in women. In comparative studies, ofloxacin single dose treatment was as effective as co-trimoxazole and was superior to amoxicillin.[47,49] Similar results were obtained when a 3-day course was compared.

Ofloxacin was also efficacious in treating complicated urinary tract infections. In comparative studies 200 to 400 mg per day ofloxacin given for 7 days was as effective as or superior to co-trimoxazole, nitrofurantoin, amoxicillin, clavulanic acid, and pipemidic acid.[47,49]

In general, bacteriological eradication in uncomplicated urinary tract infections was over 95%, whereas in complicated urinary tract infections it was around 90%, lowest being in infections due to *Pseudomonas aeruginosa* (67%).[47]

These results suggest that both oral and parenteral forms of ofloxacin do have a place in the treatment of nosocomial urinary tract infections, because of the features that have already been mentioned.

Ofloxacin has been used in the treatment of prostatitis. In several studies bacteriological cure rates were between 69–92%.[49] Although these results are promising, additional data are needed in this field.

2. Sexually transmitted diseases

a. Gonococcal urethritis. Ofloxacin, like other quinolones is highly active against both β-lactam sensitive and resistant strains of *Neisseria gonorrhoeae*. Ofloxacin in various doses has been shown to yield excellent results in the treatment of gonorrhoea. A single dose of 100, 200 or 400 mg ofloxacin therapy resulted in 100% bacteriological eradication in a number of studies.[51–54] Data for extragenital *Neisseria gonorrhoeae* infections are limited.

b. Chlamydia infections. Ofloxacin is the most active quinolone against *Chlamydia trachomatis*, in vitro. Several studies have shown that this activity may be useful in the treatment of urethritis caused by this organism.[55] Ofloxacin 200 mg twice daily for 5 days resulted in a cure rate of 90%.[56] In another study 9 days of treatment with the same dose of the drug eliminated the organism in all patients.[57] In a recent study, 7 days of therapy with 200 mg twice a day ofloxacin eradicated *Chlamydia trachomatis* in 47 patients.[58] Although these results are promising, additional studies are needed in this field.

Fig. 1 Metabolism of Ofloxacin

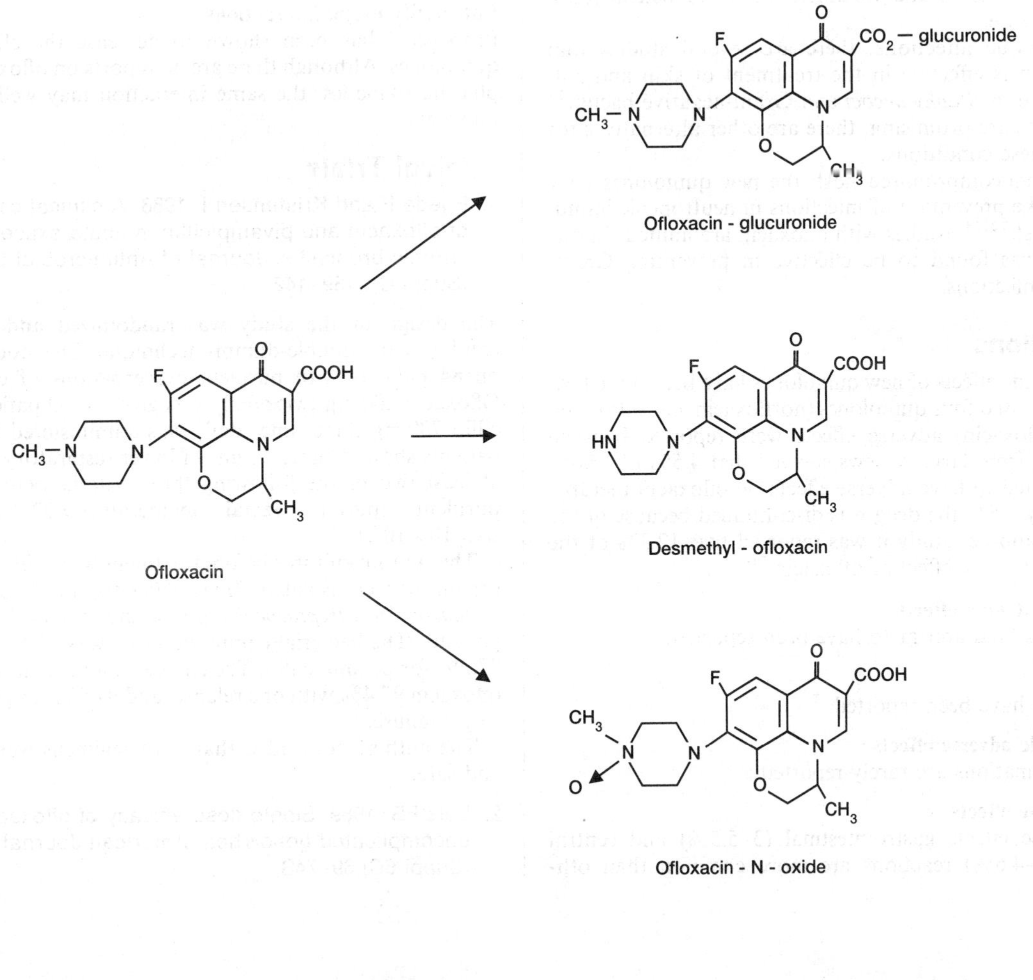

Ofloxacin

3. Gastrointestinal infections
Ofloxacin has very good in vitro activity against pathogens that cause acute bacterial diarrhoeas and enteric fever. Because of the increase in resistance to standard agents that are used in the treatment of these infections, quinolones can be added to the list of drugs for the treatment of these diseases. Ofloxacin was shown to be effective in the treatment of shigellosis when given 200 mg twice daily for five days.[13] Furthermore, single doses of 400 mg or 200 mg three times a day for only one day were also effective in achieving 100% clinical and bacteriological cures in patients with shigellosis.[59] These results with ofloxacin and the data obtained with other quinolones suggest that they will probably become the drug of choice for acute bacterial diarrhoeal diseases.[60,61]

The worldwide emergence of resistance of *Salmonella* spp to chloramphenicol, ampicillin and co-trimoxazole has made it necessary to evaluate new quinolones in the treatment of enteric fever. Available data suggest that ofloxacin is effective in the treatment of enteric fevers.[60,62] Out of 155 patients with enteric fever treated with ofloxacin, only one was not cured (cure rate of 99.4%).[62] Similar results were obtained with other quinolones. New quinolones, including ofloxacin appear to be the drugs of choice in the treatment of enteric fever, especially in infections caused by multiple-resistant strains.

4. Pulmonary infections
The major indication for the use of ofloxacin in the treatment of pulmonary infections will likely be acute exacerbations of bronchitis in patients with chronic obstructive pulmonary diseases. Several studies have been carried out to study the efficacy of ofloxacin in lower respiratory tract infections. In non-comparative studies, ofloxacin was found to be clinically satisfactory in 86% of patients.[63] The bacteriological eradication rate was 76%. In comparative studies ofloxacin was as effective as or superior to amoxicillin, pivampicillin, cefaclor or erythromycin.[63–65]

5. Other infections
Osteomyelitis: experimental data suggest that ofloxacin is effective in the treatment of *Pseudomonas aeruginosa* osteomyelitis in animals.[66] There is limited clinical data for the use of ofloxacin in the treatment of acute or chronic osteomyelitis.[67–70] These studies suggest that ofloxacin, like other quinolones may be considered as an alternative agent for the treatment of chronic osteomyelitis. Parenteral form of the drug may be useful in the treatment of acute osteomyelitis following open fracture.

Skin and soft tissue infections: there are several studies that show that ofloxacin is effective in the treatment of skin and soft tissue infections due to *Staphyloccoci* and Gram-negative bacilli.[71] Although the results are promising, there are other alternatives for the treatment of these conditions.

Use in the immunocompromised host: the new quinolones have been evaluated in the prevention of infections in neutropenic immunocompromised host.[72,73] Studies with ofloxacin are limited. In one study[74] the drug was found to be effective in preventing Gram-negative bacillary infections.

Adverse reactions

In general, clinical side effects of new quinolones have been quite low. For the most widely used four quinolones (norfloxacin, ciprofloxacin, ofloxacin and perfloxacin) adverse effects were reported between 4.5–10.2%.[75] Data from large reviews showed that 4.5% of 15,651 patients were reported to have adverse effects on ofloxacin therapy, and of these in only 1.5% the drug was discontinued because of the adverse effects. In another study it was reported that 12.3% of the patients experienced a side effect of ofloxacin.[76]

Potentially life-threatening effects
No reactions of this kind appear to have been reported.

Acute overdosage
No cases appear to have been reported.

Severe or irreversible adverse effects
Seizures and hallucinations are rarely reported.

Symptomatic adverse effects
Among the adverse effects gastrointestinal (3–5.5%) and central nervous system (1–4.6%) reactions are more common than others.[75–77] Nausea, vomiting, abdominal pain, diarrhoea and gastrointestinal distress are gastrointestinal adverse effects. Common central nervous system reactions are headache, dizziness, and insomnia.

Other effects
Laboratory abnormalities in ofloxacin treated patients are rare.[76] Granulocytopenia, eosinophilia, elevated serum glutamic pyruvic transaminase are all reported in less than 1% of patients who receive ofloxacin.

Interference with clinical pathology tests
No technical interferences of this kind appear to have been reported.

High risk groups

Neonates
Ofloxacin, like other quinolones, should not be used in the treatment of infections in neonates because of possible cartilage damage.

Breast milk. Ofloxacin may enter breast milk but data are not available.

Children
What has been said about neonates also applies to older children. There are a few studies of quinolone usage in children with cystic fibrosis.

Pregnant women
The safety of ofloxacin during pregnancy has not been established.

The elderly
In the elderly, dose alteration is necessary, if there is moderate to severe renal failure.

Drug interactions

Potentially hazardous interactions
Mineral antacids (magnesium or aluminium containing) reduce absorption of ofloxacin.[70,80,81] No interaction between ofloxacin and ranitidine was found, Sucralfate reduces absorption of some quinolones.[70] Ofloxacin inhibits GABA-receptor binding.[81] The clinical importance of this effect is not known.

Ofloxacin and its oxo-metabolite do not interfere with theophylline clearance and its major metabolic pathways.[79–81] Ofloxacin has no significant effect on caffeine metabolism and elimination.[81]

Potentially useful interactions
Probenecid has been shown to decrease the elimination of most quinolones. Although there are no reports on ofloxacin, because of its pharmacokinetics, the same interaction may well be observed with ofloxacin.

Clinical Trials

1. Egede F and Kristensen I. 1988. A clinical comparative study of ofloxacin and pivampicillin in acute exacerbations of chronic bronchitis. Journal of Antimicrobial Chemotherapy 22 (Suppl C): 139–142.

The design of the study was randomized and double-blind and employed the double-dummy technique. The study was carried out on 84 patients with purulent exacerbations of chronic bronchitis. Ofloxacin 200 mg twice daily was given to 39 patients, and pivampicillin 700 mg three times daily was administered to 42 patients. All patients showed clinical signs of lower respiratory tract infection, i.e. at least two of the following three criteria were met: macroscopic purulent sputum, rectal temperature $>37.7°$, or leukocytosis $>10 \times 10^9.1^{-1}$.

The sputum cultures before treatment were obtained and following organisms were isolated: *Hemophilus* spp in 31, *Streptococcus pneumoniae* in 19, *Streptococci* spp in 8 and seven other organisms in 13 patients. The bacterial elimination rate was 94.1% for ofloxacin and 97.2% for pivampicillin. The clinical response showed a cure rate for ofloxacin 97.4% with one relapse, and 97.6% for pivampicillin with a single failure.

The authors concluded that both regimens were equally effective and safe.

2. Lutz FB. 1989. Single-dose efficacy of ofloxacin in uncomplicated gonorrhea. American Journal of Medicine 87 (Suppl 6C):69–74S.

Ofloxacin

In this study, two multicenter trials compared single-dose oral therapy with 400 mg of ofloxacin or 3 g of amoxicillin plus 1 g probenecid in the treatment of uncomplicated gonorrhea in 160 men and 102 women. All pretreatment isolates were sensitive to ofloxacin. Posttreatment culture results showed that ofloxacin had eradicated the organism in 97.5% of 42 men and all 28 women. Amoxicillin-probenecid achieved microbiologic eradication in 92.7% of 55 men and 92.6% of 27 women.

Clinical cure rates were 84.6% in men, and 81.8% in women with ofloxacin, and 83% in men and 66.7% in women with amoxicillin-probenecid.

The author concluded that, single-dose ofloxacin was as effective as amoxicillin-probenecid in eradicating *Neisseria gonorrhaea* and relieving clinical signs and symptoms of gonococcal infections.

General review articles

Monk J P, Campoli-Richards D M 1987 Ofloxacin: A review of its antibacterial activity, pharmacokinetic properties and therapeutic use. Drugs 33: 346–391

Wise R, Knothe H (eds) 1987 First International Symposium on ofloxacin. Drugs 34 (suppl 1): 1–187

Leigh D, Finch D, Spencer B (eds) 1988 Focus on ofloxacin — a new 4-quinolone antimicrobial agent. Journal of Antimicrobial Chemotherapy 22 (suppl C): 1–179

Moellering R C, Neu H C (eds) 1989 Ofloxacin: a pharmacodynamic advance in quinolone antimicrobial therapy. American Journal of Medicine 87 (suppl 6C): 1S–81S

Wolfson J S, Murray B E (eds) 1989 value of new quinolones in the treatment and prophylaxis of infectious diseases. European Journal of Clinical Microbiology and Infectious Diseases 8: 1071–1116

Rubinstein E, Adam D, Moellering R, Waldvogel F (eds) 1988 International symposium on new quinolones. Reviews of Infectious Diseases 10 (suppl 1): S1–S271

Rubinstein E, Adam D, Moellering R, Waldvogel F (eds) 1989 Second International Symposium on new quinolones. Reviews of Infectious Diseases 11 (suppl 5): S897–S1431

References

1. Neu H C 1989 Chemical evolution of fluoroquinolone antimicrobial agents. American Journal of Medicine 87 (suppl 6C): 2S–9S
2. Cozzarelli N R 1980 DNA gyrase and the supercoiling of DNA. Science 207: 161–163
3. Hooper D C, Wolfson J S 1988 Mode of action of the quinolone antimicrobial agents. Reviews of Infectious Diseases 10 (suppl 1): S14–S21
4. Shen L 1, Kohlbrenner W E, Weigl D, Baranowski J 1989 Mechanism of quinolone inhibition of DNA gyrase. Journal of Biological Chemistry 264: 2973–2978
5. Lockley M R, Wise R, Dent J 1984 The pharmacokinetics and tissue penetration of ofloxacin. Journal of Antimicrobial Chemotherapy 14: 647–652
6. Davis J, McKenzie B E 1989 Toxicologic evaluation of ofloxacin. American Journal of Medicine 87 (suppl 6C): 43S–46S
7. Christ W, Lehrert T, Ulbrich B 1988 Specific toxicologic aspects of the quinolones. Reviews of Infectious Diseases 10 (suppl 1): S141–S146
8. Stahloman R, Merker H J, Hinz N, Chahoud I, Webb J, Heger W, Neubert D 1990 Ofloxacin in juvenile non-human primates and rats. Arthropathia and drug plasma concentrations. Archives of Toxicology 64: 193–204
9. Grünberg R N, Felmingham D, O'Hare M D et al 1988 The comparative in vitro activity of ofloxacin. Journal of Antimicrobial Chemotherapy 22 (suppl C): 9–19
10. Mitsuhashi S 1988 Comparative antibacterial activity of new quinolone-carboxylic acid derivatives. Reviews of Infectious Diseases 10 (suppl 1): S27–S31
11. Bellido F, Pechere J C 1989 Laboratory survey of fluoroquinolone activity. Reviews of Infectious Diseases 11 (suppl 5): S917–S924
12. Fuchs P C 1989 In vitro antimicrobial activity and susceptibility testing of ofloxacin. American Journal of Medicine 87 (suppl 6C): 10S–13S
13. Firat M, Akalin H E, Serin A, Baykal M 1987 In vitro activity and clinical efficacy of ofloxacin in shigellosis due to multiply-resistant strains. In: Berkarda B, Kummerle H P (eds) Progress in antimicrobial and anticancer chemotherapy, vol 2. Ecomed, FRG, p 1780–1782
14. Baykal M, Akalin H E, Firat M, Serin A 1989 In vitro activity and clinical efficacy of ofloxacin in infections due to Brucella melitensis. Reviews of Infectious Diseases 11 (suppl 5): S993–S994
15. Oriel J D 1989 Use of quinolones in chlamydial infection. Reviews of Infectious Diseases 11 (suppl 5): S1273–S1276
16. Babinchak T J, Fass R J 1989 Quinolone antibacterial agents for the treatment of genitourinary tract infections. European Journal of Clinical Microbiology and Infectious Diseases 8: 1111–1116
17. Schachter J, Moncada J V 1989 In vitro activity of ofloxacin against Chlamydia trachomatis. American Journal of Medicine 87 (suppl 6C): 14S–16S
18. Garcia-Rodriguez J A 1988 Activity of quinolones against Mycobacteria — 'in vitro' and 'in vivo' —. Quinolones Bulletin 4: 21–25
19. Felmingham D, Foxall P, O'Hare M D, Webb G, Ghosh G, Brüneberg R N 1988 Resistance studies with ofloxacin. Journal of Antimicrobial Chemotherapy 22 (suppl C): 27–34
20. Hooper D C, Wolfson J S 1989 Bacterial resistance to quinolone antimicrobial agents. American Journal of Infectious Diseases 87 (suppl 6C): 17S–23S
21. Daikos G L, Lolans V T, Jackson G G 1988 Alterations in outer membrane proteins of Pseudomonas aeruginosa associated with selective resistance to quinolones. Antimicrobial Agents and Chemotherapy 32: 785–787
22. Cheng A F, Li M K W, Ling T K W, French G L 1987 Emergence of ofloxacin-resistant Citrobacter freundii and Pseudomonas maltophilia after ofloxacin therapy. Journal of Antimicrobial Chemotherapy 20: 283–285
23. Courvalin P 1990 Plasmid-mediated 4-quinolone resistance: is it possible? Antimicrobial Agents and Chemotherapy 34: 681–684
24. Flor S 1989 Pharmacokinetics of ofloxacin. The American Journal of Medicine 87 (suppl 6C): 24S–30S
25. Wise R, Lockley M R 1988 The pharmacokinetics of ofloxacin and a review of its tissue penetration. Journal of Antimicrobial Chemotherapy 22 (suppl C): 59–64
26. Wise R, Lister D, McNulty C A M, Griggs D, Andrews J M 1986 The comparative pharmacokinetics of five quinolones. Journal of Antimicrobial Chemotherapy 18 (suppl D): 71–81
27. Wise R, Griggs D, Andrews J M 1988 Pharmacokinetics of the quinolones in volunteers: a proposed dosing schedule. Reviews of Infectious Diseases 10 (suppl 1): S83–S89
28. Wolfson J S, Hooper D C 1989 Comparative pharmacokinetics of ofloxacin and ciprofloxacin. American Journal of Medicine 87 (suppl 6C): 31S–36S
29. Fillastre J P 1988 Quinolones and renal failure. Quinolones Bulletin 4: 1–8
30. White L O, MacGowan A P, Mackay I G, Reeves D S 1988 The pharmacokinetics of ofloxacin, desmethyl ofloxacin and ofloxacin N-oxide in haemodialysis patients with end-stage renal failure. Journal of Antimicrobial Chemotherapy 22 (suppl C): 65–72
31. Fillastre J P, Leroy A, Humbert G 1987 Ofloxacin pharmacokinetics in renal failure. Antimicrobial Agents and Chemotherapy 31: 156–160
32. Norrby S R, Ljungberg B 1989 Pharmacokinetics of fluorinated 4-quinolones in the aged. Reviews of Infectious Diseases 11 (suppl 5): S1102–S1106
33. Lode H, Höffken B, Olschewski P, Sievers B, Kirsch A, Borner K, Koeppe P 1987 Pharmacokinetics of ofloxacin after parenteral and oral administration. Antimicrobial Agents and Chemotherapy 31: 1338–1342
34. Lode H 1989 Pharmacokinetics and clinical results of parenterally administered new quinolones in humans. Reviews of Infectious Diseases 11 (suppl 5): S996–S1004
35. Lode H, Höffken G, Olschewski P, Sievers B, Kirsch A, borner K, Koeppe P 1988 Comparative pharmacokinetics of intravenous ofloxacin and ciprofloxacin. Journal of Antimicrobial Chemotherapy 22 (suppl C): 73–79
36. Sörgel F, Jaehde U, Naber K, Stephan U 1989 Pharmacokinetic disposition of quinolones in human body fluids and tissues. Clinical Pharmacokinetics 16 (suppl 1): 5–24
37. Gerding D N, Hiff J A 1989 Tissue penetration of the new quinolones in humans. Reviews of Infectious Diseases 11 (suppl 5): S1046–S1057
38. Symonds J, Javaid A, Bone M, Turner A 1988 The penetration of ofloxacin into bronchial secretions. Journal of Antimicrobial Chemotherapy 22 (suppl C): 91–95
39. Stübner G, Weinrich W, Brands U 1986 Study of the cerebrospinal fluid penetrability of ofloxacin. Infection 14 (suppl 4): S250–S253
40. Stahl J P, Leduc D, Fourtillan J B, Micoud M 1986 Diffusion of ofloxacin into cerebrospinal fluid in patients with bacterial meningitis. Infection 14 (suppl 4): S254–S255
41. Wijnands W J A, Vree T B, Baars A M, Hafkenscheid J C M, Kohler B E M, van Herwaarden C L A 1988 The penetration of ofloxacin into lung tissue. Journal of Antimicrobial Chemotherapy 22 (suppl C): 85–89
42. Wittman D M, Kotthas E 1986 Further methodological improvement in antibiotic bone measurements: penetration of ofloxacin into bone and cartilage. Infection 14 (suppl 4): S270–S273
43. Naber K G, Adam D, Kees F 1987 In vitro activity and concentrations in serum, urine, prostate secretions and adenoma tissue of ofloxacin in urological patients. Drugs 34 (suppl 1): 44–50
44. Koga H 1987 High performance liquid chromatography measurement of antimicrobial concentrations in polymorphonuclear leukocytes. Antimicrobial Agents and Chemotherapy 31: 1904–1908
45. Outman W R, Nightingale C H 1989 Metabolism and fluoroquinolones. American Journal of Medicine 87 (suppl 6C): 37S–42S
46. Borner K, Lode H 1986 Biotransformation of certain gyrase inhibitors. Infection 14: 554–559
47. Malinverni R, Glauser M P 1988 Comparative studies of fluoroquinolones in the treatment of urinary tract infections. Reviews of Infectious Diseases 10 (suppl 1): S153–S163
48. Kromann-Andersen B, Sommer P, Pers C, Larsen V, Rasmussen F 1988 Ofloxacin compared with ciprofloxacin in the treatment of complicated lower urinary tract infections. Journal of Antimicrobial Chemotherapy 22 (suppl C): 143–147
49. Naber K G 1989 Use of quinolones in urinary tract infections and prostatitis. Reviews of Infectious Diseases 11 (suppl 5): S1321–S1337
50. Cox C E 1989 Ofloxacin in the management of complicated urinary tract infections, including prostatitis. American Journal of Medicine 87 (suppl 6C): 61S–68S
51. Aznar J, Prados R, Herrera A, Rodriquez-Richardo A, Perea E J 1987 Single doses of ofloxacin in uncomplicated gonorrhoea. Drugs 34 (suppl 1): 107–110
52. Richmond S J, Bhattacharyya M N, Mouti H, Chowdhury F H, Stirland R M, Tooth J A 1988 The efficacy of ofloxacin against infection caused by Neisseria gonorrhoea and Chlamydia trachomatis. Journal of Antimicrobial Chemotherapy 22 (suppl C): 149–153
53. Chan A S C 1989 Results of treatment with quinolones of sexually transmitted diseases in the Far East. Reviews of Infectious Diseases 11 (suppl 5): S1305–S1306
54. Lutz F B 1989 Single-dose efficacy of ofloxacin in uncomplicated gonorrhoea. American Journal of Medicine 87 (suppl 6C): 69S–74S

O

55. Perea E J 1989 Treatment of genital chlamydial infections with ciprofloxacin or ofloxacin. Quinolones Bulletin 5: 1–3
56. Bischoff W 1986 Ofloxacin; therapeutic results in Chlamydia trachomatis urethritis. Infection 14 (Suppl 4): S316–S317
57. Franson L, Avonts D, Piot P 1986 Treatment of genital chlamydia infection with ofloxacin. Infection 14 (suppl 4): S318–S320
58. Nayagam A T, Ridgway G L, Oriel J D 1988 Efficacy of ofloxacin in the treatment of non-gonococcal urethritis caused by Chlamydia trachomatis in men and women. Journal of Antimicrobial Chemotherapy 22 (suppl C): 155–158
59. Akalin H E, Firat M, Unal S, Serin A, Baykal M 1989 Clinical efficacy of single dose or one-day treatment with ofloxacin in shigellosis. Reviews of Infectious Diseases 11 (suppl 5): S1152–S1153
60. Murray B E 1989 Quinolones and the gastrointestinal tract. European Journal of Clinical Microbiology and Infectious Diseases 8: 1093–1102
61. Gotuzzo E 1989 Travellers' diarrhoea. Quinolones Bulletin 5: 4–8
62. Limson B M 1989 Use of quinolones in typhoid fever. Quinolones Bulletin 5: 17–19
63. Thys J P, Jacops F, Motte S 1989 Quinolones in the treatment of lower respiratory tract infections. Reviews of Infectious Diseases 11 (suppl 5): S1212–S1219
64. Stocks J M, Wallace R T, Griffith D E, Garcia J G, Hokler R B 1989 Ofloxacin in community-acquired lower respiratory infections. American Journal of Medicine 87 (suppl 6C): 52S–56S
65. Egede F, Kristensen I 1988 A clinical comparative study of ofloxacin and pivampicillin in acute exacerbations of chronic bronchitis. Journal of Antimicrobial Chemotherapy 22 (suppl C): 139–142
66. Norden C W, Niederriter K 1987 Ofloxacin therapy for experimental osteomyelitis caused by Pseudomonas aeruginosa. Journal of Infectious Diseases 155: 823–825
67. Waldvogel F A 1989 Use of quinolones for the treatment of osteomyelitis and septic arthritis. Reviews of Infectious Diseases 11 (suppl 5): S1259–S1263
68. Dellamonica P, Bernard e, Etesse H, Garroffo R, Drugen H B 1989 Evaluation of pefloxacin, ofloxacin and ciprofloxacin in the treatment of thirty-nine cases of chronic osteomyelitis. European Journal of Clinical Microbiology and Infectious Diseases 8: 1024–1030
69. Waldvogel F A 1989 Clinical role of quinolones today and in the future. European Journal of Clinical Microbiology and Infectious Diseases 8: 1075–1079
70. Ketterl R, Beckurts T, Stübinger B, Claudi B 1988 Use of ofloxacin in open fractures and in the treatment of post-traumatic osteomyelitis. Journal of Antimicrobial Chemotherapy 22 (suppl C): 159–166
71. Gentry L O, Rodriguez-Gomez G, Zeluff B J, Khosdel A, Prize M 1989 A comparative evaluation of oral ofloxacin versus intravenous cefotaxime therapy for serious skin and skin structure infections. American Journal of Medicine 87 (suppl 6C): 57S–60S
72. Grassi C, Marseglia G L 1989 The newer quinolones for infection prophylaxis in neutropenia. Quinolones Bulletin 5: 9–11
73. Rozenberg-Arska M, Dekker A W, Verhoef J 1989 Prevention of infections in granulocytopenic patients by fluorinated quinolones. Review of Infectious Diseases 11 (suppl 5): S1231–S1236
74. Kern W, Kurrle E, Vanek E 1987 Ofloxacin for prevention of bacterial infections in granulocytopenic patients. Infection 15: 427–432
75. Wolfson J S 1989 Quinolone antimicrobial agents: adverse effects and bacterial resistance. European Journal of Clinical Microbiology and Infectious Diseases 8: 1080–1092
76. Tack K J, Smith J A 1989 The safety profile of ofloxacin. American Journal of Medicine 87 (suppl 6C): 78S–81S
77. Jüngst G, Mohr R 1988 Overview of postmarketing experience with ofloxacin in Germany. Journal of Antimicrobial Chemotherapy 22 (suppl C): 167–175
78. Adam D 1989 Use of quinolones in pediatric patients. Reviews of Infectious Diseases 11 (suppl 5): S1113–S1116
79. Wijnands G J A, Vree T B, Janssen T J, Guellen P J M 1989 Drug-drug interaction with quinolones. American Journal of Medicine 87 (suppl 6C): 47S–51S
80. Davey P G 1988 Overview of drug interactions with the quinolones. Journal of Antimicrobial Chemotherapy 22 (suppl C): 97–107
81. Davies B I, Maesen F P V 1989 Drug interactions with quinolones. Reviews of Infectious Diseases 11 (suppl 5): S1083–S1090

Olsalazine sodium

Olsalazine sodium is a sulpha-free 5-aminosalicylic acid (5-ASA) based drug for the treatment of ulcerative colitis.

Chemistry

Olsalazine sodium (Dipentum)
$C_{14}H_8N_2Na_2O_6$
Disodium 3,3'-azobis(6-hydroxy-benzoate)

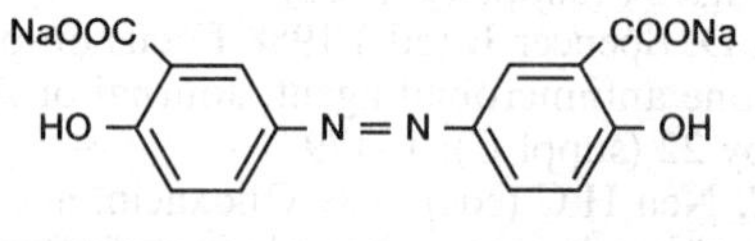

Molecular weight (free acid)	346.2 (302.2)
pKa	
pKa_1	2.07
pKa_2	2.85
pKa_3	11.2
pKa_4	12.5
Solubility	
in alcohol	1 in 10 000
in water	high
Octanol/water partition coefficient	10^{-4}

Olsalazine sodium is a yellow, tasteless, odourless crystalline powder. It is prepared by chemical synthesis. It is not used in combination with any other drug.

Pharmacology

On reaching the large intestine olsalazine is totally transformed by cleavage of the azo-bond[1] through azo-reduction achieved by colonic bacteria. As olsalazine is only minimally absorbed in the small intestine[2] two molecules of 5-aminosalicylic acid are delivered to the colon. 5-ASA exerts its anti-inflammatory effect by topical action on the intestinal mucosa. The way 5-ASA exerts its pharmacologic effect in inflammatory bowel disease is largely unknown. 5-ASA has inhibitory effects on prostaglandin metabolism but it is also a very effective scavenger of free oxygen radicals.[3]

Toxicology

Olsalazine does not appear to have mutagenic potential, and toxicological testing in animals (rat, rabbits, dogs) failed to demonstrate any results of potential clinical relevance. There was no evidence of carcinogenicity in tests lasting up to 24 months in mice or rats, and no evidence of teratological effects in rats or rabbits. Bacterial mutagenicity tests did not show any mutagenic activity.

Clinical pharmacology

The tolerance of olsalazine was evaluated on the basis of 804 patients who had received the drug in different studies.[4] The mean daily dosage was 1.2 g (0.5–4.0) and the maximum single dose was 1.0 g. The treatment period varied from 3 days to more than 12 months. 114 patients had been treated for one year or more.

88 of these 804 patients (10.9%) experienced a total of 104 side effects, most commonly diarrhoea, nausea and headache (see Adverse reactions).

The presently recommended dose for the treatment of ulcerative colitis in remission is 0.5 g twice daily and in active disease 0.75–1 g

Olsalazine sodium

two or three times daily. A slow increase of the dose is recommended to reduce the risk of diarrhoeal side effects.

As 5-ASA has no therapeutic effect on arthritis and ankylosing spondylitis it cannot be expected that olsalazine will have any effect on these extraintestinal conditions, unlike sulphasalazine. The reason is that it is the sulphapyridine moiety in sulphasalazine which is of benefit in joint conditions.[5,6] In such circumstances sulphasalazine is to be preferred if the patient can tolerate it.

Olsalazine does not affect spermatogenesis in males in contrast to sulphasalazine.

Pharmacokinetics

The preferred analytical method for both olsalazine and 5-ASA is high pressure liquid chromatography following extraction. Detection limits in serum are olsalazine > 0.5 μmol.l^{-1}, olsalazine sulphate > 0.2 μmol.l^{-1}, 5-ASA > 0.4 μmol.l^{-1} and acetyl-5-ASA > 0.4 μmol.l^{-1}.

The bioavailability of an oral dose of olsalazine is less than 3%. Of the minute amount of olsalazine absorbed more than 90% is excreted in the bile[7] as a result of an enterohepatic circulation. Thus, almost all ingested olsalazine reaches the colon. After reduction of the azo-bond, two molecules of 5-ASA are released. The absorption of 5-ASA from the large bowel has earlier been found to be about 20%, mainly in its acetylated form. Both 5-ASA and its acetylated metabolite are rapidly excreted in the urine.

During olsalazine medication steady state is reached after 20–28 days. The volume of distribution is about 6 litres. Systemic olsalazine is rapidly conjugated to sulphate ester, which is slowly eliminated. The mean residence time after discontinuation of therapy is 5.3–11 days because of the sulphated metabolite. After a single dose the plasma half life for olsalazine is 56 min and for its sulphated metabolite 7 days.

Olsalazine and its metabolites are highly protein bound: olsalazine 99.8%, olsalazine sulphate conjugate 99.8%, 5-ASA 74% and acetyl-5-ASA 81%.

Autoradiography in animals indicated that olsalazine does not pass into the brain.

Excretion of olsalazine into human breast milk has not been studied. 5-ASA and acetyl-5-ASA pass in minute quantities into the breast milk[8] which, however, does not affect the bilirubin binding.[9]

It is unlikely that renal or hepatic dysfunction, or old age, will have any important effect on the kinetics of the drug.

Oral absorption	<3%
Presystemic metabolism	—
Plasma half life	
olsalazine	56 min
olsalazine sulphate	7 days
Volume of distribution	6 l
Plasma protein binding	99.8%

Concentration–effect relationship

Olsalazine acts locally in the colon by delivery of two 5-ASA molecules after splitting of the azo-bond. Whether an increased 5-ASA concentration in the bowel is of clinical benefit is poorly studied. One study of sulphasalazine[10] showed that 2 g and 4 g of sulphasalazine daily were better than a 1 g dose. A trend in favour of the 4 g dose in comparison to the 2 g dose was found, but the difference was not statistically significant.

Another placebo-controlled study[11] of acute ulcerative colitis using olsalazine showed significantly better results the larger the dose. The dose levels compared in this study were 0.75, 1.5 and 3 g daily. It is unlikely that the plasma concentration of 5-ASA has any direct correlation with its therapeutic effect.

Metabolism

Less than 3% of an oral dose of olsalazine is absorbed before the drug reaches the colon. The absorbed olsalazine is sulphated in the liver and most of the absorbed compound is excreted again in the bile. The remainder is eliminated very slowly by routes which are incompletely known, but renal excretion is probably the most important.

Thus, almost all orally ingested olsalazine reaches the colon, where its azo-bond is reduced, delivering two molecules of 5-ASA. This is acetylated in the colonic mucosa and by the colonic bacteria. Of the 5-ASA released in the colon about 20% is absorbed as 5-ASA or acetyl-5-ASA and excreted in the urine. The remaining part is eliminated in the faeces. Of the olsalazine metabolites only 5-ASA has been found to be pharmacologically active. (Fig. 1.)

Fig. 1

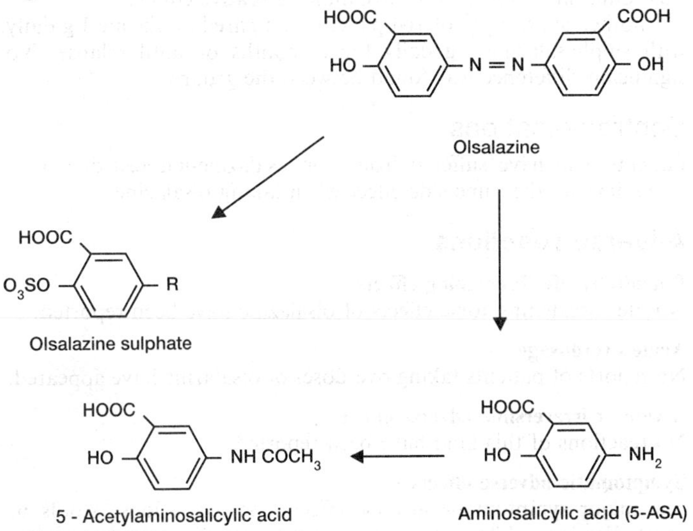

Pharmaceutics

Olsalazine is only available for oral use. Presently it is administered as opaque, beige, hard gelatin capsules, size 1, containing 250 mg olsalazine sodium. The capsules are marked with the legend 'Dipentum 250 mg' (Pharmacia, Sweden). The only other constituent is 1.25 mg magnesium stearate.

The capsules should be stored dry in a well-closed container. The container does not have to be protected from light or stored in a refrigerator. The storage time has presently been restricted to 3 years.

Therapeutic use

Indications

1. Treatment of active ulcerative colitis of mild to moderate severity with or without the concomitant use of steroids
2. Long-term maintenance treatment of patients with ulcerative colitis in remission.

Contraindications

1. Hypersensitivity to salicylates
2. Pregnancy, if not urgently needed
3. Lactation, if not urgently needed.

Mode of use

To reduce the risk of diarrhoeal side effects it is recommended that the therapy is introduced gradually during the first week, so that the full dose is not administered immediately. It is suggested that treatment is begun with one capsule the first day, increasing the dose by one capsule each day or two days until the required dose is reached.

For treatment of acute ulcerative colitis a daily dose of 1.5–3 g appears appropriate.

For treatment of ulcerative colitis in remission a daily dose of 1 g seems sufficient, although a possibility exists that a higher dose might be more effective in some patients.

Indications

1. Active ulcerative colitis

Three controlled trials of the effect of olsalazine in acute, ulcerative colitis have been performed. Two of them[11,12] showed a significantly better outcome in patients treated with olsalazine than in the placebo-treated patients. One small study[13] of 30 patients showed an insignificant advantage for the olsalazine treatment.

The largest study[11] showed that the clinical effect increased the larger the dose.

2. Ulcerative colitis in remission

In a large study,[14] 102 patients allergic or otherwise intolerant to sulphasalazine were treated with olsalazine 1 g daily or placebo for 6 months or until relapse. The relapse rate in the olsalazine group was 23% and in the placebo group 49%. The greatest benefit of olsalazine was found in patients with substantial ulcerative colitis.

Another big study[15] of 164 patients compared olsalazine 1 g daily with sulphasalazine 2 g daily for 6 months or until relapse. No significant difference was found between the groups.

Contraindications

Patients who have suffered from sulphasalazine-induced diarrhoea often develop the same side effect when taking olsalazine.

Adverse reactions

Potentially life-threatening effects

No life-threatening toxic effects of olsalazine have been reported.

Acute overdosage

No reports of patients taking overdoses of olsalazine have appeared.

Severe or irreversible adverse effects

No reactions of this kind have been reported.

Symptomatic adverse effects

The major symptomatic adverse effect reported is loose stools or overt diarrhoea. This effect of a severity which necessitates withdrawal of the drug occurs in about 6–7%.[4]

Among 804 patients the reported frequency of side effects was diarrhoea (44), nausea (11), headache (8), loose stools (7), abdominal pain (7), rash (3), alopecia (2), dizziness (2), lightheadedness (2), others (18). Of 18 others, which all occurred only once, the following are worth mentioning: nose bleed, burning sensation in the rectum, erythema nodosum, muscle stiffness, joint pain, haemolysis, anaemia, thrombocytopenia. Apart from the occurrence of loose stools or overt diarrhoea the other reported adverse events were not significantly more frequent than in the placebo-treated patients in the National Cooperative Crohn's Disease Study.[16]

Interference with clinical pathology tests

Olsalazine does not affect biochemical or other clinical pathology tests.

High risk groups

Neonates

The drug should not be used in neonates, and an indication rarely if ever exists. How olsalazine or its metabolites can affect a neonate during lactation is not known, but 5-ASA and acetyl-5-ASA appear to be harmless.

Breast milk. The drug should only be used in breast-feeding mothers if it is essential.

Children

Olsalazine has been used in children aged two years or more with the same dosages as in adults without the occurrence of harmful effects.

Pregnant women

Olsalazine should only be used during pregnancy if the indication is very strong. Sulphasalazine can safely be used during pregnancy and lactation.[17,18] Thus, if a patient is tolerant to this drug it should be the first choice in these circumstances if treatment is needed.

The elderly

No harmful effects have been observed during olsalazine treatment in elderly patients.

Drug interactions

There are no reports of olsalazine interacting with other drugs.

General review articles

Sandberg-Gertzén H 1985 Studies on the medical treatment of ulcerative colitis with special reference to olsalazine sodium (thesis)

van Hogezand R A 1986 5-aminosalicylic acid compounds. Pharmacokinetic and clinical aspects (thesis)

Järnerot G 1987 New 5-aminosalicylic acid based drugs: an evaluation of properties and possible role in the treatment of inflammatory bowel disease. In: Inflammatory bowel disease. Raven Press, New York, pp 153–164

Järnerot G 1989 Newer 5-aminosalicylic acid based drugs in chronic inflammatory bowel disease. Drugs 37: 73–86

References

1. Lauritsen K, Hansen J, Ryde M, Rask-Madsen J 1984 Colonic azodisalicylate metabolism determined by in vivo dialysis in healthy volunteers and patients with ulcerative colitis. Gastroenterology 86: 1496–1500
2. Sandberg-Gertzén H, Ryde M, Järnerot G 1983 Absorption and excretion of a single 1-g dose of azodisal sodium in subjects with ileostomy. Scandinavian Journal of Gastroenterology 18: 107–111
3. Miyachi Y, Yoshioka A, Imamura S, Niwa Y 1987 Effect of sulphasalazine and its metabolites on the generation of reactive oxygen species. Gut 28: 190–195
4. Järnerot G 1987 New 5-aminosalicylic acid based drugs: an evaluation of properties and possible role in the treatment of inflammatory bowel disease. In: Järnerot G (ed) Inflammatory bowel disease. Raven Press, New York, pp 153–164
5. Neumann V C, Grindulis K A, Hubball S, McConkey B, Wright V 1983 Comparison between penicillamine and sulphasalazine in rheumatoid arthritis: Leeds-Birmingham trial. British Medical Journal 287: 1099–1102
6. Pullar T, Hunter J A, Capell H A 1985 Which component of sulphasalazine is active in rheumatoid arthritis. British Medical Journal 290: 1535–1538
7. van Hogezand R A 1986 Biliary excretion of disodium azodisalicylate, salicylazosulphapyridine and 5-aminosalicylic acid in dogs and human volunteers. In: 5-aminosalicylic acid compounds. Pharmacokinetic and clinical aspects. Krips repro meppel, ch 6, pp 81–91 (thesis)
8. Rasmussen S N, Bondesen S, Hansen S H, Hvidberg E F 1984 5-aminosalicylic acid in amniotic fluid, cord and maternal plasma, and breast milk during sulfasalazine treatment. XII International Congress Gastroenterology Lisbon Sept. 17–22 1984 Abstract No 959
9. Järnerot G, Anderson S, Esbjörner E, Sandström B, Brodersen R 1981 Albumin reserve for binding of bilirubin in maternal and cord serum under treatment with sulphasalazine. Scandinavian Journal of Gastroenterology 16: 1049–1055
10. Azad Khan A K, Howes D T, Piris J, Truelove S C 1980 Optimum dose of sulphasalazine for maintenance treatment of ulcerative colitis. Gut 21: 232–240
11. Meyers S, Sachar D B, Present D H, Janowitz H D 1987 Olsalazine sodium in the treatment of ulcerative colitis among patients intolerant to sulfasalazine. A prospective, randomized, placebo-controlled, double-blind, dose-ranging clinical trial. Gastroenterology 93: 1255–1262
12. Selby W S, Barr G D, Ireland A, Mason C H, Jewell C P 1985 Olsalazine in active ulcerative colitis. British Medical Journal 291: 1373–1375
13. Hetzel D J, Shearman D J C, Bochner F et al 1986 Azodisalicylate (olsalazine) in the treatment of active ulcerative colitis. A placebo controlled clinical trial and assessment of drug disposition. Journal of Gastroenterology and Hepatology 1: 257–266
14. Sandberg-Gertzén H, Järnerot G, Kraaz W 1986 Azodisal sodium in the treatment of ulcerative colitis. Gastroenterology 90: 1024–1030
15. Ireland A, Mason C H, Jewell D P 1988 A controlled trial comparing olsalazine and sulphasalazine for the maintenance treatment of ulcerative colitis. Gut 29: 835–837
16. Singleton J W, Law D H, Kelley M L, Mekhjian H S, Sturdevant R A L 1979 National Cooperative Crohn's Disease Study: adverse reactions to study drugs. Gastroenterology 77: 870–882
17. Järnerot G 1982 Fertility, sterility and pregnancy in chronic inflammatory bowel disease. Scandinavian Journal of Gastroenterology 17: 1–4
18. Korelitz B I 1985 Pregnancy, fertility and inflammatory bowel disease. American Journal of Gastroenterology 80: 365–370

Omeprazole

Omeprazole is one of a new family of agents which inhibit gastric secretion.

Chemistry

Omeprazole (Losec)
$C_{17}H_{19}N_3O_3S$
5-methoxy-2-[[(4-methoxy-3,5 dimethyl-2-pyridinyl) methyl] sulphinyl]-1H-benzimidazole

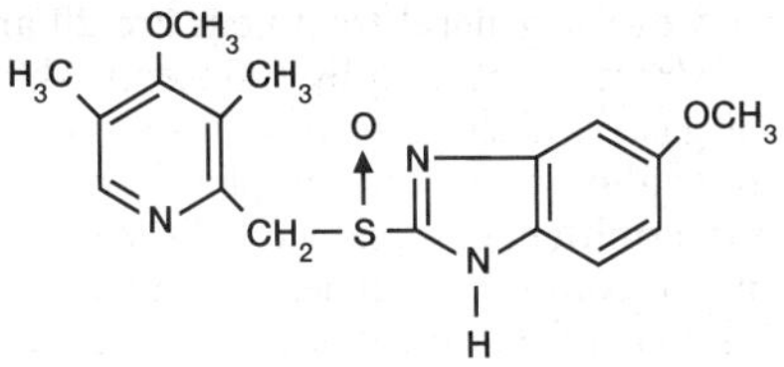

Molecular weight		345.4
pKa (pyridine, benzimidazole)		4.0, 8.7
Solubility		
in alcohol		1 in 25
in water		1 in 7700
Octanol/water partition coefficient	log Kp	2.2

Pharmacology

The exact mechanism of action of omeprazole is still not certain. However the weight of evidence suggests that its effects are mediated by specific binding to the parietal cell proton pump H^+, K^+-ATPase.[1,2] The proton pump is present in a wide variety of animal species and although it is primarily found in gastric parietal cells, there is some evidence that it also exists in the colon and jejuneum.[3,4] In gastric mucosa the enzyme is found on the apical membrane and in tubulovesicles lining the secretory canaliculi of the parietal cell.[5,6]

As a weak base, omeprazole accumulates in acid spaces and thus selectivity to the gastric H^+, K^+-ATPase is afforded in vivo, even though in vitro binding has been noted in dog kidneys.[7] The site of action of omeprazole is clearly distal to cAMP activation[8] and it seems that binding of omeprazole to the proton pump results in inhibition of acid secretion. The drug is activated at the low pH found in secretory canaliculi allowing binding with sulphydryl groups on the enzyme.[9–11] Omeprazole may bind to other ATPases,[12] but the unique acidic pH of the parietal cell tubulovesicles encourages both accumulation and activation of the drug. In vitro, the binding of omeprazole to the proton pump is reversible by washing the tissue.[13] However, in vivo the effects of omeprazole are long lasting and it is likely that the binding of omeprazole is irreversible. New synthesis of enzyme, which occurs at a normal rate[13], may be required before the effects of omeprazole wear off.[14,15]

Omeprazole virtually abolishes gastric acid secretion ($\geqslant$90%) in animal studies.[8] Plasma gastrin concentrations would be expected to rise because of the hypoacidity which may be prolonged. Studies suggest that the rise of plasma gastrin concentration is a secondary effect rather than a direct effect of the drug. Omeprazole has cytoprotective effects in rats, protecting the gastric mucosa from the effects of gastric irritants. This protective effect does not seem to be prostaglandin mediated.[16]

Omeprazole has no effect on the secretion of pepsin[17] but pepsinogen I concentrations rise during therapy with omeprazole.[18] Omeprazole has no effect on hepatic blood flow as assessed by indocyanine green clearance,[19] and also has no effect on renal tubular function.[20]

Toxicology

General tolerance is good with long-term use in doses of up to 138 mg.kg^{-1} in dogs and 414 mg.kg^{-1} in rats and mice.

Gastric mucosal cell hyperplasia has been observed in animals after 3 months high-dose therapy and these changes are prevented by antrectomy.[21] Carcinoid tumours and enterochromaffin-like (ECL) cell hyperplasia have been reported to occur in rats treated for two years with doses ranging from 14 to 140 mg.kg^{-1}. The ECL cell changes were dose-related and female rats were particularly susceptible.[22] ECL cell hyperplasia is reversible on cessation of high-dose omeprazole.[23] The development of ECL cell hyperplasia and carcinoids is thought to be related to hypergastrinaemia produced by prolonged hypochlorhydria. Support for this hypothesis is strong. Plasma gastrin levels in rats receiving omeprazole correlate directly with acid secretory inhibition. Reversible, coordinated gastric mucosal hypertrophy is related to hypergastrinaemia and does not occur in antrectomized animals. It is not clear, however, why ECL cell growth outstrips that of other mucosal constituents with subsequent development of autonomy. In man, circulating levels of gastrin rise during omeprazole treatment.[24–26] However, after four week omeprazole therapy gastrin levels in man are generally considerably lower than levels in treated rodents, in the Zollinger–Ellison syndrome or in pernicious anaemia. Mucosal ECL cell morphology appears unchanged in man following short[27] or long-term use.[28,29] Thus the relevance of gastric mucosal changes in rats and dogs to man is unclear. Drug regulatory bodies in Europe, North America and Australia have accepted this hypothesis.

Clinical pharmacology

Omeprazole decreases basal and stimulated gastric secretion independent of the stimulus. The reduction of pentagastrin-stimulated gastric secretion is dose-dependent with single oral doses between 10 and 80 mg.[30] The highest dose of omeprazole produced nearly complete inhibition of gastric secretion and this effect lasted for at least 4 hours. The duration of action of omeprazole is also known to be dose-dependent and significant inhibition of gastric acid secretion is seen 72 hours after a single dose of 40 mg. Normal gastric acid secretion has returned 3–5 days after a single oral dose[31] and with repeated administration of omeprazole increasing inhibition of gastric acid secretion is seen up to 7 days after oral administration.[32] Studies in patients with peptic ulceration have shown that maximum consistent inhibition of gastric acid secretion occurs in most patients taking 20–30 mg daily. Individual variation in response is greatest at doses lower than 20 mg. Plasma gastrin concentrations rise in patients treated with omeprazole for periods of 7 days or more[24,33,30] and return to pretreatment levels within 7–14 days of stopping treatment.

Pharmacokinetics

Omeprazole is an ampholyte (pKa 4.0 and 8.7). It is poorly soluble in water but dissolves well in alkaline solutions and is rapidly activated at low pH. Oral formulations have changed during its development and have moved from combinations of omeprazole in methylcellulose with sodium bicarbonate to enteric-coated granules. This change prevents much activation of the drug in the luminal acid of the stomach. If drug is activated in the lumen it rapidly binds to sulphydryl groups in gastric mucus and food rendering it non-available.

Formulation differences give widely variable absorption characteristics. The time to maximum plasma concentration ranges from 20 minutes for solutions, 30 minutes for uncoated granules to over 2 hours for enteric-coated granules. Erratic absorption follows administration of the enteric-coated granules as this is dependent on gastric emptying but is of doubtful importance as the plasma concentration/activity relationship is not direct. Although delayed gastric emptying affects peak concentrations, the total amount absorbed and thus available to the parietal cell is unchanged.[34] Maximal plasma concentrations are disproportionate to dosage increments[35] and also relate to the duration of administration. Significant increases in C_{max} and AUC follow repeated oral administration over 5 to 7 days.[36]

Omeprazole may increase its own bioavailability by inhibiting gastric secretion, thus decreasing pre-absorption activation. It may also saturate its own metabolic pathway.

Bioavailability is highly variable and dependent on formulation. It increases with enteric coating and dosage increments. With unbuffered solutions less than 50% is available, while enteric coating increases bioavailability to about 65%. Using buffered solutions of increasing dosage bioavailability was shown to increase from 40% with 10 mg to over 90% with 90 mg.[37] While some of these increments may reflect the saturation of some excretory pathway, they may also be due to increasing absorption following antisecretory activity. Food may delay absorption of the enteric-coated granules but overall systemic bioavailability is unaffected by food or concomitant antacid administration.[38]

Following intravenous administration, omeprazole concentrations fit a two-compartment model.[37] Autoradiographic studies in animals show rapid distribution of omeprazole to the stomach, liver, kidneys, gall bladder, hair follicles, choroid plexus and thyroid gland.[39] Omeprazole crosses the placenta in mice and sheep but in man this information is unavailable. In plasma, omeprazole is bound mainly to albumin and α_1-acid-glycoprotein.

The terminal plasma half life is between 0.5 and 1.5 hours. Accumulation of omeprazole does not occur, at least after 7 days.[24] Omeprazole clearance is not limited by renal disease or by haemodialysis[30,33]

Faecal excretion accounts for 20%, the remainder is excreted in the urine as metabolites.

Oral absorption	50–65%
Presystemic metabolism	
(faecal excretion)	20%
Plasma half life	
range	0.5–1.5 h
mean	1.0 h
Volume of distribution	0.3–0.4 $l.kg^{-1}$
Plasma protein binding	95%

Concentration–effect relationship

There is a clear dose-related inhibition of gastric acid secretion with omeprazole. However, peak concentrations of the drug in plasma are not correlated with antisecretory activity.[25,26] There is some suggestion that there may be a correlation between the area under the plasma concentration versus time curve for omeprazole and its antisecretory effect.[31,35] However, further work is needed to clarify this position.

Metabolism

Omeprazole undergoes rapid and almost complete metabolism. Unchanged omeprazole is not excreted in urine but nearly 20% of administered radiolabel is recovered in the faeces. Six inactive urinary metabolites account for the remaining 80%. There are measurable plasma concentrations of a sulphone metabolite following oral adminstration with a T_{max} delayed by nearly two hours. A sulphide metabolite and hydroxyomeprazole have also been identified in plasma. These three main metabolites are not considered to be active inhibitors of acid secretion.[37]

Pharmaceutics

Omeprazole (Losec; Astra, UK) 20 mg capsules contain white enteric-coated granules. One half of the hard gelatin capsule is dark pink and marked 'A/OM', the other half is brown and marked '20'. An intravenous preparation under investigation is presented as a white powder soluble in polyethylene glycol, and is stable for four hours after dissolution. With refrigeration it has a two-year shelf-life.

Therapeutic use

Indications

Absolute indications for omeprazole are not defined. As a potent antisecretory agent it should have a role as treatment for all the conditions presently managed by histamine H_2-receptor antagonists. Treatment with omeprazole may be considered, in the short term, for the following conditions. Long-term use for maintenance of healing is not recommended.

1. Duodenal ulcer
2. Gastric ulcer
3. Oesophagitis and ulceration
4. Zollinger-Ellison syndrome
5. Treatment of 'resistant' ulcers.

Less clear-cut indications where benefit might be expected but where data are limited include:

6. Prevention of stress ulceration
7. Prevention of the acid aspiration syndrome
8. Treatment of upper gastrointestinal bleeding.

Contraindications

None is known.

Mode of use

Adequate control of gastric acidity is achieved by once daily administration and 2–4 weeks treatment should suffice for the major indications. The doses for general treatment are 20 and 40 mg once daily. Confirmation of ulcer healing by endoscopy should be advised after treatment of gastric ulcer as in recognized practice. The once-daily regimen should allow adequate compliance but the action of the drug itself makes intermittent compliance of little importance. A non-compliant patient will continue to benefit from treatment for up to 3 days. Rapid withdrawal of treatment is also unlikely to be a problem.

Indications

1. Duodenal ulcer healing

Endoscopic healing has been confirmed after two weeks treatment with omeprazole in open and controlled blinded studies. Healing 'rates' at two weeks range from 50% (10 mg daily), 63–69% (20 mg daily), 73–78% (30 mg daily) to 91–95% (40 mg daily). At two weeks the trend certainly suggests a dose–response relationship with healing. After four weeks treatment healing rates are between 90–100% when doses of 20 mg or more are used (see General review articles). In a group of 104 patients, treatment with omeprazole 20 mg or 40 mg daily resulted in healing 'rates' at two weeks of 83%, significantly greater than 53% treated with ranitidine.[40]

Significantly higher healing rates were found when omeprazole 30 mg daily was compared with cimetidine (73% vs 46% at two weeks and 92% vs 74% at four weeks).[41]

2. Gastric ulcer healing

Omeprazole 20 mg daily healed similar numbers of gastric ulcers as ranitidine but rates were generally lower than in duodenal ulcer (43%, 81% and 95% at 2, 4 and 8 weeks).[42,43]

3. Oesophagitis

In a double-blind placebo-controlled trial, omeprazole 20 and 40 mg daily produced endoscopic healing significantly more often than placebo (81% against 6% at four weeks) and symptomatic improvement was equally impressive.[44] Another study using ranitidine as comparator showed significant advantage to omeprazole 40 mg daily. Similar success rates have been reported by numerous groups.[45–48]

4. Zollinger–Ellison syndrome

In patients whose acid hypersecretion is uncontrolled by H_2-receptor antagonists omeprazole has been shown to reduce secretion to $< 10\ mmol.h^{-1}$ in almost all patients in doses of up to 180 mg daily. Some patients have received omeprazole for longer than 5 years and the median dosage requirement is between 60 and 70 mg daily. Details of these patients are given by Lloyd-Davies and others.[49]

5–8. Minor indications

Omeprazole would be expected to prevent much stress ulceration found in acutely ill or burns patients. The rapid antisecretory action could also be useful in emergency anaesthesia to prevent acid aspiration syndromes but more data are required on effects during pregnancy. It is plausible that recurrent bleeding from gastroduodenal lesions may be limited by anacidity but data are awaited. In a recent group of 17 patients with resistant ulcers (failure to heal in 6 months on standard treatments) omeprazole 40 mg daily for up to eight weeks produced 100% healing.[50]

Adverse reactions

Potentially life-threatening effects
None has been reported. The development of carcinoid tumours in rats due to hypergastrinaemia is mentioned above. In man the relative proportions of ECL and G cells are not significantly changed during up to four years treatment.[51]

Acute overdosage
None has been reported; 200 mg intravenously over 24 hours has been given without problem. General supportive measures should be used.

Severe or irreversible adverse effects
None has been reported.

Symptomatic adverse effects
No different from placebo.

Other effects
One report of an increase in alanine aminotransferase[53] has not been confirmed in larger series. No other consistent abnormality of routine biochemical or haematological testing has been reported.[52] An increase in gastric nitrites, nitroso-compounds and bacterial counts would be expected due to hypochlorhydria.[55] Hypergastrinaemia is similarly believed to result from hypochlorhydria though some disagree.[54]

Interference with clinical pathology tests
None is known.

High risk groups

Neonates
There are no data and the drug is not recommended for neonates.
Breast milk. There are no data.

Children
No data available and the drug is not recommended.

Pregnant women
No data available and the drug is not recommended.

The elderly
There is no particular problem in clinical use to date.

Concurrent disease
Bioavailability is increased in liver cirrhosis but there are no reports of increased toxicity.[56]

Drug interactions

Omeprazole inhibits oxidative metabolism of some drugs. Significant increments in diazepam concentrations and prolongation of elimination half life was reported in a group of healthy volunteers receiving 7 days treatment with omeprazole 40 mg daily.[57] Administration of 60 mg daily for 2 weeks caused a 10–20% prolongation of aminopyrine and antipyrine half life[58] while half this dose had no significant effect. In most animal models, the effects of omeprazole on barbiturate sleeping times and antipyrine clearance are less marked than those caused by cimetidine.[59,60] Omeprazole does not interfere with theophylline or propranolol metabolism (data on file, Astra).

In one study, however, omeprazole was a more potent inhibitor of 7 ethoxycoumarin de-ethylase activity than cimetidine.[61] It is too soon to know if important drug interactions will occur with omeprazole, but in a group of 49 patients receiving long-term treatment, concomitant drug administration was not problematical.[52]

General review articles

Borg K O, Olbe L (eds) 1985 Omeprazole; a survey of preclinical data. Scandinavian Journal of Gastroenterology 20 (suppl 108)

Borg K O, Rune S J, Walan A (eds) 1986 Proceedings of the first international symposium on omeprazole. Scandinavian Journal of Gastroenterology 21 (suppl 118)

Clissold S P, Campoli-Richards D M 1986 Omeprazole: a preliminary review of its pharmacodynamic and pharmacokinetic properties and therapeutic potential in peptic ulcer and Zollinger–Ellison syndrome. Drugs 32 (suppl 1): 15–47

Omeprazole

Bader J P, Walan A (eds) 1988 The International Symposium on omeprazole. Scandinavian Journal of Gastroenterology 24 (suppl 166)

References

1. Wallmark B, Jaresten B-M, Larsson H, Ryberg B, Brandstrom A, Fellenius E 1983 Differentiation among inhibitory actions of omeprazole, cimetidine and SCN on gastric acid secretion. American Journal of Physiology 245: G64–G71
2. Wallmark B, Lorentzon P, Larsson H 1985 The mechanism of action of omeprazole — a survey of its inhibitory actions in vitro. Scandinavian Journal of Gastroenterology 20 (suppl 108): 37–52
3. Gustin M C, Goodman D B P 1981 Isolation of brush-border membrane from the rabbit descending colon epithelium. Partial characterization of a unique K^+-activated ATPase. Journal of Biological Chemistry 256: 10 651–10 656
4. White J F 1985 Omeprazole inhibits H^+ secretion by *Amphiuma* jejunum. American Journal of Physiology 248: G256–G259
5. Berglindh T, Sachs G 1985 Emerging strategies in ulcer therapy: pumps and receptors. Scandinavian Journal of Gastroenterology 20 (suppl 108): 7–14
6. Helander H F, Smolka A, Ramsay C-H, Sachs G, Fellenius E 1983 Localization of gastric K^+, H^+-ATPase. Hepato-gastroenterology 30: 74
7. Keeling C J, Fallowfield C, Milliner K J, Tingley S K, Ife R J, Underwood A H 1985 Studies on the mechanism of action of omeprazole. Biochemical Pharmacology 34: 2967–2973
8. Larsson H, Carlsson E, Syndell G 1984 Effects of omeprazole and cimetidine on gastric acid secretion and right atrial beating frequency on isolated organ preparations from the guinea pig. Digestion 29: 12–18
9. Sewing K-Fr, Hannemann H 1985 Studies on the mechanism of action of omeprazole. Naunyn-Schmiedebergs Archives of Pharmacology 239 (suppl): R65
10. Im W B, Blakeman D P, Sachs G 1985 Reversal of antisecretory activity of omeprazole by sulfhydryl compounds in isolated rabbit gastric glands. Biochimica et Biophysica Acta 845: 54–59
11. Im W B, Sih J C, Blakeman D P, McGrath J P 1985 Omeprazole, a specific inhibitor of gastric (H^+-K^+)-ATPase, is a H^+-activated oxidizing agent of sulfhydryl groups. Journal of Biological Chemistry 260: 4591–4597
12. Beil W, Sewing K-Fr 1984 Inhibition of partially purified K^+/H^+-activated oxidizing agent of sulfhydryl groups. Journal of Biological Chemistry 260: 4591–4597
13. Larsson H, Carlsson E, Ryberg B, Fryklund J, Wallmark B 1988 Rat parietal cell function after prolonged inhibition of gastric secretion. American Journal of Physiology 254: 933–939
14. Berglindh T, Hansen D, Bergqvist E 1985 Irreversible inhibition by omeprazole. The in vivo–in vitro connection. Gastroenterology 88: 1322
15. Im W B, Blakeman D P, Davis J P 1985 Irreversible inactivation of rat gastric (H^+-K^+)-ATPase in vivo by omeprazole. Biochemical and Biophysical Research Communications 126: 78–82
16. Mattson H 1986 Protective effects of omeprazole in the gastric mucosa. Scandinavian Journal of Gastroenterology 21 (suppl 118): 86–87
17. Festen H, Thijs J, Lamers C et al 1986 Effect of oral omeprazole on fasting and stimulated gastrin and serum pepsinogen I levels in healthy volunteers. Scandinavian Journal of Gastroenterology 21 (suppl 118): 160–161
18. Festen H P M, Thijs J C, Lamers C B H W et al 1984 Effect of oral omeprazole on serum gastrin and serum pepsinogen I levels. Gastroenterology 87: 1030–1034
19. Nielsen A M, Trap-Jensen J, Bonnevie O, Lech V 1986 Immediate effect of omeprazole and cimetidine on apparent liver blood flow in man. Scandinavian Journal of Gastroenterology 21 (suppl 118): 166–168
20. Howden C W, Payton C D, Meredith P A et al 1985 Antisecretory effect and oral pharmacokinetics of omeprazole in patients with chronic renal failure. European Journal of Clinical Pharmacology 28: 637–640
21. Ekman L, Hansson E, Havu N, Carlsson E, Lundberg C 1985 Toxicological studies on omeprazole. Scandinavian Journal of Gastroenterology 20 (suppl 108): 53–69
22. Carlsson E 1986 Pharmacology and toxicology of omeprazole — with special reference to the effects on the gastric mucosa. Scandinavian Journal of Gastroenterology 21 (suppl 118): 108–116
23. Stockman P, Polsch U R, Bonatz G, Wulfrath M, Creutzfeldt W 1984 Influence of a substituted benzimidazole (omeprazole) on rat gastric endocrine cells. Digestive Diseases and Sciences 29 (suppl) 83S.
24. Sharma B K, Walt R P, Pounder R E, Gomes M De F A, Wood E C, Logan L H 1984 Optimal dose of oral omeprazole for maximal 24 hour decrease of intragastric acidity. Gut 25: 957–964
25. Pounder R E, Sharma B K, Walt R P 1986 Twenty four hour intragastric acidity during treatment with oral omeprazole. Scandinavian Journal of Gastroenterology 21 (suppl 118): 108–116
26. Allen J M, Adrian T E, Webster J, Howe A, Bloom S R 1984 Effect of single dose of omeprazole on the gastrointestinal peptide response to food. Hepato-gastroenterology 31: 44–46
27. Karvonen A L, Keyrilainen O, Uusitalo A et al 1986 Effects of omeprazole in duodenal ulcer patients. Scandinavian Journal of Gastroenterology 21: 449–454
28. Lloyd-Davies K K A, Rutgersson K, Solvell L 1986 Omeprazole in Zollinger–Ellison syndrome: four-year international study. Gastroenterology 90: 1523
29. Lamberts R, Creutzfeldt W, Stockmann F, Vacubaschke U, Maas S, Brunner G 1988 Long-term omeprazole treatment in man: Effects on gastric endocrine cell populations. Digestion 39: 126–135
30. Howden C W, Reid J L 1984 Omeprazole, a gastric 'proton pump inhibitor': lack of effect on renal handling of electrolytes and ordinary acidification. European Journal of Clinical Pharmacology 26: 639–640
31. Lind T, Cederberg C, Ekenved G, Haglund U, Olbe L 1983 Effect of omeprazole — a gastric proton pump inhibitor — on pentagastrin stimulated acid secretion in man. Gut 24: 270–276

32. Cederberg C, Ekenved G, Lind T, Olbe L 1985 Acid inhibitory characteristics of omeprazole in man. Scandinavian Journal of Gastroenterology 20 (suppl 108): 105–112
33. Naesdal J, Anderson T, Bodemar G et al 1985 Pharmacokinetics of ^{14}C omeprazole in patients with impaired renal function. Scandinavian Journal of Gastroenterology 20 (suppl 113): 34
34. Prichard P J, Yeomans N D, Mihaly G W et al 1985 Omeprazole: a study of its inhibition of gastric pH and oral pharmacokinetics after morning or evening dosage. Gastroenterology 88: 64–69
35. Londong W, Londong V, Cederberg C, Steffen H 1983 Dose–response study of omeprazole on meal-stimulated gastric acid secretion and gastrin release. Gastroenterology 85: 1373–1378
36. Howden C W, Meredith P A, Forrest J A H, Reid J L 1984 Oral pharmacokinetics of omeprazole. European Journal of Clinical Pharmacology 26: 641–643
37. Regardh C-G, Gabrielsson M, Hoffman K-J, Lofberg I, Skaberg I 1985 Pharmacokinetics and metabolism of omeprazole in animals and man — an overview. Scandinavian Journal of Gastroenterology 20 (suppl 108): 79–94
38. Pilbrant A, Cederberg C 1985 Development of an oral formulation of omeprazole. Scandinavian Journal of Gastroenterology 20 (suppl 108): 113–120
39. Helander H, Ramsay C-H, Regardh C-G 1985 Localization of omeprazole and metabolites in the mouse. Scandinavian Journal of Gastroenterology 20 (suppl 108): 95–104
40. Bardhan K D, Bianch Porro G, Bose K et al 1985 Comparisons of two different doses of omeprazole versus ranitidine in duodenal ulcer (DU) healing. Gut 26: A557–A558
41. Lauritsen K, Rune S J, Bytzer P, Kelbaek H, Jensen K G et al 1985 Effect of omeprazole and cimetidine on duodenal ulcer. New England Journal of Medicine 312: 958–961
42. Barbara L, Saggioro A, Olsson J, Cisternino M, Franceschi M 1987 Omeprazole 20 mg om and ranitidine 150 mg bd in the healing of benign gastric ulcers – an Italian Multicentre Study. Gut 28: A1341
43. Walan A, Bader J P, Classen M, Lamers C B, Piper D, Rutgersoon R 1987 Omeprazole and ranitidine in the treatment of benign gastric ulcer — an international multicentre study. Gut 28: A1340
44. Hetzel D J, Dent J, Laurence B H, Reed W D, Narielvala F, Shearman D J C 1986 Omeprazole heals reflux oesophagitis: a placebo controlled trial. Gut 27: A609
45. Klinkenberg-Knol E C, Jansen J M B J, Festen H P M, Meuwissen S G M, Lamers C B H W 1987 Double-blind multicentre comparison of omeprazole and ranitidine in the treatment of reflux oesophagitis. Lancet 1: 349–351
46. Hetzel D J, Dent J, Reed W, Mitchell B, Beveridge B et al 1987 Healing of peptic oesophagitis with omeprazole: a dose–response study. Gastroenterology 92: 1434
47. Vantrappen G, Coenegrachts J L, Rutgeerts L, Schurmans P 1987 Omeprazole (40 mg) is superior to ranitidine in the short term treatment of ulcerative reflux oesophagitis. Gastroenterology 92: 1681
48. Klinkenberg-Knol M, Festen H P M, Meuwissen S G M 1987 Omeprazole compared to ranitidine in effect on 24-hour pH in the distal oesophagus of patients with reflux oesophagitis. A double-blind trial. Gastroenterology 92: 1471
49. Lloyd-Davies K A, Rutgersson R, Solvell L 1988 Omeprazole in the treatment of Zollinger–Ellison Syndrome: a 4-year international study. Aliment. Pharmacology Therapeutics 2: 13–32
50. Tytgat G N J, Lamers C B H W, Wilson J A, Hameeteman W, Jansen J B M J et al 1985 100% healing with omeprazole of peptic ulcers resistant to histamine H_2-receptor antagonists. Gastroenterology 88: 1620
51. Brunner G, Creutzfeldt W, Harke U, Lamberts R 1988 Therapy with omeprazole in patients with peptic ulcerations resistant to extended high dose ranitidine treatment. Digestion 39: 81–83
52. Soelvell L 1986 Safety aspects of omeprazole. Scandinavian Journal of Gastroenterology 21 (suppl 118): 129–134
53. Gustavsson S, Aami H-O, Loof L, Nybern O 1983 Rapid healing of duodenal ulcers with omeprazole. Lancet 2: 124–125
54. Wormsley K G 1984 Assessing the safety of drugs for the long-term treatment of peptic ulcers. Gut 25: 1416–1423
55. Sharma B K, Santana I A, Wood E C et al 1984 Intragastric bacterial activity and nitrosation before, during and after treatment with omeprazole. British Medical Journal 289: 717–719
56. Andersson T, Olsson Skanberg I, Heggelund A, Johnsson G, Lundborg P, Regardh C G 1986 Pharmacokinetics of omeprazole in patients with liver cirrhosis. Acta Pharmacologica et Toxicologica 59 (suppl 5): 203
57. Gugler R, Jensen J C 1984 Omeprazole inhibits elimination of diazepam. Lancet 1: 969
58. Henry D A, Somerville K W, Kitchingman G, Langman M J S 1984 Omeprazole: effects on oxidative drug metabolism. British Journal of Clinical Pharmacology 18: 195–200
59. Henry D A, Gerkens J F, Brent P, Somerville K 1984 Inhibition of drug metabolism by omeprazole. Lancet 2: 46–47
60. Webster L K, Jones D B, Smallwood R A 1984 How potent is the inhibition of drug metabolism by omeprazole? Lancet 2: 761
61. Gugler R, Jensen J C 1985 Omeprazole inhibits oxidative drug metabolism. Gastroenterology 89: 1235–1241

Ondansetron (hydrochloride)

Ondansetron is a selective 5-hydroxytryptamine (5HT3) receptor antagonist which was licensed for the first time in 1990 for the treatment of nausea and vomiting related to cancer chemotherapy and radiotherapy.

Chemistry

Ondansetron hydrochloride (Zofran, Zophren)
$C_{18}H_{19}N_3O$, HCl. $2H_2O$
1,2,3,9-Tetrahydro-9-methyl-3-[(2-methylimidazole-1-yl) methyl]-4H-carbazol-4-one, hydrochloride dihydrate

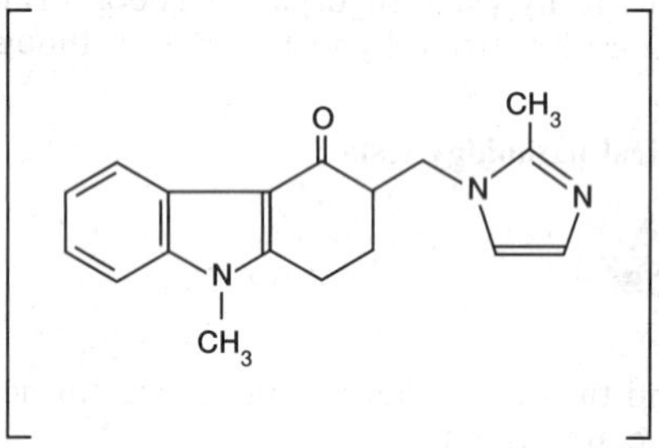

Molecular weight (free base)	365.8 (293.3)
pKa	7.4
Solubility	
in alcohol	—
in water	1 in 3
Octanol/water partition coefficient	—

Ondansetron hydrochloride is a white to off-white solid prepared by chemical synthesis. It is not present in any compound preparations.

Pharmacology

Ondansetron is a highly selective 5HT3 receptor antagonist, which inhibits nausea and vomiting caused by cytotoxic agents and radiation. Its action is believed to be mediated via antagonism of 5-hydroxytryptamine receptors located in the chemoreceptor trigger zone in the area postrema of the brain[1,2] and possibly on vagal afferents in the upper gastrointestinal tract.[3] Selective 5HT3-receptor antagonism by ondansetron has been demonstrated in ferrets[4] and guinea-pigs.[5] Ondansetron also acts to enhance gastric emptying.[5]

Ondansetron appears to have no effect on vascular dopamine receptors in the mesenteric bed of the anaesthetized dog or presynaptic dopamine receptors on sympathetic nerves in the heart.

Toxicology

Ondansetron has little acute toxicity in rodents and dogs, subdued activity, ataxia and convulsions being seen only at near lethal doses, some 30–100 times the human dose.

Serum transaminases rose by less than 50% in some rodents, but no long-term liver damage was seen. At doses less than 3 $mg.kg^{-1}$ intravenously, ondansetron has no significant cardiovascular effects in the anaesthetized cat or the conscious dog or monkey.

No teratogenic, reproductive or oncogenic effects have been identified.

Clinical pharmacology

Ondansetron is an effective anti-emetic in patients receiving chemotherapy and radiotherapy[6–11] and has been particularly useful in the

Ondansetron (hydrochloride)

control of vomiting in patients receiving cisplatin[8,9]. From studies in laboratory animals such as ferrets, the site of action of ondansetron is likely to be at 5HT3 receptor sites in the visceral afferent vagus and in the area postrema of the brain. Ondansetron causes an increase in the rate of gastric emptying both in animals[5] and in man.[12] However the gastric emptying rate appears to be increased only when the basal rate of gastric emptying is slow. Ondansetron slows gastrointestinal transit time as shown by a doubling of the whole-gut transit time in 10 healthy volunteers given 16 mg ondansetron three times daily for 7 days compared to controls.[13] Constipation may thus follow the use of ondansetron. Ondansetron is not effective in the treatment of motion sickness,[14] compared to a standard therapy such as hyoscine.

Ondansetron has no effect on normal behaviour patterns in animals, even at high dosage. In human studies there has been no evidence of any activity in the central nervous system and no evidence of dependence liability.[15] The commonest adverse effect is a mild headache and dystonic reactions are much less likely than with agents such as metoclopramide.

Pharmacokinetics

High performance liquid chromatography after solid phase extraction is the method of choice for determining the plasma concentration of ondansetron.[15] The limit of sensitivity of the assay is 1 μg. l^{-1}.

Following oral administration ondansetron is rapidly absorbed, with a lag of approximately 30 min before absorption is measurable. Maximum concentration is usually achieved after 1–1.5 h, a maximum plasma concentration of approximately 30 μg.l^{-1} being achieved after a single dose of 8 mg. After dosing at 8 mg three times daily for 6 days, a steady-state maximum concentration of 40 μg.l^{-1} was achieved. Oral bioavailability in healthy volunteers has been reported as 59%.

Ondansetron is moderately highly bound to plasma proteins, 70–76%. It is rapidly distributed throughout the body, with a volume of distribution of 163 ± 25 l.

Ondansetron is rapidly cleared from the body, almost entirely by metabolism, with less than 10% of an intravenous dose being recovered unchanged in the urine. The terminal plasma half life is approximately 3 h.

The extent to which ondansetron is excreted in breast milk or crosses the placenta is not known.

Ondansetron is extensively metabolized in the liver.

Oral absorption	59%
Presystemic metabolism	high
Plasma half life	3.3 ± 0.8 h
Volume of distribution	163 ± 25 l
Plasma protein binding	70–76%

Concentration–effect relationship

Complete blockade of 5HT3 receptors is believed to be achieved by plasma concentrations of ondansetron greater than 30 μg.l^{-1}. Pharmacokinetic modelling suggested that these levels could be achieved by ondansetron administered as an 8 mg intravenous loading dose followed by 1 mg.h^{-1} for 24 h. The results of several studies suggest complete or major control of emesis in 72–86% of patients receiving non-cisplatin chemotherapy[12], but there was no dose-related enhancement of control and no relationship between efficacy and plasma levels of ondansetron.[17]

Metabolism

The oral absorption of ondansetron is rapid. The renal clearance of the drug is low, indicating that the major route of systemic clearance is by metabolism.[18]

The major route of metabolism is hydroxylation followed by glucuronide or sulphate conjugation. N-Demethylation is a minor route of metabolism (See Table 1 and Fig. 1). The activity of the metabolites is not known. Less than 10% of the drug is excreted unchanged in urine.

Fig. 1 The metabolism of ondansetron

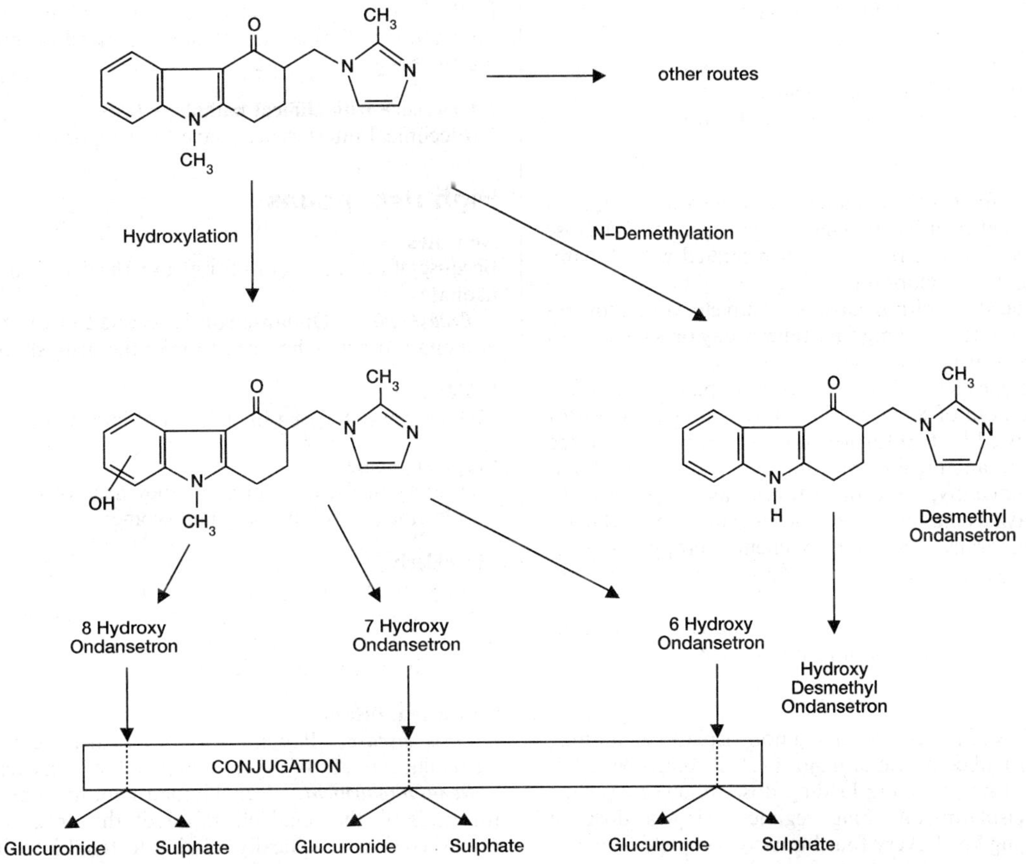

O

Table 1 Urinary recoveries of a radiolabeled dose of Ondansetron to healthy volunteers

Unchanged ondansetron	<10%
Glucuronide conjugates	45%
Sulphate conjugates	20%
Hydroxylation products N-Demmethylation products	10%
Unidentified products	15%

Pharmaceutics

Ondansetron (Zofran; Glaxo, UK) is available in both oral and parenteral forms.

1. Ondansetron tablets contain ondansetron base as the hydrochloride dihydrate, lactose, microcrystalline cellulose, starch and magnesium stearate. Tablets containing 4 mg or 8 mg are film-coated, oval, yellow and engraved '4' or '8' on one face and 'Glaxo' on the other.

The tablets have demonstrated good chemical and physical stability, with no significant change in ondansetron content after storage at 45°C/50% relative humidity for 6 months or 37°C/50% relative humidity for 12 months. If stored at temperatures below 30°C, shelf-life is 2 years.[19]

2. Ondansetron for injection is an aqueous solution containing ondansetron base as the hydrochloride dihydrate at a concentration of 2 $mg.ml^{-1}$. Sodium citrate and citric acid monohydrate are added to buffer the solution at pH 3.5 and sodium chloride is added to achieve isotonicity. The injection solution is filled into ampoules to provide dose volumes of 2 ml and 4 ml, equivalent to 4 mg and 8 mg ondansetron respectively.

Ondansetron may be diluted for administration by slow intravenous injection or infusion, and is compatible with several infusion fluids including sodium chloride BP 0.9% and glucose BP 5% w/v. Ondansetron injection should be protected from light, and should not be mixed in the same syringe or infusion with any other medication. The shelf-life is 3 years when stored below 30°C and protected from light.[20]

Therapeutic use

Indications

1. The control of nausea and vomiting associated with the treatment of cancer by radiotherapy and chemotherapy.

Contraindications

1. Hypersensitivity to any of the components.
   As yet, there are no other reported contraindications.

Mode of use

A major indication is for (a) those patients who have not achieved adequate control with alternative antiemetic regimens, and (b) those who have experienced dystonic reactions when treated with dopamine antagonists such as metoclopramide.

Radiotherapy-induced vomiting gave a complete or major response of 71–91% for a dose of 4 mg four times a day or 8 mg twice a day with no advantage at higher dose.

For highly emetogenic chemotherapy (such as cisplatin-containing regimens), a loading dose of 8 mg by slow intravenous injection or 15 min infusion followed by two further doses of 8 mg administered similarly 4 h apart or an infusion of 1 $mg.h^{-1}$ for up to 24 h is recommended. Subsequently, 8 mg three times daily may be given orally for up to 5 days as maintenance. For less emetogenic chemotherapy, either 8 mg orally 2 h prior to chemotherapy, or 8 mg intravenously immediately before chemotherapy may be given, followed by the same maintenance regimen.

During radiotherapy, 8 mg 8-hourly commencing 12 h prior to the first fraction of radiotherapy has been recommended.

Indications

In pilot studies, 92% of patients receiving non-cisplatin containing chemotherapy, either had complete or major (<1–2 vomits per 24 h) control of emesis by using an 8 mg loading dose followed by 8 mg eight-hourly[21]. In cisplatin-containing regimes using a dose of ondansetron of 0.15 $mg.kg^{-1}$ every four hours, a complete or major response was seen in 73% of patients receiving ondasetron over the first 24 h[17]. No significant reduction in vomiting or nausea was seen after the first day.

Adverse reactions

Potentially life-threatening effects
No deaths caused by ondansetron have been reported.

Acute overdosage
Four patients have been reported to have received intravenous doses up to tenfold the recommended dose, with only minor adverse effects.

Severe or irreversible adverse effects
None has been reported.

Symptomatic adverse effects
Ondansetron is generally well tolerated. Constipation is the commonest complaint, probably mediated via the 5HT3 receptors found in the gut. There is slowing of the intestinal transit time in both healthy volunteers and patients receiving both chemotherapy and radiotherapy.

An occasional complaint is of headache, but this is rarely severe. Flushing or a sensation of warmth have occasionally been noted during infusion of ondansetron.

Healthy volunteer studies have resulted in 223 volunteers receiving ondansetron on 1638 occasions until December 1988. The commonest side effect was headache occurring in 17% of patients given ondansetron in a single dose and in 31.4% of patients receiving the drug in repeated doses. These differences were not significant. Constipation occurred in 7.1% of patients receiving ondansetron in repeated doses and in none of the placebo group.

In trials comparing ondansetron and metoclopramide against cisplatin-induced emesis there was a significant increase in the incidence of headache: 19% for ondansetron. 10% for metoclopramide, and constipation: 7% and 2% respectively. However, no extrapyramidal effects were seen in the ondansetron group compared with 5% treated with metoclopramide. Flushing was more common in patients treated with metoclopramide compared with ondansetron, 2% against none. Sedation, abdominal discomfort and diarrhoea occurred equally in both groups.

Other effects
In 9/223 healthy volunteers, elevation of liver transaminases were observed. In all cases, the changes resolved promptly on discontinuing the drug.

Interference with clinical pathology tests
No technical interferences have been reported.

High risk groups

Neonates
Because of the indications for its use, the drug is unlikely to be used in neonates.

Breast milk. Ondansetron is secreted in the breast milk of rats. Nursing mothers who need to take the drug should not breast-feed.

Children
The drug may be used in children, if indicated, in appropriate doses.

Pregnant women
The safety of the drug in pregnancy has not been established and it should not be used by pregnant women.

The elderly
Studies in the elderly have demonstrated similar pharmacokinetic parameters to those in younger patients although there is a tendancy for plasma half life to be increased, 5.0 h (4.3–5.8) compared with 3.2–3.7 h for younger volunteers.

Concurrent disease
Liver disease. Patients with severe hepatic disease would be at particular risk of toxicity and have so far been excluded from studies.

Renal impairment. Renal impairment was not an exclusion factor for trials as the renal clearance of the drug is low. There is no published data specifically relating to renal impairment.

Ondansetron (hydrochloride)

Drug interactions

No interactions with other centrally acting drugs (such as diazepam, alcohol or morphine), or any interaction with concomitantly prescribed antiemetics, have yet been identified. The potential for enhanced antiemetic activity when used in conjunction with other agents, for example corticosteroids, is under active investigation.

Clinical trials

1. Marty M, Pouillart P, Scholl S et al 1990 New England Journal of Medicine 322: 816–821

The authors compare the efficacy of ondansetron with metoclopramide in a crossover study of the control of cisplatin-induced vomiting in 76 patients. Ondansetron was given as an 8 mg loading dose followed by an infusion of 1 mg.h^{-1} for 24 h. Metoclopramide was given as a 3 mg.kg^{-1} loading dose followed by a 4 mg.kg^{-1} infusion over 8 h.

A statistically significant improvement in complete or nearly complete (less than two vomits) control of vomiting was seen with ondansetron, 75% vs 42% ($p<0.001$). Ondansetron was also more effective at reducing nausea as assessed with a patient-completed visual analogue scale. There was a significant ($p=0.006$) patient preference for ondansetron rather than metoclopramide.

2. Priestman T J 1989 Clinical Studies with ondansetron in control of radiation-induced emesis European Journal of Cancer 25 (suppl 1): S29–S33

Ondansetron 8 mg three times daily orally was compared with metoclopramide 10 mg three times daily in the control of nausea and vomiting induced by radiotherapy to the upper abdomen (given as a single dose of 8–10 Gy to a 100 cm^2 field centred on T10–L2 or larger fields centred on T8–T3).

Ondansetron achieved better control of both nausea and vomiting than metoclopramide on the day of treatment. An advantage for ondansetron was also seen on days 2 and 3 following treatment, but this did not reach a statistically significant level. Only two patients experienced side effects attributed to ondansetron (one headache, and the other headache and vertigo).

Ondansetron was superior to metoclopramide in the control of vomiting (97% vs 45% absence of vomiting; $P<0.001$) and nausea (95% vs 61% none or mild nausea; $P<0.001$) on the day of treatment.

3. Bonneterre J, Chevallier B, Metz R et al 1990 Journal of Clinical Oncology 8: 1063–1069

75 previously untreated patients with breast cancer starting treatment with combination chemotherapy (cyclophosphamide, 5-fluorouracil and adriamycin or epirubicin) were randomly assigned to receive ondansetron (8 mg loading dose, and 8 mg three times daily for 3–5 days) or metoclopramide (80 mg loading dose, and 20 mg three times daily for 3–5 days) in a double-blind crossover study. In the first 24 hours, complete or major control of emesis was achieved in 86% (30 of 55) of patients receiving ondansetron compared with 42% (14 of 33) of patients receiving metoclopramide ($p<0.001$). On days 2 and 3, control of emesis was significantly better with ondansetron, but there was no statistical difference in the control of nausea. Extrapyramidal reactions were seen in two patients receiving metoclopramide, none with ondansetron. There was a significant patient preference for ondansetron (63% vs 26%, $p=0.001$).

References

1. Smith W C, Callahan E M, Alphin R S 1988 The emetic activity of centrally-administered cisplatin in cats and its antagonism by zacopride. Journal of Pharmacy and Pharmacology 40: 142–143
2. Higgins G A, Kilpatrick G J, Bunce K T, Jones B J, Tyers M B 1989 5HT$_3$ receptor antagonists injected into the area postrema inhibits cisplatin-induced emesis in the ferret. British Journal of Pharmacology 97: 247–255
3. Gunning S, Hagan R M, Tyers M B 1987 Cisplatin induces biochemical and histological changes in the small intestine of the ferret. British Journal of Pharmacology 90: 135P
4. Andrew P L R, Bailey H E, Hawthorn J, Stables R, Tyers M B 1987 GR38 032F, a novel 5HT3 receptor antagonist, can abolish emesis induced by cyclophosphamide and radiation in the ferret. British Journal of Pharmacology 91 (suppl): 1417P
5. Costall B, Gunning S J, Naylor R J, Tyers M B 1987 The effect of GR38 032F, a novel 5HT3 receptor antagonist on gastric emptying in the guinea pig. British Journal of Pharmacology 91: 263–164
6. Cunningham D, Hawthorne J, Pople A, Gazet J-C, Ford H T, Challoner T 1987 Prevention of emesis in patients receiving cytotoxic drugs by GR 38 032F, a selective 5-HT3 receptor antagonist. Lancet 1: 1461–1463
7. Kris M G, Gralla R J, Clark R A, Tyson L B 1988 Dose-ranging evaluation of the serotonin antagonist GR-C507/75 (GR 38 032F) when used as an antiemetic in patients receiving anticancer chemotherapy. Journal of Clinical Oncology 6: 659–662
8. Marty M, Droz J-P, Pouillart P, Paule B, Brion N, Bons J 1989 GR38 032F, a 5-HT3 receptor antagonist, in the prophylaxis of acute cisplatin-induced nausea and vomiting. Cancer Chemotherapy and Pharmacology 23: 389–391
9. Marty M, Pouillart P, Scholl S et al 1990 Comparison of the 5-HT3 (serotonin) antagonist ondansetron (GR38 032F) with high-dose metoclopramide in the control of cisplatin-induced emesis. New England Journal of Medicine 322: 816–821
10. Priestman T J 1989 Clinical studies with ondansetron in the control of radiation-induced emesis. European Journal of Cancer and Clinical Oncology 25(suppl): S29–S33
11. Bonneterre J, Chevallier B, Metz R et al 1990 A randomized double-blind comparison of ondansetron and metoclopramide in the prophylaxis of emesis induced by cyclophosphamide, fluorouracil and doxorubicin or epirubicin chemotherapy. Journal of Clinical Oncology 8: 1063–1069
12. Blackwell C P, Harding S M 1989 Clinical Pharmacology of Ondansetron. European Journal of Cancer and Clinical Oncology 25 (Suppl 1) S21–S24
13. Gore S, Gilmore I T, Haigh C G, Brownless S M, Stockdale H 1990. Colonic transit in man is slowed by Ondansetron (GR 38032F), a selective 5-hydroxytryptamine receptor (type 3) antagonist. Alimentary Pharmacology and Therapeutics 4: 139–144
14. Stott J R R, Barnes G R, Wright R J, Ruddock C J S 1989 The effect on motion sickness and oculomotor function of GR 38032F, a 5HT$_3$ receptor antagonist with anti-emetic properties British Journal of Clinical Pharmacology 27: 147–158
15. Smith P N 1989 Safety of Ondansetron. European Journal of Cancer and Clinical Oncology 25 Suppl 1: S47–S50
16. Colthup P V, Palmer J L 1989 The determination in plasma and pharmacokinetics of ondansetron. European Journal of Cancer and Clinical Oncology 25(suppl): S71–S74
17. Marty M 1989 Ondansetron in the prophylaxis of acute cisplatin-induced nausea and vomiting. European Journal of Cancer and Clinical Oncology 25 (suppl): S41–S46
18. Saynor D A, Dixon C M 1989 The metabolism of ondansetron. European Journal of Cancer and Clinical Oncology 25 (suppl): S75–S77
19. Leak R E, Woodford J D 1989 The pharmaceutical development of ondansetron tablets. European Journal of Cancer and Clinical Oncology 25 (suppl): S63–S66
20. Leak R E, Woodford J D 1989 The pharmaceutical development of ondansetron injection. European Journal of Cancer and Clinical Oncology 25 (suppl): S67–S70
21. Schmoll H-J 1989 The role of ondansetron in the treatment of emesis induced by non-cisplatin-containing chemotherapy regimes. European Journal of Cancer and Clinical Oncology 25 (Suppl): S35–S39

Oral rehydration salts

The discovery that simple glucose–electrolyte solutions could adequately rehydrate patients with cholera is one of the major therapeutic advances of this century and over the last 20 years has saved the lives of many thousands of children. It has become the mainstay of treatment for the dehydration and acidosis associated with acute infectious diarrhoea.

Chemistry

Oral rehydration solutions (ORS, WHO-ORS, Electrolade, Glucolyte, Rehidrat, Pedialyte). All oral rehydration solutions contain the following constituents in combination although the concentrations of each individual component may vary (see Table 1): sodium, potassium, chloride, base—bicarbonate, citrate, lactate and glucose.

ORS may be available as a colourless aqueous solution, but more usually as a white powder which is sterile and made up fresh as required in clean potable water before ingestion. Artificial flavourings are occasionally added in an attempt to make the solutions more palatable.

Pharmacology

The key constituents of ORS are sodium and glucose. The central principle of oral rehydration therapy (ORT) is the utilization of sodium-glucose co-transport in the small intestine, a phenomenon which remains largely unaffected during acute infectious diarrhoea.[1] Thus the success of ORT is largely dependent on glucose-driven sodium absorption (transcellular route) leading to passive absorption of water by the paracellular route. The clinical result is usually rapid rehydration and correction of acidosis.

Toxicology

All the constituents of oral rehydration salts are physiological and when used appropriately are not toxic.

Clinical pharmacology

The major cause of morbidity and mortality in diarrhoeal disease is the loss of water and electrolytes from the intestine with ensuing acidosis, hypovolaemia and hypoperfusion of vital organs. Cholera is the archetypal secretory diarrhoea although other bacterial and viral enteropathogens can have similar but generally milder effects. To prevent these potentially serious complications, it is imperative that the lost fluid and electrolytes are replaced rapidly. Since the 19th century it has been known that this can be accomplished via the intravenous route using physiological solutions.[2] However, clinical and physiological discoveries over the last 25 years have promoted the concept of rehydration via the oral route, so-called oral rehydration therapy (ORT). The scientific rationale for ORT is based on the phenomenon of co-transport whereby sodium ions cross the small intestinal epithelium simultaneously with hexoses and other organic molecules such as amino acids by a series of common carrier proteins.[3] The discovery that this phenomenon remains intact during diarrhoeal diseases has allowed for its clinical exploitation in ORT.

Figure 1 summarizes the major small intestinal electrolyte transport systems in man.

Sodium absorption

Sodium absorption is accomplished by three different processes, the energy required being generated by the 'sodium pump' situated on the basolateral membrane of the enterocyte. This sodium-K-ATPase is a 250-300kDa molecular weight transport protein which extrudes sodium from the cell in exchange for potassium in a stoichiometric

Fig. 1 Electrolyte transport in the enterocyte

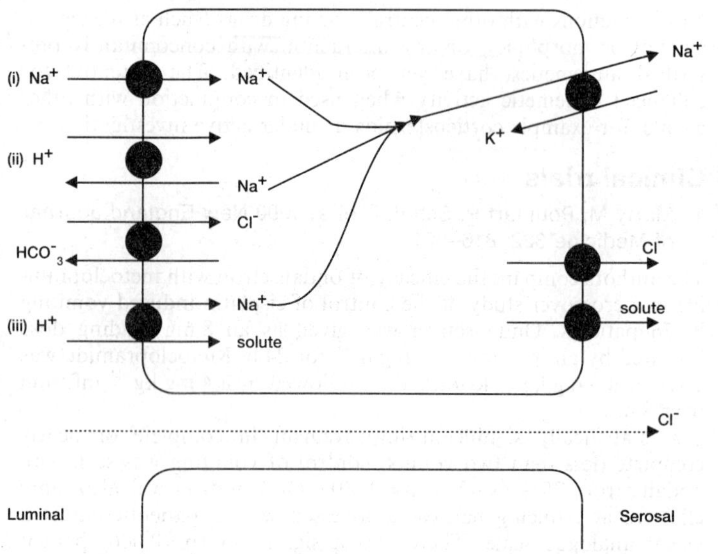

ratio of 3:2. The effect of the sodium pump is to maintain a low intracellular sodium concentration thereby keeping the interior of the cell relatively electronegative.

i. 'Electrogenic' non-nutrient coupled Na absorption appears to be present both in the small and large intestine. Sodium ions enter the cell passively through selective ion channels down the electrochemical gradient.
ii. 'Neutral' NaC1 absorption occurs mainly in the ileum and appears to be accomplished through the action of a pair of linked ion exchangers. The Na/H antiport or cation exchanger serves to maintain the intracellular pH, increasing it in the presence of extracellular sodium. In the ileum the $C1/HCO_3$ antiport is the anion exchanger which acts in consort with the Na/H antiport to maintain electroneutrality. Both of these transport systems operate with a 1:1 stoichiometry.
iii. The final mechanism of sodium entry into the enterocyte is coupled non-electrogenic sodium absorption which operates in both the jejunum and ileum and is the most important therapeutically. Sodium absorption is coupled to the absorption of a variety of organic solutes including glucose, amino acids, bile salts, water-soluble vitamins and organic acids. Carrier proteins responsible for sodium entry are situated in the brush border membrane and one of the best characterised is the Na-glucose symporter. This carrier protein utilizes the potential energy released as sodium ions enter the epithelial cells down their electrochemical gradient to drive the 'up hill' movement of glucose in the same direction. The 'down hill' electrochemical gradient for Na is, as stated above, maintained by the Na-K-ATPase of the basolateral enterocyte membrane. The configuration of the symporter is such that it is only operative when the sodium-and glucose-binding sites are occupied. Sodium efflux occurs via by the sodium pump while solute leaves the cell via means of facilitated diffusion across the basolateral membrane (Figure 2).

Chloride absorption. Chloride ions cross the epithelium transcellularly through the action of the coupled ion exchangers but are also absorbed by the paracellular route down the electrical gradient (serosa positive, lumen negative) generated by the 'electrogenic' and 'coupled' mechanisms of sodium entry. In the small intestine most net chloride absorption takes place via the coupled Na-C1 transport mechanism which is particularly active in the jejunum. However, in the distal ileum and colon, chloride absorption also occurs by a Cl/HCO_3 anion exchanger.

Potassium absorption. In the small intestine potassium ions are absorbed passively via the paracellular route. However, in the colon both passive absorption and active secretion of potassium ions have been described.

Water transport. Water absorption occurs by the passive route and is always secondary to the active transport of electrolytes or

Oral rehydration salts

Fig. 2 Solute-coupled sodium absorption

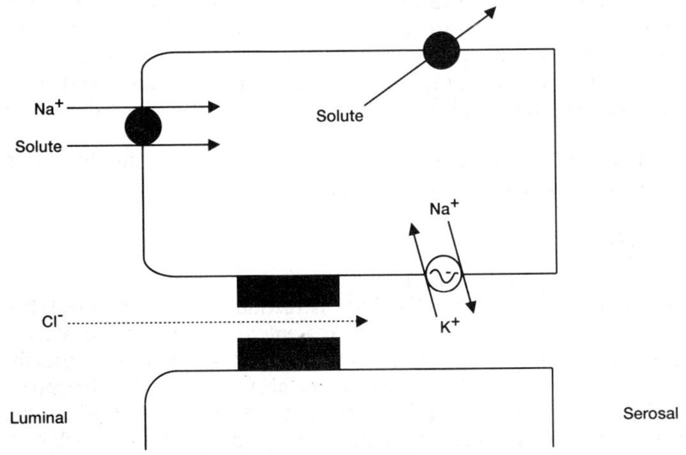

other solutes, increasing directly in proportion to the amount of solute transported.

Mechanisms of acute infectious diarrhoea.
Many infectious agents cause acute diarrhoeal disease and in the developed world rotavirus accounts for almost 50% of all cases of acute diarrhoea. Other viruses such as enteric adenoviruses (types 40 & 41) and Norwalk virus are also important while the majority of other infections are due to bacterial enteropathogens.

Rotavirus diarrhoea. After oral ingestion, virions are bound to the brush border membrane of the mature enterocytes in the region of the villus tip by specific receptors which have been shown to be present in much greater numbers in the mucosa of younger animals.[4] Once bound, the virions invade the enterocyte leading eventually to cell death, exfoliation and a progressive shortening of the villus. The crypt region responds by increasing cell production rate and the small intestinal mucosa becomes rapidly repopulated by immature cells. Thus there is a paucity of mature enterocytes resulting in a decrease in the functional mucosal surface area. In addition, nutrient and electrolyte transport functions of the damaged mucosa are perturbed because of the preponderance of immature crypt-type cells. The resulting diarrhoea therefore has two components: osmolar (resulting from the malabsorption of nutrients especially disaccharides) and secretory (due to the reduced capacity for sodium chloride absorption).

Bacterial diarrhoea. A number of bacteria are known to cause enteric infection and acute diarrhoea. To cause diarrhoeal disease the majority of bacterial enteropathogens must colonize and proliferate in the small intestine and/or colon. Despite the diversity of bacteria able to cause diarrhoea the pathogenetic mechanisms responsible can be grouped into four categories:

Adherence (enterpathogenic *Escherichia coli*)
Invasion (*Shigella, Salmonella, C. jejuni, Y. enterocolitica,* enteroinvasive *E. coli*)
Cytotoxin production (*C. difficile, Shigella,* enterohaemorrhagic *E. coli*)
Enterotoxin production (*Vibrio cholerae, Vibrio parahaemolyticus, C. jejuni, Y. enterocolitica, Aeromonas hydrophila* and enterotoxigenic *E. coli*)

Invasive enteropathogens usually affect the distal ileum and colon although *Campylobacter jejuni* has also been shown to colonize the jejunum.[5] The ensuing inflammation particularly reduces colonic absorptive function which normally absorbs over 90% of the fluid passing the ileo-caecal valve. Inflammatory mediators such as prostaglandins and kinins are also thought to have some secretagogue activity thereby providing a secretory stimulus to the damaged intestinal mucosa. Although all the bacteria need to adhere closely to the intestinal mucosa in order to exert their pathological effects, in some the adhesive property appears to be the only pathogenetic mechanism. An example of this type are those serotypes of *E. coli* which have been designated 'enteropathogenic' EPEC which during the adhesive process induce morphological changes in the mucosa.[6]

Concentration–effect relationship

Not relevant.

Metabolism

Not relevant.

Pharmaceutics

A number of formulations are available. Table 1 shows the solute composition and osmolality of ORS available in the UK.

In the USA, Resol (Wyeth-Ayerst) contains sodium 50 mmol.l^{-1} potassium 20 mmol.l^{-1}, chloride 50 mmol.l^{-1}, glucose 100 mmol.l^{-1}. This ready for use sterile solution also includes citrate, phosphate, calcium and magnesium.

WHO-ORS
The WHO has pioneered the use of a single ORS for diarrhoeal dehydration throughout the world. The ORS recommended by the Diarrhoeal Disease Control Programme of the World Health Organisation and the United Nations Childrens Fund (UNICEF), contains either bicarbonate as the base or the base-precursor citrate. These formulations are referred in the British National Formulary (BNF),

Table 1 Composition of ORS preparations available in UK

ORS	Na (m.mol.l^{-1})	K (m.mol.l^{-1})	Cl (m.mol.l^{-1})	$HC0_3$ (m.mol.l^{-1})	Citrate (m.mol.l^{-1})	Glucose (m.mol.l.$^{-1}$)	Osmolality (mOsmkg^{-1})
Powders							
WHO (Formula C)	90	20	80	—	10	111	311
WHO (Formula B)	90	20	80	30	—	111	331
Diaralyte (Formula A) (Rover UK)	35	20	37	18	—	200	310
Electrolade (Nicholas UK)	50	20	40	30	—	111	251
Gluco-lyte (Capal UK)	35	20	37	18	—	200	310
Rehidrat (Searle UK)	50	20	50	20	9	91 (also: sucrose94 & Frutose2)	336
Ready-made Fluids							
Dextrolyte (Cow & Gate UK)	35	13.4	30.5	17.7	—	200	297
Pedialyte RS (Abbott UK)	75	20	65	—	10	139	309
Pedialyte MS (Abbott UK)	45	20	35	—	10	139	249
Effervescent tablets							
Dioralyte (Rover UK)	35	20	—	—	55	200	310

1990 as Formula B and Formula C. The main reason for the alternative citrate-containing preparation is that bicarbonate ORS is relatively unstable with a short shelf-life due to the formation of furfural compounds with glucose which give rise to brown discolouration of the ORS on reconstitution with water.

Therapeutic use

Indications

1. Acute infectious diarrhoea
2. Enteral fluid therapy in ITU patients
3. Dehydration of the patient with burns
4. Fluid and electrolyte balance in the surgical patient
5. Dehydration in the elderly.

Contraindications

1. Dehydration of 10% or more
2. Continued vomiting.

Mode of use

Usually there are considered to be two treatment phases: the initial rehydration phase during which the main aim is to replace the water and electrolytes already lost as diarrhoea and vomit, followed by the maintenance phase which is started once the signs of dehydration have resolved and which is designed to replace the ongoing losses of water and electrolytes due to continuing diarrhoea and vomiting, as well as the insensible losses (respiration and sweating) which may be especially high in infants and neonates.

It should go without saying that prevention is the best cure. Therefore, in order to avoid the development of dehydration and its attendant potential complications, the first appropriate response to acute diarrhoea, particularly where children and infants are concerned should be the prompt administration of ORT.

Whatever the clinical situation, clean drinking water should be used to prepare the ORS and great care should be taken to ensure that the appropriate amount of water is used to make up the solution. The dangers of using too little water must be stressed. In developing countries the water should be boiled and allowed to cool before administration. Where young children and infants are being treated a family member, preferably the mother, should be shown how to prepare and administer the ORS correctly and that a clean feeding bottle, cup or spoon should always be used. The volume of ORS to be administered can be calculated by estimating the degree of dehydration on clinical criteria (Table 2).

Table 2 Clinical features of the dehydrated infant

Degree of dehydration	Physical signs
Mild	
2–3%	Thirst; mild oliguria
5%	Thirst; oliguria; alert & restless
Moderate	
6–9%	Marked thirst and oliguria; increasingly restless, becoming lethargic & apathetic Sunken eyes, loss of intraocular tension & sunken fontanelle; obvious loss of skin turgor, dry mucous membranes & absent tears; tachycardia but normal B.P.
Severe	
10% or more	Drowsy & limp; cold, sweaty & cyanosed peripheries; later lose consciousness; rapid feeble pulse & hypotension; sunken eyes & fontanelle; very dry mucous membranes with pinched skin retracting very slowly (>2sec); anuria

The WHO have recommended the following protocol for preventing and treating diarrhoeal dehydration in children:[7]

Plan A (prevention)

Give the child more fluids than usual
Continue giving food during the diarrhoeal illness
Watch for the signs of dehydration
Take the child to a health centre in the case of deterioration.

Plan B (treatment)

Give as much of the ORS as the dehydrated child will accept in 4–6 hours, or 50 $ml.kg^{-1}$ to the mildly dehydrated and 100 $ml.kg^{-1}$ to the moderately dehydrated patient. After 4–6 hours reassess, and if the child is rehydrated, offer breast milk (or milk formula) and clean water for continuing ORS. Continue with Plan A until the diarrhoea ceases.

There is no evidence to suggest that a normal diet should not be started as soon as the patient is ready to eat.

Indications

1. Acute infectious diarrhoea

Dehydration during acute diarrhoea is the indication where ORT has made its mark. Although rotavirus and enterotoxigenic secretory diarrhoea are the areas where ORT has proved itself to be of major benefit, it can be used in the management of any acute, dehydrating diarrhoea.

Most of the clinical trial data relating to the efficacy of ORT in the treatment of diarrhoeal dehydration has come from the developing world. The clinical value and feasibility of ORT was demonstrated by Mahalanabis et al during cholera outbreaks in Bangladeshi refugees in 1971.[8] Their work demonstrated a dramatic reduction in mortality from 30% to 1% and set the scene for extending the use of ORT worldwide. Indeed this challenge has been taken up vigorously throughout the developing world where the use of the WHO solution has been actively promoted, leading to a major decline in morbidity and mortality from acute diarrhoeal dehydration.[9] Progress in the developing world continues at a rapid pace. 18 months ago, only 30% of the world's children has access to ORT while today that figure has risen to 60%. Patients of all ages have been successfully treated with ORT including neonates.[10–12] Furthermore, ORT has been used with great success in diarrhoea of diverse aetiology[13–15] and has been shown to be effective for all but the most severe degrees of dehydration. Patients with hypernatraemia or hyponatraemia are also potentially treatable by ORT[16,17] as are those with hypokalaemia and acidosis.[18]

Despite the convincing evidence of the early trials in the developing world, developed nations were slow to implement this form of treatment. A major concern was that WHO-ORS was based on the faecal sodium losses in cholera,[19] particularly as the major cause of infectious diarrhoea in developed nations is rotavirus in which faecal sodium losses are much lower. In addition there is evidence that well-nourished children in developed nations respond differently to ORT than under-nourished children in developing countries. Several randomized controlled trials comparing oral and intravenous rehydration regimens in well-nourished, moderately dehydrated children from developed countries have dismissed these concerns.[20–25] The overall success rate for ORT was 80–90% (see Clinical trials).

2. Enteral rehydration of intensive treatment unit (ITU) patients

In some seriously ill ITU patients, particularly those who may require management over a relatively long period of time, enteral fluid support may prove beneficial. For example, septicaemia or persistent central catheter sepsis may require the catheter to be removed; trauma or burns involving the head, neck and thorax may make the insertion of the jugular or subclavian lines impractical; venous access in general may be compromised by thrombosis or phlebitis. Even though a patient may not be able to comply with oral administration of ORS, it is relatively easy to pass a finebore nasogastric feeding tube into the stomach or duodenum to administer the ORS. ORT is always worth considering even in these very sick patients.

3. Rehydration of burns victims

A severe burn injury is associated with massive inter-compartmental fluid shifts and vascular changes which are associated with very high mortality from hypovolaemic shock if not adequately treated. Initially, fluid and electrolyte replacement therapy needs to be vigorous and often large volumes of hypertonic salt solutions need to be administered, generally via a central venous catheter. Central lines may become compromised by thrombosis and sepsis. Although the infusion of hypertonic salt solutions through nasogastric feeding tubes is not currently recommended, this approach can be used for the subsequent administration of water and electrolytes.

4. Fluid therapy in the surgical patient

Although there are reports testifying to the early return of normal gastrointestinal function after abdominal surgery there is a growing body of opinion that the oral route for rehydration is greatly underused and many patients are maintained on an intravenous fluid regimen longer than is necessary. Enteral fluid support using glucose–electrolyte solutions infused via a nasogastric tube (after cholecystectomy and colonic surgery) or nasoduodenal tube (after oesophageal and gastric surgery) is currently under evaluation. Preliminary evidence indicates that enteral rehydration and early postoperative oral rehydration will be tolerated by most patients within 12–48 h after surgery. Such an outcome would clearly have beneficial implications in terms of reducing the necessity for prolonged intravenous fluid and electrolyte support which is more costly and demanding on nursing resources. The complications of prolonged intravenous infusion such as sepsis, phlebitis and thrombosis would presumably be reduced.

Contraindications

1. Severe dehydration
A patient with > 10% dehydration is not an appropriate candidate for ORT and should, at least initially, be given intravenous fluid and electrolytes for rehydration. ORT however, may be introduced subsequently as maintenance therapy to prevent further dehydration.

2. Continued vomiting
Vomiting is common in acute infectious diarrhoeal disease but is not a contraindication to ORT. It may however, continue or even be worsened when ORS is administered. To minimize vomiting ORS should be given in small amounts at 5–10 min intervals rather than as a large bolus. This cautious but persistent method of administration is usually successful. However, should vomiting continue and the signs of dehydration reappear or worsen then ORT should be abandoned. In these circumstances hospitalization and rehydration by the intravenous route should be considered.

Adverse reactions

Potentially life-threatening effects
Hyponatraemia, hypernatraemia, hypokalaemia and hyperkalaemia are all possible adverse effects of ORT, but the most important of these is hypernatraemia. Sodium overload usually occurs when high sodium ORS such as WHO-ORS (sodium 90 mmol.l^{-1}) are used inappropriately without access to free water. Those particularly at risk of hypernatraemia are neonates and young infants where the ability of the kidneys to deal with a high sodium load is impaired. Reports of occasional hypernatraemia complicated by periorbital oedema, which are known to occur with the WHO formulation, and which may be particularly troublesome in well-nourished infants and children in the developed world fed on high-solute feeds, have caused concern among some paediatricians. However, it is sometimes forgotten that after an initial relatively short period of rehydration the WHO solution is recommended to be used with ad libitum water, at least in the ratio 2.1 with ORS. The resultant sodium would be 60 mmol.l^{-1}. The reported incidents of hypernatraemia and its complication probably occurred because insufficient water was taken with the WHO-ORS. The use of an overdiluted ORS particularly in malnourished patients may be associated with hyponatraemia, particularly if the faecal sodium losses (as in cholera) are excessive. Hyperkalaemia is a very uncommon complication but has been reported in well-nourished children who were given WHO-ORS without being given free water.[26] Hypokalaemia may develop in up to a third of dehydrated, mildly malnourished children receiving ORS with potassium 20 mmol.l^{-1} although it was never observed in a group receiving a similar ORS with potassium 30 mmol.l^{-1}. Malnourished children who have recurrent episodes of diarrhoea are at greatest risk of potassium depletion. In hypernatraemic dehydration, the symptoms of dehydration may not be present. The skin may feel doughy and the fontanelle may be bulging. The peripheral circulation in these children may not become compromised until late in the illness and it is important therefore to have a high index of suspicion. Early features of hypernatraemic dehydration in a child are hyperirritability and lethargy.

Severe or irreversible adverse effects
These have already been mentioned.

Symptomatic adverse effects
Apart from minor degrees of the adverse affects mentioned above, there are none.

Oral rehydration salts

Interference with clinical pathology tests
No interferences of this kind have been reported.

High risk groups

Although any moderately dehydrated individual is at risk of adverse effects, particularly if ORS is used inappropriately there are three groups about whom there should be special concern, namely: neonates, young infants, and those who are hypernatraemic before treatment.

There are no special problems with other children, pregnant or lactating women, or the elderly.

Drug interactions

None has been described.

Major outcome trials

1. Nalin D R, Cash R A, Islam R, Molla M, Phillips R A 1968 Oral maintenance therapy for cholera in adults. Lancet 2: 370–372

This is a seminal study in that it was the first controlled trial to show that orally administered glucose–electrolyte solutions could reduce intravenous fluid requirements by 80%, and it paved the way for clinical implementation of oral rehydration therapy on a wide scale.

29 patients with acute diarrhoea due to *V. cholerae* were treated initially with intravenous therapy to correct shock and then randomly assigned such that 10 received oral therapy by intragastric infusion while another 10 were given intravenous therapy. The controlled group required an average total volume of 19.4 l of intravenous therapy compared to only 4.3 l for the orally treated group. The total volume of solution required for oral therapy (after initial rehydration) was 19.8 l. Thus, those patients receiving oral therapy required 78.8% less in terms of intravenous fluids than that required by controlled patients. Nine patients were given the oral solution to drink and tolerated it remarkably well.

2. Santosham N, Daum R S, Dillman L et al 1982 Oral rehydration therapy of infantile diarrhea. A controlled study of well nourished children hospitalized in the United States and Panama. New England Journal of Medicine 306: 1070–1076

This landmark study was instrumental in changing the clinical practice of paediatricians in the USA and other developed countries where the accepted standards for management of hospitalized patients with diarrhoea suggested intravenous rehydration as first-line therapy. The primary obstacle to widespread acceptance of the WHO formula in the USA was the fear of hyponatraemia and the lower faecal sodium concentration (< 90 mmol.l^{-1}) in cases of non-cholera acute diarrhoea was often cited as justification.

In this well-controlled, prospective, clinical trial 146 well-nourished children (3 months–2 years old) hospitalized for acute diarrhoea in North (52 USA) and South (94 Panama) America were randomized to receive standard WHO solution (90 mmol.l^{-1} sodium), or a modification of the WHO formula (where the sodium concentration was reduced to 50 mmol.l^{-1}) or standard intravenous therapy. All children with 10% or more dehydration received intravenous resuscitation (until their blood pressure and pulse normalized) before randomization.

Oral rehydration therapy with either solution was 99% successful, only one child requiring unscheduled intravenous therapy. In 89% (87 of 97 children) no intravenous therapy was required at all. All six children admitted with hypernatraemic dehydration were successfully treated with oral therapy alone. Serious complications of this study (hydrothorax and phlebitis) occurred only in the subgroup receiving intravenous treatment.

The authors concluded that not only would glucose–electrolyte solutions containing 50 and 90 mmol.l^{-1} sodium be effective and safe for the treatment of well nourished children hospitalized with acute diarrhoea but they could completely replace intravenous fluids in the majority of such children.

3. Listernick R, Zieserl E, Davies T A 1986 Outpatient oral rehydration in the United States. American Journal of Diseases in Childhood 140: 211–215

These authors bemoan the reluctance of paediatricians in industrialized nations to move away from parenteral rehydration because of unsubstantiated fears of iatrogenic hypernatraemia. They set about killing the 'sacred cow' of intravenous therapy by performing a prospective, randomized clinical trial in 29 well-nourished infants (3–24 months) presenting with acute diarrhoeal dehydration at the emergency room of a children's hospital in Chicago comparing the safety, efficacy and costs of oral versus intravenous rehydration. 13 of the 15 infants randomized to outpatient therapy with a modified WHO solution (containing 60 mmol.l^{-1} sodium instead of 90 mmol.l^{-1}) were successfully hydrated orally, only 2 requiring admission (later found to have urinary tract infections) before intravenous therapy. Moreover, these outpatients spent only 10.7 h (mean) in the holding room of the casualty compared to the 103.2 h of the hospitalized intravenous therapy group.

The authors strongly argue that oral rehydration is safe and cost effective means of treating children with diarrhoea dehydration in an outpatient setting in the United States, and therefore by extension, any industrialized or developed nation.

4. Vesikari T, Isolauri E, Baer M 1987 A comparative trial of rapid oral and intravenous rehydration in acute diarrhoea. Acta Paediatrica Scandinavica 76: 300–305

This trial presents yet more evidence to persuade recalcitrant Western paediatricians to embrace oral rehydration salts as first-line therapy in acute diarrhoeal dehydration.

In this prospective clinical trial, 37 children under 5 years of age, hospitalized for dehydration in association with acute gastroenteritis were randomized to receive oral or intravenous rehydration during 6–12 h. Dehydration, metabolic acidosis and the sodium deficit were all corrected equally satisfactory in both groups but it was easier to reintroduce normal feeding earlier in the orally rehydrated children than in the intravenous therapy group and, consequently, the former showed a 2.9% weight gain by the time of discharge, unlike the latter. Moreover, the duration of diarrhoea was shorter with oral rehydration therapy.

The authors conclude that oral rehydration therapy to be equally superior even to rapid intravenous rehydration therapy in the management of acute diarrhoea in children.

5. Pizarro D, Posada G, Mata L 1983 Treatment of 242 neonates with dehydrating diarrhea with an oral glucose–electrolyte solution. Journal of Paediatrics 102: 153–156

This very large study is a retrospective analysis of the experience of a large South American paediatric unit with oral rehydration therapy for acute diarrhoeal dehydration in neonates between 1978–1981. They showed that 96.7% of these neonates were rehydrated successfully with an oral glucose–electrolyte solution in an average time of 7.4 h. also found that vomiting did not prove to be an obstacle to complete oral rehydration. The hypernatraemia, hyponatraemia and acidosis present on admission was corrected within a few hours and they concluded that oral rehydration therapy should be the treatment of choice for uncomplicated diarrhoeal dehydration in neonates.

Other trials

Pizarro D, Pasada G, Villavicencio N, Mohs E, Levine M M 1983 Oral rehydration in hypernatraemia and hyponatraemic diarrheal dehydration. American Journal of Diseases in Children 137: 730–734

This is a clinical study directly addressing the issue of potential iatrogenic hypernatraemia following the use of oral rehydration therapy and is a significant contribution to the previously sparse published experience concerning the oral rehydration of infants with hypo- and hypernatraemic dehydration.

61 hypernatraemic and 33 hyponatraemic infants were rehydrated orally according to a regimen where two-thirds of the fluid volume was given as the WHO glucose–electrolyte solution (containing 90 mmol.l^{-1} sodium) and one-third as plain water to all the hypernatraemic infants and all but 8 of the hyponatraemic infants. These 8 were given WHO solution alone. Successful correction of fluid and electrolyte deficits was accomplished within 10 h in 92 out of 94 subjects and only 5 (8%) of hypernatraemic subjects developed seizures. This complication rate compares favourably with the 14% incidence of major seizures which the authors encountered when they previously used intravenous rehydration alone.

Oral rehydration salts

References

1. Hirschhorn N, Kinzie J L, Sachar D B, Northrup R S, Taylor J O, Ahmed S Z, Phillipas R A 1968 Decrease in net stool output in cholera during intestinal perfusion with glucose-containing solutions. New England Journal of Medicine 279: 176–181
2. Latta T 1832 Malignant cholera: Documents communicated to the Central Board of Health, London. Relative to the treatment of cholera by the copious injection of aqueous and salien fluids into the veins. Lancet 2: 274–277
3. Schultz S 1977 Sodium coupled solute transport by small intestine: A status report. American Journal of Physiology 233: E249–E254
4. Riepenhoff-Talty M, Lee P L, Carmody P L, Barrett H J, Ogra P L 1982 Age-dependent rotavirus–enterocyte interactions. Proceedings of the Society of Experimental Biology and Medicine 170: 146–154
5. Cadranel S, Rodesch P, Butzler J P, Dekeyser P 1973 Enteritis due to related Vibrio in children. American Journal of Diseases in Childhood 126: 152–155
6. Ulshen M H, Rollo J L 1980 Pathogenesis of *Escherichia coli* gastroenteritis in man — another mechanism. New England Journal of Medicine 302: 99–100
7. WHO 1986 Diarrhoeal Disease Control Programme. Fifth Programme Report 1984–1985. World Health Organisation/ Control Diarrhoeal Disease/ 86.6, Geneva
8. Kahn A, Blum D 1980 Hyperkalaemia and UNICEF type rehydration solutions. Lancet 1: 1082
9. Tamer A, Friedman L B, Maxwell S R W, Synamon H A, Perez H N, Cleveland W W 1985 Oral rehydration of infants in the large urban US medical center. Journal of Pediatrics 107: 14–19
10. Mahalanabis D, Choudhuri A B, Bagchi N G, Bhattacharya A K, Simpson T W 1973 Oral fluid therapy of cholera among Bangladesh refugees. Johns Hopkins Medical Journal 132: 197–205
11. Williams G 1987 A simple solution. UNCIEF Special Report. New York, UNICEF
12. Palmer D L, Koster F T, Islam A F M R, Rahman A S M M, Sack R B 1977 Comparison of sucrose and glucose in the oral electrolyte therapy of cholera and other severe diarrhoeas. New England Journal of Medicine 297: 1107–1110
13. Nalin D R, Levine M, Mata L et al 1978 Comparison of sucrose with glucose and oral therapy of infant diarrhoea. Lancet 2: 277–279
14. Pizarro D, Posada G, Mata L 1983 Treatment of 242 neonates with dehydrating diarrhoea with an oral glucose–electrolyte solution. Journal of Pediatrics 102: 153–156
15. Sack D A, Chowdhury A M A K, Eusof A, Ali M A, Merson M H, Islam S, Black R E, Brown K H 1978 Oral hydration in rotavirus diarrhoea: A double-blind comparison of sucrose with glucose electrolyte solution. Lancet 2: 280–283
16. Nalin D R, Levine M M, Mata L, de Cespedes C, Vargas W, Lizano C, Loria A R, Simhon A, Mohs E 1979 Oral rehydration in maintenance of children with rotavirus and bacterial diarrhoeas. Bulletin of World Health Organisation 57: 453–459
17. Black R E, Merson M H, Taylor P R, Yolken R H, Yunus M, Alim A R M A, Sack D A 1981 Glucose vs. sucrose in oral rehydration solutions for infants and young children with rotavirus-associated diarrhoea. Pediatrics 67: 79–83
18. Pizarro D, Posada G, Villavicencio N, Mohs E, Levine M M 1983 Oral rehydration in hypernatraemic and hyponatraemic diarrhoeal dehydration. American Journal of Diseases in Childhood 137: 730–734
19. Pizarro D, Posada G, Levine M M 1984 Hypernatraemic diarrhoea treated with 'slow' (12-hour) oral rehydration therapy: A preliminary report. Journal of Pediatrics 104: 316–319
20. Pizarro D 1986 Oral rehydration therapy: its use in neonates and young infants. Journal of Pediatric Gastroenterology and Nutrition 5: 6–8
21. Santosham M, Daum R S, Dillman L et al 1982 Oral rehydration therapy of infantile diarrhoea: a controlled study of well-nourished children hospitalized in the United States and Panama. New England Journal of Medicine 306: 1070–1076
22. Listernick R, Zieserl E, Davies A T 1986 Outpatient oral rehydration in the United Sates. American Journal of Diseases in Childhood 14: 211–215
23. Vesikari T, Isolauri E, Baer M 1987 A comparative trial of rapid oral and intravenous rehydration in acute diarrhoea. Acta Paediatrica Scandinavica 76: 300–305
24. Elliot E J, Armitstead J C M, Farthing M J G, Walker-Smith J A 1988 Oral rehydration therapy without bicarbonate for prevention and treatment of dehydration: a double-blind controlled trial. Alimentary Pharmacology and Therapeutics 2: 253–263
25. Elliott E J, Cunha Ferreria R M, Cameron D, Farthing M J G, Walker-Smith J A 1989 Evaluation of three oral rehydration solutions designed for use in developed communities. Alimentary Pharmacology and Therapeutics 3: 233–243
26. Molla A M, Rahman M, Sarker S A, Sack D A, Molla A 1981 Stool electrolyte content and purging rates in diarrhoea caused by rotavirus, enterotoxigenic *E coli* and *V cholerae* in children. Journal of Pediatrics 98 835–838
27. Pierce N F, Banwell J G, Mitra R C, Caranasos G J, Keimowitz R J, Mondal A, Manji P M 1968 Effect of intragastric glucose–electrolyte infusion upon water and electrolyte balance in Asiatic cholera. Gastroenterology 55: 333–343

Orciprenaline (sulphate)

Orciprenaline was the first noncatecholamine β-agonist to be used therapeutically as a bronchodilator.[1]

Chemistry

Orciprenaline sulphate (metaproterenol, Alupent, Metaprel, Novasmasol)
$(C_{11}H_{17}NO_3)_2H_2SO_4$
(RS)1-(3,5-Dihydroxyphenyl)-2-isopropylaminoethanol

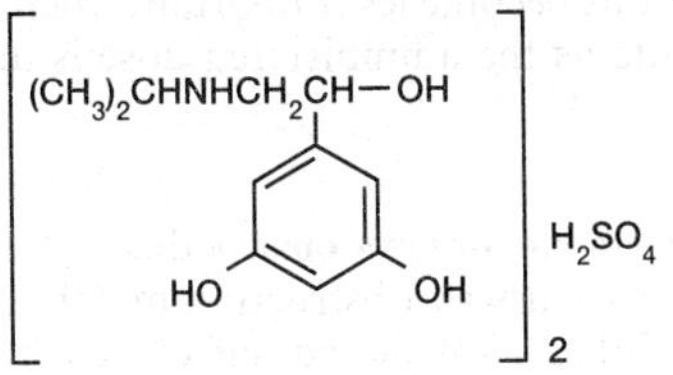

Molecular weight (free base)	520.6 (211.3)
pKa	
(OH)	10.1
(NH)	11.4
Solubility	
in alcohol	1 in 1
in water	1 in 2
Octanol/water partition coefficient	—

Orciprenaline is a white, odourless, crystalline powder with a bitter taste. It is a racemic mixture of two optically active isomers. Orciprenaline sulphate is prepared by chemical synthesis and the racemate is used clinically. It is not present in any combination products.

Pharmacology

Orciprenaline is a resorcinol derivative of isoprenaline that produces bronchodilatation and its other effects by stimulation of β-adrenoceptors. It has been shown to produce the same maximal relaxation as isoprenaline in the guinea-pig isolated trachea[2] and human isolated bronchus.[3] Experiments with tracheal (β_2) and atrial (β_1) preparations isolated from the guinea-pig have demonstrated that orciprenaline is selective for β_2-adrenoceptors.[4,5] However, it is less selective for β_2-adrenoceptors than either terbutaline or salbutamol.[1,6]

Toxicology

Toxicological tests in laboratory animals have failed to show any toxic or mutagenic effects with doses in the therapeutic range.

Clinical pharmacology

Either oral or inhaled orciprenaline has been shown to increase FEV_1, increase the maximal forced expiratory flow rate and decrease airway resistance in asthmatic patients. When a single 20 mg dose is given orally, its bronchodilator effect peaks after 1 hour and the improvement in airways function lasts for 4 hours.[7] By aerosol it is expected to act more quickly but its duration of action may be shorter. Despite orciprenaline being a selective β_2-agonist in vitro,[4] intravenous orciprenaline has been shown to increase heart rate as much as intravenous isoprenaline in asthmatic patients.[8] When orciprenaline is given by metered-dose pressurized aerosol effective bronchodilatation can be achieved without tachycardia.[9,10]

Because orciprenaline relaxes uterine smooth muscle it has been administered intravenously to manage premature labour.[11] However, it is not as β_2-selective as more recently introduced drugs such as salbutamol.[1,12]

Pharmacokinetics

A standard analytical method for the measurement of orciprenaline in plasma has not been published. It has been reported that by using tritiated orciprenaline labelled on the α-carbon atom, free orciprenaline was measured[13] to a concentration as low as 0.05 μg.l^{-1}. A high performance liquid chromatographic assay using fluorescence detection has been developed that is capable of accurately measuring orciprenaline to 0.5 mg.l^{-1} in human urine following extraction.[14]

After oral administration peak levels of the free amine are reached within 2–4 hours. The amount of drug absorbed orally was approximately 40%, and about 10% of the orciprenaline reached the systemic circulation, demonstrating a significant presystemic metabolism.[13] The enzymes in the gut wall rather than the liver are responsible for its presystemic metabolism. More than 90% of the dose of inhaled orciprenaline is swallowed[15] and it is not inactivated by COMT in the lung. Thus the metabolism of inhaled orciprenaline is similar to that of the orally administered drug.

The distribution of ^{3}H-orciprenaline in the rat after intravenous injection has been examined.[13] In the first 30 minutes the highest concentration of ^{3}H-activity was in the kidneys, liver, plasma and lungs. The other tissues exhibited less ^{3}H-activity than plasma. 240 minutes after injection, ^{3}H-activity fell considerably in all tissues and after 24 hours the ^{3}H-concentration was equal to that of plasma in most tissues. In the plasma a maximum of 20% of the total radioactivity was present as free amine while in heart, lungs, kidneys and skeletal muscle 50 to 80% was present as free amine.

When ^{3}H-orciprenaline was infused over 12 hours in man the free plasma levels of drug could be analysed according to an open two-compartment model.[13] Orciprenaline is mainly eliminated by the formation of polar conjugates and their subsequent excretion via the urine. Macgregor and his co-workers have shown that for a 20 mg oral dose of orciprenaline sulphate, most of the dose was excreted over the first 12 hours, with a biological half life of 5–6 hours, followed by a slower excretion phase with a half life of 20 hours.[14]

Oral absorption	40%
Presystemic metabolism	75%
Plasma half life	6 h, 20 h
Volume of distribution	700 l
Plasma protein binding	—

Much of the dose is metabolized presystemically, in the intestinal wall, and the metabolites are excreted largely in the urine. The fate of systemic orciprenaline has yet to be determined. It is not known whether orciprenaline crosses the placenta or enters breast milk.

Reduction in dose might be necessary in patients with severe renal impairment because of decreased elimination of the drug but there are no experimental data available. This might also be the case in the elderly subject with compromised renal function.

Concentration–effect relationship

No relationship has been established between plasma levels and clinical effects of orciprenaline. Thus the dosage should be adjusted for each individual patient according to improvements in lung function and adverse effects observed.

Metabolism

Orciprenaline is not subject to degradation by catechol-O-methyltransferase because it has a resorcinol ring structure.[16] Oral drug is presystemically metabolized, principally in the gut wall, to form polar conjugates, most probably at the phenolic hydroxyl groups.[13] In the rat the conjugates were mainly glucuronides[14] but in man the major urinary conjugated metabolite was shown to be orciprenaline-3-O-sulphate (see Fig. 1).[14] Macgregor and his co-workers found that 40% of a 20 mg oral dose was recovered in the urine as orciprenaline-

Fig. 1 Metabolism of orciprenaline

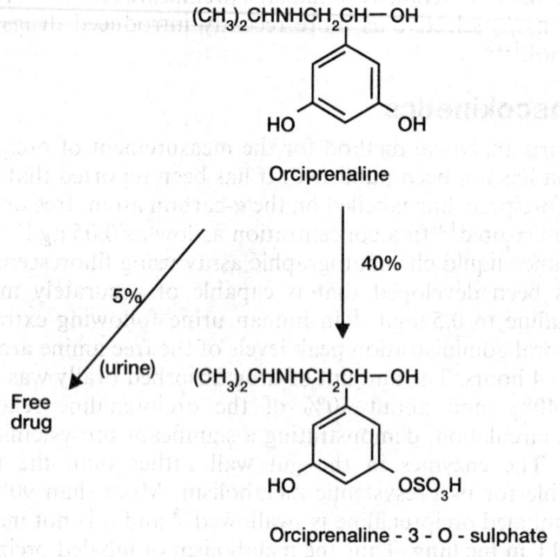

3-O-sulphate with 5% of this dose in the conjugated form. Hence, most of oral or inhaled orciprenaline is conjugated to an inactive sulphate by sulphokinase enzymes in the gastrointestinal wall. The role of the liver in metabolizing systemic orciprenaline remains to be more thoroughly investigated.

Pharmaceutics

Orciprenaline is available in oral, parenteral and inhalation forms.

1. Alupent (Boehringer Ingelheim, UK): tablets containing either 20 mg or 10 mg of orciprenaline sulphate BP. They are white, round and flat with bevelled edges and are supplied in bottles of 100. The 20 mg tables are scored and marked '20A over 20A' with the company symbol on the reverse side. The strength of the 10 mg tablets is also marked.
2. Alupent is available as a cherry-flavoured syrup in 300 ml bottles, in which the concentration of orciprenaline sulphate is 10 mg per 5 ml.
3. Alupent (Boehringer Ingelheim, UK) is available for intravenous use as a solution of orciprenaline sulphate BP in water. Each 1 ml ampoule contains 0.5 mg and there are 5 ampoules per box.
4. For the metered aerosol of Alupent, 225 mg of orciprenaline sulphate BPC is present as a fine suspension mixed with suitable aerosol propellants in a pressurized canister. The concentration is 15 $mg.ml^{-1}$ and 0.750 mg is provided in each metered dose, but approximately 0.65 mg is actually delivered from the mouthpiece. The volume of the vial is 15 ml hence it is able to provide 300 metered doses. A mouthpiece is required.
5. A 2% Alupent solution in 20 ml bottles (Germany) and a 5% inhalation solution in 10 and 30 ml bottles (USA) are available. Alupent inhalant solution is also available in unit dose vials containing colourless solutions of 0.4 and 0.6% orciprenaline sulphate. Each vial contains 2.5 ml of solution and there are 25 vials per box.

Tablets, syrup, inhalation solution and ampoules should be protected from light. Orciprenaline preparations present a minimal risk as potentially allergenic substances. However, individuals who are allergic to sulphite food preservatives may exhibit a hypersensitivity response to orciprenaline preparations containing sodium bisulphite.

Preparation maximum shelf-life
Ampoules 5 years
Syrup 4 years
Tablets 3 years
Metered aerosol 3 years
Inhalation solution 2.5 years

Therapeutic use

Indications

Indications for use of orciprenaline are asthma, bronchitis and other types of reversible airway obstruction.

Contraindications

1. Pre-existing cardiac arrhythmias associated with tachycardia
2. Recent myocardial infarction
3. Thyrotoxicosis
4. Sub-valvular aortic stenosis
5. Ischaemic heart disease
6. Hypersensitivity to orciprenaline
7. Situations requiring extra care.

a. Liver and/or kidney disease
b. Diabetes
c. Quadriplegia
d. Cystic fibrosis
e. Treatment with drugs that may enhance the adverse effects of β-agonists.

The contraindications become less important when the drugs are used by the aerosol route as the administered dose is much reduced.

Mode of use

In treatment of reversible airways obstruction
Orciprenaline reverses airway obstruction mainly by relaxing airway smooth muscle. Other β-mediated effects such as inhibition of chemical mediator release from mast cells, improvement of mucociliary transport and reduction of mucosal oedema by inhibition of increased vascular permeability may contribute to the therapeutic effect.[17] Orciprenaline has been shown to be useful for the reversal of an acute asthmatic attack, as well as for long-term therapy.

A pressurized aerosol is generally used for inhalation and it delivers 0.75 mg of orciprenaline sulphate in each dose but about 0.65 mg is actually delivered at the mouthpiece. A single dose of two to three inhalations of pressurized aerosol has a duration of action that varies from 1 to 5 hours, during which it increases the FEV_1 by 15% or more. The recommended dose is one to two inhalations three to four times daily. Metered-dose orciprenaline will provide protection against exercise-induced bronchoconstriction[18] but longer lasting protection is obtained with salbutamol, terbutaline or fenoterol.[19]

When the asthmatic attacks become more severe, orciprenaline sulphate may be inhaled in a 2% solution from a hand nebulizer, from which 10–15 inhalations may be taken three to four times daily. A 5% inhalant solution is also available, which may be administered either by an intermittent positive pressure breathing (IPPB) apparatus or a hand-bulb nebulizer to significantly improve airways function (increase FEV_1 by 15% or more) within 5 to 30 minutes of administration.

When 0.3 ml of the 5% inhalation solution is delivered by IPPB the duration of action is approximately 6 hours while when 10 inhalations are given by hand-bulb nebulizer the bronchodilator effect lasts for 2 to 3 hours (Physicians Desk Ref USA, 1984).

Orciprenaline, either in the form of tablets or syrup, may be effectively used for prophylactic or long-term therapy.[20,21,22] The bronchodilator effect of an oral dose of 20 mg starts after about 20 to 30 minutes, peaks after an hour and is maintained for about 4 hours.[7] In adults, the recommended maintenance oral dose is 20 mg of orciprenaline taken three to four times daily.

When oral orciprenaline was administered prophylactically for periods from 2 to 6 months, headache and tachycardia were observed in some patients yet no serious adverse effects were reported.[20,21,23] Significant bronchodilator tolerance does not appear to develop when the recommended doses of oral orciprenaline are used prophylactically.

If asthma becomes extremely severe, orciprenaline may be given by slow intravenous infusion, but great caution is required because intravenous orciprenaline has been reported to produce the same degree of tachycardia as intravenous isoprenaline.[8] If intravenous administration of a β-agonist is necessary, a more selective β_2-agonist such as salbutamol should be preferred in order to minimize cardiac stimulation, especially if the patient has ischaemic heart disease, pre-existing cardiac arrhythmias or is taking theophylline.

In severe asthma, where obstruction is mainly caused by mucous plugging and airway oedema, β-agonists may become relatively ineffective and a greater emphasis should be directed towards alternative modes of treatment, particularly with corticosteroids.

Contraindications

1. Pre-existing arrhythmias associated with tachycardia
β_2-agonists taken orally have been reported to exacerbate pre-existing cardiac arrhythmias.[24,25] Extra care is required when such cardiac patients require orciprenaline; the aerosol route should be preferred and the dosage may have to be reduced and cardiac function carefully monitored according to the severity and nature of the pre-existing arrythmias.

2. Recent cardiac infarction
Orciprenaline and other β-agonists should be avoided because they may increase the size of the myocardial infarct by increasing heart rate and contractility. In addition, they may exacerbate the ventricular ectopic activity that is commonly associated with a myocardial infarction. When it is considered that a β-agonist bronchodilator is necessary, a very selective β_2-agonist such as salbutamol would be theoretically preferable.

3. Thyrotoxicosis
Experiments in human subjects indicated that cardiac β-adrenoceptor sensitivity was not altered by thyroid dysfunction but resting heart rate was markedly elevated in the hyperthyroid patients.[26,27] Results have been reported which suggest that the airways in hyperthyroid subjects are less responsive to β-agonists.[28] The use of orciprenaline should be carefully appraised in hyperthyroid patients because of the elevated cardiac activity associated with this disorder and the reduced bronchodilator effectiveness.

4. Subvalvular aortic stenosis
Abnormal hypertrophy of the left ventricle causes narrowing of the left ventricular outflow below the aortic valve. The severity of obstruction is enhanced by an increase in myocardial contractility and tachycardia. Inhaled orciprenaline should be used with caution if an asthmatic has this condition.

5. Ischaemic heart disease
In susceptible patients with ischaemic heart disease the relatively large doses of β_2-agonist given by nebulizer may increase heart work sufficiently to produce anginal attacks or even myocardial infarction.[29]

6. Hypersensitivity to the β-agonist preparation
Orciprenaline presents a minimal risk as a potentially allergic substance, but an orciprenaline preparation should be stopped if an allergic response to the preparation is suspected. Hypersensitivity-mediated bronchoconstriction has been reported to be produced by sodium bisulphite present in nebulized isoetharine.[30,31] Hence in individuals who are allergic to sulphite food preservatives, it would be prudent to examine the composition of the bronchodilator preparation and use one not containing sodium bisulphite or metabisulphite. It is of interest to note that the severe bronchoconstriction believed to be due to a hypersensitivity reaction to an oral terbutaline sulphate preparation was alleviated by intravenous orciprenaline sulphate.[32]

7. Situations requiring extra care
a. Liver and/or kidney disease. The oral dose may need to be reduced in patients with impaired renal function according to the severity of the disease although the risk will be minimal if recommended aerosol doses are used.

b. Diabetes. β_2-agonists produce much greater increases in plasma glucose and ketone bodies in diabetic subjects than in healthy individuals but tolerance may develop to the metabolic effects produced by this group of drugs.[33] Thus, as β_2-agonists may produce or exacerbate hyperglycaemia and ketoacidosis in diabetics,[34,35] orciprenaline should be given with extra care to diabetic patients and plasma insulin, glucose, free fatty acids and ketone bodies should be carefully monitored.

c. Quadriplegia. Pingleton and his co-workers have reported that subcutaneous terbutaline produced very severe hypotension in two quadriplegic asthmatics with autonomic dysfunction.[36] These authors thus proposed that the unsupervised use of β_2-agonists should be discouraged in asthmatics with quadriplegia. Orciprenaline should be used with extra caution in patients with this condition.

d. Cystic fibrosis. In advanced cystic fibrosis, where the airways become severely damaged and unstable, the reduction in bronchomotor tone produced by a bronchodilator may dramatically reduce the ability of the airways to withstand dynamic compression during forced expiration.[37] The indiscriminate use of a β-agonist for cystic fibrosis may disadvantage some patients by actually reducing their end-expiratory flow rates. Thus orciprenaline should be used with extra caution in patients with this condition.

e. Treatment with drugs that may enhance the adverse effects of β-agonists. This is covered in the section on drug interactions.

Adverse reactions

Potentially life-threatening effects
Fatalities have been reported in association with excessive use of β-agonist aerosol bronchodilators.[38,39] Excessive administration carries a potential hazard both from the freon propellants and from overdosage of the β-agonist delivered, but the cause of death in such circumstances is still controversial. In several cases, cardiac arrest had been reported, although ventilatory arrest may be observed first. The possibility of fatal ventricular arrhythmia from inhalation of excessive amounts of β-agonist in susceptible individuals has never been fully excluded.

However, it is more commonly believed that the asthma rapidly deteriorated and the airway obstruction progressed to a fatal extent because the extensive mucous plugging and bronchial oedema did not, ultimately, respond to therapy with β-agonist.[39,40] Thus a major potential danger with β-agonist bronchodilators is an overestimation of their benefit as asthma becomes worse. This should be distinguished from direct toxic effects. Patients should be advised to contact their physician quickly if the response to their usual dose of orciprenaline aerosol diminishes or disappears.

As β-agonists can increase cardiac output and produce pulmonary vasodilatation, they can increase blood flow through poorly ventilated areas and worsen ventilation/perfusion mismatch to reduce arterial oxygen tension (PaO_2), even though they at the same time improve airway function.[41] Generally, the drop in PaO_2 produced by β-agonists is not a problem, but in asthmatics where the initial PaO_2 is below 60 mmHg any decrease in PaO_2 would be clinically significant.[42] If orciprenaline is used in severe life-threatening asthma, the PaO_2 should be carefully monitored and supplemental oxygen be immediately available as required.

Acute overdosage
The symptoms of β-agonist overadministration include marked tachycardia, tremor, excitement, restlessness, anxiety, headache, nausea and changes in blood pressure. Usually unwanted symptoms cease to be a problem with a simple reduction in dosage and/or frequency of administration. In rare cases where the adverse symptoms of sympathetic overactivity become very marked, admission to a hospital should be considered. Cardiac arrhythmias may be a potential danger in some patients with cardiac problems.

A suicide attempt by deliberate overdose has not been reported for orciprenaline. If it occurs, the major emphasis should be on maintaining cardiac function. In addition, PaO_2 should be carefully monitored and supplemental oxygen should be administered when required. Cautious use of a β-receptor antagonist would have to be considered but the balance of advantage would require very careful consideration if the patient had severe asthma.

Severe or irreversible adverse effects
In some individuals orciprenaline may produce extrasystoles, palpitations causing anxiety and intolerable muscle tremor but in most patients adverse effects are not severe enough to stop treatment.[20,21] If such adverse effects of orciprenaline become too severe they quickly decline when administration is stopped. There are no reports that orciprenaline produces irreversible toxic effects if it is taken over a long period of time.

Symptomatic adverse effects
The most frequent adverse effects of orciprenaline are nervousness, tachycardia, tremor and nausea. Less frequent adverse reactions are

hypertension, palpitations, vomiting, bad taste, headache, dizziness and sweating. With the recommended dosages adverse effects are not marked and most patients can continue with therapy.[20,21]

Other effects
The biochemical effects of orciprenaline are as for other β_2-agonists. Acutely, β-agonists have been shown to lower plasma potassium levels, elevate plasma glucose and insulin levels and to produce hyperlipidaemia in some subjects. All of these metabolic changes are reversible and are mediated through stimulation of β-adrenoceptors.[33]

Tolerance usually develops to these metabolic changes when β_2-agonists are given chronically and in the majority of patients they are not of major clinical importance.[33,43] Caution is advised when β-agonists are given to patients who are suffering from diabetes because the drugs may produce or exacerbate hyperglycaemia and ketoacidosis,[35,44] although this is unlikely with small doses given by aerosol.

Interference with clinical pathology tests
To our knowledge, there have been no reports published indicating that orciprenaline interferes with clinical pathology tests.

High risk groups

Neonates
It has been shown that while nebulized salbutamol reduced airways obstruction in most wheezing children over 20 months of age, it did not improve lung function or the clinical state in wheezing children between 7 and 18 months of age.[45] Thus, since a β-agonist is unlikely to improve airways function in wheezing children under 18 months of age, orciprenaline is not recommended in neonates.

Breast milk. It is not known whether β-agonists are secreted in large amounts in human milk[46] and so they should be used cautiously in nursing women. Aerosol administration is preferred as very little of the dose is delivered systemically.

Children
The safety and effectiveness of orciprenaline sulphate in the form of a metered-dose aerosol or an inhalant solution has not been established in children below the age of 12 (Physicians Desk Reference USA, 1984). For children over 12 years of age the adult dosage may be given. Children may have difficulty adequately coordinating the discharge from the metered-dose inhaler and inspiratory effort. They should be allowed to use nebulizers only if they are supervised by a knowledgeable adult; the emphasis should be towards using lower potency preparations and minimum adult doses. Oral orciprenaline is not recommended to be used by children under 6 years of age because its safety and effectiveness have not been confirmed for this age group. The recommended dosage is 10 mg of orciprenaline sulphate, three or four times daily for children who weigh less than 27 kg or are 6 to 9 years of age and 20 mg for those who weigh 27 kg or are over 9 years of age.

Pregnant women
It has been shown that oral orciprenaline at a dose of 50 mg.kg^{-1} (30 times the human oral dose) showed no teratogenic or embryocidal adverse effects in reproduction studies with mice, rats and rabbits. Although there is no evidence of human teratogenic effects, the potential benefit of orciprenaline should be weighed against the possible risks to the mother and child. Particular care should be recommended during the first trimester and the inhaled route should be preferred because of the much lower systemic dose.

The elderly
In the elderly the dosage of each agent should be adjusted to the response of the patient and the patient's general state of health. The dose may have to be reduced in those with impaired liver or renal function. Cardiovascular disorders are expected to be more prevalent in the elderly than in younger patients.

Drug interactions

Potentially hazardous interactions

Tricyclic antidepressants. Tricyclic compounds such as imipramine not only enhance the bronchodilator effects of β-agonists but also may exacerbate their adverse cardiovascular effects. They may be particularly likely to cause disturbances of cardiac rhythm in some patients. Thus patients on tricyclics who may be susceptible to cardiac arrhythmias need careful consideration if orciprenaline is to be prescribed. Once again, the aerosol route is to be preferred.

β-adrenoceptor blockers. The bronchodilatation produced by orciprenaline is antagonized by β-blockers. β-blockers are contraindicated in asthma because they exacerbate airway obstruction as well as antagonizing the effect of therapeutic β-agonists. Selective β_1-antagonists such as metoprolol are said to be less likely to cause worsening of asthmatic symptoms, but even these should be avoided in patients with chronic reversible airway obstruction as other drugs are available for the same purpose.

Sympathomimetic amines. Care is required when orciprenaline is given with adrenaline or other sympathomimetics that are potent in stimulating β-adrenoceptors because their effects will be additive and this may be dangerous in patients with cardiovascular disease.

Hydrocarbon inhalation anaesthetics. Anaesthetics such as halothane, trichloroethylene and enflurane sensitize the myocardium to the arrhythmogenic effects of β-agonists. Orciprenaline is selective for β_2-adrenoceptors but it is less β_2-selective than salbutamol, terbutaline or fenoterol.[1] In these circumstances the cautious use of more selective β_2-agonists such as salbutamol is preferable.

Digitalis glycosides. When a patient is taking digitalis glycosides, β-agonist bronchodilators may increase the risk of serious cardiac arrhythmias. Orciprenaline given by aerosol should be safe but a more selective β_2-agonist such as salbutamol should be preferred.

Other significant interactions

Salicylamide. Evidence has been provided that sulphate conjugation is an important means by which oral orciprenaline and isoprenaline are inactivated in man.[47,14] It has been demonstrated in dogs that salicylamide considerably increased the systemic availability of oral isoprenaline by competing for the pool of sulphate available for conjugation.[48,49] This suggests that concomitant administration of drugs such as salicylamide which are extensively conjugated with sulphate could enhance the effects produced by oral β-agonists or the swallowed fraction of aerosol β-agonists as they would decrease the extent of conjugation in the bowel wall.

Monoamine oxidase inhibitors. Most texts suggest that there should be a significant interaction between β-agonists and monoamine oxidase inhibitors. However, orciprenaline is not a substrate for monoamine oxidase so it would not be expected that monoamine oxidase inhibitors would enhance its effect. Hypothetically, orciprenaline could enhance the effect of tyramine by competition for sulphate conjugation enzymes but this seems unlikely.

Food. Food would be expected to retard the absorption of oral orciprenaline but would have no particular effect when it is taken by aerosol.

Alcohol. At a blood concentration of 5–11 mg.l^{-1}, alcohol produces increases in heart rate and cardiac output due to sympathoadrenal activation. These changes are slight and transient and thus the possibility that tachycardia induced by oral orciprenaline would be significantly exacerbated is unlikely. There is no evidence that there would be any interaction between inhaled preparations and alcohol.

Potentially useful interactions

Theophylline. The effects of β-agonists may be enhanced by the concomitant administration of theophylline and many asthmatics benefit from combining theophylline with β-agonist therapy. When the β-agonist is given by aerosol an additive effect in the lung but not elsewhere may be achieved. One should, of course, be alert for evidence of increased adverse reactions such as insomnia, nervousness, gastrointestinal disturbances and alterations in cardiac function when orciprenaline or other β_2-agonists are combined with theophylline.

Corticosteroids. When asthma becomes severe and airway obstruction is principally due to mucous plugging and airway oedema, orciprenaline and other β-agonists may become ineffective as bronchodilators, and corticosteroid administration becomes necessary. Corticosteroid administration can restore responsiveness to β-agonist bronchodilators.[50,51] It has been proposed that steroids can restore responsiveness to β-agonist aerosols by clearing the airways, increasing β-receptor number and inhibiting extra-neuronal catecholamine uptake.[17] The predominant mechanism is still not known.

Clinical trials

1. Chervinsky P 1975 Alupent syrup: results of a six month trial in asthmatic children. Annals of Allergy 34: 170–176

Double-blind crossover tests with Alupent syrup against placebo were performed at the beginning and at two 3-month intervals during a 6-month study period in 23 schoolchildren. Patients had to respond to two puffs of isoprenaline from a metered inhaler with at least a 20% increase in FEV_1 in order to be accepted into the study.

With Alupent therapy during the 6-month period the mean number of asthmatic attacks decreased and pulmonary function tests indicated significant improvement in FEV_1 and PEFR after Alupent syrup. No tolerance to orciprenaline was observed. In fact, the mean increase in FEV_1 produced by Alupent syrup during the final crossover was significantly greater than the drug-induced increase at the beginning of the treatment.

2. Swarts C L, Hyde J S 1976 Long-term efficacy and safety of nebulized metaproterenol solution in bronchial asthma. Chest 70: 617–620

A 5% solution of orciprenaline sulphate (Alupent) was compared with a 0.5% solution of isoprenaline in a double-blind crossover study before and after 60 days of inhalation of 5% Alupent taken at least 4 times daily by means of a hand-bulb nebulizer. 27 asthmatic patients were studied, 8 with severe asthma, 17 with moderate asthma and 2 with mild asthma.

All patients benefited during the 60-day trial with Alupent, with several being able to decrease or stop the use of other medications. Pulmonary function tests and evaluation by both patient and physician indicated that tolerance did not develop to inhaled Alupent. Inhaled orciprenaline produced a greater maximal increase in FEV_1 than isoprenaline and it also acted longer in both crossover tests.

3. Sackner M A, Silva G, Zucker C, Mark M B 1977 Long-term effects of metaproteranol in asthmatic children. American Review of Respiratory Disease 115: 945–952

Orciprenaline syrup was administered daily for 3 months to asthmatic children in a double-blind crossover design comparing orciprenaline syrup with placebo on the first and last two days of the investigation in order to test for drug-induced tolerance. The 12 boys and 6 girls were aged between 8 and 14 years and their asthma was mild to moderate. During the 3-month treatment period the frequency of attacks diminished and there were no significant side effects. The changes in FEV_1 produced by orciprenaline on the crossover pulmonary function days at the beginning of the 3-month trial period were no different from the measured changes at the end of the study, indicating that chronic administration of orciprenaline syrup did not lead to significant drug-induced tolerance.

4. Galant S P, Groncy C E, Duriseti S, Strick L 1978 The effect of metaproterenol in chronic asthmatic children receiving therapeutic doses of theophylline. Journal of Allergy and Clinical Immunology 61: 73–79

In a double-blind crossover study the effect produced by orciprenaline added to therapeutic doses of theophylline (plasma level of greater than 10 $mg.ml^{-1}$) was compared with the response produced by placebo combined with theophylline by measurement of FEV_1, an index of large-airways function, and maximum mid-expiratory flow rate (MMEFR), an index of small-airways function, in 17 asthmatic children.

Orciprenaline caused significantly greater improvement in the functioning of both the large and smaller airways than when placebo was combined with theophylline. No difference in adverse effects was observed between orciprenaline and placebo combinations and there was no evidence for tolerance developing to orciprenaline.

General review articles

Leifer K N, Wittig H J 1975 The beta-2 sympathomimetic aerosols in the treatment of asthma. Annals of Allergy 35: 69–80

Lulich K M, Goldie R G, Ryan G, Paterson J W 1986 Adverse reactions to $Beta_2$-agonist bronchodilators. Medical Toxicology 1: 286–299

Orciprenaline (sulphate)

Paterson J W, Tarala R A 1985a The treatment of asthma Part 1. Pharmacology of therapeutic agents. Medical Journal of Australia 143: 390–394

Paterson J W, Tarala R A 1985b The treatment of asthma Part 2. Practical aspects of management. Medical Journal of Australia 143: 453–455

Tattersfield A E 1982 Bronchodilator drugs. Pharmacology and Therapeutics 17: 299–313

Webb-Johnson D C, Andrews J L 1977 Bronchodilator therapy (first of two parts). New England Journal of Medicine 297: 476–482

Weinberger M, Hendeles K 1977 The pharmacologic basis of bronchodilator therapy. Rational Drug Therapy 11(6): 1–6

References

1. McFadden E R 1981 $Beta_2$ receptor agonist: metabolism and pharmacology. Journal of Allergy and Clinical Immunology 68: 91–97
2. Chahl L A, O'Donnell S R 1968 The actions of orciprenaline and protokylol on guinea-pig trachea. British Journal of Pharmacology and Chemotherapeutics 33: 552–559
3. Svedmyr N, Thiringer G 1971 The effects of salbutamol and isoprenaline on beta-receptors in patients with chronic obstructive lung disease. Postgraduate Medical Journal (suppl 47): 44–46
4. O'Donnell S R, Wanstall J C 1974 Potency and selectivity in vitro of compounds related to isoprenaline and orciprenaline on beta-adrenoceptors in the guinea-pig. British Journal of Pharmacology 52: 407–417
5. Malta E, Raper C 1974 Non-catechol phenylethanolamines; agonistic and antagonistic actions on beta adrenoceptors in isolated tissues from the guinea-pig. Clinical and Experimental Pharmacology and Physiology 1: 259–268
6. Wilson A F, McPhillips J J 1978 Pharmacological control of asthma. Annual Review of Pharmacology and Toxicology 18: 541–561
7. Wolfe J D, Yamate M, Biedermann A A, Chu T J 1985 Comparison of the acute cardiopulmonary effects of oral albuterol, metaproterenol, and terbutaline in asthmatics. Journal of the American Medical Association 253: 2068–2072
8. McEvoy J D S, Vall-Spinosa A, Paterson J W 1973 Assessment of orciprenaline and isoproterenol infusions in asthmatic patients. American Review of Respiratory Disease 108: 490–500
9. Choo-Kang Y F J, Simpson W T, Grant I W B 1969 Controlled comparison of the bronchodilator effects of three beta-adrenergic stimulant drugs administered by inhalation to patients with asthma. British Medical Journal 2: 287–289
10. Gent P N C, Nisbet I G, Hughes D T, Pearson S B, Sturgeon J G F 1968 Double-blind comparative trial of two metered bronchodilator aerosols. British Journal of Clinical Practice 22: 479–481
11. Belizan J M, Diaz A G, Abusleme C, Poseiro J J, Caldeyro-Barcia R 1975 Effects of orciprenaline on uterine contractility and maternal heart rate. Obstetrics and Gynecology 46: 385–388
12. Milner A D, Ingram D 1971 Bronchodilator and cardiac effects of isoprenaline, orciprenaline, and salbutamol aerosols in asthma. Archives of Disease in Childhood 46: 502–507
13. Dengler H J, Hengstmann J H 1976 Metabolism and pharmacokinetics of orciprenaline in various animal species and man. Archives of International Pharmacodynamics 223: 71–87
14. Macgregor T R, Nastasi L, Farina P R, Keirns J J 1983 Isolation and characterization of metaproterenol-3-O-sulphate: a conjugate of metaproterenol in human urine. Drug Metabolism and Disposition 11: 568–573
15. Davies D S 1982 Pharmacokinetic studies with inhaled drugs. European Journal of Respiratory Disease (suppl 119) 63: 67–72
16. Paterson J W, Woolcock A J, Shenfield G M 1979 Bronchodilator drugs. American Review of Respiratory Disease 120: 1149–1188
17. Paterson J W, Lulich K M, Goldie R G 1984 Drug effects on beta-adrenoceptor function in asthma. In: Morley J (ed) Perspectives in asthma 2: beta-adrenoceptors in asthma. Academic Press, London, pp 245–268
18. Konig P, Eggleston P A, Serby C W 1981 Comparison of oral and inhaled metaproterenol for prevention of exercise-induced asthma. Clinical Allergy 11: 597–604
19. Nelson H S 1985 Stepwise therapy of bronchial asthma: the role of beta-adrenergic agonists. Annals of Allergy 54: 289–293
20. Chervinsky P 1975 Alupent syrup: results of a six month trial in asthmatic children. Annals of Allergy 34: 170–176
21. Sackner M A, Silva G, Zucker C, Marks M B 1977 Long-term effects of metaproterenol in asthmatic children. American Review of Respiratory Disease 115: 945–953
22. Schuller D E, Oppenheimer P J 1982 A comparison of metaproterenol and theophylline for control of childhood asthma. Clinical Pediatrics 21: 135–142
23. Swarts C L, Hyde J S 1976 Long-term efficacy and safety of nebulized metaproterenol solution in bronchial asthma. Chest 70: 617–620
24. Banner A S, Sunderrajan E F, Agarwal M K, Addington W W 1979 Arrhythmogenic effects of orally administered bronchodilators. Archives of Internal Medicine 139: 434–437
25. Al-Hillawi A H, Hayward R, Johnson N M 1984 Incidence of cardiac arrhythmias in patients taking slow release salbutamol and slow release terbutaline for asthma. British Medical Journal 288: 367
26. Aoki V S, Wilson W R, Theilen E O 1972 Studies on the reputed augmentation of the cardiovascular effects of the catecholamines in patients with spontaneous hyperthyroidism. Journal of Pharmacology and Experimental Therapeutics 181: 362–368
27. McDevitt D G, Riddell J G, Hadden D R, Montgomery D A D 1978 Catecholamine sensitivity in hyperthyroidism and hypothyroidism. British Journal of Clinical Pharmacology 6: 297–301

28. Harrison R N, Tattersfield A E 1984 Airway response to inhaled salbutamol in hyperthyroid and hypothyroid patients before and after treatment. Thorax 39: 34–39
29. Neville E, Corris O A, Vivian J, Nariman S, Gibson G J 1982 Nebulised salbutamol and angina. British Medical Journal 285: 796–797
30. Twarog F J, Leung D Y M 1982 Anaphylaxis to a component of isoetharine (sodium bisulfite). Journal of the American Medical Association 248: 2030–2031
31. Koepke J W, Christopher K L, Chai H, Selner J C 1984 Dose-dependent bronchospasm from sulphites in isoetharine. Journal of the American Medical Association 251: 2982–2983
32. Drexel H, Regele M, Lange V 1982 Successful treatment of terbutaline-induced bronchospasm with orciprenaline sulphate. Lancet 2: 446
33. Rolf Smith S, Kendall M J 1984 Metabolic responses to beta$_2$ stimulants. Journal of the Royal College of Physicians of London 18: 190–194
34. Sanders J P, Potter D E, Ellis S, Bee D E, Grant J A 1977 Metabolic and cardiovascular effects of carbuterol and metaproterenol. Journal of Allergy and Clinical Immunology 60: 174–179
35. Wicklmayr M, Dietze G 1979 Effect of metaproterenol on ketone body metabolism of the forearm in healthy and diabetic subjects. Hormone and Metabolic Research 11: 1–6
36. Pingleton S K, Schwartz O, Szymanski D, Epstein M 1982 Hypotension associated with terbutaline therapy in acute quadriplegia. American Review of Respiratory Disease 126: 723–725
37. Zach M S, Oberwaldner B, Forche G, Polgar G 1985 Bronchodilators increase airway instability in cystic fibrosis. American Review of Respiratory Disease 131: 537–543
38. Stolley P D, Schinnar R 1978 Association between asthma mortality and isoproterenol aerosols: a review. Preventive Medicine 7: 519–538
39. Hendeles L, Weinberger M 1984 Nonprescription sale of inhaled metaproterenol - Deja Vu. New England Journal of Medicine 310: 207–208
40. Johnson A J, Nunn A J, Somner A R, Stableforth D E, Stewart C J 1984 Circumstances of death from asthma. British Medical Journal 288: 1870–1872
41. Tai E, Read J 1967 Response of blood gas tensions to aminophylline and isoprenaline in patients with asthma. Thorax 22: 543–549
42. Paterson J W, Courtenay Evans R J, Prime F J 1971 Selectivity of bronchodilator action of salbutamol in asthmatic patients. British Journal of Diseases of the Chest 65: 21–38
43. Larsson S 1977 Long-term treatment with beta$_2$-adrenostimulants in asthma. Side effects, selectivity, tolerance and routes of administration. Acta Medica Scandinavica (suppl 608) 202: 1–40
44. Gundogdu A S, Brown P M, Juul S, Sachs L, Sonksen P H 1979 Comparison of hormonal and metabolic effects of salbutamol infusion in normal subjects and insulin-requiring diabetics. Lancet 2: 1317–1321
45. Lenney W, Milner A D 1978 At what age do bronchodilators work? Archives of Disease in Childhood 53: 532–535
46. Buchanan N 1986 A guide chart to drugs in lactation. Current Therapeutics 27 (5): 67–81
47. Conolly M E, Davies D S, Dollery C T, Morgan C D, Paterson J W, Sandler M 1972 Metabolism of isoprenaline in dog and man. British Journal of Pharmacology 46: 458–472
48. George C F, Blackwell E W, Davies D S 1974 Metabolism of isoprenaline in the intestine. Journal of Pharmacy and Pharmacology 26: 265–267
49. Bennett P N, Blackwell E, Davies D S 1975 Competition for sulphate during detoxification in the gut wall. Nature 258: 247–248
50. Ellul-Micallef R, Fenech F F 1975 Effect of intravenous prednisolone in asthmatics with diminished adrenergic responsiveness. Lancet 2: 1269–1270
51. Shenfield G M, Hodson M E, Clarke S W, Paterson J W 1975 Interaction of corticosteroids and catecholamines in the treatment of asthma. Thorax 30: 430–435

Orphenadrine hydrochloride

Orphenadrine is an antagonist of muscarinic cholinergic receptors mainly used in the treatment of Parkinson's disease.

Chemistry

Orphenadrine hydrochloride (Disipal, Brocadisipal, Biorphen)
$C_{18}H_{23}NO.HCl$
N,N-Dimethyl-2-(2-methylbenzhydryloxy) ethylamine hydrochloride

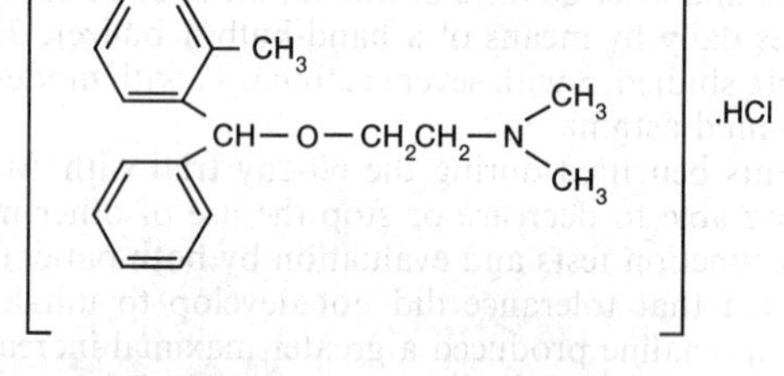

Molecular weight (free base)	305.8 (269.3)
pKa	9
Solubility	
in alcohol	1 in 1
in water	1 in 1
Octanol/water partition coefficient	—

Orphenadrine hydrochloride is a white or almost white crystalline powder, odourless, with a bitter, numbing taste. It is soluble in one part ethanol, and two parts chloroform, but insoluble in ether. Orphenadrine is prepared by chemical synthesis.

Pharmacology

Orphenadrine is an antagonist at central and peripheral muscarinic cholinergic receptors. In addition, it has a weak antihistaminic action. Orphenadrine has been shown to lower concentrations of acetylcholine in rat brain slices but the mechanism for this effect is not known.[1] In addition, orphenadrine increases rat brain concentrations of serotonin and noradrenaline,[2] and inhibits dopamine uptake in striatal synaptosome preparations.[3]

Toxicology

No teratogenic effects of orphenadrine have been observed in mice, rats or rabbits. No mutagenicity was observed in either the Ames test or the Bridges test (Brocades medical information service).

Clinical pharmacology

The main therapeutic effect of orphenadrine is thought to be derived from its antagonistic effect at muscarinic cholinergic receptors. Total daily doses of 150–400 mg of orphenadrine by mouth produce a dose-related improvement in rigidity and tremor in subjects with idiopathic Parkinson's disease, as well as in postencephalitic and drug-induced parkinsonism. In a double-blind placebo-controlled study, Onnaguluchi (see Major outcome trials) observed that orphenadrine given only in the dose of 100 mg three times daily gave a satisfactory clinical response in 15/24 subjects, and a fair response in 7/24 subjects, with peak benefit seen 2 hours after a dose. There are no reports of dose-ranging studies.

Orphenadrine has also been given orally to treat vertigo in vestibular disease.

Acute dystonia may be treated with intramuscular orphenadrine. When used for its central anticholinergic effects, the peripheral anticholinergic effects of orphenadrine may be troublesome. These unwanted effects include dryness of the mouth, blurring of vision, and micturition difficulties. However, a central therapeutic effect can generally be achieved without severe peripheral side effects.

Pharmacokinetics

Gas chromatography is the method of choice for analysing orphenadrine in the plasma.[4] It has a sensitivity of 1 μg.l^{-1}. Absorption from the gastrointestinal tract is almost complete, with presystemic metabolism of 30% following a single oral dose.[5] The half life with acute dosage is 13.7 h after oral administration and 16.1 h after intramuscular administration. However, in chronic administration, plasma levels exceeded those calculated from single-dose pharmacokinetics by a factor of 2 to 3. Elimination half life was also increased over the calculated value by a factor of 2 to 3. Experiments in dogs suggest that this is due to competition for biotransformation between orphenadrine and one of its metabolites, N-desmethylorphenadrine.[6] Plasma protein binding is 95%.

In animals, whole body autoradiography has demonstrated the following tissue distribution of orphenadrine: good penetration into the central nervous system, high concentrations in lung, thymus, lymph nodes and glandular tissue. Lower concentrations were seen in liver and bone marrow.[7]

Orphenadrine is metabolized in the liver and then eliminated in the urine. In a study by Ellison et al[8] 60.8% of a 100 mg dose of tritiated orphenadrine citrate was recovered over 72 h in the urine, and 15.6% over 72 h in the faeces. 8% of the drug was recovered unaltered in the urine. There is no evidence for enterohepatic circulation of the drug.

Oral absorption	≃100%
Presystemic metabolism	30%
Plasma half life	
range	13.7–16.1 h
Volume of distribution	—
Plasma protein binding	95%

Concentration–effect relationship

Antiparkinsonian effects are seen with a plasma concentration in the range 200–500 μg.l^{-1}, but there is no clear cut relationship between the plasma concentration of orphenadrine and its therapeutic effect.

Metabolism

The main metabolic reactions that orphenadrine undergoes in man are: N-demethylation, aromatic hydroxylation and side-chain degradation (Fig. 1).

N-desmethylorphenadrine is pharmacologically active, with anticholinergic and mood-elevating properties.

Fig. 1

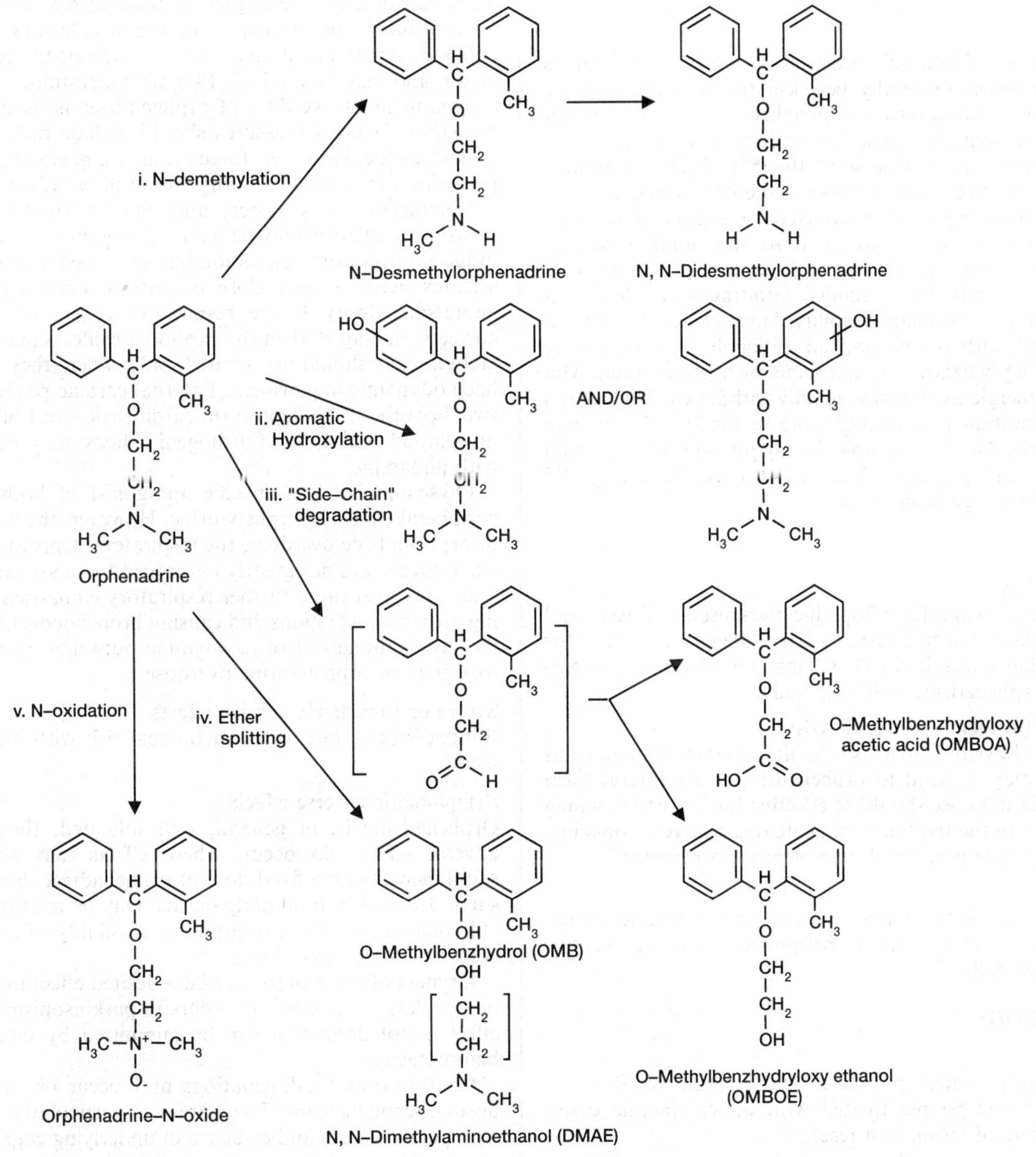

Pharmaceutics

Orphenadrine is available in oral (tablet and elixir) forms.

1. Elixir 25 mg per 5 ml; Biorphen (Bio-Medical, UK).
2. Tablets 50 mg, sugar coated, yellow, imprinted with 'Disipal' (Brocades, UK).
3. Tablets 100 mg, round white tablet: Norflex (3M Riker, USA) coded '221'.
4. Ampoules of 2 ml, 30 mg per ml^{-1} (3M Riker, USA).

Orphenadrine should be stored in airtight containers and protected from light. The shelf-life of the tablets is 3 years.

Orphenadrine citrate is available in oral dose forms for muscle spasm, but its efficacy has not been proved scientifically since it is often combined with analgesics.

Therapeutic use

Indications

1. Idiopathic Parkinson's disease
2. Postencephalitic parkinsonism
3. Drug-induced parkinsonism
4. Acute dystonia
5. Vertigo.

Contraindications

1. Glaucoma
2. Prostatic hypertrophy
3. Pyloric stenosis.

Mode of use

Beneficial and adverse effects of orphenadrine are derived from its anticholinergic properties. Generally, beneficial (i.e. central) effects are seen at a lower dose than adverse (i.e. peripheral) effects. In a recent review Quinn[9] states that all anticholinergic drugs have a modest but useful action in improving the disease by 10–25%. Rigidity is usually improved more than tremor, and akinesia is the least benefited.

An initial dose of 150 mg daily in divided doses is given, and can be increased by 50 mg every second or third day until a desired therapeutic effect is obtained. If orphenadrine needs to be stopped, this should be done gradually, as sudden withdrawal may lead to a marked increase in parkinsonian disability. Horrocks et al[10] studied 25 subjects treated with l-dopa and an anticholinergic (including some subjects taking benzhexol, benztropine, or orphenadrine), who had their anticholinergic treatment gradually withdrawn. There was a 14% mean deterioration in disability score in the 19 subjects who completed the study. All 25 were subsequently put on benzhexol, and though the clinical rating scale once more improved, the change did not reach statistically significant levels.

Indications

1, 2, 3. Parkinsonism

The optimal dosage range for idiopathic Parkinson's disease and postencephalitic parkinsonism is usually 250–300 mg daily, whilst for drug-induced parkinsonism it is 150–300 mg. The maximum recommended dose of orphenadrine is 400 mg daily.

4. Acute dystonia (including oculogyric crises)

Acute drug-induced dystonia (e.g. as seen after metoclopramide) and oculogyric crises may respond to orphenadrine in parenteral form 20–40 mg. A single stat dose should be effective for 2–4 hours, which is usually sufficient in the treatment of acute dystonic reactions due, for example, to a single parenteral dose of prochlorperazine.

5. Vertigo

Orphenadrine is useful in the management of post-traumatic vertigo and other disorders of central and/or peripheral origin. An effective dose is 50 mg twice daily.[11]

Contraindications

1. Glaucoma

Anticholinergic drugs cause pupillary dilation and paralysis of accommodation. Some people treated with anticholinergic drugs complain of blurring of vision as a result.

Anticholinergic drugs are contraindicated in narrow-angle glaucoma, as they may precipitate angle closure and raised intraocular pressure. Blindness has been reported in these circumstances with benzhexol,[12] though there are no cases described of blindness due to orphenadrine.

2. Prostatic hypertrophy

Prostatism may be exacerbated, and occasionally acute retention precipitated, by the anticholinergic effect of orphenadrine inhibiting detrusor muscle action.

3. Pyloric stenosis

Orphenadrine has an antispasmodic effect, decreasing gut motility. Pyloric stenosis may be made worse, paralytic ileus may be precipitated, and constipation made worse by orphenadrine.[11]

Adverse reactions

Potentially life-threatening effects

Potentially lethal effects are extremely rare with therapeutic doses of orphenadrine.[13]

Acute overdosage

Up to 1981, 271 cases of orphenadrine overdose were described in the literature. Of these, 37 died.[14] The lethal dose is estimated to be 2–3 g of orphenadrine.

In mild overdosage, a picture similar to that of atropine poisoning is seen, with a dry mouth, dilated pupils, fever, tachycardia and hallucinations. Larger doses cause coma, and depressed respiration which may be fatal. However, if the patient is given ventilatory support the direct cardiotoxic effects of orphenadrine may be seen. These cardiotoxic effects include bradycardia, atrioventricular conduction block, and impaired contractility, leading to cardiovascular collapse. Arrhythmias may develop, secondary to myocardial hypoxia, and may be fatal 12–18 h after ingestion.

Treatment of overdose of orphenadrine is by general supportive measures. General measures should include induced vomiting and gastric lavage. However, forced diuresis, haemodialysis and haemoperfusion are ineffective in orphenadrine overdose.[15]

Convulsions may occur, and can be treated with diazepam. Assisted ventilation may be required, not only to treat orphenadrine-induced respiratory depression but also when a patient with frequent seizures needs a large dose of anticonvulsants (i.e. a respiratory depressant dose). If the respiratory effects of orphenadrine are correctly managed, then the cardiotoxic effects may be seen. Cardiac arrhythmias should be treated only when they cause significant haemodynamic impairment. External cardiac pacing may be ineffective, because of the depressant cardiotoxic effect of orphenadrine on myocardial excitation. Cardiogenic shock may need to be treated with dopamine.

Physostigmine is a specific antagonist of both the central and peripheral effects of orphenadrine. However, the most serious effects of orphenadrine overdose, the respiratory depression and cardiovascular effects, are not greatly influenced by physostigmine. Physostigmine may also cause further respiratory embarrassment, by increasing bronchial secretions and causing bronchoconstriction. In general, the disadvantages of physostigmine outweigh its advantages in the treatment of orphenadrine overdose.

Severe or irreversible adverse effects

Blindness (see above) is a theoretical risk with orphenadrine treatment.

Symptomatic adverse effects

Orphenadrine is, in general, well tolerated, though symptomatic adverse effects do occur. These effects may sometimes resolve spontaneously on a fixed dose of orphenadrine, but if they persist, a small decrease in total daily dosage may be required.

If blurring of vision occurs, the possibility of angle-closure glaucoma should be considered.

Dryness of the mouth may be a desired effect in patients troubled by drooling, as commonly occurs in parkinsonism. However, if this effect is not desired, it can be minimized by taking orphenadrine before meals.

Confusion and hallucinations may occur on normal therapeutic doses of orphenadrine. These are seen particularly in elderly patients with parkinsonism and evidence of underlying cognitive impairment.

If orphenadrine causes confusion and hallucinations, treatment with it should be stopped.

Orphenadrine may worsen abnormal involuntary movements caused by levodopa.[16] A smaller dose of orphenadrine, or complete cessation of treatment, may be required.[16] Jenner and Marsden[17] state that cholinergic function may be altered in tardive dyskinesias; the administration of anticholinergic agents to patients receiving neuroleptic therapy can reveal or exacerbate abnormal movements. Jenner and Marsden[17] advocate the withdrawal of any anticholinergic when tardive dyskinesia is a problem.

Interference with clinical pathology tests

Orphenadrine has been reported to increase levels of protein-bound thyroxine in a dose-dependent and reversible manner.[18]

High risk groups

Neonates

There is no clinical indication for the use of orphenadrine in patients in this age group.

Breast milk. There is no information available on orphenadrine and lactation.

Children

No special precautions are required. The dose of orphenadrine should be adjusted in accordance with the weight of the child.

Pregnant women

Orphenadrine crosses the placenta, so caution must be exercised in its use during pregnancy.

The elderly

The elderly are more likely than young adults to develop confusion and hallucinations with orphenadrine. Elderly men are likely to have prostatic hypertrophy, which may produce symptoms when they are given orphenadrine.

Concurrent disease

The drug should be avoided, whenever possible, in patients with, or suspected of having, glaucoma, prostatic hypertrophy or pyloric stenosis.

Drug interactions

Potentially hazardous interactions

Alcohol. Alcohol will enhance the hepatic metabolism of orphenadrine, and thus lower blood concentrations and decrease the therapeutic effect. Alcohol should be avoided when on orphenadrine treatment.

Neuroleptics. Neuroleptic drugs have extrapyramidal adverse effects which include parkinsonism and tardive dyskinesia. Orphenadrine may be used to treat drug-induced parkinsonism, but should not be used prophylactically against extrapyramidal effects. The risk of developing a tardive dyskinesia when an anticholinergic drug is given from the start of neuroleptic therapy is greater than if the neuroleptic is given alone.[19]

An additional reason for not giving orphenadrine with chlorpromazine, for example, is that both drugs induce hepatic microsomal enzymes, and therefore enhance the metabolism of each other (and of themselves).[20] A lowered plasma concentration of chlorpromazine may be part of the mechanism for orphenadrine improving parkinsonism caused by chlorpromazine, though the central anticholinergic property of orphenadrine must also be important.

Other drugs. Orphenadrine is 95% protein-bound, and theoretically will interact with another drug bound in the same place. However, no such interactions have been described.

Other significant interactions

Orphenadrine may theoretically alter the absorption of other drugs by decreasing gastrointestinal motility.

Potentially useful interactions

In the treatment of parkinsonism, orphenadrine and levodopa may be given together, and have a synergistic beneficial effect.[21]

Major outcome trials

1. Onnaguluchi G 1963 Assessment of drug therapy in parkinsonism. British Medical Journal 1: 443–448

This is a short-term double-blind trial comparing placebo and orphenadrine 100 mg three times a day. Orphenadrine produced a satisfactory response in 15 out of 24 subjects, a fair response in 7 out of 24, and no response in 2 out of 24.

In the orphenadrine treatment period, two subjects experienced micturition difficulties, three experienced limb myoclonus (two of these only transiently), and one a feeling of 'nervousness'. Orphenadrine was also noted to have a mood elevating effect.

2. Hughes R C, Polgar J G, Weightman D, Walton J N 1971 Levodopa in parkinsonism: the effects of withdrawal of anticholinergic drugs. British Medical Journal 2: 487–491

36 patients, treated with levodopa and an anticholinergic drug (23 taking orphenadrine) were divided into two study groups. In one, anticholinergic drugs were withdrawn gradually, in the other anticholinergics were withdrawn suddenly. Both groups experienced an increase in disability: tremor, rigidity and bradykinesia all increasing. In those in whom the anticholinergic was withdrawn suddenly, increase in disability was greater than in those in whom the drug was withdrawn gradually.

Other trials

3. Capstick N, Pudney H 1976 A comparative trial of orphenadrine and tofenacin in the control of depression and extrapyramidal side effects associated with fluphenazine decanoate therapy. Journal of International Medical Research 4 (6): 435–440

Orphenadrine and tofenacin (N-desmethylorphenadrine) were compared double-blind. They were found to be equally efficacious in treating extrapyramidal side effects of fluphenazine, but orphenadrine was in addition effective against depression.

4. Johnsson D A W 1981 A double blind trial of orphenadrine against placebo. British Journal of Psychiatry 139: 96–97

This study was part of a larger study of the treatment of depression in schizophrenia. 40 subjects with schizophrenia were treated with orphenadrine in a double-blind manner. There was a small, non-statistically significant improvement in depression in the orphenadrine-treated group.

References

1. Hespe W, Ernsting M J E, Nauta W T 1969 The effect of orphenadrine hydrochloride on the acetylcholine concentration in rat brain. International Journal of Neuropharmacology 8: 471–474
2. Van der Zee P, Hespe W 1973 Influence of orphenadrine hydrochloride and its demethylated derivatives on the in vitro uptake of noradrenaline and 5-hydroxytryptamine by rat brain slices. Neuropharmacology 12: 843–851
3. Coyle J T, Snyder S H 1969 Antiparkinsonian drugs: inhibition of dopamine uptake in the corpus striatum as a possible mechanism of action. Science 166: 899–901
4. Labout J J M, Thijssen C T, Hespe W 1977 Sensitive and specific gas chromatographic and extraction method for the determination of orphenadrine in body fluids. Journal of Chromatography 144: 201–208
5. Rutiliano G, Labout J J M 1982 The bioavailability of orphenadrine hydrochloride after intramuscular and oral administration. Journal of International Medical Research 10: 447–450
6. Labout J J M, Thijssen C T, Keijser G G J, Hespe W 1982 Difference between single and multiple dose pharmacokinetics of orphenadrine hydrochloride in man. European Journal of Clinical Pharmacology 21: 343–350
7. Prins H, Hespe W 1968 Autoradiographic study of the distribution of radioactivity in mice after oral administration of tritium labelled orphenadrine hydrochloride. Archives Internationales de Pharmacodynamie et de Therapie 171: 47–57
8. Ellison T, Snyder A, Bolger J, Okun R 1971 Metabolism of orphenadrine citrate in man. Journal of Pharmacology and Experimental Therapeutics 176: 284–295
9. Quinn N P 1984 Anti-parkinsonian drugs today. Drugs 28: 236–262
10. Horrocks P, Vicary D, Rees J, Parkes J, Marsden C D 1973 Anti-cholinergic drug withdrawal and benzhexol treatment in Parkinson's disease. Journal of Neurological and Neurosurgical Psychiatry 36: 936–941
11. Camarda V, Di Carlo A 1982 A controlled study of the effect of orphenadrine hydrochloride (Disipal) on vertigo in patients with spontaneous vestibular disease. British Journal of Clinical Practice 36: 186–188
12. Friedman Z, Neumann E 1972 Benzhexol induced blindness in Parkinson's disease. British Medical Journal 1: 605
13. Daggett P, Ibrahim S Z 1976 Intestinal obstruction complicating orphenadrine treatment. British Medical Journal 1: 21–22
14. Sangster B 1982 Orphenadrine intoxication. Geneesmiddelen Bulletin 16 no. 12: 53–56
15. Sangster B, van Heijst A N P, Zimmerman A N E 1978 Vergiftiging door orfenadrine (Disipal). Nederlands Tijdschrift voor Geneeskunde 122: 988–992

16. Birket-Smith E 1975 Abnormal involuntary movements in relation to anticholinergics and levodopa therapy. Acta Neurologica Scandinavica 52: 158–160
17. Jenner P, Marsden C D 1983 Neuroleptics and tardive dyskinesia. In: Coyle J T, Enna S J (eds) Neuroleptics: neurochemical behavioural and clinical perspectives. Raven Press, New York, pp 223–253
18. Beermann B, Wester P O 1974 Effect of orphenadrine on total thyroxine. Acta Medica Scandinavica 196: 113–114
19. Gerlach J, Reisby N, Randrup A 1974 Dopaminergic hypersensitivity and cholinergic hypofunction in the pathophysiology of tardive dyskinesia. Psychopharmacologia 34: 21–35
20. Loga S, Curry J, Lader M 1975 Interactions of orphenadrine and phenobarbitone with chlorpromazine: plasma concentrations and effects in man. British Journal of Clinical Pharmacology 2: 197–208
21. Hughes R C, Polgar J E, Weightron D, Walton J N 1971 Levodopa in Parkinsonism: the effects of withdrawal of anti-cholinergic drugs. British Medical Journal 2: 487–491

Ouabain

Ouabain is an injectable cardiac glycoside with a faster onset of action than digoxin.

The term 'cardiac glycosides' encompasses compounds which contain a cardenolide moiety (the steroid-like structure illustrated below) linked to one or more glycoside (glucose-like) moieties, and which have a positive inotropic action on the heart. The term 'digitalis' strictly speaking should refer only to those cardiac glycosides which are obtained from plants of the *Digitalis* species, which ouabain is not. However, by convention the term 'digitalis' is generally used to refer to all natural and semi-synthetic cardiacglycosides, whether derived from *Digitalis* plants or not. This is the convention adopted here. When the word 'digitalis' is used it can be taken that the information refers to all cardiac glycosides. When this is not the case the term 'ouabain' is used.

Chemistry

Ouabain (G-strophanthin, Gratus strophanthin, acocantherin, Ouabaine Arnaud)
$C_{29}H_{44}O_{12}.8H_2O$
3β-[(6-Deoxy-α-L-mannopyranosyl)oxy]-1-β,5,11α,14,19-pentahydroxycard-20(22)-enolideoctahydrate
The cardenolide (or 'aglycone') is called ouabaigenin. The sugar is rhamnose.

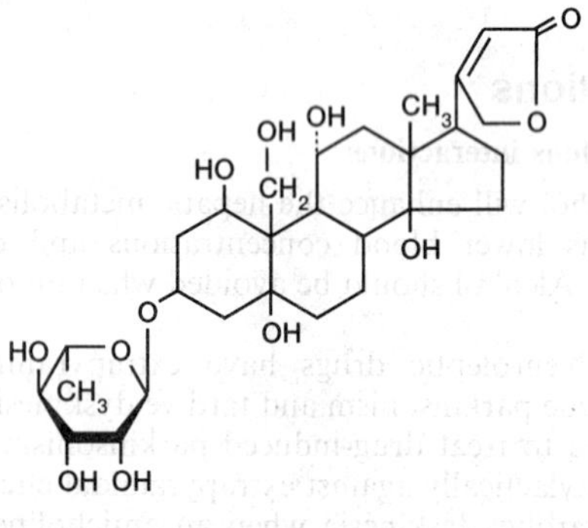

Molecular weight (anhydrous)	728.8 (584.6)
pKa (at pH 7)	not ionized
Solubility	
in alcohol	1 in 100
in water	1 in 75
Octanol/water partition coefficient	0.01

A white, odourless powder or crystals with a bitter taste. Ouabain cannot be synthesized, and is extracted from the seeds of *Strophanthus gratus* and the wood of *Acokanthera schimperi* and *A. ouabaii*.

Pharmacology

At the molecular level digitalis binds to and inhibits the membrane-bound cation transport enzyme, the magnesium-dependent sodium- and potassium-linked adenosine triphosphatase (Na^+,K^+-ATPase; EC 3.6.1.37); this is regarded as its pharmacological receptor. At the cellular level ouabain thus increases the intracellular concentration of sodium, and this in turn alters the intracellular disposition of calcium. At low concentrations (below 10^{-8}–10^{-9} M) there may also be both stimulation of Na^+,K^+-ATPase and a direct effect on calcium,[1,2] but the relevance of these actions to the therapeutic effects of digitalis is not clear.

Toxicology

Ouabain is not mutagenic and has not been shown to be carcinogenic in either man or animals. It is not known to be teratogenic in man.

Clinical pharmacology

At the physiological level digitalis has a positive inotropic effect on myocardial cells (it increases the rate of contractility of the myocardium). It also has complex direct effects on the action potentials of the conducting fibres: in ventricular muscle and Purkinje fibres it increases automaticity, decreases conduction velocity, and increases the refractory period; in the atrioventricular node it increases automaticity and shortens the refractory period, but has no effect on the conduction velocity. It has no important direct actions on the sinus node. In addition to these direct effects digitalis has indirect effects on the heart; it increases vagal input and decreases sympathetic drive, both of which effects contribute to its action in slowing the ventricular rate,[3] both in sinus rhythm and in atrial fibrillation. Digitalis also has effects on pericardial reflexes and baroreceptor reflexes, but the clinical significance of these is unclear. In arterial smooth muscle it increases tone by a mechanism as yet unknown.

At the level of the whole organ digitalis slows the ventricular rate and increases cardiac output. Its effect on vascular smooth muscle can cause hypertension during rapid intravenous administration. By its action on Na^+,K^+-ATPase in the ascending limb of the loop of Henle digitalis causes a diuresis, but in cardiac failure this effect is small by comparison with the diuresis which occurs secondary to its action on the heart.

Pharmacokinetics

Ouabain pharmacokinetics[4] have been studied by the use of radiolabelled ouabain and by radioimmunoassay with a sensitivity[5] of 5.0 µg.l^{-1}. Assay kits for routine measurement are not available, but, if necessary, the drug can be assayed by bioassay, using the concentration-dependent inhibition by digitalis of erythrocytic Na^+,K^+-ATPase, measured as an inhibition of the active transmembrane inward transport of rubidium-86.

Ouabain is poorly (no more than 5%) absorbed after oral administration, and is therefore always given parenterally. There is no presystemic metabolism.

Ouabain is not bound to plasma proteins (<5%). It is widely distributed to all body tissues except fat, and has an apparent volume of distribution of about 10 l.kg^{-1}. The apparent volume of distribution may be reduced in patients with hypothyroidism and increased in patients with hyperthyroidism.[6] Because of its high apparent volume of distribution, haemodialysis removes very little ouabain from the body.

Oral absorption	5%
Presystemic metabolism	None
Plasma half life	
range	18–25 h
mean	22 h
Volume of distribution	10 l.kg^{-1}
Plasma protein binding	<5%

Ouabain is metabolized to a very minor extent in the liver.

About 50% of an intravenous dose of ouabain is excreted unchanged via the kidneys, and about 30% in the faeces, although less than 15% is excreted via the bile. There must therefore be some intestinal excretion.

The plasma half life of ouabain when renal function is normal is about 22 hours. In patients with renal dysfunction the half life is prolonged to 50 or 60 hours, which results in a lower dosage requirement.[7] Similarly, as renal function decreases with age, some dosage adjustments may be necessary.

Concentration–effect relationship

One would expect plasma ouabain concentrations to correlate with measures of its therapeutic efficacy and of its pharmacodynamic actions, as in the cases of digoxin and digitoxin. There is no direct information on this; however, indirect evidence suggests that the plasma concentration–effect relationship for ouabain and systolic time intervals may be similar to that for digoxin and digitoxin.[8]

Ouabain

Certain factors may alter the relationship between the expected effects of ouabain and its actual effects: these factors are of two types (note that some factors appear in both groups):

Factors which alter the amount of ouabain in the body for a given dose

Decreased renal clearance[7] in renal failure and old age is the most important factor, because most of the drug is eliminated unchanged in the urine. In these cases dosage reductions will be necessary (see below).

Factors which alter the sensitivity of the tissues to a given amount of ouabain

Potassium depletion (e.g. due to diuretics)
Magnesium depletion
Calcium excess
Acidosis and hypoxia
Old age
Hypothyroidism
Cardiac disease[6]
Chronic cor pulmonale
Myocardial infarction
Cardiogenic shock
Myocarditis
Primary cardiomyopathies.

In all of these cases doses of digoxin may have to be reduced, but there is no information on the extent to which dosage reductions may be required.

A plasma potassium concentration below 3.5 mmol.l^{-1} is highly likely to result in increased sensitivity to digitalis and in such cases ouabain is better avoided until the plasma potassium is restored to normal.

Metabolism

Ouabain is metabolized to a very small extent in the liver by hydrolysis, yielding rhamnose and the aglycone ouabaigenin which is much less cardioactive than ouabain (Fig. 1).

Fig. 1 Metabolites of ouabain

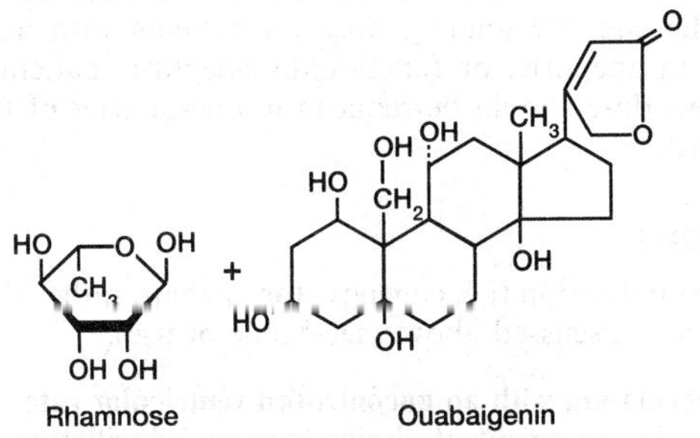

Pharmaceutics

Ouabain is available only in parenteral form — a clear solution for intravenous or intramuscular injection.

Intravenous injections contain 250 µg in 1 ml of water. The pH is usually buffered to between 6 and 7.5. Injections should be protected from light during storage.

Ouabaine Arnaud contains crystalline ouabain derived from *Strophanthus gratus.*

Therapeutic use

Indications

1. Atrial fibrillation with an uncontrolled ventricular rate
2. Atrial flutter and supraventricular tachycardia
3. Acute left ventricular failure.

Contraindications

1. Hypertrophic obstructive cardiomyopathy
2. Arrhythmias due to accessory pathways (e.g. Wolff–Parkinson–White syndrome).

Relative contraindications

1. Chronic cor pulmonale
2. Aortic valve disease
3. Acute myocarditis
4. Congestive cardiomyopathies
5. Constrictive pericarditis
6. Heart block.

Mode of use

Ouabain is so poorly absorbed that it must be given parenterally. Its faster onset of action is thus the only reason for giving ouabain in preference to digoxin, and it may be resorted to if there is urgency to treat, e.g. in a patient with severe heart failure and uncontrolled atrial fibrillation. As soon as the patient is satisfactorily digitalized with ouabain one should switch to oral digoxin if possible. Intravenous infusion of ouabain should be administered over at least 30 minutes, since a faster rate of infusion may be associated with hypertension and cardiac arrhythmias.

There are no clear-cut guidelines to what are likely to be appropriate dosages of ouabain, but one can make theoretical calculations from first principles. Assuming that ouabain has an apparent volume of distribution of $10\,l.kg^{-1}$, a total body clearance rate of $350\,ml.min^{-1}$, and a half life of 22 hours, and assuming that the unbound plasma ouabain concentration associated with a therapeutic effect is similar to that for digoxin, one would expect a daily maintenance dose of 0.5 mg to produce a steady-state plasma concentration of $1\,\mu g.l^{-1}$ (which compares with a plasma digoxin concentration of about $1.2\,\mu g.l^{-1}$, correcting for protein-binding). The corresponding loading dose would be about 1 mg (i.e. 15 μg per kg lean body weight). Thus, one can recommend a loading dose of 15 μg per kg, which, because of the more rapid onset of action of ouabain, would be given in three divided doses at intervals of two hours, watching for signs of digitalis intoxication before the second and third doses, and not giving those doses if such evidence appeared. If there was no evidence of toxicity after the third dose and it was considered that a full therapeutic effect had not yet been achieved, then a further $5\,\mu g.kg^{-1}$ could be given. In cases of extreme urgency the full loading dose of 15 μg per kg could be given as a single dose. If ouabain were continued thereafter the maintenance dose would be one-half the effective loading dose (in patients with normal renal function). In anephric, or functionally anephric, patients the daily maintenance dose should be reduced to one-quarter of the effective loading dose.

Indications

The general indication (i.e. cogency) for ouabain rather than digoxin or digitoxin is discussed above (see Mode of use).

1. Atrial fibrillation with an uncontrolled ventricular rate
Digitalis is the treatment of choice for atrial fibrillation with a fast ventricular rate, except in the following cases:

a. In patients whose atrial fibrillation is due to hyperthyroidism, digitalis may be relatively or completely ineffective, and a β-adrenoceptor antagonist may be required instead. In such cases, however, digitalis may still prove useful either in supplementing the effects of the β-blocker or in decreasing its negative inotropic effect on the left ventricle.
b. In patients with atrial fibrillation due to accessory pathways, as in the Wolff–Parkinson–White syndrome, digitalis blocks conduction through the AV node, but not through the accessory fibres. It is therefore contraindicated.
c. In the prevention of paroxysmal attacks of atrial fibrillation for which digitalis is not effective. Although this might appear inappropriate for ouabain, it is not. In some countries ouabain is given by repeated intermittent parenteral injections for a variety of reasons.

2. Atrial flutter and supraventricular tachycardia
Although digitalis can slow the ventricular rate in both atrial flutter and supraventricular tachycardia, and may restore sinus rhythm, it is generally ineffective, and it is usually better to use other drugs or cardioversion.

3. Acute left ventricular failure
The positive inotropic action of digitalis can undoubtedly be beneficial in the treatment of acute left ventricular failure, but its use has steadily declined for at least two reasons:

a. Its use in patients with acute myocardial infarction has been thought to be associated with an unacceptable risk of cardiac arrhythmias, although evidence for this is scanty.
b. Other drugs are more effective, either in the early treatment of acute left ventricular failure (e.g. opiates and diuretics), or in cases where early therapy has failed (e.g. positive inotropic drugs such as dopamine and dobutamine, or vasodilators such as nitrates).

Contraindications

1. Hypertrophic obstructive cardiomyopathy
Digitalis increases the force of contraction in the hypertrophied left ventricular outflow tract in this condition and thus impairs cardiac output.

2. Arrhythmias due to accessory pathways
Digitalis does not block conduction through most types of accessory pathways and can thus accentuate arrhythmias due to such abnormalities.

Relative contraindications

1. Chronic cor pulmonale
Perhaps because of the presence of hypoxia and acidosis there is both decreased effectiveness and an increased risk of cardiac arrhythmias in patients with chronic cor pulmonale.

2. Aortic valve disease
Digitalis increases left ventricular contractility and may therefore worsen ventricular function in patients with aortic valve disease, as it does in hypertrophic obstructive cardiomyopathy (i.e. 'subvalvular stenosis'). However, digitalis may sometimes be beneficial in cases where there is severe left ventricular dilatation.

3. Acute myocarditis
In acute myocarditis the myocardium, for reasons which are not understood, seems to be sensitized to the actions of digitalis; the risk of arrhythmias is thus increased.

4. Congestive cardiomyopathies
The effectiveness of digitalis in some congestive cardiomyopathies is reduced and the risk of arrhythmias increased. The reasons are not understood.

5. Constrictive pericarditis
The efficacy of digitalis is poor in the presence of constrictive pericarditis, because of the fixed obstruction to movement of the myocardium.

6. Heart block
Because digitalis can cause heart block care should be taken if there is pre-existing heart block. However, careful use of digitalis should not cause worsening of heart block.

Adverse reactions[10–15]

Potentially life-threatening effects
Deaths due to digitalis occur only in severe cases of toxicity, and are always due to cardiac arrhythmias, usually in combination with heart block.

Acute overdosage
Self-poisoning with ouabain is highly unlikely, since it will not generally be available to patients for self-administration. Treatment would be as for digoxin, omitting gastric lavage, but including activated charcoal, because of the excretion of ouabain via the gut. In cases where the plasma potassium concentration rises antidigoxin antibody could be tried, on the expectation that it might be effective against ouabain in man, as it is against digitoxin and lanatoside C.

Severe or irreversible adverse effects
Cardiac. The commonest cardiac adverse effects of digitalis are extra beats, usually ventricular, and these may characteristically be coupled ('pulsus bigeminus'). In more severe cases ventricular tachy-

Ouabain

cardia and fibrillation may occur. Supraventricular extra beats may also occur, and in more severe cases paroxysmal supraventricular tachycardia. Rarely, there may be worsening of atrial fibrillation. Any degree of heart block can occur as a result of toxicity, although prolongation of the electrocardiographic PR interval commonly occurs in the absence of toxicity. The combination of an ectopic arrhythmia and heart block is particularly typical of digitalis toxicity (e.g. paroxysmal supraventricular tachycardia with AV block). Sinus bradycardia can occur, but in patients at rest it is not frequently a sign of toxicity. Rarely, digitalis toxicity can cause worsening of heart failure.

The risk of digitalis-induced arrhythmias is increased when DC cardioversion is used. If elective cardioversion is to be attempted in a digitalized patient then one should start with a very low energy (10 J), increasing gradually as required. Some advise giving a single dose of an antiarrhythmic drug, such as phenytoin or lignocaine, before cardioversion in a digitalized patient, but there is no good evidence of the efficacy of this.

Gastrointestinal. The commonest symptoms of digitalis toxicity are anorexia, nausea, and vomiting. Diarrhoea sometimes occurs, particularly in the elderly.

Central nervous system. Digitalis can cause confusion, dizziness, drowsiness, bad dreams, restlessness, nervousness, agitation and amnesia. Acute psychoses and delirium can occur, particularly in the elderly. Chorea, organic brain syndrome, and epilepsy have also been reported. Digitalis affects the eyes and can cause disturbances of colour vision. The most common form of colour vision disturbance is xanthopsia (i.e. yellow vision), but many other kinds of disturbance have been reported, including rhodopsia, cyanopsia, castanopsia, leucopsia and melanopsia. Digitalis can also cause blurred vision and photophobia.

Symptomatic adverse effects
When mild, some of the adverse effects described above fall into this category.

Treatment of digitalis toxicity
In the majority of cases all that need be done is to withhold digitalis. If there is potassium depletion, this should be remedied; oral administration of potassium chloride is generally all that is required. For more severe cases, see Digoxin: Acute overdosage.

Other effects
Digitalis in overdose may cause an increase in plasma potassium concentration, because it inhibits the Na^+,K^+-ATPase and prevents the entry of potassium into cells. When given intravenously digitalis can cause rises in the activity in the serum of cardiospecific creatine kinase.

Changes in the electrocardiogram. Digitalis prolongs the PR interval and shortens the QRS duration. It causes sagging (so-called 'reverse ticking') of the ST segment, and T wave inversion. All of these changes can occur in the absence of toxicity and do not aid in its diagnosis.

Interference with clinical pathology tests
Digitalis may increase the apparent concentration of 17-hydroxycorticosteroids in the urine.

High risk groups

Neonates
There is no information on what appropriate doses of ouabain should be in children. It is probably better avoided in the young.[3]

Breast milk. There is no information on the excretion of ouabain in breast milk.

Children
What has been said about neonates also applies to older children.

Pregnant women
Ouabain crosses the placenta,[16] but fetal plasma and amniotic fluid concentrations are lower after a single dose than maternal plasma concentrations. The relevance of this observation to the use of ouabain in pregnant women is not clear.

The elderly
Partly because of reduced renal function and partly because their tissues are more sensitive to the effects of digitalis, the elderly require lower maintenance doses of ouabain than younger adults. The loading dose should be as outlined above, and maintenance doses should be adjusted according to measured (creatinine clearance) or supposed renal function. In patients over 60 years of age, renal function should be assumed to be no more than 50% of normal even if the plasma creatinine is normal.

Concurrent disease

Patients with renal impairment.[7] Doses in patients with renal impairment should be reduced; see Mode of use.

Thyroid disease.[6] For reasons which are not fully understood the pharmacokinetics and pharmacodynamics of cardiac glycosides are altered in thyroid disease. The apparent volume of distribution and renal clearance of ouabain are increased in hyperthyroidism and decreased in hypothyroidism, and the response of the tissues to digitalis is decreased in hyperthyroidism and increased in hypothyroidism. For these reasons, ouabain can be very difficult to use correctly in patients with abnormalities of thyroid function. In hyperthyroidism there may be resistance to its effects, and increasing the dose above normal in order to counteract the kinetic problems is likely to result in toxicity without any therapeutic response; conversely in hypothyroidism toxicity may readily occur at low doses.

Drug interactions[15,17]

Potentially hazardous interactions

Potassium-depleting drugs. The most common interaction with cardiac glycosides occurs with drugs which cause potassium depletion, since the effects of digitalis are increased in the absence of potassium. This can occur when, for example, diuretics or corticosteroids are given. Since hypercalcaemia increases the effects of digitalis, toxicity may occur during the co-administration of calcium salts.

Potentially useful interactions
Digitalis improves left ventricular function in patients in whom it has been impaired by β-adrenoceptor antagonists.

References

1. Schwarz A, Lindenmayer C E, Allen J C 1975 The sodium-potassium adenosine triphosphatase: pharmacological, physiological and biochemical aspects. Pharmacological Reviews 27: 3–134
2. Noble D 1980 Mechanism of action of therapeutic levels of cardiac glycosides. Cardiovascular Research 14: 495–514
3. Gillis R A, Quest J A 1980 The role of the central nervous system in the cardiovascular effects of digitalis. Pharmacological Reviews 31: 19–97
4. Greeff K, Wirth K E 1981 Pharmacokinetics of strophanthus glycosides. In: Greeff K (ed) Cardiac glycosides part II: pharmacokinetics and clinical pharmacology. Springer-Verlag, Berlin, pp 57–85
5. Selden R, Margolies M N, Smith T W 1974 Renal and gastrointestinal excretion of ouabain in dog and man. Journal of Pharmacology and Experimental Therapeutics 188: 615–623
6. Shenfield G M 1981 The influence of thyroid dysfunction on drug pharmacokinetics. Clinical Pharmacokinetics 6: 275–297
7. Aronson J K 1983 Clinical pharmacokinetics of cardiac glycosides in patients with renal dysfunction. Clinical Pharmacokinetics 8: 155–178
8. Weissler A M, Lewis R P, Leighton R F, Bush C A 1972 Comparative responses to the digitalis glycosides in man. In: Marks B H, Weissler A M (eds) Basic and clinical pharmacology of digitalis. Charles C Thomas, Springfield, Illinois, pp. 260–280
9. Ochs H R, Greenblatt D J, Bodem G, Dengler H J 1982 Disease-related alterations in cardiac glycoside disposition. Clinical Pharmacokinetics 7: 434–451
10. Chung E K 1969 Digitalis intoxication. Excerpta Medica, Amsterdam
11. Aronson J K 1983 Digitalis intoxication. Clinical Science 64: 253–258
12. Smith T W, Antman E M, Friedman P L, Blatt C M, Marsh J D 1984 Digitalis glycosides: mechanisms and manifestations of toxicity. Part I. Progress in Cardiovascular Diseases 26: 413–458
13. Smith T W, Antman E M, Friedman P L, Blatt C M, Marsh J D 1984 Digitalis glycosides: mechanisms and manifestations of toxicity. Part II. Progress in Cardiovascular Diseases 26: 495–540
14. Smith T W, Antman E M, Friedman P L, Blatt C M, Marsh J D 1984 Digitalis glycosides: mechanisms and manifestations of toxicity. Part III. Progress in Cardiovascular Diseases 27: 21–56
15. Aronson J K 1989 Cardiac glycosides and drugs used in dysrhythmias. In: Dukes M N G (ed) Meyler's side effects of drugs, 11th edn. Elsevier, Amsterdam, pp 333–358
16. Saarikoski S 1980 Placental transmission and foetal distribution of ^{3}H-ouabain. Acta Pharmacologica et Toxicologica 46: 278–282
17. Binnion P F 1978 Drug interactions with digitalis glycosides.Drugs 15: 369–380

Oxamniquine

This drug is used in the treatment of infection due to *Schistosoma mansoni.*

Chemistry

Oxamniquine (Vansil, Mansil)
$C_{14}H_{21}N_3O_3$
1,2,3,4-Tetrahydro-2-(isopropylamino)methyl-7-nitro-6-quinoline-methanol[1]

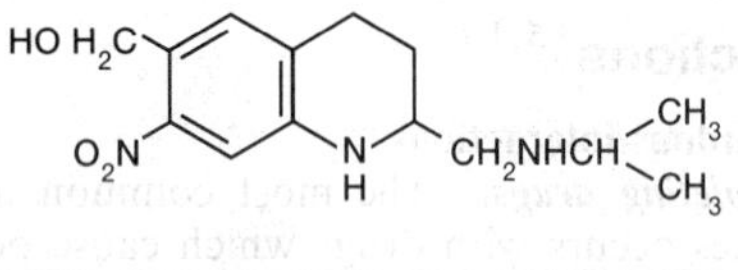

Molecular weight	279.3
pKa	—
Solubility	
in alcohol	—
in water	1 in 3300
Octanol/water partition coefficient	—

Oxamniquine is a light orange crystalline solid with melting point of 151–152°C. It is prepared from the synthetic precursor 2-isopropylamino-methyl-6-methyl-7-nitro-1,2,3,4-tetrahydroquinoline by microbiological hydroxylation catalysed by the fungus *Aspergillus sclerotiorum.*[2] It is not present in any combination preparations.

Pharmacology

Experimentally, oxamniquine is inactive against *Schistosoma japonicum* in mice, hamster and monkey models. In both animal models and in man, the drug is highly active against *S. mansoni* and produces a shift of worms from the mesenteric vessels to the liver within a few days after administration. In mice, hamsters and primates infected with *S. mansoni*, male worms proved more susceptible than females. Whereas the shift of males to the liver was irreversible since they were retained there by tissue reactions and died, surviving unpaired females returned to the mesenteric vessels. Since these surviving females ceased to lay eggs in the absence of the males, the vast majority of whom died, the basic cause of the pathological effects of schistosomiasis was removed.[3,4] Oxamniquine has weak anticholinergic effects shown by the stimulation of motor activity in *S. mansoni.* However, this is not the mechanism of action of oxamniquine in killing *S. mansoni* which remains unknown.

The drug has virtually no effect against *S. haematobium* or *S. mattheei* in man.[5–8]

Toxicology[9]

The approximate oral LD_{50} of oxamniquine in mice was 1400 mg.kg^{-1}, giving an LD_{50}/ED_{50} ratio of 65:1. The LD_{50} in mice when given intramuscularly was >2000 mg.kg^{-1}, probably due to slow absorption of poorly solubilized base from the injection site. In rats, the female was 8–10 times more sensitive in acute toxicity studies and this was reflected in the oral LD_{50} values which were 300 mg.kg^{-1} and 30–40 mg.kg^{-1} in males and females, respectively. The oral LD_{50} values in mg.kg^{-1} were 950 in male hamsters and 500–1000 in rabbits.

Clinical signs were rather non-specific in rodents and rabbits (e.g. hypomotility, malaise, mild motor incoordination and occasionally convulsions), occurring only, except in female rats, after doses above those used clinically. An atypical response to oxamniquine occurred in rats where deaths occurred up to 14 days after dosage due to hepatic failure with parenchymal necrosis and/or bile-duct proliferation.

In subacute and extended toxicity studies (manufacturer's communication to WHO), mice tolerated dose levels of 40 and 120 mg.kg^{-1} daily given in the diet. At 750 mg.kg^{-1} daily for 4 weeks, mice showed weight loss, slight anaemia and mild liver changes of fatty deposition without necrosis. In mice given 300 mg.kg^{-1} daily intramuscularly there were no abnormal findings (n=26).

In eight rabbits given 100 mg.kg^{-1} every fifth day intramuscularly for 4 weeks there were no effects, but focal hepatic necrosis and slight bile-duct proliferation occurred in 2/8 rabbits given 400 mg.kg^{-1} in a similar fashion.

Although there were no histopathological changes in dogs given a variety of regimes ranging from 8 mg.kg^{-1} daily to 50 mg.kg^{-1} daily for four weeks by the oral route, a few animals exhibited disturbances of gait, posture and behaviour lasting for up to four hours after each dose, in extended drug administration which in 30 animals lasted for 14 months at doses of 30 mg.kg^{-1} daily by mouth.

Chronic studies were conducted in mice and hamsters by giving oxamniquine in doses ranging from 25 to 150 mg.kg^{-1} daily every eight weeks, with appropriate controls, by both the oral and intramuscular routes. The mice studies were terminated at 18 months with survival rates ranging from 63% to 87% in various dosage groups; those in hamsters were ended after 19 months because of an increasing mortality in all groups, including controls; survival rates in hamsters varied between 55% and 81%. In neither species could differences in survival rates be related to drug treatment. No haematological abnormalities were detected. The overall incidence of tumours paralleled that reported in the literature and the spontaneous tumour incidence in control groups in the laboratory conducting the study. In none of the four studies could the distribution of tumours in the treatment groups be related to drug administration. There were no non-neoplastic lesions attributable to drug treatment.

Mutagenicity studies were negative in cytogenetic, host-mediated or dominant-lethal tests at doses up to 150 mg.kg^{-1} intramuscularly or intraperitoneally.[9]

In direct plate tests with or without liver microsomal enzymes, a weak response was seen in the frameshift mutant TA 1538 of *Salmonella typhimurium*. Oxamniquine was reported as having mutagenic activity in a host-mediated assay with *Salmonella TA* 100.[10] The urine of mice given oxamniquine showed low mutagenic activity.[10]

In reproduction studies pregnant mice were given doses by gavage of up to 400 mg.kg^{-1} daily from days 6 to 13 of gestation. No adverse effects on fertility or gestation were found. The drug was not embryolethal. No drug-related malformations occurred. Intramuscular injections of 100 mg.kg^{-1} every third day from day 6 through day 15 of gestation did not produce embryotoxic or teratogenic effects. At higher doses there was slight embryotoxicity, a decreased number of implantations and an increase in early resorption, but no evidence of teratogenicity.[9]

No maternal toxicity or fetal teratogenicity was found after oral treatment of rabbits with doses of up to 300 mg.kg^{-1} daily from day 6 through day 18 of gestation. Intramuscular injection of up to 400 mg.kg^{-1} every three days from day 6 through day 18 of gestation caused no drug-related maternal toxicity or teratogenicity.

Clinical pharmacology

The pharmacological actions in man, in the absence of methods for direct measurement, are assumed to parallel those in experimental animal models, i.e. the production of a hepatic shift of schistosomes residing in the blood vessels of the mesenteric plexus, their retention and subsequent resorption in the liver and the resulting cessation of egg deposition in the body and excretion in the faeces. Oxamniquine has no other clinical pharmacological effects except that the urine is occasionally coloured orange–red.

After various dose-ranging trials,[5,11–15] it became clear that there is a distinct difference in the dose–response relationship to oxamniquine of schistosome strains of South American and African origin. In *Schistosoma mansoni* infections originating in the New World, cure rates varying between 60% and over 90% in different samples were found when adult patients were given a single oral dose of 15 mg.kg^{-1} body weight. In children under 30 kg in weight, a total dose of 20 mg.kg^{-1} given in two divided portions each of 10 mg.kg^{-1} at a 4–6 h interval was the preferred regime. In *S. mansoni* infections originating in Africa, the therapeutic response to a dose of 15–20 mg.kg^{-1} is inferior to that obtained on the South American continent. Various dose regimes have been used and there is a suggestion of a gradation of responses from West Africa through East Africa to the Sudan and Egypt. While some *S. mansoni* infections in the Ivory Coast and Burkina Faso have similar responses to the dosages used in South America, those infections found in Kenya, Uganda and Ethiopia respond best to a total dose of 30 mg.kg^{-1}, usually given in two divided doses each of 15 mg.kg^{-1} in one day.[16–18] In Sudan, a total dose of 60 mg.kg^{-1} given as 15 mg.kg^{-1} twice daily for 2 days gave a 95% cure rate[14] and similar results have been obtained in South Africa and in Egypt. Total doses thus vary from 15 to 60 mg.kg^{-1} body weight and times of administration range from a single oral dose to a two-day regime. In all uncured patients the residual excretal egg count is markedly reduced — of the order of 80–90%.

These differences in schistosome strain response to oxamniquine appear to be a property of the schistosomes themselves and their origin. On investigation, neither methodological variations nor different bioavailabilities of oxamniquine appeared to be causal, since the former were broadly parallel and drug serum concentrations in patients from Brazil, and South and East Africa were very similar following equivalent doses.

In a crossover study, the serum levels of oxamniquine after the ingestion of 750 mg were determined, both in the fasting state and within 20 min of completing a large meal. Maximum serum concentrations were significantly reduced from 352 to 273 μg.l^{-1} and the mean times to peak levels were delayed from 1½ to 4 h when the drug was taken after food (manufacturer's data). As noted above, there were no significant differences in the comparison of serum levels after equivalent oral doses in different ethnic groups from Brazil, East Africa, South Africa and Sudan.

Pharmacokinetics

The preferred analytical method for the determination of oxamniquine in serum or plasma, sensitive to 10 μg.l^{-1}, is by ether extraction, derivatization with N,O-bis(trimethylsilyl) acetamide and estimation as the trimethylsilyl derivative by gas–liquid chromatography with electron-capture detection.[19]

Oxamniquine is well absorbed after an oral dose, with peak plasma concentrations at 1–1.5 h. The presence of food in the stomach and upper intestinal tract delays absorption and may limit the plasma concentrations. The plasma half life is 1–1.25 h.[20] It is not known if there is presystemic metabolism in man but it has been demonstrated in dogs.[21] There are no data on the volume of distribution, binding to plasma proteins, entry into brain or other tissues and excretion in human breast milk.

Oral absorption	good
Presystemic metabolism (CPIB acid)	possible
Plasma half life	
range	1–1.25 h
Volume of distribution	—
Plasma protein binding	—

Fig. 1 Metabolism of oxamniquine

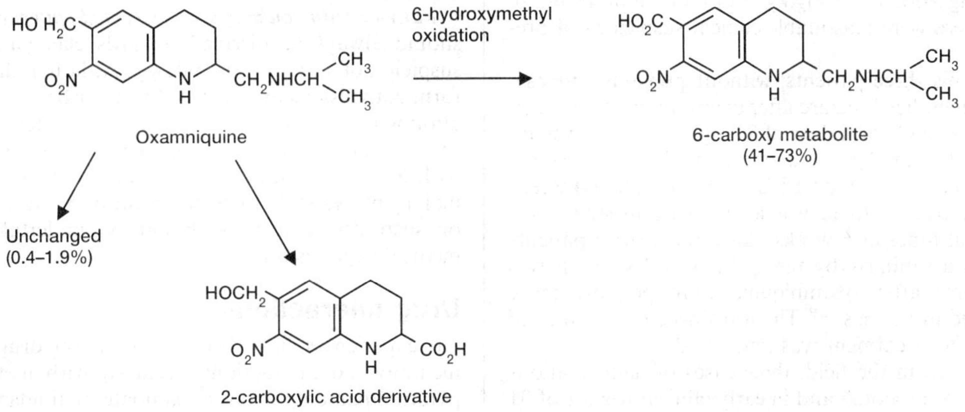

Concentration–effect relationship

No hard data exist on the relationship between the plasma concentration of oxamniquine and its therapeutic effect.

Metabolism

Oxamniquine is metabolized extensively, presumably in the liver, to inactive acidic products which are excreted largely in the urine (see Fig. 1). In human volunteer studies,[20] only 0.4–1.9% of the dose was excreted as unchanged drug in the urine and 41–73% was excreted as the 6-carboxy metabolite, with only traces of the 2-carboxylic acid derivative. Most of the dose was excreted in the first 12 hours. The metabolites were pharmacologically inactive.

There is no evidence of enterohepatic circulation.

Pharmaceutics

Oxamniquine is formulated as capsules of 250 mg or as a syrup containing 50 mg.ml^{-1} and marketed under the trade names Mansil in South America and Vansil in Africa. Both capsules and syrup are a light orange colour. In the USA Vansil (Pfizer, USA) is marketed as a 250 mg capsule with a dark green cap marked 'VANSIL' and a yellow body marked 'PFIZER 641'.

Storage conditions should be those in normal use for pharmaceutical products and no special recommendations are made. Capsules have a shelf-life of 5 years while that for the syrup is 3 years.

Therapeutic use

Indications

Oxamniquine is indicated in acute, subacute, chronic and complicated cases of *S. mansoni* infection. All stages of infection have been treated with uniformly good results.

Contraindications

Although there are no absolute contraindications to oxamniquine, there are several groups which require close medical supervision.

1. Patients with a history of any form of epilepsy should be medically supervised for 48 h after treatment
2. The drug should not be used in early pregnancy
3. Those whose work involves driving automobiles, ships, aircraft or other private or public forms of transport should be kept away from their occupation during treatment and probably for 24–48 h afterwards in case dizziness or drowsiness occur.

Mode of use

The drug was used in a major mass chemotherapeutic control programme in Brazil which began in 1976 and in which to date over 5 million doses have been given.

In the toxaemic form of *S. mansoni* infection, about 50% of a small number of patients treated with a single oral dose of 20 mg.kg^{-1} body weight were cured with no significant side effects.[22] Since early-maturing forms of schistosomiasis are usually less sensitive to chemotherapy than the stages of infection when the parasites are mature, this result is both hopeful and helpful.

Chronic and advanced cases with hepatosplenomegaly and/or ascites can now be treated successfully.[23,24] Similarly, the improvement of anaemia and protein-losing enteropathy from colonic schistosomal polyposis can be anticipated.[25]

Several rarer complications associated with *S. mansoni* infection can now be treated successfully with oxamniquine, e.g. prolonged septicaemic salmonellosis,[26] spinal cord disease,[27] or schistosome-induced glomerulonephritis.[28]

Since the therapeutic response varies with the age and hence the surface area of the patient and with the geographical origin of the infection, dose varies with these two major determinants.

In South America the recommended total dose in adults is 15 mg kg^{-1} body weight, given as a single oral dose. In children under 30 kg in weight the recommended total dose is 20 mg.kg^{-1} body weight given in two divided portions each of 10 mg.kg^{-1} in one day with an interval of 4–6 h between doses. Tolerance is improved if the drug is given after food or just before sleep.

In *S. mansoni* infections of African origin the recommended doses for both adults and children are:

West Africa: 15 mg.kg^{-1} body weight given as a single oral dose.

East Africa: A total dose of 30–40 mg.kg^{-1} body weight given either as 15 mg.kg^{-1} twice daily in one day or as 10 mg.kg^{-1} twice daily for two days.

Southern Africa: A total dose of 60 mg.kg^{-1} body weight given as 15 mg.kg^{-1} twice daily for two days or 20 mg.kg^{-1} once daily for 3 days.

North Africa: As for Southern Africa.

Patients should be followed up by stool examination for eggs of *S. mansoni* at 3, 6 and 12 months after treatment. If eggs are found, treatment should be repeated with oxamniquine or alternatively the patients may be treated with praziquantel.

Adverse reactions

In general oxamniquine is well tolerated and this is borne out by a decade of experience in many parts of the world but particularly in the large national Brazilian schistosomiasis control programme.

Potentially life-threatening effects

No effects of this kind have been reported.

Acute overdosage

There is a single report of an adult male who ingested 25 capsules (6.25 g) of oxamniquine. After 30 minutes he complained of dizziness, had a generalized convulsion and for 12 hours was semicomatose with episodes of vomiting. He recovered consciousness and was discharged from hospital after 48 hours with no neurological abnormalities. The patient had had hepatitis five months before this incident but did not develop jaundice and there were no serum enzyme alterations over two months. An EEG on the second day after ingestion showed diffuse paroxysmal abnormalities in the fronto-parietal regions. Follow-up EEGs on days 4 to 90 revealed a progressive decrease in abnormalities and a return to normal appearances (Manufacturer's literature).

Severe or irreversible adverse effects

Five occurrences of epileptiform convulsions in an estimated 250 000 treatments were reported in manufacturer's literature (Pfizer, 1978, report prepared for WHO Expert Committee on the Epidemiology and Control of Schistosomiasis). Convulsions occurred at between 10 min and 2 h after ingestion of 15 mg.kg^{-1} of oxamniquine and in four of the patients there were reasonable clinical suspicions of pre-existing epilepsy.

A recent report details three patients, without previous epilepsy, each of whom had a generalized seizure after oxamniquine treatment. One patient was given a single oral dose of 20 mg.kg^{-1} body weight, one a single oral dose of 25 mg.kg^{-1} and one 20 mg.kg^{-1} twice daily in one day. In two patients, follow-up EEGs were normal at 4 weeks and 4 months. In one patient there was an increase in slow wave activity over the frontal lobes at 6 weeks. Since these three patients were among 200 treated similarly by the authors in 2 years, it was speculated that seizures after oxamniquine were possibly more frequent than estimated in the past.[29] The warning on avoidance of driving for 24 hours after treatment was reinforced.

In 600 treatments given in the field, three cases of hallucinations and psychic excitement were noted and in early clinical trials 1 of 31 adults given a single oral dose of 15 mg.kg^{-1} and 1 of 60 children given 10 mg.kg^{-1} twice in a day developed short-lived hallucinations.[30]

Symptomatic adverse effects

The most frequent symptomatic adverse effects reported are dizziness, drowsiness and headache which have occurred, predictably, in varying proportions of patients treated in South America and Africa. These symptoms have appeared about one hour after drug ingestion and have lasted some 4–5 h. An overall estimate of frequency is not possible and the incidence has ranged from 0% to 20% of treated patients. Dizziness does not deter patients from accepting further doses. While in some studies the incidence of dizziness increased with increase in unit dosage, it was not aggravated by multiple doses. In practice, these side effects have not proved to be a constraint during large-scale or mass chemotherapy programmes.

While abdominal discomfort, vomiting and diarrhoea have all been reported in association with oxamniquine treatment, the causal relationship is not established.

Occasionally an orange–red discoloration of the urine is seen after treatment.[14] Caused by excretion of a mixture of drug and metabolites, it is short-lived and harmless.

In Egypt a characteristic fever was seen 24–72 h after a three-day course of oxamniquine. Associated with a Loeffler-like syndrome of peripheral blood eosinophilia, scattered pulmonary infiltrates, an increase in serum immune complexes and excretion of schistosomal antigens in the urine, the syndrome has not been described from other centres undertaking treatment of large numbers of patients.[31]

An eosinophilia, maximal 7–10 days after treatment, occurs frequently and represents the usual reaction to dead or dying schistosomes. The peripheral blood shows no other changes after oxamniquine.

Serial electrocardiography has not shown any consistent or significant findings.

Interference with clinical pathology tests

No technical interferences of this kind have been reported.

High risk groups

Neonates

The drug is most unlikely to be used in this age group.

Breast milk. No information is available on the secretion of the drug in breast milk. It is most uncommon for infants in the conventional breast-feeding age group to be diagnosed as having schistosomiasis but for absolute safety it is best for mothers taking oxamniquine to abstain from breast-feeding during treatment (one or two days depending on geographical location) and for some 72 hours after.

Children

The drug is used in the treatment of *S. mansoni* infections in children at the recommended dose with excellent tolerance and safety.

Pregnant women

Although evidence of teratogenicity is lacking in animal experiments, it would be wise to avoid treatment during the first 16 weeks of pregnancy.

The elderly

No special precautions are necessary in older patients.

Concurrent disease

Patients with confirmed or suspected epilepsy. The clinical history should always be directed towards clarifying the presence or the suspicion of any form of epilespy. Although the incidence of epileptiform convulsions and/or psychic disturbances encountered in association with oxamniquine treatment is very low, it would be preferable to use another schistosomicide, e.g. praziquantel, in known epileptics with *S. mansoni* infection. If oxamniquine is the only antischistosomal agent available then treatment of *S. mansoni* infection in proven or suspected epileptics should be undertaken only under close medical supervision.

Drug interactions

No experiences have been reported on drug interactions. Experimentally, no interactions occurred with metriphonate, niridazole, pyrantel pamoate, oxantel pamoate or tinidazole. The simultaneous administration of oxamniquine and metriphonate to patients with double infections with *S. mansoni* and *S. haematobium* in Egypt produced high cure rates and no adverse effects.[13]

There are a few reports from Brazil on the occurrence of resistance to multiple doses of oxamniquine but these patients are responsive to praziquantel.[32] This phenomenon is rare and, at this time, does not constitute a public health problem.

General review articles

Davis A 1982 Management of the patient with schistosomiasis. In: Jordan P, Webbe G (eds) Schistosomiasis. Epidemiology, treatment and control. William Heinemann Medical Books, London, pp 184–226

Davis A 1986 Recent advances in schistosomiasis. Quarterly Journal of Medicine NS 58: 95–110

Foster R, 1987 A review of clinical experience with oxamniquine. Transactions of the Royal Society of Tropical Medicine and Hygiene 81: 55–59.

References

1. Reynolds J E F, Prasad A B (eds) 1982 Anthelmintics and schistosomicides. Oxamniquine, Martindale. The Extra Pharmacopoeia 28th edn. The Pharmaceutical Press, London, pp 101–102
2. Foster R 1973 The preclinical development of oxamniquine. Revista do Instituto de Medicina Tropical de Saõ Paulo 15 (suppl 1): 1–9
3. Foster R, Cheetham B L 1973 Studies with the schistosomicide oxamniquine (UK-4271) I Activity in rodents and in vitro. Transactions of the Royal Society of Tropical Medicine and Hygiene 67: 674–684
4. Foster R, Cheetham B L, King D F 1973 Studies with the schistosomicide oxamniquine (UK-4271) II Activity in primates. Transactions of the Royal Society of Tropical Medicine and Hygiene 67: 685–693
5. Clarke V de V, Blair D M, Weber M C, Garnett P A 1976 Dose-finding trials of oral oxamniquine in Rhodesia. South African Medical Journal 50: 1867–1871
6. McMahon J E 1976 Oxamniquine (UK-4271) in *Schistosoma haematobium* infections. Annals of Tropical Medicine and Parasitology 70: 121–122
7. Kale O O, Lucas A O 1978 Oxamniquine (UK-4271) in the treatment of vesical schistosomiasis in Western Nigeria. Revista do Instituto de Medicina Tropical de Saõ Paulo 20: 55–63
8. Pitchford R J, Lewis M 1978 Oxamniquine in the treatment of various schistosome infections in South Africa. South African Medical Journal 53: 677–680
9. Chvedoff M, Faccini J M, Gregory M H et al 1984 The toxicology of the schistosomicidal agent oxamniquine. Drug Development Research 4: 229–235
10. Batzinger R P, Bueding E 1977 Mutagenic activities in vitro and in vivo of five antischistosomal compounds. Journal of Pharmacology and Experimental Therapeutics 200: 1–9
11. Silva L C, da Sette H Jr, Chamore D A F, Alquezar A S, Punskas J A, Raia S 1974 Clinical trials with oral oxamniquine (UK-4271) on the treatment of mansonian schistosomiasis. Revista do Instituto de Medicina Tropical de Saõ Paulo 16: 103–109
12. Katz N, Zicker F, Pedro Pereira J 1977 Field trials with oxamniquine in a schistosomiasis mansoni-endemic area. American Journal of Tropical Medicine and Hygiene 26: 234–237
13. Saif M, Gaber A, Hassanein Y S, Khameis S 1978 Efficacy of oxamniquine in treatment of *S. mansoni* in a closed community in Egypt and the concomitant administration of both metrifonate and oxamniquine in mixed infections. Journal of the Egyptian Medical Association 61: 427–481
14. Omer A H S 1978 Oxamniquine for treating schistosomiasis mansoni infections in Sudan. British Medical Journal 2: 163–165
15. Pitchford R, Lewis M 1978 Oxamniquine in the treatment of various schistosome infections in South Africa. South African Medical Journal 53: 7667–7680
16. Siongok T K, Ouma J H, Kabiri J 1976 A preliminary report on the treatment of *Schistosoma mansoni* infestation in school children with oxamniquine in Kenya. East African Medical Journal 43: 504–505
17. Ongom V L, Wamboka G W, Kadil A U K 1976 Oxamniquine (UK 4271) in the treatment of *Schistosoma mansoni* infections in Uganda. East African Medical Journal 53: 505
18. Pehrson P O, Bengtsson E 1983 Treatment of Eritrean schistosomiasis mansoni with oxamniquine. Transactions of the Royal Society of Tropical Medicine and Hygiene 77: 282
19. Woolhouse N M, Wood P R 1977 Determination of oxamniquine in serum. Journal of Pharmaceutical Sciences 66: 429–430
20. Kaye B, Woolhouse N M 1976 The metabolism of oxamniquine, a new schistosomicide. Annals of Tropical Medicine and Parasitology 70: 323–328
21. Kaye B, Roberts D 1980 The metabolism of oxamniquine in the gut wall. Xenobiotica 10: 97–101
22. Lambertucci J R, Pedroso E R P, de Souza D W C et al 1980 Therapeutic efficacy of oral oxamniquine in the toxemic form of schistosomiasis mansoni: treatment of eleven individuals from two families, an experimental study. American Journal of Tropical Medicine and Hygiene 29: 50–53
23. Bassily S, Farid Z, Higashi G I, Watten R H 1978 Treatment of complicated schistosomiasis mansoni with oxamniquine. American Journal of Tropical Medicine and Hygiene 27: 1284–1286
24. Farid Z, Higashi G I, Bassily S, Trabolsi B, Watten R H 1980 Treatment of advanced hepatosplenic schistosomiasis with oxamniquine. Transactions of the Royal Society of Tropical Medicine and Hygiene 74: 400–401

25. Abaza H H, Hammouda N, Abd Rabbo H, Shafei A Z 1978 Chemotherapy of schistosomal polyposis with oxamniquine. Transactions of the Royal Society of Tropical Medicine and Hygiene 72: 602–604
26. Lambertucci J R, Marinho R P, Ferreira das dores M, Neves J, Pedroso E R P 1985 Eficacia terapeutica da oxamniquine oral no tratamento da salmonelose septicemica prolongada. Revista do Instituto de Medicina Tropical de Saõ Paulo 27: 33–39
27. Efthimiov J, Denning D 1984 Spinal cord disease due to *Schistosoma mansoni* successfully treated with oxamniquine. British Medical Journal 288: 1343–1344
28. Ott B R, Libbey P, Ryter R J, Trebbin W M 1983 Treatment of schistosome-induced glomerulonephritis. Archives of Internal Medicine 143: 1477–1479
29. Stokvis H, Bauer A G C, Stuiver P C, Malcolm A D, Overbosch D 1986 Seizures associated with oxamniquine therapy. American Journal of Tropical Medicine and Hygiene 35: 330–331
30. Katz N, Grinbaum E, Chaves A, Zicker F, Pellegrino J 1976 Clinical trials with oxamniquine, by oral route, in schistosomiasis mansoni. Revista do Instituto de Medicina Tropical de Saõ Paulo 18: 371–377
31. Higashi G I, Farid Z 1979 Oxamniquine fever — drug induced or immune-complex reaction. British Medical Journal 2: 830
32. De Souza Dias L C, De Jesus Pedro R, Deberaldini E R 1982 Use of praziquantel in patients with schistosomiasis mansoni previously treated with oxamniquine and/or hycanthone. Transactions of the Royal Society of Tropical Medicine and Hygiene 76: 652–658

O

Oxazepam

Oxazepam is a benzodiazepine with a medium duration of action which has no pharmacologically active metabolites.

Chemistry

Oxazepam (Serax, Oxamid)
$C_{15}H_{11}ClN_2O_2$
7-Chloro-1,3-dihydro-3-hydroxy-5-phenyl-2H-1,4-benzodiazepin-2-one

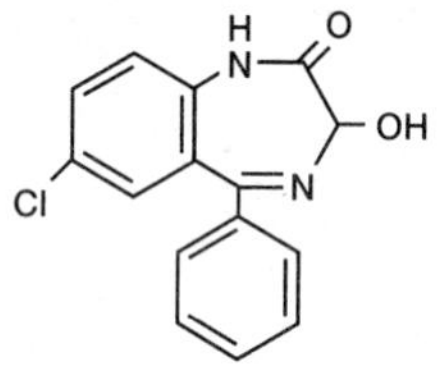

Molecular weight	286.7
pKa	1.7, 11.3[1]
Solubility	
in alcohol	1 in 220
in water	<1 in 10000
Octanol/water partition coefficient	97[2]

Oxazepam is a white or off-white odourless powder, prepared by chemical synthesis. It contains a chiral centre.

Pharmacology

Oxazepam is a sedative and anxiolytic acting by potentiation of the inhibitory effect of gamma-aminobutyrate by binding to specific receptor sites of the brain stem reticular formation and other parts of the CNS. The anxiolytic effects have been demonstrated in experimental animals and man.[3–7]

Toxicology

No significant drug-related toxic effects were seen in oxazepam-treated experimental animals in studies lasting up to a year. Tests for mutagenicity or carcinogenicity have not been carried out.

Clinical pharmacology

Studies in man indicated that oxazepam produced an anxiolytic effect with a low incidence of side effects.[7] Normal response to stress is not affected and no release of hostile or aggressive feelings, rage or drug-related irritability was observed. 'Paradoxical excitability' is rare.[8–12]

Continuous recording of EEG, ECG, ocular movements and respiration during spontaneous sleep and sleep occurring after administration of oxazepam showed no significant changes.[13] The residual effects after overnight ingestion of 45 mg oxazepam included impaired visuomotor coordination.[14]

On continued daily dosage of 15–180 mg for the treatment of anxiety, the following side effects were observed: dizziness, torpor, ebriety, drowsiness, lethargy, headache, giddiness, dreams, nausea, excitation and rashes.

Pharmacokinetics

For oxazepam the preferred analytical method for quantitative measurements in biological fluids is by gas–liquid chromatography with electron capture detection using lorazepam as the internal standard.[15,16] The limit of detection is $10\ \mu g.l^{-1}$. HPLC may also be used.

Oxazepam is completely absorbed after oral administration and peak plasma concentrations are seen at 1–5 hours. Food intake has no influence on bioavailability. The mean plasma half life is 9 hours with a range of 4–25 hours. Oxazepam is conjugated with glucuronic acid in the liver and excreted in urine as the pharmacologically inactive glucuronide.[15]

The absolute bioavailability of oxazepam has not been established because a parenteral preparation is not available. All clinical pharmacokinetic studies were carried out using the oral dosage form. Most recent studies following single-dose administration indicate that the volume of distribution may vary from 0.4 to $2.3\ l.kg^{-1}$ and the clearance from 0.52 to $2.38\ ml.min^{-1}.kg^{-1}$. Oxazepam is extensively bound to plasma proteins with a free fraction of 4–13% which is partly responsible for the large variation in the volume of distribution.[15] Data are not available on the concentration of oxazepam in the CSF or brain tissue in man. It is excreted in human milk in small amounts. It readily crosses the placental barrier and the concentration is higher in the fetus than in the mother.[17]

Oral absorption	≤98%
Presystemic metabolism	—
Plasma half life	
range	4–25 h
mean	9 h
Volume of distribution	$0.4–2.3\ l.kg^{-1}$
Plasma protein binding	95–98%

Oxazepam biotransformation involves extensive hepatic glucuronic acid conjugation with only a trace excreted unchanged in urine. Acute viral hepatitis or cirrhosis have no significant effect on absorption, distribution, biotransformation and excretion of the drug or metabolite.[18] In severely uraemic patients the total drug clearance is normal but the plasma elimination half life is significantly longer (24 to 91 hours) and plasma protein binding is reduced (83–93%). The rate of elimination of the inactive oxazepam glucuronide is prolonged. Possibly, alteration in volume of distribution and protein binding are responsible for these changes.[19] Old age has been reported to have little effect on oxazepam pharmacokinetics[19,20] and a small prolongation of elimination half life and reduction of total clearance in females, as opposed to males, was reported.[20] The plasma half life in the mother after delivery was found to be 7.8 hours but in the newborn it was considerably longer at 21.9 hours.[17]

Concentration–effect relationship

There is no suggestion of a defined range of plasma concentration required for the therapeutic effect to occur. Following multiple-dose administration steady-state concentration is attained after 2 days and the mean half life during the 'washout' period following termination of multiple-dose therapy is similar to that observed in the same subjects following single doses.[21]

There are large individual variations in plasma or serum steady state concentrations of oxazepam following the oral administration of identical doses (see Table 1).

Table 1

Dose/mg	Conc./$\mu g.l^{-1}$
5 tid	20–130
10 tid	100–350
30 hs	200–400
15 qid	300–650
30 tid	270–950
25 qid	159–808

note: hs = at bedtime
tid = three times daily
qid = four times daily

Metabolism

Oxazepam is extensively metabolized in the liver with very little of the unchanged drug excreted. Excretion is primarily in the urine (67–80%) with 3–7% in the faeces after 72 hours.[22]

The primary pathway of metabolism is glucuronic acid conjugation (Fig. 1) but additional minor metabolites such as quinazoline and dihydroxy derivatives were also identified in urine.[15]

Significant enterohepatic recirculation was found in dogs. Up to 30% of the dose was excreted in the bile as conjugate in 3 hours. Deconjugation takes place in the intestine because only 20% of the dose was found in the faeces of normal animals without a bile fistula. About 30% of the dose is metabolized during absorption following oral administration in dogs.[23]

Fig. 1 Major metabolic pathway of oxazepam in humans

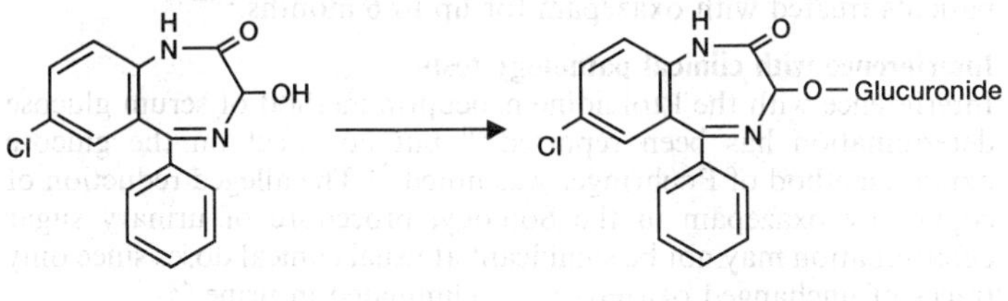

Oxazepam

No pharmacologically active metabolites have been identified. Oxazepam is a metabolite of several benzodiazepines, including chlordiazepoxide, clorazepate, demoxepam, diazepam, ketazolam, medazepam, nordazepam, prazepam and temazepam.

Pharmaceutics

Oxazepam is available in oral form only from Wyeth (UK USA).

1. Tablets containing 10 mg and 15 mg oxazepam. The 10 mg tablets are white, flat, bevel-edged, 6.5 mm in diameter, marked 'WYETH' on one face and 'WY 012' on the other. Oxazepam 10 mg (Wyeth, UK) was formerly known as Sevenid-D. The 15 mg oxazepam tablets (Wyeth, UK) are white, flat, bevel-edged, 8.0 mm in diameter, marked 'WY 013' on one face and 'WYETH' on the other.
2. Serax (Wyeth, USA) is available in three capsule strengths and one tablet strength. The 10 mg capsule is marked 'Wyeth 51' on a pink cap and 'SERAX 10' on the white base.
   The Serax 15 mg capsules are marked 'Wyeth 6' on an orange–red cap and 'SERAX 15' on a white base (Wyeth, US).
   The Serax 30 mg capsules are marked 'Wyeth 52' on a maroon cap and 'Serax 30' on a white base.
   The Serax 15 mg tablet is a yellow, five-sided tablet with a raised 'S' and '15' on one side and 'WYETH' and '317' on the other.
   Wyeth UK formerly marketed a 30 mg capsule under the name Serenid Forte.
   A number of generic alternatives are now available.

Therapeutic use

Indications

1. Treatment of the symptoms of anxiety, tension, fear, agitation, irritability and insomnia
2. Anxiety associated with depression and psychoses, e.g. as in transient situational disorder, psychoneurotic reaction and psychophysiological reaction
3. Anxiety syndrome secondary to organic disease
4. Anxiety syndrome in alcoholics and in alcohol withdrawal
5. Anxiety syndrome in elderly patients, geriatric behavioural disturbances or personality disorder.

Contraindications

1. Oxazepam should not be given to patients with a previous history of sensitivity to benzodiazepines
2. Acute pulmonary insufficiency
3. Children
4. The drug is not indicated for treatment of psychoses
5. Myasthenia gravis
6. Acute narrow-angle glaucoma.

Oxazepam

Mode of use

Recommended dosage is as follows: Mild to moderate anxiety syndromes, 10–15 mg three or four times daily.

Severe anxiety syndromes, 15–30 mg three or four times daily.

Geriatric behaviour problems, 10 mg initially three times a day, if necessary increasing cautiously to 15 mg three or four times daily.

Residual anxiety syndrome in alcoholics and alcohol withdrawal, 15–30 mg three or four times daily.

Patients with severe sleep disturbance can be given 60 mg at bedtime.

Not recommended for children.

Prolonged or excessive use of oxazepam may result in the development of psychological dependence with withdrawal symptoms on sudden discontinuation. Treatment in these cases should be withdrawn gradually. Prolonged use should be avoided in most cases. As with other drugs acting on the central nervous system, patients should be cautioned against driving or operating machinery until it is established that they do not become dizzy or drowsy while taking oxazepam.

Oxazepam should not be administered during pregnancy unless in the judgement of the physician such administration is clinically justifiable. Special care should be taken in the first and last trimester of pregnancy.

Indications

1. Treatment of anxiety

Oxazepam provides relief of anxiety at doses of 30–180 mg daily with a low incidence of side effects. The release of hostile or aggressive feelings, which is sometimes seen when anxiety is reduced, is rare with oxazepam and there appears to be little effect on the normal response to stress.

Oxazepam is completely absorbed from the gastrointestinal tract and peak serum levels are reached in 1–5 hours. Food intake appears not to affect absorption. The mean half life of elimination from plasma is relatively short. Oxazepam, like lorazepam, has the shortest possible metabolic pathway, comprising conjugation as the glucuronide, and the drug is excreted almost entirely in this form in the urine. There is no accumulation after plasma concentrations have reached a steady level and no effects from active metabolites. These pharmacokinetic properties probably explain the good tolerance of oxazepam, which allows a very flexible dosage regimen.

Prolonged or excessive use of oxazepam may result in the development of psychological dependence with withdrawal symptoms on sudden discontinuation. Treatment in these cases should be withdrawn gradually. Very careful consideration should be given to the balance between relief of anxiety and risk of dependence if prolonged use is contemplated. The drug should not be administered without proper supervision to individuals who have a history of drug abuse and the dose should not be increased to compensate for tolerance after prolonged use.

2. Anxiety associated with depression and psychoses

Oxazepam, at doses of 20–225 mg, can be used to treat anxiety and related symptoms in psychotic patients. Many patients, including those with schizophrenia and other psychoses and acute and chronic brain syndromes, respond to oxazepam therapy where they may remain refractory to other treatments. In general, side effects are mild and low in incidence. Drowsiness is the most common side effect. The use of oxazepam permits a reduction in the dose of neuroleptics, reducing the incidence of side effects with these agents. Patients suffering from phobic and compulsive behaviour disorders may be effectively treated with oxazepam.

3. Anxiety syndrome secondary to organic disease

In open and double-blind trials oxazepam was shown to be effective in reducing the anxiety associated with various physical disorders. Daily doses of 10–15 mg two to six times daily were effective, safe and dependable for the reduction of anxiety during the diagnosis and treatment of cardiovascular disease, diabetes, peptic ulcer, hypothyroidism and many other diseases. Remission was independent of age, sex, disease, dose or duration of treatment. Patients felt better generally, they slept well and had a better appetite. Side effects were minor, consisting of transient drowsiness and transient excitement which subsided after reduction of dosage. There were no cases of

O

ataxia or incoordination observed but in one case severe nausea occurred.

4. Anxiety syndrome in alcoholics and in alcohol withdrawal
Oxazepam in doses of 10–15 mg three times daily is effective in alleviating subacute stages of alcoholism by reducing postintoxication symptoms and associated anxiety. The biotransformation or plasma half life is minimally affected by disulfiram in contrast to diazepam and chlordiazepoxide. In addition to anxiety and sleep problems, postalcoholic patients suffering from tension, depression, lethargy, irritability, insomnia, autonomic and phobic reactions, obsessive thinking and compulsive behaviour may require a total daily dose of 180–240 mg oxazepam. Side effects most commonly observed are drowsiness, dizziness and, rarely, nausea and headache.

5. Anxiety syndrome in elderly patients, geriatric behavioural disturbances or personality disorder
The aging process, with a reduced ability to absorb, metabolize and excrete drugs, may result in prolongation of their effects. Treatment of elderly patients with anxiolytic agents is frequently associated with unwanted effects such as over-sedation, unsteadiness, ataxia and mental confusion. The pharmacokinetic qualities of oxazepam indicate that it is particularly suitable for treatment of the elderly and there is evidence that the elimination half life of this drug is unaffected in elderly subjects, in contrast to the three- to six-fold increase in half life with age which has been observed with diazepam and chlordiazepoxide. In several clinical trials, including elderly patients suffering from cerebral arteriosclerosis, organic brain syndrome and psychoses, oxazepam was effective in relieving symptoms of anxiety, confusion, irritability and agitation. The patients often became much more co-operative with nursing staff and the incidence of side effects was low. Few cases of ataxia, confusion or over-sedation were observed. Initial doses were usually low and increased until symptoms were reduced without unwanted sedation. Caution should be exercised if prolonged use is under consideration.

Contraindications

1. Sensitivity to benzodiazepines
Oxazepam belongs to the benzodiazepine group of drugs; therefore patients with adverse reaction to one member of this group may be expected to react similarly to all drugs with similar pharmacological characteristics.

2. Acute pulmonary insufficiency
There is no specific evidence to suggest that oxazepam has undesirable effects on respiratory function in acute or chronic pulmonary insufficiency. The warning is an extra precaution.

3. Children
The drug is not indicated for children under 6 years of age. No definite dose has been established for children between 6 and 12 years of age.

Adverse reactions

Potentially life-threatening effects
Members of the benzodiazepine group have occasionally caused blood dyscrasias, including agranulocytosis, which are potentially life-threatening.

Acute overdosage
A few cases of attempted suicide with oxazepam have been reported but none has been successful with oxazepam alone. Up to 2400 mg have been taken without long-term ill effects.[24] As with other benzodiazepines, overdosage should not present a threat to life. General supportive measures should be used. Treatment is symptomatic and gastric lavage may be of use if performed shortly after ingestion. If the patient is conscious, an emetic such as ipecacuanha may be given. The patient is likely to sleep and a clear airway should be maintained.

Severe or irreversible adverse effects
Jaundice, both hepatocellular and cholestatic, has been attributed to benzodiazepine drugs on rare occasions. Although there is no evidence to suggest that oxazepam has undesirable side effects on respiratory functions, caution should be observed in using it in acute and chronic pulmonary insufficiency.

Symptomatic adverse effects
The most commonly reported side effect in clinical trials was drowsiness in 6.1% of the patients. The others were, in decreasing order: headache, dizziness, nausea and skin rashes, and some rare or single cases of lowering of blood pressure, increase in parkinsonism, increase in arthritis, transient excitement or irritability, dry mouth and vomiting. Drowsiness appeared to be dose-related and symptoms improved or disappeared after the dose was reduced.

Other effects
Laboratory studies, including haematological tests, liver function tests and routine analysis of urine, showed no significant changes in patients treated with oxazepam for up to 6 months.[25–29]

Interference with clinical pathology tests
Interference with the l-toluidine neocuprin method of serum glucose determination has been reported,[30] but no effect on the glucose oxidase method of Boehringer was noted.[31] The alleged reduction of copper by oxazepam in the Somogyi procedure of urinary sugar determination may not be significant at usual clinical doses since only traces of unchanged oxazepam are eliminated in urine.[32]

High risk groups

Neonates
The drug should not be used in neonates.

Breast milk. Oxazepam is excreted in human milk; therefore it is not recommended during lactation and breast-feeding should be terminated during treatment of the mother.[17]

Children
Oxazepam is not recommended for children.

Pregnant women
Oxazepam should not be administered during pregnancy unless in the judgement of the physician such administration is clinically justifiable. Special care should be taken in the first and last trimesters of pregnancy.

Oxazepam should not be used in labour unless considered essential since single doses or repeated low doses of other benzodiazepines have been reported to produce hypotonia, poor sucking and hypotension in the neonate and irregularities in the fetal heart.

The elderly
No special precautions are required but an initial dose of 10–20 mg three or four times daily is recommended. Oxazepam may offer advantages in the treatment of the elderly because of its short half life and lack of accumulation.

Concurrent disease
Oxazepam pharmacokinetics in patients with liver disease differ little from those in normal subjects but caution should be observed in patients with liver damage.

Drug interactions

Potentially hazardous interactions

CNS depressants. Concomitant administration with central nervous system depressants, including alcohol, general anaesthetics, narcotic analgesics, monoamine oxidase inhibitors and antidepressants, will result in an accentuation of their effects.

Alcohol. Oxazepam significantly enhances the alcohol-induced impairment of psychomotor skills[33] but low doses of alcohol do not affect the subjects' coordination, mood or concentration any more than oxazepam alone.[34]

Potentially useful interactions
Oxazepam disposition is only minimally altered by the coadministration of disulfiram. In comparison, the plasma half life of chlordiazepoxide and diazepam is significantly prolonged by disulfiram in normal volunteers or alcoholics. Oxazepam may be the drug of choice if benzodiazepine therapy is used for patients taking disulfiram.[35]

Major outcome trials

1. Maneksha S, Harry T V A 1974 Anxiety neurosis in general practice. British Journal of Clinical Practice 28: 65–66

This double-blind, crossover study was conducted on 35 clinic patients who suffered from anxiety neuroses. The patients were randomly allocated to two groups and treated with three daily doses of 30 mg, 30 mg and 60 mg oxazepam, or placebo, for three weeks before being crossed over to the other group. Hamilton ratings were completed for each patient at 0, 1, 3, 4 and 6 weeks. The two groups were similar in initial degrees of anxiety. In the first week a significant fall in anxiety was seen in both groups, followed by a further significant fall during the second and third weeks in the oxazepam group but not in the placebo group. When crossed over from oxazepam to placebo, patients returned to their initial levels of anxiety. Assessment on the Hamilton Rating Scale at the end of the six-week study showed that oxazepam was significantly more effective than placebo. Side effects in the oxazepam group were few, consisting of drowsiness in two patients and dry mouth in one.

2. Krakowski A J 1965 Suppression of anxiety with oxazepam in a private psychiatric practice. Psychosomatics 6: 26–31

The suppression of anxiety with oxazepam in an open trial involving 94 psychiatric clinic patients is described. 38 of the patients were considered psychotic whose symptoms had proved refractory to a variety of treatments. All previous psychotropic drugs were discontinued two weeks before the commencement of the study. Doses (individually adjusted) varied from 20 to 225 mg daily and treatment continued for 4 to 112 days. 67% of the total patients received concomitant therapy, mainly antidepressants. Assessment consisted of weekly gradings on a three-point scale of the level of anxiety and other symptoms. At the start of the trial, 98% of the patients had one or more symptoms of grade three severity. The clinical response was excellent or moderate in 62% of psychotic patients (grade 0–1), a reduction in anxiety followed by a reduction in associated symptoms generally being seen within 1–4 weeks. Laboratory studies of blood and liver function showed no significant abnormalities. Side effects (mainly drowsiness) occurred in 18% of patients overall but there was no ataxia or incoordination.

3. Halpern M M 1969 The anti-anxiety activity of oxazepam in patients with multiple organic disorders. Clinical Medicine, July: 42–44

An open trial of oxazepam with 103 elderly, clinic outpatients is reported. All patients suffered from moderate to severe anxiety, which was associated in most cases with cardiovascular disease, diabetes, peptic ulcer or hypothyroidism. Ten patients suffered from multiple disorders. Previous treatment with chlordiazepoxide, meprobamate, phenothiazines, reserpine or antidepressants, had failed to suppress anxiety adequately, and was discontinued. Therapy with oxazepam commenced, together with appropriate medication for the physical disorders, at doses of 10 mg two or four times daily, and continued for 1–20 weeks. Anxiety and related symptoms were evaluated before the study and at weekly intervals on a four-point scale (0 = absent; 3 = most severe). Anxiety was satisfactorily relieved (reduced to 0 or 1) in 79% of the patients and other symptoms (tension, irritability, phobia, insomnia, agitation, lethargy, headache) in 74% of patients.

4. Bowman E D, Thiman J 1966 Treatment of alcoholism in the subacute stage. Diseases of the Nervous System 27: 342–346

In this study 99 non-psychotic alcoholic patients (ages 24–70 years) were randomly divided into four groups and treated with 50–150 mg promazine, 60–180 mg oxazepam, 60–180 mg chlordiazepoxide or placebo in a double-blind trial. Treatment continued in most cases for six weeks and was divided into inpatient and outpatient phases. The patients were assessed before treatment for the presence of anxiety, tension, depression, lethargy, irritability, insomnia, autonomic and phobic reactions, obsessive thinking and compulsive behaviour. Symptoms were evaluated again at weekly intervals and graded on a scale 0–3 (0 = none, 3 = severe). After six weeks symptoms were reduced by more than 50% in 78% of promazine patients, 68% of oxazepam patients, 65% of chlordiazepoxide patients and 40% of placebo patients. Global ratings showed a satisfactory response in 61% of promazine patients, 72% of oxazepam patients, 46% of chlordiazepoxide patients and 16% of placebo patients. All active agents were equally effective in controlling symptoms of the alcoholic debauch and were superior to placebo in this respect. One patient on promazine experienced drowsiness; one patient on oxzepam experienced slight dizziness, nausea and headache.

Oxazepam

5. Beber C R 1965 Management of behaviour in the institutionalized aged. Diseases of the Nervous System 26: 591–595

Oxazepam was compared with placebo in a double-blind trial involving 100 institutionalized geriatric patients (ages 67–94 years) suffering from neurotic anxiety associated with physical diseases. The patients had symptoms of anxiety, tension, depression, lethargy, irritability, insomnia, agitation, and autonomic and phobic reactions, but none were psychotic. 50 subjects received oxazepam at doses of 20–80 mg daily, adjusted according to individual response, and 50 received placebo. At weekly intervals, target symptoms were assessed as a percentage of the original status and nine target symptoms were also analysed by grouping in three major clusters. At the end of eight weeks of treatment, 68% of the oxazepam patients showed moderate to notable (over 50%) improvement in target symptoms, 20% showed complete elimination of symptoms and there were no cases of deterioration. In the placebo group 18% of patients improved, 2% were symptom-free and 12% deteriorated. Anxiety, tension, irritability, insomnia and agitation were the symptoms most responsive to oxazepam therapy. In the oxazepam group, 14 patients experienced side effects of drowsiness, dizziness and nausea, one patient an increase in parkinsonism and one an increase in arthritis. A reduction in dose was necessary in nine cases. In the placebo group, seven patients experienced drowsiness, dizziness, headache or excitability and one patient developed jaundice. There was no ataxia or abnormal blood pressure change. The response was significantly more satisfactory after oxazepam treatment than placebo administration.

General review articles and symposia

Ayd F J Jr (ed) 1975 Oxazepam update. Diseases of the Nervous System 36: 1–32

Greenblatt D J, Shader R I 1974 Benzodiazepines in clinical practice. Raven Press, New York

Hindmarch I, Oh H, Roth T (eds) 1984 Sleep, benzodiazepines and performance. Experimental methodologies and research prospects. Springer Verlag

Marks J 1985 The benzodiazepines, use, overuse, misuse, abuse. MTP Press Ltd

Proceedings of a symposium held in Amsterdam Holland 1982 Benzodiazepines, sleep and daytime performance. The Medicine Publishing Foundation, Symposium Series 10. Oxford, UK

Schutz H 1982 Benzodiazepines, a handbook, basic data, analytical methods, pharmacokinetic and comprehensive literature. Springer-Verlag, Heidelberg

Trimble M R 1983 Benzodiazepines divided. John Wiley and Sons

Usdin E, Skolnick P, Tallman J F Jr, Greenblatt D, Paul S M (eds) 1982 Pharmacology of benzodiazepines. MacMillan Press Ltd

References

1. Hagel R B, Debesis E M 1975 The non-aqueous reactions of some 1,4-benzodiazepines. Analytica Chimica Acta 78: 439–450
2. Greenblatt D J, Arendt R M, Abernethy D R, Giles H G, Sellers E M, Shader R I 1983 In vitro quantitation of benzodiazepine lipophilicity; relation to in vivo distribution. British Journal of Anaesthesia 55: 985–988
3. Gluckman M I 1965 Pharmacology of oxazepam (Serax) a new anti-anxiety agent. Current Therapeutic Research 7: 721–740
4. Garrattini S, Mussini E, Marcucci F, Guaitani A 1973 Metabolic studies on benzodiazepines in various animal species. In: Garrattini S, Mussini E, Randall L O (eds) The benzodiazepines. Raven Press, New York, pp 75–97
5. Randall L O, Scheckel C L, Banziger R F 1965 Pharmacology of the metabolites of chlordiazepoxide and diazepam. Current Therapeutic Research 7: 590–606
6. Geller I 1964 Relative potencies of benzodiazepines as measured by their effects on conflict behaviour. Archives Internationales de Pharmacodynamie et de Therapie 149: 243–247
7. DiMascio A, Barrett J 1965 Comparative effects of oxazepam in 'high' and 'low' anxious student volunteers. Psychosomatics 6: 298–302
8. Brown M L, Sletten I W, Kleinman K M, Korol B 1968 Effect of oxazepam on physiological responses to stress in normal subjects. Current Therapeutic Research 10: 543–553
9. DiMascio A, Shader R I, Harmatz J 1969 Psychotropic drugs and induced hostility. Psychosomatics 10: 46–47
10. Kochansky G E C, Salzman C, Shader R I, Harmatz J S, Ogeltree A M 1975 The differential effects of chlordiazepoxide and oxazepam on hostility in a small group setting. American Journal of Psychiatry 132: 861–863
11. Gardos G, DiMascio A, Salzman C, Shader R I 1968 Differential actions of chlordiazepoxide and oxazepam on hostility. Archives of General Psychiatry 18: 757–760
12. Lion J R 1979 Benzodiazepines in the treatment of aggressive patients. Journal of Clinical Psychiatry 40: 70–71

O

13. Dolce G, Kaemmerer E 1967 The effect of the benzodiazepine — Adumbran — on the rest and sleep EEG as well as the visual reaction potential in the awake person. Medizinische Welt (Stuttgart) 9: 510–514
14. Clarke C H, Nicholson A N 1978 Immediate and residual effects in man of the metabolites of diazepam. British Journal of Clinical Pharmacology 6: 325–331
15. Greenblatt D J 1981 Clinical pharmacokinetics of oxazepam and lorazepam. Clinical Pharmacokinetics 6: 89–105
16. Greenblatt D J, Franke K, Shader R I 1978 Analysis of lorazepam and its glucuronide metabolite by electron-capture gas–liquid chromatography. Use in pharmacokinetic studies of lorazepam. Journal of Chromatography 146: 311–320
17. Tomson G, Lunell N O, Sundwall A, Rane A 1979 Placental passage of oxazepam and its metabolism in mother and newborn. Clinical Pharmacology and Therapeutics 25: 74–81
18. Shull H J, Wilkinson G R, Johnson R, Shenker S 1976 Normal disposition of oxazepam in acute viral hepatitis and cirrhosis. Annals of Internal Medicine 84: 420–425
19. Odar-Cederloff I, Vessman J, Alvan G, Sjoqvist F 1977 Oxazepam disposition in uraemic patients. Acta Pharmacologica et Toxicologica 40 (suppl 1): 52–62
20. Greenblatt D J, Divoll M, Harmatz J S, Shader R I 1980 Oxazepam kinetics: effects of age and sex. Journal of Pharmacology and Experimental Therapeutics 215: 86–91
21. Alvan G, Siwers B, Vessman J 1977 Pharmacokinetics of oxazepam in healthy volunteers. Acta Pharmacologica et Toxicologica 40 (suppl 1): 40–51
22. Vessman J, Alexanderson B, Sjöqvist F, Strindberg B, Sundwall A 1977 Comparative pharmacokinetics of oxazepam and nortriptyline after single oral doses in man. In: Garattini S (ed) The benzodiazepines. Raven Press, New York, pp 165–173
23. Alvan G, Jönsson M, Sundwell A, Vessman J 1978 First pass conjugation and enterohepatic recycling of oxazepam in dogs; intravenous tolerance of oxazepam in propylene glycol. Acta Pharmacologica et Toxicologica 40 (suppl 1): 16–27
24. Solomon K 1978 Safety of oxazepam. New York State Journal of Medicine 78: 91–92
25. Sawle Thomas J C 1966 Clinical evaluation of oxazepam in an out-patient psychiatric clinic. Diseases of the Nervous System 27: 261–264
26. Tobin J M, Lorenz A A, Brousseau E R, Conner W R 1964 Clinical evaluation of oxazepam for the management of anxiety. Diseases of the Nervous System 25: 689–696
27. Krakowski A J 1965 Suppression of anxiety with oxazepam in a private psychiatric practice. Psychosomatics 6: 26–31
28. Velloso F M, Paprocki J 1967 Reduction of treatment obstructing anxiety with oxazepam. Folha Medica 54: 103–109
29. Gerz H O 1964 A preliminary report on the management of geriatric patients with oxazepam. American Journal of Psychiatry 120: 1110–1111
30. Mestman J H, Pocock D S, Kirchner A 1969 Lactic acidosis with recovery in diabetes mellitus on phenformin therapy. California Medicine 111: 181–185
31. Sharp P 1972 Interference in glucose oxidase–peroxidase blood glucose methods. Clinica Chimica Acta 40: 115–120
32. Caraway W T, Kammeyer C W 1972 Chemical interference by drugs and other substances with clinical laboratory test procedures. Clinica Chimica Acta 41: 395–434
33. Palva E S, Linnoila M 1978 Effect of active metabolites of chlordiazepoxide and diazepam alone, or in combination with alcohol, on psychomotor skills related to driving. European Journal of Clinical Pharmacology 13: 345–350
34. Molander L, Duvhok C 1976 Acute effects of oxazepam, diazepam and methylperone, alone and in combination with alcohol on sedation, co-ordination and mood. Acta Pharmacologica et Toxicologica 38: 145–160
35. MacLeod S M, Sellers E M, Giles H G et al 1978 Interaction of disulfiram with benzodiazepines. Clinical Pharmacology and Therapeutics 24: 583–589

Oxpentifylline

Oxpentifylline was the first drug approved for the treatment of intermittent claudication.

Chemistry

Oxpentifylline (Pentoxifylline, Trental, Elorgan, Tarontal, Terental, Torental)

$C_{13}H_{18}N_4O_3$

3,7-Dimethyl-1-(5-oxohexyl)xanthine

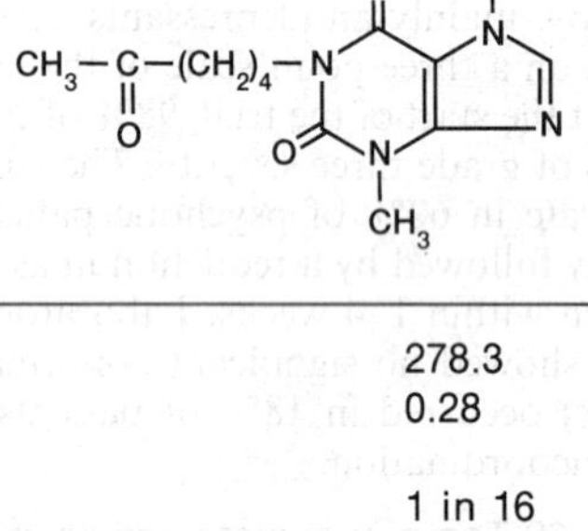

Molecular weight	278.3
pKa	0.28
Solubility	
in alcohol	1 in 16
in water	—
Octanol/water partition coefficient	1.96

Oxpentifylline is a creamy white powder, almost odourless with a bitter taste, and is prepared by chemical synthesis. It is not available in any combination products.

Pharmacology

Oxpentifylline and its metabolites are vasodilators which are also claimed to improve the flow properties of blood by decreasing its viscosity.[1] The exact mechanism of action is unknown but proposed mechanisms include increased blood cell deformability or flexibility,[2] possibly related to increased phosphorylation of red cell membrane proteins,[3] and a reduction in plasma fibrinogen levels.[4] In vitro studies also suggest that it may enhance the vascular production of prostacyclin.[5,6,]

Infusion of oxpentifylline in the rat results in an increase in cardiac output, reduction in systemic blood pressure and an increase in blood flow to heart and skeletal muscle, liver, stomach, skin and brain.[7] Vascular smooth muscle vasodilation following phosphodiesterase inhibition is the probable haemodynamic mechanism. However, the vascular effects of oxpentifylline are less marked than those produced by parenteral aminophylline.[8]

Toxicology

Oxpentifylline, in concentrations of 4.0–5000 $mg.l^{-1}$, gives a negative result in the Ames test; consequently it is unlikely to have mutagenic potential. Tests in rats and mice lasting up to 78 weeks revealed no evidence of carcinogenicity. Teratological effects were not noted in rats (12.5 $mg.kg^{-1}$ intravenously or 570 $mg.kg^{-1}$ orally) or rabbits (10 $mg.kg^{-1}$ intravenously or 265 $mg.kg^{-1}$ orally).

Clinical pharmacology

Intravenous injection of oxpentifylline in man reduces systemic vascular resistance. In addition to its vasodilator effects, oxpentifylline reduces plasma fibrinogen concentrations and blood viscosity, although the importance of these effects in therapy is not established. Increased blood flow to the extremities has been documented by Doppler techniques and oscillography, suggesting an increase in blood flow through collateral channels. Improved perfusion is supported by enhancement of muscle clearance of xenon-133, thermography, and measurements of skeletal muscle oxygen tension. The reduction in plasma fibrinogen concentration is maximal within 2–4 weeks, possibly explaining the observation that clinical improvement may be delayed until the second or even as late as the fourth to sixth week of therapy. Consequently, trial of treatment must be continued for up to 8 weeks.[9]

Although intravenous injection of oxpentifylline in man reduces systemic vascular resistance and the animal studies mentioned earlier have demonstrated increases in blood flow in many organs, there is no evidence that oxpentifylline alters the diameter of atheromatous stenoses in human blood vessels.

Pharmacokinetics

The preferred analytical method is gas–liquid chromatography of a trifluoroacetate derivative of oxpentifylline and the ethyl ester derivatives of its metabolites using a nitrogen detector. The limit of detection is approximately 10 $\mu g.l^{-1}$.[10]

Oxpentifylline is almost completely (>95%) absorbed after oral administration. It undergoes extensive presystemic metabolism (60–70%), presumably in the liver, and parent compound and metabolites appear in the plasma within 30 min of ingestion. Peak plasma levels of the parent compound (120–130 $\mu g.l^{-1}$ after 400 mg of the slow-release preparation) are reached within 1 h of ingestion. Following oral administration of the slow-release compound, pharmacokinetic indices are dose-related and non-linear, being determined mainly by the rate of release and absorption of the parent compound. The plasma half life of oxpentifylline following intravenous administration is biphasic, the α-phase half life being 8.3 min and the β-phase half life being 1.8 h. Half lives of the metabolites vary from 1 to 1.6 h and the effective plasma half life of the slow-release preparation ranges from 4 to 6 h. There is no evidence of accumulation following multiple oral doses.[11]

Excretion is almost complete (>95%) within 24 h and is primarily renal, less than 4% of the parent drug being excreted in the faeces. No parent drug is found in the urine.

Oxpentifylline is excreted in breast milk and the concentrations achieved may be sufficient to affect nursing infants. It is not known whether the drug crosses the placenta. Although oxpentifylline is extensively metabolized, the metabolites are pharmacologically active. Thus, as they are excreted primarily by the kidneys, some reduction in dose might be necessary in renal impairment and in the elderly with decreased renal function.

Oral absorption	>95%
Presystemic metabolism	60–70%
Plasma half life	
range (slow release)	4–6 h
mean	1.8 h
Volume of distribution	168±82 l
Plasma protein binding	low

Fig. 1 Major metabolites of oxpentifylline

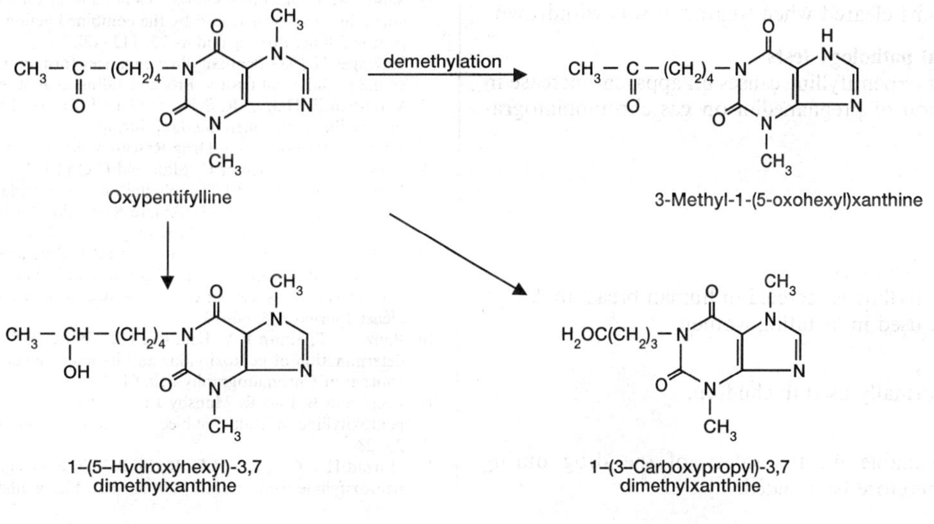

Concentration–effect relationship

There is no evidence of a relationship between the plasma concentration of oxpentifylline and its therapeutic effect.

Metabolism

Oxpentifylline is metabolized both by the red cells and the liver. Two major pathways have been described: demethylation at C7, and hydroxylation of the side-chain. Seven metabolites have been identified. Two of them, 1-(5-hydroxyhexyl)-3,7-dimethylxanthine and 1-(3-carboxypropyl)-3,7-dimethylxanthine, have been shown to be active in vitro. They are equipotent with oxpentifylline and achieve plasma levels 5–8 times greater than the parent compound, respectively. 1-(3-Carboxypropyl)-3,7-dimethylxanthine constitutes 80% of the metabolic products and contributes to the pharmacodynamic effect, although it has a shorter half life than the parent compound.[12]

Pharmaceutics

Oxpentifylline, Trental (Hoechst, UK), is available as controlled-release tablets each containing 400 mg in a slow-release formulation. These pills are pink, sugar-coated, oblong, and imprinted with 'Trental'. Oxpentifylline formulations are stable, with a shelf-life of 5 years for tablets. They do not contain allergenic components.

Therapeutic use

Indications

1. Intermittent claudication secondary to chronic occlusive vascular disease
2. Raynaud's syndrome
3. Transient ischaemic attacks.

Contraindications

1. Hypersensitivity to methylxanthine compounds, e.g. caffeine, theophylline
2. Care should be exercised in patients with coronary artery disease or orthostatic hypotension where, occasionally, the hypotensive effect of oxpentifylline may exacerbate symptoms.

Mode of use

Oral treatment is usually begun with 400 mg three times daily using the controlled-release tablets. Twice daily dosing may be adequate in some patients; however, smaller doses seem to be ineffective in the treatment of claudication.[13] Doses above 1200 mg per day have little therapeutic advantage. Clinical benefit is usually seen in 2–4 weeks, however the effects may be delayed up to 8 weeks.[9]

Intravenous administration should be used with the greatest of care and is intended for initial therapy of severe peripheral vascular disorders only. A 5 ml (100 mg) ampoule may be diluted in 250–500 ml of normal saline or dextrose and water and infused over

90–180 min. The maximum parenteral dose should not exceed 400 mg daily. Neither rebound on withdrawal nor tachyphylaxis on prolonged administration have been reported.

Indications

1. Intermittent claudication

Although many small controlled and uncontrolled studies in Europe in the 1970s suggested a clinical benefit from treatment with oxpentifylline, the strongest evidence was provided by the multi-centre, double-blind, placebo-controlled trial of Porter et al.[9] They reported that 24 weeks of treatment with oxpentifylline (1200 mg daily) doubled the initial claudication distance, measured serially on a treadmill, an improvement significantly greater than that seen in the placebo-treated group. The improvement in absolute claudication distance in the 42 actively treated patients was less striking but was significantly better than in the 40 patients treated with placebo.

2. Raynaud's syndrome

A number of small and poorly controlled studies have reported benefit in some patients with Raynaud's syndrome or Buerger's disease.[14,15]

3. Transient ischaemic attacks

A study comparing the frequency of transient ischaemic attacks during a 6-month period of treatment with acetylsalicyclic acid combined with dipyridamole in 73 patients, and oxpentifylline administered in 65 patients, reported 80 events in 19 patients of the first group compared with 19 episodes in 9 patients on oxpentifylline. These results were statistically significant. They have not, however, been confirmed.[16]

Adverse reactions

Potentially life-threatening effects

No effects of this kind have been reported in man.

Acute overdosage

There has been one case report of a deliberate overdose.[17] The main clinical features following a dose of 4–6 g included extreme bradycardia with first, and later second, degree atrioventricular block. The latter was responsive to atropine, although first degree block persisted for 16 h. No effects on the central nervous system or on metabolism were reported.

Severe or irreversible adverse effects

No effects of this kind have been reported.

Symptomatic adverse effects

Oxpentifylline is generally well tolerated although adverse effects such as dyspepsia, nausea, dizziness, headache, and vomiting have been reported. In a multi-centre, double-blind study,[9] the incidence of side effects with oxpentifylline was 57%, in comparison with 39% for placebo. Nausea was the most common adverse effect, occurring in 36%, followed by dizziness, in 21% of patients. The effects were dose-dependent and decreased when the doses were lowered. In all cases, reported symptoms cleared when treatment was withdrawn.

Interference with clinical pathology tests

A urinary metabolite of oxpentifylline causes an apparent increase in the urinary concentration of pregnanediol on gas chromomatographic assay.[18]

High risk groups

Neonates

The drug is not used in neonates.

Breast milk. Oxpentifylline is secreted in human breast milk,[4] so the drug should not be used in lactating women.

Children

Oxpentifylline is not normally used in children.

Pregnant women

No information is available on the safety of the drug during pregnancy; it should therefore be avoided.

The elderly

No clinical trials have been performed specifically to study the side-effect profile in this group.

Concurrent disease

Liver disease. A small study on patients with liver disease (metastatic, cirrhotic, or due to chronic hepatitis) reported increased hepatic blood flow caused by intravenous oxpentifylline 200 mg. There were no unexpected adverse effects but studies of chronic oral administration in patients with hepatic disease have not been reported.[19]

Renal disease. Since the active metabolites are excreted predominantly by the kidney, doses should be reduced in patients with renal dysfunction.[20]

Bleeding disorders. Oxpentifylline should be administered with care in patients with a bleeding diathesis as its potential for reducing the plasma fibrinogen concentration in these patients may be detrimental.

Drug interactions

Potentially hazardous interactions

Aspirin. Concomitant use of oxpentifylline with aspirin has been reported to cause increased bleeding in some patients.

Antihypertensive drugs. Oxpentifylline may occasionally enhance the effects of hypotensive drugs and its use may require reduction of their doses.

Hypoglycaemic agents. Parenteral oxpentifylline has been reported to enhance the hypoglycaemic effects of insulin and oral hypoglycaemic drugs.

Other significant interactions

Food may delay the absorption of oxpentifylline but the area under the plasma concentration–time curve is not changed.[21]

Potentially useful interactions

No reactions of this kind have been reported.

Major outcome trials

None are known to have been carried out.

General review articles

Dettelbach H R, Aviado D M 1985 Clinical pharmacology of pentoxifylline with special reference to its hemorheologic effect for the treatment of intermittent claudication. Journal of Clinical Pharmacology 25: 8–26

Muller R 1981 Hemorheology and peripheral vascular diseases: a new therapeutic approach. Journal of Medicine 12: 209–226

References

1. Hess H V, Franke I, Juch M 1973 Medikamentose Verbesserung der Fliesseigenschaften des Blutes. Ein Wirksames Prinzip zur Behandlung von Arteriellen Durchblutungsstorungen. Fortschritte der Medizin 91: 743–748
2. Ehrly A M 1976 Improvement of the flow properties of blood. A new therapeutical approach in occlusive arterial disease. Angiology 27: 188–196
3. Kramer J J, Swislocki N I 1983 Effects of pentoxifylline on membrane protein phosphorylation in erythrocytes. Vascular Medicine 1: 159–174
4. Witter F R, Smith R V 1985 The excretion of pentoxifylline and its metabolites into human breast milk. American Journal of Obstetrics and Gynecology 151: 1094–1097
5. Santos M T, Martinez-Sales V, Vall'es J et al 1985 Prostacyclin production by rat aorta 'in vitro' is increased by the combined action of dipyridamole plus pentoxifylline. Prostaglandins 29: 113–122
6. Sinzinger H 1983 Pentoxifylline enhances formation of prostacyclin from rat vascular and renal tissues. Prostaglandins Leukotrienes and Medicine 12: 217–226
7. Vetterlein F, Halfter R, Schmidt G 1979 Regional blood flow determination in rats by the microsphere method during i.v. infusion of vasodilating agents. Arzneimittel-Forschung/Drug Research 29: 747–751
8. Komarek J, Kartheuser C, Mansfeld C et al 1977 Der Effekt von Pentoxifyllin, Xantinol-nicotinat und Theophyllin auf das Kreislaufsystem, die myokardiale Dynamik und die linksventrikulare Kontraktilitat beim Hund im akuten Experiment. Arzneimittel-Forschung 27: 1932–1939
9. Porter J M, Cutler B S, Lee B U I et al 1982 Pentoxifylline efficacy in the treatment of intermittent claudication: multi-center controlled double-blind trial with objective assessment of chronic occlusive arterial disease patients. American Heart Journal 104: 66–72
10. Bauza M T, Smith R V, Knutson D E, Witter F R 1984 Gas chromatographic determination of pentoxifylline and its major metabolites in human breast milk. Journal of Chromatography 310: 61–69
11. Beermann B, Ings R, Mansby J et al 1985 Kinetics of intravenous and oral pentoxifylline in healthy subjects. Clinical Pharmacology and Therapeutics 37: 25–28
12. Hinzad H J, Grigoleit H G, Rethy B 1976 Bioavailability and pharmacokinetics of pentoxifylline from 'trental 400' in man. Pharmatherapeutica 1: 460–471

13. Donaldson D R, Hall T J, Kester R C et al 1984 Does oxpentiphylline have a place in the treatment of intermittent claudication? Current Medical Research and Opinion 9: 35–40
14. Galindo Planis N, Vallve C 1980 Estudio oscilografico sobre la accion de la pentoxifilina en el tratamiento de trastornos de la irrigacion periferica. Angiologia 32: 81–90
15. Schmidt C, Marrequis P, Royer R J et al 1976 Etude clinique et hemodynamique du BL 191 dans les affections vasculaires peripheriques. Annales de Medicin Nancy 15: 257–261
16. Herskovits E, Famulari A, Tamaroff L et al 1985 Preventive treatment of cerebral transient ischaemia: comparative randomized trial of pentoxifylline versus conventional antiaggregants. European Neurology 24: 73–81
17. Sznajder I, Bentur Y, Titelman U 1984 First and second degree atrial ventricular block in oxpentiphylline overdose. British Medical Journal 288: 26
18. Metcalf M G 1977 Analysis of pregnanediol in urine: Trental interference. Clinica Chimica Acta 76: 285–288
19. Koppenhagen K, Wenig H G 1979 Wirkung von pentoxifylline auf die Leberdurchblutung. Medizinische Klinik 74: 1254–1256
20. Schaefer K, von Herrath D, Hensel A et al 1977 Untersuchungen zur Pharmakokinetik von Pentoxifyllin bei chronischer Niereninsuffizienz. Medizinische Klinik 72: 204–206
21. Wills R J, Waller E S, Puri S K et al 1981 Influence of food on the bioavailability of 'Trental pentoxifylline' in man. Drug Rev Ind Pharm 7: 385–396

Oxprenolol (hydrochloride)

A non-selective β-adrenergic receptor antagonist with some partial agonist activity.

Chemistry

Oxprenolol hydrochloride (Trasicor, Apsolox, Laracor, Slow-Pren, Slow-Trasicor)
$C_{15}H_{23}NO_3HCl$
1-(2-Allyloxyphenoxy)-3-isopropylaminopropan-2-ol hydrochloride

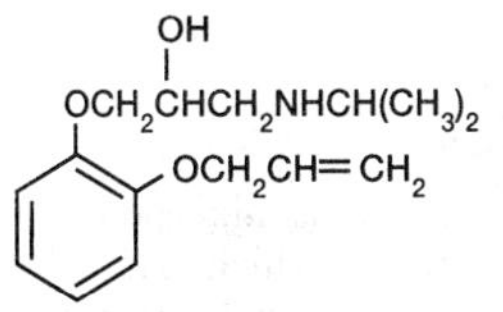

Molecular weight	301.8
pKa	9.5
Solubility	
in alcohol	high
in water	high
Octanol/water partition coefficient	1.6

A white, odourless powder with a bitter taste, it is prepared by chemical synthesis and the racemate is used clinically. Oxprenolol is also available in an oral combination product with cyclopenthiazide (Trasidrex).

Pharmacology

Oxprenolol is a competitive antagonist at both the β_1 and β_2-adrenoceptor, and therefore is not cardioselective.[1] It has some partial agonist activity, more marked than acebutolol but less marked than pindolol.[2] Oxprenolol, which is equipotent as a β-adrenoceptor antagonist to propranolol, has less membrane-stabilizing activity than propranolol and this action is unlikely to be of any significance at the concentrations achieved in clinical use.[3]

Toxicology

Prolonged administration of oxprenolol to rats, dogs and rhesus monkeys has shown no evidence of clinically relevant toxicity.

No teratogenicity was seen in mice, rats or rabbits and there was no evidence of mutagenicity or carcinogenicity.

Clinical pharmacology

Competitive β-adrenoceptor antagonism has been demonstrated in man by a parallel shift to the right in the dose heart-rate response curve or airways resistance curve to β-agonists such as isoprenaline. Because oxprenolol antagonizes both responses, it is an unselective β-adrenoceptor antagonist in man.

Daily doses in the range 20–480 mg produce a dose-related decrease in the rise in heart rate on exercise. The maximum reduction in the tachycardia which follows stepping on and off a box 46 cm high, 32 times per minute for 3 minutes is about 30%, which is less than that seen with an equivalent dose of propranolol.[4] The dose exercise heart rate response curve is flatter than for propranolol and this is probably due to the partial agonist activity.

Oxprenolol decreases maximal exercise tolerance in normal individuals but in patients with angina, exercise tolerance is usually increased, due to a reduction in total myocardial oxygen consumption. Oxprenolol lowers blood pressure in both the lying and standing positions, although the exact mechanism for this effect is still debated. Oxprenolol reduces cardiac output, and while this effect is probably not the cause of the fall in blood pressure, it can lead to the precipitation of frank heart failure in some patients. Oxprenolol in addition to reducing heart rate, particularly on exercise, slows conduction in the atria and in the A-V node and decreases the spontaneous rate of depolarization of ectopic pacemakers. These properties make the drug a useful anti-arrhythmic agent.

Oxprenolol blocks the action of adrenaline on β-adrenoceptors in other tissues. In particular airways resistance is increased by oxprenolol and this may be dangerous in asthmatic patients. Many of the somatic manifestations of thyrotoxicosis, e.g. increased heart rate, tremor and irritability, are improved by oxprenolol and the relief from anxiety induced by oxprenolol has been used successfully in the relief of short term stressful situations, such as examinations and solo instrument playing.

There are widespread metabolic and endocrine effects of β-adrenoceptor antagonism including a reduction in plasma renin, and in high density lipoprotein, an increase in total serum cholesterol, low density lipoprotein, triglycerides and very low density lipoproteins. No changes in prolactin and growth hormone are seen with chronic therapy.

Pharmacokinetics

A reliable analytical method is high-performance liquid chromatography using UV detection,[5] which has a limit of sensitivity of 10 $\mu g.l^{-1}$. Oxprenolol is well absorbed after oral administration, has a large (25–80%) pre-systemic elimination and reaches peak plasma concentrations between 0.5 and 1.5 hours.[6] The mean plasma elimination half life is 1.9 hours with a range of 1.4–4.6 hours and the volume of distribution is $1.3\ l.kg^{-1}$. Animal studies have shown accumulation of oxprenolol in liver, kidney, lung and heart. After chronic administration, concentrations of oxprenolol in human brain are an order of magnitude higher than plasma concentrations.[7] Used to treat hypertension in pregnancy, the cord/maternal blood ratio was 0.4 and the breast milk/maternal ratio was 0.5.[8] More than 95% of an orally administered dose is excreted as inactive metabolites in the urine following oxidative metabolism and glucuronidation in the liver.

Oral absorption	100%
Presystemic metabolism	25–80%
Plasma half life	
range	1.4–4.6 h
mean	1.9 h
Volume of distribution	$1.3\ l.kg^{-1}$
Plasma protein binding	70–80%

The slow release formulation of oxprenolol gives plasma concentrations which are lower at 1 and 2 hours post dose and higher at 24 hours, but with little difference between the two formulations in effect on an exercise tachycardia.[9] Oxprenolol plasma concentrations are raised in inflammatory disease, probably due to increased α_1 acid glycoprotein concentrations.[10]

Concentration–effect relationship

Increasing β-adrenoceptor antagonism[11] is seen at plasma concentrations up to 300 $g.l^{-1}$ and antagonism is still present when oxprenolol is virtually undetectable.[12] Because of the high therapeutic index of this drug, plasma concentration monitoring is unlikely to be clinically useful.

Metabolism

Oxprenolol is extensively metabolized with less than 5% of an orally administered dose excreted unchanged in urine.

The principal metabolites are oxprenolol glucuronide (40%) and ring hydroxylated metabolites and their glucuronides. These pathways are similar to propranolol elimination and would be expected to be under similar genetic control and produce an active 4-hydroxy metabolite.[13]

Pharmaceutics

Trasicor tablets (Ciba, UK) containing oxprenolol hydrochloride BP 20 mg and 40 mg are circular, flat, white, film-coated with bevelled edges having the monogram 'CIBA' impressed on one side and 'Trasicor 20' or 'Trasicor 40' on the other.

Tablets containing oxprenolol hydrochloride BP 80 mg are circular, pale yellow, slightly biconvex, film-coated having the monogram 'CIBA' impressed on one side and 'Trasicor 80' on the other.

Tablets containing oxprenolol hydrochloride BP 160 mg are circular, pale orange, slightly biconvex, film-coated having the monogram 'CIBA' impressed on one side and 'Trasicor 160' on the other.

Slow-Trasicor is a sustained release formulation containing 160 mg oxprenolol hydrochloride BP. The tablets are circular, slightly biconvex, white, film-coated having the monogram 'CIBA' impressed on one side and 'Slow-Trasicor' on the other.

Trasicor ampoules each contain 2 mg oxprenolol hydrochloride BP.

Therapeutic use

Indications

1. The treatment of hypertension
2. The management of angina pectoris
3. The control of some cardiac arrhythmias
4. The management of hypertrophic obstructive cardiomyopathy
5. The control of somatic manifestations of anxiety.

Contraindications

1. Bronchospasm
2. Low cardiac output and untreated cardiac failure
3. Bradycardia and heart block
4. Hypoglycaemia
5. Severe haemorrhage.

Fig. 1 The metabolism of oxprenolol

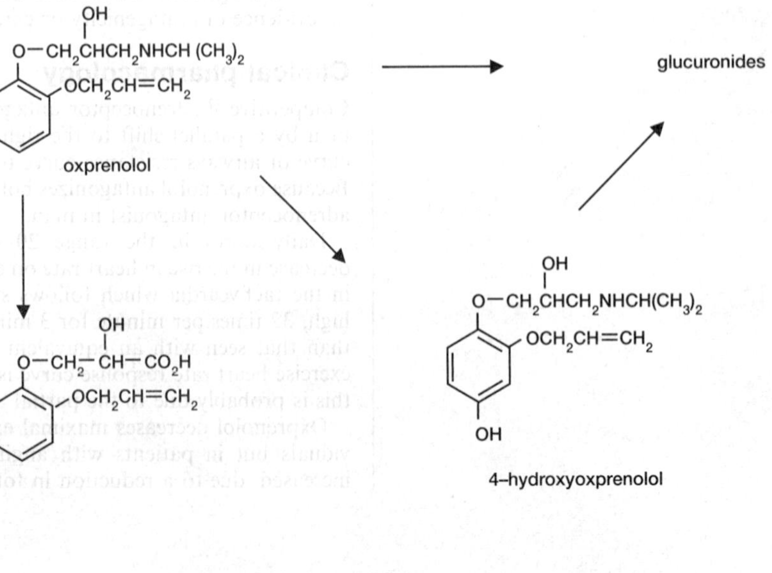

Mode of use

All the clinical uses depend upon competitive antagonism of the β-adrenoceptors.

Oral treatment is usually commenced with 20-40 mg two or three times daily and the dose is increased up to a maximum of 480 mg daily depending on the therapeutic response.

Sudden withdrawal of oxprenolol treatment can be hazardous to patients with severe ischaemic heart disease as severe exacerbations of angina or myocardial infarction may occur. This may be a lesser problem with oxprenolol than β-adrenoceptor antagonists without partial agonist activity but the rebound increase in heart rate on standing after chronic oxprenolol therapy was similar to that after propranolol.[14]

Indications

1. Hypertension

Many clinical studies have shown the safety and efficacy of oxprenolol in the treatment of hypertension as either monotherapy,[15] or in combination with diuretics or other antihypertensive agents.[16] In moderate hypertensives, systolic and diastolic blood pressure is reduced in both the supine and erect posture by 19/15 mmHg during the day and 6/7 mmHg at night[15] but there is no postural hypotension. The fall in blood pressure comes on with the absorption of the drug and there is no evidence of tolerance. Blood pressure is better controlled during the day than at night probably due to the presence of intrinsic sympathomimetic activity. No increased antihypertensive effect is seen with doses above 320 mg.

Even after 20 years of use the mode of hypotensive action is not clear. Suggested mechanisms include inhibition of renin release and reduced cardiac output.

2. Angina pectoris

Oxprenolol is an effective treatment for exercise-induced angina, increasing walking time, reducing ST depression and heart rate but the dose must be titrated to achieve optimal effect.[17] A starting dose of 40 mg three or four times daily is increased weekly depending on response up to a maximum of 480 mg daily. Near maximal effects are seen with 160 mg.[17] Treatment should not be stopped suddenly because patients with severe ischaemic heart disease on long term treatment with β adrenoceptor antagonists may suffer an exacerbation in their symptoms due to an increase in the number of β adrenoceptors during treatment.

3. Cardiac arrhythmias

β adrenoceptor antagonists reduce the potential for arrhythmias to develop in response to catecholamines but their use as a single agent in phaeochromocytoma may cause marked hypertension due to unopposed α-agonism. Oxprenolol has been shown to be effective in supraventricular arrhythmias following myocardial infarction[18] but to have little effect on the incidence of ventricular premature beats or ventricular tachycardia.[19]

4. Hypertrophic obstructive cardiomyopathy

β adrenoceptor antagonists have been shown to improve some of the haemodynamic alterations in this condition but there are no satisfactory trials and long term results are disappointing.

5. Anxiety

Acute situational anxiety has been successfully treated with oxprenolol[20] and the somatic manifestations of chronic anxiety, particularly tachycardia and tremor, are relieved.

Contraindications

1. Bronchospasm

All β adrenoceptor antagonists may cause severe bronchospasm in patients with obstructive airways disease.

2. Low cardiac output and untreated cardiac failure

β adrenoceptor antagonism reduces heart rate and myocardial contractility. In patients whose cardiac output depends on sympathetic drive oxprenolol may precipitate heart failure.

3. Bradycardia

Oxprenolol is contraindicated in patients with second and third degree atrioventricular block and sick sinus syndrome.

4. Hypoglycaemia

The normal homeostatic response to hypoglycaemia involves the production of adrenaline and β adrenoceptor mediated reflex metabolic consequences. As oxprenolol antagonizes the subjective feelings of hypoglycaemia like tremor and the metabolic reflexes, the condition may not be recognized early and may persist for longer.

5. Severe haemorrhage

The usual haemodynamic response to haemorrhage involves a sympathetically mediated tachycardia which is inhibited by oxprenolol. The signs of severe haemorrhage must be interpreted in the knowledge of the presence of a β adrenoceptor antagonist.

Adverse reactions

Potentially life-threatening effects

The β-adrenoceptor antagonists have a high therapeutic index and life-threatening effects are rare. The predictable effects of bronchospasm, hypotension, bradycardia, and hypoglycaemia may occur in susceptible patients but should be infrequent. Chronic treatment with oxprenolol increases VLDL and reduces HDL[21] which may have an adverse effect on the risk of cardiovascular events.

Acute overdosage

The β-adrenoceptor antagonists are not very toxic in overdose and patients have survived 6 g of oxprenolol. Compared with the other drugs in this class, oxprenolol is less toxic than propranolol.[22] Bradycardia may be treated with atropine and isoprenaline or glucagon may be administered if required.

Severe or irreversible adverse effects

Severe and irreversible effects are unusual with oxprenolol. The sclerosing peritonitis seen with practolol was reported with oxprenolol but this has not been confirmed.

Symptomatic adverse effects

In prospective studies, when comparison with placebo has been made, the incidence of adverse effects was similar in both groups. The incidence of lethargy is similar in patients treated with propranolol and oxprenolol. The incidence of cold extremities and wheezing is said to be lower with oxprenolol than propranolol, but there is little good evidence to support this claim.

Other effects

HDL cholesterol is decreased by chronic oxprenolol treatment and VLDL increased. Serum uric acid, urea and creatinine are little changed and plasma renin activity is decreased.

Interference with clinical pathology tests

Rado and Vegh found that oxprenolol in daily doses of 60, 120 and 180 mg gave falsely high fluorometric readings in urine cortisol determinations.[23]

High risk groups

Neonates

There is no information available on the use of oxprenolol in neonates.

Breast milk. Oxprenolol is excreted in breast milk and a child consuming 500 ml milk would receive a maximum dose of about 0.07 $mg.kg^{-1}$.

Children

There is little information available on the use of oxprenolol in children.

Pregnant women

Oxprenolol has been successfully used to treat hypertension in pregnancy, but no comparative trials are reported.

The elderly

There is little effect of age on the kinetics of oxprenolol, and little dosage adjustment is required.

Drug interactions

Potentially hazardous interactions

Hydralazine. Concurrent administration of slow-release oxprenolol and hydralazine resulted in a significant increase in the area under the blood/plasma concentration–time curve for oxprenolol.

However, the increase in mean peak plasma concentration for oxprenolol during coadministration failed to reach statistical significance and the effect is of little practical significance.[24]

Adrenaline. In the presence of a β-adrenoceptor antagonist like oxprenolol, adrenaline is essentially an α-agonist and marked rises in blood pressure can occur.

Anaesthetic agents. The vasodilating effect of some anaesthetic agents may tend to cause a fall in blood pressure and a rise in heart rate. In the presence of oxprenolol this homeostatic mechanism may be impaired but, with care, oxprenolol can be administered during anaesthesia.

Clonidine. In common with other β-adrenoceptor antagonists, oxprenolol may increase the rebound hypertension following clonidine withdrawal which is associated with high levels of circulating catecholamines.

Ergot. The vasoconstrictor effect of the ergot alkaloids is potentiated by oxprenolol, because the vasodilation mediated through the β_2 adrenoceptor is inhibited.

Lignocaine. The metabolism of lignocaine is inhibited by oxprenolol, which may lead to accumulation.

Oral contraceptives. Plasma concentrations of oxprenolol are increased in patients taking oral contraceptives but this is unlikely to be of clinical significance.

Verapamil. β-adrenoceptor antagonists administered with verapamil may cause marked bradycardia. More serious rhythm disturbance can occur in the presence of nodal dysfunction.

Other significant interactions

Indomethacin. In common with other β-adrenoceptor antagonists the hypotensive effect is lessened by the concurrent administration of indomethacin, probably due to inhibition of the synthesis of vasodilating prostaglandins.

Hypoglycaemic agents. The homeostatic response to hypoglycaemia is impaired by β-adrenoceptor antagonists.

Potentially useful interactions

Oxprenolol can reduce the reflex tachycardia which occurs with vasodilators increasing the hypotensive effect.

Major outcome trials

1. The IPPPSH Collaborative Group 1985 Cardiovascular risk and risk factors in a randomized trial of treatment based on the β-blocker oxprenolol: the international prospective primary prevention study in hypertension (IPPPSH). Journal of Hypertension 3: 379–392

This is a randomised, double-blind trial conducted in over 6000 patients with uncomplicated essential hypertension treated for 3–5 years to evaluate the effect of including oxprenolol in antihypertensive drug regimens. Non-smoking men had half the cardiac event rate of their peers. Oxprenolol treatment was associated with a lower withdrawal rate because of uncontrolled blood pressure and a lower prevalence of hypokalaemia. Oxprenolol therapy was associated with fewer complaints of anxiety, headache, dizziness, dry mouth and sexual dysfunction.

2. Petrie J C, Jeffers T A, Kobb O J, Scott A K and Webster J 1980 Atenolol, sustained-release oxprenolol, and long acting propranolol in hypertension. British Medical Journal 280: 1573–1574

This is a double-blind cross over trial involving 23 selected hypertensive patients who received treatment with atenolol 100 mg daily, slow release oxprenolol 160 mg daily and long acting propranolol 160 mg daily. After 4 weeks treatment the systolic and diastolic blood pressures were significantly reduced by all active treatments with no difference between them. There was some loss of control of blood pressure towards the end of the 24 hour period with slow release oxprenolol.

Other trials

The European Infarction Study Group 1984 European Infarction Study (E.I.S.) A secondary prevention study with slow release oxprenolol after myocardial infarction: morbidity and mortality. European Heart Journal 5: 189–202

This is a multicentre, double-blind, randomized study involving 1741 patients, 35 to 69 years old, who had survived a myocardial infarction and 14 to 36 days later commenced oxprenolol slow release 160 mg twice daily for one year.

The results failed to confirm the positive effects found in other secondary prevention trials with β-adrenergic-blocking drugs.

General review articles

Brechbuhler S, Brunner H, Meier M, Orwin J, Rogg H 1980 Oxprenolol. In: Scriabine A (ed) Pharmacology of antihypertensive drugs. Raven Press, New York, pp 209–222

Frishman W H 1982 The β-adrenoceptor blocking drugs. International Journal of Cardiology 2: 165–178

Kendall M J, John V A 1983 Oxprenolol: clinical pharmacology, pharmacokinetics, and pharmacodynamics. American Journal of Cardiology 52: 27D–33D

Russo M E, Covinsky J O 1983 Oxprenolol hydrochloride: pharmacology, pharmacokinetics, adverse effects and clinical efficacy. Pharmacotherapy 3: 68–81

Winchester J F 1974 Drug profile: Trasicor. Journal of International Medical Research 2: 448–457

References

1. Brunner H, Hedwall P R, Maier R, Meier M 1970 Pharmacological aspects of oxprenolol. Postgraduate Medical Journal 46 (November supply): 5–14
2. Bilski A, Robertson H H, Wale J L 1979 A study of the relationship between cardiac β-adrenoceptor blockade and intrinsic sympathomimetic activity in rats depleted of catecholamines. Clinical and Experimental Pharmacology and Physiology 6: 1–9
3. Yasuhara H, Sakamoto K, Ueda I 1981 Dissociation between local anaesthetic and membrane-stabilising actions in antiarrhythmic β-adrenergic blockers and local anaesthetics. Anaesthesia and Analgesia 60: 897–900
4. McDevitt D G, Brown H C, Carruthers S G, Shanks R G 1977 Observations on the influence of intrinsic sympathomimetic activity and cardioselectivity on β-adrenoceptor blockade in man. Clinical Pharmacology and Therapeutics 21: 556–566
5. Tsuei S E, Thomas J, Moore R G 1980 Quantification of oxprenolol in biological fluids using high-performance liquid chromatography. Journal of Chromatography 181: 135–140
6. Mason W D, Winer N 1976 Pharmacokintics of oxprenolol in normal subjects. Clinical Pharmacology and Therapeutics: 20, 401–412
7. Neil-Dwyer G, Bartlett J, McAinsh J, Cruickshank J M 1981 β-adrenoceptor blockers and the blood brain barrier. British Journal of Clinical Pharmacology 11: 549–553
8. Sioufi A, Hillion D, Lumbroso P et al 1984 Oxprenolol placental transfer, plasma concentrations in newborns and passage into breast milk. British Journal of Clinical Pharmacology 18: 453–456
9. Leahey W J, Neill J D, Varma M P S, Shanks R G 1980 Comparison of the activity and plasma levels of oxprenolol, slow release oxprenolol, long acting propranolol and sotalol. European Journal of Clinical Pharmacology 17: 419–424
10. Kendall M J, Quarterman C P, Bishop H, Schneider R E 1979 Effects of inflammatory disease on plasma oxprenolol concentrations. British Medical Journal 2: 465–468
11. Racine-Poon A, Moppert J 1985 Concentration–effect relationship of oxprenolol in healthy volunteers: a retrospective analysis. British Journal of Clinical Pharmacology 19: 143S–149S
12. Brunner L, Imhof P, Jack D 1975 Relation between plasma concentrations and cardiovascular effects of oral oxprenolol in man. European Journal of Clinical Pharmacology 8: 3–9
13. Riess W, Huerzeler H, Raschdorf F 1974 The metabolites of oxprenolol (Trasicor) in man. Xenobiotica 4: 365–373
14. Ross P J, Lewis M J, Sheridan D J, Henderson A H 1981 Adrenergic hypersensitivity after β-blocker withdrawal. British Heart Journal 45: 637–642
15. Millar-Craig M W, Mann S, Subramanian V B, Altman D G, Raftery E B 1983 The effects of oxprenolol on ambulatory intra-arterial blood pressure in essential hypertension. European Journal of Clinical Pharmacology 24: 713–721
16. Tarpley E L 1982 Oxprenolol hydrochloride: a long term study of efficacy, safety and tolerability, Pharmacotherapy 2: 281–284
17. Thadani U, Davidson C, Singleton W, Taylor S H 1979 Comparison of the immediate effects of five β-adrenoceptor-blocking drugs with different ancillary properties in angina pectoris. New England Journal of Medicine 300: 750–755
18. Sandler G, Pistevos A C 1971 Use of oxprenolol in cardiac arrhythmias associated with acute myocardial infarction. British Medical Journal 1: 254–257
19. The European Infarction Study Group 1985 Effect of oxprenolol on ventricular arrhythmias: the European Infarction Study experience. Journal of the American College of Cardiology 6: 963–972
20. James I M, Griffith D N W, Pearson R M, Newberry P 1977 Effect of oxprenolol on stage fright in musicians. Lancet 2: 952–954
21. Day J L, Metcalfe J, Simpson C N 1982 Adrenergic mechanisms in control of plasma lipid concentrations. British Medical Journal 284: 1145–1151
22. Henry J A, Cassidy S L 1986 Membrane stabilising activity: a major cause of fatal poisoning. Lancet 1: 1414–1417
23. Rado J P, Vegh L 1977 Interference of β-blocking drugs with cortisol determinations. International Journal of Pharmacology 15: 5–6
24. Hawkesworth G M, Dart A M, Chiang C S, Parry K, Petrie J C 1983 Effect of oxprenolol on the pharmacokinetics and pharmacodynamics of hydralazine. Drugs 25 (suppl 2): 136–140

Oxygen

Oxygen comprises 21% of the atmospheric gas. Higher concentrations are used to treat patients with serious impairment of gas exchange in the lung.

Chemistry

Oxygen
O_2

Molecular weight	31.999
Isotope composition	
^{16}O	99.79%
^{17}O	0.037%
^{18}O	0.204%
Solubility	
in alcohol (20°C)	1 vol of gas in 7 vols
in water	1 vol of gas in 32 vols
Melting point	−218°C
Boiling point	−183°C
Density at 0°C and 760 mmHg	1.429 g.l^{-1}

Oxygen is a colourless, odourless, tasteless gas which is non-flammable and supports combustion. It is prepared by liquefaction of air.

Pharmacology

Inspired oxygen diffuses across the alveolar membrane and is carried in the blood both bound to haemoglobin and dissolved in plasma. At atmospheric pressure the bulk of oxygen in the blood is carried on the ferrous iron in the haem moiety of haemoglobin, each haemoglobin molecule carrying up to four molecules of oxygen. When fully saturated with oxygen each gram of haemoglobin carries 1.34 ml of oxygen. 0.003 ml of oxygen are dissolved in each 100 ml blood per mmHg PO_2. Thus when breathing air at sea level, arterial blood usually carries around 19.8 ml oxygen per 100 ml blood, 0.3 ml in solution and 19.5 ml bound to haemoglobin.

Toxicology

The retinal changes described later under 'Adverse reactions' have been reproduced in animals. Because of the nature of this drug no teratogenicity or carcinogenicity tests have been carried out.

Clinical pharmacology

Oxygen administration will improve tissue oxygen delivery in arterial hypoxaemia, provided the hypoxaemia is not due to a true right-to-left heart shunt and that tissue blood flow is not reduced by oxygen therapy. Oxygen therapy may decrease ventilation, heart rate and cardiac output. 100% oxygen at atmospheric pressure does not alter oxygen consumption, carbon dioxide production or the respiratory quotient in normal subjects at rest.

Pharmacokinetics

Blood oxygen tensions are usually measured polarographically with silver and platinum electrodes.[1] Arterial oxygen saturation can be measured non-invasively by oximetry, but the error is around ±5%.[2,3] In normal subjects oxygen transfer across the alveolar membrane is efficient and end-pulmonary capillary blood is nearly 100% saturated with oxygen both at rest and on exercise. The delivery of oxygen to the tissues depends on arterial oxygenation, cardiac output, regional perfusion, local oxygen carriage systems and oxygen utilization. Oxygen is excreted almost entirely as carbon dioxide.

Concentration–effect relationship

A moderate reduction in arterial oxygen tension usually increases ventilation, heart rate and cardiac output and dilates coronary, cerebral and most peripheral vascular beds without changing systemic blood pressure. In contrast, hypoxia produces pulmonary vasoconstriction and pulmonary hypertension[4,5] and impairs cerebral function. When arterial PO_2 falls to around 30 mmHg normal subjects become unconscious. Severe hypoxia may produce irreversible damage to the brain, heart and other tissues. Hyperoxaemia may decrease ventilation, heart rate and cardiac output and may produce coronary, cerebral and retinal vasoconstriction but dilates the pulmonary vascular bed.

Metabolism

Oxygen is metabolized in all tissues to CO_2 which is excreted by the lungs.

Pharmaceutics

Oxygen is available either in compressed form in cylinders of varying purity, in liquid form, or can be produced on-site by oxygen concentrators. Cylinder oxygen is bulky, often inconvenient to supply and relatively expensive. Liquid oxygen is currently the form of choice for institutional supply. Portable liquid oxygen reservoirs are available for mobile patients. Oxygen concentrators use a compressor to deliver air to a molecular sieve which removes nitrogen from the air, and thus deliver 95–98% oxygen[6] at 2–3 l.min^{-1}. They are convenient, relatively cheap to run and are the form of choice for domiciliary supply to individuals.

Therapeutic use

Indications

1. Treatment of acute hypoxaemia
2. Long-term therapy of chronic hypoxaemia
3. Management of shock
4. Treatment of decreased available haemoglobin
5. To promote resorption of interstitial/intracavity gas
6. Management of local hypoperfusion
7. Treatment of sleep apnoea syndrome
8. Treatment of cluster headaches
9. To increase the radiosensitivity of tumours.

Contraindications

1. Acute carbon dioxide retention
2. Concurrent cigarette smoking
3. Oxygen-radical-induced lung injury.

Mode of use

Inspired oxygen tension can be increased by delivering oxygen by a face mask, nasal cannulae, mouthpiece, tracheal catheter or oxygen tents or by increasing atmospheric pressure.

Face masks deliver a range of inspired oxygen concentrations (21–80%) depending on the dead space of the mask and on the flow rate of oxygen addition. High-dead-space masks result in carbon dioxide rebreathing which, with the associated suppression of hypoxic drive by the high oxygen level, may result in CO_2 retention in patients with impaired ventilatory responses to chemostimuli. Patients with hypoxaemia plus carbon dioxide retention should receive low-concentration supplemental oxygen (24–35%) by specifically designed oxygen mask (e.g. Ventimask) or by nasal cannulae, and arterial blood gas tensions should be monitored. With this exception all other patients with acute hypoxaemia due to whatever cause should receive high-concentration oxygen (50–70%).

Nasal cannulae deliver 24–35% oxygen at low flow rates (1–4 l.min^{-1}) and are thus a cheap method of delivering low-concentration oxygen. They are well tolerated by patients and are the method of choice for domiciliary oxygen delivery. The amount of oxygen required, and thus the cost, can be further reduced by using either oxygen-conserving nasal cannulae[7–10] or intermittent flow devices which deliver oxygen only during inspiration.[9,11]

Indwelling percutaneous tracheal catheters may be used to improve oxygenation and to reduce the flow rate of oxygen required, and thus they will reduce the cost.[12] This system is currently under evaluation but seems to be acceptable to many patients and to be associated with few complications.[13]

The use of hyperbaric chambers to increase the amount of oxygen carried in solution in plasma is of limited value but may be useful in the early treatment of carbon monoxide poisoning.[14] Unfortunately hyperbaric oxygen often induces vasoconstriction, thereby reducing oxygen delivery despite its apparent theoretical advantage of a very high arterial PO_2.

Indications

1. Acute hypoxaemia

Oxygen is used in the routine treatment of arterial hypoxaemia of all causes. Frequent indications include pneumonia, acute severe asthma, acute exacerbations of chronic bronchitis and emphysema, pulmonary embolism, pulmonary oedema, adult and neonatal respiratory distress syndromes, and chest wall or neuromuscular diseases. In all the above, high-concentration oxygen should be administered initially unless CO_2 retention is suspected or documented. Thus in hypoxaemia secondary to chronic bronchitis and emphysema low-concentration O_2 is usually used initially.

2. Chronic hypoxaemia

Long-term oxygen therapy can improve survival in hypoxaemic patients with chronic bronchitis and emphysema.[15,16] Patients with arterial $PO_2 < 55–60$ mmHg and $PCO_2 > 45$ mmHg when in a stable clinical state should be assessed for long-term oxygen therapy. Domiciliary oxygen should be given for as much of the day as possible, certainly for more than 12 hours,[15,16] and all patients should receive oxygen at night to decrease nocturnal hypoxaemia.[17] The aim should be to increase arterial PO_2 to above 60 mmHg (8 kPa) without increasing arterial hydrogen ion (without decreasing pH). Oxygen concentrators are often the method of administration of choice, although in patients who work or are highly mobile, liquid oxygen systems have the advantage of portable reservoirs.

3. Shock

Shock is generally associated with decreased tissue oxygen delivery. High-concentration oxygen therapy is usually given, but in the absence of pulmonary abnormality, there is usually little increase in oxygen carriage as arterial haemoglobin is often fully saturated even when breathing air.

4. Decreased available haemoglobin

High concentrations of oxygen should be given as soon as possible following carbon monoxide poisoning. When hyperbaric facilities are readily available immediate compression to 2 to 2½ atmospheres oxygen may be beneficial.[14] Oxygen may also be used as an adjunct in the treatment of severe anaemia.

5. Interstitial/intracavity gas

Decreasing arterial oxygen tension by breathing high-concentration oxygen will speed reabsorption of gas which has escaped into the pleural cavity (pneumothorax) or into the mesentery (pneumatosis cystoides intestinalis). In practice the clinical significance of a pneumothorax is rarely altered by such treatment, and the indication for oxygen therapy is usually hypoxaemia. Pneumatosis cystoides intestinalis may improve with oxygen therapy[18] although the improvement may be short-lived.[19]

6. Local hypoperfusion

Oxygen may be of some value in the acute phase treatment of local ischaemia, such as myocardial infarction/ischaemia, cerebrovascular accident or peripheral vascular occlusion. The value of oxygen in such situations is debated.

7. Sleep apnoea syndrome

Oxygen has been used in the treatment of the sleep apnoea syndrome. Although oxygen may prolong some apnoeas it may decrease the total number of apnoeas and also decrease the amount of time spent apnoeic,[20] improve sleep quality[21] and raise the level of oxygenation during sleep with only a slight (<1 mmHg) rise in end apnoeic end tidal PCO_2.[21]

8. Cluster headaches

Oxygen therapy during the pain of cluster headaches may decrease the headache, according to both anecdotal reports and to a double-blind crossover study comparing compressed air with oxygen.[22]

9. Radiotherapy

There is some evidence that hyperbaric oxygen treatment may augment the effect of radiotherapy in some tumours. Oxygen at 3 atmospheres both increased the survival and improved local control of head and neck tumours and uterine cervical tumours but not lung or bladder tumours.[23]

Contraindications

1. Acute CO_2 retention

Oxygen treatment may raise arterial PCO_2, particularly in patients with impaired ventilatory responses to chemostimuli. In patients with chronic hypercapnia, low-concentration oxygen should be used, with adequate monitoring. Patients with acute CO_2 retention (increased CO_2 and increased hydrogen ion) should be given oxygen with caution and with facilities for ventilation available. The aim should be to achieve arterial PO_2 of 6–8 kPa (45–60 mmHg) depending on the patient's clinical state, without letting the hydrogen ion rise above 55 nmol.l^{-1} (pH above 7.25).[24]

2. Cigarette smoking

It is highly dangerous to smoke when receiving oxygen therapy. Serious burns and death due to burns have occurred. Further, in patients receiving long-term oxygen therapy, those who continue to smoke do not show improvement of some of the indices of hypoxic damage.[25]

3. Oxygen radical lung injury

Patients with damage to their lungs presumed due to oxygen radical effects as, for example, following paraquat ingestion, should be given as little supplemental oxygen as feasible as this may increase the availability of reactive oxygen species. This may also be the mechanism for relapse of bleomycin-induced lung disease produced by oxygen therapy.[26]

Adverse reactions

Potentially life-threatening effects

CO_2 retention. In patients with depressed respiratory drive oxygen therapy may result in CO_2 retention, leading to acidosis and ultimately death.

Pulmonary oxygen toxicity. Inspiring high-concentration (80–100%) oxygen at atmospheric pressure for over 12 hours may result in progressive damage to the lungs. Both alveolar lining cells and capillary endothelial cells become leaky with production of a protein-rich oedema fluid which may organize to form 'hyaline membranes'. There is often co-existing tracheobronchitis. These changes may be reversible if the concentration of oxygen can be reduced early, but otherwise they may progress and cause death, either acutely or later because of fibrosis. Pulmonary oxygen toxicity may result from production of oxygen-derived free radicals.[27]

Acute overdosage

Cerebral oxygen toxicity may occur with hyperbaric oxygen (see Symptomatic adverse effects).

Severe or irreversible adverse effects

High-concentration oxygen may result in decreased retinal blood flow and in preterm neonates this may cause retrolental fibroplasia. The high oxygen pressure halts the outward growth of the retinal vessels. Removal of the patient to air causes a disorderly proliferation of vessels at the growing front. There may be many other causes of retrolental fibroplasia, including hypoxaemia. Careful monitoring of oxygen therapy in neonates is mandatory.[28,29]

Symptomatic adverse effects

Breathing pure oxygen at pressures in excess of 2 atmospheres may induce mood changes, nausea, dizziness and convulsions. Full recovery is usual, although such fits can lead to death from drowning in scuba divers.

Interference with clinical pathology tests

No technical interferences of this kind are known.

Oxygen

High risk groups

Neonates

The lowest concentration of oxygen which maintains adequate oxygenation is usually advocated in neonates because of the risk of retrolental fibroplasia.

Breast milk. Oxygen may be given to women who are breast-feeding.

Children

No special precautions are required.

Pregnant women

No special precautions are required.

The elderly

No special precautions are required.

Drug interactions

Potentially hazardous interactions

Bleomycin. Oxygen therapy may cause relapse of bleomycin-induced lung disease.[25]

Alcohol. Alcohol may cause respiratory depression and this potentiates the ventilatory depression caused by oxygen.

Major outcome trials

1. Nocturnal Oxygen Therapy Trial Group 1980 Continuous or nocturnal oxygen in hypoxaemic chronic obstructive lung disease. Annals of Internal Medicine 93: 391–398

203 hypoxaemic patients ($PaO_2 < 55$ mmHg) with chronic obstructive lung disease were randomly allocated to receive oxygen therapy for 24 hours per day or 12 hours nocturnal oxygen per day and followed up for at least 12 months (mean 19.3 months). The two groups were well matched for baseline cardiorespiratory function. The patients receiving 12 hours nocturnal oxygen per day had 1.94 times the mortality of the patients receiving 24 hours oxygen per day ($p = 0.01$). The improvement in mortality with 24 hours per day oxygen was more striking in patients with carbon dioxide retention and with neuropsychiatric disturbance.

2. Medical Research Council Working Party 1981 Long term domiciliary oxygen therapy in chronic hypoxic cor pulmonale complicating chronic bronchitis and emphysema. Lancet 1: 681–686

87 hypoxic patients ($PaO_2 < 60$ mmHg) with chronic bronchitis and emphysema were randomly allocated to receive oxygen therapy for at least 15 hours per day or to a control group who received no supplemental oxygen. Follow-up was for five years. Overall mortality in the control patients receiving no supplemental oxygen (30/45) was significantly greater than that in the patients receiving oxygen for 15 hours per day (19/42).

General review articles

Flenley D C 1985 Long term home oxygen therapy. Chest 87: 99–103

Petty T L 1985 Who needs home oxygen? American Review of Respiratory Disease 131: 930–931

Lambertson C J 1978 Effect of hyperoxia on organs and their tissues. In: Robin E D (ed) Extrapulmonary manifestations of respiratory diseases. Marcel Dekker, New York, pp 239–303

Davies J C 1983 Hyperbaric oxygen therapy: a committee report. Undersea Medical Society Inc., Bethesda, Maryland

References

1. Severinghaus J W, Bradley A S 1958 Electrodes for blood PO_2 and PCO_2 determination. Journal of Applied Physiology 13: 515
2. Douglas N J, Brash H M, Wraith P K et al 1979 Accuracy, sensitivity to carboxyhaemoglobin and speed of response of the Hewlett Packard 47201A ear oximeter. American Review of Respiratory Disease 119: 311–313
3. Tweeddale P M, Douglas N J 1985 Evaluation of Biox IIa ear oximeter. Thorax 40: 825–827
4. Fishman A P 1976 Hypoxia and the pulmonary circulation: how and where it acts. Circulation Research 38: 221–231
5. Voelkel N F 1986 Mechanisms of hypoxic pulmonary vasoconstriction. American Review of Respiratory Disease 133: 1186–1195
6. Gould G A, Scott W, Hayhurst M D, Flenley D C 1985 Technical and clinical assessment of oxygen concentrators. Thorax 40: 811–816
7. Tiep B L, Nicotra B, Carter R, Belman M J, Mittman C 1984 Evaluation of a low-flow oxygen conserving nasal cannula. American Review of Respiratory Disease 130: 500–502
8. Moore-Gillon J C, George R J D, Geddes D M 1985 An oxygen conserving nasal cannula. Thorax 40: 817–819
9. Gould G A, Hayhurst M D, Scott W, Flenley D C 1985 Clinical assessment of oxygen conserving devices in chronic bronchitis and emphysema. Thorax 40: 820–824
10. Gonzales S C, Huntingdon D, Romo R, Light R W 1986 Efficiency of the oximiser pendant in reducing oxygen requirements of hypoxemic patients. Respiratory Care 31: 681–688
11. Tiep B L, Nicotra B, Carter R, Phillips R, Otsap B 1985 Low-concentration oxygen therapy via a demand oxygen delivery system. Chest 87: 636–638
12. Korcok M 1982 Delivering oxygen transtracheally may be a boon for COPD patients. Journal of the American Medical Association 248: 153–154
13. Christopher K L, Spofford B T, Brannin P K, Petty T L 1986 Transtracheal oxygen therapy for refractory hypoxemia. Journal of the American Medical Association 256: 494–497
14. Smith G, Ledingham I M, Sharp G R, Norman J N, Bates E H 1962 Treatment of coal-gas poisoning with oxygen at 2 atmospheres pressure. Lancet 1: 816–819
15. Nocturnal Oxygen Therapy Trial Group 1980 Continuous or nocturnal oxygen in hypoxaemic chronic obstructive lung disease. Annals of Internal Medicine 93: 391–398
16. Medical Research Council Working Party 1981 Long term domiciliary oxygen therapy in chronic hypoxic cor pulmonale complicating chronic bronchitis and emphysema. Lancet 1: 681–686
17. Douglas N J, Calverley P M A, Legget R J E, Brash H M, Flenley D C, Brezinova V 1979 Transient hypoxaemia during sleep in chronic bronchitis and emphysema. Lancet 1: 1–4
18. Holt S, Gilmore H M, Buist T A S, Marwick K, Heading R C 1979 High flow oxygen therapy for pneumatosis coli. Gut 20: 493–498
19. van Der Linden W 1974 Reappearance of intestinal gas cysts after oxygen treatment. Lancet 2: 1388–1389
20. Martin R J, Sanders M H, Gray B A, Pennock B E 1982 Acute and long-term ventilatory effect of hyperoxia in the adult sleep apnea syndrome. American Review of Respiratory Disease 125: 175–180
21. Smith P L, Haponik E F, Bleecker E R 1984 The effects of oxygen in patients with sleep apnea. American Review of Respiratory Disease 130: 958–963
22. Fogan L 1985 Treatment of cluster headache. Archives of Neurology 42: 362–363
23. Medical Research Council Working Party Report 1978 Radiotherapy and hyperbaric oxygen. Lancet 2: 881–884
24. Warren P M, Flenley D C, Millar J S, Avery A 1980 Respiratory failure revisited: acute exacerbations of chronic bronchitis between 1961–68 and 1970–76. Lancet 1: 467–471
25. Calverley P M A, Leggett R J E, McElderry L, Flenley D C 1982 Cigarette smoking and secondary polycythaemia in hypoxic cor pulmonale. American Review of Respiratory Disease 125: 507–510
26. Gilson A J, Sahn S A 1985 Reactivation of bleomycin lung toxicity following oxygen administration. Chest 88: 304–306
27. Fisher A B, Forman H J, Glass M 1984 Mechanisms of pulmonary oxygen toxicity. Lung 162: 255–259
28. Lucey J F, Dangman B 1984 Re-examination of the role of oxygen in retrolental fibroplasia. Pediatrics 73: 82–96
29. Phelps D L, Rosenbaum A L 1984 Effects of marginal hypoxemia on recovery from oxygen induced retinopathy in the kitten model. Pediatrics 73: 1–6

O Oxymetazoline hydrochloride

Oxymetazoline is a nasal decongestant.

Chemistry

Oxymetazoline hydrochloride (Afrazine, Iliadin, Neo-Synephrine)
$C_{16}H_{24}N_2O.HCl$
2-(4-tert-Butyl-2,6-dimethyl-3-hydroxybenzyl)-2-imidazoline hydrochloride

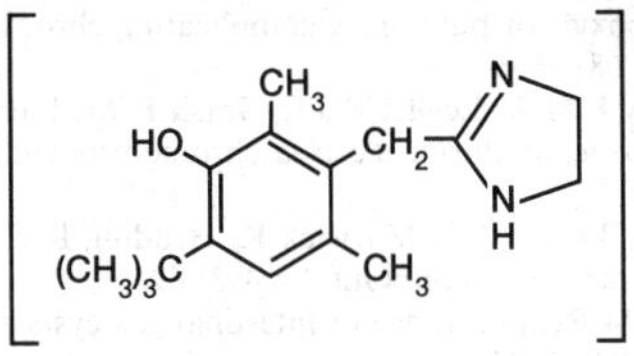

Molecular weight (free base)	296.8 (258.4)
pKa	not relevant
Solubility	
in alcohol	1 in 3.6
in water	1 in 6.7
Octanol/water partition coefficient	—

Oxymetazoline is a white or almost white, odourless, hygroscopic crystalline powder with a bitter taste.

It was also formerly available in combination with camphor and menthol as Afrazine menthol spray. This product is no longer available in the UK.

Pharmacology

Oxymetazoline is a sympathomimetic amine of the imidazoline class.[1,2] It is a direct agonist at α-adrenoceptors but has no actions on β-adrenoceptors. It is without activity on catecholamine uptake mechanisms. Unlike phenylephrine, oxymetazoline does not cause mydriasis. Given systemically, oxymetazoline has actions on the central nervous system, including sedation, dry mouth and sweating, but these are rarely seen in practice since the drug is only used as a topical agent.

Toxicology

Little is known of the toxicology of oxymetazoline. The manufacturers report no significant organ damage or general toxicity in dog, cat, rabbit or mouse at dosages close to those used in man. Nor have the manufacturers identified any teratogenic effect in rats. When administered subcutaneously in rabbits, no drug-related abnormalities or effects on the offspring were found.

In a retrospective study in man no association was found between the drug and congenital disorders.

No carcinogenicity tests have been reported.[3]

Clinical pharmacology

Oxymetazoline is used for its vasoconstrictor properties, acting on α-adrenoceptors. It produces a potent long-lasting vasoconstriction.[4] It is used as a topical agent on the nasal mucosa, when it causes vasoconstriction of the arterioles thus reducing blood flow and diminishing swelling of the mucosa. This results in improved patency of the airway and better drainage of the nasal sinuses.[5] If the eustachian tube is blocked by swelling at its nasal orifice, the use of oxymetazoline may restore patency and permit drainage from the ear.[6] Prolonged use of oxymetazoline may lead to rebound vasodilation (drug-induced rhinitis). This may be due to an inhibition of the release of noradrenaline at vasomotor adrenergic nerve endings. Given topically, oxymetazoline has no systemic effects.

Pharmacokinetics

Little information is available at present concerning the distribution, metabolism and excretion of oxymetazoline in man.

Local vasoconstriction is normally achieved within 5–10 min of intranasal administration. The full effect lasts for 5–6 h and subsides gradually over the course of the next 6 h.

Oxymetazoline enters tissues rapidly and is released slowly. (No data are available for brain.) The plasma half life is 5–8 days. 30% of any absorbed drug is eliminated in the urine in 72 h post-dose, mainly as unchanged drug, and approximately 10% in the faeces.

Oral absorption	—
Presystemic metabolism	—
Plasma half life	
range	5–8 d
Volume of distribution	—
Plasma protein binding	—

Concentration–effect relationship

Since oxymetazoline is only used topically, no correlation between the plasma concentration of the drug and its clinical effect would be expected and there are no data on the subject.

Metabolism

Little is known about the metabolism of oxymetazoline. 30% of absorbed drug is excreted unchanged in urine, and 10% in faeces.

Pharmaceutics

Oxymetazoline is available as nasal drops or spray.

1. Afrazine (Schering-Plough, UK) is available as nasal drops containing 0.05% oxymetazoline hydrochloride. The paediatric drops contain 0.025%. It is also formulated as a spray (0.05%).
2. Neo-Synephrine 12 hour (Winthrop Consumer, USA) is available in two nose-drop formulations and two squeeze bottle nasal spray preparations for over-the-counter sale: Nasal spray 0.05%, Vapor Nasal Spray 0.05%, adult strength nose drops 0.05% and children's strength nose drops 0.025%. All contain benzalkonium as one preservative, the other being phenylmercuric nitrate except in the case of the vapour nasal spray which contains thiomersol.

The maximum shelf-life for each formulation is 5 years.

For ocular use oxymetazoline is only available in sterile solution in combination with antazoline.

Therapeutic use

Indications

1. As a nasal decongestant in allergic rhinitis, with or without the addition of antazoline or sodium cromoglycate[7]
2. As a nasal decongestant in sinusitis where there is evidence of obstruction of the ostia to the sinuses
3. As a nasal decongestant in otitis media where there is evidence of obstruction of the eustachian tube, especially in subacute serous otitis media ('glue ear') and otitic barotrauma
4. As a decongestant in an infective rhinitis (e.g. an acute viral upper respiratory tract infection). Where there is a secondary bacterial infection there is no evidence of benefit
5. As an ocular decongestant in allergic conjunctivitis, whether seasonal ('hay fever') or perennial
6. To 'whiten' an inflamed ('red') eye caused by a local irritant such as dust, or following the removal of a foreign body.

Contraindications

1. As a sympathomimetic, oxymetazoline should not be used in patients being simultaneously treated with monoamine oxidase inhibitor therapy

Oxymetazoline hydrochloride

2. Narrow-angle glaucoma
3. The safety of use in pregnancy has not fully been established and administration of oxymetazoline during that time should be avoided unless absolutely essential.

Precautions
The drug should be used with caution in patients suffering from:

1. Coronary artery disease
2. Hypertension
3. Hyperthyroidism
4. Diabetes mellitus.

Mode of use

For nasal use, 2–3 drops should be instilled into each nostril twice daily. In adults a 0.05% solution (approximately 1.5 $\mu g.kg^{-1}$) should be used. The drops should be instilled into the nose, one nostril at a time, in the head-low position to reduce the risk of the patient swallowing any of the solution.

In adults a nasal spray may be used as an alternative to instilling the solution from a dropper bottle. The spray can be used with the patient in the upright position. Sprays are generally unsuitable for young children because of the small size of their nostrils. (Oxymetazoline spray is not available in the paediatric strength.)

Both in children and adults a treatment course should not normally exceed three to five days, and on no account should it be continued for longer than two weeks because of the risk of developing 'rhinitis medicamentosa'.

Before oxymetazoline drops are used in the eye it is essential to exclude any ocular pathology (e.g. an infection or glaucoma) which may indicate the need for treatment. The presence of narrow-angle glaucoma is an absolute contraindication.

Adverse reactions

Potentially life-threatening effects
None is known.

Acute overdosage
Used correctly (i.e. as an intranasal application) the local vasoconstriction produced by the drug inhibits absorption and a systemic action is unlikely. If, however, some of the drops are swallowed they can be absorbed from the gastrointestinal tract and a systemic effect can be produced.[8] In children an overdose, if swallowed and absorbed, has been reported to cause sedation. As oxymetazoline is an α_2-adrenergic agonist it might be expected to produce effects similar to those of clonidine, with a short-lived rise in pressure caused by a peripheral action, followed by more prolonged hypotension and sedation as a result of inhibition of the sympathetic outflow from the brain.

Severe or irreversible adverse effects
Overuse is associated with a more persistent rhinitis related to the rebound phenomenon — the condition known as 'rhinitis medicamentosa' (often spoken of as 'nose-drop nose' or 'Fenox-nose', so called after one of the more popular nasal decongestants).[9] It is claimed by the manufacturer of oxymetazoline that, because of its more prolonged action, it is less likely to cause rebound congestion than other decongestants.

Symptomatic adverse effects
Stinging, discomfort or a dryness locally in the nose or eye are encountered infrequently.[10] If the symptoms persist, the discomfort from the use of the drops probably outweighs any advantage they may confer.

Headache has been reported, albeit infrequently, as has tachycardia.

High risk groups

Neonates
As mentioned above, sprays are unsuitable for young children.

Breast milk. No information is available.

Children
The drug may be used in older children.

Pregnant women
As the safety of the drug has not been established, it should be avoided by pregnant women.

The elderly
No special precautions are necessary.

References

1. Hotovy R, Enenken H J, Gillissen J 1961 Zus Pharmakologie des 2(4'-test. Butyl-2',6'-dimethyl-3'-hydroxybenzyl)2-imidazolinium chlorids. Arzneimittel-Forschung 2: 1016–1022
2. Proctor D F, Adams G K 1976 Physiology of nasal function and mucus secretion. Pharmacology and Therapeutics 2: 493–509
3. Jick J, Lewis J, Hunter J R, Madsen S, Stegaduis A 1981 First trimester drug uses and congenital disorders. Journal of the American Medical Association 246: 343–346
4. 1969 Annals of Allergy 27: 541–546
5. Kameswaran S 1970 Clinical evaluation of a nasal decongestant. Indian Practitioner 23: 453–459
6. Cohen B M 1969 Relief of nasal flow obstruction. Journal of Asthma Research 7: 65–73
7. Bailey A 1969 Clinical evaluation of a topical nasal decongestant, oxymetazoline. Eye, Ear, Nose and Throat Monthly 48: 46–48
8. Soderman P, Sahlberg D, Wiholm B-D 1984 (Letter) Lancet 1: 573
9. Black M J, Remsen K A 1980 Rhinitis medicamentosa. Canadian Medical Association Journal 122: 881
10. Leitch G B 1976 A trial of Iliadin in non-specific allergic rhinitis. British Journal of Clinical Practice 30: 41–42

O

Oxytetracycline (dihydrate)

This antibiotic was introduced in 1950 two years after chlortetracycline, the first tetracycline, was discovered. It has a wide range of antibacterial activity and thus possible indications for use are numerous.

Chemistry[1–3]

Oxytetracycline dihydrate (oxytetracycline, Terramycin, Abboin Berkmycen, Imperacin, Oxymycin)
$C_{22}H_{24}N_2O_9.2H_2O$
Also available as the calcium and hydrochloride salts.
4-(Dimethylamino)-1,4,4a,5,5a,6,11,12a-octahydro-3,5,6,10,12,12a-hexahydroxy-6-methyl-1,11-dioxo-2-naphthacene carboxamide

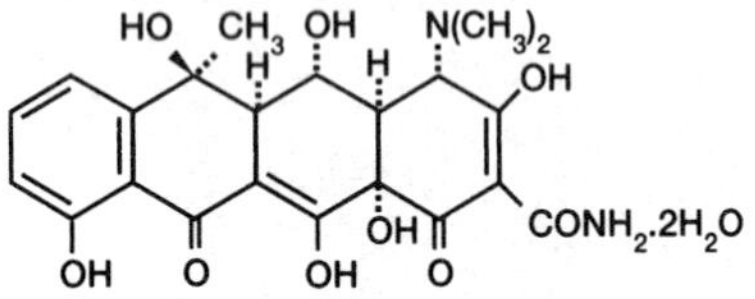

Molecular weight (anhydrous)	496.5 (464.5)
pKa	3.3, 7.3, 9.1
Solubility	
in alcohol	~1 in 80
in water	<1 in 4000
Octanol/water partition coefficient	0.025

A yellow to tan coloured, odourless, crystalline powder with a slightly bitter taste.[4] It is produced from the growth of certain strains of *Streptomyces rimosis*.

It is available in combination with hydrocortisone[2]
Terra-Cortril Ear suspension
Terra-Cortril Spray
Terra-Cortril Topical ointment
Terra-Cortril Nystatin cream
Terra-Cortril Ophthalmic ointment with Polyxin B Sulphate
Terra-Bron Syrup
Bisolvomycin (in combination with bromhexine hydrochloride)
Irimovate (with clobetasone butyrate and nystatin)

Pharmacology

Oxytetracycline is a naturally occurring tetracycline elaborated by *Streptomyces rimosis*. Like other tetracyclines it has a wide spectrum of activity. In addition to its antibiotic activity it is also a chelating agent and will chelate Ca^{2+}, Mg^{2+} or Al^{3+} ions in the gut. Oxytetracycline has its main mechanism of action on protein synthesis. An energy-dependent active transport system pumps the drug, like all tetracyclines, through the inner cytoplasmic membrane. Once inside the bacterial cell, oxytetracycline inhibits protein synthesis by binding specifically to the 30S ribosomes. The drug appears to prevent access of aminoacyl tRNA to the acceptor site on the mRNA–ribosome complex.[5] This prevents the addition of amino acids to the growing peptide chain. Oxytetracycline will impair protein synthesis in mammalian cells if used at very high concentrations. However, these cells lack the active transport system found in bacteria. There is also some evidence that tetracyclines may cause alterations in the cytoplasmic membrane thus allowing leakage of nucleotides from the cell.[6] This would explain the rapid inhibition of DNA replication that ensues when cells are exposed to concentrations of tetracycline in excess of that required for inhibition of protein synthesis.

Toxicology

There is no evidence of carcinogenicity or mutagenicity on tests lasting up to 8 weeks in dogs and rats.[7] Toxicological testing in animals failed to demonstrate any results of potential clinical relevance. Teratological effects have been shown to occur in chicks and rats.[8] The tetracyclines cross the placenta and cause fetal damage characterized by retardation of skeletal development in these animals. However, the frequency of congenital abnormalities in children of mothers who have received tetracycline is no higher than in children of mothers who received penicillin during pregnancy.[9]

Clinical pharmacology

Oxytetracycline is primarily a bacteriostatic antibiotic and has a similar spectrum of activity to other tetracyclines.[10–17]

Oxytetracycline is active against most strains of *Haemophilus influenzae* and is particularly useful for infections with *H. ducreyi*, *Actinomyces*, *Brucella* and *Vibrio cholerae*. Oxytetracycline is also active against *Nocardia*, *Chlamydia*, *Mycoplasma*, and a wide range of *Rickettsiae*. Oxytetracycline is active against spirochaetes such as *Borrelia recurrentis*, *Treponema pallidum* and *T. pertenue*.

Oxytetracycline was initially useful for the treatment of Gram-positive infections but many strains are now resistant to the drug. The overall resistance in the UK of the pneumococcus is about 13%. Oxytetracycline possesses some activity against *Staphylococcus aureus*, particularly for community acquired infections, but in hospitals the prevalence of resistance to staphylococci is high. Many Gram-negative organisms have acquired resistance to oxytetracycline and for *E. coli* more than 50% of strains may be resistant. Oxytetracycline is usually effective against *Haemophilus influenzae*. A recent nationwide survey found that 2.7% of *H. influenzae* were resistant to tetracycline although there were geographical variations.[19] Occasional reports of *Neisseria gonorrhoea* resistant to tetracycline have been described.[18,19] Oxytetracycline has no activity against *Pseudomonas aeruginosa* while most strains of *Campylobacter* are sensitive. Oxytetracycline is also active against anaerobic species of bacteria and, since concentrations of the drug are quite high in the gastrointestinal contents, the enteric flora are usually altered by the drug.

Resistance to tetracyclines develops slowly and organisms that show resistance to one tetracycline frequently show resistance to others in the group (with some exceptions for minocycline and doxycycline). Most resistance is mediated by a plasmid and is an inducible trait, appearing only after exposure of the bacteria to the drug. Resistance seems to occur because the plasmid implants genetic material in the cell for a number of proteins and this affects penetration of the cell wall by the tetracycline.[16]

Pharmacokinetics

The preferred analytical method is by spectrofluorometry involving the use of protein precipitation, solvent extraction, and alkaline degradation. It can measure oxytetracycline to better than 0.1 mg.l^{-1} of blood or plasma.[20]

Oxytetracycline is absorbed irregularly to the extent of about 60% after an oral dose, absorption mostly occurring in the stomach and upper small intestine. Peak plasma concentrations are achieved 2 to 4 hours after an oral dose.[15] After an oral dose of 500 mg oxytetracycline, serum levels are detectable after 30 minutes, and peak levels of approximately 4 μg.ml^{-1} are reached. A dose of 250 mg reaches a peak level of approximately 2 μg.ml^{-1}. The hydrochloride is reasonably soluble in water giving a highly acid solution, but in neutral or alkaline medium it tends to precipitate or not to dissolve. The calcium salt is almost insoluble in water, but it will dissolve in dilute alkali. Tetracyclines combine with divalent metals, antacids and milk products. The chelated compounds are not absorbed and pass out into the faeces. The presence of food also reduces absorption (by almost 50%) as does ferrous sulphate. Thus oxytetracycline should be given when the patient is fasting.[22] The mean plasma half life is 9.2 h.[15] Oxytetracycline is widely distributed in the body and penetrates human organs well including free secretion into the bile, with tissue/serum concentration ratios of about 1. The brain and adipose tissue, however, are relatively impermeable to tetracyclines.[2,3]

Penetration into CSF is low, giving about one-tenth of the serum concentration, whereas the concentration in breast milk is about one-half the plasma value.[2] Tetracyclines also deposits in bone (when it is being laid down) and teeth (see Adverse reactions).

Oxytetracycline is not highly protein bound (range 27–35%).[23]

Oral absorption	60%
Presystemic metabolism	negligible
Plasma half life	
mean	9.2 h
Volume of distribution	406.6 $l.kg^{-1}$
Plasma protein binding	27–35%

The drug is eliminated largely unchanged, mostly in the urine, with some in the faeces. A small amount of the drug is metabolized in the liver. As a consequence of the renal elimination of the drug, some modification of the dose may be necessary in patients with severe kidney disease, or in the elderly with reduced renal function.

Concentration–effect relationship

The therapeutic range will depend upon the minimum inhibitory concentration (MIC) of the antibiotic for the organism in question. Full susceptibility occurs when the MIC is less than 4.0 $mg.l^{-1}$ and intermediate susceptibility is said to occur when the MIC is between 4.0 and 12.5 $mg.l^{-1}$. Concentrations greater than 25 $mg.l^{-1}$ are usually required to inhibit most strains of group B and group D streptococci and strains of *Staphylococcus aureus*. The MIC for *Streptococcus pyogenes* is usually about 1.0 $mg.l^{-1}$ and for the pneumococcus it is often between 0.4 and 0.8 $mg.l^{-1}$.

Metabolism

Oxytetracycline is excreted mainly in its active form in the urine (10–35%).[24] Some is concentrated in the bile, excreted into the faeces and partially reabsorbed. Oxytetracycline is incompletely absorbed from the gastrointestinal tract, and the unabsorbed percentage increases with increasing dosage. Only relatively small amounts are metabolized to bacteriologically inactive derivatives in the liver.[2,14,20]

Pharmaceutics

Oxytetracycline is available in an oral form. Intravenous preparations are not available. Rolitetracycline should be used.

The oral forms include:

1. Terramycin (Pfizer, UK, US) yellow opaque hard gelatin capsules containing 250 mg oxytetracycline as the hydrochloride. It is printed with 'Pfizer TER250' in black ink (UK) or 'Terramycin' (cap) and 'PFIZER OT3' (base) for US formulation.
2. Terramycin (Pfizer, UK) sugar-coated light yellow tablet containing 250 mg oxytetracycline dihydrate. It is round, concave, 0.45–0.462 inches in diameter, 0.245–0.255 inches thick and bears the Pfizer logo on one side. The shelf-life of the capsules is 36 months and that of the tablets is 60 months (when stored below 25°C and protected from light).

Both products contain a potentially allergenic substance.

Other brand names each containing 250 mg oxytetracycline dihydrate include:

Berkmycen: yellow film-coated tablet engraved 'BERK 1C5' on one side (Berk, UK). The capsule form is coloured red and yellow.

Imperacin: yellow biconcave film-coated tablet marked with 'IMPERACIN' on one side (ICI, UK).

The BP requires a 70% dissolution within 45 minutes. Oxytetracycline should be stored in closed containers, protected from light, at temperatures below 30°C.

A 50 $mg.ml^{-1}$ intramuscular injection is available from Roerig, US. Marketed under the Pfizer trade name Tellamycin, it contains 2% lignocaine.

Therapeutic use

Indications

1. Respiratory infection
2. *Mycoplasma* pneumonia
3. Brucellosis
4. Cholera
5. Rickettsial infections
6. Q fever
7. Relapsing fever, tularaemia and bubonic plague
8. Gonorrhoea
9. Chlamydial infection
   a. Psittacosis
   b. Lymphogranuloma venereum
   c. Trachoma
   d. Non-specific urethritis
10. Chancroid and granuloma inguinale
11. Syphilis
12. Lyme disease
13. Actinomycosis, gas gangrene and anthrax
14. Meliodosis
15. Acne and rosacea
16. Amoebic dysentery
17. *Mycobacterium balnei (marinum)*
18. Whipple's disease
19. Malaria
20. Staphylococcal infections
21. Biliary tract infections
22. Urinary tract infections.

Contraindications

1. Hypersensitivity to tetracyclines
2. Women who are or may become pregnant
3. Patients less than 8 years of age
4. Patients who have systemic lupus erythematosus.

Mode of use

The causative organism should be isolated for oxytetracycline susceptibility testing. Patients should avoid direct sunlight if possible during treatment as a photosensitivity reaction may occur.[24]

Oxytetracycline should be administered in four equal doses and therapy should be continued for at least 24–48 hours after fever and symptoms have subsided. For mild illness 250 mg oxytetracycline 6 hourly may be sufficient, but for a more severe illness 1.5–2 g daily is required.

The drug should be taken on an empty stomach (1 hour before or 2 hours after a meal).

Indications

1. Respiratory infection

Tetracyclines are frequently used for pneumonia, bronchitis and especially for acute exacerbation of chronic bronchitis. Chemoprophylaxis should be considered in patients with chronic bronchitis with recurrent exacerbation. Patients can also be advised to begin antibiotics themselves where they develop signs of infection. Tetracyclines can be used in rotation with other drugs such as ampicillin, erythromycin, or cotrimoxazole. Patients with pneumonia or bronchitis do not always respond to tetracycline therapy because resistant strains of pneumococci (up to 40% in some areas), staphylococci, streptococci and *H. influenzae* occur.[17]

2. Mycoplasma pneumonia

Oxytetracycline is effective in the treatment of this disease.[25]

3. Brucellosis

Combination of a tetracycline and streptomycin is regarded as the best treatment for this disease administered for a 2–3 week period. Tetracyclines alone are effective but less satisfactory in severe or prolonged cases.[14]

4. Cholera

Correcting dehydration is the most important measure. Oral tetracycline therapy is effective in eradicating vibrios from stools, and in diminishing volume of diarrhoea.[26] It may also be useful for prophylactic purposes during an epidemic.[27] Unfortunately, tetracycline resistance is developing and thus the antibiotic will not be effective in these cases.

5. Rickettsial infections

Tetracyclines are drugs of choice for the treatment of epidemic typhus, murine typhus, scrub typhus, rickettsial pox and Rocky

Mountain spotted fever. Chloramphenicol is an alternative treatment for children under 8 years of age with Rocky Mountain spotted fever.[16]

6. Q fever
Tetracyclines are the best form of treatment for chronic Q fever (usually a self-limited febrile illness).

7. Relapsing fever, tularaemia and bubonic plague
A single dose of 0.5 g tetracycline is considered to be the optimum treatment of relapsing fever. A two week course is regarded as the treatment of choice for tularaemia. Tetracyclines are also effective in plague, but streptomycin is usually preferred.

8. Gonorrhoea
Usually 1.5 g followed by 0.5 g four times daily for a total of 9 g of tetracycline is recommended, for patients in whom penicillin is contraindicated, after susceptibility testing.[14]

9. Chlamydial infection
Psittacosis. A daily dose of 1 g tetracycline for 21 days has been advocated for treatment and prevention of relapse.[28]

Lymphogranuloma venereum (serotype of C. trachomatis). Treatment is usually required for 2 weeks.[28]

Trachoma (various serotypes of C. trachomatis). Hyperendemic trachoma responds to topical treatment with tetracycline eye ointment for 5–6 weeks. It also responds to oral tetracycline 0.75 g twice daily for 3 weeks.

Paratrachoma is transmitted sexually and includes TRIC ophthalmia neonatorium in the newborn. Topical tetracycline eye ointment should be used for 3 to 5 weeks, with 250 mg four times daily of oxytetracycline for 3 weeks (in neonates or pregnancy erythromycin should be used).[29]

Non-specific urethritis. 500 mg four times daily oxytetracycline for 2 weeks, or 250 mg four times daily for 3 weeks is recommended for the treatment of chlamydial infections. Sexual partners of patients with non-specific urethritis should also be treated.[29] Ureaplasma can also cause this disease, and infection with this organism usually responds to tetracycline although some strains may be resistant.

10. Chancroid and granuloma inguinale
Tetracyclines given for 2 weeks are effective in these diseases.[30] Some strains may be resistant and treatment with sulphonamides may be required.

11. Syphilis
Oxytetracycline is an alternative to penicillin. A total of 30–40 g should be given over a period of two weeks, in equally divided doses.[14]

12. Lyme disease
Tetracyclines are effective therapy for Lyme disease in patients without involvement of the central nervous system.

13. Actinomycosis, gas gangrene, and anthrax
Can be used as an alternative to penicillin in these diseases.

14. Meliodosis
Tetracycline alone, or as combination with chloramphenicol or cotrimoxazole, is effective.

15. Acne and rosacea
A twice daily dosage of 250 mg oxytetracycline reduced to a daily dose of 250 mg after 2–4 months is usually beneficial for patients with acne. Treatment may be continued for months or even years. It results in the reduction of free fatty acid concentrations in the sebum, probably by inhibiting *Cornynebacterium acnes.*[33]

16. Amoebic dysentery
Tetracyclines only have a minor place in the treatment of this infection. Oxytetracycline appears to be beneficial by interfering with the bowel flora necessary for the nutrition of these parasites. They are of no value for the treatment of systemic infection or hepatitis.

17. *Mycobacterium balnei (marinum)*
Tetracyclines have been used to treat infections caused by this organism.[31]

18. Whipple's disease
This may respond to tetracycline therapy.[31]

19. Malaria
Chloroquine resistant falciparum malaria responds slowly to tetracycline therapy alone, and is usually used in conjunction with quinine sulphate for a duration of 10 days.[34]

20. Staphylococcal infections
Minor infection may be treated by oxytetracycline if sensitivity testing indicates that the organism is susceptible.

21. Biliary tract infections
Oxytetracycline can be used if organism is susceptible.

22. Urinary tract infection
Now rarely used, and again only if organism is susceptible.

Contraindications

1. Hypersensitivity to tetracyclines
These effects are uncommon, and usually take the form of urticaria, asthma or faecal oedema.

2. Women who are or may become pregnant[35]
Oxytetracycline can cross the placenta and damage the fetus by diminishing skeletal growth.

3. Patients less than 8 years of age[35]
The tetracyclines have been found to cause permanent tooth discoloration, enamel hypoplasia and depressed bone growth in children under 8 years of age.

4. Systemic lupus erythematosus
There are some grounds for believing that tetracyclines may exacerbate this condition.[36]

Adverse reactions

Potentially life-threatening effects
These are very rare. Staphylococcal enterocolitis with severe fulminating diarrhoea has occurred, usually as a postoperative complication associated with parenteral or oral therapy. Treatment consists of stopping the tetracycline, using an antistaphylococcal agent such as cloxacillin and fluid replacement.

Acute overdosage
The case of a 4-year-old child who consumed an undetermined amount of oral oxytetracycline has been reported. The child vomited and went into coma.[7] General supportive treatment including monitoring of renal and liver function is indicated.

Severe or irreversible adverse effects
Nephrotoxicity. Aggravation of pre-existing renal failure may occur, probably due to the antianabolic effect of the tetracyclines, although the exact mechanism is difficult to determine.[37]

Renal failure may also occur in association with acute fatty liver, but usually only when high doses of intravenous tetracycline are used. It is an unusual form of renal failure characterized by the absence of oliguria.[38]

To prevent accumulation of oxytetracycline lower doses should be used. The need for prolonged therapy in patients with renal impairment is an indication for serum level monitoring.

Hepatotoxicity. Overdosage is particularly dangerous during pregnancy.[39] In fatal cases there is fatty infiltration in the liver and pathological changes in the pancreas, kidney and brain. It is probable that administration of tetracycline may be one of the aetological factors in acute fatty liver of pregnancy.

A similar picture has been seen in non-pregnant patients, when excessive doses of tetracycline are used, or when levels have been high due to renal impairment.

Symptomatic adverse effects
Gut. Gastrointestinal adverse effects are quite common, with diarrhoea in 12.5% of patients, and nausea and vomiting in 8%. Anorexia, dysphagia and enterocolitis occur less commonly (less than 0.1%).

Rare instances of oesophagitis and oesophageal ulceration have been described in patients taking oral tetracyclines, mostly occurring when taken just before going to bed. It is recommended that capsules should be taken with an adequate quantity of water not less than 1 hour before retiring. Oxytetracycline should not be given to patients with oesophageal obstruction.[40]

Skin. Dermatological effects include photosensitivity reactions and maculopapular and erythematous rashes, in less than 1% of patients. Exfoliative dermatitis occurs rarely (less than 0.1% of patients).[33]

Anaphylaxis, urticaria, angioedema, anaphylactoid purpura, pericarditis and exacerbation of systemic lupus erythematosus have been described.

Blood. Mild leucopenia can occur with tetracycline therapy, but is rare. Vascular purpura, sometimes associated with thrombocytopenia, has rarely occurred. This may be due to a lowered leucocyte ascorbic acid level.

Miscellaneous. Benign intracranial hypertension[41] in adults and bulging fontanelles in infants have been reported in patients receiving full therapeutic doses. Both were rapidly reversed on discontinuation of the drug.

Other effects

Tetracyclines have been reported to exert an antianaerobic action which may lead to an increased blood urea concentration (BUN).[42] They may also decrease plasma prothrombin activity due to inhibition of gut organisms that normally provide vitamin K.

Interference with clinical pathology tests

Oxytetracycline may produce an interfering fluorescence in the Hingerty method for measuring urinary catecholamines.[43] Oral antibiotics may reduce bacterial convertors of bilirubin to urobilinogen in the gut. This may affect urinary urobilinogen excretion test levels.[44]

High risk groups

Neonates

The drug is contraindicated in neonates because of tooth staining.

Breast milk. Breast-feeding is contraindicated as antibiotics pass to the child in the milk.

Children

What has been said about neonates also applies to older children.

Pregnant women

The drug is contraindicated because of tooth staining in the fetus and possible growth retardation effects (see above).

The elderly

Care only needs to be taken in older patients when there is severe renal or hepatic dysfunction.

Drug interactions

Potentially hazardous interactions

Tetracyclines may enhance methoxyflurane-induced nephrotoxicity. Sodium bicarbonate may inhibit dissolution of the antibiotic in the gastrointestinal tract by increasing the pH.[45,46]

Oxytetracycline may decrease the plasma prothrombin activity due to inhibition of vitamin K-producing flora in the gut.

Antacids containing divalent or trivalent cations chelate to tetracycline, impairing oral absorption. These cations are contained in foods, particularly dairy products. Some iron preparations have the same effect.[22]

The bacteriostatic action of the tetracyclines may interfere with the bactericidal effect of penicillin.[47]

Tetracyclines do not interact with alcohol or with cigarette smoking.

Potentially useful interactions

There are no therapeutically useful interactions.

General review articles

Kucers A, Bennet N Mck 1979 Tetracyclines. In: The use of antibiotics. Heinemann, London, pp 592–645

Garrod L P, Lambert H P, O'Grady F 1981 Tetracyclines. In: Antibiotics and chemotherapy. Churchill Livingstone, Edinburgh, ch 7, pp 169–182

References

1. Merck Index 1976 9th edn. Merck & Co Inc, Rahway, NJ, USA, p 6791
2. Bioavailability monograph on oxytetracycline 1975 American Pharmaceutical Association
3. Green R, Brown J R, Calvert R T 1976 The disposition of four tetracyclines in normal subjects. European Journal of Clinical Pharmacology 10: 245–250
4. Reynolds J E F (ed) 1982 Martindale: the extra pharmacopoeia, 28th edn. The Pharmaceutical Press, London, pp 1181–1191
5. Gilman A G, Goodman L S, Gilman A (eds) 1980 The pharmacological basis of therapeutics, 6th edn. Macmillan, New York, pp 1510–1514
6. Pato M L 1977 Tetracycline inhibits propagation of deoxyribonucleic acid replication and alters membrane properties. Antimicrobial Agents and Chemotherapy 11: 318–323
7. Data on file, Pfizer Inc
8. Anon 1965 Tetracyclines in pregnancy. British Medical Journal 1: 743–744
9. Carter M P, Wilson F 1963 Antibiotics and congenital malformation. Lancet 1: 1267
10. Hobby G L 1950 Antimicrobial action of Terramycin in vitro and in vivo. Proceedings of the Society of Experimental Medicine 73: 503–511
11. Kneeland Y et al 1950 Experimental and clinical studies of Terramycin. Transactions of the Association of American Physicians 63: 126–129
12. Bliss E A et al 1950 The experimental background for the clinical use of Terracyine. Bulletin Johns Hopkins Hospital 86: 419–420
13. Yow E M 1951 Laboratory and clinical studies on Terramycin. American Practitioner 2: 689–693
14. Terramycin Data Sheet
15. Milek J F, Kalfopoulos P, Merier G 1971 The kinetics of tetracyclines in man. 1. Digestive absorption and serum concentration. Schweizerischer Medizinische Wochenschrift, Journal Suisse de Medecine 101: 593–598
16. Chopra I, Howe T G B, Linton A H, Richmond M H, Speller D C E 1981 The tetracyclines: prospects at the beginning of the 80s. Journal of Antimicrobial Chemotherapy 8: 5–21
17. Pines A 1982 The tetracyclines in purulent exacerbation of chronic bronchitis. Journal of Antimicrobial Chemotherapy 9: 333–341
18. Ison C A, Terry P, Bindayna K, Gill M J, Adams J, Woodford N 1988 Tetracycline resistant gonococci in UK. Lancet 1: 651–652
19. Powell M, Koutsia-Carouzou C, Voutsinas D, Seymour A, William J D 1987 Resistance of clinical isolates of *Haemophilus influenzae* in United Kingdom 1986. British Medical Journal 295: 176–179
20. Scales B, Assider D 1973 Fluorometric estimation of oxytetracycline in blood and plasma. Journal of Pharmaceutical Science 63: 913–917
21. Jonas M, Comer J B, Cunha B A 1984 Tetracyclines. In: Ristucca A M, Cunha B A (eds) Antimicrobial therapy. Raven Press, New York, pp 219–234
22. Neuvonen P J 1976 Interactions with the absorption of tetracycline. Drugs 11: 45–48
23. Fabre J, Milek E, Kalfopoulas P, Merier G 1971 The kinetics of tetracyclines in man. II. Excretion, penetration in normal inflammatory tissues, behaviour in renal insufficiency and hemodialysis. Schweizerischer Medizinische Wochenschrift, Journal Suisse de Medecine 101: 625–633
24. Siegel D 1978 Tetracyclines. New look at old antibiotics. II. Clinical uses. New York State Journal of Medicine 78: 1115–1120
25. Foy H M, Kenny G E, McMahan R, Manhy A M, Grayson J T 1970 *Mycoplasma pneumoniae* in urban area. Journal of the American Medical Association 214: 1666
26. Leading article 1966 Antibiotics in cholera. Lancet 1: 801
27. McCormack W M, Chowdury A M, Jahangir N, Fariduddin Ahmed A B, Morby W H 1968 Tetracycline prophylaxis in families of cholera patients. Bulletin of the World Health Organisation 38: 787
28. Jawetz E 1969 Chemotherapy of chlamydial infection. Advances in Pharmacology and Chemotherapy 7: 253
29. Dunlop E M C 1977 Treatment of patients suffering from chlamydia infections. Journal of Antimicrobial Agents and Chemotherapy 3: 377
30. Willcox R R 1977 How suitable are available pharmaceuticals for the treatment of sexually transmitted diseases. 2. Conditions presenting as sores or tumours. British Journal of Venereal Disease 53: 340
31. Wilson W R, Cockerill F R III 1987 Tetracycline, chloramphenicol, erythromycin and clindamycin. Mayo Clinic Proceedings 62: 906–915
32. Acne today 1984 Drug and Therapeutics Bulletin 24: 93–96
33. Pockin P E 1970 Editorial. Antibiotics in acne. New England Journal of Medicine 294: 43
34. Leading Article 1972 Tetracyclines for malaria. British Medical Journal 3: 487
35. Cohlan S Q 1977 Tetracycline staining of teeth. Teratology 15: 127–131
36. Domz C A, McNamara D H, Holzapfel H F 1959 Tetracycline provacationing Lupus erythematosus. Annals of Internal Medicine 50 (5): 1217–1226
37. Leading Article 1972 Tetracyclines and blood urea. British Medical Journal 3: 370
38. Lew H T, French S W 1966 Tetracycline nephrotoxicity and non oliguric acute renal failure. Archives of Internal Medicine 118: 123
39. Schultz J C, Adamson J S J, Workman W W, Norman T D 1963 Fatal liver disease after intravenous administration of tetracycline in high dosage. New England Journal of Medicine 269: 999
40. Crowsin T D, Head C H, Ferrante W A 1976 Oesophageal ulcers associated with tetracyclines therapy. Journal of the American Medical Association 235: 2747
41. Mull M M 1966 The tetracyclines. A critical reappraisal. American Journal of Diseases of Children 112: 483
42. Koiekeila J 1971 Antianabolic effect of tetracyclines. Lancet 1: 974–977
43. Klotz M et al 1964 Interference by formaldehyde forming drugs in the determination of urinary catecholamines. Clinical Chemistry 10: 372–374
44. Levinson S A, MacFate R P 1969 Clinical laboratory diagnosis, 7th edn. Lea and Febiger, Philadelphia, pp 646–647
45. Mazze R I, Shue G L, Jackson S H et al 1971 Renal dysfunction associated with methoxyflurane anesthesia. A randomized, prospective clinical evaluation. Journal of the American Medical Association 216: 278–288
46. Kuzucu E Y 1970 Methoxyflurane, tetracycline and renal failure. Journal of the American Medical Association 211: 1162–1164
47. Kabins S A 1972 Interactions among antibiotics and other drugs. Journal of the American Medical Association 219: 206–212

O

Oxytocin

Oxytocin binds to specific receptors in the uterus causing uterine contraction, particularly when oestrogen levels are high.

Chemistry

Oxytocin (Syntocinon, Pitocin)

$C_{43}H_{66}N_{12}O_{12}S_2$

[3-Isoleucine, 8-Leucine]-vasopressin

Oxytocin is a naturally occurring nonapeptide produced by the supraoptic and paraventricular nuclei in the hypothalamus and stored in the posterior pituitary. Structurally it is a cyclic polypeptide with all amino acids in the L-form

HOOC — Cys — Tyr — Ile — Glu — Asp — Cys — Pro — Leu — Gly — NH_2

Molecular weight	1007
pKa	—
Solubility	
in alcohol	—
in water	soluble
Octanol/water partition coefficient	—

Oxytocin is a white powder soluble in water. Extractable from pituitary glands of larger mammals, it is prepared commercially by chemical synthesis. The colourless concentrated solution has a pH of 4.5 and is buffered with sodium acetate/acetic acid. It is also combined in solution with ergometrine maleate (Syntometrine).

Pharmacology

As a pharmacological agent, oxytocin produces effects similar to endogenous oxytocin. Oxytocin's major effect is to cause uterine muscle contraction, but the effects produced are dependent upon the hormonal state of the animal, the presence or absence of a pregnancy, and the stage of the pregnancy. In the uterus specific oxytocin receptors have been demonstrated on human myometrial cells.[1] Oxytocin binding to the receptors in the uterus causes an influx of sodium and calcium ions, lowering the transmembrane potential, increasing excitability, and causing myometrial contraction. The process may also involve a prostaglandin mediator. However, whether or not a response is elicited depends upon the relative dominance of oestrogen or progesterone. High levels of oestrogen cause the myometrium to be more responsive to oxytocin, while progesterone hyperpolarizes the myometrium, rendering it less responsive to oxytocin.

Oxytocin also binds to receptors on myoepithelial cells in the breast and stimulates contraction of these cells, causing milk to flow into the larger ducts, and facilitating the milk ejection reflex.

The drug affects vascular smooth muscle by causing vasodilation and increasing cerebral, coronary and renal blood flow. Hypotension with a reflex tachycardia, followed by a small but sustained increase in blood pressure, may be produced by a large dose or an undiluted solution.[2]

Because of a structural similarity with vasopressin, the hormone also possesses weak antidiuretic properties.

Toxicology

No relevant data are available.

Clinical pharmacology

The clinically most important action of oxytocin is to cause contraction of uterine smooth muscle. In the pregnant and puerperal uterus oxytocin has been shown to produce a dose-related increase in uterine contractile frequency and amplitude and at high doses an increase in resting uterine tone.[3] During pregnancy the sensitivity of the uterus to oxytocin increases, paralleling the increase in myometrial weight, actinomycin content, and oxytocin receptor density of uterine smooth muscle.[4] At term, the intravenous infusion of oxytocin at a rate of 1–16 $mU.min^{-1}$ produces 'physiological levels' of oxytocin with the production of contractions indistinguishable from those occurring spontaneously late in pregnancy and during labour.[3] At term, infusion rates above 16 $mU.min^{-1}$ may elevate basal uterine tone.[3]

Suckling stimulates sensory receptors in the breast which send afferent nerve impulses to the paraventricular and supraoptic nuclei in the brain, causing release of oxytocin. Circulating oxytocin stimulates the myoepithelial cells of the mammary gland causing milk ejection from the mammary gland during lactation, the so-called 'milk-ejection' reflex. Oxytocin administration prior to nursing has been shown to enhance this 'let down' reflex in lactating women.[5]

Rapid administration of 5 or 10 IU of oxytocin intravenously causes relaxation of vascular smooth muscle, resulting in a short-lived decrease in blood pressure and a reflex tachycardia.[6]

Structurally, oxytocin is related to arginine-vasopressin and has weak antidiuretic properties. Oxytocin acts directly on the distal renal tubules and causes water resorption.[7]

Pharmacokinetics

The preferred analytical method for oxytocin is radioimmunoassay[8,9] of plasma samples extracted with Fullers' earth. Methods using unextracted plasma consistently give higher values. The sensitivity of the antisera of the better oxytocin assays range from 1 pg to 5 pg. Although the sensitivity and specificity of the radioimmunoassay for oxytocin depend upon the particular antibody used, the better assays have 1–5% cross reactivity with arginine-vasopressin, vasotocin, and some analogues of oxytocin and vasopressin.[10]

Since oxytocin is a peptide it is enzymatically destroyed in the gastrointestinal tract by chymotrypsin and is not active orally. However, it is rapidly absorbed from mucous membranes.

Like vasopressin, oxytocin distributes in extracellular fluid space, and has a volume of distribution of approximately 0.3 $l.kg^{-1}$.[11] Used pharmacologically, oxytocin appears not to bind to protein.[12]

The plasma half life of oxytocin is in men 3.2–10.3 minutes;[11] in non-pregnant women 3.3–4.5 minutes; and in pregnant women 1.8–4.9 minutes.[13] Mean metabolic clearance is 21.5 ± 3.3 $ml.kg^{-1}.min^{-1}$.[11] The liver and the kidneys are primarily responsible for rapid elimination of oxytocin. In pregnancy circulating plasma oxytocinase is produced and from early pregnancy it is also capable of inactivating the hormone. Less than 1% of oxytocin is excreted in urine unchanged during pregnancy, while in the non-pregnant woman 20% is recovered in the urine.[13]

As a pharmacological agent, no data are available regarding oxytocin penetration into the CSF. Oxytocin is inactivated by the lactating mammary gland; thus breast milk should contain no active hormone.[2] There is little evidence that oxytocin can cross the placenta.

Oral absorption	—
Presystemic metabolism	—
Plasma half life	
range	2–10 min
Volume of distribution	0.3 $l.kg^{-1}$
Plasma protein binding	nil

Concentration–effect relationship

The effect that oxytocin produces on the myometrium varies with the stage of pregnancy. In early pregnancy oxytocin doses as high as 250 $mU.min^{-1}$ are required to elicit uterine contractions, while in late pregnancy and at term 1–20 $mU.min^{-1}$ of oxytocin may be all that is necessary to cause a pattern of uterine contractions which is indistinguishable from normal labour.

Oxytocin plasma levels, as measured by radioimmunoassay, have been found to be 40.3±9.8 pg.ml^{-1} during first stage spontaneous labour, 123.9±23.6 pg.ml^{-1} during second stage labour, and 64.5±13.1 pg.ml^{-1} during third stage labour.[8] No data concerning plasma levels of therapeutic doses of oxytocin are available, but it can be assumed that the range would be similar. The frequency and duration of uterine contractions and the fetal heart rate pattern are used to titrate oxytocin to the desired effect rather than a measured drug level.

Oxytocin released in response to suckling appears in a pulsatile manner and has been reported as 19.2±3.4 pg.ml^{-1} in samples drawn immediately after the initiation of breast feeding.[14] No data exist for corresponding oxytocin plasma levels after intranasal administration. However, a similar range could be assumed.

Metabolism

Metabolic inactivation of oxytocin in the liver involves an initial reduction of the disulphide group by a glutathione-dependent thiol protein disulphide oxidoreductase followed by degradation by aminopeptidase which cleaves amino acid residues from the N-terminal end.[15] This sequential system is referred to as the 'tissue oxytocinase' system, and is found in high concentration in homogenates of placental tissue.[16] The initial product of the disulphide reduction, dihydro-oxytocin, has oxytocin-like activity,[17] but it is completely inactivated by degradation by aminopeptidase.

The renal enzyme responsible for oxytocin degradation acts upon the C-terminal end of the molecule.[18]

During pregnancy another system develops to degrade oxytocin. This is plasma oxytocinase, produced by the placenta and found in increasing concentrations as pregnancy progresses. This enzyme degrades oxytocin by directly hydrolysing the peptide linkage between cysteine and tyrosine,[19] then cleaving tyrosine and subsequent residues. None of the intermediaries are active. Plasma oxytocinase seems to contribute little to the inactivation of oxytocin, and its exact role is unknown.[20]

Pharmaceutics

Oxytocin is available in parenteral formulations only. The potency of the synthetically produced oxytocin is standardized according to its vasodepressor activity in chickens, correlated closely to oxytocin activity, and expressed in posterior pituitary units. A unit is equivalent to 2.0–2.2 μg of the pure hormone. The British Pharmacopoeia specifies that it contains not more than 1 unit of vasopressor activity per 20 units of oxytocic activity.

Prepared for injection or intravenous administration as a clear solution, ampoules containing 1 IU.ml^{-1}, 5 IU.ml^{-1}, and 10 IU.ml^{-1} are available. Syntocinon Parenteral solution (Sandoz, UK) 10 IU.ml^{-1} Syntocinon Injection (Sandoz, USA)/Pitocin (Parke-Davis, USA)/generic injection (Wyeth, USA).

As a nasal spray, oxytocin is available in a concentration of 40 IU.ml^{-1}, Syntocinon Nasal Spray (Sandoz, USA).

Storage of oxytocin ampoules should be at temperatures between 4° and 25°C. Although refrigeration is recommended and may prolong shelf-life, stability is maintained when stored at room temperatures not above 25°C for approximately the same period of time. For ampoules shelf-life when stored between 2 and 8°C is approximately 5 years, and 3 years when stored at temperatures not above 22°C.

For the nasal spray, storage between 0° and 5°C is recommended. Once open the bottle should be used within one month. Shelf-life of the nasal spray is approximately 4 years when stored in a fridge.

Therapeutic use

Indications

1. The induction of labour when medically indicated
2. The augmentation of spontaneous labour
3. The management of incomplete, missed, or inevitable abortion
4. The prevention or treatment of postpartum or postabortal uterine atony and postpartum haemorrhage
5. To facilitate the milk-ejection reflex.

Other use

6. To assess fetal well-being in the oxytocin challenge test.

Contraindications

1. Any obstetrical condition in which spontaneous normal labour is not in the best interests of the mother and/or the fetus and surgical intervention offers a better risk:benefit ratio, such as those listed below. However, some of these conditions are relative rather than absolute and the final decision must rest with an experienced obstetrician.

   Cephalopelvic disproportion
   Fetal malpresentation
   Fetal distress
   Placenta praevia, vasa praevia
   Impaired strength of the uterus: grand multiparity, or prior uterine surgery where the cavity of the uterus has been entered
   A condition where vaginal delivery is contraindicated such as cord prolapse or invasive cancer of the cervix.

2. Uterine hyperactivity, especially with elevation of basal uterine tone as in placental abruption
3. Hypersensitivity to the drug
4. The nasal spray is contraindicated prior to delivery
5. Severe toxaemia. The manufacturer's package insert lists this as a contraindication. However, this is a matter of judgement and in clinical practice oxytocin is used for induction of labour and for fetal assessment in patients with severe pre-eclampsia prior to resorting to Caesarian section.

Mode of use

When used for the induction or augmentation of labour parenteral oxytocin should be considered a potentially dangerous drug, to be administered only in a hospital setting under close supervision by personnel well trained in the drug's use and potential complications. Provision must be made for continuous monitoring of uterine activity, fetal heart rate, and progression of labour during oxytocin use.

Prior to delivery oxytocin should only be administered as a dilute solution by intravenous infusion using a controlled infusion device. There are many satisfactory infusion techniques which allow safe administration of oxytocin, depending upon the particular infusion device employed and the amount of fluid which clinically can safely be used.

Oxytocin is a potent uterine stimulant which can produce uterine hyperstimulation at even a very small dose. Since the sensitivity of the pregnant uterus to oxytocin varies widely,[21] the infusion should be begun at a rate of 0.5–1.0 mU.min^{-1} and increased gradually every 15–20 minutes, 'titrating' the oxytocin infusion to the uterine contractile pattern and to the fetal heart rate response.[22] After the infusion is begun, continuous monitoring of the patient must include: observation of uterine response, in terms of contraction frequency, intensity and duration; and observation of the fetal response to labour as indicated by fetal heart rate. Good uterine activity is characterized by moderate to strong contractions every 2–3 minutes, lasting 45–60 seconds, with complete relaxation between contractions.[23] At any time, if uterine activity becomes excessive or contractions last more than 90 seconds, the infusion should immediately be stopped. Too frequent uterine contractions or excessively long contractions can interfere with uteroplacental blood flow and cause fetal hypoxia. Oxytocin's safety factor is its short half life: stopping the infusion rapidly dissipates the effect.

Uterine hypertonus or hyperstimulation can occur at any time during the progress of labour. For this reason, many advocate the use of an intrauterine pressure catheter when oxytocin is used. Although the catheter can only be used after the membranes are ruptured, it does help to prevent overt uterine tetany by showing characteristic changes in the uterine contraction wave form which precede uterine tetany, namely, the 'damping sign', a decrease in contraction amplitude and elevation of basal tone which precedes uterine tetany.[24]

The dose of oxytocin will vary during labour, necessitating careful monitoring and adjustment of the infusion rate. It is not uncommon to have the sensitivity of the uterus increase as labour progresses, requiring a lower infusion rate or no further oxytocin to continue a normal uterine contractile pattern.[23]

Indications

1. Induction of labour when medically indicated
Oxytocin is usually combined with amniotomy in the induction of labour. Amniotomy has been shown to shorten labour and has been associated with pulsatile release of endogenous oxytocin[25] and an increase in plasma prostaglandin levels.[26] At term, the physiological dose necessary to initiate labour has been found to be as low as 2 $mU.min^{-1}$ [29] and rarely exceeds 16 $mU.min^{-1}$.[28,29] Some authors have advocated the use of substantially higher infusion rates (e.g. up to 250 $mU.min^{-1}$) with the claim that this reduces the induction to delivery interval and the number of failed inductions.[30] However, high doses are associated with a higher rate of rise, a shortened time to maximum contraction, a shortened duration of maximal contraction and a higher initial pressure and these effects could have very serious adverse consequences.

A novel and more physiological approach to labour induction has been tried where oxytocin is 'pulsed' one minute in every 10 minutes,[34] mimicking the pulsatile spurts during parturition.[35] In comparison to a group induced with continuous oxytocin, there was no difference in induction-to-delivery time. However, the total dose of oxytocin was significantly less in the group administered oxytocin in a pulsatile manner, which may further reduce the risk of neonatal jaundice.

2. Augmentation of spontaneous labour
During the course of spontaneous labour patients may exhibit less than optimal uterine activity which may contribute to dysfunctional labour patterns, such as prolonged latent phase, prolonged active phase, and secondary arrest of dilatation or descent. Administration of oxytocin by dilute infusion in the manner outlined above stimulates the uterus to produce a good contractile pattern, that is, moderate to strong uterine contractions every 2–3 minutes, which last 45–60 seconds. If labour is progressing normally oxytocin is usually not indicated, although routine use is advocated by some as in the 'active management of labour'.[36]

Oxytocin augmentation of labour should not be done in the presence of excessive uterine activity, or elevation of basal uterine tone, such as in placental abruption.

Although the presence of cephalopelvic disproportion is listed by the manufacturer and some authorities[23,29] as a contraindication to oxytocin use, in current practice a trial of labour with oxytocin induction or augmentation is viewed as the only means whereby the diagnosis of cephalopelvic disproportion can be made.[37] In such cases the diagnosis should be made as quickly as possible to avoid prolonged oxytocin infusion and possible uterine rupture.

3. Management of incomplete, missed, or inevitable abortion
The uterus is relatively insensitive to oxytocin early in gestation. Therefore, oxytocin in this setting must be used in high doses for long periods of time to completely empty the uterus. To avoid water intoxication, which has particularly been reported with oxytocin use in this setting,[38] higher concentrations of oxytocin should be used so that the volume of infused fluid is not excessive and oxytocin should be infused with normal saline. Careful attention should also be given to monitoring urinary output, a declining urinary output being one of the first signs of water intoxication.

With abortifacients such as prostaglandin $F_2\alpha$ and E_2, saline, and hyperosmolar urea, oxytocin has been used in an attempt to decrease the induction-to-abortion interval. In different regimens infusion of high-dose oxytocin enhances uterine contractions and seems a useful adjunct in midtrimester abortions.[39] However, the use of oxytocin in this setting appears to increase the risk of uterine rupture[40] and cervical lacerations.[41]

4. The prevention or treatment of postpartum or postabortal uterine atony and postpartum haemorrhage
In an attempt to reduce maternal morbidity from postpartum and postabortal uterine atony oxytocin's use in the third stage of labour is advocated. The goals have been to reduce the time to placental expulsion, reduce the incidence of postpartum haemorrhage, and reduce the incidence of placental retention. Under careful obstetric supervision, 5 or 10 U of oxytocin can be administered intramuscularly or 5 U slowly intravenously after the delivery of the anterior shoulder of the fetus. When used in this manner the clinician must be absolutely sure that no multiple gestation is present, and must be willing to accept the possibility of occasionally trapping the placenta.

Since the uterotonic effect of a single injection of oxytocin is of relatively short duration, an infusion of oxytocin or use of an ergot alkaloid may be necessary for sustained action.[42]

In comparison to the use of ergometrine or methylergometrine, oxytocin is better at promoting placental separation and expulsion with no increased risk of placental trapping,[43] causes less vomiting or retching, has fewer cardiovascular side effects,[44] and causes less overall blood loss.[45]

An alternative agent, Syntometrine (0.5 mg ergometrine and 5 U oxytocin) can also be administered intramuscularly at the birth of the anterior shoulder. The agent, when compared with ergometrine seemed to cause less puerperal haemorrhage and fewer incidents of placental entrapment.[46–47]

As an alternative regimen to the use of a uterotonic agent given with the birth of the anterior shoulder, oxytocin can be given as an infusion, 10–20 $U.l^{-1}$ of intravenous solution, begun after the delivery of the placenta, given at a rate of 100–200 $ml.h^{-1}$, and continued until the risk of postpartum haemorrhage is deemed clinically past.

Although the use of uterotonic agents postpartum and postabortion has become routine, there is evidence to suggest that postpartum uterine haemostasis is independent of sustained uterine contracture,[48] rendering routine use possibly unnecessary. Nevertheless, uterotonic agents should particularly be used in patients who have factors rendering them at increased risk for postpartum haemorrhage, such as an over distended uterus (large baby, multiple gestation), high parity, history of previous postpartum haemorrhage, prolonged or precipitous labour, or use of a general anaesthetic for delivery.[42]

5. To facilitate the milk-ejection reflex
Oxytocin is indicated as a nasal spray administered as one spray into one or both nostrils just prior to nursing or pumping the breasts. Although not necessary routinely, the nasal spray is particularly helpful in patients with breast engorgement, patients using a breast pump to feed premature infants,[49] and in patients having difficulties with the let-down reflex in nursing their babies.[50]

Other use
6. To assess fetal well-being in the oxytocin challenge test
Based upon the suggestion of Hammacher[51] that the response of the fetal heart rate to oxytocin-induced contractions in late pregnancy would be a valuable method of predicting how the fetus might withstand the stress of labour, the oxytocin challenge test was developed. In actuality the test measures placental respiratory reserve or placental oxygen transfer reserve. The oxytocin challenge test has become a test of fetal well-being for patients at risk of uteroplacental insufficiency.

Reported complications related to the use of the oxytocin challenge test are hyperstimulation of the uterus occurring in approximately 3% of tests,[52] inadvertent initiation of labour, and inadvertent haemorrhage from an unsuspected placenta praevia.[53]

The test is cumbersome, requiring an intravenous line and performance on or near a delivery unit. It is also time consuming, taking an average of 90 minutes to complete.[54] The test is subject to as high as a 30–40% false positive rate,[55] generally related to the presence of good fetal heart rate variability and accelerations with fetal activity.[56] The false negative rate for the oxytocin challenge test is approximately 0.4%[57] related to fetal demise from causes other than uteroplacental insufficiency, misinterpretation of an oxytocin challenge test, and acute, rapid fetal deterioration.[58] A negative oxytocin challenge test as a test of fetal well-being is felt to be reassuring for a further week of intrauterine survival[59] provided there are no changes in maternal status.[60]

Contraindications

1. Any obstetrical condition in which normal spontaneous labour is not in the best interests of the mother or the fetus
Specific obstetrical conditions where oxytocin is contraindicated include: cephalopelvic disproportion; fetal malpresentation; fetal distress; placenta praevia or vasa praevia; impaired strength of the uterus, as in grand multiparity, or prior uterine surgery where the cavity of the uterus has been entered, e.g. myomectomy, prior caesarean section; cord prolapse; invasive cancer of the cervix; and any condition where surgical intervention offers a better risk:benefit ratio to the mother and/or fetus.

Oxytocin

Cephalopelvic disproportion is listed by the manufacturer and some authorities,[23,29] as a contraindication to the use of oxytocin. However, in current practice oxytocin induction or augmentation is used to make the diagnosis of cephalopelvic disproportion.[37] Care must be taken in such cases to make the diagnosis in as short a period of time as possible, avoiding prolonged infusions of oxytocin and possible uterine rupture.

Whether or not any of these conditions are absolute or relative contraindications to the use of oxytocin depends very much on the particular obstetrical situation, and the decision whether or not to use oxytocin must be left to the judgement of the experienced physician.

2. Uterine hyperactivity
In cases of placental abruption with uterine hyperactivity and elevation of basal uterine tone, oxytocin is particularly contraindicated because of an increased risk of uterine rupture.

3. Hypersensitivity to the drug
Hypersensitivity to oxytocin is more a theoretical than real contraindication to oxytocin use. Cases may exist, but more often than not extreme sensitivity to oxytocin is probably related to use of too high a dose of oxytocin. In such a case increasing the infusion rate by gradual increments, not doubling the infusion rate, will avoid hyperstimulating the uterus.

4. The nasal spray prior to delivery
Nasal oxytocin is unsuitable for use prior to delivery because of variable absorption and poor predictability of uterine response.

Adverse reactions

Potentially life-threatening effects
Oxytocin is an endogenous hormone which has not been reported to produce toxic effects of its own. Overdose caused by inappropriate use produces uncontrolled uterine contractions, decreased placental blood flow, fetal asphyxia and fetal death.

Life-threatening conditions associated with oxytocin use include: maternal water intoxication; tetanic uterine contractions, which can cause severe fetal hypoxia and fetal death; and rupture of the gravid uterus.

Oxytocin is structurally similar to arginine-vasopressin and possesses weak antidiuretic properties. Water intoxication caused by oxytocin is usually only seen in patients requiring high doses or prolonged infusions of oxytocin, and can be avoided by use of saline-containing intravenous fluids and careful monitoring of fluid intake and urinary output.

Tetanic uterine contractions, which can happen at any time during induction or augmentation with oxytocin, with their concomitant effects on the fetus, are best avoided by continual observation of the patient and adjustment of the oxytocin infusion rate. To aid in the early detection of tetany, use of the intrauterine pressure catheter is advocated. In cases of tetanic uterine contractions not responsive to discontinuing the oxytocin infusion, a bolus of a β_2-sympathomimetic agent, such as 0.25 mg terbutaline, or 0.01 mg hexoprenaline, has been successful in reversing uterine tetany and treating fetal distress.[62,63]

Rupture of the gravid uterus is usually caused not by the oxytocin infusion per se, but by either the failure to recognize obstructed labour or the presence of a weakened uterus, caused by a prior uterine scar or grand multiparity.

Iatrogenic premature delivery caused by inappropriate induction of labour can also be a life-threatening condition to the newborn with risk of respiratory distress, intracranial haemorrhage and death.

Severe or irreversible adverse effects
Oxytocin has been associated with an increased incidence of neonatal jaundice when used for labour induction but not for labour augmentation.[64,65] This adverse effect of oxytocin use has been found to be independent of gestational age at birth, birth weight, sex, race, anaesthesia used for delivery, and method of delivery[66,67] although another study suggests neonatal jaundice is related to fetal maturity.[70] The probability of neonatal jaundice is related to the dose of oxytocin given to the mother, with no neonatal jaundice seen when oxytocin was administered at a rate less than 20 $mU.min^{-1}$.[33] Neonatal jaundice has also been related to the duration of oxytocin administration with increases in cord bilirubin levels seen only when mothers received more than 2500 mU or 4000 mU oxytocin per kilogram birth weight of the infant.[65,66] Oxytocin is postulated to cause neonatal jaundice by inhibition of hepatic glucuronyl transferase,[68] and by causing an increased erythrocyte deformability and haemolysis particularly at high doses.[69]

Rapid administration of high doses postpartum may cause a short episode of hypotension and a reflex tachycardia.

Symptomatic adverse effects
When oxytocin is used for induction or augmentation of labour, patients sometimes complain that the oxytocin stimulated contractions are harder to tolerate than contractions of spontaneous labour.

Interference with clinical pathology tests
No significant interferences have been reported.

High risk groups

Neonates
The drug is not used in this patient group.

Breast milk. Oxytocin is inactivated by the lactating mammary gland; thus breast milk should contain no active hormone.[2]

Children
The drug is not used in this patient group.

Pregnant women
As outlined above.

The elderly
The drug is not used in this patient group.

Drug interactions

Potentially hazardous interactions
Used concomitantly with prostaglandins, the risk of uterine rupture and cervical lacerations is increased.[40,41]

Potentially useful interactions
When oxytocin is used with ergometrine, postpartum haemorrhage due to uterine atony is controlled by two different mechanisms, oxytocin producing an immediate response and ergometrine producing a sustained response.

Major outcome trials

1. Sorbe B 1978 Active pharmacologic management of the third stage of labor. Obstetrics and Gynecology 52: 694–697

This was a randomized clinical trial of intravenous use of either 10U oxytocin or 0.2 mg methylergometrine given to 1049 parturients with the birth of the anterior shoulder. The study examines duration of the third stage of labour, immediate postpartum blood loss, and the incidence of retained placenta. A large historical control group given 0.2 mg methylergometrine after delivery provides an additional comparative group.

The mean duration of the third stage of labour was not significantly different in any group. Blood loss and the incidence of postpartum haemorrhage was significantly less in the groups treated with methylergometrine or oxytocin at the birth of the anterior shoulder as compared with the control group treated only after delivery of the placenta. Postpartum haemorrhage was significantly less in patients treated with oxytocin. Methylergometrine significantly increased the incidence of retained placenta, and for this reason blood loss was slightly greater in the methylergometrine group as compared to the oxytocin group.

2. Moodie J E, Moir D D 1976 Ergometrine, oxytocin and extradural analgesia. British Journal of Anaesthesia 48: 571–574

This was a randomized clinical trial of intravenous use of either 5 U oxytocin or 0.5 mg of ergometrine given to 148 parturients with the birth of the anterior shoulder. The study examines blood loss and incidence of emesis.

There was no significant different in mean blood loss between the two groups, however nausea and emesis were only seen with the use of ergometrine.

3. Friedman E A 1967 Comparative clinical evaluation of postpartum oxytocics. American Journal of Obstetrics and Gynecology 73: 1306–1313

This study compares methylergometrine, ergometrine, oxytocin and dihydroergotamine administered randomly to parturients in the third stage of labour. Blood loss, the incidence of hypertension, and the incidence of haemorrhage were found to be equivalent for methylergometrine and ergometrine. However, oxytocin caused less blood loss, less postpartum haemorrhage, and no incidence of hypertension.

4. Bremme K, Bygdeman M 1980 A comparative study of uterine activity and fetal heart rate pattern in labor induced with oral prostaglandin E_2 or oxytocin. Acta Obstetrica Gynecologica Scandinavica (suppl) 92: 23–29

This was a randomized clinical trial of oxytocin and prostaglandin E_2 used for labour induction in 200 patients at or near term. The study examined uterine contraction patterns and perinatal outcome as measured by Apgar scores.

Although labour was initiated earlier in the oxytocin-treated group, once labour was established uterine contractility patterns, as measured by frequency and amplitude of contractions, were the same in both groups. There was a higher frequency of atypical contractility patterns in the group treated with prostaglandin E_2, and one episode of overt hypertonus, but abnormalities in fetal heart rate patterns were similar in both groups. There were no cases of perinatal mortality, and Apgar scores were similar in both groups.

5. Pavlou C, Barker G H, Roberts A, Chamberlain G V P 1978 Pulsed oxytocin infusion in the induction of labour. British Journal of Obstetrics and Gynaecology 85: 96–100

This was a randomized clinical trial of intermittent pulsed oxytocin (one minute infusion every 10 minutes) and continuous infusion of oxytocin used for labour induction in 28 patients. The study examines induction–delivery and induction-to-full-dilatation time intervals and total dose of oxytocin required.

Time intervals of induction-to-full-dilatation and induction–delivery were similar for both groups. The group treated with pulsed oxytocin required significantly higher rates of oxytocin infusion during labour induction than the group treated with continuous infusion oxytocin. However, the total dose of oxytocin necessary during the course of labour was significantly less in the group treated with pulsed oxytocin.

Other outcome trials

1. O'Driscoll K, Stronge J M, Minogue M 1973 Active management of labour. British Medical Journal 3: 135–137
2. Turnbull A C, Anderson A B M 1968 Induction of labour. Part III: Results with amniotomy and oxytocin 'titration' Journal of Obstetrics and Gynaecology of the British Commonwealth 75: 32–41
3. Embrey M P, Barber D T C, Scudamore J H 1963 Use of 'Syntometrine' in prevention of post-partum haemorrhage. British Medical Journal 1: 1387–1389
4. Chukuderbelu W O, Marshall A T, Chalmers J A 1963 Use of 'Syntometrine' in the third stage of labour. British Medical Journal 1: 1390–1391
5. Kemp J 1963 Clinical trial of 'Syntometrine' in the third stage of labour. British Medical Journal 1: 1391–1392
6. Beard R J, Bishop N L, Jones B J M 1973 A comparison of intramuscular ergometrine maleate and oxytocin with intravenous oxytocin and intramuscular ergometrine in the third stage of labour. The British Journal of Clinical Practice 27: 13–14
7. Djahanbakhch O, Vere M, Gardner N H N, Morris E C 1978 The intramuscular use of oxytocic agents for prophylactic management of the third stage of labour. The British Journal of Clinical Practice 32: 137–138

General review articles

Caldeyro-Barcia R, Heller H (eds) 1961 Oxytocin, Proceedings of an international symposium held in Montevideo, 1959. Pergamon Press, Oxford
Dawood M Y 1984 Annual Research Reviews Oxytocin, Volume 2. Eden Press, Montreal, Canada
Dawood M Y 1985 Induction of labor. In: Amico J A, Robinson A G (eds) Oxytocin: clinical and laboratory studies. Elsevier Medical Publishers, New York
Hendricks C H, Brenner W E 1970 Cardiovascular effects of oxytocic drugs used post partum. American Journal of Obstetrics and Gynecology 108: 751–760
Theobald G W 1968 Oxytocin reassessed. Obstetrical and Gynecological Survey 23: 109–131
O'Driscoll K, Stronge J M 1975 The active management of labour. Clinics in Obstetrics and Gynaecology 2: 3–16
Pauerstein C J 1973 Use and abuse of oxytocic agents. Clinical Obstetrics and Gynecology 16: 262–277
Clark J F B 1973 Medical induction of labour - a review. Clinics in Obstetrics and Gynaecology 2: 49–79
Petrie R H 1981 The pharmacology and use of oxytocin. Clinics in Perinatology 8: 35–47

References

1. Soloff M S, Schroeder B T, Chahraborty J, Pearlmutter A F 1977 Characterization of oxytocin receptors in the uterus and mammary gland. Federation Proceedings 36: 1861–1866
2. Rall T W, Schleifer L S 1980 Oxytocin, prostaglandins, ergot alkaloids, and other agents. In: Goodman A G, Gilman L S, Goodman A (eds) The pharmacological basis of therapeutics, 6th edn. Macmillan, New York, pp 935–950
3. Poseiro J J, Noriega-Guerra L 1961 Dose–response relationships in uterine effects of oxytocin infusions. In: Caldeyro-Barcia R, Heller H (eds) Oxytocin, proceedings of an international symposium held in Montevideo, 1959. Pergamon Press, Oxford, pp 158–174
4. Caldeyro-Barcia R, Sereno J A 1961 The response of the human uterus to oxytocin throughout pregnancy. In: Caldeyro-Barcia R, Heller H (eds) Oxytocin, proceedings of an international symposium held in Montevideo, 1959. Pergamon Press, Oxford, pp 177–200
5. Newton M, Egli G E, Jackson M S 1958 The effect of intranasal administration of oxytocin on the let-down of milk in lactating women. American Journal of Obstetrics and Gynecology 76: 103–107
6. Hendricks C H, Brenner W E 1970 Cardiovascular effects of oxytocic drugs used postpartum. American Journal of Obstetrics and Gynecology 108: 751–760
7. Abdul-Karim R, Assali N S 1961 Renal function in human pregnancy: effects of oxytocin on renal hemodynamics and water and electrolyte excretion. Journal of Laboratory and Clinical Medicine 57: 522
8. Dawood M Y, Raghavan K S, Pociask C 1978 Radioimmunoassay of oxytocin. Journal of Endocrinology 76: 261–270
9. Chard T 1973 The radioimmunossay of oxytocin and vasopressin. Journal of Endocrinology 58: 143–160
10. Dawood M Y 1984 Annual Research Reviews Oxytocin, Volume 2. Eden Press, Montreal, Canada, pp 48–49
11. Dawood M Y, Ylikorkala O, Trivedi D, Gupta R 1980 Oxytocin levels and disappearance rate of plasma follicle-stimulating hormone and luteinizing hormone after oxytocin infusion in men. Journal of Clinical Endocrinology and Metabolism 50: 397–400
12. Fabian M, Forsling M, Jones J J, Prior J S 1969 The clearance and antidiuretic potency of neurohypophysical hormones in man, and their plasma binding and stability. Journal of Physiology (London) 204: 653–668
13. Gonzaliz-Panizza V H, Sica-Blanco Y, Mendez-Bauer C 1961 The fate of injected oxytocin in the pregnant women near term. In: Caldeyzo-Barcia R, Heller H (eds) Oxytocin, proceedings of an international Symposium held in Montevideo, 1959. Pergamon Press, Oxford, pp 347–357
14. Leake R D, Weitzman R E 1979 Developmental pharmacokinetics of the posterior pituitary hormones. Clinics in Perinatology 6: 65–68
15. Branda L A, Ferrier B M, Celhoffer L 1972 Thiol-protein disulfide oxidoreductase activity in human placental tissue homogenates. Canadian Journal of Biochemistry 50: 507
16. Ferrier B M, Branda L A 1970 Degradation of insulin and oxytocin by human placental tissue. Proceedings of the Canadian Federation of Biology Society 13: 99
17. Branda L A, Ferrier B M 1976 Biochemistry of oxytocin. In: Goodwin J W, Godden J O, Chance G W (eds) Perinatal medicine. The basic science underlying clinical practice. Williams and Wilkins, Baltimore, Maryland, pp 481–498
18. Walter R, Shlank H 1971 In vivo inactivation of oxytocin. Endocrinology 89: 990
19. Tuppy H, Nesvadba H 1957 Uber die Aminopeptidaseaktivatat des Schwangerenserums und ihre Beziehung zu dessen Vermogen, Oxytocin zu inaktivieren. Monatsschrift Chemie 88: 977
20. Branda L A, Ferrier B M 1971 Degradation of oxytocin by human placental tissue. American Journal of Obstetrics and Gynecology 109: 943
21. Turnbull A C, Anderson A B M 1968 Uterine contractility and oxytocin sensitivity during human pregnancy in relation to the onset of labour. Journal of Obstetrics and Gynaecology of the British Commonwealth 75: 278–288
22. Turnbull A C, Anderson A B M 1968 Induction of labour III. Results with amniotomy and oxytocin 'titration'. Journal of Obstetrics and Gynaecology of the British Commonwealth 75: 32–41
23. Friedman E A 1978 Therapeutic issues. In: Friedman E A, Labor: clinical evaluation and management, 2nd edn. Appleton Century Crofts, New York, pp 329–347
24. Dawood M Y 1985 Induction of labor. In: Amico J A, Robinson A G (eds) Oxytocin: clinical and laboratory studies. Elsevier Medical Publishers, New York

25. Chard T, Gibbens G L D 1983 Spurt release of oxytocin during surgical induction of labor in women. American Journal of Obstetrics and Gynecology 147: 678–680
26. Mitchell M D, Flint A P F, Bibby J et al 1977 Rapid increases in plasma prostaglandin concentrations after vaginal examination and amniotomy. British Medical Journal 2: 1183–1185
27. Theobald G W 1955 The separate release of oxytocin and antidiuretic hormone. Journal of Physiology 149: 443
28. Caldeyro-Barcia R, Sica-Blanco Y, Poseiro J J, Gonzales-Panizza V H, Mendez-Bauer C 1957 A quantitative study of the action of synthetic oxytocin on the pregnant human uterus. Journal of Pharmacology and Experimental Therapeutics 121: 18
29. Petrie R H 1981 The pharmacology and use of oxytocin. Clinics in Perinatology 8: 35–47
30. Toaff M E, Hezroni J, Toaff R 1978 Induction of labour by pharmacological and physiological doses of intravenous oxytocin. British Journal of Obstetrics and Gynaecology 85: 101–108
31. Seitchik J, Chatkoff M L 1976 Oxytocin-induced uterine hypercontractility pressure wave forms. Obstetrics and Gynecology 48: 436–441
32. Seitchik J, Chatkoff M L, Hayashi R H 1977 Intrauterine pressure waveform characteristics of spontaneous and oxytocin or prostaglandin $F_2\alpha$ induced active labor. American Journal of Obstetrics and Gynecology 127: 223–227
33. Jeffares M J 1977 A multifactorial survey of neonatal jaundice. British Journal of Obstetrics and Gynaecology 84: 452–455
34. Pavlou C, Barker G H, Roberts A, Chamberlain G V P 1978 Pulsed oxytocin infusion in the induction of labour. British Journal of Obstetrics and Gynaecology 85: 96–100
35. Gibbens G L D, Chard T 1976 Observations of maternal oxytocin release during human labor and the effect of intravenous alcohol. American Journal of Obstetrics and Gynecology 126: 243–246
36. O'Driscoll K, Stronge J M 1975 The active management of labour. Clinics in Obstetrics and Gynaecology 2: 3–17
37. O'Driscoll K, Jackson R J A, Gallagaher J T 1970 Active management of labour and cephalopelvic disproportion. Journal of Obstetrics and Gynaecology of the British Commonwealth 77: 385–389
38. Morgan D B, Kirwan N A, Hancock K W, Robinson D, Howe J G, Ahmad S 1977 Water intoxication and oxytocin infusion. British Journal of Obstetrics and Gynaecology 84: 6–12
39. Dawood M Y 1984 Induction of abortion and labor. In: Dawood M Y 1984 Annual Research Reviews Oxytocin, Volume 2. Eden Press, Montreal, Canada, pp 93–108
40. Propping D, Stubblefield P G, Golub J, Zuckerman J 1977 Uterine rupture following midtrimester abortion by laminaria, prostaglandin $F_2\alpha$ and oxytocin: report of two cases. American Journal of Obstetrics and Gynecology 128: 689–690
41. Perry G, Siegal B, Held B 1977 Uterine trauma associated with midtrimester abortion induced by intra-amniotic prostaglandin $F_2\alpha$ with and without concomitant use of oxytocin. Prostaglandins 13: 1147–1159
42. Pauerstein C J 1973 Use and abuse of oxytocic agents. Clinical Obstetrics and Gynecology 16: 262–277
43. Sorbe B 1978 Active pharmacologic management of the third stage of labor. Obstetrics and Gynecology 52: 694–697
44. Moodie J E, Moir D D 1976 Ergometrine, oxytocin and extradural analgesia. British Journal of Anaesthesia 48: 571–574
45. Friedman E A 1957 Comparative clinical evaluation of postpartum oxytocics. American Journal of Obstetrics and Gynecology 73: 1306–1313
46. Embrey M P, Barber D T C, Scudamore J H 1963 Use of 'Syntometrine' in prevention of postpartum haemorrhage. British Medical Journal 1: 1387–1389
47. Kemp J 1963 Clinical trial of 'Syntomerine' in the third stage of labour. British Medical Journal 1: 1391–1392
48. Hendricks C H 1968 Uterine contractility changes in the early puerperium. Clinical Obstetrics and Gynecology 11: 125–144
49. Ruis H, Rolland R, Doesburg W, Broeders G, Corbey R 1981 Oxytocin enhances onset of lactation among mothers delivering prematurely. British Medical Journal 283: 340–342
50. Lawrence R A 1980 Breast-feeding. A guide for the medical profession. C V Mosby, St. Louis, pp 125–128
51. Hammacher K 1966 In: Elert R, Hüter K A (eds) Prophylaxe frühkindlicher Hirnschäden. George Thieme Verlag, Stuttgart, p 120
52. Odendaal H J 1978 Hyperstimulation of the uterus during the oxytocin stress test. Obstetrics and Gynecology 51: 380–383
53. Newton M 1979 The role of the oxytocin reflexes in three interpersonal reproductive acts: coitus, birth, and breast feeding. In: Carenza L, Pancheri P, Zichella L (eds) Clinical psychoneuroendocrinology in reproduction. Academic Press, London, pp. 411–418
54. Schifrin B S 1977 Antepartum fetal heart rate monitoring. In: Gluck L (ed) Intrauterine asphyxia and the developing fetal brain. Yearbook Medical Publishers, Chicago, pp 205–244
55. Baskett T F, Sandy E A 1977 The oxytocin challenge test and antepartum fetal assessment. British Journal of Obstetrics and Gynecology 84: 39–43
56. Trierweiler M W, Freeman R K, James J 1976 Baseline fetal heart rate characteristics as an indicator of fetal status during the antepartum period. American Journal of Obstetrics and Gynecology 125: 618–623
57. Neuhoff S D, Gal D, Tancer M L 1979 False negative oxytocin challenge test result. New York State Journal of Medicine 10: 1537–1540
58. Dawood M Y 1984 Oxytocin Challenge Test. In: Dawood M Y Annual Research Reviews Oxytocin, Volume 2. Eden Press, Montreal, Canada pp 84–92
59. Schifrin B S 1979 The rationale for antepartum fetal heart rate monitoring. Journal of Reproductive Medicine 23: 213
60. Druzin M L, Paul R H, Gratacos J 1979 Current status of the contraction stress test. Journal of Reproductive Medicine 23: 222–226
61. Scanlon J W, Suzuki K, Shea E, Tromick E 1978 Clinical and neurobehavioural effects of repeated intrauterine exposure to oxytocin: a prospective study. American Journal of Obstetrics and Gynecology 132: 294–296
62. Arias F 1978 Intrauterine resuscitation with terbutaline: a method for the management of acute intrapartum fetal distress. American Journal of Obstetrics and Gynecology 131: 39–43
63. Lipshitz J 1977 Use of a β_2 sympathomimetic drug as a temporizing measure in the treatment of acute fetal distress. American Journal of Obstetrics and Gynecology 129: 31–36
64. Chew W C, Swann I L 1977 Influence of simultaneous low amniotomy and oxytocin infusion and other maternal factors on neonatal jaundice: a prospective study. British Medical Journal 1: 72–73
65. D'Souza S W, Black P, MacFarlane T, Richards B 1979 The effect of oxytocin in induced labour on neonatal jaundice. British Journal of Obstetrics and Gynaecology 86: 133–138
66. Conway D I, Read M D, Bauer C, Martin R H 1976 Neonatal jaundice — a comparison between intravenous oxytocin and oral prostaglandin E_2. Journal of International Medical Research 4: 241–246
67. Friedman L, Lewis P J, Clifton P, Bulpitt C J 1978 Factors influencing the incidence of neonatal jaundice. British Medical Journal 1: 1235–1237
68. Schikler K N, Cohen M I, McNamara H 1976 Oxytocin administration. American Journal of Diseases of Children 130: 1377
69. Buchan P 1979 Pathogenesis of neonatal hyperbilirubinaemia after induction of labor with oxytocin. British Medical Journal 2: 1255–1257
70. Lange A P, Westergaard J G, Secher N J, Skovgard I 1982 Neonatal jaundice after labour induced or stimulated by prostaglandin E_2 or oxytocin. Lancet 1: 991–994

Pamidronate (disodium pentahydrate)

Pamidronate is an amino-substituted geminal biphosphonate (bisphosphonate) with potent inhibitory effects on bone resorption.

Chemistry

Pamidronate disodium pentahydrate (Aredia)
$C_3H_9O_7P_2NNa_2.5H_2O$
Disodium-3-amino-1-hydroxypropylidene-1,1-bisphosphonate pentahydrate

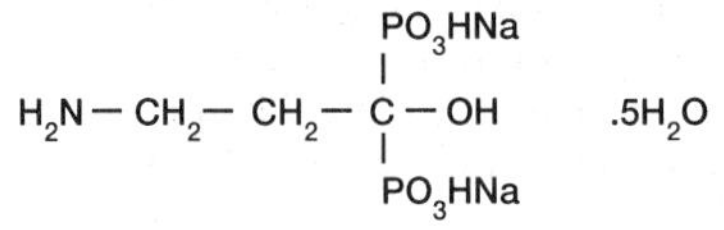

Molecular weight (anhydrate)	367 (279.04)
pKa	0.1, 6.2, 10.9
Solubility	
in alcohol	–
in water	1 in 30
Octanol/water partition coefficient	–

A white odourless crystalline powder, it is prepared by chemical synthesis. It is not available in any combination product.

Pharmacology

Biphosphonates were produced to mimic some of the actions of pyrophosphate in biological systems. Early studies had shown that pyrophosphate, present in biological fluids such as plasma and urine, inhibited calcium phosphate precipitation [1]. When given in vivo pyrophosphate inhibited ectopic calcification[2] but was inactive when given by mouth and parenterally it was hydrolysed very rapidly. Biphosphonates were synthesised since it was expected that they would have similar effects to pyrophosphate but would resist enzymic hydrolysis. The basic structure of biphosphonates contains a P-C-P backbone and substitutes a carbon atom for the oxygen atom in pyrophosphate. Many variations are possible on the basic structure. Pamidronate is an amino-substituted biphosphonate.

Biphosphonates such as pamidronate inhibit the precipitation of calcium phosphate from clear solutions[3], and block the transformation of amorphous calcium phosphate into hydroxyapatite[4]. Biphosphonates bind onto hydroxyapatite and thus ^{99m}Technetium-labelled biphosphonates are useful as skeletal markers in nuclear medicine[5]. Biphosphonates inhibit calcification in vivo and are active both parenterally and by the oral route[3]. Some of this activity is probably due to an inhibition of crystal growth.

Biphosphonates such as pamidronate inhibit bone resorption both in vivo and in vitro. The mechanism of action involves a number of processes.[6] Biphosphonates inhibit the bone-resorbing ability of osteoclasts and, within a few days of starting treatment, a decrease in osteoclast numbers can be demonstrated[7]. The effect on the osteoclast is due to a number of factors. There is a direct toxic effect of ingested biphosphonate on the resorbing osteoclast (see Fleisch General Review article) and there is an inhibition of the differentiation of osteoclast precursors into mature osteoclasts[8]. There is also a disruption of the chemotactic gradient between bone and osteoclasts, or interference with the recognition and attachment of mature osteoclasts to the bone surface[9,10]. Pamidronate is more potent than etidronate and clodronate in inhibiting osteoclast activity. While pamidronate can inhibit bone mineralisation in vivo, this effect is seen only at doses 50 times higher than those which inhibit bone resorption[11].

Toxicology

Pamidronate is not known to have mutagenic potential and no carcinogenicity has been demonstrated in mice and rats at 80 and 104 weeks respectively. At high doses (40 μmol.kg^{-1} daily) pamidronate reduces metaphyseal bone mineralization and longitudinal bone growth in rats.[11] Inhibition of bone mineralisation has not been reported at the doses which are used in clinical practice.

Clinical pharmacology

Treatment with pamidronate in man causes marked inhibition of osteoclastic bone resorption within 1–2 days of administration. Biochemically, this is reflected by a reduction in serum calcium, fasting urinary calcium and urinary hydroxyproline levels.[12–15] In conditions where bone turnover is increased (such as Paget's disease), suppression of bone formation follows the reduction in bone resorption, and this is reflected by a progressive fall in serum alkaline phosphatase levels from about 10 days post treatment onwards.[16–18] This effect is accompanied by a reduction in bone pain. The duration of pamidronate's inhibitory effect on bone turnover varies, depending on the clinical application. In normocalcaemic subjects, and in patients with cancer-associated hypercalcaemia, bone resorption remains suppressed for between 2–6 weeks after a single dose of pamidronate.[12,14,19,20] In Paget's disease however, the inhibitory effect of pamidronate on bone turnover may persist for months or years after treatment is stopped.[16–18]

Except at extremely high doses, suppression of bone formation by pamidronate is a consequence of the reduction in bone resorption, rather than a direct effect on osteoblast function.[21] Since maximal inhibition of bone resorption with pamidronate occurs rapidly and precedes the maximal inhibitory effect on bone formation by about three months (the estimated duration of the bone remodelling cycle), pamidronate treatment may result in a generalised increase in bone mass — an effect which has prompted the successful use of pamidronate in various forms of osteoporosis.[22–24]

Although its main effects are manifest on the skeleton, pamidronate also acts on the immune system. Pamidronate causes a reduction in macrophage-induced lymphocyte proliferation in vitro.[25] In vivo, approximately 30% of pamidronate-treated patients exhibit an acute-phase response (usually on first exposure to the drug) manifest by mild pyrexia and transient lymphopenia.[26,27] Gastrointestinal symptoms are the commonest dose-related side effects.

Pharmacokinetics

Two techniques are available for the assay of pamidronate in biological fluids. One involves high performance anion exchange chromatography followed by spectrophotometric detection of a phosphomolybdate complex,[28] the other utilizes high performance liquid chromatography, followed by fluorescence detection of a fluorescamine bisphosphonate derivative.[29] The limit of sensitivity of both methods is approximately 10–20 μg.l^{-1}.

The absorption of orally-administered pamidronate is poor and in rats has been estimated at approximately 0.2% of the administered dose.[30] Currently, the drug is generally available only for intravenous use. There is no presystemic metabolism. Plasma pamidronate levels reach steady-state between 1–2 hours after commencing intravenous infusions of 0.125–0.25 mg.min^{-1} in man, consistent with its half life. Levels decline rapidly when administration is terminated with a plasma half life of approximately 30 min.[31] Studies in rodents using radiolabelled pamidronate, have revealed accumulation of the drug principally in bone (approximately 50% of the administered dose), with significant uptake also in the liver, spleen and tracheal cartilage.[32,33] The proportion of pamidronate bound to plasma proteins varies with concentration but tends to be low — less than 14%. The volume of distribution approximates to that of the estimated total body water space.[32] The kidney is the principal site of elimination where it is excreted unchanged; it has been estimated that approximately 50% of an infused dose of pamidronate is excreted in the urine within 72 hours of administration.[31] The skeletal half life of pamidronate is prolonged — in the order of 1–2 years — but may be less in states of increased bone turnover.[25]

Oral absorption	poor
Presystemic metabolism	nil
Plasma half life	
mean	30 min
Volume of distribution	0.5–0.6 l.kg^{-1}
Plasma protein binding	<14

Little is known about the possible excretion of pamidronate in breast milk, but the drug is known to cross the placenta in experimental animals.

The elimination of pamidronate may be prolonged in patients with severe renal dysfunction. The effect of hepatic impairment on the kinetics of the drug are not known but it is unlikely to be of clinical significance.

Concentration–effect relationship

The biological effects of pamidronate are thought to depend on the concentrations in bone, rather than the plasma levels, although this area has not been extensively studied. In practical terms, inhibition of bone resorption starts to occur in man with doses of between 0.03–0.15 mg.kg^{-1}. Maximal effects seem to occur with doses[19,34,35] in the range 0.50–1.50 mg.kg^{-1}.

Metabolism

Pamidronate is not metabolized to any significant extent, and approximately 50% of the administered dose is excreted unchanged in the urine within 72 hours of administration.[31] Less than 0.1% of the dose appears in bile and there is no evidence of significant enterohepatic circulation.

Pharmaceutics

Pamidronate is currently available in parenteral form only for routine clinical use.

1. Aredia (Ciba, UK): for intravenous infusion containing 3 mg.ml^{-1} pamidronate disodium (anhydrous). The 5 ml ampoules contain 15 mg pamidronate disodium, 250 mg mannitol and water for Injection. The pH is approximately 6.5.

Pamidronate is stable at 4°C for 1–2 years. It should be diluted before use in calcium-free solutions (e.g. saline or dextrose) to an approximate concentration of 0.1 mg.ml^{-1}. The diluted solution should not be stored for prolonged periods before use.

Therapeutic use

Indications

1. For the treatment of accelerated bone resorption in cancer-associated hypercalcaemia
2. (Unlicensed) The treatment of accelerated bone resorption and hypercalcaemia in other malignant and non-malignant conditions.

Contraindications

1. History of allergy to bisphosphonates.

Mode of use

All the clinical indications for pamidronate depend on its action as an inhibitor of bone resorption. Intravenous treatment is given after dilution of the concentrate with an appropriate volume of a calcium-free solution (e.g. 0.9% saline or 5% dextrose) to a final concentration of 0.1 mg.ml^{-1}. Intravenous infusions of between 15 and 90 mg are administered over 2–8 hours, at a rate not exceeding 15 mg.h^{-1}. Treatment is usually given as a single slow infusion, but the dose may be divided and given on consecutive days.[19,20,35–38] Rapid rates of infusion and bolus injections should be avoided, because of the theoretical risk of nephrotoxicity as the result of deposition of calcium-bisphosphonate complexes in the kidney.[39]

Pamidronate is also active when given by mouth[13,17,23,40,41] but the oral formulation is not yet available for routine clinical use.

Indications

1. Cancer-associated hypercalcaemia

Pamidronate is usually given after an initial period of rehydration with 6–8 l of 0.9% saline over 1–2 days. Hypercalcaemia improves in virtually all patients, even with doses as low as 5 mg, but it is more usual to give doses in the range 15–60 mg.[19,37,38,42] Total doses of 90 mg have been given by single infusion in some cases.[44] The dose of pamidronate has been divided and given as separate infusions on consecutive days to a total of 150 mg,[36,45] but this offers no advantage in terms of clinical response.[20,38] The percentage of patients achieving normocalcaemia with pamidronate varies between 50–100%.[15,18–20,36,43] Some workers believe that higher doses give a more complete response,[34,44] but this has been disputed.[19,42] Those with local osteolytic hypercalcaemia (e.g. myeloma, some cases of breast carcinoma) tend to respond better than those with humoral hypercalcaemia[46,47] (e.g squamous cancer) since in the latter, the elevation in blood calcium is partly due to an increase in renal tubular calcium reabsorption.[47]

In general terms, patients with recurrent hypercalcaemia appear to require increasing doses of pamidronate to maintain an equivalent response.[19] Complete resistance to pamidronate is rare, but may occur in patients with advanced disease.[37] Pamidronate has not been used in the presence of severe renal failure, but with moderate renal impairment (serum creatinine 250–300 μmol.l^{-1}) low doses (i.e. 5–15 mg) have been successfully used without further deterioration in renal function.

2. Other uses

Both oral and intravenous pamidronate have been successfully used in the treatment of a variety of other conditions associated with increased bone resorption, including; Paget's disease of bone[16–18] steroid-induced osteoporosis,[22] post-menopausal osteoporosis,[23] hypercalcaemia due to immobilization,[48] thyrotoxicosis[49] and metastatic bone disease.[12,31,50–52] In Paget's disease, various regimens of pamidronate have been used ranging from oral treatment[11] to intravenous infusions of between 30–45 mg, divided as daily infusions for one week, or on a single occasion each week, on a three-monthly basis.[16,18] All have been successful in improving symptoms and biochemical manifestations of the disease. In patients with bone metastases due to breast cancer and prostate cancer, intravenous pamidronate (30 mg weekly or two-weekly) and oral treatment have been variously shown to improve bone pain, biochemical parameters of bone resorption and skeletal morbidity.[12,50,51,52] Oral pamidronate has also been shown to increase bone mass in steroid-induced osteoporosis and post-menopausal osteoporosis.[22,23]

At present, pamidronate is not licensed in the UK for any of the above conditions.

Adverse reactions

Potentially life-threatening effects

None has been reported.

Acute overdosage

No cases have been reported, but hypocalcaemia may occur and should be reversed by an infusion of calcium gluconate.

Severe or irreversible adverse effects

Pyrexia and acute-phase response. Between 20–30% of patients treated with pamidronate experience a mild pyrexia (38–40°C) within 24–72 hours of drug administration, usually after first exposure to the drug.[53,54] The pyrexia is usually asymptomatic and does not require treatment, but rigors may occur. Associated symptoms may include; malaise and an increase in bone pain in patients with Paget's disease of bone.[17] For reasons which are unclear, the above complication seems to be more common in patients where pamidronate is being given for benign disease (e.g. Paget's, osteoporosis)[54]. Laboratory abnormalities associated with the above include, reduced serum zinc, raised ESR and C-reactive protein levels and mild lymphopenia.[17,27] All are self-limiting and normal values are restored after a few days.

Less common adverse effects which have been described in patients

Pamidronate (disodium pentahydrate)

treated with pamidronate include thrombophlebitis in patients receiving repeated infusions[45] and seizures in hypercalcaemic cancer patients with brain metastases.[38] While it is impossible to ascribe a cause–effect relationship in these situations, the association remains. One patient with severe renal dysfunction (creatinine = 600 μmol.l^{-1}) due to myeloma has been described in whom renal failure deteriorated after treatment with low dose pamidronate.[55] Again a cause–effect relationship remains unclear, since in most pamidronate-treated patients, renal function has been unchanged or improved.[19,36,55,56]

Symptomatic adverse effects

Hypocalcaemia. Mild hypocalcaemia has been recorded in some patients treated with pamidronate,[15,43,57] but in most cases has been asymptomatic and has not required treatment. Clinically apparent hypocalcaemia is rare but may require treatment with intravenous calcium salts.[57]

Hypophosphataemia. A transient fall in serum inorganic phosphate levels typically occurs in hypercalcaemic patients within 3–5 days of starting treatment. This is self-limiting, asymptomatic and usually corrects spontaneously within 10–14 days.

Interference with clinical pathology tests

No technical interferences appear to have been reported.

High risk groups

There is almost no published experience on pamidronate's use in children, neonates, nursing or pregnancy mothers. A recent report of the use of pamidronate, 30 mg, in the last trimester of pregnancy indicated no long term adverse effects for mother or fetus. Low plasma calcium levels were observed in the child in the first week after delivery and it was suggested that plasma calcium should be monitored for 1 week after delivery.[60]

The elderly

The drug may be used provided that renal function is not severely impaired.

Drug interactions

Potentially hazardous interactions

Pamidronate has been used in combination with a variety of antineoplastic and antihypercalcaemic drugs and to date, no hazardous interactions have been documented.

Potentially useful interactions

In patients with severe hypercalcaemia, pamidronate has been successfully combined with both calcitonin[58] and mithramycin[59] to accelerate and potentiate the calcium-lowering effect.

Randomized comparative studies

1. Ralston S H, Dryburgh F J, Cowan R A et al 1985 Comparison of aminohydroxypropylidene disphosphonate, mithramycin and corticosteroids/calcitonin in treatment of cancer-associated hypercalcaemia. Lancet 2: 907–910

Pamidronate (15 mg daily intravenously for a mean of 6 days) was compared with mithramycin (25 μg.kg^{-1} on 2 consecutive days) and corticosteroids/calcitonin (prednisolone 40 mg a day, calcitonin 100 units i.v. three times daily) in 39 patients with cancer-associated hypercalcaemia. Patients were randomised into three treatment groups of 13 patients each and were rehydrated with normal saline before treatment. All three regimens lowered serum calcium values, but pamidronate-treated patients had lower serum calcium values 9 days after treatment than patients in both other treatment groups.

2. Ralston S H, Gallacher S J, Patel U et al 1989 Comparison of three intravenous bisphosphonates in cancer-associated hypercalcaemia. Lancet 2: 1180–1182

Three intravenous bisphosphonates were compared in the treatment of cancer-associated hypercalcaemia. 48 patients were randomly allocated to one of three treatment groups (each with 16 subjects)–30 mg pamidronate or 600 mg clodronate, both as single intravenous infusions; or etidronate as three infusions of 7.5 mg kg^{-1} per day for three consecutive days. Patients were rehydrated with normal saline before bisphosphonate treatment. All three bisphosphonates lowered serum calcium by inhibition of bone resorption; pamidronate was the most potent in this respect. By comparison with the other groups, more patients in the pamidronate group became normocalcaemic, and effect on serum calcium was apparent sooner and lasted longer.

General review articles

Fleisch H 1982 Bisphosphonates: mechanisms of action and clinical applications. In: Peck W A (ed) Bone and mineral research, Annual 1. Excerpta Medica, Amsterdam, pp 319–357

Bijvoet O L M 1990 Pamidronate (APD) in cancer therapy - the pharmacological background. In: Rubens R D (ed) The management of bone metastases and hypercalcaemia by osteoclast inhibition. Hogrefe and Huber, Toronto, pp 13–27

Dodwell D J, Murphy D J, Howell A 1991 Bisphosphonates for bone metastases. Proceedings of the Royal College of Physicians of Edinburgh 21: 8–15

References

1. Fleisch H, Neuman W F 1961 Mechanisms of calcification: role of collagen, polyphosphates and phosphatase. American Journal of Physiology 200: 1296–1300
2. Schibler D, Russell R G G, Fleisch H 1968 Inhibition of pyrophosphate and polyphosphate on aortic calcification induced by vitamin D in rats. Clinical Science 35: 363–372
3. Fleisch H, Russell R G G, Bisaz S 1970 The inhibitory effect of phosphonates on the formation of calcium phosphate crystals in vitro and on aortic and kidney calcification in vivo. European Journal of Clinical Investigation 1: 12–18
4. Francis M D 1969 The inhibition of calcium hydroxyapapite crystal growth by polyphosphates. Calcified Tissue Research 3: 151–162
5. Subramanian G, McAffee J G 1971 A new complex of ^{99m}Tc for skeletal imaging. Radiology 99: 192–196
6. Fleisch H, Russell RGG, Francis MD 1969 Disphosphonates inhibit hydroxyapatite dissolution in vitro and bone resorption in tissue culture and in vivo. Science 165: 1262–1244
7. Stutzer A, Trechsel U, Fleisch H 1987 Effect of diphosphonates on osteoclast number and bone resorption in the rat. Journal of Bone and Mineral Research 2 (Suppl 1): 266
8. Hughes D E, MacDonald B R, Russell R G G, Gowen M 1989 Inhibition of osteoclast-like cell formation by bisphosphonates in long-term cultures of human bone marrow. Journal of Clinical Investigation 83: 1930–1935
9. Boonekamp P M, van der Wee-Pals L J A, van Wijk-van Lennep M L L, Thesing C W, Bijvoet O L M 1986 Two modes of action of bisphosphonates on osteoclastic resorption of mineralised matrix. Bone and Mineral 1: 27–39
10. Lowik C W G M, van der Pliujm G, van der Wee-Pals L J A, van Treslong-de Groot H B, Bijvoet O L M 1988 Migration and phenotypic transformation of osteoclast precursors into mature osteoclasts: the effect of a bisphosphonate. Journal of Bone Mineral Research 3: 185–192
11. Reitsma P H, Bijvoet O L M, Verlinden-Ooms H, van der Wee-Pals L J A 1980 Kinetic studies of bone and mineral metabolism during treatment with (3-amino-1-hydroxypropylidene)-1,1-bisphosphonate (APD) in rats. Calcified Tissue International 32: 145–147
12. Dodwell D J, Howell A, Ford J 1990 Reduction in calcium excretion in women with breast cancer and bone metastases using the oral bisphosphonate, pamidronate. British Journal of Cancer 61: 123–125
13. van Breukelen F J M, Bijvoet O L M, Frijlink W B, Sleeboom H P, Mulder H, van Oosterom A T 1982 Efficacy of amino-hydroxypropylidene bisphosphonate in hypercalcemia: observations on regulation of serum calcium. Calcified Tissue International 34: 321–327
14. Ralston S H, Hacking L, Willocks L, Pitkeathly D A 1989 Clinical, biochemical and radiographic effects of aminohydroxypropylidene bisphosphonate treatment in rheumatoid arthritis. Annals of Rheumatic Disease 48: 396–399
15. Sleeboom H P, Bijvoet O L M, van Oosterom A T, Gleed J H, O'Riordan J L H 1983 Comparison of intravenous (3-amino-1-hydroxypropylidene)-1,1-bisphosphonate and volume repletion in tumour-induced hypercalcaemia. Lancet 2: 239–234
16. Cantrill J A, Buckler H M, Anderson D C 1986 Low dose intravenous 3-amino-1-hydroxypropylidene-1,1-bisphosphonate (APD) for the treatment of Paget's disease of bone. Annals of Rheumatic Disease 45: 1012–1018
17. Harinck H I J, Papapoulos S E, Blanksma H J, Moolenar A J, Vermeij P, Bijvoet O L M 1987 Paget's disease of bone: early and late responses to three different modes of treatment with aminohydroxypropylidene bisphosphonate (APD). British Medical Journal 295: 1301–1305
18. Thiebaud D, Jaeger Ph, Gobelet C, Jacquet A F, Burckhardt P 1988 A single infusion of the bisphosphonate AHPrBP (APD) as treatment of Paget's disease of bone. American Journal of Medicine 85: 207–212
19. Ralston S H, Alzaid A A, Gallacher S J et al 1988 Clinical experience with aminohydroxypropylidene bisphosphonate in the management of cancer-associated hypercalcaemia. Quarterly Journal of Medicine 69: 825–834
20. Morton A R, Cantrill J A, Craig A E, Howell A, Davies M, Anderson D C 1988 Single dose versus daily intravenous aminohydroxypropylidene bisphosphonate (APD) for the hypercalcaemia of malignancy. British Medical Journal 296: 811–814
21. Bijvoet O L M 1990 Pamidronate (APD) in cancer therapy — the pharmacological background. In: Rubens R D (ed) The management of bone metastases and hypercalcaemia by osteoclast inhibition. Hogrefe and Huber, Toronto, pp 13–27

Pamidronate (disodium pentahydrate)

22. Reid I R, King R A, Alexander C J, Ibbertson H K 1988 Prevention of steroid-induced osteoporosis with (3-amino-1-hydroxypropylidene)-1,1-bisphosphonate (APD). Lancet 1: 143–146
23. Valkema R, Vismans F J E E, Papapoulos S E, Pauwels E K J, Bijvoet O L M 1989 Maintained improvement in calcium balance and bone mineral content in patients with osteoporosis treated with the bisphosphonate APD. Bone and Mineral 5: 183–192
24. Hoeckman K, Papapoulos S E, Peters A C B, Bijvoet O L M 1985 Characteristics and bisphosphonate treatment of a patient with juvenile osteoporosis. Journal of Clinical Endocrinology and Metabolism 61: 952–956
25. de Vries E, van der Weij J P, van der Veen C J P et al 1982 In vitro effect of (3-amino-1-hydroxypropylidene)-1,1-bisphosphonic acid (APD) on the function of mononuclear phagocytes in lymphocyte proliferation. Immunology 47: 157–163
26. Gallacher S J, Ralston S H, Patel U, Boyle I T 1989 Side effects of pamidronate. Lancet 2: 42–43
27. Adami S, Bhalla A K, Dorrizi R et al 1987 The acute phase response after bisphosphonate administration. Calcified Tissue International 41: 326–331
28. Daley-Yates P T, Gifford L A, Hoggarth C R 1989 Assay of 1-hydroxy-3-aminopropylidene-1,1-bisphosphonate and related bisphosphonates in human urine and plasma by high performance ion chromatography. Journal of Chromatography and Biomedical Applications 490: 329–338
29. Flesch G, Hauffe S A 1989 Determination of the bisphosphonate, pamidronate disodium in urine by pre-collumn derivatization with fluorescamine, high performance liquid chromatography and fluorescence detection. Journal of Chromatography 489: 446–451
30. Reitsma P H, Bijvoet O L M, Potokar M, van der Wee-Pals L J A, van Wijk-van Lennep M M L 1983 Apposition and resorption of bone during oral treatment with (3-amino-1-hydroxypropylidene)-1,1-bisphosphonate (APD). Calcified Tissue International 35: 357–361
31. Dodwell D J, Howell A, Morton A, Daley-Yates P T, Hoggarth C R 1990 Pamidronate (APD) treatment of skeletal metastases from breast cancer. In: Rubens R D (ed) The management of bone metastases and hypercalcaemia by osteoclast inhibition. Hogrefe and Huber, Toronto, pp 62–75
32. Daley-Yates P T, Bennet R 1988 A comparison of the pharmacokinetics of 14C-labelled APD and 99mTc-labelled APD in the mouse. Calcified Tissue International 43: 125–127
33. Wingen F, Schmahl D 1987 Pharmacokinetics of the osteotropic diphosphonate 3-amino-1-hydroxypropane-1,1-diphosphonic acid in mammals. Arzneimittelforschung/Drug Research 37: 1037–1042
34. Thiebaud D, Jaeger Ph, Jacquet A F, Burckhardt P 1988 Dose–response in the treatment of hypercalcemia of malignancy by a single infusion of the bisphosphonate AHPrBP. Journal of Clinical Oncology 6: 762–768
35. Body J J, Pot M, Borkowski A, Sculier J P, Klastersky J 1987 Dose–response study of aminohydroxypropylidene bisphosphonate in tumor-associated hypercalcemia. American Journal of Medicine 82: 957–963
36. Harinck H I J, Bijvoet O L M, Platingh A S T et al 1987 Role of bone and kidney in tumor-induced hypercalcemia and its treatment with bisphosphonate and sodium chloride. American Journal of Medicine 82: 1133–1142
37. Coleman R E, Rubens R D (3-amino-1,1-hydroxypropylidene) bisphosphonate for hypercalcaemia of breast cancer. British Journal of Cancer 56: 465–469
38. Yates A J P, Jerums G J, Murray R M L, Martin T J A comparison of single and multiple intravenous infusions of 3-amino-1,1-hydroxypropylidene bisphosphonate (APD) in the treatment of hypercalcaemia of malignancy. Australian and New Zealand Journal of Medicine 17: 387–391
39. Bijvoet O L M, Frijlink W B, Jie K et al 1980 APD in Paget's disease of bone: role of the mononuclear phagocyte system? Arthritis and Rheumatology 23: 1193–1204
40. Thiebaud D, Portmann L, Jaeger Ph, Jacquet A F, Burckhardt P 1986 Oral versus intravenous AHPrBP (APD) in the treatment of hypercalcaemia of malignancy. Bone 7: 247–253
41. van Holten-Verzanthvoort ATh, Bijvoet O L M, Cleton F J et al 1987 Reduced morbidity from skeletal metastases in breast cancer patients during long-term bisphosphonate (APD) treatment. Lancet 2: 983–985
42. Davis J R E, Heath D A 1989 Comparison of different dose regimens of aminohydroxypropylidene -1,1-bisphosphonate (APD) in hypercalcaemia of malignancy. British Journal of Clinical Pharmacology 28: 269–274
43. Thiebaud D, Jaeger P, Gobelet C, Jacquet A F, Burckhardt P et al 1988 A single infusion of the bisphosphonate AHPrBP (APD) as treatment of Paget's disease of bone. American Journal of Medicine 85: 207–212
44. Nussbaum S R, Mallette L, Gagel R, Chapman R, Henderson G, Vandepol C 1990 Pamidronate (APD) treatment of hypercalcaemia associated with malignancy — preliminary report of a multicentre double-blind trial. In: Rubens R D (ed) The management of bone metastases and hypercalcaemia by osteoclast inhibition. Hogrefe and Huber, Toronto, pp 44–46
45. Ralston S H, Dryburgh F J, Cowan R A, Gardner M D, Jenkins A S, Boyle I T 1985 Comparison of aminohydroxypropylidene diphosphonate, mithramycin and corticosteroids/calcitonin in treatment of cancer-associated hypercalcaemia. Lancet 2: 907–910
46. Gurney H, Kefford R, Stuart-Harris R 1989 Renal phosphate threshold and response to pamidronate in humoral hypercalcaemia of malignancy. Lancet 1: 241–244
47. Ralston S H, Gardner M D, Jenkins A S, McKillop J A, Boyle I T 1987 Malignancy-associated hypercalcaemia: relationship between mechanisms of hypercalcaemia and response to antihypercalcaemic therapy. Bone and Mineral 2: 227–242
48. McIntyre H D, Cameron D P, Urquhart S M, Davies W E 1989 Immobilisation hypercalcaemia responding to intravenous pamidronate therapy. Postgraduate Medical Journal 65: 244–246
49. Tan T T, Alzaid A A, Sutcliffe N, Gardner M D, Thomson J A, Boyle I T 1988 Treatment of hypercalcaemia in thyrotoxicosis with aminohydroxypropylidene diphosphonate. Postgraduate Medical Journal 64: 224–227
50. Clarke N W, McClure J, George N J R 1990 Subjective and metabolic effects of aminohydroxypropylidene bisphosphonate (APD) in patients with advanced cancer of the prostate — preliminary report. In: Rubens R D (ed) The management of bone metastases and hypercalcaemia by osteoclast inhibition. Hogrefe and Huber, Toronto, pp 81–89
51. Coleman R E, Woll P J, Miles M, Scrivener M, Rubens R D 1988 Treatment of bone metastases from breast cancer with (3-amino-1-hydroxypropylidene)-1,1-bisphosphonate (APD). British Journal of Cancer 58: 621–625
52. Morton A R, Cantrill J A, Pillai G V et al Sclerosis of lytic bone metastases after disodium aminohydroxypropylidene bisphosphonate (APD) in patients with breast carcinoma. British Medical Journal 297: 772–773
53. Frijlink W B, Bijvoet O L M, Te Velde J, Heynen G 1979 Treatment of Paget's disease with (3-amino-1-hydroxypropylidene)-1,1-bisphosphonate (APD). Lancet 1: 799–803
54. Gallagher S J, Ralston S H, Patel U, Boyle I T 1989 Side effects of pamidronate. Lancet 2: 42–43
55. Morton A R, Dodwell D J, Howell A 1989 Disodium pamidronate (APD) for the management of hypercalcaemia of malignancy: comparative studies of single-dose versus daily infusions and of infusion duration. In: Burckhardt P (ed) Disodium pamidronate (APD) in the treatment of malignancy-related disorders. Hogrefe and Huber, Toronto, pp 85–89
56. Cantwell B M J, Harris A L 1987 Effect of single high dose infusions of aminohydroxypropylidene diphosphonate on hypercalcaemia caused by cancer. British Medical Journal 294: 467–469
57. Jodrell D I, Iveson T J, Smith I E 1987 Symptomatic hypocalcaemia after treatment with high dose aminohydroxypropylidene bisphosphonate. Lancet 1: 622
58. Ralston S, Alzaid A A, Gardner M D, Boyle I T 1986 Treatment of cancer-associated hypercalcaemia with combined aminohydroxypropylidene diphosphonate and calcitonin. British Medical Journal, 292: 1549–1550
59. Ralston S H, Gallacher S J, Dryburgh F J, Cowan Ra A, Boyle I T 1988 Treatment of severe hypercalcaemia with mithramycin and aminohydroxyproplidene bisphosphonate. Lancet, ii: 277 (letter)
60. Dunlop D J, Soukop M, McEwan H P 1990 Antenatal administration of aminopropylidene diphosphonate. Annals of Rheumatic Diseases 49: 955

Pancuronium bromide

Pancuronium has been one of the most widely used non-depolarizing neuromuscular blocking agents for over 15 years and has an excellent safety record.

Chemistry

Pancuronium bromide (Pavulon)
$C_{35}H_{60}N_2O_4.Br_2$
2β,16β-Dipiperidino-5α-androstane-3α,17β-dioldiacetate dimethobromide

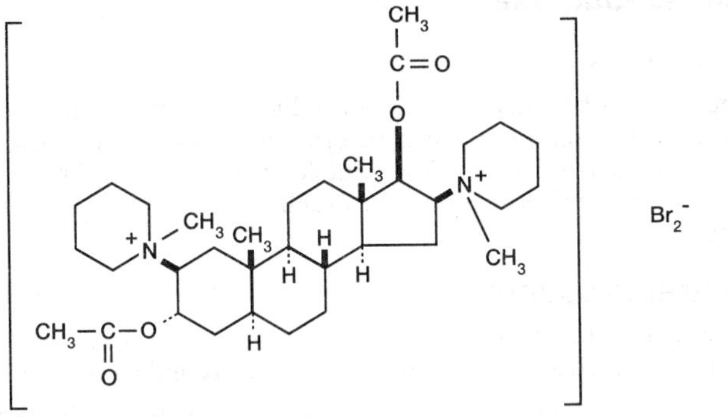

Molecular weight (free base)	732.7 (572.9)
pKa	—
Solubility	
in alcohol	1 in 5
in water	1 in 1
Octanol/water partition coefficient	low

Pancuronium bromide is an androstane-based neuromuscular blocking agent developed by Organon Laboratories in Scotland. It has two acetylcholine-like molecules in the 2-3 and the 16-17 positions on the steroid ring. The bisquaternary structure gives it its nicotinic receptor blocking properties and its strong positive charge. The muscarinic-blocking side effects are largely associated with the stereoisometric position of the 3-acetyl group.[1]

The compound is prepared by chemical synthesis, as odourless, white crystals with a bitter taste. It is dextrorotatory in water.

Pharmacology

Pancuronium is a potent neuromuscular blocking agent whose action is limited to the postsynaptic nicotinic receptors in clinical dosages.[2] Although Gergis et al[3] have demonstrated depression of acetylcholine release from stimulated frog's nerve following the administration of pancuronium in moderately high doses, it has not been shown to have any significant presynaptic effect in man. There is experimental evidence of channel block, but only in higher dosages than used clinically. The principal side effects are upon the cardiovascular system, where it causes tachycardia at four times the ED_{90} (where ED_{90} is the dose derived from log-dose response that gives 90% depression of isometric twitch response) and hypertension, especially during light anaesthesia. The tachycardia is related to a combination of muscarinic blocking action,[4] and block of the inhibitory vagal action upon resting sympathetic tone.[5] Hypertension is associated with block of noradrenaline reuptake one[6,7] (reuptake two is only blocked at high doses). It has little histamine-releasing action,[8] but antagonizes cholinesterase in doses producing neuromuscular block.[9] It has no hormonal activity.

Toxicology

Pancuronium has not been shown to have any organic system toxicity or teratogenicity as used in clinical practice. Anaphylactoid responses have been reported with pancuronium but the occurrence is rare.[10]

Clinical pharmacology

Neuromuscular activity

Pancuronium produces neuromuscular block. The onset time for neuromuscular block in the thumb adductor muscles is 60–90 seconds (depending upon dose and rate of administration), but good tracheal intubating conditions are seldom achieved in under 3 minutes. In conscious volunteers, 90% depression of grip strength is seen at a dose of $0.025\ mg.kg^{-1}$. In anaesthetized patients, the ED_{90} dose varies from 0.02 to $0.05\ mg.kg^{-1}$, depending upon the type of anaesthetic used. Isoflurane and enflurane potentiate its action to a greater extent than halothane whilst balanced or neuroleptic anaesthesia has the least effect.[11,12]

In clinical practice the usual dose range for bolus administration varies between $0.05\ mg.kg^{-1}$ and $0.15\ mg.kg^{-1}$. At low doses recovery to 90% twitch response takes 15–20 minutes whilst at doses of $0.08\ mg.kg^{-1}$, recovery takes about 65 minutes and at $0.1\ mg.kg^{-1}$ the time to 90% recovery of the twitch response is about 74 minutes.[13] There is considerable individual variation in both the amount and duration of its action.

Provided the plasma level is low and there is 10% recovery of the twitch or the first two of a train of four responses are present, reversal by neostigmine or edrophonium is readily achieved. Reports of difficulty in reversal or incomplete reversal have usually been associated with conditions that prevent adequate rapid lowering of plasma level, e.g. renal disease[14,15] or excessive use of aminoglycoside antibiotics.[16]

Cardiovascular effects

As the dose of pancuronium is increased, the vagolytic actions become more pronounced. At four times the ED_{90} complete vagal block occurs.[17] This effect has also been demonstrated in the isolated perfused rabbit heart preparation, either challenged with acetylcholine or following vagal stimulation.[18] A contributory cause of the tachycardia is the abolition of the vagal postsynaptic inhibition of sympathetic cardiac nerves.

Unlike tubocurarine, pancuronium has no effect on autonomic ganglia in doses up to 15 times the ED_{90}.

Hypertension is not uncommon following pancuronium administration during light anaesthesia, especially if stimulating manoeuvres such as endotracheal intubation are performed. This appears to be the result of a block of noradrenaline reuptake-one.[6,7] Reuptake at secondary sites is only blocked at very high plasma levels of drug.

Histamine-induced hypotension is not seen with clinical doses of the drug.

Other effects

Lebowitz and co-workers[19] demonstrated that mixing pancuronium with metocurarine had a positive synergistic effect. This has been suggested as indicating differing accessibility to the two asymmetrically placed receptor sites for non-depolarizing drugs at the cholinoceptor on the postsynaptic junction.[20]

Pancuronium has no effect on cerebral activity, on CSF pressure, on intraocular pressure or on pupil size. Peripheral resistance and cardiac output are well maintained following its administration.

Pharmacokinetics

The method of analysis most commonly used for pancuronium is spectrofluorimetry[21] It is difficult with this method to separate metabolites from the parent compound. The sensitivity is of the order of $2\ \mu g.l^{-1}$. More recently, more specific HPLC methods have been used and give very similar results. It has been estimated that in cats between 10 and 35% of an injected dose may be metabolized (probably less in man except in the case of high dose, prolonged use or poor renal function).[22]

Pancuronium is a water-soluble, lipophobic, highly ionized molecule. As a consequence it cannot be used orally. Following intravenous injection its α volume of distribution consists of the extracellular fluid, the vessel-rich areas of muscles, the kidneys, the liver and the spleen. Unlike tubocurarine, it is not taken up in the salivary

Pancuronium bromide

P

glands. Within 5 minutes of injection the greatest concentration is found in the kidney, followed by the liver and spleen. Provided renal blood flow is maintained, urinary excretion begins within minutes of injection. The distribution half life of the drug is approximately 4 minutes. During the β phase (half life 32 min) pancuronium concentration in muscle increases; at the same time there is increasing urinary loss of drug, and biliary excretion, which varies from 5 to 30% of injected dose in humans, occurs. Metabolism, which may account for up to 25% of the drug administered, produces metabolites which are excreted both in the bile and in the urine. Up to 25% of the dose is excreted unchanged in the urine. The principal metabolite is the 3-hydroxy derivative, which also has the highest neuromuscular potency of the metabolites of of pancuronium.[23] The 17-OH and 3,17-OH metabolites have only 2% of the activity of the parent compound. The Vd_{ss} for pancuronium in anaesthetized man is variously given as between 0.21 and 0.37 $l.kg^{-1}$. Vd is[24–26] between 0.28 and 0.34 $l.kg^{-1}$.

Plasma clearance at steady-state concentrations varies according to method of study and is given as 0.9–2.1 $ml.kg^{-1}.min^{-1}$.

Metabolism and biliary excretion are both depressed in liver disease, especially jaundice.[27] In patients with cirrhosis of the liver the Vd is increased by about 50% and the plasma clearance decreased.[28,29]

Plasma clearance is markedly depressed by a fall in renal blood flow, in oliguric and anuric states.

Various figures for protein binding of pancuronium have been obtained depending upon the in vitro methodology.[30,31] It is usual to consider about 30% as being bound to plasma protein but the binding is weak and of little pharmacokinetic significance. No correlation has been demonstrated between dosage or volume of distribution and any particular serum protein fraction.

Very little pancuronium crosses the placenta, as might be expected from its high water solubility. Specific information on the excretion of pancuronium in breast milk is not available but is unlikely to occur to any great extent. In patients with renal failure and in subjects with age-related reduction in renal function the half life of the drug is increased and its clearance reduced such that there may be some prolongation of the duration of action of the compound. In hepatic disease there may be an increase in the volume of distribution by up to 50%, resulting in a reduction of the effect of the drug. However, there may also be an increase in the half life, resulting in a prolongation of recovery from the drug.

Oral absorption	negligible
Presystemic metabolism	nil
Plasma half life	32 min
Volume of distribution	0.21–0.37 $l.kg^{-1}$
Plasma protein binding	30%

Concentration–effect relationship

The steady-state plasma concentration that produces good surgical relaxation is about 200 $\mu g.l^{-1}$. It is impractical to monitor the plasma level of the drug during anaesthesia, but it is recommended that the biological effect is followed using a neuromuscular block monitor, during the use of all neuromuscular blocking agents.

Metabolism

Between 5 and 25% of an injected dose of pancuronium undergoes metabolism in the liver. The principal metabolite is the 3-hydroxy derivative but 17-hydroxy and 3,17-dihydroxypancuronium are also formed (Fig. 1). The 3-hydroxy compound has significant neuromuscular blocking activity — about 40% that of the parent compound.

Pharmaceutics

The drug is soluble in water and acetic acid is added to give a solution of pH 4. It is marketed as Pavulon (Organon-Teknika, UK) presented in 2 ml ampoules containing 2 $mg.ml^{-1}$. At room temperature it has a shelf-life of over 6 months with minimal loss of potency. At 2 to 8°C, it can be stored for over 2 years.

Therapeutic use

Indications

Pancuronium bromide is used to produce neuromuscular block for muscle relaxation during surgical procedures. Due to its slow onset and prolonged action, it is less suitable for short surgical procedures than the newer short-acting drugs such as vecuronium and atracurium.

Contraindications

1. Patients with anuria
2. Hypersensitivity to pancuronium or the bromide ion.

In common with all neuromuscular blocking agents, the drug should not be administered in any situation where control of the airway and artificial ventilation cannot be ensured.

Mode of use

For intubation a bolus intravenous dose of 0.1–0.15 $mg.kg^{-1}$ is required. Adequate relaxation of the jaw usually takes three minutes to develop. This dose of pancuronium bromide will produce adequate surgical relaxation for most patients for 40–60 minutes; however, return of adequate neuromuscular conduction as judged by the train of four responses (1:4 twitch > 70% at 2 Hz) may take 90 minutes. Because of the slow recovery, it is preferable to reverse the effect of the drug using neostigmine (2.5 mg intravenously accompanied by

Fig. 1 Metabolism of pancuronium bromide

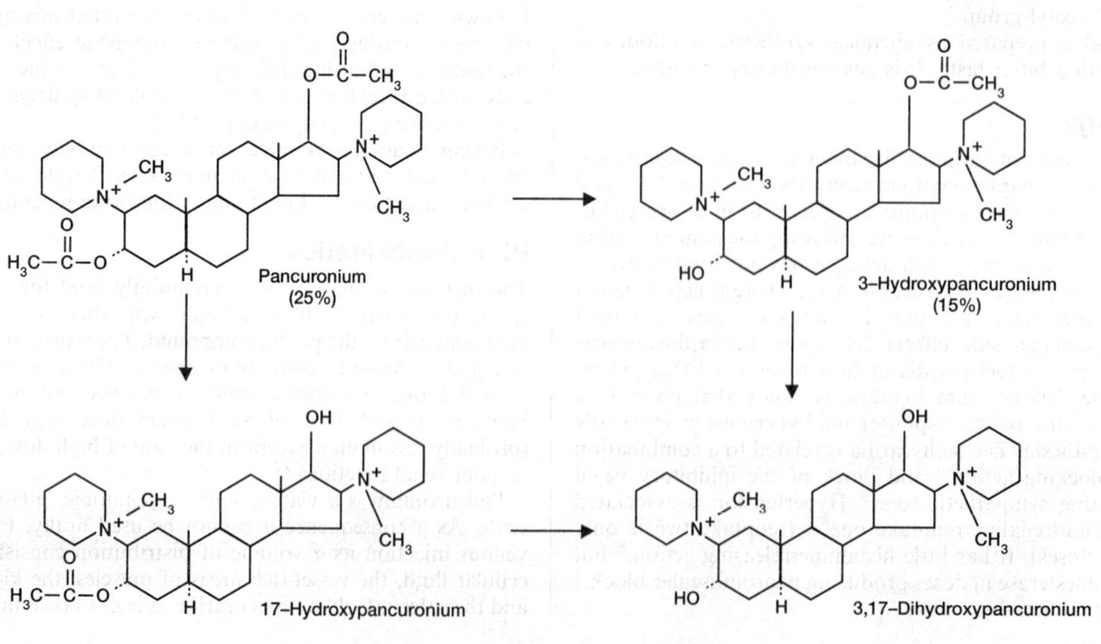

atropine 0.5–1.0 mg or glycopyrrolate 1 ml (0.2 mg drug) to prevent bradycardia).

For longer procedures and for use in the intensive care unit, repeated 'top-up' doses of 0.05 mg.kg^{-1} pancuronium are required at intervals of approximately 60 minutes but due to the marked cumulative nature of the response and individual pharmacokinetic variability, repeated administration for prolonged relaxation should be controlled using a nerve stimulator to determine the state of recovery before additional doses are administered. Unless the dose of pancuronium used has been very modest and carefully monitored, prolonged use in the ITU often results in a very slow, prolonged recovery of neuromuscular conduction.

Pancuronium is largely excreted in the urine and it should be used with caution in patients with renal disease. As with most quaternary neuromuscular blocking agents, patients with hepatic disease may require larger than normal doses.

Pancuronium is well tolerated in elderly patients and those with compromised cardiovascular systems. Because of its propensity to potentiate the action of endogenous catecholamines, it should not be administered in too light a state of anaesthesia or to patients with autonomic system instability such as occurs in some patients with tetanus.

Adverse reactions

Potentially life-threatening effects
Pancuronium is non-toxic even in very high doses, provided artificial ventilation is used to overcome respiratory paralysis. Anaphylactoid reactions have very rarely been reported and in some circumstances might be life-threatening.

Acute overdosage
Acute overdose has no meaning as the drug is always given in a paralytic, hence potentially toxic dose. Treatment is always the same: artificial ventilation until blood concentration is subtherapeutic, that is less than that which causes paralysis.

Severe or irreversible adverse effects
None has been reported.

Symptomatic adverse effects
Tachycardia may occur, due to vagal blockade and especially during light anaesthesia, mild hypertension may be observed.

Interference with clinical pathology tests

No interference of this kind has been reported.

High risk groups

Neonates
The drug may be used in neonates in appropriate doses. It should be noted that in neonates the usual sensitivity to non-depolarizing agents is also demonstrated by pancuronium.

Breast milk. It is not known whether pancuronium enter breast milk, but absorption from the gastrointestinal tract is unlikely to be sufficient to affect the breast-fed infant.

Children
The drug may be used in children in appropriate doses.

Pregnant women
The drug can be safely used in pregnant women.

The elderly
No problems are likely to be encountered in elderly patients with reasonable renal function.

Concurrent disease

Renal disease. Patients with renal disease may demonstrate delayed recovery from large doses of the drug.[32]

Patients with sympathetic overactivity. These patients may exhibit exaggerated hypertensive response to the drug due to inhibition of catecholamine reuptake.

Hypothermia and jaundice. The action of pancuronium may be prolonged in hypothermia and in patients with jaundice.

Drug interactions

Pancuronium is potentiated by volatile anaesthetics (especially diethyl ether, isoflurane and ethrane), and local anaesthetics.[11,12]

Pancuronium bromide

Its action may be prolonged by aminoglycoside antibiotics,[16] tetracycline, and lithium carbonate,[34] while the duration of action of pancuronium may be shortened by frusemide.[35]

References

1. Savage D S, Sleigh T, Carlyle I 1980 The emergence of ORG NC45 from the pancuronium series. British Journal of Anaesthesia 52: 35
2. Baird W C M, Reid A M 1967 The neuromuscular blocking properties of a new steroid compound, pancuronium bromide. British Journal of Anaesthesia 39: 775
3. Gergis S D, Dretchen L, Sokoll M D et al 1972 Effects of pancuronium bromide on acetylcholine release. Proceedings of the Society of Experimental Biology and Medicine 139: 74
4. Saxena P R, Bonta I L 1971 Specific blockade of cardiac muscarinic receptors by pancuronium bromide. Archives Internationales de Pharmacodynamie 189: 410
5. Bowman W C 1982 Non-relaxant properties of neuromuscular blocking drugs. British Journal of Anaesthesia 54: 147
6. Ivankovich A D, Miletch D J, Albrecht R F, Zahed B 1975 The effect of pancuronium on myocardial contraction and catecholamine reuptake. Journal of Pharmacy and Pharmacology 27: 837
7. Salt P J, Barnes P K, Conway C M 1980 Inhibition of neuronal uptake of noradrenaline in isolated perfused rat heart by pancuronium and its analogues Org 6368, Org 7268, NC 45. British Journal of Anaesthesia 52: 313
8. Bodman R I 1978 Pancuronium and histamine release. Canadian Anaesthetists Society Journal 25: 40
9. Stovner J, Oft et al 1964 The inhibition of cholinesterase by pancuronium. British Journal of Anaesthesia 47: 949
10. Brauer F S, Ananthanarayan C R 1978 Histamine release by pancuronium. Anesthesiology 49: 434
11. Miller R D, Eger E I II, Way W I 1971 Comparative neuromuscular effects of pancuronium, gallamine and succinylcholine during forane and halothane anesthesia in man. Anesthesiology 35: 509
12. Swen J 1985 Neuromuscular blocking agents common interactions in daily practice. University of Leiden Thesis printed ICG
13. Katz R L 1977 Clinical neuromuscular pharmacology of pancuronium. Anesthesiology 34: 550
14. Geha D G, Blitt C D, Moon B J 1976 Prolonged neuromuscular blockade with pancuronium in the presence of acute renal failure: a case report. Anesthesia and Analgesia Current Research 58: 107
15. Pooner M A, Reves J G 1975 Aortic valve replacement in a haemodialysis department patient, anaesthetic considerations — a case report. Anesthesia and Analgesia Current Research 58: 107
16. Burkett L, Bikhazi G B, Thomas, K C Jr, Rosenthal D A, Wirton M G, Foldes F F 1979 Mutual potentiation of the neuromuscular effects of antibiotics and relaxants. Anesthesia and Analgesia Current Research 58: 107
17. Hughes R, Chapple D J 1976 Effects of non-depolarizing neuromuscular blocking agents on peripheral autonomic mechanisms in cats. British Journal of Anaesthesia 48: 59
18. Goat V A, Feldman S A 1972 The effect of non-depolarizing muscle relaxants on cholinergic mechanisms in the isolated rabbit heart. Anaesthesia 27: 149
19. Lebowitz P W, Ramsey F M, Savarese J J, Ali H H, de Bros F M 1981 Combination of pancuronium and metocurine: neuromuscular and haemodynamic advantages over pancuronium alone. Anesthesia and Analgesia Current Research 60: 1
20. Waud B E, Waud D R 1985 Interactions amongst agents that block end-plate depolarization competitively. Anesthesiology 63: 4
21. Kersten U W, Meyer D K F, Agoston S 1973 Fluorimetric and chromatographic determination of pancuronium and metabolites in biological materials. Clinica Chimica Acta 44: 59
22. Agoston S, Kersten U W, Meyer D K F 1973 Fate of pancuronium bromide in cats. Acta Anesthesiologica Scandinavica 17: 129
23. Booij L H D, Miller R D, Cruil J, Agoston S, Feldman S 1981 Comparison of pancuronium and its metabolites in the isolated arm. University of Nijmegen Press
24. Agoston S, Kersten U W 1973 The fate of pancuronium in man. Acta Anesthesiologica Scandinavica 17: 267
25. Hull C J et al 1978 A pharmacodynamic model of pancuronium. British Journal of Anaesthesia 50: 1113
26. Shanks C A, Somogyi A A, Triggs E J 1979 Dose–response and plasma concentration response relationships of pancuronium in man. Anesthesiology 51: 111
27. Ward S 1982 Pharmacokinetics of pancuronium bromide in liver failure. British Journal of Anaesthesia 54: 277p
28. Dulvaldestin P et al 1978 Pancuronium pharmacokinetics in patients with liver cirrhosis. British Journal of Anaesthesia 50: 1131
29. Somogyi A A, Shanks C A, Triggs E J 1977 Disposition kinetics of pancuronium bromide in patients with biliary obstruction. British Journal of Anaesthesia 49: 1103
30. Wood M, Stone W J, Wood AJ 1983 Plasma binding of pancuronium: effect of age, sex and disease. Anesthesia and Analgesia Current Research 62: 29
31. Thompson J M 1976 Pancuronium binding by serum proteins. Anesthesia 31: 219
32. Miller R D, Stevens W C 1973 The effect of renal failure and hyperkalaemia on the duration of pancuronium blockade in man. Anesthesia and Analgesia, Current Research 52: 661
33. Westra P et al 1980 The effect of experimental cholestasis on muscle relaxants in cats. British Journal of Anaesthesia 52: 747
34. Borden H, Clarke M T 1974 The use of pancuronium bromide in patients receiving lithium carbonate. Canadian Anaesthetists Society Journal 21(i): 79
35. Cotrell J E et al 1978 Facilitated recovery of the evoked twitch response after pancuronium and frusemide. ASA Annual Meeting Report

Papaveretum

A mixture of natural alkaloids whose action is predominantly due to its morphine content

Chemistry

Papaveretum (Omnopon)
A mixture of opium alkaloid hydrochlorides standardized to contain the equivalent of anhydrous morphine 47.5–52.5%, anhydrous codeine 2.5–5%, noscapine 16–22% and papaverine 2.5–7% (with narcotine, narceine, thebaine, hydrocotarnine, codamine, laudanine, laudanidine, laudanoeine, meconidine, papaveramine, protopine, lanthopine, cryptopine, goscopine, oxynarcodine, xanthaline and tritopine).[1]

Papaveretum is an amorphous, yellowish-brown powder, resembling finely powdered crude opium.[2] It is available in combination with hyoscine (Omnopon-Scopolamine).

Pharmacology

The pharmacology of papaveretum is predominantly that of morphine since 20 mg of papaveretum contains the equivalent of 13.3 mg of morphine sulphate. However the papaverine it contains may contribute to its effect.

Morphine is a potent analgesic with competitive agonist actions at the μ receptor which is thought to mediate many of its other actions of respiratory depression, euthoria, inhibition of gut motility and physical dependence. These actions are similar in papaveretum. It is possible that analgesia, euphoria and dependence may be due to the effects of morphine on a μ-1 receptor subtype, while respiratory depression and inhibition of gut motility may be due to actions on a μ-2 receptor subtype. Morphine is also a competitive agonist at the κ receptor which mediates spinal analgesia, miosis and sedation. Morphine has no significant actions at the other two major opioid receptors, the δ and the σ receptors.

Morphine directly suppresses cough by an effect on the cough centre in the medulla. It also produces nausea and vomiting by directly stimulating the chemoreceptor trigger zone in the area postrema of the medulla. Morphine provokes the release of histamine.

Papaverine is an alkaloid unrelated to the opioids. It is a non-specific smooth muscle relaxant, perhaps achieved by inhibition of the enzyme phosphodiesterase. Large doses of papaverine depress A-V nodal and His bundle conduction in the heart. Papaverine has a weak analgesic effect.[3]

Toxicology

The toxicology is as for morphine and codeine. There is no evidence to date for nervous system damage from direct (intrathecal or intracerebroventricular) injection of morphine to the neuraxis, even when such injection is continued for months. This observation might not be valid for papaveretum in view of the additional constituents.

Clinical pharmacology

The prime clinical pharmacological effects of papaveretum are due to the effects of morphine.

The occupancy of the μ receptor by morphine results in pain relief, a feeling of calmness and respiratory depression. Morphine also induces drowsiness in subjects and this effect is paramount when the drug is given to normal pain-free individuals. Elsewhere in the central nervous system morphine suppresses cough and may cause nausea and vomiting due to stimulation of the chemoreceptor trigger zone.

Respiratory depression occurs following papaveretum due to the actions of morphine and is manifest by a reduced responsiveness of the brain stem respiratory centre to increasing concentrations of inhaled carbon dioxide.

Papaveretum has little effect on the cardiovascular system in the supine patient. However, on standing, patients given papaveretum may experience postural hypotension due to morphine-induced arteriolar and venous dilation. This vasodilation is partially blocked by the histamine (H_1)-antagonists. There is no effect on the ECG or on the cerebral circulation. Morphine may cause some decrease in gastric acid secretion, as well as in biliary and pancreatic secretions. The morphine in papaveretum may cause an increase in the pressure in the biliary tract.

The constriction of smooth muscle induced by morphine may be partially offset by the relaxation of smooth muscle induced by papaverine. However, these latter effects are rarely noted clinically. The pupils are constricted by papaveretum and tolerance and physical dependence are problems as with morphine.

Papaveretum 20 mg by injection produces analgesia clinically indistinguishable from that produced by 16.2 mg of morphine sulphate.[4] There are no precise studies of equi-analgesic dosage. The onset time of analgesic effect (20–30 min), time of peak effect (1 hour) and duration of effect (4 hours) are the same as those for morphine. These figures are derived from clinical experience rather than from controlled data.

The usual dose for an adult is 10–20 mg intramuscularly. This is equivalent to 6.6–13.3 mg morphine sulphate. The lower dose would produce barely measurable effect.

Pharmacokinetics

The kinetics of the mixture are not known. Morphine measured by either radioimmunoassay or high pressure liquid chromatography has an elimination half life of about three hours.[4] Plasma clearance varies widely, from 300 to 1000 $ml.min^{-1}$.[4] The major metabolites in man are morphine-3-glucuronide (M3G) and morphine-6-glucuronide (M6G).[4] M6G is active, with at least 10 times the potency of morphine in the central nervous system. The major site of metabolism is the liver, but there is evidence for extrahepatic metabolism. Excretion of these glucuronides via the kidney is reduced in renal dysfunction, leading to unexpected degree and duration of effect of a given dose(s).

Concentration–effect relationship

There are no studies in this field with papaveretum.

Metabolism

As for morphine.[4]

Pharmaceutics

Papaveretum is available for parenteral injection, as a colourless liquid containing 20 $mg.ml^{-1}$. Ampoules should be protected from light.

Use is restricted by the Misuse of Drugs Act.

Therapeutic use

Indications

1. Preoperative medication
2. Relief of postoperative pain
3. Relief of severe chronic pain.

Contraindications

There are no absolute contraindications, but care should be exercised as for morphine in patients with renal dysfunction,[4] hepatic disease[4] and respiratory disease. Patients with renal dysfunction may be at risk from accumulation of morphine-6-glucuronide, which may lead to unexpected degree and duration of effect.[4]

Mode of use

Papaveretum is an alternative to morphine. It has no proven specific advantage over morphine. 20 mg of papaveretum is the equivalent in analgesic potency of some 13 mg of morphine. Administration of both injection and tablets should be as for injected and oral morphine.

The dose and dosing interval should be titrated against pain. A simple rule is that while the patient is still complaining of pain and sufficient time has elapsed for absorption of the preceding dose, then it is safe to give another dose. This subsequent dose may be smaller than the first. By using regular doses and 'as necessary' doses an estimate of requirement per unit time (e.g. 40 mg per 12 hours) is established, and the regular prescription may be rewritten to take account of shortfall. Postoperatively pain decreases as time goes on; in chronic pain it may well increase. Constant assessment is necessary to achieve adequate analgesia safely in either context.

Adverse reactions

The adverse effects of papaveretum, in common with other opiate strong analgesics, are respiratory depression, nausea and vomiting, constipation, miosis and dependence. There is no comparative evidence to suggest quantitatively greater or lesser degrees of these problems occurring with papaveretum compared with either morphine or the other alternatives.

Potentially life-threatening effects

Respiratory depression may occasionally be fatal especially in the elderly and those with severe chronic respiratory disease.

Acute overdosage

Respiratory depression resulting in cyanosis and hypotension will ultimately lead to cardiac arrest. Medical management is respiratory and cardiovascular support and intravenous injection of naloxone, 0.4 mg repeated as necessary at one minute intervals. No effect after 4 mg (4 min) means that the opiate is not the cause of the problem.

Bradycardia may occur (reversible with atropine), as may muscular rigidity (manage with muscle relaxants).

The metabolism of morphine to its active metabolite morphine-6-glucuronide has the potential for producing respiratory depression.[4]

Severe or irreversible adverse effects

No relevant physical sequelae are known. Drug use for reasons other than pain relief may result in psychological dependence.

Symptomatic adverse effects

Symptomatic adverse events mediated by opiate receptor occupancy are constipation, sedation and nausea (and vomiting). Unpleasant dreams, mood alteration, itching and urinary retention are also probably opiate receptor effects, being common to all opiates. The histamine release with morphine is greater than that with fentanyl but much less than that with pethidine.

High risk groups

Neonates

Reduced glomerular filtration rate will result in reduced M6G excretion, resulting in greater degree and duration of effect of a given dose.

Breast milk. Components of papaveretum are excreted in breast milk and so breast feeding should be avoided.

Children

There is no convincing evidence for greater incidence of problems in infants or children with normal renal function than in adults.

Pregnant women

Components of papaveretum cross the placenta. There is inadequate evidence of safety, even though the drug has been used without apparent harmful effect. Administration in labour may cause respiratory depression in the new born infant.

The elderly

Older people seem to obtain greater analgesia from a given dose of morphine than do younger. The simplest explanation is diminished renal function resulting in increased elimination half life for the active metabolite.

Concurrent disease

Respiratory disease. There is no good evidence that patients with respiratory disease who are treated appropriately with opiates for opiate-sensitive pain have any greater incidence of respiratory depression.

Papaveretum

Renal disease. Decreased renal function will result in increased elimination half life for the metabolite M6G.[4] Fixed dose regimes must therefore take account of renal function.

Liver disease. There is no clinical evidence that hepatic dysfunction up to the point of pre-coma presents any problems with morphine treatment.

Drug interactions

As for morphine.

Clinical trials

There are few careful clinical studies of papaveretum. It is extremely doubtful whether there is any measurable clinical advantage in the use of papaveretum rather than morphine, in terms of either efficacy or side effect incidence. This was suggested over 50 years ago.[5]

1. Loan W B, Dundee J W, Clarke R S J 1966 Studies of drugs given before anaesthesia XII: a comparison of paraveretum and morphine. British Journal of Anaesthesia 38: 891–900

Papaveretum 20 mg (n = 200; two 'pooled' groups) was compared as a premedicant with morphine (10 mg n = 150; 13.3 mg, n = 50; 15 mg, n = 150). The study was partially double-blind (?open for some patients). The results reported suggest that there was significantly greater drowsiness with papaveretum than with 10 or 15 mg of morphine, but no significant difference in alleviating apprehension. There was no significant difference in emetic potential.

Postoperative analgesic

2. Hayman J M, Fox F 1937 Comparison of the analgesic action of pantopon and morphine sulfate. Journal of the American Medical Association 109: 1813–1814

Hayman and Fox found no significant difference in a comparison blind to nurse and patient of papaveretum 21.6 mg with morphine 16.2 mg (48 and 44 hypodermic doses respectively) although 16.2 mg morphine was more likely to provide relief than 10.8 mg morphine (53 doses).

In patients with renal colic, pleurisy, peritonitis, facial herpes and other conditions Hayman and Fox found no difference in a comparison blind to nurse and patient of papaveretum 21.6 mg with morphine 16.2 mg (22 and 28 hypodermic doses respectively) although 16.2 mg morphine was more likely to provide relief than 10.8 mg morphine (19 doses).

3. Catling J A, Pinto D M, Jordan C, Jones J G 1980 Respiratory effects of analgesia after cholecystectomy: comparison of continuous and intermittent papaveretum. British Medical Journal 281: 478–480

Most recent studies such as this one have been comparisons of administration modes (continuous versus infusion) for papaveretum rather than comparisons of papaveretum with other drugs.

References

1. Sahli H 1909 Ueber Pantopon, ein die Gesamtalkaloide des Opiums in leichtloslicher und such zu subkutaner Injecktion geeigneter Form enthaltendes Apiumparparat. Therapeutische Monatshefte 1: 1–6
2. Leipoldt C L 1911 Some remarks on pantopon anaesthesia. Lancet 1: 368–369
3. Macht D I, Herman N B, Levy C S 1916 A quantitative study of the analgesia produced by opium alkaloids, individually and in combination with each other, in normal man. Journal of Pharmacology and Experimental Therapeutics 8: 1–37
4. Moore R A, Hand C W, McQuay H J 1987 Opioid metabolism and excretion. In: Budd K (ed) Update in Opiods, Clinical Anaesthesiology (Volume 1, No. 4), Bailliere Tindall, London, pp 829–858
5. Hayman J M, Fox F 1937 Comparison of the analgesic action of pantopon and morphine sulfate. Journal of American Medical Association 109: 1813–1814

P

Papaverine (hydrochloride)

Papaverine is a smooth muscle relaxant and vasodilator. It is an alkaloid devoid of narcotic properties and was first described and extracted from opium in 1848 by Merck[1] and later synthesized in 1909 by Picket and Gams. It has been largely superseded by drugs with more specific actions such as α-adrenergic blockers and calcium slow channel antagonists but may still have a place in the treatment of vascular spasm.

Chemistry

Papaverine hydrochloride (Cardoverina; Cerebid; Cerespan; Dispamil; Lapav; Panergon; Papacon; Papital T.R.; Pavabid; Pavacap; Pavacen; Pavcla; Pavacol D; Pavadel; Pavagen; Pavakey; Pavased; Pavatest; Vasal; Vasospan)
1-[(3,4-Dimethoxyphenyl)methyl]-6,7-dimethoxyisoquinoline hydrochloride.
$C_{20}H_{21}NO_4.HCl$

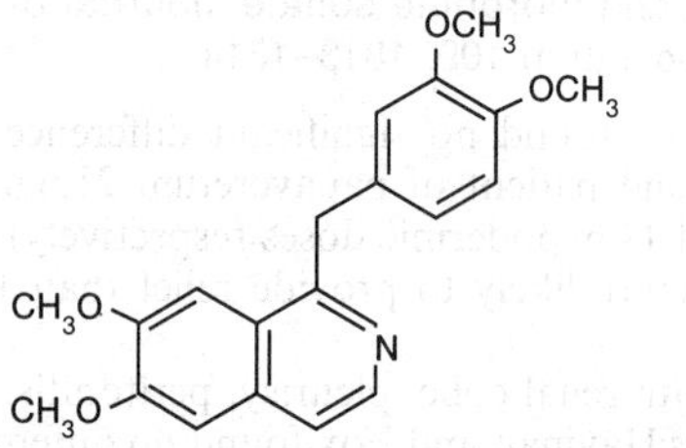

Molecular weight (free base)	375.9 (339.4)
pKa	6.4
Solubility	
in alcohol	1 in 120
in water	1 in 40
Octanol/water partition coefficient	low

Chemically it has been classed as a benzylisoquinoline like quinidine and later the chemical structure was found to be similar to that of some calcium channel blockers.

Papaverine is extracted from opium which contains 0.8–1% of it and is also synthesized chemically. Papaverine is almost insoluble in water, 1 in 40, but it is soluble in hot benzene, glacial acetic acid and acetone. Optimal pH for storage is 2.0–2.8.[2]

The hydrochloride salt of papaverine is marketed under more than 40 trade names throughout the world. It is a white crystalline powder that melts at 220–225°C with decomposition. The pH in 2% aqueous solution is 3.3. It is an ingredient of APP, Pholcomed (linctus and pastilles).

Pharmacology

The main pharmacological action[3] is that of a non-specific vasodilator acting on the smooth muscle of the arterioles and capillaries of all vascular beds including the cerebral and coronary circulation. This activity is related to the inhibition of cyclic AMP phosphodiesterase found in many tissues and has also been shown to inhibit the function of cyclic GMP phosphodiesterase.[4] As a consequence of phosphodiesterase inhibition, the myocardial cyclic AMP levels rise substantially, but without any increase in positive inotropic effects. This pharmacological contradiction is explained by the direct calcium blockade caused by papaverine,[5] which may, under some circumstances, be strong enough to negate the cyclic AMP action. Large doses may depress A–V nodal and intraventricular conduction to the point of causing conduction arrhythmias. Papaverine is an opium derivative, but it is not habit forming.

Toxicology

LD_{50} in rats was determined to be 750 mg.kg^{-1} orally, 33 mg.kg^{-1} intravenously in mice. In man no data are available. However gastrointestinal disturbances do occur as well as flushing, headache, weakness and tachycardia. There is no knowledge of human death caused by papaverine. No information exists on teratogenicity and carcinogenicity.

Clinical pharmacology

This drug is a very active, non-specific, smooth muscle depressant with consequent effects on the blood vessels and other smooth muscle systems; it may bring about hypotension and tachycardia.[6] Papaverine hydrochloride also may depress myocardial conduction and prolong the diastolic period. The cerebral blood flow is increased in most observations, but the effect is very short lived. Two possible danger points are hypotension and development of a steal phenomenon especially after an occlusive stroke or subarachnoid haemorrhage. The fact that dilatation of the vessels of the extremities has been described as very favourable to not effective, is probably related to how advanced the sclerotic process is in the wall of the arteries and arterioles. Therefore, the dilating ability is probably inversely related to the vascular pathology. Papaverine hydrochloride is more valuable in conditions where spasm is actually present or where it is to be prevented.

Papaverine hydrochloride blocks Ca^{2+} flux to some extent at the cellular membrane level,[7] which explains its anti-tachyarrhythmic activity. This blockade may vary in intensity in different vascular beds and different patients. High plasma levels and prolonged administration are more conducive to Ca^{2+} blockade. It is now clear that the widespread pharmacological actions make this compound usable and seemingly useful in a great variety of diseases affecting vessels and viscera. The activity is evident in most cases, but it is of short duration and not curative. Furthermore, chronic usage may lead to disturbing side effects.

Pharmacokinetics

Several methods have been used for the determination of papaverine in body fluids, but the most reliable seems to be HPLC[8] which is a modification of Pierson's. This method is very specific and has an excellent reproducibility. Sensitivity is 2 μg.l^{-1}.

In man, after intravenous administration, the blood level versus time curve fits an open two-compartment model, but after oral administration the curve is best described by an open one-compartment model, with peak concentrations occurring at 1 h. The half life is 1.5 to 2.2 h and the volume of distribution is 0.99–1.52 l.kg^{-1}. The drug is highly protein bound at 87%.[6–8] The oral absorption is rapid and extensive. The hepatic blood clearance is 60 ml.min^{-1}, equivalent to 69% extraction.[9] After intravenous administration a dose of 1 mg.kg^{-1} produces plasma concentrations of 1 mg.l^{-1} in 5 min.[8] The drug is extensively metabolized in the liver with 50–80% of a dose excreted in urine in 48 h. Less than 1% of the dose is present as unchanged papaverine. There is some biliary excretion.

Oral absorption	>90%
Presystemic metabolism	70%
Plasma half life	
range	1.5–2.2 h
Volume of distribution	0.99–1.52 l.kg^{-1}
Plasma protein binding	87%

Concentration–effect relationship

The concentration–effect relationship for papaverine hydrochloride is evident but has not been precisely defined. Plasma concentrations of the drug vary from 0.5 to 0.15 mg.l^{-1} during oral administration. However, the duration of action is quite short and frequent dosing is necessary. It is important to know that various vascular beds and smooth muscle performing different body functions respond differently in intensity of action and duration. Plasma papaverine levels correlate well with the increase of blood flow through the extremities and patients show a greater vasodilatation when the limb is previously sympathectomized. It seems clear, however, that a minimum papaverine plasma level of 200 $\mu g.l^{-1}$ is necessary to elicit an adequate pharmacological effect. Dosage and duration of administration may relate to incidence and intensity of side effects.

Metabolism

A dose of papaverine is 90% metabolized by the liver within a few hours. In man, less than 1% of the dose is found in the urine unchanged, more than 50% is in the urine as metabolites and the rest is eliminated through biliary excretion.[10] The metabolites are formed by glucuronic acid and sulphate conjugation of the phenolic group produced by demethylation.[11] The phosphodiesterase inhibitory activity of 4-hydroxypapaverine, one of the main metabolites, compared to the parent compound, was found present to an extent capable of sustaining clinical effects (Fig. 1).[12]

Fig. 1

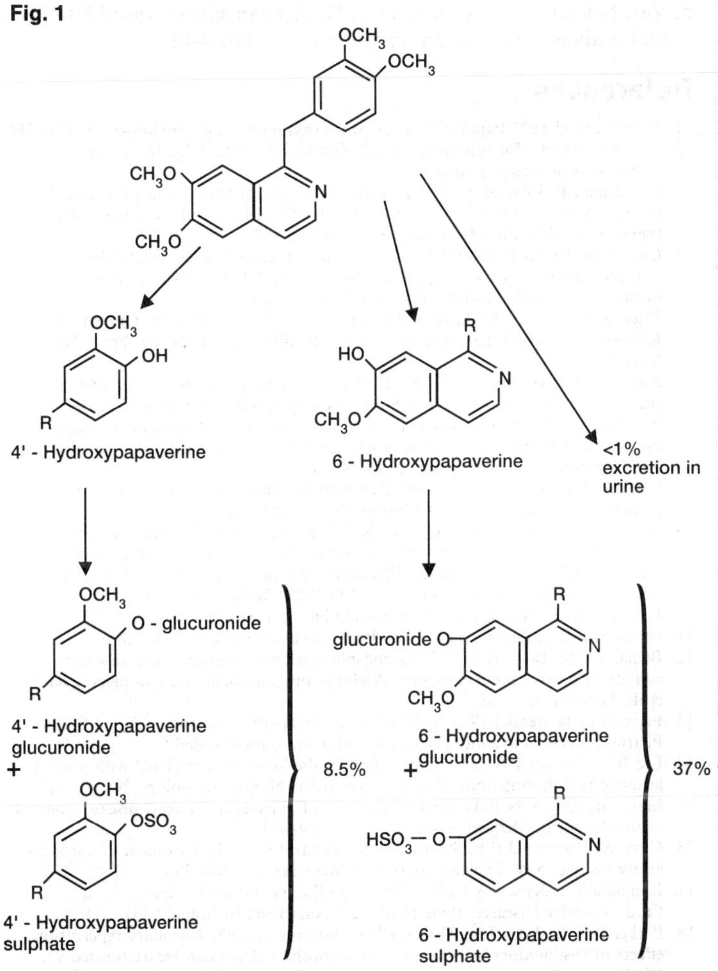

Pharmaceutics

Oral preparations are 75–100 mg tablets and the usual adult dose is 75–300 mg three to five times a day.[13] In order to reduce stomach disturbances it should be taken with food, milk or antacids. The USP requires 80% dissolution within 30 min. In the UK, clinicians feel there is little justification for using the drug orally.

Extended-release capsules are prepared in 150–200 mg and 300 mg strength. These are ingested every 12 hours starting from 150 mg and increasing to the desired level. The papaverine in the form of soft gelatin capsule produced consistently greater plasma levels and marked increase in vasodilatation up to 130% of baseline.[14]

The elixir, which is a non-alcoholic preparation, contains papaverine hydrochloride 100 mg per 15 ml.

The parenteral form is 60 mg per ampoule of 2 ml. The pH should be above 3. The dosage is 40 mg in 1–2 min intra-arterially, intramuscularly or intravenously, 30–120 mg may be injected over 1–2 min every 3 h. However, these dosages may be exceeded under special circumstances. The usual paediatric dose intramuscularly or intravenously is 1.5 $mg.kg^{-1}$ body weight four times a day. All these pharmaceutical preparations should be stored at between 15 to 40°C in darkness.

A papaverine/phentolamine injection is injected into the corpus cavernosum in males unable to achieve erection.

No dose dependency was reported after oral or intravenous administrations of tablets and solutions. Furthermore, it has been proven that chronic studies of tablets four times daily and capsules twice daily showed lack of accumulation.

Papaverine (hydrochloride)

P

Therapeutic use

Indications

Most of the indications rest on clinical experience and few, if any, have been subjected to clinical trials that would be regarded as adequate for a modern drug. The main use is as a potent intravenous vasodilator with a short duration of action. Conditions in which the drug has been used include:

1. Cerebrovascular insufficiency
2. Cerebral ischaemia
3. Myocardial ischaemia
4. Intermittent claudication
5. Visceral spasm
6. Pulmonary embolism
7. Bronchospasm
8. Spastic obstipation.

Contraindications

1. Cardiac failure
2. Glaucoma
3. Recent myocardial infarction
4. Recent stroke
5. Bradycardia and heart block
6. Liver disease.

Mode of use

Cerebral ischaemia is diminished by increasing the cerebral blood flow, without increasing oxygen consumption even in normal subjects.

Papaverine hydrochloride also dilates the vessels of the heart making it potentially useful in myocardial ischaemia especially where this is the result of arterial spasm, although nitrites are more convenient and probably more effective.[15] The administration of this drug intravenously increased the work capacity and diminished the electrocardiographic ischaemic changes. It reached a maximum effect in 5 minutes and had all but disappeared after 60 min.[16] This method of treatment seems of little clinical value to the patient except in hospital and in perioperative conditions.

Oral administration is variably effective. Recently, intra-aortic injection of papaverine has come into use before open heart procedure to prevent or treat aortocoronary graft spasm and to allow better distribution of cardioplegic solution for enhanced myocardial protection.[17] Moreover, after the graft is in place, intracoronary injection elicits up to a three-fold increase in flow in all layers of the myocardium.[18,19]

This compound has also been used in vascular spasms of the hands and legs with reported improvement; nocturnal cramps were diminished and claudication was often less severe. Oscillographic studies on these patients provided evidence of an increase in blood flow.

Visceral spasm like ureteric colic, biliary colic and gastrointestinal colic have been treated with debatable results. In most of these cases the most effective route of administration is the intravenous one.

Adverse reactions

Potentially life-threatening effects

Caution should be exercised in the presence of angina, serious myocardial depression, glaucoma, recent myocardial infarction and recent stroke. When using vasodilators, especially in cerebrovascular conditions, it is important to remember that a steal situation could develop with dire consequences; this may occur even after a non-occlusive stroke. Papaverine should not be given intravenously when atrioventricular dissociation is present, because it may enhance it. Liver disease may be a serious contraindication.

Acute overdosage
Serious severe deliberate overdose has not been reported.

Severe or irreversible adverse effects
Jaundice accompanied by symptoms of hepatotoxicity, demonstrated by increased alkaline phosphatase, AST (SGOT), LDH, cholesterol and high WBC count has been described, but on discontinuation of the drug all symptoms disappeared and the liver function tests came back to normal without residual problems. Up to 60% of patients show abnormal reactions to this drug.[20–22] Glaucoma may be precipitated or aggravated.

Symptomatic adverse effects
Such effects related to papaverine treatment do occur frequently, but are directly related to the length or mode of administration. Over a period of time in excess of several weeks, gastrointestinal symptoms may develop. They are more annoying than dangerous. However, they may occur with increasing frequency. They include also blurred vision, drowsiness and weakness, and may be considered signs of overdosage.

When papaverine is given intravenously or intra-arterially the side effects are always transient and due to too rapid and/or too large an administration.

The patient on chronic administration should be checked frequently. Hepatic function tests, blood tests, and ocular pressure measurement should be done at regular intervals. Furthermore, the patient should be advised to take the drug at meal times, to get up slowly from a lying or sitting position in order to avoid postural hypotension and to refrain from the use of tobacco so as to increase the beneficial effect.

High risk groups

Neonates
The drug is not used in this age group.

Breast milk. Even though there is no evidence of problems during lactation, caution must be used.

Children
Children do not react adversely to this drug.

Pregnant women
There is no report or evidence that pregnant patients may react adversely to papaverine; however, one must consider the risk benefit ratio.

The elderly
No special precautions are needed when using the drug in the elderly.

Concurrent disease
Hepatic or cardiac failure are contraindications to the use of this drug.

Drug interactions

Other significant interactions

Nicotine. Papaverine hydrochloride should not be used in conjunction with nicotine because its beneficial vasodilator effect will be minimized or more probably abolished.

Levodopa. Since this antispasmodic and vasodilator compound has been reported to have dopamine receptor-blocking activity it is advisable not to prescribe it in patients who are being treated with levodopa, since recurrence of extrapyramidal symptomatology would probably ensue.

Potentially hazardous interactions

Calcium blockers. It is possible that some calcium blockers may have potentiating effects because they have a similar molecular structure to papaverine. Since papaverine is a mild antiarrhythmic agent it may potentiate other similar agents as well as hypotensive drugs.

Major outcome trials

The medical literature does not contain large and well-defined studies which prove beyond a reasonable doubt the efficacy and the reliability of such therapeutic treatment. Furthermore, in the light of more recent discoveries and introduction into the clinician armamentarium of drugs like calcium blockers, α-adrenoceptor blockers and other types of vasodilators, it is likely that papaverine hydrochloride will have a secondary role in this field. This drug is probably more useful for intravenous and intra-arterial administration for acute relief of vascular spasm, rather than for chronic administration. The occurrence of side effects is common during chronic administration and the efficacy of the drug is debatable. The therapeutic value must be weighed also against the hepatotoxic action of papaverine that occurs frequently, though it is not life threatening.

General review articles

1. Cook P, James I 1981 Cerebral vasodilators. New England Journal of Medicine 305: 1508–1513
2. Coffman J D 1979 Vasodilator drugs in peripheral vascular disease. New England Journal of Medicine 300: 713–717
3. Coffman J D 1975 Vasodilator drugs in peripheral vascular disease. Journal of the Maine Medical Association 66: 262–269
4. Petrie W M, Ban T A 1978 Drugs in gerophyschiatric. Psychopharmacology Bulletin 14: 7–19
5. Van Nueten J M, Wellens D 1979 Mechanisms of vasodilatation and antivasoconstriction. Angiology 30: 440–446

References

1. Whipple G H 1977 Papaverine as an antiarrhythmic agent. Angiology 28: 737–749
2. 1976 Papaverine. In: Windholz M (ed) The Merck index, 9th edn. Merck, Rahway, New Jersey, p 6822
3. Needleman P, Johnson E M 1980 Vasodilators and the treatment of angina. In: Gilman A G, Goodman L S, Gilman A (eds) The pharmacological basis of therapeutics, 6th edn. Macmillan, New York, p 830
4. Chasin M, Harris D N 1976 Inhibitors and activators of cyclic nucleotide phosphodiesterase. In: Greengard P, Robinson G A (eds) Advances in cyclic nucleotide research. Raven Press, New York, 7: 225–264
5. Tsien R W 1977 Cyclic AMP and contractile activity in heart. In: Greengard P, Robinson G A (eds) Advances in cyclic nucleotide research. Raven Press, New York 8: 363–420
6. Ritschel W A, Hammer G V 1977 Pharmacokinetics of papaverine in man. International Journal of Clinical Pharmacology and Biopharmacy 15: 227–229
7. Nawrath H 1981 Action potential, membrane currents and force of contraction in cat ventricular heart muscle treated with papaverine. Journal of Pharmacology and Experimental Therapeutics. 218: 544–549
8. Kramer W G, Romagnoli A 1984 Papaverine disposition in cardiac surgery patients. European Journal of Clinical Pharmacology 27: 127–130
9. Garrett E R, Roseboom H, Green J R, Schuermann W 1978 Pharmacokinetics of papaverine hydrochloride and the biopharmaceutics of its oral dosage forms. International Journal of Clinical Pharmacology and Biopharmacy 16: 193–208
10. Belpaire F M, Rosseel M T, Gogaert M G 1978 Metabolism of papaverine IV. Urinary elimination of papaverine metabolites in man. Xenobiotica 8: 297–300
11. Papaverine hydrochloride 1979 The Pharmaceutical Codex, 11th edn, p 637
12. Belpaire F M, Bogaert M G 1973 Phosphodiesterase inhibition and vascular activity of papaverine metabolites. Archives Internationales de Pharmacodynamie et de Therapie 203: 388–390
13. Papaverine (systemic) 1983 In: The United States Pharmacopeia. United States Pharmacopeial Convention, Rockville, Maryland, pp 479–480
14. Lee B Y, Trainor F S 1978 Arterial flow in the lower leg correlated with plasma levels of two formulations of papaverine hydrochloride. Angiology 29: 310–319
15. Elek S R, Katz L N 1942 Some clinical use of papaverine in heart disease. Journal of the American Medical Association 120: 434–441
16. Gray W, Riseman J E F, Stearns S 1945 Papaverine in the treatment of coronary-artery disease. New England Journal of Medicine 232: 389–394
17. Romagnoli A, Koska A J 1981 Coronary dilators and cardioplegia. Cardiovascular Diseases, Bulletin of the Texas Heart Institute 8: 467–474
18. Parker P E, Bashour F A, Downey H F, Boutros I S 1977 Coronary reperfusion: effects of vasodilators (papaverine and adenosine). American Heart Journal 93: 66–72
19. Goldman S, Henry R, Friedman M J et al 1982 Increased regional myocardial perfusion after intracoronary papaverine in patients after coronary artery bypass grafting. Journal of Thoracic and Cardiovascular Surgery 84: 563–568
20. Snider G B, Gogate S A 1978 Clinical observations following papaverine therapy. Ohio State Medical Journal 74: 571–573
21. Zimmerman H J 1969 Papaverine revisited as a hepatotoxin. New England Journal of Medicine 281: 1364–1365
22. Geiger G S 1981 Elevations in serum transaminases and alkaline phosphatase secondary to papaverine hydrochloride. Drug Intelligence and Clinical Pharmacy 15: 127–129

Paracetamol

Paracetamol is a long-established non-prescription antipyretic analgesic drug.

Chemistry

Paracetamol (Acetaminophen, Panadol, Tylenol)
$C_8H_9NO_2$
N-Acetyl-p-aminophenol; 4-hydroxyacetanilide;
4-acetamidophenol

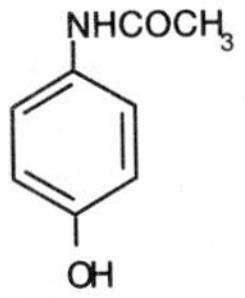

Molecular weight	151.2
pKa (–OH)	9.5
Solubility	
in alcohol	1 in 70
in water	1 in 70
Octanol/water partition coefficient	—

Paracetamol is a white odourless crystalline powder with a bitter taste prepared by chemical synthesis. It is a constituent of numerous single and combination analgesic products.

Pharmacology

Paracetamol has antipyretic and mild analgesic actions together with some anti-inflammatory activity. These effects are thought to be related to inhibition of prostaglandin synthesis. In this respect paracetamol has greater tissue selectivity than aspirin and the non-steroidal anti-inflammatory drugs. The reason for this difference is unknown.

Toxicology

In large toxic doses paracetamol causes acute centrilobular hepatic necrosis in animals[1] and man.[2] There are considerable species differences in susceptibility and acute hepatotoxic doses in hamsters, man, mice and rats are about 150, 250, 300 and 3000 mg.kg^{-1} respectively. Paracetamol causes methaemoglobinaemia and oxidative haemolysis in dogs and cats but not normally in man, even after overdosage. In chronic toxicity studies, paracetamol has less potential for nephrotoxicity (renal papillary necrosis) than aspirin and the non-steroidal anti-inflammatory analgesics.[3] Strain-dependent cataract formation and other ocular abnormalities have been described in induced mice[4] and in one study (but not in others), paracetamol produced a high incidence of liver cell tumours in 1F mice.[5]

Clinical pharmacology

In therapeutic doses paracetamol has antipyretic and mild analgesic actions comparable to those of aspirin. It has no other important pharmacological effects and does not adversely affect platelet function and haemostasis.

Pharmacokinetics

The preferred analytical method is high-performance liquid chromatography. This is highly specific and methods involving extraction have a sensitivity of about 100 µg.l^{-1}. Rapid colorimetric and spectrophotometric methods based on hydrolysis to 4-aminophenol without prior solvent extraction include conjugates and give gross overestimates of the true concentration.[6]

Paracetamol is rapidly and completely absorbed after oral administration, with peak plasma concentrations occurring between 15 minutes and 2 hours after ingestion, depending on the formulation. Dissolution and gastric emptying are rate limiting steps: the mean half time of absorption from the upper small intestine is only 7 minutes.[7] The absolute oral bioavailability is about 80% and is independent of dose in the range of 5 to 20 mg.kg^{-1}. Paracetamol is well absorbed following rectal administration, but the rate of absorption is slow. It is not bound to plasma proteins to any extent and the volume of distribution is about 0.9 l.kg^{-1}.[8] The concentrations of paracetamol in saliva are similar to those in plasma. Concentrations in whole blood are up to 20% higher and in breast milk about 20% lower.[9] Paracetamol crosses the placenta.

The mean plasma paracetamol half life after a therapeutic dose is about 2.3 hours in healthy adults with a range of 1.5 to 3.0 hours. It varies relatively little between individuals, and is not prolonged to a clinically significant extent at the extremes of age. Paracetamol is extensively metabolized in the liver and the total body clearance is about 5 ml.min^{-1}.kg^{-1}. The clearance of paracetamol is reduced and the half life increased following a hepatotoxic overdose. Prolongation beyond 4 hours usually indicates impending liver damage.[10]

Some 2 to 5% of a therapeutic dose of paracetamol is excreted unchanged in the urine. Its renal clearance is about 10 ml.min^{-1} and is weakly dependent on urine flow rate but not on pH.

Oral absorption	>95%
Presystemic metabolism	20%
Plasma half life	
range	1.5–3.0 h
mean	2.3 h
Volume of distribution	0.9 l.kg^{-1}
Plasma protein binding	<20%

The kinetics of paracetamol elimination have been investigated in patients with renal, hepatic, thyroid and gastrointestinal disease. No clinically significant changes were observed except in patients with severe acute and decompensated chronic liver disease in whom the half life was considerably prolonged. In patients with chronic renal failure there was marked accumulation of paracetamol conjugates. In epileptic patients receiving anticonvulsants which cause microsomal enzyme induction, the plasma paracetamol half life is reduced by about 20%.[8]

Concentration–effect relationship

Little is known of the concentration–effect relationship of paracetamol. As judged by pain relief scores, the onset and duration of analgesic activity corresponds approximately to the plasma concentration–time curve after oral administration of a therapeutic dose, and from such data it would appear that analgesia is associated with concentrations above 3 to 5 µg.ml^{-1}. In a study of analgesia following intravenous injection of 1000 mg of paracetamol in patients with dental pain, there was no clear relationship between pain relief and paracetamol concentrations in either central or peripheral compartments.[11]

Metabolism

Paracetamol undergoes extensive biotransformation in the liver and the major metabolites are inactive phenolic sulphate and glucuronide conjugates (Fig. 1). A minor degree of saturation of sulphate conjugation can be demonstrated within the therapeutic dose range and this pathway (but not glucuronide conjugation) is completely saturated following overdosage.[12] A small fraction of the dose is converted by cytochrome P450-dependant mixed function oxidase to N-acetyl-p-benzoquinoneimine, a reactive potentially cytotoxic arylating intermediate which is normally conjugated with glutathione (GSH) and excreted in the urine as mercapturic acid and cysteine conjugates of paracetamol. Glutathione is depleted following overdosage and the reactive metabolite binds covalently to hepatic macromolecules, causing irreversible damage and necrosis.[13]

Fig. 1

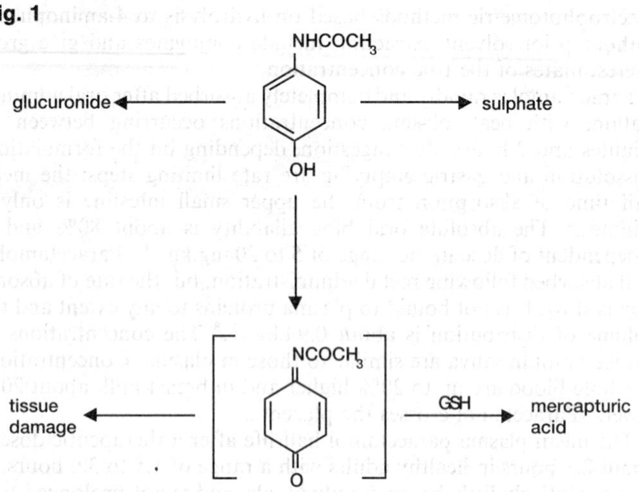

The major metabolites of paracetamol following a therapeutic dose are as follows:

	% of dose
Glucuronide conjugate	55
Sulphate conjugate	30
Mercapturic acid conjugate	4
Cysteine conjugate	4

Other minor metabolites have been identified.[14]
The glutathione conjugate may be excreted in bile but is then largely degraded by intestinal peptidases and the products reabsorbed.

Pharmaceutics

Paracetamol is available in tablet (plain and effervescent), capsule, syrup and elixir forms: suppositories are available for paediatric use. The prominent branded products are Panadol (Sterling-Winthrop, UK) and Tylenol (McNeil, US). Paracetamol is also available in combination with many drugs, including other analgesics, caffeine, antihistamines and sympathomimetics. Macrogol suppository bases give the best release/absorption characteristics. Degradation of paracetamol in aqueous solutions is catalysed by acids and bases. Maximum stability is achieved by buffering solutions at pH6.

Paracetamol preparations are generally stable, with a shelf-life of three years or more.

Therapeutic use

Indications

1. Relief of mild to moderate pain
2. Reduction of fever.

Contraindications

Known sensitivity to paracetamol.

Mode of use

1. Relief of mild to moderate pain
Paracetamol is probably the most widely used general purpose mild analgesic and it is indicated for the relief of mild to moderate pain of diverse aetiology. In equivalent dosage paracetamol is as effective as aspirin for most painful conditions, but is generally held to be less effective when pain is associated with acute inflammation. The maximum analgesic effect occurs within 30 minutes to 2 hours after administration of a dose of 0.5 to 1.0 g in adults, and some degree of pain relief persists for 4 to 6 hours. The maximum recommended adult dose is 0.5 to 1.0 g every 4 to 6 hours up to a maximum of 4 g in 24 hours. As with antipyresis, the mode of analgesic action is thought to be inhibition of prostaglandin synthesis.

2. Reduction of fever
Paracetamol is used extensively for reduction of fever associated with influenza and other infections, particularly in children. It is only effective in reducing abnormally elevated body temperature. Paracetamol and aspirin are equally effective antipyretics. The maximum lowering of temperature occurs 2 to 3 hours after a therapeutic oral dose, and the effect usually persists for at least 6 hours.

Adverse reactions

Potentially life-threatening effects
Deaths caused by paracetamol in therapeutic dosage are virtually unheard of. There have been isolated reports of blood dyscrasia (pancytopenia, agranulocytosis and thrombocytopenia) and these have usually been reversible.

It has been claimed that liver damage may occur with the therapeutic use of paracetamol. The number of cases reported is very small and most patients were chronic alcoholics who may be particularly susceptible to paracetamol-induced hepatotoxicity. The maximum recommended dose was often exceeded and some patients had clearly taken the drug in overdosage.

Acute overdosage
Because of its ready availability, paracetamol is often taken in overdosage. The major complication is acute hepatic necrosis, although without treatment fewer than 10% of unselected patients are at risk of severe liver damage (plasma aminotransferase > 1000 $\mu.l^{-1}$). About 1% develop fulminant hepatic failure which is usually fatal. Renal failure from acute tubular necrosis is a further uncommon complication which may develop in the absence of hepatic failure. There are no specific early manifestations of severe paracetamol poisoning. Consciousness is not impaired except in the occasional unusually severely poisoned patient with metabolic acidosis, and maximum abnormality of liver function tests is delayed for at least 3 days. Emergency estimation of the plasma paracetamol concentration is therefore necessary to determine the severity of intoxication and the need for specific therapy with N-acetylcysteine. Without treatment, about 60% of patients with paracetamol concentrations above a line on a semilogarithmic graph joining plots of 200 $mg.l^{-1}$ at 4 hours and 30 $mg.l^{-1}$ at 15 hours after ingestion will suffer severe liver damage while above a parallel line joining 300 $mg.l^{-1}$ at 4 hours and 45 $mg.l^{-1}$ at 15 hours the chance is more than 90%.[15] Liver damage following overdosage is relatively uncommon in young children.[16]

Paracetamol causes liver damage through its conversion to a highly reactive metabolite, and necrosis does not occur unless hepatic glutathione is depleted.[13] Early treatment with agents which facilitate glutathione synthesis, such as N-acetylcysteine and methionine, effectively prevent liver damage, renal failure and death following paracetamol overdosage. Treatment must be started within 8 to 10 hours and is ineffective if delayed beyond 15 hours. Intravenous N-acetylcysteine is the treatment of choice.[17] Oral methionine has also been used.[18] However, its absorption is unpredictable and most patients develop nausea and vomiting within a few hours of ingestion of a hepatotoxic dose of paracetamol.

Severe or irreversible adverse effects
Paracetamol may very rarely aggravate bronchospasm in patients who are sensitive to aspirin and other non-steroidal anti-inflammatory drugs. It does not normally produce methaemoglobinaemia or haemolysis, even after overdosage or in patients with glucose-6-phosphate dehydrogenase deficiency.[19] Nevertheless, there have been isolated reports of these complications. Paracetamol is not an important cause of analgesic nephropathy.[3]

Symptomatic adverse effects
Skin rashes and minor gastrointestinal disturbances have been reported.

Interference with clinical pathology tests
In the range of concentrations associated with overdosage, paracetamol may give a false positive result for plasma salicylate in tests based on the direct colour reaction with ferric ions. In the same circumstances it may induce spuriously high results for blood glucose estimated with the YSI and Yellow Springs Model 23AM glucose analysers.[20]

High risk groups

None. No special precautions are necessary in the very young or the elderly.

Paracetamol

Concurrent disease

Although some consider the use of paracetamol inadvisable in patients with liver disease, there is no evidence that it is harmful when taken in recommended doses. Paracetamol does not cause or aggravate chronic active hepatitis,[21] and there was no deterioration in liver function in patients with chronic liver disease given 4 g of paracetamol daily for 13 days.[22] Paracetamol is likely to be much safer than aspirin in patients with cirrhosis and portal hypertension.

Similarly, in patients with impaired renal function, paracetamol is less likely to cause further deterioration than the salicylates and other non-steroidal anti-inflammatory analgesics.[3] As with other analgesics which inhibit prostaglandin synthesis, regular use should be avoided in patients with analgesic nephropathy.

Drug interactions

Potentiation of paracetamol hepatotoxicity. Drugs which induce the specific microsomal isoenzyme responsible for the metabolic activation of paracetamol might be expected to increase susceptibility to its toxic effects on the liver in man, as is the case in animals.[13] Despite anecdotal reports of such interactions involving ethanol and anticonvulsants in man, the metabolic activation of paracetamol is not increased in regular heavy drinkers or induced patients taking phenobarbitone or phenytoin (diphenylhydantoin).[23] Chronic alcoholics seem to be at particular risk of liver damage following overdosage of paracetamol, but the mechanism is uncertain. Acute ingestion of ethanol markedly reduces the metabolic activation of paracetamol.

Major outcome trials

1. Skjelbred P, Lokken P 1979 Paracetamol versus placebo: effects on postoperative course. European Journal of Clinical Pharmacology 15: 27–33

Paracetamol (1 g four times daily for 2 days starting on the day of surgery, then 0.5 g four times daily for the next 2 days) was compared with placebo in a double-blind crossover study in which the identical operation of removal of impacted wisdom teeth was carried out in 24 patients on two separate occasions (one on each side). The second operation was performed about 4 weeks after the first and each treatment could thus be compared in each patient under the same conditions. Paracetamol provided significantly greater analgesia than placebo with significantly less postoperative swelling.

2. Laska E M, Sunshine A, Zighelboim I, Roure C, Marrero I, Wanderling J, Olson M 1983 Effect of caffeine on acetaminophen analgesia. Clinical Pharmacology and Therapeutics 33: 498–509

A single-dose, parallel-group, double-blind comparison of placebo and paracetamol 0.5, 1.0 and 1.5 g alone and with 65, 130 and 195 mg of caffeine respectively was carried out in a total of 1345 patients with postpartum pain. A further 173 patients with pain following dental extraction received placebo or paracetamol 1.0 or 2.0 g with or without caffeine 130 or 260 mg. Pain relief was greater with paracetamol than with placebo, and its analgesic effect was consistently potentiated by caffeine.

3. Brewer E J 1968 A comparative evaluation of indomethacin, acetaminophen and placebo as antipyretic agents in children. Arthritis and Rheumatism 11: 645–651

223 infants and children with rectal temperatures above 101°F due to common paediatric conditions were randomly allocated to treatment with placebo, indomethacin (1 $mg.kg^{-1}$) or paracetamol (approximately 6.6 $mg.kg^{-1}$). Compared with placebo, paracetamol produced a highly significant reduction in body temperature (mean maximum fall 2.6°F).

4. Other Trials

Beaver W T, McMillan D 1980 Methodological considerations in the evaluation of analgesic combinations: acetaminophen (paracetamol) and hydrocodone in postpartum pain. British Journal of Clinical Pharmacology 10 (suppl 2): 215S–223S

A double-blind comparison of placebo and paracetamol (1.0 g) alone and in combination with hydrocodone and codeine in 108 postpartum patients with discussion of the methodological problems of assessment of efficacy of analgesics and analgesic combinations. Paracetamol provided significantly greater pain relief than placebo and the effect of hydrocodone was no more than additive, suggesting a different mechanism of analgesia.

Eden A N, Kaufman A 1967 Clinical comparison of three antipyretic agents. American Journal of Diseases of Childhood 114: 284–287

150 infants and children with a minimum temperature of 102° were divided into three equal groups and received aspirin, paracetamol or salicylamide. The dose of each drug ranged from 40 to 320 mg depending on age. Aspirin and paracetamol were equally effective in lowering temperature, and both were significantly more effective than salicylamide. Peak action occurred at 3 hours and the effect was over by 6 hours.

General review articles

Koch-Weser J 1976 Acetaminophen. New England Journal of Medicine 295: 1297–1300

Prescott L F, Critchley J A J H 1983 The treatment of acetaminophen poisoning. Annual Review of Pharmacology and Toxicology 23: 87–101

References

1. Boyd E M, Bereczky G M 1966 Liver necrosis from paracetamol. British Journal of Pharmacology 26: 606–614
2. Davidson D G D, Eastham W N 1966 Acute liver necrosis following overdose of paracetamol. British Medical Journal 2: 497–499
3. Prescott L F 1982 Analgesic nephropathy: a reassessment of the role of phenacetin and other analgesics. Drugs 23: 75–149
4. Shichi H, Tanaka M, Jensen N M, Nebert D W 1980 Genetic abnormalities in cataract and other ocular abnormalities induced by paracetamol and naphthalene. Pharmacology 20: 229–241
5. Flaks A, Flaks B 1983 Induction of liver cell tumours in IF mice by paracetamol. Carcinogenesis 4: 363–368
6. Stewart M J, Adriaenssens P I, Jarvie D J, Prescott L F 1979 Inappropriate methods for the emergency determination of plasma paracetamol. Annals of Clinical Biochemistry 16: 89–95
7. Clements J A, Heading R C, Nimmo W S, Prescott L F 1978 Kinetics of acetaminophen absorption and gastric emptying in man. Clinical Pharmacology and Therapeutics 24: 420–431
8. Forrest J A H, Clements J A, Prescott L F 1982 Clinical pharmacokinetics of paracetamol. Clinical Pharmacokinetics 7: 93–107
9. Bitzen P O, Gustafsson B, Jostell K G, Melander A, Wahlin-Boll E 1981 Excretion of paracetamol in human breast milk. European Journal of Clinical Pharmacology 20: 123–125
10. Prescott L F, Wright N, Roscoe P, Brown S S 1971 Plasma-paracetamol half-life and hepatic necrosis in patients with paracetamol overdosage. Lancet 1: 519–522
11. Seymour R A, Rawlins M D 1981 Pharmacokinetics of parenteral paracetamol and its analgesic effects in post-operative dental pain. European Journal of Clinical Pharmacology 20: 215–218
12. Prescott L F 1984 Drug conjugation in clinical toxicology. Biochemical Society Transactions 12: 96–99
13. Mitchell J R, Thorgiersson S S, Potter W Z, Jollow D J, Keise H 1974 Acetaminophen-induced hepatic injury. Protective role of glutathione in man and rationale for therapy. Clinical Pharmacology and Therapeutics 16: 676–684
14. Andrews R S, Bond C C, Burnett J, Saunders A, Watson K 1976 Isolation and identification of paracetamol metabolites. Journal of International Medical Research 4 (suppl 4): 34–39
15. Prescott L F 1983 Paracetamol overdosage: pharmacological considerations and clinical management. Drugs 25: 290–314
16. Meredith T J, Newman B, Goulding R 1978 Paracetamol poisoning in children. British Medical Journal 2: 478–479
17. Prescott L F, Illingworth R N, Critchley J A J H, Stewart M J, Adam R D, Proudfoot A T 1979 Intravenous N-acetylcysteine: the treatment of choice for paracetamol poisoning. British Medical Journal 2: 1097–1100
18. Vale J A, Meredith T J, Goulding R 1981 Treatment of acetaminophen poisoning. The use of oral methionine. Archives of Internal Medicine 141: 394–396
19. Chan T K, Todd D, Tso S C 1976 Drug induced haemolysis in glucose-6-phosphate dehydrogenase deficiency. British Medical Journal 2: 1227–1229
20. Farah D A, Boag D, Moran F, McIntosh S 1982 Paracetamol interference with blood glucose analysis: a potentially fatal phenomenon. British Medical Journal 285: 172
21. Neuberger J, Davis M, Williams R 1980 Long-term ingestion of paracetamol and liver disease. Journal of the Royal Society of Medicine 73: 701–707
22. Benson G D 1983 Acetaminophen in chronic liver disease. Clinical Pharmacology and Therapeutics 33: 95–101
23. Prescott L F, Critchley J A J H 1983 Drug interactions affecting analgesic toxicity. American Journal of Medicine 75 (No 5A): 113–116
24. Critchley J A J H, Dyson E H, Scott A W, Jarvie D R, Prescott L F 1983 Is there a place for cimetidine or ethanol in the treatment of paracetamol poisoning? Lancet 1: 1375–1376
25. Miners J O, Drew R, Birkett D J 1984 Mechanism of action of paracetamol protective agents in mice in vivo. Biochemical Pharmacology 33: 2995–3000

Penicillamine

Penicillamine was discovered as a hydrolysis product of penicillin in 1943 and has been used as a copper chelator since 1956 and more recently in the treatment of rheumatoid arthritis.

Chemistry

Penicillamine (D-penicillamine D-Pen, Distamine, Perdolat, Cuprimine Pendramine)
$C_5H_{11}NO_2S$
3,3-Dimethyl-D-cysteine

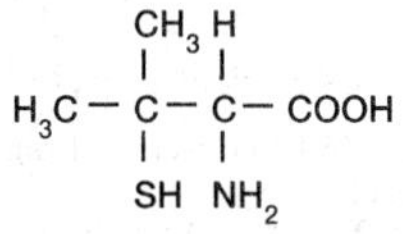

Molecular weight	149.2
pKa (COOH, NH, SH)	1.8, 7.9, 10.5
Solubility	
in alcohol	1 in 530
in water	1 in 9
Octanol/water partition coefficient	—

Penicillamine is a fine, white crystalline solid with a characteristic odour and a bitter taste.

Penicillamine may exist as the D- or L-stereoisomer but when derived from the controlled hydrolysis of penicillin is in the D-form only and this is the form available for therapeutic use. It is optically laevorotatory in aqueous solution. In aqueous solution it is readily oxidized to penicillamine disulphide.

D-penicillamine participates in three chemical reactions.

1. Metal binding (chelates mercury, lead, nickel, copper, zinc, cadmium, cobalt, iron and manganese)
2. Sulphydryl–disulphide exchange, producing penicillamine–cysteine and penicillamine–protein mixed disulphides
3. Thiazolidine formation.

Pharmacology

Penicillamine chelates metals such as copper and zinc, which:

1. interferes with cross-linking of skin collagen
2. dissociates serum macroglobulins
3. has variable effects on leucocyte function
4. may affect serum immunoglobulins and immune complexes.

Toxicology

No oral LD_{50} in animals has been recorded. Micrognathia and skull defects have been reported in offspring of mice fed D-penicillamine.

Clinical pharmacology

Heavy metal chelating activity of penicillamine has been utilized to advantage in the treatment of Wilson's disease. The mechanism of action of penicillamine in rheumatoid arthritis is still unclear but treatment reduces rheumatoid factor and circulating immune complex levels in serum and synovial fluid, possibly because of its ability to dissociate large protein molecules.[1] Penicillamine modulates activities of lymphocytes[2,3] and interferes with the destructive effects of oxygen radicals.[4] Many of these effects may be mediated through complexes of D-penicillamine with metals such as copper rather than being direct effects of D-penicillamine itself.

Pharmacokinetics

Penicillamine can be assayed by high performance liquid chromatography using an electrochemical detector[5] (sensitivity 75 μg.l^{-1}) or fluorescent derivitization (sensitivity 130 μg.l^{-1}).[6]

Penicillamine is rapidly but incompletely absorbed from the gastrointestinal tract with an apparent fraction of absorption of approximately 40% in normal fasting subjects.[3] This fraction of absorption is reduced by food.[7] In normal volunteers peak plasma concentrations after oral administration usually occur after two hours and the plasma half life is approximately 60 minutes following both intravenous and oral administration.[8]

In patients with rheumatoid arthritis plasma half life has been shown to be biphasic with a short early elimination phase (about 1 hour) and a longer β elimination phase of 5 to 7 hours. There is some suggestion of dose-dependent kinetics[9] though this is not seen in all studies.[8,10]

Penicillamine has a large mean volume of distribution (57 litres) in normal individuals.[5] Protein and tissue binding of penicillamine is extensive (in excess of 80%) but there is little known about penicillamine's distribution to deep compartments such as cerebrospinal fluid,[11,12] or the extent to which it crosses the placenta.

Oral absorption	40%
Presystemic metabolism	—
Plasma half life	
range	1–6 h
Volume of distribution	0.8 l.kg^{-1}
Plasma protein binding	up to 85%

Concentration–effect relationship

Because of the short half life, plasma concentrations vary greatly over a dosing interval and there are no data currently available to suggest a plasma concentration–effect relationship.

Metabolism

After absorption penicillamine appears in the plasma as free penicillamine, cysteine–penicillamine disulphide and penicillamine disulphide.[13] Approximately 10% of ingested penicillamine is excreted in the urine unchanged with 4% as S-methyl-penicillamine and about 25% as mixed disulphide.[14] The remainder is excreted as penicillamine disulphide with small amounts of homocysteine–penicillamine mixed disulphide.[12] Up to 50% of an oral dose is excreted in faeces but the metabolites have not yet been fully characterized.

Patients with rheumatoid arthritis, cysteinuria and Wilson's disease show varying excretion rates of these metabolites.

Pharmaceutics

Penicillamine is available in oral forms.

Distamine: (Dista, UK) film-coated tablets containing 50 mg, 125 mg, or 250 mg of D-penicillamine base. The 50 mg tablets are white-coated and scored. The 125 mg tablets are white-coated and marked DS. The 250 mg tablets are white-coated and marked DM.

Cuprimine: (MSD, USA) capsule, 125 mg light grey cap/pale yellow body, coded '672'. 250 mg yellow/yellow capsules coded '602'. All preparations should be stored in airtight containers below 25°C and have a shelf-life of approximately 2 years.

Sterilization of solutions is by membrane filtration and low concentrations (3%) stored under nitrogen lose 10% of their potency within 1.1 years.

Sterilization of solutions is by membrane filtration and low concentrations (3%) stored under nitrogen lose 10% of their potency within 1.1 years.

Therapeutic use

Indications

1. Wilson's disease
2. Cystinuria
3. Rheumatoid arthritis
4. Juvenile chronic polyarthritis

5. Palindromic rheumatism
6. Sero-negative polyarthritis
7. Progressive systemic sclerosis.

Contraindications

1. Hypersensitivity to penicillamine except in a life-threatening situation
2. Previous serious adverse reactions to penicillamine
3. Sensitivity to penicillin is not a contraindication to a trial of D-penicillamine.

Mode of use

D-penicillamine may be commenced in a relatively large dose (1.5–2 g daily) in the treatment of Wilson's disease or cystinuria. In the treatment of rheumatoid arthritis a much lower dose (125 or 250 mg daily) should be used initially and the dose increased in 125 mg or 250 mg increments at not less than 4 week intervals. Few patients now require more than 1000 mg daily as a maintenance dose. In rheumatoid arthritis, response to D-penicillamine may not be seen for six months though many patients will respond at an earlier stage.

Indications

1. Wilson's disease (hepato-lenticular degeneration)
Wilson's disease is a rare autosomal recessive condition where a deficiency of ceruloplasmin leads to excess accumulation of copper in the liver and brain. Use of penicillamine as a copper chelator to increase urinary copper excretion and produce negative copper balance has revolutionized the treatment of this previously fatal condition. Untreated patients with Wilson's disease generally excrete several hundred micrograms of urinary copper daily but this can be increased to 8 mg when 2 g of penicillamine is administered. Despite use of doses of D-penicillamine much larger than those used in rheumatoid arthritis only about 10% of patients develop drug-related side effects.[15,16]

2. Cystinuria
Cystinuria is inherited as an autosomal recessive defect characterized by failure of specific epithelial cell transport of the amino acids cystine, lysine, ornithine and arginine. The major manifestations are recurrent formation of cystine stones in the renal tract. Penicillamine undergoes a thiol–disulphide exchange with cystine reducing the quantity of plasma cystine and producing a mixed disulphide (cysteine–penicillamine disulphide) which is more soluble in aqueous solution than cystine and therefore less likely to form urinary stones. Not all patients with cystinuria require penicillamine therapy, but if urinary cystine concentrations cannot be kept below the precipitation point (less than 300 $mg.l^{-1}$) by adequate fluid intake then penicillamine in doses of up to 3 g daily may be required.[17]

The dose of penicillamine can be modified in response to the therapeutic goal, i.e. maintenance of urinary cystine concentration below 250 $mg.l^{-1}$, and penicillamine is usually given as a divided dose.[18] In some patients a single dose of 750 mg D-penicillamine once a day with a high fluid intake is adequate.[19]

3. Rheumatoid arthritis
Penicillamine now has a well-established role along with gold and anti-malarials as a second-line treatment for severe rheumatoid arthritis. D-penicillamine reduces both subjective and objective indices of disease activity but response is usually not seen within the first six weeks of treatment. Patients need to remain on treatment for up to six months before deciding that treatment failure has occurred. With continuing use of penicillamine, both initial and maintenance doses have fallen and it is now recommended that the starting and incremental dose be 125 or 250 mg per day increasing by 125 or 250 mg daily every eight to twelve weeks up to a maximum maintenance dose of 1000 mg daily.[17]

A number of clinical trials have compared penicillamine with placebo and other second- and third-line drugs such as gold, hydroxychloroquine, azathioprine and auranofin. While penicillamine is clearly significantly better than placebo there is no clear indication from clinical trials that it is significantly different from other disease-modifying agents used for severe rheumatoid arthritis. The optimal dose of D-penicillamine has not yet been determined. Doses of 600 mg daily have been shown to be significantly better than placebo,[20,21] while recent studies comparing 500 mg or 600 mg daily with 125 and 300 mg show higher doses to be slightly more effective but with an increased frequency of side effects.[22,23] The question as to whether D-penicillamine alters the course of rheumatoid arthritis in the long term is still unclear, as despite the fact that radiological deterioration may be halted[24] the majority of patients commenced on D-penicillamine have ceased treatment for a variety of reasons, including side effects and disease breakthrough if patients are followed long term.[25]

4. Juvenile chronic polyarthritis
A number of carefully conducted studies have now demonstrated efficacy of penicillamine in the treatment of juvenile chronic polyarthritis.

5. Palindromic rheumatism
Penicillamine has been shown to be efficacious in some patients with palindromic rheumatism in an uncontrolled clinical trial.

6. Sero-negative polyarthritis
Sero-negative rheumatoid arthritis seems to respond in a similar way as sero-positive disease to penicillamine but B27 associated arthropathies are usually not helped.

7. Progressive systemic sclerosis
There is some evidence that penicillamine may affect progression of both cutaneous and systemic lesions in progressive systemic sclerosis.[26,27]

Contraindications

Those who have demonstrated hypersensitivity to penicillamine or have suffered a previous severe adverse reaction such as aplastic anaemia or severe renal impairment should not be given penicillamine.

Adverse reactions

Potentially life-threatening effects
1. Aplastic anaemia
2. Neutropenia
3. Thrombocytopenia
4. Goodpasture's syndrome
5. Obliterative bronchiolitis.

Penicillamine administration was associated with the cause of death of 18 patients reported to the British Committee on Safety of Medicines between January 1964 and December 1977.[28] The majority were due to marrow aplasia. Thrombocytopenia, neutropenia, Goodpasture's syndrome and obliterative bronchiolitis have also occasionally been reported as causing death.[13]

Acute overdosage
Few reports are available, but haemolysis has occurred in a woman taking of 4 g of penicillamine by mistake. There are no data available on the management of penicillamine overdose.

Severe or irreversible adverse effects
Bullous pemphigoid-like (late) rash. The 'late' rash associated with penicillamine appears only after months or even years of treatment. Single or multiple red scaly bullous lesions develop mainly on the trunk.

Proteinuria and haematuria. Proteinuria occurs in up to 30% of R.A. patients on long-term D- penicillamine treatment and may be associated with immune-complex-mediated glomerulonephritis.[29] Proteinuria and haematuria may persist for over 2 years after D-penicillamine has been discontinued.

Thrombocytopenia. Thrombocytopenia is the most frequently reported side effect of D-penicillamine. The platelet count may fall at any time during therapy and most cases respond rapidly to withdrawal of the drug. It is standard practice to reintroduce D-penicillamine at a lower dose in these cases and patients usually tolerate this without recurrence of thrombocytopenia.

Drug-induced systemic lupus erythematosus and poly-dermatomyositis. Antinuclear antibody titres often rise during D-penicillamine treatment and some patients develop symptoms of drug-induced lupus. Other autoimmune syndromes such as poly-dermatomyositis have also been reported.

Myasthenia gravis. Myasthenia gravis is now well recognized as a complication of D-penicillamine therapy. This is sometimes associated with antibody to acetylcholine receptors.

Symptomatic adverse effects

Loss of taste. Transient loss of taste which usually occurs in the first six months of treatment is common.

Skin rashes. Early itchy skin rashes occurring in the first 10 days of therapy are less common with low-dose regimens.

Gastrointestinal disturbances. Although indigestion occasionally occurs, there is no evidence to suggest that D-penicillamine is ulcerogenic. There is no good evidence to support the contention that D-penicillamine interferes with wound healing in patients undergoing surgery.

Factors modifying the development of adverse effects to D-penicillamine

Adverse effects of penicillamine are reported more frequently in patients with arthritis than Wilson's disease or cystinuria despite the larger doses used in the latter condition. The reason for this is not clear but may be related to the 'mopping up' effect of copper–cystine complex formation.

Side effects occur more commonly in the presence of HLA-B8 and DRW3, suggesting some general predisposition.[30] There seems little evidence of cross-reactivity of gold and D-penicillamine except perhaps for proteinuria.

Monitoring for adverse reactions

Regular blood and urine tests are recommended for all patients on D-penicillamine therapy. The relatively high frequency of adverse reactions to D-penicillamine in patients with rheumatoid arthritis has led to development of fairly specific guidelines.[12] It is recommended that full blood and platelet count is checked every 2 to 4 weeks and that urine is tested for blood and protein at least monthly. It is best to record results serially on a form to reveal any progressive change.

Interference with clinical pathology tests

No changes have been reported in serum biochemistry or on chemical pathology tests.

High risk groups

Neonates

There are no data on D-penicillamine administration to neonates.

Breast milk. There are no data available on excretion of penicillamine in breast milm, though because of extensive binding the amounts are likely to be small.

Children

The starting dose of D-penicillamine is 50 mg daily increasing by 50 mg at intervals of not less than 4 weeks. Tolerance of D-penicillamine by children is similar to adults.

Pregnant women

D-penicillamine can be continued through pregnancy in Wilson's disease and cystinuria. In rheumatoid arthritis slow withdrawal may be attempted but normal pregnancies have resulted from patients taking D-penicillamine throughout gestation.

Although there are isolated cases of an Ehlers–Danlos 'type' of defect reported in children of mothers treated with D-penicillamine, many normal children have been born to mothers treated with D-penicillamine for all or part of their pregnancy.[31,32]

The elderly

No special precautions are required in elderly patients and they have been shown to respond in a similar fashion to younger patients.[33]

Drug interactions

Interactions have not been described between penicillamine and non-steroidal anti-inflammatory agents or other drugs. Food can reduce the availability of penicillamine as previously described.

Oral iron reduces D-penicillamine-induced cupruresis[34] and absorption may be similarly reduced in patients with rheumatoid arthritis.[35]

Major outcome trials

1. Multi Centre Trial Group 1973 Controlled trial of D-penicillamine in severe rheumatoid arthritis. Lancet 1: 275–280

This is a twelve-month double-blind comparison of D-penicillamine (1.5 g daily) and placebo in 105 patients with severe rheumatoid arthritis. 30 patients out of 52 on D-penicillamine and 38 of 53 on placebo completed the trial. 110 patients taking D-penicillamine for more than 6 months showed a decrease in arthritis while 17% of patients on placebo showed progression of disease necessitating withdrawal.

Adverse reactions to D-penicillamine were common (60%) requiring withdrawal in 30% of patients over the 12 month period. All measurements of disease activity, except radiographic change in the small joints of the hand, showed greater improvement on D-penicillamine.

2. Dixon A St. J, Davis J, Dormandy T L et al 1975 Synthetic D-penicillamine in rheumatoid arthritis. Annals of the Rheumatic Diseases 34: 416–421

This is a six-month comparison of D-penicillamine in doses of 600 mg and 1200 mg daily with a placebo (12 mg D-penicillamine) in 121 patients with rheumatoid arthritis. Both regimens were superior to placebo but no significant differences were seen between 600 and 1200 mg daily. Withdrawals due to adverse reactions, in particular blood dyscrasias and skin rashes, were higher on the high-dose regimen.

3. Williams H J, Ward J R, Reading J C et al 1983 Low dose D-penicillamine therapy in rheumatoid arthritis. Arthritis and Rheumatism 26: 581–592

225 patients with active rheumatoid arthritis were randomly allocated to 36 weeks of treatment with D-penicillamine 500 mg daily, D-penicillamine 125 mg daily or placebo. The 500 mg D-penicillamine group showed a statistically significant improvement over the placebo group in proximal interphalangeal joint circumference, grip strength and patient assessment. No significant differences were demonstrated between the 125 mg D-penicillamine and placebo groups or between the 125 and 500 mg D-penicillamine regimens. This study concluded that D-penicillamine in a dose of 500 mg daily is only slightly more effective than placebo in the treatment of severe rheumatoid arthritis of long duration.

4. Gibson T, Huskisson E C, Wojtulewski J A et al 1976 Evidence that D-penicillamine alters the course of rheumatoid arthritis. Rheumatology and Rehabilitation 15: 211–215

This is a comparison of gold and D-penicillamine in 87 rheumatoid arthritis patients followed for two years. Doses of gold thiomalate were 50 mg weekly to 1 g and then 50 mg monthly while D-penicillamine was increased from 250 mg daily in 250 mg increments at fortnightly intervals to 1.8 g daily and then adjusted according to response.

Equivalent clinical improvement was seen in both groups though a larger number of patients withdrew from gold therapy due to side effects.

5. Rothermich N O, Thomas M H, Phillips V K, Bergen W 1981 Clinical trial of penicillamine in rheumatoid arthritis. Arthritis and Rheumatism 24: 1473–1478

This is a descriptive study of 200 patients originally commenced on D-penicillamine at up to 1 g daily and followed for up to 5 years. Only 28% were still receiving treatment with D-penicillamine, the major reasons for drop-out being development of side effects or relapse on therapy. Over 70% of patients benefited (remission or improvement) from D-penicillamine therapy but this was not sustained in the majority of cases. This study demonstrated that while D-penicillamine is a valuable drug in the treatment of rheumatoid arthritis, its long-term value is limited by a high incidence of toxicity and relapse during treatment.

6. Situnayacke R D, Gurindulis K A, McConkey B 1987 Long term treatment of rheumatoid arthritis with sulphasalazine, gold or penicillamine; A comparison using life table methods. Annals of Rheumatic Diseases 46: 177–183

In this study a life table analysis was applied to the records of 317 patients with rheumatoid arthritis treated with sulphasalazine, 201 patients treated with sodium aurothiamalate and 163 treated with penicillamine. Between 80% and 90% of patients had ceased their

Penicillamine

treatments within five years. The risk of treatment termination due to inefficacy was slightly higher for D-penicillamine and sulphasalazine than for gold while adverse effects were a more common cause of withdrawal with gold than with penicillamine or with sulphasalazine.

General review articles

Leading article 1973 Penicillamine in the treatment of rheumatoid arthritis. British Medical Journal 2: 464

Leading article 1978 Penicillamine: its place in rheumatology. British Medical Journal 1: 131

Netter P, Bannwarth B, Péré P, Nicholas A 1987 Clinical pharmacokinetics of D-penicillamine. Clinical Pharmacokinetics 13: 317–333

Muirden K D 1986 The use of chloroquine and D-penicillamine in the treatment of rheumatoid arthritis. Medical Journal of Australia 144: 32–37

References

1. Bloch H S, Prasard A, Anastasi A, Briggs P R 1960 Serum protein changes in Waldenstroms macroglobulinaemia during administration of a low molecular thiol (penicillamine). Journal of Laboratory and Clinical Medicine 56: 212
2. Lipsky P E, Ziff M 1978 The effect of D-penicillamine on mitogen induced human lymphocyte proliferation: synergistic inhibition by D-penicillamine and copper salts. Journal of Immunology 170: 1006–1013
3. Lipsky P E 1983 Remission-inducing therapy in rheumatoid arthritis. American Journal of Medicine 75: 40–49
4. Skosey J L, Chow D C, Marbach W J, Liu S 1982 D-penicillamine and oxygen derived agent mediated inflammatory responses. Immunogenetics in Rheumatology. Amsterdam. Excerpta Medica 297
5. Saetre R, Rabenstein D L 1978 Determination of penicillamine in blood and urine by high performance liquid chromatography. Analytical Chemistry 50: 276–280
6. Miners J O, Fearnley I, Smith K J, Birkett D J, Brooks P M, Whitehouse M W 1983 The analysis of D-penicillamine in plasma by fluorescence derivitisation with N-(p-(benzoxazolyl)-phenyl) maleimide and high performance liquid chromatography. Journal of Chromatography 275: 89–96
7. Schuna A, Osman M A, Patel R B, Welling P G, Sundstrom W R 1983 Influence of food on the bioavailability of penicillamine. Journal of Rheumatology 10: 95–97
8. Wiesner R H, Dickson E R, Carlson G L, McPhaul L W, Go V L W 1981 Pharmacokinetics of D-penicillamine in man. Journal of Rheumatology 8 (suppl 7): 51–55
9. Bergstrom R F, Kay D R, Harkcom T M, Wagner J G 1981 Penicillamine kinetics in normal subjects. Clinical Pharmacology and Therapeutics 30: 404–413
10. Butler M, Carruthers G, Harth M, Freeman D, Percy J, Rabenstein D 1982 Pharmacokinetics of reduced D-penicillamine in patients with rheumatoid arthritis. Arthritis and Rheumatism 25: 111–116
11. Gibbs K, Walshe J M 1971 Studies with ^{35}S-labelled D.L.penicillamine in patients with Wilson's disease. Quarterly Journal of Medicine 158: 275–287
12. Perrett D 1981 Metabolism and pharmacology of D-penicillamine in man. Journal of Rheumatology 8 (suppl 7): 41–50
13. Brooks P M, Miners J O, Smith K O, Smith M D, Fearnley I, Birkett D J 1984 Dose, plasma concentration and response relationships of D-penicillamine in patients with rheumatoid arthritis. Journal of Rheumatology 11: 772-775
14. Perrett D, Sneddon W, Stephens A D 1976 Studies on D-penicillamine metabolism in cystinuria and rheumatoid arthritis: isolation of S-methyl-d-penicillamine. Biochemical Pharmacology 25: 259–264
15. Walshe J M 1977 Brief observations on the management of Wilson's disease. Proceedings of the Royal Society of Medicine 70 (suppl 3): 1-3
16. Scheinberg I H 1981 Wilson's disease. Journal of Rheumatology 8 (suppl 7): 90–93
17. Lyle W H 1979 Penicillamine. Clinics in the Rheumatic Diseases 5: 569–601
18. Stephens A D, Fenton J C B 1977 Serum immunoglobulins in D-penicillamine treated cystinurics. Proceedings of the Royal Society of Medicine 70 (suppl 3): 31
19. Purkiss P, Watts R W E 1977 Low dose D-penicillamine in cystinuria. Proceedings of the Royal Society of Medicine 70 (suppl 3): 27–30
20. Dixon A St J, Davies J, Dormandy T L et al 1975 Synthetic D-penicillamine in rheumatoid arthritis: double-blind controlled study of a high and low dose regimen. Annals of the Rheumatic Diseases 34: 416–427
21. Berry H, Liyanage S P, Durance R A, Barnes C G, Berger L A, Evans S 1976 Azathioprine and penicillamine in treatment of rheumatoid arthritis: a controlled trial. British Medical Journal 1: 1052–1054
22. Williams H J, Ward J R, Reading J C et al 1983 Low dose D-penicillamine therapy in rheumatoid arthritis: a controlled double blind clinical trial. Arthritis and Rheumatism 26: 581–592
23. Nissil A M, Nuotio P, Von Essen R, Makisara P 1982 Low dose penicillamine treatment of R.A. comparison of 600 mg and 300 mg regimens. Scandinavian Journal of Rheumatology 11: 161–164
24. Gibson T, Huskisson E C, Wojtulewski J A 1976 Evidence that D-penicillamine alters the course of rheumatoid arthritis. Rheumatology and Rehabilitation 15: 211–215
25. Rothermich N O, Thomas M H, Phillips V K, Bergen W 1981 Clinical trial of penicillamine in rheumatoid arthritis. Arthritis and Rheumatism 24: 1473–1478
26. Jayson M I V, Black C M, Lovell C R, Bailey A J 1976 The effects of D-penicillamine on collagen in systemic sclerosis and rheumatoid arthritis. In: Munthe E (ed) Penicillamine research in rheumatic disease. Fabritius and Sônner M S D, Oslo, pp 105–107
27. Steen V D, Medsger T A, Rodnan G P 1982 D-penicillamine therapy in progressive systemic sclerosis (Scleroderma). Annals of Internal Medicine 97: 652–659
28. Kay A G L 1979 Myelotoxicity of D-penicillamine. Annals of the Rheumatic Diseases 38: 232–236
29. Dische F E, Swinson D R, Hamilton E D, Parons V 1976 Immunopathology of penicillamine induced glomerular disease. Journal of Rheumatology 3: 145–154
30. Wooley P H, Griffin J, Panayi G S, Batchelor J R, Welsh K I, Gibson T J 1980 HLA-DR Antigens and toxic relations to sodium aurothiomalate and D-penicillamine in patients with rheumatoid arthritis. New England Journal of Medicine 303: 300–302
31. Mjolnerod O K, Dommerud S A, Rassmussen K, Gjeruldsen S T 1971 Congenital connective tissue defect probably due to D-penicillamine treatment in pregnancy. Lancet 1: 673–675
32. Lyle W H 1978 Penicillamine in pregnancy. Lancet 1: 1064
33. Kean W F, Anastassiades T P, Dwosh I, Ford P M, Kelly H G, Dok C 1982 Efficacy and toxicity of D-penicillamine for rheumatoid disease in the elderly. Journal of the American Geriatric Society 30: 94–100
34. Lyle W H, Pearcey D F, Hui M 1977 Inhibition of penicillamine induced cupruresis by oral iron. Proceedings of the Royal Society of Medicine 70 (suppl 3): 48–49
35. Harkness J A, Blake D R 1982 Penicillamine nephropathy and iron. Lancet 2: 1368–1369

Pentamidine

Pentamidine is a synthetic aromatic amidine with actions against a range of pathogenic protozoa. It is used in the treatment of pneumonia due to *Pneumocystis carinii*. Pentamidine has weak antifungal actions.

Chemistry

Pentamidine
$C_{19}H_{24}N_4O_2$
4,4′-Diamidinodiphenoxypentane

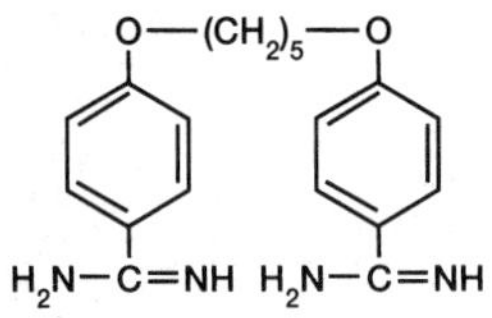

Molecular weight	340.4
pKa (amino group)	11.4
Solubility	
in alcohol	—
in water	—
Octanol/water partition coefficient	—

Pentamidine isethionate (Pentacarinat)
$C_{19}H_{24}N_4O_2.2C_2H_6O_4S$
Pentamidine di(2-hydroxyethanesulphonate)

Molecular weight	592.7
pKa	—
Solubility	
in alcohol	low
in water	1 in 10
Octanol/water partition coefficient	—

Pentamidine isothionate is an odourless white powder with a bitter taste, prepared by chemical synthesis.

Pentamidine mesylate (Lomidine)
$C_{19}H_{24}N_4O_2.2CH_3SO_3H$
Pentamidine dimethylsulphonate

Molecular weight	532.6
pKa	—
Solubility	
in alcohol	low
in water	low
Octanol/water partition coefficient	—

Pentamidine mesylate is an odourless white powder prepared by chemical synthesis.

Pharmacology

Pentamidine, like other diamidines, is effective against *Trypanosoma rhodesiense* and *T. congolense* infections in animals. The drug is also active against *Leishmania donovani* in hamsters. Pentamidine is concentrated by trypanosomes via an energy-dependent, high affinity uptake system. In drug-sensitive strains this system operates particularly rapidly. Pentamidine has a number of effects on the cells. It binds to DNA (especially extranuclear DNA); it inhibits DNA synthesis; it inhibits RNA polymerase, ribosomal synthesis of protein and synthesis of phospholipid;[1,2] and at high concentrations it damages mitochondria. Pentamidine also interferes with the uptake and function of polyamines. The drug has some antifungal properties and kills *Pneumocystis carinii* in a non-replicating state.

Toxicology

Limited unpublished data (May and Baker) are available. These are summarized below.

Pentamidine isethionate was well tolerated by rats given 5 mg.kg^{-1} daily intravenously, but higher doses caused prostration, dyspnoea, cyanosis and sedation. It was not well tolerated in dogs given 5 mg.kg^{-1} daily for 5 days intravenously. There was local irritation at the site of intravenous or intramuscular injection.

Rabbits were dosed intravenously once on each of days 5–20 post-coitum with 1, 3 or 8 mg.kg^{-1} pentamidine isethionate. Maternal toxicity, including mortality, was seen at 8 mg.kg^{-1}. Litter data remained largely unaffected by treatment, except for a mild fetotoxic effect in all dosage groups, as indicated by increased post-implantation loss and increased incidence of minor fetal skeletal abnormalities, which may be linked with maternal toxicity.

Pentamidine isethionate was not mutagenic in an Ames test (*S. typhimurium*) with or without metabolic activation (S9 rat liver fraction). From an experiment to assess mutation to 6-thioguanine resistance in the mouse lymphoma fluctuation assay, it was concluded that pentamidine isethionate displayed weak mutagenic activity in the presence, but not the absence, of liver metabolism.

The treatment of human lymphocyte cultures with toxic doses of pentamidine isethionate resulted in a small increase in chromosomal aberrations in the absence of metabolic activation (S9 rat liver fraction), which was not biologically significant; there were no induced aberrations in the presence of S9 activation.

Clinical pharmacology

Pentamidine has few clinical pharmacological effects in man, though if the drug is injected intravenously a rapid fall in blood pressure is often seen. Pentamidine is useful in the treatment of trypanosomiasis but the drug does not cross the blood–brain barrier and so melarsoprol must be given when the central nervous system is involved. Pentamidine is effective in the treatment of cutaneous and visceral leishmaniasis, although sodium stibogluconate is usually the first choice. In diffuse cutaneous leishmaniasis pentamidine is of value in some cases caused by *L. aethiopica*. It is of value in the treatment of systemic blastomycosis, although amphotericin B is usually preferred. Presently it is most often used in the treatment of pneumonia due to *Pneumocystis carinii* in the immunodeficient or immunosuppressed patient particularly in the acquired immune deficiency syndrome (AIDS) due to the human immunodeficiency virus.

Pharmacokinetics

Two assays are in use at present, a bioassay using *Candida tropicalis*[3] and high performance liquid chromatography.[4] The bioassay will measure concentrations of 80 μg.l^{-1} in serum and urine and 800 μg.l^{-1} in tissue.[3] High performance liquid chromatography (HPLC) will measure 2.29 μg.l^{-1} in plasma and 229 μg.l^{-1} in urine.[5] No data are available for the use of HPLC in assays of tissue. While bioassay is satisfactory at levels over 80 μg.l^{-1}, it is much less satisfactory than HPLC in measuring low concentrations in biological fluids.

The peak plasma level of 209 μg.l^{-1} was found about 40 min after a first intramuscular injection of 300 mg pentamidine isethionate. Intravenous infusion of this dose over 2 h produced a peak level of 612 ± 371 μg.l^{-1}, both measurements by HPLC.[5,6] No data are available for peak levels after intramuscular injection using the bioassay.

Using HPLC the kinetics of drug distribution have been followed[5] in 12 patients receiving their first doses. At 15 min after intramuscular injection of 186–270 mg of the isethionate in six patients, plasma levels ranged from 29.6 to 163 μg.l^{-1} with a further increase to 112–246 μg.l^{-1} at 1 h. At 2 h the range was 73.1–129 μg.l^{-1}, at 4 h 33.2–49.2 μg.l^{-1} and at 24 h 3.33–13.2 μg.l^{-1}. Six patients received infusions of 200–440 mg over two hours. After 20 minutes of the infusion plasma levels ranged from 91.2 to 604 μg.l^{-1} increasing to 129–876 μg.l^{-1} by one hour and 89.6–1254 μg.l^{-1} by the end of infusion. After completion of the infusion there was a progressive and fairly rapid decline in plasma levels. There is evidence of drug accumulation with repeated administration; trough concentrations[6] ranged from 4.3 to 67.5 μg.l^{-1}. The drug is rapidly cleared from circulation by tissue binding and uptake. The apparent volume of distribution in the central compartment[6] is 3.31 l.kg^{-1}.

The mean half life of the drug determined by HPLC in patients receiving their first dose is 9.36 h after intramuscular injection and 6.4 h after intravenous infusion. Where previous doses had been given, the half life was considerably prolonged to 52±89 h.[6]

This study also reported a significant correlation between half life and number of previous injections but found no correlation between half life and creatinine clearance over the range <20 to 76 ml.min^{-1}. The plasma levels and rate of decline of plasma pentamidine concentrations in patients with renal failure requiring haemodialysis were similar to those seen in patients with normal renal function.[6] Pentamidine could not be detected in peritoneal dialysis fluid. Renal excretion of the drug varied from 4.08% of the administered dose per 24 h after intramuscular injection to 2.46% after infusion.

Bioassay has been used to measure concentrations in postmortem samples of internal organs in patients dying with AIDS.[7] Highest tissue concentrations are found in liver, kidney, adrenal and spleen while lowest concentrations were consistently found in lung. In two patients who had each received two doses amounting to a total of 324 mg and 400 mg, concentrations in liver were 35 and 25 μg.g^{-1} of tissue; in spleen 40 and 33 μg.g^{-1}; kidney 9 and 13 μg.g^{-1}; and zero in the lungs of both patients. Four and five doses amounting to 1200 and 1400 mg produced concentrations of 186 and 84 μg.g^{-1} (liver); 40 and 33 μg.g^{-1} (spleen); 119 and 46 μg.g^{-1} (kidney); and 30 and 17.5 μg.g^{-1} (lung). This delay in accumulation in the lung may explain why seven or eight days' treatment are needed to produce improvement in *Pneumocystis carinii* pneumonia (PCP). After 33 doses the lung concentrations were 81 and 72 μg.g^{-1}. By 13 and 71 days after total doses of 2160 mg and 1600 mg lung concentrations had fallen to 36 and 1.5 μg.g^{-1}, while liver concentrations were 109 and 3.9 μg.g^{-1}.

When repeat courses are given, tissue concentrations appear to rise rapidly. For example, when a patient restarted pentamidine 33 days after his last course and was given two 200 mg doses, spleen concentrations were similar to those in a patient just starting on the drug, liver concentrations were considerably higher and the mean lung concentration was 29 μg.g^{-1}, a level achieved after four or five doses in a first course.[7] Pentamidine is found in the pancreas and also in the brain but only after prolonged dosing.

The delivery of pentamidine to the lung was compared in patients given either aerosolized drug or an intravenous infusion.[8] Within 24 h of receiving the drug by either route patients were bronchoscoped and the right middle lobe was lavaged. It was found that concentrations were significantly higher in patients receiving inhaled drug than in patients given infusions. Further analysis indicated that, after inhalation, pentamidine reaches the alveolar spaces which are the sites of the pneumonic process in PCP.

Oral absorption	—
Presystemic metabolism	—
Plasma half life (first dose)	
mean (i.m.)	9.36 h
mean (i.v.)	6.4 h
Volume of distribution	3.31 l.kg^{-1}
Plasma protein binding	—

Concentration–effect relationship

Little is known about this aspect of pentamidine use. Binding of the drug to affected tissues may be important in determining the response. The better response of patients with *Pneumocystis carinii* pneumonia who have received 9 or more days' treatment may reflect the slow build-up to therapeutic levels but there is no evidence of any correlation between the plasma concentration and its therapeutic effect.

Metabolism

There are no data about metabolism of pentamidine as yet, though the current interest in the drug resulting from its use in PCP may produce further studies on this aspect of it. The unaltered drug is excreted in small amounts, 2–4% over 24 h after parenteral administration, in the urine. Prolonged urinary excretion occurs after finishing a course of treatment. Unaltered drug is excreted in small amounts in the faeces.

Pharmaceutics

Pentamidine is supplied for parenteral use in vials containing 300 mg of pentamidine isethionate as a powder: Pentacarinat (Rhone Poulenc, UK); Pentam-300 LyphoMed (Aldrich Chemical Co, USA). The drug is given by intramuscular injection or intravenous infusion. Water for Injections BP, 2 or 3 ml, is added to the contents of the vial. When the contents have dissolved the appropriate dose is drawn up and injected intramuscularly. For intravenous infusion the appropriate dose of dissolved drug is added to 50–250 ml of 5% dextrose and infused over one or two hours. Bolus injections should not be given.

Pentamidine isethionate solutions, 1.0 and 2.5 mg.ml^{-1} in 5% dextrose, retain their potency for 24 h at room temperature.

Therapeutic use

Indications

1. *Pneumocystis carinii* pneumonia (PCP)
2. Leishmaniasis
3. Trypanosomiasis.

Contraindications

No information is available about its use in pregnancy and so the drug is best avoided. Otherwise there are no absolute contraindications.

Mode of use

Pentamidine isethionate is usually given in a dose of 4 mg.kg^{-1} body weight. The frequency of dosing and the number of doses to be given depend on the infection to be treated (see below). Intramuscular injection is the traditional route for administration, but this is associated with local pain at the site, inflammation and abscess formation. Slow intravenous infusion is safe.[9] Local reactions at the injection site and hypotension were less frequent than following intramuscular injection.[9] Recent studies in patients with AIDS have shown that administration of pentamidine as an aerosol is effective in the treatment of PCP.[10–12] Details are set out below.

Indications

1. *Pneumocystis carinii* pneumonia

This condition occurs in children and adults with immunodeficiency. This may be due to malnutrition, malignant disease, particularly leukaemia, cytotoxic chemotherapy, immunosuppression after organ transplantation and AIDS. The latter is now the most common condition predisposing to this infection. The standard regimen is to give pentamidine isethionate, 4 mg.kg^{-1} of the salt, by slow intravenous infusion or intramuscular injection daily for 14 to 21 days. Improvement can be expected after 5 to 7 days and survival is greatest in those receiving eight or more injections.

Recent studies in patients with AIDS have shown that inhalation of aerosolized pentamidine is an effective way of administering the drug in PCP of mild to moderate severity with fewer side effects.[10] A dose of 600 mg of pentamidine is dissolved in 6 ml of sterile water and nebulized through a suitable system such as the Respigard II (Marquest). The patient inhales the aerosol over 20 minutes daily for 21 days. Half of the nebulized dose reaches the lungs. The performance of the nebulizer is critical to the effectiveness of this method of giving the drug, as the dose of drug reaching the lungs is inversely proportional to the size of the particles generated. The Respigard II produces a mass median particle size of 1.0 μm with 79% of particles less than 2.0 μm.[9] The main adverse effects of aerosolized pentamidine are cough, bronchial irritation and bronchospasm caused by large particles settling on bronchiolar walls. The nebulizer used should have high-efficiency filters to remove pentamidine from exhaled air to prevent environmental contamination. Aerosolized pentamidine appears to be effective in the chemoprophylaxis of *Pn. carinii* pneumonia in AIDS patients,[11] giving 300 mg of drug dissolved in 4 ml of sterile water through the same sort of nebulizer once monthly. In a prospective controlled trial the incidence of PCP in AIDS patients taking zidovudine was 2 out of 22 on inhaled pentamidine prophylaxis and 16 out of 26 not receiving the drug.[12]

2. Leishmaniasis

a. Visceral leishmaniasis. Pentamidine is the second choice drug for this disease. Sodium stibogluconate is less toxic, but pentamidine is effective in cases that are resistant to sodium stibogluconate.[13] The dose used is 4 $mg.kg^{-1}$ pentamidine isethionate given on alternate days or twice weekly. The duration of treatment depends on the clinical and parasitological response. Five to six weeks is the minimum duration, while up to 39 weeks has been reported.[14] Examination of smears of bone marrow or splenic aspirate indicates the parasitological response. Fixed durations of treatment for visceral leishmaniasis contracted in particular geographical areas are no longer recommended.

b. Cutaneous leishmaniasis. Pentamidine is effective in the treatment of diffuse cutaneous leishmaniasis due to *Leishmania aethiopica* though it is not curative in all cases. The dose used in one study was 4 mg of base per kg body weight of pentamidine mesylate[15] weekly or every 2 weeks for 5 doses. Pentamidine is also effective in treatment of *Leishmania braziliensis guyanensis.*[16]

3. Trypanosomiasis

Pentamidine was used very successfully in the prophylaxis of sleeping sickness due to *Trypanosoma brucei gambiense* but this is no longer recommended.[17] It is used for treatment of blood and lymphatic infections with *T. br. gambiense* but it cannot be used when there is involvement of the central nervous system as it does not cross the blood–brain barrier. The dose is worked out at 3–4 mg pentamidine base per kg body weight. The calculated dose is given intramuscularly daily or on alternate days until 7 to 10 doses have been given. It is not recommended for *T. br. rhodesiense* infections as primary resistance is recorded. Suramin is the drug of first choice in early trypanosomiasis.

Contraindications

There are no absolute contraindications to the use of this drug. Because of its cardiovascular and renal side effects appropriate supportive care is essential to ensure normal hydration and tissue perfusion. When impairment of glucose tolerance occurs during treatment the drug should be withdrawn if the abnormalities do not resolve spontaneously.

Adverse reactions

Potentially life-threatening effects

These are uncommon. Severe hypotension and acidosis occurred in a 14-year-old boy who subsequently died. These features occurred 11 h after an intramuscular injection.[18] Irreversible hypoglycaemia causing death occurs with an incidence of 13 per 10 000 patients.[19] Myoglobinuria with nephrotoxicity has also been reported.[20]

Cardiac toxicity is potentially life-threatening. Jha reported fatal cardiac arrest in two patients.[13] The mechanism in those cases is not known but subsequent clinical studies have shown prolongation of the Q-T interval, bradycardia and *torsades de pointes*.[21–24] The latter is a polymorphic form of ventricular tachycardia with gradually changing polarity of QRS complexes producing an undulating form on ECG tracings. This arrhythmia can cause cardiac arrest.

Acute overdosage

Cases of deliberate or accidental overdosing with pentamidine have not been reported.

Severe or irreversible adverse effects

As noted above, hypoglycaemia is a serious and potentially fatal side effect. The incidence of hypoglycaemia in a large retrospective chart review was 14%.[19] Risk factors for the development of hypoglycaemia were prolonged duration of treatment, an increased total dose given, previous pentamidine treatment and azotaemia. Hypoglycaemia is the result of drug toxicity on the β-cells of the pancreas producing hyperinsulinaemia.[25] Diazoxide effectively countered hypoglycaemia in two patients.[26] In about 5% of those receiving long-term pentamidine, insulin-dependent diabetes mellitus develops.[13] This has occurred as early as the sixth and tenth days of treatment but more often in patients receiving prolonged courses, 20 days or more.[25] Pancreatitis has been reported after intravenous and inhaled pentamidine,[27,28] though it should be noted that pancreatic abnormalities are not uncommon in patients with AIDS.

Renal impairment is common, with up to 25% of patients exhibiting evidence of nephrotoxicity. This is seen in patients with normal or impaired renal function before treatment and is usually reversible after discontinuing the drug. Nephrotoxicity occurred significantly more often among those patients with diarrhoea who received the drug by the intramuscular route (32%) than by infusion (14%) whereas there was no difference in the occurrence in those without diarrhoea,[29] suggesting that adequate hydration may help to prevent this effect. Occasionally irreversible renal damage is seen.[20]

Pneumothorax has been reported in patients receiving nebulized pentamidine for prophylaxis but has not been featured in reports describing treatment of *Pn. carinii* pneumonia by inhalation.

Symptomatic adverse effects

Dizziness, hypotension and syncope are symptoms associated with cardiac toxicity. The usual clinical features occurring in hypoglycaemia are seen with pentamidine, though hypoglycaemic patients may be asymptomatic. Flushing, nausea, pruritus and maculopapular rash may occur. Inhaled pentamidine caused urticaria in one patient. Local inflammation and muscle necrosis producing a sterile abscess may develop at sites of intramuscular injection.

Inhaled pentamidine causes bronchial irritation, cough and bronchospasm. The severity of these effects appears in part to relate to the size of particles produced by the nebulizer but there is some evidence to suggest that the drug may inhibit cholinesterase.[30]

Other effects

There is some evidence of liver damage, with elevation of plasma aminotransferases. Liver failure has not been reported and the abnormalities resolve after finishing the course of treatment. Reversible neutropenia and thrombocytopenia have also occurred.

Interference with clinical pathology tests

No interference with tests has been reported.

High risk groups

Neonates

No information is available.

Breast milk. The drug is excreted in breast milk in small amounts. This was biologically effective in the chemoprophylaxis of *T. br. gambiense* infection in suckling rats and possibly in humans too (cited by Williamson[31]). It is not known if there is enough drug to cause hypoglycaemia in the infant.

Children

Children should receive the drug in standard doses.

Pregnant women

The safety of pentamidine in pregnancy has not been established and so it should not be used unless it is absolutely necessary. A World Health Organisation Expert Committee on Trypanosomiasis[32] noted that pregnancy was not a contraindication to the use of pentamidine in this infection.

The elderly

Monitoring for the occurrence of hypotension and hypoglycaemia may be advisable.

Drug interactions

Potentially hazardous interactions

Patients with *Pneumocystis carinii* pneumonia, particularly those cases occurring in leucopenic patients and in the acquired immunodeficiency syndrome, often have infections with several pathogens and may be receiving several antibiotics, including aminoglycosides. Aminoglycoside blood levels should be monitored to ensure optimal but safe levels. There is no evidence of a synergistic adverse interaction between pentamidine and aminoglycosides on the kidneys or of any adverse reaction with any antibiotic or other drug.

Pentamidine

Other significant interactions
The inhibition, in vitro, of human cholinesterase raises the possibility that pentamidine may potentiate the effects of suxamethonium and other cholinesterase-sensitive drugs.[30]

Potentially useful interactions
No reactions of this kind have been reported.

Major outcome trials

1. Hughes W T, Feldman S, Chaudhary S C, Ossi M J, Cox F, Sanyal S K 1978 Comparison of pentamidine isethionate and trimethoprim–sulfamethoxazole in the treatment of *Pneumocystis carinii* pneumonia. Journal of Pediatrics 92: 285–291

This prospective randomized controlled trial showed pentamidine to be as effective as trimethoprim–sulfamethoxazole in curing this infection in children with malignancy. Cure occurred in 75% and 77% respectively after receiving one or other drug only. Nine cases from each initial treatment group were crossed over to receive the other drug and overall cure rates were 71% and 81% respectively. Mild reversible nephrotoxicity occurred in the pentamidine group (9 cases). Hypoglycaemia occurred in 6 cases (asymptomatic in 5/6). Pentamidine was recommended as the drug of second choice to be used in those who do not respond to the more easily administered trimethoprim–sulfamethoxazole. Niegel et al[33] reported similar results.

2. Wharton J M, Coleman D L, Wofsy C B et al 1986 Trimethoprim–sulphamethoxazole or pentamidine for *Pneumocystis carinii* pneumonia in the acquired immunodeficiency syndrome. A prospective randomized trial. Annals of Internal Medicine 105: 37–44

This prospective, randomized trial examined the outcome of treatment of a proven first episode of *Pn. carinii* pneumonia with either pentamidine or trimethoprim–sulphamethoxazole. The two groups of patients were comparable with regard to a wide range of parameters. Other opportunistic infections were evenly distributed, apart from cytomegalovirus infection of the lungs which was significantly more common among the pentamidine-treated patients (14 out of 20). There was no difference in the efficacy of the two drugs with regard to survival; numbers of patients switched to the other drug because of failure to respond or major allergic reactions; decline of fever, respiratory rate or dyspnoea score; or changes in pulmonary function tests. Allergic reactions were common, occurring in half of each group. Eight out of 20 (pentamidine) and 7 out of 20 (trimethoprim–sulphamethoxazole) remained on the drug first allocated throughout the 21 days of treatment. Both drugs caused neutropenia but this was more common with pentamidine. This adverse effect of pentamidine appears to be associated with its use in this clinical setting. Hypoglycaemia occurred but did not require a change of treatment, and renal impairment necessitating a change occurred in two patients. Intravenous infusion of pentamidine was well tolerated. Despite the fact that organisms were present in the lungs of 60% of patients after treatment, none of the six deaths over the following three months were thought to be due to recurrence of PCP.

3. Montgomery A B, Debs R J, Luce J M et al 1987 Aerosolised pentamidine as sole therapy for *Pneumocystis carinii* pneumonia in the acquired immunodeficiency syndrome. Lancet 2: 480–483

Patients with AIDS presenting with their first attack of PCP were treated with inhaled pentamidine. The patients had mild or moderate attacks; patients with a PaO less than 50 mmHg were excluded. 600 mg of pentamidine isethionate were dissolved in 6 ml of sterile water and administered via a Respigard II nebulizer over 20 minutes daily for 21 days. 13 out of 15 showed a satisfactory response and did not require alternative treatment. Ten patients improved during the first week and three during the second week. Absorption of the drug occurred with serum levels of less than $10\ \mu g.l^{-1}$ in 12 out of 14 patients. Coughing was the main side effect and was particularly troublesome in smokers. Systemic toxicity due to pentamidine was not seen.

4. Girard P-M, Landman R, Gaudebout C et al 1989 Prevention of *Pneumocystis carinii* pneumonia relapse by pentamidine aerosol in zidovudine-treated AIDS patients. Lancet 1: 1348–1353

This prospective controlled trial showed that inhaled pentamidine is very effective in preventing relapse of PCP in AIDS patients on zidovudine. Pentamidine mesylate was used in this study giving 4 mg base per kg body weight every two weeks for the first month and then monthly. The drug was diluted in 0.9% sterile saline to a concentration of $10\ mg.ml^{-1}$. An ultrasonic nebulizer, Ultraneb 99 (De Vilbiss), was used and patients attended a day care centre for treatments under medical supervision. Relapse of PCP occurred in 2 out of 22 patients receiving the drug and 16 out of 26 randomized to receive no prophylaxis. This difference was highly significant ($P < 0.0002$). Side effects were those of bronchial irritation and these were very troublesome in some patients. Prophylaxis had to be withdrawn in one patient. There was no evidence of other toxicity.

Note: The United States Public Health Service has published recommendations with regard to the prophylaxis of PCP in adult patients with AIDS. These indicate that any patient who has had PCP should receive prophylaxis. Inhaled pentamidine isethionate, 300 mg every four weeks, can be given using the Respigard II jet nebulizer. The dose should be diluted in 6 ml of sterile water and delivered at $6\ l.min^{-1}$ from a 50 psi source of compressed air. Primary prophylaxis of PCP is justified in AIDS patients whose counts of CD4+ are $< 200\ mm^{-3}$ or $< 20\%$ of total lymphocyte count.

(See: Guidelines for prophylaxis against *Pneumocystis carinii* pneumonia for persons infected with human immunodeficiency virus. Morbidity and Mortality Weekly Reports 1989: No S-5, pp 1–9.)

Other trials

1. Soo Hoo G W, Mohsenifar Z, Meyer R D 1990 Inhaled or intravenous pentamidine therapy for *Pneumocystis carinii* pneumonia in AIDS. Annals of Internal Medicine 113: 195–202

Patients enrolled in this prospective study were randomized to receive intravenous or inhaled pentamidine. The infection was proven in all cases. All patients receiving intravenous pentamidine responded whereas 6 out of 11 given inhaled pentamidine deteriorated during initial treatment. The two groups were comparable on admission to the study particularly with respect to the numbers having more or less severe disease. The main criterion for outcome seemed to be severity of disease when treatment was begun. By a range of measurements indicating severity, e.g. PaO_2, $PaCO_2$, alveolar–arterial PaO_2 difference, those with more severe infections failed to respond to inhaled drug. Major toxicity required early termination of treatment more often with intravenous than inhaled therapy. Manifestations of toxicity included drug fever, hypotension, neutropenia, hypoglycaemia and azotaemia. Relapse occurred in 3 patients over a 3-month follow-up period; one had received intravenous and the other 2 inhaled pentamidine. The authors argue for the use of inhaled pentamidine in mild *Pn. carinii* pneumonia and for intravenous infusion in the remainder.

2. Conte Jr J E, Chernoff D, Feigal D W, Joseph P, McDonald C, Golden J A 1990 Intravenous or inhaled pentamidine for treating *Pneumocystis carinii* pneumonia in AIDS. Annals of Internal Medicine 113: 203–209

This paper also describes a prospective randomized study and the conclusions were that reduced-dose pentamidine by the intravenous route was more effective than aerosolized drug for treatment of mild to moderately severe *Pn. carinii* pneumonia.

3. Leoung G S, Feigal D W, Montgomery A B et al and the San Francisco County Community Consortium 1990 Aerosolized pentamidine for prophylaxis against *Pneumocystis carinii* pneumonia. New England Journal of Medicine 323: 769–775

This is a prospective, randomized unblinded study that compares the efficacy of 3 regimens of pentamidine administered by aerosol in AIDS patients; 30 mg every 2 weeks, 150 mg every 2 weeks or 300 mg every 4 weeks. In all cases the Respigard II nebulizer was used. The three groups were evenly matched with regard to patient characteristics though it should be noted that all but 3 patients were male. The proportions taking zidovudine and other drugs were similar in the groups. Overall 300 mg every 4 weeks gave the best results and was significantly better than the other 2 regimens for secondary prophylaxis. Numbers of patients in which aerosolized pentamidine was given for primary prophylaxis were low and the superiority of one regimen was not established. Respiratory side effects were common but not severe and only 2.2% had to withdraw because of these effects. There was no evidence of any adverse reaction to the simultaneous administration of pentamidine with zidovudine or other drugs. The study lasted 18 months and during this time there was no suggestion of pulmonary toxicity related to accumulation of pentamidine there. A potential area of concern in the use of this route of administration relates extrapulmonary pneumocystosis. Enteral or parenteral prophylaxis might offer the control of extrapulmonary pneumocystosis while inhaled drug with its low systemic absorption is unlikely to achieve this.[34]

4. Sattler F R, Cowan R, Nielsen D M, Ruskin J 1988 Trimethoprim–sulphamethoxazole compared with pentamidine for treatment of *Pneumocystis carinii* pneumonia in the acquired immunodeficiency syndrome. A prospective non-crossover study. Annals of Internal Medicine 109: 280–287

Leishmaniasis

5. Jha T K 1983 Evaluation of diamidine compound (pentamidine isethionate) in the treatment of resistant cases of kala azar occurring in North Bihar. Transactions of the Royal Society of Tropical Medicine and Hygiene 77: 167–170
6. Bryceson A D M, Chulay J D, Mugambi M et al 1985 Visceral leishmaniasis unresponsive to antimonial drugs II. Response to high dose sodium stibogluconate or prolonged treatment with pentamidine. Transactions of the Royal Society of Tropical Medicine and Hygiene 79: 705–714
7. Low-A-Chee R M, Rose P, Ridley D S 1983 An outbreak of cutaneous leishmaniasis in Guyana: epidemiology, clinical and laboratory aspects. Annals of Tropical Medicine and Parasitology 77: 255–260
8. Bryceson A D M 1970 Diffuse cutaneous leishmaniasis in Ethiopia: II treatment. Transactions of the Royal Society of Tropical Medicine and Hygiene 64: 369–379

References

1. Williamson J 1979 Effects of trypanocides on the fine structure of target organisms. Pharmacology and Therapeutics 7: 445–512
2. Bornstein R S, Yarbro J W 1970 An evaluation of the mechanism of action of pentamidine isethionate. Journal of Surgical Oncology 2: 393–398
3. Bernard E M, Donnelly H J, Maher M P, Armstrong D 1986 Use of a new bioassay to study pentamidine pharmacokinetics. Journal of Infectious Diseases 152: 750–754
4. Lin J, Shi R J, Lin E T 1986 High performance liquid chromatographic determination of pentamidine in plasma. Journal of Liquid Chromatography 9: 2035–2046
5. Conte J E Jr, Upton R A, Phelps R T, Wofsky C B, Zurlinden E, Lin E T 1986 Use of a specific and sensitive assay to determine pentamidine pharmacokinetics in patients with AIDS. Journal of Infectious Diseases 154: 923–929
6. Conte J E Jr, Upton R A, Lin E T 1987 Pentamidine pharmacokinetics in patients with AIDS with impaired renal function. Journal of Infectious Diseases 156: 885–890
7. Donnelly H, Bernard E M, Rothkotter H, Gold J W M, Armstrong D 1988 Distribution of pentamidine in AIDS. Journal of Infectious Diseases 157: 985–989
8. Montgomery A B, Debs R J, Luce L M et al 1988 Selective delivery of pentamidine to the lung by aerosol. American Review of Respiratory Diseases 137: 477–478
9. Narin T R, Fontaine R E 1984 Intravenous versus intramuscular injection of pentamidine. New England Journal of Medicine 311: 1701–1702
10. Montgomery A B, Debs R J, Luce J M et al 1987 Aerosolized pentamidine as sole therapy for *Pneumocystis carinii* pneumonia in patients with acquired immunodeficiency syndrome. Lancet 2: 480–483
11. Golden J A, Chernoff D, Hollander H, Feigal D, Conte J E 1989 Prevention of *Pneumocystis carinii* pneumonia by inhaled pentamidine. Lancet 2: 654–657
12. Girard P-M, Landman R, Gaudebout C et al 1989 Prevention of *Pneumocystis carinii* pneumonia relapse by pentamidine aerosol in zidovudine-treated AIDS patients. Lancet 1: 1348–1353
13. Jha T K 1983 Evaluation of diamidine compound (pentamidine isethionate) in the treatment of resistant kala azar occurring in north Bihar. Transactions of the Royal Society of Tropical Medicine and Hygiene 77: 167–170
14. Bryceson A D M, Chulay J D, Mugambi M et al 1985 Visceral leishmaniasis unresponsive to antimonial drugs. II Treatment with pentamidine. Transactions of the Royal Society of Tropical Medicine and Hygiene 79: 705–714

Pentamidine

15. Bryceson A D M 1970 Diffuse cutaneous leishmaniasis in Ethiopia: II Treatment with pentamidine. Transactions of the Royal Society of Tropical Medicine and Hygiene 64: 369–379
16. Low-A-Chee R M, Rose P, Ridley D S 1983 An outbreak of cutaneous leishmaniasis in Guyana: epidemiology, clinical and laboratory aspects. Annals of Tropical Medicine and Parasitology 77: 255–260
17. Molyneux D H 1983 Selective interventions for the control of diseases in the developing world: VII Trypanosomiasis. Reviews of Infectious Diseases 5: 945–946
18. Stark R, Crast F, Clemmer T, Ramirez R 1976 Fatal Herxheimer reaction after pentamidine in *Pneumocystis carinii* pneumonia. Lancet 1: 1193–1194
19. Waskin H, Stehr-Green J, Helmick C G, Sattler F R 1988 Risk factors for hypoglycemia associated with pentamidine therapy for *Pneumocystis carinii* pneumonia. Journal of the American Medical Association 260: 345–347
20. Sensakovic J W, Suarez M, Perez G, Johnson E S, Smith L G 1985 Pentamidine treatment of *Pneumocystis carinii* pneumonia in the acquired immunodeficiency syndrome. Association with acute renal failure and myoglobinuria. Archives of Internal Medicine 145: 2247
21. Wharton J M, Demopulos P A, Goldschlager N A 1987 Torsades de pointes during administration of pentamidine isethionate. American Journal of Medicine 83: 571–576
22. Loescher Th, Loeschke K, Niebel J 1987 Severe ventricular arrhythmia during pentamidine treatment of AIDS-associated *Pneumocystis carinii* pneumonia. Infection 15: 455
23. Boughton B J 1987 Cardiac side effects of pentamidine. British Medical Journal 294: 110
24. Pujol M, Carratala J, Mauri J, Viladrich P F 1988 Ventricular tachycardia due to pentamidine isethionate. American Journal of Medicine 84: 980
25. Bouchard Ph, Sai P, Reach G, Caubarrere I, Ganeval D, Assan R 1982 Diabetes mellitus following pentamidine induced hypoglycemia in humans. Diabetes 31: 40–45
26. Fitzgerald D B, Young I S 1984 Reversal of pentamidine induced hypoglycaemia with oral diazoxide. Journal of Tropical Medicine and Hygiene 87: 15–19
27. Salmeron S, Petitpretz P, Katlama C et al 1986 Pentamidine and pancreatitis. Annals of Internal Medicine 105: 140–141
28. Herer B, Chinet T, Labrune S, Collignon M A, Chretien J, Huchon G 1989 Pancreatitis associated with pentamidine by aerosol. British Medical Journal 298: 605
29. Sterh-Green J K, Helwick C G 1985 Pentamidine and renal toxicity. New England Journal of Medicine 313: 694–695
30. Alston T A 1988 Inhibition of cholinesterases by pentamidine. Lancet 2: 1423
31. Williamson J 1982 Chemotherapy and chemoprophylaxis in African trypanosomiasis. Experimental Parasitology 12: 274–322
32. World Health Organisation 1979 Report of an Expert Committee on Trypanosomiasis. Technical Report Series No 247
33. Niegel S F, Wolff L J, Bachner R L, Hammond D 1984 Treatment of *Pneumocystis carinii* pneumonitis. A comparative trial of sulphamethoxazole–trimethoprim versus pentamidine in pediatric patients with cancer: report from the Child Cancer Study Group. American Journal of Diseases of Children 138: 1051–1054
34. Hardy et al 1989 Fatal, disseminated pneumocystosis in a patient with the acquired immunodeficiency syndrome receiving prophylactic aerosolized pentamidine. American Journal of Medicine 87: 329–331

Pentazocine (hydrochloride)

Pentazocine is an opioid agonist–antagonist analgesic of the nalorphine type and was the first mixed agonist–antagonist to be widely used in clinical practice.

Chemistry

Pentazocine hydrochloride (Fortral, Talwin, Fortralgesic, Fortralin, Sosegon, Sosenyl, Pentgin, Liticon)
$C_{19}H_{27}NO.HCl$
1,2,3,4,5,6-Hexahydro-6,11-dimethyl-3-(3-methylbut-2-enyl)-2,6-methano-3-benzazocin-γ-ol hydrochloride

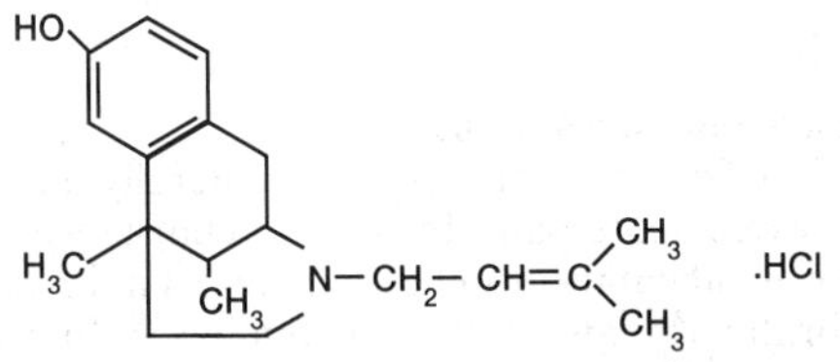

Molecular weight (free base)	321.9 (285.4)
pKa	8.7, 10.0
Solubility	
in alcohol	1 in 16
in water	1 in 30
Octanol/water partition coefficient	—

A white or cream, odourless, crystalline powder, consisting of a racemic mixture of d- and l-isomers, soluble in acidic, aqueous solutions. Pentazocine hydrochloride is also available in an oral combination product with paracetamol (Fortagesic) in some countries.

Pharmacology

Pentazocine is a potent analgesic in animal models and has both agonist and antagonist action at opioid receptors. It produces a type of analgesia that is different from that produced by morphine. Pentazocine interrupts nociceptive input in the spinal cord while morphine also acts at supraspinal sites. These analgesic effects are probably due to agonist actions at κ-receptors.[1] Pentazocine, like morphine, produces respiratory depression and it is about half as potent in this regard as morphine. The dysphoric and psychotomimetic effects seen in man which are dose-related are antagonized by naloxone and are thought to be due to agonist actions at σ-receptors.[1]

Pentazocine is a weak antagonist at μ opioid receptors with about one fiftieth the potency of nalorphine. Pentazocine does not antagonize the respiratory depression induced by morphine.

Toxicology

Testing in animals has shown no signs of acute or chronic toxicity of potential clinical relevance. Local skin reactions characterized by oedema, haemorrhage, thickening of the subcutaneous tissue and adhesions to underlying muscle have been observed after repeated injections in rats, rabbits and some dogs, but not monkeys. No evidence of teratogenicity or impaired fertility has been found in rats or rabbits.

Clinical pharmacology

The action of pentazocine is attributable principally to its l-isomer. Given parenterally it is a powerful analgesic and estimates of its potency relative to morphine range from $\frac{1}{3}$[2] to $\frac{1}{6}$[3] (30–60 mg pentazocine intramuscularly is equivalent to 10 mg morphine intramuscularly). When given by mouth the analgesic action of pentazocine is much weaker, the oral to parenteral potency ratio being about $\frac{1}{4}$ in terms of peak effect and $\frac{1}{3}$ in duration of effect.[4] Comparative studies indicate that the analgesic activity of oral pentazocine (50 mg) lies somewhere between that of the peripherally acting analgesics aspirin and paracetamol, and the weak opioids such as codeine.[5,6] The usual parenteral dose is 20 to 60 mg by subcutaneous, intramuscular or intravenous injection. The oral dose is 25–100 mg every 3–4 h. Other effects related to the opioid agonist activity of pentazocine may occur, including respiratory depression, cough suppression, miosis, reduced gastric emptying and constipation, and increased smooth muscle tone in uterus and bladder. In normal use these effects are usually of little clinical significance. Pentazocine causes an increase in renal plasma flow but no change in glomerular filtration rate is seen. In contrast to other strong opioid analgesics, haemodynamic disturbance occurs following administration of pentazocine with dose-related systemic and pulmonary hypertension, increased left ventricular end diastolic pressure and a rise in central venous pressure.[7,8] This is probably due to a rise in plasma catecholamine concentrations.

Weak opioid antagonist activity has been demonstrated in man, both postoperatively and in patients physically dependent on opioid analgesics.[3]

Pharmacokinetics

Two analytical methods are available: high performance liquid chromatography (HPLC) with ultraviolet detection of the 2-p-chlorosulphophenyl-3-phenylindone (DIS-CL) derivative;[9] and a specific radioimmunoassay which does not cross-react with pentazocine metabolites.[10] HPLC has a detection limit of 10 μg.l^{-1} and radioimmunoassay 1 μg.l^{-1}.

Pentazocine is completely absorbed after oral administration[11] but blood levels show considerable variation both within and between subjects. Peak plasma concentrations occur one to three hours after oral administration and the mean plasma half life is about 2 h. There is extensive but variable presystemic elimination, with systemic bioavailability ranging from 11% to 32% in subjects with normal hepatic function.[12] This accounts for the wide individual variations in total plasma concentrations. Peak plasma concentrations after intramuscular injections are reached in 15 min to 1 h.

Data from animal studies show rapid and widespread distribution of pentazocine in liver, lungs, kidneys, muscles and brain following intramuscular or intravenous administration.[13] Following oral administration low levels are detected in organs other than the liver because of the extensive presystemic elimination. The apparent volume of distribution varies widely from around 250 to 550 l, with a mean of 396 l indicating significant drug accumulation in some tissues. Plasma protein binding of pentazocine varies from 48% to 75%, and in whole blood up to 50% may be present in red blood cells.[14] Placental transfer occurs, with mean cord blood levels in the region of 60–70% of those in maternal blood.[15]

As a result of extensive hepatic metabolism less than 10% of an oral dose appears unchanged in the urine.[16] In patients with cirrhosis a significant reduction in body clearance and a marked increase in bioavailability are seen.[17]

Oral absorption	95%
Presystemic metabolism	up to 90%
Plasma half life	
mean	2 h
Volume of distribution	250–550 l
Plasma protein binding	48–75%

Concentration–effect relationship

As with other analgesics no consistent relationship between analgesic activity and plasma concentrations of pentazocine has been convincingly demonstrated.

Metabolism

Up to 10% of pentazocine is excreted unchanged in the urine and 1–2% is found in faeces as a result of enterohepatic circulation

P

independent of the route of administration.[16] Hepatic metabolism occurs extensively, following oral or parenteral administration, by conjugation with glucuronic acid and oxidation of the terminal methyl groups of the dimethylallyl side-chain. The two principal metabolites found in urine are the cis-alcohol metabolite (11%) and the trans-carboxylic acid metabolite (40%) (Fig. 1). Both metabolites are inactive. An increased rate of metabolism due to enzyme induction has been reported in smokers and following nitrous oxide inhalation anaesthesia.

Pharmaceutics

Pentazocine Fortral (Sterling-UK), Talwin (Winthrop-Breon, USA) is available in oral, rectal and parenteral forms. Tablets contain 25 mg pentazocine hydrochloride BP and are white, biconvex, film-coated and marked FORTRAL. Capsules contain 50 mg pentazocine hydrochloride BP which are grey with a yellow cap marked FORTRAL 50.

Combination products include pentazocine 25 mg with paracetamol 650 mg Fortagesic and Talacen (US). Talwin Compound (US) is pentazocine 12.5 mg with 325 mg aspirin. To overcome oral pentazocine being illicitly crushed and injected by drug misusers, the US formulation is now Talwin NX which contains 50 mg pentazocine and 0.5 mg naloxone. It is a yellow oblong tablet coded T51.

For rectal use a white Fortral suppository with a suppocire base contains 50 mg pentazocine BP as the lactate, weighing 1.89 g. Suppositories should be stored in a cool place.

For intravenous, intramuscular or subcutaneous use, there are 1 and 2 ml ampoules containing pentazocine BP as the lactate, 30 mg.ml^{-1} in an isotonic colourless aqueous solution. The pH is adjusted to between 4 and 5. Ampoules should be protected from light during storage.

Pentazocine preparations are stable with a long shelf-life. Tartrazine is no longer present in current formulations, with which risks from potentially allergenic substances are minimal.

Therapeutic use

Indications

1. Relief of moderate to severe pain
2. Intravenous anaesthesia and premedication.

Contraindications

1. Established respiratory depression
2. Raised intracranial pressure
3. Arterial or pulmonary hypertension
4. Individuals physically dependent on opioid analgesics

Fig. 1 Metabolism of pentazocine

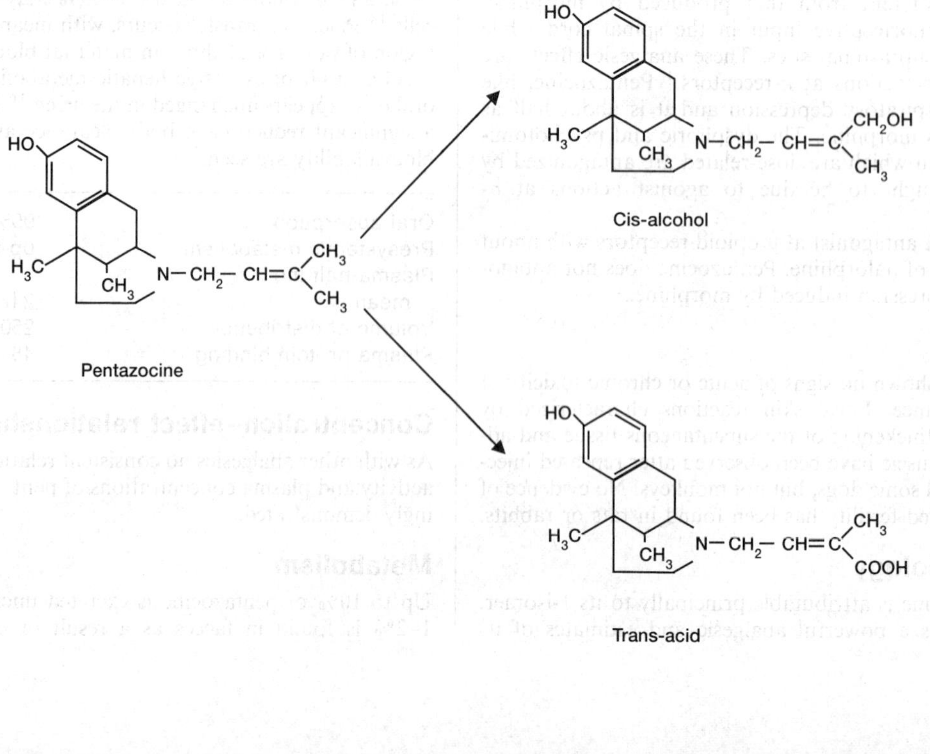

Pentazocine (hydrochloride)

5. Head injury or other conditions where clouding of consciousness is undesirable
6. Porphyria.

Mode of use

Oral administration is usually initiated in adults with a dose of 50–100 mg three- to four-hourly, titrating dose and frequency of administration to pain relief with the total daily dose not exceeding 600 mg. In children under 12 a dose of 25 mg every three to four hours is recommended. Initiation of treatment at night and frequent small doses in preference to less frequent large doses are helpful in reducing the incidence of side effects.

Rectal administration using a 50 mg suppository may give more prolonged analgesia than equivalent oral doses. For parenteral use 30 mg intravenously or 30–60 mg intramuscularly or subcutaneously is recommended initially, repeated at 3–4-hourly intervals as necessary with a total daily dose not exceeding 360 mg. In children under 12 years a dose of 0.5 mg.kg^{-1} intravenously or 1 mg.kg^{-1} intramuscularly or subcutaneously is given.

Although pentazocine has low abuse potential compared with morphine and other strong opioid agonists, dependence may develop with chronic use and withdrawal symptoms may occur if the drug is discontinued abruptly.

Indications

1. Relief of moderate to severe pain

Pentazocine is effective when given parenterally for the relief of moderate to severe acute pain. In these circumstances 30–60 mg by intramuscular or subcutaneous injection has a similar analgesic effect to 10 mg morphine[2,3] and 100 mg pethidine.[18] In comparison to morphine or pethidine the duration of action of pentazocine is slightly shorter. It has been claimed that pentazocine produces a lower incidence of side effects in postoperative patients, in particular nausea and vomiting, sedation and hypotension, compared with morphine or pethidine. However, side effects of pentazocine are dose-related and overall the incidence and severity of side effects at equianalgesic doses are similar with all three drugs.

When given by mouth pentazocine is not a strong analgesic. Whilst some comparisons have shown pentazocine (50 mg) to be as effective as codeine or dihydrocodeine[5] other studies have shown a better analgesic effect with aspirin 500–650 mg.[6] The duration of analgesia produced by pentazocine in these studies was about three hours.

The usefulness of oral pentazocine in chronic pain is limited by its weak and unpredictable analgesic activity, dose-related (particularly psychotomimetic) side effects, and its ability to antagonize the effects of pure opioid agonists if used concurrently.

Pentazocine (hydrochloride)

In obstetric use pentazocine is an effective analgesic during labour. There is some evidence that uterine activity may be increased by pentazocine and compared with pethidine the second stage of labour may be shortened.[19,20] Side effects in the mother and respiratory depression in the neonate appear to be similar with pentazocine and pethidine.

Pentazocine may be used for the relief of acute pain from renal or biliary colic and has been shown to cause less smooth muscle contraction in renal and biliary tracts than morphine.[21] A more recent study has shown significant elevations in intrabiliary pressure following pentazocine compared with buprenorphine[22] so that its use in pancreaticobiliary disease may be best avoided. In myocardial infarction pentazocine is an effective analgesic and may cause a rise in systolic blood pressure in contrast to the hypotensive effect of other opioids.[23] However, the associated increase in pulmonary artery pressure, left ventricular end diastolic pressure and left ventricular minute work which has been demonstrated[8,22] is potentially hazardous in this situation since it can lead to an increase in myocardial oxygen demand and extension of the area of ischaemia. An alternative opioid analgesic is generally preferred.[24]

2. Intravenous anaesthesia and premedication
Like other potent analgesics pentazocine has been used as a component of 'balanced' intravenous anaesthetic regimens, and also as a premedicant before general anaesthesia. However it has no particular advantages over standard drugs in these situations and is not now widely used.[25]

Contraindications

1. Established respiratory depression
In common with all drugs having opioid agonist activity, pentazocine has a respiratory depressant action which has been demonstrated to reside mainly in the l-isomer. In equipotent doses its respiratory depressant effect appears to be similar to that of morphine. Care is required in the use of pentazocine in patients with impaired respiratory drive and transient apnoea may occur in the neonate following its use in labour.

2. Raised intracranial pressure
In patients with brain damage or where intracranial pressure is already raised due to a space-occupying lesion an increase in intracranial and spinal fluid pressure occurs after administration of pentazocine. These changes are not seen in normal patients, or in patients with brain damage who are mechanically ventilated, suggesting that mild respiratory depression with an associated intracranial vasodilatation secondary to a rise in P_aCO_2 may be the underlying cause.[26]

3. Arterial or pulmonary hypertension
Pentazocine has a number of interrelated effects on the cardiovascular system, resulting in an increase in heart rate and an increase in systolic blood pressure.[7] The degree to which these changes occur varies considerably and a fall in blood pressure or no effect has also been demonstrated in some patients. Doses of 30–60 mg parenterally cause significant increases in pulmonary artery pressure with an associated increase in left ventricular end-diastolic pressure. Increased central venous pressure has also been reported but little consistent effect on systemic vascular resistance, cardiac output, stroke volume or coronary circulation has been demonstrated. Whilst these cardiovascular effects may be advantageous in certain situations, alternative opioid analgesics are preferable in patients with established arterial or pulmonary hypertension.

4. Individuals physically dependent on opioid analgesics
Withdrawal effects may occur in patients who are dependent on opioids following administration of pentazocine, due to its opioid antagonist action. Its use in these patients should therefore be avoided.

5. Conditions where clouding of consciousness is undesirable
Following head injury and in certain other acute conditions the patient's level of consciousness is an important clinical sign. Where analgesia is required, non-sedative drugs are preferable to pentazocine. Pentazocine also causes pupillary constriction[26] which, though less marked than with other opioid agonists, may further obscure signs of raised intracranial pressure.

6. Porphyria
Pentazocine has been shown to be porphyrogenic in rats and on this basis is not recommended for use in patients with porphyria.[27]

Adverse reactions

Potentially life-threatening effects
Potentially life-threatening respiratory depression may occur when pentazocine is used as an adjuvant to anaesthesia in patients with chronic respiratory insufficiency[28] and deaths have been associated with pentazocine abuse though the precise role of the drug in such cases is unclear.

Agranulocytosis due to pentazocine is recognized with a latency of 4–24 weeks from exposure to the drug. Although fatalities have been reported, most cases are reversible on withdrawing the drug.[29]

Acute overdosage
Deaths due to overdose of pentazocine alone are rare. The main clinical features are tachycardia and a rise in blood pressure, and respiratory depression. Status epilepticus, coma, respiratory depression, acidosis, profound hypotension and ventricular arrhythmias were observed in one case following ingestion of 1.5 g.[30] Treatment involves the administration of naloxone which is a competitive antagonist at the opioid receptors mediating the respiratory depression due to pentazocine, and the maintenance of respiration. Naloxone is given intravenously in a dose of 0.1 mg repeated at two-minute intervals according to the clinical state of the patient, with total doses of between 0.4 and 2 mg being sufficient in most cases. Higher doses of up to 15 or 20 mg may be required in some instances.

Severe or irreversible adverse effects
Epileptic seizures occur rarely following the administration of pentazocine. These have been predominantly associated with high-dose intravenous use during anaesthesia and patients with underlying intracranial pathology are particularly at risk.[31]

When first introduced pentazocine was not considered to be addictive. Subsequently, its abuse potential has been recognized[32] and increasing controls on prescribing have been introduced. Abuse is usually associated with parenteral use and often in association with other drugs. The combination of pentazocine with the antihistamine, tripelannamine, dissolved in water and injected intravenously ('T's and Blues') has become popular amongst addicts in some countries.[33] Withdrawal symptoms are usually mild but may include anxiety, dysphoria, tremor, sweating and musculoskeletal pains. Abuse of pentazocine has led in the United States to the introduction of a new formulation containing the specific opioid antagonist naloxone. Naloxone is inactive by mouth but is effective when injected intravenously. No formulation for oral use of pentazocine by itself is now available in the USA.

When given by injection pentazocine may be locally irritant with stinging, pruritus or flushing occurring at the injection site. Repeated intramuscular injections over long periods have resulted in local soft tissue induration, fibrosis or ulceration, hyperpigmentation in surrounding skin and a myopathy which if severe may impair movement and result in contractures. Such changes are usually associated with drug abuse rather than therapeutic use.

Symptomatic adverse effects
Psychotomimetic adverse effects may occur in up to 20% of patients receiving pentazocine, and are generally dose-related.[34] These most commonly occur as auditory or visual hallucinations, euphoria, and depersonalization. Vivid, disturbed dreams may be a further manifestation. These effects, though unpleasant, are usually mild and self-limiting but may be severe. If severe, naloxone may be effective in relieving them. Other ill effects of pentazocine are also dose-related. The most common side effect is mild sedation. In common with other opioids, nausea, vomiting, light-headedness and vertigo may occur. Other minor side effects include sweating, hot flushes, dry mouth, transient changes in blood pressure, tachycardia and urinary retention, and effects on the eye including blurred vision, nystagmus, diplopia and miosis. Headache, chills and fever have also been reported.

Other effects
No significant biochemical effects following pentazocine administration have been recognized.

Interference with clinical pathology tests
No interference with established assay methods has been reported, but in common with other intramuscular injections, elevation of creatine kinase levels following repeated administration by this route is seen.

High risk groups

Neonates
Respiratory depression in the neonate following administration of pentazocine to the mother during labour may occur. This can be reversed with naloxone. No dosage recommendations are made for children less than one year old.

Breast milk. Pentazocine has not been demonstrated in the milk of nursing mothers.

Children
Pentazocine is used as an analgesic for moderate to severe pain in children. When administered parenterally the maximum single dose should be 1 mg.kg^{-1} body weight by subcutaneous or intramuscular injection, or 0.5 mg.kg^{-1} body weight by intravenous injection. Oral administration to children under the age of six years is not recommended. The dose for children between six and twelve years of age is 25 mg every 3–4 h as required. Children over 12 years may receive an adult dose. Pentazocine suppositories are unsuitable for children under 12 years.

Pregnant women
Although pentazocine has been widely used for many years, its safety in pregnancy has not been established unequivocally, and it should be used with caution in pregnant women. Neonatal dependence with associated withdrawal symptoms which may include hyperirritability, hypertonicity and tremors have been reported in babies whose mothers have taken oral pentazocine in doses of 150–300 mg per day regularly during pregnancy.[35] Many women have received the drug during labour without significant effects upon the fetus other than occasional respiratory depression as with other opioid analgesics. There is no evidence of teratogenicity or of any adverse effects on fertility.

The elderly
No specific problems are seen in the elderly following administration of pentazocine. However, certain conditions which may be more common in the elderly, in particular impairment of hepatic or renal function, may impair handling of the drug. This may predispose to increased toxicity and care is required in these situations.

Drug interactions

Potentially hazardous interactions

Halothane anaesthesia. The use of pentazocine with halothane during anaesthesia increases the respiratory depression and hypotensive effects associated with halothane.

Anticoagulants. The use of pentazocine in patients receiving heparin or oral anticoagulants may occasionally result in an increased anticoagulant effect. Careful monitoring in such patients is necessary though in the majority of cases no significant effect is seen.

Hydroxyzine. The combination of hydroxyzine and pentazocine may reduce nausea and vomiting and enhance analgesia, but is also associated with an increase in respiratory depression.

Lignocaine. The respiratory depressant effect of pentazocine may be enhanced by prior parenteral administration of lignocaine.

Other significant interactions

CNS depressants. When pentazocine is administered with any CNS depressant increased sedation may occur.

Opioid analgesics. Withdrawal symptoms may be precipitated by pentazocine if given to patients who are physically dependent on opioid analgesics.

Monoamine oxidase inhibitors. Despite the demonstration of increased toxicity from the use of pentazocine with monoamine oxidase inhibitors in mice, a similar effect in man has not been reported. An initial small test dose is recommended in patients receiving one of these drugs.

Soluble barbiturates. When pentazocine is mixed together in solution with soluble barbiturates precipitation will occur.

Alcohol. Increased sedative effects occur when pentazocine is taken together with alcohol.

Smoking. Smokers appear to require higher doses of pentazocine and experience a shorter duration of analgesia, and this is associated with an increased rate of metabolism.[36]

Potentially useful interactions

Naloxone. The opioid agonist effects of pentazocine can be reversed by the specific competitive antagonist naloxone.

Major outcome trials

1. Paddock R, Beer E G, Belville J W, Ciliberti B J, Forrest W H, Miler E V (Veterans Administration Cooperative Analgesic Study) 1969 Analgesic and side effects of pentazocine and morphine in a large population of postoperative patients. Clinical Pharmacology and Therapeutics 10: 355–365

This is a prospective randomized double-blind study involving five hospitals into which 1074 surgical patients were entered to compare 5 mg and 10 mg morphine sulphate intramuscularly with 10 mg, 20 mg and 40 mg pentazocine intramuscularly. 1030 patients had postoperative pain and the remainder had acute pain from a variety of other causes. Response was assessed using structured interviews by nurse observers recording pain intensity and pain relief on a four point categorical scale for each parameter. Interviews were performed prior to medication and then every 45 min for 4.5 h. Side effects were only recorded if volunteered by the patient or noticed by the observer.

A dose-related analgesic effect with pentazocine was observed. In comparison to morphine, pentazocine produced an earlier peak effect but a more rapid decline of activity. Relative to 10 mg morphine sulphate, the approximate equivalent dose of pentazocine for overall analgesic effect was 36 mg, for peak analgesic effect 27 mg and for sedative effects 20 mg.

2. Beaver W T, Wallenstein S L, Houde R W, Rogers A 1966 A comparison of the analgesic effects of pentazocine and morphine in patients with cancer. Clinical Pharmacology and Therapeutics 7: 740–751

A double-blind crossover evaluation of the relative analgesic potency of graded intramuscular doses of pentazocine and morphine was carried out in patients with chronic pain due to cancer. 48 patients were involved in two sequential series, the first involving crossover comparisons of 8 and 16 mg morphine with 20 and 40 mg pentazocine, and the second 8 and 16 mg morphine with 40 and 80 mg pentazocine.

The analgesic potency of pentazocine, based on 'total' effect (including both intensity and duration of effect), is estimated to be approximately one-sixth that of morphine.

This study involved a longer observation period (6 h) compared with the study cited above and may give a better estimate of the total effects of both drugs. This may account for the difference in estimates of relative potency.

3. Beaver W T, Wallenstein S L, Houde R W, Rogers A 1968 A clinical comparison of the effects of oral and intramuscular administration of analgesics: pentazocine and phenazocine. Clinical Pharmacology and Therapeutics 9: 582–597

The relative analgesic potency of oral and intramuscular pentazocine was evaluated in a double-blind crossover comparison of graded single doses in 24 patients with chronic pain due to cancer. Oral pentazocine was one-third as potent as the intramuscular form in terms of total effect, but one-fourth as potent in peak effect.

Single oral doses of 240 mg caused psychotomimetic reactions 4 out of 23 times. These reactions were transient and not seen after the intramuscular or lower oral doses.

Other trials

Moertel C G, Ahmann D L, Taylor W F, Schwartau N 1972 A comparative evaluation of marketed analgesic drugs. New England Journal of Medicine 286: 813–815

In a double-blind placebo-controlled crossover study in 57 patients with cancer pain aspirin 650 mg was superior to pentazocine 50 mg and to several other weak opioids and peripherally acting analgesics.

The drugs were administered in single doses in randomized sequences according to a latin-square design. Patients themselves recorded the time of administration, onset of definite relief of pain

Pentazocine (hydrochloride)

and the time when pain returned, together with an estimate of the maximum degree of pain relief on a percentage basis. Specific enquiry was made regarding side effects.

Pentazocine was the only drug which produced significant side effects (gastrointestinal and CNS) compared with placebo.

General review articles

Potter D R, Payne J P 1970 Newer analgesics: with special reference to pentazocine. British Journal of Anaesthesia 42: 186–193

Brogden R N, Speight T M, Avery G S 1973 Pentazocine: a review of its pharmacological properties, therapeutic efficacy and dependence liability. Drugs 5: 1–96

Hameroff S R 1983 Opiate receptor pharmacology: mixed agonist/antagonist narcotics. Contemporary Anesthetic Practice 7: 27–43

References

1. Martin W R, Eades C G, Thompson J A, Huppler R E, Gilbert P E 1976 The effects of morphine- and nalorphine-like drugs in the nondependent and morphine-dependent chronic spinal dog. Journal of Pharmacology and Experimental Therapeutics 197: 517–532
2. Paddock R, Beer E G, Belville J W, Ciliberti B J, Forrest W H, Miller E V 1969 Analgesic and side effects of pentazocine and morphine in a large population of postoperative patients. Clinical Pharmacology and Therapeutics 10: 355–365
3. Beaver W T, Wallenstein S L, Houde R W, Rogers A 1966 A comparison of the analgesic effects of pentazocine and morphine in patients with cancer. Clinical Pharmacology and Therapeutics 7: 740–751
4. Beaver W T, Wallenstein S L, Houde R W, Rogers A 1968 A clinical comparison of the effects of oral and intramuscular administration of analgesics: pentazocine and phenazocine. Clinical Pharmacology and Therapeutics 9: 582–597
5. Kantor T G, Sunshine A, Laska E, Meisner M, Hopper M 1966 Oral analgesic studies: pentazocine hydrochloride, codeine, aspirin, and placebo and their influence on response to placebo. Clinical Pharmacology and Therapeutics 7: 447–454
6. Moertel C G, Ahmann D L, Taylor W F, Schwartau N 1972 A comparative evaluation of marketed analgesic drugs. New England Journal of Medicine 286: 813–815
7. Stephen G W, Davie I, Scott D B 1970 Circulatory effects of pentazocine and pethidine during general anaesthesia with nitrous oxide, oxygen and halothane. British Journal of Anaesthesia 42: 311–315
8. Jewitt D E, Maurer B J, Sonnenblick E H, Shillingford J P 1974 Pentazocine: effect on ventricular muscle and haemodynamic changes in ischaemic heart disease. Circulation 13/14 (suppl II): 118
9. Anderson R D, Ilett K F, Dusci L J, Hackett L P 1982 High performance liquid chromatographic analysis of pentazocine in blood and plasma. Journal of Chromatography 227: 239–243
10. Peterson J E, Graham M, Banks W F et al 1979 Plasma pentazocine radioimmunoassay. Journal of Pharmaceutical Science 68: 626–628
11. Beckett A H, Taylor J F, Kouroumakis P 1970 The absorption, distribution and excretion of pentazocine in man after oral and intravenous administration. Journal of Pharmacy and Pharmacology 22: 123–128
12. Ehrnebo M, Boreus L O, Lonroth U 1977 Bioavailability and first-pass metabolism of oral pentazocine in man. Clinical Pharmacology and Therapeutics 22: 888–892
13. El-Mazakai A M, Way E L 1971 The biologic disposition of pentazocine in the rat. Journal of Pharmacology and Experimental Therapeutics 177: 332–341
14. Ehrnebo M, Agurell S, Boreus L H, Gordon E, Lonroth U 1974 Pentazocine binding to blood cells and plasma proteins. Clinical Pharmacology and Therapeutics 16: 424–428
15. Moore J, McNabb T G, Glynn J P 1973 The placental transfer of pentazocine and pethidine. British Journal of Anaesthesia 45 (suppl): 798–801
16. Berkowitz B, Way E L 1969 Metabolism and excretion of pentazocine in man. Clinical Pharmacology and Therapeutics 10: 681–689
17. Neal E A, Meffin P J, Gregory P B, Blaschke T F 1979 Enhanced bioavailability and decreased clearance of analgesics in patients with cirrhosis. Gastroenterology 77: 96–102
18. Scott R, Barrie W, Simpson R W, Bell D 1973 The use of pentazocine as a strong analgesic in urological practice. British Journal of Urology 45: 227–232
19. Filler W W, Filler N W 1966 Effect of potent non-narcotic analgesic agent (pentazocine) on uterine contractility and foetal heart rate. Obstetrics and Gynecology 28: 224–232
20. Duncan S L, Ginsberg J, Morris N F 1969 Comparison of pentazocine and pethidine in normal labor. American Journal of Obstetrics and Gynecology 105: 197–202
21. Economou G, Ward-McQuaid J N 1971 A crossover comparison of the effect of morphine, pethidine, pentazocine and phenazocine on biliary pressure. Gut 12: 218–221
22. Staritz M, Poralla T, Manns M, Ewe K, Meyerzum Buschenfelde K-H 1985 Pentazocine hampers bile flow. Lancet 1: 573–574
23. Scott M E, Orr R 1969 Effects of diamorphine, methadone, morphine and pentazocine in patients with suspected acute myocardial infarction. Lancet 1: 1065–1067
24. Leading Article 1976 Pentazocine in myocardial infarction. Lancet 2: 888–889
25. Bailey P L, Stanley T H 1986 Pharmacology of intravenous narcotic anaesthetics. In: Miller R D (ed) Anesthesia, 2nd edn. Churchill Livingstone, New York, pp 747–776
26. Barker J, Miller J D, Johnston I H 1972 The effect of pentazocine on pupillary size and intracranial pressure. British Journal of Anaesthesia 44: 197–202
27. Parikh R K, Moore M R 1978 Effect of certain anaesthetic agents on the activity of rat hepatic δ-aminolaevulinate synthase. British Journal of Anaesthesia 50: 1099–1103
28. Reichenberg S, Pobirs F 1973 Severe respiratory depression following Talwin. American Review of Respiratory Diseases 107: 280–282
29. Sheehan M, Hyland R H, Norman C 1985 Pentazocine-induced agranulocytosis. Canadian Medical Association Journal 132: 1401
30. Stahl S M 1983 Pentazocine overdose. Annals of Emergency Medicine 12: 28–31
31. Jackson S H, Dueker C, Grace L 1971 Seizures induced by pentazocine. Anaesthesiology 35: 92–95
32. Inciardi J A, Chambers C D 1971 Patterns of pentazocine abuse and addiction. New York State Journal of Medicine 71: 1727–1733
33. Showalter C V 1980 T's and Blues: abuse of pentazocine and tripelennamine. Journal of the American Medical Association 244: 1224–1225
34. Taylor M, Galloway D B, Petrie J C, Davidson J F, Gallon S C, Moir D C 1978 Psychomimetic effects of pentazocine and dihydrocodeine tartrate. British Medical Journal 2: 1198
35. Goetz R L, Bain R V 1974 Neonatal withdrawal symptoms associated with maternal use of pentazocine. Journal of Paediatrics 84: 887–888
36. Vaughan D P, Beckett A H, Robbie D S 1976 The influence of smoking on the inter-subject variation in pentazocine elimination. British Journal of Clinical Pharmacology 3: 279–283

P

Pentobarbitone (sodium)

Pentobarbitone is a barbiturate sedative and hypnotic.

Chemistry

Pentobarbitone sodium (pentobarbital sodium, Nembutal)
$C_{11}H_{17}N_2NaO_3$
Sodium 5-ethyl-5-(1-methylbutyl) barbiturate

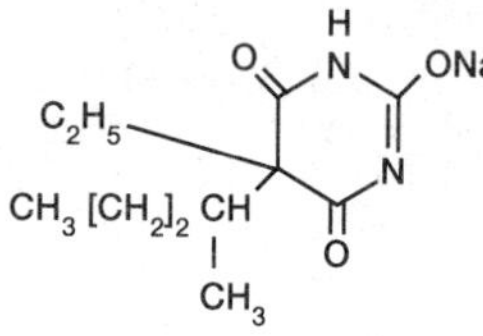

Molecular weight (free acid)	248.3 (226.3)
pKa	8.1
Solubility	
in alcohol	1 in 5
in water	very soluble
Octanol/water partition coefficient	2.03

A white, hygroscopic, crystalline powder or granules, odourless or with a slight characteristic odour and a slight bitter taste. A 10% aqueous solution has a pH of 9.6–11 and slowly decomposes. Solutions for injection can be prepared in Water for Injections and should be used immediately after preparation.

Pharmacology

The barbiturates unselectively depress the central nervous system producing dose-dependent effects ranging from mild sedation to general anaesthesia. All have anticonvulsant properties.

Toxicology

No information is available on animal toxicology.

Clinical pharmacology

Barbiturates demonstrate dose-dependent reversible depression of neurological function.[1] Part of this action may relate to interference with synaptic transmission and multineuronal connections. A direct local anaesthetic effect has also been demonstrated. Barbiturates have multiple actions including enhancement of GABAergic inhibition, reduction of glutaminergic and cholinergic excitations, reduction in presynaptic calcium entry and non-synaptic sodium and potassium conductances and blockage of repetitive firing.[2] Brain function depression is associated with a parallel dose-dependent reduction in cerebral metabolic rate and blood flow.[3] Barbiturates may improve the ratio of oxygen supply to demand by metabolic depression, and, in focal ischaemia, by redistributing blood flow.[4] Barbiturates also reduce intracranial pressure while maintaining cerebral perfusion pressure.

Pharmacokinetics

The preferred method of pentobarbitone analysis is by gas–liquid chromatography.[5,6] With nitrogen detection this has limits of detection of 80 μg.l^{-1}. More recently, attempts to quantify the drug using an enzyme-immunoassay system have been made.[7]

Pentobarbitone is completely absorbed following both oral and rectal administration.[8] The presence of food reduces the apparent rate constant of absorption but not the amount absorbed.[6] Peak plasma concentrations occur one hour after administration of the drug. Volume of distribution[9] is approximately 1 l.kg^{-1}, and the drug is 59–63% protein bound.[10] Binding is decreased in uraemic patients. The drug is biotransformed by hepatic metabolic processes with an elimination half life of between 20 and 30 hours.[6] Clearance is unchanged in renal failure[11] but is impaired in some patients with liver disease.[12,13] Increased metabolism has been reported in idiopathic systemic lupus erythematosus.[14] The half life of the drug appears shorter in children[15] and following chronic dosing,[16] the latter being due to autoinduction of metabolism.

As expected from its metabolic profile, pentobarbitone is excreted in breast milk.[17] The major route of elimination is via the kidneys with approximately 80% of the dose excreted in the urine over five days, with only 1% of the dose as unchanged drug.

Oral absorption	~100%
Presystemic metabolism	none
Plasma half life	
range	20–30 h
mean	27 h
Volume of distribution	1 l.kg^{-1}
Plasma protein binding	~60%

Concentration–effect relationship

A weak correlation between concentration and effect has been shown for pentobarbitone used rectally as premedication in children[18] and orally in healthy volunteers.[19] No threshold concentration could be identified in either study.

Metabolism

Pentobarbitone is almost completely eliminated by metabolic processes with less than 1% of an oral dose excreted unchanged.[20] Three major metabolites have been recognized and these are 3′-hydroxypentobarbitone (7% as the (d) isomer and 30% as the (l) isomer), see (Fig. 1, I), 3′-oxypentobarbitone (7–14%) (Fig. 1, II), and a 3^1-carboxy-derivative (10–15%) (Fig. 1, III).[16] An N-hydroxylated metabolite (Fig. 1, IV), suggested by some workers[20] but not others,[16] has now been identified as the N-glucoside conjugate (13%).

Fig. 1 Metabolism of pentobarbitone

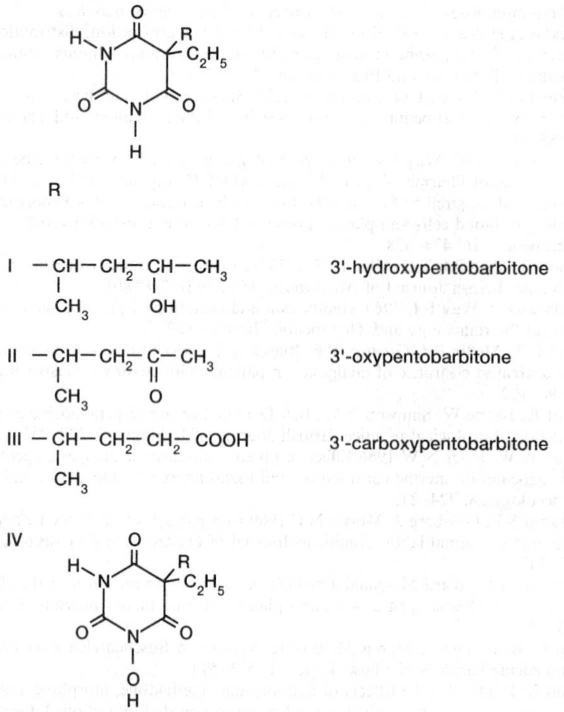

Pharmaceutics

Pentobarbitone is available as Nembutal (Abbott, US) in yellow capsules containing 100 mg of the sodium salt. They are coded 'CH' and marked with the Abbott logo. A 50 mg transparent/orange capsule is also available. Nembutal Sodium solution (Abbott, US) contains 100 mg in each 2 ml injection vial. It is formulated propylene glycol (40% v/v) and ethyl alcohol (10% v/v). It is adjusted to around pH 9.5. The injection is physically incompatible with some cephalosporins, clindamycin and pentazocine. Nembutal Sodium suppositories (Abbott, US) are available in 30 mg, 60 mg, 120 mg and 200 mg strengths.

Therapeutic use

Indications

1. The treatment of severe, intractable insomnia.

Contraindications

1. Hypersensitivity to barbiturates
2. History of porphyria
3. Presence of uncontrolled pain
4. Pregnancy and lactation.

Barbiturates should not be administered to children, young adults, patients with a history of drug or alcohol abuse, the elderly or the debilitated.

Mode of use

Pentobarbitone should be prescribed only to adults with severe intractable insomnia and then only after careful evaluation of safer alternatives such as benzodiazepines. Recommended oral doses range from 100 to 200 mg at night. For the large majority of patients a benzodiazepine should be initially preferred in view of the addictive and abuse potential of the barbiturates.[21] Pentobarbitone should be used intermittently as tolerance to its hypnotic effects rapidly develops.[22] Psychomotor performance may be impaired for up to 19 hours after a single dose[23] and rapid-eye-movement sleep is reduced.[24]

Other uses

The therapeutic effects of barbiturates have been extensively investigated in brain ischaemia but their use cannot currently be recommended.[4] Barbiturates reduce intracranial pressure in animal experimental systems and clinical studies with high doses of parenteral pentobarbitone during anaesthesia,[3] following severe head injury,[25] in Reye's syndrome[26] and in near-drowning[27] are, in the main, contradictory although benefit has been claimed for some patients. Pentobarbitone has been used orally[28] and parenterally[29] as premedication prior to surgery. Infusions of the drug have been reported to be effective in status epilepticus refractory to phenobarbitone, phenytoin and diazepam.[30]

Adverse reactions

Potentially life-threatening effects

Impaired consciousness. Because of residual or 'hangover' effects the next day[31,32] patients should be warned against driving and operating dangerous machinery. Respiratory depression can be produced and the drug should not be prescribed for patients in respiratory failure.[33]

Carcinogenesis. Chronic pentobarbitone therapy has been reported to be associated with an increased relative risk of bronchial and ovarian carcinoma but this may have been due to coincidental cigarette smoking.[34]

Acute overdosage

Symptoms of self-poisoning include respiratory and cardiac depression, hyporeflexia, pupillary constriction (or dilatation in severe cases), bradycardia, hypotension, oliguria, hypothermia and coma.[35] Muscle necrosis leading to acute renal failure has been reported.[36] Many patients require assisted ventilation and fatalities are not uncommon.[35] Treatment consists of symptomatic and supportive therapy including gastric lavage, intravenous fluids, and maintenance of blood pressure, body temperature and adequate respiratory exchange.[37]

Severe or irreversible adverse effects

Hypersensitivity. Rash can occur, but it is rare.[38] Barbiturate use may occasionally result in localized diffuse, myalgic, neuralgic and arthritic pain particularly in the neck, shoulder girdle, and upper limbs.[1] Other idiosyncratic reactions, including fever and angioneurotic oedema, may develop, particularly in atopic individuals.

Abuse. Like all barbiturates, pentobarbitone is a drug of abuse. Long-term use or use of high dosage may lead to tolerance and subsequently to physical and psychological dependence. Signs of barbiturate intoxication include nystagmus, slurred speech, ataxia, insomnia, and diminished tendon reflexes.[39] Confusion, defective judgement, and loss of emotional control may be apparent. On higher doses, semi-coma, respiratory depression, and shock can result in a fatal outcome. Withdrawal symptoms include apprehension, muscular weakness, tremor, and disturbed sleep. Nightmares are a prominent complaint. Anorexia is apparent in the early stages with fits, and delirium occurring 3–8 days after drug discontinuation. Treatment schedules involve slow reduction in pentobarbitone dosing over a number of months.[39]

Symptomatic adverse effects

Pentobarbitone is well tolerated in therapeutic doses with around 5% of patients reporting adverse effects.[38] Commonest problems relate to central nervous system symptomatology and include: drowsiness and sedation, unsteadiness and incoordination, vertigo, paradoxical excitement, confusion, and memory defects. Subtle effects on hand–eye coordination,[32] arousal[40] and reaction times[23] have been demonstrated.

High risk groups

Neonates

The drug should not be used in neonates.

Breast milk. Barbiturates are contraindicated for the nursing mother.[41]

Children

The drug should not be administered to children or adolescents.

Pregnant women

Barbiturates are contraindicated during pregnancy.[41]

The elderly

The drug should be avoided in elderly patients because of the risk of confusion and falls.

Concurrent disease

The use of barbiturates in patients with a history of drug or alcohol abuse should be avoided. Like all other barbiturates, pentobarbitone should not be prescribed for patients with porphyria as it increases haem synthesis and can precipitate or exacerbate an acute porphyric attack.[42] Caution is advised particularly in patients with impaired hepatic function.[38] Dosage reduction is not required in renal failure.

Drug interactions

Potentially hazardous interactions

Pentobarbitone, in common with other drugs in its chemical class, is an inducer of hepatic monooxygenase activity in man.[44] Pentobarbitone has been reported to increase the metabolism of cortisol,[45] quinidine,[46] and alprenolol.[47] Additionally, it may reduce the bioavailability of lipid-soluble drugs with a high hepatic extraction ratio such as metoprolol.[48] The possibility that pentobarbitone will increase the metabolism of other lipid-soluble drugs such as warfarin, systemic steroids, and phenothiazines must be borne in mind. Synergistic sedation can be anticipated when patients receiving pentobarbitone are prescribed other central nervous system depressants and, of course, ethanol.

Potentially useful interactions

No interactions of this kind have been reported.

Major outcome trials

1. Hinton J M 1963 A comparison of the effects of six barbiturates and a placebo on insomnia and motility in psychiatric patients. British Journal of Clinical Pharmacology 20: 319–325

Six barbiturates, each for 8 successive nights, were compared with placebo in a controlled double-blind trial in 24 insomniac psychiatric patients. Each of the barbiturates significantly prolonged sleep and

P

Pentobarbitone (sodium)

P

hastened its onset. Pentobarbitone (200 mg) was among the three most effective drugs.

2. Sapienza P L 1966 A double-blind comparison of methaqualone, pentobarbital and placebo in the management of insomnia. Current Therapeutic Research 8: 523–527

The effect of methaqualone (150–300 mg) and placebo, each given for 2 weeks, was compared with pentobarbitone (100–200 mg) in a double-blind, crossover study of 50 patients with insomnia. There were no clinically or statistically significant differences between pentobarbitone or methoqualone but both drugs were more effective than placebo. Side effects were not a problem.

3. Brown P J, Forrest W H, Brown C R 1975 Lorazepam compared with pentobarbitone for nighttime sedation. Journal of Clinical Pharmacology 15: 752–759

Pentobarbitone (60 and 180 mg) was compared with lorazepam (0.5, 1, 2 and 4 mg) in patients in hospital. Pentobarbitone was more effective than lorazepam for the induction and prolongation of sleep.

References

1. Harvey S C 1985 Barbiturates. In: Gilman A G, Goodman L S, Rall T W, Murad F (eds) The pharmacological basis of therapeutics, 7th edn. McMillan Publishing Co, New York, pp 351–360
2. MacDonald R L 1983 Mechanisms of anticonvulsant drug action. In: Pedley T A, Meldrum B S (eds) Recent advances in epilepsy 1. Churchill Livingstone, Edinburgh, pp 1–23
3. Shapiro H M 1985 Barbiturates in brain ischaemia. British Journal of Anaesthesia 57: 82–95
4. Deardon N M 1985 Ischaemic brain. Lancet 1: 255–259
5. MacGee J 1970 The rapid determination of diphenylhydantoin in blood plasma by gas liquid chromatography. Analytical Chemistry 42: 421–422
6. Smith R B, Dittert L W, Griffen W D, Doluisio J T 1973 Pharmacokinetics of pentobarbital after intravenous and oral administration. Journal of Pharmacokinetics and Biopharmaceutics 1: 5–16
7. Pape B E, Cary P L, Clay L C, Godolphin W 1983 Pentobarbital quantitation using EMIT serum barbiturate assay reagents: application to monitoring of high-dose pentobarbital therapy. Therapeutic Drug Monitoring 5: 467–471
8. Doluisio J T, Smith R B, Chun A H C, Dittert L W 1978 Pentobarbital absorption from capsules and suppositories in humans. Journal of Pharmaceutical Sciences 167: 1586–1588
9. Ehrnebo M 1974 Pharmacokinetics and distribution properties of pentobarbital in humans following oral and intravenous administration. Journal of Pharmaceutical Sciences 63: 1114–1118
10. Ehrnebo M, Odar-Cederlof I 1975 Binding of amobarbital, pentobarbital and diphenylhydantoin to blood cells and plasma proteins in healthy volunteers and uraemic patients. European Journal of Clinical Pharmacology 8: 445–453
11. Reidenberg M M, Lowenthal D T, Briggs W, Gasparo M 1977 Pentobarbital elimination in patients with poor renal function. Clinical Pharmacology and Therapeutics 20: 67–71
12. Held H, Von Oldershausen H F, Remmer H 1970 Der abbau von pentobarbital bei lederschaden. Klinische Wochenschrift 48: 565–567
13. Carulli N, Manenti F, Ponz de Leon M, Ferrari A, Salvioli G, Gallo M 1975 Alteration of drug metabolism during cholestasis in man. European Journal of Clinical Investigation 5: 455–462
14. Drayer D E, Lorenzo B, Lahita R G, Robbins W C, Reidenberg M M 1982 Microsomal hydroxylation as measured by pentobarbital elimination in patients with idiopathic systemic lupus erythematosus. Clinical Pharmacology and Therapeutics 32: 195–200
15. Schaible D H, Cupit G C, Swedlow D B, Rocci M L 1982 High-dose pentobarbital pharmacokinetics in hypothermic brain-injured children. Journal of Pediatrics 100: 655–660
16. Baldeo W C, Gilbert J N T, Powell J W 1980 Multidose studies on the human metabolism of pentobarbitone. European Journal of Drug Metabolism and Pharmacokinetics 5: 75–80
17. Wilson J T, Brown R D, Cherek D R et al 1980 Drug excretion in human breast milk: principles, pharmacokinetics and projected consequences. Clinical Pharmacokinetics 5: 1–80
18. Kanto J, Iisalo E, Kangas L, Valovirta E 1980 A comparative study on the clinical effects of rectal diazepam and pentobarbital on small children. Relationship between plasma level and effect. International Journal of Clinical Pharmacology, Therapy and Toxicology 18: 348–351
19. Hollister L E, Clyde D J 1968 Blood levels of pentobarbital sodium, meprobamate and tybamate in relation to clinical effect. Clinical Pharmacology and Therapeutics 9: 204–208
20. Tang B K, Inaba T, Kalow W 1977 Hydroxylation of pentobarbital in man. Drug Metabolism and Disposition 5: 71–74
21. Griffiths R R, Bigelow G E, Liebson I, Kaliszak J E 1980 Drug preference in humans: double-blind choice comparison of pentobarbital, diazepam and placebo. Journal of Pharmacology and Experimental Therapeutics 215: 649–661
22. Kales A, Kales J D, Bixler E O, Scharf M B 1976 Effectiveness of hypnotic drugs with prolonged use: flurazepam and pentobarbital. Clinical Pharmacology and Therapeutics 18: 356–363
23. Borland R G, Nicholson A N 1975 Comparison of the residual effects of two benzodiazepines (nitrazepam and flurazepam hydrochloride) and pentobarbitone sodium on human performance. British Journal of Clinical Pharmacology 2: 9–17
24. Kay D C, Jasinski D R, Eisenstein R B, Kelly O A 1972 Quantified human sleep after pentobarbital. Clinical Pharmacology and Therapeutics 13: 221–231
25. Ward J D, Becker D P, Miller J D et al 1985 Failure of prophylactic barbiturate coma in the treatment of severe head injury. Journal of Neurosurgery 62: 383–388
26. Marshall L F, Shapiro H M, Rauscher A, Kaufman N M 1978 Pentobarbital therapy for intracranial hypertension in metabolic coma: Reye's syndrome. Critical Care Medicine 6: 1–5
27. Conn A W 1979 Near-drowning and hypothermia. Canadian Medical Association Journal 120: 397–400
28. Hovi-Viander M, Kangas L, Kanto J 1980 A comparative study of the clinical effects of pentobarbital and diazepam given orally as preoperative medication. Journal of Oral Surgery 38: 188–190
29. Aleniewski M I, Bulas B J, Maderazo L, Mendoza C 1977 Intramuscular lorazepam versus pentobarbital premedication: a comparison of patient sedation, analysis and recall. Anesthesia and Analgesia 56: 489–492
30. Young R S K, Ropper A W, Hawkes D, Woods M, Yohn P 1983 Pentobarbital in refractory status epilepticus. Pediatric Pharmacology 3: 63–67
31. Von Felsinger J M, Lasagna L, Beecher H K 1953 The persistence of mental impairment following a hypnotic dose of a barbiturate. Journal of Pharmacology and Experimental Therapeutics 109: 284–291
32. Stoller K P, Belleville J P, Belleville J W 1976 Visual tracking following lorazepam or pentobarbital. Anesthesiology 45: 565–568
33. Brown C R, Forrest W H, Hayden J 1973 The respiratory effects of pentobarbital and secobarbital in clinical doses. Journal of Clinical Pharmacology 13: 28–35
34. Friedman G D 1981 Barbiturates and lung cancer in humans. Journal of the National Cancer Institute 67: 291–295
35. Greenblatt D J, Allen M D, Harmatz J S, Noel B J, Shader R I 1979 Overdose with pentobarbital and secobarbital: assessment of factors related to outcome. Journal of Clinical Pharmacology 19: 758–768
36. Clark J G, Sumerling M D 1966 Muscle necrosis and calcification in acute renal failure due to barbiturate intoxication. British Medical Journal 2: 214–215
37. Hadden J, Johnson K, Smith S, Price L, Giardina E 1969 Acute barbiturate intoxication: concepts of management. Journal of the American Medical Association 209: 893–900
38. Shapiro S, Slone D, Lewis G P, Jick H 1969 Clinical effects of hypnotics 2: an epidemiologic study. Journal of the American Medical Association 209: 2016–2020
39. Teggin A F, Bewley T H 1979 Withdrawal treatment for barbiturate dependence. Practitioner 223: 106–107
40. Bonnett M H, Webb W B, Barnard G 1979 Effect of flurazepam, pentobarbital and caffeine on arousal threshold. Sleep 1: 271–279
41. Anon 1979 Committee on the Review of Medicines: recommendations on barbiturate preparations. British Medical Journal 2: 717–720
42. Brodie M J, Goldberg A 1980 Acute hepatic porphyrias. In: Goldberg A, Moore M R (eds) Clinics in haematology: the porphyrias. W B Saunders, London, pp 253–272
43. Bennett W M, Muther R S, Parker R A et al 1980 Drug therapy in renal failure: dosing guidelines for adults. Part ii: sedatives, hypnotics and tranquillisers; cardiovascular, antihypertensive and diuretic agents; miscellaneous agents. Annals of Internal Medicine 93: 286–325
44. Danhof M, Verbeek R M A, Von Boxtel C J, Boeijinga J K, Breimer D D 1982 Differential effects of enzyme induction on antipyrine metabolite formation. British Journal of Clinical Pharmacology 13: 379–386
45. Berman M L, Green O C 1971 Acute stimulation of cortisol metabolism by pentobarbital in man. Anesthesiology 34: 365–369
46. Chapron D J, Mumford D, Pitegoff G I 1979 Apparent quinidine-induced digoxin toxicity after withdrawal of pentobarbital. Archives of Internal Medicine 139: 363–365
47. Alvan G, Piafsky K, Lind M, Von Bahr C 1978 Effect of pentobarbital on the disposition of alprenolol. Clinical Pharmacology and Therapeutics 22: 316–321
48. Haglund K, Seiderman P, Collste P, Borg K-O, Von Bahr C 1979 Influence of pentobarbital on metoprolol plasma levels. Clinical Pharmacology and Therapeutics 26: 326–329

P

Peritoneal dialysis fluids

Chemistry

Peritoneal dialysis fluids are aqueous solutions of electrolytes at concentrations similar to plasma, containing lactate or acetate as sources of bicarbonate, and dextrose as an osmotic agent. Dianeal with glucose 1.36% w/v manufactured by Travenol, contains sodium 140 mmol.l^{-1}, chloride 101 mmol.l^{-1}, calcium 1.8 mmol.l^{-1}, magnesium 0.7 mmol.l^{-1}, lactate 45 mmol.l^{-1} and anhydrous dextrose 13.6 g.l^{-1}. The pH of the solutions is between 5 and 6.

Pharmacology

The main actions of peritoneal dialysis fluids are removal, by diffusion and osmosis, of accumulated extracellular fluid water and sodium and the products of catabolism, and correction of electrolyte and acid–base imbalance.

Toxicology

All peritoneal dialysis fluids have a mild irritant action on the peritoneal membrane. Long-term use may lead to peritoneal fibrosis and loss of ultrafiltration capacity.[1] The aluminium content of fluids should be less than 0.37 μmol.l^{-1}. High concentrations of aluminium may result in acute toxicity.[2]

Clinical pharmacology

The main action of peritoneal dialysis fluid is removal of water from the extracellular fluid space by the osmotic action of dextrose. This action depends on the peritoneum acting as a dialysis membrane of surface area 1–2 m^2. The volume of fluid removed depends on the membrane permeability, dialysate flow, peritoneal blood flow, the formulation of the fluid, dialysate temperature and the duration of the dwell phase within the peritoneal cavity. Fluid is most rapidly removed during the first two hours after instillation when the osmolar gradient between the fluid and the plasma is maximal. As dextrose is absorbed the gradient falls, leading eventually to reabsorption of fluid. At the same time as the diffusion of water is occurring, there is an efflux of ions, including sodium, and dialysable substances including urea, creatinine, phosphate, drugs and poisons. Tables 1 to 3 show a comparison of clearances of various substances of different molecular weights according to dialysis technique used.

Between 0.3 and 90×10^6 cells can be obtained from a litre of peritoneal dialysis fluid, 50% of these are macrophages that retain their phagocytic capacity. However, in vitro dialysis solutions inhibit phagocytosis and the bactericidal ability of peripheral blood leucocytes, an effect attributed to the pH and high osmolality of the solution. Since it takes 30 min for the peritoneal dialysate pH to rise from 5 to 7 and 2 h for the osmolality to equilibrate, it is likely that peritoneal dialysis fluids inhibit macrophage function in vivo.

Table 1 Clearances (litres per week) for different solutes by various dialysis techniques (from Drukker, 1989)[3]

Solute	Modality				
	MW	HD (15 h)	IPD (40 h)	CAPD (168 h)	Normal kidney
Urea	60	135	60	80	604
Creatinine	113	90	28	58	1200
B_{12}	1350	30	15–16	50	1200
Inulin	5200	5	12	30	1200

MW = molecular weight
HD = haemodialysis
IPD = intermittent peritoneal dialysis
CAPD = continuous ambulatory peritoneal dialysis

Table 2 Dialysate flow rates and clearances (reproduced from Khanna and Nolph 1986[4] with permission)

	Flow rate ml.min^{-1}	Hours/ week	Urea clearance/ litres per week	Inulin clearance/ litres per week
Haemodialysis	500	12	110	5
Intermittent peritoneal dialysis	67	40	60	12
CAPD	5.5	168	70	26

Table 3 Clearance of common drugs by CAPD/IPD (adapted from Lameire, Bogaert and Belpaire 1986[5])

Drug	Dialysis clearance/ml.min^{-1}
Cefotaxime	1.7
Tobramycin	3.8
Vancomycin	1.48
Digoxin	2.74
Cimetidine	4.2

Pharmacokinetics

The pharmacokinetics of peritoneal dialysis fluids cannot be described in a conventional sense, for they are administered into the peritoneum to act locally and not for absorption by the patient. However, a number of changes in their constituents take place during the process of peritoneal dialysis.

1. Water. In the first 2–4 h of the dwell period of dialysate, ultrafiltration of sodium-free water into the peritoneal cavity occurs. This ranges from 1 l with 3.8% glucose solution to 0.2–0.4 l with 1.36% solutions. After 4 h the water is gradually reabsorbed. Were the fluid not to be drained out it would be completely reabsorbed within 24–48 h.

2. Sodium. Following the ultrafiltration of water there is equilibration of sodium between the dialysate and the plasma such that over a 24 h period of dialysis generating a 2 l negative balance (volume of peritoneal dialysis fluid administered minus volume of peritoneal fluid removed) would generate negative sodium balance of between 260 and 280 mmol.

3. Potassium. Most peritoneal dialysis fluids contain no potassium so that over a 24 h period a negative balance of 20–40 mmol of potassium occurs.

4. Bicarbonate. Since lactate uptake during peritoneal dialysis is exceeded by the dialysate bicarbonate loss, peritoneal dialysis leads to a mild metabolic acidosis.

5. Calcium. Because the calcium concentration of CAPD fluid is 1.75 mmol.l^{-1} there is a net uptake of calcium. This is balanced by the calcium loss associated with ultrafiltration which is approximately 3 mmol per day.

6. Glucose. Between 60% and 80% of the glucose in the dialysate is absorbed during a 6 h dwell period. Thus 60 g glucose are absorbed from 2 l of a 3.86% dialysate and 15–22 g from a 1.36% dialysate. Glucose absorption is increased during peritonitis and may increase with time on CAPD treatment.

7. Magnesium. The dialysate concentration of magnesium (0.75 mmol.l^{-1}) leads to positive magnesium balance and mild hypermagnesaemia.

CAPD allows significant peritoneal removal of β_2-microglobulin (average daily peritoneal output 38 mg) such that the levels of β_2-microglobulin in plasma are lower in CAPD patients than in haemodialysis patients. This may reduce the risk of development of β_2-microglobulin associated amyloidosis.[6]

Concentration–effect relationship

The osmotic effect of the CAPD fluid is proportional to the concentration of dextrose, which varies between 13.6 and 63.6 g.l^{-1}. Sodium, potassium, magnesium and calcium balance are altered by their concentrations in the dialysis fluid.

P

Metabolism

The dextrose, lactate or acetate are metabolized by the normal pathways.

Pharmaceutics

The formulations of peritoneal dialysis fluid vary with respect to concentrations of dextrose (13.6–63.6 $g.l^{-1}$), sodium (130–140 $mmol.l^{-1}$) and magnesium (0.25–0.75 $mmol.l^{-1}$), inclusion of acetate or lactate, and the addition or exclusion of potassium. The solutions are available in bags from 0.5–3 l volumes, in 10 l tanks for use with peritoneal dialysis machines and in specially adapted bags for use in continuous ambulatory dialysis. The solutions have a 24 month shelf-life and should be stored below 25°C.

Therapeutic use

Indications

1. Treatment of acute renal failure
2. Treatment of chronic renal failure
3. Peritoneal lavage
4. Treatment of poisoning
5. Correction of severe derangements of salt and water balance
6. Treatment of hypothermia.

Contraindications

There are no contraindications to peritoneal dialysis as such, but there are circumstances in which it is: impossible to perform, e.g. after major abdominal surgery; inadvisable, e.g. in hypercatabolic subjects and those with respiratory problems which would be aggravated by diaphragmatic splinting; less effective than haemodialysis, e.g. in lithium intoxication.

Mode of use

Details of regimes for various indications are given in the next section. Measures may be required to minimize pain which patients may experience during the period when the dialysate is flowing into the abdominal cavity. This is attributed to stretching of the peritoneum by the increased volume, the temperature of the fluid and the pH. It can be alleviated by slowing the rate of flow, warming the peritoneal dialysis fluid or adding lignocaine to the dialysate.

An average daily absorption of glucose of between 100 and 200 g means that a substantial part of the total energy intake of patients on CAPD comes from their dialysate. In patients with glucose intolerance this may lead to hyperglycaemia. If the diet is not modified the absorption of glucose during CAPD may lead to obesity and hyperlipidaemia.

Peritonitis may occur and may be sterile, bacterial or fungal,[7–9] though it is usually bacterial in origin, access to the peritoneum being obtained by contamination of the connection site for the peritoneal dialysis bag. The common organisms are: *Staphylococcus epidermidis*, *Staphylococcus aureus*, Enterobacteriaceae. It presents as abdominal pain, cloudly peritoneal dialysis fluid and occasionally fever. After appropriate microbiological samples are obtained, treatment with intraperitoneal antibiotics is started (see Table 4).

Indications

1. Treatment of acute renal failure

This was first described by Fine et al.[10] It is the preferred method of treatment in infants, in patients in whom heparinization is a risk and in those with cardiovascular instability.

Peritoneal dialysis fluid is administered into the peritoneal cavity via a dialysis catheter, the placement of which is critical to the safe and successful execution of treatment. The warmed fluid is administered in doses of 500–2000 ml hourly in an adult (30 $ml.kg^{-1}$ for infants and children). The fluid is run in over 10 minutes and then immediately allowed to drain out. After 20 minutes of drainage the cycle is repeated. Treatment is continued for 48–72 h or until the biochemical or fluid balance abnormality is controlled.

2. Treatment of chronic renal failure

Intermittent peritoneal dialysis. A similar regimen is used in the management of chronic renal failure by intermittent peritoneal dialysis (IPD).[11] Patients usually undergo treatment for 48 hours each week and the fluid is administered either manually or more usually by a machine which automatically controls the cycles and measures the fluid balance. A variation of this method is continuous cycling peritoneal dialysis (CCPD) in which the patient undergoes machine peritoneal dialysis overnight.[12]

Continuous ambulatory peritoneal dialysis. This was first described by Popovich and others[13] (reviewed by Gokal[14]). This requires regular (3–5 times per day) self administration of peritoneal dialysis by the patient. Specially adapted soft collapsible bags of peritoneal dialysis fluid (1.5–3 l) are attached to a giving set attached to a permanent indwelling pd catheter and the fluid is allowed to run in as fast as is comfortable. The folded empty bag is then tucked into a belt until drainage is performed. Usually there are three 4-hour cycles during the day and one overnight. The dialysis bags and giving sets are specially adapted to allow safe bag changes, minimizing the risk of bacterial contamination of the pd fluid. CAPD is now an established modality of treatment of end stage renal failure, giving comparable results to haemodialysis and transplantation in the short-term. It is the treatment of choice for diabetics,[15] children and those patients with vascular access problems making haemodialysis difficult.

3. Peritoneal lavage

When lavage of the peritoneum is performed in cases of pancreatitis, peritoneal dialysis fluids are used.[16]

4. Poisoning

Peritoneal dialysis can be used for removal of certain poisons and drugs, e.g. ethylene glycol, acetylsalicylic acid, lithium and phenobarbitol (see Table 5). In general, however, haemodialysis is preferred for

Table 4 Antibiotics useful in treatment of peritonitis in CAPD[8]

Antibiotic	Loading dose* iv or ip (mg)	Maintenance dose ip (mg/l)	Stability† in dialysis fluid at room temperature (h)	Approximate maximum safe blood level (mg.l)
Pencillins				
Ampicillin	1000	125	48	300
Cloxacillin	1000	125	24	300
Ticarcillin	2000	250	24	300
Azlocillin	2000	250	48	300
Aminoglycosides				
Gentamicin	1.7 mg/kg	4–8	48	Steady-state
Tobramycin	1.7 mg/kg	4–8	48	
Netilmicin	2.5 mg/kg	4–8	48	4
Amikacin	7.5 mg/kg	25	48	10
Cephalosporins				
Cefuroxime	750	125	24	100
Cephalothin	1000	250	24	100
Cefotaxime	1000	250	24	100
Ceftazidime	1000	125	24	100
Others				
Vancomycin	500	25	24	60–80
Antifungal agents				
Amphotericin B	—	5*	24	NK
Miconazole	—	20	NK	NK
Flucytosine	—	50	NK	80

NK = not known.
*Not recommended for routine use, see text.
†10% degradation.

Table 5 Comparison of clearances by peritoneal dialysis and haemodialysis for some common poisons (adapted from Lameire, Bogaert and Belpaire (1986)[5])

Drug	Clearance $ml.min^{-1}$	
	Peritoneal dialysis	Haemodialysis
Salicylates	20	100
Bromide	14	>150
Thiocyanate	—	>150
Barbiturates	3–10	65–110
Phenytoin	—	12
Lithium	14	75

Peritoneal dialysis fluids

its more rapid effect. The clearance of drugs by peritoneal dialysis depends upon the physicochemical properties of the drug including water solubility and protein binding, the volume of dialysis performed and the state of the peritoneum. In general peritoneal clearance of drugs is low and slow.[5]

5. Electrolyte and fluid balance problems other than those caused by renal failure
Peritoneal dialysis can be employed as a short-term means to treat hypercalcaemia, hyperuricaemia (in tumour lysis) and intractable oedema in congestive heart failure. In practice, haemodialysis is preferred in each of these circumstances and peritoneal dialysis is used only when haemodialysis or haemofiltration is not available.

6. Treatment of hypothermia[17]
Peritoneal dialysis can be used for gradual rewarming in cases of hypothermia.

Adverse reactions

Potentially life-threatening effects
Adverse effects of peritoneal dialysis can be divided into those which are the direct consequence of the action of peritoneal dialysis and those that result from its execution. Hypovolaemia, hypernatraemia and hyperkalaemia result from uncontrolled peritoneal dialysis and may occasionally be life-threatening, and the same is true of peritonitis, which may be sterile, bacterial or fungal.[7–9]

Acute overdosage
The effects would be those described above.

Severe or irreversible adverse effects
These include hyperglycaemia and hyperlipidaemia, and weight gain as a result of the calorie load of dextrose. Hypoproteinaemia may also occur: 6–12 g protein and 2–4 g of amino acids may be lost in the peritoneal dialysis fluid each day.

Increased intrabdominal pressure may lead to hernias and diaphragmatic splinting. Peritoneal fibrosis and adhesions are often a complication of recurrent infection and may lead to loss of ultrafiltration capacity.[1,18–20] It is possible that sclerosing peritonitis is caused by exposure to chlorhexidine used to sterilize the tubing connection.[21]

Symptomatic adverse effects
Pain may occur during the procedure.

High risk groups

Neonates
These are not a high risk group for treatment but extra care is required to avoid electrolyte imbalance in neonates. The peritoneal surface area is relatively large so dialysis is more efficient. This can lead to greater water losses, resulting in hypernatraemia. Glucose is more rapidly absorbed in neonates and protein losses are greater.

Breast milk. Patients requiring peritoneal dialysis are unlikely to breast feed.

Children
What has been said above about neonates also applies to children.

Pregnant women
Pregnancy is not a contraindication to peritoneal dialysis but it is very rare for patients with renal failure to become pregnant. Successful pregnancies have been reported. If delivery is to be by caesarean section, peritoneal dialysis will have to stop until the abdominal wound is healed.

The elderly
No difference in the outcome of treatment was observed when elderly patients (aged over 65) were compared to younger patients.[22]

Concurrent disease

Diabetes. CAPD has proved successful in diabetics with chronic renal failure and the complication rate of the treatment itself is no different from that of non-diabetics. Because of the high glucose load, insulin doses must be modified after institution of treatment. It is possible to administer insulin by injection into the CAPD dialysate bag. The insulin dose requirements are established after first administering one quarter of the baseline insulin requirement as soluble insulin to each of four peritoneal dialysis bags. Doses are then adjusted according to blood glucose levels and higher doses are usually required when dialysate containing higher concentrations of glucose is used.

Respiratory disease. Respiratory failure is a contraindication to intermittent peritoneal dialysis for it may lead to splinting of the diaphragm. CAPD can be used in patients with respiratory disease, for the dialysate pools in the pelvis.

Patients with ascites. CAPD should not be performed in patients with ascites because the protein losses would be excessive.

Drug interactions

A number of drugs are added to peritoneal dialysis fluid, for example heparin to prevent fibrin clot formation in the pd catheter; insulin to provide an alternative route of delivery for diabetics;[15] and antibiotics for the treatment of peritonitis. Most antibiotics in common usage for the treatment of CAPD peritonitis are stable in peritoneal dialysis fluid for 24 hours[8,23,24] (see Table 4). Peritoneal transport can be affected by a number of drugs though none is in clinical use; for example, intraperitoneal nitroprusside at doses of 3–6 $\mu g.ml^{-1}$ can increase peritoneal clearance.

Major outcome trials

There are no trials comparing peritoneal and haemodialysis directly because selection for a particular treatment is not random. Burton and Walls[25] have compared the three means of treating end stage renal failure (renal transplantation, haemodialysis and CAPD) and found no significant differences in patient survival. Whether CAPD will provide as reliable a long-term replacement therapy as haemodialysis remains to be established.

The outcome of patients started or CAPD on haemodialysis has been prospectively monitored in a collaborative study undertaken in seven different units. Although survival was similar at 2 years technique failure was slightly higher for CAPD.[26]

1. Chan M K, Baillod R A, Chuah P et al 1981 Three years experience of continuous ambulatory peritoneal dialysis. Lancet 1: 1409–1412

62 patients were treated with CAPD, 29 of whom had been followed for at least 6 months. In comparison with patients on intermittent haemodialysis or intermittent peritoneal dialysis, urea, potassium, phosphate and urate levels were significantly lower and haemoglobin levels significantly higher. There were 2.22 episodes of peritonitis per patient year. CAPD patients had significantly higher HDL/cholesterol concentrations than haemodialysis patients.

2. Gokal R, McHugh M, Fryer R, Ward M K, Kerr D N S 1980 Continuous ambulatory peritoneal dialysis: one year's experience in a UK dialysis unit. British Medical Journal 281: 474–477

32 patients were managed by CAPD. Blood urea concentrations were well controlled, mean values ranging between 10 and 20 $mmol.l^{-1}$; mean serum creatinine was between 800 and 1000 $\mu mol.l^{-1}$; peritoneal protein losses were 6–10 g per 24 h such that mean serum albumin and total protein concentrations were below the normal range. Serum ionized calcium concentrations were within the normal range. Serum phosphate remained above the normal range. The incidence of peritonitis was one episode per 20 patient weeks.

3. Gokal R, Baillod R, Bogle F et al 1987 Multicentre study on outcome of treatment in patients on continuous ambulatory peritoneal dialysis and haemodialysis. Nephrology, Dialysis and Transplantation 2: 172–178

338 patients starting CAPD were compared with 175 starting haemodialysis. Actuarial patient survival estimates at 2 years were 84% for haemodialysis and 83% for CAPD. Technique survival, i.e. continued successful use of the dialysis modality, was 92% for haemodialysis and 80% for CAPD.

General review articles

Gokal R 1987 Continuous ambulatory peritoneal dialysis (CAPD) — 10 years on. Quarterly Journal of Medicine 63: 465–472
Majorca R, Cancarini G C, Camerini C et al 1989 Is CAPD competitive with haemodialysis for long term treatment of uraemic patients? Nephrology, Dialysis and Transplantation 4: 244–253

Mion C M 1989 Practical use of peritoneal dialysis. In: Maher J F (ed) Replacement of renal function by dialysis — a textbook of dialysis, 3rd edn. Martinus Nijhoff, Boston, pp 537–589

Winchester J F 1986 CAPD systems solutions. In: Gokal R (ed) Continuous ambulatory peritoneal dialysis. Churchill Livingstone, Edinburgh, pp 94–109

References

1. Slingenmeyer A, Canaud B 1983 Permanent loss of ultrafiltration capacity of the peritoneum in long-term peritoneal dialysis: an epidemiological study. Nephron 33: 133–138
2. Cumming A D, Simpson G, Cowie J, Winney R J 1982 Acute aluminium intoxication on continuous ambulatory peritoneal dialysis. Lancet 1: 103–104
3. Drukker W 1989 Peritoneal dialysis: a historical review. In: Maher J F (ed) Replacement of renal function by dialysis. A textbook of dialysis, 3rd edn. Martinus Nijhoff, Boston, pp 476–515
4. Khanna R, Nolph K D 1986 Peritoneal morphology in microcirculation. In: Gokal R (ed) Continuous ambulatory peritoneal dialysis. Churchill Livingstone, Edinburgh, pp 14–37
5. Lameire N, Bogaert M, Belpaire F 1986 Peritoneal pharmacokinetics and pharmacological manipulation of peritoneal transport. In: Gokal R (ed) Continuous ambulatory peritoneal dialysis. Churchill Livingstone, Edinburgh, pp 56–93
6. Tielemans C, Dratwa M, Bergmann P et al 1988 Continuous ambulatory peritoneal dialysis versus haemodialysis: a lesser risk of amyloidosis? Nephrology, Dialysis and Transplantation 3: 291–294
7. Mion C, Slingeneyer H, Canaud B 1986 Peritonitis. In: Gokal R (ed) Continuous ambulatory dialysis. Churchill Livingstone, Edinburgh, ch 8, pp 163–217
8. Working Party of the British Society of Antimicrobial Chemotherapy 1987 Diagnosis and management of peritonitis in continuous ambulatory peritoneal dialysis. Lancet 1: 845–849
9. Gokal R, Ramos J M, Ward M K, Kerr D N S 1981 'Eosinophilic' peritonitis in continuous ambulatory peritoneal dialysis (CAPD). Clinical Nephrology 15: 328–330
10. Fine J, Frank H A, Seligman A M 1946 The treatment of acute renal failure by peritoneal irrigation. Annals of Surgery 124: 857–878
11. Doolan P D, Ruben R M, cited by Drukker W 1983 The first chronic case successfully treated by periodic peritoneal dialysis. In: Drukker W, Parsons F M, Maher J F (eds) Replacement of renal function by dialysis — a textbook of dialysis 2nd edn. Martinus Nijhoff, Boston, p 422
12. Diaz-Buxo J A, Walker P J, Chandler J T, Farmer C D, Holt K L, Cox P 1981 Continuous cyclic peritoneal dialysis. In: Gokal G H, Kessel M, Nolph K D (eds) Advances in peritoneal dialysis. Excerpta Medica, Amsterdam, pp 126–130
13. Popovich R P, Moncrief J W, Nolph K D, Ghode A J, Twardowski S J, Pyle W K 1978 Continuous ambulatory peritoneal dialysis. Annals of Internal Medicine 88: 449–456
14. Gokal R 1987 Continuous ambulatory peritoneal dialysis (CAPD) — ten years on. Quarterly Journal of Medicine 63: 465–472
15. Amair P, Khanna R, Leibel B et al 1982 Continuous ambulatory peritoneal dialysis in diabetics with end-stage renal disease. New England Journal of Medicine 306: 625–630
16. Mayer A D, McMahon M J, Corfield A P et al 1985 A controlled trial of peritoneal lavage for the treatment of severe acute pancreatitis. New England Journal of Medicine 312: 399–404
17. Reuler J B, Parker R A 1978 Peritoneal dialysis in the management of hypothermia. Journal of the American Medical Association 240: 2289–2240
18. Rottembourg J, Gahl G M, Poignet H L et al 1983 Severe abdominal complications in patients undergoing continuous ambulatory peritoneal dialysis. Proceedings of the European Dialysis and Transplantation Association 20: 236–241
19. Slingenmeyer A, Elie M, Mion C 1986 Sclerosing encapsulation peritonitis: results of an international survey. Nephrology Dialysis and Transplantation 1: 112
20. Henderson I, Gokal R 1986 Loss of ultrafiltration in CAPD. In: Gokal R (ed) Continuous ambulatory dialysis. Churchill Livingstone, Edinburgh, pp 218–227
21. Oulès R, Challah S, Brunner S P 1988 Case-controlled study to determine the cause of sclerosing peritoneal disease. Nephrology, Dialysis and Transplantation 3: 66–69
22. Kaye M, Pajel P A, Somerville P J 1982 Continuous ambulatory peritoneal dialysis in the elderly. Lancet 2: 270–271
23. Mion C M 1983 Practical use of peritoneal dialysis. In: Drukker W, Parsons F M, Maher J F (eds) Replacement of renal function by dialysis — a textbook of dialysis 2nd edn. Martinus Nijhoff, Boston, pp 457–492
24. Sewell D L, Golper T A, Brown S D, Nelson E, Knower M, Kimbrough R C 1983 Stability of single and combination antimicrobial agents in various peritoneal dialysates in the presence of insulin and heparin. American Journal of Kidney Diseases 3: 209–212
25. Burton P R, Walls J 1987 Selection-adjusted comparison of life expectancy of patients on continuous ambulatory peritoneal dialysis, haemodialysis and renal transplantation. Lancet 1: 1115
26. Gokal R, Baillod R, Bogle S et al 1987 Multicentre study on outcome of treatment in patients on continuous ambulatory peritoneal dialysis and haemodialysis. Nephrology, Dialysis and Transplantation 2: 172–178

Perphenazine

Perphenazine was among the first phenothiazine-neuroleptics to achieve wide therapeutic use.

Chemistry

Perphenazine (Trilafon, Fentazin, Phenazine)
$C_{21}H_{26}ClN_3OS$.
2-Chloro-10-{3-[1-(2-hydroxy)(ethyl)-4-piperazinyl]propyl} phenothiazine

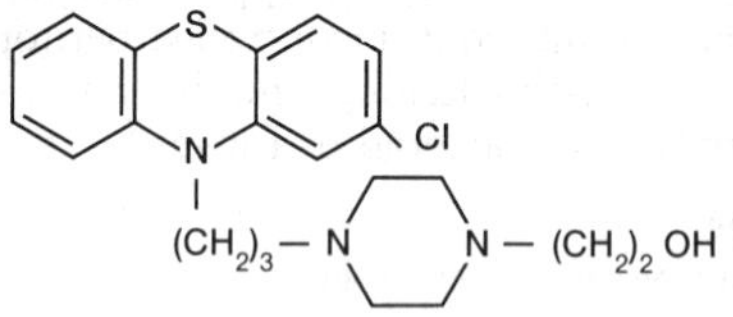

Molecular weight (free compound)	404.0
pKa	7.8
Solubility	
in alcohol	1 in 10000
in water	insoluble
Octanol/water partition coefficient	1,260

Perphenazine is a piperazinyl phenothiazine. It is prepared by the condensation of 10-(3-chloropropyl)-2-chlorophenothiazine with 1-(2-hydroxyethyl) piperazine. Perphenazine crystals are sensitive to light and are practically insoluble in water and sesame oil.

Perphenazine is available in combination with amitriptyline (Triptafen).

Pharmacology

Perphenazine, like other phenothiazines, affects many different anatomical sites of the central nervous system including the reticular lobe, the hypothalamus and the globus pallidus and corpus striatum.[2] Its mechanism of action is possibly linked to (1) antagonism of the postsynaptic dopamine-D_1 receptor, with inhibition of the activation of the dopamine D_1-sensitive adenylate cyclase and synthesis of cyclic AMP, (2) antagonism of the postsynaptic dopamine-D_2 receptor and/or (3) interactive effects between dopamine-D_1 and dopamine-D_2 receptors, e.g. antagonism on the dopamine-D_2 receptor blocks behaviour elicited by the overactivity of the dopamine-D_1 receptor. There is also inhibition of adrenergic, serotoninergic, histaminergic and cholinergic receptors.

Perphenazine belongs to the large group of piperazinyl phenothiazines. These compounds are known as high potency drugs (neuroleptics) because they exert pharmacological effects (e.g. induction of catalepsy, inhibition of spontaneous motor activity, interference with conditioned avoidance responses, suppression of apomorphine-induced behaviour) in a lower mg per kg dosage than phenothiazines with other side-chain substituents. This is particularly true for compounds, such as perphenazine, which possess a hydroxyethyl substituent. In contrast to these pharmacological effects, however, the protective action of perphenazine against the lethal effects of adrenaline and noradrenaline follows a different pattern. It is, in fact, less pronounced with piperazine neuroleptics than with their dimethyl-aminopropyl analogues.[3]

Toxicology

Perphenazine is teratogenic in pregnant mice and rats, but not in rabbits, when given orally in doses 15 to 25 times the maximum

Perphenazine

recommended human daily dose. Most of the fetuses in which cleft palate occurred also showed less prenatal growth and weight gain. In other studies, perphenazine, given orally to pregnant rats in doses 120 to 150 times the maximum recommended human daily dose, induced cleft palate, retrognathia, micromelia, hydrocephalus and anophthalmia or microphthalmia in the offspring. On the other hand, when administered orally to pregnant rats in doses only 4 to 7 times the maximum recommended human daily dose, perphenazine did not induce teratogenic changes in the fetus, although the doses were lethal to some treated dams.[4,5]

Long-term perphenazine studies in animals to evaluate carcinogenic potential have not been done; and data for studies using peripheral leucocyte cultures prepared from patients receiving perphenazine are insufficient to determine whether perphenazine can produce chromosome damage and/or has mutagenic potential.

Clinical pharmacology

Perphenazine acts primarily as an antipsychotic agent to reduce agitation and restlessness and to diminish aggression and impulsive behaviour. Perphenazine reduces initiative and interest in the environment and drowsiness often occurs. Mental confusion, delusions, hallucinations and irrational behaviour are usually improved. Perphenazine also relaxes skeletal musculature, it acts on the chemoreceptor trigger zone to relieve nausea and vomiting, and in the cardiovascular system it may produce postural hypotension. Effects on the circulation are less likely than with aliphatic phenothiazines such as chlorpromazine. Furthermore, in most patients tolerance develops to these effects over a period of days or weeks. The same does not apply to the lowering of convulsive threshold and the electrocardiographic changes which may occur in the course of perphenazine administration. The latter is characterized by prolongation of the QTc interval with widening, blunting, and notching of the T wave. At higher doses, lowering and inversion of the T wave may occur.[6] Nevertheless, such changes occur considerably less frequently with perphenazine than with thioridazine.

Perphenazine, like other phenothiazines, can cause an elevation in protein-bound iodine in serum without apparent thyrotoxicosis and/or a decrease in the secretion of adrenocorticosteroids as a result of diminished release of corticotrophin.

Perphenazine, like other phenothiazines with neuroleptic properties, elevates prolactin levels and this elevation persists during chronic administration. Although tissue culture experiments indicate that approximately one-third of human breast cancers are prolactin dependent in vitro, to-date neither clinical nor epidemiological studies have shown an association between chronic administration of perphenazine and breast cancer. Available data, however, are insufficient to draw final conclusions.

Pharmacokinetics

Perphenazine, like other phenothiazines, is readily absorbed from the gastrointestinal tract and from parenteral sites. Of an orally administered dose 60 to 70% is rapidly removed from the portal circulation by the liver, and, as a result, less unchanged drug enters the systemic circulation than when it is given parenterally.

The drug is very lipophilic and is highly bound to membranes and proteins. High concentration of the unchanged substance is found in the brain, whereas metabolites predominate in the lung, liver, kidney and spleen. Perphenazine can cross the human placental barrier and enter the fetal circulation easily.

Elimination of perphenazine from the plasma is more rapid than from sites of high lipid content and binding, e.g. central nervous system. Age is considered to be an important determinant not only in the rate of metabolism but also in the rate of excretion of the drug. Accordingly, the elderly, the fetus and the infant have diminished capacities for excretion.

The preferred analytical method studies with perphenazine is high performance liquid chromatography. By employing this method, concentrations of 0.2 µg of perphenazine per litre of whole blood can be assayed with a sufficient degree of accuracy.

In clinical pharmacological studies maximal absorption was reached 1–3 hours after oral dosage, 1 hour after 5 mg intramuscularly and 2 days after 100 mg intramuscularly. Because of the great individual variations in absorption, no definite relationship between dose and blood levels could be found. Similarly, with continuous oral medication, there was a poor systemic bioavailability of the drug.

Perphenazine was found to have a plasma half life of 9.5 h after intravenous administration.

Plasma levels of perphenazine may be elevated in patients with impaired heptic function.

Oral absorption	100%
Presystemic metabolism	60–70% in case of oral administration
Plasma half life	
mean	9.5 h
Volume of distribution	20 l.kg^{-1}
Plasma protein binding	90–93%

Concentration–effect relationship

In a recent study perphenazine plasma levels above 1.5 nmoles.l^{-1} (610 ng.l^{-1}) were associated with favourable (excellent) therapeutic effects. In the same study there was a high risk for extrapyramidal side effects at perphenazine plasma levels above 3 nmoles.l^{-1} (1200 ng.l^{-1}). Contrary to expectations perphenazine sulphoxide levels did not differ among patients with or without side effects.[7,8]

Metabolism

Perphenazine, like other phenothiazines, is extensively metabolized in the liver. The major metabolic pathways are glucuronidalion N-oxidation, axomatic hydroxylation, removal of the terminal N-alkyl group, and sulphoxide formation with conjugation to glucuronic acid of the phenolic derivatives (Fig. 1). The number of metabolites is further increased by the occurrence of oxidation and degradation of the piperazine ring. Perphenazine-sulphoxide is the major inactive metabolite; during chronic treatment, plasma levels of sulphoxide may equal or exceed free drug levels. The N-dealkyl metabolite of perphenazine may be active, but current data suggest that N-dealkylation is a minor pathway of perphenazine metabolism in man. In patients on long-term perphenazine therapy about 1% of the diurnal dose of orally administered perphenazine is excreted in urine unchanged. The main metabolites are perphenazine glucuronide and perphenazine sulphoxide of which 30% or 12% respectively of diurnal dose is excreted. Systemic bioavailability is poor with the metabolite level being much higher than that seen after parenteral administration.

A recent report (1986; personal communication) has found the following Ki values for 7-OH perphenazine for noradrenergic and dopamine receptors (corresponding values for perphenazine are given in brackets): D_2 receptor 8.7 (5.9); α_1 noradrenergic receptor 44 (24); α_2 noradrenergic receptor 1340 (683). Thus, 7-OH perphenazine has significant affinity for the D_2 dopamine receptor. Although no information on the formation of 7-OH perphenazine in man is currently available, 7-hydroxylation of similar compounds can be significant. It has therefore been recommended that 7-OH perphenazine be considered as a possible factor in the therapeutic activity of perphenazine.

Pharmaceutics

Perphenazine is available in oral and parenteral forms.[9]

Trilafon tablets (Schering, US) contain 2 mg, 4 mg, 8 mg and 16 mg of perphenazine. They are grey, sugar-coated and branded respectively in black, green, blue and red with the Schering trademark. They need to be stored between 2 and 30°C.

Fentazin tablets (A & H, UK) contain 2 mg and 4 mg in a white, round sugar coated tablet. They are coded AH/1C and AH/2C respectively.

Trilafon Repetabs (Schering, US) contain 8 mg of perphenazine — 4 mg in an outer layer for immediate release and 4 mg in an inner layer for release three to six hours later — are white, sugar-coated and branded in grey with the Schering trademark.

Concentrate, containing 16 mg of perphenazine per 5 ml in approximately 2 fluid ounces of diluent is light sensitive and dispensed in amber bottles of 4 fluid ounce (118 ml). The bottles need to be stored between 2 and 30°C in cartons until they are used.

Injection material (no longer marketed in the UK) contains 5 mg of perphenazine per ml, 24.6 mg disodium citrate, and 2 mg sodium

Perphenazine

bisulphite and water. The pH is adjusted to a range of 4.2 to 5.6. It is dispensed in 1 ml ampoules which need to be stored in the carton until used. Exposure to light may cause discoloration.

Depot preparations are perphenazine enanthate (PE) and perphenazine decanoate (PD). Perphenazine enanthate has been available since the mid-1970s in several countries in Europe, whereas perphenazine decanoate has only recently been introduced. Neither of these two depot preparations is available for clinical use in the United States and Canada.

Therapeutic use

Indications

1. In the management of psychotic disorders
2. For the control of severe nausea and vomiting in adults

Contraindications

1. In comatose or greatly obtunded patients
2. In patients receiving large doses of central nervous system depressants such as barbiturates, alcohol, narcotics, analgesics, and antihistamines
3. In the presence of blood dyscrasias, bone marrow depression, and liver damage
4. In patients who have shown hypersensitivity to perphenazine products, components of perphenazine products, and compounds related to perphenazine
5. In patients with suspected or established subcortical brain damage.

Mode of use

For both therapeutic indications, i.e. management of psychotic disorders and control of nausea and vomiting, perphenazine may be employed orally or parenterally.

Indications

1. Psychotic disorders

The primary indications for perphenazine are schizophrenic disorders, mania, organic brain syndrome with psychosis and schizoaffective disorder. It is also indicated for the treatment of paranoid disorders. In major depression with psychotic features and bipolar depressive disorders, perphenazine should be reserved for patients unresponsive to other, non-neuroleptic, therapeutic agents. It may be prescribed, however, as adjunctive medication during the initial period of treatment to control agitation and anxiety.

The target symptoms that respond favourably and consistently to perphenazine include combativeness, tension, hyperactivity, hostility, negativism, auditory hallucinations, paranoid delusions, insomnia, poor self-care, and anorexia.[10]

Dosage, formulation and routes of drug administration. The manufacturers of perphenazine recommend that the total daily dose should not exceed 24 mg, although higher doses have been described in clinical literature and are mentioned below. Dosage must be individualized and adjusted according to the severity of the condition and the observed response.

Divided doses at the onset of treatment minimize the initial impact of many unwanted pharmacological effects. Frequency of administration, however, should be reduced once the full therapeutic effect has been achieved. The goal is a single daily dose. Giving the medication in the evening promotes sleep and prevents excessive daytime sedation. Also, patients are less likely to suffer disabling extrapyramidal signs if peak concentrations of perphenazine occur while they are asleep. On the other hand frightening dreams are not infrequent, if a single daily dose of perphenazine is taken at bedtime.[11]

Recommended doses for orally administered perphenazine tablets in moderately disturbed hospitalized patients is 4–8 mg three times daily initially; and for Repetabs tablets, it is 8–16 mg twice daily. Corresponding doses for hospitalized psychotic patients are 8–16 mg two to four times daily, and 8–32 mg twice daily.

The usual dosage range of orally administered perphenazine concentrate is 8–16 mg ($\frac{1}{2}$ to 1 teaspoonful) two to four times daily in hospitalized patients. Although higher dosages have been used, a total daily dose of more than 64 mg (4 teaspoonsful) is usually not required. Perphenazine concentrate should be diluted only with water, saline, homogenized milk, carbonated orange drink, or pineapple, apricot, prune, orange, V-8, tomato or grapefruit juices. It should not be mixed with beverages containing caffeine (coffee, cola), tannins (tea), or pectinates (apple juice). The suggested dilution is

Fig. 1 The metabolism of perphenazine

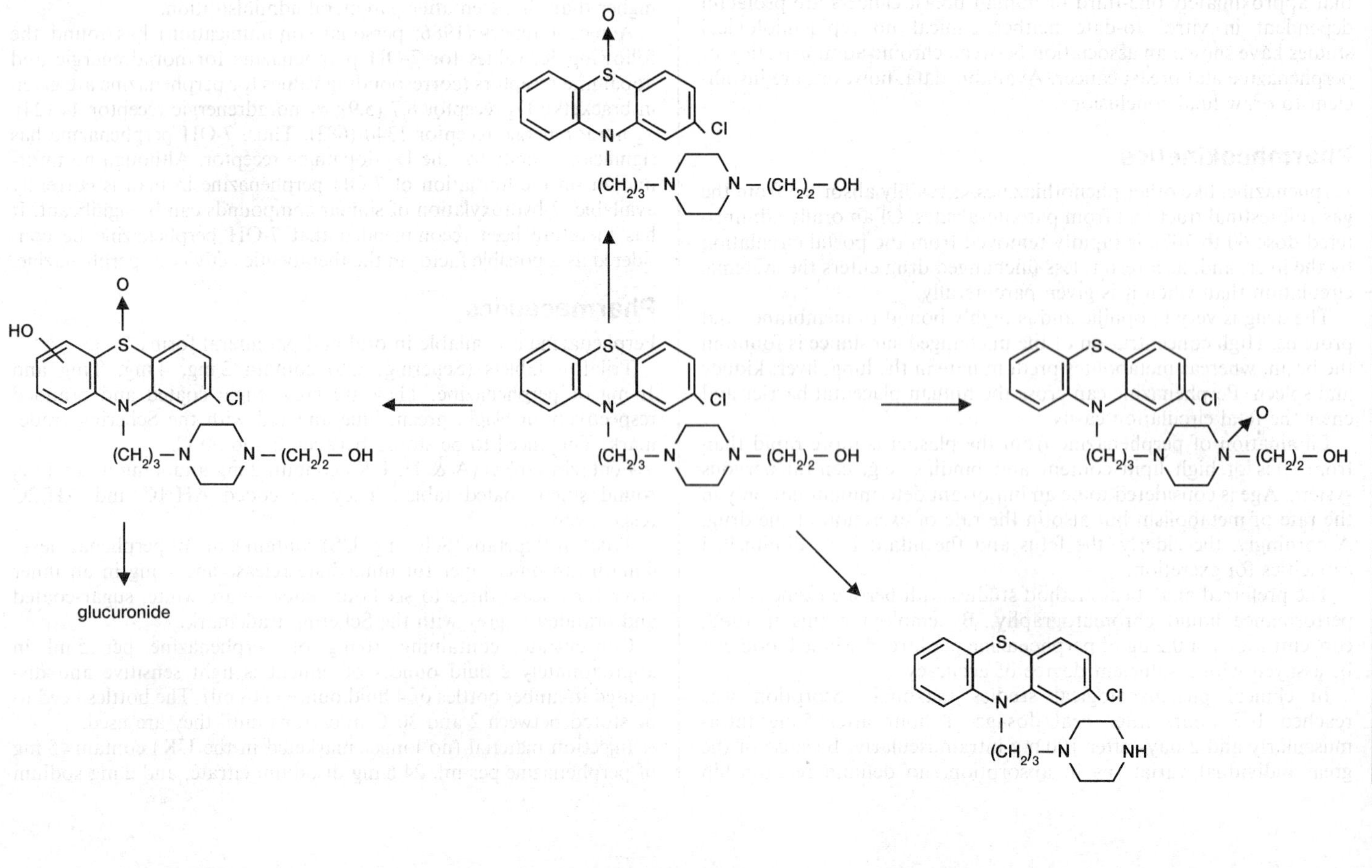

approximately two fluid ounces of diluent for each 5 ml (16 mg) of perphenazine concentrate.

Intramuscular perphenazine is indicated for patients who refuse to take medication orally or whose absorption of drugs by the intestines is compromised. In situations calling for rapid tranquillization, the intramuscular route is also preferable. This might apply to patients who present with great pressure of speech, agitation and incoherence. It would also apply to patients who endanger others with their hostility, destructiveness, or violent behaviour. Other clinical indications for intramuscular perphenazine treatment include psychotic reactions to alcohol and alcohol withdrawal, such as delirium tremens and acute alcoholic hallucinosis; psychotic reaction to drugs, such as LSD_{25} and amphetamines; psychosis with chronic brain syndrome, irrespective of the presence or absence of delirium; agitated and stuporous depression; acute delirious mania; schizophrenia with persistent and frightening hallucinations; and/or delirious and excited or inhibited catatonia.

Parenteral perphenazine should be administered by deep intramuscular injection with the patient seated or recumbent. Following the injection the patient should be observed for a short time for possible adverse effects. Therapeutic effects are seen usually within 10 min and peak effects are attained within one to two hours. The average duration of effect is 12–24 hours. The usual initial dose for psychotic conditions is 5 mg (1 ml), although when required an initial 10 mg intramuscular dose may be given. The initial 5 mg dose may be repeated every 6 hours or, in case of rapid tranquillization, hourly. It is the usual practice to replace intramuscular by oral treatment as soon as possible. In most patients this can be achieved within 24–48 hours. In some patients, however, parenteral (intramuscular) injections need to be continued for several months. Perphenazine is more potent by the parenteral route than in oral formulations. Because of this, at least equal, or higher dosages should be used when the patient is transferred to oral from parenteral treatment.

Treatment rules. As with other neuroleptics, sedative effects are evident after a single dose of perphenazine, while more specific effects take longer. Accordingly, changes in disturbed behaviour may appear within a few hours or days, but alterations in thought and delusional perceptions may take several weeks. Psychopathologic symptoms related to arousal, such as psychomotor excitement and insomnia, are expected to be controlled within two weeks; symptoms related to affectivity, such as anxiety and social withdrawal, within four weeks, and symptoms related to mental integration, such as hallucinations and delusions, within six to eight weeks. Symptomatic improvement may continue slowly for months.

There is no consensus on how long perphenazine administration should be continued if there is no therapeutic response. It is an acceptable practice, however, to continue treatment with gradually increasing doses for four to six weeks. In special, treatment-resistant cases doses up to 100 mg daily have been given. Only if no improvement occurs to maximally tolerated doses of perphenazine within three months should the patient be categorized as refractory to the compound and treated with another neuroleptic.

Long-term treatment is not indicated with perphenazine following an initial episode with a sudden onset and a short course, in a patient with a good premorbid history. For such a patient, medication may be discontinued after 6 to 12 months. For other patients, it is common practice to continue maintenance treatment with perphenazine for two years after the first schizophrenic episode, for five years after the second, and indefinitely after the third.[12]

2. Nausea and vomiting

Recommended doses for severe nausea and vomiting in adults is 8–16 mg of orally administered regular perphenazine tablets daily or 8 mg Repetabs tablets twice a day. In acute cases two (16 mg) Repetabs tablets may be given.

When given parenterally by intramuscular route the usual dose for the rapid control of vomiting is 5 mg (1 ml). Rarely, a 10 mg (2 ml) dose may be necessary although this is greater than the manufacturer's recommendation.

Intravenous administration of perphenazine is seldom required. This route of administration should be used only when absolutely necessary to control severe vomiting, or acute conditions, such as violent retching during surgery. Its use should be limited to recumbent hospitalized adults in doses not exceeding 5 mg. When employed in this manner, intravenous injection should be given as a diluted solution by either fractional injection or as a slow drip infusion. In the surgical patient, slow infusion of not more than 5 mg is preferred. When administered in divided doses, the perphenazine injection should be diluted to 0.5 $mg.ml^{-1}$ (1 ml mixed with 9 ml of physiologic saline solution), and not more than 1 mg per injection given at not less than 1–2 minute intervals. Intravenous injection should be discontinued as soon as symptoms are controlled and should not exceed 5 mg. The possibility of acute hypotensive and extrapyramidal side effects should be considered and appropriate means for management kept available.

Contraindications

1. Comatose and greatly obtunded patients

Perphenazine is contraindicated in these patients because of its depressant effects on the central nervous system.

2. Patients receiving large doses of central nervous depressants

Perphenazine is contraindicated, because of the potentiation of central nervous system depressant effects. The respiratory depressant effects of meperidine, and possibly also of other opioid analgesics, may be increased.

3. Patients with blood dyscrasias, bone marrow depression, or liver damage

Perphenazine is contraindicated, because latent pathologies can be precipitated and existing ones aggravated by the drug.

4. Hypersensitivity

In patients who have shown hypersensitivity to perphenazine, perphenazine is contraindicated. If hypersensitivity is not known, a significant rise in body temperature, which cannot be explained otherwise, may suggest individual intolerance to the drug.

5. Patients with subcortical brain damage, with or without hypothalamic damage

Perphenazine is contraindicated, because a hyperthermic reaction with temperatures in excess of 40°C may occur in these patients.

Adverse reactions

Potentially life-threatening effects

The neuroleptic malignant syndrome has been reported with perphenazine. It is a relatively uncommon, potentially lethal syndrome, characterized by severe extrapyramidal dysfunction with rigidity, stupor and coma, hyperthermia, and autonomic disturbances, including cardiovascular effects. There is no specific treatment; symptomatic treatment may include the administration of dantrolene and/or bromocriptine; perphenazine administration should be stopped immediately.[13]

Sudden death has occasionally been reported in patients who have received perphenazine. In some cases the death was apparently due to cardiac arrest; in others, the cause appeared to have been asphyxia due to failure of the cough reflex.

Acute overdosage

Manifestations of an overdosage of perphenazine primarily involves the extrapyramidal system. The severe adverse effects are extensions of the many pharmacological effects of the drug.

Patients with early or mild intolerance may experience restlessness, confusion, and excitement. Other symptoms include hypotension, tachycardia, hypothermia, miosis, tremor, muscle twitching, spasms, rigidity or hypotonia, convulsions, difficulty in swallowing and breathing, cyanosis, and respiratory and/or vasomotor collapse, possibly with sudden apnoea.

All patients suspected of having taken an overdose should be hospitalized as soon as possible.

There is no specific antidote for overdosage with perphenazine. Treatment is symptomatic and supportive. If consciousness is retained, the patient should be induced to vomit even if emesis has occurred spontaneously. Following emesis, any drug remaining in the stomach may be absorbed by activated charcoal administration. If vomiting is unsuccessful, gastric lavage should be performed. Standard measures, such as oxygen, intravenous fluids and corticosteroids should be used to manage circulatory shock or metabolic acidosis; an open airway and adequate fluid intake should be maintained; body temperature should be regulated, and cardiac function monitored.

Cardiac arrhythmias may be treated with neostigmine, pyridostigmine, or propranolol, and cardiac failure with digitalis. Hypotension should be treated with plasma expanders and, possibly, dopamine or dobutamine. Adrenaline, however, should not be used, because its pressor effects might be antagonized by perphenazine. Convulsions should be treated with anticonvulsants, such as inhalation anaesthetics, diazepam, or paraldehyde. Barbiturates, however, should not be used, because perphenazine might increase their central nervous system depressant action. Parkinson-like symptoms should be treated with benztropine mesylate, trihexyphenidyl, or diphenhydramine.

It should be noted that dialysis is of no value, because of the low plasma concentrations and high tissue binding of perphenazine. Consciousness may not be fully regained for 48 hours following a toxic overdose, despite supportive and contra-active measures.

Severe or irreversible adverse effects

Central nervous system effects. These include extrapyramidal signs, such as opisthotonus, trismus, torticollis, retrocollis, aching and numbness of the limbs; motor restlessness, oculogyric crisis; hyperreflexia; dystonia, including protrusion, discoloration, aching and rounding of the tongue, tonic spasm of the masticatory muscles; tight feeling in the throat; slurred speech; dysphagia; akathisia; dyskinesia; parkinsonism; and ataxia. They can usually be controlled by the concomitant use of antiparkinsonian drugs, such as benztropine mesylate, trihexyphenidyl, or diphenhydramine, and/or by reduction in dosage. Adolescents and young adults are most likely to develop dystonic reactions even after single doses of the drug; while these reactions may appear to be quite alarming, they respond quickly to antiparkinsonian drugs.

Other CNS effects include cerebral oedema, abnormality of cerebrospinal fluid proteins, lowering of convulsive threshold, particularly in patients with EEG abnormalities or a history of seizure disorders, and headaches.

Drowsiness may occur, particularly during the first or second week, after which it usually disappears. Hypnotic effects tend to be minimal, especially in patients who are permitted to remain active.

Adverse behaviour effects include restlessness, hyperactivity, nocturnal confusion, bizarre dreams, insomnia, paradoxical exacerbation of psychotic symptoms, catatonic-like states, paranoid reactions, lethargy, and paradoxical excitement.

As with other neuroleptics, chronic treatment with perphenazine may result in tardive dyskinesia.[14] It usually begins insidiously with exaggerated and persistent chewing movements or variations, such as sucking and smacking movements, tongue protrusion, grimacing, and grunting. The cephalic or buccolingual–masticatory part of the syndrome is frequently accompanied by widespread choreiform movements of the neck, shoulders, and arms, and occasionally the legs and trunk. The symptoms are persistent and in many patients they appear to be irreversible. There is no known effective treatment. It is suggested that perphenazine be discontinued if these symptoms appear. Neuroleptic-induced Pisa syndrome, and rabbit syndrome and withdrawal dyskinesia need to be differentiated from tardive dyskinesia.

Autonomic effects. Dry mouth or salivation, nausea, vomiting, gastric retention, diarrhoea, anorexia, constipation, obstipation, faecal impaction, urinary retention, frequency or incontinence, bladder paralysis, polyuria, nasal congestion, pallor, adynamic hypertension, and change in pulse rate may occur. Significant autonomic effects have been infrequent in patients receiving less than 24 mg of perphenazine daily.

Allergic effects. Among the reported effects of this kind are urticaria, erythema, eczema, exfoliative dermatitis (rare), pruritus, photosensitivity, asthma, fever, anaphylactoid reactions and laryngeal oedema. Angioneurotic oedema and contact dermatitis have been reported in nursing personnel administering perphenazines. In extremely rare instances, individual idiosyncrasy or hypersensitivity to perphenazine has resulted in cerebral oedema, circulatory collapse, and death.

Endocrine effects. These include lactation, galactorrhoea, moderate breast enlargement in females and gynaecomastia in males on large doses, disturbances in the menstrual cycle, amenorrhoea, changes in libido, inhibition of ejaculation, hyperglycaemia, hypoglycaemia, glycosuria and the syndrome of inappropriate ADH (antidiuretic hormone) secretion.

Perphenazine

Cardiovascular effects. Postural hypotension, tachycardia (especially with sudden marked increase in dosage), bradycardia, cardiac arrest, faintness, and dizziness may occur. Occasionally the hypotensive effect may produce a shock-like condition. ECG changes, which generally are non-specific (quinidine-like effect) and usually reversible, have been observed in some patients receiving perphenazine.

Haematological effects. Agranulocytosis, eosinophilia, leucopenia, haemolytic anaemia, thrombocytopenic purpura, and pancytopenia have been reported. Most cases of agranulocytosis have occurred between the fourth and tenth weeks of therapy. Patients should be watched closely, especially during that period, for the sudden appearance of sore throat or other signs of infection. If white blood cell counts are definitely depressed and differential cell counts show significant cellular depression of granulocytes, perphenazine administration should be discontinued. However, a slightly lowered white cell count is not in itself an indication to discontinue the drug.

Hepatic effects. Liver damage (biliary stasis) has been reported with perphenazine. Jaundice may occur, usually between the second and fourth weeks of treatment, and is regarded as a hypersensitivity reaction. The incidence is low. The clinical picture resembles infectious hepatitis but with laboratory features of obstructive jaundice. It is usually reversible; however, chronic jaundice has been encountered.

Miscellaneous effects. Pigmentation of the skin may occur during long-term therapy, chiefly in the exposed areas. Ocular changes consisting of deposition of fine particulate matter in the cornea and lens, progressing in more severe cases to star-shaped lenticular opacities, epithelial keratopathies, and retinal changes (rare) have been observed.

Also recorded are peripheral oedema, reversed adrenaline effect, parotid swelling (rare), hyperpyrexia, systemic lupus erythematosus-like syndrome, increases in appetite and weight, polyphagia, photophobia, and muscle weakness.

Other effects

Perphenazine may cause elevated serum protein-bound iodine levels.

Interference with clinical pathology tests

Urinary metabolites of perphenazine may cause urine to darken, resulting in false-positive tests for urobilinogen, amylase, uroporphyrins, porphobilinogens, and 5-hydroxy-indoleacetic acid.

Since phenothiazines may cause a decrease in the secretion of adrenocorticosteroids as a result of diminished release of corticotropin, perphenazine may interfere with metyrapone testing of the hypothalamic–pituitary complex.

Depending on the urine pregnancy test being used, false-positive or false-negative results may be reported.

High risk groups

Neonates

The fetus and the infant have diminished capacities to metabolize and excrete perphenazine.[15] In newborn infants of mothers treated with perphenazine during pregnancy, extrapyramidal reactions, including agitation, hypertonicity, opisthotonus, tremors, hyperreflexia, and bizarre motor activity have been reported. In occasional cases the movement disorders persisted for 3–12 months.

Breast milk. Perphenazine is secreted in mother's milk. Because of this, it can induce a mild degree of sedation, followed by motor excitement in the newborn. Furthermore, since even small doses of perphenazine may adversely affect the immature brain, women treated with perphenazine should not breast-feed.

Children

Perphenazine preparations are not recommended for children under 12 years of age.

Pregnant women

Early in pregnancy, fetal development may be impaired by toxic agents. For this reason, some clinicians believe that perphenazine should not be prescribed during the first trimester. However, perphenazine has no known teratogenicity, and therefore, if the risk that the psychosis will relapse seems high, continuation of the medication is not contraindicated and may even be advisable.

The elderly

The elderly, like infants, have diminished capacity to metabolize and excrete perphenazine. Because of this the dose requirements of perphenazine are lower.[16]

Perphenazine

Drug interactions

Potentially hazardous interactions

Guanethidine. Perphenazine may antagonize the antihypertensive effect of guanethidine and its congeners by blocking uptake at the site of action. Although this interaction may not be as great with perphenazine as with some other phenothiazines, if guanethidine antagonism is noted, the dose of guanethidine needs to be increased, or guanethidine needs to be substituted by another antihypertensive drug used in its place.

Clonidine. Like guanethidine, the effect of clonidine on blood pressure may be partially inhibited.

Pethidine. The respiratory depressant effects of pethidine and possibly also of other opioid analgesics is increased when perphenazine is added to the treatment regime.

Phenytoin. Inhibition of phenytoin metabolism can occur, if perphenazine is added to the treatment regime, resulting in increased plasma levels of phenytoin.

Alcohol. The use of alcohol should be avoided, since it may potentiate drug effects including hypotension. The risk of suicide and the danger of overdose may be increased in patients who use alcohol excessively, because of the potentiation of the drug's effects by alcohol.

Other significant interactions

Anaesthetics. Perphenazine may potentiate the central nervous system depressant effects of anaesthetics.

Barbiturates. Administration of single doses of barbiturates may potentiate the sedative effects of perphenazine. On the other hand, prolonged barbiturate administration decreases the serum level and consequently the therapeutic effects of perphenazine. Because the induction of drug-metabolizing enzymes can enhance the metabolism of perphenazine, the dosage of the drug may require adjustment.

Anticonvulsants. Perphenazine can lower the seizure threshold in susceptible individuals and so the dosage of the anticonvulsant may need to be increased, if perphenazine is added to the treatment regime.

Atropine. Perphenazine may potentiate the anticholinergic effects of atropine. The same applies to tricyclic antidepressants and antihistamines. Potentiation of the anticholinergic effects of organophosphorus insecticides can occur in patients receiving perphenazine.

Methyldopa. Concurrent use of perphenazine and methyldopa may result in additive hypotensive effects. The same applies to the concurrent administration of β-adrenergic receptor blocking drugs and perphenazine.

Levodopa. Concurrent use of levodopa with perphenazine may result in lessened antiparkinsonian response due to dopamine receptor blockade.

Antacids. Concomitant ingestion of perphenazine and antacids (also coffee, tea, cola beverages, and pectinates) may result in decreased absorption of perphenazine and a lessened therapeutic response.

Cigarette smoking. Cigarette smoking accelerates the metabolism of perphenazine by liver microsomal enzyme induction.

Potentially useful interactions

The use of perphenazine to treat amphetamine-like drug poisoning is based on pharmacologic evidence of antagonistic action.

Clinical trials

Pharmacokinetic studies

a. Hansen C E, Christensen T R, Elley J, Hansen L B, Kragh-Sorensen P 1976 Clinical pharmacokinetic studies of perphenazine. British Journal of Clinical Pharmacology 3: 915–923
b. Hansen L B, Larsen N E, Gulmann N 1983 Dose–response relationships of perphenazine in the treatment of acute psychoses. Psychopharmacology 78: 112–115
c. Hansen L B, Larsen N E, Vestergard P 1981 Plasma levels of perphenazine (Trilafon) related to development of extrapyramidal side effects. Psychopharmacology 74: 306–309

Therapeutic

a. Adelson D, Epstein L J 1962 A study of phenothiazines with male and female chronically ill schizophrenic patients. Journal of Nervous and Mental Disease 134: 543–554
b. Casey J F, Lasky J J, Klett C F, Hollister L E 1960 Treatment of schizophrenic reactions with phenothiazine derivatives: a comparative study of chlorpromazine, triflupromazine, mepazine, prochloperazine, perphenazine and phenobarbital. American Journal of Psychiatry 117: 97–105
c. Hanlon T E, Michaux M H, Ota K Y, Shaffer J W, Kurland A A 1965 The comparative effectiveness of eight phenothiazines. Psychopharmacologie (Berlin) 7: 89–106
d. Kurland A A, Hanlon T E, Tatom M H, Ota K Y, Simopoulos A M 1961 The comparative effectiveness of six phenothiazine compounds, phenobarbital and inert placebo in the treatment of acutely ill patients: global measures of severity of illness. Journal of Nervous and Mental Disease 133: 1–18

Depot treatment

a. Knudsen P, Hansen L, Larsen N E 1985 Perphenazine decanoate in sesame oil vs. perphenazine enanthate in sesame oil. Acta Psychologica (suppl 72) (No. 322): 11–14
b. Knudsen P, Hansen L B, Auken G, Waehrens J, Hojholdt K, Larsen N E 1984 Perphenazine decanoate vs. perphenazine enanthate: efficacy and side effects in a 6 week double-blind, comparative study of 50 drug monitored psychotic patients. Acta Psychologica (suppl 72) (322): 5–28
c. Knudsen P, Hansen L K, Hojhold K, Larsen N-E 1985 Long-term depot neuroleptic treatment with perphenazine decanoate I. Efficacy and side effects in a 12 month study of 42 drug monitored psychotic patients. Acta Psychologica (suppl 72) (No. 322): 29–40
d. Knudsen P, Hansen L B, Hojholdt K, Larsen N-E 1985 Long-term depot neuroleptic treatment with perphenazine decanoate II. Different depot intervals in the last 6 months of a 12 month study of 42 drug monitored psychotic patients. Acta Psychologica (suppl 72) (No. 322): 41–50

References

1. The Merck Index of Chemicals and Drugs 1960 Merck & Co Inc, Rahway
2. Hollister L E 1977 Antipsychotic medications and the treatment of schizophrenia. In: Barchas J D, Berger P A, Ciaranello R D, Elliott G R (eds) Psychopharmacology. From theory to practice. Oxford University Press, New York
3. Breyer V, Muller-Oerlinghausen B, Mauruschot W 1977 Phenothiazines with piperazine side chains. In: Usdin E, Forrest I S (eds) Psychotherapeutic drugs. Part II. Application. Marcel Dekker, New York
4. Beall J R 1972 A teratogenic study of chlorpromazine, orphenadrine, perphenazine and LSD_{25} in rats. Toxicology and Applied Pharmacology 21: 20–236
5. Beall J R 1973 A teratogenic study of four psychoactive drugs in rats. Teratology 8: 214–215
6. Elkayam U, Frishman W 1980 Cardiovascular effects of phenothiazines. American Heart Journal 100: 397–401
7. Ayd F J 1964 Perphenazine: a reappraisal after eight years. Diseases of the Nervous System 25: 311–317
8. Larsen M-E, Naestoft J 1973 Determination of perphenazine and fluphenazine in whole blood by gas chromatography. Medical Laboratory Technology 30: 129–132
9. Physicians Desk Reference 1986 PDR 40 Edition 1986 Medical Economics Co, Oradell, pp 1655–1657
10. Ban T A, Hollender M 1981 Psychopharmacology for everyday practice. Karger, Basel, p 49
11. Strayhorn J M, Nash J L 1978 Frightening dreams and dosage schedule of tricyclic and neuroleptic drugs. Journal of Nervous and Mental Disease 166: 878–880
12. Davis J M, Garver D L 1978 Neuroleptics: clinical use in psychiatry. In: Iversen L L, Iversen S D, Snyder S H (eds) Handbook of Psychopharmacology, vol 10. Plenum Press, New York
13. Caroff S N 1980 The neuroleptic malignant syndrome. Journal of Clinical Psychiatry 41: 79–83
14. Mallya A, Jose C, Baig M, Williams R, Cho D, Mehta D, Volavka J 1979 Antiparkinsonics, neuroleptics and tardive dyskinesia. Biological Psychiatry 14: 645–649
15. Green M, Zelson C 1976 The effect of psychotherapeutic drugs on the neonate. In: Usdin I, Forrest I S (eds) Psychotherapeutic drugs. Part I. Marcel and Dekker, New York
16. Fann W E 1976 Effects of psychotherapeutic drugs on geriatric patients. In: Usdin E, Forrest I S (eds) Psychotherapeutic drugs. Part I. Marcel Dekker Inc, New York
17. Cahn C H, Lehmann H E 1957 Perphenazine: observations on the clinical effects of a new tranquilizing agent in psychotic conditions. Canadian Psychiatric Association Journal 2: 104–112
18. Ayd F J 1964 Perphenazine: a reappraisal after eight years. Diseases of the Nervous System 25: 311–317
19. Larsen N-E, Naestoft J 1975 Determination of perphenazine and its sulphoxide metabolite in human plasma after therapeutic dose by gas chromatography. Journal of Chromatography 109: 259–264

20. Eklund K L 1972 Perphenazine enanthate and perphenazine tablets. A double-blind comparison in schizophrenic psychoses. Nordisk Psykiatr Tidsskr. 26: 474–482
21. Larsson M, Axelsoon R, Forswan A 1984 On the pharmacokinetics of perphenazine: a clinical study of perphenazine enanthate and decanoate. Current Therapeutic Research 36: 1071–1088

Pethidine (hydrochloride)

Pethidine, introduced by Eisleb and Schaumann in 1939,[1] was the first synthetic narcotic analgesic drug to achieve wide therapeutic use.

Chemistry

Pethidine (Meperidine, pethidine hydrochloride Centralgin, Demer-Idine, Demerol, Dolantin, Dolosal, Pethidine Roche, Pethoid)
$C_{15}H_{21}NO_2.HCl$
Ethyl 1-methyl-4-phenylpiperine-4-carboxylate hydrochloride

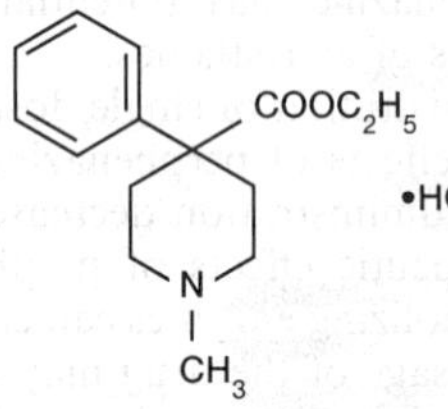

Molecular weight (free base)	283.8 (247.3)
pKa	8.6
Solubility	
in alcohol	1 in 20
in water	>1 in 2
Octanol/water partition coefficient	40 (pethidine)

A white colourless crystalline powder, with a slightly acid bitter taste. It is prepared by chemical synthesis via the reaction of dichlorodiethylmethylamine with benzylcyanide or from isonicotinic acid methochloride. Pethidine hydrochloride is also available as an injection product with an antihistamine, promethazine hydrochloride (Pamergan P100), with promethazine hydrochloride and atropine sulphate (Pamergan AP100/25) and with a narcotic antagonist, levallorphan tartrate (Pethilorfan).

Pharmacology

Pethidine, a narcotic agonist, exerts its chief pharmacological actions on the central nervous system (CNS). It binds onto the anionic site and the P-site of the opiate receptor which is conceptualized as consisting of three elementary binding sites:[5,6] The t-site which binds hydroxylated rings (as in morphine or the tyrosine residue in enkephalin), the anionic site which interacts with the piperidine nitrogen and the P-site which binds preferably non-hydroxylated aromatic rings (as in pethidine or the phenylalanine in enkephalin). Based on binding studies of opioid analgesics pethidine, like most commonly used opioids, has high affinity and high efficacy for μ-receptors and moderate affinity but high efficacy for κ-receptors. Therapeutic doses of pethidine (50–100 mg, parenterally) produce analgesia, sedation, euphoria/dysphoria, respiratory depression and other diverse CNS effects such as abolishing the corneal reflex, causing pupil constriction and inducing CNS excitation which is characterized by tremors, muscle twitches, and seizures. It possesses atropine-like activity and has a spasmogenic effect on certain smooth muscles. Pethidine causes a release of ADH and stimulates the chemoreceptor trigger zone, thereby causing nausea and vomiting. It inhibits release of ACTH and gonadotrophic hormones and also produces a rise in blood sugar.

Toxicology

The estimated minimal lethal dose in man is 1 g; a fatality has been reported following the ingestion of 1.2 g but recovery has occurred after the ingestion of 2 g. Pethidine possesses a marked addiction-producing property; doses as large as 3 or 4 g daily may be taken by addicts. There is no available information on the carcinogenic and teratological effects in animal species or in the human.

Clinical pharmacology

Pethidine is a strong narcotic agonist[2] which is widely used as a strong analgesic and as a premedicament prior to anaesthesia.[3,4] Traditionally, pethidine has been used as an analgesic for the relief of most types of moderate to severe pain including postoperative pain and the pain of labour (60 to 100 mg intramuscularly or orally, repeated every 3 to 4 h; up to 150 mg for severe pain). It is also used for preoperative medication (50 to 100 mg subcutaneously or intramuscularly). The analgesic effects of pethidine are detectable about 15 min after oral administration, reach a peak in about an hour and subside gradually over several hours (2–4 h). After intramuscular or subcutaneous administration the onset of analgesic effect is faster (10 min). Peak respiratory depression, which can be antagonized by naloxone or other related antagonists, is observed within 1 h after intramuscular administration of pethidine.

The most significant cardiovascular effects of pethidine, after intravenous injection during anaesthesia, are the decreases in cardiac output and rise in central venous pressure and there is no significant change in heart rate.[7]

Pethidine has a spasmolytic effect on certain smooth muscles. The order of spasmolytic potency, evaluated using noradrenaline-contracted pelvic strips from hydronephrotic patients, was found to be fentanyl > pethidine = papaverine > pentazocine = naloxone. Norpethidine, the only metabolite of pethidine found in the plasma, had the same relaxing potency as pethidine.[8] Clinically, pethidine does not cause as much constipation when given over a prolonged period of time as other opiates; it has, therefore, no value in the treatment of diarrhoea. After equianalgesic doses pethidine induces less spasm in the biliary tract and less rise in pressure in the common bile duct than morphine.

In the non-pregnant uterus pethidine causes mild stimulation. In later pregnancy pethidine does not alter the activity of the normally contracting uterus but increases tone, frequency and intensity of contractions in a uterus made hyperactive after the administration of oxytocics. In labour a therapeutic dose of pethidine has little effect, nor does it alter the post-partum contractions or involution of the uterus. It does not increase the incidence of post-partum haemorrhage.[9]

Pharmacokinetics

The preferred analytical method is gas–liquid chromatography with nitrogen-selective detection which can simultaneously measure pethidine and norpethidine in the same biological sample.[10] The limit of detection is 5 µg.l^{-1} for pethidine and 2.5 µg.l^{-1} for norpethidine, respectively.

Pethidine is readily absorbed after oral administration and peak plasma concentrations are observed between 1 and 2 hours. The systemic bioavailability is about 0.52 ranging between 0.47 and 0.61.[11,12] Systemic bioavailability of oral pethidine is increased in subjects with hepatic dysfunction.[13,14] Variable absorption has been observed following intramuscular administration into gluteal muscle.[11,15,16] 80% or more of a 100 mg dose of intramuscular pethidine is absorbed, with a mean time to maximum plasma concentration of approximately 24 min. Marked variations in plasma concentration of pethidine amongst different patients are observed and the duration of action is in the order of 2–4 h after intramuscular administration. In contrast, the intramuscular administration of pethidine (25 mg) into deltoid muscles of healthy volunteers resulted in complete and rapid absorption of the drug.[17] Thus, the site of injection, muscle blood flow, type of subjects and dose may influence the intramuscular absorption of pethidine.

A comparison of plasma concentration–time curves and pharmacokinetic parameters of pethidine after intravenous, intramuscular and oral administration of 26 mg.m^{-2} doses to 6 healthy volunteers showed that there was no significant difference between the curves after intramuscular and intravenous routes, and that after 2 h all 3 curves were the same.[18] The elimination $t_{\frac{1}{2}}$ were, respectively, 3.93 ± 0.33, 3.25 ± 0.71 and 3.49 ± 0.37 h after intravenous, intramuscular and oral administration. In this study blood sampling was stopped at 8 h and a biexponential elimination of pethidine was assumed. Pethidine kinetics and analgesia were studied in women in labour after intravenous, intramuscular and epidural administration.[19] Absorption of pethidine from the epidural space in pregnant women was found to be rapid and excepting the lower initial values, the average plasma concentration and area under the plasma concentration–time curve did not differ significantly from those obtained with intravenous dosage, but were significantly higher during the first 2 h after dosage than the results after intramuscular administration. The analgesia provided by the epidural route was greater than with intravenous or intramuscular administration.

Pethidine is rapidly and extensively distributed extravascularly into rapidly perfused tissues[11] with an apparent volume of distribution (V)[20] of 4.17 l.kg^{-1} following a single intravenous dose of pethidine in healthy subjects. The V is significantly reduced in women in labour (to 2.66 l.kg^{-1}) and surgical patients (2.61 l.kg^{-1}) when compared to healthy subjects, but it is increased in heavy drinkers.[21]

Using carefully controlled conditions (pH 7.4 at 37°C) the in vitro binding of pethidine to whole blood and plasma was studied.[22,23] In contrast to previously reported high values[11] the percentage of binding of pethidine in blood is around 30 to 40% and that in plasma 40 to 50%. Nation[24] investigated the determinants of pethidine binding using plasma obtained from 9 women in childbirth and their infants. The binding ratio (bound concentration to free concentration) was found to correlate strongly with α_1-acid glycoprotein concentrations. It was also observed that pethidine free fraction decreases from 0.26 at the time of surgery in surgical patients to 0.18, 3 to 5 days postoperatively.[25] α_1-Acid glycoprotein concentrations are known to be significantly elevated following infection, surgery or severe trauma. However, because of the large volume of distribution of pethidine, displacement of pethidine from plasma proteins is not likely to cause significant increase in the free pethidine concentration.

The plasma and CSF concentrations of pethidine and norpethidine in 20 patients were measured after a standard intramuscular dose of 100 mg of pethidine hydrochloride.[26] The pethidine concentration ratio of CSF/plasma was relatively stable at 0.4 to 0.5 and the drug appeared in the CSF within less than 18 min reaching a maximum after about 90 min. Norpethidine appeared in the CSF rather slowly and erratically and after 240 min the CSF/plasma ratio was similar for pethidine and its metabolite norpethidine. There is little evidence for a functionally significant blood–brain barrier for pethidine and norpethidine.

In 25 children receiving pethidine 1 mg.kg^{-1} intravenously, intramuscularly or rectally following surgery,[27] peak plasma concentrations and time to peak were, respectively: 2800 ± 462, 1609 ± 367, 531 ± 179 nmol.l^{-1} and 5 ± 1, 10 ± 2 and 60 ± 10 minutes. Area under the curve (0–240 min) was similarly reduced following rectal administration. Rectal bioavailability was 40%, with considerable interindividual variation.

The peridural administration of pethidine to 16 cancer patients with postoperative and intractable pain produced analgesia which paralleled the rise in CSF pethidine concentrations.[28] Systemic absorption of peridurally administered pethidine produced blood concentrations high enough to contribute to analgesia after approximately 20 min in the majority of patients.

The primary route of pethidine elimination is via hepatic biotransformation. Most of the dose is excreted in urine. The excretion of unchanged pethidine and its metabolite, norpethidine, in urine is pH-dependent.[17,29,30] Pethidine disposition was studied in 10 Caucasian healthy subjects under uncontrolled and controlled (acidic and alkaline) urinary pH.[30] It was observed that large variations in the 48 h recovery of pethidine and norpethidine (26.9 ± 5.9% and 23.4 ± 4.6%, 0.6 ± 0.3% and 3.6 ± 1.6%, 6.9 ± 3.2% and 17.6 ± 6.6%, respectively under acidic, alkaline and uncontrolled urinary pH) were induced by change in urinary pH, but the terminal half life (7–8 h), the area under the plasma concentration–time curves (AUC) and the plasma concentration–time curve profiles were not affected. Under all urinary conditions the elimination of pethidine from the plasma was best described by a triexponential function.[17,31]

Pethidine (hydrochloride)

Increased bioavailability and decreased clearance in cirrhotic patients were observed[13]: blood clearance was 573 ml min^{-1} (normally 850 ml.min^{-1}) in 8 patients with biopsy-proven cirrhosis and absolute bioavailability was 0.87 in the cirrhotics and 0.48 in 4 healthy volunteers. The AUC was 3 times greater in the cirrhotics after oral pethidine. Similar results of two other studies[14,32] reported clearance being reduced to 390 ml.min^{-1} and bioavailability increased to 0.83 in cirrhosis. Norpethidine elimination may also be impaired in patients with cirrhosis as norpethidine persisted much longer in the serum of patients with cirrhosis than in healthy volunteers after a single dose of pethidine.[32]

In patients with renal failure the plasma norpethidine to pethidine ratios were higher than control (cancer) patients with normal renal function. The half life of norpethidine was 14 and 21 h in 2 patients with normal renal function and 35 h in 1 patient with impaired renal function.[33] The average plasma concentration versus time profile was significantly higher in 18 patients with renal dysfunction than that of 10 healthy volunteers.[34] The AUC (1660 ± 216 ng.ml^{-1}.h^{-1}) and half life (18.6 ± 3.3 h) were significantly higher in the renal patients than the respective values (533 ± 104 ng.ml^{-1}.h^{-1}, 9.9 ± 3.2 h) in volunteer subjects. These results suggest that the elimination of pethidine and norpethidine is considerably modified in patients with renal disease and probably both renal elimination and hepatic metabolism of pethidine in these patients are impaired. The elimination of pethidine is impaired in the elderly.

No significant differences were noted in the elimination half life, renal clearance, total plasma clearance or protein binding of pethidine in Caucasian, Chinese and Indian subjects following an intravenous dose of 150 μg.kg^{-1}. However, differences in mean recovery (% dose) between the groups suggested a possible interethnic variation in oxidative demethylation of pethidine.[35]

Pethidine is excreted in breast milk although the significance of this has yet to be determined. The drug also crosses the placenta together with norpethidine. Both compounds are only slowly eliminated in the neonate.

Oral absorption	100%
Presystemic metabolism	47–61%
Plasma half life	
range	3–8 h
mean	5 h
Volume of distribution	4.2 l.kg^{-1}
Plasma protein binding	40–50%

Concentration–effect relationship

Studies in patients following abdominal surgery suggest that blood pethidine concentrations of 0.5 to 0.7 mg.l^{-1} are required for analgesia.[16,36] The concentration–analgesic response relationship for pethidine is extremely steep, with concentration differences as small as 0.05 mg.l^{-1} representing the difference between no anal-gesia and complete suppression of pain. Dosage regimens of pethidine which produce variable or fluctuating blood concentrations can be expected to achieve inconsistent relief of pain. It is suggested that the use of continuous intravenous infusions of pethidine appears to be a rational new approach to acute pain management.[25,37] For postoperative pain relief, Stapleton et al[36] designed an intravenous infusion regimen for pethidine which comprised a loading infusion followed by a standardized constant infusion of 24 mg.h^{-1}. This regimen fails to take into account the individual differences in drug kinetics and pain tolerance. Tamen and co-workers[37] used a PACAT (patient-controlled analgesic therapy) model in 20 patients, who received self-administered small intravenous doses of pethidine to relieve pain after major abdominal surgery by means of a programmable drug injector, and showed that the average pethidine consumption was 26 ± 10 mg.h^{-1} (12 to 50 mg.h^{-1}) with average plasma concentrations being 551 ± 182 μg.l^{-1} (132 to 896 μg.l^{-1}). Of the 20 patients 19 obtained subjectively satisfactory analgesia.

Metabolism

Pethidine is extensively metabolized in the liver, primarily by hydrolysis and N-demethylation (see Fig. 1). The drug and its metabol-

Fig. 1 The metabolism of pethidine

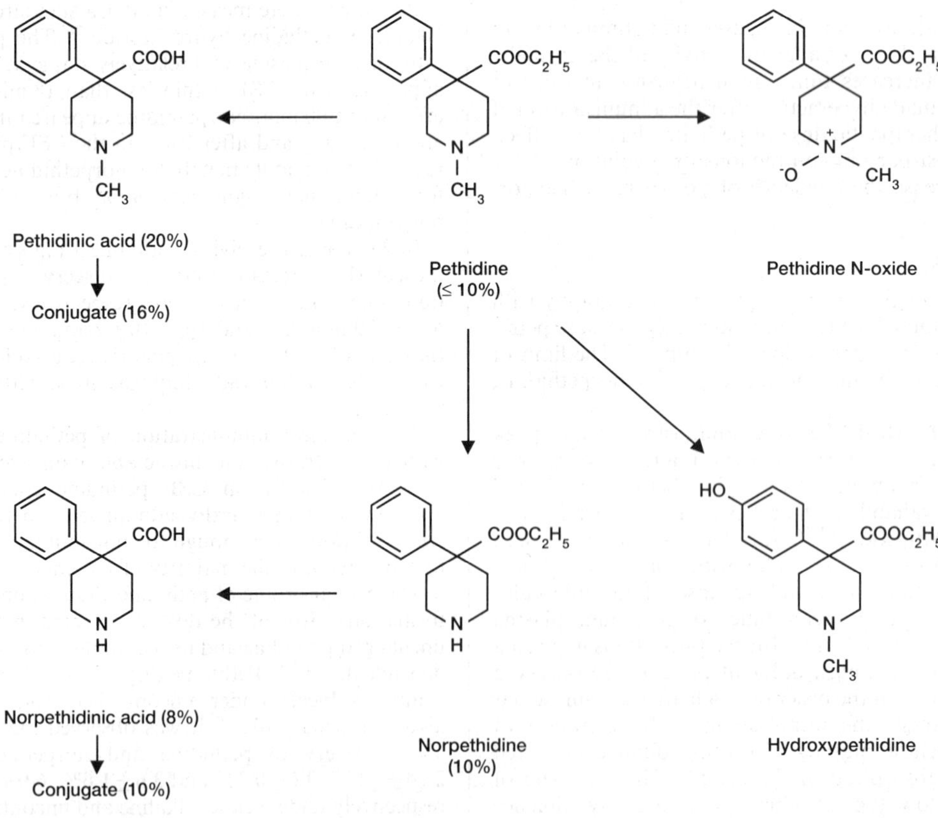

Biotransformations N-Demethylation, hydrolysis (major routes)
N-Oxidation, aromatic hydroxylation (minor routes)
(% in urine in 24 h)

Pethidine (hydrochloride)

ites are largely excreted in the urine. The amount of the dose excreted unchanged varies with urine pH, from 0.6 to 27%. The recovery of metabolites is also influenced by the urinary pH.[30] Major metabolites include pethidinic acid and its conjugates, norpethidine, norpethidinic acid and its conjugates. Minor metabolites isolated are pethidine N-oxide, the aromatic hydroxylated product (4-hydroxypethidine), the N-oxidation product of norpethidine (N-hydroxynorpethidine) and a phenyl hydroxy derivative. Norpethidine is estimated to possess half the analgesic potency of pethidine but is twice as potent as a convulsive compared to the parent drug. The other metabolites are considered to be inactive. The metabolism of pethidine is significantly reduced in the neonate when compared to the adult.[38]

Pharmaceutics

Pethidine hydrochloride is available in oral and parenteral forms: tablets contain 25 mg and 50 mg of pethidine hydrochloride BP. Pethidine Roche tablets are white, round and biconvex. Demerol tablets (Winthrop, USA) are deep pink, round and marked '31/D'. Pethidine injection is available for intravenous use as a clear solution containing pethidine hydrochloride BP 50 mg per ml. Other proprietary preparations include: Demerol syrup (Winthrop, USA), an alcohol-free, banana-flavoured syrup containing 50 mg pethidine per 5 ml; Pamergan P100 (Rhone Poulenc, UK) injection which contains 50 mg of pethidine hydrochloride and 25 mg promethazine hydrochloride per ml in a 2 ml ampoule; Pethilorfan (Roche, UK) injection which contains 50 mg of pethidine hydrochloride and 625 μg per ml of levallorphan tartrate in 1 ml or 2 ml ampoules.

Solutions are adjusted to pH 3.5 to 6.0 with sodium hydroxide or hydrochloric acid.

Most tablets and injectable forms should be stored below 25°C and protected from light. Shelf-life, in general, is 3 years. There are no physicochemical incompatibilities reported in the literature, but it would be wise to avoid mixture with high pH solutions such as sodium bicarbonate or phenytoin (diphenylhydantoin) injections.

Therapeutic use

Indications

1. Relief of severe pain (medical and surgical)
2. Pre-anaesthetic medication
3. Obstetrical analgesia.

Contraindications

1. Respiratory depression
2. Raised intracranial pressure
3. Acute bronchial asthma
4. Supraventricular tachycardias
5. Phaeochromocytoma
6. Convulsive states such as status epilepticus, tetanus and strychnine poisoning
7. Concurrent use of MAOIs, or use of MAOIs within previous 2 weeks
8. Acute alcoholism or delirium tremens
9. Diabetic acidosis where there is a danger of coma
10. Hypersensitivity to pethidine
11. Severe liver disease
12. Hypothyroidism, Addison's disease.

Mode of use

The clinical uses of pethidine for analgesia depend mainly on its action on the opiate receptors in the CNS. To relieve severe pain 25–150 mg intramuscularly 3 to 4 hourly or 25–50 mg slowly intravenously 3 to 4 hourly (up to 200 mg per day) may be used. A narcotic antagonist (e.g. naloxone) and facilities for administration of oxygen and control of respiration should be available at once during and immediately following intravenous administration of all narcotic analgesics. In obstetrics 50–100 mg intramuscularly or subcutaneously, repeated 3 to 4 times at 1 to 3 hourly intervals if necessary, but not more than 4 doses in 24 h, is suggested. In children the recommended dose is 1–2 $mg.kg^{-1}$ intramuscularly or 1 $mg.kg^{-1}$ by slow intravenous injection 4 hourly. Safety has not been established for use of pethidine in neonates; excretion and metabolism in the neonate is reduced compared with adults. Recent studies[16,36] observed that the use of continuous intravenous infusions of pethidine appears to be a rational new approach to acute pain management.

Indications

Pethidine hydrochloride is mainly used as an analgesic. Unlike morphine, it has little effect on cough or on diarrhoea.

1. Relief of pain
Pethidine can be used for the relief of most types of moderate to severe pain including postoperative pain and the pain of labour. It also has local anaesthetic and slight atropine-like actions. A dose of 60 to 100 mg of pethidine is approximately equivalent to 10 mg of morphine while the analgesic effect of pethidine is shorter and usually lasts for 2 to 4 hours after a single dose. For the relief of pain pethidine is given in a dose of 50 to 100 mg orally or by intramuscular injection which may be repeated 3 or 4 hourly. Up to 150 mg may be required for severe pain. It is suggested that for adequate pain relief, when a 4-hourly regimen is adopted, the first and last doses are linked to patient's waking and bedtimes. The best additional times during the day are usually 10 am, 2 pm and 6 pm unless the patient wakes exceptionally late.

2. Pre-anaesthetic medication
The usual dose for preoperative medication is 50 to 100 mg by subcutaneous or intramuscular injection with 0.3 mg atropine. In children, doses of 1 to 1.5 $mg.kg^{-1}$ (5–6 years, 25 mg; 7–11 years, 50 mg; 12 years and over, 75 mg) may be given orally or by intramuscular or subcutaneous injection. Pethidine 1 $mg.kg^{-1}$, diazepam 250 $\mu g.kg^{-1}$ and flunitrazepam 20 $\mu g.kg^{-1}$ intramuscularly were compared as premedicants in a double-blind study of 145 children (aged 0 to 15 years) who were undergoing otolaryngological surgery. All drugs demonstrated antianxiety effects in children 5 years and older, but diazepam was less effective in children under 5 years.[39] Pethidine has also been used in conjunction with chlorpromazine or promethazine to produce special types of basal narcosis known as 'potentiated anaesthesia' and 'artificial hibernation'.

3. Obstetrical analgesia
Pethidine is commonly used for analgesia during labour,[38] often in multiples of 50 mg by intramuscular or subcutaneous injection as soon as contractions occur at regular intervals. This dose may be repeated after 1 to 3 hours if required. Pethidine does not diminish the force of uterine contraction but it may prolong labour and cross the placenta causing neonatal depression including respiratory depression.[41] A narcotic antagonist such as naloxone may be required to reverse such depression.

Contraindications

1. Respiratory depression
Larger doses and/or rapid administration of narcotics may produce rapid onset of respiratory depression, bradycardia (as a result of stimulation of medullary vagal nuclei) or even cardiac arrest.

2. Raised intracranial pressure
Pethidine and other narcotics may obscure the diagnosis and/or mask the clinical course of patients with head injuries or acute abdominal conditions and should not be used unless absolutely necessary in these conditions. The respiratory depressant effects of pethidine may be markedly exaggerated in the presence of head injury. Hypercapnia associated with respiratory depression can itself result in elevated intracranial pressure.

3. Acute bronchial asthma
In patients with reduced respiratory reserve such as emphysema, kyphoscoliosis or even severe obesity pethidine should be used with great caution.

4. Cardiac arrhythmias and cardiac infarction
Pethidine should be used with caution if at all in patients with atrial flutter and other supraventricular tachycardias because of a possible vagolytic action which may produce a significant increase in ventricular response rate. Pethidine may cause a transient rise in blood

P

pressure and systemic vascular resistance and increased heart rate; it should not be used for pain relief in cardiac infarction.

5. Phaeochromocytoma
Use of pethidine in such patients may result in a hypertensive crisis.

6. Convulsive disorders
Pethidine may aggravate pre-existing convulsions in patients with convulsive disorders such as status epilepticus, tetanus and strychnine poisoning. If dosage is escalated substantially above recommended levels because of tolerance development, convulsions may occur in individuals without a history of convulsive disorders.

7. Concurrent use of MAOIs
The combination of monoamine oxidase inhibitors, or use of MAOIs within 2 weeks prior, and pethidine has caused hypotension, hypertension, excitation, rigidity, hyperpyrexia and/or convulsions and in some cases fatalities have been reported. However, deliberate administration of moderate doses of pethidine with MAOI has been carried out without problems. The mechanism of the interaction, if there is one, is not clear. However, because of the severity of the reactions reported, this combination should be avoided.

8. Acute alcoholism or delirium tremens

9. Diabetic acidosis where there is a danger of coma

10. Hypersensitivity to pethidine

11. Severe liver disease

12. Hypothyroidism, Addison's disease
Pethidine should be given with caution and the initial dose should be reduced in patients with hypothyroidism or Addison's disease.

Adverse reactions

Potentially life-threatening effects
Respiratory depression, coma, convulsions (due possibly to elevated levels of norpethidine) and hypotension have been reported. Treatment with a narcotic antagonist such as naloxone or nalorphine in cases of respiratory depression or loss of consciousness should be effective. Circulation should be maintained with infusions of plasma or suitable electrolyte solutions. Assisted respiration may be necessary.

Continuous administration of pethidine may produce dependence. In individuals physically dependent on pethidine, the use of narcotic antagonists should be avoided. If a narcotic antagonist must be used to treat serious respiratory depression, the antagonist should be administered with extreme care and only 10 to 20% of the usual initial dose administered otherwise an acute withdrawal syndrome will be precipitated.

Acute overdosage
The estimated minimal lethal dose in man is 1 g; a fatality has been reported following the ingestion of 1.2 g but recovery has occurred after the ingestion of 2 g. Pethidine possesses marked addiction-producing property; doses as large as 3 or 4 g daily may be taken by addicts. Overdosage usually produces CNS depression ranging from stupor to a profound coma, respiratory depression which may progress to Cheyne–Stokes respiration and cyanosis, cold clammy skin and hypothermia, flaccid skeletal muscles, bradycardia and hypotension. In patients with severe overdosage after rapid intravenous administration of a narcotic, apnoea, circulatory collapse, cardiac arrest, respiratory arrest and death may occur. Complications such as pneumonia, shock and pulmonary oedema may also prove fatal. Overdosage of pethidine, unlike that of morphine derivatives, may produce mydriasis rather than miosis. Toxic effects of pethidine may be excitatory, especially in patients who have developed tolerance to the depressant effects of the drug. These patients may exhibit dry mouth, increased muscular activity, muscle tremors and twitches, tachycardia, delirium with disorientation, hallucinations, and, occasionally, grand mal seizures.

Gastric lavage may be effective even many hours after drug ingestion because pylorospasm produced by the narcotic analgesic may cause much of the drug to be retained in the stomach for an extended period of time. A charcoal slurry may be useful to absorb excess pethidine. A saline purgative (e.g. sodium sulphate 30 g in 250 ml water) should be given to help peristalsis. In most cases of overdose, both parenteral and oral, the circulation should be maintained with infusions of plasma or suitable electrolyte solution and assisted respiration may be required.

If consciousness is impaired and respiration depressed naloxone, a pure antagonist, should be administered; naloxone (e.g. 0.4 mg), repeated at 2 to 3 min intervals if required, may be administered intravenously. For children the initial recommended dose is $0.01\ mg.kg^{-1}$; in neonates, a more rapid and improved antagonism was noted after $0.02\ mg.kg^{-1}$ intravenous naloxone.[42] A response should be apparent after 2 or 3 doses. The duration of action of naloxone is usually shorter than that of pethidine and thus the patient should be carefully observed for signs of CNS depression returning. Acidification of the urine will enhance excretion of the unchanged pethidine in the circulation.[31]

Severe or irreversible adverse effects
The parenteral route was found superior to oral administration of pethidine for pain relief but was associated with a higher incidence of serious adverse reactions in 3634 hospitalized patients. The frequency of adverse reactions increased as the unit dose, average daily dose and total dose increased. Adverse reactions were reported in 4.3% of the 366 oral recipients and 3.1% of the 3268 parenteral recipients.[43]

After oral administration gastrointestinal disturbances were the most commonly reported adverse reaction in patients including nausea and vomiting (2.0%), constipation (0.5%), neuropsychiatric disturbance (0.5%), drowsiness and malaise (0.8%) and coma (0.3%).

Among patients given the drug parenterally CNS adverse effects were the most frequent: neuropsychiatric effects (0.4%) which included disorientation, bizarre feelings, hallucinations and psychosis. Drowsiness and malaise were also observed (0.2%).

Cardiovascular effects such as hypotension (0.3% after parenteral route), tachycardia (0.03% after parenteral route) vasodilation and hypertension have been reported.[44] Inadvertent intra-arterial administration can produce severe necrosis and gangrene.[45]

CNS effects such as vertigo (0.09% after parenteral route), dizziness and coma (0.3% after oral route and 0.09% after parenteral route), headache (0.09% after parenteral route), convulsions and tremor (0.09% after parenteral route) have been observed.[46] Respiratory depression was reported in 0.09% of patients after parenteral administration.[47]

Psychiatric effects including hyperactivity or agitation (0.06% after parenteral route), depression (0.03% after parenteral route), mental clouding and dysphoria were observed.[43]

Symptomatic adverse effects
Dermatological reactions such as rash, pruritus or hives (0.09% after parenteral injection), urticaria, erythema, injection site complications such as local irritation and induration, fibrosis of muscle tissue with frequent repetition and abscesses have been reported.[21]

Gastrointestinal effects such as decreased gastric emptying were observed. Other effects such as diaphoresis (0.06% after parenteral route), addiction, dry mouth, weakness and hypersensitivity have been reported.[48]

Other effects
Pethidine elevates the serum levels of amylase and lipase due to spasm of the sphincter of Oddi induced by pethidine.[49] The serum hydroxybutyric acid dehydrogenase activity may also be raised after the administration of pethidine.[50]

Interference with clinical pathology tests
No significant interferences of this kind have been reported.

High risk groups

Pethidine should be used with caution in patients taking other CNS depressant drugs such as hypnotics and sedatives, phenothiazines, tranquillizers and anaesthetics. Patients with severe pain may tolerate very high doses of pethidine but may exhibit respiratory depression if their pain suddenly subsides.

Neonates
Pethidine, while commonly used for pain relief in obstetrics, is known to pass the placenta and may cause neonatal depression. Naloxone, a narcotic antagonist, may be required to reverse such depression. Ratios of about 0.6 to 0.8[51] to 1 or greater[52] are usually observed 120–140 min after dosing. In general, after a dose of 150 mg (intra-

venous or intramuscular) concentrations in cord blood may range from 200 to 600 mg.l^{-1}at 1 to 5 h after dosing and from 100 to 250 μg.ml^{-1} for intervals longer than 5 h. Higher concentrations (600–900 mg.l^{-1}) have been reported for shorter dosing–delivery intervals.[38,53,54] The metabolite, norpethidine, may reach about 50% of pethidine concentrations.[55] Norpethidine concentrations as high as 100 to 200 μg.l^{-1} may be present at birth after administration of pethidine at 1.5 to 3.1 mg kg^{-1} to the mother.[56]

Pethidine in the newborn is eliminated at a significantly slower rate than in the mother; respective half lives for neonate and mother were reported as 22.7 h and 2.8 h.[51] Norpethidine blood concentrations in the newborn appear to increase consistently and steadily over 12–14 h with peak levels of 80–140 μg.ml^{-1} attained 24 to 36 h after birth.[56] Thus, despite a drop in pethidine plasma concentrations in the 12 to 24 h after birth, it is possible that high and sustained levels of norpethidine would contribute to some of the adverse effects at later times.[57] The excretion of pethidine and norpethidine in the newborn is usually very limited in the first 24 h, due to the immaturity of both hepatic and renal function. About 95% of the total pethidine transferred from the mother to the fetus would be eliminated by the neonate by the second to third day following birth.[53] After placental transfer the ratio of norpethidine to pethidine (N/P) is very low during the first 24 h; the amount of norpethidine increases steadily over the next 24 to 48 h with N/P values above one.[53,56]

After multiple dosing of pethidine to the mother maximum exposure of the fetus to both pethidine and norpethidine would result because of a continued diffusion gradient from mother to fetus;[58] and over long time periods maximum accumulation of both pethidine and norpethidine resulted in fetal tissues. With long drug-to-delivery intervals the levels of norpethidine may become clinically important and the elimination of both compounds by the neonate is prolonged.[59] There are neurobehavioural responses associated with very low levels of pethidine in normal healthy infants.[60] However, earlier findings suggest that the newborn infant responds to pethidine in the same way as the adult, but the changes observed were relatively subtle, and comparison of these infants with a control group whose mothers had received no drug revealed no between-group differences in behaviour.[61]

Breast milk. The excretion of pethidine in breast milk was reported[62] and its presence in the milk would further delay the elimination of pethidine in the neonate. However, clinical data on the rate of excretion or concentration of pethidine in breast milk are not available. The significance of this finding is yet to be determined.

Children

In children the dose of pethidine by intramuscular injection for up to 1 year is 1–2 mg.kg^{-1}, 1–5 years 12.5–25 mg and 6–12 years 25–50 mg every four hours. For slow intravenous administration the dose is usually 1 mg.kg^{-1} up to 50 mg. There is very little information available for use in children. However, similar precautions to those for neonates should be given to very young children or older infants when pethidine is used.

Pregnant women

There is no available information on teratological effects in the human. The addiction-producing property of the drug, and most narcotics, will be transmitted to neonates from the addict mother. Other problems relative to pregnancy have been discussed above under neonates.

The elderly

Significantly higher plasma levels of pethidine were observed in elderly patients of over 70 and over 65 respectively after intramuscular administration[15] of 1.5 mg.kg^{-1} and after intravenous doses[63] of 1 mg.kg^{-1} than in those under 30 years old. Plasma protein binding was reduced in the elderly patients when compared with young subjects.[64] However, a subsequent in vitro study found that there was no age-related difference in the distribution of pethidine between erythrocytes and plasma and in the plasma protein binding and a slower elimination rate was proposed to be the most likely explanation of the increased plasma concentration of pethidine in the old patients.[11] A review suggests that the dose of pethidine be reduced to half the normal adult doses in the over 70s[11] but a more recent study comments that no reduction in the dose of pethidine is necessary if it is given as a single intravenous dose, while on repeated therapy it is advisable to reduce the total daily dose.[63]

Concurrent disease

Impaired liver function. Pethidine is extensively metabolized by the liver. It exhibits significant first-pass metabolism.[13] In 10 cirrhotic patients there was a 50% decrease in clearance of pethidine and a 2-fold increase in half life after an intravenous dose of 0.8 mg.kg^{-1} pethidine.[20] The area under the blood concentration–time curve after the oral administration of pethidine was 3.1 times greater in the cirrhotics than in healthy volunteers, reflecting an increased bioavailability and a decreased clearance of pethidine in the cirrhotics.[13] It is suggested[14] that because of the increased bioavailability and half life of pethidine in hepatic dysfunction, when multiple dosing is required for either parenteral or oral administration, the dosing interval should be increased (i.e. doubled) or the dosage reduced (i.e. to 50–75% for oral dosing).

Impaired renal function. Significantly higher plasma concentrations at various time-intervals after intravenous administration of 150 μg.kg^{-1} (one-tenth of the therapeutic dose) were observed in patients with varying degrees of renal dysfunction compared with healthy volunteers under 'normal' urinary pH.[34] After multiple doses of pethidine, patients with renal failure had higher plasma norpethidine to pethidine concentration ratios (1.0 to 3.0) than control groups of patients with neoplastic disease and normal renal function who had ratios of less than one.[33] The accumulation of pethidine metabolites such as norpethidine in renal failure may lead to adverse effects of CNS excitation (irritability, twitching and convulsions). Caution should be exercised when pethidine is administered to patients with renal disease, especially if pethidine is given over prolonged periods of time. There are no data available on the efficacy of dialysis in reducing plasma concentrations of pethidine or its metabolites. The urinary excretion of pethidine and norpethidine may be enhanced by acidification of the urine.[30,31,65]

Drug interactions

Potentially hazardous interactions

Alcohol. In general alcohol potentiates the CNS depressant effect of pethidine.

Monoamine oxidase inhibitors (MAOIs). Pethidine should be avoided in subjects who are receiving or who have recently received MAOIs.[66,67] This combination has resulted in both excitation and depressant effects in the CNS including hypotension, hypertension, agitation, rigidity, hyperpyrexia, hallucinations, unconsciousness, respiratory depression and death in some cases. The onset of these symptoms may occur within minutes of administration of intramuscular pethidine. Several psychopharmacological agents are potent competitive inhibitors of pethidine N-demethylase in rat liver microsomal preparations.[68,69] These include: the MAOIs phenelzine, iproniazid, amphetamine, pargyline and tranylcypromine with phenelzine being an inhibitor of hydrolysis;[66] the neuroleptics chlorpromazine and promazine; and the tricyclic antidepressants amitriptyline, desipramine and imipramine. However, the nature and rapidity of the onset of the symptoms suggest that this interaction in man is not due to inhibition of pethidine metabolism alone.

Chlorpromazine and other phenothiazines. Concomitant administration of chlorpromazine and/or promethazine with pethidine has resulted in profound respiratory depression, respiratory arrest in children and hypotension in both adults and children.[70,71] No significant difference in pethidine clearance was observed in the presence of chlorpromazine, although significantly more norpethidine and norpethidinic acid were recovered in the urine. Excessive lethargy and a larger depression in blood pressure were observed in the 10 healthy subjects when taking both active drugs.[71]

Phenobarbitone and phenytoin. The effects of phenobarbitone and other CNS depressants are, in general, additive. Exaggerated pethidine toxicity in a patient receiving phenobarbitone on a long-term basis was observed.[46] Analysis of pethidine kinetics and metabolites indicated that phenobarbitone enhanced the N-demethylation of pethidine to norpethidine in 12 healthy volunteers.[72] Similarly, norpethidine generation and metabolism of pethidine were increased in volunteers taking phenytoin.[73] These studies suggest that higher dose rates of pethidine may be required in patients taking phenobarbitone and/or phenytoin in order to attain effective blood concentrations of the drug. Although norpethidine is approximately twice as CNS-toxic as pethidine, the clinical relevance of the observed increases in norpethidine formation remains speculative.

Other significant interactions

Inhibition of gastric emptying. The potent inhibitory effect of pethidine on gastric emptying is important since Mendelsohn's syndrome is a leading cause of maternal mortality and because patients in labour are frequently given premedicants by mouth. Pethidine, by causing a decrease in gastric emptying rate, has been found to delay the absorption of paracetamol.[74] It was observed that metoclopramide was ineffective in reversing the delaying of gastric emptying by pethidine.[74] However, it is suggested that in patients requiring general anaesthesia for emergency surgery, whose stomachs may not be empty and who have been given pethidine for preoperative pain relief, it may be a useful adjunct to administer metoclopramide intravenously just before induction of anaesthesia.[75] On the other hand naloxone, a narcotic antagonist, was effective in blocking the similar effects of pentazocine (pethidine was not studied), suggesting that opiate receptors are important in the inhibition of gastric emptying.[76]

Thiopentone. The mixing of thiopentone solution with pethidine in the same solution results in the formation of a pharmacologically inactive complex.[66]

Cimetidine. During cimetidine treatment, pethidine total body clearance decreased by 22% and pethidine volume of distribution at steady state decreased by 13% in 8 healthy male volunteers.[77] A cimetidine-induced reduction in pethidine demethylation to norpethidine was observed. Caution is advised when patients are treated concurrently with these two agents.

Controlled clinical trials

At present up to 15 narcotic analgesics are included in the British National Formulary. Wide differences of opinion and practice exist concerning the choice of potent analgesics for relief of pain and new drugs continue to be introduced. However not many systematically controlled clinical trials have been conducted to evaluate or compare the efficacy of various narcotic analgesics.

1. Morrison J D, Logan W B, Dundee J W 1971 Controlled comparison of the efficacy of fourteen preparations in the relief of post-operation pain. British Medical Journal 3: 287–290

The study reported, which occupied four years, was undertaken to answer the need for the assessment of relative merits of the numerous available potent analgesics. The lack of standardized methodology makes the compiling of an overall assessment difficult.

13 analgesics, four of them at two dose levels, four analgesics in combination with antagonist or neuroleptic agents, and saline have been evaluated simultaneously in the relief of postoperative pain. The method of assessment was designed to favour drugs which provided freedom from pain with minimum depression of consciousness. Only levorphanol 2 mg proved significantly superior to pethidine 100 mg, which was used as the standard reference drug. Oxycodone 10 mg, pentazocine 20 mg, and the morphine 10 mg and cycline 50 mg combination were the most successful of the remaining drugs. None of the drug combinations was significantly better than the analgesic given alone.

2. Taylor I 1971 Clinical trial comparing pentazocine with pethidine and morphine in severe ischaemic limb pain. British Journal of Clinical Practice 25: 27–30

This double-blind trial with predetermined randomization was designed to compare the efficacy of the intramuscular administration of pentazocine 45 mg with morphine 15 mg and pethidine 100 mg in the relief of ischaemic muscle pain in 18 male patients with severe peripheral vascular disease of the lower limb. Both pentazocine and pethidine produced fewer total side effects than morphine. Whereas all patients were able to complete the course of pentazocine injections, the morphine injection needed to be stopped in 4 patients and the pethidine injections in 1 patient because of the severity of side effects (vomiting, nausea and giddiness).

3. Banister E H D A 1974 Six potent analgesic drugs, a double-blind study in post-operative pain. Anaesthesia 29: 158–162

A double-blind study of 6 intramuscular analgesics following non-emergency orthopaedic operation was conducted in 572 adult patients. Pethidine (100 mg), papaveretum (20 mg) and pentazocine (60 mg) were superior to levorphanol (2 mg), phenoperidine (1 mg) and piritramide (15 mg). Side effects were few except that all drugs produced drowsiness with pentazocine producing the highest incidence. The lowest order of drowsiness combined with the highest order of efficacy came from pethidine. One reservation about this study was that if the least effective drugs had been given at higher dosage, they might have produced similar effects to the best drugs.

4. Girvan C B, Moore J, Dundee J W 1976 Pethidine compared with pethidine–naloxone administered during labour: a study of analgesic treatment by a sequential method. British Journal of Anaesthesia 48: 563–569

In a restricted sequential trial in 121 healthy parturient women, the pain relief from pethidine 100 mg and pethidine 100 mg plus naloxone 0.4 mg was compared. Pethidine alone gave better relief. The incidence of minor side effects was higher with both treatments but dizziness was reduced slightly by naloxone. It was concluded that naloxone antagonized the analgesia without abolishing the side effects of pethidine.

5. Chakravarty K, Tucker W, Rosen M, Vickers M D 1979 Comparisons of buprenorphine (a relatively new agonist–antagonist narcotic) and pethidine given intravenously on demand to relieve post-operative pain. British Medical Journal 2: 895–897

In a double-blind study of on-demand intravenous analgesia of 29 patients buprenorphine was found to be about 600 times as potent as pethidine. The incidence of side effects was similar with both drugs. The quality of analgesia, subjectively assessed, was good with both drugs using this method of administration.

6. Slattery P J, Harmer M, Rosen M, Vickers M D 1981 Comparison of meptazinol and pethidine given intravenously on demand in the management of post-operative pain. British Journal of Anaesthesia 53: 927–931

Meptazinol, a relatively new opiate antagonist with analgesic properties, and pethidine were compared under double-blind conditions in 20 patients, using an on-demand analgesic system to provide pain relief after upper abdominal surgery. The degree of analgesia, subjectively assessed, was good with both drugs; although meptazinol produced significantly more nausea than pethidine, there was no statistically significant difference in the frequency of other side effects. Over 24 h average consumption of meptazinol was 2.4 times that of pethidine, suggesting that, when given intravenously, meptazinol is less potent than pethidine.

General review articles

Lasagna L 1964 The clinical evaluation of morphine and its substitutes as analgesics. Pharmacological Review 16: 47–83

Mather L E, Meffin P J 1978 Clinical pharmacokinetics of pethidine. Clinical Pharmacokinetics 3: 352–368

1982 Pethidine. In: Reynolds E F (ed) Martindale: the extra pharmacopoeia, 28th edn. The Pharmaceutical Press, London, pp 1026–1028

Edwards D J, Svensson C K, Visco J P, Lalka D 1982 Clinical pharmacokinetics of pethidine: 1982. Clinical Pharmacokinetics 7: 421–433

References

1. Eisleb O, Schaumann O 1939 Dolantin, ein neurartiges spasmolytikum und Analgetikum (Chemisches und Pharmakologisches). Deutsche Medizinische Wochenschrift 65: 967–968
2. Twycross R G 1984 Analgesics. Postgraduate Medical Journal 60: 876–880
3. Chan K, Edward J A 1978 The use of narcotic analgesics in hospital practice II. A survey on the use in the Mersey Region. Journal of Clinical and Hospital Pharmacy 3: 253–266
4. Chan K 1984 The use of narcotic analgesics in a regional hospital in Hong Kong. British Journal of Clinical Pharmacology 17: 225P
5. Portoghese P S, Alreja B D, Larson D L 1981 Allylprodine analogues as receptor probes. Evidence that phenolic and norphenolic ligands interact with different subsites on identical opioid receptors. Journal of Medicinal Chemistry 24: 782–787
6. Thorpe D H 1984 Opiate structure and activity — a guide to understanding the receptor. Anesthesiology and Analgesia 63: 143–151

Pethidine (hydrochloride)

7. Davies I T 1981 Respiratory and circulatory effects of pentazocine and meperidine on anesthetized patients. Mount Sinai Journal of Medicine 39: 146–157
8. Kinn A C, Boreus L O, Nergårdh A 1982 Effects of narcotic analgesics especially pethidine and norpethidine, on renal pelvic smooth muscle in patients with hydronephrosis. European Journal of Clinical Pharmacology 22: 407–410
9. Jaffe J H, Martin N R 1975 Narcotic analgesics. In: Goodman L S, Gilman A (eds) The pharmacological basis of therapeutics, 5th edn. Macmillan, New York, p 265
10. Tse J, Chan K 1981 The simultaneous determination of pethidine and norpethidine in biofluids by nitrogen selective gas chromatography. Methods and Findings in Experimental and Clinical Pharmacology 3: 99–104
11. Mather L E, Meffin P J 1978 Clinical pharmacokinetics of pethidine. Clinical Pharmacokinetics 3: 352–368
12. Kramer W G 1979 Excretion of meperidine. Journal of Clinical Pharmacology 19: 84
13. Neal E A, Meffin P J, Gregory P B, Blashke T F 1979 Enhanced bioavailability and decreased clearance of analgesics in patients with cirrhosis. Gastroenterology 77: 96–102
14. Pond S M, Tong T, Benowitz N L, Jacob P 1980 Enhanced bioavailability of pethidine and pentazocine in patients with cirrhosis of the liver. Australian and New Zealand Journal of Medicine 19: 515–519
15. Chan K, Kendall M J, Mitchard M, Wells W D E, Vickers M D 1975 The effect of ageing on plasma concentrations of pethidine. British Journal of Clinical Pharmacology 2: 297–302
16. Austin K L, Stapleton J V, Mather L E 1980 Relationship between blood meperidine concentrations and analgesic response: a preliminary report. Anesthesiology 53: 460–466
17. Verbeeck R K, Branch R A, Wilkinson G R 1981 Meperidine disposition in man: influence of urinary pH and route of administration. Clinical Pharmacology and Therapeutics 30: 619–628
18. Stambaugh J E, Wainer I W, Sanstead J K, Hemphill D M 1976 The clinical pharmacology of meperidine — comparison of routes of administration. Journal of Clinical Pharmacology 16: 245–256
19. Husemeyer R P, Cumming A J, Rosankiewicz J R, Davenport H T 1982 A study of pethidine kinetics and analgesia in women in labour following intravenous, intramuscular and epidural administration. British Journal of Clinical Pharmacology 13: 171–176
20. Klotz U, McHorse T S, Wilkinson G R, Schenker S 1974 The effect of cirrhosis on the disposition and elimination of meperidine in man. Clinical Pharmacology and Therapeutics 16: 667–675
21. Jaffe J T, Martin W R 1980 Opioid analgesics and antagonists. In: Goodman L S, Gilman A (eds) The pharmacological basis of therapeutics, 6th edn. Macmillan, New York, pp 513–517
22. La Rosa C, Morgan D J, Mather L E 1984 Pethidine binding in whole blood: methodology and clinical significance. British Journal of Clinical Pharmacology 17: 405–409
23. La Rosa C, Mather L E, Morgan D J 1984 Pethidine binding in plasma: effects of methodological variables. British Journal of Clinical Pharmacology 17: 411–415
24. Nation R L 1981 Meperidine binding in maternal and fetal plasma. Clinical Pharmacology and Therapeutics 29: 472–479
25. Tamen A, Hartvig P, Fagerlund C, Dahlstrom B 1982 Patient-controlled analgesic therapy. Part I: pharmacokinetics of pethidine in per- and post-operative periods. Clinical Pharmacokinetics 7: 149–163
26. Boreus L O, Sköldefors E, Ehrnebo M 1983 Appearance of pethidine and norpethidine in cerebrospinal fluid of man following intramuscular injection of pethidine. Acta Anaesthesiologica Scandinavica 27: 222–225
27. Jacobsen J, Flaschs H, Dich-Nielsen J O, Rosen J, Larsen A B, Hvidberg 1988 Comparative plasma concentration profiles after i.v., i.m. and rectal administration of pethidine in children. British Journal of Anaesthesia 60: 623–626
28. Glynn C J, Mather L E, Cousins M J, Graham J R, Wilson P R 1981 Peridural meperidine in human: analgesic response, pharmacokinetics, and transmission into CSF. Anesthesiology 55: 30–36
29. Asatoor A M, London D R, Milne M D, Simonhoff M H 1963 The excretion of pethidine and its derivatives. Journal of Pharmacology 20: 285–298
30. Chan K 1979 The effects of physico-chemical properties of pethidine and its basic metabolites on their buccal absorption and renal elimination. Journal of Pharmacy and Pharmacology 31: 672–675
31. Chan K, Tse J, Jennings F, Orme M L E 1985 Influence of urinary pH on pethidine kinetics in healthy volunteer subjects. Methods and Findings in Experimental and Clinical Pharmacology 7: 245–252
32. Pond S M, Tong T, Benowitz N L, Jacob P, Rigod J 1981 Presystemic metabolism of meperidine to normeperidine in normal and cirrhotic subjects. Clinical Pharmacology and Therapeutics 30: 183–188
33. Szeto H H, Inturrisi C E, Houde R, Saal S, Cheigh J, Reidenberg M M 1977 Accumulation of normeperidine an active metabolite of meperidine, in patients with renal failure or cancer. Annals of Internal Medicine 86: 738–741
34. Chan K, Tse J, Jennings F, Orme M L E 1987 Pharmacokinetics of low-dose intravenous pethidine in patients with renal function. Journal of Clinical Pharmacology 27: 516–522
35. Chan K, Tse J, Jennings F, Orme M L E 1987 Disposition of pethidine in man under acidic urinary pH: 3. A comparison of pharmacokinetics among Caucasian Chinese and Indian subjects. Methods and Findings in Experimental and Clinical Pharmacology 9: 243–250
36. Stapleton J V, Austin K L, Mather L E 1979 A pharmacokinetic approach to post-operative pain: continuous infusion of pethidine. Anaesthesia and Intensive Care 7: 25–32
37. Tamsen A, Hartvig P, Fagerlund C, Dahlstrom B 1982 Patient-controlled analgesic therapy, Part II: individual analgesic demand and analgesic plasma concentrations of pethidine in post-operative pain. Clinical Pharmacokinetics 7: 164–175
38. Caldwell J, Notarianni L J, Smith R L 1978 Impaired metabolism of pethidine in the human neonate. British Journal of Clinical Pharmacology 5: 362P–363P
39. Lindgren L, Saarnivaara L, Himberg J J 1979 Comparisons of intramuscular pethidine, diazepam and flunitrazepam as premedications in children undergoing otolaryngological surgery. British Journal of Anaesthesia 51: 321–327
40. Fishburne J I 1982 Systemic analgesia during labor. Clinical Perinatology 9: 29–53
41. Belfrage P, Boreus L O, Hartvig P, Irestedt L, Raabe N 1981 Neonatal depression after obstetrical analgesia with pethidine. The role of the injection–delivery time interval and of the plasma concentrations of pethidine and norpethidine. Acta Obstetrica Gynecologica Scandinavica 60: 43–49
42. Brice J E H, Moreland T A, Walker C H M 1979 Effects of pethidine and its antagonists on the newborn. Archives of Disease in Childhood 54: 356–361
43. Miller R R, Jick H 1978 Clinical effects of meperidine in hospitalized medical patients. Journal of Clinical Pharmacology 18: 180–189
44. Lawrence C A 1978 Pethidine-induced hypertension in phaeochromocytoma. British Medical Journal 1 (6106): 149–150
45. Browning M L 1977 Inadvertent intra-arterial administration may cause gangrene. Hospital Pharmacy 12: 404
46. Stambough J E, Wainer I W, Hemphill D M, Schwartz J 1977 A potentially toxic drug interaction between pethidine (meperidine) and phenobarbitone. Lancet 1: 398–399
47. Rigg J R A, Ilsley A H, Vedig A E 1981 Relationship of ventilatory depression to steady state blood pethidine concentrations. British Journal of Anaesthesia 53: 613–620
48. Waisbren B A, Smith M B 1978 Hypersensitivity to meperidine. Journal of the American Medical Association 239: 1395
49. Sher P D 1976 Drug interference with laboratory tests: amylase and lipase. Drug Therapy 158–160
50. Clark F 1977 Drugs and enzymes. In: Davies D M (ed) Adverse drug reaction bulletin No 66: 232–235
51. Caldwell J, Wakile L A, Notarianni L J et al 1977 Maternal and neonatal disposition of pethidine in childbirth — a study using quantitative gas chromatography–mass spectrometry. Life Sciences 22: 589–596
52. Morgan D, Moore G, Thomas J, Triggs E 1978 Disposition of meperidine in pregnancy. Clinical Pharmacology and Therapeutics 23: 288–295
53. Hogg M I J, Wiener P C, Rosen M, Mapleson W W 1977 Urinary excretion and metabolism of pethidine and norpethidine in the newborn. British Journal of Anaesthesia 49: 891–899
54. Cooper L V, Stephen G W, Aggett P J A 1977 Elimination of pethidine and bupivacaine in the newborn. Archives of Diseases of Childhood 52: 638–641
55. Barrier G, Lassner J, Morselli P L et al 1980 Pharmacokinetics of meperidine in women in labour and in the newborn. British Journal of Anaesthesia 52: 101P
56. Kuhnert B R, Kuhnert P M, Prochaska A L, Sokol R J 1980 Meperidine disposition in mother, neonate and nonpregnant females. Clinical Pharmacology and Therapeutics 27: 486–491
57. Morrison J C, Whybrew W D, Rosser S I, Bucovaz E T, Wiser W L, Fish S A 1976 Metabolites of meperidine in the fetal and maternal serum. American Journal of Obstetrics and Gynecology 126: 997–1102
58. Kuhnert B R, Philipson E H, Kuhnert P M, Syracuse C D 1985 Disposition of meperidine and normeperidine following multiple doses during labour I. mother. American Journal of Obstetrics and Gynecology 151: 406–409
59. Kuhnert B R, Kuhnert P M, Philipson E H, Sycacuse C D 1985 Disposition of meperidine and normeperidine following multiple doses during labour II. fetus and neonate. American Journal of Obstetrics and Gynecology 151: 410–415
60. Kuhnert B R, Linn P L, Kennard M J, Kuhnert P M 1985 Effects of low doses of meperidine on neonatal behaviour. Anesthesiology and Analgesia 64: 335–342
61. Belsey E M, Rosenblatt D B, Lieberman B A et al 1981 The influence of maternal analgesia on neonatal behaviour: I. Pethidine. British Journal of Obstetrics and Gynaecology 88: 398–406
62. Freeborn S F, Calvert R T, Black P, MacFarlane T, D'Souza S W 1980 Saliva and blood pethidine concentrations in the mother and the newborn baby. British Journal of Obstetrics and Gynaecology 87: 966–969
63. Holmberg L, Odar-Cederlöf I, Boreus L O, Heyner L, Ehrnebo M 1982 Comparative disposition of pethidine and norpethidine in old and young patients. European Journal of Clinical Pharmacology 22: 175–179
64. Mather L E, Tucker G T, Pflug A E, Lindop M J, Wilkerson C 1975 Meperidine kinetics in man. Clinical Pharmacology and Therapeutics 17: 21–30
65. Madan P L 1977 Effect of urinary pH on renal excretion of drugs. Journal of the American Medical Association 238: 210
66. Rawlins M D 1978 Drug interactions and anaesthesia. British Journal of Anaesthesia 50: 689–693
67. Brown T C K, Cass N M 1979 Beware — the use of MAO inhibitors is increasing again. Anaesthesia and Intensive Care 7: 65–68
68. Eade N R, Renton K W 1970 Effect of monoamine oxidase inhibitors on the N-demethylation and hydrolysis of meperidine. Biochemical Pharmacology 19: 2243–2250
69. Clark B, Thompson J W, Widdington G 1972 Analysis of the inhibition of pethidine N-demethylation by monoamine oxidase inhibitors and some other drugs with special reference to drug interactions in man. British Journal of Pharmacology 44: 89–99
70. Benusis K P, Kapaun D, Furnan L J 1979 Respiratory depression in a child following meperidine, promethazine and chlorpromazine premedication: report of case. Journal of Dentistry for Children 46: 50–53
71. Stambaugh J E, Wainer I W 1981 Drug interactions: meperidine and chlorpromazine, a toxic combination. Journal of Clinical Pharmacology 21: 140–146
72. Stambaugh J E, Wainer I W, Schwartz I 1978 The effect of phenobarbitone on the metabolism of meperidine in normal volunteers. Journal of Clinical Pharmacology 18: 482–490
73. Pond S M, Kretzschmar K M 1981 Effect of phenytoin on meperidine clearance and normeperidine formation. Clinical Pharmacology and Therapeutics 30: 680–686

74. Nimmo W S, Wilson J, Prescott L F 1975 Narcotic analgesics and delayed gastric emptying during labour. Lancet 1: 890–892
75. Hey V M F, Ostick D G, Mazumder J K, Lord W D 1981 Pethidine, metoclopramide and the gastro-oesophageal sphincter. A study in healthy volunteers. Anaesthesia 36: 173–176
76. Clements J A, Heading R C, Nimmo W S, Prescott L F 1978 Kinetics of acetaminophen absorption and gastric emptying in man. Clinical Pharmacology and Therapeutics 24: 420–431
77. Guay D R P, Meatherall R C, Chalmers J L, Grahame G R 1985 Cimetidine alters pethidine disposition in man. British Journal of Clinical Pharmacology 18: 907–914

Phenazocine (hydrobromide)

Phenazocine hydrobromide is a powerful synthetic analgesic drug of the benzomorphan group, used for the relief of severe pain, including preoperative and postoperative pain and obstetric analgesia.

Chemistry

Phenazocine hydrobromide (Narphen)
$C_{22}H_{27}NOHBr.\frac{1}{2}H_2O$
1,2,3,4,5,6-Hexahydro-6,11-dimethyl-3-phenethyl-2,6-methano-3-benzazocin-8-ol hydrobromide hemihydrate

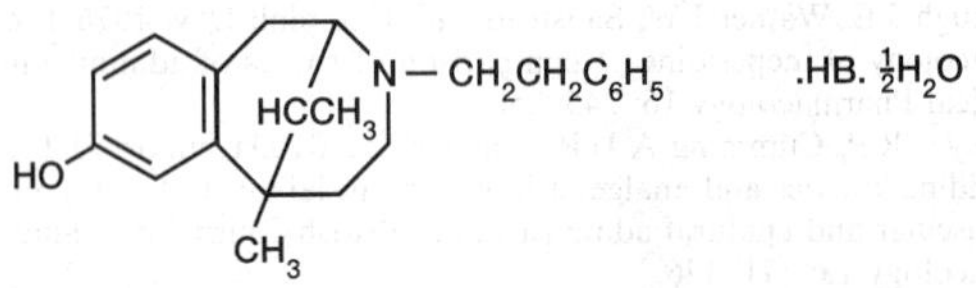

Molecular weight (free base)	411.4 (321.4)
pKa (amino group)	8.5
Solubility	
in alcohol	1 in 45
in water	1 in 350
Octanol/water partition coefficient	—

It is a white, odourless microcrystalline powder with a bitter taste, prepared by chemical synthesis.

Pharmacology

Phenazocine is a potent synthetic opiate analgesic of the benzomorphan group. At analgesic doses only agonist effects are observed, although antagonism of the effects of morphine can be demonstrated in guinea-pig ileum at low concentrations.[1] Phenazocine appears to act like morphine in pharmacological experiments in vitro. The behavioural effects of phenazocine in animals have been observed to be reversed[2] by low doses of naloxone 0.01–1 $mg.kg^{-1}$. This, and the lack of serious psychological side effects in clinical use, would support the idea that it acts primarily on μ binding sites. However, no detailed binding studies have been published. The effects of phenazocine are blocked by naloxone. Pharmacologically, phenazocine is distinct from other morphine-like drugs in not causing a rise in pressure in the common bile duct at analgesic doses.[3]

Toxicology

Cardiovascular collapse and respiratory failure have been observed in rats during chronic usage. Teratogenicity tests in rabbits, rats and mice showed no effects, with the possible exception of a mouse fetus showing a kinky tail.

Clinical pharmacology

Phenazocine is a potent analgesic in doses of 5–20 mg orally or sublingually, four to six times daily. A number of clinical trials have been performed in the past using an injectable form of the drug, which is no longer available. A dose–response relationship has been demonstrated for the oral form between single doses of 4 and 12.2 mg.[4] The duration of action is 5–6 hours.

Phenazocine appears to be about three times as potent as morphine in its analgesic effects and it is more reliably absorbed than morphine from the gastrointestinal tract. Phenazocine also has antitussive and constipating activity. Experiments in monkeys suggested that the dependence liability of phenazocine was considerably less than that of morphine. However, in man phenazocine is only slightly less potent in this regard compared to morphine.

Detailed studies on the respiratory depressive actions of oral phenazocine have not been done but normal volunteer studies examining the effects of equianalgesic doses of intramuscular morphine and phenazocine have shown similar effects on respiratory depression.[5]

Pharmacokinetics

Detection of the drug following the addition to human plasma in concentrations between 0.5 and 8.0 $\mu g.ml^{-1}$ has been achieved (approx. 100% recovery) using gas chromatography.[6] However, no method capable of measuring the drug in the low concentrations resulting from clinical use (doses in the range 0.1–0.3 $mg.kg^{-1}$) has been reported, and thus no data are available on its absorption, metabolism or excretion.

Concentration–effect relationship

There is no evidence of a relationship between the plasma concentration of phenazocine and its analgesic effects.

Metabolism

No data are available.

Pharmaceutics

Phenazocine (Narphen; Smith & Nephew, UK) is available in oral form only, as a white, biconvex compressed tablet, embossed 'SNP/2' on one side and scored on the reverse. Each tablet contains 5 mg phenazocine hydrobromide BP. No known potentially allergenic substance is included in the formulation. In the UK it is a controlled drug under the Misuse of Drugs Act.

Maximum shelf-life is 3.5 years, and the tablets should be protected from light.

Therapeutic use

Indications

1. Relief of acute pain and chronic severe pain.

Contraindications

1. Coma
2. Convulsive disorders
3. Delirium tremens
4. Myxoedema
5. Alcoholism
6. Respiratory depression
7. Obstructive airways disease
8. Concurrent use of monoamine oxidase inhibitors.

Mode of use

Phenazocine is only available in oral form, although it has been used intramuscularly (see Randomized controlled trials). It has also been reported to be effective sublingually[7] but this has not been clearly documented. Oral doses are in the range 5–20 mg and can be repeated 4–6 times daily.

Indications

1. Relief of pain

Phenazocine is a powerful analgesic for the relief of severe pain, and is indicated for the relief of preoperative and postoperative pain, and for obstetric analgesia. It has been used in the treatment of intractable pain in malignant disease. However, it should be stated that there are no clearcut advantages of phenazocine over morphine. The side effect profiles after intramuscular injection of equianalgesic doses of morphine and phenazocine in postoperative pain were very similar.[8]

Contraindications

It is contraindicated in coma, convulsive disorders and delirium tremens because it may either worsen the clinical state of the patient or make the interpretation of level of consciousness impossible.

Phenazocine (hydrobromide)

Opiates are generally contraindicated in myxoedema and alcoholism as they may precipitate coma. Because of the risk of further respiratory depression phenazocine should not be used in respiratory depression and obstructive airways disease. It should not be given concurrently with MAO inhibitors, or within two weeks of discontinuation of their use.

Adverse reactions

Potentially life-threatening effects

No life-threatening effects have been recorded at therapeutic doses.

Acute overdosage

The most important result of poisoning is respiratory depression for which naloxone should be used as an antidote.

Severe or irreversible adverse effects

Although detailed studies on tolerance and dependence have not been done there is no reason to believe that these do not occur. It should therefore be assumed that tolerance and dependence may occur.

Symptomatic adverse effects

The most serious side effect is respiratory depression, as with other narcotic drugs. Some patients may experience a feeling of lightheadedness or dizziness, which soon passes. Nausea and vomiting may be troublesome. Pruritis and occasionally dryness of the mouth and sweating have been reported. Hypotension is rare.

Interference with clinical pathology tests

Phenazocine may interfere with thin-layer chromatographic methods for measuring alkaloids and barbiturates in urine.

High risk groups

Neonates

No information is available on the use of this drug in neonates and therefore it is not recommended.

Breast milk. No information is available on the presence or absence of the drug in breast milk.

Children

Paediatric doses have not been established.

Pregnant women

There is no evidence of safety in human pregnancy, but the drug has been used for many years without apparent ill consequence, and animal studies have not shown any hazard. Administration during labour may cause respiratory depression in the newborn. No information is available on the effect of the drug in lactating women.

The elderly

Dosage should be reduced in the elderly.

Concurrent disease

The dose should be reduced in hypothyroidism or chronic hepatic disease. Care is required in the presence of renal insufficiency.

Drug interactions

Potentially hazardous interactions

MAO inhibitors. Potential interaction of phenazocine with MAO inhibitors has been demonstrated in mice but has not been reported in man. This interaction may result from an enhanced response to 5-HT.[9] Chlorpromazine antagonizes this reaction in rabbits and may theoretically be of use in this situation.

Potentially useful interactions

None is known.

Major outcome trials

There are no major outcome trials concerning the use of oral phenazocine.

Randomized controlled trials

1. Hopton D 1971 Double-blind clinical trial of the analgesic effects of phenazocine hydrobromide (Narphen) compared with morphine sulphate in patients with acute abdominal pain. Gut 12: 51–54

No randomized placebo-controlled trials have been performed on oral phenazocine but a double-blind controlled trial comparing intramuscular phenazocine (2.5 mg) with morphine (10 mg intramuscularly) in postoperative pain has been carried out. This trial had relatively small numbers of patients (27 and 22 patients in each group), but, within those limits, showed no significant difference between morphine and phenazocine-induced analgesia.

2. DeKornfeld T J, Lasagna L 1960 A controlled clinical evaluation of two new analgesics, phenazocine and phenampromid. Anesthesiology 21: 159–162

This was a well designed double-blind controlled trial comparing three different doses (0.5 mg, 2 mg, 3 mg) of intramuscular phenazocine with a standard dose of intramuscular morphine in postoperative pain. 23 patients were studied with phenazocine and 12–18 patients were studied with phenampromid. Patients were either given alternate doses of morphine and phenazocine, or morphine and phenampromid. The results were analysed on an individual patient basis and on a single dose of drug basis. 3 mg of phenazocine was found to be equivalent to 10 mg of morphine from 1–4 h after injection, whereas 25 mg and 50 mg of phenampromid did not equal or surpass the performance of 10 mg of morphine.

Other trials

Economou G, Monson R, Ward-McQuaid J N 1971 Oral pentazocine and phenazocine: a comparison in postoperative pain. British Journal of Anaesthesia 43: 486–494

Oral pentazocine (50 mg and 75 mg) was compared with oral phenazocine (5 mg) in a non-randomized, double-blind assessment of postoperative analgesia. Patients had undergone different types of operations including abdominal operations at varying time intervals prior to the administration of the trial drug. Analgesia was assessed for four hours post-administration. There was no placebo group. 5 mg of phenazocine was found to be equivalent to a dose intermediate between 50 and 75 mg of pentazocine.

References

1. Gyang E A, Kosterlitz H W 1966 Agonist and antagonist actions of morphine-like drugs on the guinea-pig isolated ileum. British Journal of Pharmacology and Chemotherapeutics 27: 514–527
2. Leander J D 1982 Effects of ketazocine, ethylketazocine and phenazocine on schedule controlled behaviour. Antagonism by naloxone. Neuropharmacology 21: 923–928
3. Hopton D S, Torrance H B 1967 Action of various new analgesic drugs on the human common bile duct. Gut 8: 296–300
4. Beaver W T, Wallenstein S L, Houde R W, Rogers A 1968 A clinical comparison of the effects of oral and intramuscular administration of analgesics: pentazocine and phenazocine. Clinical Pharmacology and Therapeutics 9: 582–597
5. Papadopoulos C N, Keats A S 1960 Studies of analgesic drugs VI. Comparative respiratory depressant activity of phenazocine and morphine. Clinical Pharmacology and Therapeutics 2: 8–12
6. Ahmad K, Medzihradsky F 1971 The determination of benzomorphan derivatives in plasma by gas chromatography. Life Sciences 10: 707–710
7. Economou G, Monson R, Ward-McQuaid J N 1971 Oral pentazocine and phenazocine: a comparison in postoperative pain. British Journal of Anaesthesia 43: 486–494
8. York J E, Campbell S M, Gordon R A 1962 Evaluation of phenazocine in postoperative patients. Canadian Anaesthetists Society Journal 9: 121–124
9. Rogers K J, Thornton J A 1969 The interaction between monoamine-oxidase inhibitors and narcotic analgesics in mice. British Journal of Pharmacology 36: 470–480

Phenelzine

Phenelzine is the most widely used hydrazine monoamine oxidase inhibitor, being effective and relatively free from side effects. Most recent drug trials that have investigated the uses of monoamine oxidase inhibitors have been carried out with this drug.

Chemistry

Phenelzine sulphate (Nardil, Nardelzine)
$C_8H_{12}N_2H_2SO_4$
β-Phenylethyl hydrazine hydrogen sulphate

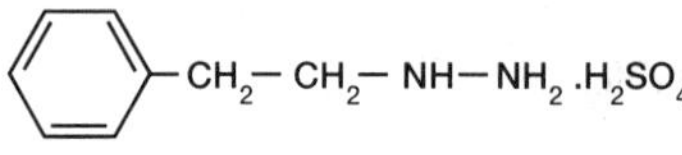

Molecular weight (free base)	234.3 (136.2)
pKa	—
Solubility	
in alcohol	practically insoluble
in water	1 in 7
Octanol/water partition coefficient	—

Phenelzine sulphate is a white or yellowish-white powder, with a pungent odour and characteristic taste. It is prepared by chemical synthesis. There are no combination products on the market.

Pharmacology

Phenelzine acts by irreversibly inhibiting monoamine oxidase (MAO) A and B. The rate of recovery depends upon resynthesis of the enzyme and is slower in the brain than in other tissues or gut. Non-methylated biogenic amines are inactivated by two main pathways involving monoamine oxidase and catechol-O-methyl transferase (COMT). Phenelzine inhibits the former, which is present on the outer membranes of neuronal mitochondria, and causes an increase in the amount of amine available for synaptic release.[1] Phenelzine has additional actions such as the inhibition of re-uptake of amines from the synaptic cleft.

Toxicology

Phenelzine has been shown to decrease the number of viable offspring of pregnant mice when given in large amounts and has not been shown to be free of mutagenic potential.

A single case report of angiosarcoma of the liver in a lady who had been taking phenelzine for six years has been reported and a similar relationship has been demonstrated in mice.

Clinical pharmacology

Two subtypes of monoamine oxidase, A and B, have been found in man. An antidepressant effect has been demonstrated[2] with drugs which selectively inhibit monoamine oxidase-A, e.g. clorgyline, but not with those selectively inhibiting monoamine oxidase-B, e.g. deprenyl. Phenelzine, however, is non-selective in action. Markers of monoamine oxidase-A activity include urine MHPG (3-methoxy-4-hydroxy phenylethanediol) and plasma DHPG (dihydroxy-phenyl ethanediol) but no completely specific method of determining inhibition of brain MAO exists in man. An 80% reduction in platelet monoamine oxidase-B activity is required for an antidepressant effect, when using non-selective inhibitors of monoamine oxidase. Similar data suggest that a > 70% reduction of urinary MHPG is required for antidepressant activity.

Phenelzine

Adverse reactions

Potentially life-threatening effects
The severe sympathomimetic crises resulting from an interaction between phenelzine and tyramine-rich foods or drugs containing indirectly acting amines such as phenylpropanolamine have been described by various authors.[28,29] All patients taking phenelzine should be given a card warning them of the dangers and care should be taken to make sure that this warning has been understood. The risk of a fatal outcome, however, is relatively small. Only 17 non-fatal cases of an adverse reaction between phenelzine and food substances have been reported over a 10-year period. The mechanism involved is release of noradrenaline from neuronal stores by the indirectly acting amine. Normally much of the noradrenaline released into the cytosol of the nerve ending would be degraded by MAO before release but in the presence of an MAO inhibitor much increased amounts are available. In the case of tyramine-containing foods and beverages an additional mechanism is inhibition of the normal extensive presystemic metabolism of tyramine by MAO in the gut wall and liver.

The main risk is from sub-arachnoid or intracerebral haemorrhage during a severe rise in blood pressure. The blood pressure elevation can be speedily reversed by intravenous injection of the α-adrenoceptor blocking agent phentolamine. Severe tachycardia or tachyarrhythmia responds quickly to small doses of β-adrenoceptor blocking drugs. These risks must be weighed up against the risks of mortality and morbidity from the untreated depressive illness.

Acute overdosage
Fatalities have been recorded when phenelzine has been taken in dosages of between 375 mg and 1500 mg. A lag period of approximately 12 hours may occur before symptoms are manifest and a prolonged observation period is recommended. The following symptoms have been recorded: neuromuscular weakness, extrapyramidal symptoms, agitation, mental confusion, tachypnoea, hyperthermia, involuntary movements, headache, dizziness, chest pain, convulsions and death.

Symptomatic treatment to correct blood pressure, body temperature and fluid balance is indicated. As gastric motility is reduced, lavage is recommended for up to several hours post-ingestion. Phenelzine is effectively removed by haemodialysis.[30] Hypertension can be controlled with intravenous phentolamine; opiates should be avoided and agitation can be treated with chlorpromazine.

Severe or irreversible adverse effects
(See also Drug interactions).

Monoamine oxidase inhibitors have been held responsible for causing hepatocellular jaundice,[17] but the early population sampled may have contained patients suffering from viral hepatitis which would give a similar histological picture. The risks are therefore less than were previously believed, but liver function should be monitored in patients at risk of liver disease, for example heavy drinkers.

Leucopenia is a rare but serious adverse effect.[31] Psychotic reactions have been reported[32] and hypomania (although not as commonly as with tranylcypromine). Peripheral neuropathy secondary to pyridoxine deficiency has been reported in one patient on long-term phenelzine therapy.

Symptomatic adverse effects
Minor ill effects are common, but most will clear up if the dose is reduced or the drug discontinued. Anticholinergic effects are common, as are drowsiness (or sometimes insomnia), tremor, dizziness, weakness, fatigue and gastrointestinal problems. Less commonly oedema, headache, peripheral neuropathy, nervousness, increased appetite and weight, skin rashes, arrhythmias, convulsions, anorgasmia, purpura and blood dyscrasias have been reported.

Other effects
A rise in central and peripheral catecholamine levels has been reported.

Interference with clinical pathology tests
No data are available.

High risk groups

Neonates
There is no indication for the use of this drug in neonates. Drowsiness and ataxia have been reported following accidental ingestion.

Breast milk. No data are available on the excretion of this drug in breast milk so women taking it should not breast-feed.

Children
What has been said about neonates applies equally to children.

Pregnant women
There is no evidence available as to the safe use of this drug in human or animal pregnancies. Its use is not advised in pregnancy, especially in the first or third trimesters.

The elderly
The elderly are more vulnerable to side effects and care should be exercised in its use.[33]

Drug interactions

Potentially hazardous interactions

Food. Reactions occur with foods rich in dopamine and tyramine, resulting in elevated blood pressure, headache, sweating, pallor, stiff neck, chest pain, palpitations and even cerebral haemorrhage. Only foods high in dopamine and tyramine, for example pickled herrings, ripe cheese, are absolutely contraindicated. There is much variation in the dopamine and tyramine content of foods in the UK and the impact of these restrictions on a person's diet should not be too great.

When a reaction occurs, hypertension should be controlled by slow intravenous administration of 5–10 mg of phentolamine. If phentolamine is not available, 75–100 mg of chlorpromazine given intramuscularly can be used.

Sympathomimetics. The effects of indirectly acting sympathomimetics, for example nasal decongestants and bronchial dilators, as well as appetite suppressants, e.g. phenylpropanolamine, fenfluramine, phentermine and levodopa, can be augmented by phenelzine. In some cases this is partly due to inhibition of their metabolism but the main effect is that such sympathomimetics act by causing the release of stored catecholamines. Severe hypertensive reactions may occur.

Tricyclic antidepressants. The use of a tricyclic antidepressant within two weeks of phenelzine use can lead to severe side effects, including hypertension.

Opiates. Phenelzine potentiates the effects of opiate analgesics, possibly through the inhibition of the liver enzymes responsible for their metabolism although a pharmacodynamic effect has also been suggested. Excitement, muscle rigidity, hyperpyrexia, flushing, sweating, hypotension, respiratory depression and unconsciousness can occur. Pethidine is absolutely contraindicated and other opiates should first be given in 5–10% of their normal dosage, with careful monitoring of vital signs, to identify susceptible patients. Phenelzine should be withdrawn two weeks before elective surgery.

Potentially useful interactions
None have been reported.

Clinical trials

1. Paykel E S, Parker R R 1982 Response to phenelzine and amitriptyline in subtypes of outpatient depression. Archives of General Psychiatry 39: 1041–1049

In a prospective double-blind trial, 131 out-patients with depression or anxiety/depression were treated with either phenelzine, amitriptyline or a placebo. Patients were included if they scored between 7 and 11 on the Raskin Three-Area Scale, but excluded if their depression was severe enough to warrant in-patient treatment. Three categories of depression were defined — atypical depression, depression with reverse functional shift and neurotic depression. Both phenelzine and amitriptyline appeared to be equally effective in comparison with the placebo. There seemed to be little difference in the effect of drug action whatever the category of depression treated. The only significant difference between phenelzine and amitriptyline was that the former was less effective in patients with personality disorder and more effective when symptoms of anxiety were present.

2. Tyrer P, Candy J, Kelly D 1973 A study of the clinical effects of phenelzine and placebo in the treatment of phobic anxiety. Psychopharmacologia 32: 237–254

In a double-blind controlled trial, phenelzine and placebo were

Phenelzine

compared in patients with agoraphobia or a social phobia. Patients were included in the trial if their primary diagnosis was a phobic disorder, their symptoms had persisted for over one year, they were between 16 and 60 years of age and they had not been previously exposed to monoamine oxidase inhibitors for more than two weeks.

40 such patients were found, matched in pairs and included in the trial; in all there were eight dropouts. Those who dropped out were more likely to have been on phenelzine. Of those who completed the trial, follow-up at two months and assessment on an adapted clinical rating scale revealed significantly more improvement in those who were treated with phenelzine compared with placebo. It did not appear that phenelzine was acting indirectly through an antidepressant effect. Follow-up over a further six months confirmed these findings.

General review articles

Daly R E 1973 In: Florey K (ed) Analytical profiles of drug substances, vol 2. Academic Press, New York, pp 383–407

Pare C M B 1985 The present status of monoamine oxidase inhibitors. British Journal of Psychiatry 146: 576–584

Robinson D S, Nies A, Ravaris L, Ives J O, Bartlett D 1978 Clinical pharmacology of phenelzine. Archives of General Psychiatry 35: 629–635

Tollefson G 1983 Monoamine oxidase inhibitors: a review. Journal of Clinical Psychiatry 44: 280–288

Tyrer P J 1982 Drugs in psychiatric practice. Butterworths, pp 249–279

Editorial 1989 Rediscovering MAOIs benefits underestimated side effects exaggerated. British Medical Journal 298: 345–346

References

1. Tollefson G D 1983 Monoamine oxidase inhibitors: a review. Journal of Clinical Psychiatry 44: 280–288
2. Murphy D L et al 1981 Selective inhibition of monoamine oxidase subtype-A. In: Youdim M B H, Paykel E S (eds) Monoamine oxidase inhibitors — the state of the art. John Wiley, Chichester, pp 189–205
3. Tyrer P, Gardner M, Lambourn J 1980 Clinical pharmacokinetic factors affecting the response to phenelzine. British Journal of Psychiatry 136: 359–365
4. Paykel E S 1979 Predictors of treatment response. In: Paykel E S, Coppen A (eds) Psychopharmacology of affective disorders. Oxford University Press, pp 193–220
5. Oswald I, Dunleavy D L F 1973 Mood and sleep changes with monoamine oxidase inhibitors. Archives of General Psychiatry 28: 353–356
6. Nies A 1982 Monoamine oxidase inhibitors. In: Paykel E S (ed) Handbook of affective disorders. Churchill Livingstone, Edinburgh
7. Caddy B, Stead A H 1977 Indirect determination of phenelzine in urine. Analyst 102: 42–49
8. Caddy B, Tilstone W J, Johnstone E L 1976 Phenelzine in urine. British Journal of Clinical Pharmacology 3: 633–637
9. Cooper T B, Robinson D S, Nies A 1978 Phenelzine measurement in human plasma. Communications in Psychopharmacology 2: 505–512
10. Tilstone W J, Margot P, Johnstone E L 1979 Acetylation of phenelzine. Psychopharmacology 60: 261–263
11. Marshall E F, Mountjoy C Q, Campbell I C, Garside R F, Leitch I N, Roth N 1978 The influence of acetylator phenotype on the outcome of treatment with phenelzine in a clinical trial. British Journal of Clinical Pharmacology 6: 247–254
12. Paykel E S, West P S, Rown P R, Parker R R 1982 Response to phenelzine and amitriptyline in subtypes of outpatient depression. British Journal of Psychiatry 141: 243–248
13. Loomer H P, Saunders J C, Kline N S 1957 A clinical and pharmacodynamic evaluation of iproniazid as a psychic energiser. Psychiatric Research Reports 8: 129–141
14. Medical Research Centre Trial 1965 Clinical trial of the treatment of depressive illness. British Medical Journal 1: 881–886
15. Blackwell B 1963 Hypertensive crisis due to monoamine oxidase inhibitors. Lancet 2: 849–851
16. Pare C M B 1964 Toxicity of psychotropic drugs. Proceedings of the Royal Society of Medicine 57: 757–778
17. Tyrer P 1984 Chemical effects of abrupt withdrawal from tricyclic antidepressants and monoamine oxidase inhibitors after longterm treatment. Journal of Affective Disorders 6: 1–7
18. Davidson J, McLeod M M N, Turnbull C D, Miller R D 1981 A comparison of phenelzine and imipramine in depressed inpatients. Journal of Clinical Psychiatry 42: 10
19. Tyrer P 1976 Towards rational therapy with monoamine oxidase inhibitors. British Journal of Psychiatry 128: 354–360
20. Davidson J, McLeod M N, Blum M R et al 1979 A comparison of E.C.T. and combined phenelzine–amitriptyline in refractory depression. Archives of General Psychiatry 35: 639–642
21. Robinson D S et al 1985 Panic attacks in outpatients with depression: response to antidepressant treatment. Psychopharmacology Bulletin 21: 562–567
22. Sheehan D V, Ballenger J, Jacobsen G 1980 Treatment of endogenous anxiety. Archives of General Psychiatry 37: 51–59
23. Pohl R, Berchou R, Rainey J M 1982 Tricyclics and monoamine oxidase inhibitors in the treatment of agoraphobia. Journal of Clinical Psychopharmacology 2: 399–401
24. Lipsedge M S, Hajioff J, Huggins P et al 1973 The management of severe agoraphobia. Psychopharmacologia 32: 67–80
25. Tyrer P, Candy J, Kelly D 1973 A study of the clinical effects of phenelzine and placebo in the treatment of phobic anxiety. Psychopharmacologica 32: 237–254
26. Annesley P T 1969 Nardil response in a chronic obsessive/compulsive. British Journal of Psychiatry 115: 748
27. Walsh B T 1984 Treatment of bulimia with phenelzine. Archives of General Psychiatry 41: 1105–1109
28. Marks J 1965 Interactions involving drugs used in psychiatry. In: Marks J, Pare C M B (eds) The scientific basis of drug therapy in psychiatry. Pergamon Press, Oxford
29. Pare C M B 1977 Monoamine oxidase inhibitors: a personal account. In: Burrows G D (ed) Handbook of studies on depression. Excerpta Medica, Amsterdam
30. Versaci A A, Nakamoto S, Kolf W J 1964 Phenelzine intoxication. Report of a case treated by haemodialysis. Ohio State Medical Journal 60: 770
31. Tipermas A, Gilman H E, Russakoff L M 1984 A case report of leukopenia associated with phenelzine. American Journal of Psychiatry 141: 806–807
32. Sheehy L M, Maxmen J S 1978 Phenelzine-induced psychosis. American Journal of Psychiatry 135: 1422–1423
33. Jenike M A 1984 The use of monoamine oxidase inhibitors in the treatment of elderly, depressed patients. Journal of the American Geriatrics Society 32: 571–575
34. Anon 1989 MOAIs. Move the menu up. Drugs and Therapeutics Bulletin 6: 3–4

Phenindione

Phenindione is a synthetic oral anticoagulant. It is not a dicoumarol derivative and its association with allergic effects makes members of the coumarin family the first choice of oral anticoagulants.

Chemistry

Phenindione (Dindevan)
$C_{15}H_{10}O_2$
2-Phenylindan-1,3-dione

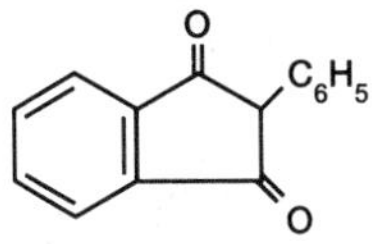

Molecular weight	222.2
pKa	4.1
Solubility	
in alcohol	1 in 125
in water	insoluble
Octanol/water partition coefficient	high

Phenindione consists of a tasteless, almost odourless, soft, white or creamy white crystals. It is readily soluble in alkaline solution.

Pharmacology

Phenindione is an indirect antagonist of vitamin K. Vitamin K is converted to vitamin K 2-3 epoxide during the activation of clotting factor precursors. The epoxide is metabolized by the enzyme vitamin K epoxide reductase to regenerate active vitamin K. Phenindione inhibits the enzyme epoxide reductase and this leads to a reduction in the amount of vitamin K available for clotting factor synthesis. Vitamin K epoxide levels rise, with the consequent inhibition of vitamin K-dependent carboxylation of the coagulation proteins. These proteins are then synthesized lacking the normal number of γ-carboxyl residues which are required to bind calcium; thus they do not function as normal clotting factors.

Toxicology

Dogs were fed 25 to 50 $mg.kg^{-1}$ of phenindione orally for periods of up to 27 months. No abnormality was noted in estimations of liver function tests or basic haematological parameters. This drug was introduced into clinical use at a time before drug regulations demanded the recent more stringent toxicological studies. This section is therefore limited in size.

Clinical pharmacology

Phenindione reduces the synthesis of the vitamin K-dependent clotting factors (II, VII, IX, X and Protein C) by the liver. The onset of action is delayed until existing clotting factors have been catabolized. Factor VII has the shortest half life and Factor II the longest half life in the body. The aim of treatment is to activate a partial inhibition of clotting factor synthesis such that the prothrombin time is prolonged by a factor of two to three times the normal rate. The normal maintenance dose is 25 to 150 mg daily.

Pharmacokinetics

Phenindione has been quantified by polarography, which has a limit of detection of 4 $mg.l^{-1}$.

Following intravenous administration of 5 $mg.kg^{-1}$ phenindione to six subjects over a period of 2–3 minutes, the rate of decline in plasma levels of the drug averaged 10% per hour, corresponding to a half life of 5–6 hours.[1]

Absorption of oral phenindione in 12 subjects was rapid, with peak plasma levels being attained in 1–3 hours. In three subjects given the same dose intravenously, plasma levels were identical to those following oral administration, indicating complete absorption.

Plasma levels of phenindione following a single 400 mg dose in 10 subjects were related to prothrombin response. There was a delay of 8–12 hours before any prothrombin response could be detected. All subjects showed a detectable prothrombin time increase within 24 hours. In 9 out of 10 subjects the prothrombin response was maximal two days after dosage, and in one subject three days after dosage. Prothrombin times in all 10 subjects did not return to control values until at least four days after dosage. Although there was no correlation among different individuals between the maximum prothrombin response and the plasma levels of phenindione, the duration of prothrombin response reflected the rate at which the drug disappeared from the plasma.

Following repeated dosage with 50–150 mg per day for periods of three weeks to five months, no accumulation of phenindione was observed, although a satisfactory maintenance of prothrombin response was obtained.

Oral absorption	rapid and complete
Presystemic metabolism	<5%
Plasma half life	
range	5–6 h
Volume of distribution	—
Plasma protein binding	>97%

Metabolism

Phenindione appears to be excreted exclusively in the urine, with no significant amounts being found in faeces. The presence of metabolites gives a reddish colour to the alkalinized urine of patients taking the drug: the parent drug does not produce this response.

In some subjects the red colour in urine is more intense on the second day after intravenous or oral administration than on the first day, this delayed renal excretion suggesting that metabolites are produced in the liver, secreted into the bile and then absorbed from the gastrointestinal tract, before finally being excreted in the urine.

The nature of the metabolites of phenindione has not been confirmed.

Pharmaceutics

Phenindione Dindevan (Duncan, Flockhart & Co., UK) is available in an oral tablet form in 10, 25 and 50 mg sizes. The 10 mg tablet is white engraved with DF/D10; the 25 mg tablet is green engraved with DF/D25; the 50 mg tablet is white engraved with DF/D50. US proprietary name: Hedulin. Careful formulation is necessary for reproducible disintegration/dissolution.

Therapeutic use

This is identical to that for warfarin sodium which is the most commonly used and preferred oral anticoagulant in the United Kingdom and North America.

Indications

1. Prevention of deep venous thrombosis after surgery in high-risk groups
2. Management of deep venous thrombosis and pulmonary embolism
3. Prevention of embolism associated with artificial cardiac valves
4. Prevention of embolism associated with rheumatic heart disease

Other uses

5. Post myocardial infarction
6. Cerebrovascular disease.

P

Contraindications

1. Groups at risk of haemorrhage
2. Pregnant women.

Precautions

The anticoagulant action of phenindione may be potentiated or inhibited by drugs (see Drug interactions).

Mode of use

Dosage and administration

Providing the prothrombin time is normal, before treatment with phenindione is commenced, a dose of 200 mg as a single dose is given on the first day, followed by 100 mg on the second day. The dose is adjusted thereafter according to the prothrombin time: usual maintenance dose range between 50 and 150 mg daily in two divided doses. When an oral anticoagulant is being introduced to a patient on heparin the two drugs should be overlapped until the prothrombin time is prolonged into the therapeutic range. In the UK a rabbit thromboplastin produced by the Manchester Thrombosis Research Foundation is used by most laboratories. The results are commonly expressed as the ratio of results obtained from patient and control plasmas using thromboplastin compared with a standard. Efforts are now being made to ensure that results from thromboplastins produced by different manufacturers are expressed with reference to an international thromboplastin standard. The relationship between the reference thromboplastin and the commercial thromboplastin allows an International Normalized Ratio (INR) to be calculated. The current recommended intensities of anticoagulation[2] depend on the indication for therapy and are as follows:

Table 1

(INR)	Indication
2.0–2.5	Prophylaxis of deep vein thrombosis.
2.0–3.0	Treatment of deep venous thrombosis and/or pulmonary embolism. Prophylaxis for hip surgery.
3.0–4.5	Recurrent deep venous thrombosis and/or pulmonary embolism. Prosthetic valves and grafts.

It is important that all patients on anticoagulant therapy are educated prior to commencing treatment regarding the potential hazards of therapy. Control should be assessed regularly and the patient interviewed to determine if any complications are being encountered.

Duration of therapy

Patients with a long-term risk of thrombosis, such as those with rheumatic heart disease or certain artificial heart valves, require long-term anticoagulation. Important members of this group are patients who have familial deficiency of the naturally occurring anticoagulants antithrombin III or Protein C which predispose them to recurrent thromboembolism.

In patients who have had a single episode of deep venous thrombosis or pulmonary embolism, there is no definite evidence that treatment for longer than 6 weeks is beneficial.[3] Although there have been reports of 'rebound' thrombosis if an oral anticoagulant is stopped abruptly, others have not documented such a risk.

Indications

1. Prevention of deep venous thrombosis

There is good clinical trial evidence to support use in venous thrombosis and embolism. (Much of the data has involved the use of warfarin but it is reasonable to expect the same results with phenindione if it is given in doses to produce the same intensity of anticoagulation.)

Controlled studies have demonstrated the effectiveness of oral anticoagulants in the prophylaxis of deep venous thrombosis in patients undergoing surgery.[4,5] The efficacy of oral anticoagulants in such high-risk situations has to be balanced against the risk of bleeding. However, conventional low dose heparin is relatively ineffective in these situations and if the intensity of treatment is in the range INR 2–3 the benefit in terms of reduction in thromboembolism would appear to outweigh the risk.[6]

2. Acute deep venous thrombosis and/or pulmonary embolism

There is clinical evidence with supportive but not conclusive trial data to recommend use here.

Prior to consideration of treatment the diagnosis should be made objectively, as clinical signs of thromboembolic disease are notoriously unreliable.[7] The use of anticoagulants became established following the randomized trial of Barritt and Jordan[8] in which a significant difference in total and recurrent embolism was documented in the placebo group, compared to the treatment group. The trial in fact was stopped before its completion and has been further criticized for its method of randomization, small number of patients, and lack of reliable objective assessments. However, recent studies comparing follow-up patients with deep venous thrombosis, treated initially with heparin and then randomized to either warfarin or heparin appear to confirm the value of oral anticoagulants.[9,10]

3. Prosthetic heart valves

No randomized controlled trials have conclusively demonstrated the role of oral anticoagulants in patients with prosthetic valves. Clinical experience, however, suggests a higher embolism rate in unprotected patients.[11] The combination of an oral anticoagulant agent and an anti-platelet drug (dipyridamole) may be a more effective form of therapy.[12] Tissue valves are less thrombogenic and there is no need for life-long anticoagulation.

4. Rheumatic heart disease

This indication for the use of anticoagulant is less common nowadays.

5. Controversial indications

Myocardial infarction. Trials conducted in the 1950s and 1960s reported conflicting results regarding the role of oral anticoagulants after myocardial infarction. These studies failed to fulfil the criteria necessary for good trial design but Douglas and McNicol[13] reviewing 12 reports considered that a small benefit did accrue from treatment. This view was supported by a 'Collaborative analysis of long-term anticoagulant administration after myocardial infarction.'[14] In this, nine soundly designed trials were re-evaluated by going back to the authors and collecting in a uniform way the simple essential data. The numbers when pooled were 2205 men and 282 women. In men under 55 years of age at the end of two years, 91% of the anticoagulant group were alive compared to 85% of the comparative group. This difference was significant at $p<0.01$. In men over 55 years of age at the end of three years, 75% of the anticoagulant group were alive compared to 69% of the comparative group. This difference was significant at $p<0.05$. Overall there was a reduction of death by about 20%: not too dissimilar to that being reported by the use of β-blockers. In the anticoagulant study when patients with no previous history of coronary heart disease were excluded, the benefit was found to be limited almost entirely to those with previous angina or a previous event of myocardial infarction. Peripheral thrombotic and embolic events did seem to be prevented but the ability of anticoagulants to prevent reinfarction or decrease mortality was not proven. The debate has been renewed following the results of a trial conducted in the Netherlands.[15] Patients on anticoagulants following infarction were randomized to stop treatment or to continue. Increased reinfarction mortality was demonstrated in the placebo group over the study period of two years. Further studies are still required to definitely define the role of anticoagulants after myocardial infarction but the balance of evidence indicated a degree of benefit from their use.

6. Cerebrovascular disease

Completed stroke. Development of new scanning techniques has helped considerably in the differentiation between a stroke caused by cerebral haemorrhage from that related to thrombosis or embolism. Anticoagulation would be contraindicated in the former situation but theoretically might be beneficial in the latter. However, trial data does not support the use of anticoagulants in thrombotic cerebral infarction although there is some evidence of benefit in the presence of embolism.[16]

Transient ischaemic attacks. Trials have again led to conflicting results and many studies have been criticized on methodological grounds.[16] Not only has there been a failure to demonstrate a definite reduction in strokes and mortality but the use of anticoagulants has been associated with a significant risk of intracranial haemorrhage. However, it must be said that the exact role of anticoagulant in transient ischaemic attacks remains to be delineated by well-designed trials.

Contraindications

Groups at risk of haemorrhage
The major complication of phenindione is haemorrhage. The use of this drug in patients considered at special risk of bleeding or in whom bleeding would be particularly catastrophic, should always be considered in comparison to the risk of thromboembolism (see also High risk groups).

Adverse reactions

Potentially life-threatening effects
Bleeding. The incidence of haemorrhage varies depending on the age of the patient, intensity of treatment and indication for using an anticoagulant. Figures are very variable and are reviewed by Mackie and Douglas.[17] In general, a 20% incidence might be expected although half of these episodes at least will be minor. More serious haemorrhage (10%) might be expected after hip surgery and with the treatment of transient ischaemic attacks. Haematuria, bruising and gastrointestinal bleeding are the commonest signs of bleeding in general medical patients. An underlying lesion is often present. Bleeding might be expected in certain sites in particular patient populations, for example, wound haematoma post surgery. The most common site of fatal haemorrhage is intracranial.

Blood dyscrasias. These are usually reversible on stopping the drug but fatalities have been reported. Agranulocytosis, anaemia and thrombocytopenia are well described, as well as leukaemoid reactions and lymphadenopathy. Agranulocytosis is potentially the most serious problem. It tends to occur during the first month of treatment and may be preceded by fever.[18] Depending on the time at which the marrow is examined, the picture may be that of myeloid hypoplasia or lack of neutrophils but plentiful myelocytes; the latter indicates incipient recovery of the peripheral neutrophil count.

Hepatitis. Hepatic derangement, usually cholestasis, can occur during treatment (fifth week of treatment). Like all complications it may be accompanied by other manifestations of hypersensitivity. Fatalities have been recorded.

Severe or irreversible adverse effects
Skin necrosis. Although this rare early complication of treatment with oral anticoagulants has been most commonly described complicating treatment with members of the coumarin family,[19] it has occurred during therapy with phenindione.[20] It usually occurs between the first and tenth days and affects predominantly females. Histologically there is thrombosis in venules and capillaries and areas of the body with abundant fat (e.g. breast, buttocks) are principally involved. The lesions may resolve spontaneously but skin grafting may be required. Intravenous heparin therapy has also been reported as beneficial. Patients with this complication should not be given further oral anticoagulant therapy as repeat episodes have occurred. There is recent evidence that this complication occurs in patients with protein C deficiency given oral anticoagulants.

Hypersensitivity reactions. Skin rashes, fever, liver and kidney problems, blood dyscrasias, myocarditis, visual disturbances and colitis have all occurred in patients taking phenindione. The reported incidence varies from 0.1–10%.[21] In an MRC trial[22] a 2.25% incidence of reactions necessitating discontinuation of phenindione occurred during the first 28 days of treatment. All these problems occurred in the higher dosage group studied. The seriousness of these reactions is variable but they may be fatal.

Skin rashes. These are the commonest manifestation of hypersensitivity. Erythematous, scarlatiniform, papular and urticarial rashes have occurred. Severe exfoliative dermatitis has also been reported. Rashes usually occur during the first month of treatment.

Fever. This is an early important sign of sensitivity and often accompanies or is followed by a skin rash. Phenindione should be stopped at this stage. Patients developing hypersensitivity reactions should not receive further courses of phenindione as the complications will recur.[23] Warfarin can usually be substituted safely.

Renal. Phenindione therapy may be complicated by a mild elevation of the urea, renal failure and nephrotic syndrome. These are usually preceded by fever and rash. Renal biopsy shows interstitial oedema with an infiltrate of eosinophils and plasma cells; tubular necrosis is also frequently seen.[24] Six cases were reported with renal problems occurring over a 5-year period.

Antidote to oral anticoagulants and management of bleeding
Vitamin K_1 is the antidote to oral anticoagulants. If excessive prolongation of the prothrombin time occurs but the patient is not bleeding then the anticoagulant should merely be withheld and the prothrombin time rechecked daily. A small oral dose of vitamin K_1 (2.5–5 mg) can also be used to hasten the return of the prothrombin time towards normal. If bleeding is present or there is very marked prolongation of the time (ratio >5) then vitamin K_1 should be given. Intravenous vitamin K_1 (10 mg) should be given slowly and this will significantly shorten the prothrombin time in 6–10 hours. The patient may well be relatively refractory to reinstitution of anticoagulant therapy after vitamin K_1. If more rapid correction is required, as in the presence of major haemorrhage, fresh-frozen plasma should be given in addition. Prothrombin concentrates (contains all vitamin K-dependent factors) should only be used with extreme caution because of reports of thromboembolic complications.

Symptomatic adverse effects
Mild skin reactions and diarrhoea may occur.

Interference with clinical pathology tests
Phenindione may impart a red colour to urine.

High risk groups

Neonates
The drug is not used in this age group.

Breast milk. The drug is secreted in breast milk and mothers taking it should not breast-feed.[25]

Children
No data is available on use in children.

Pregnant women
Phenindione can cross the placenta and this results in a risk of fetal haemorrhage during the third trimester. In addition it may be teratogenic.[26] Subcutaneous heparin should be substituted for phenindione during pregnancy.

The elderly
Elderly patients may be more susceptible to the effects of oral anticoagulants and thus require a lower dosage. This is probably related to pharmacodynamic changes.

Concurrent disease
Most severe illnesses may increase the sensitivity to oral anticoagulants and special care is required in the presence of alcoholism, cardiac failure, liver disease, renal failure, diarrhoea and thyrotoxicosis. These diseases either decrease the availability of vitamin K-dependent clotting factors, inhibit the excretion of phenindione (renal failure) or lower the dose of warfarin required (hyperthyroidism). As the disease states are brought under control, regular monitoring is required and dosage adjustments should be made accordingly.
The major complication of phenindione is haemorrhage. The use of this drug in patients considered at special risk of bleeding or in whom bleeding would be particularly catastrophic, should always be considered in comparison to the risk of thromboembolism. If anticoagulation is felt to be mandatory, measures should obviously be taken to correct, if possible, any of the following situations: presence of a congenital or acquired disorder with coagulation factor deficiency(ies) or disorders; those with abnormal renal or hepatic function; postsurgical patients; patients with a history of recent peptic ulceration; patients with severe uncontrolled hypertension; patients on other drugs which alter haemostasis.

Any severe illness may increase the sensitivity to oral anticoagulants and special care is required in the presence of alcoholism, cardiac failure, liver disease, renal failure, diarrhoea and thyrotoxicosis.

Other patients at risk
Patients in whom poor compliance is anticipated.

Drug interactions

Potentially hazardous interactions
The anticoagulant action of phenindione may be potentiated or inhibited by other drugs. The latter is usually caused by stimulation

Phenindione

P

of liver microsomal enzymes by the potentiating drug, whereas the former may be related to inhibition of metabolism.

Particular care is required when any alterations are made to the drug regimen given to a patient on phenindione. No list of interacting drugs is complete and the lists shown below require to be continuously updated.

Pharmacokinetic

Non steroidal anti-inflammatory drugs and analgesics. A number of these drugs enhance the effect of phenindione by inhibiting its metabolism; the best documented example is phenylbutazone. Corticosteroids, dextropropoxyphene and tolbutamide also increase the action of phenindione.

Sulphinapyrazone. This may enhance the effect of phenindione, probably by inhibiting its metabolism.

H2 antagonists. Cimetidine is likely to enhance the phenindione effect by inhibiting its metabolism.

Antibiotics. Cotrimoxazole and metronidazole probably interfere with the metabolism of phenindione, thus potentiating its effect.

Reduced effect. (Hepatic microsomal enzymes induction). Drugs such as phenobarbitone and carbamazepine induce enzymes to increase the metabolism of phenindione and thus reduce its anticoagulant effect. Alcohol has also been reported to decrease the activity of phenindione.

Pharmacodynamic

Vitamin K. A high vitamin K intake will tend to reduce the effect of phenindione. This may be a problem in patients receiving parenteral nutrition.

Other drugs affecting haemostasis. Anti-platelet drugs (e.g. aspirin) will have an additive effect with phenindione on haemostasis. High doses of aspirin decrease prothrombin synthesis and therefore may potentiate the effect of phenindione.

Drugs causing gastric erosions or ulceration. Drugs causing damage to the gastric wall (e.g. aspirin) may precipitate haemorrhage in patients taking phenindione.

Diuretics. The treatment of cardiac failure by diuretics may result in higher availability of vitamin K and therefore a reduction in the phenindione effect.

Antibiotics. Some of the newer cephalosporins may lead to a prolongation of the prothrombin time and thus could potentiate the phenindione effect. Broad-spectrum antibiotics in general can cause suppression of vitamin K-producing bowel flora and thus, particularly in patients with reduced dietary intake of vitamin K, potentiate the effect of phenindione.

Potentially useful interactions

No interactions of this kind have been reported.

References

1. Schulert A R, Weiner M 1954 The physiologic disposition of phenylindanedione in man. Journal of Pharmacology 110: 451–457
2. Poller L 1985 Therapeutic ranges in anticoagulant administration. British Medical Journal 290: 1683–1686
3. Sullivan E F 1972 Duration of anticoagulant therapy in venous thromboembolism. Medical Journal of Australia 2: 1104–1107
4. Sevitt S, Gallagher N G 1959 Prevention of venous thrombosis and pulmonary embolism in injured patients. Trial of anticoagulant prophylaxis with phenindione in middle-aged and elderly patients with fractured necks of femur. Lancet 2: 981–989
5. Taberner D A, Poller L, Burslem R W, Jones J B 1978 Oral anticoagulants controlled by British comparative thromboplastin versus low dose heparin prophylaxis of deep vein thrombosis. British Medical Journal 1: 272–274
6. Morris G K, Mitchell J R 1976 Warfarin sodium in prevention of deep venous thrombosis and pulmonary embolism in patients with fractured neck of femur. Lancet 2: 869
7. Gallus A S, Hirsh J 1976 Diagnosis of venous thromboembolism. Seminars in Thrombosis and Hemostasis 2: 203–231
8. Barritt D W, Jordan S C 1960 Anticoagulant drugs in the treatment of thromboembolism. A controlled trial. Lancet 1: 1309–1312
9. Hull R, Delmore T, Genton E 1979 Warfarin sodium versus low dose heparin in long term treatment of venous thrombosis. New England Journal of Medicine 301: 855–858
10. Hull R, Delmore T, Carter C 1982 Adjusted subcutaneous heparin versus warfarin sodium in the long-term treatment of venous thrombosis. New England Journal of Medicine 306: 189–194
11. Gadboys H L, Litwak R S, Neimetz J, Wisch N 1967 Role of anticoagulants in preventing embolization from prosthetic heart valves. Journal of the American Medical Association 202: 282–286
12. Sullivan J M, Harken D E, Gorlin R 1968 Pharmacologic control of thromboembolic complications of cardiac value replacement. A preliminary report. New England Journal of Medicine 279: 576–580
13. Douglas A S, McNicol G P 1970 In: Biggs R (ed) Human blood coagulation, haemostasis, and thrombosis, 2nd edn. Blackwell Scientific Publications, Oxford, pp 585–586
14. International anticoagulant review group 1970 Collaborative analysis of long term anticoagulant administration after acute myocardial infarction. Lancet 1: 203–209
15. Sixty Plus Reinfarction Group 1980 A double blind trial to assess long term oral anticoagulant therapy in elderly patients after myocardial infarction. Lancet 2: 989–994
16. Mackie M J, Douglas A S 1978 Oral anticoagulants in arterial disease. British Medical Bulletin 34: 177–183
17. Mackie M J, Douglas A S 1984 Drug induced disorders of coagulation. In: Ratnoff O D, Forbes C D (eds) Disorders of haemostasis. Grune and Stralton, London, ch 16, pp 485–510
18. Ager J A M, Ingram G I S 1957 Agranulocytosis during phenindione therapy. British Medical Journal 1: 1102–1103
19. Nalbandian R M, Mader I J, Barret J L, Pearce J F, Rupp E C 1965 Petichial, euhymosis, and necrosis of skin. Induced by coumarin congeners. Journal of the American Medical Association 192: 603–608
20. Douglas A S 1962 Haemorrhage during coumarin or indanedione therapy. In: Anticoagulant therapy. Blackwell Scientific Publications, Oxford, ch 12, pp 299–318
21. Wright J S 1970 Phenindione sensitivity with leukaemoid reaction and hepato-renal damage. Postgraduate Medical Journal 46: 452–455
22. Report of the Working Party on anticoagulant therapy in coronary thrombosis to the Medical Research Council 1969 Assessment of short-term anticoagulant administration after cardiac infarction. British Medical Journal 1: 335–342
23. Brooks R H, Calleja H B 1960 Dermatitis, hepatitis and nephritis due to phenindione (phenylindandione). Annals of Internal Medicine 52: 706–709
24. Smith K 1965 Acute renal failure in phenindione sensitivity. British Medical Journal 1: 24–26
25. Gogul M, Noel G, Giller J-Y, Muller P, Mayer G 1970 Therapeutic anticoagulants et allaitement. Revue Française Gynecologie et Obstetric 65: 409–412
26. Pettifor J M, Benson R 1975 Congenital malformations associated with the administration of oral anticoagulants during pregnancy. Journal of Paediatrics 1975 86: 459–462
27. Standing Advisory Committee for Haematology of the Royal College of Pathologists 1982 Drug interaction with coumarin derivative anticoagulants. British Medical Journal 285: 274–275
28. Co-operative Clinical Trial 1973 Anticoagulants in acute myocardial infarction. Journal of the American Medical Association 724–729

Pheniramine (maleate)

Pheniramine is a member of the alkylamine class of H_1-histamine receptor antagonists with anticholinergic and local anaesthetic properties.

Chemistry

Pheniramine maleate (Daneral-SA, Avil, Aller G, Avilettes, Fenamine)

$C_{16}H_{20}N_2.C_4H_4O_4$

NN-Dimethyl-3-phenyl-3-(2-pyridyl)propylamine hydrogen maleate

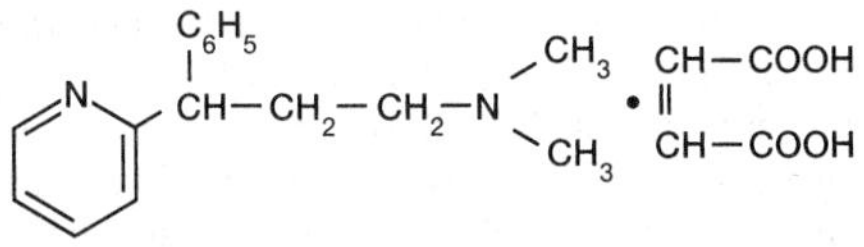

Molecular weight (free base)	356.4 (240.3)
pKa	4.2, 9.3
Solubility	
in alcohol	1 in 2.5
in water	1 in 0.3
Octanol/water partition coefficient	—

A white or almost white crystalline powder with a slight amine-like odour. It is prepared by chemical synthesis. Pheniramine maleate is also available in oral combinations with phenylpropanolamine and mepyramine maleate (Triominic), with phenylpropanolamine and paracetamol (Triotussic), with dextromethorphan hydrobromide (Syrtussar), and guaiphenesin and codeine phosphate (Robitussin), and with pentylenetetrazol and nicotinic acid (Ru-Vert). Other products marketed outside the UK (Avil, Avilettes, Aviletten) contain the p-aminosalicylate derivative of pheniramine. It is also combined with phenylephrine (Driston).

Pharmacology

Pheniramine is a competitive H_1-histamine receptor antagonist. Like other alkylamine antihistamines it is also an antagonist of muscarinic cholinergic receptors and possesses local anaesthetic properties. However, the concentration required for this latter effect is probably not achieved at therapeutic doses.

Toxicology

Pheniramine p-aminosalicylate in daily doses between 12.5 and 40 $mg.kg^{-1}$ in rats and 2.5 and 5.0 $mg.kg^{-1}$ in dogs for 6 months caused reduction in body and organ weights, slight agitation, changes in haemoglobin levels, red cell content and haematocrit, tachycardia, reduction in blood pressure and changes in ECG. In rodents pheniramine maleate does not affect the rate of implantation of embryos[1] and has no demonstrable mutagenic potential.[2] There are no data on carcinogenicity.

Clinical pharmacology

As with other alkylamines, pheniramine maleate is a competitive antagonist of histamine at its H_1-receptors. It is less potent than promethazine and has a shorter duration of action. On account of the latter, pheniramine maleate is available in the UK as a slow-release preparation, Daneral-SA. Daneral has a duration of action on inhibiting the skin wheal of approximately 8 hours while this is extended to 24 hours with Daneral-SA. A single tablet of Daneral-SA is reported to have equivalent H_1 blocking activity in the skin as standard Daneral formulation given in three divided doses.

Blockade of histamine H_1-receptors has a wide range of effects pertinent to the vasoactive effects of this mediator in diseases associated with mast cell or basophil activation.

Pheniramine antagonizes the effects of histamine on the skin that cause the 'triple response'. In particular pheniramine antagonizes the flare and the itching. Pheniramine is thus useful in the symptomatic treatment of allergic skin reactions and of allergic rhinitis. Pheniramine suppresses the histamine-evoked salivary secretions but much of the effect is due to the anticholinergic rather than the antihistamine effects of the drug. Pheniramine has weak antiemetic effects and is used for this purpose in the treatment of vertigo. The effect is due to an effect on vestibular and visual influx. Pheniramine is less effective as an antiemetic than antihistamines of the ethanolamine class (e.g. diphenhydramine or dimenhydrinate). Pheniramine, like most H_1-antihistamines, is a depressant of CNS activity and this is usually manifest as sedation. Central excitation may occur following overdosage with the drug.

Pharmacokinetics

The preferred analytical method is gas chromatography, with which the retention time for free pheniramine is 7.0 min.[3] With nitrogen detection, the limit of sensitivity is 50 $\mu g.l^{-1}$.

Like most antihistamines, pheniramine is well absorbed from the gastrointestinal tract. After oral administration peak plasma concentrations are seen at 1–2.5 hours. The terminal half life in serum ranges between 16 and 19 hours after oral ingestion.[4] After a single 75 mg oral dose of Daneril-SA (Avil Retard) in 3 healthy male volunteers, peak serum concentrations of 242–304 $\mu g.l^{-1}$ were reached after 5–8 hours with levels falling back to a mean of 117 $\mu g.l^{-1}$ at 24 h. The mean serum half life was 19 h. About 42% of the dose was excreted in the urine as pheniramine and metabolites. Only low levels of the metabolites were found in serum, although equal amounts of the native drug and N-desmethyl derivative were detected in the urine. The two metabolites, N-desmethylpheniramine and N-didesmethylpheniramine, are only present at low levels in the serum.

The mean total clearance of the drug is about 123 $ml.min^{-1}$ and the systemic volume of distribution is 230 l. No information is available on whether it is bound to plasma protein or its concentrations in the CSF and breast milk. It is not known whether the drug crosses the placenta.

Oral absorption	good
Presystemic metabolism	—
Plasma half life	
range	16–19 h
Volume of distribution	230 l
Plasma protein binding	—

The drug is eliminated both by urinary excretion of the unchanged compound and by hepatic metabolism (>25%), the metabolites being excreted in urine. The effects of hepatic and renal disease, and of old age, on the kinetics of pheniramine have not been reported, though some reduction in clearance is likely in these situations.

Concentration–effect relationship

No data are available on this topic.

Metabolism

In the urine about 33–43% of the total ingested dose of pheniramine is excreted unchanged for up to 5 days.[4] The remainder of the absorbed drug is excreted in the urine as one of the two metabolites, N-desmethylpheniramine and N-didesmethylpheniramine (Fig. 1), with the former present in approximately the same amount as the free drug and the latter making up 0.5–9% of the oral dose.[3,4] After an oral dose of 30.5 mg pheniramine as the free base, the second metabolite, N-didesmethylpheniramine, was recovered in the urine in amounts of only 0.2–0.8 mg.[4] It is not known if these metabolites are biologically active. The drug is not excreted in the bile and there is no evidence for an enterohepatic circulation.

Fig. 1

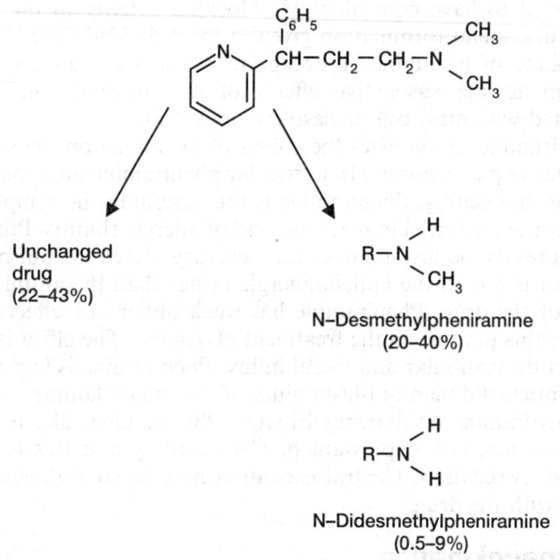

Pharmaceutics

Pheniramine is available in oral forms only. Tablets are constructed in a slow-release form in which pheniramine maleate is embedded in a matrix to allow continuous release of the drug during passage through the gastrointestinal tract. The matrix contains a wax that delays release of the active drug, which is released by diffusion and elution.

Daneral-SA (Hoechst, UK) are unmarked, pink, sugar-coated tablets of 10.3 mm in diameter. Each tablet contains 75 mg of pheniramine maleate. In Australia there is a syrup form available with each 5 ml containing 15 mg of pheniramine maleate (Fenamine syrup). In some countries pheniramine is also available as a para-aminosalicylate salt (Fenamine). In the USA it is combined with phenylephrine (Driston, Whitehall).

Pheniramine should be stored in a cool place and protected from light. The maximum shelf-life is 5 years.

Therapeutic use

Indications

1. Hay fever and perennial rhinitis
2. Vasomotor rhinitis
3. Mild uncomplicated allergic skin reactions — dermatitis, eczema, urticaria, angio-oedema and pruritis of various aetiologies
4. Vertigo.

Contraindications

1. Hypersensitivity to pheniramine
2. Newborn or premature infants. In children it may act as a CNS stimulant
3. Concomitant use of monoamine oxidase inhibitors
4. Pregnant women
5. Prostatic hypertrophy.

In common with many antihistamines, pheniramine may cause drowsiness, especially when taken together with alcohol. Those affected should not drive or operate heavy machinery. The sedative effects of other CNS depressants such as tranquillizers, sedatives and neuroleptic agents may be enhanced. In patients with narrow-angle glaucoma, treatment with pheniramine must be carried out under ophthalmological supervision.

Mode of use

All clinical use depends upon the production of histamine H_1-receptor blockade and possibly additional blockade of CNS muscarinic receptors in the treatment of vertigo.

Oral treatment is recommended as a single dose of 75 or 150 mg of pheniramine maleate at bedtime or twice daily. As there is considerable interindividual variation in effective doses, dosage must be individually adjusted in all cases.

Indications

1. Rhinoconjunctivitis

As a H_1-receptor antagonist, pheniramine maleate is recommended for the symptomatic treatment of seasonal and perennial rhinitis. An open, comparative, crossover study of pheniramine in a conventional tablet formulation and in the Daneral-SA formulation was carried out in 44 patients with symptoms of hay fever.[5] The drug was found to be effective in 42 patients and, of these, 61% expressed a preference for the Daneral-SA formulation. The remaining patients were almost equally divided between those who preferred the conventional tablets and those who expressed no preference. A second comparative, crossover study[6] was performed by the same group in order to determine whether a group of 96 patients with hay fever preferred Daneral-SA or a long-acting form of chlorpheniramine (Piriton spandets). A total of 50% patients preferred Daneral-SA and 40% preferred the chlorpheniramine spandets. The symptoms of hay fever could be controlled by the use of just a single daily dose of Daneral-SA in 24% patients but only 9% patients were controlled on one chlorpheniramine spandet daily. Its efficacy in this condition is improved with the concomitant use of certain sympathomimetic agents such as phenylpropanolamine.[7] More recently, pheniramine (as Daneral-SA) and terfenadine were compared for efficacy and tolerability for 2 weeks in 60 patients with pollinosis.[8] Efficacy was measured in terms of clinical parameters (e.g. sneezing attacks and intensity of rhinorrhoea). The treatment outcome was good or very good in 26 patients in both groups; moderate in 3 cases in the pheniramine group and 2 cases in the terfenadine group; and unsuccessful in 1 case in the pheniramine group and 2 cases in the terfenadine group. Tolerability was reported to be good in 29 cases in each group, moderate in 1 case in the pheniramine group and poor in 1 case in the terfenadine group.

A similar comparative study of Daneral-SA and terfenadine in seasonal allergic rhinitis and pollinosis is also available.[9] 15 patients were randomized to each treatment. Initial doses of two Daneral-SA tablets or 120 mg terfenadine were used. Both drugs were found to be effective in reducing or abolishing symptoms within a few days of starting therapy. Daneral-SA was discontinued by one patient after seven days due to persistent tiredness. It was not necessary to discontinue therapy in any other patients.

In summary, clinical studies of pheniramine in the Daneral-SA formulation have indicated that it is well tolerated and of comparable efficacy to other drugs used for the symptomatic relief of allergic symptoms.

Because pheniramine may cause sedation, it is recommended to take the drug at bedtime.

2. Vasomotor rhinitis

The pathophysiology of this disorder is not known, although histamine may play some role. As with other H_1-receptor antagonists, pheniramine may produce some symptomatic benefit but less than that found in allergic rhinitis. Its weak anticholinergic effect may tend to lessen rhinorrhoea.

3. Allergic skin reactions

Histamine plays an important role in the pathogenesis of urticaria and angio-oedema. By blocking H_1-receptors possibly at nerve endings and capillary endothelium, pheniramine may provide symptomatic relief in such conditions. In a randomized, crossover study,[10] 86 patients with chronic allergic dermatoses, with itching as the predominant symptom, were given pheniramine 25 mg three times daily in a conventional tablet formulation for one week and Daneral-SA once daily for one week. The dose of the slow-release preparation was doubled in 10 patients who showed an inadequate response to the first two treatments.

Both treatments relieved itching in over 90% patients. The incidence of side effects in both groups was comparable and low. The 25 mg tablet corrected sleep disturbances due to itching in 82.5% patients. Daneral-SA corrected sleep disturbances in 96.8% patients and was preferred for this reason. On doubling the dose, the preparation was effective in all 10 patients who had not responded previously, although an increased incidence of side effects was seen. No data are available on the effects of pheniramine in atopic eczema. However, as with other sedating antihistamines, the sedating effect of the drug may help to palliate the itchiness that is frequently present in such conditions.

4. Vertigo
Pheniramine 12.5 mg, in a combined preparation with 25 mg of pentylenetetrazol and 50 mg of nicotinic acid (Ru-Vert), is effective in the symptomatic relief of vertigo associated with labyrinthitis, arteriosclerosis, hypertension, Menière's disease and benign positional vertigo.[11,12]

Contraindications

1. Hypersensitivity to pheniramine
Pheniramine should not be given to patients who have previously developed a hypersensitivity reaction to the drug or any of the alkylamine class of the H_1-receptor antagonists.

2. Newborn or premature infants
Pheniramine is contraindicated in this age-group because of the higher risk of adverse effect such as convulsions.

3. On theoretical considerations, concomitant use of monoamine oxidase inhibitors (MAOI)
MAOI intensify or prolong the anticholinergic effects of antihistamines and therefore pheniramine should be avoided in patients on treatment with these drugs.

4. Pregnant women
As there are few data on the safety of pheniramine in human or animal pregnancy, this drug should be avoided in pregnant women.

5. Prostatic hypertrophy
The anticholinergic activity of pheniramine can lead to urinary retention in patients with benign prostatic hypertrophy.

Adverse reactions

Potentially life-threatening effects
No life-threatening effects related to pheniramine have been reported.

Acute overdosage
Several cases of overdosage have been reported ranging from 30 to 40 mg.kg^{-1} to 1 g in a single dose.[13–16] In some cases the drug had been taken with the aim of producing hallucinations. The majority of the cases involved overdosage in children. Apart from hallucinations the primary symptom is sedation; other expected clinical effects may include inability to concentrate, lassitude, dizziness, palpitations, muscle weakness, toxic psychosis, dryness of mouth, gastrointestinal disturbances, hyperthermia, flushing and dermatitis. There have been two published reports of convulsion in children following overdosage.[13,17]

There is no specific antidote for acute poisoning. Treatment should be symptomatic and supportive. In the case report mentioned above, the child was treated by means of gastric lavage, purgatives, forced diuresis, transperitoneal dialysis and exchange transfusions. Diazepam was given to control seizures and excessive hyperkinesis. Forced diuresis resulted in excretion of larger amounts of pheniramine, transperitoneal dialysis had little effect whereas exchange transfusions facilitated rapid reduction of the high concentration of the drug in the blood.

Severe or irreversible adverse effects
Pheniramine in doses in excess of 300 mg may have a hallucinating effect of varied duration.[17,18]

Symptomatic adverse effects
The most common adverse effect of pheniramine is sedation which varies from slight drowsiness to deep sleep. Inability to concentrate, lassitude, dizziness, muscular weakness and incoordination may also occur. It is advised that patients be cautioned against ingestion of alcohol and engaging in mechanical operations requiring mental alertness. Sedative effects may disappear after a few days if tolerance is acquired. Other CNS effects include nervousness, irritability, insomnia and tremors. Its anticholinergic effects may cause blurred vision, dry mouth, constipation, urinary retention and tachycardia.

Interference with clinical pathology tests
No interferences of this type have been reported.

High risk groups

Neonates
Pheniramine is not recommended in this age-group, because of the higher risk of adverse effects such as convulsions.

Breast milk. The drug is not recommended during breast-feeding, although the concentrations achieved in breast milk are unlikely to be of clinical significance.[19]

Children
Pheniramine is not recommended in children because of its potentially serious CNS effects.

Pregnant women
Contraindicated, since safety of pheniramine has not been thoroughly studied.

The elderly
As with other H_1-receptor antagonists with anticholinergic properties, care should be taken since adverse effects may occur more frequently. Moreover side effects such as dizziness, sedation and hypotension are more likely to occur. Since pheniramine is excreted by the kidneys, it may be necessary to reduce the dose in this age-group.

Drug interactions

Potentially hazardous interactions
Monoamine oxidase inhibitors. These drugs enhance the anticholinergic effects of pheniramine.
CNS depressants. As with other antihistamines, the sedative effect of other CNS depressants may be potentiated.

Potentially useful interactions
No interactions of this kind are known.

Major outcome trials

1. Maddison B, Clements R D, Rivett G C, Roberts R R, Holland E J, Douse F A 1970 A comparative study of two long-acting antihistamines. Journal of the Royal College of General Practitioners 19: 366–368

This is a prospective study to compare the long-acting form of chlorpheniramine (Piriton spandets) with that of pheniramine (Daneral-SA). 104 patients with typical hay fever symptoms commenced the study. In a randomized and cross-over fashion they were given one week's supply of Piriton spandets or an equivalent supply of Daneral-SA tablets. In both cases the patients were instructed to start on a dose of one daily in the morning and add another at night if required. Their comments on efficacy and side effects were recorded after one week's treatment with either of these two drugs.

Results were available on 96 subjects. 46 of them preferred Daneral-SA and of these 50% were adequately controlled on a dose of 1 tablet daily. Of the 34 subjects who preferred Piriton spandets, only 26.5% were adequately controlled on a single daily dose. There was no significant difference between the incidence of drowsiness on these two preparations, nor was there a direct relationship between side effects and dosage. The authors concluded that in the treatment of hay fever in general practice, more patients preferred the longer acting preparation of pheniramine to that of chlorpheniramine.

Other trials

Aaronson A L, Ehrlich N J, Frankel D B, Gutman A A, Aaronson D W 1968 Effective oral nasal decongestion. A double-blind, crossover analysis. Annals of Allergy 26: 145–150

Pou J W, Quinn H J 1966 A clinical study of Ru-Vert in the management of vertigo. Current Therapeutic Research 8: 494–497

References

1. Garg G P, Chaudhury R R 1971 The effect of intraluminally administered drugs on implantation in normal pregnant rats. Journal of Reproduction and Fertility 27: 287–289
2. Subramanyam S, Ganeshan S, Devi P U 1981 Action of anti-allergic agent pheniramine maleate on mammalian and meiotic chromosomes. Indian Journal of Experimental Biology 19: 516–519
3. Kabasakalian P, Taggart M, Townley E 1968 Urinary excretion of pheniramine and its N-demethylated metabolites in man — comparison with chlorpheniramine and bromopheniramine data. Journal of Pharmaceutical Sciences 57: 621–623
4. Witte P U, Irmisch R, Hajdu P 1985 Pharmacokinetics of pheniramine (Avil) and metabolites in healthy subjects after oral and intravenous administration. International Journal of Clinical Pharmacology, Therapy and Toxicology 23: 59–62

5. Maddison B, Clements R D, Rivett G C, Roberts R R, Holland E J, Douse F A 1970 A comparative study of two long-acting antihistamines. Journal of the Royal College of General Practitioners 19: 366–368
6. Maddison B, Clements R D, Rivett G C, Roberts R R, Holland E J, Douse F A 1969 A comparative study of two antihistamines. Journal of the Royal College of General Practitioners 17: 393–395
7. Aaronson A L, Ehrlich N J, Frankel D B, Gutman A A, Aaronson D W 1968 Effective oral nasal decongestion. A double-blind, crossover analysis. Annals of Allergy 26: 145–150
8. Day U, Granin G, Kuhl E D 1985 Pheniramine and terfenadine are equally effective. Arztliche Praxis 37: 841–843
9. Schata M, Hubner R 1985 Comparative study of two antihistamines in seasonal allergic rhinitis. Medizinische Welt 36: 841–843
10. Gupta B N, Gupta R N 1971 Clinical evaluation of a sustained release antihistamine, Avil Retard. Indian Journal of Dermatology and Venereology 1971: 203–208
11. Pou J W, Quinn H J 1966 A clinical study of Ru-Vert in the management of vertigo. Current Therapeutic Research 8: 494–497
12. Herndon J W, Haug O, Horowitz M J, Lynes T E 1975 Benign paradoxical positional vertigo; a clinical study. Annals of Otology, Rhinology and Laryngology 84: 218–222
13. Diekmann L, Hosemann R, Dibbern H E 1972 Pheniramine (Avil) intoxication in a young child. Archives of Toxicology 29: 317–324
14. Bobik A, Mclean A J 1976 Cardiovascular complications due to pheniramine overdosage. Australian and New Zealand Journal of Medicine 6: 65–67
15. Mendelson G 1976 Accidental poisoning: pheniramine. Medical Journal of Australia 2: 110
16. Streat S 1982 Fatal salt poisoning in a child. New Zealand Medical Journal 95: 285–286
17. Jones J H, Stevenson J, Jordan A, Connell H M, Hetherington H D, Gidney G N 1973 Pheniramine as an hallucinogen. Medical Journal of Australia 1: 382–386
18. Csillag E R, Landauer A A 1973 Alleged hallucinogenic effect of a toxic overdose of an antihistamine preparation. Medical Journal of Australia 1: 653–654
19. Catz S, Giacoia G P 1972 Drugs and breast milk. Pediatric Clinics of North America 19: 151–166

Phenobarbitone

Phenobarbitone was introduced into therapeutics over 70 years ago. In the past it was widely used as a sedative and anticonvulsant. At present it is used mainly for the treatment of epilepsy, the barbiturates now being regarded as undesirable sedatives.

Chemistry

Phenobarbitone (phenobarbital, Phenobarb, Luminal, Gardenal)
$C_{12}H_{12}N_2O_3$
5-Ethyl-5-phenylbarbituric acid

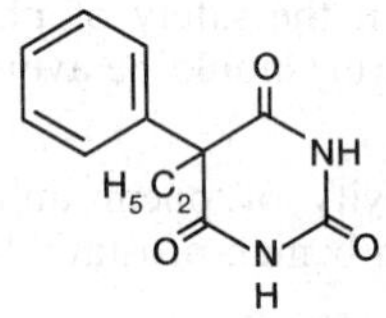

Molecular weight (sodium salt)	232.2 (254.2)
pKa	7.2
Solubility	
in alcohol	1 in 10
in water	1 in 1000
Octanol/water partition coefficient	60

Phenobarbitone is a white crystalline material with a slightly bitter taste. The sodium salt is more water soluble (1 in 3).

Phenobarbitone is marketed in some countries in a fixed-dose combination with phenytoin.

Pharmacology

Phenobarbitone has a widespread depressant action on cerebral function. It has sedative effects and has some protective action against all varieties of human partial and generalized epilepsy, with the exception of absence seizures. Phenobarbitone is also effective in preventing seizures in the corresponding experimental animal models of epilepsy. In different studies phenobarbitone appears to have had inconsistent effects in suppressing experimental epileptic foci, and epileptic after-discharges, but it inhibits synaptic transmission, at least in the spinal cord.[1] The drug's probable biochemical mechanism of action is through prolonging the opening time of Cl^- ion channels in postsynaptic neuronal membranes. This effect causes membrane hyperpolarization and thus impairs nerve impulse propagation. Phenobarbitone also decreases intraneuronal Na^+ concentrations, and inhibits Ca^{2+} influx into depolarized synaptosomes. It raises brain serotonin levels, and inhibits noradrenaline reuptake into synaptosomes. These additional biochemical actions may contribute towards the anticonvulsant effects of the drug.

Toxicology

It has not been possible to trace mutagenicity tests for this drug.

The experimental animal evidence does not establish phenobarbitone as a teratogen.[2] There have been reports that phenobarbitone is a teratogen when given to pregnant human epileptics, though the interpretation of the situation has sometimes been confounded by the intake of other potential teratogens.[3] In humans the reported abnormalities have mainly been facial clefts. One major study failed to find evidence that phenobarbitone was associated with an increased risk of teratogenesis when the drug was used as a sedative in women who did not have epilepsy, yet there appeared to be an increased risk of teratogenesis when the drug was used as an anticonvulsant in pregnant women.[4]

Over seven decades of human use, no suspicion of carcinogenetic potential seems to have become attached to phenobarbitone.

Clinical pharmacology

In humans phenobarbitone is now used mainly as an anticonvulsant. It protects against partial epilepsy, whether or not the seizures undergo secondary generalization. It also protects against convulsive seizures of generalized epilepsy and against myoclonic seizures beginning in adolescence and adult life. Phenobarbitone, if given in sufficient dosage, is an effective prophylactic for benign febrile convulsions of infancy. The drug is still used occasionally as a sedative and minor tranquillizer. It may be employed to enhance bilirubin metabolism in treating certain varieties of jaundice, particularly in neonates.

Pharmacokinetics

Phenobarbitone in biological fluids may be measured by gas–liquid chromatography, high performance liquid chromatography or various forms of immunoassay. However, the latter assays may not always distinguish between phenobarbitone and N-methylphenobarbitone, which is sometimes prescribed as an anticonvulsant and which is biotransformed to phenobarbitone in humans, and also may fail to distinguish between phenobarbitone and its metabolite p-hydroxyphenobarbitone. The limit of detection of all of these methods is 0.5–1 $mg.l^{-1}$.

Phenobarbitone appears to be absorbed completely after oral administration, though data from formal bioavailability studies are not available. Peak plasma levels occur 6–18 hours from oral intake,[5] though shorter times to peak level have been reported.[6] Phenobarbitone is also absorbed satisfactorily from intramuscular and rectal administration sites, peak plasma levels of the drug usually occurring 2–3 hours after intramuscular injection.[7]

The apparent volume of distribution of phenobarbitone[8] is 0.7–1.0 $l.kg^{-1}$, with studies in neonates providing a mean value of 0.97 ± 0.20 $l.kg^{-1}$ for this parameter.[9] Some 50%[10,11] to 59%[12] of the phenobarbitone in plasma is protein bound. The concentration of phenobarbitone in CSF averages between 43 and 52% of that in the plasma,[13] and salivary concentrations are between 30 and 38% of the plasma concentrations (a consequence of the effect of pH differences between plasma and saliva on drug ionization and of binding to plasma proteins).[13] Phenobarbitone concentrations in breast milk are approximately 45% of those in plasma.[14] Phenobarbitone appears to be uniformly distributed throughout the animal body. In humans, brain to plasma phenobarbitone concentration ratios have been in the range 0.59:1[15] to 1.13:1.[16] Neonatal umbilical cord serum phenobarbitone concentrations are 95% of maternal serum concentrations of the drug.

Phenobarbitone elimination follows linear kinetics. In adults the terminal half life is 4 days,[17] but in children it is shorter (37 hours).[18] In the newborn the mean half life is 115 hours at the end of the first postnatal week, and 67 hours by the end of the fourth postnatal week.[9] The plasma clearance of the drug declines from about 0.012 $l.kg^{-1}.h^{-1}$ in young children to 0.004 $l.kg^{-1}.h^{-1}$ in adolescents.[19] Phenobarbitone is metabolized in the liver and excreted largely in the urine. Figures vary for the percentage of the dose excreted unchanged (25%[20] to 67%[21]).

The elimination of the parent compound in urine increases with increasing pH and volume of the urine.

The half life of phenobarbitone is increased in liver disease, as a consequence of decreased metabolism. Patients with hepatic dysfunction may thus require some dosage adjustment.

Oral absorption	>90%
Presystemic metabolism	nil
Plasma half life	
range	50–150 h
mean	100 h
Volume of distribution	0.7 $l.kg^{-1}$
Plasma protein binding	50%

The clearance of phenobarbitone decreases with age and may well be reduced in renal disease.

Concentration–effect relationship

Plasma phenobarbitone concentrations below 10 $mg.l^{-1}$ (40 $\mu M.l^{-1}$) are often ineffective in controlling epilepsy of susceptible type[17] and concentrations around 20 $mg.l^{-1}$ (80 $\mu mol.l^{-1}$) may be required to prevent seizures when the disorder is severe.[22] The upper limit of the therapeutic range of plasma phenobarbitone concentration is not sharply defined, to some extent because the development of drug-induced sedation, which ultimately limits dosage, is often insidious. An upper limit to the therapeutic range of 30 $mg.l^{-1}$ (120 $\mu mol.l^{-1}$) is sometimes used, but some patients after weeks or months of intake tolerate plasma phenobarbitone concentrations of 40–50 $mg.l^{-1}$ (160–200 $\mu mol.l^{-1}$) without undue drowsiness and with improved seizure control. Plasma phenobarbitone concentrations of the order of 100 $mg.l^{-1}$ (400 $\mu mol.l^{-1}$) are likely to be associated with stupor. Plasma phenobarbitone concentrations should be interpreted in the light of the marked tolerance that is seen with this drug in long-term use.

It is clear that plasma phenobarbitone levels must be above 15 $mg.l^{-1}$ (60 $\mu mol.l^{-1}$) to prevent febrile convulsions in infants.[23,24]

Metabolism

The majority of a phenobarbitone dose cannot be accounted for in urine as unchanged drug, and is therefore probably eliminated by metabolism.[20] Known phenobarbitone metabolites fail to account for all of the outstanding fraction of the dose. Most of the identified metabolites are oxidation products, due to hepatic mono-oxygenase activity.[25] The main oxidized metabolite is a phenolic derivative, p-hydroxyphenobarbitone, arising presumably from initial arene oxide formation, but there are also catechol and a 5-hydroxyethyl derivative. A 1-N-glucoside metabolite has been identified (which was originally identified as an N-hydroxy derivative) and this may account for as much as 30% of the dose.[26] Phenobarbitone is a potent inducer of drug oxidation primarily through an increase in P450 IIIA, and glucuronidation. This can lead to interactions with other drugs increasing their elimination.

Pharmaceutics

Phenobarbitone and sodium phenobarbitone are both available in many countries as 15, 30, 60 and 100 mg tablets. Sodium phenobarbitone is available in ampoules for parenteral use: 30 mg in 1 ml, 65 mg in 1 ml and 130 mg in 1 ml (USA) and 200 mg in 1 ml (UK). The vehicle is 90% propylene glycol and should be sterilized by heating at 99°C for 30 minutes. The pH of the injection is 10–11.

The shelf-life of phenobarbitone tablets is 3 years, and that of sodium phenobarbitone ampoules 15 months, stored in the dark below 25°C.

Therapeutic use

Indications

Although phenobarbitone may sometimes still be used as a sedative and minor tranquillizer, the various benzodiazepines have largely supplanted it in these roles. The main contemporary indication for phenobarbitone is the treatment of epilepsy. The drug is effective in the prevention of

1. Partial seizures, whether or not they become secondarily generalized
2. Generalized epilepsy, if manifesting as tonic–clonic or tonic seizures, or as myoclonic seizures (but only if beginning in adolescence or later life)
3. Benign febrile convulsions of infancy.

The drug is sometimes prescribed with the aim of inducing the liver glucuronyl transferase to increase the conjugation of bilirubin. This may reduce the severity of toxicity of unconjugated bilirubin, as in neonatal jaundice or Gilbert's syndrome.

Contraindications

Absolute

1. Known hypersensitivity to phenobarbitone, or to a drug metabolized to phenobarbitone (primidone or N-methylphenobarbitone)
2. Acute intermittent porphyria

Relative
3. The elderly
4. Persons with hepatic insufficiency
5. Those in whom sedation is undesirable.

Mode of use

Phenobarbitone is usually given by mouth once or twice daily. The slow elimination of phenobarbitone means that there is little fluctuation in its steady-state plasma levels across a dosage interval of as long as 24 hours. However, it requires approximately 2 weeks after a phenobarbitone dosage change for a new steady state to apply. To allow time for the development of tolerance to sedation produced by the drug, it is often preferable to commence therapy with phenobarbitone in about half the expected daily dose, and to increase the dose after some 2 or 3 weeks, the extent of the increase being guided by plasma phenobarbitone concentration measurement. With each subsequent dose increment plasma phenobarbitone levels tend to rise more than would be expected from their behaviour in relation to the previous dose increment.[27] In treating epilepsy the initial aim of phenobarbitone therapy should be to achieve a plasma phenobarbitone concentration in the therapeutic range for the drug unless the clinical response indicates that a satisfactory therapeutic effect has already been attained. The mean phenobarbitone dose to achieve a therapeutic range plasma phenobarbitone level of 15 $mg.l^{-1}$ (60 $\mu mol.l^{-1}$) is 3.1 $mg.kg^{-1}$ (for children 1 month to 4 years old), 2–3 $mg.kg^{-1}$ (for children 4–14 years old), 1.75 $mg.kg^{-1}$ (for persons 14–40 years old) and 0.9 $mg.kg^{-1}$ (for persons over 40 years of age).[27] If epilepsy is not controlled with plasma phenobarbitone levels in the therapeutic range for the drug, the phenobarbitone dose may still be increased cautiously until seizures are controlled, or until the side effects of therapy become unacceptable or more troublesome to the patient than the seizures are.

Intramuscular phenobarbitone may be given to substitute for oral phenobarbitone, on a mg for mg basis. Phenobarbitone is not often administered intravenously, possibly because of fear of the protracted problems that might arise from accidental overdosage of a drug which is very slowly eliminated.

Adverse reactions

Several accounts of the unwanted effects of phenobarbitone are available.[28,29,30,31,32,33,34]

Potentially life-threatening effects

Widespread exfoliative dermatitis, agranulocytosis, aplastic anaemia, and hepatitis are rare but severe reported unwanted effects of phenobarbitone.

Acute overdosage

Severe phenobarbitone overdosage may cause sedation, stupor, coma and finally death through respiratory and circulatory failure.

Forced alkaline diuresis (e.g. by giving an adult 12 to 24 litres of fluid each 24 hours with enough sodium bicarbonate to keep the urine pH in the range 7.5 to 8.0), haemodialysis, or charcoal haemoperfusion may be used in treatment together with appropriate supportive measures.

Severe or irreversible adverse effects

The main consequences of chronic phenobarbitone overdosage arise from sedation. This usually causes a degree of intellectual dulling and drowsiness but some chronically overdosed patients may become depressed, or irritable and aggressive, or confused, and some develop headaches. Paradoxically children may sometimes become hyperac-

Fig. 1 Pathways of phenobarbitone metabolism

(1) phenobarbitone (5-phenyl-5-ethyl barbituric acid) (2) p-hydroxyphenobarbitone (5-(p-hydroxyphenyl)-5-ethyl barbituric acid) (3) dihydrodiol metabolite (5-(3,4-dihydroxy-1,5-cyclohexadiene-1-yl)-5-ethyl barbituric acid) (4) catechol metabolite (5-(3,4-dihydroxyphenyl)-5-ethyl barbituric acid) (5) hydroxyethyl metabolite (5-phenyl-5-hydroxyethyl barbituric acid) (6) phenobarbitone-N-glucoside (7) α-phenyl-γ-butyrolactone

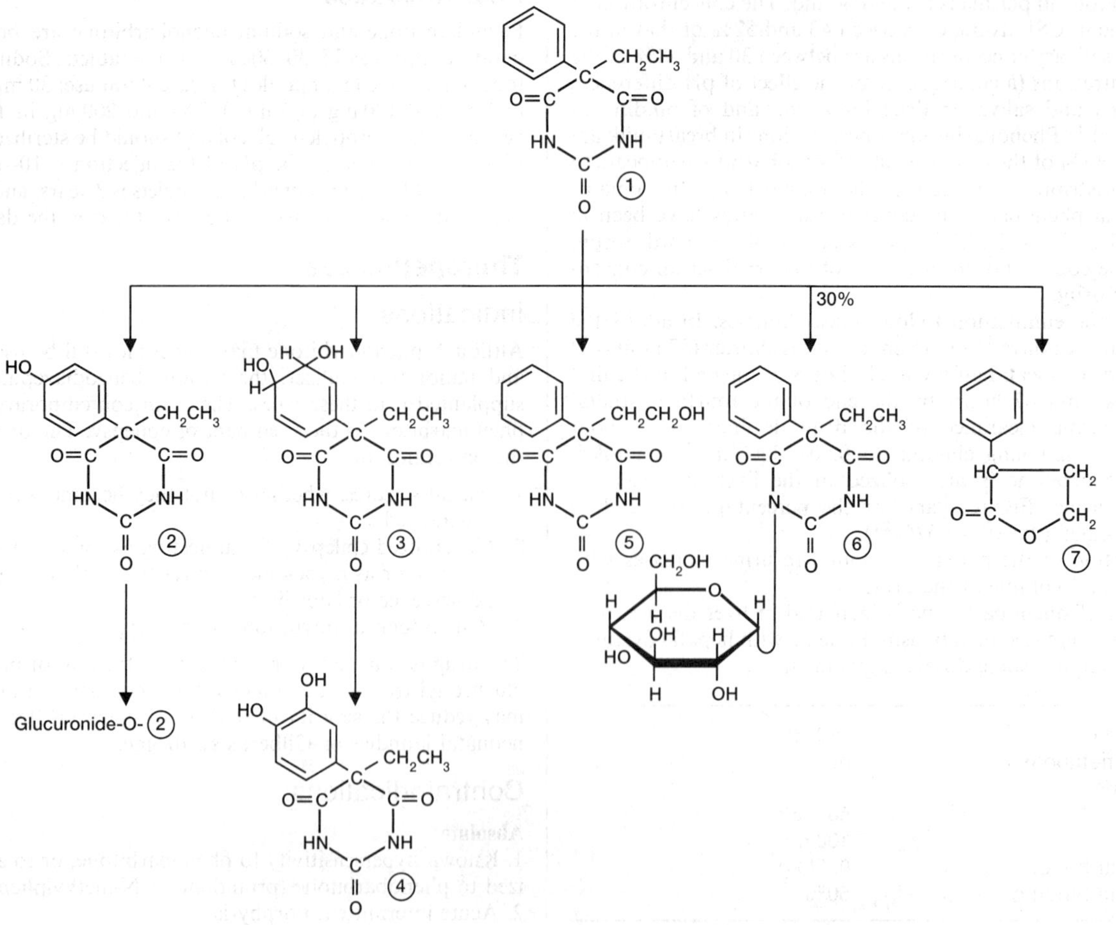

tive. Rather more severe overdosage may cause nystagmus and ataxia of gait, and increasing degrees of clouding of consciousness. The effects of severe overdosage are described above. Minimal overdosage may produce an almost unnoticed slow decline in intellectual performance, which in children is often manifested as a gradual deterioration in school results.

In continued use phenobarbitone may rarely be responsible for macrocytic anaemia, hypocalcaemia and osteomalacia, and possibly Dupuytren's contracture.

Symptomatic adverse effects

Phenobarbitone occasionally causes a variety of skin rashes, usually fine punctate erythema but sometimes morbilliform.

Other effects

Continued phenobarbitone administration induces the liver mono-oxygenase system.[35] This induction causes reduced plasma levels of bilirubin, endogenous steroids, folate, bile salts, cholesterol and lipids. Plasma gamma glutamyl transpeptidase and alkaline phosphatase activities are often raised. D-glutamic acid excretion in urine is increased. In some infants blood and CSF glutamine and ornithine levels may be raised.

Interference with clinical pathology tests

Phenobarbitone intake does not appear to interfere with commonly used laboratory methods.

High risk groups

Neonates

Neonates may require 5–6 $mg.kg^{-1}$ daily of phenobarbitone to achieve a lower limit therapeutic range plasma drug level of 15 $mg.l^{-1}$ (60 $\mu mol.l^{-1}$).[36] However, such phenobarbitone doses may produce double this plasma level in the first few postnatal days, with the drug concentrations then taking 3 weeks to decline to 15 $mg.l^{-1}$ as the clearance capacity for the drug rises in the first postnatal month.

Breast milk. Phenobarbitone is excreted in breast milk, in which its concentration averages 45% of the whole-plasma concentration of the drug. The usual maternal milk intake of an infant is unlikely to be sufficient for the phenobarbitone content to affect the infant clinically, so long as the mother is not herself overdosed with the drug.

Children

Children under 4 years of age require average phenobarbitone doses of 3.1 $mg.kg^{-1}$, and older children average doses of 2.3 $mg.kg^{-1}$, to achieve a plasma phenobarbitone level of 15 $mg.l^{-1}$ (60 $\mu mol.l^{-1}$).[27]

Pregnant women

Phenobarbitone dosage has to be increased during pregnancy to maintain plasma phenobarbitone levels at their pre-pregnancy values, and thus to decrease the risk of seizures worsening in pregnancy.[37] Intake of phenobarbitone in pregnancy may lead to hypoprothrombinaemia and a bleeding tendency in the neonate.[38] Infants born to mothers who have taken phenobarbitone during pregnancy may exhibit certain withdrawal phenomena (hypotonia, irritability and a tendency to vomit).[39]

The elderly

Phenobarbitone clearance diminishes in the elderly. Relative to body weight, the mean dose to achieve a therapeutic range plasma level of 15 $mg.l^{-1}$ (60 $\mu mol.l^{-1}$) in persons over 40 years of age is only half that required in younger adults.[27]

Drug interactions

Several accounts of the known pharmacokinetic-type interactions involving phenobarbitone are available.[13,28,40,41,42,43]

Potentially hazardous interactions

During chronic administration of phenobarbitone considerable induction of the hepatic mixed function oxidase enzymes occurs. If another drug is co-administered whose action is terminated by metabolism by these enzymes, a higher dose will be required to maintain its effect. Cessation of phenobarbitone intake allows activity of the hepatic mono-oxygenase system to decline over a period of 14–21 days. This problem has been particularly well studied with coumarin anticoagulants such as warfarin. It is commonplace for the dose requirement to change by a factor of two and much larger changes have been described. If the anticoagulant dosage is not adjusted downwards when phenobarbitone is withdrawn, serious haemorrhage may occur. A ketogenic diet (sometimes used in treating resistant myoclonic seizures in childhood) raises plasma phenobarbitone levels.[44] Excess alcohol and phenobarbitone would be expected to interact additively to cause increased sedation.

Combination of phenobarbitone with other drugs with sedative properties may occasionally produce a dangerous degree of depression of consciousness.

Other significant interactions

Hepatic mono-oxygenase induction resulting from continued phenobarbitone intake may increase the metabolism, and therefore reduce the plasma levels of cortisol, folate, aminopyrine, antipyrine, bishydroxycoumarin, carbamazepine, chloramphenicol, dicophane (DDT), digitoxin, dipyrone, doxycycline, griseofulvin, nortriptyline, phenylbutazone, phenytoin (inconsistently), valproate and warfarin. Phenytoin, phenylacetylurea and, particularly, valproate intake may cause raised plasma phenobarbitone levels, while frusemide intake raises phenobarbitone levels slightly. Administered folate, pyridoxine, dicoumarol and phenylbutazone cause lowering of plasma phenobarbitone levels.

Potentially useful interactions

Induction of glucuronyl transferase by phenobarbitone, which leads to lowered plasma bilirubin levels by enhancing bilirubin clearance, can be utilized therapeutically in the treatment of certain forms of neonatal jaundice (which are due in part to immature liver function).

Major outcome trials

Phenobarbitone has been widely used to treat epilepsy for over 60 years. Its clinical efficacy became evident long before carefully designed placebo-controlled clinical trials came into widespread use. The results of earlier clinical studies on the efficacy of phenobarbitone as an antiepileptic agent are summarized in Coatsworth J J 1971 Studies on the clinical efficacy of marketed antiepileptic drugs. NINDS Monograph No 12.

General review articles

Eadie M J, Tyrer J H 1989 Anticonvulsant therapy, 3rd edn. Churchill Livingstone, Edinburgh

Frey H-H, Janz D (eds) 1985 Antiepileptic drugs. Handbook of experimental pharmacology, vol 74. Springer, Berlin

Glaser G H, Penry J K, Woodbury D M (eds) 1980 Antiepileptic drugs: mechanisms of action. Raven Press, New York

Johanessen S I 1981 Antiepileptic drugs: pharmacokinetic and clinical aspects. Therapeutic Drug Monitoring 3: 17–37

Pippenger C E, Penry J K, Kutt H (eds) 1978 Antiepileptic drugs: quantitative analysis and interpretation. Raven Press, New York

Richens A 1976 Drug treatment of epilepsy. Henry Kimpton, London

Schneider H, Janz D, Gardner-Thorpe C, Meinardi H, Sherwin A L (eds) 1975 Clinical pharmacology of anti-epileptic drugs. Springer, Berlin

Snead O C III 1983 On the sacred disease: the neurochemistry of epilepsy. International Review of Neurobiology 24: 93–180

Levy R H, Dreifuss F E, Mattson R H, Meldrum B S, Penry J K (eds) 1989 Antiepileptic drugs, 3rd edn. Raven Press, New York

References

1. Esplin D W 1963 Criteria for assessing effects of depressant drugs on spinal cord synaptic transmission, with examples of drug selectivity. Archives of International Pharmacodynamics 143: 479–497
2. Staples R E 1972 Teratology. In: Woodbury D M, Penry J P, Schmidt R P (eds) Antiepileptic drugs. Raven Press, New York, pp 55–62
3. Meadow S R 1970 Congenital abnormalities and anticonvulsant drugs. Proceedings of the Royal Society of Medicine 63: 48–49
4. Shapiro S, Hartz S C, Siskind V et al 1976 Anticonvulsants and parental epilepsy in the development of birth defects. Lancet 1: 272–275
5. Lous P 1954 Blood serum and cerebrospinal fluid levels and renal clearance of Phenemal in treated epileptics. Acta Pharmacologica et Toxicologica 10: 166–177
6. Wilensky A J, Friel P N, Levy R H, Comfort C P, Kaluzny S P 1982 Kinetics of phenobarbital in normal subjects and epileptic patients. European Journal of Clinical Pharmacology 23: 87–92

7. Boreus L O, Jalling B, Kallberg N 1975 Clinical pharmacology of phenobarbital in the neonatal period. In: Morselli P L, Garrattini S, Sereni F (eds) Basic and therapeutic aspects of perinatal pharmacology. Raven Press, New York, pp 331–340
8. Hvidberg E F, Dam M 1976 Clinical pharmacokinetics of anticonvulsants. Clinical Pharmacokinetics 1: 161–188
9. Pitlick W, Painter M, Pippenger C 1978 Phenobarbital pharmacokinetics in neonates. Clinical Pharmacology and Therapeutics 23: 111–115
10. Waddell W J, Butler T C 1957 The distribution and excretion of phenobarbital. Journal of Clinical Investigation 36: 1217–1226
11. Johanessen S I, Strandjord R E 1975 Absorption and protein binding in serum of several anti-epileptic drugs. In: Schneider H, Janz D, Gardner-Thorpe C, Meinardi H, Sherwin A L (eds) Clinical pharmacology of antiepileptic drugs. Springer, Berlin, pp 262–273
12. McAuliffe J J, Sherwin A L, Leppik I E, Fayle S A, Pippenger C E 1977 Salivary levels of anticonvulsants: a practical approach to drug monitoring. Neurology 27: 409–413
13. Eadie M J 1984 Anticonvulsant drugs. An update. Drugs 27: 328–363
14. Kaneko S, Sato T, Suzuki K 1979 The level of anticonvulsants in breast milk. British Journal of Clinical Pharmacology 7: 624–627
15. Vajda F, Williams F M, Davidson S, Falconer M A, Breckenridge A 1974 Human brain, cerebrospinal fluid and plasma concentrations of diphenylhydantoin and phenobarbital. Clinical Pharmacology and Therapeutics 15: 597–603
16. Houghton G W, Richens A, Toseland P A, Davidson S, Falconer M A 1975 Brain concentrations of phenytoin, phenobarbitone and primidone in epileptic patients. European Journal of Clinical Pharmacology 9: 73–78
17. Buchthal F, Lennox-Buchthal M A 1972 Phenobarbital. Relation of serum concentration to control of seizures. In: Woodbury D M, Penry J K, Schmidt R P (eds) Antiepileptic drugs. Raven Press, New York, pp 335–343
18. Garrettson L K, Dayton P G 1970 Disappearance of phenobarbital and diphenylhydantoin from serum of children. Clinical Pharmacology and Therapeutics 11: 674–679
19. Guelen P J M, Van der Kleijn E, Woudstra U 1975 Statistical analysis of pharmacokinetic parameters in epileptic patients chronically treated with antiepileptic drugs. In: Schneider H, Janz D, Gardner-Thorpe C, Meinardi H, Sherwin A L (eds) Clinical pharmacology of anti-epileptic drugs. Springer, Berlin, pp 2–10
20. Whyte M P, Dekaban A S 1977 Metabolic fate of phenobarbital. A quantitative study of p-hydroxyphenobarbital elimination in man. Drug Metabolism and Distribution 5: 63–70
21. Butler T C, Makafee C, Waddell W J 1954 Phenobarbital: studies of elimination, accumulation, tolerance and dosage schedules. Journal of Pharmacology and Experimental Therapeutics 111: 425–435
22. Buchthal F, Svensmark O 1959 Aspects of the pharmacology of phenytoin (Dilantin) and phenobarbital relevant to their dosage in the treatment of epilepsy. Epilepsia 1: 373–384
23. Faero O, Kastrup K W, Lykkegaard Neilsen E, Melchior J C, Thorn I 1972 Successful prophylaxis of febrile convulsions with phenobarbital. Epilepsia 13: 279–285
24. Thorn I 1975 A controlled study of prophylactic long-term treatment of febrile convulsions with phenobarbital. Acta Neurologica Scandinavica (suppl 60): 67–73
25. Eadie M J 1968 Metabolism of anticonvulsant drugs. Reviews on Drug Metabolism and Drug Interaction 3: 317–347
26. Tang B K, Kalow W, Grey A A 1979 Metabolic fate of phenobarbital in man. N-glucoside formation. Drug Metabolism and Disposition 7: 315–318
27. Eadie M J, Lander C M, Hooper W D, Tyrer J H 1977 Factors influencing plasma phenobarbitone levels in epileptic patients. British Journal of Clinical Pharmacology 4: 541–547
28. Eadie M J, Tyrer J H 1989 Anticonvulsant therapy. Pharmacological basis and practice, 3rd edn. Churchill Livingstone, Edinburgh
29. Eadie M J 1980 Unwanted effects of anticonvulsant drugs. In: Tyrer J H (ed) The treatment of epilepsy. MTP Press, Lancaster, pp 129–160
30. Booker H E 1975 Idiosyncratic reactions to the antiepileptic drugs. Epilepsia 16: 171–181
31. Plaa G L 1975 Acute toxicity of antiepileptic drugs. Epilepsia 16: 183–191
32. Reynolds E H 1975 Chronic antiepileptic toxicity: a review. Epilepsia 16: 319–352
33. Mattson R H, Cramer J A 1982 Phenobarbital. Toxicity. In: Woodbury D M, Penry J K, Pippenger C E (eds) Antiepileptic drugs, 2nd edn. Raven Press, New York, pp 351–363
34. Schmidt D 1985 Adverse effects. In: Frey H-H, Janz D (eds) Antiepileptic drugs. Springer, Berlin, pp 791–829
35. Conney A H 1967 Pharmacological implications of microsomal enzyme induction. Pharmacology Reviews 19: 317–366
36. Pippenger C E, Rosen T S 1975 Phenobarbital pharmacokinetics in neonates. Clinics in Perinatology 2: 111–115
37. Lander C M, Edwards V E, Eadie M J, Tyrer J H 1977 Plasma anticonvulsant concentrations during pregnancy. Neurology 27: 128–131
38. Mountain K R, Hirsch J, Gallus A S 1970 Neonatal coagulation defect due to anticonvulsant drug treatment in pregnancy. Lancet 1: 265–268
39. Erith M J 1975 Withdrawal symptoms in newborn infants of epileptic mothers. British Medical Journal 3: 40
40. Richens A 1977 Interactions with antiepileptic drugs. Drugs 13: 266–275
41. Perucca E, Richens A 1980 Anticonvulsant drug interactions. In: Tyrer J H (ed) The treatment of epilepsy. MTP Press, Lancaster, pp 95–128
42. Perucca E 1982 Pharmacokinetic interactions 7: 57–84
43. Perucca E, Richens A 1985 Antiepileptic drug interactions. In: Frey H-H, Janz D (eds) Antiepileptic drugs. Springer, Berlin, pp 831–855
44. Livingstone S 1972 Comprehensive management of epilepsy in infancy, childhood and adolescence. Charles C Thomas, Springfield

Phenol

Phenol is a general protoplasmic poison that is used as a disinfectant. Although it has been used in a variety of clinical indications its toxicity is such that it should be used with extreme caution.

Chemistry

Phenol
C_6H_5OH
Hydroxybenzene

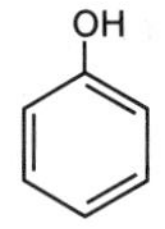

Molecular weight	94.1
pKa	10.0
Solubility	
in alcohol	very soluble
in water	1 in 15
Octanol/water partition coefficient	—

Phenol is an easily liquifiable crystal. Liquified phenol is a solution of 80% w/w phenol in water. It is a faintly coloured caustic liquid with characteristic odour. It is miscible with alcohol, ether and glycerol and with an equal volume of glycerol is miscible with water.[1]

It should be stored in an airtight container and protected from light. It may congeal or deposit crystals if stored below 4°C.

Pharmacology

When used in low concentrations, 0.5 to 1% aqueous solution, it is antipruritic through an effect on pain receptors. At higher concentrations (up to 80%) it acts as a protein precipitant when applied to body tissues.[2]

As a disinfectant it is active against vegetative Gram-positive and Gram-negative bacteria, but only slowly effective against spores and acid-fast bacilli. Its activity is affected by the presence of organic matter. Solutions up to 1% are bacteriostatic and above 1% bacteriocidal.[1] Solutions above 1.3% are fungicidal.

Toxicology

The US National Cancer Institute carried out tests for possible carcinogenicity in F344 rats and B6C3F1 mice in 1980.[3] The conclusion of the study was that under the conditions of the bioassay, phenol was not carcinogenic for either male or female B6C3F1 mice.

Teratogenicity and reproductive toxicity studies include earlier work by Heller and Pursell in 1938[4] and Minor and Becker in 1971,[5] as well as more recent and complete studies by Jones-Price et al in 1983.[6,7] In the Jones-Price studies, there was no evidence for a teratogenic effect of phenol in CD rats. Neither was there any statistically significant evidence for a teratogenic effect of phenol in the main teratology study in CD-I mice. In the preliminary range-finding study in mice, there was some evidence of an increased incidence of malformations, but only at high doses (up to 400 mg.kg^{-1}) when maternal toxicity, sometimes severe, was noted. Phenol is extremely toxic if systemic absorption occurs, and a number of deaths have been reported following its use. The toxic dose for adults has been estimated at between 8 and 15 g.[8]

Clinical pharmacology

Phenol is rarely used as a therapeutic agent today. Its use as a local caustic agent can lead to systemic toxic manifestations and even death (see refs 15 and 16). Application of concentrations above 0.5% cause a depolarizing local anaesthetic effect. Higher concentrations cause epidermal separation and necrosis. Its main use relates to its antibacterial effect.[2]

Pharmacokinetics

The preferred method of analysis in blood is by capillary column gas chromatography.[9] A semi-quantitative method for analysis in urine has also been described.[10]

Phenol is readily absorbed through intact skin, mucous membranes and the gastrointestinal tract. It is metabolized to phenyl glucuronide and phenyl sulphate. Small amounts are oxidized to catechol and quinol which are mainly conjugated. These metabolites are excreted in the urine which may turn green on standing.[1]

Phenol in vapour form can be absorbed via the respiratory tract and skin.[1] Concentrations applied locally in excess of 5% cause protein coagulation and are less readily absorbed.

Blood levels of 6.8 $mg.l^{-1}$ have been recorded one hour after application of 2 ml of 50% solution to the face and levels of 4 $mg.l^{-1}$ have been found after applications of 2% phenol in calamine lotion.[2]

99% of an absorbed dose was found to have been excreted in the urine in 24 hours.[1] The effects of hepatic and renal disease on metabolism and excretion are not documented.

Concentration–effect relationship

Not relevant.

Metabolism

In the liver, phenol is conjugated with glucuronide and sulphate, and is also oxidized in small amounts to catechol and quinol (Fig. 1). All metabolites are excreted in the urine.

Fig. 1 Metabolism of phenol

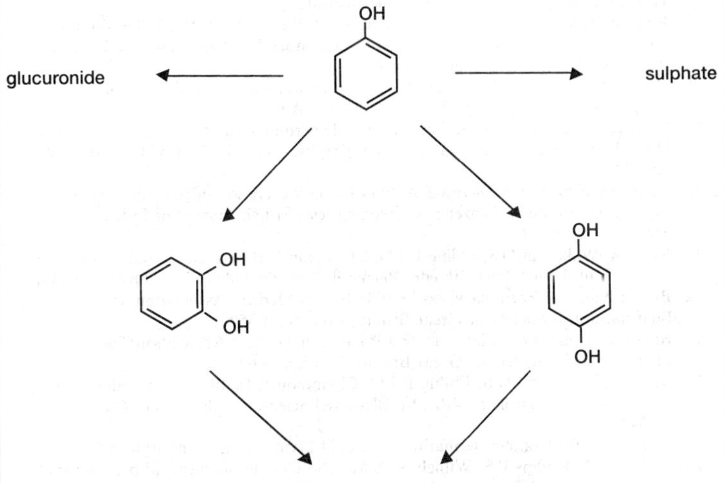

Pharmaceutics

Liquified phenol has been used in both dermatology and plastic surgery for its local caustic action.[2,11]

As a phenol gargle. Phenol glycerin 5% to be diluted with equal volumes of warm water.[12] A 1.4% solution has also been used as a mouthwash and gargle.[23]

For sclerotherapy of haemorrhoids, it is available as an oily injection phenol 5% in almond oil.[13]

It is present as a 4% aqueous solution as a constituent of Magenta paint (Castellani's paint).[2]

As a neurolytic agent it is used as a 5% w/w solution in glycerol, which has been given intrathecally. 6% aqueous solutions of phenol have been used for chemical sympathectomies.[1]

Solutions of up to 2% often in calamine lotion have been used as an antipruritic,[14] though their use has declined with the advent of antihistamines.

Phenol, when used as a preservative in cosmetics, has been responsible for a contact dermatitis.[15] This use is now restricted in the UK.[1] Phenol interacts with resorcinol and formulations should not be prepared using utensils containing iron.

Therapeutic use

Indications

The use of phenol for these indications has been largely superseded.

1. As a local caustic agent
2. As a local antiseptic and throat gargle
3. For sclerotherapy of haemorrhoids
4. For use locally in pain relief
5. As an antipruritic agent.

Contraindications

1. Children (particularly neonates)
2. Application to large areas, particularly under occlusion.

Mode of use

Varies with the intended therapeutic use.

Indications

1. Caustic agent

It is still used as a chemical peeling agent. However, there is increasing awareness of its toxicity, and it should only be used with caution by experienced personnel.[16] Diluting the application may increase its absorption. Cardiotoxicity may develop acutely during use. Rhythm disturbances including ventricular fibrillation may occur and cardiac monitoring is recommended, during and following the procedure.[17] Only small areas at a time should be treated.

Liquified phenol has been recommended for the treatment of molluscum contagiosum applied to a lesion with a sharpened stick;[18] it has also been used to ablate the nail matrix following the removal of ingrowing toe nails. Its toxicity is such that it should be used with extreme caution.[19]

2. Antisepsis and throat gargle

Its use as a topical antiseptic has decreased following reports of toxicity and deaths and it should no longer be used for this purpose.[20] Significant systemic absorption has been demonstrated and deaths have occurred in children.[2,21]

It is available as a 4% aqueous solution in Magenta paint (Castellani's paint) for the treatment of superficial mycological infection but there are now more effective and much safer alternatives. Significant absorption and urinary excretion of phenol from this has been demonstrated and its use in children is not advised.[22]

As an antiseptic mouth gargle, phenol glycerin 5% to be diluted with equal volumes of warm water[12] has been found effective when compared with placebo[23] but can no longer be recommended.

3. Sclerotherapy

In the form of a 5% phenol solution in oil (usually almond oil) it is used for sclerotherapy of haemorrhoids.[24] Complications include local ulceration and sterile abscess formation. A maximum of 10 ml at one treatment is recommended.[13]

4. Pain relief

In the relief of intractable pain, especially when due to malignant disease, it is used as a nerve-blocking and neurolytic agent.[1] It can also be given intrathecally to relieve spasticity. It is used in the relief of a variety of disorders in pain clinics.[25] There is a report of accidental paraplegia following coeliac axis block with 6% aqueous phenol solution.[26]

A 1.4% solution has been used as a gargle or spray for local relief of sore throat.[23]

5. Antipruritic

Its use has decreased with the availability of antihistamines and reports of toxicity[20] especially when applied under occlusive bandages or dressings.

Contraindications

1. Children

Significant absorption of phenol has been shown to occur in infants.[22]

P

2. Application of large areas particularly under occlusion
Application to large areas of skin, particularly wounds, has resulted in signs of toxicity, particularly if this has been done under occlusive dressings.[20]

Adverse reactions

Potentially life-threatening effects
Significant absorption of phenol has been shown to occur through the skin[2] even from small areas treated in infants[22] and death has occurred on several occasions.[20,21] When applied in dilute solutions to extensive wounds, abdominal pains, dizziness, cyanosis, methaemoglobin formation, haemoglobinuria and coma have occurred.[27] Repeated applications of 1% solutions have caused dizziness and collapse.[20]

The management of accidental spillage on the skin includes removal of all contaminated clothes and rubbing contaminated skin for at least ten minutes with swabs soaked in glycerol, a liquid macrogol or a mixture of 70% macrogol 30% methylated spirits. Water can be used initially if these are not immediately available.[1]

Acute overdosage
Symptoms of toxicity from absorption via the skin are detailed above and, apart from local measures, only symptomatic treatment is available.

Symptoms of oral ingestion include local pain and vomiting, followed by pulmonary oedema and shock. Fatal respiratory failure may rapidly occur. Cautious gastric aspiration and lavage using olive oil may remove any drug that remains in the stomach.[28] Further measures including assisted ventilation are mainly symptomatic. Activated charcoal is reported as an effective absorbent in acute poisoning.[29] Correction of fluid and electrolyte balance are crucial and peritoneal dialysis may be of value in preventing a precipitous rise in serum potassium. This will not remove significant amounts of phenol. Levels of total blood phenols greater than 10 $mg.l^{-1}$ have serious prognostic significance but no fatal levels are recorded.[30]

Severe or irreversible adverse effects
Many of the side effects of phenol have been related to its caustic activity, particularly in more concentrated solutions.

Symptomatic adverse effects
Dizziness and collapse have been recorded after applications to extensive areas or wounds.

The prolonged use of phenol-containing dressings has given rise to exogenous ochronosis with darkening of the cornea and skin of the face.[31]

Interference with clinical pathology tests
Phenol absorbed through the skin may interfere with the trihydroxyindole method of estimating plasma adrenaline and noradrenaline; the ferric chloride test for ketones or salicylates in urine (but not the Phenistix test); tests for ionized calcium in serum; measurement of sulphonamides in serum; and the Benedict test for glycosuria.

High risk groups

Neonates
The use of any phenolic preparation in neonates is contraindicated.

Breast milk. No information is available on whether or not phenol absorbed through the skin of the mother enters breast milk, but lactating mothers should either not breast-feed or should avoid the use of preparations containing phenols.

Children
What has been said about neonates also applies to older children.

Pregnant women
The use of phenol is probably best avoided during pregnancy.

The elderly
There are no specific contraindications to use of phenol in the elderly apart from its general hazards.

Drug interactions

No significant interactions have been reported.

Major outcome trials

1. Valle Jones J C 1983 Chloraseptic liquid in sore throats. Practitioner 227: 1037–1039

This was a prospective study to assess the efficacy of phenol gargle. 100 patients with non-bacterial sore throats were randomly given phenol gargle or a placebo prescribed five times a day. The treated group at three days reported a significant decrease in pyrexia, incidence of headache and degree of pain compared to the placebo group.

2. Sim A J, Mure J A, Mackenzie I 1983 Three year follow-up study on the treatment of first and second degree haemorrhoids by sclerosant injection or rubber band ligation. Surgery, Gynaecology and Obstetrics 157: 534–537

This was a review of two groups of 18 patients with first or mild second degree haemorrhoids who had been randomly treated with either sclerotherapy or rubber band ligation. At three-year follow-up, any history of further bleeding was noted. Of the 18 treated with sclerotherapy, only four had remained free of further bleeding episodes but of the 18 treated with rubber band ligation, 13 had remained free of further bleeding. The authors concluded that rubber band ligation produced better long-term results for the treatment of bleeding haemorrhoids.

References

1. Reynolds J E F (ed) 1982 Martindale, the extra pharmacopoeia, 28th edn. Pharmaceutical Press, London, pp 570–572
2. Maddin S (ed) 1982 Current dermatological therapy, 1st edn. Saunders, Philadelphia, pp 590–591
3. National Cancer Institute 1980 Bioassay of phenol for possible carcinogenicity. Bethesda, MD: US Department of Health and Human Studies; Technical Report Series No. NCI-CG-TR-203
4. Heller V G, Pursell L L 1938 Phenol-contaminated waters and their physiological actions. Journal of Pharmacology and experimental therapeutics 63: 99–107
5. Minor J L, Becker B A 1971 A comparison of the teratogenic properties of sodium salicylate, sodium benzoate and phenol. Toxicology and Applied Pharmacology 19: 373
6. Jones-Price C et al. Teratologic evaluation of phenol (CAS No. 108-95-2) in CD-I mice. Laboratory study: September 18, 1980 to January 12, 1981. Research Triangle Park, NC: Research Triangle Institute
7. Jones-Price C et al. Teratologic evaluation of phenol (CAS No. 108-95-2) in CD rats. Laboratory study: July 10, 1980 to December 19, 1980. Research Triangle Park, NC: Research Triangle Institute
8. Nater J P, De Groot A C, Liem D H 1985 Unwanted effects of cosmetics and drugs used in dermatology, 2nd edn. Elsevier, Amsterdam, p 192
9. Cline R E, Yert L W, Needhem L L 1984 Determination of germicidal phenols in blood by capillary column gas chromatography. Journal of Chromatography 307: 420–425
10. Rainsford S G, Lloyd Davies T A 1964 Urinary excretion of phenol by men exposed to vapour of benzene: a screening test. British Journal of Industrial Medicine 22: 21–26
11. Rook A, Wilkinson D S, Ebling F J G, Champion R H, Burton J L (eds) 1986 Textbook of dermatology, 4th edn. Blackwell Scientific Publications, Oxford, p 2591
12. British National Formulary, no 18 1989 British Medical Association/The Pharmaceutical Society of Great Britain, London, p 359
13. British National Formulary, no 18 1989 British Medical Association/The Pharmaceutical Society of Great Britain, London, p 69
14. Rook A, Wilkinson D S, Ebling F J G, Champion R H, Burton J L (eds) 1986 Textbook of dermatology, 4th edn. Blackwell Scientific Publications, Oxford, p 2543
15. Cronin E 1980 Contact dermatitis. Churchill Livingstone, Edinburgh, p 673
16. Farber G A, Collins P S, Wilhelmus S M 1984 Update on chemical peel. Journal of Dermatological Surgery and Oncology 10: 559–560
17. Trappmann E S, Ellenby J D 1979 Major ECG changes during chemical face peeling. Plastic and Reconstructive Surgery 63: 44–48
18. Ive F A 1973 Diseases of the skin. Treatment of skin infections and infestation. British Medical Journal 4: 475–478
19. Shepherdson A 1977 Nail matrix phenolisation, a preferred method to surgical excision. Practitioner 219: 725–728
20. Deichmann W B 1949 Local and systemic effects following skin contact with phenol — a review of the literature. Journal of Industrial Hygiene and Toxicology 31: 146–154
21. Barry B W 1983 Dermatological formulations (Drugs and the therapeutic sciences, vol 13). Marcel Dekker Inc, New York, p 142
22. Rodgers S C F, Burrows D, Neill D 1978 Percutaneous absorption of phenol and methyl alcohol in magenta pain BPC. British Journal of Dermatology 98: 559–560
23. Valle Jones J C 1983 Chloraseptic liquid in sore throats. Practitioner 227: 1037–1040
24. Goligher J C 1984 Surgery of the anus, rectum and colon, 5th edn. Balliere Tindall, London, pp 105–113
25. Churcher M D 1973 Pain clinic cases. Practitioner 210: 243–246
26. Galizia E J, Lahiri S K 1974 Paraplegia with coeliac plexus block. British Journal of Anaesthesia 46: 539–540
27. Rook A, Wilkinson D S, Ebling F J G, Champion R H, Burton J L (eds) 1986 Textbook of dermatology, 4th edn. Blackwell Scientific Publications, Oxford, pp 1267

28. Davies D M (ed) 1977 Textbook of adverse drug reactions. Oxford University Press, Oxford, p 413
29. Reynolds J E F (ed) 1982 Martindale, the extra pharmacopoeia, 28th edn. Pharmaceutical Press, London, p 79
30. Thomas B B 1969 Letter. Peritoneal dialysis and lysol poisoning. British Medical Journal III: 720
31. Wooley P B 1952 Exogenous ochronosis. British Medical Journal II: 760–761

Phenoperidine hydrochloride

Phenopendine is an opioid agonist with greater potency than morphine.

Chemistry

Phenoperidine hydrochloride (Operidine)
$C_{23}H_{29}NO_3.HCl$
Ethyl 1-(3-hydroxy-3-phenylpropyl)-4-phenylpiperidine-4-carboxylate hydrochloride

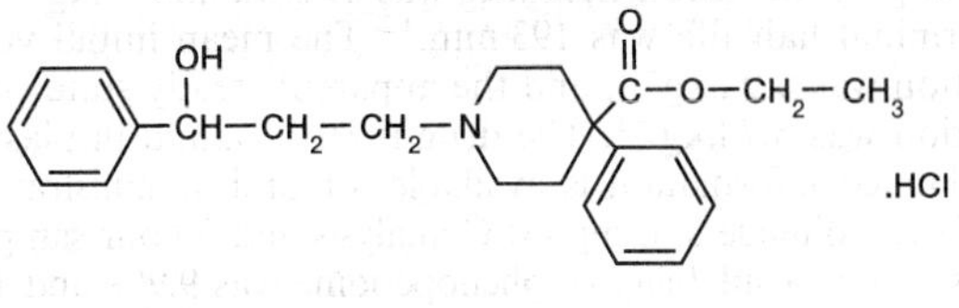

Molecular weight (free base)	403.9 (367.5)
pKa	8.01
Solubility	
in alcohol	1 in 10
in water	—
Octanol/water partition coefficient	—

Phenoperidine hydrochloride is a white, crystalline powder prepared by chemical synthesis.

Pharmacology

Phenoperidine is an opioid agonist that binds to opiate receptors.[1] It is an agonist at μ (Mu) receptors[2] and in rats subcutaneous phenoperidine was 75 times more potent than morphine in the hot plate test. In mice given the drug by the same route phenoperidine was 33 times more potent than morphine. Phenoperidine produces analgesia, respiratory depression, constipation, emesis and has vagal effects. Bronchoconstriction may occur in animals and is reversed by atropine. Phenoperidine produces a bradycardia but this is probably less than that seen with other opioids such as fentanyl. Phenoperidine has little effect on blood pressure but does reduce cardiac output.

Toxicology

Unpublished manufacturer's information from subcutaneous injection in mice (2 weeks), and intravenous injection in rats (2 weeks) and beagles (3 weeks) on dose–doubling regimes to upper doses of 40, 1.25 and 0.63 mg.kg^{-1}, respectively, showed no untoward effects.

Clinical pharmacology

Phenoperidine 1–2 mg intravenously produces analgesia equivalent to morphine 10 mg. There are no precise studies of equi-analgesic dosage. The onset time of analgesic effect is 2–3 min, peak is at 5 min, and duration of effect is 40–60 minutes. These figures are derived from clinical experience and not from controlled data. In one study, phenoperidine 2 mg per 60 kg intravenously relieved tibial pressure pain.[3]

Phenoperidine is a potent respiratory depressant,[4] and is used clinically in intensive care for this purpose. Bronchoconstriction may be reversed by atropine.

The effect of phenoperidine on pupils, sedation and nausea and vomiting is similar to that of other agonist opiates. There is no information about constipation. The drug may have less constrictive effect on the bile duct relative to morphine or pethidine.[5] Dependence may occur.

Phenoperidine hydrochloride

No gross disturbance of the cardiovascular system was reported with phenoperidine use initially.[6] Subsequent reports suggested that 2 mg intravenous phenoperidine given to ventilated patients produced a fall in blood pressure (maximum 20 mmHg), with a marginal fall in cardiac output.[7] Phenoperidine causes less bradycardia than fentanyl. In intensive care use there have been reports of severe cardiovascular collapse with phenoperidine.[8–10] The cause of the collapse in these cases is unclear.

Intracranial pressure increase with phenoperidine has been reported,[10] but was associated with hypotension.

Pharmacokinetics

The analytical methods used for phenoperidine concentrations have been gas–liquid chromatography (GLC) with a nitrogen detector,[11] with a sensitivity limit of 2 μg.l^{-1}, and radioimmunoassay (RIA),[12] with a sensitivity limit of 0.1 μg.l^{-1}.

A plasma clearance of 20 ml.min^{-1}.kg^{-1} was obtained in anaesthetized patients given a 2 mg dose, with a terminal half life of about 1.5 h.[13] Similar values were obtained for volunteers after intravenous administration of the drug by the same group, using GLC.[14,15] Using RIA on samples obtained from anaesthetized patients undergoing general surgery, the mean clearance was 24.5 ml.min^{-1}.kg^{-1}, but the mean terminal half life was 193 min.[12] The mean initial volume of distribution was 0.9 l.kg^{-1}, and the apparent steady-state volume of distribution was 5.7 l.kg^{-1}. The drug is 80% bound in plasma.

Only limited information is available for oral administration. In a study of two volunteers, using GLC analysis and 3-hour sampling, the relative systemic availability of phenoperidine was 9.9% and 13.5%.[15]

Secondary rises in plasma concentrations have been reported in all the intravenous studies. These are not unique to phenoperidine, and attempts to impute clinical significance (respiratory depression) have not been substantiated.

Oral absorption	10–14%
Presystemic metabolism	—
Plasma half life	3.2 h
Volume of distribution	5.7 l.kg^{-1}
Plasma protein binding	80%

Concentration–effect relationship

Concentrations in excess of 4 μg.l^{-1} are seen in all the kinetic studies for about an hour after a 2 mg intravenous dose. Such concentrations produce analgesia. No study of dose–response with plasma concentration measurement is available to allow further comment.

Metabolism

Studies in anaesthetized patients suggested that phenoperidine is metabolized to pethidine and norpethidine, which are eliminated with unchanged drug in the urine (Fig. 1).[13] The site of metabolism is presumed to be hepatic.

Up to 5% of a dose is excreted unchanged in the urine, with 18% as norpethidine and 2% as pethidine, over two to three days. Acidification of urine increased the urinary excretion of unchanged phenoperidine to 7%.[16] In alkaline urine the proportion excreted as norpethidine and pethidine increased.

Pharmaceutics

Phenoperidine, Operidine (Janssen, UK) is available for parenteral injection, as a colourless liquid containing 1 mg.ml^{-1} phenoperidine (as hydrochloride). Ampoules containing 2 ml (2 mg) or 10 ml (10 mg) are available. The ampoules contain no preservative.

The drug may be used without problem with 5% dextrose or normal saline. It should not be mixed with the induction agents thiopentone, propanidid or methohexitone because of the difference in pH.

Usage in the UK is restricted by the Misuse of Drugs Act.

Therapeutic use

Indications

1. Analgesia during operation

Fig. 1 The metabolism of phenoperidine

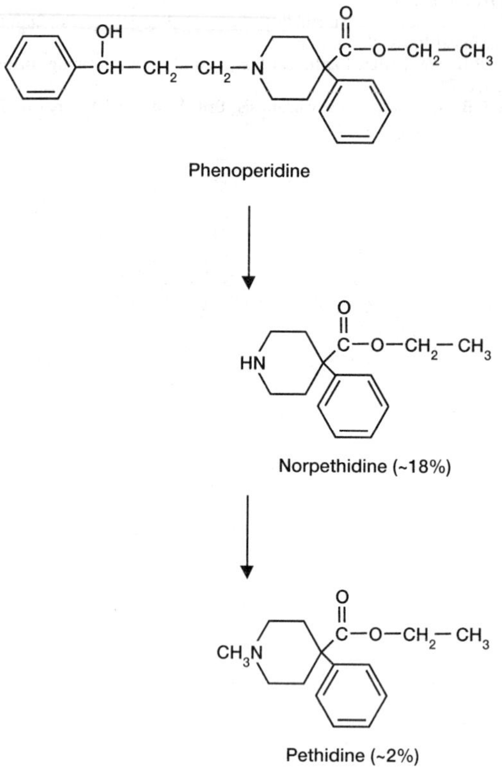

2. Neuroleptanalgesia
3. Enhancement of anaesthetics
4. Respiratory depressant in prolonged assisted respiration
5. Premedication
6. Postoperative analgesia.

Contraindications

There are no absolute contraindications, but care should be exercised as for other strong opiate agonists in patients with hepatic dysfunction,[14] respiratory disease, in the elderly and the hypothyroid. Patients with renal dysfunction may be at risk from accumulation of norpethidine, which may lead to CNS toxicity.[17] Unpredictable and ill-understood cardiovascular problems may occur in intensive care (although this is not an approved indication for use).

Mode of use

2 mg of phenoperidine is thought to be equal in analgesic potency to 10 mg of morphine.

The intravenous bolus dose size is 1 mg initially to adults breathing spontaneously; increments of 0.5 mg may be given at intervals of 40–60 min. For ventilated patients the initial dose may be 2–5 mg, and the increment 1 mg.

Indications

1–4. Anaesthetic uses

Phenoperidine is a strong opiate agonist for use in anaesthesia and intensive care. It has no specific advantage over the available alternatives, and the potential problems inherent in its metabolism to norpethidine may be a specific disadvantage, particularly in renal dysfunction.

It is also doubtful whether there is any measurable clinical advantage in the use of phenoperidine rather than any other opiate agonist, in terms of either efficacy or adverse event incidence at equi-analgesic dosage. There are few careful clinical studies of phenoperidine (see Clinical trials). Interpreting results is made more difficult because studies used different assumptions as to the dose of phenoperidine which would provide equivalent analgesia to 10 mg of morphine.

5. Premedication

Doses of 0.044 mg.kg^{-1} intramuscularly have been used in children.[20] Doses of 2 mg intramuscularly have been used in women.[21]

Phenoperidine hydrochloride

6. Postoperative analgesia
Doses of 1–2 mg intravenously or intramuscularly produced analgesia equivalent to parenteral doses of other opiates.

Adverse reactions

Potentially life-threatening effects
Severe hypotension has occurred during use in severely ill patients undergoing intensive care. As with other opiates severe respiratory depression may occur and pose a special hazard to patients with chronic lung disease.

Acute overdosage
Respiratory depression resulting in cyanosis and hypotension will ultimately lead to cardiac arrest. Medical management is by respiratory and cardiovascular support and intravenous injection of naloxone, 0.4 mg, repeated as necessary at 1 min intervals. No effect after 4 mg means that the opiate is not the cause of the problem.

Severe or irreversible adverse effects
No relevant physical sequelae are known. Drug use for reasons other than pain relief may result in psychological dependence.

Symptomatic adverse effects
Symptomatic adverse effects mediated by opiate receptor occupancy are constipation, sedation and nausea (and vomiting). Unpleasant dreams, mood alteration, itching and urinary retention are also probably opiate receptor effects, being common to all opiates. There is no comparative evidence to suggest quantitatively greater or lesser degrees of these problems occurring with phenoperidine compared with the alternatives.

Bradycardia may occur (reversible with atropine), as may muscular rigidity (manage with muscle relaxants).

The metabolism of phenoperidine to pethidine and norpethidine has the potential for CNS toxicity from the metabolite norpethidine.[18]

High risk groups

Neonates
The drug is not used in neonates.

Breast milk. The same precautions apply as with other opiate agents.

Children
The same precautions apply as with other opiate agents.

Pregnant women
The same precautions apply as with other opiate agents.

The elderly
The same precautions apply as with other opiate agents.

Concurrent disease

Respiratory disease. There is no good evidence that patients with respiratory disease who are treated appropriately with opiates for opiate-sensitive pain have any greater incidence of respiratory depression.

Renal disease. Decreased renal function may increase the plasma pethidine:norpethidine ratio. Fixed dose regimes must therefore take account of renal function.

Liver disease. Plasma clearance will be lower and elimination half life extended in liver disease.[14]

Drug interactions

Potentially hazardous interactions
The metabolic pathway of phenoperidine to pethidine suggests that phenoperidine should be avoided in patients taking monoamine oxidase inhibitors,[19] and for up to two weeks after stopping them.

Clinical trials

1. Davies D R, Doughty A G 1971 Premedication in children. British Journal of Anaesthesia 43: 65–74

Phenoperidine was used in combination with droperidol as a premedicant in 120 children (0.044 and 0.22 mg.kg^{-1} respectively, intramuscularly). The study was double-blind, and a greater proportion of patients vomited postoperatively after the combination than after the saline control (n = 120), but fewer children given the phenoperidine combination cried or were restless after surgery.

2. Morrison J D, Loan W B, Dundee J W, McDowell S A, Brown S S 1970 Studies of drugs given before anaesthesia XVIII: the synthetic opiates. British Journal of Anaesthesia 41: 987–993

Phenoperidine 2 mg was used intramuscularly as premedication in 100 women undergoing minor surgery, and was compared with other opiate premedicants in an open design and using historical controls. Phenoperidine had weak soporific activity, was judged to be an effective 'calming' agent, and was relatively less toxic (drowsiness and emesis) than other opiates studied.

3. Banister E H 1974 Six potent analgesic drugs; a double-blind study in postoperative pain. Anaesthesia 29: 158–162

Phenoperidine (n = 76) 1 mg intravenously was compared as a postoperative analgesic in adults with other opiates; doses of drugs were not equi-analgesic, but all but nine patients given phenoperidine obtained a degree of relief. Phenoperidine caused 19 patients to drop blood pressure by more than 20 mmHg, a higher proportion than with the other opiates.[23] Increasing the phenoperidine dose to 2 mg produced a greater (65%) proportion of patients with relief than the 40% relieved by 1 mg.[23]

References

1. Stahl K D, van Bever W, Janssen P, Simon E J 1977 Receptor affinity and pharmacological potency of a series of narcotic analagesic, anti-diarrheal and neuroleptic drugs. European Journal of Pharmacology 46: 199–205
2. Shephard N W 1964 The chemistry and pharmacology of droperidol, phenoperidine and fentanyl. In: Shephard N W (ed) The application of neuroleptanalgesia in anaesthetic and other practice. Pergamon, London
3. Morrison J D 1970 Alterations in response to somatic pain associated with anaesthesia XIX: studies with the drugs used in neuroleptanaesthesia. British Journal of Anaesthesia 42: 838–848
4. Jennett S, Barker J, Forrest J B 1968 A double-blind controlled study of the effects on respiration of pentazocine, phenoperidine and morphine in normal man. British Journal of Anaesthesia 40: 864
5. Hopton D S, Torrance H B 1967 Action of various new analgesic drugs on the human common bile duct. Gut 8: 296–299
6. Foldes F F, Kepes E R, Kronfeld P P, Shiffman H P 1966 A rational approach to neuroleptanalgesia. Anesthesia and Analgesia 45: 642
7. Prys-Roberts C, Kelman G R 1967 The influence of drugs used in neuroleptanalgesia on cardiovascular and ventilatory function. British Journal of Anaesthesia 41: 800–806
8. Easy W R 1982 Severe cardiovascular collapse following phenoperidine. Anaesthesia 37: 211
9. Green D W 1981 Severe cardiovascular collapse following phenoperidine. Anaesthesia 36: 617–619
10. Grummitt R M, Goat V A 1984 Intracranial pressure after phenoperidine. Anaesthesia 39: 565–567
11. Chan K, Murray G R, Rostron C, Calvey T N, Williams N E 1981 Quantitative gas–liquid chromatographic method for the determination of phenoperidine in human plasma. Journal of Chromatography 223: 213–218
12. Fischler M, Levron J C, Trang H, Vaxelaire J F, Flaisler B, Vourc'h G 1985 Pharmacokinetics of phenoperidine in anaesthetised patients undergoing general surgery. British Journal of Anaesthesia 57: 872–876
13. Milne L, Williams N E, Calvey T N, Murray G R, Chan K 1980 Plasma concentration and metabolism of phenoperidine in man. British Journal of Anaesthesia 52: 537–540
14. Isherwood C N, Calvey T N, Williams N E, Chan K, Murray G R 1984 Elimination of phenoperidine in liver disease. British Journal of Anaesthesia 56: 843–847
15. Calvey T N, Milne L A, Williams N E, Chan K, Murray G R 1983 Effect of antacids on the plasma concentration of phenoperidine. British Journal of Anaesthesia 55: 535–539
16. Milne L, Williams N E, Calvey T N, Murray G R, Chan K 1983 Effect of urine pH on the elimination of phenoperidine. British Journal of Clinical Pharmacology 16: 101–103
17. Szeto H H, Inturrisi C E, Houde R et al 1977 Accumulation of normeperidine, an active metabolite of meperidine in patients with renal failure or cancer. Annals of Internal Medicine 86: 738–741
18. Inturrisi C E, Umans J 1986 Meperidine biotransformation and central nervous system toxicity in animals and humans. In: Foley K M, Inturrisi C E (eds) Opioid analgesics in the management of clinical pain. Advances in pain research and therapy, vol 8. Raven Press, New York, pp 117–127
19. Schnieden H 1966 Prescriber's Journal 6: 82

Phenoxybenzamine (hydrochloride)

Phenoxybenzamine was discovered in the 1940s and was originally used for treating hypertension. It has significant adverse effects as well as potential mutagenicity and consequently it has largely fallen out of favour, other α -receptor antagonists being preferred. Its main use currently is in managing hypertension associated with phaeochromocytoma.

Chemistry

Phenoxybenzamine hydrochloride (Dibenyline, Dibenzyline)
$C_{18}H_{22}ClNO.HCl$
N-(2-Chloroethyl)-N-(1-methyl-2-phenoxyethyl)benzylamine

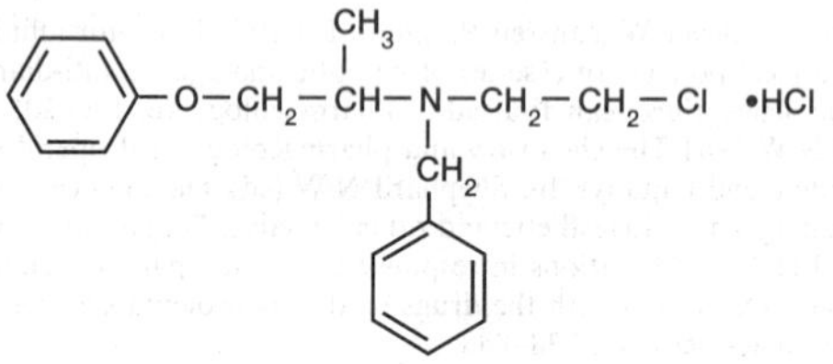

Molecular weight	340.3 (303.8)
pKa	—
Solubility	
in alcohol	1 in 9
in water	1 in 25
Octanol/water partition coefficient	—

Phenoxybenzamine hydrochloride is a white or off-white, odourless crystalline powder. It is a haloalkylamine, closely related chemically to the nitrogen mustards. The formation of a carbonium ion intermediate is considered to be responsible for receptor blockade. It is prepared by chemical synthesis. Neutral and alkaline solutions are unstable.

Pharmacology

Phenoxybenzamine is a non-competitive α-adrenoceptor antagonist. Both α_1 and α_2 receptors are blocked with only modest selectivity for the α_1-adrenoceptor. Phenoxybenzamine has a relatively slow onset of action and even after intravenous dosing the peak effect takes an hour or more to develop. Phenoxybenzamine is believed to act by conversion of the three membered ring into a highly reactive carbonium ion. The slow onset of action may be due to the time taken to form this reactive species. The carbonium ion then binds covalently to the α_1-receptor, thus producing an irreversible blockade. During the stage of development of the full α-blockade, the extent of that blockade can be reduced by a catecholamine or α-blocking drug that competes for the α-receptor. These drugs have no effect once α-blockade is fully developed. The α-blocking effects of phenoxybenzamine disappears slowly with a half life of approximately 24 h. Demonstrable α-blockade is present several days after stopping administration of phenoxybenzamine.

Phenoxybenzamine, in addition to α-blockade, increases the rate of turnover of noradrenaline in peripheral tissues. It also increases the amount of noradrenaline released by each nerve terminal which is probably due to α_2-receptor blockade.[1] Phenoxybenzamine also inhibits the uptake of noradrenaline into adrenergic nerve terminals. Phenoxybenzamine has no α-agonist activity and no action on β-receptors.[2] In high doses it inhibits the responses to 5-hydroxytryptamine and acetylcholine.

Toxicology

Phenoxybenzamine is carcinogenic in rats and demonstrates mutagenicity in the Ames test. No clinical evidence of this potential has been seen in man.

Clinical pharmacology

The α-adrenoceptor blocking action of phenoxybenzamine in humans is relatively slow in onset and wears off slowly, as is the case in animal studies. The α-blockade leads to relaxation of smooth muscle but the overall effect depends partly on the level of sympathetic activity present. The hypotensive effect is minimal in the resting supine position but there is usually a marked fall in blood pressure in the upright posture because of inhibition of the vasoconstrictor response to standing. Thus, postural hypotension is common with phenoxybenzamine, and this is exaggerated in the presence of volume depletion or in the presence of vasodilation where compensatory sympathetic vasomotor tone is in operation. This is accompanied by a reflex tachycardia and the tachycardia may be accentuated by enhanced release of noradrenaline (due to α_2-receptor blockade) and decreased inactivation of catecholamines due to reduced uptake into noradrenergic nerve endings.

Phenoxybenzamine produces a marked increase in cardiac output and a decrease in peripheral resistance in studies in healthy volunteers. Changes in organ blood flow reflect the differential effects of sympathetic tone in various tissues. Cerebral and coronary artery blood flow are not usually affected by phenoxybenzamine. Coronary artery blood flow usually increases in parallel with the increase in cardiac output. Cutaneous blood flow and blood flow to muscle are increased in low temperature environments by phenoxybenzamine. However, in warm temperatures there is little change in these blood flows. Splanchnic and renal blood flows are not affected at rest; however, in situations of increased sympathetic tone (e.g. hypovolaemia) these blood flows are increased by phenoxybenzamine. Perfusion to the outer cortex of the kidney is particularly increased in these circumstances by phenoxybenzamine. α-Adrenoceptor blockade caused by phenoxybenzamine leads to a shift of fluid from the interstitial to the vascular compartments due to differential effects on the pre and post capillary vessels.[3]

α-Adrenoceptor blockade caused by phenoxybenzamine leads to mild hyperinsulism due to blockade of the inhibitory action of adrenaline on insulin secretion. Relaxation of smooth muscle also causes miosis due to blockade of radial fibres of the iris but accommodation is not affected. Phenoxybenzamine may cause failure of ejaculation but is useful in patients with prostatic symptoms since by lowering urethral resistance phenoxybenzamine increases urine flow. Phenoxybenzamine has little effect on gastrointestinal function. In the CNS it may cause sedation after intravenous use; fatigue and lethargy may follow prolonged oral use. In larger doses given intravenously phenoxybenzamine may cause CNS stimulation resulting in vomiting, motor excitability or convulsions.

Pharmacokinetics

A high performance liquid chromatography assay is available that has a sensitivity of detection of 10 ng phenoxybenzamine.[4]

Phenoxybenzamine although effective is incompletely absorbed orally. Only 20–30% appears in the active form after an oral dose. It is effective when given parenterally but is irritant and should therefore only be given intravenously in a diluted form. Peak effect after intravenous injection is at one 1 h. The mean plasma half life is approximately 24 h. The clinical effects after a single oral dose may last for up to 3–4 days. Daily dosage can have cumulative effects with a dose response being evident for up to one week.

Oral absorption	not relevant
Presystemic metabolism	not relevant
Plasma half life	24 h
Volume of distribution	—
Plasma protein binding	—

Phenoxybenzamine has high lipid solubility and can accumulate in fatty tissue after large doses.

Concentration–effect relationship

Phenoxybenzamine is a typical example of a 'hit and run' type of drug with irreversible actions on α receptors. Thus no correlations are expected or observed between plasma concentrations of the drug and its therapeutic effects.

Metabolism

Phenoxybenzamine is metabolized in the liver and excreted in bowel and urine. The precise underlying metabolic pathways are not well understood as the drug was developed before such studies became part of the normal development process, however, the urinary metabolite N-p-hydroxyphenoxyisopropylamine has been detected in significant quantities.[5]

Pharmaceutics

Phenoxybenzamine is available as Dibenyline (SmithKline Beecham, UK) in oral and parenteral forms.

1. The 10 mg oral capsules are white with clear ruby-red caps, double marked 'SKF', the formulation being a white powder. Dibenzyline capsules (SmithKline Beecham, USA) are ruby-red capsules, double-marked 'SKF E33'.
2. The intravenous preparation is 100 mg of phenoxybenzamine hydrochloride in a 2 ml ampoule. It should be diluted in saline and given slowly over an hour. It has irritant effects when given intramuscularly.

Therapeutic use

Indications

1. Management of hypertension with phaeochromocytoma.

Other possible uses

2. Raynaud's phenomenon
3. Urinary outflow tract obstruction.

Contraindications

Any state where orthostatic hypotension is particularly undesirable, e.g. fluid depletion.

Indications

1. Hypertension associated with phaeochromocytoma

Phenoxybenzamine is especially useful in managing hypertension associated with phaeochromocytoma due to its non-competitive α-receptor antagonism. This prevents sudden surges of catecholamines from overcoming the blockade as would normally occur with a competitive antagonist. This advantage is utilized in the pre-operative preparation of patients undergoing surgery for phaeochromocytoma.[6,7]

Treatment is usually commenced with oral therapy, starting at 10 mg, and the dose is increased by 10 mg daily until an adequate response is obtained or postural hypotension supervenes. The usual dose required is 1–2 $mg.kg^{-1}$ daily in two divided doses. Only after adequate α-blockade should a β-blocker be added for control of tachycardia (if required), as partial β-blockade without adequate α blockade could provoke a hypertensive crisis.

Phenoxybenzamine can be given intravenously, but as its onset of action is slow it is not particularly useful for treating paroxysms of hypertension which occur during surgical manipulation of the tumour. Intravenous phentolamine is preferable if a rapid onset and short duration of α-blockade is required.

In patients who have inoperable or malignant phaeochromocytoma oral phenoxybenzamine is useful for longer term control of blood pressure, although CNS side effects can be troublesome.[8]

2. Raynaud's phenomenon

Phenoxybenzamine has been shown to be of some benefit in Raynaud's phenomenon and other vasospastic conditions.[9] Often the dose required for symptomatic improvement is fairly low and it should be appreciated that this is not the mainstay therapy in these conditions.

3. Urinary outflow tract obstruction

Phenoxybenzamine can improve symptoms in bladder outlet obstruction by relaxation of the internal urethral sphincter.[10] Unfortunately, hypotension and dizziness are frequent side effects limiting its usefulness.

Contraindications

Phenoxybenzamine is contraindicated in any condition where hypotension would be poorly tolerated. A history of cerebrovascular accident, recent myocardial infarction, critical angina or obstructive valvular heart disease would therefore contraindicate its use. However, in a patient with a phaeochromocytoma the need to control blood pressure might over-ride these relative contraindications.

Adverse reactions

The main adverse effects related to phenoxybenzamine use are due to excessive α-blockade. Such adverse effects are more pronounced with volume depletion, following exercise or in a hot environment.

Potentially life-threatening effects

Very severe postural hypotension can be life-threatening in some circumstances.

Acute overdosage

The treatment of overdose is mainly supportive, with fluid replacement and use of posture to maintain blood pressure. Adrenaline is absolutely contraindicated as it would tend to exacerbate hypotension by its unopposed β_2 -stimulation. Cautious volume expansion is likely to be the most effective way of preventing severe hypotension.

Severe or irreversible adverse effects

Phaeochromocytoma patients who are inadequately prepared for surgery may suffer intra- or post-operative hypotension. One possible explanation is that catecholamine excess causes a contraction of plasma volume. Careful preparation with a period of adequate α-adrenergic blockade combined with quantitative replacement of blood loss during surgery has largely obviated this problem.

Symptomatic adverse effects

Ejaculatory failure, dizziness, miosis and nasal stuffiness are also directly related to α-receptor blockade. Neurological symptoms such as sedation and lethargy are well recognized at normal dosage. However, with higher dosage nausea and vomiting can be stimulated, probably as a result of a direct action on the brain stem.

Interference with clinical pathology tests

None has been documented.

High risk groups

Neonates

Little is known about the safety of phenoxybenzamine in neonates or children.

Breast milk. No information is available on the secretion of the drug in breast milk, so mothers taking the drug should not breast-feed.

Children

See neonates above.

Pregnant women

The manufacturers advise that the drug should not be used in pregnancy unless absolutely essential. However, there are reports of successful use of phenoxybenzamine during pregnancy and labour in the management of phaeochromocytoma, which can otherwise be lethal.[11]

The elderly

The drug should be used very cautiously in elderly patients, because they are more likely to suffer hypotensive episodes.

Drug interactions

Potentially hazardous interactions

Adrenaline. Hypotension can be exacerbated due to unopposed β_2-stimulation which will also tend to exacerbate the reflex tachycardia.

Anaesthetic agents. Profound hypotension may be precipitated by this combination due to the suppression of the vasoconstrictor compensatory response. Volume replacement is helpful in correcting it.

Potentially useful interactions
The drug is used in combination with β-blockers in the management of phaeochromocytoma (see 'Mode of use').

General review articles

Gilman AG, Goodman L S, Rall TW, Murad F 1985 The pharmacological basis of therapeutics, 7th edn. Macmillan, New York, ch 9, pp 183–187

Nickerson M, Hollenberg N K 1967 Blockade of alpha adrenergic receptors, In: Root W S, Hofmann F G (eds) Physiological pharmacology Vol 4, part D. Academic Press, New York, pp 242–305

References

1. Langer S Z 1970 Presynaptic receptors and their role in the regulation of transmitter release. British Journal of Pharmacology 60: 481–497
2. Nickerson M, Goodman L S 1947 Pharmacological properties of a new adrenergic blocking agent. N,N-dibenzyl-β-chloroethylamine (dibenamine). Journal of Pharmacology and Experimental Therapeutics 89: 167–185
3. Hollenberg N, Nickerson M 1970 Changes in pre and post capillary resistance in pathogenesis of hemorrhagic shock. American Journal of Physiology 219: 1483–1489
4. Moor M J, Bickel M H 1987 Tissue distribution of phenoxybenzamine in the rat: lack of adipose tissue storage. Life Sciences 41: 2041–2046
5. Napp D R, Holcombe N H, Krueger S A, Privitera P J 1976 qualitative metabolic fate of phenoxybenzamine in rat, dog and man. Drug Metabolism and Disposition 4: 164–168
6. Ross E J, Prichard B N C, Kaufman L, Robertson A I G, Harries B J 1967 Preoperative and operative management of patients with phaeochromocytoma. British Medical Journal 1: 191–198
7. Bravo E L, Gifford R W 1984 Medical intelligence: current concepts: phaeochromocytoma: diagnosis, localization and management New England Journal of Medicine 311: 1298–1303
8. Engelman K, Joerdsma A 1964 Chronic medical therapy for phaeochromocytoma: a report of four cases. Annals of Internal Medicine 61: 229–241
9. Cleophas T J, van Lier H J, Faaber P, Fennis J F, van't Laar A 1984 Therapeutic efficacy of α-adrenoceptor blockade in primary and secondary Raynaud's syndrome. Angiology 35: 719–723
10. Abrams P H, Shah P J, Stone R, Choa R G 1982 Bladder outflow obstruction treated with phenoxybenzamine. British Journal of Urology 54: 527–530
11. van der Spuy Z M, Jacobs H S 1984 Management of endocrine disorders in pregnancy: part II pituitary, ovarian and adrenal disease. Postgraduate Medical Journal 60: 312–320

Phenoxymethylpenicillin (potassium)

Phenoxymethylpenicillin (Penicillin V) is an acid-stable penicillin developed in 1953. Since then, it has been widely used as an oral preparation of penicillin.[1–3]

Chemistry

Phenoxymethylpenicillin potassium (penicillin V potassium, Phenoxymethylpenicillinum kalicum, Apsin VK, Cystapen VK, Distaquaine V-K, Econocil VK, Ledercillin VK, Pen-Vee K, Stabilin V-K, Uticillin VK, V-Cil-K, V-cillin-K, Veetids)
$C_{16}H_{17}N_2O_5S.K$
(6R)-6-(2-Phenoxyacetamido)penicillanic acid potassium salt

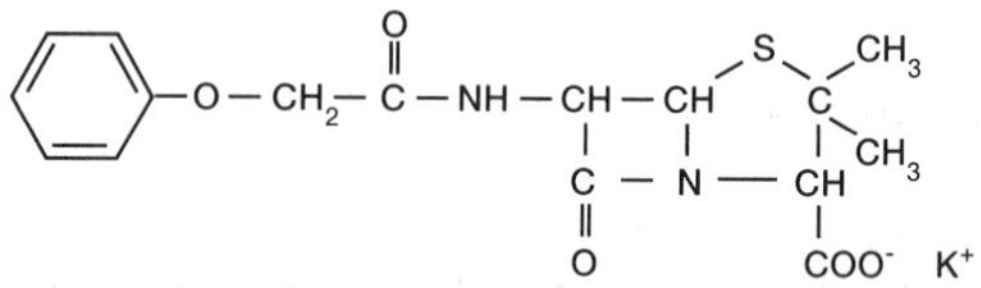

Molecular weight (free acid)	388.5 (350.4)
pKa	2.7
Solubility (potassium salt)	
in alcohol	1 in 150
in water	1 in 1.5
Octanol/water partition coefficient	very low

Phenoxymethylpenicillin and the potassium salt are both fine, white, odourless crystalline powders, produced biosynthetically. Phenoxymethylpenicillin is soluble 1 in 1700 of water and 1 in 7 of ethanol. It is optically active but only the d-isomer, which is marketed, is biologically active. One unit of phenoxymethylpenicillin was contained in 0.00059 mg of the first international standard preparation which contained 1695 units per mg. Most commercial preparations of phenoxymethylpenicillin contain the potassium salt, a white crystalline solid.

Pharmacology

Phenoxymethylpenicillin is an orally active member of the penicillin family. The discovery of penicillin by Fleming in 1928 and its exploitation by Florey and his colleagues a decade later is well known. The penicillin nucleus consists of a thiazolidine ring connected to a β-lactam ring to which is attached a side chain. The side-chain determines most of the pharmacological and antibacterial properties of the penicillin in question. Penicillin kills bacteria by interfering in the synthesis of the bacterial cell wall. Peptidoglycan is a heteropolymeric structure that provides the cell wall with mechanical stability. The final stage in the synthesis of peptidoglycan involves the completion of the cross linking and the terminal glycine residue of the pentaglycine bridge is linked to the fourth residue of the pentapeptide (d-alanine). The transpeptidase enzyme that performs this step is inhibited by penicillins and cephalosporins. As a result the bacterial cell wall is weakened, the cell swells and then ruptures.

Toxicology

Oral penicillins are of low toxicity.

Clinical pharmacology

Phenoxymethylpenicillin (also known as penicillin V) is highly active against Gram-positive cocci. This penicillin is easily destroyed by β-

Phenoxymethylpenicillin (potassium)

lactamase enzymes produced by some of these bacteria. Phenoxymethylpenicillin is less active than benzylpenicillin against streptococci and much less active against Gram-negative organisms such as *Neisseria*. Most strains of *Staphylococcus aureus* and *Staph. epidermidis* are resistant to penicillin V. Pneumococci are in general sensitive to penicillin V although some resistant strains have been described. Meningococci are quite sensitive to penicillin V, as are most strains of *Corynebacterium diphtheriae*, *Bacillus anthracis* and *Clostridia* spp. *Actinomyces israeli*, *Streptobacillus moniliformis*, *Listeria monocytogenes* and *Pasturella multocida* are also inhibited by penicillin V. *Treponema pallidum* is sensitive to penicillin V although more so to benzylpenicillin (penicillin G). Most Gram-negative bacilli are resistant to penicillin V although *Proteus mirabilis* and *Escherichia coli* may be susceptible to high concentrations. The main virtue of phenoxymethylpenicillin as opposed to benzylpenicillin is that the drug is more stable in an acid medium and is therefore better absorbed from the gastrointestinal tract. The drug goes into solution in the alkaline contents of the small intestine and is absorbed (incompletely) from the upper part of the small intestine. The peak concentration in the blood[4–5] after a 500 mg oral dose of phenoxymethylpenicillin is about 3 $mg.l^{-1}$. Peak concentrations are obtained about 30 min after dosing. Newer penicillins such as phenethicillin show higher plasma concentrations on a dose-for-dose basis compared with penicillin V.[6–8] Even so, phenoxymethylpenicillin is considered better than other phenoxypenicillins for the treatment of *Streptococcus pyogenes* infections.[9]

Pharmacokinetics

The pharmacokinetics of phenoxymethylpenicillin were studied in 12 healthy volunteers recently by Josefsson and Bergan.[10] The results showed that phenoxymethylpenicillin is rapidly but incompletely absorbed, with 40% of the drug remaining in the intestine. Peak serum concentrations occur within 0.75 h. The mean peak serum levels were 6.1, 15.0, 26.3 and 35.5 $mg.l^{-1}$ after 0.4, 1, 2 and 3 g of penicillin V administered orally, respectively. The urinary excretion over 10 h was 37–43% of the dose given, as unchanged drug and penicilloic acid. Over 24 h virtually all of the absorbable drug is recovered in the urine either unchanged or as the hydrolysis product. Very low penicillin concentrations were obtained in saliva.

The serum level of penicillin V has been compared with oral penicillin G and three other phenyoxypenicillins, namely phenoxyethylpenicillin (phenethicillin) phenoxybenzylpenicillin, and phenoxypropylpenicillin (PA-24B) by using different bioassay methods. The results showed that penicillin V was more efficiently absorbed from the gastrointestinal tract, and the urinary excretion of penicillin V was 2.6 times greater than that of penicillin G. This study also proved that oral penicillin V produced a higher and more prolonged degree of penicillinaemia than did an equivalent amount of penicillin G. When taken in a fasting state, blood levels of penicillin V are at least twice as high as that seen with an equal quantity of oral penicillin G; and when taken with food, the blood level of penicillin V is five times higher than that of penicillin G. This indicates that oral penicillin V is more resistant to destruction by gastric acid than penicillin G and less influenced by food compared with penicillin G.[3–5] Early studies showed that peak serum levels of oral phenoxypenicillins are obtained within half to one hour. Penicillin V is more highly bound by human plasma than is penicillin G. The average per cent binding of penicillin V by human plasma in 16 trials was 75.6±14% the corresponding value for penicillin G was 48.1±1.4%.[11]

Oral absorption	60%
Presystemic metabolism	—
Plasma half life	~0.5 h
Volume of distribution	0.2 $l.kg^{-1}$
Plasma protein binding	80%

Concentration–effect relationship

The results obtained from a concentration–effect relationship study in 16 normal young men showed that penicillin V provided greater serum activity than phenethicillin against the streptococci and pneumococci, at least equivalent activity against the staphylococci and *Sarcina*; and the same applied to activity in the urine.[12]

Bond et al[9] have done an excellent study on the concentration–effect relationship of four phenoxypenicillins. The results obtained after a single oral dose of 250 mg are shown in Table 1.

Although phenbenicillin has the highest serum peak level, the concentration–effect relationship study showed that phenoxymethylpenicillin is the best choice against *Strep. pyogenes*.

Table 1 Comparison of serum activity of four phenoxypenicillins against *Streptococcus pyogenes* on the basis of the ratio of total or free blood level to the appropriate MIC value

Penicillin	A Total level of antibiotic in serum $mg.l^{-1}$(1 h)	B Level of free antibiotic $mg.l^{-1}$(1 h)	C MIC in serum $mg.l^{-1}$	D MIC in broth $mg.l^{-1}$	A/C	B/D
Penicillin V	2.27	0.36	0.06	0.015	37.8	24.0
Phenethicillin	3.37	0.64	0.25	0.03	13.4	21.3
Propicillin	3.58	0.28	0.25	0.03	14.3	9.3
Phenbenicillin	5.60	0.11	1.00	0.03	5.6	33.7

Metabolism

As for benzylpenicillin, up to 35% of the dose is excreted in urine over 24 h with similar amounts of phenoxymethylpenicilloic acid (Fig. 1).

Fig. 1 Metabolism of phenoxymethylpenicillin

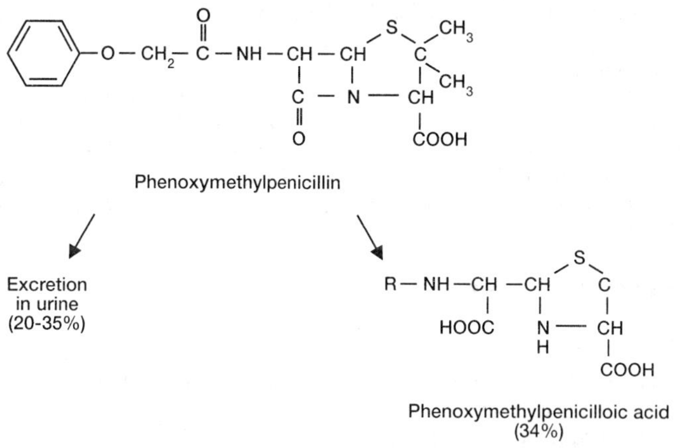

Pharmaceutics

Phenoxymethylpenicillin is available in a wide range of formulations[2]

1. Penicillin V for oral suspension: a dry mixture of phenoxymethylpenicillin and one or more suitable suspending, colouring and flavouring agents; it may contain one or more suitable buffers and preservatives. The suspension is prepared by the addition of diluent immediately before issue. Usual size: 1.5 g in a 7.5 ml container.
2. Penicillin V potassium for oral solution: a dry mixture of phenoxymethylpenicillin potassium and one or more suitable colours and flavours. It may contain one or more suitable buffers and preservatives. The solution is prepared by the addition of diluent immediately before issue. It is available in a range of strengths.
3. Phenoxymethylpenicillin capsules: capsules containing phenoxymethylpenicillin, phenoxymethylpenicillin calcium, or phenoxymethylpenicillin potassium. Penicillin V capsules usually contain 250 mg of phenoxymethylpenicillin.
4. Phenoxymethylpenicillin elixir; penicillin V elixir; phenoxymethylpenicillin solution; phenoxymethylpenicillin syrup: a solution of phenoxymethylpenicillin potassium in a suitable coloured, flavoured vehicle. It is prepared freshly by dissolving granules of the dry mixed ingredients in the specified quantity of water. Store in a cool place and use the elixir or diluted elixir within 1 week. Loses not more than 20% potency in a week at 15°C. When a dose less than 5 ml is prescribed, the

Phenoxymethylpenicillin (potassium)

P

elixir should be diluted to 5 ml with syrup. Such dilution must be freshly prepared.

5. Phenoxymethylpenicillin mixture: penicillin V mixture, a suspension of phenoxymethylpenicillin, phenoxymethylpenicillin calcium, or phenoxymethylpenicillin potassium in a suitably flavoured oily vehicle, which may be coloured. Store in a cool place. When a dose less than 5 ml is prescribed, the mixture should be diluted to 5 ml with fractionated coconut oil. Such dilutions must be freshly prepared and not used more than 2 weeks after issue.
6. Phenoxymethylpenicillin tablets: penicillin V tablets: tablets containing phenoxymethylpenicillin, phenoxymethylpenicillin calcium, or phenoxymethylpenicillin potassium. The tablets may be film-coated. Penicillin V tablets are usually available in strengths of 125, 250, 300 and 500 mg of phenoxymethylpenicillin. Penicillin V potassium tablets usually contain the equivalent of 125, 250 and 500 mg of phenoxymethylpenicillin.

In a crossover study on the relative bioavailability of 16 phenoxymethylpenicillin preparations, the results showed that the highest bioavailability was seen with the aqueous solutions and the tablets or capsules containing the potassium salt of phenoxymethylpenicillin. Two calcium salt tablet brands showed lower mean serum concentrations, but may be useful in patients who should avoid an excess of potassium. The suspensions intended for paediatric use were significantly inferior to most of the other preparations. The lowest bioavailability was observed with a suspension containing the poorly soluble benzathine phenoxymethylpenicillin.[13] Similar results from benzathine penicillin V in tablet form were also reported by Palatsi and Kaipainen.[14] Potassium penicillin V administered in the same dose to the same patients gave 3–4 times higher concentrations than benzathine penicillin V.

Stability studies showed that the degradation appeared to be by a first-order process for penicillin V potassium. Penicillin V potassium oral solution can be effectively stored for at least 50 days in a freezer at −10°C with little loss of activity.[15] Penicillin V potassium stored at 25°C (room temperature) was unstable after storage for less than 37 h.[16]

Therapeutic use

Indications

1. The treatment of mild infections caused by susceptible Gram-positive organisms
2. As a prophylactic to prevent the recurrence of rheumatic fever.

Previous uses

3. *Streptococcus viridans* endocarditis
4. *Haemophilus* infections
5. Gonorrhoea and syphilis.

Contraindications

1. A history of penicillin hypersensitivity
2. Severe acute infections.

Mode of use

Phenoxymethylpenicillin preparations are administered by the oral route. The dosage for infants is 62.5–125 mg, for children under five years 125 mg (200 000 units), and for children 6–12 years 250 mg. For children over 12 years and adults, 250–500 mg is administered every six hours. This drug should be given one hour before meals.[1,2]

Indications

1. Treatment of group-A streptococcal infections

Phenoxymethylpenicillin is effective for the treatment of mild infections caused by *Strep. pyogenes*. McLinn reported that there was no significant difference between the clinical effectiveness of cefaclor and phenoxymethylpenicillin in the treatment of streptococcal pharyngitis.[17] Colcher and Bass treated 300 children with streptococcal pharyngitis by three regimens. The first group of patients was treated with penicillin G procaine or penicillin G benzathine; the second group was treated with penicillin V, the patients of this group were given no special instructions. The third group was given the same penicillin V treatment but their parents received special counselling on the importance of taking the medication for the full ten days. The results showed that there was no significant difference between group 1 and group 3 in the number of treatment failures and in the incidence of relapse, but in respect of relapse in group 2, there was a significant difference when compared with group 1 or group 3. The results showed that oral penicillin V therapy with adequate counselling is as effective as intramuscular injection.[18]

2. Prevention of rheumatic fever

Penicillin V was recommended as one of the useful prophylactics for rheumatic fever.[19,20] The usual dose for prophylactic use is 500 mg daily given in two divided doses.[1] Patients receiving long-term penicillin V prophylaxis may carry resistant strains in the oropharynx, but resistant streptococci decreased rapidly when therapy was discontinued.[21]

Other uses

3. Treatment and prevention of penicillin-susceptible streptococcus endocarditis

27 patients with penicillin-susceptible (MIC $\leqslant 0.2\ \mu g.ml^{-1}$) *Streptococcus viridans* endocarditis treated with penicillin V 600–750 mg every 4 h orally plus 0.5–1.0 g streptomycin intramuscularly every 12 h were cured successfully. No relapse was noted in the penicillin V treatment group.[22]

Recommendations for the use of penicillin V for prophylaxis of bacterial endocarditis following dental manipulation were as follows: penicillin V 2.0 g orally 30 min to 1 hour prior to the procedure and then 500 mg orally every 6 h for eight doses.[3,23] Shanson et al reported that a 2 g oral dose of penicillin V was found to be effective in reducing the incidence of bacteraemia following dental extraction, when administered under supervision 1 hour before extraction.[24] However, prophylaxis with amoxycillin is now preferred.[33]

4. Treatment of *Haemophilus* infections

Although it has been suggested that *H. influenzae* will be inhibited by levels of penicillin in the serum which should be achieved by oral penicillin V, Garrod indicated that penicillin V was four to eight times less active against *H. influenzae* than benzylpenicillin, and 16 times less active than ampicillin. Therefore, penicillin V should not be considered as an antihaemophilus antibiotic.[25] Kamme and Lundgren reported that in the treatment of acute otitis media due to *Haemophilus influenzae*, therapeutic failure will occur in about 5% of cases in children 2–9 years of age, and in about 30% in children 0–1 year of age with penicillin V therapy at a daily dosage of 50 $mg.kg^{-1}$ body weight. It was pointed out that in the youngest age group acute otitis media caused by a typable *H. influenzae* strain should be regarded as unamenable to penicillin V therapy in the doses used.[26]

5. Treatment of gonorrhoea and syphilis

Oral penicillin V is relatively ineffective in the treatment of gonorrhoea and syphilis. The treatment of these diseases with oral penicillin V is not recommended.

Adverse reactions

Potentially life-threatening effects

The toxicity of penicillin V is low, but in a small number of patients penicillin can cause allergic reactions. Penicillin V may be cross-allergenic with penicillin G and with all other penicillins. In a patient without a past history of allergy to penicillin, penicillin V administered orally has caused anaphylactic shock.[27]

Severe or irreversible adverse effects

Goldstein described a patient who developed a syndrome resembling serum sickness, accompanied by liver damage, following a course of phenoxymethylpenicillin.[28]

Symptomatic adverse effects

Bolme and Eriksson stated that diarrhoea was evident in more than 60% of the children during treatment with penicillin V.[29] When large doses are given for a long period, penicillin V can cause gastrointestinal symptoms, such as abdominal discomfort, nausea and vomiting, and increased capillary fragility characterized by spontaneous petechial haemorrhages with a positive result on the tourniquet test in 2 of 8 patients.[4]

Interference with clinical pathology tests

The penicillins may interfere with urinary tests for fructose, aminolaevulinic acid, oestrogens, 17-hydroxycorticosteroids, protein and sugar, with serum tests for uric acid; with biological tests for serum folate; and with serum electrophoresis.

High risk groups

Neonates

There are no special precautions needed in this age group.

Breast milk. Penicillin excreted into human breast milk may lead to allergic reactions in the infant.[30]

Children

The drug may be used in children in appropriate doses.

Pregnant women

There are no contraindications to the use of penicillin in pregnancy.

The elderly

There are no special problems relating to the use of penicillin in elderly patients.

Drug interactions

Potentially hazardous interactions

The activity of penicillin V against *Staphylococcus aureus* is reduced in the presence of zinc oxide and reduced to a lesser extent in the presence of magnesium carbonate, magnesium oxide, calamine, etc.[2]

Other significant interactions

Aspirin, sulphamethoxypyridazine and sulphaethidole inhibit the serum-binding of penicillin V in vitro and in vivo.[31]

Phenoxymethylpenicillin in a dose of 653 mg orally every 8 h decreased oestrogen in six mothers 38–40 weeks pregnant.[32] It was not observed to cause any adverse effects on the fetus or during delivery.

Aminoglycosides may be inactivated by penicillins in vitro but this is unlikely to be a problem with phenoxymethylpenicillin. The excretion of phenoxymethylpenicillin in urine is retarded by probenecid, as is the case for all penicillins.

Potentially useful interactions

None is known.

General review articles

Mandell G L, Sane M A 1980 Antimicrobial agents, penicillin and cephalosporins. In: Goodman L S, Gilman A (eds) The pharmacological basis of therapeutics, 6th edn. Macmillan, New York

Garrod L P, Lambert H P, O'Grady F (eds) 1973 Antibiotics and chemotherapy, 4th edn. Churchill Livingstone, Edinburgh

Kucers A, Bennett N M 1979 The use of antibiotics, 3rd edn. William Heinemann, London

Reynolds J E F (ed) 1982 Martindale: the extra pharmacopoeia. The Pharmaceutical Press, London

AMA Division of Drugs 1983 AMA drug evaluation, 5th edn. W B Saunders, Philadelphia, pp 1563–1594

Joint Formulary Committee 1984 British National Formulary (BNF) Number 7, British Medical Association and the Pharmaceutical Society of Great Britain. Pitman Press, Bath

Edward D I 1980 Antimicrobial drug action. Macmillan Press, London, ch 6, pp 107–136

References

1. Kucers A, Bennett N M 1979 The use of antibiotics, 3rd edn. William Heinemann, London
2. Reynolds J E F (ed) 1989 Martindale: the extra pharmacopoeia, 29th edn. The Pharmaceutical Press, London
3. AMA Division of Drugs 1983 AMA drug evaluation, 5th edn. W B Saunders, Philadelphia, pp 1563–1594
4. Cox F Jr, Colville J M, Truant J, Quinn E L 1957 Further observations on the use of large doses of oral penicillin V (phenoxymethyl penicillin). Antibiotics Annual 1956–1957: 282–286
5. Heatley N G 1956 Comparative serum concentration and excretion experiments with benzyl penicillin (G) and phenoxymethyl penicillin (V) on a single subject. Antibiotic Medicine 11: 33–41
6. Carter M J, Brumfitt W, Willmott I 1962 Bacteriological and clinical studies with phenoxymethylpenicillin. British Medical Journal 1: 80–82
7. Williamson G M, Morrison J K, Stevens K J 1961 A new synthetic penicillin PA-248. Lancet 1: 847–850
8. Rollo I M, Somers G F, Burley D M 1962 Bacteriological and pharmacological properties of phenoxymethylpenicillin. British Medical Journal 1: 76–80
9. Bond J M, Lightbown J W, Barber M, Waterworth P M 1963 A comparison of four phenoxypenicillins. British Medical Journal 2: 956–961
10. Josefsson K, Bergan T 1982 Pharmacokinetics of phenoxymethylpenicillin in volunteers. Chemotherapy 28: 241–246
11. Smith C I, Levin J D, Embody D R 1957 Studies of the binding of penicillins G and V by human plasma. Antibiotics Annual 1956–1957: 306–310
12. McCarthy C G, Finland M, Wilcox C, Yarrows J H 1960 Absorption and excretion of four penicillins. New England Journal of Medicine 263: 315–326
13. Bergan T, Berdal B P, Holm V 1976 Relative bioavailability of phenoxymethylpenicillin preparations in a cross-over study. Acta Pharmacologica et Toxicologica 38: 308–320
14. Palatsi I, Kaipainen W 1971 A comparative study of blood concentrations after peroral benzathine (DBED) penicillin V and potassium penicillin V. Scandinavian Journal of Infectious Diseases 3: 71–74
15. Allen L V Jr, Lo P 1979 Stability of oral liquid penicillins in unit dose containers at various temperatures. American Journal of Hospital Pharmacy 36: 209–211
16. Grogan L J, Jensen B K, Makoid M C, Baldwin J N 1979 Stability of penicillin V potassium in unit dose oral syringes. American Journal of Hospital Pharmacy 36: 205–208
17. McLinn S E 1980 Cefaclor in treatment of otitis media and pharyngitis in children. American Journal of Diseases of Children 134: 560–563
18. Colcher I S, Bass J W 1972 Penicillin treatment of streptococcal pharyngitis. Journal of the American Medical Association 222: 657–659
19. Garrod L P 1975 Chemoprophylaxis. British Medical Journal 4: 561–564
20. Phair J P, Weihl C 1973 Penicillin phenoxymethyl. American Journal of Diseases of Children 126: 48–50
21. Sprunt K, Redman W, Leidy G 1968 Penicillin resistant alpha streptococci in pharynx of patients given oral penicillin. Pediatrics 42: 957–968
22. Tan J S, Terhune C A Jr, Kaplan S, Hamburger M 1971 Successful two-week treatment schedule for penicillin-susceptible streptococcus viridans endocarditis. Lancet 2: 1340–1343
23. Petersdorf R G 1978 Antimicrobial prophylaxis of bacterial endocarditis. American Journal of Medicine 65: 220–223
24. Shanson D C, Cannon P, Wilks M 1978 Amoxycillin compared with penicillin V for the prophylaxis of dental bacteraemia. Journal of Antimicrobial Chemotherapy 4: 431–436
25. Garrod L P 1973 Penicillins for haemophilus infections. British Medical Journal 3: 290
26. Kamme C, Lundgren K 1971 Frequency of typable and non-typable Haemophilus influenzae strains in children with acute otitis media and results of penicillin V treatment. Scandinavian Journal of Infectious Diseases 3: 225–228
27. Coates W H 1963 A case of anaphylactic shock following the administration of oral penicillin. Medical Journal of Australia 1: 967
28. Goldstein I I, Ishak K G 1974 Hepatic injury associated with penicillin therapy. Archives of Pathology 98: 114–117
29. Bolme P, Eriksson M 1975 Influence of diarrhea on the oral absorption of penicillin V and ampicillin in children. Scandinavian Journal of Infectious Diseases 7: 141–145
30. Catz C S, Giaoia G P 1972 Drugs and breast milk. Pediatric Clinics of North America 19: 151–166
31. Kunin C M 1966 Clinical pharmacology of the new penicillins. Clinical Pharmacology and Therapeutics 7: 180–188
32. Pulkkinen M, Willman K 1971 Maternal oestrogen levels during penicillin treatment. British Medical Journal 4: 48
33. Recommendations from the Endocarditis Working Party of The British Society for Antimicrobial Chemotherapy 1980 Antibiotic prophylaxis of infective endocarditis. Lancet 335: 88–89

P

Phentolamine (mesylate)

Phentolamine is a short-acting, injectable, α-adrenergic receptor blocking agent used to treat hypertension caused by excess circulating catecholamines.

Chemistry

Phentolamine mesylate (Rogitine, Regitin(e))
$C_{17}H_{19}N_3O.CH_3SO_3H$
3-[N-(2-imidazolin-2-ylmethyl)-4-toluidino]phenol methanesulphonate

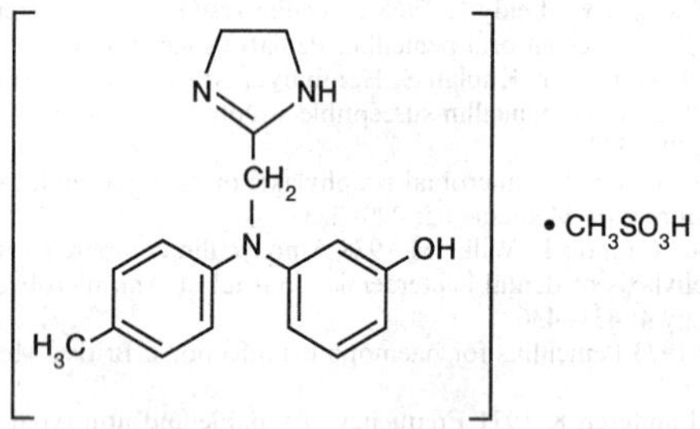

Molecular weight (free base)	377.5 (281.4)
pKa	7.7
Solubility	
in alcohol	1 in 5
in water	1 in 1
Octanol/water partition coefficient	—

Phentolamine mesylate is a white or off-white, odourless, crystalline compound which is slightly hygroscopic. Phentolamine is a 2-substituted imidazoline derivative that is prepared by chemical synthesis. It is not available in any combination preparations.

Pharmacology

Phentolamine is a competitive α-adrenoceptor antagonist acting on the α_1- and α_2-adrenoceptors with almost equal efficacy. Phentolamine also acts as a weak antagonist of 5-hydroxytryptamine and releases histamine from mast cells. It has a direct effect on smooth muscle to cause relaxation and this is independent of the α-blockade. It has been suggested that this is due to stimulation of the β-adrenoceptor, but it is unclear if this effect is due to direct receptor stimulation or is a consequence of increased catecholamine turnover following presynaptic α_2-receptor antagonism. The smooth muscle relaxation results in reduced peripheral resistance and increased venous capacitance. There is also a cardiac stimulant effect following phentolamine and cardiac arrhythmias have been seen in animal studies. These may be due to increased sympathetic activity mediated via the baroreflex.

Phentolamine causes some stimulation of lacrimal, salivary and respiratory tract secretions and has a more marked effect on gastric and pancreatic secretions. This is probably due to a direct effect on muscarinic cholinergic receptors and can be blocked by atropine.

Toxicology

No significant mutagenic potential has been demonstrated with phentolamine.

Clinical pharmacology

Phentolamine is a short-acting α-adrenoceptor antagonist in man and is usually given by intravenous or intramuscular injection. It causes a dose-related fall in both systolic and diastolic blood pressure due to α-adrenoceptor blockade coupled with a direct effect on smooth muscle. Peripheral resistance falls and venous capacitance increases. Pulmonary arterial pressure is also usually reduced by phentolamine. In a study of patients with cardiac failure a 10 μg.kg^{-1}.min^{-1} phentolamine infusion caused a 10 mmHg drop in systolic arterial pressure and a 7 mmHg drop in pulmonary artery systolic pressure, maximal effect occurring at 20 μg.kg^{-1}.min^{-1}.[1] Peak effect usually occurs within 15 min and lasts for at least one hour. Postural hypotension is sometimes a problem following phentolamine. The fall in blood pressure is accompanied by a marked tachycardia — again due both to direct stimulant effects on the heart and to α-blockade. Cardiac output is increased and phentolamine does have a weak inotropic effect.

Phentolamine increases intestinal motility and results in enhanced secretion of gastric and pancreatic secretions. These effects can be prevented with atropine, as diarrhoea can be a problem following repeated doses of phentolamine.

Pharmacokinetics

Assay by high performance liquid chromatography is sensitive to 5 ng.ml^{-1} of phentolamine in serum.[2] Although phentolamine is absorbed to some extent when it is administered orally, it has only limited activity in comparison to that after parenteral administration. With high oral dosage there have been intolerable gastrointestinal symptoms and it is therefore marketed only in a parenteral dosage form. The half life of phentolamine after intravenous administration is approximately 90 min, although the haemodynamic response is more prolonged, lasting for up to 12 h.

It is not known whether phentolamine is excreted in breast milk and there is no information on its transfer across the placenta.

Oral absorption	low
Presystemic metabolism	—
Plasma half life	90 min
Volume of distribution	
Plasma protein binding	54%

Concentration–effect relationship

There is no evidence of any correlation between the therapeutic effects of phentolamine and its concentration in biological fluids.

Metabolism

Around 70% of phentolamine is excreted in urine within the first 24 h. Only 10–13% is excreted in urine unchanged. A prominent metabolite is the carboxyphenyl derivative which constitutes 17% of the injected dose (unpublished data Ciba). Faecal excretion accounts for only 3% of the total dose. Conjugation appears to be unimportant in the metabolism of phentolamine.

Pharmaceutics

Parenteral phentolamine, Rogitine (Ciba, UK), is a colourless or slightly yellow solution containing 10 mg.ml^{-1} phentolamine mesylate.

Regitine injection (Ciba, USA) contains 5 mg lyophilized powder per vial, combined with 25 mg mannitol.

Therapeutic use

Indications

1. Diagnosis and control of hypertension secondary to a phaeochromocytoma
2. Management of hypertensive crisis secondary to overdose with sympathomimetic agents, including the 'cheese reaction' to monoamine oxidase inhibitors
3. The management of impotence.

Contraindications

1. Hypotension or any condition where sudden hypotension would be undesirable.

Mode of use

Phentolamine is usually administered as an intravenous infusion in 5% dextrose, or saline, at a rate of 0.2–2 $mg.min^{-1}$, titrating the dose to the desired blood pressure response. The initial dosage can be increased up to 5 $mg.min^{-1}$ for more rapid response and it can also be administered in 5–10 mg boluses intramuscularly.

Indications

1. Phaeochromocytoma
Phentolamine is useful in controlling paroxysms of hypertension in phaeochromocytoma. It is usually given intramuscularly for preoperative preparation although the use of phenoxybenzamine, a non-competitive α-adrenoceptor antagonist, is preferable for long-term α-adrenoceptor blockade.[3] However, due to its rapid onset of action, phentolamine is especially useful during surgery when manipulation of the tumour can lead to a massive release of catecholamine and a hypertensive crisis.[3]

Nowadays, the diagnosis of phaeochromocytoma should be based on measurements of increased production of catecholamine metabolites in the urine or free catecholamines in plasma. The use of phentolamine as a diagnostic test for phaeochromocytoma was based on its marked effect on blood pressure when hypertension is due to excessive catecholamines, in contrast to a relative lack of response with essential hypertension. Following a basal blood pressure recording, a 5 mg intravenous injection of phentolamine is administered. With a positive response there is a marked drop in systolic pressure and a drop of more than 25 mmHg in the diastolic pressure, usually maximal within 2 minutes of injection. Unfortunately, false positive hypotensive responses can occur with stress, uraemia or with sedative or narcotic administration. Equally, false negatives can occur if the tumour is not actively secreting or if there is co-existing essential hypertension.

2. Sympathomimetic-induced hypertension
Phentolamine is effective in controlling the hypertensive crisis associated with sympathomimetic overdose. It is very effective in the hypertensive crisis associated with the interaction of monoamine oxidase inhibitors with foods or rebound hypertension following abrupt clonidine withdrawal.

3. Impotence
Phentolamine in combination with papaverine injected directly into the corpus cavernosum has been used effectively in managing psychogenic as well as organic impotence.[4]

Other uses
Local infiltration of phentolamine is useful in preventing skin necrosis associated with extravasation of α-adrenergic agonists, such as noradrenaline and dopamine, during an intravenous infusion. 5–10 mg phentolamine is diluted in 10 ml 0.9% saline and infiltrated into the affected area.

Contraindications

Phentolamine is contraindicated in the presence of significant hypotension and also in any condition where hypotension and a tachycardia would be particularly undesirable. Severe coronary artery disease, hypertrophic obstructive cardiomyopathy and aortic stenosis as well as cerebrovascular disease would preclude its use.

Adverse reactions

Potentially life-threatening effects
When used in the diagnosis of phaeochromocytoma, hypotension may occasionally be very severe, and death has ensued on rare occasions. The explanation is probably that patients with very high plasma catecholamine concentrations may have a reduced plasma volume and are unable to maintain circulatory filling when the vasoconstriction is suddenly withdrawn. This is one reason why gradual introduction of α-adrenergic blockade is generally preferable as it allows plasma volume to normalize.

Acute overdosage
Phentolamine overdose is characterized by hypotension, tachycardia and arrhythmias. In addition to the adverse effects mentioned above, excessive sweating, overexcitation, headache, visual disturbances as well as hypoglycaemia can also occur.

Phentolamine (mesylate)

The treatment consists of placing the patient in the supine or head-down position and cautiously administering plasma expanders. Noradrenaline is of little value because its vasoconstrictor effects will be blocked. Adrenaline should not be used as it can precipitate further hypotension and exaggerate the tachycardia due to its unopposed β_2 action.

Severe or irreversible adverse effects
None have been reported apart from hypotension and its consequences.

Symptomatic adverse effects
Nausea, vomiting and diarrhoea may occur after intravenous administration.

Interference with clinical pathology tests
Phentolamine may interfere with colorimetric measurements of 5-hydroxyindole acetic acid, giving falsely high values.

High risk groups

Neonates
The drug is not used in this age group.

Breast milk. No information is available, so the drug is best avoided by breast-feeding mothers.

Children
Phentolamine has been used in children and 1–5 mg can be administered intravenously according to age during surgical resection of phaeochromocytoma. A 1 mg dose is used for the purpose of a diagnostic test.

Pregnant women
There is insufficient information about the use of phentolamine during pregnancy and its use should therefore be avoided if possible.

The elderly
The increased risks of hypotension in this age group should be considered carefully prior to administration of phentolamine.

Drug interactions

Potentially hazardous interactions
Phentolamine should be used with great caution in combination with other hypotensive agents. The interaction with adrenaline has already been mentioned in the overdose section.

Potentially useful interactions
None has been described.

Clinical trials

There do not appear to have been any formal randomized, placebo-controlled trials of phentolamine.

General review articles

Imhoff P R, Garnier B, Brunner L, Keller G, Rohrer T 1975 Human pharmacology of orally administered phentolamine. In: Taylor S H, Could L A (eds) 1975 Phentolamine in heart failure and other cardiac disorders. Proceedings of International Workshop, London. Hans Huber, Bern

Das P K, Parrat J R 1971 Myocardial and haemodynamic effects of phentolamine. British Journal of Pharmacology 41: 437–444

References

1. Stern M A, Gohlke H K, Loeb H S, Croke R P, Gunnar R M 1978 Haemodynamic effects of intravenous phentolamine in low output cardiac failure. Circulation 58: 157–163
2. Kerger B D, James R C, Roberts S M 1987 An assay for phentolamine using high performance liquid chromatography with electrochemical detection. Analytical Biochemistry 170: 145–151
3. Hull C J 1986 Phaeochromocytoma — diagnosis, pre-op preparation and anaesthetic management. British Journal of Anaesthesia 58: 1453–1468
4. Zorgniotti A W, Lefleur R S 1985 Auto-injection of the corpus cavernosum with a vasoactive drug combination for vasculogenic impotence. Journal of Urology 133: 39–41
5. Zenck K E 1981 Management of intravenous extravasations. Infusion 5: 77–79

P

Phenylbutazone

Phenylbutazone was the first of the many non-steroidal anti-inflammatory drugs. Synthesized in 1946, it was introduced into clinical practice soon afterwards and for 25 years was used extensively for most of the rheumatic diseases. Clinical usage has declined considerably since 1975 and in many countries it is now licensed only for very limited indications, such as ankylosing spondylitis or acute gout. In the UK it is recommended only for treatment of ankylosing spondylitis, under hospital supervision.

Chemistry

Phenylbutazone (butadione, fenilbutazona, Butacote, Butazolidin(e), Phenbutazone)
$C_{19}H_{20}O_2N_2$
1,2-Diphenyl-3,5-4-n-butylpyrazolidine

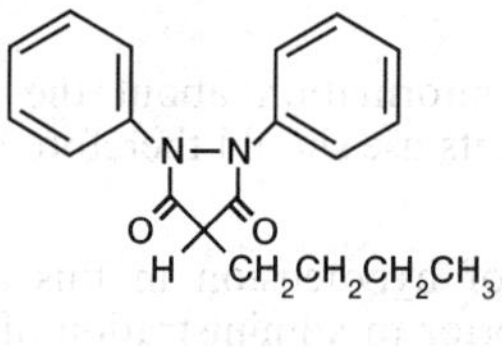

Molecular weight	308.4
pKa (N)	4.5
Solubility	
in alcohol	1 in 28
in water	1 in 11 000
Octanol/water partition coefficient	
(pH 7.4)	5

Phenylbutazone is a fine, colourless, crystalline compound, soluble in organic solvents, but only sparingly soluble in water. It is synthesized by the condensation of hydrazobenzene with the diethylester of n-butyl malonic acid. It was at one time available in combination with several analgesics, muscle relaxants and corticosteroid preparations (e.g. Parazolidin, Delta-Butazolidin).

Pharmacology

Phenylbutazone is a powerful analgesic with antipyretic and anti-inflammatory actions demonstrable with the classical pharmacological models. It causes retention of sodium and chloride ions, with consequent water retention. It has a mild but definite uricosuric action.

Its anti-inflammatory action depends upon inhibition of the cyclo-oxygenase enzyme with resultant reduction in the formation of the prostaglandins E_2 and $F_{2}\alpha$. It does not affect the leukotriene pathway. The drug also reduces platelet adhesiveness[1] with consequent prolonged platelet survival time and diminished turnover.[2]

Toxicology

The half life of phenylbutazone in small animals is only 2–4 hours. Routine toxicology tests must be interpreted with this in mind. LD_{50} doses in mice and rats are between 120 and 215 $mg.kg^{-1}$, with tetanic convulsions preceding death. Chronic toxicity studies in dogs at 10 and 100 $mg.kg^{-1}$ daily produced no gross toxicity, but 200 $mg.kg^{-1}$ daily produced weight loss, anorexia and anaemia with gastrointestinal ulceration.

Phenylbutazone has no significant mutagenic, teratogenic or carcinogenic effect.

Clinical pharmacology

In addition to the desired analgesic and anti-inflammatory effects, phenylbutazone has effects on the kidney, the thyroid gland and on the gastrointestinal tract.

The renal effect is manifest as salt and water retention and is due to increased tubular resorption. Early studies had shown that it had no effect on glomerular filtration as measured by various clearance tests (inulin,[3,4] creatinine.[5,6]) Mild hypertension may develop in the normal person and a further rise in pressure may occur in hypertensive patients. Similarly, the effectiveness of diuretic therapy for hypertension is diminished.[7,8,9] This effect is secondary to the decrease in production of renal prostaglandins, with consequent fall in aldosterone levels and plasma renin activity, as has been described with indomethacin.[10] In healthy subjects balance is restored after a few days medication when there is a compensating diuresis, but in patients with decreased cardiac output severe complications may ensue, as described below.

Phenylbutazone also has a uricosuric effect. This is also a tubular effect, preventing reabsorption of uric acid.[11,12] Although present in healthy people the fall in serum uric acid concentration is much easier to demonstrate in gouty subjects, as is the increased urinary excretion of uric acid. The uricosuric effect of phenylbutazone is much less than that of its analogue, sulphinpyrazone.

The observation of thyroid hyperplasia following treatment with phenylbutazone prompted investigations of the mechanism. Studies in man have shown that phenylbutazone inhibits the thyroid uptake of radioactive iodine.[13] The underlying mechanism is an interference with organification of iodine. This effect, though well recognized, is rarely of clinical significance.

In the gastrointestinal tract gastric mucus protects the lining cells by maintaining a physical barrier at neutral pH, maintained by diffusion of bicarbonate ions from the mucosal cells towards the stomach lumen. Prostanoids stimulate bicarbonate production and NSAIDs directly affect the mucus pH as well as inhibiting cyclo-oxygenase as already noted. This results in an impaired ability of the gastric and duodenal mucosa to resist acid attack and hence ulceration may occur.[14]

In therapeutic doses, phenylbutazone has no direct pharmacological effect on the cardiovascular system, hepatic function or the central nervous system.

Pharmacokinetics

Spectrophotometric methods (e.g. Burns et al 1953)[15] have proved useful for biological fluids, but the two main hydroxymetabolites interfere with the assay. Several gas chromatographic methods are available, which are specific for phenylbutazone, even in the presence of its metabolites.[16] With electron capture detection the limit of sensitivity is 10 $\mu g.l^{-1}$. The drug can also be determined by high pressure liquid chromatography,[17] with a limit of sensitivity of 50 $\mu g.l^{-1}$, and by chemical ionization mass spectrometry.[18]

The basic understanding of phenylbutazone kinetics and transformation was elucidated more than 30 years ago, using spectrophotometric assays.[15,19] Subsequent studies, using chromatographic[20,21] and radio-tracer[22] methods have extended this knowledge, but the picture is still not complete.

Absorption of phenylbutazone is rapid and virtually complete following oral administration, with peak plasma levels occurring in 2 to 4 hours. There is no significant presystemic metabolism. The plasma half life is very long, usually in the range 70–100 hours, although it varies from 49 to 142 hours.[23] Following a single dose, phenylbutazone may be detected in the plasma for 4 or 5 days. It takes at least 10 days, and sometimes more than 20 days, to reach steady-state plasma levels following any alteration in dosage, as would be predicted from its long half life.

Phenylbutazone is highly lipophilic, so that it readily diffuses through lipid membranes. There are high concentrations in liver, heart, lung and kidney, but low concentrations in the central nervous system. In human serum, phenylbutazone, at therapeutic concentrations (90 $mg.l^{-1}$) is 99.4% bound to plasma proteins (particularly to albumin and α-globulin fractions), but with increasing concentrations of the drug the free fraction increases rapidly, so that at 220 $mg.l^{-1}$ there is 2.6% free drug. The apparent volume of distribution is only 172 ± 21 $ml.kg^{-1}$, reflecting the very high binding to serum proteins.

Phenylbutazone

Concentrations in synovial fluid vary between 50 and 80% of the plasma concentration,[24] with a tendency to be lower in more acutely inflamed joints. The drug can be detected up to 3 weeks after cessation of treatment. Only trace amounts of phenylbutazone cross the placenta to enter the fetal circulation. Similarly, only trace quantities are present in breast milk.[25,26]

Oral absorption	>95%
Presystemic metabolism	negligible
Plasma half life	
range	49–142 h
mean	72 h
Volume of distribution	172 ± 21 ml.kg^{-1}
Plasma protein binding	99.4%

The extensive protein binding and relatively high pKa of phenylbutazone result in only 1% of the administered dose being excreted unchanged in the urine. Phenylbutazone is extensively transformed in the liver, with 60% of a single dose excreted as metabolites in urine over a period of three weeks.[22] In this interval approximately 27% of the dose is excreted in the faeces as metabolites.

The rate of elimination is determined by the rate of hepatic biotransformation. This varies from 10 to 35% per day, with a mean of 21%. Studies of identical and fraternal twins[27] and two-generation family units[28] have shown that phenylbutazone metabolism is under polygenic control. Only in extremes of liver dysfunction is metabolism impaired. There might be some prolongation of half life in renal failure and in the elderly.

Phenylbutazone can displace several drugs, including warfarin and methotrexate, from their binding sites on plasma proteins. This effect was once believed to be the cause of some of the drug interactions caused by phenylbutazone, but has since been shown to be due largely to inhibition of metabolism. Both phenylbutazone and oxyphenbutazone inhibit the oxidation of several compounds, including warfarin, specifically the more potent S-isomer, tolbutamide, acetohexamide and phenytoin. It has been suggested that phenylbutazone might induce its own metabolism and that of other drugs, but this has not been substantiated. Phenylbutazone is a weak acid and as such it can compete with other weak acids, such as methotrexate and chlorpropamide, for active renal tubular secretion. As a consequence, the elimination of such drugs is impaired and their plasma concentrations are elevated.

There is no mechanism by which highly lipophilic compounds can be excreted unchanged. Only 1% of administered phenylbutazone is excreted unchanged in urine. Phenylbutazone is transformed by the liver, 60% of a single dose can be identified as metabolites in urine.[22] Three weeks after a single dose about 90% can be identified in urine (61%) or faeces (27%).

Concentration–effect relationship

An early study[29] showed that plasma levels were related directly to dosage, and that the effective therapeutic range was 50–150 mg.l^{-1}. Subsequent studies[30] have shown that plasma concentration correlates well in the lower dose range 50–100 mg daily but at higher doses, 200–300 mg daily, plasma concentrations were lower than predicted. While this type of effect could be due to metabolizing enzyme stimulation which occurs in the hydroxylation mechanism in animals, it does not occur with the major enzyme glucuronyl transferase in man, where the mechanism is considered to be saturation of binding sites resulting in a greater proportion of free drug available for metabolism. Another study[31] confirmed the dosage/plasma concentration relationship, but neither study was able to establish a clear relationship with plasma concentration and clinical efficacy. The most recent study[32] compared eight dose levels in 30 mg steps from 90 to 450 mg daily in a double-blind study in patients with rheumatoid arthritis. The 'best' dose was 300 mg daily. Doses below this did not give full effect, and above this did not give further improvement. There was no relationship between plasma levels and either response or side effects. The wide variation of symptom severity in rheumatoid disease and the absence of a simple numerical measure of efficacy, together with the lack of correlation between dose and plasma level, make plasma level/response studies unhelpful.

Metabolism

Phenylbutazone is almost wholly metabolized in the liver, with less than 1% of the dose excreted unchanged in the urine (see Fig. 1). Initial studies[15] suggested that aromatic (metabolite I, oxyphenbutazone) and side-chain (metabolite II) oxidation were the main path-

Fig. 1 Phenylbutazone

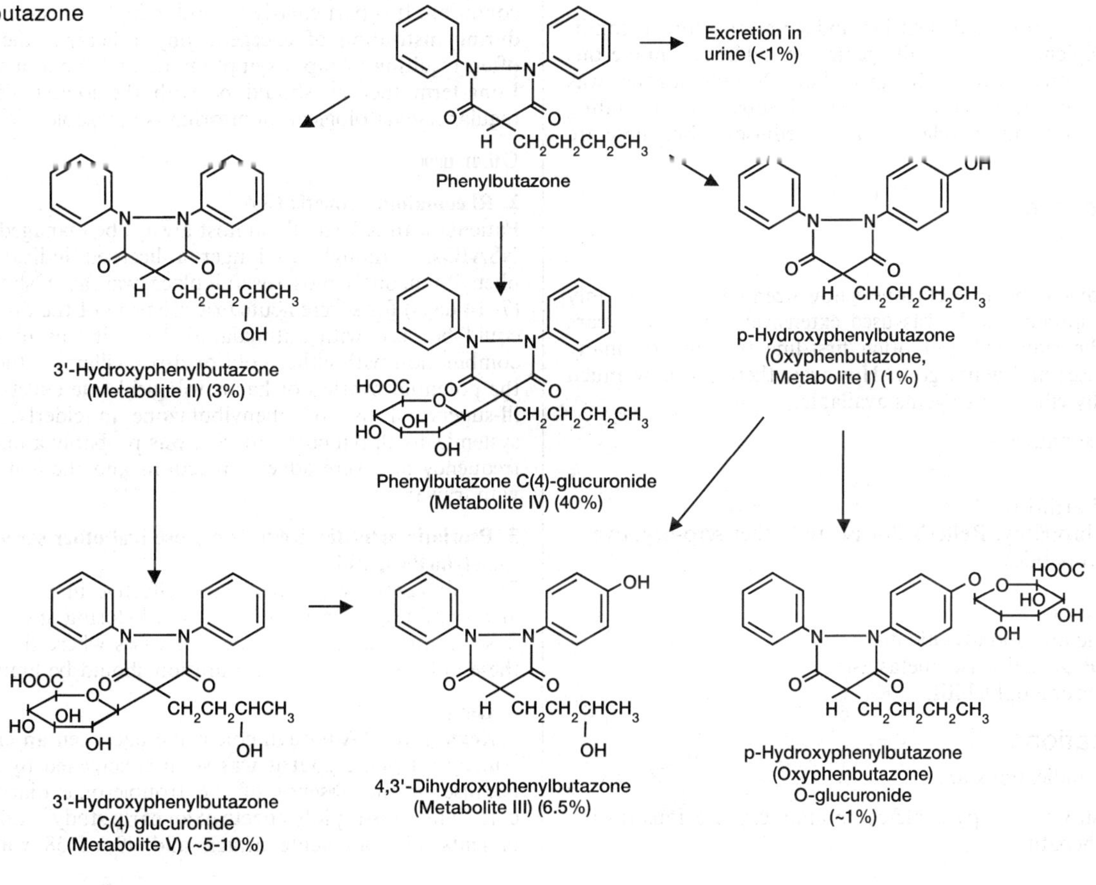

P

ways of metabolism, though these metabolites accounted for only a small percentage of the dose. Subsequent studies identified the dihydroxylated product (metabolite III). These metabolites are subsequently conjugated with glucuronic acid. Radio-label studies showed that these three metabolites, together with phenylbutazone, account for 89% of the radioactivity in plasma.[33]

However, in urine these products account for only 10% of the radioactivity present. Analysis of urine by thin-layer chromatography and autoradiography enabled the identification of metabolites IV and V. These are the C(4)-glucuronide conjugates of phenylbutazone and gamma(3')hydroxyphenylbutazone, not identifiable in urine following treatment with β-glucuronidase, because the sugar is coupled directly to the pyrazolidine ring through a C–C bond, and as such is not subject to hydrolysis.

27% of the dose is excreted in the faeces and 60% in urine, comprising (relative to the dose) 40% C(4)-glucuronide of phenylbutazone, 1% free phenylbutazone and free oxyphenbutazone, 6% 4,3'-dihydroxyphenylbutazone, 3% 3'-hydroxyphenylbutazone and 12% other metabolites, including the C-glucuronide of 3'-hydroxyphenylbutazone and the O-glucuronide of oxyphenbutazone.

The p-hydroxy (N-1 phenyl) metabolite of phenylbutazone (oxyphenbutazone) has pharmacological properties similar to those of the parent compound, and is marketed as such. It is extensively bound to plasma proteins and has a half life of 2–3 days. It accumulates in plasma and contributes to the effects of phenylbutazone. 3'-Hydroxyphenylbutazone has uricosuric properties, and is probably responsible for this effect of phenylbutazone. The half life of this metabolite is approximately 30 hours.

Pharmaceutics

Phenylbutazone is available as Butazolidin (Geigy) in the following forms:

1. 100 mg red, sugar-coated biconvex tablets, imprinted 'Geigy'
2. 200 mg white, sugar-coated biconvex tablets, imprinted 'Geigy'
3. 250 mg white, waxy suppository
4. 600 mg ampoules, phenylbutazone sodium in 3 ml, with 1% zylocaine;

and as Butacote (Geigy):

5. 100 mg pale violet sugar-coated enteric tablets imprinted 'Geigy'.

The tablets have a prolonged shelf-life under normal storage conditions. The excipients are non-allergenic. In addition, numerous generic preparations used to be available. Phenylbutazone was available in combination with a number of substances including alkalis, paracetamol, muscle relaxants and prednisone, but these are no longer available.

Therapeutic use

Indications

Because of its toxicity phenylbutazone is now licensed in the UK only for ankylosing spondylitis. It was used extensively for many years when it was the standard and often first-line therapy for many rheumatic diseases and acute gout. However, there are now much safer and equally efficacious agents available.

1. Ankylosing spondylitis

Other uses

2. Rheumatoid arthritis
3. Psoriatic arthropathy, Reiter's disease and other sero-negative spondylarthropathies
4. Gout
5. Rheumatic fever
6. Osteoarthritic and spondylotic disorders
7. Bone pain (Paget's disease, metastasis)
8. Superficial thrombophlebitis.

Contraindications

Absolute contraindications are:

1. Known sensitivity to a pyrazole compound, e.g. previous rash, leucopenia, hepatitis
2. The presence of any type of blood dyscrasia
3. Uncontrolled congestive cardiac failure or severe hypertension
4. Active peptic ulcer.

Relative contraindications are:

5. Drug-induced or idiopathic dyspepsia. Healed peptic ulcer.
6. Recent infective hepatitis
7. Controlled congestive cardiac failure or hypertension where salt and water retention would be likely to provoke failure
8. Hepatitis or renal disease of a severity sufficient to decrease metabolism or excretion.

Relative contraindication implies that the patient has symptoms of such severity that they cannot be controlled by an alternative preparation less likely to aggravate the concomitant contraindications.

Mode of use

Clinical effectiveness is dependent in the short term on the rapid analgesic effect. The anti-inflammatory features, demonstrable in inflammatory polyarthritis as reduction in joint swelling and morning stiffness, are not evident for two or three weeks.

Dosage requirements vary considerably. In very painful conditions such as acute gout, severe exacerbations of ankylosing spondylitis, or acute onset of reactive forms of polyarthritis an initial dose of 200 mg three or even four times daily would be not unreasonable, with phased reductions commencing as soon as adequate symptomatic control is achieved, reducing to the minimum satisfactory maintenance dose. For minor complaints 50 mg twice daily would be adequate.

In patients in whom prolonged medication seems likely, the sugar-coated enteric form should be used. Patients who need phenylbutazone but suffer gastric upset can often use the 100 mg suppository, once or twice daily. The intramuscular form is used very infrequently. Because of local protein binding of phenylbutazone at the injection site it is not rapidly effective. Although there are reports of both intra-articular and intravenous use, these are not recommended.

Indications

1. Ankylosing spondylitis

Phenylbutazone should be used as single drug therapy in this condition. It is particularly helpful in higher dosage (600 mg per day) during institution of energetic physiotherapy, the two treatments often resulting in rapid symptomatic and functional improvements. Long-term therapy should be with the lowest effective dose and regular haematological monitoring is advisable.

Other uses

2. Rheumatoid arthritis (RA)

Patients with RA should almost always be managed with alternative NSAIDs. Although no longer a licensed indication in the UK, phenylbutazone's most useful place was as a short-term measure (7–14 days) for severe acute exacerbation of the disease. Although it could be used with antimalarial drugs it was unwise to use it in combination with either gold or d-penicillamine therapy because of the potential overlap of haematological side effects. The long-term, ill-supervised use of phenylbutazone in elderly, frail and often systemically ill patients with RA was probably a major factor in the frequency of severe adverse reactions and the cause of its ultimate withdrawal.

3. Psoriatic arthritis, Reiter's disease and other seronegative spondylarthropathies

Phenylbutazone was particularly effective in psoriatic and Reiter's arthropathies, diseases related to ankylosing spondylitis. A similar dose regime was used. In the rare cases where the drug is used for these indications treatment duration should be limited.

4. Gout

Acute gout. Although colchicine had been an effective universal remedy for acute gout it was soon superceded by phenylbutazone, because of the absence of the troublesome diarrhoea caused by colchicine. It is rapidly effective: an early study[34] noted that 15 of 16 patients with an acute attack and 49 of 58 with acute attacks

Phenylbutazone

superimposed on chronic disease had major improvement, half having complete remission within one week and 84% being asymptomatic by 7 days. In a comparison with flufenamic acid[35] both treatments were rapidly effective, but relapses were much more frequent with flufenamic acid, a difference attributed to the uricosuric effect of the phenylbutazone.

Initial dosage should be 600–800 mg per day for 2 or 3 days, then reducing to 300 or 400 mg per day for up to 7 days. When patients are taking xanthine oxidase inhibitor or uricosuric drugs these should be continued in unchanged dosage in addition to phenylbutazone. Alternative NSAIDs are now usually used for acute gout.

Chronic gout. Phenylbutazone alone is not an effective treatment for chronic gout.

5. Rheumatic fever
Although no longer used in this now rare disease, phenylbutazone was more rapidly effective than aspirin in controlling joint pain and swelling, fever, tachycardia and ESR, and was associated with a lower relapse rate.[36]

6. Osteoarthritis and spondylotic disease
Although many studies have shown phenylbutazone to be effective in these disorders, often in low dosage, they are not recommended indications because many patients are elderly and prolonged treatment is often needed.

7. Bone pain (Paget's disease, bony metastases)
In Paget's disease, phenylbutazone has been superceded by specific therapy such as calcitonin and diphosphonates. Although no longer an officially approved indication it was very effective in relieving the pain from bony metastases and often allowed considerable reduction in opiate requirements.

8. Superficial thrombophlebitis
For many years phenylbutazone was regarded as a specific remedy for superficial thrombophlebitis, though its effect was probably due to a combination of effective analgesic, anti-inflammatory and antiplatelet properties. It is no longer used for this condition.

Contraindications

Absolute contraindications

1. Known pyrazole drug sensitivity
Many of the severe adverse drug reaction reports indicate that, for example, agranulocytosis has occurred in a patient who had previously had a phenylbutazone drug rash. Similar events have been noted in patients who have developed life-threatening or fatal skin reactions such as Lyell's syndrome (toxic epidermal necrolysis) or Stevens–Johnson syndrome.

2. Blood dyscrasia
Phenylbutazone treatment has been associated with aplastic anaemia, thrombocytopenia, leucopenia and agranulocytosis. Full blood count should always be done before instituting therapy and any suggestion of inadequate bone marrow activity is a contraindication.

3. Uncontrolled congestive cardiac failure or hypertension
The initiation of phenylbutazone is almost always associated with some degree of sodium and water retention. In healthy individuals a compensatory diuresis usually occurs within a few days. Patients with compromised cardiac function may develop extensive peripheral and pulmonary oedema which is rapidly fatal unless there is urgent medical intervention.

4. Active peptic ulcer
Most patients with active peptic ulcer develop an acute exacerbation of gastric symptoms following administration of phenylbutazone, even when administered as the enteric-coated tablet.[37] Perforation and gastric bleeding may follow. If phenylbutazone therapy is absolutely needed it may be tolerated in suppository form, particularly with concurrent H_2 antagonist therapy. Phenylbutazone cannot, however, be recommended in these patients.

Relative contraindications

5. Drug-induced or simple idiopathic dyspepsia
Many patients suffering from chronic rheumatic disorders develop dyspepsia associated with their NSAID therapy. Except that indomethacin is particularly potent in this respect there is little difference between the other preparations and a change to phenylbutazone, especially the enteric-coated tablets, is often very well tolerated.[37]

6. Recent hepatitis
Phenylbutazone hepatitis is a very rare sensitivity reaction. Although there are no reports suggesting that post-hepatitis patients are prone to this reaction it seems wise to avoid phenylbutazone in these cases.

7. Controlled congestive cardiac failure or hypertension
The effect of phenylbutazone has been noted above. Such patients treated with phenylbutazone should be under close clinical supervision in the early stages of therapy. Any increasing oedema should be treated immediately with increasing doses of diuretics or withdrawal of phenylbutazone (or both). Most NSAIDs affect the renal prostaglandin system with consequent decrease in renal blood flow and increase in blood pressure. Hypertensive patients should thus receive additional monitoring.

8. Severe hepatic and renal disease
Although phenylbutazone is metabolized in the liver and excreted as metabolites in urine it is only in gross disease that accumulation of drug occurs. Nevertheless the effect of phenylbutazone on the renal prostaglandin system may aggravate renal insufficiency.

Adverse reactions

Potentially life-threatening effects
Phenylbutazone has been withdrawn from general use in the UK mainly because of the accumulation in the records of the Committee on Safety of Medicines of many severe and fatal adverse reaction reports. While there is no controversy about the facts, it should be remembered that phenylbutazone was used extensively as the major drug for treatment of all types of rheumatic disorder for about 20 years, and that it was used indiscriminately, often in unnecessarily high dosage.

The disease being treated may affect the likelihood of adverse reaction, patients with rheumatoid arthritis being apparently more susceptible than those with osteoarthritis or ankylosing spondylitis.[38]

Blood dyscrasias. The estimate of the frequency of blood dyscrasias caused by phenylbutazone and oxyphenbutazone[39] in the years 1960–1965, was one case per 150 000 'patient-months' of treatment and one fatal case per 250 000 patient-months of treatment, and was based on a monthly dose of 9 g, market research statistics, and case reports. Subsequent estimates[40] in 1977 were one case from 33 000–99 000 prescriptions, with a mortality of 3.8 per 100 000 prescriptions for oxyphenbutazone and 2.2 per 100 000 for phenylbutazone, with confirmation of the high rate among elderly females. Although isolated reports in the past suggested that leukaemia may develop as a result of phenylbutazone therapy, the evidence is largely circumstantial and has not been substantiated.

Agranulocytosis is an acute sensitivity reaction, usually presenting within a few weeks of onset of therapy[38,39] with fever, stomal and pharyngeal ulceration, and toxaemia. It may be associated with a drug rash. Although frequent white cell counts in the early stage of treatment have been recommended for early detection of leucopenia, close clinical supervision for early symptoms is more important.

Aplastic anaemia presents as severe anaemia or haemorrhagic diathesis. It usually occurs after prolonged therapy, often of 2 or 3 years' duration, elderly females being particularly likely to be affected,[38,39] a finding which has been independently confirmed.[40]

Thrombocytopenia may occur as an isolated acute sensitivity phenomenon early in treatment or as a late complication due to an effect on the bone marrow. In the former type megakaryocytes are prominent in the marrow, in the latter they are absent.

Peptic ulceration, bleeding, and perforation. Gastric ulceration with bleeding or perforation is commonest in elderly women, who develop large ulcers on the lesser curvature. These may be painless. Duodenal ulcer problems usually occur because of exacerbation of a pre-existing lesion.

Salt and water retention with pulmonary oedema and cardiac failure. The mechanism of this reaction is based on the inhibition of the renal prostaglandin synthetase system. Its frequency and outcome obviously depend on the care taken in prescribing and subsequent supervision of patients and is clearly more a function of medical skill than a toxic effect of the drug.

P

Acute idiosyncratic reactions. Although all are very rare, the commonest are the acute severe skin reactions such as the Stevens–Johnson syndrome, Lyell's syndrome (epidermal necrolysis), and exfoliative dermatitis. They are most likely to occur soon after starting the medication. They were much commoner in the early days of phenylbutazone when much larger initial doses were used and early signs of idiosyncratic reaction were not recognized. Acute hepatocellular disease and acute interstitial nephritis have been reported with acute skin reactions. All these reactions may be rapidly fatal.

The tables of the UK Committee on Safety of Medicines for the years 1964 to 1984 give a total of 10–25 for the skin conditions with 3/24 fatalities for Stevens–Johnson syndrome and 7/10 for epidermal necrolysis. In the same period, 7 deaths from hepatic reactions were recorded.

Acute overdosage

Phenylbutazone overdose is a rare and usually accidental occurrence, mainly in young children. In adults a very large dose may be tolerated with minor disturbances only. In children overdose is often associated with consumption of other medication, particularly aspirin.

Overdose may cause encephalitic or other neurological symptoms, acute renal failure, acute hepatitis, or death from acidosis. Pulmonary oedema also occurs. A 20-year-old who consumed 40 g developed severe neurological symptoms followed by hepatitis and leucopenia, but survived. In another case, two doses of 8 and 20 g separated by 9 hours were fatal in a subject aged 45 years.

A 15-year-old survived 8 g and a 3-year-old 6 g. Both had severe neurological symptoms and the former developed jaundice. In contrast, a 19-month-old child died following 2.5 g.

Treatment should include evacuation of the stomach (induction of vomiting or gastric lavage) and use of activated charcoal. If necessary, additional measures include saline, purgatives, artificial respiration, measures to support the circulation, anticonvulsants (e.g. diazepam) and haemodialysis. Haemoperfusion and exchange transfusion may be useful.

Severe or irreversible adverse effects

Peptic ulceration. This has already been noted above. The frequency is not known. As dyspeptic symptoms are so common with NSAIDs they are an accepted hazard and thus are infrequently reported.

Acute gastric erosions. This condition usually presents as acute and often dramatic haematemesis and can be diagnosed only by endoscopy. Transfusion may be required, but healing is usually rapid once the drug is withdrawn. It may occur with any NSAID.

Hepatitis. In addition to hepatitis occurring as part of a generalized idiosyncratic reaction, jaundice may occur as an isolated reaction. Although drug reactions are among the commoner causes of jaundice, phenylbutazone is a very rare offender. Only 59 reports were received by the Committee on Safety of Medicines, with seven fatalities, in the 20 years to 1984.

In a review of 41 case reports,[41] three main types of liver damage were recognized: (a) hepatocellular damage; (b) intra-hepatic biliary cholestasis; (c) mixed. There was a 3.5:1 female preponderance and 75% of the patients were over 50 years old. In the majority, the onset of symptoms was within 4 weeks of starting treatment, but three had been treated for more than 12 months and three for 6–12 months before the onset of symptoms. The hepatocellular type of damage presented with malaise, with or without fever, or nausea and vomiting, with jaundice appearing up to 14 days after the onset of symptoms. In the cholestatic type, jaundice was usually the presenting feature. All but one of the fatal cases involved hepatitis or hepatic necrosis.

Exfoliative dermatitis. A small number of cases have been reported to the Committee on Safety of Medicines and there are at least four published reports. It appears most likely to occur when patients who have had a severe drug rash are again exposed to phenylbutazone, and confirms the importance of recording drug eruptions.

Goitre. Diffuse thyroid enlargement has been reported but is very rare. It occurs after prolonged therapy. Phenylbutazone binds to thyroxine-binding globulin (TBG) and so decreases TBG binding capacity, with consequent decrease in total T_4 and T_3 levels. If an effect is suspected, free levels of T_4 and T_3 should be measured or the free-thyroxine index calculated.

Chromosomal damage. Leucocytes from 50 patients who had been taking phenylbutazone for at least 3 months were cultured for 48 hours.[54] The frequency of cells with damaged chromosomes was higher than in controls. Nine patients tested before and after treatment confirmed that this was a drug effect. There is no direct in vitro effect. The significance of this finding is not clinically apparent.

Symptomatic adverse effects

Dyspepsia and allied symptoms. The most common cause for withdrawal of phenylbutazone therapy is dyspepsia — mainly nausea, less frequently epigastric pain or heartburn. In an early study[43] in 1958, it was reported that 20% of patients developed gastric symptoms. In a later large scale study,[44] 1.6% of patients dropped out while 12.1% of those who completed the study period had dyspeptic symptoms and in another similar study[45] the corresponding figures were 2.6% and 11.0%. In some patients with these symptoms, superficial gastric erosions have been seen.

Gastric tolerance can be considerably improved by the use of the enteric-coated formulation[46,47] or by use of the suppository[48] though both may cause symptoms via the systemic effect and the former is certainly not well tolerated by patients with a known peptic ulcer.

Minor drug rashes. Rashes of any type may occur — erythematous, macular, urticarial and petechial. The reported incidence is variable — 8% in one study,[43] but there were none in another study of 112 patients.[45] Rash usually occurs early and is a definite contraindication to further exposure.

Stomatitis. Buccal ulceration occurs early in treatment and resolves rapidly on withdrawal, but will usually recur with re-exposure.

Rectal bleeding and haematuria. Although most likely to occur with suppository medication, rectal bleeding has been reported with oral medication. Proctitis has been seen, but more often no obvious cause is detected and the symptom disappears with drug withdrawal.

Benign haematuria, with red cells identified in the urine, has also been reported. No renal lesions (including renal papillary necrosis) have been found in the majority of cases and the bleeding ceases on drug withdrawal. It may be due to uric acid crystals but this has not been proved.

Salivary gland swelling. This unusual adverse effect most commonly affects the parotid gland but any single one, or all, of the glands may be affected. It is a sensitivity reaction and settles rapidly on withdrawal of the drug. The main danger is that it goes unrecognized as a drug reaction so that the patient may be subjected to invasive investigations or even surgery.

Local reactions to suppository or injection.

(a) Suppository: local irritation or anal discharge may occur. Occasionally proctitis has been seen.

(b) Injection: induration may develop at the injection site, particularly if it is not given by deep intramuscular injection. Misplaced injections have caused severe, irreversible sciatic nerve damage.

Other effects

The effect of phenylbutazone on salt and water retention and increased uric acid excretion has already been noted.

Interference with clinical pathology tests

Plasma proteins appear to be decreased when fluid retention occurs. The effect on thyroid function tests has been noted above.

High risk groups

Neonates

Phenylbutazone is not given to neonates.

Breast milk. Phenylbutazone is excreted in small quantities in maternal milk, but the concentrations are very low — 0.063 $mg.l^{-1}$.

Children

Phenylbutazone has been used for treating children suffering from juvenile chronic arthritis, especially the subgroup with ankylosing spondylitis. It has also been extensively used for rheumatic fever, though cardiac failure has been precipitated by the water retention effect. When given at a dose of 10 $mg.kg^{-1}$ daily plasma phenylbutazone levels were in the range 90–120 $mg.l^{-1}$,[49] i.e. the accepted therapeutic range. Although it has been reported[50] that phenylbutazone has a significantly shorter biological half life in children, this

Phenylbutazone

report should be cautiously interpreted, as 8 of the 10 children suffered from plumbism.

Pregnant women
Phenylbutazone is detectable in small quantities in umbilical cord blood following administration during labour.[26] There is no convincing evidence that phenylbutazone has any teratogenic effects. In a special study[42] of 18 women who had used phenylbutazone or oxyphenbutazone during the first trimester, one had a miscarriage, six had infants with minor malformations, and one had an infant with a major malformation, but it is concluded that there is little difference in the use of analgesics between women who have normal or deformed babies.

Any indication for phenylbutazone during pregnancy must be exceedingly rare. It should certainly not be used during the third trimester, as, in common with other NSAIDs, it may cause premature closure of the fetal ductus arteriosus.

The elderly
Biological half life in subjects aged over 70 years is not significantly different to that in younger people.[51] Nevertheless, the elderly are much more susceptible to severe adverse drug reactions.[38]

Drug interactions

Potentially hazardous interactions

Warfarin and other coumarin anticoagulants. Phenylbutazone and oxyphenbutazone displace warfarin from plasma protein binding sites. This was thought to be the reason for the enhanced anticoagulant effect. Subsequent studies have shown that the effect is due to inhibition of metabolism of the S-isomer of warfarin, which is five times more potent than the R-isomer. Phenylbutazone may be given with anticoagulants provided that during initiation of therapy prothrombin time is repeatedly checked and appropriate dose adjustments are made.

Antidiabetic drugs. Phenylbutazone and oxyphenbutazone inhibit the metabolism of tolbutamide and acetohexamide so that their hypoglycaemic effect is enhanced. Concurrent treatment is best avoided.

Methotrexate. Phenylbutazone inhibits renal clearance of methotrexate and displaces it from plasma protein. They should not be used concurrently.

Other significant interactions

Phenytoin. Phenylbutazone and oxyphenbutazone inhibit the metabolism of phenytoin. Consequently dosage changes are required during introduction and withdrawal of pyrazole therapy, so that the combination is best avoided.

Antihypertensives, β-blockers, and diuretics. Because of inhibition of renal prostaglandin synthesis the vasodilator response to vasoconstriction is reduced or abolished by NSAID therapy. Thus the hypotensive effect of β-blockers may be diminished, as may the effect of diuretics.[7,8,9]

Antacids. One report[52] shows that the rate and extent of oxyphenbutazone absorption is increased by concomitant administration of aluminium hydroxide or magnesium trisilicate. Another[53] shows that phenylbutazone is not affected by the combination when administered in enteric-coated form.

Alcohol. Phenylbutazone has a minor delaying action on the metabolism of alcohol.

Potentially useful interactions
No reactions of this kind have been described.

Major outcome trials

Rheumatoid arthritis

1. Fjellström K E, Goldberg L, Lindgren G, Nillson F 1957 Phenylbutazone in active periods of rheumatoid arthritis. Acta Medica Scandinavica (suppl 320) 127: 1–49

This double-blind study compared phenylbutazone (initial dose 800 mg daily, maintenance 400 mg daily) with placebo, for one month. Phenylbutazone was significantly effective in reducing rheumatoid activity, analgesic requirements, number of tender joints and in improving functional capacity. Improvement was evident within seven days.

2. Smyth C J, Clark G M 1957 Phenylbutazone in rheumatoid arthritis. Journal of Chronic Diseases 5: 734–750

Phenylbutazone and cortisone were compared in a double-blind crossover study. Each preparation was given for five months, with one month on aspirin only between. Both trial drugs suppressed the overall inflammatory index, aspirin did not.

3. Mason R M, Steinberg V L 1960 Long-term use of phenylbutazone in rheumatoid arthritis. British Medical Journal 2: 828–830

This study follows the progress of 315 patients over a four year period, analysing the reasons for withdrawal. In one third, it was discontinued within three months, mainly because of intolerance. By three years 80% had stopped, either because of disease remission or lack of continued effectiveness.

Ankylosing spondylitis

There are numerous publications on this subject

1. Mason R M, Howes R G 1963 The treatment of ankylosing spondylitis. Proceedings of the Australian Rheumatology Congress, Sydney; Sept 1963, p 51

A survey of 342 patients over a five year period. The majority had radiotherapy, with or without drugs, but 61 had phenylbutazone or oxyphenbutazone alone. 92% of the drug-treated and 68% of the radiotherapy-treated patients obtained immediate relief, with advantages to the drug-treated group being maintained or increased as the years passed.

Gout

Kuzell W C, Shaffarzick R W 1952 Phenylbutazone and butapyrin. A study of clinical effects in arthritis and gout. Annals of California Medicine 77: 319–325

Douglas G, Thompson M 1970 A comparison of phenylbutazone and flufenamic acid in the treatment of acute gout. Annals of Physical Medicine 6: 275–280

General review articles

Von Rechenberg H J 1962 Phenylbutazone, 2nd edn. Edward Arnold, London

Fowler P D 1983 Phenylbutazone. In: Huskisson E C (ed) Antirheumatic drugs. Praeger Publishers, Eastbourne and New York, pp. 353–370

Phenylbutazone metabolism and kinetics

Aarbakke J 1978 Clinical pharmacokinetics of phenylbutazone. Clinical Pharmacokinetics 3: 369–380

Faigle J W, Dieterle W 1977 The biotransformation of phenylbutazone. Journal of International Medical Research 5 (suppl 2): 2–14

Aarbakke J, Bakke O M, Milde E J, Davies D S 1977 Metabolism of phenylbutazone in man. European Journal of Clinical Pharmacology 11: 359–366

Phenylbutazone induced blood dyscrasias and adverse reactions reviews

Fowler P D 1967 Marrow toxicity of the pyrazoles. Annals of the Rheumatic Diseases 26: 344–345

Fowler P D, Faragher E B 1977 Drug and non-drug factors influencing adverse reactions to pyrazoles. Journal of International Medical Research 5 (suppl 2): 108–120

Inman W H W 1977 Study of fatal bone marrow depression with special reference to phenylbutazone and oxyphenbutazone. British Medical Journal 1: 1500–1505

Fowler P D, Woolf D, Alexander S 1975 Phenylbutazone and hepatitis. Rheumatology and Rehabilitation 14: 71–75

Fowler P D 1987 Aspirin, paracetamol and non-steroidal anti-inflammatory drugs: a comparative review of side effects. Medical Toxicology 2: 338–366

Phenylbutazone

P

References

1. Bobek K von, Cepelak V 1958 Butazolidin as an anti-thrombitic agent. Gynaecologia (Basle) 145: 434–444
2. Packham M A, Warrior E S, Glynn M F 1967 Alteration of the response of platelets to surface stimuli by pyrazole compounds. Journal of Experimental Medicine 126: 171–191
3. Greif St 1956 Wien. Medicine Wochenschrift 106: 36–39
4. Smyth C J 1956 Proceedings of the 3rd European Congress of Rheumatology. Elsevier, Amsterdam, pp 585–586
5. Ogryzlo M A, Harrison J 1957 Annals of the Rheumatic Diseases 16 : 425–437
6. Wilkinson E L, Brown H 1953 American Journal of Medical Science 225: 153–158
7. Shafar J 1965 Phenylbutazone induced pericarditis. British Medical Journal 11: 795
8. Prescott L F 1968 Antipyretic analgesic drugs. In: Meyler L, Herxheimer A (eds) Side effects of drugs, vol VI. Associated Scientific Publishers, Amsterdam
9. Sperling L E 1969 Adverse reactions with long-term use of phenylbutazone and oxyphenbutazone. Lancet 2: 535
10. Fröhlich J, Hollifield J W, Dormios J C et al 1976 Suppression of plasma renin activity by indomethacin in man. Circulation Research 39: 447
11. Sirota J H, Yu T F 1953 Journal of Clinical Investigation 32: 605
12. Yu T F, Sirota J H, Gutman A B 1953 Journal of Clinical Investigation 32: 1121–1132
13. Linsk J A, Paton B C, Persky M, Isaacs M, Kupperman H S 1957 Journal of Clinical Endocrinology 17: 416–423
14. Horton E W 1979 Prostaglandin pharmacology. In: Davies D M, Rawlins M D (eds) Topics in therapeutics 5. Pitman Medical, London
15. Burns J J, Rose R K, Chenkin T L, Goldman A, Schulert A, Brodie B B 1953 The physiological disposition of phenylbutazone in man and a method for its estimation in biological material. Journal of Pharmacology and Experimental Therapeutics 109: 346–357
16. Aarbakke J, Bakke O M, Milde E J, Davies D S 1977 Metabolism of phenylbutazone in man. European Journal of Clinical Pharmacology 11: 359–366
17. Pound N J, McGilveray J, Sears R W 1974 Analysis of phenylbutazone in plasma by high-speed liquid chromatography. Journal of Chromatography 89: 23–30
18. Weinkam R S, Rowland M, Meffin P J 1977 Determination of phenylbutazone, tolbutamide and metabolites in plasma and urine using chemical ionisation mass spectrometry. Biochemical Mass Spectrometry 4: 42–47
19. Burns J J, Rose R K, Goodwin S, Reichental J, Horning E C, Brodie B B 1955 The metabolic fate of phenylbutazone in man. Journal of Pharmacology and Experimental Therapeutics 113: 481–489
20. Tanimura Y, Saitoh Y, Nakagawa F, Suzuki T 1975 Determination of phenylbutazone and its metabolites in plasma by gas–liquid chromatographic procedure. Chemical and Pharmaceutical Bulletin 23: 651
21. Pounds N J, Sears N 1975 Simultaneous determination of phenylbutazone and oxyphenbutazone in plasma by high-speed liquid chromatography. Journal of Pharmaceutical Science 64: 284
22. Dieterle W, Faigle J W, Frün F et al 1976 Metabolism of phenylbutazone in man. Arzneimittel-Forschung (Drug Research) 26: 275
23. Davies D S, Thorgeirsson S S 1971 Individual differences in plasma half-lives of lipid soluble drugs in man. Acta Pharmacologica et Toxicologica 29 (suppl 3): 181
24. Farr M, Willis J V 1977 Investigation of phenylbutazone in synovial fluid. Journal of International Medical Research 5 (suppl 2): 26–29
25. Leuxner E, Pulver R 1956 Verabreichung Von Irgapyrin bei Schwargeren und Wochnerinnen. München Medicine Wochenshrift 98: 84–86
26. Strobel E, Leuxner E 1957 Über die Zulassigkeit der Verabreichung von Butazolidin bei Schwangerin und Wochnerinnen. Medicine Klin 52: 1708–1710
27. Vessel E S, Page J G 1968 Genetic control of drug levels in man: phenylbutazone. Science 19: 1479–1480
28. Whittaker J A, Price Evans D A 1970 Genetic control of phenylbutazone metabolism in man. British Medical Journal 4: 323
29. Bruck E, Fearnley M E, Meanock I, Patley H 1954 Phenylbutazone therapy. Relationship between toxic and therapeutic effect and the blood level. Lancet 1a: 225
30. Orme M L'E 1977 Phenylbutazone: plasma concentrations and effectiveness in patients with rheumatoid arthritis. Journal of International Medical Research 5 (suppl 2): 40–47
31. Dick W C, Brooks P M, Buchanan W W, Fowler P D 1977 Phenylbutazone dose response in patients with rheumatoid arthritis. Journal of International Medical Research 5 (suppl 2): 48–51
32. Bird H, Leatham P A, Lowe J R, Downie W, Fowler P D, Wright V 1983 A phenylbutazone dose-finding study in rheumatoid arthritis. European Journal of Clinical Pharmacology 24: 773–776
33. Faigle J W, Dieterle W 1977 The biotransformation of phenylbutazone. Journal of International Medical Research 5 (suppl 2): 2–14
34. Kuzell W C, Schaffarzick R W 1952 Phenylbutazone and butapyrin. A study of clinical effects in arthritis and gout. California Medicine 77: 319–325
35. Douglas G, Thompson M 1970 A comparison of phenylbutazone and flufenamic acid in the treatment of acute gout. Annals of Physical Medicine 6: 275–280
36. Will G, Murdock W R 1964 Treatment of rheumatic fever: comparison of effect of aspirin and phenylbutazone. British Medical Journal 2: 281–284
37. Cardoe N, Fowler P D 1972 Enteric-coated phenylbutazone — clinical studies of effectiveness and long-term tolerance. Clinical Trials Journal 9: 23–31
38. Fowler P D, Faragher E B 1977 Drug and non-drug factors influencing adverse reactions to pyrazoles. Journal of International Medical Research 5 (suppl 2): 108–120
39. Fowler P D 1967 Marrow toxicity of the pyrazoles. Annals of the Rheumatic Diseases 26: 344–345
40. Inman W H W 1977 Study of fatal bone marrow depression with special reference to phenylbutazone and oxyphenbutazone. British Medical Journal 1: 1500–1505
41. Fowler P D, Woolf D, Alexander S 1975 Phenylbutazone and hepatitis. Rheumatology and Rehabilitation 14: 71–75
42. Kullander S, Kallen B 1976 A prospective study of drugs and pregnancy. Acta Obstetrica Gynaecologica Scandinavica 55: 287–295
43. Mason R M, Hayter R R P 1958 The present status of phenylbutazone therapy in rheumatic disease. Practitioner 181: 23–28
44. Lewis-Faning E, Fowler P D 1971 Drug treatment of rheumatic disorders in general practice. A comparative study of aspirin and an alkali-phenylbutazone preparation. British Journal of Clinical Practice 25: 123–129
45. Regalado R G, Fowler P D 1974 Butacote and Brufen in the treatment of rheumatic diseases. Journal of International Medical Research 2: 115–124
46. Rushford W A I, Fowler P D 1977 Butacote: the first assessment in general practice. Journal of International Medical Research 5 (suppl 2): 67–69
47. Cardoe N, Fowler P D 1977 Butacote: a six-year follow-up of patients with gastric intolerance to other medications. Journal of International Medical Research 5 (suppl 2): 59–66
48. McIntosh I B, Fowler P D 1977 Phenylbutazone suppositories: a multicentre general practice study. The Practitioner 219: 391–395
49. Laplane R, Debray P, Salbrenx R, Polonovski Cl 1957 The importance of phenylbutazone in rheumatic fever in children. Bulletin Soc Medicin Hôp. Paris 73: 302–314
50. Alvares P, Kapilner S, Sassa S, Kappas A 1975 Drug metabolism in normal children, lead-poisoned children and normal adults. Clinical Pharmacology and Therapeutics 18: 179–183
51. O'Malley I, Crooks J, Duke E, Stevenson I H 1971 Effect of age and sex on human drug metabolism. British Medical Journal 3: 607–609
52. Dugal R, Dupuis C, Bertrand M, Gagnon M A 1980 The effect of buffering on oxyphenbutazone kinetics and systemic availability. Biopharmaceutics and Drug Disposition 1: 307–321
53. Downie W W, Lowe J R, Pickup M E 1977 The effects of antacids on the absorption of enteric-coated phenylbutazone. Journal of International Medical Research 2 (suppl 5): 20–25
54. Stevenson A C, Patel C R, Bedford J, Hill A G S, Hill H F S 1971 Chromosomal studies in patients taking phenylbutazone. Annals of the Rheumatic Diseases 30: 487–500
55. Leza M A 1966 Agranulocytosis medicamentossas con plasmacitosis medulae & hipergammaglobulinaemia. Reuta Clin Esp 103: 316
56. Gross L 1969 Oxyphenbutazone induced parotitis. Annals of Internal Medicine 70: 1229
57. Batsakis J G, Briere R D 1967 Interpretive Enzymology. Thomas, Springfield

Phenylephrine (hydrochloride)

Phenylephrine is a relatively selective α_1-adrenoceptor agonist which is widely used as a constituent of proprietary cough and cold cure preparations for its vasoconstrictor and decongestant properties.

Chemistry

Phenylephrine hydrochloride (Neophryn)
$C_9H_{13}NO_2.HCl$
(S)-1-(3-Hydroxyphenyl)-2-methylaminoethanol hydrochloride

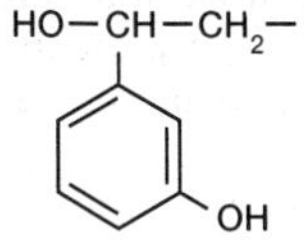

Molecular weight (free base)	203.7 (167.2)
pKa (-OH, -NH-)	8.9, 10.1
Solubility	
in alcohol	1 in 4
in water	1 in 2
Octanol/water partition coefficient	—

Phenylephrine hydrochloride is an odourless, bitter-tasting, white crystalline powder which is prepared by chemical synthesis. It is available for clinical use by oral and topical administration and also as a parenteral formulation for use in special circumstances.

It is present in a number of combination preparations, including Isopto Frin (with hydroxypropylmethylcellulose), Vibrocil (as base with dimethindene maleate and neomycin sulphate), Duo-Autohaler (as bitartrate with isoprenaline hydrochloride), Medihaler-Duo (as bitartrate with isoprenaline hydrochloride), Betnovate rectal (with betamethasone valerate and lignocaine hydrochloride), Dimotapp (with brompheniramine maleate and phenylpropanolamine hydrochloride), Bronchilator (with isoetharine mesylate) and Uniflu (with caffeine, codeine phosphate, diphenhydramine hydrochloride and paracetamol).

Pharmacology

Phenylephrine is a relatively selective α_1-adrenoceptor agonist. It has weak α_2-adrenoceptor agonist activity and some activity as a β-adrenoceptor agonist. It is also termed a sympathomimetic vasoconstrictor. Most of the α_1-stimulant activity is due to a direct action on the receptors and relatively little is due to an indirect effect via release of noradrenaline.

Toxicology

There is no evidence to indicate mutagenic potential and teratogenicity testing in the dog suggested that it was 'not likely that any sizeable amount crosses the placenta'.[1] There is no reported carcinogenicity.

Clinical pharmacology

In research studies, phenylephrine is used as a preferential α_1-agonist drug, leading to dose and concentration-dependent vasoconstriction and increases in blood pressure. The rise in blood pressure is accompanied by a profound reflex bradycardia which can be antagonized by atropine. Cardiac output is slightly decreased but there is a marked fall in blood flow to the renal, cutaneous, splanchnic and skeletal muscle vascular beds. Coronary blood flow is, however, increased by phenylephrine, and pulmonary arterial pressure is increased. There is evidence in man that the pressure effect can be competitively antagonized by selective α_1-antagonists (e.g. prazosin) with parallel shifts to the right of the pressor dose–response curves.

As a vasoconstrictor it has been administered parenterally, typically intravenously, to counteract hypotension, with dose titration up to approximately 10 mg. Sympathomimetic vasoconstriction forms the basis of its decongestant actions, for which it is most widely used, but in addition it has mydriatic activity following local instillation into the eye. As a decongestant it may be administered orally or topically: by mouth it is typically administered in divided doses up to 40 mg daily; it may be administered topically as a 0.25/0.5% solution to the nasal mucosa and as a 0.1–5.0% solution to the eye.

Pharmacokinetics

The preferred analytical method is high performance liquid chromatography with fluorescence detection at excitation and emission wavelengths of 270 and 305 nm, respectively. Phenylephrine can be quantitatively measured at levels as low as 0.5 $\mu g.l^{-1}$ and the assay precision was respectively 23.6% and 15.9% at the lower sensitivities[2] of 0.5 and 1.0 $\mu g.l^{-1}$.

Phenylephrine is readily absorbed after oral administration but is subject to extensive presystemic metabolism, much of which occurs in the enterocytes. As a consequence, systemic bioavailability is only about 40%. Following administration, peak plasma concentrations are achieved in 1–2 h. The mean plasma half life is in the range 2–3 h. Penetration into the brain appears to be minimal.

Following absorption, the drug is extensively biotransformed in the liver. Both phenylephrine and its metabolites are excreted in urine, with < 20% as unchanged drug (16% after intravenous administration). There is no evidence that any of the metabolites is pharmacologically active.

The volume of distribution is between 200 and 500 l, but there are no data on the extent of plasma protein binding. Excretion in breast milk appears to be minimal. Although the drug may not cross the placenta there are pharmacological reasons why it should be avoided in pregnancy.

Oral absorption	high
Presystemic metabolism	~60%
Plasma half life	2–3 h
Volume of distribution	~340 l
Plasma protein binding	—

Concentration–effect relationship

There are only limited data investigating the concentration dependency of the pressor response. Average rises of 3, 11, 26 and 53 mmHg in systolic blood pressure were obtained with doses of 0.5, 1.0, 2.0 and 4 $\mu g.kg^{-1}.min^{-1}$, producing average plasma concentrations of 20, 56, 118 and 308 $nmol.l^{-1}$ (4.1, 11.4, 24.1 and 62.8 $\mu g.l^{-1}$) respectively.[3,4]

Metabolism

Phenylephrine undergoes extensive biotransformation, in the intestinal wall during absorption and in the liver. Only a small amount of the drug is excreted unchanged, 16.6% following intravenous administration and less following oral administration. Both unchanged drug and its metabolites are excreted almost entirely in the urine. The principal routes of metabolism are to sulphate conjugates, which are formed largely in the gut wall, and oxidative deamination by monoamine oxidase (Fig. 1).

Sulphation gives rise to phenylephrine 3-O-sulphate and deamination to 3-hydroxymandelic acid and 3-hydroxyphenylglycol which itself is sulphated to give rise to the 3-O-sulphate. Some glucuronidation of phenylephrine also occurs. 3-Hydroxymandelic acid is excreted without further metabolism. More of the drug is sulphated after oral administration (46%) than after intravenous administration (8%) due to the contribution of the gut wall to this pathway. Conversely, more of the drug is deaminated after intravenous administration (50%) than after oral administration (24%), as most of the drug orally administered has already been metabolized by sulphation prior to reaching the liver.

Pharmaceutics

Phenylephrine is available in oral, parenteral and topical forms, in combination with other agents and as a parenteral formulation.

Compound tablets typically contain 5, 10 or 15 mg phenylephrine or as doses of 5 mg per 5 ml of syrup.

The parenteral form is a 1% solution (10 $mg.ml^{-1}$) for administration as 5 mg doses subcutaneously or intramuscularly, or as 100–500 μg by slow intravenous bolus injection.

Other dosage forms include nasal drops and nasal sprays (Neophryn; Winthrop, UK), typically 0.25/0.5% solutions, and eye drops of 2.5/10% solutions. It is also a constituent in a bronchodilator aerosol, ear drops and rectal ointment.

Therapeutic use

Indications

1. Decongestion of mucous membranes (especially nasal mucosa)
2. Mydriasis
3. To counteract hypotension — only in specialized circumstances, e.g. spinal anaesthesia.

Contraindications

1. Concurrent administration of monoamine oxidase inhibitors or tricyclic antidepressants

Relative contraindications to use, particularly with respect to systemic administration, are

2. Hypertension
3. Unstable angina and recent myocardial infarction (arbitrarily within the previous 6 months)
4. Hyperthyroidism
5. Pregnancy.

Mode of use

As a single agent, phenylephrine is administered mainly by topical application as a decongestant, but there are also compound oral preparations for this purpose. As a pressor agent it is administered parenterally, usually intravenously, by dose titration.

Indications

1. Decongestant

Phenylephrine is widely used by topical application as a decongestant in allergic rhinitis, coryza, sinusitis, etc. It is most appropriately administered topically, but this does carry some risk of local irritation, and rebound congestion on cessation of treatment. Prolonged use as a nasal decongestant may lead to chronic rhinitis.

2. Mydriatic

Local application to the conjunctiva causes mydriasis (dilation of pupil) for a few hours, with the advantage of not causing cycloplegia, or increasing intraocular pressure. This local application may also be useful in the treatment of wide-angle glaucoma, and in reducing posterior synechiae in uveitis.

3. Pressor agent

The pressor activity of phenylephrine is useful only in a few very specialized circumstances such as spinal anaesthesia and, rarely, it has been used in the intraoperative management of phaeochromocytoma.[5]

Contraindications

Absolute contraindications

Severe or unpredictable increases in blood pressure may occur if the patient is receiving concurrent treatment with a monoamine oxidase inhibitor drug, or with a tricyclic antidepressant drug.

Relative contraindications

These relate to the vasoconstrictor and pressor effects such that phenylephrine should be avoided in patients who are also suffering from hypertension, aortic aneurysm, severe or unstable ischaemic heart disease, or hyperthyroidism.

Because phenylephrine also has actions that promote smooth muscle contractility, it should be avoided in pregnancy.

Adverse reactions

Potentially life-threatening effects

Persistent and/or severe hypertension is a potentially lethal hazard of the response to phenylephrine. Severe hypertension complicated by headache, vomiting and profound reflex bradycardia has been reported, and infants and young children appear to be especially at risk. Under routine therapeutic circumstances, particularly in relation to its use as a decongestant, such effects are unlikely and this complication is exceedingly rare.

Acute overdosage

Cases of deliberate overdose have been reported, but there are no recorded fatalities. The principal clinical features are a rise in blood pressure and associated reflex bradycardia. In most cases, a severe hypertensive response can be countered by means of an α-antagonist, such as intravenous phentolamine, and, correspondingly, any reflex bradycardia may be specifically countered with atropine (but, preferably, only after the pressure has been controlled by α-adrenergic blockade).

Fig. 1 Metabolism of phenylephrine

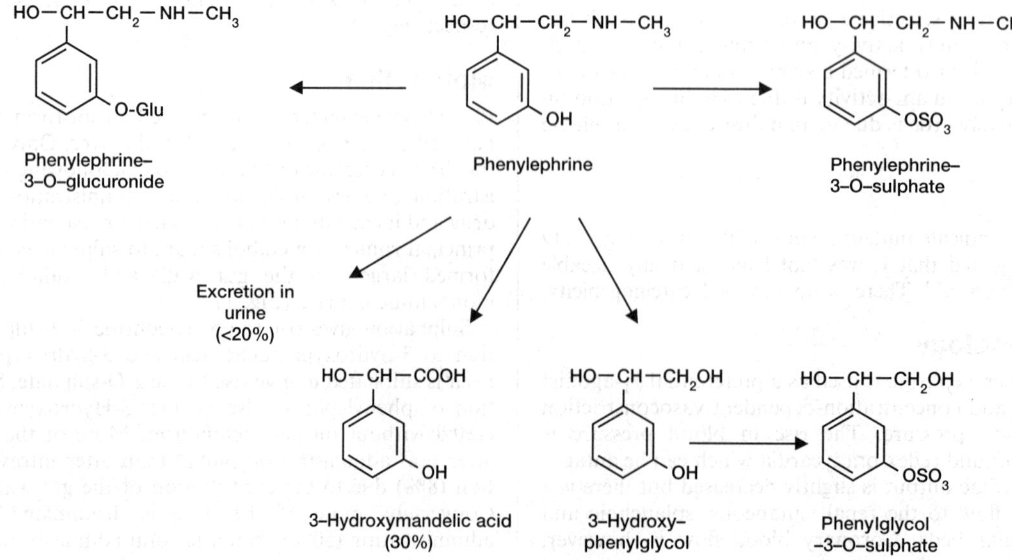

Severe or irreversible adverse effects
Apart from those already described, none has been reported.

Symptomatic adverse effects
Symptomatic adverse effects are uncommon.

Other effects
There are no reports of any biochemical or metabolic effects.

Interference with clinical pathology tests
No technical interferences of this kind have been reported.

High risk groups

Neonates
For use as a topical application it is recommended that solution strength does not exceed 2.5%.

Breast milk. Excretion of the drug in breast milk appears to be minimal.

Children
What has been said about neonates also applies to older children.

Pregnant women
Because of the potential promotion of uterine contractility and peripheral vasoconstriction, with the possibility of fetal hypoxia, phenylephrine is best avoided during pregnancy.

The elderly
Again, a 2.5% solution for topical application is preferred to avoid the risks of an exaggerated hypertensive response.

Drug interactions

Potentially hazardous interactions
Hypertension may occur when phenylephrine is given concurrently with antidepressants of both monoamine oxidase and tricyclic types, ganglion-blocking agents, adrenergic-blocking drugs, rauwolfia alkaloids, and methyldopa.

Potentially useful interactions
None has been described.

References

1. Linkie D M, Boba A, Plotz E J 1966 Fetal effects of phenylephrine injection. American Journal of Medical Science 252: 277–281
2. Chien D-S, Schoenwald R D 1985 Fluorimetric determination of phenylephrine hydrochloride by liquid chromatography in human plasma. Journal of Pharmaceutical Sciences 74: 562–564
3. Martinsson A, Bevergard S, Hjemdahl P 1986 Analysis of phenylephrine in plasma: initial data about the concentration–effect relationship. European Journal of Clinical Pharmacology 30: 427–431
4. Hengtsmann J H, Goronzy J 1988 Pharmacokinetics of ^{3}H-phenylephrine in man. European Journal of Clinical Pharmacology 21: 335–341
5. Gilman A G, Goodman L S, Rall T W, Murad F 1985 The Pharmacological basis of therapeutics, 7th edn. Macmillan, New York

Phenylpropanolamine (hydrochloride)

Phenylpropanolamine is an indirectly acting sympathomimetic amine, with mainly α_1-agonist activity but also some β_1-agonist activity, which is used in a number of compound preparations principally as a decongestant.

Chemistry

Phenylpropanolamine hydrochloride (dl-norephedrine hydrochloride)
$C_9H_{13}NO.HCl$
dl-2-Amino-1-phenylpropan-1-ol hydrochloride

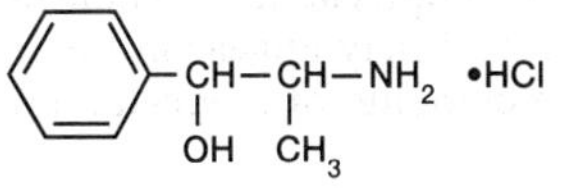

Molecular weight (free base)	187.7 (151.2)
pKa (NH_2)	9.4
Solubility	
in alcohol	1 in 9
in water	1 in 2.5
Octanol/water partition coefficient	low

Phenylpropanolamine hydrochloride is a white or off-white crystalline powder, odourless or with a slight aromatic odour, and with a bitter taste. It is prepared by chemical synthesis. It is present in a variety of nasal decongestants and cough preparations, including Dimotane Expectorant, Dimotapp, Eskornade, Triogesic, Triominic.

Pharmacology

Phenylpropanolamine is an α_1-adrenoceptor agonist, a β_1-adrenoceptor agonist and an indirect sympathomimetic agent.[1–5]

Toxicology

Phenylpropanolamine has not undergone detailed testing but there are no reports of mutagenicity, carcinogenicity or teratogenicity.

Clinical pharmacology

The use of phenylpropanolamine as a decongestant reflects its α_1-agonist activity leading to mucosal vasoconstriction. Stimulation of α_1-adrenoceptors in the smooth muscle of the urinary tract is thought to mediate its effects on bladder function, due to stimulation of the α_1-adrenoceptors in the base of the bladder and subsequent contraction of muscles in that region.

Pharmacokinetics

The preferred analytical method is gas chromatography with electron-capture detection.[6] The limit of sensitivity is 1 $\mu g.l^{-1}$.

Only limited information is available on the pharmacokinetics of phenylpropanolamine. It is rapidly and almost completely absorbed after oral administration. There is no presystemic metabolism, so that bioavailability is essentially complete. Peak plasma concentrations are achieved 1–2 h after dosing. The half life is approximately 3–4 h but there is no information on the volume of distribution or on the extent of plasma protein binding. The drug is eliminated mainly unchanged, with 90–100% recovery in the urine within 24 h.

It is not known whether the drug is excreted in breast milk, nor whether it crosses the placenta.

Oral absorption	>90%
Presystemic metabolism	negligible
Plasma half life	3–4 h
Volume of distribution	—
Plasma protein binding	—

The effects of renal impairment on the elimination of phenylpropanolamine are not known, but is highly probable that elimination will be delayed. Similarly, although the effects of old age have not been reported, some reduction in elimination might be expected in elderly people with reduced renal function. It is unlikely that hepatic disease will have any significant effect on the kinetics of phenylpropanolamine, but studies in such patients have not been reported.

Concentration–effect relationship

It is reported that therapeutic doses produce serum levels of between 60 and 200 μg.l^{-1} but there is no information on toxic plasma concentrations,[7] and there is no clear relationship between the plasma concentration of phenylpropanolamine and its therapeutic effects.

Metabolism

Most (>90%) of an oral dose is excreted unchanged in the urine within 24 h. There is no appreciable metabolism in man, though trace amounts of hippuric acid may appear in the urine. Phenylpropanolamine is an active metabolite of amphetamine, diethylpropion and ephedrine.

Pharmaceutics

Phenylpropanolamine is available only in compound preparations for oral use, typically in syrup or elixir form, but also in tablets or capsules. The compound preparation Eskornade (SmithKline, Beecham, UK) (with diphenylpyraline) is a capsule containing wax-coated pellets with different release times such that about 60% of the dose is intended for release over 6–8 hours. This compound preparation also contains tartrazine and sunset yellow so that there is the potential for allergic responses. It is also notable that Dimotapp LA (Robins, UK) contains 3 mg of wheat and it should therefore be avoided in patients known to suffer from gluten sensitivity.

There are over 70 preparations on the American market containing phenylpropanolamine. Most of these are combination products for the common cold.

Therapeutic use

Indications

1. Nasal decongestant
2. For the treatment of urinary incontinence
3. Anorectic (in the USA only).

Contraindications

1. Hypertension and severe or unstable ischaemic heart disease
2. Glaucoma
3. Prostatic hypertrophy or urinary retention
4. Intestinal obstruction
5. Patients receiving concurrent treatment with monoamine oxidase inhibitor drugs
6. Severe hyperthyroidism.

Mode of use

Phenylpropanolamine is used mainly as an oral medication, typically as a constituent of a proprietary compound preparation for decongestion of the upper respiratory tract, because of its α-adrenergic-mediated vasoconstricting effects.[8]

The recommended dose range is 25–50 mg per 4 h, or 50 mg per 12 h if a sustained-release formulation is used.

Indications

1. Nasal decongestion
Phenylpropanolamine is used in preparations for the symptomatic relief of nasal and upper respiratory congestion.

2. Urinary incontinence
Phenylpropanolamine is used in preparations for the treatment of enuresis due to bladder neck dysfunction.[9]

3. Appetite suppression
The value of phenylpropanolamine as an anorectic is debatable. Significant benefits have been reported and a dose–response relationship has been described,[10] but a lack of long-term efficacy has also been reported.[11] It is approved for use as an anorectic in the USA but not in the UK.

Adverse reactions

Potentially life-threatening effects
Severe increases in blood pressure have been reported following the ingestion of less than therapeutic doses. Such exaggerated responses are exceedingly rare, and only minimal increases in blood pressure are normally observed in otherwise healthy subjects. Life-threatening increases in blood pressure have been reported with doses of more than three times the therapeutic recommendation.

There are also isolated reports of acute renal failure due to rhabdomyolysis.

Acute overdosage
There are case reports of deliberate overdoses, with elevations of blood pressure a predominant feature. Since such toxic effects are generally short-lived, supportive measures alone are normally sufficient. Specific treatment to reduce blood pressure is indicated if myocardial ischaemia or encephalopathy is provoked.[12] CNS effects, including psychosis, hallucinations and epilepsy, have been reported.

Symptomatic adverse effects
These have not been systematically studied, but nausea and dizziness, headache, palpitation and chest tightness, and tremor have been reported.[13]

Other effects
A fall in serum potassium has been described with overdoses.[6]

Interference with clinical pathology tests
None has been reported.

High risk groups

Neonates
The toxic dose of the drug has not been established in neonates.

Breast milk. It is not known whether or not phenylpropanolamine is excreted in breast milk, so it is best for lactating mothers to avoid the drug.

Children
The toxic dose of the drug has not been established in young children.

Pregnant women
There is no specific experimental or clinical evidence of hazard to the fetus, but the usual guidelines should be followed and the drug avoided during pregnancy, especially in the first trimester.

The elderly
The drug should be used with caution in the elderly in view of the increased incidence in such patients of disorders that might be aggravated by the drug.

Drug interactions

Potentially hazardous interactions
The concomitant administration with monoamine oxidase inhibitors has been associated with very severe elevations of blood pressure. Use with the non-steroid drug, indomethacin, has been associated with hypertension,[14] and there is a report that concomitant atropine administration also promoted sustained hypertension, presumably by interfering with the hypertension-induced reflex fall in heart rate.[7,15]

References

1. Nickerson M, Nomagochi G M 1950 Responses to sympathomimetic amines after clibenamine blockade. Journal of Pharmacology and Experimental Therapeutics 107: 284–299
2. Greiner T H, Garb S 1950 The influence of drugs on the irritability and automaticity of heart muscle. Journal of Pharmacology and Experimental Therapeutics 98: 215–223

3. Trendelenburg U, De La Sierra B G A, Muskus A 1963 Modification by reserpine of the response of the atrial pacemaker to sympathomimetic amines. Journal of Pharmacology and Experimental Therapeutics 141: 301–309
4. Cameron W M, Tainter M L 1936 Comparative action of sympathomimetic compounds: bronchodilator actions in bronchial spasm induced by histamine. Journal of Pharmacology and Experimental Therapeutics 57: 152–169
5. Gilman A G, Goodman L S, Rall T W, Murad F (eds) 1985 The pharmacological basis of therapeutics, 7th edn. Macmillan, New York
6. Neelakantan L, Kostenbauder H B 1976 Electron-capture GLC determination of phenylpropanolamine as a pento-fluorophenyloxazolidine derivative. Journal of Pharmaceutical Sciences 65: 740–742
7. Pentel P 1984 Toxicity of over the counter stimulants. Journal of the American Medical Association 252: 1898–1903
8. Bende M, Anderson K E, Johansson C J, Sjögren C, Svensson G 1984 Dose–response relationship of a topical nasal decongestant: phenylpropanolamine. Acta Otolaryngologica 98: 543–547
9. Awad S A, Downie J W, Kiruluta H G 1978 Alpha adrenergic agents in urinary disorders of the proximal urethra Part 1. Sphincteric incontinence. British Journal of Urology 50: 332–335
10. Weintraub M, Ginsberg G, Stein E C et al 1986 Phenylpropanolamine OROS (Acutrim) vs. placebo in combination with caloric restriction and physician managed behaviour modification. Clinical Pharmacology and Therapeutics 39: 501–509
11. 1979 A nasal decongestant and a local anaesthetic for weight control. Medical Letters 21: 65 (357): 65–68
12. Horowitz J D, McNeil J J, Sweet B, Mendelsohn F A 1979 Hypotension and postural hypotension induced by phenylpropanolamine (Trimolets). Medical Journal of Australia 1: 175–176
13. Horowitz J D, Lang W J, Howes L G, Fennessy M R, Christophidis N, Rand M J, Louis W J 1980 Hypertensive responses induced by phenylpropanolamine in anorectic and decongestant preparations. Lancet 1: 60–61
14. Cuthbert M F, Greenberg M P, Morley S W 1969 Cough and cough remedies: a potential danger to patients on monoamine oxidase inhibitors. British Medical Journal 1: 404–406
15. Pentel P, Mikell F 1982 Reaction to phenylpropanolamine/chlorpheniramine/belladonna compound in a woman with recognized autonomic dysfunction. Lancet 2: 274

Phenytoin (sodium)

Phenytoin has been widely used as an anticonvulsant drug for some fifty years. Its clinical pharmacology has been studied extensively.

Chemistry

Phenytoin sodium (formerly diphenylhydantoin sodium in the USA, Dilantin sodium; Epanutin)
$C_{15}H_{11}N_2NaO_2$
5,5-Diphenylhydantoin; 5,5-diphenyl-2,4-imidazolidinedione sodium

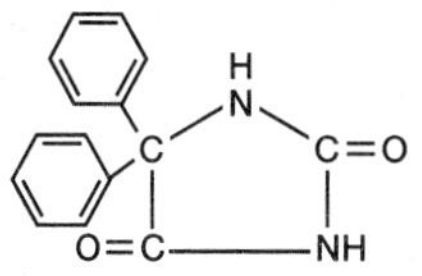

Molecular weight (free acid)	274.3 (252.3)
pKa	8.3
Solubility	
in alcohol (free acid)	1 in 10.5 (1 in 70)
in water (free acid)	1 in 66 (almost insoluble)
Octanol/water partition coefficient	high

Phenytoin is a white crystalline tasteless and odourless powder. The sodium salt also occurs as white crystals, but it is slightly hygroscopic and has a bitter soapy taste. On exposure to air it absorbs CO_2 and liberates the free acid.

Phenytoin is marketed in some countries in preparations which also contain phenobarbitone.

Pharmacology

In humans, phenytoin protects against partial epilepsy and against tonic clonic seizures of generalised epilepsy. It is also effective in animal models of generalized epilepsy manifesting as convulsive seizures (for example, maximum electroshock seizures) and in models of partial epilepsy (for example, the kindling model). The drug appears to act by limiting the spread of seizure discharges rather than by preventing their initiation.[1] Phenytoin appears to bind to specific receptors on neuronal cell membranes.[2] The drug inhibits voltage-dependent Na^+ ion channels in the neuronal cell membrane, and thus impairs the passage of trains of rapid axon potentials along axons. In this way it discriminates against epileptic activity but not against more physiological discharge patterns.[3,4] The drug may also cause neuronal hyperpolarization by increasing Na^+ extrusion from cells into extracellular fluid.[5] By interfering with Ca^{++} and calmodulin-mediated mechanisms, phenytoin may impair noradrenaline release into synaptic clefts.[6] All these molecular effects may contribute in different ways to limitation of seizure spread, though its action on voltage-gated Na^+ channels is now thought to be its main mechanism of action.

Toxicology

There is some controversy as to whether chronic phenytoin overdosage in experimental animals and humans causes cerebellar Purkinje cell degeneration.[7] Overdosage in humans has been reported to cause computerised tomographic appearances of cerebellar atrophy.[8] There is no evidence of significant mutagenicity from phenytoin. Phenytoin given to rats and mice between the 10th and the 14th day of pregnancy causes an increased incidence of fetal malformation (fetal resorption, cleft lip and cleft palate, hydronephrosis, hydrocephalus and abdominal haemorrhages).[9] In humans phenytoin very occasionally causes a reversible pseudo-lymphoma syndrome in which the enlarged lymph nodes have a histological appearance resembling that of Hodgkin's disease. There have been suggestions that the drug may occasionally be responsible for the development of malignant lymphomas and leukaemia.[11] However, one study found no association between phenytoin intake and neoplasia in humans.[12]

Clinical pharmacology

Phenytoin is reasonably effective in controlling the tonic-clonic seizures of generalized epilepsy, and in both decreasing the frequency of partial seizures and diminishing the risk of their becoming secondarily generalized, with the occurrence of bilateral convulsing. The drug also helps prevent attacks of certain forms of supraventricular cardiac arrhythmia,[13] possibly by a central nervous system effect. Phenytoin appears to inhibit the conduction of trigeminal pain impulses in tic douloureux and in certain other forms of neuralgia.[14] The drug appears to prevent certain varieties of migraine[15] through mechanisms of action which are not understood, and it appears to act on skeletal muscle to relieve myotonia,[16] perhaps by altering C1-ion transport through sarcolemmal membranes.

The drug's effects appear to correlate more closely with its plasma concentrations than with its dose (see Concentration–effect relationship).

Pharmacokinetics

Many assay methods have been described for phenytoin. However, plasma and serum phenytoin levels are now preferably measured by one of a number of different forms of immunoassay, or by gas–liquid[17] or high performance liquid chromatography with UV detection.[18] This last method may have a sensitivity as low as 100 μg.l^{-1}

Following oral administration, phenytoin is absorbed slowly but almost completely, although there have been some marketed formulations from which absorption was incomplete.[19] The rate of absorption is prolonged as the dose increases. Peak plasma concentrations of phenytoin usually occur 2–4 hours after an oral dose, with a second peak at 10–12 h.[20] There is no significant pre-systemic metabolism, hence bioavailability is usually > 0.90, but will be less than this with formulations exhibiting poor absorption characteristics. Food does not appear to have any appreciable effect on the absorption of phenytoin. Although intramuscularly administered phenytoin is eventually absorbed completely, the drug first crystallizes out at its injection site, and then slowly redissolves in tissue fluids, before entering the circulation.[20,21] As a consequence, absorption of phenytoin following intramuscular administration is too slow to produce a reliable therapeutic effect.

The apparent volume of distribution of phenytoin is approximately 0.50–0.70 l.kg^{-1}. Some 90–93% of the phenytoin in plasma is normally bound to plasma proteins, mainly albumin,[20,23] though the degree of binding is decreased in renal insufficiency, severe liver disease, and in the very young and the elderly.[24] CSF and salivary phenytoin concentrations are approximately 10% of those in plasma.[25] Phenytoin is excreted in breast milk at concentrations 25–50% of those in plasma.[26] Brain concentrations of phenytoin are generally similar to plasma concentrations of the drug.[27] Phenytoin readily crosses the placenta and has been associated with teratogenicity.

Phenytoin is eliminated from the body almost entirely by metabolism in the liver.[28] Only about 5% of the dose is excreted unchanged in urine. Up to about 15% of the dose is eliminated in the faeces, the majority of the dose being excreted in the urine as metabolites. The rate of elimination of phenytoin is dose dependent,[29] the terminal half life increasing with dose. The half life also varies considerably amongst individuals, with a range from 7 to 60 h, averaging 22 ± 9 hours.[30] Thus the elimination of phenytoin can be described by Michaelis-Menten kinetics.[31] The apparent K_m value is in the range 4–6 mg.l^{-1} (16–24 μM and the V max in the range 6–8 mg.kg^{-1} per day for adults, and around 12 mg.kg^{-1} per day for children.[32] The total body clearance of phenytoin[30] is in the range 0.016–0.042 l.kg^{-1}.h^{-1}. As a consequence of the saturable elimination of phenytoin at clinically relevant doses, consecutive dose increments of equal size produce progressively increasing increments in steady-state plasma phenytoin levels in a given subject.[33] This non-linearity becomes quite marked while plasma phenytoin concentrations are within the normal therapeutic range for the treatment of epilepsy, 20–40 mg.l^{-1}. Failure to appreciate this can lead to overdosage of patients by what would otherwise seem a reasonable and proportionate dose increment of the drug.

Severe liver disease may reduce the elimination of phenytoin,[34] and occasional instances of inherited or sporadic slow elimination due to impaired hydroxylation of the drug have been reported.[35,36] Plasma protein binding for phenytoin is reduced in the presence of renal insufficiency,[37] but this is compensated for by increased elimination. The renal clearance of phenytoin is not affected by changes in urinary pH.

Phenytoin is a potent inducer of hepatic monooxygenase activity, increasing the elimination of dicoumarol, primidone, carbamazepine, prednisolone, dexamethasone and other glucocorticoids. A large number of compounds inhibit the oxidation of phenytoin, thereby increasing plasma levels of the drug, due to competition for the capacity-limited system. Such drugs include isoniazid, tricyclic antidepressants, phenylbutazone and propoxyphene.

Phenytoin oxidation can be induced by other anticonvulsants such as phenobarbitone, primidone, carbamazepine, clonazepam and valproate, resulting in decreased concentrations of the drug.

The combination of a narrow therapeutic window and readily saturable metabolism means that even relatively modest changes in the kinetics of phenytoin can result in profound changes in the efficacy and toxicity of the drug.

Oral absorption	reasonably complete: > 90%
Presystemic metabolism	nil
Plasma half life	
range	7–60 h (dose dependent)
mean	22 ± 9 h
Volume of distribution	0.5–0.7 l.kg^{-1}
Plasma protein binding	90–93%

Concentration–effect relationship

It is rather widely accepted that plasma phenytoin concentrations in the range 10–20 mg.l^{-1} (40–80 μM.l^{-1})[38] offer the best chance of controlling epilepsy in most patients without producing an unacceptable incidence of adverse effects. Occasionally authors set the lower limit of the therapeutic range to as low as 5 mg.l^{-1} (20 μM.l^{-1}) and many patients tolerate plasma phenytoin levels up to 25 mg.l^{-1} (100 μM.l^{-1}). On the other hand occasional patients develop overdosage manifestations with plasma phenytoin levels as low as 5–6 mg.l^{-1} (20–24 μM.l^{-1}). Kutt and McDowell[38] generalized that nystagmus tended to appear when plasma phenytoin levels exceeded 20 mg.l^{-1} (80 μM.l^{-1}), diplopia and ataxia of gait when levels exceeded 30 mg.l^{-1} (120 μM.l^{-1}) and drowsiness at levels above 40 mg.l^{-1} (160 μM.l^{-1})

The therapeutic range of plasma phenytoin levels which correlates with control of susceptible cardiac arrhythmias is similar to that which applies for epilepsy. However, lower plasma phenytoin levels usually suffice to control responsive forms of migraine.

Metabolism

Phenytoin is extensively biotransformed by oxidation in the liver, with less than 5% of the dose excreted unchanged in the urine. The majority of the dose is excreted in the urine as metabolites, with up to 15% of the dose eliminated in the faeces. The major route of metabolism of phenytoin is aromatic hydroxylation of one of the benzene rings on C5 of the hydantoin ring.[39] The major metabolite is 5-p-hydroxypheny-5-phenylhydantoin (HPPH), which is subsequently glucuronidated. Between them, free and conjugated HPPH in urine account for 60–80% of the dose. p-Hydroxylation is capacity limited, so that at higher doses a smaller proportion of the dose is excreted as HPPH. A number of minor phenolic and catechol metabolites of phenytoin have been identified. Scission of the hydantoin ring and N-glucuronides of the drug have also been reported.

Phenytoin (sodium)

Inherited and sporadic instances of a decreased capacity to form the p-hydroxyphenyl metabolite, associated with abnormally reduced tolerance to normal doses of phenytoin have been reported.[35,37] None of the metabolites of phenytoin appears to be active.

Pharmaceutics

Phenytoin (Epanutin/Dilantin, Parke-Davis UK/US) is available as 50 mg chewable tablets (Infatabs) and as oral suspensions containing 30 mg per 5 ml and in parenteral formulations.

Sodium phenytoin is available as 25 mg, 50 mg (or alternatively in some countries, 30 mg) capsules, 100 mg capsules and tablets, and in ready mixed ampoules containing 100 mg per 2 ml and 250 mg per 5 ml.

Lactose is the recommended capsule excipient. Some other excipients, such as calcium sulphate, drastically reduce bioavailability. Small particle size crystals are absorbed significantly faster than large particles: Prompt Phenytoin Sodium Capsules USP achieve a peak plasma concentration between 1½ and 3 hours, compared to 4 to 12 hours with Extended Phenytoin Sodium Capsules USP.

Epanutin Ready Mixed Parenteral (Parke-Davies, UK) contains 250 mg in 5 ml propylene glycol 40% alcohol 10%. Since the pH is 12 the injection must not be mixed with infusion fluids or other drugs.

Administration must be by the IV route only, since intramuscular

Fig. 1 Pathways of phenytoin metabolism

1) phenytoin. 2) 5-(p-hydroxyphenyl)-5-phenylhydantoin. 3) 5-5-bis(4-hydroxyphenyl)hydantoin. 4) 5-(m-hydroxyphenyl)-5-phenylhydantoin. 5) postulated transient epoxide metabolite. 6) 5-(3,4-dihydroxy-1,5-cyclohexadiene-1-yl)-5-phenylhydantoin. 7) 5-(3,4-dihydroxyphenyl)-5-phenylhydantoin. 8) 5-(4-hydroxy-3-methoxyphenyl)-5-phenylhydantoin. 9) phenytoin-N-glucuronide. 10) diphenylhydantoic acid. 11) α-amino-diphenylacetic acid. 12) 5-(p-hydroxyphenyl)-5-phenylhydantoin O-glucuronide

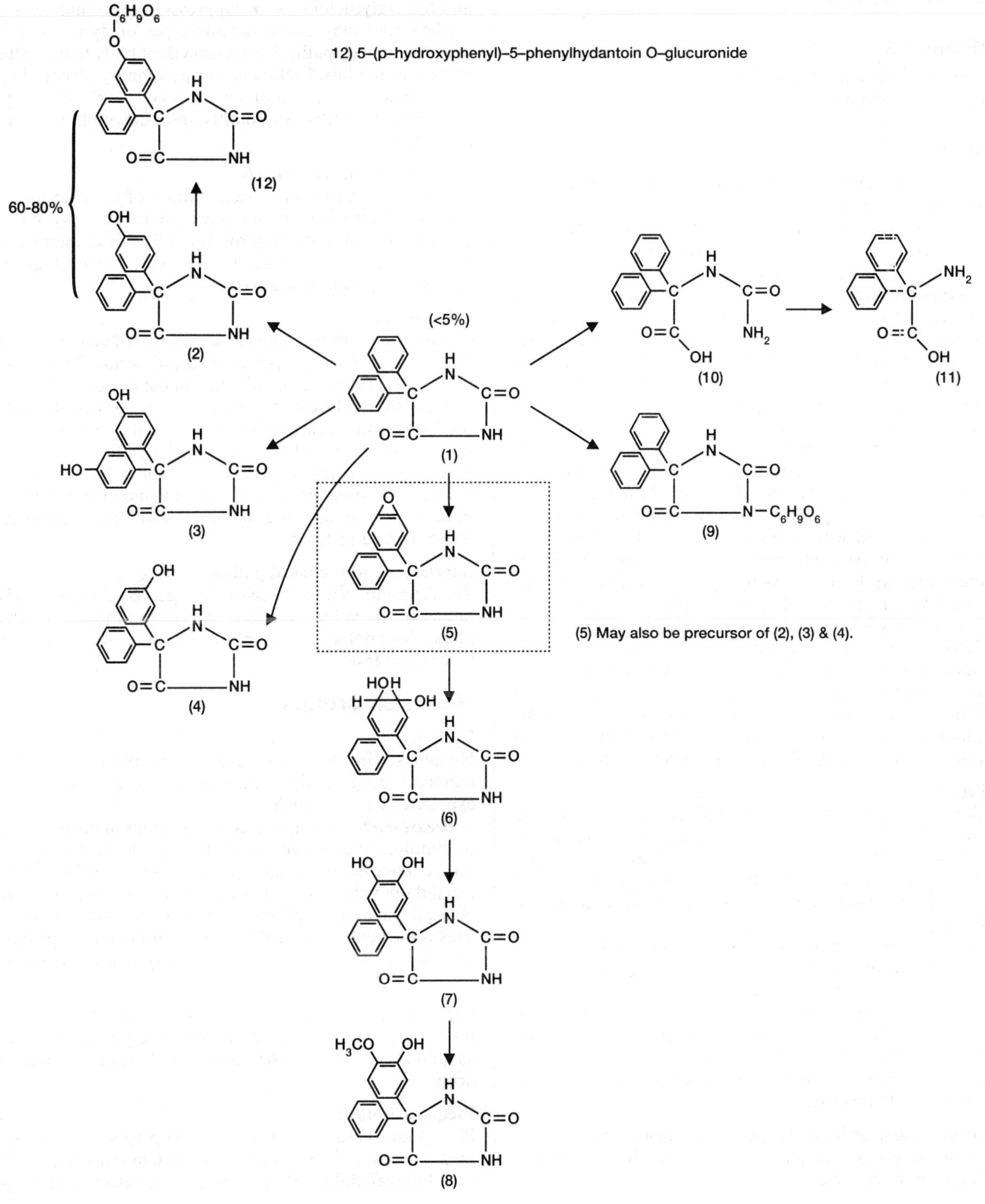

injection leads to crystallization of phenytoin in the tissues, with consequent reduced bioavailability. If short term intramuscular administration is necessary for a patient previously stabilised orally, the dosage should be increased by 50% over the oral dose.

Therapeutic use

Indications

1. The prophylactic treatment of all varieties of partial epilepsy, whether or not the seizures become secondarily generalized
2. The prophylactic treatment of convulsive seizures of generalized epilepsy
3. The treatment of status epilepticus
4. The prophylactic management of certain forms of supraventricular cardiac arrhythmia
5. The prophylactic management of certain varieties of migraine (particularly childhood, basilar artery and 'hemiplegic' migraine)
6. The treatment of tic douloureux
7. The treatment of myotonia.

Contraindications

1. Known hypersensitivity to phenytoin
2. Acute intermittent porphyria.

Mode of use

1. Prophylaxis of partial epilepsy, and 2. Prophylaxis of convulsive seizures of generalized epilepsy

Used prophylactically, for either indication, oral phenytoin need not be taken more often than twice daily, and often once daily therapy suffices to keep steady-state plasma and tissue concentrations of the drug within acceptable limits over each dosage interval. Unless a satisfactory clinical response occurs at lower plasma phenytoin levels, the aim of the initial phenytoin dose should be to achieve steady-state plasma phenytoin concentrations within the therapeutic range of 10–20 $mg.l^{-1}$ (40–80 $\mu M.l^{-1}$). The average dose to achieve such levels in adults is 5 $mg.kg^{-1}$ per day, and in children 11 $mg.kg^{-1}$ daily.[40] A slightly lower initial dose may be advisable, with subsequent dose adjustments being made in the knowledge of the non-linear relation in the individual between steady-state plasma phenytoin levels and dose increments. In adults, if plasma phenytoin concentrations are below 10 $mg.l^{-1}$ a 100 mg per dose increment will generally be tolerated, and with levels in the range 10–15 $mg.l^{-1}$ a 50 mg per day increment. At levels above 15 $mg.l^{-1}$ even a 30 mg per day dose increment may lead to toxicity after a few days. Dosage adjustments should be made, guided by plasma phenytoin concentration measurements, only when steady state conditions apply (usually 1 week or longer after the most recent dose increment). If the patient's symptoms are not controlled with plasma phenytoin concentrations in the therapeutic range, and if no significant adverse effects of therapy are present, the phenytoin dose may still be increased cautiously in the hope of relieving the disorder being treated without causing unacceptable adverse effects of therapy.

3. Status epilepticus

In status epilepticus phenytoin needs to be given parenterally. The drug is best given into the tubing of a running intravenous infusion, (because the drug is irritant to veins) at a rate of up to 50 mg per minute (in adults). The drug is so insoluble that it may precipitate out if injected into the contents of a fluid reservoir, resulting in unreliable intake of the drug.

The solvent in parenteral phenytoin preparations tends to cause hypotension,[41] a circumstance which contributes to the need for slow infusion of the drug. The adult phenytoin dose to achieve therapeutic range plasma levels in a previously untreated patient may be of the order of 1000 mg,[41] and this dose may have to be given intravenously in stages over several hours to avoid hypotension.

Intramuscular phenytoin is absorbed too slowly and too unpredictably to provide reliable therapy.[22]

4. Prophylaxis of cardiac arrhythmias and 6. tic douloureux

If used for these purposes oral phenytoin is prescribed as for the prevention of epileptic seizures.

Phenytoin (sodium)

Adverse reactions

Several reviews of the adverse effects of phenytoin are available.[24,42–46]

Potentially life-threatening effects

Very rarely phenytoin-associated hepatitis[47] or dermatitis[48] may assume life-threatening proportions. A possible association between phenytoin and a pseudo-lymphoma syndrome has been described,[10] and there has been speculation about an association between the drug and frank neoplasia.[11]

Acute overdosage

Death from acute phenytoin overdosage in humans is very uncommon.

Severe or irreversible adverse effects

Chronic phenytoin overdosage typically produces a concentration-related hierarchy of disturbances, namely nystagmus, blurred vision, diplopia and ataxia of gait, nausea, vomiting, drowsiness, stupor and finally coma with hypotension. Chronic overdosage manifestations include intellectual dulling, depression of mood, gum hypertrophy and hyperglycaemia (from suppression of insulin release).

Phenytoin may cause various types of dyskinesia,[49] sub-clinical peripheral neuropathy,[50] overgrowth of body hair,[51] altered collagen growth in the lips, heel pads and pulmonary alveoli, hypocalcaemia, osteomalacia, manifestations of folate depletion (e.g. macrocytic anaemia), hepatitis, thyroiditis, pseudolymphoma and exfoliative dermatitis.

Symptomatic adverse effects

Various skin rashes may occur. Many of the overdosage and severe adverse effects of phenytoin may be regarded as symptomatic, if they are not allowed to develop too far before drug therapy is withdrawn. This applies in particular to the typical neurological overdosage effects of diplopia and ataxia.

Other effects

Chronic phenytoin intake causes decreased serum and red blood cell folate levels, hypocalcaemia, reduced serum 25-hydroxycholecalciferol levels, raised serum alkaline phosphatase and raised γ-glutamyl transpeptidase levels, decreased serum protein-bound iodine and total thyroxine levels with increased unbound thyroxine concentrations, a shortened plasma cortisol half life, hypercholesterolaemia, raised serum caeruloplasmin and copper levels, raised serum sex-hormone-binding globulin levels (in women) and reduced concentrations of IgA in serum and saliva, with some tendency to reduced serum Ig G and Ig M levels.

Interference with clinical pathology tests

The drug-induced biochemical changes listed immediately above may influence the values obtained in certain laboratory tests. Phenytoin intake does not appear to interfere with the results of commonly used laboratory tests.

High risk groups

Neonates

Neonates who have been exposed to phenytoin in utero (due to maternal drug intake) eliminate the drug fairly rapidly if drug exposure ceases at birth.

Breast milk. Phenytoin concentrations in breast milk are 20–50% of simultaneous plasma phenytoin levels. If a mother has plasma phenytoin levels in the therapeutic range it may be calculated that the usual daily volume of milk taken by her infant is unlikely to produce clinically significant plasma phenytoin concentrations in that infant. This is particularly so if there has been in utero exposure to the drug so that the infant's mono-oxygenase system is already induced.

Children

Children eliminate phenytoin more rapidly than adults and, on a body weight basis, require approximately twice as much phenytoin as adults to achieve the same steady-state plasma levels of the drug.

Pregnant women

Phenytoin clearance increases during pregnancy, and returns to pre-pregnant values between 2 weeks and 6 months after parturition. The oral bioavailability of the drug is not decreased in pregnancy.[52]

Pholcodine

Pholcodine is one of the non-addiction-producing narcotic drugs, an amino alkyl-ether of morphine.

Chemistry

Pholcodine (morpholinylethylmorphine, Dia-Tuss, Duro-Tuss, Fectolin, Sancos, Triopaed)
$C_{23}H_{30}N_2O_4.H_2O$
3-O-(2-Morphinoethyl)morphine monohydrate

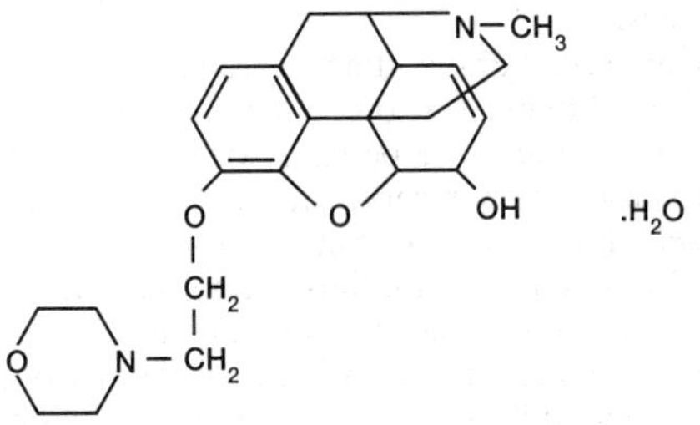

Molecular weight	416.5
(anhydrous)	(398.5)
pKa	8.0, 9.3
Solubility	
in alcohol	1 in 3
in water	1 in 50
Octanol/water partition coefficient	—

Pholcodine is a colourless, odourless crystalline powder, with a slightly bitter taste. It is prepared by chemical synthesis via substitution of the radical morpholinylethyl for the phenolic hydrogen of morphine.[1]

Available in combination with ephedrine hydrochloride (Falcodyl, Rubelix), with papaverine hydrochloride (Pholcomed, Pavacol-D, Pholcomed-D), with phenyltoloxamine (Pholtex), with cineole, menthol and terpin hydratel (Copholco, Copholcoids), with carbinoxamine maleate and ephedrine hydrochloride (Davenol) and with chlorpheniramine maleate and ephedrine hydrochloride (Expulin) and others.

Pharmacology

Pholcodine is an opioid with low affinity for opioid receptors. It has weak analgesic activity and primarily acts on the brain stem to relieve cough. It also has mild sedative actions which help to relieve local irritation in the respiratory tract.[2,3] The actions to relieve cough appear to be due to a direct effect on the cough centre.[4]

Pholcodine exerts its antitussive effect by suppressing the cough centre in the medulla at doses below those necessary to produce analgesia. It probably has very little affinity for the opioid receptors associated with analgesia and addiction and produces less constipation than codeine.[5]

Pholcodine possesses anticonvulsant activity in animals and blocks pentylenetetrazol-induced convulsions. It has mild hypotensive effects which are mediated both centrally and peripherally. The peripheral effect is due partly to a dircct vasodilating action and partly to histamine release. Pholcodine also inhibits gastrointestinal motility in animal studies.[2]

Toxicology

There is no evidence of teratological effect in animals or in man.[2] The estimated minimum lethal dose is 500 mg although a toxic dose in children is reported to be 200 mg. Nausea and vomiting occasionally occur and large doses may produce restlessness, excitement and ataxia. Pholcodine does not produce withdrawal symptoms. It is not liable to cause addiction and tolerance on prolonged use.

Clinical pharmacology

Pholcodine is almost exclusively used for its ability to relieve cough. Studies in man have shown that 80–100 mg of pholcodine can suppress the cough induced by the intravenous injection of lobeline. The antitussive effect is also more effective than codeine against coughs of various pathological origins.[1] The results of other experiments conducted in laboratory animals also indicated that pholcodine has an antitussive potency about 1.6 times that of codeine.[5,15] It has little or no analgesic effect and has no useful euphoriant activity. It has mild sedative effects and may produce constipation by its effects on gastrointestinal motility. It has weak actions on the chemoreceptor trigger zone and so may sometimes cause nausea and vomiting. It has no significant effect on the cardiovascular system in standard dosage. It may cause respiratory depression particularly if the dose used is large. Since its euphoriant activity is weak it rarely produces dependence. There is no available information on the dose–response relationship of pholcodine. It is likely that, as with codeine, the degree of relief reported by patients does not necessarily correlate with actual reduction in the frequency of coughing.[6] The duration of action is between 4 and 5 h.

Pharmacokinetics

Pholcodine in pharmaceutical preparations can be determined by high performance liquid chromatography (HPLC) or by a colorimetric method.[7,8] A radioimmunoassay is also available for the determination of codeine and pholcodine.[9] Recently an HPLC assay with fluorescence detection has been developed for the determination of pholcodine in plasma, saliva and urine.[10]

The pharmacokinetics of pholcodine are independent of the dose. Pholcodine kinetics are best described by a two-compartment model since its absorption is not well described by either first order or zero order kinetics. Maximum plasma concentrations are attained at 4–8 h after an oral dose.[11] The elimination half life ranges from 32 to 43 h, which is approximately 16 times longer than that of codeine. This may be related to the high volume of distribution of pholcodine (36–49 $l.kg^{-1}$) rather than a difference in clearance (mean 100 1 $ml.min^{-1}$). Following a single oral dose of pholcodine, its slow elimination can interfere with the radioimmunoassay of opiates in urine for 2–6 weeks. Chen and colleagues[12] recently reported a pharmacokinetic study of pholcodine after 2 single doses (20 and 60 mg) and after chronic administration (20 mg 8 hourly for 10 days) in six healthy volunteer subjects according to a balanced crossover design with an interval of 3 weeks between treatments. Plasma, saliva and urine concentrations of pholcodine were determined by an HPLC assay. After the single doses, pholcodine was absorbed rapidly ($T_{max} = 1.6 \pm 1.2$ h) and eliminated slowly with a mean half life of 50.1 ± 4.1 h with a total body clearance ranging from 400 to 600 $ml.min^{-1}$ of which about 25% was due to renal clearance (137 ± 34 $ml.min^{-1}$). The renal clearance was inversely correlated with urinary pH ($r = 0.60$) but not with urine flow rate. The urinary recovery of unchanged pholcodine was 26.2 ± 3% of the administered dose. The concentration of pholcodine in saliva was 3.6 times higher than in plasma. After chronic administration the pharmacokinetics of pholcodine were not statistically different from the single dose parameters. The plasma protein binding of pholcodine was 23.5%. No morphine (in conjugated or unconjugated form) was detected in the urine of the subjects after pholcodine administration.

Oral absorption	rapid
Presystemic metabolism	nil
Plasma half life	
range	32–43 h
mean[12]	37 h; 50.1 ± 4.1 h
Volume of distribution[11,12]	30–49 $l.kg^{-1}$
Plasma protein binding	23.5%[12]

Concentration–effect relationship

There is no evidence of any correlation between the plasma concentration of pholcodine and its antitussive effect.

Metabolism

Pholcodine is metabolized in the liver,[9,11] but undergoes little conjugation with glucuronide or sulphate. The radiolabelled drug is only slowly metabolized and eliminated.[13] Very little or no metabolically derived morphine is produced from pholcodine.[12] Two unidentified peaks which consistently appeared in all the urine and saliva chromatograms in subjects after oral pholcodine are probable metabolites.[12]

Pharmaceutics

Pholcodine is available in a large variety of preparations.[14] It is administered by mouth, usually as a linctus or syrup, in a dose of 5–15 mg for adults (5–15 ml pholcodine linctus), 5 mg for children over 2 years and 2.5 mg for children under 2 years. Pholcodine tartrate has been given in doses of 10–30 mg.

Preparations available are:
Pholcodine citrate syrup: 0.2% pholcodine citrate
Pholcodine linctus CF: 0.05% pholcodine, for children
Pholcodine linctus: 0.1% pholcodine
Strong pholcodine linctus: 0.2% pholcodine
Sugar-free linctuses are available in all strengths. Pastilles are also available containing 4 mg pholcodine.

All preparations should be stored in airtight containers in a cool place.

Therapeutic use

Indications

Pholcodine is used in the relief of unproductive cough.

Contraindications

None

Mode of use

The clinical use of pholcodine for cough suppression depends mainly on its control action on the cough centre in the medulla. It is administered orally in syrup or linctus form in a dose of 5 to 10 mg three to four times daily: children over 2 years old may be given 5 mg four times daily and those under 2 years, 1 to 2.5 mg four times daily. In view of the long elimination half life,[11,12] these current prescribing recommendations of relatively frequent dosing may need revising.

Adverse reactions

Potentially life-threatening effects
No reactions of this kind appear to have been described.

Acute overdosage
Little information is available specifically on pholcodine overdose, but respiratory depression, drowsiness, restlessness, and ataxia may occur after large doses of pholcodine. A toxic dose of pholcodine in children is about 200 mg, which causes sleep.

Severe or irreversible adverse effects
Epigastric distress or biliary colic may occur. The development of tolerance and physical dependence with chronic use is a characteristic feature of the opioid drugs in general. There is also the possibility of developing psychological dependence on the effects produced by the drug. However, pholcodine has very low euphorigenic activity and is unlikely to be a problem. It has been demonstrated that pholcodine has essentially no addiction liability and, in large doses, fails to substitute for morphine in addicts.[2,15]

Symptomatic adverse effects
The gastrointestinal effects include nausea and vomiting and constipation. However, none of the subjects after chronic dosing of 10 days experienced any of the usual opioid-like side effects such as constipation, urinary hesitancy, drowsiness, dizziness, nausea and confusion.[12]

Interference with clinical pathology tests
Pholcodine interferes with the radioimmunoassay of opiates in urine.

High risk groups

Neonates
The drug may be used in neonates in appropriate doses.

Breast milk. There is no information available as to whether the drug is excreted in breast milk but it is unlikely to be harmful to the infant.

Children
The drug may be used in children in appropriate doses.

Pregnant women
The safety of pholcodine in pregnancy has not been fully established, but its use in pregnancy has not revealed any direct evidence of teratogenicity.[2,16]

The elderly
There is no information available on the pharmacokinetics of pholcodine in the elderly. Consequently, it is not known whether a reduction in the dose is necessary.

Concurrent disease

Respiratory disease. Pholcodine depresses the respiratory centre, releases histamine, depresses the cough reflex and tends to dry secretions. It should therefore be used with caution in patients who have decreased respiratory reserve and in asthmatic patients.

Liver disease. Pholcodine is metabolized in the liver. Therefore, the dosage and frequency of administration may have to be reduced in patients with severely impaired liver function.[4]

Renal disease. No information is available of the elimination of pholcodine in renal failure. With its long elimination half life in normal subjects,[11,12] it may be necessary to adjust the dose in patients with renal failure to avoid overdosage.

Drug interactions

Potentially hazardous interactions
Phenothiazines, monoamine oxidase inhibitors and tricyclic antidepressants may exaggerate and prolong the depressant effects of some opioids,[4] but information on possible interactions of pholcodine with these drugs is not available.

Potentially useful interactions

No interactions of this type have been recorded.

Clinical trials

Clinical trials have shown that pholcodine has equal or greater potency than codeine as an antitussive agent. Most of the reports showed favourable results for pholcodine, with few side effects and no addiction liability to the drug. However, these clinical trials were not well controlled by modern standards and there were no good quantitative comparisons with codeine.

1. Snell E S, Armitage P 1957 Clinical comparison of diamorphine and pholcodine as cough suppressants by a new method of sequential analysis. Lancet 1: 860–862
2. Mulinos M G, Epstein I G 1962 Clinical investigation of antitussive properties of pholcodine. New York State Journal of Medicine 62: 2373–2377
3. Bickerman H A, Itkin S E 1960 Further studies on the evaluation of antitussive agents employing experimentally induced cough in human subjects. Clinical Pharmacology and Therapeutics 1: 180–191
4. Jaffe G, Grimshaw J J 1983 Randomized single-blind trial in general practice comparing the efficacy and palatability of two cough linctus preparations, Pholcolix and Actifed compound, in children with acute cough. Current Medical Research and Opinion 8: 594–599

These clinical studies, along with others summarized by Eddy et al.,[15] generally have shown that pholcodine is an effective antitussive, particularly with its lower toxicity, fewer side effects and no greater liability to produce dependence. These views are further substantiated by more recent comparative studies which demonstrated that pholcodine is not metabolized to morphine in man.[11,12] However, the long half life of pholcodine may require a revised prescribing recommendation of the frequency of dosing. In general, very little information on the clinical pharmacology of pholcodine is available. More studies are required on this very popular antitussive agent.

References

1. Chabrier P, Guidicelli R, Thiullier J 1950 Etude chimique, pharmacologique et clinique d'un nouveau sédatif de la toux: la morpholylethyl-morphine (MEM). Annals of Pharmacology (France) 8: 261–273
2. Cahen R 1961 The pharmacology of pholcodine. Bulletin of Narcotics 13: 19–36
3. Wade A 1977 Martindale: the extra pharmacopoeia, 27th edn. The Pharmaceutical Press, London, pp 1247–1248
4. Jaffe J H, Martin W R 1975 Narcotic analgesics and antagonists. In: Goodman L S, Gilman A (eds) The pharmacological basis of therapeutics, 5th edn. Macmillan, New York, pp 245–283
5. Findlay J W 1988 Pholcodine. Journal of Clinical Pharmacy and Therapeutics 13: 5–17
6. Sevelius H, McCoy J F, Colmore J P 1971 Dose response to codeine in patients with chronic cough. Clinical Pharmacology and Therapeutics 12: 449–455
7. Carnevale L 1983 Simultaneous determination of acetaminophen, quaifenesin, pseudoephedrine, pholcodine and paraben preservatives in cough mixture by high performance liquid chromatography. Journal of Pharmaceutical Science 72: 196–198
8. Shohet J S 1975 Analysis of pholcodine in cough preparations. Journal of Pharmaceutical Science 64: 1011–1013
9. Butz R F, Jones E C, Welch R M, Findlay J W 1983 Pharmacokinetics and O-dealkylation of morphine-3-alkyl ethers in the rat. A radioimmunoassay study. Drug Metabolism and Disposition 11: 481–488
10. Chen Z R, Siebert D M, Somogyi A A, Bochner F 1988 Determination of pholcodine in biological fluids by high performance liquid chromatography with fluorescence detection. Journal of Chromatography Biomedical Applications 424: 170–176
11. Findlay J W, Fowle A S, Butz R F et al 1986 Comparative disposition of codeine and pholcodine in man after single oral doses. British Journal of Clinical Pharmacology 22: 61–71
12. Chen Z R, Bochner F, Somogyi A 1988 Pharmacokinetics of pholcodine in healthy volunteers: single and chronic dosing studies. British Journal of Clinical Pharmacology 26: 445–453
13. Neuvonen P J, Pentikainen P J, Penttila A 1980 Pharmacokinetics of pholcodine in man. World Conference on Clinical Pharmacology and Therapeutics, London, Abstract 0488
14. Reynolds J E F 1989 Martindale: the extra pharmacopoeia, 29th edn. The Pharmaceutical Press, London, p 913
15. Eddy N B, Friebel H, Klaus-Jurgen H, Halbach H 1970 Codeine and its alternatives for pain and cough relief. World Health Organization, Geneva, pp 160–164
16. Colley D P, Gibson G T 1982 Three common Australian cough mixtures: study of their use in pregnancy. Australian Journal of Pharmacy 63: 213–217

Physostigmine

P

The calabar bean, or an extract thereof, was used by the Efik people in West Africa in witchcraft trials. The accused swallowed the beans and survival, and thus innocence, was established by early vomiting. The action of the alkaloid involved was described some hundred years ago and physostigmine has since been used to antagonize atropine poisoning[1] and in ophthalmological practice as a miotic agent.[2]

Chemistry

Physostigmine (eserine, Antilirium)

$C_{15}H_{21}N_3O_2$

(3aS,8aR)-1,2,3,3a,8,8a-Hexahydro-1,3a,8-trimethyl-pyrrolo[2,3-b]indol-5-yl methylcarbamate

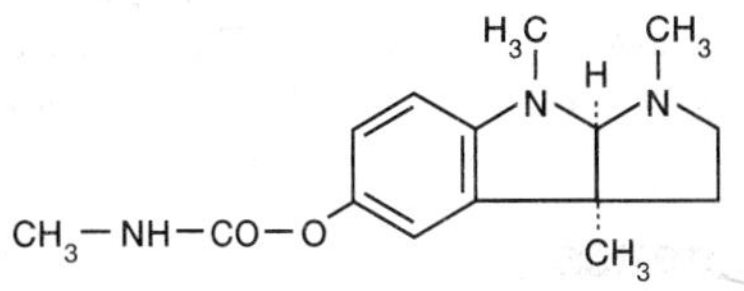

Molecular weight	275.3
	413.5 (salicylate)
	648.8 (sulphate)
pKa1	1.8
pKa2	7.9
Solubility	
in alcohol	1 in 25 (salicylate)
	1 in 1 (sulphate)
in water	1 in 90 (salicylate)
	1 in 1 (sulphate)
Octanol/water partition coefficient	40

Physostigmine, or eserine, is an alkaloid extracted from the calabar bean, the dried ripe seed of woody vine, *Physostigma venemosum*. Physostigmine salicylate consists of colourless or white crystals or powder with a slightly bitter taste. Physostigmine sulphate is also an odourless white powder. Physostigmine salts and their aqueous solutions turn red on exposure to air, light, heat or on contact with traces of metals.

Physostigmine is available in combination with pilocarpine.

Pharmacology

Physostigmine is a tertiary amine which is an inhibitor of acetylcholinesterase. Although physostigmine is almost completely ionized in the body at the pH of most tissues, there is a difference between it and quaternary compounds such that distinct differences in pharmacology are seen. Unlike neostigmine, physostigmine does cross the blood–brain barrier and central effects are seen. Physostigmineis also better absorbed across the gastrointestinal mucosa. The inhibition of cholinesterase causes accumulation of acetylcholine at the nerve synapses and cholinergic effects are enhanced. Physostigmine combines with the anionic site of cholinesterase and since it is much less readily hydrolysed than acetylcholine, it remains bound to the enzyme. Physostigmine is hydrolysed by cholinesterases but about 1 million times more slowly than acetylcholine. Physostigmine also increases the release of acetylcholine and may also have a direct cholinergic action on acetylcholine receptors.

Physostigmine

Toxicology

There is no information about mutagenic, carcinogenic or teratogenic effects of physostigmine.

Clinical pharmacology

Physostigmine has cholinergic effects on the eye, intestine and skeletal muscle. In the eye, physostigmine causes miosis due to constriction of the sphincter pupillae muscle, and in addition constriction of the ciliary muscle causes blurring of near vision. The block of accommodation is more transient than the miosis. Intraocular pressure falls, due to the enhanced flow of aqueous humour.

In the gastrointestinal tract physostigmine causes intestinal muscles to contract and increases secretion of gastric acid from the parietal cells. Both gastric emptying and intestinal transit are speeded. At the neuromuscular junction, physostigmine usually results in increased skeletal muscle contraction. Physostigmine, like neostigmine, will reverse the effects of competitive neuromuscular blocking drugs like tubocurarine. In larger (or repetitive) doses, physostigmine may itself result in depolarization of the neuromuscular junction and neuromuscular transmission may be blocked.

Physostigmine has effects on the cardiovascular system but the end results depend on the relative effects of ganglionic and postganglionic stimulation of acetylcholine. The usual effect is bradycardia with a fall in cardiac output and no effect on blood pressure, but blood pressure may fall with higher doses. Physostigmine also causes increased secretion from secretory glands and this causes salivation, lachrymation and sweating. There may be increased production of bronchial secretions, and, rarely, airways narrowing may occur due to smooth muscle contraction.

Pharmacokinetics

Analysis of physostigmine in plasma samples is based on high pressure liquid chromatography with electrochemical detection, which has a sensitivity[3,4] of 500 $ng.l^{-1}$. There is also indirect measurement of physostigmine plasma concentrations by the degree of inhibition of cholinesterases.

Physostigmine is rapidly distributed in the body after intravenous administration. The volume of distribution has a mean of 46.5 ± 19.5 l. The fraction bound to plasma proteins is not known. Plasma clearance of physostigmine is similar to other reversible cholinesterase inhibitors used clinically, with a mean of $92.5 \pm 37.7\ l.h^{-1}$. This results in a short plasma elimination half life of about 20 minutes.[3]

After intramuscular and subcutaneous administration the availability of physostigmine is of the same order as after intravenous dosage.

Oral bioavailability has also been determined, with values of 11% to 37% due to presystemic metabolism. Peak plasma concentrations are achieved in about 45 min.[5,6]

Oral absorption	readily absorbed
Presystemic metabolism	11–37%
Plasma half life	
range	12–40 min
mean	20 min
Volume of distribution	15–75 l
Plasma protein binding	—

Physostigmine readily enters the CNS.

Concentration–effect relationship

Sensitive and reliable methods for the plasma assay of physostigmine have only recently become available, which means that studies on concentration–effect relationships are sparse. An arousal effect of physostigmine was suggested at plasma concentrations exceeding 3.5 $\mu g.l^{-1}$ after intravenous administration.[3] The effect may, however, be dependent on, for example, anaesthetic technique or drugs administered concomitantly.[5]

The lowering of blood pressure has been related to physostigmine plasma concentrations after oral dosage.[7]

Metabolism

Physostigmine is rapidly metabolized in the body, mainly by hydrolytic cleavage of the carbamate ester by cholinesterases (Fig. 1). Metabolism results in the loss of pharmacological activity. With the exception of a minor metabolite, eseroline, the metabolites have not been identified in man. Metabolism may also occur in the blood.

Renal excretion obviously plays a minor role in physostigmine disposition, as very little unchanged drug is excreted in urine. Biliary excretion of physostigmine has been reported.

Pharmaceutics

Physostigmine salicylate is available for parenteral use, whereas physostigmine sulphate is used in eye drops because of its higher water-solubility and better compatibility with some preservatives.

Physostigmine, both as crystals and as aqueous solution, becomes pink to red on exposure to heat, light, and air and in contact with metals, owing to the formation of rubreserine. Solutions of physostigmine should not be used when they have turned red.

Eye drops

Physostigmine sulphate is used in 0.25–1% solution as eye drops, often in combination with 1–4% pilocarpine hydrochloride. It is not evident that combination therapy has additive effects.[8] The solution also contains 0.2% sodium bisulphite, 0.02% benzalkonium chloride and occasionally disodium edetate. Eye drops should be protected from light.

Parenteral solution

Physostigmine salicylate is available for parenteral use as Antilirium (Forest, USA) in 2 ml ampoules containing 1 $mg.ml^{-1}$ in sterile water. Sodium bisulphite 0.1% is added as antioxidant and benzyl alcohol 2.0% as a preservative. The ampoules should be protected from light.

Therapeutic use

Indications

1. Glaucoma
2. Poisoning with anticholinergic and tricyclic/tetracyclic antidepressant drugs
3. Reversal of postoperative oversedation
4. Preliminary trials in some psychiatric and neurological disorders.

Contraindications

1. Anaesthesia using depolarizing neuromuscular block agents, i.e. succinylcholine or decamethonium
2. Asthma
3. Gangrene
4. Diabetes
5. Severe cardiovascular disease
6. Mechanical obstruction of the intestine or urogenital tract or any vagotonic state
7. Parkinson's disease.

Mode of use

Physostigmine as eye drops for the lowering of intraocular pressure has a duration of some hours, similar to that of the cholinergic agonist, pilocarpine. In chronic primary glaucoma physostigmine is used primarily in patients with hypersensitivity reactions to pilocarpine. It is used in aqueous solutions in concentrations of 0.25–1% administered every 4–6 hours. Miosis is seen within 30 minutes and persists for many hours (12–36 hours). It can rarely be used for a long period of time because of irritation and follicular hypertrophy of the conjunctiva.[8]

Physostigmine by the parenteral route is administered slowly, intravenously or intramuscularly. The initial dose of 0.5–1.2 mg may be followed by a second one, if the desired effect is not seen within 30 minutes. Physostigmine has a short duration of action and continuous dosage has been suggested for a protracted effect.[5] Intravenous physostigmine should not be given at a higher rate than 1 $mg.min^{-1}$.

Physostigmine is used only in life-threatening situations in children, and the maximum parenteral dose is 0.5 mg or 0.25 mg in children below 4 years of age.

P

Indications

1. Glaucoma
Cholinergic drugs are used primarily in the therapy of glaucoma but are also used in ophthalmological practice to reverse the effects of mydriatic agents such as atropine and homatropine given locally. Physostigmine is nowadays mostly replaced by other cholinergic drugs such as pilocarpine or phospoline iodide.

Closed-angle glaucoma. In closed-angle glaucoma, agents that constrict the pupil are capable of relieving the obstructive effects of peripheral iris, blocking the trabecular meshwork. This is a consequence of the pull of the pupillary sphincter, which reduces the volume of iris in the angle and tightens the iris periphery. Constriction of the pupil increases the area of contact between the iris and lens, thus increasing the resistance between the posterior and anterior chambers. In most instances less potent cholinergic drugs such as physostigmine and pilocarpine will permit a greater access of aqueous humor to the trabecular structures.[8]

Open-angle glaucoma. In the open-angle glaucomas various cholinergic drugs improve outflow facility. This is true for both normal eyes and those suffering from glaucoma. The mechanism does not appear to depend on the effects on the sphincter of the pupil. The effectiveness of miotics relates to stimulation of the ciliary musculature, resulting in a pull on the scleral spur or trabecular meshwork, and perhaps to direct cholinergic effects on parts of the trabecular meshwork bordering Schlemm's canal, which may constitute the major resistance site.

In open-angle glaucoma miotics do not constitute a cure of the basic outflow disorder. They relieve the obstructed outflow, thus lowering intraocular pressure and avoiding optic nerve damage.[8]

2. Poisoning with anticholinergic and tricyclic/tetracyclic antidepressant drugs
Physostigmine has been used for more than a hundred years as an antidote for atropine overdoses and more recently also in poisoning with tricyclic/tetracyclic antidepressant drugs. A reversal of symptoms such as disorientation, confusion, hallucinations and unconsciousness elicited by all classes of drugs showing affinity for brain muscarinic receptors has been reported after physostigmine therapy.[1,9] The reversal of overdose symptoms of the following drugs has been reported: atropine and scopolamine, anticholinergic antiparkinson drugs, tricyclic antidepressant drugs and the phenothiazines. The inhibition of cholinesterase by the centrally acting physostigmine is probably the most important mechanism for restoration of cholinergic activity, but release of acetylcholine and a direct cholinergic receptor agonism might also be important for the effects. Most reports describe a rapid reversal of disorientation and confusion and, in cases of high overdosage, also an increased level of consciousness. Although some have reported treatment as life-saving, the value of routine physostigmine in, for example, tricyclic antidepressant overdosage has been doubted, and conservative treatment may give equally good results.

Physostigmine treatment has not been shown to affect the mortality rate in tricyclic/tetracyclic antidepressant overdosage and treatment may exacerbate the risk of grand mal seizures.[10,11] Short duration of action and manifestation of severe side effects are other obstacles to the use of physostigmine. Of these, convulsions and respiratory symptoms are particularly troublesome. Cholinergic symptoms after excessive amounts of physostigmine are hypersalivation and bronchosecretion which may interfere with the respiration and airway maintenance in the comatose patient. Also bradycardia followed by hypotension may develop and occasionally asystole has occurred.

Physostigmine should therefore be reserved for life-threatening complications of poisoning with ensuing manifest anticholinergic symptoms. There is no clinical evidence that physostigmine is effective in combating tachycardia, except supraventricular tachycardia, after overdoses of tricyclic/tetracyclic antidepressant drugs.[9]

3. Reversal of postoperative oversedation
Physostigmine has a non-specific arousal effect, demonstrated after a number of drugs including anticholinergic agents, benzodiazepines, methoprylon, ethchlorvynol, droperidol, barbiturates and ketamine. The effect has been studied most extensively for benzodiazepine drugs, although a more specific antidote is now available.[12] On the other hand the antagonistic effect of physostigmine has been attributed to the preservative benzyl alcohol in the injected preparation (Antilirium).[13] Physostigmine as such has, however, an effect of its own.

Clinically, physostigmine has been used in the early postoperative period to antagonize oversedation and the anticholinergic syndrome, characterized by delirium, coma, medullary paralysis and more mild symptoms such as disorientation, hallucinations, anxiety and excessive somnolence.[14,15] Peripheral symptoms of the syndrome include tachycardia, hyperpyrexia, mydriasis, vasodilation, diminution of gastrointestinal motility and loss of salivary and sweat secretion.

Besides the arousal effect, physostigmine has a respiratory stimulating effect[16] and analgesia is not reduced in postoperative patients treated with opioid drugs.[17] The somnolent effect of opioids is rapidly reversed and respiratory rate is increased after physostigmine, presumably by the raising of levels of acetylcholine in the brain after these had been reduced by the opioid drug. The analgesic effect of cholinergic drugs seems to potentiate and be independent of opioid analgesia.[18] Severe side effects such as convulsions have not been seen in postoperative patients. Effects are generally of short duration, however.

4. Preliminary trials in some psychiatric and neurological disorders
Dementia. There is evidence that cholinergic mechanisms are involved in memory and learning, and that deficit in cholinergic function plays a role in certain mental disorders.[19] Several trials with physostigmine have addressed the effect of memory improvement in different types of dementia. Physostigmine has consistently shown a small, but usually positive, effect on memory in Alzheimer patients. In the literature, about one-third of the studies using physostigmine have indicated no effect, while others have shown some type of positive effect. The strength of the cholinergic model and the finding of beneficial effects have kept research active into the use of physostigmine in different types of dementia. In one study, a dose-dependent increase in memory has been shown in dementia of the Alzheimer type. The effect was more pronounced for very short-term memory, which may imply that improvement involves attention rather than long-term memory and retrieval.[21] Others have shown that physostigmine infusions have significantly better effect on long-term memory and retrieval compared to placebo in patients with Alzheimer's disease, whereas short-term memory was not affected.[22] The duration of action of physostigmine was short, however.

Other psychiatric and neurological disorders. Occasional reports have appeared on the effect of physostigmine in other mental disorders. Physostigmine was claimed to suppress manic symptoms.[23] Patients with tardive dyskinesias,[24] ataxia,[25] the Tourette syndrome[26] and amyotropic lateral sclerosis[27] have been treated with physostigmine. Results were negative or inconclusive.

Contraindications

See Drug interactions.

Adverse reactions

Potentially life-threatening effects
There is one report of a patient having asystole after a large dose of physostigmine given for poisoning.[28] In Parkinson's disease rigidity and respiratory insufficiency may occur.

Fig. 1 The metabolism of physostigmine

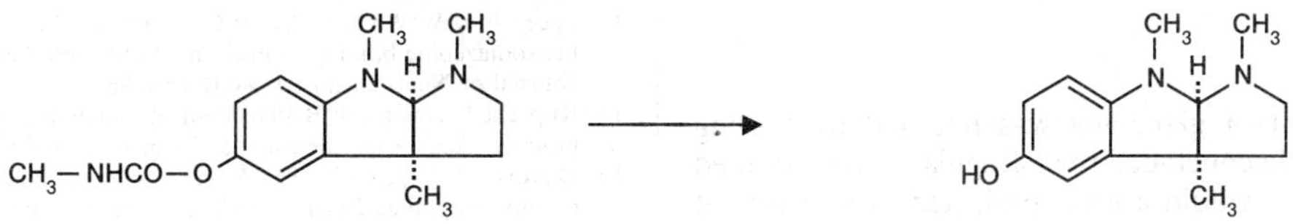

Acute overdosage
Effects after overdoses of physostigmine are all related to an excessive cholinergic action. Overdosage may cause a cholinergic crisis, including bradycardia, hypersalivation, urination, defecation and respiratory paralysis. Ventricular arrhythmia has also been reported.[29]

The antidote for physostigmine overdose is atropine. The dosage is judged by the disappearance of peripheral symptoms caused by physostigmine.

Severe or irreversible adverse effects
Convulsions may appear after an excessively rapid intravenous administration.[30]

Long-term oral administration of physostigmine for Alzheimer's disease may cause hypertension.[31]

Retinal detachment has been said to occur following local application[32] but the evidence is not conclusive.

Symptomatic adverse effects
Adverse effects after local application of eye drops occur frequently and include ciliary and conjunctival congestion, ocular and periorbital pain, twitching lids, headache and accommodation myopia.[8]

Systemic adverse effects from topical administration are rare.

Other adverse effects of physostigmine include nausea, vomiting, hypersalivation, excessive sweating, bradycardia and respiratory effects.

Other effects
Physostigmine causes a release of adrenaline which results in increased blood pressure and heart rate.[33]

Interference with clinical pathology tests
No interferences of this kind have been reported.

High risk groups

Neonates
The drug is unlikely to be used in neonates.

Breast milk. It is not known if physostigmine enters breast milk but indications for the use of the drug make it very unlikely that a breast-fed infant would ever be exposed to a significant quantity of the drug.

Children
Physostigmine has been used in children to antagonize the 'central cholinergic syndrome'. Owing to the high risk of complications, it is suggested that use of physostigmine in children should be reserved for life-threatening situations.[34]

Pregnant women
No information is available on the effect of physostigmine on the fetus.

The elderly
Cardiovascular disease, which often occurs with increasing age, is a relative contraindication for physostigmine use. Plasma clearance and volume of distribution were not related to age in postoperative patients.[3]

Drug interactions

Potentially hazardous interactions

Neuromuscular blocking agents such as suxamethonium and demecarium. Physostigmine interacts with succinylchloride to prolong its effects to 45 min from the usual 5 min duration of action. This interaction gains clinical significance in the poisoned patient who is paralysed for intubation.[9]

Cholinergic and anticholinergic drugs. Physostigmine may potentiate the action of cholinergic drugs and antagonize the action of cholinergic receptor blockers.

Potentially useful interactions
No interactions of this kind have been reported.

Clinical trials

Glaucoma
The first medical treatment of glaucoma was initiated by Ludvig Laqueur as early as 1876. He concluded that 'Regular and continued instillation of physostigmine would appear indicated in all cases of glaucoma simplex and in all cases of glaucoma in which a previous iridectomy has not been entirely successful'.[2] This first miotic was soon followed by others.

1. Aquilonius S M, Hedstrand U 1978 The use of physostigmine as an antidote in tricyclic antidepressant intoxication. Acta Anaesthesiologica Scandinavica 22: 40–45

Physostigmine was given to 10 unconscious patients because of self-poisoning with tricyclic antidepressant drugs. Before intravenous physostigmine, probantheline 30 mg was given to ascertain that peripheral cholinergic, muscarinic receptors were blocked. The following conclusions were drawn:

1. A slow intravenous injection of 2 mg increased consciousness within 15 min and is of potential diagnostic value
2. Repeated intravenous doses cause rapid shifts in the level of consciousness and are of limited practical value
3. If the test dose has a positive effect, an intravenous infusion of physostigmine 4 $mg.h^{-1}$ will raise the level of consciousness substantially
4. Intravenous injection of physostigmine increases the risk of grand mal seizures
5. No enhanced peripheral cholinergic action was seen
6. There is no evidence that physostigmine reduces mortality in cases of tricyclic antidepressant overdosage.

2. Petersson J, Gordh T E, Hartvig P, Wiklund L 1986 A double-blind trial of the analgesic properties of physostigmine in postoperative patients. Acta Anaesthesiologica Scandinavica 30: 283–288

A double-blind clinical trial of the analgesic and antisedative effects of intravenous physostigmine salicylate 2 mg was carried out in surgical patients (n = 60). Pethidine 50 mg and placebo were included for comparison. Physostigmine caused analgesia of the same magnitude as for pethidine during the first 15 min after which it decreased to the level of placebo at 30 min. An antisedative or arousal effect was recorded over a somewhat longer period; after this there was no difference between placebo and physostigmine. In contrast to pethidine, physostigmine caused no decrease in ventilatory rate. Heart rate and blood pressure did not change. Although the effects of physostigmine were of short duration, the drug may be preferred to naloxone when intermediate alertness of the patient is wanted without the increase of postoperative pain.

References

1. Aquilonius S M 1978 Physostigmine in the treatment of drug overdose. In: Jenden D J (ed) Cholinergic mechanisms and psychopharmacology. Plenum Press, New York, pp 817–825
2. Lebensohn J E 1963 The first miotic. American Journal of Ophthalmology 55: 657–659
3. Aquilonius S M, Hartvig P 1986 Clinical pharmacokinetics of choline esterase inhibitors. Clinical Pharmacokinetics 11: 236–249
4. Whelpton R 1983 Sensitive liquid chromatographic method for physostigmine in biological fluids using dual-electrode electrochemical detection. Journal of Chromatography, Biomedical Applications 23: 216–220
5. Hartvig P, Lindström B, Pettersson E, Wiklund L 1989 Reversal of postoperative somnolence using a two-rate infusion of physostigmine. Acta Anaesthesiologica Scandinavica 33: 681–685
6. Whelpton R, Hurst P 1985 Bioavailability of oral physostigmine. New England Journal of Medicine 313: 1293–1294
7. Gibson M, Moore T, Smith C M, Whelpton R 1985 Physostigmine concentrations after oral doses. Lancet 1: 695–696
8. Kolker A E, Hetherington J 1983 Mechanism of action of miotics. In: Becker-Schaffer's diagnosis and therapy of the glaucomas, Vth edn. C V Mosby, St Louis, p 373
9. Litovitz T L 1984 The anecdotal antidotes. Emergency Medical Clinics of North America 2: 145–158
10. Knudsen K, Heath A 1984 Effects of self-poisoning with maprotilene. British Medical Journal 288: 601–603
11. Aquilonius S M, Hedstrand U 1978 The use of physostigmine as an antidote in tricyclic antidepressant intoxication. Acta Anaesthesiologica Scandinavica 22: 40–45
12. Pedersen J E 1985 Fysostigmine: Antidot ved diazepamforgiftning. Ugeskrift for Laeger 147: 3586–3587
13. Speeg Jr K V, Wang S, Avant G R, Berman M L, Schenker S 1980 Antagonism of benzodiazepine binding in brain by Antilirium, benzyl alcohol and physostigmine. Journal of Neurochemistry 34(4): 856–865
14. Rupreht J, Dworacek B 1976 Central anticholinergic syndrome in anaesthetic practice. Acta Anaesthesiologica Belgica 2: 45–60
15. Duvoisin R C, Katz R 1968 Reversal of central anticholinergic's syndrome in man by physostigmine. Journal of the American Medical Association 206: 1964–1965

16. Snir-Mor I, Weinstock M, Davidson J T, Bahar M 1983 Physostigmine antagonizes morphine-induced respiratory depression in human subjects. Anaesthesiology 59: 6–9
17. Petersson J, Gordh T E, Hartvig P, Wiklund L 1986 A double-blind trial of the analgesic properties of physostigmine in postoperative patients. Acta Anaesthesiologica Scandinavica 30: 283–288
18. Weinstock M, Davidson J T, Rosin A J, Schnieden H 1982 Effect of physostigmine on morphine induced postoperative pain and somnolence. British Journal of Anaesthesia 54: 429–434
19. Davis K L, Mohs R C, Tinklenberg J R, Pfefferbaum A, Hollister L E, Kopel B S 1978 Physostigmine improvement of longterm memory processes in normal humans. Science 201: 272–274
20. Ashford J W, Sherman K A, Kumar V 1989 Advances in Alzheimer therapy: cholinesterase inhibitors. In: Neurobiology of ageing, vol. 10. Pergamon, Oxford, pp 99–105
21. Beller S A, Overall J A, Swann A C 1985 Efficacy of oral physostigmine in primary degenerative dementia. Psychopharmacology 87: 147–151
22. Davis K L, Mohs R C 1982 Enhancement of memory processes in Alzheimer's disease with multiple-dose intravenous physostigmine. American Journal of Psychiatry 139 (11): 1421–1424
23. Davis K L, Berger P A, Hollister L E, Defraites E 1978 Physostigmine in mania. Archives of General Psychiatry 35: 119–122
24. Tamminga C A, Smith R C, Ericksen R C, Davis J M 1977 Cholinergic influence in tardive dyskinesias. American Journal of Psychiatry 134: 769–774
25. Kark P R A, Blass J P, Spence A 1977 Physostigmine in familial ataxias. Neurology 27: 70–72
26. Stahl S S, Berger P A 1980 Letter. New England Journal of Medicine 302: 1311
27. Aquilonius S M, Askmark H, Eckernäs S A, Gillberg P G, Hilton-Brown P, Rydin E, Stahlberg E 1986 Cholinesterase inhibitors lack therapeutic effect in amyotropic lateral sclerosis. A controlled clinical study of physostigmine versus neostigmine. Acta Neurologica Scandinavica 73: 628–632
28. Boon J, Prideaux P R 1980 Cardiac arrest following physostigmine. Anaesthesia and Intensive Care 8: 92–93
29. Dysken M W, Janowsky D S 1985 Dose-related physostigmine induced ventricular arrhythmia: case report. Journal of Clinical Psychiatry 46 (10): 446–447
30. Stewart G O 1979 Convulsions after physostigmine. Anaesthesia and Intensive Care 7: 283
31. Cain J W 1986 Hypertension associated with oral administration of physostigmine in a patient with Alzheimer's disease. American Journal of Psychiatry 143 (7): 910–912
32. Alper J J 1979 Miotics and retinal detachment. Annals of Ophthalmology 11: 395–401
33. Janowsky D S, Risch C S, Huey L Y, Kennedy B, Ziegler M 1985 Effects of physostigmine on pulse, blood pressure and serum epinephrine levels. American Journal of Psychiatry 142 (6): 738–740
34. Slay R D 1985 Ponder physostigmine use. Editorial. Journal of Emergency Medicine 3 (6): 485–486

P

Pilocarpine (hydrochloride, nitrate)

Pilocarpine, a direct-acting muscarinic agonist, is widely used to reduce intraocular pressure in glaucoma.

Chemistry

Pilocarpine (Ocusert Pilo)
$C_{11}H_{16}N_2O_2$
3S,4R-3-Ethyldihydro-4-[(1-methyl-1H-imidazol-5-yl)methyl]-2(3H)-furanone
Pilocarpine hydrochloride (Adsorbocarpine, Akarpine, Isopto Carpine, I-Pilopine, Pilocar, Miocarpine, Almocarpine, Ocu-Carpine, Pilokair, Sno Pilo, Opulets Pilocarpine)
$C_{11}H_{16}N_2O_2.HCl$
3S,4R-3-Ethyldihydro-4-[(1-methyl-1H-imidazol-5-yl)methyl]-2(3H)-furanone hydrochloride
Pilocarpine nitrate (P.V. Carpine Liquifilm, Dulcicarpine, Marticarpine, Miopos, Pilo, Pilopos, Vistacarpine, Minims Pilocarpine Nitrate)
$C_{11}H_{16}N_2O_2.HNO_3$
3S,4R-3-Ethyldihydro-4-[(1-methyl-1H-imidazol-5-yl)methyl]-2(3H)-furanone nitrate

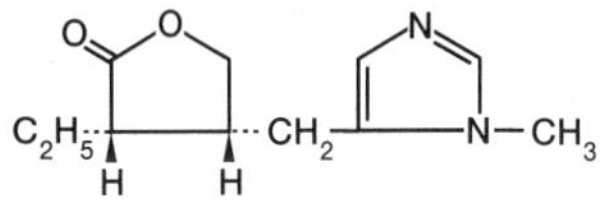

Molecular weight	208.3
hydrochloride	244.7
nitrate	271.3
pKa =N−, −N<	1.6, 7.1
Solubility	
in alcohol	>1 in 30
hydrochloride	1 in 3
nitrate	1 in 160
in water	>1 in 30
hydrochloride	>1 in 1
nitrate	1 in 8
Octanol/water partition coefficient	low

Pilocarpine is an alkaloid obtained from the leaves of *Pilocarpus microphyllus* (Rutaceae) or *P. jaborandi*. It occurs as a viscous, colourless, oily liquid or crystals that melt at about 34°C. It is hygroscopic. Pilocarpine hydrochloride occurs as colourless, odourless, translucent crystals or a white crystalline powder with a faintly bitter taste and melts at 199–205°C. It is hygroscopic and is affected by light. It is available in combination with adrenaline bitartrate (E-Pilo, PE) and with physostigmine salicylate (Isopto E-PS).

Pilocarpine nitrate exists as shining, white or colourless crystals or a white crystalline powder that melts at 170–179°C with decomposition. It is affected by light and the solutions are acidic.

Pharmacology

Pilocarpine is a direct-acting muscarinic parasympathomimetic agonist. The intrinsic muscarinic activity of pilocarpine is less than that of acetylcholine.[1,2] Imidazole-containing compounds like pilocarpine nitrate stimulate in vitro enzymatic synthesis of acetylcholine from acetyl-CoA and choline.[3] They may also be involved in non-enzymatic transfer of the acetyl group from acetyl-CoA to choline and ester hydrolysis during the production of acetylcholine.[4] It produces contraction of iris sphincter muscle leading to miosis or pupillary constriction. Pilocarpine also stimulates the ciliary muscle resulting in increased accommodation and improved outflow of aqueous humour through the trabecular meshwork.[5] The ciliary muscle is attached to the scleral spur and the displacement of the latter leads to an increased facility of aqueous outflow presumably by altering the configuration of the trabeculum, Schlemm's canal or both. It has been observed that pilocarpine produces a decrease in the depth of the anterior chamber.[6–12] This could be produced by a pupillary block resulting in the bowing of the iris (iris bombé), a change in the shape of the lens[11] or a forward displacement of the lens due to relaxation of the zonules or swelling of the ciliary body from vascular congestion. The narrowing of the anterior chamber can convert an eye with an open-angle component into one predisposed to angle closure attacks. Occasionally, a change in scleral rigidity is noted after pilocarpine therapy. This change is usually a decrease but increases have been noted.[12–15]

Toxicology

There have been no long-term studies with pilocarpine in animals to evaluate carcinogenic, mutagenic or impairment of fertility potential. Pilocarpine nitrate given subcutaneously in daily doses of 100 mg.kg^{-1} body weight affected tooth development and produced slight enlargement of the sublingual gland in rats treated throughout pregnancy.[16]

Clinical pharmacology

Pilocarpine has been used since 1877 in the treatment of glaucoma because of its effect in lowing intraocular pressure. The decrease in intraocular pressure is detected within 60 minutes and is maximal within 75 minutes. Depending on the concentration of pilocarpine used, the pressure stays reduced for 4–14 hours. Both normal and glaucomatous eyes show a similar tension-lowering response to pilocarpine.[12] The percentage tension decrease in normal subjects may range from 8 to 38%, while 12 to 40% reduction is seen in glaucomatous patients. Generally, the higher the average pretreatment tension, the greater the tension reduction produced by any strength of pilocarpine. Pilocarpine produces a marked effect on outflow facility in 2 to 4 hours. The average changes in outflow facility after pilocarpine may range from 0.03 to 0.16 µl.mg^{-1} per mmHg.[17–19] Dissipation of the effect on outflow facility is more rapid than the effect on intraocular pressure. The daily diurnal fluctuations in intraocular pressure are also reduced by pilocarpine in both normal and glaucomatous eyes.[12,20]

Pilocarpine may also influence the active transport of aqueous humour through the endothelial linings of the canal of Schlemm. Grierson and co-workers found more than twice the number of large vacuoles in the endothelium of the inner wall of Schlemm's canal in human eyes that were pretreated with pilocarpine prior to enucleation for melanoma.[21] In some patients, pilocarpine decreases secretion of aqueous humour, probably by altering the blood flow in the anterior uvea.[12,17,19,22]

Topical pilocarpine may initially increase episcleral venous pressure resulting in a transient rise in intraocular pressure lasting 20–40 minutes.[23] The ciliary muscle contraction by pilocarpine decreases the uveoscleral outflow of aqueous humour.[24] Topical 4% pilocarpine increased pseudofacility in young normotensive humans.[19] Pseudofacility is the amount of reduced aqueous humour inflow that follows each unit of rise in intraocular pressure. Using single drop response, Rothkoff and co-workers found that they could not predict which patients would have their intraocular pressures controlled consistently below 24 mmHg but they could predict who would be uncontrolled.[25]

When 1% solution of pilocarpine hydrochloride or nitrate is instilled in the lower cul-de-sac, progressive miosis begins at about 10 minutes, reaches a peak within 30 minutes and gradually decreases over a period of 4–8 hours. The pupillary reflex to light persists unless miosis is maximal.[26] Miosis improves outflow facility in eyes with angle-closure glaucoma by relieving pupillary block or by pulling the peripheral iris away from the anterior chamber angle.

The effect on accommodation begins in approximately 15 minutes and persists for 2–3 hours. When a pilocarpine ocular delivery system is placed in the conjunctival sac there is an immediate release of drug at a range of 2.5 to 3 times the projected rates (burst phenomenon).[27] At about 6 hours, the rate of release decreases to the labelled value, and may continue to decline for about a week in most patients. The average hourly release of pilocarpine from Ocusert Pilo-20 is 20 µg (range 16–24 µg) and Ocusert Pilo-40 is 40 µg (range 32–48 µg). The maximal reduction in intraocular pressure is seen within 1.5–2 hours after placement of the ocular system and is usually maintained for two days to a week. The drug-induced myopia and miosis decrease after the first several hours and then may remain constant as long as the system is functioning. The rate of release of pilocarpine from the ocular system is not affected by concurrent use of topical or systemic ocular medications like adrenaline, β-blocker ophthalmic solutions, fluorescein, anaesthetics, antibiotics, corticosteroid ophthalmic solutions, carbonic anhydrase inhibitors, or even hard and soft contact lenses. The 20 µg.h^{-1} system produces a reduction in intraocular pressure approximately equal to that produced by topical application of a 2% solution of pilocarpine hydrochloride or nitrate every 6 hours and the 40 µg.h^{-1} system produces a reduction in pressure approximately equal to that produced by topical application of a 4% solution of pilocarpine hydrochloride or nitrate every 6 hours.

Pilocarpine, when given intravenously, increases the flow from salivary and other exocrine glands. Bronchial smooth muscle and intestinal smooth muscle contract and in the brain cortical arousal occurs. In the cardiovascular system a brief fall in blood pressure is seen. However, none of these effects are likely to result from the small doses of pilocarpine usually given into the ocular sac.

Pharmacokinetics

The preferred analytical method for determining pilocarpine and its major metabolite, pilocarpic acid, concentrations in aqueous humour samples is high performance liquid chromatography.[28] The chromatographic separation is carried out on an octadecyl reverse-phase column. This method is able to detect 20 ng of pilocarpine and 10 ng pilocarpic acid in ocular tissues.

Pilocarpine, being a tertiary amine, is lipophilic and traverses the cornea well after topical application. After instillation of two drops of a 2% solution of pilocarpine in man, an aqueous humour concentration of 0.2% is achieved at 20 minutes post-instillation.[29]

The intraocular penetration of topical pilocarpine is mainly through the cornea. The human lacrimal volume is approximately 7 µl and a blinking eye can tolerate up to 10 µl of volume without overflow. Commercial medication containers dispense drops in the range of 25–75 µl. It is obvious that over 80% of the applied solution is lost through overflow. A tear turnover rate of about 16% per minute in humans further reduces the amount of drug. This portion is ultimately absorbed by ocular or extraocular tissues. The intraocular content depends on the dosage, form, concentration, volume and frequency of applications, tear production and loss through the lacrimal drainage system. With frequent and prolonged use of pilocarpine, sufficient may be absorbed through the conjunctival and nasal mucosae to cause systemic parasympathomimetic effects. Pilocarpine is bound to serum and various ocular tissues.

Studies in animals with radioactive tracers have demonstrated that the maximum concentration of pilocarpine occurs in 5-minute paracentesis samples following a single instillation of 1%, 4%, or 8% drops.[30] A soft contact lens presoaked in 1% pilocarpine produces higher aqueous humour concentrations than 1% pilocarpine drops. Higher drug concentrations resulted in higher aqueous humour concentrations. By 2 hours, the aqueous humour concentration is negligible, for all but soft lens applications. The latter maintain detectable aqueous humour levels for almost 4 hours. Pilocarpine is absorbed by iris pigment, which may act as a reservoir like the cornea.[31] Increased pilocarpine–eye contact time also enhances drug penetration.[32] After instillation of a 50 µl drop of pilocarpine on to the rabbit cornea, about 0.1% of the drug enters the aqueous humour if the vehicle is saline; 0.5% if the vehicle is viscous. The presence of benzalkonium chloride as a preservative enhances penetration by about 50%, due presumably to disruption of the corneal epithelium. Frequent application of pilocarpine drops at 5-minute intervals increases aqueous humour concentration.

Small amounts of pilocarpine may be excreted in breast milk. It is not known if it crosses the placenta. Given the normal usage of pilocarpine by an ocular application, the possible effects of old age,

Pilocarpine (hydrochloride, nitrate)

renal and hepatic disease or the kinetics of the drug are unlikely to be of any consequence.

Concentration–effect relationship

The pressure-reducing response is dose-related up to the administration of a single instillation of 4% pilocarpine.[33] Harris and Galin demonstrated that single dose loading with pilocarpine hydrochloride of 1 to 10% in patients produced no significant difference in ocular hypertensive response.[34] The chronic administration of 4% pilocarpine produces a significant improvement over a 1% solution. There was not much difference between 8% and 4% pilocarpine in duration of response. Several studies have found that Ocusert systems dispensing 50 μg.h^{-1} are more effective in open-angle glaucoma therapy than the 20 μg.h^{-1} membranes.[27,35] Higher than 40 μg.h^{-1} releasing systems were no more effective.

Metabolism

The mechanism by which pilocarpine is inactivated in the body is unclear, but human serum and secondary aqueous humour contain an enzyme that inactivates pilocarpine.[36] This enzyme is apparently an ion-dependent heat-labile esterase that is not cholinesterase. The major metabolite of pilocarpine is pilocarpic acid.

Pharmaceutics

Pilocarpine is available in the form of drops, ointments and slow-release systems. The ophthalmic solutions are sterile, buffered aqueous solutions of pilocarpine hydrochloride or nitrate with suitable antimicrobial agents, stabilizers and additives to increase the viscosity and retain full activity for almost a year. Pilocarpine hydrochloride solutions have a pH of 3.5–5.5 and are available in 0.25–10% strengths. Pilocarpine nitrate solutions have a pH of 4–5.5 and are available in 1–4% strengths. Most US manufacturers use green top containers for all miotic solutions to conform with uniform colour coding policy. Pilocarpine hydrochloride is marketed in combination with adrenaline bitartrate. Pilocarpine hydrochloride 2% and physostigmine salicylate 0.25% combinations are also available.

Pilocarpine salts may be sterilized by autoclaving. Both pilocarpine hydrochloride and nitrate are incompatible with alkalis, iodine and chlorhexidine acetate. However, chlorhexidine gluconate 0.02% and phenylmercuric borate 0.005% may be used as the preservative for pilocarpine nitrate sterilized by filtration. The latter may be used as a preservative for eye drops sterilized by steaming at 99°C for 30 minutes. Pilocarpine nitrate is incompatible with benzalkonium chloride but benzalkonium chloride 0.1% is used as the preservative for pilocarpine hydrochloride whether sterilized by filtration or 'steaming'. Chlorhexidine gluconate 0.02% is also used as a preservative for pilocarpine hydrochloride eye drops sterilized by filtration.

Pilocarpine hydrochloride ophthalmic gel is sterile and contains the drug in an aqueous gel base. The gel base contains more than 90% water and also contains carbomer 940 (3.5% w/w), a polymer of acrylic acid cross-linked with a polyfunctional agent, which provides a high viscosity for the gel. The gel also contains benzalkonium chloride as a preservative, disodium edetate and hydrochloric acid and/or sodium hydroxide to adjust the pH to 4.7–4.9.

The slow-release pilocarpine system, Ocusert (Rhone Poulenc, UK) designed by ALZA (USA), is composed of a core reservoir of pilocarpine and alginic acid surrounded by thin laminate of hydrophobic polymers that control the rate of diffusion. The ocular system that releases 20 μg of pilocarpine per hour is surrounded by a single membrane of ethylene vinyl acetate (EVA) copolymer. A second membrane consisting of dioctyl phthalate increases the rate of pilocarpine diffusion across the EVA copolymer membrane in the system that releases 40 μg.h^{-1}. Alginic acid is an inactive ingredient and is not released from the delivery unit. The system contains an excess amount of pilocarpine that is released at a constant rate over a 7-day period. The oval unit has a visible white margin to aid in placement on the cornea and retrieval. Pilocarpine ocular systems and solutions should be stored at 2–8°C, and freezing is to be avoided. Once dispensed, the gel may be stored at room temperature, but the unused portion should be discarded after 8 weeks.

Therapeutic use

Indications

1. Management of open-angle glaucoma
2. Treatment of angle closure glaucoma
3. During certain intraocular procedures
4. To counteract mydriasis
5. Diagnosis of Adie's (tonic) pupil
6. Management of accommodative esotropia.

Contraindications

1. Glaucoma secondary to inflammation
2. Hypersensitivity to ingredients.

Mode of use

Pilocarpine solutions, gels, and ocular systems are applied topically to the conjunctival sac. Eye closure and finger pressure should be applied to the lacrimal sac for 1–2 minutes following topical instillation to minimize drainage into the nasal mucosa and reduce the risk of absorption and systemic reactions. Excess solutions about the eye should be washed with a tissue and any medication on the hands should be rinsed off immediately. The concentration and dosage of pilocarpine must be adjusted to the requirement and response of individual patients and determined by tonometric and visual field findings before and during therapy.

The Ocusert system is more expensive than pilocarpine solutions and many patients may experience difficulty with insertion. The migration of the device over the cornea may produce blurred vision and pain. This may be hazardous during driving. The younger patients tend to tolerate it better because of reduced miosis and ciliary spasm. The therapy is usually begun with a 20 μg.h^{-1} system and changed to a 40 μg.h^{-1} device if needed. As the system releases a larger amount of pilocarpine during the first 6 hours, it is advisable to insert the device at bedtime. The follow-up intraocular pressure should be checked on the sixth or seventh day initially as some individuals may eventually require a change in system on the fourth or fifth day. The continued slow release may adequately depress the diurnal fluctuation of intraocular pressure and also improve patient compliance.

The usual dose of pilocarpine gel is a 0.5 inch ribbon applied to the lower cul-de-sac once daily at bedtime. Occasionally, more frequent administration may be necessary.

Indications

1. Open-angle glaucoma

Among the miotics, pilocarpine is usually the first agent used in primary open-angle glaucoma, because it provides good control of intraocular pressure with relatively few adverse effects. Reduction in intraocular pressure may decrease or prevent glaucomatous visual field loss or optic nerve damage and obviate the need for surgery. Initially, 1% or 2% solution is instilled in each eye every 6 to 8 hours. The concentration and frequency of administration may be adjusted later as needed. In patients with advanced glaucoma or with dark irides, concentrations of 6% or 8% may be necessary.[37] Higher concentrations of pilocarpine have a longer duration of effect than lower concentrations. The pressure-reducing effect of 1% pilocarpine wears off at 8 hours, whereas the effect of 4% or 8% pilocarpine may last for as long as 14 hours.

In the management of open-angle glaucoma, pilocarpine may show additive effects when used in conjunction with a carbonic anhydrase inhibitor, adrenaline and/or β-blocker ophthalmic solutions. It is doubtful that any benefit would result from simultaneous use of different miotics. In some patients concomitant instillation of a 1–2% solution of adrenaline hydrochloride or a 2.5% solution of phenylephrine hydrochloride may be used to improve visual acuity by dilating the small pupil. Use of combinations of drugs in a single preparation is generally not recommended because of the improper dosage that may result from the different durations of action. Many patients may gradually build some tolerance to pilocarpine therapy. It is advisable in such instances to substitute pilocarpine with other miotics for a period of a few weeks or months. This period of rest may make the patient respond more effectively when pilocarpine is reinstituted.

2. Angle closure glaucoma

Pilocarpine drops in conjunction with topical β-blockers, systemic carbonic anhydrase inhibitors, or hyperosmotic agents are used intensively for the management of acute angle closure glaucoma. The aim is to pull the lax iris away from the trabeculum. Initially, 2% solution is instilled frequently until the angle opens and pressure decreases. Occasionally, pilocarpine is unable to contract the paralysed iris sphincter damaged from the extremely high intraocular pressure. Stronger than 4% solutions should be avoided as they may exaggerate angle closure by further shallowing the anterior chamber.

3. Ocular surgery

Pilocarpine is used to lower intraocular pressure and to protect the lens by causing miosis prior to goniotomy and iridectomy. The miotic effect is also helpful before inserting an anterior chamber intraocular lens in an aphakic patient.

4. To counteract mydriasis

Mydriasis produced by sympathomimetic agents such as phenylephrine or hydroxyamphetamine is easily neutralized by a 1–2% pilocarpine solution.[38] The mean pilocarpine-induced recovery time after phenylephrine is 22 minutes and after hydroxyamphetamine is 14 minutes. However, it has little effect on mydriasis produced by parasympatholytic agents such as homatropine or tropicamide. Occasionally, a mydriatic-induced dilated pupil in uveitis may develop posterior synechiae. Pilocarpine may be employed especially initially to cause miosis and lysis of the adhesions.

5. Diagnosis of Adie's (tonic) pupil

The tonic pupil is a disorder in which the postganglionic parasympathetic innervation of sphincter pupillae or the ciliary muscle or both is impaired. There is supersensitivity of the cholinergic stimulation so that the pupil constricts or accommodation increases after the instillation of a low dose of pilocarpine that does not affect the normal pupil. It may occur with orbital tumours, zoster ophthalmicus, retrobulbar anaesthesia, trauma, neuropathy in diabetes mellitus or dysautonia, idiopathically with reduced tendon reflexes (Adie's syndrome) and after inferior oblique surgery. Single drops of 0.25% pilocarpine are instilled bilaterally. The test is best performed under conditions in which ambient lighting and accommodation are controlled, since both can affect pupil size. The pupil diameter is evaluated by observation, photographs or pupillography after 30–60 minutes under similar ambient surroundings.

6. Accommodative esotropia

The near reflex consists of accommodation, convergence and miosis. Decreased accommodative effort results in decreased convergence. Pilocarpine is sometimes used in reducing accommodative esotropia.[39]

Contraindications

1. Glaucoma secondary to inflammation

As pilocarpine affects the blood–aqueous barrier,[40] its use in inflammatory secondary glaucoma may worsen the clinical course of the disease. Increased protein and cellular content of the aqueous would raise intraocular pressure and stimulate adhesion of iris with lens (posterior synechiae) and the filtration angle (peripheral anterior synechiae). Moreover, both the human serum and secondary aqueous inactivate pilocarpine.[36]

2. Hypersensitivity to ingredients

Pilocarpine is to be avoided in patients known to be allergic to any component used in various pilocarpine preparations.

Adverse reactions

Among the miotics, topical pilocarpine is generally better tolerated. Adverse effects of pilocarpine are reduced if therapy is started with a low concentration of the drug and then gradually increased if necessary. Many effects often subside after the first few days of therapy.

Potentially life-threatening effects

Systemic reactions after ocular use of pilocarpine are rare. A dose of 100 mg of pilocarpine contained in 10 ml of a 1% solution is considered dangerous. Bronchiolar spasm and pulmonary oedema may cause death. Some commercially available preparations of pilocarpine contain sodium bisulphide which may cause allergic-type reactions, including anaphylaxis and life-threatening or less severe asthmatic episodes. Such sensitivity appears to occur more often in asthmatics.

Acute overdosage

The clinical symptoms may include nausea, vomiting, diarrhoea, abdominal pain and intestinal cramps. In addition, frequent urination, excessive salivation, lacrimation, sweating, pallor, cyanosis, bronchoconstriction, or increased secretion, nasal congestion, and rhinorrhoea may occur. Systemically absorbed pilocarpine may precipitate an attack in asthmatics. Severe pilocarpine toxicity may produce vertigo, tremors, muscle weakness, paraesthesia, bradycardia, cardiac arrhythmias, hypotension, syncope, increased systemic vascular resistance and central nervous system excitation, followed by depression, confusion, ataxia, seizures, and coma.

If systemic reactions to pilocarpine appear, its use should be discontinued immediately. Adequate respiration should be maintained. Tracheostomy, bronchial aspiration and postural drainage may be required to maintain adequate airway supplemented with oxygen or artificial ventilation. The antidote is 1–4 mg of atropine sulphate administered intravenously, intramuscularly, or subcutaneously. Additional doses of atropine may be given every 3–60 minutes as needed to control muscarinic symptoms and then as needed for 24–48 hours; as much as 50 mg atropine may be required in the first 24 hours. The dose of atropine sulphate in children is 0.04–0.08 $mg.kg^{-1}$ up to 4 mg intramuscularly or intravenously. The intravenous dose may be repeated every 5 minutes and the intramuscular dose every 15 minutes. Atropine should be administered with caution if the patient is cyanotic because of the risk of ventricular fibrillation. Atropine does not control the skeletal muscle effects and consequent respiratory paralysis. A short-acting barbiturate may control seizures not relieved by atropine; dosage should be carefully adjusted to avoid respiratory depression. Accidental ingestion of an overdose of pilocarpine requires the same treatment and a 0.02% solution of potassium permanganate may be employed for gastric lavage to detoxify the drug.

Severe or irreversible adverse effects

Some patients with peripheral retinal degenerative changes using pilocarpine may develop retinal detachment precipitated by ciliary spasm. Careful examination of the retinal periphery of patients treated with miotics should be done at least annually to detect impending detachment. A sudden drop in intraocular pressure may indicate that retinal detachment has occurred. Rarely, macular holes[41] or band keratopathy may appear. Prolonged pilocarpine use may interfere with lens metabolism and hasten the development of cataract. Pilocarpine-induced malignant glaucoma[42] and middle ear and eustachian tube disturbances[43] have been reported.

Symptomatic adverse effects

Topical pilocarpine therapy usually produces blurred vision or myopia, poor vision in dim light or sometimes painful ciliary or accommodative spasm. Ophthalmic ointments interfere with vision more than do solutions. Miosis may reduce the background illumination of the eye enough in some patients to make glaucomatous field defects enlarge. Such patients need visual field retesting with dilated pupils. Pilocarpine-induced spasm and myopia may respond to the clip-on minus lenses but may necessitate changing to β-blockers or adrenaline compounds.

Many patients on pilocarpine may experience ciliary or conjunctival congestion, follicular conjunctivitis, lacrimal passage stenosis, twitching of eyelids, stinging, burning, lacrimation, ocular or brow ache, headache, photophobia and increased visibility of floaters. Pain is usually relieved by analgesics such as salicylates. Hypersensitivity reactions such as allergic conjunctivitis, dermatitis or keratitis may occur either due to the drug itself or preservatives in the preparations.

Some patients may develop pupillary dilation following the use of pilocarpine. This is believed to be due to an impurity of the drug called 'jaborin' which has strong atropine-like properties.[44] This substance may be a mixture of several alkaloids, chiefly isopilocarpine, the optical isomer of pilocarpine and a small quantity of isocarpidine.

Other effects

Rarely, iris cysts or nodular excrescences of the iris pigment epithelium may form at the pupillary margin, enlarge and obscure vision following prolonged use of pilocarpine in children.

Pilocarpine is absorbed by soft contact lenses and patients using them concurrently may experience exaggerated drug response. In

Pilocarpine (hydrochloride, nitrate)

addition, preservatives used in pilocarpine preparations may have a deleterious effect on soft lenses. However, clinically, patients are not advised against the use of their soft lenses during pilocarpine therapy.

Prolonged use of pilocarpine produces loss of tone of the dilator muscle fibres and fine synechiae leading to persistent miosis. Such patients usually require lysis of synechiae and sector iridectomy during cataract extraction procedures.

About 40% of patients on pilocarpine gel may develop during the first two weeks of therapy mild to moderate superficial punctate keratitis over the lower portion of the cornea. This usually resolves even with continued therapy. During long-term gel therapy some 20% of patients may show asymptomatic, subtle, diffuse, superficial corneal changes. The aetiology of these corneal opacities is not known and they may persist for prolonged periods even after discontinuing the gel.

Interference with clinical pathology tests

No technical interferences of this kind have been reported.

High risk groups

Neonates

Prolonged pilocarpine use in some neonates may result in chronic miosis probably because of the immature state of the iris dilator muscle.

Breast milk. Topical pilocarpine is absorbed systemically and may appear in small amounts in human milk. The general health of the newborn should dictate the use of pilocarpine by the mother.

Children

Some younger patients may be significantly affected by ciliary spasm. Iris cysts and pigmented cysts of the ciliary epithelium may infrequently appear. Children with implanted Jones pyrex conjunctivodacryocystorhinostomy tubes may experience more systemic adverse effects due to rapid drug exposure to nasal mucosa.

Pregnant women

No reports of adverse outcome of pregnancy with pilocarpine use have been published. However, all due precautions of therapy during pregnancy should be adhered to.

The elderly

The miosis usually causes difficulty in dark adaptation. Elderly patients with lens opacities should avoid driving at night time. These and other factors may severely affect compliance.

Concurrent disease

Patients with trisomy 21[45] and familial dysautonomia[46] may have cholinergic neural deficiency and are more sensitive to muscarinic agonists and antagonists. Due care is needed in patients with corneal abrasions because of excessive penetration of pilocarpine.

Drug interactions

Potentially hazardous interactions

Although not proven beyond doubt it has been suggested that the miotic and/or ocular hypotensive effects of pilocarpine may be antagonized by long-term topical or systemic corticosteroid therapy, systemic anticholinergics, antihistamines, meperidine hydrochloride, sympathomimetics or tricyclic antidepressants. Concomitant administration of two miotics is not recommended because of inter-drug antagonism, and unresponsiveness may develop to both drugs. In addition, there may be an increased risk of allergic reactions and toxicity.

Other significant interactions

The miotic and intraocular pressure-lowering effects of topical anticholinesterases are competitively inhibited by pilocarpine.

Potentially useful interactions

When used in combination with topical adrenaline, β-adrenergic-blocking drugs, and/or systemically administered carbonic anhydrase inhibitors, the miotic and intraocular pressure effects of pilocarpine are additive.

Major outcome trials

1. Romano J H 1970 Double-blind cross-over comparison of aceclidine and pilocarpine in open-angle glaucoma. British Journal of Ophthalmology 54: 510–521

This is a double-blind crossover comparison of 2% aceclidine hydrochloride and 2% pilocarpine in 27 glaucoma patients (54 eyes). Patients on concurrent oral carbonic anhydrase inhibitor therapy were excluded. One eye received pilocarpine and the other aceclidine. The patients were examined at the end of the first week. Placebo was used in both eyes for the next week to eliminate the effect of previous medication. Crossover therapy was then instituted. The mean percentage fall in the pressure from placebo to pilocarpine was 24.5% and from placebo to aceclidine 19.1%. The mean increase in outflow coefficient from placebo to pilocarpine was 34.37% and that from placebo to aceclidine 31.25%. The percentage reduction in pupil diameter from placebo to pilocarpine was 47.84% and that from placebo to aceclidine was 52.43%. Browache or headache and conjunctival hyperaemia were less frequent with pilocarpine.

2. Worthen D M 1966 Effect of pilocarpine drops on the diurnal intraocular pressure variation in patients with glaucoma. Investigative Ophthalmology 15: 784–787

This study looked at the effect of pilocarpine on the diurnal pressure variation in seven glaucoma patients (14 eyes). The patients were hospitalized during the study, but sent on pass between the control and pilocarpine treatment phase. Each patient stopped adrenaline 2 weeks before admission, pilocarpine 48 hours before admission, and acetazolamide 14 hours before admission. During the 48-hour control period, the pressures measured every three hours with a non-contact tonometer had a mean value of 26 mmHg and a mean maximum diurnal variation of 18.5 mmHg. After a waiting period of another 34–36 hours, patients received pilocarpine drops every 6 hours for a day. Pressures were then again measured every 3 hours for 48 hours. During the pilocarpine treatment period, the mean pressure and maximum diurnal variation dropped to 17 and 8.5 mmHg, respectively. The period of low intraocular pressure was between 0900 h and 1800 h.

3. Kriss A E, Newell F W 1964 Effects of pilocarpine on ocular tension dynamics. American Journal of Ophthalmology 57: 34–41

This study looked at the effect of pilocarpine on the diurnal pressure variation and outflow facility in six normal subjects and 11 glaucoma patients. All glaucoma patients and three of the normal individuals were hospitalized during the period of testing. Local ocular medications were discontinued at least 4 days prior to admission. All subjects initially had baseline studies done and thereafter received 1–4% pilocarpine four times daily in one eye of five of the six normal subjects and in both eyes of all glaucomatous patients. All subjects showed a decrease in tension with pilocarpine. Generally, the higher the average pretreatment tension, the greater was the tension reduction by any strength of the drug. Except for three eyes, all the rest showed a decreased daily fluctuation in pressure with pilocarpine. It also increased the mean initial coefficient of outflow in 16 eyes from 0.03 to 0.08. In two normal eyes and five glaucomatous eyes pressure reduction occurred without corresponding changes in the outflow facility, a suggesting a possible effect of pilocarpine on the aqueous humour production.

4. Quigley H A, Pollack I P, Harbin T S 1975 Pilocarpine Ocuserts: long-term clinical trials and selected pharmacodynamics. Archives of Ophthalmology 93: 771–775

This study looked at the use of Ocuserts in 22 glaucoma patients for an average period of 10 to 12 months. Three patients were intolerant to the device and left the study. Loss of the device was a real problem as 12 patients were found without an Ocusert on two or fewer occasions. Most of the patients noted no subjective symptoms like pain or change in vision. The majority of patients (60%; 30/50 eyes) required less medications; 12% (6/50 eyes) required the same and 28% (14/50 eyes) needed more medications than pre-study therapy. Most of the patients using 0.5% and 1% pilocarpine drops were controlled with P-20 while P-40 adequately controlled the majority of patients on 2% or 4% pilocarpine drops. Concurrent use of topical adrenaline was additive.

5. Johnson D H, Epstein D L, Allen R C et al 1984 One-year multicenter clinical trial of pilocarpine gel. American Journal of Ophthalmology 97: 723–729

This is a one-year, multicentre clinical study evaluating the safety and efficacy of once-a-day 4% pilocarpine gel in 83 patients with glaucoma. Patients on long-term topical anticholinesterase therapy and those with corneal or conjunctival abnormalities, active infection or inflammation, and recent ocular surgery were excluded. The pressures following the use of pilocarpine gel were equal to or slightly better than those with eye drops. 41 patients (50%) complained of burning and/or foreign body sensation and as a result nine patients left the study. Mild blurring of vision in the mornings was mentioned by 57 patients (69%) and five stopped using the gel. Asymptomatic mild to moderate superficial punctate keratitis developed in 33 patients (40%) over the lower portion of the cornea within the first 2 weeks. This corneal change resolved spontaneously with continued therapy. A majority of patients experienced crusting of gel on the eyelids and eyelids sticking together in the mornings. Diffuse, subtle superficial corneal change was noted in 15 (20%) of patients who used the gel for more than 8 weeks. Many of these patients had developed superficial punctate keratitis earlier in the treatment period. Discontinuation of the gel did not result in disappearance of this asymptomatic corneal haze.

General review articles

Ellis P P 1971 Pilocarpine therapy. Survey of Ophthalmology 16: 165–169

Havener W H 1983 Ocular pharmacology. C V Mosby Co, St Louis, ch 12, pp 319–347

Holland M G 1974 Autonomic drugs in ophthalmology: some problems and promises. Section I: Directly and indirectly acting parasympathomimetic drugs. Annals of Ophthalmology 6: 447–461

Leopold I H, Duzman E 1986 Observations on the pharmacology of glaucoma. Annual Review of Pharmacology and Toxicology 26: 401–426

Mindel J S 1987 Cholinergic pharmacology. In: Duane T D, Jaeger E A (eds) Biomedical foundations of ophthalmology. Harper and Row, Philadelphia, vol 3, ch 26, pp 10–21

References

1. Van Rossum J M V, Cornelissen M J W J, DeGroot C T P, Hurkmans J A T M 1960 A new view on an old drug — pilocarpine. Experientia 16: 373–375
2. Furchgott R F, Bursztyn P 1967 Comparison of dissociation constants and of relative efficacies of selected agonists acting on parasympathetic receptors. Annals of the New York Academy of Sciences 144: 882–889
3. Mindel J S, Mittag T S 1978 In vitro activation of human ocular acetylcholine synthesis by pilocarpine. Investigative Ophthalmology (suppl) 188
4. Burt A M, Silver A 1973 Non-enzymatic imidazole-catalysed acyl transfer reaction and acetylcholine synthesis. Nature New Biology 243: 157–159
5. Armaly M F, Burian H M 1958 Changes in the tonogram during accommodation. Archives of Ophthalmology 60: 60–69
6. Gorin G 1966 Angle-closure glaucoma induced by miotics. American Journal of Ophthalmology 62: 1063–1067
7. Lowe R F 1966 Acute angle-closure glaucoma precipitated by miotics plus adrenaline eye drops. Medical Journal of Australia 2: 1037–1038
8. Romano J 1968 Anterior chamber depth in medically-treated open-angle glaucoma. British Journal of Ophthalmology 52: 361–367
9. Wilkie J, Drance S M, Schulzer M 1969 The effects of miotics on anterior-chamber depth. American Journal of Ophthalmology 68: 78–83
10. Abramson D H, Chang S, Coleman J 1976 Pilocarpine therapy in glaucoma. Archives of Ophthalmology 94: 914–918
11. Abramson D H, Franzen L A, Coleman D J 1973 Pilocarpine in the presbyope. Demonstration of an effect on the anterior chamber and lens thickness. Archives of Ophthalmology 89: 100–102
12. Krill A E, Newell F W 1964 Effects of pilocarpine on ocular tension dynamics. American Journal of Ophthalmology 57: 34–41
13. Drance S M 1960 The coefficient of scleral rigidity in normal and glaucomatous eyes. Archives of Ophthalmology 63: 668–674
14. Cambiaggi A, Bottino C 1962 The influence of miotic therapy on ocular rigidity. American Journal of Ophthalmology 53: 169
15. Macri F J, Wanko T, Grimes P A 1958 The elastic properties of the human eye. Archives of Ophthalmology 1021–1026
16. Kropp B N, Forward R B 1963 The effect of pilocarpine on teeth and salivary glands in the rat embryo. Anatomical Record 145: 250–251
17. Barsam P C 1972 Comparison of the effect of pilocarpine and echothiophate on intraocular pressure and outflow facility. American Journal of Ophthalmology 73: 742–749
18. DeRoetth A, Knighton W S 1952 Clinical evaluation of the aqueous-flow test: a preliminary report. Archives of Ophthalmology 48: 148–153
19. Gaasterland D, Kupper C, Ross K 1975 Studies of aqueous humor dynamics in man: IV. Effects of pilocarpine upon measurements in young normal volunteers. Investigative Ophthalmology 14: 848–853
20. Worthen D M 1976 Effect of pilocarpine drops on the intraocular pressure variation in patients with glaucoma. Investigative Ophthalmology 15: 784–787
21. Grierson I, Lee W R, Abraham S 1978 Effects of pilocarpine on the morphology of human outflow apparatus. British Journal of Ophthalmology 62: 302–313
22. Becker B, Friedenwald J S 1953 Clinical aqueous outflow. Archives of Ophthalmology 50: 557–571
23. Wilke K 1974 Early effects of epinephrine and pilocarpine on the intraocular pressure and the episcleral venous pressure in the normal eye. Acta Ophthalmologica 52: 231–241
24. Bill A, Walinder P E 1966 The effects of pilocarpine on the dynamics of aqueous humor in a primate (*Macaca irus*). Investigative Ophthalmology 5: 170–175
25. Rothkoff L, Biedner B, Biger Y, Blumenthal M 1978 A proposed pilocarpine therapeutic test. Archives of Ophthalmology 96: 1380–1382
26. Lowenstein O, Lowenfeld I E 1953 Effect of physostigmine and pilocarpine on iris sphincter of normal man. Archives of Ophthalmology 50: 311–318
27. Armaly M F, Rao K R 1973 The effect of pilocarpine Ocusert with different release rates on ocular pressure. Investigative Ophthalmology 12: 491–496
28. Wood R W, Robinson J R 1984 High-performance chromatographic determinations of pilocarpine and pilocarpic acid in ocular tissues. International Journal of Pharmaceutics 20: 285–293
29. Potts A 1961 Physiological chemistry of the eye. Archives of Ophthalmology 66: 578–595
30. Asseff C F, Weisman R L, Podos S M, Becker B 1973 Ocular penetration of pilocarpine in primates. American Journal of Ophthalmology 75: 212–215
31. Ohara K 1977 Effects of cholinergic agonists on isolated iris sphincter muscles: a pharmacodynamic study. Japanese Journal of Ophthalmology 21: 516–520
32. Green K, Downs S J 1975 Ocular penetration of pilocarpine in rabbits. Archives of Ophthalmology 93: 1165–1168
33. Drance S M, Nash P A 1971 The dose response of human intraocular pressure to pilocarpine. Canadian Journal of Ophthalmology 6: 9–13
34. Harris L S, Galin M A 1970 Dose response analysis of pilocarpine-induced ocular hypotension. Archives of Ophthalmology 84: 605–608
35. Drance S M, Mitchell D W A, Schulzer M 1975 The duration of action of pilocarpine Ocusert on intraocular pressure in man. Canadian Journal of Ophthalmology 6: 14–19
36. Scholberg S S, Ellis P P 1969 Pilocarpine inactivation. Archives of Ophthalmology 82: 351–355
37. Harris L S, Galin M A 1971 Effect of ocular pigmentation on hypotensive response to pilocarpine. American Journal of Ophthalmology 72: 923–925
38. Anastasi L M, Ogle K N, Kearns T P 1968 The effect of pilocarpine in counteracting mydriasis. Archives of Ophthalmology 79: 710–715
39. Abraham S V 1949 The use of miotics in the treatment of convergent strabismus and anisometropia. American Journal of Ophthalmology 32: 233–240
40. Stocker F W 1947 Experimental studies on the blood aqueous barrier. Archives of Ophthalmology 37: 583–590
41. Garlikov R S, Chenoweth R G 1975 Macular hole following topical pilocarpine. Annals of Ophthalmology 7: 1313–1316
42. Rieser J C, Schwartz B 1972 Miotic-induced malignant glaucoma. Archives of Ophthalmology 87: 706–712
43. Moose R M 1974 Middle ear disturbance from glaucoma medication. Journal of the American Medical Association 230: 1255
44. Lebensohn J E 1977 Spectacular adverse reactions from pilocarpine. American Journal of Ophthalmology 83: 281
45. Lejeune J, Bourdais M, Prieur M 1976 Sensibilité pharmacoligique de l'iris des enfants trisomiques 21. Thérapie 31: 447–454
46. Smith A A, Dancis J, Breimin G 1965 Ocular responses to autonomic drugs in familial dysautonomia. Investigative Ophthalmology 4: 358–361

Pimozide

Pimozide is a neuroleptic and a selective blocker of dopamine (D_2) receptors.

Chemistry

Pimozide
$C_{28}H_{29}F_2N_3O$
1-[1-[4,4-bis(4-fluorophenyl)butyl]-4-piperidyl]-2-benzimidazolin-one

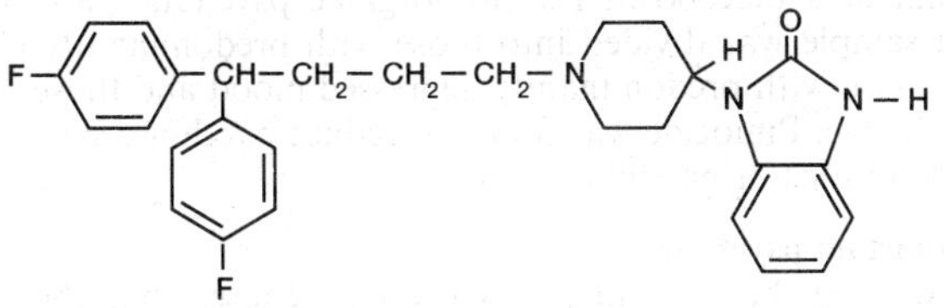

Molecular weight	461.54
pKa (piperidine group)	8.63
Solubility	
in alcohol	1 in 40
in water	insoluble
Octanol/water partition coefficient	5.56

A white to creamy white crystalline powder prepared by chemical synthesis.

Pharmacology

Pimozide is a selective blocker of dopamine D_2-receptors in the limbic system, the striatum and the pituitary. It appears to block predominantly postsynaptic dopamine receptors, although it may also block presynaptic dopamine receptor sites. It increases the turnover of dopamine but not noradrenaline, unlike most antipsychotic agents.[1] Pimozide blocks apomorphine-induced emesis, which is a dopamine-mediated response.[2] To a much lesser extent pimozide also blocks serotonin and α_1-adrenergic receptors,[3] and is a weak antagonist of muscarinic acetylcholine receptors.

Toxicology

Oral LD_{50} values for various species have been ascertained. They range from 10 g.kg^{-1} in the guinea-pig, to 40 mg.kg^{-1} in the dog and have no relevance to clinical usage. Acute toxic symptoms include tremor, sedation and convulsions. Hypothermia, a feature of chlorpromazine-treated animals, was not observed with pimozide. There is no evidence of chronic toxicity. In animal studies concerning dysmorphology and reproduction the only adverse effect noted was an increased rate of fetal resorption in rabbits treated with very high doses. There are no data on humans.

Clinical pharmacology

Pimozide is the best known of the diphenylbutylpiperidines, compounds structurally related to the butyrophenones by replacement of the carbonyl in the propylene chain by a fluorophenyl group. The biochemical basis of schizophrenia, although not fully established, is thought to be related to an abnormality in the dopamine system. The clinical effectiveness of the neuroleptics appears to be related to their ability to block dopamine receptors. Pimozide is a highly selective blocker of D_2-receptors, but this also leads to a high frequency of extrapyramidal side effects, such as akathisia, rigidity, tremor, oral dyskinesia and disturbance of gait.

Pimozide also blocks α_1-adrenoceptors and serotoninergic receptors and this may result in hypotension, particularly postural hypotension. However, such hypotensive effects are infrequent. In higher doses, prolongation of the QT interval on the ECG may occur, as with other neuroleptics. There may be anticholinergic effects, but these are unusual. Pimozide is relatively free of sedative effects due to its relatively weak antagonist effects at receptors other than D_2-receptors. The effective dose range as recorded in the literature is from 2.8 mg daily to 11.4 mg daily. No benefit is gained by increasing the dose beyond 20 mg daily. The duration of action is between 24 and 48 hours; thus a single daily dose is in common use.

Pharmacokinetics

Radioimmunoassay techniques have been used to measure pimozide plasma concentrations and have a detection limit[4] of 50 pg.ml^{-1}. After oral administration, peak plasma concentrations are reached in 8 hours (range 4–12). The plasma elimination half life following a single oral dose is approximately 53 hours.[5] There is some evidence that pimozide may accumulate in plasma over a prolonged period of high-dose administration.[6] Animal studies have indicated that the drug is widely distributed in the body, but with considerably increased concentrations in the liver.

Metabolic studies in animals suggest that the effects of pimozide are due to the unchanged drug. Pharmacological effects occurred in dogs in the absence of brain metabolites,[7] while in rats they correlate with the amount of pimozide and not with the total pimozide plus metabolites.[8] Pimozide is excreted in breast milk at a concentration of, or slightly above, that of the plasma.

Oral absorption	60–80%
Presystemic metabolism	extensive
Plasma half life	53 h
Volume of distribution	—
Plasma protein binding	—

Concentration–effect relationship

There does not appear to be any clear correlation between plasma concentration of pimozide and clinical response, and doses of pimozide need to be varied according to clinical response. Plasma concentrations among patients receiving 6 mg daily varied by as much as 17-fold, and in patients receiving a 24 mg single dose by 9-fold.[5] This wide variability in plasma concentration confirms the clinical experience and suggests that doses should be adapted individually. It is accounted for by a combination of limited absorption by the gastrointestinal tract (30–60% absorbed), and extensive presystemic metabolism by the liver.

Metabolism

Animal studies have shown that pimozide is metabolized in the liver by oxidative N-dealkylation, and excreted in the urine and in the faeces both unchanged and in the form of metabolites. The main metabolite, accounting for some 60% of the urinary excretion, is N-4-piperidyl-2-benzimidazolinone. The remaining 40% is made up of unchanged drug. Faecal excretion consists predominantly of the unchanged drug.[8] None of the metabolites is active.

Pharmaceutics

Pimozide Orap (Janssen, UK/Lemmon, USA) is available in oral form only.

Tablets containing 2 mg of pimozide are white, scored, uncoated tablets marked 'JANSSEN' on one side and 'O/2' on the obverse (UK) or imprinted 'LEMMON' on one side and 'ORAP LEMMON 2' on the obverse. They contain lactose.

Tablets containing 4 mg of pimozide, pale-green, scored, uncoated are marked 'JANSSEN' on one side and 'O/4' on the obverse. They contain two colouring agents, iron oxide (E172) and indigotine (E132). Tablets containing 10 mg of pimozide are white, scored, uncoated and marked 'JANSSEN' on one side and 'O/10' on the obverse.

All tablets have a shelf-life of 5 years and should be kept at room temperature in dry conditions.

P

P

Fig. 1 Metabolism of pimozide

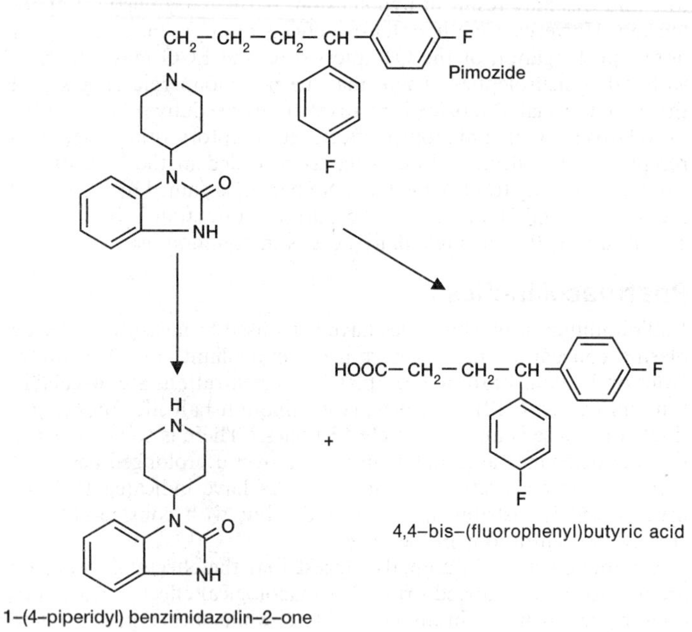

Therapeutic use

Indications

1. Acute schizophrenia
2. Chronic schizophrenia
3. Mania
4. Postpartum psychosis
5. Gille de la Tourette syndrome
6. Monosymptomatic hypochondriacal psychoses, paranoid delusional disorders and erotomania.

Contraindications

1. Known hypersensitivity to pimozide
2. Parkinson's disease
3. Endogenous depression
4. Cardiac arrhythmias and ECG abnormalities
5. Severe CNS depression
6. Congenitally prolonged QT interval.

Mode of use

All therapeutic uses of pimozide appear to depend on D_2-receptor blockade, but individual response and dosage requirements vary. Single daily doses are given in the initial treatment period and increased until adequate control of symptoms is achieved. In acute psychoses therapeutic doses are in the range of 5–50 mg, with a mean dose of 20 mg.[9] When used in a preventative capacity or in the long-term treatment of chronic psychotic conditions, the dose is in the range of 2–20 mg daily. It can also be given less frequently, up to a once-weekly schedule. Plasma levels are not routinely monitored due to the lack of a clear concentration–effect relationship.

Indications

1. Acute schizophrenia
Pimozide was shown to be effective in pilot studies.[10] The drug was slow to come into common usage due to the small doses used, and the drug's lack of sedative side effects. In a study of 46 first-episode schizophrenics,[11] pimozide was compared with flupenthixol. Both drugs were found to be effective in controlling the positive symptoms of the acute illness. As with other antipsychotic drugs there is a delay of 1–3 weeks in the onset of the therapeutic effects of pimozide, and it is during this period that its relative lack of sedative side effects is noticeable. In a comparative trial against haloperidol in which pimozide was found to be as effective, the mean pimozide dose was 20 mg, which is the maximum recommended dose, with a range of 5–50 mg.[9]

2. Chronic schizophrenia
Pimozide has been shown to be at least as effective as other long-acting neuroleptics in the maintenance treatment of schizophrenic patients.[11] It may also have a less deleterious effect on social functioning than do other neuroleptics in the treatment of the chronic schizophrenic syndrome.[13] For this purpose it can be given as a once-daily or once-weekly schedule. Daily dosage is in the range of 6–12 mg, and weekly dosage in the range of 10–40 mg. There is no strong evidence that any particular symptoms respond to pimozide and not to other neuroleptics, although it has been suggested that pimozide may be more effective in the withdrawn, autistic type of patient.[14] A recent report suggests that pimozide may preferentially treat the negative schizophrenic syndrome, but the data are still inconclusive.[15]

3. Mania
In a small double-blind trial[16] of pimozide versus chlorpromazine, a mean daily dose of 23 mg, with a range of 6–32 mg, was found to be as effective as chlorpromazine in improving clinical ratings.

In the Northwick Park 'functional' psychosis study,[17] the efficacy of pimozide, lithium and a combination of the two, was compared with that of a placebo in 120 non-organic psychotic patients. The patient sample was divided into those with predominantly elevated mood, those with predominantly depressed mood and those with no mood change. Pimozide was found to reduce psychotic symptoms in all three groups of patients.

4. Postpartum psychosis
Pimozide may be used in postpartum psychoses, but there is no evidence to suggest that it is any more effective than other antipsychotics. An uncontrolled case report describes three cases of postpartum psychosis where the patient had developed postural hypotension with other antipsychotics, and subsequently responded well to pimozide.[18] It must be noted that if the underlying illness is depressive, antidepressants may need to be combined with the antipsychotic medication.

5. Gille de la Tourette syndrome
Pimozide has been found to be as effective as haloperidol in treating the Tourette syndrome in both adults and children and to have fewer adverse side effects.[19] The same group subsequently reported that pimozide was significantly better than placebo in the treatment of this disorder.[20] Treatment is begun at a low dose (1 or 2 mg at night) and increased every week until symptoms decrease and/or adverse side effects occur.[21]

6. Monosymptomatic hypochondriacal psychoses, paranoid delusional disorders and erotomania
Pimozide has been used successfully in the treatment of many of these diverse group of conditions.[22–24] Controlled trials[25] are few, due to the rarity of the disorders, and there is no evidence to suggest that the drug has any specific or exclusive effects over and above those of other neuroleptics.

Contraindications

1. Known hypersensitivity to pimozide

2. Parkinson's disease
Because of its extrapyramidal effects pimozide is contraindicated in patients with pre-existing Parkinson's disease.

3. Endogenous depression
This is a relative contraindication, as pimozide may be used to treat delusional symptoms seen in severe depression.

4. Cardiac arrhythmias and ECG abnormalities
Pimozide is less prone than are many neuroleptics to cause hypotension or postural hypotension. It is recognized as producing prolongation of the QT interval,[26] particularly at higher doses. Therefore it should not be used in patients with known prolongation of the QT interval, with hypokalaemia or with pre-existing cardiac arrhythmias.

5. Severe CNS depression
Pimozide may potentiate the primary effects of anaesthetic drugs, analgesics and drugs with central nervous system depressant effects, such as barbiturates, antihistamines, benzodiazepines and alcohol.

Adverse reactions

Potentially life-threatening effects

Deaths due to pimozide have been recorded but have usually been associated with large doses (exact amount unknown) taken in combination with other drugs in a suicide. A report of a 17-year-old girl taking 100 mg of pimozide in a suicide attempt records that she only exhibited a slight tremor in her extremities.[27] Cases of agranulocytosis have been reported but are extremely rare. Pimozide has also been associated with the neuroleptic malignant syndrome, symptoms of which include hyperthermia, muscle rigidity, altered consciousness and coma. Treatment includes withdrawal of the neuroleptic, general support measures and administration of dantrolene sodium or bromocriptine mesylate.

Acute overdosage

Pimozide is relatively safe in overdose. Cases where doses of up to 100 mg have been taken have been reported to have no serious sequelae. Treatment of overdose should include gastric washout, intravenous fluids, ECG monitoring, and anticholinergic agents if required.

Severe or irreversible adverse effects

In common with many other neuroleptics, patients treated with pimozide may develop tardive dyskinesia. The evidence suggests that the risk of irreversible tardive dyskinesia is proportional to the cumulative dose of the neuroleptic medication received, and increases with increasing age. The syndrome often becomes more pronounced when the drug is withdrawn. Each patient should have the minimum dose necessary to keep psychotic symptoms at bay, and the need for the drug should be reviewed from time to time. There is no evidence to suggest that intermittent drug therapy has any advantage over continuous therapy, and it may even make matters worse.[28]

Pimozide reduces the threshold for epileptic seizures in susceptible patients. A review of the literature indicates that pimozide and other diphenylbutylpiperidines may be less likely to induce seizures than the phenothiazines.[29] Epilepsy is in itself not a contraindication for treatment with pimozide, and if an increase in seizure frequency occurs, the dose of anticonvulsant should be increased rather than the neuroleptic withdrawn.

Symptomatic adverse effects

The extrapyramidal syndrome or pseudoparkinsonism, is the commonest adverse effect encountered with pimozide; it is characterized by rigidity and akinesia, with tremor being less apparent.[11] This syndrome is caused by dopaminergic blockade in the basal ganglia. Acute dystonia can occur, most often early in treatment and in younger patients. This syndrome may range from clenching of jaw muscles or protrusion of the tongue, to an oculogyric crisis or opisthotonos. A further syndrome encountered is that of akathisia. This is a distressing motor restlessness which leads to constant movement and shifting of position and an inability to relax.

The prevalence of these extrapyramidal adverse effects with pimozide may be as high as 80%, occurring most frequently in patients receiving high doses. They can be treated with the concurrent administration of an anticholinergic medication, by reduction of the dose of pimozide, or by adopting both methods. The acute dystonic reactions may require intramuscular administration of an anticholinergic drug, such as procyclidine 5–10 mg.

Pimozide can itself cause anticholinergic effects but these are rare. Hyperprolactinaemia can occur, leading to galactorrhoea, gynaecomastia, and oligomennorrhoea or amenorrhoea. A range of other adverse effects have been reported including tiredness, insomnia, anxiety, mood alterations, anorexia, nausea, vomiting and constipation.

Other effects

A rise in the transaminases and lactate dehydrogenase levels has been reported following pimozide administration, but is usually transient. Occasionally, serum cholesterol levels are increased.

Interference with clinical pathology tests

No such interference appears to have been reported.

High risk groups

Neonates

Pimozide is not indicated in neonates.

Breast milk. Pimozide is excreted in breast milk and may reach concentrations higher than that in plasma. Consequently, mothers receiving pimozide should not breast-feed their infants.

Children

Pimozide is not recommended in children under 12. Older children should be started on the lowest dose possible, usually 1 mg daily, with individual dose-titration against clinical effect and body weight. The elimination half life of the drug in children appears to be shorter than that in adults.[30]

Pregnant women

Studies in animals have not demonstrated any teratogenic effects, but safety in human pregnancy has not been established; thus pimozide should be avoided in pregnancy as far as possible.

The elderly

Because of the possibility of reduced drug metabolism in the elderly, dosage should start lower and be increased in proportion to a maximum dose of 10–20 mg. There is an increased likelihood of extrapyramidal effects, and elderly patients on potassium-losing diuretics should have their potassium levels monitored in view of the known effects of pimozide on the QT interval. It is reported that pimozide may have a role in the management of senile dementia.[31]

Drug interactions

Potentially hazardous interactions

Pimozide potentiates the action of drugs possessing central nervous system depressant effects, including alcohol, anaesthetics, barbiturates, antihistamines and benzodiazepines.

Other significant interactions

Anticholinergics. These agents may act synergistically and increase anticholinergic toxicity.

Narcotic analgesics. These drugs may increase sedation, anticholinergic, and respiratory depressive effects.

Antidepressants. Antidepressants may increase sedative, hypotensive and anticholinergic effects.

Antacids, kaopectate and milk of magnesia. These drugs will delay the absorption, onset of clinical effects, and toxic effects of pimozide.

Propranolol and cimetidine. Both these drugs decrease hepatic metabolism of pimozide, and will increase clinical and toxic effects.

Potentially useful interactions

No interactions of this kind have been reported.

Major outcome trials

1. Johnstone E C, Crow T J, Frith C O, Owens D G 1988 The Northwick Park 'functional' psychosis study: diagnosis and treatment response. Lancet 2: 119–125

In this trial, the efficacy of pimozide, lithium, pimozide and lithium combined, and placebo were compared in 120 non-organic psychotic patients. The patient sample was divided into those with depressed mood, those with elated mood and those with normal mood. Pimozide was significantly superior to placebo in reducing psychotic symptoms in all groups of patients.

2. The Scottish Schizophrenia Research Group 1988 The Scottish first episode schizophrenia study. British Journal of Psychiatry 152: 470–476

In this study, patients who responded to acute treatment were compared in a double-blind trial of pimozide taken once weekly versus intramuscular flupenthixol decanoate as maintenance therapy. On follow-up after one year both medications were found to be equally effective, 9 out of 13 in each group completing 12 months without relapse.

Other trials

1. Falloom I, Watt D C, Shephard M 1978 A comparative controlled trial of pimozide and fluphenazine decanoate in the continuation therapy of schizophrenia. Psychological Medicine 8: 59–70
2. Silverstone T, Cookman J, Ball R, Chin C N, Jacobs D, Lader S, Gould S 1984 The relationship of dopamine receptor blockade to clinical response in schizophrenic patients treated with pimozide or haloperidol. Journal of Psychiatric Research 18 (3): 255–268

P

3. Regeur L, Pakkenberg B, Fog R, Pakkenberg H 1986 Clinical features and long term treatment with pimozide in 65 patients with Gilles de la Tourette's syndrome. Journal of Neurology, Neurosurgery and Psychiatry 49: 791–795

General review articles

Reynolds J E F (ed) 1982 Martindale, the extra pharmacopoeia, 28th edn. The Pharmaceutical Press, London

Pinder R M, Brogden R N, Sawer P R, Speight T M, Spencer R, Avery G S 1976 Pimozide: a review of its pharmacological properties and therapeutic uses in psychiatry. Drugs 12: 1–40

Simpson G M, Pi E H, Sramek J J 1984 Neuroleptics and antipsychotics. In: Dukes M N G (ed) Meyler's side effects of drugs, 10th edn. Elsevier Science Publishers, New York

References

1. Anden N E, Butcher S G, Corrodi H, Fuxe K, Ungerstedt U 1970 Receptor activity and turnover of dopamine and noradrenaline after neuroleptics. European Journal of Pharmacology 11: 303–314
2. Rotrosen J, Wallach M B, Angrist B, Gershon S 1972 Antagonism of apomorphine-induced stereotypy and emesis in dogs by thioridazine, haloperidol and pimozide. Psychopharmacologia (Berlin) 26: 185–194
3. Van Wielink P S, Leysen J E 1983 Choice of neuroleptic on the basis of in-vitro pharmacology. Journal of Drug Research 8: 1984–1997
4. Michiels I J, Heykants J J, Knaeps A G et al 1975 Radioimmunoassay of the neuroleptic drug pimozide. Life Science 16: 937–944
5. McCreadier R G, Heykants J J P, Chalmers A, Anderson A M 1979 Plasma pimozide profiles in chronic schizophrenics. British Journal of Clinical Pharmacology 7: 534–535
6. Givant Y, Shani J, Goldhaber G, Serebrenic R, Sulman F G 1973 Pharmacology of three mammotrophic butyrophenones in the rat. Archives Internationales de Pharmacodynamie et de Therapie 205: 317–327
7. Janssen P A J, Soudijn W, Van Wijngaarden I, Dresse A 1968 Pimozide, a chemically novel, highly potent and orally long acting neuroleptic drug. Part III. Regional distribution of pimozide and of haloperidol in the dog brain. Arzneimittel-Forschung 18: 261–279
8. Soudijn W, Van Wijngaarden I 1969 The metabolism and excretion of the neuroleptic drug pimozide (R6238) by the Wistar rat. Life Sciences 8: 291–295
9. Silverstone T, Cookson J, Ball R, Chin C N, Jacobs D, Lader S, Gould S 1984 The relationship of dopamine receptor blockade to clinical response in schizophrenic patients treated with pimozide or haloperidol. Journal of Psychiatric Research 18: 255–268
10. Garton D, Silverstone T 1979 Pimozide in acute schizophrenia: a pilot study. Current Medical Research Opinion 5: 799–806
11. The Scottish Schizophrenia Research Group 1987 The Scottish first episode schizophrenia study II. Treatment: pimozide versus flupenthixol. British Journal of Psychiatry 150: 334–338
12. Kolivakis T, Azim H, Kingstone E 1974 A double-blind comparison of pimozide and chlorpromazine in the maintenance care of chronic schizophrenic outpatients. Current Therapeutic Research 16(9): 998–1004
13. Shepherd M 1979 Medico-social evaluation of the long term pharmacotherapy of schizophrenia. Comparative study of fluphenazine and pimozide. Progress in Neuropsychopharmacology 3: 383–389
14. Denijs E L, Vereecken J L T 1973 Pimozide (Orap, R6238) in residual schizophrenia: a clinical evaluation. Psychiatria, Neurologia, Neurochirurgia 76: 47–59
15. Feinberg S S, Kay S R, Elijovich L R, Fiszbein A, Opler L A 1988 Pimozide treatment of the negative schizophrenic syndrome: an open trial. Journal of Clinical Psychiatry 49(6): 235–238
16. Cookson J C, Silverstone T, Wells B 1879 A double-blind controlled study of pimozide vs chlorpromazine in mania. Neuropharmacology 18: 1011–1013
17. Johnstone E C, Crow T J, Frith C D, Owens D G 1988 The Northwick Park 'functional' psychosis study: diagnosis and treatment response. Lancet 2: 119–125
18. Barnes T R E, Katona C L E 1986 Susceptibility to drug induced hypotension in post-partum psychosis. International Clinical Psychopharmacology 1: 74–76
19. Shapiro A K, Shapiro E, Eisenkraft G F 1984 Treatment of Gilles de la Tourette syndrome with pimozide. American Journal of Psychiatry 140: 1183–1186
20. Shapiro A K, Shapiro E 1984 Controlled study of pimozide vs. placebo in Tourette's syndrome. Journal of the Academy of Child Psychiatry 23: 161–173
21. Shapiro A K, Shapiro E, Fulop G 1987 Pimozide treatment of tic and Tourette disorders. Pediatrics 79: 1032–1039
22. Reilly T M, Jopling W H, Beard A W 1978 Successful treatment with pimozide of delusional parasitosis. British Journal of Dermatology 98(4): 457–459
23. Munro A, O'Brien J V, Ross D 1985 Two case of 'pure' or 'primary' erotomania successfully treated with pimozide. Canadian Journal of Psychiatry 30: 619–622
24. Lindskov R, Baadsgaard O 1985 Delusions of infestation treated with pimozide: a follow up study. Acta Dermatovenereologica Stockholm 65(3): 267–270
25. Ungvari G, Vladar K 1986 Pimozide treatment for delusions of infestation. Activitas Nervosa Superior (Praha) 28(2): 103–107
26. Fulop G, Philips R A, Shapiro A K, Gomes J A, Shapiro E, Nordlie J W 1987 ECG changes during haloperidol and pimozide treatment of Tourette's disorder. American Journal of Psychiatry 114(5): 673–675
27. Ayd F J 1971 Pimozide: a promising new neuroleptic. International Drug Therapy Newsletter 6: 17
28. McCreadie R G, Dingwall J M, Wiles D H, Heykants J J P 1980 Intermittent pimozide versus fluphenazine decanoate as maintenance therapy in chronic schizophrenia. British Journal of Psychiatry 137: 510–517
29. Trimble M R 1985 The psychosis of epilepsy and their treatment. In: Trimble M R (ed) The psychopharmacology of epilepsy, ch 6. John Wiley and Sons, Chichester, pp 83–94
30. Sallee F R, Pollock B G, Stiller R L, Stull S, Everett G, Peral J M 1987 Pharmacokinetics of pimozide in adults and children with Tourette's syndrome. Journal of Clinical Pharmacology 27(10): 776–781
31. Kodjian A, Barriaga C, Turcot G, Natarajan M, Engelsmann F, Ananth J 1986 Double-blind study of pimozide in senile dementia. Current Therapeutic Research 40 (4): 694–701

Pinacidil monohydrate

Pinacidil is a vasodilator drug used to treat hypertension, which acts by opening potassium channels.

Chemistry

Pinacidil monohydrate (Pindac)
$C_{13}H_{19}H_5.H_2O$
N′-Cyano-N-4-pyridinyl-N″-(1,2,2-trimethylpropyl)guanidine monohydrate

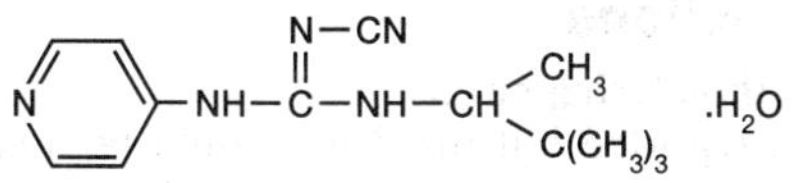

Molecular weight (anhydrous)	263.4 (245.4)
pKa	6.0, 10.8
Solubility	
in alcohol	1 in 7
in water	—
Octanol/water partition coefficient	—

It is a white crystalline odourless powder with a slight bitter taste which is prepared by chemical synthesis. It has an optically active centre but the racemic mixture is used clinically. It is not available in any combination products.

Pharmacology

The pharmacological profile of pinacidil is that of a directly acting peripheral vasodilator which causes, dose-dependent blood pressure reduction in hypertensive animals and humans. Its characteristics as a vasodilator mainly come from its ability to open potassium channels. Recent studies show that pinacidil can selectively activate the type of potassium channels which are closed by intracellular ATP, known as ATP-sensitive potassium channels. ATP-sensitive potassium channels have been found in smooth muscles, pancreatic β-cells, cardiac muscles, skeletal muscles and some neuronal cells. The sensitivity of ATP-sensitive potassium channels to pinacidil is different in vascular smooth muscles (activation threshold: 0.02–0.5 μM) from cardiac muscles (activation threshold: > 5 μM). This effect of pinacidil can be antagonized by elevation of intracellular ATP. The effect can also be eliminated by sulphonylureas such as glibenclamide and tolbutamide. The effect is temperature dependent.[1–3]

Toxicology

Adverse effects are predictable, that is hypotension and tachycardia.

There is no other evidence of acute toxicity and no reports of laboratory toxicological results which are of potential clinical significance.

Clinical pharmacology

When administered acutely or chronically, the haemodynamic and neuroendocrine profiles are those of a peripheral arterial vasodilator.[4] The drug produces a decrease in peripheral vascular resistance, and blood pressure decreases are associated with reflex increments in heart rate. When hypertensive patients were treated with pinacidil in doses ranging from 12.5 to 75 mg twice daily, 66.9% of patients had a decrease in supine diastolic blood pressure by 10 mm Hg or more, whereas only 23.9% of patients had similar falls during placebo treatment. Plasma catecholamines increased about twofold during chronic therapy, presumably due to baroreflex activation. Plasma renin activity, however, was not increased during chronic treatment with pinacidil monotherapy. During maintenance therapy with pinacidil, the average blood pressure during the daytime dosing interval was 137.8 ± 1.2/83.4 ± 0.7 mm Hg (mean ± SEM). Pinacidil monotherapy resulted in a characteristic adverse reaction profile dominated by the presence of dose-related oedema. Other features included tachycardia, palpitations and headache. When pinacidil was given to patients unresponsive to hydrochlorothiazide (25 mg twice daily) there was a fall of post-dose supine diastolic blood pressure in the pinacidil group of 13.5 ± 0.8 mm Hg compared with 7.3 ± 0.9 mm Hg in the placebo group. Under these conditions, the prevalence of oedema was reduced to 9%. A number of additional effects of pinacidil were noted which may be related to its mechanism of action, including hypertrichosis; transient, asymptomatic changes in the T wave of the electrocardiogram; and favourable trends in serum lipid concentrations. Serum potassium concentration did not appear to be affected by pinacidil given alone. These data suggest that potassium channel openers are effective antihypertensive agents when given alone at low doses, and when given in combination with diuretic.

Pharmacokinetics

Pinacidil and pinacidil pyridine-N-oxide can be assayed in serum and urine by modified HPLC.[5,6] The onset of action of pinacidil after oral administration is rapid (within 1 hour in most studies) and the mean maximum plasma concentration is linearly related to the dose administered within the range of 5 to 25 mg. The mean half life of elimination of pinacidil ranges from 1.6 to 2.9 h and is unrelated to the dose administered. No accumulation of pinacidil occurs during long term administration to healthy volunteers over a 4-week period. However, accumulation of the major metabolite pinacidil-N-oxide, which is active, does occur and this increases in patients with renal dysfunction,[7,8]

The clearance of pinacidil decreases with age. In patients with hepatic dysfunction the N-oxidation of pinacidil is reduced prolonging the elimination of the drug. In severe hepatic disease some reduction in dosage may be necessary.

Using a single dose of ^{14}C-labelled pinacidil in solution, DeLong et al[9] demonstrated that 58% of the circulating radioactivity in plasma was pinacidil, while 25% was pinacidil-N-oxide and 17% other unidentified metabolites.

The volume of distribution of pinacidil[5,9] after an intravenous infusion 0.2 mg.kg^{-1} in 2 groups of healthy volunteers has been reported as 1.4 and 1.1 l.kg^{-1}. The blood plasma concentration ratio is 0.8 to 0.9.[10] In the rat highest tissue concentrations are obtained in liver, kidney and small intestine.[6,11] High levels of pinacidil in the wall of the small intestine suggest a possible enterohepatic and/or enterogastric recirculation of the drug. Distribution to the brain in rats is minimal.[6] The extent to which pinacidil is excreted in breast milk or crosses the placenta is not known.

Pinacidil is extensively metabolized in the liver, and is excreted in the urine, only 10% of the dose as unchanged drug.

Oral absorption	high
Presystemic metabolism	—
Plasma half life	
range	1.6–2.9 h
Volume of distribution	1.1–1.4 l.kg^{-1}
Plasma protein binding	40%

Concentration–effect relationship

The antihypertensive action requires plasma concentrations in the range 100–300 μg.l^{-1}. There is a highly significant correlation between the change in mean blood pressure and the serum concentration of pinacidil in patients with essential hypertension.[12]

Metabolism

The metabolism and elimination of pinacidil involve biotransformation in the liver, via the cytochrome P450 enzyme system, followed by the renal excretion of the metabolites.[13] The major urinary excretory product over a 24-hour period after an oral dose of pinacidil has been identified as pinacidil-N-oxide which is pharmacologically active. The remainder is accounted for by a mixture of polar metabolites (29%) and unmetabolized pinacidil (10%). These metabolites have not yet been completely identified although they appear to be primarily glucuronide conjugates of pinacidil and/or pinacidil-N-oxide.[6] Because of the early appearance of pinacidil-N-oxide in the urine and its relatively low plasma concentrations the metabolism of parent compound to the active N-oxide metabolite is presumably rapid. While its contribution to the antihypertensive effect of pinacidil is probably limited in patients with normal renal function, a more pronounced effect could be anticipated in patients whose renal function is impaired. The faecal excretion of pinacidil and pinacidil-N-oxide in humans has not been reported although values in animals of 1 to 4%, indicate that this is not a significant route of elimination.[6]

Pharmaceutics

Pinacidil (Leo, UK) is available in oral forms.
Capsules containing 12.5 mg (red/dark blue), 25 mg (collarless/ dark blue) and 37.5 mg (light blue/dark blue) of pinacidil monohydrate.

Controlled-release capsules contained rapidly released pellets and slowly released pellets in the same ratio.

Pinacidil is not commercially available for intravenous use.

Therapeutic use

Indications

1. The control of essential hypertension
2. The control of secondary renal hypertension
   Other uses under study include
3. The control of bladder hyperactivity
4. The treatment of impotence.

Contraindications

1. Allergy to constituents

Relative contraindications
Caution should be used in patients with:
2. Symptomatic ischaemic heart disease
3. Cerebrovascular disease
4. Tachyarrythmias.

Mode of use

All the clinical uses depend upon smooth muscle relaxation induced by K^+ channel opening.

Oral treatment is usually begun with 12.5 mg twice daily. If there is no response to this dose, or if oedema develops, a diuretic may be added. If the response remains inadequate, the dose is increased up to a maximum of 75 mg daily depending upon the therapeutic response. Dose–response relationships for pinacidil monotherapy do not show a progressive increase in effect as the dose is increased. This may be explained by attenuated responses in patients with oedema. The incidence of oedema is clearly dose-related. It is observed in 6% of patients administered 25 mg daily rising to 30% at 150 mg daily pinacidil monotherapy. Diuretics attenuated this incidence of oedema. Caution should be exercised in dose titration in elderly patients and those with renal or hepatic dysfunction. Intravenously a dosage of 0.1–0.2 $mg.kg^{-1}$ body weight has been used as emergency treatment of severe hypertension and of cardiac failure. Pinacidil causes a marked fall of blood pressure accompanied by tachycardia. Because of this effect, it does not offer advantages over other vasodilators for emergency usage.

The clinical experience obtained so far shows absence of withdrawal syndromes and rebound effects, postural hypotension, decreased exercise tolerance, cold extremities, CNS-effects, and sexual dysfunction.

The abrupt cessation of treatment with pinacidil will not usually cause any adverse effects but in patients with oedema and associated heart failure diuretic therapy should first be initiated, followed by gradual withdrawal of pinacidil. The drug should not be used in patients with uncontrolled congestive cardiac failure.

Indications

1. Hypertension
Pinacidil is used in the treatment of high blood pressure as monotherapy or combination therapy with other antihypertensive drugs. The systolic and diastolic blood pressure in both supine and erect positions decrease, and supine heart rate increases in relation to the dosage level of pinacidil.

2. Secondary renal hypertension
A series of studies by Breen et al addressed the efficacy of pinacidil in treating renal hypertensive patients over a prolonged period. Blood pressure control was achieved with a mean daily dose of pinacidil 30 mg in patients with various types of renal disease.[14,15]

Other possible uses
3. Bladder hyperactivity
Trials have been conducted in the isolated human bladder. Pinacidil depressed contractions elicited by carbachol, low concentrations of K^+ (less than 60 mM) and electrical stimulation, in a concentration-dependent fashion. The result of clinical studies has not yet been reported.[16]

4. Impotence
A study reported that pinacidil depressed the contraction induced by low-K^+ solution in isolated human corpus cavernosum penis. There seems to be a possibility that pinacidil may be useful in the pharmacological treatment of impotence.[17]

Adverse reactions

Potentially life-threatening effects
None has been reported but the drug should be used cautiously in patients with symptomatic ischaemic heart disease, cerebrovascular disease or tachyarrhythmias, and the concomitant administration of a β-adrenoceptor blocking drug is recommended.

Acute overdosage
No cases of deliberate acute overdosage have so far been reported.

Severe or irreversible adverse effects
Pinacidil is relatively free from serious adverse effects apart from causing depedent oedema, like other vasodilators. Pinacidil (from a randomized, parallel, double-blind dose-titration study to 197 patients; 12.5 to 75 mg twice daily) caused tachycardia (15% to 20%) and palpitation (13% to 15%). Oedema was also frequent (38.2%).[5]

Symptomatic adverse effects
Symptomatic adverse effects include headache, dizziness, palpitations and tachycardia. These effects are common, occur early in treatment and are usually transient. They are dose-related and occur particularly when treatment is initiated with single dose of pinacidil above 25 mg.

There have been infrequent cases of nausea, dyspepsia and rashes. A small number of cases of hypertrichosis have been reported; this effect disappearing within 3 months of withdrawal of therapy.

Other effects
Therapeutic trials of pinacidil to date have generally reported little or no change in commonly measured biochemical parameters during therapy. Sodium retention has been reported and the excretion rate of albumin and β_2-microglobulin was reduced in the study of Krusell et al.[18]

Pinacidil reduces blood lipids. Patients treated with the drug exhibited a significant average decrease from baseline in concentrations of total and low-density lipoprotein cholesterol and triglycerides and a significant average increment in high-density lipoprotein cholesterol.[19]

Interference with clinical pathology tests
The development of antinuclear antibodies (ANA) has been reported in a number of patients,[20] but this was not accompanied by any clinically evident adverse effects.

High risk groups

Neonates
There is no experience of the use of the drug in neonates.

Breast milk. The excretion of the drug in breast milk has not been investigated, so women taking the drug should not breast-feed.

Children
There is no experience of the use of the drug in children.

Pregnant women
As there is no evidence of the safety of the drug in pregnancy, it should not be given to pregnant women.

The elderly
The plasma clearance of pinacidil was found to be significantly correlated with age in patients, being significantly reduced in older patients in Caucasians, which may indicate that lower doses will be needed.[21]

Concurrent disease
Renal disease. The plasma clearance of pinacidil-N-oxide correlates with creatinine clearance. Mean peak plasma concentrations of the metabolite are lower in patients with a creatinine clearance of > 115 ml.min than in patients with renal dysfunction (creatinine clearance < 80 ml.min). No data are available from patients with end-stage renal disease.
Liver disease. In comparison with healthy volunteers the plasma concentration of pinacidil in chronic stable cirrhosis was 2-fold higher, the clearance of pinacidil was markedly reduced (42 vs 21 $l.h^{-1}$) and the elimination half life was prolonged (3.8 vs 6.1 h). The reduced clearance of pinacidil in cirrhosis was due to a reduced ability to oxidize pinacidil to the N-oxide metabolite since urinary recovery of pinacidil-N-oxide in cirrhotic patients was only 31% compared with 52% in health volunteers.[22] Data on the long-term administration of pinacidil to patients with liver dysfunction are as yet unavailable, these findings suggest that a dose reduction may be necessary.

Drug interactions

Potentially hazardous interactions
There are no reports on hazardous interactions between pinacidil and other drugs.

Other significant interactions
Hydrochlorothiazide. In patients taking hydrochlorothiazide with pinacidil the mean peak plasma pinacidil concentration was significantly higher (203 $\mu g.l^{-1}$) than in patients taking pinacidil alone (168 $\mu g.l^{-1}$), and the clearance rate of pinacidil in the former group was 13% lower than in the latter.
Food. Generally, food intake has little influence on peak concentration of pinacidil and N-oxide. However, a report[23] on the effects of a standard breakfast meal on the bioavailability of a sustained-release tablet formulation of pinacidil, showed that concomitant food intake resulted in significantly increased maximum measured serum pinacidil concentrations and relative bioavailability with decreased terminal elimination half life.
Alcohol. Alcohol (> 28 ml daily) has no effect on the clearance of pinacidil.[22]
Cigarette smoke. In smokers the rate of pinacidil clearance was 12% higher than in non-smokers.[22]

Potentially useful interactions
The beneficial effect of using pinacidil with a diuretic in some patients has already been discussed.

Clinical trials

1. Callaghan J T, Goldberg M R, Brunelle R 1988 Double-blind comparator trials with Pinacidil, a potassium channel opener. Drugs 36 (suppl 7): 77–82

The antihypertensive effects of pinacidil, a potassium channel opener, were studied in 4, dose titration, double-blind trials. Patients had mild to severe hypertension, with supine diastolic arterial pressures between 91 and 150 mm Hg during the qualification assessment. Efficacy was assessed using an 'intention-to-treat' analysis. In one study, pinacidil-treated patients had a response rate significantly greater than placebo-treated patients. In another study, the pinacidil group had a response rate significantly greater than the prazosin group (83% vs 75%, respectively). In a third study, the response rate in the pinacidil group was marginally greater than in the hydralazine group (77% vs 73%, respectively). In a 'step 2' trial, pinacidil was as effective as methyldopa and more effective than placebo. Adverse changes occurred intermittently and may be related to its mechanism of action. These studies suggest that antihypertensive monotherapy with pinacidil was effective and generally well tolerated.

2. Goldberg M R, Sushak C S, Rockhold F W, Thompson W L 1988 Vasodilator monotherapy in the treatment of hypertension: comparative efficacy and safety of pinacidil, a potassium channel opener, and prazosin. Clinical Pharmacology and Therapeutics 44: 78–92

Antihypertensive effects of monotherapy with pinacidil (N = 197) or prazosin (N = 204) were compared in a randomized, parallel, double-blind dose-titration study in which hydrochlorothiazide or propranolol could be added for adverse events or lack of efficacy. Pinacidil (12.5 to 75 mg twice daily) was a more potent vasodilator, producing a mean decrease in supine diastolic blood pressure (baseline = 102 to 103 ±9 mm Hg) of 18.8 ±10.0 (SD) mm Hg compared with 15.5 ±9.2 mm Hg with prazosin (1 to 10 mg twice daily; p less than 0.001). Patients responding to each drug had similar average blood pressure levels during 12-hour monitoring (137/85 mm Hg). More patients taking pinacidil required hydrochlorothiazide for oedema (p = 0.008) and more taking prazosin required hydrochlorothiazide and propranolol for lack of efficacy (p less than 0.001). Tachycardia (15% to 20%) and palpitation (13% to 15%) were frequent events with both drugs. Oedema (38.2% vs 22.3%) was more frequent with pinacidil (p less than 0.001) and postural hypotension (4.7% vs 1.0%) and asthenia (20.2% vs 13.2%) were more frequent with prazosin (p = 0.025; 0.062). No significant laboratory toxicity was noted. In conclusion, both pinacidil and prazosin are effective as monotherapy for hypertension. Monotherapy with pinacidil is limited by adverse events related to vasodilatation and monotherapy with prazosin is limited by lack of efficacy.

3. Goldberg M R, Rockhold F W, Thompson W L, DeSante K A 1989 Clinical pharmacokinetics of pinacidil, a potassium channel opener, in hypertension. Journal of Clinical Pharmacology 29: 33–40

Pinacidil is a potassium channel opener that decreases blood pressure by reducing peripheral arterial resistance. In two multicenter trials, we studied the concentrations and apparent clearance of pinacidil (406 patients) and concentrations of its pyridyl-N-oxide matabolite (147 patients). Responding patients had plasma samples collected hourly for 12 hours on two occasions after weeks to months of treatment. Pinacidil dose was titrated from 12.5 to 75 mg b.i.d. The peak concentration of pinacidil and N-oxide and the area under the concentration-time curve (AUC) were proportional to the dose of pinacidil, with an average pinacidil concentration of 268 $\mu g.l^{-1}$ (1.02 μM) and N-oxide concentration of 172 $\mu g.l^{-1}$ (0.65 μM) for every 1 $mg.kg^{-1}$ pinacidil administered. Clearance of pinacidil (Clp = Dose/AUC) was 31 $l.h^{-1}$ in patients younger than 45 years and 27 $l.h^{-1}$ in those older than 60. Clp was significantly smaller in white patients compared with other races (Clp = 28 vs. 34 $l.h^{-1}$). Clp was significantly less in patients taking hydrochlorothiazide (27 vs. 31 $l.h^{-1}$) and greater in smokers (33 vs. 29 $l.h^{-1}$). Concomitant propranolol use did not influence Clp.

Other trials

1. Sterndorff B, Johansen P 1988 The antihypertensive effect of pinacidil versus prazosin in mild to moderate hypertensive patients seen in general practice. Acta Medica Scandinavica 224: 329–336

The antihypertensive effect of a new vasodilating drug, pinacidil, was compared with prazosin in a randomized, open study in general practice including 131 patients with a sitting diastolic blood pressure (DBP) between 100–115 mm Hg. At inclusion 108 patients were untreated and the remaining patients were on treatment with thiazide diuretics and/or β-blockers. The aim was to reduce the sitting DBP to less than or equal to 95 mm Hg, which was achieved in 85% of the patients treated with pinacidil and in 77% of the patients treated with prazosin (NS). In the responding patients the reductions were (mean ± SD) 16 ± 7 mm Hg (p less than 0.001) and 13 ± 6 mm Hg (p less than 0.001) in the pinacidil group (n = 60) and the prazosin group (n = 46), respectively (p less than 0.001). During 5 months of maintenance therapy no statistically significant differences in blood pressures between the two treatment groups were present. Side-effects were typical of vasodilator therapy, i.e. headache, dizziness, tachycardia and oedema, leading to discontinuation of therapy in 10 patients in each treatment group. Heart rate (HR) was increased with pinacidil and unchanged with prazosin. Oedema was frequently seen with pinacidil and dizziness with prazosin. Because of oedema a thiazide diuretic was given to nine patients in the pinacidil group and two patients in the prazosin group. No clinically significant changes in ECG and biochemical variables were observed. In conclusion, the study demonstrated that pinacidil is as effective an antihypertensive agent as prazosin. Pinacidil may be used as monotherapy. However, the study suggests that pinacidil should be used as add-on therapy to thiazide diuretics.

General review articles

Ahnfelt-Ronne I, Jurgensen H J 1989 Pinacidil (Pindac): a new antihypertensive agent. Drugs of today 25: 65–74

Ahnfelt-Ronne I 1988 Pinacidil: history, basic pharmacology, and therapeutic implications. Journal of Cardiovascular Pharmacology 12 (suppl 2): S1–S4

Friedel H A, Brogden R N 1990 Pinacidil. A review of its pharmacodynamic and pharmacokinetic properties, and therapeutic potential in the treatment of hypertension. Drugs 36: 929–967

References

1. Fan Z, Nakayama K, Hiraoka M 1990 Pinacidil activates the ATp-sensitive K^+channels in inside-out and cell-attached patch membranes of guinea-pig ventricular myocytes. Pflugers Archives 415: 387–394
2. Nakayama K, Fan Z, Marumo F, Hiraoka M 1990 Interrelation between pinacidil and intracellular ATP concentration on activation of the ATP-sensitive K+current in guinea-pig ventricular myocytes. Circulation Research 67: 1124–1133
3. Fan Z, Nakayama K, Hiraoka M 1990 Multiple actions of pinacidil on adenosine triphosphate-sensitive potassium channels in guinea-pig ventricular myocytes. Journal of Physiology 430: 273–295
4. Carlsen J E, Kardel T, Hilden T, Tango M, Trap-Jensen J 1981 Immediate central and peripheral hemodynamic effects of a new vasodilating agent pinacidil (P1134) in hypertensive man. Clinical Physiology 1: 375–384
5. Ward J W, McBurney A, Farrow P R, Sharp P 1984 Pharmacokinetics and hypotensive effect in healthy volunteers of pinacidil, a new potent vasodilator. European Journal of Clinical Pharmacology 26: 603–608
6. Eilertsen E, Magnussen M P, Petersen H J, Rastrup-Andersen N, Sorensen H, Arrigoni Martelli E 1982 Metabolism of the new antihypertensive agent pinacidil in rat, dog and man. Xenobiotica 12: 187–196
7. Kardel T, Hilden T, Carlsen J, Trap-Jensen J 1981 N'-cyano-N-4-pyridyl-N'-1,2,2-trimethyl-propylguanideine, a new vasodilating agent: acute effect on blood pressure and pharmacokinetics in hypertensive patients. Journal of Cardiovascular Pharmacology 3: 1002–1007
8. Goldberg M R, Sushak C S, Rockhold F W, Thompson W L 1988 Vasodilator monotherapy in the treatment of hypertension: comparative efficacy and safety of pinacidil, a potassium channel opener, and prazosin. Clinical Pharmacology and Therapeutics 44: 78–92
9. Laher M S, Hickey M P 1985 Pharmacokinetics and bioavailability of pinacidil capsules in human volunteers. Journal of Internal Medical Research 13: 159–162
10. DeLong A F, Oldham S W, DeSante K A, Nell G, Henry D P 1988 Disposition of [^{14}C] pinacidil in humans. Journal of Pharmacological Science 77: 153–156
11. Arrigioni-Martelli E, Finucane J 1985 Pinacidil In: Scriabine A (ed) New drugs annual. Cardiovascular Drugs, vol 3. New York: Raven Press 133–151
12. Goldberg M R, Rockhold F W, Thompson W L, DeSante K A 1989 Clinical pharmacokinetics of pinacidil, a potassium channel opener, in hypertension. Journal of Clinical Pharmacology 29: 33–40
13. Ayesh R, Al Waiz M, McBurney A, Mitchell S C, Idle J R, Ward J R, Smith R L 1989 Variable metabolism of pinacidil: lack of correlation with the debrisoquine and trimethylamine C- and N-oxidative polymorphisms. British Journal of Clinical Pharmacology 27: 423–428
14. Breen E G, Mulhall D, Keogh J A 1985 Treatment of essential hypertension and hypertension associated with renal impairment with pinacidil: a new vasodilator. European Journal of Clinical Pharmacology 28: 381–386
15. Breen E G, Mulhall D, Keogh J A 1985 Long-term effects of pinacidil in hypertensive dialysis patients. European Journal of Clinical Pharmacology 28: 375–380
16. Fovaeus M, Andersson K E, Hedlund H 1989 The action of pinacidil in the isolated human bladder. Journal of Urology 141: 637–640
17. Holmquist F, Andersson K E, Hedlund H 1990 Effects of pinacidil on isolated human corpus cavernosum penis. Acta Physiologica Scandinavica 138: 463–469
18. Krusell L R, Christensen C K, Lederballe Pedersen O 1986 Renal effects of pinacidil in hypertensive patients on chronic β-blocker therapy. European Journal of Clinical Pharmacology 30: 641–647
19. Rockhold F W, Goldberg M R, Thompson W L 1989 Beneficial effects of pinacidil on blood lipids: comparisons with prazosin and placebo in patients with hypertension. Journal of Laboratory and Clinical Medicine 114: 646–654
20. Byyny R L, Nies A S, loVerde M E, Mitchell W D 1987 A double-blind, randomized, controlled trial comparing pinacidil to hydralazine in essential hypertension. Clinical Pharmacology and Therapeutics 42: 50–57
21. Goldberg M R, Rockhold F W, Thompson W L, DeSant K A 1989 Clinical Pharmacokinetics of pinacidil, a potassium channel opener, in hypertension. Journal of Clinical Pharmacology 29: 33–40
22. Shaheen O, Patel J, Avant G R, Hamilton M, Wood A J 1986 Effect of cirrhosis and debrisoquine phenotype on the disposition and effects of pinacidil. Clinical Pharmacology and Therapeutics 40: 650–655
23. McBurney A, Farrow P R, Ward J W 1988 Effects of food on the bioavailability of sustained-release pinacidil in humans. Journal of Pharmaceutical Sciences 77: 68–69

Pindolol

A non-selective beta-adrenergic receptor antagonist with substantial partial agonist activity.

Chemistry

Pindolol (Visken, Betadren)
$C_{14}H_{20}N_2O_2$
1-(1H-Indol-4-yloxy)-3-isopropylamino-2-propanol

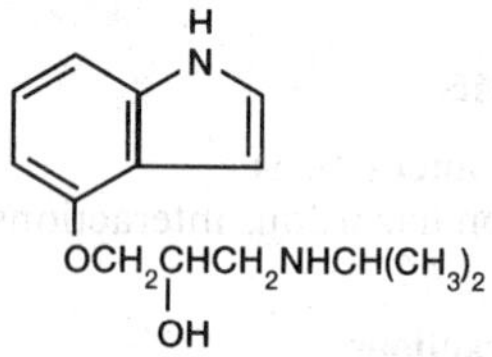

Molecular weight	248.3
pKa	6.5 and 8.3
Solubility	
in alcohol	1 in 120
in water	insoluble
Octanol/water partition coefficient	0.41

A white to pink tinged or grey tinged, odourless powder it is prepared by chemical synthesis and the racemate is used clinically. Pindolol is also available in an oral combination product (Viskaldix) with a thiazide diuretic, clopamide.

Pharmacology

Pindolol is a competitive antagonist at both the β_1- and β_2-adrenoceptor, and therefore is not cardioselective.[1] With the exception of xamoterol, pindolol has the most marked partial agonist activity of the currently available β-adrenoceptor antagonists and there is evidence that this partial agonist activity is largely at the β_2-adrenoceptor.[2] It exerts weak membrane stabilizing activity but this is unlikely to have any effect at the concentrations achieved in clinical use.

At orders of magnitude higher concentrations than those producing β antagonism, pindolol also acts as an α-adrenoceptor antagonist. This is, however, unlikely to be relevant to its therapeutic use.

Toxicology

Prolonged administration of pindolol to rats, dogs and rhesus monkeys has shown no evidence of clinically relevant toxicity.

No teratogenicity was seen in mice, rats or rabbits and there was no evidence of mutagenicity or carcinogenicity.

Clinical pharmacology

Competitive β-adrenoceptor blockade has been demonstrated in man by a parallel shift to the right in the dose heart-rate response curve to β agonists such as isoprenaline.[3] Pindolol has equal antagonist activity at the β_1 and β_2 adrenoceptors. Partial agonist activity has been demonstrated in man by increases in resting heart rate and finger tremor.[4] The effect of cumulative doses of up to 57.5 mg on a sub-maximal exercise tachycardia and resting heart rate showed no increase beyond that produced by 2.5 mg, and the effect on exercise heart rate was slightly less than metoprolol 300 mg.[5] In subjects with normal lungs, blockade of the pulmonary β-adrenoceptors by pindolol has little effect upon function. However, in patients with a history of asthma, airways resistance may increase following pindolol therapy.

Pindolol has little effect on exercise tolerance in normal individuals but in patients with angina, exercise tolerance is usually increased due to a reduction in total myocardial oxygen consumption. Pindolol lowers blood pressure in both the lying and standing positions, with little overall effect on resting heart rate. The mechanism for the fall in blood pressure is still debated. Unlike many other β-adrenoceptor antagonists, pindolol does not reduce resting cardiac output significantly in patients with normal myocardial function. However, cardiac failure can on occasion be precipitated by pindolol in patients with myocardial disease.

There are widespread metabolic and endocrine effects of β-adrenoceptor blockade, including a reduction in plasma renin, reduced breakdown of muscle glycogen and inhibition of catecholamine dependent lipolysis. However, pindolol has fewer metabolic effects than most other β-adrenoceptor antagonists, probably due to its partial agonist activity.[6] In patients receiving chronic therapy for angina pectoris with pindolol no changes were seen in lipoprotein profile.[7]

Pharmacokinetics

A reliable analytical method in plasma and urine is by high performance liquid chromatography with ultraviolet detection which has a limit of sensitivity of 1.2 ng.[8]

Pindolol is completely absorbed after oral administration, with nearly 100% bioavailability, but there is about fourfold variability in the plasma concentrations achieved after a single dose reducing to twofold on chronic dosing. Food increases plasma concentrations and rate of absorption. There is no evidence of any significant presystemic metabolism.[9] Bioavailability is reduced in patients with uraemia. Peak plasma concentrations are seen at 1–2 hours in fasting patients. The mean plasma half life is in the range of 2.5–4 hours.[10]

Protein binding of pindolol is in the range 50–70% with about 30% of this to α_1 acid glycoprotein. The volume of distribution is 1.2–2 $l.kg^{-1}$. The concentration of pindolol in the CSF approximates to the free drug concentration in the plasma. An approximate CSF:plasma ratio of 0.29 has been observed with chronic oral doses of 10–20 mg daily in man.[11]

Oral absorption	>90%
Presystemic metabolism	<10%
Plasma half life	
range	2.5–4 h
mean	3.6 h
Volume of distribution	1.2–2.0 $l.kg^{-1}$
Plasma protein binding	50–70%

About 40% of an oral dose of pindolol is excreted in the urine as the unchanged drug and the major routes of metabolism are conjugation and oxidation.[12] The elimination of the drug in patients with liver[13] and renal disease has been reported to be reduced[14] but it is probably necessary to alter pindolol dosage only in patients with severe renal or hepatic impairment. Pindolol tends to accumulate in the elderly but the magnitude of the effect is not likely to cause clinical problems.[15] The drug has been reported to cross the placenta and appear in breast milk.

Concentration–effect relationship

There is a good correlation between plasma concentrations of pindolol and β-antagonism measured as inhibition of an exercise- or isoprenaline-induced tachycardia. A correlation has also been claimed between plasma concentrations of pindolol in the range 10–70 $\mu g.l^{-1}$ and blood pressure reduction.[16] Monitoring of plasma concentrations is unlikely to be advantageous in clinical practice because of the high therapeutic index of pindolol.

Metabolism

About 40% of an oral dose of pindolol is excreted in the urine as the unchanged drug figure (see Fig. 1).[12] The major route of metabolism is oxidation accounting for about 50% of the administered dose with the remaining 10% excreted as conjugates in the urine. There are numerous oxidation products but none are pharmacologically active.

Fig. 1 The metabolism of pindolol

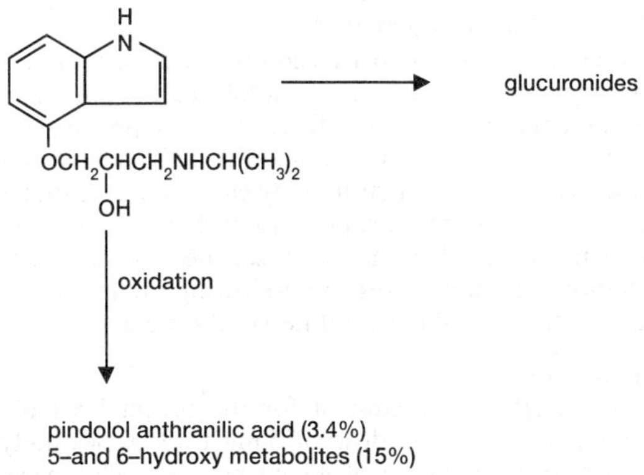

Pharmaceutics

Pindolol is available as tablets of 5 and 15 mg.

Visken (Sandoz, UK) 5 mg is a white, round, flat, bevel-edged tablet of 7 mm diameter marked Visken 5 on one side and with a single break line on the reverse. Each tablet contains 5 mg of pindolol base.

Visken 15 mg is a white, round, flat, bevel-edged tablet of 9 mm diameter branded 'Visken 15' on one side, and scored on the reverse. Each tablet contains 15 mg of pindolol base. A generic preparation, Betadren (Lagap, UK), is also available in 5 and 15 mg tablets.

Therapeutic use

Indications

1. The control of hypertension
2. The management of angina pectoris
3. The treatment of tachycardia, paroxysmal tachycardia, tachycardia in patients with atrial flutter or fibrillation, supraventricular extrasystoles.

Contraindications

1. Bronchospasm
2. Low cardiac output and untreated cardiac failure
3. Bradycardia and heart block
4. Hypoglycaemia
5. Severe haemorrhage.

Mode of use

All the clinical uses depend on β-adrenoceptor antagonism. The decrease in resting heart rate and cardiac output caused by most other β-adrenoceptor antagonists is not seen with pindolol, due to its partial agonist activity, and the peripheral vascular resistance is also reduced.

Treatment of hypertension is usually commenced with one 15 mg tablet daily or 5 mg two or three times daily. If necessary, dosage may be increased at weekly intervals up to a maximum of 45 mg daily in single or divided doses. There is little evidence of increased effect above 20 mg daily and some suggestion that reducing higher doses may reduce blood pressure. In mild and moderate hypertension pindolol alone is often sufficient. In more severe or in resistant cases additional therapy with other antihypertensive drugs may be necessary.

For the treatment of angina pectoris and cardiac arrhythmias, the daily dosage of 10-30 mg is generally divided into 2 or 3 single doses: once-a-day dosage can be used with the retard tablet.

Indications

1. The control of hypertension

Pindolol is widely used for the treatment of mild to moderate hypertension either alone or in combination with a thiazide diuretic. Blood pressure falls are seen within 2 hours of administration of the first dose and there is no evidence of tolerance with prolonged usage. A single daily dose is often effective, with both systolic and diastolic blood pressure reduction and no postural hypotension. Daytime blood pressure falls by about 15% but during the night pindolol, when given once a day, has little effect on blood pressure, probably due to its partial agonist activity.[17]

The mode of action in hypertension is not clearly understood. Of the β-adrenoceptor antagonists, pindolol has the smallest effect on plasma renin concentrations and these correlate poorly with changes in blood pressure.[18] Also, partial agonist activity at β_2-adrenoceptors on the peripheral vasculature may cause some vasodilation, but significant differences from propranolol in hypotensive efficacy have not been demonstrated.[19] Other proposed mechanisms are changes in autoregulation of blood pressure following reduction of cardiac output and actions on the central nervous system.

2. Angina pectoris
Pindolol is an effective treatment for the prophylaxis of exercise-induced angina. A starting dose of 5 mg three times daily may be increased up to a maximum of 45 mg per day. The mechanism of action is reduction of myocardial oxygen demand by reduction in heart rate. There is no evidence of tolerance to the effect of the drug and on cessation of therapy it is claimed that there is less of a 'rebound' phenomenon than with other β-adrenoceptor antagonists.[20]

Contraindications

1. Bronchospasm
Pindolol can cause severe bronchospasm in patients with asthma or other obstructive airways disease. It also antagonizes the bronchodilating effects of β_2-agonists and should not be prescribed for patients with obstructive airways disease.

2. Low cardiac output and untreated cardiac failure
While the partial agonist activity of pindolol causes a smaller reduction in cardiac output than β-adrenoceptor blocking drugs without agonist activity it should not be used in patients with untreated cardiac failure who are often dependent upon a high sympathetic drive.

3. Bradycardia and heart block
Pindolol is the least likely of the β-adrenoceptor antagonists to cause bradycardia at rest due to the presence of partial agonist activity but while this reduces, it does not eliminate, an effect on intracardiac conduction. The drug is contraindicated in patients with second or third degree heart block.

4. Hypoglycaemia
As part of the metabolic response to hypoglycaemia is mediated through the β-adrenoceptors pindolol can reduce the premonitory signs of hypoglycaemia and delay recovery.

5. Severe haemorrhage
The usual response to haemorrhage is a sympathetically mediated rise in heart rate and this is prevented by β-blockage. The absence of a marked tachycardia must be interpreted in the knowledge that a β-adrenoceptor antagonist is present.

Adverse reactions

Potentially life-threatening effects
Pindolol has a low toxicity. Like all β-adrenoceptor antagonists pindolol can cause bronchospasm, cardiac failure and hypoglycaemia in patients with preexisting organic disease. Sudden withdrawal of treatment with pindolol is not recommended in patients with severe ischaemic heart disease because of a 'rebound' effect but this seems to be less with pindolol than β-adrenoceptor antagonists without partial agonist activity.

Pindolol has little effect on total cholesterol, HDL, VLDL, LDL and plasma triglycerides.

Acute overdosage
Compared with the other β-adrenoceptor antagonists pindolol is among the least toxic in overdose,[21] and 480 mg orally caused no toxic effects. Overdose should be treated by induced emesis, if ingestion is recent, and general supportive measures. Atropine may be used to treat bradycardia, and isoprenaline may be administered if required. Large concentrations of isoprenaline may be necessary because of the presence of the β-adrenoceptor antagonist.

Severe or irreversible adverse effects
Severe or irreversible adverse effects are rare with pindolol. This may be due to the partial agonist activity which the drug possesses.

Symptomatic adverse effects
In general, pindolol is well tolerated. A survey of the adverse effects of pindolol administration in more than 1000 patients showed that the most common symptoms were headache, dizziness, insomnia, joint and muscle pain, fatigue, oedema, nervousness, and muscle cramps.[22] Compared with propranolol, only fatigue and muscle cramps were more frequent with pindolol.

Other effects
Pindolol has little effect on blood lipids or uric acid, but serum potassium rises slightly. Blood creatine phosphokinase (CPK) concentrations may be elevated, particularly in patients complaining of muscle cramps.

Interference with clinical pathology tests
Pindolol and its metabolites do not interfere with routine clinical pathology tests.

High risk groups

Neonates
The safety and efficacy of pindolol in this group has not been established.

Breast milk. Pindolol is excreted in breast milk but this is unlikely to be clinically significant.

Children
The safety and efficacy of pindolol in children has not been established.

Pregnant women
Pindolol has been used to control hypertension in pregnancy and there was no detrimental effect on fetal growth. The effect of pindolol on fetal heart rate was less than that of atenolol.

The elderly
Pindolol has a longer elimination half-life in the elderly and may tend to accumulate. This effect is unlikely to be clinically significant.

Drug interactions

Potentially hazardous interactions

Adrenaline. Blood pressure may rise markedly if adrenaline is co-administered with pindolol because the vasodilating effects of adrenaline are inhibited but the α-mediated pressor effects are unaffected.

Anaesthetic agents. Because the reflex rise in heart rate due to vasodilation caused by anaesthetic agents may be reduced by β-adrenoceptor antagonists, cardiac output may fall. However, with care, serious interactions can be avoided.

Clonidine. In common with all the β-adrenoceptor blocking drugs pindolol can exacerbate the rebound hypertension following withdrawal of clonidine therapy.

Verapamil. Verapamil in combination with pindolol has been reported to cause bradycardia, hypotension, and heart failure.

Other significant interactions

Food. When administered with food pindolol is more rapidly absorbed and achieves a higher peak plasma concentration.

Cimetidine. The plasma concentrations of pindolol are increased by 30% when co-administered with cimetidine. This is not likely to be clinically important.

Indomethacin. The antihypertensive effect of all β-adrenoceptor blocking drugs is impaired by indomethacin.

Hypoglycaemic agents. Pindolol may increase the duration and severity of hypoglycaemic reactions in diabetic patients. Due to the increase in plasma adrenaline caused by the hypoglycaemia blood pressure may rise markedly. The drug is probably best avoided in these patients.

Potentially useful interactions
The reflex tachycardia caused by vasodilating drugs may be inhibited by pindolol and the drugs may be used concomitantly to increase the hypotensive effect.

Pindolol

P

Major outcome trials

1. Gonasun L M 1982 Antihypertensive effects of pindolol. American Heart Journal 104: 374–387

This is the combined result of seven trials totalling 300 patients with mild to moderate hypertension who were treated with pindolol. The studies were double-blind, randomized, parallel group design and compared the effects of pindolol to placebo, propranolol, hydrochlorthiazide, alpha methyldopa and chlorthalidone. Pindolol, administered as monotherapy in the dosage range 5–50 mg daily, taken twice or three times daily was as effective as propranolol, hydrochlorthiazide, alpha methyldopa or chlorthalidone and more effective than placebo. Nearly 60% of all the pindolol treated patients had a reduction in supine diastolic blood pressure of at least 10 mm Hg.

2. Kostis J B, Frishman W, Hosler M H, Thorsen N L, Gonasun L M, Wienstein J 1982 Treatment of angina pectoris with pindolol: the significance of intrinsic sympathomimetic activity of β blockers. American Heart Journal 104: 496–504

This is a randomized, double-blind, parallel group study of titrated doses of propranolol and pindolol in 52 patients with angina due to proven coronary artery disease. The maximum dose of pindolol was 10 mg four times daily. Both propranolol and pindolol were shown to be effective treatments for angina with pindolol having less effect on resting heart rate, ejection fraction and left ventricular end diastolic volume than propranolol.

3. Australian and Swedish Pindolol Study Group 1983 The effect of pindolol on the two years mortality after complicated myocardial infarction. European Heart Journal 4: 367–375

The effect of oral pindolol 15 mg daily was compared with placebo in 529 patients who had electrical and/or mechanical complications after an acute myocardial infarction. No significant difference was seen between treatments in terms of mortality but in patients commenced on treatment more than five days after the infarct there was a 20% reduced mortality in the pindolol treated group. There was also a lower mortality in patients treated with digoxin who also received pindolol.

General review articles

Frishman W H 1983 Pindolol: A new β-adrenoceptor antagonist with partial agonist activity. New England Journal of Medicine 308: 940–944

Golightly L K 1982 Pindolol: a review of its pharmacology, pharmacokinetics, clinical uses and adverse effects. Pharmacotherapy 2: 134–147

Riddell J G, Harron D W G, Shank R G, 1987 Clinical pharmacokinetics of β-adrenoceptor antagonists – an update. Clinical Pharmacokinetics 12: 305–320

Weil C 1980 Pindolol. In: Scriabine A (ed) Pharmacology of antihypertensive drugs. Raven Press, New York, pp 237–246

References

1. Aellig W H 1976 β-adrenoceptor blocking activity and duration of action of pindolol and propranolol in healthy volunteers. British Journal of Clinical Pharmacology 3: 251–257
2. Clark B J, Bertholet A 1983 Effects of pindolol on vascular smooth muscle. General Pharmacology 14: 117–119
3. Aellig W H 1976 β-adrenoceptor blocking activity and duration of action of pindolol and propranolol in healthy volunteers. British Journal of Clinical Pharmacology 3: 251–257
4. McCaffrey P M, Riddell J G, Shanks R G 1987 An assessment of the partial agonist activity of Ro 31-1118, flusoxolol and pindolol in man. British Journal of Clinical Pharmacology 24: 571–580
5. Carruthers S G, Twum-Barima Y 1981 Measurement of partial agonist activity of pindolol. Clinical Pharmacology and Therapeutics 30: 581–585
6. Aellig W H 1982 Pindolol — a β-adrenoceptor blocking drug with partial agonist activity: clinical pharmacological considerations. British Journal of Clinical Pharmacology 13: 187S–192S
7. Northcote R J, Ballantyne D 1987 β-adrenoceptor blockade and plasma lipoproteins. Comparison of the effects of propranolol and pindolol on plasma lipoproteins including high-density lipoprotein subfractions. Clinical Science 72: 549–556
8. Shields B J, Lima J J, Binkley P F, Leier C V, MacKichan J J 1986 Determination of pindolol in human plasma and urine by high-performance liquid chromatography with ultraviolet detection. Journal of Chromatography 387: 163–171
9. Meier J 1982 Pindolol: a pharmacokinetic comparison with other β-adrenoceptor blocking agents. American Heart Journal 104: 364–373
10. Gugler R, Herold W, Dengler H J, 1974 Pharmacokinetics of pindolol in man. European Journal of Clinical Pharmacology 7: 17–24
11. Taylor E A, Jefferson D, Carrol J D and Turner P 1981 Cerebrospinal fluid concentrations of propranolol, pindolol and atenolol in man: evidence for central actions of β-adrenoceptor antagonists. British Journal of Clinical Pharmacology 12: 549–559
12. Schwartz H J 1982 Pharmacokinetics of pindolol in humans and several animal species. American Heart Journal 104: 357–364
13. Ohnhaus E E, Munch U, Meier J 1982 Elimination of pindolol in liver disease. European Journal of Clinical Pharmacology 22: 247–251
14. Ohnhaus E E, Heidemann H, Meier J, Maurer G 1982 Metabolism of pindolol in patients with renal failure. European Journal of Clinical Pharmacology 22: 423–428
15. Hitzenberger G, Fitscha P, Beveridge T, Nuesch E, Pacha W 1982 Effects of age and smoking on the pharmocokinetics of pindolol and propranolol. British Journal of Clinical Pharmacology 13: 217S–222S
16. Weiss Y A, Loria Y, Safar M E, Lavene D E, Simon A C, Georges D R, Milliez P L, 1977 Relationship between the antihypertensive effect and the drug plasma concentration of pindolol. Current Therapeutic Research 21: 644–655
17. Mann S, Millar Craig MW, Balasubramanian V, Raftery E B 1981 Once daily β-adrenoceptor blockade in hypertension: an ambulatory assessment. British Journal of Clinical Pharmacology 12: 223–228
18. Man in't Veld A J, Schalekamp A D H 1983 Effects of 10 different β-adrenoceptor antagonists on haemodynamics, plasma renin activity, and plasma norephinephrine in hypertension: the key role of vascular resistance changes in relation to partial agonist activity. Journal of Cardiovascular Pharmacology 5: S30–S45
19. Beaton G R, Rosendorff C, Kramer R, Simpson R D 1974 A comparison of propranolol and pindolol in the treatment of essential hypertension. Current Therapeutic Research 16: 268–274
20. Rangno R E, Langlois S 1982 Comparison of withdrawal phenomena after propranolol, metoprolol and pindolol. British Journal of Clinical Pharmacology 13: 345S–351S
21. Henry D A, Cassidy S L, 1986 Membrane stabilising activity: a major cause of fatal poisoning. Lancet 1: 1414–1417
22. Gonasun L M, Langrall H, 1982 Adverse reations to pindolol administration. American Heart Journal 104: 482–486

P

Piperacillin (sodium)

Piperacillin is a semi-synthetic penicillin, derived from d(−)-α-aminobenzylpenicillin, and belongs with mezlocillin and azlocillin to the ureidopenicillins.

Chemistry

Piperacillin sodium (Pipril, Pipracil)
$C_{23}H_{26}N_5NaO_7S$
Sodium 6-D(−)α-(4-Ethyl-2,3-dioxo-1-piperazinylcarbonylamino)-α-phenylacetamidopenicillanate

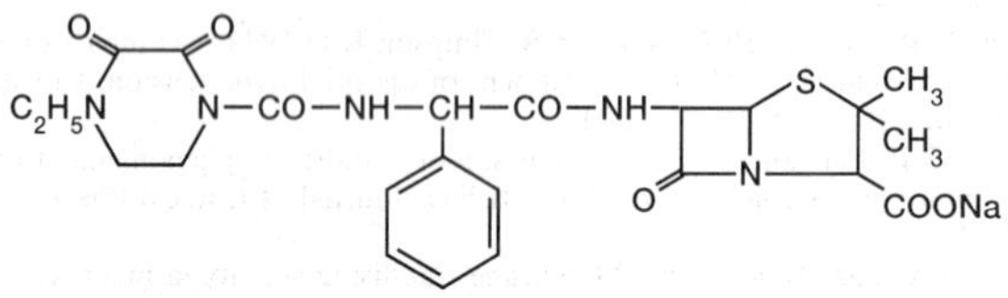

Molecular weight (free acid)	539.5 (517.6)
pKa	
Solubility	—
in alcohol	1 in 50
in water	—
Octanol/water partition coefficient	—

Piperacillin is a white crystalline powder, prepared by substituting 4-ethyl-2,3-dioxo-1-piperazinyl-carboxylic acid on the α-amino group of ampicillin. The compound is stable in the dried form, 90% of potency being maintained for 3 years at 15–30°C, but unstable in aqueous solution, 90% of potency being maintained for only 1 day at 25°C and pH 4.7.

Pharmacology

Piperacillin is an orally inactive semi-synthetic member of the penicillin family. The penicillin nucleus consists of a thiazolidine ring connected to a β-lactam ring to which is attached a side-chain. The side-chain determines most of the pharmacological and antibacterial properties of the penicillin in question. Penicillin kills bacteria by interfering in the synthesis of the bacterial cell wall. Piperacillin binds to penicillin binding proteins (PBPs) on the bacterial cell wall. It binds most strongly to PBPIII, thereby interfering with septum formation during cell division. Piperacillin also binds to PBPs Ia, Ib and II, thus interfering with peptidoglycan synthesis. Peptidoglycan is a heteropolymeric structure that provides the cell wall with mechanical stability. The final stage in the synthesis of peptidoglycan involves the completion of the cross linking and the terminal glycine residue of the pentaglycine bridge is linked to the fourth residue of the pentapeptide (d-alanine). The transpeptidase enzyme that performs this step is inhibited by penicillins and cephalosporins. As a result the bacterial cell wall is weakened, the cell swells and then ruptures.

Toxicology

Animal studies have shown that piperacillin exhibits the safety typical of all penicillins. Prolonged administration of piperacillin did not demonstrate clinically relevant adverse effects. A transient rise in serum enzymes has been noted in dogs.

No toxic effects on the proximal tubule of the kidney have been demonstrated. No teratological effects were seen in mice following administration of piperacillin before and during pregnancy. A slight decrease in fetal survival rate in rats was noted in association with the administration of three times the maximum recommended adult dose throughout pregnancy.

Clinical pharmacology

Piperacillin is a broad-spectrum antibiotic with particular uses for *Klebsiella* and *Pseudomonas* infections. Piperacillin is active against *Acinetobacter*, *Citrobacter*, *Enterobacter*, *Haemophilus influenzae*, *Klebsiella pneumoniae*, *Neisseria* spp., *Proteus* spp. (both indole-positive and indole-negative species), *Providencia* spp., *Pseudomonas aeruginosa*, *Serratia* sp. and *Shigella* spp. It is also active against certain anaerobic bacteria such as *Clostridia*, *Bacteroides fragilis*, and other *Bacteroides* spp., *Fusobacterium* sp. and *Peptococcus*. Among Gram-positive organisms, piperacillin is active against *Enterococci*, non β-lactamase producing *Staphylococci*, *Streptococcus pneumoniae* and *Strep. pyogenes*. Piperacillin has no other clinical pharmacological effect in man.

Pharmacokinetics

Concentrations of piperacillin in body fluids can be determined by the agar well method using *Bacillus subtilis* ATCC 6633 in spore suspension as test organism.[1] The sensitivity of the method is limited to 0.4 $mg.l^{-1}$. Specificity is 100%. Using a microbiological agar disc diffusion assay employing *Sarcina lutea* ATCC 9341 as the test organism, the sensitivity was 0.3 $mg.l^{-1}$.[2]

Piperacillin is poorly absorbed after oral administration, and thus can only be administered parenterally. After intramuscular administration the bioavailability of piperacillin is 70–80% (calculated as AUC i.m./AUC i.v.) with peak levels being reached within 30–50 min. Administration of piperacillin as a 15–30 min intravenous infusion produces peak serum levels of between 63.5 $mg.l^{-1}$ (2 g dose) and 450 $mg.l^{-1}$ (15 g dose).[3,4]

A property of piperacillin is its dose-dependent pharmacokinetics. Upon increasing dose sizes, initial serum concentrations, the 'area under the curve' and the serum half life increase more than in proportion to the dose increase.[1,5]

Apparent serum half lives increase from 36 min after 1 g intravenous dose to 63 min after a 6 g intravenous dose. However, a study of ill, bedridden patients showed a serum half life of 122 min following a 2 g intravenous dose. Serum half lives following intramuscular administration range from 60 min after a 0.5 g dose to 80 min after a 2 g dose.[1]

The apparent volume of distribution is between 16 and 24 l per 1.73 m^2. The serum protein binding is 16–22%. Piperacillin penetrates inflamed meninges well. Levels of piperacillin in the cerebrospinal fluid approximate 35% of those in serum.[6] Small amounts of piperacillin are excreted in breast milk. Levels of piperacillin in umbilical cord blood up to 75% of those in maternal blood have been found. Considerable amounts can be detected in amniotic fluid.

Oral absorption	poor
Presystemic metabolism	—
Plasma half life	
range	36–80 min
Volume of distribution	16–24 l/1.73 m^3
Plasma protein binding	16–22%

Piperacillin is excreted in the unchanged form by both renal (80%) and non-renal mechanisms. It is cleared by active tubular secretion in addition to glomerular filtration. 1 g of probenecid decreases the excretion rate of piperacillin, thereby increasing serum half life.[1] Non-renal clearance is through biliary excretion.[7] Concentrations of piperacillin in gallbladder and common duct bile of 30–60 times those in serum are reached.[8] Non-renal clearance is also affected by probenecid administration.[1] The serum half life of piperacillin increases to 2.6–3.9 h in patients with creatinine clearance <20 $ml.min^{-1}$.[9,10]

Concentration–effect relationship

Piperacillin is effective against a wide range of bacteria provided that the dose is high enough to exceed the minimum inhibitory concentration (MIC) for that organism.

Piperacillin (sodium)

Table 1 Total body clearance of piperacillin

	Renal (ml.min^{-1} per 1.73 m^2)	Non-renal (ml.min^{-1} per 1.73 m^2)
1 g i.v.	303.6	105.1
2 g i.v.	245.7	54.7
4 g i.v.	203.7	53.8
6 g i.v.	186.9	24.3
0.5 g i.m.	431.6	152.4
1 g i.m.	314.3	108.0
2 g i.m.	219.8	71.0

Metabolism

Piperacillin is excreted in the unchanged form both in bile and urine.

Pharmaceutics

Piperacillin, Pipril/Pipracil (Lederle, UK/USA) is available in parenteral forms only.

Vials containing 1 g, 2 g, 4 g and 6 g piperacillin sodium are available, though not in all countries. In some countries infusion bottles containing 3 g or 4 g of piperacillin as piperacillin sodium are available. Each g of piperacillin sodium contains 1.98 mEq (45.5 mg) of sodium.

For intravenous infusion each g of piperacillin should be reconstituted with at least 5 ml of Water for injection. The total dose should then be further diluted to at least 50 ml before infusion over 20–40 min. The major infusion fluids in common use are all compatible with piperacillin. Care must be taken with intravenous usage to avoid thrombophlebitis. Because of chemical instability, piperacillin should not be diluted with solutions containing only sodium bicarbonate. Piperacillin should not be added to blood products or protein hydrolysates.

Piperacillin is stable for at least 24 h at room temperature or 48 h at 4°C.

Piperacillin should not be mixed in the same solution with aminoglycosides and should be administered separately from any other drug unless compatibility is proven.[11]

For intramuscular injection each gram of piperacillin should be reconstituted with at least 2 ml of Water for injection or 0.5% lidocaine. Administration should be by deep intramuscular injection. A single dose in adults should not exceed 2 g. A single dose in children should not exceed 0.5 g.

Therapeutic use

Indications

1. Urinary tract infections
2. Respiratory tract infections
3. Abdominal infections
4. Septicaemia
5. Infections in immunocompromised patients
6. Meningitis
7. Bone and joint infections
8. Uncomplicated gonorrhoeal infections
9. Infections in paediatric patients.

Contraindications

1. Penicillin hypersensitivity or immediate type cephalosporin hypersensitivity.

Mode of use

In vitro activity

Piperacillin is a broad-spectrum penicillin with bactericidal activity against Gram-positive and Gram-negative aerobic and anaerobic bacteria. It is inactivated by β-lactamases of plasmidal origin. It has some resistance to chromosomally mediated β-lactamases.

Gram-positive bacteria

Piperacillin is not as active as penicillin against penicillin-sensitive staphylococci and not as active as the isoxazolylpenicillins (methicillin, oxacillin, cloxacillin, flucloxacillin) against penicillin-resistant staphylococci. It is inactive against methicillin-resistant staphylococci. *Streptococcus pneumoniae* and the β-haemolytic streptococci are very sensitive to piperacillin, but it is not considered to be the agent of first choice for these organisms. Activity against *Enterococcus faecalis* is fairly good but less than that of ampicillin or amoxycillin.[12–16]

Gram-negative facultatively aerobic rods, Enterobacteriaceae

Piperacillin has good activity against Enterobacteriaceae. On average, the level of its activity is as that of the other acylureidopenicillins and ticarcillin, or slightly higher. Because piperacillin is sensitive to β-lactamases it is not active against β-lactamase producing Enterobacteria. β-lactamase resistant cephalosporins, like latamoxef, cefotaxime and ceftazidime, and aminoglycosides are therefore more often active against enterobacteria than is piperacillin.[12,16,17]

Gram-negative aerobic rods, *Pseudomonas* spp

Piperacillin is more active against *Pseudomonas* species and *P. aeruginosa* than the other penicillins. It is also more effective than latamoxef and cefotaxime, but ceftazidime is slightly more active against *Pseudomonas* species than piperacillin.[13–15,18–20]

Other aerobic Gram-negative organisms, *Haemophilus* and *Neisseria* species

Piperacillin possesses marked activity against *Haemophilus influenzae* and *Neisseria gonorrhoeae* like latamoxef,[15] cefotaxime and ceftazidime, but becomes inactive when β-lactamase is produced. The cephalosporins, however, are not influenced by production of β-lactamase. *Neisseria meningitidis* is highly susceptible to piperacillin, as it is to latamoxef, cefotaxime and ceftazidime.

Anaerobic bacteria

Piperacillin is slightly more active than other penicillins against *Bacteroides* species but metronidazole, clindamycin and cefoxitin are considerably more active than piperacillin. Metronidazole is also more active against *Clostridium* species than piperacillin. Against anaerobic cocci clindamycin is the more active drug.[12]

Dosage

Dosage depends on the site and severity of the infection and the sensitivity of the bacteria. It varies between 100 and 200 mg.kg^{-1} daily.

Dosage should be reduced in patients with renal insufficiency. A suggested schedule is given in Table 2.

Table 2 Dosage in patients with renal insufficiency

Degree of renal impairment	Creatinine clearance ml.min^{-1}	Maximum daily maintenance dose/g	Dosage schedule
Mild impairment	40–80	16	4 g/6 h
Moderate impairment	20–40	12	4 g/8 h
Severe impairment	20	8	4 g/12 h
Haemodialysis		6	2 g/8 h

Duration of therapy ranges from 3 to 14 days on average. It is dependent upon the clinical and bacteriological course of the infection. It should be continued for at least 3 to 4 days after the patient becomes asymptomatic.

Indications

1. Urinary tract infections

High levels of piperacillin in the urine are achieved. In uncomplicated infections clinical response rates of 74–90% are reported, in complicated infections response rates range from 38% to 85%. Bacteriological response rates range from 33% (with *Serratia marcescens*) to 88% in *E. coli* and indole-positive *Proteus* infections, depending further on other factors such as indwelling catheters and time of assessment of response.

Piperacillin as a single agent can be effective in the treatment of urinary tract infections but comparative studies are lacking to assess its exact place in the treatment of these infections.[3,12,21–23]

2. Respiratory tract infections

Piperacillin is an effective drug in the treatment of lower respiratory tract infections, particularly those caused by *H. influenzae* and

Streptococcus pneumoniae, but good results have also been achieved in infections caused by Gram-negative aerobic rods.[24] In a comparative trial on patients with lower respiratory tract infections, including chronic infections but not cystic fibrosis, clinical response was better in patients treated with piperacillin than in those treated with ampicillin (81.5% and 64% clinical response rates respectively in acute infections, 67.5% and 47% respectively in chronic infections).[25]

Failures are more common in *Pseudomonas* infections, chronic disease states, lung abscess or empyema and infections by hospital-acquired micro-organisms.[3,12,21,23]

Cystic fibrosis. Piperacillin as a single agent is not very effective in treating the pulmonary infections in cystic fibrosis patients.[21] In a comparative trial with two penicillins and five cephalosporins the best results were achieved by ceftazidime, followed by cefsulodin. Piperacillin and cefoperazone gave intermediate results.[26]

In another study, addition of tobramycin to piperacillin improved clinical response rates from 4 out of 7 to 7 out of 7 in paediatric cystic fibrosis patients given the combination.[19]

3. Abdominal infections

Abdominal infections are usually polymicrobial in origin, with aerobic and anaerobic micro-organisms. Clinical response rates to piperacillin therapy were near 90% in gynaecological infections and between 70% and 90% in intra-abdominal sepsis.[27] In these studies failures were mostly due to lack of adequate surgical drainage, only rarely due to persistence of resistant bacteria.

In one comparative study piperacillin scored as well as cefoxitin in treating intra-abdominal infections due to perforations of the gastro-intestinal tract and acute peritonitis (91% and 92% response rates respectively).[28]

Because of the high levels of piperacillin achieved in the bile, it can be effective in treating infections of the biliary tract.[12]

4. Septicaemia

Clinical cure rates varied between 60% and 90% in different studies on patients with various types of septicaemia. Doses varied widely and sometimes an aminoglycoside was used concomitantly. Failures were largely due to serious underlying conditions.[3,12,21]

5. Infections in immunocompromised patients

Piperacillin as a single agent should not be given to immunocompromised patients, suspected of having an infection. Combination with an aminoglycoside is imperative in these instances. Comparative trials are therefore performed using combination therapy. Piperacillin combined with amikacin in one study gave an equivalent response rate (76%) as cefotaxime plus amikacin (78%) in leukaemic patients.[29] Piperacillin with netilmicin scored as well as latamoxef with netilmicin (82% and 84% response rates respectively) in another study.[30] In two studies by Wade et al piperacillin plus amikacin gave better results than ticarcillin plus amikacin. However, in a study by Winston et al no difference in response rates was found between the combination piperacillin plus amikacin and that of carbenicillin plus amikacin.

To avoid the toxicity of the aminoglycosides comparative studies were performed with double β-lactam combinations. Latamoxef in combination with amikacin gave about equal results as latamoxef plus piperacillin while toxicity was reduced.[31] Another study done by de Jongh et al with the same antibiotics gave equal results.[32]

Overall response rates for the combinations of piperacillin with another antibiotic have averaged 74% in granulocytopenic patients.

6. Meningitis

Piperacillin penetrates inflamed meninges well.[6] Not many studies are known in which piperacillin was evaluated for therapy in meningitis. *Pneumococci* and *H. influenzae* are sensitive to piperacillin and the few patients treated with this antibiotic for meningitis due to these organisms were cured, but it is not likely that it will become the drug of choice in these instances.

Piperacillin might find a place in the therapy for Gram-negative meningitis. In the few instances where it was used for meningitis due to *Pseudomonas aeruginosa* or *E. coli* results were satisfactory. However, no comparative trials have been published yet.

7. Bone and joint infections

Piperacillin was found to achieve satisfactory concentrations in bone tissue. Clinical cure rates of 84–87% and bacteriological eradication rates of 75% are reported in bone and joint infections.[3,12,23,33]

Piperacillin (sodium)

8. Uncomplicated gonorrhoeal infections

Piperacillin plus probenecid was found satisfactory in the treatment of uncomplicated gonorrhoeal infections caused by non-penicillinase producing gonococci (95–100% cure rates) but no advantage over penicillin plus probenecid was demonstrated.

Piperacillin cannot be relied upon in infections by penicillinase-producing *N. gonorrhoeae*.[12]

9. Infections in paediatric patients

In the few trials where piperacillin was used to treat infections in children good results were achieved and no specific adverse reactions in this age group were encountered.

Adverse reactions

Potentially life-threatening effects

Potentially lethal effects of piperacillin have not been described so far, but when administered to patients allergic to penicillin and/or cephalosporins anaphylactic reactions can be expected, as with all other penicillins.

Acute overdosage

No cases of overdosage with piperacillin have been described.

Severe or irreversible adverse effects

Adverse effects of piperacillin are similar to those of other penicillins. None is severe or irreversible, except those described under Potentially life-threatening effects.

Prolongation of bleeding time has occurred rarely.

Symptomatic adverse effects

Piperacillin is usually well tolerated. Thrombophlebitis has occurred in about 4% of patients treated with piperacillin intravenously. It can be minimized by adequate dilution of the piperacillin solution.

Pain at the injection site following intramuscular administration can be minimized by reconstituting the drug with 0.5% lignocaine.

In about 4% of patients vomiting, nausea, loose stools and/or diarrhoea have occurred.

Other effects

Reversible leucopenia has occurred in 4% of patients, eosinophilia in 5–6%. Transient elevations of hepatic enzymes have been observed in 2.3% of the patients.

Electrolyte and fluid disturbances can occur during piperacillin therapy. Since piperacillin is a monosodium salt (1.98 mEq Na^+ per g^{-1}) these adverse effects should be less frequent than during ticarcillin (5.2 mEq Na^+ per g) or carbenicillin (4.7 mEq Na^+ per g) use (as was indeed found in a study by Winston et al (see Clinical trials). However, no difference in the occurrence of hypokalaemia was found between patients receiving ticarcillin plus amikacin (15%) and patients receiving piperacillin plus amikacin (16%) in one study (see Clinical trials).

Only rarely were serum creatinine levels raised during piperacillin use. Renal toxicity is otherwise unknown as an adverse effect of piperacillin.

Interference with clinical pathology tests

A positive Coombs' test is sometimes found during piperacillin therapy.

High risk groups

Neonates

The only experience of using piperacillin in neonates so far published is a study in which six neonates were treated with the combination of piperacillin plus flucloxacillin during the first 48 h of life. No serious adverse effects were recorded.

Breast milk. Small amounts of the drug are secreted in breast milk, and it is probably best for mothers taking it to avoid breast-feeding as there is a possibility of sensitizing the infant, though no other adverse effects are likely.

Children

Though not used extensively in children, piperacillin did not cause serious adverse effects in those that were treated it.

Pregnant women

It is not yet known whether the drug is safe to use during pregnancy.

The elderly
No special precautions are required when the drug is used in elderly patients.

Drug interactions

Potentially hazardous interactions
No potentially hazardous interactions with other drugs are known.

Other significant interactions

Aminoglycosides. An interaction between aminoglycosides and piperacillin, resulting in inactivation of the aminoglycoside, has been observed.[11,37] It is generally accepted that this inactivation is clinically significant in patients with poor renal function in whom excretion of the drug is delayed, or when both drugs are mixed in the same infusion bottle, but Konishi[7] also found the interaction in healthy volunteers using tobramycin with carbenicillin, ticarcillin and piperacillin. The maximum serum concentration of tobramycin when used with piperacillin was reduced by approximately 11% (compared with 33% and 26% when mixed with carbenicillin and ticarcillin respectively).

Potentially useful interactions

Aminoglycosides. Results of in vitro synergism testing have been variable. Several studies showed synergy between piperacillin and an aminoglycoside against 36–100% of the bacterial strains, depending on the bacterial species tested.[34–36] Antagonism between piperacillin and aminoglycosides has also been observed, possibly due to the inactivation of the aminoglycosides by piperacillin.

Cephalosporins. Synergistic activity between piperacillin and cephalosporins has been reported.[19,34,35] Piperacillin combined with latamoxef was reported to be synergistic, as was the combination of piperacillin and cefoperazone in a small percentage of strains tested. However, indifference and antagonistic action were observed in several other studies, for example, the combination of cefoxitin and piperacillin showed evidence of antagonism in vitro, as did the combination of latamoxef and piperacillin against *Enterobacter cloacae* and *Proteus mirabilis*.

Probenecid. Probenecid blocks the renal tubular secretion of piperacillin, thereby slowing its clearance. Peak serum concentrations of piperacillin and the serum half life increased by 30% when 1 g of probenecid was given orally before administration of piperacillin.

Major outcome trials

1. Winston D J, Murphy W, Young L S, Hewitt W L 1980 Piperacillin therapy for serious bacterial infections. The American Journal of Medicine 69: 255–261

This is a prospective study of 59 patients in severely compromised condition (48% with a rapidly fatal underlying disease, 52% in critical or poor condition and 63% with renal failure) with serious bacterial infections. Piperacillin as single-agent therapy was evaluated in these patients. Piperacillin was used at a dosage of 200–300 mg.kg^{-1} daily intravenously, or adjusted to renal function.

The overall response rate (clinical and bacteriological) was 89%. Treatment failures only occurred in patients with rapidly or ultimately fatal diseases, superinfections occurred in five patients, all were severely immunosuppressed. In three organisms (two *Pseudomonas aeruginosa* strains, one *Serratia marcescens*) resistance developed during piperacillin therapy. No serious side effects occurred.

The authors conclude that piperacillin as a single agent can be a useful drug in the therapy of serious bacterial infections. However, because of the possibility of the emergence of resistant strains one must be cautious, especially in immunocompromised patients.

2. Wade J C, Schimpff S C, Newman K A, Fortner C L, Standiford H C, Wiernik P H 1981 Piperacillin or ticarcillin plus amikacin, a double-blind prospective comparison of empiric antibiotic therapy for febrile granulocytopenic cancer patients. American Journal of Medicine 71: 983–990

This is a double-blind prospective comparative study on the efficacy of piperacillin plus amikacin (P+A) versus ticarcillin plus amikacin (T+A) in 121 infections in 92 febrile (38.3°C), granulocytopenic (1000 granulocytes.l^{-1}) patients.

Of the 34 evaluable infections in the T+A group, 19 (56%) improved, compared to 22 (58%) of 38 evaluable infections in the P+A group. There was no difference in the occurrence of superinfections between the two groups. However, patients in the T+A group acquired more Gram-negative bacteria resistant to the penicillin in their routine surveillance cultures than those in the P+A group. Despite the difference in sodium content of the two penicillins, no difference was found in the occurrence of hypokalaemia between the two groups of patients.

The authors conclude that although piperacillin has a wider in vitro antibacterial spectrum than ticarcillin, the clinical efficacy and toxicity of the combination of piperacillin plus amikacin were similar to those of ticarcillin plus amikacin.

3. Winston D J, Ho W G, Young L S, Hewitt W L, Gale R P 1982 Piperacillin plus amikacin therapy v. carbenicillin plus amikacin therapy in febrile, granulocytopenic patients. Archives of Internal Medicine 142: 1663–1667

This is a prospective randomized comparative study on the efficacy of piperacillin plus amikacin (P+A) versus carbenicillin and amikacin (C+A) in 297 infections in 244 febrile (38°C), granulocytopenic (1000 granulocytes.mm^{-3}) patients.

The overall response rates were 79% for the P+A group and 75% for the C+A group, even though significantly more Gram-negative bacilli isolated from initial cultures were susceptible to piperacillin than to carbenicillin. Hypokalaemia was found less often in the P+A group in this study (26 or 143 versus 56 of 154).

The authors conclude that the overall efficacy of piperacillin plus amikacin is similar to carbenicillin plus amikacin and that piperacillin plus amikacin may be associated with less hypokalaemia.

General review articles

Fortner C L, Finley R S, Schimpff S C 1982 Piperacillin sodium: antibacterial spectrum, pharmacokinetics, clinical efficacy, and adverse reactions. Pharmacotherapy 2: 287–299

Beran T 1981 Overview of acylureidopenicillin pharmacokinetics. Scandinavian Journal of Infectious Diseases (suppl 29): 81–86

Klastersky J 1982 Treatment of severe infections in patients with cancer. The role of new acyl-penicillins. Archives of Internal Medicine 142: 1984–1987

Eliopoulos G M, Moellering R C 1982 Azlocillin, Mezlocillin and Piperacillin: New broad-spectrum penicillins. Annals of Internal Medicine 97: 755–760

References

1. Tjandramaga T B, Mullie A, Verbesselt R, de Schepper P J, Verbist L 1978 Piperacillin: human pharmacokinetics after intravenous and intramuscular administration. Antimicrobial Agents and Chemotherapy 14: 829–837
2. Marlin G E, Burgess K R et al 1901 Penetration of piperacillin into bronchial mucosa and sputum. Thorax 36: 774–780
3. Drusano G L, Schimpff S C, Hewitt W L 1984 The acylampicillins: mezlocillin, piperacillin and azlocillin. Reviews of Infectious Diseases 6: 13–32
4. Meyers B R, Hirschman S Z, Strougo L, Srulevitch E 1980 Comparative study of piperacillin, ticarcillin and carbenicillin pharmacokinetics. Antimicrobial Agents and Chemotherapy 17: 608–611
5. Bergan T, Williams J D 1982 Dose dependence of piperacillin pharmacokinetics. Chemotherapy 28: 153–195
6. Dickinson G M, Draller D G, Greenman R L, Hoffman T A 1981 Clinical evaluation of piperacillin with observations on penetrability into cerebrospinal fluid. Antimicrobial Agents and Chemotherapy 20: 481–486
7. Giron J A, Meyers B R, Hirschman S Z 1981 Biliary concentrations of piperacillin in patients undergoing cholecystectomy. Antimicrobial Agents and Chemotherapy 19: 309–311
8. Russo J, Thompson M I B, Russo M E, Saxon B A, Matsen J M, Moody F G, Rikkers L F 1982 Piperacillin distribution into bile, gallbladder wall, abdominal skeletal muscle, and adipose tissue in surgical patients. Antimicrobial Agents and Chemotherapy 22: 488–492
9. Giron J A, Meyers B R, Hirshman S Z, Srulevitch E 1981 Pharmacokinetics of piperacillin in patients with moderate renal failure and in patients undergoing hemodialysis. Antimicrobial Agents and Chemotherapy 19: 279–238
10. Welling P G, Craig W A, Bundtzen R W, Kwok F W, Gerber A U, Madsen P O 1983 Pharmacokinetics of piperacillin in subjects with various degrees of renal function. Antimicrobial Agents and Chemotherapy 23: 881–887
11. Konishi H, Goto M, Nakamoto Y, Yamamoto I, Yamashina H 1983 Tobramycin inactivation by carbenicillin, ticarcillin and piperacillin. Antimicrobial Agents and Chemotherapy 23: 653–657
12. Holmes B, Richards D M, Brogden R N, Heel R C 1984 Piperacillin. A review of its antibacterial activity, pharmacokinetic properties and therapeutic use. Drugs 28: 375–425
13. White G W, Malow J B, Zimelis V H, Pahlavanzadeh H, Pamvalker A P, Jackson G G 1973 Comparative in vitro activity of azlocillin, ampicillin, mezlocillin, piperacillin and ticarcillin. Alone and in combination with an aminoglycoside. Antimicrobial Agents and Chemotherapy 15: 550–543

14. Machka K, Dickert H, Braveny I 1980 In vitro activity of piperacillin compared with that of ampicillin, ticarcillin, azlocilin and mezlocillin. Arzneimittel Forschung/Drug Research 30 (I): 304–307
15. Reimer L G, Mirrett S, Reller L B 1980 Comparison of in vitro activity against moxalactam (LY 127 935) with cefaxolin, amikacin, tobramycin, carbenicillin, piperacillin and ticarcillin against 420 blood culture isolates. Antimicrobial Agents and Chemotherapy 17: 412–416
16. Reeves D S, Path F R C 1982 In vitro activity of piperacillin and other microbials on 491 bacterial isolates. Archives of Internal Medicine 142: 2023–2032
17. Gordon R C, Tack K J, Haddy R I, Fechner L, Wofford R 1984 Antibiotic susceptibility of community hospital blood culture isolates of gram-negative bacilli. Chemotherapy 30: 40–43
18. Sobel J D, Levison M E, Kaye D 1980 Comparison of mezlocillin, piperacillin, Bay K 4999 with carbenicillin and ticarcillin against Enterobacteriaceae and *Pseudomonas aeruginosa*. Infection 8: 121–122
19. Hoogkamp-Korstanje J A A, Westerdaal N A C 1982 Activity and synergy of ureido penicillins and aminoglycosides against *Pseudomonas aeruginosa*. Infection 10 (suppl 3): S247–S261
20. Norrby R 1981 Current status of *Pseudomonas* infections and antibiotics. Scandinavian Journal of Infectious Diseases (suppl) 29: 81–86
21. Pancoast S, Prince A S, Francke E L, Neu H C 1981 Clinical evaluation of piperacillin therapy for infection. Archives of Internal Medicine 141: 1447–1450
22. Lutz B, Mogabgab W, Holmes B, Pollock B, Beville R 1982 Clinical evaluation of the therapeutic efficacy and tolerability of piperacillin. Antimicrobial Agents and Chemotherapy 22: 10–14
23. Eron L J, Goldenberg R I, Poretz D M, Park C H 1983 Piperacillin therapy for *Pseudomonas* infections. Southern Medical Journal 76: 859–862
24. Valenti S, Crimi P, Scordamaglia A 1983 The use of piperacillin in bacterial infections of the respiratory system. Current Therapeutic Research 33: 745–750
25. Nakagawa K, Kabe J, Watanabe K, Kihara N, Koyama M, Kato Y 1978 Comparative test of the effectiveness of T 1220 (piperacillin) and ampicillin on respiratory tract infection by double blind method. Chemotherapy 26: 124–166
26. Agostini M, Barlocco G, Bonomi U et al 1983 Alternative antibiotica against *Pseudomonas* infections in cystic fibrosis. In vitro activity, pharmacokinetics and double-blind randomized clinical trial with azlocillin, piperacillin, cefoperazone, ceftazidime, cefsulodin, cefotaxime and moxalactam. Preliminary results. Drugs under Experimental and Clinical Research 9: 671–686
27. Privitera G, Scalambrino S, Ortisi G, Milani R, Mangioni C, Morini M 1983 Clinical evaluation of piperacillin in the treatment of severe infections in obstetrics and gynaecology. Current Therapeutic Research 33: 881–885
28. Najem A Z, Kaminski Z S, Spillert C R, Lazaro E J 1983 Comparative study of parental piperacillin and cefoxitin in the treatment of surgical infections of the abdomen. Surgery, Gynaecology and Obstetrics 157: 423–425
29. Duprez P, Michaux Y L 1982 Piperacillin or cefotaxime plus amikacin: results of empirical antibiotic therapy for febrile episodes in granulocytopenic patients. In: Periti, Grassi, (eds) Current chemotherapy and immunotherapy. Proceedings of the 12th International Congress of Chemotherapy. American Society for Microbiology, pp 699–700
30. Wade J C, Schimpff S, Newman K A, Fortner C L, Standiford H C, Young V, Wiernik P 1980 Piperacillin, moxalactam or ticarcillin plus amikacin: double blind comparisons of emperic antibiotic therapy for febrile granulocytopenic patients. Program and Abstracts 20th Interscience Conference of Antimicrobial Agents and Chemotherapy no 485. New Orleans Sept 22–24
31. Barnes R C, Winston D J, Ho W G, Yang L, Hewitt W, Champlin R E, Gale R P 1982 Comparative efficacy and toxicity of moxalactam/piperacillin versus moxalactam/amikacin in febrile granulocytopenic patients. Program and Abstracts 22nd Interscience Conference of Antimicrobial Agents and Chemotherapy. Miami Beach, p 66
32. Jongh C de, Joshi J, Newman K et al 1982 Moxalactam plus piperacillin or amikacin: empiric antibiotic therapy for febrile neutropenic cancer patients. Program and Abstracts 22nd Interscience Conference of Antimicrobial Agents and Chemotherapy. Miami Beach, p 233
33. Thadepalli H, Rao B, White D, Bach V T 1980 Clinical evaluation of piperacillin. Chemotherapy 26: 377–383
34. Chanbusarakum P, Murray P R 1978 Analysis of the Interactions between piperacillin, ticarcillin or carbenicillin and aminoglycoside antibiotics. Antimicrobial Agents and Chemotherapy 14: 505–506
35. Daschner F, Langmaack H, Grehn M, Steffens A, Just M 1981 Combination effect of piperacillin with four aminoglycosides on nonfermenting Gram-negative bacteria. Chemotherapy 27: 39–43
36. Hoogkamp-Korstanje J A A, Laag J van der 1983 Piperacillin and tobramycin in the treatment of Pseudomonas lung infections in cystic fibrosis. Journal of Antimicrobial Chemotherapy 12: 175–183
37. Thompson M I B, Russo M E, Saxon B J, Atkin-Thor E, Matsen J M 1982 Gentamicin inactivation by piperacillin or carbenicillin in patients with end-stage renal disease. Antimicrobial Agents and Chemotherapy 21: 268–273

Piperazine

Piperazine is very effective for the treatment of ascariasis and enterobiasis. It does not have any significant action against other nematodes that infest man.

Chemistry

Piperazine (citrate, phosphate or hexahydrate) (Antepar, Helmezine)
$C_4H_{10}N_2$
Diethylenediamine

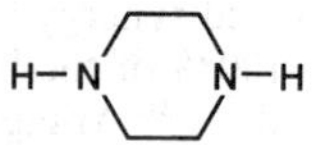

Molecular weight (hydrate)	86.14 (194.2)
pKa	4.2
Solubility	
in alcohol (hydrate)	1 in 10–1 in 30 (1 in 1)
in water	1 in 10–1 in 30
Hydrate Octanol/water partition coefficient	0.06

Piperazine citrate: fine, white, almost odourless, granular powder with an acid taste.
Piperazine phosphate: white, odourless, crystalline powder, with slightly acid taste.
Piperazine hydrate: colourless, glassy, crystals with faint characteristic odour and saline taste that liquefy upon exposure to moisture.
Pripsen (Westminster, Reckitt & Colman Pharmaceuticals) is the name of a fixed combination product of piperazine phosphate and sennosides.

Pharmacology

Piperazine acts in mammalian tissues to increase the tone of isolated smooth muscle. In addition, a dose-dependent contraction of isolated smooth muscle is produced. These effects appear to be mediated by muscarinic cholinergic receptors, since the effects are blocked by atropine.[1] These effects are however only seen at relatively high doses of piperazine (10^{-4}M). In frogs, piperazine produces an initial increase in muscular activity, but this is followed by a two-stage blockade, firstly on neuromuscular transmission and then later, directly on muscle. This later effect has been likened to the effect of tubocurarine on mammalian smooth muscle.

The predominant effect of piperazine in helminths such as *Ascaris lumbricoides* is to cause a flaccid paralysis of the worm that results in the worm being expelled from the gut by normal peristaltic activity.[2] This paralysis is reversible, since the worm recovers if placed in a drug-free medium. Acetylcholine causes a contraction of smooth muscle in *Ascaris* and this effect is blocked competitively by piperazine. Piperazine seems to alter the permeability of the cell wall to ions that are responsible for the maintenance of the resting potential. The differing effects in mammalian and helminth tissues seem to be due to fundamental differences in the myoneural receptors in the two species.[2]

Toxicology

Piperazine has very low toxicity in mammals, and in the doses used clinically there is no specific organ damage or general toxicity. No adequate teratogenicity studies have been conducted but one-dose studies did not produce evidence of fetal malformation in the rat and rabbit. No carcinogenicity tests have been performed.

Clinical pharmacology

In the doses used clinically piperazine has very little effect on the human organs. It may stimulate gastrointestinal motion or sometimes cause tremors as a result of central nervous stimulation. Very occasionally CNS stimulation may result in ataxia or choreiform movements particularly if the patient also has renal impairment.

The main action of the drug is to cause flaccid paralysis of *Ascaris* and *Enterobius spp.* so that the worms can be expelled from the gut during normal faecal excretion.

Pharmacokinetics

The preferred analytical method of urinary levels of piperazine is by gas chromatography.[3] The sensitivity is 50 $mg.l^{-1}$.

The absorption from the gastrointestinal tract is rapid but variable. Between 5–30% of the total single dose is found in the urine as piperazine within the first 24 hours.

No data are available on half life, volume of distribution, plasma protein binding and tissue distribution.

Concentration–effect relationship

There is no data to link therapeutic effect with plasma levels, and monitoring of blood levels is not needed.

Metabolism

No detailed studies have been done on the metabolism of piperazine. N-Mononitrosopiperazine has been found in the stomach and urine of volunteers,[4] while the dinitroso derivative which is a carcinogen, has not been detected in gastric juice, blood or urine. No data are available on whether the metabolites are active.

Pharmaceutics

Piperazine is available as yellow scored chewable tablets from Wellcome, UK (with 'Antepar' embossed on one side) each containing piperazine phosphate BP equivalent to 500 mg piperazine hydrate, and the elixir contains piperazine hydrate BP and piperazine citrate BP in a stable combination (equivalent to 750 mg piperazine per 5 ml). The tablets contain tartrazine which may be potentially allergenic. 'Helmezine' tablets (Allen and Hanburys) contain 260 mg piperazine phosphate. 'Helmezine' elixir contains 550 mg piperazine citrate in each 4 ml.

The tablets and elixir should be protected from light. Both have a shelf-life of 5 years.

Piperazine and the anthelmintic pyrantel are mutually antagonistic.

Therapeutic use

Indications

Piperazine is used for the treatment of infestations with *Ascaris lumbricoides* and *Enterobius vermicularis* (pinworm).

Contraindications

Piperazine is contraindicated in epileptic patients because of the possibility that the drug may induce neurotoxic effects[5] of a transitory nature. Therefore the drug should be used cautiously in patients with impaired renal and hepatic functions[6,7] because they will be more likely to suffer from these side effects. Furthermore, piperazine tablets should not be given to individuals who are known to be allergic to tartrazine, an inactive constituent of 'Antepar' chewable tablets.

Mode of use

Piperazine can be given any time of the day and no fasting period is required. When tablets are given these should preferably be chewed before swallowing.

Ascariasis

A single dose is usually sufficient to treat ascariasis; the worm(s) will be expelled by normal defaecation, flaccidly paralysed. A dose of 75 $mg.kg^{-1}$ bodyweight with a maximum of 3.5 g can be given as a single dose; some authorities advocate a two-day treatment to improve cure rate. Children should be given the same regimen.

Piperazine

Enterobiasis

A 7-day treatment is required for elimination of *Enterobius*. This is partly due to the lesser sensitivity of the drug against the larval stages, and the easy transmittability among family members. Furthermore autoinfection is common with pinworm infestation. Therefore strict measures of hygiene are required in order to minimize reinfection. The anal orifice may be covered with a tape when the patient retires at night to prevent eggs from being spilled in bed when the mature female worm creeps out of the anus. The tape may be removed in the morning and the perianal skin and also the finger nail beds should be cleaned with copious water.

The dose is 65 $mg.kg^{-1}$ body weight with a maximum of 2.5 g given as a single dose for 7 consecutive days. The cure rate on this regimen is about 95–100%.

Adverse reactions

Potentially life-threatening effects

Piperazine in usual recommended doses is a safe drug. Neurotoxicity is rare, but one death has occurred in a child with epilepsy given piperazine. The principal manifestations of piperazine neurotoxicity include ataxia, muscle hypotonia, clonic convulsions, somnolence, and impaired consciousness. In general, withdrawal of the drug will result in recovery without sequellae.

Acute overdosage

No reports of acute overdosage have been published. In the event of poisoning, the most likely symptoms will be convulsion with coma. Treatment with diazepam or another anticonvulsant drug would seem to be the best approach to management.

Severe or irreversible adverse effects

With the exception of those already discussed no reactions of this degree of severity have been reported.

Symptomatic adverse effects

Rarely, gastrointestinal upset accompanies piperazine intake, and allergic reactions such as urticaria may be seen. Neurological adverse effects mentioned above seem dose-dependent and are often the result of aggravation of a pre-existing disease.

Single case reports of purpura,[8] acute hepatitis,[9] and acute haemolysis in a G-6-PD-deficient individual[10] have appeared in the literature.

Interference with clinical pathology tests

Piperazine interferes with the estimation of serum uric acid.

High risk groups

Neonates

The drug is not given to neonates.

Breast milk. No information is available on the presence of piperazine in breast milk, so mothers taking the drug should not breast-feed.

Children

The use of piperazine in children does not differ from the mode of use in adults. Often they are involved in mass treatment of schoolchildren and in this case they will most likely receive a fixed dose not adjusted to their body weights, resulting in higher or lower doses for some. There is no special risk when the drug is given to this age-group, except that unnecessarily high doses may precipitate neurotoxicity.

Pregnant women

Piperazine has been given to pregnant women without ill effect. Although piperazine is not contraindicated in pregnancy it would be quite acceptable to postpone treatment until after delivery, unless there is a real urgency for immediate treatment.

The elderly

Renal, hepatic, and central nervous system impairment are quite common in elderly patients, and therefore the drug should be used cautiously in these patients.

Concurrent disease

As mentioned earlier, the drug should be avoided in epileptics, and used cautiously in those with renal or hepatic disease.

Drug interactions

Potentially hazardous interactions

Care should be taken in administration of piperazine to patients receiving phenothiazines as it has been suggested that a high blood concentration of piperazine potentiates the extrapyramidal effects of chlorpromazine in man.[11]

Other significant interactions

Bephenium and pyrantel may antagonize the activity of piperazine on *Ascaris* preparations in vitro.[12]

Potentially useful interactions

It is controversial whether laxatives will interact favourably by expelling the paralysed worm from the colon, but perhaps this may be beneficial only when there is constipation. Fixed combination preparations containing senna give high cure rates in single doses, although no controlled studies have been done to compare its relative efficacy.

Major outcome trials

1. Goodwin L G, Standen O D 1958 Treatment of ascariasis with various salts of piperazine. British Medical Journal 1: 131–133

This paper discusses two trials carried out in Gambia on a total of 770 schoolchildren where piperazine was used to treat ascariasis. In the first trial different salts of piperazine were compared; they were the citrate, adipate, phosphate, sebacate, and stearate. The drug was given as a single oral dose equivalent to 3 or 4 g piperazine hexahydrate. Cure as measured by the total absence of eggs in the stools, varied from 76 to 89%; the higher rates were for the 4 g dose. No significant difference was shown among the various salts used.

The second part of the trial compared piperazine citrate in tablet and syrup form in a dose equivalent to 4 g piperazine hexahydrate. Cure rates were between 84 and 88% and thus showed no difference between the treatment groups. Also there was no difference in the results when the drug was freshly prepared or was stored under high temperature (50°C for 6 months). Only two cases of nausea and vomiting were reported.

2. Brown H W, Chan K F, Hussey K L 1956 Treatment of enterobiasis and ascariasis with piperazine. Journal of the American Medical Association 161: 515–520

Sixty patients weighing from 18.5 to 72 kg with pinworm infestation were treated with piperazine citrate for seven days with a daily dose of 1 and 2 g as the hexahydrate form. Cure rate was 97%. Extending the course of treatment to 10–14 days did not alter the outcome.

Ascariasis was treated in 46 patients with a single dose of piperazine citrate. The doses used were 2, 3 and 3.5 g depending on the body weight. One-day treatment cured 74%, but when a two-day regimen was used the cure rate was 94%.

References

1. Mason P A, Sturman G 1972 Some pharmacological properties of piperazine. British Journal of Pharmacology 44: 169–176
2. Saz H J, Bueding E 1966 Relationship between anthelmintic effects and biochemical and physiological mechanisms. Pharmacology Review 18: 871–894
3. Fletcher K A, Evans D A P, Kelly J A 1982 Urinary piperazine excretion in healthy caucasians. Annals of Tropical Medicine and Parasitology 76: 77–82
4. Bellander T, Osterdahl B G, Hagmar L 1985 Formation of N-mononitrosopiperazine in the stomach and its excretion in the urine after oral intake of piperazine. Toxicology and Applied Pharmacology 80: 193–198
5. Berger J R, Globus M, Melamed E 1979 Acute transitory cerebellar dysfunction associated with piperazine adipate. Archives of Neurology 36: 180–181
6. Graf W, Haldimann B, Flury W 1978 Piperazinintoxikation bei Langzeithämodialyse. Schweizerische Medizinische Wochenschrift 108: 177–181
7. Belloni C, Rizzoni G 1967 Neurotoxic side effects of piperazine. Lancet 2: 369
8. Shanker A, Gulati J 1960 Purpura after administration of piperazine. British Medical Journal 1: 1622
9. Hamlyn A N, Morris J S, Sarkany I, Sherlock S 1976 Piperazine hepatitis. Gastroenterology 70: 1144–1147
10. Buchanan N, Cassel R, Jenkins T 1971 G-6-PD deficiency and piperazine. British Medical Journal 2: 110
11. Sturman G 1974 Interaction between piperazine and chlorpromazine. British Journal of Pharmacology 50: 153–155
12. Aubry M L, Cowell P, Davey M J et al 1970 Aspects of the pharmacology of a new antihelmintic: pyrantel. British Journal of Pharmacology 38: 332–344
13. Report of a WHO Expert Committee on Control of Ascariasis 1967 Technical Report Series 379
14. Greenberg G L, Gilman R H, Shapiro H et al 1981 Single dose piperazine therapy for *Ascaris lumbricoides*: an unsuccessful method to promote growth. American Journal of Clinical Nutrition 34: 2508–2516
15. Gupta M C, Urrutia J J 1982 Effect of periodic antiascaris and antigiardia treatment on nutritional status of preschool children. American Journal of Clinical Nutrition 36: 79–86
16. Messer J, Solano C, Romeu J, Dave P B 1984 An unusual case of obstructive jaundice. American Journal of Gastroenterology 79: 152–153
17. Schulman A 1977 Biliary ascariasis presenting in the United States. American Journal of Gastroenterology 68: 167–170
18. Mathies A W, Burlington V T 1961 Enterobis Vermicularis infection: certain aspects of the host-parasite relationship. American Journal of Diseases in Children 101: 174–177

P

Pipothiazine

Pipothiazine is a phenothiazine with general properties similar to those of chlorpromazine. Pipothiazine palmitate and undecenoate are esters of pipothiazine.

Chemistry

Pipothiazine (Pipothiazine, Piportil)
$C_{24}H_{33}N_3O_3S_2$
10-{3-[4-(2-Hydroxyethyl)piperidino]propyl}-NN-dimethylphenothiazine-2-sulphonamide

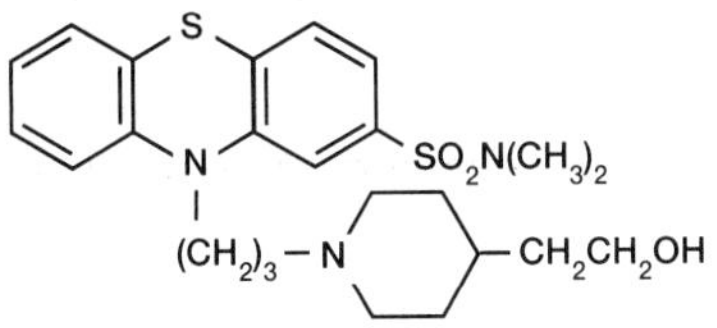

Pipothiazine palmitate (Pipotiazine Palmitate, Piportil Depot)
$C_{40}H_{63}N_3O_4S_2$

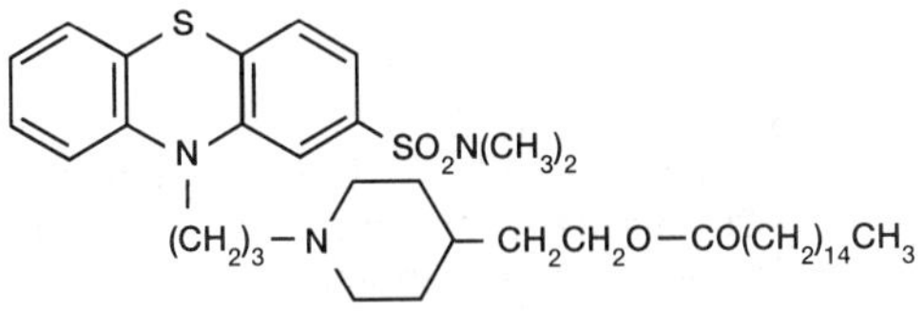

Molecular weight of palmitate	714.1
(free compound)	(475.7)
pKa	—
Solubility	
in alcohol	1 in 100
in water	<1 in 10 000
Octanol/water partition coefficient	—

Pipothiazine undecenoate (Pipotiazine Undecenoate, Pipothiazine Undecylenate)
$C_{35}H_{51}N_3O_4S_2$

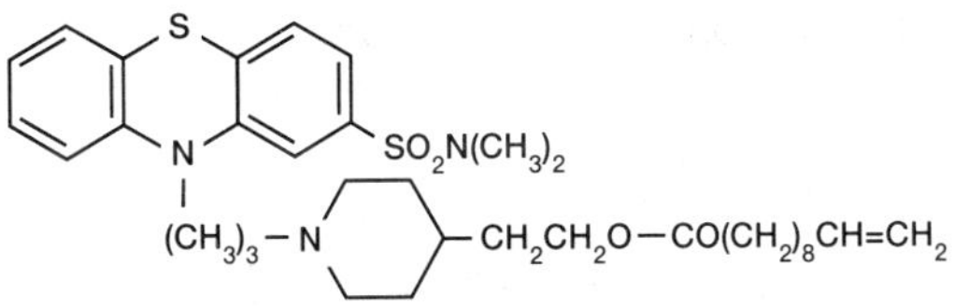

Chemically, pipothiazine differs from the other major phenothiazine neuroleptics, such as thioproperazine and fluphenazine, by the presence of a piperidine ring instead of a piperazine ring in its side-chain. The esterification with fatty acids of the primary alcohol function of pipothiazine gives the long-acting injectable esters, pipothiazine palmitate and pipothiazine undecenoate. The palmitate is a pale yellow crystalline powder. Pipothiazine and its esters are not marketed in any combination preparations.

Pharmacology

Pipothiazine is a potent neuroleptic agent. It suppresses spontaneous movements and complex behaviour while spinal reflexes and unconditional nociceptive behaviour remain unaffected. Pipothiazine achieves most of its effects via antagonism of dopamine-mediated neurotransmission. It also has antihistaminic and antiserotonin properties. It has relatively little anticholinergic effect. Pipothiazine also has α-blocking effects and in animal studies induces hypotension with progressive recovery over 3 hours. In the dog it has no effect on the electrocardiogram.

Toxicology

In the mouse via the intraperitoneal route, pipothiazine has acute toxicity including sedation and catalepsy. Via the subcutaneous route, pipothiazine is about twice as toxic as thioproperazine and fluphenazine (LD_{50}); via the oral route, pipothiazine has about the same toxicity (behavioural toxicity as well as LD_{50}) as fluphenazine and is about twice as toxic as thioproperazine.[1]

In humans, no toxic effects have been seen on the liver, the bone marrow (blood) or the kidneys, nor has photosensitivity or allergy developed.[1]

Clinical pharmacology

Pipothiazine shows the usual neuroleptic effects in humans. It reduces initiative and reduces displays of emotion. At first, there is often drowsiness and slowness in response to external stimuli. Psychotic patients become less agitated and withdrawn individuals become more responsive. Psychotic symptoms of hallucinations, delusions and incoherent thinking tend to lessen. Pipothiazine is a relatively weak sedative agent. Pipothiazine causes some relaxation of skeletal muscle in spastic conditions, probably mediated via an action in the basal ganglia. Like all phenothiazines, pipothiazine causes an elevation of the plasma prolactin concentration. Pipothiazine has no effect on the respiratory system, but hypotension may occur due to its α-blocking effect. Pipothiazine has extrapyramidal effects and these may be manifest as Parkinsonism, acute dystonic reactions, akathisia or tardive dyskinesia.

Pharmacokinetics

Pipothiazine is quantified in plasma (limit of detection 250 $ng.l^{-1}$) and urine (limit of detection 2 $\mu g.l^{-1}$) by HPLC with fluorescence detection.[2] Pipothiazine is readily absorbed, but is subject to extensive presystemic metabolism. As a consequence, plasma concentrations following oral administration are much lower than those following intramuscular administration.[1,3–8] It is only slowly absorbed from the site of injection.

Although the plasma half life of pipothiazine has been reported to be only a few hours, it has a very prolonged terminal elimination phase of up to about 3 weeks. Its duration of therapeutic effect can range from a few days to several weeks or possibly longer.[3–8]

After injection of 0.75 $mg.kg^{-1}$ intramuscularly of pipothiazine palmitate, an amount close to the minimal dose per kg used clinically, pipothiazine palmitate and free pipothiazine are found in the brain as well as in the plasma (free pipothiazine is derived by the enzymatic hydrolysis of the ester). The maximal plasma and brain levels of pipothiazine palmitate and free pipothiazine are, however, very low, and hardly exceed 100 $ng.l^{-1}$ in the plasma and 200 $ng.kg^{-1}$ in the brain.[9]

In the plasma, the decrease of the level of pipothiazine palmitate appears very early. After the fourth day, it corresponds to a half life of about 15 days. After a slight initial increase, the level of free pipothiazine remains nearly constant until the tenth day. It then decreases with a half life close to 16 days.[9] This is due to the slow absorption of the ester from its site of injection.

In the brain, the variations with time of the levels of pipothiazine palmitate and free pipothiazine follow a similar pattern to those in the plasma.

In the rat, 45 days after an injection of 4.5 $mg.kg^{-1}$ intramuscularly of tritium-labelled pipothiazine palmitate, the cumulative urinary and faecal elimination of total radioactivity represents only about 65% of the injected radioactivity; moreover, faecal elimination is about 10 times higher than urinary elimination. Similar results are obtained after administration of 0.75 $mg.kg^{-1}$ intramuscularly of the undecylenic ester.[1]

Pipothiazine is metabolized in the liver, and only 1% of the dose is excreted unchanged in the urine in 24 hours. The metabolites are excreted in both urine and faeces.

	Pipothiazine	Pipothiazine palmitate
Oral absorption	readily absorbed	—
Presystemic metabolism	extensive:	—
Plasma half life	a few hours (but very prolonged terminal elimination phase)	15–16 days
Volume of distribution	—	—
Plasma protein binding	—	—

Concentration–effect relationship

There is very wide intersubject variation in plasma concentrations of pipothiazine; no simple correlation has been found between plasma concentrations of pipothiazine and its metabolites, and their therapeutic effect.[3–8]

Metabolism

Pipothiazine is subject to presystemic metabolism in the gut wall. Systemic availability of drug is approximately the same after oral and parenteral doses, but there are wide variations both within individuals and between individuals (ten-fold). These do not always explain variations in clinical response. It is also extensively metabolized in the liver and is excreted in the urine and faeces in the form of numerous active and inactive metabolites; there is evidence of enterohepatic recycling. Paths of metabolism of pipothiazine include hydroxylation and conjugation with glucuronic acid (most important for inactivation of the drug), N-oxidation, oxidation of a sulphur atom, and dealkylation (see Fig. 1). Following oral administration, less than 1% of the drug is excreted unchanged in the urine in 24 hours.

Studies performed in vitro have shown that rat plasma and brain as well as liver homogenates contain enzymes which are capable of hydrolysing pipothiazine palmitate and undecenoate.[1]

In the rat, 15 to 20 days after administration of a dose of 0.75 mg.kg^{-1} intramuscularly of either pipothiazine undecenoate or palmitate, 40–50% of the injected radioactivity remains in the organism. However, 80 days after injection of the palmitic ester, only about 10% of the administered radioactivity remains in the organism; furthermore, at any moment during the 80 days of observation, about 95% of the radioactivity present in the organism is found at the site of injection.

The prolonged duration of action of the palmitic and undecanoic esters of pipothiazine after injection in oily solution results primarily from their slow release from the injection site; this is due to the increase of the lipophilic character of the products from which they are derived. It is likely that the role of secondary deposit of the esters in other tissues is negligible.

Pharmaceutics

Pipothiazine is formulated in oral and parenteral forms in Europe.

Pipothiazine itself is usually administered by mouth. The longer-acting palmitate and undecenoate esters are given by intramuscular injection. The latter are very slowly absorbed from the site of injection, gradually releasing pipothiazine into the body; they are thus suitable for use as depot injections.

Pipothiazine palmitate, Piportil Depot (Rhone Poulenc, UK) is available for intramuscular use as a straw-coloured viscous liquid containing pipothiazine palmitate 5.0% w/v (50 mg.ml^{-1}) in sesame oil. Both 1 ml and 2 ml ampoules are marketed.

Pipothiazine should be protected from light and can be stored at room temperature. Maximum shelf-life is five years.

Therapeutic use

Indications

1. Psychotic disorders
2. To control aggressive symptoms in mentally handicapped patients.

Contraindications

1. Coma caused by CNS depressants
2. Bone marrow depression
3. Narrow angle glaucoma.

Mode of use

The usual dose of pipothiazine for the treatment of psychoses is 10–20 mg daily in a single dose.[10–30] The maximum dose which is generally given is 200 mg daily. In severe psychoses, higher doses have been given for brief periods. In acute conditions treatment is sometimes started with intramuscular injections of 10–20 mg daily in one or two injections. In doses of 30–60 mg daily, the activating effect of pipothiazine is most pronounced; in doses of 60–100 mg daily its antipsychotic effect is good, and in doses of 100–200 mg daily a marked sedative effect is observed.

Fig. 1 Metabolism of pipothiazine

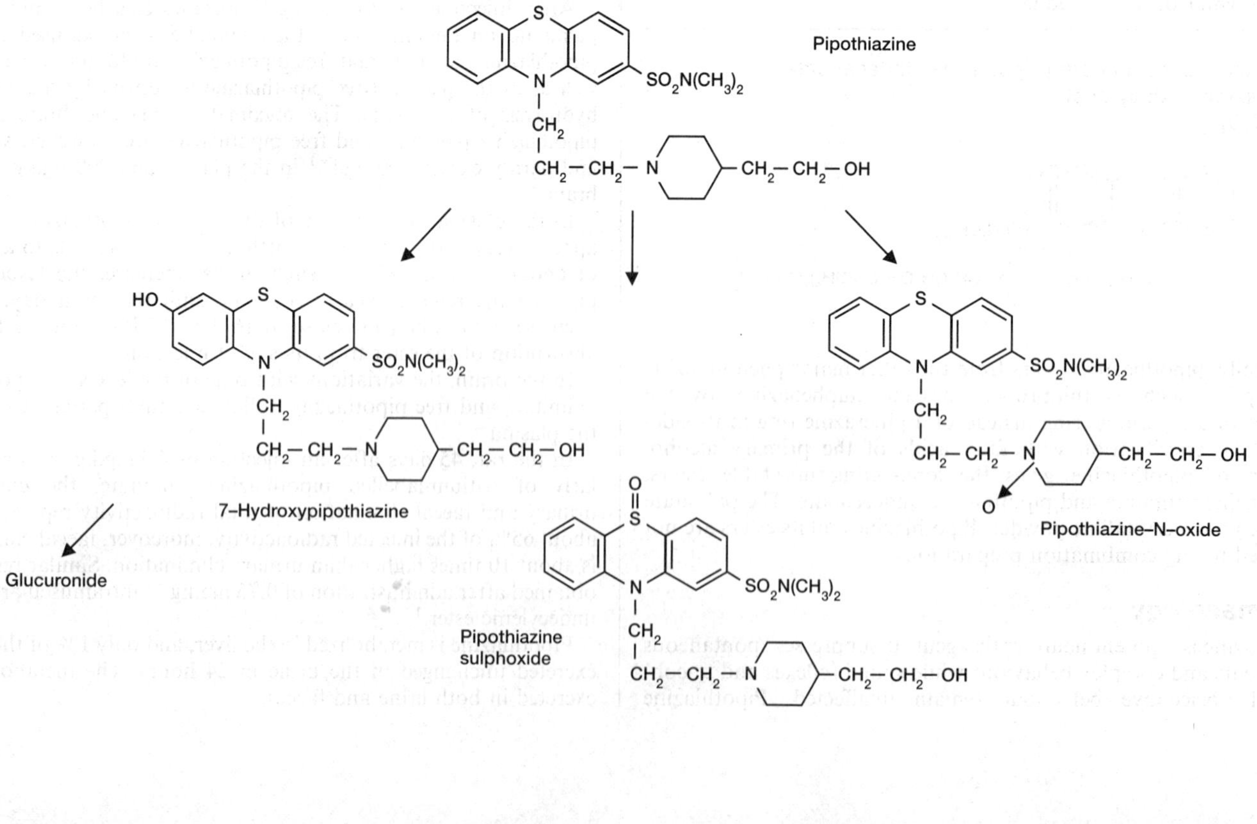

For pipothiazine palmitate, 25 mg (0.5 ml) should be given initially to assess the response of the patient to the drug. If this dose is tolerated and higher subsequent doses are needed, the dose should be raised gradually. Further doses should be administered at appropriate intervals, increasing by increments of 25 or 50 mg until a satisfactory response is obtained. These small incremental doses provide the opportunity to weigh clinical effects against side effects. High starting doses, particularly if administered at close intervals, may cause a higher-than-usual incidence of relatively severe striopallidal reactions, some of which may not respond readily to antiparkinsonian drugs.

In clinical practice pipothiazine palmitate has been shown to have a long duration of action, allowing intervals of 4 weeks between injections for maintenance therapy.[10–30] The duration of action depends on the dose administered, allowing dosage intervals to be varied to suit individual circumstances. Most patients respond favourably to a dose of 50–100 mg (1–2 ml) every 4 weeks. The maximum recommended dose is 200 mg (4 ml) every 4 weeks.

The usual dose of pipothiazine undecenoate is 75 mg intramuscularly given at an average interval of 2 weeks. The amount required may range from 25 to 200 mg. A one week washout period is recommended for patients being switched from oral neuroleptics to pipothiazine palmitate, to avoid superimposing depot pipothiazine on the accumulated oral neuroleptic. This lessens the likelihood of inadvertent overdosage and severe side effects, especially extrapyramidal reactions.

Pipothiazine should not be administered to patients with marked cerebral atherosclerosis, phaeochromocytoma, renal or liver failure, severe cardiac insufficiency or hypersensitivity to other phenothiazine derivatives.

Indications

1. Psychotic disorders
Pipothiazine is indicated primarily for chronic psychosis,[10–30] especially schizophrenia with a predominance of the following symptoms: difficulty in socializing, aggressiveness, agitation, irritability, perceptual defects, and conceptual disorganization and bizarre thought content. Pipothiazine can also be given to newly admitted acute schizophrenics, and patients with other acute psychoses. Pipothiazine (palmitate) can also be an alternative for some patients' unresponsiveness to or intolerance of other neuroleptics. Care should be taken with schizo-affectives whose mood swings might be set in motion. Compared to all presently available depot neuroleptics, pipothiazine palmitate has the longest duration of action. This is advantageous since most patients can be treated with many fewer injections.

2. To control aggressive symptoms in mentally handicapped patients
In severely mentally handicapped patients who present with overt aggressiveness, drug treatment is usually required on a long-term basis. Difficulties of patient compliance may be overcome by the use of a depot neuroleptic. Pipothiazine palmitate controls aggressive symptoms in schizophrenics and this action is also reproduced in aggressive mentally handicapped patients.

Contraindications

1. Coma caused by CNS depressants
Most neuroleptics can potentiate the sedative effects of CNS depressants, including alcohol, barbiturates, narcotics, and anaesthetics.

2. Bone marrow depression
Various neuroleptics can rarely cause bone marrow depression.

3. Narrow-angle glaucoma
Pipothiazine may occasionally cause mydriasis, and should not be used in patients with narrow-angle glaucoma.

Adverse reactions

Potentially life-threatening effects
Months and years of pipothiazine palmitate, even in high doses, have not produced hepatotoxicity or toxic changes in the haematopoietic system.[10–30] However, pipothiazine palmitate is theoretically subject to the adverse effects generally seen with neuroleptics. Although not specifically reported for pipothiazine, neuroleptics as a class can induce the rare condition, neuroleptic malignant syndrome — a potentially fatal syndrome characterized by fever, muscular rigidity, elevated creatine phosphokinase and coma.

Acute overdosage
This should be treated symptomatically with full supportive therapy. Extrapyramidal reactions should be treated with oral or parenteral antiparkinsonian drugs. Should severe hypotension occur, procedures for the management of circulatory shock should be instituted. Noradrenaline may be relatively ineffective as a vasoconstrictor because of α-adrenergic blockade, and adrenaline may well lower the blood pressure even further through actions on β-receptors.

Severe or irreversible adverse effects
Extrapyramidal symptoms (reversed by dose reduction or anticholinergic drugs) and, on prolonged administration, occasionally tardive dyskinesia may occur. Like all potent oral and injectable neuroleptics, pipothiazine can evoke extrapyramidal symptoms. Clinical experience, however, has substantiated that piperidine phenothiazines (like pipothiazine) cause a much lower incidence of extrapyramidal symptoms than aliphatic, piperazine, and other high potency neuroleptics. In addition, antiparkinsonian medication can sometimes be discontinued or lowered in patients switched from oral neuroleptics to depot pipothiazine.

Although not specifically reported for pipothiazine, the following adverse effects of phenothiazine neuroleptics might be expected to occur: hypothermia (occasionally pyrexia), cardiovascular symptoms such as hypotension and arrhythmias, and sensitivity reactions such as agranulocytosis, leucopenia, leucocytosis, and haemolytic anaemia, photosensitization, contact sensitization, rashes and jaundice.

Prolonged high dosage may induce corneal and lens opacities, and purplish pigmentation of the skin, cornea, conjunctiva and retina. Intramuscular injection may be painful, cause hypotension and tachycardia, and give rise to nodule formation.

Symptomatic adverse effects
These include drowsiness, apathy, pallor, nightmares, insomnia, depression, and, more rarely, agitation, asthenia, nausea and hyperhidrosis.

Anticholinergic symptoms, such as dry mouth, nasal congestion, constipation, difficulty with micturition and blurred vision may occur, as may endocrine effects such as menstrual disturbances (amenorrhoea), galactorrhoea, impotence and weight gain.

Other effects
Biological tolerance is good and changes in laboratory findings have only been seen in a very few cases. Slight increases in alkaline phosphatase and prothrombin time have been reported.[1]

With pipothiazine, there are no changes in red or white blood cell counts. Blood, liver and kidney function tests did not show any change.

With pipothiazine undecanoate, blood, liver and kidney function tests showed no change. Slight eosinophilia has been reported during the first few months of administration.

Interference with clinical pathology tests
Although pipothiazine has not been specifically implicated, other phenothiazines are known to interfere with the Frings TLC procedure for estimating urinary alkaloids and barbiturates, the Trinder method for measuring urinary salicylate, and some urinary tests for pregnancy.

High risk groups

Neonates
The drugs are not recommended for use in neonates.

Breast milk. The drugs should not be used during lactation unless the physician considers it essential.

Children
The drugs are not recommended for use in children.

Pregnant women
The drugs are not recommended for use in pregnant women. There is inadequate evidence of safety of pipothiazine palmitate in human pregnancy, although animal studies have shown no evidence of hazard. The drug should only be used if the physician considers it essential. Of two patients who received pipothiazine palmitate during pregnancy, one was delivered six weeks before term, and the other at term. Both children are normal.

Pipothiazine

P

The elderly
Pipothiazine should be used with caution in the elderly, and a reduced starting dose is recommended. The elderly tend to be less tolerant than younger patients. The risk of extrapyramidal symptoms is highest in this population, and concomitant physical disorders frequently require patients to take other medication. Low depot pipothiazine dosages and frequent monitoring reduce the likelihood of harmful effects and adverse interactions with other drugs. Experience with this treatment regimen in the elderly has verified that it is safe and well tolerated.

Drug interactions

Potentially hazardous interactions
Pipothiazine should be given with caution in conjunction with CNS sedative drugs, drugs which suppress the bone marrow, or those that can lead to respiratory depression.

Cigarette smoking. Interactions of cigarette smoking and pipothiazine have not been reported. However, cigarette smoking may lower the incidence of hypotension after administration of some neuroleptics.

Alcohol. Alcohol can potentiate the sedative effects of neuroleptics, leading to respiratory depression.

Potentially useful interactions
None has been reported.

Controlled trials

1. Albert J M, Elie R, Cooper S F 1980 Long-term double-blind evaluation of pipothiazine palmitate and fluphenazine enanthate. Current Therapeutic Research, vol 27, no 6, section 2: 897–907

33 male chronic schizophrenic patients were selected for a double-blind evaluation of pipothiazine palmitate and fluphenazine enanthate, two long-acting injectable neuroleptics. Following a two month drug standardization period, the patients received either 100 or 150 mg pipothiazine palmitate per month, or 50 mg fluphenazine enanthate every 2 weeks.

At intervals throughout the 39 weeks of observation, the patients were evaluated using a battery of psychological rating scales. The results of testing revealed that both drugs provided stable control of symptoms over the duration of the study. However, pipothiazine palmitate, particularly with the 100 $mg.month^{-1}$ dose, provided significant improvement in several target symptoms, such as emotional withdrawal and social behaviour.

Both drugs were found to be well tolerated. Extrapyramidal reactions occurred, but were readily controlled and never necessitated any interruption of therapy.

2. Singh A N, Saxena B 1979 A comparative study of prolonged action (depot) neuroleptics: pipothiazine palmitate versus fluphenazine enanthate in chronic schizophrenic patients. Current Therapeutic Research 25: 121–133

30 adult chronic schizophrenic patients participated in a 44 week double-blind evaluation of pipothiazine palmitate and fluphenazine enanthate. Half the patients received monthly intramuscular injections of pipothiazine palmitate in dosages ranging from 100 to 175 mg. The other 15 patients were given fluphenazine enanthate every 2 weeks, in dosages ranging from 25 to 75 mg intramuscularly.

Both drugs provided good control of psychotic symptoms throughout the treatment period. Pipothiazine palmitate was favoured, however, as it produced a significant degree of clinical improvement from 4 to 8 weeks faster than fluphenazine enanthate. Pipothiazine palmitate also appeared to be effective against a wider range of symptoms. An analysis of variance comparing the Brief Psychiatric Rating Scale (BPRS) scores for each drug group revealed significantly more improvement with pipothiazine palmitate for the overall cumulative scores as well as for several individual symptoms.

Side effects appeared with both drugs only at more elevated doses. The incidence of side effects with fluphenazine enanthate was twice that of pipothiazine palmitate; however, none of the patients had to be withdrawn from the study because of side effects.

Pipothiazine palmitate represents one of the better choices in the long-acting armamentarium of antipsychosis, as it has an activity of 4–5 weeks' duration, and it belongs to the piperidine derivatives, and thus may, as suggested by this study, be predisposed to produce less extrapyramidal effects.

3. Schlosberg A, Shadmi M 1978 A comparative controlled study of two long-acting phenothiazines; pipothiazine palmitate and fluphenazine decanoate. Current Therapeutic Research 23: 642–655

75 chronic schizophrenics received at random, after a washout period, fluphenazine, pipothiazine and placebo in a double-blind trial. At first, drugs were administered orally, when optimal results were seen; the patients were then given monthly long-acting injections for 15 months. Finally, the group of improved patients was divided, one half continuing to receive their medication, and one half receiving placebo for a further 3 months.

Regular evaluations were made starting from the pre-washout period, by the Brief Psychiatric Rating Scale (BPRS), Nursing Observation Scale of Inpatient Evaluation (NOSIE), social functioning, five major symptoms for each patient, global clinical evaluation, and whenever possible, an evaluation by the patient's family.

Blood counts, urinalysis, liver function tests, EKG, EEG, and eye fundus examination were performed to detect any toxicity. Untoward clinical reactions were evaluated according to the National Institute of Mental Health (NIMH) scale. Results were discussed evaluating the nature of the patient's schizophrenia and its symptoms; non-pharmacological factors were stressed in relation to the final results.

Two patients receiving placebo, nine patients receiving fluphenazine decanoate and nine patients receiving pipothiazine palmitate improved. Analysis of these results was made as to favourable relative indications of each psychoactive drug for the specific psychiatric population and illness involved. Of the two drugs, pipothiazine seems to be more active.

4. Steinert J, Neder A, Erba E, Pugh C R, Robinson C, Priest R G 1986 A comparative trial of depot pipothiazine. Journal of International Medical Research (England) 14 (2): 72–77

39 chronic schizophrenic patients were selected for a 12 month double-blind evaluation of the effectiveness of pipothiazine palmitate (PPT) and flupenthixol decanoate (FPX) in the maintenance management of their illness. Allocation was at random and, in order to allow constant injection intervals, the patients typically received every 2 weeks either 40 mg of flupenthixol decanoate or alternating injections of 100 mg of pipothiazine palmitate and placebo.

At monthly intervals the patients were assessed using both a battery of rating scales — which included the Brief Psychiatric Rating Scale (BPRS) and the Extrapyramidal Symptoms Rating Scale (EPS) — and a general side effects evaluation. At three-monthly intervals they were in addition rated on the Comprehensive Psychiatric Rating Scale (CPRS) and the Zung Depression Scale. Haematological and biochemical tests were also performed every 3 months. Both drugs provided good control of psychotic symptoms and side effects were not troublesome. No substantial difference was detected on the CPRS or the Zung scales. There was a trend in favour of PPT on the BPRS survey, detectable at 6 months. The authors conclude that the PPT regime is at least as effective as the FPX treatment and probably more so. It is possible that even longer periods of control could be obtained with PPT.

Other trials

1. Gerlach J, Nyeborg O, Prieto R 1973 General evaluation of pipothiazine palmitate (19.552) in hospitalized schizophrenic patients. Acta Psychiatrica Scandinavica 241 (suppl): 69–71

26 schizophrenic patients in hospital were treated in an open study with the parenteral depot neuroleptic, 19.552 R.P. After 4 months' treatment, 11 patients improved, 11 were unchanged and four had deteriorated in comparison with their condition during previous neuroleptic treatment. After completion of this study, 19.552 R.P. was included among the depot neuroleptics available in the ward, on an equal footing with the previously established preparations.

2. Lynch D M, Eliatamby C L S, Anderson A A 1985 Pipothiazine palmitate in the management of aggressive mentally handicapped patients. British Journal of Psychiatry 146: 525–529

The efficacy of intramuscular pipothiazine palmitate in the management of aggressive mentally handicapped patients was examined in a double-blind, placebo-controlled, crossover study, in which 30 patients received each treatment for 13 weeks. Patients were rated on a target symptom scale of aggressiveness and a clinical global impression scale of efficacy at monthly intervals, and on an extrapyramidal side effects scale weekly. The patients showed marked improvement during treatment with pipothiazine palmitate, which was assessed as superior to placebo. Individual and total target symptom scale of aggression scores were also reduced compared to placebo.

References

1. May and Baker Limited 1987 Document GM 86/2723G. Pipothiazine palmitate
2. Le Roux et al 1982 Journal of Chromatography 230, Biomedical Applications 19: 401–408
3. Villeneuve A, Pires A, Jus A et al 1972 A long-term pilot study of pipotiazine in chronic schizophrenia. Current Therapeutic Research 14: 696–706
4. Jain R C, Ananth J V, Klinger A et al 1973 Uncontrolled study with pipotiazine palmitate. International Journal of Clinical Pharmacology, Therapeutics and Toxicology 7: 32–36
5. Gerlach J, Nyeborg O, Prieto R 1973 General evaluation of pipotiazine palmitate in hospitalized schizophrenic patients. Acta Psychiatrica Scandinavica 241 (suppl): 69–74
6. Imlah N W, Murphy K P 1975 A preliminary evaluation of pipothiazine palmitate in schizophrenia. Current Medical Research and Opinion 3: 169–174
7. Simpson G M, Varger V 1975 Pipotiazine palmitate — a new depot neuroleptic. Current Therapeutic Research 17: 276–280
8. Johnston R E, Niesink F 1979 A versatile new sustained-action neuroleptic pipotiazine palmitate. Journal of International Medical Research 7: 187–193
9. Blanc M, Girard M, Grainier F et al 1986 Pharmacocinetique de l'ester palmitique de pipotiazine apres administration intramusculaire chez des malades schizophrenes. Therapie 41: 27–30
10. Brown-Thomsen J 1973 Pipotiazine, pipotiazine undecylenate and pipothiazine palmitate. Acta Psychiatrica Scandinavica 241 (suppl): 119–138
11. Julou L, Bourat G, Ducrot R et al 1973 Pharmacological study of pipotiazine and its undecylenic and palmitic esters. Acta Psychiatrica Scandinavica 241 (suppl): 9–30
12. Julou L, Bourat G, Ducrot R et al 1973 Correlations between the results of pharmacokinetic and pharmacological studies on some pipotiazine esters. Therapie 28: 491–499
13. Albert J M, Elie R, Cooper S F 1980 Long-term double blind evaluation of pipotiazine palmitate and fluphenazine enanthate. Current Therapeutic Research 27: 897–907
14. St Laurent J, Carle R, Dumais B et al 1974 Monthly intermittent chemotherapy of chronic schizophrenic outpatients with pipothiazine palmitate. Canadian Psychiatric Association Journal 19: 583–591
15. Burch E, Ayd F J 1983 Depot pipotiazine 1970–1982: a review. Journal of Clinical Psychiatry 44: 242–247
16. Singh A N, Saxena B 1979 A comparative study of prolonged action (depot) neuroleptics: pipothiazine palmitate versus fluphenazine enanthate in chronic schizophrenic patients. Current Therapeutic Research 25: 121–132
17. Schlosberg A, Shadmi M 1978 A comparative controlled study of two long-acting phenothiazines; pipothiazine palmitate and fluphenazine decanoate. Current Therapeutic Research 23: 642–654
18. Lynch D M, Eliatamby C L S, Anderson A A 1985 Pipothiazine palmitate in the management of aggressive mentally handicapped patients. British Journal of Psychiatry 146: 525–529
19. Imlah N W, Murphy K P 1985 Ten year follow-up of schizophrenic patients on pipothiazine palmitate. Current Medical Research and Opinion 9: 449–453
20. Villeneuve A, Fontaine P 1980 A near-decade experience with pipotiazine palmitate in chronic schizophrenia. Current Therapeutic Research 27: 411–418
21. Woggan B, Dick P, Fleischaur H et al 1977 The efficacy of pipothiazine palmitate and fluphenazine decanoate compared in a multicentre double blind trial. International Pharmacopsychiatry 12: 192–209
22. Steinert J, Neder A, Erba E, et al 1986 A comparative trial of depot pipothiazine. Journal of International Medical Research 14: 72–77
23. Itil T M, Reisberg B, Patterson C et al 1978 Pipotiazine palmitate, a long acting neuroleptic — clinical and computerised EEG affects. Current Therapeutic Research 24: 689–707
24. Ayd F J 1983 Depot pipotiazine palmitate — thirteen years later. International Drug Therapy News 18: 5–8
25. Salvesan C, Vaksdal K 1973 General evaluation of pipotiazine palmitate in hospitalised and open ward patients with functional psychosis. Acta Psychiatrica Scandinavica 241 (suppl): 67
26. Elley J H, Peterson J H 1973 Clinical evaluation of 19 552 R.P. used on patients in an acute reception ward. Acta Psychiatrica Scandinavica 241 (suppl): 75–82
27. Imlah N W, Murphy K P 1973 The clinical use of long-acting psychotropic drugs. Therapie 28: 595–602
28. Dencker S J, Frankenberg K, Malm U et al 1973 A controlled one year study of pipothiazine palmitate and fluphenazine decanoate in chronic schizophrenic syndromes. Acta Psychiatrica Scandinavica 241 (suppl): 101–118
29. Aref M A, Guindy E A 1980 Pipotiazine palmitate in the long term treatment of schizophrenia. Journal of International Medical Research 8: 293–294
30. Albert J M, Elie R, Cooper S F 1980 Long-term double-blind evaluation of pipotiazine palmitate and fluphenazine enanthate. Current Therapeutic Research 27: 897–907

Pirenzepine (dihydrochloride)

Pirenzepine is a muscarinic cholinergic receptor antagonist used for its antisecretory action in the stomach.

Chemistry

Pirenzepine dihydrochloride (Gastrozepin)
$C_{19}H_{21}N_5O_2.2HCl$
5,11-Dihydro-11-(4-methylpiperazin-1-yl-acetyl)-6H-pyrido-(2,3-b) (1,4)-benzodiazepin-6-one dihydrochloride

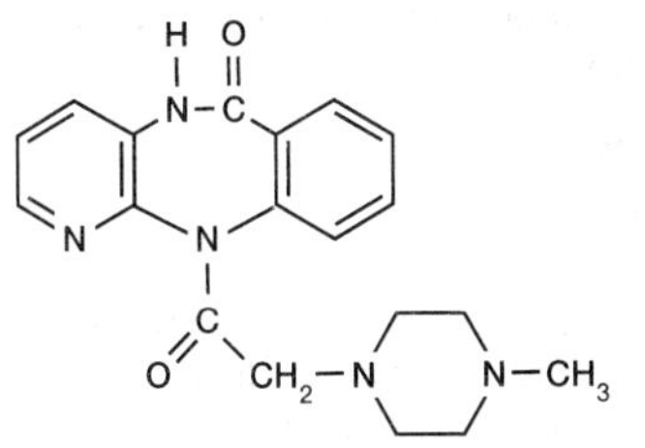

Molecular weight (free base)	424.3 (351.4)
pKa	2.1, 8.1
Solubility	
in alcohol	1 in 105
in water	~1 in 5
Octanol/water partition coefficient	0.23

Pirenzepine is a white to slightly yellow crystalline substance, virtually insoluble in ether but slightly more soluble in methanol. It is hydrophilic at pH 7.4. It is not available in any combined preparations.

Pharmacology

Pirenzepine is a selective antagonist of muscarinic acetylcholine receptors.[1] There are now known to be two types of muscarinic receptor: receptors that show high affinity for pirenzepine are known as M_1 receptors and those receptors that have low affinity for pirenzepine are known as M_2 receptors. M_1 receptors are predominantly found in the CNS and in ganglia while M_2 receptors are largely found in postganglionic effector organs such as the heart and ileum. The M_1 receptor may be involved in the regulation of calcium homeostasis and in the generation of phosphoinositol. Pirenzepine's antimuscarinic effects are chiefly felt in the stomach and intestine. Pirenzepine inhibits salivary secretion, weakly inhibits the emptying of the stomach, mildly stimulates bile and pancreatic flow and increases heart rate.[3–5]

Toxicology

Acute toxicity in mice (after 1000 times the usual clinical dose) includes tachycardia, ataxia and tremor; rats develop spasms and pupillary dilation; dogs develop severe vomiting. Chronic toxicity in rats and dogs is minimal. Pirenzepine is not teratogenic in rats and rabbits at high doses. It is not mutagenic in the Ames test. A nitrosation product of pirenzepine is not mutagenic.

Clinical pharmacology

Pirenzepine selectively blocks muscarinic receptors which control gastric acid and pepsin secretion.[2] It inhibits gastric acid secretion induced by insulin hypoglycaemia, pentagastrin and histamine. It diminishes the volume of gastric juice rather than the concentration of acid.

In fasted healthy subjects, therapeutic doses of pirenzepine inhibit basal gastric acid output by more than 50%. Pirenzepine inhibits submaximal and maximal pentagastrin stimulation to a similar degree (about 30%) and is thus a non-competitive inhibitor of the muscarinic receptor. It inhibits nocturnal gastric acid secretion by 44%. In patients with duodenal ulcer, oral or intravenous pirenzepine produces dose-related reduction of basal acid secretion. Pirenzepine does not raise gastrin levels following sham feeding, but a small rise in basal gastrin level occurs after multiple dosing.

Salivation is reduced by pirenzepine 100 mg daily, causing a dry mouth. This is usually not a problem, unless the dose is increased further. Oesophageal peristalsis is slightly reduced in the recumbent and sitting positions. Intravenous pirenzepine decreases lower oesophageal pressure. Gastric emptying and pancreatic function are unaffected by pirenzepine. Intravenous pirenzepine has little or no effect on basal and postprandial levels of insulin, glucagon and gastric inhibitor peptide (GIP).

Parenteral pirenzepine reduces colonic motility. In clinical trials using pirenzepine 100 mg daily for 4–6 weeks, constipation has occasionally been reported. At doses of 100 to 150 mg daily, pirenzepine does not usually produce any signs of mental impairment, difficulty with accommodation or change in pupil diameter and intraocular pressure. Bladder function is not altered by pirenzepine 25 mg three times a day.

Pharmacokinetics

The method of analysis for pirenzepine is HPLC,[5] which has a sensitivity of 100 μg.l^{-1}.

Pirenzepine absorption after oral administration is limited. Bioavailability in man is low, approximately 26% of the dose administered orally reaching the peripheral circulation.[6] There is little or no presystemic metabolism. The absorption of the drug is reduced by food.

Despite the low bioavailability, there is little interindividual variation in serum levels. The variability in plasma pirenzepine levels after a single oral dose of 50 mg has been investigated in ten countries in a total of 87 volunteers. Plasma profiles were similar in every country, reaching a peak of about 50 μg.l^{-1} within two hours of the dose.

Steady-state plasma concentrations are reached within 2-3 days of treatment, consistent with the half life. The similarity of plasma profiles throughout the test population confirms that the rates of absorption and of disposition of pirenzepine show little intersubject variation. The volume of distribution is 14 litres in normal subjects.

The area under the plasma concentration–time curve and the peak levels of pirenzepine are linearly related to dose. This indicates that over the usual clinical dose range the amount of pirenzepine absorbed is directly proportional to the dose administered.

Over the dosage range 12.5–150 mg, the elimination half life of pirenzepine is constant, with a mean of 12.5 hours.[6]

After intramuscular injection pirenzepine is rapidly and completely absorbed. The plasma level reaches a peak of approximately 90 μg.l^{-1} 50 minutes after the administration of 8 mg pirenzepine intramuscularly.

Intravenous (^{14}C) pirenzepine given to rats is detectable in skeletal muscles and internal organs, but not in the brain to any significant extent. In addition, in other animals given ten times the therapeutic dose, there is very limited penetration of the blood–brain barrier.[7]

In man, the ratio of the pirenzepine concentration in the cerebrospinal fluid to peripheral blood serum is about 0.095:1, i.e. a ten-fold difference.[8] Movement across the placental barrier is also very limited. Pirenzepine appears in breast milk in minimal quantities, thought unlikely to affect the infant.

In vitro, pirenzepine is only about 10% bound to plasma proteins. This binding is independent of pirenzepine concentration in the range 10–160 μg.l^{-1}. Since protein binding is low, the concentration of pirenzepine in the extravascular space is similar to that in the circulation.

Pirenzepine has no appreciable effect on the mixed function oxidase enzyme system in rats. Its effects on drug oxidation in man are not known.

Renal impairment results in a modest increase in the plasma concentration of pirenzepine, not such that any adjustment of dose is necessary.

Pirenzepine is excreted largely as the unchanged compound in both urine and faeces, with minor amounts of the hepatic metabolite desmethylpirenzepine present in urine.

It is unlikely that liver disease has any effect on the kinetics of pirenzepine.

Oral absorption	20–30%
Presystemic metabolism	negligible
Plasma half life	
mean	11 h
Volume of distribution	14 l
Plasma protein binding	10%

Concentration–effect relationship

There is no information on plasma pirenzepine concentrations and inhibition of gastric acid secretion in patients with peptic ulceration. In normal subjects, pirenzepine concentrations of 200 and 300 μg.l^{-1} are required to produce 50% and 80% inhibition of meal-stimulated acid secretion. At these concentrations there is an appreciable incidence of dry mouth and blurred vision. These anticholinergic side effects tend to be low at plasma pirenzepine concentrations of 70 to 165 μg.l^{-1} though gastric acid inhibition is not maximal.[4,9,10]

Metabolism

Pirenzepine is metabolized only to a slight extent; at least 80% of the dose administered is excreted unchanged (80% in faeces and 10% in urine). The primary metabolite, desmethylpirenzepine, occurs in small amounts accounting for no more than 10% of the dose. This metabolite has little pharmacological activity.

In man, following oral administration of ^{14}C-pirenzepine the cumulative urinary excretion (over 96 hours) is 7–12% (mean 10%). Over the same period, 90% of the radioactivity appears in faeces. Via both routes, most (90%) of the radioactivity is due to unchanged pirenzepine. After intravenous and intramuscular injection of radiolabelled pirenzepine the cumulative 96 hour excretion in urine and faeces is 48% and 50%, respectively.

Renal and hepatic elimination of pirenzepine is about equal, the total plasma clearance being 255 ml.min^{-1}. Hepatic clearance is due almost entirely to biliary excretion.

Pharmaceutics

Pirenzepine dihydrochloride is available in oral form.

Gastrozepin tablets (Boots, UK) contain the equivalent of 50 mg of anhydrous substance. The tablets are scored on one face and impressed with 'G' on one side of the score and '50' on the other. The obverse is impressed with the manufacturer's symbol.

Tablets should be stored in a cool dry place.

Therapeutic use

Indications

1. Duodenal ulcer
2. Benign gastric ulcer.

Contraindications

1. Renal failure.

Mode of use

For most patients the total daily dose is 100 mg, given as one 50 mg tablet twice per day. Symptomatic relief in peptic ulcer disease usually occurs after a few days but treatment should be given for a total of 4–6 weeks to try and achieve complete ulcer healing. If symptoms are severe the total daily dosage may be increased to 150 mg, one tablet taken three times a day. Pirenzepine may be given continuously for up to three months. The tablets are best taken half an hour or more before meals with a little liquid.

Indications

1. Duodenal ulcer

Pirenzepine is used as single agent in the healing of duodenal ulcer or in combination with an H_2 antagonist in 'resistant' duodenal ulcer. The usual dose is 50 mg two or three times per day. Doses lower than

Pirenzepine (dihydrochloride)

100 mg per day do not significantly improve the rate of healing of duodenal ulcers.

In randomized double-blind controlled trials, pirenzepine has been compared with placebo, cimetidine and other ulcer-healing agents. A dose of 100 mg per day, when compared with placebo, causes healing in 70–80% of patients, whereas 30–50% of patients heal on placebo.[11,12] In studies where pirenzepine has been compared with cimetidine, the healing rate has favoured those given cimetidine (70–84% at four weeks, versus 64–80% for pirenzepine), but the difference was not significant.[13,14] In one study comparing pirenzepine 100 mg per day with ranitidine 300 mg per day, each given for four weeks, the duodenal ulcer healing rates were 80% and 87%, respectively.[14]

2. Benign gastric ulcer

The doses for healing of gastric ulcer are the same as those for duodenal ulcer (see above), but the results (18–64%) are less impressive than those achieved in duodenal ulcer. The duration of treatment is usually longer, i.e. 6 to 8 weeks.

Contraindications

1. Renal failure

In patients with renal failure, plasma pirenzepine concentrations are 30–40% higher than in normal subjects, though still within the suggested therapeutic range.

Adverse reactions

Potentially life-threatening effects

Deaths from pirenzepine have not been reported.

Acute overdosage

There are insufficient data regarding clinical features of overdose with pirenzepine. Anticholinergic (antimuscarinic) effects are to be expected, along with sedation.

There is no specific antidote to pirenzepine and the treatment of overdose is entirely symptomatic. Haemodialysis does not remove significant amounts of pirenzepine.

Severe or irreversible adverse effects

No effects of this kind have been reported.

Symptomatic adverse effects

Pirenzepine is usually well tolerated. Occasionally dry mouth and accommodation difficulties may occur, but these are usually transient and rarely of sufficient severity to warrant discontinuation of therapy.

Interference with clinical pathology tests

No technical interferences of this kind have been reported.

High risk groups

Neonates

Pirenzepine is not recommended for use in neonates.

Breast milk. Pirenzepine appears in breast milk in small amounts after therapeutic doses but is unlikely to adversely affect the infant.

Children

There is no information on the use of pirenzepine in children.

Pregnant women

Pirenzepine is not recommended for use during pregnancy.

The elderly

No specific dosage adjustment is specified. The information on the use of pirenzepine in the elderly is limited; therefore caution is warranted in the administration of the standard dose of 100–150 mg per day.

Drug interactions

Potentially hazardous interactions

None has been recorded.

Other significant interactions

Food. Food reduces the absorption of pirenzepine from the gastrointestinal tract when the tablet is taken after a meal.

Smoking. The pharmacological interaction between pirenzepine and smoking is not known; however, smokers are likely to show reduced rate of healing of duodenal and gastric ulceration compared with non-smokers.

Potentially useful interactions

Antacids. The antacid sodium bicarbonate and the combination of magnesium trisilicate with aluminium hydroxide increase pirenzepine absorption from 14.2% to 20.3%.

H_2 antagonists. There appears to be synergy between pirenzepine and H_2 antagonists such as cimetidine and ranitidine, such that in combination greater gastric acid inhibition is achieved than with either given alone. This has been used to achieve achlorhydria in the Zollinger–Ellison syndrome, although pirenzepine is not indicated for Zollinger–Ellison syndrome.

Major outcome trials

Brunner H, Dittrich H, Kratochvil et al 1985 Treatment of duodenal ulcer with pirenzepine and cimetidine. Gut 25: 206–210

This Austrian multi-centre study, conducted single-blind, randomized duodenal ulcer patients to 4 weeks treatment with pirenzepine 100 mg daily (n = 126) or cimetidine 1 g daily (n = 128). Endoscopic healing after 4 weeks was 64.3% with pirenzepine and 73.4% with cimetidine, but this difference was not significant. Pain relief was achieved equally rapidly with both drugs. Adverse effects such as dry mouth and blurred vision were commoner in the pirenzepine group, but were reversible on dosage reduction or treatment withdrawal.

General review articles

Anonymous, undated. Gastrozepin: pirenzepine; technical and clinical review. The Boots Company PLC, Nottingham, pp 1–41

Dotevall G (ed) 1982 Symposium: advances in gastroenterology with the selective antimuscarinic compound — pirenzepine. Proceedings of the Stockholm Symposium, 17 June 1982 Excerpta Medica, Amsterdam

Baron J H, Londong W (eds) 1980 Advances in basic and clinical pharmacology of pirenzepine; proceedings of the second international symposium on pirenzepine. Scandinavian Journal of Gastroenterology 15 (suppl 66): 1–114

Dotevall G, Jaup B H, Stockbrugger R W (eds) 1982 On the selectivity of antimuscarinic compounds: proceedings of the third international symposium on pirenzepine. Scandinavian Journal of Gastroenterology 17 (suppl 72): 1–273

Carmin A A, Brogden R N 1985 Pirenzepine: a review of its pharmacodynamic and pharmacokinetic properties and therapeutic efficacy in peptic ulcer disease and other allied diseases. Drugs 30: 85–126

Londong W, Londong V, Meierl A, Voderholzer U 1987 Telenzepine is at least 25 times more potent than pirenzepine — a dose response and comparative secretory study in man. Gut 28: 888–895

Richardson C T, Barnett C C, Walsh J H, Feldman M 1987 Comparison of two antimuscarinic drugs, pirenzepine and propantheline, on gastric acid secretion, serum gastrin concentration, salivary flow and heart rate in patients with duodenal ulcer disease. Alimentary Pharmacology and Therapeutics 1: 281–291

Procacciante F, Citone G, Montesani C, Ribotta G 1984 Antisecretory activity of pirenzepine versus cimetidine in man: a controlled study. Gut 25: 178–182

Etienne A, Fimmel C J, Bron B A, Loizeau E, Blum A L 1985 Evaluation of pirenzepine on gastric acidity in healthy volunteers using ambulatory 24 hour intragastric pH monitoring. Gut 26: 241–245

Williams J G, Deakin M, Ramage J K 1986 Effect of cimetidine and pirenzepine in combination on 24 hour intragastric acidity in subjects with previous duodenal ulceration. Gut 27: 428–432

References

1. Hammer R, Berrie C P, Birdsall N J M, Burgen A S V, Hulme E C 1980 Pirenzepine distinguishes between different subclasses of muscarinic receptors. Nature 283: 90–92
2. Browning J G, Heathcote B V 1983 A comparison of pirenzepine and cimetidine inhibition of centrally-mediated gastric acid and pepsin secretion in the gastric-fistula cat. Archives Internationales de Pharmacodynamie et de Therapie 263: 288–296
3. Konturek S J, Obtulowics W, Kwiecien N, Dobrzanska M, Swierczek J 1980 Effect of pirenzepine and atropine on gastric secretory and plasma hormonal responses to sham-feeding in patients with duodenal ulcer. Scandinavian Journal of Gastroenterology 15 (suppl 66): 47–50

4. Baldi F, Ferrarini F, Cassan M, Brunetti G, Borionin D, Miglioli M 1983 Pirenzepine inhibits prostigmine stimulated sigmoid motility in man. Current Therapeutic Research 33: 802–806
5. Meineke I, Witsch D, Brendel E 1986 Journal of Chromatography 375: 369–375
6. Bolzer G, Hammer R 1980 An international pharmacokinetic study on pirenzepine following a single oral dose. Scandinavian Journal of Gastroenterology 15 (suppl 66): 27–33
7. Kobayashi S, Kyui S, Yoshida T, Nagakura A, Oiwa Y, Matsumura R, Kohei H 1981 Absorption, distribution and excretion of ^{14}C-pirenzepine in rats. Arzneimittel-Forschung 31: 679–690
8. Jaup B H, Blomstrand C 1980 Cerebrospinal fluid concentrations of pirenzepine after therapeutic dosage. Scandinavian Journal of Gastroenterology 15 (suppl 66): 35–37
9. Jaup B H, Dotevall G 1981 The effect of pirenzepine and L-hyoscyamine on gastric emptying and salivary secretion in healthy volunteers. Scandinavian Journal of Gastroenterology 16: 769–773
10. Jaup B H, Stockbrugger R W, Dotevall G 1982 Comparison between the effects of pirenzepine and L-hyoscyamine in man. Scandinavian Journal of Gastroenterology 15 (suppl 66): 89–94
11. Barbara L, Belasasso E, Bianchi Porro G, Blasi A, Caenazzo E 1979 Pirenzepine in duodenal ulcer. A multicentre double-blind controlled trial. Scandinavian Journal of Gastroenterology 14 (suppl 57): 11–19
12. Do D, Martelli S, Daniotti S 1982 Pirenzepine in duodenal ulcer: a six week double blind study. Scandinavian Journal of Gastroenterology 17 (suppl 72): 211–214
13. Brunner H, Dittrich H, Kratochvil P, Brandstatter G, Hentschel E, Schutze K 1984 Treatment of duodenal ulcer with pirenzepine and cimetidine. Gut 25: 206–210
14. Giacosa A, Cheli R, Molinari F, Parodi M C 1982 Comparison between ranitidine, cimetidine, pirenzepine and placebo in the short term treatment of duodenal ulcer. Scandinavian Journal of Gastroenterology 17 (suppl): 215–219

Piroxicam

This is a member of the oxicam series of compounds being a non-steroidal anti-inflammatory agent with analgesic and anti-pyretic properties and a particularly long half life.

Chemistry

Piroxicam (Feldene)
$C_{15}H_{13}N_3O_4S$
4-Hydroxy-2-methyl-(2-pyridyl)-2H-1,2-benzothiazine-3-carboxamide-1,1-dioxide

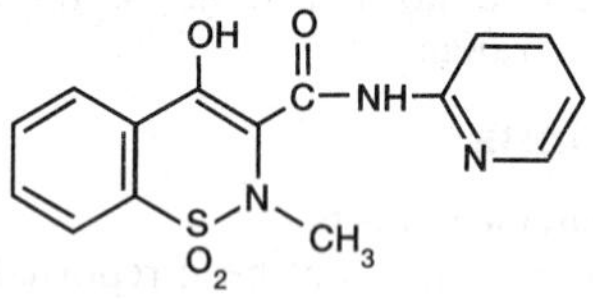

Molecular weight	331.3
pKa (4-hydroxyl)	6.3
Solubility	
in alcohol	slightly soluble
in water	slightly soluble
Octanol/water partition coefficient	—

Piroxicam is a crystalline compound prepared by chemical synthesis.

Pharmacology

Piroxicam has potent anti-inflammatory effects in addition to having antipyretic and analgesic effects. It has a potency in these effects similar to that of indomethacin. It is effective in inhibiting pyrexia induced by the intramuscular injection of *Escherichia coli* lipopolysaccharide in mice.[1] Piroxicam's main mechanism of action, like that of other non-steroidal anti-inflammatory drugs, is by inhibition of the enzyme cyclo-oxygenase, resulting in reduced prostaglandin synthesis. Piroxicam inhibits prostaglandin (thromboxane) synthesis in the platelet and thus inhibits the secondary phase of platelet aggregation. Since platelets can be involved in the inflammatory process, this action may contribute to the effectiveness of piroxicam.

Toxicology

Piroxicam appears to have a lesser ulcerogenic effect in starved rats than indomethacin, while in 4-day human studies it has caused fewer gastric erosions, less gastritis and a lower mean daily faecal blood loss than aspirin. There has been no effect on reproductive performance studied in rats and rabbits, and a lack of dysmorphogenic effects. However, in rats there has been a tendency to increased gestation and prolonged labour, with increased fetal mortality. No such information is available for pregnant women.[2] In laboratory animals, intravenous piroxicam does not significantly affect blood pressure or heart rate or modify pressure responses to exogenous or endogenous catecholamines. It also appears to have very limited CNS activity.[1] In vitro piroxicam does not adversely affect the function of cartilage cells from dogs or humans.

Clinical pharmacology

Piroxicam is effective in relieving pain and reducing temperature in febrile patients. Since the drug has useful anti-inflammatory activity it is not used primarily as an analgesic. In patients with rheumatoid arthritis piroxicam relieves pain and reduces joint swelling but rarely affects the ESR or other measures of disease activity. Piroxicam inhibits prostaglandin (thromboxane) synthesis in the platelets, rendering them less sticky. Like other NSAIDs, it acts as a uterotropic agent by inhibiting the synthesis of prostaglandins in the uterus which are normally increased in amount in the hours before parturition.

Piroxicam has little effect on renal function in normal individuals but may worsen renal function in patients who depend upon the vasodilatory action of prostaglandins (e.g. PgE_2) to maintain renal blood flow. This may be seen in patients with hypertension, diabetes mellitus or cirrhosis of the liver. Piroxicam also helps to promote salt and water retention by interfering with the prostaglandin-induced inhibition of both chloride reabsorption and of the action of ADH. Prostaglandins, particularly E_1 and E_2, are synthesized by the gastric mucosa and seem to promote integrity of that mucosa by stimulating the secretion of cytoprotective mucus. Piroxicam, by inhibiting the synthesis of these prostaglandins may lead to gastric erosions and ulceration.

Pharmacokinetics

Piroxicam is measured in serum by HPLC which has a sensitivity of 300 μg.l^{-1}.[3] The drug is readily absorbed after oral or rectal administration. Absorption is not influenced by either food or antacids. In healthy subjects or patients following the administration of a single oral dose, the pharmacokinetics of piroxicam are linear, with the maximum plasma concentration usually being obtained in about 2 h, but this can vary from 1 to 6 h in different subjects. It has a low clearance rate of approximately 45 h, but the half life can vary from 30 to 60 h.[4] After repeated doses of 20 mg daily, steady-state concentrations are generally achieved in 7 to 12 days, with a peak plasma concentration ranging from 4.5 to 7.2 mg.l^{-1}. When a loading dose of 40 mg daily is administered for 2 days, on the second day the plasma concentration is 75% that of the steady state. Omission of one day's dosage after 7 days of continual medication results in only a minimal fall in the plasma concentration of piroxicam.[5]

Piroxicam plasma concentrations do not appear to be significantly influenced by concomitant aspirin[4] or iron[6] or antacids.[4] In man it penetrates into the synovial fluid of patients with rheumatoid arthritis, osteoarthritis and reactive synovitis, where mean concentrations are approximately 40% of those in the plasma; it is also demonstrable in synovial tissues.[7] Concentrations of piroxicam in breast milk are about 1% of those in the maternal plasma at the same time. Overall piroxicam is 99% bound to plasma protein.[4]

Pharmacokinetics do not appear to be age related, and renal function has only a limited influence on the elimination of piroxicam, but plasma concentrations are increased in patients with severe liver dysfunction.[8,9]

Oral absorption	~100%
Presystemic metabolism (CPIB acid)	
Plasma half life	
range	30–60h
Volume of distribution (CPIB acid)	0.1 l.kg^{-1}
Plasma protein binding (CPIB acid)	99%

Concentration–effect relationship

Piroxicam has a metabolite, a hydroxylated derivative, with very weak anti-inflammatory activity, and this could influence the relationship between piroxicam plasma concentrations and the clinical effects of the drug. There is a suggestion that pain relief with piroxicam is greater in patients with higher concentrations of piroxicam. Siegmeth[10] found plasma concentrations of piroxicam to be greater than 6.7 mg.l^{-1} in patients experiencing adequate pain relief. However, as with most other NSAIDs plasma concentration of piroxicam does not necessarily correlate with its adverse or therapeutic effects.[11]

Metabolism

Piroxicam is eliminated largely by biotransformation in the liver. The major route is hydroxylation, with the resultant product being excreted alone or as a glucuronide in urine and faeces (Fig. 1).[12] The metabolites of piroxicam have little or no anti-inflammatory activity in animal models. Approximately 10% of an oral dose is excreted as unchanged drug in 10 days.

Fig. 1 The metabolism of piroxicam

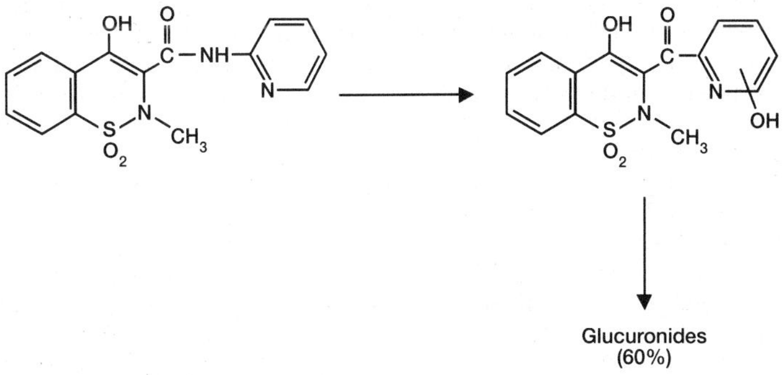

Pharmaceutics

Piroxicam (Feldene; Pfizer, UK/USA) is available as:

1. 10 mg maroon and blue capsules coded 'Fel 10', or 20 mg maroon capsules, coded 'Fel 20' in the UK and '322' and '323' respectively in the USA.
2. In the UK the following are also marketed. Dispersible tablets: 10 mg and 20 mg; the 10 mg tablets are scored.
3. Suppositories containing 20 mg piroxicam.
4. Feldene gel for local application, 0.5% strength (i.e. 5 mg.g^{-1} gel).

Therapeutic use

Indications

1. Rheumatoid arthritis
2. Osteoarthritis
3. Ankylosing spondylitis
4. Acute gout
5. Acute musculoskeletal disorder
6. Juvenile chronic arthritis.

Contraindications

1. Active peptic ulceration
2. Hepatic dysfunction
3. Previous known hypersensitivity to piroxicam
4. Asthma, rhinitis, angio-oedema or urticaria induced by other NSAIDs.

Relative contraindications

5. Pregnancy
6. Nursing mothers
7. Anticoagulant therapy
8. Inflammatory lesion of rectum or anus if suppository is to be used.

Mode of use

Piroxicam is a potent NSAID in the management of rheumatoid arthritis, ankylosing spondylitis and juvenile chronic arthritis. The once daily dosage is welcomed by patients. Care should be taken not to exceed 20 mg daily for long-term use and to watch for gastrointestinal side effects.

Indications

1. Rheumatoid arthritis

The recommended starting dose is 20 mg given as a single morning dose; however, in severe inflammatory arthritis it is wise to start with 40 mg daily for 2 days in order to get good blood levels quickly. They can then be maintained on 20 mg daily; although there is no absolute correlation between the effect of the inflammatory process and the blood level, those patients who do well tend to have a level between 5 and 8 mg.l^{-1}. In general it takes 5 to 7 days to get maximum clinical benefit from this treatment.

Original placebo-controlled studies showed piroxicam to be superior to placebo in alleviating pain, decreasing morning stiffness, increasing functional activity and improving sleep. This was so in a parallel study of 18 patients[13] over 12 weeks with 20 or 30 mg daily, while in another study adequate pain relief occurred in 24 of 30 patients treated for 6 weeks with piroxicam, but in only 7 of 30 patients treated with placebo.

In comparison with aspirin, piroxicam produced improvement comparable with aspirin as regards pain, walking time, duration of morning stiffness and the patients' global evaluation. In general, side effects were more troublesome with aspirin than with piroxicam, although gastrointestinal upset occurred in a similar proportion of patients with enteric-coated aspirin and piroxicam.[14] Comparing 20 mg of piroxicam with indomethacin 75 mg daily, Davies et al[15] found a tendency for piroxicam to be more effective, while in two other multi-centre trials piroxicam 20 mg daily was preferred to 75 mg of indomethacin daily as it was better tolerated and more effective. Other comparisons include those with 400 mg of phenylbutazine daily, 600–1200 mg and 2400 mg daily of ibuprofen, as well as naproxen at 500 mg daily, ketoprofen at 300 mg daily, diclofenac at 75 mg daily and sulindac at 400–800 mg daily. In all these studies piroxicam proved more effective, with relatively little more in the way of adverse effects. Under double-blind conditions piroxicam was found to be more effective than ketoprofen 300 mg daily in improving the articular index.[16]

Long-term open trials proved a valuable assessment of its efficacy and tolerability.[17]

2. Osteoarthritis

In a double-blind crossover study involving 591 patients, piroxicam 20 mg daily was superior to placebo in alleviating pain, decreasing morning stiffness, increasing physical activity and improving joint mobility.[18] It has also been shown to be more effective than aspirin in improving mobility in patients with osteoarthritis.[19] In a 12-week multi-centre trial, the efficacy of piroxicam 10–20 mg daily was not significantly different from that of indomethacin 75–100 mg daily, while there was a similar overall efficacy with piroxicam 20 mg daily as compared to diclofenac 150 mg daily.[16] The gel preparation has been shown to be more effective than placebo in the management of osteoarthritis of the knee.[20]

Apart from the use of the gel for local application to the knees, oral use should be reserved for the more severe cases of osteoarthritis who do not respond to simple analgesics.

3. Ankylosing spondylitis

A double-blind, multi-centre, crossover trial in 87 patients found 20 mg of piroxicam was more effective than 75 mg of indomethacin over a 4 week period.[21] Other studies noted that piroxicam 20 mg or 40 mg daily compared favourably with phenylbutazone 300 mg and was better tolerated. An open study in ankylosing spondylitis indicates that piroxicam at 10–30 mg daily reduces pain and morning stiffness and improves chest expansion and other objective criteria of assessment within 2 to 4 weeks of treatment. The effectiveness of piroxicam in the long term for this condition is reviewed by Schattenkirchner et al.[22]

4. Acute gout

Piroxicam 40 mg daily given as a single dose on the first day followed by 40 mg in divided doses for 3 to 4 days has been effective in alleviating pain and swelling and restoring of movement.[23] There have been no trials comparing piroxicam with other commonly used drugs.

5. Acute musculoskeletal conditions

Piroxicam has been compared with placebo, indomethacin, phenylbutazone and ibuprofen in acute musculoskeletal disorders. Certainly piroxicam is better than placebo, but studies comparing piroxicam with other non-steroidal anti-inflammatory drugs have usually not included a placebo control group and have seldom been double-blind. It is therefore difficult to compare the effect of piroxicam with other non-steroidal anti-inflammatory drugs. Having said that, Santilli et al[24] noted piroxicam once daily to be more effective than ibuprofen 900 mg daily and placebo in 30 patients with minor sports injuries. Studies currently in progress suggest that the gel will have an important role in the management of muscle and tendon pain as well as traumatic lesions.[25]

6. Juvenile chronic arthritis

The pharmacokinetics of piroxicam in children aged 5–16 years was no different from adults.[26] At a dosage of 0.3–0.5 $mg.kg^{-1}$ body weight daily it proved to be an effective and well tolerated non-steroidal.

The number of non-steroidal anti-inflammatory drugs which are currently available for children and have had appropriate studies performed is small. Thus the report of Garcio Morteo et al,[27] suggesting that piroxicam was more effective than naproxen in its usual dose in such children and also well tolerated, was very valuable. Williams et al,[28] using a higher dosage of naproxen, showed both drugs to be effective and well tolerated. The dispersible form of piroxicam allows minor modifications of dosage to be undertaken easily; its once daily dosage is particularly liked by parents or children with arthritis.

Adverse reactions

Potentially life-threatening effects

The major adverse effect of piroxicam is due to its effect on the gastrointestinal tract. Peptic ulceration and gastrointestinal haemorrhage may occur and call for the withdrawal of treatment in about 4% of patients, and may occasionally be life-threatening.

Renal damage has been observed and has occasionally been fatal. Aplastic anaemia and purpura (thrombocytopenic and non-thrombocytopenic) have occurred.

One fatal case of pemphigus vulgaris[29] has been reported. Presumably because of its inhibition of prostaglandin biosynthesis, piroxicam can contribute to a variety of renal syndromes, notably oedema, interstitial nephritis and very occasionally irreversible azotaemia.[30] Bronchoconstriction in asthmatic patients with aspirin hypersensitivity has also been reported.[31]

Acute overdosage

A moderate number of cases of self-poisoning with piroxicam have been reported. Poisoning may damage the gut, causing nausea, vomiting, diarrhoea and gastrointestinal bleeding; the kidney, causing proteinuria, haematuria and acute renal failure; the liver, causing hypoprothrombinaemia and other evidence of hepatic dysfunction; and the central nervous system, causing hyperreflexia, convulsions and coma. Hyperventilation is also a feature.

Treatment should include induced vomiting or gastric lavage, if indicated by the amount of the drug ingested and the time of ingestion, and the administration of activated charcoal in doses of 50–100 g, repeated if necessary. Diazepam, 5–10 mg intravenously, should be used to control convulsions. Forced diuresis, haemodialysis and haemoperfusion are all ineffective. Other measures are supportive.

Severe or irreversible adverse effects

Skin irritation and erythema multiforme have been reported. There appears to be no direct correlation between plasma concentration and the frequency of adverse effects, but administration of 30 mg or 40 mg daily for long periods appears to increase the gastrointestinal risks.[32] Gastrointestinal adverse effects have been reported in about 13% of 73 000 patients studied in a post-marketing surveillance programme, but not all these were of serious importance. Despite Boardman's comments[33] that the incidence of adverse effects does not appear to increase in elderly patients, several reports of upper gastrointestinal bleeding in elderly patients receiving piroxicam 20 mg daily have been published. In general, however, piroxicam does not appear to produce more gastrointestinal problems than other non-steroidal anti-inflammatory drugs.[34]

Adverse effects other than those affecting the gastrointestinal tract have been infrequent.

Symptomatic adverse effects

Headaches, dizziness, insomnia, depression, mood alteration, mental confusion, paraesthaesia and vertigo have also been reported, but extremely rarely. Other adverse effects tend to be anecdotal, namely, palpitations, impaired hearing, hypoglycaemia, swollen eyes and irritation.

Other effects

As with other non-steroidal anti-inflammatory agents, some patients may develop increases in serum transaminases. Changes in other liver function tests are also occasionally observed.

Piroxicam

Interference with clinical pathology tests
No interference of this kind has been reported.

High risk groups

Neonates
The drug is not used in neonates.

Breast milk. The drug enters breast milk at a concentration of about 1% of maternal plasma levels. It is not recommended for use in nursing mothers.

Children
As mentioned earlier, the drug has been used in children with juvenile chronic arthritis and is said to be well tolerated.

Pregnant women
The safety of the drug in pregnancy has not been established.

The elderly
There have been several reports of upper gastrointestinal bleeding in elderly patients taking piroxicam.

Concurrent disease
The diseases which contraindicate the use of piroxicam have been listed earlier under Contraindications.

Drug interactions

Potentially hazardous interactions
Piroxicam has been reported to potentiate the anticoagulant effect of dicoumarol because of its effect on platelets.[35] It can cause sodium, potassium and fluid retention, and may interfere with the natriuretic action of diuretic agents and thus aggravate or precipitate heart failure.

Other significant interactions
Piroxicam has not been shown to interact pharmacokinetically with digoxin or antacids containing aluminium hydroxide alone or combined with magnesium hydroxide, or with aspirin. However, the concomitant use of aspirin and piroxicam has been shown to produce a reduction in the plasma levels of piroxicam. It is highly protein bound and therefore might be expected to displace other protein-bound drugs.

Potentially useful interactions
None has been reported.

Major outcome trials

1. Lochead J A, Baragar F D, Tetreault L L 1985 A double blind comparison of piroxicam and enteric coated ASA in rheumatoid arthritis: a co-operative multicentre Canadian trial. Journal of Rheumatology 12: 68–77

The co-operative multi-centre Canadian trial provides one of the best studies in rheumatoid arthritis. 145 patients from 10 centres, aged between 21 and 70, were entered into it, with 71 receiving piroxicam and 74 receiving enteric-coated aspirin. The medication was dispensed using a double placebo technique, with piroxicam being administered once daily and aspirin in four doses. An adequate wash-out period was required before starting therapy. Initially the two groups were well matched for age, sex, weight and duration of disease. The duration of the study was 12 weeks.

81.7% of those patients treated with piroxicam and 67.6% of those receiving aspirin completed the full 12-week period. Nine patients in each group discontinued due to lack of effect, while 4 piroxicam patients and 13 enteric coated aspirin patients discontinued because of adverse effects. Prompt improvement occurred in both groups and, in particular, the once daily dosage of piroxicam was as effective as aspirin in controlling disease symptoms. Side effect profiles of the two drugs were similar except for tinnitus, and decreased hearing, which were only observed with enteric-coated aspirin. There was a slightly greater frequency of heartburn in the piroxicam group, but the overall frequency of gastrointestinal side effects compares favourably to enteric-coated aspirin. In neither group did alterations in laboratory values necessitate discontinuation of therapy, except for one aspirin patient who had to discontinue because of an elevation in serum SGOT. Needless to say, piroxicam did not alter the ESR. Thus it was concluded that both enteric-coated aspirin and piroxicam were effective in modifying the signs and symptoms of rheumatoid arthritis, but piroxicam was better tolerated by patients, with fewer drop outs and good compliance to the single daily dosage regime.

2. Husby G, Holme I, Rugstad H E, Herland O B, Giercksey K E 1986 A double-blind multicentre trial of piroxicam and naproxen in osteo-arthritis. Clinical Rheumatology 5: 84–91

A multi-centre, double-blind comparison of 20 mg of piroxicam with 750 mg of naproxen in more than 2000 patients with osteoarthritis, 43% of whom were over 70 years of age, showed that over 12 weeks both drugs had similar efficacy with regard to pain, patient acceptability and effectiveness; side effects were similar in both groups, with no increased risk of serious gastrointestinal side effects with piroxicam.

References

1. Wiseman E H 1978 Review of preclinical studies with piroxicam: pharmacology, pharmacokinetics and toxicology. Royal Society of Medicine International Congress and Symposium Series No 1, pp 11–23
2. Perrand J, Stadler J, Kessedjian M J, Munro A M 1984 Reproductive studies with the anti-inflammatory agent, piroxicam: modification of classical protocols. Toxicology 30: 59–63
3. Fraser A D, Noordbary J F L 1983 Therapeutic Drug Monitor 5: 239–242
4. Hobbs D C, Twomey T M 1979 Piroxicam pharmacokinetics in man: aspirin and antacid interaction studies. Journal of Clinical Pharmacology 19: 270–281
5. Fourtillan J B, Dubourg D 1984 Pharmacokinetics of piroxicam with multiple dosing. Comparison between two dosage regimens. In: The rheumatological disease process: focus on piroxicam. Royal Society of Medicine, International Congress and Symposium Series No 67, pp 85–89
6. Tilstone W J, Lawson D H, Omara F, Cunningham F 1981 The steady-state pharmacokinetics of piroxicam: effects of food and iron. European Journal of Rheumatology and Inflammation 4: 309–313
7. Bontoux D, Xavier Phelip A G, Fourtillan J B 1984 Pharmacokinetics of piroxicam in synovial fluid, synovial membrane and cartilage. In: The rheumatological disease process: focus on piroxicam. Royal Society of Medicine, International Congress and Symposium Series No 67, pp 91–94
8. Woolf A D, Rogers H J, Bradbrook I D, Corless D 1983 Pharmacokinetic observations on piroxicam in young adult, middle-aged and elderly patients. British Journal of Clinical Pharmacology 16: 433–437
9. De Schepper P J, Heynen G 1984 Pharmacokinetics of piroxicam in man. In: The rheumatological disease process: focus on piroxicam. Royal Society of Medicine, International Congress and Symposium Series No 67, pp 77–84
10. Hobb D C 1986 Piroxicam pharmacokinetics: recent clinical results relating kinetics and plasma levels to age, sex and adverse effects. American Journal of Medicine 81 (suppl 5b): 22–27
11. Siegmeth W 1980 Serum concentrations of piroxicam in relation to its clinical effect in patients with chronic polyarthritis. Weiner Medizinischer Wochenschrift (special issue): 31–35
12. Twomey T M, Hobbs D C 1978 Biotransformation of piroxicam by man. Federation Proceedings 37: 271
13. Weintraub M, Jacox R F, Angevine C D, Atwater E C 1977 Piroxicam (CP 16 171) in rheumatoid arthritis: a controlled clinical trial with novel assessment techniques. Journal of Rheumatology 4: 393–404
14. Wilkens R F, Ward J R, Louie J S, McAdam L P 1982 Double-blind study comparing piroxicam and aspirin in the treatment of rheumatoid arthritis. American Journal of Medicine 72 (2A): 23–26
15. Davies J, Dixon A St J, Ring E F J 1981 A double-blind crossover comparison of piroxicam and indomethacin in the treatment of rheumatoid arthritis. European Journal of Rheumatology and Inflammation 4: 314–317
16. Brogden R N, Heel R C, Speight T M, Avery G S 1984 Piroxicam: a reappraisal of its pharmacology and therapeutic efficacy. Drugs 28: 292–323
17. Weintraub M, Jacox R F, Angevine C D, Atwater E C 1978 Piroxicam and rheumatoid arthritis: an 18-month open-label continuation of a double-blind study. Royal Society of Medicine, International Congress and Symposium Series No 1, pp 53–58
18. Heynen G 1984 A double-blind placebo-controlled trial of piroxicam in 591 patients with osteoarthritis. In: The rheumatological disease process: focus on piroxicam. Royal Society of Medicine, International Congress and Symposium Series No 67, pp 19–22
19. Abruzzo J L, Gordon G V, Meyers A R 1982 Double-blind study comparing piroxicam and aspirin in the treatment of osteoarthritis. American Journal of Medicine 72 (2A): 45–49
20. Kageyama T 1987 A double blind placebo controlled multicentre study of piroxicam 0.5% gel in osteoarthritis of the knees. European Rheumatology and Inflammation 8: 114–115
21. Romberg O 1982 Comparison of piroxicam with indomethacin in ankylosing spondylitis. A double-blind crossover trial. American Journal of Medicine 72 (2A): 58–62
22. Schattenkirchner M, Muller-Fassbender H, Melzer H, Henze K 1982 Effectiveness of piroxicam in the treatment of patients with ankylosing spondylitis. An open long-term study. American Journal of Medicine 72 (2A): 54–57
23. Bluestone R H 1982 Safety and efficacy of piroxicam in the treatment of gout. American Journal of Medicine 72 (2A): 66–69
24. Santilli G, Tuccimei U, Cannistra F M 1980 Comparative study with piroxicam and ibuprofen versus placebo in the supportive treatment of minor sports injuries. Journal of International Medical Research 8: 265–269
25. Kroll, Hess 1989 A clinical evaluation of piroxicam gel: an open comparative trial with diclofenac gel in the treatment of acute musculo-skeletal disorders. Clinical Therapeutics 2: No 3

26. De Vere-Tyndall A G, Ansell B M, Piper S 1980 Piroxicam in juvenile chronic arthritis. In: Boyle (ed) Rheumatology in the eighties: an advance in therapy — piroxicam. Excerpta Medica, Princeton, pp 45–51
27. Garcio Morteo O, Maldonado-Cocco J A, Cuttica R, Garay S M 1987 Piroxicam in juvenile rheumatoid arthritis. European Journal of Rheumatol Inflamm 8: 49–53
28. Williams P L, Ansell B M, Bell A et al 1986 Multicentre study of piroxicam versus naproxen in juvenile chronic arthritis, with special reference to problem areas in clinical trials of nonsteroidal anti-inflammatory drugs in childhood. British Journal of Rheumatology 25: 67–71
29. Martin R L, McSweeney G W, Schneider J 1983 Fatal pemphigus vulgaris in a patient taking piroxicam. New England Journal of Medicine 309: 795–796
30. Mitnick P D, Klein W J 1984 Piroxicam-induced renal disease. Archives of Internal Medicine 144: 63–64
31. Spector S L, Morris H G, Selner J C 1981 Clinical response and serum prostaglandin levels in aspirin idiosyncrasy. Effect of aspirin and a new nonsteroidal anti-inflammatory agent. Chest 80: 676–681
32. Pisko E J, Rahman M A, Turner R A, Agudelo C A 1980 Long term efficacy and safety of piroxicam in the treatment of rheumatoid arthritis. Current Therapeutic Research 27: 852–859
33. Boardman P L, Burke M J, Camp A V et al 1983 Treatment of osteoarthritis with piroxicam. European Journal of Rheumatology and Inflammation 6: 73–83
34. Gierksey K E 1986 Piroxicam and gastrointestinal bleeding. American Journal of Medicine 81 (suppl 5B): 2–5
35. Jacotot B 1980 Interaction study of piroxicam with oral anti-coagulants. Proceedings of a symposium organized by Academy Professional Information Services Inc., and presented at the IXth European Congress of Rheumatology, September 4 1979. Academy Professional Information Services, New York, pp 46–48

Pivmecillinam (hydrochloride)

Pivmecillinam (BAN; INN) is an esterified form of mecillinam rendering the drug suitable for administration by mouth. It is available as the hydrochloride (tablets) and the base (suspension). The US Adopted Name (USAN) is amdinocillin pivoxyl.

Chemistry

Pivmecillinam hydrochloride (Selexid, Melicin, Maxibiol, Selecid, Tindacillin)
$C_{21}H_{33}N_3O_5S.HCl$
Pivaloyloxymethyl-6β[(hexahydro-1H-1-yl)-methyleneamino] penicillanic acid hydrochloride

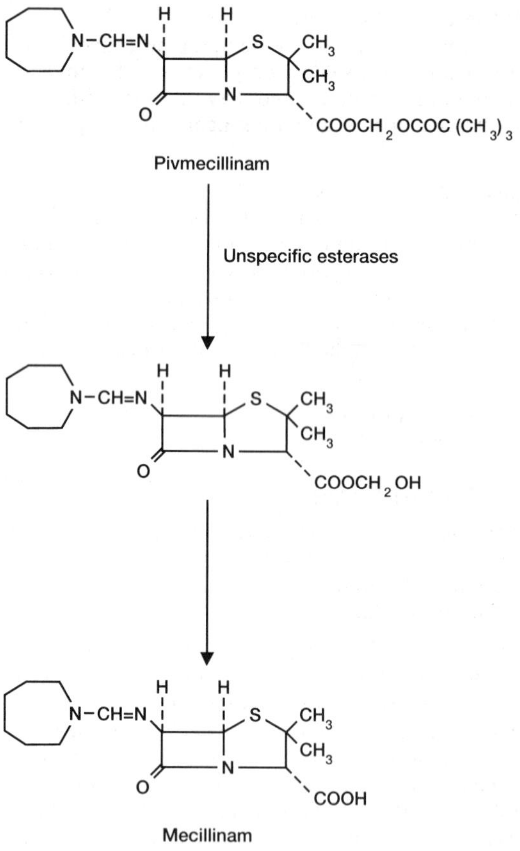

Molecular weight (free base)	476.0 (439.6)
pKa	8.9
Solubility	
in alcohol	1 in 4 (base 1 in 40)
in water	1 in 4 (base 1 in 20 000)
Octanol/water partition coefficient	—

A white crystalline odourless powder with a bitter taste; 1.35 g pivmecillinam base, or 1.46 g pivmecillinam hydrochloride is approximately equivalent to 1 g mecillinam. Pivmecillinam is also available as an oral combination product with pivampicillin (Miraxid).

Pharmacology

Pivmecillinam is a prodrug formulation of mecillinam which allows the drug to be administered by mouth. The prodrug form lacks

Pivmecillinam (hydrochloride)

antibacterial activity, but the active drug is liberated by enzymic hydrolysis during absorption in the gastrointestinal tract. Tissue esterases split off pivalic acid with formation of the hydroxymethyl ester of mecillinam; this product spontaneously decomposes to mecillinam and formaldehyde.[1]

Mecillinam is active primarily against Enterobacteriaceae. Although it is a penicillin derivative its mechanism of action is different from that of most penicillins. The antibiotic acts in *Escherichia coli* by interfering with bacterial cell wall synthesis through inhibition of one of the high molecular weight penicillin-binding proteins (PBP-2) located in the bacterial cell membrane; the mode of action in other susceptible organisms is probably the same. PBP-2 is involved in the maintenance of cell shape and susceptible Gram-negative bacilli exposed to mecillinam assume a spherical appearance and eventually succumb to lysis unless osmotic protection is given. Bacterial growth is not prevented by mecillinam (in contrast to other β-lactam antibiotics) so that bacteria surviving osmotic lysis continue to grow in the presence of the antibiotic. In this way, phenotypically resistant variants are readily selected from large bacterial populations. Acquired resistance is otherwise usually due to β-lactamase production, but mecillinam is less susceptible to some of the common enterobacterial β-lactamases than is ampicillin, partly because of low affinity for the enzymes.

Toxicology

Toxicological studies in animals failed to reveal any adverse effect of potential clinical relevance. The LD_{50} of pivmecillinam for rats and mice is > 2000 mg.kg^{-1}. No reactions were observed in rats and mice given up to 630 mg.kg^{-1} orally, nor were adverse effects on embryogenic or fetal development seen (information supplied by manufacturers).

Clinical pharmacology

Pivmecillinam is hydrolysed to mecillinam during the process of absorption through the gastrointestinal wall. Thus the activity of the drug is manifested through mecillinam. Mecillinam has poor activity against Gram-positive organisms. However, it is very active against Enterobacteriaceae. It is active against *E. coli*, *Klebsiella*, *Proteus*, *Enterobacter*, *Salmonella*, *Shigella* and *Yersinia*. Mecillinam has poor activity against *Pseudomonas aeruginosa* and has practically no activity against *Enterococcus faecalis*. Mecillinam has no other clinical pharmacological effects in man.

Pharmacokinetics

For assay in body fluids, assay methods applicable to mecillinam are appropriate (q.v.). If required, pivmecillinam can be assayed as mecillinam after hydrolysis with mouse serum; if both pivmecillinam and mecillinam are present, pivmecillinam can be separated from the mixture by ether extraction and the residue, after evaporation, dissolved in phosphate buffer.[1]

Hydrolysis of pivmecillinam after oral administration is extremely rapid: although mecillinam can be detected in the bloodstream within 5 minutes of ingestion of the prodrug, concentrations of pivmecillinam rarely achieve detectable levels (limit of detection = 0.02 mg.l^{-1}) at any time.[1] Any residual pivmecillinam in the bloodstream is rapidly hydrolysed there.

About 75% of an oral dose of pivmecillinam is absorbed in the form of the active compound and about 45% of the dose is recoverable from urine within 6 h.[1] In the most comprehensive study of the pharmacokinetics of pivmecillinam[1] it was found that 400 mg doses of pivmecillinam hydrochloride (273 mg mecillinam) administered by mouth to healthy volunteers achieved peak plasma concentrations of approximately 5 mg.l^{-1} 50 min after ingestion. However, other investigators have found somewhat lower values.[2–4] The natural instability of mecillinam in solution may have contributed to these discrepancies.

The fate of the pivalic acid (syn. trimethylacetic acid) and formaldehyde byproducts of pivmecillinam do not appear to have been investigated. The formaldehyde may be presumed to be metabolized to formic acid in the liver, with subsequent excretion in the urine or further metabolism to labile methyl groups.[5]

Other pharmacokinetic parameters are identical to those of mecillinam.

Oral absorption	>75%
Presystemic metabolism	~75%
Plasma half life	—
Volume of distribution	—
Plasma protein binding	—

Concentration–effect relationship

The efficacy of pivmecillinam depends on adequate concentrations of mecillinam being achieved at the site of the infection. Bacteria that are inhibited in vitro by 1 mg.l^{-1} or less of mecillinam are generally regarded as being fully susceptible. Organisms inhibited by 1–8 mg.l^{-1} show reduced susceptibility to mecillinam while if more than 8 mg.l^{-1} of the drug is required in vitro the organisms are regarded as being resistant to mecillinam.

Metabolism

Once it is de-esterified, pivmecillinam behaves as mecillinam. Mecillinam is not metabolized in the accepted sense and over 60% of a dose is eliminated unchanged. However, the compound is inherently unstable and the amidino side-chain and the β-lactam ring are both susceptible to aqueous hydrolysis. The products of hydrolysis are N-formyl-6-aminopenicillanic acid (which exhibits modest antibacterial activity) and the penicilloic acid derivatives of mecillinam and its N-formyl metabolite (which display no antibacterial activity).

Pharmaceutics

Pivmecillinam (Selexid; Leo, UK) is available as tablets or as granules for the preparation of suspensions.

Tablets contain 200 mg pivmecillinam hydrochloride; they are white, film-coated, biconvex tablets marked '137' on one face and with an Assyrian lion on the obverse.

The granules are presented in unit-dose foil sachets containing 100 mg pivmecillinam as white granules.

Pivmecillinam tablets and granules are also available as a combined preparation with pivampicillin (Miraxid, Fisons, UK; Pondocillin Plus, Leo, UK). Tablets (white, film-coated) contain 100 mg pivmecillinam hydrochloride and 125 mg pivampicillin or 200 mg pivmecillinam hydrochloride and 250 mg pivampicillin; granules are presented as unit-dose foil sachets containing 46.2 mg pivmecillinam and 62.5 mg pivampicillin.

It is recommended that tablets should be stored below 25°C and granules below 15°C in a dry place. The shelf-life of the tablets is three years, and of the granules 2 years. Suspensions prepared from the granules should be used immediately.

Therapeutic use

Indications

1. Urinary tract infection
2. Salmonellosis (including enteric fever).

Contraindications

1. Hypersensitivity to penicillins or cephalosporins.

Mode of use

For the treatment of uncomplicated cystitis, a loading dose of 400 mg pivmecillinam is followed by eight 200 mg doses given at 8-hourly intervals. In chronic or recurrent bacteriuria a dose of 400 mg may be administered 3 or 4 times a day. For children weighing < 40 kg, a dose of 20–40 mg.kg^{-1} daily is administered in 3 or 4 divided doses.

For the treatment of salmonellosis (including enteric fever) a dose of 1.2–2.4 g daily is administered for 14 days; to eliminate salmonella carriage therapy may be prolonged for 2–4 weeks. Children weighing < 40 kg should receive 30–60 mg.kg^{-1} daily in 3 or 4 divided doses.

Indications

1. Urinary tract infection

The spectrum of activity of mecillinam encompasses most Gram-negative urinary tract pathogens;[6] although Gram-positive organisms lie outside the conventional antibacterial spectrum, some, notably micrococci, may be susceptible to the very high concentrations of active drug achievable in the urine.[7] Mecillinam is less susceptible than ampicillin to enterobacterial β-lactamase[8] and many ampicillin-resistant strains of enterobacteria remain sensitive to mecillinam. These features suggest a useful role for pivmecillinam in the treatment of frequency/dysuria syndrome in domiciliary practice.

The role of pivmecillinam in the treatment of pyelonephritis, or of complicated urinary infection associated with urinary tract abnormalities or urinary catheters, is less clear. Some of the more resistant organisms that may be encountered in such infections, including *Klebsiella* spp., *Enterobacter* spp., *Proteus* spp. and *Pseudomonas aeruginosa*, are as resistant to mecillinam as to other oral β-lactam antibiotics. Furthermore, conditions of urinary stasis such as may be provided by anatomical abnormalities or urinary catheters may be conducive to the emergence of bacterial variants that are phenotypically resistant to mecillinam.[6,9] Nevertheless, pivmecillinam, especially when combined with pivampicillin, has been successfully used in the treatment of urinary infection in elderly catheterized patients.[10]

2. Salmonellosis
Antibiotic treatment is not usually indicated in salmonella infection that is restricted to the intestinal tract so that, although mecillinam is very active against most strains of *Salmonella* spp., the agent would not normally be used. In invasive infection with *Salmonella*, pivmecillinam and parenteral mecillinam are both effective, but no more so than co-trimoxazole, chloramphenicol or amoxycillin; Ball and Geddes[11] found that patients treated with mecillinam responded more slowly and continued to excrete the organism for a longer period of time.

Claims for the efficacy of pivmecillinam in the eradication of chronic carriage of *Salmonella* appear to be based on a single study in which 12 *Salmonella* carriers were treated.[12] The organism was eradicated in 8 of the 12 patients, but in three of the cases that were successfully treated, cholecystectomy was also performed.

Adverse reactions

Reported adverse effects of pivmecillinam therapy are mild and similar to those of parenteral mecillinam (q.v.). No adverse reactions attributable to the pivaloyloxymethyl side-chain, or its degradation products, have been reported. Pivmecillinam tablets may cause oesophageal ulceration if they get stuck in the oesophagus and it is recommended that tablets should be taken with at least half a glass of water.

Acute overdosage
No cases of this kind have been reported.

Severe or irreversible adverse effects
No reactions of this kind appear to have been reported.

Symptomatic adverse effects
None has yet been reported.

Other effects
A transient increase in alkaline phosphatase and transaminase levels has been caused by mecillinam and it can be assumed that this might happen with pivmecillinam. Short-term administration of pivmecillinam (or pivampicillin) has been shown to result in a reduction in serum carnitine and a correspondingly increased excretion of acylcarnitine in urine).[13]

Interference with clinical pathology tests
No technical interferences of this kind appear to have been reported.

High risk groups

Neonates
Mecillinam appears to be safe in neonates, so it may be presumed that pivmecillinam is also safe.

Breast milk. The drug does not enter breast milk.

Children
Pivmecillinam has been given to small numbers of children without ill effects.[14]

Pregnant women
The drug has been used in pregnant women without apparent ill effect,[15,16] but is probably best avoided in the first trimester.

The elderly
No special precautions are necessary in older people.[10,17]

Concurrent disease
In patients with impaired renal function a normal loading dose should be given, but subsequent doses should be reduced as follows.

Mild to moderate impairment (glomerular filtration rate 10–50 $ml.min^{-1}$): half the normal dose.

Severe impairment (glomerular filtration rate <10 $ml.min^{-1}$): one-quarter the normal dose. However, the dose should not be reduced below 200 mg 8-hourly in adults, or below 10 $mg.kg^{-1}$ in children.

Drug interactions

The following comments relate to mecillinam, but can also be applied to pivmecillinam.

Potentially hazardous interactions
Hazardous interactions between pivmecillinam and other drugs have not been reported.

Potentially useful interactions
Simultaneous administration of probenecid delays excretion of mecillinam by competition for renal tubular secretion.[11]

Potential useful synergy between mecillinam and ampicillin or other β-lactam antibiotics against some strains of enteric bacteria have been demonstrated in vitro[18,19] and in experimental animals.[20,21] The basis of the interaction probably rests on differential inhibition of the penicillin-binding proteins (PBPs) located in the bacterial cell membrane. Mecillinam binds exclusively to PBP-2 and bactericidal synergy is most evident when the compound is combined with β-lactam agents like cephalexin and cephradine, which preferentially inhibit PBP-3.[22]

Major outcome trials

Most large trials of the use of pivmecillinam have been in urinary tract infection; results of the two biggest trials were presented in the context of a symposium on mecillinam sponsored by the manufacturers.

1. Bresky B 1977 Controlled randomized study comparing amoxycillin and pivmecillinam in adult out-patients presenting with symptoms of acute urinary tract infection. Journal of Antimicrobial Chemotherapy 3 (suppl B): 121–127

A total of 298 patients were randomly allocated to receive 400 mg pivmecillinam or 375 mg amoxycillin three times a day for 10 days. Of the patients enrolled, 43 were excluded from analysis because of non-attendance (14 patients), in vitro resistance to the antibiotic (5 patients), unsatisfactory bacteriological control (11 patients), and interruption of treatment because of side effects (6 patients treated with amoxycillin and 7 patients treated with pivmecillinam). Of the remainder, 142 patients were treated with amoxycillin and 113 with pivmecillinam, but only 94 patients in the amoxycillin group and 78 patients in the pivmecillinam group were subsequently found to have significant bacteriuria ($>10^5$ organisms per ml of urine). Eradication of bacteriuria was achieved in 82% of patients treated with amoxycillin and 90% of patients treated with pivmecillinam as judged by follow-up 10 days post-treatment.

2. Ishigami J 1977 Clinical evaluation of pivmecillinam in acute simple cystitis: a comparative study with amoxycillin by a randomized double-blind technique. Journal of Antimicrobial Chemotherapy 3 (suppl B): 129–135

Patients with significant bacteriuria ($>10^5$ organisms per ml or urine) or those with bacterial counts $<10^4$ per ml, but with severe symptoms of cystitis, were randomly allocated to receive 50 mg pivmecillinam (calculated as mecillinam) or 250 mg amoxycillin 3 times a day for 7 days. One day after completion of treatment, 82 of 94 patients receiving pivmecillinam and 63 of 96 receiving amoxycillin were bacteriologically cured. Clinical assessment of the response by a urologist also favoured pivmecillinam. The difference in efficacy was associated with a higher level of resistance to amoxycillin than to mecillinam in the infecting organisms. Both treatments were well tolerated.

Other trials

1. Verrier Jones E R, Asscher A W 1975 Treatment of recurrent bacteriuria with pivmecillinam (FL 1039). Journal of Antimicrobial Chemotherapy 1: 193–196

30 schoolgirls aged 6–12 years, suffering from recurrent infection with *Escherichia coli*, were treated with 400 mg pivmecillinam 3 times a day for a week. Of 23 children infected with mecillinam-sensitive organisms 16 (70%) were cured on follow-up after 3 months; 3 of 7 (43%) children harbouring mecillinam-resistant strains were also cured. The same group of children had previously been treated with co-trimoxazole or amoxycillin for earlier infections; these drugs had achieved cure rates of 53% and 40% respectively.

2. Bint A, Bullock D, Reeves D, Wilkinson P 1979 A comparative trial of pivmecillinam and ampicillin in bacteriuria of pregnancy. Infection 7: 290–293

100 pregnant women with significant bacteriuria ($>10^5$ bacteria per ml of urine) were randomly allocated to receive 400 mg pivmecillinam or 500 mg ampicillin, four times a day for seven days. 65 patients were available for assessment after 2 weeks and 54 patients after 6 weeks. Cure rates at 2 and 6 weeks were: 88% and 76% (pivmecillinam); 85% and 64% (ampicillin). Side effects (chiefly nausea and vomiting) were significantly more common in patients treated with pivmecillinam, but in a follow-up study of 20 patients treated with a lower dose of 200 mg pivmecillinam, side effects were reduced without loss of therapeutic efficacy.

3. Damsgaard T, Jacobsen J, Korner B, Tybring L 1979 Pivmecillinam and trimethoprim/sulfamethoxazole in the treatment of bacteriuria. A bacteriological and pharmacokinetic study. Journal of Antimicrobial Chemotherapy 5: 267–274

Pivmecillinam (600 mg) or co-trimoxazole (80 mg trimethoprim plus 400 mg sulphamethoxazole) was administered twice a day for six days to 46 elderly patients. One day post-treatment, 2 of 23 patients treated with pivmecillinam and none of 23 patients treated with co-trimoxazole still had significant bacteriuria ($>10^5$ bacteria per ml of urine). Five patients in the pivmecillinam group and six patients in the co-trimoxazole group relapsed within 6–8 weeks. Nausea and vomiting was the only side effect noted (one patient in each group).

4. Tanphaichitra D, Srimuang S, Chiaprasittigul P, Menday P, Christensen O E 1984 The combination of pivmecillinam and pivampicillin in the treatment of enteric fever. Infection 12: 381–383

39 patients suffering from invasive infection with *Salmonella* (*Salmonella typhi* in 30 cases) were treated in an open non-comparative trial with a combination of 200 mg pivmecillinam and 250 mg pivampicillin four times a day for 14 days. Treatment was successful in all but two cases of typhoid fever. Treatment was well tolerated.

5. Bukh N 1983 Double-blind comparison of pivmecillinam plus pivampicillin ('Miraxid') with pivampicillin alone in chronic bronchitis: a Danish multi-centre study. Pharmatherapeutica 3: 422–428

64 patients with acute exacerbations of chronic bronchitis were given a combination of 100 mg pivmecillinam plus 125 mg pivampicillin, or 250 mg pivampicillin alone three times a day for 7–14 days. Response was assessed on clinical grounds and by sputum examination. 29 of 32 patients receiving combination therapy and 27 of 30 receiving pivampicillin alone were considered 'improved', but there were more relapses in the pivampicillin group (5 versus 1).

General review articles

Editorial 1976 Mecillinam. Lancet 2: 503–505

Symposia

Geddes A M, Wise R (eds) 1977 Mecillinam. Journal of Antimicrobial Chemotherapy 3 (suppl B): 1–160

Moellering R C, Nelson J D, Neu H C 1983 An international review of amdinocillin: a new beta-lactam antibiotic. American Journal of Medicine 75 (2A): 1–138

Pivmecillinam (hydrochloride)

References

1. Roholt K, Nielsen B, Kristensen E 1975 Pharmacokinetic studies with mecillinam and pivmecillinam. Chemotherapy 21: 146–166
2. Williams J D, Andrews J, Mitchard M, Kendall M J 1976 Bacteriology and pharmacokinetics of the new amidino penicillin — mecillinam. Journal of Antimicrobial Chemotherapy 2: 61–69
3. Wise R, Reeves D S, Symonds J M, Wilkinson P J 1976 A clinical investigation of pivmecillinam. Chemotherapy 22: 335–339
4. Mitchard M, Andrews J, Kendall M J, Wise R 1977 Mecillinam serum levels following intravenous injection: a comparison with pivmecillinam. Journal of Antimicrobial Chemotherapy 3 (suppl B): 83–88
5. Reynolds J E F (ed) 1982 Martindale: the extra pharmacopoeia 28th edn. The Pharmaceutical Press, London, p 563
6. Greenwood D, Linton Brooks H, Gargan R, O'Grady F 1974 Activity of FL 1060, a new β-lactam antibiotic, against urinary tract pathogens. Journal of Clinical Pathology 27: 192–197
7. Anderson J D, Adams M A, Wilson L C, Shepherd C A 1977 Studies on the effect of mecillinam upon Micrococcaceae and faecal streptococci under conditions simulating urinary tract infection. Journal of Antimicrobial Chemotherapy 2: 351–361
8. Richmond M H 1977 In vitro studies with mecillinam on *Escherichia coli* and *Pseudomonas aeruginosa*. Journal of Antimicrobial Chemotherapy 3 (suppl B): 29–39
9. Greenwood D, O'Grady F 1973 FL 1060: a new beta-lactam antibiotic with novel properties. Journal of Clinical Pathology 26: 1–6
10. Thoerner Andersen B, Joergensen M, Lorenzen J 1980 Pivmecillinam in the treatment of therapy resistant urinary tract infections. A comparison with pivmecillinam, pivampicillin and their combination. Infection 8: 27–31
11. Ball A P, Geddes A M 1983 Management of enteric fever with amdinocillin. American Journal of Medicine 75 (2A): 130–133
12. Jonsson M 1977 Pivmecillinam in the treatment of *Salmonella* carriers. Journal of Antimicrobial Chemotherapy 3 (suppl B): 103–107
13. Holme E, Greter J, Jacobson C-E, Lindstedt S, Nordin I, Kristiansson B, Jodal U 1989 Carnitine deficiency induced by pirampicillin and pivmecillinam therapy. Lancet 2: 469–473
14. Verrier Jones E R, Asscher A W 1975 Treatment of recurrent bacteriuria with pivmecillinam (FL 1039). Journal of Antimicrobial Chemotherapy 1: 193–196
15. Bint A, Bullock D, Reeves D, Wilkinson P 1979 A comparative trial of pivmecillinam and ampicillin in bacteriuria of pregnancy. Infection 7: 290–293
16. Sanderson P, Menday P 1984 Pivmecillinam for bacteriuria in pregnancy. Journal of Antimicrobial Chemotherapy 13: 383–388
17. Damsgaard T, Jacobsen J, Korner B, Tybring L 1979 Pivmecillinam and trimethoprim/sulfamethoxazole in the treatment of bacteriuria. A bacteriological and pharmacokinetic study. Journal of Antimicrobial Chemotherapy 5: 267–274
18. Cleeland R, Squires E 1983 Enhanced activity of beta-lactam antibiotics with amdinocillin in vitro and in vivo. American Journal of Medicine 75 (2A): 21–29
19. Neu H C 1976 Synergy of mecillinam, a beta-amidino-penicillanic acid derivative combined with beta-lactam antibiotics. Antimicrobial Agents and Chemotherapy 10: 535–542
20. Grunberg E, Cleeland R, Beskid G, DeLorenzo W S 1976 In vivo synergy between 6β-amidinopenicillanic acid derivatives and other antibiotics. Antimicrobial Agents and Chemotherapy 9: 589–594
21. Gordin F M, Sande M A 1983 Amdinocillin therapy of experimental animal infections. American Journal of Medicine 75 (2A): 48–53
22. Greenwood D, O'Grady F 1973 The two sites of penicillin action in *Escherichia coli*. Journal of Infectious Diseases 128: 791–794

Pizotifen (hydrogen malate)

Pizotifen succeeded methysergide in the prophylactic treatment of vascular headaches of the migraine type.

Chemistry

Pizotifen hydrogen malate (Pizotyline, Pizotifan, Sandomigran, Sanomigran, Sandomigrin, Sanmigran)
$C_{19}H_{21}NS.C_4H_6O_5$
4-(9,10-Dihydro-4H-benzo[4,5]cyclohepta[1,2-b]thien-4-ylidene)-1-methylpiperidine hydrogen malate

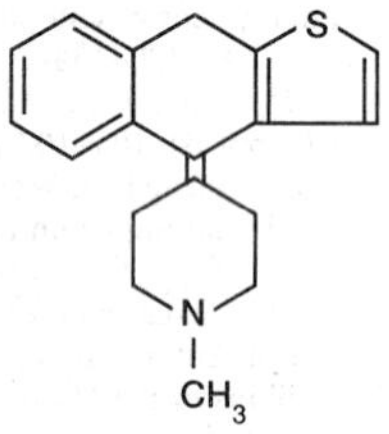

Molecular weight	429.5
pKa	8.7 ± 0.10
Solubility	
in alcohol	1 in 25
in water	—
n-octanol/0.1M HCl partition coefficient	8:1
n-octanol/phosphate buffer (pH 6.8)	55:1

Pizotifen is a colourless crystalline solid prepared by chemical synthesis.

Pharmacology

Pizotifen is a tricyclic (benzocycloheptathiophene) compound possessing structural similarities to cyproheptadine and the tricyclic antidepressants. Routine pharmacological screening in experimental animals shows the medication to possess strong antiserotoninergic and antihistaminergic effects, together with a weak anticholinergic action, but little or no activity on kinins or their liberators. At low concentrations pizotifen may potentiate the actions of serotonin. It was described for the treatment of the vascular headaches of the migraine type by Sicuteri et al. in 1967.[1]

Toxicology

Routine screening for acute, subacute and chronic toxicity up to 6 months in mice, rats, rabbits and dogs reveals little of potential clinical relevance. Toxic symptoms are sedation, impaired weight gain, tachycardia, hypotension, vomiting, diarrhoea and ataxia. In rats and rabbits the administration of pizotifen induces no evidence of embryotoxic or dysmorphogenic effects in either species.

Clinical pharmacology

The pathogenesis of the vascular headaches of the migraine type is not well understood. Dilation of cranial non-cerebral blood vessels in addition to a decrease in pain threshold of peripheral and/or central nature have been implicated.[2] The aura, which characterizes classic migraine, is currently attributed to a neuronal mechanism related to Leão's spreading depression.[3] The autonomic symptoms, which tend to be systemic in migraine and localized in cluster headache, have been explained by sympathetic activation[4] and a localized shift in autonomic balance[5] respectively.

How pizotifen affects the pathogenesis of the migraine headache is unknown. It was introduced because of its antiserotoninergic activity at a time when an excess of serotonin in the body was thought to play a major role in the pathogenesis of migraine.[6] Currently serotonin agonists are receiving more attention and agonistic effects have been demonstrated with pizotifen in lower concentrations.[7] An involvement of the central serotoninergic system in the pathogenesis of migraine has been postulated and pizotifen may potentiate this system at times of relatively low activity. Low activity of the central serotoninergic system is associated with dysinhibition of central pain transmission[8] and sympathetic nervous system activity.[9]

Pizotifen is devoid of vasoconstrictor activity although it has been reported to decrease vasomotor lability;[10] in high doses it may have a slight lowering effect on blood pressure and may mildly elevate heart rate. On the electroencephalogram it induces changes characteristic of those seen in the early stages of sleep,[11] compatible with a decrease in wakefulness as being its most common adverse effect.

Pharmacokinetics

Measurement of pizotifen in body fluids by gas chromatography–mass spectrometry gives a sensitivity of 0.1 μg.l^{-1} for the unchanged medication in urine and 0.3 μg.l^{-1} for its main N-glucuronide metabolite in plasma.[12] Pizotifen measured by the total radioactivity method has a sensitivity of 0.01 μg.l^{-1} in both plasma and urine.[13] However, this method does not allow the distinction between the unchanged medication and its metabolites. Using the latter method, after single oral doses of 1 mg ^{3}H-pizotifen in normal human subjects, radioactivity in the plasma is first noted after 2 hours. Peak concentrations are observed after 5 to 7 hours and lie in the order of magnitude of 9 μg.l^{-1}, which is, however, mostly metabolite as unchanged medication remains largely undetectable.[12] Then the plasma concentration decreases very slowly and small but significant amounts are still present in the plasma after 96 hours. Total excretion of pizotifen in the first 24 hours accounts for only 36% of the administered radioactivity.[13]

Following the multiple administration of ^{3}H-pizotifen at doses of 0.5 and 1 mg three times daily, the plasma radioactivity level increases progressively and levels off around the 5th day at 4 and 8 μg.l^{-1}, respectively.[13]

Oral administration of ^{3}H-pizotifen to rats is followed by a wide distribution of the radioactivity throughout the body. The plasma levels are lower than the concentrations found in most other organs. The highest concentrations of radioactivity are found in the lungs and liver. The concentration in these organs is about 10 times higher than that in plasma; in milk the level of radioactivity is about twice that in blood.

The total volume of distribution of pizotifen in man is 485 ± 45 l; the total binding of pizotifen to plasma proteins and erythrocytes is 91%. The biological half life as the time taken for 50% elimination of the absorbed doses determined from the urinary excretion averages 26 hours.

Oral absorption	80%
Presystemic metabolism	—
Plasma half life	26 h
Volume of distribution	485 ± 45 l
Plasma protein binding	91%

Concentration–effect relationship

The steady-state concentration for pizotifen in the plasma is 7 to 9 μg.l^{-1} at a dose of 1 mg three times daily as measured by the total radioactivity method. A relationship between the plasma concentration of pizotifen and its antimigraine effect has not been established.

Metabolism

The metabolism of pizotifen is extensive with less than 1% excreted unchanged in the urine. The main metabolite of pizotifen in the urine is the quaternary N-glucuronide. Of a single dose of 1 mg, 62% is excreted in the urine and 24% in the faeces over a period of 120 hours; only 36% is excreted in the first 24 hours.

Clinical pharmacology

Podophyllum is primarily useful as a caustic agent in dermatology practice. It is applied locally to the lesion (e.g. wart) and causes destruction of the tissues locally. Podophyllum is also caustic to normal skin if applied to it and can be absorbed into the systemic circulation with resultant toxic effects, in particular nausea, vomiting and thrombocytopenia.

Pharmacokinetics

After topical application, podophyllin is absorbed through the skin, particularly when used in the intertrigenous areas. Due to its high lipid solubility, it is distributed throughout the body including the central nervous system. This explains its high neurotoxicity. No data are available about the rate of percutaneous absorption.

Concentration–effect relationship

The therapeutic effect of podophyllin depends on its local concentration, not on systemic absorption of the drug.

Metabolism

No data are available on the metabolism of podophyllin resin.

Pharmaceutics

Podophyllum resin is commonly available in strengths of 5–25% w/v in compound benzoin tincture or alcohol and is used as a paint, e.g. Pod-Ben-25 (C & M Pharmacal, USA) contains 25% podophyllum resin (Indian) in Tincture of Benzoin, USP.

A proprietary ointment is available that combines podophyllum resin BP 20% with 25% salicylic acid BP in a fatty base as Posalfilin (Norgine, UK).

A topical liquid including 30% salicylic acid is available with 5% podophyllum. Cantharone-Plus or Verrusol also include 1% cantharidin (Seres, USA/C & N, USA). 10% podophyllum with 30% salicylic acid is marketed as Verrex (C & M, USA).

Preparations should be stored in a cool place in airtight containers and protected from light.

Extemporaneous compounding of podophyllum should be made in accordance with local guidelines for the handling of cytotoxics (e.g. using an isolator or cytotoxic HEPA cabinet, together with protective clothing including a respirator and protective goggles).

Purified podophyllotoxin is available as a 0.5% w/v acidic ethanolic solution (Warticon) and as a 0.5% alcoholic solution (Condyline).

Therapeutic use

Indications

1. Anogenital warts
2. Non-facial warts.

Contraindications

1. Due to its colour and staining of the skin, podophyllin is not recommended for use on the face
2. Pregnant and lactating women should avoid its use
3. Bleeding and friable warts should also be avoided due to the increased risk of systemic absorption.

Mode of use

Podophyllin remains the first-line treatment of choice for anogenital warts. Newer preparations of purified podophyllotoxin are now superseding the older podophyllin resin preparations as they cause less irritation and can be used for self-treatment.

Anogenital warts. Surrounding skin should be protected with vaseline, and the podophyllin paint applied with a cotton bud to all lesions and allowed to dry. The paint should be left in place for 6–8 hours and then carefully washed off with soap and water. Podophyllin is an irritant and if left on for too long will cause acute inflammation and burning at the site. A low initial concentration of 15% should be used which can be increased, depending on the therapeutic effect, to 30%. Lesions should be treated on a weekly basis.

If one of the newer purified podophyllotoxin preparations is used (Condyline or Warticon) the preparation can be used twice daily for 3 days each week until the warts have resolved.

Podophyllum

Other non-facial warts. The wart should be rubbed down with a pumice stone and the surrounding skin protected with vaseline before applying the podophyllin paint. This should be repeated on a daily basis, increasing the concentration from 15% to 30% depending on the response.

Indications

1. Anogenital warts

Podophyllin remains the first-line treatment for anogenital warts, but efficacy trials and comparative trials against other therapeutic modalities have shown that it has only a moderate success rate and a high recurrence rate.[1–4] Studies report cure rates of 22% to 98%, with 50% being about average.

2. Non-facial warts

Podophyllum preparations have been generally superseded by salicylic acid preparations and cryotherapy for the treatment of non-facial viral warts. Uncontrolled trials have shown cure rates of over 80% with plantar warts treated with podophyllin paint[5,6] but such studies are difficult to evaluate due to the high spontaneous remission rate for plantar warts.

Contraindications

Podophyllin is contraindicated in bleeding and friable warts, facial warts and in pregnant and lactating women.

Adverse reactions

Potentially life-threatening effects

Application of podophyllin ointment to extensive condyloma acuminata[7] and the oral intake of podophyllum[8] have been reported to have had fatal outcomes.

Acute overdosage

Acute overdosage may follow topical application or oral ingestion, presenting with abdominal pain, nausea, vomiting and diarrhoea. If seen within 4 hours of ingestion, the podophyllin must be eliminated from the stomach by lavage, charcoal and carthartics. If the resin was used externally, the treated area must be washed with soap and water. It is recommended that not more than 2 ml of a 20% podophyllin resin be applied to the skin. One patient who had 3 ml of a 20% podophyllin resin paint applied to anogenital warts suffered severe toxic effects with bone marrow suppression and severe sensorimotor neuropathy.

Haemodialysis is of no value due to the low water solubility of podophyllin, but charcoal haemoperfusion[9] has been reported to be of some benefit. No specific measures are indicated apart from support of vital functions. Patients with systemic toxicity must be observed for at least 24 hours.

Severe or irreversible adverse effects

These may follow topical application of podophyllin resin or oral ingestion of podophyllin extracts and can be split into neurological, gastrointestinal and haematological effects. Neurological effects are: diminished deep tendon reflexes, lethargy, confusion, delirium, sensorimotor peripheral neuropathy and coma. Gastrointestinal effects are: abdominal pain, vomiting, diarrhoea, nausea and paralytic ileus. Haematological effects include: leucopenia and thrombocytopenia, but there have been at least two reports[10,11] of an initial leucocytosis attributed to an acute bone marrow response.

Miscellaneous systemic adverse effects have been reported including hepatotoxicity with transient elevation of liver enzymes, tachycardia, tachypnoea,[12] fever and renal toxicity.

Symptomatic adverse effects

Podophyllum resin is highly irritant to the skin and mucous membranes and may cause pain on application. Occasional cases of apparent allergic, as well as unexpectedly intense irritant, reactions have been reported.

Inadvertent contact with the eye causes intense chemosis and conjunctivitis.

If the resin gains entry through cuts or an application to excessively pared verrucae, pain and swelling may occur ('podophyllin foot').

Interference with clinical pathology tests

No technical interferences of this kind have been reported.

P

High risk groups

Podophyllin does not have a particularly good safety profile and should only be used under close supervision. No particular age group is at higher risk of toxicity.

Neonates
The drug is not indicated in neonates.
Breast milk. Mothers using the drug should not breast-feed.

Children
The drug should be used with great care in children and only under close supervision.

Pregnant women
Podophyllin is teratogenic and its use is contraindicated in pregnancy.[13,14]

The elderly
No special hazards exist for the elderly.

Drug interactions

Potentially hazardous interactions
No drug interactions of this kind have been reported.

Potentially useful interactions
No useful drug interactions have been reported.

Major outcome trials

1. Stone K M, Becker T M, Hadgu A et al 1990 Treatment of external genital warts: a randomised clinical trial comparing podophyllin, cryotherapy and electrodesiccation. Genitourinary Medicine 66: 16–19

In this study 450 patients with external genital warts, both male and female, were randomized into treatment with podophyllin paint, cryotherapy or electrodesiccation. At the end of 6 weeks, 41% of the podophyllin-treated group, 79% of the cryotherapy group and 94% of the electrodesiccation group had cleared completely. Relapses occurred in 25% of all patients.

Duration and extent of warts did not influence outcome. Women responded better than men in all treatment groups.

Cryotherapy and electrodesiccation were thus shown to be more effective than podophyllin paint.

Other controlled trials

1. Douglas J M, Eron L J, Judson F N et al 1990 A randomised trial of combination therapy with intralesional interferon alpha 2b and podophyllin versus podophyllin alone for the treatment of anogenital warts. Journal of Infectious Diseases 162: 52–59

In this trial, 97 patients were randomized into receiving weekly treatment with podophyllin alone or podophyllin and intralesional interferon α 2b at a dose of 1.5×10^6 iu in three warts.

Maximal responses were seen at 2 weeks. The combination treatment resulted in 67% clearing of the warts compared to 42% for the podophyllin-alone group.

Relapse rates were 67% for the combination therapy and 65% for the podophyllin-only therapy.

2. Kirby P, Dunne A, King D H et al 1990 Double blind randomised clinical trial of self administered Podofilox solution versus vehicle in the treatment of genital warts. American Journal of Medicine 88: 465–469

In this trial 38 men with penile warts were randomized for treatment with 0.5% podophyllotoxin (Podofilax) solution or vehicle. Treatment was twice daily for three days per week, for 4 weeks. After this time a further 4 weeks course of active open labelled treatment was given to the 11 Podofilox and 15 placebo recipients with residual warts. Treatment with the active drug reduced numbers of warts to 15.9% of baseline and the area of the warts to 5.1% of baseline compared with vehicle which gave values of 97.4% and 92.9% respectively. Warts relapsed in all patients.

References

1. Culp O S, Magid M A, Kaplan I W 1944 Podophyllin treatment of condyloma acuminatum. Journal of Urology 51: 655–659

Podophyllum

2. Von Krogh G 1981 Podophyllotoxin for condyloma acuminatum eradication. Acta Dermato Venereologica (suppl) 98: 1–48
3. Simmons P D 1981 Podophyllin 10% and 25% in the treatment of ano-genital warts. British Journal of Venereological Diseases 57: 208–209
4. Gabriel G, Thin R N T 1983 Treatment of ano-genital warts. British Journal of Venereological Diseases 59: 124–126
5. Bunney M H, Nolan M W, Williams D A 1976 An assessment of methods of treating viral warts by comparative trials based on a standard design. British Journal of Dermatology 94: 667–679
6. Coskey R J 1984 Treatment of plantar warts in children with a salicylic acid — podophyllin — cantharidin product. Paediatric Dermatology 2: 71–73
7. Ward J W, Clifford W S, Monaco A R 1954 Fatal systemic poisoning following podophyllin treatment of codyloma acuminata. Southern Medical Journal 47: 1204–1206
8. West W M, Ridgway N A, Morris A J et al 1982 Fatal podophyllin ingestion. Southern Medical Journal 75: 1269–1270
9. de Torrente A, Rumack B H, Blair D T et al 1979 Fixed-bed uncoated charcoal hemoperfusion in the treatment of intoxications: animal and patient study. Nephron 24: 71–77
10. Montaldi D H, Giambrone J P, Courey N G et al 1974 Podophyllin poisoning associated with the treatment of condyloma acuminata. American Journal of Obstetrics and Gynecology 119: 1130–1131
11. Slater G E, Rumack B H, Peterson R G 1978 Podophyllin poisoning. Systemic toxicity following cutaneous application. Obstetrics and Gynecology 52: 94–96
12. Rate R G, Leche L, Chervenak C 1979 Podophyllin toxicity. Annals of Internal Medicine 90: 723
13. Cullen J E 1962 Congenital deformities and herbal 'slimming' tablets. Lancet 2: 511
14. Chamberlain M J, Reynalds A L, Yeoman W B 1972 Toxic effect of podophyllin application in pregnancy. British Medical Journal 3: 391–392

9. Langley P F, Lewis J D, Mansford K R L, Smith D 1966 Biochemical studies on poldine methyl methosulphate. Biochemical Pharmacology 15: 1821–1829
10. Wilson R, Long C 1960 Nacton and milk treatment of duodenal ulcer. Journal of the Irish Medical Association 47: 117–120
11. Seidelin R 1961 Effect of poldine methosulphate on gastric secretion of acid. British Medical Journal 1: 1079–1080
12. Kaye M D, Rhodes J, Sweetnam P M 1968 Clinical evaluation of three long-acting anticholinergic compounds. Gut 9: 590–596
13. Cook H B, Lennard-Jones J E 1966 Effect of antisecretory drugs on gastric hypersecretion in endocrine-adenoma syndrome. Lancet 2: 247–250
14. Colin-Jones D G, Copping R M L, Gibbs D D, Sharr M M 1969 Malignant Zollinger–Ellison syndrome with gastrin containing skin metastases. Lancet 1: 492–494
15. Lawrie R S, Williamson A W R, Hunt J N 1962 Zollinger–Ellison syndrome treated with poldine methyl methosulphate. Lancet 1: 1002–1004
16. Cartlidge M, Burton J L, Shuster S 1972 The effect of prolonged topical application of an anti-cholinergic agent on the sebaceous glands. British Journal of Dermatology 86: 61–63
17. Grice K, Sattar H, Baker 1972 Treatment of idiopathic hyperhidrosis with iontophoresis of tap water and poldine methosulphate. British Journal of Dermatology 86: 72–78
18. Cunliffe W J, Johnson C E, Williamson D M 1972 Localized unilateral hyperhidrosis — a clinical and laboratory study. British Journal of Dermatology 86: 374–378
19. Grice K A, Bettley F R 1966 Inhibition of sweating by poldine methosulphate. British Journal of Dermatology 78: 458–464

Polymyxin B (sulphate)

Polymyxin B is one of a family of polypeptide antibiotics produced by various *Bacillus polymyxa* strains.

Chemistry

Polymyxin B sulphate (polymyxin B sulphate, Aerosporin) is a mixture of the sulphates of polymyxin B_1 and polymyxin B_2.
Polymyxin B_1 $C_{56}H_{98}N_{16}O_{13}$
Polymyxin B_2 $C_{56}H_{96}N_{16}O_{13}$

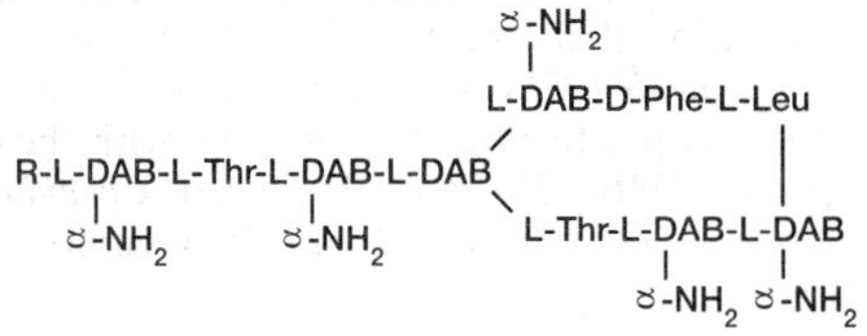

DAB = diaminobutyric acid
Thr = threonine
Leu = leucine
Phe = phenylanine

Molecular weight	
Polymyxin B_1	1202
Polymyxin B_2	1188
pKa	8.9
Solubility	
in alcohol	slight
in water	high
Octanol/sodium phosphate buffer partition coefficient	<0.05

Polymyxin B sulphate is a white or buff-coloured hygroscopic powder. It is produced from culture of certain strains of *Bacillus polymyxa*. Polymyxin B sulphate is also used in combination with a variety of other antimicrobials; generally for topical usage:
Gregoderm (ointment): polymyxin B sulphate, neomycin sulphate, nystatin, hydrocortisone.
Maxitrol (eye drops): polymyxin B sulphate, neomycin sulphate, dexamethasone, hypromellose.
Neosporin (eye drops): polymyxin B sulphate, gramicidin, neomycin sulphate.

Pharmacology

Polymyxin B sulphate is a cationic cyclic decapeptide that is surface active. It intercalates into the bacterial cell membrane binding to the lipid A region of lipopolysaccharides, in particular to phosphatidylethanolamine, and renders the osmotic barrier ineffective. This leads to loss of cell contents and bacterial cell death.

Toxicology

There is no information on mutagenicity, carcinogenicity or teratogenicity testing in animals. Polymyxin B sulphate produces neuromuscular blockade following intravenous administration in cats (ED_{95}, 10.8 $mg.kg^{-1}$) and hypotension (ED_{50} for 50% fall in arterial pressure is 6–12 $mg.kg^{-1}$). The latter has been attributed to a combination of ganglionic blockade, direct depression of the heart and histamine release. Polymyxin B sulphate also causes renal tubular epithelial damage (e.g. in the dog a dose of 2.5 $mg.kg^{-1}$ results in marked proteinuria, loss of renal concentrating power and reduced glomerular filtration). There is some evidence that polymyxin B sulphate may have ototoxic effects when applied directly to the middle ear.

Clinical pharmacology

Polymyxin B sulphate has been found to be effective in treating serious infections due to sensitive bacteria. In particular, before the advent of the newer aminoglycosides, penicillins and cephalosporins, polymyxin B sulphate and colistin were the antibiotics of choice for treatment of infections due to *Pseudomonas aeruginosa*. Infections treated successfully include septicaemia, meningitis, urinary tract infection and superficial skin and eye infections.[1–4] In systemic infections the usual dose is 1.5 to 2.0 $mg.kg^{-1}$ daily by slow intravenous infusion. For intrathecal use, doses up to 10 mg daily have been used.

Spectrum of activity

Polymyxin B sulphate is rapidly bactericidal for a variety of Gram-negative bacteria. It is active at clinically achievable concentrations against bacteria such as *Escherichia coli*, *Klebsiella pneumoniae* and *Ps. aeruginosa* (Table 1). However, it is not clinically active against *Proteus*, *Providencia*, *Brucella*, *Serratia* and Gram-negative cocci such as *Neisseria meningitidis* or *N. gonorrhoeae*. It is not clinically active against Gram-positive bacteria or fungi with the exception of *Candida tropicalis* (MIC 30–75 $mg.l^{-1}$) and *Coccidiodes immitis* (MIC 5–10 $mg.l^{-1}$). The range of MICs for common organisms is shown in Table 1.

Table 1 Minimum Inhibitory Concentration/$mg.l^{-1}$. (Data accumulated from references 5, 9, 13, 15, 33, 36, 37.)

Escherichia coli	0.02–12.0
Enterobacter spp.	0.02–12.0
Klebsiella pneumoniae	0.02–0.5
Serratia marcescens	12.0
Proteus spp.	>100
Providencia spp.	0.02
Salmonella typhi	0.02
Salmonella typhimurium	0.02
Shigella sonnei	0.02
Pseudomonas aeruginosa	0.02–4.0

Plasmid-encoded resistance has not been encountered nor do bacteria usually sensitive to polymyxin B sulphate become readily resistant.

Interactions

Complex interactions occur with polymyxin B sulphate in serum. The natural bactericidal activity of serum is enhanced but Ca^{2+} and Mg^{2+} ions inhibit the activity of polymyxins.

Pharmacokinetics

The preferred analytical method for polymyxin B is an agar plate diffusion method using *Bordetella bronchiseptica* ATCC 4617.[5] The sensitivity of the assay is said to be 0.2 $mg.l^{-1}$ but serum estimations may not always be reliable. Polymyxin B sulphate is very poorly absorbed after oral administration except in the neonate,[2] and therefore systemic therapy is achieved only by intramuscular or intravenous injection. Absorption of polymyxin B sulphate is negligible following topical administration to the intact skin, burns, granulating wounds, mucous membranes or the bladder.[2,6] However absorption does occur through the pleura and peritoneum[2] and may occur following inhalation into the bronchial tree.[7] There is no evidence of presystemic metabolism.

The plasma half life of polymyxin B is about 6 h.[8] The peak serum level is achieved 2 hours after a single intramuscular dose but is subject to considerable individual variation. For example, after an intramuscular injection of 500 000 units (50 mg) peak levels can be as high as 8 $mg.l^{-1}$ or as low as 1–2 $mg.l^{-1}$. The volume of distribution is unknown but it is known that polymyxin B does not pass readily from blood into joint spaces, the cerebrospinal fluid or aqueous humor even when there is inflammation.[1,2] Polymyxin B is bound to a very limited extent to plasma proteins[8] but binds strongly to mammalian cell membranes thus producing some accumulation.

Excretion of polymyxin B into breast milk has not been documented nor has its placental transfer.

Oral absorption	negligible
Presystemic metabolism	—
Plasma half life	
mean	6 h
Volume of distribution	—
Plasma protein binding	very low

Concentration–effect relationship

The therapeutic effect of polymyxin B sulphate is dependent upon the minimum inhibitory concentration of the infecting bacterium (see Table 1). However, during parenteral therapy serum levels should be monitored[9] and kept below 10 $mg.l^{-1}$. It should be noted that polymyxin B sulphate appears to be less effective in vivo than in vitro.

Metabolism

Polymyxin B sulphate is excreted mainly by the kidneys but there is a time lag with only 0.1% of the dose being excreted in the first 12 hours. Overall about 60% of the injected dose is excreted in the urine.[2] The drug is not excreted in bile and is not removed in appreciable amounts by peritoneal dialysis. Polymyxin B is not known to undergo metabolic change in the body.

Pharmaceutics

Polymyxin B sulphate, Aerosporin (Burroughs Wellcome, USA/Wellcome, UK), is available for parenteral use as a white or buff-coloured, freeze-dried powder in rubber-stoppered, aluminium-capped vials. There are no oral preparations. The intravenous or intramuscular dosage forms consist of sterile powder in vials containing 500 000 units (50 mg of free base equivalent).

There is no slow-release formulation and the parenteral form does not contain any other potentially allergenic substance. The vials should be stored in a dry place below 25°C and protected from light. Excess product should be discarded after reconstitution since it contains no preservative and resistant microorganisms would not be killed. When stored correctly polymyxin B sulphate has a shelf-life of 5 years.

Polymyxin B sulphate is also available as a mixture with other components for topical use and formulated as ear drops, dusting powders, sprays for wounds, ointments and suppositories.

Therapeutic use

Indications

1. Serious infection (meningitis, urinary tract infection, bacteraemia and superficial infections) caused by sensitive strains of *Ps. aeruginosa*
2. Serious infection due to other Gram-negative bacteria resistant to all other available antimicrobials but sensitive to polymyxin B sulphate
3. Topical therapy in combination with other antimicrobials.

Contraindications

Known hypersensitivity to the polymyxin group of antibiotics.

Mode of use

The clinical use of polymyxin B sulphate depends upon achieving concentrations in excess of the minimum inhibitory concentration of the microorganism at the site of infection. Since it is relatively toxic it is recommended that peak levels are kept below 10 $mg.l^{-1}$, thus only the most sensitive bacteria are amenable to this therapy.

Indications

Although polymyxin B sulphate is approved for treatment of serious infection due to a wide range of susceptible Gram-negative bacteria and particularly *Ps. aeruginosa*, it is not the antibiotic of choice.

Polymyxin B (sulphate)

Normally it would be reserved for cases where the bacteria were resistant to all other less toxic antibiotics.

Meningitis

Polymyxin B sulphate has been used to treat meningitis due to *Ps. aeruginosa*.[1,3] Since the antibiotic does not cross the blood–brain barrier it is given by the intrathecal or intraventricular routes. The usual dose for adults and children of 2 years and over is 5 mg diluted in 1–2 ml sterile 0.9% NaCl. This is given as a single injection daily until the CSF is sterile and then on alternate days for 1–3 weeks. The dose may if necessary be increased to 10 mg per day but must never be exceeded. For children under 2 years the daily dose is 2 mg per day diluted and given as for older patients. The dose may, if necessary, be increased to 4 mg per day.

Bacteraemia and urinary tract infection

Polymyxin B sulphate has been used to treat both bacteraemia and urinary tract infection due to *Ps. aeruginosa* and other susceptible Gram-negative bacteria.[1,2,4,10] It may be given intramuscularly or as an infusion intravenously.

The intramuscular dose for adults and children is from 1.5 mg to 2.5 $mg.kg^{-1}$ per day and for neonates 1.5 mg to 4.5 $mg.kg^{-1}$ per day in four equally divided doses at 6-hourly intervals. The powder is reconstituted in 1–2 ml of sterile water, 0.9% sterile NaCl or 1% sterile procaine hydrochloride solution. The latter diluent is used because intramuscular injections of polymyxin B sulphate are frequently painful. The intravenous dose for adults and children is 1.5 to 2.5 $mg.kg^{-1}$ per day. This dose is dissolved in 300–500 ml of sterile 5% dextrose in water and given either as a continuous infusion or two infusions per day each for 1–2 h with an interval of at least 12 h between doses. Treatment is maintained according to clinical judgement but is generally in the range 7–10 days.

There are no clinical trials to demonstrate optimal duration of treatment. The total daily dosage should not exceed 200 mg. There is no specific dosage information for neonates.

Joint infections

Joint infection by *Ps. aeruginosa* has been treated by injection into the joint space.[11] Polymyxin B sulphate (in 5 ml sterile water) was injected at a dose of 5 mg and continued until clinical resolution.

Superficial infections

Superficial conjunctival infections or corneal ulcerations due to sensitive *Ps. aeruginosa* or other sensitive Gram-negative bacteria have been treated by subconjunctival injection or by eye drops containing polymyxin B sulphate. For subconjunctival infection, up to 0.2 ml of a 50 $mg.ml^{-1}$ solution in sterile water or 0.9% NaCl (i.e. 10 mg) is injected each day until there is clinical resolution.[12,13] If eye drops are used, 3 drops of a 1.0 $mg.ml^{-1}$ solution in sterile water or 0.9% NaCl are administered hourly.[1]

Superficial infections of the skin including burns[14,15,16] and otitis externa[1,13,17] due to *Ps. aeruginosa* have been successfully treated with topically applied polymyxin B sulphate either in aqueous solution or ointment form (1 $mg.ml^{-1}$). In the latter case, since oxotoxicity has been described in animals following direct application to the middle ear, care must be taken to exclude possible perforation of the tympanic membrane.[18] Because of its disinfectant-like activity, the negligible development of resistance, lack of absorption and very infrequent parenteral usage combined with rapid and high bactericidal activity, polymyxin B sulphate is ideal for topical application. It is frequently combined with other antimicrobials for treatment of superficial infection (vide supra). There are few trials indicating superior efficacy but for example a trimethoprim, polymyxin B solution, has been compared with either neomycin, polymyxin B, gramicidin or a chloramphenicol solution in bacterial conjunctivitis.[19] Both the polymyxin-containing solutions were found to be more effective than chloramphenicol and there were no adverse reactions. Similarly, the efficacy of a cream containing a mixture of trimethoprim and polymyxin B sulphate was compared with fusidic acid cream in treating pyoderma in the tropics and the former combination proved superior.[20] Inhalation of nebulized polymyxin B sulphate has been employed in treating lower respiratory tract infections due to *Ps. aeruginosa*[21] as well as prophylactically in ventilated patients.[22,23] Although some success was reported initially one study demonstrated an increased incidence of infection due to polymyxin-resistant bacteria including *Serratia*, *Ps. maltophilia* and *Ps. cepacia*.[24] In addition acute respiratory failure following inhalation of polymyxin B has been observed.[25–27]

Contraindications

The only absolute contraindication is known hypersensitivity to the polymyxin group of antibiotics.

Adverse reactions

Potentially life-threatening effects

Deaths caused by polymyxin B administration are rare. However, the polymyxins are a relatively toxic group of antibiotics, although polymyxins B and E are less toxic than the others. In general, the sulphated derivatives are more toxic than the sulphomethyl derivatives, but this is counterbalanced by the higher intrinsic antibacterial effect of the sulphates, which means that lower doses are administered. Potentially lethal toxic effects include nephrotoxicity, neurotoxicity and hypersensitivity. These follow parenteral administration but the occurrence of each is rare.

Nephrotoxicity. This effect is dose-related and rarely a clinical problem in patients with adequate renal function. With a parenteral dose of 2.5 $mg.kg^{-1}$ per day, proteinuria, microscopic haematuria and cast formation are not uncommonly encountered.[13] For example, 33 of 66 children given intramuscular polymyxin B sulphate (2.5 $mg.kg^{-1}$) developed proteinuria and haematuria.[7] This is generally reversible but occasionally and especially with higher doses, glomerular filtration diminishes with nitrogen retention.[1,13] This occurs more readily in patients with pre-existing renal impairment.

Neurotoxicity. Respiratory paralysis leading to apnoea due to neuromuscular blockade is a rare but serious toxic effect of polymyxin B sulphate.[25,28] It is often preceded by dyspnoea and restlessness. It is not antagonized by neostigmine or reliably by calcium ions[28] as has been claimed previously.[25] The only reliable way to manage the problem is to initiate mechanical ventilation until recovery occurs. Apnoea is a rare problem and occurs when there is excessive accumulation of polymyxin B sulphate, for example in overdosage, renal impairment or in patients with myasthenia gravis. Respiratory paralysis has been reported following irrigation of surgical wounds or the peritoneal cavity.[28,29]

Hypersensitivity. Two patients developed respiratory distress after inhaling polymyxin B; it was considered that this was due to bronchospasm consequent upon histamine release.[27]

Acute overdosage

No specific cases of deliberate overdose have been recorded. There is some evidence that haemodialysis, but not peritoneal dialysis, can lower serum levels of polymyxin B.[30] This will not, however, greatly affect the levels of antibiotic bound in the tissue.

Severe or irreversible adverse effects

Neurotoxicity. Polymyxin B can cause neurotoxicity especially during the first four days of treatment; this is more likely to occur with serum levels of 5 $mg.l^{-1}$ or higher.[2] Features vary from dizziness, paraesthesiae (circumoral), and muscle weakness to ataxia, confusion and drowsiness to psychoses, convulsions and coma. The latter occur more frequently in patients receiving large doses or with renal impairment, but all are reversible.

Neuromuscular blockade. This effect can also occur with varying severity, from diplopia, ophthalmoplegia, ptosis and slurred speech to generalized weakness and generalized areflexia.[31] Intrathecal polymyxin B is irritative and produces meningism with headache, neck stiffness and fever.[13] This occurs very rarely with daily doses of 5 mg and doses greater than 10 mg should never be given intrathecally.[13] Local pain on intramuscular or subconjunctival injection can be a problem. This may be immediate or delayed. The immediate pain is prevented by inclusion of procaine hydrochloride in the intramuscular injection. The delayed type occurs one hour or more after the injection and is not prevented by the presence of a local anaesthetic.

Nephrotoxicity. An acute interstitial nephritis unrelated to dose has rarely been associated with polymyxin B sulphate therapy.[32] In this case a renal biopsy taken seven days after starting polymyxin B sulphate therapy showed interstitial oedema with an infiltrate consisting of eosinophils, plasma cells, lymphocytes and very occasionally neutrophils. The findings were interpreted as showing both acute tubular damage and acute diffuse interstitial nephritis.

Hypersensitivity reactions. These are rare when polymyxins are used orally or topically. After intramuscular administration urticarial and macular rashes and drug fever may occur rarely.[2,4] This may be potentiated in immune suppressed patients perhaps because suppressor T-cells no longer affect B-cell synthesis of IgE.[33]

Symptomatic adverse effects
Nausea and vomiting can occur following parenteral administration of polymyxin B sulphate. Topically applied polymyxin B very rarely causes ill effects nor does it readily sensitize patients.

Other effects
Electrolyte imbalance, in particular hyponatraemia, hypochloraemia, hypokalaemia and hypocalcaemia, has been reported, especially in patients with serious underlying malignancy.[34]

Interference with clinical pathology tests
No technical interferences of this kind are known.

High risk groups

Neonates
In general infants tend to tolerate polymyxin B better than adults.

Breast milk. Excretion of polymyxin B sulphate into breast milk has not been demonstrated, but as oral absorption is negligible no harm is likely to come to a breast-fed baby.

Children
Polymyxin B sulphate can be used in children as described in the section on Therapeutic use.

Pregnant women
The safety of polymyxin B sulphate in pregnancy has not been established.

The elderly
No specific information is available on the use of the drug in older patients.

Concurrent disease

Renal failure. The dosage should be modified according to the creatinine clearance (Table 2). However, it should not be used unless there is no other alternative, especially in chronically uraemic patients.

Other diseases. Polymyxin B sulphate is contraindicated in patients with myasthenia gravis.

Table 2 Polymyxin B sulphate dosage in renal impairment

Creatinine clearance	Dose
Normal or >80% of normal	2.5 mg.kg^{-1} per day
<80% to >30% Normal	First day: 2.5 mg.kg^{-1} per day Daily thereafter: 1.0–1.5 mg.kg^{-1} per day
<25% Normal	First day: 2.5 mg.kg^{-1} per day Every 2–3 days thereafter: 1.0–1.5 mg.kg^{-1} per day
Anuria	First day: 2.5 mg.kg^{-1} per day Every 5–7 days thereafter: 1.0 mg.kg^{-1} per day

Drug interactions

Potentially hazardous interactions

Nephrotoxic drugs. Concomitant use of other nephrotoxic drugs, such as cephalothin and aminoglycosides, should be avoided.

Anaesthetics and muscle relaxants. Neuromuscular blockade has been potentiated by ether anaesthesia, sedatives, muscle relaxants and antibiotics such as aminoglycosides that have muscle-relaxant activity.[31,35]

Potentially useful interactions
In vitro synergy between trimethoprim and polymyxin B has been demonstrated for a variety of multi-drug-resistant Gram-negative bacteria.[36] Combinations of polymyxin B sulphate and rifampicin[37] or co-trimoxazole[38] have been used to treat a variety of infections including septic thrombophlebitis, urinary tract infections, pneumonia and osteomyelitis due to multi-resistant *Serratia*[37] and endocarditis due to *Ps. cepacia*.[38]

Major outcome trials

There are no high quality controlled randomized clinical trials to provide evidence of efficacy. Most of the information available comes from a review of cases where polymyxin B sulphate was used.[1–3,10,11,13,15–17,21]

References

1. Jawetz E 1961 Polymyxin B, colistin and bacitracin. Pediatric Clinics of North America 8: 1057–1065
2. Hoeprich P D 1970 The polymyxins. Medical Clinics of North America 54: 1256–1265
3. Biehl J P, Hamburger M 1954 Polymyxin B therapy of meningitis following procedures on the central nervous system. Archives of Internal Medicine 93: 367–378
4. Weinstein L 1975 Polymyxin B. In: Goodman L S, Gilman A (eds) The pharmacological basis of therapeutics. Macmillan, London, pp 1230–1232
5. Sullman S F 1978 Polymyxins. In: Reeves D S, Phillips I, Williams J D, Wise R (eds) Laboratory methods in antimicrobial chemotherapy. Churchill Livingstone, Edinburgh, ch 37, pp 232–234
6. Chamberlain G, Needham P 1976 The absorption of antibiotics from the bladder. Journal of Urology 116: 172–173
7. Kaplan S, Fischer A E, Kohn J L 1949 Treatment of pertussis with polymyxin B (Aerosporin). Journal of Pediatrics 35: 49–57
8. Kunin C M 1976 Tissue binding of antibiotics. Chemotherapy 4: 1–5
9. Ball A P, Gray J A, Murdoch J M 1975 Antibacterial drugs today Part III. Medical Programs 2: 63–80
10. Pulaski E J, Rosenberg M L 1949 Use of polymyxin in Gram-negative urinary tract infections. Journal of Urology 62: 564–573
11. Tindel J R, Crowder J G 1971 Septic arthritis due to *Pseudomonas aeruginosa*. Journal of the American Medical Association 218: 559–561
12. Ainslie D 1962 Chemotherapy in ophthalmology. Practitioner 188: 45–52
13. Jawetz E W 1968 Polymyxins, colistin bacitracin, ristocetin and vancomycin. Pediatric Clinics of North America 15: 85–94
14. Jackson D M, Lowbury E J L, Topley E 1951 Pseudomonas pyocyanea in burns. Lancet 2: 137–147
15. Pulaski E J, Baker H J, Rosenberg M L, Connell J F 1949 Laboratory and clinical studies of polymyxin B and E. Journal of Clinical Investigation 28: 1028–1031
16. Swift P N 1956 Polymyxin. Practitioner 176: 47–55
17. Farrar D A T 1954 Use of polymyxin B in the external ear. British Medical Journal 2: 629
18. Editorial 1976 Ear drops. Lancet 1: 896–897
19. Gibson J R 1983 Trimethoprim–polymyxin B ophthalmic solution in the treatment of presumptive bacterial conjunctivitis: a multicentre trial of its efficacy versus neomycin–polymyxin B–gramicidin and chloramphenicol ophthalmic solutions. Journal of Antimicrobial Chemotherapy 11: 217–221
20. Jaafar R B, Pettit J H S, Gibson J R, Harvey S G, Marks P, Webster A 1987 Trimethoprim–polymyxin B sulphate cream versus fusidic acid cream in the treatment of pyodermas. International Journal of Dermatology 26: 60–63
21. Jawetz E 1952 Infections with *Pseudomonas aeruginosa* treated with polymyxin B. Archives of Internal Medicine 89: 90–98
22. Greenfield S, Teres D, Bushnell L S, Hedley-Whyte J, Feingold D S 1973 Prevention of Gram-negative bacillary pneumonia using aerosol polymyxin as prophylaxis. Journal of Clinical Investigation 52: 2935–2940
23. Klick J M, du Moulin G C, Hedley-Whyte J, Teres D, Bushnell L S, Feingold D S 1975 Prevention of Gram-negative bacillary pneumonia using polymyxin aerosol as prophylaxis. Journal of Clinical Investigation 55: 514–519
24. Feeley T W, du Moulin G C, Hedley-Whyte J, Bushnell L S, Gilbert J P, Feingold D S 1975 Aerosol polymyxin B and pneumonia in seriously ill patients. New England Journal of Medicine 293: 471–475
25. Levine R A 1969 Polymyxin B induced respiratory paralysis reversed by intravenous calcium chloride. Mount Sinai Journal of Medicine 36: 380–387
26. Wilson F E 1981 Acute respiratory failure secondary to polymyxin B inhalation. Chest 79: 237–238
27. Marschke G, Sarauw A 1971 Polymyxin inhalation a therapeutic hazard. Annals of Internal Medicine 74: 144–145
28. Lindesmith L A, Baines R D, Bigelow D B, Petty T L 1968 Reversible respiratory paralysis associated with polymyxin therapy. Annals of Internal Medicine 68: 318–327
29. Frogdall R P, Miller R D 1974 Prolongation of pancuronium-induced neuromuscular blockage by polymyxin B. Anaesthesiology 40: 84–87
30. Whelton A 1974 Antibacterial chemotherapy in renal insufficiency. Antibiotics and Chemotherapy 18: 1–48
31. McQuillen M P, Cantor H E, Rourke J R 1968 Myasthenic syndrome associated with antibiotics. Archives of Neurology 18: 402–406
32. Beirne G J, Hansing C E, Octaviano G N, Burns R O 1967 Acute renal failure caused by hypersensitivity to polymyxin B sulphate. Journal of the American Medical Association 202: 156–158
33. Lakin J D, Strong D M, Sell K W 1975 Polymyxin B reactions, IgE antibody and T-cell deficiency. Annals of Internal Medicine 83: 204–206
34. Rodriguez V, Green S, Bodey G P 1969 Serum electrolyte abnormalities associated with the administration of polymyxin B in febrile leukemic patients. Clinical Pharmacology and Therapeutics 11: 106–111
35. Hemmer M 1973 Anesthésie générale et antibiotiques. Médecine et Hygiene 1076: 1630–1631
36. Rosenblatt J E, Stewart P R 1974 Combined activity of sulphamethoxazole, trimethoprim and polymyxin B against Gram-negative bacilli. Antimicrobial Agents and Chemotherapy 6: 84–92

37. Ostenson R, Fields B T, Nolan C M 1977 Polymyxin B and rifampicin: new regimen for multiresistant *Serratia marcescens* infections. Antimicrobial Agents and Chemotherapy 12: 655–659
38. Noriega E R, Rubinstein E, Simberkoff M S, Rahal J J 1975 Subacute and acute endocarditis due to *Pseudomonas cepacia* in heroin addicts. American Journal of Medicine 59: 29–36

Polythiazide

Polythiazide is a diuretic of the benzothiadiazine group.

Chemistry

Polythiazide (Nephril)
$C_{11}H_{13}ClF_3N_3O_4S_3$
6-Chloro-3,4-dihydro-2-methyl-3-(2,2,2-trifluoroethylthiomethyl)-2H-1,2,4-benzothiadiazine-7-sulphonamide-1,1-dioxide

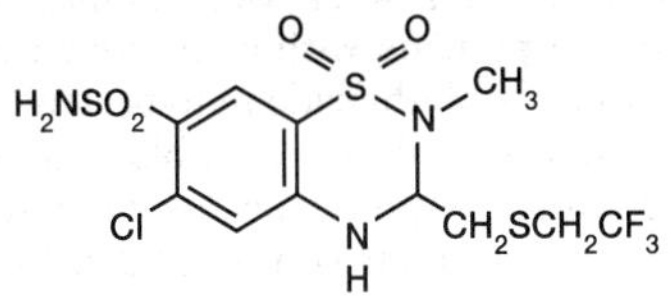

Molecular weight	440
pKa	9.1
Solubility	
in alcohol	1 in 17
in water	<1 in 10 000
Octanol/water partition coefficient	relatively lipid soluble

It is a white crystalline powder, soluble in alkaline solutions. Polythiazide is prepared by chemical synthesis. It is not available in any combination preparations.

Pharmacology

The benzothiadiazine (thiazide) diuretics were developed as a result of studies investigating the metabolic and diuretic properties of sulphanilamide and acetazolamide, both powerful carbonic anhydrase inhibitors. These studies resulted in the development of a series of substituted derivatives that were much less potent as carbonic anhydrase inhibitors, and hence less prone to induce significant metabolic acidosis.[1] The principal site of action of all the thiazide diuretics is in the early distal convoluted tubule (cortical diluting segment).[2] Although their mechanism of action at the molecular level is still poorly understood, they inhibit the transport of sodium and chloride across the epithelium from the tubular lumen. Delivery of drug in the urine to its site of action on the tubular epithelium is necessary and this partly accounts for the loss of efficacy of thiazides in renal failure. Natriuretic activity is negligible[3] once glomerular filtration rate falls below 20 $ml.min^{-1}$.[1] Thiazides inhibit free water clearance when the subject is fluid replete[4] and enhance water reabsorption during experimental dehydration.[5] Increased delivery of sodium to the collecting duct results in an increased urinary loss of potassium, and also magnesium. The secondary aldosteronism that accompanies the natriuresis may accentuate the loss of potassium and may predispose to a metabolic alkalosis. Thiazides also enhance the renal tubular reabsorption of calcium.

In both pituitary and nephrogenic diabetes insipidus thiazide diuretics increase the reabsorption of water from the distal tubule. The initial effect may be secondary to salt depletion and to a reduced delivery of sodium chloride to the distal nephron and can be abolished by salt loading. In the longer term a beneficial antidiuretic effect is maintained without evidence of sustained sodium depletion.

It remains to be established whether or not thiazides have other direct actions on blood vessels, independent of sodium loss, that contribute to their antihypertensive effect.

Toxicology

No data are available from mutagenicity, carcinogenicity or teratogenicity tests.

Clinical pharmacology

Polythiazide exhibits its diuretic effect predominantly as a result of inhibition of sodium reabsorption from the distal convoluted tubule (cortical diluting segment). Because most of the filtered sodium is reabsorbed before it reaches the distal tubule, the natriuretic effect of polythiazide is relatively modest. Maximal fractional excretion of sodium approaches 10%.[6] Polythiazide was developed with the aim of producing a drug that would have a greater natriuretic action and a lesser kaliuretic action than other thiazide diuretics.[7] Its relative natriuretic potency among drugs of this group is not in doubt, nor its prolonged action, but there is less certain evidence in clinical practice that it minimizes potassium loss. A single oral dose of 4 mg polythiazide had a more prolonged natriuretic effect than a single dose of 100 mg hydrochlorothiazide. After polythiazide the peak natriuretic response occurred between 12 and 36 hours and the increased renal sodium excretion lasted for 72 hours.[8] However, the relative efficacy of the two drugs given for a week were similar when expressed in terms of weight loss in patients with congestive cardiac failure.

The mode of action of polythiazide in hypertension is incompletely understood but is considered to resemble that of other thiazide diuretics. A rapid initial response occurs (2–3 days) that may be related to the fall in extracellular volume and reduced cardiac output secondary to the natriuresis. In the longer term (months) plasma volume is restored and the net haemodynamic effect is a reduction in total peripheral resistance.[9] Thiazide diuretics reduce vascular reactivity to both angiotensin II[10] and to noradrenaline[11] but it remains unclear if this is as a result of a direct or indirect effect on blood vessels. It had appeared that the ability of the kidneys to excrete sodium was essential to the antihypertensive effect of thiazides[12] but a subsequent study in patients with chronic renal failure suggested the possibility of a mechanism independent of sodium loss.[13] Indomethacin is known to attenuate the antihypertensive effect of bendrofluazide[14] but the hypothesis that thiazides reduce total peripheral resistance and blood pressure by enhanced synthesis, release or activity of vasodilator prostanoids[15] remains to be confirmed.

It is possible that thiazides have a direct, though as yet undefined action on resistance vessels. It has been claimed that polythiazide is a more potent antihypertensive than other thiazides[16] but the observations in this report were entirely uncontrolled, as were so many reports at this period of drug discovery. Another study, double-blind but otherwise unsophisticated, showed that polythiazide was equipotent to chlorthalidone 100 mg daily in respect to its effects on blood pressure.[17]

The dose–response relationship for polythiazide is unclear, either for its diuretic or for its antihypertensive effect. However, the dose–response curve is almost certainly flat and lower doses than currently used are likely to be effective. The recommended dose range is 0.5 to 4 mg daily. Diuresis begins within 2 hours and lasts for 24–48 hours. Polythiazide reduces the renal excretion of calcium as do other thiazides, and this may be of value in patients with renal stones due to idiopathic hypercalciuria. Polythiazide, like other thiazides, increases the LDL lipid fraction in the blood. However, this effect is dose-related, is small at low doses and of uncertain clinical importance, especially in long-term treatment.

Pharmacokinetics

A gas–liquid chromatographic method of analysis with electron capture detection and a lower limit of sensitivity of 0.2 $\mu g.l^{-1}$ has been used for analysis of polythiazide concentrations in plasma.[18] Polythiazide is well absorbed after oral administration. Plasma concentration peaks at 5 hours. No data are available on the metabolic pathways of polythiazide in man. Volume of distribution is 4 $l.kg^{-1}$ and 85% is bound to plasma albumin. About 25% is excreted unchanged in the urine with an elimination half life of 26 hours. The clearance ratio of polythiazide to creatinine in urine is only 5% that of hydrochlorothiazide.[19] This may be due to its greater degree of lipid solubility and reabsorption from the glomerular filtrate and may explain its longer duration of action. No data are available on its penetration into the CSF, breast milk or across the placenta although these are likely to occur given the lipid solubility and volume of distribution of the drug. The effect of old age or disease states on the kinetics of polythiazide are not known, but renal disease is unlikely to reduce elimination to any significant extent.

Oral absorption	100%
Presystemic metabolism	negligible
Plasma half life	25 h
Volume of distribution	4 $l.kg^{-1}$
Plasma protein binding	85%

Concentration–effect relationship

No data specific to polythiazide are available. There is no evidence of any correlation between the plasma concentration of polythiazide and its therapeutic effects.

Metabolism

About 25% of an oral dose of polythiazide is excreted in the urine unchanged. The fate of the remainder of the compound is not known, but is presumably eliminated by metabolism.

Pharmaceutics

Polythiazide (Nephril; Pfizer, UK) is available in oral form as tablets containing 1 mg. Tablets are white, round, flat, film-coated and scored, with 'Pfizer' on one side and 'NEP/1' on the reverse. Tablets contain corn starch. Maximum shelf-life is 5 years. In the USA Pfizer market three strengths of polythiazide tablets as Renese: 1 mg round white tablet coded '375'; 2 mg round yellow tablet coded '376'; and 4 mg round white tablet coded '377'.

Therapeutic use

Indications

1. Peripheral oedema
2. Cardiac failure
3. Hypertension
4. Calcium balance
5. Diabetes insipidus.

Contraindications

1. Hypokalaemia
2. Hyperuricaemia
3. Diabetes mellitus
4. Pregnancy.

Indications

1. Peripheral oedema

The underlying cause should be established and the need for and type of diuretic selected accordingly. Cardiac oedema is discussed below. Peripheral oedema and ascites due to cirrhosis responds to polythiazide but great care must be taken to avoid hypokalaemia and severe intravascular volume depletion, both of which may precipitate hepatic encephalopathy. In oedema secondary to cirrhosis it is often desirable to use polythiazide together with the aldosterone antagonist spironolactone. Polythiazide may be used to treat oedema due to renal disease although in practice the control of severe oedema secondary to nephrotic syndrome or to end-stage renal failure necessitates the use of loop diuretics. The diuretic efficacy of thiazides declines rapidly when glomerular filtration rate falls below 20 $ml.min^{-1}$. In practical terms this means that when serum creatinine rises above the upper limit of normal, consideration should be given to replacing thiazide with a loop diuretic.

An increasingly prevalent form of peripheral oedema that may not respond well to diuretic therapy is that induced by treatment with dihydropyridine calcium antagonists.[20] It is suggested that this form of oedema is largely a local phenomenon due to relaxation of precapillary sphincters. The more severe oedema caused by the most powerful vasodilator drugs such as minoxidil does respond to diuretic therapy but loop diuretics are usually required, often in large doses.

Polythiazide

The value of diuretic therapy for the treatment of swollen legs in venous incompetence or occlusion, lymphatic obstruction, non-renal hypoalbuminaemia, premenstrual oedema and so-called idiopathic oedema is uncertain. Severe chronic persistent oedema, whatever the cause, may justify an attempt at treatment with polythiazide with the aim of alleviating discomfort, improving cosmetic appearance and preventing stasis ulceration. Cyclical oedema presents a much more difficult problem since treatment may substitute an intermittent cosmetic symptom with a chronic dependence on drug therapy. Long-term therapy with polythiazide results in stimulation of the renin-angiotensin system with secondary aldosteronism. One important consequence of this is rebound oedema on withdrawal of diuretic treatment.[21] This is especially problematic in women prescribed diuretics for premenstrual oedema who may find themselves condemned to a lifetime of diuretic therapy (with all its biochemical and metabolic consequences) as a result of oedema developing on attempted cessation of therapy. Such rebound oedema commonly lasts 3–4 weeks and patients need considerable encouragement to remain off treatment until the secondary aldosteronism subsides. The possibility of an underlying psychiatric disturbance should be considered in women presenting with 'idiopathic oedema'.[22]

2. Cardiac failure

Diuretics are very widely used as first line treatment for cardiac failure and for pulmonary congestion secondary to valvular heart disease. The aim is to improve symptoms; there is little evidence that they improve morbidity or mortality. Thiazide diuretics such as polythiazide are used when symptoms are mild and renal function normal.

Other drugs are frequently used in conjunction with polythiazide in heart failure. Digoxin now tends to be reserved for patients also in rapid atrial fibrillation but it is especially important in this context to avoid potassium depletion from the diuretic. Angiotensin converting enzyme (ACE) inhibitors are increasingly used together with diuretics. It is important to take precautions to avoid first dose hypotension when such drugs are added to background therapy even with small doses of polythiazide. In brief, the rationale for combining diuretics with ACE inhibitors in the treatment of heart failure is that diuretics alleviate symptoms of oedema and also reduce the preload on the heart whereas ACE inhibitors reduce the afterload by blocking production of angiotensin II that is stimulated by both the heart failure and by the diuretic treatment.

3. Hypertension

Polythiazide is also used in the treatment of hypertension either as monotherapy or as combination with most other antihypertensives. It lowers systolic and diastolic blood pressure in both supine and erect positions. Some patients experience postural hypotension on treatment with polythiazide although this is very unusual at the recommended starting dose of 0.5 mg once daily. The effective dose range is from 0.5 to 4 mg daily. It is widely claimed that the dose–response is flat but a comprehensive dose–response study has never been carried out, despite the widespread use of thiazides for this purpose for over 25 years.[23] As with most other antihypertensives the magnitude of the blood pressure response varies directly with the pretreatment level of blood pressure. In mild to moderate hypertension, say at a pretreatment blood pressure of 165/105 mmHg, most thiazide diuretics may be expected to reduce the blood pressure by 15/10 mmHg. A reduction in blood pressure occurs within a few days of starting treatment and the response is sustained after several months, although the mechanism of action may change with time. After cessation of long-term therapy with polythiazide it may take several weeks or months for the blood pressure to return to its pretreatment level.

In the long term the treatment of moderate to severe hypertension results in a reduction in morbidity and mortality, especially with respect to stroke, heart failure and renal failure. In such patients thiazide diuretics such as polythiazide are generally used as part of combination therapy regimens and it is difficult to identify the contribution of individual drugs to the improvement in prognosis. In mild hypertension the MRC trial showed that bendrofluazide prevents stroke.[24] The principal overall finding of this study was that the combined active treatments (one group on bendrofluazide, the other on propranolol) prevented about one stroke per 850 patient years of treatment. Bendrofluazide may have been rather more effective at preventing stroke than propranolol. Although the benefit was small in relation to the number of patients treated no other antihypertensive drug has yet been shown to match even this degree of efficacy in primary prevention in mild hypertension. It has been widely assumed that other thiazide diuretics share the beneficial effects shown in this study but it is unlikely that this assumption will ever be tested.

4. Calcium balance

All thiazides inhibit the renal tubular secretion of calcium by about 50%. This effect has been utilized in the prophylaxis of renal calculi,[25] especially those associated with idiopathic hypercalciuria.[26] Chronic thiazide treatment is often accompanied by a mild degree of hypercalcaemia — this is usually not harmful, though it occasionally raises the suspicion of hyperparathyroidism. Thiazides have been shown to improve calcium balance in osteoporosis[27] and thiazide treatment of hypertension has been shown in one study in Japanese men to enhance the mineral content of bone.[28] Two recent independent studies have suggested that the use of thiazide diuretics is associated with a reduction in the risk of hip fracture.[29,30] These studies indicate that the risk of such fractures may be reduced by as much as one-third and the benefit may be even greater with increasing duration of drug use. These potentially beneficial effects have certainly not been widely adopted in clinical practice, but may represent a 'hidden bonus' of long-term thiazide treatment.

5. Diabetes insipidus

In 1960 it was reported that chlorothiazide had a paradoxical effect in decreasing urine volume and thirst in both pituitary and nephrogenic forms of diabetes insipidus.[31] Polythiazide has also been used in the treatment of patients with diabetes insipidus of pituitary origin.[32] With sustained therapy urinary volumes were reduced by about 50% at daily doses of 4 mg. The authors suggested that whereas the acute effects may be related to the induction of a negative sodium balance, long-term therapy was not associated with any detectable alteration in sodium balance or glomerular filtration rate. Hypokalaemia persisted in spite of oral potassium supplements but may be corrected by the addition of a potassium-sparing diuretic.

Contraindications

1. Hypokalaemia

All thiazide diuretics increase the renal elimination of potassium, principally as a result of enhanced tubular flow and delivery of sodium to the distal sites of potassium excretion. The urinary loss of potassium may be greater after acute than after chronic administration. Total body depletion of potassium may be present even when serum potassium levels remain normal whereas chronic hypokalaemia (serum potassium <3.5 mmol.l^{-1}) may occur in the absence of a substantial total body deficit of potassium.

Potassium replacement therapy is not routinely necessary in hypertension, when low doses of thiazides are now preferred. At the 10 mg daily dose of bendrofluazide used in the MRC trial, severe hypokalaemia was observed in some patients and may have contributed to some of the ventricular ectopic activity observed.[33] Similar considerations might reasonably be expected to apply to high dose polythiazide used for similar purposes. Hypokalaemia may be more of a problem in the treatment of heart failure, especially if digoxin is also being prescribed, as hypokalaemia enhances the cardiotoxic effects of cardiac glycosides. In this context there is a very much stronger case for the routine co-administration of a potassium conserving diuretic. Potassium chloride supplementation in conventional dosage may be relatively inefficient in patients with thiazide-induced hypokalaemia.[34]

Polythiazide should be used with caution in patients with pre-existing hypokalaemia as the potassium deficit may be aggravated. Profound hypokalaemia developing in response to diuretic therapy in hypertension should raise suspicion of the diagnosis of primary aldosteronism.

Even in the presence of a normal total body and serum potassium, serum potassium may fall sharply in response to stimulation of β_2-adrenoceptors. This is partly a direct effect, mediated via activation of cell membrane-bound Na^+,K^+-ATPase, partly an indirect effect mediated by insulin release that activates the same enzyme and also drives glucose into the cells accompanied by potassium. This mechanism accounts for the acute hypokalaemia that accompanies the administration of adrenaline.[35] This phenomenon may also be important in the context of acute myocardial infarction when endogenous adrenaline release may provoke dangerously low levels of serum potassium, especially if the patient is pretreated with diuretics.[36]

2. Hyperuricaemia

All thiazides in common use cause retention of urate. There is evidence that thiazide diuretics, like salicylates and ethacrynic acid, have a paradoxical effect on uric acid secretion by the kidney. At low doses and after intravenous administration thiazides may have a uricosuric effect, whereas prolonged oral dosage causes urate retention. It has been suggested that low doses block urate reabsorption in the proximal tubule whereas high doses block both reabsorption and secretion. Since the former has a greater capacity, urate retention results.[37] Both probenecid and sulphinpyrazone prevent the rise in serum uric acid in such patients without inhibiting the natriuresis.[38]

Occasionally, the hyperuricaemia results in precipitation of acute gout. Thiazides should be avoided in patients with pre-existing hyperuricaemia unless prophylactic therapy such as allopurinol is being administered concurrently.

3. Diabetes mellitus

Long-term therapy with thiazide diuretics may result in impaired glucose tolerance, occasionally with the emergence of frank diabetes mellitus and, rarely, ketoacidosis or hyperosmolar non-ketotic coma.[39] The time course of deterioration in glucose tolerance may be many years[40] and careful monitoring is required, especially in high risk patients such as the obese and those with a familial predisposition. In pre-existing diabetes, thiazides may impair the response to oral hypoglycaemic drugs and in particular may antagonize the effects of sulphonylureas. Dose adjustment may be required and the patient may even require a change to insulin unless the diuretic is stopped. One of the likely mechanisms for thiazide-induced diabetes is by inhibition of insulin release from the pancreatic islet cells, either by a direct effect or via an effect of chronic hypokalaemia. A number of other mechanisms have been proposed, including impaired tissue sensitivity to insulin,[41] and it is possible that these may all contribute to the effect. There is some evidence that correction of hypokalaemia restores glucose tolerance towards normal.[42] A more recent study provides convincing evidence that glucose intolerance due to thiazides can be prevented by adequate potassium supplementation and that the mechanism of the diabetogenic effect is mediated via a hypokalaemic impairment of β cell response to glucose.[43] Impaired glucose tolerance was observed in the EWPHE trial even when hydrochlorothiazide was combined with the potassium sparing drug triamterene, although in this study the impairment of glucose tolerance occurred mainly in the first year and was greatest in patients in whom serum potassium decreased.[44] A recent report of a randomized comparison between bendrofluazide and propranolol in mild hypertension found that glucose tolerance improved in both groups over a ten year follow-up and that diabetes developed in fewer patients in the bendrofluazide group.[45] The results of this study are very reassuring but apply only to middle aged men with mild hypertension and to treatment with low doses of bendrofluazide (2.5–5 mg daily) that were not accompanied by a severe degree of hypokalaemia.

In insulin-dependent diabetes co-administration of thiazides seldom has an important influence on insulin requirements or in the quality of metabolic control.

4. Pregnancy

Oedema is common during pregnancy but there are several reasons why diuretics should not be used routinely to deal with this.

Oedema is not harmful to either the mother or fetus.[46] There is little evidence that treatment of oedema with diuretics improves the fetal prognosis. An overview of many clinical trials, individually lacking sufficient power, suggested that diuretic therapy may prevent the development of gestational hypertension.[47] These authors also concluded from their analysis that adverse effects of thiazides in pregnancy may have been exaggerated in the past as a result of selected case reporting. However, it has been argued that a further reduction in plasma volume, already contracted in gestational hypertension, may be undesirable.[48] Diuretic therapy in pregnancy should be reserved for the control of heart failure and for the treatment of hypertension in patients whose blood pressure is refractory to conventional therapy with methyldopa, β-adrenoceptor antagonists and calcium channel antagonists.

Adverse reactions

Potentially life-threatening effects

Fatal idiosyncratic reactions to polythiazide have not been recorded. Thiazide diuretics may cause devastating and sometimes fatal hyponatraemia.[49,50] Numerous examples have been reported — those at greatest risk are frail elderly females.

It is certainly possible that thiazide-related hypokalaemia may precipitate fatal cardiac arrhythmias in some patients but many of these patients have either pre-existing hypertension or heart failure and may be liable to sudden cardiac death unrelated to drug therapy. The MRC trial in mild hypertension showed that although bendrofluazide (10 mg daily) was associated with an increased incidence of ventricular ectopic beats and arrhythmias related to hypokalaemia, the overall cardiovascular mortality was not adversely affected. Nevertheless, it is generally considered now that low doses of thiazides should be used and that these maintain the haemodynamic effect while minimizing the potentially adverse electrolyte and metabolic effects.

Long-term therapy with thiazides may result in an abnormal lipid profile. However, the average reported elevations in both cholesterol (6%) and triglyceride (15%) are small, may not be sustained over many years,[51] and may be prevented by a cholesterol-lowering diet.[52] It remains uncertain if this predisposes to atheroma and fatal cardiac and cerebrovascular disease. One major study (MR FIT) suggested that treatment of hypertension with a diuretic-based regimen might be associated with an increase in cardiovascular events.[53] However, this still controversial conclusion was based on a subgroup analysis of patients with abnormal prestudy electrocardiograms and a subsequent statistical review[54] suggested that the evidence was inconclusive. The MRC trial utilized a high dose of bendrofluazide by current standards, so that if there was a true arrythmic effect then this should have been identified. On the other hand, the overall cardiac event rate in this study was low and some uncertainty must remain about the applicability of these results to patients with a higher risk of coronary artery disease.

Acute overdosage

Doses of polythiazide at the top of the accepted normal range may occasionally precipitate severe volume depletion, hypotension, hyponatraemia and hypokalaemia. Deliberate or accidental overdosage with polythiazide has been reported in one 14-year-old girl who took 18 to 24 mg without fatal consequences. Serum potassium levels were 2.5–3.0 mEq.l^{-1} for a week. No additional toxic effects were recorded. Renal failure may result from severe volume depletion, whatever the cause, and renal function should be monitored. Overdosage may result when two or more diuretics are prescribed simultaneously, for example by the use of proprietary medications that include a thiazide. Unfortunately, many proprietary names give no indication of the nature of the active constituents — a powerful argument in favour of generic prescribing. Overdosage is managed by withdrawal of the diuretic, potassium supplementation and in severe cases by parenteral rehydration.

Diuretics are also subject to a more insidious form of abuse by subjects who misuse them as slimming aids or by athletes who use them to control weight. They may be combined with laxatives. Electrolyte disturbances and rebound oedema may occur.

Severe or irreversible adverse effects

The main concern in this context has been that long-term treatment of asymptomatic patients with thiazide diuretics for hypertension may predispose to the development of atherosclerosis, possibly as a result of adverse effects on carbohydrate and lipid metabolism. It has to be said that there is very little good evidence that this is the case. Indeed, the results of several major trials reported over the past five years prove conclusively that thiazides do not increase the morbidity or mortality from ischaemic heart disease.

Symptomatic adverse effects

Reported symptoms may be more frequent when a patient is being treated for a normally asymptomatic condition (e.g. hypertension) than when treated for troublesome symptoms (e.g. heart failure). In the MRC trial of mild hypertension bendrofluazide was most com-

Polythiazide

monly associated with nausea, dizziness and headache (women) and gout and impotence (men).[55]

The mechanism by which thiazide diuretics induce impotence is unknown but this is a serious limitation in men with otherwise asymptomatic hypertension. The prevalence in the MRC trial was 23% on bendrofluazide and 10% on placebo at 2 years. The problem is usually reversible although some men that suffer this may have sexual difficulties on other drugs and may have persistent problems in this respect. This symptom remains one of the unsolved mysteries of the MRC trial and many clinicians remain to be convinced that the true prevalence is as high as that reported.

There is no comparable data base on which to judge the side effect profile of polythiazide. Weakness and dizziness have been reported in less than 3% of patients. Numerous other symptoms have been reported, although in most of these the proof of a causative drug effect is lacking. These include: nausea, vomiting, cholestatic jaundice, pancreatitis; maculopapular rash, photosensitivity, necrotizing vasculitis; fatigue, headache, vertigo, paraesthesia, xanthopsia, cramps, restlessness; aplastic anaemia, neutropenia, thrombocytopenia.

Polyuria and thirst may occasionally be inconvenient after a few days of diuretic therapy. The symptoms often subside with time, partly as a result of patients adapting to the symptoms.

Other effects

Biochemical disturbances caused by thiazide diuretics include metabolic alkalosis, hypercalcaemia, hyperglycaemia, hyperlipidaemia, hyperuricaemia, hypokalaemia, hypomagnesaemia and hyponatraemia. A minor elevation in plasma urea is common, reflecting a degree of volume depletion. Established renal failure is uncommon, although thiazides may enhance the nephrotoxicity of other drugs such as non-steroidal anti-inflammatory drugs and angiotensin converting enzyme inhibitors.

Diuretics stimulate the renin–angiotensin–aldosterone system. This tends to conserve salt and water and tends to offset the beneficial effects of thiazides in both hypertension and heart failure. Long-term stimulation of this system is not known to be harmful although one important consequence is that sudden cessation of thiazide treatment results in a state of secondary aldosteronism that may result in rebound oedema for a few weeks before a new state of salt and water equilibrium is achieved.

Interference with clinical pathology tests

No information is available on any direct interference with biochemical assays.

Diuretic therapy may result in apparent polycythaemia with an elevated haematocrit. Formal isotope studies will, however, reveal the underlying cause to be a reduction in plasma volume rather than a true increase in red cell mass.

High risk groups

Neonates

The drug is not normally used in neonates.

Breast milk. Thiazide diuretics may inhibit lactation, and some have been used therapeutically for this purpose. However, it is no longer considered good practice to subject patients to the risk of electrolyte disturbances, haemoconcentration and hyperuricaemia in the puerperium. No information is available on excretion of the drug in breast milk.

Children

Little information is available on the use of the drug in children.

Pregnant women

Factors relating to this topic have been outlined above, under Contraindications.

The elderly

Extra caution is required in order to avoid severe volume depletion, postural hypotension, syncope, renal failure and adverse interactions with other drugs, all of which are more likely in the elderly. Dietary intake of potassium may be poor and the patient more prone to hypokalaemia. Severe hyponatraemia may occur in previously well patients given modest doses of thiazides.

Concurrent disease

Renal failure. Polythiazide should not be given to patients with severe renal impairment or anuria as the drug is ineffective, may further worsen renal function and may produce cumulative effects. The long elimination half life of polythiazide may be a disadvantage in patients with impaired renal function because of the risk of accumulation.

Drug interactions

Potentially hazardous interactions

Antidiabetic drugs. Polythiazide antagonizes the action of sulphonylureas in particular, with potential loss of diabetic control.

Antihypertensive drugs. The antihypertensive effect of all commonly used antihypertensive drugs is enhanced by treatment with thiazide diuretics. It remains difficult to prove whether or not the enhanced response represents an additive or synergistic effect. In some patients the result may be profound hypotension. An exaggerated 'first dose' effect is observed after the addition of other drugs. This has been highlighted recently with respect to the introduction of angiotensin converting enzyme inhibitors[56] but many other antihypertensives share this problem.

Renal insufficiency in patients on ACE inhibitors is a serious problem but is seldom observed unless the patient is also receiving a diuretic. It is probable that the influence of angiotensin on the kidney is enhanced by diuretic treatment, especially in heart failure and in the presence of renovascular disease. In these circumstances autoregulatory failure in the kidney is more likely, when the production of angiotensin II is inhibited.

β-Adrenoceptor agonists. The hypokalaemic effect of adrenaline has been referred to previously. Exogenous agonists such as ritodrine, salbutamol and terbutaline all result in a similar effect, especially when given parenterally in high doses. A dangerous degree of hypokalaemia may develop if such drugs are given to patients on diuretics.

Corticosteroids. Potassium loss may be enhanced by the combination of corticosteroid and diuretic.[57]

Curare. The effects of curare-like drugs such as tubocurarine, gallamine, alcuronium and pancuronium may be enhanced by hypokalaemia and prolonged neuromuscular blockade may result.

Cardiac glycosides. The cardiotoxicity of digoxin is enhanced by potassium depletion[58] and possibly also by hypomagnesaemia, although these electrolyte disturbances often coexist. Total body depletion of potassium, in the presence of normal plasma concentrations, may predispose to digoxin toxicity.

Lithium. Thiazide diuretics inhibit the tubular elimination of lithium. This results in an elevated plasma lithium concentration, with a resultant risk of toxicity.[59] It is essential to monitor plasma lithium concentrations when these drugs are prescribed concurrently.

Non-steroidal anti-inflammatory drugs (NSAIDs). The nephrotoxicity of these drugs is increased by concomitant therapy with diuretics, especially in the elderly. NSAIDs attenuate both the diuretic and antihypertensive effects of thiazides.[60]

Quinidine. Thiazides increase the tubular reabsorption of quinidine, leading to higher plasma concentrations and the possible risk of adverse cardiac effects.

Uricosuric drugs. By causing retention of urate by the kidney, thiazides may antagonize the action of uricosuric drugs such as probenecid and also of the xanthine oxidase inhibitor allopurinol. Dosages of both may need to be adjusted if diuretic treatment is continued.

Other significant interactions

Food. No definite pharmacokinetic interaction has been demonstrated. A high intake of liquorice will tend to negate the beneficial effects of thiazide diuretics and enhance the hypokalaemia.

Alcohol. Excessive alcohol intake is now recognized as an important contributory factor in hypertensive patients whose blood pressure control is inadequate. This appears to be a non-specific effect and applies to patients treated with diuretics as well as those treated with other antihypertensives.

Potentially useful interactions

The benefit of combining a thiazide with another antihypertensive drug has already been discussed.

Cigarette smoking. The potential of thiazides to prevent stroke in mild hypertension may be preserved even in cigarette smokers, whereas some doubt exists as to whether other drugs such as propranolol are equally effective.

Porcine insulin

P

metabolized in a single pass through the liver. Very little free insulin is excreted in the urine. Some is excreted in the bile.

Concentration–effect relationship

A sigmoidal dose–response relationship for the utilization of glucose and for inhibition of glucose production in response to insulin has been demonstrated in normal subjects.[26] However, whilst concentrations of insulin required to suppress ketogenesis and stop hepatic glucose production are within the physiological range (4–80 mU.l^{-1}), maximal glucose utilization is only reached at pharmacological insulin concentrations. Effects on amino acids show half-maxima within the physiological range.[29] Insulin infusion rates of 4–6 units per hour achieve circulating insulin concentrations at the upper end of the physiological range in diabetic adults.

Metabolism

Insulin is metabolized[30] in the liver and kidney;[31] small amounts are metabolized in muscle and fat. In the fasting state, the liver accounts for 40% of insulin clearance, and the kidneys for 20%.[31] Insulin binds to cell surface receptors, is taken into the cells and is then degraded by intracellular insulin-specific proteases. There is little evidence for altered insulin metabolism in diabetes, except in very rare instances of increased degradation of subcutaneous insulin in situ.[32]

Pharmaceutics

All insulins are available as sterile solutions for injection, and the standard concentration of all commercial preparations in the UK is 100±10 IU.ml^{-1}. Only 'highly purified' porcine insulins are available in the UK at present. Preparations may contain a modifier which slows the absorption of insulin administered subcutaneously, and thus prolongs its duration of action. All contain one or more preservatives, and may contain a pH buffer (see Table 1).

Insulin is administered by subcutaneous or sometimes intramuscular injection, and 0.5 or 1.0 ml syringes calibrated in units of insulin for U100 insulin (100 IU.ml^{-1}) are generally used. Soluble insulins (but not others) may be given by intravenous injection or infusion.

When kept at 4°C, insulin zinc preparations retain potency for at least 2 years; at 20–25°C, potency falls by about 20% each year,[33] so it is wise to store insulin in a refrigerator at 2–8°C, but there is no significant loss of potency in insulin kept at room temperature for a few days. Freezing or direct exposure to sunlight causes inactivation of insulin.

Insulin is adsorbed onto plastics. In practice, allowing 40 ml of soluble insulin solution to run through plastic infusion tubing before the tubing is connected to the patient overcomes the problem. Alternatively, adsorption may be reduced by adding albumin to the solution.

Therapeutic use

Indications

1. The treatment of insulin-requiring diabetes mellitus
2. The acute treatment of hyperkalaemia.

Contraindications

1. Hypoglycaemia
2. Severe systemic allergic reactions to porcine insulins.

Mode of use

1. The treatment of insulin-requiring diabetes mellitus
All patients with diabetic ketoacidosis require insulin, and in addition, patients with diabetes whose symptoms are not controlled by other treatment, who continue to lose weight or who have persistent hyperglycaemia without symptoms (especially in pregnancy), may require insulin. Insulin treatment also allows satisfactory control of blood glucose concentration during major surgery[34] or intercurrent illness.

In acute diabetic ketoacidosis, treatment should be started with soluble insulin, given by continuous intravenous infusion at a rate of 6 IU.h^{-1} initially, or by intramuscular injection (20 IU intramuscularly initially, then 6 IU intramuscularly hourly), together with potassium chloride and 0.9% sodium chloride infusions. Frequent measurements of blood glucose and potassium concentrations are essential.[35,36]

Hyperosmolar, non-ketotic diabetic coma is managed similarly, except that larger volumes of fluid are commonly needed and hypernatraemia may be present, when 0.45% sodium chloride solution is used.[37]

Treatment in insulin-requiring diabetics who are not ketoacidotic may begin with subcutaneous injections of insulin. Circumstances will dictate the regime used: commonly two subcutaneous injections a day, one about 30 minutes[38] before breakfast, and one about 30 minutes before the evening meal, are used.[39] Whilst at first only intermediate-acting insulin may be needed, it is later necessary to inject both short- and intermediate-acting insulins together. Doses are adjusted by monitoring blood (or less satisfactorily, urine) glucose concentrations. The aim of treatment in the younger diabetic patient is to render him as near metabolically normal as possible, in the hope that this will reduce the chances of developing the long-term complications of diabetes. Blood glucose concentration therefore should ideally fall in the range 4–7 mmol.l^{-1}. Usual intravenous insulin requirements in diabetic subjects are around 0.1–0.4 U.kg^{-1} daily. In states of insulin resistance,[40] subcutaneous doses in excess of 10 U.kg^{-1} daily may have to be used.

2. Hyperkalaemia
Life-threatening hyperkalaemia may be treated acutely by intravenous injection of soluble insulin with glucose (to prevent hypoglycaemia). It is satisfactory to give 5 g of glucose for every 1 IU of soluble insulin, for example as 50 ml of 50% dextrose strong solution BP, containing 5 IU soluble insulin. This measure is only temporarily effective in lowering serum potassium concentration.

Adverse reactions

Potentially life-threatening effects
Hypoglycaemia[41] is the most common adverse effect of treatment with insulin, and occurs with all insulin preparations. It is more likely when meals are missed, after exercise, and if inappropriately large doses of insulin are used. Symptoms of hypoglycaemia include hunger, unsteadiness and sweatiness. Signs include sweating, pallor, irrational behaviour, aggression, unconsciousness, focal neurological deficit and convulsions. Hypoglycaemia should be recognized and treated promptly, so all outpatients treated with insulin should carry a card, or wear a necklace or bracelet, bearing a suitable warning message.

Table 1 Porcine insulins

Manufacturer	Name	Form	Modifier	Preservative	pH
Nordisk & Wellcome	Velosulin	soluble	—	*m*-cresol	7.3
	Insulatard	isophane	protamine	*m*-cresol + phenol	7.3
	Mixtard 30/70	30% soluble 70% isophane	protamine	*m*-cresol + phenol	7.3
	Initard 50/50	50% soluble 50% isophane	protamine	*m*-cresol + phenol	7.3
Novo (Squibb-Novo, US)	Semitard MC	IZS: amophous	zinc	methylparabens	

*Insulin zinc suspension

If the patient is conscious, treatment of hypoglycaemia is the administration of rapidly absorbed carbohydrate by mouth. The traditional carbohydrate to give is warm milk and sugar (sucrose), but chocolate bars, glucose tablets, raisins or sugary carbonated drinks are also effective. If the patient is unconscious, glucose should be given intravenously as 50% dextrose strong solution. Rectal administration is probably ineffective.[42] The effects of insulin may also be counteracted briefly by the intramuscular injection of glucagon 1 mg. This may allow sufficient recovery for the patient to take oral carbohydrate. In the absence of permanent brain damage, which is rare,[41] or of other illness, increasing blood glucose concentration to normal rapidly restores consciousness.

Acute overdosage
The cardinal features and management of overdosage with porcine insulin are as for other types of insulin-induced hypoglycaemia.[43] Prolonged release of large doses of insulin from subcutaneous tissues demands prolonged glucose infusion, measurement of blood glucose concentrations, and awareness of possible hypokalaemia. In patients who have injected vast amounts of insulin subcutaneously, excision of the insulin-containing tissue may be useful.[44]

Severe or irreversible adverse effects
Apart from those already described, there are none.

Symptomatic adverse effects
Porcine insulin is intrinsically less antigenic in man than bovine insulin, and highly purified insulins are much less antigenic than the older recrystallized insulins.[45] Systemic allergic reactions[46] to the new preparations are very rare. Insulin resistance, due to circulating insulin-binding antibodies, and lipoatrophy, due to immune-complex deposition,[47] are also rare.[45]

Lipohypertrophy, which is probably due to the metabolic effects of high local concentrations of insulin, can occur with highly purified insulins.[48]

High risk groups

Neonates
In the very rare instances in which it would be required in neonates there would be no contraindication to its use.

Breast milk. As insulin is destroyed in the stomach there is no adverse effect on the breast-fed infant of a mother receiving insulin therapy.

Pregnant women
In pregnant women, hyperglycaemia is associated with fetal abnormalities, especially macrosomia, so good diabetic control is especially important.[49,50] Insulin requirements tend to fall during the first trimester, but steadily increase during the second and third trimester. Immediately after placental separation, insulin requirements are markedly reduced, and the dose of insulin, including that in intravenous infusions, should then be halved.

The elderly
In the elderly, insulin clearance may be reduced as renal function declines, and so the duration of action may be prolonged.

Concurrent disease
Renal disease. Insulin clearance is reduced when renal function is impaired, so elimination is slower and the duration of action of standard preparations is prolonged.

Other diseases. Patients with diabetes secondary to pancreatic disease and those with Addison's disease or hypopituitarism in addition to diabetes, are very insulin-sensitive and generally require very small doses of insulin.

Insulin may aggravate hypokalaemic myopathy in susceptible patients.[51]

Drug interactions

Potentially hazardous interactions
Although several drugs may interact with insulin, such interactions are often of theoretical rather than practical importance.[52] The actions of insulin may be augmented by monoamine oxidase inhibitors,[53] β-blocking drugs, which also suppress the tachycardia which accompanies hypoglycaemia (but not the sweating),[54] ganglion-blocking drugs,[55] captopril,[56] clonidine,[57] and, perhaps most importantly, ethanol.[58] In patients with residual pancreatic function, sulphonylureas and salicylates[59] may increase endogenous insulin secretion and so interact with exogenous insulin.

The effects of insulin may be antagonized by adrenaline,[60] thyroid hormones, corticosteroids, oestrogens, isoniazid, chlorpromazine, and cyclophosphamide.

Potentially useful interactions
It has been suggested that sulphonylureas, by their ability to enhance insulin sensitivity, may be of benefit when given with insulin to insulin-dependent patients.[61] Metformin may improve insulin sensitivity in similar fashion.[62]

Major outcome trials

No outcome trials have been published but the UK Multicentre Study 1983 (UK prospective study of therapies of maturity onset diabetes. Diabetologia 24: 404–411) and the Diabetes Complication and Control Trial 1987 (Effects of age, deviation and treatment of insulin-dependent diabetes mellitus on residual β-cell function: observations during eligibility testing for the DCCT. Journal of Clinical Endocrinology and Metabolism 65: 30–36) should in time make it clear whether treatment affects the long-term complication rate in non-insulin-dependent diabetes and insulin-dependent diabetes respectively.

Other studies

1. Home P D, Mann N P, Hutchison A S et al 1984 A fifteen month double-blind cross-over study of the efficacy and antigenicity of human and pork insulins. Diabetic Medicine 1: 93–98

This was a five-centre trial of patients already receiving insulin. Of 100 selected, 96 were randomized and 87 completed the study. A three-month run-in period was followed by treatment with soluble and zinc suspensions of insulin of highly purified porcine or human (emp) type, with crossover to the alternative preparations after 4 and 8 months. Monthly assessment of blood glucose series, glycosylated haemoglobin and 24 h urinary glucose excretion showed significantly lower fasting blood glucose in patients treated with porcine insulin, after 1 month's treatment. However, other statistically significant differences between insulins are not large enough to be clinically significant, and multiple significance tests are used where analysis of variance or time-series methods might be better. The authors conclude of human insulin '... no definite preference for its clinical use has emerged except in rare instances of insulin allergy, and for biosynthetic human insulin in vegans'.

2. Clark A J L, Adenyi-Jones R O, Knight G et al 1982 Biosynthetic human insulin in the treatment of diabetes. Lancet 2: 354–357

This was a five-centre double-blind crossover trial of patients already receiving insulin. Of 94 recruited, half were receiving bovine and half porcine insulins; six patients failed to complete the study. After a six-week run-in period, patients received their usual insulins or human (crb) insulins for 6 weeks and then crossed over to the alternative. Blood glucose series showed significantly higher fasting glucose concentrations on human insulin than on either beef or pork insulin, by analysis of variance. The M-value, a summary measure of blood glucose concentration, was significantly greater on human insulin than on porcine insulin. The study may not have lasted long enough to establish optimum doses of human insulin for blood glucose control, but three patients withdrew because of hypoglycaemia when taking human insulin. The authors note that 'higher glucose levels on human insulin (crb) may be due to its slightly different pharmacokinetic properties'.

3. Mann N O, Johnston D I, Reaves W G, Murphy M A 1983 Human insulin and porcine insulin in the treatment of diabetic children: comparison of metabolic control and insulin antibody production. British Medical Journal 287: 1580–1582

In this single-centre study, 21 insulin-dependent diabetic children received their usual insulin during a three-month run-in and were then randomized to highly purified porcine or human (emp) insulins in double-blind fashion. After 4 and 8 months, patients crossed over

Porcine insulin

P

to the alternative preparation. There were significantly higher glycosylated haemoglobin and fasting glucose concentrations during human insulin treatment, but statistical analysis was by repeated t-tests. The authors conclude: 'We have shown that semisynthetic human insulin is a safe and effective preparation in children with established diabetes. Further work is needed to determine optimal regimens for human insulin... '.

4. Olczak S A, Greenwood R H 1985 A clinical comparison of purified porcine and purified bovine insulins. Postgraduate Medical Journal 61: 15–18

24 patients with established diabetes treated with standard soluble and isophane bovine insulins were randomized to receive either purified bovine insulins (11) or purified porcine insulins (12 subjects). All subjects were studied for 2 months before randomization, and tests of control improved markedly during that period. There were no significant improvements in glucose control during six months of treatment with either species of purified insulin. Anti-insulin antibodies did fall significantly in the group treated with porcine insulins, and this may represent a benefit. The main conclusion is that diabetic control improves most when the patient is carefully supervised by a motivated doctor.

Reviews

Bliss M 1983 The discovery of insulin. Paul Harris Publishing, Edinburgh

References

1. Hodgson A J, Rogers M L 1985 North East Thames Region U100 Insulins Chart 5th edn. The London Hospital, Whitechapel
2. Home P D, Alberti K G M M 1982 The new insulins. Their characteristics and clinical indications. Drugs 24: 401–413
3. Brown H, Sanger F, Kitai R 1955 The structure of pig and sheep insulin. Biochemical Journal 60: 556–565
4. British Pharmacopoeia 1980 Addendum 1986 Insulin. Her Majesty's Stationery Office, London, p 413 (1986)
5. United States Pharmacopoeia 1985 21st edn. Insulin. United States Pharmacopeial Convention, Inc, Rockville, Maryland, p 534 (1984)
6. Best C H, Scott D A 1923 The preparation of insulins. Journal of Biological Chemistry 57: 709–723
7. Hagedorn H C, Jensen B N, Krarup N B, Wodstrup I 1936 Protamine insulinate. Journal of the American Medical Association 106: 177–180
8. Hallas-Moller K 1954 Chemical, biological and physiological background of the new insulin-zinc suspensions. Lancet 2: 1029–1034
9. Felig P 1983 Physiologic action of insulin. In: Ellenberg M, Rifkin H (eds) Diabetes mellitus. Theory and practice, 3rd edn. Medical Examination Publishing Co Inc, New York
10. Cox M, Sterns R H, Singer I 1978 The defense against hyperkalemia: the roles of insulin and aldosterone. New England Journal of Medicine 299: 525–532
11. Banting F G, Campbell W R, Fletcher A A 1923 Further clinical experience with insulins (pancreatic extracts) in the treatment of diabetes mellitus. British Medical Journal 1: 8–12
12. Gammeltoft S 1984 Insulin receptors: binding kinetics and structure–function relationship of insulin. Physiological Reviews 64: 1321–1378
13. Bangham D R, de Jonge H, van Noordwijk J 1978 The collaborative assay of the European Pharmacopoeia Biological Reference preparation for insulin. Journal of Biological Standardization 6: 301–314
14. Fingel M, Volund A, Sorensen E, Collins J E, Dieters C T 1985 Biological potency of porcine, bovine and human insulins in the rabbit bioassay system. Diabetologia 28: 862–869
15. Starr J I, Horwitz D L, Rubenstein A H, Hako M B 1979 Insulin, proinsulin and C-peptide. In: Jaffe B M, Behrman H R (eds) Methods of hormone radioimmunoassay, 2nd edn. Academic Press, New York, pp 613–642
16. Kurt A B, Mustaffa B E, Daggett P R, Nabarro J D N 1977 Effects of insulin antibodies on free and total plasma-insulin. Lancet 2: 56–58
17. Lauritzen T, Pramming S, Gale E A M, Deckert T, Binder C 1982 Absorption of isophane (NPH) insulin and its clinical implications. British Medical Journal 285: 159–162
18. Hildebrandt P, Madsbad S 1984 Smoking and insulin absorption. British Medical Journal 289: 1077
19. Berger M, Cuppers H J, Hegner H, Jorgens V, Berchtold P 1982 Absorption and biologic effects of subcutaneously injected insulin preparations. Diabetes Care 5: 77–91
20. Koivisto V A, Felig P 1980 Alterations in insulin absorption and in blood glucose control associated with varying insulin injection sites in diabetic patients. Annals of Internal Medicine 92: 59–61
21. Heine R J, Bilo H J G, Fonk T, van der Veen E A, van der Meer J 1984 Absorption kinetics and action profiles of mixtures of short and intermediate-acting insulins. Diabetologia 27: 558–562
22. Heine R J, Bilo H J G, Sikkenk A C, van der Veen E A 1985 Mixing short and intermediate acting insulins in the syringe: effect on post prandial blood glucose concentrations in type 1 diabetics. British Medical Journal 290: 204–205
23. Anonymous 1982 Which insulin? Drug Therapy Bulletin 2(23): 89–92
24. Home P D, Massi-Benedetti M, Sheppard G A A, Hanning I, Alberti K G M M, Owens D R 1982 A comparison of the activity and disposal of semi-synthetic human insulins and porcine insulin in normal man by the glucose clamp technique. Diabetologia 22: 41–45
25. Gerlis L S, Adenyi-Jones R, Jones R H, Sonksen P H, Barnes G D 1982 The metabolism and distribution of human monocomponent insulin in man. Minerva Endocrinologica 7 (suppl 1): 49–54
26. Binder C 1984 Insulin pharmacokinetics. Diabetes Care 7: 188–199
27. Owen O B, Reichard C A J, Boden G, Shuman C R 1974 Comparative measurements of glucose, beta-hydroxybutyrate, acetoacetate and insulin in blood and cerebrospinal fluid during starvation. Metabolism 23: 7–14
28. Rizza R A, Mandarino L J, Gerich J B 1981 Dose–response characteristics for effects of insulin on production and utilization of glucose in man. American Journal of Physiology 240: E630–639
29. Fukagawa N K, Minaker K L, Young V R, Rowe J W 1986 Insulin dose-dependent reductions in plasma amino acids in man. American Journal of Physiology 250: E13–E17
30. Duckworth W C, Kitabchi A B 1981 Insulin metabolism and degradation. Endocrine Reviews 2: 210–233
31. Henriksen J H, Tronier B, Bülow J B 1987 Kinetics of circulating insulin, c-peptide and proinsulin in fasting nondiabetic man. Metabolism 36: 463–468
32. Anonymous 1980 Subcutaneous injections and absorption of insulin. Lancet 1: 1005–1006
33. Stephenson N R, Romans R G 1960 Thermal stability of insulin made from zinc insulin crystals. Journal of Pharmacy and Pharmacology 12: 372–376
34. Alberti K G M M, Gill G V, Elliott M J 1982 Insulin delivery during surgery in the diabetic patient. Diabetes Care 5: 65–77
35. Alberti K G M M, Hockaday T D R 1977 Diabetic coma: a reappraisal after five years. Clinics in Endocrinology and Metabolism 6 (2): 421–455
36. Kitabchi A B, Fisher J N 1981 Insulin therapy of diabetic ketoacidosis: physiologic versus pharmacologic doses of insulin and their routes of administration. In: Brownlee M (ed) Handbook of diabetes mellitus. Vol 5. Current and future therapies. Garland STPM Press, New York
37. Mather H M 1980 Management of hyperosmolar coma. Journal of the Royal Society of Medicine 73: 134–138
38. Lean M B J, Ng L L, Tennison B R 1985 Interval between insulin injection and eating in relation to blood glucose control in adult diabetics. British Medical Journal 290: 105–108
39. Alberti K G M M, Hockaday T D R 1987 Diabetes Mellitus. In: Weatherall D J, Ledingham J G G, Warrell D A (eds) Oxford Textbook of Medicine. Oxford University Press, Oxford, pp 9.51–9.101
40. Flier J S, Kahn C R, Roth J 1979 Receptors, antireceptor antibodies and mechanisms of insulin resistance. New England Journal of Medicine 300: 413–419
41. Malouf R, Brust J C M 1985 Hypoglycaemia: causes, neurological manifestations, and outcome. Annals of Neurology 17: 421–430
42. Attvall S, Kager I, Smith U 1985 Rectal glucose administration cannot be used to treat hypoglycaemia. Diabetes Care 8: 412–413
43. Critchley J A J H, Proudfoot A T, Boyd S G, Campbell I W, Brown N S, Gordon A 1984 Deaths and paradoxes after intentional insulin overdosage. British Medical Journal 289: 225
44. Campbell I W, Ratcliffe J G 1982 Suicidal insulin overdose managed by excision of insulin injection site. British Medical Journal 285: 408–409
45. Deckert T 1985 The immunogenicity of new insulins. Diabetes 34 (suppl 2): 94–96
46. Wiles P G, Guy R, Watkins S M, Reeves W G 1982 Allergy to purified bovine, porcine and human insulins. British Medical Journal 287: 531
47. Reeves W G, Allen B R, Tattersall R B 1980 Insulin-induced lipoatrophy: evidence for an immune pathogenesis. British Medical Journal 280: 1500
48. Campbell J W, Duncan C, Anani A R 1984 Paradoxical lipodystrophic changes due to conventional porcine and highly purified porcine/bovine insulins. Postgraduate Medical Journal 60: 439–441
49. Stowers J M 1981 Assessment and management of diabetic pregnancy. In: Brownlee M (ed) Handbook of diabetes mellitus. Vol 5. Current and future therapies. Garland STMC Press, New York
50. Coustan D R, Imarah J 1984 Prophylactic insulin treatment of gestational diabetes reduces the incidence of macrosomia, operative delivery and birth trauma. American Journal of Obstetrics and Gynecology 150: 836–842
51. Ruff R L 1979 Insulin-induced weakness in hypokalemic myopathy. Annals of Neurology 6: 139–140
52. Shinn A F, Shrewsbury R F 1985 Hypoglycaemia drug interactions. In: Evaluations of drug interactions, ch 14. C V Mosby Co, St Louis, pp 552–592
53. Adnitt P I 1968 Hypoglycemic action of monoamine oxidase inhibitors. Diabetes 17: 628–633
54. Seltzer H S 1972 Drug-induced hypoglycemia. Diabetes 21: 955–966
55. Gupta K K, Lillicrap C A 1968 Guanethidine and diabetes. British Medical Journal 2 (5606): 697–698
56. Ferriere M, Lachkar H, Richard J-L, Bringer J, Orsetti A, Mirouze J 1985 Captopril and insulin sensitivity. Annals of Internal Medicine 102: 134–135
57. Hedeland H, Dymling J F, Hokfelt B 1972 The effect of insulin induced hypoglycaemia on plasma renin activity and urinary catecholamines before and following clonidine (Catapresan) in man. Acta Endocrinologica 71: 321–330
58. Arky R A, Veverbrandts E, Abramson E A 1968 Irreversible hypoglycemia. A complication of alcohol and insulin. Journal of the American Medical Association 206: 575–578
59. Prince R L, Larkins R G, Alford F F 1981 The effect of acetylsalicylic acid on plasma glucose and the response of glucose regulatory hormones to intravenous glucose and arginine in insulin treated diabetics and normal subjects. Metabolism 30: 293–298
60. Berk M A, Clutter W E, Skor D et al 1985 Enhanced glycaemic responsiveness to epinephrine in insulin-dependent diabetes mellitus is the result of the inability to secrete insulin. Journal of Clinical Investigation 75: 1842–1851
61. Rizza R A 1985 Combined sulfonylurea and insulin therapy in insulin-dependent diabetes: research or clinical practice. Diabetes Care 8: 511–514
62. Gin H, Messerschmitt C, Brottier E, Aubertin J 1985 Metformin improves insulin resistance in type 2, insulin-dependent, diabetic patients. Metabolism 34: 923–925

Potassium canrenoate

Potassium canrenoate is one of the few spironolactones in current clinical use. Together with its metabolites, it acts as a competitive antagonist of the sodium-retaining properties of the mineralocorticoids.

Chemistry

Potassium canrenoate (Spiroctan-M injection, Aldactone pro Infusion, Spiroctan pro Infusion)
$C_{22}H_{29}KO_4$
Potassium 17β-hydroxy-3-oxo-17α-pregna-4,6-diene-21-carboxylate

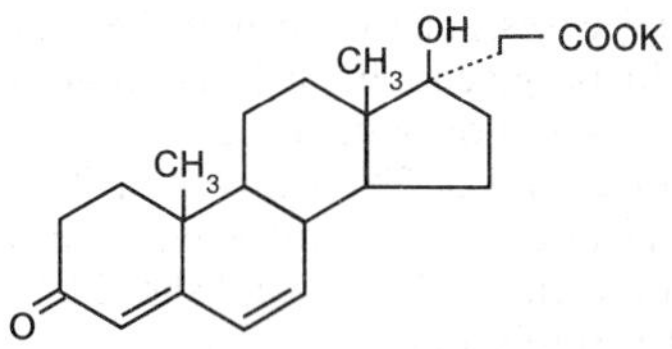

Molecular weight	396.2
pKa	5.2[1]
Solubility	
in alcohol	so – luble
in water	soluble
Octanol/water partition coefficient	—

Canrenoic acid is a yellow–brown powder with a faint characteristic odour. The potassium salt is prepared during product manufacture only and is presented as a clear yellow aqueous solution.

In the Federal Republic of Germany, potassium canrenoate is available in combination with frusemide for injection (potassium canrenoate 200 mg and frusemide 20 mg: Aldactone-Diurapid Ampullen).

Pharmacology

The spironolactones compete with aldosterone for binding to specific peripheral aldosterone receptors. Potassium canrenoate has one-tenth the affinity for cytoplasmic receptors of its chief metabolite canrenone. This difference has been attributed to opening of the γ-lactone ring which occurs during the formation of the water-soluble potassium salt.[2–4]

Aldosterone receptors are present in many tissues (e.g. salivary glands and colon) but the kidney is the most important site. Aldosterone receptors are soluble cytoplasmic proteins that appear to exist in two allosteric forms. The spironolactones bind with aldosterone receptors and thus inhibit the cascade of subcellular events which result from interaction of the active hormone–receptor complex with the genome.[2,3]

Potassium canrenoate has antihypertensive effects and promotes a diuresis.[5] In addition, it appears to have antiarrhythmic effects in dogs which may be the indirect result of changes in electrolyte balance.[6]

In experimental myocardial infarction, the use of potassium canrenoate is associated with an increase in dp/dt_{max} and maximum cardiac output. Possible mechanisms include a non-specific effect of reduction in interstitial and cellular oedema.[7]

Toxicology

Myelocytic leukaemia and other neoplastic changes were observed in rats following administration of potassium canrenoate orally for two years.

Clinical pharmacology

Potassium canrenoate promotes a diuresis with an increase in urinary sodium excretion.[8] The drug has been used in the treatment of primary hyperaldosteronism[9] and in various fluid-retaining states associated with secondary aldosteronism, e.g. cardiac failure, hepatic dysfunction, nephrotic syndrome, ascites associated with neoplasia.[10,11] 80% of patients with fluid retention because of hepatic cirrhosis improved symptomatically following use of potassium canrenoate given either singly or in combination with a thiazide diuretic.[10]

In normal volunteers, a single dose of potassium canrenoate had only one-third the potency of a single dose of spironolactone of the same weight. By comparison, in a multiple-dosing study potassium canrenoate had two-thirds the potency of spironolactone. These differences have been attributed to the observation that canrenone, which binds well to mineralocorticoid receptors and which is a common metabolite of both spironolactone and potassium canrenoate, accumulates in plasma to a greater extent than other active metabolites because of its long half life. However, recently doubt has been cast on this interpretation because the canrenone levels were determined using a fluorimetric method which is less specific than the currently favoured HPLC assay.[12–14]

In conjunction with increased urinary sodium excretion, intravenous potassium canrenoate causes a marked increase in plasma renin activity and slight increases in plasma aldosterone levels and aldosterone excretion, raising the possibility that canrenone has a direct inhibitory effect on aldosterone secretion.[9,15]

There is also evidence that potassium canrenoate reduces the incidence of ventricular arrhythmias due to digoxin toxicity, an effect attributed to changes in electrolyte balance.[16] In an uncontrolled study of acute myocardial infarction during which potassium canrenoate was administered, ventricular arrhythmias were less frequent and the incidence of ventricular fibrillation was 1.1% by comparison with quoted figures of 3–10%.[17,18]

Evidence regarding the positive inotropic effect of potassium canrenoate is conflicting. The drug improved stroke volume and cardiac output in healthy volunteers and also in patients with cardiac failure,[19,20] but there was no discernible effect in patients undergoing cardiac catheterization because of coronary artery disease.[21] The mechanism of any inotropic effect is uncertain and is apparently independent of changes in pre-load and after-load.[22] Some authors suggest that potassium canrenoate has a direct effect on myocardial fibres similar to that of adrenal steroids, whereas others postulate a hypothetical inotropic receptor for which potassium canrenoate and digoxin compete.[20] Beneficial effects of single-dose potassium canrenoate on ventilatory function have been described in patients with chronic lung disease and cor pulmonale.[23,24] The recommended intravenous daily dose is 200–800 mg with the highest quoted dose being 1400 mg. The majority of patients with biventricular or left-sided cardiac failure responded symptomatically to 400 mg per day (70%), whereas a few patients responded to 200 mg per day (20%) and a smaller number (10%) required 400–600 mg per day.[25] Patients with cor pulmonale responded satisfactorily to 200 mg per day.

There is no apparent effect on glucose metabolism or on the control of diabetes mellitus. The drug has less antiandrogenic effect than spironolactone on a weight basis and may reverse the gynaecomastia produced during treatment with spironolactone.[26,27]

Pharmacokinetics

Following intravenous administration of potassium canrenoate there is rapid lactonization to canrenone, a conversion which is enzymatically controlled because the in vitro half life of the canrenone ⇔ canrenoic acid conversion at physiological pH is approximately 24 days.[1]

Originally canrenone was assayed using a spectrofluorimetric method but neither this nor its later modifications were specific for

P

canrenone. Recently more sensitive and specific assay methods using gas–liquid or high pressure liquid chromatography (HPLC) have been developed.[28] The limit of sensitivity for canrenone by HPLC is approximately 5 μg.l^{-1}.

The mean plasma half life of canrenone measured using the fluorimetric assay is 17 hours (range 10–35). Data for half life are not available at present for the HPLC assay.

Canrenoic acid is 98% protein bound and its volume of distribution is unknown. Whether there is tissue accumulation of drug and whether it crosses the blood–brain barrier is not known.

Because of its high degree of protein binding, only traces of canrenone have been detected in the breast milk of lactating females taking oral spironolactone.[29] No information is available about the use of potassium canrenoate during lactation.

Oral absorption	not relevant
Presystemic metabolism	not relevant
Plasma half life	
range	10–35 h
mean	17 h
Volume of distribution	
Plasma protein binding	98%

Concentration–effect relationship

The major therapeutic effect depends on the relative affinities of potassium canrenoate, canrenone and various glucuronide and sulphur-containing metabolites for mineralocorticoid receptors so that there is no clear relationship between concentration of any single metabolite in plasma and therapeutic effect.[30] The drug has a shorter latency than spironolactone.

Metabolism

Following intravenous injection, potassium canrenoate becomes ionized to yield free canrenoic acid which is rapidly protein-bound and which exists in equilibrium with canrenone (Fig. 1). Canrenoic acid is metabolized to a glucuronide ester which is excreted in urine. Canrenone itself is metabolized to a variety of hydroxylated, polyhydroxylated and reduced metabolites, all of which have been identified in urine. The excretion of metabolites of potassium canrenoate is almost entirely in the urine (88%) but a small amount of canrenone is metabolized in the liver and excreted in bile[31] (Fig. 1).

Canrenone is thought to be the major active metabolite and the contribution of other metabolites to therapeutic effect is not fully understood.

Pharmaceutics

Potassium canrenoate is available for parenteral use as Spiroctan-M injection (Boehringer Mannheim UK (Pharmaceuticals) Ltd, UK). It is an aqueous solution containing 200 mg of potassium canrenoate per 10 ml ampoule. The drug should be protected from light and has a shelf-life of 24 months. It is compatible with dextrose 5% or sodium chloride 0.9%.

Therapeutic use

Indications

1. The diagnosis and treatment of primary hyperaldosteronism
2. The treatment of oedema associated with secondary aldosteronism, e.g. cardiac failure, hepatic dysfunction, nephrotic syndrome
3. The additional treatment of oedema refractory to other diuretic agents given orally or intravenously
4. Correction of potassium and/or magnesium deficiency resulting from prior use of potassium-wasting diuretics.

Contraindications

1. Hyperkalaemia
2. Hyponatraemia
3. Renal impairment.

Mode of use

The dose of potassium canrenoate should be titrated to the clinical response, starting at 200–400 mg per day and increasing to 800 mg daily in exceptional cases. The drug may be administered without dilution but should be given into a large vein slowly over 2 to 3 minutes to avoid irritation or pain at the injection site. Alternatively, it may be diluted in 250 ml of 5% dextrose or 0.9% sodium chloride solution and administered by slow intravenous infusion. The diluted drug should be used within 12 hours and should be discarded if there is any evidence of precipitation.

Indications

1. Primary hyperaldosteronism

Potassium canrenoate has been infused in a dose of 200–400 mg per day in patients with primary hyperaldosteronism. Changes were similar to those observed after oral administration of spironolactone, namely an increase in urinary volume and sodium excretion and serum potassium and plasma renin activity, together with a reduction in body weight and blood pressure.

2. Secondary aldosteronism

The use of potassium canrenoate in cardiac failure depends on its diuretic and antimineralocorticoid properties and to a lesser extent on its postulated positive inotropic effects. Potassium canrenoate may have some advantages in the treatment of hepatic cirrhosis because of its lesser antiandrogenic effects by comparison with spironolactone.

3. Intractable oedema

Potassium canrenoate may be used in the short term in combination with other diuretics to treat intractable fluid retention.

Fig. 1 The metabolism of potassium canrenoate

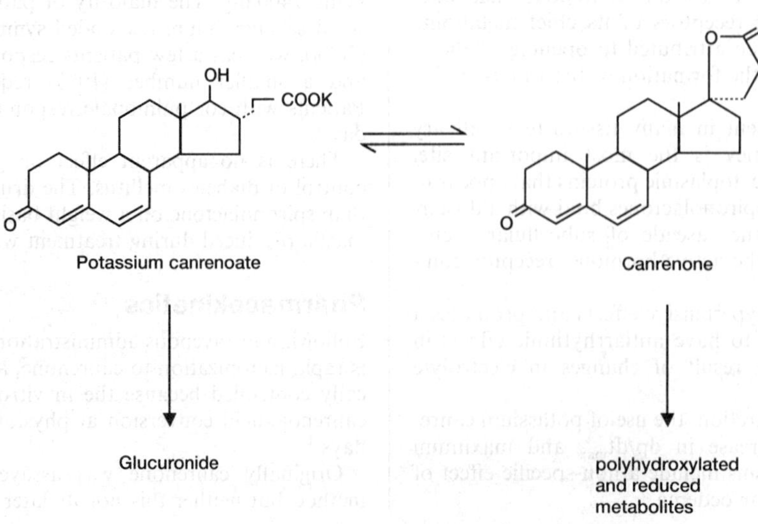

Contraindications

Pre-existing hyperkalaemia and hyponatraemia are contraindications to the use of potassium canrenoate. The drug should not be used if there is evidence of renal impairment, i.e. creatinine clearance less than 30 ml.min^{-1} or serum creatinine greater than 175 mmol.l^{-1}.

Adverse reactions

Potentially life-threatening effects
In rare instances hyperkalaemia may occur, particularly if other potassium-sparing diuretics or large supplements of potassium are in use concurrently.

Acute overdosage
At doses of 1000 mg daily, nausea, vomiting, transient confusion, restlessness and hallucinations have been described. Life-threatening hyperkalaemia in association with deterioration in renal function has been observed in occasional patients given therapeutic doses of potassium canrenoate.

All these adverse effects resolved with cessation of treatment together with use of antiemetic drugs and control of hyperkalaemia where appropriate.

Severe or irreversible adverse effects
In rare cases, changes in the voice have been described and consist of the development of hoarseness and deepening of the voice in women or raising of the pitch in men. These side effects may not regress even after withdrawal of the drug so that the use of potassium canrenoate should be considered carefully in all cases.

Symptomatic adverse effects
If undiluted potassium canrenoate is administered too rapidly, irritation and pain at the injection site may occur. Treatment is usually of short duration but if chronic therapy is undertaken, there may be antiandrogenic effects such as nipple sensitivity and gynaecomastia in men and mastodynia or menstrual disturbances in women.

Interference with clinical pathology tests
Potassium canrenoate has been reported to interfere with measurement of serum digoxin levels by radioimmunoassay. Its close relative spironolactone is known to interfere with the same test and also with tests for the measurement of corticosteroids, 17-ketosteroids, 17-hydroxycorticosteroids and 11-hydroxycorticosteroids in blood and urine.

High risk groups

Neonates
Potassium canrenoate is not recommended for use in neonates.

Breast milk. Because of its protein binding, transfer of canrenone to breast milk is low. The amount of canrenone ingested by a human infant in a mother's milk is estimated at 0.2% of the mother's daily dose of spironolactone which is insufficient to affect the infant's serum sodium and potassium. Nevertheless use of potassium canrenoate is not advised during lactation.

Children
The drug is not recommended for use in children.

Pregnant women
Potassium canrenoate should not be used during pregnancy.

The elderly
The drug may be used in the elderly, provided renal function is normal.

Drug interactions

Potentially hazardous interactions
Potassium canrenoate should be used cautiously in the presence of other potassium-sparing drugs such as amiloride, triamterene and converting-enzyme inhibitors. If chronic therapy is considered, regular checks of electrolyte balance are necessary.

Other significant interactions
Drugs with fluid-retaining properties may reduce the efficacy of the drug. Potassium canrenoate may antagonize the effect of carbenoxolone.

Potassium canrenoate

Potentially useful interactions
The antihypertensive effect of potassium canrenoate may be potentiated in the presence of other antihypertensive agents.

References

1. Garrett E R, Won C M 1971 Prediction of stability in pharmaceutical preparations XVI: kinetics of hydrolysis of canrenone and lactonization of canrenoic acid. Journal of Pharmaceutical Sciences 60: 1801–1809
2. Funder J W, Feldman D, Highland E, Edelman I S 1974 Molecular modifications of antialdosterone compounds: effects on affinity of spironolactones for renal aldosterone receptors. Biochemical Pharmacology 23: 1493–1501
3. Sakauye C, Feldman D 1976 Agonist and antimineralocorticoid activities of spirolactones. American Journal of Physiology 231: 93–97
4. Rossier B C, Claire M 1978 Mechanism of action of spirolactones in the toad bladder. In: Addison G M, Wirenfeldt Asmussen N, Corvol P et al (eds) Aldosterone antagonists in clinical medicine. Excerpta Medica, Amsterdam, pp 10–17
5. Hofmann L M 1976 Spironolactone and its metabolite canrenone: anti-aldosterone activity in the rhesus monkey. Federation Proceedings 35: 224
6. Dupuis B, Gagnol JP 1978 Antiarrhythmic action of canrenoate in experimental infarction in dogs. In: Addison G M, Wirenfeldt Asmussen N, Corvol P et al (eds) Aldosterone antagonists in clinical medicine. Excerpta Medica, Amsterdam, pp 371–372
7. Kotter V, von Leitner E, Kuhlmann J, Schröder R 1978 Effects of canrenoate-K in experimental myocardial infarction. In: Addison G M, Wirenfeldt Asmussen N, Corvol P et al (eds) Aldosterone antagonists in clinical medicine. Excerpta Medica, Amsterdam, pp 329–333
8. Cherie Ligniere T L, Ghizzi A 1974 Clinical findings on the use of a new injectable aldosterone antagonist. Terapia Antiboitica e ChemioTerapia 24: 33–50
9. Mantero F, Armanini D, Opocher G 1978 Effect of spironolactone and potassium canrenoate on plasma renin activity and plasma and urinary aldosterone in primary aldosteronism. In: Addison G M, Wirenfeldt Asmussen N, Corvol P et al (eds) Aldosterone antagonists in clinical medicine. Excerpta Medica, Amsterdam, pp 428–437
10. Siegel C, Bauer J 1969 Advances in the treatment of oedema with intravenously administered spirolactone. Die Medizinische Welt 39: 2129
11. Ceremuzynski L, Budaj A, Michorowski B 1983 Single-dose i.v. Aldactone for congestive heart failure. International Journal of Clinical Pharmacology, Therapy and Toxicology 21: 417–421
12. Ramsay L, Shelton J, Harrison I, Tidd M, Asbury M 1976 Spironolactone and potassium canrenoate in normal man. Clinical Pharmacology and Therapeutics 20: 167–177
13. Ramsay L, Asbury M, Shelton J, Harrison I 1977 Spironolactone and canrenoate-K: relative potency at steady-state. Clinical Pharmacology and Therapeutics 21: 602–609
14. Peile E B 1986 Relative potencies of spironolactone, canrenone and potassium canrenoate. In: Brunner H R et al (eds) Contemporary trends in diuretic therapy. Excerpta Medica, Amsterdam, pp 47–57
15. Erbler H C, Wernze H, Hilfenhaus M 1976 Effect of the aldosterone antagonist canrenone on plasma aldosterone concentration and plasma renin activity and on the excretion of aldosterone and electrolytes by man. European Journal of Clinical Pharmacology 9: 253–257
16. Yeh B K, Chiang B N, Sung P-K 1976 Anti-arrhythmic activity of potassium canrenoate in man. American Heart Journal 92: 308–318
17. Denis B, Machecourt J, Denis M C et al 1978 Anti-arrhythmic action of canrenoate in patients with acute myocardial infarction. In: Addison G M, Wirenfeldt Asmussen N, Corvol P et al (eds) Aldosterone antagonists in clinical medicine. Excerpta Medica, Amsterdam, pp 364–370
18. Denis B, Denis M C, Machecourt J et al 1986 Potassium canrenoate in the prophylaxis of ventricular fibrillation in acute myocardial infarction. In: Brunner H R et al (eds) Contemporary trends in diuretic therapy. Excerpta Medica, Amsterdam, pp 183–186
19. Marco J, Alibelli J M, Dardenne P 1978 The influence of canrenoate on left ventricular performance and contractility in healthy patients. In: Addison G M, Wirenfeldt Asmussen N, Corvol P et al (eds) Aldosterone antagonists in clinical medicine. Excerpta Medica, Amsterdam, pp 321–327
20. De Divitiis O, Fazio S, Petitto M et al 1984 Potassium canrenoate in the treatment of heart failure. Current Therapeutic Research 35: 40–47
21. Coltart D J, Koblic M, Signy M 1986 Central heamodynamic effects of potassium canrenoate. In: Brunner H R et al (eds) Contemporary trends in diuretic therapy. Excerpta Medica, Amsterdam, pp 176–182
22. Schroder R, Schuren K P, Biamino G, Meyer V, Sadee W 1971 Positive inotropic cardiac effect of potassium aldadiene (Aldactone pro Injectione). Klinische Wochenschrift 49: 1093–1096
23. Huttemann U, Schuren K P 1972 The treatment of chronic cor pulmonale with Aldactone (spironolactone, Potassium Canrenoate). Deutsche Medizinische Wochenschrift 97: 1533–1535
24. Ramdohr B, Schuren K P, Schröder R 1975 The treatment of heart failure with spironolactone potassium canrenoate. Therapiewoche 35: 4598–4606
25. Widmann L, Glocke M, Muller W 1980 The action of potassium canrenoate on patients with left heart failure, global heart failure and pulmonary heart disease. Herz 12: 435–441
26. Dupont A 1985 Disappearance of spironolactone-induced gynaecomastia during treatment with potassium canrenoate. Lancet 2: 731
27. Bellati G, Ideo G 1986 Gynaecomastia after spironolactone and potassium canrenoate. Lancet 1: 626
28. Karim A 1978 Pharmacokinetics and metabolism of aldosterone antagonists: a review. In: Addison G M, Wirenfeldt Asmussen N, Corvol P et al (eds) Aldosterone antagonists in clinical medicine. Excerpta Medica, Amsterdam, pp 115–131

Drug interactions

No particular adverse drug interactions are known, but explosions may occur after contact with organic materials or other easily oxidizable substances.

Major outcome trials

Although potassium permanganate has been used for centuries,[1] no formal clinical trials have been performed with it.

General review articles

Reynolds J E F (ed) 1982 Potassium permanganate. In: Martindale The extra pharmacopoeia, 28th edn. The Pharmaceutical Press, London, p 1233

Remington J P (ed) Potassium permanganate USP. In: Remington's pharmaceutical sciences, 14th edn. Mack Publishing Co, USA, pp 1186–1187

References

1. Redwood, Warrington (eds) 1867 Potassaa Permanganas, Permanganate of Potash. In: British pharmacopoeia, Medical Council. Spottiswoode & Co, London, p 254
2. Reynolds J E F (ed) 1982 Potassium permanganate. In: Martindale The extra pharmacopoeia, 28th edn. The Pharmaceutical Press, London, p 1233
3. Barry B W 1983 Skin structure, function, diseases and treatment. In: Swanbeck J (ed) Dermatological formulations. Vol 18, Drugs and pharmaceutical sciences. Dekker, New York, ch 1, pp 26–27
4. Maddin S (ed) 1982 The therapeutic agents of special interest to dermatologists. In: Current dermatologic therapy. W B Saunders, Philadelphia, p 594
5. Remington J P (ed) Potassium permanganate USP. In: Remington's pharmaceutical sciences, 14th edn. Mack Publishing Co, USA, pp 1186–1187
6. Medicines Commission 1980 Potassium permanganate. In: British Pharmacopoeia. HMSO, London, p 361
7. European Pharmaceutical Commission 1971 Kalii permanganas. In: European Pharmacopoeia. Council of Europe, 57 Sainte Ruffine, Maisonneuve, pp 279–280
8. Arndt K A (ed) 1978 Treatment principles and formulary. In: Manual of dermatological therapeutics, 2nd edn. K A Brown & Co, Boston, ch 37, p 332
9. Wilkinson D S 1979 Topical therapy. In: Rook A, Wilkinson D S, Ebling F J G (eds) Textbook of Dermatology, vol 2, 3rd edn. Blackwell, Oxford, ch 69, p 2312
10. Sulzberger M B, Wolf J (eds) 1952 Principles of topical medication. In: Dermatology essentials of diagnosis and treatment. The Year Book Publishers, Chicago, ch 1, p 42
11. McClure J 1980 The production of heterotopic calcification by certain chemical salts. Journal of Pathology 131: 21–33
12. Waisman M (ed) 1968 Treatment of bullous dermatoses. In: Pharmaceutical therapeutics in dermatology. Charles C Thomas, Springfield, Illinois, ch 17, p 142
13. Canizares O (ed) 1982 External medications. In: A manual of dermatology for developing countries. Oxford University Press, ch 1, p 15
14. Pillsbury M, Shelley W B, Kligman A M (eds) 1956 Diseases of the eccrine sweat gland. In: Dermatology. W B Saunders, Philadelphia, section V, ch 36, pp 833, 854
15. 1986 Potassium permanganate. In: Official information sheet, Lothian Regional Drug Information Centre, Royal Infirmary of Edinburgh
16. Mahomedy M C, Mahomedy Y H, Canham P A S, Downing J W, Jeal D E 1975 Methaemoglobinaemia following treatment dispensed by witch doctors. Anaesthesia 30: 190–193
17. Wong A L, Morran C G, McGeorge A, Abel B J 1985 Accidental urethrocutaneous fistula. British Journal of Urology 57: 239
18. Lustig S, Pitlik S D, Rosenfeld J B 1982 Liver damage in acute self-induced hypermanganemia. Archives of Internal Medicine 142: 405–406

Potassium salts

Potassium salts, usually chloride, are available for oral or intravenous use to correct and maintain plasma and total body levels.

Chemistry

Potassium chloride (Kay-Cee-L, K-Contin Continus, Leo K, Micro-K, Nu-K, Slow-K)
KCl

Molecular weight	74.6
pKa	—
Solubility	
in alcohol	1 in 400
in water	1 in 2.8
Octanol/water partition coefficient	very low

1 g of potassium chloride contains 13.4 mmol of potassium and chloride ions. It is a white crystalline substance with a bitter aftertaste, to some people. It is present in a number of compound preparations including Kloref, Kloref-S, Sando-K and in combination with glucose and/or sodium chloride.

Potassium bicarbonate
$KHCO_3$

Molecular weight	100.1
pKa	—
Solubility	
in alcohol	practically insoluble
in water	1 in 2.8
Octanol/water partition coefficient	very low

1 g of potassium bicarbonate contains 10 mmol of potassium and bicarbonate ions. Its appearance is colourless, transparent crystals, white granules or powder. It is present in several compound preparations including effervescent potassium tablets, Kloref, Kloref-S, Sando-K.

Potassium gluconate
$K(C_6H_{11}O_7)$

Molecular weight	234.2
pKa	—
Solubility	
in alcohol	practically insoluble
in water	freely soluble
Octanol/water partition coefficient	very low

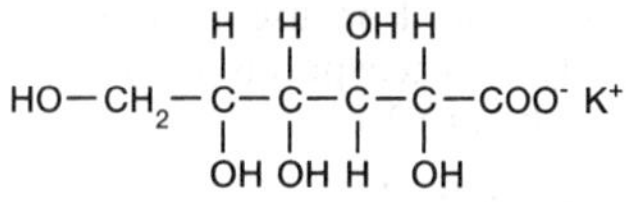

1 g of potassium gluconate contains 4.3 mmol of potassium. It is a yellowish-white crystalline solid, with a mild, slightly saline taste.

Pharmacology

The potassium ion is essential to life, being the predominant intracellular cation. It plays a major role in maintaining a normal

Potassium salts

transmembrane potential, which is fundamental to neuromuscular cell function, particularly automaticity and conduction in the heart. Both deficiency and excess of potassium have adverse cardiac effects and, if severe, also affect skeletal and smooth muscle function. The normal serum potassium concentration is 3.5–5.0 $mmol.l^{-1}$ while the intracellular concentration is about 150 $mmol.l^{-1}$. Potassium is accumulated by cells using an energy-dependent mechanism that pushes sodium out of the cell.

Toxicology

Potassium salts are not known to have mutagenic or carcinogenic effects.

Clinical pharmacology

Cardiac myocytes have an intracellular potassium concentration of approximately 150 $mmol.l^{-1}$ compared to an extracellular concentration of around 3.5–5.0 $mmol.l^{-1}$. In the resting state the cell membrane of cardiac myocytes is most permeable to potassium and much less so to sodium. Potassium ions tend to diffuse down the concentration gradient until limited by the negative intracellular potential; its magnitude is very close to that calculated from the Nernst equation.[1]

An increase in the extracellular potassium concentration will affect this system, tending to make the potential less negative; this may result in heart block or cardiac arrest. Hypokalaemia causes hyperpolarization of the cell membranes and an increase in excitability. In hypokalaemia the ECG may show prolongation of the QT interval and depression of the ST segment, while in hyperkalaemia the T-waves become increased in height and the PR interval lengthens. If potassium concentrations rise further (8–9 $mmol.l^{-1}$) asystole or ventricular fibrillation may ensue.

Pharmacokinetics

Plasma or serum potassium concentrations are conveniently measured by flame photometry — normal range 3.5–5.0 $mmol.l^{-1}$ in plasma. Spuriously high levels commonly occur as a result of haemolysis, and occasionally secondary to a very high peripheral white cell count.[2] Total body potassium may be measured non-invasively using a whole body radiation counter. This method, which is suitable for research purposes, relies on the fact that the majority of the natural radioactive emission from the human body is derived from the decay of the ^{40}K isotope. This isotope makes up 0.01% of natural potassium.

The human body contains 50–55 mmol potassium per kg body weight, which is concentrated in the intracellular compartment with only 2% in the extracellular space. In uncomplicated deficiency or retention of potassium, the plasma levels tend to reflect the total body status. However, it is essential to be aware that plasma potassium concentrations can be very misleading in predicting total body status, because the proportional distribution between intra- and extracellular spaces is affected by alterations in acid–base status and endocrine function.

No specific control mechanisms limit absorption of potassium, which is usually complete. An isolated dietary deficiency is unusual because of its ubiquitous occurrence in foods, but in malnutrition hypokalaemia is common.

When interpreting plasma potassium measurements, other factors, which are known to alter distribution, must be considered. Several hormones have the capacity to profoundly affect this balance, the most significant being insulin and adrenaline. Insulin induces cellular uptake of potassium by stimulation of the sodium/potassium pump.[3] This effect is exploited clinically to reduce plasma potassium in an emergency. It is also of great importance in the management of diabetic ketoacidosis, when large amounts of potassium may be required to prevent life-threatening hypokalaemia during the administration of insulin. Circulating adrenaline also induces a transfer of potassium into the intracellular space, via a β_2 effect.[4] This function can be affected by β-adrenoceptor blocking drugs; for example, propranolol has been shown to reduce tolerance to potassium loading[5] and to potentiate the normal rise in plasma potassium on exercise.[6] Alterations in acid–base balance also alter the intra- to extracellular distribution of potassium; an acidosis tends to raise extracellular potassium, and treatment of this with alkali will tend to reduce plasma potassium levels.

Potassium is excreted largely by the kidneys, though 10% is excreted by the colonic mucosa.

Potassium excretion is reduced in patients with renal impairment and in the elderly, so that extreme caution should be used in treating such patients with potassium salts.

Concentration–effect relationship

The effects of potassium are clearly related to its concentration in plasma, with both hypokalaemia (<3.0 $mmol.l^{-1}$) and hyperkalaemia (>5.0 $mmol.l^{-1}$) having deleterious effects.

Metabolism

A normal response to changes in potassium intake is essential to maintain normal total body level. The kidney is essential to potassium homeostasis, though in fact around 10% of potassium is actively excreted by colonic mucosa under the partial control of aldosterone. This alternative route of excretion may be of importance in the adaptation to chronic renal failure. Normal renal function includes a large reserve in its ability to respond to a potassium load. This homeostatic system makes it difficult to significantly increase total body potassium with oral loading, though it is, of course, possible to induce a temporary hyperkalaemia. The body is not so adept at responding to a restriction in intake and, despite an established deficiency, with hyperkalaemia, will continue to lose 15 to 20 mmol daily.

Potassium is freely filtered at the glomerulus and 80–90% is reabsorbed in the proximal tubule. Distal tubular cells have a substantial capacity to actively excrete potassium in response to an increase in plasma levels. The major part of this response is via aldosterone, which is released from the adrenal cortex as plasma potassium rises and stimulates potassium secretion in the distal tubules. However, it is clear that if plasma aldosterone is held constant then increases in plasma potassium are in themselves kaliuretic.[7]

The potassium-wasting effects of aldosterone are most marked in states of pure mineralocorticoid excess such as Conn's syndrome. The hypervolaemia in this condition tends to suppress proximal tubular solute reabsorption, so a greater volume of fluid is presented to the distal tubule. This in turn allows an increase in potassium secretion. An analogous situation is created when patients with secondary hyperaldosteronism are treated with thiazide or loop diuretics, e.g. for heart failure or cirrhosis. Before therapy, proximal sodium reabsorption is high and the flow rate into the distal tubule is low. This tends to limit the effect of excess aldosterone on potassium secretion, but when the distal inflow is increased by these diuretics then substantial potassium loss is generated.

Pharmaceutics

Potassium salts are available in oral forms, and in parenteral forms for addition to infusion fluids.

1. Oral preparations include wax matrix or microencapsulated formulations containing 8 mmol (8 mEq) potassium and effervescent tablets containing between 6 and 12 mmol (6–12 mEq). Potassium chloride is also produced as an effervescent powder and in various liquid preparations for oral use. Such preparations should be diluted for administration orally or via a nasogastric tube.
2. Ready prepared intravenous solutions:
   5% dextrose
   0.9% sodium chloride
   4% dextrose, 0.18% sodium chloride
   Available with potassium chloride 20–40 $mmol.l^{-1}$
3. For addition to infusion solutions:
   Potassium chloride solution strong 2.0 $mmol.ml^{-1}$
   Potassium chloride 10% 1.5 $mmol.ml^{-1}$
   Potassium chloride 20% 3.0 $mmol.ml^{-1}$
   It is essential that adequate mixing takes place before the infusion is commenced.

Potassium salts

P

Therapeutic use

Indications

1. Replacement of potassium deficit
2. Diuretic-induced hypokalaemia
3. Hypokalaemia from renal potassium wasting
4. Hypokalaemia from gastrointestinal losses
5. Prevention of hypokalaemia during diuretic therapy.

Contraindications

1. Acute or chronic renal failure
2. Oesophageal dysfunction (slow-release preparations)
3. Hyperkalaemic periodic paralysis
4. Adrenocortical insufficiency.

Mode of use

A reduction of plasma potassium from 4.0 to 3.0 mmol.l^{-1} in the absence of factors which influence the distribution of potassium, represents a 10% reduction in total body potassium, that is approximately 300 mmol. Similarly, a fall in plasma potassium to 2.0 mmol.l^{-1} indicates a deficit of 600 mmol or more. Therefore the correction of losses requires a relatively high daily dose of potassium, 50–100 mmol. This should be given after meals to minimize gastric irritation.

Severe potassium deficiency, particularly when associated with other illness, may need more urgent correction with parenteral preparations. It is preferable to use ready prepared solutions which are available with between 10 and 40 mmol.l^{-1} of potassium chloride. If potassium is added manually then care should be taken that the final solution is completely mixed; adverse effects have occurred when a dense potassium solution has been added to a container and not fully dispersed.[8] The usual maximum potassium concentration should be 40 mmol.l^{-1} administered at not more than 20 mmol.h^{-1}. It may be necessary, at the discretion of the physician, to exceed these limits, for example in the treatment of diabetic ketoacidosis. If concentrations of more than 40 mmol.l^{-1} are used, then extreme caution is essential; the infusion should be rigorously controlled into a large vein. Extravasation of such solutions is likely to be highly irritant to the tissues. Additionally, continuous ECG monitoring is advisable.

Indications

1. Replacement of a potassium deficit
It is obviously important to consider the cause of a potassium deficit and take measures to limit further losses in addition to instituting replacement therapy.

2. Diuretic-induced hypokalaemia
Oral supplements are appropriate to correct an established deficiency, but if the diuretic is to be continued then the addition of a potassium-retaining diuretic should be considered after the deficit is corrected and supplements of potassium discontinued. It is probably not necessary to treat mild hypokalaemia unless there are other reasons to do so, for example digoxin therapy or ischaemic heart disease.[9] Opinion has been divided on this point.[10,11]

3. Hypokalaemia from renal potassium wasting
Severe degrees of hypokalaemia can arise from renal losses in several circumstances:

a. Primary hyperaldosteronism
b. Bartter's syndrome
c. Renal tubular acidosis.

More modest, but significant losses occur in:

d. Secondary hyperaldosteronism
e. Cushing's syndrome
f. Carbenoxalone therapy
g. Magnesium deficiency.

In these situations therapy should be directed toward the underlying cause of potassium loss, in addition to replacement. Potassium chloride is the therapy of choice,[12] except in renal tubular acidosis when there is usually a combination of hyperchloraemia, acidosis and hypokalaemia. This is best corrected with potassium bicarbonate, which will correct the acidosis without worsening the hypokalaemia. Patients with reimplantation of the ureters into the sigmoid colon also develop hypokalaemia with hyperchloraemic acidosis and would be best treated with potassium bicarbonate, but they do usually have normal kidney function and can thus tolerate a combination of potassium chloride and sodium bicarbonate.

4. Hypokalaemia from gastrointestinal losses
Prolonged vomiting induces hypokalaemia, not by direct loss from the stomach but secondary to renal losses consequent upon the hypovolaemia and alkalosis. A combination of sodium chloride and potassium chloride will correct this situation. Diarrhoea and fluid from gastrointestinal fistulae may contain up to 100 mmol.l^{-1} of potassium. Villous adenoma of the colon can cause large losses of potassium.

5. Prevention of hypokalaemia
Thiazides, carbonic anhydrase inhibitors and loop diuretics all increase potassium excretion from the kidney. It is a matter of much debate as to whether it is necessary to give regular potassium supplements (or retaining diuretics) routinely to patients taking these drugs.[9–11] On balance, they should probably be reserved for patients who are likely to suffer important effects from hypokalaemia — i.e. those taking digoxin, with ischaemic heart disease or hepatic cirrhosis. When thiazides are used to treat uncomplicated hypertension the risk of hypokalaemia is probably slight: the initial suggestion that hypokalaemia may have contributed to an increased risk of sudden death[13,14] has not been borne out in the MRC trial in a much larger group of patients.[15,16] In addition, the continuing trend to reduce the dose of diuretics used for hypertension should further reduce their hypokalaemic potential.[17] When diuretic therapy is initiated in states of secondary hyperaldosteronism such as cirrhosis and heart failure, the risk of serious hypokalaemia is much greater. However, the routine use of potassium supplements is no substitute for regular monitoring of plasma potassium, and the use of potassium-retaining diuretics may prove much easier.

Contraindications

1. Renal failure
Potassium should not be routinely prescribed to patients with a glomerular filtration rate of less than 50% normal. It is more appropriate to follow plasma levels and reserve therapy for cases when levels fall below 3.0 mmol.l^{-1}. The risk of inducing serious hyperkalaemia is much greater in patients with renal failure, so frequent measures of plasma potassium are mandatory.

2. Oesophageal dysfunction
Patients with enlarged hearts have been shown to have delayed passage of barium tablets in the oesophagus.[18] Delayed passage of wax matrix potassium preparations has been reported to cause strictures and haemorrhage.[19]

3. Hyperkalaemic periodic paralysis
An acute increase in potassium intake has been reported to initiate an attack of paralysis.[20]

4. Adrenocortical insufficiency
Subjects with Addison's disease do not respond normally to a potassium load; similarly, hyporeninaemic hypoaldosteronism, a rare condition found most often in elderly type II diabetes, presents with unexpected hyperkalaemia.[21] Care is required in such patients.

Adverse reactions

Potentially life-threatening effects
Hyperkalaemia occurs in a small percentage of subjects treated with potassium. The greatest risk is in the use of intravenous preparations, when administration at a rate greater than clearance from the plasma can cause serious disturbances of cardiac rhythm and even cardiac arrest. In addition to this risk, hyperkalaemia may cause muscle weakness and, in extreme cases, chest pain and paralysis.

Acute overdosage
Significant hyperkalaemia has been reported soon after the ingestion of slow-release preparations.[22] The first priority in treatment of potassium overdosage is to ensure stability of cardiac rhythm.

10–30 ml of 10% calcium gluconate will reduce the effect of hyperkalaemia on the heart and can be given immediately. Continuous ECG monitoring is essential and if there is clinical evidence of hyperkalaemia then insulin and dextrose should be administered. Gastric lavage should be undertaken and 60 g of Calcium Resonium left in the stomach. The prolonged release of potassium from an overdose should be noted, and plasma potassium will need to be monitored for several hours. Severe and unresponsive hyperkalaemia is very effectively treated with haemodialysis.

Severe or irreversible adverse effects
Oesophageal stricture or haemorrhage have been reported with wax matrix preparations.[18,19] Ulceration of the small intestine has also been reported with the wax matrix formulation, presenting with stricture, bleeding or perforation.[23–26]

Symptomatic adverse effects
Nausea and vomiting are very common and evidence of gastritis has been observed, which is claimed to be less severe with the microencapsulated forms.[27]

Interference with clinical pathology tests
Potassium salts may interfere with flame photometric methods of measuring sodium and calcium if the instrument is of poor quality.

High risk groups

Neonates
Potassium may be given to neonates if indicated, in suitable preparations.

Breast milk. There are no contraindications to breast-feeding while taking potassium salts.

Children
No special precautions are required.

Pregnant women
Solid oral preparations should be avoided during pregnancy, because of reduced gastrointestinal motility.

The elderly
Renal function should be considered before prescription. Elderly patients are more likely to have disordered upper gastrointestinal motility.

Drug interactions

Potentially hazardous interactions

Potassium-retaining diuretics. Concurrent prescription of potassium and potassium-retaining diuretics is very likely to result in hyperkalaemia.[28] Occasionally this combination may prove useful if hypokalaemia is profound.

Angiotensin converting enzyme inhibitors. This combination has been reported to cause hyperkalaemia during the therapy of heart failure.[29]

Non-steroidal anti-inflammatory drugs. A potential for interaction exists in that these drugs have occasionally been reported to cause hyperkalaemia.[30]

β-adrenoceptor blockers. β-blockers reduce tolerance to a potassium load and therefore increase the risk of hyperkalaemia when given with potassium supplements.

Potentially useful interactions
The very occasional therapeutic usefulness of combining treatment with potassium salts and potassium-retaining diuretics (normally a potentially dangerous combination) has been mentioned above.

References

1. Nernst W 1908 Zur theori des elektrischen reizes. Pflugers Archive 122: 275–314
2. Ringelham B, Laszlo E, Vajda L 1974 Pseudohyperkalaemia in acute myeloid leukaemia. Lancet 2: 928
3. Andres R, Baltzan M A, Cader G, Zierler K L 1962 Effect of insulin on carbohydrate metabolism and on potassium in the forearm of man. Journal of Clinical Investigation 41: 108–114
4. Silva P, Spokes K 1981 Sympathetic system in potassium homeostasis. American Journal of Physiology 241: F151–F155
5. Rosa R M, Silva P, Young J B, Landsley L, Brown R S, Rose J W, Epstein F H 1980 Adrenergic modulation of extrarenal potassium disposal. New England Journal of Medicine 302: 431–434

6. Carlsson E, Fellenius E, Lundorg P, Svensson L 1978 β-adrenoceptor blockers plasma potassium and exercise. Lancet 2: 424–425
7. Field M J, Giebisch G J 1985 Hormonal control of potassium excretion. Kidney International 27: 379–387
8. Williams R H P 1973 Potassium overdosage. A potential hazard of non-rigid parenteral fluid containers. British Medical Journal 1: 714
9. Harrington J T, Isner J M, Kassirer J P 1982 Our national obsession with potassium. American Journal of Medicine 73: 155–159
10. Kaplan N M 1984 Our appropriate concern about hyperkalaemia. American Journal of Medicine 77: 1–4
11. Morgan D B, Davison C 1980 Hypokalaemia and diuretics: an analysis of publications. British Medical Journal 280: 905–908
12. Kassirer J P, Berkman P M, Lawrenz D R 1965 The critical role of chloride in the correction of hypokalaemic alkalosis in man. American Journal of Medicine 38: 172–189
13. Hollifield J W, Slaton P E 1981 Thiazide diuretics, hypokalaemia and cardiac arrhythmias. Acta Medica Scandinavica suppl 647: 67–73
14. Morgan T, Adam W, Hodgson M 1984 Adverse reactions to long term diuretic therapy for hypertension. Journal of Cardiovascular Pharmacology suppl 1: S269–S271
15. Medical Research Council Working Party 1985 MRC trial of treatment of mild hypertension, principal results. British Medical Journal 291: 97–104
16. Editorial 1985 Treatment of hypertension, the 1985 results. Lancet 2: 645–647
17. Medical Research Council Working Party on Mild to Moderate Hypertension 1983 Ventricular extrasystoles during thiazide treatment; sub-study of MRC mild hypertension trail. British Medical Journal 287: 1249–1253
18. Howie A D, Strachan R W 1975 Slow release potassium chloride treatment. British Medical Journal 2: 176
19. McCall A J 1975 Slow K ulceration of the oesophagus with aneurysmal left atrium. British Medical Journal 3: 230–231
20. Egan T J, Klein R 1959 Hyperkalaemic familial periodic paralysis. Pediatrics 24: 761
21. Williams G H 1986 Hyporeninemic hypoaldosteronism. New England Journal of Medicine 314: 1041–1042
22. Illingworth R N, Proudfoot A T 1980 Rapid poisoning with slow release potassium. British Medical Journal 2: 485
23. Weiss S M, Rutenberg H L, Paskin D L, Zaren H A 1977 Gut lesions due to slow release potassium chloride tablets. New England Journal of Medicine 296: 111–112
24. Farquarson-Roberts M A, Giddings A B, Nunn A J 1975 Perforation of the small bowel due to slow release potassium chloride (Slow-K). British Medical Journal 3: 206
25. Brower R A 1986 Jejunal perforation possibly induced by slow release potassium in a patient with Chron's disease. Digestive Diseases and Sciences 31: 1387–1390
26. Barloon T J 1986 A case of stenotic obstruction of the jejunum secondary to slow-release potassium. American Journal of Gastroenterology 81: 192–194
27. McMahon F G, Akdaman K, Ryan J R 1982 Upper gastrointestinal lesions after potassium chloride supplements. A controlled clinical trial. Lancet 2: 1059–1060
28. Lawson D H 1974 Adverse reactions to potassium. Quarterly Journal of Medicine 171: 433
29. Dzau V J, Colucci W S, Williams G H, Curfman G, Meggs L, Hollenberg N K 1980 Sustained effectiveness of converting enzyme inhibition in patients with severe heart failure. New England Journal of Medicine 302: 1373
30. Ponce S P, Jennings A E, Madias N E, Harrington J T 1985 Drug induced hyperkalaemia. Medicine 64: 357–370

P

Practolol

Practolol was the first cardioselective β-adrenoceptor blocking drug to be marketed. However, a severe practolol-induced adverse reaction, the oculomucocutaneous syndrome, has been recognized and because of this practolol tablets have been withdrawn from the market. This syndrome has not been reported following short-term intravenous therapy and the injection formulation has been available until recently. This formulation has also been withdrawn.

Chemistry

Practolol (Eraldin, Dalzic)
$C_{14}H_{22}N_2O_3$
(dl)-4′-(2-Hydroxy-3-isopropylaminopropoxy)acetanilide

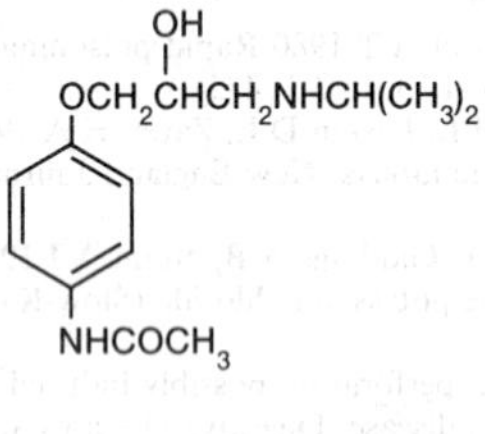

Molecular weight	266.3
pKa	9.5
Solubility	
in alcohol	1:40
in water	1:400
Octanol/water partition coefficient	0.060

A colourless, stable, fine crystalline solid, prepared by chemical synthesis; the racemate is used clinically. Practolol was also available in an oral combination product with clofibrate (Eramid).

Pharmacology

Practolol is a competitive β_1-selective antagonist with a higher affinity for β_1-adrenoceptors than for β_2-adrenoceptors, and is therefore cardioselective. It has no membrane-stabilizing activity but possesses intrinsic sympathomimetic activity with approximately 15–20% of the activity of isoprenaline.[1–4]

Toxicology

Practolol does not have mutagenic potential, and toxicological testing in animals failed to demonstrate any results of potential clinical relevance. There is no evidence of teratological effects in rats and rabbits. In spite of toxicity tests done to full current international standards, no evidence for the practolol syndrome appeared in animals.[67]

Clinical pharmacology

Studies in healthy volunteers and patients have shown that practolol reduces the heart rate at rest[5–9] and attenuates the increase in heart rate produced by exercise,[6–8,10–13] catecholamine administration[5,10,14] and tilting.[8,10] Although some reductions both in systolic and diastolic blood pressure have been reported in healthy subjects at rest after single doses of practolol, they were not considered to be of any significance.[8,15–16] As expected, the increase in blood pressure due to exercise is reduced by practolol.[8,16]

In general, pulmonary arterial pressure is not significantly affected by the administration of practolol[11] and haemodynamic studies, in both patients and normal subjects, have shown that practolol either has no effect or causes slight increases in peripheral resistance.[11,13,16] The response of stroke volume and cardiac output to practolol varies. In some studies stroke volume in cardiac patients did not change or only decreased slightly after practolol.[17,18] In other studies stroke volume was actually seen to increase both at rest and during exercise and, in spite of a fall in heart rate, cardiac output was often unchanged.[11,19]

Practolol is a β_1-selective (cardioselective) β-blocker. It has been shown to block cardiac β-receptors more effectively than peripheral vascular β-receptors at the same dose levels in man.[10,14] Practolol used to be the cardioselective standard but was later shown in asthmatic patients to be somewhat less selective than atenolol,[20] about as selective as metoprolol[21,22] and somewhat more selective than acebutolol.[23] The Formgren study[21] demonstrated very clearly that the benefits of both metoprolol and practolol were diminished at higher dosage.

Practolol, like propranolol, inhibits catecholamine-induced lipolysis but the inhibition following practolol is much smaller than that seen with propranolol.[24] Practolol does not appear to affect the increase in blood glucose due to catecholamines[24] and in man practolol has no effect on adrenaline-induced increases in lactate in doses which blocked the rise in free fatty acids.[25]

Pharmacokinetics

The preferred analytical method is by gas–liquid chromatography. This method depends on the conversion of practolol to the deacetylated amine followed by its reaction with trifluoroacetic anhydride.[26] The limit of sensitivity is 10 μg.l^{-1}. It can also be measured by HPLC with UV detection. In man, practolol is completely absorbed after oral administration and maximum blood levels are reached between 1 and 3 hours after a single oral dose.[7] These levels after 2 hours are usually in the range 0.5–0.9 mg.l^{-1} and 1.5–3 mg.l^{-1} after single oral doses of 100 mg and 200 mg, respectively.[7,27,28] Chronic oral dosing, with a preliminary dose of 200 mg, followed at 12-hourly intervals with a maintenance dose of 100 mg, gives moderately ascending blood levels which level off by the third day. At this time the blood levels vary between 1.8 and 2.6 mg.l^{-1} at 2 hours and 0.8 and 1.3 mg.l^{-1} at 12 hours after the last dose. There is no first-pass metabolism. The plasma half life of practolol following oral administration in man has been reported as 10 hours[7] and 13 hours[29] and the kidney is the main eliminating organ. The urinary excretion pattern of practolol was studied by Fitzgerald and Scales[7] and by Reeves et al,[30] and on average 74–100% of the drug is excreted unchanged, 80% within the first 24 hours and the remainder in the second 24-hour period. The excretion of practolol after chronic dosage was studied by Bodem and Chidsey.[29] The results show that the amount of practolol found in the urine equalled the amount of drug administered. These observations indicate that practolol is eliminated by renal excretion with little or no detectable metabolic transformation.

The distribution of practolol has been studied in rats, mice and dogs after oral, intraperitoneal and intravenous injections.[26] The drug is rapidly absorbed from the blood, the highest level being found in the bile. Most tissue levels, except in the brain, are at least five times higher than in the blood. The lowest level of practolol is found in the brain. In man the volume of distribution is 1.6 l.kg^{-1}. Plasma protein binding is negligible (<5%).

Oral absorption	>95%
Presystemic metabolism	<5%
Plasma half life	
range	10–13 h
mean	11.5 h
Volume of distribution	1.6 l.kg^{-1}
Plasma protein binding	<5%

Practolol passes into breast milk to give concentrations four times those of the expected maternal blood level. It is highly unlikely that this blood level will have any adverse effects on the baby, as blood levels as high as 20 mg.l^{-1} are well tolerated in adults.

The excretion of practolol is markedly impaired in advanced chronic renal failure. The plasma half life is markedly prolonged but can be significantly shortened by haemodialysis.[31] The pharmacokinetics of practolol were similar in young and elderly subjects with normal renal function.[65]

Concentration–effect relationship

There is no clear-cut therapeutic range. Reduction of exercise-induced tachycardia is proportional to the logarithm of the plasma concentration.[32]

Practolol produces near maximum effects on exercise heart rate so long as blood levels of 1.0–1.4 $mg.l^{-1}$ are maintained. The duration of action of practolol effect depends on dose. Thus 400 mg exerts some effect up to 96 hours. There is no disparity between oral and intravenous blood levels of practolol and pharmacological effect once a steady state is obtained. This is consistent with the absence of metabolism in man. The oral route provides a reasonably fast and highly predictable means of achieving therapeutic blood levels.

There is no apparent relationship between blood levels of practolol and antihypertensive activity or antianginal activity.

Metabolism

In man practolol is not metabolized to any degree, with 74–100% of the drug excreted unchanged in the urine.[30,32] Furthermore, in animals at least 85% of the administered drug is excreted unchanged in the urine with the remainder as 18 metabolites. The major metabolite accounts for about 9% of the dose in rats and dogs and has been identified as 2-hydroxy-4′-(2-hydroxy-3-isopropylaminopropoxy)acetanilide.[26]

Pharmaceutics

Practolol was available in oral and parenteral forms but now both have been withdrawn.

Tablets contained 100 mg practolol BP. The tablets were blue, round, biconvex, film-coated and printed with the name Eraldin in black.

Practolol was available for intravenous use as a clear solution in 5 ml ampoules each containing 10 mg of practolol BP in 5 ml of a buffered aqueous solution.

The Eraldin injection (ICI, UK) was stable with a reasonable shelf-life but had to be stored in a cool place and protected from light.

Eramid was presented as bilateral yellow/black soft gelatin capsules each containing 500 mg clofibrate BP and 100 mg practolol BP. This formulation has been withdrawn.

Therapeutic use

Indications

1. The management of angina pectoris
2. The control of cardiac dysrhythmias caused or maintained by excessive sympathetic activity and particularly those associated with (i) organic cardiac disease including post-infarction tachyarrhythmias, (ii) functional disorders such as anxiety tachycardia, (iii) the unwanted effects of sympathetic stimulating bronchodilators, (iv) endocrine disturbances such as thyrotoxicosis and (v) anaesthesia and surgery.

Contraindications

1. Second- or third-degree heart block
2. Metabolic acidosis
3. Digitalis refractory heart failure
4. Severe bradycardia
5. Cardiogenic shock.

Mode of use

All the clinical uses depend upon production of β-adrenoceptor blockade, usually of β_1-receptors in the heart, and the advantages of cardioselectivity have been described by Kendall.[33]

Oral treatment was usually begun with 100–200 mg two or three times daily and the dose increased to an upper limit of 1.2 g depending upon the therapeutic response.

Intravenous doses are intended for the emergency treatment of cardiac dysrhythmias and thyrotoxic crisis. Although this route bypasses the liver, the dose is no more effective than the oral one. A 5 mg intravenous dose should be given slowly and if no response occurs the dose may be repeated. Doses of more than 20 mg are not normally required.

Practolol

Indications

1. Angina pectoris

Practolol was an effective prophylactic drug for the relief of classical exercise-induced angina although the dose required had to be adjusted for optimal effect.

In results from many clinical trials involving thousands of patients, approximately 82% of all patients responded to treatment with practolol by improvement in the number or severity of anginal attacks, exercise tolerance, nitrate consumption or ischaemic ECG changes. In particular, Wiseman[34] showed that intravenous practolol improved effort tolerance in anginal patients and, in comparison with placebo, was significantly more effective in decreasing anginal frequency and glyceryl trinitrate consumption and increasing effort tolerance. Similar results were obtained by Backman and Martikainen.[35]

A number of studies have shown that the antianginal efficacy of practolol is similar to that of propranolol[36–39] and oxprenolol[37–41] but inferior to the other cardioselective β-blockers atenolol[42] and metoprolol.[36,37,43] The calcium antagonist verapamil has also been shown to be superior to practolol in decreasing anginal frequency and glyceryl trinitrate consumption and in increasing effort tolerance.[44]

Eraldin tablets were prescribed as one to two tablets two or three times daily, adjusted according to response. The usual dose range was two to six tablets per day. Clinical experience was limited to an upper dosage of 12 tablets (1.2 g) daily.

Eramid was used in the treatment of both the acute and chronic aspects of angina. It reduced the frequency of anginal attacks and increased exercise tolerance. It protected the heart against excessive or inappropriate sympathetic nervous stimulation, thus reducing myocardial oxygen demand and increasing cardiac efficiency.

Eramid was recommended for the treatment of angina pectoris where both clofibrate and practolol were indicated. The product had lipid-lowering and antithrombogenic properties. The combination capsule contained 500 mg clofibrate BP and 100 mg practolol BP and the dose was one capsule three times daily, or two capsules given twice daily.

2. Cardiac dysrhythmias

The place of practolol in the treatment of dysrhythmias is well established. Analysis of clinical trial data showed that 78% of supraventricular dysrhythmias and 69% of all ventricular dysrhythmias responded to intravenous doses of between 5 and 60 mg and oral doses in the range 50–800 mg daily.

Patients with sinus tachycardia respond well to treatment.[45–47] In atrial fibrillation, flutter or tachycardia, administration of practolol will slow ventricular rate, usually by increasing conduction time through the atrioventricular node due to blockade of the sympathetic activity on the node.[48–49] Practolol is also a very effective drug in atrial tachycardia[49] and provides an effective treatment in paroxysmal supraventricular dysrhythmias.[47] Useful results have also been obtained in ventricular dysrhythmias[49] and those occurring in the first 24 hours after resuscitation from ventricular fibrillation have also been treated successfully with practolol.[50]

Practolol has also been found useful in the treatment of drug-induced dysrhythmias, particularly digitalis toxicity,[49] those resulting from overdoses of tricyclic antidepressants,[51] those following the administration of isoprenaline[52] and those arising from the use of pacemakers.[53] The combination of practolol and digitalis in atrial fibrillation and atrial flutter is highly beneficial.[49]

Practolol has proved useful in both the treatment and prevention of dysrhythmias, without untoward haemodynamic effects, in the early stages of myocardial infarction,[49,50,54–56] suggesting that the prevention and treatment of dysrhythmias following myocardial infarction with practolol may lead to an improved prognosis in these patients.

Practolol provides a safe, efficient way of controlling the dysrhythmias which occur due to anaesthesia.[57–59]

It is recommended that for the treatment of cardiac dysrhythmias 5 mg practolol (2.5 ml) should be given slowly intravenously, and if no response occurs the dose may be repeated. Doses of more than

20 mg (10 ml) are not normally required. The oral dose depends on the extent to which sympathetic stimulation is responsible for the dysrhythmia. The usual dose is 100 mg twice daily, but higher doses may be necessary.

Adverse reactions

Potentially life-threatening effects
Some of the disorders described below under the heading practolol-induced syndrome resulted in death on rare occasions.

Acute overdosage
A 39-year-old man with rheumatic mitral disease and mental depression took 90 tablets (9000 mg) of Eraldin during a depressive mood. His general condition remained good although after three hours his heart rate was 70 beats per minute and his blood pressure 90/70 mmHg. There were no signs of cardiac decompensation. After a further two hours his blood pressure and heart rate increased and he later recovered without special treatment.[60]

Excessive bradycardia can be countered, however, with atropine 1–2 mg intravenously, followed, if necessary, by a β-adrenoceptor stimulant such as isoprenaline 25 μg initially, or orciprenaline 0.5 mg, given by slow intravenous injection. Care must be taken to ensure that the blood pressure does not fall too low if the dose of β-adrenoceptor agonist has to be increased. Glucagon has been reported to be useful as a cardiac stimulant in a dose of 10 mg intravenously.

Severe or irreversible adverse effects

Practolol-induced syndrome. Practolol had been generally available in the UK since June 1970 before its unique toxicity came to light in the middle of 1974. At that time patient exposure was estimated to be approximately 1 million patient years.

The chief features of the oculomucocutaneous syndrome are:

1. A psoriasiform rash with hyperkeratosis of the palms and soles and fissuring along the sides of the digits. In some cases it was extensive and required hospitalization. It invariably recovered completely within three to four months of cessation of therapy.
2. An unusual form of keratoconjunctivitis sicca with characteristic and unique subconjunctival fibrotic changes, mainly in the fornices, and leading to shallowing of the fornices and occasionally symblepharon. Corneal ulceration leading to opacification and loss of vision occurred in some cases. In some instances these changes were permanent and did not resolve on cessation of therapy.
3. A bilateral secretory otitis media causing deafness and requiring treatment by myringotomy and the insertion of grommets: some patients also had a sensorineural type of deafness from cochlear involvement.
4. A unique type of sclerosing peritonitis in which the visceral peritoneum became thickened and enclosed the bowel in a cocoon of fibrous tissue leading to repeated attacks of subacute high intestinal obstruction and sometimes requiring laparotomy. The definitive treatment was to strip the thickened peritoneum from the whole length of the bowel and this was generally successful.
5. In a small number of cases there was also a bilateral sclerosing pleuritis with or without effusion in the costophrenic angles.
6. Very rarely, a form of sclerosing pericarditis of a constrictive nature.

The fact that no dose relationship or abnormality in metabolism or kinetics has been observed in patients developing the practolol syndrome argues against both a pharmacological and a conventional toxicological mechanism for the reaction. If a toxicological process were involved, it would have been expected that the toxicity would have been demonstrated in animals, but this has not been so. An immunological mechanism has its attractions, but has not been established categorically. Certainly, a number of immunological events did occur in some patients. An antibody to the intercellular region of epidermal tissue was found to be present in serum of patients with the practolol syndrome. Some patients with the syndrome had a positive test for antinuclear factor (ANF), but there was no correlation between clinical evidence of practolol toxicity and the presence of ANF.

About 50% of patients had skin reactions; about 73% had some eye involvement; 14% had ear damage; 17% had peritoneal involvement; 4% had a pleural reaction; and only about 1% had a pericardial reaction. The figures given above add up to more than 100 because many patients had more than one feature of the syndrome.

This syndrome has arisen only during or after oral treatment following a mean duration of treatment of 24 months[61] and has not been reported following short-term intravenous therapy. In view of the serious and unusual nature of these reactions, Eraldin tablets have been withdrawn from sale.

SLE-like syndrome. A drug-induced SLE-like syndrome, sometimes characterized by skin rashes associated with fever and with joint pains, has also been reported in a few patients.

Symptomatic adverse effects
The oculomucocutaneous syndrome, which caused withdrawal of oral dosage forms of practolol, comprised serious adverse reactions including conjunctival scarring, psoriasiform rash, and peritoneal fibrosis when taken by mouth. No such adverse reactions have been reported following intravenous administration of practolol.

Other common side effects are nausea, paraesthesia, constipation, bradycardia, hypotension, heart failure, bronchospasm, sleep disturbance, dizziness, tiredness of legs, feeling of heat in arms and AV block. In many cases these effects have been transient and have disappeared after a reduction in dosage.

High risk groups

Neonates
Practolol is not recommended for therapeutic use in neonates. In mothers treated with practolol, fetal heart rate was not significantly changed.[62]

Breast milk. Practolol enters breast milk, but it is not considered that a breast-fed baby will be harmed in consequence.

Children
Practolol is not recommended for children as the safety and efficacy have not been established.

Pregnant women
Practolol is not recommended during pregnancy. However, several reports have been received of women treated with practolol during part of or throughout pregnancy. In none of these cases were there any adverse effects on the mother or fetus.[63,64] There is no evidence to suggest that practolol is teratogenic.

The elderly
No special precautions are required as doses are adjusted according to patient response. The elimination of practolol is similar in elderly subjects with normal renal function and young subjects.[65]

Concurrent disease
Heart disease. Practolol need not necessarily be withheld from patients with signs of heart failure. For such patients, however, myocardial contractility must be maintained and signs of failure controlled with digitalis and diuretics.

Lung disease. Practolol may be used with caution in patients with chronic obstructive airways disease, and β_2-mediated reversal with a bronchodilator is permitted. However, occasionally some increase in airways resistance may occur in asthmatic patients.

Renal disease. The excretion of practolol is markedly impaired in advanced chronic renal failure.[31] The plasma half life was markedly prolonged but could be significantly shortened by haemodialysis. Therapeutic drug levels were achieved by the administration of 200 mg of the drug orally at the beginning and end of each dialysis.

Diabetes. Practolol modifies the tachycardia of hypoglycaemia. In insulin-dependent and labile diabetes it may be necessary to adjust the hypoglycaemic therapy.

Drug interactions

Potentially hazardous interactions
Disopyramide. β-adrenoceptor blocking agents may enhance the negative inotropic action of antiarrhythmic agents. Two cases of severe bradycardia, one of them having a fatal outcome, followed the intravenous injection of practolol and disopyramide in the treatment of supraventricular tachycardia.[66] Thus care should be taken in

Practolol

prescribing a β-adrenoceptor blocking drug with Class I antidysrhythmic agents such as disopyramide.

Verapamil. Serious myocardial depression can result from the concurrent use of verapamil and β-blocking agents in those with impairment of left ventricular function.[66] Hence β-adrenoceptor blocking agents should be used with caution in combination with verapamil in patients with impaired ventricular function. The combination should not be given to patients with conduction abnormalities and neither drug should be administered intravenously within 48 hours of discontinuing the other.

Clonidine. The rebound hypertension following abrupt withdrawal of clonidine may be potentiated by a β-blocker such as practolol. If β-adrenoceptor blocking drugs and clonidine are given concurrently, clonidine should not be discontinued until several days after withdrawal of the β-adrenoceptor blocking drug.

General anaesthesia. Anaesthesia may proceed safely under β-adrenoceptor blockade provided that the patient is protected against bradycardia by the intravenous administration of atropine 1–2 mg, and provided that anaesthetic agents causing myocardial depression, such as ether, chloroform, cyclopropane, and trichloroethylene, are avoided.

Practolol is compatible with light anaesthesia using halothane. Ether, chloroform, cyclopropane and possibly trichloroethylene depend for their safety on increased circulating levels of endogenous catecholamines and it is possible that they are therapeutically incompatible with β-adrenoceptor blocking drugs. Vagal dominance, if it occurs, may be countered with atropine.

Potentially useful interactions
None has been described.

Major outcome trials

1. Westerlund A 1973 Three years experience with Eraldin (practolol) in angina pectoris. Klin Aspekter pa β-Receptor Blockad, Linkoping Symposium: 117–122

Westerlund carried out a double-blind trial investigating the effects of practolol in 14 patients with angina pectoris. Treatment with practolol was continued after the trial in 13 of these patients and exercise tests were undertaken at intervals. The study was continued for nearly three years, during which time exercise tolerance increased from an average of 70% seen in the double-blind study to at least 300% in the 8 patients who were still taking practolol at the end of the study. A subjective improvement of more than 50% was also seen. The author found it possible to lower the average daily dose from 700 mg to 400 mg during the study.

2. Green K G, Chamberlain D A, Fulton R M et al 1975 Improvement in prognosis of myocardial infarction by long-term β adrenoceptor blockade using practolol. British Medical Journal 3: 735–740

In a large-scale double-blind controlled trial of practolol (200 mg twice daily) in the long-term prophylactic treatment of 3038 patients recovering from acute myocardial infarction treatment was started 1–4 weeks after the acute attack. The trial was originally planned to include 4000 patients treated for at least a year but had to be terminated prematurely because of the serious oculocutaneous and peritoneal reactions reported elsewhere.

The practolol-treated group showed a significant reduction in overall mortality and in sudden deaths. However, this reduction was indecisive if the data were analysed on an 'intention to treat' basis. It was concluded that practolol used in the long-term treatment of patients who have survived the acute phase of myocardial infarction reduces the death rate when the original infarct is sited anteriorly. Since practolol produces severe side effects in long-term use, it was recommended that an alternative β-adrenoceptor blocking agent should be used.

3. Van Durme J P, Bossaert L, Vermeire P, Pannier R 1972 One hundred and fifty cases of cardiac arrythmias treated with practolol (ICI 50,172). Acta Cardiology (suppl XV): 285–291

150 cases of cardiac tachyarrhythmias were treated with practolol. Return to normal sinus rhythm or slowing of the heart rate below 100 beats/min were obtained in 118 cases of supraventricular tachyarrhythmias. Comparison between the patients receiving only practolol and those where it was combined with digitalis indicates a potentiating effect of digitalis on the antiarrhythmic effectiveness of practolol. Ventricular tachyarrhythmias (32 cases) did not respond as well, and constitute only a secondary indication for practolol. In 59 patients with congestive heart failure and in 17 patients with chronic obstructive lung disease the therapeutic results were excellent.

4. Evemy K L, Pentecost B L 1978 Intravenous and oral practolol in the acute stages of myocardial infarction. European Journal of Cardiology 7/5-6: 391–396

The influence of routine administration of practolol on the outcome of acute myocardial infarction was studied in 94 patients under the age of 70 experiencing their first myocardial infarction. An initial dose of intravenous practolol 15 mg was followed by five oral doses of practolol 200 mg at 12-hour intervals. There was a significant reduction in the incidence of atrial fibrillation among those patients receiving practolol compared with the control group. However, at seven months there was no difference between the treated and control groups in the incidence of cardiac failure, death or reinfarction.

References

1. Dunlop D, Shanks R G 1968 Selective blockade of adrenoceptive beta receptors in the heart. British Journal of Pharmacology and Chemotherapy 32: 201–218
2. Kofi Ekue J M, Shanks R G, Zaida S A 1970 Observations on the sub-division of β-adrenoceptor in the circulation of the dog. British Journal of Pharmacology 39: 184–185
3. Levy B, Wilkenfeld B E 1969 An analysis of selective beta receptor blockade. European Journal of Pharmacology 5: 223–234
4. Barrett A M, Carter J 1970 Comparative chronotropic activity of β-adrenoceptive antagonists. British Journal of Pharmacology 40: 373–381
5. Brick I, Hutchison K H, Roddie I C, Shanks R G 1968 Cardiac adrenergic blockade by 4-(2-hydroxy-3-isopropylamino propoxy) acetanilide (ICI 50,172). Archives of Pharmacology and Experimental Pathology 259: 156–157
6. Areskog N H, Adolfsson L 1969 Effects of a cardioselective β-adrenergic blocker (ICI 50, 172) at exercise in angina pectoris. British Medical Journal 2: 601–603
7. Fitzgerald J D, Scales B 1968 Effect of a new adrenergic β- blocking agent (ICI 50, 172) on heart rate in relation to its blood levels. International Journal of Clinical Pharmacology 1: 467–474
8. Kirchhoff H W, Kuemmerle H P, Dusterlho J C 1969 Vergleichende Untersuchungen uber den Einfluss von Beta-Rezeptoren-blockern auf verschiedene Kreislaufparameter. I — Untersuchungsergebnisse vor, wahrend und nach Belastung. II — Untersuchungsergebnisse bei Stehbelastung. International Journal of Clinical Pharmacology 2: 229–245, 300–314
9. Macdonald A G, McNeill R S 1968 A comparison on the effect on airway resistance of a new β-blocking drug ICI 50, 172 and propranolol. British Journal of Anaesthesia 40: 508–510
10. Brick I, Hutchison K J, McDevitt D G, Roddie I C, Shansk R G 1968 Comparison of the effects of ICI 50, 172 and propranolol on the cardiovascular responses to adrenaline, isoprenaline and exercise. British Journal of Pharmacology 34: 127–140
11. Gibson D, Sowton E 1968 Effects of ICI 50, 172 in man during erect exercise. British Medical Journal 1: 213–215
12. Wilson A G, Brooke O G, Lloyd H J, Robinson B F 1969 Mechanism of action of β-adrenergic receptor blocking agents in angina pectoris. Comparison of action of propranolol with dexpropranolol and practolol. British Medical Journal 4: 399–401
13. Shinebourne E, Fleming J, Hamer J 1968 Haemodynamic responses to exercise in hypertension. Place of the sympathetic nervous system evaluated by a new selective cardiac β-adrenergic blocking agent ICI 50, 172. Cardiovascular Research 4: 379–383
14. Harrison J, Turner P 1969 Comparison of propranolol and ICI 50, 172 on isoprenaline-induced increase in skin temperature in man. British Journal of Pharmacology 36: 177–178
15. Baumgartl P, Knapp E, Raas E, Aigner A 1971 Hamodynamische Wirkungen von Practolol (ICI 50, 172). Medizinische Klinik 66: 597–601
16. Leon D F, Thompson M E, Shaver J A, McDonald R H 1972 Hemodynamic effects of practolol at rest and during exercise. Circulation 45: 46–54
17. Dagenais G R, Blouin S, Marquis Y, Moisan A 1972 Effects of practolol on exercise tolerance and on cardiac hemodynamics and metabolism. Canadian Medical Journal 107: 638
18. Finegan R E, Marlon A M, Harrison D C 1972 Circulatory effects of practolol. American Journal of Cardiology 29: 315–322
19. Sowton E, Balcon R, Cross D 1968 Haemodynamic effects of ICI 50, 172 in patients with ischaemic heart disease. British Medical Journal 1: 215–216
20. Vilsvik J S, Schaanning J 1976 Effect of atenolol on ventilatory and cardiac function in asthma. British Medical Journal 2: 453–455
21. Formgren H 1976 The effect of metoprolol and practolol on lung function and blood pressure in hypertensive asthmatics. British Journal of Clinical Pharmacology 3: 1007–1014
22. Thiringer G, Svedmyr N 1976 Interaction of orally administered metoprolol, practolol and propranolol with isoprenaline in asthmatics. European Journal of Clinical Pharmacology 10: 163–170
23. Skinner C, Gaddie J, Palmer K N V 1975 Comparison of intravenous AH 5158 (Ibidomide) and propranolol in asthma. British Medical Journal 2: 59–61
24. Cash J D, Woodfield D G, Allan A G E 1970 Adrenergic mechanisms in the systemic plasminogen activator response to adrenaline in man. British Journal of Haematology 18: 487–494

Practolol

25. Sirtori M D, Azarnoff M D, Shoeman D W 1972 Dissociation of the metabolic and cardiovascular effects of the β-adrenergic blocker practolol. Pharmacological Research Communications 4: 123–133
26. Scales B, Cosgrove M B 1970 The metabolism and distribution of the selective adrenergic beta blocking agent, practolol. Journal of Pharmacology and Experimental Therapeutics 175: 338–346
27. Schenk D W, Kroetz F W 1972 Correlation of beta blockade with serum practolol levels after oral administration. Clinical Pharmacology 13: 685–693
28. Alderman E L, Davis R O, Friedman J P, Graham A F, Matlof H J, Harrison D C 1973 Practolol in patients with angina pectoris. Clinical Pharmacology and Therapeutics 14: 175–181
29. Bodem G, Chidsey C A 1973 Pharmacokinetic studies of practolol, a beta adrenergic antagonist, in man. Clinical Pharmacology and Therapeutics 14: 26–29
30. Reeves P R, Case D E, Jepson H T et al 1978 Practolol metabolism. II Metabolism in human subjects. Journal of Pharmacology and Experimental Therapeutics 205: 489–498
31. Eastwood J B, Curtis J R, Smith R B 1973 Pharmacodynamics of practolol in chronic renal failure. British Medical Journal 4: 320–322
32. Carruthers S G, Kelly J G, McDevitt D G, Shanks R G 1974 Blood levels of practolol after oral and parenteral administration and their relationship to exercise heart rate. Clinical Pharmacology and Therapeutics 15: 497–509
33. Kendall M J 1981 Are selective β-adrenoceptor blocking drugs an advantage? Journal of Royal College of Physicians, London 15: 33–40
34. Wiseman R A 1972 Practolol — an analysis of clinical trials in angina pectoris. Acta Cardiology (suppl 16): 29–42
35. Backman H, Martikainen T 1974 Practolol in angina pectoris: a double-blind ergometric study. Annals of Clinical Research 6: 347–355
36. Thadani U, Davidson C, Singleton W, Taylor S H 1979 Comparison of the immediate effects of five beta-adrenoreceptor-blocking drugs with different ancillary properties in angina pectoris. New England Journal of Medicine 300: 750–755
37. Thadani U, Davidson C, Singleton W, Taylor S H 1980 Comparison of five beta-adrenoreceptor antagonists with different ancillary properties during sustained twice daily therapy in angina pectoris. American Journal of Medicine 68: 243–250
38. Coltart D J 1972 Observations of exercise tolerance in anginal patients treated with β-blockers. New perspectives in Beta Blockade Symposium (Ciba), May 1972, Denmark
39. Thadani U, Sharma B, Meeran M K, Majid P A, Whitaker W, Taylor S H 1973 Comparison of adrenergic β-receptor antagonists in angina pectoris. British Medical Journal 1: 136–142
40. Sowton E, Das Gupta D S, Baker I 1975 Comparative effects of β-adrenergic blocking drugs. Thorax 30: 9–18
41. Forrest W A 1975 A double-blind clinical trial in angina pectoris. British Journal of Clinical Practitioners 29: 343–346
42. Roy P, Day L, Sowton E 1975 Effect of new beta-adrenergic blocking agent, atenolol (Tenormin) on pain frequency, trinitrin consumption, and exercise ability. British Medical Journal 3: 195–197
43. Keyrilainen O, Uusitalo A 1978 A comparitive study of three beta-1-adrenoreceptor blocking drugs with different degree of intrinsic stimulating activity (metoprolol, practolol and H 87/07) in patients with angina pectoris. Annals of Clinical Research 10: 185–190
44. Fagher B, Svensson S E, Persson S 1977 Double-blind comparison of verapamil and practolol in the treatment of angina pectoris. Postgraduate Medical Journal 53: 61–65
45. Vohra J K, Dowling J T, Sloman G 1970 Practolol (ICI 50, 172), a β-adrenergic receptor blocking agent in the management of cardiac arrhythmias. Medical Journal of Australia 2: 228–231
46. Bracchetti D, Russo F, Accorsi A G 1971 L'impiego clinico del practololo nelle aritmie cardiache. Clinical Medicine 52: 446–474
47. Rymaszewski Z, Polawska W, Preibisz J, Januszewica W 1972 Clinical evaluation of practolol in acute arrhythmias. British Heart Journal 34: 260–262
48. Jewitt D, Croxson R 1972 Practolol in the management of cardiac dysrhythmias following myocardial infarction and cardiac surgery. Postgraduate Medical Journal 47: 25–29
49. Van Dume J P, Bossaert L, Vermiere P, Pannier R 1972 One hundred and fifty cases of cardiac arrhythmias treated with practolol (ICI 50, 172). Acta Cardiology XV: 285–291
50. Allen J D, Pantridge J F, Shanks R G 1972 Practolol in the treatment of ventricular dysrhythmias in acute myocardial infarction. Postgraduate Medical Journal 47: 29–35
51. Brown K G E, McMichen H U S, Briggs D S 1972 Tachyarrhythmia in severe imipramine overdose controlled by practolol. Archives of Disease in Childhood 47: 104–106
52. Powles R, Shinebourne E, Hamer J 1969 Selective cardiac sympathetic blockade as an adjunct to bronchodilator therapy. Thorax 24: 616–618
53. Jachuk S J 1973 Implanted-pacemaker-induced dysrhythmia and its management. Postgraduate Medical Journal 49: 14–17
54. Jewitt D E, Burgess P A, Shillingford J P 1970 The circulatory effects of practolol (ICI 50, 172) in patients with acute myocardial infarction. Cardiovascular Research IV: 188–193
55. Epois A, Rocha P, Roudy G, Bardet J, Bourdaris J P, Mathivat A 1972 Haemodynamic effects of selective β-adrenergic blockade during acute stage of myocardial infarction. British Heart Journal 34: 1295–1301
56. Jewitt D, Croxson R 1972 Practolol in the management of cardiac dysrhythmias following myocardial infarction and cardiac surgery. Postgraduate Medical Journal 47: 25–29
57. Johnstone M 1971 Haemodynamic effects of oxprenolol and practolol during halothane anaesthesia. British Journal of Anaesthesia 43: 820–821
58. Jenkins A V 1970 Adrenergic β-blockade with ICI 50, 172 (practolol, Eraldin) during bronchoscopy. British Journal of Anaesthesia 42: 59–63
59. Mathias J A, Payne J P 1970 Practolol in the management of cardiac dysrhythmias in patients anaesthetized with halothane. British Journal of Pharmacology 40: 572–573
60. Karhunen P, Hartel G 1973 Suicidal attempt with practolol. British Medical Journal 2: 178–179
61. Nicholls J T 1978 The practolol syndrome: a retrospective analysis. In: Post-marketing surveillance of adverse reactions to new medicines. Medico-Pharmaceutical Forum, No 7, The Royal Society of Medicine, London
62. Beveridge H, Wood C 1970 Du 21 220 — A new β-mimetic drug: a pilot trial to determine its use as a uterine relaxant in conjunction with the beta-blocking drug practolol. Australian and New Zealand Journal of Obstetrics and Gynaecology 10: 252–255
63. Goodwin J F, Oakley C M 1972 The cardiomyopathies. British Heart Journal 34: 545–552
64. Robards G J, Saunders D M 1973 Refractory supraventricular tachycardia complicating pregnancy. Medical Journal of Australia 2: 278–280
65. Castleden C M, George C F, Short M D 1978 Contribution of individual differences in gastric emptying to variability in plasma propranolol concentrations. British Journal of Clinical Pharmacology 5: 121–122
66. Stockley I H 1981 Drug interactions. Blackwell Scientific Publications 61
67. Cruickshank J M, Fitzgerald J D, Tucker M 1984 β-adrenoceptor blocking drugs: pronethalol, propranolol and practolol. In: Safety testing of new drugs 1984 615: 70LA

Pralidoxime

Pralidoxime is a cholinesterase reactivator used to treat poisoning with certain cholinesterase inhibitors. It has been administered as the chloride, iodide, lactate, mesylate and methylsulphate salts.

Chemistry

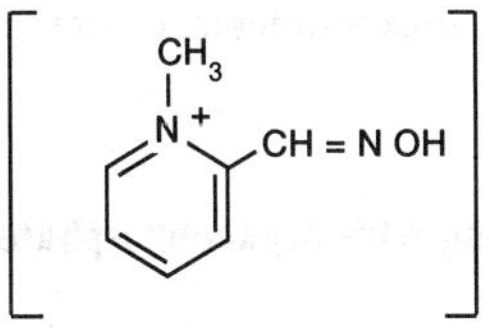

Pralidoxime chloride (2-PAM chloride, 2-pyridine aldoxime methochloride, Protopam Chloride)
$C_7H_9ClN_2O$
2-Hydroxyiminomethyl-1-methylpyridinium chloride

Molecular weight (free compound)	172.6 (137.1)
pKa	8.0
Solubility	
in alcohol	1 in 100
in water	~1 in 20
Octanol/water partition coefficient	very low

A white or pale yellow crystalline powder.

Pralidoxime iodide (PAM, P-2-AM, 2-PAM iodide, 2-pyridine aldoxime methiodide)
$C_7H_9IN_2O$

Molecular weight	264.1
pKa	8.0
Solubility	
in alcohol	<1 in 10 000
in water	1 in 20
Octanol/water partition coefficient	very low

A yellow hygroscopic crystalline powder. Aqueous solutions are unstable.

Pralidoxime mesylate (P2S, 2-PAMM, 2-pyridine aldoxime methyl mesylate)
$C_8H_{12}N_2O_4S$

Molecular weight	232.3
pKa	8.0
Solubility	
in alcohol	1 in 12
in water	1 in 2
Octanol/water partition coefficient	very low

A colourless or white, hygroscopic powder that is crystalline or granular.

Pralidoxime methylsulphate (2-pyridine aldoxime methylsulphate, Contrathion)
$C_8H_{12}N_2O_5S$

Molecular weight	248.3
pKa	8.0
Solubility	
in alcohol	soluble
in water	>1 in 1
Octanol/water partition coefficient	very low

A white crystalline powder.

The salts of pralidoxime are all prepared by chemical synthesis. None is available in combination preparations.

Pharmacology

Pralidoxime is a cholinesterase reactivator. Following poisoning by certain agents, acetylcholinesterase is inactivated by a process of alkylphosphorylation. This leads to the accumulation of acetylcholine and the development of the characteristic signs of poisoning (see below under Indications). Pralidoxime is used for its effect as a reactivator of acetyl cholinesterase. The nucleophilic oxime binds to the phosphate to form an oxime–phosphate complex which splits off from the acetyl cholinesterase to leave the regenerated enzyme.

The speed of this reactivation varies, depending on the nature of the phosphoryl group, so that pralidoxime is a more potent reactivator of acetyl cholinesterase after some poisons than others.[1] Also phosphorylated acetyl cholinesterase undergoes a process called ageing.[2] This probably results from the loss of an alkyl or alkoxy group to produce the much more stable monoalkyl — or monoalkoxy–phosphoryl–acetyl cholinesterase complex. This ageing process results in almost complete resistance to the effect of pralidoxime.

Toxicology

Extensive toxicity studies have not been performed. The LD_{50} of pralidoxime chloride has been estimated in mice as 136 mg.kg^{-1} when given by the intraperitoneal route, as 140 mg.kg^{-1} after subcutaneous injection[3] and as 4100 mg.kg^{-1} after oral administration.[4] The LD_{50} in rats by the intravenous route[5] was 96 mg.kg^{-1}.

Clinical pharmacology

Observations in man have confirmed that the expected symptomatic effects of pralidoxime are accompanied by increases in levels of both plasma cholinesterase (pseudo-cholinesterase) and red blood cell cholinesterase. The latter has shown better correlation with the effect of pralidoxime.[6] Comparative studies in workers exposed to organophosphates showed that those receiving pralidoxime maintained more nearly normal levels of cholinesterase than those not receiving the drug.[7] Pralidoxime in high doses can cause neuromuscular blockade and inhibition of acetylcholinesterase but such effects are minimal at standard doses.

Animal data demonstrate that maximal recovery of neuromuscular blockade is achieved with serum levels of pralidoxime[8] of 4 mg.l^{-1} with a flat dose–response curve at higher levels. Dose–response to pralidoxime has not been formally studied in humans, for obvious reasons, but the data accumulated are in agreement with the animal findings. The duration of action is one and a half to two hours after parenteral administration, persisting only as long as adequate serum levels are maintained in the presence of the poison.

Pharmacokinetics

The assay methods used in the majority of studies of pralidoxime have utilized ultraviolet spectrophotometry.[9] However, methods utilizing high performance liquid chromatography are now available[10] for which the sensitivity is 10 μg.l^{-1}.

Most forms of pralidoxime are poorly soluble in water, so that the usual route of administration is by parenteral injection. Pralidoxime mesylate (30% w/w) and methylsulphate (60% w/w) are more soluble in water and have been given orally and by intramuscular injection. Absorption after oral administration is slow, peak levels occurring between two and three hours,[11–13] and incomplete. Approximately 30% of a dose of the mesylate is absorbed after oral administration, less of the chloride.

Pralidoxime is not bound to plasma proteins and, being a quaternary ammonium compound, would not be expected to penetrate the blood–brain barrier to any significant extent. However, there have been reports of symptomatic improvement following its use in patients suffering from the central side effects of organophosphate poisoning suggesting that, on occasions at least, sufficient may pass into the central nervous system to be of clinical benefit.[6,14] Its volume of distribution is 0.6 l.kg^{-1}, corresponding to total body water. It is not significantly bound to plasma proteins.

Elimination is rapid, with a half life of 75 min and a clearance of approximately 7 ml.min^{-1}.kg^{-1}. The majority of the compound is recovered unchanged in the urine, with 80.4% and 91% of intravenous and intramuscular doses, respectively, being recovered unchanged in the urine 12 hours after administration.[15–17] Thus, pralidoxime is eliminated by renal secretion as well as filtration. It is metabolized to a minor extent. Pralidoxime is unlikely to be excreted in breast milk. It is not known whether it crosses the placenta. The elimination of the drug is decreased in renal disease and with declining renal function with age. Liver disease is unlikely to have any effect on the kinetics of the drug.

Oral absorption	<30%
Presystemic metabolism	—
Plasma half life	75 min
Volume of distribution	$0.6\ l.kg^{-1}$
Plasma protein binding	negligible

Concentration–effect relationship

There is no specific evidence of a correlation between the plasma concentration of pralidoxime and its therapeutic effect.

Metabolism

Pralidoxime is excreted in the urine largely unchanged. A small fraction of the dose is metabolized, possibly to an aldehyde. 1-Methyl-2-cyanspyridinium ion has been detected in urine.

Pharmaceutics

Pralidoxime is an infrequently used drug and is usually available only at specific centres used to dealing with these emergencies. In the UK the whereabouts of centres holding the drug (as the mesylate) can be obtained from the National Poisons Centres.

1. Pralidoxime chloride tablets (USP) contain 500 mg of pralidoxime chloride.
2. Sterile pralidoxime chloride (USP) in containers for sterile solids is usually available in 1 g amounts to be made up in 20 ml of sterile water or given as a saline infusion.
   Proprietary name Protopam chloride (Ayerst, Canada/USA)

Therapeutic use

Indications

1. As an adjunct to atropine in the treatment of poisoning with organophosphate acetylcholinesterase inhibitors.
2. Pralidoxime has also been used in the treatment of overdosage with the reversible acetyl cholinesterase drugs used in the treatment of myasthenia gravis. It is not as effective as an antidote to these drugs as it is to the organophosphates and its use may precipitate a myasthenic crisis so that it has little role in the management of these patients.

Contraindications

Pralidoxime should be avoided in cases of carbamate toxicity since there is no reason to suppose that it is of benefit and on theoretical grounds pralidoxime may exacerbate the situation. Similarly, pralidoxime is relatively ineffective in the treatment of excessive doses of acetyl cholinesterase used in patients with myasthenia gravis in whom it may precipitate a myasthenic crisis.

Mode of use

Pralidoxime is used for its effect as a reactivator of acetyl cholinesterase. The nucleophilic oxime binds to the phosphate to form an oxime–phosphate complex which splits off from the cholinesterase to leave the regenerated enzyme.

There are two circumstances in which this fails to work. Firstly with the passage of time (after poisoning has occurred) the phosphorylated enzyme undergoes a process of 'ageing' which renders it almost completely resistant to regeneration. This ageing process probably occurs as a result of the loss of an alkyl or alkoxy group to leave the more stable monoalkyl- or mono-alkoxy-phosphoryl-acctyl cholinesterase and the rate of ageing varies with different organophosphates.[2] As a result the drug should be given as soon as possible after exposure. Secondly, there is no beneficial effect of pralidoxime in poisoning with carbamyl ester inhibitors since the oxime complex so formed does not hydrolyse rapidly to leave the regenerated enzyme. Indeed this process is slower for the oxime complex formed than for the carbamate alone. Further, it has been observed in animal studies that the carbamate–oxime complex formed when pralidoxime is given to treat carbamate poisoning is actually a more potent inhibitor of acetylcholinesterase than the carbamate alone.[1] In the absence of observed benefit in cases of human poisoning, its use should therefore be avoided in carbamyl poisoning.

Agents against which pralidoxime has been reported as effective include the following: amiton, demeton-methyl, diazinon, dichlorvos, disulfoton, dyflos, fenthion, malathion, mevinphos, parathion, parathion-methyl, phosphamidon and TEPP.

Agents against which pralidoxime appears less effective include: dimefox, dimethoate, methyl diazinon, mipafos and schradan.

Pralidoxime appears to be only slightly effective against the reversible cholinesterase inhibitors used in the treatment of myasthenia gravis.

In carbamate toxicity pralidoxime appears unlikely to be beneficial and may, on the basis of animal experiments, exacerbate the situation.

Indications

1. Treatment of acute poisoning with organophosphate inhibitors of acetylcholinesterase

Exposure may result from accidents in those involved in their manufacture or application; it may follow accidental ingestion by children or deliberate overdose in adults. These chemicals have also been developed as agents of warfare (nerve gases).

The patient presents with the combined muscarinic and micotinic signs of acetylcholine accumulation caused by the antagonism of acetyl cholinesterase activity. The muscarinic effects are nausea, vomiting, diarrhoea, abdominal cramps, increased sweating, lacrimation, increased tracheobronchial secretion and salivation, meiosis and bradycardia. Nicotinic effects are skeletal muscle weakness, fasciculations, paralysis and central effects of confusion, dysphonia, seizures and coma. Mortality results from respiratory failure secondary to pulmonary oedema, skeletal muscle paralysis and cardiorespiratory depression.

In each case the general principles of treatment must be applied. These include the clearing of secretions and maintenance of an airway and, when necessary, artificial ventilation of the patient. Steps to avoid the continuing absorption of the poison must be taken as appropriate: removal of contaminated clothing, washing of skin or irrigation of the eyes, gastric aspiration and lavage. Atropine sulphate must be administered so as to reduce the volume of secretions and maintain the patency of the airways. Doses (given intramuscularly or intravenously) are from 1 to 5 mg depending on the severity of symptoms, and may be repeated frequently (every 3–30 minutes), the dose being titrated to stop salivation. It is advised to continue atropine for 24 hours or until symptoms no longer recur on its withdrawal.

Pralidoxime should be administered as soon as possible in severe cases to reverse the nicotinic effects of poisoning, in particular the problem of skeletal muscle paralysis which can lead to respiratory arrest in the fully atropinized patient. The drug combination of pralidoxime and atropine is complementary and superior to either used alone.[14] Pralidoxime may be given in doses of 1–2 g either by intramuscular injection or by slow intravenous infusion as a 5% solution in Water for Injection at rates of $100–300\ mg.min^{-1}$ (not exceeding $500\ mg.min^{-1}$), or as an infusion in 100 ml of saline over 15–30 minutes. The suggested dose for children is $20–40\ mg.kg^{-1}$ body weight.

Second or third doses may be administered at intervals of one hour if indicated by the persistence of muscular weakness. When the facility is available it is desirable to monitor the effects of treatment by determinations of cholinesterase levels. These are measured as pseudo-cholinesterase levels in the plasma and, more appropriately, as red blood cell cholinesterase levels.

If pralidoxime is not administered within 24–48 hours of exposure to the poison its beneficial action tends to disappear due to the ageing process which, as mentioned above, results in the irreversible binding of the organophosphate to acetyl cholinesterase. However, clinical benefit may result from the administration of pralidoxime as late as 2–5 days after the toxic exposure, probably due to prolonged absorption of toxin from the gastrointestinal tract. In a reported case of poisoning with a fat-soluble organophosphate — fenthion — symptoms were reported at up to 30 days after poisoning, both atropine and pralidoxime being continued to that time.[18]

Prophylaxis of organophosphate poisoning
It has been suggested that pralidoxime has a role in the prophylaxis of organophosphate poisoning. While it can be effective in maintaining acetyl cholinesterase activity, as has been shown,[2] this role is indicated only under exceptional circumstances. It is usually possible, and certainly preferable, to take adequate steps to avoid contamination in those at risk of exposure.

Long-term sequelae consisting of neuromuscular weakness occasionally follows poisoning with organophosphates. It has been suggested that the chance of this occurring may be reduced by the early use of pralidoxime[19] but there is no significant supportive evidence for this actually occurring in man.

Adverse reactions

Potentially life-threatening effects
Adverse effects are usually regarded as being mild[14] and have been difficult to ascribe to pralidoxime as distinct from the toxicity of the poison being treated and from the adverse effects of the concurrently administered atropine. No potentially life-threatening effects of pralidoxime have been identified.

Acute overdosage
No reports of deliberate overdose have been reported with this antidote.

Severe or irreversible adverse effects
Manic behaviour and excitement, occurring on recovery of consciousness, have been reported in several cases.

Symptomatic adverse effects
When given parenterally to normal volunteers,[13] symptoms of heaviness of the eyes, blurred vision, and difficulty in accommodation were noted. Stinging at the injection site occurred after intramuscular injection, and looseness of the stools after oral administration. Iodism affected subjects who received pralidoxime iodide, and doses of 1 g per 70 kg of pralidoxime dibromide resulted in a reduction of acetyl cholinesterase activity of 20%.[12] A hot feeling in the facial area together with a feeling of coldness in the nasopharynx, impaired concentration and dizziness were reported by other investigators.[20]

The following suspected adverse reactions have been associated with the use of pralidoxime in the treatment of organophosphate poisoning: dizziness, blurred vision, diplopia and impaired accommodation, headache, drowsiness, nausea, tachycardia, hyperventilation and muscular weakness.

Interference with clinical pathology tests
No technical interferences of this kind appear to have been reported.

High risk groups

Neonates
The drug is unlikely to be used in neonates, but if required, the doses used in children should be administered.

Breast milk. A woman requiring treatment with pralidoxime would not be in a fit state to breast-feed until recovery, by which time breast-feeding would be safe.

Children
Appropriate doses are 20–40 $mg.kg^{-1}$ body weight, and no other special precautions are recommended.

Pregnant women
There are no significant human data. In studies in animals oximes have been reported as reducing fetal abnormalities resulting from organophosphates and physostigmine.[18]

The elderly
There are no specific precautions regarding the use of pralidoxime in the elderly, although it must be remembered that many elderly patients will have reduced renal function (see below).

Concurrent disease
Pralidoxime should be used with caution in patients with impaired renal function as it is excreted by the kidney. The initial dose should be reduced and repeat doses titrated against the patient's symptoms. Specific studies to determine the degree of dosage reduction required in varying degrees of renal failure have not been performed.

Drug interactions

The mechanism of action involves drug interaction with the organophosphate, as has been described. Unwanted interactions are generally not severe and are (other than with atropine), uncommon.

Potentially hazardous interactions
Interactions may occur with the following drugs which should be avoided when pralidoxime is given: morphine, theophylline, aminophylline, suxamethonium, reserpine and phenothiazine-like tranquillizers.

Other significant reactions
Atropine. When given together with atropine, pralidoxime may be expected to result in the signs of atropinization occurring earlier than would be found with atropine alone.[13]

Potentially useful interactions
Barbiturates. These drugs may be used to control convulsions in organophosphate toxicity. Their action is potentiated by pralidoxime.

General review articles

Thompson D F, Thompson D G, Greenwood R B, Trammel H L 1987 Therapeutic dosing of pralidoxime chloride. Drug Intelligence and Clinical Pharmacy 21: 590–593

References

1. Sterri S H, Rognerud B, Fiskum S E, Lyngaas S 1979 Effect of toxigonin and P2S on the toxicity of carbamates and organophosphorus compounds. Acta Pharmacologica et Toxicologica 45: 9–15
2. Berry W K 1966 Factors influencing the rate of 'ageing' of a series of alkyl methyl phosphonyl-acetyl cholinesterases. The Biochemical Journal 100: 572–576
3. Kewitz H 1956 Specific antidote against lethal alkyphosphate intoxication. Archives of Biochemistry 60: 261–262
4. Ellin R I, Willis J H 1964 Oximes antagonistic to inhibitors of cholinesterase. Part 2. Journal of Pharmaceutical Sciences 53: 1143–1150
5. Fleischer J H, Harris L W, Miller G R, Thomas N C, Cliff W G 1970 Antagonism of savin poisoning in rats and guinea pigs by atropine oximes and mecamylamine. Toxicology and Applied Pharmacology 16: 40
6. Namba T, Nolte C T, Jackrel J, Grob O 1958 PAM (pyridine-2-aldoxime methiodide) therapy for alkylphosphate poisoning. Journal of the American Medical Association 166: 1834–1839
7. Quinby G E 1968 Feasibility of prophylaxis by oral pralidoxime. Archives of Environmental Health 16: 812–820
8. Sundwall A 1961 Minimum concentrations of N-Methylpyridinium-2-Aldoxime methane sulphonate (P2S) which reverse nueromuscular block. Biochemical Pharmacology 18: 413–417
9. Goff W A 1969 A new and rapid determination of pyridinium aldoximes in blood and urine. Clinical Chemistry 15: 72–83
10. Prue D, Johnson B N, Kho B T 1983 High performance liquid chromatographic determination of pralidoxime chloride and its major decomposition products in injectable solutions. Journal of Pharmaceutical Sciences 72: 751–756
11. Sundwall A 1960 Plasma concentration curves of N-methylpyridinium-2-aldoxime methane sulphonate (P2S) after intravenous, intramuscular and oral administration in man. Biochemical Pharmacology 5: 225–230
12. Kronditzer A A Zvirbliss P, Goodman A, Papanus S H 1968 Blood plasma levels and elimination of salts of 2-PAM in man after oral administration. Journal of Pharmaceutical Science 57: 1142–46
13. Holland P, Parkes D C 1976 Plasma concentrations of the oxime pralidoxime mesylate (P2S) after repeated oral and intramuscular administration. British Journal of Industrial Medicine 33: 43–46
14. Namba T 1971 Poisoning due to organophosphate insecticides. American Journal of Medicine 50: 475–492
15. Siddell F R, Groff W A 1971 Intramuscular and intravenous administration of small doses of 2-pyridinium aldoxime methochloride to man. Journal of Pharmaceutical Sciences 60: 1224–1228
16. Jager B V, Stag G N, Green N, Jager L 1958 Studies on distribution and disappearance of pyridine-2-aldoxime methiodide (PAM) and of diacetyl monoxime (DAM) in man and in experimental animals. Bulletin of the Johns Hopkins Hospital 102: 225–234
17. Calesnick B, Christensen J A, Richter M 1967 Human toxicity of various oximes. Archives of Environmental Health 15: 599–608
18. Merrill D 1982 Prolonged toxicity of organophosphate poisoning. Critical Care Medicine 10: 50–551
19. Wecker L, Kiauta T, Deltbasn W-D 1978 Relationship between acetylcholinesterase inhibition and the development of a myopathy. The Journal of Pharmacology and Experimental Therapeutics 206: 97–104
20. Vojvodic V, Boskiwic B 1976 A comparative study of pralidoxime, obidoxime, and trimedoxime in healthy men volunteers and in rats. In: Stoores J (ed) Medical protection against chemical-warfare agents. Almquist and Wilsell International, Stockholm International Peace Research Institute, Stockholm, Sweden, ch 5, pp 65–73
21. Landauer W 1976 Cholinomimetic teratogens V. The effect of oximes and related cholinesterase reactivators. Teratology 15: 33–42

P

Pravastatin (sodium)

Pravastatin (CS-514, eptastatin, SQ31,000) is a hydrophilic competitive inhibitor of 3-hydroxy-3-methylglutaryl coenzyme A (HMG-CoA) reductase, the rate-limiting enzyme of cholesterol synthesis. The drug lowers plasma cholesterol levels in normal heterozygous familial, familial combined, and non-familial hypercholesterolaemic subjects.

Chemistry

Pravastatin sodium (CS-514, eptastatin, SQ31,000, Pravachol, Pravacor, Lipostat)
$C_{23}H_{35}O_7.Na$
[1S-[1α(βS,δS,2α,6α8β-(R),8aα]]-1,2,6,7,8,8a-hexahydro-β,δ, 6-trihydroxy-2-methyl-8-2-(methyl-1-oxobutoxy)-1-napthalene heptanoic acid, monosodium salt

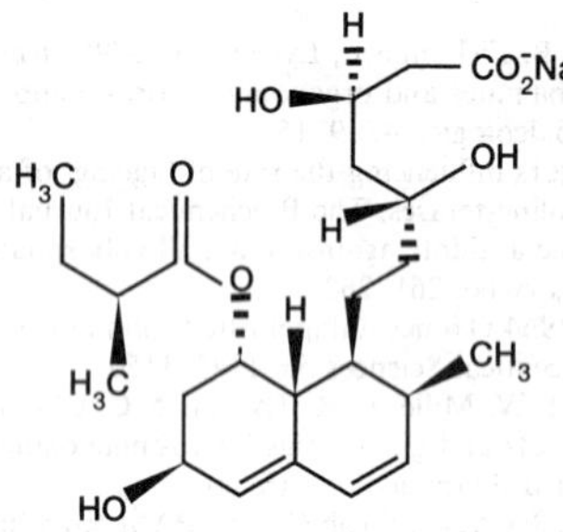

Molecular weight (free acid)	446.5 (423.4)
pKa	
Solubility	
in alcohol	readily soluble
in water	readily soluble
Octanol/water partition coefficient	—

Pravastatin is a white crystalline powder prepared by microbial transformation of the parent compound mevastatin. It is not available in any combination preparations.

Pharmacology

The lipid-lowering effects of pravastatin appear to result from the specific inhibition of HMG-CoA reductase in the liver.[1] This enzyme catalyses the conversion of HMG-CoA to mevalonate which is the major rate-limiting step in the cholesterol synthetic pathway. The resultant decrease in endogenous hepatic cholesterol synthesis leads to compensatory upregulation of hepatic low density lipoprotein (LDL) receptors which promotes LDL and apoB catabolism. LDL production is also decreased due to the associated impaired synthesis and/or secretion of its precursor, very low density lipoprotein (VLDL).

There has been considerable debate about the degree of liver selectivity of different HMG-CoA reductase inhibitors. Reported studies are not easy to interpret because they have used a range of isolated tissues from different species and widely varying concentrations. In Hep-G2 cells (a human liver cell line) none of the drugs tested, including lovastatin and pravastatin, showed tissue selectivity when compared with human fibroblasts.[2] In contrast all the drugs caused equal and potent inhibition in primary cultures of rat hepatocytes, and pravastatin was more than 100 times more potent in these cells than it was in human fibroblasts. In mice, an oral dose of 20 $mg.kg^{-1}$ of pravastatin caused 90% inhibition of synthesis of cholesterol in ileum and liver but only 14% in kidney, spleen, adrenal, testis and brain.[3] In rat liver slices the active acid forms of lovastatin, simvastatin and pravastatin were all of similar potency with IC_{50} values of 20–50 nM. In explants of weanling rat lenses the IC_{50} values for lovastatin acid, simvastatin acid and pravastatin were 4.5, 5.2 and 469 nM respectively.[4] The low potency of pravastatin in the intact lens appeared to be due to inability to enter the tissue because pravastatin and lovastatin acid were equally effective inhibitors of HMG-CoA reductase activity in lens homogenates.

It has been suggested that the hydrophilic property of pravastatin contributes to differential effects on cholesterol synthesis in various tissues. However, simvastatin is subject to extensive presystemic metabolism in the liver leading to the formation of the active open acid in the hepatocytes so the question of relative tissue selectivity of drugs in this class (and, if there is one, its mechanism) is still an open one.[5]

Although cholesterol synthesis is inhibited in vitro in rat tissues, when the drug is administered to rodents in vivo there is no fall in the plasma cholesterol concentration, unlikc other species such as dogs. Cholesterol synthesis in vivo in the rat is inhibited by other products of the cholesterol synthetic pathway (e.g. dolichol and ubiquinone) through feedback regulation and during pravastatin therapy this feedback is removed. The net result therefore in the rat is an increase in HMG-CoA reductase and mevalonate kinase activity (and an increase in its mRNA) and no fall in plasma cholesterol.[6]

Inhibition of HMG-CoA reductase activity does not lead to a build-up of intermediary metabolites since this enzyme is involved early in the synthetic pathway of cholesterol. The precursor, HMG-CoA, is readily metabolized back to acetyl-CoA which is involved in many biosynthetic processes throughout the tissues of the body.

Pravastatin, combined with cholestyramine, has been shown to lower serum cholesterol and retard formation of atheromatous lesions in Watanabe heritable hyperlipidaemic (WHHL) rabbits.[7]

Toxicology

A 21-month study with doses of 10 to 100 $mg.kg^{-1}$ daily in mice failed to show any evidence of carcinogenic potential. In a 2-year oral study in rats, using doses of 10 to 100 $mg.kg^{-1}$ daily, a statistically significant increase in the incidence of hepatocellular carcinomas was observed in male rats given 100 $mg.kg^{-1}$ daily (over 75 times the maximum human dose) of pravastatin. These changes were not seen in male rats given 40 $mg.kg^{-1}$ daily (over 30 times the recommended human dose) or less, nor in female rats at any dose level. Beagle dogs tolerated 25 $mg.kg^{-1}$ daily for 2 years without developing toxicity.[8] Cynomolgus monkeys given doses of up to 400 $mg.kg^{-1}$ daily for 5 weeks developed severe hepatic and renal toxicity with doses of 200 and 400 $mg.kg^{-1}$ day (and one at 100 $mg.kg^{-1}$ daily). The no-effect dose was estimated to be 50 $mg.kg^{-1}$ daily.[9]

No evidence of mutagenicity was observed in vitro, with or without rat liver metabolic activation, in microbial mutagen tests using mutant strains of *Salmonella typhimurium* or *Escherichia coli*, in a forward mutation assay in L5178Y Tk+/−mouse lymphoma cells, in a chromosomal aberration test in hamster cells, or in a gene conversion assay using *Saccharomyces cerevisiae*. In addition, there was no evidence of mutagenicity in either a dominant lethal test in mice or a micronucleus test in mice.

In a study in rats, with daily doses as high as 500 $mg.kg^{-1}$, pravastatin did not produce any adverse effects on fertility or general reproductive performance.

Clinical pharmacology

Pravastatin is highly effective in reducing total and LDL cholesterol in patients with heterozygous familial, familial combined, and non-familial (non-FH) forms of hypercholesterolaemia.[10–15] A marked response is seen within 1 week, and the maximum therapeutic response usually occurs within 4 weeks. The response is maintained during extended periods of therapy. Single daily doses administered in the evening are as effective as the same total daily dose given in two divided doses. Single daily doses given in the morning are also effective, with only a marginal decrease in efficacy compared with the evening or twice-daily schedules of administration.

In addition to a fall in LDL cholesterol of 25–30% there is usually a modest reduction in VLDL and in triglycerides, as well as a small

Pravastatin (sodium)

increase in high density lipoprotein (HDL) cholesterol. Apolipoprotein B concentrations fall by 20–40%. Both species of HDL (Lp A-II:A-I and Lp A-I) are increased by pravastatin.[16] Dose–response relationships for pravastatin's effects on some of these parameters are shown in Table 1.

Table 1 Dose–response results (% change)

Daily dose of pravastatin	Total cholesterol	LDL cholesterol	HDL cholesterol	TG
5 mg	−14	−19	+5	−14
10 mg	−16	−22	+7	−15
20 mg	−24	−32	+2	−11
40 mg	−25	−34	+12	−24

At therapeutic doses in man HMG-CoA reductase activity is not completely inhibited by pravastatin and thus necessary amounts of mevalonate are produced for intermediary metabolism. Pravastatin has no effect on steroidogenesis in man. A group of 10 patients awaiting cholecystectomy were treated with pravastatin, 20 mg twice daily, for 3 weeks before cholecystectomy, at which a liver biopsy was taken. Twenty further patients served as controls. Pravastatin therapy reduced LDL cholesterol by 39%. Serum levels of lathosterol fell by 63%. Microsomal HMG-CoA reductase activity, in the absence of the inhibitor, was increased nearly 12-fold by the active treatment. Expression of LDL receptors was increased 1.8 times in actively treated patients.[17] A reduction in cholesterol saturation of fasting gall bladder bile was demonstrated in 9 patients with heterozygous familial hypercholesterolaemia treated with pravastatin 40 mg daily.[18]

Pharmacokinetics

The preferred assay procedure involves extraction and purification of the drug or its metabolites with C_{18} disposable solid phase columns. Following derivatization, pravastatin and metabolite concentrations are determined by a capillary gas chromatography–mass spectrometry technique.[19] The limit of sensitivity is 0.5 µg.l^{-1}.

Pravastatin is administered orally in the active form. Following oral ingestion it is rapidly absorbed, with peak plasma levels attained at about 1 to 1.5 hours. Average oral absorption of pravastatin, based on urinary recovery of total radioactivity after oral and intravenous dosing of carbon-14 labelled pravastatin, is 34%.[20] After an intravenous dose, 60% was recovered in urine and 34% in faeces over 96 h, indicating substantial biliary excretion. Corresponding figures for the oral dose are 20% in the urine and 71% in the faeces over the same time period. Average systemic bioavailability of pravastatin is 17% based on the plasma AUC and urinary excretion data. These figures indicate that approximately half of the absorbed drug is subject to presystemic metabolism. The presence of food in the gastrointestinal tract reduces the bioavailability by about 35–40%; however, the therapeutic response to pravastatin is similar whether taken with meals or one hour prior to meals.

The LDL cholesterol response to 10 mg twice daily of pravastatin administered within 15 minutes of eating a meal is about 25% and administered one hour or more prior to eating a meal about 26%.

Oral absorption	34%
Presystemic metabolism	—
Plasma half life range	1.5–2 h
Volume of distribution	0.5 l.kg^{-1}
Plasma protein binding	50%

Pravastatin plasma concentrations show dose proportionality for both areas under the concentration–time curve (AUC) and maximum and steady-state plasma levels. Steady-state areas under the plasma concentration–time curves and maximum blood concentrations show no evidence of pravastatin accumulation following twice-daily administration of pravastatin tablets. Approximately 50% of the circulating drug is bound to plasma proteins. The volume of distribution is about 0.5 l.kg^{-1}.

The plasma elimination half life of pravastatin is between 1.5 and 2 hours. It is not known whether pravastatin crosses the placenta. Although the drug is not excreted to any significant extent in breast milk, its use in lactating women is not advisable. The average renal clearance of 400 ml.min^{-1} indicates that tubular secretion is an important mechanism of elimination. The kinetics of the drug may be influenced by severe renal or hepatic dysfunction but the availability of two different paths of elimination means that significant accumulation is unlikely if only one route is impaired.

Concentration–effect relationship

No information is available.

Metabolism

Unlike other HMG-CoA reductase inhibitors pravastatin is administered in the active form and therefore does not need to be activated by metabolism. However when it is metabolized its major degradation product is the 3-α-hydroxy isomer (SQ 31,906) which has 1/40 the inhibitory activity of the parent on HMG-CoA reductase. This metabolite is excreted in the urine and faeces. Its concentration in the plasma is 50–80% of that of pravastatin. A further metabolite, 3-α,5-β,6β-trihydroxypravastatin, has been identified. It is inactive and present in plasma at concentrations 10% to 25% of those of pravastatin.

Pharmaceutics

Pravastatin sodium (Lipostat: Bristol-Myers-Squibb, UK) is produced only in tablet form. The tablets are pink, oblong and biconvex and available in 10 and 20 mg doses. The drug is marketed in a number of countries including Canada, Japan and Italy.

Therapeutic use

Indications

1. Pravastatin is efficacious for the treatment of patients with phenotypes IIa and IIb hypercholesterolaemia when total cholesterol ⩾7.8 mmol.l^{-1} and LDL cholesterol levels remain elevated despite restriction of total dietary fats, cholesterol and, if warranted, total calories.

Contraindications

1. Active liver disease
2. Patients with a history of serious adverse reaction to prior administration of HMG-CoA reductase inhibitors
3. Pregnancy and breast-feeding
4. Women of child-bearing potential unless protected by adequate contraception.

Mode of use

Before initiating therapy with pravastatin, secondary causes for elevated cholesterol values, such as obesity, poorly controlled diabetes mellitus, hypothyroidism, nephrotic syndrome, obstructive liver disease, or drug therapy, should be excluded. It is important to determine whether increased levels of total cholesterol are due to increased LDL cholesterol before initiating treatment. In primary hyperalphalipoproteinaemia (elevated HDL cholesterol) serum levels of total cholesterol may be elevated. Treatment with cholesterol-lowering agents in this instance is not indicated. When total cholesterol is elevated along with marked hypertriglyceridaemia (>5 mmol.l^{-1}), the intermediate density lipoprotein (IDL) fraction may be increased. The efficacy of pravastatin has not been evaluated in such patients. However, in a Japanese study, hypertriglyeridaemic patients experienced a 40% decrease in triglycerides.

Prior to starting pravastatin therapy patients should be placed on a cholesterol-lowering diet which should be maintained during treatment. Fasting lipids should be measured and, as part of on-going safety assessment procedures, liver function tests, creatine phosphokinase, urine microscopy and slit-lamp examination of the lens should be performed. Pravastatin is administered initially as a 10 mg dose once daily at bedtime. The maximum effect of a given dose is evident within 4 weeks. Measurement of the lipid profile and biochemical safety tests should be repeated after one month and, if necessary, the dose may be increased. The maximum recommended

Prazepam

Prazepam is a prodrug whose active principle is desmethyldiazepam which has typical benzodiazepine anxiolytic effects.

Chemistry

Prazepam (Centrax, Demetrin, Lysanxia, Prazene, Sedapran, Trepidan)
$C_{19}H_{17}ClN_2O$
7-Chloro-1-(cyclopropylmethyl)-1,3-dihydro-5-phenyl-2H-1,4-benzodiazepin-2-one

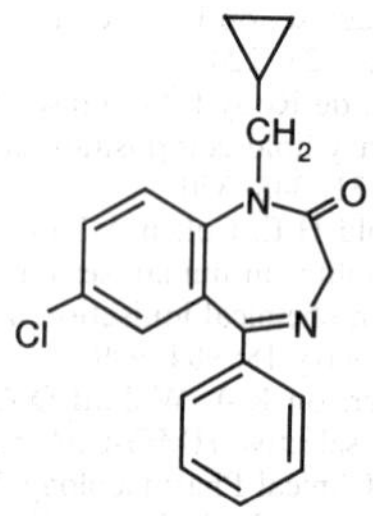

Molecular weight	324.8
pKa (amino)	2.7
Solubility	
in alcohol	>1 in 30
in water	insoluble
Octanol/water partition coefficient	5000

Prazepam is a white to off-white crystalline powder prepared by chemical synthesis.

Pharmacology

Prazepam is a pharmacologically inactive benzodiazepine derivative. Levels of intact prazepam in the blood reach at best only trace amounts. Its major metabolite, desmethyldiazepam, is responsible for the drug's neuropharmacological properties.[1,2] These properties, which include sedation, anxiolysis, impaired memory acquisition, muscle relaxation and anticonvulsant effects, are mediated via specific benzodiazepine receptors situated in the limbic system, cerebral cortex and thalamic nuclei.[3] Prazepam results in blockade of EEG arousal from stimulation of the brain stem reticular formation. The drug, via its metabolite, acts as a CNS depressant on spinal reflexes. It is anxiolytic in animal test systems such as fear of electric shock. Prazepam also has sedative effects and is active as a muscle relaxant acting via spinal reflexes.

Toxicology

Prazepam given intravenously to animals can cause convulsions.[4] Intraperitoneal, intramuscular and oral administration causes sedation and ataxia with increasing dosage. There is no evidence of carcinogenicity. There is no information concerning teratogenicity in man or animals.

Clinical pharmacology

The pharmacological effects of prazepam are those of its clinically active metabolite, desmethyldiazepam (nordiazepam).[5] These include sedation, anxiolysis, impaired memory acquisition, muscle relaxation, anticonvulsant effects and, rarely, a paradoxical reaction of increased arousal. Prazepam offers a slow onset of effect (4–48 hours) due to the delayed delivery of the active metabolite, desmethyldiazepam, by hepatic dealkylation, and a long duration of activity due to the long elimination half life (40–100 hours) of this metabolite.[2]

While these characteristics offer a potential measure of protection against its abuse (delayed onset of action), a lessening of the adverse effects of rapid withdrawal (slow elimination) and a suitability for single daily dosing, the same characteristics also serve to provide the potential for clinically significant drug accumulation over a period of weeks. Prazepam has no significant effects on the cardiovascular system; however, respiratory depression may be seen following large doses or in sensitive individuals (e.g. chronic obstructive airways disease).

Pharmacokinetics

Prazepam, and its active metabolite desmethyldiazepam (nordazepam), can be detected in plasma by gas chromatography with a sensitivity[6] of 1 $\mu g.l^{-1}$. Prazepam is approximately 90% absorbed after oral administration but only negligible amounts can be detected in the blood. This is because the drug undergoes nearly complete presystemic dealkylation in the liver, yielding the major metabolite, desmethyldiazepam. The peak blood level of this metabolite occurs at about six hours with a range of 4–48 hours following oral administration. Its plasma half life exhibits considerable interindividual variation (30–200 hours).[7] Desmethyldiazepam is the only pharmacologically active unconjugated compound detectable in blood in quantitatively important amounts; 3-hydroxyprazepam is found in the blood only as a glucuronide conjugate. The major urinary metabolites of prazepam are glucuronide conjugates of 3-hydroxyprazepam and oxazepam.

Desmethyldiazepam is a highly lipid-soluble drug and is rapidly and widely distributed throughout the body. It has an apparent volume of distribution of 0.5 to 2.5 litres per kg and is highly bound (97%) to plasma proteins. The volume of distribution is increased in elderly subjects, leading to a longer half life.

Oral absorption	>95%
Presystemic metabolism (prazepam)	>95%
Plasma half life (desmethyldiazepam)	
range	30–200 h
mean	60 h
Volume of distribution (desmethyl)	0.5–2.5 $l.kg^{-1}$
Plasma protein binding (desmethyl)	97%

Desmethyldiazepam crosses the placenta and is excreted in breast milk.

Concentration–effect relationship

Following the administration of a standard dose of prazepam to healthy subjects, considerable variation of plasma desmethyldiazepam has been noted.[2] Dosage is adjusted according to the clinical response. Despite extensive accumulation of desmethyldiazepam during the first few weeks of multiple-dose prazepam therapy, the sedative effects of the drug are not similarly cumulative. The central nervous system appears to adapt to the depressant effects of this metabolite.[8] There is no evidence of any correlation between the plasma concentration of desmethyldiazepam and its clinical effects.

Metabolism

Prazepam shares with diazepam its main metabolites, oxazepam and the desalkyl compound which is called either desalkylprazepam or desmethyldiazepam. Both prazepam and desmethyldiazepam have 3-hydroxyl derivatives, namely 3-hydroxyprazepam and oxazepam. These compounds are rapidly inactivated by glucuronide conjugation and have little persistent clinical effect (see Fig. 1). They are present in relatively minor quantities and have short elimination half lives compared to their parent compounds. The main metabolites are excreted in the urine as glucuronide conjugates. No significant amounts of free prazepam or desmethyldiazepam are found in the urine.

Prazepam

Fig. 1 The metabolism of prazepam

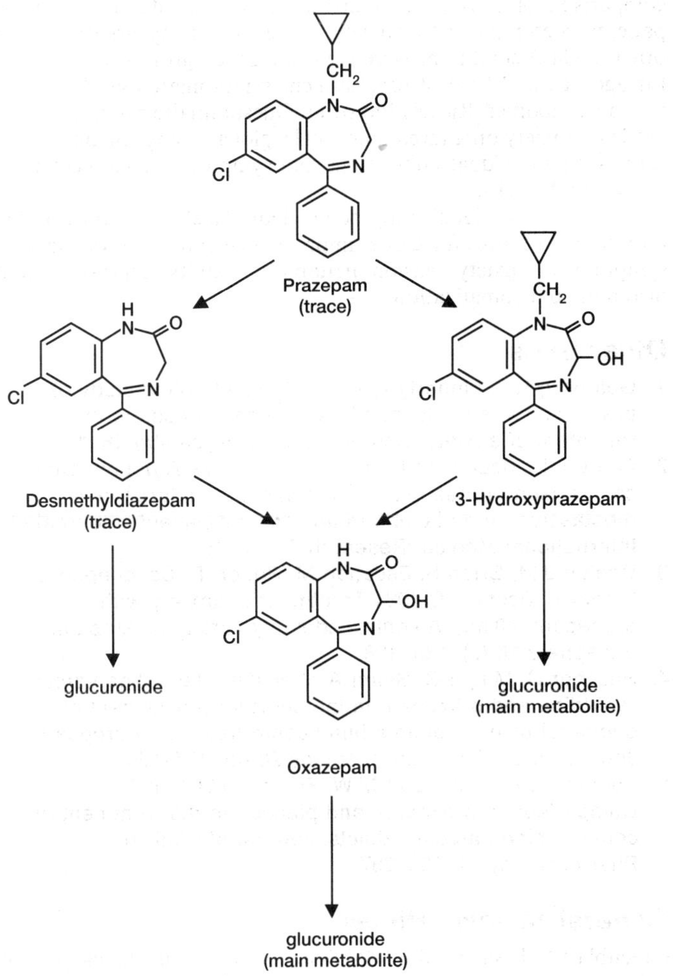

Pharmaceutics

Prazepam is available in oral form as Centrax (Warner, UK). Tablets containing 10 mg of prazepam are blue, slightly mottled, circular and biconvex, having a single breakline on one face.

Therapeutic use

Indications

1. The symptomatic relief of anxiety tension states
2. As an adjunct in other disease states in which anxiety is manifested
3. As a sedative and premedicant
4. For the control of muscle spasm
5. In the management of alcohol withdrawal symptoms.

Contraindications

1. Acute pulmonary insufficiency
2. Respiratory depression
3. Phobic or obsessional states
4. Chronic psychosis
5. Known sensitivity to benzodiazepines.

Mode of use

The dosage range for prazepam is 20–60 mg in a single dose at bedtime or in divided doses. Clinical trials have shown prazepam to be effective and well tolerated in the management of patients with anxiety states and comparable in efficacy to diazepam. In one study[9] prazepam had fewer and milder side effects than diazepam in the early treatment period, and especially in a divided-dose regimen.

Indications

1. The symptomatic relief of anxiety–tension states
Non-blind clinical evaluations of prazepam for its anxiolytic effect have in general reported good symptom relief in both out-patients and in-patients.[10,11] Double-blind controlled trials on neurotic out-patients[12,13] have found prazepam to be superior to placebo and comparable to chlordiazepoxide in comparable doses. In a double-blind, randomized, multi-centre comparison of prazepam vs. placebo,[14] prazepam was significantly superior to placebo as shown by final on-treatment scores for global improvement and for target symptoms including anxiety, tension and insomnia.

The dose is usually between 10 mg and 60 mg and is adjusted according to the response of the patient. The modal dose is 10 mg three times a day. If dizziness is a problem then a single dose at night may be more acceptable. However, a double-blind trial[15] comparing 40 mg of prazepam in divided doses with 40 mg at night showed a clear superiority of the divided-dose schedule with better anxiolytic efficacy on the Hamilton Anxiety scale.

2. As an adjunct in other disease states in which anxiety is manifested
Prazepam has been reported as being useful in treating anxiety associated with depressive neurosis and depressive reactions.[16] It may be useful in the symptomatic relief of anxiety in endogenous or psychotic depressions while awaiting the onset of the therapeutic effects of antidepressants. It has also been shown to be useful in the management of anxiety associated with acute alcoholism.[17]

3. As a sedative and premedicant
Prazepam has been found to provide good preoperative sedation prior to anaesthetic induction,[18] but there is no evidence to suggest that it is any better than any other benzodiazapine, some of which can provide a more rapid onset of their sedative effects, which is usually preferable.

4. For the control of muscle spasm
A series of non-blind trials has shown positive results in the treatment of children with cerebral palsy and in adults with various types of spastic paresis. It is claimed that a reduction in rigidity, spasticity and reflex muscle spasms was obtained without pronounced fatigue or oversedation.[19] One double-blind study found prazepam to be useful in the treatment of muscle spasms associated with multiple sclerosis.[20] Prazepam in doses of 5–25 mg significantly reduced muscle spasms associated with multiple sclerosis in 9 out of 16 patients.

5. In the management of alcohol and drug withdrawal symptoms
Prazepam has been used in the treatment of both the acute withdrawal phase and the convalescent phase of alcoholism. One study reported a stronger tranquillizing effect with chlordiazepoxide 25 mg than with prazepam 15 mg, with both being significantly better than placebo.[21] Prazepam 10–15 mg three times daily caused greater symptomatic improvement than a placebo in the first two weeks of a double-blind trial involving 50 patients suffering from anxiety following the withdrawal of narcotic drugs.

Contraindications

1, 2. Acute pulmonary insufficiency or respiratory depression
In common with other benzodiazepines prazepam can produce moderate hypoventilation with increased pCO_2 and is thus contraindicated in situations where respiratory function is already compromised.

Adverse reactions

Potentially life-threatening effects
There are no reports of any lethal toxic effects of prazepam.

Acute overdosage
Serious poisoning following large doses of benzodiazepines is rare. No data specific to prazepam are recorded but blood levels of up to 100 times the therapeutic level of diazepam have been recorded in overdosed cases.[22] Clinical features of benzodiazepine overdose include impaired level of consciousness, dizziness, ataxia, slurred speech and respiratory depression. Early gastric lavage or emesis may be useful; otherwise treatment consists of general supportive therapy.

Severe or irreversible adverse effects
The dependence potential for prazepam is similar to that of other long-acting benzodiazepines. It is exacerbated when high doses are used, especially over long periods, in patients with a history of alcoholism or drug abuse, and in patients with severe personality

disorder. Routine repeat prescriptions in such patients should be avoided, and the indications for commencing therapy in the first instance should be carefully considered. In such cases where dependence is likely, withdrawal should be gradual. Symptoms such as depression, nervousness, rebound insomnia, irritability, sweating and diarrhoea have been reported following abrupt cessation of therapy, even in patients receiving normal therapeutic doses. Acute withdrawal symptoms following excessive doses include confusion, toxic psychosis and convulsions.

Symptomatic adverse effects
Drowsiness, sedation, ataxia and blurring of vision have been recorded. These effects may follow single or repeated doses, and can last for well over 24 hours. The incidence may be reduced by starting treatment with a low dose and gradually increasing it. Performance at skilled tasks and alertness may be impaired and patients should be advised not to drive or operate machinery, particularly during the early phase of treatment. Abnormal psychological reactions to benzodiazepines have been reported, including paradoxical aggressive outbursts, excitement and confusion,[23] although a review of other studies stated that there is little conclusive evidence to show that the benzodiazepines are associated with an increase in aggression.[24]

Other effects
There is no evidence to suggest that prazepam causes any abnormalities in blood biochemistry.

Interference with clinical pathology tests
Prazepam is not known to interfere with any clinical pathology tests.

High risk groups

Neonates
Prazepam is not recommended in neonates.

Breast milk. Desmethyldiazepam is excreted in breast milk and is absorbed by the infant and metabolized by conjugation. Babies should not be breast-fed if the mother is receiving prazepam.

Children
In open trials prazepam has been found to be of some use in treating rigidity and spasticity in children with cerebral palsy.[25]

Pregnant women
The major metabolite of prazepam, desmethyldiazepam, is known to cross the placenta and may accumulate in the infant's serum even if the mother is taking a low dose.[26] This could lead to problems with withdrawal in the neonate.

The elderly
Caution should be observed when giving prazepam to elderly or debilitated patients as they are likely to be sensitive to the adverse effects; approximately one-half to one-third of the usual dose should be given.[26] Prazepam should not be prescribed for patients with acute closed-angle glaucoma.

Drug interactions

Potentially hazardous interactions
In general there are few reports of commonly encountered hazardous interactions but the concurrent use of phenothiazines, narcotics, barbiturates, alcohol and other CNS depressant drugs will potentiate any adverse effects of the benzodiazepine.

Other significant interactions
There are few reports of interactions specifically with prazepam. The half lives of other benzodiazepines are prolonged by drugs such as disulfiram[27] and cimetidine.[28] Absorption of diazepam is increased by the concurrent intramuscular administration of metoclopramide, morphine, pethidine or atropine.[29]

Nicotine, a hepatic enzyme inducer, may increase the metabolism of prazepam, but there is conflicting clinical evidence.

Potentially useful interactions
No interactions of this kind have been reported.

Major outcome trials

1. Weir J H 1978 Prazepam in the treatment of anxiety: a placebo-controlled multicenter evaluation. Journal of Clinical Psychiatry 39: 842–847

This was a double-blind, randomized, multicentre parallel-group comparison of prazepam in divided doses vs. placebo. Over 800 patients presenting with anxiety alone or anxiety associated with other medical conditions were included. Study groups were matched for age, sex and level of pretreatment symptomatology. Evaluation was by a modified Rickels Physician Questionnaire rating the global grade of anxiety on a three-point scale, global change in anxiety, and ratings for individual target signs and symptoms. Treatment varied from 2 to 4 weeks.

Prazepam was significantly better than placebo as shown on final on-treatment scores for global improvement ratio and for the target symptoms of anxiety, tension, irritability/hostility, depressive mood, insomnia and somatization.

Other trials

1. Goldberg H L, Finnerty R J 1977 A double-blind study of prazepam versus placebo in single daily doses in the treatment of anxiety. Comprehensive Psychiatry 18: 147–155
2. Fabre L F, McLendon D M, Mallette A 1979 A double-blind comparison of prazepam with diazepam, chlorazepate dipotassium and placebo in anxious out-patients. Journal of International Medical Research 7: 147–151
3. Danion J M, Brion S, Escande M, Robert R, Sacquepee L, Singer L, Scotto J C 1984 Treatment of anxiety with prazepam, 40 mg. A controlled study versus lorazepam. Encephale 10 (3): 135–138
4. Huscher C, Magni G, Salmi A et al 1985 Ranitidine versus ranitidine and prazepam in the short-term treatment of duodenal ulcer: a double-blind controlled trial. European Journal of Clinical Pharmacology 28 (2): 177–180
5. Sugerman A A, Miksztal M W, Freymuth H W 1971 Comparison of prazepam and placebo in the treatment of convalescing narcotic addicts. Journal of Clinical Pharmacology 11: 383–387

General review articles

Greenblatt D J, Shader R I 1974 Benzodiazepines in clinical practice. Raven Press, New York

Reynolds J E F 1982 The extra pharmacopoeia (Martindale) 28th edition. The Pharmaceutical Press, London

References

1. Allen M D, Greenblatt D J, Harmatz J S, Shader R I 1979 Single dose kinetics of prazepam, a precursor of desmethyldiazepam. Journal of Clinical Pharmacology 19: 445–450
2. Ochs H R, Greenblatt D J, Verburg-Ochs B, Locniskar B S 1984 Comparative single dose kinetics of oxazolam, prazepam, and chlorazepate: Three precursors of Desmethyldiazepam. Journal of Clinical Pharmacology 24: 446–451
3. Mohler H, Okada T 1970 Benzodiazepine receptors: Demonstration in the central nervous system. Science 198: 849–851
4. Robichaud R C, Gylys J A, Sledge K L 1970 The pharmacology of prazepam, a new benzodiazopine derivative. Archives Internationales de Pharmacodynamie et de Therapie 185: 213–227
5. Greenblatt D J, Shader R I 1978 Prazepam, a precursor of desmethyldiazepam. Lancet 2: 720
6. Nau H et al 1978 Journal of Chromatography 146. Biomedical Applications 3: 227–239
7. Greenblatt D J, Shader R I 1978 Pharmacokinetic understanding of anti-anxiety drug therapy. Southern Medical Journal 71s: 3–9
8. Greenblatt D J, Shader R I 1978 Prazepam and lorazepam, two new benzodiazepines. New England Journal of Medicine 299: 1342–1344
9. Dorman T 1983 A multicentre comparison of prazepam and diazepam in the treatment of anxiety. Pharmatherapeutica 3: 433–440
10. Kingstone E, Villeneuve A, Kossatz I 1966 Prazepam in the treatment of anxiety and tension: a clinical study of a new benzodiazepine derivative. Current Therapeutic Research 8: 159–163
11. Dunlop E, Weisberg J 1966 Use of prazepam for treatment of patients with anxiety: a pilot study. Journal of Psychopharmacology 6: 75–78
12. Dunlop E, Weisberg J 1968 Double-blind study of prazepam in the treatment of anxiety. Psychosomatics 9: 235–238
13. Kingstone E, Villeneuve A, Kossatz I 1969 Double-blind evaluation of prazepam, chlordiazepoxide and placebo in non-psychotic patients with anxiety and tension: some methodological considerations. Current Therapeutic Research 11: 106–114
14. Weir J H 1978 Prazepam in the treatment of anxiety: a placebo-controlled multicenter evaluation. Journal of Clinical Psychiatry 39: 841– 847
15. Ansseau M, Doumont A, Von-Frenckell R, Collard J 1984 Duration of benzodiazepine clinical activity: lack of direct relationship with plasma half-life. A comparison of single vs. divided dosage schedules of prazepam. Psychopharmacology, Berlin 84 (3): 293–298

16. Koufen J, Schulte P W, Consbruch U 1973 Hospital treatment of neurotic and reactive depression using a new benzodiazepine derivative. Medizinische Klinik (Munich) 68: 1701–1705
17. Rickels K, Sablosky L, Silverman H et al 1977 Prazepam in anxiety: a controlled clinical trial. Comparative Psychiatry 18: 239–249
18. Pyszko J 1974 Clinical investigation with demetrin in clinical surgery. Medizinische Welt (Stuttgart) 25: 1004–1006
19. Jelasic F 1974 The medical treatment of spasticity. Muench Medizinische Wochenschrift 116: 851–854
20. Levine I M, Jossman P S, Friend D G 1969 Prazepam in the treatment of spasticity: a quantitative double-blind evaluation. Neurology 19: 510–516
21. Shaffer J W, Yeganch M L, Foxwell N H 1968 A comparison of the effects of prazepam, chlordiazepoxide and placebo in the short-term treatment of convalescing alcoholics. Journal of Clinical Pharmacology 8: 392–399
22. Greenblatt D J, Allen M D 1978 Intramuscular injection site complications. Journal of the American Medical Association 240: 542–544
23. Hall C W, Joffe J R 1972 Abberant response to diazepam: A new syndrome. American Journal of Psychiatry 129: 738–743
24. Bond A, Lader M 1979 Benzodiazepines and aggression. In: Sandler M (ed) Psychopharmacology of aggression. Raven Press, New York, p 173
25. Morselli P L, Principi N, Tognoni G et al 1973 Diazepam elimination in premature and full-term infants and children. Journal of Perinatal Medicine 1: 133–141
26. Allen M D, Greenblatt D J, Harmatz J S, Shader R I 1980 Desmethyldiazepam kinetics in the elderly after oral prazepam. Clinical Pharmacology and Therapeutics 28: 196–202
27. Klotz U, Reimann I 1980 Delayed clearance of diazepam due to cimetidine. New England Journal of Medicine 302: 1012–1014
28. MacLeod S M, Sellers E M, Giles H G, Billings B J, Martin P R, Greenblatt D J, Marshman J A 1978 Interaction of disulfiram with benzodiazepines. Clinical Pharmacology and Therapeutics 24 (5): 583–589
29. Gamble J A S, Gaston J H, Nair S G 1976 Some pharmacological factors influencing the absorption of diazepam following oral administration. British Journal of Anaesthesia 48: 1181–1185

Praziquantel

Praziquantel is the first anthelmintic drug to fulfil the WHO requirements for population-based chemotherapy of a broad range of parasitic infections.

Chemistry

Praziquantel (Biltricide, Droncit, Cesol, Cysticide)
$C_{19}H_{24}N_2O_2$
2-Cyclohexylcarbonyl-1,2,3,6,7,11b-hexahydro-4H-pyrazino[2,1-*a*]-isoquinolin-4-one

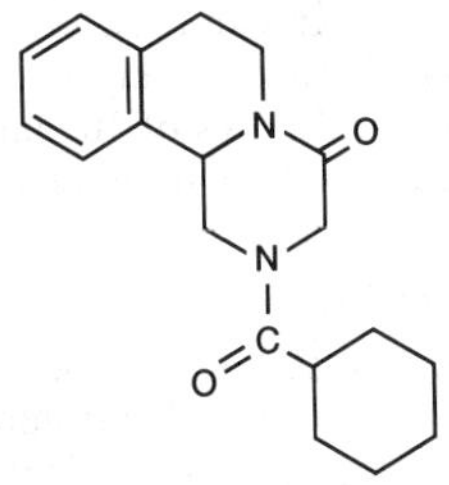

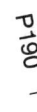

Molecular weight	312.4
pKa	>3
Solubility	
in alcohol	soluble
in water	very slight
Octanol/water partition coefficient	2.67

Praziquantel is a joint development of the German pharmaceutical manufacturers Bayer AG, Leverkusen, and E. Merck, Darmstadt. It is a white of nearly white crystalline powder, prepared by chemical synthesis,[1] and is stable under normal conditions. The active substance is hygroscopic.

Pharmacology

Praziquantel is effective against a wide range of cestode and trematode infections. The drug is rapidly and reversibly taken up by helminths in vitro. It has two main mechanisms of action. Firstly, at low concentrations it causes increased muscular activity[2] followed by contraction and spastic paralysis. It is this mode of action that causes parasites such as *Schistosoma mansoni* to loosen its grip on the wall of mesenteric veins and to migrate to the liver. Almost immediately after exposure to it, praziquantel causes vacuolization and vesiculation of the tegument of the parasite.[3] Through these lesions, host phagocytic cells enter the interior of the parasite eating up its contents within a few days. At the molecular level praziquantel causes the parasite membrane to be more permeable to certain cations such as sodium and calcium.[2]

Praziquantel has no relevant pharmacological effects in animals. At high dose levels, signs of non-specific CNS irritation are seen.[4] At concentrations of 10^{-4}–10^{-6} M, praziquantel causes an increase in the rate of force development of rat atria. This effect dependent and is blocked by verapamil bu phentolamine.[5] Praziquantel also produces on guinea-pig ileal muscle that is appro produced by muscarinic receptor stimulati calcium-dependent.

Toxicology

Because praziquantel represented a novel che mintics, particular attention was paid to thoro compound's profile in acute and subacute toxicity as the drug is intended only for short-term use. Acute toxicity tested in rats, mice, rabbits, and dogs was very low. Daily doses of up to 1 g.kg^{-1} given to rats over 4 weeks and up to 180 mg.kg^{-1} given daily to dogs for 13 weeks were well tolerated without any organ damage or impairment of vital functions. There was no effect whatsoever on male and female fertility, on parturition, on the newborn, on lactation, weaning, or postnatal development and the reproductive ability of the F_1 generation and development of the F_2 generation in rats was not adversely affected. No embryotoxic or teratogenic effects could be detected. No mutagenic activity was demonstrated in tissue-, host-, and urine-mediated assays (including healthy and schistosome-infected patients) with *Salmonella typhimurium* TA 98 and TA 100 strains.[7] Furthermore, there was no induction of point mutation, gene conversion, damage to DNA-repair mechanisms, sister chromatid exchanges, and/or X-linked recessive lethals.[8] Only one group of investigators claims to have observed mutagenic urinary metabolites in their modified Ames test.[9] These results, however, could not be reproduced by any other laboratory.

Praziquantel was also tested in different in vivo mammalian assays such as the dominant lethal test on male and female mice, the mononucleus test on male and female mice, and spermatogonial chromosome investigations in Chinese hamsters. All results were negative for mutagenicity.[10] In carcinogenicity tests, rats were given oral doses of 250 mg.kg^{-1} once weekly for 104 weeks and Syrian golden hamsters received oral doses of 100 mg.kg^{-1} once weekly for 80 weeks. In neither species were carcinogenetic effects detected.[11]

Clinical pharmacology

Healthy volunteers and schistosome-infected patients with a light parasitological and clinically complicationless course of infection were subjected to a broad range of medical, neurological, clinico-physiological, clinico-psychological and laboratory examinations including ECG, EEG, blood chemistry, haematology, coagulation physiology and urinalysis. The possible occurrence of parasite-related impairments had been considered in the investigational protocol, e.g. cerebral involvement due to infection by *S. mansoni* or *S. japonicum*. The doses tested against placebo ranged from 1 × 20 mg.kg^{-1} to 3 × 10 mg.kg^{-1} up to 3 × 25 mg.kg^{-1}. Regardless of a few small variations within the normal range in medical, neurological and clinico-physiological examinations, no changes attributable to the substance tested were observed. The evaluation of EEG and urinalysis did not reveal drug-related changes either. Subjective statements and objective observations of tiredness to sleepiness, dizziness, nausea and hangover occurred in some cases, but only after the highest daily dose (3 × 25 mg.kg^{-1} = 75 mg.kg^{-1}). These effects can be regarded as substance-specific and are supported by EEG findings as well as by psychological tests and pharmacokinetic data. This impairment of general well-being was rather transient and of minor intensity and was felt more subjectively than could be demonstrated objectively. Thus, tolerability of praziquantel has been described generally as good to very good. This has been confirmed virtually in all therapeutic trials that were conducted consequently.[12] None of all observations made in this respect could be regarded as serious enough to prevent starting of clinical trials on a larger scale.

Pharmacokinetics

Analytical methods available include GLC and fluorometry.[13–15] The concentration and fate of ^{14}C-labelled praziquantel and its metabolites have been determined in a number of species, including rats, beagle dogs, rhesus monkeys and sheep.[16–18] In these studies it was shown that after oral administration, praziquantel is almost completely absorbed in the gastrointestinal tract. Maximum serum concentrations were reached within 30 min to 1 h. However, the serum concentrations of unchanged praziquantel are very low, due to extensive presystemic metabolism in the liver. The pharmacokinetics of ^{14}C-praziquantel in man are very similar to those determined in animals.[19]

The distribution of praziquantel, after oral and intravenous admin-[illegible]ation (in rats and mice), is rapid and extensive. ^{14}C-labelled [illegible]rial tended to accumulate in the liver and kidneys. This might [illegible] the rapid elimination of the drug via the urine and bile.

Praziquantel is bound 80% to plasma proteins. No irreversible binding of labelled material to body constituents has been observed.

In man, praziquantel crosses the blood–brain barrier. Its concentration in the CSF of rats was, however, only $\frac{1}{5}$ to $\frac{1}{7}$ of that in plasma,[20] whilst in the CSF of rabbits[19] it was only $\frac{1}{10}$. Unchanged praziquantel is excreted in human milk, its concentration changing in parallel with that of the plasma.[20] On average, concentrations in milk are only 22% of those in plasma, so that only 0.0008% of an oral dose is excreted by this route. This indicates that transfer to milk is not due to active secretion, but rather to passive diffusion from the plasma. It is not known to what extent praziquantel crosses the placenta.

Oral absorption	>90%
Presystemic metabolism	extensive
Plasma half life	
unchanged praziquantel	1.5 h
total metabolites	4 h
total of unchanged praziquantel and all metabolites	3–8 h
Volume of distribution	—
Plasma protein binding	80%

Praziquantel is almost completely metabolized, probably largely in the liver. In animals, renal excretion of ^{14}C-labelled material accounts for 80–85% of the dose within 4 days, and over 90% of this is eliminated within the first 24 h, leaving only traces of radioactivity in the serum after that time. The fraction of ^{14}C-activity not excreted in the urine is eliminated via the bile to appear in the faeces. No unmetabolized praziquantel could be detected by qualitative thin layer chromatography in the urine, bile or faeces of rats treated either intravenously or orally. Comparable findings have been reported in man.[19]

The effect of liver disease on the pharmacokinetics of praziquantel is not known, but it is likely to result in impaired metabolism, with consequent increases in bioavailability and higher plasma concentrations. Old age and renal disease do not appear to alter the pharmacokinetics of praziquantel significantly.[21]

Concentration–effect relationship

There are no data available in this respect.

Metabolism

Praziquantel is eliminated almost entirely by metabolism, in part if not entirely in the liver. Thin-layer separation of extracts from urine and serum of man and monkey, faeces from monkey, rat, dog, and of the bile from rat revealed a variety of metabolites.[18] The most polar fraction was identified by enzymatic hydrolysis as a mixture of glucuronic and sulphuric acid conjugates that proved to be at least 400-fold less effective in inducing contraction in schistosomes than the parent compound. The metabolites of intermediate polarity were hydroxylation products of praziquantel.[19] The major metabolite in the serum of man and all animals studied so far has been identified as the 4-hydroxycyclohexylcarbonyl analogue of praziquantel. This metabolite retains some of the biological activity of the parent compound. In urine, metabolites with two hydroxyl groups prevail. There is no doubt that praziquantel itself is the active molecule requiring no biotransformation to become effective. Such transformations always result in less active or inactive metabolites.[1] Remarkable in this context is the fact that in none of the very many parasites that can be treated successfully with praziquantel have studies in vitro or in vivo revealed any ability to metabolize praziquantel.

Pharmaceutics

The compound for use in human therapy is available as tablets for oral administration. A 600 mg tablet, 'Biltricide' (Bayer, West Germany/UK; Miles, USA), is oblong, white and has three scores thus forming four segments of 150 mg each. 500 mg 'Cysticide' and 150 mg 'Cesol' tablets (E. Merck, West Germany) are white. The tablets are coated and are taken unchewed with liquid preferably after a meal. In case of repeated intake on the same day the interval between the individual doses should not be less than 4 h and not more than 6 h.

Praziquantel is not allergenic.

Therapeutic use

Indications

Antiparasitic therapy of infections due to

1. Trematodes infecting man, e.g.
a. Schistosome species such as *S. haematobium*, *S. intercalatum*, *S. japonicum*, *S. mansoni*, *S. mekongi*
b. Lungfluke species such as *Paragonimus westermani*, *P. heterotremus*, *P. africanus*, *P. ecuadoriensis*, *P. uterobilateralis*
c. Liverfluke species such as *Clonorchis sinensis*, *Opisthorchis viverrini*, *Opisthorchis felineus*, *Fasciola hepatica*, *Dicrocoelium dendriticum*
d. Intestinal fluke species such as *Fasciolopsis buski*, *Heterophyes heterophyes*, *Metagonimus yokogawai*, *Phanoropsolus bonnei*, *Haplorchis* spp., *Echinostomum* spp.
2. Cestodes infecting man, e.g.
a. Diphyllobothridae such as *Diphyllobothrium latum* and *D. pacificum*
b. Hymenolepididae such as *Hymenolepis nana* and *H. diminuta*
c. Taenidae (adult worms) such as *Taenia saginata* and *T. solium*
d. Taenidae (larval forms) such as *Cysticercus cellulosae* (*T. solium*).

Contraindications

In the supervised treatment of over 25 000 patients no contraindications came to light except in a few cases with ocular cysticercosis, a condition that deteriorated under praziquantel treatment.

Mode of use

Concerning this antiparasitic drug, there are no special remarks to be made in addition to those already included in the sections describing the pharmacology and/or those dealing with the indications in particular.

Indications

1. Trematode infections

Schistosomiasis

Jointly standardized trial designs and agreed technical protocols adapted to particularities of the schistosome species were used through collaboration with WHO Parasitic Diseases Programme and to local constraints.[22] Multi-centre trials were started, in part double-blind, simultaneously in Africa,[23] South America,[24] and Asia.[25,26] These trials aimed in particular at assessing the drug's usefulness for delivery in community healthy care projects to control schistosomiasis by reducing morbidity and eventually transmission. Results obtained furnished clear evidence of good to very good tolerability. No changes of biological significance in a battery of haematological and biochemical monitoring tests or in serial electrocardiograms and electroencephalograms could be detected.

Parasitological cure was achieved at six months between 75 and 100% in the various samples of patients treated.[27] Virtually no differences in tolerability and efficacy were found considering sex, age of patients and origin of parasite.[28] These results were confirmed time and again in series of further trials[29] including successful treatment of *S. intercalatum*[30,31] and *S. mekongi*.[32] In addition, special trials were performed to study cerebral involvement due to *S. japonicum*[26] and *S. mansoni*.[33,34]

Table 1 Control of schistosomiasis

	Days	No. of single doses per day	Dose ($mg.kg^{-1}$)	Total drug ($mg.kg^{-1}$)
S. haematobium	1	1	40	40
S. intercalatum	1	1	40	40
Hybrids of *S. haematobium* and *S. intercalatum*	1	1	40	40
S. mansoni	1	2	20	40
S. haematobium and *S. mansoni*	1	2	20	40
S. japonicum	1	2	30	60
S. mekongi	1	2	30	60

No adverse reactions could be observed in either condition. No hint at development of resistance against praziquantel has been reported so far. It could be demonstrated, however, that infections by *S. mansoni* sub-strains resistant against oxamniquine could be treated successfully with praziquantel.[35] The dosages recommended for the control of schistosomiasis are shown in Table 1.

In conclusion, these results, obtained irrespective of parasite species, of geographical occurrence and of age and sex of ethnically different patients, came so near to the fulfillment of requirements that praziquantel has been highly favoured by WHO[36] for all projects of schistomiasis control.

Lung fluke infections (paragonimiasis)

Various sub-species have been described in Southeast and East Asia, West Africa and South America. Often the diagnosis of this infection is rendered more difficult because of the similarity of symptoms with those of pulmonary tuberculosis. Up to now therapy has been time consuming (e.g. with bithionol) or drugs had been used which cause serious adverse reactions such as hetol. Significant improvement of treatment has been demonstrated with praziquantel in trials conducted in Korea,[37] Thailand,[38] Cameroon[39] and Ecuador.[40] Table 2 shows the recommended dosage for the control of lung fluke.

Table 2 Control of lung fluke

	Days	No. of single doses per day	Dose ($mg.kg^{-1}$)	Total drug ($mg.kg^{-1}$)
Paragonimus spp. (irrespective of geographical origin)	2	3	25	150

Liver fluke infections

Similar to schistosomiasis, infection with *C. sinensis* or *O. viverrini* affects a great part of the populations in, for example, Korea, Thailand and the People's Republic of China. Before the advent of praziquantel there was no satisfactory treatment, reports of its effectiveness coming from Korea,[41] Thailand[42] and Southeast Asia.[43]

In *Fasciola hepatica* infestations therapeutic efficacy can be achieved only by prolonging the time of exposing the parasite to drug influence; failures being due to short term application.[46,47] Table 3 shows the recommended dosages for the control of liver fluke.

Table 3 Control of liver fluke

	Days	No. of single doses per day	Dose ($mg.kg^{-1}$)	Total drug ($mg.kg^{-1}$)
C. sinensis[44]	1	3	25	75
O. viverrini[45]	1	1–3	40–25	40–75
F. hepatica	3–5	5	15	225–375

In vitro and in mice, rats and sheep the parasite was refractory to the compound.[48]

Intestinal fluke infections

Out of the great number of intestinal flukes that have been found in man there are only a few species invading man as final host, while many infections occur only accidentally. In any case, pathogenicity depends on the intensity of infection. *Fasciolopsis buski* may be considered the most important of these parasites affecting 10–20 million individuals, mainly children and juveniles in all countries from India to China.

Infection with *Metagonimus yokogawai* in Korea[49] also represents a public health problem; treatment became safe and effective only recently with the advent of praziquantel. The recommended dosages of praziquantel for the control of intestinal flukes are shown in Table 4.

2. Cestode infections (cestodiasis)

Infections due to fish tapeworms (Diphyllobothridae)
With a single-dose one-day application of praziquantel the therapy of *Diphyllobothrium latum* can be shortened remarkably in comparison to earlier treatment. More drug is required for cure of this species, however, than needed for *Diphyllobothrium pacificum* (see Table 5).[50,51]

Table 4 Control of intestinal flukes

	Days	No. of single doses per day	Dose (mg.kg^{-1})	Total drug (mg.kg^{-1})
Fasciolopsis buski	1	1	15–20	15–20
Metagonimus yokogawai	1	2	20	40
Heterophyes heterophyes	1	1	25	25
Other intestinal flukes	1	1	25	25

Table 5 Control of fish tapeworms

	Days	No. of single doses per day	Dose (mg.kg^{-1})	Total drug (mg.kg^{-1})
Diphyllobothrium latum	1	1	25	25
D. pacificum	1	1	10	10

Infection due to dwarf tapeworms (hymenolepiasis)
In the case of this parasitosis, treatment with praziquantel is regarded by all investigators as a considerable improvement over previous therapy because of nearly 100% cure rates after administering one single dose. However, patients harbouring very recent infections in which the cystericercoids are not yet fully developed may need a second treatment given 4 days after the first one.[52,53] See Table 6 for the dosage recommendations.

Table 6 Control of dwarf tapeworms

	Days	No. of single doses per day	Dose (mg.kg^{-1})	Total drug (mg.kg^{-1})
Hymenolepis nana	1(+1)	1	15–25	15–25
H. diminuta	1	1	25(?)	25(?)

Though human infection with *H. diminuta* seems to be not uncommon in poor communities plagued by rodents (Iran, Papua New Guinea),[54] no therapeutic experience with praziquantel is available. Regarding experimental therapy in laboratory animals, 100% efficacy was observed with 20 mg.kg^{-1} for *H. nana* and with 5 mg.kg^{-1} for *H. diminuta* in rats.[52]

Infections due to tapeworms (taeniasis)
In therapeutic studies where the differential diagnosis between *T. saginata* and *T. solium* could be made with certainty the former appeared more susceptible to praziquantel than the latter. Since very often differential diagnosis can be rather difficult, however, a uniform dosage has been established that provides 100% cure in both species (see Table 7).[53]

Table 7 Control of tapeworms

	Days	No. of single doses per day	Dose (mg.kg^{-1})	Total drug (mg.kg^{-1})
Taenia saginata	1	1	10	10
T. solium	1	1	10	10

Infections due to larval tapeworms (cysticercosis)
There are two species of metacestodes affecting man: hydatide cysts originating from *Echinococcus granulosus*; and *Cystericercus cellulosae* developing from *Taenia solium*.

As regards hydatid cysts, experimental chemotherapy using many animal species did not reveal any curative efficacy of praziquantel. Results were so hopeless that investigators concluded that no consideration should be given to its use in the treatment of hydatid disease in man.[52,53] Concerning the larval stage of *T. solium*, however, the therapeutic prospect for cysticercosis using praziquantel is quite favourable.[55] From 1977 onwards several thousand patients mainly affected by neurocysticercosis have been treated successfully, thus substituting in many cases for the risky neurosurgical intervention that had been the only previous treatment. Since modern diagnostic tools such as computerized tomography facilitate diagnosis and assessment of eventual therapeutic progress, it was established that particular cysts located within the parenchyma of the brain respond very well to praziquantel and much better than intraventricular cysticercosis. No general recommendation can be given regarding concomitant corticosteroid treatment,[56] which has been recommended as a precautionary measure to prevent or at least relieve cerebral pressure that, in rare cases, may result from reaction to parasite proteins released from a cyst disintegrating under praziquantel influence. However, undiagnosed infections such as tuberculosis, amoebiasis, trypanosomiasis and some fungal infections may be exacerbated if corticosteroids are given over a long period. In the case of giant cysts, praziquantel should be administered for about 4 weeks.

Subsequently, different dosage schemes have been tested. Investigators recommending concomitant corticosteroid application favoured shorter treatment with higher single doses, e.g. 25 mg.kg^{-1} three times daily for 7–10 days.[57,58] Treatment with praziquantel alone at a lower dosage level for a prolonged application period also resulted in very favourable parasitological and clinical results with less unwanted adverse effects,[59] and this regime is now recommended by the manufacturer (E. Merck) (see Table 8). Calcified cysts do not respond to treatment.

Table 8 Control of cysticercosis

	Days	No. of single doses per day	Dose (mg.kg^{-1})	Total drug (mg.kg^{-1})
Dermal cysticercosis	3–7	3	25	225–525
Neurocysticercosis	15	3	16.67	750
Gaint cells	28	3	16.67	1400

For the indications described above cure rates in the range of 70–100% have been achieved depending on the population sample treated. The only exceptions reported were for *Fasciola hepatica* (cure rate 25–40%; optimum dosage still under investigation) and *Cysticercus cellulosae* (cure rate 40–87%).[56]

Adverse reactions

Potentially life-threatening effects
No effects of this kind were detected in comprehensive toxicological studies,[11] though a single dose as high as 70 mg.kg^{-1} had been used and tolerated in a trial.

Acute overdosage
No case of deliberate, negligent, or inadvertent overdosing has been observed and reported so far.

Severe or irreversible adverse effects
Severe adverse reactions are very rare. In general, they consist of colicky abdominal pain occurring from about 30 minutes to 1–2 hours after drug intake, which may require spasmolytics for relief. Severe pain of this kind, accompanied by bloody diarrhoea, was observed in 23% and 56% respectively of the patients involved in a clinical trial of the drug in the treatment of *S. mansoni* infection in Maniema, Zaire. No explanation could be found for the frequency

and severity of adverse effects encountered in this trial, when compared with experience of thousands of courses of treatment for *S. mansoni* infection elsewhere.

Praziquantel is not ovicidal, and therefore it is not expected to provoke serious cerebral reactions when parasitic eggs have found their way into the brain, as may be the case in infections due to *S. japonicum* and *S. mansoni*. If, however, adult parasites susceptible to praziquantel reach the cerebrum, serious and even dangerous adverse reactions such as raised intracranial pressure may occur immediately. This applies in particular to infections due to *Paragonimus* spp. and to *F. hepatica*. Where clinical symptoms already point to cerebral involvement in these infections it is mandatory to make arrangements for immediate intervention.

A very small number of cases of jaundice have been reported. However, jaundice has not been observed in animals with a liver already damaged by infection; nor was jaundice observed in about 200 patients selected for treatment of advanced hepatosplenic schistosomiasis with already impaired liver function. In six cases of abnormal transaminases and concomitant jaundice, liver biopsy was performed and a pre-existing viral hepatitis B of recognizable chronicity was detected. In patients thought to have progressive liver damage, actual improvement was observed after praziquantel treatment.[33,34]

Symptomatic adverse effects

In general, these are mild and transient and do not require additional treatment. They begin about 30 minutes after drug intake and usually disappear spontaneously after a few hours.

Three main groups of adverse reactions can be distinguished.

1. Those affecting the intestinal tract. However, it should be noted that in schistosomiasis due to *S. haematobium* these are virtually non-existent.
2. Reactions involving the central nervous system, including dizziness and sleepiness.
3. Reactions, such as fever, skin manifestations, and eosinophilia, that develop after medication and disappear spontaneously a few days later. If these reactions were drug-related they should appear after treatment in all types of schistosome infections, but it is not the case, and there is reason to believe that these reactions are due to foreign protein released by parasites killed by praziquantel.

In assessing tolerability, the very rapid elimination of the compound from the human body should be considered (see Pharmacokinetics). In the light of this observation, it is debatable whether events such as fainting, hallucinations, psychotic symptoms, and excitement, occurring about 15 days after medication, can be attributed to the drug treatment. In such cases concomitant cerebral schistosomiasis must be taken into account.

In general, the frequency and intensity of untoward effects of praziquantel appear to depend less on the amount of drug applied than on the intensity of infection (i.e. on the amount of parasite protein released due to drug efficacy).

It may sometimes be difficult to decide whether an effect observed after praziquantel medication is caused by the infection or by the drug or by both.

Other effects

Hyperglycaemia of varying degree was observed in 33 out of 100 Mexican patients who were treated with 50 $mg.kg^{-1}$ daily for 15 days because of cerebral cysticercosis.[63] This observation could not be confirmed, however, in any other therapeutic trial, even though blood glucose concentrations were monitored.

Interference with clinical pathology tests

Glucose-6-phosphate dehydrogenase deficiency (G-6-PD deficiency) and haemoglobinopathies have to be taken into account for chemotherapy in parts of Asia and particularly in many African population groups. In a WHO-sponsored study group in Zambia[61] 40 out of 151 individuals were detected by targeted screening showing H_b genotype AS in 20, genotype AC in 9, and G-6-PD deficiency in 11 cases. No measurable changes occurred after praziquantel medication and tolerability was not influenced by any of the dosages administered. Corresponding observations were made in another trial conducted in Mali.[62]

High risk groups

Neonates

There are no data available. Infection of neonates by one of the parasites in question must be regarded as extremely rare.

Breast milk. Excretion of praziquantel into the milk was studied in lactating women. The concentrations of unmetabolized praziquantel increased and decreased in parallel with the concentrations in plasma. On average, concentrations in milk were only 22% of those in the plasma and only 0.0008% of the oral dose taken. This indicates that the drug is not secreted into the milk but passively equilibrates between serum and milk.[63] Despite the small amount likely to be absorbed by a breast-fed infant, the manufacturer recommends that the mother should not breast-feed on the day of treatment or during the subsequent 72 hours.

Children

In early therapeutic trials, children of six years and above were included. When no evidence of unfavourable age-related reactions was found, the age limit of children entering trials was less rigorously maintained, and only children under the age of two years remained excluded from treatment.[42] There was no difference in dosages between those administered to adults and those given to children, and no adverse reactions were observed.

Pregnant women

Though comprehensive animal experiments revealed no harmful effects on either pregnant women or their unborn children,[11] the manufacturer recommends withholding praziquantel during the first three months of pregnancy. Since this compound has been used in many large-scale treatment projects one may be justified in assuming, however, that some pregnant women may have been treated inadvertently. There are no reports of any critical observations in this respect.

The elderly

No special precautions are required in the elderly.

Concurrent disease

Severe renal insufficiency can be one of the final consequences of infection with *S. haematobium*. Whether individuals suffering from such a condition and undergoing haemodialysis may be hopefully subjected to praziquantel treatment can hardly be decided for every case. Observations made in an uraemic patient revealed unchanged kinetics of praziquantel in blood and only slightly changed renal elimination of unmetabolized praziquantel.[21]

Drug interactions

Potentially hazardous interactions

Consumption of alcohol may aggravate the drug related adverse reactions of dizziness and may render such patients unfit for driving a car or operating machinery on the day of treatment and the following day.

Potentially useful interactions

No reactions of this kind have been detected during comprehensive pharmacological studies and worldwide clinical use of praziquantel.

Major outcome trials

Schistosomiasis

1. In: World Health Bulletin 1979 57(5): 5 articles dealing with tolerability in first application to patients infected with *S. haematobium* (WHO conducted trial: Davis A, Biles J E, Ulrich A M 1979, pp 773–779), *S. mansoni* and *S. japonicum*

These describe first steps of determining optimum dosages on the bases of tolerability and efficacy, conducted double-blind (investigational phase IIa). The trial design obligatory for these studies was elaborated and agreed upon in close cooperation with WHO Parasitic Diseases Programme.

2. In: Arzneimittelforschung/Drug Research 1981 31(I) (3a) special issue with the proceedings of a Biltricide symposium on African schistosomiasis held in Nairobi, February 1980

Contains 4 articles on preclinical studies; 5 articles on the treatment of *S. haematobium*, including one WHO conducted trial (Davis A, Biles

Praziquantel

P

J E, Ulrich A M, Dixon H 1981 pp 568–574); 7 articles on the treatment of *S. mansoni* and *S. intercalatum*; 5 articles on the treatment of mixed infections including a large scale project following the trial protocol of CDC San Juan, Puerto Rico, USA.

3. Prata A, Castro C N, Silva A E, Paiva M, Macedo V, Junqueira Jr L F 1982 Praziquantel no tratamento da esquistossomose mansoni. Revista do Instituto da Medicina Tropical, São Paulo 24, 2: 95–103

This study complements the results obtained in Africa for Latin America, i.e. Brazil. 135 patients were allocated to 3 strata according to intensity of infection: I. 95–500 eggs per gram faeces (epg) II. 500–1000 epg III. over 1000 epg. Cure rates were highest by administering 2×25 mg.kg^{-1} to all 3 strata (other dosages 1×30 and 1×40 mg.kg^{-1}) and were better, too, in cases with lower intensity: I. 86.7% II. 73.3% and III. 46.7% at 6 months follow-up. In comparison similar studies in Africa did not show such significant differences within the strata with I. 74% II. 70% and III. 76%, but reported also the best antischistosomal efficacy to the split dosage[63] of 2×20 mg.kg^{-1}.

For trematode infections other than schistosomiasis

4. Arzneimittelforschung/Drug Research 1984, 34(II), 9b

Special issue with symposium proceedings on trematode infections and chemotherapy in Southeast and East Asia, Kyongju, Korea, Oct. 1984. Out of 39 contributions, 19 deal with successful praziquantel therapy of clonorchiasis, opisthorchiasis, paragonimiasis, fasciolopsiasis, metagonimiasis and other intestinal fluke infections.

Cestode infections

Major outcome trials paving the way for further studies that enlarged the number of patients treated but did not bring to light any new aspects are reported in Boletín Chileno de Parasitología 1977, 32 with 8 studies covering all cestode species pathogenic to man.

Other trials

For neurocysticercosis

1. Botero D, Castaño S 1982 Treatment of cysticerosis with praziquantel in Colombia. American Journal of Tropical Medicine and Hygiene 31, 4: 810–821

31 patients suffering from neurocysticercosis, one with ocular cysticercosis and three with subcutaneous cysticercosis were treated with praziquantel at a dosage of 10 mg.kg^{-1} given three times daily to 27 patients for 6 days. This treatment was repeated after 1–2 months, not however for the three cases with dermal cysticercosis who were cured after the first course. The remaining five patients received 50 mg.kg^{-1} bodyweight daily divided into 3 single doses for 10 consecutive days. Intracranial hypertension and headache disappeared in 13 out of 15 cases, 2 further cases improved. Epilepsy came under control in 14 of 19 cases. In 7 out of 11 cases with cerebral lesions diagnosed by computerized tomography, the lesions disappeared and were reduced in number and/or in size in a further 2. Two cases remained unchanged as did also the ocular infection. One patient died, i.e. a mortality rate of 3.2% contrasting significantly with the previous case fatality rate of 50–80% in the same Colombian institution.

2. Spina-França A, Nobrega J P S, Livramento J A, Machado L R 1982 Administration of praziquantel in neurocysticercosis. Tropenmedizin und Parasitologie 38, 1: 1–68

Praziquantel was given to four groups of 10 patients each as follows: I, II & III: two series of 6 days with one month interval between I = 20 mg.kg^{-1} daily; II & III: 30 mg.kg^{-1} daily; IV 50 mg.kg^{-1} daily for 21 consecutive days. Some of the patients received concomitantly dexamethasone. Transient exacerbation in 31/40 patients was interpreted as drug action on the cysts. 34/40 had intracranial hypertension, 10 of them were cortico-dependent. No improvement occurred in 6 cases, 2 patients died and 3 others had to undergo extracranial ventricular derivation. Cortico-dependence disappeared in all cases concerned. Also ventricular dilatation disappeared in 4 out of 6 and no new intracranial hypertension periods were observed in 15 out of 20.

3. Sotelo J, Escobero F, Rodriguez-Carbajal J, Torres B, Rubio-Donnadieu F 1984 Therapy of parenchymal brain cysticercosis with praziquantel. The New England Journal of Medicine 310, 16: 1002–1007

26 patients were given praziquantel 50 mg.kg^{-1} daily in 3 single doses for 15 consecutive days. Initially a strong inflammatory reaction occurred with exacerbation of neurological symptoms as evidenced by increased protein and cells in the cerebrospinal fluid. In 9 out of 26 patients total remission of cysts was observed and CT scans of 25 out of 26 improved since the number of cysts decreased from initially 152 to 51. These results indicate efficacy of praziquantel for treatment of cysticercosis of the brain parenchyma.

General review articles

Wegner D H G, Snellen W 1981 Aperçu généal des résultats cliniques obtenus avec le Biltricide dans le traitement de la schistosomiase humaine. Bulletin de la Société de Pathologie Exotique 74: 583–589

Davis A 1982 Available chemotherapeutic tools for the control of Schistosomiasis. Behring Institut, Mitteilungen Nr 71: 90–103

Davis A 1982 Management of the patient with schistosomiasis. In: Jordan P, Webbe G (eds) Schistosomiasis, William Heinemann Medical Books Ltd, London, pp 184–226

Andrews P, Thomas H, Pohlke R, Seubert J 1983 Praziquantel. Medicinal Research Review 3, 2: 177

Wegner D H G 1984 The profile of the trematodicidal compound praziquantel. Arzneimittel/Drug Research 34(II), 9b: 1132–1136

World Health Organization 1985 The control of schistosomiasis. Technical Report Series 728: 55 cont'd.

For trematode infections other than schistosomiasis

Andrews P, Thomas H, Pohlke R, Seubert J 1983 Praziquantel. Medicinal Research Review 3, 2: 181–185

Wegner D H G 1984 The profile of the trematodicidal compound praziquantel. Arzneimittelforschung/Drug Research 34(II), 9b: 1132–1136

Wegner D H G 1986 Zur Therapie der nicht durch Schistosomen bedingen Trematodeninfektionen des Menschen. Mitteilungen der Österreichischen Gesellschaft für Tropenmedizin und Parasitologie. Band 8, Wien. In press.

Cestode infections

Gemmell M A, Johnstone P D 1981 Cestodes. Antibiotics Chemotherapy 30: 54–114

Andrews P, Thomas H, Pohlke R, Seubert J 1983 Praziquantel. Medicinal Research Review 3, 2: 185–189

Groll E 1984 Praziquantel. Advances in Pharmacology and Chemotherapy 20: 219–238

Pawlowski Z S 1984 Cestode infections: Taeniasis, diphyllobothriasis, hymenolepiasis, and others. In: Warren K S, Mahmoud A A F Tropical and Geographical Medicine. McGraw Hill, New York, ch 55, pp 471–486

Cestode infections

Groll E 1982 Chemotherapy of human cysticercosis with praziquantel. In: Cysticercosis, present state of knowledge and perspectives. Academic Press, New York, pp 207–218

References

1. Andrews P, Thomas H, Pohlke R, Seubert J 1983 Praziquantel. Medicinal Research Review 3: 147–200
2. Pax R, Bennett J L, Fetterer R 1978 A benzodiazepine derivate and praziquantel: effects on musculature of Schistosoma mansoni and Schistosoma japonicum. Naunyn Schmiedebgerg's Archives of Pharmacology 304: 309–315
3. Mehlhorn H, Becker B, Andrews P, Thomas H, Frenkel K J 1981 In-vivo and in-vitro experiments on the effects of praziquantel on Schistosoma mansoni. Arzneimittelforschung/Drug Research 31(I),3a: 544–554
4. Frohberg H, Schulze Schenking M 1981 Toxicological profile of praziquantel, a new drug against cestode and schistosome infections, as compared to some other schistosomicides. Arzneimittelforschung/Drug Research 31(I),3a: 555–565
5. Chubb J M, Bennett J L, Akera T, Brody T M 1978 Effects of praziquantel, a new anthelmintic, on electromechanical properties of isolated rat atria. Journal of Pharmacology and Experimental Therapeutics 207: 284–293
6. Jim K, Triggle D J 1979 The actions of praziquantel and 1-methyladenine in guinea pig ileal longitudinal muscle. Canadian Journal of Physiology and Pharmacology 57: 1460–1462
7. Obermeier J, Frohberg H 1977 Mutagenicity studies with praziquantel, a new anthelmintic drug: tissue-, host- and urine-mediated assays. Archives of Toxicology 38: 149–161
8. Bartsch H, Kuroki T, Malaveille C et al 1978 Absence of mutagenicity of praziquantel, a new effective antischistosomal drug, in bacteria, yeasts, insects and mammalian cell. Mutation Research 58: 133–142

Concentration–effect relationship

Most studies with orally administered prazosin have shown a poor correlation between plasma concentration of the drug and blood pressure reduction: a better correlation has been observed when prazosin has been administered intravenously.

Metabolism

The major route for prazosin metabolism is via 6- and 7-O-dealkylation to products I & II in Figure 1 followed by hepatic conjugation.[17]

Fig. 1 Metabolites of prazosin

I

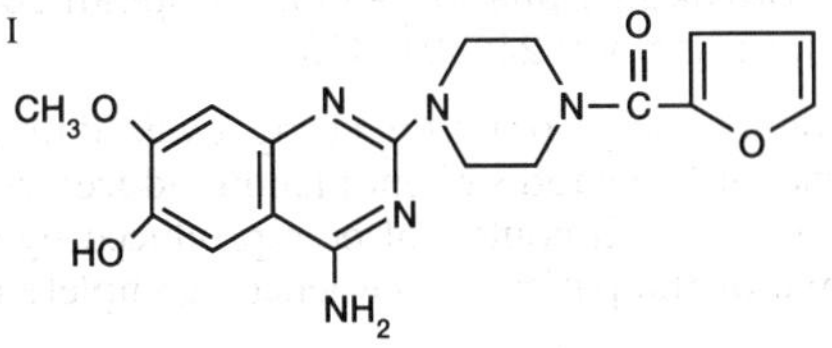

II

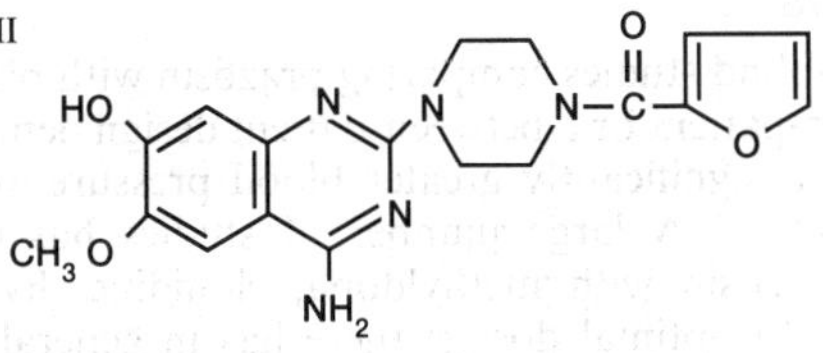

Approximately 50% of the drug is metabolized during each pass through the liver. Some of the metabolites of prazosin are active. Three of four metabolites identified in one study had 10–25% of the antihypertensive activity of prazosin.[5]

Pharmaceutics

Prazosin is available in four tablet formulations in the UK and as three capsule formulations in the USA.

1. Hypovase (Pfizer, UK) 0.5 mg: white, 0.282 inch diameter oval, unscored tablet with Pfizer logo on one side.
2. Hypovase (Pfizer, UK) 1 mg: orange, 0282 inch diameter oval, scored tablet marked HYP/1 on one side.
3. Minipress (Pfizer, US) 1 mg white capsule marked 'MINIPRESS' on the body and 'Pfizer 431' on the cap.
4. Hypovase (Pfizer, UK) 2 mg: white, 0.312 inch diameter oval, scored tablet bearing HYP/2 on one side and 'Pfizer' on the other.
5. Minipress (Pfizer, US) 2 mg: capsule with white body marked 'MINIPRESS' and a pink cap marked 'PFIZER 437'.
6. Minipress (Pfizer, US) 5 mg capsule with white body marked 'MINIPRESS' and a blue cap marked 'PFIZER 438'.

The only potentially allergenic component of the tablets is corn starch. The maximal shelf-life of tablets is 24 months when they are stored in either an opaque polypropylene container (Securitainer) or a blister pack. Three fixed-dose thiazide combinations are available in the USA, all containing 0.5 mg polythiazide (Minizide 1', Minizide 2' and Minizide 5' - Pfizer, US).

Therapeutic use

Indications

1. All grades of hypertension
2. Moderate to severe congestive heart failure
3. Raynaud's phenomenon and disease.

Contraindications

The only absolute contraindication is sensitivity to prazosin.

Mode of use

1. Hypertension

Prazosin can be used either alone or in combination with other antihypertensive drugs. Treatment is started with a dose of 0.5 mg twice daily or three times daily for 3–7 days. Patients should be advised to take the first dose before going to bed at night because the first dose of prazosin may cause a marked postural hypotension, although this is unusual with a starting dose of 0.5 mg. The dose may then be increased to 1 mg twice daily or three times daily over the next 3–7 days. Thereafter the dose should be gradually adjusted according to the patient's individual blood pressure response. Daily doses greater than 20 mg are not recommended. The antihypertensive efficacy of prazosin can be potentiated by adding a mild diuretic such as a thiazide.

The above dosage schedule may be employed when prazosin is added to other antihypertensive drugs (such as β-adrenoceptor blockers or angiotensin-converting enzyme inhibitors) which have not adequately controlled blood pressure. In this case the dose of the first agent is sometimes reduced to a maintenance level before adding prazosin.

2. Congestive cardiac failure

Prazosin may be added to the therapeutic regimen in those patients who have not shown a satisfactory response or who have become refractory to conventional therapy with cardiac glycosides and diuretics. Treatment is started with a dose of 0.5 mg three or four times daily, with ambulatory patients, taking the first dose before going to bed. The dose is titrated every two or three days according to the clinical response under close medical supervision. In severely ill, decompensated patients, rapid dose titration over 1 to 2 days may be indicated. The maximal recommended daily dose is 20 mg.

3. Raynaud's phenomenon and Raynaud's disease

The recommended starting dose is 0.5 mg twice daily for 3-7 days. The dose is adjusted according to the patient's response. The usual maintenance dose is 1–2 mg twice daily.

Adverse reactions

Potentially life-threatening effects

The hypotension occasionally observed with prazosin is rarely life threatening (see below).

Acute overdosage

Accidental ingestion of at least 50 mg of prazosin resulted in profound drowsiness and depressed reflexes. No decrease in blood pressure was noted and recovery was uneventful. The stomach should be emptied by aspiration and lavage. Hypotension should be treated by lying the patient supine: if this is inadequate, plasma volume expanders should be administered. Pharmacological vasoconstrictor agents (such as metaraminol) may then be given if blood pressure is not maintained. Because of the high degree of protein binding prazosin is not dialysable.

Severe or irreversible adverse effects

Shortly after prazosin was introduced there were reports of acute symptoms 30–90 minutes following the first dose of the drug.[22] In milder cases these symptoms took the form of dizziness and palpitations on standing upright: in more severe cases the patient lost consciousness. The mechanism appears to be acute reduction in venous return to the heart, hypotension and bradycardia. This probably explains the fact that pre-existing sodium depletion aggravates the first-dose phenomenon.[23] The first-dose phenomenon appears have been due to the high starting dose (2 mg) which was originally recommended. It is rarely seen in clinical practice with a starting dose of 0.5 mg and the recommendation that the first tablet is taken in the evening.[24]

Symptomatic adverse effects

Orthostatic hypotension and dizziness have frequently been reported in clinical trials although the prevalence has varied from 1% to 75% of patients exposed to the drug. Most studies report about 20%.[7] Other adverse effects which have been less frequently encountered include headache, drowsiness, lack of energy, weakness, palpitations, impotence and nausea. Whilst it has been claimed that there is a high incidence of antinuclear antibodies in patients treated with prazosin[25] there is no convincing evidence demonstrating conversion from negative to positive tests in patients followed longitudinally.

Other effects

Some studies have reported an increase in the HDL/LDL cholesterol ratio.[8]

P

Interference with clinical pathology tests
Prazosin may cause a rise in circulating and urinary catecholamines, giving false positive results when these tests are used for diagnosing phaeochromocytoma.

High risk groups
Neonates
No clinical experience is available with the use of prazosin in neonates.

Breast milk. Prazosin is excreted in small amounts in human breast milk.

Children
As in neonates, no data on the use of the drug in children are available.

Pregnant women
Although no teratogenic effects were seen in animal testing, the safety of prazosin in pregnancy has not been established. However, prazosin has been used successfully in several studies of hypertension of pregnancy without apparent harm to mother or fetus.[7]

The elderly
Although the elimination half life of the drug is slightly prolonged in the elderly, this does not usually seem to be clinically significant. However, small doses of the drug should be used initially and dose titration should be performed carefully. Baroreflex function is often impaired in the elderly and this may exacerbate postural hypotension.

Drug interactions
Potentially hazardous interactions
The only known drug interaction is the excessive hypotensive response observed when prazosin is administered to patients on other antihypertensive therapy. Patients who are sodium depleted as a result of diuretic therapy are probably at particular risk.

Other significant interactions
Food and alcohol have no effect upon the absorption or pharmacological response to prazosin.

Major outcome trials
1. Veterans Administration Cooperative Study Group 1981 Comparison of prazosin with hydralazine in patients receiving hydrochlorothiazide. A randomised, double blind clinical trial. Circulation 64: 772–779

The Veterans Administration Cooperative Study Group compared prazosin and hydralazine in a randomized double-blind trial of 232 patients with diastolic blood pressures of 95–114 mmHg. After an initial pre-randomizing period patients were followed for 6 months. There were no significant differences between regimens in the percentage of patients who attained the goal blood pressure (reduction of diastolic blood pressure to 90 mmHg or less) although there was a slightly better response of systolic blood pressure to prazosin at 3 and 6 months. Both agents were given in addition to hydrochlorothiazide and doses ranged up to 150 mg daily hydralazine and 15 mg daily prazosin. Orthostatic dizziness and sexual dysfunction were more frequent with prazosin than with hydralazine. These differences persisted with time, although they were less marked after one month.

2. Stokes G S, Frost G S, Graham R M, MacCarthy E P 1979 Indoramin and prazosin as adjuncts to beta adrenoceptor blockade in hypertension. Clinical Pharmacology and Therapeutics 25: 783–789

Stokes et al compared indoramin with prazosin, using a double-blind crossover design in 15 patients. Patients were already receiving a β-adrenoceptor blocker with or without a diuretic. Dosage of prazosin was 6–12 mg per day and of indoramin 60–120 mg per day. Dosage was titrated for optimal effect. Equal degrees of blood pressure control were observed except that only prazosin reduced exercise systolic and diastolic pressures at the end of the 8-week treatment period.

3. Colucci W S, Wynne J, Holman B L, Braunwald E 1980 Long term therapy of heart failure with prazosin. A randomized double blind trial. American Journal of Cardiology 45: 337–344

22 patients with severe left ventricular failure (New York Heart Association) Class III or IV treated with digoxin and diuretics were randomized to prazosin (10 patients) or placebo (12 patients). Dose of prazosin was titrated up to 16 mg daily. After 8 weeks the prazosin-treated patients showed significant improvement in function and classification (mean 3.7 falling to 2.3), treadmill exercise duration, echocardiographic and radionuclide ejection fraction and velocity of circumferential fibre shortening. Placebo-treated patients showed no change. Nevertheless there was clinical evidence for attenuation of the prazosin response at 2 months.

4. Nielsen S L, Vitting K, Rasmussen K 1983 Prazosin treatment of primary Raynaud's phenomenon. European Journal of Clinical Pharmacology 24: 421–423

In a double-blind study, prazosin (1 mg twice daily) reduced the reported attacks of Raynaud's phenomenon induced by cold in 5 out of 7 patients. The benefit could not be reproduced by cold provocation tests. None of the patients experienced complete relief.

Other trials
Early double-blind studies comparing prazosin with placebo utilizing either a within-patient or a between-patient design demonstrated that prazosin had a significantly greater blood pressure-lowering action than placebo.[26,27] A large number of studies has compared the efficacy of prazosin with methyldopa, clonidine, hydralazine and indoramin.[5,7] In optimal dosage there has in general been little to choose between the blood pressure-lowering effect of prazosin and its comparator drug.

General review articles
Graham R M, Pettinger W A 1979 Prazosin. New England Journal of Medicine 300: 232–236

References

1. Patel P, Bose D, Greenway C 1981 Effect of prazosin and phenoxybenzamine and alpha-and beta-receptor mediated response in intestinal resistance and capacitance vessels. Journal of Cardiovascular Pharmacology 3: 1050–1059
2. Wood A J, Phelan E L, Simpson F O 1975 Cardiovascular effects of prazosin in normotensive and genetically hypertensive rats. Clinical Pharmacology and Physiology 2: 297
3. Cambridge D, Davey M J, Massingham R 1977 Prazosin, a selective antagonist of post-synaptic alpha adrenoceptors. British Journal of Pharmacology 59: 514p–515p
4. Hornung R, Presek P, Glassmann H 1979 α-adrenoceptors in rat brain: direct identification with prazosin. Archives of Pharmacology 308: 223–230
5. Brogden R N, Heel R C, Speight T M, Avery G S 1977 Prazosin: a review of its pharmacological properties and therapeutic efficacy in hypertension. Drugs 14: 163–197
6. Ram C V, Anderson R J, Hart G R, Crumpler C P 1981 α-adrenergic blockade by prazosin in therapy of essential hypertension. Clinical Pharmacology and Therapeutics 29: 719–722
7. Stanaszek W F, Kellerman D, Brogden R N, Romankiewicz J A 1983 Prazosin — pharmacological properties and therapeutic use in hypertension and congestive heart failure. Drugs 25: 339–384
8. Scriabine A 1980 Prazosin. In: Scriabine A (ed) Pharmacology of Antihypertensive Drugs. Raven Press, New York, pp 151–160
9. Chatterjee K, Rubin S A, Ports T A, Parmley W W 1981 Influence of oral prazosin therapy on exercise hemodynamics in patients with severe chronic heart failure. American Journal of Medicine 7: 140–146
10. Weidmann P, Uehlinger De, Gerber A 1985 Anti-hypertensive treatment and serum lipoproteins. Journal of Hypertension 3: 297–306
11. Twomey T M, Hobbs D C 1978 Analysis of prazosin in plasma by a sensitive high-performance liquid chromatographic-fluorescence method. Journal of Pharmaceutical Sciences 67: 1468–1469
12. Rubin P C, Scott P J W, Reid J L 1981 Prazosin disposition in young and elderly subjects. British Journal of Clinical Pharmacology 12: 401–404
13. Bateman D N, Hobbs D C, Twomey T M, Stevens E A, Rawlins M D 1979 Prazosin pharmacokinetics and concentration effect. European Journal of Clinical Pharmacology 16: 177–181
14. Verbesselt R, Mullie A, Tjandramaga T B 1976 The effect of food intake on the plasma kinetics and toleration of prazosin. Acta Therapeutica 2: 27-31
15. Jaillon P 1980 Clinical pharmacokinetics of prazosin. Clinical Pharmacokinetics 5: 365–376
16. McEvoy G K (ed) 1984 American Hospital Formulary Service, Drug Information. American Society of Hospital Pharmacists, Bethesda MD, p 542
17. Taylor L A, Twomey T M, Schuch von Wintenau M 1977 The metabolic fate of prazosin. Xenobiotica 7: 357–364
18. Jaillon P, Rubin Y, Yee Y G et al 1979 Influence of congestive heart failure on prazosin kinetics. Clinical Pharmacology and Therapeutics 26: 790–794
19. Baughman R A Jr, Arnold S, Benet L Z 1980 Altered prazosin pharmacokinetics in congestive heart failure. European Journal of Clinical Pharmacology 17: 425–428

20. Stokes G S, Monaghan J C, MacCarthy E P, Oates H F 1979 Responsiveness to prazosin in renal failure. Clinical Science 57: 383s–385s
21. Chaignon M, LeRoux E, Aubert P et al 1981 Clinical pharmacology of prazosin in hypertensive patients with chronic renal failure. Journal of Cardiovascular Pharmacology 3: 151–160
22. Graham R M, Thornell I R, Gain J M, Bagnoli C, Oates H F, Stokes G S 1977 A controlled study in hypertensive patients of the 'first dose phenomenon' observed with prazosin therapy. Australian and New Zealand Journal of Medicine 7: 211–212
23. Stokes G S, Graham R M, Gain J M, Davis P R 1977 Influence of dosage and dietary sodium on the first-dose effects of prazosin. British Medical Journal 1: 1507–1508
24. Fauchald P, Helgeland A, Storm-Mathiasen H 1979 Treatment of hypertension with prazosin. An open study in general practice. In: Rawlins M D et al (eds) Proceedings of European Prazosin Symposium, Vienna, 24–25th November 1978 International Congress Series no 475. Excerpta Medica, Amsterdam, pp 85–93
25. Marshall A J, McGraw M E, Barritt D W 1979 Positive antinuclear factor tests with prazosin. British Medical Journal 1: 165–166
26. Mroczek W J, Finnerty F A 1974 Prazosin — a double blind evaluation. In: Cottan et al (ed) Prazosin — evaluation of a new antihypertensive agent. Excerpta Medica, Amsterdam
27. Bolli P, Wood A J, Phelan E L, Lee D R, Simpson F O 1975 Prazosin: preliminary clinical and pharmacological observations. Clinical Science and Molecular Medicine 48: 177s–179s

Prednisolone and prednisone

Prednisolone and prednisone were amongst the earliest of the synthetic steroid drugs used in therapeutics. They are analogues of the natural corticosteroid cortisol and belong to a group of compounds known as 'glucocorticoids'.

Chemistry

Prednisolone is 1,2-dehydrocortisol which by dehydrogenation at the C-11 hydroxyl group is converted to prednisone. In dealing with the biological and clinical aspects of these two steroid drugs, in this monograph the names prednisone and prednisolone will often be used interchangeably.

Prednisolone (Codelcortone, Delta Phoricol, Deltacortril Enteric, Deltacortone, Deltalone, Deltastab, Marsolone, Precortisyl)

$C_{21}H_{28}O_5$

11β,17α,21-Trihydroxypregna-1,4-diene-3,20-dione

Prednisone (Decortisyl, Deltacortone, Econasone, Marsone)

$C_{21}H_{26}O_5$

17α,21-Dihydroxypregna-1,4-diene-3,11,20-trione

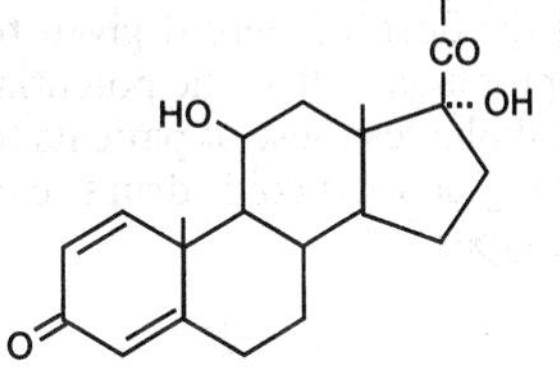

(Prednisolone)

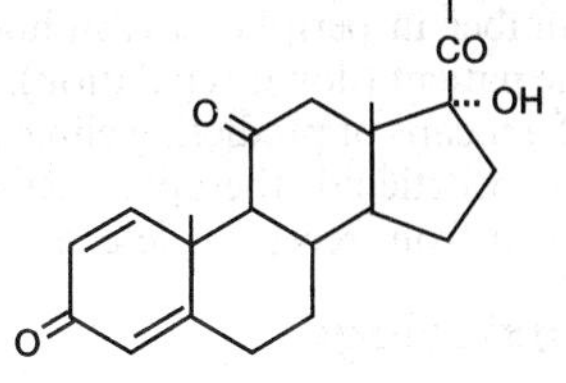

(Prednisone)

Prednisolone (Prednisone)	
Molecular weight	360.4 (358.4)
pKa	not ionizable (not ionizable)
Solubility	
in alcohol	1:35 (1:20)
in water	1:1300 (<1:10 000)
Octanol/water partition coefficient	high (high)

Both compounds are white or almost white, odourless, crystalline powders with a bitter taste. While the tablets for oral ingestion usually contain the parent steroid, preparations of prednisolone for parenteral and topical uses often contain an esterified derivative such as 21-acetate, hexanoate, pivolate, metasulphobenzoate and phosphate.

It is also available in a number of combination preparations, with hexachlorophane, Laureth '9' and heparinoid in Anacal, and as the hexanoate with cinchocaine hydrochloride in Scheriproct.

Pharmacology

Modification of cortisol structure to prednisone and prednisolone leads to enhanced biological potency in regard to metabolic actions, involution of lymphoid tissue and anti-inflammatory effect, while the mineralocorticoid property declines. Parallel increases in these activities may be multifactorial in origin, encompassing protein binding, rate of metabolic degradation and excretion, interaction with membranes, cellular transport of Ca^{2+} and action at the intracellular receptor level. Prolonged exposure to large doses of prednisolone can be diabetogenic with increased hepatic gluconeogenesis and glycogen storage. Peripheral utilization of glucose is curtailed and there is resistance to insulin. As a result of antianabolic and catabolic action

Prednisolone and prednisone

on proteins in peripheral tissues, there is raised amino acid availability to the liver and a negative nitrogen balance. Glucocorticoids may also induce calcium loss by affecting bone resorption and more importantly renal excretory mechanisms.

The major therapeutic uses of prednisolone and prednisone are based on the anti-inflammatory and immunosuppressive activities of glucocorticoids. The suppression of inflammatory response is independent of the initiating stimulus and the action is mainly local. Some important components of the mechanism underlying the anti-inflammatory effects of corticosteroids are (i) inhibition of the adherence of neutrophils and monocyte-macrophages to the capillary endothelial cells of the inflamed area, (ii) blocking of the effect of macrophage migration inhibitory factor, (iii) decreased activation of plasminogen to plasmin, and (iv) inhibition of phospholipase A_2 activity thereby lowering the formation of prostaglandins, leukotrienes and related compounds.

This suppression of inflammatory response by corticoids may also be a key feature of the way they counteract complications that arise from cell-mediated immune reactions. An acute effect of such steroids is sequestration of lymphocytes from blood although lysis of tissues also occurs, e.g. in lymphatic malignancies. At therapeutic dose levels corticoids do not seem to have any significant effect on circulating antibodies or on the metabolism of complement.

The two major targets of glucocorticoids, such as prednisolone, would be the liver (induction of enzymes, e.g. those involved in gluconeogenesis and amino acid degradation) and the lymphatic system (growth inhibitory actions which ultimately may result in cell death). The central feature of these hormonal actions is the combination of the steroid with an intracellular receptor, producing conformational changes that expose the DNA-binding domain on the receptor. The binding of the steroid–receptor complex to specific sequences, known as hormone response elements, brings about transcriptional activation or repression of specific genes. A significant negative correlation was shown between glucocorticoid receptor number in peripheral lymphocytes and the dose of steroid given to the patient (down-regulation). This receptor assay offers the potential of a means of predicting clinical and metabolic response of patients to glucocorticoid therapy.[1] Resistance to glucocorticoid drugs can result from receptor defects of different types.[2]

Toxicology

Teratogenic effects of glucocorticoids have not been demonstrated in the human. Although malignancies are known to arise in patients undergoing immunosuppression with corticosteroids, any role of these compounds in the induction of tumours remains uncertain. The classic toxic effects of prednisolone-like drugs are given under Adverse reactions.

Clinical pharmacology

Prednisone is almost quantitatively converted into the biologically more active form, prednisolone, in the liver; a fact that must be borne in mind when selecting one of these two steroids for patients with hepatic insufficiency. The plasma half life of prednisone is around 3.3 hours, whereas that of prednisolone is generally shorter. The anti-inflammatory activity and hypothalamic–pituitary–adrenal (HPA) suppression produced by prednisolone-like steroids, given orally, parallel each other in terms of degree and duration. The HPA axis thus provides a means of quantitating the therapeutic effects of such drugs. The very large differences (Table 1) between, for example, prednisone plasma half life and the duration of its biological actions imply that it is not the presence of the drug per se but the continuation of complex receptor-mediated events, initiated by prednisolone, which produces the result in the end.

The reasonable anti-inflammatory potency of prednisolone together with its low sodium-retaining activity allows, in general terms, a greater margin of safety in man. As the relevance of plasma prednisolone levels to its therapeutic efficacy still remains unproven, the use of this drug is largely empirical, aimed to give sufficient benefit with minimum complications.

Table 1 Approximate relative activity[3]

	Anti-inflammatory potency[a]	Daily dose (mg) above which HPA axis suppression possible[b]	Plasma half-life (min)	Biological half-life[c] (h)
Cortisol	1	20–30	90	8–12
Prednisone	3.5	7.5–10	200 or >	18–36
Prednisolone	4	7.5–10	200 or >	18–36
Betamethasone	25	1–1.5	300 or >	36–54

a. Potency is defined as a mg for mg equivalence with cortisol.
b. Intended as a general guide only.
c. Based on HPA axis suppression.

Pharmacokinetics

For the determination of prednisolone or prednisone levels in body fluids radioimmunoassay is the method of choice.[4,5] The limit of sensitivity is 10 μg.l^{-1}. An alternative is high performance liquid chromatography with u.v. detection at 254 nm. This procedure allows for the simultaneous analysis of the required combination of cortisol, prednisone, prednisolone and 6β-hydroxyprednisolone.[6,7] The limit of sensitivity is 5–10 μg.l^{-1}.

Both prednisone and prednisolone are readily absorbed from the gastrointestinal tract, producing peak plasma concentrations at approximately 1 to 2 hours after an oral dose. The availability of prednisolone in plasma after taking prednisone by mouth is usually in the region of 70–80% in healthy volunteers but can vary more widely in patients,[8,9] reflected in pronounced individual differences in peak plasma prednisolone levels and the areas under the plasma concentration versus time curves (AUC). For example, the mean peak plasma prednisolone levels after a 10 mg oral dose can range between 116 and 248 μg.l^{-1}. Food in the stomach or the use of some form of enteric-coated tablets may delay and reduce peak plasma drug levels but bioavailability may not be affected much. A sustained-release preparation of prednisolone may offer the advantage of a lesser degree of hypothalamic–pituitary–adrenal axis suppression than with standard tablets.[10]

Plasma prednisolone is mostly bound to albumin (low affinity, high capacity) and corticosteroid-binding globulin (CBG, high affinity, low capacity). The free concentrations of prednisolone can be affected by the plasma concentrations of these proteins, the concentration of total prednisolone and the presence of certain drugs. This ultimately can have serious implications for the disposition kinetics of the drug and the patient response to prednisolone.[7,11–14] The volume of distribution and clearance of both total and unbound prednisolone are concentration (and therefore dose) dependent and this has been attributed to saturable protein binding of the drug over the therapeutic plasma concentration range.[11]

The plasma half life of prednisolone, after a single dose of prednisolone, falls between 2.1–3.5 hours, whereas following prednisone it is generally longer, 3.4–3.8 h. A reduction in prednisolone metabolism by impairment of hepatic or renal function or by drugs such as cyclosporine and oral contraceptives prolongs the elimination half life[14–17] whilst acceleration of metabolism in hyperthyroidism and by enzyme-inducing drugs such as anticonvulsants and rifampicin will shorten the plasma elimination half life markedly.[18–22] Tuberculosis patients under rifampicin therapy had plasma prednisolone half lives of 1.4 ± 0.2 h (mean ± SD) compared with 2.5 ± 0.7 found in normal subjects.[18] The corresponding metabolic clearance rates (MCR) were 141 ± 53 l.m^{-2} daily and 75 ± 25 l.m^{-2} daily. Rifampicin therapy for 3 weeks reduced the area under the time–plasma concentration curve (AUC) of total prednisolone by 48% and of free prednisolone by 57%.[19] In children the elimination of plasma prednisolone tends to be more rapid than in adults, whereas in older, post-menopausal women elimination is slower.

The relationship between salivary and plasma total or unbound prednisolone concentration has yet to be resolved. On current evidence, saliva levels cannot replace those in plasma for prednisolone pharmacokinetic studies.[4,23]

Oral absorption	rapid (rapid)
Presystemic metabolism	5–20%
Plasma half life	
range	2.1–3.5 hours (3.4–3.8 hours)
mean	2.8 hours (3.6 hours)
Volume of distribution	30–44 l
Plasma protein binding	70–90%

Prednisolone and prednisone

Prednisolone is excreted in breast milk to a small extent, concentrations reaching 5–25% of those in plasma. Two hours after an oral dose of 10 mg prednisolone (when plasma prednisolone level would be expected to be between 150 and 200 $\mu g.l^{-1}$), breast milk was found to contain prednisone and prednisolone at 26.7 and 1.6 $\mu g.l^{-1}$ respectively.[24] Prednisolone can cross the placenta and give significant fetal concentrations.

Prednisolone is extensively metabolized, mainly in the liver. Over 90% of the dose is excreted in the urine, with 11–30% as free prednisolone and small amounts of prednisone.

Concentration–effect relationship

There does not appear to be a clear relationship between prednisolone pharmacokinetics or plasma (total or unbound) concentration and its therapeutic effect.[25–27]

Correlation, however, was observed between prednisolone pharmacokinetic values and the Cushingoid side effects of the drug.[28] Patients who showed these side effects also had significantly higher peak serum prednisolone concentrations, a longer elimination half life and a larger area under the time–concentration curve of total and free prednisolone.

Metabolism

The metabolic pathways of prednisolone and prednisone are far from clearly defined. The reactions concern oxidation–reduction at the C-11 position, reduction of the 20-keto group, cleavage of the dihydroxyacetone side chain, reduction of A ring double bonds and hydroxylation at the C-6 carbon. Over 90% of administered prednisolone is excreted in the urine within 48 hours, mostly as conjugated steroids. The 24-hour urinary free steroids comprise intact prednisolone (11–30% of dose), 6β-hydroxyprednisolone (2–10%), 20-dihydro metabolite and small amounts of prednisone.[4,29,30] There is an association between an enhanced non-renal clearance of prednisolone and the fractional excretion of 6β-hydroxyprednisolone in the urine. This metabolite might, therefore, be of some predictive value for plasma concentrations of prednisolone and thereby for adjusting its dosage in patients who fail to respond to treatment or develop side effects.

Pharmaceutics

Prednisolone is available in forms suitable for oral, parenteral and topical uses. While the tablets for oral ingestion usually contain the parent steroid, preparations for parenteral and topical uses often contain a derivative such as 21-acetate, hexanoate, pivolate, metasulphobenzoate and phosphate.

Prednisolone-21-acetate (tablet and injection, Deltastab).

Prednisolone-21-pivolate (injection, Ultracortesol).

Prednisolone-21-hexanoate (ointment and suppositories, Scheriproct).

Prednisolone-21-metasulphobenzoate (retention enema, Predenema).

Prednisolone-21-phosphate (oral tablets, injection, retention enema, eye and ear drops, Predsol, Prednesol, Codelsol, Minim Prednisolone). Predsol-N also contains 0.5% neomycin sulphate and 0.005% thiomersal.

Standard generic tablets are usually white and scored, containing 1 and 5 mg of prednisolone. Prednisolone disodium phosphate, Prednesol (Glaxo, UK) tablets are soluble, pink, scored tablets marked with 'PREDNESOL' and 'GLAXO'. Deltacortril (Pfizer, UK) are enteric-coated tablets 2.5 mg (brown) and 5 mg (red) and marked 'PFIZER'. Some tablets contain lactose and are therefore unsuitable for lactose-intolerant individuals.

Prednisolone (25 $mg.ml^{-1}$) in acetate form is used for intra-articular and intramuscular injections. The disodium phosphate ester, containing prednisolone equivalent to 16 $mg.ml^{-1}$, Codelsol (MSD, UK)/Hydeltrasol (MSD, US), is suitable for parenteral purposes. It is compatible with glucose 5% and sodium chloride 0.9% and may be given by intermittent or continuous infusion.

Prednisolone preparations for application to the colon or rectum include 20 mg retention enemas (phosphate and metasulphobenzoate), 5 mg suppositories (phosphate) and ointment (0.19% prednisolone hexadecanoate, 0.5% cinchocaine HCl and 1% clemizole undecanoate). Prednisolone sodium phosphate is also applied topically as eye drops at 0.5% concentrations either alone or with 0.5% neomycin sulphate. It is also available as a sterile ophthalmic ointment in the USA.

All preparations should be protected from light and stored in a cool place. The maximum shelf-life for most formulations is thought to be 3 years but for tablets it could be up to 5 years.

Therapeutic use

Indications

1. Glucocorticoid replacement therapy
2. Diseases of connective tissue
3. Asthma and other respiratory diseases
4. Diseases of the liver and gastrointestinal tract
5. Renal diseases
6. Ocular diseases
7. Blood disorders and malignancies
8. Miscellaneous diseases.

Contraindications

Except where its use may be life-saving prednisolone must be used with great caution in patients with the following conditions.

1. Peptic ulcer
2. Osteoporosis
3. Infections
4. Diabetes mellitus
5. Psychological disturbances.

Mode of use

For systemic therapy, prednisolone is generally used within the dose range of 5–60 mg given as a single dose early in the morning, in divided doses or as a double dose on alternate days. Large doses, given orally or as injections, used for a strictly limited period of time, may not produce serious complications, but treatment must be re-evaluated from time to time and in the long term the objective would be to reduce gradually the dose of oral prednisolone to a maintenance level of not more than 7 mg daily whenever possible. Further reduction may be possible depending on clinical circumstances. In conditions that are not life-threatening, starting doses should be small and increased step-wise as may be appropriate to obtain an acceptable response. It is important to define what response is to be monitored. While an alternate early morning regimen tends to produce less suppression of cortisol production, its effectiveness in a given clinical situation has to be established prior to use. Dose-spacing can also lower the prevalence of abnormal plasma lipids associated with the use of corticosteroids.[31]

Indications

1. Replacement therapy

Prednisolone/prednisone can be given by mouth, in physiological doses (ca. 5 mg daily) to patients with adrenal insufficiency or with congenital adrenal hyperplasia. For this condition, however, cortisone or hydrocortisone are more commonly used.

2. Diseases of connective tissue

Rheumatoid arthritis: in patients with progressive rheumatoid arthritis, corticosteroids should be considered only when all other forms of management fail or as an interim measure until another non-steroidal drug has taken effect. Steroids provide symptomatic relief, but to what extent the actual course of the disease is altered is uncertain. It seems likely that the suppression of inflammation in the synovial lining of the joints will protect the articular cartilage from further destruction.

The starting dose is usually 5 mg of prednisolone daily, given as a single dose in the morning or on alternate days; the dosage regimen is adjusted to individual patient response. In the absence of adequate improvement, steroid dose may be raised by 1 mg increments, at intervals of a few weeks, up to a maximum of 10 mg daily. It is essential to attempt a gradual reduction in the dose, say in 1 mg steps every month, as soon as the disease appears to have gone into remission. Intra-articular injection of 20 mg prednisolone or an equivalent dose of longer-acting corticosteroids is also used in the treatment of affected joints in rheumatoid arthritis and sometimes in osteoarthritis. Repeated injection, however, carries a significant risk of joint damage. Corticosteroid injections given locally can also ease pain in patients with frozen shoulder and tennis elbow.

Rheumatic carditis: corticosteroids are indicated in patients who fail to respond to salicylates or cannot tolerate them in high doses. The dose usually is 1 $mg.kg^{-1}$ body weight per day given in a single or divided doses for 7–10 days, thereafter reduced by 2.5 mg daily every 5–7 days.

Other diseases: corticosteroids have a role in the treatment of patients with polymyositis, polyarteritis nodosa and the granulomatous-polyarteritis group (Wegener's granulomatosis, temporal-cranial arteritis and polymyalgia rheumatica). In temporal (giant-cell) arteritis a high starting dose (80–200 mg prednisolone) is recommended in order to avoid more serious complications, particularly eye damage. Normally treatment may begin with 20–40 mg prednisolone daily, gradually reduced to not less than 7.5 mg. In polymyalgia rheumatica smaller doses of 10–12 mg of prednisolone brought down to a maintenance level of not less than 5 mg may be adequate. Patients with polymyositis should be given, as soon as diagnosis is confirmed, prednisolone at about 60 mg daily together with potassium supplement to prevent further weakening of muscle. A fall in plasma creatine kinase activity tends to precede symptomatic improvement, and can therefore be used to adjust steroid dosage to the maintenance level of around 12.5 mg. In systemic lupus erythematosus (SLE), small daily doses, 5–10 mg of prednisolone, may be beneficial if the symptoms are mainly articular. With renal involvement, larger doses, such as 60 mg, are more appropriate. Patients with SLE of the central nervous system require extremely high doses, between 100 and 150 mg, or even greater amounts, of prednisolone.

3. Asthma and other respiratory diseases

Corticosteroid therapy can be a valuable form of treatment for chronic asthma but the decision to use the systemic, rather than the inhaled, route must be taken with great caution. Prednisolone 5–10 mg orally as a single daily dose or in divided doses can be effective. Alternatively, an equivalent intermittent regimen may be preferred. Larger doses may be required temporarily during exacerbations.

During weaning from steroid therapy, there is some risk of relapse in which case steroid therapy may have to be resumed.

In status asthmaticus, large doses of corticosteroids may be given intravenously until the acute attack is under control. The patient is then put on 10 mg prednisolone, twice daily for a few days, before reducing the amount in steps. Corticosteroids, at a starting dose such as 20 mg prednisolone daily, may produce some response in acute cases of fibrosing alveolitis but only when the lung biopsy shows little fibrosis.

4. Diseases of the liver and gastrointestinal tract

There is a place for corticosteroid therapy in the management of some forms of subacute hepatic necrosis and chronic active hepatitis and acute hepatic failure due to viral and alcoholic hepatitis. The initial oral dose tends to vary between 40 and 100 mg daily and it may be followed, for example, in chronic active hepatitis by daily administration of up to 10 mg prednisolone in combination with an immunosuppressive agent such as azothioprine. As usual in corticosteroid therapy, the tapering of the dose to a maintenance regimen depends on the need of the individual patients.

Corticosteroids are useful adjuncts to the management of patients with inflammatory bowel diseases where the object is to induce a remission or control acute attacks before giving non-steroid drugs. Ulcerative colitis patients who are unresponsive to conservative treatment or have systemic features such as weight loss, fever and arthritis are likely to benefit from prednisolone therapy. Symptomatic response can also be achieved in Crohn's disease with extensive small bowel involvement. Prednisolone suppositories or enemas may be used when ulcerative colitis is confined to the rectum or the descending colon. Systemic therapy in these inflammatory bowel diseases usually consists of 20–60 mg of prednisolone, taken by mouth daily, although severely ill patients may need more before showing any sign of improvement. In certain situations combined systemic and topical modalities might be found most effective. Failure to show remission within the first few days of drug therapy can be an indication for surgery. Cases of idiopathic steatorrhoea which do not respond to a gluten-free diet can be treated with prednisolone daily at 7–10 mg doses per day.

5. Renal diseases

Corticosteroids may have some use in patients with some forms of nephrotic syndrome attributable to SLE or to glomerulonephritis, but not in those due to diabetes mellitus, renal vein thrombosis or amyloidosis. The doses vary; in lupus nephritis, for example, oral prednisolone dose is usually maintained at 10–25 mg daily and, in severe cases, given in combination with an immunosuppressive agent such as azothioprine. Administration of corticosteroids at a daily dose of about 60 mg prednisolone will induce remission in most patients with minimal change glomerulonephritis. The steroid dose is usually continued at around 20 mg dose level for periods up to 8 weeks. Subsequent relapses can also be treated with corticosteroids or with a cytotoxic agent such as cyclophosphamide. Short-term treatment with prednisolone as a single dose of 100–150 mg on alternate days can be beneficial in adult idiopathic nephrotic syndrome with membranous nephropathy.

6. Ocular diseases

Prednisolone is used to suppress inflammation in the eye. It is given locally as a lotion or ointment for diseases of the outer eye and anterior segment, whereas for disorders involving the posterior segment an oral dose of about 30 mg, given in divided amounts, is used.

Intraocular pressure should be monitored when prednisolone or any other such steroid is applied to the eye for more than 2 weeks.

7. Blood disorders and malignancies

Corticosteroid therapy is the treatment of choice for idiopathic warm autoimmune haemolytic anaemia. The starting dose is normally 60 mg prednisolone gradually reduced to 30 mg over a few weeks and then, if needed, to a maintenance level of about 15 mg daily. If the condition is associated with lymphoma or chronic lymphatic leukaemia the response is less certain. In thrombocytopenic purpura, a daily dose of 60–100 mg prednisolone usually reduces the amount of antibody on the platelets and raises the platelet count within 2 or 3 weeks. Subsequently the dose can be decreased to the lowest level, no more than 10–15 mg, that will keep the platelet count at the near-normal level.

Various antineoplastic combination regimens used in the management of acute leukaemias and lymphomas include prednisolone at levels of 40–100 $mg.m^{-2}$ per day. Short courses of prednisolone, 1–2 $mg.kg^{-1}$ body weight used alone or intermittently with a cytotoxic drug, are used to induce remission of multiple myeloma. High doses of the corticosteroid may also counteract hypercalcaemia and provide relief from pain in this and other malignant conditions with bone metastases.

Some modalities of combination chemotherapy for malignancies, e.g. of the breast, lung and prostate, include prednisone, given by mouth in amounts between 20 and 60 mg daily.

8. Miscellaneous diseases

Corticosteroids are used in various neurological disorders. For example, a favourable response may be expected in Bell's palsy to a short course of prednisolone, the dose starting at about 60 mg daily tapered off to 5 mg over a fortnight. Alternate-day dosage of 100 mg has been used in multiple sclerosis. Prednisolone therapy, 40–150 mg per day initially, has also been indicated in subacute demyelinating neuropathy.

In sarcoidosis, corticosteroids are used at doses of between 20 and 30 mg prednisolone daily but only in patients with extensive pulmonary infiltration causing severe complications. Long-term therapy may be required.

Doses of prednisolone, 5–10 mg or more daily depending on serum calcium levels, can relieve hypercalcaemia.

In transplantation of heart, liver and kidney, large amounts (1–1.5 $mg.kg^{-1}$ body weight) of prednisolone are given daily at the time of surgery, usually together with immunosuppressive agents. A small maintenance dose at the level of 7–10 mg per day has to be continued indefinitely. Doses of 0.5–1 g of steroid may need to be given intravenously at 12–24 hour intervals to overcome the threat of graft rejection.

Contraindications

1. Peptic ulcer

Disruption of the gastric mucosal barrier resulting in peptic ulceration had always been suspected to be an occasional complication of corticosteroid therapy. However, an association between peptic ulcers and corticosteroid drugs, especially when given at standard doses, is by no means clearly established. In one survey it was concluded that corticosteroids approximately doubled the risk of peptic ulcer.[32]

2. Osteoporosis
Derangement of calcium metabolism by corticosteroids and catabolic effects on bone matrix pose potential hazards to patients with pre-existing osteoporosis. In suspected cases and in postmenopausal females it may be advisable to obtain lumbo-sacral spine films prior to initiating prolonged steroid treatment.

3. Infections
The possibility of a pre-existing infection, bacterial, viral or fungal, can have serious implications in corticosteroid therapy. At high doses, especially when used in conjunction with other immunosuppressive agents, these steroids tend to aggravate such infections and activate quiescent foci, e.g. tuberculosis. Prophylactic measures must be taken in these circumstances. Corticosteroids are also likely to mask the symptoms of infection until an advanced stage has been reached with the consequence that, for example, severe irreversible damage to the cornea can result from the use of corticoid drugs in herpes simplex infection of the eye.

Corticosteroids can also cause the spread of certain infections in an unusual way, at times in aberrant forms, such as in disseminated parasitic disease. Children who have been vaccinated with live organisms should not be treated with corticosteroids.

4. Diabetes mellitus
Prolonged corticosteroid therapy can unmask latent diabetes mellitus or aggravate pre-existing disease. These patients are also vulnerable to corticosteroid-mediated glaucoma.

5. Psychological disturbances
Patients with known emotional instabilities or psychotic tendencies may experience adverse responses of glucocorticoids, ranging from insomnia to schizophrenia and suicide attempts. Unfortunately, there is no way to predict how individual patients may react to treatment.

Adverse reactions

As a corticosteroid drug of modest potency, the adverse effects of prednisolone are usually to be found only when used in large doses, and to a greater extent, with prolonged use. These complications generally arise from, (a) suppression of the hypothalamic–pituitary–adrenal axis, (b) exaggerated actions of the steroid drug and (c) interference with immune defence mechanisms.
The incidence of adverse effects of prednisolone rises markedly with increases in the dosage above 10 mg per day.

Potentially life-threatening effects
Acute adrenal insufficiency may be precipitated by an infection, surgery or trauma in patients on long-term corticosteroid therapy or following cessation of steroid use. Failure to institute adequate corticosteroid cover during such crises may cause death.

Acute overdosage
Massive doses of corticosteroids, given intravenously as a 'pulse' in emergencies, tend to be free from hazardous consequences. As the 'therapeutically effective dose' of a corticosteroid varies according to the indications for it and the requirements of individual patients, to define an excessive dose is hardly possible. However, with continued use of large doses, often necessary to achieve a clinical response, in cases where the dose is not reduced to a more modest maintenance regimen exaggeration of usual corticosteroid-related problems is inevitable.

Severe or irreversible adverse effects
Major severe side effects arise from suppression of adrenal function and immune defence mechanisms, and from iatrogenic hyperadrenocorticism (Cushing's syndrome). These complications include growth retardation in children, osteoporosis and aseptic bone necrosis, peptic ulceration, ocular hypertension, subcapsular cataract, pancreatic disturbances and myopathy.

Other Cushing-like features characteristic of glucocorticoid excess include truncal obesity, moon-face, oedema, delayed wound healing, glaucoma, benign intracranial hypertension and psychiatric syndromes. These are reversible. Growth retardation in children receiving long-term oral corticosteroid treatment involves both linear bone growth and epiphysial closure. Accelerated growth may be seen when steroids are discontinued. Osteoporosis and vertebral compression fractures are often encountered in corticosteroid therapy. Ribs and vertebrae, bones with a high degree of trabecular structure, are usually the most seriously affected. Intra-articular injections of corticosteroids have also been implicated in the aetiology of aseptic necrosis of the bone. Corticosteroids have been associated with a high incidence of peptic ulcer involving haemorrhage and perforation. Raised intraocular pressure may be seen in up to 40% of patients receiving ocular or systemic steroids. It is reversible but in certain genetically predisposed subjects and in diabetics, irreversible glaucoma and blindness can occur. Intraocular pressure should, therefore, be checked routinely in patients receiving corticosteroids. Pancreatitis or disturbance of pancreatic endocrine secretion can appear at any time during long-term corticosteroid use.

Symptomatic adverse effects
Standard low-dose therapy with prednisolone is generally free from untoward symptoms. On a long-term basis, however, minor gastrointestinal disturbances, such as nausea and vomiting, may occur. Nocturia is fairly common during corticosteroid treatment.

Increased appetite, obesity, facial-rounding and fragility of skin are some of the prime indicators of glucocorticoid overactivity. Even low-dose steroid treatment can produce such effects if the duration of treatment is long enough.

Behavioural and personality changes can be caused by corticosteroids especially at higher doses. The symptoms range from nervousness, insomnia and euphoria to serious psychotic episodes.

Other effects
Hyperglycaemia and a low renal threshold to glucose develop in a large proportion of patients on prednisolone therapy. This reversible, mild form of diabetes appears to develop more frequently in those who have HLA-A28 antigens and are older than 40 years; it, however, has no adverse effects on graft or patient survival in renal transplant recipients.[33] Insulin requirements of diabetes patients are increased. Another related feature of corticoid therapy is hyperlipidaemia, which may be a contributory factor in post-transplant arteriosclerotic vascular disease. Among other changes, increased excretion of uric acid, calcium and phosphate are important because of their association with renal disorder and bone diseases. Plasma testosterone may be suppressed by long-term use of prednisolone which may contribute to the development of osteoporosis and soft tissue atrophy.[34]

Interference with clinical pathology tests[35]
Both prednisone and prednisolone can interfere with the measurement of plasma cortisol due to cross-reactivity in the competitive protein binding and some immunoassay methods. Other changes are primarily biological in origin, for example, high blood glucose and impaired glucose tolerance tests, reduced T_3 and TBG, increased reverse T_3 and thyroxin-binding prealbumin. In women, prednisolone reduces LH and FSH response to LHRF.

High risk groups

Neonates
Corticosteroids should be avoided in babies under 1 year.

Breast milk. Prednisolone is excreted in small amounts in the breast milk of nursing mothers receiving the drug. The concentration of the steroid in milk can be between 5 and 25% of those in serum and the two roughly parallel one another after an oral dose. Breast-feeding may be permitted at maternal prednisolone doses of up to 20 mg once or twice daily. At higher doses feeding should be avoided within at least 4 hours after a dose of prednisolone.[36]

Children
The use of corticosteroid drugs carries much greater risk in children than in adults. The principal hazards, especially in long-term oral use, are obesity and growth retardation.

Pregnant women
Despite a previously postulated connection between corticosteroid ingestion during pregnancy and an increased incidence of abortions, placental insufficiency and congenital malformations in the offspring, no noticeable rise in maternal or fetal complications was observed in

Prednisolone and prednisone

P

asthmatic mothers who were given 2.5–30 mg prednisolone daily.[37] Corticosteroid drugs taken during the late stages of pregnancy are more likely to have direct effects on the fetus leading to problems of infection and adrenal insufficiency in the child. Another potential source of danger would be maternal steroid-induced diabetes.

The elderly

The achievement of symptomatic relief with drugs like prednisolone may be justified at an earlier stage in elderly patients than would be considered in younger subjects. By using low doses a correct balance can be struck between sufficient therapeutic response and the adverse effects of steroids.

In the elderly subjects to 65–89 years of age, clearance of unbound prednisolone was found to be lower than in the younger ones; but the suppression of their plasma cortisol was relatively smaller.[38]

Drug interactions

Potentially hazardous interactions

Anticonvulsant drugs. The actions of prednisolone are blunted in patients receiving concomitant therapy with drugs like barbiturates or phenytoin.[20,21,39] The reason is the stimulation of hepatic drug-metabolizing enzymes by these drugs, resulting in enhancement of prednisolone clearance from circulation. As the extent of this effect appears to vary with the anticonvulsant drug used, it has been suggested that different pathways for prednisolone metabolism may be implicated.[20]

Rifampicin. Non-responsiveness to prednisolone has been attributed to concurrently administered rifampicin which is a known inducer of drug metabolism.[40–42] This effect is reversed when rifampicin is discontinued.

Rifampicin accelerates prednisolone metabolism which causes a marked reduction in the bioavailability of total and especially free prednisolone (see section on Pharmacokinetics).

Other significant interactions

Cyclosporine. Cyclosporine decreases the metabolism of prednisolone in the early phase of the combination therapy. Accordingly, plasma half lives are prolonged and clearance reduced.[17,43] Prednisolone dosage in such cases may, therefore, require adjustment.

Corticosteroids. Previous long-term treatment with other corticosteroids may reduce plasma prednisolone half life.

Oral contraceptives and oestrogens. Alterations in the plasma protein binding and metabolism of prednisolone caused by these drugs can result in exposure of women to increased levels of unbound prednisolone for prolonged periods of time. This is likely to have therapeutic implications.

Non-steroidal anti-inflammatory drugs. Concurrent administration of corticosteroids and large doses of aspirin may cause changes in salicylate plasma protein binding and its rate of metabolism, thereby lowering plasma salicylate levels.

Other drugs. Patients with Graves' disease receiving carbimazole or methimazole have enhanced prednisolone metabolism; this results in significant increases in the clearances of both protein-bound and unbound prednisolone and decreases in plasma half lives.[44] The antifungal drug ketoconazole was reported to cause impairment of metabolic and renal clearances of total and unbound prednisolone.[45]

Antacids. Prednisolone absorption may be impaired if a small amount of it is taken with large doses of antacids.

Insulin. In patients receiving corticosteroid drugs, the requirement of insulin is generally increased.

Food. Food delays the peaking of plasma prednisolone concentration but does not affect overall bioavailability.

Potentially useful interactions

Combination of relatively low cyclosporine doses with low prednisolone can improve graft survival in renal transplant patients. Attempt to withdraw prednisolone altogether, even one year after transplant, could lead to high incidence of rejection.[46]

Major outcome trials

1. Million R, Kellgren J H, Poole P, Jayson M I 1984 Long-term study of management of rheumatoid arthritis. Lancet 1: 812–816

This was a 10-year comparative study of two rheumatoid arthritis treatment programmes involving prednisolone. One modality consisted of rest and anti-inflammatory and antirheumatic drugs and the other comprised maintenance activity, anti-inflammatory and antiheumatic drugs and, when necessary, systemic steroids, up to a maximum of 20 mg prednisolone per day. Those patients remaining for assessment at the end of the 10 years, 29 in the first group and 37 in the second, showed little difference in terms of morning stiffness, number of inflamed joints, functional capacity, grip strength, number of American Rheumatic Association criteria present and rheumatic factor.

However, in those who started in the steroid group, the condition of several joints tended to be better clinically and radiologically than in those of the other group during and at the end of the treatment period. Both groups had as many complications of disease and treatment, and adverse effects attributable to disease seemed to be restricted to those with severe disease who had not responded to the original programme. These findings suggested that in the long term, the maintenance of mobility with judicious use of steroids, when necessary, were at least as effective and possibly better than the outcome observed with bedrest and no steroids.

2. Mitchell D M, Gildeh P, Rehahn M et al 1984 Effects of prednisolone in chronic airflow limitation. Lancet 2: 193–196

Prednisolone was given at dose levels of 40 mg daily for 14 days to 43 patients with chronic airflow limitation (mean age, 60 years, mean forced expiratory volume FEV_1 1.02 litres, FEV_1/forced vital capacity FVC ratio 43.7%) in a double-blind, randomized, placebo-controlled crossover trial. Compared with the placebo effects, a significant improvement of general well-being, exercise performance, peak expiratory flow, FEV_1, FVC and relaxed vital capacity was seen with prednisolone.

It was concluded that a proportion of patients with chronic airflow limitation derived benefit from oral steroids, but the findings did not produce any useful way of predicting steroid responsiveness.

3. Johns L J, Schonfeld S A, Scott P P, Zachary J B, MacGregor M I 1986 Longitudinal study of chronic sarcoidosis with low-dose maintenance corticosteroid therapy. Outcome and complications. Annals of the New York Academy of Science 465: 702–711

A group of 181 patients (78% black) with chronic persistent sarcoidosis for more than 5 years were reviewed with a mean follow-up period of 14 years. Treatment was usually initiated with prednisone 40 mg daily reduced at 2-week intervals to 30, 25, 20 and then to 10 mg daily. One of the objectives of the study was to evaluate the effects and complications of corticosteroid treatment.

Of the 91% of patients receiving prednisone, 53% required continued treatment, two thirds of them with doses of no more than 10 mg daily. Relapses were frequent as prednisone was withdrawn. However, the benefit of treatment greatly exceeded the infrequent complications.

4. Kemeter P, Feichtinger W 1986 Prednisolone supplementation to Clomid and/or gonadotrophin stimulation for in vitro fertilisation — a prospective randomised trial. Human Reproduction 1 (7): 441–444

A daily 7.5 mg dose of prednisolone was given, in addition to Clomid and/or gonadotrophins, to the test group in a prospective and randomized trial involving a total of 146 patients. Significantly more clinical pregnancies occurred after in vitro fertilization in the prednisolone group. A lowering of adrenal and ovarian androgen production by prednisolone was implicated.

5. Lai K N, Lai F M, Ho C P, Chan K W 1986 Corticosteroid therapy in IGA nephropathy with nephrotic syndrome: a long-term controlled trial. Clinical Nephrology 26: 174–188

The use of corticosteroids was assessed in a randomized prospective study of 34 patients with IGA nephropathy. Prednisolone or prednisone was given for 4 months to 17 patients and the rest of the group acted as controls. Judging by changes in renal function, there was an overall lack of therapeutic value of the steroids in IGA nephropathy with nephrotic syndrome. However, in 80% of the patients with mild glomerular histopathological changes, corticosteroid treatment produced excellent remission of nephrotic syndrome.

Prednisolone and prednisone

6. Smerdon D L, Hung S O, Akingbehin T 1986 Double-blind controlled trial to compare anti-inflammatory effects of tolmetin 2%, prednisolone 0.5% and placebo in post-cataract extraction eyes. British Journal of Opthalmology 70: 761–763

In a double-blind clinical trial involving 120 patients, the potencies of prednisolone and tolmetin in controlling post-cataract inflammation were evaluated. The treatment with prednisolone was found to be more effective than with tolmetin or placebo.

7. Storr J, Barrell B, Barry W, Lenney W, Hatcher G 1987 Effect of a single oral dose of prednisolone in acute childhood asthma. Lancet 1: 879–882

In a randomized double-blind trial, 140 children with acute asthma took part; the aim was to compare oral prednisolone (30 mg in children under 5 years, otherwise, 60 mg) with placebo given soon after admission to hospital. All patients received solbutamol.

On the basis of fitness for discharge within a few hours after prednisolone dose, the duration of stay in the hospital and the requirement of further steroid therapy, the authors concluded that in acute asthma, the prompt use of a single dose of oral prednisolone could reduce morbidity and need for hospitalization. No steroid side effect was observed, but then the progress after discharge was not closely monitored.

8. Strang J I, Kazaka H H, Gibson D C et al 1987 Controlled trial of prednisolone as adjuvant in treatment of tuberculous constrictive pericarditis in Transkei. Lancet 2: 1418–1422

This was a study of 143 patients with active tuberculous constrictive pericarditis without significant pericardial effusion. In it assessment was made of the use of prednisolone or placebo for 11 weeks prior to a common 6-month long antituberculous regimen including isoniazid and rifampicin therapy.

In the 114 patients assessed double-blind for periods of up to 24 months, improvement, as indicated by the rate of fall in the mean pulse rate and the rate at which jugular venous pressure and level of physical activity returned to normal, was more rapid in the prednisolone group. Regarding the symptoms and signs of constriction, by 24 months, 94% of the prednisolone group and 85% of the placebo group had a favourable status: 77% and 62% respectively had achieved this by 6 months.

9. Shiner RJ, Nunn AJ, Chung AF, Geddes DM 1990 Randomised, double-blind, placebo-controlled trial of methotrexate in steroid dependent asthma. Lancet 336: 137–140.

69 patients with steroid-dependent asthma (mean daily prednisolone dose 14.2 mg) took part in a randomized study in which methotrexate or a matched placebo, 15 mg weekly was given for 24 weeks. The patients were seen every 4 weeks by a physician who reduced the prednisolone dose in accordance with diary card responses and lung function test results.

After 24 weeks the prednisolone dose had been reduced by 50% in the methotrexate group and only 14% in the placebo group. Six patients who took methotrexate were weaned off all steroids. Abnormalities of liver function tests occurred in 12 of 38 patients given methotrexate and three of them were withdrawn because the serum aminotransferase activities were more than 4 times the baseline value. In two others, who continued, aminotransferase values were still deteriorating at 24 weeks. Gastrointestinal symptoms (heartburn, nausea, bloated abdomen, diarrhoea) were reported by 8 of the methotrexate-treated patients and two patients were withdrawn because of them. The authors comment that many questions still remain about methotrexate therapy, in its own right or as a steroid-sparing agent, in asthma.

General review articles

Axelrod L 1976 Glucocorticoid therapy. Medicine 55(1): 39–65

Haynes R C, Murad F 1985 Adrenocorticotrophic hormone: adrenocortical steroids and their synthetic analogs. In: Gilman A G, Goodman L S, Rall T W, Murad F (eds) Gilman's the pharmacological basis of therapeutics, 7th edn. Macmillan Publishing Company, New York, ch 63, pp 1459–1489

Melby J C 1974 Systemic corticosteroid therapy: pharmacology and endocrinologic considerations. Annals of Internal Medicine 81: 505–512

Morris H G 1985 Mechanisms of action and therapeutic role of corticosteroids in asthma. Journal of Allergy and Clinical Immunology 75 (1): 1–14

Myles A B, Daly J R 1974 Corticosteroid and ACTH treatment. Edward Arnold, London

Pickup M E 1979 Clinical pharmacokinetics of prednisone and prednisolone. Clinical Pharmacokinetics 4: 111–128

Reynolds J E F (ed) 1982 Corticosteroids. In: Martindale the extra pharmacopoeia, 27th edn. The Pharmaceutical Press, London, pp 446–485

References

1. Oshima H 1986 Studies on the glucocorticoid receptor in human peripheral lymphocytes. III Correlation between receptor number and clinical response to glucocorticoids. Nippon Naibunpi Gakkai Zasshi 62: 1306–1314
2. Gehring U 1988 Glucocorticoid receptor actions. In: Cooke B A, King R J B (eds) Hormones and their actions, Part I. Elsevier Science Publishers BV (Biomedical Division), Oxford
3. Swartz S L, Dluty R G 1978 Corticosteroids: clinical pharmacology and therapeutic use. Drugs 16: 238–255
4. Chakraborty J, Hayes M, English J, Baylis E M, Marks V 1981 Prednisolone concentration in plasma, saliva and urine. European Journal of Clinical Pharmacology 19: 79–81
5. Olivesi A, Smith D S, White G W, Pourfarzaneh M 1983 Specific microradioimmunoassay for prednisolone in serum. Clinical Chemistry 29: 1358–1362
6. Scott N R, Chakraborty J, Marks V 1980 Determination of prednisolone, prednisone and cortisol in human plasma by high-performance liquid chromatography. Analytical Biochemistry 108: 266–268
7. Renner E, Horber F F, Gost G, Frey B M, Frey F J 1986 Effect of liver function on the metabolism of prednisone and prednisolone in humans. Gastroenterology 90: 819–828
8. Davis M, Williams R, Chakraborty J et al 1978 Prednisone or prednisolone for the treatment of chronic acute hepatitis? A comparison of plasma availability. British Journal of Clinical Pharmacology 5: 501–505
9. Henderson R G, Wheatley T, English J, Chakraborty J, Marks V 1979 Variation in plasma prednisolone concentration in renal transplant recipients given enteric-coated prednisolone. British Medical Journal 1: 1534–1537
10. English J, Chakraborty J, Marks V, Trigger D J, Thomson A G 1975 Prednisolone levels in the plasma and urine: a study of two preparations in man. British Journal of Clinical Pharmacology 2: 327–332
11. Legler U D, Frey F J, Benet L Z 1982 Prednisolone clearance at steady state in man. Journal of Clinical Endocrinology and Metabolism 55: 762–767
12. Legler U D, Benet L Z 1986 Marked alterations in dose-dependent prednisolone kinetics in women taking oral contraceptives. Clinical Pharmacology and Therapeutics 39: 425–429
13. Reece P A 1985 Protein binding in renal transplant patients. British Journal of Clinical Pharmacology 20: 159–162
14. Gustavson L E, Legler U F, Benet L Z 1986 Impairment of prednisolone disposition in women taking oral contraceptives or conjugated estrogens. Journal of Clinical Endocrinology and Metabolism 62: 234–237
15. Frey B M, Frey F J 1985 The effect of altered prednisolone syndrome in women taking oral contraceptive steroids on human mixed lymphocyte cultures. Journal of Clinical Endocrinology and Metabolism 60: 361–369
16. Kawai S, Ichikawa Y, Homma M 1985 Differences in metabolic properties among cortisol prednisolone and dexamethasone in liver and renal diseases: accelerated metabolism of dexamethasone in renal failure. Journal of Clinical Endocrinology and Metabolism 85: 848–854
17. Ost L 1987 Impairment of prednisolone metabolism by cyclosporine treatment in renal graft recipients. Transplantation 44: 533–535
18. Kawai S 1985 A comparative study of the accelerated metabolism of cortisol, prednisolone and dexamethasone in patients under rifampicin therapy. Nippon Naibunpi Bakkai Zasshi 61: 145–161
19. Bergrem H, Refvem O K 1983 Altered prednisolone pharmacokinetics in patients treated with rifampicin. Acta Medica Scandinavica 213: 339–343
20. Bartoszek M, Brenner A M, Szefler S J 1987 Prednisolone and methylprednisolone kinetics in children receiving anticonvulsant therapy. Clinical Pharmacology and Therapeutics 42: 424–432
21. Jubiz W, Meikle A W 1979 Alterations of glucocorticoid actions by other drugs and disease states. Drugs 18: 113–121
22. Frey F J, Horber F F, Frey B M 1988 Altered metabolism and efficacy of prednisolone and prednisone in patients with hyperthyroidism. Clinical Pharmacology and Therapeutics 44: 510–521
23. Al-Habet S M, Rogers H J 1985 Prednisolone elimination in human saliva. International Journal of Clinical Pharmacology and Therapeutic Toxicology 23: 485–487
24. Katz E H, Duncan B E 1975 Entry of prednisone into human milk. New England Journal of Medicine 293: 1154
25. Naik R B, Chakraborty J, English J, Marks V, Slapak M, Lee H A 1980 Serious renal transplant rejection and adrenal hypofunction after gradual withdrawal of prednisolone two years after transplantation. British Medical Journal 280: 1337–1340
26. Hayes M, Alam A F M S, Bruckner F E et al 1983 Plasma prednisolone studies in rheumatic patients. Annals of Rheumatic Diseases 42: 151–154

27. Greenburger P A, Chew M J, Atkinson A J, Ambre J J, Patterson R 1986 Comparison of prednisolone kinetics in patients receiving daily or alternate-day prednisone for asthma. Clinical Pharmacology and Therapeutics 39: 163–168
28. Bergrem H, Jervell J, Flatmark A 1985 Prednisolone pharmacokinetics in cushingoid and non-cushingoid kidney transplant patients. Kidney International 27: 459–464
29. Sandberg A A, Slannwhite W R 1957 Differences in metabolism of prednisolone-C^{14} and cortisol-C^{14}. Journal of Clinical Endocrinology 17: 1040–1050
30. Frey F J, Frey B M 1983 Urinary 6 β-hydroxyprednisolone excretion indicates enhanced prednisolone catabolism. Journal of Laboratory and Clinical Medicine 101: 593–604
31. Curtis J J, Galla J H, Woodford J Y, Lucas B A, Luke R G 1982 Effect of alternate-day prednisone on plasma lipids in renal transplant patients. Kidney International 22: 42–47
32. Messer J, Reitman D, Sacks S R, Smith H, Chalmers T C 1983 Association of adrenocorticosteroid therapy and peptic ulcer disease. New England Journal of Medicine 309: 21–24
33. David D S, Cheigh J S, Braun D W, Folino H, Stenzel K H, Rubin A L 1980 HLA-A28 and steroid-induced diabetes in renal transplant patients. Journal of the American Medical Association 243: 532–533
34. Reid I R, Ibbertson H K, France J T, Pybus J 1985 Plasma testosterone in asthmatic men treated with glucocorticoids. British Medical Journal 291: 574
35. Salway J G (ed) 1989 Drug test interactions handbook. Chapman Hall Medical, London, Raven Press, New York
36. Ost L, Wettrell G, Bjorkhem I, Rane A 1985 Prednisolone excretion in human milk. Journal of Pediatrics 106: 1008–1011
37. Schartz M, Patterson R, Zeitz S, O'Rourke J, Melam H 1975 Corticosteroid therapy for the pregnant asthmatic patients. Journal of the American Medical Association 233: 804–807
38. Stuck A E, Frey B, Frey F J 1988 Kinetics of prednisolone and endogenous cortisol suppression in the elderly. Clinical Pharmacology and Therapeutics 43: 354–362
39. Petereit L B, Meikle A N 1977 Effectiveness of prednisolone during phenytoin therapy. Clinical Pharmacology and Therapeutics 22: 912–916
40. Hendrickse W, Mckierman J, Pickup M, Lowe J 1979 Rifampicin induced steroid non-responsiveness in the nephrotic syndrome. British Medical Journal 1: 306
41. Powel I, Jackson P R, Grey B J et al 1983 Adverse effects of rifampicin administration on steroid-dependent asthma. American Review of Respiratory Diseases 128: 307–310
42. McAllister W A, Thompson P J, Al-Habet S M, Rogers H J 1983 Rifampicin reduces effectiveness and bioavailability of prednisolone. British Medical Journal 286: 923–925
43. Langhoff E, Madsens S, Olgaard K, Ladefoged J 1985 Clinical results and cyclosporine effect on prednisolone metabolism of cadaver kidney transplanted patients. Proceedings European Dialysis Transplant Association European Renal Association 21: 963–968
44. Legler U F 1987 Enhanced prednisolone elimination: a possible cause for failure of glucocorticoid therapy in Graves ophthalmology. Hormone Metabolism and Disposition 19: 168–170
45. Zurcher R M, Frey B M, Frey F J 1989 Impact of ketoconazole on the metabolism of prednisolone. Clinical Pharmacology and Therapeutics 45: 366–372
46. Brown M W, Forwell M A 1986 Rejection reaction after stopping prednisolone in kidney-transplant recipients taking cyclosporine. New England Journal of Medicine 314: 183

Prilocaine (hydrochloride)

Prilocaine hydrochloride is an amide-type local anaesthetic. It has the highest therapeutic ratio of any drug in that group.

Chemistry

Prilocaine hydrochloride (Citanest, Xylonest)
$C_{13}H_{20}N_2O.HCl$
2-Propylaminopropriono-o-toluidide hydrochloride

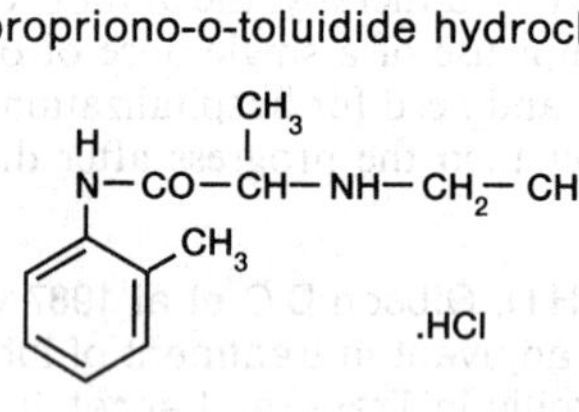

Molecular weight (free base)	256.8 (220.3)
pKa (amino)	7.9
Solubility	
in alcohol	1 in 6
in water	1 in 5
Octanol/water partition coefficient	high

Prilocaine is a white, odourless, crystalline powder with a bitter, numbing taste. It is prepared by chemical synthesis.[1]

The hydrochloride salt is available only in solution. It can be obtained in combination with felypressin as a dental preparation (Citanest with Octapressin). In some countries the free base of the anaesthetic is available mixed with lignocaine base for topical application — the eutectic mixture of local anaesthetics (EMLA).[2]

Pharmacology

Prilocaine is used primarily as a local anaesthetic drug, but it has a stabilizing action on all excitable membranes. Like other local anaesthetic agents it has both antiarrhythmic and weak neuromuscular blocking actions.[3]

Toxicology

Little data is available on potential mutagenic or carcinogenic effects. Studies in rabbits[4] and rats[5] have failed to show a teratogenic effect. Recent studies[6] showed no evidence of mutagenic potential in Ames test (with or without metabolic activation) or in mouse micronucleus test. The parent compound does not have any specific adverse actions, but one metabolite reduces haemoglobin (see 'Metabolism').

Clinical pharmacology

The nerve-blocking characteristics of prilocaine are similar to those of lignocaine. Its lower partition coefficient (indicating lower lipid solubility) and the results of in vitro studies[7] suggest that it is less potent, but in clinical use the two drugs are considered to be equipotent. Prilocaine lacks the vasodilator action of lignocaine[8] so that higher concentrations of the drug are maintained around the nerve for longer and this compensates for its inherently weaker action. The rate of onset is similar to lignocaine, but the duration of action is longer.[9,10]

Prilocaine is rapidly absorbed from the site of injection, the rate of

Pharmacokinetics

The preferred analytical method, gas–liquid chromatography with flame ionization detection, has a limit of sensitivity of 0.5 $mg.l^{-1}$ and a coefficient of variation of 7%.[11]

Prilocaine (hydrochloride)

Prilocaine is rapidly absorbed from the site of injection, the rate of rise in plasma concentration, and the peak, depending on the particular local anaesthetic technique used. There is also a degree of interindividual variation, and peak plasma concentrations occur between 5 and 30 minutes after administration. The addition of a vasoconstrictor will delay absorption and result in lower plasma concentrations. The plasma half life of prilocaine is 1–2 h, with a mean of 93 min.[12] The major site of metabolism is the liver, but unlike other amide local anaesthetics extrahepatic sites may contribute significantly to the biotransformation of this drug.[13]

Prilocaine has the largest volume of distribution (261 litres) of any of the amide local anaesthetics.[12] As a result, plasma concentrations of prilocaine are lower than those of similar drugs, regardless of the route of administration.[14,15] The combination of these two features means that the risk of toxic concentrations being produced systemically is less than with other amide local anaesthetics. At the concentrations of prilocaine achieved therapeutically, 40–55% of the drug is bound to plasma proteins,[12] mainly α_1 acid glycoprotein.

It is not known if the drug is excreted in breast milk.

Oral absorption	—
Presystemic metabolism	—
Plasma half life	
range	1–2 h
mean	93 min
Volume of distribution	261 l
Plasma protein binding	50%

Prilocaine is extensively metabolized, largely in the liver, with less than 3% of the dose excreted unchanged in the urine.

Concentration–effect relationship

Concentrations in the range 0.5–2% (depending on the size of the nerve to be blocked) are required to produce nerve block clinically. Although it is difficult to correlate the appearance of toxic symptoms with plasma concentrations, those in excess of 5–6 mg.l^{-1} are likely to produce subjective and objective systemic effects. The concomitant administration of sedative and general anaesthetic agents will raise this threshold figure considerably.

Metabolism

Only a small proportion of the drug (2–3%) is excreted unchanged in the urine and the rest is metabolized.[16] The major site of metabolism is the liver, although studies in vitro[16] have shown that renal tissue can metabolize the drug. The contribution, if any, of such metabolism to the biotransformation of the drug in vivo has yet to be determined. There is also some, as yet unsubstantiated, evidence for metabolism in the lung.[13]

The main route of metabolism of prilocaine is enzymic hydrolysis of the amide linkage. One of the products is *o*-toluidine. However, only 1% of the dose is excreted in the urine as this compound, most of it being *f*-hydroxylated before excretion in the urine (35% of the dose). There is a minor amount of 6-hydroxylation to give 6-hydroxy-*o*-toluidine, which is also excreted in the urine (3% of the dose). The other product of hydrolysis is L-N-*n*-propylalanine. This undergoes a number of reactions, including decarboxylation (see Fig. 1).

p-Hydroxytoluidine can reduce haemoglobin,[17] and methaemoglobinaemia is a recognized complication of the use of large doses of prilocaine. This may, however, be avoided by the introduction of EMLA cream (a topical lignocaine formulation).

Pharmaceutics

1. Citanest (Astra, Sweden/UK): 0.5%, 1% and 2% prilocaine hydrochloride injection.
   All injectable preparations of prilocaine are clear, isotonic solutions. The 0.5% and 1% concentrations are available in multi-dose vials (20 ml and 50 ml) and contain methylhydroxybenzoate as preservative (not used in the 2% preparation). Similar preparations containing 2% or 3% prilocaine are marketed in some countries. The 0.5% solution is also produced in a single-use 50 ml vial free of preservative, specifically for intravenous regional anaesthesia.
2. Citanest with Octapressin (Astra, Sweden/UK): For dental use standard and self-aspirating 2 ml cartridges containing prilocaine 4% plain or 3% with felypressin (Octapressin) 0.03 iu/ml, both without preservative, are available.
   Preparations of prilocaine are very stable and have a long shelf life (3 years; 2 years if with felypressin). Proven allergy to prilocaine has not been recorded, but the preservative may be the cause of a very occasional reaction.
3. EMLA (cream, 5%) (Astra, Sweden/UK): When the crystals of the base forms of prilocaine and lignocaine are mixed they form an emulsion by dissolving in one another. This eutectic mixture contains 80% of active local anaesthetic substance[2] and can penetrate intact skin. It will produce dermal anaesthesia in 45–60 min.

Fig. 1 Metabolism of prilocaine

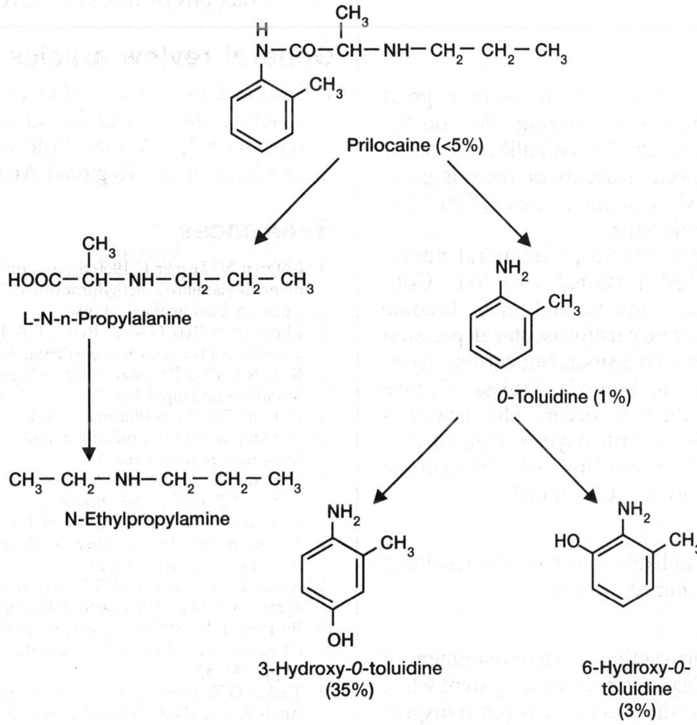

Therapeutic use

Indications

Local anaesthesia.

Mode of use

Prilocaine has been used for all forms of local anaesthesia and is particularly indicated in situations where the risk of systemic toxicity is high. Recommended concentrations are as follows:

Subcutaneous infiltration: 0.5%
Intravenous regional: 0.5% (without either vasoconstrictor or preservative)
Minor nerve block: 1.0%
Major nerve block: 1.0–1.5%
Epidural block: 1.5–2.0%

It is the agent of choice for intravenous regional anaesthesia and has been advocated[18] as the most suitable local anaesthetic for the less experienced practitioner.

The safe dose will depend on the route of administration and a recognized text on local anaesthesia should be consulted before use. The standard dose for intravenous regional anaesthesia of the upper limb is 200 mg (40 ml of 0.5%),[19] but this should be modified in the light of the size of the arm and the general status of the individual. For other uses the generally recommended maximum dose for an adult is 400 mg (600 mg if a vasoconstrictor is added). Doses in excess of 1 g have been used without adverse effect,[20] although there is one published report[21] of a major, but successfully treated, toxic reaction occurring 30 minutes after the epidural administration of 600 mg (without any vasoconstrictor) and another report[22] of death occurring after the administration of 864 mg.

Contraindications

Contraindications to prilocaine, as opposed to local anaesthesia, are few and relate to the risk of methaemoglobinaemia. Over 600 mg of prilocaine have to be given before it becomes a significant risk[23] and this dose will be exceeded only if the drug is used repeatedly as in continuous epidural analgesia. Fetal haemoglobin is more sensitive to reduction so prilocaine should be avoided in the obstetric patient. Anaemia has been considered a contraindication, but it is more appropriate to make an overall assessment of risks. There is no evidence that anaemic patients are more prone to methaemoglobinaemia, but should any occur the overall effect on oxygen carrying capacity would be greater.

Adverse reactions

Potentially life-threatening effects

Such effects may occur if plasma concentrations become great enough for the drug to exert its membrane-stabilizing effect on the central nervous system and the myocardium. This is unlikely to occur unless an accidental intravascular injection occurs or there is gross overdosage. All local anaesthetics have very similar toxic effects, but severe reactions are very rare with prilocaine.

Initial features may include anxiety, tinnitus, circumoral numbness, a metallic taste in the mouth and irrational behaviour. Consciousness is then lost, the patient may convulse and finally become apnoeic. The dose which will cause severe cardiovascular depression is much higher than that which causes convulsions, but cardiac arrest may occur and is usually secondary to hypoxia. Unless effective supportive therapy is instituted, death may occur. The airway is maintained and the lungs are ventilated with oxygen. Convulsions should be controlled with small increments of thiopentone (25–50 mg) or diazepam (2.5–5 mg) given intravenously.

Acute overdosage

Self-poisoning with this drug is most unlikely to occur. The results of accidental overdosage are described immediately above.

Severe or irreversible adverse effects

Methaemoglobinaemia. The factors leading to the development of this side effect have been described. Cyanosis becomes apparent when 1 g.dl^{-1} of haemoglobin is reduced so the effect on oxygen transport is usually small. Treatment with intravenous methylene blue (0.5–1 mg.kg^{-1}) will reverse the methaemoglobinaemia within 15 minutes.[23] It may also be used to prevent this complication.[24]

Symptomatic adverse effects

Hypersensitivity rashes may occur but are very rare.

Interference with clinical pathology tests

Prilocaine is a potent inhibitor of plasma cholinesterase[25] so its presence in a blood sample would interfere with the measurement of that enzyme.

High risk groups

Neonates

No information is available on the use of the drug in neonates.

Breast milk. It is not known if the drug is excreted in breast milk, but it is likely that the drug may be given to lactating women in normal doses without risk to the infant.

Children

Prilocaine may be used quite safely in children. The dose must, of course, be related to the age and size of the child.

Pregnant women

For reasons outlined above prilocaine should not be used in the obstetric patient.

The elderly

Studies of local anaesthetic kinetics in the elderly imply that there is no increased risk of toxicity.[26]

Concurrent disease

There is no evidence that epileptic patients are more prone to develop convulsions after the administration of local anaesthetics. On theoretical grounds, very severe hepatic disease may result in slower metabolism, but this would perhaps be less of a problem than with the other amide local anaesthetics, since it is likely that the elimination of prilocaine is not entirely dependent on liver metabolism.

Drug interactions

Potentially hazardous interactions

Interactions with other drugs rarely give rise to clinical problems. The systemic toxicity of prilocaine is additive with that of other amide local anaesthetics. Since prilocaine is a potent inhibitor of plasma cholinesterase it may increase the toxicity of drugs (including the ester local anaesthetics) which are metabolized by that enzyme.[25]

Potentially useful interactions

No interactions of this kind have been reported.

General review articles

1. Covino B G, Vassallo H G 1976 Local anesthetics: mechanisms of action and clinical use. Grune & Stratton, New York
2. Wildsmith J A W 1986 Prilocaine — an underutilised local anesthetic agent. Regional Anesthesia 10: 155

References

1. Lofgren N, Tegner C 1960 Studies on local anesthetics. XX. Synthesis of some α-monoalkylamino-2-methylproprionanilides. A new useful local anesthetic. Acta Chemica Scandinavica 14: 486
2. Ehrenstrom Reiz G M E, Reiz S L A 1982 EMLA — a eutectic mixture of local anaesthetics for topical anaesthesia. Acta Anaesthesia Scandinavica 26: 596
3. Katz R L 1965 Pharmacological effects of prilocaine. Acta Anaesthetica Scandinavica (suppl 16): 29
4. Data on file, Astra Pharmaceuticals
5. Wiedling S 1965 Reproduction study of citanest and xylocaine. Acta Anaesthetica Scandinavica (suppl 16): 45
6. Data on file, 1987, 1988. Astra Pharmaceuticals
7. Truant A P 1965 Local anesthetic and toxicologic properties of citanest. Acta Anaesthetica Scandinavica (suppl 16): 19
8. Astrom A 1965 Factors affecting the action of citanest in vivo. Acta Anaesthetica Scandinavica (suppl 16): 23
9. Albert J, Lofstrom B 1965 Effects of epinephrine in solutions of local anaesthetic agents. Acta Anaesthetica Scandinavica (suppl 16): 71
10. Bromage P R 1965 A comparison of the hydrochloride and carbon dioxide salts of lidocaine and prilocaine in epidural analgesia. Acta Anaesthetica Scandinavica (suppl 16): 55
11. Tucker G T, Lennard M S 1984 Analysis of local anaesthetics. In: Curry A S (ed) Analytical methods in human toxicology. Macmillan, London, Ch 7

12. Arthur G R, Wildsmith J A W, Tucker G T 1987 Pharmacology of local anaesthetic drugs. In: Wildsmith J A W, Armitage E N (eds) Principles and practice of regional anaesthesia. Churchill Livingstone, Edinburgh, Ch 4
13. Arthur G R 1981 Distribution and elimination of local anaesthetic agents: the role of lung, liver and kidneys. PhD thesis, University of Edinburgh
14. Scott D B 1965 Plasma levels of lignocaine (Xylocaine) and prilocaine (Citanest) following epidural and intercostal nerve block. Acta Anaesthetica Scandinavica (suppl 16): 111
15. Wildsmith J A W, Tucker G T, Cooper S, Scott D B, Covino B G 1977 Plasma concentrations of local anaesthetics after interscalene brachial plexus block. British Journal of Anaesthesia 49: 461
16. Geddes I C 1965 Studies of the metabolism of Citanest C^{14}. Acta Anaesthetica Scandinavica (suppl 16): 37
17. Akerman B, Petersson S A, Wistrand P 1966 Methemoglobin forming metabolites of prilocaine. Proceedings of the Third International Pharmacological Meeting 237
18. Tucker G T 1984 Pharmacokinetics of local anaesthetic agents. In: Scott D B, McClure J H, Wildsmith J A W (eds) Regional anaesthesia 1884–1984. ICM AB, Sodertalje
19. Thorn-Almquist A-M 1979 Intravenous regional anaesthesia. In: Eriksson E (ed) Illustrated handbook in local anaesthesia, 2nd edn. Lloyd-Luke, London
20. Lund P C, Cwik J C 1965 Citanest, a clinical and laboratory study. Current Researches in Anesthesia and Analgesia 44: 623
21. Fortuna A, Brusarosco F F 1965 Clinical evaluation of Citanest in peridural anesthesia. Acta Anaesthetica Scandinavica (suppl 16): 223
22. Kaliciak H A, Chan S C 1986 Distribution of prilocaine in body fluids and tissues in lethal overdose. Journal of Analytical Toxicology 10: 53
23. Crawford O B 1965 Methemoglobin in man following prilocaine. Acta Anaesthetica Scandinavica (suppl 16): 183
24. Bromage P R 1978 Epidural analgesia. W B Saunders, Philadelphia
25. Zsigmond E K 1978 In vitro inhibitory effect of amide-type local analgesics on normal and atypical human plasma cholinesterases. Regional Anesthesia 3,4: 7
26. Tucker G T, Mather L E 1980 Absorption and disposition of local anesthetics: pharmacokinetics. In: Neural blockade in clinical anesthesia and management of pain. L B Lippincott, Philadelphia, Ch 4, p 45

Primaquine (phosphate)

The 8-aminoquinolines were the first drugs to be synthesized for use against malaria.

In the course of an extensive research programme to find antimalarial drugs better than mepacrine, some 8-aminoquinolines were synthesized and screened. Three of these, namely pentaquine, isopentaquine and primaquine held some promise. Primaquine was found to be the most active and least toxic of the three and remains the most commonly used 8-aminoquinoline in malaria chemotherapy.

Primaquine was introduced for the treatment of malaria in 1950 when it emerged as the drug of choice for the treatment of exoerythrocytic stages of *Plasmodium vivax* and *P. ovale*.[1]

Chemistry

Primaquine phosphate (Primachin phosphate)
$C_{15}H_{21}N_3O.2H_3PO_4$
8-(4-Amino-1-methylbutylamino)-6-methoxyquinoline diphosphate

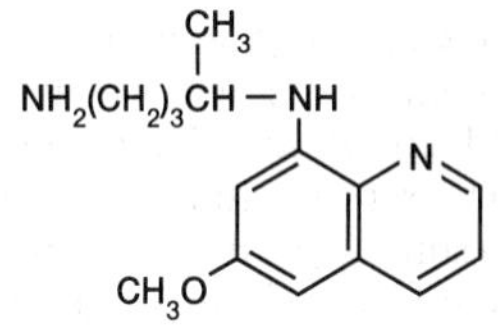

Molecular weight phosphate (free compound)	455.3 (259.4)
pKa	—
Solubility	
in alcohol (phosphate)	insoluble
in water (phosphate)	1 in 16
Octanol/water partition coefficient	—

An orange-red, odourless or almost odourless crystalline powder, primaquine is prepared by chemical synthesis as a racemate. The enantiomers have similar antimalarial activity. Clinically the drug is used as primaquine diphosphate. Primaquine is relatively unstable and easily oxidized. It is available in combination with chloroquine phosphate as Aralen in the USA.

Pharmacology

Primaquine is active at a number of stages in the development of the malaria parasites:

a. It is active against the primary exoerythrocytic stages of *Plasmodium vivax* and *P. falciparum*.
b. It has activity against the asexual erythrocytic forms of *P. vivax* and *P. falciparum*, but only at dangerously high doses.[4] It is not used as a blood schizontocide, high doses are needed and this action has little practical value.
c. It is active against the gametocytes of all four plasmodia that infect man.
d. Primaquine is highly effective against the latent exoerythrocytic stages of *P. vivax* and *P. ovale* and is the best drug for radical cure of relapsing malaria.[1,2]
e. Primaquine inhibits development of *P. falciparum* in the mosquito.

The mechanisms of action of primaquine are not fully elucidated. Both primaquine and its oxidized metabolites have antiplasmodial activity and in man it is likely that much of the antimalarial activity follows metabolism in the liver.[2] It has been suggested from evidence obtained in rodent models, that some or all of the 8-aminoquinolines formed from primaquine might be the main compounds acting against gametocytes, sporogonic stages and pre-erythrocytic stages. In contrast primaquine itself might affect the asexual and possibly the sexual intraerythrocytic parasites.[2,3,5]

In in vitro studies with *P. berghei* primaquine acts on the exoerythrocytic stages and causes poor nuclear staining with the formation of cytoplasmic vacuoles,[6] and similar changes have been shown in vivo in rats.[7] Primaquine affects the parasite mitochondrial activity with inhibition of mitochondrial respiration[6–10] but mitochondrial respiration is probably not important for the erythrocytic stages of mammalian malaria parasites.[11]

Primaquine inhibits protein synthesis in bacteria and indirectly inhibits polymerization of aminoacids by plasmodia,[12,13] but high concentrations are required for this action. Primaquine also disrupts pyrimidine synthesis and this may be the main mechanism of action of primaquine.

Primaquine binds weakly to DNA in vitro but its oxidized metabolites appear to bind to DNA more strongly.[14] Primaquine has a quinidine-like effect on the myocardium and in animal studies proved more effective than quinidine in protecting against experimentally-induced atrial fibrillation.[15,16] Primaquine also has a weak antimuscarinic effect on the guinea pig gall bladder and is synergistic with atropine on intestinal musculature in guinea pigs.[17]

Toxicology

In mice, Schmidt et al[45] obtained oral LD_{50} values for primaquine of 100 mg.kg^{-1} base while Page[46] obtained a figure of 177 mg.kg^{-1} A 5-second bolus intravenous injection of primaquine 10 mg.kg^{-1} was lethal in the anaesthetized dog model.[47]

Subacute toxicity testing of 8-aminoquinolones in the rat has produced rough hair coat; decreased weight gain; elevated reticulocyte count, white cell count and haematocrit; decreased platelet count; elevated SGOT (serum glutamic oxaloacetic transaminase) and SGPT (serum glutamic pyruvic transaminase). The main target organs for toxicity were heart, skeletal muscle, liver and kidney.

In the dog, subacute toxicity testing of 8-aminoquinolones revealed cyanosis, decreased weight gain, elevated methaemaglobin levels, elevated reticulocyte count and haptoglobins and decreased platelet count. The main target organs were heart, liver and lymphoid tissue.[47]

Clinical pharmacology

Primaquine is well absorbed in man from the gastrointestinal tract and peak concentrations of the drug in plasma are seen within 2 h of an oral dose. Primaquine is rapidly metabolized, with a half life of about 6 h[18], to several metabolites which have some antimalarial activity. The antimalarial activity of carboxyprimaquine, 5 hydroxyprimaquine and 5 hydroxy-6 desmethylprimaquine is considerably less than that of primaquine itself. Primaquine has been shown to inhibit the liver microsomal drug metabolizing enzymes[19,20] both in vitro and in vivo. However, only some isozymes of cytochrome P450 are inhibited — the half life of antipyrine is prolonged but that of ethinyloestradiol is not affected.[20] Primaquine may cause cyanosis due to methaemoglobinaemia, particularly in larger doses (60–240 mg daily). Primaquine promotes the conversion of haemoglobin to methaemoglobin and this is particularly seen in individuals with congenital deficiency of nicotinamide adenine dinucleotide (NADH) methaemoglobin reductase.

In normal erythrocytes, primaquine has been shown to stimulate the oxidative pathway of glucose metabolism. In normal erythrocytes there are mechanisms to protect against such oxidative stress but in individuals with G6PD deficiency these mechanisms are overcome and haemolysis may result.[21] It seems that the hydroxymetabolites of primaquine are more potent producers of haemolysis than primaquine itself.

Primaquine has immunosuppressive activity, but there is no evidence that it interferes with the normal immune response to malaria.[22,23] Primaquine and other 8-aminoquinolines reduce blood pressure by causing a reduced sympathetic tone.[24] These drugs have been tried in patients with hypertension but their toxicity precludes their use as hypotensive agents.[25] The quinidine-like activity and antimuscarinic activity seen in animal studies are not manifest in humans at standard doses.

Pharmacokinetics

Several methods are available for the determination of primaquine in various biological fluids. Some of these methods include thin layer chromatography, gas liquid chromatography, mass spectrometry and high performance liquid chromatography (HPLC). HPLC is the more frequently used method of analysis for both primaquine and its metabolites. The assay has a limit of sensitivity of 75 μg.l^{-1} for carboxyprimaquine and 10 μg.l^{-1} for N-acetylprimaquine.[26,27] An HPLC with electrochemical detection has also been described.[28]

Primaquine is absorbed rapidly from the gastrointestinal tract. It is also rapidly metabolized and excreted. In man, peak plasma concentrations are reached about 2 h after a single oral dose of 45 mg base giving a peak plasma concentration of about 150 μg.l^{-1}. Plasma levels fall mono-exponentially to half the peak levels in 6 h.[29] The terminal phase elimination half life is about 4–10 h. Primaquine has a large volume of distribution, about 205 l, which is the result of its extensive tissue distribution.[18,20,29] Plasma protein binding is high.[29] Primaquine is widely distributed in the tissues but it may be concentrated in some tissues more than in others. The concentrations in various tissues change significantly in relatively short time spans in animal models. Hence, it would seem that there is extensive recirculation of primaquine through the intestine following intravenous and intraperitoneal administration of the drug in animals. After oral administration a different tissue distribution of the drug was observed, indicating that a major portion of primaquine reaches the liver but that metabolism and excretion reduce systemic availability. Consequently, although primaquine is well absorbed orally it has poor bioavailability due to presystemic metabolism and to the enterohepatic circulation it appears to undergo.[18,20,29]

Regardless of the route of administration, about the same amount of primaquine is excreted in the faeces.[30,31] The amount of unchanged primaquine excreted in urine in 24 h is less than 4% of the dose administered. Renal clearance is therefore not an important mode of removal of primaquine from the body.[29,31]

Primaquine undergoes rapid side chain metabolism to its main metabolite which has been identified as carboxyprimaquine. In animal models an estimated 20% of primaquine is converted to carboxyprimaquine following intravenous and intraperitoneal administration. After oral administration however, only 4% of the dose appears as carboxyprimaquine in the plasma.[31,32]

The peak plasma levels of the carboxylic acid metabolite of primaquine are about 10 times those of the parent drug and reached in 3–12 h after oral administration of primaquine.[29] The levels of carboxyprimaquine remain high then begin to decline[29] when the concentration of primaquine falls below 100 μg.l^{-1}. However, the levels of carboxyprimaquine are well maintained for more than 24 h — at which time its concentration is about 50 times that of the parent drug.[20] Unlike primaquine, carboxyprimaquine remains detectable 120 h after oral administration.

The half life of carboxyprimaquine is about 16 h. The much higher and sustained concentrations of carboxyprimaquine in the plasma, as compared to that of primaquine, may be due to its longer half life and, perhaps more importantly, to a lower tissue affinity than primaquine.

Carboxyprimaquine is not detected in urine in man, suggesting that it undergoes further metabolism before excretion as other, as yet undefined, compounds.

Animal studies show that in the liver, where primaquine exerts its tissue schizontocide effect, it is concentrated 10 times more than in plasma, while the concentration of carboxyprimaquine is 10 times lower than it is in plasma.[31]

Different doses of primaquine do not yield widely different pharmacokinetic profiles, suggesting that the drug has linear pharmacokinetic properties. However, large pharmacokinetic variations have been observed between human subjects.

Oral absorption	readily absorbed
Presystemic metabolism	extensive
Plasma half life	
range	4–10 h
mean	6 h
Volume of distribution	3–4 l.kg^{-1}
Plasma protein binding	high

Concentration–effect relationship

There is no evidence of any useful correlation between the plasma concentration of primaquine (or carboxyprimaquine) and its therapeutic effects.

Metabolism

Primaquine is probably metabolized mainly in the liver (Fig. 1). Several urinary metabolites have been identified in animal studies, including the 5-hydroxy, 6-methoxy and 6-hydroxy derivatives of primaquine.[33] In microbes, n−acetyl primaquine has also been identified as a metabolite. In man, the principal metabolite of primaquine has been identified as carboxyprimaquine, obtained by metabolism of the side chain of the parent drug. N-acetyl primaquine has also been identified in human urine.[18] Present evidence suggests that metabolites of primaquine may be more active than the parent compound in causing haemolysis.[34]

Fig. 1 The metabolism of primaquine

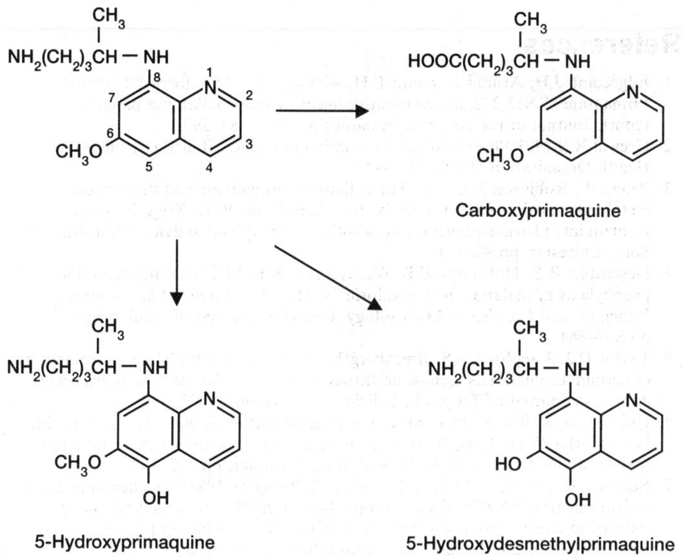

Pharmaceutics

Primaquine phosphate (ICI, UK) are brown, biconvex, sugar- coated tablets containing 7.5 mg primaquine base.

Therapeutic use

Indications

1. Terminal prophylaxis after leaving a malarious area
2. Radical cure of vivax and ovale malaria
3. As a gametocytocidal drug in *P. falciparum infections*.

Contraindications

1. Pregnancy and lactation
2. In acute exacerbations of systemic diseases, having a tendency to granulocytopenia, e.g. rheumatoid arthritis and lupus erythematosus
3. Concomitant use with other drugs which might cause haemolysis or bone marrow depression

Caution should be used in patients with:

4. Systemic disease with a tendency to granulocytopenia
5. Known or suspected G6PD deficiency.

Mode of use

Primaquine is used primarily for terminal prophylaxis after leaving a malarious area and for radical cure of vivax and ovale malaria. Its tissue schizontocidal activity depends more upon cumulative dose than on duration of treatment.[35,36] Primaquine is also effective as a gametocytocidal drug in *P. falciparum* infections. The dosage used in clinical practice is limited by drug toxicity and at the levels normally attained, primaquine does not have a clinically useful blood schizontocidal effect.

Primaquine (phosphate)

P

The dose of primaquine deployed depends upon the indication for use (prevention of relapse in benign tertian malaria, or destruction of gametocytes in *P. falciparum* infection) and the glucose-6-phosphate dehydrogenase (G6PD) status of the patient.[37]

The patient's G6PD status should be determined before administration of primaquine, especially in those ethnic groups with a significant incidence of G6PD deficiency.

Terminal prophylaxis with primaquine is indicated only for selected groups of travellers e.g. those who have had prolonged exposure in malaria endemic areas.[42] In the radical cure of vivax and ovale malaria, primaquine should be given after appropriate therapy with chloroquine. The conventional adult dose for prevention of relapse is 15 mg base daily for 14 days.[37,38] Higher doses, 30 mg base daily for 14 days, can be given to deal with less sensitive strains of the parasites, provided the patients G6PD is normal; however, the higher dosage regimen should not be used routinely.[36]

In patients with G6PD deficiency haemolysis due to primaquine is less when the drug is administered at intervals rather than on a daily basis, so that the preferred regimen is 45 mg base once weekly for 8 weeks, or 30 mg base once weekly for 15 weeks, according to the type of G6PD deficiency.[37,38] Strict medical supervision is essential. For use as a gametocytocide in *P. falciparum* primaquine is given as a sample dose of 30–40 mg base for adults.[44] Appropriate drug treatment of the acute infection must precede primaquine therapy.

Precautions and contraindications

It is recommended that primaquine be taken after a meal as abdominal pain or cramps are common if the drug is ingested on an empty stomach. Anorexia, nausea and vomiting can also occur.[37] Severity of the side effects is dose-related.

Cyanosis due to methaemoglobinaemia can develop when primaquine is used at higher doses, especially in patients with methaemoglobin reductase deficiency. If methaemoglobinaemia occurs, primaquine therapy should be stopped.

Primaquine-induced haemolysis in patients with G6PD deficiency can be made worse by:

a. liver or renal disease, which may delay elimination of the drug
b. the presence of quinacrine which enhances the toxicity of primaquine and the other 8-aminoquinolines by increasing their plasma concentrations 5 to 10 fold and extends their half life by interfering with their metabolic degradation — even when the 8-aminoquinolines are given within three months of quinacrine administration.[2]
c. the presence of other oxidant drugs such as sulphonamides which can cause a haemolytic crisis. Concurrent treatment with other oxidant drugs should be avoided.
d. the presence of other infections which may make erythrocytes more susceptible to haemolysis. If haemolysis occurs, primaquine therapy should be stopped.

It is recommended that primaquine is avoided in patients with an underlying condition compromising bone marrow function or on medication which might compromise the bone marrow.

Adverse reactions

Primaquine is well tolerated at the doses used for the treatment of recurrent malaria.[37] However, it has many adverse effects when it is used at higher doses.

Potentially life-threatening effects

Primaquine has adverse effects on the formed elements of blood and bone marrow, manifested as leucopenia, anaemia, methaemoglobinaemia and suppression of bone marrow activity. All the above adverse effects are known to disappear in most cases when the drug is discontinued.[37,38]

The most important ill effect of primaquine is the intravascular haemolysis it can cause in glucose-6-phosphate dehydrogenase (G6PD) deficiency, which may lead to anaemia.[39] Intravascular haemolysis can be precipitated by primaquine in patients with this deficiency even at therapeutic doses. The severity of the haemolysis depends on the dose of primaquine as well as the degree of the enzyme deficiency. It is estimated that about 200–300 million people have G6PD deficiency, many of them living in malarious areas of the world.[21]

The gene which determines G6PD deficiency is carried on the X chromosome so that the deficiency is seen in a more severe form in males than in females. There are 2 variants of the G6PD enzyme, classified according to electrophoretic mobility. Variant A moves fast on electrophoresis and is the variant deficient in blacks. Variant A deficiency is associated with a milder manifestation of primaquine-induced haemolysis. An estimated 10% of black males may have variant A deficiency. Variant B is slower on electrophoresis. Deficiency of variant B is associated with severe intravascular haemolysis. It is present in some blacks and in people of East Mediterranean and Asian descent.[39]

Intravascular haemolysis induced by primaquine occurs due to the fact that erythrocytes deficient in G6PD have a low reducing capacity, and reducing capacity is essential for maintenance of membrane integrity. In the presence of oxidant drugs like the 8-aminoquinolines, 4-aminoquinolines, sulphonamides, sulphones, antipyretics, analgesics and nitrofurans there is increased fragility of the deficient erythrocytes, leading to mechanical rupture of their membranes. Primaquine-induced intravascular haemolysis is not usually fatal if the drug is stopped and supportive treatment given as required. In primaquine poisoning, whether acute or chronic, the administration of folinic acid, 10–20 mg daily is recommended.[38]

If primaquine is given to patients with G6PD deficiency daily it must be done under very close medical supervision, urine and blood examination should be carried out, and the drug stopped if there is a marked darkening of urine or a significant decrease in haemoglobin levels.[38,39]

The toxicity of primaquine may be caused by the parent drug as well as some of its metabolites,[41] but how much of the toxic effect of primaquine can be attributed to the parent drug versus its metabolites is still not known.

Acute overdosage

Features of acute overdosage include anorexia, nausea, vomiting, weakness, cyanosis, haemolytic anaemia, jaundice, bone marrow depression and methaemoglobinaemia. There is no specific antidote and treatment is symptomatic.

Severe or irreversible adverse effects

Primaquine, like other oxidant drugs, causes the conversion of haemoglobin to methaemoglobin. Cyanosis can develop when the concentration of methaemoglobin reaches 10% of the haemoglobin level. This is, however, rare at the relatively small doses of primaquine used in clinical practice. Primaquine can induce cyanosis in normal people and more so in those with nicotinamide adenine dinucleotide methaemoglobin reductase deficiency.[37,38] Depression and confusion have been reported on rare occasions. Hypertension and cardiac arrhythmias have been attributed to the drug, the mechanisms involved being obscure.

Symptomatic adverse effects

These include nausea, vomiting, anorexia, epigastric discomfort, generalized abdominal pain and cramps, cyanosis, vague chest pain and discoloration of the urine.

Interference with clinical pathology tests

Primaquine may interfere with thin-layer chromatographic tests for the presence of barbiturates and alkaloids in urine.

High risk groups

Neonates

Chongsuphajaisiddhi advises that primaquine should not be given to children under one year of age in view of its relative toxicity.[43]

Breast milk. Primaquine enters breast milk, and mothers taking the drug should not breast-feed. Alternatively primaquine therapy should be delayed until breast-feeding has been completed.

Children

The drug may be given to children in appropriate doses. The dose for radical cure or terminal prophylaxis is 0.3 $mg.kg^{-1}$ base by mouth, daily for 14 days.[42] Chongsuphajaisiddhi advises that in view of the relative toxicity of primaquine, it should not be given to children under one year of age.[43] Older children can receive primaquine, under careful medical supervision.

Primaquine (phosphate)

Pregnant women

The drug is contraindicated in pregnancy, because it may be passed transplacentally to a G6PD-deficient fetus and cause haemolytic anaemia in utero.[42]

The elderly

No special precautions are required in elderly patients.

Drug interactions

Potentially hazardous interactions

Primaquine inhibits hepatic drug oxidation[20] and is reported to inhibit the metabolism of chloroquine.[19]

Potentially useful interactions

No interactions of this type have been reported.

Clinical trials

There are no recent major trials of the efficacy of primaquine. The literature on current usage has been reviewed by Peters.[44]

References

1. Edgecomb J H, Arnold J, Yount E H, Alving A S J, Eichelberger L 1950 Primaquine, SN13 272, a new curative agent in vivax malaria: a preliminary report. Journal of the National Malaria Society 9: 285–292
2. Grewal R S 1981 Pharmacology of 8-aminoquinolines. Bulletin of the World Health Organisation 59 (3): 397–406
3. Peters W, Robinson B L 1987 The activity of primaquine and its possible metabolites against rodent malaria. In: Wernsdorfer W H, Trigg P I (eds) Primaquine: pharmacokinetics, metabolism, toxicity and activity. John Wiley and Sons, Chicester, pp 93–101
4. Desjardins R E, Doberstyn E B, Wernsdorfer W H 1988 The treatment and prophylaxis of malaria. In Wernsdorfer W H and McGregor I (Eds) Malaria: Principles and Practice of Malariology. Churchill Livingstone. Edinburgh pp 827–864
5. Taylor D J, Josephson E S, Breenberg J, Coatney G R 1952 The in vitro activity of certain antimalarials against erythrocytic forms of *Plasmodium gallinaceum.* American Journal of Tropical Medicine and Hygiene 1: 132–139
6. Hollingdale M R 1987 In vitro testing of antimalarial tissue schizontocides. In: Wernsdorfer W H, Trigg P I (eds) Primaquine: pharmacokinetics, metabolism, toxicity and activity. John Wiley and Sons, Chicester, pp 129–138
7. Boulard Y, Landau I, Miltgen F, Ellis D S, Peters W 1983 The chemotherapy of rodent malaria, XXXIV. Causal prophylaxis part III: ultrastructural changes induced in exoerythrocytic schizonts of *Plasmodium yoelii yoelli* by primaquine. Annals of Tropical Medicine and Parasitology 77: 555–568
8. Aikawa M, Beaudoin R L 1969 Morphological effects of 8-aminoquinolines on the exoerythrocytic stages of *Plasmodium fallax.* Military Medicine 134 (suppl): 986–999
9. Howells R E, Peters W, Fullard J 1970 The chemotherapy of rodent malaria XIII. Fine structural changes observed in the erythrocytic stages of *Plasmodium berghei berghei* following exposure to primaquine and menoctone. Annals of Tropical Medicine and Parasitology 64: 203–207
10. Aikawa M, Beaudoin R L 1970 *Plasmodium fallax*: high resolution autoradiography of exoerythrocytic stages treated with primaquine in vitro. Experimental Parasitology 27: 454–463
11. Homewood C A 1977 Carbohydrate metabolism of malarial parasites. Bulletin of the World Health Organisation 55: 229–235
12. Olenick J G, Hahn F E 1972 Mode of action of primaquine: preferential inhibition of protein biosynthesis in *Bacillus megaterium.* Antimicrobial Agents and Chemotherapy 1: 259–262
13. Sherman I W, Tanigoshi L 1972 Incorporation of ^{14}C-amino acids by malaria (*Plasmodium lophurae* V. Influence of antimalarials on the transport and incorporation of amino-acids. Proceedings of the Helminthological Society of Washington 39 (suppl): 250–260
14. Whichard L P, Morris C R, Smith J M, Holbrook D J 1968 The binding of primaquine, pentaquine, pamaquine and plasmocid to deoxyribonucleic acid. Molecular Pharmacology 4: 630–639
15. Holland E L, McCutcheon R S 1962 Some antiarrhythmic actions of primaquine, amodiaquin and quinidine. Journal of Pharmaceutical Sciences 51: 791–793
16. Marshall R J, Ojewole J A O 1978 Comparative effects of some antimalarial drugs on isolated cardiac muscle of the guinea pig. Toxicology and Applied Pharmacology 46: 759–768
17. Seidel E R, Mundy R L, Teague R S 1978 Antimuscarinic activity of the 8-aminoquinoline antimalarial drug primaquine. Toxicology and Applied Pharmacology 45: 258 (abstract)
18. Greaves J, Price-Evans D A, Gilles H M, Fletcher K A, Bunnag D, Harinasuta T 1980 Plasma kinetics and urinary excretion of primaquine in man. British Journal of Clinical Pharmacology 10: 399–405
19. Gaudette L E, Coatney G R 1961 A possible mechanism of prolonged antimalarial activity. American Journal of Tropical Medicine and Hygiene 10: 321–326
20. Breckenridge A, Back D J, Edwards I G et al 1987 The clinical and biochemical pharmacology of primaquine. In: Wernsdorfer W H, Trigg P I (eds) Primaquine: pharmacokinetics, metabolism, toxicity and activity. John Wiley and Sons, Chicester, pp 65–76
21. Carson P E, Hohl R, Nora M V et al 1981 Toxicology of the 8-aminoquinolines and genetic factors associated with their toxicity in man. Bulletin of the World Health Organisation 59: 427–437

22. Thong Y H, Ferrante A, Rowan-Kelly B 1978 Primaquine inhibits mitogen-induced human lymphocyte proliferative responses. Transactions of the Royal Society of Tropical Medicine and Hygiene 72 (5): 537–539
23. Thong Y H 1979 Immunosuppression caused by primaquine. Transactions of the Royal Society of Tropical Medicine and Hygiene 73: 474 (letter)
24. Richardson A P, Walker H A, Miller B S 1947 Effect of pentaquine on cardiovascular system of unanaesthetised dogs. Proceedings of the Society for Experimental Biology and Medicine 65: 258–261
25. Fries E D, Wilkins R W 1947 Effect of pentaquine in patients with hypertension. Proceedings of the Society for Experimental Biology and Medicine 64: 455–458
26. Ward S A, Edwards G, Orme M, Breckenridge A M 1984 Determination of primaquine in biological fluids by reversed-phase high-performance liquid chromatography. Journal of Chromatography 305: 239–243
27. Mihaly G W, Ward S A, Edwards G et al 1984 Pharmacokinetics of primaquine in man: identification of the carboxylic acid derivative as a major plasma metabolite. British Journal of Clinical Pharmacology 17: 441–446
28. Nora M V, Parkhurst G W, Thomas R T, Carson P E 1984 High performance liquid chromatographic–electrochemical assay method for primaquine in plasma and urine. Journal of Chromatography 307: 451–456
29. Nora M V, Thomas R W, Parkhurst G W et al 1987 Pharmacokinetics of primaquine in man after single oral doses. In: Wernsdorfer W H, Trigg P I (eds) Primaquine: pharmacokinetics, metabolism, toxicity and activity. John Wiley and Sons, Chicester, pp 77–89
30. Holbrook D J, Griffin J B, Fowler L, Gibson B R 1981 Tissue distribution of primaquine in the rat. Pharmacology 22: 330–336
31. McChesney J D, Baker J K, Clark A M, Hufford C D 1987 Primaquine: studies of mammalian metabolism. In: Wernsdorfer W H, Trigg P I (eds) Primaquine: pharmacokinetics, metabolism, toxicity and activity. John Wiley and Sons, Chicester, pp 3–26
32. Baker J K, McChesney J D, Hufford C D, Clark A M 1982 High performance liquid chromatographic analysis of the metabolism of primaquine and the identification of a new mammalian metabolite. Journal of Chromatography 230: 69–77
33. Strother A, Fraser I M, Allahyari R, Tilton B E 1981 Metabolism of 8-aminoquinoline antimalarial agents. Bulletin of the World Health Organisation 59: 413–425
34. 1985 Primaquine. In: Goodman, Gilman (eds) The pharmacological basis of therapeutics. Macmillan, pp 1038–1041
35. Schmidt L H, Fradkin R, Vaughan D, Rasco J 1977 Radical cure of infections with *Plasmodium cynomolgi*: a function of total 8-aminoquinoline dose. American Journal of Tropical Medicine and Hygiene 26: 1116–1128
36. Clyde D F, McCarthy V C 1977 Radical cure of Chesson strain vivax malaria in men by 7, not 14, days of treatment with primaquine. American Journal of Tropical Medicine and Hygiene 26: 562–563
37. Clyde D F 1981 Clinical problems associated with the use of primaquine as a tissue schiontocidal and gametocytocidal drug. Bulletin of the World Health Organisation 59: 391–395
38. Bruce-Chwatt L J 1986 Chemotherapy of malaria, revised 2nd edn. WHO Monograph series No 27, Geneva, pp 61–65, 142–143
39. Chan T K, Todd D, Tso S C 1976 Drug-induced hemolysis in glucose-6-phosphate dehydrogenase deficiency. British Medical Journal 2: 1227–1229
40. Alving A S, Johnson C F, Tarlov A R, Brewer G J, Kellermeyer R W, Carson P E 1960 Mitigation of the haemolytic effect of primaquine and enhancement of its action against exoerythrocytic forms of the Chesson strain of *Plasmodium vivax* by intermittent regimens of drug administration. Bulletin of the World Health Organization 22: 621–631
41. Fletcher K A, Price-Evans D A, Gilles H M, Greaves J, Bunnag D, Harinasuta T 1981 Studies on the pharmacokinetics of primaquine. Bulletin of the World Health Organization 59: 407–412
42. Centers for Disease Control 1990 Recommendations for the prevention of malaria among travellers. Morbidity and Mortality Weekly Report 39(No-RR-3): 1–10
43. Chongsuphajaisiddhi T 1988 Malaria in paediatric practice. In: Wernsdorfer W H and McGregor I (Eds) Malaria: Principles and Practice of Malariology. Churchill Livingstone, Edinburgh p 896
44. Peters W 1987 Chemotherapy and drug resistance in malaria. 2nd Edition Academic Press, London pp 577–589
45. Schmidt L H et al 1977 Comparison of the curative antimalarial activities and toxicities of primaquine and its d and l isomers. Antimicrobial Agents and Chemotherapy 12: 51–60
46. Page J G 1985 Preclinical toxicology of new drugs. Annual Report. US Army Medical Research and Development Command Report BATT-8740-85-13
47. Heiffer M H, Davidson D E Jr, Corte D W I 1984 Preclinical testing. In: Peters W and Richards W H G (Eds) Antimalarial Drugs Handbook of Experimental Pharmacology 68(1): 351–373

Primidone

Primidone is the 2-deoxy analogue of phenobarbitone, to which it is partly metabolized. Primidone is used mainly for the treatment of patients with partial seizures and generalized convulsive seizures.

Chemistry

Primidone (Mysoline, Mylepsin, Mylepsinum, Mylepsine, Majsolin, Prosoline)
$C_{12}H_{14}N_2O_2$
5-Ethylperhydro-5-phenylpyrimidine-4,6-dione

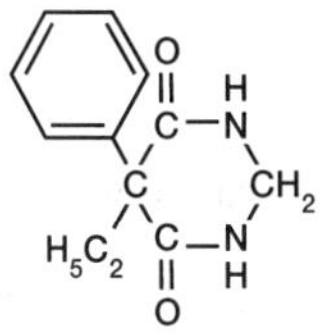

Molecular weight	218.3
pKa	N/A
Solubility	
in alcohol	1 in 170
in water	1 in 2000
Octanol/water partition coefficient	low

A white/colourless, odourless crystalline powder, with a slightly bitter taste, it is prepared by chemical synthesis.

Pharmacology

In animal models, the anticonvulsant activity appears to be mediated partly by primidone itself and partly by its metabolites phenobarbitone and phenylethylmalonamide (PEMA). The relative contribution of the metabolites to the observed pharmacological effect(s) varies depending on both the type of test and the time interval elapsed between drug administration and testing. As compared to phenobarbitone, primidone is approximately equipotent against maximal electro-shock seizures (MES) but much weaker against pentylentetrazole-induced seizures.[1] In the MES test, PEMA is less effective than either primidone or phenobarbitone, although it may potentiate the anticonvulsant action of the latter.[2]

The precise mechanism responsible for the antiepileptic effect at the molecular level is unknown. The postsynaptic depressant effects of primidone in the neuromuscular junction of the frog appear to be weak compared with those of barbiturates.

Enhancement of release of inhibitory transmitters could explain at least in part the pharmacological effects. The effects of primidone are similar to those of phenobarbitone.

Toxicology

The neurotoxic dose 50 (NTD_{50}) of primidone in the mouse is greater than 250 mg.kg^{-1}; this compares favourably with the value of 76 mg.kg^{-1} reported for phenobarbitone.[3] In animal models, susceptibility to seizures may be enhanced above baseline values after withdrawal of primidone treatment; this is indicative of the development of physical dependence.

After an attempt to induce chromosome changes in human lymphocytes Foerst and others[4] concluded that primidone and phenobarbitone are not highly mutagenic. Teratogenicity studies have shown that primidone increases the incidence of cleft palate in mice.[5]

Primidone is known to induce the hepatic microsomal drug metabolizing enzymes in animals and in man.

Clinical pharmacology

Primidone is a centrally active drug which is effective in the treatment of patients with partial seizures (with or without secondary generalization) and convulsive generalized seizures. The activity of the drug is mediated at least in part by its metabolite phenobarbitone; the potential therapeutic efficacy of PEMA in human epilepsy has not been established. Primidone is *not* indicated for the treatment of absence seizures.

Being partly converted to phenobarbitone, primidone shares all the pharmacological properties of the latter, including a sedating action. When starting treatment, transient manifestations of intolerance (which are due to unchanged primidone and not to phenobarbitone) are common. Long-term treatment usually results in tolerance to the sedative effect whereas the antiepileptic activity generally is maintained. Sudden withdrawal of treatment may precipitate rebound seizures and status epilepticus.

Primidone is effective in the treatment of essential tremor. The molecular mechanism responsible for this effect is unknown.

Primidone is a potent inducer of the hepatic microsomal enzymes. This effect could be mediated by metabolically derived phenobarbitone.

Pharmacokinetics

Methods for the specific determination of primidone and its metabolite phenobarbitone in plasma include enzyme multiplied immunoassay (EMIT),[6] substrate-labelled fluorescence immunoassay (SLFIA) and fluorescence polarization immunoassay (FPIA). These methods allow accurate measurements down to at least 2 $mg.l^{-1}$ (primidone) and 5 $mg.l^{-1}$ (phenobarbitone), which is adequate for therapeutic drug monitoring. Primidone, phenobarbitone and the other metabolite PEMA can be detected with greater sensitivity in plasma and other body fluids by gas–liquid chromatography and high performance liquid chromatography, the latter technique having a limit of detection[7] of 550 $\mu g.l^{-1}$.

Primidone is absorbed relatively rapidly from the gastrointestinal tract, peak plasma levels being attained between 0.5 and 7 h following a single oral dose. Studies based on the urinary recovery of unchanged drug and metabolites indicate that at least 75% of the administered dose is absorbed.[8,9] Primidone has no significant presystemic metabolism. The liver is assumed to be the major site of metabolism.

Primidone is well distributed in all organs and tissues; the apparent volume of distribution[10] is approximately 0.6 $l.kg^{-1}$. Brain concentrations have been found to be approximately 90% of the plasma concentrations.[11] Brain/plasma concentration ratios for phenobarbitone vary depending on plasma and tissue pH but they are usually in the range of 0.6–1.1. According to Baumel et al[2] primidone is not bound to plasma proteins, while McAuliffe et al[12] reported a protein binding value of 35%. The plasma protein binding of the metabolite, phenobarbitone, is approximately 50%.

Salivary and CSF/plasma concentration ratios for primidone are in the range of 0.7–1. For phenobarbitone, the CSF/plasma ratio is about 0.5 while the saliva/plasma ratio varies depending on salivary pH, being around 0.35 on average. Both primidone and phenobarbitone cross the placental barrier and distribute in fetal tissues. Both compounds are also excreted in breast milk: the ranges of milk/plasma concentration ratios are 0.6–1.0 for primidone and 0.2–0.6 for phenobarbitone.[13]

Oral absorption	≥75%
Presystemic metabolism	negligible
Plasma half life	
range	4–22 h
mean	10 h
Volume of distribution	0.6 $l.kg^{-1}$
Plasma protein binding	0–35%

Primidone is partly excreted unchanged in urine (15–65%) and partly metabolized to phenobarbitone and PEMA, both of which have anticonvulsant activity. More than >5% of a dose is excreted in urine as unchanged drug and metabolites. The half life of primidone ranges from 4 to 22 h. Cloyd et al[14] found that in patients receiving concurrent therapy with other enzyme-inducing anticonvulsants (phenytoin, carbamazepine) primidone half life values (8±3 h) were shorter than in patients given a single dose of primidone in the absence of associated therapy (15±5 h). In the same study clearance values estimated after a single oral dose were reported to average 35 $ml.kg^{-1}.h^{-1}$ and 52 $ml.kg^{-1}.h^{-1}$ respectively. The half life of the metabolite, phenobarbitone, is much longer (50–160 h). Following administration of primidone the half life of PEMA ranges from 17 to 36 h; these values are overestimates of the real elimination half life, since the metabolite is still being formed during the time of sampling. The half life of PEMA given as such is 10 to 25 h.[15]

Since PEMA and phenobarbitone have longer half lives than primidone, they accumulate to a greater extent during chronic dosing. Steady-state plasma levels of parent drug and metabolites in different patients are poorly correlated with the prescribed daily dose and show a wide interindividual variability. Although the plasma concentration of phenobarbitone is always greater than that of primidone, the ratio between the two varies from one patient to another depending on time of sampling and influence of associated therapy. In patients treated with primidone alone plasma phenobarbitone levels at steady state are usually 35–65% higher than those of the parent drug, while in patients treated with phenytoin and carbamazepine in combination, phenobarbitone/primidone ratios are between 2 and 4.[10] PEMA/primidone ratios are in the order of 0.5–1.

The plasma levels of primidone tend to decrease during pregnancy, but this phenomenon is inconsistent.

Neonates of mothers taking primidone have at birth plasma levels of primidone, phenobarbitone and PEMA comparable to those observed in the mother. The half life of transplacentally transferred primidone in 6 newborns was reported to be 23±10 h.[16] The rate of elimination of phenobarbitone may be reduced in newborns, especially if premature. As compared to adults, children have lower plasma level/dose ratios for both primidone and phenobarbitone.

Renal disease is likely to be associated with decreased elimination of primidone, but this possibility has not been formally investigated. There is evidence that liver disease can impair at least some of the metabolic pathways of both primidone[17] and phenobarbitone.[18]

Concentration–effect relationship

The evaluation of the relationship between plasma primidone levels and clinical effects is complicated by the presence of the active metabolite phenobarbitone, which is largely responsible for the pharmacological activity. The issue is further complicated by the possibility that the other metabolite PEMA also contributes to the pharmacological activity. In spite of these limitations, there is evidence that plasma primidone levels above 12–15 $mg.l^{-1}$ are more frequently associated with clinical signs of toxicity. In most cases, however, primidone therapy can be monitored by measuring the plasma concentration of the metabolite phenobarbitone (for the relevant concentration–effect relationship see Phenobarbitone). There seem to be no clear indications for measuring unchanged primidone, apart from patients with suspected impairment of primidone elimination and patients who develop signs of toxicity in the presence of low plasma phenobarbitone concentrations. Even then, the upper limit of the therapeutic range must be viewed flexibly and interpreted differently depending on whether peak or trough concentrations are being measured.[19]

Metabolism

Primidone is partly excreted unchanged in urine and partly metabolized. The most important metabolic pathways are conversion to PEMA and to phenobarbitone (Fig. 1). The latter, in turn, is partly converted to p-hydroxyphenobarbitone. The conversion to phenobarbitone is especially important because this metabolite is largely responsible for therapeutic and toxic effects. Minor primidone metabolites include 2-phenylbutyramide, hydroxy-primidone and alpha-phenyl-gamma-butyrolactone. Of course, phenobarbitone is further metabolized in part to various metabolites (see Phenobarbitone).

After administration of radiolabelled primidone to patients not taking other anticonvulsants, an average 64% of the oral dose was recovered in urine as unchanged drug while the amounts recovered as

Primidone

Fig. 1

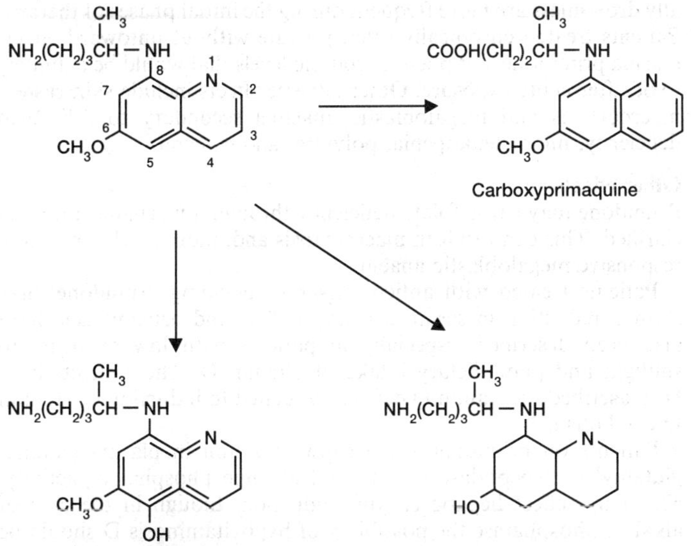

PEMA and phenobarbitone were 7% and 2% respectively. In patients chronically treated with primidone itself, barbiturates or phenytoin, the percentages of the dose recovered as unchanged drug, PEMA and phenobarbitone were 40%, 28% and 3% respectively.[9] Unidentified metabolites accounted for 3–7% of the administered dose. Studies based on the urinary recovery of primidone and its metabolites in children receiving chronic therapy indicated that 15–65% of the dose was excreted unchanged in urine, 16–65% was converted to PEMA and only 1–8% was converted to phenobarbitone.[8] Although only a minor proportion of primidone is converted to phenobarbitone, the latter accumulates markedly in the plasma of treated patients, because of its long half life. At steady state the serum concentration of phenobarbitone is greater than that of primidone, but the precise ratio between the two varies greatly from one patient to another and also within the same patient, depending on time of sampling and the influence of associated therapy. In patients treated with primidone alone, for example, phenobarbitone levels at steady state are on average 35–60% higher than those of parent drug, whereas in patients taking phenytoin and carbamazepine in combination the levels of phenobarbitone may be two to four times higher than those of primidone. Primidone is an inducer of hepatic monooxygenase activity and its own metabolism is increased by inducing agents such as phenytoin.

Pharmaceutics

Primidone is available only as tablets or suspension for oral use.

Mysoline 250 mg tablets (ICI, UK) are round, white biconvex, marked with a parallel line on each side of the bisecting line on one face, with 'ICI' on the obverse.

Mysoline oral suspension (ICI, UK) is a white, pleasantly flavoured aqueous suspension which contains 250 mg primidone BP per 5 ml. The preparation is preserved with parabens. A carboxymethyl (1%) syrup (sucrose 20%) is recommended as the diluent, with hydroxybenzoate preservatives.

Tablets are stable for 2 years (3 years in temperate climate) if packed in blisters or 4 years (5 years in temperate climate) if packed in aluminium containers or HDPE bottles. Suspensions are stable for 3 years (tropical conditions) or 5 years (temperate conditions). No special protection from light is required.

Therapeutic use

Indications

1. The treatment of partial seizures and generalized convulsive seizures
2. The treatment of essential tremor.

Contraindications

1. Known hypersensitivity to primidone or barbiturates
2. Acute intermittent porphyria.

Mode of use

Treatment should be started with a very low dose to minimize the manifestations of intolerance (nausea, vomiting, malaise, drowsiness, vertigo, ataxia) frequently encountered during the early phases of therapy.

In epilepsy, the initial dosage for adults and children over 9 years can be 100–125 mg at bedtime for days 1–3 followed by 100–125 mg b.i.d. for days 4–6, 100–125 mg t.i.d. for days 7–9 and 250 mg t.i.d. (most common maintenance regimen) thereafter. Some patients (including those with essential tremor) require smaller initial doses and slower dosage increments. Patients already receiving barbiturates conversely tolerate relatively high initial doses reasonably well. The maintenance dosage is adjusted according to clinical response but should not exceed 2 g daily in adults.

In children under 9 years, treatment may be started with 50 mg at bedtime for days 1–3 followed by 50 b.i.d. for days 4–6, 100 mg t.i.d. for days 7–9 and 125 to 250 mg t.i.d. thereafter. Maintenance dosage in children is usually 10 to 25 $mg.kg^{-1}$ daily in divided doses (750–1000 mg daily between 6 and 9 years; 500–750 mg daily between 2 and 5 years and 250 500 mg daily up to 2 years of age). When it is necessary to give 125 mg of primidone suspension to a small child, it is advisable to dilute the suspension and administer a 5 ml dose. A suitable diluent is: sodium carboxymethylcellulose (50 cp) 1% w/v, sucrose 20%, methylhydroxybenzoate 0.15%, propylhydroxybenzoate 0.015% and water to 100%.

Abrupt or too rapid withdrawal of primidone may result in status epilepticus and increased frequency of seizures.

Indications

1. Epilepsy

Primidone is still a valuable anticonvulsant, even though its tolerability profile is less favourable than that of some of the other available antiepileptic drugs. For this reason, primidone cannot be generally recommended as a first-choice drug, and is more frequently used in patients who failed on first-line treatment.

Primidone is effective in the treatment of patients with partial seizures (with or without secondary generalization) and convulsive generalized seizures.[20–23] In these conditions primidone may be used alone (though seldom as first-choice therapy) or in combination with other anticonvulsants such as phenytoin, carbamazepine and valproic acid. The median maintenance dosage in adults is about 750 mg daily but treatment should be started with much lower dosages and increased gradually. Following an adjustment in primidone dosage, steady-state plasma levels of the active metabolite phenobarbitone are not reached until 2–4 weeks; therefore, a full assessment of clinical effects can be made only after several weeks.

Available evidence suggests that in partial and convulsive generalized seizures the efficacy of primidone is comparable to that of phenytoin, phenobarbitone and carbamazepine.[20,23]

In view of the marked accumulation of metabolically derived phenobarbitone, it has not been possible to ascertain to what extent (if any) unchanged primidone and the other metabolite PEMA contribute to the overall clinical efficacy. Although primidone does not appear to be consistently superior to phenobarbitone in reducing seizure frequency, it is possible that occasional patients show greater benefit from primidone than from phenobarbitone doses producing equivalent plasma phenobarbitone levels.[24,25]

2. Essential tremor

Primidone is effective for the treatment of essential tremor.[26] A typical response in a patient population treated with dosages up to 750 $mg.d^{-1}$ would be a 50–60% average reduction in tremor amplitude, but there is a wide interindividual variability in the degree of clinical benefit.[27] The improvement affects both limbs and head tremor, while an effect on voice tremor has not been consistently observed in all studies. The therapeutic effect of primidone in essential tremor is due to a combined action of unchanged drug and metabolically derived phenobarbitone, while a possible contribution of the other metabolite PEMA has been excluded.[28] In a recent double-blind study, primidone was found to be superior to phenobarbitone in reducing essential tremor.[29]

Although on average the efficacy of primidone in essential tremor is superior to that of phenobarbitone[29] and comparable to that of

P

propranolol, primidone is not recommended as first-choice treatment because of its lower tolerability. Side effects such as nausea, ataxia and vertigo are commonly seen after the first doses of primidone in tremor patients, even when therapy is started at a low dosage (62.5 $mg.d^{-1}$).[27] It has been suggested that these patients are more sensitive to primidone toxicity than patients with epilepsy: this is probably explained by the fact that in the latter patients previous therapy with other anticonvulsants resulted in cross-tolerance to the side effects of primidone.

Contraindications

1. Known hypersensitivity to primidone or barbiturates
These patients should not be started on primidone.

2. Acute intermittent porphyria
Primidone can precipitate attacks of acute intermittent porphyria. This effect is probably related to microsomal enzyme induction.

Adverse reactions

Potentially life-threatening effects
Potentially lethal effects are usually the result of hypersensitivity to primidone or its metabolites. Severe dermatological reactions have been occasionally reported, including one fatal case of dermatitis bullosa. At least one case of systemic lupus erythematosus has been linked to primidone. Severe hypersensitivity reactions to phenobarbitone include hepatitis, systemic lupus erythematosus and various dermatological conditions. Serious haematological toxicity in response to primidone is extremely rare.

Acute overdosage
Clinical findings in primidone overdose consist of CNS depression, flaccidity and depression of deep tendon reflexes. Crystalluria may be prominent. Plasma primidone levels of about 100 $\mu g.ml^{-1}$ are associated with ataxia, dysarthria, vertigo, nausea, sleepiness and lethargy. These symptoms appear to be caused by primidone and not by its metabolites PEMA or phenobarbitone, the plasma levels of which often increase as the patient improves.[30] Although primidone poisoning may be fatal, the safety margin of the drug appears to be relatively high. One patient survived ingestion of as much as 22 g.

Overdose should be treated with gastric lavage and supportive measures. Forced diuresis and dialysis may be useful.[31] Analeptics are *not* recommended.

Severe or irreversible adverse effects
Patients receiving their initial doses of primidone may experience marked drowsiness, weakness, vertigo, ataxia, feeling of intoxication, nausea and vomiting. These symptoms, which may be highly incapacitating, are due to unchanged primidone since they occur at a time when little or no phenobarbitone or PEMA are detectable in blood. These effects are usually absent or attenuated in patients already receiving barbiturates.[32] To minimize this intolerance, patients should be started on a very low dose and warned about the possible appearance of transient adverse effects. The mechanism underlying this reaction is unknown. Within a few days, most patients develop tolerance to these effects.

Sudden or too rapid discontinuation of primidone may result in increased fit frequency and status epilepticus and other withdrawal symptoms such as sleeplessness, irritability and tremor.[31]

Symptomatic adverse effects
The most common adverse effects of primidone therapy are signs of CNS toxicity, which may be experienced by 40–80% of patients receiving therapeutic doses of the drug.[33] These side effects appear to be mediated at least in part by the metabolite phenobarbiturate.

The manifestations of intolerance after the first few doses of primidone are described above. During chronic therapy the most common symptom is drowsiness, reported by 30–70% of patients. Other CNS side effects include ataxia, nystagmus, impotence, decreased libido, difficulties with memory and concentration and impaired fine motor performance. Paradoxical hyperactivity and irritability may be seen, especially in children. Mental and personality changes have been described and include acute confusional states, depression and psychotic reactions. Rare adverse effects include external ophthalmoplegia, polyradiculitis and tremor.

Most of the symptoms described above are dose-dependent and reversible after reduction of dosage. CNS adverse effects and especially drowsiness are more frequent during the initial phases of therapy. Patients treated chronically often tolerate without untoward effects plasma primidone and phenobarbitone levels that would be definitely toxic after acute exposure. Other adverse effects include skin rashes, macrocytosis and megaloblastic anaemia secondary to folic acid deficiency, minor leukopenia, polyuria, and oedema.

Other effects
Primidone may cause folate deficiency through a mechanism not yet clarified. This can result in macrocytosis and, more rarely, in folate-responsive megaloblastic anaemia.

Patients treated with anticonvulsants, including primidone, may show a reduction in serum calcium; rickets and osteomalacia have also been described, especially in patients with low exposure to sunlight and poor dietary intake of vitamin D. These effects have been ascribed to vitamin D deficiency related to induction of vitamin D catabolism.[34]

Patients on primidone often show elevation in plasma gamma-glutamyl transpeptidase (GGT) and alkaline phosphatase activity. This may reflect hepatic enzyme induction, though in the case of alkaline phosphatase the possibility of hypovitaminosis D should be considered. Treatment with primidone may lower plasma bilirubin levels as a result of increased glucuronidation in the liver.[34]

Interference with clinical pathology tests
Urinary pregnanediol cannot be measured by a gas-chromatographic method using an internal standard with the same retention time as primidone.[35]

High risk groups

Neonates
Little information is available on primidone absorption in newborns. The elimination half life of transplacentally acquired drug is longer in newborns than in adults, probably due to decreased renal and metabolic function. The elimination of phenobarbitone is also known to be relatively slow in newborns especially if born prematurely. If primidone is used in neonates and infants, therapy should be monitored by measuring plasma levels of parent drug and its metabolite phenobarbitone.

Neonates of primidone-treated mothers may show withdrawal symptoms such as irritability, hypotonia and vomiting.[31]

Newborns of mothers treated with primidone during pregnancy are at risk of developing a serious haemorrhagic disorder. Prophylactic use of vitamin K is indicated in these women during pregnancy or in their newborns immediately after birth.[36]

Breast milk. Although primidone and phenobarbitone are excreted in breast milk, breast-feeding should not be discouraged. If signs of poor suckling or sedation are found, early weaning must be considered.[31]

Children
Primidone/phenobarbitone ratios are lower in children than in adults receiving equivalent weight-adjusted dosages.

Pregnant women
The plasma levels of primidone may decrease during pregnancy.

There is evidence that epileptic women are at greater risk of delivering a malformed baby and that this effect may be at least in part related to intake of anticonvulsant drugs. Discontinuation of anticonvulsant drug therapy during pregnancy, however, is unwarranted because of the possible serious side effects of repeated seizures on maternal and fetal health.

Newborns from mothers treated with primidone during pregnancy may develop a fatal haemorrhagic disorder.[36] To minimize this risk vitamin K_1 supplements should be given for the last month of pregnancy. In the absence of such pretreatment then 10 mg vitamin K_1 may be given to the mother at the time of delivery and 1 mg should be given immediately to the neonate at risk.

The elderly
The disposition of primidone does not appear to be grossly altered in old age, although a reduction in renal clearance of parent drug and its metabolites can be expected. Monitoring of plasma primidone and phenobarbitone levels should help in individualizing dosage.

Primidone

Concurrent disease

Hepatic and renal disease. Impaired renal function may result in accumulation of primidone and/or its metabolites PEMA and phenobarbitone. Measurement of plasma concentrations of all three substances may be necessary in order to accurately assess and possibly prevent primidone intoxication in uraemic patients.[18]

Severe hepatic disease may be associated with reduced elimination of phenobarbitone and possibly with altered conversion of primidone to its metabolites. Again it is recommended that serum primidone and phenobarbitone levels are measured as a guide to dosage adjustment in these patients. Coma has been reported in a patient on phenobarbitone and primidone who developed acute hepatitis.[37]

Drug interactions

Potentially hazardous interactions

Alcohol. Alcohol may potentiate the CNS depressant effects of barbiturates and related drugs.

Oral anticoagulants. Primidone and/or phenobarbitone may stimulate the metabolism of oral anticoagulants such as dicoumarol and warfarin. This may increase the dosage requirement of the anticoagulant. Haemorrhage may occur if anticoagulant dosage is not readjusted after withdrawal of the anticonvulsant.

Other significant interactions

Valproic acid. Valproic acid inhibits the catabolism of metabolically derived phenobarbitone, thereby increasing plasma phenobarbitone levels. This may result in excessive sedation and other signs of toxicity. Primidone, in turn, may accelerate the metabolism and decrease the plasma levels of valproic acid.

Carbamazepine. Carbamazepine may stimulate the conversion of primidone to phenobarbitone. Conversely, primidone and/or phenobarbitone may stimulate carbamazepine metabolism and reduce plasma carbamazepine levels to a clinically important extent.

Phenytoin. Phenytoin may stimulate the conversion of primidone to phenobarbitone. Phenytoin may also stimulate or inhibit phenobarbitone metabolism. Phenobarbitone, in turn, can increase phenytoin levels by inhibiting its metabolism.

Isoniazid, nicotinamide. These drugs may inhibit primidone metabolism and precipitate clinical signs of primidone intoxication.

Dicoumarol, methylphenidate, chloramphenicol, propoxyphene. These drugs may elevate plasma phenobarbitone levels and cause phenobarbitone intoxication.

Acetazolamide. There is suggestive evidence that acetazolamide may impair primidone absorption.

Oral contraceptives. Primidone and phenobarbitone induce the metabolism of oral contraceptives, thereby reducing their prophylactic efficacy.

Glucocorticoids and metyrapone. Induction of metabolism of these agents can decrease their effectiveness when they are used for therapeutic or diagnostic purposes.[38]

Urine alkalinizing agents. These agents enhance the renal clearance of phenobarbitone, a phenomenon that can be exploited in cases of phenobarbitone intoxication.

Other drugs. Patients treated with primidone and/or other enzyme-inducing anticonvulsants may show an increased rate of metabolism of various concurrently administered drugs, including doxycicline, metronidazole, various cardioactive and psychotropic drugs, and other agents.[38]

Potentially useful interactions

Primidone is sometimes used in combination with other anticonvulsants (see Indications).

Major outcome trials and other trials

1. White P T, Plott D, Norton J 1966 Relative anticonvulsant potency of primidone. Archives of Neurology 14: 31–35

This trial in 20 patients with focal or psychomotor seizures was performed according to a 10 × 10 Latin square design and compared 10 treatment schedules including full doses of primidone (1500 mg daily), phenytoin (600 mg daily) and phenobarbitone (300 mg daily), half-doses, combination of half-doses and a placebo, each given for a 2-week period. Clinical efficacy was assessed by using a 'demerit points' score calculated according to the number of seizures, with statistical comparison by analysis of variance. Serum drug levels were not measured, which is regrettable in view of the unusually high doses used, especially of phenytoin. All drugs were found to be superior to placebo without statistically significant differences among them, although there was a trend for phenytoin being the most effective treatment.

2. Oxley J, Hebdige S, Richens A 1979 A comparison of phenobarbitone and primidone in the control of seizures in chronic epilepsy. British Journal of Clinical Pharmacology 7: 414P

21 epileptic patients who had been taking primidone or phenobarbitone for at least one year, usually in combination with other anticonvulsants, entered a within-subject comparison of seizure control on either primidone or phenobarbitone in a dose tailored to yield a serum phenobarbitone concentration similar to that observed during the primidone period. The changeover from primidone to phenobarbitone or vice versa was carried out abruptly and the median duration of each treatment period was 12 months.

16 patients took primidone in the first period while 5 took phenobarbitone first. 14 of the 21 patients had fewer tonic-clonic seizures on primidone than on phenobarbitone, 4 had more frequent attacks and the remainder showed no change: the difference in favour of primidone was statistically significant but interpretation of this finding should be cautious in view of the non-balanced order of treatments. No significant differences in the frequency of minor (partial and absence) attacks were seen on the two treatments.

3. Mattson R H, Cramer J A, Collins J F et al 1985 Comparison of carbamazepine, phenobarbital, phenytoin and primidone in partial and secondarily generalized tonic-clonic seizures. New England Journal of Medicine 313: 145–151

In a multicentre double-blind trial, 622 patients with previously untreated or undertreated partial or secondarily generalized tonic-clonic seizures were randomly assigned to monotherapy with carbamazepine, phenytoin, phenobarbitone or primidone. Patients were then followed up for two years or until the drug failed to control seizures or caused unacceptable side effects. In the 421 patients available for evaluation, overall success rate was highest in the groups treated with carbamazepine or phenytoin, intermediate in the group taking phenobarbitone and lowest in the group assigned to primidone ($p<0.002$). Control of tonic-clonic seizures did not differ significantly with the 4 drugs, whereas carbamazepine was significantly superior to primidone and phenobarbitone in controlling partial seizures ($p<0.03$). The overall highest failure rate with primidone was due to intolerable acute toxic effects such as nausea, vomiting, dizziness and sedation. Reduced libido and impotence were more common with primidone, whereas phenytoin caused more dysmorphic effects and hypersensitivity reactions.

General review articles

Eadie M G 1984 Anticonvulsant drugs: an update. Drugs 27: 328–363

References

1. Bourgeois B F D, Dodson W E, Ferrendelli J A 1983 Primidone, phenobarbital and PEMA. I Seizure protection, neurotoxicity and therapeutic index of individual compounds in mice. Neurology 33: 283–290
2. Baumel I P, Gallagher B B, Mattson R H 1972 Phenylethylmalonamide (PEMA): an important metabolite of primidone. Archives of Neurology 27: 34–41
3. Schäfer H 1985 Chemical constitution and pharmacological effect. In: Frey H H, Janz D (eds) Antiepileptic drugs. Handbook of experimental pharmacology, vol 74. Springer-Verlag, Berlin, pp 200–243
4. Foerst D 1972 Chromosomenuntersuchungen nach der Einwirkung von Primidon (Mylepsinum) und seiner Abbauprodukte Phenobarbital und Phenylethylmalondiamide in vitro. Acta Genetica Medica Gemellologica (Rome) 21: 305–318
5. McElhatton P R, Sullivan F M, Toseland P A 1977 Teratogenic activity and metabolism of primidone in the mouse. Epilepsia 18: 1–11
6. Bergmeyer H U (ed) 1986 Methods of enzymatic analysis. VCH Verlaggesellschaft mBH, Weinheim, FRG
7. Frey H H 1985 Primidone. In: Frey H H, Janz D (eds) Antiepileptic drugs. Springer-Verlag, Berlin, pp 449–477
8. Kauffmann R E, Habersang R, Lansky L 1977 Kinetics of primidone metabolism and excretion in children. Clinical Pharmacology and Therapeutics 22: 200–205
9. Zavadil P, Gallagher B B 1976 Metabolism and excretion of ^{14}C-primidone in epileptic patients. In: Janz D (ed) Epileptology. Georg Thieme, Stuttgart, pp 129–138

10. Perucca E, Richens A 1985 Clinical pharmacokinetics of antiepileptic drugs. In: Frey H H, Janz D (eds) Antiepileptic drugs. Handbook of experimental pharmacology, vol 74. Springer Verlag, Berlin, pp 661–723
11. Houghton G W, Richens A, Toseland P A, Davidson S, Falconer M A 1975 Brain concentrations of phenytoin, phenobarbitone and primidone in epileptic patients. European Journal of Clinical Pharmacology 9: 73–78
12. McAuliffe J J, Sherwin A L, Leppik I E, Fayle S A, Pippenger C E 1977 Salivary levels of anticonvulsants: a practical approach to drug monitoring. Neurology 27: 409–413
13. Kaneko S, Sato T, Suzuki K 1979 The levels of anticonvulsant in breast milk. British Journal of Clinical Pharmacology 7: 624–627
14. Cloyd J C, Miller K W, Leppik I E 1981 Primidone kinetics: effects of concurrent drugs and duration of therapy. Clinical Pharmacology and Therapeutics 29: 402–407
15. Cottrell P R, Streete J M, Berry D J et al 1982 Pharmacokinetics of phenylethylmalonamide (PEMA) in normal subjects and in patients treated with antiepileptic drugs. Epilepsia 23: 307–313
16. Nau H, Rating D, Häuser I, Jäger E, Koch S, Helge H 1980 Placental transfer and pharmacokinetics of primidone and its metabolites phenobarbital, PEMA and hydroxyphenobarbital in neonates and infants of epileptic mothers. European Journal of Clinical Pharmacology 18: 31–41
17. Pisani F, Perucca E, Primerano G et al 1984 Single-dose kinetics of primidone in acute viral hepatitis. European Journal of Clinical Pharmacology 27: 465–469
18. Asconapé J J, Penry J K 1982 Use of antiepileptic drugs in the presence of liver and kidney disease: a review. Epilepsia (suppl 1) 23: 65S–79S
19. Fincham R W, Schottelius D D 1982 Primidone. Relation of plasma concentration to seizure control. In: Woodbury D M, Penry J K, Pippenger C E (eds) Antiepileptic drugs. Raven Press, New York, pp 429–440
20. White P T, Plott D, Norton J 1966 Relative anticonvulsant potency of primidone. A double-blind comparison. Archives of Neurology 14: 31–35
21. Millichap J G, Aymat F 1968 Controlled evaluation of primidone and diphenylhydantoin sodium. Comparative anticonvulsant efficacy and toxicity in children. Journal of the American Medical Association 204: 738–739
22. Cereghino J J, Brock J T, Van Meter J C, Penry J K, Smith L D, Fisher P, Ellenberg J 1964 Evaluation of albutoin as an antiepileptic drug. Clinical Pharmacology and Therapeutics 15: 406–416
23. Rodin E A, Rim C S, Kitano H, Lewis R, Rennick P M 1976 A comparison of the effectiveness of primidone versus carbamazepine in epileptic outpatients. Journal of Nervous and Mental Disease 163: 41–46
24. Olesen O V, Dam M 1967 The metabolic conversion of primidone (Mysoline) to phenobarbitone in patients under long-term treatment. Acta Neurologica Scandinavica 43: 348–356
25. Oxley J, Hebdige S, Richens A 1979 A comparison of phenobarbitone and primidone in the control of seizures in chronic epilepsy. British Journal of Clinical Pharmacology 7: 414P
26. O'Brien M D, Upton A R, Toseland P A 1981 Benign familial tremor treated with primidone. British Medical Journal 282: 178–180
27. Findley L J, Calzetti S, Cleeves L 1984 Primidone in essential tremor. In: Findley L J, Capildeo R (eds) Movement disorders: tremor. Macmillan Press Ltd, London, pp 271–282
28. Calzetti S, Findley L J, Pisani F, Richens A 1981 Phenylethylmalonamide in essential tremor. A double-blind controlled study. Journal of Neurology, Neurosurgery and Psychiatry 44: 932–934
29. Sasso E, Perucca E, Calzetti S 1988 Double-blind comparison of primidone and phenobarbital in essential tremor. Neurology 38: 808–810
30. Brillman J, Gallagher B B, Mattson R H 1974 Acute primidone intoxication. Archives of Neurology 30: 255–258
31. Schmidt D 1985 Adverse effects. In: Frey H H, Janz D (eds) Antiepileptic drugs. Handbook of experimental pharmacology, vol 74. Springer Verlag, Berlin, pp 661–723
32. Leppik I E, Cloyd J C, Miller K 1984 Development of tolerance to the side effects of primidone. Therapeutic Drug Monitoring 6: 189–191
33. Leppik I E, Cloyd J C 1982 Primidone toxicity. In: Woodbury D M, Penry J K, Pippenger C E (eds) Antiepileptic Drugs. Raven Press, New York, pp 441–447
34. Perucca E 1978 Clinical consequences of microsomal induction by antiepileptic drugs. Pharmacology and Therapeutics 2: 285–314
35. Phillipou G, Bigham D A, Farrant R K, Seamark R F, Cox L W 1976 Interference by primidone in the analysis of urinary pregnanediol by gas-chromatography. Australian and New Zealand Journal of Obstetrics and Gynecology 16: 224
36. Bleyer W A, Skinner A L 1976 Fatal neonatal hemorrhage after maternal anticonvulsant therapy. Journal of the American Medical Association 235: 626–627
37. McColl K E L, Fletcher C D, Thompson T J 1978 Hepatitis and anticonvulsant therapy. Lancet i: 1201–1202
38. Perucca E 1982 Pharmacokinetic interactions with antiepileptic drugs. Clinical Pharmacokinetics 7: 57–84

Probenecid

At a time when penicillin was expensive and in short supply, probenecid was introduced as a therapeutic adjunct to retard renal elimination of the antibiotic.[1] It is a classical competitive inhibitor of organic acid transport in both the kidney and other organs.

Chemistry

Probenecid (Benemid, Probalan, Probenimead, SK-Probenicid)
$C_{13}H_{19}NO_4S$
4-(Dipropylsulphamoyl)benzoic acid

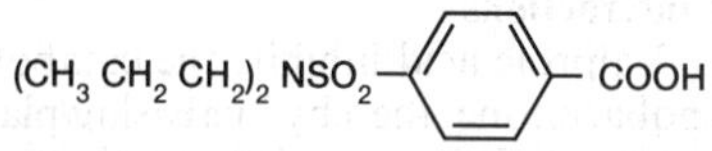

Molecular weight	285.4
pKa	3.4
Solubility	
in alcohol	1 in 25
in water	almost insoluble
Octanol/water partition coefficient	very high

Probenecid is a white or nearly white fine crystalline powder with a slightly bitter taste and pleasant after-taste.

Pharmacology

Probenecid is a competitive inhibitor of renal tubular transport, whose cellular mechanism of action is unknown. The transporter contained in renal tubular membranes functions as an anion exchanger and thus probenecid inhibits both the secretion of one anion (penicillin for example) and the reabsorption of another anion (uric acid) by inhibiting transport in the luminal membrane.[2–5] It should be noted that there is marked species variation in renal tubular handling of uric acid. In man, net reabsorption of uric acid is found invariably. In those animals that demonstrate net secretion of uric acid, probenecid inhibits secretion rather than reabsorption.

Toxicology

The acute toxicity of probenecid in animals is shown in Table 1.

Table 1

Species	Route	LD_{50} mg.kg^{-1} (95% fiducial limits)
Mouse	Intravenous	458 (433–485)
	Subcutaneous	1156 (1073–1245)
	Oral	1666 (1522–1824)
Rat	Intraperitoneal	394 (377–413)
	Subcutaneous	611 (557–671)
	Oral	1604 (1257–2050)
Rabbit	Intravenous	304 (270–343)
Dog	Intravenous	270 (234–312)

Signs of toxicity in these animals include increased respiratory rate, muscular twitching, vomiting, defaecation, micturition and clonic and tonic convulsions at the highest doses.

Chronic toxicity studies in the rat administered 0, 100, 200 and 400 mg.kg^{-1} daily on 5 days per week for 12 weeks resulted only in a reduction in weight gain at the two highest dose levels. Drug-induced

Probenecid

changes were not observed on post mortem examination. Chronic toxicity studies in the dog following the administration of 0, 50, 100, and 200 $mg.kg^{-1}$ daily on 5 days per week for 8 weeks resulted in transient anorexia and weight loss, followed by increased food consumption with a return to baseline after 3 weeks. Decreased haemoglobin, haematocrit values, and erythrocyte counts occurred in drug-treated dogs. These changes were not dose-related and may have been related to anorexia. A non-fermentable reducing substance appearing in the urine was shown to be probenecid glucuronate. There were no other drug-related changes in any of the other clinical tests or post mortem studies.

Clinical pharmacology

Probenecid will lower serum urate concentrations when given in daily doses of 0.5–3.0 g. Serum urate concentrations will fall within a few days of starting therapy. Since urinary urate concentrations rise, the urine may need to be kept alkaline to prevent the formation of urate crystals. Probenecid will only work effectively if renal function is normal. Probenecid also inhibits the tubular secretion of a number of other compounds. It will inhibit the secretion of indomethacin, methotrexate and nitrofurantoin which causes a drug interaction, beneficial in the former case but detrimental with the latter two drugs. Probenecid also inhibits the transport of 5-hydroxyindole acetic acid and other cerebral monoamines from the subarachnoid space to the plasma. This has not yet been shown to be of clinical use but has aroused psychopharmacological interest.[6]

Daily doses of 1–2 g of probenecid are employed to decrease the clearance of antibiotics such as penicillin, whether given in single or multiple dose regimes. This may be useful in reducing the very large doses of penicillin that may sometimes be needed (e.g. to treat SBE) and to minimize the amount of potassium given to the patient.

Pharmacokinetics

The analytical methods available for probenecid are spectrophotofluorometric,[7] HPLC[8], GC with electron capture detection[9] and radioimmunoassay. The limit of detection by HPLC with UV detection is 0.5 $\mu g.l^{-1}$ and by GC with ECD[10] it is 20 $\mu g.l^{-1}$. ^{14}C can be incorporated into the phenol ring of probenecid and radiolabelled drug has been used in pharmacokinetic studies in man; 10 μCi may be safely administered to humans for investigational purposes.[11,12] Gastrointestinal absorption of probenecid is rapid and complete and no presystemic metabolism occurs.[13] Following a single 1 g oral dose, plasma concentrations reach 25 $mg.l^{-1}$ at 30 minutes, peak in 2–4 hours and remain above 30 $mg.l^{-1}$ for 8 hours.

Following a single 2 g oral dose, peak concentrations of 150–200 $mg.l^{-1}$ are reached in 4 hours and remain above 50 $mg.l^{-1}$ for the next 8 hours. Maximal renal clearance of uric acid usually occurs 30 minutes post-administration of probenecid, while its effect on plasma penicillin concentration is maximal after 2 hours. Serum uric acid concentration should be used to monitor therapy. Probenecid dosage is adequate to inhibit penicillin secretion when phenolsulphonphthalein (PSP) excretion is reduced to approximately 20% of the normal rate.

Probenecid distributes rapidly after intravenous administration with a volume of distribution of approximately 11 l. The drug is bound extensively to plasma proteins (mainly albumin).[13] The CSF/plasma concentration ratio of probenecid[9,14,15] ranges between 0.2 and 0.6 at plasma levels of 220–571 $mg.l^{-1}$.

In man, considerable interindividual variation and dose-dependence has been observed in the elimination half life of probenecid. The plasma concentration decline is most rapid at lower doses ($t_{\frac{1}{2}}$ = 2–6 hours after 0.5–1.0 g, and 4–12 hours after 2 g).[13] Clearance is mainly by hepatic metabolism. Renal clearance is independent of dose, but dependent on both urinary pH and flow rate. Net tubular secretion of probenecid occurs in alkaline urine while net tubular reabsorption occurs in acid urine. The renal clearance of probenecid (corrected for binding) is 6.8–16.9 $ml.min^{-1}$ at pH 6.

Probenecid is extensively metabolized, mainly in the liver. It is largely eliminated in the urine (≃90%), with only 5–10% as the unchanged drug, although this will vary with urine pH.

No information is available on the excretion of the drug into breast milk.

The elimination of probenecid is impaired in renal dysfunction. It is likely that with increasing age, decreasing renal function will result in some reduction in the elimination of the drug.

Oral absorption	100%
Presystemic metabolism	nil
Plasma half life	
range	4–17 h
Volume of distribution	11 l
Plasma protein binding	90%

Concentration–effect relationship

Plasma probenecid concentrations of 40–60 $mg.l^{-1}$ produce maximal inhibition of renal penicillin excretion. Concentrations of 100–200 $mg.l^{-1}$ produce a uricosuric effect.[16]

Metabolism

In man, probenecid undergoes glucuronidation and side-chain oxidation/dealkylation.[17] As shown in Fig. 1 this gives rise to probenecid mono-acylglucuronide (a), two monohydroxylated compounds (b, c), a carboxylated metabolite (d) and an N-depropylated compound (e).[13] All but the former are actively uricosuric. Probenecid is metabolized slowly by the liver and after single oral doses of 0.5–2 g, 75–88% of the drug is recovered in the urine in 4 days, with only a small amount (5–11%) as intact drug. The major metabolic product is excreted as probenecid acylglucuronide, with the remainder recovered in approximately equal amounts of the four other metabolites. It is not known whether probenecid and its metabolites are excreted in bile and undergo enterohepatic recirculation in man, nor whether hepatic dysfunction reduces clearance.

Fig. 1 Metabolites of probenecid

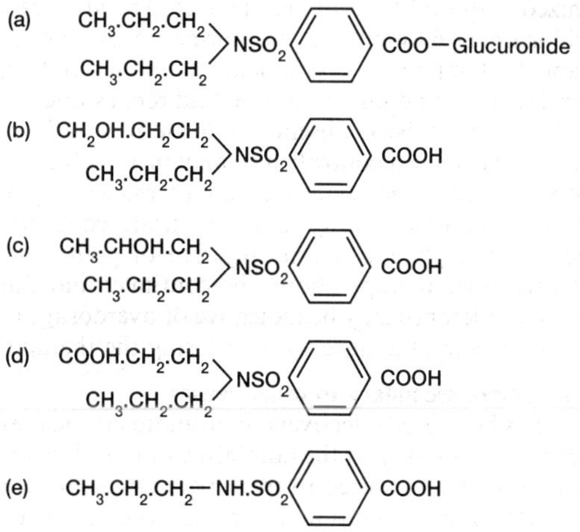

Pharmaceutics

Tablets containing 500 mg of probenecid are the form in which it is principally available. Benemid (MSD, UK) are white, round scored tablets marked 'MSD 501'. Benemid (MSD, US) are yellow elongated scored tablets also marked 'MSD 501'. Probenecid is also available in combination with colchicine (500 mg/0.5 mg) (ColBenemid; MSD, US; white, elongated scored tablet, marked 'MSD 614') or ampicillin (1 g/3.5 g) (Polycillin-PRB; Bristol, US; a single dose oral suspension to be reconstituted with water before use). Probenecid tablets should be stored in well-closed containers at a temperature less than 40°C, preferably between 15–30°C and protected from light. Commercially available tablets have an expiration date of 3–5 years depending upon packaging.

Therapeutic use

Indications

1. Hyperuricaemia associated with gout
2. Hyperuricaemia secondary to other causes
3. Adjunctive therapy with antibiotics.

Contraindications

1. Hypersensitivity
2. Acute gout attack
3. History of uric acid kidney stones
4. Blood dyscrasia
5. Young children
6. History of peptic ulcer disease
7. Renal impairment
8. Use of salicylates.

Indications

1. Hyperuricaemia associated with gout

Probenecid may be employed in patients with gout and hyperuricaemia who do not have increased urinary uric acid excretion (i.e. > 700 mg daily on a general diet).[18–20] Probenecid has no analgesic or anti-inflammatory activity and will exacerbate and prolong inflammation during an acute attack of gout. Therefore, it should be started 2–3 weeks after an acute attack, in an initial dose of 250 mg twice daily. This dose may be increased over a period of several weeks to a level which will maintain the serum urate below 7 mg per 100 ml, the minimum concentration at which urate saturates the extracellular fluid. A total dose of 1 g daily is appropriate for half of patients; the maximum dose should not exceed 3 g daily. When therapy with probenecid is initiated, negative urate balance commences, serum urate drops and urinary uric acid excretion is elevated above pretreatment levels. As therapy continues, urate is mobilized and eliminated, serum urate falls, and uric acid excretion returns to pretreatment levels. The transient increase in uric acid excretion which usually lasts for only a few days, may lead to the development of kidney stones in as many as 9% of patients treated. This complication may be minimized by initiating therapy at low doses with the gradual increases previously described. Ample urine flow should be maintained with adequate hydration and the urine should be alkalinized with oral sodium bicarbonate. The ideal candidate for probenecid is under 60 years old, has normal renal function (creatinine clearance > 80 $ml.min^{-1}$), uric acid excretion < 700 mg per 24 h on a general diet, and no history of uric acid renal stones. After acute attacks of gout have been absent for 6 months and serum urate concentrations have been controlled, it may be possible to reduce the dosage of probenecid. Daily dosage may be reduced by 500 mg per day every 4–6 months as long as serum urate concentrations are controlled and the patient is clinically free of gout attacks. Some degree of uricosuric therapy should be continued indefinitely however. Gastric intolerance may be indicative of overdosage and may be corrected by reducing the dose without losing the therapeutic effect.

2. Hyperuricaemia secondary to other causes

Probenecid has been used effectively to promote uric acid excretion in hyperuricaemia secondary to the administration of thiazide and loop diuretics. It should *not* be used to treat hyperuricaemia secondary to cancer chemotherapy, radiation or myeloproliferative disease, because it may increase the risk of uric acid nephropathy.

3. Adjunctive therapy with antibiotics

The co-administration of both probenecid and acidic antibiotics causes a decrease in the clearance of the antibiotic, and the earliest clinical application of probenecid was as an adjunct to high-dose penicillin therapy and in the treatment of tuberculosis with PAS. Detailed clinical studies have revealed that the renal tubular blocking action of probenecid is not sufficient to account for the decrease in clearance of antibiotics. Although a scientific explanation for this phenomenon has not been found, it is assumed that enhanced tissue levels will follow when plasma levels of the antibiotic are increased. Probenecid has been co-administered with many antibiotics of short biological half life to prolong their plasma concentrations, but this strategy is most commonly employed today as part of the US Centers for Disease Control (CDC) recommended treatment schedule for gonococcal infections. For single dose treatment of acute uncomplicated gonorrhoea, the CDC recommends that 1 g of probenecid be administered orally with 3 g of amoxycillin, 3.5 g of ampicillin, or 4.8 million units of procaine penicillin intramuscularly (at two injection sites). When amoxycillin or ampicillin is used for the treatment of disseminated gonococcal infections (arthritis–dermatitis syndrome) the CDC recommends that an initial oral loading dose of 3 or 3.5 g of amoxycillin or ampicillin respectively, be administered concurrently with 1 g of probenecid orally. Therapy is then continued according to different schedules without probenecid. For the treatment of acute pelvic inflammatory disease in ambulatory patients, the CDC suggests that adults receive a single 1 g oral dose of probenecid with a 2 g intramuscular dose of cefoxitin, a 3 g oral dose of amoxycillin, or a 3.5 g oral dose of ampicillin, followed by an oral doxycycline dosage of 100 mg twice daily for 10–14 days. When procaine penicillin is used for treatment of neurosyphyllis in adults, the CDC suggests 500 mg of probenecid orally and 2.4 million units of procaine penicillin intramuscularly be administered concurrently every six hours for ten days, followed by 2.4 million units of benzathine penicillin intramuscularly weekly for three doses without probenecid. The manufacturer recommends that the drug is given at least 30 minutes before a parenteral antibiotic.

Contraindications

1. Hypersensitivity

Patients with a history of known hypersensitivity to probenecid should not receive this drug.

2. Acute gout attack

Since probenecid has no analgesic or anti-inflammatory activity, it is of no value in the treatment of acute gout. It will exacerbate and prolong inflammation during the acute phase.[18] Probenecid should not be started until 2–3 weeks after an acute gout attack.

3. History of uric acid kidney stones

Patients with a history of uric acid nephrolithiasis and/or a daily urinary excretion of greater than 700 mg of uric acid should be treated with allopurinol instead of probenecid.

4. Blood dyscrasia

Patients with blood dyscrasia should not receive probenecid.

5. Young children

Because of lack of experience, probenecid is contraindicated in children younger than two years of age.

6. History of peptic ulcer disease

Probenecid should be used cautiously in patients with a history of peptic ulcer.

7. Renal impairment

Probenecid may be effective in gouty patients with mild renal impairment, but varied doses may be required. In patients with a creatinine clearance less than 50 $ml.min^{-1}$, the drug is not effective. The manufacturer recommends that the drug should not be used with β-lactam antibiotics in patients with renal impairment.

8. Use of salicylates

Salicylates are contraindicated in patients taking probenecid as acetylsalicylic acid antagonises its uricosuric action.

Adverse reactions

Potentially life-threatening effects

Both hepatic necrosis and aplastic anaemia have occurred rarely. Mild to moderately severe haemolytic anaemia which may be related to genetic deficiency of glucose-6-phosphate dehydrogenase has also been reported. Anaphylactic reactions have occurred following the administration of probenecid.

Acute overdosage

In one report, following ingestion of 47.5 g of probenecid, copious vomiting, stupor, and coma followed.[21] Several tonic–clonic seizures occurred, each lasting approximately 30 seconds and were treated with intravenous phenobarbitone and phenytoin. Serum urate decreased to very low concentrations. In the face of acute probenecid overdosage, induction of emesis or gastric lavage is recommended. Short-acting barbiturates may be administered if signs of CNS stimulation occur. Seizures may be treated with intravenous phenobarbitone and/or phenytoin.[22]

Severe or irreversible adverse effects

No reactions of this kind, other than those mentioned above, have been reported.

Probenecid

Symptomatic adverse effects
Therapy with probenecid is usually well tolerated and has a low incidence of adverse effects, the most frequent of which include headache, anorexia, nausea, vomiting, dermatitis, and pruritis. Other reported ill effects are dizziness, fever, sore gums, flushing, and urinary frequency. Probenecid may promote the development of uric acid nephrolithiasis which may cause renal colic, haematuria, and costovertebral pain. This is most likely to occur when probenecid therapy is initiated. Maintenance of a large volume of alkaline urine increases the solubility of uric acid and thus reduces the risk of stone formation in the kidneys.

Other effects
Probenecid both reduces serum uric acid concentrations and increases urinary concentration and excretion of uric acid. It may also cause a reduction in total plasma tryptophan and an increase in the free amino acid.

Interference with clinical pathology tests
Probenecid interferes with the determination of urinary 17-ketosteroids, and may give a false-positive result with both the Benedict and Clinitest tests for urinary glucose.

High risk groups

Neonates
The drug should not be used in neonates.

Breast milk. No data are available, so that it is best avoided by women who breast-feed their infants.

Children
The use of probenecid in children younger than two years old is contraindicated. In β-lactam therapy, probenecid can be given as 25 $mg.kg^{-1}$ initially, followed by 40 $mg.kg^{-1}$ a day in divided doses. For children weighing more than 50 kg, the adult dosage is recommended.

Pregnant women
Safety for use during pregnancy has not been established; probenecid crosses the placental barrier and appears in cord blood. With the exception of the death of one neonate not definitely related to probenecid, the drug has been used in pregnancy without adverse effect to mother or child. The use of probenecid during pregnancy should be limited to the treatment of gout with hyperuricaemia.

The elderly
No special precautions are required in the elderly provided there is no renal impairment.

Drug interactions

Potentially hazardous interactions

Sulphonylureas. The renal clearance of sulphonylureas (e.g. chlorpropamide) is reduced by probenecid and hypoglycaemia could therefore result.[23]

Methotrexate. Probenecid inhibits renal elimination of methotrexate and may possibly precipitate toxicity.[24] If the drugs are given together, the dose of methotrexate should be reduced, the patient should be carefully monitored for signs of methotrexate toxicity, and serum levels may need to be monitored. Probenecid may also enhance the effect of methotrexate in central nervous system malignancies by inhibiting its removal from the cerebrospinal fluid.[25]

Other significant interactions

Pyrazinamide and salicylates. These drugs antagonize the uricosuric effect of probenecid.[26,27] Alternatively, paracetamol may be employed.

Allopurinol. Probenecid promotes excretion of allopurinol's active metabolite,[28] but it is agreed that the effect of both in combination is additive.

Nitrofurantoin. Probenecid blocks renal secretion of this drug and therefore reduces its therapeutic efficacy in renal infections and increases its toxic potential. Their co-administration should be avoided.

Loop diuretics. Natriuresis induced by frusemide or ethacrynic acid is attenuated by probenecid.[29] The uricosuric effect of probenecid is decreased by loop diuretics.

Thiazide diuretics. Probenecid increases urinary excretion of calcium, magnesium, and citrate during thiazide therapy. Natriuresis by thiazides is unopposed or increased by probenecid.[30] The uricosuric effect of probenecid is inhibited by thiazides.

Sulphonamides. Probenecid decreases the renal excretion of conjugated sulphonamides and the total sulphonamide plasma levels should be determined from time to time if both drugs are given together over a long period.

Phosphorus. The renal tubular reabsorption of phosphorus is inhibited in hypothyroid but not in euparathyroid individuals.

Potentially useful interactions

Penicillin and cephalosporins. The renal excretion of these antibiotics is inhibited, thereby potentiating their anti-infective action.[31] It has been suggested that probenecid also reduces the volume of distribution of antibiotics.[32] In the presence of renal insufficiency, the co-administration of probenecid and penicillin or a cephalosporin is not recommended.

Indomethacin. The clearance of indomethacin is decreased by probenecid, although the mechanism is unknown.[33–35] The clinical importance of this interaction is unclear, but it has been suggested that reduced doses of indomethacin may produce a beneficial clinical response when probenecid is co-administered. Increases in indomethacin doses should also be made in small increments. Similar interactions with other non-steroidal anti-inflammatory drugs probably occur.[36]

Probenecid increases the mean plasma half life of a number of other drugs including acetaminophen, naproxin, ketoprofen, meclofenamate, lorazepam and rifampin. The clinical significance of this is not known; however, adjustment in the usual dosages of these drugs may be required.

References

1. Yu T-F 1974 Milestones in the treatment of gout. American Journal of Medicine 56: 676–685
2. Kelley W N, Weiner I M 1978 Uric acid. Springer-Verlag, Berlin, pp 1–639
3. Krakoff I H 1967 Clinical pharmacology of drugs which influence uric acid production and excretion. Clinical Pharmacology and Therapeutics 8: 124–138
4. Weiner I M, Washington J A, Mudge G H 1960 On the mechanism of action of probenecid on renal tubular secretion. Bulletin of the Johns Hopkins Hospital 106: 333–346
5. Poulsen H 1955 Inhibition of uric acid excretion in rabbits given probenecid or salicylic acid. Acta Pharmacologica Toxicologica 11: 277–286
6. Van der Poel F W, Van Praag H M, Korf J 1977 Evidence for a probenecid-sensitive transport system of acid monoamine metabolites from the spinal subarachnoid space. Psychopharmacology 52: 35–40
7. Cunningham R F, Israili Z H, Dayton P G 1978 New spectrofluorometric assay for probenecid. Journal of Pharmaceutical Sciences 67: 434
8. Harle R K, Cowen T 1978 Determination of probenecid in serum by high performance liquid chromatography. The Analyst 103: 492
9. Roos B E, Wickstrom C, Hartvig P, Nilsson J L G 1980 Quantitation of CSF concentrations and biological activity of probenecid metabolites. European Journal of Clinical Pharmacology 7: 223–226
10. Mu J Y, Faraj B A, Israili Z H, Dayton P G 1974 Studies of the specificity of an antibody directed against probenecid. Investigations with probenecid analogs. Life Sciences 14: 837
11. Dayton P G, Perel J M 1973 The metabolism of probenecid in man. Annals of the New York Academy of Sciences 226: 172
12. Perel J M, Cunningham R F, Fales H M, Dayton P G 1970 Identification and renal excretion of probenecid metabolites in man. Life Sciences 9: 1337
13. Dayton P G, Yu T F, Chen W, Berger L, West L A, Gutman A B 1963 The physiological disposition of probenecid, including renal clearance, in man, studied by an improved method for its estimation in biological material. Journal of Pharmacology and Experimental Therapeutics 140: 278–286
14. Perel J M, Levitt M, Dunner D L 1974 Plasma and cerebrospinal fluid concentrations as related to accumulation of acidic biogenic amine metabolites in man. Psychopharmacologica 35: 83
15. Sjostrom R 1972 Steady state levels of probenecid and their relation to acid monoamine metabolites in human cerebrospinal fluid. Psychopharmacologica 25: 96
16. Perel J M, Dayton P G 1971 Studies of the renal excretion of probenecid acyl glucuronide in man. European Journal of Clinical Pharmacology 3: 106–112
17. Cunningham R F, Israili Z H, Dayton P G 1981 Clinical pharmacokinetics of probenecid. Clinical Pharmacokinetics 6: 135–151
18. Goldfinger S E 1971 Drug therapy treatment of gout. New England Journal of Medicine 285: 1303–1306
19. Gutman A B 1966 Uricosuric drugs, with special reference to probenecid and sulfinpyrazone. Advances in Pharmacology 4: 91–142
20. Zarro V J 1978 Pharmacology of gout. In: Lowenthal, Major (eds) Clinical therapeutics. Grune and Stratton, New York, pp 343–346
21. Rizzuto V J, Inglesby T V, Grace W J 1965 Probenecid (Benemid) intoxication with status epilepticus. American Journal of Medicine 38: 646
22. McKinney S E, Peck H M, Bochey J M, Byham B B, Schuchardt G S V, Beyer K H 1951 Benemid, p-(di-n-propyl-sylfamyl)-benzoic acid: toxicologic properties. Journal of Pharmacology and Experimental Therapeutics 102: 208–214

23. Hansen H M, Christensen L K 1977 Drug interactions with oral sulphonylurea hypoglycaemic drugs. Drugs 13: 24–34
24. Aherne G W, Piall E, Marks V, Mould G, White W F 1978 Prolongation and enhancement of serum methotrexate concentrations by probenecid. British Medical Journal 1: 1097–1099
25. Howell S B, Olshen R A, Rice J A 1979 Effect of probenecid on cerebrospinal fluid methotrexate kinetics. Clinical Pharmacology and Therapeutics 26: 641–646
26. Diamond H S, Meisel A D 1977 Effect of pharmacological inhibitors on urate transport during induced uricosuria. Clinical Science and Molecular Medicine 53: 133–140
27. Fanelli G M Jr, Weiner I M 1979 Urate excretion: drug interactions. Journal of Pharmacology and Experimental Therapeutics 210: 186–195
28. Elion G B, Yu T F, Gutman A B, Hitchings G H 1968 Renal clearance of oxipurinol, the chief metabolite of allopurinol. American Journal of Medicine 45: 69–77
29. Honari J, Blair A D, Cutler R E 1977 Effects of probenecid on furosemide kinetics and natriuresis in man. Clinical Pharmacology and Therapeutics 22: 395–401
30. Brater D C 1978 Increase in diuretic effect of chlorothiazide by probenecid. Clinical Pharmacology and Therapeutics 23: 259–265
31. Boger W P, Beatty J P, Pitts F W, Flippin H F 1950 The influence of a new benzoic acid derivative on the metabolism of para-aminosalicylic acid (PAS) and penicillin. Annals of Internal Medicine 33: 18–31
32. Gibaldi M, Schwartz M A 1968 Apparent effect of probenecid on the distribution of penicillins in man. Clinical Pharmacology and Therapeutics 9: 345–349
33. Duggan D E, Hooke K F, White S D, Noll R M, Stevenson C R 1977 The effects of probenecid upon the individual components of indomethacin elimination. Journal of Pharmacology and Experimental Therapeutics 201: 463–470
34. Skeith M D, Simkin P A, Healey L A 1968 The renal excretion of indomethacin and its inhibition by probenecid. Clinical Pharmacology and Therapeutics 9: 89–93
35. Baber N, Halliday L, Sibeon R, Littler T, Orme M 1978 The interaction between indomethacin and probenecid. A clinical and pharmacokinetic study. Clinical Pharmacology and Therapeutics 24: 298–307
36. Runkel R, Mroszczak E, Chaplin M, Sevelius H, Segre E 1978 Naproxen–probenecid interaction. Clinical Pharmacology and Therapeutics 24: 706–713

Probucol

Probucol is used to lower serum lipids. Theories concerning the mechanism of action of the drug have changed substantially since it was discovered and, currently, it seems probable that the antiatheromatous effects depend mainly upon its antioxidant properties.

Chemistry

Probucol is a sulphur-containing bisphenol (Lorelco, Lesterol, Lurselle, Perfenebid, Sinlestol)

$C_{31}H_{48}O_2S_2$

4,4′-(Ioopropylidenedithio)bis[2,6-di-tert-butylphenol]

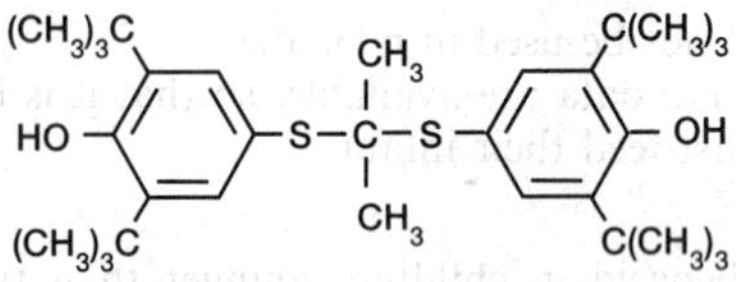

Molecular weight	516.9
pKa	
Solubility	
in alcohol	soluble
in water	insoluble
Octanol/water partition coefficient	

Pharmacology

The drug was originally developed as a cholesterol-lowering agent. More potent drugs to lower cholesterol are now available but there is considerable interest in the antiatheromatous action which is greater than would be predicted from the relatively modest reduction of cholesterol. Probucol has three separate pharmacological properties (i) antioxidant activity, (ii) stimulation of cholesterol ester transfer from high density lipoprotein (HDL) to very low density lipoprotein (VLDL) and (iii) prolongation of myocardial repolarization.

(i) The mechanisms of the hypocholesterolaemic effect of probucol was not known when the drug was first investigated, although there was some evidence that it could enhance bile acid excretion. The observation that it is an inhibitor of low density lipoprotein (LDL) oxidation opened a new line of enquiry which is still being explored.[1]

Low density lipoprotein may become atherogenic if it undergoes oxidation. Several lines of evidence indicate that such oxidative reactions occur in vivo and that oxidized LDL accumulates in atheromatous lesions. Probucol is undoubtedly a powerful antioxidant and inhibits lipid peroxidation in rat liver microsomes.[2] Sophisticated studies of the effects of probucol on LDL shape and structure have been carried out. These experiments indicated that the apoprotein B-100 structure is significantly disrupted by oxidation and that probucol can inhibit these changes.[3] When LDL is oxidized in vitro with cupric ions its binding to the fibroblast LDL receptor is diminished and uptake by macrophages is greatly increased. LDL taken from animals pretreated with probucol is relatively resistant to oxidation by cupric ions and the enhanced uptake by macrophages is prevented.

This hypothesis gained support when it was shown that probucol could substantially inhibit atheroma deposition in Watanabe heritable hyperlipidaemic rabbits at doses which caused little or no change in the concentration of plasma lipids.[4] When WHHL rabbits aged 2 months were fed 1 g daily of probucol and killed 6 months later the percentage of the surface area of the total thoracic aorta with visible

Probucol

plaque was 54.2% in controls vs. 7.0% in treated animals. In cholesterol-fed rabbits, administration of probucol decreased the thoracic aortic surface area covered by gross atherosclerotic lesions from 55.6 to 11.6%[5] and it has been proposed that probucol pretreatment inhibited the scavenger receptor pathway.[6] However, in a study in cholesterol-fed rabbits in which dietary adjustments were made to keep plasma cholesterol constant in probucol-treated and control animals there was no difference in aortic cholesterol content.[7] Thus, there is still discussion about the mechanism involved, although the data gained in WHHL rabbits is probably a better predictor for man than cholesterol feeding in the rabbit.

Enhanced oxidation of VLDL and LDL in alloxan diabetic animals has been correlated with the in vitro toxicity of this lipoprotein fraction to proliferating fibroblasts. Insulin treatment of diabetic animals inhibited both oxidation and cytotoxicity of VLDL + LDL. Treatment of diabetic rats with the antioxidants vitamin E or probucol, after diabetes was established, also inhibited both the in vivo oxidation and in vitro cytotoxicity of diabetic VLDL + LDL, but did not alter hyperglycaemia.[8]

(ii) Other studies have demonstrated that probucol affects LDL synthesis and HDL catabolism.[9,10] Probucol lowers the plasma concentration of both LDL and HDL. The proposed mechanism of reduction of HDL is that probucol stimulates cholesterol ester transfer protein (CETP) and thereby facilitates transfer of cholesterol from HDL to VLDL.

(iii) The precise mechanism of the prolongation of myocardial repolarization (QT) has not been defined.

Toxicology

Probucol is almost free of toxicological effects in normal experimental animals. In monkeys or dogs made severely hypercholesterolaemic, high doses of probucol have been shown to produce fatal cardiac arrhythmias, associated with QT prolongation.

Clinical pharmacology

The ability of probucol to prevent peroxidation of LDL was investigated in 20 hypercholesterolaemic individuals taking part in the Probucol Quantitative Regression Swedish Trial (PQRST). The effect of Cu^{2+}-induced oxidation of LDL on degradation by macrophages, binding to LDL receptors on fibroblasts and LDL thiobarbituric acid reactive substances (TBARS) content was analysed. With LDL isolated from patients on diet alone, in vitro oxidation led to a 44.3% decreased binding to fibroblasts, a nine-fold increased uptake in macrophages and a 20-fold increase in TBARS content as compared to native LDL. During treatment with probucol plus cholestyramine, exposure of LDL to Cu^{2+} resulted in an increase in TBARS which was less than 50% of that observed during the other treatment period. Furthermore, probucol treatment abolished more than 70% of the decrease in B,E receptor binding to fibroblasts and more than 90% of the increased degradation by macrophages.[11] The ability of probucol to prevent the Cu^{2+}-induced oxidation of human plasma low density lipoproteins is related to its concentration in LDL. In the absence of probucol, 3 μM Cu^{2+} induced half maximal LDL lipid oxidation. Oxidation caused loss of apolipoprotein B-100 and the appearance of higher molecular weight forms of the protein. In the presence of 0.6 mol% probucol (relative to phospholipid) the time required to obtain half maximal LDL lipid oxidation increased from 130 to 270 min and was explained by an increase in the lag time prior to LDL lipid oxidation. At a probucol concentration of 4.2 mol%, the antioxidant prevented the oxidation of LDL lipids. Moreover, probucol does not interfere with macrophage uptake of acetylated LDL.[12]

Probucol also stimulates reverse cholesteryl ester transfer in vivo apparently by mechanisms unrelated to lipoprotein binding.[13] In hyperlipidaemic patients probucol, 500 mg twice daily, lowers LDL by 10–20% and HDL by 20–30%. The HDL reduction is mainly of HDL2 and HDL3. The effect on HDL cholesterol concentrations appears to be due to inhibition of the synthesis of apolipoprotein A-1 — the major protein component of HDL. Probucol promotes the transfer of cholesteryl esters from HDL to lower density lipoproteins. In a study of 12 patients with stable type II hyperlipidaemia, probucol lowered LDL cholesterol by 9.1% and HDL cholesterol by 30%. By rate zonal ultracentrifugation, a marked reduction of HDL2 cholesterol (−68%) was shown, whereas changes in HDL3 were less significant (−21%). Polyacrylamide gradient gel electrophoresis showed a reduction or disappearance of HDL2b particles and the prevalence of particles in the HDL3a range. Cholesteryl ester transfer from HDL to lower density lipoproteins was significantly increased (30%) in all patients. These findings suggest that, in addition to prevention of LDL peroxidation and macrophage uptake, probucol modifies HDL particle distribution in vivo, and is associated with a significant increase of cholesteryl ester transfer activity (CETA).[14] However, in a patient with familial hyperalphalipoproteinaemia probucol lowered LDL and HDL without any change in CETA.[15]

In most clinical studies the maximum effect on plasma lipids is seen after 1–3 months of therapy. A reduction of HDL would be expected to have an adverse effect upon the reuptake of cholesterol from atheromatous deposits[16] but animal studies suggest that an anti-atheromatous action predominates as a result of inhibition of oxidation of LDL.

Probucol has very few other effects on physiological systems in man, apart from prolongation of the QT interval in the electrocardiogram, by a mean of about 24 milliseconds.[17]

Pharmacokinetics

An automated HPLC method for determination of the drug in plasma and lipoprotein fractions has been published.[18] Pharmacokinetic information about the drug is incomplete. Although highly lipophilic, less than 10% of the oral dose is absorbed. The largest elimination is through faeces, after biliary excretion.

The highest gastrointestinal absorption takes place when the drug is given with food. Probucol accumulates slowly in adipose tissue and it may be present and bound to fat for up to 6 months while it is slowly released into blood and excreted through bile. Renal elimination is negligible. The drug is not bound to albumin but it is incorporated into LDL.

Concentration–effect relationship

The hypocholesterolaemic effect is maximum at the usual dose of 1 $g.d^{-1}$ and does not increase with increasing dose.

There is no known correlation between blood levels and therapeutic and/or toxic effects. Plasma levels with therapeutic doses range between 10 and 75 $mg.l^{-1}$ — mean therapeutic blood level is 22 $mg.l^{-1}$.

Metabolism

Probucol is poorly absorbed and what is absorbed is mainly excreted in bile. Metabolism of the drug is negligible. However, a hypothesis of the drug's action in the LDL particle has been proposed which involves probucol interaction with free radicals. The hydroxyl radical is the most potent agent in oxidizing LDL lipids. If OH· is responsible it may extract two phenolic hydrogen atoms from probucol to form an unstable intermediate. This substance would break down to form the stable product spiroquinone which could undergo homo- or heterolytic scission to form diphenoquinone. If this substance is also a potent antioxidant, diphenoquinone and bisphenol may form a regenerative free radical scavenging cycle (Fig. 1).[19]

Pharmaceutics

Probucol/Lurselle (Merrelle Dow, UK) is available in 250 mg tablets. The round white tablets are stable and have a reasonably long shelf-life.

In the USA a 500 mg tablet (Lorelco/Merrelle Dow, USA) is also available, it is a white, oblong tablet with rounded ends.

Therapeutic use

Indications

1. Hypercholesterolaemia
2. Severe heterozygous familial hypercholesterolaemics.

Contraindications

1. Chronic diarrhoea syndrome
2. Severe cardiac arrhythmias.

Fig. 1 Metabolism of probucol

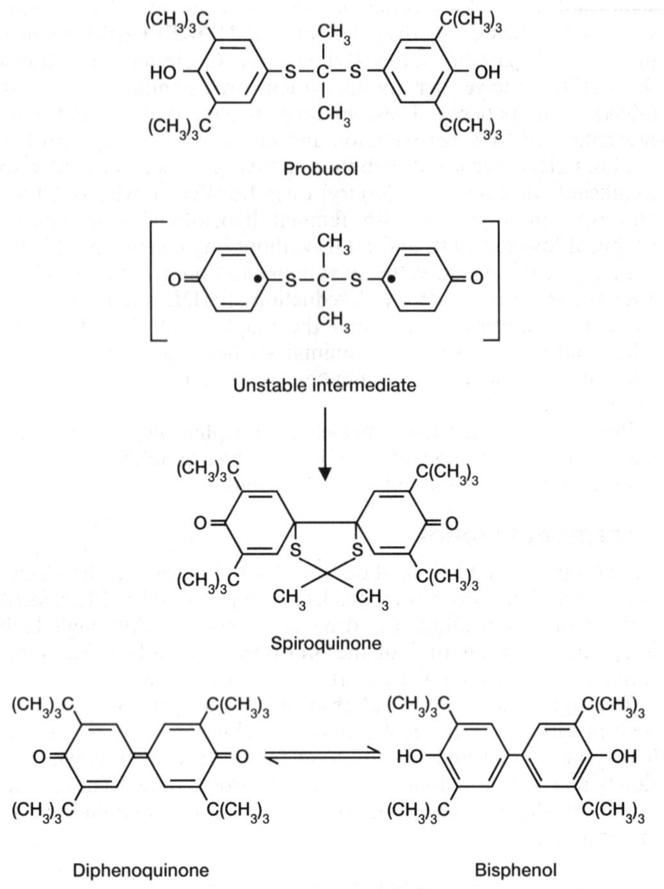

Mode of use

1. Hypercholesterolaemia

Abnormally elevated levels of total blood cholesterol or low density lipoprotein cholesterol (LDLC) at or above the 90th percentile for respective age and sex is an indication for administration of hypocholesterolaemic drugs if dietary intervention does not reduce blood levels to or below the 75th percentile for the age and sex of the patient.[20] Probucol is indicated for this use as a single drug or in combination with resins.[21–24] The usual dose is 500 mg twice daily. In most studies the reduction in LDL has been relatively small, 8% to 20%, and the reduction in HDL is larger, 20–30%. The effect may be greater in older people. Probucol treatment for 10 months caused significant reductions in the serum levels of total cholesterol, LDL-cholesterol, HDL-cholesterol, and apoprotein AI, AII, B, and CIII in both young/middle-aged and elderly patients. The decreases in the levels of LDLC and apolipoprotein B were greater in the elderly group than in the young/middle-aged group (LDLC: −17.0%, and −35.4% (elderly); apoprotein B: −12.3%, and −28.1% (elderly)). The serum probucol concentrations in the two groups were not significantly different.[25]

Comparison with the HMG-CoA reductase inhibitors lovastatin and simvastatin has shown that probucol causes a substantially smaller reduction in cholesterol, 8% versus 25–40%. Probucol also caused a substantial reduction in HDL whereas lovastatin and simvastatin caused a small increase.[26] Purely in terms of LDL reduction the HMG-CoA reductase inhibitors are much more effective and it still remains to be established whether probucol's antioxidant properties convey added advantage in human atheromatous disease.

2. Severe heterozygous familial hypercholesterolaemics

These are individuals with extreme elevation of serum cholesterol levels resulting in early, accelerated arteriosclerotic cardiovascular disease. They often have cutaneous xanthelasma and tendinous xanthomata due to excessive accumulation of tissue cholesterol. Treatment with probucol has shown to result in significant reduction of serum cholesterol and decrease in size or disappearance of xanthomatous cutaneous lesions in many of these patients.

Probucol

Recent work has demonstrated that these effects on decreasing cholesterol deposits in tissues are directly correlated with not only the reduction of LDLC but also the reduction in HDLC levels in blood. This is intriguing and difficult to explain given the known inverse relationship between HDLC levels and the incidence of coronary morbidity and mortality in most epidemiological studies.[16] Nevertheless it may help to dispel the concern shared by many regarding the HDLC-lowering effects of this drug.

Contraindications

1. Chronic diarrhoea syndrome

Probucol has a choleretic effect which may result in increased frequency of bowel movements or frank diarrhoea. This tends to be a transitory effect that disappears spontaneously in 2–4 weeks.[11] Nevertheless, on theoretical grounds, caution should be exercised when giving this drug to patients prone to bile acid diarrhoea syndromes.

2. Severe arrhythmias

Because of the common occurrence of QT prolongation in the ECG following probucol administration it is prudent not to give probucol to patients who have marked bradycardia or have an ECG showing severe myocardial conduction abnormality of the ECG prior to drug administration. However, there have been no proven clinical or electrocardiographic manifestations of significant toxic effects in man by probucol administration under any circumstances.[15]

Adverse reactions

Potentially life-threatening effects

Prolongation of the QT interval at the electrocardiogram occurs in about 50% of the patients receiving this drug at the usual dose of 500 mg twice a day. Probucol administration for 4 weeks produced torsades de pointes associated with further increased QT interval prolongation in a 36-year-old woman with Romano-Ward syndrome. When probucol was stopped the QTc interval shortened from 620 ms to 500 ms and ventricular ectopic beats disappeared completely.[27]

Acute overdosage

No cases of this kind have been reported.

Severe or irreversible adverse effects

No cases of this type have been reported.

Symptomatic adverse effects

Temporary looseness of the stools or diarrhoea occurs in a minority of patients when drug therapy is initiated. It is due to a choleretic effect of the drug which results in slight irritative effect of bile acids on the gastrointestinal mucosa and subsequent increase in motility and fluid secretion in the intestine.

Interference with clinical pathology test methods

There are no known effects of this kind.

High risk groups

Neonates

The drug is not recommended for use in neonates, and no information is available.

Breast milk. The drug should be avoided by nursing mothers for the reasons given below under Pregnant women.

Children

No information is available, but it is theoretically possible that the drug could be used in severe hypercholesterolaemic heterozygous children who do not respond to, or cannot tolerate treatment with, resins.

Pregnant women

Because of the unusually long half life and prolonged accumulation in tissues, it is advisable to discontinue probucol 2 to 3 months before pregnancy and not to give it to pregnant women.

The elderly

There is no known contraindication in the elderly, and no evidence of a different drug absorption if it causes diarrhoea.

Probucol

Drug interactions

Potentially hazardous interactions

No interactions of this kind have been reported.

Other significant interactions

Because of its effects on prolonging the QT interval in the ECG, it is theoretically possible, but not proven, that probucol might enhance intramyocardial conduction delay caused by antiarrhythmic drugs such as quinidine and procainamide.

Gastrointestinal absorption of probucol is enhanced with the presence of food, hence the recommendation of intake of the drug with meals.

Potentially useful interactions

Probucol given concomitantly with resins (cholestyramine or colestipol) may potentiate their hypocholesterolaemic effects and alleviate their constipating action.

Clinical trials

No outcome trials have yet been completed but a trial on regression of atheroma (PQRST) is in progress in Sweden.

1. The Lovastatin Study Group IV 1990 A multicenter comparison of lovastatin and probucol for treatment of severe primary hypercholesterolemia. American Journal of Cardiology 66: 22B–30B

290 patients taking lipid-lowering diets were randomly assigned to 14 weeks treatment with: lovastatin, 40 mg once a day with the morning meal; lovastatin, 40 mg once a day with the evening meal; lovastatin, 80 mg daily in the evening; lovastatin, 40 mg twice daily, or probucol, 500 mg twice daily. One-third of the patients received probucol, and the other two-thirds were equally divided between the 4 lovastatin treatment groups. The mean reductions in low density lipoprotein cholesterol were 25, 32, 37, 40 and 8%. High density lipoprotein cholesterol increased by 9 to 12% in all the lovastatin groups, but decreased by 23% in the probucol group.

General review articles

Buckley M M T, Goa K L, Price A H, Brogden R N 1989 Probucol. A reappraisal of its pharmacological properties and therapeutic use in hypercholesterolaemia. Drugs 37: 761–800

Zimetbaum P, Eder H, Frishman W 1990 Probucol: pharmacology and clinical application. Journal of Clinical Pharmacology 30: 3–9

References

1. Parthasarathy S, Young S G, Witztum, Pittman R C, Steinberg D 1986 Probucol inhibits oxidative modification of low density lipoprotein. Journal of Clinical Investigation 77: 641–644
2. Aruoma O I, Evans P J, Kaur H, Sutcliffe L, Halliwell B 1990 An evaluation of the antioxidant and potential pro-oxidant properties of food additives and of trolox C, vitamin E and probucol. Free Radicals Research Communications 10(3): 143–157
3. Bellamy M F, Nealis A S, Aitken J W, Bruckdorfer K R, Perkins S J 1989 Structural changes in oxidised low-density lipoproteins and of the effect of the anti-atherosclerotic drug probucol observed by synchrotron X-ray and neutron solution scattering. European Journal of Biochemistry 183: 321–329
4. Ishii K, Kita T 1990 Prevention of atherosclerosis using an antioxidant. Nippon Ronen Igakkai Zasshi 27: 177–181
5. Daugherty A, Zweifel B S, Schonfeld G 1989 Probucol attenuates the development of aortic atherosclerosis in cholesterol-fed rabbits. British Journal of Pharmacology 98: 612–618
6. Shankar R, Sallis J D, Stanton H, Thomson R 1989 Influence of probucol on early experimental atherogenesis in hypercholesterolemic rats. Atherosclerosis 78: 91–97
7. Stein Y, Stein O, Delplanque B, Fesmire J D, Lee D M Alaupovic P 1989 Lack of effect of probucol on atheroma formation in cholesterol-fed rabbits kept at comparable plasma cholesterol levels. Atherosclerosis 75: 145–155
8. Morel D W, Chisolm G M 1989 Antioxidant treatment of diabetic rats inhibits lipoprotein oxidation and cytotoxicity. Journal of Lipid Research 30: 1827–1834
9. Kesaniemi Y A, Grundy S M 1984 Influence of probucol on cholesterol metabolism in man. Journal of Lipid Research 25: 780–790
10. Nestel P J, Billington T 1981 Effects of probucol on low density lipoprotein removal and high density lipoprotein synthesis. Atherosclerosis 38: 203–209
11. Regnstrom J, Walldius G, Carlson L A, Nilsson J 1990 Effect of probucol treatment on the susceptibility of low density lipoprotein isolated from hypercholesterolemic patients to become oxidatively modified in vitro. Atherosclerosis 82: 43–51
12. Ku G, Schroeder K, Schmidt L F, Jackson R L, Doherty N S 1990 Probucol does not alter acetylated low density lipoprotein uptake by murine peritoneal macrophages. Atherosclerosis 80: 191–197
13. Chiesa G, Franceschini G, Sirtori C R 1990 In vitro activity of probucol on cholesteryl ester transport. Biochimica Biophysica Acta 1045: 302–304
14. Franceschini G, Sirtori M, Vaccarino V et al 1989 Mechanisms of HDL reduction after probucol. Changes in HDL subfractions and increased reverse cholesteryl ester transfer. Arteriosclerosis 9: 462–469
15. Takegoshi T, Haba T, Kitoh C, Tokuda T, Mabuchi H 1988 Decreased serum cholesterol-ester transfer activity in a patient with familial hyperalphalipoproteinaemia. Japanese Journal of Medicine 27: 295–299
16. Gordon T, Castelli W P, Hjortland M C, Kannel W B, Dawber T R 1977 Density lipoprotein as a protective factor against coronary heart disease: the Framingham study. American Journal of Medicine 62: 707–714
17. Dujovne C A, Atkins F, Wong B, DeCoursey S, Krehbiel P, Chernoff S B 1984 Electrocardiographic effects of probucol. A controlled prospective clinical trial. European Journal of Clinical Pharmacology 26: 735–739
18. Schoneshofer M, Heilmann P, Schmidt L, Schwartzkopff W 1989 Automated column liquid chromatographic determination of probucol in human serum and lipoprotein fractions. Journal of Chromatography 490: 230–235
19. Barnhart R L, Busch S J, Jackson R L 1989 Concentration-dependent antioxidant activity of probucol in low density lipoproteins in vitro: probucol degradation precedes lipoprotein oxidation. Journal of Lipid Research 30: 1703–1710
20. Consensus Conference 1985 Lowering blood cholesterol to prevent heart disease. Journal of the American Medical Association 253: 2080–2086
21. Dujovne C A, Krehbiel P, DeCoursey S et al 1984 Probucol plus colestipol in treatment of hypercholesterolemia. Annals of Internal Medicine 100: 477–482
22. Dujovne C A, Chernoff S, Krehbiel P, Jackson B, DeCoursey S, Taylor H 1984 Low dose colestipol plus probucol for hypercholesterolemia. American Journal of Cardiology 53: 1515–1518
23. Dujovne C A, Krehbiel P, Chernoff S 1986 Controlled studies of the efficacy and safety of combined probucol–colestipol therapy. American Journal of Cardiology 57 (16): 36H
24. McCaughan D 1981 Long term effects of probucol on serum lipids. Archives of Internal Medicine 141: 1428–1432
25. Morisaki N, Mori S, Kobayashi J 1990 Effects of long-term treatment with probucol on serum lipoproteins in cases of familial hypercholesterolemia in the elderly. Journal of American Geriatric Society 38: 15–18
26. Pietro D A, Alexander S, Mantell G, Staggers J E, Cook T J 1989 Effect of sivastatin and probucol in hypercholesterolaemia. American Journal of Cardiology 63: 682–686
27. Matsuhashi H, Onodera S, Kawamura Y et al 1989 Probucol-induced QT prolongation and torsades de pointes. Japanese Journal of Medicine 28: 612–615

Procainamide (hydrochloride)

Procainamide is a Class 1 agent used to treat ventricular arrhythmias.

Chemistry

Procainamide hydrochloride (Pronestyl, Procainamide Durules)
$C_{13}H_{21}N_3O.HCl$
4-Amino-N-(2-diethylaminoethyl)benzamide hydrochloride

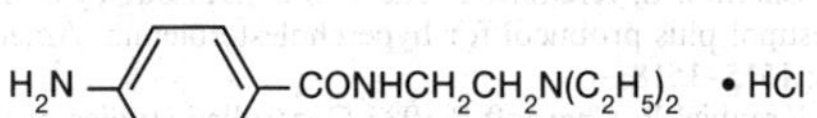

Molecular weight (free base)	271.8 (235.3)
pKa	9.2
Solubility	
in alcohol	1 in 2
in water	1 in 0.25
Octanol/water partition coefficient	low

Procainamide is a white to tan-coloured, odourless, hygroscopic, crystalline powder, synthesized chemically. A sterile solution of the drug in water, adjusted to a pH of 4–6, is available for parenteral use. An extended-release preparation is available which contains the drug in a wax matrix. Procainamide is not available in any combination preparations.

Pharmacology

Procainamide is a Class I antiarrhythmic agent,[1] reducing the rate of diastolic depolarization (phase 4) in cardiac Purkinje fibres and the rate of rise of the cardiac action potential. Procainamide also slows conduction down the bundle of His and suppresses automaticity in the His–Purkinje system.[2,3] Procainamide prolongs the effective refractory period of cardiac muscle and has a negative inotropic effect on the muscle cells.[4] Its actions are very similar to those of quinidine, and like that drug it has an anticholinergic effect (although this is weaker than with quinidine), which may modify its therapeutic effect. Procainamide has a local anaesthetic effect of similar magnitude to, but longer duration than, that of procaine itself. Procainamide is metabolized to N-acetylprocainamide (NAPA) which is particularly important in fast acetylators.[5] The NAPA metabolite has antiarrhythmic activity but its electrophysiological effects are slightly different from those of procainamide. In the dog, NAPA has little effect on automaticity or on the size of the action potential but it does prolong the duration of the action potential.[6]

Toxicology

There is no information on animal toxicology.

Clinical pharmacology

Procainamide is an effective antiarrhythmic agent in man. It is effective in a wide range of cardiac arrhythmias but it has been particularly used in the treatment of ventricular arrhythmias. The effect on the ECG is similar to that caused by quinidine, with prolongation of the PR, QRS and QT intervals. The negative inotropic effect of procainamide may precipitate cardiac failure, particularly when combinations of antiarrhythmic drugs are given. Hypotension is not unusual after procainamide therapy, particularly if the drug is given intravenously. Procainamide may produce anticholinergic effects but these effects are more common following quinidine therapy. The local anaesthetic effects of procainamide are rarely noted, but following intravenous dosing, central nervous system stimulation may occur, with hallucinations and psychosis, followed by CNS depression.

After intravenous doses of 100 mg every 5 minutes a linear correlation was found between plasma concentration and cumulative dose[7] such that:

$$\text{plasma concentration } (mg.l^{-1}) = 0.84 + 0.73\ x$$

where x = cumulative procainamide dose ($mg.kg^{-1}$ body weight). The effective plasma concentration for control of ventricular arrhythmias varied from 4 to 10 $mg.l^{-1}$, mean $= 6.4 \pm 5.3\ mg.l^{-1}$.

There was a dose-dependent fall in systolic arterial blood pressure up to a total dose of 1 g, reaching significance at a cumulative dose of 700 mg. The dose required to abolish the arrhythmia varied from 300 to 1000 mg.

Following a 1 g oral dose the absorption half time is approximately 20 min, peak plasma concentration averages 4.5 $mg.l^{-1}$ and is achieved within 1 h and the plasma half time is 2.9 h.[8] Approximately four doses of 0.5 g 3-hourly are required to reach 90% of the equilibrium state concentration. In a study of oral procainamide for the treatment of ventricular arrhythmias,[9] the plasma concentration required for 85% suppression of ventricular extrasystoles was $5 \pm 0.5\ mg.l^{-1}$ in patients with acute myocardial infarction and $9.3 \pm 0.7\ mg.l^{-1}$ in patients with chronic ischaemic heart disease. Prevention of ventricular tachycardia required $9.3 \pm 3.4\ mg.l^{-1}$.

Pharmacokinetics

The preferred analytical method is HPLC with UV detection. Various methods have been reported, with a limit of sensitivity[10] as low as 50 $\mu g.l^{-1}$.

Between 75% and 95% of orally administered procainamide is absorbed from the gastrointestinal tract, but not from the stomach, and the proportion does not appear to be affected by food. Presystemic metabolism is negligible. Peak plasma levels occur 1–2 h after oral administration but the relationship between plasma concentration and dosage varies considerably between patients. After intramuscular administration peak plasma levels occur within 15 and 60 minutes. Rapid initial distribution into the tissues, particularly heart, kidney, liver and lungs, is followed by elimination via both hepatic metabolism and renal excretion. Up to 80% of a dose is excreted in the urine in 24 h with 50–60% as unchanged drug. The apparent volume of distribution (2 $l.kg^{-1}$) is reduced in patients with heart failure.

15% of the drug is bound to plasma proteins. The half life is relatively short, at approximately 3 h,[11] whilst that of its active metabolite N-acetylprocainamide is longer, at 6–9 h. The clearance of procainamide is 5–15 $ml.min^{-1}.kg^{-1}$.

As might be expected from the large fraction of the dose excreted unchanged in the urine, renal failure prolongs the half life of procainamide to 13.9 ± 4.5 h.[12] Increasing age also prolongs the half life. Procainamide can be removed from the circulation by haemodialysis, but not by peritoneal dialysis, with a clearance of approximately 54 $ml.min^{-1}$ across the dialysis membrane.

Procainamide crosses the placental barrier and is excreted in human breast milk in small amounts.

Oral absorption	75–90%
Presystemic metabolism	negligible
Plasma half life	~3 h
N-acetyl procainamide	6–9 h
Volume of distribution	2 $l.kg^{-1}$
Plasma protein binding	15%

Concentration–effect relationship

The effective antiarrhythmic plasma concentration[13,14] is between 4 and 8 $mg.l^{-1}$. Toxic effects become apparent at 12 $mg.l^{-1}$. These figures relate primarily to procainamide itself and the contribution of NAPA to the antiarrhythmic effect is not clear. (See Clinical pharmacology.)

Metabolism

Acetylation is the major metabolic route to N-acetylprocainamide, and occurs in the liver (Fig. 1). Acetylation is genetically polymorphic. However, the clinical significance of the difference in acetylation rate between the fast and slow acetylator phenotypes is unclear.[5,15] After intravenous administration the terminal half life of procainamide is 2.5–4.7 h and that of N-acetylprocainamide is 7 h. The antiarrhythmic potency of N-acetylprocainamide is the same as that of procainamide and contributes to its therapeutic and toxic effects. Approximately 50–60% of the drug is excreted unchanged in the urine with a variable proportion as N-acetylprocainamide (≤30% in 24 h). Acetylation may be impaired in patients with severe liver disease.[16]

Pharmaceutics

Procainamide is available in oral and parenteral forms.

1. Pronestyl (Squibb/Princeton, UK/USA): White, scored tablets each containing 250 mg procainamide hydrochloride.
2. Pronestyl (Squibb/Princeton, UK/USA): Injection, procainamide 500 $mg.ml^{-1}$.
3. Procainamide Durules (Astra, UK): Yellow, sustained-release tablets, each containing 500 mg procainamide hydrochloride.

Many generic preparations are also available.

All preparations can be stored at room temperature. The maximum shelf-life of the solution is 24 months but it should be discarded if its colour is darker than light amber. The maximum shelf-life of the tablets is 36 months.

Therapeutic use

Indications

1. Treatment and prevention of ventricular arrhythmias
2. Maintenance of sinus rhythm after conversion by drugs or DC shock of atrial fibrillation, atrial flutter, supraventricular or junctional tachycardia
3. Conversion of supraventricular arrhythmias to sinus rhythm and dystrophia myotonica.[17,18] *Note*: Procainamide has been used for the treatment of hyperthermia.[19]

Contraindications

1. 1st, 2nd or 3rd degree heart block; bi- or tri-fascicular block
2. Heart (myocardial) failure
3. Myasthenia gravis
4. Digitalis intoxication
5. Known hypersensitivity to procainamide
6. Known hypersensitivity to sulphiting agents
7. Systemic lupus erythematosus (SLE)
8. Torsade de Pointes.

Special precautions

1. Impaired ventricular function
2. Unifascicular block
3. Renal disease
4. Liver disease.

Mode of use

Conversion of supraventricular arrhythmias

A single oral dose of 1.25 g should be given followed by a further 750 mg 1 hour later if there is no change in the ECG. Additional doses of 500 mg can be administered up to 2-hourly thereafter, until conversion to sinus rhythm occurs or toxic effects appear.

Daily total doses of up to 50 $mg.kg^{-1}$ in divided doses can be given to younger patients with normal renal function. If patients are elderly or have renal, hepatic or cardiac insufficiency lesser amounts or longer dosage intervals may promote adequate blood levels.

Conversion of ventricular tachycardia

A single oral dose of 1 g is administered, followed by 6.25 $mg.kg^{-1}$ every 3 hours. In urgent situations the initial loading dose can be given intramuscularly.

Maintenance dose

The oral maintenance dose is 250 mg 4 to 6-hourly or 500 mg to 1 g of the sustained-release preparation 8 to 12-hourly. Alternatively, 100–250 mg may be administered intramuscularly, 4 to 6-hourly.

Note: maintenance therapy should be controlled by estimation of plasma levels, where possible, with the aim of maintaining levels between 4 and 8 $mg.l^{-1}$.

Urgent treatment

In emergencies procainamide can be administered intravenously but must be diluted prior to use with a suitable intravenous infusion fluid such as 5% dextrose. The rate should not exceed 25–50 $mg.min^{-1}$. It is mandatory to monitor the blood pressure and the ECG continuously and adjust the dose accordingly. If a fall in blood pressure, prolongation of the PR interval, widening of the QRS complex greater than 50% or other adverse effect should occur, the infusion should be temporarily discontinued. In malignant hyperthermia the intravenous dose has ranged from 200 to 900 mg, usually followed by a maintenance infusion.

Paediatric dosage

Although generally not recommended for children, its use may be necessary for serious refractory arrhythmias. 50 $mg.kg^{-1}$ per 24 hours divided into 4 to 6 doses has been effectively used. In critically ill paediatric patients an intravenous dose of 3–6 $mg.kg^{-1}$ has been given over 5 minutes followed by an intravenous infusion of 0.02–0.08 $mg.kg^{-1}.min^{-1}$ to maintain sinus rhythm. The total dose should not exceed 1 g.

Indications

1 and 3. Conversion of arrhythmias to sinus rhythm[7,9,20]

In the case of atrial fibrillation, and particularly in the case of atrial flutter, the ventricular rate should be controlled with digoxin prior to

Fig. 1 Metabolism of procainamide

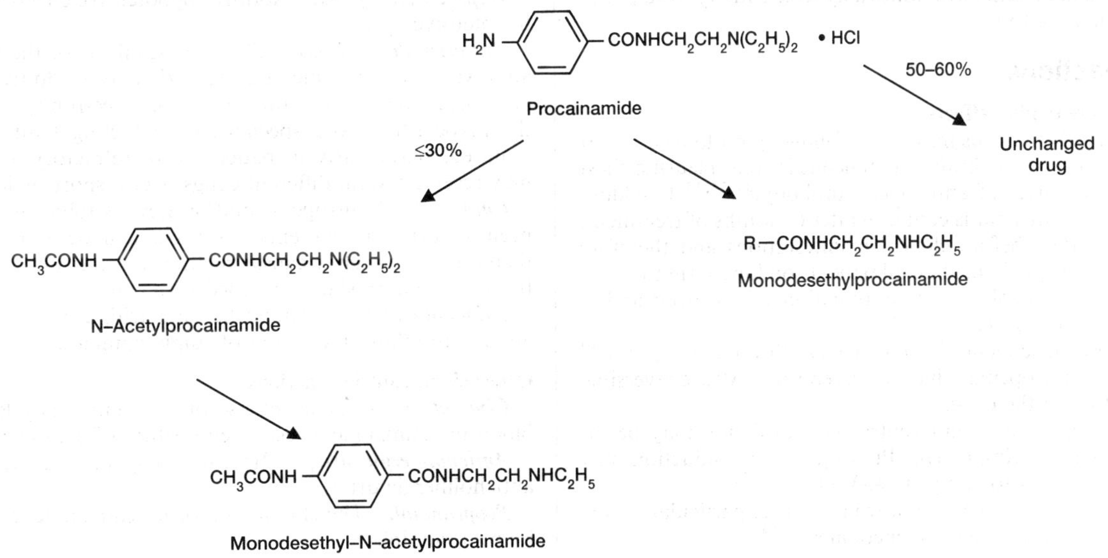

P

Procaine penicillin

Procaine pencillin is a long-acting form of benzylpenicillin (Penicillin G) used for the treatment of gonorrhoea, syphilis and other conditions caused by penicillin-sensitive organisms where a long acting compound is required.

Chemistry

Procaine penicillin (penicillin G procaine, Aquaicaine G, Aquacillin, Ayercillin, Wycillin, Megacillin, Penidural AP, Bicillin, Crysticillin AS)
$C_{16}H_{18}N_2O_4S.C_{13}H_{20}N_2O_2.H_2O$
Penicillin G compound with 2-(diethylamino)ethyl *p*-aminobenzoate

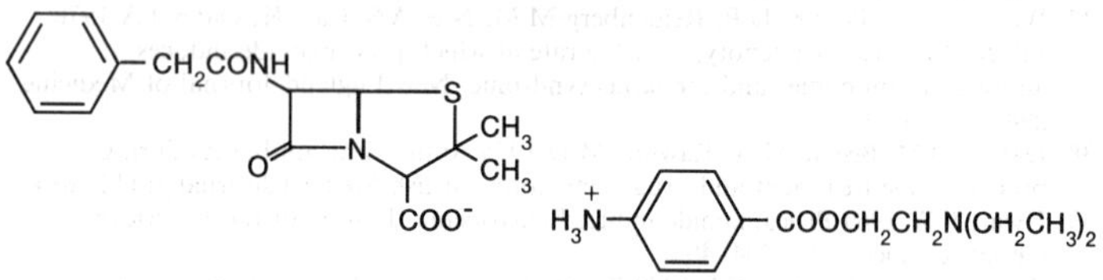

Molecular weight	588.7
pKa	—
Solubility	
in alcohol	1 in 30
in water	1 in 200
Octanol/water partition coefficient	—

Procaine penicillin is a white crystalline powder which is hydrolysed by degradation of the β-lactam ring by a range of β-lactamases produced by Gram-positive and Gram-negative bacteria, and is also inactivated by increased temperature or low pH in aqueous solution.

Pharmacology

Procaine penicillin is a long-acting form of benzylpenicillin. The penicillin nucleus consists of a thiazolidine ring connected to a β-lactam ring to which is attached a side chain. The side chain determines most of the pharmacological and antibacterial properties of the penicillin in question.

Penicillin kills bacteria by interfering in the synthesis of the bacterial cell wall. Peptidoglycan is a heteropolymeric structure that provides the cell wall with mechanical stability. The final stage in the synthesis of peptidoglycan involves the completion of the cross-linking and the terminal glycine residue of the pentaglycine bridge is linked to the fourth residue of the pentapeptide (d-alanine). The transpeptidase enzyme that performs this step is inhibited by penicillins and cephalosporins.[1] As a result the bacterial cell wall is weakened, the cell swells and then ruptures and this process appears to follow interaction of penicillin with penicillin binding proteins.[2,3] Endogenous hydrolases[4] also play a part in bacterial lysis by penicillin and those strains of bacteria that become tolerant to penicillin appear to lack these endogenous hydrolases.[5,6]

Toxicology

Procaine penicillin is virtually non–toxic, except in guinea-pigs where a single dose can cause death. Most side effects results from hypersensitivity reactions.

Clinical pharmacology

Procaine penicillin has the same spectrum of activity as benzylpenicillin. It is active against most Gram-positive bacteria and a few Gram-negative species, notably *Neisseria meningitidis* and *Neisseria gonorrhoeae*. The enterococci are relatively resistant. It is also active against spirochaetes such as *Treponema pallidum*. Mycoplasmas, chlamydiae and rickettsiae are resistant.

Over the past two decades *N. gonorrhoeae* has shown increasing resistance to procaine penicillin. This resistance can result from either plasmid-mediated production of TEM-1 β-lactamase or from chromosomal mutation at the *pen* A *pen* B *pem* and *mtr* loci producing changes to the gonococcal cell envelope.[7–11] In other Gram-positive species resistance and tolerance to procaine penicillin result from alteration in the affinity of individual PBPs to penicillin and from absence of cell wall autolysins. Other Gram-negative species are resistant to procaine penicillin.

Pharmacokinetics

Penicillin in serum and other body fluids can be measured by a plate bioassay using *Bacillus subtilis* (National Collection of Type Culture NCTC 8236) or *Sarcina lutea* (NCTC 8340).

Procaine penicillin is only suitable for intramuscular administration. Oral administration is ineffective as the combination is destroyed by stomach acid. Intravenous administration is contraindicated.

Following intramuscular administration of aqueous procaine penicillin penicillin G is released slowly. Peak serum levels of penicillin G in adults are reached at about 2 h after administration and detectable levels maintained for at least 24 h. Following a dose of 300 000 units (300 mg), a peak level of 160 $U.l^{-1}$ was obtained.[12] In neonates a dose of 50 000 units (50 mg) per kg body weight gave a mean serum level of 7 $mg.l^{-1}$, achieved between 2 and 12 h, with a level of 1.5 $mg.l^{-1}$ at 24 h.[13,14]

After administration penicillin penetrates most tissues and serous cavities. This is greater in the presence of acute inflammation. A minimum dose of 2.4 g intramuscularly daily plus 0.5 g probenecid is needed to produce effective treponemocidal levels in the CSF.[15] In neonates penicillin can be detected in CSF after 50 000 units procaine penicillin intramuscularly, peak levels of 0.7 ± 0.35 $mg.l^{-1}$ occurring after 12 h.

Oral absorption	—
Presystemic metabolism	—
Plasma half life	30 min
Volume of distribution	—
Plasma protein binding	60%

With normal renal function 70% of procaine penicillin is excreted via the kidneys. Only 10% is excreted by glomerular filtration, the majority by tubular secretion. The latter can be inhibited by probenecid. Penicillin G crosses the placenta and enters breast milk.

Concentration–effect relationship

The best predictor of cure of gonorrhoea by penicillin appears to be the time the serum concentration of penicillin exceeds the minimum inhibitory concentration (MIC) of penicillin for the infecting strain by a factor of three to four.[16] Serum concentrations of penicillin were significantly higher among those cured than in those where treatment failed. MIC values for sensitive organisms are usually less than 0.1 $mg.l^{-1}$.

Metabolism

Procaine penicillin is slowly released in the body as penicillin G and does not circulate as the procaine salt. Penicillin G is partly metabolized in the liver to inactive penicilloic acid[17] by hydrolysis of the β-lactam ring (see Benzylpenicillin). Less than 30% is metabolized. The rest is excreted unchanged mainly through the kidney, with a small amount being excreted in the bile.

Pharmaceutics

Procaine penicillin is only available for intramuscular injection.

1. Wycillin (Wyeth, USA): 1.5 g (0.6 MU), 3 g (1.2 MU) and 6 g (2.4 MU) procaine penicillin

2. Bicillin (Brocades, UK): procaine penicillin 1.8 g (1.8 MU) with benzyl penicillin sodium 360 mg (0.6 MU). Combinations of various strengths are available in the USA (e.g. Wyeth's Bicillin range).

Formulations may include parabens.

Therapeutic use

Indications

1. Syphilis
2. Gonorrhoea caused by penicillin-sensitive organisms
3. Treatment or prevention of any infection caused by penicillin-sensitive bacteria where a long-acting penicillin is required.

Contraindications

1. Penicillin hypersensitivity
2. History of penicillin allergy
3. History of adverse reactions to procaine penicillin specifically or to procaine.

Mode of use

Intramuscular injection is the only route of administration. For general purposes a common adult dosage is 1.0 g (1 000 000 units) intramuscularly once or twice a day. The dose should be reduced in neonates and when renal disease is present.

Indications

1. Syphilis
T. pallidum remains sensitive to penicillin G and it continues to be the treatment of choice for syphilis. Procaine penicillin 0.6 g daily for ten days has been recommended[18] although treatment failure has been observed. Procaine penicillin 1.0 g for 10–14 days has therefore been preferred.[19] A 10-day course of procaine penicillin 1.0 g is used for treating neurosyphilis and there has been only one reported case of progressive neurosyphilis after such treatment. This regimen can be given during pregnancy. Congenital syphilis can also be treated with 10 days intramuscular procaine penicillin. The standard treatment for gonorrhoea (see below) is thought to be effective treatment for incubating syphilis.

2. Gonorrhoea
Procaine penicillin 4.8 MU with 1 g probenecid to inhibit tubular excretion is the standard therapy for uncomplicated anogenital gonorrhoea caused by penicillin-sensitive gonococci. It is also effective against pharyngeal infection.

Penicillin-resistant gonococci are common in many parts of the world, particularly the Far East and Africa. Resistant strains may contain plasmids that code for the production of TEM-1 β-lactamase.[9] Alternatively, they may have undergone chromosomal mutation leading to changes in the cell envelope.[11]

Alternative therapy recommended for infections caused by penicillin-resistant gonococci is either spectinomycin 2 g intramuscularly or a β-lactamase-stable cephalosporin such as cefotaxime or ceftriaxone.

Other indications
Procaine penicillin can be used in any situation where penicillin G is indicated and where a long-acting preparation is considered suitable. It may be particularly useful in the later stages of infection being treated with penicillin G. Injections are less painful and are required less often. However, serum levels will be lower and it must be remembered that procaine penicillin can only be given intramuscularly. It has been used in pneumococcal pneumonia[20] and in streptococcal endocarditis.[21]

Adverse reactions

Potentially life-threatening effects

Anaphylaxis
This occurs very rarely in previously sensitized patients. It can cause death very rapidly. The features of anaphylaxis include pallor, tachycardia, urticaria, bronchospasm and peripheral vascular collapse. The main antibody class involved in this hypersensitivity reaction is IgE. Anaphylaxis occurs in 0.004–0.04% of all patients receiving penicillin G.[22] Figures are not available for procaine penicillin alone. Mortality is approximately 10%.[23]

Treatment for anaphylaxis involves 0.5–1.0 ml of a 1:1000 solution of adrenaline intramuscularly, repeated every 15 minutes.[24] Corticosteroids may be of value and even though their role in the early phase of treatment is doubtful, 100 mg hydrocortisone should be given if there is no immediate response to adrenaline.[24] The patient should be positioned with the head slightly down, a clear airway provided, aminophylline given to relieve bronchospasm and positive pressure oxygen administered. Cardiac arrhythmias may also need treatment.[25] Speed is essential.

Convulsions
The blood–brain barrier normally protects against direct cerebral toxicity of penicillins. However, intrathecal injections of systemic doses, in error, will produce convulsions and death (see also below).

Intravascular injection
Intravenous injection can cause convulsions, hypotension and cardiorespiratory arrest.[26] Intra-arterial injection has also caused transverse myelopathy[27] and ischaemic gangrene of the upper limb.[28]

Acute overdosage
Acute self-poisoning is only likely to occur with oral preparations, which are unlikely to cause serious harm. Accidental overdoses of intramuscular preparations in single doses are unlikely to produce ill effects, except in the circumstances mentioned above.

Severe or irreversible adverse effects
These include serum sickness,[23] the Jarisch–Herxheimer reaction, seen in the treatment of syphilis;[29] haemolytic anaemia[30] and other haematological disturbances, and renal impairment.

Symptomatic adverse effects
These include skin rashes, pain and abscesses after injection, and contact dermatitis. Procaine penicillin may also induce feelings of extreme anxiety, bouts of tachycardia and hypertension. The patient's mental state may remain labile for some time, a phenomenon more pronounced in those with previous evidence of mental instability.[31]

Interference with clinical pathology tests
Procaine B liberated after the injection of procaine penicillin can interfere with the measurement of 17-hydroxycorticosteroids, 17-ketosteroids and 17-ketogenic steroids to give false high results. It may also affect thyroid function tests.

High risk groups

Neonates
No special precautions are necessary in neonates. A reduced dosage should be used.

Breast milk. Penicillin is excreted in breast milk and may cause allergic reactions in infants.

Children
No special precautions are necessary in children.

Pregnant women
No special precautions are necessary during pregnancy.

The elderly
No special precautions are necessary.

Concurrent disease
Dosage should be reduced in renal disease.

Drug interactions

Potentially hazardous interactions
In vitro penicillin inactivates aminoglycosides, so that they should not be mixed in infusion fluids.

Potentially useful interactions
Probenecid delays tubular excretion of penicillin and is used to enhance its therapeutic effect in treatment of syphilis and gonorrhoea.

General review articles

Kucers A, Bennett N M 1987 The use of antibiotics, 4th edn. Heinemann, London

P

References

1. Schockman G D, Daneo-Morre L, Cornett J B, Mychajlonka M 1979 Does penicillin kill bacteria? Reviews of Infectious Diseases 1: 787–796
2. Spratt B G 1975 Distinct penicillin binding proteins involved in the division, elongation, and shape of Escherichia coli K12. Proceedings of the National Academy of Sciences of the USA 72: 2999–3003
3. Ogawara H 1981 Antibiotic resistance in pathogenic and producing bacteria with special reference to β-lactam antibiotics. Microbiological Reviews 45: 591–619
4. Handwerger S, Tomasz A 1985 Antibiotic tolerance among clinical isolates of bacteria. Reviews of Infectious Diseases 7: 368–386
5. Tomasz A, Albino A, Zanati E 1970 Multiple antibiotic resistance in a bacterium with suppressed autolytic system. Nature 227: 138–140
6. Sabath L D, Wheeler N, Laverdiere M 1977 A new type of penicillin resistance of Staphylococcus aureus. Lancet 1: 443–477
7. Phillips I 1976 B-lactamase producing, penicillin resistant gonococcus. Lancet 2: 656–657
8. Percival A, Rowlands J, Corkhill J E et al 1976 Penicillinase-producing gonococci in Liverpool. Lancet 2: 1379–1382
9. Bergström S, Norlander L, Norqvist A, Normark S 1978 Contribution of a TEM-1-like β-lactamase to penicillin resistance in Neisseria gonorrhoeae. Antimicrobial Agents and Chemotherapy 13: 618–623
10. Sparling P F, Sarubi F A, Blackman E 1975 Inheritance of low-level resistance to penicillin, tetracycline and chloramphenicol in Neisseria gonorrhoeae. Journal of Bacteriology 124: 740–749
11. Johnson S R, Morse S A 1988 Antibiotic resistance in Neisseria gonorrhoeae: genetics and mechanisms of resistance. Sexually Transmitted Diseases 15: 217–224
12. Welch H 1954 Principles and Practice of Antibiotic Therapy Medical Encyclopedia Inc., New York, pp 46, 66, 74
13. McCracken G H Jr, Ginsberg C, Chrane D F et al 1973 Clinical pharmacology of penicillin in newborn infants. Journal of Pediatrics 82: 692–698
14. Speer M E, Mason E O, Scharnberg J T 1981 Cerebrospinal fluid concentrations of aqueous procaine penicillin G in the neonate. Paediatrics 67: 387–388
15. Dunlop E M C, Al-Egaily S S, Houang E T 1981 Production of treponemicidal concentrations of penicillin in cerebrospinal fluid. British Medical Journal 283: 646
16. Jaffe H W, Schroeter A L, Reynolds Gladys H, Zaidi A A, Martin J E, Thayer J D 1979 Pharmacokinetic determinants of penicillin cure of gonococcal urethritis. Antimicrobial Agents and Chemotherapy 15: 587–591
17. Cole M, Kenig M D, Hewitt V A 1973 Metabolism of penicillins to penicilloic acids and 6-aminopenicillanic acid in man and its significance in assessing penicillin absorption. Antimicrobial Agents and Chemotherapy 3: 463–468
18. Willcox R R 1981 Treatment of syphilis. Bulletin of the World Health Organization 59: 655–663
19. Kucers A, Bennett N McK 1987 The use of antibiotics, 4th edn. Heinemann, London, p 53
20. Brewin A, Arango L, Hadley W K, Murray J F 1974 High-dose penicillin therapy and pneumococcal pneumonia. Journal of the American Medical Association 230: 409–413
21. Wilson W R, Thompson R L, Wilkowske C J et al 1981 Short-term therapy for streptococcal infective endocarditis. Combined intramuscular administration of penicillin and streptomycin. Journal of the American Medical Association 245: 360–363
22. Porter J, Jick H 1977 Drug-induced anaphylaxis convulsions, deafness and extra pyramidal symptoms. Lancet 1: 587–588
23. Polk I J 1982 Penicillin allergy skin tests. Journal of the American Medical Association 247: 1745
24. Leading article 1981 Treatment of anaphylactic shock. British Medical Journal 282: 1011–1012
25. Sullivan T J 1982 Cardiac disorders in penicillin-induced anaphylaxis. Association with intravenous epinephrine therapy. Journal of the American Medical Association 248: 2161–2162
26. Galpin J E, Chow A W, Yoshikawa T T, Guzè L B 1974 "Pseudoanaphylactic" reactions from inadvertent infusion of procaine penicillin G. Annals of Internal Medicine 81: 358–359
27. Atkinson J P 1969 Transverse myelopathy secondary to injection of penicillin. Journal of Pediatrics 75: 867–869
28. Sengupta S 1976 Gangrene following intra-arterial injection of procaine penicillin. Australian and New Zealand Journal of Medicine 6: 71–73
29. Bryceson A D M 1976 Clinical pathology of the Jarisch–Herxheimer reaction. Journal of Infectious Diseases 133: 696–704
30. White J M, Brown D L, Hepner G W, Worlledge S M 1968 Penicillin-induced haemolytic anaemia. British Medical Journal 3: 26–29
31. Menke H E, Pepplinkhuizen L 1974 Acute non-allergic reaction to aqueous procaine penicillin. Lancet 2: 723–724

Procarbazine hydrochloride

A cytotoxic agent useful in combination chemotherapy of tumours, especially lymphomas.

Chemistry

Procarbazine hydrochloride (Ibenzmethyzin, Matulane, Natulan, Natulanar)
$C_{12}H_{19}N_3O.HCl$
N-Isopropyl-α-(2-methylhydrazino)-4-toluamide hydrochloride

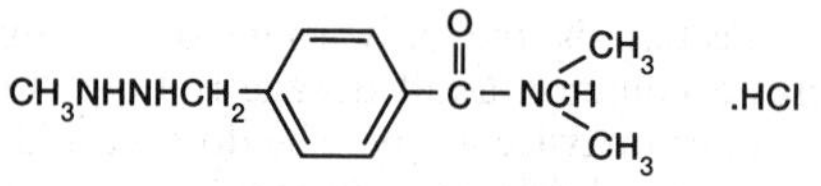

Molecular weight (free base)	257.8 (221.3)
pKa	6.8
Solubility	
in alcohol	>1 in 100
in water	>1 in 10
Octanol/water partition coefficient	low

A white to pale yellow crystalline powder with a slight odour. It is prepared by chemical synthesis. Solutions in water are unstable. Procarbazine is not available in any combination preparations.

Pharmacology

The exact cytotoxic mode of action of procarbazine is unclear. Several metabolites are active, inhibiting protein, RNA and DNA synthesis.[1] In vitro depolymerization of DNA by procarbazine-produced hydrogen peroxide has also been reported.[1] Three pathways of metabolic action have been described ultimately yielding highly reactive free radicals including hydrogen peroxidase, formaldehyde, and free hydroxide radicals. These final products are thought to comprise the alkylating and methylating metabolites[2] and a major role for the microsomal (P-450) enzyme fraction in this metabolic oxidation and subsequent activation of procarbazine has been demonstrated.[3]

The final interaction with DNA produces alterations typical of ionizing radiation and the classical bifunctional alkylating agents. However, in experimental animal tumour models procarbazine does not demonstrate alkylating agent cross-resistance and Kreiss[4] has proposed that it causes abnormal selective transmethylation of the N-7 guanine on transfer RNA. Inhibition of RNA, DNA, and protein synthesis have been noted both in vitro and in vivo.

Procarbazine inhibits mitosis by prolonging interphase. It appears to be cell cycle-phase specific with marked cytotoxic activity in S-phase.

Toxicology

As is the case with other neoplastic agents, particularly those with an alkylating action, procarbazine is known to be teratogenic[5] and carcinogenic.[7]

Clinical pharmacology

Procarbazine is an effective antitumour agent, usually given in combination with other drugs in the treatment of Hodgkin's disease. In most regimes procarbazine has been used orally at a dose of 100 mg.m^{-2} daily for 14 days each cycle of chemotherapy. There

Procarbazine hydrochloride

have been no systematic studies of dose response but a retrospective analysis of dose intensity has suggested that survival increased as the dose of nitrogen mustard, vincristine and procarbazine increased. Little is known about the duration of action. Procarbazine is rapidly metabolized in man, the oxidative degradation products having cytotoxic activity. Resistance to procarbazine develops rapidly in clinical usage, but the mechanism of this effect is unclear. Procarbazine is a potent immunosuppressive agent as well as being teratogenic, mutagenic and carcinogenic. Procarbazine is a weak monoamine oxidase inhibitor (MAOI) and thus hypertensive reactions may occur if the drug is given concurrently with sympathomimetic agents, tricyclic antidepressants and foods with a high tyramine content.

Pharmacokinetics

Procarbazine can be quantified in plasma or urine by HPLC with electrochemical detection. The limit of sensitivity[6] is 10 μg.l^{-1}. After oral administration procarbazine is rapidly and completely absorbed from the gastrointestinal tract with peak plasma levels at 0.5–1 h. It quickly equilibrates between the blood and cerebrospinal fluid.[8] Peak CSF levels are achieved 30–90 minutes after oral or parenteral administration. Procarbazine is rapidly metabolized in man with a plasma half life of 7 minutes after parenteral administration. About 70% of an oral or parenteral dose is excreted in the urine in the first 24 hours after administration.[9] The major metabolite present is the inactive N-isopropyl-terephthalamic acid (25–42% in 24 hours); about 5% of the drug in urine is the parent compound. Pretreatment with phenobarbitone increases hepatic monooxygenase activity and increases the rate of conversion of procarbazine to active forms.[10] Compromised renal function (serum creatinine > 2.0 mg per 100 ml) or depressed hepatic function (bilirubin > 17) results in delayed elimination and are an indication for dose reduction.

It is not known whether the drug is excreted in breast milk but it is likely that both procarbazine and its active metabolites are excreted in this way. Procarbazine can cross the placenta and is teratogenic.

Oral absorption	almost complete
Presystemic metabolism	—
Plasma half life	
(intravenous injection)	7 min
Volume of distribution	—
Plasma protein binding	—

Concentration–effect relationship

There are no good studies examining dose–response effects for procarbazine. Phase I and II studies have used a variety of dose regimes. The drug is usually given orally daily at a dose of 50–200 mg daily continuously for periods of 10–14 days. Dose is governed by side effects, especially marrow suppression. Continuous low-dose regimes (50–100 mg daily) have also been tested but are not recommended because of marrow suppression and an increased risk of carcinogenesis. High-dose intravenous regimes (300–1000 mg.m^{-2}) have been tested[11] but doses greater than 1 g.m^{-2} were associated with severe CNS and gastrointestinal toxicity. There is no clear evidence of any correlation between the plasma concentration of procarbazine and its cytotoxic effect.

Metabolism

Procarbazine is extensively metabolized in the liver. Over 75% of the dose is excreted in the urine, but with only 5% as unchanged drug. Several active metabolites are formed which contribute substantially to the cytotoxic effects of the drug (Fig. 1). Oxidation of procarbazine by hepatic endoplasmic reticular enzymes yields the corresponding azo compound and hydrogen peroxide. NADPH-independent conversion of procarbazine to azo-procarbazine by monoamine oxidase accounts for 25–40% of the total. Hydroxyl radicals, generated from the hydrogen peroxide, attack and degrade DNA. Azo-procarbazine then undergoes at least four biotransformations (i–iv, Fig. 1) catalysed by P450 enzymes, to yield four unstable metabolites. These unstable metabolites then either collapse, or undergo further metab-

Fig. 1 The metabolic pathway of procarbazine activation

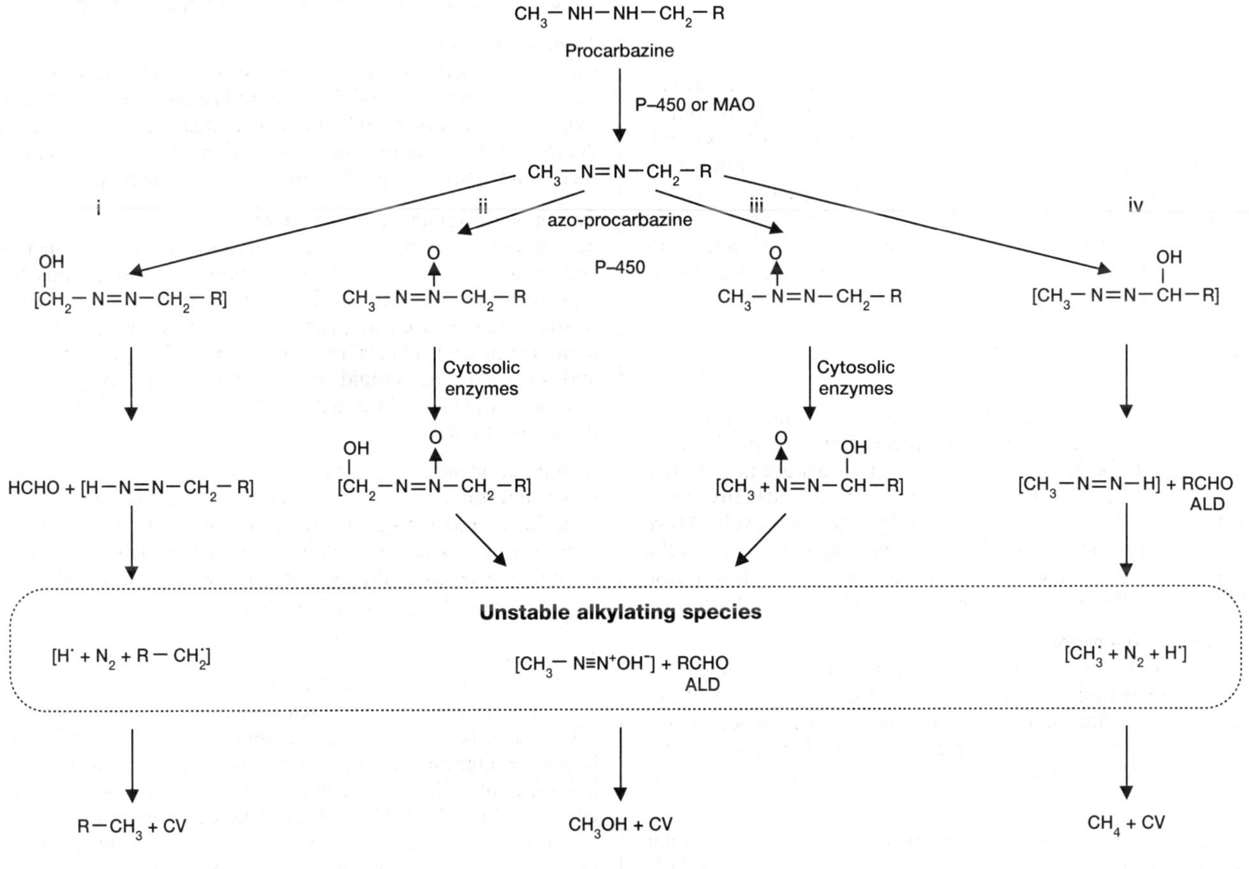

CV, covalent binding; R=—C_6H_4—CO—NH—CH$(CH_3)_2$

olism to produce a variety of unstable alkylating species, which bind covalently to DNA and protein. By-products of these processes include formaldehyde, carbon dioxide and methane. An alternative, less important, mechanism of activation involves the formation of mono-methylhydrazine and generation of methyldiazene free radicals.[2]

Pharmaceutics

Procarbazine 50 mg is available orally as the hydrochloride salt in opaque pale yellow-coloured capsules Natulan (Roche UK) with ROCHE printed in red–brown along both cap and body or Matulane (Roche, USA) with MATULANE ROCHE printed in black. The capsules should be stored in air-tight containers protected from light. Maximum storage temperature is 25°C and capsules should be stored in a dry place. Capsules are supplied in blister packs of 50. The manufacturers do not give a recommended shelf-life.

Therapeutic use

Procarbazine is generally used in combination with other cytotoxic drugs in the treatment of neoplastic diseases.

Indications

1. Hodgkin's disease[12]
2. Non-Hodgkin's lymphoma[13]
3. Lung cancer
4. Brain tumours
5. Malignant melanoma
6. Multiple myeloma
7. Polycythemia rubra vera.

Only in Hodgkin's and non-Hodgkin's lymphoma does procarbazine in combination with other cytotoxic drugs have sufficient activity to produce long-term survival.

Contraindications

1. Marrow suppression
2. Pregnancy
3. Prior lung hypersensitivity
4. Breast-feeding mothers.

Mode of use

Procarbazine should, in general, only be used as part of a proven treatment for cancer. Its main role is in the treatment of lymphomas. It is usually given daily (at a dose of 150 $mg.m^{-2}$) for 14 days with each treatment cycle. The dose of procarbazine used in combination with other cytotoxic agents will depend on the expected degree of marrow suppression from the other drugs. Procarbazine should only be used at the dose recommended in a particular combination of cytotoxic drugs and dose reductions should be made according to the patient's blood count at the time of treatment.

Indications

1. Hodgkin's disease
Procarbazine was one of the four drugs in the regime known as MOPP (mustard, vincristine [oncovin], procarbazine and prednisone) which was shown to be highly active in advanced disease in the early 1970s. In this and similar regimes, procarbazine is usually given orally at a dose of 100 $mg.m^{-2}$ daily for 14 days each cycle. More recently, it may be included in so-called hybrid regimes using cyclic combinations of drugs. These various approaches yield high response rates (80%) with 50% or more of patients surviving long term.

2. Non-Hodgkin's lymphoma
Procarbazine may be used in the same way in a similar combination to MOPP in which cyclosphosphamide is substituted for mustard. Intensive cyclic multidrug combinations which include procarbazine have also been reported. Such therapy yields high response rates (80%) with up to 50% of patients surviving long term.

3. Lung
Procarbazine has been used alone or in combination with other cytotoxic drugs in the treatment of small cell lung cancer. Oral daily doses of 100 mg have been used for up to 14 days. High response rates are reported in small cell lung cancer (70%) but long-term survival is rare.

4. Brain
Since it crosses the blood–brain barrier it has been used alone and in combination with other cytotoxics in the treatment of a variety of brain tumours. It is usually given orally at a daily dose of 100 $mg.m^{-2}$ for up to 14 days. Minor responses only are seen.

5. Malignant melanoma
Procarbazine is usually used in combination with other drugs, such as dacarbazine, when it is given orally (100 $mg.m^{-2}$) for up to 14 days. Responses are generally of a minor nature and short-lived.

6. Multiple myeloma
Although procarbazine has some activity in this disease it is now rarely used.

7. Polycythemia rubra vera
Although chronic low-dose procarbazine (50 $mg.m^{-2}$ daily) can be used to lower the haemoglobin level, this approach is rarely used.

Adverse reactions

Because procarbazine is usually given in combination with other cytotoxic drugs it is sometimes difficult to ascribe a particular side effect to one of the drugs used.

Potentially life-threatening effects
The major dose-limiting effect of procarbazine, at conventional doses, is bone marrow suppression. Infection during a period of neutropenia is potentially extremely serious and parenteral broad-spectrum antibiotics should be started as soon as possible whilst culture and sensitivity reports are awaited. Thrombocytopenia may result in bleeding and platelet transfusions may be needed until recovery of the platelet count. Patients receiving cytotoxic therapy, especially those with leukaemia and lymphoma, are especially prone to develop atypical infections as well as bacterial, viral and fungal infections.

Procarbazine is carcinogenic and an increased incidence of acute myelogenous leukaemia has been reported in patients receiving MOPP chemotherapy for Hodgkin's disease.[14] The risk is highest in patients receiving both chemotherapy and radiotherapy. A similar increased risk of leukaemia also exists in patients with other tumours.

Acute overdosage
Cases of deliberate overdose are rare. The main effects are protracted marrow suppression and CNS complications. The duration of neutropenia is closely correlated with increasing risk of infection and death. Tremors, coma and convulsions have been reported with increasing frequency as the dose of procarbazine is increased.[11]

Severe or irreversible adverse effects
Severe central nervous system adverse effects are uncommon at conventional doses, but tremor, coma and convulsions have been reported. Azoospermia and cessation of menstrual function are nearly always caused by procarbazine; in many cases this is permanent. Teratogenic effects have been reported in experimental animals and procarbazine should be avoided during pregnancy, though normal infants have been delivered to women receiving procarbazine in the third trimester.

Symptomatic adverse effects
Gastrointestinal complaints are relatively common and include nausea, vomiting and diarrhoea. Anorexia and stomatitis are less common. An influenza-like syndrome, with fevers, chills, lethargy, myalgia and arthralgia is occasionally reported, as are an allergic rash and pruritis. The rash may be prevented by concomitant steroids (often already included in combination chemotherapy for lymphomas). More severe hypersensitivity reactions with angioedema, urticaria and a precipitous drop in serum complement have been reported rarely.[15]

Central nervous system toxicity is not uncommon. A wide variety of effects have been described, including paraesthesia, ataxia, dizziness, headache, nightmares, depression, insomnia, nervousness, mania and hallucinations. Rarely, at standard doses, coma and convulsions may occur. At high doses CNS effects may be dose-limiting.[11]

Alopecia is rare, as are ophthalmic adverse effects which include nystagmus, diplopia, papilloedema, photophobia and, in the presence of thrombocytopenia, retinal haemorrhages. Pulmonary toxicity has been reported, rarely, and is probably caused by a hypersensitivity reaction.[16]

It has been suggested that procarbazine may play a role in the development of hepatic angiosarcoma.[17]

Other effects
Patients with exquisitely sensitive tumours (high grade lymphomas in the main) may on treatment with chemotherapy develop a tumour lysis syndrome. Breakdown of proteins result in a rapid rise in serum urate and potassium.

Interference with clinical pathology tests
No technical interferences of this kind have been reported.

High risk groups

Neonates
None of the currently recommended cytotoxic regimes for common neonatal tumours contain procarbazine.

Breast milk. Few data are available, but the parent compound and active metabolites are likely to be excreted in breast milk.

Children
Procarbazine may form part of drug regimes in the treatment of childhood Hodgkin's disease or non-Hodgkin's lymphoma. Dose is, as in adults, based on surface area.

Pregnant women
Procarbazine is teratogenic and should be avoided during pregnancy, especially the first trimester. There have been reports of normal infants delivered after the use of procarbazine in the third trimester. It has been suggested that ingestion of procarbazine and alcohol during pregnancy may induce the fetal-alcohol syndrome.[18]

The elderly
The elderly generally tolerate the marrow suppressive effects of chemotherapy less well and dose reductions should be considered in elderly and frail patients, though few proper guidelines are available.

Drug interactions

Potentially hazardous interactions[19,20]

CNS depressants. Procarbazine may augment the effect of CNS depressants which should therefore be administered cautiously in patients receiving procarbazine. Respiratory depression has been reported with narcotic analgesics, antihistamines, phenothiazines, barbiturates and some hypotensives.

Antidepressants. Hypertensive crisis, tremors, agitation, palpitations and angina have occasionally been reported.

Other significant interactions

Sympathomimetics. Although sympathomimetics may potentially interact with procarbazine, because it is an MAOI, there is little evidence that this is clinically significant.

Food. Procarbazine is a weak MAOI and restriction of tyramine-containing foodstuffs has been recommended[19] though the potential for hypertensive crises appears low.

Alcohol. A disulfiram-like reaction may occur following ingestion of alcohol and central nervous system depression may be accentuated.

Potentially useful interactions
No interactions of this kind have been reported.

Major outcome trials

1. DeVita V T, Serpick A A, Carbone P P 1970 Combination chemotherapy in the treatment of advanced Hodgkin's disease. Annals of Internal Medicine 73: 881–896

   DeVita V T, Simon R M, Hubbard S M et al 1980 Curability of advanced Hodgkin's disease with chemotherapy: long term follow-up of MOPP treated patients at NCI. Annals of Internal Medicine 92: 587–595

DeVita and his colleagues published their initial experience of a four drug combination (nitrogen mustard, vincristine, procarbazine and prednisolone — MOPP) in 1970. In 1980 they presented data with a 15 year follow-up. The overall complete remission rate was 80% for patients with advanced (stage III and IV) disease. 68% of those achieving a complete remission have remained continuously disease-free for more than 10 years. These results are significantly better than any reported prior to the introduction of MOPP and no randomized trials have compared this therapy with simpler treatments. Attempts to reduce the toxicity of the MOPP regime have led to the development of a large number of variations on the MOPP theme, many of which still include procarbazine.[18]

General review articles

Brunner K W, Young C W 1965 A methylhydrazine derivative in Hodgkin's disease and other malignant neoplasms: therapeutic and toxic effects studied in 51 patients. Annals of Internal Medicine 63: 69–86

Carter S (ed) 1971 Proceedings of the chemotherapy conference on procarbazine (Matulane:NSC-77 213): development and application. US Government Printing Office, Washington DC

DeConti R C 1971 Procarbazine in the management of Hodgkin's disease. Journal of the American Medical Association 215: 927–930

Weinkam R J, Shiba D A 1978 Metabolic activation of procarbazine. Life Sciences 22: 937–946

Weiss H D, Walker M D, Wiernik P 1974 Neurotoxicity of commonly use anti-neoplastic agents. New England Journal of Medicine 291: 127–133

References

1. Barneis K, Kofler M, Bollag W 1963 The degradation of deoxyribonucleic acid by new tumour inhibiting compounds: the intermediate formation of hydrogen peroxide. Experientia 19: 132–133
2. Reed D J 1974–75 Procarbazine. In: Sartorelli A C, Johns D G (eds) Antineoplastic and immunosuppressive agents Part II (Handbook of Experimental Pharmacology. New Series vol 38/2). Springer Verlag, Berlin
3. Dorr R, Fritz W 1980 Cancer chemotherapy handbook. Elsevier, New York, pp 593–601
4. Kreiss W 1971 Mechanism of action of procarbazine. In: Carter S (ed) Proceedings of the chemotherapy conference on procarbazine (Matulane:NSC-77 213): development and application. US Government Printing Office, Washington DC
5. Chambers S, Murphy M L 1969 Fetal malformation produced in rats in N-isopropyl-α-(2-methylhydrazine)-p-tolumide hydrochloride (procarbazine). Teratology 2: 23–32
6. Rucki R J, Moros S A 1980 Journal of Chromatography 190: 359–365
7. Kelly M G, O'Gara G W, Gadehar K, Yancy S T, Oliveirio V T 1964 Carcinogenic activity of a new antitumour agent, N-isopropyl-8-(2-methylhydrazine)-p-tolumide, hydrochloride (NSC-77 213). Cancer Chemotherapy Reports 39: 77–80
8. Schwartz D E, Bollag W, Obrecht P 1967 Distribution and excretion studies of procarbazine in animals and man. Arzneimittel Forschung 17: 1384–1393
9. Oliverio V T, Denham C, DeVita V T, Kelly M G 1964 Some pharmacologic properties of a new antitumour agent N-isopropyl-d (2-methylhydrazino)-p-tolamide, hydrochloride (NSC 77 213). Cancer Chemotherapy Reports 42: 1–7
10. Shiba D A, Weinkam R J, Levin V A 1979 Metabolic activation of procarbazine: activity of the intermediates and the effects of pretreatment. Proceedings of the American Association for Cancer Research 20: 139
11. Chabner B A, Sponzi R, Hubbard S 1973 High-dose intermittent infusion of procarbazine (NSC-77 213) Cancer Chemotherapy Reports 57: 361–363
12. DeVita V T, Serpick A A, Carbone P P 1970 Combination chemotherapy in the treatment of advanced Hodgkin's disease. Annals of Internal Medicine 73: 881–895
13. Fisher R I, DeVita V T, Hubbard S M et al 1980 Pro-MACE-MOPP combination chemotherapy: treatment of diffuse lymphomas. Proceedings of the American Society of Clinical Oncology 21: 468
14. Coleman C N, Williams C J 1977 Haematologic neoplasia in patients treated for Hodgkin's disease. New England Journal of Medicine 297: 1249–1252
15. Glorvky M M, Braunwald S, Opele G, Alentry A 1976 Hypersensitivity to procarbazine associated with angioedema, urticaria and low serum complement activity. Journal of Allergy and Clinical Immunology 57: 134–140
16. Lokich J J, Maloney W C 1972 Allergic reaction to procarbazine. Clinical Pharmacology and Therapeutics 13: 573–574
17. Daneschmend K, Bradfield J W B 1979 Hepatic angio-sarcoma associated with androgenic–anabolic steroids (letter). Lancet 2: 1249
18. Dunn P 1979 Metronidazole and the fetal alcohol syndrome (letter). Lancet 2: 144
19. Warren R D, Bender R A 1977 Drug interactions with antineoplastic agents. Cancer Treatment Reports 61: 1231–1241
20. ABPI Data Sheet Compendium (1985–1986) Datapham Publications Ltd, London, pp 1269–1270
21. Coltman C A 1980 Chemotherapy of advanced Hodgkin's disease. Seminars in Oncology 7: 155–173

P

Prochlorperazine

Prochlorperazine is a potent phenothiazine antipsychotic, now largely used as an antiemetic and to treat vertigo.

Chemistry

Prochlorperazine maleate/mesylate/edisylate (Temetil, Stemetil, Compazine, Nipodal)
$C_{20}H_{24}N_3SCl$
2-Chloro-10-[3-(4-methyl-1-piperazinyl)-propyl]-phenothiazine

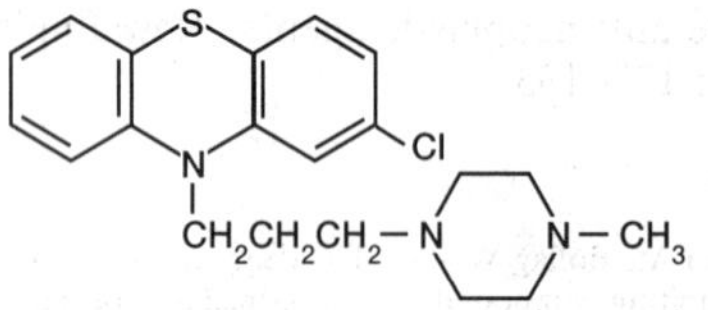

Molecular weight	373.9
pKa (maleate)	8.1
Solubility	
in alcohol	slight
in water	slight
Octanol/water partition coefficient	5000

Prochlorperazine is a clear, pale yellow liquid, the edisylate mesylate and maleate salts are white or pale yellow crystalline powders with a slightly bitter taste. It is almost odourless and is prepared by chemical synthesis.

Pharmacology

Prochlorperazine is a phenothiazine derivative of the piperazine group and has the same basic pharmacological actions as do other phenothiazines. The effects of these compounds are apparent at all levels of the nervous system. Although the mechanism of action of antipsychotic agents remains unknown, theories are based mainly upon their ability to antagonize the actions of dopamine. In rat brain there are three anatomically well-defined dopamine systems. Cell bodies are present in the substantia nigra, in the ventral tegmental area, and in the arcuate nucleus of the hypothalamus. The neurones project to the neostriatum and the amygdaloid nucleus, to the nucleus accumbens and olfactory tubercles, and to the median eminence. The antipsychotic potency of the phenothiazine derivatives appears best correlated with their ability to interact with dopamine-containing neurones. It is not understood how dopamine antagonism translates into the antipsychotic activity. In electrophysiological studies chlorpromazine has been found to increase acutely the firing rate of dopamine cells in certain areas of the brain. There are several possible interpretations of such findings, but the complexity of neuronal circuits prevents a definitive explanation. Some investigators link antipsychotic activity to an antagonism at the postsynaptic dopamine D_1 receptor, with inhibition of the activation of dopamine D_1-sensitive adenylate cyclase and synthesis of cyclic AMP. However, there is also antagonism of D_2 receptors which do not activate adenyl cyclase. Furthermore, phenothiazines inhibit pre- and postsynaptic adrenoceptors, and acetylcholine, serotonin and histamine receptors. These various pharmacodynamic actions combine to produce not only antipsychotic, but also central antiemetic and sedative effects.

The physiology and pharmacology of vomiting was advanced greatly by the work of Wang and Borison in the late 1950s. They found, in the floor of the fourth ventricle, an area sensitive to the emetic action of apomorphine and other drugs, separate from but close to the vomiting centre proper. Destruction of this area abolished vomiting in response to apomorphine without affecting vomiting elicited by other causes, such as gastric infusion of copper sulphate.[1,2] They named this area the chemoreceptor trigger zone (CTZ).

The antiemetic effect of phenothiazines has been demonstrated to be linked to interference with dopaminergic transmission[3] and is attributed to an action on the CTZ. In contrast to antihistamines and anticholinergics, which also have antiemetic activity, phenothiazines antagonize apomorphine-induced vomiting.[4] Halogenated phenothiazines, like prochlorperazine, have greater antiemetic activity and a lower incidence of sedation and hypotension, and are therefore preferred as antiemetic agents.[5]

Toxicology

Prochlorperazine, like other antipsychotic drugs, has a high safety margin.

Toxicological testing in animals, including monkeys, has not shown general organ toxicity, or teratogenic, mutagenic, or carcinogenic effects of clinical relevance.

Clinical pharmacology

Prochlorperazine is one of many phenothiazine derivatives that have been found effective in the treatment of human psychotic conditions of the schizophrenic type. This type of drug action was novel when it was first described for chlorpromazine. It is now named neuroleptic or antipsychotic. Prochlorperazine, like other antipsychotic agents, reduces the signs and symptoms of psychotic patients, such as mental confusion and delusions, hallucinations, psychomotor agitation, and aggressive and combative irrational behaviour. Patients are quietened and rendered unresponsive because there is emotional indifference to inner and external events. This emotional flatness is called an ataractic state.

No difference in therapeutic efficacy (maximal therapeutic benefit obtainable regardless of dose) has been demonstrated in controlled studies comparing drugs of this class. There are, however, marked differences in potency (dose required for maximal therapeutic benefit). Prochlorperazine is of medium potency, requiring oral doses between 20 and 100 mg daily (given in three or four divided doses).

Other central effects shared by antipsychotic drugs are: hypotension, inhibition of emesis, of vertigo resulting from vestibular dysfunction, of temperature regulation, and of hiccough, and increased prolactin release.

Prochlorperazine is used for control of nausea and vomiting, for the symptomatic treatment of vertigo, as an antipsychotic (in the management of schizophrenia) and as short-term treatment of severe non-psychotic anxiety.

Pharmacokinetics

The preferred analytical method for determination of prochlorperazine in plasma is high pressure liquid chromatography with electrochemical detection.[6,7] The specificity of the method (which has become available only recently) is adequate; its sensitivity is 1 μg.l^{-1} plasma.[8] This is insufficient for pharmacokinetic studies after low-dose oral administration.[8] Results of the one study of the pharmacokinetics of prochlorperazine in eight healthy volunteers were compatible with a two-compartment model. Intravenous doses of 6.25 mg and 12.5 mg and an oral dose of 25 mg were studied. Only the parenteral doses gave plasma levels that could be used to calculate pharmacokinetic parameters. The apparent volume of distribution was 23 l.kg^{-1}. Plasma clearance was 166 and 148 l.min^{-1}, and elimination half life was 6.7 ± 0.7 and 6.8 ± 0.8 hours, respectively. After oral administration, plasma levels were detectable in only half the subjects, with peak concentration at between 1.5 and 5 hours. Calculated bioavailability was between 0 and 16%. The chromatogram showed a second peak which was presumed to be a metabolite, but its identity was not established.

Thus, what is known about the pharmacokinetics of prochlorperazine is fully in keeping with what is known about the pharmacokinetics of other phenothiazines, especially chlorpromazine, the drug studied most widely by far. After oral administration, the predominant clinical route of administration, absorption is variable and presystemic (first-pass) metabolism is extensive. Great variability is seen even after intravenous administration. Tissue distribution is wide, as is evident from the high volume of distribution, but no direct evidence exists for prochlorperazine. There is no specific evidence regarding protein binding.

In view of the high lipid solubility and the high apparent volume of distribution, entry into the brain and other tissues must be high.

For all antipsychotic drugs plasma concentrations show wide variability with time and between patients. Correlation between plasma concentration and therapeutic or side effects has been found to be poor. Thus, plasma concentration monitoring as a guide to clinical therapy is not rational. On the other hand, such monitoring is not essential in view of the large therapeutic margin of these drugs.

Oral absorption	variable
Presystemic metabolism	high
Plasma half life	6.7±6.8 h
Volume of distribution	23 $l.kg^{-1}$
Plasma protein binding	high

Concentration–effect relationship

No data are available.

Metabolism

No confirmed information on prochlorperazine metabolism is available; sulphoxidation has been suggested.[8] By analogy with other phenothiazine derivatives and on the basis of general principles of drug metabolism, it can be postulated that metabolism by the microsomal enzyme system is extensive. Likely mechanisms are: oxidation, especially sulphoxide formation, and hydroxylation followed by conjugation.

There is no information on possible pharmacological activity of metabolites.

Pharmaceutics

Prochlorperazine is available in oral and parenteral forms and as suppositories.

1. Stemetil (Rhone Poulenc, UK) tablets are cream, uncoated, indented on the face with name and strength. They contain prochlorperazine maleate equivalent to 5 mg or 25 mg prochlorperazine.
2. Compazine (Smithkline Beecham, USA) tablets are yellow–green, coated, imprinted 'SKF'. They contain prochlorperazine maleate equivalent to 5 mg, 10 mg or 25 mg prochlorperazine and are coded 'C66', 'C67' and 'C69' respectively.
3. Compazine sustained-release capsules (Smithkline Beecham, USA) have black caps and opaque bodies, are imprinted with 'SKF' and strength information. The 10 mg, 15 mg, and 30 mg strengths are coded 'C44', 'C46' and 'C47' respectively.
4. Vertigon sustained-release capsules (Smithkline Beecham, USA) are purple/clear capsules containing 10 mg and 15 mg prochlorperazine (as maleate).
5. Stemetil Syrup (Rhone Poulenc, UK): this is a clear fruit-flavoured, orange syrup containing 5 mg prochlorperazine per 5 ml and 68% sucrose.
6. Prochlorperazine is now also available as an effervescent powder in sachets, each containing 5 mg of prochlorperazine, which can be taken as a fizzy drink after addition to a glass of water.
7. In the UK the parenteral form is a colourless solution containing 12.5 mg prochlorperazine mesylate per ml in ampoules of 1 and 2 ml. In the USA the parenteral form is available as solution containing 5 $mg.ml^{-1}$ prochlorperazine edisylate, sodium sulphite, sodium bisulphite, sodium phosphate and biphosphate in ampoules of 2 ml, in multiple-dose vials of 10 ml containing 0.75% benzyl alcohol, and in disposable syringes of 2 ml.
8. Buccastem (Reckitt & Colman, UK) is a pale yellow buccal tablet coded 'J1' and containing 3 mg prochlorperazine maleate.

Prochlorperazine

All preparations should be protected from light. The maximum shelf-life is 5 years for tablets, 3 years for solutions and suppositories, and 2 years for the syrup.

P

Therapeutic use

Prochlorperazine is a potent phenothiazine antipsychotic. These agents have a high therapeutic index and a flat dose–response curve and can be used over a wide range of dosages without acutely life-threatening effects. However, all these drugs have potentially severe side effects and should be used with restraint.

Prochlorperazine has questionable utility as an antipsychotic agent and frequently produces acute extrapyramidal reactions. It is thus not commonly employed in psychiatry, but it is used as an antiemetic and in the treatment of vertigo.

Indications

1. Nausea and vomiting
2. Vertigo and Ménière's syndrome
3. Management of psychotic disorders.

Contraindications

1. Pregnancy
2. CNS depression
3. Children under 2 years
4. History of hypersensitivity to phenothiazines.

Mode of use

When given by mouth, as is rational if nausea and vomiting are anticipated, the dose should be 5–10 mg 3 to 4 times per day, or 10 mg of the sustained-release form given twice daily. As a suppository the 25 mg preparation is recommended twice a day.

Parenteral administration is 5–10 mg intramuscularly twice a day (maximal dose 40 mg daily). It has been reported that prochlorperazine given slowly (the rate of injection should not exceed 5 mg over 1 minute) intravenously has proved effective in doses of 2.5–5 mg.[9] This type of emergency treatment of nausea and vomiting reduced the time to take effect from 35 minutes to 8.5 minutes. If time permits, the injection solution should be diluted (20 $mg.l^{-1}$ of isotonic solution) to avoid irritation of the vein.

Indications

1. Nausea and vomiting

Nausea and vomiting are symptoms that may be due to many causes. Sometimes they are diagnostic and suppression by drug therapy may obscure the diagnosis. Typical examples are nausea and vomiting associated with subacute intestinal obstruction or nausea and vomiting as symptoms of digitalis overdose. In such cases rational therapy is based on identification of the underlying cause, and symptomatic treatment with an antiemetic drug would be harmful.

However, nausea and vomiting are frequently encountered when the cause has no diagnostic importance or cannot be dealt with. Such is the case in uraemia, in radiation sickness, and secondary to other drug treatment, such as with cytostatic agents, opiates, some antibiotics, oestrogens, potassium chloride, aminophylline and general anaesthetics.[10] No antiemetic drug is accepted as clearly superior, which is in itself proof that the ideal antiemetic drug does not exist. (For a review stressing emesis in chemotherapy see reference 5.)

Prochlorperazine has been found to be a very potent antiemetic, especially when a central mechanism, such as stimulation of the chemoreceptor trigger zone,[5,10,11] is the likely cause.[4,5] However, it produces an appreciable incidence of dystonias (0.3%) and hence should be used with caution.

2. Vertigo and Ménière's syndrome

Vertigo (dizziness) is often a secondary symptom of central or peripheral pathology. For this reason symptomatic drug treatment is frequently not rational or final. However, prochlorperazine is frequently used in this fashion and has been reported to be effective in small uncontrolled studies.[12] There is no definitive evidence that prochlorperazine is more effective than placebo.

3. Management of psychotic disorders

Prochlorperazine has not been shown to possess greater efficacy in the management of psychotic states than other antipsychotic drugs in use. Thus, only advantages of lower incidence and severity of side effects would justify its recommendation. No such advantage has been claimed on the basis of controlled studies. Prochlorperazine is not a rational choice for the treatment of psychotic disorders.[13]

Contraindications

1. Pregnancy
No evidence of adverse effects of prochlorperazine on fetal development has been reported since its introduction. However, safety in pregnancy has not been established either. There seems to be no reason to take any risks not balanced by clear benefits.

2. CNS depression
Since all phenothiazine derivatives are known to potentiate CNS depressant drugs of any type, they are contraindicated in the presence of existing CNS depression.

3. In children under two years
Prochlorperazine is more frequently associated with dystonic reactions in this age group and is contraindicated on this basis.

4. History of hypersensitivity to phenothiazines
Although the verification of reported hypersensitivity reaction is often deficient, there is rarely a reason to warrant the risk of repetition.

The parenteral solution available in the USA contains sodium sulphite and sodium bisulphite. Sulphites have been reported to cause allergic reactions, including anaphylactic, life-threatening and severe asthmatic episodes in susceptible individuals. The incidence is unknown.

Adverse reactions

Potentially life-threatening effects
In view of the large therapeutic ratio of all antipsychotic drugs, life-threatening events resulting from administration of prochlorperazine alone are rare. On the other hand, administration of prochlorperazine in combination with other CNS depressant drugs may have fatal consequences. No documented numerical information is available.

Prochlorperazine has been reported to be responsible for rare cases of aplastic anaemia. However, proof of a causal relationship has not been obtained. Thus, bone marrow depression, while possible, must be very rare.

Acute overdosage
Overdose of phenothiazine drugs may cause symptoms, including severe drowsiness to unconsciousness. The most serious adverse effect is orthostatic hypotension, which may result in syncope. Piperazine analogues, such as prochlorperazine, are less likely to cause hypotension than phenothiazines with aliphatic side-chains. If hypotension is severe, reflex tachycardia is present. ECG changes, reported mainly after chlorpromazine, may be due to a quinidine-like effect or to a local anaesthetic effect. The changes include prolongation of the Q-T and P-R intervals, blunting of T waves, and depression of the S-T segment. Hyper- or hypothermia, and severe extrapyramidal symptoms and convulsions, have also been seen after acute overdoses.

If the time interval between ingestion and presentation is short, gastric lavage may be done, but there is a risk of aspiration and low expectation of benefit. Activated charcoal should be given by mouth or stomach tube.

There is no specific antidote, and treatment is symptomatic and supportive.

Hypotension is often sufficiently treated by intravenous administration of fluids. If circulatory function remains inadequate, directly acting sympathomimetic agents should be considered (though opinions differ on such use in poisoning with a phenothiazine), but adrenaline should be avoided because the α-adrenergic block produced by prochlorperazine may unmask its vasodilator component. Cardiac arrhythmias may respond to correction of hypothermia, hypotension and metabolic disturbances. Antiarrhythmic drug therapy has to take into account that myocardial depression may be present, and drugs with a negative inotropic effect should be avoided.

Convulsions should be treated with an intravenous dose of a benzodiazepine.

Respiratory depression, usually indicative of the presence of other agents with CNS depressant activity, should be treated by assisted ventilation including tracheal intubation if necessary.

Neuroleptic malignant syndrome (hyperthermia, rigidity, autonomic dysfunction and altered consciousness) may occur with any antipsychotic. Dantrolene administration should be considered.

Dystonias and extrapyramidal syndrome: see Table 1.

Severe or irreversible adverse effects
Phenothiazine derivatives in general have been reported to have occasional severe and potentially irreversible adverse effects, but no information regarding prochlorperazine specifically has been reported. Toxic effects reported for this class of drugs include: cholestatic jaundice, pigmentary retinopathy, cardiac arrhythmias and a quinidine-like effect, leucopenia, and thrombocytopenia.

The most frequently reported adverse effects are a range of extrapyramidal effects. Most of them are transitory and/or treatable. Tardive dyskinesia is serious, and no treatment is known. Since tardive dyskinesia is usually (but not always) seen after prolonged treatment and high dosage, it is rare after prochlorperazine, which is no longer used for long-term antipsychotic therapy. The use of prochlorperazine by non-psychiatrist physicians in the treatment of nausea and vomiting, and of vertigo, especially in elderly patients and

Table 1 Neurological side effects of neuroleptic-antipsychotic drugs

Reaction	Features	Period of maximum risk	Proposed mechanism	Treatment
Acute dystonia	Spasm of muscles of tongue, face, neck, back; may mimic seizures: *not* hysteria	1–5 days	Dopamine excess? Acetylcholine excess?	Antiparkinsonism agents are diagnostic and curative (i.m. or i.v., then p.o.)
Parkinsonism	Bradykinesia, rigidity, variable tremor, mask-facies, shuffling gait	5–30 days (may persist)	Dopamine blockade	Antiparkinsonism agents (p.o.); dopamine agonists risky?
Akathisia	Motor restlessness; patient may experience anxiety or agitation	5–60 days (commonly persists)	Unknown	Reduce dose or change drug; low doses of propranolol;* antiparkinsonism agents or benzodiazepines may help
Tardive dyskinesia	Oral-facial dyskinesia; choreo-athetosis, sometimes irreversible, rarely progressive	6–24 months (worse on withdrawal)	Dopamine excess?	Prevention best; treatment unsatisfactory; slow spontaneous remission
'Rabbit' syndrome	Perioral tremor (late parkinsonism variant?); usually reversible	Months or years	Unknown	Antiparkinsonism agents; reduce dose of neuroleptic
Malignant syndrome	Catatonia, stupor, fever, unstable pulse and blood pressure myoglobinaemia; can be fatal	Weeks	Unknown	Stop neuroleptic; antiparkinsonism agents usually fail; bromocriptine often helps; dantrolene variable; general supportive care crucial

* There may be an increased risk of hypotension on interacting high doses of propranolol with some antipsychotic agents; clonidine may also be effective at doses of 0.2–0.8 mg.day^{-1}, but carries a high risk of hypotension. From: Baldessarini R J 1985 Chemotherapy in Psychiatry. Harvard University Press, Cambridge, Mass. & London. With permission from the author and publisher.

in nursing home settings, has been reported to result in the occurrence of extrapyramidal adverse effects.[14,15] Since these effects may be misdiagnosed and treatment is often possible, a summary description (Table 1) is included. Epidemiological information[16,17] is inadequate.

Symptomatic adverse effects
The basic pharmacological effects of prochlorperazine may result in symptoms that are simply manifestations of these effects: anticholinergic (dry mouth, blurred vision, aggravation of glaucoma, urinary retention, constipation), anti-α-adrenergic (hypotension, sometimes orthostatic; failure of ejaculation), antidopaminergic (increased release of prolactin — leading to galactorrhoea, gynaecomastia, amenorrhoea, and impotence). Photosensitivity and skin rashes are not specific adverse effects.

Interference with clinical pathology tests
Prochlorperazine may interfere with measurements of 17-oxo steroids and 17-oxygenic steroids. Presence of phenothiazines may produce false positives in phenylketonuria (PKU) tests.

High risk groups

Neonates
Prochlorperazine should not be given to neonates.

Breast milk. There is evidence that phenothiazines are excreted in breast milk.

Children
The drug should be not used in children younger than 2 years of age.

Pregnant women
Safety of prochlorperazine in pregnancy has not been established. Thus, prochlorperazine should be given during pregnancy only for severe nausea and vomiting, with recognition of the potential risk.

The elderly
Elderly patients are more sensitive to prochlorperazine, and lower doses may suffice. Hypotension and hypothermia are more likely to be seen and patients should be watched accordingly.

Drug interactions

Potentially hazardous interactions
The original indication for chlorpromazine was potentiation of general anaesthetics and opioid analgesics. Thus, prochlorperazine potentiates sedative hypnotic agents or CNS depressants of all types, including alcohol and over-the-counter sedatives.

Other significant interactions
In view of the spectrum of pharmacological effects of phenothiazines, prochlorperazine can interact with many drugs. A prime example is the additive effect of the anticholinergic effect of prochlorperazine with that of other drugs with anticholinergic properties, such as many antihistaminics, central anticholinergics used in the treatment of parkinsonism, and tricyclic antidepressants. Many nonprescription drugs and drug combinations have anticholinergic properties. It can be postulated that the central effect of anticholinergic agents, the so-called central anticholinergic syndrome, may complicate the symptomatology of the central effects of prochlorperazine when used as an antiemetic or for vertigo.

Potentially useful interactions
Although the initial use of chlorpromazine was for the purpose of utilizing the therapeutically desirable interaction of several drugs ('lytic cocktail'), the present use of prochlorperazine (or of the phenothiazines as a group) does not include an example of such therapeutically useful interactions.

General review articles

Prochlorperazine is included in the description of antipsychotic drug trials published in several monographs and textbooks.

Usdin E, Efron D H 1972 Psychotropic drugs and related compounds. 2nd edn. US Public Health Service Publications Nr. 72-9074, US Government Printing Office, Washington, D.C.

Clark W G, del Giudice J (eds) 1978 Principles of psychopharmacology, 2nd edn. Academic Press, New York

Iversen L L, Iversen S, Snyder S H (eds) 1978 Handbook of psychopharmacology, vol.10. Neuroleptics. Plenum Press, New York

Baldessarini R G 1990 Drugs and the treatment of psychiatric disorders. In: Gilman A G, Nies A S, Rall T W, Taylor P (eds) The pharmacological basis of therapeutics, 8th edn. Pergamon, New York

References

1. Borison H L, Wang S C 1953 Physiology and pharmacology of vomiting. Pharmacological Reviews 5: 193–230
2. Wang S C 1965 Emetic and antiemetic drugs. In: Root W S, Hofmann F G (eds) Physiological pharmacology, vol II, part B. Academic Press, New York, pp 255–328
3. Perutka S J, Snyder S H 1982 Antiemetics: neurotransmitter receptor binding predicts therapeutic actions. Lancet 1: 658–659
4. Wyant G M 1962 A comparative study of eleven antiemetic drugs in dogs. Canadian Anaesthetists Society Journal 9: 399–407
5. Seigel L J, Longo D L 1981 The control of chemotherapy-induced emesis. Annals of Internal Medicine 95: 352–359
6. Fowler A, Taylor W, Bateman D N 1986 Plasma prochlorperazine assay by high performance liquid chromatography–electrochemistry. Journal of Chromatography 380: 202–205
7. Sankey M G, Holt J E, Kaye C M 1982 A simple and sensitive HPLC method for assay of prochlorperazine in plasma. British Journal of Clinical Pharmacology 13: 578–580
8. Taylor W B, Bateman D N 1987 Preliminary studies of the pharmacokinetics and pharmacodynamics of prochlorperazine in healthy volunteers. British Journal of Clinical Pharmacology 23: 137–142
9. Ordog G J, Vann P W, Owashi N D, Wasserberger J, Herman L S, Balasubramaniam S 1984 Intravenous prochlorperazine for the rapid control of vomiting in the emergency department. Annals of Emergency Medicine 13: 253–258
10. Loeser E A, Bennett G, Stanley T H, Machin R 1979 Comparison of droperidol, haloperidol, and prochlorperazine as postoperative antiemetics. Canadian Anaesthetists Society Journal 26: 125–127
11. Cunningham D, Forrest G J, Soukop M, Gilchrist N L, Calder I T, McAdrle C S 1985 Nabilone and prochlorperazine: a useful combination for emesis induced by cytotoxic drugs. British Medical Journal 291: 864–865
12. Aantaa E, Skinhoj A 1976 Controlled clinical trial comparing the effect of betahistine hydrochloride and prochlorperazine maleate on patients with Ménière's disease. Annals of Clinical Research 8: 284–287
13. Baldessarini R G 1985 Drugs and the treatment of psychiatric disorders. In: Gilman A G, Goodman L S, Rall T W, Murad F (eds) The pharmacological basis of therapeutics, 7th edn. Macmillan, New York, p 402
14. Baker F M, Cook P 1981 Compazine complications: a review. Journal of the National Medical Association 73: 409–412
15. Stephen P J, Williamson J 1984 Drug induced Parkinsonism in the elderly. Lancet 2: 1082–1083
16. Bateman D N, Rawlins M D, Simpson J M 1985 Epidemiology of acute dyskinetic–dystonic reactions to metoclopromide and prochlorperazine. British Journal of Clinical Pharmacology 20: 258P
17. Porter J, Jick H 1977 Drug-induced anaphylaxis, convulsions, deafness, and extrapyramidal symptoms. Lancet 1: 587–588

P

Procyclidine (hydrochloride)

Anticholinergic drugs were first used to treat parkinsonism in the middle of the last century when Charcot used belladonna alkaloids.[1] More recently, synthetic drugs have replaced natural alkaloids. Procyclidine was first tried in parkinsonism because of its antimuscarinic properties and its antagonism of nicotine-induced tremor.[2] It is chemically related to another antiparkinsonian drug, benzhexol.[2]

Chemistry

Procyclidine hydrochloride (Kemadrin, Arpicolin)
$C_{19}H_{29}NO.HCl$
1-Cyclohexyl-1-phenyl-3-(pyrrolidin-1-yl)propan-1-ol hydrochloride

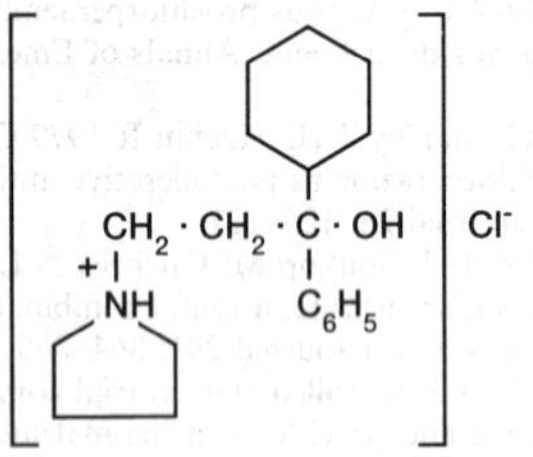

Molecular weight (free base)	323.9 (287.4)
pKa	10.7
Solubility	
in alcohol	1 in 15
in water	1 in 40
Octanol/water partition coefficient	250

Procyclidine hydrochloride is a white crystalline powder with a characteristic odour and bitter taste. It melts at 225–227°C with decomposition. It is prepared by chemical synthesis. There are no combination products containing this drug. It posesses a chiral centre.

Pharmacology

Procyclidine is a competitive inhibitor of the peripheral actions of acetylcholine at muscarinic sites. The potency has been described as approximately one-seventh that of atropine. The activity resides largely in the laevo-isomer.[3] It antagonizes effects associated with stimulation of central receptors such as nicotine-induced tremor. Prior injection of 1 $mg.kg^{-1}$ reduced, and 5 $mg.kg^{-1}$ largely eliminated, tremor produced by 0.3 $mg.kg^{-1}$ of nicotine.[2]

Toxicology

There is no information about the oncogenicity or mutagenicity of procyclidine. The adverse effects of procyclidine are largely due to its anticholinergic action. However, unlike atropine, procyclidine does not cause tachycardia.[4] Repeated-dose toxicity studies in animals have shown no morphological change in any of the major organs attributable to drug treatment. When pregnant rats were given the drug no fetal abnormalities were found.

Clinical pharmacology

Single doses of procyclidine (10 mg) give maximal autonomic effects within 0.5 h of intravenous administration and 1 to 2 h of oral dosing. Significant autonomic effects are still detectable 12 hours after both forms of treatment.[5] Subjective feelings are experienced within 15 minutes of injection. In one study, the human pharmacology of oral procyclidine and atropine was compared.[4] Surprisingly, in view of its anticholinergic action, procyclidine caused moderate cardiac slowing lasting for 7 hours. Salivary secretion was rapidly reduced by atropine, maximal after 1 h 45 min, and the drug effect disappeared by 7 h 45 min, but procyclidine produced a much smaller effect. Both drugs produced increasing pupillary dilation up to 7 h 45 min. Procyclidine 10 mg increased the visual near point maximally at 1 h 30 min and was associated with the majority of complaints of blurred vision. Atropine did not affect this. The different effect of the two drugs at different sites can be explained on the basis of cholinergic antagonist and agonist activity and local pharmacokinetic differences.

The efficacy of procyclidine in the treatment of naturally occurring parkinsonism[6] and pseudo-parkinsonism induced by neuroleptic drugs[7] has been established in placebo-controlled trials. The usual dose is 2.5 mg to 10 mg three times daily, but pharmacodynamic studies suggest that a twice-daily dosage schedule could be just as suitable.[5]

Pharmacokinetics

Plasma procyclidine can be determined by gas–liquid chromatography.[5] This method detects plasma levels down to 10 $\mu g.l^{-1}$ and when used routinely to analyse procyclidine in plasma and urine is sufficiently sensitive for bioavailability and pharmacokinetic studies.

Procyclidine is rapidly and completely absorbed after oral administration and peak plasma concentrations are seen at 1–2 h in fasting subjects. The systemic bioavailability is 75% (range 52–97) due to presystemic metabolism. Procyclidine is lipid soluble and at physiological pH migrates preferentially from water into less polar solvents. Penetration of the blood–brain barrier is therefore likely and may be inferred from its effects on the central nervous system. There is no information about the excretion of procyclidine in breast milk although some is likely. Only a small fraction of procyclidine appears in urine as the parent compound; therefore care is advisable in patients with hepatic dysfunction. The mean elimination half life after oral administration is 12.6 h (SD ±4.8): the plasma clearance is 67.5 $ml.min^{-1}$ (SD ±27.5).[5] The volume of distribution, after both intravenous and oral administration, is about 1 $l.kg^{-1}$. Procyclidine is probably moderately extensively protein-bound in plasma, but accurate figures are not available.[5]

Oral absorption	100%
Presystemic metabolism	25%
Plasma half life	
mean	12.6 h
Volume of distribution	1 $l.kg^{-1}$
Plasma protein binding	moderate

Concentration–effect relationship

The effects on pupil diameter, visual near point and salivary secretion rate are all in the direction expected for an anticholinergic drug, and maximum effect correlates well with plasma concentration.[5] In one study[5] mean maximum plasma concentration after 10 mg orally was 116 $\mu g.l^{-1}$. Clinical observations on the duration of the effect of the drug in parkinsonism are consistent with the plasma half life of the drug.

Metabolism

Little is known about the metabolism of procyclidine: when given orally about one-fifth appears as two metabolites. The principal pathway seems to involve hydroxylation of the cyclohexane ring. Some of this metabolite is then further oxidized. The hydroxylated metabolite is present in urine as glucuronide. The biological activity of these metabolites is unknown. There may also be oxidation of the benzyl ring. Figure 1 shows a metabolic scheme which has been proposed for the metabolism of procyclidine in man.[8]

Procyclidine (hydrochloride)

Fig. 1 Proposed metabolic scheme for procyclidine

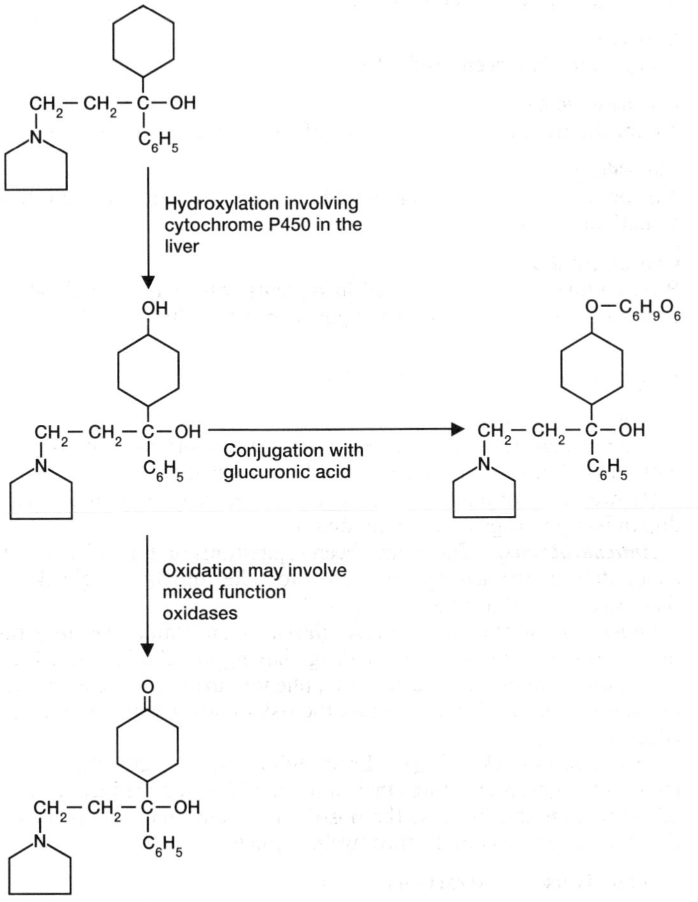

Pharmaceutics

Procyclidine hydrochloride is available in oral and parenteral forms:

1. Kemadrin (Wellcome, UK/Burroughs-Wellcome, USA): Tablets containing 5 mg. The tablets are white, round, scored and coded 'S3A' above the score line, with 'Wellcome' impressed below the score line
2. Arpicolin (RP Drugs, UK): A liquid oral preparation containing procyclidine hydrochloride 2.5 mg in 5 ml in a red-coloured syrup base containing sucrose and sorbitol
3. Kemadrin injection (Wellcome, UK): An injection containing 10 mg in 2 ml clear aqueous vehicle adjusted to pH 3.9–4.5 suitable for intravenous use.

The tablets and injection carry only a minimal risk from potentially allergenic substances. The syrup, however, contains amaranth as the colouring agent, and has a relatively high concentration of sucrose (35%).

Therapeutic use

Indications

1. The treatment of naturally occurring parkinsonism
2. The treatment of pseudo-parkinsonism induced by neuroleptic drugs
3. The treatment of oculogyric crises
4. The treatment of acute dystonic reactions.

Contraindications

1. Tardive dyskinesia in patients undergoing treatment with neuroleptic drugs

Mode of use

The initial use of anticholinergic drugs in parkinsonism was based on mistaken theories about the aetiology of the disease. However, more recent experimental work[9] supports the hypothesis that the clinical efficacy of the anticholinergic drugs employed in the treatment of parkinsonism is due entirely to a central anti-acetylcholine effect.

Oral treatment of parkinsonism is usually started at 2.5 mg three times daily, increasing by 2.5–5 mg daily at intervals of two or three days until the optimum clinical response is achieved. The usual maximum total daily dose is 30 mg. However, where appropriate, this total may be as high as 60 mg.[2] Sudden withdrawal of procyclidine in patients receiving benefit from this drug can result in a distressing exacerbation of parkinsonian symptoms and should be avoided. In acute dystonic reactions, 5 mg is given intravenously and is usually effective within 5 min. Occasionally a patient may need 10 mg or more.

Indications

1. The treatment of naturally occurring parkinsonism

Progressive degeneration of pigment-containing cells in the substantia nigra leads to deficiency of the neurotransmitter, dopamine. This in turn leads to an imbalance between the inhibitory effects of dopamine and the excitory effects of acetylcholine in the basal ganglia. Treatment aims to restore this balance, by giving either dopaminergic drugs or anticholinergic drugs. Generally, the degree of benefit obtained from dopaminergic drugs far exceeds that which can be obtained from anticholinergics; therefore in disabled patients dopaminergic drugs are the first choice in treating parkinsonism. However, in many patients taking adequate doses of dopaminergic drugs additional benefit can be obtained by adding anticholinergics.[10] It has been suggested that intravenous physostigmine can be used to predict which patients, taking levodopa, will benefit from additional anticholinergic therapy: levodopa-treated patients whose parkinsonism is not aggravated by intravenous physostigmine do not benefit from the addition of anticholinergic drugs.[11]

In view of the finite span of effective control of symptoms before long-term complications occur, it has been suggested that dopaminergic drugs should be withheld from patients with minimal disease. In such patients anticholinergics alone may give adequate improvement. The use of anticholinergics alone is particularly appropriate in patients whose only significant symptom is tremor. Other symptoms which may be improved include rigidity and leg cramps but akinesia is not helped. Drooling saliva, a troublesome symptom, is caused by poor swallowing due to akinesia but anticholinergics may give symptomatic improvement by reducing salivary flow.

Anticholinergic agents such as procyclidine have an important role in patients who are unable to tolerate dopaminergic drugs because of side effects or contraindications. While certain patients may prefer procyclidine, in general clinical use there is little to choose between the various anticholinergic agents and there is no advantage in prescribing more than one simultaneously.

The above remarks which apply particularly to idiopathic parkinsonism are also valid for postencephalitic forms of the disease; the first use of procyclidine was in postencephalitic patients.[2] Traditionally it is said that postencephalitic patients require higher doses of anticholinergic drugs than others, but this traditional view has been challenged.[12] Procyclidine is also used in parkinsonism due to other causes.

2. The treatment of pseudo-parkinsonism induced by neuroleptic drugs

In this type of parkinsonism, dopaminergic agents are not appropriate; therefore anticholinergics are the first choice.

The efficacy of procyclidine in such patients has been confirmed in a double-blind, crossover placebo-controlled trial.[7] Procyclidine helps reversible drug-induced extrapyramidal syndromes such as pseudo-parkinsonism, akathisia and dystonia, which can be caused by neuroleptics. However, routine administration of anticholinergics during neuroleptic therapy is not justified because not all patients are affected and because tardive dyskinesia is made worse by them. If an anticholinergic is prescribed, one must be aware of the possibility that its anticholinergic effect will summate with that of the neuroleptic, resulting in a toxic confusional state.

3. The treatment of oculogyric crises

Intravenous procyclidine is effective in this condition. In instances where intravenous injection is difficult the drug may be administered intramuscularly.

4. The treatment of acute dystonic reactions

If acute dystonic reactions are precipitated by neuroleptic drugs they usually occur during the first few days of treatment. Intravenous (or intramuscular) procyclidine effectively controls these reactions. In doses of 5 to 7.5 mg intravenously it has been safely and effectively given to children aged 3 to 11 years, suffering from dystonia due to metoclopramide.[13] Occasionally there may be difficulties in distinguishing acute dystonic reactions due to neuroleptics from the symptoms of tetanus; in such cases the intravenous injection of an anticholinergic is a useful diagnostic tool.

Contraindications

1. Tardive dyskinesias

Tardive dyskinesia is particularly important because it may not be reversible on withdrawing neuroleptic therapy: procyclidine will not help and may make it worse. Three possible explanations for this effect on tardive dyskinesia have been suggested: anticholinergics may (i) change the plasma levels of neuroleptic, thus increasing the severity of tardive dyskinesia, (ii) reduce muscle tone, thus worsening hyperkinetic dyskinesia, (iii) reduce central cholinergic activity, so changing the central dopaminergic/cholinergic balance which is thought to be the pathophysiological mechanism underlying tardive dyskinesia. It seems that the best explanation is the third.[14]

Adverse reactions

Potentially life-threatening effects

Chronic overdose (especially in conjunction with other anticholinergic drugs) may give a toxic confusional state. This is an indication for admission to hospital, withdrawal of anticholinergic therapy and, if necessary, parenteral administration of an anticholinesterase which gains access to the central nervous system, such as physostigmine 1–4 mg.[15]

Acute overdosage

Reports of overdosage are relatively rare. If procyclidine has been ingested within the previous two hours (or possibly longer in view of its likely effects on gastric motility) then gastric lavage is probably indicated. Most symptoms are due to anticholinergic actions. Dry mouth, blurred vision, constipation, urinary retention, agitation, restlessness and confusion with severe sleeplessness, visual hallucinations, auditory hallucinations and convulsions have been reported. Convulsions should be controlled by intravenous diazepam. With adequate supportive therapy, complete clinical and electroencephalographic recovery is likely.

Severe or irreversible adverse effects

Procyclidine may aggravate the symptoms of narrow-angle glaucoma, obstructive disease of the gastrointestinal tract or prostatic hypertrophy.

Abuse of anticholinergic drugs, including procyclidine, is apparently quite common[16] and this should be considered in patients who develop new and unusual symptoms such as excitability, dizziness, visual hallucinations, or other features of a toxic confusional state. The risk of true dependence is still unknown. Abusers seem to find the euphoriant and stimulant effects pleasurable. Although procyclidine seems to be less abused than other antiparkinsonian anticholinergic drugs, it is uncertain whether this represents a real difference in its mood-elevating properties or simply current prescribing patterns and therefore availability.

Symptomatic adverse effects

All the adverse effects due to anticholinergic activity such as dry mouth, blurred vision, constipation, urinary retention, agitation, restlessness, confusion and convulsions, are reversible on withdrawal of the drug.

Other effects

No clinically significant biochemical effects have been reported.

Interference with clinical pathology tests

No significant problems have been reported.

High risk groups

Neonates

There is no information on the use of procyclidine in neonates.

Breast milk. No data are available on the secretion of this drug in breast milk. However, since infants are particularly sensitive to anticholinergic agents, breast-feeding should probably be stopped if this drug is given to the mother.

Children

Procyclidine has been used effectively and safely in children.[13]

Pregnant women

No information is available on the safe use of this drug in pregnancy.

The elderly

No special precautions are required, as doses are adjusted according to patient response.

Concurrent disease

Procyclidine should be avoided in patients with narrow-angle glaucoma, obstructive disease of the gut or prostatic hypertrophy.

Drug interactions

Potentially hazardous interactions

Phenothiazines. Hyperpyrexia may occur if procyclidine is used with phenothiazines during hot and humid weather.[17]

(However, procyclidine can be used effectively and safely with dopaminergic drugs and amantadine.)

Anticonvulsants. There have been suggestions that if patients with adequately controlled epilepsy start to take anticholinergic drugs these may exacerbate their seizures.[18]

Other drugs with anticholinergic effects. Concomitant administration of procyclidine with other drugs having anticholinergic effects (e.g. antihistamines, opiate agonists, phenothiazines, tricyclic antidepressants, quinidine) may increase the risk of adverse anticholinergic effects.

Miscellaneous other drugs. Procyclidine reduces peristaltic movement of the gut, preventing efficient mixing. This may reduce the rate of absorption and increase the possibility of enzymic drug inactivation (e.g. hydrolysis of erythromycin, penicillin).

Potentially useful interactions

None is known.

Clinical trials

1. Strang R R 1965 The treatment of parkinsonism: a double-blind and one year follow-up study. Current Medicine and Drugs 5: 27–32

Procyclidine was introduced in the treatment of Parkinsonism on the basis of uncontrolled open studies. Definitive evidence for its efficacy was obtained by Strang who studied 70 patients (including 15 with a history of encephalitis). A double-blind comparison with placebo lasting 2 months showed improvement in 2 of the 35 patients receiving placebo and 26 of the 35 patients receiving procyclidine.

2. Mindham R H S, Lamb P, Bradley R 1977 A comparison of piribedil, procyclidine and placebo in the control of phenothiazinc-induced parkinsonism. British Journal of Psychiatry 130: 581–585

In the treatment of Parkinsonism due to neuroleptic drugs procyclodine was shown to be more effective than the placebo when given in a double blind crossover placebo trial in 16 patients with chronic schizophrenia receiving fluphenazine deconoate.

References

1. Ordenstein L 1867 M.D. thesis: sur la paralysie agitante et la sclérose en plaques généralisee. Martinet, Paris
2. Montuschi E, Phillips J, Prescott F 1952 Kemadrin in post-encephalitic Parkinsonism. Lancet 1: 583–585
3. Duffin W M, Green A F 1955 The pharmacological properties of the optical isomers of benzhexol, procyclidine, tricyclamol and related compounds. British Journal of Pharmacology 10: 383–386
4. Hamilton M, Peck A W, Smith P 1982 Procyclidine and atropine: comparison of anticholinergic effects in man. British Journal of Clinical Pharmacology 13: 614P
5. Whiteman P D, Fowle A S E, Hamilton M J et al 1985 Pharmacokinetics and pharmacodynamics of procyclidine in man. European Journal of Clinical Pharmacology 28: 73–78
6. Strang R R 1965 The treatment of parkinsonism: a double-blind and one year follow-up study. Current Medicine and Drugs 5: 27–32
7. Mindham R H S, Lamb P, Bradley R 1977 A comparison of piribedil, procyclidine and placebo in the control of phenothiazine-induced parkinsonism. British Journal of Psychiatry 130: 581–585

8. Dean K, Bye A, Land G, Whiteman P 1981 Metabolism of procyclidine in humans. Internal Group Research and Development Document. The Wellcome Foundation Ltd.
9. Duvoisin R C 1967 Cholinergic–anticholinergic antagonism in Parkinsonism. Archives of Neurology 17: 124–136
10. Hughes R C, Polgar J G, Weightman D, Walton J N 1971 Levodopa in Parkinsonism: the effects of withdrawal of anticholinergic drugs. British Medical Journal 2: 487–491
11. Weintraub M I, Van Woert M H 1971 Reversal by levodopa of cholinergic hypersensitivity in Parkinson's disease. New England Journal of Medicine 284: 412–415
12. De Jong D 1966 Medical therapy in Parkinson's disease. Journal of Neurosurgery 24: 342–348
13. Gatrad A R 1976 Dystonic reactions to metoclopramide. Developmental Medicine and Child Neurology 18: 767–769
14. Greil W, Haag G R, Rüther E 1984 Effects of anticholinergics on tardive dyskinesia. British Journal of Psychiatry 145: 304–310
15. Greenblatt D J, Shader R I 1973 Drug therapy: anticholinergics. New England Journal of Medicine 288: 1215–1219
16. Pullen G P, Best N R, Maguire J 1984 Anticholinergic drug abuse: a common problem? British Medical Journal 289: 612–613
17. Westlake R J, Rastegar A 1973 Hyperpyrexia from drug combinations. Journal of the American Medical Association 225: 1250
18. Aucamp A K, Meyer C J 1979 Epileptic seizures exacerbated by anti-cholinergic drugs. South African Medical Journal 56: 423

Progesterone

Progesterone is the major steroid secreted by the corpus luteum.

Chemistry

Progesterone (Inteal hormon, Inteine, Gestone, Cyclogest, Progestasert)
$C_{21}H_{30}O_2$
Pregn-4-ene-3,20-dione

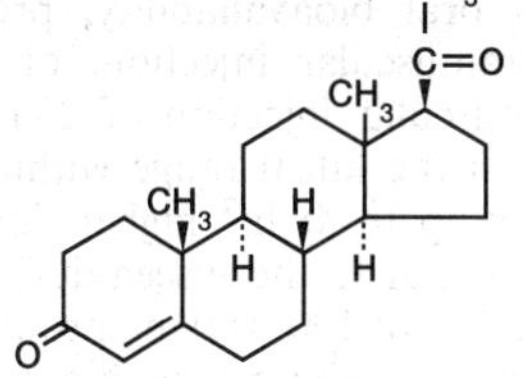

Molecular weight	314.5
pKa	not relevant
Solubility	
in alcohol	1 in 8
in water	<1 in 10 000
Octanol/water partition coefficient	high

Progesterone exists as colourless crystals, or as a colourless or yellow–white odourless, tasteless powder. It has two forms, with melting points at 126–131°C, and approximately 121°C. It is prepared commercially from diosgenin or stigmasterol, which are obtained from plant sources.

Pharmacology

Progesterone is a naturally-occurring progestogen. It also has anti-oestrogenic activity.

Toxicology

There is limited evidence that progesterone is carcinogenic in some laboratory species, and that it has mutagenic potential in some short-term tests, but there appear to be no epidemiological studies in humans.[1] Progesterone does not appear to be teratogenic in humans.[2]

Clinical pharmacology

Progesterone acts via specific receptors in target cells. The steroid–receptor complex binds to DNA in the nucleus, thereby inducing the synthesis of specific proteins. Progesterone receptor concentrations are low in the absence of oestrogens, and increase following oestrogen administration. For this reason, most of the pharmacological effects of progesterone require prior oestrogen 'priming'.[3]

The progestational actions of progesterone include the development of a glandular endometrium in an oestrogen-primed uterus and the postponement of menstruation, the maintenance of pregnancy, inhibition of uterine motility and delay in parturition. Sudden withdrawal of progesterone during the luteal phase leads to withdrawal bleeding irrespective of whether oestrogens are present or not;[4] conversely, excessively high levels during progesterone therapy may lead to intermittent breakthrough bleeding. Progesterone suppresses pituitary gonadotrophin secretion, and promotes lobuloalveolar development in the breast. It has a thermogenic effect, which is responsible for the increased basal body temperature seen during the luteal phase.

P

Progesterone also has antioestrogenic activity, being capable of inhibiting oestrogen-induced growth and motility. These actions are probably due to suppression of oestrogen receptor synthesis.

Unlike most synthetic progestogens, progesterone has virtually no androgenic or oestrogenic properties.

Pharmacokinetics

Progesterone is normally measured by radioimmunoassay, which has high sensitivity (10–20 pg) and specificity.

After oral administration, progesterone is absorbed from the gastrointestinal tract, but is rapidly metabolized by the small intestine and liver. Oral administration of 100 mg progesterone produces peak plasma concentrations of 12–43 nmol.l^{-1} after 2 h, followed by a rapid fall in concentration over 8 h; progesterone is undetectable after 24 h.[5] Daily ingestion of 100 mg produces plasma concentrations of 22–35 nmol.l^{-1}, comparable to those occurring during the normal luteal phase.[6] Peak concentrations occur within 4 h, and concentrations are elevated for up to 96 h. The bioavailability of oral progesterone has been estimated to be approximately 25%, based on a comparison of the daily production rate of endogenous progesterone and the dose required to produce physiological plasma concentrations.[6]

Owing to its low oral bioavailability, progesterone is usually administered by intramuscular injection, or as rectal or vaginal suppositories. Intramuscular injection of 25 mg or more produces peak concentrations in the luteal range within 8 h, and concentrations are elevated for up to 48 h;[7] higher doses produce transient peak concentrations similar to those seen during pregnancy.[7] Rectal or vaginal administration of 100–400 mg produces concentrations in the luteal range which are maximal within 1–8 h and then decline over 24 h:[7–9] concomitant oestrogen treatment has been reported to enhance vaginal absorption of progesterone,[8] although such concurrent treatment is seldom used clinically.

The half life of progesterone in blood is short, but published data vary widely. Progesterone has a distribution phase half life of between 3–6 minutes, followed by an elimination phase half life which has been reported to be 19–95 minutes, depending on the means of measurement. Its metabolic clearance rate is between 1800 and 2500 l daily, and does not change during the menstrual cycle. The apparent volume of distribution is 17–29 l.[10] Progesterone is taken up by fat, from which it is slowly released. Circulating progesterone is extensively bound to plasma proteins, especially albumin and corticosteroid-binding globulin. Only small amounts are associated with erythrocytes or platelets. Concentrations in cerebrospinal fluid are about 10% of those in plasma.

Oral absorption	extensive
Presystemic metabolism	~75%[6]
Plasma half life	
distribution	3–6 min
elimination	19–95 min
Volume of distribution	17–29 l
Plasma protein binding	~95–98%

Progesterone undergoes extensive biotransformation, mainly in the liver (approximately 66%) and in tissues such as the kidneys, brain, uterus and skin. The metabolites of progesterone are conjugated in the liver with glucuronic acid and excreted primarily in the urine; between 19 and 40% of a dose of labelled progesterone appears in the urine within 24 h.[11] A smaller quantity (8–17%) is excreted in the faeces, and there is extensive enterohepatic circulation of metabolites.[12]

Concentration–effect relationship

Progesterone concentrations similar to those occurring during the normal luteal phase (10–45 nmol.l^{-1}) are readily achieved after oral administration of 100 mg or more,[5,6] or by parenteral administration.[7–9] Such regimes are therefore capable of reproducing the progestational actions seen during the luteal phase. There is some evidence that the effects of progesterone on the endometrium are dose-dependent; daily oral administration of 300 mg consistently caused a secretory transformation in oestrogen-treated postmenopausal women, whereas lower doses were less effective.[13] Plasma concentrations were not however recorded in this study.

Progesterone

At high concentrations, progesterone has anaesthetic and hypnotic properties; concentrations greater than 127 nmol.l^{-1} have been associated with drowsiness,[14] but this effect has no clinical application. The hypnotic effect of progesterone is dose-dependent.

Metabolism

Progesterone is metabolized, mainly in the liver, by reduction of the A-ring, hydroxylation and conjugation (Fig. 1). The principal metabolite is pregnanediol, which accounts for up to 30% of an injected dose of progesterone.[11] Other metabolites, notably 20α-dihydroprogesterone, which is present in small concentrations in plasma, and 5α-pregnane-3,20-dione, themselves have weak progestational activity. Metabolites of progesterone are mainly excreted in the urine as glucuronide conjugates.

Fig. 1 Major routes of progesterone metabolism

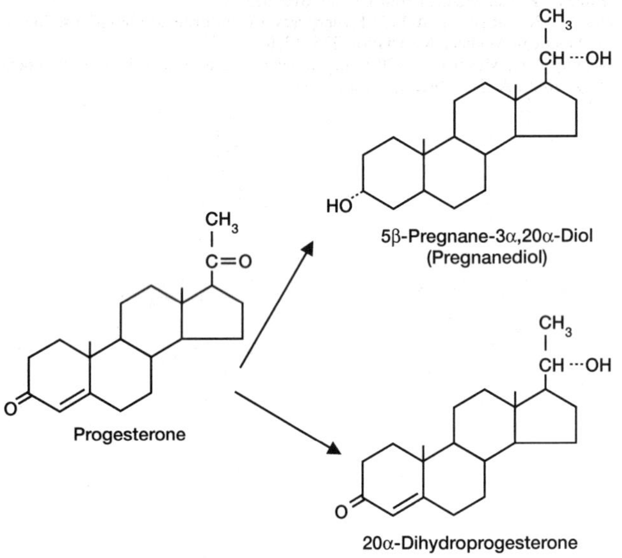

Pharmaceutics

Progesterone is available as a solution for intramuscular injection, in suppository form, and in an intrauterine device.

The solution contains 10, 25 or 50 mg.ml^{-1} in ethyl oleate or another suitable ester, in a fixed oil, or in a combination of these. Alcohols such as benzyl alcohol may be added as preservatives. The solution is sterilized by dry heat (150°C, 1 h). Solid material may separate on standing, and may be redissolved by warming. The solution should be protected from light.

Suppositories are white bullet-shaped cylinders containing 200 or 400 mg progesterone dissolved in inert wax to give a final weight of 1.85 g. They should be protected from warmth and moisture.

Progestasert (Alza, USA) is an intrauterine device containing 38 mg progesterone. It consists of a 36 mm tubular vertical stem with 32 mm horizontal cross-arms. The progesterone is contained in the stem, and released at an average rate of 65 μg daily. This preparation is no longer available outside France and the USA. In the USA it is the only IUD still on the market, due to an apparently high incidence of ectopic pregnancy in users,[15] a problem common to all IUDs.

Progesterone preparations are stable with long shelf-lives (e.g. 2 years for suppositories). There is little risk from potentially allergenic substances.

Therapeutic use

Indications

1. Treatment of dysfunctional uterine bleeding
2. Maintenance of pregnancy in cases of habitual or threatened abortion
3. Treatment of premenstrual syndrome
4. Prophylaxis of postnatal depression.

Contraindications

1. Undiagnosed vaginal bleeding

2. Abnormal liver function; history of idiopathic jaundice in pregnancy
3. Persistence of HCG levels after removal of hydatidiform mole; incomplete abortion
4. Hormone-dependent carcinoma.

Mode of use

The therapeutic uses of progesterone depend mainly upon its progestational, rather than its antioestrogenic, properties. Due to its low oral bioavailability, it is usually administered by intramuscular injection or as suppositories. Dosage depends on the intended use (see below), but is usually 50–100 mg daily when given intramuscularly and 200–400 mg daily when given in suppository form. Since progesterone is absorbed more quickly from suppositories than from an intramuscular injection,[7] it may be necessary to use two or more suppositories each day. Intramuscular injections require sufficient fat tissue to allow formation of a depot, and so are usually given into the buttock. Suppositories may be inserted into either the rectum or the vagina; the same formulation is used in each case. Rectal suppositories should not be used if there is a history of colitis, and vaginal administration should be avoided if there is a history of vaginal infection or recurrent cystitis.

Sudden withdrawal of progesterone will lead to menstrual bleeding.

Indications

1. Dysfunctional uterine bleeding

Dysfunctional uterine bleeding may occur in anovulatory cycles in which progesterone secretion is reduced or absent, or in ovulatory cycles in which no endocrine disturbance is identified.[16,17] A short or insufficient luteal phase may also be associated with menstrual disturbances.[16] Progesterone can be used to induce a withdrawal bleed which will be self-limiting. Doses of 5–10 mg daily are given intramuscularly, starting 5–10 days before the anticipated day of menstruation. The resulting bleeding usually ceases within 1–2 days. Treatment can be repeated at monthly intervals to produce regular cycles.

Although progesterone treatment of dysfunctional uterine bleeding is long established, it has not been subjected to detailed clinical trials. Due to the low oral bioavailability of oral progesterone, orally active progestogens such as norethisterone are now preferred.

Progesterone treatment has been reported to increase the number of pregnancies carried to term in patients with luteal phase insufficiency.[18]

2. Threatened or habitual abortion

Progesterone can be used prophylactically in cases of threatened abortion preceded by symptoms such as hyperemesis. The initial dose is 25–50 mg intramuscularly daily for four days, followed by 10–25 mg twice weekly until the fourth month of pregnancy. This regime maintains progesterone concentrations until adequate amounts are produced by the placenta: the shift from ovarian to placental progesterone synthesis appears to develop around the ninth week.

Progesterone has been used to maintain pregnancy in women with previous histories of spontaneous abortion, accompanied by severe pregnancy symptoms. Doses of 10–20 mg are given intramuscularly twice weekly for the first four months of pregnancy. Treatment should be started as soon as pregnancy has been detected, and before there is any blood loss. The mechanism of action involves development of the endometrium, allowing successful implantation, and hormone replacement until placental progesterone production is established.[19] It should be noted, however, that there is conflicting evidence for a correlation between low progesterone concentrations and habitual abortion;[19,20] evidence for the usefulness of progesterone in preventing habitual abortion is based largely on empirical grounds.

The use of progesterone during pregnancy does not appear to increase the risk of fetal abnormalities.[2,21]

3. Premenstrual syndrome

Progesterone has been widely used in the treatment of the premenstrual syndrome, where symptoms interfere with normal activities or where there is the possibility of domestic stress. Uncontrolled studies suggest that progesterone treatment is highly beneficial.[22] There is, however, a powerful placebo effect, and double-blind crossover studies have yielded conflicting evidence for the efficacy of progesterone.[23,24] Progesterone has been reported to be more effective at relieving some symptoms, such as measures of stress and anxiety, than others such as menstrual headaches.[24]

Treatment should be started before symptoms are expected, and hence an accurate record of previous cycles is necessary. The dose required varies widely between patients. A typical dose is 50–100 mg intramuscularly daily, or 200 or 400 mg once or twice daily by suppository, from the 12th to the 14th day of the cycle (i.e. from the time of ovulation) until menstruation begins. The precise timing of the course depends on the length of the cycle and the duration of symptoms (for details, see the reviews by Norris and Dalton). Once optimal relief has been achieved, treatment is continued for three cycles and the dosage is then gradually reduced. This can be done either by starting the course two days later each month, or by reducing the amount of progesterone and continuing treatment for 14 days. If symptoms recur, the next course should be at the lowest dose compatible with symptomatic relief. Parous or slim women tend to require higher doses, and it may be necessary to increase the dosage after pregnancy.

4. Postnatal depression

Progesterone is used in the prophylaxis of postnatal depression, the aim being to compensate for the sudden fall in progesterone concentrations at delivery, and to restore concentrations to those seen in non-pregnant women. The relationship between changes in progesterone concentrations and mood is however tenuous,[25] and the rationale for progesterone treatment is based largely on empirical grounds.

Injections of 100 mg or 200–400 mg suppositories are given daily for 7 days after delivery. Alternatively, Dalton has recommended initial high doses of 200 mg by injection or 400 mg by suppository every 2 h, the dose being gradually reduced over several days to 100 or 400 mg every 4 h. Psychotropic drugs may also be required.

Progesterone is ineffective against established postnatal depression. It may, however, be used to prevent exacerbation of depression during the first subsequent menstrual cycle. Treatment is given daily until the first menstruation, and then continued as for the premenstrual syndrome.

Contraindications

1. Undiagnosed vaginal bleeding

Irregular menstruation may be due to local pelvic disease rather than to endocrine disturbance,[16] and this possibility must be excluded before commencing progesterone treatment.

2. Acute or chronic liver disease

Progesterone may alter hepatic function, and rare cases of jaundice, similar to that occurring in pregnancy, have been reported.

3. Persistence of HCG after removal of hydatidiform mole

Elevated concentrations of human chorionic gonadotrophin occurring more than a few weeks after removal of a hydatidiform mole may indicate persistence of the tumour. Under these circumstances, progestogens may stimulate mitosis of the trophoblast.[26]

4. Hormone-dependent carcinoma

There is some evidence that progesterone is carcinogenic in animals. Evidence in humans is limited, although it is probably advisable to avoid progesterone administration in the presence of carcinoma. Progesterone has, however, been used with limited success in the treatment of endometrial and cervical cancer.

Adverse reactions

Potentially life-threatening effects

Progesterone appears to have no such effects.

Acute overdosage

Overdose is unlikely since plasma progesterone concentrations occurring during pregnancy are between 20 and 30 times higher than those produced therapeutically. Some women may, however, show symptoms related to high concentrations, such as euphoria, faintness, or uterine cramps.

P

Severe or irreversible adverse effects

Menstrual irregularities may occur. If the cycle is lengthened, progesterone may be stopped at the anticipated time of menstruation, whereupon bleeding should occur within 48 h. In shortened cycles, subsequent courses should be started slightly later. Amenorrhoea may develop with prolonged use, in which case the dosage may be reduced.

Symptomatic adverse effects

Progesterone has been associated with weight gain or loss, and with various skin conditions, such as acne. Intramuscular injections may be painful, and may lead to the formation of sterile abscesses. A generalized urticarial rash has sometimes been observed after progesterone injection; this appears to be a reaction to the solvent rather than to progesterone itself. Anal soreness, diarrhoea and flatulence may occur after rectal administration.

Other effects

Glucose tolerance may be slightly impaired by progesterone treatment, but consequent diabetes is unlikely. Progesterone has antimineralocorticoid activity, and natriuresis and diuresis have been reported to accompany elevated progesterone concentrations.[27] Fluid retention in the premenstrual syndrome has been attributed to progesterone deficiency, or to conversion of progesterone to the mineralocorticoid deoxycorticosterone.[28]

Interference with clinical pathology tests

Progesterone does not appear to interfere in any clinical laboratory test.

High risk groups

Neonates

There are no indications for the use of progesterone in neonates.

Breast milk. Progesterone is excreted into breast milk in low concentrations, which are unlikely to have any effect on the infant.

Children

There are no indications for the use of progesterone in children.

Pregnant women

Progesterone is secreted, initially by the corpus luteum and subsequently by the placenta, in large quantities during pregnancy, plasma concentrations reaching approximately 500 $nmol.l^{-1}$. These physiological concentrations are thus far higher than are achieved therapeutically. Progesterone appears to have no adverse effect on the fetus.[2,21]

The elderly

There are no indications for use in elderly patients.

Drug interactions

Potentially hazardous interactions

No such interactions have been reported.

Other significant interactions

None.

Potentially useful interactions

Progesterone can be given concurrently with synthetic progestogens, for example in women with endometriosis who are receiving norethisterone.

Major outcome trials

1. Dennerstein L, Spencer-Gardner C, Gotts G, Brown J B, Smith M A, Burrows G D 1985 Progesterone and the premenstrual syndrome: a double blind crossover trial. British Medical Journal 290: 1617–1621

This is a double-blind, randomized, crossover study of 23 women who received oral progesterone (300 mg daily) or placebo for 2 months for treatment of premenstrual symptoms, which were evaluated by appropriate questionnaires. Progesterone treatment was associated with significant improvements in measures of stress, anxiety and concentration, and the effects were distinguishable from those of placebo. Adverse effects were slight, the most serious being a single attack of migraine during progesterone treatment. The authors conclude that oral progesterone is effective in alleviating many of the symptoms of the premenstrual syndrome. They do not, however, conclude that progesterone deficiency is the cause of premenstrual syndrome.

Other trials

The use of progesterone in dysfunctional uterine bleeding and habitual abortion is based largely on empirical grounds, and has not been subjected to detailed clinical trials. Similarly, evidence for its efficacy in premenstrual syndrome and postnatal depression comes largely from uncontrolled studies: double-blind controlled studies have usually failed to demonstrate any significant effect. Problems involved in the design of such studies have been discussed by Dalton (see below).

General review articles

Aufrere M B, Benson H 1976 Progesterone: an overview and recent advances. Journal of Pharmaceutical Sciences 65: 783–800

Brenner P F 1982 The pharmacology of progestogens. Journal of Reproductive Medicine 27 (suppl 8): 490–497

Dalton K 1984 The premenstrual syndrome and progesterone therapy 2nd edn. Heinemann, London

Fotherby K 1979 Progesterone II: Clinical aspects. In: Gray C H, James V H T (eds) Hormones in blood, 3rd edn. Academic Press, London, vol 3, ch 9, pp 439–491

Neumann F 1978 The physiological action of progesterone and the pharmacological effects of progestogens — a short review. Postgraduate Medical Journal 54 (suppl 2): 11–24

Norris R V 1983 Progesterone for premenstrual tension. Journal of Reproductive Medicine 28: 509–516

References

1. World Health Organization 1979 International Agency for Research on Cancer Monographs on the Evaluation of the Carcinogenic Risk of Chemicals to Humans. Vol 21 Sex hormones (11). IRAC, Lyon, pp 491–515
2. McDonough P G 1985 Progesterone therapy: benefit versus risk. Fertility and Sterility 44: 13–16
3. Toft D O, O'Malley B W 1972 Target tissue receptors for progesterone: the influence of estrogen treatment. Endocrinology 90: 1041–1045
4. Speroff L, Glass R H, Kase N G 1983 Dysfunctional uterine bleeding. In: Clinical gynecologic endocrinology and infertility, 3rd edn. Williams and Wilkins, Baltimore, ch 8, pp 225–242
5. Kincl F A, Ciaccio L A, Benagino G 1978 Increasing oral bioavailability of progesterone by formulation. Journal of Steroid Biochemistry 9: 83–84
6. Whitehead M I, Townsend P T, Gill D K, Collins W P, Campbell S 1980 Absorption and metabolism of oral progesterone. British Medical Journal 280: 825–827
7. Nillius S J, Johansson E D B 1971 Plasma levels of progesterone after vaginal, rectal or intramuscular administration of progesterone. American Journal of Obstetrics and Gynecology 110: 470–477
8. Villaneuva B, Casper R F, Yen S S C 1981 Intravaginal administration of progesterone: enhanced absorption after estrogen treatment. Fertility and Sterility 35: 433–437
9. Glazener C M A, Bailey I, Hull M G R 1985 Effectiveness of vaginal administration of progesterone. British Journal of Obstetrics and Gynaecology 92: 364–368
10. Tait J F, Burstein S 1964 In vivo studies of steroid dynamics in man. In: Pincus G, Thimann K V, Astwood E B (eds) The hormones. Academic Press, New York, vol 5, ch 4, pp 441–557
11. Collins W P, Koullapis E N, Sommerville I N 1971 The effect of chlormadinone acetate on progesterone secretion and metabolism. Acta Endocrinologica 68: 271–284
12. Sandberg A A, Slaunwhite W R 1958 The metabolic fate of ^{14}C-progesterone in human subjects. Journal of Clinical Endocrinology 18: 253–265
13. Lane G, Siddle N C, Ryder T A, Pryse-Davies J, King R J B, Whitehead M I 1983 Dose dependent effects of oral progesterone on the oestrogenized postmenopausal endometrium. British Medical Journal 287: 1241–1245
14. de Lignieres B, Vincens M 1982 Differential effects of exogenous oestradiol and progesterone on mood in postmenopausal women: individual dose/effect relationship. Maturitas 4: 67–72
15. Anonymous 1982 Intrauterine devices now. Drug and Therapeutics Bulletin 20: 69–72
16. Baird D T, Abel M H, Kelly R W, Smith S K 1981 Endocrinology of dysfunctional uterine bleeding: the role of endometrial prostaglandins. In: Crosignani P G, Rubin B L (eds) Endocrinology of human infertility: new aspects. Academic Press, London, pp 399–417
17. Smith S K 1985 Dysfunctional uterine bleeding. British Journal of Hospital Medicine 34: 351–354
18. Wentz A C, Herbert C M, Maxson W S, Garner C H 1984 Outcome of progesterone treatment of luteal phase inadequacy. Fertility and Sterility 41: 856–862
19. DeCherney A, Polan M L 1984 Evaluation and management of habitual abortion. British Journal of Hospital Medicine 31: 261–268
20. Glass R H, Golbus M S 1978 Habitual abortion. Fertility and Sterility 29: 257–265

21. Dalton K 1981 The effect of progesterone and progestogens on the foetus. Neuropharmacology 20: 1267–1269
22. Greene R, Dalton K 1953 The premenstrual syndrome. British Medical Journal 1: 1007–1014
23. Sampson G A 1979 Premenstrual syndrome: a double-blind controlled trial of progesterone and placebo. British Journal of Psychiatry 135: 209–215
24. Dennerstein L, Spencer-Gardner C, Gotts G, Brown J B, Smith M A, Burrows G D 1985 Progesterone and the premenstrual syndrome: a double blind crossover trial. British Medical Journal 290: 1617–1621
25. Nott P N, Franklin M, Armitage C, Gelder M G 1976 Hormonal changes and mood in the puerperium. British Journal of Psychiatry 128: 379–383
26. Begent R H J, Bagshawe K D 1983 Treatment of advanced trophoblastic disease. In: Griffiths C T, Fullar A F (eds) Gynecologic oncology. Martinus Nijhoff, Boston, ch 5, pp 155–186
27. O'Brien P M S, Selby C, Symonds E M 1980 Progesterone, fluid, and electrolytes in premenstrual syndrome. British Medical Journal 280: 1161–1163
28. Ottosson U-B 1984 Oral progesterone and estrogen/progestogen therapy. Acta Obstetricia et Gynecologica Scandinavica 127 (suppl): 1–37

Proguanil (hydrochloride)

Proguanil is a prodrug that is used for malaria prophylaxis and acts through its main metabolite, cycloguanil.

Chemistry

Proguanil hydrochloride (chlorguanide hydrochloride, proguanide hydrochloride, Balusil, Biguanide, Biguanil, Bigumal, Chlorguanide, Diguanyl, Paludrine, Palusil, Proguanide, Tiriam, WR 3091)

$C_{11}H_{16}ClN_5.HCl$

1-(4-Chlorophenyl)-5-isopropylbiguanide hydrochloride

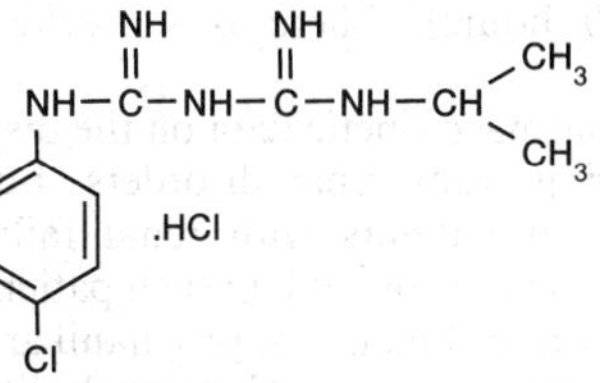

Molecular weight (free base)	290.2 (253.7)
pKa (biguanide group)	2.3; 10.4
Solubility	
in alcohol	1 in 40
in water	1 in 110
Octanol/water partition coefficient	—

A white crystalline bitter tasting powder. Proguanil is prepared by chemical synthesis. In general the hydrochloride salt is employed for malaria prophylaxis. There is also a lactate formulation (Chloriguane).

Pharmacology

Proguanil itself is a weak inhibitor of plasmodial dihydrofolate reductase, but its main metabolite, cycloguanil, is a strong inhibitor of the same enzyme. The affinity to mammalian dihydrofolate reductase of both proguanil and cycloguanil is relatively low, approximately 10^{-3}–10^{-2} of that to the parasite's enzyme. The main metabolite, cycloguanil, usually becomes detectable within 2 hours of the ingestion of proguanil. Its antiplasmodial activity is ascribed to the inhibition of plasmodial dihydrofolate reductase, especially in the late trophozoite phase and during early schizont formation, of both pre-erythrocytic and intra-erythrocytic parasites. Proguanil has no other known pharmacological properties except for an effect in rabbits to decrease the specific effect of heparin on coagulation processes.[5]

Toxicology

Proguanil is one of the safest antimalarial drugs. In experimental animals oral dosing was generally three to fivefold less toxic than intramuscular or intraperitoneal administration. Protracted administration of high oral doses in rats, mice, dogs and monkeys caused reversible gastrointestinal effects.[2] There is no evidence of mutagenic, embryotoxic or teratogenic effects at clinically relevant dose levels.[3] In man the toxicity of proguanil at the usual prophylactic doses is low.

Clinical pharmacology

In the absence of disorders interfering with their elimination, neither proguanil nor its main metabolite, cycloguanil, are known to exert major pharmacological activity on neural, cardiovascular, metabolic or endocrine function in man.

While proguanil does not interfere with human lymphocyte proliferation, its active metabolite, cycloguanil, was found to reduce or block endogenous thymidine incorporation in stimulated human lymphocytes in vitro. At the concentration achieved in normal malaria prophylaxis, cycloguanil decreased the number of mitogen- and antigen-stimulated cells. Cycloguanil concentrations corresponding to the intralymphocytic levels achieved in clinical practice permanently suppressed the growth of lymphocytes, but the effect could be reversed by low concentrations of folic acid.[4]

Pharmacokinetics

The preferred analytical method for proguanil and its main metabolite cycloguanil is high-performance liquid chromatographic (HPLC) assay with UV detection,[6] preceded by solid phase extraction.[7] This method has a detection limit of 5 μg.l^{-1}.

In the absence of a formulation for intravenous administration, there is no way of measuring absolute bioavailability of oral proguanil, but it is readily absorbed, becoming detectable within 15 minutes of ingestion. Following the administration of 100 or 200 mg proguanil hydrochloride peak plasma concentrations were reached within 2–4 hours (mean 2.88 ± 0.72 hours) in fasting adult subjects.[7] The plasma half life of proguanil varied between 11.8 and 23.4 hours (mean 16.5 ± 3.50 hours). There is no evidence of pre-systemic metabolism.

There are no pharmacokinetic data on the disposition of proguanil in persons suffering from renal disorders, but the occurrence of adverse reactions in patients with renal failure[11,12] points to a disturbed elimination of proguanil in such patients. Data on the effect of hepatic disease on the kinetics of proguanil are not available, but it is likely that conversion to the active metabolite will be impaired in such patients.

For malaria prophylaxis, proguanil is commonly administered on a daily (24-hourly) basis, using an adult dose of 100 mg or 200 mg of the hydrochloride salt. With 100 mg daily, steady state is reached within 4 days; with 200 mg daily it is reached one day earlier. The steady state mean peak concentration was 647 ± 73 nmol.l^{-1}, and the mean trough concentration 228 ± 25 nmol.l^{-1} with the 100 mg regimen. The corresponding values for the 200 mg regimen were 1258 ± 130 nmol.l^{-1} for the mean peak concentration and 354 ± 53 nmol.l^{-1} for the mean trough concentration.[13] Thus the peak/trough ratios were 2.84 for the 100 mg and 3.56 for the 200 mg regimen.

Proguanil is a prodrug that is metabolically transformed to the active compound cycloguanil, a triazine. Only a part of proguanil is converted to cycloguanil. After normalizing for differences in molecular weight, and accounting for biotransformation, a comparison of the area under the concentration–time curve (AUC) shows that the bioavailability of cycloguanil is about 19% that of proguanil.[7]

Table B

Oral absorption	>90%
Presystemic metabolism	negligible
Plasma half-life	
range	11.8–23.4 h
mean	16.5 h
Volume of distribution	—
Plasma protein binding	75%

Cycloguanil usually becomes detectable 2 hours after the administration of proguanil, reaching peak concentration within 4–9 hours (mean 6.2 ± 1.5). There is important individual variation in the extent to which cycloguanil is formed. Recent evidence suggests that this reaction is catalysed by the same isoenzyme of P450 that is responsible for the genetic polymorphism in mephenytoin oxidation, a member of the P450 IIC sub-family. The mean half life of cycloguanil formation is 3.6 ± 2.3 hours, and half life of elimination is relatively short (mean 2.1 ± 0.7 hours). The cycloguanil concentrations will thus rarely, if ever, exceed those of the parent compound.[7]

Cycloguanil	
Mean metabolic conversion	
from proguanil	19.2%
Half life of formation	1.4–8.4 h
(t 1/2 form)	mean 3.6 h
Half life of elimination	1.3–3.3 h
	mean 2.1 h

Steady state for cycloguanil is usually reached within 4 days from the start of daily administration of 100 mg or 200 mg proguanil hydrochloride. With the 100 mg regimen the mean peak concentration of cycloguanil was 186 ± 30 nmol.l^{-1}, the mean trough level 115 ± 22 nmol.l^{-1}, and the peak/trough ratio 1.62. The 200 mg regimen yielded a cycloguanil mean peak level of 293 ± 45 nmol.l^{-1}, a mean trough concentration of 142 ± 37 nmol.l^{-1} and a peak/trough ratio of 2.07.[13] Since the cycloguanil trough concentration is likely to determine the prophylactic activity and reliability of proguanil, it appears that only modest advantage is derived from doubling the daily dose. However, 12-hourly dosing with 100 mg proguanil produced smoother profiles of proguanil and cycloguanil and consistently higher trough levels of both. The steady state mean peak concentration of proguanil was 1202 ± 132 nmol.l^{-1}, the mean trough level 650 ± 58 nmol.l^{-1}, and the peak/trough ratio 1.85. The cycloguanil mean concentrations were 317 ± 44 nmol.l^{-1} for the peak and 231 ± 35 nmol.l^{-1} for the trough; the peak trough ratio was 1.37.[13]

Concentration–effect relationship

As with all antimalarial drugs, there is a marked concentration–effect relationship. With proguanil, however, this relates essentially to the active metabolite, cycloguanil. Malaria parasite populations are usually a mixture of individuals with different degrees of sensitivity to a specific drug. A prophylactic compound should be present at a concentration that either prevents pre-erythrocytic development of the parasite in the hepatocyte, or suppresses intra-erythrocytic schizogony. Both mechanisms are believed to apply to proguanil/cycloguanil, whereas 4-aminoquinoline and 4-quinoline methanol compounds only possess blood schizontocidal activity. If the drug does not reach the minimum inhibitory concentration (MIC) which for sensitive *P. falciparum* is usually in the range of 50–200 nmol cycloguanil per litre or if it is not maintained above this level, prophylaxis is likely to fail. The parasites emanating after such failure usually have low drug sensitivity. In the presence of overt resistance it may not be feasible to attain and maintain prophylactically effective drug concentrations.

Metabolism

Proguanil is only partially metabolized; some 60% is excreted in the unchanged form, almost entirely in the urine. The two main metabol-

Fig. 1 The metabolism of proguanil

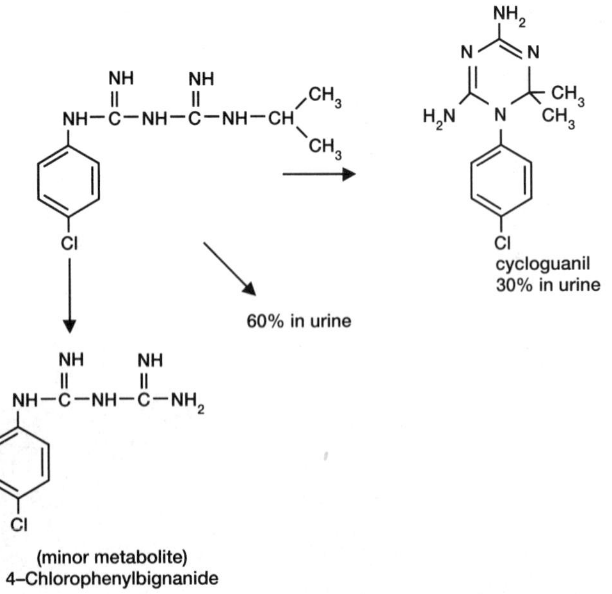

Proguanil (hydrochloride)

ites are cycloguanil, the active principle, and 4-chlorophenyl-biguanide, the antimalarial activity of which has not yet been determined but is likely to be low (Fig. 1). 4-chlorophenyl biguanide appears later than cycloguanil. It also reaches peak concentration later, but the steady state concentrations remain only slightly below those of cycloguanil.[8]

Cycloguanil is formed from proguanil by the conversion of the biguanide moiety into a triazine ring, while 4-chlorophenyl biguanide is produced by oxidation at the end of the biguanide moiety. Apart from the antimalarial effect of cycloguanil, the two metabolites are not known to exert pharmacological effects at the observed concentration levels.

In vitro studies indicate that cycloguanil is formed by a form of hepatic cytochrome P450 which is a member of the P450IIC subfamily. The precise chemical mechanism involved in the oxidative cyclization reaction remains to be established.

Metabolism of proguanil is subject to wide individual variation. There are persons who do not show any transformation of proguanil to cycloguanil.[7] Studies have shown that in persons who did produce cycloguanil the peak concentrations following an oral dose of 200 mg proguanil hydrochloride varied between 144.6 and 512.5 nmol.l^{-1}, and the AUC for cycloguanil was 0.9774–5.5542 nmol.ml^{-1}.h^{-1}. Proguanil will obviously fail to protect poor metabolizers and non-metabolizers from malaria.

Proguanil is metabolized in hepatocytes. Since hepatocytes are also the site of pre-erythrocytic schizogony it is plausible that cycloguanil may exert its greatest activity in this environment, especially against relatively young pre-erythrocytic schizonts located in hepatocytes which have not yet suffered functional damage.

Pharmaceutics

Proguanil is available in the form of tablets for oral administration. Each tablet contains 100 mg proguanil hydrochloride. The ICI brand, Paludrine (UK), is formulated in the form of white, round, flat cross-scored tablets.

The preparation should be protected from light. It has a reasonably long shelf-life and carries a minimum risk from potentially allergenic impurities or decomposition products. Generic preparations may vary in these respects.

Therapeutic use

Indications

1. Short- and long-term prophylaxis of falciparum malaria and associated malaria species
2. Long-term prophylaxis of vivax malaria.

Contraindications

1. Renal failure/impairment
2. Known resistance of local *Plasmodium* species to proguanil.

Mode of use

The use of proguanil depends on the antimalarial activity of its main metabolite, cycloguanil. This activity is directed against plasmodial dihydrofolate reductase in the pre-erythrocytic and intra-erythrocytic forms. In order to be effective, adequate cycloguanil concentrations should be established before the first exposure to infection and maintained throughout the period of exposure and for four weeks after cessation of the risk of infection in order also to eliminate any residual blood forms. The whole period of exposure and the subsequent four weeks should thus be covered by a steady state of adequate cycloguanil concentrations. This is achieved by the daily administration of an adult dose of 200 mg proguanil hydrochloride corresponding to approximately 3 mg.kg^{-1} body weight or, better, by the twice daily (roughly 12-hourly) administration of 100 mg proguanil hydrochloride; the latter will ensure higher cycloguanil trough concentrations and safeguard against a drop below the MIC. The drug administration should start one week before the first exposure to malaria risk in order to ensure steady state in the large majority of individuals.

Doses for lower age groups are as follows:

Under 1 year (3–10 kg): $\frac{1}{4}$ tablet (25 mg) daily
1–4 years (11–16 kg): $\frac{1}{2}$ tablet (50 mg) daily or $\frac{1}{4}$ tablet (25 mg) 12-hourly
5–8 years (17–27 kg): 1 tablet (100 mg) daily or $\frac{1}{2}$ tablet (50 mg) 12-hourly
9–14 years (28–50 kg): $1\frac{1}{2}$ tablets (150 mg) daily or $\frac{3}{4}$ tablet (75 mg) 12-hourly

Although the drug is well tolerated, even on an empty stomach, it is preferable always to give it with the same meal(s) in order to establish a reliable routine. When a twice-daily scheme is followed, the medicament should be taken with breakfast and dinner.

Failures of regular chemoprophylaxis with the above mentioned doses of proguanil may occur if the malaria parasites are resistant to cycloguanil, if prophylaxis has been started too late or discontinued too early, or if metabolic conversion of proguanil to cycloguanil is inadequate. Some individuals are poor metabolizers; a few fail to produce cycloguanil altogether[7] in spite of otherwise normal hepatic function. There is no simple test procedure for checking cycloguanil concentrations in blood or urine, or to screen for metabolizer state.

After withdrawing proguanil at the end of the scheduled period of prophylaxis, attention should be paid to eventual recrudescences of falciparum or quartan malaria and relapses of vivax or ovale malaria.

Indications

1. Short- and long-term prophylaxis of falciparum malaria and associated malaria species

The prophylactic activity of proguanil is due to its main metabolite, cycloguanil. The effect is primarily directed against the pre-erythrocytic intrahepatocytic forms of *Plasmodium falciparum*, thus preventing blood infection. Cycloguanil also possesses activity against the asexual intra-erythrocytic forms of all species of human malaria parasites. This may serve as a backup in the case of incomplete action against pre-erythrocytic schizogony.

In its early days, proguanil has also been used for treating falciparum malaria,[14] but the clinical response was slow. Therapeutically the drug did not offer advantages over other antimalarial compounds, which were easier to use and faster acting.

With the advent and the wide spread of chloroquine resistance in *Plasmodium falciparum*, proguanil has regained its importance for short-term prophylaxis, the more so as reports from East Africa suggested that the drug has maintained its efficacy when daily adult doses of 200 mg are administered.[15] Earlier reports of resistance to cycloguanil and breakthrough of infection under proguanil prophylaxis may be ascribed in part to a less than adequate drug regimen, e.g. 100 mg daily.

There is no doubt that cycloguanil resistance of *P. falciparum* exists in parts of the species' geographical distribution, especially in south-eastern Asia and adjacent islands;[16–18] however, on the whole, the drug has maintained a reasonably high level of efficacy when it is used in keeping with pharmacokinetic principles. The prophylactic effect also extends to other species of human malaria parasites.

Proguanil is the only drug that can be used for long-term prophylaxis exceeding 6 years since chloroquine, the only other compound suitable for medium-term prophylaxis, should be discontinued after a cumulative dose of 100 g base, an amount usually reached within 6 years.

For short-term prophylaxis in areas with considerable exposure to falciparum malaria, the use of proguanil (200 mg hydrochloride daily) and chloroquine (5 mg base per kg body weight weekly) in parallel has been suggested.[19] While this may be acceptable for the short term, it would not be wise to extend such a regimen beyond 6 months in the absence of careful, specific drug interaction studies.

Although combinations of proguanil or cycloguanil with dihydropteroate synthetase inhibitors, such as sulphonamides and sulphones, have yielded experimental evidence of synergism[20] and satisfactory results in groups exposed to high malaria risk,[21] their use cannot be recommended as long as there is no detailed toxicological documentation. However, such combinations hold considerable promise for the future.

2. Long-term prophylaxis of vivax malaria

In areas where *Plasmodium vivax* is the only, or the highly predominant, malaria parasite species, such as in many areas of western and central southern Asia, central and South America, chloroquine is usually employed for short- and medium-term prophylaxis. Proguanil is suitable for long-term prophylaxis, but its use may also be envisaged for the short and medium term if local *P. vivax* is sensitive to cycloguanil and chloroquine-resistant *P. falciparum* occurs in the same area. Experimental evidence obtained with a species closely related to *P. vivax* suggests that proguanil also acts against the pre-erythrocytic schizonts of *P. vivax*.[22] However, it has no effect on the dormant intrahepatocytic hypnozoite forms which are responsible for relapses. If there was substantial exposure to infection, such relapses are likely to occur some time after the cessation of prophylaxis, as with any other type of chemoprophylaxis. These relapses, the first manifesting as a primary attack, require radical treatment with chloroquine and primaquine.

Contraindications

1. Renal impairment/failure

Megaloblastic anaemia and pancytopenia due to proguanil were reported in two patients with chronic renal failure.[12] In these patients, the serum proguanil concentrations were grossly elevated on account of reduced renal elimination. The haematological manifestations were obviously caused by the inhibition of the hosts' dihydrofolate reductase. Patients requiring haemodialysis are usually unfit for travel to the tropics; conditions of marginal compensation require special attention, as chemoprophylaxis with any drug and, even more so, treatment in the event of an infection may result in major adverse events.

2. Known resistance of local *Plasmodium* species to proguanil

Cycloguanil resistance of local malaria parasites is a contraindication to the use of proguanil. This contraindication is relative if the occurrence of resistance is limited, but obviously becomes absolute if the majority of the parasite population is resistant. The decision for or against the use of proguanil for chemoprophylaxis in a given area should be based on practical experience and not on in vitro tests, since these reflect only the response of the erythrocytic forms, not the activity against the pre-erythrocytic parasites.

Adverse reactions

Potentially life-threatening effects

There is no record of a fatal adverse reaction caused by proguanil or cycloguanil. Potentially life-threatening adverse reactions affecting the haemopoietic system may arise in persons with impeded elimination of proguanil and/or cycloguanil, e.g. patients suffering from serious renal impairment.[12]

Acute overdosage

There is no record of fatal poisoning with proguanil. The highest overdose on record (14.5 g, corresponding to approximately 70 times the daily prophylactic dose) was followed by complete recovery.[23] Gross overdosage gives rise to abdominal pain, vomiting, diarrhoea and haematuria. There is no specific antidote and symptoms should be treated as they arise.[24]

Severe or irreversible adverse effects

All adverse reactions so far observed with proguanil have been totally reversible. With the exception of the above-mentioned haematological disturbances in persons with renal impairment, normal prophylactic doses do not cause severe adverse reactions.

Symptomatic adverse effects

Proguanil is probably the best-tolerated antimalarial drug. The only (and rare) adverse effects observed in healthy individuals taking normal prophylactic doses are mouth ulcers and stomatitis,[25–27] together with mild epigastric discomfort. Mild skin reactions and hair loss have also been reported, but their occurrence is not substantiated and may be due to climatic factors rather than the drug. The mechanism underlying the formation of mouth ulcers and stomatitis is not known.

Other effects

Folate-deficient persons may be susceptible to an aggravation of such deficiency while under malaria prophylaxis with proguanil. This type of deficiency occurs especially during pregnancy and may be aggravated by a temporary reduction of drug elimination. This may be prevented by a replenishment of the folate stores.

Interference with clinical pathology tests

Proguanil and its main metabolites are not known to interfere with clinical chemical and haematological tests. They may, however, disturb the performance of blood and urine cultures of bacteria and distort the results of drug sensitivity tests with *P. falciparum*.

High risk groups

Neonates

There is no contraindication to the use of proguanil in infants with normal renal function (for dosage see Mode of use). Malaria chemoprophylaxis will usually be restricted to infants born to non-immune mothers temporarily residing in malarious areas. Indigenous infants with the prospect of permanent residence in malarious areas will only exceptionally be put under malaria chemoprophylaxis, since compliance is generally poor and the clinical impact of malaria only delayed, not averted. Exceptions are infants with diseases or pathological conditions warranting intensive protection against malaria. In these cases it should be ascertained whether the underlying condition interferes with drug tolerance.

Breast milk. Proguanil and cycloguanil are excreted in the breast milk of nursing mothers in concentrations similar to those in plasma. This is not adequate to ensure reliable protection of the infant.

Children

There is no contraindication to the use of proguanil for malaria prophylaxis in children with normal renal function (for dosages see above). For indications and limitations see Neonates.

Pregnant women

Since its introduction, proguanil has been used for malaria prophylaxis in pregnant women. There has been not a single untoward effect or teratogenic event in which proguanil could be incriminated as a cause. Proguanil has therefore to be considered as the safest malaria prophylactic drug in pregnancy. As a precaution, pregnant women with folate deficiency should receive a replenishment of their folate stores at monthly intervals.

Malaria prophylaxis is indicated not only in non-immune pregnant women exposed to malaria risk but also in indigenous primiparae and secundiparae, especially during the second and third trimester of pregnancy and for approximately four weeks after delivery. Compliance is usually satisfactory in this group.

The elderly

No special precautions are required apart from screening for renal impairment.

Drug interactions

Potentially hazardous interactions

Hazardous interactions of proguanil with other drugs are not known. In the absence of information on the influence of potentiating agents such as sulphonamides and sulphonylureas, it would be prudent to monitor for eventual haematological/haemopoietic disturbances when proguanil is used concurrently with dihydropteroate synthetase inhibitors.

Other significant interactions

Smoking. There are no studies on the influence of smoking on the tolerance of proguanil nor ad hoc observations suggesting any such influence. However, by analogy to other drugs, it is conceivable that smoking may enhance the production of the active metabolite cycloguanil.

Potentially useful interactions

None has been reported.

Major outcome trials

Recent

1. Nevill C G, Watkins W M, Carter J Y, Munafu C G 1988 Comparison of mosquito nets, proguanil hydrochloride, and placebo to prevent malaria. British Medical Journal 297: 401–403

This was a prospective study involving 190 students aged 6 to 18 years at a boarding school 120 km west of Nairobi, Kenya. After treatment for the elimination of pre-existing infections the students were divided into three groups. One group slept under mosquito nets, one group received proguanil hydrochloride daily (100 mg or 200 mg according to weight), and the third group received matching placebo tablets daily (1 or 2 tablets). Malaria infections occurring during the trial were treated with sulphadoxine/pyrimethamine. The study extended over one school term, 188 students completed the observation. One infection was found in the mosquito net group (3893 follow-up days), eight infections occurred under proguanil (3667 follow-up days) and 35 in the placebo group (3677 follow-up days). It was concluded that both the use of mosquito nets and chemoprophylaxis with proguanil provide effective protection from malaria.

2. Fogh S, Schapira A, Bygbjerg I C et al 1988 Malaria chemoprophylaxis in travellers to East Africa: a comparative prospective study of chloroquine plus proguanil with chloroquine plus sulfadoxine–pyrimethamine. British Medical Journal 296: 820–822

In a prospective study involving 767 adult Scandinavian travellers to Kenya and Tanzania (i.e. areas with chloroquine resistant *P. falciparum*) 384 persons were given chloroquine phosphate weekly (300 mg base) and proguanil hydrochloride 200 mg daily. The other group of 383 persons followed the same chloroquine regimen and received in addition 500 mg sulphadoxine plus 25 mg pyrimethamine weekly. Malaria occurred in four persons of the chloroquine/proguanil group, and in three members of the chloroquine/sulphadoxine/pyrimethamine group. None of the infections manifested itself earlier than 7 weeks after first exposure. Side effects were observed in 36 subjects of the chloroquine/proguanil group, and in 55 subjects of the chloroquine/sulphadoxine/pyrimethamine group ($P = 0.043$). It was concluded that both regimens are probably equally effective, but the chloroquine/proguanil regimen was recommended for routine prophylaxis on account of a lesser incidence of side effects.

3. Limsomwong N, Pang L W, Singharaj P 1988 Malaria prophylaxis with proguanil in children living in a malaria-endemic area. American Journal of Tropical Medicine and Hygiene 38: 231–236

In an area with almost universal and high resistance of *P. falciparum* to chloroquine and sulphadoxine/pyrimethamine, 170 children were given either daily prophylaxis with proguanil corresponding to a daily adult dose of 200 mg (85 children) or weekly prophylaxis with chloroquine with 5 mg base per kg body weight (85 children). Blood samples were examined weekly. In the proguanil group (524 human-weeks) 17 infections occurred with *P. falciparum* and 11 with *P. vivax*, as compared to 24 *P. falciparum* infections and 1 *P. vivax* infection in the chloroquine group (537 human-weeks). It was concluded that proguanil may have some causal prophylactic action against local *P. falciparum*, but against *P. vivax* it was significantly less effective than chloroquine. Side effects were infrequent, mild and comparable in both groups.

References

1. Tester Dalderup C B M 1984 Antiprotozoal drugs. In: Dukes (ed) Meyler's side effects of drugs, 10th edn. Elsevier Science Publishers, Amsterdam, pp 525–537
2. Ferone R 1984 Dihydrofolate reductase inhibitors. In: Peters W, Richards W H G (eds) Antimalarial drugs II. Current antimalarials and new drug developments. Springer-Verlag, Berlin
3. Chebotar N A 1974 Embryotoxic and teratogenic action of proguanil, chlorproguanil, and cycloguanil on albino rats. Bulletin of Experimental Biology and Medicine 77: 646
4. Bygbjerg I C 1985 Effect of proguanil and cycloguanil on human lymphocytes in vitro. European Journal of Clinical Pharmacology 28: 287–290
5. Kremneva V F, Ushkalova E A, Shcheglova N V 1986 Influence of bigumal on the blood coagulation system and on the anticoagulant effect of heparin. Farmakologija i Toksikologija 49: 43–45 (in Russian)
6. Bygbjerg I C, Flachs H 1986 Effect of oral proguanil on human lymphocyte proliferation. European Journal of Clinical Pharmacology 30: 249–251
7. Jamaludin A, Mohamad M, Navaratnam V, Tan S C, Yeoh P Y, Wernsdorfer W H 1990 Single and multiple dose pharmacokinetics of proguanil and its principal metabolite cycloguanil. (in print)
8. Bygbjerg I, Ravn P, Rønn A, Flachs H, Hvidberg E F 1987 Human pharmacokinetics of proguanil and its metabolites. Tropical Medicine and Parasitology 38: 77–80
9. Armstrong V L, Smith C C 1974 Cyclisation and N-dealkylation of chlorguanide by rabbit and rat hepatic microsomes. Toxicology and Applied Pharmacology 29: 90
10. Moffat A C, Jackson J V, Moss M S, Widdop B, Greenfield E S (eds) 1986 Clarke's isolation and identification of drugs, 2nd edn. The Pharmaceutical Press, London

Proguanil (hydrochloride)

11. Tattersall J E, Greenwood R N, Baker L R, Cattel W R 1987 Proguanil poisoning in a haemodialysis patient. Clinical Nephrology 28: 104
12. Boots M, Phillips M, Curtis J R 1982 Megaloblastic anaemia and pancytopenia due to proguanil in patients with chronic renal failure. Clinical Nephrology 18: 106–108
13. Jamaludin A, Mohamad M, Navaratnam V, Yeoh P Y, Wernsdorfer W H 1990 Multiple-dose pharmacokinetic study of proguanil and cycloguanil following 12-hourly administration of proguanil hydrochloride (100 mg). Tropical Medicine and Parasitology 41: (in print)
14. Bruce-Chwatt L J, Black R H, Canfield C J, Clyde D F, Peters W, Wernsdorfer W H 1986 Chemotherapy of malaria. WHO Monograph Series no 27. World Health Organization, Geneva, pp 72–73
15. McLarty D G, Webber R H, Jaatinen M et al 1984 Chemoprophylaxis of malaria in non-immune residents in Dar es Salaam, Tanzania. Lancet 2: 656–659
16. Edeson J F B, Field J W 1950 Proguanil-resistant falciparum malaria in Malaya. British Medical Journal 1: 147–151
17. Wilson T, Munro D S, Richard D R 1952 Proguanil-resistance in Malayan strains of Plasmodium vivax. British Medical Journal 1: 564–568
18. Henderson A, Simon J W, Melia W 1986 Failure of malaria chemoprophylaxis with a proguanil-chloroquine combination in Papua New Guinea. Transactions of the Royal Society of Tropical Medicine and Hygiene 80: 838–840
19. World Health Organization 1990 International travel and health. Vaccination requirements and health advice. World Health Organization, Geneva
20. Black R H, Ray A P 1977 Experimental studies of the potentiation of proguanil and pyrimethamine by dapsone using Plasmodium berghei in white mice. Annals of Tropical Medicine and Parasitology 71: 131–139
21. Black R H 1973 Malaria in the Australian army in South Vietnam: successful use of a proguanil-dapsone combination for chemoprophylaxis of chloroquine-resistant falciparum malaria. Medical Journal of Australia 1: 1265–1270
22. Jiang J B, Bray R S, Krotowski W A et al 1988 Transactions of the Royal Society of Tropical Medicine and Hygiene 82: 56–58
23. Rollo I M 1980 Drugs used in the chemotherapy of malaria. In: Goodman, Gilman (eds) The pharmacological basis of therapeutics, 6th edn. Macmillan, New York, p 1044
24. World Health Organization 1988 Proguanil. WHO Drug Information 2: 92
25. Mulley G 1974 Letter: proguanil and mouth ulcers. Lancet 2: 873
26. Davidson N M 1986 Mouth ulceration associated with proguanil. Lancet 1: 384
27. Daniels A M 1986 Mouth ulceration associated with proguanil. Lancet 1: 269

P

Promazine (hydrochloride)

Promazine is a phenothiazine of the aliphatic subgroup. The major clinical use of this drug relates to its central antihallucinatory and calming activity.

Chemistry

Promazine hydrochloride (Sparine, Prazine, Protactyl, Talofen)
$C_{17}H_{20}N_2S.HCl$
10-(3-Dimethylaminopropyl)phenothiazine hydrochloride

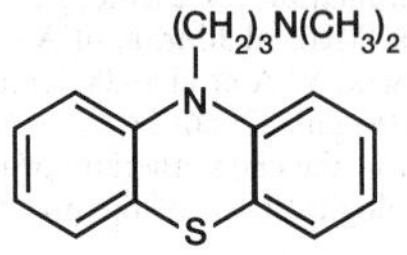

Molecular weight (free base)	320.9 (284.4)
pKa	9.4
Solubility	
in alcohol	1 in 2
in water	1 in 2
Octanol/water partition coefficient	320

Aqueous solutions are slightly acidic. Promazine hydrochloride is a white to yellowish, slightly hygroscopic crystalline powder. It is affected by air, light and heavy metals, decomposing to a blue or pink compound. Promazine is prepared by chemical synthesis. It is not present in any compound preparations.

Pharmacology

Promazine is a phenothiazine with a propylamine side-chain. In common with other phenothiazines it has a wide range of pharmacological properties. Promazine is an antagonist at dopamine (D_2) receptors, although of relatively low potency.[1,2] The Ki for promazine-mediated inhibition of dopamine-stimulated increase in adenosine cyclic 3′,5′-monophosphate in rat neostriatum and limbic forebrain was 6×10^{-5} M while the Ki for chlorpromazine was 1×10^{-6} M and for trifluoperazine it was 4×10^{-7} M.[3] Phenothiazines can adopt a conformation that mimics dopamine.[4] Promazine has considerable α_1-adrenoceptor blocking activity and this may lead to postural hypotension and tachycardia. This action may contribute to the sedative effects of the drug. Promazine, like chlorpromazine, has antimuscarinic and antiserotoninergic actions but these are weaker than with chlorpromazine.[5]

Promazine shows weak blockade of noradrenaline reuptake and open channel block of NMDA receptors.[6,7] It is a weak antagonist of monoamineoxidase with a Ki against platelet MAO of 124 μM. [8] The drug, in common with other phenothiazines, is also a calmodulin antagonist.[9]

The main pharmacological activity is that of a tranquillizer and sedative and the drug has been used extensively as a component of tranquillizer darts used to immobilize wild animals (see review by Jones). The drug passes readily across the placenta and causes sedation in the newborn.[10,11]

Toxicology

Little specific information is available regarding the toxicological profile of promazine. When promazine was given as a dietary mixture to rats at a dose level of approximately 400 $mg.kg^{-1}$ or to dogs at a level of 800 mg orally daily for a period not greater than 12 months, no outstanding adverse effects were seen.

The most profound effects of neuroleptic agents on reproductive studies result from their effects on the endocrine system. Most of the phenothiazine derivatives produce a delay in oestrus in treated rats and mice as a result of the production of a permanent dioestrus: this marked decrease in conception rate is thought to be related to an effect on the hypothalamic–pituitary axis. This effect was also observed when the neuroleptic agent was given to pregnant animals during gestation, producing a prolongation of the gestation period consequent on delayed parturition. The delay in parturition is, in turn, due to a delay in implantation of the fertilized ovum. Other effects resulting from the administration of neuroleptic agents to pregnant rats, mice or rabbits include a decreased litter size, increased number of resorptions, increased number of still-births and increased neonatal mortality. However, these effects are produced at doses which are many times in excess of the recommended clinical dose. No evidence of teratogenesis has been observed in many studies performed with various phenothiazines in the mouse, rabbit or rat.

The only report of a carcinogenicity study pertaining to a neuroleptic agent involves chlorpromazine in which it was given at a dose level of 5 $mg.kg^{-1}$ orally every 2 days for 2 years to mice with no adverse effect. Photo-excited promazine derivatives can induce breaks in DNA in vitro and this phenomenon has been the subject of extensive study.[12–14] Photosensitive cross-linking of other proteins, including lens proteins, has been demonstrated in vitro with promazine but the in vivo significance of this mechanism is not clear.[15]

Clinical pharmacology

The main effects of promazine are as a sedative and tranquillizing agent.[16] Its neuroleptic activity is relatively weak. Promazine is a CNS depressant and thus may cause respiratory depression, particularly in patients with severe respiratory disease. Prolonged administration of promazine may produce extrapyramidal symptoms related to dopamine antagonism. Thus parkinsonian symptoms and, rarely, tardive dyskinesia, may occur. Promazine, like chlorpromazine, lowers the seizure threshold and fits may be induced in patients with epilepsy.[17] Anticholinergic effects may produce dry mouth, blurred vision, difficulty in micturition (in men) and constipation. Promazine induces liver microsomal enzymes in animal studies but this effect has not been noted in man. Promazine may cause postural hypotension and tachycardia due to its α-blocking action and this is more likely after parenteral dosing.

Pharmacokinetics

The preferred method of analysis is high pressure liquid chromatography with ultraviolet or electrochemical detection. The latter has a lower limit of detection of 0.1 $\mu g.l^{-1}$.

Promazine is lipid soluble[18] and achieves a brain to plasma concentration ratio of about 4.7:1. Other tissues with a high concentration include lung, liver and kidney.[19] After oral administration, a total of 33% of the dose is excreted in the urine. Promazine is excreted in breast milk and crosses the placenta. No data are available on the half life of promazine.

Concentration–effect relationship

There are no data available concerning any correlation between the plasma concentration of promazine and its clinical effects.

Metabolism

Promazine is a major plasma metabolite of chlorpromazine in man, although not in the rat.[20] The plasma concentration of promazine exceeds that of chorpromazine during chronic dosing with the latter, but it is a much less potent substance. Like other phenothiazines, promazine is extensively metabolized to a large number of different products. Important pathways of metabolism include sulphoxidation, N-oxidation, 3-hydroxylation (followed by conjugation) and demethylation (Fig. 1). One metabolic reaction can be followed by another, e.g. to form promazine sulphoxide, N-oxide and over 20 different metabolites which have been identified.[21–23] Different species vary in the amounts of different products but the pathways are similar.[24]

Promazine (hydrochloride)

Fig. 1 The metabolism of promazine

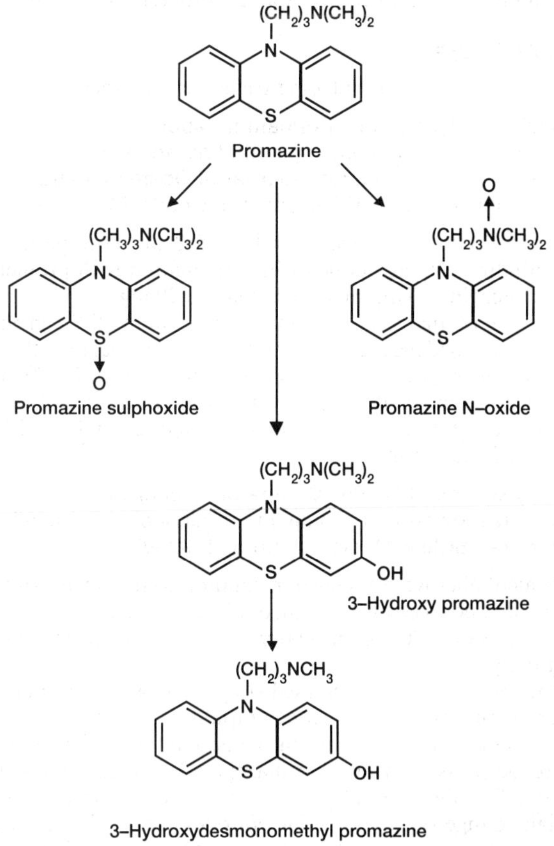

Pharmaceutics

Promazine is available in oral and parenteral forms:
Promazine tablets are available as generic tablets containing 25 mg, 50 mg and (hospitals only) 100 mg.
Suspension: each 5 ml suspension of Sparine (Wyeth, UK) contains promazine embonate equivalent to 50 mg promazine hydrochloride presented as a yellow suspension with an odour of pineapple.
Parenteral: the injectable form Sparine (Wyeth, UK) is a clear colourless aqueous solution containing 50 mg promazine hydrochloride per ml. The American presentation is a pre-filled syringe.

Therapeutic use

Indications

Promazine was patented in 1950 and its clinical investigation was less complete than would be required today. When it was first introduced it was widely used as a tranquillizer, particularly in obstetric practice,[24] in management of alcohol withdrawal[25] and as an adjunct to analgesia. Following evidence that it caused sedation in the baby after delivery its use in obstetric practice declined. Studies in patients with pain suggested that promazine had no specific action in enhancing analgesic effects and this use too declined. Promazine is widely used in veterinary practice as a component of tranquillizer pellets used to immobilize wild animals such as wolves, lions etc. The approved uses of promazine in man are now very limited.

1. As an adjunct to the short-term management of moderate to severe psychomotor agitation
2. Agitation and restlessness in the elderly
3. Treatment of intractable hiccup.

Contraindications

1. The use of promazine is contraindicated in comatose patients and is best avoided if other central nervous depressants such as alcohol, opiates and barbiturates are being used
2. If severe liver dysfunction is present, the use of promazine should be avoided
3. In patients with cardiac insufficiency, modification or restriction of the use of promazine may be advisable. If other medication is being taken which is likely to cause postural hypotension, careful dosage adjustment may be required
4. Use in patients hypersensitive to the active ingredient or other phenothiazines
5. It should not be used during pregnancy or lactation
6. Because of its anticholinergic activity the drug is contraindicated in narrow-angle glaucoma.

Mode of use

As an adjunct to the treatment of psychotic episodes with severe agitation, promazine is usually given in doses of 50–100 mg 4 times daily.[26] Larger doses have been given and a maximum daily dose of 1 g has been specified. The recommended intramuscular dose is 50 mg which may be repeated after 6 to 8 h. It is likely that oral doses undergo substantial presystemic metabolism so a 50 mg parenteral dose may be equivalent to a much higher oral dose and thus is more likely to cause hypotension. In children the recommended parenteral dose is 0.7 $mg.kg^{-1}$. In intractable hiccup larger parenteral doses have been used, up to 100 mg 4-hourly in adults. Recommended dosage schedules should be reduced in the elderly and the manufacturers stipulate that the suspension formulary is not recommended for children.

Because of its adverse reaction profile promazine is not a first choice for prolonged use and safer agents, such as the benzodiazepines, are preferable initial choices if the desired effect is to calm an agitated patient.[27]

Adverse reactions

Promazine is a phenothiazine and its adverse reaction profile resembles that of chlorpromazine, which has been much more widely used.

Potentially life-threatening effects
Agranulocytosis and transient leucopenia have been reported in patients treated with promazine. There are insufficient data available to make a reliable comparison of incidence with other phenothiazines.

Acute overdosage
Promazine overdose is characterized by deep sleep, with or without a pronounced fall in blood pressure. Respiratory rate may be slow due to sedation. Coma may be preceded by an initial period of excitement, which may on occasions be followed by grand mal seizures. In the absence of a specific antidote, treatment should be based on ordinary therapeutic principles with special emphasis on the following measures:[26]

1. Gastric lavage and instillation of activated charcoal
2. Treatment of convulsions with intravenous diazepam
3. Correction of acute hypotension by posture or volume expansion if necessary
4. Treatment of hypothermia
5. Maintenance of the airway and respiration
6. ECG monitoring.

Severe or irreversible adverse effects
Promazine rarely causes obstructive jaundice associated with stasis in biliary canaliculi;[28,29] transient abnormalities of liver function may occur without jaundice. Some individuals may be unusually susceptible to the drug in low dosage and show paradoxical effects of excitement, agitation or insomnia. Prologed use of promazine at high doses may induce extrapyramidal side effects including dyskinesia, akathisia and dystonia which are particularly likely to be severe in children. In view of its relatively low potency it may be less likely to cause dykinesia than related agents.[30] Patients may develop a parkinsonian-like syndrome which responds to withdrawal of the drug or concurrent administration of an antiparkinsonian drug. Tardive dyskinesia may supervene after longer periods of treatment which may persist particularly in the elderly. Antiparkinsonian agents should not be prescribed routinely with promazine because of the risk of aggravating the anticholinergic effects of the drug, precipitating toxic confusional states or impairing its therapeutic efficacy. Phenothiazines may impair body temperature regulation and caution should be observed in very hot weather.

Administration of promazine by the intravenous route may induce local vascular spasm or thrombophlebitis: hence the preparation must be diluted before use. Arteriolar spasm and gangrene have been reported following accidental intra-arterial injection of high concentrations.[31–32]

Symptomatic adverse effects
Promazine is usually well tolerated. Drowsiness usually occurs at the start of treatment but rapidly decreases. Patients should be cautioned about driving, operating machinery and ingestion of alcohol. Dry mouth, nasal stuffiness, blurred vision, constipation and urinary hesitancy or retention and other atropine-like effects occur. Postural hypotension with tachycardia may occur, particularly in patients treated parenterally. A photosensitive skin rash may develop. It has been suggested that the rash is caused by photo-activated promazine cation radicals.[33]

Breast enlargement and pseudolactation may occur due to high prolactin levels.

Confusional states or epileptic fits can occur and sexual function may be impaired.

Interference with clinical pathology tests
The drug may interfere with some methods used for the estimation of alkaloids, barbiturates, 17-ketosteroids, 17-hydroxycorticosteroids, 5-hydroxyindoleacetic acid, protein and salicylates in urine.

High risk groups

Neonates
Children born of mothers administered promazine during labour may be sedated by it.[34] It has been suggested that the the incidence of neonatal hyperbilirubinaemia may be increased.[35]

Breast milk. The drug enters breast milk and use in lactating mothers is not recommended.

Children
The drug has been used in children but extrapyramidal side effects such as dyskinesia, akathisia and dystonia are more common in this age group.

Pregnant women
There are insufficient animal or human data to be confident that the drug is free of hazard, although the drug was once fairly widely used as a tranquillizer in labour. It crosses the placenta readily.

The elderly
The elderly are particularly susceptible to side effects of the drug, especially to sedation, hypotension and disturbance of temperature regulation. Patients with a predisposition to Parkinson's disease may have their condition worsened.

Concurrent disease

Liver disease. As phenothiazines may cause obstructive jaundice their use is not recommened in patients with liver disease, although there is little evidence that the risk is increased.

Heart disease. The α-adrenergic blocking effect could cause severe hypotension in a patient with a low cardiac output, particularly after a parenteral dose.

Renal disease. Promazine is extensively metabolized and so should not accumulate in patients with renal failure.

Drug interactions

Potentially hazardous interactions
The most important interaction is an additive effect with other CNS depressants (including alcohol, hypnotics and anaesthetics). The α-blocking action may have an additive effect with antihypertensive drugs. Combination with other anticholinergic agents will result in accentuation of these effects. Potentiation of phenothiazine action with MAO inhibitors has been suggested but the mechanism is unclear. Glycaemic control in diabetes mellitus may be adversely affected by promazine. Phenothiazines and tricyclic antidepressants when used together can raise plasma levels of both drugs.

Other significant interactions
Antiparkinsonian anticholinergics used to counteract the extrapyrimidal effects of neuroleptics may also reduce their therapeutic effect. Tea and coffee can reduce the systemic bioavailability of phenothiazines. Phenothiazine metabolism is reduced if the drug is given concomitantly with oral contraceptives, progesterone or stilboestrol.

Clinical trials

No data from long-term outcome trials are available.

1. McQuitty F M 1967 Relief of pain in labour. A controlled double-blind trial comparing pethidine and various phenothiazine derivatives. Journal of Obstetrics and Gynaecology of the British Commonwealth 74: 925–928

This was a double-blind trial in which 512 obstetric patients were given pethidine 100 mg, alone or in combination with promethazine 50 mg, promazine 50 mg or propriomazine 20 mg.

The degree of analgesia was almost identical in all the groups and there was no evidence of potentiation by promazine. Promazine significantly increased the incidence of tachycardia (15/132) and also increased the number of patients with hypotension (5/132) although this was not significant. The incidence of nausea and vomiting was similar in all the groups.

2. Sereny G, Kalant H 1965 Comparative clinical evaluation of chlordiazepoxide and promazine in alcohol withdrawal syndrome. British Medical Journal 1: 92–97

58 male alcoholics were assigned in rotation to treatment with one of five regimes upon cessation of alcohol intake. These were placebo, chlordiazepoxide 200 mg or 400 mg daily, promazine 400 mg or 800 mg daily.

All four active regimes increased sleep. Promazine was initially the most active but tolerance developed rapidly. The effect of chlordiazepoxide was maintained. Promazine caused an immediate and abrupt fall in blood pressure while chlordiazepoxide caused a more gradual reduction. The high dose of promazine caused the largest number of potentially dangerous hypotensive episodes, although there was also an increase with the high dose of chlordiazepoxide. Four patients given promazine suffered grand mal seizures versus none on chlordiazepoxide.

General review articles

McGee J L, Alexander M R 1979 Phenothiazine analgesia — fact or fantasy? American Journal of Hospital Pharmacy 36: 633–640
Davis J M 1976 Recent developments in the drug treatment of schizophrenia. American Journal of Psychiatry 133: 208–214
Jones R S 1972 A review of tranquillisation and sedation in large animals. Veterinary Record 90: 613–617

References

1. Palmer G C, Manian A A 1976 Actions of phenothiazine analogues on dopamine-sensitive adenylate cyclase in neuronal and glial-enriched fractions from rat brain. Biochemical Pharmacology 25: 63–71
2. Meck W H 1986 Affinity for the dopamine D2 receptor predicts neuroleptic potency in decreasing the speed of an internal clock. Pharmacology, Biochemistry and Behavior 25: 1185–1189
3. Miller R J, Horn A S, Iversen L L 1974 The action of neuroleptic drugs on dopamine-stimulated adenosine cyclic 3',5'-monophosphate production in rat neostriatum and limbic forbrain. Molecular Pharmacology 10: 759–766
4. Feinberg A P, Snyder S H 1975 Phenothiazine drugs: structure–activity relationships explained by a conformation that mimics dopamine. Proceedings of the National Academy of Sciences of the USA 72: 1899–1903
5. Snyder S, Greenberg D, Yamamura H I 1974 Antischizophrenic drugs and brain cholinergic receptors. Affinity for muscarinic sites predicts extrapyramidal effects. Archives of General Psychiatry 31: 58–61
6. Richelson E, Pfenning M 1984 Blockade by antidepressants and related compounds of biogenic amine uptake into rat brain synaptosomes: most antidepressants selectively block norepinephrine uptake. European Journal of Pharmacology 104: 277–286
7. Sernagor E, Kuhn D, Vyklicky L Jr, Mayer M L 1989 Open channel block of NMDA receptor responses evoked by tricyclic antidepressants. Neuron 2: 1221–1227
8. Suzuki O, Seno H, Kumazawa T 1988 In vitro inhibition of human platelet monoamine oxidase by phenothiazine derivatives. Life Science 42: 2131–2136
9. Tallant E A, Wallace R W 1985 Calmodulin antagonists elevate the levels of 32P-labeled polyphosphoinositides in human platelets. Biochemical and Biophysical Research Communications 131: 370–377
10. Ayromlooi J 1985 Hemodynamic and acid-base effects of promazine on unanesthetized pregnant sheep and fetus. Developmental Pharmacology and Therapeutics 8: 302–310
11. Cottle M K, Van Petten G R, van Muyden P 1983 Maternal and fetal cardiovascular indices during fetal hypoxia due to cord compression in chronically cannulated sheep. II. Responses to promazine. American Journal of Obstetrics and Gynecology 146: 686–692

12. Decuyper J, Piette J, Merville Louis M P, van de Vorst A 1987 Photosensitization of SV 40 DNA mediated by promazine derivatives and 4′-hydroxymethyl-4,5′,8-trimethylpsoralen. Inhibition of the in vitro transcription. Biochemical Pharmacology 36(7): 1069–1076
13. Merville M P, Piette J, Lopez M, Decuyper J, van de Vorst A 1984 Termination sites of the in vitro DNA synthesis on single-stranded DNA photosensitized by promazines. Journal of Biological Chemistry 259: 15 069–15 077
14. Decuyper J, Piette J, Lopez M, Merville M P, van De Vorst A 1984 Induction of breaks in deoxyribonucleic acid by photoexcited promazine derivatives. Biochemical Pharmacology 33: 4025–4031
15. Merville M P, Decuyper J, Piette J, Calberg Bacq C M, Van de Vorst A 1984 In vitro cross-linking of bovine lens proteins photosensitized by promazines. Investigative Ophthalmology and Visual Science 25: 573–580
16. Corke B C 1977 Neurobehavioural responses of the newborn. The effect of different forms of maternal analgesia. Anaesthesia 32: 539–543
17. Degen R, Degen H E 1983 The diagnostic value of the sleep EEG with and without sleep deprivation in patients with atypical absences. Epilepsia 24: 557–566
18. Gescher A, Li Wan Po A 1978 Correlation of physicochemical properties with absorption and metabolism of some tricyclic drugs. Journal of Pharmacy and Pharmacology 30: 353–358
19. Hu O Y, Curry S H 1989 Stability, human blood distribution and rat tissue localization of promazine and desmonomethylpromazine. Biopharmaceutics and Drug Disposition 10: 537–548
20. Sgaragli G, Ninci R, Della Corte L et al 1986 Promazine. A major plasma metabolite of chlorpromazine in a population of chronic schizophrenics. Drug Metabolism and Disposition 14: 263–266
21. Essien E E, Cowan D A, Beckett A H 1975 Metabolism of phenothiazines: identification of N-oxygenated products by gas chromatography and mass spectrometry. Journal of Pharmacy and Pharmacology 27: 334–342
22. Beckett A H, Navas G E, Hutt A J 1988 Metabolism of chlorpromazine and promazine in vitro: isolation and characterization of N-oxidation products. Xenobiotica 18: 61–74
23. Walkenstein S S, Seifter J 1959 Fate, distribution and excretion of S35 promazine. Journal of Pharmacology and Experimental Therapeutics 125: 283
24. Dewey E A, Maylin G A, Ebel J G, Henion J D 1981 The metabolism of promazine and acetylpromazine in the horse. Drug Metabolism and Disposition 9: 30–36
25. Schwarz L, Schmidt H Jr, Stern J A 1968 A double-blind trial of the efficacy of promazine in the treatment of alcohol withdrawal syndrome. Diseases of the Nervous System 29: 173–177
26. Barry D, Meyskens F L Jr, Becker C E 1973 Phenothiazine poisoning. A review of 48 cases. Californian Medicine 118: 1–5
27. Davis J M 1976 Recent developments in the drug treatment of schizophrenia. American Journal of Psychiatry 133: 208–214
28. Ishak K G, Irey N S 1972 Hepatic injury associated with the phenothiazines. Clinicopathologic and follow-up study of 36 patients. Archives of Pathology 93: 283–304
29. Clarke A E, Maritz V M, Denborough M A 1972 Phenothiazines and jaundice. Australian and New Zealand Journal of Medicine 2: 376–382
30. Boston Collaborative Drug Surveillance Program 1973 Drug-induced extra-pyramidal symptoms. Journal of the American Medical Association 224: 889
31. Hager D L, Wilson J N 1967 Gangrene of the hand following intra-arterial injection. Archives of Surgery 94: 86–89
32. Bounameaux H, Schneider P A, Huber Sauteur E, Jolliet P 1990 Severe ischemia of the hand following intra-arterial promazine injection: effects of vasodilation, anticoagulation, and local thrombolysis with tissue-type plasminogen activator. Vasa 19: 68–71
33. Chignell C F, Motten A G, Buettner G R 1985 Photoinduced free radicals from chlorpromazine and related phenothiazines: relationship to phenothiazine-induced photosensitization. Environmental Health Perspectives 64: 103–110
34. Corke B C 1977 Neurobehavioural responses of the newborn. The effect of different forms of maternal analgesia. Anaesthesia 32: 539–543
35. John E 1975 Promazine and neonatal hyperbilirubinaemia. Medical Journal of Australia 2: 342–344

Promethazine (hydrochloride)

Promethazine is one of several H_1-receptor antagonists developed during the 1940s, which achieved wide therapeutic use due to its potency and length of action. It is now used predominantly for its central sedative effect.

Chemistry

Promethazine hydrochloride (Phenergan, Sominex)
$C_{17}H_{20}N_2S.HCl$
10-(2-Dimethyl aminopropyl) phenothiazine hydrochloride

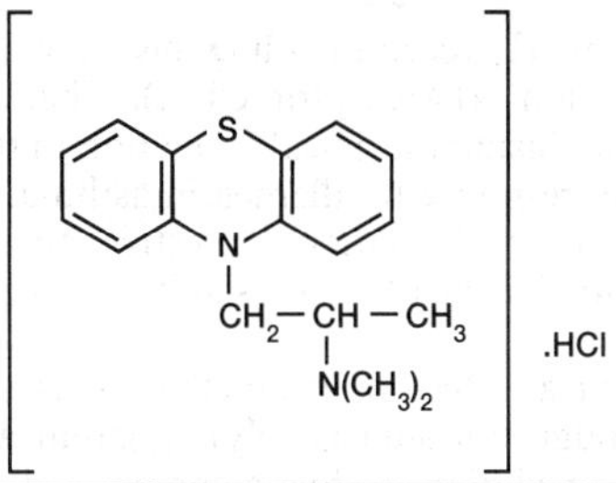

Molecular weight	320.9 (284.4)
pKa	9.1
Solubility	
in alcohol	1 in 0.6
in water	1 in 9
Octanol/water partition coefficient	—

Promethazine hydrochloride is a white or faintly yellow, odourless or almost odourless, crystalline powder with a very bitter taste. It is slowly oxidized, particularly when moistened, on prolonged exposure to air, turning blue in colour. It is prepared by chemical synthesis and in view of its tendency to oxidation should be stored in airtight, heat-resistant containers. Depending on the manufacturer and dosage form it has a shelf-life of 2–5 years.

Promethazine hydrochloride is also available as a compound preparation, with pethidine (Pamergan P100), for intramuscular and intravenous (dilution required) administration, with paracetamol (Medised), marketed in tablet or suspension form, as a 2% solution for topical application, and in a number of cough linctuses not now available on NHS prescription (Phensedyl, Tixylix).

Promethazine is also available as the theoclate (Avomine).

Pharmacology

Promethazine is a competitive antagonist of histamine at the H_1-receptor, having no influence on H_2-receptor mediated events. It is a phenothiazine H_1-antihistamine and, as such, also exhibits anticholinergic, local anaesthetic and weak α-adrenoceptor antagonistic actions. This latter property is only clinically relevant with rapid intravenous administration. Promethazine is an antiemetic and, in contrast to other phenothiazines, is effective in the treatment of motion sickness. It has weak antitussive activity and is a sedative H_1-receptor antagonist.

As histamine's regulatory effects on cellular and immunological function are predominantly mediated via H_2-receptors, promethazine would be expected to have little action in this respect. While this is so in the adult, promethazine has been found to influence the developing immune system in the fetus. Ex vivo studies indicate that promethazine depresses cell-mediated immunity, inhibits platelet aggregation, inhibits the hexose–monophosphate shunt in polymorphonuclear leucocytes and the phagocytosis and lysis of fetal rhesus positive erythrocytes by leucocytes and lymphocytes, inhibits the ability of fetal macrophages to bind to rhesus positive erythrocytes and appears to stabilize the erythrocyte membrane against haemolysis.[1–3] A number of these effects on fetal red cells have been applied to the treatment of haemolytic disease of the newborn.[4]

Toxicology

In common with all H_1-receptor antagonists, promethazine would be expected to reduce uterine blood flow and thus, when used in the first trimester, be associated with an increased incidence of spontaneous abortion. While studies in rats, utilizing high doses (25 mg.kg^{-1}), given intraperitoneally throughout pregnancy support such an embryotoxic effect,[5] this is not documented in man.

Several human studies have not shown any evidence of teratogenicity with first-trimester use of promethazine, consistent with animal data. In vitro studies identify a low level of genotoxicity and some cytotoxicity,[6,7] which is a function of both the concentration of and duration of exposure to promethazine, but no evidence of carcinogenicity.

Clinical pharmacology

Promethazine is an H_1-receptor antagonist having no influence on gastric acid secretion (H_2-receptor effect). There is a dose-related protective effect on histamine wheal formation in the skin and on the immediate airway response to allergen in asthma. It is not possible, however, to attribute the latter protective effect to H_1-receptor antagonism. Promethazine offers no significant therapeutic benefit in asthma.

The major clinical effect of promethazine is sedation, which is objectively (although not subjectively) apparent at doses as low as 10 mg in adults.[8] Sedation is thus common with therapeutic doses (25–75 mg) and, between individuals, ranges in intensity from mild drowsiness to deep sleep. Within subjects, a weak correlation has been reported between promethazine blood concentration levels and CNS effects, as reflected by impairment of rotary pursuit and simple force choice reaction time.[9]

Promethazine has considerable anticholinergic effects in clinical usage and this property may explain its use as an antiemetic, particularly for motion sickness. The anticholinergic actions give rise to unwanted dry mouth and blurred vision and, in men, the risk of urinary retention if prostatic hypertrophy is present.

Pharmacokinetics

The preferred analytical method is high performance liquid chromatography.[10] This has a sensitivity of 0.2 μg.l^{-1}.

Promethazine is well absorbed, but undergoes extensive first-pass metabolism, only 25% of the oral dose reaching the systemic circulation unchanged.[11,12] After oral therapy therapeutic effects are identifiable at 15–30 min and peak plasma concentrations at 2–3 h (5.5 μg.l^{-1}).[12] The peak plasma concentration is four times higher after intramuscular administration[12] and is delayed to 8 h with rectal suppository administration.[13] There is a large volume of distribution, 13.4 $\pm$ 3.6 l.kg^{-1},[11] consistent with a wide body tissue distribution. Compared with other organs, the brain concentration is lower, but still exceeds the plasma concentration. Promethazine is extensively plasma protein bound.[11,12]

There is no data available which applies specifically to the theoclate salt.

The major route of elimination is faecal via biliary excretion, only 0.6% of the parent compound and 10.3% as the sulphoxide being excreted in the urine within 72 hours.[11] The sulphoxide excretion approaches the glomerular filtration rate (90 ml.min^{-1}) while promethazine itself has an excretion of only 5.9 ml.min^{-1}, indicative of significant tubular reabsorption. There is a biexponential decline after intravenous administration, with a terminal half life of 7–14 h and a clearance of (1.140 l.$^{-1}$min).

Promethazine rapidly crosses the placenta at term. After intravenous administration, levels are detectable in cord blood at 1½ minutes and fetal and maternal blood concentrations are at equilibrium by 15 minutes.[14] No measurements have been made of breast milk concentrations, but it is known that some secretion of phenothiazines in breast milk occurs.

Oral absorption	>80%
Presystemic metabolism	75%
Plasma half life	
range	
mean	7–14 h
Volume of distribution	13.4$\pm$3.6 l.kg^{-1}
Plasma protein binding	76–93%

Concentration–effect relationship

This is not well defined for promethazine, but a significant correlation has been found between promethazine levels and impairment of motor performance tasks.[9]

Metabolism

Promethazine undergoes extensive first-pass metabolism, probably within the liver, only 0.6% of the unchanged drug being excreted in the urine after oral administration.[11]

Two primary pathways of metabolism have been described: sulphoxidation and N-dealkylation (Fig. 1)
The major metabolite, promethazine sulphoxide, is inactive as an H_1-receptor antagonist.

Fig. 1 The metabolism of promethazine

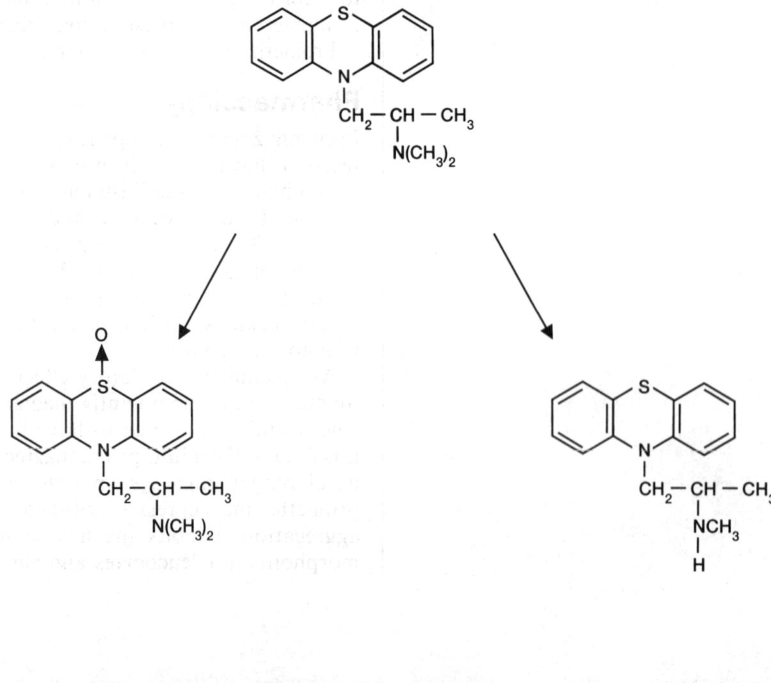

Pharmaceutics

Promethazine, Phenergan (Rhone Poulenc, UK), is available in oral, parenteral and topical forms:

1. Tablets, which contain either 10 mg or 25 mg promethazine hydrochloride BP, are blue, round, biconvex and film-coated with 'M & B' (10 mg) or 'Phenergan 25' (25 mg) on one side. No slow-release preparation is available.
2. The elixir, a clear bright golden syrupy liquid, contains 5 mg promethazine hydrochloride in 5 ml.
3. The injectable preparation for intravenous or intramuscular use, a colourless solution, contains 2.5% w/v promethazine hydrochloride BP (25 $mg.ml^{-1}$).
4. The cream, for topical administration, contains 2% w/w promethazine base. It is white or off-white in colour, but is no longer available in the UK.

None of the preparations contains tartrazine and all preparations should be protected from light.

The tablets and injectable preparations both have shelf-lives of 5 years, while the elixir and cream formulations have shelf-lives of 3 and 1 years respectively.

Sominex tablets (SmithKline Beecham, UK) are white, scored tablets, containing 20 mg promethazine and marked 'S' on one side. Phenergan (Wyeth, USA) is available as tablet, injection, syrup and suppository formulations:

1. 12.5 mg tablets are round, biconcave, coloured orange and marked 'WYETH' on one side and coded '19' on the other. 25 mg tablets are round, flat, white and marked 'WYETH' on one side and '27' on the other. 50 mg tablets are round, biconcave, coloured pink and marked 'WYETH' on one side and coded '227' on the other.
2. 25 mg in 1 ml and 50 mg in 1 ml injections include disodium edetate, calcium chloride, sodium metabisulphite, phenol and a sodium acetate/acetic acid buffer.
3. Phenergan Syrup Plain contains 6.25 mg in 5 ml whilst Phenergan Syrup Fortis contains 25 mg in 5 ml. Both are fruit-flavoured and include alcohol and sodium benzoate.
4. Rectal suppositories are in 12.5 mg, 25 mg and 50 mg strengths in a theobroma base.
5. Avomine (Rhone-Poulenc, UK) tablets contain 25 mg promethazine theoclate, impressed 'AVOMINE' on one face with a break line on the reverse.

Promethazine is also available in a number of compound preparations.

Therapeutic use

Indications

1. Symptomatic treatment of allergic conditions of the respiratory tract and skin, including anaphylaxis
2. Non-allergic skin conditions; urticaria, dermatographism and insect bites
3. For sedation, hypnosis, insomnia, premedication
4. In obstetrics
5. For motion-sickness
6. In Parkinson's syndrome and drug-induced parkinsonism
7. Haemolytic disease of the newborn.

Contraindications

1. Hypersensitivity reaction to promethazine
2. Patients in charge of vehicles or machinery who have not received the drug before or who have exhibited a sedative effect with previous administration of promethazine
3. Ventilatory impairment

In addition to the absolute contraindications there are a number of situations where caution with prescribing is necessary, which can be considered as relative contraindications.

4. Pregnancy
5. Concomitant use of other sedatives, hypnotics or alcohol
6. Glaucoma
7. Prostatic hypertrophy
8. Epilepsy.

Promethazine (hydrochloride)

Mode of use

The range of clinical uses for promethazine depends not only upon its peripheral H_1-receptor antagonistic properties but also on its anti-cholinergic, local anaesthetic and central H_1-receptor antagonistic properties.

Oral therapy is usually initiated with one 25 mg tablet at night in view of promethazine's sedative effect and long half life. The dose may be increased up to 75 mg at night if required. In allergic conditions, more frequent administration, twice or three times daily, may be necessary, starting with one or two 10 mg tablets and increasing as required. The dosage ceiling is determined by the sedative and anticholinergic effects and will vary from individual to individual.

For parenteral administration, the usual adult dose is 25–50 mg by deep intramuscular injection or, in emergency, by slow intravenous injection after dilution of the 2.5% solution to 10 times its volume with water for injection. Too rapid administration of the intravenous preparation may lead to hypotension as a result of of promethazine's α-adrenoceptor antagonistic property. Plasma levels of promethazine after parenteral administration are approximately four times greater than those obtained after an equivalent oral dose, as the effective dose is greater due to the avoidance of first-pass metabolism in the liver. The maximum parenteral dose is 100 mg.

Children may find the elixir, containing 5 mg per 5 ml, easier to take than tablets. In the treatment of allergic disorders, 5–15 mg is the recommended dose for children of 1–5 years and 10–25 mg for children of 5–10 years. If two doses are required in a 24-hour period then the lower dose option should be taken. When used as a sedative/hypnotic in children, the recommended doses of promethazine for the 1–5 and 5–10 year olds is 15–20 mg and 20–25 mg, respectively. Similar doses are used in the prophylaxis of motion-sickness, given 90 minutes before the intended journey. Promethazine is not now advised for infants less than 1 year old.

Indications

1. Allergic disorders/anaphylaxis

Allergic rhinitis and conjunctivitis are commonly treated with H_1-receptor antagonists. As rhinorrhoea, sneezing and itching respond better than nasal stuffiness, H_1-antihistamines are of greater clinical benefit in seasonal rather than perennial rhinitis. Treatment taken before exposure is likely to be more effective than if taken after exposure when symptoms are present. The therapeutic benefit of promethazine in these conditions is offset by sedation. As such it has tended to be superseded by the newer non-sedative H_1-receptor antagonists.

Although promethazine partially inhibits the immediate airway response to allergen[15] it has no significant benefit in clinical asthma and therefore, in common with other H_1-receptor antagonists, is not advocated as treatment for this condition.[16]

Promethazine has been used in the treatment of atopic dermatitis to reduce itch. Its beneficial effects in treating this symptom are likely to be related to sedation rather than H_1-receptor antagonism.[17] The preferred route of administration is thus oral. Topical treatment is of questionable benefit and may induce sensitization and produce an eczematous reaction.[18,19]

Intravenous promethazine is of value in the treatment of acute anaphylaxis, as an adjunct to subcutaneous adrenaline.

2. Urticaria, dermatographism, insect bites

As histamine promotes vasodilation and increases vascular permeability, it will produce oedema formation. These effects are predominantly mediated via H_1-receptors. H_1-receptor antagonists have therefore been used to treat histamine-related wheal formation in the skin in urticaria, dermatographism, following insect bites and with sensitization to foreign proteins. Topical therapy with promethazine is of symptomatic relief if used early after insect bites, possibly related to its local anaesthetic action as much as to its H_1-receptor antagonism. The preferred route of treatment for all whealing conditions is, however, oral. The limiting effect of promethazine by this route is sedation. Thus less sedating H_1-receptor antagonists are generally used.

3. Sedation, hypnosis, insomnia, premedication

The central sedative effects of promethazine have been utilized in the treatment of insomnia and for premedication where sedation is required.[20] Promethazine (25 mg) at bedtime produces significant improvement in sleep quality and ease of getting to sleep. There is a dose-related reduction in REM sleep with doses of promethazine from 50–200 mg. For anaesthesia premedication, the antiemetic and antisialagogic effects of promethazine are added benefits and offer advantages over benzodiazepines.[21] Promethazine is commonly used for premedication in children by the oral route (as tablets or liquid) at a dose of 1 mg.kg^{-1} 1½ hours preoperatively. Subjectively it is reported to reduce anaesthetic maintenance doses.[20]

The CNS sedative effect has also been used to diminish respiratory drive in patients with oxygenation failure associated with chronic obstructive airways disease (type I respiratory failure), whose excessive respiratory drive gives rise to unpleasant breathlessness (pink puffers).[22] Promethazine should, however, be used with caution in this instance.

4. Obstetrics

The sedative and antiemetic properties of promethazine have been commonly used as an adjunct narcotic analgesics during labour.[20,23] Promethazine itself has no analgesic property. Although marketed in combination with pethidine (Panergan P100) it has been suggested that the analgesic effect of pethidine is reduced when used with promethazine (25 mg) as compared to metoclopramide (10 mg) and that drowsiness persists for longer in promethazine-treated patients.[24] Effects on uterine activity during labour are variable, with both increases and decreases in uterine contractions being reported.

The antiemetic properties of promethazine are also used in first-trimester pregnancy, it being the most commonly used antiemetic in one survey.[25] Several large studies have not identified any association between promethazine used during the first trimester and teratogenicity.[25–28] However, the manufacturer recommends that promethazine should be avoided during pregnancy unless considered essential by the supervising physician.

5. Motion-sickness

Unlike other phenothiazines, promethazine is effective in the prevention of motion-sickness due to its central H_1-receptor and cholinergic antagonistic properties. Comparisons of combination therapy identified that promethazine (25 mg) given with dexamphetamine (10 mg) gives consistently good results in preventing motion-sickness, although this would not be a clinically recommended combination due to the addictive properties of d-amphetamine.[29] The combination of promethazine (25 mg) and ephedrine hydrochloride (25 mg) offers therapeutic advantages over many other anti-motion-sickness drugs.[30] Treatment should be taken 1½–2 h before the intended journey. It is advised that promethazine should be avoided in persons with driving or mechanical responsibility, due to possible drowsiness. The combination of promethazine (25 mg) and d-amphetamine (10 mg) has, however, been found to have no adverse effect on dynamic tracking performance, optokinetic nystagmus or visual fixation during motion.[31,32]

6. Parkinson's syndrome

Prior to the introduction of levodopa, the central anticholinergic properties of promethazine were utilized in the treatment of parkinsonism. The development of more potent central anticholinergics and levodopa have obviated the need for promethazine in the treatment of this condition. Paradoxically, although used in the treatment of parkinsonism, promethazine may be associated with extrapyramidal side effects due to dopamine receptor antagonism.[20] Restlessness, akathisia and athetoid movements have also been reported with promethazine.

7. Haemolytic disease of the newborn

Promethazine has been reported to ameliorate the effects of haemolytic disease of the newborn, when given in conjunction with exchange transfusions to rhesus-sensitized women during pregnancy.[4,33] The reports are uncontrolled but based on in vitro studies indicating a mechanism for the protective effect of promethazine in rhesus incompatibility.[3] Treatment is usually initiated after the sixteenth week of gestation with 3.7–5 mg.kg^{-1} daily in four divided doses, although up to 6.5 mg.kg^{-1} have been used.[34] Controlled studies are required to critically evaluate the benefit of this treatment.

Contraindications

Absolute contraindications

1. Hypersensitivity

Dermal application of promethazine cream, especially to eczematous skin, carries a risk of sensitization.[18,19] Further topical administration may then lead to atopic or photosensitive dermatitis.[18,35] Subsequent oral administration carries the risk of anaphylaxis. There is a case report of a 30-year-old woman experiencing stridor, wheeze and urticaria 1 hour after oral administration of promethazine hydrochloride 25 mg.[36] As there is cross reactivity with ethylenediamine found in dyes, rubber materials and other pharmacological agents,[37] promethazine should be avoided in patients known to be sensitive to ethylenediamine.

H_1-receptor antagonists have occasionally been associated with reversible agranulocytosis or neutropaenia, particularly phenothiazine antihistamines. Isolated reports of promethazine causing aplastic anaemia or agranulocytosis exist.[38] Previous haematological side effects would be a contraindication to use, as would previous jaundice with a phenothiazine.

2. Use of machinery or vehicles

As promethazine produces drowsiness and a delay in stimulus–response reaction time, patients receiving promethazine should not take charge of vehicles, other means of transport or machinery, as there is an increased risk of accidents occurring.[39] This is pertinent to all patients taking promethazine for the first time or who on previous administration have experienced disorientation, confusion or drowsiness.

3. Ventilatory impairment

Promethazine is a CNS sedative. In normal infants promethazine 1 mg.kg^{-1} has been reported to increase sleep time, decrease the duration and number of awakenings, increase non-REM sleep and increase the occurrence of central and obstructive apnoeas.[40] Such effects would have fatal consequences if promethazine was given to patients with type II respiratory failure who have hypoxaemia and hypercapnoea due to diminished ventilatory drive. Promethazine is thus contraindicated in any patient with ventilatory impairment.

Relative contraindications

4. Pregnancy

The manufacturers recommend that promethazine should be avoided in early pregnancy, unless the physician considers it necessary. While there is a theoretical risk of embryotoxicity, several large studies have identified no risk of teratogenicity[25–28] and promethazine has been widely used in first-trimester pregnancy as an antiemetic. The avoidance of any unnecessary first-trimester medication is, however, advisable.

5. Concomitant use of sedatives, hypnotics or alcohol

Promethazine is a CNS sedative and is additive with or may potentiate the sedative effects of other centrally acting drugs such as opiates, barbiturates, antihistamines, tranquillizers or alcohol. Caution should be exhibited if such drugs are co-administered with promethazine. Four out of 95 paediatric patients experienced respiratory depression (1 respiratory arrest) when given promethazine (0.65 mg.kg^{-1}) with pethidine (2.5 mg.kg^{-1}) and chlorpromazine (0.65 mg.kg^{-1}) as a premedication for cardiac catheterization.[41]

6. Glaucoma

The anticholinergic action of promethazine may lead to an increase in intraocular pressure in patients with untreated glaucoma or a predisposition to this disease. Promethazine has no effect on intraocular pressure in the normal eye.

7. Prostatic hypertrophy

Anticholinergic agents relax the detrusor muscle and decrease bladder tone. This has no effect on micturition in healthy males but leads to micturition difficulty in those with overt or latent prostatic hypertrophy. Promethazine should thus be used with caution in patients with symptoms of prostatism or in elderly males, in whom prostatic hypertrophy is more common.

8. Epilepsy

Promethazine may induce seizures at therapeutic doses in patients not previously experiencing epilepsy as well as in known epilep-

Promethazine (hydrochloride)

tics.[20,42] Promethazine should thus be avoided in patients with known epilepsy or predisposing factors such as pre-eclampsia and space-occupying cerebral lesions.

Adverse reactions

Potentially life-threatening effects
Fatalities with promethazine are exceptionally rare, occurring in 1 in 3×10^6 patients during a 3-year period of reporting to the UK Committee on Safety of Medicines. The major cause has been respiratory depression, particularly if taken with other CNS sedatives, although there is one report of death following laryngeal obstruction due to a promethazine-related dystonic reaction.

Recent concern and speculation over the role of promethazine in sudden unexpected infant death was based on the finding that in 23% of sudden deaths (n = 52) and 22% of near-miss sudden death infants (n = 36) the patients had been given a phenothiazine though not specifically promethazine within 2 days compared with only 2% of controls (n = 175). When those infants with nasopharyngitis were selected out of each group, the percentages for sudden infant death, near-sudden infant death, and the control group were 71%, 57% and 8% respectively.[43] The subsequent identification that promethazine at a dose of 1 $mg.kg^{-1}$ in four normal full-term infants with a mean age of 15.8 ± 4.6 weeks (± SEM) produced an increase in sleep time, a decrease in duration and number of awakenings, an increase in non-REM sleep, and an increase in central and obstructive apnoea[40] has led to the manufacturers elevating the initial recommended age for promethazine treatment from 6 months to 1 year.

Acute overdosage
Minor overdoses in adults may result in deep sleep. Cardiovascular effects, such as hypotension and tachycardia, are not marked, but respiratory depression and seizures can occur. Paradoxically, in children, CNS stimulation is a feature, with restlessness, akathisia, hyperexcitability, anxiety and hallucinations. In such patients the commonest neurological findings are ataxia, dysarthria, and exaggerated tendon reflexes.[44] Anticholinergic effects lead to dry mouth, blurred vision, dilated pupils, and delirium, sometimes with pyrexia. Psychosis was a feature following self-ingestion of 1250 mg in a 19-year-old girl,[44] and 575 mg in a 1.7-year-old boy.[45] Both patients recovered.

Treatment is symptomatic and supportive. Gastric lavage is of value but haemodialysis is not, in view of the large volume of distribution of promethazine. Analeptics should be avoided as they may induce seizures; mechanical ventilation may therefore be required. Seizures are best treated with benzodiazepines. Anticholinergic adverse effects have been successfully treated with intravenous physostigmine[46] and extrapyramidal symptoms with anticholinergic agents.

Severe or irreversible adverse effects
While hypotension is usually only a feature of rapid intravenous administration, there has been one report of fatal shock in a pregnant woman receiving promethazine.[47] Post mortem examination revealed the presence of an undiagnosed phaeochromocytoma, and the severe drop in blood pressure was considered to be secondary to the unmasking of hypovolaemia. Rarely leucopenia or bone marrow depression have been encountered with promethazine,[38] as has obstructive jaundice, which usually resolves on discontinuing treatment. One 9-year-old boy experienced dystonic jaw movements 5 minutes after intramuscular injection of 50 mg of promethazine.[48] Such extrapyramidal effects are rare at therapeutic doses, only being identified in 1 out of 1194 patients receiving promethazine in the Boston Collaborative Drug Surveillance Programme.[49] Seizures have been associated with promethazine at therapeutic doses.[20,42]

Promethazine use during labour impairs platelet aggregation in the newborn, to a level comparable to that associated with bleeding disorders.[50] Fortunately no haemorrhagic complications have been reported, but this is a potentially serious effect.

Intravenous administration has been associated, in one instance, with venous thrombosis, and severe chemical irritation and ulceration can occur with subcutaneous administration, and severe arteriospasm with intra-arterial administration, leading to gangrene and possibly amputation. Extreme caution should therefore be taken with parenteral administration so that inadvertent perivascular extravasation and intra-arterial administration does not occur.

Promethazine cream may stain clothing, bed linen, etc. These stains may only become evident after laundering and can be irreversible.

Symptomatic adverse effects
Promethazine commonly produces some degree of CNS depression ranging from mild sedation through disorientation to deep sleep. A feeling of fatigue and tiredness is not uncommon and may be associated with incoordination, confusion, and very rarely psychotic behaviour. CNS excitation with anxiety, nervousness, insomnia and hallucinations can paradoxically occur, most commonly in children. The anticholinergic action is associated with dry mouth, blurred vision, and rarely dizziness. Individual sensitivities vary and these effects resolve on discontinuing treatment or reducing the dose. Similar effects have been reported from dermal use of promethazine cream, although this is unusual.

Interference with clinical pathology tests
A number of immunological urinary pregnancy tests may give false results in the presence of promethazine.

Although promethazine will reduce the wheal response to allergen on skin prick testing,[51] this is not complete inhibition, as mediators other than histamine are involved in the wheal response. Thus promethazine does not interfere with skin prick testing in the diagnosis of atopy.

High risk groups

Neonates
Promethazine is not advocated as treatment for neonates. This is on two accounts. Firstly, the bioavailability of promethazine will be increased, due to the immaturity of the liver with respect to first-pass hepatic metabolism, and no dosage regime has been established to take account of this. Secondly, there is recent suspicion that promethazine may be involved in some cases of sudden infant death syndrome due to its respiratory depressant effect.[40,43] In view of these considerations the manufacturers recommend that promethazine should not be used in children less than 1 year of age.

Breast milk. Breast milk levels of promethazine have not been measured.

Children
Promethazine has been extensively used in children as a premedication sedative.

Pregnant women
Epidemiological studies indicate that promethazine is safe in pregnancy. Three studies investigating first-trimester use of promethazine in 114, 165 and 63 women, respectively, found no evidence of major or minor malformations or individual defects.[26–28] In the collaborative perinatal project, 50 282 mother–child pairs were monitored and 746 exposures to promethazine throughout pregnancy recorded, without any evidence of teratogenicity.[52] Consistent with these findings, first-trimester use of promethazine was no greater in 836 infants born with congenital malformations as compared to 836 controls.[53]

The elderly
No specific manufacturer's recommendations exist about use in older patients. However, as glaucoma and prostatic hypertrophy are commoner in the elderly, the interaction between promethazine and these diseases should be borne in mind when prescribing.

Drug interactions

Potentially hazardous interactions

CNS sedatives. Concomitant use of promethazine with other CNS sedatives such as opiates, barbiturates, tranquillizers or antihistamines may lead to an additive or potentiating effect.[54]

Alcohol. Alcohol enhances the CNS sedative effects of promethazine and the Committee on Safety of Drugs recommended that patients be warned not to take alcohol while taking antihistamine therapy.

Other significant interactions

Hydroxyzine. Regular use of hydroxyzine reduces the antihistaminic action of subsequently administered promethazine possibly due to H_1 antihistaminic tachyphylaxis.[55]

Promethazine (hydrochloride)

P

Pethidine. The possibility that promethazine may diminish the analgesic action of pethidine, when the two drugs are co-administered, has been suggested.[24]

Intravenous incompatibilities. Promethazine tends to be incompatible with alkaline solutions, such as chloramphenicol, heparin, hydrocortisone, methicillin, pentobarbitone and thiopentone, and forms precipitates with aminophylline, carbenicillin, chlorthiazide, methohexital, and the X-ray contrast media, iothalamate meglumine (Conray and Angio-Conray), and iodipamide meglumine (Cholografin).

Potentially useful interactions

Promethazine's beneficial effects in preventing motion-sickness are enhanced if given with dexamphetamine[29] or ephedrine hydrochloride.[30] As antihistamines tend to be ineffective in treating nasal blockage, combination therapy with pseudoephedrine improves global symptom control,[56] although alternative therapy may be preferable.

Clinical trials

Double-blind randomized studies have compared promethazine with lorazepam as anaesthetic premedication[21] and promethazine and metoclopramide during labour.[24] Adelman et al reported on their experience with promethazine in 5000 surgical and obstetric patients with ages ranging from 3 to 75.[20]

Major outcome trials

1. Adelman M H, Jacobson E, Lief P A, Miller S A 1959 Promethazine hydrochloride in surgery and obstetrics. Journal of the American Medical Association 169: 73–75

This is a report of the authors' experience with promethazine, as either a premedicant, an antiemetic or a sedative, in 5000 surgical and obstetric patients ranging from 3 to 75-years-old prior to the clinical trial era. Promethazine 25–75 mg was given intramuscularly with pethidine and scopolomine as a pre-anaesthetic medication (0.5 mg per lb in children) and in labour and 25 mg intravenously used as a sedative prior to spinal anaesthesia.

The authors concluded that promethazine was an effective antiemetic, produced safe sedation without respiratory or cardiovascular depression and appeared to facilitate the induction and maintenance of anaesthesia. Adverse effects were noted in only a small number of patients ($<1\%$) including restlessness, muscle twitching, athetoid movements, epilepsy and transient hypertension. These mainly occurred after intravenous administration.

Other trials

1. Dodson M E, Eastley R J 1978 Comparative study of two long-acting tranquilizers for oral premedication. British Journal of Anaesthesia 56: 1959–1964

In a double-blind, randomized study, lorazepam 2.5 mg ($n=67$) was compared to promethazine 50 mg ($n=71$) as an oral anaesthetic premedication in 124 women undergoing a total of 138 anaesthetics. Both premedicants were equally effective in relieving anxiety and no significant difference was found between their sedative effects. There was, however, significantly greater salivation and more frequent vomiting in the lorazepam-treated patients as compared to those receiving promethazine, both during and after anaesthesia. Lorazepam had a greater amnesic effect and was associated with fewer side effects.

2. Vella L, Francis D, Houlton P, Reynolds F 1985 Comparison of the antiemetics metoclopramide and promethazine in labour. British Medical Journal 290: 1173–1175

The efficacy of metoclopramide (10 mg) and promethazine (25 mg) as antiemetics when given with pethidine during labour were compared in a double-blind, randomized, placebo-controlled study involving 477 mothers. All medications were given intramuscularly with saline acting as the placebo control.

Both metoclopramide and promethazine were found to be effective antiemetics as compared to placebo, with no difference existing in this respect between the two active treatments. Sedation was more prominent in the promethazine group than in either of the other two groups ($p<0.001$), with 65% of mothers still noticing drowsiness post delivery. The analgesic effect of pethidine was less in the promethazine group than in either metoclopramide or placebo treated patients ($p<0.05$), with greater use of Entonox and a shorter interval between the first and subsequent pethidine injections in those patients receiving promethazine. This study raised the possibility of promethazine having an antianalgesic effect.

General review articles

Pearlman D S 1976 Antihistamines: pharmacology and clinical use. Drugs 12: 258–273

Schuller D E, Turkewitz D 1986 Adverse effects of antihistamines. Postgraduate Medicine 79 (2): 75–86

Wood C D 1979 Antimotion sickness and antiemetic drugs. Drugs 17: 471–479

References

1. Gusdon J P, Moore V, Myrvik Q N, Holyfield P A 1972 Promethazine HCl as an immunosuppressant. Journal of Immunology 108: 1340–1346
2. DeChatelet L R, Qualliotine-Mann D, Caldwell R, McCall C E, Gusdon J P 1973 Effects of promethazine hydrochloride on human polymorphonuclear leucocytes. Infection and Immunity 7: 403–407
3. Gusdon J P, Caudle M R, Herbst G A, Iannuzzi N P 1975 Phagocytosis and erythroblastosis: 1 modification of the neonatal response by promethazine hydrochloride. American Journal of Obstetrics and Gynaecology 125: 224–226
4. Charles A G, Blumenthal L S 1982 Promethazine hydrochloride therapy in severely Rh-sensitized pregnancies. Obstetrics and Gynecology 60: 627–630
5. West G B 1962 Drugs and rat pregnancy. Journal of Pharmacy and Pharmacology 14: 828–830
6. De-Mol N J, Becht A B, Koenen J, Lodder G 1986 Irreversible binding with biological macromolecules and effects in bacterial mutagenicity tests of the radical cation of promethazine and photoactivated promethazine. Comparison with chlorpromazine. Chemical and Biological Interactions 57: 73–83
7. Goethals F, Krack G, Deboyser D, Vossen P, Roberfroid M 1984 Critical biochemical functions of isolated hepatocytes as sensitive indicators of chemical toxicity. Fundamental Applied Toxicology 4: 441–450
8. Clark C H, Nicholson A N 1978 Performance studies with antihistamines. British Journal of Clinical Pharmacology 6: 31–35
9. Kotzan J A, Honigberg I L, Francisco G E, Zaman R, Stewart J T, Brown W J 1986 Rotary pursuit, a measure of human performance, and plasma concentrations of promethazine. Biopharmaceutics and Drug Disposition 7: 293–300
10. Taylor G, Houston J B 1982 Simultaneous determination of promethazine and 2 of its circulating metabolites by high performance liquid chromatography. Journal of Chromatography 230: 194–198
11. Taylor G, Houston J B, Shaffer J, Mawer G 1983 Pharmacokinetics of promethazine and its sulphoxide metabolite after intravenous and oral administration in man. British Journal of Clinical Pharmacology 15: 287–293
12. DiGregorio G J, Ruch E 1980 Human whole blood and parotid saliva concentrations of oral and intramuscular promethazine. Journal of Pharmaceutical Sciences 69: 1457–1459
13. Schwinghammer T L, Dittert L W, Melechil S K, Kroboth F J, Chungi V S 1984 Comparison of the bioavailability of oral, rectal and intramuscular promethazine. Biopharmaceutics and Drug Disposition 5: 185–194
14. Moya F, Thorndike V 1963 The effects of drugs used in labour on the fetus and newborn. Clinical Pharmacology and Therapeutics 4: 628–653
15. Crews S J, Herxheimer H 1952 The protective influence of graded doses of promethazine on induced asthmatic attacks of graded intensity. Internal Archives of Allergy 3: 329–333
16. Editorial 1955 Lancet 2: 1182
17. Krause L, Shuster S 1983 Mechanism of action of antipruritic drugs. British Medical Journal 287: 1199–1200
18. Epstein S 1960 Allergic photocontact dermatitis from promethazine (Phenergan). Archives of Dermatology 81: 175–177
19. Kligman A M 1966 The identification of contact allergens by human assay. Journal of Investigative Dermatology 47: 393–409
20. Adelman M H, Jacobson E, Lief P A, Miller S A 1959 Promethazine hydrochloride in surgery and obstetrics. Journal of the American Medical Association 169: 73–75
21. Dodson M E, Eastley R J 1978 Comparative study of two long-acting tranquillizers for oral premedication. British Journal of Anaesthesia 50: 1059–1064
22. Woodcock A A, Gross E, Geddes D M 1981 Drug treatment of breathlessness: contrasting effects of diazepam and promethazine in pink puffers. British Medical Journal 283: 343–346
23. Carroll J J, Moir R S 1958 Use of promethazine (phenergan) hydrochloride in obstetrics. Journal of the American Medical Association 168: 2218–2224
24. Vella L, Francis D, Houlton P, Reynolds F 1985 Comparison of the antiemetics metoclopramide and promethazine in labour.British Medical Journal 290: 1173–1175
25. Nelson M M, Forfar J O 1971 Association between drugs administered during pregnancy and congenital abnormalities of the fetus. British Medical Journal 1: 523–527
26. Heinonen O P, Slone D, Shapiro S 1977 Birth defects and drugs in pregnancy. Littleton, Publishing Services Group, pp 323–324
27. Wheatley D 1964 Drugs and the embryo. British Medical Journal 1: 630
28. Aselton P, Hershel J, Milunsky A, Hunter J, Stergachis A 1985 First trimester drug use and congenital disorders. Obstetrics and Gynaecology 65: 451–455

29. Wood C D, Graybiel A 1968 Evaluation of sixteen anti-motion-sickness drugs. Aerospace Medicine 39: 1341–1344
30. Graybiel A, Wood C D, Knepton J, Hoche J P, Perkins G F 1975 Human assay of antimotion sickness drugs. Aviation, Space and Environmental Medicine 46: 1107–1118
31. Schroeder D J, Collins W E, Elam G W 1985 Effects of some motion sickness suppressants on static and dynamic tracking performance. Aviation, Space and Environmental Medicine 56: 344–350
32. Collins W E, Schroeder D J, Elam G W 1982 Comparison of some effects of three antimotion sickness drugs on nystagmic responses to angular accelerations and to optokinetic stimuli. Aviation, Space and Environmental Medicine 53: 1182–1189
33. Bierme S, Bierme R 1967 Antihistamines in hydrops foetalis. Lancet 1: 574
34. Gusdon J P 1981 The treatment of erythroblastosis with promethazine hydrochloride. Journal of Reproductive Medicine 26: 454–458
35. Newill R G D 1960 Photosensitivity caused by promethazine. British Medical Journal 2: 359–360
36. Adverse Drug Reactions Advisory Committee 1982 Seven case studies. Medical Journal of Australia 1: 522
37. Connolly S M 1983 Allergic contact dermatitis. Postgraduate Medicine 74: 227–235
38. Girdwood R H 1976 Drug-induced anaemias. Drugs 11: 394–404
39. Skegg D C G, Richards S M, Doll R 1979 Minor tranquillisers and road accidents. British Medical Journal 1: 917–919
40. Kahn A, Hassaerts D, Blum D 1985 Phenothiazine-induced sleep apnoeas in normal infants. Pediatrics 75: 844–847
41. Nahata M C, Clotz M A, Krogg E A 1985 Adverse effects of meperidine, promethazine and chlorpromazine for sedation in pediatric patients. Clinical Pediatrics 24: 558–560
42. Waterhouse G 1967 Epileptiform convulsions in children following premedication with Pamergan SP100. British Journal of Anaesthesia 39: 268–270
43. Kahn A, Blum D 1982 Phenothiazines and sudden infant death syndrome. Pediatrics 70: 75–78
44. Cottraux J, Vedrinne J 1969 Particularités cliniques des intoxications au phénergan. Bulletin Médicale (Paris) 12: 300–306
45. Cliche F 1961 Poisoning by promethazine. Union of Medicine Canada 90: 625–626
46. Lee J H, Turndorf H, Poppers P J 1975 Physostigmine reversal of antihistamine-induced excitement and depression. Anaesthesiology 43: 683–684
47. Montminy M, Terres D 1983 Shock after phenothiazine administration in a pregnant patient with phaeochromocytoma: a case report and literature review. Journal of Reproductive Medicine 28: 159–162
48. Okojie V G 1972 Acute dystonia due to phenothiazines. British Medical Journal 4: 796
49. Porter J, Jick H 1977 Drug-induced anaphylaxis, convulsions, deafness and extrapyramidal symptoms. Lancet 1: 587–588
50. Corby D G, Shulman I 1971 The effects of antenatal drug administration on aggregation of platelets of newborn infants. Journal of Pediatrics 79: 307–313
51. Cook T J, McQueen D M, Wiftig H J, Thornby J I, Lantos R L, Virtue C M 1973 Degree and duration of skin test suppression and side effects with antihistamines. Journal of Allergy and Clinical Immunology 51: 71–77
52. Heinonen O P, Stone D 1977 Birth defects and drugs in pregnancy. Littleton, Publishing Sciences Group, p 437
53. Greenberg G, Inman W H, Weatherall J A C, Adelstein A M, Hasky J C 1977 Maternal drug histories and congenital abnormalities. British Medical Journal 2: 853–856
54. Winter C A 1948 Potentiating effect of antihistaminic drugs upon sedative action of barbiturates. Journal of Pharmacology and Experimental Therapeutics 94: 7–11
55. Long W F, Taylor R J, Leavengood D C, Nelson H S 1985 Skin test suppression by antihistamines and the development of subsensitivity. Journal of Allergy and Clinical Immunology 76: 113–117
56. Empey D W, Bye C, Hodder M, Hughes D T D 1975 A double-blind crossover trial of pseudoephedrine and triprolidine, alone and in combination for the treatment of allergic rhinitis. Annals of Allergy 34: 41–46

Propafenone (hydrochloride)

Propafenone is a Class I antiarrhythmic drug for the management of ventricular rhythm disorders.

Chemistry

Propafenone hydrochloride (Arythmol, Rytmonorm, Rythmol, Normorytmin, Ritmonorm)
$C_{21}H_{27}NO_3.HCl$
2-[2-Hydroxy-3-(propylamino)propoxy]-3-phenyl-propiophenone hydrochloride

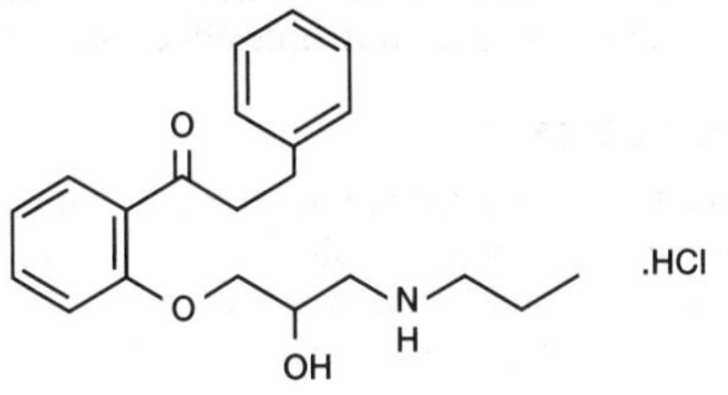

Molecular weight (free base)	377.9 (341.4)
pKa	8.8
Solubility	
in alcohol	1 in 100 to 1 in 1000
in water	low
Octanol/water partition coefficient	40

Colourless crystals or white crystalline powder with a very bitter taste and faint odour; it is prepared by chemical synthesis and the racemate is used clinically.

Pharmacology

Propafenone blocks the fast inward sodium current in all cardiac tissues and in other excitable tissues, like the central nervous system. It thus causes a dose-related, use-dependent reduction of the maximum rate and amplitude of depolarization, phase 0 of the action potential.[1,2] Propafenone can be classified in Class Ic of antiarrhythmic drugs, since it prolongs P-R and QRS electrocardiographic intervals, with little or no effect on QTc.[3,4] However, the classification is not straightforward, since propafenone prolongs action potential duration, like Class III drugs. It also has some β-blocking action, much less than that of propranolol, and a weak calcium-channel-blocking effect.[3–5] The l-isomer of propafenone has been shown to have a much higher binding affinity than the d-isomer for β-adrenoceptors from rat brain cortex and cerebellum.[6] The reversed order of potency was shown for human lymphocyte β_2-adrenoceptors.[7]

Toxicology

Propafenone does not have mutagenic potential, as shown by current in vitro tests. The drug does not have teratological effects in rabbits and rats treated with doses 10 to 40 times higher than the effective clinical doses on a $mg.kg^{-1}$ body weight basis. The highest doses were toxic to the dams. There is no evidence of carcinogenicity in tests lasting up to 25 months in rats and rabbits.

Clinical pharmacology

Propafenone has several electrophysiological actions in man. It has variable effects, but generally slows the activity of the sinoatrial node and prolongs sinoatrial conduction time (AH interval). Propafenone slows atrioventricular conduction by prolonging intranodal and intraventricular conduction times (HV interval). P-Q and QRS intervals are significantly increased with little change in the QTc interval.[3,4] Propafenone significantly increases atrial effective and functional refractory periods and, to a lesser extent, atrioventricular node effective refractory period. Effective refractory periods of the ventricle and of the accessory pathways, antegrade and retrograde (Wolff–Parkinson–White syndrome), are increased by propafenone.[8–11] Suppression of premature ventricular beats, another action of propafenone, lasts 2 to 4 hours after single oral doses, but 8 to 12 hours during multiple dosing.[12] Duration of arrhythmia suppression is proportional to the dose.[13] Most patients respond to doses of 300 mg two or three times daily; higher doses are seldom used, due to higher risk of adverse drug reactions.[13–16]

β-Blocking activity has been demonstrated in man by a shift to the right of the dose–heart rate response curve to isoprenaline in healthy volunteers, with a potency relative to propranolol of 1:40.[5] Blood pressure at rest and during exercise is not greatly affected by propafenone. Duration of this effect, after single oral doses of 150–300 mg, ranged from 1 to 3 hours. Basal heart rate did not change significantly, but it was slightly decreased at exercise.[5,17] The clinical relevance of this action seems low,[18] at least at concentrations[19] lower than 1 mg.l^{-1}. Like other Class I antiarrhythmic drugs, propafenone exerts a negative inotropic effect on the myocardium.[20]

Pharmacokinetics

The preferred method for assaying unchanged drug in plasma is high performance liquid chromatography,[21] which has a sensitivity of 50 μg.l^{-1}. Other assays have become available which allow simultaneous determination of the active metabolite, 5-OH-propafenone.[22–24]

Propafenone is absorbed almost completely after oral administration and peak plasma concentrations occur 2 to 3 hours later; in some cases, a lag of 0.5 to 2 hours is observed. Propafenone undergoes extensive presystemic metabolism and bioavailability is dose-related. Food increases propafenone bioavailability.[25] Bioavailability of single oral doses of 150, 300 and 450 mg were found to be 13%, 32% and 55%, respectively, in healthy volunteers.[26] In patients, a rise in the daily dose from 300 to 900 mg caused a ten-fold increase in average steady-state plasma concentrations of the drug.[14]

Oral absorption	>95%
Presystemic metabolism	30–90% dose dependent
Plasma half life	
mean	3.6 h
range	2.4–10 h
Volume of distribution	3.6 l.kg^{-1}
Plasma protein binding	≥80%

Plasma elimination half life is about 3.6 hours in healthy volunteers,[26] but longer in patients, about 6 hours, ranging from 2.4 to more than 10 hours, after multiple doses.[27] Plasma half life and bioavailability of propafenone markedly increase during chronic treatment.[12] The large volume of distribution of about 3.6 l.kg^{-1} body weight indicates high tissue affinity.[27] In fact, the drug shows accumulation in lung and liver samples obtained at autopsy; very low concentrations were found in brain. The metabolite, 5-OH-propafenone, reaches concentrations comparable to those of the parent drug.[28,29] About 10% of the Caucasian population are poor 5-hydroxylators of propafenone and this characteristic can be predicted from their oxidative capacity for debrisoquine, as shown in vitro[41] and in vivo.[18,38] These patients eliminate propafenone with a half life 3-4 times longer than the rest of the population and seem to require higher plasma concentrations of propafenone for the same response.[19] This suggests that therapeutic action depends also upon the metabolite 5-OH-propafenone. Plasma protein binding, in the therapeutic concentration range, is about 80%.[30]

Atrium/plasma concentration ratio of propafenone in surgical patients has been found to be 10, while that of 5-OH-propafenone is 20.[31] Propafenone and, probably, 5-OH-propafenone cross the placental barrier.[32]

Since propafenone is extensively metabolized in the liver, it is expected that hepatic cirrhosis reduces its clearance and increases its bioavailability.[33] Limited data are available on the effect of renal failure on propafenone disposition kinetics.[34,35]

Concentration–effect relationship

A good correlation was found between propafenone plasma concentrations and atrioventricular conduction time.[36] The correlation between premature ventricular beat suppression and propafenone concentration shows marked interindividual variability; concentrations ranging from 64 to 1044 μg.l^{-1} (mean 588 μg.l^{-1}) suppressed isolated premature ventricular beats in all patients who responded to propafenone (11/13), while slightly lower levels (mean 443 μg.l^{-1}) were needed for couplet suppression.[14,19] Similar results were obtained following protocols not expressly designed for thorough evaluation of concentration–response curves in individual patients.[15,16,37,38] The wide interindividual variability in concentration–response relationship and the presence of at least one active metabolite, 5-OH-propafenone, in plasma, make it difficult or even impossible to use propafenone plasma concentrations as guidelines for effective treatment.

Metabolism

Propafenone is extensively metabolized in the liver and excreted almost exclusively (90% of an oral dose) as metabolites in faeces (53%) and urine (18–38%).[39] Six pathways of metabolism have been described: conjugation of the alcohol group with glucuronic acid, ether cleavage, oxidation reactions at the aromatic rings, cleavage to phenylpropionic acid, oxidative deamination and dealkylation (Fig. 1). Seven patients (extensive metabolizers) on propafenone 150 mg three times daily excreted in urine, during a dosing interval, 20 mg of unchanged drug, 54 mg as 5-OH-propafenone and 4 mg as N-depropyl-propafenone.[40]

Fig. 1 Metabolism of propafenone

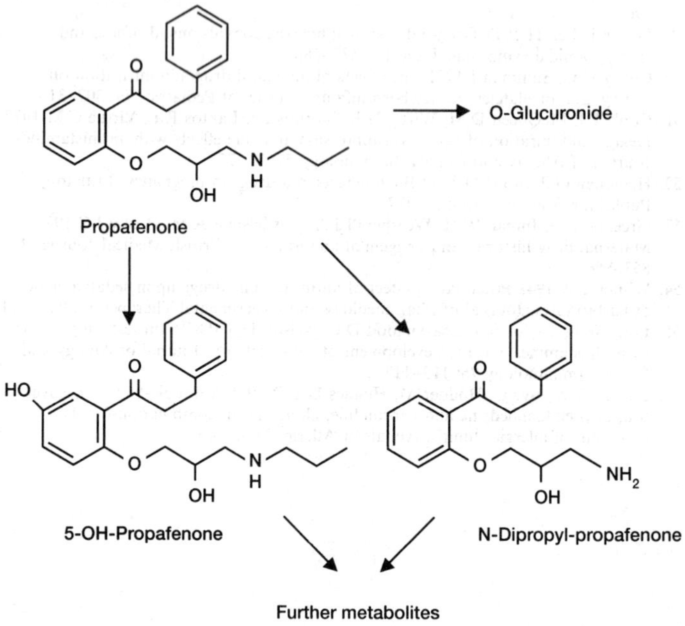

The polymorphic oxidative pathway to 5-OH-propafenone in man is saturable and seems to be the rate-limiting step of propafenone metabolism.

Two metabolites, 5-OH-propafenone and N-depropylpropafenone, are found in plasma of patients chronically treated with propafenone.[23] They seem to have negative inotropic effects but a much lower β-blocking effect than the parent compound.[42–44] The antiarrhythmic activity of 5-OH-propafenone against ventricular arrhythmias in dogs and in rats has been shown to be higher than that of propafenone and N-depropylpropafenone.[42,43]

Pharmaceutics

Propafenone Arythmol (Knoll, UK) is available in oral form, as tablets containing 150 and 300 mg of propafenone hydrochloride. The tablets are white and film-coated. The maximum shelf-life of propafenone tablets is 5 years. The intravenous formulation is not available on the market in the UK, but is available on a named-patient basis. It has been launched in several countries including Italy, West Germany, Ireland and the Netherlands.

Therapeutic use

Indications

1. Treatment and prophylaxis of ventricular arrhythmias
2. Treatment and prophylaxis of supraventricular arrhythmias, including Wolff–Parkinson–White syndrome.

Contraindications

1. Severe congestive heart failure, cardiogenic shock (except arrhythmia-induced) and marked hypotension
2. Severe bradycardia, uncontrolled electrolyte disturbance, sinus node dysfunction, atrial conduction defects, second degree or greater AV block, bundle branch block or distal block (unless adequately paced)
3. Severe obstructive pulmonary disorders.

Mode of use

The individual maintenance dose should be determined under cardiological surveillance including ECG and blood pressure monitoring. Daily doses from 450 to 900 mg (150 to 300 mg three times daily) are generally recommended and therapy initiated under hospital conditions. Initially 150 mg three times daily increasing at a minimum of three day intervals to 300 mg twice daily and, if necessary to a maximum of 300 mg three times daily. A reduction in total daily dose is recommended for patients below 70 kg body weight.

Indications

1. Ventricular hyperkinetic arrhythmias
Treatment and prophylaxis of various types of ventricular arrhythmias is the main therapeutic indication of propafenone. The efficacy of propafenone in suppressing isolated, frequent premature ventricular beats is shown by several studies. Most of them were short term (less than 6 months), some were open,[12–16,37,38,45,46] and in others propafenone was compared to placebo or to other antiarrhythmic drugs. Propafenone was reported to have a variable efficacy similar or higher than quinidine,[47] disopyramide,[48] mexiletine, flecainide, amiodarone[49] and lorajmine.[50] Propafenone also prevents the recurrence of ventricular tachycardia or fibrillation[9,37,51] and ventricular tachycardia reinduction on electrophysiological study.[9,52] The drug is effective in patients with ventricular arrhythmias in the presence of cardiac disease, impaired ventricular function or coronary heart disease.[9,15,20,53] Few data are available on the long-term efficacy of propafenone in a large number of patients. However, in one study, 80% of patients continued to respond to propafenone after two years of treatment.[46]

2. Supraventricular arrhythmias
The drug has been used with some success in patients with Wolff–Parkinson–White syndrome, complicated by atrial fibrillation or bypass tract tachycardia although this indication is not licensed in the UK.[10] The partial or total suppression of recurrences of symptomatic tachycardias has been shown over an average follow-up of more than two years; some cases of tachycardia, reinducible after propafenone administration during the acute electrophysiologic study, responded in the long term.[10] The drug is effective in terminating re-entry Wolff–Parkinson–White tachycardias when given intravenously.[54] Propafenone seems to be effective in atrial flutter or fibrillation, but experience is limited.[55–57] In some cases, when the adrenergic tone has a pathogenetic role, the β-blocking action of propafenone may contribute a small component of its antiarrhythmic action.[55]

Contraindications

1. Severe congestive heart failure, cardiogenic shock and marked hypotension
Propafenone has some negative inotropic effect, which is why it should be used with caution in patients with severe congestive heart failure or low cardiac output in general. Reports on negative inotropism of propafenone are contradictory, but it seems that this adverse effect is more likely to occur at total daily doses of 900 mg or more, in patients with low left ventricular ejection fraction.[11,20,45,51] Therapy for control of symptomatic cardiac heart failure should be continued after the patient is put on propafenone, while uncontrolled cardiac heart failure is an absolute contraindication to propafenone treatment.

2. Conduction abnormalities and bradycardias
Propafenone may produce dangerous bradycardias and conduction abnormalities most often in patients with underlying abnormalities of the sinoatrial or atrioventricular node or intraventricular conduction. Its β-blocking effect probably contributes to this action.

3. Severe obstructive pulmonary diseases
Propafenone, having a β-blocking action, can cause bronchoconstriction and possibly worsen symptoms of dyspnoea in patients with severe obstructive pulmonary disease. However, this adverse effect is reported only rarely in cardiac patients.[38,49] Propafenone has been shown to slightly decrease the dose of methacholine required to reduce FEV_1 by 20%.[58]

Adverse reactions

Potentially life-threatening effects
Propafenone can cause bradycardia, sinoatrial, atrioventricular or intraventricular blocks, or severe hypotension, particularly in the elderly, and worsen heart failure in patients with pre-existing organic heart disease. Like most antiarrhythmic drugs, propafenone has been reported to worsen or cause new severe ventricular arrhythmias, like ventricular tachycardia or fibrillation, in a limited number of patients.[9,14,59] The drug can also aggravate electrically induced ventricular tachycardia in some patients.[60] All these effects seem unrelated to dose or plasma concentration.

Acute overdosage
In cases of acute intoxication, emesis should be attempted if ingestion is recent; haemodialysis is not useful because of the large volume of distribution of propafenone. The usual emergency measures for cardiovascular resuscitation should be applied, like atropine and isoprenaline for bradycardia and sinoatrial or atrioventricular block, and inotropic agents for myocardial insufficiency. No specific antidotes are available. Convulsions should be treated with intravenous diazepam.

Severe or irreversible adverse effects
The adverse effects described immediately above can also be listed here as well, since they may often occur with less severity.

Symptomatic adverse effects
Neurological adverse effects include dizziness, headache, visual disturbances, vertigo, blurred vision, and dry mouth, and are similar to those reported for other Class I antiarrhythmic drugs reflecting inhibition of the fast inward sodium current in neural tissue. They occur occasionally, but generally do not necessitate drug withdrawal. Nausea, constipation, diarrhoea and alteration of taste have also been reported. All the above-mentioned effects generally disappear on prompt dose reduction or discontinuation of the drug. Average leucocyte count decreased significantly from 6800 ± 1800 to $5900 \pm 1500\ mm^{-3}$ in 45 patients over a mean follow-up of 12.4 months;[15] the clinical relevance is unknown. Other laboratory tests are usually not altered. Allergic skin reactions such as reddening, pruritus, exanthema or urticaria may occur infrequently. Rare cases of individual hypersensitivity reactions (cholestatis, blood dyscrasias, lupus syndrome) and seizures have been reported. All were reversible on discontinuation of treatment.

Interference with clinical pathology tests
No technical interferences of this kind have been reported.

High risk groups

Neonates
Propafenone is not recommended for use in this age-group because a suitable dose has still to be established (also see Children).

Breast milk. It is probably best if women who have to be given the drug do not breast-feed.

Children
Limited experience on children aged 1 to 15 has indicated as safe and

effective oral doses of 12–22 mg.kg^{-1} daily, divided in 3–4 individual doses.[61] The drug has been given intravenously to 7 patients aged 11 days to 4 years in order to control ventricular rate in postoperative junctional ectopic tachycardia.[62]

Pregnant women

Although animal studies have not shown any teratogenic effects, propafenone should not be used during pregnancy unless, in the clinician's judgement, it is essential for the welfare of the patient.

The elderly

Higher plasma levels of propafenone have been noted in chronically treated elderly people, so these patients may respond to a lower dose.[63,64]

Concurrent disease

Impaired renal function. Although the elimination of propafenone and its major metabolite is not affected by renal, impairment, propafenone should be administered cautiously in these patients.[34,35]

Impaired liver function. Propafenone is extensively metabolized via a saturable hepatic oxidative pathway. In view of the increased bioavailability and elimination half life of propafenone, a reduction in the recommended dose may be necessary.[3]

Cardiac pacemakers. Propafenone has been shown to alter pacing sensitivity and pacing threshold. In patients with pacemakers, appropriate adjustments may be required.

Drug interactions

Potentially hazardous interactions

Digoxin steady-state plasma concentrations rose in all five patients treated with propafenone, with an average increase of 83%.[6,45] No patient had evidence of digitalis toxicity.

The effect of propafenone may be potentiated if given in combination with local anaesthetics or other drugs which inhibit the heart rate and/or contractility, e.g. β-blockers. In particular, propafenone has been shown to raise steady-state concentrations of metoprolol, causing adverse effects in 2/8 patients,[66] and of proprandol. Dose reduction of these β-blockers may be required. Concomitant intravenous infusion of lignocaine and propafenone resulted in a mild additive negative inotropic effect.[68] The combination of propafenone with procainamide or quinidine allows a reduction of the propafenone doses, compared to monotherapy, maintaining the same antiarrhythmic effects.[69] Quinidine has been shown to increase more than two-fold propafenone steady-state concentrations in extensive metabolizers, but not in poor metabolizers. Propafenone potentiates the anticoagulant effect of warfarin.[70]

Other significant interactions

Cimetidine. Cimetidine caused significant increases in the maximum serum concentration, steady-state serum concentration and area-under-curve of propafenone in 12 volunteers,[71] although the increased propafenone levels did not appear to be clinically important. In addition, propafenone caused an acceleration in the gastrointestinal absorption of cimetidine and increased its maximum plasma concentration; elimination half life and steady-state concentrations of cimetidine were unchanged.

Potentially useful interactions

No interactions of this type appear to have been reported.

Clinical trials

Many clinical studies have been published on propafenone, involving up to 226 patients,[13] some of them including a long-term follow-up of 2–3 years (see references under the heading Therapeutic uses). None fulfils all the requisites of a high quality trial in a restrictive sense (i.e. randomized, controlled, hard end-points, long term).

General review articles

Harron D W G, Brogden R N 1987 Propafenone. A review of its pharmacodynamic and pharmacokinetic properties, and therapeutic use in the treatment of arrhythmias. Drugs 34: 617–647

Salerno D M, Hodges M 1985 New therapy focus: propafenone. Cardiovascular Reviews and Reports 6: 924–931

Seipel L, Breithardt G 1980 Propafenone. A new antiarrhythmic drug. European Heart Journal 1: 309–313

Somberg J C, Tepper D, Landau S 1988 Propafenone: a new antiarrhythmic agent. American Heart Journal 115: 1274–1279

Zipes D P 1984 Recent advances in antiarrhythmic therapy: symposium on propafenone. American Journal of Cardiology 54: 9

References

1. Thompson K A, Iansmith D H S, Siddoway L A et al 1988 Potent electrophysiologic effects of the major metabolites of propafenone in canine Purkinje fibers. Journal of Pharmacology and Experimental Therapeutics 244: 950–955
2. Kohlhardt M, Seifert C 1980 Inhibition of V_{max} of the action potential by propafenone and its voltage-, time-and pH-dependence in mammalian ventricular myocardium. Naunyn-Schmiedeberg's Archives of Pharmacology 315: 55–62
3. Dukes I D, Vaughan Williams E M 1984 The multiple modes of action of propafenone. European Heart Journal 5: 115–125
4. Ledda F, Mantelli L, Manzini S, Amerini S, Mugelli A 1981 Electrophysiological and antiarrhythmic properties of propafenone in isolated cardiac preparations. Journal of Cardiovascular Pharmacology 3: 1162–1173
5. McLeod A A, Stiles G L, Shand D G 1984 Demonstration of beta adrenoceptor blockade by propafenone hydrochloride: clinical pharmacologic, radioligand binding and adenylate cyclase activation studies. Journal of Pharmacology and Experimental Therapeutics 228: 461–466
6. Burnett D M, Gal J, Zahniser N R, Nies A S 1988 Propafenone interacts stereoselectively with β_1 and β_2-adrenergic receptors. Journal of Cardiovascular Pharmacology 12: 615–619
7. Kroemer H K, Funck-Brentano C, Silberstein D J et al 1989 Stereoselective disposition and pharmacologic activity of propafenone enantiomers. Circulation 79: 1068–1076
8. Seipel L, Breithardt G 1980 Propafenone. A new antiarrhythmic drug. European Heart Journal 1: 309–313
9. Connolly S J, Kates R E, Lebsack C S, Echt D S, Mason J W, Winkle R A 1983 Clinical efficacy and electrophysiology of oral propafenone for ventricular tachycardia. American Journal of Cardiology 52: 1208–1213
10. Breithardt G, Borggrefe M, Weibringhaus E, Seipel L 1984 Effect of propafenone in the Wolff–Parkinson–White syndrome: electrophysiologic findings and long-term follow-up. American Journal of Cardiology 54: 29D–39D
11. Shen E N, Sung R J, Morady F et al 1984 Electrophysiologic and hemodynamic effects of intravenous propafenone in patients with recurrent ventricular tachycardia. Journal of the American College of Cardiology 3: 1291–1297
12. Giani P, Landolina M, Guidici V et al 1988 The pharmacokinetics and pharmacodynamics of propafenone during acute and chronic administration. European Journal of Clinical Pharmacology 34: 187–194
13. Singh B N, Kaplinsky E, Kirsten E et al 1988 Effects of propafenone on ventricular arrhythmias: double-blind, parallel, randomized, placebo-controlled dose-ranging study. American Heart Journal 116: 1542–1551
14. Connolly S J, Kates R E, Lebsack C S, Harrison D C, Winkle R A 1983 Clinical pharmacology of propafenone. Circulation 68: 589–596
15. Hammill S C, Sorenson P B, Wood D L et al 1986 Propafenone for the treatment of refractory complex ventricular ectopic activity. Mayo Clinic Proceedings 61: 98–103
16. Frabetti L, Marchesini B, Capucci A et al 1986 Antiarrhythmic efficacy of propafenone: evaluation of effective plasma levels following single and multiple doses. European Journal of Clinical Pharmacology 30: 665–671
17. Muller-Peltzer H, Greger G, Neugebauer G, Hollmann M 1983 Beta-blocking and electrophysiological effects of propafenone in volunteers. European Journal of Clinical Pharmacology 25: 831–833
18. Cheriex E C, Krijne R, Brugada P, Heymeriks J, Wellens H J J 1987 Lack of clinically significant beta-blocking effect of propafenone. European Heart Journal 8: 53–56
19. Zoble R G, Kirsten E B, Brewington J and the Propafenone Research Group 1989 Pharmacokinetic and pharmacodynamic evaluation of propafenone in patients with ventricular arrhythmia. Clinical Pharmacology and Therapeutics 45: 535–541
20. Baker B J, Dinh H, Kroskey D, de Soyza N D B, Murphy M L, Franciosa J A 1984 Effect of propafenone on left ventricular ejection fraction. American Journal of Cardiology 54: 20D–22D
21. Harapat S R, Kates R E 1982 High-performance liquid chromatographic analysis of propafenone in human plasma samples. Journal of Chromatography 230: 448–453
22. Brode E, Kripp U, Hollmann M 1984 Simultaneous determination of propafenone and 5-hydroxypropafenone in plasma by means of high pressure liquid chromatography. Arzneimittelforschung 34: 1455–1460
23. Kates R E, Yee Y G, Winkle R A 1985 Metabolite cumulation during chronic propafenone dosing in arrhythmia. Clinical Pharmacology and Therapeutics 37: 610–614
24. Latini R, Sica A, Marchi S, Chen Z, Gavinelli M, Benfenati E 1988 High-performance liquid chromatographic separation and mass spectrometric identification of propafenone, 5-hydroxypropafenone and N-depropylpropafenone. Journal of Chromatography 424: 211–214
25. Axelson J E, Chan G L-Y, Kirsten E B, Mason W D, Lanman R C, Kerr C R 1987 Food increases the bioavailability of propafenone. British Journal of Clinical Pharmacology 23: 735–741
26. Hollmann M, Brode E, Hotz D, Kaumeier S, Kehrhahn O H 1983 Investigations on the pharmacokinetics of propafenone in man. Arzneimittelforschung 33: 763–770
27. Connolly S, Lebsack C, Winkle R A, Harrison D C, Kates R E 1984 Propafenone disposition kinetics in cardiac arrhythmia. Clinical Pharmacology and Therapeutics 36: 163–168

28. Blanke H, Aschbrenner B, Karsch K R, Kreuzer H 1979 Plasmaspiegel-wirkungs-beziehung und organverteilung von propafenon. Deutsche Medizinische Wochenschrift 104: 587–591
29. Latini R, Marchi S, Riva E et al 1987 Distribution of propafenone and its active metabolite, 5-hydroxypropafenone, in human tissues. American Heart Journal 113: 843–844
30. Higuchi S, Urano C, Kawamura S 1985 Determination of plasma protein binding of propafenone in rats, dogs and humans by highly sensitive gas chromatography–mass spectrometry. Journal of Chromatography 341: 305–311
31. Latini R, Barbieri E, Castello C et al 1989 Propafenone and 5-hydroxypropafenone concentrations in the right atrium of patients undergoing heart surgery. American Heart Journal 117: 497–498
32. Brunozzi L T, Meniconi L, Chiocchi P, Liberati R, Zuanetti G, Latini R 1988 Propafenone in the treatment of chronic ventricular arrhythmias in a pregnant patient. British Journal of Clinical Pharmacology 26: 489–490
33. Lee J T, Yee Y G, Dorian P, Kates R E 1987 Influence of hepatic dysfunction on the pharmacokinetics of propafenone. Journal of Clinical Pharmacology 27: 384–389
34. Burgess E, Duff H, Wilkes P 1989 Propafenone disposition in renal insufficiency and renal failure. Journal of Clinical Pharmacology 29: 112–113
35. Burgess E D, Duff H J 1989 Hemodialysis removal of propafenone. Pharmacotherapy 9: 331–333
36. Keller K, Meyer-Estorf G, Beck O A, Hochrein H 1978 Correlation between serum concentration and pharmacological effect on atrioventricular conduction time of the antiarrhythmic drug propafenone. European Journal of Clinical Pharmacology 13: 17–20
37. Naccarella F, Bracchetti D, Palmieri M, Marchesini B, Ambrosioni E 1984 Propafenone for refractory ventricular arrhythmias: correlation with drug plasma levels during long-term treatment. American Journal of Cardiology 54: 1008–1014
38. Siddoway L A, Thompson K A, McAllister D B et al 1987 Polymorphism of propafenone metabolism and disposition in man: clinical and pharmacokinetic consequences. Circulation 75: 785–791
39. Hege H G, Hollmann M, Kaumeier S, Lietz H 1984 The metabolic fate of ^{2}H-labelled propafenone in man. European Journal of Drug Metabolism and Pharmacokinetics 9: 41–55
40. Funk-Brentano C, Kroemer H K, Pavlou H et al 1989 Genetically-determined interaction between propafenone and low dose quinidine: role of active metabolites in modulating net drug effect. British Journal of Clinical Pharmacology 27: 435–444
41. Kroemer H K, Mikus G, Kronbach T et al 1989 In vitro characterization of the human cytochrome P-450 involved in polymorphic oxidation of propafenone. Clinical Pharmacology and Therapeutics 45: 28–33
42. Philipsborn G V, Gries J, Hofmann H P et al 1984 Pharmacological studies on propafenone and its main metabolite 5-hydroxypropafenone. Arzneimittelforschung 34: 1489–1497
43. Malfatto G, Zaza A, Forster M, Sodowick B, Danilo P Jr, Rosen M R 1988 Electrophysiologic, inotropic and antiarrhythmic effects of propafenone, 5-hydroxypropafenone and N-depropylpropafenone. Journal of Pharmacology and Experimental Therapeutics 246: 419–426
44. Valenzuela C, Delgado C, Tamargo J 1987 Electrophysiological effects of 5-hydroxypropafenone on guinea pig ventricular muscle fibres. Journal of Cardiovascular Pharmacology 10: 523–529
45. Salerno D M, Granrud G, Sharkey P, Asinger R, Hodges M 1984 A controlled trial of propafenone for treatment of frequent and repetitive ventricular premature complexes. American Journal of Cardiology 53: 77–83
46. Dinh H A, Baker B J, de Soyza N, Murphy M L 1988 Sustained therapeutic efficacy and safety of oral propafenone for treatment of chronic ventricular arrhythmias: a 2-year experience. American Heart Journal 115: 92–96
47. Dinh H A, Murphy M L, Baker B J, de Soyza N, Franciosa J A 1985 Efficacy of propafenone compared with quinidine in chronic ventricular arrhythmias. American Journal of Cardiology 55: 1520–1524
48. Naccarella F, Bracchetti D, Palmieri M, Cantelli I, Bertaccini P, Ambrosioni E 1985 Comparison of propafenone and disopyramide for treatment of chronic ventricular arrhythmias: placebo-controlled, double-blind, randomized crossover study. American Heart Journal 109: 833–840
49. Harron D W G, Brogden R N 1987 Propafenone. A review of its pharmacodynamic and pharmacokinetic properties, and therapeutic use in the treatment of arrhythmias. Drugs 34: 617–647
50. Sanna G, Meoli P, Bianchini C, Rovelli F 1983 Antiarrhythmic effectiveness of propafenone compared to lorajmine in ventricular arrhythmias. Giornale Italiano Cardiologia 13: 145–151
51. Podrid P J, Lown B 1984 Propafenone: a new agent for ventricular arrhythmia. Journal of the American College of Cardiology 4: 117–125
52. Heger J J, Hubbard J, Zipes D P, Miles W M, Prystowsky E N 1984 Propafenone treatment of recurrent ventricular tachycardia: comparison of continuous electrocardiographic recording and electrophysiologic study in predicting drug efficacy. American Journal of Cardiology 54: 40D–44D
53. Brodsky M A, Allen B J, Abate D, Henry W L 1985 Propafenone therapy for ventricular tachycardia in the setting of congestive heart failure. American Heart Journal 110: 794–799
54. Shen E N, Keung E, Huycke E et al 1986 Intravenous propafenone for termination of reentrant supraventricular tachycardia: a placebo-controlled, randomized, double-blind, crossover study. Annals of Internal Medicine 105: 655–661
55. Coumel P, Leclercq J-F, Assayag P 1984 European experience with the antiarrhythmic efficacy of propafenone for supraventricular and ventricular arrhythmias. American Journal of Cardiology 54: 60D–66D
56. Hammill S C, Wood D L, Gersh B J, Osborn M J, Holmes D R Jr 1988 Propafenone for paroxysmal atrial fibrillation. American Journal of Cardiology 61: 473–474
57. Kerr C R, Klein G J, Axelson J E, Cooper J C 1988 Propafenone for prevention of recurrent atrial fibrillation. American Journal of Cardiology 61: 914–916

58. Hill M R, Gotz V P, Harman E, McLeod I, Hendeles L 1986 Evaluation of the asthmogenicity of propafenone, a new antiarrhythmic drug: comparison of spirometry with methacholine challenge. Chest 90: 698–702
59. Buss J, Neuss H, Bilgin Y, Schlepper M 1985 Malignant ventricular tachyarrhythmias in association with propafenone treatment. European Heart Journal 6: 424–428
60. Stavens C S, McGovern B, Garan H, Ruskin J N 1985 Aggravation of electrically provoked ventricular tachycardia during treatment with propafenone. American Heart Journal 110: 24–29
61. Dressler F, Gravinghoff I, Grutte E et al 1985 Die behandlung von herzrhythmusstorungen mit propafenon bei sauglingen und kindern. Monatsschrift Kinderheilkunde 133: 154–157
62. Moak J P, Smith R T, Garson A Jr 1987 Newer antiarrhythmic drugs in children. American Heart Journal 113: 179–185
63. Lachnit K S, Rieder L 1985 Die bedeutung von herzrhythmusstorungen im alter und ihre behandlung mit propafenon unter kontrolle des plasmaspiegels. Zeitschrift Gerontologie 18: 343–352
64. Camovs J P, Benoit P, Vrancea F et al 1987 Propafenone in ventricular extrasystoles of elderly patients. Annals of Cardiology and Angiology 36: 179–182
65. Calvo M V, Martin-Suarez A, Luengo C M, Avila C, Cascon M, Dominguez-Gil Hurlé A 1989 Interaction between digoxin and propafenone. Therapeutic Drug Monitoring 11: 10–15
66. Wagner F, Kalusche D, Trenk D, Jahnchen E, Roskamm H 1987 Drug interaction between propafenone and metoprolol. British Journal of Clinical Pharmacology 24: 213–220
67. Kowey P R, Kirsten E B, Fu C-H J, Mason W D 1989 Interaction between propranolol and propafenone in healthy volunteers. Journal of Clinical Pharmacology 29: 512–517
68. Feld G K, Nademanee K, Singh B N, Kirsten E 1987 Hemodynamic and electrophysiologic effects of combined infusion of lidocaine and propafenone in humans. Journal of Clinical Pharmacology 27: 52–55
69. Klein R C, Huang S K, Marcus F I et al 1987 Enhanced antiarrhythmic efficacy of propafenone when used in combination with procainamide or quinidine. American Heart Journal 114: 551–558
70. Kates R E, Yee Y-G, Kirsten E B 1987 Interaction between warfarin and propafenone in healthy volunteer subjects. Clinical Pharmacology and Therapeutics 42: 305–311
71. Pritchett E L C, Smith W M, Kirsten E B 1988 Pharmacokinetic and pharmacodynamic interactions of propafenone and cimetidine. Journal of Clinical Pharmacology 28: 619–624

P

Propantheline bromide

Propantheline is a synthetic quaternary ammonium compound and is one of the most widely used synthetic antimuscarinics.

Chemistry

Propantheline bromide (Pro-Banthine, Pantheline, Ercoril)
$C_{23}H_{30}Br\ NO_3$
Di-isopropylmethyl [2-(xanthen-9-ylcarbonyloxy)ethyl]ammonium bromide

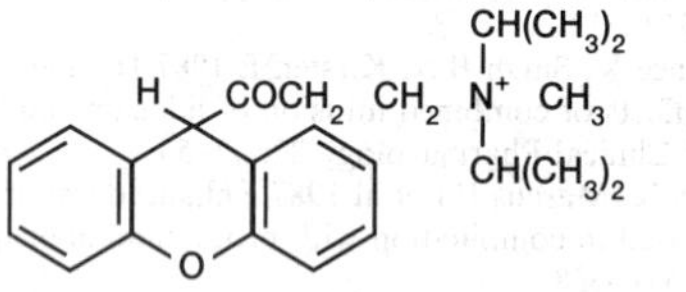

Molecular weight	448.5
pKa	—
Solubility	
in alcohol	high
in water	high
Octanol/water partition coefficient	—

Propantheline is a white or yellowish-white, odourless, hygroscopic powder with a very bitter taste, prepared by chemical synthesis. The isopropyl group replacing the ethyl group of methantheline (Banthine) makes it two to five times more potent.

Pharmacology

Propantheline has similar pharmacological properties to methantheline but is more potent. It has a much higher ratio of ganglion-blocking to antimuscarinic properties than atropine, i.e. it has greater potency at nicotinic receptors. It can therefore cause ganglion blockade at high dose and neuromuscular blockade with a large overdose.

Toxicology

Reproduction studies have not been carried out in animals. Cohort data on parasympatholytics indicate a possible association with minor malformations.

Clinical pharmacology

Propantheline has similar peripheral (muscarinic) effects to atropine. As it is poorly absorbed from the conjunctiva it is of little value in ophthalmology. As it is highly polar it is also unreliably absorbed by the oral route, does not readily cross the blood–brain barrier and so has little central effect.

Propantheline's major muscarinic action and main therapeutic indication is to inhibit gastrointestinal motility and, to a lesser extent, gastric secretion. It has long been believed that these effects were produced only at doses associated with side effects due to muscarinic block.[1] It was therefore recommended that doses should be individually titrated to the 'optimal' dose, just below that at which the undesirable side effects of dry mouth and blurred vision occurred. It has been shown, however, that food-stimulated gastric acid secretion is reduced to the same extent at the low dose of 15 mg orally as after near toxic doses (mean 48 mg).[2] These workers also showed that low-dose propantheline potentiated cimetidine-inhibited gastric acid secretion.

Propantheline delays gastric emptying two-fold in almost all subjects at an oral dose of 30 mg.[3] At this dose salivary flow decreased ten-fold and heart rate increased by 25% at one hour, but blurring of vision did not occur. These findings, using gamma camera counting of a radioisotope-labelled test meal, confirm previous studies on gastric emptying, measuring paracetamol and ethanol absorption.[4,5]

It has been suggested that the antispasmodic action of quaternary ammonium compounds is enhanced by a relatively specific ganglion-blocking action in the gut.

Pharmacokinetics

A simple and sensitive high performance liquid chromatographic (HPLC) method has been developed for assay in biological fluids.[6] This method can detect as little as 2 pmol per injection. Other methods are complex and lengthy or require gas chromatography–mass spectrometry.

Because of the low lipid solubility of propantheline (like that of the other quaternary ammonium compounds) systemic bioavailability is little more than 10%,[7] so that parenteral propantheline is ten times as effective in suppressing salivation as an identical oral dose. There is great individual variation in oral dose response, reflecting erratic and widely varying absorption. Propantheline is partly metabolized in the gut, further reducing the amount of active drug absorbed. Absorption is also delayed by food and by antacids, and peak plasma concentration may not be achieved for several hours. It appears to undergo enterohepatic circulation. No reliable data are available on the plasma half life or volume of distribution of propantheline.

Oral absorption	10%
Presystemic metabolism	—
Plasma half life	—
Volume of distribution	—
Plasma protein binding	—

Concentration–effect relationship

There is no evidence yet of a concentration–effect relationship with this drug.

Metabolism

Metabolism is largely by hydrolysis on exposure to bile and duodenal contents, to free xanthene carboxylic acid, which has no pharmacological activity (Fig. 1).[8] After an oral dose, about 10% is excreted unchanged in the urine and 20% as xanthene carboxylic acid, 3–18% in faeces and the remainder in urine as unidentified metabolites. After an intravenous dose about 50% is excreted unchanged in the urine in 24 h, 3% in the faeces, only 10% as xanthene carboxylate and the rest as the unidentified metabolites.

Fig. 1 The metabolism of propantheline

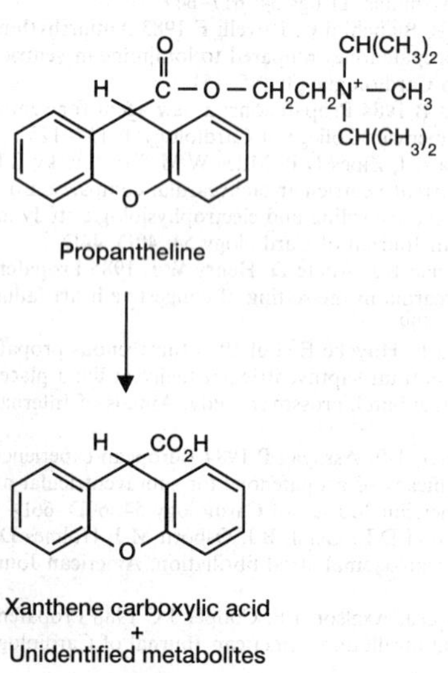

Pharmaceutics

Propantheline bromide is available in oral and parenteral formulations.

1. Pro-Banthine (Gold Cross, UK/Searle USA): small, pink, sugar-coated 15 mg tablets for oral use, with the name 'SEARLE' on one side and, for the US market, also bears the number '601' on the other. A 7.5 mg tablet is also available in the USA; it is white, sugar-coated and carries the number '611' on one side and Searle on the reverse.

Tablets are marketed and stored in foil in dry conditions.

Therapeutic use

Indications

1. Gastric and duodenal ulceration
2. Intestinal hypermotility, diverticular disease
3. Menetrier's disease
4. Reactive hypoglycaemia
5. Urinary incontinence
6. Hyperhidrosis
7. Use in radiology
8. Other uses.

Contraindications

1. Glaucoma
2. Chronic lung disease
3. Unstable cardiac rhythm
4. Prostatic hypertrophy
5. Reflux oesophagitis
6. Generally, in the elderly who are more likely to have contra-indicated conditions.

Mode of use

Propantheline is given orally or intramuscularly. It has also been used topically.

1. Gastric and duodenal ulceration

Use of anticholinergics in treating peptic ulceration was based on demonstrable inhibition of gastric acid secretion (basal, postprandial and nocturnal)[11] and on the theory that reduction of gastric emptying would prolong the effect of antacids. Yet 'in spite of several hundred published studies, anticholinergics have to be classified as unproven for the treatment of peptic ulcer disease'.[12] Although they augment acid inhibition by cimetidine, the role of the combination has not been established,[13] except in some cases of Zollinger–Ellison syndrome.[14]

Propantheline, like the other quaternary ammonium compounds, is more slowly absorbed and has a longer action than atropine or belladonna mixtures. Although it is now regarded as second-line therapy (after H_2 antagonists and antacids) in treatment of peptic ulceration, its cost may be as little as one twentieth to one fifteenth the cost of an H_2 antagonist. Low cost may therefore weigh in its favour either in combination or as alternative therapy.

As in the case of atropine or belladonna, night-time dosage may minimize side effects. A dose of 15 mg may be adequate in the majority of patients.[2]

2. Intestinal hypermotility, diverticular disease

Anticholinergics have been extensively used in irritable bowel syndrome, diverticular disease, oesophageal spasm and in abdominal cramps of miscellaneous and uncertain causes.[15–17] Propantheline 15 mg three times daily has been recommended, in addition to increased dietary fibre, in the treatment of diverticular disease,[18] but dose and frequency should be tailored individually. The addition of an antianxiety agent may be useful in some patients with irritable bowel syndrome, in blocking stress-induced hypermotility.[19] It has been said that 'anyone in a tight squeeze may benefit from the sporadic use of an anticholinergic'.[17]

3. Menetrier's disease

Short-term studies have demonstrated an acute decrease in gastric protein loss with atropine treatment,[20] while high-dose propantheline (105 mg daily) has produced long-term reduction of protein loss.[21] The mechanism is not understood, but there are several possible explanations, including reduced hydrogen ion production (thus reducing the possibility of damage to blood vessels) and reduction of mucosal blood flow.[21]

4. Reactive hypoglycaemia

A dose of 30 mg of propantheline, 45 minutes before glucose to stimulate insulin release, prevented hypoglycaemic symptoms in all of seven patients with reactive hypoglycaemia.[22] A dose of 7.5 mg was recommended, to be taken just before each meal, which should be small and low in free sugar, but again individual tailoring of dose is necessary.

5. Urinary incontinence

Propantheline blocks parasympathetic cholinergic overactivity of the detrusor muscle of the bladder, associated with the uninhibited neurogenic bladder. It is the most commonly used anticholinergic in treatment of urge incontinence due to the neurogenic bladder. Average doses are 15 mg every four to six hours.[28]

6. Hyperhidrosis

Hyperhidrosis has been treated with local application of propantheline in lotion and aerosol form.[23]

7. Use in radiology

Propantheline may be used in radiology for better visualization of the duodenum and colon at endoscopy, the biliary tract, the urinary tract, and oesophageal varices.[24,25] As this is usually a 'one off' procedure, high concentrations were achieved for brief periods using a parenteral dose of 10–30 mg (parenteral form is no longer available). By the same principle, it may be used to relieve the acute pain of biliary and renal colic.

8. Other possible uses

Propantheline has been used in treating the short-bowel syndrome, pancreatitis and enuresis. Convincing evidence of efficacy in enuresis is lacking, in spite of several studies with large numbers of children. Nevertheless, the current practice of using tricyclic antidepressants assumes efficacy through their anticholinergic effect.

Adverse reactions

Adverse reactions are similar to those of atropine except in two respects. Because it does not readily cross the blood–brain barrier, adverse effects on the central nervous system are rare. Because of its ganglion-blocking properties, orthostatic hypotension and impotence in males can occur.

Potentially life-threatening effects

Peripheral antimuscarinic effects may be less marked than with atropine, but cardiac arrhythmias remain the greatest risk. The danger of misdiagnosis in gastrointestinal disorders increases the risk of propantheline causing tragic consequences, for example, precipitating a toxic megacolon in ulcerative colitis.

Acute overdosage

As for atropine, except for minimal central nervous system toxicity. Ganglion blockade may produce neuromuscular blockade and respiratory arrest.

Treatment is as for atropine overdose, that is, physostigmine, 1–4 mg intravenously, repeated as necessary, and avoidance of the upright posture until the effects are reversed and the clinical state stable. The stomach should be emptied or activated charcoal given.

Severe or irreversible adverse effects

These are as for atropine; acute glaucoma, urinary retention, and tachycardia may occur. Orthostatic hypotension, especially in the elderly, may limit its use.

Symptomatic adverse effects

These are as for atropine, except for the absence of effects on the central nervous system. Impotence due to ganglion blockade is not uncommon.

Interference with Clinical pathology tests

No technical interferences of this kind have been reported.

High risk groups

Neonates

The drug is not normally used in patients in this age-group.

Breast milk. Propantheline has not been detected in milk of lactating mothers[26] and suppression of lactation may occur with parasympatholytus.

Children
Children appear to tolerate relatively high bedtime doses in attempts to treat enuresis. A long-recommended children's dose is $0.375\ mg.kg^{-1}$ four times daily,[27] although a major manufacturer (Searle) states that safety and efficacy have not been established.

Pregnant women
Urinary retention and constipation are a particularly great risk during pregnancy. Although marketing experience has revealed no serious adverse effects on mother or foetus, cohort data on parasympatholytics indicate a possible association with minor malformations.

The elderly
Elderly patients are more likely than others to suffer the conditions described above under severe or irreversible adverse effects.

Drug interactions

Potentially hazardous interactions
None has been reported.

Other significant interactions
Pharmacodynamic. Peripheral anticholinergic action is additive to other drugs which have anticholinergic effects, for example, tricyclic antidepressants, phenothiazines and disopyramide.

Pharmacokinetic. By delaying gastric emptying, propantheline may delay absorption of other drugs; it may both delay and reduce the peak concentration. Bioavailability may be reduced if, as in the case of paracetamol, there is a high first-pass clearance.[4] On the other hand, drugs which usually have poor bioavailability may be better absorbed if intestinal transit time is prolonged, for example, slow dissolving digoxin and nitrofurantoin, and some enteric-coated preparations.

Potentially useful interactions
None has been reported.

Clinical trials

There are no major outcome trials demonstrating unequivocal efficacy of propantheline for its major indications, e.g. peptic ulceration, and efficacy remains unproven.[12] Because it is so cheap and its use hallowed by tradition, major trials are unlikely to be forthcoming. Although the selective antimuscarinics will probably replace it ultimately for peptic ulceration, low cost will continue to be an important factor for a long time in the use of propantheline, for treating peptic ulcer, urinary incontinence and hypermotility syndromes.

General review articles

Greenblatt D J, Shader R I 1973 Drug Therapy: anticholinergics. New England Journal of Medicine 288: 1215–1219

Lewis J H 1973 Treatment of gastric ulcer. What is old and what is new? Archives of Internal Medicine 143: 265–274

Longman M J S 1977 Drugs in the treatment of gastric and duodenal ulcer. Drugs 14: 105–115

References

1. Ivey K J 1975 Anticholinergics: do they work in peptic ulcer? Gastroenterology 68: 154–166
2. Feldman M, Richardson C T, Peterson W L, Walsh J H, Fordtran J S 1977 Effect of low-dose propantheline on food-stimulated gastric acid secretion. New England Journal of Medicine 297: 1427–1430
3. Hurwitz A, Robinson R G, Herrin W F 1977 Prolongation of gastric emptying by oral propantheline. Clinical Pharmacology and Therapeutics 22: 206–210
4. Nimmo J, Heading R C, Tothill P, Prescott L F 1973 Pharmacological modification of gastric emptying: effects of propantheline and metoclopramide on paracetamol absorption. British Medical Journal 1: 587–589
5. Gibbons D O, Lant A F 1975 Effects of intravenous and oral propantheline and metoclopramide on ethanol absorption. Clinical Pharmacology and Therapeutics 17: 578–583
6. Saitoh H, Kobayashi Y, Miyazaki K, Arita T 1987 A highly sensitive HPLC method for the assay of propantheline used to measure its uptake by rat intestinal brush border membrane vesicles. Journal of Pharmacy and Pharmacology 39: 9–12

Propantheline bromide

7. Moller J, Rosen A 1968 Comparative studies on intramuscular and oral effective doses of some anticholinergic drugs. Acta Medica Scandinavica 184: 201–209
8. Barowsky H 1955 American Journal of Gastroenterology 23: 557
9. Barowsky H, Greene L, Paulo D 1965 Cinegastroscopic observations on the effect of anticholinergic and related drugs on gastric and pyloric motor activity American Journal of Digestive Diseases 10: 506–513
10. Beerman B, Hellstrom K 1972 On the metabolism of propantheline in man. Clinical Pharmacology and Therapeutics 13: 212–220
11. Mikhell R D, Hunt J W, Grossman M I 1962 Inhibition of basal and postprandial gastric secretion by poldine and atropine in patients with peptic ulcer. Gastroenterology 43: 400–406
12. Schiller L R, Feldman 1981 Medical therapy of peptic ulcer disease. In: Baron J H, Moody F F G (eds) Gastroenterology 1: Foregut. Butterworths, London
13. Peterson W L 1979 Reduction of 24-hour gastric acidity with combination drug therapy in patients with duodenal ulcer. Gastroenterology 77: 1015–1020
14. McCarthy D M, Hyman P E 1979 Cholinergic influence on gastric acid secretion in the Zollinger–Ellison Syndrome. Gastroenterology 76: 1198–2002
15. Ivey K J 1975 Are anticholinergics useful in irritable bowel syndrome? Gastroenterology 68: 1300–1307
16. Snape W J, Wright S A, Battle W M, London R, Sun E A, Cohen S 1981 Successful treatment of the irritable colon syndrome with high doses of an anticholinergic. Gastroenterology 80: 1289
17. Spiro H M 1983 Clinical Gastroenterology 3rd edn. Macmillan, New York
18. Smith A N 1983 Diverticular disease: medical and surgical management. In: Alexander-Williams J, Binder H J (eds) Gastroenterology 3: Large intestine. Butterworths, London
19. Narducci F, Nape W J, Battle W M, London R, Cohen S 1982 Stimulation of colonic myoelectric activity by emotional stress in healthy subjects and irritable bowel syndrome. Gastroenterology 82: 1137
20. Russell I J, Smith J, Dozois R R, Wahner H W, Bartholomew L G 1977 Menetrier's disease. Effects of medical and surgical vagotomy. Mayo Clinic Proceedings 52: 91–96
21. Smith R C, Powell D W 1978 Prolonged treatment of Menetrier's disease with an oral anticholinergic drug. Gastroenterology 74: 903–906
22. Permutt M A, Keller D, Santiago J 1977 Cholinergic blockade in reactive hypoglycaemia. Diabetes 26: 121
23. Frankland J C, Seville R H 1972 The treatment of hyperhidrosis with topical propantheline — a new technique. British Journal of Dermatology 85: 577–581
24. Merlo R B, Stone M, Barrgus P, Martin M 1978 The use of Pro-Banthine to induce gastrointestinal hypotonia. Radiology 127: 61–62
25. Dalinka M K, Smith E H 1972 Pharmacologically-enhanced visualization of oesophageal varices by Pro-Banthine. Radiology 102: 281–282
26. Takyi B E 1970 Journal of Hospital Pharmacy 28: 317
27. Martingdale — The Extra Pharmacopoeia, 1982 Ed: Reynolds J E F, Pharmaceutical Press, London
28. Holmes D M, Montz F J, Stanton S L 1989 Oxybutinin versus propantheline in the management of destrusor instability. British Journal Obstetrics and Gynaecology 96: 607–612

Propofol

Propofol is a short-acting rapidly metabolized intravenous anaesthetic agent.

Chemistry

Propofol (Diprivan)
$C_{12}H_{18}O$
2,6-Diisopropylphenol

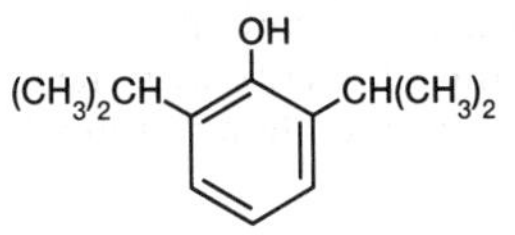

Molecular weight	178
pKa	11
Solubility	
in alcohol	very soluble
in water	slightly soluble
Octanol/water partition coefficient	5000

Propofol is a white, sterile, odourless and isotonic oil-in-water emulsion, prepared by chemical synthesis. The emulsion vehicle contains soyabean oil and purified egg phosphatide.

Pharmacology

Propofol is a short-acting, rapidly metabolized intravenous anaesthetic agent that can be used to induce and maintain general anaesthesia.[1,2,3] It is a general central nervous system depressant.

Toxicology

Propofol has not been found to have mutagenic activity in the *Salmonella* mutation test, and no potential to cause gene mutation or gene conversion was found in the yeast *Saccharomyces cerevisiae*. There is no evidence of clastogenic effects on the bone-marrow cells of the Chinese hamster and no clastogenic effects or action as a spindle poison in CCB F_1 mice micronucleus test. No evidence of teratological effects has been observed in the rat or rabbit, at dose levels of 5, 10 or 15 $mg.kg^{-1}$ daily.

Clinical pharmacology

Propofol is a non-barbiturate, rapidly acting intravenous induction agent, producing a dose-related depression of the level of consciousness. Its induction characteristics are similar to those of the barbiturate thiopentone with a dose-related depression of the central nervous system,[5,6] cardiovascular system[7,8] and respiratory system.[9,10] A dose of 1 mg of propofol is equivalent to 1.6 mg of thiopentone.[11]

In unpremedicated adult patients up to 55 years of age[6,12] 2.0–2.5 $mg.kg^{-1}$ is usually satisfactory for induction of anaesthesia, and infusion rates of 6–12 $mg.kg^{-1}.h^{-1}$ usually maintain satisfactory anaesthesia for surgery.[13] This dose requirement is reduced in the elderly.[14]

Pharmacokinetics

The preferred analytical method for detection of the drug in blood is by high performance liquid chromatography following coupling with Gibb's reagent and fluorescence detection. The limit of quantification[15] is about 2 $\mu g.l^{-1}$.

Propofol is so rapidly metabolized that extremely large doses would be required orally or rectally to achieve pharmacological effects. It is thus administered intravenously either as a bolus dose or by continuous infusion. The redistribution half life of a single bolus dose is 2–4 minutes with a half life for metabolic clearance of 30–60 minutes, and a half life for return from poorly perfused regions of 184–502 minutes.[16] The volume of distribution of the central compartment is 22–41 l and the volume of distribution at equilibrium is 297–1101 l.[16–18]

It is 97–98% bound to plasma proteins and is widely and rapidly distributed throughout the body as would be expected of a highly lipid-soluble drug. Studies using whole body autoradiography in rats have shown the highest level of total radioactivity to be detected at early time points in the liver, brown fat, nasal tissues, bile-collecting ducts and preputial glands. At 24 hours, radioactive material was detected in preputial glands of both sexes of rat, the liver and kidney of males and the fat of females.

As it is highly lipid soluble, it is likely to be excreted in breast milk and to cross the placenta in a similar fashion to other highly lipid-soluble drugs. Although these points are under investigation no data are yet available.

Oral absorption	—
Presystemic metabolism	extensive
Plasma half life	30–60 min
Volume of distribution	297–1100 l
Plasma protein binding	97–98%

Concentration–effect relationship

Plasma concentrations of 1.64–6.38 $mg.l^{-1}$ have been recorded in volunteers when falling asleep and concentrations of 1.0 to 2.19 $mg.l^{-1}$ when waking from anaesthesia.[19]

Metabolism

Propofol is conjugated in the liver with less than 0.3% excreted unchanged.[17] Conjugation is to the glucuronide (40%) of 2,6-diisopropylphenol or to the 1- and 4-glucuronides and the 4-sulphate of the quinol (2,6-diisopropylphenol-1,4-quinol) (see Fig. 1). 88% of the conjugated drug is excreted via the kidney. There is evidence of enterohepatic circulation in the rat but none of the metabolites are pharmacologically active.

Pharmaceutics

Propofol is available as Diprivan (ICI, UK) in 20 ml ampoules, containing 10 mg per ml of propofol in a white, oil-in-water, ready to use emulsion (with soyabean oil and purified egg phosphatide), for intravenous use only.

The emulsion should be stored at room temperature and must not be frozen. Each ampoule should be shaken before use. Maximum shelf-life is 3 years.

Therapeutic use

Indications

1. Induction of anaesthesia
2. Maintenance of general anaesthesia for surgical procedures which generally do not exceed 1 hour
3. Sedation by the use of continuous infusion.

Contraindications

1. General precautions as for all intravenous anaesthetic agents
2. Disorders of fat metabolism.

Mode of use

The dose of drug is titrated at a rate of approximately 4 ml (40 mg) every 10 seconds (less in the frail or elderly) intravenously until loss of consciousness occurs.[4,20] In patients of ASA Grades 3 and 4, lower rates of administration should be used (up to 2 ml every 10 seconds).

P

Fig. 1 Metabolism of propofol

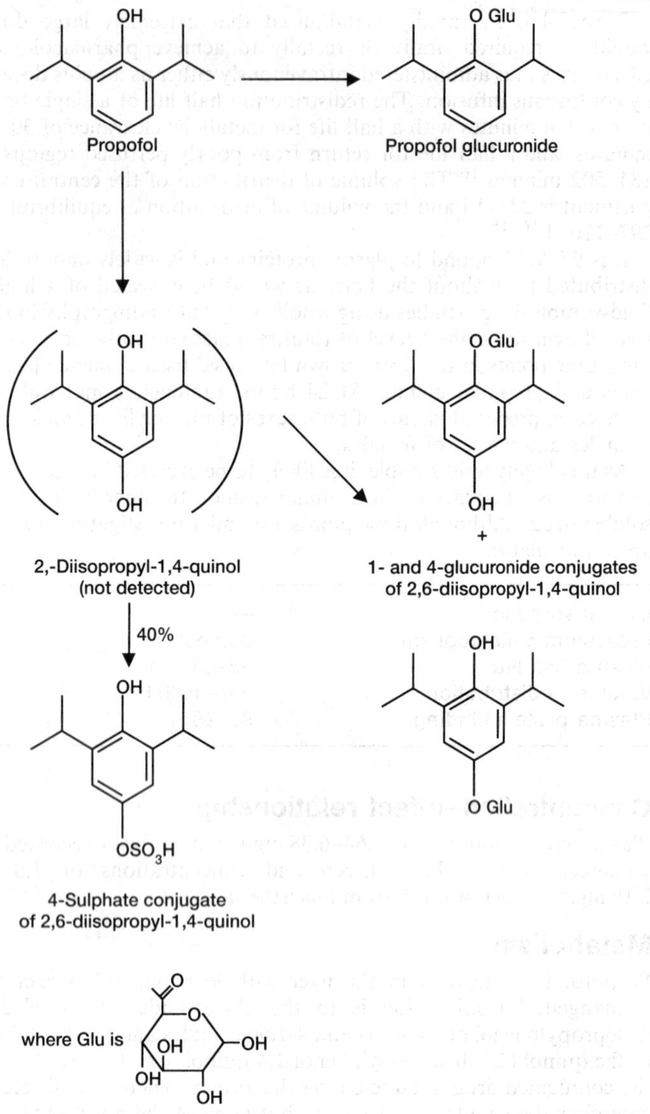

Thereafter, anaesthesia can be maintained either by administration of bolus doses of 20–50 mg or by continuous infusion at a rate[12,13] of 6–12 $mg.kg^{-1}.h^{-1}$ depending on age and prior premedication.

Indications

1. Induction of anaesthesia

Propofol has been used for induction of anaesthesia for a wide range of surgical procedures, including general surgery,[21–23] gynaecology,[24] ophthalmic surgery,[25] coronary artery surgery,[7] hepatobiliary surgery,[8] orthopaedics,[24] and ENT surgery.[25]

It has also been widely used and may have specific advantages for a range of day-stay surgical procedures including dental and oral surgery,[26] gynaecological surgery[27] and urology.[28]

2. Maintenance of general anaesthesia

Propofol may be used for maintenance of anaesthesia by intermittent bolus doses or by continuous infusion and has been used for both in-patient and day-stay surgery using both techniques.[25,27–31]

3. Sedation by use of continuous infusion

Propofol has provided background sedation in patients with an established local anaesthetic block.[24,29] Infusions of propofol have also been used as a sedative technique for colonoscopies[32] and it has been used for the prolonged sedation of patients requiring intermittent positive pressure ventilation in an Intensive Care Unit.[33,34]

Recovery from anaesthesia with propofol is rapid,[35] markedly more clear-headed than after other agents, and accompanied by fewer unwanted side effects such as postoperative nausea, vomiting and headache.[36] Unlike the barbiturates, propofol has been shown not to cause enzyme induction, which suggests it may be used in patients with porphyria.[37,38]

Contraindications

1. General precautions

As with all intravenous anaesthetic agents, propofol should be used with caution in patients with cardiac, respiratory, renal or hepatic insufficiency, and in hypovolaemic or debilitated patients.

2. Disorders of fat metabolism

Appropriate care should be exercised in patients with disorders of fat metabolism or in other conditions where lipid emulsions must be used cautiously.

Adverse reactions

Potentially life-threatening effects

As with other intravenous anaesthetic agents, accidental intravenous overdosage will result in a dose-related depression of the cardiovascular and respiratory systems. This depression should be treated symptomatically with pharmacological support of the cardiovascular system (including plasma volume expanders and pressor agents) and artificial ventilation where appropriate.

Idiosyncratic reactions or allergy with the use of propofol are rare. There is a single report in the literature in which a patient had 1 gE antibodies to propofol.[39]

Acute overdosage

No case of deliberate overdose has yet been reported.

Severe or irreversible adverse effects

Apart from the dose-related depression of the cardiovascular, respiratory and central nervous systems already discussed, no other severe or irreversible effects have so far been noted.

Symptomatic adverse effects

Systemic. A dose-related depression of the cardiovascular, central nervous and respiratory systems, common to most intravenous anaesthetic agents, is to be expected. There have also been reports of transient bradycardia with minimal heart rates usually in the range 40–50 $beats.min^{-1}$. A number of these occurred during periods of vagal stimulation, such as by instrumentation and specific surgical procedures, and all responded rapidly to the intravenous use of anticholinergic agents, such as atropine.

Local. Pain on injection has been noted. The reported incidence of pain varies from 28.5% when injected into small veins on the dorsum of the hand to only 6% when injected into larger veins in the antecubital fossa.[36] Despite this, the incidence of thrombophlebitis is very low, only 0.5%.[36]

Approximately 14% of patients will have some manifestations of excitation at induction;[36] however this will only be of a transitory nature. Up to 23% may have manifestations of excitement during anaesthesia maintained with propofol, the most common being spontaneous movement.[36]

Other effects

The drug is not known to cause any modification of body biochemistry.[40] It is currently being evaluated for its effects on body biochemistry when used for long-term infusion in an Intensive Care Unit.

Interference with clinical pathology tests

Propofol is not known to interfere with any clinical pathological measurements.

High risk groups

Neonates

The drug is not recommended in neonates.

Breast milk. The drug is likely to enter breast milk, but no data are yet available. In view of the relatively large amount that would have to be taken orally to have a pharmacological effect, a breast-fed baby would not be likely to come to harm.

Children

The drug is not yet licensed for use in children, but clinical trials have been completed.[41]

Pregnant women

The drug is not recommended in pregnancy.

Propofol

The elderly

The dose should be reduced and titrated cautiously against response in the elderly.

Drug interactions

Potentially hazardous interactions

No interactions of this kind have been reported.

Potentially useful interactions

None has been described.

General review articles

1985 Postgraduate Medical Journal 61 (suppl 3)
Dundee J W and Clarke R S J 1989 Propofol. European Journal of Anaesthesia 6: 5–22
Langley M S and Heal R C 1988 Propofol. Drugs 35: 334

References

1. Glen J B 1980 Animal studies of the anaesthetic activity of ICI 35, 868. British Journal of Anaesthesia 52: 731–742
2. Glen J B, Hunter S C 1984 Pharmacology of an emulsion formulation of ICI 35, 868. British Journal of Anaesthesia 56: 617–626
3. Glen J B, Hunter S C, Blackburn T P, Wood P 1985 Interaction studies and other investigations of the pharmacology of propofol (Diprivan). Postgraduate Medical Journal 61 (suppl 3): 7–14
4. Cummings G C, Dixon J, Kay N H et al 1984 Dose requirements of ICI 35 868 (propofol, Diprivan) in a new formulation for induction of anaesthesia. Anaesthesia 39: 1168–1171
5. Thornton C, Konieczko M, Knight A B, Kanl B, Jones J G, White D C 1986 The effect of 'Diprivan' on the auditory evoked response. In: Bergmann H, Kramar H and Steinbereithner K (eds) VII European Congress of Anaesthesiology 201 (Abstract 358)
6. McCollom J S C, Dundee J W 1986 Comparison of the induction characteristics of four intravenous anaesthetic agents. Anaesthesia 41: 995–1000
7. Patrick M R, Blair I J, Feneck R O, Sebel P S 1985 A comparison of the haemodynamic effects of propofol (Diprivan) and thiopentone in patients with coronary artery disease. Postgraduate Medical Journal 61 (suppl 3): 23–27
8. Grounds R M, Twigley A J, Carli F, Whitwam J G, Morgan M 1985 The haemodynamic effects of intravenous induction. Comparison of the effects of thiopentone and propofol. Anaesthesia 40: 735–740
9. Taylor M B, Grounds R M, Mulrooney P D, Morgan M 1986 Ventilatory effects of propofol during induction of anaesthesia. Comparison with thiopentone. Anaesthesia 41: 816–820
10. Grounds R M, Maxwell D L, Taylor M B, Aber V, Royston D 1987 Acute ventilatory changes during intravenous induction of anaesthesia with thiopentone or propofol in humans using inductance-plethysmography. British Journal of Anaesthesia 59: 1098–1102
11. Grounds R M, Moore M, Morgan M 1986 The relative potencies of thiopentone and propofol. European Journal of Anaesthesiology 3: 11–17
12. Kay N H, Uppington J, Sear J W, Allen M C 1985 Use of an emulsion of ICI 35, 868 (propofol) for the induction and maintenance of anaesthesia. British Journal of Anaesthesia 57: 736–742
13. Spelnia K R, Coates D P, Monk C R, Prys-Roberts C, Norley J, Turtle M J 1986 Dose requirements of propofol by infusion during nitrous oxide in anaesthesia in man. I: Patients premedicated with morphine sulphate. British Journal of Anaesthesia 56: 1080–1084
14. Dundee J W, Robinson F P, McCollom J S C, Patterson G C 1986 Sensitivity to propofol in the elderly. Anaesthesia 41: 482–485
15. Plummer G F 1987 Improved method for the determination of propofol in blood by high-performance liquid chromatography with fluorescence detection. Journal of Chromatography 421: 171–176
16. Cockshott I D 1985 Propofol (Diprivan) pharmacokinetics and metabolism — an overview. Postgraduate Medical Journal 61 (suppl 3): 45–50
17. Simons P J, Cockshott I D, Douglas E J, Gordon E A, Hopkins K, Rowland M 1985 Blood concentrations, metabolism and elimination after a sub-anaesthetic intravenous dose of ^{14}C-propofol (Diprivan) to male volunteers. Postgraduate Medical Journal 61 (suppl 3): 64
18. Kay N H, Sear J W, Uppington J, Cockshott I D, Douglas E J 1986 Disposition of propofol in patients undergoing surgery. A comparison in men and women. British Journal of Anaesthesia 58: 1075–1079
19. Schuttler J, Stoeckel H, Schwilden H 1985 Pharmacokinetic and pharmacodynamic modelling of propofol (Diprivan) in volunteers and surgical patients. Postgraduate Medical Journal 61 (suppl 3): 53–54
20. McCollom J S C, Dundee J W, Halliday N J, Clarke R S J 1985 Dose response studies with propofol (Diprivan) in unpremedicated patients. Postgraduate Medical Journal 61 (suppl 3): 85–87
21. Rolly G, Versichelen L 1985 Comparison of propofol and thiopentone for induction of anaesthesia in premedicated patients. Anaesthesia 40: 945–948
22. Briggs L P, White M 1985 The effects of premedication of anaesthesia with propofol (Diprivan). Postgraduate Medical Journal 61 (suppl 3): 35–37
23. Mirakhur R K, Shepherd W F I 1985 Intraocular pressure changes with propofol 'Diprivan': comparison with thiopentone. Postgraduate Medical Journal 61 (suppl 3): 41–44
24. Mackenzie N, Grant I S 1985 Comparison of propofol with methohexitone in the provision of anaesthesia for surgery under regional blockade. British Journal of Anaesthesia 57: 1167–1172
25. Rolly G, Versichelen L, Herregods L 1985 Cumulative experience with propofol (Diprivan) as an agent for the induction and maintenance of anaesthesia. Postgraduate Medical Journal 61 (suppl 3): 96–100
26. Valanne J, Kortilla K 1985 Comparison of methohexitone and propofol (Diprivan) for induction of enflurane anaesthesia in outpatients. Postgraduate Medical Journal 61 (suppl 3): 138–143
27. Mackenzie N, Grant I S 1985 Comparison of the new emulsion formulation of propofol with methohexitone and thiopentone for induction of anaesthesia in day cases. British Journal of Anaesthesia 57: 725–731
28. Kay B, Healy T E J 1985 Propofol (Diprivan) for outpatient cystoscopy. Efficacy and recovery compared with Althesin and methohexitone. Postgraduate Medical Journal 61 (suppl 3): 108–114
29. Jessop E J, Grounds R M, Morgan M, Lumley J 1985 Comparison of infusions of propofol and methohexitone to provide light general anaesthesia during surgery with regional blockade. British Journal of Anaesthesia 57: 1173–1177
30. De Grood P M R M, Ruys A H C, Van Egmond J, Booij L D H J, Crul J F 1985 Propofol (Diprivan) emulsion for total intravenous anaesthesia. Postgraduate Medical Journal 61 (suppl 3): 65–69
31. Lees N W, McCollock M, Mair W B 1985 Propofol (Diprivan) for induction and maintenance of anaesthesia. Postgraduate Medical Journal 61 (suppl 3): 88–89
32. Gepts E, Claeys M A, Camu F, Smekens L 1985 Infusion of propofol (Diprivan) as a sedative technique for colonoscopies. Postgraduate Medical Journal 61 (suppl 3): 120–126
33. Aitkenhead A R, Pepperman M L, Willatts S M et al 1989 Comparison of propofol and midazolam for sedation in critically ill patients. Lancet ii: 704–709
34. McMurray T J, Collier P S, Carson I W, Lyons S M, Elliott P 1990 Propofol sedation after open heart surgery. A clinical and pharmacokinetic study. Anaesthesia 45: 322–326
35. Grant I S, Mackenzie N 1985 Recovery following propofol (Diprivan) anaesthesia — a review of three different anaesthetic techniques. Postgraduate Medical Journal 61 (suppl 3): 133–137
36. Stark R D, Binks S M, Dutka V N, O'Connor K M, Arnstein M J A, Glen J B 1985 A review of the safety and tolerance of propofol (Diprivan). Postgraduate Medical Journal 61 (suppl 3): 152–156
37. Parikh R K, Moore M 1985 A comparison of the porphyrinogenicity of diisopropylphenol (propofol) and phenobarbitone. Proceedings Biochemical Society Transactions (616th meeting) London 14: 726–727
38. Mitherschiffthaler G, Theiner A, Hetzel H, Frith L C 1988 Safe use of propofol in a patient with acute intermittent porphyria. British Journal of Anaesthesia 60: 109–111
39. Laxenaire M C, Gueant J L, Bermejo E, Mouton C, Navez M T 1988 Analphylactic shock due to propofol. Lancet ii: 739–740
40. Sear J W, Uppington J, Kay N H 1985 Haematological and biochemical changes during anaesthesia with propofol (Diprivan). Postgraduate Medical Journal 61 (suppl 3): 165–168
41. Purcell-Jones G, Yates A, Baker J R, James I G 1987 Comparison of the induction characteristics of thiopentone and propofol in children. British Journal of Anaesthesia 59: 1431–1436

P

Propranolol (hydrochloride)

Propranolol was the first β-adrenoceptor blocking drug to achieve wide therapeutic use in angina and hypertension. It is not selective between β_1 and β_2 receptors and has no agonist activity.

Chemistry

Propranolol hydrochloride (Inderal, Avlocardyl, Dociton, Sumerial)
$C_{16}H_{21}NO_2.HCl$
1-Isopropylamino-3-(1-naphthyloxy)-propan-2-ol hydrochloride

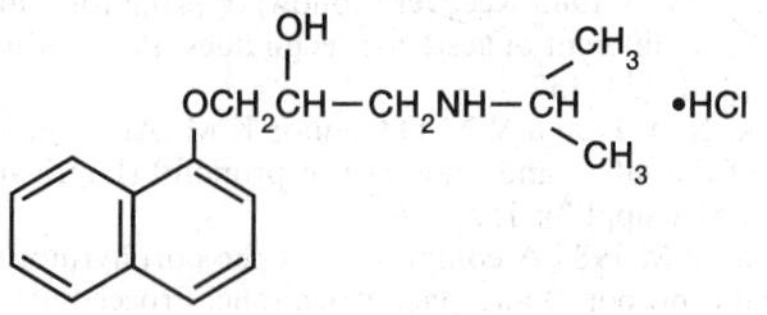

Molecular weight (free base)	295.8 (259.3)
pKa	9.5
Solubility	
in alcohol	1 in 20
in water	—
Octanol/water partition coefficient	3.65

A white or off-white odourless powder with a bitter taste, it is prepared by chemical synthesis and the racemate is used clinically. Propranolol hydrochloride is also available in an oral combination product with bendrofluazide (Inderetic, Inderex).

Pharmacology

Propranolol is an optically active compound. The β-adrenergic receptor blocking activity resides entirely in the l-isomer, although the d-isomer has equivalent membrane stabilizing activity. l-Propranolol is a competitive antagonist at both the β_1 and β_1 adrenoceptors, and therefore is not cardioselective although it has slightly greater activity at the β_1 than the β_2 receptor. It has no agonist activity at the β-adrenoceptor but has membrane stabilizing activity at concentrations exceeding 1–3 mg.l^{-1}, though such concentrations are rarely, if ever, achieved during oral therapy.

Acute administration of propranolol to animals causes a fall in heart rate and cardiac output. The blood pressure does not usually fall immediately as the fall in output is counterbalanced by peripheral vasoconstriction. Blood flow is reduced in most vascular territories, particularly the skin and the portal circulation.

If adrenaline is administered to an animal which has been pretreated with propranolol the pressor action is potentiated because the α-adrenergic, vasoconstrictor, action is not impaired but the β_2, vasodilator, action is blocked.

Toxicology

Propranolol does not have mutagenic potential, and toxicological testing in animals failed to demonstrate any results of potential clinical relevance. There is no evidence of carcinogenicity in tests lasting up to 18 months in rats, mice and dogs, and no evidence of teratological effects in rats and rabbits.

Clinical pharmacology

Competitive β-adrenoceptor blockade has been demonstrated in man by a parallel shift to the right in the dose–heart rate response curve to β-agonists such as isoprenaline. Propranolol has slightly greater activity at the β_1 receptor than the β_2.

Administration of a 10 mg intravenous dose of propranolol causes immediate slowing of the heart rate but a fall in blood pressure is usually delayed for about 2 hours.[1] Oral doses in the range 40–320 mg produce a reduction of resting heart rate and cardiac output with reduced flow to the skin, skeletal muscle, coronary circulation, splanchnic circulation and kidney. Similar doses produce a dose-related decrease in the rise in heart rate and systolic blood pressure on exercise. At maximum effect a heart rate of > 160 beats/min with a load of 150 watt might be reduced to 115 beats/min and the peak systolic blood pressure from 200 mmHg to 140 mmHg. In individuals with normal lungs, blockade of pulmonary β-adrenoceptors has little effect upon function.

There are widespread metabolic and endocrine effects of β-adrenoceptor blockade, including a reduction in plasma renin, reduced breakdown of muscle glycogen and inhibition of catecholamine-dependent lipolysis. However, during heavy exercise plasma glucose and free fatty acid concentrations are not much altered by treatment with propranolol. The effect of prolonged inhibition of β-receptors upon cells such as adipocytes, lymphocytes and mast cells is not known.[1–3]

Pharmacokinetics

The preferred analytical method is by high performance liquid chromatography with a sensitivity of about 2 µg.l^{-1}. A variety of stationary phases have been used[4,5] some of which are capable of resolving the enantiomers, which have slightly different kinetic properties.

Propranolol is completely absorbed after oral administration, and peak plasma concentrations are seen at 1–2 h in fasting patients, though the systemic bioavailability ranges between 5% and 50%. The mean plasma half life is 3.9 h with a range of 3–6 h. Presystemic metabolism by the liver removes up to 95% of an oral dose, and for any given dose there is a large variation in total plasma concentration between individuals due to this presystemic elimination. In consequence, plasma clearance is high, being a substantial fraction of the liver blood flow.[6] Presystemic metabolism is increased by induction of drug metabolizing enzymes, for example by cigarette smoking, and may be reduced by enzymatic inhibition, for example by concurrent administration of cimetidine.

Propranolol is widely and rapidly distributed throughout the body as would be expected in a highly lipid-soluble drug. The apparent volume of distribution is approximately 3 l.kg^{-1}, indicating drug accumulation in some tissues. Animal studies have demonstrated that the highest levels occur in the lungs, liver, kidney, brain and heart after oral and intravenous administration.[5,6] Propranolol is highly bound (80–95%) to proteins in plasma, and the major binding protein at therapeutic propranolol concentrations is α_1-acid glycoprotein.

The concentration of propranolol in the CSF approximates to the free drug concentration in the plasma. An approximate CSF/plasma ratio of 0.07, and an approximate brain/plasma ratio of 26 have been observed with oral doses of 80–160 mg in man.[7,8] Propranolol is excreted in breast milk in concentrations similar to those found in plasma. The high lipid solubility means that placental transfer of propranolol must occur though it is not documented. In the presence of porto-systemic shunting the systemic bioavailability of an oral dose may be markedly increased.[9]

Oral absorption	> 95%
Presystemic metabolism	50–95%
Plasma half life	
range	3–6 h
mean	3.9 h
Volume of distribution	2.3–5.5 l.kg^{-1}
Plasma protein binding	80–95%

Propranolol undergoes extensive hepatic biotransformation with only 1–4% excreted unchanged in urine and faeces. The effects of acute hepatic disease have not been documented, though cirrhosis has been shown to increase oral bioavailability, reduce systemic clearance and reduce plasma protein binding, resulting in higher steady-state blood propranolol concentrations.[9]

Propranolol (hydrochloride)

Investigations of the disposition of propranolol in renal patients have given conflicting results, though Wood et al (1980)[10] compared renal patients on dialysis and not on dialysis with age-matched controls and suggested there was no difference in steady-state pharmacokinetics. Old age has been reported to have little effect on propranolol pharmacokinetics,[11] though higher plasma propranolol concentrations were achieved in elderly compared with young adults following oral administration.[11] These effects may be complicated by changes in smoking habit with age.

Plasma concentrations may show large fluctuations during an acute illness, as the major binding protein, α_1-acid glycoprotein, is an acute phase protein whose concentration may increase several fold during an infection.

Since propranolol has a wide therapeutic range, and the dosage requirement varies widely, the clinical significance of altered pharmacokinetics appears to be quite small. However, research on propranolol pharmacokinetics has greatly improved understanding of the kinetics of drugs with high presystemic metabolism.

Concentration–effect relationship

Concentrations in the range 1 to 300 μg.l^{-1} produce increasing blockade of exercise induced tachycardia. The antianginal action correlates with blockade of exercise tachycardia and usually requires plasma concentrations in the range 10 to 100 μg.l^{-1}. There is no apparent relationship between plasma levels of propranolol and antihypertensive activity, as the antihypertensive action may persist for 24 h after a single dose, when the plasma concentration is very low.

Metabolism

Propranolol is extensively metabolized in the liver, with very little of the unchanged drug excreted. Excretion is almost entirely (>90%) in the urine with less than 5% in the faeces.

Three primary pathways of metabolism have been described:

a. Oxidative dealkylation which accounts for an average of 42% of the dose; the pricipal product is naphthoxylactic acid.
b. 4-Hydroxylation which accounts for a further 41% of the dose. 4-Hydroxypropranolol is subsequently conjugated with either sulphate or glucuronic acid before excretion in the urine.
c. Primary glucuronic acid conjugation which accounts for about 17% of the dose.[12]

These metabolic reactions can take place successively and over 20 different metabolites have been identified. One of these, 4-hydroxypropranolol has β-adrenergic blocking properties. It is equipotent with propranolol, but does not appear to contribute much to the pharmacodynamic effect, as it has a shorter half life and is mainly present in the plasma as inactive conjugates. There is evidence that two of these pathways are each subject to a different genetic polymorphism of drug metabolism, the formation of 4-hydroxypropranolol being catalysed by the form of cytochrome P-450 responsible for debrisoquine 4-hydroxylation and the formation of naphthoxylactic acid by oxidative dealkylation being due to the S-mephenytoin 4-hydroxylase form of cytochrome P-450.[13]

Pharmaceutics

Propranolol is available in oral and parenteral forms.

1. Inderal (ICI, UK): tablets containing 10 mg, 40 mg, 80 mg and 160 mg of propranolol hydrochloride BP. The tablets are pink, round, biconvex, film-coated and impressed with the legend 'INDERAL' and the strength on one face, with 'ICI' on the obverse. The impressions are highlighted in white.
2. Half-Inderal LA and Inderal-LA (ICI, UK): slow-release capsules containing 80 mg and 160 mg, respectively, of propranolol hydrochloride BP in a spheroid formulation. The gelatin capsules have a clear pink body and opaque lavender cap, marked 'ICI' and 'Half-Inderal LA' or 'Inderal LA' in black ink.
3. Inderal tablets (Wyeth-Ayerst, USA) are hexagonal scored tablets embossed with 'I' on one side and the proprietary name and strength on the obverse. The strengths are: 10 mg (orange), 20 mm (pale blue). 40 mg (green), 60 mg (pink) 80 mg (yellow) and 90 mg (lavender).
4. Inderal LA capsules are marketed in four strengths, each bearing one broad band around the circumference of the cap and three narrow bands around the base. The proprietary name is printed on the broad band. 60 mg are white/pale blue, 80 mg are pale blue, 120 mg are mid-blue/pale blue and 180 mg are mid-blue. Peak levels occur at about 6 h and the apparent plasma half life is around 10 h. The blood levels achieved will be lower dose for dose, than standard propranolol formulations. A need for upward retitration should be considered when switching a patient from the standard to the LA formulation.
5. Propranolol is available for intravenous use as a clear solution containing propranolol hydrochloride BP 1 mg.ml^{-1}.

In the USA Inderide is a fixed dose combination with hydrochlorothiazide. The LA capsules have a different ratio of active ingredients. In the UK Inderetic is a fixed-dose combination with bendrofluazide. Inderex is a double strength version of Inderetic.

All preparations should be protected from light.

Not all indications for propranolol are appropriate for the slow-release preparation.

Propranolol preparations are stable with a reasonable shelf-life, and carry a minimal risk from potentially allergenic substances, although these factors may vary between different generic preparations.

Therapeutic use

Indications

1. The control of essential and renal hypertension
2. The management of angina pectoris

Fig. 1 Metabolism of propanol

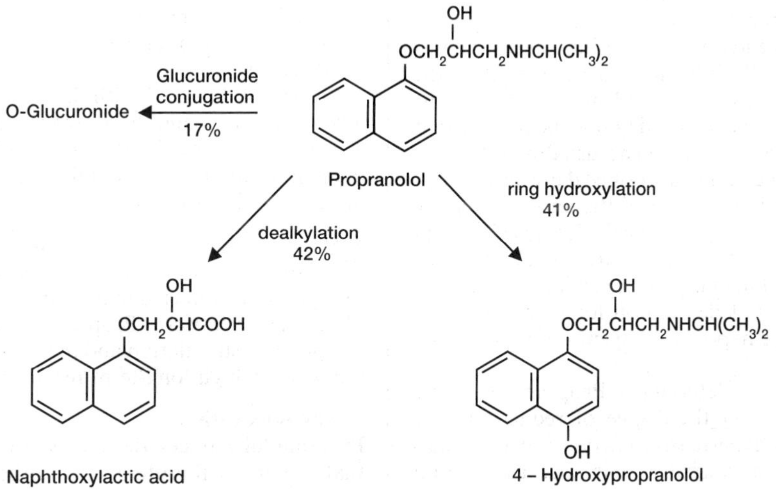

P

3. Long-term prophylaxis following acute myocardial infarction
4. The control of some forms of cardiac arrhythmias
5. The management of hypertrophic obstructive cardiomyopathy
6. The adjunctive management of thyrotoxicosis
7. The control of somatic manifestations of anxiety
8. To reduce tremor of the limbs
9. The prophylaxis of migraine
10. The management of catecholamine excess and phaeochromocytoma
11. To reduce the risk of gastrointestinal haemorrhage in patients with portal hypertension.

Contraindications

1. Bronchospasm
2. Cardiogenic shock and untreated cardiac failure
3. Second or third degree heart block
4. Hypoglycaemia or prolonged fasting
5. Metabolic acidosis
6. Severe haemorrhage.

Mode of use

All the clinical uses depend upon production of β-adrenoceptor blockade, usually of β_1 receptors in the heart. Only treatment of migraine and essential tremor make use of β_2 blockade.

Oral treatment is usually begun with 10–40 mg two or three times daily and the dose is increased up to a maximum of 320 mg daily depending upon the therapeutic response. Doses of several grams daily have been used in clinical trials but CNS side-effects increase with higher doses and they have little therapeutic advantage in most patients. Intravenous doses should be administered with the greatest care, and are intended for the emergency treatment of cardiac dysrhythmias and thyrotoxic crisis only. This route bypasses the liver so the effective dose is proportionately higher than an oral one. Rapid intravenous injection should not be used because of the additional hazard of a high concentration having a membrane-stabilizing effect upon the heart.

Sudden withdrawal of propranolol can be hazardous for patients who have ischaemic heart disease. Severe exacerbations of angina and fatal myocardial infarction have occurred. The mechanism is up-regulation of β-adrenoceptors during prolonged blockade which leads to a period of 7–10 days of hypersensitivity when the drug is suddenly stopped.[14] The degree of hypersensitivity is moderate ($\times 2$) and can be inhibited by a low dose of propranolol. There is no apparent need to reduce the dose slowly, provided the patient is treated with a low dose (e.g. 10 mg twice daily) for 2 weeks before the drug is finally stopped. The equivalent dose of an alternative β-blocking agent may be substituted.

Indications

1. Hypertension

Propranolol is widely used both as a single agent in the treatment of high blood pressure, and in combination with thiazide diuretics and vasodilators in 'step-care' procedures for control of hypertension. It lowers the systolic and diastolic blood pressure in both supine and erect positions, and minimizes the rise in pressure on exercise, though its use is not associated with postural hypotension. The degree of reduction in blood pressure depends upon the initial level. Patients with a pretreatment pressure of 180/100 mmHg achieve a fall in the systolic pressure of 12–20 mmHg and of 6–12 mmHg in diastolic pressure. The starting dose of 40 mg twice a day may be increased at weekly intervals according to the response. The usual maintenance dose is 80–320 mg per day in divided doses, or once daily administration of the slow-release preparation.[15] Most of the antihypertensive effect occurs within 6–8 h after starting at a particular dose level but there is a small further reduction following 7–10 days treatment. The resting pressure can be controlled in many patients with a single daily dose. Significant tolerance does not develop on long-term use. The efficacy of propranolol as a single hypotensive agent is similar to that of thiazide diuretics.

The mode of action has not been determined. Propranolol lowers the plasma renin concentration but the degree of reduction does not correlate well with the antihypertensive effects.[16] Autoregulatory reduction of the peripheral vascular resistance as a result of the reduced cardiac output, has been suggested. Other proposed sites of action include the CNS and an interaction with vasodilator prostanoids, but there is no direct evidence to support these hypotheses.

Black patients are less responsive to propranolol than caucasians and they usually have a lower plasma renin concentration. A small study in Chinese patients suggested that they are more sensitive to the bradycardic and hypotensive effect of propranolol than caucasians.[17]

In the MRC Hypertension Trial of treatment of mild hypertension, propranolol appeared to be less effective in preventing stroke in cigarette smokers although it was as effective as a thiazide diuretic in non-smokers. This result may have been a a random fluctuation as other controlled trials with β-adrenergic blocking drugs have not shown the same effect. There has been much debate about whether use of β-adrenergic blocking drugs in the treatment of male hypertensives reduces mortality from coronary disease. Although uncontrolled studies have suggested that there is a protective action, particularly in non-smokers, the MRC trial did not show a statistically significant reduction of coronary events.

2. Angina pectoris

Propranolol is an effective prophylactic drug for the relief of classical exercise-induced angina although the dose required must be adjusted for optimal effect.[18] A starting dose of 40 mg two or three times daily may be increased by the same amount at weekly intervals according to patient response. Patients with severe angina may require high doses, though an adequate response is usually seen in the range 120–240 mg daily in divided doses.[16] Treatment should not be stopped suddenly, as discussed earlier. As the therapeutic response depends upon the inhibition of exercise-induced rise in heart rate and myocardial contractility, it is necessary to maintain a high degree of β-receptor blockade. The mode of action appears to be due to a reduction in left ventricular work.[19]

3. Long-term prophylaxis following acute myocardial infarction

Propranolol is one of several β-adrenoceptor blocking drugs that have been shown to reduce mortality in the first two or three years after myocardial infarction. In the β-blocker heart attack (BHAT) trial (see Major outcome trials) mortality was reduced by 25% regardless of patient age or the site of infarction with an initial dose of 40 mg four times daily for 2–3 days, then given as 80 mg twice a day. Although the BHAT trial suggested that the beneficial effect was most pronounced in the first 12–18 months, some benefit continued for at least three years. The mode of action is unknown but may involve the prevention of cardiac arrhythmias. Sudden cardiac death showed a peak in the mid-morning and this peak was blunted by propranolol.

4. Cardiac arrhythmias

Both supraventricular and ventricular arrhythmias may respond to propranolol, but only in catecholamine-induced arrhythmias is it clearly the drug of first choice.[20] In the re-evaluation of antiarrhythmic therapy with type 1 agents following the disappointing results of the CAST trial, there has been renewed interest in regimens that include β-adrenergic blockade.[21] Propranolol is highly effective in controlling arrhythmias in patients with phaeochromocytoma (after α-adrenergic blockade) or with arrhythmias occurring during the use of volatile anaesthetics.[20] Some patients with ventricular extrasystoles or more serious ventricular arrhythmias[22] may also show a good response.

Propranolol is used with digoxin to reduce the ventricular rate in atrial fibrillation and flutter which are refractory to digoxin alone. It is usually effective in the control of arrhythmias associated with digoxin intoxication, though it should be used with caution as marked bradycardia may occur.

5. Hypertrophic obstructive cardiomyopathy

This condition is due to asymetrical hypertrophy of the heart such that pressure gradients may form, during systole, within the chamber of the left ventricle. Propranolol inhibits the inotropic effect of sympathetic stimulation and may reduce the intraventricular pressure gradient, though long-term results are disappointing.[23]

6. Thyrotoxicosis

Propranolol reduces the tachycardia and increased cardiac output that occur in thyrotoxicosis, although not usually to normal.[24]

Tremor is diminished, myopathy may improve and weight loss is halted but not reversed.[25] Treatment of thyrotoxicosis with propranolol is useful in reducing symptoms while antithyroid treatment is taking effect. Propranolol also reduces the concentration of reverse T3 but the clinical significance of this effect is unclear.

7. Anxiety
Propranolol may be useful in the alleviation of the somatic signs of anxiety such as palpitations, tachycardia and tremor.[26] A double-blind comparison of propranolol versus chlordiazepoxide in 212 patients demonstrated similar efficacy of the two drugs. Interestingly, there was a positive dose–response curve for chlordiazepoxide 30, 45 and 75 mg daily but a negative one with propranolol, the greatest improvement being with the lowest dose of 80 mg daily.[27]

8. Tremor of the limbs
Propranolol is highly effective in reducing the hand tremor that accompanies anxiety and fear and stress. It has been used by musicians, public orators, billiards players and pistol shooters to diminish palpitations and hand tremor, although use in some competitive sports is banned.[28,29] Propranolol also has some effect on the anxiety-provoked component of essential tremor and in parkinsonian and lithium-induced tremor.

9. Migraine
The use of propranolol is generally confined to prophylaxis[30] although there are isolated reports of it being used in the management of established headaches. The efficacy of propranolol has been established in randomized controlled trials.[31] The degree of benefit varies but some patients are almost completely free of attacks while being treated with 80–160 mg daily.

10. Catecholamine excess and phaeochromocytoma
Propranolol inhibits the tachycardia and tachyarrhythmias caused by excessive circulating catecholamines, and may be used preoperatively daily for 3 days, and 30 mg daily for long-term treatment. Propranolol must only be used in conjunction with an α-receptor blocking drug as it also inhibits the β_2 vasodilator effects.[32]

11. To reduce the risk of gastrointestinal haemorrhage in patients with portal hypertension
Bleeding from oesophageal varices is a common complication of portal hypertension. Several studies of patients with stable portal hypertension have demonstrated that propranolol causes a reduction of portal blood flow by 20–25% and a similar reduction of the gradient between portal venous pressure and free hepatic venous pressure.[33,34] Randomized controlled trials suggest that treatment with propranolol reduces the risk of serious gastrointestinal haemorrhage in these patients (see Major outcome trials).

Contraindications

1. Bronchospasm
Propranolol may cause bronchospasm in patients with asthma, allergic rhinitis or chronic obstructive airways disease. It also renders them unresponsive to normal doses of β-adrenergic bronchodilator drugs. If a β-adrenoceptor blocking agent is essential in such a patient, a β_1-selective agent should be used.

2. Low cardiac output and untreated cardiac failure
β-Blockade depresses myocardial contractility and may precipitate cardiac failure, bradycardia and atrioventricular block in patients in whom sympathetic activity is maintaining cardiac function. Therefore propranolol should not be given to patients with untreated congestive heart failure, right ventricular failure secondary to pulmonary hypertension or significant right ventricular hypertrophy. Treatment with propranolol may also be hazardous in patients with aortic regurgitation because slowing the heart increases the regurgitant flow. Patients who have suffered an acute myocardial infarction may be treated with propranolol in an attempt to limit the size of the infarct, but they should only be treated by experts who have injectable inotropic agents and resuscitation facilities available.

3. Bradycardia
Propranolol may produce dangerous bradycardia in a patient with second or third degree heart block, or sinus bradycardia (less than 45–55 beats/min). Marked sinus bradycardia may also occur in the presence of vagal overactivity or in athletically trained individuals, although in the latter case it does not seem to be hazardous. Atropine 1–2 mg intravenously should be used to correct severe bradycardia if necessary. A slow heart rate in an otherwise well (normal ECG) patient on propranolol need not cause great concern.

4. Hypoglycaemia
The metabolic response to impending hypoglycaemia involves the mobilization of free fatty acid and lactate, both of which are reduced by propranolol, so that a hypoglycaemic tendency is enhanced. The premonitory signs of hypoglycaemia such as tachycardia may also be masked. Recovery from hypoglycaemia induced by insulin, oral hypoglycaemic agents or prolonged fasting may be considerably retarded in propranolol-treated patients.

5. Severe haemorrhage
The clinical signs of severe internal haemorrhage may be masked by propranolol. Despite life-threatening blood loss the patient may have only a moderate tachycardia, often accompanied by torrential sweating.

Adverse reactions

Use of propranolol has been very extensive and the variety of suspected adverse reactions reported is large. In a number of cases the association may have been due to chance and where the probability that the drug caused the effect is low the reaction has not been included.

Potentially life-threatening effects
Deaths caused by propranolol are rare and almost all reported cases appear to have been a consequence of β blockade and not of idiosyncrasy. Those which result directly from the pharmacodynamic action include hypotension, severe bronchospasm, hypoglycaemia and bradyarrhythmias, usually in patients with pre-existing organic heart disease. Severe bradycardia, hypotension or cardiogenic shock may occur in patients who have a low cardiac ouput prior to the drug being given. Sudden withdrawal of propranolol may be dangerous in patients with ischaemic heart disease, as severe angina and fatal myocardial infarction have occurred.

Acute overdosage
In early clinical studies doses of up to 4 g daily of propranolol were used but severe toxic effects were seen if the dose was increased abruptly to that level. 31 cases of deliberate overdose have been reported.[35,36] Seven were found dead, 22 recovered and 2 died in hospital in cardiogenic shock (neither had been given glucagon). The main clinical features of massive overdose include bradycardia, hypotension and cardiogenic shock followed by coma, convulsions and seizures. In mild overdose, bradycardia and first degree heart block are seen with the disappearance of P-waves, atrial asystole and widening of QRS complex. The highest fatal dose was 9.6 g. The highest plasma concentration recorded in a survivor was 3010 $\mu g.l^{-1}$.[36] Bronchospasm, respiratory arrest and hypoglycaemia may occur.

In most cases of overdose, medical treatment has been successful. If ingestion is recent, further absorption may be prevented by induced emesis. Haemodialysis is not helpful because of the large volume of distribution. Excessive bradycardia may be countered with intravenous atropine in doses of 1–2 mg. β-Adrenoceptor stimulants are unlikely to be effective unless given in very high doses but there are several reports of successful use of glucagon 5–10 mg intravenously as a cardiac stimulant, followed by a maintenance glucagon infusion.[37] Bronchospasm may respond to inhalation of high doses of β_2-stimulants such as terbutaline or salbutamol. Intravenous diazepam is usually effective in controlling seizures.

Severe or irreversible adverse effects
There have been several publications suggesting a link between treatment with β-adrenergic blocking drugs and Peyronie's disease. In a review of 98 patients with this disease there were only five in whom β-blockers had been taken before the onset.[38]

Prolonged treatment with propranolol modifies plasma lipids with moderate elevation of triglycerides and reduction of HDL.[39,40] In the β-blocker heart attack trial (BHAT) there was no change in the most atherogenic component, LDL, but a 17% increase in triglycerides and a 6% reduction of HDL. These changes could predispose to deposition of atheroma, although they did not appear to affect the beneficial results in the BHAT study.

Spontaneous hypoglycaemia may occur in patients treated with propranolol, particularly during prolonged fasting.

A reaction similar to a psychotic episode, with visual hallucinations, has been reported in a small number of patients treated with propranolol, particularly those on high doses.

Patients with very severe Raynaud's disease (e.g. in systemic sclerosis), may experience worsening of their condition, even with necrosis of finger tips, if treated with propranolol.

There have been a very small number of reports of agranulocytosis, thrombocytopenia and eosinophilia in patients treated with propranolol.

Suggestions that propranolol, and other β-adrenergic blocking drugs may cause retroperitoneal fibrosis are not clearly substantiated.

Atopic individuals may notice a worsening of wheezing during the pollen season, but be free of problems at other times. Adverse effects of propranolol due to β-adrenoceptor blockade are most likely to occur after the first dose, even if this is low.

Symptomatic adverse effects

Propranolol is generally well tolerated, though side effects such as cold extremities, insomnia, lassitude, nausea, constipation, diarrhoea and impotence are all recognized. A report from the Boston Collaborative Drugs Surveillance Program (1974)[41] revealed the most common adverse effects to be gastrointestinal disturbances (11.2% of patients).

Disturbances in the central nervous system are also common, though they become more prominent at higher doses (>240 mg daily). These include fatigue, dizziness, insomnia, vivid dreams, alterations in mood and thought, and in a few cases daytime visual hallucinations. Cold hands and legs are experienced by many patients taking propranolol, who live in colder climates. Skin rashes and impotence have been associated with the use of β-adrenergic blocking drugs.

In most cases the symptoms clear when treatment is withdrawn, though the incidence may be reduced by starting treatment with a low dose and gradually increasing.

Other effects

β-Adrenergic blocking agents have been reported to cause a slight elevation of serum potassium and uric acid. After cardiopulmonary bypass more serious elevations of serum potassium have occurred. Plasma dextrose, urea and creatinine values may also be raised slightly as a result of reduced renal blood flow. The latter effects are not of great clinical significance.

Interference with clinical pathology tests

A propranolol metabolite may interfere with bilirubin measurements when made by the diazo method[42] and with the determination of metanephrines by the Pisano method.[43]

High risk groups

Neonates

Doses of propranolol used in neonates are as recommended for older infants, but there is very little information available.

Breast milk. Propranolol is excreted in the breast milk of nursing mothers in concentrations similar to those in plasma.[44] The child should be observed for bradycardia or hypoglycaemia.

Children

Propranolol is used in children for the treatment of dysrhythmias, phaeochromocytoma and thyrotoxicosis. The doses used should be determined according to the cardiac status of the child, and the circumstances necessitating treatment. The following are given as a guide only: oral 0.025–0.5 $mg.kg^{-1}$ three or four times daily as required; intravenous 0.025–0.5 mg injected slowly under ECG control, and repeated three or four times daily as required.

For the prophylaxis of migraine, under the age of 12, 20 mg is given two or three times daily, and the adult dose may be given to children over the age of 12.

Pregnant women

The safety of propranolol in pregnancy has not been completely established, although it has been widely used. It has been suggested that propranolol use during pregnancy may result in adverse effects in the fetus such as growth retardation, hypoglycaemia, hypocalcaemia, bradycardia and respiratory depression,[45,46] although hypertension in pregnancy may itself be associated with growth retardation and its complications. Fetal bradycardia may confuse the diagnosis of intrauterine hypoxia, but does not appear to cause any other problems. There have been no reports of teratogenicity or decreased fertility with propranolol in women.

The elderly

No special precautions are required as doses are adjusted according to patient response. β-blockers are slightly less effective hypotensive agents than diuretics in older patients.

Drug interactions

Potentially hazardous interactions

Adrenaline. Marked increases in blood pressure and severe bradycardia can occur following the administration of adrenaline to patients on non-selective β-blockers such as propranolol.

Anaesthetic agents. The heart rate and output may fall during anaesthesia in patients taking β-blockers. If precautions are taken, concurrent use is not contraindicated and intravenous injection of atropine (1–2 mg) will correct excessive vagal dominance.

Clonidine. The rebound hypertension following abrupt withdrawal of clonidine is potentiated by a β-blocker such as propranolol.

Digitalis glycosides. Propranolol is sometimes used to assist in controlling heart rate in patients with atrial fibrillation who are incompletely responsive to cardiac glycosides. Severe bradycardia may occur and great care with dosage should be exercised.

Verapamil (and other calcium antagonists). There was concern that concurrent treatment with calcium antagonists, particularly verapamil, in patients with impaired left ventricular function might be dangerous because both agents have a negative inotropic effect. However, provided care is taken to avoid excessive bradycardia the combination appears to be safe.

Other significant interactions

There are numerous reports of interactions in which moderate changes in the presystemic metabolism of propranolol take place when it is coadministered with drugs that are inhibitors or inducers of drug metabolism. The magnitude of most of these effects is not sufficient to cause clinically important modification to propranolol dosage.

Chlorpromazine. The concurrent use of propranolol and chlorpromazine results in a rise in the blood levels of both drugs, which may lead to additive hypotensive effects.

Cimetidine. The concurrent use of propranolol and cimetidine results in elevated blood propranolol levels and the possibility of enhanced β-blocking effects.

Indomethacin. The hypotensive effects of propranolol may be reduced by the concurrent use of indomethacin and other non-steroidal drugs.

Hypoglycaemic agents. Propranolol may increase the incidence and severity of hypoglycaemic episodes in some diabetic patients, which may be accompanied by a rise in blood pressure. The incidence of this reaction is thought to be low, but is potentially serious as the premonitory signs of hypoglycaemia, such as tachycardia, may be masked.

Smoking. Cigarette smoking increases the presystemic metabolism of propranolol and may partly explain the apparently reduced efficacy in smokers.

Potentially useful interactions

Propranolol inhibits baroreflex mediated tachycardia and for this reason it is widely used in combination with vasodilators such as hydralazine and minoxidil.

Propranolol has an additive effect with many other antihypertensive drugs and is widely used combined with diuretics in the control of mild to moderate hypertension.

Major outcome trials

Hypertension

Medical Research Council Working Party 1985 MRC trial of treatment of mild hypertension: Principal results. British Medical Journal 291: 97–104

Propranolol (hydrochloride)

The aim of this single-blind, placebo-controlled, study was to determine whether drug treatment of men and women aged 35–64 years with phase V diastolic pressures in the range 90–109 mmHg reduced stroke and other morbid hypertensive events. 17 354 patients were recruited and 85 572 patient years of observation were accumulated. Half the patients on active treatment were given propranolol, usually 240 mg daily, with supplementary methyldopa if required. The other half of the actively treated patients were given bendrofluazide, 10 mg daily, again with supplementary methyldopa. There were 60 strokes in the treated group and 109 in the untreated, a highly significant difference. However, in a post hoc analysis, propranolol appeared to be less effective than bendrofluazide in preventing stroke, apparently due to lack of efficacy in cigarette smokers. Total mortality was unaffected; there were 248 deaths in the actively treated group and 253 in the placebo group.

A number of additional analyses of this study have been published:

Miall W E, Greenberg G 1987 Mild hypertension: is there pressure to treat? Cambridge University Press, Cambridge

This book contains a great deal more tabulated data on the MRC trial than appears in the journal articles. It reviews the propranolol results in a somewhat more favourable light by demonstrating a significant reduction of ECG evidence of infarction. The book also points out that all cardiovascular events were reduced, 352 in controls and 286 on active treatment ($p = 0.01$), with an almost equal percentage reduction with each regime — a 20% overall reduction on bendrofluazide and 18% on propranolol.

Medical Research Council Working Party 1988 Stroke and coronary heart disease in mild hypertension: risk factors and the value of treatment. British Medical Journal 296: 1565–1570

Medical Research Council Working Party 1988 Coronary Heart Disease in the MRC trial of treatment of mild hypertension. British Heart Journal 59: 364–378

These papers presents further analyses of the coronary events in the MRC trial.

Coronary disease

2. Beta-Blocker Heart Attack Trial Research Group 1982 A randomized trial of propranolol in patients with acute myocardial infarction. 1. Mortality results. Journal of the American Medical Association 247: 1707–1714

This was a multi-centre, randomized, double-blind and placebo-controlled trial sponsored by the National Heart, Lung and Blood Institute. Over 27 months, 3837 patients (aged 30–69) were randomized to either propranolol (180–240 mg daily) or placebo within 5 to 21 days after a myocardial infarction. Total mortality over the study period was 25% less in the propranolol group, with the beneficial effect being most pronounced in the first 12 to 18 months. The benefit was seen in all patient subgroups regardless of the number of infarcts or complications. Propranolol was well tolerated in patients without contraindications, and the authors recommended its use for at least three years following a myocardial infarction.

A number of subsidiary analyses of the BHAT data have also been published of which some of the more important are:

Beta-Blocker Heart Attack Trial Research Group 1983 A randomized trial of propranolol in patients with acute myocardial infarction. 1. Morbidity results. Journal of the American Medical Association 250: 2814–2818

The incidence of definite non-fatal infarction was lowered by 15.6% in the treated group. In patients without a prior history of angina the incidence of angina was 35.7% in the propranolol group and 34.4% in the placebo group.

Chadda K, Goldstein S, Bybington R, Curb J D 1986 Effect of propranolol after acute myocardial infarction in patients with congestive heart failure. Circulation 73: 503–510

This was a subgroup analysis of 365 patients randomized to placebo and 345 randomized to propranolol in the BHAT trial. In patients with a history of congestive failure before randomization, 14.8% in the propranolol group and 12.6% in the placebo group developed congestive failure during an average of 25 months of follow-up.

Peters R W, Bybington R, Arensberg D et al 1987 Mortality in the beta blocker heart attack trial: circumstances surrounding death. Journal of Chronic Diseases 40: 75–82

There were no striking differences in the circumstances preceding death in the active and placebo groups. An unexpected finding was that the protective effect of propranolol appeared to occur during the hours 10 p.m. to 7 a.m.

Peters R W, Muller J E, Goldstein S, Byington R, Friedman L M 1989 Propranolol and the morning increase in sudden death (BHAT study). American Journal of Cardiology 63: 1518–1520

Gastrointestinal haemorrhage

3. Pascal J-P, Gales P, and a Multicenter Study Group 1987 Propranolol in the prevention of first upper gastrointestinal tract haemorrhage in patients with cirrhosis of the liver and oesophageal varices. New England Journal of Medicine 317: 856–861

230 patients with large oesophageal varices (90% due to alcohol) were randomized to propranolol or placebo. The cumulative percentage of patients free of bleeding after 2 years was 74% on propranolol and 39% in the placebo group. Cumulative 2 year survival was 72% in the propranolol group and 51% in the placebo group ($p < 0.05$).

The Italian Multicenter Project for Propranolol in Prevention of Bleeding 1988 Propranolol for prophylaxis of bleeding in cirrhotic patients with large varices: a multicenter, randomized clinical trial. Hepatology 1: 1–5

174 patients with large varices were randomized to propranolol or placebo. After a mean follow up of 22 months neither the proportion free of bleeding, propranolol 74%, placebo 63%, or survival, propranolol 59%, placebo 74%, were significantly different. Post hoc analysis suggested that propranolol might have been of value in preventing bleeding in patients without ascites and in Child–Pugh class A.

General review articles

Conolly M E, Kersting F, Dollery C T 1976 The clinical pharmacology of beta-adrenoceptor blocking drugs. Progress in Cardiovascular Diseases 19: 203–234

Conway J 1975 Beta adrenergic blockade and hypertension. In: Oliver M F (ed) Modern trends in cardiology, vol 3. Butterworths, London, ch 13, pp 376–403

Fitzgerald J D 1980 Propranolol. In: Scriabine A (ed) Pharmacology of antihypertensive drugs. Raven Press, New York, pp 195–208

Gibson D G 1977 Pharmacodynamic properties of beta-adrenoceptor blocking drugs in man. In: Avery G S (ed) Cardiovascular drugs vol 2. Adis Press, Sydney, ch 1, pp 1–39

Routledge P A, Shand D G 1979 Clinical pharmacokinetics of propranolol. Drugs 4: 73–90

References

1. Tarazi R C, Dustan H P 1972 Beta-adrenergic blockade in hypertension. American Journal of Cardiology 29: 633–640
2. Prichard B N C, Shinebourne E, Fleming J, Hamer J 1970 Haemodynamic studies in hypertensive patients treated with oral propranolol. British Heart Journal 32: 236
3. Smith R S, Warren D J 1982 Effects of acute oral beta-adrenergic blockade on muscle blood flow in man. Cardiovascular Research 16: 205–208
4. Belolipetskaja V G, Piotrovskii V K, Metelitsa V I, Pavlinov S A 1989 Ion-exchange high-performance liquid chromatography in drug assay in biological fluids. V Propranolol and metabolites. Journal of Chromatography 491: 507–512
5. Takahashi H, Kanno S, Ogata H, Kashiwada K, Ohira M, Someya K 1988 Determination of propranolol enantiomers in human plasma and urine and in rat tissues using stationary phase liquid chromatography. Journal of Pharmaceutical Science 77: 913–915
6. Hayes A, Cooper R G, 1971 Studies on the absorption, distribution and excretion of propranolol in various species. Journal of Pharmacology and Experimental Therapeutics 176: 302–311
7. Myers M G, Lewis P J, Reid J L, Dollery C T 1975 Brain concentration of propranolol in relation to hypotensive effect in the rabbit with observations on brain propranolol levels in man. Journal of Pharmacology and Experimental Therapeutics 192: 327–335
8. Neil-Dwyer G, Bartlett J, McAinsh J, Cruickshank J M 1981 Beta-adrenoceptor blockers and the blood brain barrier. British Journal of Clinical Pharmacology 11: 549–553

Propranolol (hydrochloride)

9. Wood A J J, Kornhauser D M, Wilkinson G R, Shand D G, Branch RA 1978 The influence of cirrhosis on steady-state blood concentrations of unbound propranolol after oral administration. Clinical Pharmacokinetics 3: 478–487
10. Wood A J J, Vestal R C, Spannuth C L, Stone W J, Wilkinson G R, Shand D G 1980 Propranolol disposition in renal failure. British Journal of Clinical Pharmacology 10: 561–566
11. Schneider R G, Bishop H, Yates R A, Quarterman C P, Kendall M J 1980 Effect of age on plasma propranolol levels. British Journal of Clinical Pharmacology 10: 169–170
12. Walle T, Walle U K, Olanoff L S 1985 Quantitative account of propranolol metabolism in the urine of normal man. Drug Metabolism and Disposition 13: 204
13. Ward S A, Walle T, Walle U K, Wilkinson G R, Branch R A 1989 Propranolol's metabolism is determined by both mephenytoin and debrisoquine hydroxylase activities. Clinical Pharmacology and Therapeutics 45: 72–79
14. Nattel S, Rango R E, Van Loon G 1979 Mechanism of propranolol withdrawal phenomenon. Circulation 59: 1158–1164
15. Serlin M J, Orme M Le, MacIver M, Green R G, Sibeon R G, Breckenridge A M 1983 The pharmacodynamics and pharmacokinetics of conventional and long-acting propranolol in patients with moderate hypertension. British Journal of Clinical Pharmacology 15: 519–527
16. Leonetti G, Mayer G, Terzoli L et al 1975 Hypotensive and renin suppressing activities of propranolol in hypertensive patients. Clinical Science and Molecular Medicine 48: 491–499
17. Zhou H H, Koshakji R P, Silberstein D J, Milkinson G R, Wood A J J 1989 Racial differences in drug response. Altered sensitivity to and clearance of propranolol in men of Chinese descent as compared with American whites. New England Journal of Medicine 320: 565–570
18. Prichard B N C, Gillam P M S 1971 Assessment of propranolol in angina pectoris clinical dose response curve and effect on the electrocardiogram at rest and on exercise. British Heart Journal 33: 473–480
19. Miller R R, Olson H G, Pratt C M, Amsterdam E A, Macon D T 1975 Efficacy of beta-adrenergic blockade in coronary heart disease: propranolol in angina pectoris. Clinical Pharmacology and Therapeutics 18: 598–605
20. Gibson D, Sowton E 1969 The use of beta-adrenergic receptor blocking drugs in dysrrhythmias. Progress in Cardiovascular Disease 12: 16–39
21. Friehling T D, Lipschutz H, Marinchak R A, Stohler J L, Kowey P R 1990 Effectiveness of propranolol added to a type-1 antiarrhythmic agent for sustained ventricular tachycardia secondary to coronary artery disease. American Journal of Cardiology 65: 1328–1333
22. Myerburg R J, Kessler K M, Cox M M et al 1989 Reversal of proarrhythmic effect of flecainide acetate and encainide hydrochloride by propranolol. Circulation 80: 1571–1579
23. Oakley G D G, McGarry K, Limb D G, Oakley C M 1979 Management of pregnancy in patients with hypertrophic cardiomyopathy. British Medical Journal 1: 1749–1750
24. McDevitt D G, Shanks R G 1977 Beta-adrenoceptor blocking drugs in hyperthyroidism. Cardiovascular Drugs 2: 161–178
25. Murchison L E, How J, Bewsher P D 1979 Comparison of propranolol and metoprolol in the management of hyperthyroidism. British Journal of Clinical Pharmacology 8: 581–587
26. Tyrer P J, Lader M H 1974 Response to propranolol and diazepam in somatic and psychic anxiety. British Medical Journal 2: 14–16
27. Meibach R C, Dunner D, Wilson L G, Ishiki D, Dager S R 1987 Comparative efficacy of propranolol, chlordiazepoxide and placebo in the treatment of anxiety: A double-blind trial. Journal of Clinical Psychiatry 48: 355–358
28. Brantigan C O, Brantigan T A, Joseph N 1982 Effect of beta-blockade and beta-stimulation on stage fright. American Journal of Medicine 72: 88–94
29. Siitonen L, Sonck T, Janne J 1977 Effect of beta-blockade on performance: use of of beta-blockade in bowling and in shooting competitions. Journal of International Medical Research 5: 395–366
30. Weber R B, Reinmuth O 1972 The treatment of migraine with propranolol. Neurology (Minneap) 22: 366–369
31. Ziegler D K, Hurwitz A, Hassanein R S, Kodanaz H A, Preskorn S H, Mason J 1987 Migraine prophylaxis: A comparison of propranolol and amitriptyline. Archives of Neurology 44: 486–489
32. Delarue N C, Morrow J D, Kerr J H, Colapinto R F 1978 Phaeochromocytoma in the modern context. Canadian Journal of Surgery 21: 387–394
33. Garcia-Tsao G, Grace N D, Groszmann R J et al 1986 Short-term effects of propranolol on portal venous pressure. Hepatology 6: 101–106
34. Onishi K, Nakayama T, Saito M et al 1985 Effects of propranolol on portal haemodynamics in patients with chronic liver disease. American Journal of Gastroenterology 80: 132–153
35. Frishamn W, Jacob H, Eisenberg E, Ribner H 1979 Clinical pharmacology of the new beta-adrenergic blocking drugs. Part 8. Self poisoning with beta-adrenoceptor blocking agents: recognition and management. American Heart Journal 98: 798–811
36. Prichard B N C, Battersby L A, Cruickshank J M 1984 Overdose with beta-adrenergic blcoking agents. Adverse Drug Reactions and Acute Poisoning Review 3: 91–111
37. Agura E D, Wexler L F, Witzburg R A C 1985 Massive propranolol overdose — successful treatment with high dose isoproterenol and glucagon. American Journal of Medicine 80: 755–757
38. Owen J H, Williams C A, Rees A D 1982 Is Peyronie's disease iatrogenic. Journal of the Royal College of General Practitioners 32: 499–500
39. Day J L, Simpson N, Metcalfe J, Page R L 1979 Metabolic consequence of atenolol and propranolol in treatment of essential hypertension. British Medical Journal 1: 77–80
40. Byington R P, Worthy J, Craven T, Furberg C D 1990 Propranolol-induced lipid changes and their prognostic significance after a myocardial infarction; the beta-blocker heart-attack trial experience. American Journal of Cardiology 65: 1287–1290
41. Greenblatt D J, Koch-Weser J 1974 Adverse reactions to beta-adrenergic receptor blocking drugs: a report from the Boston Collaborative Drug Surveillance Program. Drugs 7: 118–129
42. Al-Dam Iuji S, Meek J H 1980 Interference of a propranolol metabolite and serum bilirubin estimation in chronic renal failure. British Medical Journal 280: 1414
43. Chou D, Tsuru M, Holtzman J C, Eckfelt J H 1980 Interference by the 4-hydroxylated metabolite of propranolol with determination of metanephrines by the Pisano method. Clinical Chemistry 26: 776–778
44. Bauer J H, Pape B, Zajicek J, Groshong T 1979 Propranolol in human plasma and breast milk. American Journal of Cardiology 43: 860–862
45. Rubin P C 1981 Beta-blockers in pregnancy. New England Journal of Medicine 305: 1323–1326
46. Pruyn S C, Phelan J P, Buchanon G C 1979 Long-term propranolol therapy in pregnancy: maternal and fetal outcome. American Journal of Obstetrics and Gynaecology. 135: 485–489

Propyliodone

Propyliodone is an organic iodinated radio-opaque compound used for bronchography and laryngography.

Chemistry

Propyliodone (Propyliodonum)
$C_{10}H_{11}I_2NO_3$
Propyl-1,4-dihydro-3,5-di-iodo-4-oxo-1-pyridylacetate

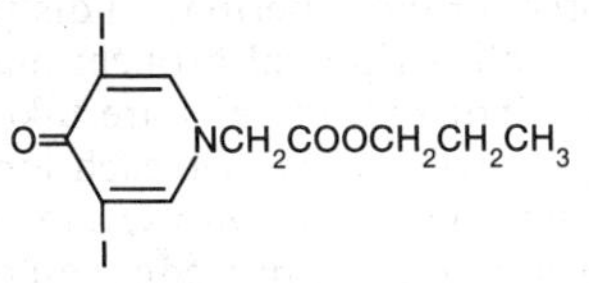

Molecular weight	447.0
pKa	—
Solubility	
in alcohol	1 in 500
in water	<1 in 5000
Octanol/water partition coefficient	high

A white or almost white, tasteless or almost tasteless crystalline powder with iodine content 56.8%. It is prepared by chemical synthesis and is available in both aqueous and oily suspensions. Propyliodone is not available in any combined preparations.

Pharmacology

The radiological use of propyliodone depends not on any conventional pharmacological properties but, rather, on its radio-opacity and its distribution in the bronchial tree.

Toxicology

Intratracheal administration of aqueous and oily suspensions of propyliodone (0.4 $ml.kg^{-1}$ body weight) to anaesthetized rabbits, repeated at 15-minute intervals, showed toleration of up to four doses before asphyxiation.[1] Up to 18 $g.kg^{-1}$ body weight administered orally to mice produced no immediate toxic symptoms and long-term growth was unaffected.[1] The intravenous (LD_{50}) dose of aqueous propyliodone for mice is 300 $mg.kg^{-1}$; death is due to blood vessel occlusion. Doses of up to 120 $mg.kg^{-1}$ produced temporary disorientation, but recovery was complete. Subcutaneous, intramuscular and intraperitoneal injection of large doses of Dionosil produced no toxic effects in mice and rabbits.[1] No data are available on mutagenicity, carcinogenicity or teratogenicity.

Both aqueous and oily forms of the agent are irritant, stimulating coughing, the former more than the latter. In animal studies, both are associated with macroscopic signs of pulmonary infiltration apparent by 16 hours and maximal at three days. After two weeks, there is a return to normal. Microscopically, there are scattered foci of round-cell infiltration in the interstitial tissues which persist up to one month. Evidence on chronic effects is contradictory (see Adverse reactions).

Clinical pharmacology

Propyliodone has no conventional clinical pharmacological effects and, unlike other iodine-containing contrast media, there is little evidence of histamine release from mast cells or anticholinesterase effects.

Pharmacokinetics

The distribution of propyliodone preparations in the bronchial tree depends on the technique used, patient position, amount and quality of bronchial secretions, inspiratory effort by the patient and whether or not he coughs. The distribution in the main airways is determined largely by gravity, but in the smaller airways more by inspiration and coughing. The object is to coat the small bronchi; this is usually achieved with these preparations, but if too high a dose is used, or too rapid an instillation, complete filling of the small airways may be the result with consequent pulmonary collapse. This is more likely to occur with the oily suspension than with the aqueous suspension. The latter is also thought, on the whole, to yield better coating.[2]

Propyliodone may be cleared from the large airways by coughing and subsequent expectoration or swallowing, but this has little effect on movement in the small airways which appears to depend principally on ciliary activity.

Following instillation of propyliodone suspension, visualization of the bronchial tree is achieved for some 20–45 minutes. Propyliodone is usually cleared from the bronchial tree within four days by enzymatic hydrolysis and absorption into the circulation,[1] and by ciliary activity and coughing with expectoration or swallowing. Some may persist for a considerable period in the abnormal lung, in cystic bronchiectasis for example.

The hydrolysed derivative is readily absorbed into the blood from the small bronchi. Propyliodone coughed up and swallowed is similarly readily hydrolysed enzymatically in the gastrointestinal tract and absorbed. The hydrolysed derivative is excreted by glomerular filtration.[1] In man, approximately 50% of an intratracheal dose appears in the urine in 72 hours.[1] Up to 50% of an intratracheal dose may be expectorated. The oily preparation clears more slowly than the aqueous preparation by all routes. The arachis oil used for the oily suspension in commercial formulations is retained in the lungs and phagocytosed and removed by ciliary activity and expectoration, or absorbed into the lymphatics. It is not known whether propyliodone or its metabolite cross the placenta or are excreted in human milk.

Oral absorption	Hydrolysed before absorption
Presystemic metabolism	Extensive
Plasma half life	—
Volume of distribution	—
Plasma protein binding	—

Concentration–effect relationship

Too large a dose, or one administered too rapidly, may result in complete filling of the smaller airways and consequent occlusion of segmental bronchi with atelectasis. Alveolarization may also occur in these circumstances, this being more likely with the oily preparation.

Metabolism

Propyliodone is hydrolysed in the lungs or gut wall to 3,5-di-iodo-4-pyridone-N-acetate which is absorbed and excreted in the urine (Fig. 1).[1]

Fig. 1 Metabolism of propyliodone

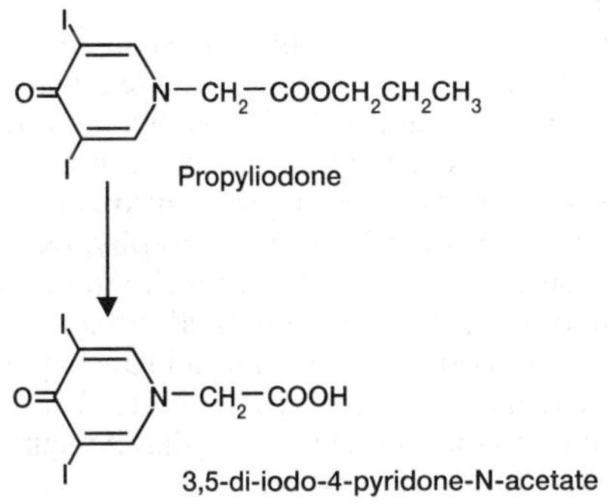

P

Pharmaceutics

Propyliodone crystals are milled to a 5–14 mm range.[3] Commercial preparations are available in two formulations:

1. Dionosil Oily (Glaxo, UK) As a 60% w/v sterile suspension in arachis oil (iodine content 28.4% w/v).
2. Dionosil Aqueous (Glaxo, UK) As a sterile 50% w/v suspension in sterile water (iodine content 34.1% w/v).

The aqueous preparation contains suspending and dispersing agents, a sodium citrate buffer, sodium chloride to render it isotonic and benzyl alcohol as an antimicrobial preservative agent. A little carboxymethyl cellulose is added as a viscosity-controlling factor.[4,5,]

Preparations are stable with a good shelf-life, but should be protected from heat and bright light as these may liberate iodine from the propyliodone. It is claimed that there is minimal risk from potentially allergenic substances used in the aqueous suspension.

Therapeutic use

Indications

1. Laryngography
2. Bronchography
3. Sinography and fistulography

Contraindications

1. Hypersensitivity to propyliodone or other iodinated contrast agents
2. Allergy to other drugs
3. Asthma
4. Chronic obstructive airways disease with an element of bronchospasm
5. Bronchiectasis in patients in whom surgery is contraindicated
6. Acute infection
7. Severe cardiac disease.

Mode of use

A variety of techniques are used for the introduction of propyliodone in oily or water suspension into the pharynx, larynx, bronchial tree, sinus tracts and fistuli.

Indications

1. Laryngography

Contrast studies of the larynx and pharynx using an oily suspension of propyliodone may be used to outline the anatomical structures.

A patient is premedicated with one milligram of atropine subcutaneously in order to suppress mucus formation. The patient sucks an anaesthetic lozenge, and a topical spray of 1% lignocaine is then used to achieve local anaesthesia. 15–20 ml of suspension are then dripped over the posterior aspect of the tongue from a curved laryngeal syringe during quiet inspiration. Radiographs are obtained in the anterior, posterior and lateral projections during inspiration, valsalva manoeuvre and phonation.

The whole of the larynx and hypopharynx may be visualized during the examination, and early mucosal changes may be evaluated. However, the advent of computed tomography (CT) has diminished the need for this examination and it should not in any case be carried out in any patients with large lesions in view of the danger of precipitating an airway obstruction.

2. Bronchography

The role of bronchography has diminished in recent years. In the diagnosis of bronchiectasis most patients have a plain chest film and CT has been shown to be useful. Occasionally, a bronchogram is still necessary to establish the diagnosis, and the surgeon may require one as a mapping procedure prior to surgery. Unexplained haemoptysis is still an occasional indication for bronchography, but the yield of the examination in such patients is low. Bronchography may occasionally be required to delineate congenital abnormalities prior to surgery, and may be used to demonstrate a bronchopleural fistula. As regards the latter, however, it is usually more fruitful to instill the contrast medium into the pleural space so that it might be sucked into the bronchial tree during respiration.

Bronchography may be performed under local anaesthesia in most patients but a few will require general anaesthesia, particularly children. Patients should be prepared by physiotherapy, antibiotic treatment of any infection, and a premedication of diazepam and atropine, and should take nothing by mouth for the previous 12 hours. Both the aqueous and oily solutions of propyliodone may be used. The aqueous form appears to give a better coating of the mucosa,[2] while the oily form tends to achieve better filling of the small bronchi. It is also more likely to produce alveolarization. One advantage of the aqueous suspension is that it may be diluted with either water or a local anaesthetic. Such a dilute suspension may be helpful in obtaining good peripheral filling. The contrast agent may be introduced into the bronchial tree: under direct vision through the fibreoptic bronchoscope through a tube introduced by the nasal route after a suitable local anaesthetic has been introduced; by the cricothyroid route, in which case, after local anaesthetic, a tube is introduced in the mid-line through the thyroid membrane; or during fibreoptic bronchoscopy. Positioning of a tube introduced by whichever route should be controlled under fluoroscopy. Patient-positioning and gravity are used to ensure that contrast medium is distributed to the main lobar bronchi. Patient inspiration is the principal driving force for more peripheral distribution of contrast. Delineation of the small peripheral bronchi may only be achieved by deep inspiration. Spot radiographs are taken at suitable intervals. Some radiologists will catheterize each lobe selectively before administering contrast. In patients with severe pulmonary disease it may be necessary to carry out the procedure on one lung only and to study the other side at a different session. Even in patients with unimpaired pulmonary function, a 15-minute interval should be allowed between bronchography of the two sides. Contrast agent should be removed from one lung as far as is possible before introducing more into the other.

3. Sinography and fistulography

The use of propyliodone as a contrast agent may be sensible in the study of sinus tracts and fistulae in the thorax if any communication with the airways is suspected. The new low-osmolality water-soluble intravascular iodinated contrast agents may now also safely be used in these circumstances. Indeed recent studies suggest they are to be preferred.[6–8]

Contraindications

1. Hypersensitivity to propyliodone or other iodinated contrast agents

Idiosyncratic anaphylactoid reactions following the systemic absorption of the contrast medium are very rare events in bronchography, but a previous episode constitutes an absolute contraindication to the repeat use of propyliodone. There appears to be cross-reactivity between different iodinated contrast agents as regards sensitivity reactions, and it might therefore be argued that a significant adverse reaction to any other iodinated contrast agent administered by any other route may constitute a contraindication to the use of propyliodone. The contraindication in these circumstances is probably only a relative one, but caution should be exercised.

2. Allergy to other drugs

This is a risk factor in general with regard to iodinated radiological contrast agents but evidence for the case of these agents in particular is not available.

3. Asthma

Bronchospasm is a well-recognized complication of bronchography. It may be related to either contrast medium or to catheter manipulation in the bronchial tree. Bronchography should therefore be performed on asthmatics only when absolutely necessary. Administration of corticosteroids and bronchodilators is indicated.

4. Chronic obstructive airways disease with an element of bronchospasm

Similar considerations apply in the case of these patients. If lung function is very poor, it may be wise to study one lung per session.

5. Bronchiectasis in patients in whom surgery is contraindicated

If surgery is contraindicated in a patient with bronchiectasis, then bronchography is best not performed. Complications may occur, and the information to be obtained from a bronchogram is rarely necessary for the management of such patients.

Propyliodone

6. Acute infection
Bronchography should not be performed in patients with acute pneumonia or acute or chronic bronchitis both because of the potential pulmonary complications, and because repeated coughing may impair the quality of the examination.

7. Severe cardiac disease
Patients with severe cardiac disease may be unable to tolerate a reduction in pulmonary function engendered by the examination; it should therefore not be performed unless absolutely necessary.

Adverse reactions

Approximately 30% of patients having bronchography suffer some sort of adverse effect. The incidence is higher with propyliodone aqueous than with propyliodone oily. Factors generally associated with adverse effects are a high contrast volume (>20 ml), and the amount radiologically apparent after 24 hours.

Potentially life-threatening effects
Anaphylactoid reactions to the absorbed drug have been reported but are very rare. Contrast laryngography in the presence of bulky disease may precipitate respiratory obstruction. Severe bronchospasm may be precipitated by catheter manipulation in a reactive bronchial tree, by the introduction of the fluid agent as a non-specific effect or, possibly, as an idiosyncratic reaction to the contrast agent itself. It is more common in asthmatics. The most effective treatment is intravenous aminophylline. The use of too large a dose of contrast agent may result in the blocking of small airways with segmental or lobar collapse; this may be catastrophic for some patients with impaired pulmonary function. This complication is frequently seen in children.[9,10] Several factors have been implicated in segmented or lobular collapse: the lack of peripheral interbronchial communications and the use of halothane with 50% oxygen/50% nitrous oxide mixture for general anaesthesia.[9,10] Local anaesthetic overdose during the procedure is a possible complication. Lignocaine is rapidly absorbed from the nasopharynx and bronchial mucosa and if an excess is used, high blood levels may be achieved.[11] The total dose should be limited to 12 ml of 2% lignocaine for an adult patient and lower concentrations of lignocaine are preferred since they are absorbed more slowly. Overdose of lignocaine may result in respiratory and cardiac depression.[12] Hypersensitivity to lignocaine has been described.[13]

All patients suffer a worsening of respiratory function tests.[14,15] A fall in vital capacity is not surprising since 40 ml propyliodone may be used for bilateral bronchography, and the total volume of the bronchial tree is only 150 ml. A reduction in diffusion capacity is also the norm for up to 72 hours. These changes may be very serious for patients with already severely impaired lung function or poor cardiac function. Isotope studies show that both ventilation and perfusion defects are routinely found following bronchography.[16] The oil has been reported as producing foreign body granulomata in the lungs,[17] but other work has disputed this, reporting only transient inflammatory reactions.[1,15,18] It has been claimed that the changes in resected human specimens are no different from those expected as a result of the underlying lung abnormality.[19] Most investigations have considered the carboxyl methylcellulose (CMC) in the aqueous preparation to be harmless,[14,18] while others have cautioned that large amounts may produce a chronic inflammatory reaction.[20] Pulmonary fibrosis is said not to occur as a result of the inflammatory effects.[21] A case of cerebral dye embolization has been reported during selective bronchography following transbronchial biopsy.[22]

Acute overdosage
Overdose in the conventional sense does not occur but, as has been indicated, too high a dose may result in blockage of small airways with segmental or lobar collapse.

Overdose of local anaesthetic is a significant danger. A maximum dose of 200 mg is recommended (10 ml of 2% or 5 ml of 4%). Lower concentrations are to be preferred as they are absorbed more slowly. Absorption through the alveoli is very rapid, a point to be remembered when sprays are used. Maximum blood concentrations are achieved after 5–25 minutes. The excretion half life is 2 hours. 73% is still in the circulation after 1 hour, hence the danger of repeated doses. As the local anaesthetic is metabolized in the liver there is thus a need for caution in patients with liver disease.

Severe or irreversible adverse effects
The mucosa of the nasopharynx or the vocal cords may be damaged during the introduction of the tube. When the cricothyroid route is used, subcutaneous emphysema or extravasation of contrast medium in the soft tissues may be a complication in inexperienced hands. There may be bleeding (necessitating tracheostomy), infected haematoma or laryngeal perichondritis. Extravasated agent may invoke a local inflammatory reaction, with oedema, pain, hoarseness and even stridor. Pyrexia and dysphagia occasionally occur. Contrast may track into the mediastinum giving a pericarditis-like condition; corticosteroids and antibiotics usually cure this condition in less than two weeks.[24,25] Propyliodone engenders a local inflammatory reaction in the lungs,[7,23] and a post-procedure pneumonitis with pyrexia is an occasional adverse effect.[26] Interference with lung surfactant has been reported.[25]

Symptomatic adverse effects
Fever, sometimes associated with malaise and aching joints, is an occasional problem following bronchography with propyliodone and other media.[28] Mechanisms are unclear, but the symptoms usually subside spontaneously within 48 hours without treatment. Headache (10–20%), abdominal pain, nausea and vomiting (10–15%) may also occur, as may a variety of skin eruptions, presumably related to systemic absorption of the iodinated contrast agent. A 'flu-like' illness, with sore throat, conjunctivitis, skin eruptions, bone pain and enlargement of the salivary glands, has been labelled 'Iodism'.[28] Severe pneumonitis has been described and ascribed to an idiosyncratic reaction.[29]

Interference with clinical pathology tests
Thyroid function tests based on measurement of iodine may be invalidated for some weeks following the procedure, as is the case with all iodinated contrast agents.[31] Thyroid function tests not based on iodine measurements are unaffected. Although no data are available, contrast agents excreted in the urine may interfere with the sulphosalicylic acid test for urinary protein[32] and it may be that the propyliodone hydrolysis metabolite can do the same.

High risk groups

Neonates
Bronchography should never be performed in children less than one year old.

Breast milk. No information is available on the appearance of propyliodone in human milk.

Children
Caution should always be exercised in children in whom general anaesthesia may be necessary. The total dose of propyliodone used should be limited to as little as possible, as the child's bronchial tree is of small volume and may be readily compromised by the use of too much, or too concentrated, a contrast medium. Dilution of the aqueous propyliodone with sterile water may help avoid these difficulties.

Pregnant women
No information is available on mutagenic or teratogenic effects of propyliodone, but all radiological investigations should be avoided in pregnancy unless it is clear that the information to be derived offsets the risk of radiation exposure to the fetus.

The elderly
Because of the higher probability of impaired pulmonary and cardiac function, caution should be exercised in the performance of bronchography in the elderly.

Concurrent disease
Some of the high risk groups are discussed above; they include those who have had previous adverse reactions to propyliodone or to other iodinated contrast agents, asthmatics, patients with chronic obstructive airways disease with a spastic element, or any patients with severely impaired pulmonary or cardiac function. Patients with bronchiectasis rarely need bronchography as clinical management is rarely affected in patients with severe cardiac disease.

Drug interactions

No significant drug interactions are known.

General review articles

Honse A J S 1977 Iodinated bronchographic agents. In: Miller R E, Skucos J (eds) Radiographic contrast agents. University Park Press, Baltimore, pp 389–401

Ansell G 1976 Bronchography. In: Ansell G (ed) Complications in diagnostic radiology. Blackwell Scientific Publications, Oxford, pp 278–300

References

1. Tomich E G, Basil B, Davis B 1953 The properties of n-propyl 3:5-di-iodo-4-pyridone-N-acetate (propyliodone). British Journal of Pharmacology 8: 166–170
2. Walker H G, Ma H 1971 Oily and aqueous propyliodone (Dionosil) as bronchographic contrast agents. Journal of the Canadian Association of Radiologists 22: 148–153
3. Holden W S, Crone R S 1953 Bronchography using dionosil oily. British Journal of Radiology 26: 317–332
4. Shelenski H O, Clark A M 1948 Physiological action of sodium carboxymethyl cellulose on laboratory animals and humans. Food Research 13: 29–35
5. Light J P, Oster W F 1966 Clinical and pathological reactions to the bronchographic agent Dionosil aqueous. American Journal of Roentgenology 98: 468–473
6. Ginai A Z 1986 Experimental evaluation of various available contrast agents for use in the gastrointestinal tract in case of suspected leakage. Effect on pleura. British Journal of Radiology 59: 887–894
7. Ginai A Z, Ten-Kate F J W, Ten-Berg R G M, Horrnstra K 1987 Experimental evaluation of various available contrast agent for use in the upper gastrointestinal tract in cases of suspected leak. Effects on lung. British Journal of Radiology 57: 895–901
8. Ginai A Z, Gen-Kate F J W, Ten Berg R G M, Hoornstra K 1985 Experimental evaluation of various available contrast agents for use in the upper gastrointestinal tract in cases of suspected leakage. Effects on mediastinum. British Journal of Radiology 58: 585–592
9. Robinson A E, Hall K D, Yokoyama K N, Capp M P 1971 Paediatric bronchography. The problem of segmental pulmonary loss of volume I. A retrospective survey of 165 paediatric bronchograms. Investigative Radiology 6: 89–94
10. Robinson A E, Hall K D, Yokoyama K N, Capp M P 1971 Paediatric bronchography: the problem of segmental pulmonary loss of volume II. An experimental investigation of the mechanism and prevention of pulmonary collapse during bronchography under general anaesthesia. Investigative Radiology 6: 95–100
11. Bromage P R, Robson J G 1961 Concentration of lignocaine in the blood after intravenous, intramuscular and endotracheal administration. Anaesthesia 16: 461–478
12. Steinhaus J E 1962 Toxic reactions to local anaesthetics. Journal of the American Medical Association 32: 168–172
13. Lehner T 1971 Lignocaine hypersensitivity. Lancet 1: 1245–1246
14. Bhargava R K, Woolf C R 1967 Changes in diffusion capacity after bronchography. American Review of Respiratory Diseases 96: 827–829
15. Christoforidis A J 1973 Bronchography. In: Meaney T F, Lalli A F, Alfidi R J (eds). Complications and legal implications of radiologic special procedures. Mosby, St Louis, pp 102–116
16. Suprenant E, Wilson A, Bennett L, O'Reilly R, Webber M 1968 Changes in regional pulmonary function following bronchography. Radiology 91: 736–741
17. Bjork L, Lodin H 1957 Pulmonary changes following bronchography with dionosil oily (animal experiments). Acta Radiologica Diagnostica 47: 177–180
18. Greenberg S D, Spjut H J, Hallman G I 1966 Experimental study of bronchographic media on lung. Archives of Otolaryngology 83: 276–282
19. Holden W S, Cowdell R H 1958 Late results of bronchography using Dionosil oily. Acta Radiologica Diagnosis 48: 105–112
20. Clement J G 1969 Inhalation bronchography — methods and results in the experimental animal. Journal of the Canadian Association of Radiologists 20: 106–113
21. Johnson P M, Montclair W J, Benson W R, Sprunt W H, Dunnagon W A 1960 Toxicity of bronchographic contrast media. Annals of Otology, Rhinology and Laryngology 69: 1103–1113
22. Oldenberg F A, Newhouse M T 1978 Cerebral dye embolus. A complication of selective bronchography following transbronchial biopsy. Chest 73: 872–873
23. Light J P, Oster W F 1966 Clinical and pathological reactions to the bronchographic agent Dionosil aqueous. American Journal of Roentgenology 98: 468–473
24. Wright F W 1970 Accidental injection of dionosil into the neck during bronchography. Clinical Radiology 21: 384–389
25. Zucherman S D, Jacobron G 1962 Transtracheal bronchography. Complications of injection outside the trachea. American Journal of Roentgenology 87: 840–843
26. Kawabrata Y, Mori J, Iwai K 1985 Pathology of dionosil pneumonia. Journal of Thoracic Diseases 23: 674–678
27. Schurch S F, Roach R M 1976 Interference of bronchographic agents with lung surfactant. Respiratory Physiology 28: 99–117
28. Rayl J E 1965 Clinical reactions following bronchography. Annals of Otology, Rhinology and Laryngology 74: 1121–1132
29. Wardman A F, Willey R F, Cook N J 1983 Unusual pulmonary reaction to oily propyliodone in bronchography. British Journal of Diseases of the Chest 77: 98–103
30. Benker G, Vosskuhler A, HJoff H G 1983 Thyroid function after bronchography with propyliodone. Hormone Research 17: 121–127
31. Salkin D, Lawrence H S, Kingsley G R 1957 Effect of dionosil bronchography on blood iodine. American Review of Tuberculosis 77: 181–183
32. Young D S, Pestaner L C, Gibberman V G 1975 Effects of drugs on clinical laboratory tests. Clinical Chemistry 21: 1D–482D

Propylthiouracil

Propylthiouracil (PTU) has been in general use for over 40 years as a treatment for thyrotoxicosis. It is a member of the thioureylene class of drug.

Chemistry

Propylthiouracil (Propycil, Procasil, Propyl-Thyracil, Prothyran, Thyreostat II)
$C_7H_{10}N_2OS$
2,3-Dihydro-6-propyl-2-thioxopyrimidin-4(1H)-one

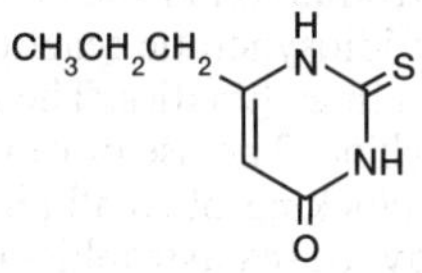

Molecular weight	170.2
pKa	7.5
Solubility	
in alcohol	1 in 900
in water	1 in 60
Octanol/water partition coefficient	—

Propylthiouracil is a white crystalline powder with a bitter taste. It is prepared by condensation of ethyl B-oxocaproate with thiourea. It is available only in tablet form, as a single product.

Pharmacology

Propylthiouracil (PTU) is an antithyroid drug that depresses the formation of thyroid hormone. This is effected by interference both with the incorporation of iodine into tyrosyl residues, and with the coupling of such residues to form iodothyronines. Propylthiouracil achieves these actions by the inhibition of the enzyme peroxidase. Propylthiouracil only binds to and inhibits peroxidase when the haem of the enzyme is in the oxidized state. In addition propylthiouracil causes a blockade of the peripheral conversion of T_4 to T_3[1,2] and also causes a gradual reduction in the circulating level of thyroid-stimulating immunoglobulins in Grave's disease.[3,4] This latter effect is also demonstrable in vitro.[5,6]

Toxicology

There have been no systematic long-term animal toxicology studies. Some short-term highly selective studies were performed 45 years ago on the introduction of this class of drugs.

The information available concerns the following:

Autoimmune phenomena. Several studies have demonstrated the production of an SLE-like syndrome in cats treated with therapeutic doses of PTU. Anti-DNA antibodies can be demonstrated but the cats rapidly recover on withdrawal of the drug.[7]

Neoplasia. Rats and other rodents treated with high doses of PTU, thiourea, thiouracil or other goitrogens and made markedly hypothyroid will frequently develop thyroid hyperplasia, adenomas, carcinoma, pituitary adenomas and parathyroid hyperplasia (there are no human counterparts for the induction of thyroid neoplasia by therapeutic doses of PTU or other drugs in this class).[8,9]

Teratogenesis. There have been small-scale studies of the effect of PTU treatment on the fetus.[10] These demonstrate effects on fetal growth rate, the production of thyroid enlargement and changes in cerebral development when the fetus is rendered hypothyroid. There is no evidence of malformations unrelated to the hypothyroid state.

Clinical pharmacology

Propylthiouracil is an effective drug in the therapy of hyperthyroidism. Its effects are only manifest after a latent period of up to 3 or 4 weeks. This is because all preformed hormone has to be utilized before circulating concentrations will fall. In some patients with large goitres or with nodular goitres the delay in onset of effect may be even longer. The main clinical pharmacological effects of propylthiouracil are the declining evidence of hyperthyroidism. Hypothyroidism is occasionally induced, particularly if the dose of drug is large, or treatment is unduly prolonged. In animal studies propylthiouracil seems to become a substrate for iodination, thereby diverting oxidized iodine away from the thyroglobulin. This mechanism of action of propylthiouracil has yet to be confirmed in man.[12]

Pharmacokinetics

The assay of the drug in biological fluids is by gas–liquid chromatography, high performance liquid chromatography, and, as currently preferred, by radioimmunoassay, the lower limit of detection[13] being about 8.5 μg.l^{-1}. Only 20% is free for diffusion.[12] No alteration in pharmacokinetics is seen in pregnancy[14] and clearance is unchanged in the elderly.[12]

Absorption from the gut is rapid, with average peak blood levels of 9.1 mg.l^{-1} about 1 hour after an oral dose of 400 mg, in a study in seven normal humans;[15] between half and three-quarters of the dose was bioavailable, the remainder appearing in the faeces due to incomplete absorption or rapid first-pass metabolism by the liver. Following intravenous administration, the average half life of the initial distribution phase was 6.3 min and the elimination half life was 1.3 h. Despite this short half life in the circulation, retention in the thyroid gland is at least 24 h.[16] The total volume of distribution is about 30 l, and about 80% is protein bound.[12]

Studies with ^{35}S-PTU demonstrate localization in normal thyroids, and in goitres, whether toxic or not.[17] The peak intrathyroidal level occurs at 1 hour after a single dose.[16] In rats given an intraperitoneal dose, the drug accumulated in the thyroid, whilst the radioactivity disappeared rapidly from plasma and liver.[17] The half life of PTU in the human thyroid is not known, but must be considerably longer than in the serum.[12]

Placental transfer of PTU occurs rapidly. In pregnant rats, intravenously administered ^{35}S-PTU appeared in a few minutes in the fetal circulation, reaching about half the maternal concentration at about an hour; in human studies, localization in the fetal thyroid has been shown.[18,19] Fetal hypothyroidism with goitre clearly could result, and has done so.[20]

Transfer of propylthiouracil into breast milk is well documented in man, the concentration reaching about 10% of the serum level.[12] An oral dose of 400 mg only gave the infant a dose of 99 μg, a dose that is unlikely to, and indeed did not, affect neonatal thyroid function. Another study based on measurement of ^{35}S in milk following an oral dose of radiolabelled drug showed the milk/serum non-protein bound ^{35}S ratio to be 0.55; 0.077% of the dose was excreted in the milk in 24 h.[21]

Oral absorption	50–75%
Presystemic metabolism	—
Plasma half life	
range	1–3 h
Volume of distribution	~30 l
Plasma protein binding	~80%

Concentration–effect relationship

The plasma concentrations of propylthiouracil have been studied in patients with thyrotoxicosis.[22] After three weeks on treatment there is a fair correlation (r=0.7) between the plasma concentration of propylthiouracil and the decrease in serum T_3 concentrations. Whether such an approach would contribute usefully to clinical management is yet to be explored. A peak concentration of over 4 mg.l^{-1} appears to be needed[11] and a single oral dose of 300 mg

Propylthiouracil

given to normal subjects usually results in a mean concentration of 5 mg.l^{-1} after one hour.[23] There is no evidence of tolerance, at least in animal studies.[24]

Metabolism

Metabolism and excretion of orally administered ^{35}S-PTU has been studied in man.[25,26] Most of the isotope was excreted in the urine in the first few hours, with 83% lost in the first 24 hours. Most was excreted as the glucuronic acid conjugate of PTU (Fig. 1) and very little as the unchanged drug. Negligible amounts appeared in the faeces.

Fig. 1 The metabolism of propylthiouracil

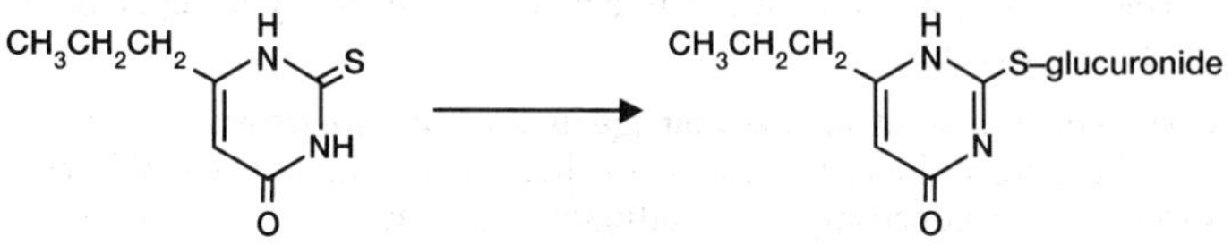

Pharmaceutics

The only available preparation of PTU is a small white 50 mg generic tablet. In the event of treatment being urgently required for a patient unable to swallow, the tablet can be crushed and administered by stomach tube.

Therapeutic use

Indications

1. Thyrotoxicosis

Contraindications

1. Previous severe hypersensitivity reaction, e.g. agranulocytosis, hepatitis, vasculilitis
2. In renal failure where urinary excretion is reduced, a lower dose than usual is needed

Mode of use

A typical course of treatment with PTU starts with a dose of 100 mg thrice daily, or for a severe case with a large goitre, up to 200 mg 6-hourly, dropping to 50 mg thrice daily as a maintenance dose once the patient is clinically and biochemically euthyroid, which usually takes 4 to 8 weeks. The effect of an overdose is to cause a subnormal serum level of thyroid hormone, which in turn stimulates an increase in release of TSH by the pituitary, and this causes thyroid hypertrophy with an increasing goitre. After a total of 18 months of treatment, the drug is stopped and the patient placed on long-term surveillance against the risk of relapse.

Major differences from the above system have been proposed and results from illustrative series will be presented later. Some authorities[27,28] have employed a much larger blocking dose throughout the treatment period, in order to achieve greater suppression of circulating thyroid-stimulating antibody levels, and T_4 or T_3 is simultaneously administered to maintain the patient euthyroid. This combined system has the advantage of not requiring as much care in adjusting the dose of antithyroid drug, and obviates the risk of transient hypothyroidism, which is believed (but unproven) to lead to exacerbation of eye signs.

The length of the treatment course has also been varied significantly. Short-term therapy has had varying success.[29,30] A relationship has been shown between duration of therapy and relapse rate.[31]

Once-daily regimes have been advocated as being equally efficacious as divided doses, and with the advantage of better compliance.[27,32] Against this idea is the fact that in rats the drug level in the thyroid was much more variable when the daily dose was given all together rather than divided in a thrice-daily regime.[33] However, intrathyroidal retention of the drug in Graves' disease has been shown to last for 24 hours.[16,17] The efficacy of a single daily dose in man is still debated.[11] If a once-daily regime were a high priority, carbimazole with its longer intrathyroidal residence and longer duration of inhibitory effect would be a better choice than propylthiouracil.

Use of ancillary drugs
Propranolol, a competitive antagonist at both the β_1-adrenoceptor and β_2-adrenoceptor, is highly effective in reducing the anxiety, tremor, sweating and tachycardia of thyrotoxicosis and is widely used with a thioureylene, at the start of therapy. The effect is immediate, and gives symptomatic relief before the antithyroid drug takes full effect.

Indications

The only indication for PTU is to control thyrotoxicosis, and it is effective whether the thyrotoxicosis is due to a hypersecreting hot nodule, a multinodular goitre, or Graves' disease, but is ineffective in the treatment of thyrotoxicosis caused by the release of thyroid hormone from a gland that has become involved by an episode of subacute thyroiditis.

Choice of treatment for the management of thyrotoxicosis
Possible choices include a course of therapy with an antithyroid drug, subtotal thyroidectomy, and radioactive iodine.

The attraction of an antithyroid drug is that it is almost certain to control the condition in the medium term, serious side effects are rare, supervision is relatively easy and infrequent, and subsequent hypothyroidism is very rare.[34] About half the patients[35] will remain in long-term remission after therapy is discontinued. Favourable factors are a small gland and a moderately elevated T_3,[36] but this cannot be predicted with any certainty.[37] Relapse usually occurs within 2 years. Then it is usual practice[34] to employ an alternative strategy such as surgery or ^{131}I.

The choice of surgery as the elective first treatment, following preparation with a short course of an antithyroid drug, is made on the grounds that there is no problem of medical supervision or patient non-compliance with a lengthy period of drug therapy and relapse is infrequent (about 5%[38]) although hypothyroidism, whether immediate or delayed, may occur. The incidence of hypothyroidism in a series of 2141 operated patients followed for a mean of 21 years was substantial at about 37%.[39,40] The other disadvantage is the inherent surgical risk, and several days of hospitalization.

The third option is ^{131}I therapy. Here the main attraction is simplicity, but disadvantages are considerable: even if a large dose is employed, not all patients are relieved. For example, in one series, about two-thirds of 215 cases became hypothyroid at one year while 5% remained hyperthyroid.[41] Again, in those rendered euthyroid with modest doses, if follow-up is long enough, hypothyroidism nearly always occurs. Thus, lifelong follow-up is mandatory. The risk of cancer can now be regarded as having been excluded by the massive clinical series already reported.[42]

A selection of therapeutic options
A selection of therapeutic options for the various circumstances in which thyrotoxicosis occurs has not yet been generally accepted. Local availability will clearly be a determinant. Beyond this, the following recommendations are offered.

Adults under 40
These constitute the largest group of patients and are generally treated with a course of 12 to 18 months of antithyroid drugs, but others would recommend surgery or ^{131}I.

Juvenile thyrotoxicosis
Here the risks of hypothyroidism or recurrence after surgery are substantial.[43,44] The difficulty of guaranteeing freedom from carcinogenic risk and ensuring a lifetime of follow-up argues against ^{131}I, so antithyroid drug therapy is usually the initial choice. If relapse occurs after a first course, either a second course or an ablative treatment is employed. As only 50% achieve a lasting remission, a case has been put forward for the use of ^{131}I.[44]

Thyrotoxicosis in pregnancy
The usual clinical problem is that the patient conceives shortly after becoming euthyroid, and when well established on a maintenance dose of an antithyroid drug. The simplest management is to carry on with the minimal dose required, until several months postpartum. A rise in dose requirement during pregnancy is not normally seen, while a dose reduction towards the end of pregnancy[45] is sometimes feasible, probably due to lower levels of circulating thyroid-stimulating antibody.

So long as a maintenance dose of 50 mg thrice daily is not exceeded, a goitre is usually not seen in the neonate. The relationship between dose and fetal goitre is imprecise.[46] The fetal outcome has been generally satisfactory in drug-treated pregnancies.[47,48] With modern free thyroid hormone assays available to guide dose titration, there would seem to be little necessity for combination treatment using both an antithyroid drug and thyroxine. Thyroxine crosses the placenta very poorly[49] and so would not protect the fetus from getting a goitre if the mother were overtreated with antithyroid drug.

In the event that a woman first manifests thyrotoxicosis during the course of pregnancy, minimum doses of PTU are advocated, for example, starting with 100 mg thrice daily, and dropping swiftly to 50 mg thrice daily as soon as a definite clinical response is seen.

Although the quantity of PTU appearing in breast milk is very small and breast-feeding has been advocated as safe,[11] some regard this as contraindicated. The antithyroid drug can be conveniently withdrawn about 6 months postpartum.

The alternative strategy of surgery, particularly advocated in the second trimester, would appear needlessly meddlesome at this particular time of a woman's life. The positive attraction of maintaining antithyroid drugs throughout the pregnancy is that it minimizes the risk of transient fetal or neonatal thyrotoxicosis[50] caused by the transfer of thyroid-stimulating immunoglobulins from mother to fetus.[51]

Thyrotoxicosis in the older or infirm patient
Here the priority is for simplicity, and first choice is ^{131}I therapy with, if need be, a second or even a third dose to achieve control. A reasonable cut-off point for the age criterion might be 40 years. In the very elderly and infirm, with but limited life expectancy, it can be simplest to use antithyroid drugs indefinitely.

Thyrotoxicosis from a hot nodule
Both surgery and ^{131}I are effective. Our bias is in favour of ^{131}I, based on its simplicity, safety and preferential uptake into the hyperfunctioning nodule with but little uptake into the suppressed normal gland tissue.

Thyrotoxicosis with a large disfiguring goitre
This is usually best treated surgically; substantial shrinkage after a course of antithyroid drugs is not to be expected.

Preparation for surgery or ^{131}I
This involves initially rendering the patient euthyroid with drugs. Continuation of drug treatment after ^{131}I treatment may be needed to maintain the patient euthyroid until the effects of irradiation become evident.

Failure of surgery to control thyrotoxicosis
Whether failure occurs initially or from subsequent relapse, it is undoubtedly best treated with ^{131}I.

Thyroid storm
This occurs very rarely. Thyrotoxicosis can become suddenly so severe that an apparently acute illness occurs, with all the usual clinical features of thyrotoxicosis, along with fever, incessant apprehension, restlessness, disorientation, diarrhoea and vomiting. It is usually precipitated by an event such as infection or trauma. For emergency treatment,[52] the swiftest possible reduction in the high circulating free thyroid hormone levels is required. Propylthiouracil is probably the antithyroid drug of choice, for although its action in blocking the synthesis of hormone in the thyroid and its action in reducing the circulating levels of thyroid-stimulating immunoglobulins are common to the other thioureylenes, it has the special property (see above) of immediately inhibiting the conversion of T_4 to the metabolically active metabolite T_3 in the periphery. A high dose of PTU is used, 600–1200 mg daily, using a gastric tube if the patient is unconscious. Two hours after the first dose of PTU, iodide is commenced, to reduce the release of stored hormone. Five drops of saturated solution of potassium iodide is given, and repeated 4-hourly. Also propranolol cover is used judiciously. High doses of glucocorticoids are traditionally used.

Choice of antithyroid drug
The thioureylenes are undoubtedly the drugs of choice for medical treatment of thyrotoxicosis. Among the thioureylenes,[34] there seems little to choose between PTU, carbimazole and methimazole; the

latter is a natural metabolic product from carbimazole. PTU is used at 10 times the dose of carbimazole. The incidence of side effects seems similar, and all three are highly effective in blocking thyroid hormone synthesis in almost all hyperthyroid patients[52] and give similar remission rates. The one real difference is that only PTU has the peripheral blocking effect on the conversion of T_4 to T_3, and so should be marginally faster in achieving control.

All three thioureylenes (and also potassium perchlorate)[4] have the beneficial effect of reducing the circulating levels of thyroid-stimulating immunoglobulins in Graves' disease. The choice of which thioureylene to use is largely a matter of physician preference.

Adverse reactions

Potentially life-threatening effects

Serious adverse effects are rare. Agranulocytosis, occurring as an autoimmune phenomenon[53] with antineutrophil antibodies, has been reported as occurring in 1 in 500 patients.[54] However, a recent reassessment of this problem indicates that its frequency has been greatly overestimated. Reversible leucopenia is very common but agranulocytosis is probably less frequent than 1 in 3000.[55] It appears mainly in the first few weeks of treatment, and develops so swiftly that prediction by regular leucocyte counts is impractical. Warning the patient to automatically cease the medication in the event of a sore throat or fever, will minimize the severity of this complication. The risk appears to be greater in those aged over 40 years,[56] and when larger doses are used.[57] Second courses are no more prone to induce agranulocytosis than are first courses.[56]

There have been very rare instances of hepatitis attributable to PTU.[58] Other very rare side effects and the mechanisms involved have been recently reviewed.[59] These include LE-like syndromes, cutaneous vasculitis, aplastic anaemia and thrombocytopenia. In addition hypoprothrombinaemia can cause a severe clotting disorder in patients receiving PTU.[11]

No teratogenic or carcinogenic effects have been identified.

Acute overdosage

The case has been reported[60] of a 12-year-old girl who ingested at least 5 g of propylthiouracil, without acute side effects. There was a temporary reduction in serum T_3. In general, overdosage is said[61] to produce vomiting, epigastric distress, headache, fever, arthralgia, pruritis and pancytopenia.

Severe or irreversible adverse effects

Apart from those mentioned immediately above, there are none.

Symptomatic adverse effects

Mild papular skin rashes occur in about 3% of patients,[62] usually in the first few weeks of therapy, are often pruritic, and usually are self-limiting. Urticaria, arthralgia and fever are also quite common. Antihistamines may relieve the symptoms. If persistent, changing to another drug of the thioureylene class is usually, but not always, effective.

Interference with clinical pathology tests

The drug may cause interference with the measurement of serum glucose and serum uric acid by the sequential multiple analyser (Technicon).

High risk groups

Neonates

The only indication for propylthiouracil at this age is for the treatment of an infant born with thyrotoxicosis due to the effect of persisting maternal thyroid-stimulating antibodies. Relatively high doses are started, such as 10 mg 8-hourly. This is a self-limiting condition, and drug control is usually needed for a few weeks only. Propranolol cover is often used.[63]

Breast milk. As reviewed above, only very small quantities of propylthiouracil reach the milk, and some authorities advocate continuing with breast-feeding despite the continuation of propylthiouracil medication,[11,12] subject to availability of frequent infant monitoring. A theoretical risk is the occurrence of an adverse reaction in the infant.[11]

Children

There are no special problems with the use of this drug in children.

Propylthiouracil

Pregnant women

As reviewed above, there is a good case for antithyroid drug therapy as the preferred treatment option during pregnancy. Some argue a case for the choice of PTU,[11] as its placental transfer is only one quarter that of methimazole.

The elderly

There are no particular problems with the drug in this age group.[12,56]

Concurrent disease

In renal failure a lower dose than usual is required to effect a euthyroid status.[12] It has been recommended[64] that when GFR is 10–50 $ml.min^{-1}$, the dose should be reduced to 75%, and when < 10 $ml.min^{-1}$, to 50%. Likewise, patients with hepatic disease have a prolonged disappearance curve[24,64,65] and may need lower doses. No significant interaction between other diseases and this drug is known to the authors.

Drug interactions

No important problems have emerged in 40 years of clinical experience.

Potentially hazardous interactions

None has been described.

Other significant interactions

A high iodine intake may impair the response of the thyroid to antithyroid drugs, both by increasing the thyroidal stores of preformed hormones, and by altering the thyroid's metabolism of antithyroid drugs.[66]

Potentially useful interactions

No interactions of this type have been reported.

Clinical trials

Being a widely used drug for 40 years, results of numerous clinical trials have emerged. Broadly, the remission rate is usually about 50%,[11] with wide variation reported, but the longer the follow-up, the higher the relapse rate reported,[67] and also the later the year of the report. Some very low remission rates of 14% to 44% were cited by Romaldini et al.[27] Some current questions involving more clinical trials concern the following:

(i) What is the optimum (i.e. minimum) duration of a course of antithyroid drugs? Reports have varied widely, and sizeable series with long-term follow-up are still needed. Greer et al[32] reported that a course lasting just as long as it takes to render the patient euthyroid, and comprising a single daily dose, produced a remission rate similar to a one-year course. On the other hand, Tamai et al[31] reported that a course of six months of therapy gave a remission rate of 31% in comparison with two years of therapy which gave an 82% remission rate. Again, Sugrue et al[67] reported a 10% remission rate after one year of treatment in comparison with 51% after at least two years' treatment.

(ii) Is there an advantage in using a high dose of antithyroid drug, covered with thyroxine? Romaldini et al[27] reported a series of 113 patients who were randomized into a high-dose with T_4 group (mean 693 mg PTU per day), and a low-dose group (mean 180 mg per day), and treated for a mean of 15 and 13 months respectively. The remission rates of 75% and 42% respectively were significantly different ($P < 0.001$). Possibly the superiority of the high-dose regime was due to a greater immunosuppressive effect. Few other such reports have been published, but more recently Weetman et al[6] in a clinical and biochemical review, made the point that the immunosuppressive effect would be greatest with larger doses and longer courses.

(iii) Is there an advantage in the use of a divided-dose regime in comparison with a single daily dose? A report by Greer et al[32] showed that a single dose of PTU of 300 mg or less achieved remission in 18 out of 31 patients. Again, Kammer and Srinivasan[68] reported that 9 patients were successfully treated with a single-dose regimen throughout and 30 out of 41 were initially treated with divided doses and successfully maintained in remission with a single daily dose.

PTU, methimazole and carbimazole, introduced over 40 years ago, remain the mainstay of drug therapy of thyrotoxicosis with few side effects.

General review articles

Cooper D S 1984 Antithyroid drugs. New England Journal of Medicine 311: 1353–1362

Halnan K E 1985 Radio-iodine treatment of hyperthyroidism — a more liberal policy. Clinics in Endocrinology and Metabolism 14: 467–489

Kampmann J P, Hansen J M 1981 Clinical pharmacokinetics of antithyroid drugs. Clinical Pharmacokinetics 6: 401–428

Marchant B, Lees J F H, Alexander W D 1979 Antithyroid drugs. In: Hershman J M and Bray G A (eds) The thyroid: physiology and treatment of disease. Pergamon Press, Oxford, pp 209–252

Weetman A P, McGregor A M, Hall R 1984 Evidence for an effect of antithyroid drugs on the natural history of Graves' disease. Clinical Endocrinology 21: 163–172

Wing S S, Fantus I F 1987 Adverse immunologic effects of antithyroid drugs. Canadian Medical Association Journal 136: 121–127

References

1. Geffner D L, Azukizawa M, Hershman J M 1975 Propylthiouracil blocks extrathyroidal conversion of thyroxine to triiodothyronine and augments thyrotropin secretion in man. Journal of Clinical Investigation 55: 224–229
2. Saberi M, Sterling F H, Utiger R D 1975 Reduction in extrathyroidal triiodothyronine production by propylthiouracil in man. Journal of Clinical Investigation 55: 218–223
3. Bliddal H, Bech K, Petersen P H, Siersbaek-Nielsen K, Friis T 1982 Evidence of a correlation between thyrotropin receptor binding inhibition and thyroid adenylate cyclase activation by immunoglobulins in Graves' disease before and during long-term antithyroid treatment. Acta Endocrinologica (Copenhagen) 101: 35–40
4. Wenzel K W, Lente J R 1984 Similar effects of thionamide drugs and perchlorate on thyroid-stimulating immunoglobulins in Graves' disease: evidence against an immunosuppressive action of thionamide drugs. Journal of Clinical Endocrinology and Metabolism 58: 62–69
5. Weiss I, Davies T F 1981 Inhibition of immunoglobulin-secreting cells by antithyroid drugs. Journal of Clinical Endocrinology and Metabolism 53: 1223–1228
6. Weetman A P, McGregor A M, Hall R 1984 Evidence for an effect of antithyroid drugs on the natural history of Graves' disease. Clinical Endocrinology 21: 163–172
7. Aucion D P, Peterson M E, Hurvitz A I et al 1985 Propylthiouracil-induced immune-mediated disease in the cat. Journal of Pharmacology and Experimental Therapeutics 234: 13–18
8. Purves H D, Griesbach W E 1947 Studies on experimental goitre VIII: thyroid tumours in rats treated with thiourea. British Journal of Experimental Pathology 28: 46–53
9. Malcolm J, Griesbach W E, Bielschowski F, Hall W H 1949 Hyperplasia of the parathyroids associated with osteitis fibrosa in rats treated with thiouracil and other compounds. British Journal of Experimental Pathology 30: 17–23
10. Goldsmith E D, Gordon A S, Charipper H A 1945 An analysis of the effects of continued thiourea treatment in pregnancy and on the development of the offspring in the rat. American Journal of Obstetrics and Gynecology 49: 197–206
11. Cooper D S 1984 Antithyroid drugs. New England Journal of Medicine 311: 1353–1362
12. Kampmann J P, Hansen J M 1981 Clinical pharmacokinetics of antithyroid drugs. Clinical Pharmacokinetics 6: 401–428
13. Cooper D S, Saxe V C, Maloof F, Ridgway E C 1981 Studies of propylthiouracil using a newly developed radioimmunoassay. Journal of Clinical Endocrinology and Metabolism 52: 204–213
14. Sitar D S, Abu-Bakare A, Gardiner R J 1982 Propylthiouracil disposition in pregnant and post-partum women. Pharmacology 25: 57–60
15. Kampmann J, Skovsted L 1974 The pharmacokinetics of propylthiouracil. Acta Pharmacologica et Toxicologica 35: 361–369
16. Lazarus J H, Marchant B, Alexander W D, Clark D H 1975 ^{35}S-antithyroid drug concentration and organic binding of iodine in the human thyroid. Clinical Endocrinology 4: 609–615
17. Marchant B, Alexander W D, Robertson J W K, Lazarus J M 1971 Concentration of ^{35}S-propylthiouracil by the thyroid gland and its relationship to anion trapping mechanism. Metabolism 20: 989–999
18. Brownlie B E W, Marchant B, Alexander W D 1971 Placental transfer of ^{35}S-methimazole in the rat. In: Fellinger K, Hofer R (eds) Further advances in thyroid research. Verlag der Wien Medizinischen Akademie, Vienna, p 143
19. Marchant B, Brownlie B E W, McKay Hart C, Horton P W, Alexander W D 1977 The placental transfer of propylthiouracil, methimazole and carbimazole. Journal of Clinical Endocrinology and Metabolism 45: 1187–1193
20. Ibbertson H K, Seddon R J, Croxson M S 1975 Fetal hypothyroidism complicating medical treatment of thyrotoxicosis in pregnancy. Clinical Endocrinology 4: 521–523
21. Low L C K, Lang J, Alexander W D 1979 Excretion of carbimazole and propylthiouracil in breast milk. Lancet 2: 1011
22. Kampmann J P, M lholm Hansen J E 1981 Correlation between antithyroid effect and serum concentrations of propylthiouracil in patients with hyperthyroidism. British Journal of Clinical Pharmacology 12: 681–686
23. McMurray J F, Gilliland P F, Ratliff R, Bourland P D 1975 Pharmacodynamics of propylthiouracil in normal and hyperthyroid subjects after a single oral dose. Journal of Clinical Endocrinology and Metabolism 41: 362–364
24. Desbrats-Schönbaum M L, Endrenyi L, Koves E, Schönbaum E, Sellers E A 1972 On the action and kinetics of propylthiouracil. European Journal of Pharmacology 19: 104–111
25. Alexander W D, Evans V, Macaulay A, Gallagher T F, Londono J 1969 Metabolism of ^{35}S-labelled antithyroid drugs in man. British Medical Journal 2: 290–291
26. Marchant B 1971 The metabolism of ^{35}S-labelled antithyroid drugs. PhD thesis, University of Glasgow, UK
27. Romaldini J H, Bromberg N, Werner R S et al 1983 Comparison of effects of high and low dosage regimens of antithyroid drugs in the management of Graves' hyperthyroidism. Journal of Clinical Endocrinology and Metabolism 57: 563–570
28. Wise P H, Marion M, Pain R W 1973 Single-dose 'block-replace' drug therapy in hyperthyroidism. British Medical Journal 4: 143–145
29. Greer M A, Kammer H, Bouma D J 1977 Short-term antithyroid drug therapy for the thyrotoxicosis of Graves' disease. New England Journal of Medicine 279: 173–176
30. Burr W A, Fitzgerald M G, Hoffenberg R et al 1979 Relapse after short-term antithyroid therapy of Graves' disease. New England Journal of Medicine 300: 200
31. Tamai H, Nakawaga T, Pukino O et al 1980 Thionamide therapy in Graves' disease: relation of relapse rate to duration of therapy. Annals of Internal Medicine 92: 488–490
32. Greer M A, Meihoff W C, Studer H 1965 Treatment of hyperthyroidism with a single daily dose of propylthiouracil. New England Journal of Medicine 272: 888–891
33. Pharmakiotis A D, Alexander W D 1975 Effect of frequency of administration on the accumulation and metabolism of ^{35}S-propylthiouracil by the rat thyroid. Endocrinology 96: 1324–1328
34. Marchant B, Lees J F H, Alexander W D 1979 Antithyroid drugs. In: Hershman J M, Bray G A (eds) The thyroid: physiology and treatment of disease. Pergamon Press, Oxford, pp 209–252
35. Holm L-E, Alinder I 1982 Relapses after thionamide therapy for Graves' disease. Acta Medica Scandinavica 211: 489–492
36. Young E T, Steel N R, Taylor J J et al 1988 Prediction of remission after antithyroid drug treatment in Graves' disease. Quarterly Journal of Medicine 66: 175–189
37. van Ouwerkerk B M, Krenning E P, Docter R et al 1987 Cellular and humoral immunity in patients with hyperthyroid Graves' disease before, during and after antithyroid drug treatment. Clinical Endocrinology 26: 385–394
38. Toft A D, Irvine W J, Sinclair I, McIntosh D, Seth J, Cameron E D H 1978 Thyroid function after surgical treatment of thyrotoxicosis. A report of 100 cases treated with propranolol before operation. New England Journal of Medicine 298: 643–647
39. Hoffman D A, McConaghey W M, Diamond E L, Kurland I T 1982a Mortality in women treated for hyperthyroidism. American Journal of Epidemiology 115: 243–254
40. Hoffman D A, McConaghey, Fraumeni J F, Kurland L T 1982b Cancer incidence following treatment of hyperthyroidism. International Journal of Epidemiology 11: 218–224
41. Kendall-Taylor P, Keir M J, Ross W M 1984 Ablative radioiodine therapy for hyperthyroidism: long term follow up study. British Medical Journal 289: 361–363
42. Halnan K E 1985 Radio-iodine treatment of hyperthyroidism — a more liberal policy. Clinics in Endocrinology and Metabolism 14: 467–489
43. Hales A B 1972 Problems of childhood Graves' disease. Mayo Clinic Proceedings 47: 850–853
44. Hamburger J I 1985 Management of hyperthyroidism in children and adolescents. Journal of Clinical Endocrinology and Metabolism 60: 1119–1024
45. Salenkow H A, Burnbaum M D, Hollander C S 1973 Thyroid function and dysfunction during pregnancy. Clinics in Obstetrics and Gynecology 16: 66–108
46. Burrow G N 1965 Neonatal goiter after maternal propylthiouracil therapy. Journal of Clinical Endocrinology and Metabolism 25: 403–408
47. Chahal P, Sidhu R, Joplin G F, Hawkins D F 1981 Treatment of thyrotoxicosis in pregnancy. Journal of Obstetrics and Gynaecology 2: 11–19
48. Ramsay I, Kaur S, Krassas G 1983 Thyrotoxicosis in pregnancy: results of treatment by antithyroid drugs combined with T_4. Clinical Endocrinology 18: 73–85
49. Myant N B 1958 Passage of thyroxine and tri-iodothyronine from mother to foetus in pregnant women. Clinical Science 17: 75–79
50. McGregor A M, Hall R, Richards C 1984 Autoimmune thyroid disease and pregnancy. British Medical Journal 288: 1780–1781
51. Zakarija M, McKenzie J M 1983 Pregnancy-associated changes in the thyroid-stimulating antibody of Graves' disease and the relationship to neonatal hyperthyroidism. Journal of Clinical Endocrinology and Metabolism 57: 1036–1040
52. Rabin D, McKenna T J 1982 Clinical endocrinology and metabolism: principles and practice. Grune and Stratton, New York, p 284
53. Weitzman S A, Stossel T P, Desmond M 1978 Drug-induced immunological neutropenia. Lancet 1: 1068–1072
54. Haynes R C, Murad F 1985 Thyroid and antithyroid drugs. In: Gilman A G, Goodman L S, Rall T W, Murad F (eds) The pharmacological basis of therapeutics. Macmillan, New York, p 1403
55. International Agranulocytosis and Aplastic Anaemia Study 1988 Risk of agranulocytosis and aplastic anaemia in relation to use of antithyroid drugs. British Medical Journal 297: 262–265
56. Cooper D S, Goldmin D, Levin A A et al 1983 Agranulocytosis associated with antithyroid drugs: effects of patient age and drug dose. Annals of Internal Medicine 98: 26–29
57. Wiberg J J, Nuttall F Q 1972 Methimazole toxicity from high doses. Annals of Internal Medicine 77: 414–416
58. Hanson J S 1984 Propylthiouracil and hepatitis. Two cases and a review of the literature. Archives of Internal Medicine 44: 994–996
59. Wing S S, Fantus I G 1987 Adverse immunologic effects of antithyroid drugs. Canadian Medical Association Journal 136: 121–127

60. Jackson G L, Flickinger F W, Weils L W 1979 Massive overdose of propylthiouracil. Annals of Internal Medicine 91: 418–419
61. Lees J F H, Alexander W D 1974 The effect of phenobarbital on the metabolism of methimazole in the rat. Endocrinology 95: 875–881
62. Van der Laan W P, Storrie V M 1955 A survey of the factors controlling thyroid function, with especial reference to newer views on antithyroid substances. Pharmacological Reviews 7: 301–334
63. Smith C S, Howard N J 1973 Propanolol in treatment of neonatal thyrotoxicosis. Journal of Pediatrics 83: 1046–1048
64. Bennett W M, Muther S, Parker R A et al 1980 Drug therapy in renal failure: dosing guidelines for adults. Part II: sedatives, hypnotics, and tranquilizers; cardiovascular, antihypertensive, and diuretic agents, miscellaneous agents. Annals of Internal Medicine 93: 286–325
65. Cooper D S, Bode H H, Nath B, Saxe V, Maloof F, Ridgway E C 1984 Methimazole pharmacology in man: studies using a newly developed radioimmunoassay for methimazole. Journal of Clinical Endocrinology and Metabolism 58: 473–479
66. Hall R, Lazarus J H 1987 Changing iodine intake and the effect on thyroid disease. British Medical Journal 295: 721
67. Sugrue D, McEvoy M, Feely J, Drury M I 1980 Hyperthyroidism in the land of Graves: results of treatment by surgery, radio-iodine and carbimazole in 837 cases. Quarterly Journal of Medicine 49: 51–61
68. Kammer H, Srinivasan K 1969 The use of antithyroid drugs in a single dose. Treatment of diffuse toxic goitre. Journal of the American Medical Association 209: 1325–1327

Protamine (sulphate)

Protamine is a heparin antagonist.

Chemistry

Protamine is a purified mixture of simple protein principles that yield basic amino acids on hydrolysis (arginine, proline, serine and valine) and are obtained from the sperm of the mature testes of fish belonging to the family *Clupeidae* or *Salmonidae*.

Molecular weight	~4500
pKa	—
Solubility	
in alcohol	very low
in water	sparing
Octanol/water partition coefficient	—

Protamine is a white or faintly grey-yellow, odourless, hygroscopic, amorphous or crystalline powder. It has a slightly acid or astringent taste.

Pharmacology

Although protamine is the potent antidote for heparin, its precise mechanism of action is unknown. However, when the strongly basic protamine combines with the strongly acid heparin, a stable salt is formed lacking in anticoagulant activity. One milligram of protamine sulphate neutralizes between 80 and 120 units of heparin.[1,2] However, methods of standardization[2] and the use of heparin from different sources (mucosal, lung) may produce different responses to protamine.[3]

Toxicology

No data are available.

Clinical pharmacology

Protamine appears to exert its effect through an acid–base interaction. When insufficient protamine is administered (protamine:heparin ratio 0.56) a heparin rebound occurs within 5 hours of neutralization, which may be associated with clinical bleeding.[4] This phenomenon has been described mainly in patients undergoing extracorporeal circulation in arterial and cardiac surgery or in dialysis procedures.

The mechanism for this rebound effect is unknown but may result from release of heparin from the protamine–heparin complex or release of heparin from extravascular compartments.

Although protamine is itself a weak anticoagulant, this is clinically unimportant.

Pharmacokinetics

Assays for the components of protamine have not been developed and applied to pharmacokinetic analysis.

The onset of action of protamine occurs within 30–60 seconds following intravenous administration. The fate of the protamine–heparin complex is unknown, but it may be partially degraded, thus freeing heparin.

Concentration–effect relationship

This relationship has to be viewed in terms of the protamine–heparin interaction discussed above.

Protamine (sulphate)

P

Metabolism

Unknown.

Pharmaceutics

The BP injection is a simple solution of protamine sulphate in Water for Injections, with a pH of 2.5–3.5, presented as 10 mg.ml^{-1}. The injection is stored below 25°C. In some formulations protamine is available for parenteral use; the injection is made isotonic with 0.9% sodium chloride. Sodium phosphate and/or sulphuric acid may have been added to adjust the pH to 6.5–7.5. The injection should be stored at 2–8°C.

Although protamine is intended for injection without further dilution, it is compatible with normal saline or 5% dextrose in water.

Therapeutic use

Indications

Antidote to heparin.

Contraindications

Previous allergic reaction to protamine resulting in life-threatening consequences.

Mode of use

Protamine is administered slowly by intravenous injection or infusion at concentrations of 10 mg.ml^{-1} over 1–3 minutes. No more than 50 mg of the drug should be administered in a 10-minute period and the rate of administration should probably not exceed 5 mg.min^{-1}. Too rapid administration of the drug can cause anaphylactoid-like reactions or anaphylaxis.

1 mg protamine will neutralize approximately 90 units of heparin sodium from bovine lung tissue, 100 units of heparin calcium from porcine intestinal mucosa or 115 units of heparin sodium from porcine intestinal mucosa.[1,2]

Because of the short half life of heparin (1–2 hours) the dose of protamine should be adjusted on the basis of the time elapsed since the heparin was discontinued. The rate and route of administration of heparin will also influence the dose of protamine selected.

Dose

Heparin bolus.

Table 1

Time elapsed	Protamine dose/100 units heparin
30 min	1–1.5 mg
30–60 min	0.5–0.75 mg
2 h	0.25–0.375 mg

Heparin infusion. 25–50 mg protamine after stopping infusion.

Subcutaneous injection. 1–1.5 mg protamine per 100 units heparin. 25–50 mg can be administered by slow intravenous injection and the rest of the calculated dose can be given by slow intravenous infusion over 8–16 hours or the expected duration of absorption of heparin. Alternatively, protamine can be administered in aliquots every two hours in amounts calculated to neutralize the twelve-hourly dose divided into two-hourly amounts (i.e.: 20 000 U in 12 hours = 1666 in 1 hour = 3333 in 2 hours = 33 mg protamine every two hours). This should be monitored by measuring sequential APTTs.

Heparin administration during extracorporeal circulation. 1.5 mg per 100 units heparin. Sequential activated coagulation times and a dose response curve may be required to guide dosage of protamine. Ellison et al have recommended that in cardiopulmonary bypass procedures for pumps with small primes, an amount of protamine equal to the total dose of heparin should be administered; for pumps with large primes, an amount equal to half the dose of heparin should be administered.[5]

Indications

Because of the short half life of heparin (1–2 hours) protamine is only indicated in the presence of severe heparin overdose. Bleeding from heparin administration is occasionally an indication for the use of protamine.

Contraindications

Protamine should be avoided in patients who have demonstrated anaphylaxis, anaphylactoid reactions or catastrophic pulmonary vasoconstriction following cardiac bypass.[6–12]

Although protamine is not thought to be allergenic, hypersensitivity to residual fish antigens that remain after purification occurs in sensitive individuals.[6]

Adverse reactions

Potentially life-threatening effects

Anaphylaxis. Although protamine is not thought to be allergenic, hypersensitivity to residual fish antigens that remain after purification occurs in allergic individuals.[6] Anaphylaxis has been reported and may be mediated by a complement-dependent IgG skin-sensitizing agent.[7]

Protamine may rarely be responsible for producing severe cardiovascular collapse, bronchospasm and death.[8–10] This is probably due to an allergic mechanism resulting in anaphylaxis. Two patients in whom anaphylaxis occurred[8,9] had been previously exposed to protamine zinc insulin, one having experienced a local reaction at the site of injection.[9]

Stewart and associates surveyed 866 consecutive patients undergoing cardiac catheterization of whom 655 received protamine.[13] Of these patients, 2.3% were diabetics on isophane insulin (containing protamine). The incidence of severe anaphylactic reactions was 27% (4/15) in the isophane-insulin group and 0.5% (3/636) in those with no history of isophane insulin use. One patient in the latter group had an allergy to fish. This represents a 50-fold increase in risk of a major reaction to protamine if the patient was receiving isophane insulin. Doolan and associates have reported positive results from skin-testing with protamine patients who had demonstrated anaphylaxis and who had all previously received protamine. The skin tests were negative for concomitant medications.[9]

There are fewer than 20 cases reported of severe allergic reactions.[11]

Too rapid administration of the drug can cause anaphylactoid-like reactions or anaphylaxis.

Catastrophic pulmonary vasoconstriction. It is not clear if the pulmonary oedema associated with the use of protamine to neutralize heparin following cardiac surgery[10,12] is a separate entity from the anaphylactic reactions reported above.[6–9]

Acute overdosage

In one study, overdoses of 600–800 mg protamine resulted in no serious sequelae; there was a notable absence of an anticoagulant effect.[5]

Severe or irreversible adverse effects

Hypersensitivity reactions — see life-threatening adverse reactions section above.

Symptomatic adverse effects

Rapid intravenous injection has caused acute hypotension, bradycardia, transient flushing and a feeling of warmth. These ill-effects are minimized when the injection is administered slowly (50 mg over 10 minutes).

Urticaria and other hypersensitivity reactions occur rarely.

Interference with clinical pathology tests

Protamine interferes with the fluorescence method of estimating plasma catecholamines.[14]

High risk groups

Neonates

No information is available.

Breast milk. Information not available but potential adverse effects may be avoided by withholding breast-feeding for several hours after the drug is administered.

Children

Information is not available.

Pregnant women
No information is available. Reproduction studies have not been performed in animals.

The elderly
Information is not available.

Drug interactions
None reported.

Major outcome trials
None reported.

References

1. Deykin D 1972 Regulation of heparin therapy. New England Journal of Medicine (editorial) 287: 355–356
2. Graham D T, Pomeroy A R, Smythe S B 1979 Measurement of the heparin neutralizing capacity of protamine. Thrombosis and Haemostasis (Stuttgart) 41: 583–589
3. Abbott W M, Warnock D F, Austen W G 1977 The relationship of heparin source to the incidence of delayed haemorrhage. Journal of Surgical Research 22: 593–597
4. Ellison N, Beatty P, Blake D R, Wurzel H A, MacVaugh H III, 1974 Heparin rebound. Studies in patients with volunteers. The Journal of Thoracic and Cardiovascular Surgery 67: 723–729
5. Ellison N, Ominsky A J, Wollman H 1971 Is protamine a clinically important anticoagulant? Anesthesiology 35: 621–629
6. Caplan S N, Berkman E M 1976 Protamine sulfate and fish allergy. New England Journal of Medicine (letter) 295: 172
7. Lakin J D, Blocker T J, Strong D M, Yocum M W, 1978 Anaphylaxis to protamine sulfate mediated by a complement-dependent IgG antibody. Journal of Allergy and Immunology 61: 102–107
8. Moorthy S S, Pond W, Rowland R G 1980 Severe circulatory shock following protamine (an anaphylactic reaction). Anesthesia and Analgesia 59: 77–78
9. Doolan L, McKenzie I, Kratchek J, Buxton S 1981 Protamine sulfate hypersensitivity. Anaesthesia and Intensive Care 9: 147–149
10. Olinger G N, Becker R M, Bonchek L I 1980 Non-cardiogenic pulmonary edema and peripheral vascular collapse following cardiopulmonary bypass: rare protamine reaction? Annals of Thoracic Surgery 29: 20–25
11. Horrow J C 1985 Protamine: a review of its toxicity. Anaesthesia and Analgesia 64: 348–361
12. Lowenstein E, Johnston W E, Lappas D G et al 1983 Catastrophic pulmonary vascoconstriction associated with protamine reversal of heparin. Anesthesiology 59: 470–473
13. Stewart W J, McSweeney S M, Kellett M A, Faxon D P, Ryan T J 1984 Increased risk of severe protamine reactions in NPH insulin-dependent diabetics undergoing cardiac catheterization. Circulation 70: 788–792
14. Carruthers M, Taggart P, Conway N, Bates D, Somerville N 1970 Validity of plasma-catecholamine estimations. Lancet 2: 62

Prothionamide

Prothionamide is a second-line drug used against tuberculosis and leprosy.

Chemistry
Prothionamide (Ektebin, Peteha, Trevintix)
$C_9H_{12}N_2S$
2-Propyl-4-pyridinecarbothioamide

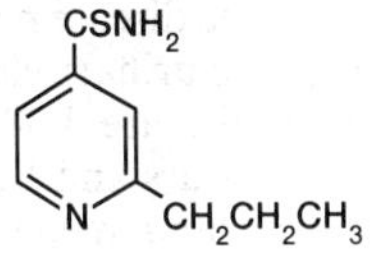

Molecular weight	180.29
pKa	—
Solubility	
in alcohol	soluble
in water	insoluble
Octanol/water partition coefficient	—

Prothionamide consists of white crystals with a mild sulphide-like odour. It is prepared by chemical synthesis via dehydration of 2-propylisonicotinamide and reaction with hydrogen sulphide, and is available only in oral form. It is not marketed in the UK.

Pharmacology
The drug is bactericidal to *Mycobacterium tuberculosis* and *Mycobacterium leprae* at a minimum inhibitory concentration of 0.6 $mg.l^{-1}$ and 0.05 $mg.l^{-1}$, respectively. Its suspected mechanism of action is inhibition of mycolic acid synthesis.

Toxicology
Unfortunately, no information exists in the literature concerning the teratogenic effects of this agent in animal models or man. It might be suspected, however, of having the potential for such effects, as its synthetic analogue ethionamide is known to cause abortions and malformations in animals and possibly man.[1]

Clinical pharmacology
Prothionamide is related to isoniazid in chemical structure, but it is less effective and more toxic, and there is usually no cross-resistance with isoniazid-resistant mycobacteria. Cross-resistance is noted between prothionamide and ethionamide.

In vitro studies of this agent indicate inhibition of multiplication of human strains of *Mycobacterium leprae* at a concentration[2] of 0.05 $mg.l^{-1}$. Summary studies of both prothionamide and ethionamide have revealed that although the antimicrobial activity and therapeutic efficacy are approximately the same, prothionamide is better tolerated and less toxic than its predecessor ethionamide.[3]

Pharmacokinetics
The preferred analytical method is by high performance liquid chromatography utilizing a normal phase column packing with ultraviolet detection at 280 nm.[4] This method allows for quantitative analysis of ethionamide and prothionamide and the sulphoxide metabolites of both compounds in one chromatographic run. Other analytical methods are also available and have been described.[5]

P

Prothionamide is well absorbed after oral administration. Peak plasma concentrations of 1.0–1.4 $mg.l^{-1}$ are noted 2 hours following a 250 mg dose.[3] The mean plasma half life is 1.8 hours. Unfortunately, the apparent volume of distribution, tissue distribution and protein binding data are unknown for this compound. Measurable quantities of this agent have not thus far been detected in cerebrospinal fluid, human breast milk or placental transfer.[6–8]

Oral absorption	>90%
Presystemic metabolism	—
Plasma half life	
range	1.5–2.1h
mean	1.8 h
Volume of distribution	—
Plasma protein binding	—

Prothionamide undergoes extensive biotransformation with only 0.08% of the drug and 0.4% of its sulphoxide metabolite, respectively, excreted unchanged in urine.[4] Less than 0.1% of the unchanged thioamide was observed by the faecal elimination route. Effects of acute or chronic hepatic disease have not been documented. The mean overall half lives of the urinary elimination of prothionamide and its sulphoxide metabolite are 1.38 and 1.63 hours, respectively, with a range of 1.3–1.4 hours and 1.5–1.8 hours, respectively. Pharmacokinetics of this drug and metabolite in renal disease or elderly patients have not been reported.

Concentration–effect relationship

Concentrations in the range of 0.05 $mg.l^{-1}$ in vitro inhibit multiplication of human strains of *Mycobacterium leprae.*[2] Peak serum concentrations of prothionamide are about 3 $mg.l^{-1}$ following a 500 mg dose. This suggests that, at this dose, peak serum concentrations of this agent would exceed the minimum inhibitory concentration of *Mycobacterium leprae* by a factor of approximately 60-fold. Taking the half life as 1.8 hours, by 24 hours the serum concentrations would be of the same order as the minimum inhibitory concentrations for this organism.[2,9]

Metabolism

Extensive interconversion takes place between the drug and its sulphoxide metabolite in vivo.[10] Excretion is almost entirely in the urine with less than 0.1% of the free drug found in the faeces.

Three primary pathways of interconversion and metabolism have been described: sulphate conjugation, desulphuration, oxidative deamination.

Of the metabolites, prothionamide sulphoxide has exhibited approximately equal antimycobacterial activity in vitro.[11] The corresponding amounts of prothionamide metabolites were 28% for the acid and 17% for the amide.[4] It is suspected that the therapeutic activity of the thioamide following administration may result from the action of both the parent drug and its sulphoxide.[11]

Pharmaceutics

Prothionamide is available in oral form only. Because it is generally supplied as a powder to developing countries, it is not encapsulated in any particular form. It was formerly marketed under the proprietary names Ektebin and Trevintex.

Therapeutic use

Indications

1. Failure after adequate treatment with primary drugs in any forms of active tuberculosis. Prothionamide should only be given with other effective antituberculosis agents.
2. Prothionamide (and ethionamide) remain the only alternatives to clofazimine in patients requiring triple drug therapy who will not accept clofazimine because of its hyperpigmentation effect upon the skin.[12]

Contraindications

1. Severe hypersensitivity
2. Severe hepatic damage.

Mode of use

The clinical use for *Mycobacterium tuberculosis* depends on when therapy with primary agents is ineffective or contraindicated. Oral treatment is usually begun with 250 mg once or twice a day with meals and this may be increased to a maximum of 1 g daily depending upon the therapeutic response. Optimum dosage for children has not been established.

Clinical use for *Mycobacterium leprae* was specified by the World Health Organization's Study group findings in 1982.[13] It was suggested that the multibacillary regimen (100 mg dapsone plus 50 mg clofazimine daily, unsupervised, with 600 mg rifampicin and 300 mg clofazimine once monthly under supervision) might be supplemented by the addition of a supervised dose of 500 mg of prothionamide (or ethionamide) once monthly; however, the efficacy of this has not been established. Also, if patients refuse to take clofazimine, it is recommended that it be replaced by 250–375 mg of prothionamide (or ethionamide) daily.[14]

Indications

1. Treatment failure with primary drugs for tuberculosis

Prothionamide is cross-resistant to thioureas and thiosemicarbazones and causes loss of acid-fastness in tubercle bacilli. Its mode of action is believed to be by the inhibition of mycolic acid synthesis in mycobacteria.

Prothionamide affects dehydrogenase activity in tubercle bacilli in

Fig. 1 The metabolism of prothionamide

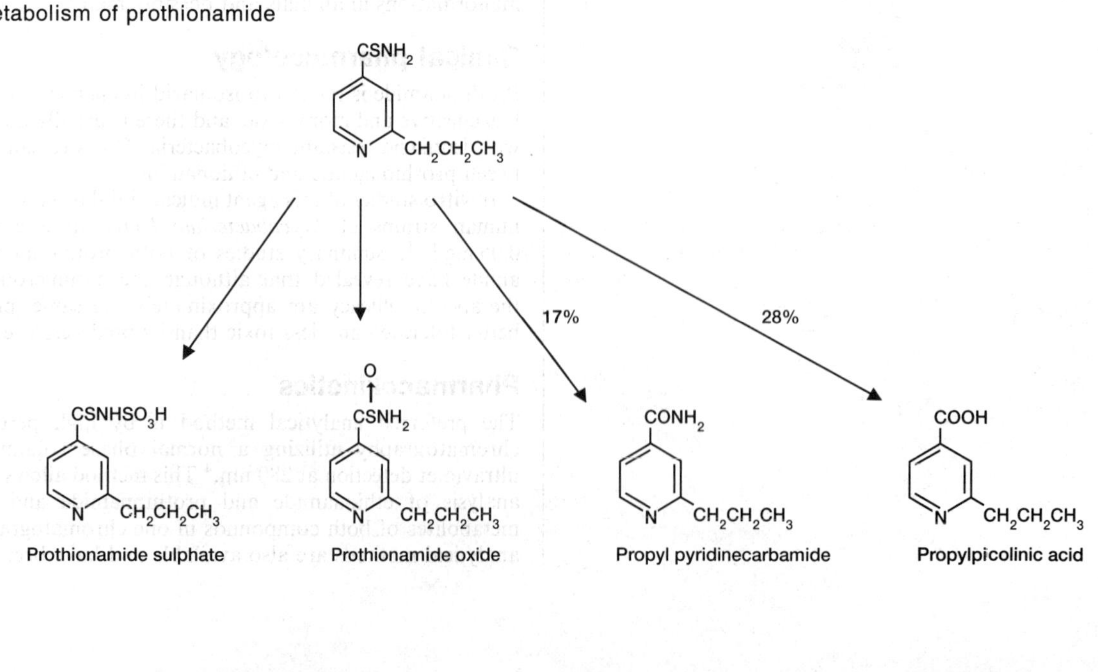

that it is converted to a substituted isonicotinic acid in the cell. It is postulated that this substituted moiety is incorporated into NAD, therefore, disturbing the NAD and NADP dehydrogenase systems.[15]

2. Alternative drug to clofazimine for leprosy
Side effects of clofazimine that lead to its unacceptability in patients are hyperpigmentation of the skin, gastrointestinal discomfort, and anticholinergic actions which result in diminished tear formation and sweating. When these become unacceptable to patients, prothionamide (or ethionamide) is recommended.

Contraindications

1. Severe hypersensitivity
Prothionamide may cause severe hypersensitivity reactions in a few individuals with the most common features being rash and fever. A scheme of challenge doses for detecting cutaneous or generalized hypersensitivity to this and other antituberculosis drugs has been proposed along with desensitization under steroidal cover.[16–18] However, as prothionamide is a secondary drug for treatment of tuberculosis, this side effect may best be controlled by discontinuation of the agent from the therapeutic regimen.

2. Severe hepatic damage
It is not known whether hepatotoxicity is due to a hypersensitivity reaction or to a direct toxic effect of the drug upon the liver. In the advent of hepatic damage, it may not be metabolized and is known to increase the plasma concentration of co-administered isoniazid, thus possibly contributing to isoniazid's toxic effects as well.

Cartel et al[19] noted a 13% incidence of hepatitis in patients with multibacillary leprosy treated during the first year with a daily three-drug combination of dapsone, rifampicin and a thioamide (either prothionamide or ethionamide at $10\,mg.kg^{-1}$). Discontinuing treatment with rifampicin and the thioamide, but not dapsone, resulted in recovery. Because the majority of the patients remained hepatitis B-antigen negative, and because no cases of hepatitis were observed in paucibacillary patients treated with rifampicin and dapsone without a thioamide, the hepatitis appeared toxic in nature and related to the administration of the thioamide in combination with rifampicin. A later study by Cartel et al[20] with $5\,mg.kg^{-1}$ prothionamide in combination with $10\,mg.kg^{-1}$ rifampicin observed a hepatitis rate of 16.5% among 110 multibacillary leprosy patients. A decrease in thioamide dosage, with performance of monthly assessments of liver function, did not decrease the incidence of hepatotoxicity but did decrease its severity. Baohong et al[21] noted liver injury in 56% of 39 leprosy patients treated with combinations of dapsone, prothionamide and isopiprazinylrifamycin SV. It has been concluded by one group of investigators that prothionamide should not be used in daily combination with rifampicin unless the daily dose is $5\,mg.kg^{-1}$ and monthly assessments of liver functions are performed routinely.[20]

Adverse reactions

Potentially life-threatening effects
Deaths caused solely by prothionamide have not been documented in the literature. However, Pattyn and others[22] have reported that when it is used in combination with rifampicin, there is a 4.5% incidence of hepatitis, with a mortality rate as high as 26% in the patients with hepatitis. In their study, the daily dose of prothionamide was 500 mg and the diagnosis of hepatitis was made mainly on clinical grounds. Baohong et al[21] have also reported two deaths from severe liver damage following combined use of prothionamide and rifampicin. Sudden withdrawal of the drug does not have any known adverse effects. As previously stated, prothionamide may intensify the adverse effects of other antituberculosis agents administered concomitantly. Convulsions have rarely been observed when its analogue ethionamide was administered with cycloserine, but a reaction of this kind has not been recorded during treatment with prothionamide.[23]

Acute overdosage
Examples of deliberate overdose have not been reported in the literature. Pellagra-like encephalopathy after ethionamide ingestion has been noted in three patients who improved with withdrawal of the compound and administration of group B vitamins, which were believed to have aided recovery.[24] Although it has not been substantiated, group B vitamins may be of some benefit in overdosage with prothionamide.

Severe or irreversible adverse effects
Most severe adverse effects involve liver and gastrointestinal dysfunction, the incidence of hepatitis (when used in combination with other antimycobacterial drugs) ranging from 13% to 56%.[19,20,21] Symptoms occasionally require cessation of antibiotic treatment. Gupta and others[25] commented that gastrointestinal disturbances were encountered more frequently with ethionamide (90.9%) than with prothionamide (78.1%) when given in a daily dosage of 0.75–1.0 g.

Symptomatic adverse effects
Various types of neuropsychotoxic effects, such as headache, insomnia, sleepiness, paraesthesia and depression, have been reported in patients using this antibiotic.[25] Other rare reactions have included cutaneous acneiform lesions,[17,25] facial pruritis[25] and excessive salivation.[26]

Other effects
AST (SGOT) has been reported to rise in patients with hepatotoxicity.[19–21]

Interference with clinical pathology tests
No interference with clinical pathology tests has been reported in the literature.

High risk groups

Neonates
Optimum dosage for neonates has not been established.

Breast milk. As far as can be determined from the literature, there are no published data indicating the secretion of prothionamide in breast milk in measurable quantities.[6]

Children
Optimum dosage for children has not been established.

Pregnant women
The safety of prothionamide has not been established in pregnancy. However, there is conflicting evidence of teratogenic effects in children born to mothers who received its analogue ethionamide during pregnancy. Therefore, it is suggested that prothionamide be avoided during pregnancy or in women of childbearing potential unless the benefits outweigh its possible hazard.[1]

The elderly
No special precautions are required as doses are adjusted according to patient response.

Drug interactions

Potentially hazardous interactions
Rifampicin. In the subgroup of patients who develop hepatitis, mortality as high as 26% has been reported when prothionamide was used in combination therapy with rifampicin.[22] Other studies have refuted this high incidence of fatal reactions associated with combined prothionamide/rifampicin therapy but have observed high incidences of hepatitis-related complications.[19–21] Hepatotoxicity is considerably increased when used in combination therapy with rifampicin and thiacetazone.[19–21]

Other significant interactions
Isoniazid. Prothionamide (and ethionamide) have the potential to increase serum concentrations of isoniazid due to an inhibition of the latter's metabolism.[6]

Rifampicin. Prothionamide has no significant effect upon the pharmacokinetics of rifampicin.[27]

Dapsone. Prothionamide has no significant effect upon the pharmacokinetics of dapsone.[27]

Potentially useful interactions
There are no therapeutically useful interactions as far as can be determined from the literature, apart from those with other antituberculous drugs.

Major outcome trials

1. Gupta D K, Mital O P, Agarwal M C, Kansal H M, Nath S 1977 A comparison of therapeutic efficacy and toxicity of ethionamide and prothionamide in Indian patients. Journal of the Indian Medical Association 68: 25–29

This was a double-blind study to assess the therapeutic efficacy and toxicity of a daily dose of 500 mg of ethionamide and prothionamide in the treatment of resistant cases of advanced pulmonary tuberculosis over a period of 6 months. Both groups also received 300 mg isoniazid and 800–1000 mg ethambutol once daily in addition to the thioamides. The ethionamide group consisted of 82 patients and the prothionamide group of 80 patients. Therapeutic efficacy was assessed by clinical improvement, sputum conversion and radiographic examination. At the end of 6 months, clinical improvement was noticed in 90.4% and 92.3% of the ethionamide and prothionamide groups, respectively. Corresponding rates of sputum conversion and radiographic regression of disease were 80.3% and 30.8% for ethionamide and 74.3% and 35.9% for prothionamide. Side effects were reported more often in the ethionamide patients with 64.6% having ill effects as opposed to 42.5% of the prothionamide group. It was concluded that prothionamide possesses almost equal therapeutic value and is a better tolerated drug than ethionamide.

Other trials

1. Cartel J L, Naudilion Y, Artus J C, Grosset J H 1985 Hepatotoxicity of the daily combination of 5 $mg.kg^{-1}$ prothionamide plus 10 $mg.kg^{-1}$ rifampicin. International Journal of Leprosy 53: 15–18

This was a prospective study with 110 multibacillary patients treated with a three-drug regimen (dapsone 100 mg plus rifampicin 10 $mg.kg^{-1}$ body weight daily for 2 years supplemented during the first year with daily prothionamide of 5 $mg.kg^{-1}$ body weight). A 16.5% incidence of hepatotoxicity was observed among the 110 patients. This was in approximate agreement with the 13% hepatotoxicity previously observed in a similar study by these authors using the same regimen with the dose of prothionamide being 10 $mg.kg^{-1}$ body weight.[19] However, jaundice was observed in only 2 out of 18 cases of hepatotoxicity (11%); whereas it was noted in 5 out of 7 cases of hepatotoxicity (71%) in the former study.[19] The decrease in thioamide dosage and performance of monthly assessments of liver functions did not decrease the incidence of hepatotoxicity but did decrease its severity. It was concluded by the authors that prothionamide should not be used in daily combinations with rifampicin unless the daily dose was 5 $mg.kg^{-1}$ and monthly assessments of liver functions were routinely performed.

General review articles

Girling D J 1982 Adverse effects of antituberculosis drugs. Drugs 23: 56–74

Holdiness M R 1984 Clinical pharmacokinetics of the antituberculosis drugs: a review. Clinical Pharmacokinetics 9: 511–544

Holdiness M R 1985 Chromatographic analysis of antituberculosis drugs in biological samples: a review. Journal of Chromatography Biomedical Applications 340: 321–359

Holdiness M R 1985 Adverse cutaneous reactions to antituberculosis drugs: a review. International Journal of Dermatology 24: 280–285

Holdiness M R 1985 Cerebrospinal fluid pharmacokinetics of the antituberculosis drugs. Clinical Pharmacokinetics 10: 532–534

Holdiness M R 1986 Contact dermatitis to antituberculosis drugs: a review. Contact Dermatitis 15: 282–288

Holdiness M R 1987 Neurological manifestations and toxicities of the antituberculosis drugs: a review. Medical Toxicology 2: 33–51

Holdiness M R 1987 Transplacental pharmacokinetics of the antituberculosis drugs. Clinical Pharmacokinetics 13: 125–129

Holdiness M R 1987 A review of iatrogenic nutritional deficiencies induced by antituberculosis drugs. Nutrition Research 7: 891–900

Holdiness M R 1988 A review of blood dyscrasias induced by the antitubercular drugs. Tubercle 68: 301–309

References

1. Holdiness M R 1987 Teratology of the antituberculosis drugs: a review. Early Human Development 15: 61–74
2. Colston M J, Ellard G A, Gammon P T 1978 Drugs for combined therapy: experimental studies on the antileprosy activity of ethionamide and prothionamide and a general review. Leprosy Review 49: 115–126
3. Gupta D K, Mital O P, Agarwal M C, Kansal H M, Nath S 1977 A comparison of therapeutic efficacy and toxicity of ethionamide and prothionamide in Indian patients. Journal of the Indian Medical Association 68: 25–29
4. Jenner P J, Ellard G A, Gruer P J K, Aber V R 1984 A comparison of the blood levels and urinary excretion of ethionamide and prothionamide in man. Journal of Antimicrobial Chemotherapy 13: 267–277
5. Holdiness M R 1985 Chromatographic analysis of antituberculosis drugs in biological samples: a review. Journal of Chromatography Biomedical Applications 340: 321–359
6. Holdiness M R 1984 Clinical pharmacokinetics of the antituberculosis drugs: a review. Clinical Pharmacokinetics 9: 511–544
7. Holdiness M R 1985 Cerebrospinal fluid pharmacokinetics of the antituberculosis drugs. Clinical Pharmacokinetics 10: 532–534
8. Holdiness M R 1987 Transplacental pharmacokinetics of the antituberculosis drugs. Clinical Pharmacokinetics 13: 125–129
9. Jenner P J, Ellard G A 1981 High performance liquid chromatographic determination of ethionamide and prothionamide in body fluids. Journal of Chromatography Biomedical Applications 225: 245–251
10. Johnson J P, Kane P O, Kibly M R 1967 The metabolism of ethionamide and its sulphoxide metabolite. Journal of Pharmacy and Pharmacology 19: 1–9
11. Matsuo Y, Tatsukawa H, Murry J F, Peters J H 1981 Prothionamide and prothionamide-S-oxide in experimental leprosy. International Journal of Leprosy 49: 302–306
12. Waters M F R 1983 The treatment of leprosy. Tubercle 64: 211–232
13. World Health Organization Study Group 1982 Chemotherapy of leprosy for control programmes. World Health Organization Technical Report Series Number 675
14. Hastings R C 1985 Leprosy. Churchill Livingstone, London, pp 208–209
15. Rist N, Grumbach F, Liberman D 1959 Experiments on the antituberculosis activity of alpha-ethylthioisonicotinamide. American Review of Tuberculosis 79: 1–5
16. Girling D J 1982 Adverse effects of antituberculosis drugs. Drugs 23: 56–74
17. Holdiness M R 1985 Adverse cutaneous reactions of antituberculosis drugs: a review. International Journal of Dermatology 24: 280–285
18. Holdiness M R 1986 Contact dermatitis to antituberculosis drugs: a review. Contact Dermatitis 15: 282–288
19. Cartel J L, Millan J, Guelpa-Lauras C C, Grosset J H 1983 Hepatitis in leprosy patients treated by a daily combination of dapsone, rifampicin, and a thioamide. International Journal of Leprosy 51: 461–465
20. Cartel J L, Naudilon Y, Artus J C, Grosset J H 1985 Hepatotoxicity of the daily combination of 5 $mg.kg^{-1}$ prothionamide plus 10 $mg.kg^{-1}$ rifampicin. International Journal of Leprosy 53: 15–18
21. Baohong J, Jiakun C, Chenmin W, Guang X 1984 Hepatotoxicity of combined therapy with rifampicin and daily prothionamide. Leprosy Review 55: 283–289
22. Pattyn S R, Janssens L, Bourland J et al and The Collaborative Study Group for the Treatment of Leprosy 1984 Hepatotoxicity of the combination of rifampicin–ethionamide in the treatment of multibacillary leprosy. International Journal of Leprosy 52: 1–6
23. Holdiness M R 1987 Neurological manifestations and toxicities of the antituberculosis drugs: a review. Medical Toxicology 2: 33–51
24. Swash M, Roberts A H, Murnyaghan D J 1972 Reversible pellagra-like encephalopathy with ethionamide and cycloserine. Tubercle 53: 132–136
25. Gupta D K, Mital O P, Agarwal M C, Kansal H M, Nath S 1977 A comparison of therapeutic efficacy and toxicity of ethionamide and prothionamide in Indian patients. Journal of the Indian Medical Association 68: 25–29
26. Stanley J N, Pearson J M H, Ellard G A 1986 Ethionamide, prothionamide and thiacetazone self-administration. Studies of patient compliance using isoniazid-marked formulations. Leprosy Review 57: 9–18
27. Mathur A, Venkatesan K, Girdhar B K, Bharadwaj V P, Girdhar A, Bagga A K 1986 A study of drug interactions in leprosy — 1. Effect of simultaneous administration of prothionamide on metabolic disposition of rifampicin and dapsone. Leprosy Review 57: 33–37

Protriptyline (hydrochloride)

Protriptyline is the most potent, on a weight basis, of the series of tricyclic antidepressants.

Chemistry

Protriptyline hydrochloride (Concordin, Concordia, Maximed, Vivactil)
$C_{19}H_{21}N.HCl$
N-Methyl-5*H*-dibenzo[*a,d*]cycloheptene-5-propylamine hydrochloride

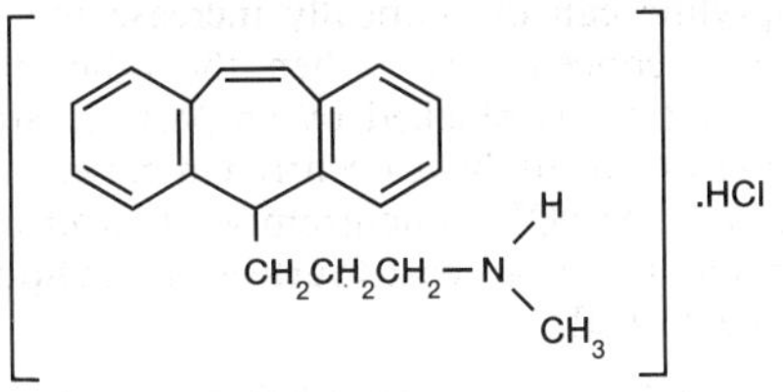

Molecular weight (free base)	299.8 (263.4)
pKa	—
Solubility	
in alcohol	1 in 3.5
in water	1 in 2
Octanol/water partition coefficient	16

Protriptyline hydrochloride is a white to yellowish, almost odourless powder with a bitter taste, prepared by chemical synthesis. It is not available in combination with any other drugs.

Pharmacology

Protriptyline is a relatively selective and potent inhibitor of noradrenaline uptake into central and peripheral noradrenergic neurons. In comparison to most other tricyclic antidepressants it is a less potent antagonist of α_1, histaminic and cholinergic receptors.[1,2] Like other tricyclic antidepressants, at higher concentrations it is a membrane stabilizer with a similar profile of activity to quinidine.

Toxicology

Protriptyline is not reported to produce tissue toxicity in animals of potential clinical relevance. Teratogenicity tests in mice, rats and rabbits are negative. Results of mutagenicity and carcinogenicity tests are not available.

Clinical pharmacology

Protriptyline is an effective antidepressant and like most drugs of this class its effects take time to develop. Some two to three weeks elapse before the full therapeutic effects are evident. Protriptyline tends to produce less sedation than drugs like imipramine. It decreases the amount of time spent in REM sleep and increases stage 4 sleep, in keeping with most tricyclic antidepressants. Protriptyline will produce some blockade of muscarinic cholinergic receptors, particularly at high dosage. Some patients may thus experience dry mouth, blurred vision and urinary retention. Protriptyline will affect the cardiovascular system, partly via vagal inhibition and partly by noradrenaline uptake blockade. Tachycardia and postural hypotension may be seen and on the ECG, T-wave inversion may occur.

In overdosage, cardiac arrhythmias are commonly seen and care must be exercised when giving protriptyline in patients with ischaemic heart disease or impairment of left ventricular function. Oral doses are usually in the range of 20–40 mg[3] although up to 80 mg daily may be required in some patients.

Both elevation and lowering of blood sugar in patients on protriptyline have been reported although not established as directly caused by the drug. Effects of long-term treatment are unknown.

Pharmacokinetics

Two analytical methods form the basis of reports in the literature: fluorimetry[4] and gas chromatography–mass fragmentography, the latter being very specific[5] with a lower level of sensitivity of 10 μg.l^{-1}. Both GC and HPLC can also be used for the analysis of the compound.

Protriptyline is slowly, but almost completely absorbed following oral administration, with essentially none being recovered in faeces. Metabolic transformation is extensive and takes place primarily in the liver. Direct estimates of presystemic metabolism of unchanged drug comparing oral and parenteral administration are not available. Some estimate that presystemic metabolism accounts for 10–25% of the dose. Peak plasma levels occur eight to twelve hours after a single oral dose. Plasma half life ranges from 54 to 158 hours if disappearance rates after chronic administration are included.[6,7] This is consistent with the observation that it can require four weeks or more to achieve steady-state. As with other lipophilic antidepressants which are extensively metabolized, it is to be expected that presystemic metabolism can be both induced, for example by cigarette smoking, and reduced by competitive inhibition, for example by concurrent administration of phenothiazines.

Protriptyline is unusually widely distributed and sequestered throughout the body with an apparent volume of distribution of 15–31.2 l.kg^{-1}, with rapid penetration and storage in lipophilic tissues such as brain. It is highly bound (92%) to plasma proteins[8] and probably preferably to α_1-acid glycoprotein as are other drugs with similar physiochemical properties. The extent to which protriptyline is excreted in breast milk is unknown.

Oral absorption	>95%
Presystemic metabolism	probably extensive
Plasma half life	
range	54–124 h
mean	74 h
Volume of distribution	15–31.2 l.kg^{-1}
Plasma protein binding	91–93%

The elimination of protriptyline is likely to be reduced in hepatic disease, although no specific information is available on this. Similarly, the clearance of the metabolites would be expected to be decreased in renal dysfunction, although no specific studies have been reported. The effect of renal impairment on the kinetics of protriptyline have not been reported, but it is likely that the excretion of potentially active metabolites will decline with decreasing renal function.

Concentration–effect relationship

Protriptyline appears to have an effective antidepressant concentration range from 70 to around 200 μg.l^{-1} although an upper limit is not well demonstrated.[3] It is assumed that like other tricyclic antidepressants it produces significant prolongation of the P-R interval at concentrations between 500 and 1000 μg.l^{-1}. A dose of 20 mg daily after four weeks produces concentrations ranging from 22 to 167 μg.l^{-1}, although many subjects are still not at steady-state. Thus, if individuals were on 60 mg a day or more they might ultimately reach concentrations of over 500 μg.l^{-1}.

Metabolism

Protriptyline is extensively metabolized in the liver, with almost no drug being excreted unchanged. Excretion of metabolites is almost wholly in urine. There is no evidence of significant enterohepatic circulation, the cumulative faecal excretion over a ten-day period after a single radiolabelled dose being 2%.[9]

Protriptyline is metabolized by oxidation to form the 10-hydroxy and 10,11-dihydro-10,11-dihydroxy derivative and 5,10-dihydro-10-formylanthracen-5-ylpropylamine; glucuronic acid conjugation also occurs.

P

N-Demethylation of protriptyline has been demonstrated in dogs and may occur in man.[10] The biological activity of the metabolites is not known, although the unconjugated 10-hydroxy metabolite might be expected to show activity similar to that of the parent compound as has been found for other hydroxy metabolites of other secondary amine tricyclic antidepressants.

Fig. 1 Metabolism of protriptyline

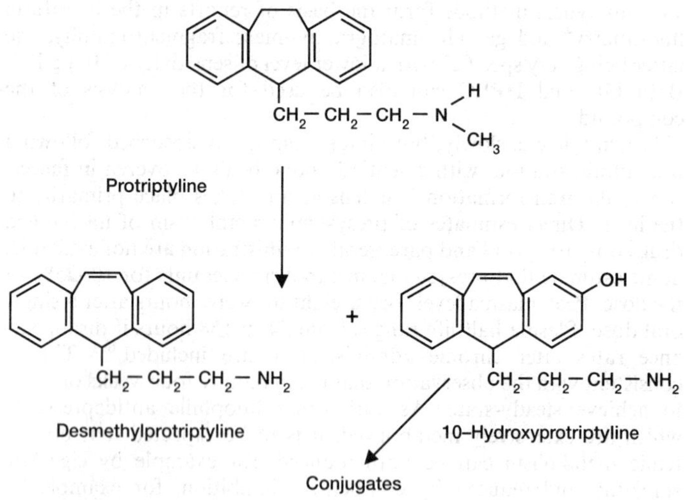

Pharmaceutics

Protriptyline is available only in oral form:
Concordin/Concordia (MSD, UK/USA): 5 mg and 10 mg tablets of protriptyline hydrochloride.
5 mg tablets are salmon-red (UK)/orange (USA), oval, film-coated, coded 'MSD 26'; 10 mg tablets are white (UK)/yellow (USA), oval, film-coated, coded 'MSD 47'.

Tablets should be stored in a cool place away from light.

Protriptyline has a long shelf-life of up to 5 years and contains no known additional substances that are potentially allergic in its formulated forms.

Therapeutic use

Indications

1. Treatment of depression.

Contraindications

1. Concomitant use of monoamine oxidase inhibitors
2. Acute recovery phase following myocardial infarction
3. Heart block or other arrhythmias
4. Previously demonstrated hypersensitivity.

Mode of use

In an otherwise healthy patient, oral treatment is begun with 15 mg a day in divided doses increasing up to 30 or 40 mg over a week if there are no significant side effects. The last dose should be given by early evening. One should then wait for two to three weeks before considering an increase in dose since at least this long is required to achieve steady-state, a period during which more pronounced side effects may emerge, and since there is a possibility that antidepressant response may be reduced at high plasma concentrations. If there is no response by four weeks, the dose can be increased up to 60 mg daily. One should wait at least two weeks, however, between 10 mg dosage increases. It is suggested that dosage increases be made in the morning dose since protriptyline may increase anxiety or agitation. If satisfactory improvement is achieved before steady-state is likely to have been reached, i.e. within less than three weeks of the last dose increase, a dose reduction to the previous level is appropriate.

Indications

1. Depression

Protriptyline, consistent with the fact that it is a weak inhibitor of α-adrenergic and histaminergic receptors,[1,2] is non-sedating. It is reported to have activating properties and may therefore be suitable for patients who are withdrawn and anergic. Since it is non-sedating, any improvement which patients experience in sleep is likely to be delayed and a direct consequence of its antidepressant effects. Moreover, effects can occur before a steady-state is achieved so that an apparently effective dose may ultimately turn out to be too high as reflected by either an increase in side effects or a worsening of the depression. Thus, before discontinuing the drug because of a reversal of response, the dose should be systematically lowered to see if response can be re-established.

There are no reported problems with stopping protriptyline suddenly. Its long half life provides for a gradual withdrawal.

The mode of action of protriptyline is presumably a secondary consequence of noradrenaline uptake inhibition. The drug is very potent in this regard[11] and is relatively weak in terms of interaction at either other neurotransmitter uptake sites or pre- or postsynaptic receptors. From a theoretical and preclinical viewpoint, it is one of the 'cleanest' antidepressants in that its major effects are on one system.

Contraindications

1. Use with monoamine oxidase inhibitors (MAOIs)

Presumably because it is such a potent inhibitor of noradrenaline uptake, protriptyline can dramatically increase the neurotransmitter's intrasynaptic concentration when the other major route of clearance, deamination, is blocked by an MAOI. Stroke, hyperpyrexia, convulsions and death have occurred in patients taking tricyclic antidepressants and MAOIs concurrently. If protriptyline is to be substituted for an MAOI, at least fourteen days should elapse after discontinuing the MAOI.

2. Recovery phase following a myocardial infarction

Protriptyline can be expected to increase the heart rate and will sometimes produce substantial tachycardia which should be avoided under conditions of cardiac vulnerability. Recent data, however, shows that tricyclic antidepressants do not directly impair left ventricular function, even in patients with pre-existing heart disease.[12] Such patients may nonetheless be at significant risk of drug-induced aggravation of orthostatic hypotension, presumably secondary to α-receptor blockade although this is most clearly a problem with tertiary amine tricyclic antidepressants (e.g. imipramine) when used at therapeutic doses.[13]

3. Heart block or other arrythmias

Protriptyline may produce dangerous bradycardia in a person with pre-existing heart block depending on its degree of severity. Like other tricyclics it possesses quinidine-like membrane-stabilizing effects which are roughly proportional to blood levels and result in widening of the QRS complex and P-R interval and some flattening of the T wave.[14] Since required therapeutic levels are lower than for more commonly used tricyclics, protriptyline may emerge as less likely to induce prolongation of conduction time when used clinically.

4. Previously demonstrated hypersensitivity

Hypersensitivity to protriptyline is rare but it is important to consider it since allergic reactions may be markedly intensified on subsequent administration and the drug is relatively slowly cleared from the body. Cross-sensitivity to other tricyclic antidepressants has been reported to occur although there are instances in which patients have shown hypersensitivity to protriptyline and been switched to another tricyclic without difficulty.

Adverse reactions

Potentially life-threatening effects

Deaths associated with the use of protriptyline or other tricyclic antidepressants used in standard therapeutic doses are currently very rare since it is now appreciated that these drugs should be avoided in individuals with significant pre-existing heart block or who are receiving monoamine oxidase inhibitors.

The major toxic effect which occurs most frequently and which may lead to dangerous or even lethal behaviour is the induction of mania in individuals with underlying manic–depressive illness or worsening of psychosis in already psychotic individuals. The drug should be stopped at the first sign of mania and/or emergence of psychosis and the patient carefully monitored.

Protriptyline (hydrochloride)

Acute overdosage
Deliberate overdose with all tricyclic antidepressants, including protriptyline, is frequent and often lethal.[15] Depending on the amount of drug ingested, the clinical features of overdose include drowsiness and stupor or coma; tachycardia and ECG evidence of impaired conduction are invariably present, and the latter may be useful in monitoring the return to non-toxic levels; altered temperature regulation involving either hypothermia or hyperpyrexia may be present; seizure threshold is lowered and convulsions may occur. Congestive heart failure, mydriasis, muscle rigidity, hyperactive reflexes, agitation and vomiting may also occur. Death may occur after as little as 2000 mg of a tricyclic antidepressant and is common if over 3000 mg has been ingested.

Management of acute overdosage
Treatment is symptomatic and supportive, especially if more than a few hours have elapsed since ingestion of the drug. Patients should be admitted to hospital and the stomach emptied by inducing emesis in the hope of eliminating any unabsorbed drug if consciousness is clear or by gastric lavage. Although the efficacy of the treatment is not that clear, it is recommended that 20 to 30 g of activated charcoal may be given every four to six hours during the first 24 to 48 hours after ingestion. An ECG should be taken and close monitoring of cardiac function instituted if there is any sign of abnormality. An open airway should be maintained, an adequate fluid intake ensured, and body temperature regulated.

The intravenous administration of 1–3 mg of physostigmine salicylate is reported to reverse the symptoms of poisoning with other tricyclic antidepressants in humans. Because physostigmine is rapidly metabolized, it should be given repeatedly if required, particularly if life-threatening signs, such as arrhythmias, convulsions and deep coma, recur and persist after the initial dose of physostigmine. Physostigmine itself may cause bronchospasm, increased respiratory secretion, bradycardia, hypotension and seizures, and so it should be used with extreme caution.

Standard measures should be used to manage circulatory shock and metabolic acidosis. Cardiac arrhythmias may be treated with neostigmine, pyridostigmine or propranolol. Should cardiac failure occur, the use of digitalis should be considered. Close monitoring of cardiac function for not less than five days is advisable.

Anticonvulsants may be given to control convulsions.

Dialysis is of no value, because of low plasma concentrations of the drug and poor partition into the dialysate.

Severe or irreversible adverse effects
A wide range of central nervous system and neuromuscular adverse reactions is possible, although they are unlikely at lower doses. Agitation and increased psychomotor activity, however, may be more marked after protriptyline than after other tricyclic antidepressants at therapeutic doses and may occur in 10–25% of patients. As already mentioned, induction of mania and worsening of psychosis, delusions, and/or hallucinations is relatively likely. Confusion, disorientation, nightmares, numbness, tingling and paresthesiae of the extremities, peripheral neuropathy, ataxia, tremors, seizures, alterations in EEG patterns, extrapyramidal symptoms, tinnitus, dizziness, weakness, fatigue, headache and drowsiness are reported after this class of drugs and may occur after protriptyline.

There are very rare reports of bone marrow depression and/or agranulocytosis with drugs of this class.[16] Endocrinological effects are minimal, although modest effects of some tricyclic antidepressants on prolactin regulation have been noted,[17] and the possibility of gynaecomastia in males or heart enlargement and galactorrhoea in females should be considered.

Symptomatic adverse effects
Protriptyline is likely to cause some degree of sympathomimetic effect, reflected in increased pulse in most patients, hyperhidrosis in many, and some initial increased insomnia if used as the sole agent. Since, in common with other tricyclics, it inhibits α_1, muscarinic and histaminergic receptors, but less potently, it can also produce dry mouth, blurred vision, disturbed accommodation, mydriasis, constipation, and urinary retention and/or delayed micturition. Dry mouth is the most frequent complaint and occurs in over 25% of patients.

Feelings variously described as 'weakness', 'dizziness' or 'giddiness' in the absence of orthostatic hypotension occurred in approximately 15% of patients in early studies which employed doses in the upper therapeutic range.

Weight gain is possible on tricyclic antidepressants, especially women, although the mechanism for this effect is not clear.

Other effects
Biochemical studies on the effects of protriptyline itself are not available. As noted above, drugs of this class may alter prolactin regulation. They also reduce growth hormone release, although this has no known clinical effects. It is probable that protriptyline raises levels of circulating noradrenaline consistent with its sympathomimetic effects. Alterations of blood chemistry, directly attributable to tricyclics, have not been noted.

Interference with clinical pathology tests
There are no recorded instances of interference with standard tests.

High risk groups

Neonates
The safety of protriptyline in neonates is not established and there are no known indications for use of tricyclic antidepressants in this group.

Breast milk. It is not known if the drug enters breast milk, so mothers taking it should not breast-feed.

Children
Studies on the use and safety of protriptyline itself in children are not available. Tricyclic antidepressants are, however, used by some in the management of enuresis and attention-deficient disorder (hyperactivity), as well as depression.[18,19]

Children may metabolize tricyclics more rapidly than adults and typically are treated with somewhat higher doses on a $mg.kg^{-1}$ basis (3–5 $mg.kg^{-1}$) than would be used for a typical 70 kg adult.[19] The potentially lethal dose in children, however, is much lower than in adults so the total amount of drug available to a child should be restricted so as to avoid fatal intentional or accidental overdose.

Pregnant women
The safety of protriptyline in pregnancy is not established, although neither it nor other tricyclic antidepressants has been specifically implicated in teratogenicity. Common practice would be to either taper dosage so as to be drug-free for two weeks prior to becoming pregnant or to stop medication if an unexpected pregnancy were to occur. In the event of relapse into a severe depression during pregnancy, the decision whether to resume protriptyline is made in the absence of adequate data.

The elderly
There is conflicting data on the impact of age on tricyclic antidepressant metabolism.[20] Specific studies with protriptyline are not available but, since it is a secondary amine tricyclic like desipramine and nortriptyline, it may be less likely to demonstrate altered clearance than would imipramine or amitriptyline. The elderly are clearly more sensitive to the anticholinergic effects of tricyclics and may also be more sensitive to the therapeutic effects, although blood concentration vs outcome studies in this population are not available. Renal clearance of hydroxylated active metabolites of tricyclics does decrease with age, and selective increases of the hydroxy metabolites of desipramine and nortriptyline have been detailed in the elderly. It is therefore recommended that initial doses be 30–50% of the recommended dose for similar younger individuals (i.e. begin with 5 mg twice-daily of protriptyline). Ordinary adult doses, however, should not be ruled out in this population since they may be necessary to achieve therapeutic effect and may be well tolerated.

Concurrent disease
Heart disease. As described above, pre-existing heart block may render an individual susceptible to potentially fatal effects.

Prostatic and eye disease. Patients with a history of urinary retention or those who have increased intraocular pressure are at special risk of aggravation of these conditions secondary to the anticholinergic effects of all tricyclic antidepressants, although protriptyline is relatively less likely to produce extensive cholinergic blockade.[21]

Thyrotoxicosis. Protriptyline should be used with great caution in patients with hyperthyroidism because of its sympathomimetic effects.

Hepatic disease. Severe liver disease is likely to reduce the metabolism of protriptyline so that an individual will be at risk of those multiple effects described above usually associated with tricyclic overdose.

Renal disease. Since the drug can be metabolized to inactive conjugated forms in the liver, it is not so dependent on renal clearance to avoid toxicity. Renal failure therefore does not contribute greatly to toxicity.

Drug interactions

Potentially hazardous interactions

Monoamine oxidase inhibitors (MAOIs). As discussed above under 'Contraindications', the addition of protriptyline to individuals on MAOIs may produce stroke, hyperpyrexia, convulsions and death although the occurrence of such severe adverse effects is unpredictable.

Noradrenaline and adrenaline. Following administration of these biogenic amines, unexpectedly large increases in blood pressure and a greater incidence of arrhythmias may occur in individuals on tricyclic antidepressants.

Phenothiazines. Additive anticholinergic effects may occur which may be manifested as appearance of psychosis and/or agitation, especially in elderly patients.

Other significant reactions

Barbiturates. Barbiturates can increase the metabolism of tricyclic antidepressants and presumably protriptyline, so that higher than usual doses are necessary.

Cimetidine. This can block the metabolism of both tertiary and secondary amine tricyclic antidepressants so that lower doses may be appropriate in patients on this H_2-receptor antagonist.

Clonidine. The effects of clonidine are reduced or blocked by desipramine, presumably secondary to its noradrenaline-uptake-inhibiting potency, and protriptyline can be expected to have a similar effect.

Guanethidine. Protriptyline should block any antihypertensive effects of guanethidine by inhibiting its uptake into nerve endings.

Haloperidol. This drug can block the metabolism of tricyclic antidepressants, depending on the dose and sequence of administration, thereby potentially raising plasma concentrations of protriptyline into a toxic or non-therapeutic range.

Food. Food has not been implicated in alteration of the effects or metabolism of protriptyline or of tricyclic antidepressants in general.

Alcohol. Specific studies with protriptyline are not available. Chronic heavy drinking, however, may induce the metabolism of at least tertiary amine tricyclics, and acute alcohol loading may impair clearance of this class of compounds.[22] CNS effects of alcohol are clearly enhanced by concomitant administration of tertiary amine tricyclics and presumably would be affected by high enough doses of secondary amine forms such as protriptyline.

Smoking. Smoking cigarettes is reported to induce the metabolism of tricyclic antidepressants, although the data are not consistent and do not include studies on protriptyline itself.

Potentially useful interactions

There are no known therapeutic interactions of protriptyline with other drugs although other tricyclic antidepressants have been combined with analgesics in the management of pain.

Major outcome trials

1. Daneman E A 1965 Clinical experience and a double-blind study of a new antidepressant, Vivactil hydrochloride. Psychosomatics 6: 342–346

This was a two-stage study of depressed outpatients who were treated under double conditions in the first phase with protriptyline (45 patients) vs placebo (47 patients) and in the second with protriptyline (48 patients) vs amitriptyline (43 patients). Patients were treated with 5 to 10 mg of protriptyline three to four times a day, placebo, or 25 to 50 mg of amitriptyline three to four times a day, so as to maintain a 1:5 ratio between protriptyline and amitriptyline. Patients were begun on one tablet (5 or 25 mg) three times a day and increased to the maximum (40 mg of protriptyline or 200 mg of amitriptyline) depending on response and/or side effects. Response was evaluated after at least four weeks of treatment.

Outcome in patients treated with protriptyline was markedly superior to that in those treated with placebo (and marginally better than following amitriptyline). The side effects of agitation and increased psychomotor activity were specific to higher doses of protriptyline. In contrast, amitriptyline produced sedation in almost 50% of patients. At none of the doses studied did protriptyline produce sedation. The author recommends limiting the dose of protriptyline in outpatients to 35–40 mg daily.

2. Williams E J 1968 Protriptyline: a double-blind clinical trial. The Medical Journal of Australia 1: 537–540

This is a double-blind comparison of protriptyline (20–80 mg daily) vs amitriptyline (75–200 mg daily) in 37 hospitalized severely depressed patients free of other significant illness. Patients who were not significantly improved after 28 days were treated with ECT. Patients responded equally well but protriptyline produced both initial and maximal clinical improvement earlier than did amitriptyline. The 8 out of 19 patients treated with protriptyline who required ECT required only 2 to 5 sessions to produce remission. In this study in which 10 out of 19 patients were on 60 or 80 mg daily of protriptyline, no significant difference in side effects between treatments could be discerned.

General review articles

Baker J M, Dewhurst W G 1985 Tricyclic antidepressants. In: Dewhurst W G, Baker G B (eds) Pharmacotherapy of affective disorders. Croom Helm, London, ch 8, pp 262–285

DeVane C L 1980 Tricyclic antidepressants. In: Evans W E, Shentag J J, Jusko W J (eds) Applied pharmacokinetics: principles of therapeutic drug monitoring. Applied Therapeutics Inc, Spokane, WA, pp 549–585

Potter W Z, Bertilsson L, Sjoqvist F 1981 Clinical pharmacokinetics of psychotropic drugs: fundamental and practical aspects. In: van Praag H M, Rafaelson O, Lader M, Sachar A (eds) The handbook of biological psychiatry: Part VI, Practical applications of psychotropic drugs and other biological treatments. Marcel Dekker, New York, pp 71–134

References

1. Maggi A, U'Prichard D C, Enna S A 1980 Differential effects of antidepressant treatment on brain monoaminergic receptors. European Journal of Pharmacology 61: 91–98
2. Kanof P D, Greengard P 1978 Brain histamine receptors as targets for antidepressant drugs. Nature 272: 329–333
3. Biggs J T, Ziegler V E 1977 Protriptyline plasma levels and antidepressant response. Clinical Pharmacology and Therapeutics 22: 269–273
4. Moody J P, Whyte S F, Naylor G J 1973 A simple method for the determination of protriptyline in plasma. Clinica Chimica Acta 43: 355–359
5. Biggs J T, Holland W H, Chang S S, Hipps P P, Sherman W R 1976 The electron beam ionization mass fragmentographic analysis of tricyclic antidepressants in human plasma. Journal of Pharmaceutical Sciences 65: 261–268
6. Moody J P, Whyte S F, MacDonald A J, Naylor G J 1977 Pharmacokinetic aspects of protriptyline plasma levels. European Journal of Clinical Pharmacology 11: 51–56
7. Ziegler V E, Biggs J T, Wylie L T et al 1978 Protriptyline kinetics. Clinical Pharmacology and Therapeutics 23: 580–584
8. Borga O, Azarnoff D L, Forshell G P, Sjoqvist F 1969 Plasma protein binding of tricyclic antidepressants in man. Biochemical Pharmacology 18: 2135–2143
9. Charalampous K D, Johnson P C 1967 Studies of C^{14}-protriptyline in man: plasma levels and excretion. Journal of Clinical Pharmacology and New Drugs 7: 93–96
10. Lisenwine S F, Tio C O, Shrader S R, Ruelius H W 1970 The biotransformation of protriptyline in man, pig and dog. The Journal of Pharmacology and Experimental Therapeutics 175: 51–59
11. Carlsson A, Corrodi H, Fuxe K, Hokfelt T 1969 Effects of some antidepressant drugs on the depletion of intrapersonal brain catecholamine stores caused by 4-d-dimethyl-meta-tyramine. European Journal of Pharmacology 5: 367–373
12. Veith R C, Raskind M A, Caldwell J H, Barnes R F, Gumbrecht G, Ritchie J L 1982 Cardiovascular effects of tricyclic antidepressants in depressed patients with chronic heart disease. New England Journal of Medicine 306: 954–959
13. Glassman A H, Bigger J T Jr 1981 Cardiovascular effects of therapeutic doses of tricyclic antidepressants: a review. Archives of General Psychiatry 38: 815–820
14. Giardina E G, Bigger J T Jr, Glassman A H, Perel J M, Kantor S J 1979 The electrocardiographic and antiarrhythmic effects of imipramine hydrochloride at therapeutic plasma concentrations. Circulation 60: 1045–1052
15. Bailey D N, Van Dyke C, Langou R A, Jatlow P I 1978 Tricyclic antidepressants: plasma levels and clinical findings in overdose. American Journal of Psychiatry 135: 1325–1328
16. Klein D F, Gittelman R, Quitkin F, Rifkin A 1980 Review of the literature on mood-stabilizing drugs. In: Diagnosis and drug treatment of psychiatric disorders: adults and children, 2nd edn. Williams & Wilkins, Baltimore, pp 268–303

17. Calil H M, Lesieur P, Gold P W, Zavadil A P, Brown G M, Potter W Z 1984 Hormonal responses to zimelidine and desipramine in depressed patients. Psychiatry Research 13: 231–242
18. Huessy H, Wright A 1970 The use of imipramine in children's behavior disorders. Acta Paedopsychiatrica 37: 194–199
19. Garfinkel B D 1984 The use of antidepressant medication in children and adolescents. In: Stancer H C, Garfinkel P E, Rakoff U M (eds) Guidelines for the use of psychotropic drugs. Spectrum Publications, New York, pp 31–62
20. Rudorfer M V, Potter W Z 1985 Metabolism of drugs used in affective disorders. In: Dewhurst W G, Baker G B (eds) Pharmacotherapy of affective disorders. Croom Helm, London, ch 12, pp 382–448
21. Snyder S H, Peroutka S J 1984 Antidepressants and neurotransmitter receptors. In: Post R M, Ballenger J C (eds) Neurobiology of mood disorders. Williams & Wilkins, Baltimore, pp 686–697
22. Dorian P, Sellers E M, Warsh J J, Reed K L, Hamilton C, Fan T 1982 Decreased hepatic first-pass extraction of oral drugs: mechanism of ethanol–amitriptyline interaction. Clinical Pharmacology and Therapeutics 31: 219

Pseudoephedrine hydrochloride

Pseudoephedrine is a stereoisomer of ephedrine with similar but less potent pharmacological activity. It is widely used as a constituent in proprietary nasal and bronchial decongestant preparations.

Chemistry

Pseudophedrine hydrochloride (d-ψ-ephedrine hydrochloride, d-isoephedrine hydrochloride, Sudafed, Galpseud)
$C_{10}H_{15}NO.HCl$
(1S,2S)-2-Methylamino-1-phenylpropan-1-ol hydrochloride

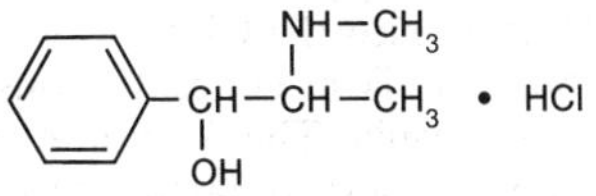

Molecular weight (free base)	201.7 (165.2)
pKa (N-H)	9.8
Solubility	
in alcohol	1 in 4
in water	1 in 1.6
Octanol/water partition coefficient	high

Pseudoephedrine hydrochloride is an almost colourless white crystalline powder with a bitter taste and faint characteristic odour. It is a naturally occurring alkaloid from the *Ephedra* species. Pseudoephedrine is an ingredient of a variety of cough preparations and nasal decongestants, including Actifed, Benylin Decongestant, Dimotane, Expulin, Sudafed linctus, Sudafed Expectorant, Congesteze, Sudafed Plus, Sudafed-Co.

Pharmacology

Pseudoephedrine is a sympathomimetic agent with direct and indirect effects on adrenergic receptors. It has direct agonist activity, particularly on cardiac β-adrenoceptors and peripheral α_1-adrenoceptors, and indirect sympathomimetic activity because it displaces noradrenaline from the cytoplasmic pool. It also has a weak central nervous system stimulant action.

Toxicology

There are no data on pseudoephedrine to suggest any mutagenic potential. Similarly, there is no evidence of teratogenicity or carcinogenicity.

Clinical pharmacology

Pseudoephedrine appears to have less pressor activity and weaker central nervous system effects than ephedrine. It has agonist activity at both β_1- and β_2-adrenoceptors, leading to increased cardiac output and to relaxation of bronchial smooth muscle.[1] Its actions on α-adrenoceptors in the mucosa of the respiratory tract produce a degree of vasoconstriction which leads to a reduction in mucosal oedema.[1] It has mild CNS stimulant activity, especially in patients sensitive to the effects of sympathomimetic drugs,[2] and its action on peripheral vascular α_1-adrenoceptors leads to an increase in systolic blood pressure.[3]

The studies designed to evaluate human tolerance and dose–response relationships are limited and incomplete.[4,5]

The drug is widely available in different compound preparations for the symptomatic relief of upper respiratory tract and similar common infections and inflammations. It can be used as adjunctive therapy in association with antibiotic treatment for acute and serious otitis media.

It reputedly has fewer pressor effects than ephedrine and, similarly, has fewer CNS excitatory effects than ephedrine.

Pharmacokinetics

Pseudoephedrine may be quantified in plasma by gas–liquid chromatography with electron-capture detection,[6] sensitivity 20 μg.l^{-1}, or by radioimmunoassay, sensitivity 0.2–2.5 μg.l^{-1}, depending on the method.[7]

Pseudoephedrine is readily and completely absorbed from the gastrointestinal tract following oral administration, with no presystemic metabolism. It achieves peak plasma concentrations between 1 and 3 h after oral dosing and a dose of 180 mg, for example, produces peak levels at 2 h after dosing of between 500 and 900 μg.l^{-1}. It is eliminated largely unchanged in the urine (55–90%) in 24 h, although there is some metabolism in the liver (< 1%) by N-demethylation. It has a plasma half life of 5–8 h following oral dosing, but its urinary elimination, and hence half life, is pH dependent such that elimination will be increased in subjects with acidic urine and decreased in subjects with alkaline urine.

Pseudoephedrine is rapidly distributed throughout the body. Its volume of distribution is 2–3 l.kg^{-1} body weight but there are no reports of the extent of plasma protein binding and similarly, although CNS effects are observed, there is no specific information concerning its penetration into the CNS.

It is excreted in breast milk at concentrations consistently higher than those in maternal plasma. The fraction of the dose excreted in milk has been estimated at approximately 0.5% of a single oral dose over 24 h.[8] Pseudoephedrine is likely to cross the placenta.

Oral absorption	>95%
Presystemic metabolism	negligible
Plasma half life	5.4–8 h
Volume of distribution	2–3 l.kg^{-1}
Plasma protein binding	—

The elimination of pseudoephedrine is reduced in renal impairment and with deteriorating renal function in the elderly. Hepatic dysfunction is unlikely to affect the pharmacokinetics of the drug.

Concentration–effect relationship

This has not been studied in detail. There is a single report of a study in which an oral dose of 180 mg produced a peak plasma concentration of 600 μg.l^{-1} in comparison to a plasma concentration of 400 μg.l^{-1} following a dose of 180 mg of a sustained-release formulation.[9] The conclusion from this study was that effect was not related closely to plasma concentration.

Metabolism

Pseudoephedrine is resistant to the actions of monoamine oxidase and is excreted essentially unchanged in the urine (⩽90% of the dose in 24 h). Less than 1% is eliminated by hepatic metabolism, by N-demethylation to norpseudoephedrine (cathine) (Fig. 1).

Fig. 1 Metabolism of pseudoephedrine

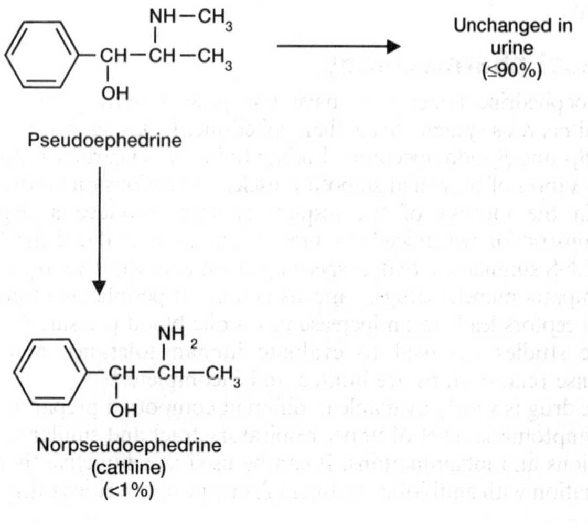

Pharmaceutics

Pseudoephedrine is available in a variety of oral forms but there is no commercially available parenteral form.

1. Both 30 mg and 60 mg tablets are available in the USP. Galpseud tablets (Galen, UK) contain 60 mg of pseudoephedrine and are white and scored.
2. Galpseud linctus (Galen, UK) is a yellow-red colour and contains 30 mg pseudoephedrine in 5 ml. Lederle manufacture an equivalent strength in the USA.
3. Sudafed SA (Calmic, UK) is a slow-release formulation, a red capsule containing a mixture of instant and sustained-release pellets.

There is a wide range of combination products.

Therapeutic use

Indications

1. Decongestant, particularly for the upper respiratory tract
2. Bronchodilator.

Contraindications

1. Cardiovascular disease including hypertension
2. Endocrine disorders, hyperthyroidism, diabetes mellitus
3. Prostatic enlargement
4. Concurrent use of monoamine oxidase inhibitor drugs
5. Nursing mothers.

Mode of use

As a decongestant and symptomatic treatment for upper respiratory tract infections the recommended daily dosage is 60 mg per 6 hours, or per 4 hours as maximum. For children, the dose is 30 mg per 4–6 hours for those aged 6–12 years and 15 mg per 4–6 hours for those aged 2–5 years. For children less than 2 years of age the drug is not advised unless specifically recommended by a physician.

Contraindications

1. Cardiovascular disease, including hypertension
Pseudoephedrine may cause tachycardia, palpitations and multifocal premature ventricular ectopic beats, particularly if administered in large doses. Patients with pre-existing cardiac disease, or those who have demonstrated a previous sensitivity to the myocardial effects of sympathomimetics, should avoid these agents.

The effects of standard antihypertensive drug treatment may be compromised by psuedoephedrine.

2. Endocrine disorders
Since tachycardia and palpitations may be exacerbated by sympathomimetics it is recommended that these agents be avoided in patients with uncontrolled hyperthyroidism, particularly if a β-adrenoceptor antagonist is not being used. Since the metabolic effects of pseudoephedrine promote hyoglycaemia, hyperlacticacidaemia and hyper-lipaemia, the use of these agents in diabetes mellitus is relatively contraindicated.

3. Prostatic hypertropy
Difficulties in initiating micturition have been reported.

4. MAOI drugs
Pseudoephedrine should not be administered in combination with monoamine oxidase inhibitor drugs because the noradrenaline it releases may lead to severe hypertension and potentially to a hypertensive crisis. It has been recommended that patients should wait at least 14 days after stopping monoamine oxidase inhibitors before using the drug.

5. Nursing mothers
Pseudoephedrine is transferred through breast milk and the infant may be exposed to sympathomimetic effects. Therefore its use is best avoided by women who are breast-feeding.

Adverse reactions

Potentially life-threatening effects
These are thought to be very rare at normal doses. There is a case report of a 17-year-old who developed transient hypertension and

Pseudoephedrine hydrochloride

loss of consciousness following a single 60 mg oral dose.[10] There are no reports of irreversible side effects.

Acute overdosage

The fatal dose is thought to be greater than 2 g in adults and greater than 200 mg in a child under 13 years. The main clinical features are similar to those of ephedrine poisoning, with central nervous system stimulation leading to excitement, restlessness, rapid speech, hallucinations, hypertonicity and hyperreflexia, dilated pupils and tachycardia. In severe poisoning the tachycardia may lead to cardiac arrhythmias which may be further potentiated by the development of hypokalaemia. There is no specific treatment for the CNS effects, but general supportive measures are recommended and, if necessary, diazepam should be administered as a sedative/anticonvulsant. β-Blockers may be administered to control the tachycardia, arrhythmia and hypokalaemia. Potassium supplements may also be required.

Severe or irreversible adverse effects

None has been reported.

Symptomatic adverse effects

There is no detailed account of the frequency or severity of symptomatic adverse effects. Dry mouth, anorexia, insomnia, anxiety, tension, tremor, restlessness and palpitation were reported to be 'commonly occurring' in a case study of 34 males given standard doses.[5] Small increases in systolic blood pressure and heart rate have been reported at 2 h after dosing with 60 mg when there was no evidence of CNS effects.[4] Paranoid psychosis and skin rash (erythematous eruption) have also been the subject of case reports.[11,12]

Interference with clinical pathology tests

None has been reported.

High risk groups

Neonates

Neonatal infants are thought to be more sensitive to pseudoephedrine.[13]

Breast milk. There is no published report of any adverse reaction in the infants of nursing mothers unless these infants had poor kidney function.[8] However, pseudoephedrine does pass into breast milk, so it should not be given to breast-feeding women.

Children

The clearance of pseudoephedrine is more rapid in children, reflecting a smaller volume of distribution and a more rapid intrinsic clearance. The mean half life has been quoted as 4.6 h for children.[14]

Pregnant women

There have been isolated reports of fetal maldevelopment in animal studies but there has been no convincing account of teratogenesis from specific studies. Teratogenicity has not been reported in humans but there have been no studies and the drug is best avoided in pregnancy.[15]

The elderly

Sustained-release preparations are not recommended for elderly patients since overdosage, perhaps reflecting underlying renal impairment, may lead to central nervous system effects with CNS depression, hallucinations, convulsions and death.[1]

Concurrent disease

Renal impairment, including renal tubular acidosis, increases the risk of drug accumulation and adverse effects.[16]

Drug interactions

Potentially hazardous interactions

Concurrent administration of other sympathomimetics may lead to additive CNS or CVS effects.[9] Interference with the antihypertensive efficacy of reserpine, methyldopa and β-blockers has been reported and similarly an exaggerated pressor effect has been reported with concurrent monoamine oxidase inhibitor administration.[1]

Other significant interactions

Increased absorption has been reported with the concurrent administration of aluminium hydroxide.[18]

Potentially useful interactions

Combination with antihistamines may reduce their sedative effects and, similarly, the combination product with tripolidine is said to give better symptomatic response than either preparation alone.[2]

References

1. American Society Hospital Pharmacy 1976 American Society Formulation Service 12–12, 17–19
2. Bye C, Dewsbury D, Peck A W 1974 Effects on the human central nervous system of the two isomers of ephedrine and triprolidine and their interaction. British Journal of Clinical Pharmacology 1: 71–78
3. Drew C D M, Knight G T, Hughes D T D, Bush M 1978 Comparison of the effects of D-(−)-ephedrine and L-(+)-pseudoephedrine on the cardiovascular and respiratory systems in man. British Journal of Clinical Pharmacology 6: 221–225
4. Empey D W, Young G A, Letley E et al 1980 Dose–response study of the nasal decongestant and cardiovascular effects of pseudoephedrine. British Journal of Clinical Pharmacology 9: 351–358
5. Dickerson J, Perrier D, Mayersohn M, Bressler R 1978 Dose tolerance and pharmacokinetic studies of L(+)pseudoephedrine capsules in man. European Journal of Clinical Pharmacology 14: 253–259
6. Lo L Y, Land G, Bye A 1981 Sensitive assay for pseudoephedrine and its metabolite, norpseudoephedrine in plasma and urine using gas–liquid chromatography with electron capture detection. Journal of Chromatography 222: Biomedical Applications 11: 297–302
7. Findlay J W A, Warren J T, Hill J A et al 1981 Stereospecific radioimmunoassays for d-pseudoephedrine in human plasma and their application to bioequivalency studies. Journal of Pharmaceutical Science 70: 624–631
8. Findlay J W A, Butz R F, Sailstad J M, Warren J T, Welch R M 1984 Pseudoephedrine and triprolidine in plasma and breast milk of nursing mothers. British Journal of Clinical Pharmacology 18: 901–906
9. Bye C, Hill H M, Hughes D T D, Peck A W 1975 A comparison of plasma levels of L(+)pseudoephedrine following different formulations, and their relation to cardiovascular and subjective effects in man. European Journal of Clinical Pharmacology 8: 47–53
10. 1978 International Journal of Clinical Pharmacology 16: 63–67
11. Rutstein H R 1963 Ingestion of pseudoephedrine. Hypertension and unconsciousness following report of a case. Archives of Otolaryngology 77: 145–147
12. Leighton K M 1982 Paranoid psychosis after abuse of Actifed. British Medical Journal 284: 789–790
13. Brater D C, Kaojarern S, Benet L Z et al 1980 Renal secretion of pseudoephedrine. Clinical Pharmacology and Therapeutics 28: 690–694
14. Boyd J R 1986 Non-prescription drug screening. Pseudoephedrine. American Pharmacy NS26: 22–24
15. Augitt 1981 Annals of Allergy 47: 139 Abstract No 10
16. Frankland A W 1973 Allergy to pseudoephedrine. Practitioner 211: 828–829
17. Kastrup E K, Olin B R (eds) 1986 Drug facts and comparisons. Lippincott, St Louis, p 692
18. Lucarotti R L, Colaizzi J L, Barry H, Poust R I 1972 Enhanced pseudoephedrine absorption by concurrent administration of aluminium hydroxide gel in humans. Journal of Pharmaceutical Sciences 61: 903–905

P

Pyrantel embonate

Pyrantel pamoate (synonymous with Pyrantel embonate) is a neuromuscular blocking agent used as an anthelminthic.

Chemistry

Pyrantel embonate (Pyrantel pamoate, Combantrin, Antiminth, Helmex, Trilombrin)
$C_{11}H_{14}N_2S.C_{23}H_{16}O_6$
1,4,5,6-Tetrahydro-1-methyl-2-[(E)2-(2-thienyl)vinyl]pyrimidine 4,4-methylenebis [3-hydroxy-2-naphthoate](1:1)

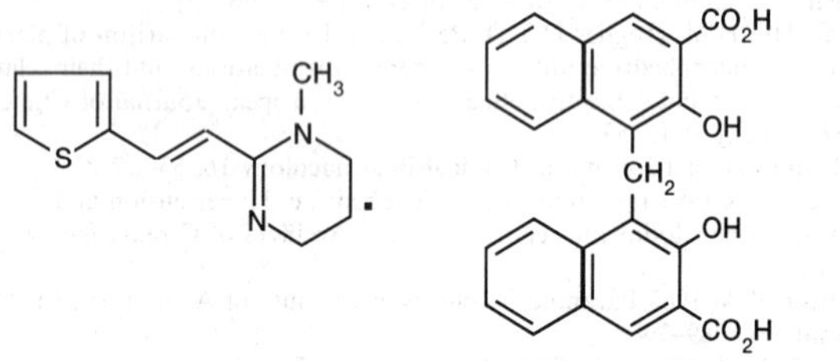

Molecular weight (free base)	594.7 (206)
pKa	206.3
Solubility	
in alcohol	insoluble
in water	insoluble
Octanol/water partition coefficient	—

Pyrantel embonate is a yellow to tan powder that is tasteless and free of characteristic odour. It is prepared by chemical synthesis.[1] The compound is soluble in dimethyl sulphoxide.

It is available in combination products: pyrantel pamoate plus oxantel pamoate. Trademarks used are Quantrel and Combantrin-Plus.

Pharmacology

Pyrantel pamoate acts as a depolarizing neuromuscular blocking agent. It causes marked nicotinic activation at the neuromuscular junction, which results in spastic paralysis of the worm. Pyrantel is 100 times more active than acetylcholine itself in producing contractures of *Ascaris* preparations. In single muscle cells of *Ascaris*, increased spike-discharge frequency is seen which is accompanied by a rise in muscle tension. In addition to its action on the neuromuscular junction, pyrantel is also an inhibitor of acetylcholinesterase which contributes to its neuromuscular effects.

Toxicology

Oral doses up to 2000 $mg.kg^{-1}$ have produced no evidence of toxicity in mice and rats. Oral doses of up to 1000 $mg.kg^{-1}$ have produced no evidence of toxicity in dogs.[2]

Pregnant rabbits were treated with up to 1000 $mg.kg^{-1}$ daily and pregnant rats were treated with up to 3000 $mg.kg^{-1}$ daily during the period of organogenesis. There was no evidence of drug-related teratogenesis or fetal toxicity in their offspring.[3,4]

Chronic toxicity studies in rats receiving up to 200 $mg.kg^{-1}$ daily for 93 weeks showed no evidence of carcinogenicity.[5]

Clinical pharmacology

Pyrantel pamoate produces neuromuscular blockade in susceptible helminths and the subsequent spastic paralysis results in their expulsion from the intestinal tract.[6,7] Pyrantel has little effect on the neuromuscular junction of skeletal muscle, primarily because of its poor absorption in man. Pyrantel is effective against *Enterobius vermicularis, Ascaris lumbricoides, Ancylostoma duodenale, Necator americanus, Trichostrongylus colubriformis* and *T. orientalis.* It is, however, ineffective against *Trichuris trichiura.* The drug is antagonistic to piperazine.

Pharmacokinetics

There is no simple analytical method available for the drug in plasma, and therefore little is known about its pharmacokinetics. Absorption from the gastrointestinal tract is very low; less than 4% of a single oral dose is recovered in the urine 48 to 96 hours after administration.[8,9]

Concentration–effect relationship

No information is available on this subject.

Metabolism

Pyrantel is thought to undergo the following metabolic degradation (Fig. 1).[9]

Fig. 1 Metabolism of pyrantel

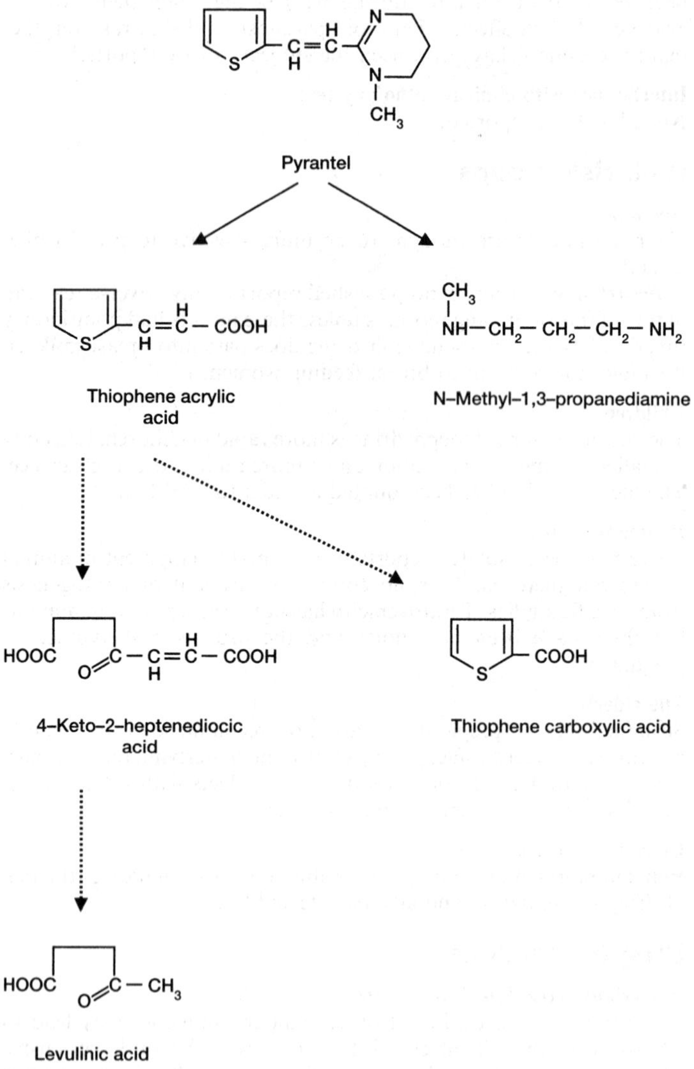

Pharmaceutics

Pyrantel is available only in oral forms.

1. Combantrin (Pfizer, UK): orange tablets containing 125 mg pyrantel as pyrantel embonate
2. Antiminth (Pfizer, USA): caramel-flavoured suspension containing 50 mg pyrantel per ml as pyrantel pamoate

3. Combination (Pfizer, Latin America): tablets and suspension containing 250 mg per tablet and per 5 ml of pyrantel pamoate

The formulations contain no potentially allergenic substances. They should be stored below 25°C.[10] Maximum shelf-life is 4 years.

Therapeutic use

Indications

Pyrantel pamoate is specifically indicated for the treatment of infection with any of the following intestinal parasites when these are present either alone or as a mixed infection.

1. *Enterobius vermicularis* (threadworm, pinworm)
2. *Ascaris lumbricoides* (roundworm)
3. *Ancylostoma duodenale* (hookworm)
4. *Necator americanus* (hookworm)
5. *Trichostrongylus colubriformis* and *T. orientalis*.

Pyrantel pamoate should be used for the treatment of infection with one or more of these parasites in both adults and children.

Contraindications

None is known.

Mode of use

The recommended dose of pyrantel pamoate for the treatment of infections with *Enterobius vermicularis, Ascaris lumbricoides, Ancylostoma duodenale, Necator americanus, Trichostrongylus colubriformis* and *T. orientalis* is 10 mg of base per kg of patient body weight, administered orally as a single dose.

For more severe infections of *Necator americanus*, the recommended dosage is 20 mg (base) per kg body weight administered as a single dose on each of two consecutive days, or 10 mg (base) per kg body weight administered as a single dose on each of three consecutive days.

Infection due to *Ascaris lumbricoides* alone can be successfully treated with a dose of 5 mg (base) per kg body weight administered as a single dose.

In mass treatment programmes directed against *Ascaris lumbricoides* a single dose of 2.5 mg (base) per kg body weight can be used.

The highest known dose used is 100 $mg.kg^{-1}$ in a single dose.[11]

Adverse reactions

Potentially life-threatening effects
None is known.

Acute overdosage
No cases of this kind have been described.

Severe or irreversible adverse effects
None is known.

Symptomatic adverse effects
The most commonly reported symptomatic effects are nausea, vomiting, diarrhoea, abdominal cramps and headache. These are usually of mild to moderate severity and have been reported in 4% of patients or less. Other, less commonly reported effects include anorexia, gastralgia, tenesmus, dizziness, drowsiness, and rash. These have been reported in less than 1% of patients.[8,12]

Other effects
Transient increases in AST (SGOT) levels have been reported in some patients.[8,12–14]

Interference with clinical pathology tests
None is known.

High risk groups

Neonates
The drug is not used in neonates.

Breast milk. The amount of the drug entering breast milk is unknown, but as absorption of the drug from the gut is low, infants of breast-feeding mothers taking the drug are unlikely to be at risk of adverse effects.

Children
The drug may be used in children.

Pregnant women
Although animal reproductive studies have not demonstrated any teratogenic effects, pyrantel pamoate has not been studied in the pregnant patient. Accordingly, it should not be used during pregnancy unless in the judgement of the physician it is essential for the welfare of the patient.

The elderly
No special precautions are required in elderly patients.

Concurrent disease
Pyrantel pamoate should be used with caution in patients with preexisting hepatic dysfunction, as minor transient elevations of the AST (SGOT) have occurred in a small percentage of patients.[10]

Drug interactions

Potentially hazardous interactions
Pyrantel pamoate and piperazine appear to be mutually antagonistic.[15,16]

Potentially useful interactions
None is known.

Major outcome trials

1. Bell W J, Gould G C 1971 Preliminary report on pyrantel pamoate in the treatment of human hookworm infection. East African Medical Journal 48 (4): 143–151

This dose-finding trial involved 55 adult East African males suffering hookworm infection, mainly due to *A. duodenale*. Pyrantel pamoate was administered as a single oral dose of five different dosages, 2.2 $mg.kg^{-1}$ being the lowest and 34.8 $mg.kg^{-1}$ the highest. Egg reductions varied from 71.8% to 93.5%. It was concluded that the most effective practical dose was around 17.4 $mg.kg^{-1}$ single dose. No significant toxic or side effects were observed.

2. Botero D, Castano A 1973 Comparative study of pyrantel pamoate, bephenium hydroxynaphthoate and tetrachloroethylene in the treatment of *Necator americanus* infections. American Journal of Tropical Medicine and Hygiene 22 (1): 45–52

A comparative trial of pyrantel pamoate, bephenium hydroxynaphthoate and tetrachloroethylene in the treatment of *Necator americanus* infections, performed in Colombia in 105 patients, revealed superior results with pyrantel. This drug was evaluated in four different dose schemes: 10 and 20 $mg.kg^{-1}$ for 2 or 3 days. The author recommended the dosage of 10 $mg.kg^{-1}$ for 3 consecutive days as the preferred dosage. This treatment scheme and that of 20 $mg.kg^{-1}$ for 2 days showed a cure rate of 73%. Of 45 cases presenting ascariasis 41 were cured. Pyrantel was tolerated well and no toxic effects were demonstrated.

3. Pitts N E, Migliardi J R 1974 Antiminth (pyrantel pamoate): the clinical evaluation of a new broad-spectrum anthelminthic. Clinical Pediatrics 13 (1): 87–94

Pyrantel pamoate was evaluated in 1506 patients, mainly children from the United States and several tropical countries, using several dosages. Single doses of 5 mg per pound showed cure rates of 97.2% and 97.5% for *E. vermicularis* and *A. lumbricoides* respectively. In tropical locations 10 mg per pound for 3 consecutive days achieved a cure rate of 86.4% for *N. americanus*. Tolerance was evaluated in all groups and mild gastrointestinal symptoms were reported in less than 5% of the cases. Headache was also found in 2.9% of the patients. No effects of significance on haematological, renal or hepatic functioning were recognized.

4. Bell W J, Nassif S 1971 Comparison of pyrantel pamoate and piperazine phosphate in the treatment of ascariasis. American Journal of Tropical Medicine and Hygiene 20 (4): 584–588

A comparison of pyrantel pamoate and piperazine phosphate was done in Egypt during an investigation that involved 182 persons, 119 being treated with pyrantel using three different dosages (2.5,

5.0 and 10 mg.kg^{-1}), 41 treated with piperazine and 22 receiving a placebo. Cure rate with the higher dose of pyrantel was 100% on day 10 after treatment, while those receiving the standard dose of piperazine achieved a cure rate of only 71%. Other than transient abdominal colic in a few patients, no obvious drug-related symptoms were observed. No trend of abnormality was noted in the serum transaminase or alkaline phosphatase levels after pyrantel treatment.

5. Farahmandian I, Sahba G H, Jalali H, Arfaa F 1972 A comparative evaluation of the therapeutic effect of pyrantel pamoate and bephenium hydroxynaphthoate on *Anclyostoma duodenale* and other intestinal helminths. Journal of Tropical Medicine and Hygiene 75: 205–207

This investigation is a comparison of the efficacy of pyrantel pamoate and bephenium hydroxynaphthoate against *A. duodenale*, *A. lumbricoides* and *Trychostrongylus* done in an Iranian village, where 500 persons were treated. The effects on *A. duodenale* and *Trichostrongylus* were not statistically different, showing cure rates of 96% and 45.4% with pyrantel and 92% and 56% with bephenium. An important difference was observed in the cases with ascariasis, in which 90.2% were cured with pyrantel and only 52.9% were cured with bephenium.

6. Farahmandian I, Arfaa F, Reza M 1977 Comparative studies on the evaluation of the effects of new anthelminthics on various intestinal helminths in Iran. Chemotherapy 23: 98–105

This comparative study of pyrantel, levamisole, mebendazole, thiabendazole and bephenium done by investigators of Teheran University, found that all the drugs used, except bephenium, were highly effective against *Ascaris*. For *A. duodenale* cure rates of 100%, 90% and 85% were observed with levamisole, pyrantel and bephenium respectively. Mebendazole and thiabendazole produced 35% and 51% cure rates. For *Trychostrongylus* the highest cure rate was achieved with levamisole, followed by thiabendazole and mebendazole. Side effects were rather low for all drugs, thiabendazole and bephenium producing more side effects.

7. Anthelmintic Study Group on Enterobiasis 1984 A comparative evaluation of mebendazole, piperazine and pyrantel in threadworm infection. Indian Journal of Pediatrics 21: 623–628

   National Anthelminthic Study Group. Relative efficacy of mebendazole and pyrantel in hookworm infection. Tropical Gastroenterology 5 (2): 92–97

   National Anthelmintic Study Group 1984 Efficacy of levamisole, mebendazole, piperazine and pyrantel in roundworm infection. Journal of Postgraduate Medicine 30 (3): 144–152

These three papers produced by the National Anthelmitic Study Group in India published in 1984 involved around 2500 cases and compared pyrantel, mebendazole, levamisole and piperazine in the treatment of intestinal nematodes. Pyrantel was superior to mebendazole and piperazine for *E. vermicularis* and superior to mebendazole for hookworms. Similar results were observed in the treatment of *A. lumbricoides* for which pyrantel was significantly better than mebendazole and levamisole. Although the results with pyrantel were better than those with piperazine, the difference was not statistically significant. These multi-centre studies are recent and used a good parasitological methodology, including Kato's method and the zinc sulphate flotation for ascaris and hookworms and an improved device of the scotch tape technique for pinworms. Tolerance to the treatments was good in general for all drugs, since drug-related symptoms were uncommon and of low intensity. The presence of side effects was more frequent in the piperazine group.

Other trials

1. Desowitz R S, Bell T, Williams J et al 1970 Anthelmintic activity of pyrantel pamoate. American Journal of Tropical Medicine and Hygiene 19 (5): 775–778

School children from Cook Islands were treated for ascaris with pyrantel pamoate, using a single dose of 5 mg per pound or the same dose for 2 days with cure rates of 85.5% and 97.4%. The same daily dose for 3 consecutive days cured 83.7% of the hookworm cases. From a total of 156 patients that received the drug, side effects occurred in 31 cases, always transient and of low intensity. The complaint most commonly elicited was abdominal cramp when ascaris worms were being passed. No blood or renal abnormal changes were seen after the treatment.

2. Haleem M A, Lari F A, Rahimtoola R J 1972 Comparative efficacy and toxicity of pyrantel pamoate and piperazine citrate in pediatric ascariasis. Journal of Pakistan Medical Association 22: 276–282

A comparison between 10 and 20 mg.kg^{-1} of pyrantel pamoate and 120 mg.kg^{-1} of piperazine citrate, all as single dose, revealed that all of 20 children were cured with pyrantel, while only 9 of the 10 children treated with piperazine were cured. Although the number of cases was small in this study from Pakistan, the results are in accordance with those reported elsewhere. Four patients in the group of 20 treated with pyrantel referred mild abdominal pain, while 4 out of 10 children treated with piperazine reported side effects, consisting of constipation, abdominal pain, dyspnoea and vomiting. One of these symptoms was presented by each of the 4 patients in the last group. No significant changes in blood and urine examinations were observed.

3. Pandey K N, Sharathchandra S G, Sarin G S et al 1971 Pyrantel embonate in the treatment of hookworm infestation. British Medical Journal 4: 399–400

In 60 cases of hookworm infestation studied in India (mainly due to *A. duodenale*), six different single doses of pyrantel embonate were administered, varying from 10 mg.kg^{-1} to 100 mg.kg^{-1}. All cases were negative in the post-treatment stool examinations and no toxic effects were found. Only two patients receiving the higher dosages presented nausea and vomiting. The authors recommend the dose of 10 mg.kg^{-1} as the optimum dose for *A. duodenale* infestations.

4. Bumbalo T S, Fugazzotto D J, Wyczalek J V 1969 Treatment of enterobiasis with pyrantel pamoate. American Journal of Tropical Medicine and Hygiene 18 (1): 50–52

The efficacy of pyrantel pamoate was studied in 69 retarded children in New York, using 10 mg.kg^{-1} single dose. The cure rate was 96.4% and the only side effects observed were loose stools, nausea and vomiting of 1 day duration in a few cases. In 5 children elevated SGOT levels were observed after treatment, which returned to normal 12 weeks later.

5. Carney D E, O'Reilly B J, Twedell E D Pyrantel embonate in the treatment of enterobiasis. Medical Journal of Australia 2: 254–256

Comparative studies between pyrantel pamoate and pyrvinium embonate were performed in South Wales in 100 cases of enterobiasis using a single dose of 10 mg.kg^{-1} for pyrantel and 5 mg.kg^{-1} for pyrvinium. Cure rates were 94% and 70% respectively, pyrantel being better tolerated and free of staining, a defect associated with the use of pyrvinium.

6. Islam N, Chowdhury N A 1976 Mebendazole and pyrantel pamoate as broad-spectrum anthelmintics. SE Asian Journal of Tropical Medicine and Public Health 7 (1): 81–84

The efficacy of mebendazole and pyrantel pamoate was studied in two groups of polyparasitized patients in Bangladesh. The two drugs cured over 90% of the ascariasis cases and close to 80% of the hookworm cases. Mebendazole was effective for trichuriasis and strongyloidiasis, although the results on the latter helmintic infection should be questioned, on the basis of more recent studies using multiple and careful laboratory techniques required for an accurate diagnosis of *S. stercoralis*. Pyrantel did not show significant effects on *T. trichiura* and *S. stercoralis*. None of the drugs had any effects on *T. saginata*.

General review articles

Pitts N E, Migliardi J R 1974 Antiminth (pyrantel pamoate): the clinical evaluation of a new broad-spectrum anthelminthic. Clinical Pediatrics 13 (1): 87–94

References

1. Gennaro A R (ed) 1985 Remington's Pharmaceutical Sciences. Mack, Easton, PA, p 1237
2. Otsuki S, Ishiko J, Sakai M et al 1971 Pharmacologic effects of pyrantel pamoate, a new broad-spectrum anthelmintic. Pharmacometrics 5 (2): 289–304
3. Owaki Y, Sakai F, Momiyama H 1971 Teratologic studies on pyrantel pamoate in rabbits. Pharmacometrics 5 (1): 33–39
4. Owaki Y, Sakai F, Momiyama H 1971 Teratologic studies on pyrantel pamoate in rats. Pharmacometrics 5 (1): 41–50
5. Data on file
6. Aubry M L, Cowell P, Davey M J, Shevde S 1970 Aspects of the pharmacology of a new anthelmintic: pyrantel. British Journal of Pharmacology 38: 332–344
7. Eyre P 1970 Some pharmacodynamic effects of the nematocides: methyridine, tetramisole and pyrantel. Journal of Pharmacy and Pharmacology 2: 26–36
8. Pitts N E, Migliardi J R 1974 Antiminth (pyrantel pamoate): the clinical evaluation of a new broad-spectrum anthelminthic. Clinical Pediatrics 13 (1): 87–94
9. Kimura Y, Kume M 1971 Absorption, distribution, excretion and metabolism of pyrantel pamoate. Pharmacometrics 5 (3): 347–358
10. Combantrin Data Sheet, in the ABPI Data Sheet Compendium 1986–87
11. Pandey K N, Sharathchandra S G, Sarin G S et al 1971 Pyrantel embonate in the treatment of hookworm infestation. British Medical Journal 4: 399–400
12. Botero D, Castano A 1973 Comparative study of pyrantel pamoate, bephenium hydroxynaphoate and tetrachloroethylene in the treatment of *Necator americanus* infections. American Journal of Tropical Medicine and Hygiene 22 (1): 45–52
13. Haleem M A, Lari F A, Rahimtoola R J 1972 Comparative efficacy and toxicity of pyrantel pamoate and piperazine citrate in pediatric ascariasis. Journal of Pakistan Medical Association 22: 276–282
14. Bumbalo T S, Fugazzotto D J, Wyczalek J V 1969 Treatment of enterobiasis with pyrantel pamoate. American Journal of Tropical Medicine and Hygiene 18 (1): 50–52
15. Pyrantel pamoate 1985 In: Gilman A G, Goodman L S, Rall T W, Murad F (eds) The pharmacological basis of therapeutics, 7th edn. Macmillan, New York, pp 1020
16. 1984 In: Dukes (ed) Meyler's side effects of drugs, 10th edn. Elsevier, New York, pp 594

Pyrazinamide

Pyrazinamide is bactericidal against intracellular *Mycobacterium tuberculosis* only and should always be used in combination with other antituberculosis drugs. It is particularly useful as part of short-course regimes (6 months or less).

Chemistry

Pyrazinamide (Zinamide, Piraldina, Pyrafat, Tebrazid)
$C_5H_5N_3O$
Pyrazine-2-carboxamide

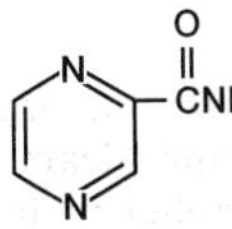

Molecular weight	123.1
pKa	0.5
Solubility	
in alcohol	1 in 110
in water	1 in 60
Octanol/water partition coefficient	—

A white, odourless crystalline powder with a slightly bitter taste. Prepared by chemical synthesis. It is available in combination (300 mg) with rifampicin (120 mg) and isoniazid (50 mg) as Rifater.

Pharmacology

Pyrazinamide is probably bactericidal to *Mycobacterium tuberculosis* at acid pH values (found inside cells) but not at neutral pH. To be bactericidal requires an enzyme, pyrazinamidase. This intrabacterial enzyme removes the amide to produce active pyrazinoic acid.[1] The susceptibility of a strain of *Mycobacterium tuberculosis* to pyrazinamide varies with the activity of this enzyme[2] which can be assayed in vitro to assess for sensitivity. In vitro MIC values of 20 $mg.l^{-1}$ have been demonstrated at an acid pH.[3] Pyrazinamide and rifampicin kill best the slowly or intermittently metabolizing semi-dormant bacilli. A recent study has questioned the intracellular action of pyrazinamide and thus its true mode of action should be regarded as unsettled.[4]

Toxicology

No adequate studies have been carried out, but there is no evidence of mutagenicity or teratogenic effect, or of carcinogenicity.

Clinical pharmacology

Daily doses of 20 to 35 $mg.kg^{-1}$ body weight (up to 3 g daily maximum) increase the efficacy of other antituberculosis drugs.[5,6] Its addition early on (in the first 2 months) to other drug regimes probably shortens the length of drug therapy required to sterilize and reduces the later relapse rate. Pyrazinamide is inactive against atypical myocobacteria. Resistance develops rapidly if pyrazinamide is used as the sole antituberculosis agent. Convenient doses are 1.5 g daily, 2 g daily or 2.5 g daily for small, medium and large adults respectively.

Pharmacokinetics

Pyrazinamide and its metabolites can be accurately quantified by gas chromatography which has a limit of sensitivity of 10 $\mu g.l^{-1}$ or by MPLC[16] down to 0.2 $mg.l^{-1}$, in which the piperazine peak is clearly separated from antituberculous drugs that might be simultaneously present.

Pyrazinamide is completely absorbed from the gastrointestinal tract with peak blood levels at 1–2 hours.[7–9] After 1.5 g orally the serum concentration[10] has been reported to reach 33 $mg.l^{-1}$ and 65 $mg.l^{-1}$ after 20 $mg.kg^{-1}$.[10] The half life is between 10 and 24 hours and the drug is widely distributed throughout the body.[8,9,11] CSF levels are almost identical to those in the blood[12] and thus this drug is useful in tuberculous meningitis.[13–15]

Oral absorption	Extensive
Presystemic metabolism	
Plasma half life	10–24 h
Volume of distribution	—
Plasma protein binding	50%

Concentration–effect relationship

There is no evidence of any in vivo correlation between plasma concentrations of pyrazinamide and its therapeutic effect.

Metabolism

Pyrazinamide is converted to the major active metabolite pyrazinoic acid[9] by an endoplasmic reticular deaminase (the rate-limiting step). Of the dose, 30–40% is excreted in urine as pyrazinoic acid and 3–4% as unchange pyrazinamide (see Fig. 1).[11,17,18] Peak levels of this active metabolite occur about 6 hours after ingestion of pyrazinamide.[11] 5-Hydroxypyrazinoic acid is a further metabolite and is produced by xanthine oxidase.[19] It is assumed that the majority of the metabolism occurs in the liver.[9,18] Pyrazinamide can be measured in the urine in order to check compliance.[20]

Fig. 1 The metabolism of pyrazinamide

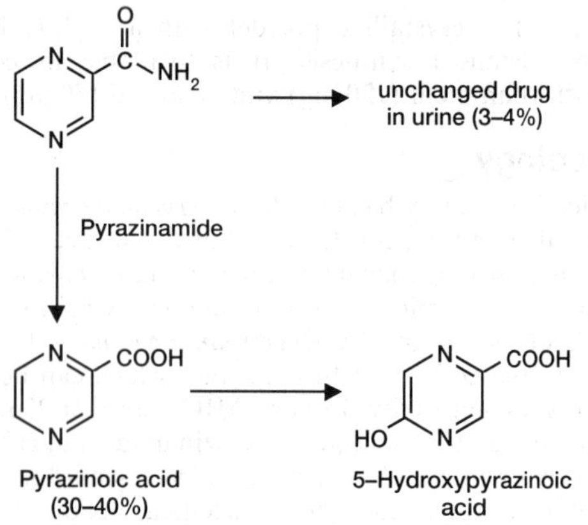

Pharmaceutics

Pyrazinamide is available as white, half-scored tablets marked either 'P/36' (Lederle, US) or 'MSD 504' (MSD, UK). Each contains 500 mg pyrazinamide BP. Pure pyrazinamide powder is available for sensitivity tests. Stable indefinitely at room temperature.

Therapeutic use

Indications

1. *Mycobacterium tuberculosis* infection.

Contraindications

1. Hepatic disease
2. Hyperuricaemia and/or gout
3. Hypoglycaemia
4. Diabetes
5. Impaired renal function
6. Hypersensitivity.

Pyrazinamide

Mode of use

Pyrazinamide is only used to treat *Mycobacterium tuberculosis* in combination with other antituberculosis drugs such as isoniazid, rifampicin, ethambutol, streptomycin, cycloserine, ethionamide and para-aminosalicylic acid.

Indications

1. *Mycobacterium tuberculosis* infection

Pyrazinamide has not been widely used until recently because of its frequent hepatotoxic effects when used at higher doses than now recommended. These may have been over-emphasized and its use with three other drugs (rifampicin, isoniazid, ethambutol) has recently been advocated because this regime seems to allow shorter courses of therapy, six months instead of nine months or more, without increased liver toxicity.[21–23] The recommended dose is 20–35 $mg.kg^{-1}$ body weight (up to 3 g total) per day divided into three or four daily doses although twice or even once daily is probably adequate. Careful monitoring of liver function (liver en zymes and bilirubin) and uric acid levels is recommended although in combination with isoniazid it is often difficult to decide which drug is to blame for any developing abnormalities.

Adding pyrazinamide to a drug regime does not in practice alter the doses of the other drugs required.

Pyrazinamide is not thought to be active against other mycobacteria (e.g. *M. bovis*, *M. intracellulare*, *M. fortuitum*, *M. scrofulaceum*, *M. xenopi*, *M. kansasii* and *M. avium*). However in vitro sensitivity testing does not always coincide with apparent in vivo sensitivity.

For a further discussion of antituberculous therapy see under rifampicin.

Contraindications

1. Hepatic disease

Because of the liver toxicity of pyrazinamide its use in patients with pre-existing liver disease is best avoided although no evidence exists to suggest absolute contraindication and no specific liver disease has been shown to be particularly sensitive.

2. Gout

Pyrazinamide raises uric acid levels by inhibiting renal urate excretion[19,24–26] and may precipitate an attack of gout in those with an already raised level. This inhibition of urate excretion occurs at pyrazinoic acid levels[19] of 3 $mg.l^{-1}$, well below the MIC[3] of 20 $\mu g.ml^{-1}$. Probenecid remains uricosuric in the presence of pyrazinamide.[18,27]

3. Hypoglycaemia

Pyrazinamide has been reported to increase the difficulty of blood sugar control in diabetics (see below).

4. Diabetes

Pyrazinamide has been shown to lower blood sugar probably by increasing glucose uptake by adipose tissue.[28] In practice this does not seem to be a problem.

5. Renal failure

Because of its renal elimination pyrazinamide should probably be reduced or avoided in patients with renal failure. No data exists on how to adjust dosage schedules in renal failure.

Adverse reactions

Potentially life-threatening effects

Severe liver damage with fulminant hepatitis can occur if pyrazinamide continues to be administered in the face of rising levels of liver enzymes,[29,20] particularly at doses in excess of 40 $mg.kg^{-1}$. Because it is always used in combination it is difficult to be sure of the relative hepatotoxicity of each antituberculosis agent.[32] Small rises in liver enzymes are sometimes seen with a spontaneous return to normal. A rise in bilirubin is generally regarded as more important. The likelihood of liver toxicity appears to increase with dose and length of use. At 3 g daily up to 15% of patients show evidence of liver damage. Withdrawal of the drug leads to prompt resolution of the abnormal enzyme levels.

Acute overdosage

No cases of this kind appear to have been reported.

Pyrazinamide

Severe or irreversible adverse effects
Gout can be precipitated by the effect of pyrazinamide on uric acid excretion. Treatment of the gout is the same as usual and stopping the drug will resolve the problem. If it is essential to continue the pyrazinamide, then probenecid will increase uric acid excretion again.[18,27] Sideroblastic anaemia has been reported.

Symptomatic adverse effects
As expected from a liver toxic agent anorexia, nausea and vomiting can occur and may sometimes be indications of liver damage. Other reported adverse effects are arthralgia, malaise and fever. The arthralgia may be related to elevation of serum uric acid but is not classical gout and does not require drug withdrawal.[33,34] The incidence of arthralgia is less in patients also taking rifampicin[35] which may be due to the increased hepatic P450 microsomal oxidase system metabolizing pyrazinoic acid. Photosensitivity and skin rashes have been reported rarely.[32]

Other effects
A rise in blood uric acid levels and abnormal liver function tests may occur. Raised plasma fibrinogen levels have been reported.

Interference with clinical pathology tests
Pyrazinamide may interfere with acetest and ketostix qualitative urine tests for ketones, producing a pinky-brown colour.[36]

High risk groups

Neonates
No information is available on use of pyrazinamide in neonates.

Breast milk Pyrazinamide is probably excreted in milk but the amounts administered to the infant are likely to be small and well below therapeutic doses.[40] No data exist as to safety but the manufacturers recommend that breast feeding is stopped.

Children
Little data is available on the use of pyrazinamide in children and thus its safety in this group is not established. It has been used without causing any problems differing from those encountered in adults.[37] If considered essential then the dose should be between 25 and 30 $mg.kg^{-1}$ daily in divided doses.[37,38]

Pregnant women
No data are available on the safety and teratogenicity of pyrazinamide in pregnancy.[39]

The elderly
No special problems have been reported.

Drug interactions

Potentially hazardous interactions
No interactions of this type have been reported.

Other significant interactions
Pyrazinamide slightly reduces serum levels of isoniazid more so in slow isoniazid acetylators but this is not thought to be of any clinical significance.[41]

Potentially useful interactions
The drug is used in combination with other agents in the treatment of tuberculosis.

Major outcome trials

Pyrazinamide has always been used in combination with other drugs and the relevant trials[21–23] with rifampicin, isoniazid, ethambutol and streptomycin are described under rifampicin.

General review articles

American Thoracic Society 1986 Treatment of tuberculosis and tuberculosis infections in adults and children. American Review of Respiratory Disease 134: 355–363

Chemotherapy of pulmonary tuberculosis in Britain 1988 Drugs and Therapeutics Bulletin 26: 1–4

Steele M A, DesPrez R M 1988 The role of pyrazinamide in tuberculosis chemotherapy. Chest 94: 842–844

References

1. Konno K, Feldmann F M, McDermott W 1967 Pyrazinamide susceptibility and amidase activity of tubercle bacilli. American Review of Respiratory Disease 95: 461–469
2. Trivedi S 1987 Pyrazinamidase activity of *Mycobacterium tuberculosis* — a test of sensitivity to pyrazinamide. Tubercle 68: 221–224
3. Stottmeier K D, Beam R E, Kubica G P 1967 Determination of drug susceptibility of mycobacteria to pyrazinamide in 7H10 agar. American Review of Respiratory Disease 96: 1072–1075
4. Rastogi N, Potar M C, David H L 1988 Pyrazinamide is not effective against intracellularly growing *Mycobacterium tuberculosis*. Letter. Antimicrobial Agents and Chemotherapy 32: 287
5. American Thoracic Society/Centers for Disease Control. Medical Section of the American Lung Association 1986 Treatment of tuberculosis and tuberculosis infection in adults and children. American Review of Respiratory Disease 134: 355–363
6. Singapore Tuberculosis Service/British Medical Research Council 1979 Clinical trial of six-month and four-month regimens of chemotherapy in the treatment of pulmonary tuberculosis. American Review of Respiratory Disease 134: 355–363
7. Ellard G A, Ellard D R, Allen B W et al 1986 The bioavailability of isoniazid, rifampicin and pyrazinamide in two commercially available combined formulations designed for use in the short-course treatment of tuberculosis. American Review of Respiratory Disease 133: 1076–1080
8. Ellard G A 1969 Absorption, metabolism, and excretion of pyrazinamide in man. Tubercle 50: 144–158
9. Lacroix C, Phan Hoang T, Nouveau J, Guyonnaud C, Laine G, Duwoos H, Lafont O 1989 Pharmacokinetics of pyrazinamide and its metabolites in healthy subjects. European Journal of Clinical Pharmacology 36: 395–400
10. Stottmeier K D, Beam R E, Kubica G P 1968 The absorption and excretion of pyrazinamide. American Review of Respiratory Disease 98: 70–74
11. Bareggi S R, Cerutti R, Rirola R, Riva R, Cisternino M 1987 Clinical pharmacokinetics and metabolism of pyrazinamide in healthy volunteers. Arzneimittel-Forschung 37: 849–853
12. Holdiness M R 1985 Cerebrospinal fluid pharmacokinetics of the anti-tuberculosis drugs. Clinical Pharmacokinetics 10: 532–534
13. Ellard G A, Humphries M J, Gabriel M, Teoh R 1987 Penetration of pyrazinamide into the cerebrospinal fluid in tuberculous meningitis. British Medical Journal 294: 284–285
14. Woo J, Humphries M, Chan K, O'Mahony G, Teoh R 1987 Cerebrospinal fluid and serum levels of pyrazinamide and rifampicin in patients with tuberculous meningitis. Current Therapeutic Research 42: 235–242
15. Forgan-Smith R, Ellard G A, Newton D, Mitchison D A 1973 Pyrazinamide and other drugs in tuberculous meningitis. Lancet 2: 374
16. Chan K, Wong C L, Lok S 1986 High performance liquid chromatographic determination of pyrazinamide in the cerebrospinal fluid and plasma in the rabbit. Journal of Chromatography 380: 367–373
17. Holdiness M R 1984 Clinical pharmacokinetics of the anti-tuberculosis drugs. Clinical Pharmacokinetics 9: 511–544
18. Ellard G A, Haslam R M 1976 Observations on the reduction of the renal elimination of urate in man caused by the administration of pyrazinamide. Tubercle 57: 97–103
19. Weiner I M, Tinker J P 1972 Pharmacology of pyrazinamide: metabolic and renal function studies related to the mechanism of drug-induced urate retention. Journal of Pharmacology and Experimental Therapeutics 180: 411–434
20. Pines A, Richardson R J 1964 A simple tablet test for the detection of pyrazinamide in the urine. Tubercle 45: 166–167
21. Snider D E, Graczyk J, Bek E, Rogowski J 1984 Supervised six-months treatment of newly diagnosed pulmonary tuberculosis using isoniazid, rifampicin and pyraxinamide with and without streptomycin. American Review of Respiratory Disease 130: 1091–1094
22. British Thoracic Association 1984 A controlled trial of 6 months chemotherapy in pulmonary tuberculosis. Final report: results during the 36 months after the end of chemotherapy and beyond. British Journal of Diseases of the Chest 78: 330–336
23. 3rd East African/British Medical Research Council study 1980 Controlled clinical trial of four short course regimes of chemotherapy for two durations in the treatment of pulmonary tuberculosis: 2nd report. Tubercle 61: 59–69
24. Yu T F, Berger L, Stone D J, Wolf J, Gutman A B 1957 Effect of pyrazinamide and pyrazinoic acid on urate clearance and other discrete renal functions. Proceedings of the Society for Experimental Biology and Medicine 96: 264–267
25. Jenner P J, Ellard G A 1981 Serum uric acid concentrations and arthralgia among patients treated with pyrazinamide-containing regimens in Hong Kong and Singapore. Tubercle 62: 175–179
26. Fanelli G M Jr, Weiner I M 1973 Pyrazinoate excretion in the chimpanzee. Relation to urate disposition and the actions of uricosuric drugs. Journal of Clinical Investigation 52: 1946–1957
27. Sommers D K 1987 Drug interactions with urate excretion in man. European Journal of Clinical Pharmacology 32: 499–502
28. Dulin W E, Gerritsen G C 1969 Effects of pyrazinamide on carbohydrate and fat metabolism. Metabolism 18: 214–225
29. Hepatic toxicity of pyrazinamide used with isoniazid in tuberculous patients; a United States Public Health Service tuberculosis therapy trial 1959 American Review of Respiratory Disease 80: 371–387
30. Danan G, Pessayre D, Larrey D, Benhamou J P 1981 Pyrazinamide fulminant hepatitis: an old hepatotoxin strikes again. Lancet 2: 1056–1057
31. Parthasarathy R, Raghupati Sarma G, Janardhanam B et al 1986 Hepatic toxicity in South Indian patients during treatment of tuberculosis with short-course regimens containing isoniazid, rifampicin and pyrazinamide. Tubercle 67: 99–108
32. Girling D J 1982 Adverse effects of anti-tuberculosis drugs. Drugs 23: 56–74
33. Zierski M, Bek E 1980 Side effects of drug regimens used in short-course chemotherapy for pulmonary tuberculosis. A controlled clinical study. Tubercle 61: 41–49

P

34. Cullen J H, Early L J, Fiore J M 1956 The occurrence of hyperuricemia during pyrazinamide–isoniazid therapy. American Review of Tuberculosis 74: 289–292
35. Sarma R G, Archarlulu C S, Kannapiran M, Krishna Murthy P V, Gurumurthy P, Tripathy S P 1983 Role of rifampicin in arthralgia induced by pyrazinamide. Tubercle 64: 93–100
36. 1972 Pyrazinamide in urine test. Drugs and Therapeutics Bulletin 10: 69
37. Jacobs R F, Abernathy R S 1985 The treatment of tuberculosis in children. Pediatric Infectious Disease 85: 513–517
38. Smith M H D 1982 What about short course and intermittent chemotherapy for tuberculosis in children? Pediatric Infectious Disease 82: 298–303
39. Snider D E, Layde R M, Johnson M W, Lyle M A 1980 Treatment of tuberculosis during pregnancy. American Review of Respiratory Disease 122: 65–79
40. Snider D E, Powell K E 1984 Should women taking anti-tuberculosis drugs breast feed? Archives of Internal Medicine 144: 589–590
41. Venho V M K, Koskinen R 1971 The effect of pyrazinamide, rifampicin and cycloserine on the blood levels and urinary excretion of isoniazid. Annals of Clinical Research 3: 277–280

Pyridostigmine (bromide)

Pyridostigmine is a potent reversible inhibitor of acetylcholinesterase, mainly used to treat myasthenia gravis.

Chemistry

Pyridostigmine bromide (Mestinon)
$C_9H_{13}BrN_2O_2$
3-Dimethylcarbamoyloxy-1-methylpyridinium bromide

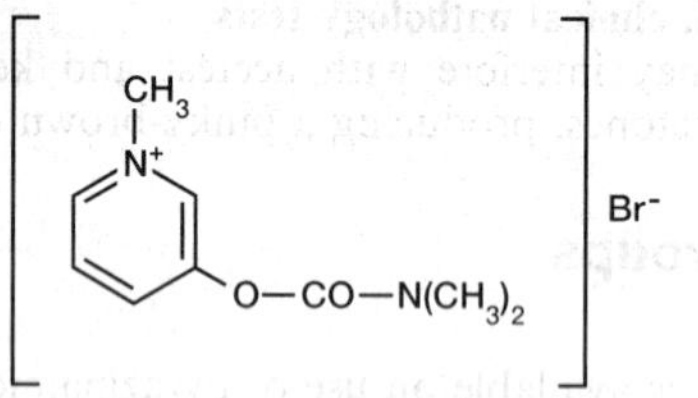

Molecular weight	261.1
pKa	strongly basic
Solubility	
in alcohol	>1 in 1
in water	>1 in 1
Octanol/water partition coefficient	low

Pyridostigmine is a quaternary ammonium compound which is prepared as a white or almost white, deliquescent, crystalline powder with an agreeable characteristic odour and a bitter taste. It is prepared by chemical synthesis. Pyridostigmine is not available in any combination preparations.

Pharmacology

Pyridostigmine is a potent reversible inhibitor of acetylcholinesterase, the enzyme responsible for destroying acetylcholine. Acetylcholinesterase exists in two molecular forms: one is of simple oligomers of 70 000 dalton subunits and the other is a complex elongated structure with a molecular weight of 10^6. The active centre of acetylcholinesterase consists of a negative subsite and an esteric subsite where nucleophilic attack occurs on the acyl carbon of the substrate. Pyridostigmine has a carbonyl ester linkage that is hydrolysed by acetylcholinesterase but much more slowly than is acetylcholine itself. The enzyme is thus carbamylated at the active centre. The duration of inhibition of acetylcholinesterase is somewhat longer than that produced by neostigmine and the onset of action is also slower.

Pyridostigmine thus intensifies both the nicotinic and muscarinic effects of acetylcholine. In addition to the effects on acetylcholinesterase, it also probably has a direct action on acetylcholine receptors. Pyridostigmine has a weaker effect on muscarinic effects than neostigmine.

Toxicology

There are no reports of mutagenic or carcinogenic effects of pyridostigmine. Although the safety of this drug has not been established in pregnancy, no untoward effects have been described of its effects on the course of pregnancy.

Clinical pharmacology

Pyridostigmine is an effective cholinesterase inhibitor with about one quarter the potency of neostigmine. The onset of action is seen within

Pyridostigmine (bromide)

one hour and the duration of action is usually 3–6 h. Pyridostigmine produces miosis and although the pupil is small, it usually reacts further to light. Accommodation is also blocked temporarily and intraocular pressure is reduced, although a transitory rise in the intraocular pressure may be seen initially.

Pyridostigmine acts on the gastrointestinal tract to increase gastric and intestinal contractions, which may result in gastrointestinal colic. The secretion of gastric acid is increased.

Pyridostigmine affects skeletal muscle by increasing skeletal muscle contraction, both directly and by inhibiting cholinesterase activity. In standard doses this is primarily due to the effects of acetylcholine in initiating a propagated muscle action potential. However, in high dosage for prolonged periods, depolarization of the motor end-plate may occur, leading to decreased muscle activity and paralysis. Pyridostigmine will reverse the effects of competitive neuromuscular blocking drugs such as tubocurarine, but it is rarely used for this purpose because of its slow onset and prolonged effects.

Pyridostigmine causes increased secretion by secretory glands innervated by postganglionic cholinergic fibres. This results in increased salivation, increased intestinal secretions which may lead to diarrhoea, and increased bronchial secretions. The predominant effect of pyridostigmine on the heart is bradycardia due to the peripheral accumulation of acetylcholine. Blood pressure is usually not affected although the cardiac output may fall. In the central nervous system, pyridostigmine may initially cause stimulation but this is followed by depression and depression of respiration with anoxia may be seen, particularly with higher doses than usual. The usual dose of pyridostigmine is 300–1200 mg daily but larger doses are sometimes needed in the treatment of myasthenia gravis. The longer duration of action of pyridostigmine compared to neostigmine is useful when the drug is taken just before retiring to bed.

Pharmacokinetics

Determination of blood levels of pyridostigmine is complicated by its ready hydrolysis in blood, plasma and buffer solutions. In addition, some decomposition of pyridostigmine occurs in samples stored at −20°C for less than one month.[1]

The preferred methods of analysis involve gas chromatography with nitrogen or mass spectrometric detection, or high pressure liquid chromatography.[2,3] The limit of sensitivity is 5 µg.l^{-1} for nitrogen detection and 40 µg.l^{-1} for HPLC. Pyridostigmine is poorly and variably absorbed from the gastrointestinal tract with a bioavailability of between 10% and 20%.[4] Following the administration of a single 60 mg oral dose of pyridostigmine, peak plasma concentrations in the range of 40 to 60 µg.l^{-1} occur at 1–2 h.[4] The time to reach the peak plasma concentration is delayed by about 90 minutes by the ingestion of food, although the area under the plasma concentration–time curve is unaffected. There have been reports of secondary plasma concentration peaks at variable times after the administration of pyridostigmine by mouth.[5] It has been suggested that this is due to the formation of ion pairs with intestinal components such as mucin or bile salts which are then absorbed because of their higher lipophilicity. Another possibility is enterohepatic recirculation of the drug, which has been found to occur with other quaternary ammonium compounds.

Plasma concentrations between oral doses of pyridostigmine do not vary much in the individual patient. However, when pyridostigmine is given by mouth to patients with myasthenia gravis there is a four- to seven-fold variation in the blood levels achieved, even amongst patients receiving the same daily dose.[6] There is no clear relationship between dose of pyridostigmine and steady-state plasma concentrations. In myasthenic patients treated with only oral pyridostigmine, there is a linear relationship between dose and AUC, but there is no such relationship in patients treated with both pyridostigmine and neostigmine,[7] the former drug being undetectable in the plasma of most such patients. It has been suggested[5] that neostigmine might inhibit the absorption of pyridostigmine but this has not been confirmed.[6]

The α-phase plasma half life of pyridostigmine after intravenous administration is between 0.015 and 0.14 h,[1,8] whilst estimates for the β-phase half life vary between 0.38 and 1.86 h.[8,9] The apparent volume of distribution of pyridostigmine[6,8] is between 0.53 and 1.76 l.kg^{-1}. There is some evidence that pyridostigmine is sequestered in a tissue compartment.[10] Pyridostigmine and its main metabolite, 3-hydroxy-N-methylpyridinium, are not bound to plasma proteins nor to red blood cells.[11]

Renal impairment results in a prolongation of the half life of pyridostigmine. In functionally anephric patients, the clearance of pyridostigmine is greatly diminished, from 0.52 l.h^{-1}.kg^{-1} to 0.12 l.h^{-1}.kg^{-1}. Both glomerular filtration and tubular secretion contribute to urinary clearance. About 16% of the dose is recovered unchanged in the urine following oral administration. This increases to 90% after intravenous administration.

The concentration of pyridostigmine in breast milk is 36–113% of that of the plasma of the nursing mother, implying that a breast-fed infant would receive only a very low dose. Pyridostigmine can undergo placental transfer. In myasthenic patients, the interindividual variation in trough plasma levels of pyridostigmine was greater in older patients who were receiving higher doses (but had more severe disease). Neither myasthenia gravis nor thymectomy appear to affect the pharmacokinetics of pyridostigmine. Liver disease is unlikely to affect the kinetics of the drug.

Oral absorption	low
Presystemic metabolism	—
Plasma half life	
range	0.38–1.9 h
mean	
Volume of distribution	0.53–1.8 l.kg^{-1}
Plasma protein binding	negligible

Concentration–effect relationship

Poorly controlled myasthenic patients have somewhat higher plasma concentrations of pyridostigmine than those who are well controlled.[6,12]

Metabolism

Up to 16% of an oral dose of pyridostigmine is excreted unchanged in the urine. The main pyridostigmine metabolite is the hydrolysis product 3-hydroxy-N-methylpyridinium which is promptly glucuronidated (Fig. 1).[13] Other metabolites have been detected in the plasma and urine and these have been tentatively identified as the hydroxy, quinone and demethylated derivatives and their corresponding glucuronides.[14] Thus, the elimination of pyridostigmine depends on both extrarenal and renal mechanisms, of which the former shows indications of being saturable. There is evidence for enterohepatic recycling. In the 24 h period following its administration, pyridostigmine is excreted in the urine with its metabolites in a ratio of 4:1.[15] After intravenous injection of ^{14}C-pyridostigmine, about 90% of the radioactivity is recovered in the urine, largely as the unchanged drug.[10]

Fig. 1 Metabolism of pyridostigmine

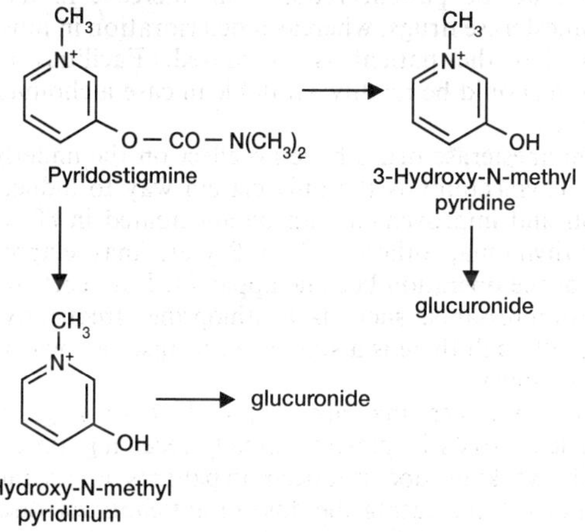

Pharmaceutics

Pyridostigmine bromide (Mestinon; Roche, UK/USA) is available in oral and parenteral forms. The tablets are white and round, containing 60 mg, with 'ROCHE' imprinted across one face and being quarter-scored on the other. In the USA a 180 mg Timespan tablet is available, together with a syrup containing 60 mg per 5 ml. The syrup vehicle contains 5% alcohol and colouring agents FD & C Red no 40 plus FD & C Blue no 1.

The parenteral preparation, Pyridostigmine injection, is available in 1 ml ampoules as a sterile solution of pyridostigmine bromide in Water for Injections, suitable for autoclaving. It contains 1 $mg.ml^{-1}$.

The maximum recommended temperature at which the tablets and ampoules should be stored is 25°C. The tablets should be protected from light and moisture.

Therapeutic use

Indications

1. Myasthenia gravis
2. Paralytic ileus
3. Retention of urine.

Contraindications

1. Intestinal obstruction
2. Urinary obstruction
3. Hypersensitivity.

Mode of use

1. Myasthenia gravis

The primary action of anticholinesterase drugs is to reduce the hydrolysis of acetylcholine by the enzyme acetylcholinesterase. Although these drugs have no effect on the underlying disease process, which is the loss of acetylcholine receptors as the result of immunological damage, they do allow the acetylcholine released by the nerve ending to act over a longer time. This permits the total number of interactions between acetylcholine and its receptor to be increased.

The dosage must be determined empirically. Patients with myasthenia gravis require widely differing doses of anticholinesterase drugs, and although it was originally presumed that variability in absorption and metabolism were responsible,[7] the blood levels in fact vary greatly among both well and poorly controlled patients.[12] It is important to establish the dose of anticholinesterase which gives the maximum therapeutic response. This often does not restore muscle strength to normal and many patients have to live with some degree of disability. If the dose is increased above the maximum response level in an attempt to improve physical activity, the opposite effect will be produced and progressive muscular weakness may end in cholinergic crisis. The short-acting anticholinesterase, edrophonium (Tensilon), may be used to decide whether a patient is under- or over-dosed. 2 mg are injected intravenously initially and if there is no deterioration in muscle strength a further 3–8 mg may then be injected. An increase in muscle strength suggests that the patient requires an increase in medication of anticholinesterase drugs, whereas a deterioration in muscle strength suggests that the patient is overdosed. Facilities for artificial ventilation should be readily available in case a cholinergic crisis is precipitated.

Anticholinesterase drugs have no effect on the underlying disease process. Thymectomy is the only certain way to induce permanent remission and improvement can be anticipated in 80% of patients without thymoma, although 3 to 5 years may elapse before the benefits of the operation become apparent. Both corticosteroids and immunosuppressants, such as azathioprine, frequently induce remission, although there is a significant relapse rate when these drugs are discontinued.

Profound weakness may accompany the early stages of treatment with corticosteroids in patients already receiving anticholinesterase drugs. The weakness does not occur in patients not on anticholinergic preparations.[16] Increasing the dose of anticholinesterase aggravates the weakness and it has been found that reducing the dose of anticholinesterase drugs in patients starting corticosteroids avoids this initial deterioration. It seems probable that steroids render the patient more sensitive to anticholinergic drugs and thus produce in effect a cholinergic crisis.

2, 3. Paralytic ileus and urinary retention

Cholinesterase inhibitors are used in the management of paralytic ileus and retention of urine. Anticholinergic drugs are used in the form of eye drops in the management of glaucoma. There is no indication for oral or systemic treatment. Physostigmine eye drops are the favoured preparation, usually in combination with pilocarpine.

Adverse reactions

Potentially life-threatening effects

With normal and appropriate doses there are none (but see Acute overdosage).

Acute overdosage

Excessive doses may impair neuromuscular transmission by causing a depolarizing block. This may precipitate a state of profound weakness described as a cholinergic crisis. Clinically this may be difficult to distinguish from a myasthenic crisis. Usually, however, in a cholinergic crisis there is evidence of muscarinic signs of parasympathomimetic action, such as sweating, abdominal pain, diarrhoea, hypersalivation and bradycardia. The Tensilon test (see Mode of use) helps to differentiate myasthenic from cholinergic weakness.

Severe or irreversible adverse effects

There is a rare syncopal reaction in which the patient feels dizzy after the injection of an anticholinergic drug. There may be transient loss of consciousness but recovery without treatment is the rule.

Central toxic effects occur with anticholinesterase preparations that cross the blood–brain barrier, such as physostigmine. These include anxiety, disorientation, hallucination and epilepsy.

Symptomatic adverse effects

Muscarinic side effects are not uncommon in patients with myasthenia gravis receiving treatment with anticholinergic drugs. These usually take the form of abdominal pain and diarrhoea. Hypersalivation is not uncommon and occasionally patients complain of sweating.

Interference with clinical pathology tests

No technical interferences of this kind have been reported.

High risk groups

Neonates

No special problems occur in neonates. Neonatal myasthenia occurs in 20% of the babies of myasthenic patients. The delay in onset of the weakness in the baby has been attributed to the passage of the mother's anticholinesterase drugs across the placenta. The half life of this is much shorter than that of the acetylcholine receptor antibody, so that children of myasthenic mothers tend to develop muscular weakness at 12 h after birth and the transient myasthenia persists for 4 to 6 weeks.[17]

Breast milk. As only relatively small amounts are secreted in breast milk, and because the drug is poorly absorbed from the gut, there appears to be no contraindication to breast-feeding.

Children

The drug may be used in children.

Pregnant women

There is no contraindication to the use of the drug during pregnancy.

The elderly

There are no special problems in this age group.

Drug interactions

Potentially hazardous interactions

Quaternary ammonium ions are poorly absorbed and their absorption may be completely inhibited by bulk laxatives such as methylcellulose.[12] Drugs that interfere with neuromuscular transmission will antagonize the effects of anticholinesterase preparations and this is particularly important in patients with myasthenia gravis where a serious relapse may occur when such preparations are used. The aminoglycoside antibiotics inhibit the release of acetylcholine. These include neomycin, streptomycin, kanamycin and gentamicin. The polypeptide antibiotics polymixin and colistin may have effects similar to those of the aminoglycosides. Oxytetracycline has also been reported to aggravate myasthenia gravis and both lincomycin and clindamycin as a result of their curare-like action may also aggravate myasthenia.

Antiarrhythmic drugs such as quinidine and procainamide and even propranolol block the acetylcholine receptor and may aggravate myasthenia gravis. Indeed, quinidine was once used as a provocative diagnostic test for myasthenia gravis. A myasthenic syndrome may develop in patients on long-term treatment with penicillamine. It tends to occur in those patients receiving penicillamine for rheumatoid arthritis and is rarely encountered in patients receiving penicillamine for Wilson's disease. The patients also develop acetylcholine receptor antibodies and the myasthenia usually remits when the penicillamine is withdrawn. Lithium and chlorpromazine also interfere with neuromuscular conduction and there are reports of the development of myasthenia gravis as a result.[18]

Potentially useful interactions
None has been reported.

Major outcome trials

The immediate effects of anticholinesterase drugs are so dramatic that there is no need for a controlled trial to be convinced of their benefit. This is the reason that there are no published controlled trials of cholinesterase inhibitors in myasthenia gravis. Indeed, most physicians would regard the therapeutic response as part of the definition of the disease. Nor have there been comparative trials to compare the relative effects of pyridostigmine and neostigmine. Most patients tend to choose pyridostigmine as there are less muscarinic side effects. Otherwise there is no convincing evidence that one drug is better than the other, or that one drug can be effective when the other has failed.

References

1. Breyer-Pfaff U, Maier U, Brinkmann A M, Schumm F 1985 Pyridostigmine kinetics in healthy subjects and patients with myasthenia gravis. Clinical Pharmacology and Therapeutics 37: 495–501
2. Nowell P T, Scott C A, Wilson A 1962 Determination of neostigmine and pyridostigmine in the urine of patients with myasthenia gravis. British Journal of Pharmacology 18: 617
3. Aquilonius S M, Hartvig P 1986 Clinical pharmacokinetics of cholinesterase inhibitors. Clinical Pharmacokinetics 11: 236–249
4. Aquilonius S M, Eckernas S A, Hartvig P, Lindstrom B, Osterman P O 1980 Pharmacokinetics and oral bioavailability of pyridostigmine in man. European Journal of Clinical Pharmacology 48: 423–428
5. Chan K, Davison S C, Dehghan A, Hyman N 1981 The effect of neostigmine and pyridostigmine bioavailability in myasthenic patients after oral administration. Methods and Findings in Experimental Clinical Pharmacology 3: 291–296
6. Aquilonius S M, Eckernas S A, Hartvig P, Linstrom B, Osterman P O 1983 Clinical pharmacology of neostigmine and pyridostigmine in patients with myasthenia gravis. Journal of Neurology, Neuro-surgery and Psychiatry 46: 929–935
7. Calvey T N, Chan K 1977 Plasma pyridostigmine levels in patients with myasthenia gravis. Clinical Pharmacology and Therapeutics 21: 187–193
8. Calvey T N, Deghan A, Williams N E 1981 Kinetics of intravenous pyridostigmine in man. British Journal of Clinical Pharmacology 11: 406–407
9. Cronnelly R, Stansky D R, Miller R D 1980 Pyridostigmine kinetics with and without renal failure. Clinical Pharmacology and Therapeutics 28: 78–81
10. Kornfeld P, Wolf R L, Samuels A J, Osserman K E 1971 The effect of chronic pyridostigmine administration on pyridostigmine ^{14}C metabolism in myasthenia gravis. Neurology 21: 530–532
11. Kornfeld P, Mittag T N, Genkins G, Horovitz S, Papastestas A E 1975 Studies in myasthenia gravis. Pyridostigmine-^{14}C metabolism after thymectomy. Neurology 25: 998–999
12. White M C, de Silva P, Havard C W H 1981 Plasma pyridostigmine levels in myasthenia gravis. Neurology 31: 145–150
13. Kornfeld P, Samuels A J, Wolf R L, Osserman K E 1970 Metabolism of ^{14}C-labelled pyridostigmine in myasthenia gravis. Evidence for multiple metabolites. Neurology 20: 634–640
14. Somani S M, Roberts J B, Wilson A 1972 Pyridostigmine metabolism in man. Clinical Pharmacology and Therapeutics 13: 393–399
15. Nowell P T, Scott C A, Wilson A 1962 Hydrolysis of neostigmine by plasma cholinesterase. British Journal of Pharmacology and Chemotherapy 19: 498–502
16. Warmolts J R, Engel W K 1972 Benefit from alternate day prednisolone in myasthenia gravis. New England Journal of Medicine 286: 17–20
17. Buckley G A, Roberts D V, Roberts J B, Thomas B H, Wilson A 1986 Drug induced neonatal myasthenia. British Journal of Pharmacology 34: 203P–204P
18. Granacher R P 1977 Neuromuscular problems associated with lithium. American Journal of Psychiatry 134: 702

Pyridoxine (hydrochloride)

Vitamin B_6, traditionally referred to as pyridoxine, covers a group of compounds that are metabolically interchangeable. Three members of this group (vitamers) are pyridoxine $C_8H_{11}NO_3$, pyridoxal $C_8H_9NO_3$ and pyridoxamine $C_8H_{12}N_2O_2$. In the body they are transformed to pyridoxal phosphate, through the action of pyridoxine kinase, pyridoxine oxidase and transaminase (Fig. 1).

Fig. 1 Metabolic interconversion of pyridoxine vitamers

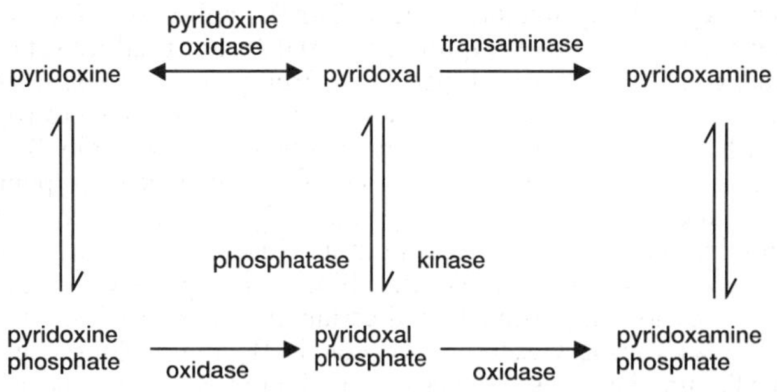

Chemistry

Pyridoxine hydrochloride (Hexa-Betalin, Hexavibex, Pyridipca, Pyridex, Becilan, Benadon, Hexermin, Compoviton, Comploment Continus, Paxadon)
$C_8H_{11}NO_3.HCl$
3-Hydroxy-4,5-bis(hydroxymethyl)-2-methylpyridine hydrochloride

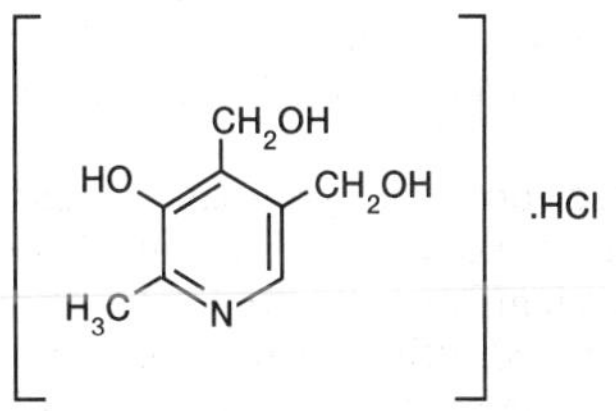

Molecular weight (free base)	205.6 (169.2)
pKa (-NO, phenolic OH)	5.0, 9.0
Solubility	
in alcohol	1 in 115
in water	1 in 5
Octanol/water partition coefficient	low

The only form in which vitamin B_6 is commercially available is pyridoxine hydrochloride, a white, crystalline, birefringent powder which is stable in air, and melts with decomposition at 204–206°C. It undergoes rapid photodecomposition in neutral or alkaline solution but remains photostable in 0.1N HCl. It is commercially synthesized by the method of Harris and Folkers.[1] It has a bitter saline taste and is odourless.

In addition to synthetic preparations, vitamin B_6 is present in a wide variety of foods from animals and plants. Very good sources are yeast, liver and cereals, which also contain the glucoside. There are also differences in vitamin bioavailability in various food sources.[2]

Pyridoxine hydrochloride is an ingredient of various multivitamin preparations such as Neurobion, Polybion and B-plex fort.

Pyridoxine (hydrochloride)

P

Pharmacology

Vitamin B_6 has two main active analogues, i.e. pyridoxal and pyridoxamine, whereas the inactive analogues are norvitamin B_6, 4-pyridoxic acid, and 5-pyridoxic acid. Vitamin B_6 is antagonized by various drugs such as 4-deoxypyridoxine, 4-methoxypyridoxine, toxopyrimidine, penicillamine, semicarbazide, isoniazid, oestrogen and Fe^{3+}. Pyridoxal phosphate is mainly involved as a coenzyme, especially in the metabolic transformation of amino acids including decarboxylation, transamination and racemization.

In the metabolism of tryptophan, vitamin B_6 is involved in a number of enzymatic reactions. In vitamin B_6-deficient humans and animals, a number of metabolites of tryptophan, especially xanthurenic acid, are excreted in urine in abnormally large quantities. Pyridoxine deficiency in rats is accompanied by a lowered threshold for electroshock-induced tonic–clonic seizures. This is reversed by pyridoxine. The tryptophan loading test has been used to assess vitamin B_6 status. This test is based on the reduction in kynureninase activity due to a deficiency of its cofactor, pyridoxal phosphate. The excretion, specifically of xanthurenic acid and possibly also of kynurenine and hydroxy-kynurenine is measured before and after administration of a dose of tryptophan (l-tryptophan 10 g or 100 $mg.kg^{-1}$ body weight) using a 24-hour collection of urine. A lower suggested dose of tryptophan (2 g) does not produce sufficient challenge to the pathway tested. The tryptophan load test is not a reliable indicator of vitamin B_6 status in persons receiving oestrogens or with increased secretion of glucocorticoids.[3,4] Vitamin B_6 is a cofactor in the conversion of tryptophan to 5-hydroxytryptamine (5HT) and of methionine to cysteine.[5] Pyridoxine is capable of modifying the action of steroid hormones in vivo by interacting with the steroid–receptor complexes.[6] Biochemical interaction occurs between pyridoxal phosphate and certain drugs and toxins.[7] Isoniazid increases urinary excretion of vitamin B_6 and prolonged use of penicillamine has caused deficiency of vitamin B_6. The drugs cycloserine and hydralazine are also antagonists of vitamin B_6. Administration of the vitamin reduces the neurological side effects associated with the use of these agents.

Toxicology

Beagles receiving a daily dose of 300 $mg.kg^{-1}$ of pyridoxine hydrochloride developed a swaying gait within 9 days. They eventually became unable to walk, but were not weak.[8] Hoover and others[9] reported a similar observation in beagles. Pyridoxine in doses of 150 $mg.kg^{-1}$ body weight given daily for 100 days caused degeneration of the central tracts arising from the spinal and trigeminal ganglia.

Rats receiving large doses of pyridoxine developed gait ataxia, that subsided after vitamin B_6 was withdrawn. Axonal degeneration of the sensory fibre system was observed. The fibres derived from the ventral root were spared although the degeneration approached the dorsal root ganglia. Neurones in the ganglia did not degenerate.[10]

Clinical pharmacology

Pyridoxine deficiency syndromes have been produced in all mammalian species including man. Incidence of vitamin B_6 deficiency among alcoholics is high.[11] Alcoholics have lower than normal mean circulating levels of pyridoxal phosphate because of reduced dietary intake or malabsorption or an abnormal hepatic handling of vitamin B_6 both in terms of storage and metabolism. Beneficial effects of vitamin B_6 on neurological and haematological disorders of alcoholics have been reported. Important features of vitamin B_6 deficiency observed in man and other species are related to the skin, nervous system and erythropoiesis. In man, seborrhoeic skin lesions about the eyes, nose and mouth accompanied by glossitis and stomatitis are produced within a few weeks by feeding a diet poor in vitamin B-complex and supplemented with the pyridoxine antagonist, 4-deoxypyridine. The lesions clear rapidly after administration of pyridoxine, but do not respond to other members of the B-complex family.[12]

In man, peripheral neuritis, associated with synovial swelling and tenderness especially in the carpal synovia (carpal tunnel disease), has been attributed to pyridoxine deficiency. The syndrome is reversible on treatment with high doses of the vitamin.[13]

The central feature of moderate pyridoxine deficiency is the decrease in the concentration of the neurotransmitters γ-aminobutyric acid[14] and 5-hydroxytryptamine[15] in the central nervous system. Generally, the levels of catecholamines are not decreased. The consequences of the non-parallel changes in the catecholamines and indolamines include neuroendocrine disturbances such as hypothyroidism.

Although no untoward effects have been noted in clinical studies from daily doses of 130 mg to more than 7 g given for periods of 6 to 21 days, long-term use may result in paraesthesia, somnolence, and low folic acid levels. Deterioration in acne vulgaris was associated with pyridoxine or cyanocobalamin therapy in a study of 14 patients.[16] Lactation was not suppressed when pyridoxine (300 mg) was given twice daily to 11 postpartum women.[17] The prolactin-inhibiting properties of pyridoxine, seen in hyperprolactonaemics, were not demonstrated in normal individuals.

Daily requirements of pyridoxine vary with the nutritional status, disease state, sex and age of the individual, and with the bioavailability of vitamin B_6 from foods. Recommendations for daily intake of vitamin B_6 are as follows:

(i) Adult (male) 2.2 mg daily
(ii) Adult (female) 2.0 mg daily
(iii) Pregnancy 2.6 mg daily
(iv) Lactation 2.5 mg daily
(v) Infant (up to 6 months) 300 μg daily
(vi) Children (from 6 months to 1 year) 600 μg daily
(vii) Older children 2.0 mg daily
(ix) Therapeutic dose 25–100 mg daily

For treatment of dietary deficiency 10–20 mg daily for 3 weeks followed by a maintenance dose of 2–5 mg pyridoxine is recommended.

Pharmacokinetics

Pyridoxal phosphate has been determined enzymatically using tyrosine apodecarboxylase.[18] Fluorimetric methods have also been used for its determination.[19] The preferred, highly sensitive, analytical method is high pressure liquid chromatography (HPLC) for determination of vitamin B_6 analogues. Limits of detection are about 100 pg pyridoxine vitamers per injection.[20,21]

All three forms of vitamin B_6 (pyridoxine, pyridoxal and pyridoxamine) are readily absorbed from the gastrointestinal tract. In tissue, they are present primarily as 5-phosphorylated derivatives of pyridoxal and pyridoxamine. Muscle seems to be a major storage site for pyridoxal phosphate in the body. About 50% of total body pyridoxal phosphate is present in the muscle, bound to glycogen phosphorylase. Pyridoxic acid is the major excretory metabolite in urine.

All three forms of vitamin B_6, i.e. pyridoxine, pyridoxal and pyridoxamine, are converted to the active form pyridoxal phosphate in the body. The half life of the pyridoxine ranges from 15 to 20 days. It is degraded in the liver to 4-pyridoxic acid which is excreted by the kidney.

5% of the ingested dose of vitamin B_6 is excreted as follows:
urine (4-pyridoxic acid 0.6–11.2 mg daily)
pyridoxal (0.005–0.04 mg daily)
pyridoxamine (0.003–0.20 mg daily)
faeces (0.003–0.20 mg daily).
Pyridoxine is not significantly bound to plasma proteins. The phosphorylated vitamers appear to bind to plasma proteins and haemoglobin.[22] Uptake of pyridoxine by brain appears to be by a saturable process.

Pooled samples of human breast milk contained 15–20 $\mu g.l^{-1}$ of vitamin B_6.

Oral absorption	high
Presystemic metabolism	negligible
Plasma half life	
range	15–20 d
Volume of distribution	—
Plasma protein binding	nil

Concentration–effect relationship

There is evidence of binding of all derivatives of vitamin B_6 to plasma proteins.[23] In man, plasma levels of pyridoxine vitamers have been shown to reflect closely its concentration in the liver.[24] Normal levels of vitamin B_6 are 46–72 μg.l^{-1} (serum) and 31–43 μg.l^{-1} (blood). Milder forms of vitamin B_6 intoxication are found among women taking considerably lower doses of vitamin B_6 but over a prolonged time period. However, pyridoxine overdose neuropathy is limited to those taking higher vitamin B_6 doses over a long time period. High potency vitamin B_6 preparations are available as non-prescription food supplements. There is a danger of toxicity due to self-prescription in doses exceeding 500 mg per day.

Metabolism

The liver plays a major role in the metabolism of pyridoxine, pyridoxal and pyridoxamine, which are all phosphorylated by pyridoxal kinase (Fig. 1).[25] Pyridoxine phosphate is oxidized to the active coenzyme form, pyridoxal 5-phosphate, by an enzyme found mainly in liver. Pyridoxal 5-phosphate interconverts with pyridoxamine

Fig. 2 Analogues and metabolites of pyridoxine

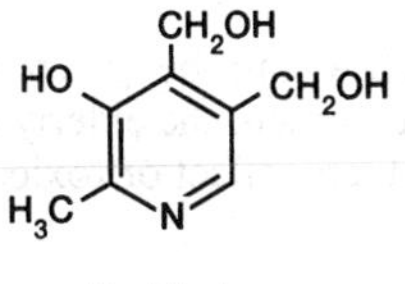

3-Hydroxy-4,5-bis(hydroxymethyl) 2-methylpyridine

Pyridoxine

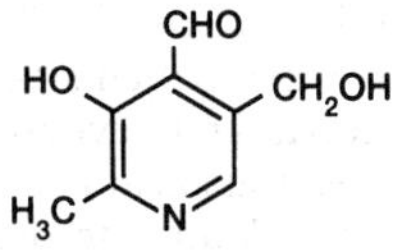

3-Hydroxy-4-formyl-5-hydroxymethyl 2-methylpyridine

Pyridoxal

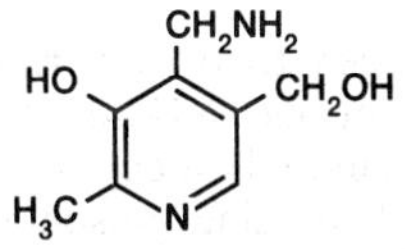

3-Hydroxy-4-aminomethyl-5-hydroxy-methyl-2-methylpyridine

Pyridoxamine

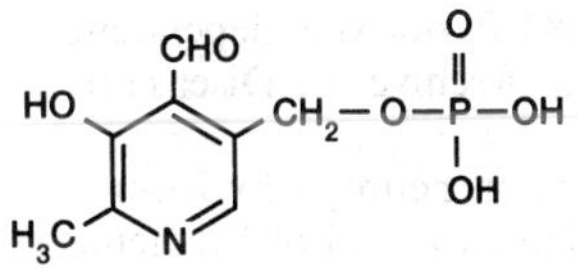

Pyridoxal 5-phosphate (PLP)
(coenzyme) biologically active vitamin

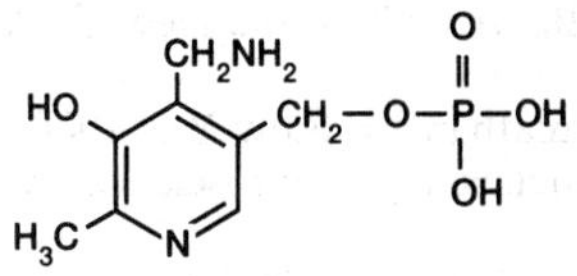

Pyridoxamine phosphate

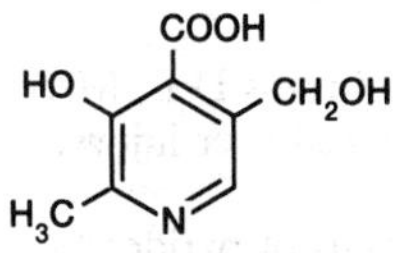

4-Pyridoxic acid
(metabolically inert, excreted in urine)

5-phosphate through enzymatic transamination. The phosphorylated forms are hydrolysed by phosphatases. Plasma levels of vitamin B_6 reflect the liver concentrations.[24]

Pyridoxal is oxidized in the liver to pyridoxic acid, the main excretory form of pyridoxine. Pyridoxal 5-phosphate (PLP) is the coenzyme for more than 100 enzymes,[15,26] with vital roles in intermediary metabolism. Therefore, at first sight, it seems unlikely that a mutation affecting formation or accumulation of PLP would be compatible with life. However, such a possibility cannot yet be excluded, since a partial reduction of available PLP may lead to reduced activity of a few enzymes due to the widely varying degrees of binding of the pyridoxal phosphate to pyridoxine apoenzymes.[27]

Pharmaceutics

Dosage forms

Pyridoxine hydrochloride is available in oral dosage forms, as tablets or soft elastic gelatin capsules. An improved bioavailability from the capsule dosage form has recently been documented.[2]

1. Pyridoxine tablets contain 10, 20 or 50 mg pyridoxine hydrochloride
2. Benadon (Roche, UK): tablets containing 20 or 50 mg pyridoxine hydrochloride
3. Paxadon (Steinhard, UK): 50 mg scored tablets
4. Complement Continus (Napp, UK): yellow, slow-release tablets containing 100 mg of pyridoxine hydrochloride
5. Tex Six TR (Schering, Canada): 100 mg timed-release capsules.

Pyridoxine hydrochloride is also available combined with other vitamins in injectable form:

6. Vitamins B and C injection: contains ascorbic acid, nicotinamide, pyridoxine hydrochloride, riboflavin and thiamine hydrochloride. It is available in two strengths for intramuscular injection and one strength for intravenous use.

The formulations do not include potentially allergenic substances.

Pyridoxine hydrochloride should be kept in a tightly closed container, protected from light. The white crystalline powder is stable, but its shelf-life is reduced when dissolved in water. Thus, even in the absence of light, pyridoxine is gradually degraded on exposure to a humid atmosphere, the decomposition being faster at higher temperatures. Vitamin B_6 is also degraded when exposed to irradiation (dose dependent); in the solid state, pyridoxine loses hydrogen atoms on irradiation.[28]

It is quite stable at room temperature and refrigeration may not be necessary. When vitamin B_6 is an ingredient of a multivitamin preparation, it may require refrigeration.

Pyridoxine hydrochloride is incompatible with alkaline solutions, iron salts and oxidizing solutions.[29]

Food processing and storage reduce vitamin B_6 activity. Vitamin C also degrades a considerable amount of B_6 in canned food preparations. Overcooking destroys vitamin B_6 content.

Therapeutic use

Indications

1. Prophylaxis and treatment of pyridoxine deficiencies
2. Vitamin B_6 dependency syndrome
3. In the treatment of various conditions, e.g. premenstrual syndrome, pregnancy sickness, carpal tunnel syndrome, pyridoxine-dependent errors of metabolism.

Contraindications

1. Concomitant administration of levodopa.

Mode of use

The preferred route of administration depends on the requirement for pyridoxine and the clinical condition of the patient. In general, the oral route of administration is preferred. Solutions for injection containing 100 mg.ml^{-1} in 10 ml vials are also available for use, especially in cases of pyridoxine deficiency. Pyridoxine hydrochloride should be injected slowly. It may produce slight momentary burning and a painful sensation at the site of injection. No untoward side effects have been reported.

The dosage recommended for infants is 2–15 mg daily, and for children 50–200 mg daily. For prophylaxis in patients taking drugs that affect pyridoxine disposition 25–50 mg daily is recommended. For treatment of deficiency in adults and children a dose of 5–25 mg daily for 3 weeks is recommended, followed by 1.5–2.5 mg daily in a multivitamin preparation for maintenance. During pregnancy and lactation, the same dose as for treatment of deficiencies can be used.

Indications

1. Prophylaxis and treatment of pyridoxine deficiencies
This vitamin is of value in patients taking anovulatory steroids, in the treatment of nausea and vomiting of pregnancy, and in the prevention of peripheral neuritis which may accompany isoniazid therapy. The toxic effects of large doses of cycloserine on the CNS have been prevented or controlled by pyridoxine alone or in combination with anticonvulsants, tranquillizers or sedatives.

2. Vitamin B_6 dependency syndrome
Treatment of this condition may require doses as high as 60 mg daily for 3 weeks, and a daily intake of 50 mg for life.

3. Other uses
Pyridoxine is used in the treatment of a wide variety of conditions which include depression and other symptoms associated with premenstrual syndrome (100–400 mg per day), pregnancy sickness as well as idiopathic carpal tunnel syndrome. Pyridoxine has been used in the management of various pyridoxine-dependent inborn errors of metabolism such as seizures, primary hyperoxaluria (type 1), homocystinuria and hereditary sideroblastic anaemia. Pyridoxine is also used in the treatment of isoniazid-induced peripheral neuritis and acute isoniazid toxicity. To prevent drug-induced (penicillamine, cycloserine, hydralazine or isoniazid) pyridoxine deficiency a daily supplement of 10–50 mg pyridoxine is recommended.

Contraindications

1. Concomitant administration of levodopa
Pyridoxine supplements should not be given to patients receiving levodopa (in Parkinson's disease) as the action of levodopa is antagonized (dopa is converted to dopamine peripherally). However, this vitamin may be used along with a preparation containing both carbidopa and levodopa. Pyridoxine (80–400 mg daily) has been reported to enhance the hepatic metabolism of phenobarbitone or phenytoin by 40–50% in some patients. This reduces the serum drug concentration.

Adverse reactions

Potentially life-threatening effects
No effects of this kind have been reported.

Acute overdosage
Toxic effects of massive doses of pyridoxine were reported in the early literature.[30] Hypervitaminosis leading to sensory neuropathy was observed only in those individuals consuming considerably more than 500 mg daily for very long periods.

Severe or irreversible adverse effects
Sensory neuropathy has been described in people who consumed more than 200 mg daily on a chronic basis.[31] Doses of pyridoxine greater than 500 mg daily for prolonged periods of time can result in sensory nerve damage. Two factors, daily dose and duration of intake, are critical for the assessment of the risk of neuropathy. Doses of 500 mg and less per day taken for up to two years have not been associated with neuropathy. Daily doses exceeding 1000 mg or total doses of 1000 g or more over years appear to represent high risk. There seems to be minimal risk of permanent adverse changes in sensory nerve function if pyridoxine supplementation is stopped when adverse changes in neurological functions are first noted. Use of pyridoxine in doses exceeding 500 mg daily should be avoided.[32,33]

A neurotoxic syndrome due to pyridoxine overdose has been reported in women. The symptoms included paraesthesia, hyperaesthesia, bone pain, muscle weakness and numbness. A raised serum vitamin B_6 level was present in these women. The neurological symptoms disappeared when pyridoxine was withdrawn and reappeared when it was readministered. There was a significant difference in the average duration of ingestion of B_6 in the neurotoxic group of 2.9 ± 1.9 years compared with 1.6 ± 2.1 years in controls.

Doses less than 500 mg daily appear to be safe on the basis of literature reports. In these cases the vitamin was administered for periods ranging from 6 months to 6 years.[34]

Symptomatic adverse effects
Temporary burning or stinging pain may be experienced at the site of injection. Although no untoward effects have been noted in clinical studies in which daily doses of from 130 mg to more than 1 g were given for periods of 6 to 21 days, longer-term use may result in paraesthesia and somnolence.

Other effects
Excessive doses of pyridoxine may lower serum folate concentrations.

Interference with clinical pathology tests
No such interference has been reported.

High risk groups

Pyridoxine in doses about ten times the RDA can be given to neonates, breast-fed infants, children, pregnant women, the elderly or women using oral contraceptive steroids. No adverse effect or toxicity has been reported at this level.

Drug interactions

Potentially hazardous interactions
Pyridoxine reduces the therapeutic effect of levodopa by stimulating the decarboxylation of dopa to dopamine in peripheral tissues. The antagonistic effect of pyridoxine does not occur when patients take the peripheral decarboxylase inhibitor, carbidopa, and levodopa concomitantly. Various other drugs, such as isonicotinic acid hydrazide, cycloserine, penicillamine, hydrazine and anovulatory steroids, may also increase the requirement for pyridoxine.

Potentially useful interactions
None has been reported.

Clinical trials

Vitamin B_6 (pyridoxine hydrochloride) has been tried in various clinical conditions including deficiencies due to chronic INH administration in alcoholics, epilepsy, anaemia, renal failure, homocysteinuria, hyperoxaluria, depression, neuropathies, hydrazine poisoning, and pregnancy. In all the above clinical situations variable beneficial effects of vitamin B_6 therapy have been reported.

General review articles

Bankier A, Turner M, Hopkins I J 1983 Pyridoxine-dependent seizures — a wider clinical spectrum. Archives of Disease in Childhood 58: 415–418

Berger A, Schaumberg H H 1984 More on neuropathy from pyridoxine abuse (letter). New England Journal of Medicine 311: 986–987

Cohen M, Bendich A 1986 Safety of pyridoxine — a review of human and animal studies. Toxicology Letters 34: 129–139

Dakshinamurti K 1982 Neurobiology of pyridoxine. Advances in Nutritional Research 4: 143–179

Dakshinamurti K (ed) 1990 Vitamin B_6. Annals of the New York Academy of Sciences 585: 1–570

Dakshinamurti K, Paulose C S, Viswanathan M, Siow Y L 1988 Neuroendocrinology of pyridoxine deficiency. Neuroscience and Behavioural Reviews 12: 189–193

Dalton K, Dalton M J 1987 Characteristics of pyridoxine overdose. Neuropathy syndrome. Acta Neurologica Scandinavica 76 (1): 8–11

Dastur D K, Dave U P 1987 Effect of prolonged anticonvulsant medication in epileptic patients. Serum lipids, vitamin B_6, B_{12} and folic acid, proteins and fine structures of liver. Epilepsia 28: 147–159

Diehl A M, Chacon M A, Potter J J, Rolfes D, Cruess D F, Mezey E 1987 Pyridoxine deficiency and ethanol induced liver injury. Alcoholism (New York) Aug 11 (4): 385–391

Flower B 1985 Recent advances in the mechanisms of pyridoxine responsive disorders. Journal of Inherited Metabolic Disorders 8 (suppl 1): 76–83

Pyridoxine (hydrochloride)

Hoyumpa A M 1986 Mechanisms of vitamin deficiencies in alcoholism. Alcoholism (New York) Dec 10 (6): 573–581

Krinke G, Schaumberg H H, Specer P S, Suter J, Thomann P, Hess R 1980 Pyridoxine megavitaminosis produces degeneration of peripheral sensory neurons. (Sensory neuropathy in the dog). Neurotoxicology 2: 13–24

Manyam B V, Ferraro T N, Hare T A 1987 Isoniazid-induced alteration of CNS neurotransmitter amino acids in Huntington's disease. Brain Research 408: 125–130

Paulose C S, Dakshinamurti K, Packer S, Stephens N L 1988 Sympathetic stimulation and hypertension in the pyridoxine-deficient adult rat. Hypertension 11: 387–391

Rose R C 1985 Intestinal transport of vitamins. Journal of Inherited Metabolic Disorders 8 (suppl 1): 13–16

Scriver C R 1967 Vitamin B_6 deficiency and dependency in man. American Journal of Diseases of Children 113: 109–114

Sebrell W H, Harris R S 1968 The vitamins, chemistry, physiology, pathology. Methods, vol II. Academic Press, New York

Viswanathan M, Siow Y L, Paulose C S, Dakshinamurti K 1988 Pineal indolamine metabolism in pyridoxine-deficient rats. Brain Research 473: 37–42

Waterston J A, Gilligan B S 1987 Pyridoxine neuropathy. Medical Journal of Australia 146: 640–642

Windebank A J, Low P A, Blexrud M D, Schmelzer J D, Schaumburg H H 1985 Pyridoxine neuropathy in rats. Neurology 35: 1617–1622

References

1. Harris S A, Folkers K 1939 Synthesis of vitamin B_6. Journal of the American Chemical Society 61: 1245–1247
2. Thakker K M, Sitren H S, Gregory J F, Schmidt J L, Baumgartner T G 1987 Dosage form and formulation effects on the bioavailability of vitamin E, riboflavin and vitamin B_6 from multivitamin preparations. American Journal of Clinical Nutrition 45: 1472
3. Sauberlich H E, Caham J E, Baker E M, Raica N Jr, Herman Y F 1972 Biochemical assessment of the nutritional status of vitamin B_6 in the human. American Journal of Clinical Nutrition 25: 629–642
4. Coon W W, Nagla E 1969 The tryptophan load test as a test for pyridoxine deficiency in hospitalized patients. Annals of the New York Academy of Sciences 166: 30–43
5. Sturman J A 1978 Vitamin B_6 and the metabolism of sulfur amino acids. In: Human vitamin B_6 requirements. National Academy of Sciences, Washington, DC, pp 37–60
6. Disorbo D M, Phelps D S, Ohl V S, Litwack G 1980 Pyridoxine deficiency influences behaviour of the glucocorticoid receptor complex. Journal of Biological Chemistry 255: 3866–3870
7. Bauernfeind J C, Miller O N 1978 Vitamin B_6, nutritional and pharmaceutical usage, stability, bioavailability, antagonists and safety. In: Human vitamin B_6 requirements. National Academy of Sciences, Washington, DC, pp 78–110
8. Krinke G, Schaumburg H H, Specer P S, Suter J, Thomann P, Hess R 1980 Pyridoxine megavitaminosis produces degeneration of peripheral sensory neurons (sensory neuropathy) in the dog. Neurotoxicology 2: 13–24
9. Hoover D M, Carlton W W 1981 The subacute neurotoxicity of excess pyridoxine hydrochloride and clioquinol (5-chloro-7-iodo-8-hydroxyquinoline) in beagle dogs. I. Clinical disease. Pathology and Veterinary Pathology 18: 745–756
10. Windebank A J, Low P A, Blexrud M D, Schmelzer J D, Shaumburg H H 1985 Pyridoxine neuropathy in rats. Specific degenerations of sensory axons. Neurology 35: 1617–1622
11. Li T 1978 Factors influencing vitamin B_6 requirements in alcoholism. In: Human vitamin B_6 requirements. National Academy of Sciences, Washington, DC, pp 210–225
12. Mueller J F, Vilter R W 1950 Pyridoxine deficiency in human beings induced with desoxypyridoxine. Journal of Clinical Investigation 29: 193–201
13. Ellis T, Folkers K, Walanabo T et al 1979 Clinical results of a cross-over treatment with pyridoxine and placebo on the carpal tunnel syndrome. American Journal of Clinical Nutrition 32: 2040–2046
14. Roberts E 1963 Some thoughts about the γ-aminobutyric acid system in the nervous tissue. Nutrition Review 21: 161–165
15. Dakshinamurti K 1977 B vitamins and nervous system function. In: Wurtman R J, Wurtman J T (eds) Nutrition and the brain, vol 1. Raven Press, New York, pp 219–318
16. Braun-Falco O, Lincke H 1976 The problem of vitamin B_6/B_{12} acne, a contribution on acne medicamentosa. Munchen Medizin Wochenschrift 118 (6): 155–160
17. Lande N I 1979 More on dangers of vitamin B_6 in nursing mothers. New England Journal of Medicine 300 (16): 926–927
18. Dakshinamurti K, Stephens N L 1969 Pyridoxal phosphate is determined enzymatically using tyrosine apodecarboxylase. Journal of Neurochemistry 16: 1515–1522
19. Durko I, Yukhonovska Y V, Ivanor Ch P 1973 A new fluorimetric method for the determination of vitamin B_6 in blood. Clinica Chimica Acta 49: 407–414
20. Gregory J F 1980 Determination of pyridoxal 5-phosphate as the semicarbazone derivative using high performance liquid chromatography. Analytical Biochemistry 102: 374–379
21. Hollins B, Henderson J M 1986 Analysis of B_6 vitamins in plasma by reversed phase column liquid chromatography. Journal of Chromatography 380: 67–75
22. Mehansho M, Buss D D, Hamm M W, Henderson L M 1980 Transport and metabolism of pyridoxine in rat liver. Biochimica Biophysica Acta 631: 112–123
23. Anderson B B, Newmark P A, Rawlins M 1974 Plasma binding of vitamin B_6 compounds. Nature 250: 502–504
24. Lumeng L, Lui A, Li T 1980 Plasma content of B_6 vitamins and its relationship to hepatic vitamin B_6 metabolism. Journal of Clinical Investigation 66: 688–695
25. Lui A, Lumeng L, Li T 1981 Metabolism of vitamin B_6 in rat liver mitochondria. Journal of Biological Chemistry 256: 6041–6046
26. Lipson M H, Kraus J, Solomon L R, Rosenberg L E 1980 Depletion of cultured human fibroblasts of pyridoxal 5′-phosphate. Effect on activity of aspartate aminotransferase, alanine aminotransferase and cystathionine B synthetase. Archives of Biochemistry and Biophysics 204: 486–493
27. Meister A 1965 Biochemistry of the amino acids. Academic Press, New York, pp 380–411
28. Galatzeanu I, Antoni E 1967 Radiosterilization of medical products. International Atomic Energy Agency, Vienna, p 33
29. Pramer W et al 1971 Some physical and chemical incompatibility of drugs for intravenous administration. Drug Intelligence and Clinical Pharmacy 5: 211
30. Antopol W, Tarlor I M 1942 Experimental study of effects produced by large doses of vitamin B_6. Neuropathology and Experimental Neurology 1: 330–336
31. Schaumburg H H et al 1983 Sensory neuropathy from pyridoxine abuse. New megavitamin syndrome. New England Journal of Medicine 309: 445–448
32. Raskin N H, Fishman R A 1965 Pyridoxine-deficiency neuropathy due to hydralazine. New England Journal of Medicine 273: 1182–1185
33. Bendich A, Cohen M 1990 Vitamin B_6 safety issues. Annals of the New York Academy of Sciences 585: 321–330
34. Cohen M, Bendich A 1986 Safety of pyridoxine. A review of human and animal studies. Toxicology Letters 34: 129–139

P Pyrimethamine

The drug is an antifolate used in human medicine to treat malaria and toxoplasmosis.

Chemistry

Pyrimethamine (Daraprim)
$C_{12}H_{13}N_4Cl$
5(4-Chlorophenyl)-6-ethyl pyrimidine-2,4,diamine

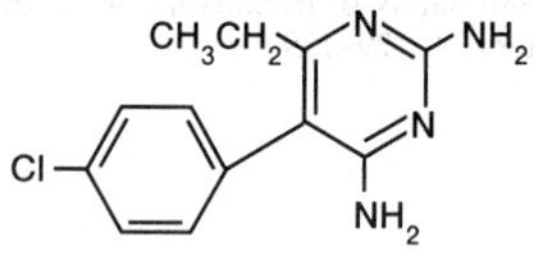

Molecular weight	248.7
pKa	7.3
Solubility	
in alcohol	1 in 200
in water	practically insoluble
Octanol/water partition coefficient	2.69

A white, odourless, tasteless crystalline powder prepared by chemical synthesis.

Pyrimethamine is also available in the UK in two oral combination products with dapsone (Maloprim) and sulphadoxine (Fansidar).

Pharmacology

Pyrimethamine inhibits dihydrofolate reductase (DHFR) (EC 1.5.1.4): its selectivity of action depends upon differential affinity for DHFR in different species. Thus the IC_{50} for DHFR from *Plasmodium berghei* is 0.5 nmol whilst that for rat liver DHFR is 700 nmol.[1]

Toxicology

The principal toxic effect in all species is bone marrow depression during high-dose, chronic daily treatment. This is prevented by concurrent administration of folinic acid.[2] Given during pregnancy it is teratogenic and causes fetal death and abnormalities consistent with folate deficiency, which are reversed by concurrent administration of folinic acid. In animal species such effects occur at doses of >2 mg.kg^{-1} daily in the rat and mini-pig, 20 mg.kg^{-1} daily in the golden hamster and 100 mg.kg^{-1} daily in the rabbit.

In vitro mutagenesis has been demonstrated at high pyrimethamine concentrations in the presence of low folinate concentrations since profound DHFR inhibition prevents chromosome repair. Chromosome abnormalities were observed in metaphases of bone marrow cells examined in 3 of 5 patients receiving total doses of 200–300 mg pyrimethamine.[3] Toxic doses in mice (100 mg.kg^{-1}) produced cytogenetic lesions in bone marrow but not germ cells. A study performed by the National Cancer Institute showed no excess of tumours in mice given 500 and 1000 p.p.m. pyrimethamine in the diet or in rats given 200–400 p.p.m. for 78 weeks. However, an approximately three-fold increase in lung tumours over control animals was seen in strain A mice treated with intraperitoneal doses of pyrimethamine to a total dose of 0.125 g.kg^{-1}.[4]

Clinical pharmacology

Within the usual dose range pyrimethamine has few effects in man. In one study no significant toxic effects were noted when 25 mg was administered weekly to 81 men for 6 months.[5] However, 25 mg given daily for 49 days induced megaloblastic anaemia in 50% of a group of normal volunteers.[6] With high doses, megaloblastic anaemia, leucopenia, thrombocytopenia, pancytopenia and atrophic glossitis are more likely. Very large doses cause nausea, vomiting, exfoliative dermatitis, dizziness and convulsions in addition to bone marrow depression.[7]

Pharmacokinetics

The preferred analytical method is high performance reverse phase liquid chromatography with ultraviolet detection which has a limit of sensitivity 1 μg.l^{-1}.[8]

Pyrimethamine is well absorbed after oral administration to healthy volunteers, although the absolute bioavailability in man is not known. In monkeys the bioavailability of oral pyrimethamine was virtually complete.[9] The mean absorption rate constant in man was 3.03 h^{-1} ($t_{\frac{1}{2}}$ absorption approximately 15 minutes). Plasma concentrations peak at 2–6 hours in healthy human subjects and the maximum plasma concentration following a single 25 mg dose is 234 ± 21 μg.l^{-1}.[10] The mean elimination half life in several studies is 85 hours with a reported range of 35–175 hours.[10,11,12] Total body clearance is 25 ± 4 ml.h^{-1}.kg^{-1}.[10] Pyrimethamine is lipid soluble and has a high apparent volume of distribution of 2.9 ± 0.5 l.kg^{-1}.[10,12]

Protein binding is 87% in the therapeutic range.[13] Animal studies[13] have demonstrated high drug concentrations relative to plasma level in lung (8:1) and brain (3:1). The erythrocyte:plasma ratio is approximately 1:2 at all plasma concentrations. The CSF:plasma ratio is 0.1–0.25 in animals but data are not available for humans. The drug is also found in human saliva in concentrations reflecting the free fraction of drug in plasma.[14] Pyrimethamine enters human breast milk: 6 hours after a 75 mg dose approximately 3 μg.l^{-1} of the parent compound and/or metabolite were detected in milk, which fell to 1.5 μg.l^{-1} at 24 hours. No adverse reactions have been seen in breast-fed babies of mothers receiving pyrimethamine.[15] The lipid solubility suggests that placental transfer of pyrimethamine would occur although this has not been documented.[16]

Of a single 100 mg oral dose 16–32% is excreted in the urine over 40 days.

Oral absorption	good
Presystemic metabolism	—
Plasma half life	
range	35–175 h
mean	85 h
Volume of distribution	2.9 ± 0.5 l.kg^{-1}
Plasma protein binding	87%

Concentration–effect relationship

The in vitro efficacy of pyrimethamine against the malaria parasite is dependent upon culture conditions and no therapeutic range of concentration has been established.

Metabolism

Pyrimethamine undergoes extensive hepatic metabolism to unknown metabolites: the 3-N-oxide has recently been identified as a metabol-

Fig. 1 Metabolism of pyrimethamine

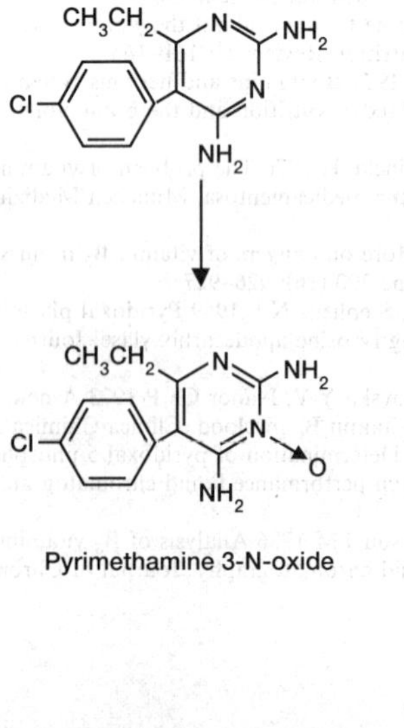

Pyrimethamine 3-N-oxide

Pyrimethamine

ite in the rat (Fig. 1). It is not known if pyrimethamine metabolites have pharmacological activity.

Pharmaceutics

Pyrimethamine (Daraprim; Burroughs Wellcome, UK/USA) is available as white, scored 25 mg tablets marked 'WELLCOME A3A'.

They should be stored in airtight containers below 35°C and protected from light. The shelf-life is 5 years.

It is also present in two combination preparations:
Sulfadoxine 500 mg + pyrimethamine 25 mg (Fansidar; Roche UK/USA): white quarter-scored tablets marked 'ROCHE' in a hexagon.
Dapsone 100 mg + pyrimethamine 12.5 mg (Maloprim; Burroughs Wellcome, UK/USA): white scored tablets marked 'WELLCOME - H9A'.

Therapeutic use

Indications

1. Malaria prophylaxis
2. Malaria treatment
3. Treatment of toxoplasmosis.

Contraindications

1. Hypersensitivity to pyrimethamine
2. Folate deficiency anaemia.

Mode of use

1. Malaria prophylaxis

The dose of pyrimethamine is 25 mg once weekly for adults (12.5 mg for children 5–16 years). There is no suitable formulation in the UK for children aged less than 5 years. Dosage should begin on or before arrival in an endemic area and continue until 4 weeks after leaving the malarious area. The geographical area where pyrimethamine alone can be used to prevent malaria has been greatly restricted by the development of resistance by *Plasmodium*, particularly in South East Asia, South America and East Africa. In these areas the folate antagonist activity of pyrimethamine can be augmented by producing a 'sequential blockade' of folic acid synthetic pathways using a sulphone or a sulphonamide. Current recommendations are for weekly therapy using the combination pyrimethamine 12.5 mg with 100 mg dapsone (Maloprim) or 25 mg pyrimethamine with 500 mg sulphadoxine (Fansidar) although the occurrence of Stevens–Johnson syndrome due to the sulphadoxine makes the latter less advisable. Chloroquine is also added in areas of high *P. vivax* exposure. On pharmacokinetic grounds twice weekly dosing with Maloprim would be logical to ensure persistence of both components in the plasma throughout the dose interval (the half life of dapsone is only about 24 hours). In practice, however, good protection is provided in most areas by once weekly dosing. It is important to obtain up-to-date advice on prophylaxis from the various centres whose addresses and telephone numbers are published in the British National Formulary (Chapter 5.4) since resistance patterns and advice change frequently. Patients with a previous history of sulphonamide hypersensitivity should avoid Fansidar.

2. Malaria treatment

Uncomplicated attacks of falciparum malaria in semi-immune patients may be treated with two tablets of Fansidar (50 mg pyrimethamine + 1 g sulphadoxine).[17] Fansidar is rarely the treatment of choice since chloroquine will usually be preferred. In areas of chloroquine resistance quinine will usually be given.

3. Toxoplasmosis

Due to lack of controlled trials and the variable course of the infection the efficacy of various treatment regimens is difficult to evaluate. The following are accepted guidelines.[18]

a. Immunologically deficient patients (e.g. Hodgkin's disease, AIDS) with widely disseminated acute infection including CNS involvement require treatment with a loading dose of pyrimethamine of 15 $mg.m^{-2}$ twice daily for two days followed by 15 $mg.m^{-2}$ alternate days (or daily for the first few weeks in severe disease). Sulphadiazine is given in addition in a loading dose of 75 $mg.kg^{-1}$ (up to 4 g) followed by 100 $mg.kg^{-1}$ daily (up to 6 g daily) in two divided doses. Treatment should continue for 4–6 weeks after complete resolution of signs and symptoms and in AIDS, treatment is given for 6 months or longer. Toxic effects are common at these doses and may contribute to mortality. Folinic acid 5 mg daily may be given to mitigate side effects.[18,19]

b. Immunologically deficient patients with chronic infection and immunologically normal patients with acquired lymphadenopathic toxoplasmosis should not be treated unless symptoms are severe.

c. Acute infection during pregnancy should be treated with two week courses of pyrimethamine and sulphonamide followed by three to four weeks of treatment until term.[20]

Pyrimethamine is potentially teratogenic in man and if possible should not be used during the first 16 weeks of pregnancy although such treatment has reduced fetal infection from 64 to 14%.[21]

d. Congenital toxoplasmosis: evidence for efficacy of treatment is meagre but it may have a protective effect against development of new ocular lesions.[22] Courses of pyrimethamine, 0.5–1 $mg.kg^{-1}$ daily, plus sulphadiazine, 50–100 $mg.kg^{-1}$ daily, are given for 21 days followed by spiromycin 100 $mg.kg^{-1}$ daily for 35–45 days are given 3–4 times in the first year of life. Prednisolone 1–2 $mg.kg^{-1}$ daily is also given whilst there are signs of an acute inflammatory process. Folinic acid 5 mg twice weekly will be required during pyrimethamine therapy.

Adverse reactions

Potentially life-threatening effects

Only two cases in this category have been reported with pyrimethamine alone. In one a severe pustular cutaneous eruption developed 24 hours after a single dose of 25 mg pyrimethamine. In the other, a patient on several drugs including pyrimethamine developed disseminated intravascular coagulation. Agranulocytosis has been reported following the use of of Maloprim (pyrimethamine plus dapsone) for malaria prophylaxis. Data from Sweden suggests a prevalence figure of about 1 in 2000.[23]

Acute overdosage

There have been several cases of acute overdosage, usually in young children. Although the major sign in a very few individuals was severe vomiting,[24] the majority suffered convulsions[25] after ingestion of 14 or more tablets. Coma, hyperpyrexia, tachycardia, dyspnoea, and reversible blindness and deafness have also been reported.[26] Gastric lavage is suitable only within the first 2 hours of ingestion. Treatment is supportive and diazepam will control the seizures. Folinic acid 15 mg daily is given to counteract the effects of DHFR inhibition until the signs of toxicity have subsided. Blood transfusion may be needed to counteract blood dyscrasias.

Severe or irreversible adverse effects

Megaloblastic anaemia may occur during long-term treatment, especially in individuals taking diets with a low folate content.

Symptomatic adverse effects

Photosensitive rashes have been observed which disappear when pyrimethamine is discontinued.[27]

Interference with clinical pathology tests

No technical interferences of this kind have been reported.

High risk groups

Neonates

No data are available for neonates, and the formulation available in the UK is unsuitable for children under the age of 5 years.

Breast milk. The drug enters breast milk (see Pharmacokinetics), but no adverse effects on the infant have been observed.

Children

The drug may be used in children in the reduced dosage mentioned earlier.

Pregnant women

The teratogenic effects of pyrimethamine in animals are dose-dependent and reduced by administration of folinic acid. Teratogenesis has not been a major problem in practice, although isolated cases have been reported.[28] It is generally considered that malaria presents a greater risk to the fetus than antimalarial prophylaxis,[29] but the risk of teratogenesis following administration in early pregnancy must be recognized. More important is the risk of exacerbating folate deficiency during pregnancy: it is recommended that pregnant women taking pyrimethamine should also receive folinic acid supplements.

The elderly
No information is available on the treatment of the elderly.

Concurrent disease
Renal disease. Pyrimethamine excretion remains unchanged in severe renal failure. It is not established whether it is removed by haemodialysis.[30]
Hepatic disease. No information is available on treatment in patients with liver disease.
Heterozygous β-thalassaemia. Perhaps because of the secondary folic acid deficiency, administration of pyrimethamine may occasionally produce pancytopenia and a megaloblastic bone marrow.[31]

Drug interactions

Potentially hazardous interactions
The antifolate properties of pyrimethamine may exacerbate those of other antifolates such as co-trimoxazole, trimethoprim, and methotrexate.[32] It has also been reported that 2 mg lorazepam given with pyrimethamine for a week was associated with abnormalities of liver function in 2 of 5 normal volunteers. It is not known if other benzodiazepines produce this effect.[33]

Potentially useful interactions
Sequential blockade of folate pathways by sulphone or sulphonamide plus pyrimethamine results in considerable potentiation in the treatment of malaria[34] and toxoplasmosis[18] in man.

Major outcome trials

1. Covell G, Shute P G, Maryon M 1953 Pyrimethamine (Daraprim) as a prophylactic against a West African strain of *P. falciparum*. British Medical Journal 1: 1081–1083

An experimental study in patients receiving malaria therapy for neurosyphilis. This was the first study to demonstrate that a weekly 25 mg dose of pyrimethamine offered complete protection against overt malarial attack. Thus, pyrimethamine was established as a true causal prophylactic against *Plasmodium*.

2. Shute P G, Maryon M 1954 The effect of pyrimethamine (Daraprim) on the gametocytes and oocysts of *Plasmodium falciparum* and *Plasmodium vivax*. Transactions of the Royal Society of Tropical Medicine and Hygiene 48: 50–63

This is a study of the gametocidal effect of pyrimethamine when administered to patients with circulating male gametocytes in the blood. They found that for *Plasmodium vivax* when 5 mg or less was given the percentage of mosquitoes infected after feeding on the patient was similar to control mosquitoes feeding on untreated subjects but a small number of the oocysts showed degeneration suggesting that this is the threshold dose for effect on the parasite. After a single 50 mg dose there was a striking reduction in the number of oocysts/mosquito gut suggesting that the drug sterilizes the gametocytes in the blood. A similar reduction in *Plasmodium falciparum* oocysts was found after administration of 25 mg pyrimethamine to the human host. This study showed that pyrimethamine was not gametocidal in the sense that the gametocytes were unable to fertilize or be fertilized but that it affects oocyte formation. They suggested the use of a weekly dose of gametocytocidal drug like pyrimethamine as a way of interrupting the completion of the sporogony cycle in populations living in endemic areas with high density of mosquitoes and gametocyte carriers.

3. Jeffery G M 1958 Infectivity to mosquitos of Plasmodium vivax following treatment with chloroquine and other anti-malarials. American Journal of Tropical Medicine and Hygiene 7: 207–211

This is a report of studies on patients undergoing malaria therapy for neurosyphilis and confirmed the previous study of Shute and Maryon (above) by showing that 25 mg pyrimethamine rendered a case of *Plasmodium vivax* non-infectious to mosquitoes within 4 hours. Subsequent feedings at 8, 12 and 24 hours showed no viable oocysts although viable gametocytes and asexual forms persisted in the peripheral blood for 6 and 8 days. It was also demonstrated that where *Plasmodium* has become resistant to pyrimethamine the resistance is also operative for infectivity to mosquitoes.

4. Bray R S, Burgess R W, Fox R M, Miller M J 1959 Effect of pyrimethamine upon sporogony and pre-erythrocytic schizogony of *Laverania falciparum*. Bulletin of the World Health Organization 21: 233–238

This study was carried out in gametocyte carriers of *Plasmodium (Laverania) falciparum* in Liberia who were treated with 25 or 50 mg pyrimethamine. These regimes rendered the malarial gametocytes uninfective to mosquitoes for up to 28 days. Mosquitoes feeding upon a malaria-free pyrimethamine-treated subject before or after feeding on a non-treated gametocyte carrier became infected showing that the effect of pyrimethamine is exerted in the carrier not the mosquito. This implies that if during mass prophylactic chemotherapy some carriers remain untreated, the presence of pyrimethamine in the remaining population gives no protection for the whole community. They also showed that pyrimethamine administered before sporozoite infection of chimpanzees will prevent the development of hepatic pre-erythrocytic schizonts of *Plasmodium falciparum*.

References

1. Ferone R, Burchall J J, Hitchings G H 1969 *Plasmodium berghei* dihydrofolate reductase. Isolation, properties and inhibition by antifolates. Molecular Pharmacology 5: 45–59
2. Castles T R, Kintner L D, Lee C C 1971 The effects of folic or folinic acid on the toxicity of pyrimethamine in dogs. Toxicology and Applied Pharmacology 20: 447–459
3. Bottura C, Coutinho V 1965 The effect of pyrimethamine on the human chromosome. Brazilian Biological Review 25: 145–147
4. Stoner G D, Shimkin M B, Kniazeff A J, Weisburger J G, Weisburger E K, Gori G B 1973 Test for carcinogenicity for food additives and chemotherapeutic agents by the pulmonary tumor response in strain A mice. Cancer Research 33: 3069–3085
5. Dern R J, Beutler E, Arnold J, Lorinez A, Block M, Alving A S 1955 Toxicity studies of pyrimethamine (Daraprim). American Journal of Tropical Medicine and Hygiene 4: 217–220
6. Myatt A V, Hernandez T, Coatney G P 1953 Studies in human malaria XXXIII. The toxicity of pyrimethamine (Daraprim) in man. American Journal of Tropical Medicine and Hygiene 2: 788–795
7. Ragah A H 1973 Pyrimethamine in central nervous system leukaemia. Lancet 1: 1061
8. Midskov C 1984 High performance liquid chromatographic assay of pyrimethamine, sulfadoxine and its N^4-acetyl metabolite in serum and urine after ingestion of Suldox. Journal of Chromatography 308: 217–227
9. Smith C C, Schmidt L H 1963 Observations on the absorption of pyrimethamine from the gastrointestinal tract. Experimental Parasitology 13: 178–185
10. Ahmad R A, Rogers H J 1980 Pharmacokinetics and protein binding interactions of dapsone and pyrimethamine. British Journal of Clinical Pharmacology 10: 519–524
11. Jones C R, Ovenall S M 1978 Determination of plasma concentrations of dapsone, monoacetyldapsone and pyrimethamine in human subjects dosed with Maloprim. Journal of Chromatography 163: 179–185
12. Weidekarum E, Plozza-Notterbrack H, Fargo I, Dubach V C 1982 Plasma concentrations of pyrimethamine and sulfadoxine and evaluation of pharmacokinetic data by computerized curve fitting. Bulletin of the World Health Organization 60: 115–122
13. Cavallito J C, Nichol C A, Brenckman W D et al 1978 Lipid soluble inhibitors of dihydrofolate reductase I kinetics, tissue distribution and extent of metabolism of pyrimethamine, metoprine and etoprine in the rat, dog and man. Drug Metabolism and Disposition 6: 329–337
14. Ahmad R A, Rogers H J 1981 Salivary elimination of pyrimethamine. British Journal of Clinical Pharmacology 11: 101–102
15. Clyde D F, Shute G T 1956 Transfer of pyrimethamine in human milk. Journal of Tropical Medicine and Hygiene 59: 277–284
16. Smith C C, Ihrig J 1959 Persistent excretion of pyrimethamine following oral administration. American Journal of Tropical Medicine and Hygiene 8: 60–62
17. Gilles H M 1981 Malaria. Medicine International 4: 153–156
18. MacCabe R E, Remington J E 1983 The diagnosis and treatment of toxoplasmosis. European Journal of Clinical Microbiology 2: 95–104
19. Hakes T B, Armstrong D 1983 Toxoplasmosis. Problems in diagnosis and treatment. Cancer 52: 1535–1540
20. Kraubig H 1963 Erste praktische Erahrungen mit der prophylaxe der konnatelen toxoplasmose. Medizinische Klinik 58: 1361–1364
21. Hengst P 1982 Zur Effektivitat einer gnerellen Testung auf *Toxoplasma-gondii*-Infektion im der Schwangerschaft. Zentralblatt Gynakologie 104: 949–956
22. Couvreur J, Desmonts G, Aron-Rosa D 1985 Le prognostic oculaire de la toxoplasmose congenitale: rôle du traitement. Semaines de l'Hôpital Paris 61: 1734–1737
23. Friman G, Nyström-Rosander, Jonsell G et al 1983 Agranulocytosis associated with malaria prophylaxis and maloprim. British Medical Journal 286: 1244–1245
24. Abbott P H, Hamdi M A 1953 British Medical Journal 1: 884–885
25. Voorhoeve H W, Meuwissen J H E Th 1963 A case of pyrimethamine intoxication in a Papuan child Tropical and Geographical Medicine 15: 82–85

26. Akinyanju O, Goddell J C, Ahmed I 1973 Pyrimethamine poisoning. British Medical Journal 4: 147–148
27. Craven S A 1974 Photosensitivity to pyrimethamine. British Medical Journal 2: 556
28. Harpey J, Darbois Y, Lefebvre G 1983 Teratogenticity of pyrimethamine. Lancet 2: 399
29. Peters W 1983 Pyrimethamine combinations in pregnancy. Lancet 2: 1005–1007
30. Bennett W M, Muther R S, Parker R A et al 1980 Drug therapy in renal failure: dosing guidelines for adults. Part I Antimicrobial agents, analgesics. Annals of Internal Medicine 93: 62–65
31. Malacarne P, Zavagli G, Castaldi G, Piffanelli A 1974 2,4-Diaminopyrimidines and heterozygous beta-thalassaemia. Lancet 2: 904–905
32. Ansdell V E, Wright S G, Hutchinson D B A 1976 Megaloblastic anaemia associated with combined pyrimethamine and cotrimoxazole administration. Lancet 2: 1257
33. Briggs M, Briggs M 1974 Pyrimethamine toxicity. British Medical Journal 1: 40
34. Hurly M G D 1959 Potentiation of pyrimethamine by sulphadiazine in human malaria. Transactions of the Royal Society of Tropical Medicine and Hygiene 53: 412–413

Quinalbarbitone (sodium)

Quinalbarbitone is a barbiturate sedative and hypnotic.

Chemistry

Quinalbarbitone sodium (secobarbitone sodium, secobarbital sodium, seconal sodium)
$C_{12}H_{17}N_2NaO_3$
Sodium 5-allyl-5-(1-methylbutyl)barbiturate

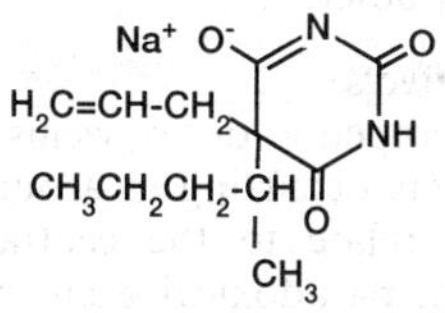

Molecular weight (free acid)	260.3 (238.3)
pKa	7.9
Solubility	
in alcohol	1 in 5
in water	1 in 3
Octanol/water partition coefficient	high

Quinalbarbitone is a white, odourless hygroscopic powder with a bitter taste, prepared by chemical synthesis; a 3.9% solution is iso-osmotic with serum.

Quinalbarbitone sodium is also available in combination of equal parts with amylobarbitone sodium (Tuinal).

Pharmacology

The barbiturates unselectively depress the central nervous system, producing dose-dependent effects ranging from mild sedation to general anaesthesia. All have anticonvulsant properties.

Toxicology

No information is available on animal toxicology.

Clinical pharmacology

Barbiturates, including quinalbarbitone, demonstrate dose-dependent reversible depression of neurological function. Part of this action relates to interference with synaptic transmission and multineuronal connections. A direct local anaesthetic effect on cell membranes has also been demonstrated.[1] Barbiturates have multiple actions including enhancement of GABAergic inhibition, reduction of glutaminergic and cholinergic excitation, increase in chloride ion conductance, reduction in presynaptic calcium entry and non-synaptic sodium and potassium conductances and blockage of repetitive firing.[2] Associated with brain function depression is a parallel dose-dependent reduction in cerebral metabolic rate and blood flow.[3] The specific mechanisms responsible for the observed clinical sedative, anaesthetic and anticonvulsant effects of the barbiturates remain uncertain. Quinalbarbitone also increases θ activity on the electroencephalogram.[4]

Pharmacokinetics

Quinalbarbitone can be assayed using gas–liquid chromatography[5] or high pressure liquid chromatography[6] with limits of detection of 30–40 μg.l^{-1}. More recently, attempts to quantify the drug using an enzyme-immunoassay system have been made.[7]

Oral absorption	>85%
Presystemic metabolism	minimal
Plasma half life	
range	19–34 h
mean	25 h
Volume of distribution	1.5 l.kg^{-1}
Plasma protein binding	65–75%

Quinalbarbitone is completely absorbed after oral administration with peak blood concentrations occurring around 3 hours after dosing.[5] The drug undergoes minimal first-pass metabolism. Its volume of distribution approximates 1.5 l.kg^{-1} and it is 65–75% protein bound in plasma. It is largely metabolized in the liver, mainly by hydroxylation, with a half life varying between 19 and 34 hours in the adult. The half life appears shorter in children[6] and in drug abusers,[7] the latter finding being consistent with auto-induction of metabolism. As expected with a lipid-soluble drug, quinalbarbitone is excreted in breast milk.[9] Quinalbarbitone readily crosses the placenta and achieves fetal concentrations of 70% of those in the mother. The kinetics of quinalbarbitone are not altered in patients with renal dysfunction. It is likely that plasma concentrations will be elevated in patients with hepatic disease.

Concentration–effect relationship

Toxicity, consisting of drowsiness, slurred speech, ataxia and nystagmus, occurs at concentrations over 6 mg.l^{-1} following subacute dosing.[8] Marked central nervous system symptomatology occurs at higher levels after acute overdose.[10]

Metabolism

Quinalbarbitone is largely metabolized in the liver, mainly by hydroxylation, and the metabolites are excreted in the urine.[11] There

Fig. 1 Metabolites of quinalbarbitone

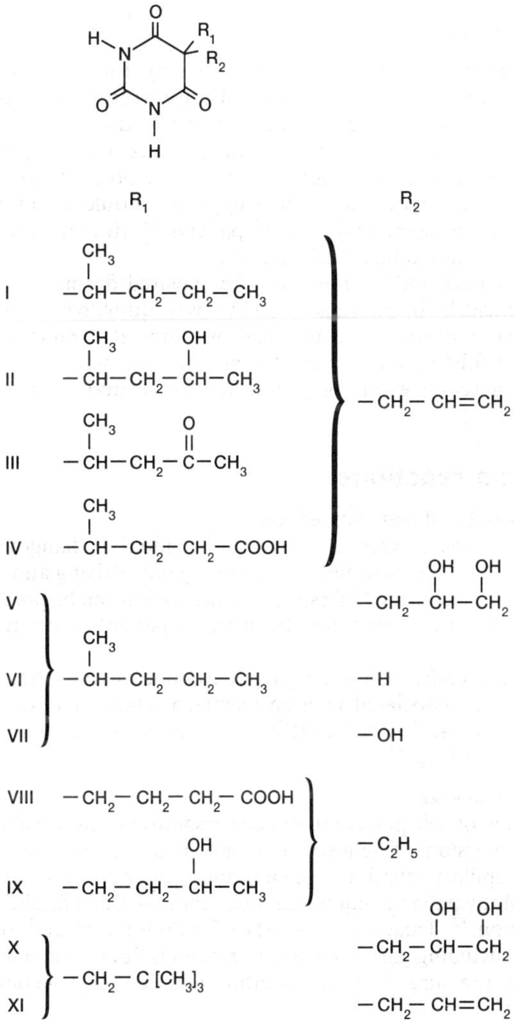

are no active metabolites. Urinary metabolites include two diastereoisomeric forms of 5-allyl-5-(3′-hydroxy-1′-methylbutyl) barbituric acid, 5-allyl-5-(3′-oxo-1′-methylbutyl) barbituric acid, 5-allyl-5-(1′-methyl-3′-carboxypropyl) barbituric acid and 5-(2′,3′-dihidroxypropyl)-5-(1′-methylbutyl) barbituric acid. Amylobarbitone is an inducer of hepatic metabolism.

Pharmaceutics

1. Seconal (Lilly, UK/USA): orange capsules containing 50 mg (coded 'F42') or 100 mg (coded 'F40') of quinalbarbitone sodium.
2. Tuinal (Lilly, UK/USA): orange/blue capsules containing 50 mg each of quinalbarbitone sodium and amylobarbitone sodium, coded 'F65'.

Containers should be kept tightly closed and the contents stored below 25°C. Maximum shelf-life for each preparation is 5 years.

Therapeutic use

Indications

1. The treatment of severe, intractable insomnia.

Contraindications

1. Hypersensitivity to barbiturates
2. History of porphyria
3. Presence of uncontrolled pain
4. Pregnancy and lactation
5. Marked impairment of liver function
6. Respiratory disease in which dyspnoea or obstruction is evident.

Barbiturates should not be administered to children, young adults, patients with a history of drug or alcohol abuse, the elderly or the debilitated.

Mode of use

Quinalbarbitone should be prescribed only for severe intractable insomnia and then only after careful consideration of safer alternatives such as benzodiazepines. Normal dosing ranges from 50–100 mg nightly, although some patients may require up to 200 mg. Because of the addictive and abuse potential of barbituric acid derivates, a benzodiazepine hypnotic should be initially preferred for the large majority of patients.[12] Intermittent use may prevent the development of tolerance.[13]

Performance and alertness may be impaired during the first week of treatment.[14] In pharmacological doses, quinalbarbitone reduces rapid eye movement sleep[15] and withdrawal symptoms can be produced following treatment for as little as a week.[16] It has been used as a sedative during parturition but cannot now be recommended.[17]

Adverse reactions

Potentially life-threatening effects

Impaired consciousness. Because of residual or 'hangover' effects the next day,[18] users should be warned against driving and operating dangerous machinery.[19] Respiratory depression can be produced and quinalbarbitone should not be used in patients with respiratory failure.

Carcinogenesis. Chronic quinalbarbitone therapy has been reported to be associated with an increased relative risk of bronchial and ovarian carcinoma but this may have been due to coincidental cigarette smoking.[21]

Acute overdosage

Symptoms of self-poisoning include respiratory and cardiac depression, depression of reflexes, pupillary constriction and, in severe cases, pupillary dilation, hypotension, oliguria, hypothermia and coma. Many patients require assisted ventilation and fatalities are not uncommon.[22] Treatment consists of symptomatic and supportive therapy including gastric lavage, intravenous fluids, and maintenance of blood pressure, body temperature and adequate respiratory exchange.[23]

Severe or irreversible adverse effects

Hypersensitivity. Rarely, the use of barbiturates results in localized diffuse, myalgic, neuralgic and arthritic pain, particularly in the neck, shoulder girdle and upper limbs.[1] Allergic reactions including rashes, angioneurotic oedema and fever may occur, particularly in atopic individuals.

Abuse. Like all barbiturates, quinalbarbitone has a high dependence potential and is commonly abused. Signs of barbiturate intoxication include nystagmus, ataxia, slurred speech, somnolence and diminished tendon reflexes.[24] On higher doses semi-coma, respiratory depression and shock can result in a fatal outcome. Intra-arterial injection may produce tissue necrosis[25] which can be reversed by injection of 1% procaine into and around the artery together with intra-arterial heparin.[26] Withdrawal symptoms include apprehension, muscular weakness, tremor and disturbed sleep. Anorexia is apparent in the early stages with fits and delirium occurring 3–8 days after drug discontinuation. Passive addiction can occur in utero in infants exposed to quinalbarbitone during pregnancy.[27] Combination barbiturate preparations such as Tuinal appear to have greater abuse potential than quinalbarbitone alone.[28] A treatment schedule for withdrawal using pentobarbitone in decreasing doses over a six-month period has been described.[24]

Symptomatic adverse effects

Quinalbarbitone in therapeutic doses seems remarkably well tolerated, with adverse effects occurring in around 2–3% of patients.[29] Commonest problems relate to the central nervous system and include excess sedation, paradoxical excitement, euphoria, vertigo, ataxia, restlessness, confusion and irritability. Subtle effects on memory,[30] task integration[31] and reaction times[32] have been reported.

High risk groups

Neonates

The drug should not be used in neonates.

Breast milk. The drug should not be used by nursing mothers.

Children

Barbiturates should not be administered to children or adolescents.

Pregnant women

Barbiturates are contraindicated in pregnancy,[33] as there may be an increased risk of cardiovascular malformation in the fetus.[34] Respiratory depression has been noted in infants born following the use of barbiturates during labour.

The elderly

Barbiturates should not be used in elderly patients because of the greater risk of confusion and falls.

Concurrent disease

The use of barbiturates in patients with a history of drug or alcohol abuse should be avoided. Barbiturates should not be prescribed for patients with porphyria as they increase haem synthesis and can precipitate or exacerbate an acute porphyria attack.[35] Caution is advised in patients with impaired hepatic or cardiac function.

Interference with clinical pathology tests

No technical interferences of this kind have been reported.

Drug interactions

Potentially hazardous interactions

Barbiturates are the classical inducers of hepatic monooxygenase activity in man and increase the metabolism of a number of endogenous substances and exogenously administered drugs. Quinalbarbitone has been reported to increase the metabolism of thyroid hormones,[36] vitamin D,[37] warfarin[38] and theophylline.[39] Other similar interactions can be expected and those affecting drugs with a narrow therapeutic ratio, such as steroids and cardiac antiarrhythmics, are most likely to be clinically relevant. Synergistic sedation can be anticipated when the drug is used in combination with other central nervous system depressants such as ethanol.

Potentially useful interactions

No interactions of this kind have been reported.

Quinalbarbitone (sodium)

Major outcome trials

1. Hinton J M 1963 A comparison of the effects of six barbiturates and a placebo on insomnia and motility in psychiatric patients. British Journal of Pharmacology 20: 319–325

Six barbiturates, each for 8 successive nights, were compared with placebo in a controlled double blind trial in 24 insomniac psychiatric patients. All the barbiturates significantly prolonged sleep and hastened its onset. Quinalbarbitone (100–200 mg) was among the three most effective drugs.

2. Linnoila M, Erwin C W, Logue P E 1980 Efficacy and side effects of flurazepam and a combination of amobarbital and secobarbital in insomniac patients. Journal of Clinical Pharmacology 20: 117–123

The barbiturate combination (100 mg of each drug) was more effective in inducing and maintaining sleep than flurazepam (30 mg) and placebo in 10 patients with severe insomnia. Tuinal was still effective on the fourteenth night of treatment and did not produce significant impairment of psychomotor function.

3. Okawa K K, Allen G S 1978 A clinical comparison of triazolam with placebo and with secobarbital in insomniac patients. Journal of International Medical Research 6: 343–347

Triazolam (0.5 mg) was preferred to quinalbarbitone (100 mg) by 76 outpatient insomniacs in a double-blind crossover trial. No differences were observed with regard to side effects and alertness the next morning.

References

1. Harvey S C 1985 Barbiturates. In: Gilman A G, Goodman L S, Rall T W, Murad F (eds) The pharmacological basis of therapeutics, 7th edn. Macmillan, New York, pp 351–360
2. Macdonald R L 1983 Mechanisms of anticonvulsant drug action. In: Pedley T A, Meldrum B S (eds) Recent advances in epilepsy 1. Churchill Livingstone, Edinburgh, pp 1–23
3. Shapiro H M 1985 Barbiturates in brain ischaemia. British Journal of Anaesthesia 57: 82–95
4. Montagu J D 1971 Effect of quinalbarbitone (secobarbital) and nitrazepam on the EEG in man: quantitative investigations. European Journal of Pharmacology 14: 238–249
5. Clifford J M, Cookson J H, Wickham P E 1974 Absorption and clearance of secobarbital, heptabarbital, methoqualone and ethinamate. Clinical Pharmacology and Therapeutics 16: 376–389
6. Levine H L, Cohen M E, Duffner P K, Lacey D J, Karpynec R, Shen D D 1982 Rectal absorption and disposition of secobarbital in epileptic children. Paediatric Pharmacology 2: 33–38
7. Pape B E, Cary P L, Clay L 1983 Reactivity of EMIT serum barbiturate assay reagents: potential application for the quantitation of selected barbiturates. Therapeutic Drug Monitoring 5: 473–477
8. Faulkner T P, McGinity J W, Hayden J H, Martinez M, Comstock E G 1978 Pharmacokinetic studies on tolerance to sedative-hypnotics in a poly-drug abuse population 1. Secobarbital. Clinical Pharmacology and Therapeutics 23: 36–46
9. Wilson J T, Brown R D, Cherek D R et al 1980 Drug excretion in human breast milk: principles, pharmacokinetics and projected consequences. Clinical Pharmacokinetics 5: 1–80
10. Broughton P M G, Higgins G, O'Brien J R P 1956 Acute barbiturate poisoning. Lancet 1: 180–184
11. Gilbert J N T, Hetherington W L, Powell J W, Whalley W B 1975 Metabolism of quinalbarbitone. Journal of Pharmacy and Pharmacology 27: 343–347
12. Okawa K K, Allen G S 1978 A clinical comparison of triazolam with placebo and with secobarbital in insomniac patients. Journal of International Medical Research 6: 343–347
13. Kales A, Hauri P, Bixler E O, Silberfarb P 1976 Effectiveness of intermediate term use of secobarbital. Clinical Pharmacology and Therapeutics 20: 541–545
14. Roth T, Piccione P, Salis P, Kramer M, Kaffeman M 1979 Effects of temazepam, flurazepam and quinalbarbitone on sleep: psychomotor and cognitive function. British Journal of Clinical Pharmacology 8 (suppl 1): 47S–54S
15. Lester B K, Coulterer J D, Cowden L C, Williams H L 1968 Secobarbital and nocturnal physiological patterns. Psychopharmacologia (Berlin) 13: 275–286
16. Hartmann E, Lindsley J G, Spinweber C 1983 Chronic insomnia: effects of tryptophan, flurazepam, secobarbital and placebo. Psychopharmacology 80: 138–142
17. Moya F, Thorndike V 1964 The effect of drugs used in labour on the foetus and newborn. Clinical Pharmacology and Therapeutics 4: 628–653
18. Kornetsky C, Vates T S, Kessler E K 1959 A comparison of hypnotic and residual psychological effects of single doses of chlorpromazine and secobarbital in man. Journal of Pharmacology and Experimental Therapeutics 127: 51–54
19. McKenzie R E, Elliot L L 1965 Effect of secobarbital and d-amphetamine on performance during a simulated air mission. Aerospace Medicine 36: 774–779
20. Brown C R, Forrest W H, Hayden I 1973 The respiratory effects of pentobarbital and secobarbital in clinical doses. Journal of Clinical Pharmacology 13: 28–35
21. Friedman G D 1981 Barbiturates and lung cancer in humans. Journal of the National Cancer Institute 67: 291–295
22. Greenblatt D J, Allen M D, Harmatz J S, Noel B J, Shader R J 1979 Overdose with pentobarbital and secobarbital: assessment of factors related to outcome. Journal of Clinical Pharmacology 19: 758–768
23. Hadden J, Johnson K, Smith A, Price L, Giardina E 1969 Acute barbiturate intoxication: concepts of management. Journal of the American Medical Association 209: 893–900
24. Teggin A F, Bewley T H 1979 Withdrawal treatment for barbiturate dependence. Practitioner 223: 106–107
25. Morgan N R, Waugh T R, Boback M D 1970 Volkmann's ischaemic contracture after intra-arterial injection of secobarbital. Journal of the American Medical Association 212: 476–478
26. Lazarus H M, Hutto W, Ellerston D G 1977 Therapeutic prevention of ischaemia following intra-arterial barbiturate injection. Journal of Surgical Research 22: 46–53
27. Bleyer W A, Marshall R E 1972 Barbiturate withdrawal syndrome in a passively addicted infant. Journal of the American Medical Association 221: 185–186
28. Dymock R B, James R A, Lokan R J 1980 Tuinal as a drug of abuse. Medical Journal of Australia 2: 214–215
29. Shapiro S, Slone D, Lewis G P, Jick H 1969 The clinical effects of hypnotics 2: an epidemiologic study. Journal of the American Medical Association 209: 2016–2020
30. Evans W O, Davis K E 1969 Dose–response effects of secobarbital on human memory. Psychopharmacologia (Berlin) 14: 46–61
31. William H L, Rundell D H Secobarbital effects on recall and recognition in a levels-of-processing paradigm. Psychopharmacology 80: 221–225
32. Fishkin V, Lovallo W R, Fishkin S M, Shurley J T 1980 Residual effects of temazepam and other hypnotic compounds on cognitive function. Journal of Clinical Pharmacology 41: 358–363
33. Anon 1979 Committee on the Review of Medicines: recommendations on barbiturate preparations. British Medical Journal 2: 719–720
34. Guay D P 1982 Sedative-hypnotics and teratogenesis. Canadian Journal of Hospital Pharmacy 35: 42–60
35. Brodie M J, Goldberg A 1980 Acute hepatic porphyrias. In: Goldberg A, Moore M R (eds) Clinics in haematology: the porphyrias. W B Saunders, London, pp 253–272
36. Hoffbrand B I 1979 Barbiturate/thyroid hormone interaction. Lancet 2: 903–904
37. Young R E, Ramsay L E, Murray T S 1977 Barbiturates and serum calcium in the elderly. Postgraduate Medical Journal 53: 212-215
38. Udall J A 1975 Clinical implications of warfarin interactions with five sedatives. American Journal of Cardiology 35: 67–71
39. Paladino J A, Blumer N A, Maddock R R 1983 Effect of secobarbital on theophylline clearance. Therapeutic Drug Monitoring 5: 135–139

Q

Quinidine (bisulphate and sulphate)

Quinidine is a dextrorotatory distereoisomer of quinine,[1] and is available as the bisulphate (Kinidin, Kiditard) or the sulphate (Quinicardine) salt.

Chemistry

Quinidine bisulphate (Kinidin, Kiditard)
$C_{20}H_{24}N_2O_2.H_2SO_4$
(8R, 9S)-6′-Methoxycinchonan-9-ol bisulphate
Quinidine sulphate (Quinicardine, Quinora, Quinidex)
$(C_{20}H_{24}N_2O_2)_2.H_2SO_4.2H_2O$
(8R, 9S)-6′-Methoxycinchonan-9-ol acid hemisulphate monohydrate

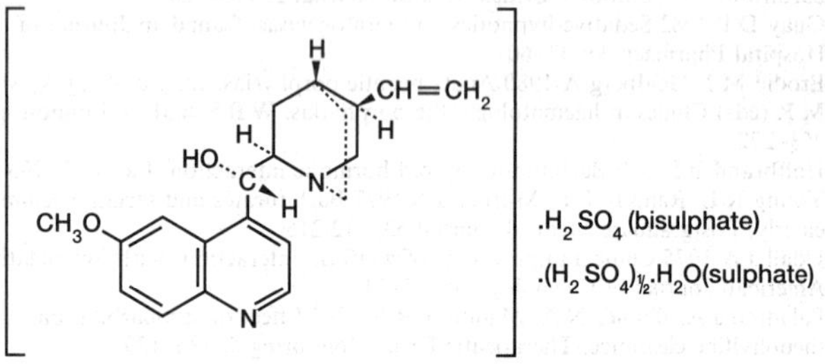

BISULPHATE	
Molecular weight (free base)	422.5 (324.5)
pKa	4.2; 8.8
Solubility	
in alcohol	1 in 3
in water	1 in 8
Octanol/water partition coefficient	high

SULPHATE	
Molecular weight (free base)	782.92 (324.5)
pKa	4.2; 8.8
Solubility	
in alcohol	1 in 10
in water	1 in 80
Octanol/water partition coefficient	high

Quinidine is a vegetable alkaloid obtained from the bark of species of *Cinchona* tree (Rubinceae) and appears as colourless, odourless crystals with an intensely bitter taste. The free base is highly lipid soluble. It usually contains 20–30% of hydroquinidine. Quinidine is the dextrorotory stereoisomer of quinine, it is highly fluorescent. The bisulphate appears as colourless crystals. The sulphate is a white odourless, fine crystalline substance with a very bitter taste.

Quinidine is not available in any combination preparations.

Pharmacology

Quinidine is a class I anti-arrhythmic agent[2] which induces use-dependent block of the sodium channel[3] in Purkinje cells and myocardial cells. Its membrane-stabilizing effect reduces automaticity. It decreases the rate of diastolic depolarization (phase 4) in cardiac Purkinje fibres. Quinidine slows conduction down the bundle of His, produces a small increase in action potential duration and prolongs the effective refractory period. Quinidine has negative inotropic effects on myocardial cells and relaxes skeletal muscle. Quinidine also has significant anti-cholinergic effects and some α adrenoceptor blocking activity.

Toxicology

Quinidine gluconate 200 mg.kg^{-1} causes myocardial necrosis in rats when injected intramuscularly or subcutaneously[4] and high doses induce acute electron microscopic changes in myocardial cells.[5]

Clinical pharmacology

Quinidine is an effective anti-arrhythmic agent in man. Its action to prolong the effective refractory period may be particularly useful in the treatment of re-entrant rhythms. The effect on the E.C.G. is to increase the P-R, QRS and QT intervals. The most obvious effect is usually a prolongation of the QT interval with inversion of the T wave. The negative inotropic effect of quinidine may precipitate heart failure, particularly when combinations of anti-arrhythmic drugs are given. Quinidine usually causes a small increase in the sinus rate, enhances A-V nodal conduction[6] and may cause a small fall in blood pressure due to the anticholinergic effect and the α-blocking effect. Quinidine, like quinine, has been shown to be effective in the treatment of falciparum malaria.

Pharmacokinetics

The preferred analytical method for quinidine, dihydroquinidine and the metabolites 3′-oxoquinidione and 3-hydroxyquinidine in plasma is assay by high performance liquid chromatography.[7] The limit of detection for quinidine is 10 μg.l^{-1}. Assay by dichloroethane and benzene extraction followed by fluorometry[8] gives values which are 2.3-fold too high due, to inclusion of metabolites.

Greater than 95% of administered quinidine bisulphate is absorbed from the gastrointestinal tract, 20–30% of which is metabolized before entering the systemic circulation.[9] When quinidine is taken with food the appearance of quinidine in the plasma is slowed due to delayed absorption and this is associated with a reduction in frequency and severity of side effects.[10]

Quinidine distributes rapidly to most tissues except brain, where accumulation is slower, with a volume of distribution of 2–3 l.kg^{-1} and a plasma half life of 5–12 hours in healthy men although there is evidence for a prolonged elimination phase with a half-life of 12–15 h. Peak plasma concentrations occur within 1–1.5 hours of oral administration.

70 to 95% of the drug is bound to plasma protein and this proportion is increased post-operatively and decreased by hepatic insufficiency or cirrhosis.[11] The binding is unchanged in renal insufficiency, respiratory insufficiency, hyperlipoproteinaemia and in the elderly.

Plasma levels are increased in congestive heart failure[12–14] due to a reduction in volume of distribution. Being a weak base, the renal clearance of quinidine is reduced by 50% when the pH of the urine increases from 6/7 to 7/8 (in renal tubular acidosis or acetazolamide administration) and the plasma concentration consequently rises.

It is excreted in small quantities in human breast milk. Quinidine is likely to cross the placenta.

Quinidine is extensively metabolized in the liver. The majority of a dose is excreted in the urine, 15-40% of the dose being recovered as the unchanged drug.

The plasma clearance of quinidine is reduced in the elderly and in hepatic disease. Although the elimination of the drug is virtually unaltered in renal failure, that of its metabolites, some of which are pharmacologically active, may be slowed. There is no evidence for enterohepatic circulation.

Oral absorption	>95%
Presystemic metabolism	20–30%
Plasma half life	
range	4–12 h
mean	7 h
Volume of distribution	2–3 l.kg^{-1}
Plasma protein binding	70–95%

Concentration–effect relationship

Therapeutic plasma concentrations are in the range of 6–12 μmol.l^{-1} (2–4 mg.l^{-1}). Following a single dose of 500 mg (Kinidin durule) given to 7 healthy volunteers, QTc prolongation was found to correlate with the rate of rise of plasma quinidine concentration but not with peak concentration; no blood pressure recordings were made.[15]

Peak plasma concentrations occur between 60 and 90 minutes following oral administration (3–4 hours in the case of quinidine gluconate). The oral administration of 250 mg quinidine bisulphate 6–8 hourly gives rise to a steady state in 24 hours with less than 50% variation in plasma concentration.

Plasma concentrations are of value to check the effectiveness of maintenance therapy for both treatment and prophylaxis of arrhythmias.

In the dog, between plasma concentrations of 1 and 5.7 $mg.l^{-1}$, there is a relationship between the logarithm of the plasma concentration and reduction in heart rate, increase in sinus node recovery time, increase in atrial to His bundle time and increase in His to ventricle conduction time.[16]

A study of the effect of quinidine on the electrocardiogram and systolic time intervals in healthy humans showed good correlation of plasma quinidine concentration and QT interval in the range 0 to 3.5 $mg.l^{-1}$ but no correlation with systolic time intervals, the results indicating activity of metabolites.[17]

Metabolism

Metabolism, mainly by the liver, accounts for the elimination of 60–85% of the drug from the body. 15 to 40% of the dose is excreted unchanged in the urine and less than 5% is excreted in the faeces.

Metabolism is predominantly by hydroxylation or dihydroxylation, the relative proportions varying amongst individuals. The major metabolites are 3-hydroxyquinidine[18] and 2′-oxoquinidione, both of which are equipotent to quinidine in their anti-arrhythmic activity and enter the hepatic venous blood in unconjugated form. O-desmethyl quinidine is less active, is produced mainly as the glucuronide conjugate and almost entirely accounts for the total biliary excretion of quinidine metabolites.[18] The unbound component of 3-hydroxyquinidine in plasma averages 26% and that of 2′-oxoquinidine 54%.[18] Other metabolites that have been detected include the 10,11-dihydrodiol and an N-oxide. Preparations of quinidine used clinically contain up to 30% hydroquinidine as a contaminant. This has similar pharmacological activity to quinidine.

During chronic oral dosing (25 patients, 12.3 ± 4.3 $mg.kg^{-1}$ daily) the 3-hydroxy/quinidine ratio was 0.61 ± 0.31 (SD) and the 2-oxo/quinidine ratio was 0.39 ± 0.44. There was marked variation between individuals, frequently with ratios of 1 or more. The ratios in patients with renal failure were not significantly different from those with normal renal function.[19]

Quinidine is a potent inhibitor of the form of P-cytochrome 450 that metabolizes debrisoquine to 4-hydroxy-debrisoquine (P450IID6). Drugs extensively metabolized by this route (e.g. metoprolol, nortriptyline) may have their effect increased.

Pharmaceutics

Quinidine is available in oral and parenteral forms.

Quinidine Sulphate (BP): Tablets, each containing 200 mg quinidine sulphate.

Quinidine Sulphate (USP): Quinora (Key, US) round flat white 300 mg tablets debossed 'QUINORA 300' on one side.

Kinidin Durules (Astra, UK). Film-coated, white, oval sustained-release tablet each containing 250 mg quinidine bisulphate, equivalent to 200 mg quinidine sulphate BP. They must not be dispensed in a metal container, but have a maximum shelf-life of 5 years in a glass bottle.

Kiditard (Delandale, UK). Light blue/dark blue sustained-release capsules each containing 250 mg quinidine bisulphate, equivalent to 200 mg quinidine sulphate BP.

Quinidex Extentabs (Robins, US), white sugar coated 300 mg tablets marked 'QUINIDEX/AHR'. 100 mg is released in the stomach, whilst 200 mg incorporated in the core is released gradually into the small and large intestine over a 6 to 8 hour period.

Quinidine sulphate. Injection. Ampoules containing 200 mg quinidine sulphate per ml.

Therapeutic use

Indications

1. Treatment or prophylaxis of:
   a. Atrial fibrillation
   b. Atrial flutter
   c. Extrasystolic atrial tachycardia
   d. Extrasystolic nodal tachycardia
   e. Ventricular tachycardia.
2. Facilitation of D.C. cardioversion and maintenance of sinus rhythm following D.C. cardioversion.

Note: (i) in atrial fibrillation and flutter it is effective mainly when the onset of the arrhythmia has been recent;
(ii) amiodarone is being used with increased frequency for the treatment of these acute arrhythmias.

Contraindications

1. Myocardial failure
2. Bi- or tri-fascicular block
3. 1st, 2nd or 3rd degree A-V block
4. Long Q-T syndrome
5. Myasthenia gravis
6. Thrombocytopenia or history of it
7. Known hypersensitivity to quinidine.

Special precautions

1. Pregnancy
2. Lactation
3. Impaired left or right ventricular function.
4. Quinidine is not the preferred drug for the treatment of arrhythmias due to digitalis toxicity because it can have adverse effects on the cardiac rhythm in this situation.[32,33]

Mode of use

A test dose of a single tablet of quinidine sulphate should be given to ascertain whether there is hypersensitivity.

A 12-lead ECG should be used to monitor the effects of quinidine. A small increase in heart rate, P-R, QRS and Q-T intervals[20] is seen with therapeutic plasma levels. The prolongation of the P-R interval is due to slowing of His-Purkinje conduction as evidenced by an increase in the H-V interval on the His bundle electrogram.[21] A-V nodal conduction may increase slightly due to the anticholinergic effect and this is seen as a reduction in the A-H interval on the His bundle electrogram. The degree of widening of the QRS complex is directly related to plasma concentration and can therefore be used as an indicator of impending toxicity;[22] it correlates better with plasma levels than does the QTc interval. The normal QRS interval is less than 80 msec. Administration of quinidine should be stopped if this interval exceeds 100 msec.

Blood pressure should also be monitored during acute administration of quinidine, hypotension due to myocardial failure being a feature of toxicity.

Acute treatment of the above-mentioned arrhythmias

Oral treatment. 200 mg quinidine sulphate orally every 2–3 hours for five to eight doses, with subsequent increase of the individual dose until sinus rhythm is restored or until early signs of toxicity appear. The tablets should be swallowed whole with water. The total daily dose should not exceed 3–4 g.

Parenteral treatment. 100–200 mg quinidine sulphate, depending on age, body weight, renal and hepatic function etc, intramuscularly every 2–3 hours, until sinus rhythm returns or signs of toxicity appear.

N.B. (a) continuous electrocardiographic monitoring and frequent (every 15 minutes) blood pressure recording is necessary in all cases in which quinidine is used in such high doses.
(b) patients with atrial fibrillation, atrial extrasystolic tachycardia and those with atrial flutter should be digitalized prior to quinidine administration. This is particularly important in the case of atrial flutter as, when the quinidine reduces the flutter rate, one-to-one conduction through the A-V node can occur leading to a very fast ventricular rate; this may profoundly reduce cardiac output and induce ventricular fibrillation.

Prophylaxis of the above-mentioned arrhythmias
200 mg quinidine sulphate 6 hourly, or 500 mg sustained release quinidine bisulphate 12 hourly. For the suppression of paroxysmal ventricular tachycardia[23,24] the maintenance dose should be adjusted according to the findings on continuous 48 hour ambulatory ECG (Holter) monitoring.[25] The aim should be to suppress all runs of three or more extrasystoles, particularly when the tachycardia rate is greater than 120 per minute.

Indications

1. Arrhythmias
Atrial fibrillation.[29,30] Quinidine's effect is by reduction of the inhomogeneity of repolarisation consequent on increasing the effective refractory period. In a controlled study of quinidine and flecainide, 30 patients with atrial fibrillation of more than 3 days duration were given 1200 mg quinidine per day. Conversion to sinus rhythm occurred in 60% of patients, in 80% when the duration of atrial fibrillation was less than 10 days and in 40% of patients when it was greater than 10 days. There were more adverse effects with quinidine but they were less severe than those encountered with flecainide.[31]

Atrial flutter. Its effect is related to both the increased effective refractory period and the prolongation of intra-atrial conduction.

Atrio-ventricular reciprocating tachycardia. Its effect is by slowing conduction and prolonging the effective refractory period, reducing responsiveness to stimulation and converting one-way to two-way block in re-entry loops. However, a number of more effective drugs are now available for the treatment of such tachycardias.

2. Facilitation of D.C. cardioversion and maintenance of sinus rhythm[26–28]

A. If 400 mg quinidine sulphate is administered orally 6 hourly for 48 hours prior to planned D.C. cardioversion, approximately one third of patients will have reverted to sinus rhythm, obviating the need for D.C. cardioversion. In the remainder D.C. cardioversion is facilitated, requiring lower energies with a greater success rate than for D.C. cardioversion alone.

B. After successful cardioversion the maintenance dose should be adjusted using the above guidelines to achieve a maintenance plasma level of 2–5 $mg.l^{-1}$.

Adverse reactions[34]

Potentially life-threatening effects
Hypersensitivity. Particularly in patients with a history of hypersensitivity, there is a risk of serious adverse effects such as granulomatous hepatitis,[35] exfoliative dermatitis, fever and thrombocytopenia. This last condition can be precipitated in those with a tendency or history of the condition. It usually occurs after several weeks or months of therapy and is mediated by antibodies, most commonly IgG, which cause platelet damage and in vivo sequestration only in the presence of the drug. The antibodies are heterogeneous and may be directed toward different epitopes on major platelet glycoproteins.[36]

Heart failure. Although adverse effects are not usually seen with therapeutic oral doses in those patients without evidence of heart failure, its negative inotropic effect will make heart failure worse.[37] In those patients with a history of heart failure and in those with treated heart failure it should be used with caution, and not until full clinical and two-dimensional echocardiographic evaluation has been performed.

Heart block. By its class 1 membrane-stabilizing activity, quinidine reduces ventricular automaticity and can therefore cause asystole in patients with complete heart block. If its use is essential, prior insertion of a temporary pacemaker is required. Because it reduces conduction velocity, it should be used with caution in patients with 1st and 2nd degree heart block and in those with fascicular block.

Cardiac arrhythmias. Premature beats, ventricular tachycardia, ventricular fibrillation or asystole can occur and are usually associated with high plasma levels. Quinidine-induced syncope with ventricular arrhythmia but normal plasma levels has been reported. In patients with the long Q-T syndrome, quinidine may precipitate ventricular tachycardia or fibrillation.[38]

Acute overdosage
Quinidine poisoning has been reported. The lethal dose is 8–15 g but a dose of 20 g has been survived. The symptoms in mild cases are those of cinchonism, i.e. impaired hearing, blurred vision, dizziness, headache and vomiting. In more severe cases abdominal pain, diarrhoea, anxiety delirium, hypotension due to myocardial failure and peripheral vasodilatation and cardiac arrhythmias occur. There is bradycardia with Q-T prolongation and QRS widening and ventricular arrhythmias. Ventricular fibrillation and asystole may occur with a fatal outcome.

Treatment of overdose. There is no specific antidote. Careful electrocardiographic, haemodynamic and respiratory monitoring is essential. Gastric lavage should be performed using charcoal 5-30 g, or sodium sulphate 20–30 g, in 25 ml water. Acidification of the urine will increase elimination, as will forced diuresis with mannitol. Severe cases will require haemodialysis. Dobutamine infusion and glucagon can be used for hypotension, and isoprenaline or pacing for bradycardia, heart block or asystole. Ventricular arrhythmias can be treated with lignocaine, phenytoin or D.C. cardioversion. Hypokalaemia should be corrected.

Severe or irreversible adverse effects
Myasthenia gravis. Quinidine may exacerbate myasthenia gravis by its depressant action on neuromuscular transmission.

Symptomatic adverse effects
Gastrointestinal irritation. Nausea and vomiting or diarrhoea are the most frequent adverse effects occurring during quinidine therapy. They have a tendency to resolve as therapy continues. Quinidine-induced diarrhoea can be ameliorated by aluminium hydroxide gel administered orally.[39]

Central nervous system symptoms
These are primarily associated with overdosage and disappear on reduction of the dosage. Known collectively as cinchonism, they include impaired hearing, blurred vision, headache, dizziness and vomiting.

Skin. Hypersensitivity reactions may cause urticaria, an exacerbation of psoriasis and lichenoid reactions.

There is evidence that adverse effects, particularly gastrointestinal, are less frequent and severe when sustained release preparations of quinidine are administered.

Interference with clinical pathology tests
Quinidine might interfere with fluorometric estimations of urinary catecholamines and with measurements of urinary 17-hydroxycorticosteroids.

High risk groups

Neonates
Quinidine is not recommended in neonates as its safety and efficacy have not been established in this group.

Breast milk. Breast-feeding is not recommended if the mother is receiving treatment with quinidine as the drug appears in breast milk.

Children
The drug is not recommended for use in children.

Pregnant women
There is a theoretical possibility that quinidine may affect the uterus and induce abortion since such an effect has been reported with quinine. Although satisfactory use of quinidine has been reported in pregnancy,[40] its use is not recommended if alternative therapy is available.

The elderly
Plasma clearance of quinidine is reduced in the elderly.

Concurrent disease
Hepatic insufficiency. It should be noted that the half life of quinidine may be significantly longer in patients with cirrhosis.[11]

Renal failure. Although the elimination of unchanged quinidine may be virtually normal in renal failure, that of metabolites may be delayed.[15]

Drug interactions

Potentially hazardous interactions

Digoxin. Quinidine may increase the plasma concentration of digitalis by up to 100%.[41–44]

Cimetidine. Cimetidine increases plasma concentrations of quinidine.

Other drugs. Quinidine may enhance the effects of antihypertensive agents, vasodilators, oral anticoagulants[45] and non-depolarizing skeletal muscle relaxants.

Drugs such as rifampicin, with enzyme-inducing effects, may enhance the metabolism of quinidine and thus reduce its effect.[46] Anticonvulsants, such as phenytoin and phenobarbitone, reduce the half life of quinidine by 50%.[47]

The negative inotropic effect of quinidine will be additive to that of calcium antagonists and β-blockers, particularly when they are given intravenously, and may induce myocardial failure in those with impaired ventricular function.

Potentially useful interactions

Quinidine can safely be combined with orally administered β adrenoceptor blocking agents[48–50] and verapamil.

Antacids containing aluminium hydroxide reduce gastrointestinal motility but do not affect the bioavailability of quinidine and therefore may be useful in countering quinidine side effects.[39]

Major outcome trials

1. Morganroth J, Somberg J C, Pool P E, Hsu P-H, Lee I K, Durkee J 1986 Comparative study of encainide and quinidine in the treatment of ventricular arrhythmias. Journal of the American College of Cardiology 7: 9–16

A nine centre, double-blind, crossover study in 187 outpatients, each with at least 30 ventricular premature complexes per hour on Holter monitoring. Following a 2 week period on placebo, they were randomized to encainide 25 mg four times daily or quinidine 200 mg four times daily for 2 weeks and these were continued for a further 2 weeks if greater than 70% reduction in frequency of the premature complexes occurred, otherwise encainide was increased to 50 mg four times daily and quinidine to 400 mg four times daily for 2 weeks. This was followed by a second 2 week placebo period with crossover. Both drugs produced a significant reduction in the frequency of premature ventricular complexes compared to placebo. Encainide produced a greater reduction than quinidine with fewer adverse effects.

2. Dinh H, Murphy M L, Baker B J, de Soyza N, Franciosa J A 1985 Efficacy of propafenone compared with quinidine in chronic ventricular arrhythmias. American Journal of Cardiology 55: 1520–1524

A single centre, double-blind, randomized, parallel study of propafenone compared with quinidine in 60 patients for the suppression of premature ventricular complexes and ventricular tachycardia. Two drug regimens were tested: propafenone 300 mg 12 hourly and 8 hourly, quinidine 200 mg and 400 mg 6 hourly. The drugs were equally effective in the suppression of premature ventricular complexes. With the lower dose regimen 100% suppression of ventricular tachycardia was obtained in 60% of patients in the quinidine group and in 56% of patients in the propafenone group. With the higher dose regimen 100% suppression was obtained in 80% of patients on quinidine and in 67% of patients on propafenone.

3. Arif M, Laidlaw J C, Oshrain C et al 1983 A randomized, double-blind, parallel group comparison of disopyramide phosphate and quinidine in patients with cardiac arrhythmias. Angiology 34: 393–400

A multicentre, randomized, double-blind, parallel group study of the efficacy of disopyramide 150 mg 6 hourly in 124 patients with more than 60 supraventricular or ventricular ectopic beats per hour on Holter recording, compared with that of quinidine 325 mg 6 hourly. The drugs had similar efficacy, with 55.4% of patients on disopyramide and 67.5% of patients on quinidine experiencing greater than 75% reduction in ectopic frequency. 22 of 62 patients on quinidine and 6 of 62 patients on disopyramide discontinued therapy due to side effects. Mean blood levels were 2.9 $mg.l^{-1}$ for disopyramide and 2.5 $mg.l^{-1}$ for quinidine.

Quinidine (bisulphate and sulphate)

Q

General review articles

Vaughan-Williams E M 1970 Classification of antiarrhythmic drugs. In: Sandoe E, Flensted-Jensen E, Olesen K H (eds) Symposium on cardiac arrhythmias, Elsinore, Denmark. AB Astra, Sodertalje, Sweden, pp 449–501

Wellens H J, Bar F W, Gagels A P, Muncharaz J F 1978 Electrical management of arrhythmias with emphasis on tachycardias. American Journal of Cardiology 41: 1025–1034

Hoffman B F, Rosen M R, Wit A L 1975 Electrophysiology and pharmacology of cardiac arrhythmias. vii. Cardiac effects of quinidine and procainamide. B. American Heart Journal 90: 117–122

Almeyda J, Levantine A 1973 Cutaneous reactions to cardiovascular drugs. British Journal of Dermatology 88: 313–319

References

1. Carroll F I, Blackwell J T 1974 Optical isomers of acyl-2-piperidyemethanol antimalarial agents. Preparation, optical purity, and absolute stereochemistry. Journal of Medical Chemistry 17: 985–987
2. Singh B N, Vaughan Williams E M 1972 A fourth class of antidysrhythmic action? Effect of verapamil on ouabain toxicity, on atrial and ventricular intracellular potentials, and on other features of cardiac function. Cardiovascular Research 6: 109–119
3. Lee K S, Hume J R, Giles W, Brown A M 1981 Sodium current depression by lidocaine and quinidine in isolated ventricular cells. Nature 291: 325–327
4. Benoit P W, Yagiela J A, Ferrel Fort N 1980 Pharmacologic correlation between local anaesthetic-induced myotoxicity and disturbance of intracellular calcium distribution. Toxicology and Applied Pharmacology 52: 187–198
5. Hiott D W, Howell R D 1971 Acute electron microscopic changes in myocardial cells induced by high doses of quinidine. Toxicology and Applied Pharmacology 18: 964–970
6. Mason J W, Winkle R A, Rider A K, Stinson E B, Harrison D C 1977 The electrophysiologic effects of quinidine in the transplanted human heart. Journal of Clinical Investigation 59: 481–489
7. Guentert T W, Coates P E, Upton R A, Coombs D L, Reigelman S 1979 Determination of quinidine and its major metabolites by high performance liquid chromatography. Journal of Chromatography 162: 59–70
8. Cramer G, Issaksson B 1963 Quantitative determination of quinidine in plasma. Scandinavian Journal of Clinical Investigation 15: 553–556
9. Mahon W A, Mayersohn M, Inaba T 1976 Disposition kinetics of 2 oral forms of quinidine. Clinical Pharmacology and Therapeutics 19: 566–575
10. Woo E, Greenblatt D J 1980 Effect of food on enteral absorption of quinidine. Clinical Pharmacology and Therapeutics 27: 188–193
11. Kessler K M, Humphries W C, Black M, Spann J F 1978 Quinidine pharmacokinetics in patients with cirrhosis or receiving propranolol. American Heart Journal 96: 627–635
12. Kessler K M, Lowenthal D T, Warner H, Gibson T, Briggs W, Reidenberg M M 1974 Quinidine elimination in patients with congestive heart failure or poor renal function. New England Journal of Medicine 290: 706–709
13. Conrad K A, Molk B L, Chidsey C A 1977 Pharmacokinetic studies of quinidine in patients with arrhythmias. Circulation 55: 1–7
14. Ueda C T, Dzindzio B S 1978 Quinidine kinetics in congestive heart failure. Clinical Pharmacology and Therapeutics 23: 158–164
15. Edwards J R, Hancock B W, Saynor R 1974 Correlation between plasma quinidine and cardiac effect. British Journal of Clinical Pharmacology 1: 455–459
16. Jaillon P, Heckle J, Juliard J-M, Aubry J-P, Weissenburger J, Cheymol G 1982 Relations entre les concentrations plasmatiques et les effets electrophysiologiques cardiaques de la quinidine chez le chien anesthesie. Journal of Pharmacology (Paris) 13: 227–289
17. Holford N H G, Coates P E, Guentert T W, Riegelman S, Sheiner L B 1981 The effect of quinidine and its metabolites on the electrocardiogram and systolic time intervals: concentration–effect relationships. British Journal of Clinical Pharmacology 11: 187–195
18. Yu V C, de Lamirande E, Horning M G, Pang K S 1982 Dose-dependent kinetics of quinidine in the perfused rat liver preparation. Kinetics of formation of active metabolites. Metabolism and Disposition 10: 568–572
19. Drayer D E, Restivo K, Reidenberg M M 1977 Specific determination of quinidine and (3S)-3-hydroxyquinidine in human serum by high pressure liquid chromatography. Journal of Laboratory Clinical Medicine 90: 816–822
20. Fieldman A, Beebe R D, Sing Sum Chow M 1977 The effect of quinidine sulphate on QRS duration and QT and systolic time intervals in man. Journal of Clinical Pharmacology 17: 134–139
21. Josephson M E, Seides S F, Batsford W P et al 1974 The electro-physiological effects of intramuscular quinidine on the atrioventricular conducting system in man. American Heart Journal 87: 55–64
22. Heissenbuttel R H, Bigger J T Jr 1970 The effect of oral quinidine on intraventricular conduction in man. Correlation of plasma quinidine with changes in QRS duration. American Heart Journal 80: 453–462
23. Bloomfield S, Romhilt D W, Te-Chuan Chou, Fowler N O 1971 Quinidine for prophylaxis of arrhythmias in acute myocardial infarction. New England Journal of Medicine 285: 979–1025
24. Jones D T, Kostuk W J, Grunton R W 1974 Prophylactic quinidine for the prevention of arrhythmias after acute myocardial infarction. American Journal of Cardiology 33: 655–660

25. Winkle R A, Gradman A H, Fitzgerald J W 1978 Antiarrhythmic drug effect assessed from ventricular arrhythmia reduction in the ambulatory electrocardiogram and treadmill test: comparison of propranolol, procainamide and quinidine. American Journal of Cardiology 42: 473–480
26. Byrne-Quinn E, Wing A J 1970 Maintenance of sinus rhythm after D.C. reversion of atrial fibrillation. A double-blind controlled trial of long-acting quinidine bisulphate. British Heart Journal 32: 370–376
27. Sodermark T, Jonsson B, Olsson H et al 1975 Effect of quinidine on maintaining sinus rhythm after conversion of atrial fibrillation or flutter. A multicentre study from Stockholm. British Heart Journal 37: 486–492
28. Bekes M, Bajkay G, Gulyas A, Maklari E, Torok E 1972 A cross-over trial of long and short acting quinidine preparations for the maintenance of sinus rhythm after defibrillation. European Journal of Clinical Pharmacology 4: 245–247
29. Stern S 1971 Treatment and prevention of cardiac arrhythmias with propranolol and quinidine. British Heart Journal 33: 522–525
30. Rosketh R, Storstrein O 1963 Quinidine therapy of chronic auricular fibrillation. Archives of Internal Medicine 111: 184–189
31. Borgeat A, Goy J-J, Maendly R, Kaufman U, Grbic M, Sigwart U 1986 Flecanide versus quinidine for conversion of atrial fibrillation to sinus rhythm. American Journal of Cardiology 58: 496–498
32. Ejvinsson G 1978 Effect of quinidine on plasma concentrations of digoxin. British Medical Journal 1: 279–280
33. Leahy E B Jr, Reiffel J A, Drusin R E, Heissenbuttel R H, Lovejoy W P, Bigger J T Jr 1978 Interaction between quinidine and digoxin. Journal of the American Medical Association 240: 533–534
34. Cohen I S, Jick H, Cohen S I 1977 Adverse reactions to quinidine in hospitalized patients: findings based on data from the Boston Collaborative Drug Surveillance Program. Progress in Cardiovascular Disease 20: 151–163
35. Geltner D, Chajek T, Rubinger D, Levij I S 1976 Quinidine hypersensitivity and liver involvement: a survey of 32 patients. Gastroenterology 70: 650–652
36. Pfueller S L, Bilston R A, Logan D, Gibson J M, Firkin B G 1988 Heterogeneity of drug-dependent platelet antigens and their antibodies in quinine — and quinidine — induced thrombocytopenia: involvement of glycoproteins Ib, IIb, IIIa and IX. Blood 72: 1155–1162
37. Crawford M H, White D H, O'Rourke R A 1979 Effects of oral quinidine on left ventricular performance in normal subjects and patients with congestive cardiomyopathy. American Journal of Cardiology 44: 714–718
38. Di Segni E, Klein H O, David D, Libhaber C, Kaplinsky E 1980 Overdrive pacing in quinidine syncope and other long CT syndromes. Archives of Internal Medicine 140: 1036–1040
39. Romankiewicz J A, Reidenberg M, Drayer D, Franklin J E 1978 The non-interference of aluminium hydroxide gel with quinidine sulfate absorption: an approach to control quinidine-induced diarrhoea. American Heart Journal 96: 518–520
40. Hill I M, Malkasian G D Jr 1979 The use of quinidine sulfate throughout pregnancy. Obstetrics and Gynecology 54: 366–368
41. Manolas E G, Hunt D, Sloman G 1980 Effects of quinidine and disopyramide on serum digoxin concentrations. Australian and New Zealand Journal of Medicine 19: 426–429
42. Leahy E B Jr, Reiffel J A, Giardina E G, Bigger J T Jr 1980 The effect of quinidine and other oral antiarrhythmic drugs on serum digoxin. A prospective study. Annals of Internal Medicine 92: 605–608
43. Dahlqvist R, Efvinsson G, Schenck-Gustafsson K 1980 Effect of quinidine on plasma concentration and renal clearance of digoxin. A clinically important drug interaction. British Journal of Clinical Pharmacology 9: 413–418
44. Schenck-Gustafsson K, Dahlqvist R 1981 Pharmacokinetics of digoxin in patients subjected to the quinidine–digoxin interaction. British Journal of Clinical Pharmacology 11: 181–186
45. Koch-Weser J 1968 Quinidine-induced hypoprothrombinemic hemorrhage in patients on chronic warfarin therapy. Annals of Internal Medicine 92: 605–608
46. Twum-Barima Y, Carruthers S G 1981 Quinidine–rifampicin interaction. New England Journal of Medicine 304: 1466–1469
47. Data J L, Wilkinson G R, Nies A S 1976 Interaction of quinidine with anticonvulsant drugs. New England Journal of Medicine 294: 699–702
48. Hillestad L, Storstein O 1969 Conversion of chronic atrial fibrillation to sinus rhythm with combined propranolol and quinidine treatment. American Heart Journal 77: 137–139
49. Fenster P, Perrier D, Mayersohn H, Marcus F I 1980 Kinetic evaluation of the propranolol–quinidine combination. Clinical Pharmacology and Therapeutics 27: 450–453
50. Ochs H R, Greenblatt D J, Woo E, Franke K, Smith T W 1978 Effect of quinidine on pharmacokinetics and acute electrocardiographic changes following intravenous quinidine in humans. Pharmacology 17: 301–306

Quinine

Quinine (in Jesuits' Bark) was the first antimalarial drug. Its use was firmly established long before the discovery of the malaria parasite.

Chemistry

Quinine (Chininum, used in the form of bisulphate, dihydrobromide, dihydrochloride, ethylcarbonate, formiate, hydrobromide, hydrochloride, salicylate, sulphate salts). It is a laevorotatory stereo-isomer of quinidine.
$C_{20}H_{24}N_2O_2.3H_2O$.
6-Methoxy-α-(5-vinyl-2-quinuclidinyl)-4-quinoline-methanol

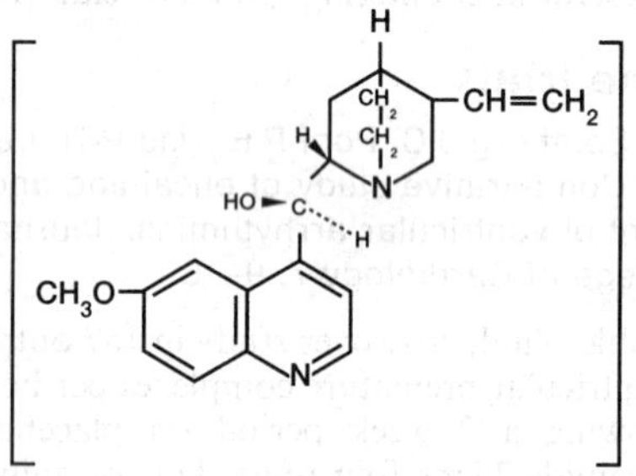

Molecular weight	378.5
pKa (quinuclidinyl group, quinoline group)	4.1, 8.5
Solubility	
in alcohol	1 in 1
in water	very low
Octanol/water partition coefficient	—

Quinine, a quinolinemethanol, is a white, flaky, granular or micro-crystalline powder with a bitter taste. It is laevorotary stereoisomer of quinidine. It is extracted from the bark of various species of *Cinchona* (Rubiaceae), where it occurs together with its dextrorotatory stereo-isomer quinidine and two other main alkaloids, namely cinchonine and cinchonidine. Chemical synthesis has been achieved but is uneconomic. Clinically, quinine is used in the form of salts, highly water-soluble ones especially for parenteral administration:

quinine bisulphate (Biquin, Biquinate, Dentojel, Myoquin, Quinbisan)
quinine ethylcarbonate (Euquinine, Equinina)
quinine hydrochloride (Kinin)
quinine sulphate (Adquin, Kinine, Quinamm, Quinate, Quine, Quinoctal, Quinsan)
quinine formiate (Quinoforme)
cinchona alkaloids (Quinimax).

Most of the salts have an intense bitter taste with the exception of the nearly water-insoluble ethylcarbonate.

It is also available in a mixture of several cinchona alkaloids.

Pharmacology

Quinine is believed to interfere with protein metabolism in malaria parasites. It is a potent and fast-acting antimalarial drug which has its most important indication in the treatment of potentially fatal severe and complicated falciparum malaria. Its numerous, mostly non-target, pharmacological effects in the human host, and its specific pharmacokinetics, necessitate the observation of very precise dose schedules.

Quinine has effects on the motor end plate of skeletal muscle to prolong the refractory period. It also has local anaesthetic activity, sensory nerves being briefly stimulated and then paralysed by the drug. The local anaesthetic effect is long lasting. Quinine is markedly irritant to local tissues, causing nausea and vomiting after an oral dose, and venous thrombosis after intravenous injection.

Toxicology

There is relatively little toxicological information on quinine in animal models, since the compound was introduced long before the creation of modern drug evaluation procedures. At clinical doses, which are usually close to toxic levels, there is no indication of mutagenic, carcinogenic or teratogenic effects. However, a multitude of pharmacological effects has been observed, some of which are used in the treatment of conditions other than malaria.

Clinical pharmacology

Erythrocytes infected by malaria parasites show active uptake of quinine. The antiplasmodial effect is related to the quinine concentration in the parasite. It affects the parasite's intra-erythrocytic mobility, and leads to a cessation of haemozoin pigment formation as a result of disturbed or arrested protein metabolism.[1] At concentrations considerably above therapeutic levels, quinine intercalates into parasite DNA and may thus inhibit nucleic acid biosynthesis.

Quinine decreases the excitability of the motor end plate and prolongs the refractory period hence its use against nocturnal muscle cramps.

The oxytocic effect of quinine on the smooth muscle of the uterus has long been overestimated. This effect is almost wholly confined to the gravid uterus, and only becomes important towards the end of pregnancy.

The cardiovascular effects of quinine are less marked than those of its dextrorotatory diastereoisomer, quinidine. Sinus arrest, junctional rhythms, AV-block, ventricular bradycardia, ventricular fibrillation and sudden death may occur with overdoses. However, apart from a prolonged QT interval, therapeutic concentrations of quinine are unlikely to produce cardiotoxicity.[2]

Quinine stimulates insulin secretion by the Langerhans islets in the pancreas; this may lead to hypoglycaemia which may confuse and/or aggravate the clinical picture of malaria.[3] Quinine has an analgesic and antipyretic effect which is advantageous in malaria treatment.

Pharmacokinetics

Of the non-chromatographic assays, a double extraction method with fluorescence measurement[4] is the most commonly used, but it does not differentiate between quinine and its metabolites. HPLC methods are more selective, sensitive and precise. Several reliable HPLC methods are available.[5,6,7] All employ fluorescence detection and have a sensitivity of 50 ng.ml^{-1}.

Between 80% and 90% of quinine is absorbed after the oral administration of quinine dihydrochloride, quinine hydrochloride, quinine bisulphate or quinine sulphate. Systemic bioavailability is of the same order as there is little presystemic metabolism. Peak concentrations are seen at 2–3 hours in fasting subjects. Following intravenous administration of quinine dihydrochloride (5 mg.kg^{-1}), the mean plasma half life in healthy adult males was 11.1$\pm$2.1 hours.[8] In another study involving oral administration of quinine hydrochloride (7.5 mg quinine base per kg), the mean half life was 8.7$\pm$1.3 hours, with a range of 7.0 to 10.7 hours.[7] However, in malaria patients plasma half life is longer, with a mean of 16.0 hours (range 8.1–31.2 hours) in uncomplicated malaria and 18.2 hours (range 5.8–47.2 hours) in cerebral malaria.[9]

Quinine is rapidly distributed throughout the body, with an apparent volume of distribution of 1.49$\pm$0.31 l.kg^{-1}.[7] In another study, in healthy adult subjects, the volume of distribution was found to be 1.80$\pm$0.37 l.kg^{-1}; that of the central compartment was 0.57$\pm$0.32 l.kg^{-1}.[8] There is a contraction of the volume of distribution in malaria that is most marked in cerebral forms, with a mean of 1.2 l.kg^{-1}.

Some 70–90% of plasma quinine is protein-bound. Protein binding is increased in severe malaria, with 92.8%$\pm$3.5% in cerebral malaria.[10] Acute phase reactant α_1-acid glycoprotein is likely to be the principle plasma binding protein.[11] The quinine concentration in erythrocytes of healthy subjects is one-fifth of that in plasma,[12] but higher concentrations are found in the erythrocytes of malaria patients.[13] This phenomenon is due in part to selective uptake by infected red blood cells, but uninfected erythrocytes are also involved, and concentrations slowly revert to normal after successful treatment.

The concentration of quinine in the CSF was found to be 7$\pm$3% of the corresponding plasma concentrations.[9] A CSF/free quinine ratio of 0.55$\pm$0.33 suggests that quinine does not freely traverse the blood–brain barrier.[10] Quinine is excreted in the breast milk in concentrations well below those found in plasma. The milk/plasma ratios varied between 0.11 and 0.53, with a mean of 0.31; the colostrum/plasma ratios were also within this range.[14] Quinine crosses the placenta. The cord blood plasma concentrations correlated significantly with the maternal plasma levels, with a mean ratio of cord plasma/maternal plasma quinine concentrations of 0.32$\pm$0.14.[14]

Quinine undergoes extensive hepatic biotransformation to hydroxylated metabolites, with less than 20% of the drug excreted unchanged in the urine. A small fraction (~5%) of the drug is eliminated through the faeces. There is evidence of enterohepatic circulation. Hepatic function is disturbed in acute malaria, and the degree of hepatic impairment is somewhat related to the severity of the disease. This explains the higher steady state plasma concentrations of quinine and prolongation of the elimination half-life during acute and severe malaria which tend to normalize rapidly under successful treatment. Significant renal impairment is also often associated with acute falciparum malaria. Although renal clearance of quinine is usually decreased with malaria infection, there is no apparent correlation between the severity of the disease and the reduction of renal clearance.[9] Renal excretion of quinine seems to be effected through both, glomerular filtration and tubular secretion.[9] Urinary excretion is increased when the urine is acidic.

With the standard regimen of 8-hourly intravenous infusions of 10 mg quinine hydrochloride per kg body weight, peak blood concentrations are usually reached on the third day of a seven or ten-day treatment course.[10] Peak values are usually in the range of 25–45 µmol.l^{-1}.

Pharmacokinetic parameters of quinine in children are significantly different from those in adults. The contraction of the volume of distribution during acute illness is more marked in children, but the elimination half life of quinine is shorter than that seen in adults,[15,16] especially after fever clearance. A marked contraction of the volume of distribution of quinine is also seen in acutely malarious pregnant women.[14]

The treatment of severe and complicated falciparum malaria requires the rate-controlled, intravenous infusion of a suitable quinine salt at 8-hourly intervals. A loading dose has proved useful for the fast establishment of effective quinine levels.[17] This is of particular importance in areas where the minimum effective concentration (MIC) of quinine against *Plasmodium falciparum* is close to the therapeutically attainable drug levels.

Oral absorption	>80%
Presystemic metabolism	<10%
Plasma half life	
range (healthy subjects)	7–11 h
range (severe malaria)	6–47 h
mean (healthy subjects)	8.7 h
mean (severe malaria)	18.2 h
Volume of distribution	
(healthy subjects)	1.5 l.kg^{-1}
(severe malaria)	1.2 l.kg^{-1}
Plasma protein binding	70–90%

Intramuscular administration of suitable quinine formulations may be the only means of treating comatose malaria patients in conditions where intravenous infusion is not feasible. The time to peak concentration tends to be longer than with oral administration,[18] and the area under the concentration time curve (AUC_{0-12}) 70% of that obtained with an identical quinine dose given by slow intravenous infusion.[19]

Absorption after oral administration is best with quinine hydrochloride, followed by quinine bisulphate and sulphate.[20] The absorption of the tasteless ethylcarbonate salt was almost equivalent to that of quinine sulphate.[21]

Concentration–effect relationship

There is a clear concentration–effect relationship with regard to the antimalarial activity of quinine. In severe and complicated falciparum malaria, fever and parasites cleared significantly faster where high quinine concentrations were established early in treatment by a loading dose and maintained at high level, as compared to cases where uniform standard doses were administered.[15] The concentration–effect relationship is also seen with the erythrocytic forms of *P. falciparum* in vitro, where it shows a log dose normal distribution.[22] In order to achieve parasitological cure, the quinine concentrations need to be maintained above the MIC for a period of at least 7 days. The MIC in vitro for *P. falciparum* is usually less than 1 mg.l^{-1} but resistant forms may have MIC values of 8 mg.l^{-1} or greater. This meets with compliance problems so that, in practice, short courses of quinine are usually given for rapid clinical improvement, followed by a radically curative drug that is better tolerated and simpler to use.

The non-target pharmacological effects also show concentration dependence; these include the stimulation of insulin secretion and resultant hypoglycaemia, cardiovascular effects and oxytocic effects. After an overdose of quinine, blindness and/or severe cardiac arrhythmias are likely to occur if the plasma concentration is above 20.0 mg.l^{-1}. Patients with severe malaria appear to tolerate high quinine plasma concentrations better than do non-infected patients.

Metabolism

Quinine is largely metabolized in the liver; less than 20% is eliminated unchanged in the urine. Less than 5% of a quinine dose is excreted in the faeces in the form of unchanged drug and metabolites. Metabolism is by oxidation to hydroxylated compounds. The 2-hydroxyquinoline and 6-hydroxyquinoline derivatives, 3-hydroxyquinine and the corresponding dihydro compounds are the most frequent metabolites. Quinine-10,11-epoxide and quinine-10,11-dihydrodiol have also been found in urine (Fig. 1).[23] All metabolites have less

Fig. 1 The metabolism of quinine

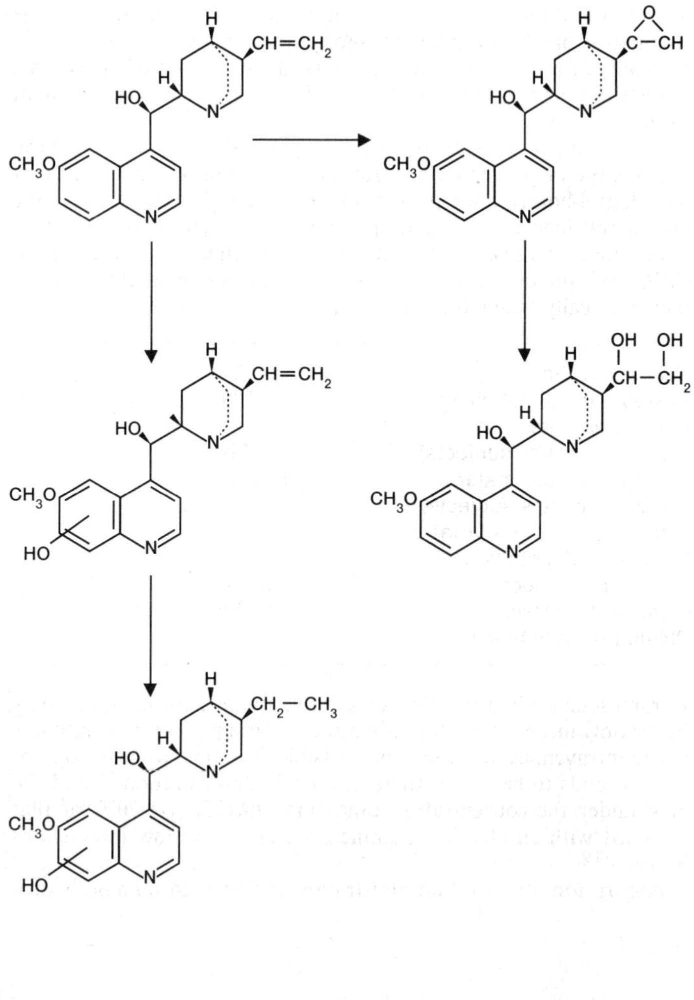

antimalarial activity than quinine. Their toxicological properties are largely unknown. Quinine may contain up to 10% hydroquinon as an impurity.

Pharmaceutics

Quinine is available in oral and parenteral forms. The various salts have different base contents, but it has not yet become customary to express doses as quinine base although this would render medication more reliable.

Tablets contain 300 mg quinine dihydrochloride, quinine hydrochloride or quinine bisulphate, or 125 mg, 200 mg or 300 mg quinine sulphate. These formulations are also available as enteric coated tablets and sugar-coated tablets. Quinine is also available in tablets containing 300 mg quinine ethylcarbonate, and in capsules containing 125 mg, 200 mg or 300 mg quinine sulphate.

Quinine is available for use by slow, rate-controlled intravenous infusion as a clear solution containing quinine dihydrochloride BP in the following formulations:

500 mg quinine dihydrochloride in 1 ml bidistilled water
600 mg quinine dihydrochloride in 2 ml bidistilled water
1000 mg quinine dihydrochloride in 2 ml bidistilled water.

These formulations are less suitable for intramuscular injection since they are not neutral and have a marked tendency to cause tissue necrosis. However, quinine formiate is better tolerated by this route.

A solution of several Cinchona alkaloids, Quinimax, is also well tolerated by the intramuscular route. It consists of 385 mg quinine-resorcin bichlorhydrate, 10 mg quinidine–resorcin bichlorhydrate, 2.7 mg cinchonin–resorcin bichlorhydrate and 2.7 mg cinchonidine–resorcin bichlorhydrate in 4 ml bidistilled water. Related to base content this formulation is at least as effective as other quinine salts, since both quinidine and cinchonine have an intrinsically higher antimalaria activity than quinine. If protected against light, quinine preparations are very stable and have a long shelf-life. They carry a minimal risk from potentially allergenic substances if they are produced under GMP. Most of the quinine formulations contain equally active hydroquinine in concentrations of up to 10%, and low concentrations of quinidine, cinchonine and cinchonidine.

Therapeutic use

Indications

1. Treatment of severe and complicated falciparum malaria
2. Treatment of falciparum malaria resistant to 4-aminoquinolines and sulfadoxine/pyrimethamine
3. Prevention of nocturnal muscle cramps
4. Alleviation of muscle cramps in Thomsen's disease (myotonia congenita).

Contraindications

1. Hypersensitivity to quinine and other cinchona alkaloids
2. Concurrent use with cimetidine, amiodarone, digoxin and other digitalis glycosides
3. Therapeutic administration of mefloquine within the preceding 14 days
4. Resistance of *P. falciparum* to quinine.

Mode of use

The uses against falciparum malaria depend upon the specific activity of quinine against the asexual erythrocytic forms of *Plasmodium falciparum*.

In falciparum malaria quinine is usually given at 8-hourly intervals in doses of 10 mg quinine salt per kg body weight.

In severe and complicated falciparum malaria this is given by slow, rate-controlled intravenous infusion of a solution of quinine dihydrochloride. A loading dose may be considered in such cases. The parenteral medication is replaced by oral administration as soon as the patient's condition has sufficiently improved and oral quinine is tolerated. If neither intravenous infusion nor oral medication are feasible, quinine may be given by the intramuscular route (deep, anterior thigh). Again, this is replaced by oral medication as soon as the patient's condition has sufficiently improved to tolerate it. This in

Quinine

turn is usually followed by another suitable medication in order to effect radical cure.

If quinine is used for treating multiresistant falciparum malaria of lesser severity, the drug is given by the oral route for 7 days. The quinine is accompanied or followed by a 7-day course of 250 mg tetracycline qds adult dose (or 4 $mg.kg^{-1}$ qds); this is contraindicated in pregnant women and in children below 8 years of age.

For the prevention of nocturnal muscle cramps, quinine is given orally at night in doses of 200 mg–300 mg of a suitable salt. Its effect is due to a decrease in the excitability of the motor end plate. The same specific pharmacological activity is used in alleviating muscle spasms in Thomsen's disease (myotonia congenita), where 2 or 3 doses daily of 4 $mg.kg^{-1}$ body weight are given.

Indications

1. Severe and complicated falciparum malaria

Quinine is the drug of choice for treating severe or complicated falciparum malaria, a condition defined by one or more of the following conditions associated with infection by *P. falciparum*: hyperparasitaemia > 5%, cerebral malaria, severe anaemia, renal failure, pulmonary oedema, circulatory collapse, shock, spontaneous bleeding, repeated generalized convulsions, acidaemia, haemoglobinuria, hyperpyrexia.

Administration of quinine dihydrochloride by slow, rate-controlled intravenous infusion is the route of choice for initiating the treatment of these conditions. The medicament is administered in doses of 10 mg quinine dihydrochloride per kg body weight diluted in isotonic infusion fluid or 5% dextrose solution (10 $ml.kg^{-1}$). The first infusion should run over 2 hours, the subsequent infusions over 4 hours each. The interval between infusions (start to start) is 8 hours.

In patients from areas where *P. falciparum* has a high MIC, such as the Indochinese Peninsula, a loading dose may be used if the patient has not been given quinine during the preceding 12 hours or mefloquine during the preceding 4 weeks. The loading dose of quinine dihydrochloride is 20 $mg.kg^{-1}$ body weight given as the first infusion, running over 4 hours.

In patients requiring more than 48 hours of parenteral therapy the maintenance dose of quinine dihydrochloride should be halved to 5 $mg.kg^{-1}$ in order to avoid undue cumulation of the drug.

When the patient's condition has improved sufficiently to accept and tolerate oral drugs, the parenteral administration is replaced by oral dosing of quinine dihydrochloride at 10 $mg.kg^{-1}$ every 8 hours. In areas with multiresistant *P. falciparum*, the treatment with quinine is conducted over 7 days and followed by a 7-day course of tetracycline, 250 mg qds (four times daily) adult dose. Medication with tetracycline may commence concurrently with quinine as soon as oral medication has become feasible again. Children below 8 years of age and pregnant women should not be given tetracycline.

In areas with chloroquine-sensitive *P. falciparum* the treatment with quinine may be discontinued when the patient is safely out of danger, and a standard course of chloroquine, total dose of 25 $mg.kg^{-1}$ body weight over 3 days, given for the elimination of the infection.

In areas with chloroquine-resistant but sulfadoxine–pyrimethamine-sensitive *P. falciparum* terminal treatment consists of a single dose of 25–30 mg sulfadoxine plus 1.25–1.50 mg pyrimethamine per kg body weight (with the exception of pregnant women).

Where rate-controlled intravenous infusion is not feasible, quinine may be used as intramuscular injection, following the same dose levels and intervals, with due attention to sterility of syringes and sound disinfection of the skin at the injection site. The injection is administered deep intramuscularly in the anterior thigh, using divided sites if a loading dose is given. The use of neutral quinine solutions reduces the risk and extent of tissue necrosis. Substitution by oral administration should be effected as soon as is possible without risk to the patient.

In children doses of quinine for parenteral administration are the same as those in adults, but for the subsequent oral treatment the 8-hourly doses are adjusted to 10 mg quinine base per kg.

Contrary to earlier fears and poorly documented anecdotal reports the doses of quinine used for malaria chemotherapy proved to be well tolerated during pregnancy.[14]

Quinine treatment may induce hypoglycaemia as a result of a stimulation of the Langerhans islets in the pancreas. This, together with a tendency to hypoglycaemia in hyperparasitaemic patients, may lead to dangerously low glucose levels which require continuous attention and correction as part of the complex ancillary management of severe and complicated malaria.[24,25,26]

2. Treatment of multiresistant falciparum malaria

Quinine is being used in the treatment of ordinary cases of falciparum malaria in areas with resistance to chloroquine and sulfadoxine/pyrimethamine, such as parts of the Indochinese Peninsula and South America. Quinine dihydrochloride is more suitable for this purpose than the commonly prescribed quinine sulphate which has a lesser bioavailability.[21]

The typical treatment course consists of the 8-hourly administration of quinine salt 10 $mg.kg^{-1}$ body weight for 7 days. Except in children of less than 8 years of age and pregnant women, this should be accompanied or followed by a 7-day course of tetracycline 250 mg qds adult dose (4 $mg.kg^{-1}$ qds for adolescents and juveniles) in order to effect a complete elimination of parasitaemia.

This regimen is feasible under hospital conditions, but meets with poor compliance among outpatients[22] on account of the side effects of quinine which tend to manifest themselves when the clinical symptoms of malaria have already subsided. It is therefore simpler and more efficient to use a single dose treatment with mefloquine.

In paediatric practice, the oral administration of quinine poses a problem on account of the intensely bitter taste of most quinine formulations. Coated tablets tend to vary with regard to the bioavailability of their quinine content and hence their therapeutic reliability. However, quinine ethyl carbonate is practically tasteless and its bioavailability comparable to that of quinine sulphate.[21]

3. Prevention of nocturnal muscle cramps

For the prevention of nocturnal muscle cramps quinine dihydrochloride or quinine sulphate is given at an adult dose of 200–300 mg approximately one hour before going to bed. In these conditions, quinine should only be given if a sound clinical and neurological examination fails to identify a cause other than a non-specifically increased excitability of the motor end plate.

4. Alleviation of muscle spasms in myotonia congenita

In myotonia, muscle contractions are prolonged and relaxation slow due to an abnormally high excitability of the muscle cell membrane. In Thomsen's disease (myotonia congenita) this is the sole symptomatology. It becomes manifest in early childhood and does not lead to dystrophic changes. Quinine hydrochloride, quinine sulphate or quinine ethyl carbonate are given at 4–6 $mg.kg^{-1}$ body weight three times daily. Monitoring of blood glucose levels is required.

Contraindications

1. Hypersensitivity to quinine or other Cinchona alkaloids

Hypersensitivity reactions to quinine are relatively rare and consist of fever, skin rash and also, occasionally, asthma and thrombocytopenia. Such reactions seem to be more frequent with quinidine, small amounts of which are also present in most quinine preparations. Cross-hypersensitivity between quinine and the other three main Cinchona alkaloids may also occur.

Hypersensitivity to quinine necessitates alternative medication. In the management of severe and complicated falciparum malaria, chloroquine may be used by slow, rate-controlled intravenous infusion. If there is resistance to chloroquine, mefloquine may be administered by nasogastric tube, once hypersensitivity to mefloquine, which is structurally related to quinine, has been excluded.

2. Concurrent use with cimetidine, amiodarone, digoxin and other digitalis glycosides

Quinine concentrations are increased if the drug is concurrently given with cimetidine. This may result in adverse reactions.[27] It is conceivable that amiodarone will also unduly increase the quinine concentrations since this effect has been observed with quinidine.[28] Quinine enhances the toxicity of digoxin and other digitalis glycosides both through reducing their renal clearance and by an interaction in the myocardium.[2]

3. Therapeutic administration of mefloquine within the preceding 14 days

Mefloquine on its own has an intrinsic cardiovascular toxicity which may enhance that of quinine when both drugs are present. Since mefloquine has a half life of 2–3 weeks, such situations may arise in areas where mefloquine is available for treatment. The major risk is with unconscious patients whose condition has continued to deteriorate in spite of medication with tablets of unknown nature. Under these conditions it may be difficult to withhold treatment with quinine, but this should be given very carefully by slow, rate-controlled intravenous infusion under continuous cardiovascular monitoring.

Quinine should not be used for the treatment of uncomplicated and non-severe falciparum malaria if the patient has received a therapeutic dose of mefloquine within the preceding 2 weeks. In such patients little may be expected from quinine in any case, in view of cross-resistance.

4. Resistance of *P. falciparum* to quinine

Substantial resistance of *P. falciparum* to quinine is quite rare. Low grade resistance is of little importance in the management of severe and complicated malaria since the main role of quinine in such cases is the fast suppression of malaria parasites and to expedite improvement of the patient's condition. This will usually be followed by complementary curative chemotherapy when oral medication has become possible.

Adverse reactions

Potentially life-threatening effects

When quinine is correctly used and at the normal therapeutic doses, life-threatening effects are rare and are only exceptionally due to hypersensitivity. They are almost exclusively of cardiovascular nature, namely sinus arrest, junctional rhythms, AV block, ventricular tachycardia, ventricular fibrillation and sudden death.[2] The risk of such cardiovascular accidents is high when quinine is given by ordinary intravenous injection, even if it is administered very slowly, and this procedure is now considered to be malpractice. Potentially fatal toxic effects of the same nature may also occur if an intravenous infusion is allowed to run too fast, especially when a loading dose is being used. This calls for careful, continuous monitoring of infusion speed.

Acute overdosage

Deliberate overdosing of quinine was and still is a frequent occurrence; it is only rarely with suicidal intentions, but mostly for the induction of abortion. Such an induction is however rarely successful, since the oxytocic effect in early pregnancy is relatively weak. However, toxic effects are marked in both mother and fetus. The most frequent result of acute quinine poisoning is visual disturbance, leading in some cases to permanent visual deficit or blindness, cardiotoxic manifestations, and lesions of the auditory nerve with hearing deficits and deafness. Nerve blindness and deafness were reported in infants of mothers who had taken toxic doses of quinine during pregnancy. The incidence and severity of quinine intoxication is related to the quinine plasma levels. Concentrations higher than 10 $\mu g.ml^{-1}$ are closely correlated with visual toxicity.[2]

Unintentional overdosing may result from disturbances of quinine metabolism and elimination which are usually observed in severe and complicated malaria. This is the reason for reducing the 8-hourly maintenance dose from 10 mg to 5 $mg.kg^{-1}$ when parenteral treatment needs to be extended beyond 48 hours. Such a situation indicates that the patient is in a clinical state likely to be associated with reduced quinine elimination. The toxic manifestations resulting from excessive quinine concentrations are similar to those seen with deliberate overdosing.

There is no specific antidote to quinine. Forced acid diuresis, stellate ganglion block and vasodilatator therapy have been suggested for treating quinine poisoning but were found to be without benefit.[2]

Severe or irreversible adverse effects

Such effects may occur under correctly conducted medication with quinine. These pertain mainly to visual disturbances and partial or complete loss of hearing, to cardiac conduction disturbances and arrythmia, and to hypersensitivity reactions. Among the latter, allergic thrombocytopenia and asthma are the most frequent, but circulatory collapse may also occur and lead to renal failure. Myopathy is a rare event. The occurence of haemolytic anaemia, the characteristic manifestation of blackwater fever, has been ascribed to a hypersensitivity reaction to quinine, but the role of quinine in the causation of this syndrome remains unclear.

Symptomatic adverse effects

Adverse effects of quinine are frequently seen and are the rule rather than the exception in correctly dosed malaria treatment. Most of the ill effects are part of a complex called cinchonism. The milder forms of cinchonism consist of tinnitus, headache, nausea and slight visual disturbances. More pronounced forms of cinchonism are characterized by vertigo, hearing deficiency/loss, and various manifestations of visual disturbances, such as blurred vision, reduced colour perception, diplopia, night blindness, narrowed peripheral vision and central scotomata.[2] Most of these manifestations are reversible, but permanent damage does occasionally occur.

Quinine may cause a prolongation of the QT interval, but cardiovascular manifestations are rare at quinine concentrations below 20 $\mu g.ml^{-1}$.

Mild cinchonism may also occur at the doses employed for alleviating muscle cramps in Thomsen's disease.

Other effects

Quinine has a marked tendency to stimulate insulin production. This may lead to dangerously low blood glucose levels, since falciparum malaria also often leads to hypoglycaemia. Infusion of 5% glucose may not suffice for correcting abnormally low glucose levels; intravenous injection of 50% glucose may be required. A synthetic somatostatin analogue was found to counteract quinine-induced hypoglycaemia.[29]

Interference with clinical pathology tests

Quinine may interfere with some methods of measuring urinary alkaloids, corticosteroids, 17-ketogenic steroids, 17-hydroxy corticosteroids and heroin, and may impart a brownish colour to the urine.

The drug may slow the erythrocyte sedimentation rate; and it may interfere with tests for plasma catecholamines.

High risk groups

Neonates

There is rarely occasion to treat neonates with quinine. Should the need arise, the dose regimens are as recommended on a drug/bodyweight basis. The treatment should be conducted under intensive care conditions.

Breast milk. Quinine is excreted in the breast milk of nursing mothers in concentrations similar to those of free quinine in plasma. The correlation between milk and maternal plasma quinine concentrations is significant.[14] The quantities of quinine taken up by the infant are below the threshold of antimalarial activity but they may suffice for causing sensitization or hypersensitivity reactions.

Children

Children tolerate quinine relatively well. There is also less risk of drug interaction in children, since the use of cardiovascular drugs is quite limited in this group. Malaria treatment follows the same principles as in adults.

Children receiving quinine for the alleviation of muscle cramps in Thomsen's disease are a special risk group, since the administration of quinine is continuous, albeit at a lower dose than in malaria treatment. Nevertheless, cinchonism may occur and necessitate a course with a suitable alternative medication.

Pregnant women

Until a few years ago, pregnancy was listed as a contraindication to the use of quinine for malaria treatment. However, recent studies provided no evidence that the quinine regimen used for the management of severe and complicated malaria stimulated uterine contractions or fetal distress. On the contrary, both frequency and amplitude of uterine contractions and fetal distress decreased under quinine medication, along with a drop of core temperature.[14] Thus it appears that malaria in pregnancy is responsible for the bulk of the manifestations previously wrongly ascribed to quinine.

Quinine medication in pregnant women is likely to provoke marked hypoglycaemia, since pancreatic β-cell response in pregnancy is amplified. This calls for the regular monitoring of the blood glucose levels.

Quinine

The elderly
The only potential special risks of quinine in the elderly stem from its interaction with cardiovascular drugs, especially digoxin and other digitalis glycosides (see Drug interactions).

Drug interactions

Potentially hazardous interactions
Digitalis glycosides. Quinine increases the toxicity of digoxin and other digitalis glycosides through both a reduction of renal clearance and interaction in the myocardium.[30]

Warfarin. Since quinidine is known to increase the hypoprothrombinaemic effect of warfarin[31] it can be assumed that quinine does the same, the more so as quinine exerts a hypoprothrombinaemic activity on its own.[2]

Other significant interactions
Rifampicin. The concurrent use of quinine and enzyme-inducing agents such as rifampicin may lead to increased metabolism of quinine and thereby hamper the achievement of effective levels; this is analogous to the effects of such agents on quinidine levels.[2]

Cimetidine. The concurrent use of cimetidine, which inhibits microsomal oxidation of quinine, increases quinine concentrations, which may therefore reach toxic levels.[27]

Other drugs. Quinine, like other quinoline derivatives, is a general inhibitor of drug metabolism by cytochrome P-450. This may result in higher than usual concentrations and an increased risk of adverse effects of concurrently administered drugs.[2] This field has not yet been sufficiently explored.

Hypoglycaemic agents. Since quinine is a potent stimulator of pancreatic β-cells, it can be expected to interact with antidiabetic medication and to play havoc with a pre-existing stabilization. Falciparum malaria is likely to do the same. Diabetic patients with malaria therefore require careful blood glucose monitoring during both the malarious episode and quinine treatment, and new adjustment of antidiabetic medication after these events.

Potentially useful interactions
None has been reported.

Major outcome trials

The four main alkaloids of Cinchona bark were isolated and purified during the first half of the 19th century. Quinine sulphate became a part of the second edition of the US Pharmacopoeia in 1830, and by 1832 the sulphates of the other three main alkaloids had also found their place in the sixth edition of the US Pharmacopoeia.[32]

The first major outcome trial was conducted in 1866–1868, with 3617 patients suffering from malarial fever. Identical dose regimens with quinine, quinidine, cinchonine and cinchonidine confirmed the high efficacy of these drugs. Fever clearance was not less than 97.6% in any one of the regimens.[33]

Many hospital- and field-based studies were subsequently conducted which served to elucidate suitable drug regimens for quinine. After the advent of potent synthetic antimalarial drugs, which are both simpler to use and generally better tolerated, the use of quinine gradually became restricted to the management of severe and complicated falciparum malaria.

The occurrence of resistance to chloroquine and sulfadoxine/pyrimethamine of *P. falciparum* in parts of southeastern Asia and South America stimulated new interest in quinine as an alternative drug for treating multiresistant falciparum malaria. At the same time modern technology and methodology were applied to the improvement of the use of quinine and quinidine in the management of severe and complicated malaria. This experience is summarized in a series of publications,[11,14,34–38] which indicate that quinine is currently the drug of choice for treating severe and complicated malaria. This is in spite of reductions in the quinine sensitivity of *P. falciparum* in areas where quinine has been extensively used.

References

1. Warhurst D C 1973 Chemotherapeutic agents and malaria research. In: Taylor A E R, Muller R (eds) Chemotherapeutic agents in the study of parasites. Blackwell, Oxford, pp 1–28
2. Orme M 1987 Side effects of quinine and derivatives. Acta Leidensia 55: 77–86
3. White N J, Warrell D A, Chanthavanich P et al 1983 Severe hypoglycaemia and hyperinsulinaemia in falciparum malaria. New England Journal of Medicine 309: 61–66
4. Cramer G, Isaksson B 1963 Quantitative determination of quinidine in plasma. Scandinavian Journal of Clinical Laboratory Investigation 15: 553–556
5. Edstein M, Stace J, Shann F 1983 Quantification of quinine in human serum by high-performance liquid chromatography. Journal of Chromatography 278: 445–451
6. Mihaly G W, Hyman K M, Smallwood R A, Hardy K J 1987 High-performance liquid chromatographic analysis of quinine and its diastereoisomer quinidine. Journal of Chromatography 415: 177–182
7. Jamaludin A, Mohamed M, Navaratnam V, Mohamed N, Yeoh E, Wernsdorfer W H 1988 Single-dose comparative kinetics and bioavailability study of quinine hydrochloride, quinidine sulfate and quinidine bisulfate sustained-release in healthy male volunteers. Acta Leidensia 57: 39–46
8. White N J, Chanthavanich P, Krishna S, Bunch C, Silamut K 1983 Quinine disposition kinetics. British Journal of Clinical Pharmacology 16: 399–404
9. White N J, Looareesuwan S, Warrell D A, Warrell M J, Bunnag D, Harinasuta T 1982 Quinine pharmacokinetics and toxicity in cerebral and uncomplicated falciparum malaria. American Journal of Medicine 73: 564–572
10. Silamut K, White N J, Looareesuwan S, Warrell D A 1985 Binding of quinine to plasma proteins in falciparum malaria. American Journal of Tropical Medicine and Hygiene 34: 681–686
11. White N J 1987 The pharmacokinetics of quinine and quinidine in malaria. Acta Leidensia 55: 65–76
12. World Health Organization 1984 Advances in malaria chemotherapy. WHO Technical Report Series no 711. World Health Organization, Geneva
13. White N J, Looareesuwan S, Silamut K 1983 Red cell quinine concentrations in falciparum malaria. American Journal of Tropical Medicine and Hygiene 32: 456–460
14. Looareesuwan S, White N J, Silamut K, Phillips R E, Warrell D A 1987 Quinine and severe falciparum malaria in late pregnancy. Acta Leidensia 55: 115–120
15. Chongsuphajaisiddhi T, Sabcharoen A, Attanath P 1981 In vivo and in vitro sensitivity of falciparum malaria in Thai children. Annals of Tropical Paediatrics 1: 21–26
16. Sabcharoen A, Chongsuphajaisiddhi T, Attanath P 1982 Serum quinine concentrations following the initial dose in children with falciparum malaria. Southeast Asia Journal of Tropical Medicine and Public Health 13: 556–662
17. White N J, Looareesuwan S, Warrell D A et al 1983 Quinine loading dose in cerebral malaria. American Journal of Tropical Medicine and Hygiene 32: 1–5
18. Wattanagoon Y, Phillips R E, Warrell D A et al 1986 Intramuscular loading dose of quinine for falciparum malaria: pharmacokinetics and toxicity. British Medical Journal 293: 11–13
19. Hall A P, Hanchalay S, Doberstyn E, Bumnetphund S 1975 Quinine dosage and serum levels in falciparum malaria. Annual report of the SEATO Medical Research Laboratories. SEATO, Bangkok
20. Garnham J C, Raymon D, Shotton E, Turner P 1976 The bioavailabilty of quinine. Journal of Tropical Medicine and Hygiene 70: 264–269
21. Tan S C, Navaratnam V, Mohamad M, Selliah K, Yuen K H, Wernsdorfer W H 1988 Comparative bioavailability of quinine hydrochloride, quinine sulfate and quinine ethyl carbonate. British Journal of Clinical Pharmacology 25: 261–264
22. Suebsaeng L, Wernsdorfer W H, Rooney W 1986 Sensitivity to quinine and mefloquine of Plasmodium falciparum in Thailand. Bulletin of the World Health Organization 64: 759–765
23. Moffat A C, Jackson J V, Moss M S, Widdop B, Greenfield E S 1986 Clarke's isolation and identification of drugs, 2nd edn. The Pharmaceutical Press, London, pp 954–955
24. World Health Organization 1990 Severe and complicated malaria. Transactions of the Royal Society of Tropical Medicine and Hygiene 84 (suppl 2): 1–65
25. White N J, Warrell D A 1988 The management of severe malaria. In: Wernsdorfer W H, McGregor I A (eds) Malaria. Principles and practice of malariology. Churchill Livingstone, Edinburgh, pp 865–888
26. Chongsuphjaisiddhi T 1988 Malaria in paediatric practice. In: Wernsdorfer W H, McGregor I A (eds) Malaria: principles and practice of malariology. Churchill Livingstone, Edinburgh, pp 889–902
27. Wanwimolruk S, Sunbhanich P, Pongmaruta M, Patamasucon P 1986 Effects of cimetidine and ranitidine on the pharmacokinetics of quinine. British Journal of Clinical Pharmacology 22: 346–350
28. Tartini R, Steinbrunn W, Kappenberger L, Meyer U A 1982 Dangerous interaction between amiodarone and quinidine. Lancet 1: 1327–1329
29. Phillips R E, Looareesuwan S, Bloom S R et al 1986 Effectiveness of SMS 201-995, a synthetic long acting somatostatin analogue in treatment of quinine-induced hyperinsulinaemia. Lancet 1: 713–715
30. Pederson K E, Madson J L, Klitgaard N A, Kjaer K, Hvidt S 1985 Effect of quinine on plasma digoxin concentration and renal digoxin clearance. Acta Medica Scandinavica 218: 229–232
31. Koch-Weser J 1986 Quinidine-induced hypoprothrombinaemic haemorrhage in patients on chronic warfarin therapy. Annals of Internal Medicine 68: 511–517
32. Dawson W T 1932 Antimalarial value of Cinchona alkaloids other than quinine. Southern Medical Journal 25: 529–533
33. Madras Cinchona Commission 1870 Return East India (Cinchona cultivation). Her Majesty's Stationery Office, London
34. Warrell D A 1987 Clinical management of severe falciparum malaria. Acta Leidensia 55: 99–113
35. Delacollette C, Cibanguka J, Buregea H, Nkera J 1987 Compared response to chloroquine, Fansidar, quinine and quinidine slow release of infections with Plasmodium falciparum in the Kivu region of Zaire. Acta Leidensia 55: 159–162
36. Bunnag D, Harinasuta T 1987 Quinine and quinidine in malaria in Thailand. Acta Leidensia 55: 163–166
37. Salako L A 1987 Quinine and malaria: the African experience. Acta Leidensia 55: 167–180
38. Wernsdorfer W H 1987 Quinine in health care in the tropics. Acta Leidensia 55: 197–208

Ramipril

Ramipril is a potent long-acting oral converting enzyme inhibitor, a pro-drug, which requires metabolism to its diacid, ramiprilat, for activity.

Chemistry

Ramipril (Tritace)
$C_{23}H_{32}N_2O_5$
2-(N-((S)-1-Ethoxycarbonyl-3-phenylpropyl)-l-alanyl)-(1S,3S,5S)-2-azabicyclo(3.3.0)octane-3-carboxylic acid

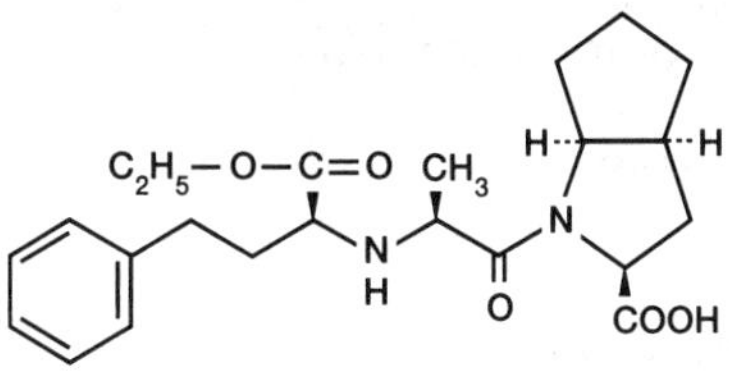

Ramipril

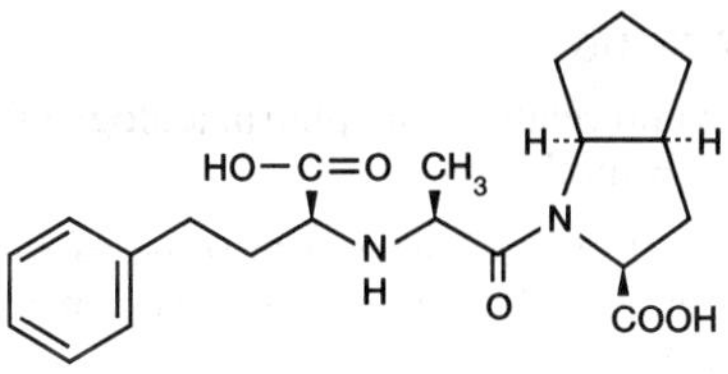

Ramiprilat

Molecular weight (ramiprilat)	416.5 (388.2)
pKa (ramiprilat)	3.1, 5.6 (1.55, 3.44)
Solubility	
in alcohol	soluble
in water	low
Octanol/water partition coefficient (ramiprilat)	0.06 (0.006)

Ramipril is a colourless crystalline substance poorly soluble in water. It is a pro-drug which requires cleavage of an ester group to form the active metabolite, the diacid, ramiprilat. Ramipril is prepared by chemical synthesis.[1]

Pharmacology

Ramipril (after conversion to ramiprilat) is a competitive antagonist of angiotensin-converting enzyme (ACE). Ramiprilat binds rapidly to form an initial enzyme–inhibitor complex which then slowly undergoes isomerization to give complete inhibition. The subsequent low dissociation rate contributes to the high potency and long duration of action of the drug. The overall inhibitory constant for ramiprilat is 7 pmol.l^{-1} compared with other inhibitors; e.g. enalaprilat (50 pmol.l^{-1}), and captopril (330 pmol.l^{-1}).[2,3] The enzyme renin cleaves the decapeptide angiotensin I from its substrate. The cleavage of the terminal two amino acids from angiotensin I by converting enzyme (which is widely distributed throughout the endothelium of blood vessels and within other tissues) produces the active octapeptide angiotensin II. ACE is a peptidyl peptide hydrolase identical with kininase-II and also therefore breaks down the vasodilator, bradykinin. Inhibition of this enzyme results therefore in vasodilation.

The characteristic result of inhibition of ACE is the loss or attenuation of the pressor response to angiotensin I. The pressor response to angiotensin II is not affected. In animal models of renal hypertension, such as the Goldblatt hypertensive rat, or the spontaneously hypertensive rat, ramipril effectively lowers systemic arteriolar resistance and both systolic and diastolic blood pressures.[4–6]

Toxicology

Ramipril and its metabolites have not been shown to have a mutagenic effect. Long-term toxicity studies, including carcinogenicity tests, have shown no untoward effects.

In common with other converting enzyme inhibitors, and therefore related to the mechanism of action of the drug, large doses will cause a reversible electrolyte deficiency which can damage the renal tubules. Ramipril may also cause fetal damage. However, in rats and rabbit embryotoxicity studies no intrauterine deaths were seen. Similarly in rat fertility studies using doses up to 500 mg.kg^{-1} there was no evidence of intrauterine death caused by ramipril.

Clinical pharmacology

Ramipril is rapidly absorbed after oral ingestion and converted in the liver to its active diacid, ramiprilat. Ramiprilat binds competitively with ACE, initially forming an enzyme–inhibitor complex, which then undergoes isomerization to a complex with a slow rate of dissociation.[2,3]

Ramipril is an effective drug for the treatment of hypertension. A single daily dose of 5 mg will reduce blood pressure for 24 h in chronic treatment. Doses as low as 1.25 mg may be effective for some patients. The dose–response curve seems flat between 10 and 20 mg, which is the average daily dose.[7–10] Although in theory it should be more effective in patients with high renin hypertension, in practice it lowers blood pressure in the long term and this is unrelated to the initial renin level. Blood flow in the coronary and cerebral beds is well maintained and renal blood flow is often increased following ACE inhibitors such as ramipril. Cardiac output and stroke volume are usually well maintained following ramipril, although a small fall may be seen. Aldosterone levels are usually reduced by ramipril but the output is maintained to near normal levels by ACTH.

Ramipril reduces afterload in patients with heart failure, due to systemic arteriolar dilation. As a result cardiac index and cardiac output increase and the drug, like other ACE inhibitors, is useful for the treatment of patients with heart failure.[11,12]

Measurement of components of the renin–angiotensin system in the circulation in man show that a single oral dose of 5 mg of ramipril, producing plasma concentrations of ramiprilat of 2 μg.l^{-1}, can suppress ACE activity to less than 20% of basal activity and angiotensin II concentrations for up to 24 hours (see General review articles). Tissue concentrations of ACE activity and angiotensin II may be more relevant to the drug's long-term effects; lower doses may provide 24-hour inhibition.

Ramiprilat is excreted largely through the kidney and the dose should be reduced in patients with impaired renal function.

Pharmacokinetics

The preferred analytical method for ramipril and ramiprilat in plasma is radioimmunoassay.[13] The drug and its metabolites in urine are assayed using a capillary gas–liquid chromatography technique.[14]

In fasting subjects peak concentrations of the inactive native drug ramipril are reached on average within 1 hour. Peak concentrations of the active ramiprilat are observed usually within 2 hours.[15] Delay of absorption with food is small and clinically unimportant. Ramipril is rapidly hydrolysed mainly in the liver to ramiprilat; some hydrolysis may occur across the intestinal wall.[16] With radioactive labelling of ramipril, 56±6% of a single dose was recovered in the urine and 39±5% in the faeces,[16] indicating 60% absorption. The drug and its metabolites may also be excreted in the bile, leading to an underestimate of absorption. This drug is widely distributed with a volume of distribution of approximately 91.5 l (430 l for ramiprilat).

Animal studies indicate that the drug may have differential effects on ACE inhibition in different tissues. Organs concerned with cardiovascular control, brain, kidney, vascular wall and heart, may be particular targets for the drug; its effects at these sites may be longer lasting than in the serum.[6,17]

R

In man both ramipril and ramiprilat are protein bound, 73±2% and 56±2% respectively, over a wide concentration range (0.01 to 10 mg.l^{-1}).[15]

Limited data indicate that ramipril and ramiprilat do not readily pass into the CSF (data on file Hoechst).

Animal studies suggest placental transfer of the drug is small. Although ramipril and its metabolites may be present in milk in concentrations of one-third those found simultaneously in blood, less than 1% of the dose given to lactating rats was excreted through this route.

	Ramipril	*Ramiprilat*
Oral absorption	~60%	—
Presystemic metabolism	occurs	
Plasma half life		
range	0.3–1 h	1.1–4.5 h
mean	0.6 h	3 h
Volume of distribution	91.5 l	430 l
Plasma protein binding	65–80%	50–60%

Witte et al[18] measured serum concentrations of ramiprilat up to 14 days after ingestion of a single 10 mg dose of ramipril in 10 normal healthy volunteers. A terminal half life of 110 hours was calculated. This is probably caused by the slow dissociation of ramiprilat from the enzyme–drug complex.[2,3] Accumulation of the drug does not occur with 20 mg daily, the maximum likely to be used clinically. At lower doses a steady state is reached within 1–2 days.[19]

Renal impairment results in elevated levels of the active metabolite, ramiprilat, so that some adjustment of dosage may be necessary. In patients with severe hepatic dysfunction there may be reduced conversion to ramiprilat, resulting in elevated levels of ramipril. It is suggested that lower initial doses should be used.

Concentration–effect relationship

Ramipril, after absorption, is rapidly converted to ramiprilat. Circulating concentrations of ramiprilat of 2 μg.l^{-1} or more will cause more than 80% inhibition of plasma ACE activity. Circulating concentrations of renin and angiotensin I rise and angiotensin II concentrations fall rapidly at this point. A dose of 10 mg will achieve circulating concentrations of ramiprilat of 2 μg.l^{-1} or more within 1–2 hours; this level will be reached sooner by larger doses and later by smaller doses. A dose of 5 mg or more will suppress circulating ACE activity to less than 20% of basal activity and angiotensin II levels for up to 24 hours (see General review articles).

The initial fall in blood pressure in patients relates well to circulating angiotensin II concentrations and therefore, if the levels are high, substantial falls in pressure may occur, usually 1–4 hours after dosing depending on the amount administered. Long-term pressure reduction does not relate well to the initial circulating concentrations of angiotensin II or to their reduction by treatment.

Metabolism

Three major metabolites of ramipril have been identified (see first review). The most important is the active diacid ramiprilat. The two diketopiperazine derivatives (of both drug and ramiprilat) are inactive. Conjugation with glucuronic acid accounts for a small proportion only of metabolism of ramipril and ramiprilat.

Excretion of ramiprilat throughout the kidney is the major route of elimination. Of the total urinary excretion of ramipril and its metabolites, 2% occurs as the unchanged drug ramipril, 3% as its glucuronide, 35% as ramiprilat, 3% as ramiprilat glucuronide, 35% as the diketopiperazine acid, and 8% as its ester. (Fig. 1.)

Pharmaceutics

Ramipril is available as Tritace (Astra, Hoechst, UK) capsules for oral administration. Capsule sizes are 1.25 mg (yellow/white) 2.5 mg (orange/white) and 5 mg (red/white). A parenteral form of ramiprilat may become available.

Ramipril has a shelf-life of 3 years.

Therapeutic use

Indications

1. Control of hypertension
2. Treatment of heart failure (this is not a licensed indication for ramipril in the UK).

Contraindications

These are relative and relate to the pharmacology of the drug and are relevant to all ACE inhibitors.

1. Bilateral renal artery stenosis and in some cases of unilateral renal artery stenosis when treatment may jeopardize the kidney with the stenosed vessel
2. Low blood pressure
3. High-dose diuretic therapy
4. Salt-depleted states
5. Renal impairment
6. Pregnancy
7. Use of potassium-sparing diuretics.

Fig. 1 Metabolism of ramipril

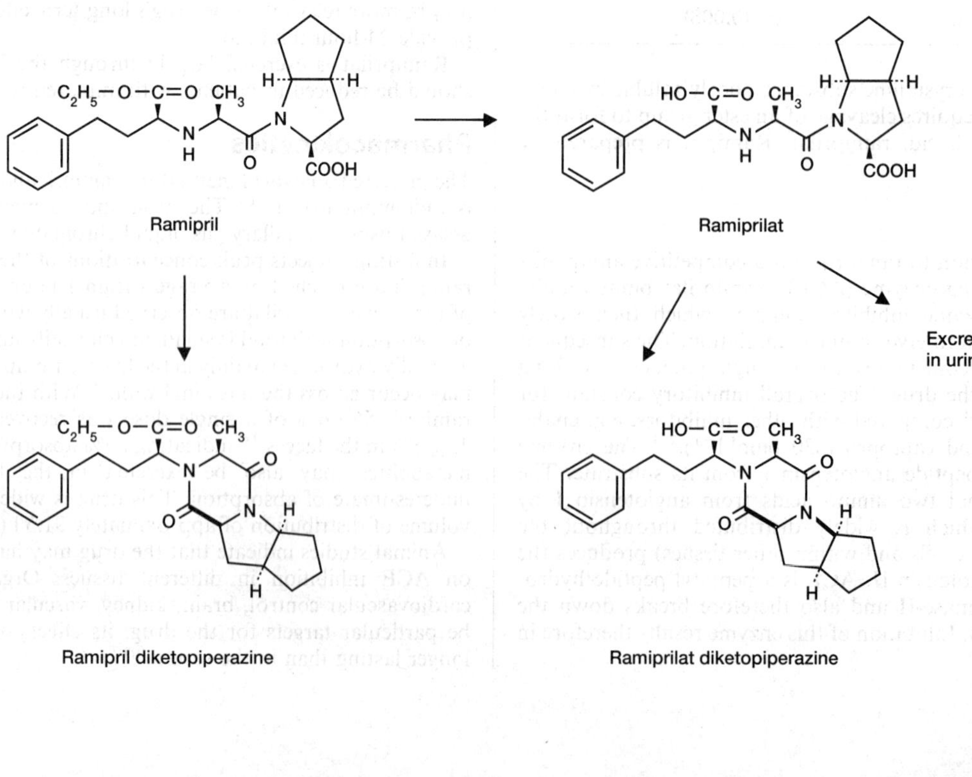

Ramipril

Mode of use

This depends on the indication for treatment. A low initial dose, 1.25–5 mg, is used, increasing to a maximum of 10 mg daily in those with normal renal function; lower maintenance doses are required for patients with renal impairment.[20–23] There seems little advantage in using the drug more than once daily. Sudden withdrawal of the drug is not associated with untoward effects. Tolerance does not appear to be a problem.

Dosage adjustment in renal impairment[20–23]

The usual dose of ramipril is recommended for patients with a creatinine clearance > 30 ml.min^{-1} (serum creatinine < 165 µmol.l^{-1}). For patients with a creatinine clearance < 30 ml.min^{-1} (serum creatinine > 165 µmol.l^{-1}) the initial dose is 1.25 mg ramipril once daily and the maximum dose 5 mg ramipril once daily.

In patients with severe renal impairment (creatinine clearance < 10 ml.min^{-1} and serum creatinine of 400–650 µmol.l^{-1}), the recommended initial dose is also 1.25 mg ramipril once a day but the maintenance dosage should not exceed 2.5 mg ramipril once a day.

Dosage adjustment in liver impairment

In patients with markedly impaired liver function the metabolism of the parent compound ramipril, and therefore the formation of the bioactive metabolite ramiprilat, is reduced due to a diminished activity of esterases in the liver, resulting in elevated plasma ramipril levels. Lower initial doses are recommended.

Indications

1. Hypertension

ACE inhibitors are effective antihypertensive agents with efficacy similar to other drugs currently available for reducing blood pressure[24,25] (see also review by Todd and Benfield). In patients with contraindications to the use of β-antagonists or diuretics they make a sensible initial choice. Ramipril is long-acting and can be given once daily to produce 24-hour control.[7–10,26,27] It combines particularly effectively with diuretics[28,29] (but see Contraindications) and the dihydropyridine calcium antagonists, challenging the traditional 'step-care' approach with one, two then three drugs. ACE inhibitors when combined with β-antagonists reduce blood pressure further than either alone, though some regard this as a less effective combination than that with vasodilating antihypertensive drugs. Postural hypotension is not a problem unless patients are 'salt-depleted' (see Contraindications). Apart from any immediate fall in pressure the maximal effect on blood pressure is likely to be reached 1–3 months after starting dosing.

Ramipril, like other ACE inhibitors, does not appear to adversely affect plasma lipids of patients with raised blood pressure.

A few anecdotal reports suggest that ACE inhibition may be useful in certain situations is patients with phaeochromocytoma, although α-adrenergic blockade in clearly the preferred treatment.

The mode of blood pressure reduction is not understood. The drug affects bradykinin and probably, indirectly, prostaglandin metabolism as well as interfering with the renin–angiotensin–aldosterone system and centrally or peripherally with the function of the sympathetic nervous system. The outcome is reduction of peripheral resistance without compensatory increase in heart rate, and therefore reduction of blood pressure. 25% of patients considered to have essential hypertension are usually classed as 'low renin' and probably respond equally as well to the drug in the long term as those with high circulating renin concentrations.

Renovascular hypertension. In the presence of unilateral renal artery stenosis, the kidney distal to the obstruction becomes ischaemic and secretes renin. ACE inhibitors would be expected to be particularly effective in reducing pressure in this group. Ramipril is no exception. However, concern exists over the fate of the kidney distal to the stenosis as the fall in pressure associated with removal of angiotensin II entering or being formed within the kidney may lead to a serious decline in glomerular filtration in this kidney. It has been suggested that renal artery occlusion may also be precipitated but the reported cases are not clearly drug-related. More seriously, if stenosis is bilateral, or if only one kidney is present, renal failure may develop, particularly in those on concomitant diuretic therapy. This is reversible if recognized early enough. Concomitant diuretic therapy may exacerbate the renal impairment.

2. Heart failure

Ramipril, in common with other ACE inhibitors, has been found to be effective in treating patients with heart failure[12,30,31] whose symptoms are not adequately controlled by digoxin and diuretics (but see Contraindications). The drug is renally excreted and therefore its dosage should be reduced in patients with this condition as invariably they have some degree of renal impairment. Patients with severe forms of heart failure may also benefit from the addition of ramipril to diuretic therapy; some of the benefit may accrue from blocking the stimulating effects of diuretics on the renin–angiotensin–aldosterone system. The initial dose should be low and great care is required in patients on high doses of loop diuretics.

Ischaemic heart disease. Although the majority of patients who have benefited from ramipril therapy for heart failure have underlying ischaemic disease, the role of ACE inhibition in the setting of ongoing ischaemia manifesting as chest pain is unclear. Since these agents venodilate and reduce afterload and, at least when circulating angiotensin II levels are high, reduce coronary tone, they might be expected to benefit those with angina. Alternatively, they could impair perfusion across a critical stenosis by reducing blood pressure too much, though the simultaneous decrease of pressure within the ventricle and vasodilation of the small distal resistance vessels would be expected to compensate initially and allow adequate blood flow to the myocardium. Current evidence indicates that those with stable angina do not suffer worsening of symptoms or exercise capacity when taking ramipril.

Contraindications

1. Renal artery stenosis

See above — renovascular hypertension.

2, 3, 4, 5. Salt- and water-depleted states

The initial fall in pressure on administration of an ACE inhibitor relates to the prevailing circulating concentration of angiotensin II. Patients who are 'salt depleted' through therapy with diuretics or illness, for example diarrhoea and vomiting, may have markedly elevated plasma angiotensin II levels and maintenance of blood pressure is critically dependent upon it. These individuals may experience precipitous falls in blood pressure when angiotensin II concentrations are reduced after the first dose of an inhibitor. The drug should be used with extreme caution in such individuals and fluid replacement or 'diuretic holiday' before starting therapy may be indicated. Interestingly ACE inhibitors may 're-set' autoregulation of cerebral blood flow and marked pressure falls may be tolerated without CNS symptoms. An appropriate reflex tachycardia often fails to occur in response to the fall in pressure induced by ACE inhibitors and thereby compounds the problem. Rarely syncope, with marked bradycardia, may ensue.

Patients who have low initial blood pressure through a cardiovascular disorder, for example those in cardiac failure who are often also taking large doses of loop diuretics, may be particularly susceptible and the initial dose should be small, 1.25 to 2.5 mg. Hypertensive patients on small doses of diuretics may also occasionally exhibit symptomatic hypotension with initial dosing.

Similarly symptomatic hypotension may occur with long-term therapy in such patients, necessitating reduction of the diuretic therapy.

The combination of low blood pressure and removal of the renal actions of angiotensin II may lead to renal impairment and even renal failure. This appears to be reversible if recognized at an early stage.

6. Pregnancy

Insufficient data are available to allow use of this drug in patients of child-bearing potential. ACE inhibitors have caused intrauterine death in animals, possibly due to disturbed blood pressure regulation in the fetus.

7. Potassium-sparing diuretics

ACE inhibitors reduce the formation of angiotensin II and consequently also aldosterone. Combination with potassium-sparing diuretics may lead to dangerous hyperkalaemia, especially if renal function is impaired. The combination may be clinically useful provided frequent monitoring of renal function and serum potassium is undertaken.

R

Adverse reactions

Potentially life-threatening effects
Deaths related to the drug have not been reported. The major concerns are severe hypotension and renal failure. Administration of any ACE inhibitor may lead to renal failure in some situations. These are discussed under Contraindications.

Acute overdosage
No reports have yet been published, but prolonged hypotension is the most likely immediate difficulty, with renal impairment developing in certain situations. Restoration of pressure by increasing blood volume should suffice; this can be achieved by elevating the patient's legs and infusion of plasma volume expanders/saline. Vasoconstrictor therapy is unlikely to be necessary. ACE inhibitors, possibly through removing angiotensin II, appear to 'switch off' sympathetic nerve activity and judicious infusion of noradrenaline (10 ng.kg^{-1}.min^{-1} increasing according to pressure and ECG response) may restore the circulation through its inotropic and chronotropic effects as well as its α-agonist properties. In extreme cases infusion of angiotensin II can be undertaken but this peptide is not readily available.

If restoration of blood volume and pressure with appropriate correction of any electrolyte abnormality fails to restore renal function then the management becomes that of acute renal failure.

Severe or irreversible adverse effects
The most serious adverse effects are hypotension and renal failure (see Contraindications). Severe angioedema leading to airway obstruction has been reported with ACE inhibitors. As with other ACE inhibitors some patients in stable mild renal failure have had rapid deterioration of renal function when non-steroidal anti-inflammatory drugs have been added to their treatment.

Symptomatic adverse effects
Headache, dizziness, nausea and vomiting, diarrhoea and rash have been reported. A mild dry cough is a well recognized side effect common to all ACE inhibitors. Rarely (1:1000) angioedema may occur with ACE inhibitors, usually in the first day or two of treatment. If angioedema involves the tongue, pharynx or larynx prompt treatment with adrenaline is required. Small increases in urea, creatinine and potassium may occur (see Contraindications).

Interference with clinical pathology tests
When ACE inhibitors are administered renin concentrations rise markedly. Absolute concentrations of renin in the circulation are therefore difficult to interpret but renal blood renin sampling may still be undertaken with the expectation of particularly high circulating levels for analysis.

High risk groups

Neonates
No information is yet available on the use of the drug in neonates.

Breast milk. Ramipril should not be used during lactation.

Children
No information is yet available on the use of the drug in children.

Pregnant women
Insufficient data on the use of ramipril during pregnancy and lactation in humans are available to permit assessment of the possible risk. From animal experiments it is known that use of ramipril may cause decreased utero-placental perfusion. There is also a potential risk of a fetal or postnatal effect as ACE inhibitors also influence the local renin–angiotensin system. Pregnancy should be excluded before start of treatment with ramipril and avoided during treatment; ramipril should not be used during lactation.

The elderly[32,33]
Renal function deteriorates with age and lower doses are appropriate. Cardiovascular reflexes may be more impaired and elderly patients therefore more at risk of hypotension than younger individuals.

Concurrent disease

Patients with collagen vascular disease. Agranulocytosis and bone marrow depression have been seen rarely in patients on ACE inhibitors, particularly high doses of captopril. This is more frequent in patients with renal impairment, especially if they also have a collagen vascular disease. No cases of agranulocytosis and neutropenia have been reported to date with ramipril. However, regular monitoring of white blood cell counts and protein levels in urine should be considered in patients with collagen vascular disease (e.g. lupus erythematosus and scleroderma), especially associated with impaired renal function and concomitant therapy with drugs, particularly corticosteroids and antimetabolites.

Renal impairment. See Dosage adjustment

Drug interactions

Potentially hazardous interactions

Diuretics and potassium-sparing diuretics. Concomitant administration may lead to serious hypotension with the former and in addition dangerous hyperkalaemia with the latter (see Contraindications).

Lithium. Serum lithium concentrations may rise if patients are receiving an ACE inhibitor in addition to lithium.

Alcohol. When first administered the reduction in blood pressure may affect the ability to drive and operate machinery and this may be exacerbated by alcohol.

Other significant reactions

Non-steroidal anti-inflammatory drugs. This type of drug, for example indomethacin, may reduce the antihypertensive effects of ramipril and cause deterioration of renal function.

Potentially useful interactions
ACE inhibitors inhibit baroreflex-mediated tachycardia and can be used with vasodilator drugs.

General review articles

1987 A symposium: ramipril — a new angiotensin converting enzyme inhibitor. American Journal of Cardiology 59 (10): 1D–177D

Todd P A, Benfield P 1990 Ramipril — a review of its pharmacological properties and therapeutic efficacy. Drugs 39 (i): 110–135

References

1. Teetz V, Geiger R, Henning R, Urbach H 1984 Synthesis of a highly active angiotensin converting enzyme inhibitor: 2-(N-((S)-1-Ethoxycarbonyl-3-phenylpropyl)-L-alanyl)-1S,3S,5S)-2-azabicyclo(3.3.0)octane-3-carboxylic acid (HOE 498). Arzneimittelforschung/Drug Research 34 (II): 1399–1401
2. Bunning P 1984 Inhibition of angiotensin converting enzyme by 2-(N-((SS)-1-carboxy-3-phenylpropyl)-L-alanyl)-1S,3S,5S)-2-azabicyclo(3.3.0)octane-3-carboxylic acid (HOE 498 diacid): comparison with captopril and enalaprilat. Arzneimittel-Forschung 34(II): 1406–1410
3. Bunning P 1987 Kinetic properties of the angiotensin converting enzyme inhibitor ramiprilat. Journal of Cardiovascular Pharmacology 10 (suppl 7): S31–S35
4. Scholkens B A, Becker R H A, Kaiser J 1984 Cardiovascular and antihypertensive activities of the novel non-sulfhydryl converting enzyme inhibitor 2-(N-((S)-1-ethoxycarbonyl-3-phenylpropyl)-L-alanyl)-1S,3S,5S)-2-azabicyclo(3.3.0)octane-3-carboxylic acid (HOE 498). Arzneimittel-Forschung 34: 1417–1425
5. Unger T, Fleck T, Ganten D, Lang R E, Rettig F 1984 2-(N-((S)-1-ethoxycarbonyl-3-phenylpropyl)-L-alanyl)-1S,3S,5S)-2-azabicyclo(3.3.0)octane-3-carboxylic acid (HOE 498): antihypertensive action and persistent inhibition of tissue converting enzyme activity in spontaneously hypertensive rats. Arzneimittel-Forschung 34: 1426–1430
6. Unger T, Ganten D, Lang R E, Scholkens B A 1985 Persistent tissue converting enzyme inhibition following chronic treatment with HOE 498 and MK421 in spontaneously hypertensive rats. Journal of Cardiovascular Pharmacology 7: 36–41
7. Walter U, Forthofer R, Witte P U 1987 Dose–response relation of the angiotensin converting enzyme inhibitor ramipril in mild to moderate essential hypertension. American Journal of Cardiology 59: 125D–132D
8. Villamil A S, Cairns V, Witte P U, Bertolas C A 1987 A double-blind study to compare the efficacy, tolerance and safety of two doses of the angiotensin converting enzyme inhibitor ramipril with placebo. American Journal of Cardiology 59: 110D–114D
9. Karlberg B E, Lindstrom T, Rosenqvist U L F, Ohman K P 1987 Efficacy, tolerance and hormonal effects of a new oral angiotensin converting enzyme inhibitor ramipril (HOE 498), in mild to moderate primary hypertension. American Journal of Cardiology 59: 104D–109D
10. Heber M E, Brigden G S, Caruana M P, Lahiri A, Raftery E B 1988 First dose response and 24-hour antihypertensive efficacy of the new once-daily angiotensin converting enzyme inhibitor, ramipril. American Journal of Cardiology 62: 239–245
11. de Graeff P A, Kingma J H, Dunselman P H J M, Wesseling H, Lie K I 1987 Acute hemodynamic and hormonal effects of ramipril in chronic congestive heart failure and comparison with captopril. American Journal of Cardiology 59: 164D–170D
12. de Graeff P A, Kingma J H, Viersma J W, Wesseling H, Lie K I 1989 Acute and chronic effects of ramipril and captopril in congestive heart failure. International Journal of Cardiology 23: 59–67

13. Eckert H G, Munscher G, Oekonomopulos H, Strecker H, Urbach H, Wissman H 1985 A radioimmunoassay for the angiotensin converting enzyme inhibitor ramipril and its active metabolite. Drug Research 35 (II) 8: 1251–1256
14. Schmidt D, Keller A, Fresenius Z 1985 Sensitive determination of the ACE inhibitor (HOE 498) and its metabolites in human urine by capillary gas chromatography. Analytical Chemistry 320: 731
15. Ball S G, Robertson J I S 1987 Clinical pharmacology of ramipril. American Journal of Cardiology 59/10: 23D–27D 16
16. Eckert H-G, Badian M J, Gantz D, Kellner H M, Voltz M 1984 Pharmacokinetics and biotransformation of 2-(N-((S)-1-carboxy-3-phenylpropyl)-L-alanyl)-1S,3S,5S)-2-azabicyclo(3.3.0)octane-3-carboxylic acid (HOE 498 Diacid) in rat, dog and man. Arzneimittelforschung/Drug Research 34: 1435–1447
17. Unger T, Ganten D, Lang R E, Scholkens B A 1984 Is tissue converting enzyme inhibition a determinant of the antihypertensive efficacy of converting inhibitors? Studies with the two different compounds. Hoe 498 and MK421, in spontaneously hypertensive rats. Journal of Cardiovascular Pharmacology 6: 872–880
18. Witte P U, Irmisch R, Hajdu P, Metzger H 1984 Pharmacokinetics and pharmacodynamics of a novel orally active angiotensin converting enzyme inhibitor (HOE 498) in healthy subjects. European Journal of Clinical Pharmacology 27: 577–581
19. Kondo K, Ohashi K, Saruta T, Shimura M, Toyodera K 1986 Tolerability, pharmacodynamics and pharmacokinetics of HOE 498 after multiple administration of 5 mg for 15 days in healthy male subjects. Japanese Pharmacology and Therapeutics 14: 339–359
20. Debusmann E R, Pujadas J O, Lahn W et al 1987 Influence of renal function on the pharmacokinetics of ramipril (HOE 498). American Journal of Cardiology 59: 70D–78D
21. Aurell M, Delin K, Herlitz H et al 1987 Pharmacokinetics and pharmacodynamics of ramipril in renal failure. American Journal of Cardiology 59: 65D–69D
22. Shionoiri H, Ikeda Y, Kimura K, Miyakawa T, Kaneko Y 1986 Pharmacodynamics and pharmacokinetics of single-dose ramipril in hypertensive patients with various degrees of renal function. Current Therapeutic Research 40: 74–85
23. Harada A, Inenaga T, Washio M 1988 Pharmacokinetics of ramipril in chronic renal failure. Current Therapeutic Research 44: 200–212
24. Zabludowski J, Rosenfeld J, Akbary M A, Rangoonwala B, Schinzel X 1988 A multi-centre comparative study between ramipril and enalapril in patients with mild to moderate essential hypertension. Current Medical Research and Opinion 11: 93–106
25. Witte P U, Walter U 1987 Comparative double-blind study of ramipril and captopril in mild to moderate essential hypertension. American Journal of Cardiology 59: 115D–120D
26. Kaneko Y, Omae T, Yoshinaga K et al 1987 Effect of ramipril, a new angiotensin converting enzyme inhibitor, on diurnal variations of blood pressure in essential hypertension. American Journal of Cardiology 59: 86D–91D
27. Tochikubo O, Asahina S, Kaneko Y 1987 Effect of ramipril on 24-hour variability of blood pressure and heart rate in essential hypertension. American Journal of Cardiology 59: 83D–85D
28. Weinberger M H 1989 Angiotensin converting enzyme inhibitors enhance the antihypertensive efficacy of diuretics and blunt or prevent adverse metabolic effects. Journal of Cardiovascular Pharmacology 13 (suppl 3): S1–S4
29. Bauer B, Lorenz H, Zahlten R 1989 An open multicenter study to assess the long-term efficacy, tolerance, and safety of the oral angiotensin converting enzyme inhibitor ramipril in patients with mild to moderate essential hypertension. Journal of Cardiovascular Pharmacology 13 (suppl 3): S70–S74
30. Manthey J, Osterziel J, Rohrig N et al 1987 Ramipril and captopril in patients with heart failure: effects on hemodynamics and vasoconstrictor systems. American Journal of Cardiology 59: 171D–175D
31. Crozier I G, Ikram H, Nicholls M G, Jans S 1989 Global and regional hemodynamic effects of ramipril in congestive heart failure. Journal of Cardiovascular Pharmacology, 14: 688–693
32. Gilchrist W J, Beard K, Manhem P et al 1987 Pharmacokinetics and effects on the renin–angiotensin system of ramipril in elderly patients. American Journal of Cardiology 59: 28D–32D
33. Meyer B H, Muller F O, Badian M et al 1987 Pharmacokinetics of ramipril in the elderly. American Journal of Cardiology 59: 33D–37D

Ranitidine

Ranitidine is a histamine H_2 receptor antagonist which was the second such drug (with cimetidine) to become generally available.

Chemistry

Ranitidine hydrochloride (Zantac, Zantic, Ranidil)
$C_{13}H_{22}N_4O_3S.HCl$
NN-Dimethyl-5-[2-(1-methylamino-2-nitrovinylamino)ethylthiomethyl]furfurylamine

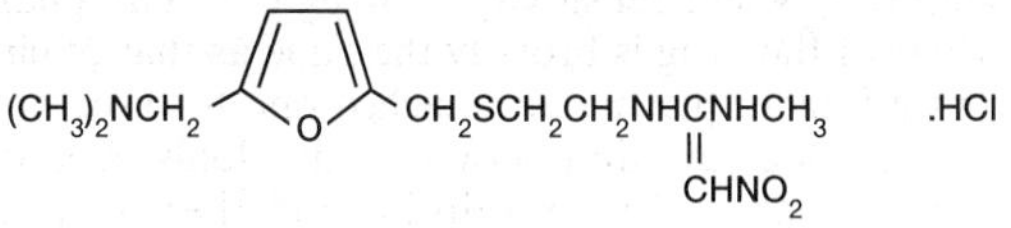

Molecular weight (free base)	350.9 (314.4)
pKa	2.3, 8.2
Solubility	
in alcohol	—
in water	>1 in 10
Octanol/water partition coefficient	—

An off-white solid with a melting point of 133–134°C and a slightly bitter taste.

Pharmacology

Ranitidine is a potent histamine H_2 antagonist. Thus it antagonizes the effects of histamine in vitro upon isolated guinea pig atrium and rat uterine horn, which possess H_2 receptors, but not guinea pig ileum which has H_1 receptors.[1] There is displacement to the right of the histamine dose–response curve indicating that ranitidine is a competitive antagonist. It is about five times more potent than cimetidine in these tests on a molar basis. It is a potent inhibitor of gastric secretion induced in response to histamine, pentagastrin, bethanechol and test meals.[2–4]

Toxicology

No significant toxicological abnormalities have been reported during extensive testing. The drug has proved neither mutagenic nor teratogenic. No carcinogenicity has been demonstrated during prolonged testing with high doses, such as 2000 mg.kg^{-1} daily for 2 to 2½ years in rats and mice.

Clinical pharmacology

The drug has been extensively tested in human volunteers and ulcer patients. When given in doses of 0.12–0.15 mg.kg^{-1}.h^{-1} intravenously there was approximately 50% inhibition of acid output in response to histamine, sham feeding, test meals and pentagastrin. Similarly, 50% or greater inhibition of acid output has been achieved in response to the same stimuli when oral doses of 50–150 mg were employed, the degree of inhibition varying according to the time after drug dosage. Effects have still been demonstrable after five hours but not after ten hours when conventional clinical doses (150 mg) have been employed. Ranitidine has been found to be at least five times as potent as cimetidine on a molar basis.[2–4]

Total pepsin output has been reduced in association with reduced gastric secretory volume but concentrations of pepsin were unaltered. No consistent changes in serum gastrin levels, in gastric mucus production or in pancreatic secretory output have been noted. Gastric mucosal damage in response to aspirin test meals is reduced.

Ranitidine

R

No consistent effects on gastrointestinal motility have been noted.

Ranitidine tends to form a ligand complex with hepatic cytochrome P450 but more weakly than cimetidine.[5] It does not, in contradistinction to cimetidine, inhibit the elimination of warfarin, theophylline or phenytoin, drugs with narrow margins between toxic and therapeutic doses, nor does it appear to retard the metabolism of diazepam, propranolol, aminopyrine or amidopyrine all of which are inactivated by the cytochrome P450 system.[6–9] Effects upon the metabolism of other drugs notably metoprolol are contested.[10,11]

Renal clearances of procainamide, carbamazepine and sodium valproate are modestly reduced.[12,13]

Ranitidine neither displaces dihydrotestosterone from androgen receptor binding sites nor reduces rodent seminal vesicle weight when given in high doses. Serum testosterone levels in man are unaffected nor have serum prolactin levels been affected except when intravenous doses are given, when effects are small.[14] A claimed association with gynaecomastia[15] has been contested.

No specific changes in immune function have been noted.

Pharmacokinetics

The preferred method of analysis is by high performance liquid chromatography[16] where sensitivity is 10 μg.l^{-1}. The pharmacokinetic behaviour of the drug is broadly the same as that of cimetidine. Peak concentrations in plasma are reached one to three hours after oral dosing with wide variation between individuals. About 50% of the drug is bioavailable after oral dosing and there is a significant first-pass effect. The area under the plasma concentration–time curve is not greatly affected by food. Plasma concentrations above 150 μg.l^{-1}, a value associated with a useful therapeutic effect, are maintained for three to five hours after a 150 mg oral dose. The drug is about 15% protein bound.[17–19]

The apparent volume of distribution[50] is between 1 and 2 l.kg^{-1} after intravenous injection with a total volume of about 100 l. Drug is detectable in cerebrospinal fluid at rather less than a twentieth of concentrations found in plasma, and the drug is detectable in breast milk and in semen. It does not affect spermatozoal motility.

Plasma clearance is in the range between 600 and 800 ml.min^{-1} after intravenous dosing, with unchanged drug forming the greatest fraction in the urine (70-80%). Most of the drug is excreted unchanged, 30–70% following oral dosing and 70–86% after intravenous dosing over the first 24 h. The elimination half life is between 1.5 and 2 hours after intravenous dosing, and slightly longer after oral dosing. As might be expected, elimination is considerably delayed in patients with renal failure; the drug is removed during haemodialysis.

Oral absorption	incomplete
Presystemic metabolism	—
Plasma half life	
range	2–3 h
Volume of distribution	1–2 l.kg^{-1}
Plasma protein binding	~15%

Concentration effect relationship

Although a dose-response relationship is evident, there is no clear relationship between plasma concentration and effect and thus there is little value in clinical practice is measuring plasma ranitidine concentrations. Useful therapeutic effects are usually seen when the plasma concentration is above 150 μg.l^{-1}.

Metabolism

Excretion of the drug and its metabolites is largely in urine. Unchanged ranitidine, the S- and N-oxides and desmethylranitidine are detectable in urine within 24 hours of dosing.

Pharmaceutics

Ranitidine (Zantac; Glaxo, UK/USA) is available in oral and parenteral forms as tablets syrup or dispersible tablets of 150 or 300 mg of the hydrochloride.

It is available in a strength of 25 mg per ml as a clear solution in ampoules for intravenous use.

Preparations are stable, have a reasonable shelf-life (tablets three years, injection three years) and are, for all practical purposes, unlikely to be allergenic. The injection should be protected from light, stored below 30°C and should not be autoclaved. It should be infused intermittently in glucose 5%, sodium chloride 0.9% or sodium lactate compound.

Therapeutic use

Indications

Those which are uncontested are:

1. The healing and maintenance treatment of gastric, duodenal and stomal ulceration, prophylaxis of NSAID-associated duodenal ulcers
2. Reduction of acid secretion in reflux oesophagitis
3. Control of acid hypersecretion in the Zollinger–Ellison syndrome
4. Prevention of Mendelsons syndrome
5. Prevention of acid-peptic digestion of pancreatic supplements in patients treated for chronic pancreatic insufficiency
6. Prevention of peptic ulceration in patients with renal disease after transplantation or undergoing dialysis.

Controversy exists over the true place of the drug in treating

7. Haematemesis and melaena
8. Stress ulcer prophylaxis
9. Functional possibly acid-related dyspepsia
10. Non-steroidal anti-inflammatory agent related dyspepsia

Contraindications

There are no clear contraindications to drug use other than known hypersensitivity.

Indications

Ranitidine is, in general, an effective drug in all conditions where inhibition of acid-peptic digestion is indicated.

1. The healing and maintenance treatment of gastric, duodenal and stomal ulceration

Oral treatment in doses of 100–150 mg twice daily or 300 mg at night promotes duodenal ulcer healing more rapidly and more often than during placebo treatment.[20–22] Healing properties are broadly equivalent to those of cimetidine and to those of other standard ulcer-healing remedies including chelated bismuth, sucralfate and pirenzepine. The increase in proportions of ulcers which heal varies from community to community according, inter alia, to the placebo healing rate and to patient compliance. Thus in the UK a placebo healing rate of 30% is raised to about 80% following one month's treatment and to 90% or more if treatment is prolonged. Resistance to treatment is uncommon and depends upon a variety of factors which probably include poor compliance, reduced responsiveness in smokers, and genuine reduced inhibitory effect in a few individuals.

Generally similar considerations apply for gastric ulcer healing to those which operate for duodenal ulcer disease. Drug dosage is similar, and healing responses are much the same in rate and proportion as in duodenal ulcer.[23,24] Treatment (as in duodenal ulcer) is somewhat less effective than with the proton pump inhibitor omeprazole although ultimately healing rates are high[43,44]. Ranitidine will also prevent nonsteroidal-induced mucosal damage and duodenal but not gastric ulcer[45,46,47].

Ranitidine treatment is effective in reducing the rate of both duodenal and gastric ulcer recurrence. In general terms recurrence rates can be expected to be reduced to about 10 to 20% when 150 mg of ranitidine is taken daily at night for 6 to 12 months instead of being 50 to 80% when placebo tablets are taken.[23,25] Direct comparison between 150 mg of ranitidine and 400 mg of cimetidine in duodenal ulcer disease suggests that ranitidine may be more effective in keeping with the generally greater potency but the differences are not great. Parallel comparisons of efficacy in gastric ulcer maintenance are not available.[25]

2. Reflux oesophagitis

Treatment ameliorates symptoms of heartburn and odynophagia but may (by analogy with cimetidine) have little influence upon any

Ranitidine

tendency to stricture formation although the endoscopic appearances of oesophagitis are improved by treatment. Treatment is more effective in minor grades of disease and less effective than omeprazole in severe erosive disease[48].

3. Zollinger–Ellison syndrome
Ranitidine like cimetidine is effective but high doses, several times those used for duodenal ulcer, may be necessary. In addition, concurrent treatment with an antimuscarinic agent like pirenzepine may be necessary.[26]

4. Protection against Mendelson's syndrome
Ranitidine and cimetidine are effective in reducing the volume of gastric secretion and in raising the pH of secretions in surgical and obstetric patients requiring urgent operations, and so protect against aspiration damage to the lungs.[27] Doses of 50–100 mg intravenously or 150 mg orally are required.

5. Treatment of chronic pancreatitis
Pancreatic supplements are susceptible to acid-peptic digestion. Antisecretory treatment reduces this and can therefore ameliorate steatorrhoea when pancreatic supplements on their own are apparently ineffective.

6. Treatment of patients with renal disease
Patients undergoing dialysis, or with renal transplants, are susceptible to peptic ulceration and H_2 antagonists can prevent this. Doses may need reducing as the drug is ordinarily eliminated by the kidneys.

7. Haematemesis and melaena
Small case series have been reported in which evidence of benefit has been claimed, for instance in duodenal ulcer. No trial is of sufficient size to stand on its own and give a clear indication that treatment is valuable, but combined analysis of all available trials of H_2 antagonists suggests that there may be a useful clinical effect.[28]

8. Prevention of haemorrhage from stress ulceration
Though theoretically treatment might be expected to be effective, good supportive trial data are lacking except on managing patients with fulminant hepatic failure (with cimetidine). Difficulties in establishing that drug treatment is of value in stress ulceration or in haematemesis and melaena may stem from the failure of clinicians to determine what is the right dose of drugs to give parenterally. Recommended doses, such as 50 mg twice daily by injection, may be too low if analogy with cimetidine holds[29] given the expected rate of drug elimination.

9. Functional possibly acid-related dyspepsia
The place of antisecretory drug treatment is unclear, basically because the condition is ill defined and heterogeneous and because a high placebo response rate is to be expected. The drug is nevertheless widely used and may be effective in some patients.[49].

10. Non-steroidal anti-inflammatory agent-related dyspepsia
There is widespread clinical suspicion that this condition is associated with undue susceptibility to acid-peptic attack. H_2 antagonists are therefore commonly prescribed in the hope of ameliorating symptoms and preventing overt ulceration[46].

Adverse reactions

Potentially life-threatening effects
None has been reported.

Acute overdosage
No specific effects of gross drug overdosage are to be expected.

Severe or irreversible adverse effects
Abnormal liver function tests have been reported in patients taking ranitidine but a clear causal relationship has not been established, and the occurrence of toxic hepatitis has not therefore been clarified although recurrence on rechallenge is reported.[30,31] Likewise toxic haematological effects have not been firmly established.

Symptomatic adverse effects
Headache, dizziness, rash, constipation, diarrhoea and nausea have been reported in very small proportions of patients taking ranitidine, and placebo.[23,32] Headache and rash have recurred in some of those rechallenged with active drug. The drug is not antiandrogenic. Isolated reports of drug-induced gynaecomastia or impotence are poorly supported. The drug does, however, enter the cerebrospinal fluid and confusion, which reverses rapidly on stopping treatment, has been reported.[33–35]

Other effects
Spurious healing can be induced in malignant ulcers which delays the true diagnosis: this occurs as with any other effective antiulcer drug. Severe rebound recurrence of benign ulceration, though postulated, has not proved to be a clinical problem.

Reduced intrinsic factor production and retarded absorption of cobalamins from food have been demonstrated.[36,37] Whether these short-term effects have any practical consequences in ordinary use is doubtful.

Inhibition of cholinesterases has been demonstrated as has interference with aldosterone secretion.[38,39] These do not seem to be of such a degree as to have practical consequences.

Interference with clinical pathology tests
No technical interferences of this kind have been reported.

High risk groups

Neonates
There is no indication for drug use in this age-group.

Breast milk. Drug is detectable in breast milk in concentrations roughly equivalent to those in plasma. No adverse effects are to be expected.

Children
Doses of 50–150 mg daily by mouth or 0.5–1.0 $mg.kg^{-1}$ intravenously have been used uneventfully in treating childhood ulcer.

Pregnant women
Safety has not been completely established although many will have received the drug. No fetal effects are recognized.

The elderly
There is a theoretical risk that high doses might precipitate confusion but it does not seem to be a practical risk during ordinary oral treatment.

Concurrent disease
Elimination of the drug is delayed in patients with renal failure, but this delay does not appear to have clinical significance.

Drug interactions

Potentially hazardous interactions
None is described.

Other significant interactions
Despite the observable binding of ranitidine in vitro to hepatic microsomal cytochrome P450,[5] there is no good evidence that clinically significant retardation of metabolism of drugs by the mixed function oxidase system occurs. Isolated reports[40] of apparent interaction are difficult to place in general context. No coherent body of evidence exists to suggest that the drug can induce carcinoma either directly through nitrosated products or indirectly through bacterial nitrosamine formation in the hypoacidic stomach.[41]

Drug absorption does not seem to be significantly altered by concurrent food intake. Smoking does however reduce the clinical effectiveness of H_2 antagonists, about 10% less ulcers healing than in non-smokers.[42]

Potentially useful interactions
None has been described.

Clinical trials

In acute ulcer, healing results are generally uniform with high rates of ulcer healing in randomized controlled trials compared with the outcome in individuals given placebo. No particular study is pre-eminent. A fair and detailed analysis has been presented in the following review.

1. Grant S M, Langtry H D, Brogden R N 1989 Ranitidine: an updated review of its pharmacodynamioc and pharmacokinetic properties and therapeutic use in peptic ulcer disease and other allied diseases. Drugs 37: 801–70

R

Ranitidine

R

2. Gough K R, Korman M G, Bardhan K D, Lee F I, Crowe J P, Reed P I 1984 Ranitidine and cimetidine in prevention of duodenal ulcer relapse. Lancet 2: 659–662

In maintenance treatment, direct comparison with cimetidine suggests a marginal advantage to ranitidine. In this very large study 484 patients with healed duodenal ulcers were randomly allocated to bedtime treatment with ranitidine 150 mg (n=243) or cimetidine (n=241). As calculated using life tables relapse was less frequent in ranitidine recipients (cimetidine 37% at 12 months compared with ranitidine 21%). The difference may in part be explainable by the compliance with treatment method which, whilst using a double-dummy technique, required patients to take two 200 mg cimetidine tablets or one 150 mg ranitidine tablet to be effective. However, differences were manifest at all levels of compliance. Given the five times greater potency of ranitidine a difference was to be expected, although it is likely to be of minor importance in clinical practice where in acute healing the drugs are for practical purposes equivalent, and where prolonged maintenance treatment is less likely to be undertaken than intermittent therapy.

References

1. Woodings E P, Dixon G T, Harrison C, Carey P, Richards D A 1980 Ranitidine — a new H_2 receptor antagonist. Gut 21: 187–191
2. Sewing K Fr, Billian A, Malchow H 1980 Comparative study with ranitidine and cimetidine on gastric secretion in normal volunteers. Gut 21: 750
3. Walt R P, Male P J, Rawlings J, Hunt R, Milton Thompson G J, Misiewicz J J 1981 Comparison of the effects of ranitidine, cimetidine and placebo on the 24 hour intragastric acidity and nocturnal acid secretion in patients with duodenal ulcer. Gut 22: 49–54
4. Gledhill T, Howard O M, Buck M, Paul A, Hunt R H 1983 Single nocturnal dose of an H_2 receptor antagonist for the treatment of duodenal ulcer. Gut 24: 904–908
5. Rendic S, Alebic-Kolbah T, Kajtez F, Rug H-H 1982 Interaction of ranitidine with liver enzymes. Xenobiotica 12: 9
6. Serlin M J, Sibeon R G, Breckenridge A M 1981 Lack of effect of ranitidine on warfarin action. British Journal of Clinical Pharmacology 12: 791–794
7. Henry D A, Macdonald I A, Kitchingman G, Bell G D, Langman M J S 1980 Cimetidine and ranitidine: comparison of effects on hepatic drug metabolism. British Medical Journal 281: 775
8. Powell R J, Rogers J F, Wargin W A, Cross R E, Eshelman F N 1984 Inhibition of theophylline clearance by cimetidine but not ranitidine. Archives of Internal Medicine 144: 484–486
9. Breen K J, Bury R, Desmond P V et al 1982 Effects of cimetidine and ranitidine on hepatic drug metabolism. Clinical Pharmacology and Therapeutics 31: 297–300
10. Kirch W, Ramsch K, Janisch H D, Ohnhaus E E 1984 The influence of two histamine H_2 receptor antagonists, cimetidine and ranitidine, on the plasma levels and clinical effect of nifedepine and metoprolol. Archives of Toxicology (suppl 7): 256
11. Kelly J G, Shanks R G, McDevitt D G 1983 Influence of ranitidine on plasma metoprolol concentrations. British Medical Journal 287: 1218–1219
12. Somogyi A, Bocher F 1984 Dose and concentration dependent effect of ranitidine on procainamide disposition and renal clearance in man. British Journal of Clinical Pharmacology 8: 175
13. Webster L K, Mihaly G W, Jones D B 1984 Effect of cimetidine and ranitidine on carbamazepine and sodium valproate pharmacokinetics. European Journal of Clinical Pharmacology 27: 341
14. Delitala G, Devilla L, Pende A, Canessa A 1982 Effects of the H_2 receptor antagonist ranitidine on anterior pituitary hormone secretion in man. European Journal of Clinical Pharmacology 22: 207–211
15. Bianchi Porro G, Cheli R 1984 Gynaecomastia and ranitidine. Italian Journal of Gastroenterology 16: 56
16. Carey P F, Martin L E, Evans M B 1984 High-performance liquid chromatographic methods for the determination of ranitidine and its metabolites in biological fluids. Chromatographia 19: 200–6
17. Lebert P A, MacLeod S M, Mahon W A, Soldin S J, Vandenberghe H M 1981 Ranitidine kinetics and dynamics. I. Oral dose studies. Clinical Pharmacology and Therapeutics 30: 539
18. Lebert P A, Mahon W A, MacLeod S M, Soldin S J, Fenje P, Vandenberghe H M 1981 Ranitidine kinetics and dynamics. II. Intravenous dose studies and comparison with cimetidine. Clinical Pharmacology and Therapeutics 30: 545
19. McNeil J J, Mihaly G W, Anderson A, Marshall A W, Smallwood R W, Louis W J 1981 Pharmacokinetics of the H_2 receptor antagonist ranitidine in man. British Journal of Clinical Pharmacology 12: 411
20. Peden N R, Boyd E J S, Saunders J H B, Wormsley K G 1981 Ranitidine in the treatment of duodenal ulceration. Scandinavian Journal of Gastroenterology 16: 325
21. Langman M J S, Henry D H, Bell G D, Burnham W R, Ogilvy A 1980 Cimetidine and ranitidine in duodenal ulcer. British Medical Journal 281: 473
22. Ireland A, Colin Jones D G, Gear P et al 1984 Ranitidine 150 mg twice daily or 300 mg nightly in treatment of duodenal ulcers. Lancet 2: 274–276
23. Brogden R N, Carmine A, Heel R C, Speight T M, Avery G S 1982 Ranitidine. A review of its pharmacology and therapeutic use in peptic ulcer disease and other allied diseases. Drugs 24: 267–303
24. Ashton M G, Holdsworth C D, Ryan R P, Moore M 1982 Healing of gastric ulcers after one, two and three months ranitidine. British Medical Journal 284: 467
25. Gough K R, Korman M G, Bardhan K D, Lee F I, Crowe J P, Reed P I 1984 Ranitidine and cimetidine in prevention of duodenal ulcer relapse. Lancet 2: 659–662
26. Mignon M, Vallot T K, Mayeur S, Bonfils S 1980 Ranitidine and cimetidine in Zollinger–Ellison syndrome. British Journal of Clinical Pharmacology 10: 173
27. Andrews A D, Brock-Utne J G, Downing J W 1982 Protection against pulmonary acid aspiration with ranitidine. Anaesthesia 37: 22
28. Collins R, Langman M J S 1985 Treatment with histamine H_2 antagonists in acute upper gastrointestinal hemorrhage. Implications of randomized trials. New England Journal of Medicine 313: 660–666
29. Peterson W L, Richardson C T 1985 Sustained fasting achlorhydria: a comparison of medical regimens. Gastroenterology 88: 666–679
30. Lauritsen K, Havelund T, Rask Madsen J, Fenger C 1984 Ranitidine and hepatotoxicity. Lancet 2: 1471
31. Souza Lima M A 1984 Hepatitis associated with ranitidine. Annals of Internal Medicine 101: 207
32. Zimmerman R W 1984 Problems associated with medical treatment of peptic ulcer disease. American Journal of Medicine 77 (suppl 58): 51–56
33. Epstein C M, Silverstone P H 1984 Ranitidine and confusion. Lancet 1: 1071
34. Walt R P, La Broay S J, Avgerinos A, Oehr T, Riley A, Misiewicz J J 1981 Investigation of the penetration of ranitidine into the cerebro-spinal fluid and a comparison of the effects of cimetidine and ranitidine on male sex hormones. Scandinavian Journal of Gastroenterology (suppl 69): 19–24
35. Hughes J D, Reed W D, Serjeant C S 1981 Mental confusion associated with ranitidine. Medical Journal of Australia 2: 12–13
36. Belaiche J, Zitoun J, Marquet J, Nurit Y, Yvart J 1983 Effet de la ranitidine sur la secretion de facteur intrinsique gastrique et sur l'absorption de la vitamine B_{12}. Gastroenterologie Clinique et Biologique 7: 381–384
37. Hamborg B, Kittang E, Schjonsby H 1985 The effect of ranitidine on the absorption of food cobalamins. Scandinavian Journal of Gastroenterology 20: 756–758
38. Hansen W E, Berth S 1983 Inhibition of cholinesterases by ranitidine. Lancet 1: 235
39. Sancho J M, Robles R G, Mancheno E 1984 Interference by ranitidine with aldosterone secretion in vivo. European Journal of Clinical Pharmacology 27: 495
40. Gardner M E, Sikorski G W 1985 Ranitidine and theophylline. Annals of Internal Medicine 102: 559
41. Wormsley K G 1984 Assessing the safety of drugs for the long term treatment of peptic ulcers. Gut 25: 1416–1423
42. Korman M G, Hansky J, Merrett A C, Schmidt G T 1982 Ranitidine in duodenal ulcer: incidence of healing and effect of smoking. Digestive Diseases and Sciences 27: 712–715
43. McFarland R J, Bateson M C, Green J R B, O'Donoghue D P Dronfield M W 1989 Omperazole provides quicker symptom relief and duodenal ulcer healing than ranitidine. Gastroenterology 98: 278–83
44. Walan A, Bader J P, Classen M, Lamers C B H W, Piper D W et al 1989 Effect of omeprazole and ranitidine on ulcer healing and relapse rates in patients with benign gastric ulcer. New England Journal of Medicine 320: 69–79
45. Robinson M G, Griffin J W Jr, Bowers J, Kogan F J et al 1989 Effect of ranitidine on gastroduodenal mucosal damage induced by non steroidal anti-inflammatory drugs. Digestive Diseases and Sciences 34: 424–428
46. Ehsanullah R S B, Page M C, Tildesley G, Wood J R 1988 Prevention of gastroduodenal induced by non-steroidal anti-inflammatory drugs: controlled trial of ranitidine. British Medical Journal 297: 1017–1021
47. Ryan F P, Jorde R, Ehsanullah R S B, Summers K, Wood J R 1986 A single night time dose of ranitidine in the acute treatment of gastric ulcer: a European multicentre trial. Gut 27: 784–8
48. Havelund, Laursen L S, Skoubo Kristiansen G, Andersen B N, Pedersen S A et al 1988 Omeprazole and ranitidine in the reflux oesophagitis: double-blind comparative trial. British Medical Journal. 296: 89–92
49. Saunders J H, Oliver R J, Higson D L 1986 Dyspepsia: incidence of non-ulcer disease in a controlled trial of ranitidine in general practice. British Medical Journal 292: 665–668
50. Mitchard M, McIsaac R L, Bell J A. 1989 H_2-receptor antagonists. In: Damani (ed), Sulphar-containing drugs and related organic compounds. Vol 3, part A. Ellis Horwood pp. 53–86

Rauwolfia-reserpine

The genus *Rauwolfia*, which comprises a large number of species, is widely distributed in tropical countries. *Rauwolfia serpentina* (L) Benth. is a small shrub indigenous to India and neighbouring countries where crude extracts of the plant, particularly the root, have been used medicinally for centuries. *Rauwolfia serpentina* contains some 20 alkaloids.[1] The most potent is reserpine. The other analogous alkaloids have effects which are qualitatively similar to those of reserpine, as have extracts of the whole root.[2]

Chemistry

Reserpine (serpasil)
$C_{33}H_{28}N_2O_9$
11,17α-Dimethoxy-18β-(3,4,5-trimethoxybenzoyl)oxy-3β,20α-yohimban-16β-carboxylic acid methyl ester

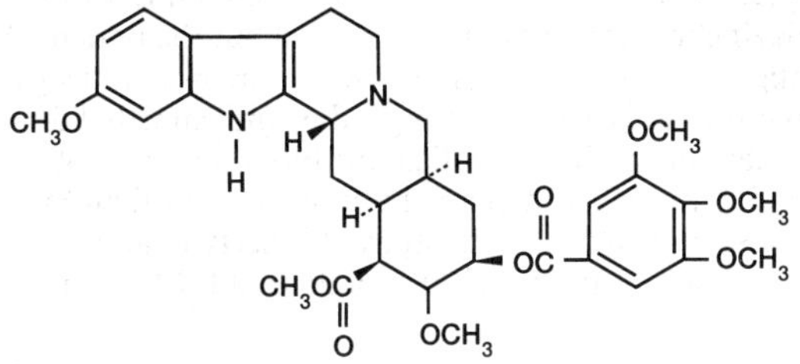

Extracts of whole root contain, in addition to reserpine, other indole alkaloids including rescinnamine (reserpinine) deserpidine (recanescine), yohimbine (rauwolscine) and ajmaline (rauwolfine).

Molecular weight	608.7
pKa	6.6
Solubility	
in alcohol	1 in 1800
in water	virtually insoluble
Octanol/water partition coefficient	high

The free alkaloid is a white to slightly yellow crystalline solid prepared by extraction of *Rauwolfia serpentina*. It is available in combination with hydrochlorothiazide (Serpasil-Esidrex) and with amylobasbitone (Hypercal-B). A mixture of Rauwolfia alkaloids is available as Hypercal.

Pharmacology

Reserpine impairs the function of the granular noradrenaline storage vesicles in the postganglionic sympathetic nerve endings allowing the noradrenaline to become accessible to monoamine oxidase in the neuronal cytoplasm. Destruction of noradrenaline is accompanied by impairment of synthesis within the degranulated vesicles. Depletion of noradrenaline and also of adrenaline, dopamine and serotonin also involves other tissues, in particular the brain, heart and to a lesser extent the adrenal medulla. Impairment of peripheral adrenergic nerve function due to depletion of the neurotransmitter, noradrenaline, is thought to be mainly responsible for its antihypertensive effect rather than its action on the CNS.[3] Cardiac output is also diminished. CNS effects are thought to be due to the depletion of catecholamine and serotonin stores in the brain. Platelets are depleted of serotonin, because reserpine binds to their granular storage vesicles and impairs their uptake of the amine.[4]

Toxicology

There are great variations in the dose toxic to animals depending on species and route of administration. However, the LD_{50} intravenously is of the order of 10–20 $mg.kg^{-1}$, the intramuscular, intraperitoneal and subcutaneous LD_{50} 50–100 $mg.kg^{-1}$, and the oral LD_{50} 100–500 $mg.kg^{-1}$. Carcinogenic hazard status is equivocal. Tumours have been induced in rats and mice at doses 100–300 times the human dose.[5]

Clinical pharmacology

After large (e.g. 2.5 mg) parenteral doses a transient rise in blood pressure may be evident followed by a slow fall over 2 or 3 hours accompanied by bradycardia. If further parenteral doses are given within this period blood pressure may fall excessively. With oral administration of usual therapeutic doses of reserpine alone (0.1–0.25 mg daily), no more than a minor fall in blood pressure is to be expected. The extent of this is fully evident only after several weeks. However, the hypotensive effect is substantially increased when reserpine is used in combination with a diuretic. Postural hypotension is not marked but is present in a proportion of patients. Congestion of nasal mucous membranes is frequent and on higher dosage there is overt cutaneous vasodilatation with flushing of the face. Cardiac output is diminished, and there may be fluid retention. Responses to indirect-acting vasopressor amines, e.g. ephedrine, are diminished while those to direct-acting agents (e.g. noradrenaline) are enhanced.

Central nervous effects vary from mild sedation to severe depression. A relative preponderance of parasympathomimetic effects causes hypermotility of the gut. Gastrin release is enhanced. Bronchospasm is promoted in susceptible people.

Pharmacokinetics

The most important feature of the kinetics of reserpine and other rauwolfia alkaloids is their extremely long elimination half life. That of reserpine is of the order of 1–2 weeks.[6]

Of the analytical methods available the most satisfactory data have been obtained by the use of tritium-labelled reserpine. Methods of quantitation in pharmaceutical materials and body fluids are referred to in the review by Stitzel.[7]

Absorption after oral administration is rapid, peak plasma levels being reached in 1–2 h.[6] Oral absorption is incomplete, some 30% only being accountable in the body after the administration of ^{3}H-reserpine and some 60% in the faeces.

Following intramuscular administration absorption is prompt but even when given by this or the intravenous route, significant amounts appear in the faeces, presumably as a result of biliary excretion.

Distribution is extensive because of the high lipid solubility of the alkaloids. However, no satisfactory quantitative data are available.

Reserpine crosses the placenta and affects the fetus in utero. Since it is excreted in the milk of mothers on reserpine, breast-fed infants may develop reserpine-induced effects.

After oral or parenteral reserpine the plot of plasma (or whole blood) concentration versus time is exponential with an initial relatively steep decline over the first 12 hours (α half life 4.5 hours) and a very flat terminal portion with a β half life of some 1–2 weeks.[7,8] Plasma protein binding is 96%,[9] with a significant amount bound to plasma lipoproteins, the latter fraction varying with the plasma lipoprotein concentration and being much increased in hyperlipoproteinaemia patients. The major fraction in normals was bound to albumin, but this was relatively less in hyperlipoproteinaemic patients, although the total bound fraction was the same in both groups.

Elimination is mainly by metabolism and faecal excretion. After tritium-labelled reserpine, 60% of radioactivity, mainly as reserpine, could be collected in the faeces in 96 hours.[6] Even after parenteral (intramuscular) ^{3}H-reserpine, 30% of administered radioactivity appeared in the faeces, presumably from biliary excretion. Some 4–6% of administered radioactivity was found in the urine,[6,8] most of it as trimethoxybenzoic acid and its conjugates.

In patients with severely impaired renal function given ^{3}H-reserpine, the elimination half life of radioactivity was markedly increased,[8] probably by accumulation of trimethoxybenzoic acid and its conjugates. No concomitant increase of pharmacological effects was observed. The half-life of reserpine is likely to be prolonged in the elderly.

Oral absorption	30%
Presystemic metabolism	—
Plasma half life	
range	1–2 weeks
Volume of distribution	—
Plasma protein binding	96%[9]

Concentration–effect relationship

As a consequence of the extremely long terminal elimination half life, cumulation occurs on daily dosage, the body burden only reaching a plateau after some 4–8 weeks. At this time the amount in the body would be 10–20 times that after the initial dose.

Metabolism

Metabolism is largely by hydrolysis of the ester linkage to the trimethoxybenzoyl group and excretion of methyl reserpate and related compounds (Fig. 1).[7]

O-Desmethylation is also an important route of metabolism. Other metabolites include reserpic acid, syringomethyl reserpate and syringic acid. The phase 1 metabolite may be further transformed to the corresponding glucuronide or sulphate conjugates.

Fig. 1

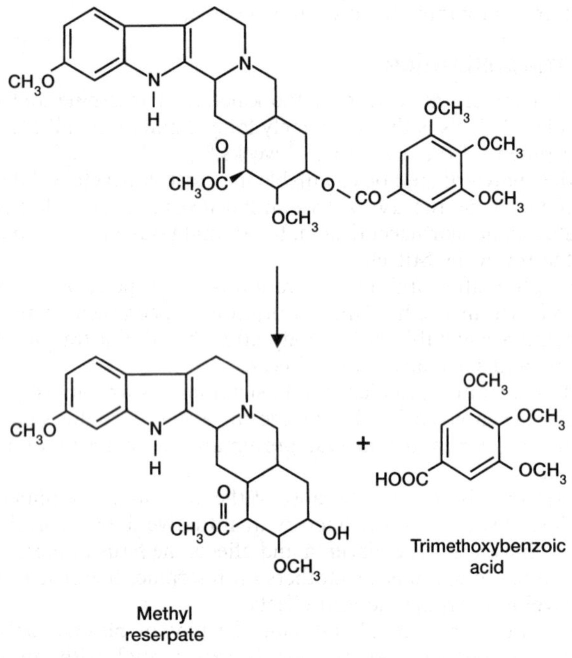

Pharmaceutics

Reserpine is marketed in oral and injectable forms by several manufacturers in the USA including CIBA (Serpasil). Deserpidine for oral use is marketed in some countries, e.g. Harmonyl (Abbott, US). An extract of total alkaloids (alseroxylon fraction) is also available for oral use as are preparations of whole root of *Rauwolfia serpentina*.[5,10]

Reserpine 0.1 mg is approximately equivalent to 1 mg of alseroxylon fraction and to 50 mg of whole root of *Rauwolfia serpentina*.

Reserpine is marketed in combination with a range of diuretics as also is deserpidine and a preparation of whole root.[5,10]

Therapeutic use

Indications

1. Control of mild to moderate hypertension
2. Management of hypertensive emergencies in pregnancy
3. Management of cerebrovascular accidents associated with severe hypertension
4. Treatment of agitated psychoses.

Other uses

5. Treatment of peripheral vasospasm.

Contraindications

1. Depression
2. Severe renal failure.

Relative contraindications

3. Peptic ulceration or ulcerative colitis
4. Bronchial asthma.

Indications

1. Hypertension

In the treatment of hypertension there is little to be gained by using a rauwolfia alkaloid as the sole form of therapy. For it to be effective it should be used in association with a diuretic. A thiazide or analogous diuretic should be given initially and reserpine added after one or two weeks if the response to the diuretic alone is inadequate.

The maintenance dose should be no more than 0.1 mg reserpine or 1 mg alseroxylon fraction per day. However, in order to attain an effective body burden reasonably quickly the initial dose should be 0.25 mg per day for 1 week. As a result of the prolonged half life and consequent accumulation, even a dose of 0.1 mg per day may be inappropriately high after a month of continuous daily use and a trial might be made of 0.1 mg on alternate days only. If a regime of diuretic plus rauwolfia is inadequate a direct-acting vasodilator such as hydralazine might be considered as well but the patient should not be too long denied the benefits of newer more potent drugs. In trials, a combination of reserpine 0.05 mg a day and chlorthalidone 50 mg a day succeeded in producing a diastolic blood pressure of less than 90 mmHg and 5 mmHg less than the level of chlorthalidone alone in 58% of those allocated to that study. Finnerty et al. also obtained a satisfactory result in 19 out of 20 on a dose of 0.125 mg reserpine (see Major outcome trials).

2. Treatment of peripheral vasospasm

In the treatment of peripheral vasospasm benefit has been claimed in Raynaud's syndrome from reserpine given intra-arterially.[11] However, other workers[12] observed no benefit. Nevertheless, reserpine given orally in dosage as for hypertension, may produce a worthwhile increase in skin blood flow.

Contraindications

1. Depression

Reserpine or rauwolfia extracts are absolutely contraindicated in the presence of depression or a history of pre-existing depression.

2. Severe renal failure

Severe renal failure (creatinine clearance < 10 ml.min^{-1}) is a contraindication.

3. Relative contraindications

Relative contraindications are a history of peptic ulceration or of ulcerative colitis or bronchial asthma.

Adverse reactions

Potentially life-threatening adverse effects

The toxic effect of crucial importance in patients under treatment with rauwolfia alkaloids is depression. This may be severe enough to cause suicide. However, failure in the past to appreciate the cumulative property of rauwolfia and use of inappropriately high doses must have enhanced the severity of the depression in many cases.

Allegations of an association of reserpine with breast cancer have not been substantiated.[12] Angioimmunoblastic lymphadenopathy has been reported following long-term use of reserpine.[13]

Acute overdosage

Consciousness is impaired and coma may supervene fairly rapidly. Bradycardia is usual but there may be ectopic beats and, in patients still conscious, complaints of palpitations. Progressive lowering of blood pressure with extreme cutaneous vasodilatation is usual, but in a significant proportion of cases there may be a period of grossly

Rauwolfia-reserpine

raised blood pressure. In severe cases there is respiratory depression and this, together with intractable vasodilation and reduced cardiac output, is the cause of death when this occurs. Bronchospasm may contribute to the respiratory inadequacy. Tremor and dystonic movements may be evident. Hypothermia is a possible complication.

Treatment is by gastric lavage with a large-bore tube to ensure that all drug remaining in the stomach is removed. To diminish the ill effects of inhalation of gastric contents 200 mg cimetidine should be given intramuscularly. If consciousness has been lost, lavage requires insertion of a cuffed endotracheal tube as a preliminary.

An intravenous line should be set up and a plasma expander infused. An additional line with the catheter tip in a central vein should be used for an infusion of dobutamine, or, if this is ineffective, noradrenaline. Atropine should be given in full dosage, and frusemide 40 mg intravenously. Urinary output should be monitored.

Severe or irreversible adverse effects

Apart from depression, serious adverse effects include bronchospasm and occasionally exacerbation of pre-existing congestive cardiac failure or precipitation of incipient failure. Extrapyramidal sequelae of dopamine depletion of the basal ganglia include parkinsonism, dyskinesia, and dystonia. Aggravation of peptic ulcer may occur.

Symptomatic adverse effects

These include diurnal drowsiness but nocturnal restlessness with disturbed sleep and nightmares; weight gain from either increased appetite or fluid retention; nasal obstruction from mucosal congestion; dyspepsia, looseness of the bowels; loss of libido and impotence; menstrual irregularity or amenorrhoea and galactorrhoea. Ocular palsies have been reported.[14]

Other effects

Catecholamine excretion is elevated, as is prolactin secretion, the latter though apparently only at doses greater than 0.25 mg per day.[15]

Interference with clinical pathology tests

By interfering with the Porter-Silber reaction, rauwolfia alkaloids may cause a falsely high reading in tests for urinary corticosteroids or falsely low readings for urinary 17-hydroxycorticosteroids; and either falsely high or low readings in measurement of urinary 17-ketosteroids, by interference with the Zimmerman reaction.

A false-positive result may occur in the Rogers spot-test screening method for urinary VMA or other guaicols.

High risk groups

Neonates and children

There is no indication for the use of rauwolfia alkaloids in neonates or children.

Breast milk. Reserpine appears in breast milk, and breast-feeding is contraindicated in mothers taking the drug.

Pregnant women

In the management of hypertension during pregnancy, when a rauwolfia alkaloid is already in use it may be continued. However, the alkaloids cross the placenta and may cause complications in the neonate. The major untoward effects are respiratory, particularly nasal obstruction, which may contribute to anoxia. Bradycardia and hypothermia may also be significant.

In the management of hypertensive emergencies due to pregnancy toxaemia, intramuscular reserpine 2.5 mg usually produces a small fall in blood pressure. However, reserpine would not now be considered the drug of choice in this context.

The elderly

The already long half life of the rauwolfia alkaloids is likely to be further increased with advancing age. In patients over 70 a dose of 0.05 mg per day may well be the highest consistent with freedom from risk of depression.

Concurrent disease

See Contraindications.

Drug interactions

Potentially hazardous interactions

The effect of alcohol may be enhanced both on the central nervous system and the cardiovascular system with enhanced peripheral vasodilatation and possible hypotension.

Other vasodilating agents may produce unexpected falls in blood pressure, e.g. glyceryl trinitrate. So also may drugs used in other contexts but having effects in lowering blood pressure, e.g. levodopa, fenfluramine, phenothiazine tranquillizers.

Per contra, the pressor effects of phenylephrine and of catecholamines are potentiated, but those of indirect-acting amines such as ephedrine are diminished.

Interaction with monoamine oxidase inhibitor antidepressants may produce excessive CNS excitation. Reserpine lowers the convulsive threshold of epileptic patients and if reserpine is to be used in such patients, dosage of anticonvulsants may have to be revised.

Digitalis-induced bradycardia may be enhanced. The negative inotropic effects of antiarrhythmic agents such as disopyramide and quinidine may be increased. Halothane anaesthesia may cause a more marked degree of myocardial depression than usual.

Increased prolactin secretion with breast enlargement and secretion may accompany the use together of oral contraceptives and reserpine.

Potentially useful interactions

None has been reported.

Major outcome trials

1. Veterans Administration Medical Centres 1982 Low doses vs. standard dose of reserpine. A randomized, double-blind, multi-clinic trial in patients taking chlorthalidone. Journal of the American Medical Association 248: 2471–2477

This trial was performed on men aged 30–69 (mean 55) with diastolic pressures untreated of 95–114. Slightly more than 50% were black. Patients with major cardiovascular complications or a history of depression or of prior intolerance to reserpine were excluded. Of 3205 patients screened, 646 were admitted to the trial and started on a placebo which they continued for up to 8 weeks. At the end of that time 505 subjects in whom blood pressure remained elevated were started on chlorthalidone 50 mg per day. On this regime some attained a satisfactory blood pressure and did not continue further. The remaining 329 were admitted to the reserpine trial proper. These were assigned in random, double-blind fashion to regimes including chlorthalidone (C), and reserpine (R) in the following amounts: C 50 mg, R 0.25 mg; C 50, R 0.05; and C 25, R 0.125. The goal was a diastolic blood pressure of less than 90 mmHg and 5 mmHg less than their level on C alone.

On C 50, R 0.25, 65% achieved the goal; on C 50, R 0.125 69%; on C 50, R 0.05 58%; and on C 25, R 0.125, 56%. The numbers achieving the goal increased at each 4 week period up to 12 weeks. The proportion of patients with side effects was greatest on C 50, R 0.25, least on C 50, R 0.05, and consisted of depression, lethargy, nasal obstruction, nightmares, sexual dysfunction, and gastrointestinal symptoms.

Other trials

1. Veterans' Administration Co-operative Study Group on antihypertensive agents 1977 Propranolol in the treatment of essential hypertension. Journal of the American Medical Association 237: 2303–2310

This study was primarily designed to assess the efficacy of propranolol, used either alone or with hydrochlorothiazide and/or hydralazine in the treatment of mild hypertension. However the study compared these regimes with reserpine (R) 0.3 mg per day plus hydrochlorothiazide (T) 105 mg per day. The 450 male hypertensives were distributed between 5 regimes. The R+T regime was effective in achieving a diastolic blood pressure of less than 90 mmHg and a reduction of 5 mmHg or more in 72% at 6 months, 62% at 12 months and 65% at 18 months. This result was comparable with those of the propranolol regimes. The dose of reserpine was inappropriately high at 0.1 mg three times a day but even then the frequency of adverse effects, including depression, was no greater than that with the regimes including propranolol.

2. Finnerty F A, Gyftopoulos A, Berry C, McKenney A 1979 Step 2 regimes in hypertension — an assessment. Journal of the American Medical Association 241: 579–581

This was a single-blind trial in which the effects of hydroflumethiazide 50 mg plus reserpine 0.125 mg given once daily were compared

R

R

with those of the thiazide plus propranolol or methyldopa. There were 20 patients in each group. After a preliminary week on hydroflumethiazide 50 mg the dose was increased to 100 mg for 2 weeks. The reserpine (0.125 mg) was then added and the thiazide cut back to 50 mg. A clinically satisfactory result was obtained in 19 of the 20 patients in the reserpine group on the above dose and in the 20 when the dose was doubled. The regime including reserpine was considered the most satisfactory of the 3 assessed. It was continued for a further 6 months when all patients were satisfactorily controlled.

3. Finnerty F A 1980 Chlorthalidone plus reserpine versus hydrochlorothiazide plus reserpine in a stepped-care approach to the treatment of essential hypertension. Journal of Clinical Pharmacology 20: 357–363

A very satisfactory blood pressure control was established after the addition of reserpine to a regime of either diuretic. The dose of reserpine for most patients was 0.25 mg per day but 37% of them were satisfactorily controlled on 0.125 mg per day and it was noteworthy that the blood pressure was still falling at the end of the 6 week observation period.

General review articles

McMahon F G 1978 Management of essential hypertension. Futura Publishing Company Inc, Mount Kisco, New York, pp 318–354

References

1. Woodsen R E, Youngken H W, Schlittler E, Schneider J A 1957 Rauwolfia: botany, pharmacognosy, chemistry and pharmacology. Little Brown & Co, Boston
2. Schlittler E, Bein H J 1967 Rauwolfia alkaloids. In: Schlittler E (ed) Antihypertensive agents. Academic Press, New York, pp 191–221
3. Gilman A G, Goodman L S, Rall T W, Murad F (eds) 1985 The pharmacological basis of therapeutics, 7th edn. Macmillan Co, New York, pp 207–210
4. Da Prada M, Pletscher A 1969 Storage of exogenous monoamines and reserpine in 5-hydroxytryptamine organelles of blood platelets. European Journal of Pharmacology 7: 45–48
5. 1984 Drug information for the health care provider, vol 1. United States Pharmacopeial Convention Inc, Rockville, Maryland, pp 966–976
6. Maas A R, Jenkins B, Shen Y, Tannenbaum B 1969 Studies on absorption, excretion, and metabolism of ^{3}H-reserpine in man. Clinical Pharmacology and Therapeutics 10: 366–371
7. Stitzel R E 1976 The biological fate of reserpine. Pharmacological Review 28: 179–205
8. Zsoter T T, Johnson G E, De Veber G A, Paul H 1973 Excretion and metabolism of reserpine in renal failure. Clinical Pharmacology and Therapeutics 14: 325–330
9. Chen Z, Danon A 1979 Binding of reserpine to plasma albumin and lipoproteins. Biochemical Pharmacology 28: 267–271
10. Reynolds J E F, Prasad A B 1982 Martindale. The extra pharmacopoeia, 28th edn. Pharmaceutical Press, London
11. Nelson K H, Jayson M I V 1980 Cutaneous microcirculation in systemic sclerosis and response to intraarterial reserpine. British Medical Journal 1: 1408–1411
12. Shapiro S, Parsells J L, Rosenberg L et al 1984 Risk of breast cancer in relation to the use of Rauwolfia alkaloids. European Journal of Clinical Pharmacology 26: 143–146
13. Entrican J H, Denburg J A, Gauldie J, Kelton J G 1984 Angioimmunoblastic lymphadenopathy associated with reserpine. Lancet 2: 820–821
14. Davies D M 1984 Textbook of adverse drug reactions, 2nd edn. Oxford University Press, Oxford, p 458
15. Brass E P 1984 Effects of antihypertensive drugs on endocrine function. Drugs 27: 447–458

Retinol

Retinol is one of the four oil-soluble vitamins and has wide therapeutic uses.

Chemistry

Retinol (axerophthol, vitamin A, Ro-A-Vit tablets, as acetate; ampoules as palmitate)
$C_{20}H_{30}O$
3,7-Dimethyl-9-(2,6,6-trimethyl-1-cyclohexen-1-yl)-2,4,6,8-nonantetraen-1-ol

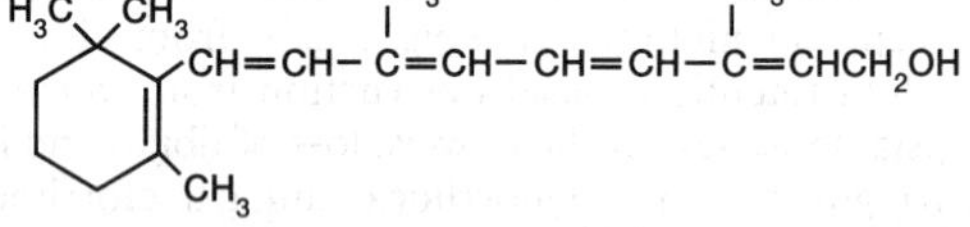

Molecular weight	286.46
pKa	—
Solubility	
in alcohol	soluble
in water	practically insoluble
Octanol/water partition coefficient	high

Retinol is a yellow crystalline solid with a low melting point (62–64°C) which is prepared by chemical synthesis.

Various esters are used clinically, including the acetate in tablets and the palmitate in the parenteral form. Apart from the one commercially available, single-substance product, Ro-A-Vit, retinol is contained at various dose levels in a multitude of multivitamin, multivitamin–mineral and general nutritional products available through pharmacists and other sales outlets. Retinol is also used to supplement various foods.

Retinol, if kept under dry, cool, dark anaerobic conditions, is stable for long periods. However, in both the alcohol and ester form it is very sensitive to oxidation, particularly when also exposed to light. In consequence, commercial forms usually consist of beadlets in a gelatin–carbohydrate matrix with antioxidants — particularly alphatocopherol.

Pharmacology

Retinol has several biochemical functions.

1. Retina

The derivative 11-*cis* retinaldehyde (11-*cis* retinene) is bound to a protein (photopsin) in the visual pigment (rhodopsin) in the rods. Exposure to light changes the 11-*cis* form to all-*trans* retinal via a series of intermediates.[1] All-*trans* retinal no longer forms a stable complex with photopsin. The generation of energy in the optic nerves which is interpreted by the occipital cortex of the brain as scotopic vision is the result of a decrease in the sodium dark current. There is no proven current explanation for this energy generating mechanism.[2]

In the dark the all-*trans* retinaldehyde is re-isomerized to the 11-*cis* form which conjugates again with photopsin.

Retinol esters are also found in high concentrations in other sensory receptors and retinol deficiency is associated with reduced sensitivity of these receptors.[3] Hence retinol or a metabolite may be an important component of receptors for various special senses.

2. Growth

Whereas visual activity depends on retinol, animal growth can be maintained by the related retinoic acid as well as retinol. The fact that growth occurs rapidly when retinoic acid is administered and slowly when retinol is given suggests that retinol is the storage form and retinoic acid is the tissue active form for growth. Loss of appetite with impaired taste is an early feature of retinol deficiency and may be an important cause of the depressed growth.[4]

3. Tissue differentiation
Many mucus-secreting tissues become keratinized, while most epithelial tissues (e.g. skin, cornea, trachea, testis) show gross degeneration in retinol deficiency. The cornea is particularly sensitive and in retinol deficiency corneal ulceration is a major cause of childhood blindness. One current hypothesis for an effect on tissue differentiation is that retinol serves as, or leads to the formation of, a carrier of sugars in the synthesis of some specific glycoproteins.[5]

4. Immunological responses
Many aspects of the animal immune response, including non-specific components (e.g. mucus production and phagocytosis) as well as humoral and cell-mediated immunity are sensitive to retinol levels.[6]

5. Anti-cancer activity
There is increasing recent epidemiological and experimental evidence[7] that retinol and its precursor β-carotene have anti-cancer activity. This may be due to blocking of free radical activity[8] or to effects on cell adhesion.[5]

Toxicology

Retinol was first introduced into clinical medicine and animal nutrition in the 1940s; hence most of the information about toxicity is based on earlier style experimental studies, coupled with some four decades of clinical experience. Hypervitaminosis A has been demonstrated in many animal species including fowls, pigs, cattle, monkeys and rats. In general, toxic manifestations in animals appear only at doses some 10–50 times the recommended daily requirement for the species. This safety ratio is less than that for most of the vitamins.[9]

The toxic reactions are similar to those described for human adverse effects which are described later. In animal studies high doses of vitamin A are teratogenic but the significance of this for humans is in dispute.[9,10]

Clinical pharmacology

Since retinol intake is required for the maintenance of health, the clinical pharmacology can best be considered in relation to the clinical manifestations of deficiency. Although retinol deficiency has been reported in otherwise healthy adults, deficiency is usually seen in children, associated with protein calorie malnutrition, a low intake of essential fatty acids and intercurrent infections. Hence it is often difficult to define the signs of pure deficiency.

The only unequivocal signs of vitamin deficiency are in the eyes. Depletion of retinene leads to poor dark adaptation while corneal degeneration — xerophthalmia — represents a more serious deficiency. The exact signs depend not only on the severity of the deficiency but on concurrent local infection. In xerosis there is a dry wrinkled corneal surface with pearly white Bitot's spots. Xerosis can progress to keratomalacia with extensive eye destruction. Skin keratinization (toad skin) may be due to retinol deficiency or essential fatty acid deficiency.

Pharmacokinetics

The best analytical method for the estimation of retinol in body fluids is high pressure liquid chromatography. The handling of orally administered retinol as a therapeutic agent is similar to that taken in from food or derived from the precursor β-carotene. Hence it will be dealt with under metabolism.

Parenterally administered retinol in oily form is gradually absorbed from the injection site and then stored in depots as is the orally administered dose. A single large parenteral dose maintains protective plasma levels for several weeks at least — perhaps as long as six months.

Oral absorption of retinol is dependent on several factors, including the integrity of the bile salt system and intestinal mucosa, the level of fat in the diet, and the pharmaceutical dosage form. About 80% of dietary retinol is absorbed at normal intake, less with higher doses. The remaining 20% is excreted in the faeces within 1–2 days. At high doses the proportion of retinol absorbed is less.

Retinol is excreted in breast-milk and readily crosses the placenta.

Intestinal parasites reduce the absorption of retinol, whereas liver flukes and schistosomes impair liver storage.

Concentration–effect relationship

No relevant information is available.

Metabolism

The metabolism of administered retinol is complicated by the ability of the body to produce this substance from natural carotenoids in the normal diet. Beta-carotene is the main source and for this substance one-sixth (on a weight basis) is estimated to be converted within the body into retinol. For other carotenoids about one-twelfth is converted to retinol.[11]

Dietary or pharmaceutical esters of retinol are hydrolysed in the intestinal lumen and unless the intestinal tract is abnormal about 80% of the retinol is absorbed, probably associated with a specific all-*trans* retinol binding protein in the enterocytes. This process is influenced by the level of bile salts present. The remaining 20% is excreted in the faeces in 1–2 days.[12] The major part of the retinol is converted to retinyl ester and carried in the chylomicrons, and ultimately reaches the liver parenchymal cells. There they are removed from the circulation by receptor-mediated endocytosis.[13]

A substantial portion of the retinol is transferred to hepatic perisinusoidal stellate cells and stored there. The remainder is carried in the plasma in association with retinol binding protein.[14] The level of retinol binding protein and hence plasma retinol is elevated in chronic renal disease but is depressed in the severe protein calorie malnutrition which is the usual clinical situation in which retinol therapeutic administration is most likely to occur. The retinol ligand is bound by cell surface receptors on target cells. The retinol is transferred from the retinol binding protein across the cellular membrane by an undefined mechanism to be bound by specific binding proteins in the cell cytoplasm (CRBP) which carry retinol to its intracellular site of action. An alternative intracellular binding protein is specific for retinoic acid.

Of the 80% retinol which is absorbed from the intestinal tract, 20–50% is either conjugated or oxidized to various products and excreted over a matter of days after ingestion in the urine and faeces, while the remainder is stored. This stored retinol is gradually metabolized by liver and peripheral tissues, mainly by oxidation to retinaldehyde and retinoic acid. Those derivatives with an intact carbon side-chain tend to be excreted in the bile, whereas acidic chain-shortened products are usually excreted in the urine (see Fig. 1).

Pharmaceutics

Retinol is available in both oral and parenteral form.

1. Ro-A-Vit tablets (Roche, UK) contain 15 mg retinol equivalent (50 000 IU vitamin A). The sugar-coated tablets are round, cream coloured with 'ROCHE' printed in red on one face.
2. Ro-A-Vit (Roche, UK) for deep intramuscular injection only, is available as a 1 ml solution containing retinol palmitate (90 mg retinol equivalent; 300 000 IU vitamin A).
3. Aquasol A (Armour, USA) capsules contain 25 000 IU (7.5 mg) or 50 000 IU (15 mg) retinol solubilized with polysorbate 80. The capsules are dark red, soft gelatin.
4. Over-the-counter products include cream formulations for dry, sensitive skin. Pedi-Vit A Creme (Pedinol, USA) contains 100 000 IU per 28 g.

The tablets should be stored below 25°C in well-closed containers. The ampoules should be protected from light and stored below 25°C.

The tablets contain no known allergenic substances. However reactions may occur in sensitive subjects after deep intramuscular injection of the oily injection formulation.

Retinol is available as a component of numerous multivitamin and multivitamin/mineral preparations. The dosage of retinol is very variable in these combination preparations.

Therapeutic use

Indications

1. Prevention and treatment of vitamin A deficiency
2. Defined skin disorders

Other uses
3. Experimentally as prophylaxis against cancer.

Contraindications

1. Hypersensitivity to retinol
2. Pregnancy.

Retinol

Mode of use

Treatment is normally undertaken in developed countries by daily oral dosage. However when intestinal malabsorption disorders complicate absorption, infrequent deep intramuscular injection of high doses may be substituted, relying on the extensive storage of retinol which results. For a like reason, therapy and prophylaxis in third

Fig. 1 Metabolism of retinol

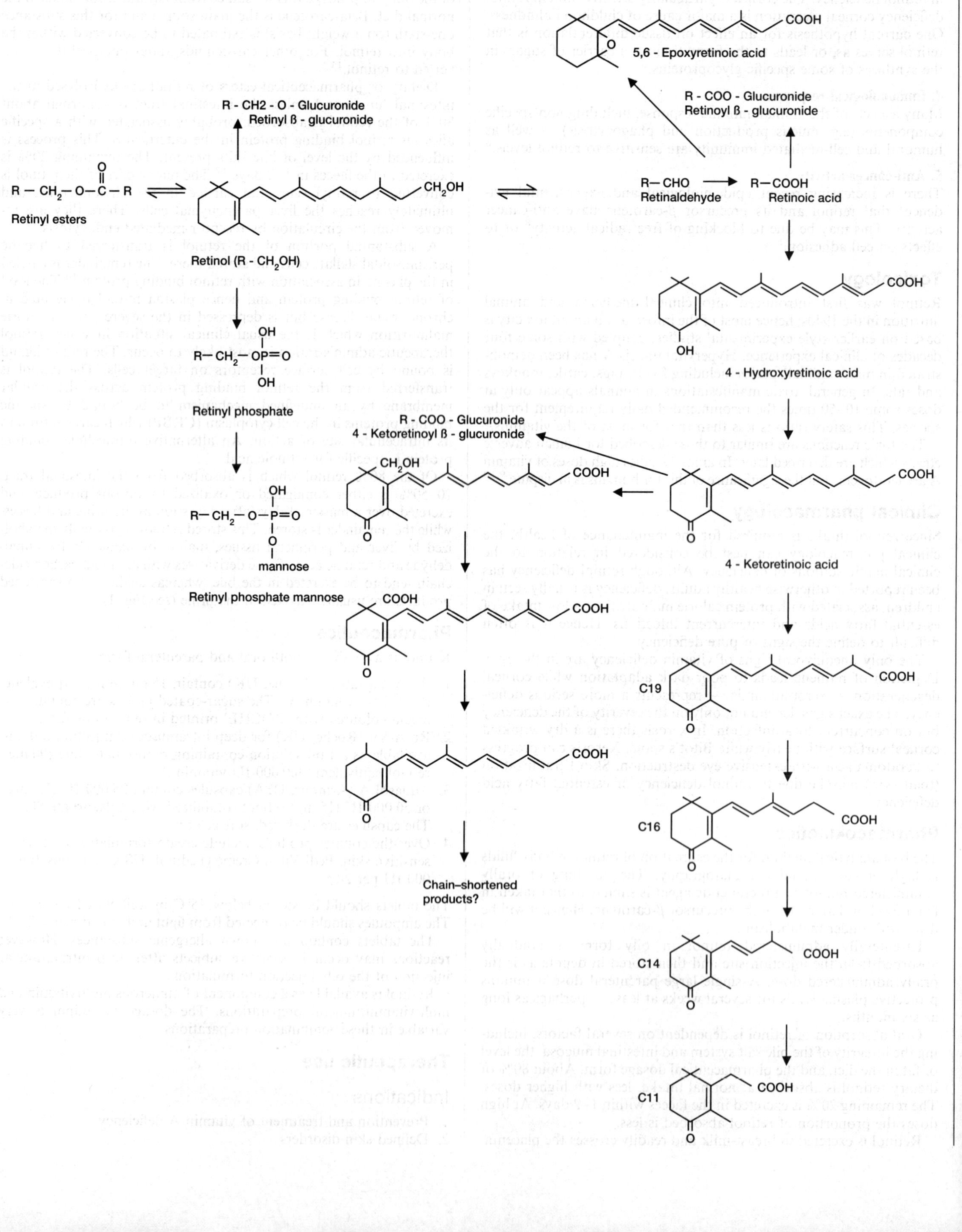

world communities can conveniently be by intermittent, higher oral or parenteral dosage. The advised daily dose depends on the degree of deficiency and the age, namely:
for children — oral doses up to 5 mg per day
parenteral doses up to 15 mg per month
for adults — oral doses 15–60 mg per day for short periods
parenteral doses 45 mg monthly.

Indications

1. Prevention and treatment of vitamin A deficiency
Deficiency states should be treated as soon as they are diagnosed (on clinical or biochemical grounds) with relatively high doses of retinol (5–60 mg daily according to age). When minor grades of vitamin A deficiency are suspected (e.g. in malabsorption syndrome, post gastrectomy, etc.) doses of 2–10 $mg.d^{-1}$ are normally regarded as adequate.
Due to retinol storage, these doses do not need to be given on a daily basis but equivalent higher dosage can be given less regularly.

An interesting recent development has been the use of very high doses (of the order of 90 mg oil-miscible retinol) at intervals of say 6 months for the prophylaxis of deficiency states in areas where hypovitaminosis A is endemic. Studies have demonstrated that in preschool children given such prophylactic retinol the death rate from intercurrent infections (particularly measles) is substantially reduced. Although retinol has been used extensively in the past for the prevention of infections in industrially developed communities there is no clear evidence of such an effect, except when there is a deficiency.

2. Defined skin disorders
High doses of retinol have been administered in a wide range of dermatological and epithelial disorders, including acne, though with rather mixed results. Topical retinoic acid has also been used for certain skin disorders, but for such disorders the retinoids, etretrinate and isotretinoin, are now preferred, though their toxicity precludes their use other than with very careful precautions.

Other uses

3. Experimental use in the prevention of cancer
Based upon experimental and epidemiological evidence retinol and, or perhaps more importantly, the precursor β-carotene, is being used in experimental studies for the prevention of cancer. While this use cannot yet be regarded as proven, it would be inappropriate to ignore the possibility for the future.

Contraindications

1. Hypersensitivity to retinol
The nature of the manifestations of hypervitaminosis A are described later and the acute or chronic dosage which leads to these adverse effects is now reasonably well defined. However, the possibility of occasional cases of hypersensitivity to retinol cannot be ignored, though the author has personally never encountered a case.

2. Pregnancy
Whether excessively high dosage of retinol during pregnancy can give rise to fetal defects in humans is uncertain. The related retinoids are clearly teratogenic. In common with all other forms of medication, caution should be exercised during early pregnancy. Standard dosage (i.e. the recommended daily allowance of 1 mg retinol equivalents) should not be exceeded during early pregnancy.

Adverse reactions

Potentially life-threatening effects
It is very doubtful whether any human has died from retinol intoxication alone.

Acute overdosage
No cases of this kind appear to have been reported.

Severe or irreversible adverse effects
Severe toxicity is itself very rare despite the use of inappropriately high intakes by a substantial number of people.[9,16,17]

The toxic effects which are encountered are normally reversible and an irreversible toxic effect is effectively unknown.
Chronic overdosage can lead to peeling and redness of the skin, disturbed hair growth, loss of appetite, and sickness. Cases of liver derangement have been reported in adults but these have been seen mainly in patients with impaired renal function. Renal failure causes depressed levels of retinol-binding protein in the plasma and excessive levels (higher than 3 $mg.g^{-1}$) of retinol in the liver tissue.

Symptomatic adverse effects
Some 500–600 cases of retinol-related adverse reactions have been recorded in the literature.

Adverse reactions due to acute administration of high doses of retinol include headache, nausea, vomiting and irritability. In infants, acute toxicity may lead to transient hydrocephalus. All these effects disappear within about 24 hours of discontinuing retinol.

Safe dosage
In view of the level of storage of retinol in the body it is very difficult to assess the safe dose. If retinol is given *every day*, adverse effects are extremely rare at doses below 9 mg daily, and the majority of patients with adverse reactions were taking amounts substantially above this level. The maximum safe level for daily use has been stated variously as 9 mg[17] and 15 mg.[18] The maximal safe single dose is of the order of 150 times the recommended dietary allowance. Thus retinol is one of the very few vitamins (the others are cholecalciferol and pyridoxine) for which the safety margin is relatively limited.

Interference with clinical pathology tests
High levels of retinol do not appear to interfere with biochemical observations or clinical pathology tests.

High risk groups

Neonates
There is no contraindication to the use of retinol in neonates in appropriate doses.

Breast milk. High doses of retinol are best avoided by breast-feeding mothers.

Children
Retinol may be given to children in appropriate doses. As has already been described, the appropriate dose depends on age.

Pregnant women
High dosage should not be given in pregnancy.

Concurrent disease
Renal disease. Caution should be exercised in those with chronic renal failure or during renal dialysis.

Drug interactions

Potentially hazardous interactions
None is known.

Other significant reactions
Food and alcohol. Acute protein malnutrition interferes both directly and indirectly with retinol metabolism, increasing the retinol requirements. Fat in the diet, on the other hand, enhances the absorption of retinol. Alphatocopherol acts as an antioxidant for retinol and therefore reduces its destruction, iron, on the other hand, is a pro-oxidant and increases retinol need. Zinc deficiency also increases retinol requirements.

The main effect of alcohol ingestion on retinol requirements occurs when cirrhosis results in a limitation of retinol storage and hence dosage must be given daily.

Heavy metals. Both cadmium and copper decrease retinol plasma levels.

Antibiotics. Neomycin and bleomycin reduces the absorption of retinol.

Major outcome trials

1. Reddy V 1987 Vitamin A deficiency and blindness in Indian children. Indian Journal of Medical Research 68: 26–37

Large doses of retinol in oily form (60 mg of retinol in the form of retinyl palmitate) have been administered each 6 months to children between 1 and 5 years of age. The incidence of hypovitaminosis A fell dramatically. The study involved over 20 million children treated annually over the period.

R

2. Tarwotjo I, Sommer A, West K P, Djunaedi E, Mele L, Hawkins B and Aceh Study Group 1987 Influence of participation on mortality in a randomised trial of vitamin A prophylaxis. American Journal of Clinical Nutrition 46: 1466–1471

This is a further report from the Sommer group. In the previous studies (the references are given in the above paper) the relationship of mortality to retinol deficiency is stressed and the beneficial effect of prophylactic retinol determined. The present report confirms the previous observations but demonstrates some of the difficulties of such epidemiological studies in third world communities.

General review articles

Bauernfeind J C (ed) 1981 Carotenoids as colorants and vitamin A precursors: technological nutritional applications. Academic Press, San Diego
Bauernfeind J C (ed) 1986 Vitamin A deficiency and its control. Academic Press, San Diego
Marks J 1985 The vitamins: their role in medical practice. MTP Press, Lancaster, pp 111–122
Maddy K H 1978 Vitamin A. BASF Wyondotte Corp, New York
Vitamin A deficiency and xerophthalmia 1976 Technical Report No 590. World Health Organization, Geneva
International vitamin A consultative group 1977 Guidelines for the eradication of vitamin A deficiency and xerophthalmia. The Nutrition Foundation, New York
The control of vitamin A deficiency and xerophthalmia 1982 Technical Report No 672. World Health Organization, Geneva
International vitamin A consultative group 1981 The symptoms and signs of vitamin A deficiency and their relationship to applied nutrition. The Nutrition Foundation, New York
International vitamin A consultative group 1981 Biochemical methodology for the assessment of vitamin A status. The Nutrition Foundation, New York

References

1. Honig B 1978 Light energy transduction in visual pigments and bacteriorhodopsin. Annual Review of Physical Chemistry 29: 31–57
2. Fung B K, Stryer L 1980 Photolyzed rhodopsin catalyzes the exchange of GTP for bound GTP in retinol rod outer segments. Proceedings of the National Academy of Sciences USA 77: 2500–2504
3. Biesalski K 1985 Aspects of vitamin A metabolism in sensory epithelia. In: Hanck A, Hornig D (eds) International Journal for Vitamin and Nutrition Research, suppl 27. Vitamins: nutrients and therapeutic agents. Huber, Bern, pp 224–246
4. Anzano M A, Lamb A J, Olson J A 1979 Growth, appetite, sequence of pathological signs and survival following the induction of rapid, synchronous vitamin A deficiency in the rat. Journal of Nutrition 109: 1419–1431
5. De Luca L M, Bhat P V, Sasak W, Adamo S 1979 Biosynthesis of phosphoryl and glycosyl phosphoryl derivatives of vitamin A in biological membranes. Federation Proceedings 38: 2535–2539
6. Chandra S, Chandra R K 1986 Nutrition, immune response and outcome. Progress in Food and Nutrition Science 10: 1–65
7. Bertram J S, Kolonel L N, Meyskens F L 1987 Rationale and strategies for chemoprevention of cancer in humans. Cancer Research 47: 3012–3031
8. Sies H (ed) 1985 Oxidative stress. Academic Press, London
9. Marks J 1989 The safety of the vitamins. In: Walter P, Brubacher G, Stähelin H (eds) Elevated dosages of vitamins; benefits and hazards. Huber, Bern, pp 12–20
10. Stange L, Carletrom K, Erickson A 1978 Hypervitaminosis A in early human pregnancy and malformations of the central nervous system. Acta Obstetrica et Gynecologica Scandinavica 57: 289–291
11. Helgerud P, Saarem K, Norum K R 1981 Acyl-CoA: cholesterol acyltransferase in human small intestine: its activity and some properties of the enzymic reaction. Journal of Lipid Research 22: 271–277
12. Ong D E 1984 A novel retinol-binding protein from rat. Journal of Biological Chemistry 259: 1476–1482
13. Windler E, Chao T, Havel R 1980 Determinants of hepatic uptake of triglyceride-rich lipoprotein and their remnants in the rat. Journal of Biological Chemistry 255: 5475–5480
14. Blomhoff R, Berg T, Norum K R 1987 Absorption, transport and storage of retinol. Chemica Scripta 27: 109–177
15. De Luca H F 1979 Retinoic acid metabolism. Federation Proceedings 38: 2519–2523
16. Olson J A 1984 Vitamin A. In: Machlin L J (eds) Handbook of vitamins: nutritional, biochemical and clinical aspects. Marcel Dekker, New York
17. Bauernfeind J C 1980 The safe use of vitamin A. International vitamin A consultative group. The Nutrition Foundation, New York
18. Korner W F, Vollin J 1975 New aspects of the tolerance of retinol in humans. International Journal of Vitamin and Nutritional Research 45: 363–372

Ribavirin

Ribavirin is a broad-spectrum antiviral agent. It has been developed for the treatment of respiratory syncytial virus (RSV) infections by an aerosol route of administration and has shown considerable efficacy in the treatment of influenza A and B by this aerosol route of administration. It has also been administered intravenously in the effective treatment of Lassa fever and epidemic haemorrhagic fever with renal syndrome.

Chemistry

Ribavirin (Tribavirin, Virazole, Vilona, Virazide, Virazid)
$C_8H_{12}N_4O_5$
1-β-D-Ribofuranosyl-1,2,4-triazole-3-carboxamide

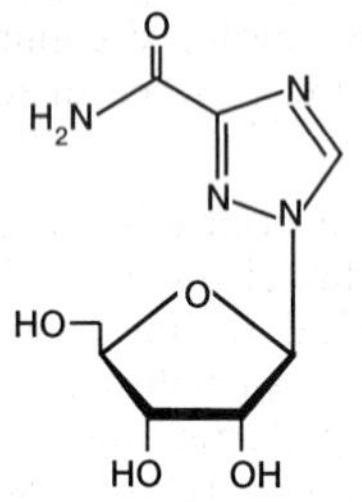

Molecular weight	244.2
pKa	—
Solubility	
in alcohol	poor
in water	1 in 7
Octanol/water partition coefficient	low

Ribavirin is a colourless, odourless, tasteless, crystalline compound prepared by chemical synthesis.
It is supplied as a sterile lyophilized powder to be reconstituted in sterile water at a final concentration of 20 g.l^{-1}. Ribavirin is not available in any combination preparations.

Pharmacology

Ribavirin is a broadly effective antiviral agent which has shown virustatic activity against a wide range of DNA and RNA viruses in vitro.[1] It has been approved for human use in an aerosol formulation for the treatment of lower respiratory disease caused by RSV and is being explored in the treatment of influenza A and B. It has also been employed in an injectable formulation for the treatment of Lassa fever and epidemic haemorrhagic fever with renal syndrome caused by the Hantaan virus. Its use in the treatment of early stages of human immunodeficiency virus infection is currently under investigation.

Ribavirin is taken up by cells and phosphorylated intracellularly to ribavirin 5′-monophosphate and quite rapidly to ribavirin 5′-triphosphate.[2,3] Ribavirin 5′-monophosphate is a powerful inhibitor of inosine monophosphate dehydrogenase,[4] which in turn causes considerable perturbation of both the ribonucleoside triphosphate and deoxyribonucleoside triphosphate pool sizes.[5,6] What effect this change in pool sizes may have on viral replication is unknown at present.

Ribavirin triphosphate both inhibits the guanylation reaction in formation of the 5′ cap on messenger RNA[7,8] and is an effective inhibitor of the viral RNA (guanine-7) methyltransferase. Messenger RNA isolated from Venezuelan equine encephalitis virus grown in BHk-21 cells exposed to low levels of ribavirin was only able to support protein synthesis at a very reduced efficiency.[8]

Although ribavirin triphosphate is a powerful inhibitor of influenza virus RNA polymerase,[9] it has no effect on a wide array of animal cell RNA polymerases.[10] Ribavirin is a powerful inhibitor of thymidine phosphorylation but has no effect on DNA synthesis at normal therapeutic levels,[11] nor is it incorporated into nucleic acids.[5]

Toxicology

A wide range of toxicology testings with ribavirin were performed in animal studies using different animal species to evaluate the possible adverse effects of the drug. The results of these studies, where a variety of parameters were investigated, have shown that ribavirin does not induce any serious effects if administered at a dose level close to that used in man under clinical conditions.

In general, adverse effects occurred only at dose levels which were many-fold greater than the intended human dose. There were variations in the degree of toxicity, attributable to the biological differences between the animal species and sexes used in these studies.

Some drug-related effects were noted in animals treated with doses close to the human therapeutic dose, which might have clinical relevance in the treatment of humans. Most of these changes were mild and reversible after cessation of drug administration, others were not evaluated for reversibility, because of minor significance.

Haematology and bone marrow

Studies of the haematological and bone marrow effects of ribavirin were conducted in groups of four Rhesus monkeys, given 30 and 100 mg.kg^{-1} ribavirin daily for 10 days by intramuscular injection.[12] The low-dose group developed a mild, and the high-dose group a more severe, normochromic, normocytic anaemia by the tenth day of treatment. Red cell counts, haematocrit and haemoglobin values decreased during drug administration. The anaemia was reversible and normal values were obtained by about 32 days post-dosing.

Dose-related thrombocytosis occurred on day 15–22 in both groups; platelet counts returned to control levels on day 42. Platelet function was not affected by treatment. Myeloid/erythroid ratio of bone marrow aspirates increased in both groups by day 10 and returned to baseline by day 22. The increase was not significant in the low-dose group. Myeloid precursors were not affected. Megakaryocytes were increased on day 10 in both groups. Blood and bone marrow effects were completely reversed when treatment was discontinued.

Short-term repeated dose studies

Short-term repeated dose studies of ribavirin have been conducted in rats, monkeys, dogs, and ferrets. As was observed in the acute studies, the dog is abnormally sensitive as compared to rodents or monkeys.

Groups of beagle dogs were given 0, 15, 30 or 60 mg.kg^{-1} ribavirin daily by oral gavage for 28 days.[13] Dose-related clinical findings included diarrhoea with soft, mucoid stools, anorexia, depression, and emesis in the high- and mid-dose animals, but symptoms were limited to diarrhoea and soft, mucoid stools in the low-dose group. Upon microscopic examination, only mild changes were noted in the gastrointestinal tract of the low-dose animals.

Effects on the developing mammalian lung

A study of inhaled ribavirin aerosols in the developing mammalian lung (ferrets) demonstrated lactation failure in the nursing mothers,[14] but only in the high- and mid-dose animals. Groups of jill (mother) ferrets and their litters were given whole body inhalation exposures for 6 hours a day for 10 or 30 consecutive days at concentrations of 0 (vehicle control), 162, 355 or 620 μg.l^{-1}. The effects, including special lung observations in suckling kits, were evaluated after exposures, at weaning and at puberty. The lung DNA analyses (DNA to protein ratios) indicated the possible presence of a mild proliferative response in smaller animals. This effect was no longer present after the 120 to 140 day of recovery. At the low dose level, which represents a dose 4 to 7 times that used clinically in man, there was a slight body-weight decrease, otherwise it appeared to be a no-effect level.[15]

Chronic studies

Two chronic studies of ribavirin were performed in rats. In the first study,[16] doses of 0, 30, 60 or 120 mg.kg^{-1} ribavirin daily were administered in the feed for two years. Regarding non-neoplastic lesions, a treatment-related increase in small testes was reported in males dying between 3 and 5 months on test. An increased incidence of mammary galactocoeles in females and testicular atrophy in males were noted at interim sacrifice at 15 months.

Reproduction and teratogenicity

Reproduction and teratogenicity studies have been conducted in rats, mice, rabbits and baboons.

Rats were administered doses of 0.1, 1.0 or 10 mg.kg^{-1} ribavirin daily orally from day 6 through 15 or gestation.[17] An increased incidence of terata, including gastroschisis and adactylia, was seen at the highest dose but not the lower doses. A marginal increase in embryo lethality was found in rabbits treated with 1.0 mg.kg^{-1} or ribavirin daily by the oral route, from day 6 through 18 of gestation,[17] but not in those treated with 0.1 or 0.3 mg.kg^{-1}. Thalidomide was utilized as a positive control.

No terata or embryotoxicity was found in baboons given up to 120 mg.kg^{-1} ribavirin orally during gestation in 4-day periods ranging from day 20 to day 39, corresponding to the major stages of organogenesis.[18]

Mutagenicity

Genetic toxicity studies on ribavirin have been carried out using a wide variety of organisms and cultured cells. No genotoxicity has been reported with the exception of a marginal and non-dose-related response in a cell transformation assay in BALB 3T3 cells and a response at the thymidine kinase locus in mouse lymphoma cells. The thymidine kinase locus is an inappropriate site for studying ribavirin's mutagenicity since the compound inhibits thymidine kinase activity at the genetic locus being studied.

Carcinogenicity

Two carcinogenicity studies of ribavirin in rats were performed. In the first study, only two tumour types occurred at an incidence of greater than two in any of the treatment groups: pituitary adenomas in males and females, and mammary fibroadenomas in females. In neither case was the tumour incidence increased by a statistically significant amount in the treated as compared to the control animals. Pituitary adenomas occurred at a higher incidence in the low- and mid-dose males, but the probability values were insignificant at the $p = 0.025$ level as required by the Bonferroni multiple comparison methodology customarily employed in analysing carcinogenicity studies.

In the second study tumours occurred at incidences great enough for statistical analyses for only five tumour types: pituitary gland adenomas and adrenal phaeochromocytomas in males and females; and mammary papillary cyst adenomas, mammary gland adenomas, and mammary fibroadenomas in females. The above findings occurred in lower incidence or at the same rate in the high-dose group compared with the controls, if adjustments were made for mortality. An increased mammary adenoma incidence with increasing dose was detected by the Cochran–Armitage and Incidental tumour tests ($p < 0.05$). However, this trend was not confirmed by comparisons of treatment groups to control, with all results non-significant at the Bonferroni significance level of incidence of mammary adenoma. In summary, there did not appear to be a statistically significant increase in tumours at any organ site in any of the treated as compared to control groups.

Clinical pharmacology

Ribavirin has antiviral activity against a range of DNA and RNA viruses in culture as shown in Table 1.

When given as an aerosol for 8 hours at a dose of 0.82 mg.kg^{-1}.h^{-1}, ribavirin achieves plasma concentrations of 0.8–1.5 mg.l^{-1}, corresponding to 3.3–6.1 μM (1 μg.ml^{-1} = 4.1 μM), whereas concentrations achieved in respiratory secretions are approximately 1000-fold higher (0.24–2.0 g.l^{-1}).[19] When ribavirin is administered intravenously in doses of 1000 mg four times daily, concentrations (not necessarily peak) in plasma vary from 21.5 to 24 mg.l^{-1}, whereas after 500 mg doses given four times daily concentrations in plasma are approximately 16 mg.l^{-1}. However, concentrations ranging from 1.1 to 16.8 mg.l^{-1} are observed 2.5 hours after 1000 mg doses of ribavirin given intravenously four times daily. Following multiple oral doses of ribavirin (1000 mg daily given in three divided doses), mean peak plasma ribavirin concentrations are in the range of 0.4 to 1.3 mg.l^{-1}.

The only approved route of administration in the USA is by

Table 1

Virus	Cells	Minimum inhibitory concentration ($mg.l^{-1}$)
DNA viruses		
Herpes simplex type I strain HF	KB	1
Herpes simplex type II strain HF	VERO	100
Herpes simplex type II strain MS	RK-13	3.2
RNA viruses		
Rhinovirus type 1A strain 2060	KB	10
Parainfluenza virus type 1 Sendai strain	CE	3.2
Coxsackie B virus type 1 strain Conn-S	KB	100
Measles virus strain Edmonston	VERO	32
Respiratory syncytial virus. Long strain	HEP-2	3.2
Lassa fever virus strain Josiah	RAM	10

aerosol for the treatment of RSV. Ribavirin may be given by small particle aerosol for 12 h or more per day for approximately three days for influenza disease in young adults, and for 18 h or more per day for 3–5 (or more) days in the treatment of RSV infection in children. For Lassa fever, intravenous ribavirin doses used ranged from 500 mg three times daily to 1000 mg four times daily.[20] Studies with oral and intravenous ribavirin for a variety of viral infections are currently ongoing.

Pharmacokinetics

Early studies were performed with radiolabelled drug.[21] Ribavirin concentrations have also been determined both by HPLC[22] and RIA.[23] However, the availability of the antiribavirin antibody is extremely limited. Therefore, the ability to measure ribavirin by this method is limited to only a few laboratories as a research tool for performing pharmacokinetic studies. The HPLC methodology, though not widely available, is technically feasible for many laboratories.

Ribavirin is incompletely absorbed from the gastrointestinal tract, with peak concentrations occurring at about 1.5 h (range, 1–2 h) after an oral dose.[24] The average bioavailability of ribavirin is approximately 45% (range 0.36–0.52). Ribavirin exhibits dose-independent kinetics when administered either orally or intravenously over the range of 600–2400 mg.[24] The drug has a very complex kinetic profile and following intravenous administration the decay of plasma ribavirin concentration appears to have at least three phases. In single-dose intravenous studies,[24] the terminal (γ) phase half life was 35.5 h (range 22.1–63.6 h). However, after multiple oral doses of ribavirin,[25] the drug persisted in plasma for weeks, with an average terminal half life of almost two weeks, with a range of 1–3 weeks. The β phase half life is approximately 2 h. The volume of distribution of ribavirin at steady state is extremely large (647 l with a range of 379–1138 l). This is somewhat unexpected for a water-soluble drug, and appears to be due to intracellular trapping of the drug as its phosphorylated forms in erythrocytes and perhaps other tissues. Ribavirin does not bind to plasma proteins (0%–7%).

Ribavirin is eliminated by both metabolism and by renal excretion.[21] Renal clearance ($99\ ml.min^{-1}$) accounts for approximately 35% of the elimination of the drug.[24] The total body clearance of ribavirin is $283\ ml.min^{-1}$. Because of its very long terminal half life, ribavirin will accumulate with any of the standard dosing intervals commonly used. Based on the terminal half life obtained from the chronic dosing studies (half life of approximately 2 weeks), and since it takes 4–5 half lives to obtain steady state, a loading dose is necessary. Because of the complex pharmacology of ribavirin, how loading should be accomplished has not yet been established.

The concentration of ribavirin in CSF is on average slightly less than that found in plasma. The CSF/plasma ratio ranges from 0.66 to 1.15.[26,27] Ribavirin is concentrated in erythrocytes as mentioned above. The mean erythrocyte to plasma ribavirin concentration ratio at steady state is approximately 9:1.[24] The decay of ribavirin from erythrocytes is very slow (half life of 40 days),[21] and probably plays a major role in the complex nature of ribavirin's pharmacokinetic profile.

Studies of ribavirin pharmacokinetics in patients with organ dysfunction are lacking. However, because only one-third of a dose is eliminated renally, it is unlikely that any modifications of the dose of ribavirin will be necessary in patients with renal dysfunction. This, of course, assumes that non-renal clearance of the drug is unaffected by renal insufficiency and that any renally excreted metabolites are non-toxic. The effects of hepatic dysfunction on the kinetics of ribavirin are unknown. No dose adjustment appears to be necessary in the elderly. It is not known whether the drug crosses the placenta, nor to what extent it is excreted in breast milk.

Oral absorption	~45%
Presystemic metabolism	—
Plasma terminal half life	
range	1–3 weeks
mean	2 weeks
Volume of distribution	647 l
Plasma protein binding	<10%

Concentration–effect relationship

There is no evidence of a correlation between the plasma concentration of ribavirin and its antiviral effects. However the in vitro minimum inhibitory concentration (MIC) values for some viruses in culture are shown in the Clinical pharmacology section.

Metabolism

Ribavirin is normally absorbed through the gut, or when administered by the aerosol route is readily absorbed through the endothelial tissues of the respiratory system. The only metabolite observed in human urine in single-bolus studies using ^{14}C-labelled ribavirin is deribosylated triazole carboxamide. The site of this deglycosylation is thought to be the liver, although the kidney may also possess this activity.[5]

The active intracellular form of ribavirin is the 5′-triphosphate which results from the combined action of adenosine kinase and other kinases on the absorbed nucleoside. Human red blood cells, which are poor in triphosphatases, tend to accumulate ribavirin while turnover in other tissues is considerably greater.[5]

Pharmaceutics

Ribavirin (Virazole; ICN Pharmaceuticals, USA/Virazid, Brittania, UK) is supplied for aerosol use as a 6 g lyophilized powder for reconstitution with water for injection to a final volume of 300 ml. The powder does not contain preservatives but once reconstituted may be stored for up to 24 hours at room temperature. Administration is by nebulization using a small particle aerosol generator such as a SPAG-2 or Bird respirator. Virazole is also available as a 200 mg capsule in some countries.

An injection formulation is not available commercially.

Therapeutic use

Indications

1. Treatment of bronchiolitis, pneumonia and other manifestations of RSV infection in infants.

Other uses

Ribavirin has recently been approved for the management of CDG stage III and IV a patients infected with human immunodeficiency virus by the Government of the Republic of Ireland.

Contraindications

There are no specific contraindications to the use of ribavirin small-particle aerosol in treatment of RSV infection. It is the only specifically active agent available for treatment of this disease.[28,29] In adult patients some deterioration in pulmonary function occurred during 215 min experimental exposures to usual therapeutic dosage of ribavirin aerosol.[30] These studies were performed, however, 24 h after stopping maintenance bronchodilator treatment. Pulmonary function returned to pretreatment levels spontaneously or following reinstitution of medication. One asthmatic female, age 5, was treated for 5 days for viral pneumonia from which she recovered promptly while receiving intravenous and inhalation bronchodilator medications.[31] Her asthma was improved following treatment during a follow-up period of several months.

Though not approved in the USA, ribavirin aerosol treatment of patients receiving mechanical ventilation has been performed regularly with favourable results.[32,33] One report, however, describes the occurrence of tension pneumothorax in an infant following fouling of positive end expiratory pressure valves by aerosol particles.[34] This can be avoided by inserting an air filter (BB-50T breathing circuit filter, Pall Biomedical Products Corp., East Hills, NY, USA) in the expiratory loop from the patient. The filter should be inspected for fouling and changed every 2 to 4 h.

The mild, reversible anaemia that may follow oral and intravenous treatment has not been observed following aerosol treatment, and no respiratory irritation has been associated with ribavirin aerosol treatment of babies. No untoward respiratory effects on adult patients treated with ribavirin aerosol are known.

Mode of use

The recommended concentration is 20 mg.ml^{-1} of ribavirin in the liquid reservoir of the aerosol generator to deliver 200 µg.l^{-1} of ribavirin, average concentration during a 12 h period of operation. The aerosol has a flow-rate of about 12.5 l.min^{-1} and the average adult will deposit about 50 mg hourly in the respiratory tract or 0.8 mg.kg^{-1} hourly.[31] This dose was arbitrarily adopted based on therapeutic studies in mice with the same dosage. Infants inhaling this aerosol will deposit about 1.7 times the amount deposited by adults, or about 1.4 mg.kg^{-1} hourly.[35]

The original dosage recommendations were for 12 h daily of treatment. With the observation of no apparent pulmonary or systemic intolerance, dosage periods were increased to 18–22 h daily for up to 5–6 days for severely ill patients. No intolerance was observed at these dosage levels, and such regimens have been used for more seriously ill patients. Dosage titration in human illness is logistically challenging and has not been formally undertaken. In mice, tripling the concentration to 60 mg.kg^{-1} in the liquid reservoir with a corresponding increase in concentration of ribavirin to about 600 µg.l^{-1} in the aerosol, and reducing the treatment period to 4 h daily from 12 or more hours daily with the lower concentration, gives protection from mortality equivalent to that with the longer treatment with the lower concentration.[36,37]

The concentration of ribavirin in the aerosol described above is used for infants and adults since actual dosage is controlled by the patient's minute volume. Rate and depth of breathing also affect the location and the extent of deposition of particles but these effects have not been adequately quantitated. The two major ways in which dosage may be changed are altering the duration of treatment or by increasing or decreasing the amount of drug in the liquid reservoir.

Indications

1. Treatment of bronchiolitis, pneumonia, and other manifestations of RSV infection

Ribavirin aerosol has been used successfully in the treatment of influenza A and B infections and is probably active in parainfluenza virus infections.[38–41] Current approval is for treatment of RSV infections and approval for influenza A and B is sought. Treatment for the above infections consists of two to six day courses of treatment as described above. The criterion for duration of treatment is severity of illness and once recovery has been substantially accomplished, treatment may be discontinued because relapse of illness with the above infections has not been observed. In some studies with RSV infection treatment has been limited to three days for economic reasons, with the expectation that any residual mild illness will resolve. There are no known untoward effects of stopping treatment suddenly other than insufficient treatment.

Contraindications

At present pregnancy is a contraindication to treatment (see below). The cost of the drug can be a limiting factor but not a contraindication. Any patient with RSV infection and any degree of illness should benefit by treatment with ribavirin. It seems logical not to treat milder cases however, since the vast majority recover quickly. The reversal of hypoxaemia more promptly in treated patients raises the question as to whether treatment with earlier resolution of the pulmonary lesion might diminish the possibility of chronic pulmonary disease subsequently.[32,33] No answer is available to this question at this time.

Ribavirin

It is most unlikely that local or systemic intolerance will occur and this possibility should not constitute a contraindication to treatment. As with all medication, close supervision of treated patients is advised to detect as early as possible any unexpected complication of the disease or of the treatment.

Adverse reactions

When ribavirin is administered by aerosol, no clinically significant toxicity was observed. When given by oral or intravenous route, adverse reactions were dose-related.[25] Significant adverse reactions are seen when ribavirin doses of greater than 600 mg daily are given.

Potentially life-threatening effects

No adverse effects of this kind appear to have been reported.

Acute overdosage

No case of this kind appears to have been reported.

Severe or irreversible adverse effects

No effects of this kind appear to have been reported.

Symptomatic adverse effects

The adverse reactions of ribavirin have included metallic taste, increased thirst, gastrointestinal complaints, fatigue and irritability, mood changes, headache, insomnia and a decrease in erythrocytes. At oral doses of ribavirin of 600, 1200 and 2400 mg daily, the mean decrease in the haematocrit was 0%, 4.4% and 12.1%, respectively.[25,27] This dose-related fall in haematocrit was associated with a reticulocytosis and an increase in the serum bilirubin.

The haematological changes have not occurred following ribavirin aerosol treatment.[42]

Beyond the occasional complaint of eye irritation due to deposited drug, which is infrequent and inconsequential, no other symptoms have been attributed to the use of ribavirin aerosol.

Other effects

Deposited drug has also been observed on the tip of endotracheal catheters. Periodic rinsing of catheters or replacing them will obviate the problem. Note the earlier report of reduction of pulmonary function in COPD patients and transient wheezing in asthma patients challenged after stopping maintenance bronchodilator treatment.[30]

No modifications of body biochemistry are known to result from ribavirin aerosol treatment and none are known to follow parenteral treatment.

Interference with clinical pathology tests

No such interference is known.

High risk groups

Neonates

At one time it was suggested that excess water was deposited in the lungs of neonates treated with ribavirin aerosol. Calculation reveals that a baby would deposit less than 0.25 ml of water in drug aerosol per hour. In addition, about 0.5 ml of water vapour would be inhaled during this time, but this would equilibrate with the high relative humidity of air or air–oxygen mixtures used in care of babies.[43] These amounts of water would not cause harm. Iatrogenic water loading through parenteral infusion is a common problem in care of infants receiving mechanical ventilation. This event needs to be distinguished from the inconsequential effect of pulmonary deposition of water from ribavirin aerosol.

Breast milk. It is not known whether the drug enters breast milk, so mothers taking it should not breast-feed.

Children

No special precautions appear to be necessary.

Pregnant women

There is no evidence of fetal toxicity in pregnant women in a very limited experience[44] but the drug has been shown to be teratogenic and embryocidal to rodents.[45] In a study in primates, pregnant baboons exposed to the drug during the period of organogenesis delivered normal offspring.[45]

The drug is therefore contraindicated in pregnant women unless its safety in this circumstance can be demonstrated in the future. The drug has been used on one patient at term with influenzal pneumonia with a favourable clinical result and a normal baby.[31] Pregnant

Ribavirin

R

women, however, have a worse prognosis from influenzal pneumonia than other patients, and it is reasonable to consider treating such patients with ribavirin aerosol after full and detailed disclosure of hazards to the patient and her family.

The elderly

Many elderly patients have been treated with ribavirin aerosol for influenza without toxicity or intolerance. No special precautions are required.

Concurrent disease

Clinical experience to the present has not revealed hazards in relation to ribavirin aerosol treatment in common systemic diseases. Renal failure would necessarily reduce renal excretion of the drug, but the short duration of ribavirin aerosol treatment probably makes reducing treatment unnecessary. About one-third of the drug is excreted unchanged in the urine and the disposition of the remaining portion is not known.[24] An early report of slight increases in serum bilirubin after oral medication with ribavirin probably represented excess destruction of red cells in treated patients and not liver disease or toxicity resulting from ribavirin treatment.[46]

Drug interactions

No interactions between ribavirin and other drugs have been reported.

References

1. Viratek, Inc. Virazole 1986: Ribavirin. Lyophilized for Aerosol Administration. Canadian Label, ICN, Montreal, Quebec, Canada, 28 July
2. Zimmerman T P, Deeprose R D 1978 Metabolism of 5-amino-2-beta-D-ribofuranosyl-imidazole-4-carboxamide and related five-membered heterocycles to 5′-triphosphates in human blood and L51 784 cells. Biochemical Pharmacology 27: 709–716
3. Willis R C, Carson D A, Seegmiller J E 1978 Adenosine kinase initiates the major route of ribavirin activation in a cultured human cell line. Proceedings of the National Academy of Sciences USA 75: 3042–3044
4. Streeter D G, Witkowski J T, Khare G P et al 1973 Mechanism of action of 1-beta-D-ribofuranosyl-1,2,4-triazole-3-carboxamide (Virazole), a new broad-spectrum antiviral agent. Proceedings of the National Academy of Sciences USA 70: 1174
5. Smith R A, Wade M J 1973 Ribavirin: a broad-spectrum antiviral agent. In: Stapleton T (ed) Studies with a broad-spectrum antiviral agent. Royal Society of Medicine Services, London, pp 3–23
6. Lowe J K, Brox L, Henderson J F 1977 Consequences of inhibition of guanine nucleotide synthesis by mycophenolic acid and Virazole. Cancer Research 37: 736–743
7. Goswami B B, Borek E, Sharma O K, Fujitaki J, Smith R A 1979 The broad-spectrum antiviral agent ribavirin inhibits capping of mRNA. Biochemical and Biophysical Research Communications 89: 830–836
8. Canonico P G, Little J S, Jahrling P B, Stephen E L 1980 Molecular aspects of the antiviral activity of ribavirin on Venezuelan Equine Encephalomyelitis virus. In: Proceedings of the 11th ICC and 19th ICAAC, American Society of Microbiology. Current Chemotherapy of Infectious Diseases, pp 1370–1372
9. Wray S K, Gilbert B E, Noall M W, Knight V 1985 Mode of action of ribavirin: effect of nucleotide pool alterations on influenza virus ribonucleoprotein synthesis. Antiviral Research 5: 29–37
10. Smith R A, Sidwell R W, Robins R K 1980 Antiviral mechanisms of action. Annual Review of Pharmacology and Toxicology 20: 259–284
11. Drach J C, Shipman C Jr 1977 The selective inhibition of viral DNA synthesis by chemotherapeutic agents: an indicator of clinical usefulness. Annals of the New York Academy of Science 284: 396–409
12. United States Army Medical Institute of Infectious Diseases, 1981
13. Hazelton, 1982
14. Litton Bionetics Institute, Kensington, Maryland, USA 1984
15. Hoffmann S H, Staffa J H, Smith R A, Craig D K, Parker G 1987 Inhalation toxicity of ribavirin in suckling ferrets. Journal of Applied Toxicology 7: 343–351
16. Industrial Biotest Laboratories, Northbrook, Illinois, USA 1975
17. Industrial Biotest Laboratories, Northbrook, Illinois, USA 1973
18. Inverness Research Institute, Inverness, Scotland 1977
19. Connor J D, Hintz M, Van Dyke R, McCormick J B, McIntosh K 1984 Ribavirin pharmacokinetics in children and adults during therapeutic trials. In: Smith R A, Knight V, Smith J A D (eds) Clinical applications of ribavirin. Academic Press, New York, pp 107–123
20. McCormick J B, King I J, Webb P A et al 1986 Lassa fever. Effective therapy with ribavirin. New England Journal of Medicine 314: 20–26
21. Catlin D H, Smith R A, Samuels A I 1980 ^{14}C-ribavirin: Distribution and pharmacokinetic studies in rats, baboons and man. In: Smith R A, Kirkpatrick W (eds) Ribavirin: a broad-spectrum antiviral agent. Academic Press, New York, pp 83–98
22. Smith R H A, Gilbert B E 1987 Quantification of ribavirin in biological fluids and tissues by high-performance liquid chromatography. Journal of Chromatography 414: 202–210
23. Austin R K, Trefts P E, Hintz M, Connor J D, Kagnoff M F 1983 Sensitive radioimmunoassay for the broad-spectrum antiviral agent ribavirin. Antimicrobial Agents and Chemotherapy 24: 696–701
24. Laskin O L, Longstreth J A, Hart C C et al 1987 Ribavirin disposition in high-risk patients for acquired immunodeficiency syndrome. Clinical Pharmacology and Therapeutics 41: 543–555
25. Roberts R B, Laskin O L, Laurence J et al 1987 Ribavirin pharmacodynamics in high-risk patients for acquired immunodeficiency syndrome. Clinical Pharmacology and Therapeutics 42: 365–373
26. Crumpacker C, Bubley G, Lucey D, Hussey S, Connor J 1986 Ribavirin enters cerebrospinal fluid (letter). Lancet 2: 45–46
27. Roberts R B, Laskin O L 1988 Phase 1 clinical studies of ribavirin in high risk patients for the acquired immunodeficiency syndrome. In: Smith R A (ed) HIV and other highly pathogenic viruses. Academic Press, New York, pp 95–112
28. Taber L H, Knight V, Gilbert B E et al 1983 Ribavirin aerosol treatment of bronchiolitis associated with respiratory syncytial virus infection in infants. Pediatrics 72: 613–618
29. Hall C B, McBride J T, Walsh E E et al 1983 Aerosolized ribavirin treatment of infants with respiratory syncytial virus infection. New England Journal of Medicine 308: 1443–1447
30. Light B, Aoki F Y, Serrette C 1984 Tolerance of ribavirin aerosol inhaled by normal volunteers and patients with asthma or chronic obstructive airways disease. In: Smith R A, Knight V, Smith J A D (eds) Clinical applications of ribavirin. Academic Press, New York, pp 97–105
31. Knight V, Gilbert B E, Wilson S Z 1986 Ribavirin small-particle aerosol treatment of influenza and respiratory syncytial virus infections. In: Stapleton T (ed) Studies with a broad-spectrum antiviral agent. Royal Society of Medicine Services, London, pp 37–56
32. Hall C B, McBride J T, Gala C L, Hildreth S W, Schnabel K C 1985 Ribavirin treatment of respiratory syncytial viral infection in infants with underlying cardiopulmonary disease. Journal of the American Medical Association 254: 3047–3051
33. Hall C B, Powell K R, MacDonald N E et al 1986 Respiratory syncytial viral infection in children with compromised immune function. New England Journal of Medicine 315: 77–86
34. Conrad D A, Christensen J C, Waner J L, Marks M I 1987 Aerosolized ribavirin treatment of respiratory syncytial virus infection in infants hospitalized during an epidemic. Pediatric Infectious Disease Journal 6: 152–158
35. Knight V, Gilbert B E 1987 Ribavirin aerosol treatment of influenza. Infectious Disease Clinics of North America, vol 1, no 2: 441–457
36. Wyde P R, Wilson S Z, Gilbert B E, Smith R H A 1986 Protection of mice from lethal influenza virus infection with high dose–short duration ribavirin aerosol. Antimicrobial Agents and Chemotherapy 30: 942–944
37. Wyde P R, Wilson S Z, Petrella R, Gilbert B E 1987 Efficacy of high dose–short duration ribavirin aerosol in the treatment of respiratory syncytial virus infected cotton rats and influenza B virus infected mice. Antiviral Research 7: 211–220
38. Knight V, Wilson S Z, Quarles J M et al 1981 Ribavirin small-particle aerosol treatment of influenza. Lancet 2: 945–949
39. McClung H W, Knight V, Gilbert B E, Wilson S Z, Quarles J M, Divine G 1983 Ribavirin aerosol treatment of influenza B virus infection. Journal of the American Medical Association 249: 2671–2674
40. Wilson S Z, Gilbert B E, Quarles J M et al 1984 Treatment of influenza A (H1N1) virus infection with ribavirin aerosol Antimicrobial Agents and Chemotherapy 26: 200–203
41. Gilbert B E, Wilson S Z, Knight V et al 1985 Ribavirin small-particle aerosol treatment of infections caused by influenza virus strains A/Victoria/7/83 (H1N1) and B/Texas/1/84. Antimicrobial Agents and Chemotherapy 27: 309–313
42. Canonico P G 1983 Ribavirin. A review of efficacy, toxicity and mechanisms of antiviral activity. In: Hahn F E (ed) Antibiotics vol VI: modes and mechanisms of microbial growth inhibitors. Springer-Verlag, Berlin, pp 161–186
43. Knight V, Gilbert B E, Wilson S Z 1986 Ribavirin aerosol treatment of influenza and respiratory syncytial virus infections. In: de la Maza L M, Peterson E M (eds) Medical virology. Academic Press, New York, Lawrence Erlbaum Assoc, Hillsdale, New Jersey (USA), pp 445–466
44. Fernandes U 1987 Personal Communication
45. Hillyard I W 1980 The preclinical toxicology and safety of ribavirin. In: Smith R A, Kirkpatrick W (eds) Ribavirin: a broad-spectrum antiviral agent. Academic Press, New York, pp 59–71
46. Smith C B, Charette R P 1980 Double-blind evaluation of ribavirin in naturally occurring influenza. In: Smith R A, Kirkpatrick W (eds) Ribavirin: a broad-spectrum antiviral agent. Academic Press, New York, pp 147–164

Riboflavin

Riboflavin is a vitamin of the B complex.

Chemistry

Riboflavin (Riboflavine, vitamin B_2 Beflavit, Beflavin, Flavin, Ribipca, Beflavina, Berivine)
$C_{17}H_{20}N_4O_6$
(7,8-Dimethyl-10(D-ribo-2-3,4-5-tetrahydroxypentyl)-isoalloxazine-

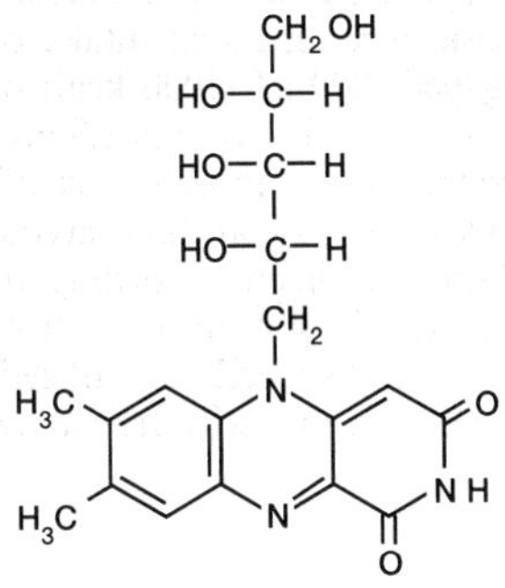

Molecular weight	376.4
pKa	1.9, 10.2
Solubility	
in alcohol	<1 in 10 000
in water	1 in 3000–20 000
Octanol/water partition coefficient	—

Lactoflavin is an isoalloxazine derivative with a ribitol side-chain. The vitamin was designated as riboflavin because of the presence of ribose in its structure.

Riboflavin is a yellow or orange crystalline powder, with a slight odour and persistent bitter taste, prepared by chemical synthesis. It is present in yeast, milk, egg, malted barley, liver, kidney, heart, and green leafy vegetables, and in minute amounts in plant and animal cells. It occurs in the free form only in retina, in whey and in urine. Its principal biologically active forms are flavin mononucleotide (FMN) and flavin adenine dinucleotide (FAD).

When dry, it is not affected by diffuse light, but when in solution, riboflavin deteriorates rapidly, deterioration being accelerated by light. Three different crystal forms have different solubilities in water, due to differences in the crystal structure. Riboflavin is more soluble in NaCl solution, less soluble in alcohol than in water. The aqueous solution is neutral to litmus and is yellow in colour, showing green fluorescence with an absorption maximum at 565 nm. Optimal fluorescence is obtained at pH 6–7. Although sensitive to alkalis, riboflavin is quite stable to mineral acids in the dark. Riboflavin is soluble in physiological saline and 10% urea solution.

Various multivitamin preparations (B-complex group) contain an active ingredient of riboflavin (vitamin B_2) in the form of tablets, capsules, injections and pills. They are also sold over the counter as nutritional supplements in the form of syrups and elixirs.

Pharmacology

Riboflavin is inactive until phosphorylated. Flavin mononucleotide (FMN) and flavin adenine dinucleotide (FAD) are its active forms and these are involved as coenzymes in the respiratory chain. FAD and FMN influence hydrogen transport in oxidative enzyme systems such as cytochrome C reductase, succinic dehydrogenase and xanthine oxidase. Riboflavin is converted to FMN and FAD by two enzyme-catalysed reactions:[1,2]

Riboflavin + ATP → FMN + ADP
FMN + ATP → FAD + PP

FMN and FAD are coenzymes for a wide variety of respiratory flavoproteins, some of which also require metals.

Thyroid hormones, corticotrophins and aldosterone enhance the formation of FMN and FAD, while phenothiazines and tricyclic antidepressants inhibit FAD formation. Boric acid increases the excretion of riboflavin.[3]

The requirement for riboflavin depends on the carbohydrate intake and is increased during pregnancy, lactation and in women taking oral contraceptive agents. Riboflavin requirement is also increased by prolonged administration of drugs such as phenothiazines. Riboflavin reduces the antibacterial activity of solutions of streptomycin, erythromycin, tyrothricin, carbomycin and tetracycline. In the case of tetracyclines, the reaction is a photochemical oxidation. Inactivation also occurs with chloramphenicol, penicillin or neomycin.[4,5]

Toxicology

Riboflavin has been found to be practically non-toxic. LD_{50} in mice and rats is 340–560 mg.kg^{-1} intraperitoneally. Daily administration of riboflavin (10–25 mg.kg^{-1} body weight) to rats and dogs for up to 4 months produced no toxic effect.

There is no report of a teratogenic effect resulting from either riboflavin deficiency or excess. Mutagenicity and carcinogenicity tests have not been carried out.

Clinical pharmacology

Simple riboflavin deficiency is rare. It is associated with the combined vitamin B-complex deficiencies.[3] Riboflavin deficiency symptoms include angular stomatitis, glossitis, cheolosis, red denuded lips, and seborrhoeic dermatitis over the trunk and extremities, followed by anaemia, neuropathy, corneal vascularization, cataract formation and normochromic anaemia. Anaemia of riboflavin deficiency is also due to a disturbance in folic acid metabolism. Certain features of riboflavin deficiency such as glossitis and dermatitis are common to deficiencies of other vitamins. Recognition of early riboflavin deficiency in human beings is difficult as it rarely occurs in isolation. Assessment of riboflavin status is made by correlating dietary history with clinical and laboratory findings. Excretion of less than 50 mg of riboflavin daily is indicative of deficiency. Although the concentration of flavins in blood is not of diagnostic value, an enzyme activation assay that utilizes glutathione reductase from erythrocytes correlates well with riboflavin status.[6]

Patients with hepatitis and cirrhosis of the liver and those given probenecid have reduced intestinal absorption of riboflavin.[7,8]

Riboflavin could cause discoloration of urine.[9] No overt pharmacological effect follows after oral or parenteral administration of riboflavin.

NRC has recommended a riboflavin intake of 0.6 mg per 1000 kcal (4200 kJ). This is equivalent to 1.6 mg daily for young adult males and 1.2 mg daily for young adult females. Intake for elderly persons should not be less than 1.2 mg daily even when caloric intake falls below 2000 kcal (8400 kJ). See Table 1.

Table 1 Recommended dietary intake of riboflavin

	Age (years)	Dose per day (mg)
Infants	0–1	0.4–0.6
Children	1–10	0.6–1.2
Males	10–75	1.3–1.7
Females	10–75	1.3–1.5
Pregnancy		1.8–2.0
Lactation		2.0

Pharmacokinetics

Riboflavin and its coenzymes (FMN and FAD) can be detected with high sensitivity using high pressure liquid chromatography which has a sensitivity[10] of 50 μg.l^{-1}.

R

Riboflavin is readily absorbed from the gastrointestinal tract, and in circulation it is bound to plasma proteins. Although riboflavin is widely distributed to all tissues, little is stored in the body.[11] Amounts in excess of the body's requirement are excreted in the urine. Riboflavin excretion in the faeces represents biosynthesis of this vitamin by microorganisms in the large intestine. There is little evidence of its reabsorption from the large intestine.[7]

Renal clearance of riboflavin involves renal tubular secretion as well as glomerular filtration and exceeds endogenous creatine clearance by up to three times. Clearance is reduced at low serum concentrations of riboflavin. Sixty per cent of the riboflavin in serum is bound to serum proteins. Prior administration of probenecid decreases the renal clearance of riboflavin but does not affect its protein binding.[8]

Riboflavin is readily absorbed from the upper gastrointestinal tract by a specific transport mechanism involving phosphorylation of the vitamin to FMN.[12] Here, as in other tissues, riboflavin is converted to FMN by flavokinase, a reaction that is sensitive to thyroid hormone status and inhibited by chlorpromazine and by tricyclic antidepressants.[3] The riboflavin content of human milk[13] is 300 $\mu g.l^{-1}$.

Oral absorption	good
Presystemic metabolism	—
Plasma half life	~1 h
Volume of distribution	—
Plasma protein binding	60%

Concentration–effect relationship

Though the concentration of flavin in blood is not of diagnostic value, an enzyme activation assay that utilizes glutathione reductase from erythrocytes correlates well with riboflavin status.[6]

Metabolism

When riboflavin is ingested in amounts approximating the minimum daily requirement most of it is utilized in various tissues with only 9% appearing in the urine. Larger doses of riboflavin are excreted in the urine largely unchanged. It is not stored in body tissues to any great extent. Riboflavin is converted to FMN and FAD in the liver after its absorption through the gastrointestinal tract (Fig. 1). Patients with hepatitis and cirrhosis of liver and those given probenecid have reduced absorption of riboflavin.[7] Riboflavin in the form of FMN and FAD is phosphorylated in the intestinal mucosa during absorption and stored in small quantities in liver, spleen, kidney and heart muscle. FMN and FAD are mainly involved in the electron transport chain, and form a link between the pyridine nucleotide system and the cytochrome system. Xanthine oxidase flavoprotein, which converts hypoxanthine to uric acid, and amino acid oxidases, which convert amino acids to ammonia and keto acids, require riboflavin coenzymes. The flavoproteins are mainly concerned with hydrogen transport (oxidation). Excess riboflavin is excreted in urine as such and there is no known metabolite with pharmacological activity.

Fig. 1 The metabolism of riboflavin

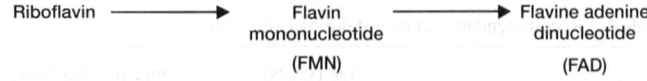

Riboflavin ⟶ Flavin mononucleotide (FMN) ⟶ Flavine adenine dinucleotide (FAD)

Pharmaceutics

Vitamin B_2 is available in oral, parenteral and intravenous preparations. It is usually administered by mouth. If for any reason it cannot be absorbed or utilized by the oral route, it may be injected.

Tablets and capsules of 1 mg, 2 mg, 5 mg are available. Vitamin B_2 is available in the form of a mixture with other vitamins.

Sterile solutions containing 5 mg of riboflavin with stabilizer which is dissolved in 2.3 ml sterilized distilled water before use. Solutions are sterilized by autoclaving or by filtration.

Riboflavin is incompatible with alkali and salts of heavy metals. It should be stored in airtight containers and protected from light. When dry it is not appreciably affected by diffuse light, but in solution, especially in the presence of alkali, it deteriorates rapidly. The decomposition is enhanced by light. Liver, kidney, egg, milk, yeast and green vegetables are rich dietary sources of this vitamin. There is little loss of riboflavin from these foods during cooking.

Under cool, airtight, watertight and light-protected conditions, riboflavin can be stored for 2–3 years without any degradation.

Therapeutic use

Indications

1. Arabinoflavinosis
2. Multiple nutritional vitamin deficiency.

Contraindications

None is known.

Mode of use

Riboflavin requirement is related to the energy intake but it appears to be more closely related to resting metabolic requirement. A normal adult requires 1.3–1.8 mg daily. Requirements are increased during pregnancy and lactation. The basic recommended intake of riboflavin has been reported to be 550 μg per 4200 kJ (1000 kcal) of diet, so that a man requires 1.8 mg of riboflavin and a woman 1.3 mg of riboflavin per day.

There is little evidence that riboflavin is of specific therapeutic value except in the treatment of arabinoflavinosis (rare) for which doses of 2–10 mg daily are given according to the severity of the condition. It is administered by mouth but it may be injected if for any reason it cannot be absorbed or utilized by the oral route. Riboflavin does not produce any withdrawal symptoms.

Indications

1. Arabinoflavinosis

2. Multiple nutritional vitamin deficiency

Riboflavin is used to prevent or treat diseases caused by deficiency. Arabinoflavinosis seldom occurs as a distinct or discrete deficiency but may accompany other nutritional disorders. Specific therapy with riboflavin 5 to 10 mg daily is recommended for treating multiple nutritional deficiencies.

Adverse reactions

Riboflavin is reported to be completely safe and no toxic symptoms have been reported so far.

Interference with clinical pathology tests

No technical interferences of this kind have been reported.

High risk groups

No special precautions are required in any healthy patient.

Concurrent disease

Patients with hepatitis and cirrhosis of the liver and those given probenecid have reduced absorption of riboflavin.

Drug interactions

Potentially hazardous interactions

None has been described.

Other significant interactions

Prior administration of probenecid decreases the renal clearance of riboflavin but does not affect its binding with proteins.

Riboflavin reduces the antibiotic activity of solutions of streptomycin, erythromycin, tyrothricin, carbomycin and tetracyclines. At least in the case of tetracyclines the reaction is a photochemical oxidation. No inactivation occurs with chloramphenicol, penicillin or neomycin.[7]

Thyroid hormones, corticotrophin and aldosterone enhance the formation of FMN and FAD, while phenothiazines and possibly tricyclic antidepressants inhibit FAD formation. Boric acid increases the excretion of riboflavin.[3]

Potentially useful interactions

None has been described.

General review articles

Adelekan D A, Thurnham D J 1986 The influence of riboflavine deficiency or absorption and liver storage of iron in the growing rat. British Journal of Nutrition 56: 171–179

Bates C J, Fuller N J 1986 The effect of riboflavine deficiency on methylene tetrahydrofolate reductase and folate metabolism in the rat. British Journal of Nutrition 55(2): 455–464

Botticher B, Botticher D 1987 A new HPLC method for the simultaneous determination of B_1, B_2 and B_6 vitamers in serum and whole blood. Journal of Vitamin and Nutrition Research 57(3): 273–278

Brodfuehrer J I, Zannoni V G 1987 Flavin containing monooxygenase and ascorbic acid deficiency. Qualitative and quantitative differences. Biochemical Pharmacology 36: 3161–3167

Cimino J A, Noto R A, Fusco C L, Cooperman J M 1988 Riboflavin metabolism in the hypothyroid new born. American Journal of Clinical Nutrition 47(3): 481–483

Danas J, Lehanka J, Levitz M 1988 Placental transport of riboflavin, differential rates of uptake at the maternal and fetal surfaces of the perfused human placenta. American Journal of Obstetrics and Gynecology 158: 204–210

Lane M, Smith F E, Alfrey C P 1975 Experimental dietary and antagonist induced human riboflavin deficiency. In: Rivlin R S (ed) Riboflavin. Plenum Press, New York, pp 245–277

Lavingne C, Zee J A, Simard R E, Gosselin C 1987 High performance liquid chromatographic diode array determination of ascorbic acid, thiamine and riboflavin in goat's milk. Journal of Chromatography 410: 201–205

Lucas A, Bates C J 1987 Occurrence and significance of riboflavin deficiency in preterm infants. Biology of the Neonate 52: 113–118

Moore G L, Fishman R M 1987 High performance liquid chromatographic analysis of ascorbate-2-phosphate, adenine and hypoxanthin in stored human blood. Journal of Chromatography 419: 95–102

Pinto J T, Rivlin R S 1987 Drugs that promote renal excretion of riboflavin. Drug Nutrient Interactions 5: 143–151

Roe D A, Kalkwarf H, Stevens J 1988 Effect of fibre supplements on the apparent absorption of pharmacological doses of riboflavin. Journal of the American Dietetic Association 88(2): 211–213

Ross N S, Hoppel C L 1987 Acyl-CoA dehydrogenase activity in the riboflavin-deficient rat, effects of starvation. Biochemical Journal 244: 387–391

Visweswariah S S, Adiga P R 1987 Isolation of riboflavin carrier proteins from pregnant human and umbilical cord serum. Similarities with chicken egg riboflavin carrier protein. Biological Science Reports 7(7): 563–571

Visweswariah S S, Karande A A, Adiga P R 1987 Immunological characterization of riboflavine carrier proteins using monoclonal antibodies. Molecular Immunology 24(9): 969–974

References

1. Wagner-Jauregg T 1972 Riboflavin (chemistry). In: Sebrell W H, Harris R S (eds) The vitamins, 2nd edn, vol V. Academic Press, New York, pp 3–43
2. McCormick D B 1975 Metabolism of riboflavin. In: Rivlin R S (ed) Riboflavin. Plenum Press, New York, pp 153–198
3. Rivlin R S 1979 Hormones, drugs and riboflavin. Nutrition Reviews 37: 241–246
4. Leeson L J, Weidenheimer J F 1969 Stability of tetracycline and riboflavin. Journal of Pharmaceutical Sciences. 58: 355–357
5. Dony T, Devleeschouwer M J 1976 Etude de la d'egradation photochemique de macrolides en presence de riboflavine. Journal de Pharmacie Belgique 31(5): 479–484
6. Prentice A M, Bates C J 1981 A biochemical evaluation of the erythrocyte glutathione reductase test for riboflavine status. British Journal of Nutrition 45: 37–52
7. Rivlin R S 1976 Riboflavin metabolism. New England Journal of Medicine 283: 463–472
8. Jusko W J, Levy G, Yaffe S J, Gorodisc R 1970 Effect of probenecid on renal clearance of riboflavin in man. Journal of Pharmaceutical Sciences 59: 473–477
9. Baran R B, Rowles B 1973 Factors affecting coloration of urine and feces. Journal of the American Pharmacy Association 13: 139–142
10. Lopez-Anaya A, Mayersohn M 1987 Quantification of riboflavin, riboflavin 5 phosphate and flavin adenine dinucleotide in plasma and urine by high performance liquid chromatography. Journal of Chromatography 423: 105–113
11. Horwitt M K, Harvey C C, Rothwell W S, Cutler J L, Hafforn D 1956 Tryptophan–niacin relationship in man. Journal of Nutrition 60 (suppl 1): 1–43
12. Jusko W J, Levy G 1975 Absorption, protein binding and elimination of riboflavin. In: Rivlin R S (ed) Riboflavin. Plenum Press, New York, pp 99–152
13. Committee on Medical Aspects of Food Policy 1980 Report on Health and Social Subjects 18, London, HM Stationary Office

Rifampicin

Rifampicin (rifampin) is a synthetic derivative of a natural antibiotic rifamycin B produced by *Streptomyces mediterranei*, and belongs to the class of naphthalenic ansamycins.[1,2] Its principal uses are for the treatment of tuberculosis and leprosy. It is a potent inducer of microsomal liver enzymes.

Chemistry

Rifampicin (rifampin, Rifamycin AMP, Rifaldazine, Rifampicinium, Rifadin, Rimactane)

$C_{43}H_{58}N_4O_{12}$

3-(4-Methy-1-piperazinylaminomethyl)rifamycin SV

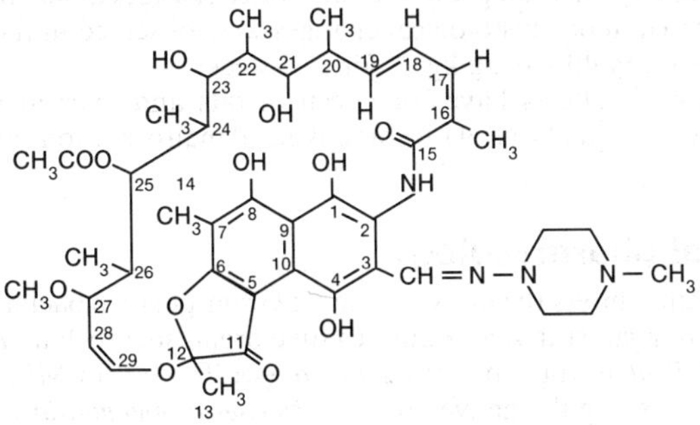

Molecular weight	822.9
pKa (4-OH, 3-piperazine N)	1.7, 7.9
Solubility	
in alcohol	1 in 200
in water	1 in 300
Octanol/water partition coefficient	—

Rifampicin is a brick red crystalline powder with little odour, freely soluble in chloroform. It is also soluble in ethyl acetate and methanol. It is relatively insoluble in water but solubility increases at low values of pH. There are combination products with isoniazid (Rifinah, Rimactizid) and with pyrazinamide plus isoniazid (Rifater).

Pharmacology

In vitro, rifampicin is bactericidal against a wide range of organisms, including *Mycobacteria*.[3–7] The minimum inhibiting concentrations (MIC mg.l^{-1}) against some important groups are given in Table 1. Despite this broad spectrum of activity, the antibiotic has been principally used in the management of tuberculous infections at all sites, and more recently in leprosy. The mode of action is by inhibition of DNA-dependent RNA polymerase, inhibiting transcription. This occurs in bacteria in low concentrations, much higher ones being required to inhibit mammalian RNA synthesis.[8,9] In tuberculosis rifampicin is bactericidal for both intracellular and extracellular microorganisms. Microbial resistance to rifampicin can develop, although certain rifampicin-resistant bacteria have decreased virulence. It is unusual to encounter initial resistance in a white patient.

Against acute organisms resistance develops more readily, and therefore it is usual to give rifampicin in combination with other agents, as in tuberculosis and leprosy. Rifampicin has been shown to inhibit certain DNA viruses such as herpes, adenovirus and pox virus, but at concentrations 500–1000 times higher than those required to inhibit the growth of bacteria.[10,11]

Table 1

Organism	MIC/ $mg.l^{-1}$
Strep. aureus	0.002–0.005
Strep. pyogenes	0.01–0.5
N. gonorrhoeae	0.02
H. influenzae	0.02
Legionella pneumophilia	0.01
E. coli	5–10
Proteus vulgaris	5
Pseudomonas aerogenes	10
Mycobacteria tuberculosis	0.005–0.2

Toxicology

Acute and subacute toxicity tests in rodents show good tolerance at well above therapeutic doses. The LD_{50} in the mouse following oral administration is approximately 1250 $mg.kg^{-1}$ in 24 h. In the rat the LD_{50} values are 1700 $mg.kg^{-1}$ for oral administration, 550 $mg.kg^{-1}$ for intraperitoneal administration and 330 $mg.kg^{-1}$ for intravenous administration. Rats given 50 and 100 $mg.kg^{-1}$ daily for 26 weeks showed no notable toxicity, but at doses over 100 $mg.kg^{-1}$ there were dose-related histological changes in the liver. Rabbits also given doses over 100 $mg.kg^{-1}$ for 4 weeks or more showed progressive hepatotoxicity, including jaundice and fatty changes at 400 $mg.kg^{-1}$. Dose-related minor histological changes were observed in the liver of monkeys given 40–80 $mg.kg^{-1}$ for 2–4 weeks.

Teratogenic effects have been seen in rats and mice at doses of 150 $mg.kg^{-1}$ and above, with some skeletal malformations and spina bifida.[12]

Clinical pharmacology

Rifampicin inhibits the growth of most Gram-positive bacteria and is also active against many Gram-negative organisms such as *Escherischia coli, Proteus* spp. and *Pseudomonas* (see Table 1 for MIC values). The drug is highly active against *Neisseria meningitidis* and *N. gonorrhoeae*. Rifampicin is very active against *Legionella* species in cell cultures and is used as a second line agent for *Legionella* infections in man. Rifampicin inhibits the growth of *Mycobacterium tuberculosis* and has some activity against the atypical mycobacteria such as *M. kansasii, M. scrofulaceum* and *M. intracellulare* with MIC values of under 4 $mg.l^{-1}$. Rifampicin increases the in vitro activity of streptomycin and isoniazid but not that of ethambutol.

Bacterial resistance may develop rapidly to rifampicin and occurs as a one-step process. One of every 10^7–10^8 tubercle bacilli is resistant to rifampicin so the drug should not be used on its own. Rifampicin is generally administered in a dose of 450–600 mg on an empty stomach.

Pharmacokinetics

High performance liquid chromatography is the usual method of assay for both rifampicin and its two major metabolites in serum and urine,[13–15] although bioassay techniques may be easier to perform in some hospital situations. The precision of the assay is $\pm$1.3–4% for values up to 20 $mg.l^{-1}$

Rifampicin is well absorbed from the gastrointestinal tract although food may delay absorption.[16–19] Also, gastric pH is of importance and acidification of gastric juice increases absorption and serum concentrations. Following a typical 600 mg dose peak concentrations in the region of 7–10 $mg.l^{-1}$ are reached in 2–4 h and this is well above therapeutic levels for tuberculosis, leprosy and some acute infections. There is considerable individual variability, and concurrent administration of para-aminosalicylic acid may delay absorption.[20]

Rifampin readily diffuses into most organs, tissues, bone and body fluids, including exudates into tuberculous lung cavities.[21] High concentrations appear in the lachrymal glands and tears. The urine is coloured orange to brick-red. The volume of distribution is approximately 1 $l.kg^{-1}$.

On first-dose administration on an empty stomach of 300 mg rifampicin, the serum concentration curves are similar to those following intravenous dosing, indicating little presystemic metabolism,[22,23] but repeated administration induces hepatic endoplasmic reticular enzymes, including deacetylation with reduction in serum half life and AUC; typical figures are given in Table 2.

Table 2 Effect of repeated doses on half life and AUC

	$t_{\frac{1}{2}}$/h	AUC 0–12 h
Day 1	3.4	131.4
Day 2	2.9	84.6
Day 6	2.5	100.5
Day 14	2.1	87.7

Serum binding has been estimated at 60–80%[24] with approximately 30% with the serum albumin fraction where it may compete, for instance, with warfarin anticoagulants. Tissue distribution occurs at a relatively fast rate. At physiological pH only about 25% of the drug is ionized while the molecule as a whole is lipid soluble.[24] Levels of rifampicin in the cerebrospinal fluid are approximately one tenth of those achieved in the blood, although this may be increased in inflammatory states.[25,26]

The principal excretion pathway is the bile (with enterohepatic circulation), with the urine as a secondary pathway. Although the kidney is not the main excretion pathway for rifampicin or its metabolites, urinary concentrations increase with doses above 450 mg when the biliary excretion pathway is more saturated. With a dose of 900 mg, 25% of rifampicin may be excreted in the urine.[27,28]

Oral absorption	extensive
Presystemic metabolism	< 10%
Plasma half life	
range	1–6 h
mean	3.4 h
Volume of distribution	1 $l.kg^{-1}$
Plasma protein binding	60–80%

Patients with impaired renal function are not at risk but impaired hepatic function or biliary excretion may require modification of dosage and careful monitoring. In infants where hepatic mechanisms are less fully developed, more rifampicin is excreted in the urine and there is less change with time because enzyme induction is low at this age. Over the age of one year, metabolism is similar to that in adults. There is evidence that rifampicin can cross the placenta.

Concentration–effect relationship

Doses of 450–600 mg rifampicin daily give blood levels substantially in excess of the MICs for *M. tuberculosis* and *M. leprae* and are effective over a period of 18 h (see Table 1). Similarly, for both coagulase-positive and -negative staphylococci there is substantial excess in the serum for bactericidal effect. Good penetration into exudates, caseous material and bronchial secretions aids destruction of bacilli remote from blood supply.

Metabolism

The principal pathways of metabolism are by desacetylation and hydrolysis as indicated in Fig. 1. Desacetylation at the C25 position results in a more polar compound with increased capacity for biliary excretion.[29] Depending on the dose of rifampicin, one-third to one-eighth may be excreted in the bile, either as a desacetylrifampicin which is still bacteriologically active or as unchanged rifampicin. The unchanged rifampicin is reabsorbed, creating an enterohepatic circulation, whereas the 25-O-desacetyl derivative is poorly absorbed.[30] Enzyme induction increases the metabolism of rifampicin and the biliary excretion of desacetylrifampicin. The rifampicin-induced increase in hepatic monoxygenase activity enhances the metabolism of other concomitantly administered drugs such as digitoxin, corticosteroids, methadone, oral contraceptives, dapsone and 25-hydroxycholecalciferol a major circulating metabolite of vitamin D.[31] Rifampicin is an inducer of P400IIIA, and this would be expected to increase the metabolism of substrates for this isoenzyme, including phenytoin, glucocorticoids, macrolide antibiotics and cyclosporin.

Rifampicin

Fig. 1 Metabolism of rifampicin

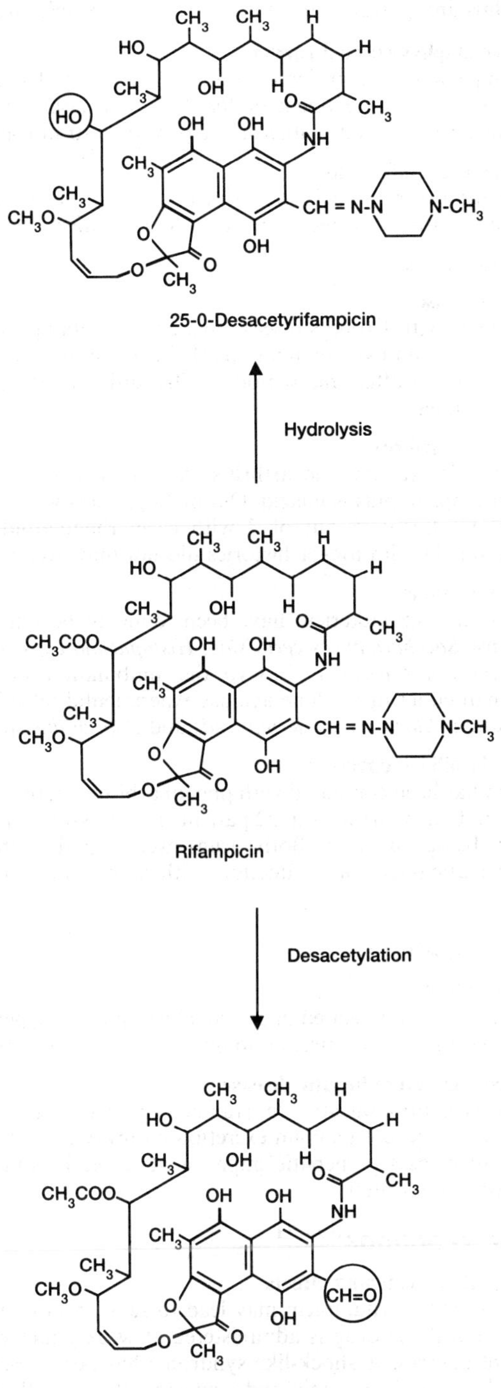

Pharmaceutics

Rifampicin is available for oral and parenteral use.

1. Rimactane (Ciba, UK/USA): red capsules coded 'J2150' containing 150 mg rifampicin and red/brown capsules coded 'CS300' (UK) or '154' (USA) containing 300 mg.
2. Rifadin (Merrell Dow, UK): capsules marked 'LEPETIT', blue/red ones containing 150 mg rifampicin and red/red ones 300 mg. In the USA the capsules are both red, marked with the proprietary name and strength.
3. There is also a syrup containing 100 mg per 5 ml (Rimactane, Rifadin).
4. A combination of isoniazid and rifampicin is available as a tablet containing either 100 mg isoniazid with 150 mg rifampicin (Rimactazid 150; Ciba, UK/Rifinah 150; Merrell Dow, UK) or 150 mg isoniazid with 300 mg rifampicin (Rimactazid 300; Ciba, UK/Rifinah 300; Merrell Dow, UK/Rifamate capsule; Merrell Dow, USA).
5. Rifater (Merrell Dow, UK) is a tablet containing rifampicin 120 mg, isoniazid 50 mg and pyrazinamide 300 mg.
6. An intravenous infusion, Rimactane Infusion (Ciba, UK) is available as 300 mg rifampicin in a 10 ml vial (a red lyophilized powder) accompanied by 5 ml ampoule of Water for Injection BP with sodium formaldehyde sulphoxylate. Rifadin-Infusion (Merrell Dow, UK) is available in 600 mg vials.

Therapeutic use

Indications

1. Infections with *Mycobacterium tuberculosis* at all sites
2. Prophylaxis in tuberculin-positive children
3. Opportunist mycobacterial infections
4. Leprosy
5. Prophylaxis of meningococcal meningitis.

Although rifampicin is largely preserved for use in the above indications, it has also been used with success, usually in combination with other antibiotics, in the following:

6. Brucellosis
7. Gonorrhoea
8. Legionnaires' disease
9. Severe staphylococcal infections, including endocarditis
10. Chronic staphylococcal nasal carriers and chronic furunculosis
11. Urinary tract infections.

Indications under investigation are:

a. Crohn's disease
b. Rheumatoid arthritis
c. Fungal infections
d. Pruritis.

Contraindications

1. Hypersensitivity
2. Jaundice and severe hepatic disease.

Mode of use

The standard dose of rifampicin in tuberculosis is 600 mg daily in adults (450 mg in patients under 50 kg) and 10 $mg.kg^{-1}$ in children. In leprosy it is 600 mg a month. It should always be used in combination with other antituberculous and antileprosy drugs. In tuberculosis, the standard regimen in addition to rifampicin includes isoniazid, pyrazinamide and ethambutol, in leprosy clofazamine and dapsone. The optimal duration of therapy in tuberculosis is now considered to be 6 months and in paucibacillary leprosy, 6 months and multibacillary leprosy, 2 years. In many areas of the world, particularly in developing countries, considerations of drug availability, cost, compliance and the need for close supervision may dictate alternative regimes to optimize eradication of the two diseases.

An intravenous infusion is available for patients who are unconscious or cannot swallow. The 10 ml vial containing 300 mg rifampicin (a red lyophilized powder) is accompanied by a 5 ml ampoule of water for injection BP and sodium formaldehyde sulphoxylate. This solvent can be added to the powder and after vigorous shaking for 30 s the completely dissolved powder can be immediately diluted into 250 ml of an infusion fluid such as 5% glucose and administered over a period of 2–3 h.

Indications

1. Tuberculous infections

Many countries have issued guidelines for the management of tuberculous infections through various official bodies. In the UK, the Joint Tuberculosis Committee of the British Thoracic Society, in emphasizing the importance of the correct prescription and patient compliance, have recommended a 6 month regimen for pulmonary tuberculosis in adults, with an initial phase of 2 months treatment with rifampicin 450 mg daily (<50 kg), 600 mg daily (⩾50 kg), isoniazid 300 mg daily, pyrazinamide 1.5 g (<50 kg), 2.0 g (⩾50 kg) and ethambutol 25 $mg.kg^{-1}$, followed by a continuation phase of 4 months therapy with rifampicin 450 mg (<50 kg) or 600 mg (≥50 kg) daily and isoniazid 300 mg daily.[32–34]

Similar dosage schedules should be used for tuberculosis at other sites, but ethambutol may be omitted in tuberculous meningitis, lymph node and bone joint tuberculosis, and the continuation phase extended in tuberculus meningitis to 10 months (12 months therapy altogether).[35–38]

In children, the daily dose of rifampicin is 10 mg.kg^{-1} given with isoniazid 10 mg.kg^{-1} and pyrazinamide 35 mg.kg^{-1} for 2 months, followed by rifampicin 10 mg.kg^{-1} and isoniazid 10 mg.kg^{-1} for a further 4 months. Ethambutol is usually omitted because of the difficulty in testing eyesight in young children. If pyrazinamide is omitted from the regimen, rifampicin and isoniazid should be continued for a total of 9 months.

In developing countries, a variety of short course daily and intermittent regimens have been investigated in Hong Kong, Singapore, East Africa and Madras.[39–41] Whether rifampicin is used intensively or intermittently will depend on local considerations and whether therapy can be fully supervised. The situation has been well reviewed by Fox.[42,43]

Mycobacterial resistance to all or some of the agents above may require the substitution of second or third line agents. The advent of AIDS has increased the problem of susceptibility to tuberculosis.[44]

2. Prophylaxis tuberculin-positive children

Regimens of rifampicin and isoniazid given for 3 months have been used in the UK with good effect in children under 16 who have strongly positive tuberculin skin test response without evidence of disease.[32,45]

3. Opportunist mycobacterial infections

Rifampicin is effective against other strains of mycobacteria such as *M. kansasii* and some avian strains.[46] However, some newer rifamycins are being developed which may be more effective against such infections.[47]

4. Leprosy

The World Health Organization has recommended the following regimes in leprosy.

Multibacillary leprosy:

Rifampicin 600 mg monthly fully supervised.

Clofazamine 300 mg monthly fully supervised plus clofazamine 50 mg daily.

Dapsone 50–100 mg daily (1–2 mg.kg^{-1}).

Paucibacillary leprosy:

As above for 6 months but dapsone can be omitted. If rifampicin is omitted the clofazamine and dapsone should be continued for 12 months.[48–50]

5. Prophylaxis of meningococcal meningitis contacts

Rifampicin prophylaxis is recommended for intimate household or institutional contacts of cases of meningococcal meningitis. Adults should be given 600 mg every 12 h for four doses. Children should be given 10 mg.kg^{-1} every 12 h for four doses and infants 5 mg.kg^{-1}.[51–53]

6. Brucellosis

The World Health Organization recommended regime is rifampicin 600–900 mg daily with doxycycline 200 mg daily for 6 weeks, the drugs being given together as a single dose.[54]

Co-trimoxazole has been used with rifampicin in children.[55]

7. Gonorrhoea

Single doses of 900 mg–1.2 g rifampicin have been used to treat gonorrhoea, although in order to avoid emergence of resistant strains, coadministration of 1 g erythromycin has been recommended.[56,57]

8. Legionnaires' disease

Although erythromycin is usually considered to be the treatment of choice, rifampicin has been added when response has been poor.[58,59] Oxytetracycline and co-trimoxazole have been used with rifampicin in patients not responding to erythromycin and rifampicin.[60]

9. *Staphylococcus aureus* infections

These usually respond well to rifampicin although resistance may develop if the antibiotic is used alone. However, rifampicin is usually reserved for severe infections and septicaemia as part of a hospital antibiotic policy. A completed course of the combination of rifampicin and ciprofloxacin cured 10 out of 10 intravenous drug users with right sided *Staph. aureus* endocarditis.[61]

Rifampicin with lincomycin was used to treat 12 patients with acute osteomyelitis and postoperative infections due to *Staph. aureus*.[62]

10. Chronic staphylococcal carriers

Since rifampicin appears in high concentrations in nasal secretions, it has been used in the treatment of *Staph. aureus* nasal carriers with methicillin-resistant strains, either alone or with co-trimoxazole.[63]

11. Urinary tract infections

A combination of rifampicin and trimethoprim can be effective and safe for the treatment of recurrent urinary tract infections.[64]

Under investigation

a. Crohn's disease

Of 20 patients with Crohn's disease treated with rifampicin, ethambutol, isoniazid and pyrazinamide (or clofazamine) for 9 months, 10 were in remission after this period.[65] The authors suggest further controlled studies.

b. Rheumatoid arthritis

20 patients with rheumatoid arthritis were treated with rifampicin alone or rifampicin plus isoniazid. Out of 18 patients who completed 3 months' treatment, 6 out of 7 with early rheumatoid arthritis improved, but 11 with longer histories did not improve.[66]

c. Fungal infections

Rifampicin and amphotericin have been found to be synergistic in vitro against *Saccharomyces cerevisiae*, *Histoplasma capsulatum* and several species of *Aspergillus*. In vivo, the combination proved more effective than either drug alone against experimental infections with *H. capsulatum*, *Blastomyces dermatitidis* and *Aspergillus* spp.[67]

d. Pruritis in biliary cirrhosis

Rifampicin has been compared with phenobarbitone in the treatment of pruritis in biliary cirrhosis in 22 patients in a crossover study, with rifampicin being superior. Both drugs were equally effective in inducing hepatic microsomal function, with rifampicin also reducing cholestasis.[68]

Contraindications

1. Hypersensitivity

Rifampicin is contraindicated in patients known to be hypersensitive to any of the rifamycin series, although desensitization is possible.

2. Jaundice and severe hepatic disease

Rifamycin is contraindicated in jaundiced patients and in severe hepatic disease because its main excretion pathway is via the biliary tract. In other cases of hepatic impairment, careful monitoring of liver function is essential.

Adverse reactions[69–71]

Potentially life-threatening effects

Used intermittently, rifampicin may lead to sensitization and this is more common if the drug is administered at weekly intervals or as intermittent courses. A shock-like syndrome has been described, as has acute haemolytic anaemia and acute renal failure. Risk can be minimized by reintroducing the drug gradually, in small increasing daily doses.

Acute overdosage

29 overdose cases have been reviewed, in which the drug produced cutaneous pigmentation, described as the 'red-man syndrome'.[72] In addition to pigmentation, periorbital or facial oedema is described, as well as pruritis, nausea, vomiting and abdominal tenderness. In adults, cardiovascular/pulmonary arrest may occur after a total dose of 14 g.[73] There are no specific antidotes or resuscitative measures, but rifampicin is dialysable.

Severe or irreversible adverse effects

Severe reactions to rifampicin are not common and when they occur, are usually related to sensitization or enzyme induction effects on the liver and consequent effects on the metabolism of other drugs.[74] Sensitivity to rifampicin is commoner with intermittent therapy (as mentioned above) and this may result in the 'flu syndrome' (fever, chills and headache) or produce thrombocytopenic purpura.[75] If purpura occurs during rifampicin administration, the drug should be discontinued and not administered again.

Rifampicin

Hepatic reactions may occur in patients with chronic liver disease, including alcoholism, and such patients need careful monitoring.[76] Associated drugs such as isoniazid and pyrazinamide may aggravate the situation.[77–79] Enzyme induction may decrease the clinical efficacy of drugs such as digitoxin, corticosteroids, coumarin anticoagulants and oral antidiabetic agents which could lead to life-threatening events. Also, oral contraceptives may not work[90] and certain analgesics and narcotics have a reduced effect. Dapsone may also have reduced activity.

An increased risk of venous thrombosis in patients receiving rifampicin has also been reported.[80]

Symptomatic adverse effects
Gastrointestinal reactions, including anorexia, nausea and abdominal discomfort, occur from time to time, and occasionally vomiting may be severe. Taking rifampicin with meals usually reduces these effects, although not always. Diarrhoea is less frequent.

Patients should be warned about highly coloured (red, orange or pink) urine and pink tears while on rifampicin. The high concentration in tears may tint some varieties of contact lenses.

Other effects
Rifampicin can affect both haem and bilirubin metabolism in man.[81] The serum unconjugated bilirubin concentration increases two to three-fold during the first 24 h of administration, but subsequently falls to below pretreatment values after 3–4 weeks.[82,83] Liver enzyme values often rise at the same time. Unless liver function tests continue to deteriorate, these changes are not an indication for discontinuing treatment.

ALA synthetase activity also increases markedly during the first week of therapy.[81]

Interference with clinical pathology tests
Rifampicin interferes with many colorimetric tests, including bromsulphthalein tests of liver function and assays of bilirubin. Erroneously low estimates of vitamin B_{12} or folate may occur if rifampicin is being taken.[84–86]

High risk groups

Neonates
If required for tuberculosis in the first year of life, the dose of 10 $mg.kg^{-1}$ should not be exceeded.

Breast milk. Rifampicin is excreted in breast milk but not in amounts likely to cause harm.[32]

Children
Doses of 10–20 $mg.kg^{-1}$ are safe.

Pregnant women
Standard treatment of tuberculosis should be given to pregnant women, although concomitant streptomycin should be avoided.[12] If pregnancy occurs in a woman taking rifampicin, it is not an indication for termination.[32]

The elderly
The patient should be monitored for hepatic insufficiency which may require dosage adjustment.

Drug interactions

Potentially hazardous interactions

Antidiabetic agents. Rifampicin reduces serum half life and clinical efficacy of some oral antidiabetic agents (sulphonylureas and biguanides).[87]

Antiepileptic drugs. Rifampicin may reduce the efficacy of antiepileptic drugs and induce fits.[88]

Corticosteroids. Rifampicin may reduce the efficacy of corticosteroids in Addison's disease and induce an Addisonian crisis.[89]

Anticoagulants. Rifampicin can reduce the efficacy of coumarin anticoagulants, and also its withdrawal can precipitate bleeding in patients.[31]

Other significant interactions
Like antipyrine, rifampicin enhances the metabolism of diazepam.[91] Interactions have also been described with enalapril,[92] theophylline,[93–94] pirmenol,[95] digoxin[96] and vitamin D.[97]

Through microsomal liver enzyme induction, rifampicin has also been variously reported to affect the metabolism of a wide range of drugs apart from those mentioned above, including chloramphenicol, clofibrate, corticosteroids, cyclosporin, dapsone, digitoxin, disopyramide, hexobarbitone, ketoconazole, lorcarnide, methadone, mixiliteine, oral contraceptives, quinidine, sulphasalazine and verapamil.

Potentially useful interactions
None is known.

Major outcome trials

1. British Thoracic Association 1981 A controlled trial of six months chemotherapy in pulmonary tuberculosis. First report: results during chemotherapy. British Journal of Diseases of the Chest 75: 141–153

This study compared two 6-month courses of chemotherapy for pulmonary tuberculosis with one 9-month course as follows:

a. Isoniazid and rifampicin for 6 months, with streptomycin and pyrazinamide added during the first 2 months (the SHRZ6 regimen)
b. Isoniazid and rifampicin for 6 months, with ethambutol and pyrazinamide during the first 2 months (the EHRZ6 regimen)
c. Isoniazid and rifampicin for 9 months plus ethambutol for the first 2 months (the EHR9 regimen).

The doses used were isoniazid (H) 300 mg daily; rifampicin (R) 600 mg daily or 450 mg daily if the patient weighed less than 50 kg; streptomycin (S) 0.75 g on 6 days a week; pyrazinamide (Z) 1.5 g daily if the patient weighed less than 50 kg; 2 g if the patient weighed between 50 kg and 74 kg and 2.5 g if the patient weighed 75 kg or more; and ethambutol (E) 25 $mg.kg^{-1}$ body weight.

Eligible patients were males and females between 18 and 60 years who had culture-positive pulmonary tuberculosis and who had not received more than two weeks antituberculosis therapy at any time. Pregnant patients and those with impaired hepatic or renal function, gout or impaired vision were excluded.

593 patients were recruited and 511 started chemotherapy; 170 on SHRZ6, 164 on EHRZ6 and 177 on EHR9. All patients were sputum-negative at the end of chemotherapy, but conversion was quicker in those receiving pyrazinamide in the first two months.

Of the 334 patients on SHRZ6 and EHRZ6 14 (4%) developed hepatitis and the incidence was the same in the EHR9 group. The incidence of other side effects, notably skin rash, was greater in the pyrazinamide-containing regimens. 444 patients completed chemotherapy.

2. British Thoracic Association 1982 A controlled trial of six months chemotherapy in pulmonary tuberculosis. Second report: results at 24 months. American Review of Respiratory Disease 126: 460–462

All 444 patients completing chemotherapy in the study described above had negative sputum culture at the end of treatment. In the subsequent 24 months, 393 were able to be followed up and of these 1 of 125 on SHRZ6 had relapsed, 3 of 132 on EHRZ6 and 2 of 136 on EHR9.

These two studies taken together are important because they established that two alternative 6-monthly regimens were as effective as a 9-month regimen previously recommended, and they form the basis of current recommendations in the UK for the management of pulmonary tuberculosis using a short, cheap and well tolerated regimen.

General review articles

Rifampicin: a review 1971 Drugs 1: 354–398
Acocella G 1978 Clinical pharmacokinetics of rifampicin. Clinical Pharmacokinetics 3: 108–127
Kenny M T, Strates B 1981 Metabolism and pharmacokinetics of the antibiotic rifamipicin. Drug Metabolism Reviews 12: 159–218
Farr B, Mandell G L 1982 Rifampin. Medical Clinics of North America 66: 157–167
Reviews of Infectious Diseases 1983 5 (suppl 3): July–August

References

1. Maggi N, Pallanza R, Sensi P 1965 New derivatives of rifamycin SV. Antimicrobial Agents and Chemotherapy 5: 765–769
2. Sensi P 1983 History of the development of rifampin. Reviews of Infectious Diseases 5 (suppl 3): S402–S406

3. Atlas E, Turck M 1968 Laboratory and clinical investigation of rifampin. American Journal of the Medical Sciences 256: 247–254
4. McCabe W R, Lorian V 1968 Comparison of the antibacterial activity of rifampicin and other antibiotics. American Journal of the Medical Sciences 256: 255–265
5. Kunin C M, Brandt D, Wood H 1969 Bacteriological studies of rifampin, a new synthetic antibiotic. Journal of Infectious Diseases 119: 132–137
6. Ariola V, Pallanza R et al 1967 Rifampicin: a new rifamycin. Arzneimittel-Forschung 17: 523–529
7. Thornsberry C, Hill B C et al 1983 Rifampicin: spectrum of antibacterial activity. Reviews of Infectious Diseases 5 (suppl 3): S412–S417
8. Zillig W, Zechel K et al 1970 The role of different sub-units of DNA-dependent RNA polymerase form E. coli in the transcription process. Cold Spring Harbor Symposia on Quantitative Biology 35: 47
9. Wehrli W 1983 Rifampin: mechanisms of action and resistance. Reviews of Infectious Diseases 5 (suppl 3): S407–S411
10. Heller E, Argeman M et al 1969 Selective inhibition of vaccinia virus by the antibiotic rifampicin. Nature 222: 273–274
11. Subak-Sharpe J, Timbury M C, Williams J F 1969 Rifampicin inhibits the growth of some mammalian viruses. Nature 222: 341–345
12. Steen J S, Stainton-Ellis D M 1977 Rifampicin in pregnancy. Lancet 2: 604–605
13. Ratti B, Parenti R et al 1981 Quantitative assay of rifampicin and its main metabolite 25-desacetyl rifampicin in human plasma. Journal of Chromatography 225: 526–531
14. Weber A, Opheim K E et al 1983 High pressure liquid chromatographic quantitation of rifampicin and its two major metabolites in urine and serum. Reviews of Infectious Diseases 5 (suppl 3): S433–S439
15. Woo J, Wong C L et al 1987 Liquid chromatographic assay for the simultaneous determination of pyrazinamide and rifampicin in serum samples from patients with tuberculous meningitis. Journal of Chromatography 420: 73–80
16. Keberle H, Schmid K, Meyer-Brunot H 1968 The metabolic fate of rimactane in animal and man. Ciba Symposium on Rimactane, Basle
17. Keberle H 1970 Physio-chemical factors of drugs affecting absorption, distribution and excretion. Acta Pharmacologica suppl 3: 30–47
18. Verbist L, Gyselen A 1968 Antituberculous activity of rifampicin in vitro and in vivo and the concentrations obtained in the blood. American Review of Respiratory Disease 98: 923–932
19. Siegler D I, Burley D M et al 1974 Effect of meals on rifampicin absorption. Lancet 2: 197–198
20. Boman G, Hannegren A et al 1971 Drug interaction: decreased serum concentrations of rifampicin when given with PAS. Lancet 1: 800
21. Acocella G, Nicolis F B, Lamarina A 1967 A study of the kinetics of rifampicin in man. Chemotherapia 5: 87
22. Keberle H, Riess W et al 1969 Pharmacokinetic studies in the field of rifamycins. Proceedings of the Congress of Chemotherapy. University of Tokyo Press 1970, pp 905–913
23. Keberle H 1971 Physicochemical factors of drugs affecting absorption, distribution and excretion. Acta Pharmacologica 29 (suppl 3): 30–47
24. Acocella G, Pagani V et al 1971 Kinetic studies on rifampicin. Chemotherapy 16: 356–370
25. Nahata M C, Fan-Havard P et al 1990 Pharmacokinetics, cerebrospinal fluid concentration and safety of intravenous rifampicin in pediatric patients undergoing shunt placements. European Journal of Clinical Pharmacology 38: 515–517
26. Reubi F, Sackmann W, Pluecke 1970 La clearance renale de la rifampicine. Journal de Urologie et de Nephrologie 76: 829–833
27. Acocella G 1978 Clinical pharmacokinetics of rifampicin. Clinical Pharmacokinetics 3: 108–127
28. Brufani M, Fedeli W et al 1964 The X-ray analysis of the structure of rifamycin Biologica Experientia 20: 339–344
29. Loos U, Musch E et al 1985 Pharmacokinetics of oral and intravenous rifampicin during chronic administration. Klinische Wochenschrift 63: 1205–1211
30. Teunissen M W, Bakker W et al 1984 Influence of rifampicin treatment on antipyrine clearance and metabolite formation in patients with tuberculosis. British Journal of Clinical Pharmacology 18: 701–706
31. Burley D M 1977 Rifampicin, enzyme induction, oestrogens and the 'pill'. In Grahame-Smith D J (ed) Drug interactions. Macmillan Press, London.
32. Ormerod L P (for the subcommittee of the Joint Tuberculosis Committee) 1990 Chemotherapy and management of tuberculosis in the United Kingdom: recommendations of the Joint Tuberculosis Committee of the British Thoracic Society. Thorax 45: 403–408
33. British Thoracic Association 1981 A controlled trial of 6 months chemotherapy in pulmonary tuberculosis. First report: results during chemotherapy. British Journal of Diseases of the Chest 75: 141–153
34. British Thoracic Association 1982 A controlled trial of 6 months chemotherapy in pulmonary tuberculosis. Second report: results during the 24 months after the end of chemotherapy. American Review of Respiratory Disease 126: 460–462
35. British Thoracic Society Research Committee 1985 Short course chemotherapy for lymph node tuberculosis. British Medical Journal 290: 1106–1108
36. British Thoracic Society Research Committee 1988 Short course chemotherapy for lymph node tuberculosis: final report at 5 years. British Journal of Diseases of the Chest 82: 282–284
37. Girling D J, Darbyshire J H, O'Mahoney G 1988 Extra-pulmonary tuberculosis. British Medical Bulletin 44: 738–756
38. Leading Article 1989 The treatment of tuberculous meningitis. Tubercle 70: 79–82
39. Hong Kong Chest Service 1989 A controlled trial of 3 month, 4 month and 6 month regimens of chemotherapy for sputum smear-negative tuberculosis. American Review of Respiratory Disease 139: 871–876
40. Singapore Tuberculosis Service 1988 Five-year follow-up of a clinical trial of three month and six month regimens of chemotherapy given intermittently in the continuation phase in the treatment of pulmonary tuberculosis. American Review of Respiratory Disease 137: 1147–1150
41. East and Central African/British MRC STudy 1986 Controlled clinical trial (three 6-month and one 8-month) for pulmonary tuberculosis. Final report. Tubercle 67: 5–15
42. Fox W 1981 Whither short-course chemotherapy. Bulletin of the International Union against Tuberculosis 56: 135–159
43. Fox W 1988 Tuberculosis case finding and treatment programmes in tuberculosis. British Medical Bulletin 44: 717–737
44. Chaisson R E, Schechter G F, Thever C P 1987 Tuberculosis in patients with acquired immunodeficiency syndrome, clinical features, response to therapy and survival. American Review of Respiratory Disease 136: 570–574
45. Citron K M 1988 Control and prevention of tuberculosis in Great Britain. British Medical Bulletin 44: 704–716
46. Editorial 1989 Treatment of pulmonary disease caused by opportunist mycobacteria. Thorax 44: 449–454
47. Traxler P, Vischer W A, Zac O 1988 New rifamycins. Drugs of the future 13: 845–856
48. Editorial 1988 Chemotherapy of leprosy. Lancet 2: 487–488
49. Ellard G A 1988 Chemotherapy of leprosy. British Medical Bulletin 44: 775–790
50. Venkatesan K 1989 Clinical pharmacokinetic considerations in the treatment of patients with leprosy. Clinical Pharmacokinetics 16: 365–386
51. Hendeles L, Kagan B M 1978 The prevention of meningococcal disease. Reviews of Infectious Diseases 5 (suppl 3): 451–458
52. Schwartz B, Al-Ruwais A et al 1988 Comparative efficacy of cefriaxone and rifampicin in eradicating pharyngeal carriage of Group A Neisseria meningitidis. Lancet 1: 1239–1242
53. Devine L F, Johnson D P 1970 Rifampicin: levels in serum and saliva and effect on meningococcal carrier state. Journal of the American Medical Association 214: 1055–1059
54. Sixth report of Joint FAO/WHO Expert Committee on Brucellosis. Series World Health Organization Number 740
55. Llorens-Terol J, Busquets R M 1980 Brucellosis treatment with rifampicin. Archives of Disease in Childhood 55: 486–488
56. Cobbold R J, Morrison G D, Willcox R R 1968 Treatment of gonorrhoea with a single oral dose of rifampicin. British Medical Journal 4: 681–682
57. Boakes A J, Loo P S et al 1984 Treatment of uncomplicated gonorrhoea in women with a combination of rifampicin and erythromycin. British Journal of Venereal Disease 60: 309–311
58. Gibson D H, Fitzgeorge R B, Baskerville A 1983 Antibiotic therapy of experimental airborne Legionnaires' disease. Journal of Infection 7: 210–217
59. Medical Letter 1986 Drugs for Tuberculosis 28: 6–8
60. Dodds L 1986 Treatment of legionnaires' disease. Pharmacology Journal 236: 728
61. Dworkin R J, Lee B L et al 1989 Treatment of right-sided Staphylococcus aureus endocarditis in intravenous drug users with ciprofloxacin and rifampicin. Lancet 2: 1071–1073
62. Gilbert V E, Fardon D F, Brown F F 1990 Combined use of rifampicin and lincomycin in the treatment of acute osteomyelitis and post-operative infections due to Staphylococcus aureus. Current Therapeutic Research 47: 367–378
63. Wheat L J, Kohler R B et al 1983 Long-term studies on the effect of rifampicin on nasal carriage of coagulase-positive staphyloccoci. Reviews of Infectious Diseases 5 (suppl 3): S459–S462
64. Brumfitt W, Dixon S, Hamilton-Miller J M 1983 Use of rifampicin to treat urinary tract infections. Reviews of Infectious Diseases 5 (suppl 3): S573–S581
65. Hampson S J, Parker M C et al 1989 Quadruple antimycobacterial chemotherapy in Crohn's disease: results at 9-months of a pilot study. Alimentary Pharmacology and Therapeutics 3: 343–352
66. McConkey B, Situnayke R D 1988 Effects of rifampicin with and without isoniazid in rheumatic arthritis. Journal of Rheumatology 15: 46–50
67. Medoff G 1983 Antifungal action of rifampicin. Reviews of Infectious Diseases 5 (suppl 3): S614–S619
68. Bachs L, Pares A et al 1989 Comparison of rifampicin with phenobarbitone for the treatment of biliary cirrhosis. Lancet 1: 574–576
69. Grosset J, Leventis S 1983 Adverse effects of rifampicin. Reviews of Infectious Diseases 5 (suppl 3): S440–S446
70. Girling D J 1982 Adverse effects of antituberculosis drugs. New Ethicals, September: 123–147
71. Nariman S 1988 Adverse reactions to drugs used in the treatment of tuberculosis. Adverse Drug Reactions and Acute Poisoning Reviews 4: 207–227
72. Holdiness M R 1989 A review of the Redman syndrome and rifampicin overdosage. Medical Toxicology Adverse Drug Exp 4: 444–451
73. Plomp T A, Battista H J et al 1981 A case of fatal poisoning by rifampicin. Archives of Toxicology 48: 245–252
74. Girling D J 1977 Adverse reactions to rifampicin in anti-tuberculosis regimens. Journal of Antimicrobial Chemotherapy 3: 115–132
75. The Hong Kong Tuberculosis Service 1976 Adverse reactions to short-course regimens containing streptomycin, isoniazid, pyrazinamide and rifampicin in Hong Kong. Tubercle 57: 81–95
76. Lesobre R, Ruffino J et al 1969 Jaundice during treatment with rifampicin. Review de la Tuberculose et de Pneumologie 35: 393–403
77. Girling D J 1978 The hepatic toxicity of antituberculous regimens containing isoniazid, rifampicin and pyrazinamide. Tubercle 59: 13–32
78. Jenner P J, Ellard G A 1989 Isoniazid related hepatotoxicity: a study of the effect of rifampicin administration on the metabolism of acetylisoniazid in man. Tubercle 70: 93–101
79. Lees A W, Alan G W et al 1971 Toxicity from rifampicin plus isoniazid and rifampicin plus ethambutol therapy. Tubercle 52: 182–190
80. White N W 1989 Venous thrombosis and rifampicin. Lancet 2: 434–435
81. McColl K E, Thompson E et al 1987 Effect of rifampicin on haem and bilirubin metabolism in man. British Journal of Clinical Pharmacology 23: 553–559
82. Baron D N, Bell J L 1974 Serum enzyme changes in patients receiving anti-tuberculosis therapy with rifampicin or para-amino-salicylic acid, plus isoniazid and streptomycin. Tubercle 55: 115–120

83. Drugs and abnormal liver function test. Adverse Drug Reactions Bulletin 139: 520–523
84. Capelle P, Dhumeaux D 1972 Effect of rifampicin on liver function in man. Gut 13: 366
85. Meisel S, Pupkoff R, Svaan J 1980 In vitro effects of rifampicin on serum bilirubin determinations. Antimicrobial Agents and Chemotherapy 18: 206
86. Stanford C F, Bittles A 1982 Vitamin B12 estimation and rifampicin. Tubercle 62: 236–238
87. Self T H, Fowler J W 1989 Interaction of rifampicin and glyburide. Chest 96: 1443–1444
88. Kay L, Kampman J P, Svendsen T L 1985 Influence of rifampicin and isoniazid on the kinetics of phenytoin. British Journal of Clinical Pharmacology 20: 323–326
89. Elansary E H, Earis J E 1983 Rifampicin and adrenal crisis. British Medical Journal 286: 1861–1862
90. Black D J, Orme M L'E 1990 Pharmacokinetic drug interactions with oral contraceptives. Clinical Pharmacokinetics 18: 472–484
91. Ohnhaus E E, Brockmeyer N et al 1987 The effect of antipyrine and rifampicin on the metabolism of diazepam. Clinical Pharmacology and Therapeutics 42: 148–156
92. Kandiah D, Penny W et al 1988 A possible drug interaction between rifampicin and enalapril. European Journal of Clinical Pharmacology 35: 431–432
93. Boyce E G, George E et al 1986 The effect of rifampicin on theophylline pharmacokinetics. Journal of Clinical Pharmacology 26: 696–699
94. Powell-Jackson P R, Jamieson A P et al 1985 Effect of rifampicin administration on theophylline pharmacokinetics in humans. American Review of Respiratory Disease 131: 939–940
95. Stringer K A, Cetnarowski A B et al 1988 Enhanced pirminal elimination by rifampicin. Journal of Clinical Pharmacology 28: 1094–1097
96. Rodin S M, Johnson B F 1988 Pharmacokinetic interactions with digoxin. Clinical Pharmacokinetics 15: 227–244
97. Williams S E, Wardman A G et al 1985 Long term study of the effect of rifampicin and isoniazid on vitamin D metabolism. Tubercle 66: 49–54

Rimiterol hydrobromide

Rimiterol is a β_2-adrenoceptor agonist used in the treatment of reversible airways obstruction.

Chemistry

Rimiterol hydrobromide (Pulmadil)
erythro-α-(3,4-Dihydroxyphenyl)-2-piperidyl-methanol-hydrobromide
$C_{12}H_{17}.NO_3.HBr$

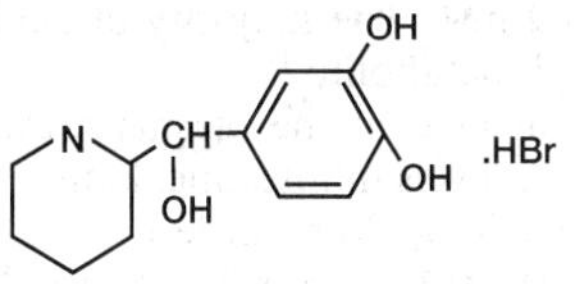

Molecular weight (free base)	304.2 (223.3)
pKa	8.7, 10.3
Solubility	
in alcohol	1 in 20
in water	1 in 10
Octanol/water partition coefficient	unknown

A white or pale grey crystalline powder. It is prepared by chemical synthesis and possesses two asymmetric carbon atoms. Rimiterol is a catecholamine with a high degree of β_2 selectivity.

Pharmacology

Rimiterol is a β-adrenoceptor agonist with selectivity for the β_2 receptor. On the isolated guinea-pig trachea rimiterol has about 55% of the potency of isoprenaline. However, on the guinea-pig atrium, isoprenaline is about 250 times more potent than rimiterol.[1] As it is a catechol it is metabolized by catechol-O-methyl transferase, and therefore has a short duration of action.[2] In animal studies it is less potent than isoprenaline and has about the same potency as salbutamol at causing bronchodilatation and suppressing bronchoconstriction due to 5-hydroxytryptamine and histamine.[3] Its duration of action is, however, shorter than salbutamol. The 3-O-methyl rimiterol metabolite is able to inhibit the effect of the parent compound in vitro and it is theoretically possible that this β-antagonist could be involved in the development of tolerance to rimiterol.[4] However, this has not been reported. When given systemically rimiterol has similar β_2-actions to isoprenaline; these include vasodilatation associated with reduction in blood pressure, reduction in serum potassium and an elevation in plasma insulin. Rimiterol will also relax uterine smooth muscle at doses which produce higher plasma concentrations. Rimiterol is less likely to stimulate β_1-receptors on cardiac muscle.

Toxicology

The toxicity of rimiterol is low compared with other sympathomimetic amines. Intravenous LD_{50} values are 120 $mg.kg^{-1}$ in mice and rats and over 160 $mg.kg^{-1}$ in dogs. Animal studies have shown no hazard to reproduction.[3]

Clinical pharmacology

Rimiterol appears to be an effective bronchodilator in patients with airways obstruction,[5] and is capable of inhibiting bronchoconstriction due to inhaled challenges.[6] It has a similar bronchodilating potency to isoprenaline when given by inhalation. It is, however, 3.5

times less potent than salbutamol on a weight basis.[7] Its duration of action is also significantly less than that of salbutamol.[8] In one study nebulized salbutamol increased forced expiratory volume at 1 second (FEV_1) for between 210 and 240 minutes; however, the bronchodilatation due to rimiterol declined after 30 minutes.[3] After intravenous administration rimiterol was more potent than salbutamol at protecting histamine-induced bronchoconstriction, and produced less increase in heart rate than isoprenaline.[9] After inhalation at bronchodilating doses equivalent to isoprenaline, there was no alteration in heart rate with rimiterol. However, increased cardiac output and tachycardias may occur in clinical use, perhaps due to reflex mechanisms. There was also little or no tremor.[10] Tremor may occur after intravenous dosing.

Pharmacokinetics

Rimiterol can be measured by monitoring its ultraviolet absorption at 280 nm. However, most pharmacokinetic studies were performed using ^{14}C rimiterol. The pharmacokinetics of rimiterol are very similar to those of isoprenaline. Intravenous administration demonstrated a plasma half-life of about 3 minutes. Peak plasma levels following aerosol administration were observed at 2 hours, levels ranging from 8.7-28.9 nM. The majority of rimiterol in the plasma was as its 3-O-methyl metabolite.[11]

Rimiterol is concentrated in the plasma rather than erythrocytes and distributed in high levels in intestine, kidney and liver with lesser amounts in heart and lung. Very little crosses into the brain. ^{14}C rimiterol crosses the placenta in rats but the total content in the fetus was small, <0.01% of the dose.[12]

Oral absorption	high
Presystemic metabolism	extensive
Plasma half life	
mean	<5 minutes
Volume of distribution	unknown
Plasma protein binding	unknown

Concentration–effect relationship

The concentration of rimiterol at its site of action following inhalation is unknown. However, alteration in the amount reaching the site of action due to poor technique in using the metered dose aerosol or due to the pulmonary pathology may explain differences in clinical effects between patients.

Metabolism

The main route of metabolism of rimiterol is by catechol-O-methyltransferase (COMT), forming 3-O-methyl-rimiterol which may be conjugated in the liver by sulphate or glucuronide conjugation. (see Fig. 1)

Fig. 1 The metabolism of rimiterol

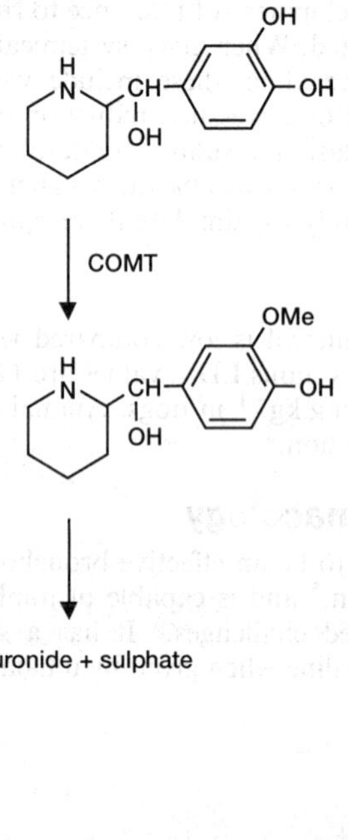

Most of the drug is excreted in this form. After oral administration rimiterol is readily absorbed and subject to rapid first pass metabolism by conjugation, 50% of the drug being excreted in the urine as conjugates. After inhalation, most of the drug is swallowed and subject to conjugation but it is also readily absorbed from the lungs. After intrabronchial administration about 70% of the dose is excreted in the urine in 24 hours, mainly as free and conjugated 3-O-methyl rimiterol together with some free unconjugated rimiterol.

Pharmaceutics

Rimiterol is only available in inhaled forms:

Metered dose inhaled vials contain rimiterol hydrobromide 10 mg.ml^{-1} and carrier freons.[11,12,114] Each metered dose delivers 200 µg of rimiterol. The vial contains 300 metered doses. The vial is contained in a turquoise blue plastic holder bearing the inscription 'Pulmadil' (Riker, UK).

Rimiterol is also available in a breath actuated pressurized aerosol. The vial contains a suspension of rimiterol hydrobromide 10 mg.ml^{-1} and will delivery 300 metered dose inhalations each containing 200 µg. The aerosol is triggered by the patient sucking at the mouthpiece. The vial is contained in a light grey plastic holder with similar coloured mouthpiece and has the inscription 'Pulmadil Auto' (Riker, UK).

Both Pulmadil inhaler and Pulmadil Auto should be stored in a cool place and protected from frost and direct sunlight. The aerosols should not be incinerated or opened, even when empty. The shelf life of rimiterol preparations is 3 years.

Therapeutic use

Indications

1. Treatment of chronic reversible airways obstruction due to asthma or chronic bronchitis.
2. Diagnostic bronchodilator tests.

Contraindications

Absolute
Known hypersensitivity to rimiterol

Relative
1. Known sensitivity to other β_2 stimulants
2. Thyrotoxicosis
3. Hypertension
4. Cardiac disease.

Mode of use

1. Chronic reversible airways disease
Rimiterol 1–3 puffs 0.2–0.6 mg can be used on an as required basis for the treatment of episodic bronchoconstriction in patients with mild asthma and as a prophylactic in exercise-induced asthma. In patients with more severe symptoms doses up to 3 puffs (0.6 mg) can be taken 4 hourly. It is recommended that doses should not be repeated in less than 30 minutes and no more than 8 treatments should be taken in any 24 hour period. This may indicate the onset of severe asthma.

Patients on regular inhaled β-sympathomimetic agents who still have episodes of bronchospasm, especially at night, should have therapy with an inhaled prophylactic agent such as sodium cromoglycate or inhaled corticosteroids or oral xanthine. Patients who notice a reduction in effectiveness of inhaled β-adrenergic agents or reduction in duration of the effect associated with increasing symptoms of asthma should normally be treated with high dose inhaled corticosteroids or oral corticosteroid agents.

2. Diagnostic bronchodilator tests
Rimiterol is an ideal drug for use in the lung function laboratory for testing bronchodilator responses in patient because it is available in an activated metered dose aerosol, has a rapid onset and relatively few side effects.

Contraindications

2. Thyrotoxicosis
β-sympathomimetic agents may increase the symptoms of elevated

plasma thyroxine and potentiate its cardiotoxic effects. Patients with thyrotoxicosis should therefore be treated with caution.

3. Hypertension

Theoretically increased cardiac output following high doses of β-sympathomimetic agents could worsen hypertension, although this is rarely seen in practice.

4. Cardiac disease

Caution is necessary in the presence of cardiac disease.

Adverse reactions

Potentially life-threatening effects

Idiosyncratic reactions of rimiterol are rare. High doses in patients with myocardial disease can, as mentioned previously, lead to dysrhythmias and sudden death.

Acute overdosage

As rimiterol is rapidly eliminated from the blood, it carries little risk of accumulation, even if used repeatedly. No cases of overdose have been reported. However, possible consequences of overdose would be fall in blood pressure, tremor, anxiety, and tachycardia, as well as a fall in serum potassium and increase in plasma glucose and insulin. These effects should be treated symptomatically. It is unlikely that the patient will require use of β-blockade.

Severe or irreversible adverse effects

Potentially serious hypokalaemia has been reported in patients taking β_2-agonist therapy. Hypokalaemia may also occur in hypoxic patients and those treated with xanthine derivatives, steroids, diuretics and long-term laxatives. Extra care should therefore be taken if β_2-agonists are used in these groups of patients and serum potassium levels should be monitored.

Symptomatic adverse effects

Excessive use might be expected to cause anxiety, tremor, and tachycardia in some patients.

Interference with clinical pathology tests

No interferences of this kind appear to have been reported.

High risk groups

Neonates

There are few data on the use of this drug in neonates.

Breast milk. It is unlikely that sufficient drug would be excreted in breast milk to affect the infants.

Children

Rimiterol should be administered to children only under supervision of a responsible adult. The same doses given to adults should be used.

Pregnant women

There is no animal evidence or evidence from prolonged use in humans that rimiterol has teratogenic effects. Regular use in pregnant patients with asthma could theoretically delay the onset of labour.

The elderly

No specific precautions are required in older patients.

Drug interactions

Potentially hazardous interactions

No significant interactions of this kind have been reported during trials of rimiterol. However, theoretically interactions with monoamine oxidase inhibitors and tricyclic antidepressants require that caution should be used in the treatment of patients taking these drugs.

Potentially useful interactions

No reactions of this kind appear to have been described.

Clinical trials

No large group clinical trials have been reported. From small clinical trials it appears to have no advantage over other β-stimulants and its relatively short duration of action may be a disadvantage in some patients with chronic reversible airways obstruction. However, some patients have found its breath activated metered dose aerosol to be an advantage.

Rimiterol hydrobromide

References

1. Carney I, Daly M J, Lightowler J E, Pickering R W 1971 The comparative pharmacology of WG 253 (rimiterol hydrobromide), a new bronchodilator. Archives International Pharmacodynamie and Therapeutics 194: 334–345
2. McFadden E R 1987 Beta$_2$ receptor agonist: metabolism and pharmacology. Journal of Allergy and Clinical Immunology 68: 91–97
3. Pinder R M, Brogden R N, Speight T M, Avery G S 1977 Rimiterol: a review of its pharmacological properties and therapeutic efficacy in asthma. Drugs 14: 81–104
4. Hornsey P A, Gailer K A J, Turner P, Griffin J P 1971 Studies of the 3-methoxy derivatives of isoprenalin, isoetharine and WG 253 on isolated human tissue. Archives International Pharmacodynamie and Therapeutics 191: 357–364
5. Mallin G E, Hartnett B J S, Bergend N 1977 Comparative potencies and β_2-adrenoreceptor selectivities of rimiterol and salbutamol aerosols. British Journal of Clinical Pharmacology 4: 77–79
6. Phillips E M, Woolnough M, Marinova U M, Turner P 1972 A comparison of isoprenaline, salbutamol and rimiterol inhalation on skin temperature, heart rate and respiration in man. Journal of Clinical Pharmacology 12: 158–168
7. Shenfield G M, Paterson J W 1973 Clinical assessment of bronchodilator drugs delivered by aerosol. Thorax 28: 124–128
8. Madsen B W, Tandon M K, Patterson J W 1979 Cross-over study of the efficacy of four β_2-sympathomimetic bronchodilator aerosols. British Journal of Clinical Pharmacology 8: 75–82
9. Mallin G E, Turner P 1975 Comparison of the β_2-adrenoreceptor selectivity of rimiterol, salbutamol and isoprenalin in asthmatic subjects by the intravenous route in man. British Journal of Clinical Pharmacology 2: 41–48
10. Griffin J P, Turner P 1971 Preliminary studies of a new bronchodilator (WG 253) in man. Journal of Clinical Pharmacology 11: 280–287
11. Evans M E, Shenfield G M, Thomas N, Walker S R, Paterson J W 1974 The pharmacokinetics of rimiterol in man. Xenobiotica 4: 681–692
12. Griffin J P, Williams J R B, Maughan E 1974 The metabolism of rimiterol hydrobromide at different intravenous dose levels in the rat. Xenobiotica 4: 755–764

Ritodrine (hydrochloride)

Ritodrine is a β-adrenergic stimulant used in the treatment of premature labour.

Chemistry

Ritodrine hydrochloride (Yutopar, Pre-par, Utopar, Utemerin)
$C_{17}H_{21}NO_3.HCl$
(R*,S*)-2-(4-Hydroxyphenethylamino)-1-(4-hydroxyphenyl)propan-1-ol hydrochloride

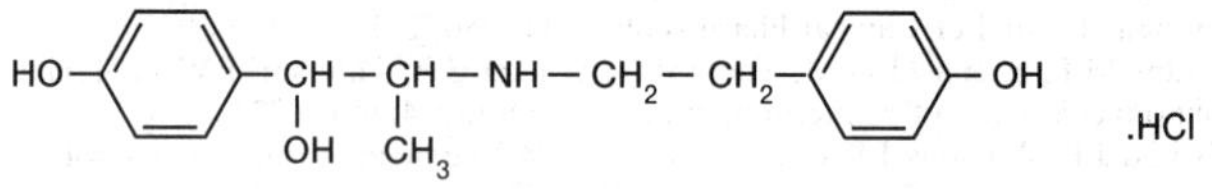

Molecular weight (free base)	323.8 (287.3)
pKa	8.6
Solubility	
in alcohol	>1 in 10
in water	>1 in 10
Octanol/water partition coefficient	low

A white, odourless, slightly bitter, crystalline powder, ritodrine hydrochloride is prepared by chemical synthesis. Ritodrine possesses two chiral carbon atoms in the relative configuration (R*,S*)

Pharmacology

Ritodrine is a selective β_2-adrenoceptor agonist that was developed specifically for its uterine effects. However, some chronotropic cardiac effects and peripheral vasodilation are also seen at therapeutic doses. By its effects on β_2-receptors in the periphery it causes metabolic effects including a rise in blood glucose, and free fatty acids and a decrease in serum potassium.[1–3]

Toxicology

The toxic effects of ritodrine are largely the result of excessive β-adrenergic stimulation. Ritodrine has no adverse effects on reproduction and fertility. Experiments in animals have shown that even at high dosage riodrine has no teratogenic effects. No short-term mutagenicity or long-term carcinogenicity tests have been carried out.

Clinical pharmacology

The main effect of ritodrine is to relax uterine muscle. Nevertheless, by its action as a β_2 agonist it, like other drugs of this class, has a number of other effects. Mean arterial blood pressure does not change very much but there is often a dose-related tachycardia in both mother and fetus. This is due to both direct stimulant and reflex mechanisms. There is also an increase in cardiac output. The secretion of renin is increased and this probably leads to decreased renal excretion of salt and water leading to oedema. Hyperglycaemia has been recorded, and persistent hyperglycaemia in the mother may lead to reactive hypoglycaemia in the infant. Hypokalaemia may occur[4] due to the movement of potassium into cells. Bronchial muscle dilatation may occur but this is unlikely to be noted clinically in the situation in which the drug is used.

The effective dosage of ritodrine usually lies between 150 and 350 $\mu g.min^{-1}$, and infusion should be continued for 12–48 hours after uterine contractions have ceased.

Pharmacokinetics

The preferred analytical method is by specific radioimmunossay (sensitivity 100 $ng.l^{-1}$).[6]

Ritodrine is rapidly and almost completely absorbed after oral administration, with 90% of a dose of radioactive ritodrine being excreted in the urine irrespective of route of administration. Although it is almost completely absorbed, the oral bioavailability of ritodrine is only 30–40%, presumably due to first-pass metabolism.

Following oral administration, peak plasma concentrations are achieved in 20–40 min. Plasma elimination of ritodrine is apparently triphasic. Following discontinuation of a 1-hour infusion at 150 $\mu g.min^{-1}$, plasma ritodrine levels fell rapidly, with a half life of 6–9 minutes. Thereafter, the half life increased to 1.7–2.6 hours for the next 4–5 hours, becoming even longer thereafter.

The volume of distribution of ritodrine has been calculated in man as 0.6–0.9 $l.kg^{-1}$. Ritodrine is approximately 30% bound to plasma protein at therapeutic concentrations. No information is available regarding entry of ritodrine into brain or other tissues, and it is not known if the drug is excreted in breast milk. Ritodrine crosses the placenta.

Oral absorption	>95%
Presystemic metabolism	60–70%
Plasma half life	
phase 1	6–9 min
phase 2	1.7–2.6 h
phase 3	15–20 h
Volume of distribution	0.6–0.9 $l.kg^{-1}$
Plasma protein binding	~30%

The effects of hepatic and renal disease on the kinetics are not known, though some increase in bioavailability might be expected in hepatic dysfunction. Ritodrine is extensively metabolized by conjugation, the major route of excretion being the urine. Only about 5% of the dose is excreted unchanged in the urine.

Concentration–effect relationship

The maximal infusion rate and the concentration of ritodrine in maternal serum after 4 hours of treatment have been reported[4] to be significantly correlated to the frequency of uterine contractions prior to infusion rate, i.e. the higher the rate of uterine contraction, the larger the dose of ritodrine required to suppress it. Plasma concentrations of 15–31 $\mu g.l^{-1}$ were effective in suppressing labour in 10 out of 17 women.

Metabolism

Approximately 90% of an administered dose of ritodrine is excreted in the urine, regardless of route of administration. In rats whose bile was diverted, urinary excretion was approximately 50% of the dose with about 25% recovered in the bile, compared to 60–75% urinary excretion in control rats, suggesting enterohepatic recirculation.

Following oral administration, 67% of urinary radioactivity is associated with a sulphuric acid ester and 25% with a glucuronic acid conjugate. After intravenous administration, the same metabolites are found but the proportion of the sulphuric acid ester is halved in favour of unchanged drug. It is not known if any of the metabolites are pharmacologically active.

Pharmaceutics

Ritodrine (Yutopar; Astra, USA/Duphar, UK) is available in oral and parenteral forms.

Tablets are round, buff coloured, with the inscription '177' on one face, 'Duphar' on the reverse, each containing 10 mg ritodrine hydrochloride.

Ritodrine for injection is a clear aqueous solution containing 10 $mg.ml^{-1}$ ritodrine hydrochloride.

A sustained-release preparation has been developed, but is not available for use in the UK. It consists of capsules containing a granulate coated with a layer of drug surrounded by a barrier layer of acrylic resin that swells but does not dissolve in digestive juices, thus allowing the drug to diffuse only gradually. The rate of diffusion varies inversely with the thickness of the barrier layer.

Both ritodrine tablets and solution for injection should be stored in a cool dry place, protected from light. The maximum shelf-life for tablets is 5 years and for injection solution 3 years.

Therapeutic use

Indications

1. Management of uncomplicated premature labour
2. Management of fetal asphyxia in labour where desired.

Contraindications

1. Antepartum haemorrhage which requires immediate delivery
2. Eclampsia and severe pre-eclampsia
3. Intrauterine fetal death
4. Chorioamnionitis
5. Maternal cardiac disease
6. Maternal hyperthyroidism
7. Cord compression.
8. Abnormal ECG.

Mode of use

The recommended dose of ritodrine is 50 $\mu g.min^{-1}$ by intravenous infusion, gradually increasing at 10-minute intervals by 50 $\mu g.min^{-1}$ increments. It is recommended that in healthy patients, no further increases in dosage should be made when the maternal heart rate reaches 140 beats per minute. The effective dosage lies between 150 and 350 $\mu g.min^{-1}$ min. Alternatively, 1 ml of the 10 $mg.ml^{-1}$ solution supplied, equivalent to 10 mg ritodrine hydrochloride, may be administered every 3–8 hours by intramuscular injection. This regimen should be continued for 12–48 hours following arrest of labour. For oral maintenance therapy, one 10 mg tablet may be given 30 minutes before termination of intravenous therapy, followed by 10 mg every 2 hours for the first 24 hours. Thereafter, dosage is usually maintained at 10–20 mg every 4–6 hours, depending on uterine activity and side effects. The total daily dosage of oral ritodrine should not exceed 120 mg.

To improve the condition of the baby prior to assisted delivery, 50 $\mu g.min^{-1}$ ritodrine may be administered by intravenous infusion, increasing the rate rapidly until uterine activity is suppressed or until the maternal heart rate reaches 140 beats per minute. If fetal acid–base balance is satisfactory, the infusion can be continued for a further 15–30 minutes with observation, before proceeding with the delivery.

Maternal pulmonary oedema has been reported. Care should be taken not to overhydrate. Dextrose rather than saline is the preferred infusion vehicle. Respiratory signs should be monitored carefully.

As ritodrine may lower serum potassium or increase blood glucose, the metabolic status of the patient should be considered, particularly with diabetics and patients on potassium-depleting diuretics.

Indications

1. Management of uncomplicated premature labour
Ritodrine hydrochloride was first used for the treatment of premature labour in the early 1970s. It acts by suppressing uterine contractions by a β-sympathomimetic action. Doses of between 50 and 200 $\mu g.min^{-1}$ are effective in approximately 80% of cases,[7,8] although individual titration of dose to the patient's requirements has been found to produce a higher success rate.[10] Administration of ritodrine has been reported to produce a significantly reduced incidence of neonatal death and respiratory distress syndrome and a significantly higher proportion of infants reaching 36 weeks' gestation or birth weight greater than 2500 g. There was also a significant improvement in gestational age at delivery and in the number of days gained in utero among ritodrine-treated patients compared to controls.[9]

2. Management of fetal asphyxia in labour
Ritodrine produced a significant improvement in the number of infants born with respiratory distress syndrome, compared to untreated controls, when administered to the mother either unsuccessfully to prevent labour or prior to planned premature delivery.[9,11] Respiratory distress syndrome in neonates has been described as arising from pulmonary vasoconstriction resulting from hypoxia, which results in damage to the alveolar epithelial cells responsible for surfactant synthesis. By counteracting the vasoconstriction, ritodrine could prevent cell damage and aid production of surfactant. It has also been postulated that stress may stimulate lung maturation, and thus administration of ritodrine, by mimicking the β-adrenergic effects of the 'fight or flight' responses, may evoke this response.[11]

Contraindications

1. Antepartum haemorrhage
When this condition is sufficiently severe to make immediate delivery essential, ritodrine administration is contraindicated. In addition, the increase in heart rate and vasodilatation resulting from ritodrine treatment could aggravate the bleeding.

2. Eclampsia and severe pre-eclampsia
In these conditions it would be inadvisable for both mother and baby to postpone delivery, since the effects of continued pregnancy are likely to carry a greater risk than those of premature delivery.

3. Intrauterine fetal death
If the fetus is dead, or has major malformations incompatible with survival, labour should not be postponed.

4. Intrauterine infection
Intrauterine infection represents a greater threat to fetal well-being than premature delivery, and therefore ritodrine should not be administered.

5. Maternal cardiac disease
Since many patients receiving ritodrine develop palpitations and increased heart rate, ritodrine is usually contraindicated in maternal cardiac disease.

6. Maternal hyperthyroidism
Again, the side effects of nervousness, tremor and palpitations encountered during intravenous infusion of ritodrine contraindicate its use in patients with hyperthyroidism.

7. Cord compression
Cord compression may lead to oxygen lack and possible death of the fetus. If this condition is confirmed, immediate delivery is desirable.

8. Abnormal ECG
Because of its cardiostimulatory effects, ritodrine is contraindicated in the presence of an abnormal ECG.

In general, ritodrine should not be used to delay labour if this would result in risk to the baby, nor should it be used in situations where its known pharmacology would constitute a danger to the mother.

Adverse reactions

Potentially life-threatening effects
Cardiopulmonary complications, including pulmonary oedema, angina-like complaints, cardiac arrhythmias, and maternal death in association with the use of ritodrine have been reported, although their incidence is rare.

Among all patients treated with ritodrine (estimated as approximately 480 000 in 1980), only two maternal deaths have been reported,[12] neither directly attributable to the drug.

Acute overdosage
Deliberate overdose with ritodrine has not been reported. Accidental overdosage during intravenous infusion produces symptoms resulting from β-adrenoceptor stimulation. If cessation of the infusion does not produce a rapid enough improvement, it can be treated with a non-selective β-blocking drug.

Severe or irreversible adverse effects
Metabolic disturbances, including an increase in blood glucose, serum insulin and free fatty acids, and a fall in serum potassium, may occur, and particular caution is necessary when administering the drug to diabetic patients.

Symptomatic adverse effects
The usual clinical adverse effects of ritodrine are related to its inherent pharmacology as a β-mimetic drug. Although selected for its action on β_2-adrenoceptors, ritodrine administered by intravenous infusion uniformly causes an elevation of maternal heart rate and a widening of pulse pressure. Many patients receiving ritodrine develop palpitations (approximately 33%), tremor, nausea, vomiting, head-

ache, erythema (10–15%), restlessness, and anxiety (5–10%).[12] These symptoms generally resolve when the dose of ritodrine is reduced.

Other effects
Ritodrine causes increases in blood glucose, serum insulin and free fatty acids, and a fall in serum potassium.[12]

Interference with clinical pathology tests
No interference of ritodrine with urinalysis using Bili Labstix (Ames) or Combur-8 (Boehringer) has been observed.

High risk groups

Neonates
The drug is not used in neonates.

Breast milk. No information is available regarding the excretion of ritodrine in breast milk.

Children
The drug is not used in children.

Pregnant women
Ritodrine is used only in pregnant women.

The elderly
Ritodrine is not used in patients in this age-group.

Concurrent disease
Ritodrine should not be given to mothers with pre-existing cardiac disease, hyperthyroidism, or uncontrolled hypertension unless the physician considers that the benefits clearly outweigh the risks. In diabetic patients, glucose levels should be closely monitored and insulin requirements adjusted accordingly during intravenous therapy.

Drug interactions

Potentially hazardous interactions

Monamine oxidase inhibitors (MAOIs). By inhibiting the destruction of catecholamines, MAOIs may potentiate the β-adrenergic effects of ritodrine, leading to a higher incidence and severity of side effects.

Tricyclic antidepressants. Tricyclic antidepressants inhibit reuptake of noradrenaline into nerve endings and may increase uterine contractions.

Corticosteroids. Several cases of severe pulmonary oedema have been described in patients receiving corticosteroids in conjunction with ritodrine.[12]

Sympathomimetic amines. These may potentiate the β-adrenergic effects of ritodrine, leading to increased toxicity. α-Agonists may increase uterine contractions.

β-Blocking drugs. These will inhibit the effects of ritodrine on uterine β-adrenoceptors.

Anaesthetics. General anaesthetics may sensitize the heart to circulating adrenaline and noradrenaline released from cardiac sympathetic nerve endings, leading to the development of arrhythmias. Since ritodrine causes an increase in heart rate, sometimes leading to palpitations, the co-administration of general anaesthetics and ritodrine is contraindicated.

Potassium-depleting diuretics. Ritodrine causes a fall in plasma potassium levels which would be additive with that induced by potassium-depleting diuretics, leading to the development of cardiac arrhythmias.

Potentially useful interactions
Non-selective β-sympatholytic agents can be used as antidotes to ritodrine overdosage.

Major outcome trials

1. Wesselius-De Casparis A, Thiery M, Yo Le Sian A et al 1971 Results of double-blind, multicentre study with ritodrine in premature labour. British Medical Journal 3: 144–147

This is a double-blind, placebo-controlled, multicentre study of 91 patients in premature labour. Criteria for inclusion in the trial were that the patient must present between the 20th and 36th weeks of pregnancy, with a diagnosis of premature labour. No patients were excluded because of membranes, toxaemia or other maternal or fetal complications. All patients were treated according to a fixed dosage scheme consisting of an intravenous infusion followed by oral tablets for a total of 7 days. Ritodrine arrested premature labour in 80% of patients (placebo, 48%), although this course of treatment was not usually sufficient to prolong gestation until term. No serious side effects were observed. Of 17 patients in whom ritodrine failed to arrest labour, 11 had complications such as membrane rupture or toxaemia. The authors concluded that ritodrine was a well-tolerated uterine relaxant that could arrest premature labour in most cases.

2. Merkatz I R, Peter J B, Barden T P 1980 Ritodrine hydrochloride: a β-mimetic agent for use in preterm labour. II. Evidence of efficacy. Obstetrics and Gynecology 56: 7–12

This is a multicentre, randomized, double-blind controlled study, in which ritodrine hydrochloride was compared with either ethanol or placebo in the treatment of idiopathic preterm labour. Compared to controls, there was a significantly reduced incidence of neonatal death and respiratory distress syndrome ($P<0.05$) among offspring of ritodrine-treated mothers, and a significantly higher proportion of infants achieved 36 weeks' gestation ($P<0.05$) or birth weight greater than 2500 g ($P<0.05$). There was also a significant improvement in gestational age at delivery ($P<0.05$) and in the number of days gained in utero ($P<0.001$) among ritodrine-treated patients compared with controls.

3. Frolich H 1973 Clinical experience of the treatment of threatened premature labour with a β-mimetic drug. Zeitschrift fur Geburtshilfe und Perinatologie 177: 251–262 (English translation)

This paper describes the results of ritodrine treatment for premature labour in 104 patients between 1970 and 1971. Compared with a similar group of 82 patients studied in 1968, the proportion of premature deliveries was reduced from 72 to 62%. Perinatal mortality was 13.6% in the treated group and 25.6% in the untreated patients. The author concluded that ritodrine should be used routinely in the treatment of threatened premature labour.

4. Thiery M, Baumgarten K, Brosens I et al 1972 A multicentre trial with ritodrine in the treatment of premature labour in patients with intact membranes. Paper given at the International Symposium on the Treatment of Fetal Risks, Baden, Austria, May

This study describes two clinical trials of ritodrine in the treatment of premature labour, one double-blind and the other variable dose. Some of the centres involved in the clinical trial reported by Wesselius-De Casparis and colleagues (see 1 above) participated. 97 patients were studied, 25 each in the fixed-dose ritodrine and placebo groups, and 47 in the variable dose trial. In the double-blind trial, 200 $\mu g.min^{-1}$ ritodrine was administered intravenously for 24–48 hours, followed by an oral course of treatment consisting of 10 mg ritodrine 4 times daily for 7 days. In the variable dose study the starting infusion rate was between 50 and 200 $\mu g.min^{-1}$, the dose being increased or decreased according to response and continued for as long as necessary, at least until 12 hours after contractions had ceased. Oral treatment was then commenced at a dose of 10–20 mg, 4–8 times daily, depending on the response to the infusion and the cervical status, and was continued until 36–38 weeks of pregnancy. The authors concluded that (1) with intact membranes, ritodrine could postpone premature labour more efficiently than placebo; and (2) by individual adjustment of the dose according to each patient's response, the efficacy of treatment could be increased.

General review articles

Gonik B, Creasy R K 1986 Preterm labor: its diagnosis and management. American Journal of Obstetrics and Gynecology 154: 3–8

Martin A J 1981 Treatment of premature labour. Severe unwanted effects associated with β-sympathomimetics: causes, incidence and preventive measures. British Journal of Intravenous Therapy, December: 14–21

Melchior J, Bernard N 1975 Current methods of prevention and treatment of threatened premature delivery, clinical appearances, results and general consequences. Symposium on Recent Advances in β-mimetic Drugs in Obstetrics, Rome, October

References

1. Landesman R, Wilson K H, Coutinho E M, Klima I M, Marcus R S 1971 The relaxant action of ritodrine, a sympathomimetic amine, on the uterus during term labor. American Journal of Obstetrics and Gynecology 110: 111–114
2. Siimes A S I, Creasy R K 1980 Maternal and fetal metabolic responses to ritodrine in the sheep. Acta Obstetrica et Gynecologica Scandinavica 59: 181–186
3. Kleinman G, Nuwayhid B, Rudelstorfer R et al 1984 Circulatory and renal effects of β-adrenergeric-receptor stimulation in pregnant sheep. American Journal of Obstetrics and Gynecology 149: 865–874
4. Caritis S N, Lin L S, Toig G, Wong L K 1983 Pharmacodynamics of ritodrine in pregnant women during preterm labour. American Journal of Obstetrics and Gynecology 147: 752–759
5. Ingels F, Thiery M, Belpaire F, Bogaert M 1985 Search for rational ritodrine dose regimen in preterm labour. IRCS Medical Science 13: 205–206
6. Gandar R, de Zoeten L W, van der Schoot J B 1980 Serum level of ritodrine in man. European Journal of Clinical Pharmacology 17: 117–122
7. Thiery M, Baumgarten K, Brosens I et al 1972 A multicentre trial with ritodrine in the treatment of premature labour in patients with intact membranes. Paper given at the International Symposium on the Treatment of Foetal Risks, Baden, Austria, May
8. Wesselius-De Casparis A, Thiery M, Yo Le Sian A et al 1971 Results of double-blind, multicentre study with ritodrine in premature labour. British Medical Journal 3: 144–147
9. Merkatz I R, Peter J B, Barden T P 1980 Ritodrine hydrochloride: a β-mimetic agent for use in preterm labour. II. Evidence of efficacy. Obstetrics and Gynecology 56: 7–12
10. Frolich H 1973 Clinical experience of the treatment of threatened premature labour with a β-Mimetic drug. Zeitschrift fur Geburtshilfe und Perinatologie 177: 251–262 (English translation)
11. Boog G, Ben Brahim M, Gandar R 1975 β-mimetic drugs and possible prevention of respiratory distress syndrome. British Journal of Obstetrics and Gynaecology 82: 285–288
12. Barden T P, Peter J B, Merkatz I R 1980 Ritodrine hydrochloride: a β-mimetic agent for use in preterm labour. I. Pharmacology, clinical history, administration, side effects, and safety. Obstetrics and Gynecology 56: 1–6

Salbutamol

Salbutamol is a β_2-adrenoceptor agonist used in the treatment of asthma and other forms of diffuse airways obstruction.

Chemistry

Salbutamol (albuterol, Ventolin, Proventil, Salbulin, Cobutolin, Asmaven)
$C_{13}H_{21}NO_3$
1-(4-(RS)-Hydroxy-3-hydroxymethylphenyl)-2-(t-butylamino)ethanol

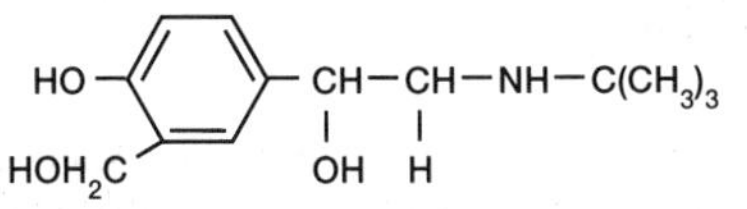

Molecular weight (sulphate)	239.3 (288.4)
pKa	9.3, 10.3
Solubility	
in alcohol	1 in 25
in water	1 in 70 (1 in 4)
Octanol/water partition coefficient	—

The racemic mixture is used clinically. A white, odourless, almost tasteless crystalline powder prepared by chemical synthesis. Products other than metered-dose aerosol contain salbutamol sulphate. It is an ingredient of Ventide with bectomethasone dipropionate.

Pharmacology

Salbutamol is a selective β_2-adrenoceptor agonist[1,2] with effects on smooth and skeletal muscle. These include bronchodilatation, relaxation of uterine muscle and tremor. Smooth muscle relaxation is dose-dependent and is thought to occur via the adenyl cyclase-cyclic adenosine monophosphate (cAMP) system, with binding of the drug to the β-adrenergic receptor in the cell membrane causing conversion of ATP to cAMP, which activates protein kinase. This leads to phosphorylation of proteins which ultimately increase bound intracellular calcium; the consequent reduced availability of ionized intracellular calcium inhibits actin–myosin linkage thus causing relaxation of smooth muscle.

β_2-agonists such as salbutamol also have an antiallergic effect on mast cells causing inhibition of release of bronchoconstrictor mediators including histamine, neutrophil chemotactive factor (NCF) and prostaglandin D_2 (PGD_2). This effect has been shown with human lung mast cells in vitro[3] and with inhibition of circulating mediators following antigen provocation testing in vivo.[4] As with β-receptors on bronchial smooth muscle, it is likely that the cAMP system acts as the second messenger in regulating the mast cell response.

Toxicology

In common with other selective β_2-agonists, salbutamol has been shown to induce benign mesovarian leiomyomas in certain strains of rat susceptible to this type of tumour.[5] There is no evidence of carcinogenicity or teratogenicity.

Clinical pharmacology

Bronchodilatation occurs after administration of salbutamol in normal subjects and in patients with asthma or chronic obstructive pulmonary disease (COPD). Asthmatic subjects usually show the largest responses but the magnitude of effect depends on pretreatment airway calibre, dose, route and method of administration. Study of human bronchial smooth muscle in vitro has suggested that, in comparison with isoprenaline, salbutamol is only a partial agonist,[6] but measurements in vivo indicate that similar maximal effects can be achieved with each drug given by inhalation.[7] The effect is dose-dependent, both in asthma[7,8] and in COPD;[9] larger doses result in a more sustained effect.

Other actions on the respiratory system include enhanced mucociliary clearance which has been demonstrated in patients with COPD and in normal subjects[10] and an antiallergic effect due to inhibition of mediator release.[3,4] The clinical relevance of these actions is not established.

Salbutamol has a relaxant effect on smooth muscle at other sites, including the myometrium, where its inhibitory effect is put to therapeutic use,[11] and peripheral blood vessels. Stimulation of β_2-receptors on vascular smooth muscle leads to vasodilatation and a reflex increase in heart rate with little effect on stroke volume.[12] The chronotropic effect of salbutamol is considerably less than that of a β_1-stimulant such as isoprenaline, which acts directly on cardiac β-receptors.

Stimulation of β_2-receptors results in widespread metabolic effects, including rises in free fatty acid, insulin, lactate and glucose levels and a fall in serum potassium concentration.[13,14] The hypokalaemia is not clearly related to hyperinsulinaemia and may be due to direct stimulation of β_2-adrenoceptors linked to a membrane-bound Na^+K^+-ATPase.[15]

Studies of tolerance during long-term treatment with β_2-stimulants have produced conflicting results. Although tachyphylaxis is readily demonstrable in non-airway receptors in vivo[16–18] and in non-asthmatic bronchial smooth muscle in vitro,[19] it is unlikely that a clinically important loss of therapeutic effect occurs in airway receptors in patients with asthma using regular treatment in moderate[20] or high[18] doses.

Pharmacokinetics

Early studies involving salbutamol assay were performed using tritium-labelled drug administered orally, intravenously or by inhalation and assaying plasma or urine for salbutamol and its metabolites using a liquid scintillation spectrometer.[21] Subsequently, gas chromatography–mass spectrometry became the technique of choice.[22,23] Recently, a method using high performance thin-layer chromatography has been developed, with a sensitivity of approximately 20 μg.l^{-1} in urine and 1 μg.l^{-1} in plasma.[24] A specific radioimmunoassay with sensitivity sufficient to measure 0.5 μg.l^{-1} has also been described.[25]

Salbutamol is well absorbed from the gastrointestinal tract with between 58 and 78% of a radiolabel appearing in the urine within 24 hours and 65–84% in 72 hours.[26] Presystemic metabolism is considerable. The major metabolite is a sulphate conjugate,[27] which is probably formed in the bowel mucosa and is inactive. After conventional tablets peak plasma levels are seen at 2–3 hours and at that time the ratio of free drug to metabolite is about 1:5.[28] Peak plasma concentrations after a single oral dose of 4 mg salbutamol are reported[28] to range from 10 to 16.9 μg.l^{-1}. The plasma half life varies between 2.7 and 5 hours; 34–47% of a radiolabel appears in the urine as the conjugate and approximately half this amount as unchanged drug.[26]

The absolute bioavailability of oral preparations and the effects of food are not known. After ingestion of a slow-release preparation (Spandet), peak plasma levels are seen at 5–6 hours and are lower than after the same dose of conventional formulation; however, the areas under the curves of plasma concentration versus time are similar, indicating equivalent bioavailability of the two formulations.[23]

Following intrevenous infusion most of the infused drug circulates unchanged and plasma concentration of drug exceeds that of the conjugate at all times after injection.[21] Between 75 and 81% of the radiolabel appears in the urine within 72 hours, but compared with oral administration the ratio of free drug to metabolite is reversed. The average proportion of the dose excreted unchanged in two studies was 50%[21] and 64%;[28] the corresponding proportions excreted as the metabolite were 27%[21] and 12%.[28]

In general, only 10% or less of an inhaled drug from a pressurized aerosol is deposited in the airways and the remainder is swallowed. The profile of plasma radioactivity and proportions circulating as free drug and metabolite are similar after inhalation of labelled drug from a pressurized aerosol and after oral administration, with peak plasma levels at 3–5 hours and a ratio of free drug to metabolite of approximately 1:4, strongly suggesting that the detectable drug represents the portion absorbed after swallowing.[26] The maximal therapeutic effect is, however, seen much sooner after inhalation, suggesting a local action and little therapeutic effect may be detectable by the time peak plasma concentrations are achieved. When larger doses are given by wet nebulization, either with or without IPPB (intermittent positive pressure breathing), a second plasma peak representing mainly free salbutamol is seen at 30 minutes, which is presumed to reflect absorption of drug from the bronchial tree.[30,31] Also, when the drug is instilled via a bronchoscope, the peak plasma concentration is seen early and most circulates unchanged, indicating no significant metabolism of the drug by the lung.[32] The lower plasma concentrations achieved after inhalation compared with oral or parenteral administration are associated with correspondingly less severe non-respiratory side effects.

The proportion of circulating drug that is protein-bound is approximately 10%. The mean volume of distribution after intravenous infusion calculated from the data of Fairfax and others[33] is 3.4 ± 0.6 l.kg^{-1}; in a later study a mean distribution volume of 156 l was reported.[28] This high volume implies extensive uptake into the tissues. In the rat, salbutamol shows almost uniform distribution in the majority of tissues, with the notable exception of the brain where the concentration is only approximately 5% of that in plasma[34,35] Transfer across the placenta has been demonstrated both in vitro[36] and in vivo.[37]

Oral absorption	85%
Presystemic metabolism	considerable
Plasma half life	
range	2.7–5 h
Volume of distribution	3.4 ± 0.6 l.kg^{-1}
Plasma protein binding	10%

Concentration–effect relationship

Temporal relationships between bronchodilatation and plasma levels of radioactivity have been shown after oral administration.[26] A therapeutically effective oral dose of 4 mg gives peak plasma concentrations[22,23], as determined by GC–MS, of 5–15 µg.l^{-1} but the full therapeutic range is not clearly defined. After steady-state dosing with the newer osmotically controlled release preparation (Volmax) a dose of 4 mg twice daily gives average plasma concentrations between a minimum of 4.5 and maximum of 8.5 µg.l^{-1}; the corresponding values reported during treatment with 8 mg twice daily[29] are 8.7 and 16.1 µg.l^{-1}. An intravenous infusion rate of 8 µg.kg^{-1}.h^{-1}, which in chronic asthma produces near maximal bronchodilatation with minimal cardiovascular side effects,[38] results in steady-state plasma levels[33] of 20.3 (SD 3.2) µg.l^{-1}. Plasma concentrations are of no relevance to the effects of administration by inhalation. Assay in clinical practice is unnecessary, except possibly in monitoring patient compliance.[39]

The therapeutic concentration which completely inhibits uterine contractions during premature labour is reported[40] to vary between 8 and 33 µg.l^{-1}.

Metabolism

Unlike isoprenaline, salbutamol is not a substrate for catechol-O-methyl-transferase or for monoamine oxidase.[32] Metabolism is by conjugation: the major metabolite was for some time in doubt but has now been identified as the 4′-0-sulphate ester (Fig. 1).[27] Earlier failure to hydrolyse the metabolite using arylsulphatase[26] has subsequently been shown to be due to poor substrate specificity.[27]

Total plasma clearance after intravenous infusion, calculated from the data of Fairfax and others[33] is 6.6 ± 1.0 ml..min^{-1}.kg^{-1}; a later study[28] reported a similar mean value of 7.72 ml.min^{-1}.kg^{-1}. Excretion is mainly via the kidneys and the ratio of unchanged drug to metabolite depends on the route of administration, with the metabolite dominating after oral treatment and the unchanged drug after intravenous dosing. After inhalation via conventional aerosol the pattern of excretion is similar to that after oral treatment, while with larger inhaled doses a relatively higher excretion of unchanged drug reflects greater pulmonary absorption.

Fig. 1 Metabolism of salbutamol

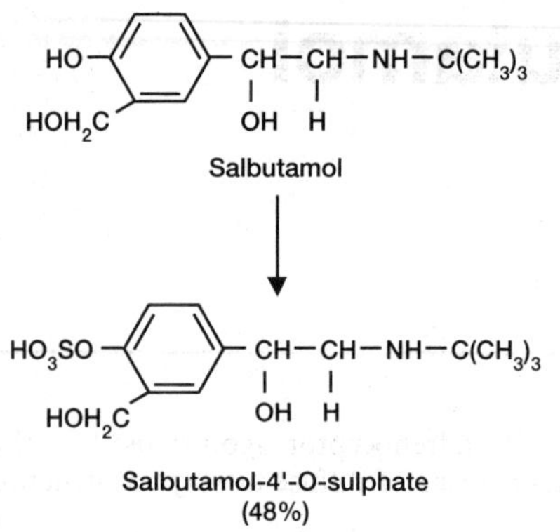

Pharmaceutics

Oral preparations

Ventolin tablets (as salbutamol sulphate) (Allen and Hanbury's, UK/Glaxo, USA): 2 mg pink, round scored tablets; 4 mg pink, round scored tablets; 8 mg Spandets pink/white, slow-release tablets (no longer available in USA or UK); 4 mg, 8 mg controlled-release tablets with osmotic core containing salbutamol and sodium chloride surrounded by a semi-permeable membrane punctured by a single laser drilled pore of 250 µm diameter (Volmax, Duncan Flockhart, UK).

Proventil tablets (Schering, USA): 2 mg white round tablets marked ‘2’ on one side and ‘252’ on the other; 4 mg white round tablets marked ‘4’ on one side and ‘573’ on the other.

Syrup (elixir) (as salbutamol sulphate): 400 µg.ml^{-1} in sugar-free, orange–yellow coloured, strawberry flavoured syrup for dilution with water, life of diluted syrup 28 days (Ventolin Syrup).

Parenteral preparations

As salbutamol sulphate: 50 µg.ml^{-1} in 5 ml ampoules; 500 µg.ml^{-1} in 1 ml ampoules; 1 mg.ml^{-1} in 5 ml ampoules to dilute for infusion.

Inhaled preparations

Metered dose aerosol (as salbutamol base): 100 µg per puff (UK); 90 µg per puff (USA) (‘volumatic’ large spacer device is available)

The following are unavailable in the USA (Allen & Hanbury's).

Insufflation cartridges (salbutamol sulphate) (Rotacaps): 200 µg light blue/clear cartridges inhaled by Rotahaler.

Insufflation cartridges (salbutamol sulphate) (Rotacaps): 400 µg dark blue/clear cartridges inhaled by Rotahaler.

Ventodisks: powder for inhalation in blister disks; each disk contains 8 doses of 200 µg or 400 µg.

Respirator solution (salbutamol sulphate): 5 mg.ml^{-1} in 20 ml bottles to be diluted with saline; 1 mg.ml^{-1} in 2.5 ml ampoules, 2 mg.ml^{-1} in 2.5 ml ampoules (‘nebules’).

The various preparations have a quoted shelf-life of 2–3 years. Parenteral and respirator solutions should be protected from light. The respirator solution contains benzalkonium chloride as a preservative; no preparations contain tartrazine.

Therapeutic use

Indications

1. Bronchodilator for use in asthma, chronic bronchitis, emphysema and other conditions associated with airways obstruction
2. In management of premature labour.

Contraindications

1. Hypersensitivity to salbutamol, or other ingredients of the preparations.

There are no absolute contraindications in the treatment of airways obstruction. Care is required in patients with thyrotoxicosis or ischaemic heart disease. Inhaled preparations are unlikely to cause problems unless large doses are used.

In management of premature labour, antepartum haemorrhage or toxaemia of pregnancy are contraindications and caution is necessary in the presence of cardiac disease.

Mode of use

1. Bronchodilatation
Selective β_2-agonists given by inhalation are the bronchodilators of first choice in patients with asthma and other forms of reversible airways obstruction. For the relief of occasional symptoms, one or two inhalations from a metered-dose aerosol as necessary may suffice. An inhaler may be used in similar fashion before exercise in subjects prone to exercise-induced asthma. In patients with asthma or COPD who have persistent symptomatic airways obstruction, the drug should be inhaled regularly four times a day. The need for treatment and its effects should be monitored by measurements of peak expiratory flow rate (PEF) and/or FEV_1. The magnitude of improvement after inhalation helps in defining the optimal dose but a small or unrecordable increase on a single occasion does not necessarily imply the absence of a useful therapeutic effect. For patients who find difficulty with pressurized aerosols, the insufflation cartridges (Rotacaps) provide a useful alternative.[41]

If regular inhaled treatment is insufficient to control chronic asthmatic symptoms the effect of an increased dose may be tried or alternative therapy added, e.g. inhaled steroid or slow-release theophylline. Troublesome nocturnal symptoms are usually improved by more regular daytime inhaled treatment (with or without the addition of an inhaled steroid) and can also be helped by the addition of the sustained-release oral preparation before retiring. A few asthmatic subjects with markedly variable airway function consistently show large increases in PEF or FEV_1 with large doses of β-stimulants; in these individuals the domiciliary use of a nebulizer and compressor pump with doses of salbutamol respirator solution up to 5 mg four times daily may be necessary to maintain symptomatic control. Such patients will almost inevitably also be taking inhaled or oral steroids, possibly together with a sustained-release theophylline preparation. Patients using these large doses should also monitor PEF and should be advised to take additional oral steroids or seek medical help if the nebulized drug appears to be losing its effect. Nebulizers are also particularly valuable in small children who may be unable adequately to use a pressurized aerosol.

Oral preparations other than the sustained-release tablets are indicated only for patients unable to use the inhaled route.

In severe asthma a selective β-stimulant should be given by nebulization, e.g. salbutamol respirator solution 2.5–5 mg two to four hourly, preferably driven by oxygen. Parenteral β-agonists are now rarely used in the management of severe asthma, as a similar degree of bronchodilatation can be obtained after nebulized drug with less severe tachycardia and the effect of nebulized drug is more prolonged.[42,43] Cardiac monitoring is advisable if parenteral treatment or large doses of nebulized salbutamol are given to a patient with ischaemic heart disease.

2. Prevention of premature labour
Salbutamol, like other selective β_2-stimulants, has an inhibitory effect on the myometrium, producing a demonstrable decrease or abolition of uterine contractions in advanced labour in a dose-dependent manner.[11,40,44]

Its efficacy in prolongation of labour beyond 37 weeks' gestation has, however, been doubted.[45] The drug is infused at increasing rates from 10 to 50 $\mu g.min^{-1}$ until contractions cease and then titrated down to the lowest effective dose. Treatment may be continued by oral administration. This type of treatment is contraindicated after antepartum haemorrhage or in the presence of toxaemia of pregnancy.

Adverse reactions

Potentially life-threatening effects
Salbutamol is generally well tolerated and serious toxic effects are few. Electrocardiographic evidence of myocardial ischaemia was reported in one apparently healthy pregnant woman after withdrawal of salbutamol infused for premature labour.[46]

Acute overdosage
Overdose of oral salbutamol with doses between 5 and 240 mg in 40 patients produced no fatalities.[50] The commonest symptoms were tremor, flushing, agitation and palpitations due to sinus tachycardia. Usually no specific treatment is necessary. Administration of a cardioselective β-sympathetic antagonist may be appropriate but is best avoided if the subject is asthmatic. A volume expanding agent may be given if the patient is hypotensive and in premature labour a loop diuretic should be given. Hypokalaemia can be expected and should be monitored and treated, if necessary. Occasionally patients have developed psychotic reactions while taking excessive doses of salbutamol.[51]

Severe or irreversible adverse effects
Ventricular ectopic beats have been reported during infusion of salbutamol in one pregnant women receiving the drug for treatment of premature labour.[47] An increase in ectopic activity during nebulized salbutamol in domiciliary use has been record in patients with COPD.[48] Angina accompanied by ECG changes was reported in three patients with ischaemic heart disease and either asthma or COPD during oxygen-driven nebulization in hospital.[49]

Symptomatic adverse effects
These are mainly predictable, dose-related and less likely with inhaled than with oral or parenteral treatment. They include tremor, anxiety, muscle cramps, headache and palpitations. Tolerance develops to many of these effects with regular treatment.

Interference with clinical pathology tests
No technical interferences of this kind have been reported.

High risk groups

Neonates
The drug is rarely indicated in the neonatal period.

Breast milk. Salbutamol probably enters breast milk, but the concentrations are unknown. However, no adverse effects have been reported in the breast-fed babies of mothers taking the drug by inhalation.

Children
Children may have difficulties using pressurized aerosols in which case syrup or nebulized solution is appropriate. Suitable oral doses for children under 7 years are:[52] syrup/tablets 2 mg three times daily; slow-release tablets 4 mg at night; respirator solution 1 mg four times daily.

Pregnant women
Although there is no evidence that salbutamol is teratogenic, it should be used in the first trimester only if absolutely essential. Its use in premature labour has been discussed earlier.

The elderly
Inability to use a pressurized aerosol is more common in the elderly and alternative inhalation devices, for example Rotacaps or spacers, may be needed. In older patients, oral or high-dose inhaled treatment may be more likely to provoke angina, cardiac arrhythmias or, in patients with prostatism, urinary retention.

Concurrent disease
Impaired renal or hepatic function. Significant renal or hepatic impairment is unlikely to modify the kinetics of the unchanged drug after an oral dose. No modification is necessary if the drug is given by inhalation.

Drug interactions

Potentially hazardous interactions
No interactions of this kind have been described.

Other significant interactions
Treatment with diuretics may augment the hypokalaemia that occurs with large doses of salbutamol. There are no other significant adverse interactions but the effects of salbutamol are inhibited by β-antagonists, especially those without $beta_1$-receptor selectivity.

Potentially useful interactions
The theoretical synergism of β-stimulants and theophylline as bron-

Salbutamol

chodilators is not borne out in practice where their effects are at best additive.

Major outcome trials

The short-term efficacy of salbutamol has precluded any long-term placebo-controlled studies in patients with symptomatic airways obstruction.

Evidence on β-receptor tolerance after chronic treatment has been conflicting: while tolerance is readily demonstrable in other tissues, there is no evidence for clinically significant tachyphylaxis of the airway response in asthmatic subjects taking regular oral or inhaled salbutamol.[18,20,54]

References

1. Warrell D A, Robertson D G, Newton Howes J et al 1970 Comparison of cardiorespiratory effects of isoprenaline and salbutamol in patients with bronchial asthma. British Medical Journal 65–70
2. Paterson J W, Courtenay Evans R J, Prime F J 1971 Selectivity of bronchodilator action of salbutamol in asthmatic patients. British Journal of Diseases of the Chest 65: 21–38
3. Church M K, Young K D 1983 The characteristics of inhibition of histamine release from human lung fragments by sodium cromoglycate, salbutamol and chlorpromazine. British Journal of Pharmacology 78: 671–679
4. Howarth P H, Durham S R, Lee T H, Kay B, Church M K, Holgate S T 1985 Influence of albuterol, cromolyn sodium and ipratropium bromide on the airway and circulating mediator responses to allergen bronchial provocation in asthma. American Review of Respiratory Disease 132: 986–992
5. Poynter D, Harris D M, Jack D 1978 Salbutamol: lack of evidence of tumour induction in man (letter). British Medical Journal 1: 46–47
6. Davis C, Conolly M E, Greenacre J K 1980 β Adrenoceptors in human lung, bronchus and lymphocytes. British Journal of Clinical Pharmacology 10: 425–432
7. Barnes P J, Pride N B 1983 Dose response curves to inhaled β adrenoceptor agonist in normal and asthmatic subjects. British Journal of Clinical Pharmacology 15: 677–682
8. Ruffin R E, Obminski G, Newhouse M T 1978 Aerosol salbutamol administration by IPPB: lowest effective dose. Thorax 33: 689–693
9. Corris P A, Neville E, Nariman S, Gibson G J 1983 Dose response study of inhaled salbutamol powder in chronic airflow obstruction. Thorax 38: 292–296
10. Lafortuna C L, Fazio F 1984 Acute effect of inhaled salbutamol on mucociliary clearance in health and chronic bronchitis. Respiration 45: 111–123
11. McDevitt D G, Wallace R J, Roberts A, Whitfield C R 1975 The uterine and cardiovascular effects of salbutamol and practolol during labour. British Journal of Obstetrics and Gynaecology 82: 442–448
12. Gibson D G, Coltart D J 1971 Haemodynamic effects of intravenous salbutamol in patients with mitral valve disease: comparison with isoprenaline and atropine. Postgraduate Medical Journal 47 (suppl): 40–44
13. Goldberg R, Van As M Joffe B I, Krut L, Bersohn I, Seftel H C 1975 Metabolic responses to selective β-adrenergic stimulation in man. Postgraduate Medical Journal 51: 53–58
14. Nogrady S G, Hartley J P R, Seaton A 1977 Metabolic effects of intravenous salbutamol in the course of acute severe asthma. Thorax 32: 559–562
15. Whyte K F, Addis G J, Whitesmith R, Reid J L 1987 The mechanism of salbutamol-induced hypokalaemia. British Journal of Clinical Pharmacology 23: 65–71
16. Holgate S T, Stubbs W A, Wood P, McCaughey E S, Alberti K G M M, Tattersfield A E 1980 Airway and metabolic resistance to intravenous salbutamol: a study in normal man. Clinical Science 59: 155–161
17. Harvey J E, Baldwin C J, Wood P J, Alberti K G M M, Tattersfield A E 1981 Airway and metabolic responsiveness to intravenous salbutamol in asthma: effect of regular inhaled salbutamol. Clinical Science 60: 579–585
18. Lipworth B J, Struthers A D, McDevitt D 1989 Tachyphylaxis to systemic but not to airway responses during prolonged therapy with high dose inhaled salbutamol in asthmatics. American Review of Respiratory Disease 140: 586–592
19. Davis C, Conolly M E 1980 Tachyphylaxis to β adrenoceptor agonists in human bronchial smooth muscle: studies in vitro. British Journal of Clinical Pharmacology 10: 417–423
20. Harvey J, Tattersfield A E 1982 Airway response to salbutamol: effect of regular salbutamol inhalations in normal, atopic and asthmatic subjects. Thorax 37: 280–287
21. Evans M E, Walker S R, Brittain R T, Paterson J W 1973 The metabolism of salbutamol in man. Xenobiotica 3: 113–120
22. Martin L E, Rees J, Tanner R J N 1976 Quantitative determination of salbutamol in plasma as either its trimethylsilyl or t-butyldimethylsilyl ether using a stable isotope multiple ion recording technique. Biomedical Mass Spectrometry 3: 184–190
23. Maconochie J G, Fowler P 1983 Plasma concentrations of salbutamol after an oral slow release preparation. Current Medical Research and Opinion 8: 634–639
24. Colthup P V, Dallas F A A, Saynor D A, Carey P F, Skidmore L F, Martin L E 1985 Determination of salbutamol in human plasma and urine by high performance thin-layer chromatography. Journal of Chromatography 345: 111–118
25. Loo J C K, Beaulieu N, Jordan N, Brian R, McGilveray I J 1987 A specific radio-immunoassay for salbutamol (albuterol) in human plasma. Research Communications in Chemical Pathology and Pharmacology 55: 283–286
26. Walker S R, Evans M E, Richards A J, Paterson J W 1972 The clinical pharmacology of oral and inhaled salbutamol. Clinical Pharmacology and Therapeutics 13: 861–867
27. Lin C, Li Y, McGlotten J et al 1977 Isolation and identification of the major metabolite of albuterol in human urine. Drug Metabolism and Disposition: The biological fate of chemicals 5: 234–238
28. Morgan D J, Paull J D, Richmond B H, Wilson-Evered E, Ziccone S P 1986 Pharmacokinetics of intravenous and oral salbutamol and its sulphate conjugate. British Journal of Clinical Pharmacology 22: 587–593
29. Lipworth B J, Clark B A, Dhillon D P, Charter M K, Palmer J B D, McDevitt D G 1989 Single dose and steady-state pharmacokinetics of 4 mg and 8 mg oral salbutamol controlled-release in patients with bronchial asthma. European Journal of Clinical Pharmacology 37: 49–52
30. Shenfield G M, Evans M E, Walker S R, Paterson J W 1973 The fate of nebulized salbutamol (albuterol) administered by intermittent positive pressure respiration to asthmatic patients. American Review of Respiratory Disease 108: 501–505
31. Shenfield G M, Evans M E, Paterson J W 1974 The effect of different nebulizers with and without intermittent positive pressure breathing on the absorption and metabolism of salbutamol. British Journal of Clinical Pharmacology 1: 295–300
32. Shenfield G M, Evans M E, Paterson J W 1976 Absorption of drugs by the lung. British Journal of Clinical Pharmacology 3: 583–589
33. Fairfax A J, McNabb W R, Davies H J, Spiro S G 1980 Slow release oral salbutamol and aminophylline in nocturnal asthma: relaxation of overnight changes in lung function and plasma drug levels. Thorax 35: 526–530
34. Martin L E, Hobson J C, Page J A, Harrison C 1971 Metabolic studies of salbutamol-^{3}H: a new bronchodilator, in rat, rabbit, dog and man. European Journal of Pharmacology 14: 183–199
35. Caccia S, Fong M H 1984 Kinetics and distribution of the beta-adrenergic agonist salbutamol in rat brain. Journal of Pharmacy and Pharmacology 36: 200–202
36. Nandakumaran M, Gardey C L, Challier J C, Richard M O, Panigel M, Olive G 1981 Transfer of salbutamol in the human placenta in vitro. Developmental Pharmacology and Therapeutics 3: 88–98
37. Arnold J D, Badcock N R, Pollard A C, Chapman M G 1979 Umbilical cord and maternal plasma salbutamol levels in two patients. Australian Paediatric Journal 15: 207
38. May C S, Paterson J W, Spiro S G, Johnson A J 1975 Intravenous infusion of salbutamol in the treatment of asthma. British Journal of Clinical Pharmacology 2: 503–508
39. Horn C R, Essex E, Hill P, Cochrane G M 1989 Does urinary salbutamol reflect compliance with the aerosol regimen in patients with asthma? Respiratory Medicine 83: 15–18
40. Hutchings M J, Paull J D, Wilson-Evered E, Morgan D J 1987 Pharmacokinetics and metabolism of salbutamol in premature labour. British Journal of Clinical Pharmacology 24: 69–75
41. Hartley J P R, Nogrady S G, Gibby O M, Seaton A 1977 Bronchodilator effects of dry salbutamol powder administered by rotahaler. British Journal of Clinical Pharmacology 4: 673–675
42. Lawford P, Jones B J M, Milledge J S 1978 Comparison of intravenous and nebulized salbutamol in initial treatment of severe asthma. British Medical Journal 1: 84
43. Hetzel M R, Clark T J H 1976 Comparison of intravenous and aerosol salbutamol. British Medical Journal 2: 919
44. Dawson A M, Davies H J 1977 The effect of intravenous and oral salbutamol on foetus and mother in premature labour. British Journal of Obstetrics and Gynaecology 84: 348–353
45. Sims C D, Chamberlain G V P, Boyd I E, Lewis P J 1978 A comparison of salbutamol and ethanol in the treatment of premature labour. British Journal of Obstetrics and Gynaecology 85: 761–766
46. Whitehead M I, Mander A M, Hartogs K, Rothman M T 1979 Myocardial ischaemia after withdrawal of salbutamol for pre-term labour. Lancet 2: 904
47. Chew W C, Lew L G 1979 Ventricular ectopics after salbutamol infusion for pre-term labour. Lancet 2: 1383–1384
48. Cookson W O C M, John S, McCarthy G, McCarthy S, Lane D J 1985 Nebuliser therapy and cardiac dysrhythmias in patients with COAD. Thorax 40: 704–705
49. Neville E, Corris P A, Vivian J, Nariman S, Gibson G J 1982 Nebulized salbutamol and angina. British Medical Journal 285: 796–797
50. Prior J G, Cochrane G M, Raper S M, Ali C, Volans G N 1981 Self-poisoning with oral salbutamol. British Medical Journal 282: 1932
51. Whitehouse A M, Novosel S 1989 Salbutamol psychosis. Biological Psychiatry 26: 631–633
52. Milner A D 1984 Bronchodilators in childhood asthma. In: Clark T J H, Cochrane G M (eds) Bronchodilator therapy. ADIS Press, Auckland, New Zealand, pp 93–111
53. Lipworth B J, McDevitt D G, Struthers A D 1989 Prior treatment with diuretic augments the hypokalaemic and electrocardiographic effects of inhaled salbutamol. American Journal of Medicine 86: 653–657
54. Tattersfield A E 1985 Tolerance to beta-agonists. Clinical Respiratory Physiology 21: 1S–5S

Salicylic acid

Salicylic acid is a much used component of topical medicaments which assists in desquamation (keratolytic) and in addition possesses some antimicrobial activity. It is also used for its ability to enhance percorneal penetration of other topically applied substances.

Chemistry

Salicylic acid
$C_7H_6O_3$
2-Hydroxybenzoic acid

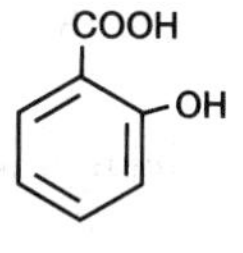

Molecular weight	138.1
pKa	3.0, 13.4
Solubility	
in alcohol	1 in 4
in water	1 in 550
Octanol/water partition coefficient	—

It is available in many combination preparations.

Pharmacology

Topical salicylic acid is keratolytic, bacteriostatic and fungistatic. Its main clinical use is as a keratolytic and as an agent that increases percutaneous absorption of combined drugs by removing the strateum corneum.[2] The keratolytic activity results from solubilisation of the intercellular ground substance in the stratum corneum and shedding of the scales which are bound by it.

Toxicology

Salicylic acid has a relatively low toxicity. Toxicity depends on the dose, oral doses of 150–300 $mg.kg^{-1}$ giving mild to moderate toxic reactions, 300–500 $mg.kg^{-1}$ giving serious toxic reactions and doses over 500 $mg.kg^{-1}$ being potentially fatal.[3] The LD_{50} for oral administration in rats is 890 $mg.kg^{-1}$.

No specific effects on the gastrointestinal tract, kidneys or liver have been reported with topical application.

Salicylates cross the placental barrier in rodents, rabbits, dogs and ferrets and are teratogenic when used at high doses. Teratogenicity in humans has not been proven.

Clinical pharmacology

Salicylic acid is a very effective keratolytic and, depending on the concentration used, is used for the treatment of warts and corns, for the treatment of dry skin problems such as ichthyosis and is used in combination creams to increase penetration of the other ingredients through normal or thickened skin.

At concentrations of 6%, salicylic acid significantly reduces the thickness of the stratum corneum and increases shedding of corneocytes in normal human skin.[4] In scaly skin conditions, such as ichthyosis, 3% salicylic acid in white soft paraffin or aqueous cream has been shown to be effective in reducing the scaling.

Salicylic acid applied topically to human skin has no effect on the underlying epidermis and no effect on the mitotic index of the epidermis. Salicylic acid is therefore not atrophogenic to the epidermis.[1,4] Topical salicylic acid has an antiinflammatory activity. In a UV induced dermatitis inhibition test,[5] 0.5% to 5% w/w salicylic acid showed antiinflammatory activity that was equivalent to 0.5% hydrocortisone. This antiinflammatory activity is not of therapeutic importance. Salicylic acid is bacteriostatic to various species of *Streptococcus*, *Staphylococcus*, *Escherischia coli* and *Pseudomonas aeroginosa*. It is also fungistatic to species of *Trichophyton* and *Candida*. These effects are seen at low concentrations (2–3 $g.l^{-1}$) which is considerably below the concentration found in most commercial preparations[6–7], 1 to 5% i.e. 10–50 $g.kg^{-1}$. When used in combination with topical corticosteroids, salicylic acid has been shown to increase the absorption of the corticosteroid through membranes, and clinical studies have shown the increased efficacy of combination creams compared with the corticosteroid cream alone.

Pharmacokinetics

Salicylic acid is absorbed percutaneously with maximal plasma levels achieved after 6–12 hours.[8] In man, 65–85% of the administered dose is absorbed. The rate of absorption of salicylic acid depends on the level of hydration of the skin, the frequency of application of the preparation and the presence of occlusion. Absorption of the drug should theoretically be higher in diseased skin as diseased epidermis is a poor barrier to the passage of topically applied substances. In adults, 1 g of a topical 6% salicylic acid preparation (i.e. 60 mg of salicylic acid) increases the serum salicylate level by not more than 5 $mg.l^{-1}$ of plasma.[9]

Following percutaneous absorption, salicylic acid is distributed in the extracellular space, 58% is protein bound to albumin and as such, free salicylate levels will be increased in hypoalbuminaemia and salicylates may compete for albumin binding sites with other drugs and modify their activity.

Concentration–effect relationship

Therapeutic effect depends on the local concentration of the salicylic acid not on the systemic absorption of the drug.

Metabolism

Salicylates are metabolized in the liver by microsomal enzymes and either conjugated with UDP-glucuronic acid to form phenyl or acyl glucuronides or hydroxylated into gentisic acid. In the liver and kidneys, the carboxyl groups are conjugated in the mitochondria to form salicylates or gentisurates (see Sodium salicylate).

65–85% of topically administered salicylates are recoverable from the urine, 52% of which are in the form of salicyluric acid, 42% as phenolic glucuronides of salicylic acid and the rest as salicylic acid. Of a single dose 95% is excreted within 24 hours of its entry into the extracellular space.[9]

Pharmaceutics

1. Cuplex (Smith & Nephew, UK): salicylic acid 11% w/w, lactic acid 4% w/w and copper acetate in the viscous gel.
2. Salactol (Dermal Laboratories, UK): salicylic acid 16.7% w/w lactic acid 16.7% w/w in collodion.
3. Salatac gel (Dermal Laboratories, UK): salicylic acid 12% w/w lactic acid 4% w/w in a clear viscid gel.
4. Duofilm (Stiefel Laboratories, UK): salicylic acid 16.7%, lactic acid 16.7% in flexible collodion.
5. Salicylic acid adhesive plasters 20% or 40%.
6. Salicylic acid collodion. Salicylic acid 12% in flexible collodion.
7. Verrugon (Pickles & Son, UK): salicylic acid 50% in a paraffin base.
8. Salicylic acid ointment. Salicylic acid 2% in wool alcohol ointment.
9. Zinc and salicylic acid paste (Lassar's paste): zinc oxide 24% salicylic acid 2%, starch 24% in white soft paraffin.

Combination creams are also available.

Salicylic acid preparations should be stored in a cool place. Many of the preparations are flammable and should not be placed near naked flames.

Therapeutic use

Indications

1. Treatment of warts and corns
2. Treatment of scaly skin conditions such as psoriasis and ichthyosis
3. Treatment of hyperkeratotic eczema.

Contraindications

1. Sensitivity to salicylic acid
2. Neonates
3. Use in pregnant and breast-feeding women.

Mode of use

In the treatment of warts and corns, the lesion should be pared down with a foot file or pumice stone and the paint or ointment should be carefully applied, avoiding contact with normal skin. If an ointment is being used, surrounding skin can be protected with a prior application of petroleum jelly. The preparations should be applied daily.

In the treatment of dry and scaly skin conditions, concentrations of 0.5 to 6% salicylic acid are usually employed. The creams are best applied to maximally hydrated skin and are thus recommended for use after a bath. Creams can be used twice daily, used sparingly and rubbed well into the skin.

Indications

1. Warts and corns

The most widespread use of salicylic acid as a topical preparation is for the treatment of warts and corns. This makes use of the keratolytic activity of the drug. The mode of action is unclear but it has been suggested that it affects the adhesive bonds between corneocytes. For warts and corns it is usually used in concentrations in excess of 12% and is often formulated in paints, flexible quick-drying films or in adhesive plasters. Salicylic acid preparations compare very favourably with other local destructive methods in the treatment of viral warts with cure rates of 65–70%.[10]

2. Scaly skin conditions

Salicylic acid used as a cream of 0.5 to 6% is an effective treatment of ichthyosis, particularly of the less severe ichthyosis vulgaris and X-linked ichthyosis. In psoriasis and hyperkeratotic eczema, salicylic acid appears to enhance desquamation and removes abnormal scale, and is also used in combination creams with dithranol, tar and corticosteroids to enhance penetration of the active drug.

Contraindications

Salicylic acid is contraindicated in those who are known to be sensitive to the drug. Salicylic acid is teratogenic in animal models, and although this has not been demonstrated in man, it is not advised to use the drug in pregnancy. Salicylic acid should not be used in neonates and young children, and because of passage in milk, should not be used by breast-feeding women.

Adverse reactions

Potentially life-threatening effects

Salicylate intoxication[11–16] and death[12,16] has resulted from the topical use of salicylic acid and methyl salicylate. Large doses need to be applied to induce toxic reactions but certain factors increase this risk. These are the age of the patient (the risk is higher in young children due to the high relative surface area in childhood); amount applied (absorption depends on the dose applied); frequency of application and presence of occlusion, either natural in skin folds or as occlusive dressings.

Salicylate toxicity from topical application gives clinical symptoms of thirst, tinnitus, headache, lethargy, confusion, vomiting, depression and disorientation. In one reported case, a patient died 28 hours after treating 50% of his body surface with 20% salicylic acid alcoholic lotion.[16]

Acute overdosage

The effects are described above. Treatment is described fully in the Aspirin monograph.

Severe or irreversible adverse effects

Severe systemic toxicity results in central excitation manifest as irritability, restlessness, incoherent speech, excitement, hallucinations, delusions, delirium and mania. Respiratory depression and metabolic acidosis may occur and more severe toxicity may be followed by stupor and coma.[17] Allergic responses to salicylic acid may occur, including urticaria, anaphylaxis and erythema multiforme.

Symptomatic adverse effects

When used at high concentration, local irritation or inflammation may occur. This may happen during the treatment of warts or corns. Often a hyperkeratotic arm becomes sodden and appears white. When treatment is stopped the condition rapidly resolves. Contact allergic dermatitis may occur.[18] Systemic absorption may result in tinnitus, nausea, thirst, sweating, hypernoea, fatigue, fever and confusion.

Interference with clinical pathology tests

When applied locally in normal amounts the drug is unlikely to interfere with such tests (but see Aspirin).

High risk groups

Neonates

The drug should not be used in neonates.

Breast milk. The drug appears in breast milk, and mothers applying large quantities topically should not breast-feed.

Children

Salicylic acid may be used in children in appropriate doses.

Pregnant women

There has been conflicting evidence on whether or not salicylates are teratogenic; but when used late in pregnancy they may cause haemorrhage in the newborn. Consequently, topical application of large amounts during pregnancy is best avoided.

The elderly

No special precautions are necessary in elderly patients.

Drug interactions

Potentially hazardous interactions

Topical salicylic acid may be absorbed and cause adverse interactions with a number of drugs. Toxicity of some drugs may be increased — acetazolamide, anticoagulants, dipyridamole, heparin, hypoglycaemics, methotrexate, moxalactam. The efficacy of some drugs may be decreased — bumetanide, captopril and probenecid.

Potentially useful interactions

The keratolytic activity of salicylic acid is used to potentiate the effect of certain topical drugs by increasing the penetration of the drug into the skin. Topical corticosteroids and dithranol and tar are available in combination with salicylic acid, with clinical increase efficacy.

Clinical trials

1. Bart B J, Biglow J, Corwin Vance J et al 1989 Salicylic acid in Karaya gum patches as a treatment for verruca vulgaris. Journal of the American Academy of Dermatology 20: 74–76

In this trial, 61 healthy volunteers with warts on the hands of less than one year's duration were entered into a double-blind randomized study to compare 15% salicylic acid in medicated patches with the patches alone. The control group showed a high cure rate of 28% which was attributed to natural resolution. The active treatment gave a significantly higher cure rate of 69% ($p<0.01$). This study shows that 15% salicylic acid in a Karaya gum patch was a safe and effective treatment of verruca vulgaris.

2. Steele K, Shirodaria P, O'Hare M et al 1988 Monochloracetic acid and 60% salicylic acid as a treatment for simple plantar warts: effectiveness and mode of action. British Journal of Dermatology 118: 537–544

This double-blind study compared the efficacy of monochloracetic acid crystals and 60% salicylic acid ointment with sodium sulphate crystals as a control in 57 patients with simple plantar warts.

After 6 weeks treatment 18% of the placebo-treated patients had responded with clearing of the warts. In the active treatment group, a significantly higher response rate was observed, 66% ($p=0.002$). This study shows the efficacy of the salicylic acid and monochloracetic acid crystals in treating plantar warts.

3. Elie R, Durocher L P, Kavalec E C 1983 Effect of salicylic acid on the activity of betamethasone-17,21-dipropionate in the treatment of erythematous squamous dermatoses. Journal of International Medical Research 11: 108–112

40 adult with scaly scalp disorders (psoriasis, seborrhoeic dermatitis or neurodermatitis) were entered into a double-blind study comparing four treatment regimes — 2% salicylic acid in alcoholic lotion, 0.05% betamethasone-17,21-diproprionate plus 2% salicylic acid, 0.05% betamethasone-17,21-diproprionate alone, and vehicle. The results showed that the salicylic acid potentiated the effectiveness of the topical steroid with better responses to the combination than to either active treatments alone or to the vehicle.

References

1. Davies M, Marks R 1976 Studies on the effects of salicylic acid on normal skin. British Journal of Dermatology 95: 187–192
2. Fridricksson T 1976 Studies with betamethasone diproprionate plus salicylic acid (Diprosalic) in psoriasis. Pharmatherapeutica 1: 277–285
3. Temple A R 1981 Acute and chronic effects of aspirin toxicity and their treatment. Archives of Internal Medicine 141: 366–370
4. Roberts D L, Marshall R, Marks R 1980 Detection of the action of salicylic acid on the normal stratum corneum. British Journal of Dermatology 103: 191–196
5. Weirich E G, Longauer J F, Kirkwood A H 1976 Dermatopharmacology of salicylic acid. III. Topical contra-inflammatory effects of salicylic acid and other drugs in animal experiments. Dermatologica 152: 87–99
6. Angelillo B, Boccia A 1977 Betamethasone diproprionate ointment with salicylic acid: a report of antibacterial and anti-fungal activity. Pharmatherapeutica 1: 434–438
7. Rainsford K D 1984 In: Aspirin and the salicylates. Butterworths
8. Miller R L, Insel P A, Melmon K L 1978 Drugs used in inflammatory disorders. In: Melmon K L, Morrelli H F (eds) Clinical pharmacology
9. Robertson D M, Maibach H I 1987 Dermatological pharmacology. In: Katzung B G (ed) Basic and clinical pharmacology. Lange
10. Bunney M H, Nolan M W, Williams D A 1976 An assessment of methods of treating viral warts by comparative treatment trials based on standard design. British Journal of Dermatology 94: 667–679
11. Shupp D Y, Schroeter A L 1986 An unusual case of salicylate toxicity. Journal of the American Academy of Dermatology 15: 300–301
12. von Weiss J F, Lever W F 1964 Percutaneous salicylic acid intoxication in psoriasis. Archives of Dermatology 90: 614–619
13. Cawley E P, Peterson N T, Wheeler C E et al 1953 Salicylic acid poisoning in dermatological therapy. Journal of the American Academic Association 151: 372–374
14. Davies M G, Vella Briffa D, Greaves M W 1979 Systemic toxicity from topically applied salicylic acid. British Medical Journal 1: 661
15. Aspinall J B, Goel K M 1978 Salicylate poisoning in dermatological therapy. British Medical Journal 2: 1373
16. Lindsey C P 1968 Two cases of fatal salicylate poisoning after topical application of an anti-fungal solution. Medical Journal of Australia 1: 353–354
17. de Groot A C, Nater J P 1988 Dermatological drugs and cosmetics. In: Meyler's side effects of drugs, 11th edn
18. Rasmussen J E, Fisher A A 1976 Contact allergic dermatitis to a salicylic acid plaster. Contact Dermatology 2: 237–238

Selegiline (hydrochloride)

Selegiline — also known as deprenyl — was the first selective inhibitor of B-type MAO and is still the only one in therapeutic use.

Chemistry

Selegiline hydrochloride (l-deprenyl) (Jumex, Eldepryl, Movergan)

$C_{13}H_{17}N.HCl$

(R) (-)-N,α-Dimethyl-N-(2-prop-2-inyl)-phenethylamine hydrochloride

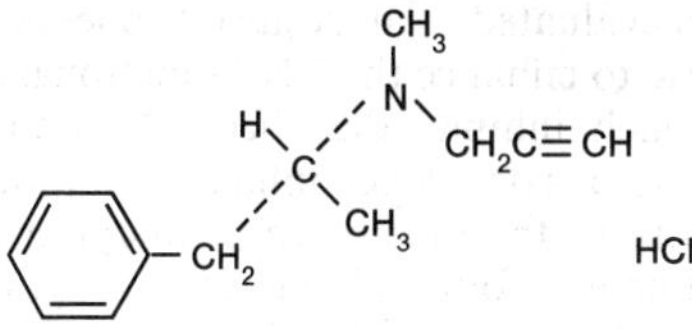

Molecular weight (free base)	223.7 (187.3)
pKa (>N–)	6.88
Solubility	
in alcohol	1 in 3
in water	1 in 3
Octanol/water partition coefficient	low

A white odourless crystalline powder, with a slightly bitter taste, it is prepared by chemical synthesis and the l-isomer is used clinically. It is not available in any combination preparations.

Pharmacology

Selegiline has the following properties:

1. It is a highly potent, selective irreversible inhibitor of the monoamine oxidase (MAO) (EC 1.4.3.4) type B enzyme.[1] MAO, a spherical protein widely distributed in the brain and peripheral tissues, is bound to the outer mitochondrial membrane and exists in two forms: MAO-A, which preferentially deaminates serotonin, is localized in the brain, mainly within the neurones, and is selectively inhibited by clorgyline; and MAO-B, which preferentially deaminates phenylethylamine (PEA), is mainly localized in the neuroglia and is selectively inhibited by selegiline.
2. Inhibits the uptake of tyramine, noradrenaline and dopamine into the catecholaminergic nerve endings, an effect which is reversible and independent of MAO-B inhibition.
3. Increases the turnover rate of dopamine and facilitates the release of dopamine in the rat striatum, with no substantial effect on the postsynaptic dopaminergic receptor.
4. Prevents the neurotoxic effect of 6-hydroxydopamine on the striatum.
5. Prevents the selective neurotoxicity of 1-methyl-4-phenyl-1,2,5,6-tetrahydropyridine (MPTP) (causing parkinsonism in man and parkinson-like symptoms in animals) on the nigrostriatal dopaminergic system.
6. Enhances superoxide dismutase activity in the striatum, an effect independent of MAO-B inhibition.

Toxicology

Selegiline does not have mutagenic potential, and toxicological testing in animals failed to demonstrate any results of potential clinical relevance to selegiline treatment, or the selegiline–levodopa combination. There is no evidence of teratological effects in rats and rabbits.

Clinical pharmacology

Selective inhibition of the MAO-B activity has been demonstrated with therapeutic doses of selegiline in man.

Two hours after the oral administration of 10 mg selegiline, platelet MAO activity (type B enzyme) is almost completely inhibited and this inhibition is maintained for up to 8 h. When the MAO-B inhibition approaches 90% a substantial, 30 to 90-fold increase of urinary phenylethylamine (PEA, the preferential substrate of the B enzyme) output occurs. The increased PEA output returns to normal within a few days of stopping the drug. Platelet enzyme activity rises to pretreatment levels after a period of approximately 3 weeks. The recovery of platelet MAO activity is linear at a rate of approximately 10% per day. Selegiline inhibits human platelet MAO activity at concentrations approximately 500-fold less than those required for inhibition by clorgyline, a selective MAO-A inhibitor, in vitro.

The selective inhibitor of brain MAO-B by selegiline has also been demonstrated. In man, dopamine is primarily metabolized by the B form of MAO,[2] which is selectively inhibited by selegiline.

The selective inhibition of MAO-B in the human caudate was estimated to give a 63% decrease in total dopamine oxidation.[3]

Selegiline, the first MAO inhibitor which could be given concurrently with levodopa without provoking a dangerous hypertensive reaction, has been evaluated as an adjuvant to levodopa treatment of Parkinson's disease to enhance the CNS functional stores of dopamine. Selegiline, which inhibits the effect of tyramine on vascular smooth muscle,[4] is a safe MAO inhibitor without provoking an enhanced sensitivity to the pressor effect of tyramine, an indirectly acting sympathomimetic found abundantly in the diet. This 'cheese effect' is the most dangerous side effect of commonly used MAO inhibitors.[5]

Selegiline applied in the usual, recommended doses induces little or no change in sensitivity to the pressor effect of tyramine in man.[6–8]

Pharmacokinetics

Selegiline is assayed by HPLC with a limit of sensitivity of 10 μg.l^{-1}. Selegiline is rapidly ($t_{\frac{1}{2}}$ of absorption 0.39 h) and completely absorbed after oral administration in fasting patients. Food does not appear to affect the bioavailability of the drug. Peak plasma concentrations of the drug, from 37 to 45 μg.l^{-1}, are achieved at between 0.5 and 2 h.[9]

The decline in plasma concentrations of ^{14}C labelled material are best described by a two compartment open model.

The drug is rapidly distributed throughout the body, the volume of distribution of the central compartment being high, at 137 l. The volume of distribution at steady state is 4.7 l.kg^{-1}, indicating accumulation of drug or its metabolites in some tissues. Selegiline is highly bound (94%) to plasma proteins.

It is not known whether selegiline is excreted in breast milk or whether it is subject to placental transfer.

Selegiline is extensively metabolized, most likely in the liver. An average of 52% of the dose (40 to 66%) is excreted in urine in 24 hours and 73% (59 to 86%) in 72 hours, mostly as metabolites. Only 15% (3-26%) of the dose is excreted in faeces.

The half life of the β-phase, which is considered the biological half life of the drug and metabolites is 39 hours. The plasma clearance is 1.7 ml.min^{-1}.kg^{-1}.

The elimination of the drug is unlikely to be affected by renal dysfunction or old age.

Oral absorption	100%
Presystemic metabolism	—
Plasma half life	
range	16–69 h
mean	39 h
Volume of distribution	4.7 l.kg^{-1}
Plasma protein binding	94%

Concentration–effect relationship

Selegiline administered in the usual therapeutic dose of 5–10 mg per day produces a selective maximal inhibition of the MAO-B enzyme in different tissues. Treatment with substantially higher doses (30 and 60 mg per day) for periods of 3 weeks or longer results in a significant decrease of the deaminated noradrenaline metabolite MHPG indicating the inhibition of the type A enzyme as well. Therapeutic trials with selegiline as an adjuvant to levodopa observed no more benefit for the parkinsonian patients by increasing the selegiline dose above 10 mg per day.

Metabolism

Selegiline is extensively metabolized in the body with little of the unchanged drug excreted (Fig. 1). Approximately 75% of the dose is excreted in the urine and 15% in the faeces. Urinary excretion of the metabolites is increased at acid pH.

The primary route of metabolism is oxidative dealkylation and 7 metabolites have been identified in the plasma and urine. The main metabolites are desmethylselegiline, l-metamphetamine, l-amphetamine.

Although the amphetamine metabolites are pharmacologically active do not contribute to the therapeutic benefit conferred by selegiline.[10]

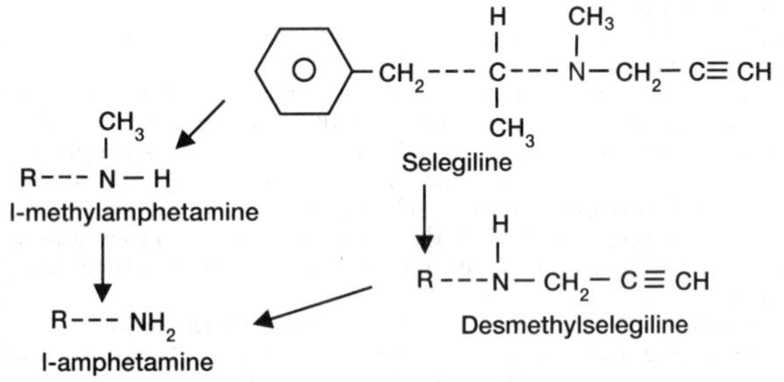

Pharmaceutics

Selegiline is available in oral form.

Jumex (Chinoin, Hungary) tablets contain 5 mg selegiline hydrochloride. The tablets are almost white, round shaped, flat, rimmed with impressed 'JU' letters on one face, the other face being smooth, diameter 7 mm, height 2.8–3.2 mm, average weight 150 mg.

Eldepryl (Britannia, UK) tablets contain 5 mg selegiline hydrochloride. Presentation: white, scored, uncoated tablets of 6 mm diameter.

Movergan (Asta Pharm, FRG) tablets contain 5 mg selegiline hydrochloride. Presentation: white, scored, uncoated tablets, 6 mm diameter.

All preparations should be protected from heat, moisture and light.

Selegiline preparations are stable with a five year shelf-life and carry a minimal risk from potentially allergenic substances.

Therapeutic use

Indications

1. The adjunctive management of Parkinson's disease
2. The control of some forms of 'on-off' response fluctuations.

Contraindications

1. Extrapyramidal movement disorders which are associated with increased dopaminergic receptor sensitivity, or neurotransmitter function in the brain, like tardive dyskinesia, adult-onset Huntington's disease, etc.
2. Levodopa pyschosis.

Mode of use

The initial dose of selegiline is one tablet (5 mg) in the morning. Since selegiline is an adjuvant to levodopa replacement therapy it should be administered concurrently with levodopa, or levodopa and peripheral decarboxylase inhibitor treatment.

When added to established levodopa therapy, if the known side effects of levodopa develop then the dose of levodopa should be reduced. Usually, it is possible to reduce the levodopa dosage when selegiline is added to the regimen. If the symptoms of levodopa failure are severe, or little therapeutic benefit is achieved with one tablet (5 mg) selegiline, the dose of selegiline can be increased to 10 mg (two tablets) in the morning.

Indications

1. The adjunctive management of Parkinson's disease
Selegiline is widely used in the adjunctive management of Parkinson's disease, or symptomatic parkinsonism treated with levodopa, or levodopa and peripheral decarboxylase (l-aromatic amino acid decarboxylase) inhibitor (PDI), like carbidopa and benserazide.

The conclusion from clinical trials is that selegiline as a primary adjuvant to levodopa or levodopa and peripheral decarboxylase inhibitor, is a safe MAO inhibitor, it can be administered without dietary restrictions and there is no risk of a hypertensive crisis, i.e. 'cheese effect' arising from food–drug interaction.

Selegiline in conjunction with levodopa-containing medication is effective in alleviating primarily akinesia and rigidity, leaving tremor the least affected.

Overall disability improves on selegiline treatment, while in general a dose reduction of 0–30% is possible, or necessary. Selegiline also prolongs the duration, and enhances the therapeutic effect, of a single dose of levodopa, or levodopa-containing medication, which may result in an effective levodopa sparing. Selegiline is effective in the early as well as the late phase of Parkinson's disease.

2. The control of some forms of 'on-off' fluctuations
Selegiline has been shown to provide therapeutic benefit in the control of primarily dose-related 'on-off' response fluctuation, particularly wearing-off, end-of-dose deterioration, nocturnal and early morning akinesia and other periods of apparent refractoriness to levodopa containing medication in the late phase of Parkinson's disease and late levodopa treatment syndrome.[11–16]

Since the drug prolongs and enhances the therapeutic effect of levodopa, the 'on' periods are longer and the 'off' periods are shorter on combined selegiline adjuvant treatment with an obvious tendency to decrease the frequency of 'on-off' switches.[14]

Some of the patients who gradually lose therapeutic benefit on maximally tolerated doses of levodopa could recoup at least part of this loss while on combination with selegiline.[12]

The favourable smoothing of response fluctuations is usually maintained for years in the late levodopa treatment syndrome.

Hyperkinetic type 'on-off' symptoms, non-dose related, random oscillations (apart from sporadic observations[34]) are usually not improved by the addition of selegiline to the levodopa regimen.

Adverse reactions

Potentially life-threatening effects
Death, or fatal idiosyncrasy to selegiline; selegiline–levodopa; or selegiline, levodopa and peripheral decarboxylase inhibitor combination have not been reported.

Acute overdosage
Cases of deliberate overdose with death, or serious clinical consequences have not been reported.

In animal experiments selegiline has a remarkably wide safety margin, the LD_{50} in a number of species is approximately 300 to 500-fold higher than that required for complete, selective MAO-B inhibition.[17] A therapeutic trial in depressed patients[18] using up to 60 mg selegiline daily for at least 3 weeks did not reveal intolerance.

Severe or irreversible adverse effects
No severe complications of selegiline treatment have been reported.

Symptomatic adverse effects
Selegiline is generally well tolerated. When an optimal levodopa dose has been established, the adverse effects of treatment with selegiline–levodopa, or selegiline and levodopa plus peripheral decarboxylase inhibitor combination, are usually less frequent and severe than with levodopa alone.[19,20] This finding can be interpreted on the basis of the recognized levodopa-sparing property of selegiline. In general the adverse reactions observed during concurrent treatment with levodopa-containing medication are consistent with an overdosage of levodopa.

Hypertension following ingestion of tyramine-containing foods or drinks has not been observed after the usual 5 to 10 mg per day of selegiline.

Selegiline (hydrochloride)

Other effects

No clinically significant alterations in the laboratory values including haematology, liver and renal function tests, blood chemistry, serum electrolytes and urinalysis have been associated with selegiline treatment.

Interference with clinical pathology tests
No interference of this kind has been reported.

High risk groups

Neonates
Selegiline is neither indicated nor recommended for neonates.

Breast milk. Safety of the drug during breast-feeding has not been established.

Children
What has been said about neonates applies also to older children.

Pregnant women
Safety of selegiline for use during pregnancy has not been established.

The elderly
No special precautions are required in this age group.

Drug interactions

Potentially hazardous interactions
Tyramine. Treatment with selegiline (in a dose of 60 mg per day), which is six to twelve times higher than the usual therapeutic dose and no more selective in inhibiting B type MAO, was shown to potentiate the tyramine pressor response.[18]

Other significant interactions
Opiates. Selegiline in selective doses has been shown to potentiate the opiate-induced analgesia in rats.[21] The clinical relevance of this finding has not been established.

Phenothiazines and butyrophenones. These drugs block striatal dopamine receptors and agonize the effects of levodopa and the adjuvant effect of selegiline, thus aggravating parkinsonism.

2-Methyl-paratyrosine. This compound, a competitive inhibitor of tyrosine hydroxylase, will decrease dopamine production and can be expected to antagonize selegiline action.

Reserpine and tetrabenazine. These drugs can be expected to interfere with the effects of levodopa and the adjuvant selegiline.

Amantadine and centrally acting cholinergics. Such compounds increase the anti-parkinsonian action of levodopa and adjuvant selegiline, due to a pharmacodynamic interaction.

Major outcome trials

1. Birkmayer W, Knoll J, Riederer P, Youdim M B H, Vera Hars, Marton J 1985 Increased life expectancy resulting from addition of l-deprenyl to Madopar treatment in Parkinson's disease: a long term-study. Journal of Neural Transmission 64: 113–127

This is a retrospective study over a period of 15 years of a total of 941 patients of which 377 were treated with Madopar (the 4 to 1 combination of l-dopa and benserazide), while 564 were treated with selegiline plus Madopar combination. The daily dose of selegiline was 5 or 10 mg and all patients were monitored at regular visits one to four times a year, when the Madopar dosage was adjusted according to the patient's needs assessed by the rating of disability. The average length of selegiline treatment was about 4 years.

A better control of disability was achieved in selegiline treated patients than in the Madopar group without selegiline. Selegiline was well tolerated with low incidence and severity of side effects.

Survival analysis of the data revealed that the life expectancy of the selegiline-Madopar treated group was significantly longer than that of the Madopar treated group. The authors conclude, that selegiline is a useful and important adjuvant to levodopa substitution and its use is indicated in the early as well as long term treatment of Parkinson's disease.

S

2. Yahr M D, Mendoza M R, Moros D, Bergmann K H 1983 Treatment of Parkinson's disease in early and late phases. Use of pharmacological agents with special reference to deprenyl (selegiline). Acta Neurologica Scandinavica (suppl) 93: 95–102

This is a retrospective study over a period of 6 years of 79 selected patients. The patients were in the late, decompensated phase of parkinsonism which comes after 3–5 years when the therapeutic response diminishes and more of the complications due to the use of levodopa begin to occur. All patients were receiving optimal doses of levodopa to which selegiline 5 mg twice daily was added. During selegiline administration it was possible to decrease the levodopa dose by 25–30%. Many of the side effects diminished when the levodopa dose was reduced. The authors concluded that the major usefulness of selegiline has been demonstrated in patients under treatment with levodopa which has become complicated by fluctuating responses, particularly those of the end-start-dose variety. In such patients, it is possible to achieve an increase in 'on' time and a decrease in the severity of parkinsonism. In most patients, such a response can be maintained for a period of two years or longer.

Randomized, controlled trials

3. The Parkinson Study Group 1989 Effect of deprenyl on the progression of disability in early Parkinson's disease. New England Journal of Medicine 321: 1364–1371

Eight hundred patients were admitted to a study with a factorial design involving use of placebo, tocopherol or deprenyl. The end point was the onset of sufficient disability to require use of levodopa. During an average of 12 months of follow-up, 97 patients on deprenyl reached this end point against 176 patients not receiving deprenyl. The difference was very highly significant statistically. The patients who received deprenyl also had a significant reduction of the risk of having to give up full time employment. The authors conclude that their findings support the prescription of deprenyl 10 mg daily to otherwise untreated patients who are in the early stages of Parkinson's disease.

4. Presthus J, Hajba A 1983 Deprenyl (selegiline) combined with levodopa and a decarboxylase inhibitor in the treatment of Parkinson's disease. Acta Neurologica Scandinavica (suppl) 95: 127–133

This is a short-term, double-blind, randomized trial comparing two parallel groups (selegiline vs placebo control) with stepwise dose escalation of the adjuvant (5 and 10 mg per day) over two subsequent 4–week treatment periods together with a symptom limited dose reduction of levodopa containing medication, involving 40 parkinsonian patients. Only patients with a minimum of 3 (on average 9–10) years of history have been selected and most of them (36) were presenting with 'on-off' symptoms.

Disability was unchanged in the placebo but significantly decreased in the selegiline treated group. There was an overall positive change of 'on-off' symptoms during the study period.

5. Tetrud J W, Langston J W 1989 The effect of deprenyl (Selegiline) on the natural history of Parkinson's disease. Science 245: 519–522

Fifty-four patients were randomly assigned to deprenyl (10 mg/day) or placebo treatment groups and followed until levodopa therapy was indicated or until the patient had been in the study for 3 years. Analysis of Kaplan-Meier survival curves for each group showed that deprenyl delayed the need for levodopa therapy; the average time until levodopa was needed was 312.1 days for patients in the placebo group and 548.9 days for patients in the deprenyl group. Disease progression, as monitored by five different assessment scales, was slowed (by 40 to 83% per year) in the deprenyl group compared to placebo. Therefore, early deprenyl therapy delays the requirement for antiparkinsonian medication, possibly by slowing progression of the disease.

Other trials

Csanda E, Antal J, Antony M, Csanaky M 1978 Experience with l-deprenyl in Parkinsonism. Journal of Neural Transmission 43: 263–269

This is a report of an uncontrolled trial of selegiline treatment of 152 parkinsonian patients for a minimum of one year conducted at three clinics. The mean age of the patients was 64 years and 114 of them had a history of more than 5 years and only 16 with a history of less than one year.

Treatment with selegiline dose of 2.5 to 5 mg per day in addition to levodopa brought about a clinical improvement of the motor performance in about two thirds of the patients. The levodopa dose could be reduced by 30%.

General review articles

Knoll J 1976 Analysis of the pharmacological effects of selective monoamine oxidase inhibitors. In: Wolstenholme G E W, Knight J (eds) Monoamine oxidase and its inhibition. Ciba Foundation symposium 39 (new series). Elsevier-Excerpta Medica North-Holland, Amsterdam, ch 7, pp 135–161

Editorial 1982 Deprenyl in Parkinson's disease. Lancet 2: 695–696

Knoll J 1983 Deprenyl (selegiline): the history of its development and pharmacological action. Acta Neurologica Scandinavica (suppl) 95: 57–80

Birkmayer W, Riderer P 1983 Parkinson's disease. Biochemistry, clinical pharmacology and treatment. Springer–Verlag, Wien, p 194

Knoll J 1986 Role of monoamine oxidase inhibitors in the treatment of Parkinson's disease: an update. In: Donald A G, Shah N S (eds) Movement disorders. Plenum Press, New York, ch 2, pp 53–80

Knoll J 1987 R-Deprenyl (Selegiline, Movergan) facilitates the activity of the nigrostriatal dopaminergic neuron. Journal of Neural Transmission (suppl) 25: 45–66

Riederer P, Prunztek H (eds) 1987 MAO-B-inhibitor selegiline (R(-)Deprenyl). A new therapeutic concept in the treatment of Parkinson's disease. Proceedings of the International Symposium in Berlin, January 23–25, 1987. Journal of Neural Transmission (suppl) 25, Springer-Verlag, Wien

Knoll J 1988 The striatal dopamine dependency of life span in male rats. Longevity study with (-)deprenyl. Mechanism of Ageing and Development 46: 237–262

References

1. Knoll J, Magyar K 1972 Some puzzling effects of monoamine oxidase inhibitors. Advances in Biochemical Psychopharmacology 5: 393–408
2. Glover V, Sandler M, Owen F, Riley G J 1977 Dopamine is a monoamine B substrate in man. Nature 265: 80–81
3. Oreland L, Arai Y, Senstrom A 1983 The effect of deprenyl (selegiline) on intra- and extraneuronal dopamine oxidation. Acta Neurologica Scandinavica (suppl) 95: 81–85
4. Knoll J, Vizi E S, Somogyi G 1968 Phenylisopropylmethylpropinylamine (E-250), a monoamine oxidase inhibitor antagonizing effects of tyramine. Arzneimittel Forschung 18: 109–112
5. Blackwell B 1963 Hypertensive crisis due to monoamine oxidase inhibitors. Lancet 2: 849–851
6. Elsworth J D, Glover V, Reynolds G P et al 1978 Deprenyl administration in man: a selective monoamine oxidase B inhibitor without the 'cheese effect'. Psychopharmacology 57: 33–38
7. Stern G M, Lees A J, Sandler M 1978 Recent observations on the clinical pharmacology of (-)deprenyl. Journal of Neural Transmission 43: 245–251
8. Pickar D, Cohen R M, Jimerson D C, Murphy D L 1981 Tyramine infusions and selective monoamine oxidase inhibitor treatment. I. Changes in pressor sensitivity. Psychopharmacology 74: 4–7
9. Benakis A 1981 Pharmacokinetic study in man of ^{14}C-Jumex. Report from the Laboratoire du metabolisme des medicaments, de l'Universite de Geneve Department de Pharmacologie
10. Elsworth J D, Sandler M, Lees A J, Ward C, Stern G M 1982 The contribution of amphetamine metabolites to its antiparkinsonian properties. Journal of Neural Transmission 54: 105–110
10. Rinne U K, Siirtole T, Sonninen V 1978 L-deprenyl treatment of on-off phenomena in Parkinson's disease. Journal of Neural Transmission 43: 253–262
11. Yahr M D 1978 Overview of present day treatment of Parkinson's disease. Journal of Neural Transmission 43: 227–238
12. Lader C M, Lees A J, Stern G M 1979 Oscillations in performance in levodopa-treated parkinsonians: treatment with bromocriptine and l-deprenyl. Clinical and Experimental Neurology 6: 197–203
13. Goldstein L 1980 The 'on-off' phenomena in Parkinson's disease – treatment and theoretical considerations. Mount Sinai Journal of Medicine 47: 80–84
14. Antony M, Toth G, Szëplaki Z 1982 Klinikopharmakologische Erprobung der Arzneimittelkombination Jumex + Depaflex in der Dauertherapie des Parkinson-Syndromes. Therapia Hungarica 30: 185–189
15. Csanda E, Tärczy M, Takäts A, Mogyoros I, Koves, Katona G 1983 L-deprenyl in the treatment of Parkinson's disease. Journal of Neural Transmission (suppl) 19: 265–272

16. Trebinin F, Daniele D, Gilio S, Scarzella L 1985 Clinical evaluation of selegiline (l-deprenyl) in the long-term l-dopa treatment syndrome. Acta Neurologica (New Series) 7: 432–439
17. Knoll J 1978 The possible mechanism of action of (-)deprenyl in Parkinson's disease. Journal of Neural Transmission 43: 177–198
18. Sunderland T, Mueller E A, Cohen R M, Jimerson D C, Pickar D, Murphy D L 1985 Tyramine pressor sensitivity changes during deprenyl treatment. Psychopharmacology 86: 432–437
19. Birkmayer W 1978 Long-term treatment with l-deprenyl. Journal of Neural Transmission 43: 239–244
20. Birkmayer W 1983 Deprenyl (selegiline) in the treatment of Parkinson's disease. Acta Neurologica Scandinavica (suppl) 95: 95–102
21. Garzön J, Moratalla R, del Rio J 1980 Potentiation of the analgesia induced in rats by morphine or (D-Ala^2)-met-enkephalin-amide after inhibition of type B monoamine oxidase: the role of phenylethylamine. Neuropharmacology 19: 723–729
22. Birkmayer W, Riederer P, Ambrozi L, Youdim M B H 1977 Implications of combined treatment with 'Madopar' and l-deprenyl in Parkinson's disease. Lancet 1: 439–443
23. Csanda E, Tärczy M 1983 Clinical evaluation of deprenyl (selegiline) in the treatment of Parkinson's disease. Acta Neurolgoica Scandinavica (suppl) 95: 117–122
24. Eisler T, Teräväinen H, Nelson R et al 1981 Deprenyl in Parkinson disease. Neurology 31: 19–23
25. Gerstenbrand F, Ransmayr G, Poewe W 1983 Deprenyl (selegiline) in combination treatment of Parkinson's disease. Acta Neurologica Scandinavica (suppl) 95: 123–126
26. Giovannini P, Grassi M P, Scigliano G, Piccolo I, Soliver P, Caraceni T 1985 Deprenyl in Parkinson disease: personal experience. Italian Journal of Neurological Sciences 6: 207–212
27. Gyimoti G, Csanaky A, Leposa D 1983 Observations made with l-deprenyl (Jumex) in the long-term treatment of outpatients with Parkinson's syndrome. Therapia Hungarica 31: 26–30
28. Lees A J, Kohout L J, Shaw K M, Stern G M, Elsworth J D, Andlre M, Youdim M B H 1977 Deprenyl in Parkinson's disease. Lancet 2: 791–795
29. Rinne U K 1983 Deprenyl (selegiline) in the treatment of Parkinson's disease. Acta Neurologica Scandinavica (suppl) 95: 107–111
30. Schacter M, Marsden C D, Parkes J D, Jenner P, Testa B 1980 Deprenyl in the management of response fluctuations in patients with Parkinson's disease on levodopa. Journal of Neurology, Neurosurgery and Psychiatry 43: 1016–1021
31. Stern G M, Lees A J, Hardie R J, Sandler M 1983 Clinical and pharmacological problems of deprenyl (selegiline) treatment in Parkinson's disease. Acta Neurologica Scandinavica (suppl) 95: 113–116
32. Streifler M, Vardi J, Borenstein N, Rabey M J, Fletcher S 1980 Beta-type monoamine oxidase inhibitors in long-term levodopa treated parkinsonism: A combined clinical trial with l-deprenyl. Current Therapeutic Research 27: 643–648
34. Trebim F, Daniele D, Gilio S, Searzella L 1985 Clinical evaluation of selegiline (L-deprenyl) in the long-term l-dopa treatment syndrome. Acta Neurologica (New Series) 7: 432–439

Selenium sulphide

Selenium sulphide has been used widely in dermatology in the treatment of scaling scalp disorders and pityriasis versicolor.

Chemistry

Selenium sulphide (Lenium, Selsun)
SeS, SeS_2, S, Se

Molecular weight, SeS_2	143.1
pKa	not relevant
Solubility	
in alcohol	1 in > 10 000
in water	1 in > 10 000
Octanol/water partition coefficient	—

Selenium sulphide is formed by chemical synthesis giving rise to selenium monosulphide and elemental forms of selenium and sulphur. Contrary to some reports only trace amounts of selenium disulphide are formed. The mixture formed is a reddish-brown insoluble powder with a faint hydrogen sulphide-like odour. The formulated preparation Lenium is an orange-brown cream with a lavender odour. Selenium sulphide is not present in any topical combination preparations.

Selenium is included in some parenteral nutrition (hyperalimentation) regimens and in combination with other trace elements in oral vitamin/trace element supplements.

Pharmacology

Selenium sulphide has a number of actions. It has antibacterial[1] and antifungal[2] activity. In particular it is known to be active against *Pityrosporum ovale*,[3] a yeast-like fungus, found on the normal scalp. Selenium sulphide also has antimitotic activity.[4] The mode of action is unknown but may be related to incorporation of selenium into epithelial cell enzyme systems. Its residual adherence to skin structures after a shampoo and rinse (known as substantivity) help to explain its efficacy as an anti-dandruff agent.

Toxicology

No evidence of carcinogenicity was observed after application of selenium to the skin of mice.[5] However, when rats were fed selenium sulphide by gavage at a dose of 100 $mg.kg^{-1}$ daily approximately 40% developed hepatocellular carcinoma. A raised incidence of lung tumours was also recorded. These tumours were not observed at the lower dose of 20 $mg.kg^{-1}$.[5] Further animal studies are currently under evaluation.

There is no evidence of teratogenicity.

The apparent lack of toxicity when applied topically contrasts sharply with the highly toxic soluble selenites, selenates and organic selenium compounds.

Clinical pharmacology

Both an anti-dandruff effect and effectiveness against pityriasis versicolor of topical selenium sulphide has been demonstrated in man.[6] Its anti-dandruff effect may be related to its activity against *Pityrosporum ovale* which has been implicated in the pathogenesis of seborrhoeic dermatitis. Protracted use can lead to an irritant dermatitis, particularly of flexural skin.

It is only used in the UK as a lotion containing 2.5% selenium sulphide. It is not available for oral or systemic administration.

Pharmacokinetics

The method of analysis for selenium is atomic absorption spectroscopy of the hydride. This is performed after removal of organic selenium by mixed acid digestion. Sensitivity depends on the precise method used, but for 1% absorption it is 0.5 mg.ml^{-1} in an air acetylene flame. Using the hydride generation technique[7] the detection limit is improved to 0.002 g.l^{-1}.

Selenium sulphide is not absorbed through normal skin, but can be through inflamed or damaged epithelium, leading to systemic toxicity.[8] Selenium is then detectable in plasma and urine. Urinary coproporphyrins and uroporphyrins may be elevated after systemic absorption. Selenium is excreted in humans in three elimination phases. Phase 1 lasts approximately one day, phase 2 lasts 20 days and phase 3 lasts 65–116 days. Selenium is able to bind to lipoprotein in plasma. Since selenium is an essential trace element it must cross the placenta but in physiological concentrations would cause no problems. No information is available on excretion in breast milk.

Concentration–effect relationship

Selenium sulphide is only available in various bases as a 2.5% solution, used topically. Since the drug is not absorbed through normal skin a concentration–effect relationship is not apparent.

Metabolism

Selenium sulphide is practically insoluble and easily washed off the skin. Following systemic absorption it is excreted mainly via the urine but also via the faeces. Conversion to methyl selenite occurs, probably in the liver.[9] Selenium is very rapidly oxidized to methyl selenite and none appears in the urine as selenium.

Pharmaceutics

Selenium sulphide is available in five preparations for external use.

Scalp application (BPC): 2.5% solution in liquid base
Exsee Lotion (Herbert, US): 2.5% solution in liquid base
Lenium (Janssen, UK): 2.5% cream
Selsun (Abbot UK/US): 2.5% suspension in detergent base
Selsun Blue (Ross, US): 1.0% suspension in detergent base

All should be stored in air-tight containers and protected from heat. They have a long shelf-life. Incidence of contact sensitivity is very low, though as mentioned, protracted use can lead to an irritant dermatitis.

Therapeutic use

Indications[10]

1. Control of dandruff and seborrhoeic dermatitis of the scalp
2. Eradication and control of pityriasis versicolor.

Contraindications

1. Inflamed or damaged skin
2. Young infants and children.

Mode of use

All clinical uses depend on its antifungal and anti-dandruff activity.

Dandruff and seborrhoeic dermatitis of the scalp[11]
After the scalp is washed, up to 10 ml of solution should be added to the scalp and massaged in. After 2 to 3 minutes the application should be washed off and then reapplied. Care should be taken to ensure all traces are removed from the hair and fingernails. The eyes should be avoided. Applications should be twice a week for two weeks, then weekly for two weeks then only as required.

Pityriasis versicolor
Several regimes exist for treatment, as the incidence of recurrence is high. It is therefore recommended that the lotion be applied nightly to the body from the neck to the knees, excluding the genitalia, before washing off in the morning. This should be repeated daily for a week.

Subsequently, monthly applications should be applied for six months to minimize the chances of recurrence.

Selenium sulphide

Adverse reactions

Potentially life-threatening effects
No reactions of this severity have occurred from local application.

Acute overdosage
If accidentally taken by mouth selenium sulphide is highly toxic. Symptoms include anorexia, vomiting and tremor.[12]

Investigations may reveal anaemia and fatty degeneration of the liver. Treatment should include gastric lavage. Ascorbic acid orally may increase the rate of urinary excretion.

Chronic toxicity of selenium was seen at whole blood concentration 1.3–7.5 μg.ml^{-1} (non-toxic normal range 0.35–0.58 μg.ml^{-1}). Serum levels are approximately 30% of whole blood levels. Urine levels for these patients were 0.88–6.63 μg.ml^{-1} (toxic) and 0.04–0.33 μg.ml^{-1} (normal).[13]

Severe or irreversible adverse effects
Long-term topical use on damaged skin has led to systemic absorption. Symptoms included a garlic-like odour on the breath, metallic taste, anorexia, vomiting, weakness, fatigue, hyperreflexia and tremor. Biochemical abnormalities included anaemia, abnormal porphyrins and raised urinary selenium. All parameters had returned to normal one month after cessation of therapy with selenium sulphide.[8]

Symptomatic adverse effects
Protracted use of selenium sulphide has been associated with a primary irritant dermatitis, although in some instances this may be due to the base. Contact with the eyes can cause irritation. Diffuse hair loss and onychodystrophy has been reported though this is reversible with cessation of selenium.

Other effects
Discoloration of natural and dyed hair has been recorded. 48 hours should be allowed between application of selenium sulphide and hair-tinting agents. All jewellery should be removed prior to application of selenium, as it may damage metals.

Interference with clinical pathology tests
No technical interference of this type has been reported.

High risk groups

Selenium sulphide may be absorbed through broken skin and those with excoriations of the scalp or infections of the scalp should avoid its use. It is not recommended for use in infants and children, but the reasons for this are unclear.

Drug interactions

Potentially hazardous interactions
No drug interactions of this kind have been reported.

Potentially useful interactions
No useful interactions have been reported with this drug.

References

1. Spoor H J 1955 A study of antidandruff agents. Drug and Cosmetic Industry 77 (11): 44–45
2. Matson E J 1956 Selenium sulphide as an antidandruff agent. Journal of the Society of Cosmetic Chemistry 7: 459–465
3. McEvoy G K 1989 Selenium sulphide. American Hospital Formulary Service. American Society Hospital Pharmacists, Bethesda, pp 1967–1968
4. Flesch P 1953 Mode of action of selenium sulfide. Journal of Investigative Dermatology 21: 233–235
5. National Institute of Health Selenium Sulphide Survey: US Department Health and Human Services. No. NIH/80/1750
6. Sanchez J L, Torres V M 1984 Double-blind efficacy study of selenium sulfide in tinea versicolor. Journal of the American Academy of Dermatology 11: 235–238
7. Thompson K D, Reynolds P J 1978 Atomic absorption fluorescence and flame emission spectroscopy: a practical approach, 2nd edn. Wiley, New York, p 79
8. Ransome J W, Scott N M, Knoblock E C 1961 Selenium sulfide intoxication. New England Journal of Medicine 264: 384–385
9. Klevay L M 1976 Pharmacology and Therapeutics I: 211
10. Reynolds J E F (ed) Martindale: the extra pharmacopoeia, 28th edn. The Pharmaceutical Press, London, p 502
11. Kligman A M, Marples R R, Lantis L R, McGinley K J 1974 Appraisal of efficacy of antidandruff formulations. Journal of the Society of Cosmetic Chemistry 25: 73–91
12. Fishbein L 1977 Toxicology of selenium and telenium. In: Boyer R A, Mehlman M A (eds) Advances in modern toxicology (Toxicology of trace elements). Wiley, London, p 191–240
13. Yang G, Wang S, Zhou R, Sun S 1983 Endemic selenium intoxication. American Journal of Clinical Nutrition 37: 872–881

Sennosides

Sennosides are plant glycosides with laxative actions.

Chemistry

Sennosides A + B (Senokot, X-Prep)
$C_{42}H_{38}O_{20}$
5,5′-Bis(β-D-glucopyranosyloxy)-9,9′10-10′-tetrahydro-4,4′-dihydroxy-10,10′-dioxo(9,9′-bianthracene)-2,2′-dicarboxylic acid

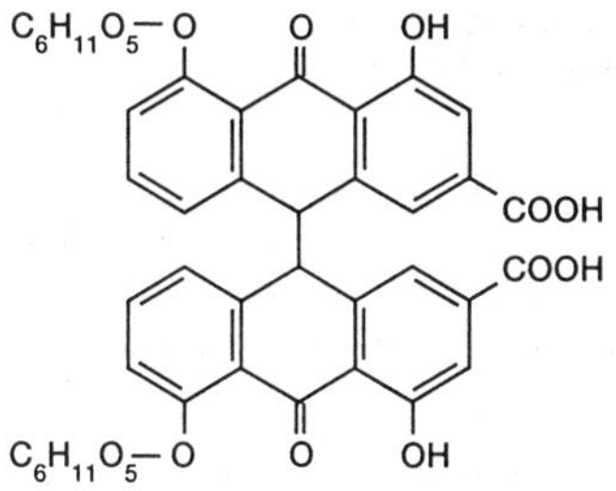

Molecular weight	862.7
pKa	—
Solubility	
in alcohol	sparingly soluble
in water	insoluble
Octanol/water partition coefficient	—

A yellowish brown powder (Senokot) with a slight odour and taste, or chocolate flavoured brown liquid (X-Prep). Anthroquinine glucosides are found in senna in equal amounts and in the rhubarbs, where sennoside A predominates. Sennoside A can be isomerized to sennoside B in sodium bicarbonate solution at 80°C.

Sennosides are extracted from the pericarp of senna pods, which are powdered and standardized for sennosides. They are also available in combination with Plantago ovata (Agiolax) and with piperazine phosphate (Pripsen).

Pharmacology

Senna compounds are laxative by virtue of the anthraquinone derivatives they contain. They are pro-drugs that produce an effect on the large intestine, having first been partly metabolized by gastrointestinal microflora. Peristalsis is stimulated via an increase in propulsive activity in the left and sigmoid colon.

Toxicology

Sennosides have been shown to have no mutagenic or teratogenic effects. No carcinogenicity studies have been reported.

Clinical pharmacology

Senna compounds in doses of 15–30 mg produce a laxative effect after about 6 h, since the drug has to reach the colon via the digestive tract and to a limited extent by recirculation after intestinal absorption. Induction of peristalsis has been demonstrated in man[1] and the drug often causes griping abdominal pain. Stimulation of the intestinal secretions in both small and large intestines also occurs,[2] and in larger doses an increased laxative effect is seen due to increased water content of the faeces.

Pharmacokinetics

The preferred analytical method is by HPLC after alkali infusion.[3] The sensitivity is 1 $\mu g.l^{-1}$. A rapid urine test for qualitative detection is also available.[4] Sennosides are pro-drugs requiring metabolic action by colonic bacteria to produce the active metabolites, rhein-9-anthrone and rhein. Systemic bioavailability is $<5\%$. Sennosides in the colon require bacterial degradation because they are pharmacologically inactive.

Sennoside distribution outside body water is not known and likely to be small. Sennosides are not excreted in human breast milk in significant amounts.

There is no known effect of altered disease states on sennoside kinetics, but where the colon is sterile a reduction in active metabolite formation may be expected.

Concentration–effect relationship

There is no information available on this subject and a correlation between the blood concentration of senna and its laxative effect would be unlikely.

Metabolism

Sennosides are extensively metabolized within the gut lumen.[5] Excretion is almost entirely as metabolites in faeces. Unchanged faecal excretion is slight ($<5\%$) as is urinary elimination ($<5\%$).

Sennosides are hydrolysed at the glycoside linkages to give sennidin A + B which in turn are hydrolysed at the C–C linkage, possibly by free radicals in the colon, to rhein and rhein-9-anthrone (Fig. 1). Rhein is conjugated to a sulphate and a glucuronide. The main pharmacological activity of the sennosides may lie in the rhein-9-anthrone metabolite.

Fig. 1 Metabolism of sennosides

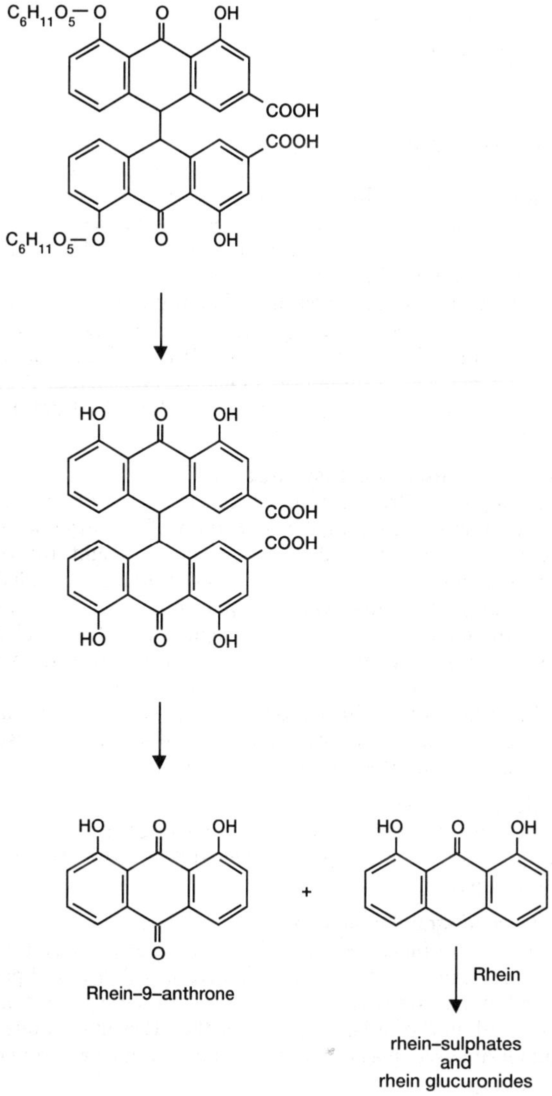

Pharmaceutics

Sennosides are available only in oral forms.

1. Senokot (Reckitt & Colman, UK/Purdue Frederick, USA): tablets containing standardized senna equivalent to 7.5 mg total sennosides. The tablets are small, brown and impressed on one side only with the legend 'Senokot' and have a shelf-life of 5 years.
2. Senokot granules: each 5 ml (2.73 g) contains standardized senna equivalent to 15 mg total sennosides. The granules are brown and chocolate flavoured.
3. Senokot syrup: each 5 ml contains standardized senna extract equivalent to 7.5 mg total sennosides. The syrup is brown and fruit flavoured. It has a shelf-life of two years.
4. X-Prep (Napp, UK/Gray, USA) contains 72 mg total sennosides in 72 ml for use as two divided doses prior to bowel radiology. It contains alcohol 7% w/v.

Sennoside preparations contain no potential allergens such as tartrazine. No special storage conditions are required.

Therapeutic use

Indications

1. Simple constipation
2. As a laxative prior to gut investigation
3. Constipation in the elderly, pregnancy and puerperium, slow transit constipation (idiopathic)
4. Avoidance of straining at stool with haemorrhoids, after surgery and in cerebral cardiovascular disease
5. As an adjunct to antihelminth therapy.

Contraindications

1. Intestinal obstruction
2. Undiagnosed acute or chronic abdominal symptoms.

Mode of use

1. Simple constipation

Clinical use depends on the production of an adequate catharsis. The lowest dose needed for the desired effect varies between individuals. Oral treatment usually starts with 5 ml of the granules or syrup, or 2 tablets daily. The dose is best taken at bedtime by adults and in the morning by children. The tablets can be taken with fluids, and the granules stirred into hot milk, sprinkled on food or eaten as they are.

The dose can be increased by half the initial dose daily until a comfortable formed motion is produced. If after 3 days no effect is seen, further medical examination should be considered. Prolonged high-dose use should be avoided because of the risk of developing a 'cathartic colon'.

2. As a laxative prior to gut investigation

The senna liquid (X-Prep) is administered as a drink on the day prior to either barium or endoscopic examination of the large bowel. The dose is 1 ml (1 mg sennosides) per kg body weight for patients weighing less than 72 kg. Heavier patients should take the full dose of 72 ml (72 mg). The dose can be split into two equal volumes separated by one hour, or taken as a single drink. The ideal time of administration is between 2 and 4 p.m. Each administration should be followed by at least half a pint of water and similar volumes should be drunk hourly throughout the afternoon and evening. The large purgative dose and accompanying fluid intake results in thorough purgation after six to eight hours.

3. Constipation in special cases

Sennosides may be helpful in the management of constipation in the elderly, pregnant women, puerperium and in patients with slow transit constipation.

4. Avoidance of straining at stool

Straining at stool increases intra-abdominal and intracerebral pressure and may cause fluctuations in circulating volume, and potential risk to abdominal sutures and anastomoses. In these patients it seems rational to administer a laxative. As for the other indications, senna compounds are used in as low a dose and for as short a period of time as is necessary.

5. As an adjunct to antihelminth therapy

Sennosides are included in a piperazine preparation (Pripsen) for the elimination of threadworms and roundworms. After administration the worms are effectively paralysed by the piperazine and are then evacuated before recovery by the cathartic effect of the senna.

Contraindications

1. Intestinal obstruction

The pharmacological effects of sennosides administration, an increase in intraluminal fluid and electrolyte content and an increase in muscular contractions, are likely to exacerbate the effects of any intestinal obstruction.

2. Undiagnosed intestinal symptoms

Because of the known effects on gut fluid balance and motility, sennosides have the potential to exacerbate a number of acute intestinal conditions, e.g. acute diverticulitis, peritonitis, high-output diarrhoea.

Adverse reactions

Potentially life-threatening effects

No effects of this kind are known.

Acute overdosage

The major adverse effect consequent on senna overdose is diarrhoea leading to dehydration. Conservative measures by an increase in fluid intake are usually sufficient to reverse the loss of fluid and electrolytes. It is rarely necessary to resort to intravenous therapy.

Severe or irreversible adverse effects

Prolonged high-dose senna ingestion involves the risk of inducing the 'cathartic colon'. Initially patients use sennosides to provide a regular bowel movement. They then develop dependence on such laxatives to provide an effective catharsis, requiring increasing laxative doses with time. Chemically this chronic overusage can be recognized by the presence of a brown–black melanin-like pigment in the large bowel (melanosis coli). The pigment usually appears a year or more after the start of ingestion and takes 3–4 months to disappear on laxative withdrawal.[6] Other contact laxatives such as aloes and cascara can also be responsible.[7]

More significant changes are seen with increased or more prolonged use. The sennosides can act as neurotoxins, damaging the myenteric plexus. Schwann cell proliferation develops, with depletion due to death of the overstimulated neurones and axons. The intestinal smooth muscle cells atrophy, the muscularis mucosae hypertrophies (secondary to overstimulation) and submucosal depletion of adipose tissue gives rise to an inert, dilated aperistaltic colon. The barium enema appearance of the cathartic colon shows smooth, regular dilated bowel wall with loss of colonic haustral pattern. Pseudo-strictures caused by neuromuscular incoordination are often transient and variable in site and position. Such characteristic changes in radiological appearances may be absent despite habitual use.[8]

Symptomatic adverse effects

Sennosides in conventional doses are well tolerated, with adverse effects being only occasional abdominal pain. In sennoside laxative abuse, patients may have multiple symptoms including disturbed bowel habits, abdominal pain, weakness, nausea and vomiting, weight loss, fever, bone pain, tetany and finger clubbing.[9]

Other effects

Habitual laxative abuse has been associated with dehydration, hypotension and uraemia secondary to excessive losses of sodium and water.[10] Hypokalaemia is a characteristic feature of excessive use. It has a multifactorial aetiology: alteration in intestinal electrolyte transport, increased plasma renin, secondary aldosteronism and decreased intake.[11,12] These changes are usually reversible on laxative withdrawal.

Interference with clinical pathology tests

No interferences of this kind have been reported.

High risk groups

Neonates

These drugs are not recommended in neonates.

Breast milk. Sennosides are not excreted in breast milk in significant quantities and conventional doses have no effects on the infants.[13]

Children

Children over 6 years old require half the adult dosage, whilst those of 2–6 years should take 2.5–5 ml of the syrup (3.75–7.5 mg total sennosides). As with adults, sennosides should be administered for the shortest possible period.

Pregnant women

The drug is widely used in pregnancy as self-medication. No specific precautions are required.

The elderly

In frail elderly patients the starting dose should be at the lower end of the range.

Drug interactions

No major drug interactions have been described.

General review articles

Godding E W 1976 Therapeutics of laxative agents with special reference to the anthraquinones. Pharmacology 14 (suppl): 78–101

Avery Jones F 1974 The management of constipation. Prescribers Journal 14: 85–92

Cummings J H 1974 Laxative abuse. Gut 15: 758–766

Cummings J H 1976 The use and abuse of laxatives. In: Bouchier E D (ed) Recent advances in gastroenterology, vol 3. Churchill Livingstone, Edinburgh

1980 Natural anthraquinone drugs. Pharmacology 20 (suppl 1)

1988 First International Symposium on Senna. Pharmacology 36 (suppl 1)

References

1. Hardcastle J D, Wilkins J L 1970 The action of sennosides and related compounds on human colon and rectum. Gut 11: 1038–1042
2. Fingl E 1980 Laxatives and cathartics. In: Goodman L S, Gilman A (eds) The pharmacological basis of therapeutics, 6th edn Macmillan, New York, pp 1002–1012
3. Hietula P, Lainonen H, Marvata M 1988 New aspects on the metabolism of the sennosides. Pharmacology 36 (suppl 1): 138–143
4. Kaspi T, Royds R B, Turner P 1978 Qualitative determination of senna in urine. Lancet 1: 1162
5. Lenl J, Lemmens 1980 Metabolism of sennosides and rhein in the rat. Pharmacology 20 (suppl): 50–57
6. Hattori M, Kim G, Motoike S, Kobashi K, Namba T 1982 Metabolism of sennosides by intestinal flora. Chemical and Pharmaceutical Bulletin 30: 1338–1346
7. Wittoesch J H, Jackman R J, McDonald J R 1958 Melanosis coli: general review and a study of 887 cases. Diseases of the Colon and Rectum 1: 172–180
8. Bockus H L, Willard J H, Bank J 1933 Melanosis coli the aetiologic significance of the anthracene laxatives: a report of 41 cases. Journal of the American Medical Association 101: 1–6
9. Cummings J H, Sladen G E, James O F W, Sarner M, Misiewicz J J 1974 Laxative-induced diarrhoea: a continuing clinical problem. British Medical Journal 1: 537–541
10. Morris A I, Turnberg L A 1979 Surreptitious laxative abuse. Gastroenterology 77: 780–786
11. Fordtram J S, Ingelfinger F J 1968 Absorption of water electrolytes and sugars from the human gut. In: Code C F (ed) Intestinal absorption (Handbook of physiology, vol. 3). American Physiological Society, Washington DC, pp 1457–1496
12. Schwartz W B, Relman A S 1953 Metabolic and renal studies in chronic potassium depletion resulting from overuse of laxatives. Journal of Clinical Investigation 32: 258–271
13. Faber P, Strenge-Hesse A 1988 Relevance of rhein excretion in breast milk. Pharmacology 36 (suppl 1): 212–221

Silver nitrate

Silver nitrate, the most frequently used of the inorganic silver salts in medicine, exhibits antibacterial, astringent, escharotic and caustic activity.

Chemistry

Silver nitrate (*Argenti Nitras*, nitric acid silver salt)
$AgNO_3$

Molecular weight	169.9
pKa	—
Solubility	
in alcohol	1 in 30
in water	1 in 0.4
Octanol/water partition coefficient	very low

Silver nitrate is an odourless, white, crystalline powder or large transparent colourless crystals, with a bitter metallic taste. It melts at 212°C, and decomposes at 444°C to metallic silver, nitrogen, oxygen and nitrous oxides. Solubility in both water and alcohol increases with temperature. The pure compound is not photosensitive. However, silver nitrate becomes grey or greyish black on exposure to air or light in the presence of organic matter due to photoreduction to metallic silver. It is incompatible with organic material, alkalis, halogen acids and their salts, tannins, phosphates and benzalkonium chloride. Silver nitrate is not present in any combination preparations.

Pharmacology

Silver nitrate, in common with other heavy metal salts, is cytotoxic. The silver ion is responsible for most of the pharmacological effects as it readily combines with sulphydryl, carboxyl, phosphate, amino and other biologically important chemical groups. When these interactions involve proteins, their physical properties are altered; at high silver ion concentrations, the protein may be denatured and precipitation usually occurs. At low concentrations, the silver ion causes substantial damage to the cell membrane by binding to sulphydryl and other active groups of the membrane proteins. Silver ion concentrations of 10^{-7} to 10^{-4} M increase membrane permeability to cations in both the renal proximal tubule[1] and the corneal epithelium of rabbit,[2] induce haemolysis in red blood cells[3] and inhibit DNA replication in human lymphoid cells.[4]

Similar effects occur in bacterial cells. The broad antibacterial activity of silver nitrate is attributed to the interaction of silver ions with bacterial DNA as well as with sulphydryl groups in the microbial enzymes responsible for cell growth and replication.[5] A number of bacterial metabolic processes, including substrate oxidation and solute transport, are also inhibited.[6]

Toxicology

The primary toxic effects of silver in animals are exerted on the cardiovascular, hepatic and haematopoietic systems. Repeated administration of silver nitrate to animals in their drinking water may produce anaemia, growth retardation, degenerative changes of the liver, cardiac enlargement and ventricular hypertrophy. Deposits of silver are found in the liver, spleen, muscle, brain and skin.[7,8]

Clinical pharmacology

Solutions of silver nitrate ranging in concentration from 0.01% to 10% and solid (toughened) forms are used clinically for local application to the skin and mucous membranes. Concentrations of up to 1% are antibacterial and astringent, and higher concentrations caustic and escharotic. The astringent and caustic effects are due to the ability of silver nitrate to combine with and precipitate proteins at the site of application, causing scab and sloughing. At low concentrations, precipitation is confined to proteins in the interstitial space and an astringent effect occurs, whereas at higher concentrations membrane and intracellular junctions are also damaged, and caustic and escharotic action ensues.

The broad antibacterial spectrum of silver nitrate in vitro covers common bacterial and fungal pathogens such as *Staphylococcus*, *Streptococcus*, *Pseudomonas* and *Klebsiella* species, and penicillinase and non-penicillinase producing strains of *Neisseria gonorrhoeae*.[9] Consequently, it is used clinically as a bacteriostatic agent for non-specific infections of the eye, genito-urinary tract and skin. Silver nitrate (0.5%) has proved to be an effective bacteriostatic agent to prevent burn wound sepsis in the severely burned patient, and a single application of a 1% ophthalmic solution prevents gonococcal eye infections in the newborn. The onset of action is immediate and there is little absorption as silver nitrate rapidly binds with chloride ions, proteins and enzymes in the tissue at the site of action. The prophylactic effect will depend on the high concentration of silver ions immediately after application, thus the compound must be reapplied repeatedly for continuing therapeutic benefit.

Pharmacokinetics

The preferred analytical method for the drug in biological fluids is a radiolabelled technique. Using Ag-110m a sensitivity of 10^{-10}g can be achieved.[10]

The absorption of silver nitrate from the skin or mucous membranes of the lungs or gastrointestinal tract is limited by its rapid binding to the various nucleophilic groups in proteins and its precipitation as silver chloride. In animals, between 1% and 10% of silver is absorbed following ingestion of radiolabelled silver nitrate.[10] The small quantities of absorbed silver are distributed diffusely throughout the body and deposited in the tissues and organs, possibly bound as silver sulphides and selenides.[11] It is not clear how the silver ion is transported to the tissues; available data suggest that it is bound in the plasma to transferrin rather than albumin.[7] The highest concentrations were found in the liver and spleen, with lower concentrations in the muscle, skin and brain. The biological half life of silver in the liver of humans has been estimated to be approximately 50 days. The half life of silver in the skin is possibly much longer as argyria can persist for years after administration of silver nitrate.[8]

After eyedrop application of radioactive silver nitrate to albino rabbits, silver was located mainly in the cornea and conjunctiva, with high uptake by the optic nerve.[12]

It is unlikely that the kinetics of silver nitrate would be affected by concurrent disease such as renal or hepatic impairment. Similarly, no significant change in the kinetics is anticipated in the elderly. The amount of silver nitrate excreted in the breast milk or that crosses the placenta is not known. However, it is unlikely that either route is of significance.

Oral absorption	low
Presystemic metabolism	—
Plasma half life	—
Volume of distribution	—
Plasma protein binding	high

Concentration–effect relationship

The action of silver nitrate depends on both the concentration and the length of time that it is allowed to act. It has a narrow therapeutic range. Concentrations above 2% are caustic and a 0.1% solution is astringent, with only slight bacteriostatic properties. Bacteriocidal concentrations are toxic to tissues.

Metabolism

Silver does not occur regularly in animal or human tissues. There is little information about its metabolism and excretion in man; in animals the main excretory route for silver is in the bile, possibly by a glutathione-dependent mechanism,[13] and by faecal elimination. Over 90% of the silver absorbed in animals given radioactive silver nitrate by oral, intravenous or intraperitoneal routes is eliminated via the faeces.[10] Some silver is deposited in the body for long periods of time in chemically stable and essentially inert forms and retention is greatest in the reticuloendothelial organs.[11]

Pharmaceutics

Clear solutions of silver nitrate are available for bladder irrigation and as topical and ophthalmic forms for application to the conjunctiva, skin and mucous membranes. Concentrations range from approximately 0.01% to 15% w/v silver nitrate.

1. Toughened silver nitrate, formed by fusing together 95 parts of silver nitrate and 5 parts of potassium nitrate (BP), sodium chloride or hydrochloric acid (USP) and moulding into pencils or cones, is available for topical use. The tip of the preparation should be moistened by dipping in water and applied carefully to the lesion, avoiding contact with normal skin.
2. Silver nitrate ophthalmic solutions (0.2–1% w/v) are clear, colourless and have a pH of 4.5–6. The solutions may contain sodium acetate as buffer. They are preferably dispensed from unit dose wax ampoules designed to prevent evaporation that might result in increased solution concentration. Phenylmercuric borate 0.005% may be used as a preservative and the solution sterilized by filtration. A decreasing trend in the use of eye drops is noted in the Indications section below.
3. Silver Nitrate Lotion BNF contains 0.5% w/v silver nitrate in distilled water.

All preparations should be protected from light. The solutions have a short shelf-life, as silver is readily reduced to elemental silver. Solutions should be freshly prepared, supplied in alkali-free amber bottles, used undiluted, and discarded after use. Such solutions may be sterilized by autoclaving.

Silver nitrate is incompatible with most preservatives and many organic compounds, plus alkalis, phosphates and halogen acids.

Contact with normal skin and tissues should be avoided, as silver nitrate may cause black stains on skin, tissues and fabric.

Therapeutic use

Indications

1. The management of infection in burn wounds
2. The prophylaxis of gonococcal ophthalmia neonatorum
3. The management of epidermal necrolysis
4. Cauterization of warts and other abnormal epithelium or granulation tissue
5. Miscellaneous and occasional uses include the treatment of eczematous reaction and suppurative wounds; prophylaxis of genito-urinary tract infections; the management of interstitial cystitis; control of haematuria and massive bladder haemorrhage; treatment of aphthous and herpetic ulcers; treatment of epistaxis and allergic and vasomotor rhinitis; pleurodesis to prevent recurrence of primary spontaneous pneumothorax; the surgical treatment of hydatid cysts and as a surgical skin marker.

Contraindications

None is known.

Mode of use

The concentration of silver nitrate used in therapy depends upon the indication. Weaker preparations utilize the astringent and antibacterial action: stronger solutions and solid applicators are used as caustics.

Indications

1. Burn wounds

Aqueous silver nitrate solution, 0.5% w/v in distilled water, has been used effectively since 1965 as a prophylactic agent to control bacterial infection within the burn wound.[14,15] When applied as a wet dressing, the solution is particularly useful in suppressing bacterial growth in moderate to major burns involving up to 50% of body

Silver nitrate

surface area. For lesser burns, 0.5% silver nitrate cream may be more convenient.[16] The compound delays eschar removal and is unable to penetrate the burn tissue appreciably due to the precipitation of silver on the wound surface. Therapy should be initiated, therefore, on the first day, before bacterial growth is established; treatment has proved to be less effective if it is begun later, when significant microbial growth is already underway in the tissues.[17]

The solution is used to saturate gauze dressings which are then applied to the burn wound, previously cleansed to remove necrotic tissue which would render silver nitrate ineffective. Resaturation is necessary at two hour intervals and the dressings should be totally changed twice a day. Thorough debridment should be made with each change. The dressings are sometimes covered with light cotton blankets to reduce both heat and evaporative water losses. This has been shown to maintain a lower metabolic rate and an improved state of nutrition in patients so managed.[18]

Silver nitrate is the therapy of choice when the use of occlusive dressings is required. Other advantages of silver nitrate include negligible bacterial resistance among common infecting organisms, rare patient sensitivity, painless application and ease of use. A major disadvantage is that it stains organic matter black, making it difficult to differentiate between necrotic and healing tissues of the wound. Other disadvantages include electrolyte depletion and the occasional development of significant methaemoglobin.[19]

Silver nitrate is often compared to silver sulphadiazine, a compound first introduced by Fox in 1968[20] specifically to combine the antibacterial activity of sulphadiazine with that of silver. Although electrolyte disturbances and staining do not occur with sulphadiazine therapy, the incidences of bacterial resistance to sulphadiazine are increasing with the widespread use of the drug.

2. Ophthalmia neonatorum prophylaxis

Ophthalmia neonatorum, an acute conjunctivitis in the newborn, has been associated with several organisms, including *Chlamydia trachomatis*, *Staphylococcus aureus* and *Neisseria gonorrhoeae*. The organisms are usually transmitted to the conjunctivae of the neonates during passage through the birth canal of infected mothers. The most serious form of neonatal conjunctivitis is due to *N. gonorrhoeae*, because if untreated, it can lead to corneal ulceration and permanent blindness. Silver nitrate prophylaxis against gonococcal ophthalmia neonatorum was introduced by Credé in 1880[21] and is considered one of the triumphs of preventative medicine; there were dramatic reductions in the incidence of blindness due to the disease after Credé's prophylaxis was adopted by legislation in many parts of the world early this century.[22]

Prior to administration the neonate's eyes are cleaned, then two drops of the 1% solution are instilled into the lower conjunctival sac, a single ampoule being used for each eye. The closed eyelids can be gently massaged to help spread the solution to all areas of the conjunctival sac. After one minute any excess solution is wiped from the eyelids and the surrounding skin to prevent staining. This prophylaxis should be performed no later than one hour and preferably immediately after delivery, since delayed application may reduce efficacy. Irrigation of the eyes following application is not recommended currently by the Canadian Paediatric Society or by the American Academy of Pediatrics.[23,24]

Credé's prophylaxis is still a legal requirement in some European countries and North American states, although the practice has long been abandoned in the UK because of the low prevalence of maternal gonococcal infection and better methods of prenatal diagnosis and treatment. Although the incidence of gonococcal neonatal conjunctivitis in developing countries, where there is no regulatory prophylaxis, is high,[25] in many industrial nations ocular infections due to *Chlamydia trachomatis* occur more often than gonococcal infections and silver nitrate is not effective against this agent. In addition, reservations that silver nitrate does not prevent all cases of gonococcal ophthalmia neonatorum and that it causes chemical conjunctivitis, pain and visual impairment which may interfere with the mother–infant bonding process have led to several recent critical reviews on the subject,[26–29] and many authorities in Canada and the USA are currently reviewing their policies of statutory silver nitrate prophylaxis with a view to either using other agents or abandoning prophylaxis altogether. In areas of the world where chlamydial infection is common and is a greater concern than gonococcal infection, erythromycin or tetracycline ophthalmic preparations are considered a suitable alternative to silver nitrate for prophylaxis against gonococcal ophthalmia neonatorum. Ophthalmic penicillin preparations have been abandoned for the prophylaxis because of concern about drug sensitization and the emergence of penicillinase-producing *N. gonorrhoea* strains.

3. Epidermal necrolysis

Epidermal necrolysis may be treated by continuous dressings of 0.25–0.5% silver nitrate solution. The principles of burn wound management discussed above apply to the treatment which involves continual debridement, careful monitoring of serum electrolytes and awareness of the possibility of significant methaemoglobin developing.[30]

4. Warts and other skin growths

Applicators of toughened silver nitrate are used to destroy warts and other abnormal skin growths. Granulomatous lesions secondary to isotretinoin therapy have been successfully treated with silver nitrate.[31]

5. Miscellaneous occasional uses

Eczematous reaction and suppurative wounds. Silver nitrate lotion (0.5%) when applied to the skin is mildly astringent and assists in the sealing of exudating wounds by the precipitation of proteins. The lotion is now rarely used, as it stains the skin black and chronic use may lead to argyria.

Aphthous and herpetic ulcers. Silver nitrate applicators have been used in the oral cavity to cauterize aphthous and herpetic ulcerations and inflamed lymphoid follicles. They relieve pain by forming a crust and combat infection. However, it is difficult to retain the drug in contact with the ulcer, and tissue damage may delay the healing process. Silver nitrate is not effective in vitro or in vivo against herpes simplex virus type 2.

Genito-urinary tract prophylaxis. Very dilute solutions (0.01–0.1%w/v) of silver nitrate are bacteriostatic and astringent. In the pre-antibiotic era such solutions were widely used as bladder irrigants to control non-specific cystitis and by urethral or vaginal instillation as a venereal prophylactic. They are still used occasionally today. A recent study of children with neurogenic bladders indicated that silver nitrate instilled into the bladder after intermittent catheterization effectively decreases bacteriurea, and is less expensive and easier to use than other effective (neomycin–polymyxin) irrigants.[32]

Interstitial cystitis. Instillation of dilute silver nitrate solution (0.05%) to distend the bladder for a short time period has proved useful for the treatment of chronic interstitial cystitis,[33] although it is possibly less effective than intravesical instillation of dimethylsulphoxide.[34]

Haematuria and massive bladder haemorrhage. Stronger silver nitrate solutions (concentrations ranging from approximately 0.25% to 1% w/v) are used as bladder and urethral irrigants to control massive bladder haemorrhage (haemorrhagic cystitis) and haematuria of diverse causes. The therapy has been used successfully to treat haematuria from sickle cell haemoglobinopathy,[35] benign renal haematuria[36] and haemorrhage secondary to complications of current treatments of cancer, in particular irradiation and cyclophosphamide therapies.[37,38] Silver nitrate irrigation is also an effective palliative to relieve haematuria in advanced bladder cancer.

Nasal epistaxis. The common sites of bleeding in the nasal cavity are the anterior inferior septum, the prominence of a septal deviation and the posterior inferior meatus. If packing fails to staunch the haemorrhage, strong caustic solutions of silver nitrate applied at the bleeding point, with simultaneous use of suction to remove blood, occludes the open blood vessel wall by a coagulum of tissue necrosis, and a clot forms. A second application of silver nitrate may be made more accurately when the bleeding is partially stopped.

Allergic and vasomotor rhinitis. Strong silver nitrate solution (15%) has been presented as a simple and effective caustic treatment for intractable allergic and vasomotor rhinitis.[39] However, such a destructive treatment would only be contemplated in extreme cases.

Recurrent primary spontaneous pneumothorax. Pleurodesis provoked by instillation of 15% silver nitrate solution to prevent recurrence of primary spontaneous pneumothorax has been used successfully for many years. However, a large number of side effects occur and tetracycline pleurodesis is now considered by some to be the treatment of choice.[40]

Hydatid cysts. Intrahepatic cysts of *Echinococcus granulosus* may be treated by freezing the operation area then administering 0.5% silver nitrate to destroy the scolices.[41]

Surgical skin-marking. Silver nitrate (20% solution) applied with a sharpened applicator stick several days before surgery leaves a distinct mark for 10–14 days that is not affected by bathing.[42]

Adverse reactions

Potentially life-threatening effects

Electrolyte depletion. Silver nitrate solutions applied to extensive burns can cause severe electrolyte derangement by depleting the serum of chloride, sodium, potassium and calcium ions. Hypochloraemia occurs when the silver ion combines with chloride in the serum and wound exudates to yield insoluble silver chloride. Hyponatraemia and sometimes hypokalaemia or hypocalcaemia follow when the cations that accompany chloride are lost in the exudate. The problem may be exacerbated by the absorption of large volumes of the distilled water vehicle, which cause osmolar dilution of the circulating blood.[17] Depletion can occur rapidly, especially in children and in patients with extensive areas of burn injury, and this iatrogenic complication has sometimes proved to be fatal when not recognized and corrected with electrolyte supplements.[14,15]

Methaemoglobinaemia. Methaemoglobinaemia is a rare but potentially serious complication of topical silver nitrate burn therapy and there have been occasional reports of death.[43] This condition is believed to occur when the nitrate ion is converted to nitrite by *Aerobacter cloacae* and other specific bacteria of the burn wound. Systemic absorption of the nitrite, enhanced by the presence of large areas of damaged skin or granulating wounds, may lead to the formation of significant methaemoglobinaemia. The treatment varies according to the severity of the condition. Discontinuation of silver nitrate is sufficient for serum methaemoglobulin concentrations of up to 30%. For higher methaemoglobulin concentrations, 1–2 $mg.kg^{-1}$ of intravenous methylene blue accelerates the normal metabolic conversion of methaemoglobin to haemoglobin and rapidly reverses the toxic symptoms.[44,45]

Acute overdosage

Acute toxic effects of silver nitrate are due to the corrosive action of the compound, for it severely irritates the skin, eyes and mucosae. Cases of accidental overdose have occurred when toughened silver nitrate, used in the oral cavity, has been inadvertently swallowed, or after mistaken administration of strong solutions (5–50% w/v) or solid forms to the eye. Death followed rapidly after intrauterine administration of 7% silver nitrate.[8]

Ingestion of significant amounts of silver nitrate corrodes the mucosae of the digestive tract. The fatal oral dose ranges between 10 and 30 mg and death results from local trauma, haemorrhagic gastroenteritis and shock. Toxic symptoms include a metallic taste and pain in the mouth, sialorrhoea, diarrhoea, vomiting, coma and convulsions; the tissues and vomit are black. Treatment of these effects involves the repeated administration of a 1% solution of sodium chloride as soon as possible after ingestion to precipitate insoluble silver chloride. Copious draughts of demulcents, such as milk or white of egg, are recommended and analgesics such as morphine or pethidine may be required if the pain is severe. The stomach may be emptied by aspiration and lavage, although great care is needed if there is extensive corrosion. Plasma volume expansion may be required if fluid loss into tissues is extensive.

Accidental large doses to the eye can cause severe ocular injury including permanent corneal opacification and cataracts. These effects may also result from repeated ocular application of silver nitrate solution. Treatment by lavage should be started immediately.

Severe or irreversible adverse effects

The long-term application of small amounts of silver nitrate to the mucous surfaces or open wounds leads to the gradual accumulation of high concentrations of silver in the body. The absorbed silver is widely distributed through the organs and tissues, and large amounts in the subepithelial layers of the skin can impart either local or generalized areas of grey-blue pigmentation, especially in those regions exposed to light. The condition, known as argyria, also occurs as a result of chronic industrial or medical exposure to other silver compounds.[46] There is controversy over the chemical form of the silver deposits.[47] Chloride, sulphide and selenide complexes have been identified[11,48] as well as metallic silver produced by the photoactivated reduction of silver salts in the tissues. The eye is particularly prone to pigmentation after either local use or systemic absorption from other sites. The conditions giving rise to argyria are not well defined. The dose required to induce argyrosis by ingestion of soluble salts appears to be between 2 and 4 g.[47]

Although argyria is generally considered to be only of cosmetic relevance, there have been attempts to link the condition with clinical symptoms, including liver and kidney dysfunction, vertigo, progressive disturbances of taste and smell and epicritic sensitivity.[8,47] However, since the few reported cases have not been evaluated in comparison with reference groups, it is not clear whether there is a casual relationship between argyria and the symptoms.

The reduced use of silver compounds in recent times has dramatically lowered the incidence of this iatrogenic condition, for which there is no recognized treatment. Argyria can persist through life although the pigmentation remains relatively stable after discontinuation of the therapy. Chelating agents are not effective, possibly because the considerable deposits of the inert form of silver, silver selenide Ag_2Se, is relatively resistant to their action.[49] Repeated intradermal injections of potassium ferrocyanide (1%) and sodium thiosulphate (6%) to the entire pigmented area to reduce the coloration are painful and not of proven effectiveness. Most cases of generalized argyria reported recently are secondary to use on the oral mucosae; few cases have been reported after burn wound therapy.

Symptomatic adverse effects

Chemical conjunctivitis. Mild chemical conjunctivitis may occur in up to 90% of neonates during the first six hours following ocular silver nitrate prophylaxis, although the condition rarely lasts more than 24 h. The silver ions irritate the conjunctiva by binding with epithelial cell protein and the chloride in tears. The American Academy of Pediatrics and the Canadian Paediatric Society do not recommend saline irrigation after silver nitrate instillation as there is insufficient evidence that it reduces the incidence of conjunctivitis, and it may reduce the efficacy of the prophylaxis.[23,24,50]

Maternal–infant bonding. Chemical conjunctivitis secondary to silver nitrate prophylaxis may interfere with the eye-to-eye contact with the mother and therefore impede the bonding process. In a recent study, the degree of 'eye openness' in the newborn did not significantly affect the attention of the mother toward the baby immediately postpartum.[51] Sometimes prophylaxis is delayed for one hour to allow maternal–infant bonding, but further study is required to determine effects on both the prophylaxis and the bonding process.

Interference with clinical pathology tests

Silver compounds have interfered with protein-bound iodine estimations of thyroid function.[52]

High risk groups

Neonates

The drug may be used in neonates, as described above.

Breast milk. The drug should not be used in breast-feeding women.

Children

The drug may be used in children.

Pregnant women

The drug is best avoided during pregnancy.

The elderly

The drug may be used in the elderly.

Drug interactions

Few interactions have been reported, although silver nitrate is incompatible with many substances. Silver interacts with selenium, copper and vitamin E.

In animals, selenium antagonizes the toxicity of silver ions; addition of selenium to the diets of rats exposed to silver in their drinking water prevented growth retardation but increased hepatic and renal concentrations of silver.[8,13]

Silver nitrate administered in the food of rats modulates the effect of oestradiol administered simultaneously through its interaction with copper from the ferroxidase molecule in the blood.[53]

The clinical relevance of these findings is not clear.

Clinical trials

1. Laga M, Plummer F A, Piot P et al 1988 Prophylaxis of gonococcal and chlamydial ophthalmia neonatorum: a comparison of silver nitrate and tetracycline. New England Journal of Medicine 318: 653–657

This controlled clinical trial compares 1% silver nitrate eye drops and 1% tetracycline ointment in the prevention of gonococcal and chlamydial ophthalmia neonatorum in a population with a high prevalence of infection with *C. trachomatis* and multiresistant strains of *N. gonorrhoeae*. This multinational funded study, involving 2732 newborns in Nairobi, Kenya, appears to be the only large controlled clinical trial of these prophylactic agents. Previous trials are critically evaluated in the article; most were of a retrospective case note nature and did not involve comparison with reference groups not receiving the prophylaxis.

The authors conclude that ocular prophylaxis at birth should be directed against neonatal gonococcal infection, not chlamydial infection, and that tetracycline ointment is as effective as silver nitrate eye drops in preventing gonococcal ophthalmia neonatorum.

Other trials

1. Hick J F, Block D J, Ilstrup D M 1986 A controlled study of silver nitrate prophylaxis and the incidence of nasolacrimal duct obstruction. Journal Ophthalmology and Nursing Technology 5: 61–62

This is a controlled double-blind study of a possible casual relationship between the use of silver nitrate prophylaxis in the newborn and the subsequent development of nasolacrimal duct obstruction. The trial involved 145 newborns randomized either to 1% silver nitrate or 1% tetracycline hydrochloride ophthalmic solutions. There was no significant difference in the incidence of nasolacrimal duct obstruction between the two groups at either two weeks or two months, and it was concluded that silver nitrate prophylaxis does not predispose to nasolacrimal duct obstruction in the newborn.

2. Lowbury E L, Babb J R, Bridges K, Jackson D M 1976 Topical chemoprophylaxis with silver sulphadiazine and silver nitrate chlorhexidine creams: emergence of sulphonamide-resistant Gram-negative bacilli. British Medical Journal 1: 493–496

This controlled trial involving 186 patients, of 0.5% silver nitrate compresses, 1% silver sulphadiazine cream and a cream containing 0.5% silver nitrate and 0.2% chlorhexidine digluconate, showed that all were comparably effective in protecting burns from infection. Silver nitrate compresses were much less active against miscellaneous Gram-negative bacilli than the other preparations, and the mean morning and evening temperature and respiration rates in the patients treated with the compresses were higher than those treated with silver sulphadiazine. *P. aeruginosa* and other *Pseudomonas* spp., although rare in all groups, were less often found in patients treated with silver nitrate. Sulphonamide-resistant Gram-negative bacilli became predominant during the trial of silver sulphadiazine cream on extensive burns and the prophylactic effectiveness of that preparation was thus reduced in the later stages of the trial.

General review articles

Armstrong J H, Zacarias F, Rein M F 1976 Ophthalmia neonatorum: a chart review. Pediatrics 57: 884–892

Bernstein G A, Davis J P, Katcher M L 1982 Prophylaxis of neonatal conjunctivitis. Clinical Pediatrics 21: 545–550

Cason J S 1981 Some aspects on prevention and treatment of infection in burns. Progress in Pediatric Surgery 14: 3–18

Dillon H C 1986 Prevention of gonococcal ophthalmia neonatorum. New England Journal of Medicine 315: 1414–1415

Friendly D S 1983 Ophthalmia neonatorum. Pediatric Clinics of North America 30: 1033–1042

Gennaro A R (ed) 1985 Remington's pharmaceutical sciences, 17th edn. Mack Publishing Co, USA

Holmes K K 1976 Gonococcal infection. In: Remington J S, Klein J O (eds) Infectious diseases of the fetus and newborn infant. Saunders and Co, London, ch 14, pp 616–636

Kendray J C 1984 Investigation of the microbial activity of silver salts with particular reference to burn wound therapy. PhD Thesis, University of Strathclyde, Glasgow, UK

Silver nitrate

MacMillan B G 1981 The control of burn wound sepsis. Intensive Care Medicine 7: 63–69

Reynalds J E (ed) 1982 Martindale: The extra pharmacopoeia, 28th edn. The Pharmaceutical Press, London

Richards R M E, Mahlungu G N 1981 Therapy for burn wound infection. Journal of Clinical and Hospital Pharmacy 6: 233–243

S

References

1. Kone B C, Kaleta M, Gullans S R 1988 Silver ion (Ag^+)-induced increases in cell membrane K^+ and Na^+ permeability in the renal proximal tubule: reversal by thiol reagents. Journal of Membrane Biology 102: 11–19
2. Klyce S D, Marshall W S 1982 Effects of Ag^+ on ion transport by the corneal epithelium of the rabbit. Journal of Membrane Biology 66: 133–144
3. Ribarov S, Benov L, Benchev I 1986 On the mechanism of $AgNO_3$-induced lipid peroxidation in erythrocytes. Biomedica Biochimica Acta 45: 321–330
4. Norlind K 1986 Further studies on the ability of different metal salts to influence the DNA synthesis of human lymphoid cells. International Archives of Allergy and Applied Immunology 79: 83–85
5. Richards R M E 1981 Antimicrobial action of silver nitrate. Microbios 31: 83–91
6. Schreurs W J, Rosenberg H 1982 The effect of silver ion on transport and retention of phosphate by *Escherischia coli*. Journal of Bacteriology 152: 7–13
7. Matuk Y, Ghosh M, McCulloch C 1981 Distribution of silver in the eyes and plasma proteins of the albino rat. Canadian Journal of Ophthalmology 16: 145–150
8. Fowler B A, Nordberg G F 1979 Silver. In: Friberg L, Nordberg G F, Vouk V B (eds) Handbook on the toxicology of metals. Elsevier, Oxford, ch 34, pp 579–586
9. Peeters M, Vanden-Berghe D, Meheus A 1986 Antimicrobial activity of seven metallic compounds against penicillinase-producing and non-penicillinase-producing strains of *Neisseria gonorrhoeae*. Genitourinary Medicine 62: 163–165
10. Furchner J E, Richmond C R, Drake G A 1968 Comparative metabolism of radionuclides in mammals — 1. Retention of silver-110 m in the mouse, rat, monkey, and dog. Health Physics 15: 505–514
11. Aaseth J, Olson A, Halse J, Hovig T 1981 Argyria-tissue deposition of silver as selenide. Scandinavian Journal of Clinical Laboratory Investigation 41: 247–251
12. Lambrecht R M, Packer S 1985 Distribution of 110-silver nitrate prophylaxis solutions following eyedrop application to the albino rabbit. Nuclear Medicine Communications 6: 245–247
13. Alexandria J, Aaseth J 1981 Hepatobiliary transport and organ distribution of silver in the rat as influenced by selenite. Toxicology 21: 179–186
14. Moyer C A, Brentano L, Gravens D L, Margraf H W, Monafo W W 1965 Treatment of large human burns with 0.5% silver nitrate solution. Archives of Surgery 90: 812–867
15. Mofano W W, Moyer C A 1965 Effectiveness of dilute aqueous silver nitrate in the treatment of major burns. Archives of Surgery 91: 200–210
16. Cason J S, Jackson D M, Lowbury E J L, Ricketts C R 1966 Antiseptic and aseptic prophylaxis for burns: use of silver nitrate and of isolators. British Medical Journal 11: 1288–1294
17. Moncrief J A 1969 Topical therapy of burn wound. Present status. Clinical Pharmacology and Therapeutics 10: 439–448
18. MacMillan B 1975 The management of burns in children. In: Shirkey H C (ed) Pediatric therapy, 5th edn. pp 1171–1185
19. Davis S K, Bennett R W 1984 Topical treatment of burn wounds. U.S. Pharmacist 9: 39–53
20. Fox C L 1968 Silver sulphadiazine — a new topical therapy for *Pseudomonas* in burns. Archives of Surgery 96: 184–188
21. Forbes B F, Forbes G M 1971 Silver nitrate and the eyes of the newborn. Credé's contribution to preventative medicine. American Journal of Diseases of Children 121: 1–4
22. Barsam P C 1966 Specific prophylaxis of gonorrheal ophthalmia neonaturum. New England Journal of Medicine 274: 731–734
23. Infectious Diseases and Immunisation Committee of the Canadian Paediatric Society 1983 Recommendations for prevention of neonatal ophthalmia. Canadian Medical Association 129: 554–555
24. 1986 Report of the Committee on Infectious Diseases, 20th edn. American Academy of Pediatrics, Illinois, USA
25. Frasen L, Nsanze H, Klauss V et al 1986 Ophthalmia neonatorum in Nairobi, Kenya: the roles of *Neisseria gonorrhoeae* and *Chlamydia trachomatis*. Journal of Infectious Diseases 153: 862–869
26. Rothenberg R 1979 Ophthalmia neonatorum due to *Neisseria gonorrhoeae*: prevention and treatment. Sexually Transmitted Diseases 2: 187–191
27. Oriel J D 1984 Ophthalmia neonatorum: relative efficiency of current prophylactic practices and treatment. Journal of Antimicrobial Chemotherapy 14: 209–220
28. Zola E M 1984 Evaluation of drugs used in the prophylaxis of neonatal conjunctivitis. Drug Intelligence and Clinical Pharmacy 18: 692–696
29. Schneider G 1984 Silver nitrate prophylaxis. Canadian Medical Association Journal 131: 193–196
30. Ortiz J E, Horn M S, Peterson H D 1982 Toxic epidermal necrolysis — case report and review of the literature. Annals of Plastic Surgery 9: 249–253
31. Robertson D B 1984 Excess granulation tissue responses associated with isotretinoin therapy. British Journal of Dermatology 111: 689–704
32. Wolraich M L, Hawtrey C, Mapel J, Henderson M 1983 Results of clean intermittent catheterization for children with neurogenic bladders. Urology 22: 479–482
33. DeJuana C P, Everett J C 1977 Interstitial cystitis: experience and review of recent literature. Urology 10: 325–329
34. Editorial 1985 Chronic interstitial cystitis. Lancet 2: 134–135
35. Bahnson R R 1987 Silver nitrate irrigation for hematuria from sickle cell hemoglobinopathy. Journal of Urology 137: 1194–1195

S

36. Diamond D A, Jeffs R D, Marshall F F 1981 Control of prolonged, benign, renal hematuria by silver nitrate instillation. Urology 18: 337–341
37. Kumar A P M, Wrenn E L, Jayalakshmamma B, Conrad L, Quinn P, Cox C 1976 Silver nitrate irrigation to control bladder hemorrhage in children receiving cancer therapy. Journal of Urology 116: 85–86
38. Jerkins G R, Noe H N, Hill D E 1986 An unusual complication of silver nitrate treatment of hemorrhagic cystitis: case report. Journal of Urology 136: 456–458
39. Bhargava K B, Abhyankar U S, Shah T M 1980 Treatment of allergic and vasomotor rhinitis by the local application of silver nitrate. Journal of Laryngology and Otology 94: 1025–1036
40. Weid U, Halkier E, Hoeier-Madson K, Plucnar B, Ramussin E, Sparup J 1983 Tetracycline versus silver nitrate pleurodesis in spontaneous pneumothorax. Journal of Thoracic and Cardiovascular Surgery 86: 591–593
41. Saidi F, Nazarian M D 1971 Surgical treatment of hydatid cysts by freezing of cyst wall and instillation of 0.5% silver nitrate solution. New England Journal of Medicine 284: 1346–1350
42. Hoffman S 1987 Silver nitrate for skin marking. Plastic and Reconstructive Surgery 80: 755–756
43. Ternberg J L, Luce E 1968 Methemoglobinemia: complication of silver nitrate treatment of burns. Surgery 63: 328–330
44. Strauch B, Buch W, Grey W, Laub D 1969 Successful treatment of methemoglobinemia secondary to silver nitrate therapy. New England Journal of Medicine 281: 257–258
45. Geffner M E, Powars D R, Choctaw W T 1981 Acquired methemoglobinemia. The Western Journal of Medicine 134: 7–10
46. Hill W R, Pillsbury D M 1939 Argyria. The pharmacology of silver. Balliere, Tindall and Cox, London
47. Westhofen M, Schafer H 1986 Generalized argyrosis in man: neurological, ultrastructural and X-ray micro-analytical findings. Oto-Rhino-Laryngology 243: 260–264
48. Marshall J P, Schneider R P 1977 Systemic argyria secondary to topical silver nitrate. Archives of Dermatology 113: 1077–1079
49. Aeseth J, Halse J, Falch J 1986 Chelation of silver in argyria. Acta Pharmacologica et Toxicologica (Copenhagen) 59: 471–474
50. Nishida H, Risemberg H M 1975 Silver nitrate ophthalmic solution and chemical conjunctivitis. Pediatrics 56: 368–373
51. Butterfield P M, Emde R N, Svejda M J 1981 Does the early application of silver nitrate impair maternal attachment? Pediatrics 67: 737–738
52. Anon 1972 Adverse Drug Reaction Bulletin 6: 104
53. Pribyl T, Jahodova J, Schreiber V 1980 Partial inhibition of oestrogen-induced adenohypophyseal growth by silver nitrate. Hormone Research 12: 296–303

Silver sulphadiazine

Silver sulphadiazine is an antimicrobial agent for the topical prophylaxis of burn wound infection.

Chemistry

Silver sulphadiazine (Silvadene, Flamazine, Flammazine)
$AgC_{10}H_9N_4O_2S$
Argentum-N[1]-pyrimidin-2-yl-sulphanilamide

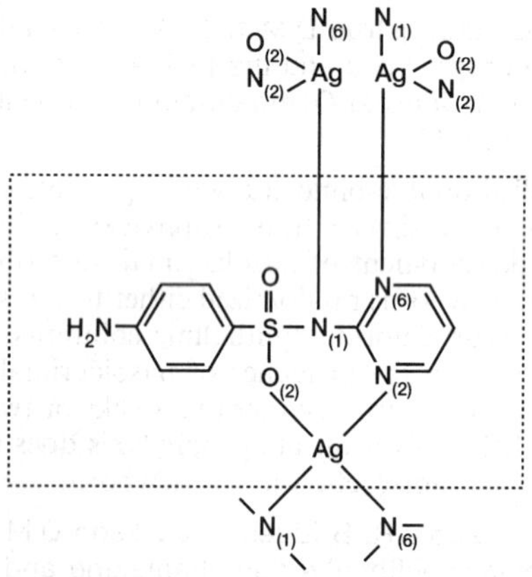

Molecular weight	357.1
pKa	—
Solubility	
in alcohol	—
in water	<1 in 10 000
Octanol/water partition coefficient	—

Silver sulphadiazine is a white, microcrystalline powder, practically insoluble in water. Upon synthesis from sodium sulphadiazine and silver nitrate, the two moieties form a crystalline structure in which each silver atom coordinates to three sulphadiazine molecules, and each sulphadiazine molecule coordinates to three silver atoms.[1] It is available as a combination product Silvazine (silver sulphadiazine and chlorhexidine) in Australia.

Pharmacology

After application of silver sulphadiazine cream onto the burn wound surface the compound acts as a reservoir of silver ions.[2] During continuous dissociation of the molecule most of the released silver is bound to tissue proteins, while unbound silver ions (Ag^+) exert a bactericidal effect on prevalent bacteria. The antibacterial action of silver sulphadiazine is not blocked by para-aminobenzoic acid.

When susceptible bacteria are exposed to silver sulphadiazine, structural changes and weakening of the bacterial cell wall and cell membrane result, leading to distortion and enlargement of the cell, and loss of viability due to interference with macromolecular synthesis.[3–5] Such cell alterations are not exhibited by bacteria resistant to silver sulphadiazine.[5] It has not been clarified whether silver remains bound to the cell surface,[6] or if it also penetrates into the cell and binds to DNA,[7] thereby inhibiting its replication.

Toxicology

In mice, the LD_{90-100} within 24 hours was $\geqslant 550\ mg.kg^{-1}$ when given by a single intraperitoneal injection. Oral or subcutaneous administration of 1050 $mg.kg^{-1}$ per day during 30 days did not result in acute or subacute toxicity or pathological changes in kidney, intestine, liver, or spleen.[8] In rabbits, silver was deposited in the renal pyramids after daily application of silver sulphadiazine (5–15 $mg.kg^{-1}$) for 100 days, while no other structural damage to the kidney or renal impairment was found.[9] Similar effects in humans have not been reported.

Burned mice given mixed Gram-negative infections and treated topically with silver sulphadiazine cream had a lower total white blood cell count, a lower percentage of actively phagocytosing polymorphonuclear leucocytes, and a reduced bactericidal capacity, as compared with cream-base treated controls.[10]

Silver sulphadiazine is not mutagenic in a mutagenicity assay using *Salmonella typhimurium*.[11] There are no published observations of mutagenicity or teratogenicity in animals or man.

Clinical pharmacology

At concentrations of 50 $mg.l^{-1}$ (or less) silver sulphadiazine is active against > 95% of the strains of many bacterial species, including *Pseudomonas aeruginosa, Escherichia coli, Enterobacter cloacae, Proteus morganii, Staphylococcus aureus*, and *Staph. epidermidis*.[12] However, with *Ps. aeruginosa*, in vitro sensitivity does not consistently predict therapeutic efficacy in experimentally infected burned rats.[13,14] Emergence of silver sulphadiazine resistant strains has been reported (see below). The susceptibility of bacteria to silver sulphadiazine is not related to their sulphonamide susceptibility.[12]

The drug is also active against *Candida albicans* and certain other fungi,[15] dermatophytes,[16] and *Herpesvirus hominis*.[17]

Daily application of silver sulphadiazine cream offers a significantly better protection against bacterial colonization of human burn wounds than application every three or four days.[18] The efficacy is higher against colonization than against established infection.[10] There is no systemic antibacterial efficacy.

Pharmacokinetics

Up to 10% of the topically applied amount of sulphadiazine is absorbed. The absorption is higher from deep partial thickness burn wounds than from full thickness burn wounds,[19] due to the avascularity of the latter. Reported serum sulphadiazine levels during therapy are generally in the range of 10–50 $mg.l^{-1}$, although levels of 100–150 $mg.l^{-1}$ occasionally may occur. The concentration of absorbed sulphadiazine can be measured in serum or urine by the Bratton and Marshall method.[20] The specific determination of the parent sulphadiazine as well as its metabolites requires the use of high performance liquid chromatography.[20] The limit of detection of sulphadiazine in plasma using this method is 400 $\mu g.l^{-1}$. For the determination of antimicrobial sulphonamide activity in body fluids, biological assays using suitable bacterial test strains will suffice. The concentration of silver in body fluids can be assayed by atomic absorption spectrophotometry.[9,21]

After a single application of silver sulphadiazine cream to scalds in pigs, less than 1% of the silver is absorbed during the following 48 hours.[22] In humans who had silver sulphadiazine cream applied daily to partial and full thickness burns covering a mean of 47% of the total body surface area, the overall mean serum silver concentration was approximately 300 $\mu g.l^{-1}$ and was twice as high in patients with > 60% burns (upper limit of normal range 200 $\mu g.l^{-1}$). The mean daily urinary excretion of silver was approximately 100–400 μg (normal range < 1 μg), sometimes exceeding 1000 μg in patients with > 60% burns.[21]

Absorbed silver has never been reported as the cause of serious toxic manifestations. No silver deposits were demonstrable by light microscopy or electron microscopy of renal tissue specimens obtained at necropsy of two patients who died from 80% and 90% partial and full thickness burns who had been treated with extensive amounts of silver sulphadiazine cream (up to 12 kg daily) for three weeks.[23] Silver deposits have been demonstrated in the cytoplasm of epidermal cells and sweat glands in a patient who had silver sulphadiazine cream applied for 21 days to a 12% mixed superficial and deep dermal burn.[24] Reversible silver deposits in the buccal mucosa were diagnosed in 2% of the patients in a burns centre, where silver sulphadiazine was applied as an extraordinary highly concentrated suspension (20 or 50%).[25]

Silver sulphadiazine

Absorbed sulphadiazine is excreted in the urine, peak concentrations ranging from 150 to 350 $mg.l^{-1}$.

Oral absorption	
sulphadiazine	⩽10%
silver	< 1%
Presystemic metabolism	
Plasma half life	
range (sulphadiazine)	10–12 h
mean	
Volume of distribution (sulphadiazine)	0.36 $l.kg^{-1}$
Plasma protein binding (sulphadiazine)	29–45%

Sulphadiazine is excreted in breast milk, at concentrations 15–35% of those in serum. Absorbed sulphadiazine may also cross the placenta. Both renal and hepatic disease may reduce the elimination of absorbed sulphadiazine.

Concentration–effect relationship

There are no published studies of a possible association between the in situ concentration of the two moieties during treatment of burns with silver sulphadiazine cream and the effect on the number of colonizing or infecting bacteria.

Metabolism

Absorbed sulphadiazine is metabolized in the liver by N_4-acetylation and by 5-hydroxylation (see Fig. 1).[20] About 50% of the absorbed material is excreted as unchanged drug, with up to 40% as the acetylated metabolite. Absorbed silver, if any, may remain in the body, predominantly in the liver, for long periods of time, being slowly excreted via the bile.

Fig. 1 Metabolism of silver sulphadiazine

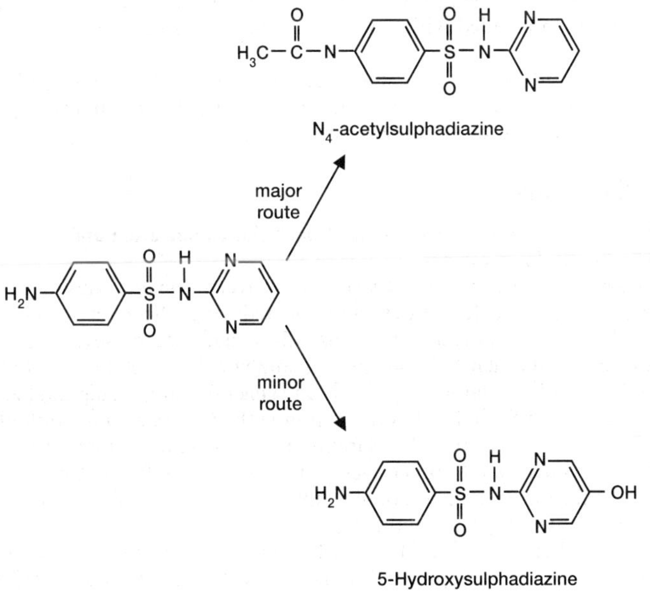

Pharmaceutics

Silver sulphadiazine is commercially available as a 1% (w/w) white cream:

1. Flamazine (S+N, UK)
2. Flint SSD (Boots-Flint, USA)
3. Silvadene (Marion, USA).

In Australia, a 1% cream supplemented with chlorhexidine gluconate 0.2% is available (Silvazine)

Some formulations contain cetyl alcohol and propylene glycol; most formulations contain 0.3% methylparaben. Silver sulphadiazine cream has a shelf-life of three years. It should be stored at 4–8°C.

S

Therapeutic use

Indications

1. The topical prophylaxis against bacterial colonization and infection in burn wounds
2. The topical antibacterial management of certain contaminated or infection-prone wounds, other than burns.

Contraindications

1. A known hypersensitivity against sulphonamides
2. Neonates
3. Lactation
4. Pregnancy.

Mode of use

If early excision and grafting of exposure-treated burns is performed (i.e. on day 3–5 post-burn), topical chemoprophylaxis can be omitted. Many burn centres, however, advocate an observation period of 2–3 weeks before surgical intervention, and under these circumstances topical antibacterial prophylaxis should be initiated as soon as possible after the injury.[10,26]

Silver sulphadiazine cream is applied as a thick layer (1.5–2 mm) onto the burn wound, using a sterile spatula or the sterilely gloved hand. The treated areas should not be covered with occlusive dressings. Alternatively, the cream may be applied onto sheets of tulle gras, which subsequently are placed onto the burn wound.[27] Preferably, the cream should be re-applied daily after cleaning off old cream, or even more frequently, as needed. The period of silver sulphadiazine treatment should extend until spontaneous re-epithelialization has occurred, or until surgical excision and skin grafting is performed.

The burned hand may be treated by daily application of silver sulphadiazine cream, and enclosure in plastic bags or plastic gloves, even on an outpatient basis.[28]

A 75% reduction in nursing time was achieved by spray application of silver sulphadiazine cream.[29] The use of various synthetic dressings, preloaded with silver sulphadiazine, is in an experimental stage.[30]

Treatment with silver sulphadiazine cream does not lead to electrolyte disturbances or acid–base shifts. It is painless upon application, and does not stain bed linen.

Indications

1. The topical prophylaxis against bacterial colonization and infection in burn wounds

In burn patients, the protective effect of silver sulphadiazine cream on bacterial colonization rates, and the reducing effect on infectious morbidity and mortality rates usually equal that of several other topical agents such as silver nitrate, sulphamylon acetate, povidone-iodine, and gentamicin.[19,31–34] In general, silver sulphadiazine cream effectively reduces colonization with *Ps. aeruginosa*, while the effect against various other Gram-negative bacilli is more variable. Against *Staph. aureus* other agents are often more effective than silver sulphadiazine cream, although supplementation of the latter with chlorhexidine appears useful.[35]

Like other agents, the efficacy of silver sulphadiazine in preventing local burn wound sepsis is lower the greater the burn size.[19] The efficacy is also lower in deep burns than in superficial burns.

Accompanying an increasing usage of topical silver sulphadiazine in burns units, clinically significant bacterial resistance may develop, especially in *Enterobacter cloacae*,[45] but also in *Ps. aeruginosa*,[46] and *Providencia stuartii*.[47] The emerging silver sulphadiazine–resistant bacterial strains may also achieve resistance towards sulphonamides in general;[33,34] in one case, the withdrawal of all sulphonamide treatment in the particular ward led to the reappearance of normal sulphonamide sensitivity levels.[48] Reintroduction of the drug, however, was followed by an increase in the rate of sulphonamide-resistant strains.[48] Silver sulphadiazine–resistant strains may carry plasmids capable of transferring multiple antibiotic resistance to other strains,[34,49] while transfer of resistance to silver sulphadiazine has never been identified.

2. The topical antibacterial management of certain contaminated or infection-prone wounds, other than burns

Silver sulphadiazine cream used for prophylactic antiseptic cord care in newborn infants reduced the colonization rate with group B streptococci and Gram-negative rods, but not with *Staph. aureus*.[36]

A reduction of bacterial colonization was found in chronic pressure ulcers treated with silver sulphadiazine cream, as compared with saline dressings.[37] In uncontrolled studies, a similar effect was found in leg ulcers.[38]

Contraindications

1. Known hypersensitivity against sulphonamides

The incidence of possible cross-hypersensitivity between silver sulphadiazine and other sulphonamides has not been determined. In case of a well-documented hypersensitivity towards sulphonamide compounds in a burn patient, the potential risk of provoking allergic manifestations must be weighed against the benefits of using silver sulphadiazine. Apparently, the risk is low. By skin patch testing of 10 subjects having contact allergy to a sulphonamide, none were found to react to the silver sulphadiazine compound.[39]

Adverse reactions

Adverse effects during treatment with silver sulphadiazine cream are rare. They are usually due to absorbed sulphadiazine.

Potentially life-threatening effects

None has been reported.

Acute overdosage

No cases of this kind have been reported.

Severe or irreversible adverse effects

A nephrotic syndrome developed in a 62-year-old male after treatment for a total of eight weeks with silver sulphadiazine cream for a 78% acid burn. A renal biopsy revealed membranoproliferation and interstitial glomerulonephritis. The clinical condition was eventually relieved by immunosuppressive therapy.[40]

Acute leucopenia (total white blood cell counts $<5.0 \times 10^9\ l^{-1}$ or $<3.5 \times 10^9\ l^{-1}$), most probably due to absorbed sulphadiazine, occurs in 3–5% of burn patients treated with silver sulphadiazine cream.[41] In most cases, levels of $2.0–3.0 \times 10^9\ l^{-1}$ were reported, the lowest value being $1.1 \times 10^9\ l^{-1}$, which was temporally associated with a serum sulphadiazine level of 150 $mg.l^{-1}$.[42] The leucopenia is due to neutropenia. The condition is almost exclusively reported for patients with relatively large burns (>30% burned body surface area), and is usually diagnosed after 2–4 days of silver sulphadiazine cream therapy. Spontaneous resolution occurs within 2–3 days, whether silver sulphadiazine is continued or discontinued. No infectious or other complications ascribable to this condition have been reported. An ability of concomitant cimetidine to augment the incidence of leucopenia during silver sulphadiazine therapy has been claimed, but has not been adequately documented.

Crystalluria occurred in none of 345 patients treated with silver sulphadiazine.[19]

Symptomatic adverse effects

Skin rashes have been reported to occur in 2.3% of the patients treated with silver sulphadiazine cream.[19] Hypersensitivity testing of 14 patients allegedly allergic to a silver sulphadiazine cream revealed the cause to be vehicle constituents (cetyl alcohol and propylene glycol) rather than the silver sulphadiazine compound.[39]

Interference with clinical pathology tests

Hyperosmolality with an increased osmolar gap may follow the absorption of propylene glycol; the vehicle of some formulations of silver sulphadiazine cream contains 77 $mg.g^{-1}$ propylene glycol.[43] The condition has been reported only for patients having at least a 35% skin loss, often considerably more; the incidence appears to be 6%.[23,43,44] Renal biopsies, when performed, showed no evidence of specific changes.[23]

High risk groups

Neonates

In the rare case of thermal injuries in neonates, the benefits of using silver sulphadiazine should be weighed against the risk of inducing hyperbilirubinaemia as a consequence of the possible absorption of high amounts of sulphadiazine. In the case of small burns, this risk is negligible.

Breast milk. The sulphonamide concentration in mother's milk is 15–35% of the concomitant level in serum. Females with burns so large that a significant amount of sulphadiazine can be absorbed are usually not able to breast-feed their infants.

Children
Silver sulphadiazine cream can be used safely in children.

Pregnant women
High maternal serum levels of absorbed sulphadiazine during the last week of pregnancy may cause kernicterus in the newborn infant. In case of large burn injuries in a pregnant woman, the threat imposed on the fetus by the burn itself, even if uninfected, and especially if infected, outweighs the risk of inducing kernicterus.

The elderly
Silver sulphadiazine cream can be used safely in elderly people.

Concurrent disease
Silver sulphadiazine should be used with caution in patients with hepatic or renal dysfunction, especially in the case of large burns.

Drug interactions

Potentially hazardous interactions
Absorbed sulphadiazine is a competitive inhibitor of enzymes in the hepatic metabolism of diphenylhydantoins and tolbutamide.

Other significant interactions
In vitro studies have provided discrepant results as to whether topically applied cerium nitrate exerts synergism or antagonism to the antibacterial action of silver sulphadiazine.[50–52] Certain animal experiments[51,53] and clinical trials in burned patients[54] failed to document a superiority of cerium nitrate/silver sulphadiazine cream over silver sulphadiazine cream alone. However, a significantly better protection against bacterial colonization of burn wounds was achieved with a cream containing silver sulphadiazine and cerium nitrate, compared with 0.05% chlorhexidine baths, and the resulting dry firm burn eschar remained intact for several weeks, thereby providing a satisfactory wound cover until tangential excision eventually could be carried out.[55]

The addition of trimethoprim to silver sulphadiazine cream has been shown not to increase the prophylactic effect of the latter.[56]

Potentially useful interactions
The clinical efficacy of silver sulphadiazine cream against colonization, especially with *Staph. aureus*, can be increased by the incorporation of chlorhexidine digluconate 0.2%.[35]

A synergistic action of silver sulphadiazine and topical sodium piperacillin has been demonstrated in vitro and in animal experiments,[57] but has so far not been evaluated in clinical trials.

Major outcome trials

1. Inman R J, Snelling C F T, Roberts F J, Shaw K, Boyle J C 1984 Prospective comparison of silver sulfadiazine 1 per cent plus chlorhexidine digluconate 0.2 per cent (Silvazine) and silver sulfadiazine 1 per cent (Flamazine) as prophylaxis against burn wound infection. Burns 11: 35–40

This is a prospective, randomized, comparative study of the prophylactic efficacy of a 1% silver sulphadiazine cream with or without chlorhexidine digluconate 0.2% (Silvazine and Flamazine, respectively). The patients (54 and 67, respectively) were treated topically for at least 7 days, and the two groups were comparable as to age, and mean (31% and 33%) and range (1–85% and 1–80%) of total body surface burned. The mortality was 6% in both groups. The bacterial colonization rate was significantly lower in patients receiving chlorhexidine (65%) than in those not given this supplementation (88%). Significantly fewer patients in the Silvazine group became colonized with *Staph. aureus* (41%) than in the Flamazine group (64%), while colonization with *Ps. aeruginosa* was diagnosed with nearly equal frequency (15% and 18%, respectively). The overall rate of wound infection did not differ in the two groups (14% and 18%), while wound infection with *Staph. aureus* tended (insignificantly) to occur more frequently in the Flamazine group (7%) than in the Silvazine group (2%).

2. Snelling C F T, Ronald A R, Waters W R, Yaworski D S, Drulak K, Sunderland M 1978 Comparison of silver sulfadiazine and gentamicin for topical prophylaxis against burn wound sepsis. Canadian Medical Association Journal 119: 466–470

This is a prospective trial in which patients having sustained burns > 10% of the total body surface area within 24 hours before admission were randomized on an alternate case basis to receive topical prophylaxis with either 1% silver sulphadiazine cream (38 patients) or 0.1% gentamicin cream (33 patients). Eligible for analysis were 49 adults and 22 children, who all had been treated topically for at least 7 days.

The mortality was 11% and 9%, respectively. Colonization rates with Gram-negative bacilli, Gram-positive bacteria, and *Candida* sp. were 47%, 64%, and 11%, respectively, in the silver sulphadiazine group, and 34%, 25%, and 58% in the gentamicin group. *Pseudomonas aeruginosa* colonized the wounds of 14 patients (37%) in the former group, and in 10 patients (30%) in the latter group; in 2 and 7 of these patients, respectively, the strains were gentamicin resistant. Burn wound infection and septicaemia were diagnosed in 11 (29%) and 4 (11%) of the patients in the silver sulphadiazine group, and in 7 (23%) and 2 (7%) in the gentamicin group. It was concluded that for most burn patients silver sulphadiazine is a safe and effective antibacterial agent.

Other trials

1. Pegg S P, Ramsay K, Meldrum L, Laundy M 1979 Clinical comparison of maphenide and silver sulphadiazine. Scandinavian Journal of Plastic and Reconstructive Surgery 13: 95–101

General review articles

Bult A 1982 Silver sulfadiazine and related antibacterial metal sulfanilamides: facts and fancy. Pharmacy International 3: 400–404

Hoffmann S 1984 Silver sulfadiazine: an antibacterial agent for topical use in burns. A review of the literature. Scandinavian Journal of Plastic and Reconstructive Surgery 18: 119–126

Moncrief J A 1979 Topical antibacterial treatment of the burn wound. In: Artz C P, Moncrief J A, Pruitt B A Jr (eds) Burns. A team approach. W B Saunders, Philadelphia, pp 250–269

Nangia A K, Hung C T, Lim J K C 1987 Silver sulfadiazine in the management of burns — an update. Drugs of Today 23: 21–30

References

1. Cook D S, Turner M F 1975 Crystal and molecular structure of silver sulphadiazine (N^1-Pyrimidin-2-ylsulphanilamide). Journal of the Chemical Society (Perkin Transactions) II: 1021–1025
2. Fox C L Jr, Modak S M 1974 Mechanism of silver sulfadiazine action on burn wound infections. Antimicrobial Agents and Chemotherapy 5: 582–588
3. Coward J E, Carr H S, Rosenkranz H S 1973 Silver sulfadiazine: effect on the ultrastructure of *Pseudomonas aeruginosa*. Antimicrobial Agents and Chemotherapy 3: 621–624
4. Coward J E, Carr H S, Rosenkranz H S 1973 Silver sulfadiazine: effect on the growth and ultrastructure of Staphylococci. Chemotherapy 19: 348–353
5. Coward J E, Rosenkranz H S 1975 Electron microscopic appearance of silver sulfadiazine-treated *Enterobacter cloacae*. Chemotherapy 21: 231–235
6. Rosenkranz H S, Carr H S 1972 Silver sulfadiazine: effect on the growth and metabolism of bacteria. Antimicrobial Agents and Chemotherapy 2: 367–372
7. Modak S M, Fox C L Jr 1973 Binding of silver sulfadiazine to the cellular components of *Pseudomonas aeruginosa*. Biochemical Pharmacology 22: 2391–2404
8. Wysor M S 1975 Orally-administered silver sulfadiazine: chemotherapy and toxicology in CF-1 mice; *Plasmodium berghei* (malaria) and *Pseudomonas aeruginosa*. Chemotherapy 21: 302–310
9. Grabowski B F, Haney W G Jr 1972 Characterization of silver deposits in tissue resulting from dermal application of a silver-containing pharmaceutical. Journal of Pharmaceutical Sciences 61: 1488–1490
10. Roe E A, Jones R J 1977 Leucocyte responses of burned mice given mixed Gram-negative infections and treated topically with creams containing silver compounds. Burns 3: 72–79
11. McCoy E C, Rosenkranz H S 1978 Silver sulfadiazine: lack of mutagenic activity. Chemotherapy 24: 87–91
12. Carr H S, Wlodkowski T J, Rosenkranz H S 1973 Silver sulfadiazine: in vitro antibacterial activity. Antimicrobial Agents and Chemotherapy 4: 585–587
13. McManus A T, Denton C L, Mason A D Jr 1983 Mechanisms of in vitro sensitivity to sulfadiazine silver. Archives of Surgery 118: 161–166

Silver sulphadiazine

14. Modak S M, Fox C L Jr 1981 Sulfadiazine silver-resistant *Pseudomonas* in burns. Archives of Surgery 116: 854–857
15. Wlodkowski T J, Rosenkranz H S 1973 Antifungal activity of silver sulphadiazine. Lancet 2: 739–740
16. Speck W T, Rosenkranz H S 1974 Activity of silver sulphadiazine against dermatophytes. Lancet 2: 895–896
17. Chang T-W, Weinstein L 1975 In vitro activity of silver sulfadiazine against *Herpesvirus hominis*. Journal of Infectious Diseases 132: 79–81
18. Lowbury E J L, Jackson D M, Lilly H A et al 1971 Alternative forms of local treatment for burns. Lancet 2: 1105–1111
19. Baxter C R 1971 Topical use of 1.0% silver sulfadiazine. In: Polk H C Jr, Stone H H (eds) Contemporary burn management. Little, Brown & Co, Boston, pp 217–225
20. Vree T B, Hekster Y A 1987 Sulfadiazine. In: Clinical pharmacokinetics of sulfonamides and their metabolites. An encyclopedia. Antibiotics and chemotherapy, vol 37. Series ed Schönfeld H. Karger, Basel, pp 1–9, 16–24
21. Boosalis M G, McCall J T, Ahrenholz D H, Solem L D, McClain C J 1987 Serum and urinary silver levels in thermal injury patients. Surgery 101: 40–43
22. Lazare R, Watson P A, Winter G D 1974 Distribution and excretion of silver sulphadiazine applied to scalds in the pig. Burns 1: 57–64
23. Bekeris L, Baker C, Fenton J, Kimball D, Bermes E 1979 Propylene glycol as a cause of an elevated serum osmolality. American Journal of Clinical Pathology 72: 633–636
24. Akahane T, Tsukada S 1982 Electron-microscopic observation on silver deposition in burn wounds treated with silver sulphadiazine cream. Burns 8: 271–273
25. Wang X-W, Wang N Z, Zhang O Z, Zapata-Sirvent R L, Davies J W L 1985 Tissue deposition of silver following topical use of silver sulphadiazine in extensive burns. Burns 11: 197–201
26. Salisbury R E, Bevin A G, Steinkraus G E, Enterline D S 1980 Burn wound sepsis: effect of delayed treatment with topical chemotherapy on survival. Journal of Trauma 20: 120–122
27. Lawrence J C 1977 An experimental and clinical evaluation of a tulle gras dressing medicated with silver sulphadiazine. Burns 3: 186–193
28. Sykes P J, Bailey B N 1976 Treatment of hand burns with occlusive bags: a comparison of 3 methods. Burns 2: 162–168
29. Denny A D, Twomey J A, Hitchcock C R 1978 A preliminary report on the spray application of topical silver sulfadiazine to burn wounds. Journal of Trauma 18: 730–731
30. Robb E C, Nathan P 1981 Control of experimental burn wound infections: comparative delivery of the antimicrobial agent (silver sulfadiazine) either from a cream base or from a solid synthetic dressing. Journal of Trauma 21: 889–893
31. Hummel R P, MacMillan B G, Altemeier W A 1970 Topical and systemic antibacterial agents in the treatment of burns. Annals of Surgery 172: 370–384
32. Ollstein R N, Symonds F C, Crikelair G F, Pelle L 1971 Alternate case study of topical sulfamylon and silver sulfadiazine in burns. Plastic and Reconstructive Surgery 48: 311–317
33. Lowbury E J L, Babb J R, Bridges K, Jackson D M 1976 Topical chemoprophylaxis with silver sulphadiazine and silver nitrate chlorhexidine creams: emergence of sulphonamide-resistant gram-negative bacilli. British Medical Journal 1: 493–496
34. Babb J R, Bridges D M, Jackson D M, Lowbury E J L, Ricketts C R 1977 Topical chemoprophylaxis: trials in silver phosphate chlorhexidine, silver sulphadiazine and povidone iodine preparations. Burns 3: 65–71
35. Clarke A M 1975 Topical use of silver sulphadiazine and chlorhexidine in the prevention of infection in thermal injuries. Medical Journal of Australia 1: 413–415
36. Speck W T, Driscoll J M, O'Neil J, Rosenkranz H S 1980 Effect of antiseptic cord care on bacterial colonization in the newborn infant. Chemotherapy 26: 372–376
37. Kucan J O, Robson M C, Heggers J P, Ko F 1981 Comparison of silver sulfadiazine, povidone–iodine and physiologic saline in the treatment of chronic pressure ulcers. Journal of the American Geriatrics Society 29: 232–235
38. Melotte P, Hendrickx B, Melin P, Mullie A, Lapiere C M 1985 Efficacy of 1% silver sulfadiazine cream in treating the bacteriological infection of leg ulcers. Current Therapeutic Research 37: 197–202
39. Degreef H, Dooms-Goosens A 1985 Patch testing with silver sulfadiazine cream. Contact Dermatitis 12: 33–37
40. Owens C J, Yarbrough D R III, Brackett N C Jr 1974 Nephrotic syndrome following topically applied sulfadiazine silver therapy. Archives of Internal Medicine 134: 332–335
41. Gbaanador G B M, Policastro A J, Durfee D, Bleichner J N 1987 Transient leukopenia associated with topical silver sulfadiazine in burn therapy. Nebraska Medical Journal 72: 83–85
42. Wilson P, George R, Raine P 1986 Topical silver sulphadiazine and profound neutropenia in a burned child. Burns 12: 295–296
43. Fligner C L, Jack R, Twiggs G A, Raisys V A 1985 Hyperosmolality induced by propylene glycol. A complication of silver sulfadiazine therapy. Journal of the American Medical Association 253: 1606–1609
44. Kulick M I, Lewis N S, Bansal V, Warpeha R 1980 Hyperosmolality in the burn patient: analysis of an osmolal discrepancy. Journal of Trauma 20: 223–228
45. Gayle W E Jr, Mayhall C G, Lamb V A, Apollo E, Haynes B W Jr 1978 Resistant *Enterobacter cloacae* in a burn center: the ineffectiveness of silver sulfadiazine. Journal of Trauma 18: 317–323
46. Heggers J P, Robson M C 1978 The emergence of silver sulphadiazine-resistant *Pseudomonas aeruginosa*. Burns 5: 184–187
47. Wenzel R P, Hunting K J, Osterman C A, Sande M A 1976 *Providencia stuartii*, a hospital pathogen: potential factors for its emergence and transmission. American Journal of Epidemiology 104: 170–180
48. Bridges K, Lowbury E J L 1977 Drug resistance in relation to use of silver sulphadiazine cream in a burns unit. Journal of Clinical Pathology 30: 160–164
49. Markowitz S M, Smith S M, Williams D S 1983 Retrospective analysis of plasmid patterns in a study of burn unit outbreaks of infection due to *Enterobacter cloacae*. Journal of Infectious Diseases 148: 18–23
50. Rosenkranz H S 1979 A synergistic effect between cerium nitrate and silver sulphadiazine. Burns 5: 278–281
51. Saffer L D, Rodeheaver G T, Hiebert J M, Edlich R F 1980 In vivo and in vitro antimicrobial activity of silver sulfadiazine and cerium nitrate. Surgery, Gynecology and Obstetrics 151: 232–236
52. Holder I A 1982 In vitro inactivation of silver sulphadiazine by the addition of cerium salts. Burns 8: 274–277
53. Fox C L Jr, Monafo W W, Ayvazian V H et al 1977 Topical chemotherapy for burns using cerium salts and silver sulfadiazine. Surgery, Gynecology and Obstetrics 144: 668–672
54. Bowser B H, Caldwell F T Jr, Cone J B, Eisenach K D, Thompson C H 1981 A prospective analysis of silver sulfadiazine with and without cerium nitrate as a topical agent in the treatment of severely burned children. Journal of Trauma 21: 558–563
55. Boeckx W, Focquet M, Cornelissen M, Nuttin B 1985 Bacteriological effect of cerium–flamazine cream in major burns. Burns 11: 337–342
56. Lowbury E J L, Jackson D M, Ricketts C R, Davis B 1971 Topical chemoprophylaxis for burns: trials of creams containing silver sulphadiazine and trimethoprim. Injury 3: 18–24
57. Modak S, Fox C L Jr 1985 Synergistic action of silver sulfadiazine and sodium piperacillin on resistant *Pseudomonas aeruginosa* in vitro and in experimental burn wound infections. Journal of Trauma 25: 27–31

Simvastatin

Simvastatin is a lactone prodrug which is metabolized after oral ingestion to the dihydroxy open acid form which inhibits 3-hydroxy-3-methylglutaryl coenzyme A (HMG-CoA) reductase, an enzyme which catalyses an early rate-limiting step in the biosynthesis of cholesterol.

Chemistry

Simvastatin (synvinolin, MK-733, Zocor)
(1S,3R,7S,8S,8aR)-1,2,3,7,8,8a-Hexahydro-3,7-dimethyl-8-(2-[(2R,4R)-tetrahydro-4-hydroxy-6-oxo-2H-pyran-2-yl]ethyl)-1-naphthyl-2,2-dimethylbutanoate
$C_{25}H_{38}O_5$

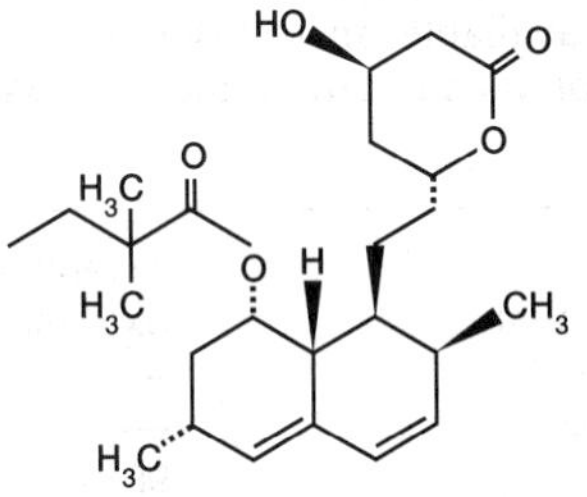

Molecular weight	418.6
pKa	—
Solubility	
in alcohol	freely soluble
in water	almost insoluble
Octanol/water partition coefficient	high

Simvastatin is a white crystalline powder. It is prepared by replacing the 2-methy-butyryl side chain of lovastatin with a 2,2-dimethy-butyryl group. It is not present in any combination preparations.

Pharmacology

Simvastatin is a γ-lactone obtained by chemical modification of lovastatin. Hydrolysis of the lactone by esterases results in the dihydroxy open acid originally designated by the manufacturer as L654,969, now known as simvastatin acid or SVA, which is the active form of the compound. This active metabolite is a competitive inhibitor of HMG-CoA reductase, a key rate-limiting enzyme in the cholesterol biosynthetic pathway. The Ki of inhibition of the solubilized HMG-CoA reductase preparation obtained from rat liver microsomes is approximately 1×10^{-10} M. The enzyme HMG-CoA reductase catalyses the conversion of HMG-CoA to mevalonate.

The main mechanism of reduction of low density lipoprotein (LDL) cholesterol is that, following inhibition of HMG-CoA reductase activity, the LDL receptor density on the liver cells is increased (up regulation) and this leads to an increased removal of LDL cholesterol from the plasma and increased catabolism of LDL cholesterol. In addition there is a reduction in the very low density lipoprotein (VLDL) cholesterol and reduced formation of LDL from VLDL. Inhibition of HMG-CoA reductase does not lead to a build up of intermediary metabolites since this enzyme step is involved early in the synthetic pathway for cholesterol. The precursor HMG-CoA is readily metabolized back to acetyl CoA which participates in many biosynthetic processes throughout the tissues of the body. Two systems have been utilized to demonstrate that simvastatin is an inhibitor of cholesterol synthesis; mammalian cells grown in culture and in vivo studies in various species.

In cultured mammalian cells simvastatin inhibited the incorporation of radiolabelled acetate into sterols with IC_{50} values of 20 nM or less. In Hep-G2 cells simvastatin inhibited cholesterol formation from acetate in a dose-dependent fashion without inhibiting its formation from mevalonate. HMG-CoA reductase activity was increased and the specific binding of LDL to the cells was increased, suggesting increased expression of the LDL receptor.[1] In the rat the drug blocked cholesterol synthesis after a single oral dose with ID_{50} values of less than 0.2 $mg.kg^{-1}$.

Studies have been carried out in the dog to assess the effects of simvastatin on serum total lipoprotein cholesterol. The drug effectively lowers circulating cholesterol in this species, both in the presence and absence of cholestyramine, whereas in rats it has no sustained effect on cholesterol levels. In rodents in vivo other products of the cholesterol synthetic pathway (e.g. oxysterols) inhibit cholesterol synthesis by feed back regulation and during simvastatin therapy this feed back is diminished or removed. The net result in the rat is that HMG-CoA reductase activity is increased so greatly that no fall in serum cholesterol takes place. In dogs treated with 12 g daily of cholestyramine, cholesterol is decreased by an average of 35%. Treatment of these animals with 1 and 2 $mg.kg^{-1}$ daily of simvastatin resulted in an additional 29.1% and 37.6% decrease respectively from the cholestyramine baseline. These effects of simvastatin are primarily on LDL cholesterol in spite of the fact that approximately 70–80% of circulating cholesterol in the dog is in the form of high density lipoprotein (HDL). In the cholestyramine-primed dogs, LDL cholesterol decreased by 57–72% with a 19–38% increase in HDL.

In cholesterol fed (0.25% of diet) rabbits[2] there was a dose dependent inhibition of the increase in serum cholesterol over the range 0.7 $mg.kg^{-1}$ to 6 $mg.kg^{-1}$.

Ancillary pharmacology studies to assess effects on organ systems and biological parameters were conducted with L654,969. No major changes were seen. Minor effects were noted on acid secretion and respiratory parameters in dogs.

Toxicology

The oral LD_{50} of simvastatin in mice is approximately 3.8 $g.kg^{-1}$ and in rats approximately 5 $g.kg^{-1}$.

Hepatic changes have been detected in several species used in toxicity tests. In the rat these changes appeared to be due to proliferation of the smooth endoplasmic reticulum consequent upon induction of HMGCo-A reductase. They were reversible by mevalonate. In the rabbit a dose of 50 $mg.kg^{-1}$ caused a 50% mortality and a high incidence of centrilobular necrosis in the liver and tubular necrosis in the kidney. These changes were prevented by mevalonate feeding. In the dogs there were elevations of transaminases without histological changes and there were no hepatic changes in the monkey.[3] Acanthosis and hyperkeratosis in the rat forestomach and testicular degeneration in the dog appear to be species specific changes.

At very high doses simvastatin causes cataracts in dogs.[4] The amounts of drug in the lenses of animals developing cataracts (<500 $mg.l^{-1}$) were low and there was no change in cholesterol content or sterol composition in these lenses. While there is no clear correlation between the magnitude of serum lipid-lowering and the development of cataracts, a consistent relationship has been observed between high serum levels of drug and cataract development with simvastatin and related HMG-CoA reductase inhibitors. A suggested mechanism is that high concentrations of the drug in the aqueous humor inhibit cholesterol synthesis in the outer cortical region of the lens. There appears to be a wide margin of safety for the human lens, based on either dose or on plasma concentration.

At maximally tolerated doses in both the rat and the rabbit, simvastatin produced no fetal malformations and had no effects on fertility, reproductive function or neonatal development. Other related inhibitors of HMG-CoA, however, including the open acid form of simvastatin (L-654,969) have produced treatment- related skeletal malformations in the fetus. This is thought to be a result of a decrease in the availability of mevalonic acid to the developing fetus.

In vitro and in vivo genetic toxicity tests provided no evidence of an interaction of simvastatin or L-654,969 with genetic material.

In mouse carcinogenicity studies conducted with simvastatin at doses from 1 mg.kg^{-1} daily to 25 mg.kg^{-1} daily, there was no evidence of a treatment-related incidence of tumour types in any tissue. In similar studies in rats a statistically significant increased incidence of thyroid follicular cell adenomas was observed in females receiving 25 mg.kg^{-1} day^{-1} (31 times the maximum human dose). No other statistically significant increased incidence of tumour types was found in any tissues.

Clinical pharmacology

Simvastatin lowers both total and LDL cholesterol in patients with heterozygous familial, familial combined, familial dysbetalipoproteinemia and non-familial (non-FH) forms of hypercholesterolaemia[9] Simvastatin has been shown to reduce both normal and elevated LDL cholesterol concentrations by 25–40% in a dose-dependent manner with doses in the range 10–40 mg daily. Simvastatin also causes a modest reduction (10–15%) of VLDL cholesterol and a rise in HDL cholesterol of similar magnitude. There is a small reduction in concentration of triglycerides in plasma. Apolipoprotein B also falls substantially during treatment with simvastatin. Since each LDL particle contains one molecule of apolipoprotein B, and since little apolipoprotein B is found in other lipoproteins, this strongly suggests that simvastatin does not merely cause cholesterol to be lost from LDL, but also reduces the concentration of circulating LDL particles. As a result of these changes the ratio of total to HDL cholesterol and LDL to HDL cholesterol are reduced. However, Lp(a) levels are not reduced by treatment with this drug or other inhibitors of HMG-CoA reductase[10] Female FH patients with the apoE3E3 phenotype appear to respond better to simvastatin than male patients with the same phenotype.[11]

In a study in 7 normolipidaemic volunteers given simvastatin 20 mg daily for a month, 125-I-labelled LDL and 131-I-labelled cyclohexanedione-treated LDL were used to quantify the receptor pathway. Simvastatin did not modify the synthetic rate of LDL-apo B but increased the catabolic rate of the receptor-dependent pathway and the contribution of this pathway to overall catabolism. It appeared that the fall in LDL could be entirely explained by enhanced fractional removal by the receptor route.[12]

Simvastatin is a specific competitive inhibitor of HMG-CoA reductase. At therapeutic doses, however, the enzyme is not completely blocked, thereby allowing biologically necessary amounts of mevalonate to be available. Steroidogenesis is unaffected although a small rise in ACTH levels has been noted[13] Platelet hyperreactivity in untreated FH patients is decreased by treatment with simvastatin.[14]

Pharmacokinetics

Most pharmacokinetic studies with the drug have been carried out using radioactive tracer doses supplemented by HPLC with UV detection or FAB mass spectrometry.[15] Simvastatin is an inactive lactone which is readily hydrolysed in vivo to the corresponding β-hydroxy acid, L-654,969 a potent inhibitor of HMG-CoA reductase. In some species conversion of the lactone to the open acid occurs in plasma but this 'lactonase' activity is not present in human plasma and the conversion takes place, mainly in the liver. Inhibition of HMG-CoA reductase is the basis for an assay used in pharmacokinetic studies for the β-hydroxy acid metabolites (active inhibitors) and, following base hydrolysis, active plus latent inhibitors (total inhibitors). Both are measured in plasma following administration of simvastatin.

When the availability of L-654,969 to the systemic circulation following an oral dose of simvastatin was estimated using an intravenous reference dose of L-654,969, the value was found to be less than 5% of the dose. By analogy with the dog, simvastatin appears to be well absorbed and undergoes extensive first- pass extraction in the liver, its primary site of action, with subsequent excretion of metabolites in the bile. Availability of active drug to the general circulation is low. Maximum plasma concentrations of inhibitors occur 1.3–2.4 hours post-dose.

In dose-proportionality studies using doses of simvastatin of 5, 10, 20, 60, 90 and 120 mg there was no substantial deviation from linearity of area under the curve (AUC) of inhibitors in the general circulation with increasing dose. The plasma profile of inhibitors is not affected when simvastatin is administered immediately before a test meal rather than in the fasting state.

Pharmacokinetic studies of single and multiple doses of simvastatin showed that no accumulation of drug occurs during multiple dosing.

Both simvastatin and L-654,969 are highly bound to plasma proteins (98%).

In a disposition study with ^{14}C-labelled simvastatin, 100 mg (20 µCi) of drug was administered as capsules (5 × 20 mg), and blood, urine and faeces collected. 13% of the radioactivity was recovered in the urine and 60% in the faeces. Most of the urinary and faecal radioactivity was from metabolites, not simvastatin or the open acid. This suggests that the drug is well absorbed but subject to extensive biliary excretion as the drug is unlikely to be metabolised by gut flora. Less than 0.5% of the dose was recovered in the urine as HMG-CoA reductase inhibitors. In plasma, inhibitors account for 14% and 28% (active and total inhibitors) of the AUC of total radioactivity, indicating that the majority of metabolites are inactive or weak inhibitors.

Tissue distribution studies 4 h after a 1 mg.kg^{-1} intravenous dose in the rat showed high concentrations in intestinal contents and moderate amounts in the liver and kidneys. In dogs given a 60 mg.kg^{-1} radiolabelled dose by mouth the highest concentration 4 h after the dose was in bile (2389 mg equiv.l^{-1}) with substantial amounts in the liver (15.6 µg equiv.g^{-1}) and kidney (8.2 µg equiv.g^{-1}). Amounts in the lens (0.08 µg equiv.g^{-1}) aqueous humor and CSF were very low. Although it is not known whether simvastatin crosses the placenta or is excreted in breast milk, it seems likely that this will occur, given the lipid solubility of the parent compound. No information is available on transfer of the active metabolites. Little simvastatin or its inhibitory metabolites is excreted in the urine.

Oral absorption	extensive
Presystemic metabolism	extensive
Plasma half life	—
Volume of distribution	—
Plasma protein binding	98%

The effects of liver disease on the kinetics of simvastatin are not known.

Concentration–effect relationship

There is insufficient data in man to establish concentration–effect relationships.

Metabolism

Simvastatin (SV) is extensively metabolized in the liver which is also the main site of action of the drug.[16] The paths of metabolism are shown in Figure 1. Metabolite I, 6′-OH-SV, is formed by microsomal oxidation in liver. It is a major metabolite in microsomal preparations. Metabolite II is an allylic rearrangement product of 1 with the with the 6′-OH group moving to the 3' position and double bond rearrangement. Metabolite III is a second oxidation product but with the hydroxyl group in the 3' position of the acyl side chain. It is formed by rat microsomes. Metabolite IV is the triene, 6′- exomethylene-SV. It is a microsomal product and it may be formed by a double hydrogen abstraction catalysed by cytochrome P-450. Microsomal metabolism of these compounds is stereoselective.[17] Formation of simvastatin acid (SVA) occurs as a result of the activity of both microsomal and plasma esterases.

The major metabolites present in human bile are the hydroxy acid form of 3′-OH-SV, and two products of 6′-exomethylene-SV (M-IV), 6′-COOH-SV (M-VI) and 6′-beta-CH2OH-SV (M-V). The acid form of M-II was inactive but M-V and M-VI were active with about 90% and 40% of the activity of SVA respectively. The main product in plasma is simvastatin acid but the main biliary metabolites have also been identified in plasma.

Pharmaceutics

Simvastatin is available only in tablet form.

1. Zocor (MSD, UK) tablets containing 10 mg simvastatin are peach coloured, oval film-coated and marked 'ZOCOR 10' on one side. Tablets containing 20 mg simvastatin are tan-coloured, oval, film-coated and are marked 'ZOCOR 20' on one side.

Simvastatin

Simvastatin is currently marketed in Europe, Australia and South Africa.

Therapeutic use

Indications

1. Primary hypercholesterolaemia in patients who have a cholesterol level in excess of 7.8 $mmol.l^{-1}$.

Contraindications

1. Hypersensitivity to any component of the preparation
2. Acute liver disease or unexplained persistent elevations of serum transaminases
3. Pregnancy and breast feeding
4. Women of child-bearing potential unless adequately protected by barrier contraceptive methods
5. In patients with the homozygous form of familial hypercholesterolaemia, in whom there is a complete absence of LDL receptors, therapy with simvastatin is unlikely to result in clinical benefit
6. As simvastatin has only a moderate triglyceride-lowering effect it is not indicated where hypertriglyeridaemia is the abnormality of most concern (i.e. hyperlipidaemia types I, IV and V).

S

Fig. 1 The metabolism of simvastatin

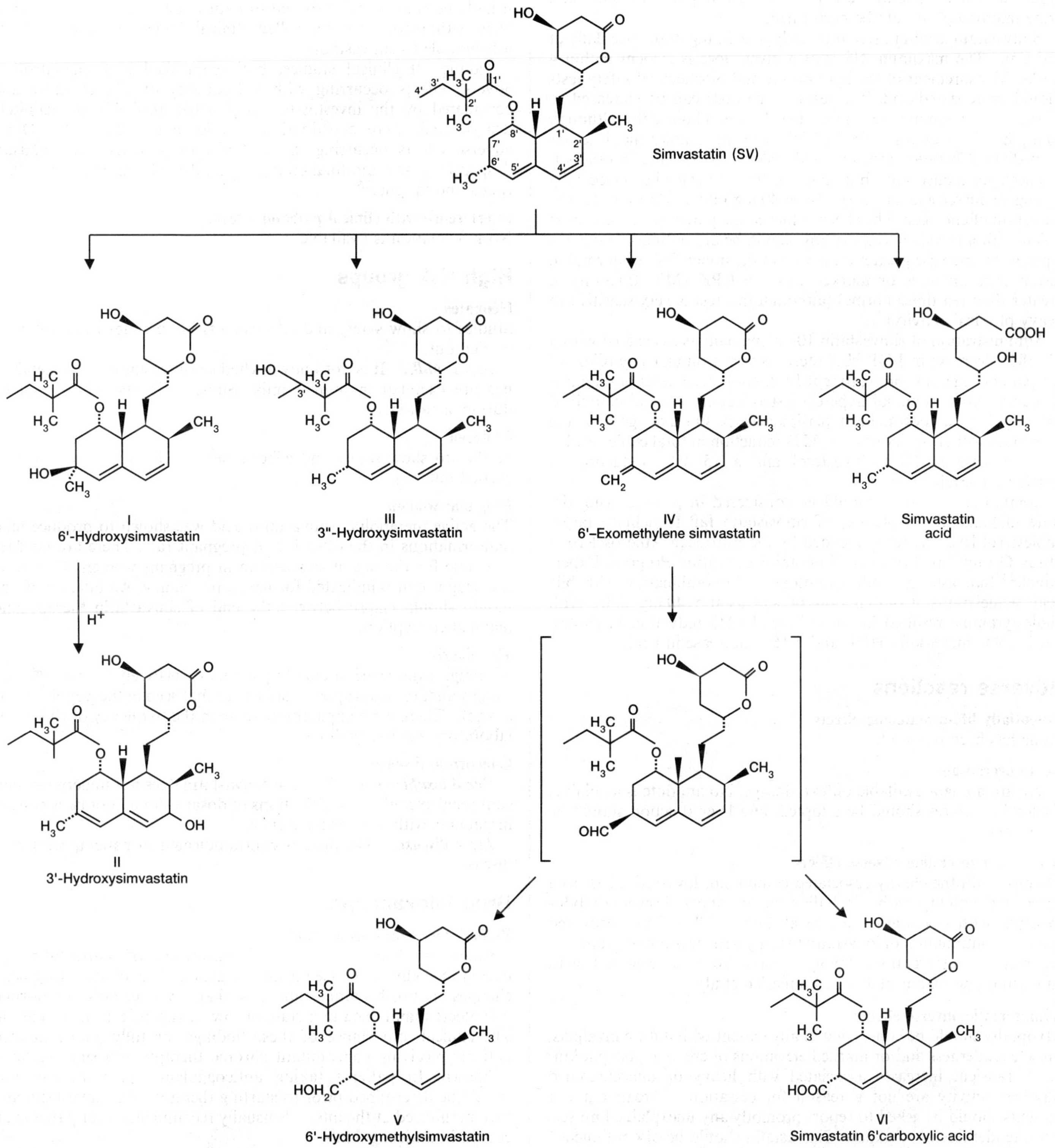

Mode of use

Before initiating therapy with simvastatin, secondary causes for elevated cholesterol values, such as obesity, poorly controlled diabetes mellitus, hypothyroidism, nephrotic syndrome, obstructive liver disease, or drug therapy, should be excluded. It is important to determine whether increased levels of total cholesterol are due to increased LDL cholesterol before initiating treatment. In primary hyperalphalipoproteinaemia (elevated HDL cholesterol), serum levels of total cholesterol may be elevated. Treatment with cholesterol-lowering agents in this instance is not indicated. When total cholesterol is elevated along with marked hypertriglyceridaemia (>5.0 mmol.l^{-1}), the intermediate density lipoprotein (IDL) fraction may be increased. The efficacy of simvastatin has not been evaluated in such patients.

Prior to starting treatment with the drug, patients should be placed on a cholesterol-lowering diet and maintained on it during treatment. Fasting lipids should be measured and, as part of safety assessment procedures, liver function test, plasma creatine phosphokinase and urine microscopy should be performed.

Simvastatin is administered initially as a 10 mg dose once daily at bed time. The maximum effect of a given dose is evident within 4 weeks. Measurement of the lipid profile and biochemical safety tests should be repeated and, if necessary, the dose can be increased to 20 mg. The maximum recommended dose is 40 mg daily although 80 mg has been used in clinical trials. In some studies the dose has been divided between morning and evening doses[8] and in others it has been given once a day but there is little to be gained by twice daily dosing or increasing the dose above 40 mg daily. Once the desired reduction of cholesterol has been achieved the patients can be seen at 2–3 month intervals. Drug therapy should be discontinued if there is a persistent increase greater than 3 times the upper limit of normal in serum transaminases or marked elevated CPK (MM fraction) of greater than ten times normal (although this test is very sensitive to heavy physical activity).

Administration of simvastatin 10–40 mg daily is associated with a 23–38% decrease in LDL cholesterol which is similar regardless of the patients age, sex, pretreatment LDL-cholesterol level or diagnostic classification (familial hypercholesterolaemia, familial combined hyperlipidaemia, polygenic hyperlipidaemia). On average a 40 mg daily dose will bring about a 25–35% reduction in total cholesterol, a 15% increase in HDL-cholesterol and a 15–25% reduction in triglyceride levels.[18–22]

Combination therapy should be considered in patients who, despite maximal doses (40 mg) of simvastatin fail to achieve target cholesterol levels as recommended by the European Atherosclerosis Study Group[23] or National Cholesterol Education Program Expert Panel.[24] Simvastatin is effective alone or in combination with bile acid sequestrants. Combination of simvastatin 40 mg daily with cholestyramine resulted in an additional 12% reduction in cholesterol, a 9% increase in HDL and a 16% decrease in triglycerides.[19]

Adverse reactions

Potentially life-threatening effects
None has been reported.

Acute overdosage
There are no data available on overdosage. No antidote is available. General measures should be adopted, and liver function should be monitored.

Severe or irreversible adverse effects
Therapy with the closely associated compound, lovastatin, has been associated with myopathy, including rare instances of severe rhabdomyolysis with secondary acute renal failure. All patients recovered upon discontinuation of lovastatin therapy with appropriate supportive medical intervention. Myolysis has also been reported with simvastatin (see Clinical Trials, Emmerich et al).

Symptomatic adverse effects
Myopathy should be considered in any patient with diffuse myalgias, muscle tenderness and/or marked elevations of creatine phosphokinase. Transient increases associated with heavy or unaccustomed physical activity are not a reason for cessation of treatment but patients should be asked to report promptly any unexplained muscle pain, tenderness or weakness. Simvastatin should be discontinued if markedly elevated CPK levels occur or if myopathy is diagnosed. Minor asymptomatic transient rises in serum transaminases may occur soon after initiation of treatment. These do not require the drug to be discontinued. There is no evidence of hypersensitivity.

It is recommended that liver function tests be performed before treatment begins, every 4–6 weeks during the first 12 months of therapy and periodically thereafter in all patients. Special attention should be paid to patients who develop elevated serum transaminase levels and in such patients measurements should be repeated promptly and then performed more frequently. If the transaminase levels show evidence of progression, particularly if they rise to three times the upper limit of normal and are persistent, the drug should be discontinued. Liver biopsy should be considered if elevations persist after the drug has been stopped.

Simvastatin should be used with caution in patients who consume substantial quantities of alcohol.

Simvastatin is generally well tolerated and adverse effects have usually been mild and transient in nature. Less than 2% of patients were withdrawn from controlled clinical studies because of effects attributable to simvastatin.

Taking all clinical studies, both controlled and uncontrolled, adverse effects occurring with a frequency of 1% or more and considered by the investigator as possible, probably or definitely drug-related, were constipation, flatulence and headache. Other adverse effects occurring in 0.5–0.9% of patients were: nausea, dyspepsia, gastrointestinal cramps and other abdominal pains, diarrhoea and fatigue.[25]

Interference with clinical pathology tests
No information is available.

High risk groups

Neonates
Studies to show safety and effectiveness in neonates have not been carried out.

Breast milk. It is not known whether simvastatin or its metabolites are excreted in human milk. Simvastatin should be avoided during lactation.

Children
Studies to show safety and effectiveness in children have not been carried out.

Pregnant women
The active metabolite, simvastatin acid was shown to produce fetal malformations in the offspring of pregnant rats. There are no data available for the use of simvastatin in pregnant women. Therefore, the drug is contraindicated for use in pregnancy. An interval of one month should elapse between the end of simvastatin therapy and planned conception.

The elderly
Although experience in elderly patients is relatively limited, efficacy using standard doses appears similar to that seen in the population as a whole. There is no apparent increase in the frequency of clinical or laboratory adverse findings.

Concurrent disease

Renal insufficiency. Because simvastatin does not undergo significant renal excretion, modifications of dosage should not be necessary in patients with renal insufficiency.

Liver disease. The drug is contraindicated in patients with liver disease.

Drug interactions

Potentially hazardous interactions

Coumarin derivatives. The administration of simvastatin appeared to slightly enhance the anticoagulant effect of warfarin (mean changes in prothrombin time less than two seconds) in normal volunteers maintained in a state of low therapeutic anticoagulation. The clinical importance of these findings for fully anticoagulated patients receiving concomitant chronic therapy with simvastatin is unknown. In patients taking anticoagulants, prothrombin time should be determined prior to starting therapy with simvastatin and then monitored at the intervals usually recommended for patients on coumarin anticoagulants.

Simvastatin

Other significant interactions
In clinical studies, simvastatin was used concomitantly with β-blockers, calcium channel blockers, diuretics and non-steroidal anti-inflammatory drugs (NSAIDs) without evidence of clinically significant adverse interactions.

Potentially useful interactions
No information yet available.

Clinical trials

No outcome trial results are available. Many short term studies on hypercholesterolaemic patients have been undertaken.

1. Jones P H 1990 Lovastatin and simvastatin prevention studies. American Journal of Cardiology 66: 39B–43B

An outline of the design of two proposed outcome trials.

2. Emmerich J, Aubert I, Bauduceau B et al 1990 Efficacy and safety of simvastatin (alone or in association with cholestyramine). A 1-year study in 66 patients with type II hyperlipoproteinaemia. European Heart Journal 11: 149–155

The effects and safety of simvastatin were investigated alone or in combination with cholestyramine in 66 patients with hypercholesterolaemia, in a 1-year open study.

In type IIa hypercholesterolaemia (n=41), the association was more effective than simvastatin used alone in lowering total cholesterol (37% vs 29%) and LDL-cholesterol (45% vs 37%). In type IIb hypercholesterolaemia (n=23), combined treatment did not appear more effective than simvastatin used alone. The most serious side-effect was myolysis in two patients.

3. Stein E, Kreisberg R, Miller V, Mantell G, Washington L, Shapiro D R 1990 Effects of simvastatin and cholestyramine in familial and nonfamilial hypercholesterolemia. Multicenter Group I. Archives of Internal Medicine 150: 341–345

Simvastatin was compared with cholestyramine in a randomized open 12-week multi centre study of 251 patients with familial or nonfamilial hypercholesterolemia. Simvastatin, 20 mg and 40 mg daily, produced mean reductions in total cholesterol of 26% and 33%, respectively, and reductions in low-density lipoprotein cholesterol level of 32% and 40%. Cholestyramine resin, 4 to 12 g twice daily, reduced total cholesterol and low-density lipoprotein cholesterol levels 15% and 21%, respectively. High-density lipoprotein cholesterol levels were increased 8% to 10% by all treatments. Plasma triglyceride levels were moderately decreased by simvastatin treatment, while triglyceride levels increased with cholestyramine treatment. Simvastatin was better tolerated than cholestyramine, which caused many gastrointestinal tract side effects. No patient had a serious drug-related adverse event.

4. Tikkanen M J, Bocanegra T S, Walker J F, Cook T 1989 Comparison of low-dose simvastatin and gemfibrozil in the treatment of elevated plasma cholesterol. A multicenter study. The Simvastatin Study Group. American Journal of Medicine 87(4A): 47S–53S

This was a 12-week, randomized, double-blind, multicentre study to compare the efficacy and safety of simvastatin and gemfibrozil in 290 patients with primary hypercholesterolemia. Patients were stratified into those with initial LDL cholesterol level less than 195 mg daily (I)and stratum II with initial LDL at least 195 mg daily. Simvastatin was given as a dose of 5 to 20 mg once daily, gemfibrozil in a constant dosage of 600 mg twice daily. Simvastatin reduced LDL cholesterol levels by 26 and 34 percent in strata I and II, respectively. The corresponding reductions brought about by gemfibrozil were 18 and 17 percent. Both were well tolerated.

General review articles

Maher V M, Thompson G R 1990 HMG CoA reductase inhibitors as lipid-lowering agents: five years experience with lovastatin and an appraisal of simvastatin and pravastatin. Quarterly Journal of Medicine 74: 165–75

Walker J F, Shapiro D R 1990 Hydroxymethylglutaryl coenzyme A reductase inhibitors as monotherapy in the treatment of hypercholesterolemia. American Journal of Cardiology 65: 19F–22F

Walker J F 1989 Simvastatin: the clinical profile. American Journal of Medicine 87: 44S–46S

Todd PA, Goa K L 1990 Simvastatin: a review of its pharmacological properties and therapeutic potential in hypercholesterolaemia. Drugs 40: 583–607

References

1. Nagata Y, Hidaka Y, Ishida F, Kamei T 1990 Effect of simvastatin (MK-733) on the regulation of cholesterol synthesis in Hep G2 cells. Biochemical Pharmacology 40: 843–850
2. Ishida F, Watanabe K, Sato A et al 1990 Comparative effects of simvastatin (MK-733) and pravastatin (CS-514) on hypercholesterolemia induced by cholesterol feeding in rabbits. Biochimica Biophysica Acta 1042: 365–373
3. Gerson R J, MacDonald J S, Alberts A W et al 1989 Animal safety and toxicology of simvastatin and related hydroxy-methylglutaryl-coenzyme A reductase inhibitors. American Journal of Medicine 87: 28S–38S
4. Gerson R J, MacDonald J S, Alberts A W et al 1990 On the etiology of subcapsular lenticular opacities produced in dogs receiving HMG-CoA reductase inhibitors. Experimental Eye Research 50: 65–78
5. Mol M J T M, Erkelens D W, Gevers-Leuven J A, Schouten J A, Stalenhoef A 1986 Effects of synvinolin (MK 733) on plasma lipids in familial hypercholesterolaemia. Lancet 2: 936–939
6. Hagemenas F C, Pappu A S, Illingworth D R 1990 The effects of simvastatin on plasma lipoproteins and cholesterol homeostasis in patients with heterozygous familial hypercholesterolaemia. European Journal of Clinical Investigation 20: 150–157
7. Molgaard J, Von Schencer H, Olsson A G 1988 Effects of simvastatin on plasma lipid, lipoprotein and apolipoprotein concentrations in hypercholesterolaemia. European Heart Journal 9: 541–555
8. Stuyt P M, Mol M J, Stalenhoef A F, Demacker P N, Van 't Laar A 1990 Simvastatin in the effective reduction of plasma lipoprotein levels in familial dysbetalipoproteinemia (type III hyperlipoproteinemia). American Journal of Medicine 88: 42N–45N
9. Bard J M, Luc G, Douste Blazy P et al 1989 Effect of simvastatin on plasma lipids, apolipoproteins and lipoprotein particles in patients with primary hypercholesterolaemia. European Journal of Clinical Pharmacology 37: 545–550
10. Kostner G M, Gavish D, Leopold B, Bolzano K, Weintraub M S, Breslow J L 1989 HMG CoA reductase inhibitors lower LDL cholesterol without reducing Lp(a) levels. Circulation 80: 1313–1319
11. De Knijff P, Stalenhoef A F, Mol M J 1990 Influence of apo E polymorphism on the response to simvastatin treatment in patients with heterozygous familial hypercholesterolemia. Atherosclerosis 83: 89–97
12. Malmendier C L, Lontie J F, Delcroix C, Magot T 1989 Effect of simvastatin on receptor-dependent low density lipoprotein catabolism in normocholesterolemic human volunteers. Atherosclerosis 80: 101–109
13. Mol M J, Stalenhoef A F, Stuyt P M, Hermus A R, Demacker P N, Van 'T Laar A 1989 Effects of inhibition of cholesterol synthesis by simvastatin on the production of adrenocortical steroid hormones and ACTH. Clinical Endocrinology Oxford 31: 679–689
14. Schror K, Lobel P, Steinhagen Thiessen E 1989 Simvastatin reduces platelet thromboxane formation and restores normal platelet sensitivity against prostacyclin in type IIa hypercholesterolemia. Eicosanoids 1989, 2: 39–45
15. Vickers S, Duncan C A, Chen I W, Rosegay A, Duggan D E 1990 Metabolic disposition studies on simvastatin, a cholesterol-lowering prodrug. Drug Metabolism and Disposition 18: 138–145
16. Vickers S, Duncan C A, Vyas K P et al 1990 In vitro and in vivo biotransformation of simvastatin, an inhibitor of HMG CoA reductase. Drug Metabolism and Disposition 18: 476–483
17. Vyas K P, Kari P H, Pitzenberger S M 1990 Regioselectivity and stereoselectivity in the metabolism of HMG-CoA reductase inhibitors. Biochemical Biophysical Results and Communication 166: 1155–1162
18. Simons L A, Nestel P J, Calvert G D, Jennings G L 1987 Effects of MK-733 on plasma lipid and lipoprotein levels in subjects with hypercholesterolaemia. Medical Journal of Australia 147 (2): 65–68
19. Mol M J, Stuyt P M, Demacker P N, Stalenhoef A F 1990 The effects of simvastatin on serum lipoproteins in severe hypercholesterolaemia. Netherlands Journal of Medicine 36: 182–190
20. Antonicelli R, Onorato G, Pagelli P, Pierazzoli L, Paciaroni E 1990 Simvastatin in the treatment of hypercholesterolemia in elderly patients. Clinical Therapeutics 12: 165–171
21. Bach L A, Cooper M E, O'Brien R C, Jerums G 1990 The use of simvastatin, an HMG CoA reductase inhibitor, in older patients with hypercholesterolemia and atherosclerosis. Journal of the American Geriatric Society 38: 10–14
22. Schulzeck P, Bojanovski M, Jochim A, Canzler H, Bojanovski D 1988 Comparison between simvastatin and bezafibrate in effect on plasma lipoproteins and apolipoproteins in primary hypercholesterolaemia. Lancet 1: 611–613
23. European Atherosclerosis Society Study Group 1988 The recognition and management of hyperlipidaemia in adults: A policy statement of the European Atherosclerosis Society. European Heart Journal 9: 571–600
24. The Expert Panel. Report of the National Cholesterol Education Program Expert Panel on detection, evaluation, and treatment of high blood cholesterol in adults. Archives of Internal Medicine 148: 36–69
25. Stalenhoef A F, Mol M J, Stuyt P M 1989 Efficacy and tolerability of simvastatin (MK-733). American Journal of Medicine 87: 39S–43S

S

Sodium bicarbonate

Sodium bicarbonate is a systemic alkalinizing agent. It increases plasma bicarbonate, buffers excess hydrogen ion concentration and raises blood pH, thereby reversing the clinical manifestations of acidosis. It can also be used to replenish electrolyte imbalance as a treatment adjunct for severe diarrhoea where the loss of bicarbonate can be significant.[1,2]

Chemistry

Sodium bicarbonate (sodium hydrogen carbonate carbonic acid, monosodium salt, monosodium carbonate)
$NaHCO_3$

Molecular weight	84.0
pKa	—
Solubility	
in alcohol	insoluble
in water	1 in 10
Octanol/water partition coefficient	—

A white, crystalline powder that is odourless. It has a saline and slightly alkaline taste. It is prepared by the ammonia–soda process, or Solvay process. Carbon dioxide is passed into a solution of common salt in ammonia water, sodium bicarbonate is precipitated and ammonium chloride, being much more soluble, remains in the solution.

It can also be prepared from sodium carbonate.

Pharmacology

Sodium bicarbonate is a salt which on reaction with acid will raise the pH by lowering the concentration of hydrogen ions $[H^+]$:
$NaHCO_3 + HCl = CO_2 + NaCl + H_2O$
Thus sodium bicarbonate is used as an antacid in the stomach or as an agent to increase the pH of the urine or of the whole body.

Toxicology

There is no toxicological data from animal or human studies available. Teratogenicity tests have not been conducted nor have mutagenicity or carcinogenicity tests.

Clinical pharmacology

The bicarbonate buffer system in the body is quantitatively the most important extracellular fluid buffer.

$$H^+ + HCO_3^- \underset{\text{ionic dissociation}}{\rightleftharpoons} H_2CO_3 \underset{\text{carbonic anhydrase}}{\rightleftharpoons} CO_2 + H_2O \text{ (renal)} \downarrow CO_2 \text{ (respiratory)}$$

Alterations in alveolar ventilation can compensate rapidly for metabolic abnormalities, while renal mechanisms operate over a long time course and can compensate for respiratory disturbances.

The Henderson–Hasselbalch equation quantifies the bicarbonate buffer system.

$$pH = 6.1 + \log \frac{[HCO_3^-]}{PaCO_2 \times 0.03}$$

$PaCO_2$ can therefore be plotted against hydrogen ion activity (H^+ or pH) and the various acid–base disturbances described. The total or actual bicarbonate is defined as the concentration of biocarbonate circulating in the blood. The actual bicarbonate is influenced by alterations in the amount of CO_2 and by the metabolic changes in the amounts of acid and alkali in the blood. Measurement of the standard bicarbonate is of more use in acid–base determination. Standard bicarbonate is the concentration of bicarbonate in plasma at a $PaCO_2$ of 5.3 kPa with the haemoglobin fully saturated, at 38°C.

To aid in the correction of acid–base imbalance it is more convenient to calculate the base deficit. The base deficit is defined as the amount of base which would be needed to add to, or subtract from, one litre of extracellular fluid to return the pH value to 7.4 at a $PaCO_2$ of 5.3 kPa at 38°C. As a rough guide, the following formula is used to calculate this correction:

Sodium bicarbonate (mmol) = 0.3 × body weight (kg) × base deficit (8.4% sodium bicarbonate, ml)

In clinical practice half of this value is given and a further acid–base determination made before a further dose of bicarbonate is administered.

There are two types of lactic acidosis, A and B. Type A is commonly caused by hypoxia or anaerobic glycolysis. The clinical management is directed to reversing the tissue hypoxia.

Type B occurs in the absence of tissue hypoxia. It may result from the administration of phenformin in patients in renal or hepatic failure. Other notable causes are diabetic ketoacidosis, severe liver disease, intravenous infusion of fructose or sorbitol, ethanol or methanol ingestion or glucose-6-phosphate dehydrogenase deficiency. Treatment again is directed at removing the primary cause and to the administration of sodium bicarbonate. Large quantities of bicarbonate are required, up to 1000 mmol. The initial therapy is 2–3 l 1.26% (isotonic) sodium bicarbonate followed by the 8.4% solution. These large fluid volumes may precipitate volume overload and pulmonary oedema, making type B lactic acidosis very difficult to treat.

As a systemic alkalinizer the rationale for use of sodium bicarbonate infusions after cardiac arrest was to reduce the metabolic acidosis caused by release of lactic acid. However, over-enthusiastic, blind, administration of sodium bicarbonate may do more harm than good. Where possible, sodium bicarbonate should be administered according to results of arterial/venous blood pH and CO_2 and the calculation of base deficit. If these are not available then 1 $mEq.kg^{-1}$ body weight (1 $ml.kg^{-1}$ 8.4% solution) can be given if deemed necessary. The need for bicarbonate is negligible where proper artificial ventilation and circulation (basic life support) has been initiated early in the arrest and continued effectively. Sodium bicarbonate should never be given to a hypoventilating patient.

In other metabolic acidotic situations an intravenous infusion of 2–5 $mEq.kg^{-1}$ body weight may be given over a period of four to eight hours with frequent reassessment of the metabolic status. Sodium bicarbonate has been used to maintain a neutral pH or alkalosis in the prevention of a sickle cell crisis. Recent studies have shown that such therapy does not significantly reduce the incidence of crisis.[3,4]

Urinary alkalinization can enhance the elimination of drugs such as salicylates and phenobarbitone; 2–5 $mEq.kg^{-1}$ body weight of intravenous sodium bicarbonate given over four to eight hours will raise the urinary pH.[5,6] Alternative formulae for dosage calculation are as follows:
0.5 × body weight (kg) × desired increase in serum $HCO_3^- = HCO_3^-$ dose ($mEq.l^{-1}$)
0.5 × body weight (kg) × base deficit = HCO_3^- dose ($mEq.l^{-1}$)
Give one half of the above calculated estimate and determine the clinical response by pH and blood gas analysis

Sodium bicarbonate has been used as an antacid in patients with peptic ulceration or indigestion but there are now many preferable alternatives. Large amounts of sodium bicarbonate may be needed to alter the pH of the stomach significantly; thus 4.4 g of sodium bicarbonate are needed to raise the pH of 50 mmol of HCl to pH 4.5. The relief of pain is rapid but the release of CO_2 may itself cause gastric discomfort and belching. Excess sodium intake in these patients may be harmful since after absorption it may precipitate oedema and heart failure, particularly in patients with cardiac or renal disease.

Systemic alkalosis can ensue following sodium bicarbonate use (see above).

Sodium bicarbonate

Pharmacokinetics

There is little pharmacokinetic information available. The volume of distribution depends on the acid–base status of the individual. For the purpose of calculation of dosage, it has been assumed that the value of distribution is 50% of body weight (kg). However, on correction, this volume diminishes accordingly.

Once it has entered the body, the action and fate of sodium bicarbonate is identical to that of endogenous sodum and bicarbonate ions. The kinetics are therefore determined by the physiological state of the patient at the time. A sodium depleted patient or one with heart failure or renal failure will retain sodium. A replete patient with normal renal function will eliminate an excess in the urine.

Concentration–effect relationship

The normal physiological range of bicarbonate in plasma is 20–30 mmol.l^{-1} depending on the laboratory standards.

Metabolism

The bicarbonate ion, at a normal concentration of hydrogen ion, is converted to carbonic acid and then to carbon dioxide which is excreted from the lungs. Less than 1% is excreted in the urine.

Pharmaceutics

Sodium bicarbonate is available in oral or intravenous forms.

Oral formulations are tablets or powder containing 300 mg or 600 mg or capsules containing 500 mg.

In its intravenous formulations the following solutions are available (see Table 1).

Table 1

Concentration (% w/v)	Volume (ml)	HCO_3[1] (mtq.ml^{-1} or mmol. ml^{-1})	mσsmol. ml^{-1}
1.26	500	0.15	0.30
2.74	500	0.33	0.65
4.2	10 or 200	0.50	1.00
7.5	50	0.89	1.79
8.4	10, 50 or 200	1.00	2.00

An eye lotion and 5% ear drop preparation are also available. The parenteral dosage form is a sterile, pyrogen-free preparation in the above concentrations. Solutions have an approximate pH of 7.8, which may have been adjusted by means of added carbon dioxide. It is recommended that storage be at 15–30°C and the solution protected from freezing. The optimal shelf-life is 36 months.

There is a sodium bicarbonate mixture, paediatric BPC which contains sodium bicarbonate 50 mg.

Therapeutic use

Indications

1. Management of acidosis in cardiac arrest
2. Management of metabolic acidosis in:
a. severe renal disease
b. uncontrolled diabetes
c. circulatory insufficiency from shock or dehydration
d. severe primary lactic acidosis
3. Alkalinization of urine
4. Local applications for the eye and ear.

Contraindications

1. In hypoventilatory states
2. Chloride depletion due to continuous gastric fluid loss
3. Metabolic or respiratory alkalosis
4. Hypocalcaemia
5. Diuretics known to produce hypochloraemic alkalosis
6. Hyperosmolar states in:

Anuria or oliguria
Oedematous sodium-retaining conditions
Hypertension.

Mode of use

In oral administration the tablet should be allowed to dissolve in the mouth.

Parenteral administration is by the intravenous route either slowly as a bolus or by infusion. Responses should be repeatedly monitored and doses reassessed.

Indications

1. Cardiac arrest

Cardiac arrest is often associated with a systemic acidosis with both respiratory and metabolic components. It was believed that this acidosis exacerbated electrolyte disturbances, antagonized the effects of catecholamines[7–9] and reduced the threshold for ventricular fibrillation.[10] This provided the rationale for the aggressive use of sodium bicarbonate during cardiopulmonary resuscitation.

There have been many measurements of the degree of acidosis following cardiopulmonary arrest. The results have varied widely for although the respiratory component can be estimated, it is impossible to forecast the metabolic component. Thus the dosage schedules for sodium bicarbonate in resuscitation have remained empiric.

Recent studies have indicated that the over-administration of sodium bicarbonate may adversely affect the outcome of resuscitation.[11] Intracellular carbon dioxide, an important factor in myocardial cell function, can be reduced simply by hyperventilation.[12] The administration of sodium bicarbonate will generate more carbon dioxide and may worsen the situation. Furthermore, carbon dioxide may cross the blood–brain barrier inducing a paradoxical central nervous system acidosis.[13] Another detrimental effect from the administration of sodium bicarbonate includes a shift in the oxyhaemoglobin saturation curve with an increase in pH, so as to inhibit the release of oxygen.[14] The induced metabolic alkalosis can itself induce malignant arrhythmias,[15] cause hyperosmolality and hypernatraemia,[16] inactivate simultaneously administered catecholamines,[14] and depress myocardial cell function,[8,12,17] In outcome studies, only one study supports the administration of sodium bicarbonate to improve results.[9] There are several studies that show it does not.[18,19] Current recommendations both from the USA[20] and the UK[21] recommend a decrease in the use of bicarbonate. The suggested initial dose is 1 mEq.kg^{-1} body weight and further administration is to be guided by the measurement of arterial/venous blood pH and carbon dioxide levels; 0.5 mEq.kg^{-1} body weight can be administered every 10 minutes if pH measurements are not available. Sodium bicarbonate should never be given to patients who are not ventilating adequately.

Following administration intravenous lines must be flushed.

Sodium bicarbonate solutions are hypertonic, hyperosmolar and may produce an undesirable rise in plasma sodium concentration. Excessive or too rapid administration may result in the overcorrection of the acidosis resulting in an alkalosis . Severe alkalosis may be accompanied by hyperirritability or tetany.

2. Metabolic acidosis

In other less acute forms of metabolic acidosis, sodium bicarbonate may be added to other intravenous fluid infusions. Parenteral solutions containing calcium ions should be avoided as precipitation may result. The recommended dose is one-half of the calculated requirement followed by reassessment of the acid–base status. If severe symptoms have abated, the frequency and dosage should be reduced. It is unwise to attempt full correction of a low total carbon dioxide content during the first 24 hours, since this may accompany an unrecognized alkalosis due to a delayed readjustment of ventilation to normal. Thus, achieving a total carbon dioxide content of about 20 mEq.l^{-1} at the end of the first 24-hour period will usually be associated with a normal blood pH. Further modification of the acidosis to completely normal values usually occurs in the presence of normal renal function. Total carbon dioxide brought to normal or above normal within the first day may be associated with a grossly elevated blood pH.

3. Forced alkaline diuresis

The elimination of weak acids (e.g. salicylates) by forced alkaline diuresis relies on the principle that the urinary excretion of such drugs is enhanced by altering the pH of the urine in order to increase the degree of ionization of the substance and reduce its lipid solubility.

A regimen of 500 ml sodium bicarbonate 1.26% or 1.4%, 1 l 5%

dextrose, and 500 ml normal saline and potassium chloride 20 mmol is administered over three successive hours and repeated until either the patient regains consciousness or, in salicylate overdosage, the blood level falls to below 500 $mg.l^{-1}$ (3.6 $mmol.l^{-1}$) for adults or 300 $mg.l^{-1}$ (2.2 $mmol.l^{-1}$) for children.

The technique is subject to considerable risk of fluid overload and pulmonary oedema. It is essential to monitor plasma electrolytes, urinary electrolyte and urinary pH repeatedly for it to be effective.

The method has now been superseded by haemodialysis or peritoneal dialysis.

Contraindications

1. Hypoventilation
The respiratory acidosis from hypoventilation should be corrected by improving the ventilation of the patient. Bicarbonate should never be given if the patient is not breathing normally or is not able to respond to a rise in arterial carbon dioxide tension.

2. Chloride depletion
Bicarbonate should not be used in patients losing chloride due to vomiting or a continuous gastrointestinal suction. There is an increased risk of severe metabolic alkalosis.

3. Metabolic and/or respiratory alkalosis
These conditions may be exacerbated by administration of more alkali.

4. Hypocalcaemia
There is an increased risk that alkalosis may induce tetany.

5. Diuretics known to produce hypochloraemic alkalosis
Bicarbonate may exacerbate this alkalosis.

6. Hyperosmolar states
8.4% bicarbonate has a high osmolar value, so use of sodium bicarbonate should be carefully considered in:

a. Anuria or oliguria — because of the increased risk of sodium retention.
b. Oedematous sodium-retaining conditions such as hepatic cirrhosis, congestive heart failure, impaired renal function, toxaemia of pregnancy.
c. Hypertension.

Adverse reactions

Potentially life-threatening effects
The rapid and total correction of acidosis is usually unnecessary and can be accompanied by the following:

1. Compensatory hyperventilation, which may persist for as long as 48 hours, placing the patient at risk of respiratory alkalosis. Should the patient not be able to respond to a raised carbon dioxide level or should respiratory function be compromised then a potentially serious metabolic problem will result.
2. Paradoxical acidosis in the cerebrospinal fluid.
3. Severe hypokalemia, due to the redistribution of potassium.
4. Tetany, from the rapid shifts of free ionized calcium or to serum protein alterations due to pH changes.
5. Volume overload and pulmonary oedema.

The potential lethality of the above is purely a function of the amount administered and the method of use of sodium bicarbonate in a particular patient.

Acute overdosage
Overdosage can occur due to excessive or too rapid administration and will result in a metabolic alkalosis. Severe alkalotic states will be accompanied by hyperirritability and/or tetany.

The management of overdosage is to discontinue the administration of bicarbonate. The control of symptoms can be temporarily alleviated by rebreathing expired air or, if more severe, by the administration of calcium gluconate. In severe alkalosis, an intravenous infusion of 2.14% ammonium chloride is recommended, except in patients with pre-existing hepatic disease.

Relative overdosage occurs frequently, especially when sodium bicarbonate is administered without frequent and constant checking of blood gas and pH results.

Severe or irreversible adverse effects
These have already been described above.

Symptomatic adverse effects
Extravasation of this hypertonic solution may cause a chemical cellulitis, with tissue necrosis, ulceration or sloughing at the extravasation site.

Elevation, local warmth and the local injection of lignocaine or hyaluronidase will limit cellular damage.

Interference with clinical pathology tests
By producing a high urinary alkalinity, bicarbonate may produce a false-positive Labstix test for urinary protein.
Sodium bicarbonate may antagonize the effect of pentagastrin in the evaluation of gastric acid secretory function.

High risk groups

Neonates
Rapid injection (10 $ml.min^{-1}$) of hypertonic sodium bicarbonate may produce hypernatraemia, decrease in cerebrospinal fluid pressure and possible intracranial haemorrhage. A maximum dose of 8 $mEq.kg^{-1}$ daily is suggested, administered slowly in a 4.2% w/v solution (8.4% solution diluted 50:50 with 10% dextrose).

Breast milk
Patients requiring intravenous infusions of sodium bicarbonate are unlikely to be in a fit condition to breast feed. In those receiving the drug orally or in local preparations, no harm is likely to come to the infant.

Children
There are no special precautions except in children under two years of age (see Neonates)

Pregnant women
Safe use during pregnancy has not been established.

The elderly
Sodium retention may result especially if there is concomitant impaired cardiac or renal function.

Concurrent disease
Impaired renal function. This may result in sodium retention.
Congestive heart failure. Cautious administration is necessary as the sodium ion may increase sodium retention and oedema.
Potassium depletion. This may predispose to metabolic acidosis, and co-existent hypocalcaemia may be associated with carpopedal spasm as the plasma pH rises. Chloride loss from vomiting or gastrointestinal tract fluid loss may predispose patients to cardiac arrhythmias due to intracellular shifts of potassium. In these patients careful administration, repeated electrolyte measurements and cardiovascular monitoring may be required.

Drug interactions

Potentially hazardous interactions
Corticosteroids and corticotrophin. Use caution when giving parenteral fluids, especially those containing high sodium ion concentrations. This is especially relevant in patients receiving corticosteroids or corticotrophin.
Alkalis. Urinary alkalinization will increase renal clearance of tetracyclines especially doxycycline.
Calcium. Precipitant haze will occur when added to parenteral solutions containing calcium.
Diuretics. Hypochloraemic alkalosis may occur if used in conjunction with potassium-depleting diuretics such as bumetamide, ethacrynic acid, frusemide and thiazides.
Potassium. Concurrent use in patients taking potassium supplements decreases serum potassium concentrations by promoting an intracellular ion shift.
Other drugs. Sodium bicarbonate increases the half lives and duration of action of basic drugs such as quinidine, amphetamines, ephedrine and pseudoephedrine by alkalinizing the urine.

Potentially useful interactions
Potassium. Sodium bicarbonate reduces serum potassium concentrations by inducing a shift of the potassium ion into the cell.
Other drugs. Alkalinization of the urine by sodium bicarbonate is

used in the management of certain drug overdoses (barbiturates, salicylates, lithium, methanol). It is used in haemolytic reactions to diminish the nephrotoxicity of blood pigments. Similarly, it is used in methotrexate therapy to prevent nephrotoxicity.

References

1. Olin B R (ed) 1986 Intravenous nutrition therapy. Facts and comparisons, Drug information. J B Lippincott, St Louis, Missouri, p 45
2. USP 1987 D I for the health care provider, 7th edn. Easton Pennsylvania Printing Co, p 1576
3. Mann J R, Stuart J 1974 Sodium bicarbonate prophylaxis of sickle cell crisis. Pediatrics 53: 414–416
4. Co-operative Urea Trials 1974 Journal of the American Medical Association 228: 1120
5. Ferrand R J, Green J H, Haworth C 1975 Enteric-coated aspirin overdosage and gastric perforation. British Medical Journal 4: 85–86
6. Smith M J, Dawkins P D 1971 Salicylate and enzymes. Journal of Pharmacy and Pharmacology 23: 729–744
7. Cancy R L, Cingolani H E, Taylor R R, Graham T P, Gilmore J P 1967 Influence of sodium bicarbonate on myocardial performance American Journal of Physiology 212: 917–919
8. Cingolani H E, Mattiazzi A R, Blesa E S, Gonzales N C 1970 Contractility in isolated mammalian heart muscle after acid base changes. Circulation Research 26: 269–278
9. Redding J S, Pearson J W 1968 Resuscitation from ventricular fibrillation. Journal of the American Medical Association 203: 255–260
10. Gerst P H, Flemming W H, Malm J R 1966 Increased susceptibility of the heart to ventricular fibrillation during metabolic acidosis. Circulation Research 19: 63–65
11. Bishop R L, Weisfeldt M L 1976 Sodium bicarbonate administration during cardiac arrest. Journal of the American Medical Association 235: 506–509
12. Weisfeldt M L, Bishop R L, Green H L 1975 Effects of pH and PCO_2 on performance of ischaemic myocardium. In: Roy P, Rona G (eds) International study group of research in cardiac metabolism. University Park Press, Baltimore, vol X
13. Berenyi K J, Wolk M, Killip T 1975 Cerebrospinal fluid acidosis complicating therapy of experimental cardiopulmonary arrest. Circulation 52: 319–324
14. McIntyre K M, Lewis A J 1981 Textbook of advanced cardiac life support. American Heart Association, pp VIII-1–16
15. Lawson N W, Butler G H, Ray C T 1973 Alkalosis and cardiac arrhythmias. Anesthesia and Analgesia 52: 951–964
16. Mattar J A, Weil M H, Shubin H, Stein L 1974 Cardiac arrest in the critically ill. Hyperosmolal states following cardiac arrest. American Journal Medicine 56: 162–168
17. Ostrea E M, Odell G B 1972 The influences of bicarbonate administration on blood pH in a closed system. Clinical implications. Journal of Pediatrics 80: 671–680
18. Telivuo L, Maamies T, Siltanem P, Tala P 1968 Comparison of alkalization agents in resuscitation of the heart after ventricular fibrillation. Annales Chirurgiae et Gynaecologiae 57: 221–224
19. Minuck M, Shamea G P 1977 Comparison of THAM and sodium bicarbonate in resuscitation of the heart after ventricular fibrillation in dogs. Anesthesia and Analgesia 56: 38–45
20. American Heart Association 1986. Standards and guidelines for cardiopulmonary resuscitation and emergency cardiac care. Journal of the American Medical Association 255: 2841–3044
21. Evans T R (ed) 1990 ABC of resuscitation. British Medical Publishers, London, 2nd edn
22. Acid–base balance 1976 In: Weldy N J (ed) Body fluids and electrolytes. C V Mosby Company, St Louis, Missouri, pp 45–46, 52, 115
23. AMA Division of Drugs 1983. Agents used in acid–base disturbances. In: Bennett R (ed) The AMA drug evaluations 1983 5th edn. American Medical Association, Chicago, Illinois, pp 1107, 1110
24. British Pharmacopoeia 1980 (Addendum 1986) Published on the recommendation of the Medicines Commission pursuant to the Medicines Act 1968. HMSO, p 44
25. Cali Thomas J 1983 Acid–base disorders. In: Koda-Kimble M A (ed) Applied therapeutics, the clinical use of drugs, 3rd edn. Applied Therapeutics Inc, Spokane, Washington, pp 622–623
26. Committee of Revision 1985 United States Pharmacopoiea XXI Rev. US Pharmacopoeial Convention, Inc, Mack Printing Company, Easton, Pennsylvania
27. Mudge G H 1980 Agents affecting volume and composition of body fluids. In: Goodman L S, Gilman A G (eds) The pharmacological basis of therapeutics, 6th edn. Macmillan Publishing Co Inc, New York, pp 863–867
28. Swinyard E A 1985 Gastrointestinal drugs. In: Gennaro A (ed) Remington's pharmaceutical sciences — 100 years. Mack Publishing Co, Easton, Pennsylvania, p 796

Sodium calciumedetate

Sodium Calciumedetate is a chelating agent.

Chemistry

Sodium calciumedetate (calcium disodium edetate, Ledclair, Sequestrene)
$C_{10}H_{12}CaN_2\ Na_2O_8.2H_2O$
Calcium disodium ethylenediaminetetraacetate dihydrate

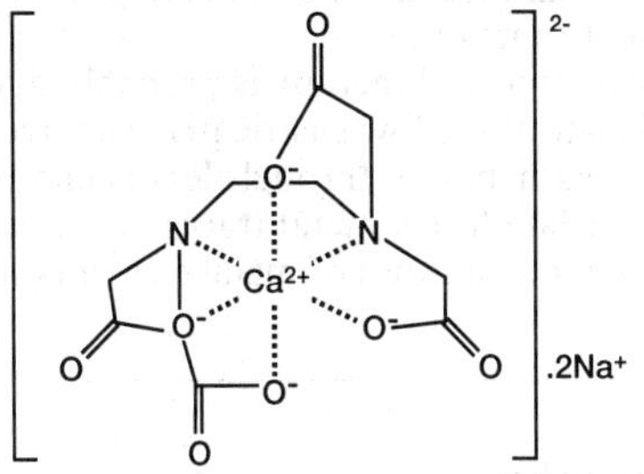

Molecular weight (anhydrous)	410.3 (374.3)
pKa	—
Solubility	
in alcohol	almost insoluble
in water	1 in 2
Octanol/water partition coefficient	very low

Sodium calciumedetate is a white or creamy-white, slightly hygroscopic, tasteless crystalline powder or granules, odourless or with a slight odour and a faint saline taste.

Pharmacology

Sodium calciumedetate is a chelating agent with an ability to combine with metal ions to form anionic, water-soluble complexes or chelates.

Toxicology

Sodium calciumedetate is well tolerated in both single and multiple doses. Experimental animals have tolerated up to 3000 $mg.kg^{-1}$ (mice) intraperitoneally in a single dose, without death, and up to 2000 $mg.kg^{-1}$ (rats) in multiple doses.[1]

The LD_{50} for rats is quoted as 3 $g.kg^{-1}$ by intraperitoneal injection. High values are also obtained in other animals.[2] Death in all cases is characteristic. Animals in their terminal days become anorexic and refuse water with subsequent severe dehydration.

A human with beryllium poisoning has tolerated a total of 99 g in doses up to 10 g per day.[1]

The most important toxic effect is renal tubular destruction which is dose-related, reversible and rarely occurs at doses < 1500 $mg.kg^{-1}$.[1,3]

EDTA is reported to be teratogenic in rats.[4,5] However, this is likely to be a result of zinc deficiency which can be prevented by using zinc supplements.[5] No data are available on carcinogenicity.

Clinical pharmacology

At the pH of the body fluids, EDTA combines with polyvalent metallic ions to form a non-ionized water-soluble complex or chelate which is comparatively stable.[6] When the complex is given either by injection or orally, the calcium is exchanged for metallic ions and the chelate enters all body fluids. EDTA does not enter erythrocytes. EDTA will instantly chelate the metals circulating in the extracellular compartment and those in the parts of the intracellular compartment that it can reach. The rest of the intracellular compartment will then gradually lose its metallic ions as they migrate back into the extracellular fluid across the gradient. The chelate is rapidly and almost completely excreted via the kidneys. Heavy metals can be removed in this way from the plasma, the gastrointestinal tract, soft tissues and bone deposits.

Pharmacokinetics

Oral EDTA is poorly absorbed from the gastrointestinal tract with over 90% usually eliminated in the faeces.[6,7]

EDTA administered intravenously, intramuscularly or subcutaneously becomes rapidly distributed throughout the extracellular fluid. Red cells are impervious to EDTA and it seems likely that many other cell membranes are also.[6,8]

After initial distribution, EDTA appears to become preferentially bound to bone, with delayed release subsequently. It passes slowly into the spinal fluid compartment.[9] Elimination is almost entirely via the kidneys by glomerular filtration and tubular secretion. About 60 to 70% of the drug is excreted within two hours and 90 to 90% within six hours when given intravenously.[9] Estimated half life is 20 to 60 minutes.[3] Renal clearance is approximately 1.5 ml.min^{-1} but is dependent on renal function.

Poor absorption after oral therapy is probably due to dissociation of the calcium chelate at the low gastric pH. The free acid-precipitate slowly redissolves as it passes through less acidic parts of the gut. EDTA will then chelate heavy metal traces in the gut, and may lead to absorption of large quantities of metal elements such as lead from the gut.[7]

Oral absorption	⩽10%
Presystemic metabolism	nil
Plasma half life range	20–60 min
Volume of distribution	—
Plasma protein binding	—

Concentration–effect relationship

One molecule of EDTA is capable of binding one molecule of lead, therefore in theory 0.5 g of EDTA is capable of producing the excretion of about 260 mg of lead. However, the efficiency appears to be low, i.e. less than 0.7% since only 1.8 mg of lead is excreted after 0.5 g of EDTA intravenously.[10] This is probably because EDTA is excreted rapidly into urine whilst the release of lead from its binding sites is slow. A prolonged intravenous infusion may be logical, but does not appear to have been tried.

Metabolism

Calciumedetate is not metabolized, the unchanged drug being eliminated in the urine.

Pharmaceutics

Sodium calciumedetate is available as an injection, in tablet form, as a cream and as eye-drops (Moorfields Eye Hospital, UK).[11]

1. The injection — Ledclair (Sinclair, UK)/Calcium disodium edetate (Riker, USA) — contains the equivalent of 18 to 22% of anhydrous sodium calciumedetate, pH 6.5 to 8, and should be diluted with sodium chloride or dextrose injection before use
2. Tablets contain the equivalent of 500 mg of anhydrous sodium calciumedetate
3. The cream contains 10% EDTA in a water-miscible base.

All preparations must be stored in airtight containers which are lead-free.

Therapeutic use

Indications

1. Acute or chronic lead poisoning
2. Chrome ulceration of the skin
3. Removal of radioactive nuclear fission products.

Contraindications

1. Renal insufficiency.

Indications

1. Acute or chronic lead poisoning

The object in treating patients with sodium calciumedetate is to mobilize lead from the tissues and promote its excretion. Adults and children have been treated successfully in both symptomatic and asymptomatic lead poisoning.

Acute lead poisoning occurs from ingestion of acid-soluble lead compounds, e.g. lead acetate, which have a sweet taste. Nausea, vomiting and diarrhoea may result. Severe abdominal pain is characteristic and stools may be black due to the presence of lead sulphide. With a large ingestion, shock may develop rapidly. Paraesthesias, pain and muscle weakness may occur, sometimes with an acute haemolytic crisis, causing anaemia and haemoglobinuria. Kidney damage with oliguria can precede death within one or two days. Emergency treatment includes gastric lavage/emesis followed by magnesium sulphate to speed passage through the gut. Shock should be treated conventionally. Chelation therapy may then be introduced, as described below.

Chronic lead poisoning (plumbism) may lead to headache, malaise, muscle discomfort and constipation in adults. Persistent metallic taste is an early symptom. Severe exposure may lead to distressing abdominal pain, rigidity of abdominal muscles and tenderness around the umbilicus; muscle weaknesses/palsy may develop after exercise, with wrist drop or foot drop. The most serious manifestation of lead poisoning is lead encephalopathy which is common only in children. First signs may include clumsiness, vertigo, ataxia, headache, insomnia, restlessness and irritability. As encephalopathy develops, excitement and confusion may lead to grand mal convulsions, lethargy and coma. Meningitis, oedema, gliosis and focal necrosis develop. Mortality rate at this stage is 45%; 40% of survivors have permanent cerebral damage.

Commonly, basophilic stippling and microcytic hypochromic anaemia are haematological manifestations.

Blood lead measurements will give a good indication of recent absorption.

Normal values in adults and children in whole blood: 50–250 μg.l^{-1}.

Asymptomatic: 230–400 μg.l^{-1}
Non-specific, mild symptoms: 400–700 μg.l^{-1}
Clear symptoms: >700 μg.l^{-1}
Lead encephalopathy: >1200 μg.l^{-1}

Exposure to lead which occurred six months or more previously may not lead to specific symptoms or increased blood levels. However, it is desirable to estimate the body burden of lead in such individuals. Lead stores are primarily held in the trabecular structure of the skeleton and early evidence suggests that many forms of acute stress can lead to the release of skeletal lead and give rise to symptoms of lead poisoning.[6]

The usefulness of disodium calciumedetate challenge resting in diagnosing subacute lead poisoning has been well documented.[3,12,13] In this test, the total amount and concentration of lead excreted in the urine following drug administration is determined. The output of a normal child after treatment averages 165 μg.l^{-1}. Concentrations in excess of 500 μg.l^{-1} indicate the presence of potentially toxic amounts of lead in the body, and the patient should be investigated further. The diagnostic test is as follows:[14] 75 mg.kg^{-1} of sodium calciumedetate is given intramuscularly with procaine as described therapeutically. The dose is divided into three equal parts given at 8-hourly intervals. Urine is collected for the following 24 hours and the lead content measured.

Once lead poisoning has been diagnosed, using either the challenge test or other conventional methods, and chelation therapy is indicated, the protocol outlined below is initiated.

1 g (5 ml) sodium calcium EDTA is diluted with 250 to 500 ml of sodium chloride BP or injection of dextrose BP 5% and the solution administered slowly by intravenous infusion over a period of one hour. The dose is 60 to 80 mg.kg^{-1} per day given in two equal doses with 8 to 12 hours between each treatment. The therapy is continued for up to five days then repeated after a break of at least 48 hours if

Sodium calciumedetate

necessary. The 48 hour break is necessary to allow redistribution of the lead, thus increasing the amount of lead available for chelation.

Intramuscular injection may be indicated if the patient shows increased intracranial pressure, or if lead encephalopathy is present, thus avoiding excess fluid load. The dosage is as for intravenous therapy. Procaine (without preservative) should be added to give a final concentration of 1.5% of anaesthetic. The total daily dose should be divided into two or four injections.

It is important not to exceed the maximum daily dose of 80 $mg.kg^{-1}$ or to give more than a total of 800 $mg.kg^{-1}$ in the two five-day treatment periods.

Symptoms usually abate rapidly. Abdominal pains may disappear within two hours, muscular weakness and tremor after four to five days. Haematological changes resolve after four to nine days. Urinary excretion of lead is greatest after the first infusion. Adequate renal function is vital and must be maintained throughout therapy.

Oral administration of EDTA is contraindicated in any case of suspected lead poisoning, or indeed prophylactically. There is good evidence[7,17] to suggest that EDTA binds available lead readily in the intestines with the calcium–edetate–lead complex then being absorbed.[17] Thus symptoms of poisoning may be precipitated or increased.[7]

2. Chrome ulceration of the skin

Calcium disodium EDTA has been used successfully to treat chrome ulcers of the skin and nasal septum.[18,19]

Chrome ulcertaion results from penetration of the skin or mucous membranes by chromium in the hexavalent form only. Such chromium compounds are used in the tanning industry.

EDTA cream should be applied to affected parts immediately signs of irritation are present. On the skin, the ointment is applied to the lesion and bandaged. After 24 hours the chrome deposit is shrunk and peeled back from the base where it can be removed, intact by means of splinter forceps. Additional applications may be needed until this is possible. When the nasal septum is involved, ointment ensures healing without perforation. Treatment should be continued until irritation has subsided. Sodium calciumedetate can be applied prophylactically to the nares to prevent subsequent injury.

3. Removal of radioactive nuclear fission products

Early reports of increased urinary excretion of yttrium in rats following administration of calciumedetate has led to speculation on the usefulness of EDTA therapy in accidental ingestion of radioactive yttrium, if given within 24 hours.[20] This suggestion does not appear to have been tested further.

Adverse reactions

Potentially life-threatening effects

Apart from renal failure, described below, no reactions of this kind have been reported.

Severe or irreversible adverse effects

Unlike the closely related compound disodiumedetate, the calcium chelate does not present a hazard to calcium homeostasis. However, transient hypercalcaemia has been observed.[21]

Sodium calciumedetate has been described as relatively non-toxic.[22] Its main toxic actions are on the kidney. Tubular destruction can be produced with very large doses of EDTA.[23] Severe hydropic degeneration of proximal tubules has been observed in rats and man, in some cases with almost total destruction of the proximal tubular epithelium.[3,12] Changes in distal tubules and glomeruli are less conspicuous.

Renal toxicity is dose-related, reversible and only occurs at doses well above those recommended.[24] It may be reduced by adequate diuresis. Sodium calciumedetate should never be given in cases of renal insufficiency.

During chelation therapy, blood and urea creatinine concentrations and liver function tests should be carefully monitored. Increased blood urea and creatinine concentrations signify impending renal failure and treatment should be discontinued. Renal toxicity may be related to the large amounts of chelated metals passing through the tubules in a short period of time. Both dissociation of the chelated metals due to competition or pH changes and the depletion of essential metals from the tubular cells have been suggested as the mechanism of toxicity.[3, 22]

These claims, however, have not been substantiated.

Symptomatic adverse effects

A febrile systemic reaction has been observed in patients 4 to 8 hours post infusion. Characteristically there is an onset of malaise, fatigue, excessive thirst, followed by sudden appearance of chills and fever. This may progress to severe myalgia, frontal headache, nausea, vomiting and rarely, increased urinary frequency and urgency.

Other toxic side effects have included a histamine-like reaction, with sneezing, nasal congestion and lacrimation, glycosuria, anaemia, dermatitis, with lesions very similar to those of vitamin B_6 deficiency, transitory lowering of systolic and diastolic blood pressure, prolonged prothrombin time and inversion of the T-wave of the ECG. The minimal dose required to produce these effects lies between 3 and 5 $mg.kg^{-1}$ body weight, the drug being given intramuscularly at 4-hourly intervals.[21]

Intramuscular injection is extremely painful and therefore a local anaesthetic is included in the formulation.

Patients given long-term courses of disodium calcium edetate may suffer from symptoms of zinc deficiency.[17] EDTA is likely to chelate other trace metals it comes into contact with, but zinc appears to be preferentially chelated and excreted in urine.[7] This may lead to depletion of zinc stores from within cells, bone and tissue stores. If oral EDTA is administered, dietary zinc will also be chelated.

Various mucocutaneous lesions have been described in patients after prolonged administration of EDTA[25] and this has been attributed to zinc deficiency.

References

1. Conference Report 1953 Use of ethylenediamine tetraacetate in treating heavy metal poisoning. American Medical Association, Archives of Industrial Hygiene and Occupational Medicine 7: 137–147
2. Bauer R O, Rullo F R, Spooner C, Woodman E 1952 Acute and subacute toxicity of EDTA salts. Federation of American Societies of Experimental Biology 2: 321
3. Klaasen C D 1980 Heavy metals and heavy metal antagonists. In: Gilman A G, Goodman L S, Gilman A (eds) The pharmacological basis of therapeutics 6th edn. MacMillan, New York, ch 69, pp 1615–1622
4. Hurley L S 1979 Zinc in prenatal and neonatal development. In: Kharash N (ed) Trace metals in health and disease. Raven Press, New York, pp 171–175
5. Swenerton H, Hurley L S 1971 Teratogenic effects of a chelating agent and their prevention by zinc. Science 173: 62–64
6. Leckie W J H, Tompsett S L 1958 The diagnostic and therapeutic use of edathamil calcium disodium in excessive inorganic lead absorption. Quarterly Journal of Medicine 27: 65–82
7. Lilis R, Fischbein A 1976 Chelation therapy in workers exposed to lead. A critical review. Journal of American Medical Association 235, No. 26: 2823–2824
8. Foreman H 1960 The pharmacology of some useful chelating agents. In: Seven M J, Johnson L A (eds) Metal binding in medicine. Lippincott, Philadelphia, ch 9, pp 82–94
9. Foreman H, Tryjillo, B S, Los Alamos N M 1954 The metabolism of C14 labelled ethylenediaminetetraacetic acid in the human being. Journal of Laboratory and Clinical Medicine 43: 566–571
10. Locket S 1957 Antibiotics and antidotes. Clinical Toxicology. Henry Kimpton, London, chapter 7, p 163
11. Reynolds J E F (ed) 1982 Martindale, the extra pharmacopoeia 28th edn. Pharmaceutical Press, p 391
12. Saenger P, Rosen J G, Markowitz M 1982 Diagnostic significance of edetate disodium calcium testing in children with increased lead absorption. American Journal of Diseases in Childhood 136: 312–315
13. Brangstrup Hansen J P, Dossing M, Pauley P E 1981 Chelatable lead body burden and blood lead concentration in man. Journal of Occupational Medicine 23: 39–43
14. Sinclair Pharmaceuticals Ltd. 1985
15. Piomelli S, Rosen J F, Chisolm J C, Graef J W 1984 Management of childhood lead poisoning. Journal of Pediatrics 105: 523–532
16. Chisholm J J 1968 The use of chelating agents in the treatment of acute and chronic lead intoxication in children. Journal of Pediatrics 73: 1
17. Meyboom R H B 1984 Metal antagonists. Dukes M N G (ed) Meylers side effects of drugs, 10th edn. Elsevier Science, Amsterdam, Chapter 24, p 417
18. Maloof C C 1965 The use of edathamil calcium in the treatment of chronic ulcers of the skin. American Medical Association Archives of Industrial Health 2: 123–125
19. British Medical Journal 1963, Chrome ulceration of the nasal septum 1: 1364
20. Vaughan J M, Tutt M L 1953 The use of ethylene diamine tetraacetic acid for removing fission products from the skeleton. Lancet 265: 856
21. Chisolm J 1970 Treatment of acute lead intoxication. Clinical Toxicology 3: 527–540
22. Whitaker A, Austin W, Nolson J D 1962 Edathamil calcium disodium diagnostic test for lead poisoning 29: 381–388
23. Dudley H R, Ritchie A C, Schilling A, Baker W H 1955 Pathological changes associated with the use of sodium ethylene diamine tetra acetate in the treatment of hypercalcaemia. New England Journal of Medicine 252: 331–337
24. Moel D I, Kumar K 1982 Reversible nephrotoxic reactions to combined 2,3-dimercapto-1-propanol and $CaNa_2$ EDTA regimen in asymptomatic children with elevated blood lead levels. Pediatrics 70: 259–262
25. Perry H M, Shroeder H A 1957 Lesions resembling vitamin B complex deficiency and urinary loss of zinc produced by ethylenediamine tetra-acetate. American Journal of Medicine 22: 168

Sodium chloride

Administration of sodium chloride in order to maintain the extracellular fluid volume and to correct any pre-existing losses is a widely available, inexpensive and, when correctly administered, effective and life-saving treatment.

Chemistry and pharmacology

Sodium chloride (salt, common salt)
NaCl

Molecular weight	58.5
pKa	not relevant
Solubility	
in alcohol	slight
in water	1 in 3
Octanol/water partition coefficient	very low

Sodium chloride consists of odourless, colourless cubic crystals or a white crystalline powder with a distinctive taste ('salty' or 'briny'). It is freely soluble in water and slightly soluble in alcohol. The molecular weight of sodium chloride is 58. One gram consists of 17.1 mmol of sodium and chloride. Thus a 0.9% solution of sodium chloride (9 g per litre) contains 154 mmols of sodium and 154 mmol of chloride per litre. This solution is isosmotic with human serum with an osmolality of 308 $mOsm.l^{-1}$. Such solutions are termed 'normal' saline but the less confusing term is 'physiological' saline. By analogy a 0.45% solution is hypotonic compared to human serum and contains 77 $mmol.l^{-1}$ of sodium and 77 of chloride with an osmolality of 154 $mOsm.l^{-1}$. Other solutions available are 3% (513 mmol) and 5% (855 mmol) preparations. Sodium chloride injections are now prepared so that they are sterile, without the need to add preservatives. Sodium chloride is found in a variety of combination preparations.

Solutions are sterilized by autoclaving or by filtration. Domestic or table salt may contain sodium iodide and magnesium carbonate added as an anti-caking agent.

Toxicology

No formal toxicological studies in animals appear to have been carried out at any time.

Pharmacokinetics

Sodium chloride is readily absorbed from the gastrointestinal tract. After absorption there is equilibration with extracellular fluid. The regulation of the extracellular fluid and plasma volume is carried out by the kidney.[1] Under conditions of sodium balance the excretion of sodium in the urine will match intake.[2] This mechanism is under hormonal control and while many hormones may be involved a major role in sodium balance is exerted by the renin–angiotensin–aldosterone system.[3]

Gut absorption of sodium chloride, particularly in the jejunum, is enhanced by the addition of dextrose.[4] This simple aspect of the pharmacokinetics of sodium chloride, and its application by administering glucose or dextrose in oral electrolyte mixtures, has improved enormously the effectiveness of the oral route in correcting electrolyte losses in children with gastroenteritis and in enteric infections, particularly the cholera epidemics still prevalent in the developing countries.[5,6]

Metabolism

Sodium chloride is not metabolized. When in sodium balance, the sodium absorbed is matched by excretion in the urine.

Pharmaceutics

Sodium chloride is available in oral and parenteral forms. Oral forms include sodium chloride tablets and oral rehydration solutions.

Tablets
Sodium chloride tablets: 300 mg (5 mmol)
Slow sodium: enteric-coated slow release tablets contain 600 mg (10 mmol)

Parenteral forms
There is a variety of strengths of sodium chloride for parenteral administration.

Sodium chloride. 0.45%; 76 mmol of sodium and chloride
0.9%; 153 mmol of sodium and chloride (physiological or normal)
3%; 513 mmol of sodium and chloride
5%; 855 mmol of sodium and chloride
20% injection

Irrigation solutions
Sodium chloride eye lotion. A 0.9% solution (900 mg per 100 ml) that is sterile and used to irrigate the eye.

Therapeutic use

Indications

1. The maintenance of daily electrolyte requirements
2. The correction of pre-existing deficits in the extracellular fluid compartment
3. The correction of continuing losses from excessive gastrointestinal (vomiting or diarrhoea) or renal losses
4. The correction of losses from pyrexia or sweating
5. To correct sodium losses in diabetic ketoacidosis
6. In the treatment of hyponatraemic or hypernatraemic states
7. To induce diuresis in poisoning from iodides, bromides, salicylates or barbiturates
8. To alleviate muscle cramps resulting from sodium deficiency
9. As a priming fluid for haemodialysis procedures and in the solutions used in dialysis
10. To maintain intravenous cannulae patency for drug or blood administration
11. As a sterile irrigation solution in cleaning wounds and also in eye lotions
12. To induce abortion by the intra-amniotic injection of a 20% solution.

Contraindications

1. Cirrhosis of the liver
2. Congestive cardiac failure
3. Nephrotic syndrome
4. Acute renal failure
5. Ischaemic heart disease
6. Patients on sodium-retaining drugs e.g. corticosteroids, non-steroidal anti-inflammatory drugs, carbenoxolone
7. Hypertension, including pre-eclampsia.

Mode of use

The method and rate of administration depends on the indications for use and the clinical state of the individual patient. The total amount of sodium chloride to be given over the period of replacement (hourly in small children and seriously depleted adults and over 24 hours in adults) is best given continuously. Thus if 4 litres of sodium chloride containing 600 mmol of sodium are the assessed needs, then a regime of 1 litre in 6 hours is established.

Oral forms such as tablets are best given in divided doses throughout the replacement period.

Indications

1. The maintenance of daily electrolyte requirements
In man there is a wide variety of intakes of salt in the diet. In normal subjects the dietary intake of salt can range from 10 to 200 mmol of

sodium chloride per day.[7] The replacement values that are adopted are thus highly arbitrary. Thus for adults the normal intake of sodium chloride is empirically assumed to be about 100–150 mmol daily. Sodium is lost in sweat but unless this is marked it only accounts for 5–10 mmol per day.

Most normal subjects require between 1 and 3 litres of water in 24 hours. In conditions where the subject cannot eat or drink and cannot be fed by nasogastric tube these daily requirements can be given parenterally. Where food cannot be tolerated but the patient can still drink the necessary sodium and chloride can be administered in a solution. This mode is an important route in children with gastroenteritis.[6]

Sodium chloride solutions can be administered rectally via the appropriate tube if there is no vascular access or the equipment is not available for intravenous use. This route is seldom necessary today but is occasionally of use in paediatric practice and in areas with restricted medical facilities.

The need to provide daily electrolyte replacement exists in patients who are unable to eat a normal diet. Most commonly this is due to recent anaesthesia or bowel surgery in clinical practice. Recurrent vomiting and inability to tolerate fluids is another common indication. Where the gut is functioning normally it is often preferable to use nasogastric or fine-bore tube feeding to provide daily requirements of electrolytes. This avoids the need to use the intravenous route and the potential complications that the cannulae can cause.

2. The correction of pre-existing deficits in the extracellular fluid compartment

The term dehydration strictly implies a loss of water but by convention the crucial loss is that of the extracellular fluid and thus chloride which is the cation that governs the state of the extracellular fluid volume. The mechanisms that regulate osmolarity in man ensure that the balance of water loss to sodium loss is maintained and it is rare for plasma sodium to be altered even when there is marked sodium deficit. Indeed abnormalities of plasma sodium suggest that there is a derangement in the hormonal control of osmolarity or renal sodium handling.

The extracellular fluid volume is regulated by the kidney and if changes do not occur too rapidly for the necessary adjustments an exact balance is maintained.[12] Deficits can only occur if these mechanisms of balance are disrupted due to rapid extrarenal losses or due to a disturbance of renal function.

The extracellular fluid volume together with the intracellular fluid (cell volume) comprise the total body water. This accounts for between 50 and 70% of body weight depending on the composition of that weight. Thus as adipose tissue is relatively free of water there is a lower water content in fat people as opposed to thin and in females compared to males.

In the adult male there is approximately 42 l of total body water and 25 l of this is intracellular while 17 l consists of the extracellular portion. Of this 17 l of extracellular fluid the plasma volume accounts for 3.5 l.[8] As sodium is the major cation of the extracellular fluid it can easily be calculated that if the concentration is 140 $mmol.l^{-1}$ then in the 70 kg lean man there is a total of 2380 mmol of sodium in this compartment. Thus 16 l of 0.9% sodium chloride would replace the total extracellular fluid of the average man.

The basic knowledge of physiology is vital in correctly assessing the losses and pre-existing deficits in the patient who is clinically 'dehydrated'. Under many circumstances the knowledge of actual losses can guide replacement and careful fluid balances and charting of all losses from secretions that are accurately measured needs to be achieved.

The 'clinical' assessment of the degree of dehydration or extracellular fluid contraction can be very difficult and is often imprecise. Just as plasma sodium is well regulated, so is the plasma volume, so that considerable losses of extracellular fluid need to exist before this is reduced.

The best method of assessment of the state of the extracellular fluid volume is the weight of the patient. This presumes, however, that a previous weight is known and that the readings are accurate. Serial weights are an important guide to the replacement of the extracellular fluid.

In hospital practice, and in particular in the intensive care situation, the measurement of central venous pressure (CVP) is another method.[9] This measurement is particularly useful in assessing the relative fullness of the central blood volume as it measures right-atrial pressure. A low reading suggests a diminished plasma volume and thus extracellular fluid volume. A high reading may suggest that there is an already over-expanded extracellular fluid volume or that cardiac function is impaired leading to higher pressures. Unfortunately the measurement of central venous pressure requires the insertion of a catheter and this has its own risks.

In clinical practice at the bedside the measurement of the jugular venous pressure remains the most useful manometer of central pressures. A raised jugular venous pressure (JVP) suggests either cardiac disease or an expanded extracellular space, while an absent JVP is compatible with a reduced extracellular space. By careful observation of the venous pressure during fluid replacement overfilling of the extracellular space can be avoided. This danger is particularly likely to occur in the elderly undergoing forced alkaline diuresis, and in these circumstances extensive monitoring using central pressures and accurate fluid balance is advised.

Clinically mild 'dehydration' or extracellular fluid loss can be manifested by decreased skin turgor and dry mucous membranes. Moderate extracellular fluid volume contraction is marked by an increased severity of these signs together with a reduced intra-ocular pressure, tachycardia, oliguria and postural hypotension. Severe extracellular fluid volume contraction is characterized by a marked increase in the severity of the above signs, with in addition drowsiness and both supine and postural hypotension.

There are many formulae for replacing deficits but the assessment of extracellular fluid volume contraction remains very crude. Two useful rules are:

1. that where there is moderate or severe dehydration it is likely that a deficit of as much as 50% of the extracellular fluid exists and as much as 8–10 litres will need to be replaced and
2. if electrolytes and the clinical state including weight and jugular venous pressure or CVP are serially measured excessive replacement will be avoided.

If the kidneys are healthy then any slight over-estimation will be corrected in time by sodium excretion.

Formulae based on the plasma sodium can be extremely misleading as they often result in inappropriate replacement of sodium when there is only excess water, i.e. dilutional hyponatraemia. In severe contraction of the extracellular fluid, plasma sodium will lower but it can in these circumstances also be high. The plasma sodium is only a measure of the amount of body water that exists relative to the sodium, and cannot be used on its own as a guide to absolute sodium amounts.

3. The correction of continuing losses from excessive gastrointestinal secretions (vomiting or diarrhoea) or renal losses

The most sensible approach is to measure directly where this is possible, or estimate where this is not, the losses from the gastrointestinal tract and in the urine. In hospitals with trained staff, carefully kept fluid balances are very important. To check the accuracy of these charts weighing should be performed. This is essential where fluid balance is critical, especially in patients with renal failure.

In surgical practice, drains into the abdomen are a further means of assessing continuing losses and in medical practice any paracentesis needs to be included. If the bowel is not emptying, large amounts of fluid may remain in the lumen and estimates need to include this. Replacement needs to be with fluid of the same composition of electrolytes. For sodium the compositions of gastrointestinal secretions are:

gastric 20–80 $mmol.l^{-1}$
small bowel 100–140 $mmol.l^{-1}$
bile/peritoneal 120–140 $mmol.l^{-1}$
colostomy 60 $mmol.l^{-1}$
diarrhoea 40 $mmol.l^{-1}$

The replacement of renal losses is best carried out with a knowledge of the urinary sodium concentration analysed in the laboratory. This is extremely variable, depending on the avidity of tubular sodium retention. In general the urine is hypotonic to plasma. Even when patients are treated with diuretics it is very unusual for the urinary sodium to be greater than 150 $mmol.l^{-1}$. Most urines have concen-

Sodium chloride

trations between 20 and 60 mmol.l^{-1}. Correction of renal losses using dextrose and the appropriate amount of saline is particularly important in the polyuric phase of recovery from acute tubular necrosis. Many patients with chronic renal failure also excrete large quantities of urine and these losses need to be replaced to avoid extracellular fluid contraction and acute deterioration in renal function due to this.

4. The correction of losses from pyrexia and excess sweating

The so called insensible losses calculated at 500–700 ml daily for the average adult include respiratory losses and loss from sweating. It is important to remember, particularly in small children with a relatively large surface area compared to body weight, that persistent fever increases fluid requirements by about 12% for each degree centigrade rise.[10] The other aspect of losses with fever is the fact that the vasodilation increases the venous capacitance so that adequate fluid replacement is essential to avoid hypovolaemia. Sweat contains about 30 mmol.l^{-1} sodium. Often replacement in pyrexial subjects is with 0.9% saline to replace not only total sodium losses but the relative deficiency in the vascular compartment because of the associated vasodilation. It may seem logical in severe pyrexia-induced hypovolaemia to use either plasma or a substitute colloid but all of these contain similar amounts of sodium (e.g. Haemaccel, HPPF).

5. The correction of sodium chloride losses in diabetic ketoacidosis

The hyperglycaemia and ketosis of diabetes mellitus when poorly controlled can lead to excessive losses of sodium and water. The coexistence of acidosis has led in the past to the practice of replacement of sodium using sodium bicarbonate. Most clinicians do not use sodium bicarbonate now unless the pH is less than 7.0. Replacement should take place using 0.9% saline. The assessment of the total deficit can be difficult. As a general rule the apparent degree of sodium loss based on the clinical signs discussed above tends to underestimate the true losses particularly in previously fit young adults. In general, in adults in ketoacidosis as much as 8–10 l of extracellular fluid may have been lost. Most regimes advise rapid replacement. It is important to do this in very severe cases but in milder cases a more gradual regimen should be adopted. For severe cases, for example those in coma or about to become comatose, approximately 2 litres of 0.9% (150 mmol.l^{-1} of saline) should be given in the first 2 hours. After this a further litre should be given every 2 hours until about half of the estimated deficit is reached, then the rate should be slowed to 1 l every 4 hours. Once blood glucose has returned to between 10 and 13 mmol.l^{-1} it is important to be able to continue low-dose insulin therapy, and so dextrose/saline can be used to provide glucose yet continue saline replacements.[11] Once the deficit has been replaced it is important to remember that the patient will still require replacement of maintenance sodium chloride.

In diabetic ketoacidosis if the plasma sodium on admission is greater than 150 mmol.l^{-1} or rises above 155 mmol.l^{-1} with replacement, then hypotonic sodium chloride (77 mmol.l^{-1}) needs to be used. Hyponatraemia may be false and reflect an effect of high lipids. Early and regular electrolyte estimations are important in diabetic ketoacidosis. Fluctuation in plasma potassium must be monitored and controlled by appropriate replacement. Most regimes advise waiting until electrolytes are available (within 30 minutes of admission) then giving 20 mmol.l^{-1} with each saline litre adjusting according to electrolytes. There is normally a total body deficit of potassium which needs to be replaced but initially plasma potassium can be high, but will fall often to hypokalaemic levels with saline replacement and insulin therapy.

A recently described complication of diabetic ketoacidosis and its treatment is cerebral oedema.[12] This is probably due to osmotic disequilibrium secondary to the rapid falls in blood glucose. After the initial resuscitation the more gentle correction of fluid and electrolyte deficits and the hyperglycaemia may help to reduce the incidence of this side effect. The cause of this side effect is unknown but it is commoner in children.[13]

6. In the treatment of hyponatraemic or hypernatraemic states

Hyponatraemia implies a decrease in the serum sodium concentration below the normal range of 135–145 mmol.l^{-1} and usually implies an excess of water relative to sodium in the extracellular space. This excess of water can occur with a normal total amount of sodium and chloride and indeed this is the most common cause — 'dilutional hyponatraemia'. There can also be in addition to excess water an excess of total body sodium and chloride in the extracellular fluid which can manifest as oedema and is seen in some subjects with cirrhosis of the liver, congestive cardiac failure, nephrotic syndrome and toxaemia of pregnancy. It is readily apparent in all these dilutional hyponatraemic states, which are often associated with inappropriately high levels of ADH, that the treatment should be water restriction or attempts to produce water loss.

Severe sodium depletion can produce a hyponatraemic state, particularly if there is replacement of sodium losses with water on its own. The most common cause of this type of hyponatraemia is the over-zealous use of diuretics. Treatment of this group involves correcting the extracellular fluid deficit. This may be done by simply stopping the diuretics. If the deficiency is severe, replacement with saline is indicated. A hypertonic solution (3%) is logical in this group although many correct with an isotonic solution combined with water restriction.

Hypertonic solutions are used in clinical situations where symptoms of water intoxication are apparent. These usually do not occur until serum sodium falls below 120 mmol.l^{-1}. The amount of sodium sufficient to raise the serum sodium concentration to about 120–125 mmol.l^{-1} should be given over 12 hours.[14] The rate of replacement should be gradual and most experts advise that it should never exceed 0.7 mmol.l^{-1} per hour, as there have been suggestions that too rapid correction can contribute to the long-term neurological deficits that can follow these cases. To work out the amount of sodium (mmol.l^{-1}) necessary to raise the serum level to 125 mmol.l^{-1} the deficit (125 − measured plasma Na) can be multiplied by the total body water (60% of body weight in kg). In severe hyponatraemia with symptoms, where there is concomitant ECF expansion, the use of hypertonic sodium chloride should be combined with frusemide.

Hypernatraemia represents an elevation of the serum sodium concentration above the normal range and indicates a deficit of body water relative to sodium. The mechanisms of thirst normally protect from this, so that those at risk are infants, the elderly and confused or comatose patients. Urine tends to be hypotonic so excess losses with inadequate water intake can lead to this state. This is rarely seen in ADH deficiency, the polyuric phase of the recovery from acute renal failure and in hypercalcaemic and hypokalaemic states. Probably the commonest cause in clinical practice is the syndrome of hyperglycaemic (hyperosmolar) non-ketotic diabetic pre-coma and coma. In this circumstance there is a loss of total body sodium and chloride but greater losses of water due to the glycosuria.

Treatment consists of water replacement and, if there is an associated sodium depletion, restoration of the extracellular fluid. In the hyperglycaemic hyperosmolar syndrome 0.45% sodium chloride solutions should be used. The hypernatraemia should be corrected slowly over a period of 24–48 hours, otherwise the osmotic shifts can cause cerebral oedema.[15]

7. To induce diuresis in poisoning from salicylates, barbiturates, iodides and bromides

Standard treatment for these poisonings is to use a forced alkaline diuresis.[16] Indications are salicylates with levels > 500 mg.l^{-1} or barbiturates[17] if severe and the patient is unconscious and only if barbitone or phenobarbitone has been taken. This procedure involves using large volumes of fluid intravenously and has inherent danger in patients with heart failure, impaired renal function, or the elderly. In all cases regular examination of the patient, with accurate records of fluid intake and urine output and pH, needs to be maintained. In many circumstances it is appropriate to carry out this process in the intensive care unit or with the provision of an experienced nurse if this is to be attempted in the ward setting. Patients should be catheterized only if unconscious.

Many regimes are proposed. One simple regime is to infuse 500 ml 1.4% sodium bicarbonate, 500 ml 0.9% saline and 500 ml 5% dextrose in rotation at a rate of 2 litres per hour for 3 hours, then 1 litre per hour. Add 15 mmol of potassium chloride to each 500 ml of fluid after the first hour. Urine output and urine pH need to be assessed hourly. If the output is below 4 ml per min in the first hour the state of hydration should be reassessed. It is probably important at this stage to consider monitoring using a CVP line to do this accurately. If the patient is dehydrated and CVP is low, increase the

Sodium chloride

rate of saline infusion. If CVP is normal or high, frusemide, 40 mg intravenously can be tried but if there is no response the infusion should be stopped. At this stage in those with very high levels (>900 mg.l^{-1}) if the facilities for haemodialysis are available this may be the most appropriate method of treatment.

In forced alkaline diuresis it is very important to actually achieve alkalinization of the urine above 7.5, preferably 8.0–8.5. In the regime substitute 1.4% sodium bicarbonate for 0.9% saline until this is achieved. The forced diuresis should be continued until salicylate levels are below 400 mg.l^{-1} or, in phenobarbitone overdose, until the patient has recovered. Plasma electrolytes should be monitored at 2 hours and then 4 hourly during these procedures. When giving large amounts of bicarbonate and increasing blood pH it is important to correct for any potassium deficit, and often the administration of potassium will allow the development of satisfactory urinary alkalinization.[16]

8. To alleviate muscle cramps resulting from sodium deficiency

In hot climates where sweating can result in losses that are then not replaced, sodium deficiency has been implicated as a cause of muscle cramps. Slow-release sodium tablets (enteric-coated) can be used to supplement sodium intake if this cannot be taken adequately in the diet. Adequate sodium replacement has been found to be particularly important in athletes in hot climates. Adequate sodium replacement is important during haemodialysis to prevent muscular cramps.[18]

9. As a priming fluid for haemodialysis procedures and in solutions used in renal dialysis

Because of its similar composition to plasma sodium concentrations, 0.9% saline is often used to start infusions and to prime equipment before haemodialysis, peritoneal dialysis or haemofiltration procedures. Sodium chloride solutions also form part of the dialysis fluid used and the concentration is altered according to the assessment of the extracellular space of the patient undergoing dialysis.

10. To maintain intravenous cannulae patency for drug or blood administration

A common use of sodium chloride (0.9% or 150 mmol.l^{-1}) is to maintain the patency of intravenous cannulae prior to their use for drug or blood administration or where frequent blood sampling is necessary. Mixtures of heparin and saline are used where long periods between sampling or administration occur.

11. As a sterile irrigation solution in cleaning wounds and as an irrigation solution for eye lotions

0.9% saline is used because it is isosmotic with plasma, as an irrigation fluid for cleaning wounds and burns. It is also available for bathing the eyes. Salt baths remain a recommended treatment after surgery. Domestic salt suffices for this mild antiseptic purpose.

12. To induce abortion by the intra-amniotic injection of a 20% solution

Injections of 20% sodium chloride have been used by transabdominal intra-amniotic installation to induce abortion late in the second trimester of pregnancy (beyond the sixteenth week of gestation). This method is effective and abortion could be produced in about 91% of patients within 72 hours. It has been used in conjunction with oxytocin infusion. It has largely been replaced in modern practice by the use of prostaglandins to induce second trimester abortions.

Contraindications

1. Cirrhosis of the liver

Sodium retention in cirrhosis may be apparent in those decompensated with ascites or oedema. Administration of further sodium chloride will just further increase the extracellular space. Hypovolaemia in patients with cirrhosis should be corrected with blood, plasma or salt-free albumin solutions. Hyponatraemia does not reflect a reduced amount of sodium, and is a reflection of increased total body water and a dilutional effect despite the excess body sodium.

2. Congestive cardiac failure

Oedema in patients with congestive cardiac failure implies an expanded extracellular fluid space. Further sodium chloride administration will make this situation worse. Hyponatraemia is common in congestive cardiac failure and is particularly seen when diuretics have been used. The fact that it often co-exists with peripheral oedema shows that it is not reflecting a reduced total body sodium and is a reflection of an increased total body water. This problem can be particularly difficult in the elderly with apparently 'dry' membranes or loss of skin turgor, yet in whom there is congestive failure with high venous pressures and oedema. In this group, saline replacement given inappropriately can often precipitate worsening of left ventricular failure.

3. Nephrotic syndrome

The increased extracellular fluid space in this condition, and the marked oedema, represent a contraindication to the further administration of sodium and chloride. Renal tubular sodium retention is an important patho-physiological feature of this disease.

4. Acute renal failure

In established renal failure, when it is certain that the extracellular fluid and plasma volume are normal, further sodium chloride cannot be eliminated and should not be given. In practical terms it is often necessary to check that the extracellular fluid volume is replete by the measurement of central venous pressure.

5. Ischaemic heart disease

Impaired cardiac function and left ventricular performance increases pulmonary capillary pressures and can lead to oedema. Excess sodium chloride administration will aggravate these processes and can lead to pulmonary oedema. Caution should be used in fluid replacement in all subjects with ischaemic heart disease. Where there is a recognized deficit in extracellular fluid volume that needs to be corrected it is safest to use central venous pressure monitoring or, where this facility is not available, to replace any deficits slowly with careful clinical observation of signs of rises in the jugular venous pressure or pulmonary oedema.

6. Patients on sodium-retaining drugs

The administration of sodium chloride to patients on drugs which cause sodium retention can lead to excessive accumulation of extracellular fluid and oedema. Non-steroidal anti-inflammatory drugs and steroids are the most commonly used sodium-retaining drugs.

7. Hypertension

The role of sodium chloride in the pathogenesis of hypertension is much debated. There is evidence to support a link between high salt intake and prevalence of hypertension. It is sensible advice to be cautious in sodium chloride replacement in subjects with hypertension. If renal disease is the cause of the hypertension then sodium retention is often the patho-physiological mechanism that sustains it.

Adverse reactions

Potentially life-threatening effects

Sodium chloride is a major constituent of the human body so that any toxic effects are simply due to inappropriate and excessive replacement. The contraindications include disease states with an already expanded extracellular fluid volume and those with inability to excrete sodium rapidly due to kidney dysfunction.

Acute overdosage

Excess ingestion of sodium chloride is occasionally seen in suicidal patients as an attempted overdose. More commonly, it is a paediatric presentation as accidental ingestion. On occasions it is due to the mistaking of salt for sugar.[19] Hyperosmotic solutions are irritant to the gastrointestinal mucosa and can cause nausea, vomiting and diarrhoea. This function was the basis of a now obsolete practice of using salt solutions to induce emesis. This practice has been associated with the occasional death and has now been replaced by safer emetics. The use of hyperosmotic saline solutions to induce abortion has been associated with many severe complications including cardiovascular shock, CNS disorders, haemolysis and renal necrosis. Other adverse effects include disseminated intravascular coagulopathy with marked haemorrhage.[21]

Severe or irreversible adverse effects

Other than those described earlier, none has been described.

Symptomatic adverse effects

The administration of sodium chloride via the intravenous route requires the insertion of a cannula. This can lead to bruising and infection at the site of insertion. Thrombophlebitis in the superficial

S

veins can be a complication and is relatively common. Bacteraemia and septicaemia are further complications of cannula insertion.[21]

Interference with clinical pathology tests
No technical interferences of this kind have been reported.

Drug interactions

Potentially life-threatening effects
It is sometimes assumed that any drug to be administered intravenously may be added to isotonic saline for this purpose, but this is not true, and the manufacturer's literature and published tables of compatible drugs (e.g. in the British National Formulary) should be consulted before adding a drug to a saline solution.

Potentially useful interactions
No interactions of this kind have been reported.

References

1. McCance R 1936 Experimental sodium chloride deficiency in man. Proceedings of the Royal Society (London) 119: 245–249
2. Strauss M B, Lamdin E, Smith W P, Bleifer D J 1958 Surfeit and deficit of sodium. Archives of Internal Medicine 102: 527–530
3. Earley L E, Daugharty T M 1969 Sodium metabolism. New England Journal of Medicine 281: 72–76
4. Gray G M 1975 Carbohydrate digestion and absorption. Role of the small intestine. New England Journal of Medicine 292: 1225–1230
5. Favin M N, McMurty M E 1983 Oral rehydration therapy. World Federation of Public Health Associations, Geneva
6. Pierce N F, Hirschorn N 1977 Rehydration therapy. Chronicle of the World Health Organisation 31: 87–92
7. Fregly M J 1984 Sodium and potassium. In: Olsen R E (ed) Nutrition reviews' present knowledge in nutrition. The Nutrition Foundation, Washington, DC, pp 439–458
8. Ganong W F 1985 Review of medical physiology, 12th edn. Lange Medical Publications, Los Altos, California, pp 14–15
9. Riordan J F, McLay W D, Walters G 1969 The significance of central venous pressure and cardiac output measurements in shock. Postgraduate Medical Journal 45: 506–510
10. Wood B 1977 A paediatric vade-mecum, 9th edn. Lloyd-Luke, London, pp 47–53
11. Page M B, Alberti K G M, Greenwood R et al 1974 Treatment of diabetic coma with continuous low dose infusion of insulin. British Medical Journal 2: 687–691
12. Young E, Bradley R F 1967 Cerebral oedema with irreversible coma in severe diabetic ketoacidosis. New England Journal of Medicine 276: 665–669
13. Krane E J, Rockoff M A, Wallman J K, Wolsdorf J I 1985 Subclinical brain swelling in children during treatment of diabetic ketoacidosis. New England Journal of Medicine 312: 1147–1151
14. Arieff A I 1986 Hyponatraemia, convulsions, respiratory arrest and permanent brain damage after elective surgery in healthy women. New England Journal of Medicine 314: 1529–1535
15. Gerich J, Martin M, Recant L 1971 Clinical and metabolic characteristics of hyperosmolar non-ketotic coma. Diabetes 20: 228–232
16. Lawson A, Proudfoot A, Brown J et al 1968 Salicylate poisoning in adults. Quarterly Journal of Medicine 138: 31–38
17. Linton A, Luke R, Briggs J 1967 Methods of forced diuresis and their application in barbiturate poisoning. Lancet 2: 337–340
18. Catto G R D, Smith F W, MacLeod M 1973 Treatment of muscle cramps during maintenance haemodialysis. British Medical Journal 3: 389–390
19. Calvin M E, Knepper R, Robertson W O 1964 Hazards to health. Salt poisoning. New England Journal of Medicine 270: 625–626
20. Tietze C, Lewit S 1973 Studies in Family Planning 4: 133–138
21. Maki D G 1973 Infection control in intravenous therapy. Annals of Internal Medicine 79: 867–871

Sodium cromoglycate

Sodium cromoglycate is an antiallergic drug mainly used in the prophylaxis of asthma.

Chemistry

Sodium cromoglycate (cromolyn sodium, Intal, Nalcrom, Opticrom, Rynacrom)
$C_{23}H_{14}Na_2O_{11}$
Disodium 4,4′-dioxo-5,5′-(2 hydroxytrimethylenedioxy) di(4H-chromene-2-carboxylate).
Sodium cromoglycate is a moderately large molecule whose structure consists of two chromone rings with two strongly polar carboxylic acid groups, joined by a flexible linking chain

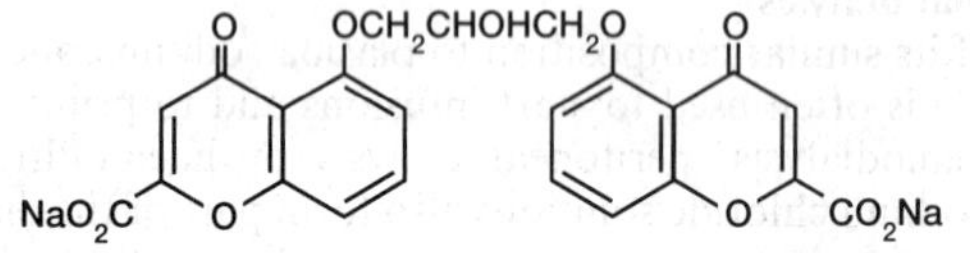

Molecular weight (free acid)	512.3 (468.3)
pKa (acid)	1.9
Solubility	
in alcohol	insoluble
in water	1 in 20
Octanol/water partition coefficient (salt)	22.39

(The more lipophilic free acid is too insoluble to provide a measured value)

Sodium cromoglycate is a white, odourless, hygroscopic crystalline powder freely soluble in water up to approximately 5%. The compound is prepared by chemical synthesis and possesses a slightly bitter after taste.

Sodium cromoglycate is available in combination with isoprenaline sulphate for inhalation, and in combination with xylometazoline hydrochloride for nasal application (Intal compound and Rynacrom compound).

Pharmacology

Sodium cromoglycate (SCG) is among the most active of the bischromones in its ability to inhibit certain anaphylactic reactions in animals and to inhaled allergens in man. SCG is neither an adrenergic agonist nor an anticholinergic agent. It has no direct bronchodilator action and no antihistaminic or corticosteroid-like properties. Further, it does not antagonize the effects of leukotrienes, serotonin or bradykinin.[1,2] Early research suggested that SCG inhibited the release of chemical mediators from sensitized mast cells[3] and was capable of rapid phosphorylation of mast cell protein.[4] However, SCG also causes inhibition of bronchoconstriction resulting from non-specific or irritant stimuli to the airways including exercise and sulphur dioxide[5,6,7] in which there is little evidence for mast cell involvement. The exact mechanism of action of the drug remains to be elucidated but SCG appears to modulate the allergic response to antigen–antibody interaction in a way which prevents the subsequent formation or release of toxic or inflammatory mediators. In addition there is also evidence to suggest that sodium cromoglycate may inhibit bronchoconstriction following stimulation of irritant receptors by acting on the nervous reflex arc.[7] Again the exact mechanism remains to be determined.

Sodium cromoglycate

Toxicology

Subcutaneous injections of sodium cromoglycate administered daily over a 90-day period have been shown to cause dose-related impairment of renal function and/or death in rats. However, at a low dose of 30 mg.kg^{-1} no histological changes were found in any organ, nor were there disturbances in hepatic or renal function or on biochemical testing.[8] In addition, no damage was reported in rhesus monkeys injected with an intravenous dose of 50 mg.kg^{-1} daily for a period of six months.[8]

Teratogenicity tests in both mice and rabbits, using large doses of 500–540 mg.kg^{-1} during pregnancy, produced no fetal abnormalities, despite being lethal to some rabbits and producing renal lesions in all survivors. Treatment of both male and female rats for 14 days prior to mating had no effect on either mating or fertility.[8]

There is no published information on either mutagenicity or carcinogenicity testing for this drug.

Clinical pharmacology

The most impressive demonstration of the clinical pharmacological action of sodium cromoglycate in the lungs relates to the inhibitory effect of pretreatment with the drug on the immediate asthmatic response to inhalation of a specific antigen, which has been confirmed many times since Altounyan's first report of this effect in 1967.[9] The protective effect of 20 mg of SCG lasts for several hours if it is inhaled together with, or shortly before, the antigen. However, the drug is ineffective if taken even a short time after challenge. Following an immediate reaction to bronchial challenge many patients develop a late reaction 4–12 hours later. If the immediate reaction to challenge is successfully inhibited by the prior inhalation of sodium cromoglycate the late reaction is also blocked in most cases without further inhalation of the drug.[10]

There is no indication that SCG affords more protection against any particular antigen. Inhibition of the asthmatic response to inhalation of toluene diisocyanate (TDI), piperazine, platinum salts, flux fumes, and detergent enzymes have all been reported.[11]

Sodium cromoglycate has also been shown to inhibit the immediate bronchial response to non-specific stimuli such as exercise[5] or airway cooling.[12] In addition, Harries and co-workers[7] have reported that SCG is effective in inhibiting increased airway reactivity provoked by inhalation of sulphur dioxide. This increased reactivity could also be partly inhibited by atropine, suggesting that SCG, in addition to its ability to modulate responses involving the mast cell, may also act on bronchial irritant receptors or directly on smooth muscle in asthmatic patients.

Investigations of the long-term effect of sodium cromoglycate on levels of bronchial hyperreactivity have produced conflicting results. Both Altounyan[13] and Dickson[14] showed that several weeks therapy with SCG reduced the level of hypersensitivity to inhaled histamine but this effect was not observed by Ryo and co-workers[15] following two weeks' therapy. However, it is probable that any change in airway responsiveness after prolonged treatment with SCG is an indirect result of the suppression of the asthmatic response to allergen by the drug rather than a direct action of SCG itself.

Since sodium cromoglycate has no bronchodilator or direct anti-inflammatory activity the drug is not suitable for the relief of acute asthmatic attacks and is essentially a prophylactic agent in asthma. There is clear indication of which patients may benefit from prophylactic treatment with sodium cromoglycate. There are tendencies to more frequent responses in younger patients in whom allergy is a dominant factor of their asthma or patients in whom the drug can be shown to produce marked inhibition of exercise-induced asthma. However, the absence of demonstrable allergy does not preclude a good response to therapy.

In concordance with the effect of SCG in the lung, intranasal application of SCG has been demonstrated to prevent nasal blockage following allergen provocation testing in 70–80% of hayfever patients.[16] However, in clinical use there have been conflicting results as to its efficacy.[17,18,19] Although both SCG powder and solution reduce nasal symptoms in seasonal rhinitis, the degree of symptom amelioration has not demonstrated that SCG is of significant clinical benefit in the majority of adult hayfever patients. SCG appears to be more efficient in the lower than in the upper airways of pollen-sensitive individuals.

In the treatment of perennial rhinitis, both allergic and non-allergic, a series of controlled studies have shown SCG powder and solution to be significantly more effective than placebo.[20,21,22] The degree of response appears to depend on the selection of patients. Mygind[23] has reported that no effect of SCG could be found in patients with large nasal polyps or those without demonstrable nasal eosinophilia on smear testing. In patients who respond to SCG administered intranasally the drug rarely gives complete freedom from symptoms and the relative protection obtained may be of clinical significance only in patients with moderately severe symptoms.

The exact mode of action of SCG in the eye and gastrointestinal tract remains to be elucidated although its efficacy has been demonstrated in both sites. SCG is effective in reducing symptoms of acute seasonal conjunctivitis,[24] chronic allergic conjunctivitis[25] and vernal kerato conjunctivitis.[26] In its oral formulation SCG has also been shown to be of some benefit in food allergy where sensitivity to one or more ingested allergens can be clearly demonstrated.[27]

Pharmacokinetics

The preferred analytical method for sodium cromoglycate in biological fluids is radioimmunoassay as described by Brown and co-workers in 1983.[28] Using this method direct analysis of sodium cromoglycate levels in plasma samples collected several hours after administration of single therapeutic doses of the compound is possible. The assay employs an antiserum raised in sheep, labelled with iodine-125, and a second antibody technique for the separation of bound and free radioligand. To encompass the concentration range of 0.93–139 nmol.l^{-1} encountered in plasma samples from patients both 0.01 and 0.1 ml volumes of plasma must be analysed, since the range of the assay is limited. The inter-assay coefficient of variation is less than 14% and the intra-assay coefficient of variation less than 9%. This method is specific for sodium cromoglycate as indicated by a low cross-reactivity of the anti-cromoglycate antiserum with a number of drugs. Sodium cromoglycate may now be quantified in urine by HPLC, limit of detection 50 μg.l^{-1}.

Sodium cromoglycate is poorly absorbed from the gastrointestinal tract, less than 1% being absorbed by this route.[29] For this reason the main routes of administration are by inhalation to the lungs or by topical application to the nose or eyes. When SCG is inhaled approximately 10% penetrates deep into the lungs and is absorbed into the blood, where its half life is approximately 90 minutes. Following intravenous administration plasma half lives are 9 minutes ($t\frac{1}{2}\alpha$) and 63 minutes ($t\frac{1}{2}\beta$).

The volume of distribution of the drug is 0.32 l.kg^{-1}. Sodium cromoglycate undergoes no systemic or presystemic metabolism in man and plasma levels fall due to excretion of the unchanged drug from the body, about half in the urine and half in the bile. There is no excretion into human breast milk and the drug is not capable of crossing the blood–brain barrier.

Sodium cromoglycate belongs to a large group of acidic drugs which are reversibly associated with plasma albumin in a non-specific way (57–69% being protein-bound in human plasma). Binding in human plasma appears to be largely independent of the drug concentration. The highly polar nature of the compound results in the binding being relatively weak. This being so, SCG would not be expected to displace other protein-bound drugs from albumin and is therefore unlikely to result in adverse effects during clinical use due to this type of interaction.[30]

Oral absorption	<1%
Presystemic metabolism	nil
Plasma half life	
range	60–90 min
Volume of distribution	0.32 l.kg^{-1}
Plasma protein binding	57–69%

Concentration–effect relationship

There is no evidence to suggest that the therapeutic effect of sodium cromoglycate occurs within a defined range of plasma concentrations.

Metabolism

Sodium cromoglycate does not undergo any metabolic reactions in man. The drug is eliminated unchanged in urine ($\sim 50\%$) and faeces ($\sim 50\%$) after intravenous administration. After inhalation more is excreted in the faeces ($\sim 87\%$) due to the large amount of the dose that is swallowed with correspondingly less appearing in the urine ($< 10\%$).

Pharmaceutics

Formulations of the drug available from Fisons (UK) include:

1. Intal: administration by inhalation. 20 mg of sodium cromoglycate as micronized powder in yellow/colourless transparent hard gelatin capsules. Printed 'FISONS INTAL P'. Store in a moisture-proof container in a cool dry place, protected from light.
2. Intal Compound: administration by inhalation. 20 mg of sodium cromoglycate as micronized powder and 0.1 mg of isoprenaline sulphate powder in orange/colourless transparent hard gelatin capsules. Printed 'FISONS INTAL P-C'. Storage conditions as above.
3. Intal Inhaler: administration by inhalation. Metered dose pressurized aerosol delivering 5 mg of sodium cromoglycate per actuation. Store in a cool place. The canister should be protected from direct sunlight and must not be punctured or burnt even when empty.
4. Intal Nebuliser Solution: ampoules containing 20 mg of sodium cromoglycate in 2 ml of clear, colourless, sterile aqueous solution for inhalation via a nebulizer. Store in a cool place and protect from sunlight.
5. Nalcrom: for oral administration. 100 mg of sodium cromoglycate in clear/clear hard gelatin capsules printed 'FISONS 101'. Store in a dry place.
6. Opticrom eye drops: drops for ocular application. A colourless aqueous solution of sodium cromoglycate (2% w/v) and benzalkonium chloride (0.01% w/v). Store below 25°C and protect from direct sunlight. The contents should be discarded 4 weeks after opening.
7. Opticrom eye ointment: cream coloured opaque sterile ointment for ocular application containing 4% w/w of sodium cromoglycate. Store below 25°C and protect from direct sunlight. The contents should be discarded 4 weeks after opening. Maximum shelf-life 2 years.
8. Rynacrom: for nasal application. 10 mg of sodium cromoglycate powder, in pink, transparent, hard gelatin capsules printed 'RYNACROM', for use with insufflator. Store below 30°C in a dry place protected from light.
9. Rynacrom nasal spray: for nasal application. A metered dose formulation containing sodium cromoglycate (2% w/v) in aqueous solution. Delivery approximately 2.6 mg per metered dose. Store below 30°C and protect from direct sunlight. A 4% w/v solution is available in the USA as Nasalcrom (Fisons, USA). Delivery approximately 5.2 mg per metered dose.
10. Rynacrom nasal drops: for nasal application. Plastic dropper bottle containing aqueous solution of sodium cromoglycate (2% w/v). Store below 30°C and protect from direct sunlight.
11. Rynacrom Compound: for nasal application. Metered dose presentation containing an aqueous solution of sodium cromoglycate (2% w/v) and xylometazoline hydrochloride (0.025% w/v). Delivery approximately 2.6 mg of sodium cromoglycate and 0.0325 mg of xylometazoline hydrochloride per metered dose. Store below 30°C and protect from direct sunlight. Maximum shelf-life 2 years.

Rynacrom nasal drops and spray and Rynacrom Compound contains benzalkonium chloride as a preservative. All formulations have a maximum shelf-life of 3 years except where indicated otherwise.

Therapeutic Use

Indications

1. Management of bronchial asthma
2. Prophylactic treatment of seasonal and/or perennial rhinitis
3. Allergic rhinitis
4. Food allergy
5. Acute and chronic allergic conjunctivitis.

Contraindications

There are no specific contraindications for products containing sodium cromoglycate only. Known hypersensitivity to benzalkonium chloride is a contraindication for the use of formulations of which it is a constituent.

Benzalkonium chloride is a surfactant and there is a risk that its detergent effect may break up the tear film and promote friction between a contact lens and the cornea. The preservative binds to the lens material and is subsequently released into the eye, therefore being continuously present. Bound benzalkonium chloride may also modify the hydrophilic properties, and hence the refractive index, of the lens. For these reasons benzalkonium chloride solution and soft contact lenses are regarded as incompatible, and these should not be worn during treatment with Opticrom eye drops.

Mode of use

Intal products. For preventative treatment of bronchial asthma due to a variety of causes including allergy, exercise, cold air and chemical or occupational irritants. Since Intal acts prophylactically it is important to continue treatment in those patients who benefit. Intal should be withdrawn progressively if necessary to reduce the risk of worsening of asthma symptoms.

1. Intal and Intal Compound spincaps.
   One spincap (Intal — 20 mg sodium cromoglycate, Intal compound — 20 mg sodium cromoglycate and 0.1 mg isoprenaline sulphate) 4 times a day. May be increased to 6–8 times a day in more severe cases and additional doses may be taken prior to exercise.
2. Intal inhaler.
   Initially two (5 mg) inhalations 4 times a day. May be reduced to a maintenance dosage of one inhalation 4 times a day once adequate control of symptoms has been achieved. Additional doses may be taken prior to exercise.
3. Intal nebulizer.
   Contents of one ampoule (20 mg) 4 times a day. May be increased to 5–6 times a day in severe cases. Additional doses may be taken prior to exercise.

Rynacrom products. Rynacrom cartridges, nasal spray and drops are recommended for the prophylactic treatment of seasonal and/or perennial rhinitis. Patients should be instructed to maintain regular dosage as distinct from using the drug intermittently to relieve symptoms.
Recommended dosage:

1. Rynacrom nasal spray.
   One squeeze (2.6 mg approx) to each nostril 4 times a day.
2. Rynacrom cartridges.
   Contents of one cartridge (10 mg) to be insufflated into each nostril 4 times daily.
3. Rynacrom drops.
   Instil 2 drops into each nostril 6 times a day.
4. Rynacrom Compound.
   This is recommended for the treatment of allergic rhinitis, both seasonal and perennial, where accompanied by nasal congestion. Regular dosage should be maintained as above. One squeeze (2.6 mg sodium cromoglycate and 0.0325 mg xylometazoline hydrochloride) into each nostril 4 times daily.

Nalcrom. For food allergy where sensitivity to one or more ingested allergens has been adequately demonstrated. Use in conjunction with restriction of the main causative allergens.
Recommended dosage:
Initial dose for adults: 2 (100 mg) capsules 4 times a day before meals.
Initial dose for children (2–14 years): 1 (100 mg) capsule 4 times a day before meals.
For adults and children if satisfactory control is not achieved within 2–3 weeks the dosage may be doubled but should not exceed 40 $mg.kg^{-1}.d^{-1}$.

Opticrom eye drops and ointment. For the relief and treatment of acute and chronic allergic conjunctivitis.
Recommended dosage:

1. Opticrom eye drops.
   1 or 2 drops applied to each eye 4 times a day.
2. Opticrom eye ointment.
   To be applied to the eye 2–3 times daily.

Adverse reactions

Potentially life-threatening effects
In extremely rare cases severe bronchospasm has resulted immediately following administration when the drug is inhaled. The incidence of this reaction is much less than one case per million patients, although exact figures are not available.

Acute overdosage
Two reports of deliberate overdosage have been documented and there are no published reports. No abnormal symptoms have been reported, and no action other than medical observation should be necessary.

Severe or irreversible adverse effects
None has been reported.

Symptomatic adverse effects
Local irritation of the target organ, which is usually mild and transient, sometimes occurs. No published estimates of the incidence of local irritation exist. However, cumulative experience suggests a figure of 5–10%.

Interference with clinical pathology tests
None has been reported.

High risk groups

Neonates
Most formulations appear safe for use in neonates, although the safety of the oral preparation Nalcrom in the treatment of children under two years of age has not been established.

Breast milk. Sodium cromoglycate is not excreted in breast milk.

Children
What has been said about neonates also applies to older children.

Pregnant women
Sodium cromoglycate has been used in treating pregnant women since its introduction in 1968. There is currently no evidence to suggest that such administration has been associated with an increase in the incidence of foetal abnormalities. A prospective study, over a 10-year period, of 296 asthmatic women treated throughout pregnancy with 20 mg of SCG three times daily published by Wilson in 1982 reported a neonatal malformation rate of 1.35% representing a frequency less than that reported for the population as a whole (2–3%). Maternal tolerance was good, with no side effects reported during the course of normal pregnancies with delivery at term.[31]

Drug interactions

Sodium cromoglycate has no known drug interactions.

Major outcome trials

Inhaled preparations

Adults

1. Brompton Hospital/Medical Research Council Collaborative Trial 1972 Long-term study of disodium cromoglycate in treatment of severe extrinsic or intrinsic bronchial asthma in adults. British Medical Journal 4: 383–388

In 1972 the results of the first long-term study of sodium cromoglycate in adult asthma were published. The year-long, double-blind study included 103 patients with severe extrinsic or intrinsic asthma randomly allocated to receive treatment with SCG, SCG and isoprenaline, isoprenaline alone or placebo. The difference between the placebo group and the two SCG regimens in terms of treatment failures attained significance after four weeks and remained significant thereafter. In those patients who continued on SCG or SCG/isoprenaline statistically significant improvements in the forced expiratory volume in one second (FEV1) were seen at 24 and 52 weeks. This was not seen in patients receiving placebo therapy. There was no significant factor from which a satisfactory response to SCG could be predicted. However, in those patients on SCG therapies only one failure occurred in 14 patients with multiple skin reactions to common inhalant allergens compared with 8 of 21 patients who had weak single, or absent, skin prick test responses.

Children

2. Silverman M, Connolly N M, Balfour-Lynn L, Godfrey S 1972 Long-term trial of disodium cromoglycate and isoprenaline in children with asthma. British Medical Journal 3: 378–381

This year-long, double-blind study of 53 asthmatic children compared the effect of sodium cromoglycate with placebo by means of diary card scores and clinical and physiological investigations. The treatment group inhaled SCG with isoprenaline (Intal compound) four times daily whereas the placebo group received lactose with isoprenaline. After one year 76% of the placebo group were treatment failures compared with only 29% of the group receiving active therapy ($p<0.001$). In both groups diary scores improved significantly compared with pre-trial levels, but the improvement was significantly greater in the SCG group. By contrast, mean daily peak flow rates improved only in the treatment group due to an improvement in both morning and evening recordings and a smaller diurnal swing. There was no significant change in bronchial hyperreactivity to exercise or histamine in either group. As in adults none of the pre-trial characteristics of the patients predicted a good response to SCG.

Nasal preparations

3. Resta O, Foschino Babaro M P, Carnimeo N 1982 A comparison of sodium cromoglycate nasal solution and powder in the treatment of allergic rhinitis. British Journal of Clinical Practice 36 (3): 94–98

A double-blind, randomized comparison of sodium cromoglycate nasal solution and powder in the treatment of allergic rhinitis was reported by Resta and co-workers in 1982. The 28-day study included 39 symptomatic rhinitic patients. No therapy other than sodium cromoglycate was permitted. Active therapy was a 2% solution of sodium cromoglycate applied to each nostril six times daily or sodium cromoglycate powder at a dose of one 20 mg capsule equally divided between nostrils four times a day. Two drops of an aqueous solution applied to each nostril four times a day acted as a placebo control.

Response to therapy was assessed subjectively by daily records of severity of sneezing, blocking, itching and rhinorrhoea and objectively by measurement of specific airways resistance in the nasal cavities (sGaw N) using a body plethysmograph.

There was a significant improvement in sGaw N with both active preparations but not in the placebo group. Symptomatically sodium cromoglycate powder was significantly better than placebo for all four variables measured. Sodium cromoglycate solution was significantly better than placebo in reducing sneezing and rhinorrhoea. Assessment of weekly changes in symptom scores showed a more rapid improvement in sneezing and rhinorrhoea, during treatment with the two active formulations, than was the case for blockage.

It is suggested that both sodium cromoglycate powder and solution are effective in the treatment of allergic rhinitis, with patients whose predominant symptoms are sneezing and rhinorrhoea showing a clinical response within two weeks. In patients whose predominant symptom is nasal obstruction, however, maximum therapeutic benefit may not be obtained for at least four weeks.

Ocular preparations

Sodium cromoglycate eye drops have been studied in the treatment of both seasonal, allergic and chronic conjunctivitis.

Seasonal allergic conjunctivitis

4. Lindsay-Miller A C M 1979 Group comparative trial of 2% sodium cromoglycate (Opticrom) with placebo in the treatment of seasonal allergic conjunctivitis. Clinical Allergy 9: 271–275

A double-blind study of 50 patients with seasonal allergic conjunctivitis was reported by Lindsay-Miller in 1979. Over a four week period

Sodium cromoglycate

S

2% sodium cromoglycate eyedrops or placebo were applied to each eye at the rate of two drops four times a day. Active therapy was found to be significantly more effective than placebo when assessed subjectively by both patients and physicians ($p<0.05$), 90% of patients on active treatment reporting improvement. Diary card scores indicated that a beneficial effect was obtained within only 1–3 days of commencing treatment.

Chronic conjunctivitis

5. Van Bijsterveld O P 1984 A double-blind crossover study comparing sodium cromoglycate eye drops with placebo in the treatment of chronic conjunctivitis. Acta Ophthalmologica 69: 479–484

A double-blind, placebo-controlled, crossover study of the efficacy of sodium cromoglycate eye drops in the treatment of 60 patients with chronic, non-infective conjunctivitis, was reported by Van Bijsterveld in 1984. Patients were treated with sodium cromoglycate or placebo, one drop to each eye four times daily, for four-week periods. After four weeks of active treatment symptom scores for photophobia and hyperaemia were significantly lower than after placebo treatment. A similar trend was seen for symptoms of itching and discharge. Significantly more patients responded to the active treatment than the placebo treatment in the opinions of both the patients and clinicians.

Oral preparation (Nalcrom)

There are no major studies of the efficacy of Nalcrom in man.

General review articles

Cox J S G, Altounyan R E C 1970 Nature and modes of action of disodium cromoglycate (Lomudal R). Respiration 27: 292–309

Cox J S G, Beach J E, Blair A M J N et al 1970 Disodium cromoglycate (Intal R). Advances in Drug Research 5: 115–196

Cox J S G 1971 Disodium cromoglycate. Mode of action and its possible relevance to the clinical use of the drug. British Journal of Diseases of the Chest 65: 189–204

Brogden R N, Speight T M, Avery G S 1974 Sodium cromoglycate (Cromolyn Sodium): a review of its mode of action, pharmacology, therapeutic efficacy and use. Drugs 7: 164–282

Cox J S G 1977 Cromolyn sodium. In: Goldberg M E (ed) Pharmacological and biochemical properties of drug substances. American Pharmacological Association, Washington, pp 277–310

Berman B A 1983 Cromolyn: past, present and future. Paediatric Clinics of North America 30 (5): 915–930

References

1. Cox J S G 1967 Disodium cromoglycate, FPL 670, (Intal). A specific inhibitor of reaginic antibody–antigen mechanisms. Nature 216: 1328–1329
2. Cox J S G 1970 Review of chemistry, pharmacology, toxicity, metabolism, specific side effects, anti-allergic properties in vitro and in vivo of disodium cromoglycate. In: Pepys J, Frankland A W (eds) Disodium cromoglycate in allergic airways disease. Butterworths, London, pp 13–25
3. Orr T S C 1977 Mode of action of disodium cromoglycate. Acta Allergologica 32 (suppl 13): 9–27
4. Wells E, Mann J 1983 Phosphorylation of a mast cell protein in response to treatment with anti-allergic compounds. Implications for the mode of action of sodium cromoglycate. Biochemical Pharmacology 32 (5): 837–842
5. Davies S E 1968 Effect of disodium cromoglycate on exercise-induced asthma. British Medical Journal 3: 593–594
6. Silverman M, Turner-Warwick M 1972 Exercise induced asthma: response to disodium cromoglycate in skin-test positive and skin-test negative subjects. Clinical Allergy 2: 137–142
7. Harries M G, Parkes P E G, Lessof M H 1981 Role of bronchial irritant receptors in asthma. Lancet 3: 5–7
8. Cox J S G, Beach J E, Blair A M J N et al 1970 Disodium cromoglycate (Intal R). Advances in Drug Research 5: 115–196
9. Altounyan R E C 1967 Inhibition of experimental asthma by a new compound — disodium cromoglycate 'Intal'. Acta Allergolica 22: 487
10. Booij-Nord H, Orie N G M, de Vries K 1971 Immediate and late bronchial obstructive reactions to inhalation of housedust and protective effects of disodium cromoglycate and prednisolone. Journal of Allergy 48: 344–354
11. Pepys J, Hutchcroft B J 1975 Bronchial provocation tests in etiologic diagnosis and analysis of asthma. American Review of Respiratory Disease 112: 829–859
12. Latimer K M, Roberts R, Morris M M, Hargreave F E 1984 Inhibition by sodium cromoglycate of bronchoconstriction stimulated by respiratory heat loss: comparison of pressurized aerosol and powder. Thorax 34 (4): 277–281
13. Altounyan R E C 1970 Changes in histamine and atropine responsiveness as a guide to diagnosis and evaluation of therapy in obstructive airways disease. In: Pepys J, Frankland A W (eds) Disodium cromoglycate in allergic airways disease. Butterworths, London, pp 47–53
14. Dickson W 1970 A one year's trial of Intal Compound in 24 children with severe asthma. In: Pepys J, Frankland A W (eds) Disodium cromoglycate in allergic airways disease. Butterworths, London, pp 105–119
15. Ryo U Y, Kang B, Townley R G 1971 Effect of disodium cromoglycate on inhalation challenge with allergen, histamine and methacholine in subjects with bronchial asthma. Journal of Allergy 47: 96
16. Orie N G M, Booij-Nord H, Pelikan Z et al 1970 Protective effect of disodium cromoglycate on nasal and bronchial reactions after allergen challenge. In: Pepys J, Frankland A W (eds) Disodium cromoglycate in allergic airways disease. Butterworths, London, pp 33–41
17. Frankland A W, Walker S R 1975 A comparison of intranasal betamethasone valerate and sodium cromoglycate in seasonal allergic rhinitis. Clinical Allergy 5: 295–300
18. Holopainen E, Backman A, Salo O P 1971 Effect of disodium cromoglycate on seasonal allergic rhinitis. Lancet 1: 55–57
19. Taylor G, Shivalkar P R 1971 Disodium cromoglycate: laboratory studies and clinical trial in allergic rhinitis. Clinical Allergy 1: 189–198
20. Mygind N, Viner A S, Jackman N 1974 The influence on nasal mucosa of unpreserved and preserved nasal sprays containing disodium cromoglycate. Rhinology 12: 49
21. Brain D J, Singh K P, Trotter C M, Viner A S 1974 Sodium cromoglycate 2% solution in perennial rhinitis. Journal of Laryngology and Otology 88: 1001–1017
22. Hopper I, Dawson J P 1972 The effect of disodium cromoglycate in perennial rhinitis. Journal of Laryngology and Otology 86: 725–730
23. Mygind N, Hansen I, Jorgensen M B 1972 Disodium cromoglycate nasal spray in adult patients with perennial rhinitis. Acta Allergolica (Kbh) 27: 372–380
24. Lindsay-Miller A C M 1979 Group comparative trial of 2% sodium cromoglycate (Opticrom) with placebo in the treatment of seasonal allergic conjunctivitis. Clinical Allergy 9: 271–275
25. Van Bijsterveld O P 1984 A double-blind crossover study comparing sodium cromoglycate eye drops with placebo in the treatment of chronic conjunctivitis. Acta Ophthalmologica 69: 479–484
26. Hennawi M 1980 Clinical trial with 2% sodium cromoglycate (Opticrom) in vernal keratoconjunctivitis. British Journal of Ophthalmology 64: 483–486
27. Ortolani C, Pastorello E, Zanussi C 1983 Prophylaxis of adverse reactions in foods. A double-blind study of oral sodium cromoglycate for the prophylaxis of adverse reactions to foods and additives. Annals of Allergy 50: 105–109
28. Brown K, Gardner J J, Lockley W J S, Preston J R, Wilkinson D J 1983 Radioimmunoassay of sodium cromoglycate in human plasma. Annals of Clinical Biochemistry 20: 31–36
29. Walker S R 1972 The fate of [14c] disodium cromoglycate in man. Journal of Pharmacy and Pharmacology 24: 525–531
30. Clark B, Moss G F, Neale M G 1978 The degree of plasma protein binding of sodium cromoglycate. Journal of Pharmacy and Pharmacology 30: 386–387
31. Wilson J 1982 Utilisation du cromoglycate de sodium au cows de la grossesse. Resultats sur 296 femmes asthmatiques. Acta Therapeutica 8 (2): 45–51

Sodium nitrite

Sodium nitrite is employed as an antidote in acute cyanide poisoning, almost always in conjunction with sodium thiosulphate. It has also been suggested as an antidote for hydrogen sulphide poisoning, though this indication remains controversial. Sodium nitrite has also been used as a rust inhibitor and it is employed as a preservative in foods such as cured meats.

Chemistry

Sodium nitrite (Sodium nitrite injection)
$NaNO_2$

Molecular weight	69.0
pKa	—
Solubility	
in alcohol	1 in 160
in water	1 in 1.5
Octanol/water partition coefficient	—

Sodium nitrite is prepared as odourless, deliquescent, colourless or slightly yellow crystals or crystalline powder, melting point 271°C. Solutions in water are alkaline.

Acids will decompose sodium nitrite and cause evolution of brownish N_2O_3 fumes. Sodium nitrite is incompatible with oxidizing agents, phenazone, acetanilide and morphine.

Pharmacology

Sodium nitrite is nowadays primarily used as an antidote for cyanide poisoning.[1] It shows synergy with sodium thiosulphate.[2–4] The mechanism of action of nitrite was first thought to be mediated by an in vivo induction of methaemoglobin.[5,6] The trivalent iron of methaemoglobin has a high affinity for cyanide which is sequestered within the erythrocyte in the form of cyanmethaemoglobin, with the result that the concentration of cyanide in the plasma falls, in turn reducing the concentration of cyanide in the tissues.

Cyanide-inhibited cytochrome oxidase can be reactivated by methaemoglobin[7] Methaemoglobin does not have a higher affinity for cyanide than cytochrome oxidase, but there is a much larger potential source of methaemoglobin than there is of cytochrome oxidase. The induction of methaemoglobin results in a loss of oxygen-carrying capacity of the red blood cells with resultant impairment of oxygen transport to cells.

Recently it has been suggested that this methaemoglobin induction hypothesis does not explain all the beneficial effects of sodium nitrite in cyanide poisoning.[8,9] While the antidotal effect of sodium nitrite in this condition is rapid, the formation of methaemoglobin by nitrite is slow and there are indications of a mechanism of action not mediated by methaemoglobin.

Sodium nitrite has been shown to be effective in the treatment of dogs with experimental cyanide poisoning[4,5] and the LD_{50} of cyanide is raised by a factor of 5.[10] If nitrite and thiosulphate are given together the LD_{50} is increased by a factor of 18.[10]

Sodium nitrite is effective in the experimental treatment of acute sulphide poisoning.[11,12] It is thought that sulphide is trapped as sulphmethaemoglobin — a complex in which hydrosulphide anions are complexed with the ferric haem group of methaemoglobin.[13] Recent evidence, however, suggests that this is a very short-lived effect and nitrite can only be effective in the early stages of sulphide poisoning.[14]

Sodium nitrite is a potent, directly acting vasodilator and it has been suggested that the effects in cyanide poisoning may be due to an effect on blood flow.[15]

Toxicology

Acute toxicity data via a variety of routes are given in Table 1. Of the various species in which the LD_{50} has been estimated, the dog is closest to man in sensitivity to sodium nitrite, whilst the mouse is of low sensitivity. Death is probably due to anoxia, since methaemoglobin cannot carry oxygen.

Table 1 Acute lethality of sodium nitrite

Species	Route	LD_{50}/mg.kg^{-1}	References
Dog	i.v.	40	16
	s.c.	50–70	17
Mouse	i.v.	135	16
	i.p.	193	18
		159	19
		200	20
	Oral	214–216	21

In addition to methaemoglobinaemia, the acute toxic effects of sodium nitrite include vasodilation, hypotension, reduction of vitamin A stores in the liver and disturbances of thyroid function.[22]

Dogs given a single dose of 1–2 mg.kg^{-1} sodium nitrite showed a rise in respiration and heart rate, change in ECG, methaemoglobinaemia within one to two hours, a rise in serum sodium, a fall in serum potassium and a rise in aspartate aminotransferase activity.[23]

As sodium nitrite is administered in a clinical setting on only one or two occasions, chronic and subacute animal toxicity studies are not of great relevance.

Sodium nitrite is listed by the International Agency for Research on Cancer as a non-carcinogen but as being mutagenic in the Ames test.[24] It can react with secondary amines in vivo to produce potentially carcinogenic nitrosamines,[25] though a cohort of workers chronically exposed to sodium nitrite and various amines in cutting fluid did not show an increased incidence of cancer.[26]

Although sodium nitrite was not teratogenic in several species in one study,[27] there are other reports that indicate that high-dose sodium nitrite administration (100 mg.kg^{-1}) may be teratogenic.[25] However, methaemoglobin-inducing chemicals may be teratogenic because of the anoxia they induce.

Clinical pharmacology

Sodium nitrite is chiefly used as an antidote in cyanide poisoning, and is usually given with oxygen and sodium thiosulphate. The rationale for this combination is that as the methaemoglobinaemia induced by sodium nitrite is short-lived, the cyanide sequestered inside the erythrocyte as cyanmethaemoglobin might be expected to diffuse out of the red cell as the methaemoglobin content falls producing a recrudescence of symptoms. However, although there is experimental work in favour of this combination[3,4,10] there are no clinical trial data in man. The use of 100% oxygen,[28] but not hyperbaric oxygen,[29] increases the benefit of this combination.

Sodium nitrite is also used in the treatment of hydrogen sulphide poisoning since sulphide is an even more potent inhibitor of cytochrome oxidase than cyanide.[30,31] However, more recent work[14] suggests that in the presence of oxygen the sulphmethaemoglobin complex produced is short-lived and leads directly to the oxidation of sulphide by molecular oxygen. Thus it has been argued that nitrite can only be effective in the first few minutes after hydrogen sulphide exposure, at which time resuscitation and/or ventilation of the victim is likely to produce conditions in which nitrite actively slows sulphide removal. Although there are a few case reports suggesting benefit in the clinical situation[32,33] further work is required since reservations remain.[34]

Sodium nitrite is a potent vasodilator and has been used in the past in the treatment of angina. It is relatively ineffective in this role and may cause postural hypotension.

Pharmacokinetics

Nitrite can be determined in biological fluids by a sulphanilic acid–α-naphthylamine colorimetric diazotization technique, directly[35] or following isolation of the ion by dialysis, protein precipitation or steam distillation.[36] The use of an ion-selective electrode[37] and an HPLC technique[38] have also been reported.

In man, sodium nitrite is rapidly absorbed from the gut following oral administration. About 40% of absorbed nitrite is excreted unchanged in the urine but the fate of the remaining 60% is not known accurately, though it is thought to be metabolized partially to ammonia.[39] No kinetic studies following intravenous use have been reported.

Concentration–effect relationship

An intravenous injection of 400 mg sodium nitrite in humans produced a peak methaemoglobin concentration of 10.1%, while 600 mg intravenously produced a 17.5% peak methaemoglobin concentration.[40] In another case, 450 mg sodium nitrite intravenously produced a 20% concentration of methaemoglobin 1.25 h later.[41]

Metabolism

See Pharmacokinetics.

Pharmaceutics

The BPC preparation is a sterile solution of sodium nitrite 3% in water for injection. It is supplied in single-dose containers by production units with a 'specials' licence.

The USP preparation is similar and is supplied by Lilly (USA) as a component of their Cyanide Antidote Package.

The shelf-life of sodium nitrite solutions is in excess of 5 years (more than 20 years in one study[10]).

Therapeutic use

Indications

1. Cyanide poisoning.

Contraindications

1. Glucose-6-phosphate dehydrogenase deficiency
2. Hereditary methaemoglobinaemia
3. Combined carbon monoxide and cyanide intoxication.

Mode of use

Sodium nitrite is usually administered intravenously in an initial dose of 300 mg (10 ml of a 3% solution). Hypotension may occur and this may be prevented by diluting the solution with normal saline and infusing it over a 20 min period; the infusion rate may be increased if hypotension does not develop. The average paediatric dose is 0.33 $ml.kg^{-1}$ of a 3% solution (about 10 $mg.kg^{-1}$). If there is inadequate clinical improvement a second dose of sodium nitrite may be given 30 min after the first dose; customarily one-half the initial amount administered. Excessive methaemoglobinaemia may occur and, ideally, patients should therefore have methaemoglobin levels monitored to avoid this occurrence. However, reliance on methaemoglobin measurement to detect excessive methaemoglobin levels is generally not possible as neither the method of Evelyn and Malloy[42] nor the 1L 282 CO-oximeter measure cyanmethaemoglobin as methaemoglobin[43] so that such measurements can be grossly misleading. An accurate indication of the oxygen-carrying capacity of blood can only be obtained if cyanmethaemoglobin is also measured and, at present, there is no technique, that is likely to be available clinically, for doing so.

Sodium nitrite is usually administered with oxygen and sodium thiosulphate, though the efficacy of sodium nitrite alone or in combination with sodium thiosulphate is unknown because, in the absence of controlled clinical trials, anecdotal reports are all that can be evaluated. Moreover, particularly in Europe, dicobalt edetate is often preferred to methaemoglobin-inducing agents or, alternatively, the more potent methaemoglobin-inducer 4-DMAP is administered preferentially.

Indications

1. Cyanide poisoning

The only established indication for the use of sodium nitrite is cyanide poisoning. It should not be employed unless there is evidence of severe poisoning such as coma, deteriorating vital functions and metabolic acidosis. Preferably, the clinical diagnosis should be confirmed analytically.

Only one case of acute cyanide poisoning treated with sodium nitrite alone has been reported;[44] all other reported patients have been given more than one antidote, which is appropriate in the light of the known synergism with sodium thiosulphate.[10]

The first reported cases of acute cyanide poisoning in man treated with sodium nitrite and sodium thiosulphate were described by Viana et al.[45] The first patient ingested approximately 5 g potassium cyanide but recovered after being given 1500 mg sodium nitrite and 18 g sodium thiosulphate. The second patient ingested approximately 2 g potassium cyanide and recovered after being given 750 mg sodium nitrite and 12 g sodium thiosulphate. No cyanide concentrations were measured.

A series of patients with acute cyanide poisoning treated with the amyl nitrite/sodium nitrite/sodium thiosulphate combination was assembled by Chen and Rose[10,46] and comprised a total of 49 patients; only one patient, who was moribund before treatment, did not recover. Unfortunately, no analytical confirmation of the diagnosis is available in any of these cases. Further reports have indicated the value of sodium nitrite and sodium thiosulphate in cyanide poisoning due to potassium and sodium cyanide,[47–53] cyanogenic plants[54–57] and laetrile.[58–60] However, not all patients with severe cyanide poisoning who have been given the sodium nitrite/sodium thiosulphate antidote combination have survived.[10,52,61]

Administration of the sodium nitrite/sodium thiosulphate antidote combination has also been reported in five smoke inhalation victims[62] with combined carbon monoxide and cyanide intoxication and mean blood cyanide levels of 16.2 $mg.l^{-1}$. These five patients also received hyperbaric oxygen therapy; there were four survivors and one fatality. This indication for sodium nitrite remains controversial, partly on the grounds that the combination of methaemoglobinaemia and carboxyhaemoglobinaemia might result in increased hazard.

Contraindications

Glucose-6-phosphate dehydrogenase deficient individuals are at great risk from sodium nitrite therapy because of the possibility of severe haemolysis, whilst patients with hereditary methaemoglobinaemia will develop very high levels of methaemoglobin.

Patients with combined carbon monoxide and cyanide intoxication, for example after a fire, should not be given nitrite unless under treatment in a hyperbaric oxygen chamber. Alternative antidotal therapy, e.g. sodium thiosulphate and cobalt edetate, may be preferred.

Adverse reactions

Potentially life-threatening effects

Excessive methaemoglobinaemia may occur, especially when large doses of sodium nitrite are administered, particularly to children, and this can be treated with methylene blue or toluidine blue (see Acute overdosage). Hypotension may also follow the rapid intravenous infusion of sodium nitrite.

Acute overdosage

Poisoning has occurred when sodium nitrite has been ingested instead of table salt,[63–65] food has been contaminated with motor vehicle cooling fluid[66] and a solution containing sodium nitrite has been added to a cold water system rather than the hot water system. Sodium nitrite has also been ingested with suicidal intent[67] though, more usually, intoxication has followed food accidents such as the ingestion of sausage cured with sodium nitrite.[68]

In a tragic error, a 17-month-old child died with 90% methaemoglobinaemia after being given 450 mg sodium nitrite in the mistaken impression that acute cyanide poisoning was present.[69]

If no treatment is given the mean lethal oral dose is of the order of 1 g sodium nitrite.

In symptomatic patients with methaemoglobin concentrations of more than 40%, an intravenous infusion of methylene blue

1–2 mg.kg^{-1} body weight (0.1 ml of 1% solution per kg body weight) should be given.

Severe or irreversible adverse effects
Lesser degrees of the signs and symptoms described under potentially life-threatening effects may occur.

Symptomatic adverse effects
See above.

Interference with clinical pathology tests
No technical interferences of this kind have been reported.

High risk groups

Neonates
The drug is not likely to be used in this age group.

Breast milk. A lactating mother treated with this drug is unlikely to breast-feed.

Children
See Potentially life-threatening effects above.

Pregnant women
Animal experiments indicate that sodium nitrite crosses the placenta and fetal methaemoglobinaemia may be induced. It may, therefore, be more appropriate to use an alternative antidote such as dicobalt edetate in pregnant patients severely poisoned with cyanide.

The elderly
No special precautions are needed in this age group.

Concurrent disease
Individuals with glucose-6-phosphate dehydrogenase deficiency are at great risk from sodium nitrite therapy because of the likelihood of severe haemolysis.

Individuals with hereditary methaemoglobinaemias would be expected to develop high, and possibly lethal, levels of methaemoglobin.

Drug interactions

None has been described.

References

1. Mladoveanu C, Gheorghiu P 1929 Le nitrite de soude comme antidote de l'empoisonnement expérimental par le cyanure de potassium. Comptes Rendus des Séances de la Societé de Biologie 102: 164–166
2. Hug E 1932 L'intoxication par l'acide cyanhydrique. Action antidote du bleu de méthylène, du nitrite de sodium et du sulfure de sodium. Comptes Rendus des Séances de la Societé de Biologie 111: 89–90
3. Hug E 1933 Action combinée du nitrite de sodium et de l'hyposulfite de sodium dans le traitement de l'intoxication cyanhydrique chez le lapin. Comptes Rendus des Séances de la Societé de Biologie 114: 87–89
4. Chen K K, Rose C L, Clowes G H A 1933 Methylene blue, nitrites, and sodium thiosulphate against cyanide poisoning. Proceedings of the Society of Experimental Biological Medicine 31: 250–251
5. Chen K K, Rose C L, Clowes G H A 1934 Comparative values of several antidotes in cyanide poisoning. American Journal of Medical Science 188: 767–781
6. Hug E, Marenzi A-D 1933 Mecanisme de l'action antidote du nitrite de sodium vis-a-vis de l'intoxication par l'acide cyanhydrique. Comptes Rendus des Séances de la Societé de Biologie 114: 86–87
7. Albaum H G, Tepperman J, Bodansky O 1946 A spectrophotometric study of the competition of methaemoglobin and cytochrome oxidase for cyanide in vitro. Journal of Biological Chemistry 163: 641–647
8. Holmes R K, Way J L 1982 Mechanism of cyanide antagonism by sodium nitrite. Pharmacologist 24: 182 (abstract)
9. Way J L 1984 Cyanide intoxication and its mechanism of antagonism. Annual Review of Pharmacology and Toxicology 24: 451–481
10. Chen K K, Rose C L 1952 Nitrite and thiosulfate therapy in cyanide poisoning. Journal of the American Medical Association 149: 113–119
11. Smith R P, Gosselin R E 1964 The influence of methemoglobinemia on the lethality of some toxic anions. II Sulfide. Toxicology and Applied Pharmacology 6: 584–592
12. Smith R P, Gosselin R E 1966 On the mechanism of sulfide inactivation by methemoglobin. Toxicology and Applied Pharmacology 8: 159–172
13. Smith R P, Kruszyna R, Kruszyna H 1976 Management of acute sulfide poisoning: effects of oxygen thiosulfate and nitrite. Archives of Environmental Health 31: 166–169
14. Beck J F, Bradbury C M, Connors A J, Donini J C 1981 Nitrite as an antidote for acute hydrogen sulfide intoxication? American Industrial Hygiene Association Journal 42: 805–809
15. Way J L, Leung P, Sylvester D M, Burrows G, Way J L, Tamulinas C 1987 Methaemoglobin formation in the treatment of acute cyanide intoxication. In: Ballantyne B, Marrs T C (eds) Clinical and experimental toxicology of cyanides. Wright, Bristol, pp 402–412
16. Paulet G 1960 L'intoxication cyanhydrique et son traitement. Masson et Cie, Paris, pp 48–51
17. Dossin F 1911 Contribution à l'étude expérimentale de la médication hypotensive. Archives Internationales de Pharmacodynamie et de Therapie 21: 425–465
18. Paulet G 1961 Nouvelles perspectives dans le traitement de l'intoxication cyanhydrique. Archives des Maladies Professionelles de Medecine du Travail et de Securité Sociale 22: 120–127
19. Smith R P, Layne W R 1969 A comparison of the lethal effects of nitrite and hydroxylamine in the mouse. Journal of Pharmacology and Experimental Therapeutics 165: 30–35
20. Terzic M, Milosevic M 1963 Action protectrice de l'éthylène-diamine-tétra-acétate-dicobaltique dans l'intoxication cyanée. Thérapie 18: 55–61
21. Riemann H 1950 On the toxicity of hydroxylamine. Acta Pharmacologica 6: 285–292
22. WHO 1974 Food Additive Series No 5. Nitrite, potassium and sodium salts. Geneva: WHO, pp 97–109
23. Myasnikov S P, Pravosudov V P 1966 Electrocardiographic changes in dogs produced by nitrites and nitrates contained in sausages. Sig Sanit 31: 38–42
24. Kuroki T, Abbondandola A, Drevon C, Huberman E, Laval F 1980 Mutagenesis assays with mammalian cells: In: Long-term and short-term screening assays for carcinogens: a critical appraisal. IARC Monographs, suppl 2. International Agency for Research on Cancer, Lyon, pp 107–133
25. Izmerov N F 1982 Nitrites. In: Scientific reviews of Soviet literature on toxicity and hazards of chemicals. International Register of Potentially Toxic Chemicals. Centre of International Projects, Moscow
26. Jarvholm B, Lavenius B, Sallsten G 1986 Cancer morbidity in workers exposed to cutting fluids containing nitrites and amines. British Journal of Industrial Medicine 43: 563–565
27. Schardein J L 1985 Chemically-induced birth defects. Marcel Dekker Inc, New York, pp 74, 759, 810–824
28. Sheehy M, Way J L 1968 Effect of oxygen on cyanide intoxication. III Mithridate. Journal of Pharmacology and Experimental Therapeutics 161: 163–168
29. Way J L, End E, Sheehy M H et al 1972 Effect of oxygen on cyanide intoxication IV Hyperbaric oxygen. Toxicology and Applied Pharmacology 22: 415–421
30. Nicholls P 1975 The effect of sulphide on cytochrome aa_3 isoteric and allosteric shifts of the reduced peak. Biochimica et Biophysica Acta 396: 24–35
31. Smith L, Kruszyna H, Smith R P 1977 The effect of methaemoglobin on the inhibition of cytochrome c oxidase by cyanide, sulfide or azide. Biochemical Pharmacology 26: 2247–2250
32. Peters J W 1981 Hydrogen sulfide poisoning in a hospital setting. Journal of the American Medical Association 246: 1588–1589
33. Huang C-C, Chu N-S 1987 A case of acute hydrogen sulfide (H_2S) intoxication successfully treated with nitrites. Journal of the Formosan Medical Association 86: 1018–1020
34. Burnett W W, King E G, Grace M, Hall W F 1977 Hydrogen sulfide poisoning: review of 5 years experience. Canadian Medical Association Journal 117: 1277–1280
35. Baselt R C 1980 Analytical procedures for therapeutic drug monitoring and emergency toxicology. Biochemical Publications, Davis, California, pp 182–183
36. Shechter H, Gruener N, Shuval H I 1972 A micromethod for the determination of nitrite in blood. Analytica Chimica Acta 60: 93–99
37. Choi K K, Fung F W 1980 Determination of nitrate and nitrite in meat products by using a nitrate ion-selective electrode. Analyst 105: 241–245
38. Thayer J R, Huffaker R C Determination of nitrate and nitrite by high pressure liquid chromatography: comparison with other methods for nitrite determination. Analytical Biochemistry 102: 110–119
39. Reynolds J E F 1989 Martindale: the extra pharmacopoeia. The Pharmaceutical Press, London
40. Moser P 1950 Zur Wirkung von Nitrit auf rote Blutzellen des Menschen. Archiv für experimentelle Pathologie und Pharmakologie 210: 60–70
41. Ingegno A P, Franco S 1937 Cyanide poisoning: successful treatment of two cases with intravenous sodium nitrite and sodium thiosulfate. Industrial Medicine 6: 573–576
42. Evelyn K A, Malloy H T 1938 Microdetermination of oxyhemoglobin, methemoglobin and sulfhemoglobin in a single sample of blood. Journal of Biological Chemistry 126: 655–662
43. Marrs T C 1988 Antidotal treatment of acute cyanide poisoning. Adverse Drug Reactions and Acute Poisoning Reviews 4: 179–206
44. Mota M M 1933 Sobre un caso de intoxicacion por cianuro de potasio tratado con exito por el nitrito de sodio. Rev Med del Rosario 23: 670–674
45. Viana C, Cagnoli H, Cendan J 1934 L'action du nitrite de sodium dans l'intoxication par les cyanures. Comptes Rendus des Séances de la Societé de Biologie 115: 1649–1651
46. Chen K K, Rose C L 1956 Treatment of acute cyanide poisoning. Journal of the American Medical Association 162: 1154–1155
47. De Busk R F, Seidl L G 1969 Attempted suicide by cyanide: a report of two cases. California Medicine 110: 394–396
48. Stewart R 1974 Cyanide poisoning. Clinical Toxicology 7: 561–564
49. Feihl F, Domenighetti G, Perret C 1982 Intoxication massive au cyanure avec evolution favorable. Etude hemodynamique. Schweizerische Medizinische Wochenschrift 112: 1280–1282
50. Peters C G, Mundy J V B, Rayner P R 1982 Acute cyanide poisoning: the treatment of a suicide attempt. Anaesthesia 37: 582–586
51. Wood G C 1982 Acute cyanide intoxication: diagnosis and management. Clinical Toxicology Consultant 4: 140–149
52. Litovitz T L, Larkin R F, Myers R A M 1983 Cyanide poisoning treated with hyperbaric oxygen. American Journal of Emergency Medicine 1: 94–101
53. Wesson D E, Foley R, Sabatini S, Wharton J, Kapusnik J, Kurtzman N A 1985 Treatment of acute cyanide intoxication with hemodialysis. American Journal of Nephrology 5: 121–126
54. Sayre J W, Kaymakcalan S 1964 Cyanide poisoning from apricot seeds among children in central Turkey. New England Journal of Medicine 270: 1113–1115
55. Rubino M J 1978 Cyanide toxicity: report of a case. Connecticut Poison Information Bulletin 3: 1–6

56. Lasche E E, El Shawa R 1981 Multiple cases of cyanide poisoning by apricot kernels in children from Gaza. Paediatrics 68: 5–7
57. Shragg T A, Albertson T E, Fisher C J Jr 1982 Cyanide poisoning after bitter almond ingestion. Western Journal of Medicine 136: 65–69
58. Moss M, Khalil N, Gray J 1981 Deliberate self-poisoning with laetrile. Canadian Medical Association Journal 125: 1126–1128
59. Beamer W C, Shealy R M, Prough D S 1983 Acute cyanide poisoning from laetrile ingestion. Annals of Emergency Medicine 12: 449–451
60. Hall A H, Linden C H, Kulig K W, Rumack B H 1986 Cyanide poisoning from laetrile ingestion: role of nitrite therapy. Pediatrics 78: 269–272
61. Braico K T, Humbert J R, Terplan K L, Lehotay J M 1979 Laetrile intoxication: report of a fatal case. New England Journal of Medicine 300: 238–240
62. Hart G B, Strauss M B, Lennon P A, Whitcraft M D 1985 Treatment of smoke inhalation by hyperbaric oxygen. Journal of Emergency Medicine 3: 211–215
63. McQuiston T A C 1936 Fatal poisoning by sodium nitrite. Lancet 2: 1153–1154
64. Padberg L R, Martin T 1939 Three fatal cases of sodium nitrite poisoning. Journal of the American Medical Association 113: 1733
65. Aquanno J J, Chan K-M, Dietzler D N 1981 Accidental poisoning of two laboratory technologists with sodium nitrite. Clinical Chemistry 27: 1145–1146
66. Ten Brink W A G, Wiezer J H A, Luijpen A F M G, van Heijst A N P, Pikaar S A, Seldenrijk R 1982 Nitrite poisoning caused by food contaminated with cooling fluid. Clinical Toxicology 19: 139–147
67. Standefer J C, Jones A M, Street E, Inserra R 1979 Death associated with nitrite ingestion: report of a case. Journal of Forensic Sciences 24: 768–771
68. Bakshi S P, Fahey J L, Pierce L E 1967 Sausage cyanosis — acquired methemoglobinemic nitrite poisoning. New England Journal of Medicine 277: 1072
69. Berlin C M Jr 1970 The treatment of cyanide poisoning in children. Pediatrics 46: 793–796

Sodium nitroprusside

It is a vasodilator used to control blood pressure.

Chemistry

Sodium nitroprusside (Nipride)
$Na_2Fe(CN)_5NO.2H_2O$
Disodiumnitrosylpentacyanoferrate

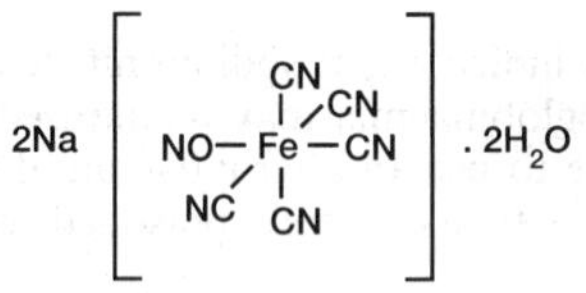

Molecular weight	298
pKa	—
Solubility	
in alcohol	poor
in water	1 in 2.5
Octanol/water partition coefficient	—

Sodium nitroprusside is an inorganic salt, which as the dihydrate forms rhomboid bipyramidal crystals of ruby-red colour. The structural unit is the nitroprusside radical which consists of one iron atom linked to one nitrosyl and 5 cyanide groups. Sodium nitroprusside is unrelated chemically to any other drug available for hypertension.

Sodium nitroprusside is commonly prepared by the oxidation of potassium ferrocyanide with dilute nitric acid and subsequent neutralization of the liquid with sodium carbonate.[1] The reaction scheme is as follows:[2]

$$K_4[Fe(CN)_6].3H_2O + 6HNO_3 \rightleftarrows H_2[(NO)Fe(CN)_5] + 4KNO_3 + NH_4NO_3 + CO_2$$

$$H_2[(NO)Fe(CN)_5] + Na_2CO_3 \rightleftarrows Na_2[(NO)Fe(CN)_5].2H_2O + H_2O + CO_2$$

The pharmaceutical preparation consists of reddish-brown crystals which are soluble in water, relatively stable and resistant to oxidation at a neutral or slightly acidic pH. On heating, the compound dehydrates between 98 and 115°C and decomposes above this temperature. One part of nitroprusside dissolves in 2.5 parts of water at 16°C; in alcohol the compound is slightly soluble. An aqueous solution is photosensitive and, upon exposure to light, there is a reduction of the ferric ion to the ferrous ion.

Pharmacology

Sodium nitroprusside is a potent, rapid-acting and short-lasting vasodilating drug. The action of sodium nitroprusside was first described in 1880 and confirmed later by Johnson in 1929.[3] Its clinical use was first reported by Page in 1955.[4]

The action of sodium nitroprusside is both on arterial and venous smooth muscle, and recently it has also been shown to act on the lower oesophageal sphincter. The vasodilating action is exerted on various vascular beds and the regional distribution of blood flow is little affected. Both systolic and diastolic blood pressures are decreased in a dose-dependent fashion.[5]

Sodium nitroprusside is active in vitro and therefore the vasodilating action is due to the molecule itself, not to breakdown products. The action probably depends on the nitrosyl group, which is 30–1000 times more powerful than nitrites. Sodium nitroprusside does not

Sodium nitroprusside

interfere with α- and β-adrenergic receptors and probably has no effect on calcium influx. Sodium nitroprusside does not increase ATP, but increases GMP levels up to 50-fold. Nitroprusside probably acts as a vasodilator by affecting the cell membrane of the vascular smooth cell, but the mechanism of this action remains to be established.[6]

Sodium nitroprusside decreases systemic blood pressure by reducing total peripheral resistance, and increasing venous capacitance. Cardiac output is unchanged or slightly increased, heart rate only slightly increased. There is a concomitant massive rise in plasma noradrenaline and adrenaline and in plasma renin activity.[7]

Toxicology

Degradation and toxicity are linked together in that the breakdown products, rather than the unchanged product, are responsible for the toxic effects, which consist of the development of metabolic acidosis. Cyanide, the principal metabolic product of sodium nitroprusside, inhibits tissue oxidation processes by blocking the action of cytochrome oxidase and possibly of other enzymes: pyruvate metabolism is converted to lactate metabolism, resulting in so-called histotoxic hypoxia.[6]

Through an enzymatic reaction cyanide is converted to thiocyanate. The latter is 150 times less toxic than cyanide, but has a long half life of elimination (8 days) through the kidneys.

In small rodents, LD_{50} of sodium nitroprusside varies between 8.0 and 12.0 $mg.kg^{-1}$ body weight.[6] In baboons, severe acidosis was found in those animals that received high doses of nitroprusside and did not recover normal blood pressure after discontinuation of the infusion: there was also a reduction in cerebral oxygen uptake.[8] The acute toxicity of sodium nitroprusside is not affected by exposure of the solution to light for 14–32 hours, in spite of the degradation of the solution.

An intramuscular irritation study showed that 0.1 and 1.0 ml doses of 0.1% solution of sodium nitroprusside in 5% dextrose injected intramuscularly into the sacrospinalis muscle of rabbits produced moderate haemorrhage, but no sign of swelling, oedema or necrosis.[4] No haemolysis was demonstrated in dogs following acute intravenous administration of 0.1% solution of sodium nitroprusside.[4]

A two-week intravenous toxicity study in dogs with three different doses of sodium nitroprusside (0.125, 0.5 and 2.0 $mg.kg^{-1}$ daily infused over 2 minutes) showed no adverse reactions related to vasodilatation and hypotension. Blood glucose was temporarily elevated after injection of doses of 0.5 and 2.0 $mg.kg^{-1}$ daily and there were very slight increases in the relative weights of liver, kidney, spleen and adrenal glands, probably related to vasodilatation.[4]

No results of teratogenicity or mutagenicity tests are available.

Clinical pharmacology

Three different types of response to intravenous administration of sodium nitroprusside have been described:

1. normal response, that is blood pressure reduction
2. resistance, that is no significant reduction in blood pressure; and
3. tachyphylaxis, that is transient blood pressure reduction in spite of a continuous sodium nitroprusside injection.

The first response is the usual one, while the second and third ones are very rare. In man the most likely cause of resistance to the drug is reflex increase in heart rate, which is often found in young patients who generally need higher doses of sodium nitroprusside to lower their blood pressure.[9]

Tachyphylaxis only rarely develops in hypertensive patients, while it occurs in normotensive subjects receiving sodium nitroprusside for controlled hypotension during surgery. Tachyphylaxis has been suggested to result from an abnormality of the metabolism of cyanide to thiocyanate as a consequence of thiosulphate depletion, since responsiveness is restored by the administration of thiosulphate. Leber's optic atrophy, a rare inherited disease, tobacco amblyopia and vitamin B_{12} deficiency are conditions in which a fault in cyanide metabolism occurs and these patients may therefore easily develop tachyphylaxis to sodium nitroprusside.[9]

Doses necessary to produce a satisfactory hypotensive response are highly variable and depend upon the patient and the degree of hypertension. However, within the same subject, there is a clear dose–response relation between the blood pressure reductions and the doses of the drug. Effective dose ranges reported in the literature are from 20 to 400 $\mu g.min^{-1}$; the average dose suggested [4,6,9–13] is between 0.5 and 8.0 $\mu g.kg^{-1}.min^{-1}$.

When the infusion has to be administered for a long time (not exceeding 72 h), safety should be monitored by periodic measurement of plasma bicarbonate, lactate and lactate/pyruvate ratio, and of mixed venous blood oxygen tension rather than by measurement of plasma concentrations of thiocyanate and cyanide. The therapeutic index (dose inducing effective reduction of blood pressure vs dose accompanied by lethal events) varies widely.

The longest duration of sodium nitroprusside infusion known in the literature is 45 days. Doses employed in elderly patients should be lower than those employed in adult subjects. Patients receiving other antihypertensive drugs also appear to be more sensitive and may require lower doses.

Intravenous infusion of sodium nitroprusside in man significantly lowers blood pressure: the hypotensive response is immediate, with a rapid fall of blood pressure when the infusion is started or the infusion rate is increased, and rapid disappearance of the effect when the infusion rate is reduced or stopped. The blood pressure reduction is due to a decrease in total peripheral resistance, whereas cardiac output is unchanged or slightly decreased. The percent reductions in systolic and diastolic blood pressures are very similar. In normotensive patients the percent decreases in mean arterial pressure ranged from 15 to 56% and in hypertensive patients from 16 to 64%. The average change in cardiac output is a 12% decrease, as a result of a decrease in some patients and a rise in others.[4–6,9,10,14]

Sodium nitroprusside has a dilating effect on capacitance vessels resulting in a reduction in central venous pressure; this effect is particularly evident in patients with cardiac failure who show a decrease in left ventricular filling pressure proportional to the degree of cardiac failure.[14]

It has been shown that sodium nitroprusside stimulates renal release of renin in normotensive subjects when mean arterial pressure is reduced below 70–75 mmHg; in patients with renal artery stenosis the increase in renin secretion from the affected kidney occurs when the mean arterial pressure is considerably higher (97–137 mmHg).[15]

Pharmacokinetics

The concentration of sodium nitroprusside in solution used for infusion (50–200 $\mu g.ml^{-1}$) can be determined photometrically by a reaction between sodium nitroprusside and alkalinized sodium sulphide (pH > 12), resulting in a red–purple colour with a maximum absorbance at 540 nm. Another colorimetric method for small amounts of sodium nitroprusside is based on the drug's reaction with isophorene (3,5,5-trimethyl-2-cyclohexane-1-one), giving a red complex with maximum absorbance at 495 nm.[16] This method[16] has a sensitivity of 25 $\mu g.ml^{-1}$. Whereas the sensitivity of these methods is limited, a procedure for the determination of minute amounts of sodium nitroprusside in blood and plasma has been described by Rodkey and Collison.[17] By incubation with cysteine, sodium nitroprusside is quantitatively converted to cyanide, which is then bound by adding methaemoglobin. On subsequent acidification, HCN is released and isolated by gas transfer into a sodium hydroxide trap. Then cyanide is chlorinated with chloramine T-phosphate reagent, and a pyridine–pyrazolone solution is added. The resulting colour, as determined spectrophotometrically at 620 nm, is a measure of the total cyanide content; after subtraction of free cyanide measured by the same method, but with the cysteine reaction omitted, the cyanide derived from sodium nitroprusside present in the sample is calculated. Although this method is useful to measure the plasma level of sodium nitroprusside in animals receiving high doses, it is not yet sufficiently sensitive for the determination of plasma levels in patients receiving sodium nitroprusside in the therapeutic range.

In the face of the technical difficulties encountered with direct measurement of sodium nitroprusside in biological fluids, the easier determinations of cyanide and thiocyanate resulting from the in vivo breakdown of sodium nitroprusside are recommended for practical purposes.

There are no human studies available on the biological half life and volume of distribution. Animal experiments only provide information on the half life of the hypotensive effect; on starting an infusion the half time for the fall in blood pressure is about 40 s; after cessation of an infusion of sodium nitroprusside in the therapeutic range, the reduced blood pressure returns to pre-infusion levels with a half time of 32 s. In a study in rats employing subtoxic doses, the volume of distribution was 236 ± 39 ml.kg^{-1} body weight, indicating a distribution of sodium nitroprusside in the extracellular space.[6]

Concentration–effect relationship

In any given patient the hypotensive effect of sodium nitroprusside is dose-dependent over a wide range of concentrations; this makes it likely that a concentration–effect relationship exists, but direct evidence is lacking because of the difficulty, discussed above, of measuring sodium nitroprusside in plasma.

Metabolism

The main route of excretion of sodium nitroprusside, cyanide and thiocyanate is through the kidney, and acute renal failure almost doubles the hypotensive response. Only negligible amounts of sodium nitroprusside are excreted through the faeces.[6]

There is no evidence of enterohepatic circulation of sodium nitroprusside, but its metabolite, thiocyanate, is subjected to repeated enterohepatic recirculation prior to being eliminated via the kidney.

The pathway for sodium nitroprusside breakdown in vivo starts with a non-enzymatic cleavage of sodium nitroprusside as a first step; then, the major part of released cyanide reacts with thiosulphates under the influence of the enzyme rhodanase to form the final product, thiocyanate.[18] Several other metabolic pathways are known for cyanide, but they do not appear to play a very important role. Little is known of the fate of the other constituents of sodium nitroprusside, but a transformation of NO groups to NO_2 ions and the binding of iron atoms to transferrin with subsequent uptake into reticuloendothelial cells are likely to occur. Thiocyanates are eliminated through the kidneys, and the other products through both kidneys and lungs.[6]

The metabolic products of sodium nitroprusside are not active on the cardiovascular system.

Pharmaceutics

Injectable sodium nitroprusside is supplied either as Nipride (Roche, UK/USA) in 5 ml amber-coloured vials containing the equivalent of 50 mg sodium nitroprusside dihydrate or Nitropress (Abbott, USA) as 50 mg of sodium nitroprusside to be first reconstituted with 2 or 3 ml of sterile dextrose 5% in water: no other diluent should be used. Depending on the desired concentration of the infusion, all the available solutions should be added to 250–1000 ml of sterile 5% dextrose in water. The freshly prepared solution for infusion has a faint orange–brown tint: if it is highly coloured it should not be used. The infusion solution should be promptly wrapped in aluminium foil or other opaque materials to protect it from light. Once prepared the solution should not be stored, or administered for a period longer than four hours.

If sodium nitroprusside is stored in 5 ml ampoules at 4°C, the shelf-life is approximately 3 months, although other authors claim that 1% solutions of sodium nitroprusside are stable for at least 6 months to 2 years, when kept in the dark at no more than 25°C. The oxidative decomposition of the solution is shown by a colour change from orange or reddish-brown to a deep blue.

Therapeutic use

As sodium nitroprusside is only available for intravenous use, and its hypotensive action has a rapid onset and short duration, the compound is used for rapid and flexible control of blood pressure in different clinical conditions. More recently, it has also been used to lower afterload in patients with congestive heart failure. A disadvantage of sodium nitroprusside therapy, however, is that because of the potent hypotensive effect of the drug, its administration calls for careful and continuous monitoring of the patient's blood pressure.

Indications

1. Hypertensive emergencies
2. Hypotensive anaesthesia
3. Dissecting aortic aneurysm
4. Acute myocardial infarction, acute congestive heart failure
5. Miscellaneous indications.

Contraindications

1. Sodium nitroprusside should not be used in the treatment of hypertension due to coarctation of aorta or an arteriovenous shunt.
2. Cyanide and thiocyanate interfere with the metabolism of cyanocobalamin (vitamin B_{12}), and therefore sodium nitroprusside should not be administered to patients who are vitamin B_{12} deficient.
3. Sodium nitroprusside is also contraindicated in patients who have severely impaired liver function, suffer from Leber's optic atrophy or tobacco amblyopia.

Mode of use

Sodium nitroprusside is given as an intravenous infusion only; other routes or methods of administration are not recommended. The infusion rate has to be determined for each individual patient by continuous monitoring of blood pressure. Sodium nitroprusside should preferably be administered using a microdrip regulator, an infusion pump or a similar device allowing a precise flow rate control. Especially in young patients, the dose of sodium nitroprusside should be increased slowly until the desired effect occurs, in order to prevent or reduce compensatory reactions (a sharp rise in plasma catecholamines and renin, tachycardia and subsequent tachyphylaxis). The infusion should not be terminated abruptly, but over a period of 10–30 minutes, in order to prevent an excessive rebound rise in blood pressure.

The dose required to achieve a given reduction in blood pressure decreases with the age of patient. If therapy is required for several days, which is rarely advisable, blood and plasma cyanide levels should be monitored regularly to ensure that concentrations of 1 mg.l^{-1} and 80 µg.l^{-1}, respectively in blood and plasma, are not exceeded. If an infusion is administered for more than three days serum thiocyanate concentration should also be monitored and should not exceed 60–100 µg.l^{-1}. A simpler method to evaluate toxicity is the evaluation of plasma bicarbonate and lactate, as toxicity is associated with development of acidosis.

Indications

1. Hypertensive emergencies

The clinical conditions called 'hypertensive emergencies' are numerous and are characterized by a sudden and marked elevation in blood pressure, which must be lowered without too much delay in order to prevent serious cardiovascular complications. A hypertensive emergency can be due to malignant hypertension, acute and chronic renal parenchymal diseases, phaeochromocytoma, renal artery stenosis, primary hyperaldosteronism, pregnancy-induced hypertension, etc. The most frequent complications are hypertensive encephalopathy, intracranial haemorrhage, acute left ventricle failure and aortic dissection. The advantages of sodium nitroprusside in these conditions are its rapid onset of action, by which blood pressure is lowered without delay, its dose–response relationship, by which the required blood pressure lowering can be achieved by varying the drug infusion rate, and the brief duration of action, that allows excessive hypotension to be rapidly corrected by stopping the infusion or reducing its rate.

Nitroprusside is consistently effective and has been proven effective when other conventional forms of antihypertensive therapy have failed.

In patients who are not receiving any antihypertensive drug, treatment with sodium nitroprusside should be instituted with a dose of 0.3–1.0 µg.kg^{-1}.min^{-1} and the dose should be gradually increased until the desired blood pressure reduction is obtained. This will normally occur at doses of 0.5–6.0 µg.kg^{-1}.min^{-1}, with an average dose of 3.0 µg.kg^{-1}.min^{-1}. In most patients an average of 200 µg.min^{-1} (range 20–400 µg.min^{-1}) is sufficient to maintain blood pressure at a level 30–40% lower than pretreatment blood pressure.

The rate of administration should be adjusted to maintain the desired antihypertensive effect, as evaluated by frequent blood pressure measurements or, preferably, by continuous intra-arterial blood pressure monitoring.

In order to avoid excessive levels of cyanide, an end-product of sodium nitroprusside metabolism, and to lessen the possibility of a precipitous fall in blood pressure, the maximum recommended dose during short-term use (several hours) is 8 μg.kg^{-1}.min^{-1}. If the desired blood pressure reduction is not obtained within 10 min with the maximum dose, the administration of sodium nitroprusside should be stopped and other methods of blood pressure lowering tested.

2. Hypotensive anaesthesia
When sodium nitroprusside is used for induction of deliberate hypotension during anaesthesia, lower doses than those employed in hypertensive emergencies should be administered. Indeed, the intrinsic hypotensive action of many anaesthetic agents must be borne in mind. The dose should not exceed 1.5 μg.kg^{-1}.min^{-1} and the usual practices and precautions employed in hypertensive emergencies should be observed.

3. Dissecting aortic aneurysm
A significant reduction in blood pressure provides a temporary control of a dissecting aneurysm and gives time to perform diagnostic procedures for a better surgical approach.

4. Acute myocardial infarction and acute congestive heart failure
Preliminary studies by Franciosa and others[19] have suggested that vasodilator therapy by sodium nitroprusside may provide considerable improvement in the abnormal haemodynamics during the early stage of acute myocardial infarction, by decreasing left ventricle filling pressure without important reduction in arterial pressure and clinically significant changes in heart rate. The final result is a reduction in oxygen consumption (reduction in heart rate–pressure product and in diastolic wall tension), although there is the possibility of decreased coronary perfusion pressure and of a 'steal phenomenon'.

Acute reduction in preload and afterload in patients with acute congestive heart failure can be achieved by infusion of sodium nitroprusside with resultant increase in cardiac output, stroke work and urinary sodium excretion. However, an increase in cardiac arrhythmias and ECG signs of myocardial injury have been described.

Sodium nitroprusside infusion should be started at a low rate (0.15–0.20 μg.kg^{-1}.min^{-1}, i.e. approximately 10–15 μg.min^{-1}) and the dosage raised in increments of 10–15 μg.min^{-1} every 5 or 10 minutes until an initial clinical response is obtained. Then the dose should be adjusted until the optimal therapeutic effect is obtained. The therapeutic range is between 10 and 200 μg.min^{-1} and doses larger than 400 μg.min^{-1} should not be exceeded. Sodium nitroprusside must be stopped if no significant improvement is achieved at these high doses. Blood pressure must be monitored at frequent intervals (or intra-arterially), and if excessive hypotension or signs of hypoperfusion occur the infusion rate should be reduced or treatment discontinued. Changes in mental status, neurological signs, oliguria, further chest pain and arrhythmias, nausea and vomiting are indications for dose reduction. In the case of a favourable response, the infusion should be continued until the patient can be stabilized on appropriate oral therapy, but administration should not last longer than 72 hours.

5. Miscellaneous indications
Sodium nitroprusside has been employed for a variety of other clinical situations such as during renal arteriography to improve visualization of renal vessels, in severe pre-eclampsia, and to counteract peripheral vasospasm due to an overdose of ergotamine tartrate.

Sodium nitroprusside can be administered in all these cases by starting at low doses (for instance 0.15–0.20 μg.kg^{-1}.min^{-1} as in cardiac failure) and increasing the dose at 5–10 minute intervals until the desired clinical effect has been obtained. Doses higher than 400–600 μg.min^{-1} should not be used unless under strict control of blood pressure and careful monitoring for possible adverse reactions.

Adverse reactions

Potentially life-threatening effects
Five deaths associated with the use of sodium nitroprusside for induction of hypotension during surgery have been reported. In all these cases doses of sodium nitroprusside larger than usual were required to maintain the desired hypotension. In the only patient in whom cyanide levels were measured in blood and urine, these were very high; a pronounced base deficit, indicative of increased anaerobic metabolism, and elevated mixed venous blood oxygen tension were found in two other patients.[10]

Acute overdosage
There are three recorded suicides with sodium nitroprusside and in each case free cyanide was found in the stomach. The toxicity of sodium nitroprusside is due to an insufficient conversion of cyanide (derived from non-enzymatic decomposition of sodium nitroprusside) to thiocyanate. This conversion is catalysed by the mitochondrial enzyme rhodanase, which facilitates transfer of a sulphur group to the cyanide molecule in the presence of a sulphur donor. The goal of prevention or treatment of cyanide toxicity is to decrease cyanide binding to cytochrome C and to remove cyanide from the blood.

After discontinuation of sodium nitroprusside the following antidotes can be employed:

1. Sodium thiosulphate (12.5 g in 25 or 50 ml of 5% dextrose), as intravenous injection in 10 minutes, which can be repeated if necessary.
2. Dicobalt edetate (300 mg in 20 ml) injected intravenously over about one minute, followed by 50 ml of 50% dextrose injection. These doses can be repeated immediately if the response is inadequate and a third dose given after 5 minutes if necessary.
3. Hydroxocobalamin has been suggested as an alternative antidote, but it is impractical in the acute treatment of cyanide poisoning because of the large dosage required. However, prophylactic infusions of lower doses (1.5 mg.kg^{-1}) have been used to reduce plasma cyanide concentrations in patients receiving sodium nitroprusside doses close to the recommended maximum.

Since haemodialysis removes thiocyanate ions, intermittent haemodialysis may be used to treat thiocyanate toxicity or to allow higher doses of sodium nitroprusside to be employed.

Severe or irreversible adverse effects
Hypothyroidism probably due to interference by thiocyanate with iodine uptake and binding by the thyroid gland seems to be an infrequent adverse effect of sodium nitroprusside administration.[20]

Symptomatic adverse effects
The most frequent adverse effects of sodium nitroprusside are nausea, retching, diaphoresis, apprehension, headache, restlessness, muscle twitching, retrosternal discomfort, palpitations, dizziness, and abdominal discomfort. They are associated with too rapid lowering of blood pressure and quickly disappear when the rate of infusion is reduced or the infusion is temporarily stopped. They generally do not reappear at a slower rate of administration.

Other effects
Metabolic acidosis is the only relevant biochemical alteration due to cyanide toxicity. Unexplained cyanosis during sodium nitroprusside infusion may be due to methaemoglobinaemia.

Interference with clinical pathology tests
No such interference has been reported in the literature available.

High risk groups

Neonates
The drug is not used in neonates

Breast milk. It is probably best for mothers who have received the drug to avoid breast-feeding their infants.

Children
For the treatment of hypertensive emergencies in children an infusion rate between 0.3 and 1.4 μg.kg^{-1}.min^{-1} has been found necessary to reduce blood pressure.

Pregnant women
The safety of sodium nitroprusside in pregnancy has not been established, but it is known that the drug crosses the placental barrier.

The elderly
Elderly people are more sensitive to the hypotensive effect of sodium nitroprusside and therefore should receive lower doses than those given to younger subjects.

Concurrent disease

Sodium nitroprusside is contraindicated in patients with severe impairment of liver function, with Leber's optic atrophy, or tobacco amblyopia.

Precautions must be taken in patients with known disturbances of cerebral blood flow, in order to avoid too rapid lowering of blood pressure. Because thiocyanate inhibits both iodine uptake and binding by the thyroid, caution must be exercised in treating patients with hypothyroidism. In patients with renal failure the excretion of thiocyanate is decreased and care must be exerted when sodium nitroprusside is administered for long periods.

Drug interactions

Potentially hazardous interactions

No such interactions have been reported in the available medical literature.

Potentially useful interactions

Hypertensive patients who are already on treatment with other antihypertensive agents are more sensitive to the effects of sodium nitroprusside and therefore require smaller doses. The association with ganglion-blocking agents and β-blockers may be useful, but the pharmacological action of sodium nitroprusside is compatible with all other drugs commonly used to treat hypertension.

In patients with cardiac failure, sodium nitroprusside infusions may be given in conjunction with diuretics, inotropic agents or other measures conventionally used in the management of cardiac failure.

References

1. Ephraim F 1954 Inorganic chemistry, 6th edn. Interscience, New York, p 332
2. Braver G 1962 In: Enke F (ed) Handbuch der Preparation anorganischen Chemie, 2nd edn. Stuttgart, p 1530
3. Johnson C C 1929 The actions and toxicity of sodium nitroprusside. Archives Internationale de Pharmacodynamie et de Therapie 35: 480–496
4. Page I A, Corcoran A C, Dustan H P, Koppanyi T 1955 Cardiovascular actions of sodium nitroprusside in animals and hypertensive patients. Circulation 11: 183–198
5. Cohn N, Burke P 1979 Nitroprusside. Annals of Internal Medicine 91: 752–757
6. Volker A, Kreye W 1980 Sodium nitroprusside. In: Scribner A (ed) Pharmacology of antihypertensive drugs. Raven Press, New York, pp 373–396
7. Stanek B, Zimpfer M, Fitzal S, Roberger G 1981 Plasma catecholamines, plasma renin activity and haemodynamics during sodium nitroprusside-induced hypotension and additional beta-blockade with bunitrolol. European Journal of Clinical Pharmacology 19: 317–322
8. McDowall D G, Keaney N P, Turner J M, Lane J R, Okuda Y 1974 The toxicity of sodium nitroprusside. British Journal of Anaesthesia 46: 327–332
9. Cole P 1978 The safe use of sodium nitroprusside. Anaesthesia 33: 473–477
10. Tinker J H, Michenfelder J D 1976 Sodium nitroprusside: pharmacology, toxicology and therapeutics. Anesthesiology 15: 340–354
11. Davies D W, Kadar D, Steward D J 1975 A sudden death associated with the use of sodium nitroprusside for induction of hypotension during anaesthesia. Canadian Anaesthetists Society Journal 22: 547–552
12. Davies D W, Greiss L, Stewart D J 1975 Sodium nitroprusside in children: observations on metabolism during normal and abnormal responses. Canadian Anaesthetists Society Journal 22: 553–560
13. Palmer R F, Lasseter K D 1975 Sodium nitroprusside. New England Journal of Medicine 293: 294–297
14. Guiha N A, Cohn J N, Mikulic E, Franciosa J A, Limas C J 1974 Treatment of refractory heart failure with infusion of nitroprusside. New England Journal of Medicine 291: 587–592
15. Kaneko Y, Ikeda T, Takeda T, Ueda H 1967 Renin release during acute reduction of arterial pressure in normotensive subjects and patients with renovascular hypertension. Journal of Clinical Investigation 46: 705–716
16. Vesey C J, Batistoni G A 1977 The determination and stability of sodium nitroprusside in aqueous solutions. Journal of Clinical Pharmacology 2: 105–117
17. Rodkey F L, Collison H A 1977 Determination of cyanide and nitroprusside in blood and plasma. Clinical Chemistry 23: 1969–1975
18. Vernier I R 1974 Sodium nitroprusside: theory and practice. Postgraduate Medical Journal 50: 576–581
19. Franciosa J A, Guiha N H, Limas C J, Rodriguera E, Cohn J N 1972 Improved left ventricular function during nitroprusside infusion in acute myocardial infarction. Lancet 1: 650–654
20. Nourok D S, Glassock R J, Solomon D H, Maxwell M H 1964 Hypothyroidism following prolonged sodium nitroprusside therapy. American Journal of Medical Sciences 248: 129–138

Sodium salicylate

An antipyretic analgesic.

Chemistry

Sodium salicylate (Entrosalyl)
$C_7H_5NaO_3$
Sodium 2-hydroxybenzoate
Each gram contains 6.25 mmol of sodium

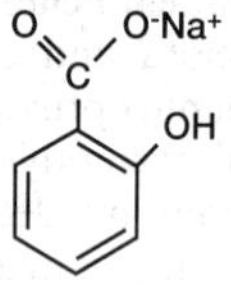

Molecular weight (free acid)	160.1 (138.1)
pKa (–COO, –OH)	2.9, 13.4
Solubility	
in alcohol	1 in 11
in water	1 in 1
Octanol/water partition coefficient	low

Colourless crystals or a white to faintly pink powder with a sweetish saline taste. It is synthesized by the neutralization of salicylic acid with sodium hydroxide. Sodium salicylate is available in combination with a variety of compounds including other analgesics, antitussives, decongestants, expectorants and antihistamines.

Pharmacology

Sodium salicylate is analgesic, antipyretic and anti-inflammatory. These effects are probably achieved by an inhibition of the enzyme cyclooxygenase and a subsequent reduction in tissue prostaglandins.[1,2] Salicylate is a much weaker inhibitor of cyclooxygenase than aspirin,[1,2] and yet in vivo it appears to be of comparable efficacy as an anti-inflammatory drug.[3] Salicyclate is formed rapidly from acetysalicylic acid in vivo, although effects on prostaglandin synthesis in platelets and the vascular endothelium appear to be entirely due to the ability of aspirin to acetylate the cyclooxygenase enzyme. Salicylate may also act via inhibition of eicosapentaenoic acid metabolism or by scavenging free oxygen radicals. Salicylate, unlike aspirin, does not inhibit platelet aggregation. Salicylate stimulates respiration by a direct effect on the medulla, and at high concentrations it uncouples oxidative phosphorylation in muscle increasing oxygen consumption and carbon dioxide production. Hyperventilation causes a respiratory alkalosis, which is compensated for by a renal excretion of bicarbonate. Subsequent events cause an accumulation of lactic and pyruvic acids causing a metabolic acidosis. Salicylate is directly toxic to the gastric mucosa and in high doses ($\geqslant$5 g daily) it is uricosuric.

Toxicology

Salicylates are teratogenic in animals, but no mutagenic potential has been demonstrated in man. There is no evidence of carcinogenicity.

Chronic intoxication (salicylism) can present with tinnitus, impaired hearing, headache, dimness of vision, dizziness, confusion, lethargy, drowsiness, sweating, thirst, hyperventilation, tachycardia, nausea, vomiting and sometimes diarrhoea. Metabolic acidosis and respiratory alkalosis usually develop. Adults most often develop auditory effects whereas children develop hyperventilation or CNS manifestations.

Acute intoxication usually results from an overdose (see Acute overdosage).

Sodium salicylate

Clinical pharmacology

The precise mechanisms of action of its analgesic and anti-inflammatory effects are unresolved but some of these activities may be associated with reduction of prostaglandin synthesis by the selective inhibition of cyclooxygenase. However, in comparison to aspirin, salicylate is a relatively weak inhibitor of prostaglandin production in vitro[1,2] but equipotent in suppressing in vivo models of inflammation.[3] In contrast to opiates the site of the analgesic effect of salicylate is peripheral.

Salicylates inhibit reabsorption of uric acid in the proximal renal tubule at high dosage and will increase urinary excretion of uric acid and decrease serum uric acid. However, they are rarely used for this indication today.

Pharmacokinetics

The preferred analytical method for salicylate is high pressure liquid chromatography with UV detection.[4] The limit of sensitivity is 50 μg.l^{-1}. It is highly sensitive and can also be used to quantify salicylurate. In the past, salicylate has been determined in biological fluids by spectrofluorimetry[5] and colorimetrically from the purple colour developed on the reaction of o-carboxyphenols with ferric ions in weak acid solution.[6]

Oral absorption	80–100%
Presystemic metabolism	—
Plasma half life	
low dose	2–3 h
anti-inflammatory dose	12 h
Volume of distribution	0.15–0.2 l.kg^{-1}
Plasma protein binding	90–95%

Sodium salicylate is rapidly absorbed by passive diffusion from the stomach and proximal small intestine at a rate greater than that for aspirin. Absorption is reduced by the concomitant use of alkalis. Peak plasma levels occur at between 40 minutes and 6 hours, depending on dosage and formulation used.

Salicylate is widely and rapidly distributed into most tissues and body fluids with an apparent volume of distribution of 0.15–0.2 l.kg^{-1} at usual therapeutic concentrations. This increases with increasing dose, due probably to decreased protein binding.

Salicylate is highly protein bound, principally to albumin. The percentage bound depends on salicylate concentration, albumin concentration, age and disease state. It is 90–95% bound at usual therapeutic levels in healthy adults but may be only 25–60% bound at high salicylate levels and more is available to distribute into tissues. Distribution is also pH dependent.

Salicylate readily penetrates synovial fluid with 50–75% of peak serum concentration following a single dose and equal concentrations at steady state. It crosses the placenta and fetal serum levels may be greater than maternal levels. Only small amounts appear to be distributed into milk.

Sodium salicylate dissociates to salicylate in vivo. It is excreted in the urine as such and is metabolized in the smooth endoplasmic reticulum of hepatocytes. The extent of metabolism depends on the rate of renal excretion of unchanged salicylate, which is both concentration and pH dependent. The extent of renal excretion increases rapidly with pH above 6.5 and, at a urine pH of 8, up to 85% of a single dose may be excreted unchanged. At low doses the elimination of salicylate is first order, with a half life of 2–3 h. However, elimination at higher concentrations is capacity limited by glycine conjugation, with the half life becoming as long as 15–30 h.[7]

The elimination of salicylate can be considerably delayed in renal failure and with deteriorating renal function associated with old age.

Concentration–effect relationship

Therapeutic effects are determined by total plasma salicylate. Plasma levels of 30–100 mg.l^{-1} are analgesic and antipyretic, but levels of 150–300 mg.l^{-1} are required for anti-inflammatory activity in rheumatic diseases. The dose required varies between individuals and needs to be tailored in each case. It may often be high enough to produce tinnitus. Most show toxicity at levels above 300 mg.l^{-1}, greater than 350 mg.l^{-1} producing hyperventilation, and acidosis occurs over 460 mg.l^{-1}.

Metabolism

Salicylate is rapidly excreted in the urine, either unchanged or as metabolites; 80–100% of a single dose is excreted in the urine within 24–72 h. Within the normal urinary pH range, less than 25% of salicylate is excreted unchanged, but this may rise to 85% in alkaline urine. The proportion that remains to be metabolized thus varies depending on the concentration and urine pH. Salicylate is metabolized by hepatic endoplasmic reticular enzymes. The principal metabolite is the glycine conjugate, salicyluric acid. Other metabolites are the phenolic glucuronide, salicylphenolic glucuronide, the ester glucuronide, salicylacylglucuronide and the hydroxylation product, gentisic acid (Fig. 1). Salicylic acid and salicylphenolic glucuronide are formed by capacity-limited processes. With increasing single doses or long-term therapy the proportions excreted as these therefore decreases. Gentisic acid is the only active metabolite. It is a potent inhibitor of prostaglandin synthesis but insufficient is formed to make a significant contribution to the pharmacological effects of salicylate.

Unchanged salicylate is excreted by glomerular filtration and by a carrier-facilitated transport mechanism for weak organic acids in the proximal tubule. If the urine is acidic, salicylate is partly reabsorbed in the distal tubule in the non-ionized lipid-soluble form. Salicylate metabolites also pass through the glumerulus and the proximal tubule. The glycine and glucuronide conjugates are not readily reabsorbed in the renal tubule and their excretion is unaffected by urinary pH. Renal clearance of salicylate can therefore be increased by alkaline diuresis.

Fig. 1 Metabolism of salicylate

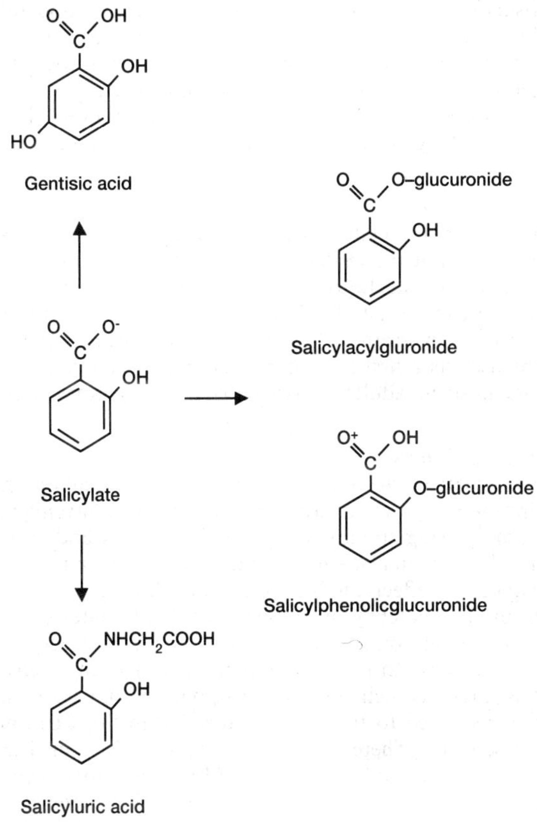

Pharmaceutics

Sodium salicylate is available in oral and parenteral forms.

Tablets contain 325, 500 or 650 mg of drug. With the exception of Pabalate (enteric-coated), they should be dissolved before administration.

Enteric-coated tablets contain 325 mg (Uracel 5; Vortech, UK), 500 mg (Entrosalyl; Cox-Continental, UK/Pabalate; Robins, USA), or 650 mg (Double-Sal; Vale, UK).

S

Sodium salicylate mixture BP contains 250 mg of drug in 5 ml and sodium salicylate mixture, strong BP contains 500 mg of drug in 5 ml.

Sodium salicylate is available for parenteral use as 100 mg.ml^{-1}.

Therapeutic use

Indications

1. Pain
2. Fever
3. Arthritic conditions.

Sodium salicylate, introduced 100 years ago, was the first orally tolerated salicylate to be developed, but it was soon followed by aspirin, which rapidly dominated the market. Few modern controlled studies have been performed with sodium salicylate alone or in comparison with aspirin, other non-steroidal anti-inflammatory agents or simple analgesics. Its effectiveness as an analgesic, antipyretic and anti-inflammatory agents appears to be similar to aspirin.

Contraindications

1. Children under 12 years of age (except juvenile chronic arthritis)
2. Aspirin or non-steroidal anti-inflammatory agent sensitivity
3. Active or history of recent erosive gastritis or peptic ulceration
4. Renal insufficiency
5. Pyruvate kinase deficiency
6. G-6-PD deficiency
7. Congestive cardiac failure (because of high sodium content)
8. Rheumatic fever (because of high sodium content).

Indications

1. Pain

Sodium salicylate is effective in the relief of mild to moderate pain, especially when associated with inflammation. It is used in the treatment of simple headache, migraine, minor postoperative pain, dental pain, post-partum pain and dysmenorrhoea.

The usual dose in adults is 325–650 mg orally every 4 hours as required, or 500 mg intravenously by slow infusion but not exceeding 1 g daily.

2. Fever

Sodium salicylate is an effective antipyretic agent, although aspirin is 1.5 times more potent.[7] Salicylates have long been used to reduce fever in childhood infectious illnesses, but due to the epidemiological evidence that aspirin may be a contributory factor in causing some cases of Reye's syndrome[8,9] a non-salicylate such as paracetamol should be used as a first-line antipyretic in children under 12 years. The usual dose in adults is 325–650 mg orally every 4 hours as required.

3. Arthritic conditions

Sodium salicylate is effective in the long-term treatment of inflammatory joint disease such as rheumatoid arthritis, juvenile chronic arthritis, ankylosing spondylitis, psoriatic arthritis and reactive arthritis. It relieves pain and stiffness and reduces swelling of joints, but has no apparent effect on the underlying disease process and its progression. The potency of non-acetylated salicylates is similar to aspirin[10] and other non-steroidal anti-inflammatory drugs.[11] Sodium salicylate is effective in the symptomatic treatment of osteoarthritis, in soft-tissue lesions such as capsulitis or bursitis, in back pain and in gout. It is also used to treat the various features of SLE: arthritis, fever and serositis. There is a risk of hepatotoxicity in SLE[12] and hepatic function should be monitored. Although it does have a useful uricosuric effect at high dose, it is not of sufficient potency to be of first choice in acute gouty inflammation. Salicylates have long been first choice in the treatment of rheumatoid arthritis, but with the advent of other non-steroidal anti-inflammatory agents, the use of salicylates has declined although similar in efficacy and side effects.

The choice of salicylates above other non-steroidal anti-inflammatory agents in juvenile chronic arthritis should be carefully considered due to the association with Reye's syndrome.[8,9] In the event of a known local epidemic of chickenpox or influenza, an alternative non-steroidal anti-inflammatory agent should be substituted.

Since sodium salicylate appears to be as potent as aspirin but less ulcerogenic[13] it should perhaps be used more often,[14] although the data comparing their efficacy and toxicity is limited. Lack of palatability is a problem.

The usual dose in the treatment of inflammatory arthritic conditions is 3.6–5.4 g daily in adults and 80–100 mg.kg^{-1} daily in children. This should be taken continuously to maintain high serum levels and the dose titrated to symptomatic response, tolerance and serum salicylate concentration. Symptoms of toxicity such as tinnitus may occur at these high dosages.

Adverse reactions

Potentially life-threatening effects

Hypersensitivity reactions. Hypersensitivity reactions to salicylates other than aspirin is extremely rare and cross-sensitivity is unusual. There is little data to the incidence with sodium salicylate. Urticaria, angioedema, severe rhinitis, bronchospasm or occasionally vasomotor collapse may occur within 3 h of administration. Very small doses of salicylate may precipitate a sensitivity reaction. Sensitivity is more common in patients with chronic urticaria or asthma. Salicylate sensitivity in asthmatics is usually associated with nasal polyps. There appears to be a relationship between in vitro cyclooxygenase inhibition and the bronchospasm-producing activity of various anti-inflammatory drugs.[15] Patients with aspirin-induced bronchospasm may therefore be able to tolerate sodium salicylate, as it is a poor inhibitor of cyclooxygenase in vitro, and cross-sensitivity has seldom been noted.[15] Sodium salicylate should, however, be used with caution in patients with a history of sensitivity to aspirin or other non-steroidal anti-inflammatory agents.

Reye's syndrome. Reye's syndrome is an acute encephalopathic illness with fatty degeneration of the viscera, in particular the liver, that may follow an acute viral illness, typically influenza or chickenpox.[16] It is frequently fatal. Its aetiology is unknown but epidemiological studies indicate that the use of aspirin during the preceding illness may be a contributory factor.[8,9] There are no data concerning the use of other salicylates including sodium salicylate. The Committee on Safety of Medicines has recommended the use of alternative effective remedies such as paracetamol in children under 12 years of age. No specific recommendation has been made concerning sodium salicylate. Children with juvenile chronic arthritis may be dependent on aspirin therapy and it is reasonable to continue except during known local epidemics of chickenpox or influenza.

Acute overdosage

Death has occurred from 10–30 g of sodium salicylate. Severe toxicity usually occurs with the ingestion of 300–500 mg.kg^{-1}.

Mild overdose may just cause epigastric pain and gastric erosion. The effects of more severe acute overdose are similar to those seen with chronic intoxication, principally gastrointestinal irritation, direct central respiratory stimulation and metabolic effects that include acid–base and electrolyte disturbance.

Children usually develop a metabolic acidosis and adults a respiratory alkalosis. Hyperglycaemia, hypoglycaemia, hyperpyrexia, oliguria and acute renal failure may also occur. CNS stimulation causes irritability, disorientation and confusion but progresses to depression and coma. Respiratory insufficiency or cardiovascular collapse may lead to death.

Treatment is to prevent further absorption, increase the clearance of salicylate and to correct the metabolic disturbances. Absorption can continue during the first 6 hours and serum salicylate levels may increase during the first 24 hours with very large overdosages. An early estimate of serum salicylate may underestimate the magnitude of overdose. Emesis or gastric lavage are effective for up to 4 hours or longer with large overdosages, and activated charcoal reduces absorption.

Correction of acidosis, fluid and electrolyte replacement, and cooling may be required. Urea, electrolytes, acid–base balance and glucose and urine output need to be monitored. If salicylate concentration exceeds 500 mg.l^{-1} at 6 hours following ingestion and the clinical picture suggests severe overdosage, forced alkaline diuresis is often used. The urinary pH should be in excess of 7.5, ideally between 8.0 and 8.5. One regime used comprises the infusion of 0.5 l 0.9% saline, 0.5 l 5% dextrose and 0.5 l 1.26% sodium bicarbonate, in rotation up to a maximum of 1.5–2.0 l per hour usually to a total of 6 l. The bicarbonate or saline may need substituting for each other to maintain the urinary pH. Alkalinization of urine is probably more important than the diuresis.

If the salicylate concentration is 900–1300 $mg.l^{-1}$ or more at 6 hours or if the manifestations are severe, then haemodialysis, haemoperfusion, peritoneal dialysis, or exchange transfusion may be used.

Severe or irreversible adverse effects

Gastrointestinal effects. Sodium salicylate may cause gastric irritation and mucosal lesions, ranging from erythema to ulceration and gastric blood loss which may be major. Sodium salicylate causes fewer gastrointestinal effects than aspirin, with little blood loss and a lower incidence of gastric ulceration.[12,17] Gastrointestinal symptoms can be reduced by taking sodium salicylate with food.

Cardiac effects. Sodium salicylate, because of its high sodium content, can precipitate or worsen pre-existing heart failure. It is not recommended for use in rheumatic fever.

Hepatic effects. Salicylates may cause hepatotoxicity,[18] but there are no reports of its occurrence with sodium salicylate. Patients with SLE or juvenile chronic arthritis are particularly at risk of developing hepatotoxicity with salicylates, notably aspirin.[13] Often the only manifestation is an elevation of serum aminotransferase and occasionally of alkaline phosphatase, but hepatic failure and death has rarely occurred.

Symptomatic adverse effects

Rashes are uncommon and are usually only found following chronic use or overdose. They can be varied but most often are of a pustular acneiform character.

Chronic salicylate intoxication, or 'salicylism', may develop with the use of high dosages for prolonged periods. Symptoms are headache, dizziness, tinnitus, impaired hearing, dimness of vision, mental confusion, drowsiness, lassitude, sweating, thirst, nausea, vomiting and diarrhoea. They may also develop tachycardia and hyperventilation. Metabolic acidosis and respiratory alkalosis develop, which are worse with higher dosage and longer duration of therapy. Salicylates uncouple oxidative phosphorylation and the resultant increased production of CO_2, with the direct effect of high levels of salicylates on the medulla, stimulates respiration to produce a respiratory alkalosis, which is compensated for by renal excretion of bicarbonate. Metabolic acidosis also occurs due to salicylate itself and the accumulation of other acids because of impaired excretion or salicylate-induced formation. Acidosis usually predominates. Salicylism usually develops when the serum salicylate level is more than 300 $mg.l^{-1}$. Adults most frequently develop tinnitus and impaired hearing, children hyperventilation or CNS effects.

Interference with clinical pathology tests

Salicylates may interfere with some tests for urinary glucose, oestrogens, 17-hydroxycorticosteroids, and ketones, and some tests for serum uric acid.

High risk groups

Neonates

Salicylates may displace bilirubin from albumin and should be avoided.

Breast milk. Salicylates are found in milk and long-term high dosage should be avoided when breast-feeding.

Children

Salicylates should be avoided in children under 12 years of age because of the association with Reye's syndrome.

Pregnant women

Fetal abnormalities have not been demonstrated at conventional doses, although chronic ingestion has been associated with an increased incidence of stillbirth, decreased birth weight, and increases in neonatal mortality, ante- and post-partum haemorrhages and complicated deliveries. Gestation and spontaneous labour are also prolonged. There may be an association with premature closure of the ductus arteriosus. Salicylates should therefore, if possible, be avoided in the last 3 months of pregnancy, in particular the last 2 weeks.

The elderly

The elderly are more susceptible to adverse reactions associated with salicylates and the lowest dose possible should be used.

Concurrent disease

Renal failure. Sodium salicylate should be used cautiously in renal impairment and avoided if significant as excretion is almost entirely in the urine.

Cardiac failure. Sodium salicylate should be avoided because of the high sodium content.

Hepatic failure. Liver function should be monitored during the use of high-dose salicylates since there is an increased risk of toxicity.

Drug interactions

Potentially hazardous interactions

Salicylate is highly protein bound and displaces, or is displaced by, other protein-bound drugs such as warfarin, sulphonylureas, hydantoins, penicillins and sulphonamides.

Concurrent use of salicylates with methotrexate may increase the serum concentration of methotrexate and the risk of toxicity.

Alcohol taken with salicylates increases the risk of gastric mucosal lesions and bleeding.

Other significant interactions

The uricosuric effects of salicylates, probenecid and sulphinpyrazone are antagonistic.

Potentially useful interactions

Drugs that alter urinary pH will alter urinary excretion of salicylate.

Clinical trials

Although probably as effective as aspirin as an analgesic, antipyretic and anti-inflammatory agent and with less gastrointestinal side effects, there have been no recent high quality controlled clinical trials comparing it to other non-steroidal anti-inflammatory agents.

References

1. Vane J R 1971 Inhibition of prostaglandin synthesis as a mechanism of action for aspirin-like drugs. Nature 231: 232–235
2. Bray M A, Gordon D 1978 Prostaglandin production by macrophages and the effect of anti-inflammatory drugs. British Journal of Pharmacology 63: 635–642
3. Higgs G A, Bunting S, Moncada S, Vane J R 1976 Polymorphonuclear leucocytes produce thromboxane A_2 like activity during phagocytosis. Prostaglandins 12: 749–757
4. Buskin J N, Upton R A, Williams R L 1982 Improved liquid-chromatography of aspirin, salicylate, and salicyluric acid in plasma, with a modification for determining aspirin in urine. Clinical Chemistry 28: 1200–1203
5. Lange W E, Bell S A 1966 Fluorometric determination of acetylsalicylic acid and salicylic acid in blood. Journal of Pharmaceutical Sciences 55: 386–389
6. Trinder P 1954 Rapid determination of salicylate in biological fluids. Biochemical Journal 57: 301–303
7. Seed J C 1965 A clinical comparison of the antipyretic potency of aspirin and sodium salicylate. Clinical Pharmacology and Therapeutics 6: 354–358
8. Editorial 1986 Reye's syndrome and aspirin. British Medical Journal 292: 1543–1544
9. CSM Update 1986 Reye's syndrome and aspirin. British Medical Journal 292: 1590
10. The multicenter Salsalate/Aspirin comparison study group 1989 Does the acetyl group of aspirin contribute to the antiinflammatory efficacy of salicylic acid in the treatment of rheumatoid arthritis. Journal of Rheumatology 16: 321–327
11. Furst D E, Blocka K, Cassell S et al 1987 A controlled study of concurrent therapy with a non-acetylated salicylate and naproxen in rheumatoid arthrits. Arthritis and Rheumatism 30: 146–154
12. Cuthbert M F 1974 Adverse reactions to non-steroidal anti-rheumatic drugs. Current Medical Research and Opinion 2: 600–610
13. Rainsford K D 1984 Aspirin and the salicylates. Butterworths, London, pp 172–176
14. Paulus H E 1989 Editorial. Aspirin versus nonacetylated salicylate. Journal of Rheumatology 16: 264–265
15. Weinberger M 1978 Analgesic sensitivity in children with asthma. Pediatrics 62: 910–915
16. Reye R D K, Morgan G, Baral J 1963 Encephalopathy and fatty degeneration of the viscera. Lancet 2: 749–752
17. Leonards J R, Levy G 1973 Gastrointestinal blood loss from aspirin and sodium salicylate tablets in man. Clinical Pharmacology and Therapeutics 14: 62–66
18. Rainsford K D 1984 Aspirin and the salicylates. Butterworths, London, pp 233–236

S

Sodium stibogluconate

Pentavalent antimonials (Sb(V)) were introduced for the treatment of leishmaniasis more than 50 years ago following observations of the efficacy but marked toxicity of trivalent antimonials (Sb(III)). Two compounds are available for clinical use, sodium stibogluconate (Pentostam) and methylglucamine antimoniate (Glucantime).

Chemistry

Sodium stibogluconate (Pentostam, Solistibosan, Stiheike)
$C_6H_9Na_2O_9Sb$

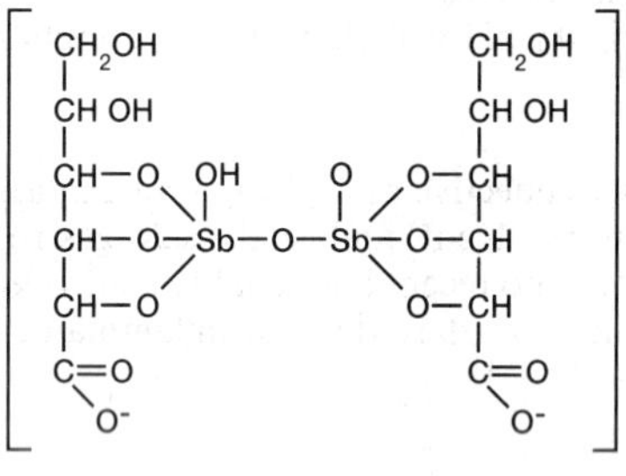

Molecular weight (digluconate)	392.8 (745.5)
pKa	acidic
Solubility	
in alcohol	poor
in water	freely soluble
Octanol/water partition coefficient	low

Pentavalent sodium stibogluconate is a mixture of ionic antimony compounds of ill defined composition containing 30–34% antimony when dried. Sodium stibogluconate is a derivative of antimonic acid with antimony attached to carbon atoms via oxygen atoms. There are usually less than two sodium atoms for each antimony atom.[1] The uncertainty about the composition is due to the complex reactive and polymeric properties of antimonic acid. Sodium stibogluconate is a crystalline solid.

Pharmacology

Sodium stibogluconate is primarily used for the treatment of leishmaniasis. *Leishmania* in vertebrate hosts including man are obligatory intramacrophage organisms. Amastigotes live and multiply in macrophages within the reticulo-endothelial system and infection in man gives rise to either visceral, cutaneous or mucocutaneous disease. In vector species and in vitro culture systems, amastigotes transform into motile, flagellated promastigotes, the form eventually infective to man following inoculation by an infected sandfly.

In vitro models employing promastigote cultures in cell-free media are simple to develop but show variable activity to existing chemotherapeutic agents. In particular, pentavalent antimonials show little effect in such systems when used in achievable serum concentrations of pentavalent antimony.

In vitro cultivation of amastigotes in macrophages provides a more satisfactory model. Two systems have been examined in experimental chemotherapy studies. In infected mouse peritoneal macrophages, *L. donovani* amastogites were susceptible to 7 days exposure to achievable serum levels of pentavalent antimony (less than 20 $mg.l^{-1}$).[2] In infected human monocyte derived macrophages exposed to achievable serum levels of Pentostam, Pentamidine and amphotericin B, more than 90% of both cutaneous and visceral amastigotes were eliminated within 6 days, compared to controls.[3] The exact mechanism of action is unknown but antimonial compounds readily react with sulphydryl groups.

In vivo models have also been used for both cutaneous and visceral infections. None are at present ideal or directly comparable to the clinical situation biologically, chemotherapeutically or immunologically. Models have been developed in hamsters, mice and, more recently, dogs and primates.[3]

Toxicology

Sodium stibogluconate has not been studied in detail for toxicological activity, nor is information available relating to carcinogenicity or mutagenicity.

Limited studies in rats treated with sodium stibogluconate for 30 days with 100–150 $mg.kg^{-1}$ daily produced a two-fold rise in SGOT and alkaline phosphatase and slight increase in organ weights of liver and kidney. These changes were not observed in rats given 50 $mg.kg^{-1}$ daily for 30 days or mice given up to 934 $mg.kg^{-1}$ daily for 7 days.

Clinical pharmacology

Pentavalent antimonial compounds are the treatment of choice for leishmanial infection especially visceral leishmaniasis, cutaneous leishmaniasis and mucocutaneous leishmaniasis.

Limited comparative studies of sodium stibogluconate and methylglucamine antimoniate suggest similar pharmacokinetic profiles and clinical efficacy when used in antimony equivalent dosages.[4] However, the manufacturers' recommended dose of Glucantime provides up to 2.8 times the amount of antimony compared to the recommended dose of sodium stibogluconate.

The choice of pentavalent antimonial is more dependent on the geographical location of patients than on differing therapeutic or pharmacokinetic properties. Sodium stibogluconate (Pentostam) has been used mainly in India, China, East Africa and North America, whilst methylglucamine antimoniate (Glucantime) has been used predominantly in South America, francophone Africa and Europe.

Therapeutic regimes were evolved without access to pharmacokinetic information and with caution resulting from the high toxicity observed with trivalent antimonials. This resulted in the concept of daily treatment courses of 6–10 days, with repeat courses only after periods of rest, still reflected in the manufacturer's dosage recommendations.

There is little information on host response to sodium stibogluconate. Intravenous administration may cause cough, nausea, vomiting or substernal pain. In one clinical study sodium stibogluconate 600 mg daily for 10 days had no effect on blood pressure, heart rate, left ventricular contractile function or rhythm.[5]

Pharmacokinetics

Until recently there was little information available on the pharmacokinetics of sodium stibogluconate. Current analytical methods depend on assays of antimony and do not differentiate between pentavalent and trivalent forms. Two methods have been reported. Anodic stripping voltametry[6] has been used to measure whole blood antimony concentrations. Separation by deposition on to copper has been used for semi-quantitative estimation of urinary antimony.[7]

Goodwin et al[8] reported blood antimony levels of 10–15 $mg.l^{-1}$ up to 1 h after intravenous sodium stibogluconate (50–100 mg Sb). 77–92% of the dose was excreted in the urine within 24 h and up to 84% excreted within 6 h. Rees[7] reported peak antimony levels of 12–15 $mg.l^{-1}$ 1 h after intravenous administration (10 mg Sb per kg). Virtually all the administered antimony was recovered in the urine within 12–14 h and 80% within 6 h.

Following intramuscular injection of sodium stibogluconate or methylglucamine antimoniate, peak antimony concentrations, of approximately 10 $mg.l^{-1}$, occur within 2 h of dosing and then fall rapidly.[4] Trough antimony concentrations rise slowly during the 30 days of treatment, from 0.04–0.06 $mg.l^{-1}$ to 0.19–0.33 $mg.l^{-1}$ after the 30th dose. A two-compartment, three-term pharmacokinetic model gives the best fit to the data, with an initial absorption phase, half life 0.85 h; a rapid elimination phase, half life 2.02 h; and a slow elimination phase, half life 76 h.

Pharmacokinetic studies have demonstrated the rapid excretion of pentavalent antimony via the kidneys, with virtually all of the dose excreted by that route, 80% within the first 6 h. Concentrations in the residual compartment rise slowly during treatment but this may be in the trivalent form. Limited studies indicate that sodium stibogluconate and methylglucamine antimoniate do not differ markedly when used at equivalent dosage for antimony.

The elimination of pentavalent antimony is delayed in renal impairment. It is not known whether sodium stibogluconate crosses the placenta.

Concentration–effect relationship

There are no data on this subject for sodium stibogluconate.

Metabolism

Pentavalent antimony is eliminated almost entirely by urinary excretion, with 80% of the administered antimony recovered within 6 h.

Pharmaceutics

Sodium stibogluconate (Pentostam; Wellcome, UK) is available as a sterile solution containing the equivalent of 100 mg.ml^{-1} pentavalent antimony for intravenous or intramuscular use. It is presented in rubber capped bottles containing 100 ml. It has a shelf-life of 3 years and should be stored below 25°C and protected from light.

Therapeutic use

Indications

Therapeutic uses are restricted to the treatment of various infections with leishmania species, notably:

1. Visceral leishmaniasis
2. Post kala-azar dermal leishmaniasis due to *L. donovani* spp.
3. Cutaneous leishmaniasis, due to *L. tropica*, *L. major*, *L. mexicana* spp.
4. Mucocutaneous leishmaniasis, due to *L. braziliensis* spp.

Contraindications

There are no absolute contraindications, but caution should be observed in:

1. Renal disease
2. Myocardial disease
3. Hepatic disease
4. Pneumonia
5. Previous antimonial therapy
6. Pregnancy
7. Complicating secondary infections.

Mode of use

Administration is by slow intravenous injection or deep intramuscular injection. Cutaneous leishmaniasis has been treated by local infiltration of cutaneous lesions.

The manufacturer's recommendations are 6 ml daily for 7–10 days by intravenous or intramuscular injection. Two or three further courses separated by an interval of 10 days may be necessary. The dosage for children is 0.1 ml.kg^{-1} body weight for 21 days or 0.25 ml.kg^{-1} for 12–14 days by intravenous or intramuscular injection up to a maximum daily dose of 6 ml.

It is now more commonly used in continuous courses of daily intravenous or intramuscular injections of 10–20 mg.kg^{-1} daily for 15 days initially. Intravenous injections should be given slowly over 5–10 min and discontinued if cough, nausea, vomiting or substernal pain occur. Thrombophlebitis may develop, especially with poor injection technique. Intramuscular injection is usually given deep into the gluteal muscles and is commonly associated with pain at the injection site lasting up to an hour.

Dosage and duration of treatment vary depending on the species of *Leishmania* and also between different geographical regions even with the same *Leishmania* species. Chemotherapy is currently undergoing review in the light of recent pharmacokinetic findings. The standard dose is 10 mg Sb per kg body weight daily ranging from 10 to 30 days initially. In children, most authorities recommend 15 mg.kg^{-1} per day. Although still included in the manufacturer's recommendations, 10 day courses separated by rest periods have been largely replaced with continuous courses, a rationale supported by pharmacokinetic studies and less likely to lead to the emergence of parasite resistance.

Indications

1. Visceral leishmaniasis

Infection with *Leishmani donovani* gives rise to a severe infection, with amastigote-laden macrophages proliferating, especially in the liver, spleen and bone marrow. Accompanying the often massive hepatomegaly and splenomegaly there is fever, anaemia, neutropenia and thrombocytopenia. This chronic infection is associated with immune depression and a variety of secondary infections which commonly lead to the fatal outcome.

Geographical variation in clinical features and response to treatment with sodium stibogluconate occur and have led to differing treatment schedules, ranging from India where parasites are usually responsive to short courses of treatment, to East Africa where prolonged courses are needed.

Recent pharmacokinetic[4,9] studies demonstrating the rapid elimination of pentavalent antimonials have led to trials in Kenya of twice and thrice daily injections for correspondingly shorter periods. These trials suggest that therapeutic efficacy is not reduced and parasite clearance from splenic aspirates was most rapid in those treated 8-hourly with sodium stibogluconate.[10] There appeared to be no increase in toxicity using these shorter regimens, although in India such regimes were abandoned due to cardiotoxicity.[11]

Relapse and non-response

In all geographic areas a variable proportion of patients fail to respond to a single course of sodium stibogluconate and a further proportion relapse after apparent clinical recovery. Such patients may respond to further courses of treatment and recently higher dosage regimens have been effectively used to promote clinical cure. Resistance to treatment has been studied especially in Kenya, where a series of studies have investigated the use of high-dose sodium stibogluconate. Antimony resistance is related to inadequate initial chemotherapy and increases progressively following further exposure to sodium stibogluconate.

Bryceson et al[12,13] studied the response of ten patients previously treated with sodium stibogluconate 16–20 mg.kg^{-1} daily for 30–98 days. All were treated with 20 mg 8-hourly. In six, treatment was modified or abandoned because of confirmed or suspected toxicity. Two were cured and four showed a partial clinical response, whilst four failed to respond. One patient died from a presumed ventricular arrhythmia. Recommendations for treatment in East Africa resulting from this study stress the need for initial adequate chemotherapy of 20 mg.kg^{-1} daily for 4 weeks (max. 850 mg Sb daily).

Relapse after chemotherapy with sodium stibogluconate should be treated aggressively. Sodium stibogluconate 20 mg.kg^{-1} twice daily for 60 days should be accompanied by monitoring parasites in splenic aspirates. Unresponsive patients are extremely difficult to manage. High-dose sodium stibogluconate is usually well tolerated and may be effective. Pentamidine may also be effective and both drugs may be given in combination. Combination therapy with allopurinol and sodium stibogluconate has given preliminary encouraging results.[13]

In India, parasites appear more sensitive. Most published information suggests that one or two 6–10 day courses of sodium stibogluconate will cure a high proportion of patients. Sanyal,[14] studying 14 371 patients, found that 36.7% required a second course of treatment whilst 7.6% required subsequent pentamidine. Thakur,[15] using 20 mg.kg^{-1} daily for 15 days in Bihar, India, had only 0.5% relapses in 603 treated patients.

2. Post kala-azar dermal leishmaniasis

Post kala-azar dermal leishmaniasis may occur several years after apparently successful treatment of visceral leishmaniasis and is especially frequent in Indian forms of the disease. It usually responds to courses of sodium stibogluconate although relapses are common and several courses are commonly required. Continuous therapy has not been assessed.

3. Cutaneous leishmaniasis

Cutaneous leishmaniasis is due to *L. tropica* and *L. major* in the Old World and *L. mexicana* in the New World. Early lesions may be treated with intralesional injections of sodium stibogluconate. The

Sodium stibogluconate

indications for systemic treatment include lesions on sites where scarring will produce disfigurement, large, ulcerated, or multiple lesions. Sodium stibogluconate should be given by daily injection of 10–20 mg.kg^{-1} until clinical healing and parasitological cure is achieved.

Diffuse cutaneous leishmaniasis (DCL) is due to *L. aethiopica* in the Old World and members of the *L. mexicana* group in the Americas. It is resistant to sodium stibogluconate at conventional doses. Therapy with pentamidine is currently the treatment of choice in Ethiopia. In South America response has been achieved with pentavalent antimonials at high dose over prolonged periods.[16]

4. Mucocutaneous leishmaniasis
South American mucocutaneous leishmaniasis due to *L. braziliensis* is indistinguishable clinically in the early stages from other forms of cutaneous leishmaniasis. All *L. braziliensis* infections should be considered capable of leading to mucocutaneous disease (espundia) and treated with prolonged courses of sodium stibogluconate for a minimum of 30 days initially.

In established mucocutaneous leishmaniasis chemotherapy must also be prolonged and monitored both clinically and parasitologically. During initial chemotherapy, enlargement of the lesion with localized oedema and haemorrhage has been described in mucocutaneous leishmaniasis.[17] Treatment failures may require alternative therapy with amphotericin B or pentamidine.

Serological monitoring can be used and failure of IFAT titres to fall or a subsequent rise in titre suggest the need for further treatment courses.

Contraindications

There are no absolute contraindications, especially in the treatment of visceral leishmaniasis which untreated is virtually always fatal. In cutaneous leishmaniasis the self-healing nature of the disease and the availability of alternative approaches to treatment permit greater discretion in the use of systemic pentavalent antimony compounds.

Visceral leishmaniasis is frequently treated in remote rural health facilities where accurate monitoring of treatment is not possible. Hepatic, renal or myocardial disease would indicate the need for referral. In cutaneous leishmaniasis, similar concurrent disease might well indicate that pentavalent antimonials should be avoided, whereas in visceral leishmaniasis the severity of the disease and absence of alternative non-toxic chemotherapeutic agents leaves little choice.

1. Renal disease
Renal impairment and renal failure impair the elimination of sodium stibogluconate. This leads to retention of antimony and increased toxicity which may prove fatal. Where treatment is required dosage should be reduced and, where possible, monitored by blood antimony estimations and clinical monitoring for toxicity, especially serial ECGs. In moderate to severe renal failure sodium stibogluconate should be avoided or given in reduced daily dosage. Impaired renal excretion may lead to high plasma concentrations and increased cardiotoxicity as well as potential renal toxicity.

2. Myocardial disease
The cardiotoxicity of sodium stibogluconate suggests a cautious approach to chemotherapy when associated myocardial disease coexists with leishmaniasis.

3. Hepatic disease
The infrequent reporting of elevation of liver enzymes suggests that sodium stibugluconate should be used with caution in patients with pre-existing liver disease.

4. Pneumonia
As with other antimonial drugs, pneumonia has been described as a complication of therapy with sodium stibogluconate in up to 7% of treated patients. Pneumonia is a common manifestation of profound immunosuppression associated with visceral leishmaniasis.

5. Previous antimonial therapy
Previous therapy with antimony should be carefully assessed prior to commencing sodium stibogluconate in view of the potential cumulative toxicity.

6. Pregnancy
In view of the lack of information concerning teratogenicity, sodium stibogluconate should not be used in pregnancy unless maternal health demands it. Sodium stibogluconate has, however, been given in pregnancy without untoward effect on the fetus.

7. Complicating secondary infections
Severe secondary infections are frequent in visceral leishmaniasis. They demand urgent specific chemotherapy and some authorities delay antileishmanial therapy until the patient's general condition has improved.

Adverse reactions

Potentially life-threatening effects
Potentially life-threatening cardiotoxicity, renal toxicity and hepatotoxicity may occur with high-dosage regimes or in the presence of renal impairment. Sodium stibogluconate, in common with trivalent antimonials, rarely induces a potentially fatal shock-like or anaphylactic syndrome with hypotension, sweating and apprehension.

Whilst trivalent antimonials invariably produce cardiac toxicity early in the course of treatment, pentavalent antimonials are less associated with either clinical or electrocardiographic evidence of toxicity using a standard dose regimen. Early reports of ECG abnormalities were described.[18,19] More recently, a study of 22 soldiers treated with sodium stibogluconate (600 mg daily for 10 days) found no clinical effect on blood pressure, heart rate, LV function or rhythm.[5] Serial ECGs showed a reversible reduction of T-wave amplitude.

Chulay et al[20] studied 65 patients with visceral leishmaniasis with serial ECGs using doses of sodium stibogluconate ranging from 10 mg.kg^{-1} body weight to 60 mg.kg^{-1} body weight per day. ECG changes occurred in 54% of treatment courses and there was close correlation with the total daily antimony and duration of treatment. Abnormalities observed were T-wave flattening, T-wave inversion, prolongation of QT_c interval (13 patients all treated with more than 20 mg.kg^{-1} body weight for more than 30 days). Three patients died during treatment — all showed QT_c prolongation, ST concavity and T-wave inversion. One patient was presumed to have developed a fatal ventricular arrhythmia and two had presumed measles infections.

Sodium stibogluconate in standard dosage, whilst associated with ECG changes, is rarely associated with clinical cardiotoxicity. At higher dosage or after prolonged chemotherapy, cardiotoxicity is more frequent and includes premature nodal or ventricular beats, ventricular tachycardia and ventricular fibrillation. ECG changes consist of T-wave flattening or inversion; ST concavity and prolongation of QT_c. Dosage in excess of 20 mg.kg^{-1} body weight per day should be monitored by twice-weekly ECGs.

Acute overdosage
Overdosage has not been described with sodium stibogluconate. Relative overdosage has been observed in patients with renal impairment, who develop features of antimony toxicity including malaise, nausea, vomiting, drowsiness, convulsions and cardiotoxicity.

There is little experience in the use of chelating agents such as dimercaprol in the treatment of overdosage.

One case report documents overdosage with methylglucamine antimoniate in a patient treated with up to 900 mg.kg^{-1} daily for 11 days. Early proteinuria was followed by elevated enzymes, disseminated intravascular coagulation, renal failure and fatal circulatory collapse.[21]

Severe or irreversible adverse effects
Intravenous injection may be associated with venous thrombosis. Intramuscular injection is painful and may be associated with abscess formation.

Renal toxicity has been reported, including a reversible defect in concentrating capacity and proteinuria.[22]

Symptomatic adverse effects
Mild anorexia, nausea, vomiting, general malaise, myalgia and arthralgia are relatively common, especially with prolonged periods of treatment. Skin reactions are unusual and include erythema, pruritis and herpes zoster.

Other effects
Minor elevation of hepatic enzymes has been reported in several studies.

Sodium stibogluconate

High risk groups

Neonates

There is no information regarding special risk in neonates.

Breast milk. Infants should not be breast-fed by mothers on sodium stibogluconate.

Children

Children require higher dosage regimens of sodium stibogluconate for the treatment of visceral leishmaniasis than adults. When estimated on a basis of body weight, a dose of 15 $mg.kg^{-1}$ per day is recommended.

Pregnant women

Whilst there are no reports of adverse effects on the fetus, sodium stibogluconate should not be given in pregnancy except for the treatment of visceral leishmaniasis, where the maternal condition requires therapy.

The elderly

Whilst there are no specific risks in the elderly, the increased frequency of cardiovascular, renal and hepatic disease requires that patients are closely monitored during therapy.

Concurrent disease

Concurrent infections are common in visceral leishmaniasis. Severe infection such as pneumonia may be treated prior to specific therapy. Relative contraindications to therapy include pre-existing cardiac, renal and hepatic disease, including myocarditis and nephritis.

Drug interactions

There are no known drug interactions apart from cumulative toxicity associated with previous antimonial therapy.

General review articles

Kirk R, Sati M H 1947 Observations on the use of sodium antimony gluconate (sodium stibogluconate) in the treatment of kala azar. Annals of Tropical Medicine and Parasitology 41: 14–21

McGreevy P B, Marsden P D 1986 American trypanosomiasis and leishmaniasis 3. In: Campbell W C, Review R S (eds) Chemotherapy parasitic diseases. Plenum Press, pp 118–127

Manson Bahr P E C 1959 East African kala azar with special reference to pathology, prophylaxis and treatment. Transactions of the Royal Society of Tropical Medicine and Hygiene 53: 123–136

Maru M 1979 Clinical and laboratory features and treatment of visceral leishmaniasis in hospitalised patients in north east Ethiopia. American Journal of Tropical Medicine and Hygiene 28: 15–18

Oster C N, Chulay J D, Lowray D et al 1985 American cutaneous leishmaniasis: a comparison of three sodium stibogluconate treatment schedules. American Journal of Tropical Medicine and Hygiene 34: 856–860

Van Peenan P F D, Reid T P 1962 Leishmaniasis in the Sudan Republic. Clinical and laboratory aspects of kala azar in hospitalised patients from Upper Nile Province. American Journal of Tropical Medicine and Hygiene 11: 723–730

Rees P H, Kager P, Wellde B T, Hockmeyer W 1984 The response of Kenyan kala azar to treatment with sodium stibogluconate. American Journal of Tropical Medicine and Hygiene 33: 357–361

Tuckman E 1949 Treatment of Chinese kala azar with sodium antimony gluconate. Journal of Tropical Medicine and Hygiene 52: 199–204

Wijers D J B 1971 A ten year study of kala azar in Tharaka (Meru District — Kenya) II. Relapses. East African Medical Journal 48: 537–558

References

1. Steck E A 1975 Chemotherapy of protozoan diseases division of medical chemistry. Walter Reed Army Institute of Research vol 2. 7.82
2. Neal R A, Mathews P J 1982 Transactions of the Royal Society of Tropical Medicine and Hygiene 76: 284
3. Burman J D 1985 Experimental chemotherapy of leishmanias. A critical review 11–138
4. Chulay J D, Fleckenstein, Smith D H 1988 Pharmacokinetics of antimony during treatment of visceral leishmaniasis with sodium stibogluconate or meglumine antimoniate. Transactions of the Royal Society of Tropical Medicine and Hygiene 82: 69–72
5. Henderson A, Joliffe D 1985 Cardial effects of sodium stibogluconate. British Journal of Clinical Pharmacology 19: 73–77
6. Anonymous 1979 Antimony in blood. In: Taylor D G (ed) NIOSH Manual of analytical methods. US Government Printing Office, Washington, DC, pp 191-1-193-7
7. Rees P H, Keating M I, Kager P A, Hockmeyer H T 1980 Renal clearance of pentavalent antimony (sodium stibogluconate). Lancet 2: 226–229
8. Goodwin L G, Page J E 1943 A study of the excretion of organic antimonials using a polarographic procedure. Biochemical Journal 37: 198–209
9. Pamplin C L, Desjardins R, Chulay J, Trammt E, Hendricks L, Canfeld C 1985 Pharmacokinetics of antimony during sodium stibogluconate therapy for cutaneous leishmaniasis. American Society for Clinical Pharmacology and Therapeutics 29: 270–271
10. Chulay J D, Soubhatt R, Mingai M H, Sachihi J B O, Chunge, Bryceson A D M 1985 A comparison of three dosage regimes of sodium stibogluconate in the treatment of visual leishmaniasis in Kenya. Journal of Infectious Diseases 148–155
11. Thakur C P 1986 Harmful effect of high stibogluconate treatment of kala azar in India 1986. Transactions of the Royal Society of Tropical Medicine and Hygiene 80
12. Bryceson A D M, Chulay J P, Mugambe M et al 1985 Response to high dosage sodium stibogluconate or prolonged treatment with Pentamidine. Transactions of the Royal Society of Tropical Medicine and Hygiene 79: 705–711
13. Bryceson A D M, Chulay J P, Ho M et al 1985 Visceral leishmaniasis unresponsive to antimonial drugs. 1. Clinical and immunological studies. Transactions of the Royal Society of Tropical Medicine and Hygiene 79: 700–704
14. Sanyal R K, Arora R R 1979 Assessment of drug therapy of kala azar in current epidemics in Bihar. Journal of Communicable Diseases 11: 198–202
15. Thakur C P 1984 Epidemiological, clinical and therapeutic features of Bihar kala azar (including post kala azar dermal leishmaniasis. Transactions of the Royal Society of Tropical Medicine and Hygiene 78: 391–398
16. Bryceson A D M 1970 Diffuse cutaneous leishmaniasis in Ethiopia II. Treatments. Transactions of the Royal Society of Tropical Medicine and Hygiene 64: 369–379
17. Marsden P D, Sampai R N R, Connah E M, Veiga J P T, Costa J L M, Llanar C 1985 High continuous antimony therapy in two patients with unresponsive mucosal leishmaniasis. American Journal of Tropical Medicine and Hygiene 34: 719–713
18. Dempsey J 1965 Leishmaniasis in the Sudan Republic 26. Electrocardiographic findings in Sudanese kala azar. East Africa Medical Journal 42: 131–134
19. Kaplan R J, Wilkin J K, Hartman P L 1979 Treatment of leishmaniasis with sodium antimony gluconate: transient ECG finding. South African Medical Journal 71: 469–470
20. Chulay J D, Spencer H C, Mugambi M 1985 Electrocardiographic changes during treatment of leishmaniasis with pentavalent antimony (sodium stibogluconate). American Journal of Tropical Medicine and Hygiene 34 (4): 702–709
21. Katlama C, Regnier B, Ben Salah N 1985 Toxicité de Glucantime. Annales de Médicine Interne 136–321
22. Veiga J P, Rosa T T, Kimachi et al 1985 Função renal em pacientes com leishmaniose muco-cutanea tratados com antimonias pentavalentes. Revista do Instituto de Medicina Tropical de São Paulo 27–298

S

Sodium thiosulphate

Sodium thiosulphate is employed as an antidote for acute cyanide poisoning, almost always in conjunction with sodium nitrite. Sodium thiosulphate can also be used to treat poisoning by cyanogenic compounds, including sodium nitroprusside, the nitriles and laetrile. Occasionally it is used topically in the treatment of pityriasis versicolor.

Chemistry

Sodium thiosulphate pentahydrate, (CAS 10 102-17-7, sodium thiosulfate, sodium hyposulphite, Sodothiol, Sulphothiorine $Na_2S_2O_3.5H_2O$

Molecular weight anhydrous (pentahydrate)	158.1 (248.2)
pKa	1.6
Solubility	
in alcohol	insoluble
in water	1 in 0.5
Octanol/water partition coefficient	—

Sodium thiosulphate pentahydrate is an odourless crystalline substance, solutions of which have a salty taste.

Pharmacology

Sodium thiosulphate acts as a substrate for the enzyme rhodanese (thiosulphate:cyanide sulphurtransferase EC 2.8.1.1.), which converts cyanide to the much less toxic thiocyanate ion.[1] Rhodanese is distributed widely in the body, notably in the liver mitochondria. The enzyme requires an adequate source of sulphane sulphur (divalent sulphur bonded to another sulphur atom), the availability of which is normally rate-limiting. Although thiosulphate is almost certainly not a physiological substrate for rhodanese, it acts as a source of sulphane sulphur.

Toxicology

Although the value of sodium thiosulphate was first documented in 1895 and experience of use is consequently relatively long, toxicological data are few. The main toxic properties appear to be osmotic effects, which result from the sodium load, together with acid–base disturbance. Such effects include metabolic acidosis, hypoxaemia and hypernatraemia.[2]

The intravenous LD_{50} in mice[3] is 1.19 g.kg $^{-1}$, while the median lethal dose in dogs[2] is 3 g.kg^{-1}. The lethal dose injected into the flank of rabbits was estimated by Verbrugge et al[4] to be 4 g.kg^{-1}.

Clinical pharmacology

Although sodium thiosulphate is used alone to counter the toxicity caused by the therapeutic use of sodium nitroprusside, in most other circumstances it is used as an adjunct to treatment with a methaemoglobin-forming agent such as sodium nitrite or 4-dimethylaminophenol (DMAP). In the management of poisoning with hydrogen cyanide or salts of hydrocyanic acid, the use of sodium thiosulphate in this way has a basis that is both theoretical and experimental. The theoretical basis is that the methaemoglobinaemia caused by sodium nitrite is short-lived, so that the cyanide, sequestered inside the erythrocyte as cyanmethaemoglobin, might be expected to diffuse out of the red cell as the methaemoglobin content falls, producing a recrudescence of symptoms. This, it might be supposed, could be prevented by sulphur detoxification catalysed by the enzyme rhodanese, for which the thiosulphate ion is cosubstrate. Furthermore, the work of Hug[5] and Chen and colleagues[6,7] suggests that sodium nitrite and sodium thiosulphate potentiate one another. Thus, in dogs it was found that sodium thiosulphate alone raised the LD_{50} of sodium cyanide by a factor of 3, sodium nitrite by a factor of 5, whilst the two antidotes together raised the LD_{50} 18-fold.[7]

Rhodanese is a mitochondrial enzyme and sodium thiosulphate is thought to cross cell membranes only slowly.[1] For this reason, sodium thiosulphate has been assumed to be a slow-acting cyanide antidote and therefore it has been used almost invariably in conjunction with other agents in severe poisoning. However, some studies[8–10] have suggested that thiosulphate may act very rapidly. Sylvester et al[10] undertook a pharmacokinetic analysis of cyanide distribution and metabolism, with and without sodium thiosulphate, in mongrel dogs. The mechanism of thiosulphate protection appeared to be due to extremely rapid formation of thiocyanate in the central compartment, thereby limiting the amount of cyanide distribution to sites of toxicity. Sodium thiosulphate increased the rate of transulphuration 30-fold. Christel et al[11] noted a similar and considerable increase in the rate of cyanide transulphuration after administration of sodium thiosulphate to dogs but also observed that the blood cyanide concentration fell somewhat slowly. The conflict in these data is more apparent than real: the data of Christel[11] imply that even a 13 to 30-fold increase in the rate of transulphuration will not produce a fall in cyanide concentrations that is rapid in the context of the timescale of events in acute cyanide poisoning. The use of sodium thiosulphate as a secondary antidote is therefore probably correct.

Pharmacokinetics

Ivankovich et al[8] described a method suitable for the estimation of thiosulphate in blood and urine which is sensitive to 1 mg.l^{-1}. Potassium iodide, potassium bromide and monobasic potassium phosphate are added to the plasma or urine. Potassium borohydride (in sodium hydroxide) and acetone are then added, followed by ferric sulphate and N,N-dimethyl-*p*-phenylenediamine sulphate in sulphuric acid. A blue colour develops and the absorbance is measured at 665 nm. A more sensitive HPLC method has been described by Newton and others[12] and, in modified form, by Shea and coworkers.[13]

Oral absorption	poor
Presystemic metabolism	—
Plasma half life	
α	0.3 h
β	3.0 h
Volume of distribution	0.15 l.kg^{-1}
Plasma protein binding	—

Sodium thiosulphate is not well absorbed by mouth,[14] as it is broken down in the acidic gastric juices to form sulphite and sulphur. It is therefore administered intravenously. Following injection, it is distributed throughout the extracellular fluid and renal excretion occurs by glomerular filtration and secretion.[15] Ivankovich et al[8] have studied the available thiosulphate pool and the pharmacokinetics of thiosulphate administered to normal volunteers. In 26 healthy volunteers the mean plasma thiosulphate concentration was 11.3 ± 1.1 mg.l^{-1} and the mean urine concentration was 2.8 ± 0.2 mg.l^{-1} (n=24). After administration of sodium thiosulphate 150 mg.kg^{-1} intravenously to five normal male volunteers, peak thiosulphate concentrations of 1012 ± 88.5 mg.l^{-1} were attained after 5 min. The half life of the distribution phase was 23 min and that of the elimination phase 182 min. The calculated volume of distribution was 0.15 l.kg^{-1} body weight. Urine concentration, clearance and the rate of thiosulphate excretion increased markedly after injection. At 180 minutes, the total amount excreted was $42.6 \pm 3.5\%$ and by 18 h, it had only risen to $47.4 \pm 2.4\%$. Therapeutic doses of thiosulphate therefore elevate the plasma concentration about 100 times and it is possible that this may facilitate penetration of the cell membrane to allow detoxification of cyanide by rhodanese.

When sodium thiosulphate was administered during sodium nitroprusside therapy, the plasma half life of thiosulphate was approximately 15 min.[16,17] In children, the elimination half life has been calculated to be about 40 min.[18]

Concentration–effect relationship

The relationship between concentration of thiosulphate and effect has not been studied in man. In dogs it has been reported that sodium thiosulphate considerably increases the rate of cyanide biotransformation. Christel et al[11] noted that 500 mg.kg^{-1} increased the rate of biotransformation 13-fold. An increase in the rate of transulphuration in dogs was also observed by Sylvester and colleagues.[10]

Metabolism

In normal man, some sodium thiosulphate would be expected to enter the sulphane sulphur pool, but much is excreted unchanged. In cyanide poisoning, thiosulphate acts as cosubstrate for the enzyme rhodanese and converts cyanide to the much less toxic thiocyanate ion, which is excreted in the urine.

Pharmaceutics

Preparations of sodium thiosulphate for intravenous injection are solutions in water. Individual pharmacopeias give solutions of varying concentrations between 20% and 50%. Sterilization is by autoclaving.[12] The widely used Lilly antidote kit contains a 25% aqueous solution of sodium thiosulphate as well as sodium nitrite.[19] Similarly, the cyanide poisoning emergency kit used in the UK (Cuxson Gerrard) contains four ampoules, each containing 50 ml sodium thiosulphate as a sterile 25% solution.

The sodium thiosulphate solution is stated to have a shelf-life of one year, if stored away from the light and below 25°C. Sodium thiosulphate solutions are incompatible with many other substances, including the cyanide antidote, hydroxocobalamin.[20] In the absence of information on the compatibility of sodium thiosulphate solutions with many other drugs and intravenous fluids, and bearing in mind the chemistry of the thiosulphates, it is unwise to coadminister sodium thiosulphate injection premixed with any other substance.

Sodium thiosulphate is available in various lotion formulations such as Komed and Tinver (Barnes-Hind division of Revlon, USA). The former is an acne lotion containing sodium thiosulphate 8% together with salicylic acid 2%, isopropyl alcohol 25% and other ingredients. Tinver is used for pityriasis versicolor and contains sodium thiosulphate 25%, salicylic acid 1%, isopropyl alcohol 10%. For silver nitrate burns, a sterile solution of sodium thiosulphate 12% freshly mixed with a sterile solution of potassium ferricyanide 0.5% is used. The solutions are sterilized by autoclaving.

Therapeutic use

Indications

1. Treatment of acute poisoning with hydrogen cyanide and cyanide salts
2. Treatment of poisoning with compounds metabolized to cyanide in vivo, for example sodium nitroprusside and certain nitriles
3. Treatment of certain skin diseases (pityriasis versicolor).

Contraindications

There are no absolute contraindications to the use of sodium thiosulphate.

Mode of use

1. Acute cyanide poisoning

Sodium thiosulphate, 12.5 g (approximately 200 mg.kg^{-1} body weight; 50 ml of 25% solution) is administered by slow intravenous injection[19] at a rate which should not exceed 5 ml.min^{-1}. In children relatively high doses (e.g. 400 mg.kg^{-1}) have often been administered, although the rationale is not clear. Sodium thiosulphate is usually given in conjunction with sodium nitrite.

2. Poisoning with cyanogenic substances

Certain substances are capable of releasing cyanide in sufficient quantities to produce subacute cyanide poisoning. They include sodium nitroprusside and nitriles. Thiosulphate has been used to treat some of these poisonings.[21,22]

Sodium nitroprusside

Toxicity problems with sodium nitroprusside may arise in two situations. The first is when sodium nitroprusside is used as a hypotensive agent and the second is acute accidental or suicidal poisoning with sodium nitroprusside.

Sodium thiosulphate is probably more effective than hydroxocobalamin in experimental nitroprusside intoxication[24] and prevents the accumulation of toxic quantities of cyanide when given as a concomitant infusion with sodium nitroprusside.[16,23,25] Alternatively, but less desirably, sodium thiosulphate may be given as a bolus dose once the cyanide has accumulated.[26] Schultz and colleagues[27] have recommended that the ratio (w/w) between sodium thiosulphate and sodium nitroprusside should be at least 4:1, preferably between 5:1 and 6:1. These findings have particular relevence to the management of patients with renal impairment who are treated with sodium nitroprusside. Schultz et al studied the kinetics of thiocyanate in healthy subjects and in patients with renal failure. The elimination half life of thiocyanate after oral dosing of healthy subjects was 1–5 days (mean 3 days), whereas the average half life in patients with renal failure was 9 days: the elimination constants increased in a parallel manner with the creatinine clearance.

In acute sodium nitroprusside poisoning, sodium thiosulphate may, as above, be used alone. Intravenous infusion should be considered and, if bolus doses are used, more than one dose may be required.

Other cyanogenic compounds

In the case of other cyanogenic compounds, for example the nitriles, there is less experimental evidence upon which to base dosing schedules. Nevertheless, Willhite and Smith[28] showed that in mice, times to death after lethal doses of certain nitriles, particularly malononitrile, succinonitrile and acetonitrile were very prolonged. Indeed, in the case of proprionitrile the time was about 20 h. These data may explain the observation, made in the same study, that single injections of sodium thiosulphate produced little therapeutic benefit and suggest that nitrile intoxication should be treated with multiple sodium thiosulphate injections or by thiosulphate infusion. It should be noted that certain nitriles, particularly acrylonitrile and methylacrylonitrile, have a component of toxicity which appears to be unrelated to cyanogenesis. Sodium thiosulphate can only be expected to counter the cyanide produced from these nitriles and other antidotes may be indicated.[29]

3. Skin diseases

When applied daily for several weeks, 10% sodium thiosulphate solution is reported to be effective in pityriasis versicolor.[30,31]

Adverse reactions

Adverse effects are mainly minor and certainly unimportant in comparison to the effects of acute cyanide poisoning.[32]

Potentially life-threatening effects

Rapid intravenous injection of sodium thiosulphate solution may produce hypotension[33] which in very rare instances might be life-threatening.

Severe or irreversible adverse effects

Apart from hypotension there are none.

Symptomatic adverse effects

Sodium thiosulphate 3 g, administered orally, daily to humans is reported to depress arterial oxygen saturation.[34] No adverse effects are to be expected when sodium thiosulphate is used topically.

Interference with clinical pathology tests

No information is available.

High risk groups

No patient group has been identified where the risk of the drug is commensurate with the risk of cyanide poisoning. The sodium load may be deleterious in those suffering from congestive cardiac failure, although such considerations are unlikely to weigh heavily in acute cyanide poisoning.

Drug interactions

Potentially hazardous interactions

Interactions of this type have not been described.

Potentially useful interactions

With sodium nitrite and probably 4-dimethylaminophenol, advantageous potentiation of antidotal efficacy occurs. Many combinations of cyanide antidotes have been tried and the advantages of the combination of hydroxocobalamin and sodium thiosulphate have been pointed out.[35,36] These combinations should not, of course, be administered with their components premixed.

Major outcome trials

None has been reported, although there are several case reports of successful usage of the sodium nitrite/thiosulphate combination and these are reviewed by Hall et al.[37]

See also Sodium nitrite.

General review articles

Westley J 1987 Cyanide and sulfane sulfur. In: Vennesland B, Conn E E, Knowles C J, Westley J, Wissing F (eds) Cyanide in biology. Academic Press, London, pp 61–76

Holland M A, Kozlowski L M 1986 Therapy reviews, clinical features and management of cyanide poisoning. Clinical Pharmacy 5: 737–741

Isom G E, Johnson J D 1987 Sulphur donors in cyanide intoxication. In: Ballantyne B, Marrs T C (eds) Clinical and experimental toxicology of cyanides. John Wright, Bristol, ch 18, pp 413–426

Bhatt H R, Linnell J C 1987 The role of rhodanese in cyanide detoxification: its possible use in acute cyanide poisoning of man. In: Ballantyne B, Marrs T C (eds) Clinical and experimental toxicology of cyanides. John Wright, Bristol, ch 20, pp 440–450

Westley J 1988 Mammalian detoxification with sulphane sulphur In: Evered D, Harnett S (eds) Cyanide compounds in biology. Ciba Foundation Symposium, pp 201–218

References

1. Westley J 1988 Mammalian detoxification with sulphane sulphur. In: Evered D, Harnett S (eds) Cyanide compounds in biology. Ciba Foundation Symposium, pp 201–218
2. Dennis DL, Fletcher WS 1966 Toxicity of sodium thiosulfate (NSC-45 624) a nitrogen mustard antagonist, in the dog. Cancer Chemotherapy Reports 50: 255–257
3. Frankenberg L 1980 Enzyme therapy in cyanide poisoning: effect of rhodanese and sulfur compounds. Archives of Toxicology 45: 315–323
4. Verbrugge K 1899 Toxicité des mononitriles gras et aromatiques et action antitoxique de l'hyposulfite de soude vis à vis de ces mononitriles. Archives de Pharmacodynamie 5: 161–196
5. Hug E 1933 Acción del nitrito de sodio y del hiposulfito de sodio en el tratamiento de la intoxicación provocada por el cianuro de potasio en el conejo. Revuta de la Sociedád Argentiniana de la Biologia 9: 91–97
6. Chen K K, Rose R L, Clowes G H A 1933 Methylene blue, nitrites and sodium thiosulphate against cyanide poisoning. Proceedings of the Society for Experimental Biology and Medicine 31: 250–252
7. Chen K K, Rose R L 1952 Nitrite and thiosulfate therapy in cyanide poisoning. Journal of the American Medical Association 149: 113–119
8. Ivankovich A D, Braverman B, Kanuru R P, Heyman, Paullisian R 1980 Cyanide antidotes and methods of their administration in dogs. Anesthesiology 53: 210–216
9. Krapez J, Vesey C J, Adams L, Cole P V 1981 Effects of cyanide antidotes used with sodium nitroprusside infusions: sodium thiosulphate and hydroxocobalamin given prophylactically to dogs. British Journal of Anaesthesia 53: 793–803
10. Sylvester D M, Hayton W L, Morgan R L, Way J L 1983 Effects of thiosulfate on cyanide pharmacokinetics in dogs. Toxicology and Applied Pharmacology 69: 265–271
11. Christel D, Eyer P, Hegemann M, Kiese M, Lörcher W, Weger N 1977 Pharmacokinetics of cyanide poisoning of dogs, and the effect of 4-dimethylaminophenol or thiosulfate. Archives of Toxicology 38: 177–189
12. Newton G L, Dorian R, Fahey R C 1981 Analysis of biological thiols: derivatization with monobromobomane and separation by reverse-phase high performance liquid chromatography. Analytical Biochemistry 114: 383–387
13. Shea M, Koziol J A, Howell S B 1984 Kinetics of sodium thiosulfate, a cisplatin neutralizer. Clinical Pharmacology and Therapeutics 35: 429–425
14. Reynolds J E F (ed) 1989 Martindale The extra pharmacopoeia, 28th edn. Pharmaceutical Press, London, p 855
15. Bucht H 1949 On the tubular secretion of thiosulfate and creatinine under the influence of caronamide. Scandinavian Journal of Clinical and Laboratory Investigation 1: 270–276
16. Schulz V, Gross R, Passch T, Busse J, Loeschke G 1982 Cyanide toxicity of sodium nitroprusside in therapeutic use with and without sodium thiosulphate. Klinische Wochenschrift 60: 1393–1400
17. Schulz V 1984 Clinical pharmacokinetics of nitroprusside cyanide thiosulphate and thiocyanate. Clinical Pharmacokinetics 9: 239–251
18. Gladtke E 1966 Der Thiosulfatraum des Kindes. Archiv für Kinderheilkunde 54: 101–103
19. Hall A, Rumack B H, Schaffer M I, Linden C H 1987 Clinical toxicology of cyanides. North American clinical experiences. In: Ballantyne B, Marrs T C (eds) Clinical and experimental toxicology of cyanides. John Wright, Bristol, ch 12, pp 312–333
20. Evans C L 1964 Cobalt compounds as antidotes for hydrocyanic acid. British Journal of Pharmacology 23: 455–475
21. Vesey C J 1987 Nitroprusside cyanogensis. In: Ballantyne B, Marrs T C (eds) Clinical and experimental toxicology of cyanides. John Wright, Bristol, ch 7, pp 184–208
22. Willhite C C 1981 Inhalation toxicology of acute exposure to aliphatic nitriles. Clinical Toxicology 991–1003
23. Höbel M, Engeser P, Nemeth L, Pill J 1980 The antidote effect of thiosulphate and hydroxocobalamin in formation of nitroprusside intoxication of rabbits. Archives of Toxicology 46: 207–213
24. Schultz V. Bonn R, Kindler J 1979 Kinetics of elimination of thiocyanate in 7 healthy subjects and 8 subjects with renal failure. Klinische Wochenschrift 57: 243–247
25. Schultz V, Roth B 1982 Detoxification of cyanide in a new-born child. Klinische Wochenschrift 60: 527–528
26. Perschau R A, Modell J H, Bright R W, Shirley P D 1977 Suspected sodium nitroprusside-induced cyanide intoxication Anesthesia and Analgesia 56: 533–537
27. Schultz V, Bonn R, Kammerer H, Kriegel R, Ecker N 1979 Counteraction of cyanide poisoning by thiosulphate when administering sodium nitroprusside as a hypotensive agent. Klinische Wochenschrift 57: 5889–602
28. Willhite C C, Smith R P 1981 The role of cyanide liberation on the acute toxicity of aliphatic nitrites. Toxicology and Applied Pharmacology 59: 589–602
29. Ballantyne B 1987 Toxicology of cyanides In: Ballantyne B, Marrs T C (eds) Clinical and experimental toxicology of cyanides. John Wright, Bristol, ch 3, pp 41–126
30. Roberts S O B, Lachapelle J M 1969 Confluent and reticulate papillomatosis (Gougerot–Carteaud) and *Pitysporum orbiculare*. British Journal of Dermatology 81: 841–845
31. Ive F A 1973 Diseases of the skin: treatment of skin infections and infestations. British Medical Journal 4: 475–478
32. Marrs T C 1987 The choice of cyanide antidotes. In: Ballantyne B, Marrs T C (eds) Clinical and experimental toxicology of cyanides. John Wright, Bristol, ch 16, pp 383–401
33. Done A K 1961 Clinical pharmacology of systemic antidotes. Clinical Pharmacology and Therapeutics 2: 750–787
34. Shigiya R, Ozawa Y 1956 The influence of internally used sodium thiosulphate upon the oxygen equilibrium of haemoglobin. Tohoku Journal of Experimental Medicine 63: 383–388
35. Marrs T C 1988 Antidotal treatment of acute cyanide poisoning. Adverse Drug Reactions and Acute Poisonings Reviews 4: 179–206
36. Hall A H, Rumack B H 1987 Hydroxocobalamin/thiosulfate as a cyanide antidote. Journal of Emergency Medicine 5: 115–121
37. Hall A H, Doutre W H, Ludden T, Kulig K W, Rumack K W 1987 Nitrite/thiosulfate treated acute cyanide poisoning: estimated kinetics after antidote. Clinical Toxicology 25: 121–133

Sodium valproate

The anticonvulsant activity of sodium valproate was identified in 1964 and it has been in therapeutic use as an antiepileptic drug in the UK since 1973.

Chemistry

Sodium valproate (Epilim, Depakine, Deprakine, Depakene, Ergenyl, Convulex, Convulexette, Logical, Orfiril, Propymal)
$C_8H_{15}NaO_2$
Sodium 2-propylvalerate, sodium di-n-propylacetate or sodium 2-propylpentanoate

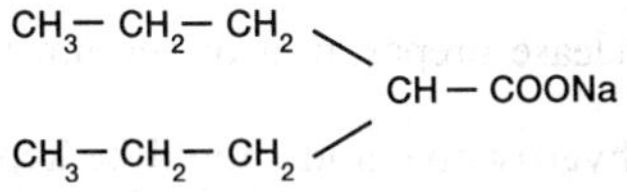

Molecular weight (sodium salt)	166.2
pKa	4.95
Solubility	
in alcohol	1:5
in water	1:5
Octanol/water partition coefficient	562

The acid (valproic acid), the magnesium salt, the amide (dipropylacetamide) and the sodium hydrogen divalproate salt are also marketed as anticonvulsants.

It is a white, odourless, deliquescent, crystalline powder with a saline or burning taste. It is prepared by chemical synthesis. It is not produced in combination form with other drugs.

Pharmacology

Valproate has been shown to have anticonvulsant properties in a variety of experimental animal models of epilepsy.[1] It has also been shown to be effective in the treatment of epilepsy in man. A number of hypotheses have been advanced to account for the anticonvulsant properties of valproate but a satisfactory explanation has yet to be provided. The suggestions include:

1. Valproate increases the levels of the inhibitory neurotransmitter, gamma-aminobutyric acid (GABA) in the brain.[2]
2. Valproate potentiates postsynaptic responses to GABA.[3]
3. Valproate has a direct effect on neuronal membranes, e.g. affects potassium ion conductance.[4,5]
4. Valproate reduces brain levels of the excitatory neurotransmitter, aspartate.[6,7]

Toxicology

Valproate does not appear to have mutagenic or carcinogenic potential and toxicological testing in animals has failed to demonstrate specific organ damage or general toxicity. However, teratogenic tests in mice, rats and rabbits have shown various congenital abnormalities including renal and skeletal defects.

Clinical pharmacology

Sodium valproate is a drug with anticonvulsant activity against a wide range of seizure types in man and appears to be well tolerated at therapeutic doses. It appears to have no significant hypnotic effect, nor does it have any significant effect on respiration, blood pressure, renal function or body temperature. Its mechanism of action is not fully established. Like many other anticonvulsants it appears to have teratogenic effects.

Pharmacokinetics

Valproic acid in plasma or serum may be measured by gas–liquid chromatography, high performance liquid chromatography and immunoassay systems which utilize differing technologies to monitor antibody–antigen reaction such as enzyme immunoassay and fluorescence immunoassay. A recent assessment of the different techniques from data derived from measurement of external quality assurance samples showed no significant differences between the techniques within or above the therapeutic range.[8] At a concentration below 350 $\mu mol.l^{-1}$ fluorescence polarization immunoassay and high performance liquid chromatography were the more precise techniques.[8] The sensitivity of the commercial kits is around 70 $\mu mol.l^{-1}$.

Valproate has been shown to be completely absorbed following oral administration of the plain tablets, enteric-coated tablets or the liquid preparations.[9–11,12] Peak plasma concentrations are achieved 1–2 hours after liquid or plain tablets and 2–8 hours after enteric-coated tablets. Absorption may be delayed by the presence of food in the stomach.[13]

The plasma half life varies between 9 and 21 hours, with a mean of 12–13 hours.[9–13] It tends to be shorter in patients who are taking other anticonvulsant drugs, consistent with the inducibility of valproate metabolism.[14] The half life varies with age, being longer in neonates (20–67 hours) but it usually falls in the first few weeks of life so that in older infants it reaches adult values.[15] The elderly also have a reduced capacity to metabolize valproate.[16] There is no evidence of autoinduction of valproate metabolism or saturation of metabolism.[12]

The distribution of valproate in adults is largely confined to the circulation and extracellular fluid with little penetration into tissues.[9,10] Values for the apparent volume of distribution have been reported as 0.1–0.4 $l.kg^{-1}$. There may be more extensive distribution in epileptic children and adults than in healthy volunteers.[14]

At plasma levels of valproate within the accepted therapeutic range, sodium valproate is highly bound ($\simeq$90%) to the plasma proteins but there is inter- and intrasubject variability. Binding is mainly to albumin and two different binding sites have been described.[17] The degree of protein binding is important as it is only the free component which is available for therapeutic action. The binding of valproate is concentration dependent and the free fraction has been shown to increase as total plasma valproate concentrations rise. This may explain the curvilinear dose plasma concentration relationship and affects the interpretation of total plasma valproate concentrations during therapeutic drug monitoring. Free fatty acids affect the protein binding of valproate both in vivo[18] (due to diurnal variations in endogenous free fatty acids) and in vitro[19] (during equilibrium dialysis). Hypoalbuminaemia, liver disease[20] and renal disease[17] all reduce valproate binding and in elderly patients there is a high free fraction, probably due to reduced albumin concentrations.[16] In patients with significant renal impairment the free fraction was increased to 20.3$\pm$4.7% compared with 8.4$\pm$2.5% in normal controls.[17] In pregnancy the free fraction of valproate was also raised, probably primarily due to a reduction in albumin concentration.[21] The administration of other drugs does not usually affect the protein binding of valproate but there is evidence that salicylate can decrease valproate binding.

Valproate levels in brain and CSF are much lower than plasma levels and appear to be related to free drug concentration in plasma. In man the brain concentration of valproate has been shown to be 6.8–27.9% of plasma concentrations.[22] Because of sodium valproate's low pKa it is secreted into saliva in small amounts which do not reflect the free plasma concentration.

Placental transfer of valproate and its metabolites has been demonstrated, with reports of higher concentrations in cord than in maternal blood.[23] Small amounts of the drug are secreted into breast milk, with levels reported as 0.17–5.4% of maternal plasma concentrations and therefore unlikely to adversely affect the baby.

Oral absorption	>95%
Presystemic metabolism	very low
Plasma half life	
range	9–21 h
mean	12 h
Volume of distribution	0.1–0.4 l.kg^{-1}
Plasma protein binding	80–94%

Concentration–effect relationship

The relationship between plasma concentration of valproate and therapeutic effect is complex. A therapeutic range for seizure control of 350–700 μmol.l^{-1} was first suggested by Schobben et al[24] but many subsequent studies have failed to show such a relationship. Studies are particularly difficult to interpret in patients on polytherapy. Some of the toxic effects of valproate such as tremor appear to be related to plasma concentrations of the drug and are more common with levels[25,26] greater than 700 μmol.l^{-1}.

Besides interindividual variations in valproate plasma concentrations when patients are given the same dose, there are large intraindividual fluctuations in plasma concentrations throughout the day depending on the frequency and time of drug administration.[27] Thus standardization of sampling times is necessary. Furthermore, the extent of protein binding is very variable due to concentration-dependent binding and disease states which alter binding. Thus perhaps it would be more relevant to attempt to relate free valproate concentration to clinical effect.

Sodium valproate has been demonstrated to have a prolonged pharmacological effect in animals[28] and humans[29] with delayed onset of action and carryover of effect. This could be due to accumulation of the drug or its metabolites in the brain or to a pharmacological effect which outlasts the presence of drug in the brain. Thus theoretically one would not expect to be able to relate single plasma drug determinations to seizure control in a direct fashion.

Metabolism

Valproate is almost completely metabolized prior to excretion (see Fig. 1). Only 1–3% of the ingested dose was found to be excreted unchanged in the urine.[12] The metabolism of valproate is complex and identification and quantification of the many metabolites has proved difficult.[30] The major elimination pathway is via conjugation with glucuronic acid. The remainder is largely metabolized via oxidative pathways (*β*, *ω*, and *ω*-1), particularly *β*-oxidation. In some animal species a small proportion of the drug dose is eliminated as CO_2 in the expired air and enterohepatic circulation of valproate has been demonstrated in the rat.

Knowledge of the pharmacological activity of the metabolites of valproate is incomplete but animal studies have shown that some of the metabolites have an anticonvulsant effect, although mostly less than that of the parent compound; the most active compounds being the 2-en and 4-en unsaturated metabolites.[31] The clinical significance of the anticonvulsant activity of these metabolites is uncertain but it has been calculated that valproate itself is responsible for >90% of the therapeutic effect.[32]

Pharmaceutics

Sodium valproate is available in oral forms as Epilim (Sanofi, UK)

200 mg lilac-coloured enteric-coated tablet
500 mg lilac-coloured enteric-coated tablet
100 mg white, scored, crushable tablet
syrup: red, cherry-flavoured syrup, containing 200 mg per 5 ml
liquid: red, cherry-flavoured sugar-free liquid, containing 200 mg per 5 ml

There is no slow-release preparation of sodium valproate currently available.

The tablets are hygroscopic and should be kept in the protective foil until taken. The syrup and liquid should be kept cool and away from direct sunlight. The syrup may be diluted with diluent syrups, such as syrup BP, which do not contain sulphur dioxide as preservative but should then be used within 14 days. The Epilim liquid preparation should not be diluted. Sodium valproate preparations are stable with a shelf-life of 2 years.

An intravenous preparation, Epilim Intravenous, 400 mg per vial is available for administration to patients in whom oral therapy is temporarily not possible.

Depakote (Abbott, USA) is in three oral forms:

125 mg salmon-coloured tablets, coded 'NT'
250 mg peach-coloured tablets, coded 'NR'
and 500 mg lavender-coloured tablets, coded 'NS'

Fig. 1

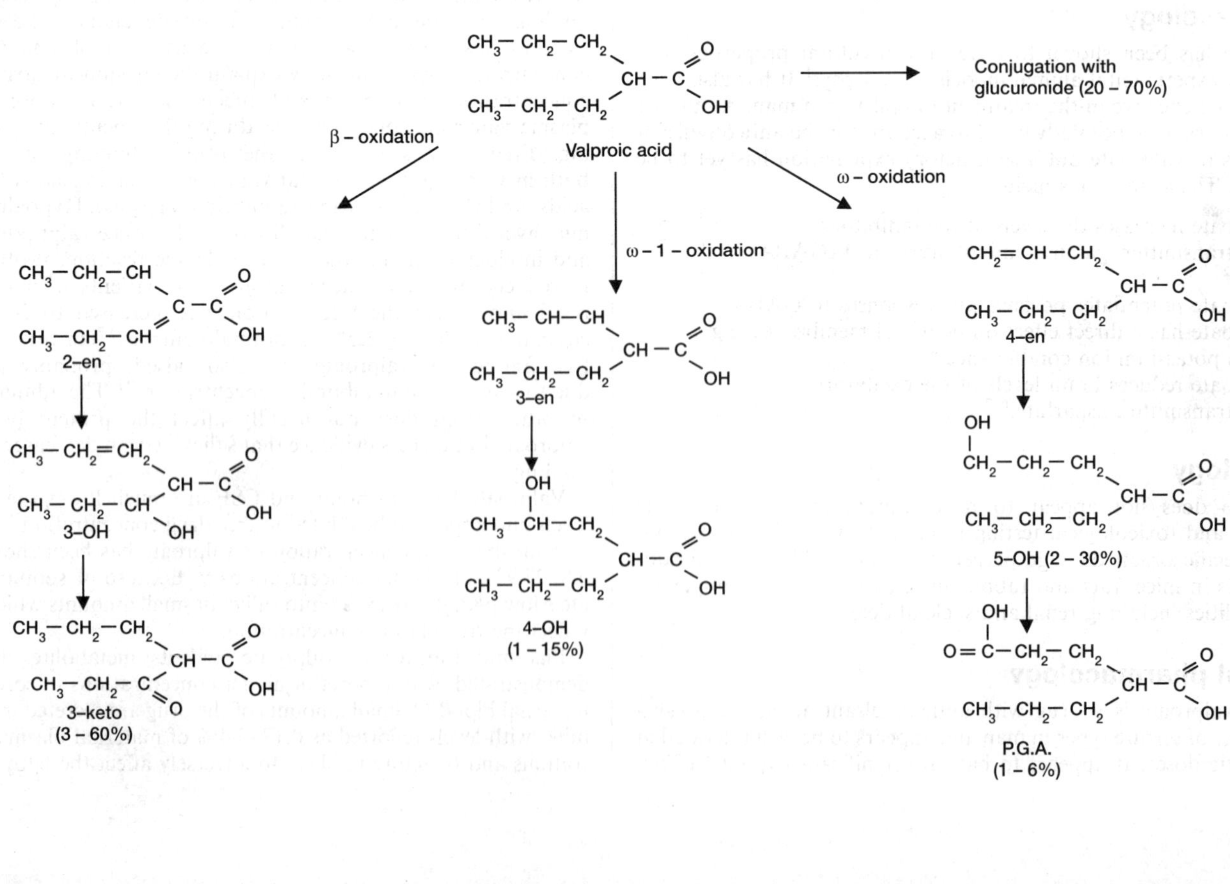

Therapeutic use

Indications

The major therapeutic indication is in the treatment of generalized, partial and other epilepsy. It has occasionally been used experimentally in a variety of other neurological and endocrine disorders.

1. Primary generalized seizures
2. Partial seizures
3. Prophylaxis of febrile convulsions
4. Prophylaxis of post-traumatic epilepsy
5. Status epilepticus
6. Miscellaneous uses.

Contraindications

Sodium valproate should not be given to patients with liver disease. Care should be exercised when prescribing sodium valproate in women of child-bearing age.

Mode of use

The daily dosage requirement varies with the age and weight of the patient. In adults treatment is started at a dose of 600 mg daily, increasing by 200 mg at 3-day intervals until control of seizures is achieved. The usual maintenance dosage lies within the range of 1000 mg to 2000 mg per day or 20–30 $mg.kg^{-1}$ body weight. Occasionally some patients may require as much as 2500 mg daily for seizure control. In children over 20 kg, the initial dose is 400 mg daily, irrespective of weight, and in children under 20 kg the dose is 20 $mg.kg^{-1}$ body weight daily. In refractory patients it is occasionally necessary to use doses of 40–60 $mg.kg^{-1}$ daily but this should only be considered in patients in whom there is no evidence of toxicity and where it is possible to monitor plasma valproate concentrations, clinical chemistry and haematological parameters.

Where possible valproate should be administered as monotherapy which prevents unwanted drug interactions, and results in lower dosage and fewer adverse reactions. If sodium valproate is to be used concurrently with antiepileptic drugs which induce liver enzyme activity, e.g. phenobarbitone, phenytoin and carbamazepine, it may be necessary to raise the dose of sodium valproate by 5–10 $mg.kg^{-1}$ daily. If there is concurrent administration of barbiturate the dose of barbiturate should be reduced if sedation develops.

Because of its short half life, especially when patients are on polytherapy, valproate is usually administered twice daily in order to minimize fluctuations in serum levels. However, due to its possible non-reversible effects this practice has been questioned. Indeed several studies have shown the equivalence or even superiority of a single daily dose over a divided dosing schedule.[33,34] In most patients there is no greater incidence of toxicity and administration once daily obviously improves compliance.

The effective range of plasma valproate levels in monotherapy is reported to be 350–700 $\mu mol.l^{-1}$ (50–100 $\mu g.ml^{-1}$) although with increasing experience of valproate some authorities would extend the range to 1000 $\mu mol.l^{-1}$ (150 $\mu g.ml^{-1}$). As previously discussed, there is controversy about the validity of recommending a therapeutic range of plasma drug concentrations for sodium valproate.

Indications

Sodium valproate is indicated for use in a wide range of seizure disorders. Its main use has been in the treatment of primary generalized epilepsies but recent evidence supports its efficacy in partial epilepsies as well.

1. Primary generalized seizures

i. Absence seizures. Sodium valproate has proved to be very effective therapy for absence seizures with a success rate approaching 100% in uncomplicated previously untreated absence seizures.[31,35] It has been suggested that the combination of ethosuximide with valproate may be particularly effective in those patients whose absence seizures do not respond to either drug alone.[36] The results in atypical absence attacks or Lennox–Gastaut Syndrome are less impressive. Since, unlike ethosuximide, valproate will also suppress tonic-clonic seizures it is the preferred treatment for absence seizures associated with tonic-clonic fits.

ii. Tonic-clonic seizures. Sodium valproate has been shown to improve seizure control in patients with generalized tonic-clonic seizures.[37,38] Valproate compared very favourably in comparative studies against phenytoin and carbamazepine in the control of tonic-clonic seizures. Sodium valproate is the drug of choice in patients with photosensitive epilepsy.[39]

iii. Myoclonic seizures. Myoclonic epilepsy is a miscellaneous group of seizure types with different aetiologies and different responses to treatment but there is evidence that in their management, particularly those associated with primary generalized epilepsy syndromes such as juvenile myclonic epilepsy,[40,41] sodium valproate is beneficial. It has also been used in the treatment of children with infantile spasms and resulted in fewer adverse effects than corticotrophin.[41]

2. Partial seizures

Experience has shown that partial seizures, particularly complex partial seizures, are relatively more resistant to drug treatment than generalized epilepsy and in common with other anticonvulsants sodium valproate is less effective for the treatment of partial seizures than it is in primarily generalized seizures.[42] It has compared favourably with phenytoin and carbamazepine in the therapy of partial seizures[47] and with carbamazepine.[44–46]

3. Prophylaxis of febrile convulsions

Valproate has been compared with phenobarbitone in several studies and has been found to be equally or more effective in the prophylaxis of febrile convulsions.[44] It is also less likely to provoke behavioural problems in children. However, because of the rare but potentially very serious hepatotoxicity which occasionally develops with sodium valproate the decision about which drug to use in this clinical situation is a difficult one.

4. Prophylaxis of post-traumatic epilepsy and use in neurosurgical practice

Sodium valproate has been used to prevent epilepsy in patients with head injury and has also been used to prevent epilepsy due to tumours and intracranial haemorrhage.[48]

5. Status epilepticus

Although there have been case reports of successful treatment with oral sodium valproate of status epilepticus which has been refractory to the usual emergency therapy, because of the delay in reaching peak drug levels with oral or rectal administration and the delayed onset of action which has been described, sodium valproate is theoretically an unsuitable drug for the routine treatment of status epilepticus.[49,50]

6. Miscellaneous uses

Successful treatment of mania with sodium valproate has been reported and it has also been used to treat alcohol withdrawal. There has been mixed success when it has been used to treat various movement disorders. Single case reports describe benefit in hemiballismus, Sydenham's chorea, post-traumatic choreoathetosis and post-anoxic action myoclonus. Several reports describe improvement in tardive dyskinesias with sodium valproate therapy. Sodium valproate has been used by endocrinologists to reduce ACTH levels and improve symptoms in patients with Nelson's Syndrome following adrenalectomy for Cushing's Disease.

Special considerations

Sodium valproate has minimal effects on cognitive function and for this reason may be the preferred antiepileptic treatment particularly in children. Because it does not induce hepatic microsomal enzyme activity it is less likely to cause oral contraceptive failure than other antiepileptic drugs.

Contraindications

Sodium valproate should not be given to patients with liver disease. Rarely severe hepatic dysfunction, including fatal hepatic failure, has occurred in patients whose treatment has included sodium valproate. Minor asymptomatic elevations in serum levels of liver enzymes are observed fairly frequently but they do not appear to be related to serious liver damage and usually resolve spontaneously or after temporary reduction in valproate dosage. The patients who seem to be most at risk include those with a prior history of liver disease and children with severe epilepsy associated with mental retardation, structural brain damage or metabolic disorder, especially when on multiple antiepileptic drug therapy. Such patients should have close

Sodium valproate

clinical supervision. Any patient on sodium valproate who develops an acute illness, including anorexia, vomiting, lethargy, drowsiness, jaundice or loss of seizure control, particularly during the first 6 months, should have valproate immediately withdrawn. The routine measurement of liver function is probably unnecessary except for those patients most at risk and there is no test available to predict the occurrence of this adverse event (see section on hepatotoxicity).

Patients about to undergo major surgery should have an estimation of platelet count and coagulation studies performed in view of the possibility of thrombocytopenia and prolongation of the bleeding time.

Valproate has been shown to be teratogenic in animals and embryotoxicity has been reported in humans. Therefore in women of child-bearing age the benefits of sodium valproate must be weighed against the possible risk of teratogenicity in the event of pregnancy.

The elimination of the metabolites of valproate in the urine as ketones may give rise to false positives in the testing of urine for diabetes.

The safety of sodium valproate in patients with porphyria is uncertain, with some case reports describing attacks precipitated by the drug and one report of improvement of the patient's clinical status while taking sodium valproate.

Adverse reactions

Potentially life-threatening effects

Liver damage. Severe hepatotoxicity, occasionally with a fatal outcome, is extremely rare.[51,52] It appears to be due to an idiosyncratic reaction and usually occurs during the first 6 months of valproate therapy. The liver histology in fatal cases is variable; some showing centrilobular necrosis, severe fatty change or cholestasis. Most of the cases have occurred in children and often they had already been noted to have developmental delay or associated neurological disease. Most were taking more than one antiepileptic drug and in some of the cases the causative role of sodium valproate was not clear cut. It has been suggested that normally valproate is not hepatotoxic but in the presence of a metabolic abnormality (e.g. an inborn error of metabolism) it may become so. The incidence of liver toxicity is very low but the risk increases when treating children with severe epilepsy, progressive neurological disease or in those taking several antiepileptic drugs.

Hyperammonaemia. Valproate also causes various metabolic disturbances because it inhibits several enzymes involved in intermediary cell metabolism. Moderate elevations in blood ammonia levels are fairly common during treatment with sodium valproate,[53,54] but there have been a small number of reports of encephalopathy and loss of seizure control. In a few instances the illness has been fatal.

Pancreatitis. Pancreatitis has recently been reported in association with valproate therapy and death has rarely occurred.[55] In some of the patients rechallenge with valproate after recovery led to recurrence of the pancreatitis.

Acute overdosage

Cases of accidental and suicidal overdose have been reported. With minor overdose, nausea, vomiting and dizziness occur but with massive overdose deep coma occurs and death has been reported. However, recovery has occurred with plasma valproate concentrations greater than 2000 $\mu g.ml^{-1}$. Hameodialysis and haemoperfusion have been used to lower valproate serum concentrations and naloxone has been administered to reverse the central nervous system depression. However, the efficacy of these treatments is unproven and supportive measures are probably all that is necessary.

Severe or irreversible adverse effects

Thrombocytopenia. There have been several studies reporting a fall in platelet count in patients taking sodium valproate. There have also been reports of abnormal platelet function including inhibition of the second phase of platelet aggregation. These abnormalities are reversible on withdrawing the drug or reducing the dose. The clinical risk of serious bleeding appears to be small but in patients about to undergo surgery, a full blood count and coagulation studies should be performed.

Symptomatic adverse effects

The incidence of adverse effects of sodium valproate is difficult to gauge exactly because many patients are taking several drugs concurrently and the method of determining adverse effects varies between the different studies. Schmidt estimated the incidence of adverse reactions based on analysis of 16 trials in a total of 1140 patients to be 26% but in only 2% were reactions severe enough to make discontinuation of therapy necessary.[56]

Gastrointestinal disorders. Reactions include anorexia, dyspepsia, nausea, vomiting, diarrhoea and constipation. The incidence of such effects has fallen since the introduction of an enteric-coated preparation. These adverse effects can be minimized by starting with a low dose of valproate and gradually increasing it and by taking the drug with food and in divided doses.

Weight gain. An increase in weight in patients taking valproate has been reported quite frequently, although the quoted incidence varies in different studies.[57] It is thought that weight gain may be due to increased appetite resulting from hypothalamic stimulation by a GABAergic effect of sodium valproate.

Skin and hair. Rashes are a rare occurrence with valproate. However, hair loss is a well-recognized phenomenon, with a reported incidence of between 2.6 and 12%.

Haematological disorders. Besides effects on platelets, valproate has been reported to lower the erythrocyte sedimentation rate and mild neutropenia has also been described.

Neurological. Tremor is a recognized adverse effect of sodium valproate. It is usually of the benign essential type and is probably dose-related and reversible. Reports on the effects of sodium valproate on cognitive function are conflicting. This is probably due to difficulties in interpretation due to multiple drug therapy and to variation in seizure frequency. In normal volunteers impairment in decision making was found but the adverse effects were much less than with phenytoin.[58] Sedation is most marked when patients are taking valproate combined with other antiepileptic drugs. Cases of coma and stupor have also been described, some of which were probably a result of drug interactions. In some reports continuing seizures may have accounted for the abnormal mental state.

Other effects

Asymptomatic transient elevations of hepatic transaminases are not uncommonly found and usually respond to dose reduction. Similarly asymptomatic hyperammonaemia may also occur but is probably of no significance.

Interference with clinical pathology tests

Metabolites of sodium valproate in the urine can give rise to positive tests for ketones and cause confusion in diabetic patients.

High risk groups

Neonates

Because of the long half life of sodium valproate in neonates, reduction in dosage is recommended in this group.

Breast milk. Breast-feeding by a mother taking sodium valproate is probably without risk to the child.

Children

Because of the chance of hepatotoxicity those children particularly at risk should be closely supervised, particularly during the first 6 months of sodium valproate therapy.

Pregnant women

As with other anticonvulsant drugs, animal studies provide evidence of a teratogenic effect of sodium valproate.

Recently reports of abnormalities in the offspring of epileptic mothers taking sodium valproate have been published and one from the Rhone-Alps region of France first drew attention to a possible causal relationship between sodium valproate and spina bifida.[59] In women in whom valproate is administered in pregnancy, serum α-fetoprotein estimation and amniocentesis should be offered.

The elderly

It has been reported that there may be an increase in the free valproate plasma concentrations in the elderly corresponding to a decrease in plasma protein binding and a reduction in clearance by the liver.[16] However, these pharmacokinetic modifications are unlikely to cause significant clinical problems.

Concurrent disease

Sodium valproate should not be prescribed to patients with active liver disease. Lower doses may be required by patients with impaired renal function.

Sodium valproate

Drug interactions

As polytherapy is common in the treatment of epilepsy there is great potential for interactions between the antiepileptic drugs. Unlike most of the other anticonvulsants in common use, sodium valproate does not induce hepatic metabolism[60] but rather appears to act as a non-specific inhibitor of drug metabolism. Most of the significant interactions which have been documented so far are pharmacokinetic.

Potentially hazardous interactions

Phenobarbitone. Serum phenobarbitone concentrations may increase when sodium valproate is introduced concurrently and result in excessive sedation. This interaction is thought to arise because of the inhibition of the metabolism of phenobarbitone by valproate increasing the elimination half life.[61]

Phenytoin. The interaction between phenytoin and valproate is more complex.[62] Valproate displaces phenytoin from its binding site on albumin and also inhibits the metabolism of phenytoin and thus reduces the intrinsic clearance of phenytoin. This results in increased free levels of phenytoin and either increased or unchanged total levels. Because of these conflicting effects on phenytoin pharmacokinetics, in some circumstances it may be necessary to measure free rather than total phenytoin concentrations in patients taking phenytoin and valproate concurrently.

Primidone. The metabolism of primidone may also be inhibited by valproate.

Carbamazepine. There have been conflicting reports about possible interactions between carbamazepine and valproate.

Ethosuximide. Most studies have shown no interaction between the drugs but one reported an increase in ethosuximide concentrations.

Antiepileptic drugs. Several antiepileptic drugs can reduce serum concentrations of sodium valproate by increasing the intrinsic clearance of valproate by enzymatic induction of metabolism. Such an interaction is seen with phenytoin, carbamazepine and phenobarbitone.

Salicylates. Salicylates have been reported to displace valproate from plasma protein binding sites.

CNS depressants. Valproate may enhance the effects of central nervous system depressants (including alcohol) and may reduce the patient's ability to drive or operate machinery.

Anticoagulants. Caution is recommended when valproate is administered with other drugs liable to interfere with blood coagulation such as warfarin or aspirin.

Potentially useful interactions

None has been described.

Major outcome trials

Most of the studies on the use of new drugs in epileptic patients has involved fairly short-term studies of the drug added on to existing antiepileptic drug therapy in patients with chronic drug-resistant epilepsy. However, within recent years several long-term studies have compared valproate monotherapy with monotherapy with other drugs in the treatment of newly diagnosed epileptic patients and children with febrile seizures.

Epilepsy

1. Callaghan N, O'Hare J, O'Driscoll D, O'Neill B, Daly M 1982 Comparative study of ethosuximide and sodium valproate in the treatment of typical absence seizures (petit mal). Developmental Medicine and Child Neurology 24: 830–836

In this study 28 children with newly diagnosed typical absence seizures were treated with valproate or ethosuximide, both drugs being dosed according to clinical effect. Clinical response was assessed at 6 months and based on 6-hour telemetry recordings and reports from parents and teachers. No significant difference between the two drugs was established following observation periods ranging from 18 to 48 months.

2. Turnbull D M, Rawlins M D, Weightman D, Chadwick D W 1983 Longterm comparative study of phenytoin and valproate in adult onset epilepsy. British Journal of Clinical Practice (Symposium Supplement) 27: 3–5

This large-scale comparative study recruited 116 newly diagnosed previously untreated adult patients with generalized tonic-clonic or partial seizures, who were randomly assigned to treatment with phenytoin or sodium valproate, and both drugs were dosed according to seizure control or the occurrence of adverse effects. There was no significant difference between the number of seizure-free patients taking each drug at 2-year follow-up.

3. Callaghan N, Kenny R A, O'Neill B, Crowley M, Goggin T A 1985 A prospective study between carbamazepine, phenytoin and sodium valproate as monotherapy in previously untreated and recently diagnosed patients with epilepsy. Journal of Neurology, Neurosurgery and Psychiatry 48: 639–644

This three-drug comparative study evaluated carbamazepine, phenytoin and sodium valproate in 181 previously untreated patients with partial or generalized seizures. The drugs were equally effective in the treatment of generalized or partial seizures.

Febrile convulsions

There have been several studies to compare the efficacy of valproate and phenobarbitone in the treatment of patients with febrile convulsions. They show that valproate seems to be at least comparable and possibly superior to phenobarbitone in the prophylactic treatment of recurrences of febrile convulsions.

1. Wallace S J, Smith J A 1980 Successful prophylaxis against febrile convulsions with valproic acid or phenobarbitone. British Medical Journal 1: 353–354
2. Minagawa K, Miura H 1981 Phenobarbital, primidone and sodium valproate in the prophylaxis of febrile convulsions. Brain Development 3: 385–393
3. Mamelle J C, Mamelle N, Plasse J C, Revol M, Gilly R 1982 Efficacité du dipropylacetate de sodium comparé au phénobarbital et á un placebo dans la prévention des récidives des convulsions fébrile. Pédiatrie 37: 433–445

General review articles

Chapman A, Keane P E, Meldrum B S, Simiand J, Vernieres J C 1982 Mechanism of anticonvulsant action of valproate. Progress in Neurobiology 19: 315–359

Gugler R, Von Unruh G E 1980 Clinical pharmacokinetics of valproic acid. Clinical Pharmacokinetics 5: 67–83

Levy R H, Koch K M 1982 Drug interactions with valproic acid. Drugs 24: 543–556

Turnbull D M 1983 Adverse effects of valproate. Adverse Drug Reactions and Acute Poisoning Reviews 2: 191–216

Schmidt D 1984 Adverse effects of valproate. Epilepsia 25 (suppl): S44–S49

Jeavons P M 1984 Non-dose-related effects of valproate. Epilepsia 25 (suppl): S50–S55

Anonymous 1981 Febrile convulsion: long term treatment. (Editorial) British Medical Journal 282: 673–674

Anonymous 1982 Valproate and malformations. (Editorial) Lancet 2: 1313–1314

Anonymous 1980 Sodium valproate and the liver. (Editorial) Lancet 11: 1119–1120

Levy R H (ed) 1984 Valproate. Modern Perspectives. Epilepsia 25 (suppl 1). Raven Press, New York

Woodbury D M, Penry J K and Pippenger C E (eds) 1982 Antiepileptic drugs. 2nd edn. Valproate. Chapters 44–50. Raven Press, New York, pp 549–611

References

1. Hammond E J, Wilder B J, Bruni J 1981 Central actions of valproic acid in man and in experimental models of epilepsy. Life Sciences 29: 2561–2574
2. Godin Y, Heiner L, Mark J, Mandel P 1969 Effects of di-n-propylacetate, an anticonvulsant compound, on GABA metabolism. Journal of Neurochemistry 16: 869–873
3. MacDonald R L, Bergey G K 1979 Valproic acid augments GABA-mediated postsynaptic inhibition in cultured mammalian neurones. Brain Research 107: 558–562
4. Slater G E, Johnston G D 1978 Sodium valproate increases potassium conductance in aplasia neurones. Epilepsia 19: 379–384
5. Hackman J C, Grayson V, Davidoff R A 1981 The presynaptic effects of valproic acid in the isolated frog spinal cord. Brain Research 220: 269–285
6. Schechter P J, Tranier Y, Grove J 1978 Effect of n-dipropylacetate on amino acid concentrations in mouse rain: correlation with anticonvulsant activity. Journal of Neurochemistry 31: 1325–1327

7. Chapman A G, Riley K, Evans M C, Meldrum B S 1982 Acute effects of sodium valproate and -vinyl GABA on regional amino acid metabolism in the rat brain: incorporation of 2-(^{14}C)-glucose into amino acids. Neurochemical Research 7: 1089–1105
8. Wilson J F, Tsanaclis L M, Williams J, Tedstone J E, Richens A 1989 Evaluation of assay techniques for the measurement of antiepileptic drugs in serum. A study based on external quality assurance measurements. Therapeutic Drug Monitoring 11: 185–195
9. Perucca E, Gatti G, Frigo G M, Crema A 1978 Pharmacokinetics of valproic acid after oral and intravenous administration. British Journal of Clinical Pharmacology 5: 313–318
10. Klotz U, Antonin K H 1977 Pharmacokinetics and bioavailability of sodium valproate. Clinical Pharmacology and Therapeutics 21: 736–743
11. Levy R H, Cenraud B, Loiseau, Akbaraly R, Brachet-Liermain A, et al 1980 Meal-dependent absorption of enteric-coated sodium valproate. Epilepsia 21: 273–280
12. Gugler R, Schell A, Eichelbaum M, Froscher W, Schulz H U 1977 Disposition of valproic acid in man. European Journal of Clinical Pharmacology 12: 125–132
13. Chun A H C, Hoffman D F, Friedmann N, Carrijan P J 1980 Bioavailability of valproic acid under fasting/non fasting regimens. Journal of Clinical Pharmacology 20: 30–36
14. Perucca E, Gatti G, Frigo G M, Crema A, Calzetti S et al 1978 Disposition of sodium valproate in epileptic patients. British Journal of Clinical Pharmacology 5: 495–499
15. Morselli P L, Franco-Morselli R, Bossi L 1980 Clinical pharmacokinetics in newborns and infants. Clinical Pharmacokinetics 5: 485–527
16. Perucca E, Grimaldi R, Gatti G, Piracchio S, Crema F et al 1984 Pharmacokinetics in valproic acid in the elderly. British Journal of Clinical Pharmacology 17: 665–669
17. Gugler R, Mueller G 1978 Plasma protein binding of valproic acid in healthy subjects and in patients with renal disease. British Journal of Clinical Pharmacology 5: 441–446
18. Marty J J, Kilpatrick C F, Moulds R F W 1982 Intra-dose variation in plasma protein binding of sodium valproate in epileptic patients. British Journal of Clinical Pharmacology 14: 399–404
19. Albani F, Riva R, Procaccianti G, Baruzzi A, Perucca E 1983 Free fraction of valproic acid: in vitro time-dependent increase and correlation with free fatty acid concentration in human plasma and serum. Epilepsia 24: 65–73
20. Klotz U, Rapp T, Muller W A 1978 Disposition of valproic acid in patients with liver disease. European Journal of Clinical Pharmacology 13: 55–60
21. Riva R, Albani F, Contin M, Baruzzi A, Altomare M et al 1984 Mechanism of altered drug binding to serum proteins in pregnant women: studies with valproic acid. Therapeutic Drug Monitoring 6: 25–30
22. Vajda F J E, Donnan G A, Phillips J, Bladin P F 1981 Human brain, plasma and CSF concentration of sodium valproate after 72 hrs of therapy. Neurology 31: 486–487
23. Nau H, Rating D, Koch S, Hauser I, Helge H 1981 Valproic acid and its metabolites: placental transfer, neonatal pharmacokinetics, transfer via mother's milk and clinical status in neonates of epileptic mothers. Journal of Pharmacology and Experimental Therapeutics 219: 768–777
24. Schobben F, Van der Kleijn E, Gabreels F J M 1975 Pharmacokinetics of di-n-propylacetate in epileptic patients. European Journal of Clinical Pharmacology 8: 97–105
25. Turnbull D M, Rawlins M D, Weightman D, Chadwick D W 1983 Plasma concentrations of sodium valproate; their clinical value. Annals of Neurology 14: 38–42
26. Chadwick D W 1985 Concentration effect relationship of valproic acid. Clinical Pharmacokinetics 10: 155–163
27. Riva A, Albani F, Cortellie P, Gobbi G, Perucca E et al 1983 Diurnal fluctuations in free and total plasma concentrations of valproic acid at steady state in epileptic patients. Therapeutic Drug Monitoring 5: 191–196
28. Lockard J S, Levy R H 1976 Valproic acid: reversibly acting drug? Epilepsia 17: 477–479
29. Rowan A J, Binnie C D, Warfield C A, Meinardi H, Meijer J W A 1979 The delayed effect of sodium valproate on the photoconvulsive response in man. Epilepsia 20: 61–68
30. Nau H, Loscher W 1984 Valproic acid and metabolites pharmacological and toxicological studies. Epilepsia 25 (suppl 1): S14–S22
31. Callaghan N, O'Hare J, O'Driscoll D, O'Neill B, Daly M 1982 Comparative study of ethosuximide and sodium valproate in the treatment of typical absence seizures (petit mal). Developmental Medicine and Child Neurology 24: 830–836
32. Loscher W 1981 Anticonvulsant activity of metabolites of valproic acid. Archives Internationales de Pharmacodynamie et de Therapie 249: 158–163
33. Covanis A, Jeavons P M 1980 Once daily sodium valproate in the treatment of epilepsy. Developmental Medicine and Child Neurology 22: 202–204
34. Gjerløff I, Arentsen J, Alving J, Secher B G 1984 Monodose versus 3 daily doses of sodium valproate: a controlled trial. Acta Neurologica Scandinavica 69: 120–124
35. Sato S, White B G, Penry J K, Dreifuss F E, Sackellares J C et al 1983 Valproic acid versus ethosuximide in the treatment of absence seizures. Neurology 32: 157–163
36. Rowan A J, Meier J W A, de Beer-Pawlikowski N, van der Geest P, Meinardi H 1983 Valproate–ethosuximide combination therapy for refractory absence seizures. Archives of Neurology 40: 797–802
37. Shakir R A, Johnson R H, Lambie D G, Melville I D, Nanda R N 1981 Comparison of sodium valproate and phenytoin as single drug treatment in epilepsy. Epilepsia 22: 27–33
38. Turnbull D M, Rawlins M D, Weightman D, Chadwick D W 1982 A comparison of phenytoin and valproate in previously untreated adult epileptic patients. Journal of Neurology, Neurosurgery and Psychiatry 45: 55–59
39. Harding G F A, Herrick C G, Jeavons P M 1978 A controlled study of the effect of sodium valproate on photosensitive epilepsy and its prognosis. Epilepsia 19: 555–565
40. Bourgeois B, Beaumanoir A, Blajev B et al 1987 Monotherapy With Volproate in Primary Generalized Epilepsies. Epilepsia 28: (Suppl 2) S8–S11
41. Ckement M J, Wallace S J 1988 Juvenile Myoclonic Epilepsy Archives of Disease in Childhood 63: 1049–1053
42. Jeavons P M, Clark J E, Maheshwari M C 1977 Treatment of generalised epilepsies of childhood and adolescence with sodium valproate. Developmental Medicine and Child Neurology 19: 9–25
43. Simon D, Penry J K 1975 Sodium di-N-propylacetate (DPA) in the treatment of epilepsy. Epilepsia 16: 549–573
44. Turnbull D M, Howel D, Rawlins M D, Chadwick D W 1985 Which drug for the adult epileptic patient: phenytoin or valproate? British Medical Journal 290: 815–819
45. Callaghan N, Kenny R A, O'Neill B et al 1985 A propective study between carbamazepine, phenytoin and sodium valproate as monotherapy in previously untreated and recently diagnosed patients with epilepsy. Journal of Neurology, Neurosurgery and Psychiatry 48: 639–644
46. Dean J C, Penry J K 1988 Valproate Monotherapy in 30 Patients With Partial Seizures. Epilepsia 29:(2) 140–144
47. Wallace S J, Aldridge-Smith J 1980 Successful prophylaxis against febrile convulsions with valproic acid or phenobarbitone. British Medical Journal 281: 353–354
48. Price D J 1980 The efficacy of sodium valproate as the only anticonvulsant administered to neurosurgical patients. In: Parsonage M J, Caldwell A D S (eds) The place of sodium valproate in the treatment of epilepsy. Academic Press, London, pp 23–24
49. Manhire A R, Espir M 1974 Treatment of status epilepsy with sodium valproate. British Medical Journal 3: 808
50. Vajda F J E, Symington G R, Bladin P F 1977 Rectal valproate in intractable status epilepticus. Lancet 1: 359–360
51. Zimmerman H J, Ishak K G 1982 Valproate-induced hepatic injury: Analyses of 23 fatal cases. Hepatology 2: 591–597
52. Zafrani E S, Berthelot P 1982 Sodium valproate in the induction of unusual hepatotoxicity. Hepatology 2: 648–649
53. Zaret B S, Beckner R R, Marini A M, Wagle W, Passarelli C 1982 Sodium valproate induced hyperammonaemia without clinical hepatic dysfunction. Neurology 32: 206–208
54. Marescaux C H, Warter J M, Laroye M, Rumbach L, Micheletti G et al 1983 Sodium valproate: a hyperammonaemic drug-study in epileptics and normal subjects. Journal of Neurological Sciences 58: 195–209
55. Parker P H, Hellineck G L, Chishon F K, Greene H L 1981 Recurrent pancreatitis induced by valproic acid. A case report and a review of the literature. Gastroenterology 80: 826–828
56. Schmidt D 1984 Adverse effects of valproate. Epilepsia 25 (suppl 1): S44–S49
57. Egger J, Brett E M 1981 Effects of sodium valproate in 100 children with special reference to weight. British Medical Journal 283: 577–581
58. Thompson P J, Trimble M R 1981 Sodium valproate and cognitive function in normal volunteers. British Journal of Clinical Pharmacology 12: 819–824
59. Robert E, Guibaud P 1982 Maternal valproic acid and congenital neural tube defects. Lancet 2: 937
60. Oxley J, Hedges A, Makki K A, Monks A, Richens A 1979 Lack of hepatic enzyme inducing effect of sodium valproate. British Journal of Clinical Pharmacology 2: 189–190
61. Kapetanovic I M, Kupferberg H J, Porter R J, Theodore W, Schilmar E et al 1981 Mechanism of valproate–phenobarbital interaction in epileptic patients. Clinical Pharmacology and Therapeutics 29: 480–486
62. Perucca E, Hebdige S, Frigo G M, Gatti G, Lecchini S, Crema A 1980 Interaction between phenytoin and valproic acid: plasma protein binding and metabolic effects. Clinical Pharmacology and Therapeutics 28: 779–789

Somatropin

Somatropin is synthetic human growth hormone (GH, somatotropin) for the treatment of states of growth hormone deficiency or insufficiency.

Chemistry

Somatropin (Genotropin, Humatrope, Norditropin, Saizen)
A synthetic 191 amino-acid polypeptide with an amino-acid sequence and 2 internal disulphide bridges identical to that of the major (molecular weight 22 000) component of human pituitary growth hormone (hGH)

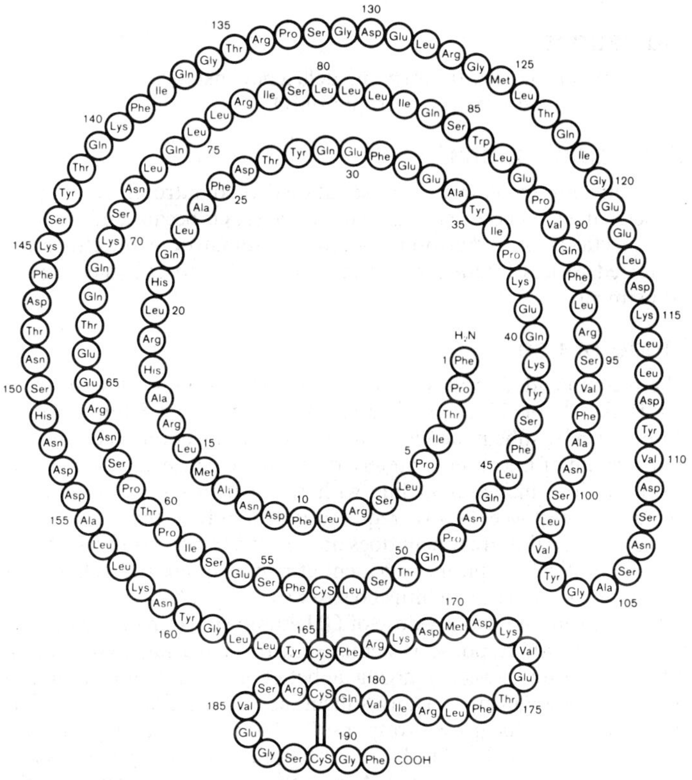

Molecular weight	22 000
pKa at pH 7	6.0–7.5
Solubility	
in alcohol	—
in water	—
Octanol/water partition coefficient	—

A white, sterile, lyophilized powder, somatropin is prepared by biosynthesis. For Genotropin, Humatrope and Norditropin this is carried out in *Escherichia coli* bacteria, which act as hosts to recombinant plasmids containing the human GH gene.[1,2] Saizen is prepared in a mammalian (mouse) tumour cell line.

Somatropin is not available as a component of any combination product.

Pharmacology

Somatropin stimulates skeletal and soft tissue growth by promoting cell division, amino-acid uptake and protein synthesis.[3] It has an immediate, brief, insulin-like effect followed by more significant anti-insulin-like actions which include decreased glucose utilization and lipolysis. GH action on tissues is mediated through specific GH receptors. These receptors do not recognize GH from other animal species, although human GH is active in lower order species, when its metabolic effects differ from those in humans. The human GH receptor, recently characterized and cloned,[4] occurs as disulphide linked oligomers of a sialoglycoprotein (MW 110 000) and may exist as several sub-types. Its distribution and expression are modulated by numerous factors.[5–7] The receptor is present in chondrocytes and osteoblasts, hepatocytes, adipocytes and fibroblasts in particular, yet is also found in many other tissues (such as the brain and gastrointestinal tract) where the role of GH is not clear. Receptor expression is dependent on developmental status. In man, receptor expression is very low or absent in fetal tissues and rises progressively during infancy. This explains why the impact of GH-deficiency on linear growth is not very marked until later infancy. Receptor expression or activity is enhanced by insulin and sex steroids, and reduced by fasting and renal insufficiency. Little is known of the mechanisms of post-receptor signal transduction, but there is data suggesting tyrosine kinase activity as one possibility. The receptor has a short half life (about 45 minutes) and few are recycled to the cell surface membrane. GH can directly influence the expression of specific genes, including those for the GH receptor, somatostatin, growth hormone releasing hormone, insulin-like growth factor-I, albumin and myosin heavy chain.[8] Individuals with abnormalities of the gene encoding the GH receptor show deficient GH binding, do not respond to hGH or somatropin, and have growth failure (Laron type dwarfism).[9]

Toxicology

Somatropin does not have toxic effects in animals at doses close to those used in man. Teratogenicity tests have not been performed on somatropin (Genotropin), but extracted human pituitary GH (hGH) and biosynthetic methionyl-GH (somatrem) have shown no mutagenic potential in Ames' bacterial test or in bone marrow cells of the Chinese hamster.[10]

Clinical pharmacology

Somatropin does not differ significantly from hGH in its metabolic actions.[11–14] These effects are both acute (within 2 hours) and long term. In GH-deficient patients, an immediate transient period of hypoglycaemia may be observed, but this is of little clinical significance and does not occur in normal subjects.[3,15] Anti-insulin-like actions are observed after 2 to 4 hours, and include inhibition of glucose utilization and lipolysis with an increase in serum free fatty acid levels. This lipolytic effect is reflected in GH-deficient children by a loss of subcutaneous fat during the early months of GH treatment.[16] In short children who are not GH-deficient, GH may provoke hyperinsulinaemia without impairment of glucose tolerance.[17]

The growth-promoting effects of GH (i.e. cell replication and differentiation) are mediated predominantly by the insulin-like growth factors/somatomedins (IGF 1 and IGF 2). These polypeptides, which are produced by most body tissues in response to GH, are of approximate molecular weight 7500. Serum IGF levels are low in GH deficiency and can rise to normal within a few days of starting somatropin treatment. This is accompanied by retention of sodium, potassium and phosphate, with an increase in intestinal absorption of calcium although serum calcium levels are unaffected since urinary calcium excretion increases.[3]

Glomerular filtration rate is increased unless impairment of renal function is already present. The serum IGF-I response to GH is dose dependent. A somatropin dose of 1.5 IU.m^{-2} daily was insufficient to maintain normal diurnal serum IGF-I levels after 14 days of treatment at this dose,[18] although the optimum dose above this level has yet to be determined. The effect of a single dose of GH on IGF-I generation does not last significantly beyond 24 hours.

Pharmacokinetics

Growth hormone can be measured by single-antibody radioimmunoassay (RIA), double-antibody immunoradiometric assay (IRMA), enzyme linked immunosorbent assay (ELISA) or immunochemiluminometric assay. Most assays have a sensitivity of 0.5–2 mU.l^{-1} GH.

IRMA techniques are usually more sensitive than RIA and a typical working range is of the order of 0.5–200 $mU.l^{-1}$ for IRMA although ELISA systems can increase the sensitivity 100-fold. Specificity can vary according to the antisera or monoclonal antibodies employed (n.b. 1 mg somatropin is equivalent to 2.6 units (approx) GH).[19] These techniques do not distinguish somatropin from endogenous GH.

Somatropin is administered either by intramuscular or subcutaneous injection. Peak serum levels of somatropin are achieved 2 to 8 hours after intramuscular injection and return to baseline after 8 to 16 hours.[13,15,20] This does not differ significantly from hGH but there is considerable variation both in and between individuals with respect to the timing and magnitude of the rise in serum somatropin levels. In one study (n = 12) the mean peak serum concentration of hGH was about 150 $mU.l^{-1}$ after either 4 or 8 IU intramuscularly.[20] Subcutaneous administration produces lower, but more consistent, serum hormone levels with a peak at 4 to 8 hours after injection and returning to baseline after 11 to 20 hours.[13,20] Subcutaneous injection of hGH (1.2 or 1.7 IU) produced a mean peak serum somatropin level of 30 to 40 $mU.l^{-1}$.[20] Although less hormone reaches the systemic circulation after subcutaneous as compared with intramuscular injection, these modes of administration give similar observed metabolic effects.[13] The fate of subcutaneously administered somatropin not reaching the systemic circulation is unknown, but may undergo degradation in adipocytes.

Somatropin is not absorbed in an active form from the gastrointestinal tract.

Somatropin has a biphasic clearance curve with a half disappearance time in normal subjects of 9.0 ± 3.5 min (mean ± SD; n = 8) for the first phase over 60 mins, and 30.7 ± 10.8 min (n = 8) for the second phase between 60 and 120 min after intravenous injection.[21] Metabolic clearance rate ranged from 82 to 139 $ml.min^{-1}.m^{-2}$ body surface area. When given by subcutaneous injection the serum half life was increased to 248 ± 55 min, reflecting the presumably rate-limiting absorption phase. Clearance does not appear to be influenced by age or sex but may be reduced in hypothyroidism and diabetes mellitus.[3]

The distribution volume for somatropin and its partitioning within the body are not known. Binding to plasma proteins is highly variable, being dependent to some extent on the presence or absence or GH-binding antibodies (see biochemical effects) and specific GH-binding proteins of high and low affinity. The high affinity GH-binding protein is homologous to the extracellular domain of the GH receptor although the physiological significance has not been defined.[5,22]

Oral absorption	—
Presystemic metabolism	—
Plasma half life	α 9.0 ± 3.5 min β 30.7 ± 10.8 min
Volume of distribution	—
Plasma protein binding	variable

Concentration–effect relationship

Physiological secretion of GH occurs in a pulsatile manner, predominantly during the night, with a pulse frequency of approximately 2–3 hours. The 24 hour secretion rate in young men is about 0.6–1.5 $mg.24\,h^{-1}$ (equivalent to 1.3–3.0 $IU.24\,h^{-1}$).[23] Animal studies suggest optimal growth is achieved by simulation of the physiological GH pulse frequency,[24] but the optimum treatment regimen for GH-deficient children has yet to be determined, even after 30 years of clinical experience.

There is no role for the measurement of serum somatropin levels in the routine management of patients. If non-compliance is suspected, serum IGF 1 levels may be of some value.

Metabolism

Routes of elimination of somatropin are undetermined. Less than 0.01% is excreted in urine.[25] It is presumed that most GH is metabolized by hydrolysis in its target tissues after receptor-binding and internalization of the GH molecule.[26]

Pharmaceutics

Somatropin is available for parenteral use only.

Genotropin (Kabi Pharmacia, UK) is available as a combined package containing 4 IU human growth hormone and in a multidose pack containing 12 IU human growth hormone and m-Cresol preservative.

Humatrope (Eli Lilly) is available as a 5 mg vial in the USA and as 4 IU vial in the UK. Both include a diluent ampoule with phenolic preservatives.

Norditropin (Nordisk, UK) is a 12 IU multidose vial, whilst Saizen (Serono, UK) is a 4 IU vial.

A clear solution (approx. pH 7.5) is prepared by addition of 1–2 ml diluent to each 4 IU somatropin with a gentle, slow, swirling motion. Vigorous shaking should be avoided as this might denature the hormone. Once reconstituted the refrigerated solution is stable for up to 14 days.

The preparation should be stored at +2 to +8°C and protected from light. Freezing should be avoided. The shelf life is approximately 24 months.

New delivery systems, comparable to the pen-like devices used for subcutaneous insulin administration, are currently under development.

Therapeutic use

Indications

1. Treatment of growth hormone deficiency/insufficiency
2. Turner's syndrome (Genotropin only).

Contraindications

There are no absolute contraindications to somatropin therapy. If diabetes mellitus co-exists, care should be taken because of the anti-insulin effects of somatropin; once-daily somatropin injections are preferred to less frequent regimens and insulin dosage may require adjustment.

Mode of use

The recommended total weekly dose of somatropin is at least 0.5 to 0.7 $IU.kg^{-1}$, or 12 $IU.m^{-2}$, divided into daily or 3-times-weekly doses given by subcutaneous or intramuscular injection. The subcutaneous route of injection is preferred for convenience and safety. The absolute dose increases in line with the patient's growth, and the maximum total weekly dose required is probably in the range 20–30 IU. Withdrawal of treatment does not produce adverse effects, except possibly in the hypopituitary patient at risk of spontaneous hypoglycaemia, or if diabetes mellitus coexists (see above).

For a given total weekly dose of GH administered in divided doses, a better growth response is achieved with increasing frequency of injections, 3-times-weekly giving a better growth response than a twice-weekly regimen.[27] Daily subcutaneous injections appear further to improve the growth response[20,28,29] and this policy has now been widely adopted.[30] The benefits of more than one injection per 24 hour period are being assessed. Administration of the hormone in the evening is preferred; this reduces the impact of anti-insulin effects on carbohydrate metabolism in relation to meals. Patients with symptomatic hypoglycaemia associated with GH deficiency should receive at least daily injections of somatropin.

The total weekly dose of somatropin should be determined by the patient's size (body weight or surface area). Standard regimens worldwide have used about 12 IU per week, or 0.3 to 0.5 $IU.kg^{-1}$ per week given in divided doses (from twice weekly up to daily). Long-term results suggest these doses are inadequate for optimal growth in the older child, particularly during puberty. Increased availability of somatropin is allowing reassessment of higher (2–3-fold) dose schedules which were not practicable with the previously limited supplies of hGH.

Indications

1. Treatment of growth hormone deficiency/insufficiency

Somatropin has replaced hGH as the preferred treatment for GH deficiency. hGH was withdrawn almost worldwide in 1985 when its association with the 'slow virus' infection Creutzfeldt-Jakob disease was recognized[31] although a few countries delayed withdrawal of hGH until biosynthetic preparations were more widely available.

Treatment should begin as early as possible after the diagnosis is established. Accurate monitoring of the growth response is essential to confirm the diagnosis. The response to treatment should be assessed by regular (3–6-monthly) measurements of stature and related auxological indices, which should include an appropriate measure of skeletal maturation/bone age (e.g. by the Tanner-Whitehouse II method).[32] Care should be taken to ensure that structural lesions responsible for impaired hypothalamo-pituitary function are excluded at presentation and during subsequent management. The dose of somatropin should be increased regularly in relation to body size. If the growth response is poor, re-evaluation of the clinical situation should be considered, with particular regard to other associated endocrine disorders (such as secondary hypothyroidism or ACTH insufficiency) and the possible, but infrequent, development of GH-binding antibodies. Treatment is usually continued until statural growth is complete or a satisfactory height has been achieved. A role for somatropin in adult life, after completion of growth, has not yet been established.

2. Turner's syndrome
Genotropin and methionyl-GH (somatrem) have product licences for the treatment of short stature in Turner's syndrome; this may be extended to other preparations of somatropin. Although the basis of the growth failure associated with Turner's syndrome may be a combination of a skeletal dysplasia with relative GH deficiency, particularly when puberty progresses abnormally in the Turner's girl, GH treatment will accelerate growth in this condition.[33] Several major studies of the effects of GH (somatrem and somatropin) in Turner's syndrome are under way, but the ultimate effect on final adult height of these girls will not be known for several years. One study, using somatrem, reports an increase in predicted final height of 4–5 cm after three years of somatrem treatment.[34,35] Doses of GH under assessment in Turner's syndrome are generally 1.5–2-fold higher than for classical GH deficiency.

Adverse reactions

Potentially life-threatening effects
None is known.

Acute overdosage
No hazard is to be expected from acute overdose, except loss of glycaemic control in diabetes mellitus.

Severe or irreversible adverse effects
None is known.

Symptomatic adverse effects
Lipo-atrophy has occurred with somatrem and somatropin when the site of subcutaneous injection was not varied.[36] This recovers when the injection site is changed.

Local urticarial reactions have rarely been reported at the injection site.[37]

Other effects
Serum free fatty acid and plasma glucose levels may be slightly elevated according to the relative times of hormone dose and blood collection.
Somatropin-binding antibodies have developed in less than 5% of patients, usually after 3–6 months of treatment.[37–41] These antibodies were of low binding capacity and their long-term significance is unknown. GH-binding antibodies developed in 30–70% of patients treated with somatrem (methionyl-GH)[42–44] and in less than 20% of patients receiving the purest preparations of hGH.[45] Only rarely were these antibodies associated with inhibition of the growth response, and attenuation of growth response has not been reported after treatment with somatropin. Antibodies have developed almost invariably after GH treatment of those rare patients in whom GH deficiency has arisen through deletion of the GH gene.[46]

Interference with clinical pathology tests
Endogenous GH is generally not distinguishable from somatropin by immunoassay.

Somatropin

S

High risk groups

Neonates
Neonates with congenital hypopituitarism are at risk of spontaneous hypoglycaemia. Somatropin treatment should be given at least once daily. An initial dose of 1–2 IU.24 h^{-1} is recommended but higher doses may be required.

Breast milk. There are no indications for the use of the drug in lactating women.

Children
See Therapeutic use.

Pregnant women
There are no indications for use during pregnancy.

The elderly
There are no indications for using the drug in elderly patients.

Concurrent disease
The problem of concurrent disease is discussed above under Contraindications.

Drug interactions

Potentially hazardous interactions
Insulin. Antagonism of the effects of insulin may necessitate an increase or adjustment of the insulin dose. Somatropin should be given on a daily regimen in patients with diabetes mellitus.

Potentially useful interactions
No interactions of this type are known.

Major outcome trials

As yet there are no reported long-term studies to final height using the various preparations of somatropin. Several preliminary reports show somatropin to have equivalent bioactivity to hGH but the efficacy of GH treatment in the long-term must be assessed from previous studies in which hGH was used.

1. Ranke M, Weber B, Bierich J R 1979 Long-term response to human growth hormone in 36 children with idiopathic growth hormone deficiency. European Journal of Pediatrics 132: 221–238

12 of these patients had isolated GH-deficiency (IGHD) and 24 had multiple pituitary hormone deficiency (MPHD). The dose of hGH was 4 IU, 2 or 3 times weekly (equivalent to 12.4 $\pm$ 3.9 (SD) IU.m^{-2} body surface area per week). Treatment was for between 1 and 6 years and few patients had reached final height. There was no significant difference in growth response between IGHD and MPHD patients. Pretreatment height velocity (mean $\pm$ SD) was 3.7 $\pm$ 1.1 cm.$year^{-1}$ and increased to 7.7 $\pm$ 2.4 cm.$year^{-1}$ during the first year. Subsequent yearly height velocities showed a progressive decline: 6.0 $\pm$ cm.$year^{-1}$ (2nd year), 5.1 $\pm$ 2.2 cm.$year^{-1}$ (3rd year), 5.1 $\pm$ 2.2 cm.$year^{-1}$ (4th year), 4.1 $\pm$ 1.6 cm.$year^{-1}$ (5th year) and 4.6 $\pm$ 2.0 cm.$year^{-1}$ (6th year).

This fall in height velocity after the initial first year of rapid 'catch-up' growth is typical of reversible growth failure, irrespective of the cause, but may represent, in part, a waning of response to GH because the dose of GH was not increased in line with body size. Other studies have shown similar results and are reviewed by the authors.

2. Burns E C, Tanner J M, Preece M A, Cameron N 1981 Final height and pubertal development in 55 children with idiopathic growth hormone deficiency, treated for between 2 and 15 years with human growth hormone. European Journal of Pediatrics 137: 155–164

60 patients were treated for GHD. 39 had IGHD, 10 had GHD and gonadotrophin deficiency (GnD), 6 had MPHD and 5 were retrospectively diagnosed as 'transient' pubertal GHD. The majority of patients started hGH treatment at a relatively late age (mean 11 years, range 9 to 14 years) and this may largely explain their failure to achieve normal stature. Final height for patients with IGHD averaged 2.0 SD below their mid-parent mean, or 2.3 SD below the population mean. Half of the boys and 15% of girls were above the population 3rd centile. This represents a height gain with treatment

S

of 2 SD, and amelioration of further height loss, since untreated GHD patients reach a mean final height about 6 SD below the population mean. Patients with GHD and GnD had final heights averaging 1.5 SD below the population mean and those with MPHD only 1.0 SD below. This apparently better outcome was considered to be due to their relatively late pubertal development, allowing disproportionately greater growth in the legs.

3. Burns E C, Tanner J M, Preece M A, Cameron N 1981 Growth hormone treatment in children with craniopharyngioma: final growth status. Clinical Endocrinology 14: 587–595

30 patients with hypopituitarism secondary to craniopharyngioma were treated with hGH for a mean period of 4.5 years, starting at mean age 14.8 years (range 9.8 to 18.7). All but 3 patients achieved a final height between the 3rd and 50th population centiles (none higher) but only 12 patients ended within 2 SD of their mid-parent mean. These heights were achieved, as with idiopathic MPHD patients, by having long legs relative to their sitting heights (final mean subischial leg length SD score+0.2 SD against mean sitting height SD score -3.0. This was again considered to be a consequence of what would now be considered late pubertal induction.

Most patients in this, and the previously cited, study received 15–20 IU hGH per week in 2 or 3 divided doses.

Further studies are awaited to define the long-term benefits of more recently adopted treatment schedules using higher doses of GH, and daily subcutaneous injection regimens.

General review articles

1. Davidson M B 1987 Effect of growth hormone on carbohydrate and lipid metabolism. Endocrine Reviews 8 (2): 115–131
2. Isaksson O G P, Lindahl A, Nilsson A, Isgaard J 1987 Mechanism of the stimulatory effect of growth hormone on longitudinal bone growth. Endocrine Reviews 8 (4): 426–438
3. Ranke M B, Bierich J R 1986 Treatment of growth hormone deficiency. In: Savage M O, Randall R A (eds) Clinics in endocrinology and metabolism. W B Saunders Co, London 15 (3): 495–510

References

1. Flodh H 1986 Human growth hormone produced with recombinant DNA technology: development and production. Acta Paediatrica Scandinavica (suppl) 325: 1–9
2. Fryklund L 1987 Production of authentic recombinant somatropin. Acta Paediatrica Scandinavica (suppl) 331: 5–8
3. Daughaday W H 1985 The anterior pituitary. In: Wilson J D, Foster D W (eds) Williams textbook of endocrinology 7th edn. W B Saunders Co, Philadelphia, ch 18, pp 577–583
4. Leung D W, Spencer S A, Cachianes G et al 1987 Growth hormone receptor and serum binding protein: purification, cloning and expression. Nature 330: 537–543
5. Waters M J, Barnard R T, Lobie P E et al 1990 Growth hormone receptors — their structure, location and role. Acta Paediatrica Scandinavica (suppl) 366: 60–72
6. Hughes J P, Friesen H G 1985 The nature and regulation of the receptors for pituitary growth hormone. Annual Reviews of Physiology 47: 469–482
7. Gluckman P D, Breier B H, Sauerwein H 1990 Regulation of the cell surface growth hormone receptor. Acta Paediatrica Scandinavica (suppl) 336: 73–78
8. Norstedt G, Enberg B, Moller C, Mathews L S 1990 Growth hormone regulation of gene expression. Acta Paediatrica Scandinavica (suppl) 336: 79–83
9. Amselem S, Duquesnoy P, Attree O et al 1989 Laron dwarfism and mutations of the growth hormone-receptor gene. New England Journal of Medicine 321: 989–995
10. Fryklund L M, Bierich J R, Ranke M B 1986 Recombinant human growth hormone. In: Savage M O, Randall R A (eds) Clinics in endocrinology and metabolism. W B Saunders Co, London, vol 15 (3): 511–535
11. Hintz R L, Rosenfeld R G, Wilson D M et al 1982 Biosynthetic methionyl human growth hormone is biologically active in adult man. Lancet 1: 1276–1279
12. Rosenfeld R G, Aggarwal B B, Hintz R L, Dollar L A 1982 Recombinant DNA-derived methionyl human growth hormone is similar in membrane binding properties to human pituitary growth hormone. Biochemical and Biophysical Research Communications 106: 202–209
13. Jorgensen J O L, Flyvbjerg A, Dinesen J, Lund H, Alberti K G M M, Orskov H, Christiansen J S 1987 Serum profiles and short term metabolic effect of pituitary and authentic biosynthetic human growth hormone in man. Acta Endocrinologica (Copenhagen) 116: 381–386
14. Van Vliet G, Bosson D, Craen M, Du Caju M V L, Malvaux P, Vanderschueren-Lodeweyckx M 1987 Comparative study of the lipolytic potencies of pituitary-derived and biosynthetic human growth hormone in hypopituitary children. Journal of Clinical Endocrinology and Metabolism 65: 876–879
15. Wilton P, Sietniks A 1987 An open-labelled study of the safety, acute metabolic activity and pharmacokinetic profile of a short term course of recombinant human growth hormone in healthy volunteers. Clinical Endocrinology 26: 125–128
16. Tanner J M, Hughes P C R, Whitehouse R H 1977 Comparative rapidity of response of height, limb muscle and limb fat to treatment with human growth hormone in patients with and without growth hormone deficiency. Acta Endocrinologica (Copenhagen) 84: 681–696
17. Hindmarsh P C, Brook C G D 1987 Effect of growth hormone on short normal children. British Medical Journal 295: 573–577
18. Jorgensen J O L, Flyvbjerg A, Lauritzen T, Alberti K G M M, Orskov H, Christiansen J S 1988 Dose–repsonse studies with biosynthetic human growth hormone (GH) in GH-deficient patients. Journal of Clinical Endocrinology and Metabolism 67: 36–40
19. Reiter E O, Morris A H, MacGillivray M H, Weber D 1988 Variable estimates of serum growth hormone concentrations by different radioassay systems. Journal of Clinical Endocrinology and Metabolism 66: 68–71
20. Albertsson-Wikland K, Westphal O, Westgren U 1986 Daily subcutaneous administration of human growth hormone in growth hormone deficient children. Acta Paediatrica Scandinavica 75: 89–97
21. Wilton P, Widlund L, Guilband O 1988 Pharmacokinetic profile of an i.v. and s.c. dose of recombinant human growth hormone. Pediatric Research 23: 117
22. Baumann G, Shaw M A 1990 A second, lower affinity growth-hormone binding protein in human plasma. Journal of Clinical Endocrinology and Metabolism 70: 680–686
23. Kowarski A, Thompson R G, Migeon C J, Blizzard R M 1971 Determination of integrated plasma concentrations and true secretion rates of human growth hormone. Journal of Clinical Endocrinology and Metabolism 32: 356–360
24. Clark R G, Jansson J O, Isaksson O, Robinson I C A F 1985 Intravenous growth hormone: growth responses to patterned infusions in hypophysectomized rats. Journal of Endocrinology 104: 53–61
25. Baumann G, Abramson E C 1983 Urinary growth hormone in man: evidence for multiple molecular forms. Journal of Clinical Endocrinology and Metabolism 56: 305–311
26. Roupas P, Herington A C 1987 Processing of growth hormone by rat adipocytes in primary culture: diffentiation between release of intact hormone and degradative processing. Endocrinology 121: 1521–1530
27. Preece M A, Tanner J M, Whitehouse R H, Cameron N 1976 Dose dependence of growth response to human growth hormone in growth hormone deficiency. Journal of Clinical Endocrinology and Metabolism 42: 477–483
28. Russo L, Moore W V 1982 A comparison of subcutaneous and intramuscular administration of human growth hormone in the therapy of growth hormone deficiency. Journal of Clinical Endocrinology and Metabolism 55: 1003–1006
29. Kastrup K W, Christiansen J S, Koch Andersen J, Orskov H 1983 Increased growth rate following transfer to daily s.c. administration from three weekly i.m. injections of hGH in growth hormone deficient children. Acta Endocrinologica (Copenhagen) 109: 163–168
30. Raiti S 1987 Statistical aspects of hGH therapy for hypopituitarism. Pediatric and Adolescent Endocrinology 16: 1–12
31. Preece M A 1986 Creutzfeldt-Jakob disease: implications for growth hormone deficient children. Neuropathology and Applied Neurobiology 12: 509–515
32. Tanner J M, Whitehouse R H, Cameron N, Marshall W A, Healy M J R, Goldstein H 1983 Assessment of skeletal maturity and prediction of adult height (TW2 method). Academic Press, London
33. Buchanan C R, Law C M, Milner D G 1987 Growth hormone in short, slowly growing children and those with Turner's syndrome. Archives of Disease in Childhood 62: 912–991
34. Rosenfeld R G, Hintz R L, Johanson A J et al 1988 Three-year results of a randomized prospective trial of methionyl human growth hormone and oxandrolone in Turner syndrome. Journal of Pediatrics 113: 393–400
35. Rosenfeld R G 1989 Update on growth hormone therapy for Turner's syndrome. Acta Paediatrica Scandinavica (suppl) 356: 103–108
36. Flodh H 1987 Update on the clinical use and experience of Somatonorm (somatrem). Acta Paediatrica Scandinavica (suppl) 337: 130–133
37. Gunnarsson R, Wilton P 1987 Clinical experience with Genotropin worldwide: an update March 1987. Acta Paediatrica Scandinavica (suppl) 337: 147–152
38. Zachmann M, Muritano M, Torresani T, Rasmussen L H 1988 Results of treatment with recombinant human growth hormone without methionine (r-hGH) in patients (pts) with growth hormone deficiency (GHD). Pediatric Research 23: 116
39. Sportsman J R, Winely C W, Heisserman J A, Frank B H 1987 Methionyl-human growth hormone provokes elevated levels of antibodies to human growth hormone relative to natural sequence human growth hormone. Abstracts of 69th Annual Meeting of the Endocrine Society, Indianapolis, Abstract no 297
40. Stubbe P, Stahnke N and study group 1988 R-HGH of mammalian cell origin for the treatment of growth hormone (GH) deficiency in children. Pediatric Research 23: 116
41. Buzi F, Buchanan C R, Morrell D J, Preece M A 1989 Antigenicity and efficacy of authentic sequence recombinant human growth hormone (somatropin): first-year experience in the United Kingdom. Clinical Endocrinology 30: 531–538
42. Tyllström J, Karlen B, Guilbaud O 1986 Somatonorm (somatrem): immunological aspects. In: Milner R D G, Flodh H (eds) Immunological aspects of human growth hormone. Medical Education Services, Oxford, pp 19–31
43. Thompson R G, Draper M W 1987 Somatropin is less immunogenic than somatrem (met-GH) in growth hormone (GH) deficient children. 1st European Congress of Endocrinology, Copenhagen, June 1987. Abstract no 21–612
44. Milner R D G, Barnes N D, Buckler J M H et al 1987 United Kingdom multicentre clinical trial of somatrem. Archives of Disease in Childhood 62: 776–779
45. Preece M A 1986 Experience of treatment with pituitary derived human growth hormone with special reference to immunological aspects. In: Milner R D G, Flodh H (eds) Immunological aspects of human growth hormone. Medical Education Services, Oxford, pp 9–16
46. Phillips J A III, Ferrandez A, Frisch H, Illig R, Zuppinger K 1986 Defects of growth hormone genes: clinical syndromes. In: Raiti S, Tolman R A (eds) Human growth hormone. Plenum Publishing Corporation, New York, ch 11, pp 211–226

Sorbitol

Sorbitol is a natural sugar which is present in a number of berries and fruits. Sorbitol is also used as a precursor of sorbose in the synthesis of vitamin C.

Chemistry

Sorbitol (D-Glucitol)
$C_6H_{14}O_6$

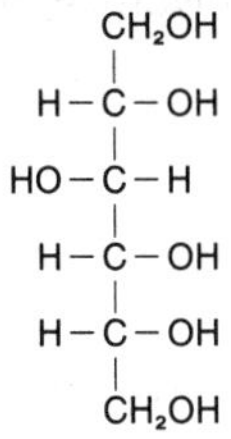

Molecular weight	182.2
pKa	13.7
Solubility	
in alcohol	1 in 25
in water	1 in 0.5
Octanol/water partition coefficient	—

Sorbitol is a white, slightly hygroscopic, odourless, crystalline powder with a sweet taste. A 10% solution has a pH of about 6.7.

Pharmacology

Sorbitol has a sweet taste and is about 60% as sweet as sucrose.

Toxicology

The main interest of sorbitol in animal and human toxicology has concerned the possible role that its formation may play in the neuropathy and vasculopathy of diabetes. The enzyme aldose reductase, which forms sorbitol in vivo, is present in the pericytes of the retinal capillary vasculature and in nerves. Once formed, sorbitol accumulates because it diffuses out of cells extremely slowly and is only very slowly catabolized.

Clinical pharmacology

The data available are limited. In three normal volunteers who received an intravenous bolus of 3.25 g 30% sorbitol over 3 minutes, injection was followed by severe epigastric pain, tachycardia, nausea and faintness lasting 15–20 minutes.[1]

Pharmacokinetics

Sorbitol concentrations in biological fluids can be measured by a microcolorimetric method.[2]

Data in humans relating to bolus administration are limited. The mean loss of sorbitol in the urine in normal adults after a five-hour infusion of 500 ml 30% sorbitol was 13.8 g $\pm$9.3 S.D. or 9.1% $\pm$6.2 S.D.).[1]

About 3% of an ingested dose of 35 g appears in the urine and at least 75% is metabolized to carbon dioxide.[3]

Oral absorption	slower than glucose
Presystemic metabolism	—
Plasma half life	20.3 min
Volume of distribution	—
Plasma protein binding	—

Concentration–effect relationship

No data are available.

Metabolism[1,4]

Sorbitol is converted, mainly by a hepatic polyol dehydrogenase, to fructose before further metabolism. Its metabolism then is as for fructose and for most tissues utilization is dependent upon its further conversion to glucose. In rats more than 85% of ^{14}C-sorbitol is converted to ^{14}C-glucose within 30 minutes of injection and this conversion is independent of insulin. Subsequent handling of the glucose is insulin-dependent. 1 g yields 3.994 kcal (16.72 kJ).

Pharmaceutics

Sorbitol solutions (30%) are available for parenteral feeding:

1. Sorbitol infusion BP
2. Sorbitol (EGIC, France).

It is present in combination with amino acids and electrolytes in some solutions available for parenteral nutrition containing amino acids:

3. Synthamin 7s (Travenol, UK): 150 g.l^{-1}
4. Aminofusin (Merck, UK): L600 100 g.l^{-1}; L1000 100 g.l^{-1} with ethanol 5%
5. Aminoplex 5 (Geistlich, UK): 125 g per litre with ethanol 5%.

Solutions are sterilized by autoclaving and are incompatible with oxidizing agents.

Therapeutic use

Indications

1. As an energy source in parenteral nutrition.

Contraindications

1. Liver failure
2. Renal failure
3. Inborn errors of metabolism affecting fructose metabolism.

Mode of use

Fructose and sorbitol infusion produce lower blood sugar levels and less hyperinsulinaemia than isocaloric glucose infusion. There is insufficient information to decide whether the nitrogen-sparing effect is different for these three carbohydrates.[5] As insulin has been proposed as a major cause of the sodium retention seen after glucose feeding[6] it might be thought that fructose (or sorbitol) could avoid such an effect. However, studies using oral glucose and fructose do not suggest any difference between the sugars in their antinatriuretic effect.[7]

Contraindications

1. In liver failure

As would be expected from the hepatic conversion of sorbitol to fructose, there is poor utilization of sorbitol in liver failure. Urinary losses of sorbitol during infusions of 0.5 g.min^{-1} were 16%, which is nearly twice normal.[1] Similarly, serum levels at the end of a five-hour infusion at the same rate were 17.58 µg.l^{-1} compared with 8.9 µg.l^{-1} in normals.[1]

2. Renal failure

Very variable peak concentrations were noted following infusions of sorbitol in patients with renal failure, though impairment of clearance was not directly related to the degree of renal impairment and could be slight even in anuric patients.[1]

S

3. **Inborn errors of fructose metabolism**
As sorbitol is mainly converted to fructose before further metabolism, deficiencies in fructose metabolism will also cause serious problems with sorbitol administration. These include hereditary fructose intolerance caused by lack of fructose biphosphate aldolase, essential fructosuria and fructose-1,6-diphosphatase deficiency.

Adverse reactions

See Fructose.

High risk groups

In the absence of adequate studies, using sorbitol as an energy source in neonates, children, pregnant and nursing mothers and the elderly cannot be recommended.

References

1. Lee H A, Morgan A G, Waldram R, Bennett J 1972 Sorbitol: some aspects of its metabolism and role as an intravenous nutrient. In: Wilkinson A W (ed) Parenteral nutrition. Churchill Livingstone, Edinburgh, pp 121–137
2. Bailey J M 1959 A microcolourimetric method for the determination of sorbitol, mannitol and glycerol in biologic fluids. Journal of Laboratory and Clinical Medicine 54: 158
3. Sorbitol for parenteral use. Martindale 28th edn, pp 59–60
4. Froesch E R, Keller U 1972 Review of energy metabolism with particular reference to the metabolism of glucose, fructose, sorbitol and xylitol and of their therapeutic use in parenteral nutrition. In: Wilkinson A W (ed) Parenteral nutrition. Churchill Livingstone, Edinburgh, pp 105–120
5. Hessov I 1981 Intravenous administration of glucose and fructose in the uncomplicated postoperative period. Danish Medical Bulletin 28: 45–63
6. Gozansky D M, Herman R H 1971 Water and sodium retention in the fasted and refed human. American Journal of Clinical Nutrition 24: 869–871
7. Rebello T, Hodges R E, Smith J L 1983 Short term effects of various sugars on antinatriuresis and blood pressure changes in normotensive young men. American Journal of Clinical Nutrition 38: 89–94

Sotalol

Sotalol, first described in 1965, is an adrenergic β-receptor blocking agent which also has Class III antiarrhythmic properties. Its antiarrhythmic properties are the main focus of current therapeutic interest.

Chemistry

Sotalol hydrochloride (Sotacor, Beta-Cardone)
$C_{12}H_{20}N_2O_3S.HCl$
4'-(2-Isopropylaminoethyl-1-hydroxy) methanesulphonanilide hydrochloride

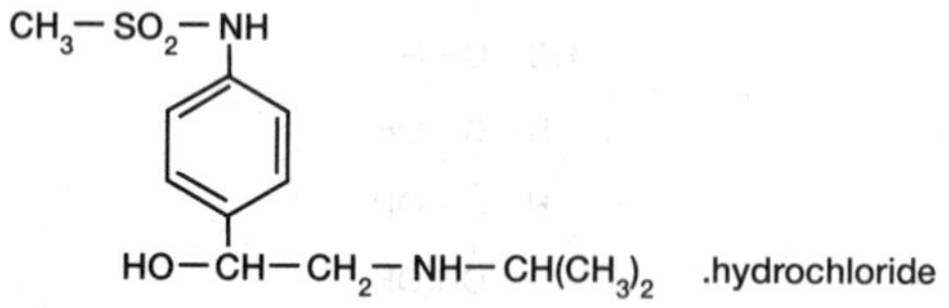

Molecular weight (free base)	308.8 (272.4)
pKa (sulphonamide, aminogroup)	8.3 9.8
Solubility	
in alcohol	insoluble
in water	freely soluble
Octanol/water partition coefficient	0.79

Sotalol hydrochloride is prepared chemically and is a racemic mixture of d- and l-sotalol, which is an off-white solid. The drug may also be combined with hydrochlorothiazide 25 mg (Sotazide, Tolerzide).

Pharmacology

Sotalol is a β-adrenoceptor blocking drug with about one third the β-blocking potency of propanolol. The β blocking property resides in the l isomer. Sotalol is devoid of intrinsic sympathomimetic activity, is not cardioselective and also lacks membrane-stabilizing properties. Unlike other β-adrenergic blocking drugs sotalol prolongs the duration of the myocardial action potential and the QT interval, effects that indicate class III antiarrhythmic properties in the Vaughan Williams classification.[1]. The class III action depends upon lengthening of repolarization due to prolongation of the slow outward potassium current. This activity is present in the d and l isomers.

There has been debate about the relative importance of the β adrenergic blocking action and the class III action in the antiarrhythmic effect in various experimental situations. In the anaesthetised dog concentrations of 0.8 $mg.l^{-1}$ were associated with a half-maximal β-blocking action but concentrations of 6.8 $mg.l^{-1}$ were required for half-maximal effects upon ventricular refractoriness[2]. In a study of changes in ventricular fibrillation threshold with d- and dl-sotalol in acutely ischaemic cat hearts, d-sotalol was much less effective than the (β-blocking) racemate[3] in preventing ventricular fibrillation. These results suggest that the class III action is only likely to be prominent at high doses and β-blocking activity is predominant with lower doses. There is evidence of an 'use dependent' action in prolongation of the refractory period in isolated papillary muscles. At slow driving rates sotalol produced a more marked prolongation of the action potential than at higher rates[4]. Class III agents may confer some protection to mitochondria against experimental ischaemic damage[5]. Like many antiarrhythmic drugs, sotalol also has a proarrhythmic action. In conscious dogs with complete A-V block, a model of torsades de pointe (polymorphic ventricular tachycardia), a

4.5 mg bolus of sotalol or infusion of 1.5 $mg.kg^{-1}.h^{-1}$ provoked torsades in 5 of 8 animals.[6]

Toxicology

Sotalol, like propanolol, lacks carcinogenicity in both mice and rats.[7] Animal tests have shown no evidence of teratogenicity.

Clinical pharmacology

These effects are dominated by the β-blocking actions of the drug on the one hand and by its ability to prolong the action potential of myocardial cells on the other.

Administration of oral doses of 40–320 mg in man is accompanied by a reduction in heart rate and cardiac output as well as an increase in systemic vascular resistance.[8]

Sotalol decreases the rise in heart rate on exercise and maximal exercise tolerance in normal individuals is reduced. In patients with angina, exercise tolerance is increased due to a reduction in total myocardial oxygen consumption. Sotalol lowers blood pressure in both the lying and standing positions although the exact mechanism for this effect is still debated. Sotalol reduces cardiac output and while this effect is probably not the cause of the fall in blood pressure, it can precipitate heart failure in some patients with severly impaired ventricular function or valvar incompetence.

Sotalol blocks the action of adrenaline on β-adrenoceptors and the unopposed α effect can produce a large rise in blood pressure. Airways resistance is increased by sotalol and this may be dangerous in patients with chronic bronchitis, or with a history of asthma. Many of the somatic manifestations of hyperthyroidism-increased heart rate, irritability and tremor are improved by β-blockers, such as sotalol and the relief from anxiety induced by sotalol has been used successfully in the relief of short-term stressful situations, such as examinations and solo instrument playing.

These findings refer to the administration of dl-sotalol; d-sotalol has the same electrophysiological action but is devoid of β-blocking effect[9]. The electrophysiological properties include lengthening of the PR and AH intervals, prolongation of the refractory periods of the atrium, atrioventricular node and ventricle, with prolongation of the QT interval, and also prolongation of accessory pathway refractoriness.[10]

Several studies have addressed the question of the dose and plasma concentration required to produce β-adrenergic blockade compared with that required to produce prolongation of the QT interval. These show that plasma concentrations of about 0.8 $\mu g.l^{-1}$ produce substantial β-blockade but concentrations in the range 2.6 $\mu g.l^{-1}$ are required for the class III effects[11]. These findings, which are in broad agreement with animal studies, suggest that substantially higher doses are needed to produce the class III effects than those producing a substantial degree of β-blockade in man.

Pharmacokinetics

Sotalol can be measured in plasma by HPLC[12] which has a limit of detection of 20 $\mu g.l^{-1}$.

Sotalol is completely absorbed after oral administration and has an absolute bioavailability of 100%. First-pass hepatic metabolism and metabolic destruction are negligible.[13] The time to maximum plasma concentration is 2–3 h and, although the absorption of the drug is not significantly affected by antacids[14] it may be reduced by food, especially milk. The volume of distribution is about 1–2 $l.kg^{-1}$ and protein binding is negligible. Unlike other β-blocking agents sotalol is excreted mostly unchanged in the urine and this takes place by glomerular filtration. The terminal elimination half life ranges from 7–18 h. The elimination half life increases in the elderly[15] and, predictably, in renal failure.[16] Elimination half life and bioavailability remain unchanged in pregnancy.[17] Some sotalol is excreted in breast milk[18]

Oral absorption	100%
Presystemic metabolism	nil
Plasma half life	
range	7–18 h
Volume of distribution	1–2 $l.kg^{-1}$
Plasma protein binding	—

Concentration–effect relationship

The degree of β-blockade is correlated with the plasma concentration of sotalol, but as with most β-adrenoceptor antagonists there is no clear relationship in the case of hypotensive effect. There is no indication for therapeutic drug monitoring. Plasma concentrations have been correlated with the different pharmacological actions and 0.8 $\mu g.l^{-1}$ appears sufficient to produce substantial β-adrenergic blockade but concentrations 3 to 5 times higher are required to invoke the class III effect.[11]

Metabolism

Sotalol is excreted in the urine without undergoing metabolism.

Pharmaceutics

Sotalol is available in oral and parenteral forms. Sotacor tablets (Bristol Myers, Squibb UK) are both 80 mg (pink) and 160 mg tablets (blue). Beta-Cardone (Duncan Fockhart, UK) is available in 40 mg, 80 mg and 200 mg tablets. Sotazide blue contains 160 mg of sotalol hydrochloride and 25 mg of hydrochlorothiazide. Tolerzide contains 80 mg sotalol hydrochloride and 12.5 mg hydrochlorothiazide (lilac).

The intravenous preparation of sotalol hydrochloride (Sotacor) is available in 2 strengths, 2 $mg.ml^{-1}$ in 5 ml ampoules or 10 $mg.ml^{-1}$ in 10 ml ampoules, the latter available on special order.

The tablets should be protected from light.

Therapeutic use

Indications

1. Cardiac arrhythmias
2. Hypertension
3. Ischaemic heart disease
4. Adjunctive therapy in thyrotoxicosis
5. Post-myocardial infarction.

Contraindications

1. Atrioventricular block
2. Cardiac failure
3. History of bronchospasm
4. Diabetic ketoacidosis, metabolic acidosis.

Mode of use

Sotalol tablets may, when given orally, be administered either in single or divided doses. Oral treatment is often begun with 80 mg twice daily but may commence with 160 mg daily. Doses of 400–600 mg daily may be used in the treatment of both hypertension and angina although slightly lower doses are usually successful in the treatment of thyrotoxicosis (120-240 mg daily in single or divided doses). In clinical studies doses of up to 960 mg daily have been used. The usual dosage for hypertension is 160–320 mg daily and for angina 160 mg daily.

Sotacor injection should be given over 2–3 minutes in doses of 20–60 mg intravenously. Larger doses may be given but should be injected over longer periods of time and continuous electrocardiographic monitoring is recommended during injection. Sotalol is propably safer than more lipid-soluble β-blockers when given by the intravenous route because it has no membrane stabilising effects.

Indications

1. Cardiac arrhythmias

Interest in this use has been fueled by the disappointing results with class I anti-arrhythmics in the CAST study and the desire to match the efficacy of amiodarone with a less toxic alternative. Because of its Class III electrophysiological actions, as well as its potent β-adrenoceptor blocking actions, sotalol is effective in the treatment of a wide spectrum of arrhythmias, both supraventricular and ventricular.

Atrial fibrillation. In patients with atrial flutter and fibrillation the drug may bring about conversion to sinus rhythm but, even if this is not achieved, it may allow better control of the ventricular response. In one study[19] 83% of patients with either reentrant or ectopic supraventricular tachycardias were converted to sinus rhythm

S

following the injection of 20 mg of intravenous sotalol. In a recent study, 109 patients with atrial fibrillation or flutter who had failed to respond to one or more other drugs were treated with propafenone and subsequently with sotalol. Maintenance doses of sotalol ranged from 160 to 960 mg daily. The cumulative proportion successfully treated with sotalol was 55%[20]. In the treatment of supraventricular tachycardia, sotalol may be more effective than other β-blocking agents.[21] In a comparison with amiodarone both drugs stopped some arrhythmias by blockade at the AV node and were of similar efficacy[22]

Ventricular arrhythmias. Sotalol has been shown to be effective for the suppression of chronic ventricular extrasystoles and the prevention of inducible ventricular tachycardia. Oral sotalol in daily doses of 160–480 mg was used successfully in the treatment of patients with serious ventricular arrhythmias including ventricular tachycardia and fibrillation.[23] In a comparison with propranolol in patients with chronic symptomatic ventricular arrhythmias sotalol was more effective in suppression of extrasystoles (65%) than propranolol (44%) but this difference did not achieve statistical significance[24]. In patients with complex ventricular arrhythmias only 10% responded to placebo, 75% to sotalol 320 mg daily and 88% to sotalol 640 mg daily[25–27]. At these high doses class III effects may have been important. A comparison of intravenous (mean dose 150 mg) and oral sotalol (mean dose 583 mg) in 16 patients undergoing electrophysiologic study for sustained ventricular tachycardia confirmed this view. β-blocking effects included prolongation of sinus cycle length and AH interval. The drug, by both routes of administration, also prolonged repolarization and refractoriness with significant increase in the QT interval (from a mean of 338 ms to 417–450 ms)[28].

2. Hypertension
Sotalol has been shown to be effective in the management of hypertension in a number of studies both alone[29] and in combination with hydrochlorothiazide.[30] Both systolic and diastolic blood pressures are reduced but the degree of reduction may be variable and may be further enhanced by an increase in dose. Although apparently effective, sotalol has never enjoyed wide use for this indication.

Sotalol has also been shown to be effective as a hypotensive agent in pregnancy but in common with other β-adrenergic blocking drugs it may cause foetal bradycardia[31].

3. Ischaemic heart disease
Sotalol has been shown to have been of use in reducing the number of episodes of chest pain in patients with chronic stable angina pectoris.[32] In the long term, sotalol has been given for the treatment of ischaemic heart disease.[33]

4. Thyrotoxicosis
Sotalol has also been shown to be of use in the management of thyrotoxicosis to control tachycardia and tremor before antithyroid therapy takes effect. The values of free thyroxine and tri-iodothyronine did not change in the serum.[35]

5. Post-myocardial infarction
In a group of patients surviving acute myocardial infarction, sotalol 320 mg once daily was compared with placebo using 12 month mortality and reinfarction rates as end points.[34] Although the 12 month mortality rate in the sotalol group was lower than in the placebo group this difference was not statistically significant. However, there was a greater than 40% reduction in the reinfarction rate in the patients treated with sotalol. The mechanism of this action is uncertain.

Adverse reactions

Potentially life-threatening effects
Because of its ability to prolong the QT interval, sotalol has been associated with the appearance of polymorphic ventricular tachycardia[36] and even ventricular fibrillation. There has been some discussion of whether a uniform drug-induced prolongation of the QT interval is less hazardous than a more dispersed prolongation in patients with severe heart disease[37] but the risk of torsades de pointe is real, if small.

Acute overdosage
A number of cases of sotalol poisoning have been described in the literature. Prichard et al[38] reviewed 13 such patients. One died after taking 3.2 g and 8 recovered after doses ranging from 2.4 to 16 g. The patient who took 2.4 g had a serum sotalol concentration of 16.8 μg.l^{-1} 13 h after ingestion and another patient, who took 8 g, had a serum concentration of 7.5 μg.l^{-1} 22 h after the dose.

Sotalol overdosage has features in common with poisoning from other β-blockers but some features of its own. The former include bradycardia, hypotension and cardiac failure. The latter include cardiac arrhythmias related to the prolongation of repolarization such as torsades de pointe and ventricular fibrillation[39].

Severe bradycardia should be treated with atropine, 0.5 mg, given intravenously as one or two bolus doses. Glucagon may be a useful cardiac stimulant. The initial doses should be 5 to 10 mg intravenously in dextrose or saline followed by infusion of 4 mg.h^{-1}, increasing the dose as necessary to maintain the cardiac output. Isoprenaline infusion may also be useful but the dose required is high and difficult to predict. A dose of 4 μg.min^{-1} intravenously, increasing the speed of infusion every 1 to 3 minutes until a heart rate response occurs, can be used.

Cardiac arrhythmias can be difficult to treat. Electrical defibrillation and/or use of intravenous lignocaine should be tried.

Severe or irreversible effects
There are rare reports of retroperitoneal fibrosis associated with use of the drug but a causal relationship has not been established[40]

Sotalol may reduce or mask the warning signs attendant upon hypoglycaemia. Prior to surgery, withdrawal of the drug if thought necessary should be undertaken over a period of a week because of the possible effect of rebound angina, arrhythmias or possibly even myocardial infarction. Caution is advised in the use of anaesthetic agents such as ether, cyclopropane etc in patients receiving sotalol.

Symptomatic adverse effects
The incidence of adverse effects due to β-blockade is similar to that of other β-blocking agents. At the recommended dosage levels, however, nausea, insomnia, lassitude and diarrhoea may be seen, which are often transient and will usually remit on reduction of the dose or, if necessary, on cessation of therapy.

Other effects
Although some studies have shown alterations in plasma lipid profile[41] this has not been found by others even after long-term treatment.[42]

Interference with clinical pathology tests
No technical interferences of this kind appear to have been reported.

High risk groups

Neonates
The drug is not used in neonates.

Breast milk. The drug enters breast milk, and mothers taking the drug should not breast feed.

Children
Sotalol is not intended for administration to children.

Pregnant women
Although sotalol is effective as a hypotensive agent in pregnancy[14] it crosses the placental barrier and does not offer any advantage, therefore, over other hypotensive agents in this respect. Although there is no evidence of teratogenicity, the drug should be used only when absolutely necessary. Foetal bradycardia may occur.

The elderly
Since the serum concentrations of the drug are greater, a more marked action for a given dose may be seen.

Drug interactions

Potentially hazardous interactions
Anaesthetic agents. General anaesthetics, e.g. ether, cyclopropane, trichloroethylene, methoxyflurane and enflurane) may cause impaired myocardial contractility in the presence of β-adrenoceptor blocking agents. Caution is, therefore, necessary when the use of these drugs is being considered.

Other drugs. In view of the reported cases of torsades de pointe (polymorphic ventricular tachycardia) patients treated concomitantly with drugs known to be associated with this arrhythmia should be observed closely. This includes treatment with antidepressant agents, Class 1 antiarrhythmic agents such as quinidine.

Other significant interactions

Food. Food, especially milk, has been reported to reduce the bioavailability of sotalol.[14]

Potentially useful interactions

The drug may be given in combination with a thiazide for treatment of hypertension.

Major outcome trials

1. Astrom M, Edhag O, Nyquist O, Vallin H 1990 Electrophysiological effects of intravenous sotalol in acute myocardial infarction: a double-blind placebo-controlled study. European Heart Journal 11: 35–42

20 patients recovering from acute myocardial infarction were randomised to sotalolol or placebo infusion for 12 hours. Programmed electrical stimulation was performed from the right atrium. The A-V nodal effective refractory period was prolonged by 15% and the QT interval by 10% by the sotalol infusion.

2. Amiodarone vs Sotalol Study Group 1989 Multicentre randomized trial of sotalol vs amiodarone for chronic malignant ventricular tachyarrhythmias. European Heart Journal 10: 685–694

This was an open, randomized study in patients with ventricular tachycardia or fibrillation not associated with acute myocardial infarction. 16 of 30 patients allocated to amiodarone completed 12 months on therapy. Five were withdrawn because of ventricular tachycardia and 9 because of adverse reactions or protocol violations, of whom 4 died. 16 of 29 patients in the sotalol group completed 12 months treatment. One was with withdrawn because of ventricular tachycardia and 9 because of adverse effects or protocol violations. Three died while on treatment and two after it was withdrawn. There was no significant difference between the results on the two drugs.

3. Cobbe S M, Alexopoulos D, Winner S J, McCaie C P, Cobbe P C, Johnston J 1988 A comparison of the long term effects of sotalol and atenolol on QT interval and arrhythmias after myocardial infarction. European Heart Journal 9: 24–31

This was a double-blind crossover study in 103 patients followed for a year after they had suffered an acute myocardial infarction. Patients received either atenolol 50 mg twice daily or sotalol 160 mg twice daily Sotalol increased the QT interval by a mean of 43 ms (9%). Marked lengthening of the QTc (>500 ms) was observed on 29 occasions in sotalol treated patients, but no episode of polymorphic ventricular tachycardia occurred. Overall there was no significant difference in the frequency of arrhythmias recorded on ambulatory monitoring.

General review articles

Singh B N, Deedewania P, Nademanee K, Ward A, Sorkin E M 1987 Sotalol: a review of its pharmacodynamic and pharmacokinetic properties and therapeutic use. Drugs 34: 311–349

Singh B N 1990 Expanding clinical role of unique class III antiarrhythmic effects of sotalol. American Journal of Cardiology 65: 84A–88A

Kehoe R F, Zheutlin T A, Dunnington C S, Mattioni T A, Yu G 1990 Safety and efficacy of sotalol in patients with drug refractory sustained ventricular tachyarrhythmias. American Journal of Cardiology 65: 58A–64A

References

1. Vaughan Williams E M 1980 Antiarrhythmic action and the puzzle of perhexiline. Academic Press, London, pp 1–35
2. Nattel S, Feder Elituv R, Matthews C, Nayebpour M, Talajic M 1989 Concentration dependence of class III and beta adrenergic blocking effects of sotalol in anesthetized dogs. Journal of the American College of Cardiology 13: 1190–1194
3. Kwan Y W, Solca A M, Gwilt M, Kane K A, Wadsworth R M 1990 Comparative antifibrillatory effects of d and dl sotalol in normal and ischaemic ventricular muscle of the cat. Journal of Cardiovascular Pharmacology 15: 233–285

4. Hafner D, Berger F, Borchard U, Kullmann A, Scherlitz A 1988 Electrophysiological characterization of the class III activity of sotalol and its enantiomers. New interpretation of use dependent effects. Arzneimittelforschung 38: 231–236
5. Sano T, Sugiyama S, Taki K, Hanaki Y, Shimada Y, Ozawa T 1990 Effects of antiarrhythmic agents classified as class III group on ischaemia-induced myocardial damage in canine hearts. British Journal of Pharmacology 99: 577–581
6. Davy J M, Weissenburger J, Ertzbischoff O et al 1988 Torsades de pointe experimentales avec le sotalol chez le chien vigile en bloc auriculo ventriculaire. Role de l'hypokaliemie. Archives de Maladies du Coeur 81: 1117–1124
7. Weikal J H, Kelly W A 1979 Tumorgenicity assays of sotalol hydrochloride in rats and mice. Journal of Clinical Pharmacology 19: 591–604
8. Hutton I, Lorimer A R, Hillis W S, McCall D, Reid J M, Lawrie T D V 1972 Haemodynamics and myocardial function after sotalol. British Heart Journal 34: 787–790
9. Nathan A W, Hellestrand K J, Bexton R S, Ward D E, Spurrell R A J, Camm A J 1982 Electrophysiological effects of sotalol — just another β-blocker? British Heart Journal 47: 575-207
10. Rowland E 1985 Clinical electrophysiological effects of D-sotalol — a new class 3 antiarrhythmic drug. Journal of the American College of Cardiology 5: 498
11. Woosley R L, Barbey J T, Wang T, Funck Brentano C 1990 Concentration/response relations for the multiple antiarrhythmic actions of sotalol. American Journal of Cardiology 65: 22A–27A
12. Lefevre et al 1980 Journal of Pharmacological Science 69: 1216–1217
13. Anttila A, Arstila M, Pfeffer M, Tikkanen R, Vallinkoski V, Sundquist H 1976 Human pharmacokinetics of sotalol. Acta Pharmacologica et Toxicologica 39: 118–128
14. Kahela P, Anttila M, Tikkanen R, Sundquist H 1979 Effects of food and food constituents and fluid volume on the bioavailability of sotalol. Acta Pharmacologica et Toxicologica 44: 7–12
15. Ishizaki T, Hirayama H, Tawara K, Nakaya H, Sato M, Sato K 1980 Pharmacokinetics and pharmacodynamics in young, normal and elderly hypertensive subjects: a study using sotalol as a model drug. Journal of Pharmacology and Experimental Therapeutics 212: 173–181
16. Blair A D, Burgess E D, Maxwell B M, Cutler R E 1981 Sotalol kinetics in renal insufficiency. Clinical Pharmacology and Therapeutics 29: 457–463
17. O'Hare M F, Leahey W, Murnaghan G A, McDevitt D G 1983 Pharmacokinetics of sotalol during pregnancy. European Journal of Clinical Pharmacology 24: 521–524
18. Hackett L P, Wojnar Horton R E, Dusci L J, Ilett K F, Roberts M J 1990 Excretion of sotalol in breast milk. British Journal of Clinical Pharmacology 29: 277–278
19. Fogelman F, Lightman S L, Sillett R W, McNicol M W 1972 The treatment of cardiac arrhythmias with sotalol. European Journal of Clinical Pharmacology 5: 72
20. Antman E M, Beamer A D, Cantillon C, McGowan N, Friedman P L 1990 Therapy of refractory symptomatic atrial fibrillation and atrial flutter: a staged care approach with new antiarrhythmic drugs. Journal of the American College of Cardiology 15: 698–707
21. Schofield P M, Reid F, Bennett D H 1987 A comparison of atenolol and sotalol in the treatment of patients with paroxysmal supraventricular tachycardia. British Heart Journal 57: 105
22. Waleffe A, Nzayinambaho K, Rodriguez L M, Dehareng A, Kulbertus H E 1989 Mechanisms of termination of supraventricular tachycardias by intravenous class III antiarrhythmic agents. A comparison of amiodarone and sotalol. European Heart Journal 10: 1084–1089
23. Steinbeck G, Back P, Haberl R 1986 Electrophysiologic and antiarrhythmic efficacy of oral sotalol for sustained ventricular tachyarrhythmias: evaluation by programmed stimulation and ambulatory electrocardiogram. Journal of the American College of Cardiology 8: 949–958
24. Kubac G, Klinke W P, Grace M 1988 Randomized double-blind trial comparing sotalol and propranolol in chronic ventricular arrhythmia. Canadian Journal of Cardiology 4: 355–921
25. Kuchar D L, Garan H, Venditti F J et al 1989 Usefulness of sotalol in suppressing ventricular tachycardia or ventricular fibrillation in patients with healed myocardial infarcts. American Journal of Cardiology 64: 33–36
26. Ruder M A, Ellis T, Lebsack C, Mead R H, Smith N A, Winkle R A 1989 Clinical experience with sotalol in patients with drug refractory ventricular arrhythmias. Journal of the American College of Cardiology 13: 145–152
27. Anderson J L 1190 Effectiveness of sotalol for therapy of complex ventricular arrhythmias and comparisons with with placebo and class 1 antiarrhythmic drugs. American Journal of Cardiology 65: 37A–42A
28. Kopelman H A, Woosley R L, Lee J T, Roden D M, Echt D S 1988 Electrophysiologic effects of intravenous and oral sotalol for sustained ventricular tachycardia secondary to coronary artery disease. American Journal of Cardiology 61: 1006–1011
29. Reynaert J 1979 Sotalol in mild to severe hypertension: twice- and once-daily administration: a long term study. Current Therapeutic Research 26: 799–812
30. Jaattela A 1981 Fixed combination of sotalol and hydrochlorothiazide in the treatment of uncomplicated hypertension. European Journal of Clinical Pharmacology 19: 395–401
31. O'Hare M F, Murnaghan G A, Russell C J, Leahey W J, Varma M P S, McDevitt D G 1980 Sotalol as a hypotensive agent in pregnancy. British Journal of Obstetrics and Gynaecology 87: 814–820
32. Gooding P G, Berman E 1974 An evaluation of sotalol, a beta-blocking agent, in patients with angina pectoris. Postgraduate Medical Journal 50: 736–737
33. Zelasco J F, Milei J, Fortunato M R 1974 Long term sotalol therapy in patients with angina pectoris. Proceedings of advances in adrenergic blocking therapy. Excerpta Medica 2: 47–50
34. Julian D G, Jackson F S, Prescott R J, Szekely P 1982 Controlled trial of sotalol for one year after myocardial infarction. Lancet 1: 1142–1147
35. Wahlberg P, Wennstrom J, Ekelund P 1976 Control of thyrotoxicosis with sotalol. Annals of Clinical Research 8: 415–417

S

36. Kontopoulos A, Filindris A, Manoudis F, Metaxas P 1981 Sotalol-induced torsade de pointes. Postgraduate Medical Journal 51: 321–323
37. Day C P, McComb J M, Campbell R W 1990 QT dispersion: an indication of arrhythmia risk in patients with long QT intervals. British Heart Journal 63: 342–344
38. Prichard B N C, Battersby L A, Cruickshank J M 1984 Overdosage with beta adrenergic blocking agents. Adverse Drug Reactions and Poisoning Review 3: 91–108
39. Elonen E, Neuvonen P J, Tarssanen L, Kala R 1979 Sotalol intoxication with prolonged QT Interval and severe tachyarrhythmias. British Medical Journal 1: 1184
40. Laakso M, Arvala I, Tervonen S, Sotarauta M 1982 Retroperitoneal fibrosis associated with sotalol. British Medical Journal 285: 1085–1086
41. Lehtonen A, Viikari J 1979 Long-term effect of sotalol on plasma lipids. Clinical Science 57: 405s–407s
42. Northcote R J, Packard C J, Ballantyne D 1986 The effect of sotalol on plasma lipoproteins and apolipoproteins. Clinica Chimica Acta 158: 187–192

Spectinomycin (hydrochloride)

Spectinomycin is an aminocyclitol antibiotic acting upon bacterial protein synthesis. It is used primarily for the treatment of anogenital gonococcal infection.

Chemistry

Spectinomycin, dihydrochloride pentahydrate (Trobicin)
$C_{14}H_{24}N_2O_7.2HCl.5H_2O$
(2R,4a,R,5aR,6S,7S,8R,9S,paR,10aS)-Decahydro-4a,7,9-trihydroxy-2-methyl-6,8-bis-(methylamino)-4H-pyrano[2,3-b][1,4]-benzodioxin-4-one dihydrochloride pentahydrate

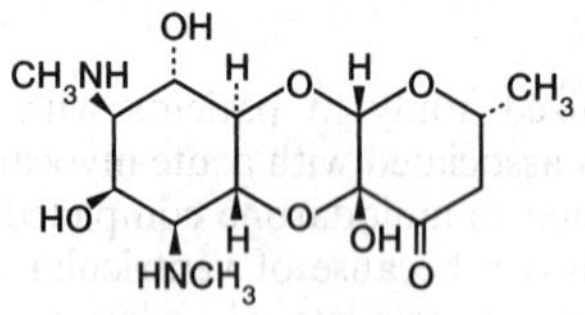

$.2HCl. 5H_2O$

Molecular weight (free base)	495.4 (332.4)
pKa	6.88, 8.84
Solubility	
in alcohol	<1 in 10 000
in water	>1 in 10
Octanol/water partition coefficient	low

A white to pale buff crystalline powder with slight, characteristic odour and taste.

Pharmacology

Spectinomycin is a bacteriostatic antibiotic derived from *Streptomyces spectabilis.* It inhibits protein synthesis in susceptible microorganisms by binding to and acting on the 30S ribosomal subunit. Its mode of action is similar to that of the aminoglycoside antibiotics but spectinomycin is not bactericidal and misreading of the genetic code due to incorrect codon–anticodon interaction does not occur. The movement of peptidyl-tRNA associated with translocation is inhibited and the osmotic integrity of the bacterial cell is impaired.

Toxicology

The acute LD_{50} for mice is 5724 mg.kg^{-1} and for rats 7500 mg.kg^{-1}, both given intraperitoneally. There is no evidence of carcinogenicity or mutagenicity, or of teratological effects in rats. No ototoxicity has been observed in animals.

Clinical pharmacology

Spectinomycin is inferior as an antibiotic to many other drugs to which the susceptible organisms are sensitive. Spectinomycin is effective against *Neisseria gonorrhoeae* in vitro and in vivo.[1] Gonococci are inhibited by concentrations of 8–32 mg.l^{-1} which are readily obtained in man. The antibiotic has no other clinically useful effects. It has minor effects on the central nervous system which lead to dizziness and fever in some patients, and occasional nausea may result from gastric irritation.

Resistance

In vitro studies show no cross-resistance between spectinomycin and other antibiotics in the treatment of gonorrhoea (e.g. penicillin and

Spectinomycin (hydrochloride)

cephalosporins). Resistance does develop to spectinomycin in the *N. gonorrhoeae* population[9,10] and minimum inhibitory concentrations (MICs) may be 500 mg.l^{-1}. Resistance develops from mutation at the SPC locus on the chromosome, leading to structural changes in the 30S ribosomal subunit. No spectinomycin inactivating enzymes have been described in *N. gonorrhoeae* as occurs with *E. coli.*[11]

Pharmacokinetics

Spectinomycin can be assayed either by a microbiological plate assay using *Escherichia coli* UC 527 as test organism and *Streptomycin* Assay Agar with Yeast Extract (BBL) (2) or by a radioenzymatic assay.[2] The sensitivity of the bioassay is 1 mg.l^{-1}.

Spectinomycin is poorly absorbed when given orally. It is rapidly absorbed after intramuscular injection, with peak serum concentrations achieved 1 h after injection of 2 g and 2 h after a 4 g dose. The mean half life for loss of bioactivity from the serum is 1.9 h, with a range from 1.25 to 2.8 h.

Following a 2 g intramuscular dose the C_{max} is approximately 103 mg.l^{-1} with a concentration of 15 mg.l^{-1} at 8 h. Corresponding figures for a dose of 4 g are C_{max} at 2 h, 160 mg.l^{-1}; concentrations at 8 h, 31 mg.l^{-1}.

The volume of distribution of spectinomycin ranges[3,4] between 10.0 and 13.4 l.kg^{-1}. There is no significant binding to plasma proteins and it is not metabolized. Between 80 and 100% is excreted in the urine within 48 h of administration in a biologically active form. Spectinomycin penetrates genital tract tissues.[5] However, penetration of ocular tissues is poor and spectinomycin does not appear to reach the CSF in man, although it does cross inflamed meninges in the rabbit.[6] Spectinomycin crosses the placental barrier. There are no human data on its excretion in milk although there is limited accumulation in cows and ewes consistent with its low lipid solubility.

Excretion is entirely via the kidney. In patients with significant renal impairment the half life ranged from 4.7 to 29.3 h after a 2 g intravenous dose.[7] There are no data on the influence of hepatic damage on elimination of spectinomycin, but this is unlikely to be of any significance. Some delay in elimination is likely in the elderly with decreased renal function.

Since spectinomycin is used almost exclusively as single-dose therapy for gonorrhoea, the importance of any impairment of excretion is minor.

Oral absorption	poor
Presystemic metabolism	nil
Plasma half life	
range	1.2–2.8 h
mean	1.93
Volume of distribution	10.0–13.4 l
Plasma protein binding	< 10%

Concentration–effect relationship

Spectinomycin is active against most strains of *N. gonorrhoeae*, with minimum inhibitory concentrations (MICs) ranging from < 8 mg.l^{-1} to 32 mg.l^{-1}, well below the serum concentration seen after a single 2 g dose.[8]

Metabolism

Spectinomycin is not metabolized. 70–100% of the administered dose is excreted unchanged in the urine over 48 hours.

Pharmaceutics

Spectinomycin Trobicin (Upjohn, UK/USA) is provided as 2 g sterile powder for injection and is reconstituted with 3.2 ml water for injection with benzyl alcohol 0.945% w/v as preservative. This is for intramuscular injection. A 4 g vial is also available in some countries and this should be reconstituted with 6.2 ml of the same solution. Vials should be shaken vigorously immediately after adding the diluent and again before withdrawing the dose. There is no oral or intravenous preparation. The sterile powder should be stored at 15–30°C. The reconstituted suspension should be stored at the same temperature and used within 24 hours.

Therapeutic use

Indications

1. Acute gonococcal urethritis, proctitis and cervicitis caused by susceptible strains of *N. gonorrhoeae*. Men and women with known exposure to gonorrhoea should be treated on this basis without waiting for specific diagnosis. Spectinomycin is particularly recommended for the treatment of gonorrhoea caused by penicillin-resistant isolates or in areas where the prevalence of such strains is high (> 5%).

Contraindications

1. Gonococcal infection with spectinomycin-resistant strains
2. Pharyngeal gonorrhoea — is ineffective
3. Complicated gonococcal infection, e.g. gonococcaemia, or pelvic inflammatory disease. Not suitable for prolonged therapy.

Mode of use

Single 2 g intramuscular injection. May be repeated once if necessary where the infecting strain is known to be sensitive.

Disadvantages
It is expensive compared to penicillin and causes mild to moderate pain at the injection site. It can mask symptoms of concurrent syphilis against which it is inactive.

It will not cure concurrent chlamydial infection.

Adverse reactions

Potentially life-threatening effects
Rare anaphylactic reactions have been reported.

Acute overdosage
No specific symptoms are known and consequently there is no specific therapy or prevention described. Given the way in which spectinomycin is used, self-administered overdosage would be difficult.

Severe or irreversible adverse effects
None has been described.

Symptomatic adverse effects
Soreness at injection site, urticaria, dizziness, nausea, chills, and fever have been reported during single-dose clinical trials. Reductions in urine output have been noted, but these have been temporary and not extensive. Renal function studies have shown no toxicity.

Interference with clinical pathology tests
Temporary decreases in haematocrit and haemoglobin have been reported as well as in creatinine clearance. Also increases in alkaline phosphatase, BUN and SGPT have been observed in multiple dose tolerance studies in healthy volunteers.

High risk groups

Neonates
Safety for use in neonates has not been established.

Breast milk. No human data on excretion into breast milk are available, so it is probably best for mothers not to breast-feed while taking the drug.

Children
Spectinomycin has been used at a dose of 40 mg.kg^{-1} in children.

Pregnant women
The safety of the drug for mother and fetus has not been established.[7]

The elderly
No special dose requirements are necessary.

Drug interactions

Potentially hazardous interactions
None has been reported.

Other significant interactions
Possible interaction with lithium in a manic depressive patient has been reported; its significance is unclear.

S

Potentially useful interactions
None has been reported.

Major outcome trials

1. Duncan W C, Holder W R, Roberts D P, Knox J M 1972 Treatment of gonorrhoea with spectinomycin hydrochloride — comparison with standard penicillin schedules. Antimicrobial Agents and Chemotherapy 1: 210–214

353 men and 314 women with culture proven gonorrhoea. Single-dose spectinomycin at 2 g and 4 g produced cure rates of >90%. Comparable with standard penicillin therapy.

2. Karney W W, Pedersen A H B, Nelson M et al 1977 Spectinomycin versus tetracycline for treatment of gonorrhoea. New England Journal of Medicine 296: 889

Minimum cure rate of 94% in culture proven anogenital gonorrhoea. Failure to eradicate pharyngeal infection in 6/11 men and 1/13 women.

General review articles

Garrod L P, Lambert H P, O'Grady F 1981 Antibiotic and Chemotherapy, 5th edn. Churchill Livingstone, Edinburgh, ch 24, p 425

Kucers A, Bennett N M 1987 The use of antibiotics. 4th edn. Heinemann, London, pp 971–978

McCormack W M, Finland M 1976 Spectinomycin. Annals of Internal Medicine 84: 712–716

References

1. Davies J, Anderson P, Davis B D 1965 Inhibition of protein synthesis by spectinomycin. Science 149: 1096–1098
2. Kawabe H, Tanaka T, Mitsuhashi S 1978 Streptomycin and spectinomycin resistance mediated by plasmids. Antimicrobial Agents and Chemotherapy 13: 1031–1035
3. Wagner J G, Novak E, Leslie L G, Metzler C M 1967 Absorption, distribution and elimination of spectinomycin dihydrochloride in man. International Journal of Clinical Pharmacology, Therapy and Toxicology 1: 261–285
4. Ksiezyk M, Danek A 1973 Studies on absorption and elimination of drugs. V Fitting of a double exponential curve to the observed concentration after a single IV injection. International Journal of Clinical Pharmacology, Therapy and Toxicology 8: 222–227
5. Elder M G, Bywater M J, Reeves D S 1977 Pelvic tissue and serum concentrations of various antibiotics given as pre-operative medication. British Journal of Obstetrics and Gynaecology 84: 887–893
6. Delgado D G, Brau C J, Avent C K 1980 Penetration of spectinomycin into cerebrospinal fluid during experimental meningitis. Antimicrobial Agents and Chemotherapy 17: 286–287
7. Kusumi R, Metzler C, Fass R 1981 Pharmacokinetics of spectinomycin in volunteers with renal insufficiency. Chemotherapy 27: 95–98
8. Barry J M, Koch R 1963 Actinospectacin serum levels and clinical data. Antimicrobial Agents and Chemotherapy 1962: 538–542
9. Ashford W A, Potts O W, Adams H J U 1981 Spectinomycin resistant penicillinase producing *Neisseria gonorrhoeae*. Lancet 2: 1035–1037
10. Easmon C S F, Ison C A, Bellinger C M, Harris J W 1982 Emergence of resistance after spectinomycin treatment for gonorrhoea due to β-lactamase producing strains of *Neisseria gonorrhoeae*. British Medical Journal 284: 1604–1605
11. Benveniste R, Yamada T, Davies J 1970 Enzymatic adenylylation of streptomycin and spectinomycin by R-factor-resistant *Escherichia coli*. Infection and Immunity 1: 109–119

Spiramycin

Spiramycin is a complex of 16-membered macrolide antibiotics with a spectrum of activity similar to that of erythromycin.

Chemistry

Spiramycin (Rovamycin, Rovamycine, Selectomycin, Sequamycin).
$C_{43}H_{74}N_2O_{14}$ (Spiramycin 1)
$C_{45}H_{76}N_2O_{15}$ (Spiramycin 2)
$C_{46}H_{78}N_2O_{15}$ (Spiramycin 3)
6-[O-2,6-Dideoxy-3-C-methyl-α-L-*ribo*-hexapyranosyl)-(1→4)-(3,6-dideoxy-3-dimethylamino-β-D-glucopyranosyl)-oxy]-7-formylmethyl-4-hydroxy-5-methoxy-9,16-dimethyl-10-[(2,3,4,6-tetradeoxy-4-dimethylamino-D-*erythro*-hexopyranosyl)oxy]-oxacyclohexadeca-11,13-dien-2-one

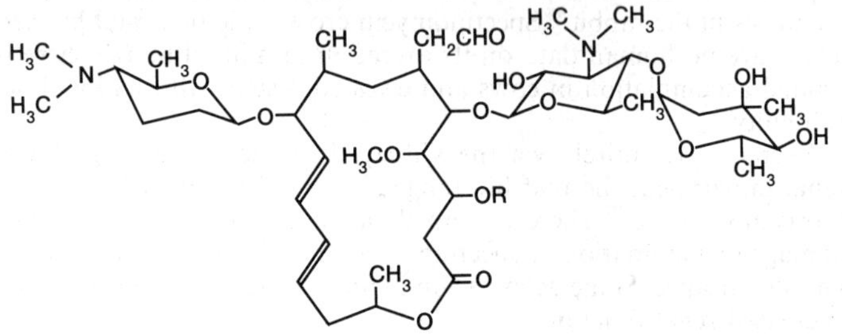

Molecular weight	
Spiramycin 1	843
Spiramycin 2	885
Spiramycin 3	899
pKa [$N(CH_3)_2$]	8.0
Solubility	
in alcohol	>1 in 1
in water	1 in 50
Octanol/water partition coefficient	high

Spiramycin was first isolated in 1954 from cultures of *Streptomyces ambofaciens*.[1] It comprises a mixture of antimicrobial substances, consisting of three closely related compounds: spiramycin 1 (about 63%), spiramycin 2 (about 24%) and spiramycin 3 (about 13%).

Spiramycins 2 and 3 are the corresponding monoacetate ester and monopropionate ester derived from the 4-position of the hexadecadiene ring.

Spiramycin is a white or off-white amorphous powder with a slight odour and a bitter taste. In its dry form spiramycin is stable to light and air. It is produced by the growth of *S. ambofaciens*.

In addition to the base preparation, spiramycin is also available for clinical use as the acetyl derivative, in a combination preparation with metronidazole (Rodogyl) and as the spiramycin salt of difetasarone (Difetasarone-Spiramycin). In veterinary practice spiramycin adipate is used widely.

Pharmacology

The precise mode of action of spiramycin is unknown. Like other macrolide antibiotics spiramycin binds to the 50s subunit of prokaryotic ribosomes and perturbs protein synthesis. It has been postulated that by binding at a site closely related to the peptidyl transferase centre of the ribosome, polypeptide elongation is disrupted.[2] At therapeutic doses spiramycin is bacteriostatic.

Toxicology

Animal studies fail to show any clinically relevant toxicity related to the administration of spiramycin. Mutagenicity has not been shown either in vitro or in vivo and in studies lasting up to two years in rats there is no evidence of carcinogenicity. Spiramycin is neither embryotoxic nor teratogenic when administered in normal doses to pregnant mice, rats and rabbits; however, at high doses in rabbits embryotoxicity may occur — an effect thought to be related to a change in gastrointestinal bacterial flora.

Clinical pharmacology

The only known effect of spiramycin in humans is the antibacterial effect. Spiramycin's spectrum of antimicrobial activity closely resembles that of erythromycin. Although the in vitro activity of spiramycin is 8–32 times less than that of erythromycin, in vivo efficacy of the two drugs is similar.[3,4] Spiramycin, more than any other macrolide, accumulates in the tissues where it persists for long periods and it is this property that is thought to account for its unpredictably good in vivo activity.

Spiramycin is active against almost all streptococci (including *Streptococcus pneumoniae* and most anaerobic strains) but has limited activity against group D streptococci (e.g. *Streptococcus faecalis*). It is active against *Neisseria meningitidis*, *Branhamella catarrhalis*, *Bordetella pertussis*, *Corynebacterium diphtheriae*, *Listeria monocytogenes*, *Bacteroides melaninogenicus*, clostridia, *Legionella pneumophila*, *Chlamydia* and *Mycoplasma pneumoniae* (*Mycoplasma hominis* is resistant); 75% of strains of staphylococci are sensitive. Although most gonococci are sensitive, resistant strains have emerged at a frequency ranging from less than 10%, to 35% in countries where spiramycin has been widely used. Most strains of *Haemophilus* are resistant in vitro (MICs 16–32 mg.l^{-1}) but tissue levels of spiramycin may well be effective. Whilst many anaerobes are sensitive, *B. fragilis* and fusobacteria are not. Aerobic Gram-negative bacilli are resistant. Activity, in vitro[5] and in vivo,[6] has been demonstrated against *Toxoplasma gondii* and there is circumstantial evidence that spiramycin is effective against cryptosporidia.[7] In vitro sensitivities of a number of common organisms are shown in Table 1. MIC breakpoints for spiramycin are 2 and 8 mg.l^{-1}.

Table 1 In vitro activity of spiramycin

Bacteria	MIC (mg.l^{-1})
Streptococcus pyogenes	0.125–1
S. viridans group	0.3–3
S. faecalis	1–5
S. pneumoniae	0.125–0.3
Staphylococcus aureus	<1–>50
S. epidermidis	0.5–4
Neisseria meningitidis	0.3–3
N. gonorrhoea	0.125–8
Hemophilus influenzae	16–32
Escherichia coli	31
Klebsiella pneumoniae	33
Proteus vulgaris	>1500
Pseudomonas aeruginosa	>1500
Bacteroides fragilis	4–16
Peptostreptococcus	0.5–2
Clostridium perfringens	2–8
Legionella pneumophila	1–5
Chlamydia trachomatis	0.5–1
Mycoplasma pneumoniae	0.016–1

Resistance to spiramycin generally develops in parallel with the development of resistance to other macrolide, lincosamide and streptogramin (MLS) antibiotics.[8] Resistance to erythromycin (which has high activity as an inducer of resistance) is not always accompanied by cross-resistance to spiramycin. For example, some staphylococci show varying degrees of resistance to erythromycin but remain sensitive to spiramycin.[9] Two mechanisms of resistance are proposed: target site alteration and antibiotic detoxification.[10] Plasmid-mediated alteration in 23S ribosomal RNA is thought to be the commonest mechanism.

The daily recommended dose in adults is 6–9 MIU daily or 2–3 g daily (1 unit is contained in 0.3125 µg of the 1st International Reference Preparation which contains 3200 U.mg^{-1}). The highest dose known to have been used therapeutically in man is 12 MIU given as a single dose for the treatment of acute gonorrhoea.

Spiramycin

Pharmacokinetics

Spiramycin may be assayed in biological fluids either by microbiological assay[11] or by high pressure liquid chromatography (HPLC).[12] Excellent correlation between these two methods has been shown. The microbiological assay in common use is an agar well diffusion assay with *Sarcina lutea* as the test organism. This method has a sensitivity of 62 µg.l^{-1} compared with 50 µg.l^{-1} for HPLC.

Spiramycin is irregularly absorbed after oral administration, systemic bioavailability varying from 10–60% (mean 39%). Factors responsible for this variation have not been fully determined. Gastric acid appears to have minimal effect on spiramycin; however, recent studies at Rhone-Poulenc show that co-administration with food significantly reduces bioavailability (by 50%) and delays the time to peak concentration (from 4 to 6 hours). Presystemic metabolism has not been reported. Peak serum levels of 1–3 mg.l^{-1} are attained 2–3 hours after an oral dose of 1.5 g and about 2–4 mg.l^{-1} following a 500 mg intravenous infusion.[13] The mean plasma half life of spiramycin is 5 hours with a range of 3–7 hours.

Spiramycin is widely distributed and persists for long periods in many tissues. Its pharmacokinetics are best described by a two-compartment open model with a high volume peripheral compartment. The large volume of distribution (mean 383 l, range 268–516 l) and tissue volume (mean 308 l, range 225–413 l) are indicative of the particularly high tissue affinity of spiramycin.

Concentrations many times those found in serum have been reported in lung, liver, kidney, spleen, prostate, placenta, muscle, bone and tonsillar tissue of man. High levels may persist for as long as 72 hours following a single oral dose. Spiramycin levels have also been measured in a variety of human secretions and high concentrations have been found in bile, saliva, lacrimal fluid and breast milk. Intracellular concentrations in phagocytic cells are markedly elevated over prolonged periods and this is likely to account for the efficacy of spiramycin against a number of intracellular organisms (*Chlamydia*, *Toxoplasma*, *Legionella*).[14] In contrast to the high levels found in most tissues and body fluids, spiramycin does not penetrate into the cerebrospinal fluid. Placental transfer is poor and only 9–16%[15] of the maternal blood concentration appears in the amniotic fluid. Spiramycin binds poorly to serum proteins, only 15% being bound to serum albumin. Spiramycin is extensively biotransformed in the tissues, with only 14% of the dose excreted unchanged in urine. Metabolites are eliminated in both bile and urine. Neither impaired renal nor hepatic function appears to markedly affect the kinetics of spiramycin.

Oral absorption	variable
Presystemic metabolism	—
Plasma half life	
range	3–7 h
mean	5 h
Volume of distribution	383 l
Plasma protein binding	15%

Concentration-effect relationship

The minimum inhibitory concentrations (MICs) for spiramycin against a range of organisms are shown in Table 1.

Metabolism

Spiramycin is eliminated from the body slowly, the majority being inactivated in the tissues. Only 14% (range 5–20%) of the dose is recovered in the urine unchanged. Biliary secretion is thought to be significant but no quantitative data are available. In man, 72 hours after a 2 g oral dose, the biliary concentration is 60 mg.l^{-1}. Enterohepatic circulation may occur but has not been proven. Although pathways of metabolism have not been delineated, the formation of active metabolites appears unlikely. In the rat, spiramycin is not transformed by liver homogenate enzymes.[16]

Pharmaceutics

Until recently spiramycin was only marketed in oral form. Now both oral and parenteral forms are available in some countries.

Oral dosage forms: (Rhone Poulenc, France) include: varnished tablets marketed under the trade name Rovamycin contain 0.75 MIU or 1.5 MIU of spiramycin base; Rovamycin syrup contains 0.375 MIU spiramycin base per 5 ml.

Parenteral dosage forms: a lyophilized injection containing 1.5 MIU of spiramycin has recently been registered. This formulation is for administration by intravenous infusion.

None of the formulations contain potentially allergenic substances.

All preparations are stable in light; however, the syrup and injectable forms must not be stored at high temperature. Tablets have a shelf-life of 4 years, whilst the syrup and injectable form have a shelf-life of 18 months.

Therapeutic use

Indications

1. Infections due to susceptible bacteria
2. Toxoplasmosis in pregnancy
3. Prophylaxis of meningococcal meningitis
4. Cryptosporidial diarrhoea in the immunocompromised host.

Contraindications

1. Known allergy to spiramycin
2. Meningitis.

Mode of use

Oral dose recommendations are as follows: adults, 6–9 MIU (2–3 g) per day; children and neonates, 150 000–300 000 IU.kg^{-1} (50–100 mg.kg^{-1} body weight) daily. All daily doses should be given in 2–3 divided doses.

The intravenous dose is administered as an infusion: 1.5 MIU 3 times daily in adults. There is no dose recommendation available for children.

Indications

1. Infections due to susceptible bacteria

Spiramycin has been used extensively in Europe for the treatment of localized bacterial infections, particularly upper respiratory tract, bronchopulmonary, cutaneous and genital infections. The recommended treatment schedule is 6–9 MIU daily for 5 days. Single dose therapy may be prescribed for gonococcal urethritis; however, success rates are variable (65–84%).[17] Although said to be useful in the management of periodontal infections, the combination preparation with metronidazole (Rodogyl) is likely to be of greater efficacy than spiramycin alone.[18] Spiramycin has shown considerable efficacy in treating systemic and localized chlamydial infections in animal models and in man.[17,19] Using 6 MIU daily for 5 days, 19/21 patients with non-gonococcal urethritis were cured. A number of authors have also indicated the potential of spiramycin therapy in mass treatment campaigns of trachoma. Recent reports of the successful use of intravenous spiramycin in an experimental model of guinea pig legionellosis and subsequently in adult patients with Legionnaire's disease suggest that this is a safe and effective alternative to therapy with erythromycin.[20] A dose of 1 g intravenously 8 hourly was used in this latter study.

Patients allergic to penicillin may safely be prescribed spiramycin in its place.

2. Toxoplasmosis in pregnancy

Spiramycin is undoubtedly less effective than the combination of pyrimethamine–sulphadiazine or trimethoprim–sulphamethoxazole in the treatment of established toxoplasmosis.[21] Where efficacy has been shown, however, is in the prevention of maternal–fetal transmission of toxoplasmosis. During a prospective study of 378 pregnant women with high initial *Toxoplasma* antibody titres or seroconversion during pregnancy,[22] treatment with spiramycin decreased the frequency of certain and probable fetal abnormalities. Spiramycin had no effect on the clinical picture of fetal abnormalities appearing before the beginning of treatment however. There are a number of explanations for this. Firstly, despite attaining good placental levels, penetration to the fetal circulation is poor. Secondly, spiramycin has only moderate activity against established infection.[23] Lastly spiramycin does not cross the blood–brain barrier and is ineffective against neurotoxoplasmosis.[24]

3. Prophylaxis of meningococcal meningitis

In France spiramycin is officially recommended for the prophylaxis of meningococcal meningitis. Being an effective, well tolerated, inexpensive antibiotic which does not penetrate the cerebrospinal fluid, it meets the necessary criteria for use as a prophylactic agent in this setting.

MICs for *N. meningitidis* are 0.3–3.0 mg.l^{-1} (higher if cultures are performed in 5–10% CO_2).[25] Despite relatively low serum levels, the high salivary concentrations of spiramycin are thought to be an important factor in the eradication of meningococci from the rhinopharynx.[26,27] The recommended prophylactic regimen is 6 MIU daily in adults and 150 000 IU.kg^{-1} daily in children for 5 days.

4. Cryptosporidial diarrhoea in the immunocompromised host

Enteric coccidial infections due to *Cryptosporidium* species and *Isospora belli* are becoming an increasing problem in immunosuppressed patients, particularly those with AIDS. There is anecdotal evidence that spiramycin is effective in reducing diarrhoea due to cryptosporidiosis in some patients[7] but it appears ineffective against *Isospora belli.*[28] A multi-centre placebo-controlled trial of spiramycin for the treatment of chronic cryptosporidiosis in AIDS patients is currently being carried out in the USA. Prolonged treatment is required in those patients who show a response, as there is a high incidence of recurrence. The usual dose is 9 MIU in 3 divided doses daily. In non-immunosuppressed patients *Cryptosporium*-associated diarrhoea is usually an acute self-limiting illness which does not warrant specific therapy. In infancy, however, cryptopsoridiosis is associated with significant morbidity and mortality. In this group of patients a double-blind, placebo-controlled study of spiramycin has shown no benefit.[29]

Contraindications

1. Allergy to spiramycin

Allergic reactions to spiramycin are rare and have never been associated with fatality, but as a general precaution spiramycin should not be prescribed in any patient with a prior history of allergy to spiramycin or to any other macrolide antibiotic.

2. Meningitis

Spiramycin penetrates the cerebrospinal fluid poorly even in the presence of meningeal inflammation and therefore should not be used in the treatment of meningitis.

Adverse reactions

Potentially life-threatening effects

Spiramycin is one of the best tolerated antibiotics used in man. In over 30 years of clinical use, there have been no reported instances of death, life-threatening toxicity or irreversible organ damage attributable to the use of spiramycin.

Acute overdosage

Significant overdosage has not been described. In the event of accidental or deliberate overdose induced emesis may prevent further absorption if ingestion is recent. No other specific treatment can be recommended.

Severe or irreversible adverse effects

There are few reports of severe adverse effects related to the use of spiramycin. Two cases of colitis[30,31] (one pseudomembranous) have been documented following its use therapeutically and occupational exposure has occasionally been associated with the development of asthma, rhinitis and dermatitis.[32,33] Workers in the pharmaceutical industry, veterinary surgeons, farmers and animal breeders are amongst those in whom such effects have been reported.

Symptomatic adverse effects

Spiramycin is well tolerated by most patients. Gastrointestinal adverse effects occur with varying frequency and more often when the dose is high. Unlike erythromycin, spiramycin has no effect on gastrointestinal motility[34] which may explain the lower incidence of

Spiramycin

gastrointestinal adverse effects associated with the administration of spiramycin as opposed to erythromycin. Nausea, vomiting, abdominal pain and diarrhoea occur in 1–10% of patients. Cutaneous reactions (urticaria, pruritis, macular rashes) have been occasionally reported (<1%) and very rarely paraesthesia has been described,[25] appearing 1–2 hours after dosing and usually of short duration. Two cases of benign hepatitis have been reported but serious hepatotoxicity is not a recognized problem. Spiramycin does not form the cytochrome P450–nitrosalkane complexes which are associated with the production of hepatitis by other macrolides.

Other effects

No clinically relevant biochemical changes have been noted following the use of spiramycin.

It has been suggested on the basis of in vitro studies that high levels within phagocytic cells may have a detrimental effect on host immunity but there is no in vivo data to support this.[35]

Interference with clinical pathology tests

This has not been reported.

High risk groups

Although pharmacokinetic data for patients in high risk groups are limited, clinical use over many years has demonstrated the excellent safety of spiramycin in patients of all ages, regardless of underlying disease and including pregnant and lactating women.

Neonates

No specific data are available: however, there are no reports of adverse effects occurring in neonates receiving spiramycin at the recommended dose of 150 000–300 000 $IU.kg^{-1}$ daily (50–100 $mg.kg^{-1}$ daily).

Breast milk. There is no specific contraindication to the use of spiramycin in lactating women. Spiramycin levels in breast milk are 2–40 times those present in serum.

Children

Spiramycin may safely be prescribed to infants and children of all ages.

Pregnant women

Spiramycin has been widely used in France for the treatment of toxoplasmosis during pregnancy. No adverse effects on mother or fetus have been reported. Forestier[36] studied 20 women with toxoplasmosis diagnosed between 3 and 10 weeks of gestation, who received spiramycin 3 g daily throughout the remaining pregnancy. Maternal plasma concentrations were respectively 0.682 ± 0.132, 0.618 ± 0.102 and 1.015 ± 0.22 $mg.l^{-1}$ after 1 month's therapy, during 20–24 weeks of pregnancy and at 6 months gestation. The mean fetal concentration was approximately 50% that of maternal values at 20–24 weeks. At birth, placental levels were four times that of maternal blood concentrations and 6.5 times that of cord blood.

The elderly

A recent study shows that the clearance of spiramycin is significantly lower in the elderly compared with younger adult subjects.[37] However, as there is no evidence of dose-related toxicity it is probably unnecessary to reduce the dose in elderly patients.

Concurrent disease

No special precautions are advocated where renal or hepatic function is impaired.

Drug interactions

There are no significant interactions of spiramycin with other drugs used in man. Unlike erythromycin and troleandomycin, spiramycin has no structural affinity with cytochrome P450 and so does not interfere with the metabolism of drugs such as theophylline, carbamazepine, cyclosporin A, ergotamine derivatives or oral contraceptives.

Potentially hazardous interactions

None has been described.

Potentially useful interactions

When used in combination with metronidazole, synergism against anaerobes may be found.[17,38]

Clinical trials

1. Desmonts G, Coeuvre J 1974 Congenital toxoplasmosis: a prospective study of 378 pregnancies. New England Journal of Medicine 290: 1110–1116

This is a prospective study of 378 pregnant women with high initial *Toxoplasma* antibody titres or seroconversion during pregnancy. Of the 378 women, 183 acquired the infection during pregnancy; 98 (54%) were treated with spiramycin 6–9 MIU daily in 3–4 week courses separated by 2 week intervals until delivery, the remainder received no treatment. Treatment with spiramycin during pregnancy reduced the overall frequency of fetal infections but not of overt disease. 76% of children born to treated mothers were normal as opposed to 44% among the untreated. The authors suggest that spiramycin is effective at reducing overall cases of congenital toxoplasmosis because it concentrates in the placenta; however, an already infected infant is unlikely to be cured because spiramycin crosses the placenta poorly.

2. Couvrer J, Desmonts G, Thulliez Ph 1988 Prophylaxis of congenital toxoplasmosis. Effects of spiramycin on congenital infection. Journal of Antimicrobial Chemotherapy 22 (suppl B): 193–200

In this study, placentas from 223 cases of documented congenital toxoplasmosis were studied parasitologically then analysed according to whether the mother had been treated, or not, with spiramycin during pregnancy. Placental culture was negative in only 10–11% of untreated women versus 25% of women receiving spiramycin alone and 50% of women treated with a combination of spiramycin, pyrimethamine and a sulphonamide. These data suggest that spiramycin treatment may decrease duration and/or severity of placental infection and consequently, if used early, might prevent materno-fetal transmission of *Toxoplasma*. The authors recommend the use of spiramycin in all infected pregnant women at a dose no lower than 3 g daily. Where fetal abnormality is diagnosed during pregnancy they recommend the addition of pyrimethamine and a sulphonamide.

3. Wittenberg D F, Miller N M, van den Ende J 1989 Spiramycin is not effective in treating *Cryptosporidium* diarrhoea in infants: results of a double-blind randomised trial. Journal of Infectious Diseases 159: 131–132

Cryptosporidium-associated diarrhoea in infants and young children is associated with significant morbidity and mortality. This is a concise report of a double-blind, placebo-controlled trial evaluating the use of spiramycin (75 $mg.kg^{-1}$ daily for 5 days) in infants and young children with *Cryptosporidium*-associated diarrhoea admitted to King Edward VIII Hospital (Durban, South Africa) between March and May 1987. 39 patients were enrolled; 21 received spiramycin and 18 were treated with placebo. The two groups were similar in all other respects. No clinical benefit from the use of spiramycin in the dose and duration chosen for the study could be demonstrated. The results of this study do not support the use of spiramycin in treating intestinal cryptosporidiosis in children with diarrhoea.

4. Mayaud C, Dournon E, Montagne V, Denis M, Rossert J, Akoun G 1988 Efficacy of intravenous spiramycin in the treatment of severe Legionnaire's disease. Journal of Antimicrobial Chemotherapy 22 (suppl B): 179–182

The efficacy and tolerability of intravenous spiramycin was evaluated in 10 patients (7 immunocompromised) with severe Legionnaire's disease admitted to the respiratory care unit of Tenon Hospital, Paris. No patient died of active infection; 3 died from the underlying disease or intercurrent complications. Spiramycin was well tolerated and no treatment had to be stopped because of adverse effects. Intravenous spiramycin appears to be a useful and safe alternative to erythromycin in the treatment of Legionnaire's disease.

General review articles

Barker B M, Prescott F 1973 Antimicrobial agents in medicine. Blackwell, Oxford

Davey P, Pechere J C, Speller D, Daly P J (eds) 1988 Spiramycin reassessed. Journal of Antimicrobial Chemotherapy 22 (suppl B)

Garrod L P, Lambert H P, O'Grady F (eds) 1981 Macrolides and lincosamides. In: Antibiotics and chemotherapy, 5th edn. Churchill Livingstone, Edinburgh, ch 8, pp 183–202

Spiramycin

Kernbaum S 1982 La spiramycine: utilisation en therapeutique humaine. Seminaire des Hopitaux Paris 58: 289–297
Kucers A, McK Bennett N (eds) 1979 Spiramycin, oleandomycin and kitasamycin. In: The use of antibiotics, 3rd edn. William Heinemann Medical Books Ltd, London, pp 517–521
McCabe R E, Remington J S 1983 The diagnosis and treatment of toxoplasmosis. European Journal of Clinical Microbiology 2: 95–104
Osono T, Umezawa H 1985 Pharmacokinetics of macrolides, lincosamides and streptogramins. Journal of Antimicrobial Chemotherapy 16 (suppl A): 151–166
Pessayre D, Larrey D, Funck-Bretano C, Benhamou J P 1985 Drug interactions and hepatitis produced by some macrolide antibiotics. Journal of Antimicrobial Chemotherapy 16 (suppl A): 181–194
Reynolds J E F 1982 Martindale, the extra pharmacopoeia, 28th edn. The Pharmaceutical Press, London
Soave R, Armstrong D 1986 *Cryptosporidum* and cryptosporidiosis. Reviews of Infectious Diseases 8: 1012–1023
Windholz M 1983 The Merck Index, 10th edn. Merck and Co Inc, USA

References

1. Pinnert-Sindico S, Ninet L, Preud'Homme J, Cosar C 1954 A new antibiotic — spiramycin. Antibiotics Annual 1954–1955: 724–727
2. Menninger J R 1985 Functional consequences of binding macrolides to ribosomes. Journal of Antimicrobial Chemotherapy 16 (suppl A): 23–34
3. Sutherland R 1962 Spiramycin: a reappraisal of its antibacterial activity. British Journal of Pharmacology 19: 99–110
4. Sekrawinata T, Ibrahim T, Driyatno E 1984 Spiramycin and erythromycin in the treatment of acute tonsillo-pharyngitis: a comparative study. Current Medical Research and Opinion 9: 296–300
5. Niel G, Videau D 1981 Activite de la spiramycine in vitro sur *Toxoplasma gondii*. Chimiotherapie Anti-infectieuse Reunion Interdisciplinaire, Paris 121: 8
6. Beverley J K A, Freeman A P, Henry L, Whelan J P K 1973 Prevention of pathological changes in experimental congenital *Toxoplasma* infections. Lyon Medical 230: 491–498
7. Portnoy D, Whiteside M E, Buckley E, Macleod C L 1984 Treatment of intestinal cryptosporidiosis with spiramycin. Annals of Internal Medicine 101: 202–204
8. Duval J 1985 Evolution and epidemiology of MLS resistance. Journal of Antimicrobial Chemotherapy 16 (suppl A): 137–149
9. Garrod L P 1957 Erythromycin group of antibiotics. British Medical Journal 3: 57–63
10. Courvalin P, Ounissi H, Arthur M 1985 Multiplicity of macrolide–lincosamide–streptogramin antibiotic resistance determinants. Journal of Antimicrobial Chemotherapy 16 (suppl A): 91–100
11. Bennett J V, Brodie J L, Benner E J, Kirby W M M 1966 Simplified accurate method for antibiotic assay of clinical specimens. Applied Microbiology 14: 170–177
12. Dow J, Lemar M, Frydman A, Gaillot J 1985 Automated high-performance liquid chromatographic determination of spiramycin by direct injection of plasma, using column-switching for sample clean-up. Journal of Chromatography 344: 275–283
13. Le Roux Y, Desmottes J F, Frydman A, Kaplan P, Gaillot J, Blanchard J C 1985 Pharmacokinetics of spiramycin after single and multiple administrations of a one-hour 500 mg IV infusion in healthy volunteers. Proceedings of the 14th International Congress of Chemotherapy, June 23–28, Kyoto, Japan
14. Pocidalo J J, Albert F, Desnottes J F, Kernbaum S 1985 Intraphagocytic penetration of macrolides: in-vivo comparison of erythromycin and spiramycin. Journal of Antimicrobial Chemotherapy 16 (suppl A): 167–173
15. Quentin C F, Besnard R M, Bonnard O et al 1983 Etudes preliminaire in vitro du passage transplacentaire de la spiramycine. Pathologie et Biologie (Paris) 31: 425–428
16. Inoue A, Deguchi T 1983 Biosynthesis and the metabolic fate of carbon-14 labelled spiramycin 1. Journal of Antibiotics 36: 442–444
17. Williams J 1975 Treatment of gonorrhoea. Journal of the Royal Navy Medical Service 61: 44–47
18. Quee T C, Roussou T, Chan E C 1983 In vitro activity of Rodogyl against putative periodontic bacteria. Antimicrobial Agents and Chemotherapy 24: 445–447
19. Treharne J D, Squires S 1982 Evaluation of topical spiramycin and other antibiotics for the treatment of experimental chlamydial ocular infection. Journal of Antimicrobial Chemotherapy 9: 125–132
20. Mayaud C, Dournon E, Montagne V, Denis M, Rossert J, Akoun G 1988 Efficacy of intravenous spiramycin in the treatment of severe Legionnaire's disease. Journal of Antimicrobial Chemotherapy 22 (suppl B): 179–182
21. Nguyen B T, Stadtsbaeder S 1983 Comparative effects of cotrimoxazole (trimethoprim–sulphamethoxazole), pyrimethamine–sulphadiazine and spiramycin during a virulent infection with *Toxoplasma gondii* (Beverley strain) in mice. British Journal of Pharmacology 79: 923–928
22. Desmonts G, Couvreur J 1974 Congenital toxoplasmosis: a prospective study of 378 pregnancies. New England Journal of Medicine 290: 1110–1116
23. Thiermann E, Apt W, Atias A, Lorca M, Olguin J 1978 A comparative study of some combined treatment regimens in acute toxoplasmosis in mice. American Journal of Tropical Medicine and Hygiene 27: 747–750
24. Leport C, Vilde J L, Saimot A G 1986 Failure of spiramycin to prevent neurotoxoplasmosis in immunosuppressed patients (letter). Journal of the American Medical Association 255: 2290
25. Dabernat H, Delmas C, Lareng M B 1984 Sensibilite aux antibiotiques de meningocoques isoles chez des malades et chez des porteurs. Pathologie et Biologie (Paris) 32: 532–535
26. Kamme C, Kahlmeter G, Melander A 1978 Evaluation of spiramycin as a therapeutic agent for elimination of nasopharyngeal pathogens. Scandinavian Journal of Infectious Diseases 10: 135–142
27. Engelen F, Vandepitte J, Verbist L, de Maeyer-Cleempoel S 1981 Effect of spiramycin on the nasopharyngeal carriage of *Neisseria meningitidis*. Chemotherapy 27: 325–333
28. Gaska J A, Tietze K J, Cosgrove E M 1985 Unsuccessful treatment of enteritis with spiramycin: a case report. Journal of Infectious Diseases 152: 1336–1338
29. Wittenberg D F, Miller N M, van den Ende J 1989 Spiramycin is not effective in treating *Cryptosporidium* diarrhoea in infants: results of a double-blind randomised trial. Journal of Infectious Diseases 159: 131–132
30. Decaux G M, Devroede C 1978 Acute colitis related to spiramycin (letter). Lancet 2: 993
31. Di Febo G, Milazzo G, Biasco G, Miglioli M 1982 Antibiotic-associated colitis: always pseudomembranous? Endoscopy 14: 128–130
32. Moscato G, Naldi L, Candura F 1984 Bronchial asthma due to spiramycin and adipic acid. Clinical Allergy 14: 355–361
33. Hjorth N, Roed-Petersen J 1980 Allergic contact dermatitis in veterinary surgeons. Contact Dermatitis 6: 27–29
34. Zara G P, Qin X Y, Pilot M A, Thomson H H, Maskell J P 1987 Erythromycin and gastrointestinal motility (letter). Lancet 2: 1036
35. Roche Y, Gougerot-Pocidalo J J 1986 Macrolides and immunity: effects of erythromycin and spiramycin on human mononuclear cell proliferation. Journal of Antimicrobial Chemotherapy 17: 195–203
36. Forestier F, Daffos F, Rainaut M, Desnotte J F, Gaschard J C 1987 Suivi therapeutique feto-maternel de la spiramycine en cours de grossesse. Archives Francaises de Pediatrie 44: 539–544
37. Frydman A M, Le Roux Y, Desnottes J F et al 1988 Pharmacokinetics of spiramycin in man. Journal of Antimicrobial Chemotherapy 22 (suppl B): 93–103
38. Brook I 1986 In vitro and in vivo activity of metronidazole and spiramycin on *Bacteroides* species and *Staphylococcus aureus*. Abstracts of the 1986 ICAAC: 197

Spironolactone

Spironolactone is probably the most important steroidal lactone in clinical use; it acts as a diuretic and antihypertensive agent by antagonizing the sodium-retaining effects of aldosterone, and also in part by inhibiting the adrenocortical biosynthesis of aldosterone.

Chemistry

Spironolactone (Aldactone, Diatensec, Spiroctan, Spirolone)
$C_{24}H_{32}O_4S$
7-α-Acetyl-thio-3-oxo-17α-pregn-4-ene-21-17β-carbolactone acid-γ-lactone

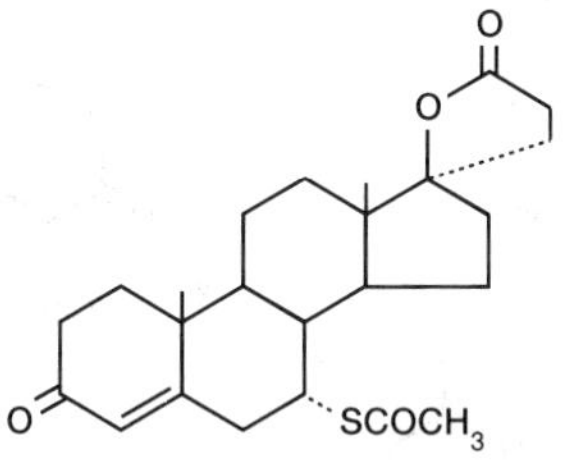

Molecular weight	416.1
pKa	not relevant
Solubility	
in alcohol	1 in 80
in water	insoluble
Octanol/water partition coefficient	—

Spironolactone is a white to light tan powder with a slightly bitter taste and is usually odourless or has a slight odour of thioacetic acid. It is prepared by chemical synthesis.

Spironolactone is also available in oral combination with frusemide (Lasilactone = frusemide 20 mg and spironolactone 50 mg) and with hydroflumethiazide (Aldactide 25 = hydroflumethiazide 25 mg and spironolactone 25 mg).

Pharmacology

The antimineralocorticoid properties of the spirolactones were first recognized more than 30 years ago.[1] Spironolactone is a competitive inhibitor of the binding of aldosterone to its receptor. Its most important site of action is the distal portion of renal tubules where it combines with soluble cytoplasmic aldosterone receptors to form complexes which are inactive and which do not bind to nuclear-acceptor sites, thus preventing a chain of biochemical events leading to the synthesis of physiologically active proteins.[2,3] Thus it promotes a diuresis and acts as an antihypertensive agent. Administration of spironolactone is associated with reversal of the electrolytic changes attributed to aldosterone and with a dose-dependent increase in plasma renin activity in rats.[4]

A separate but less important effect is direct inhibition of adrenal synthesis of aldosterone.[5]

Toxicology

The acute toxicity of spironolactone is low in rats, mice and rabbits, so that there is a high potential therapeutic ratio.

During chronic testing histological changes were noted in rat liver, thyroid gland and male genitalia. There were also changes in monkey testes and male mammary glands. In a 78-week study in rats, a number of malignant tumours occurred, mainly affecting skin and connective tissue, liver, thyroid and kidney. However, by comparison with a control group it was not clear that the incidence of tumours was greater than would be expected in any ageing rat population. Thus, whether spironolactone predisposes to tumour formation remains an unresolved question.[6]

Clinical pharmacology

Spironolactone is a competitive inhibitor of aldosterone through binding at receptor sites, the most important of which lie in the late distal renal tubules and the renal collecting system. Thus urinary sodium and water loss and retention of potassium and hydrogen result and the clinical effects are a diuresis and lowering of blood pressure.[7]

Spironolactone also inhibits adrenocortical aldosterone biosynthesis in patients with primary hyperaldosteronism, of which 'spironolactone bodies' identified in the adrenal tumour cells of treated patients are thought to be a morphological expression.[8] Theoretically, such a mechanism could enhance diuretic activity but its therapeutic importance is uncertain.

Spironolactone is primarily useful as a diuretic in patients with hyperaldosteronism. Thus it is effective in patients with ascites due to liver failure, and in patients with resistant heart failure (i.e. where other diuretics have failed). It is less useful as a first-line diuretic. Its antihypertensive effects are relatively modest in essential hypertension but it is of value in the treatment of hypertension due to primary hyperaldosteronism where other definitive treatments (e.g. surgery) are not feasible.

Single-dose studies in normal volunteers in the range 50–800 mg produced a dose-dependent reversal of aldosterone-induced sodium retention and/or decrease in the plasma Na/K ratio.[9] In essential hypertension no difference in antihypertensive effect was found between daily doses of 100, 200 or 400 mg[10] and a maximum dose of 75–100 mg per day has been recommended.[11] However, there was a dose relationship with plasma sodium, potassium and weight.[10] By comparison, spironolactone in doses of up to 400 mg per day may be necessary in the treatment of primary hyperaldosteronism.[7,12] Because of the prolonged duration of activity of its metabolites, spironolactone may be administered in a single daily dose.

Spironolactone causes a number of electrolyte changes, notably a reduction in plasma sodium and bicarbonate, together with dose-dependent elevations in plasma renin, potassium and creatinine. Fasting blood sugar, cholesterol and triglycerides are not significantly affected.[11,13]

Spironolactone was thought to increase calcium excretion through a direct effect on tubular transport, but this was later refuted.[14]

Pharmacokinetics

In the past spironolactone has been assayed using a spectrophotofluorimetric method[15] but now a HPLC assay is in more common use which has a sensitivity[16,17] of 5 $\mu g.l^{-1}$. However, because the drug is extensively metabolized to canrenone and other metabolites which are also competitive antagonists of aldosterone, pharmacokinetic studies focus on the metabolic pathways.

Oral absorption of spironolactone is variable because of its low aqueous solubility. In rhesus monkeys almost complete absorption of the drug was obtained from an aqueous ethanolic solution, and in man, absorption is enhanced by micronization of the drug in the tablet.[18,19] There is improved absorption if the drug is taken after food, probably because by delaying gastric emptying, food promotes disintegration of the tablet and improves dissolution of the drug.

Furthermore, bile acids secreted in response to the meal may dissolve spironolactone, which is very lipophilic.[20] The peak plasma concentration was observed at 1 hour in normal volunteers after a standardized meal. Systemic bioavailability has been estimated at 60–70% and the plasma half life is 1.3 ± 0.3 (SD) hours. The drug can still be detected up to 8 hours after ingestion but it is extensively metabolized so that the free drug is not detected in urine.[21–23]

Spironolactone is 98% protein bound but its volume of distribution is unknown.[24] The extent of tissue accumulation of the drug and its ability to cross the blood–brain barrier are not known. In lactating women taking spironolactone, levels of canrenone in milk were low and it was estimated that the maximum quantity of canrenone ingested daily by the human infant via milk was 0.2% of the maternal daily dose of spironolactone.[25]

Oral absorption	variable
Presystemic metabolism	—
Plasma half life	
range	1.3±0.3 h
mean	—
Volume of distribution	—
Plasma protein binding	98%

Concentration–effect relationship

Spironolactone has an active metabolite, canrenone, which contributes much to the biological effect of the drug. There is no evidence of any correlation between the plasma concentration of spironolactone or of its metabolite canrenone and the biological activity of the drug.

Metabolism

The major site of biotransformation of spironolactone is thought to be the liver.[26] The pathways are complex and some metabolites remain to be identified. The initial step is rapid deacetylation leading to formation of a 7α-thiol derivative. Thereafter elimination of hydrogen sulphide yields canrenone, which exists in enzymatic equilibrium with canrenoic acid (Fig. 1). Canrenone can also be formed from various sulphur-containing metabolites of spironolactone by cleavage of the C-7 sulphur-containing moiety (Fig. 2). Canrenone itself may undergo reduction or hydroxylation and polyhydroxylated metabolites have been identified in urine.[27,28]

Fig. 1

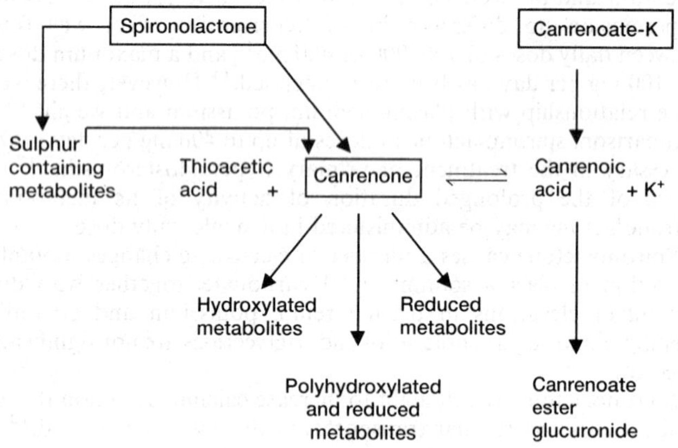

A separate metabolic pathway involves S-methylation of the 7α-thiol spironolactone derivative and further degradation and urinary excretion.[29] Many of the metabolites of spironolactone have biological activity with varying affinity for aldosterone receptors.

Pharmaceutics

In the UK spironolactone is available as Aldactone (Searle). The 25 mg and 100 mg tablets are buff-coloured round tablets, coded '39' and '134' respectively; the 50 mg tablet is off-white, and coded '916'. In the USA Aldactone is available as follows: 25 mg tablet is light yellow, and coded '1001' on one side and 'Aldactone 25' on the other; 50 mg tablet is light orange, and coded '1041' on one side and 'Aldactone 50' on the other; 100 mg tablet is peach-coloured, and coded '1031' on one side and 'Aldactone 100' on the other. Spironolactone is not available for parenteral use. All preparations should be protected from light. The shelf-life is generally several years but varies depending on the preparation.

In the UK, spironolactone is available formulated with hydroflumethiazide (Aldactide), and Frusemide (Lasilactone). Elsewhere it is available formulated with althiazide, hydrochlorothiazide, thiabutazide and isobutylhydrochlorothiazide.

Therapeutic use

Indications

1. The diagnosis and treatment of primary hyperaldosteronism (aldosterone-secreting adrenal adenoma, bilateral adrenal hyperplasia)

Spironolactone

Fig. 2 Metabolism of spironolactone

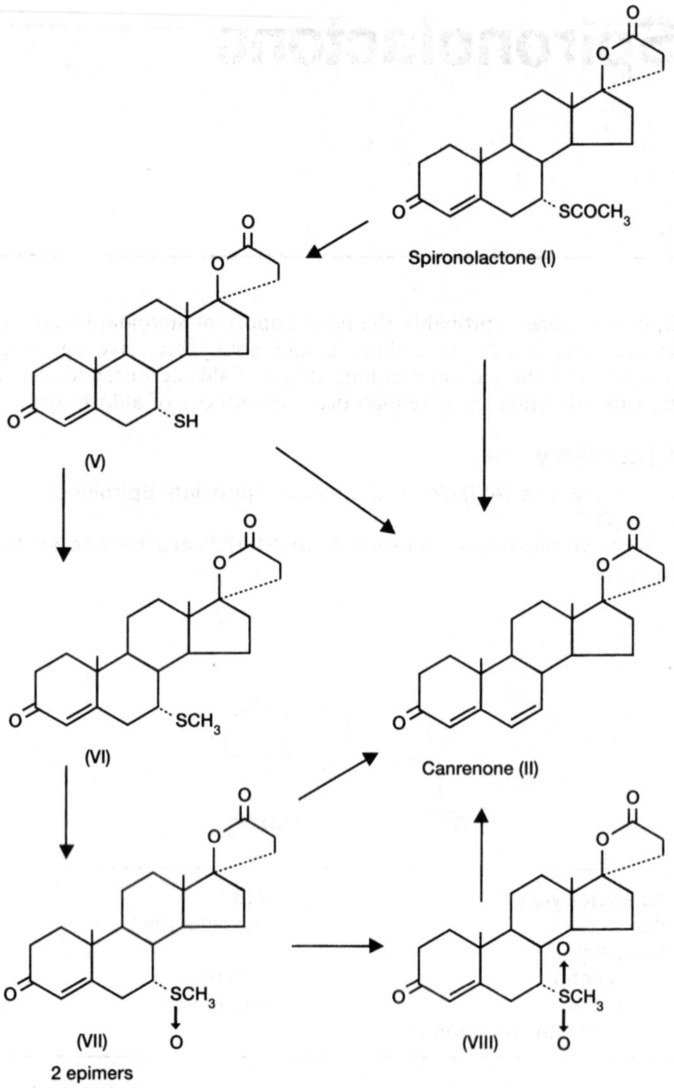

2. The treatment of essential hypertension
3. The treatment of oedema associated with secondary aldosteronism
4. The treatment of oedema refractory to other diuretics given orally or intravenously
5. Correction of potassium and/or magnesium deficiency resulting from prior use of potassium-wasting diuretics
6. The treatment of hirsutism (not licensed for this in the UK or USA).

In the United Kingdom the licences for all products containing spironolactone have been amended so that the drug is no longer indicated for essential hypertension and idiopathic oedema.

Contraindications

1. Hyperkalaemia
2. Hyponatraemia
3. Renal impairment
4. Pregnancy, breast-feeding, childhood
5. Peptic ulceration.

Mode of use

The dose of spironolactone varies depending on the clinical situation. In secondary aldosteronism and essential hypertension, a daily dose of 50–100 mg may be sufficient, whereas in the diagnosis and treatment of primary hyperaldosteronism, it may be necessary to prescribe up to 400 mg daily. Maximum drug effect may take several days to achieve.

To increase bioavailability, it is recommended that spironolactone be taken with meals.

Spironolactone

Indications

1. Primary hyperaldosteronism
Spironolactone has been used as a diagnostic test to provide presumptive evidence of primary hyperaldosteronism (aldosterone-secreting adenoma). In patients in whom surgery is either contraindicated or not appropriate, spironolactone may be used in long-term treatment. In this condition, use of spironolactone is associated with an increase in plasma active renin and angiotensin II, together with a fall in plasma sodium and bicarbonate and a rise in plasma potassium and urinary sodium excretion.[7] In patients with aldosterone-producing adrenal adenoma treated with spironolactone, there is no increase in plasma or urinary aldosterone even when plasma renin and potassium rise to normal; whereas in similar circumstances in adrenal hyperplasia, plasma and urinary aldosterone rise. This observation suggests that spironolactone blocks the potassium–aldosterone stimulatory mechanism in adrenal adenoma and could be useful in diagnosis in ambiguous cases.[30]

2. Essential hypertension
Spironolactone has been used in the treatment of essential hypertension. Its antihypertensive effect appears to be independent of the level of plasma renin.[31]

3. & 4. Secondary aldosteronism and refractory oedema
Spironolactone has been used either alone or in combination with other diuretics to treat fluid retention in cardiac failure, hepatic cirrhosis, the nephrotic syndrome, malignant ascites, idiopathic oedema and intractable fluid retention.

5. Electrolyte disturbances
Because of its potassium-sparing properties, spironolactone may be useful as an adjunct to treatment with other diuretics, thus avoiding hypokalaemia and extracellular alkalosis.

6. Hirsutism
Spironolactone has been used in the treatment of hirsutism with beneficial effect but its mode of action is uncertain. There is evidence both for impaired testosterone biosynthesis and for peripheral inhibition of androgen action.[32,33]

Contraindications

Pre-existing hyperkalaemia and hyponatraemia are contraindications to the use of spironolactone. The drug should not be prescribed in acute renal failure, or rapidly deteriorating or severe impairment of renal function. In addition, spironolactone should not be administered concurrently with other potassium-sparing diuretics, and should be given with great caution in conjunction with agents lowering plasma aldosterone, such as ACE inhibitors.

Adverse reactions

Potentially life-threatening effects
Development of breast cancer has been reported in patients taking spironolactone chronically, but a causal relationship has never been established and it seems likely that the original observation was a chance event.[34,35] Isolated cases of development of agranulocytosis or eosinophilia during treatment with spironolactone have been recorded; these may be idiosyncratic reactions and have resolved following withdrawal of the drug.[36,37]

Spironolactone may cause hyperkalaemia and hyponatraemia, and deterioration in renal function may occur, particularly in those with pre-existing renal impairment. Fatal hyperkalaemia has occurred when spironolactone has been used in combination with ACE inhibitors in hypertensive or heart failure patients with moderate renal impairment.

Hyperchloraemic metabolic acidosis has been reported in advanced hepatic cirrhosis, usually in the presence of hyperkalaemia with normal renal function.

Gastrointestinal disturbances have been described, including peptic ulceration and haematemesis.[38]

Acute overdosage
Overdosage with spironolactone may cause drowsiness, mental confusion, nausea, vomiting, dizziness and diarrhoea. Hyperkalaemia and hyponatraemia are unlikely to occur acutely.

Symptoms usually respond to withdrawal of the drug, fluid and electrolyte replacement and treatment of hyperkalaemia if appropriate.

Severe or irreversible adverse effects
Spironolactone causes a number of endocrine changes including gynaecomastia, menstrual irregularity, impotence and loss of libido. Breast enlargement relates to the dosage and duration of treatment; it is normally reversible following drug withdrawal, but, rarely, may persist. These effects have been attributed to interference with testosterone biosynthesis but this does not provide a complete explanation and it may be that there is an antiandrogen action at receptor sites. Finally, lichen planus has been described in a patient taking spironolactone.[39]

Symptomatic adverse effects
Other adverse effects include drowsiness, mental confusion, ataxia and headache.

Other effects
Use of spironolactone is associated with lowering of serum magnesium in some patients with cirrhosis,[40] but not inevitably so.[41]

Interference with clinical pathology tests
Spironolactone interferes with the fluorometric tests for measuring plasma cortisol and corticosteroids; immunoassays for serum digoxin levels; the Zimmerman reaction for 17-ketosteroids and 17-ketogenic steroids; and the Porter-Silber reaction for urinary 17-hydroxycorticoids.

High risk groups

Neonates
The drug is unlikely to be used in neonates.

Breast milk. Spironolactone is contraindicated in lactation although less than 0.2% of canrenone in maternal serum is detected in breast milk of lactating women taking spironolactone.

Children
The drug may be used in children in appropriate doses.

Pregnant women
Ideally, the drug should not be used in pregnancy because it crosses the placental barrier.

The elderly
Spironolactone should be used carefully in elderly patients with renal impairment who may develop acidosis and hyperkalaemia, although it has no effect on carbohydrate metabolism.

Concurrent disease
The drug should be avoided in diabetics with renal impairment, because it may predispose to hyperkalaemia.

Drug interactions

Potentially hazardous interactions

Aspirin. Aspirin reduces urinary excretion of canrenone.[42]

Digoxin. Patients taking both spironolactone and digoxin show an increase in plasma digoxin because spironolactone inhibits the tubular secretion of digoxin.[43]

Other drugs. Combination with ACE inhibitors, amiloride, triamterene, and carbenoxolone should be avoided. Spironolactone has synergy with lithium in manic patients.[44]

Potentially useful interactions
In some of the disorders discussed earlier, the combination of spironolactone with another diuretic may be more effective than either drug used alone.

References

1. Kagawa C M, Cella J A, Von Arman C G 1957 Action of new steroids in blocking effects of aldosterone and deoxycorticosterone on salt. Science 126: 1015–1016
2. Marver D, Stewart J, Funder J W, Feldman D, Edelman I S 1974 Renal aldosterone receptors: studies with [^{3}H]-aldosterone and the antimineralocorticoid [^{3}H]-spironolactone (SC-26 304). Proceedings of the National Academy of Science of the United States of America 71: 1431–1435
3. Corvol P, Claire M, Oblin M E, Geering K, Rossier B 1981 Mechanism of the antimineralocorticoid effects of spironolactones. Kidney International 20: 1–6

Spironolactone

4. Erbler H C 1978 Acute and chronic effects of spironolactone and canrenone on plasma aldosterone concentration, plasma renin activity, aldosterone excretion rate and electrolytes in rats. In: Addison G M, Wirenfeldt Asmussen N, Corvol P et al (eds) Aldosterone antagonists in clinical medicine. Excerpta Medica, Amsterdam, pp 77–83
5. Aupetit B, Bastien C, Aubry-Marais F, Legrand J C 1978 Effect of aldosterone antagonists on aldosterone synthesis. In: Addison G M, Wirenfeldt Asmussen N, Corvol P et al (eds) Aldosterone antagonists in clinical medicine. Excerpta Medica, Amsterdam, pp 36–40
6. Lumb G, Newberne P, Rust J H, Wagner R 1978 Effects in animals of chronic administration of spironolactone. A review. In: Addison G M, Wirenfeldt Asmussen N, Corvol P et al (eds) Aldosterone antagonists in clinical medicine. Excerpta Medica, Amsterdam, pp 132–150
7. Ferriss J B, Beevers D G, Boddy K et al 1978 The treatment of low-renin ('primary') hyperaldosteronism. American Heart Journal 96: 97–109
8. Conn J W, Hinerman D L 1977 Spironolactone-induced inhibition of aldosterone biosynthesis: morphological and functional studies. Metabolism 26: 1293–1307
9. Casals-Stenzel J, Schmalbach J, Losert W 1978 Acute effects of aldosterone antagonists in volunteers. In: Addison G M, Wirenfeldt Asmussen N, Corvol P et al (eds) Aldosterone antagonists in clinical medicine. Excerpta Medica, Amsterdam, pp 207–216
10. Zacharias F 1978 Spironolactone in essential hypertension: a dose–response study. In: Addison G M, Wirenfeldt Asmussen N, Corvol P et al (eds) Aldosterone antagonists in clinical medicine. Excerpta Medica, Amsterdam, pp 503–507
11. Jeunemaitre X, Chatellier G, Kregt-Jais C et al 1987 Efficacy andd tolerance of spironolactone in essential hypertension. American Journal of Cardiology 60: 820–825
12. Spark R F, Melby J C 1968 Aldosteronism in hypertension. The spironolactone response test. Annals of Internal Medicine 69: 685–691
13. Schersten B, Thulin T, Kuylenstierna J et al 1980 Clinical and biochemical effects of spironolactone administered once daily in primary hypertension. Hypertension 2: 672–679
14. Prati R C, Alfrey A C, Hull A R 1972 Spironolactone-induced hypercalciuria. Journal of Laboratory and Clinical Medicine 80: 224–230
15. Sadee W, Dagcioglu M, Riegelman S 1972 Fluorimetric microassay for spironolactone and its metabolites in biological fluids. Journal of Pharmaceutical Sciences 61: 1126
16. Overdiek J W P M, Hermens W A J J, Merkus F W H M 1985 Determination of the serum concentrations of spironolactone and its metabolites by high-performance liquid chromatography. Journal of Chromatography 341: 279–285
17. Merkus F W H M, Overdiek J W P M, Cilissen J, Zuidema J 1983 Pharmacokinetics of spironolactone after a single dose: evaluation of the true canrenone serum concentrations during 24 hours. Clinical and Experimental Hypertension 5: 239–248
18. Levy G 1962 Availability of spironolactone given by mouth. Lancet 2: 723–724
19. Bauer G, Rieckmann P, Schaumann W 1962 Influence of particle size and detergents on the absorption of spironolactone from the gastrointestinal tract. Arzneimittel-Forschung 12: 487–489
20. Melander A, Schersten B, Thulin T, Wahlin E 1978 Influence of food intake on the bioavailability of spironolactone and other antihypertensive drugs In: Addison G M, Wirenfeldt Asmussen N, Corvol P et al (eds) Aldosterone antagonists in clinical medicine. Excerpta Medica, Amsterdam, pp 218–226
21. Sadee W, Dagcioglu M, Schroder R 1973 Pharmacokinetics of spironolactone, canrenone and canrenoate-K in humans. Journal of Pharmacology and Experimental Therapeutics 185: 686–695
22. Karim A, Zagarella J, Hribar J, Dooley M 1976 Spironolactone: disposition and metabolism. Clinical Pharmacology and Therapeutics 19: 158–169
23. Overdiek H W P M, Hermens W A J J, Merkus F W H M 1985 New insights into the pharmacokinetics of spironolactone. Clinical Pharmacology and Therapeutics 38: 469–474
24. Chien Y W, Hofmann L M, Lambert H J 1976 Binding of spironolactones to human plasma proteins. Journal of Pharmaceutical Sciences 65: 1337–1340
25. Phelps D L, Karim A 1977 Spironolactone: relationship between concentration of dethioacetyl metabolite in human serum and milk. Journal of Pharmaceutical Sciences 66: 1203
26. Gerhardt E, Engelhardt R 1963 The metabolism of 3-(3-oxo-7-acetylthio-17-hydroxy-4-androstene-17-yl)-propionic acid lactone. Arzneimittel-Forschung 13: 972–977
27. Karim A 1978 Pharmacokinetics and metabolism of aldosterone antagonists: a review. In: Addison G M, Wirenfeldt Asmussen N, Corvol P et al (eds) Aldosterone antagonists in clinical medicine. Excerpta Medica, Amsterdam, pp 115–131
28. Karim A 1986 Spironolactone metabolism in man revisited In: Brumner H R et al (eds) Contemporary trends in diuretic therapy. Excerpta Medica, Amsterdam, pp 22–37
29. Gardiner P, Schrode K, Quinlan D et al 1989 Spironolactone metabolism: steady-state serum levels of the sulfur containing metabolites. Journal of Clinical Pharmacology 29: 342–347
30. Kater C E, Biglieri E G, Schambelan M, Arteaga E 1983 Studies of impaired aldosterone response to spironolactone-induced renin and potassium elevations in adenomatous but not hyperplastic primary aldosteronism. Hypertension 5 (suppl V): V115–V121
31. Karlberg B E, Tolagen K 1978 The predictive value of renin profiling in the choice of treatment in primary hypertension, with special reference to patients with low-renin values. In: Addison G M, Wirenfeldt Asmussen N, Corvol P et al (eds) Aldosterone antagonists in clinical medicine. Excerpta Medica, Amsterdam, pp 457–465
32. Dorrington-Ward P, McCartney A, Holland S, Scully J, Carter G, Alaghband-Zadeh J, Wise P 1985 The effect of spironolactone on hirsutism and female androgen metabolism. Clinical Endocrinology and Metabolism 23: 161–167
33. Barth J H, Cherry C A, Wojnarow S K A F, Dawber R P R 1989 Spironolactone is an effective and well-tolerated systemic antiandrogen therapy for hirsute women. Journal of Clinical Endocrinology and Metabolism 68: 966–970
34. Loube S D, Quirk R A 1975 Breast cancer associated with administration of spironolactone. Lancet 1: 1428–1429
35. Jick H, Armstrong B 1975 Breast cancer and spironolactone. Lancet 2: 368–369
36. Stricker B H C, Oei T T 1984 Agranulocytosis caused by spironolactone. British Medical Journal 289: 731
37. Wathen C G, Macdonald T, Wise L A, Boyd S M 1986 Eosinophilia associated with spironolactone. Lancet 1: 919–920
38. Mackay A, Stevenson R D 1977 Gastric ulceration induced by spironolactone. Lancet 1: 481
39. Downham T F 1978 Spironolactone induced lichen planus. Journal of the American Medical Association 240: 1138
40. Campra J L, Reynolds T B 1978 Effectiveness of high-dose spironolactone therapy in patients with chronic liver disease and relatively refractory ascites. American Journal of Digestive Diseases 23: 1025–1030
41. Wheeler P G, Smith T, Golindan O et al 1977 Potassium and magnesium depletion in patients with cirrhosis on maintenance diuretic regimes. Gut 18: 683–687
42. Ramsay L E, Harrison I R, Shelton J R, Vose C W 1976 Influence of acetylsalicylic acid on the renal handling of a spironolactone metabolite in healthy subjects. European Journal of Clinical Pharmacology 10: 43–48
43. Waldorff S, Andersen J D, Heeboll-Nielsen N et al 1978 Spironolactone induced changes in digoxin kinetics. Clinical Pharmacology and Therapeutics 24: 162–167
44. Gillman M A, Lichtigfeld F J 1986 Synergism of spironolactone and lithium in mania. British Medical Journal 292: 661–662

Stanozolol

Stanozolol is an orally active anabolic steroid.

Chemistry

Stanozolol (Stromba, Stromba Simplex, Winstroid, Winstrol; Strombaject and Stromba Winject have been used)
$C_{21}H_{32}N_2O$
17β-Hydroxy-17α-methylandrostano(3,2-c)pyrazole

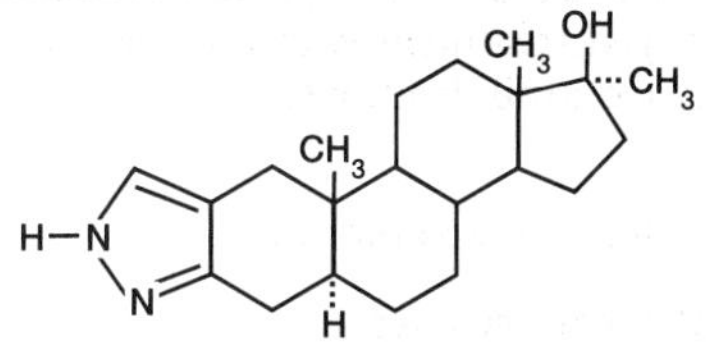

Molecular weight	328.5
pKa	not relevant
Solubility	
in alcohol	1 in 40
in water	insoluble
Octanol/water partition coefficient	—

A white, odourless powder prepared by chemical synthesis which can exist in two crystalline forms: needles and prisms.

Pharmacology

Stanozolol, like other anabolic steroids, is a structural analogue of testosterone.[1] The anabolic effects of androgens are most readily demonstrated in castrate or female animals where they promote skeletal muscle growth and cause retention of nitrogen. The receptor for the anabolic effects of androgens appears to be the same as that for the other hormonal effects of these substances[2] so androgenic effects are an inevitable accompaniment of their use.

Stanozolol increases collagen production and decreases the anti-anabolic action of cortisone,[3–5] and it has also been reported to reduce fibrin deposition.[6] Stanozolol has been shown to stimulate the incorporation of thymidine into DNA of human bone cells and increase proliferation.[7,8]

There is evidence that stanozolol activates and enhances fibrinolytic activity,[8,9]

Stanozolol has been reported to correct the formation of kinin or factors with kinin-like activity which may be associated with oedema and swelling seen in hereditary angio-oedema (HAE).[10,11]

Toxicology

Stanozolol does not appear to have teratogenic activity. Pregnant New Zealand white rabbits which received oral doses of 0.2, 1.0 or 5.0 $mg.kg^{-1}$ stanozolol from the 8th to the 16th day of gestation, showed no adverse effects. There were no malformations in the offspring attributable to the stanozolol. Rats, mice and another series of rabbits which received similar doses in pregnancy also showed no signs of teratogenicity. Rats receiving daily stanozolol 2.5 to 20 $mg.kg^{-1}$ or methyltestosterone 2.5 to 25 $mg.kg^{-1}$ by mouth, produced fetuses with increased anogenital distance indicating an androgenic effect. Otherwise, the fetuses appeared normal on gross examination.

Clinical pharmacology

Stanozolol is used chiefly for its anabolic effects. When administered in a dose of 10 mg daily for 14–21 days an increase in size of the type 1 fibres of the rectus abdominis muscle has been demonstrated.[12] The drug has androgenic effects and this may lead to greasy skin and acne, fluid retention, weight gain and ankle swelling. Masculinization of the female with growth of facial hair, acne, deepening of the voice and menstrual irregularity may develop. Stanozolol may also be useful in the treatment of hereditary angioneurotic oedema. The drug has fibrinolytic activity but its use in man is limited in this regard.

Pharmacokinetics

A gas chromatography assay method has been developed for suspensions of stanozolol[13] and colorimetric assay for stanozolol in solution,[14] but there are difficulties associated with the determination of stanozolol in biological fluids.[15] Stanozolol and its metabolite can be measured in urine by gas chromatography/mass spectrometry.[16] Studies have not been undertaken to determine tissue penetration, placental transfer or excretion into breast milk.

Concentration–effect relationship

There is no data available concerning any correlation between the plasma concentration of stanozolol and its therapeutic effects.

Metabolism

Using stanozolol in which the methylene group of the pyrazole ring has been labelled with tritium,[17] it has been shown in calves and rats that the radioactivity is slowly eliminated, partly in the urine, but mostly in the faeces.

Twelve metabolites, including conjugated stanozolol, have been detected in urine[18] and a number of the aglycones synthesized.[19] However, to date, very little quantitative data have been reported. 16α-Hydroxystanozolol, 17-epistanozolol, stanozolol and 3-hydroxy-17-epistanozolol are the most abundant in the unconjugated fraction in urine. 16α- and 16β-hydroxystanozolol, stanozolol, 3β-hydroxystanozolol and 4β-hydroxystanozolol are the most abundant in the aglycone fraction.

Pharmaceutics

Stanozolol is available in an oral form: Stromba tablets (Sterling Winthrop, UK) contain 5 mg stanozolol. The tablets are flat white, 9 mm diameter, marked 'Stromba' on one side and scored in quarters on the other side. Winstrol tablets (Winthrop-Breon, USA) are round pink scored tablets containing 2 mg stanozolol and coded 'W53'.

Stanozolol tablets are stable and carry a minimal risk from potentially allergenic substances.

Therapeutic use

Indications

1. The prevention and control of attacks of hereditary angio-oedema
2. The control of vascular manifestations of Behcet's syndrome.

Other uses
The drug has also been tried in the following condition.

3. The prevention and management of recurrent deep vein thrombosis
4. The management of postmenopausal and senile osteoporosis
5. The management of anorexia, asthenia or chronic debilitating diseases.

Contraindications

1. Cancer of the prostate
2. Pregnant women
3. Enhancement of athletic ability
4. Stanozolol should be used with caution in patients with impaired renal, hepatic or cardiac function.

Mode of use

Adults
Daily oral doses of up to 10 mg is recommended for treatment of vasculitis in Behcet's syndrome.

S

For the treatment of hereditary angio-oedema, an initial dose of 2.5–10 mg daily may control attacks. Thereafter the dose may be reduced according to patient response. Maintenance doses as low as 2.5 mg, three times a week, have been achieved in selected cases.

Children
Stanozolol is not recommended in children of less than one year old; 1–6 years: 2.5 mg daily, 6–10 years: 2.5–5 mg daily. It is suggested that tablets should be administered to children in short courses of six to eight weeks. More than one course may be given with an interval of one month between courses.

Indications

The current approved indications for stanozol are very limited and vary by country.

1. The prevention and control of attacks of hereditary angio-oedema
Stanozolol tablets have been shown to be effective in the prevention and control of attacks of heredity angio-oedema. Once control has been achieved, the lowest dose possible that maintains freedom from attacks should be used.

2. The control of cutaneous vasculitis in Behcet's syndrome
Stanozolol has been shown to increase plasminogen activator activity and plasma plasminogen, as well as significantly reducing plasma fibrinogen and macroglobulin, a plasmin inhibitor.[20] Stanozolol tablets may, therefore, be used for the control of the vascular symptoms of cutaneous vasculitis especially in Behcet's disease.

Other uses

3. The prevention and management of recurrent and deep vein thrombosis
Because of its action on plasminogen activator and plasminogen, stanozol has been tried for the prevention of recurrent venous thrombosis as occurs with antithrombin III deficiency and the treatment of the complications of deep vein thrombosis as in venous lipodermatosclerosis.

4. The management of postmenopausal and senile osteoporosis
Osteoporosis is a very common clinical problem and its treatment is unsatisfactory. Anabolic steroids are one of several types of therapy that have been tried[21] but their androgenic action and adverse effects upon hepatic function make them unsuitable.

5. The management of anorexia, asthenia or chronic debilitating diseases
Stanozolol has been used for its anabolic effect in patients suffering from anorexia, asthenia or chronic debilitating diseases where dietary measures alone have proved unsuccessful. There is little evidence of efficacy and it is better to make an aetiological diagnosis and treat the cause.

Contraindications

Stanozolol should not be used in cases of cancer of the prostate because the condition is androgen-dependent. Because of possible virilizing effects on a female fetus, stanozolol should not be administered to pregnant women.

Stanozolol should be used with caution in the presence of impaired renal or cardiac function as it may encourage sodium and water retention.

Care should be taken in administering stanozolol in patients with liver dysfunction. Such patients should be monitored by means of routine liver function tests and treatment discontinued if signs of deterioration are observed.

Tumours of the liver have been reported occasionally in patients subjected to prolonged treatment with androgenic anabolic steroids, especially patients with Fanconi's syndrome and aplastic anaemia. These tumours, however, are not typical of primary hepatocellular carcinoma and in some cases discontinuation of steroids has resulted in tumour regression without other therapy. The possibility that these compounds may induce or enhance the development of hepatic tumours should be considered when the use of this product is proposed for long-term treatment, particularly in patients who are not suffering from life-threatening disorders.

The use of stanozolol preparation may result in an alteration in the ratio of high to low density lipoprotein but the effect upon predisposition to atheroma has not been established.

Anabolic steroids may increase sensitivity to anticoagulants; therefore, the dose of the latter may have to be decreased in order to maintain the prothrombin time at the desired therapeutic level.

Prolonged use in children may lead to premature closure of the epiphyses.

Abuse of anabolic steroids by athletes
Use of anabolic steroids, because they are believed to enhance performance, has become a serious problem, particularly among weight lifters and sprinters. The evidence that anabolic compounds do enhance muscular strength in normal males is not convincing although they undoubtedly can do so in castrates or females.[21] Because of serious side effects, anabolic steroids should not be used to enhance athletic ability. Their use contravenes the rules of most governing bodies of sports.

Adverse reactions

Potentially life-threatening effects
Tumours of the liver have been reported occasionally in patients subjected to prolonged treatment with androgenic anabolic steroids as described under Contraindications.

Acute overdosage
No reports of overdose have appeared.

Severe or irreversible adverse effects
Care should be taken in administering stanozolol to patients with liver dysfunction. Such patients should be monitored by means of routine liver function tests and treatment discontinued if signs of deterioration are observed. Jaundice due to cholestasis has been reported.

Stanozolol should be used with caution in the presence of impaired renal or cardiac function, as it may encourage sodium or water retention.

Symptomatic adverse effects
Stanozolol causes androgenic effects in females depending upon the dose and duration of treatment. These include acne, voice change, amenorrhoea, hirsutism, clitoral hypertrophy and frontal baldness. Fluid retention as evidence by ankle oedema may also occur. Marked tiredness and muscle cramps are usually transitory but may be a troublesome problem. The incidence of migrainous attacks may be increased in patients with a history of migraine.

Other effects
AST (SGOT) is often raised in patients taking stanozolol. Stanozolol appears to affect fibrinolysis, coagulation, and blood lipid levels.[20,22]

Interference with clinical pathology tests
No technical interferences of this kind appear to have been reported.

High risk groups

Neonates
The drug is not used in neonates.

Breast milk. No information is available, but it is assumed that the drug enters breast milk. Consequently, lactating mothers should not breast-feed while taking it.

Children
Prolonged use in children may lead to premature closure of the epiphyses as a direct result of the androgenic effect. Use is not recommended in children less than one year old.

Pregnant women
The drug should not be given to pregnant women as there is a possibility that female fetuses will be virilized.

The elderly
In elderly males, stanozolol should not be used in cases of prostate cancer, as the condition is androgen-dependent.

Concurrent disease
The effects of hepatic, renal, and cardiac disease have been described above.

Drug interactions

Potentially hazardous interactions

Anticoagulants. The sensitivity of anticoagulants may be increased. Stanozolol sensitizes patients to warfarin, necessitating a reduction in dosage of warfarin by 30–50%.

Interaction with cytochrome P450. Stanozolol forms a high-affinity ligand complex with cytochrome P450 and may reduce the substrate interaction of other drugs, especially with such compounds which bind with low affinity to the enzyme.[23]

Clinical trials

1. Burnand K, Clemenson G, Morland M, Jarrett P E M, Browse N L 1980 Venous lipodermatosclerosis: treatment by fibrinolytic enhancement and elastic compression. British Medical Journal 280: 7–11

Thirty-four legs of 23 patients in whom other treatments had failed were studied. The patients were randomly divided into two groups who were treated with either stanozolol plus elastic stockings or placebo plus elastic stockings for three months, and then vice versa, in a double-blind cross-over trial. Treatment with or without stanozolol caused the area of lipodermatosclerosis to decrease, but the authors conclude that the rate of healing was double when patients took stanozolol compared with placebo. Stanozolol also reduced the incidence of extravascular fibrin detected in skin biopsy specimens.

2. Chestnut C H, Ivey J L, Gruber H E, Matthews M, Nelp W B, Sisom K, Baylingk D J 1983 Stanozolol in postmenopausal osteoporosis: therapeutic efficacy and possible mechanisms of action. Metabolism 32: 571–580

A 29-month double-blind study was performed in 23 patients treated with stanozolol and 23 control postmenopausal osteoporotic women. Total body calcium (TBC) increased 4.4% from baseline values ($P<0.01$) in the treated group and remained unchanged in the control group; the difference in the change in TBC between the treated and control groups was significant ($P=0.03$). The effect of the drug on TBC persisted throughout the 29-month period. In contrast to TBC, measurements of regional bone mass (RBM) indicated no significant difference between the treated and placebo group, suggesting a possible differential response to therapy at various skeletal sites.

Other studies

1. Jarrett P E M, Morland M, Browse N L 1978 Treatment of Raynaud's phenomenon by fibrinolytic enhancement. British Medical Journal 2: 523–525
2. Ayres M L, Jarrett P E M, Browse N L 1981 Blood viscosity, Raynaud's phenomenon and the effect of fibrinolytic enhancement. British Journal of Surgery 68: 51–54
3. Sheffer A L, Fearon D T, Austen K F 1981 Clinical and biochemical effects of stanozolol therapy for hereditary angioedema. Journal of Allergy and Clinical Immunology 68: 181–187

General review articles

Burnand K G, Browse N L 1982 The post phlebitic leg and venous ulceration. In: Recent Advances in Surgery No. 11, Russell RCG (ed). pp. 225–246

Burnand K G, Browse N L 1983 Use of fibrinolytic enhancement in the treatment and prevention of recurrent venous ulceration. Practical Cardiology 9: 229–237

Chesnut C H, Baylink D J 1983 The role of anabolic steroids in the treatment of osteoporosis. Geriatric Medicine Today, May 1983

Burge J J 1983 C1-inhibitor deficiency (Hereditary angioedema): case report and review. Virginia Medical 110(12): 706–711

Lowe G D O, Forbes C D (ed) 1980 Anabolic steroids and the fibrinolytic defence system against thrombosis. Scottish Medical Journal: S1–S104

Jarrett P E M, Morland M, Browse N L 1979 The complications of stanozolol and their clinical management. In: Progress in Chemical Fibrinolysis and Thrombolysis IV. Davidson J F (ed), pp 317–321

Stanozolol

Browse N L 1983 Venous ulceration. British Medical Journal 286: 1920–1922

Kluft C, Preston F C, Malia R G, Wijngaards G 1982 Characterization of the effect of stanozolol in fibrinolytic parameters in healthy volunteers. Progress in Fibrinolysis, 6

Davidson J F, Bachman F, Bouvier C A, Kruitof E K O 1982 Progress in Fibrinolysis 6: 513–518

References

1. Gribbin H R, Flavell Matts S G 1976 Mode of action and use of anabolic steroids. British Journal of Clinical Practice 30(1): 3–9
2. Saartok T, Dahlberg E, Gustafsson J 1984 Relative binding affinity of anabolic-androgenic steroids: comparison of the binding to the androgen receptors in skeletal muscle and in prostate, as well as to sex-hormone binding globulin. Endocrinology 114: 2100–2106
3. Beyler A L et al 1960 Reversal by androstanozol of catabolic actions of cortisone acetate. First International Congress of Endocrinology Session VIII f.No. 416: 829
4. Bates P C, Chew L F, Millward D J 1987 Effects of the anabolic steroid stanzolol in growth and protein metabolism in the rat. Journal of Endocrinology 114: 373–381
5. Kowalewski K, Yong S 1968 Effect of growth hormone, an anabolic steroid and cortisone upon various fractions of skin and bone hydroxyproline in mice. Canadian Journal of Physiology and Pharmacology 46: 591–594
6. Jarrett P E M et al 1975 The effect of anabolic steroids on wound healing. Third International Conference on Synthetic Fibrinolytic Thrombolytic Agents. Progress in Fibrinolysis. Glasgow, 28th, 29th and 30th September
7. Vaishnav R, Beresford J N, Gallagher J A, Russell R G G 1988 Effects of the anabolic steroid stanozolol on cells derived from human bone. Clinical Science 74: 455–460
8. Preston F E, Burakowski B K, Porter N R, Malia R G 1981 The fibrinolytic response to stanozolol in normal subjects. Thrombosis Research 22(5/6): 543–551
9. Kluft C, Preston F E, Malia R G et al 1984 Stanozolol-induced changes in fibrinolysis and coagulation in healthy adults. Thrombosis and Haemostastasis (Stuttgart), 51(2):157–164
10. Warin A P et al 1980 Treatment of hereditary angio-oedema by low dose attenuated androgens: dissociation of clinical response from levels of C1 esterase inhibitor and C4. British Journal of Dermatology 103: 405
11. Sheffer A L, Fearon D T, Austen K F 1981 Clinical and biochemical effects of stanozolol therapy for hereditary angioedema. Journal of Allergy and Clinical Immunology 68: 181–187
12. Hosegood J L, Franks A J 1988 Response of human skeletal muscle to the anabolic steroid stanazol. British Medical Journal 297: 1028–1029
13. Magin D F 1975 Gas chromatographic determination of stanozolol in veterinary suspensions. Journal of Chromatography 115: 687–689
14. Shingbal D M Barad U G 1985 Colorimetric determination of stanozolol in pharmaceutical formulations. Journal of the Association of Official Analytical Chemists 68: 98–101
15. Ward R J et al 1975 Gas chromatographic–mass spectrometric methods for the detection and identification of anabolic drugs. British Journal of Sports Medicine 9: 93–97
16. Choo H Y, Kwon O S, Park J 1990 Quantitative determination of stanozolol and its metabolite in urine by gas chromatography/mass spectrometry. Journal of Analytical Toxicology 14: 109–112
17. Conway W D 1963 Metabolic studies on carbon[14]-tagged stanozolol in calves. Data from the files of Sterling-Winthrop Research Institute
18. Massē R, Ayotte C, Bi H G, Dugal R 1989 Studies on anabolic steroids III. Detection and characterization of stanozolol urinary metabolites in humans by gas chromatography mass spectrometry. Journal of Chromatography 497: 17–37
19. Schänzer W, Opfermann G, Donike M 1990 Metabolism of stanozolol: identification and synthesis of urinary metabolites. Journal of Steroid Biochemistry 36: 153-174
20. Small M, McArdle B M, Lowe G D O, Forbes C D, Prentice C R M 1982 The effect of intramuscular stanozolol on fibrinolysis and blood lipids. Thrombosis Research 28: 27–36
21. Chesnut C H, Ivey J L, Gruber H E 1983 Stanozolol in postmenopausal osteoporosis: therapeutic efficacy and possible mechanisms of action. Metabolism 32: 571–580
22. Wilson J D, Griffin J E 1980 The use and misuse of androgens. Metabolism 29: 1278–1295
23. Rendic S, Ruf H H 1988 Interaction of stanozolol with cytochrome p-450 Biochemical Pharmacology 37: 766–768
24. Kluft C 1984 Pharmacological stimulation of endogenous fibrinolysis. Haemostasis 14: 35

Stilboestrol

Stilboestrol was the first synthetic, non-steroidal oestrogen with actions and uses similar to those of oestradiol.

Chemistry

Stilboestrol (diethylstilboestrol, stilbestrol, diethylstilbestrol, DES, Desma, Dicorvin, Stibilium, Stilbol, Distilbene)
$C_{18}H_{20}O_2$
(E)-$\alpha\beta$-Diethylstilbene-4-4′-diol
The *trans* form is the active form

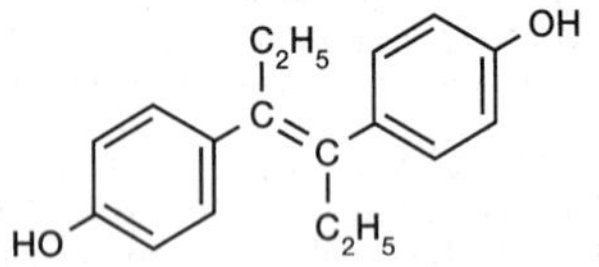

Molecular weight	268.4
pKa	—
Solubility	
in alcohol	1 in 5
in water	<1 in 10 000
Octanol/water partition coefficient	high

Stilboestrol is an almost white, odourless, tasteless, crystalline powder prepared by chemical synthesis. It is also available in combination with a lactic acid base in vaginal pessary form (Tampovagan Stilboestrol and Lactic Acid).

Pharmacology

Stilboestrol has oestrogenic effects affecting sexual characteristics, development of the uterus, fallopian tubes, vagina and breasts. In low concentrations it stimulates gonadotrophins and lactogenic activities of the anterior pituitary, and in high concentrations depresses these activities.

It has an antiandrogenic effect due to the inhibition of pituitary luteinizing hormones, and increases the levels of sex-hormone-binding globulin.

Toxicology

Administration of stilboestrol to laboratory animals has been shown to lead to tumours of endocrine/hormone-dependent sites, such as ovary, testes and breast.[1] Stilboestrol administration to golden hamsters leads to the development of adenocarcinoma of the kidney.[2]

Clinical pharmacology

Stilboestrol, when given orally, has approximately three to five times the oestrogenic potency of oestrone, a metabolite of oestradiol. Oestrone, C17 ketone, has only 10% of the activity of oestradiol.[3] The recommended dose of stilboestrol is 1–3 mg daily but doses up to 100 mg twice daily have been used for carcinoma of the prostate and 10–20 mg daily for carcinoma of the breast, though doses of 1500 mg daily have been used.

The following pharmacological actions have been demonstrated.

1. Sexual characteristics
Stilboestrol stimulates secondary sexual characteristics in the female: growth of axillary and pubic hair; maturation of skin; alterations in body contour; hypertrophy of breasts; closure of long-bone epiphyses and changes in the voice.

2. Uterus, fallopian tubes, vagina and breasts
Stilboestrol induces proliferation of the vaginal epithelium with an increase in the thickness of the superficial stratified layers, and a great increase in their glycogen content. Doderlein's bacilli convert the glycogen into lactic acid, making the vaginal environment acidic and resistant to pathogenic microorganisms.

Secretion of mucus by the cervical glands is augmented. In puberty, hypertrophy of the uterus, fallopian tubes and lower genital tract occurs due to the effect of oestrogen. Stilboestrol induces endometrial proliferation.

In pregnancy, stilboestrol stimulates proliferation of the mammary glands, endometrial hypertrophy and vascularity.[3]

3. Action on the pituitary
Stilboestrol in low concentrations stimulates the gonadotrophic and lactogenic activities of the pituitary, and in large amounts, depresses these activities.

4. Antiandrogen effect
Stilboestrol is a potent inhibitor of pituitary LH release, and thus inhibits the release of testosterone. It also increases the levels of sex-hormone-binding globulin, thus decreasing the circulating, free testosterone.

5. Cytostatic properties
Stilboestrol is cytostatic to fertilized sea urchin eggs[4,5] and also to the rat Walker carcinosarcoma;[6] however, cytostatic effects of stilboestrol on androgen-dependent tissues in man have not been convincingly demonstrated.

There are widespread metabolic and endocrine effects, including increased bony calcification, increased plasma renin and angiotensin, increased thyroid-binding globulin, and cortisol-binding globulin. Increases are also seen in cholesterol, triglyceride and high density lipoproteins,[7] and in factors seven to ten of the clotting mechanism,[8] together with a decrease in fibrinolysis, and an increase in sodium retention.[9,10]

Pharmacokinetics

Quantification is by gas chromatography with flame ionization detection, or by HPLC with UV detection.[11]

Stilboestrol is almost completely absorbed after oral administration. It is also readily absorbed through the skin, vaginally, and rectally. Peak levels in plasma are observed within the first two hours after administration. Most of an oral dose is excreted by the liver, and the drug is subject to presystemic metabolism. The main metabolite is the stilboestrol monoglucuronide.

Oral absorption	>90%
Presystemic metabolism	High
Plasma half life	—
Volume of distribution	$5\ l.kg^{-1}$
Plasma protein binding	—

Presystemic elimination by the liver can be increased by induction of drug-metabolizing enzymes.[12]

Stilboestrol is distributed throughout the body to most tissues, including liver, fat, kidneys, prostate, bladder, spleen and lungs.[13,14]

In monkeys, stilboestrol has a volume of distribution at steady state of approximately $5\ l.kg^{-1}$, and is subject to enterohepatic circulation.

In plasma stilboestrol is bound to sex-hormone-binding-globulin and, to a lesser extent, to albumin. Placental transfer of stilboestrol occurs, as evidenced by an increase in genital cancer in the offspring of women receiving the drug. Stilboestrol is likely to be excreted in breast milk.

The kinetics of the drug are unlikely to be affected by renal dysfunction or old age. The elimination of stilboestrol is likely to be impaired in hepatic dysfunction.

Concentration–effect relationship

Information on concentration–effect relationships is not available. However, an oral dose of less than 1 mg a day does not produce any suppression of plasma testosterone. A dose of 1 mg per day produces incomplete suppression of plasma testosterone, but not into the castrate range. A dose of 3–5 mg per day produces complete suppression.

Metabolism

Stilboestrol is extensively metabolized in the liver by conjugation, either to the glucuronides or, to a lesser extent, sulphates. The conjugated metabolites are excreted into the bile and pass into the intestinal lumen, where they are extensively hydrolysed by the gut flora. The deconjugated compounds are reabsorbed and returned to the liver by the enterohepatic circulation (Fig. 1).[15]

Fig. 1 Enterohepatic circulation of stilboestrol

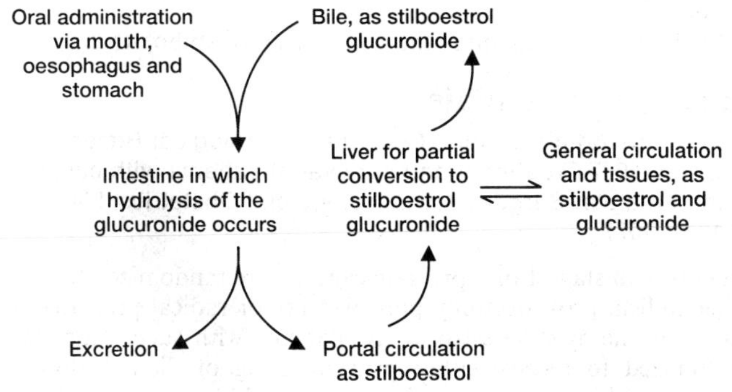

In man, 70% of the oestrogenic metabolites are excreted in the urine, and 30% in the faeces. Any disturbance of liver function or of intestinal flora can alter the metabolism of the drug.

Pharmaceutics

Stilboestrol is available as oral tablets and as vaginal pessaries in the UK.

1. Tablets containing 1 mg and 5 mg of stilboestrol BP. There are two presentations: plain, round, bi-convex, white tablets available in the two strengths; and plain, round, bi-convex pink sugar-coated tablets available in the two strengths.
2. Tampovagan Stilboestrol and Lactic Acid (Norgine, UK): Vaginal pessaries, each containing stilboestrol 500 µg with lactic acid 5% in a macrogel base. The pessaries are off-white in colour.

The tablets should be stored in an airtight container in a dry place below 25°C and protected from light. Pessaries should be stored in a cool, dry place.

In the USA there are also stilboestrol injection preparations: diethylstilbestrol injection, a sterile solution of stilboestrol in a suitable vegetable oil (these should be protected from light); and diethylstilbestrol suppositories (store in a cool, dry place in airtight containers).

For the diphophonate see Fosfestrol.

Therapeutic use

Indications

In 1971 stilboestrol was shown to have carcinogenic potential and its use is now restricted to the management of:

1. Patients with metastatic malignant disease of the prostate
2. Postmenopausal carcinoma of the breast.

Prior to 1971, stilboestrol was used for:

3. Menopausal symptoms
4. Secondary amenorrhoea due to ovarian insufficiency
5. Senile vaginitis and kraurosis vulvae
6. Inhibition of lactation
7. Post-coital contraception
8. Genital hypoplasia
9. Infantilism
10. Management of pregnancy in diabetes
11. Prevention of miscarriages and premature births
12. Management of toxaemia of pregnancy
13. Carcinoma of the breast
14. Carcinoma of the prostate.

Stilboestrol

Contraindications

1. Pregnant women
2. Children
3. Porphyria
4. Severe hypertension
5. Active liver disease
6. A history of thromboembolism and conditions predisposing to it, for example, sickle cell anaemia, untreated polycythaemia, pulmonary hypertension
7. Family history or previous history of neoplastic disease of the genital tract
8. Premenopausal carcinoma of the breast
9. Undiagnosed vaginal bleeding
10. Recent surgery.

Mode of use

Clinical use is based on the suppression of androgenic hormonal activity in the management of carcinoma of the prostate. Its use in carcinoma of the breast is dependent on its binding to the cytoplasmic oestrogen receptor and interfering with genetic programming in the nucleus of the malignant cell.

Doses for the treatment of carcinoma of the prostate are from 1–3 mg daily, and for carcinoma of the breast, 10–20 mg daily.

Stilboestrol therapy is long-term. Patient compliance is important. It has been shown that suppressed testosterone levels can return to within normal range within 12 hours of neglecting to take a daily 1 mg dose of stilboestrol.[16]

Indications

1. Prostatic carcinoma

Stilboestrol is losing popularity for the treatment of carcinoma of the prostate because of the associated cardiovascular side effects. Though a study of low-dose stilboestrol versus orchidectomy has never been performed, it is unlikely that there will be significant differences between these forms of treatment. The recent availability of LHRH analogues which produce a medical orchidectomy without the side effects of stilboestrol therapy significantly reduces the role of stilboestrol in the treatment of prostatic cancer.[26]

When stilboestrol is used in the treatment of patients with advanced metastatic prostate cancer there is no evidence that it prolongs the patient's survival, and there is probably no advantage in treating the asymptomatic patient. The dose used is 1–3 mg daily. This should be continued for as long as the tumour shows evidence of response.

Mode of action. Between 40–60% of malignant prostatic tumours are dependent on androgens for their continued growth. Stilboestrol suppresses pituitary luteinizing hormone secretion, resulting in a fall in testosterone concentrations equivalent to that of castration. It also increases the level of sex-hormone-binding globulin, which results in a lowering of the concentration of free testosterone.

2. Breast cancer

Stilboestrol is only indicated in patients with postmenopausal breast carcinoma who have not responded to the anti-oestrogen tamoxifen. Dose used is 10–20 mg daily.

Mode of action. Its mode of action is not fully understood but there is a higher percentage response rate in patients whose tumour is oestrogen-receptor positive.

Contraindications

1. Pregnancy

An increased incidence of genital tract cancer in the female offspring and in urethral abnormalities in male offspring has been reported.[17–19] A higher incidence of sub-fertility in males in later life has been reported when their mothers were treated with oestrogens during pregnancy.[20]

2. Children

Stilboestrol inhibits growth,[21] inhibits sexual characteristics in male children and leads to feminization.

Two children with muscular dystrophy developed acanthosis nigricans when treated with stilboestrol.[22]

3. Porphyria
Stilboestrol may precipitate attacks of porphyria.

4–6. Cardiovascular abnormalities
Stilboestrol has been associated with an increased risk of cardiovascular complications from pulmonary emboli, cerebrovascular accidents, myocardial infarction, and congestive cardiac failure. [9,10,23–26] It has been reported that oestrogen administration decreases antithrombin-3 levels into the hypercoagulable range.[27–29] It also causes an increased tendency for platelet aggregation.[30]

5. Active liver disease
Elevations of liver enzymes have been reported at the beginning of therapy with stilboestrol.[31] It has been associated with the development of cholestatic jaundice, and reduces liver excretory function.[32] Excessive lipid deposition has been found in the livers of animals treated with oestrogen.[3]

8. Premenopausal carcinoma of the breast
Stilboestrol accelerates the course of the carcinoma of the breast in premenopausal women and should be avoided.

Adverse reactions

Potentially life-threatening effects
Deaths due to stilboestrol are a consequence of its thromboembolic (see below) or hepatotoxic effects and not of idiosyncrasy.

Acute overdosage
There is no specific antidote to stilboestrol.

The commonest symptoms of overdosage are nausea and vomiting.

Management is by gastric lavage together with adequate monitoring of electrolytes and appropriate symptomatic relief.

Severe or irreversible adverse effects
Thromboembolic effects, including cerebral and coronary thrombosis, have been frequently associated with the use of stilboestrol. Other severe reactions include testicular atrophy and impotence.

Symptomatic adverse effects
These are related to its oestrogenic activities, and include breast discomfort, breast enlargement and nipple tenderness. Nausea and vomiting are also common.

Other effects
Stilboestrol has been reported to cause transient abnormalities of liver function tests.[31] High-dose stilboestrol elevates serum triglyceride concentrations as well as pre-beta lipoproteins.[10]

Increases in renin, angiotensin II, and aldosterone have also been reported.[10]

Interference with clinical pathology tests
The drug may interfere with some methods of measuring oestrogens in urine.

High risk groups

Neonates
Stilboestrol is not indicated in view of the carcinogenic potential.

Breast milk. A decreased milk volume may occur if diethylstilboestrol is used during lactation. The drug is not indicated in lactating mothers in view of the carcinogenic potential.

Children
Stilboestrol is not indicated in view of the carcinogenic potential.

Pregnant women
Stilboestrol is not indicated in view of the carcinogenic potential.

The elderly
Stilboestrol is contraindicated in the elderly if any cardiovascular abnormalities are present.

Concurrent disease
As mentioned under Contraindications the drug should not be used in patients with hypertension, heart disease, liver disease, thromboembolic disease or conditions, or conditions predisposing to these disorders, neoplasma of the breast or vagina, or porphyria.

Drug interactions

Potentially hazardous interactions
Concomitant administration of hepatotoxic drugs and stilboestrol may result in increased hepatotoxicity.

Other significant interactions
Antibiotics. The gut-sterilizing effect of antibiotics shortens the half life of stilboestrol by affecting the enterohepatic circulation.[33]

Liver microsomal enzyme inducers. Phenobarbitone and rifampicin enhance glucuronidation and an increased biliary excretion of conjugated stilboestrol, resulting in a lowered clinical effect.[12]

Food. The dissolution of stilboestrol crystals is inhibited by most permitted food colorants. Cationic dyes have a greater effect than anionic dyes.

Tobacco. This enhances the metabolism of stilboestrol.

Major outcome trials

1. Veterans Administration Cooperative Urological Research Group 1967 Treatment and survival of patients with cancer of the prostate. Surgery, Gynaecology and Obstetrics 124: 1011–1077

Patients with stage 1 or 2 prostate cancer were randomized to receive either radical prostatectomy plus placebo, or radical prostatectomy plus 5 mg diethylstilboestrol daily. Patients with stage 3 or 4 were randomized to receive either placebo, 5 mg of diethylstilboestrol daily, or orchidectomy plus placebo, or orchidectomy plus 5 mg of diethylstilboestrol.

The results of this study showed that overall survival was significantly worse in patients with stage 1 tumours who received 5 mg of diethylstilboestrol but no significant differences were observed in those with stage 2 tumours. Survival was also significantly worse in patients with stage 3 tumours who received orchidectomy plus 5 mg of diethylstilboestrol daily than in those who received the placebo alone, or orchidectomy plus placebo. No statistical differences were observed among patients with stage 4 tumours. Survival curves constructed for cause of death showed that patients with the advanced tumours who received 5 mg of diethylstilboestrol had a significantly higher cardiovascular death rate. Most deaths occurring during the first year of therapy were in patients with an underlying cardiovascular disease, and a correspondingly significantly lower death rate from prostate cancer.

2. Byar D P 1973 The Veterans Administration Cooperative Urological Research Group Studies of Cancer of the Prostate. Cancer 32: 1126–1130

Patients with stage 3 or 4 tumours were randomized to receive either placebo, 0.2 mg of diethylstilboestrol daily, 1 mg of diethylstilboestrol daily, or 5 mg of diethylstilboestrol daily. The results of this study showed that a 1 mg dose of diethylstilboestrol was as effective as a 5 mg dose, and significantly more effective than the 0.2 mg dose or placebo in preventing cancer deaths, and was not associated with an increased incidence of cardiovascular deaths.

This study also demonstrated that both 5 mg and 1 mg doses of stilboestrol significantly retarded the rate of progression from stage 3 to stage 4 cancer.

3. Peeling W B 1989 Phase III studies to compare goserelin (Zoladex) with orchidectomy and with diethylstilboestrol in the treatment of prostatic carcinoma. Urology 33 (suppl): 45–52

Two multi-centre, open, randomized Phase III clinical trials compared the effectiveness and safety of the depot formulation of a luteinizing hormone, releasing hormone agonist, goserelin 3.6 mg subcutaneously over each 28th day with orchidectomy and with diethylstilboestrol 1 mg three times a day in the treatment of prostatic carcinoma.

In the goserelin versus diethylstilboestrol trial, subjective and objective responses, response duration and survival were similar. However, there was a more rapid response in the depot goserelin group.

Side effects from goserelin, such as flare symptoms during the initial stages of treatment, required no discontinuation of therapy, whereas 15% of the patients receiving diethylstilboestrol required

Stilboestrol

cessation of therapy during the first three months because of side effects, which were mainly of a cardiovascular nature.

4. Carter A C, Sedransk N, Kelly K et al 1977 Diethylstilboestrol: recommended dosages from different categories of breast cancer patients. Report of the Cooperative Breast Cancer Group. Journal of the American Medical Association 237: 2079–2085

A total of 523 postmenopausal breast cancer patients with progressive disease were entered in a randomized, double-blind study of four dosages of diethylstilboestrol, 1.5, 15, 150 or 1500 mg daily. Sixteen centres were involved. Diethylstilboestrol was used as the first hormonal therapy following diagnosis of recurrent metastatic or inoperable carcinoma of the breast.

The study was designed to determine the dose–response relationships for stilboestrol and to assess menopausal age and site of metastatic disease as factors affecting responsiveness to oestrogen therapy.

Therapy was continued for a minimum of 12 weeks unless compelling progression of disease intervened.

Results

1. Regression. Higher dosages produced significantly ($p<0.05$) higher regression rates:
21% for 1500 mg daily dosage
17% for 150 mg
15% for 15 mg
10% for 1.5 mg.
High dose of 1500 mg daily was shown to be the treatment of choice in three groups of patients:

i. those one to five years postmenopausal with local disease
ii. those one to five years postmenopausal with visceral disease
iii. those ten or more years postmenopausal with local disease.

A daily dosage of 1.5 mg was the treatment of choice in those who were at least 5 but less than 10 years postmenopausal with osseous disease and local disease.

A daily dosage of 15 mg was found to be the treatment of choice in those with osseous disease and one to five years or more than ten years postmenopausal.

A daily dosage of 150 mg was to be recommended for those more than five years postmenopausal with visceral disease.

If, after six weeks, there is a definite progression of the malignant disease, the patients should be treated with 1500 mg daily of stilboestrol.

Side effects

Both gastrointestinal and the usual oestrogen-related adverse effects were worse at the highest dosage. However, cardiovascular complications were seen most frequently with the 15 mg dosage.

References

1. Lacassagne A 1936 Tumeurs malignes apparues au cours d'un traitement hormonal combiné, chez des souris appartenant à des lignées réfractaires au cancer spontane. Comptes Rendus, Societé de Biologie (Paris) 121: 607–609
2. Matthews V S, Kirkman H, Bacon R L 1947 Kidney damage in the golden hamster following chronic administration of diethylstilbestrol and sesame oil. Proceedings of the Society of Experimental Biology 66: 195–196
3. White A, Handler P, Smith E 1973 Principles of biochemistry, 5th edn. McGraw-Hill, London, pp 1062–1067
4. Druckrey H, Raabe S 1952 Organspezifische Chemotherapie des Krebs (Prostata-Karzinom). Klinische Wochenschrift 30: 882–884
5. Druckrey H, Danneberg P, Schmähl D 1952 Mitosegist-wirkung von Oestrogenen. Zjournals Naturwissen Schaften, Berlin 39: 381–382
6. Schmähl D 1954 Zytotoxische Wirkungen des Stilbostrols auf die Zellen des Walker-carcinoms der ratte. Arzneimittel Forschung 4: 479–481
7. Kontturi M, Sotaniemi E 1971 Thromboembolism during estrogen therapy of prostatic cancer. Report on two cases. Scandinavian Journal of Urology and Nephrology 5: 108–110
8. Daniel D G, Bloom A L, Giddings J, Campbell H, Turnbull A C 1968 Increased Factor IX levels in puerperium during administration of diethylstilboestrol. British Medical Journal 1: 801–803
9. Dignam W S, Voskian J, Assali N S 1956 Effects of estrogens on renal hemodynamics and excretion of electrolytes in human subjects. Journal of Clinical Endocrinology 16: 1032–1042
10. Blyth B, McRae C U, Espiner E A, Nicholls M G, Conglaen J V, Gilchrist N 1985 Effect of stilboestrol on sodium balance, cardiac state and renin–angiotensin–aldosterone activity in prostatic carcinoma. British Medical Journal 291: 1461–1464
11. Clarke's Isolation and Identification of Drugs 1986 Stilboestrol, Moffat A C, Jackson J V, Moss M S and Wigldop B, eds. The Pharmaceutical Press, London pp 975–976
12. Levine W G, Millburn P, Smith R L, Williams R T 1970 The role of hepatic endoplasmic reticulum in the biliary excretion of foreign compounds by the rat. The effect of phenobarbitone and SKF 525-A. Biochemical Pharmacology 19: 235–244
13. Perklev T 1964 Distribution of excretion of radioactivity after parenteral administration of radioactive polydiethylstilbestrol phosphate to rats and cows. Proceedings of the Society for Experimental Biology and Medicine 117: 394–398
14. Johnson W, Jasmin R, Corte G 1961 Enzymic hydrolysis of stilbestrol diphosphate in vitro and in vivo. Proceedings of the Society for Experimental Biology and Medicine 106: 327–330
15. Fischer L J, Kent T H, Weissinger J L 1973 Absorption of diethylstilbestrol and its glucuronide conjugate from the intestines of five and twenty-five day old rats. Journal of Pharmacology and Experimental Therapeutics 185: 163–170
16. Beck B H, McAnish J W, Coebel J L, Stutzman R E 1978 Plasma testosterone in patients receiving diethylstilbestrol. Urology 11: 157–160
17. Greenwald P, Barlow J J, Nasca P C, Burnett W S 1971 Vaginal cancer after maternal treatment with synthetic estrogen. New England Journal of Medicine 285: 390–392
18. Herbst A L, Kurman R J, Scully R E, Poskanzer D C 1972 Clear cell adenocarcinoma of the genital tract in young females. New England Journal of Medicine 287: 1259–1264
19. Herbst A L, Kurman R J, Scully R E 1972 Vaginal and cervical abnormalities after exposure to stilbestrol in utero. Obstetrics and Gynecology 40: 287–298
20. Gill W B, Schumacher G L B, Bibbo M, Straus F H, Schoenberg H W 1979 Association of diethylstilbestrol exposure in utero with cryptorchidism, testicular hypoplasia, and semen abnormalities. Journal of Urology 122: 36–39
21. Norman H, Wettenhall B, Cahill C, Roche A 1975 Tall girls: a survey of 15 years of management and treatment. Journal of Paediatrics 86: 602–610
22. Banuchi S R, Cohen L, Lorincz A L, Morgan J 1974 Acanthosis nigricans following diethylstilboestrol therapy: occurrence in patients with childhood muscular dystrophy. Archives of Dermatology 109: 545–546
23. Byar D R 1973 The Veterans Administration Cooperative Urological Research Group's Studies of Cancer of the Prostate. Cancer 32: 1126–1130
24. Glashan R W, Robinson M R G 1981 Cardiovascular complications in the treatment of prostatic carcinoma. British Journal of Urology 53: 624–627
25. Daniel D G, Campbell H, Turnbull A C 1967 Puerperal thromboembolism and suppression of lactation. Lancet 2: 287–289
26. Peeling W B 1989 Phase III studies to compare goserelin (Zoladex) with orchiectomy and with diethylstilboestrol in the treatment of prostatic carcinoma. Urology 33 (suppl): 45–52
27. Dobbs R M, Barber J A, Weigel J W, Bergin J E 1980 Clotting predisposition in carcinoma of the prostate. Journal of Urology 123: 706–709
28. Varenhorst E, Wallentin L, Risberg B 1981 Re: Clotting predisposition in carcinoma of the prostate (letter). Journal of Urology 126: 419
29. Buller H R, Boon T A, Henny C P, Dabhoiwala N Y, Ten Cate J W 1982 Estrogen-induced deficiency and decrease in antithrombin III activity in patients with prostatic cancer. Journal of Urology 128: 72–74
30. Eisen M, Napp H E, Vock R 1975 Inhibition of platelet aggregation caused by oestrogen treatment in patients with carcinoma of the prostate. Journal of Urology 114: 93–97
31. Kontturi M, Sotaniemi E 1969 Effect of oestrogen on liver function of prostatic cancer patients. British Medical Journal 4: 204–205
32. Clinch J, Tindall V R 1969 Effect of oestrogens and prostogens on liver function in the puerperium. British Medical Journal 1: 602–605
33. Clarke A G, Fischer L J, Millburn P, Smith R L, Williams R T 1969 The role of gut flora in the enterohepatic circulation of stilboestrol in the rat. Biochemical Journal 112: 17P 18P

S Streptokinase

Streptokinase is a plasminogen activator and is the most widely used thrombolytic agent.

Chemistry

Streptokinase (Streptase, Kabikinase).

Molecular weight	47 408
pKa	—
Solubility	
in alcohol	denatured
in water	>1 in 10
Octanol/water partition coefficient	low

Streptokinase is a single-chain protein obtained from certain strains of group Cβ haemolytic streptococci. It is a hygroscopic white powder or friable solid. It is freely soluble in water. but unstable in solutions of less than 10 000 IU.ml^{-1}. It is available in combination with streptodornase (Varidase).

Pharmacology

Streptokinase induces fibrinolysis by activating plasminogen. The first step in this process is the formation of an equimolar complex of plasminogen with streptokinase. This induces conformational changes in the plasminogen which promote the conversion of circulating uncomplexed plasminogen into plasmin. The streptokinase/plasminogen complex is itself rapidly converted to a streptokinase/plasmin complex which also has the ability to convert plasminogen to plasmin. Plasmin then promotes fibrinolysis by digesting fibrinogen and fibrin in the thrombus and in the circulation. The fibrinogen and fibrin degradation products produced by this process may, themselves, have an anticoagulant effect.[1,2]

Toxicology

Very little toxicology work has been performed in animals.

Clinical pharmacology

The administration of streptokinase produces a fall in circulating plasminogen concentrations and an increase in circulating plasmin concentrations. High plasmin concentrations induce fibrinolysis and can also produce a coagulation defect, due partly to reduced levels of fibrinogen, factor V and factor VIII, and partly to the presence of fibrinogen–fibrin degradation products.[3]

An international unit (IU) of streptokinase, which is equivalent to a Christensen or US unit, is the quantity of streptokinase that will lyse a standard blood clot completely in 10 minutes.

Clinical studies have demonstrated that intravenous streptokinase can promote thrombus dissolution in arterial and venous thromboembolic disease. The extent and rate of thrombolysis depend on the structure of the thrombus, particularly its plasminogen content,[4] as well as on the intensity of the fibrinolytic state.[5] Thrombi that are more than 5 to 7 days old are more resistant to thrombolytic therapy.[3,6]

A variety of dosage regimens have been used for systemic thrombolytic therapy. In the past most regimens have utilized an initial loading dose of between 250 000 and 600 000 IU followed by an initial maintenance dose of 100 000 IU.h^{-1}. The maintenance dose is then adjusted according to tests of plasma thrombolytic activity such as the thrombin time or the activated partial thromboplastin time.[7]

The purpose of the loading dose is to neutralize circulating anti-streptokinase antibody present as the result of previous streptococcal infection. Such antibodies can be detected in most people, and may be present in amounts equivalent to as much as 400 IU streptokinase per ml of plasma.[8] Although the loading dose can be individually tailored using the streptokinase resistance test,[9] a loading dose of 250 000 IU will neutralize all antibody in about 90% of patients.[10] Hence, standard dosage regimens will produce rapid and sustained thrombolysis in the vast majority of patients.[3,5]

More recently, an alternative dose regimen for systemic thrombolytic therapy has been introduced, in which a single very high dose (e.g. 1.5 million IU) of streptokinase is given intravenously over a period of 30 to 60 minutes. In theory, this strategy should promote thrombolysis by ensuring high concentrations of streptokinase in the region of the thrombus, and may reduce the incidence of haemorrhagic complications by avoiding a prolonged generalized fibrinolytic state.[11]

In some situations thrombolysis may be achieved by infusing lower doses of streptokinase directly into the affected vessel. This strategy has obvious logistic and technical drawbacks but may help to prevent some of the complications associated with systemic therapy. An example of this approach is the use of intracoronary streptokinase for the treatment of acute coronary thrombosis, where an initial dose of 10 000 to 30 000 IU has been infused, followed by between 2000 and 4000 IU.min^{-1}, up to a maximum of 500 000 IU.

Pharmacokinetics

Plasma concentrations of streptokinase are seldom measured because it is easier and more appropriate to monitor indices such as the thrombin time, activated partial thromboplastin time, and plasma concentrations of plasminogen activator complex, plasminogen, plasmin and fibrinogen.[5]

Plasma streptokinase concentrations reach a peak at 2 to 3 minutes after intravenous administration,[12] and peak fibrinolytic activity occurs at approximately 30 minutes, depending on the dose.

Streptokinase is cleared from the plasma in two phases.[13] The first phase has an average half time of 18 minutes, and is due to the presence of anti-streptokinase antibody which combines with streptokinase to produce a complex that is cleared rapidly from the circulation.[13] The second phase is slower, with a half time of approximately 80 minutes,[4] and reflects the rate at which streptokinase combines with plasminogen. Hence, the clearance rate will vary, according to the availability of plasminogen and the dose regimen used.[4]

Oral absorption	negligible
Presystemic metabolism	—
Plasma half life	
phase I	18 min
phase II	80 min
Volume of distribution	—
Plasma protein binding	—

Concentration–effect relationship

The therapeutic and toxic effects of a given dose of streptokinase depend on several factors, including the amount of anti-streptokinase antibody present and the availability of plasminogen. In the presence of a normal plasminogen concentration a large loading dose of streptokinase will result in the rapid production of plasmin. If the rate at which plasmin is formed exceeds the availability of neutralizing antiplasmins, a coagulation defect will occur. However, the rate of plasmin production will fall as plasminogen is consumed, so that any coagulation defect is likely to be short-lived.

The effects of maintenance streptokinase therapy are dependent on the concentration of circulating plasminogen during the infusion. Hence, if the loading dose is too large, maintenance therapy may be ineffective because there is not enough plasminogen for the streptokinase to act on. On the other hand, if the loading dose is too small, plasminogen will be freely available and maintenance therapy may result in an unwanted coagulation defect due to excessive plasmin production. The optimum circulating plasminogen concentration during maintenance therapy appears to be approximately 5% of the normal value.[3] The thrombolytic effects of streptokinase may also depend on the concentration of plasminogen in the clot itself.

Streptokinase

Clearly there is a complicated relationship between dose and effect during maintenance streptokinase therapy. Accordingly, many authorities advocate monitoring therapy by measuring the thrombin time, which should be kept between two and five times the normal value.[4] Although this will confirm activation of the fibrinolytic system, it cannot be used to predict clot lysis or haemorrhagic complications.[14] If there is no increase in the thrombin time this may be due to either excess antibody (detectable by the streptokinase resistance test), in which case the dose should be increased, or insufficient plasminogen, when the dose should be reduced. If the thrombin time becomes greatly prolonged, therapy should be discontinued until it returns to the normal range, when therapy can be restarted at a lower dose.[2] An alternative, and potentially hazardous, strategy is to increase the maintenance dose in the expectation that this will lead to increased consumption of plasminogen, thereby reducing the amount of free plasminogen available for conversion to plasmin.

Metabolism

The metabolism of streptokinase in man is intricately linked to its mode of action. A proportion of the initial dose will be inactivated by circulating anti-streptokinase antibody (see above), while the remainder binds to plasminogen, producing an active complex which catalyses the conversion of circulating plasminogen to plasmin. During this process the streptokinase is proteolytically degraded into several low molecular weight fragments.[2,15]

Pharmaceutics

1. Streptase (Hoechst UK/USA): a sterile lyophilized powder in vials containing 100 000 (UK), 250 000 and 750 000 and 1 500 000 (USA) IU of purified streptokinase.
2. Kabikinase (KabiVitrum UK/Smithkline Beecham USA): a sterile straw coloured lyophilized powder in vials containing 100 000, 250 000, 600 000, 750 000 (USA) IU of streptokinase.
3. Varidase (Lederle, UK/US): a sterile powder in vials containing 100 000 IU of streptokinase, 25 000 IU of streptodornase and 2 mg of thiomersal; for topical use only.

1. and 2. above contain sodium L-glutamate and human albumin as stabilizers. Lyophilized streptokinase is stable for three years at room temperature. The powder is freely soluble in water and may be reconstituted for infusion in 5% dextrose, physiological saline, or polygeline.[16] Maximum activity occurs in neutral solutions; all activity is lost below pH 5 and above pH 9. Streptokinase is unstable in dilute solution; accordingly, reconstituted material should be discarded if not used immediately.

Therapeutic use

Indications

1. Acute myocardial infarction
2. Acute pulmonary embolism
3. Acute deep-vein thrombosis
4. Other acute venous or arterial thrombosis
5. Thrombosis on prosthetic materials (e.g. arteriovenous shunts, heart valves and vascular grafts)
6. Desloughing wounds (topical use: Varidase).

Contraindications

1. Bleeding diathesis
2. Recent trauma (e.g. surgery, head injury, resuscitation)
3. Severe hypertension
4. Recent peptic ulcer
5. Stroke
6. Other conditions associated with increased risk of bleeding
7. Known allergy to streptokinase
8. Streptokinase treatment within last 12 months.

Mode of use

All the clinical uses depend on the ability of streptokinase to lyse thrombi. Several dosage regimens are in use. Streptokinase may be given locally or systemically. When used systemically, thrombolysis may be achieved with either a single large intravenous dose given over a short period (for example, 1.5 million IU in one hour) or an intravenous loading dose followed by intravenous maintenance therapy for several days (for example, 250 000 IU in 30 minutes followed by 100 000 IU.h^{-1}).

Indications

1. Acute myocardial infarction

Angiographic studies have shown that, in the acute phase of myocardial infarction, a substantial proportion of patients have coronary artery occlusion, and that recanalization can be achieved by using either intracoronary or intravenous thrombolytic agents. Intravenous therapy can be given far more easily — and perhaps an hour or so more promptly — than intracoronary therapy can. An overview of several trials of prolonged intravenous infusion and several large multi-centre trials of high-dose short-term infusions (see 'Major outcome trials') have shown that intravenous thrombolytic therapy improves left ventricular function, and reduces mortality in acute myocardial infarction. Currently the best established — and perhaps simplest — regimen involves a single one-hour intravenous infusion of 1.5 million IU of streptokinase, but other regimens are being studied. Although it has been suggested that, in order to prevent reocclusion, thrombolysis should be followed by some other intervention (such as anticoagulant or antiplatelet therapy, coronary angioplasty, or coronary artery bypass surgery), only antiplatelet therapy (with low-dose aspirin) has been shown to produce added benefit after streptokinase.[17]

2. Acute pulmonary embolism

Streptokinase is used to treat patients suffering from life-threatening pulmonary embolism, with the aim of lysing clots in the pulmonary circulation (thereby reversing any haemodynamic disturbance) and lysing clots in the deep veins (thereby avoiding further embolism). Most authorities recommend an initial loading dose of 250 000 IU infused in 30 minutes, followed by an infusion of 100 000 IU.h^{-1} given into a peripheral vein or into the pulmonary artery via an indwelling catheter; both routes of administration have been shown to be effective.[18,19] Successful therapy is usually followed by a period of anticoagulation with heparin and/or warfarin. If therapy is not successful, embolectomy may be indicated.

Pulmonary angiography, right heart pressure studies, and radioisotope lung scanning have shown that, in massive embolism, the rate of dissolution of pulmonary emboli is greater in patients treated with streptokinase or urokinase than in patients treated with heparin alone.[14,18,19,20] There is no clear evidence, however, that thrombolytic therapy has any greater effect on mortality than does heparin. For, although it has been reported that patients in shock (systolic blood pressure $<$ 100 mmHg) have a lower mortality when treated with streptokinase, this result derives from a retrospective analysis of a non-randomized study.[20]

3. Acute deep-vein thrombosis

Intravenous streptokinase, starting with an initial loading dose of about 500 000 IU and followed by a maintenance infusion of about 100 000 IU.h^{-1}, has been compared with heparin anticoagulation in six randomized trials of the treatment of phlebographically demonstrated acute proximal deep-vein thrombosis.[21] Overall, thrombolysis was achieved about four times more often with streptokinase than with heparin (61.5% vs 17.6%; $2P < 0.0001$). However, treatment with streptokinase was associated with a significant excess of haemorrhage (14.0% vs 3.4%; $2P < 0.05$). More recently, even better rates of thrombolysis have been reported in uncontrolled studies of an ultra-high dosage streptokinase regimen, involving infusion of 6–9 million IU over six hours.[22]

4. Other acute venous or arterial thrombosis

Streptokinase has been used in a wide variety of thromboembolic conditions in which it may be of benefit. These include central retinal vein occlusion[23] and partial peripheral arterial occlusion.[24] However, more information is required before these can be regarded as definite indications.

5. Thrombosis on prosthetic materials

Local administration of between 50 000 and 100 000 IU streptokinase has been shown to be an effective method for relieving obstruction in arteriovenous shunts.[25] Systemic therapy with either streptokinase or urokinase has been used to treat patients with acute thrombotic obstruction of prosthetic heart valves with good results in approximately 70% of cases.[26,27]

Contraindications

Since streptokinase therapy can induce a profound coagulation defect it should be avoided in patients with a bleeding diathesis or active internal bleeding. For the same reason, conditions in which serious haemorrhagic complications may occur constitute a relative contraindication to thrombolytic therapy. These include recent trauma, surgery, cardiopulmonary resuscitation, active peptic ulceration, severe hypertension, stroke and diabetic retinopathy.

Adverse reactions

Potentially life-threatening effects

The unwanted effects of streptokinase therapy fall into two categories: those due to bleeding and those due to allergy. Hypotension and arrhythmias may occur in patients with myocardial infarction.

Bleeding. Major, life-threatening haemorrhage occurs in 0.2–0.3% of patients.[28–31] Less severe bleeding has been reported in about 10% of patients.[17,28–31] In the event of serious haemorrhage, streptokinase therapy should be stopped. Antifibrinolytic therapy (tranexamic acid, aminocaproic acid or aprotinin) should be considered if there is evidence of persistent fibrinolytic activity in the blood. Transfusions of blood (preferably fresh), cryoprecipitate, or fresh frozen plasma may be necessary.[7]

There may also be an excess incidence of cerebral haemorrhage (perhaps 2 per 1000) in patients treated with systemic thrombolytic agents,[17,28–31] but there does not appear to be an increase in *total* strokes — perhaps due to a reduction in ischaemic strokes.[17]

Allergic reactions. The incidence of allergic reactions appears to have fallen with the introduction of more highly purified forms of streptokinase. The incidence of anaphylactic shock is 0.1%.[28,30,31] Less severe allergic phenomena, such as chills, rigors, nausea, vomiting and high fever, have been reported in between 2 and 20% of patients.[17,28,30,31] All these reactions usually respond well to withdrawal of therapy, intravenous hydrocortisone and antihistamines. Although some authorities recommend the use of prophylactic intravenous hydrocortisone, there is no good evidence that this is of value.[17]

Acute overdosage

Overdosage will lead to haemorrhage.

Severe or irreversible adverse effects

These have been described immediately above.

Symptomatic adverse effects

Minor examples of the allergic reaction described above fall into this category.

High risk groups

Neonates

The drug is rarely if ever used in neonates.

Breast milk. No information is available on the presence of streptokinase in breast milk but it is very unlikely to be excreted in it.

Children

In children the initial dose of streptokinase should be determined by means of the streptokinase resistance test; the recommended maintenance dose is 20 $IU.ml^{-1}$ of blood volume per hour.[3]

Pregnant women

Streptokinase has been used successfully,[32] although pregnancy constitutes a relative contraindication.

The elderly

Although old age is often regarded as a relative contraindication to thrombolytic therapy there is no good evidence to support this idea. Indeed, in patients with myocardial infarction the absolute benefit of thrombolytic therapy was greater in elderly subjects.[17,28]

Drug interactions

Anticoagulant therapy

Following thrombolysis, recanalized vessels (for example, coronary arteries) may be prone to reocclusion, particularly if a tight stenosis remains in the vessel. Hence, some authorities state that anticoagulant therapy should be used routinely after thrombolysis. But data from the randomized trials of thrombolytic therapy in acute myocardial infarction suggest that the effects of thrombolytic therapy on mortality and on reinfarction are about the same, whether or not anticoagulant therapy is used.[17,28–31] Furthermore, anticoagulant therapy appears to increase the risk of haemorrhage following fibrinolytic therapy.[17,31]

Antiplatelet therapy

The efficacy of antiplatelet therapy, such as low-dose aspirin, following thrombolysis has recently been demonstrated.[17] Such therapy — which is far easier to give than anticoagulants (see above) — does not appear to be associated with an increased incidence of bleeding when used after thrombolytic therapy.[17,31]

Major outcome trials

1. Yusuf S, Collins R, Peto R et al 1985 Intravenous and intracoronary fibrinolytic therapy in acute myocardial infarction: overview of results on mortality, reinfarction and side-effects from 33 randomized controlled trials. European Heart Journal 6: 556–585

During the past 25 years, 22 randomized trials of prolonged intravenous fibrinolytic treatment have been reported, involving a total of some 6000 patients in the acute phase of myocardial infarction. In the past few years, two small high-dose short-term intravenous trials and nine small intracoronary trials, involving a total of about 1000 patients, have been reported. Because all these intravenous and intracoronary trials were small, their separate results appear contradictory and unreliable. But an overview of the data from these trials indicates that the prolonged intravenous regimen produces a highly significant ($22\% \pm 5\%$, $2P < 0.001$) reduction in the odds of death, and a frequency of side effects that is small in comparison with the absolute reduction in mortality. The apparent size of the reduction in mortality in the intravenous trials was similar whether anticoagulants were compulsory or optional, and, surprisingly, whether treatment was started early (<6 h from onset of symptoms) or late (generally 12–24 h). In addition, there was no evidence that urokinase was more effective than the less expensive streptokinase, or that, despite their technical complexity, the new intracoronary regimens were more effective than the intravenous regimens. But these prolonged intravenous schedules were quite complex, which may partly explain why they are not widely used.

2. The ISAM Study Group 1986 A prospective trial of intravenous streptokinase in acute myocardial infarction (ISAM). Mortality, morbidity, and infarct size at 21 days. New England Journal of Medicine 314: 1465–1471

1741 patients were randomized within six hours of the onset of symptoms of myocardial infarction to receive either a widely practicable fibrinolytic regimen (a one hour intravenous infusion of 1.5 million IU of streptokinase) or placebo. The effects of streptokinase on cumulative release of cardiac enzyme (MB isomer of creatine kinase) and on global and regional ejection fractions were significantly better than placebo. Although there were fewer deaths among patients allocated to streptokinase (6.3% vs 7.1%), this difference was not statistically significant. Despite full anticoagulation (starting with immediate intravenous heparin and continuing with phenoprocoumon for at least 3 weeks) there was an apparent excess of reinfarction in the streptokinase group (2.3% vs 1.1%; $2P < 0.06$).

3. Gruppo Italiano per lo Studio della Streptochinasi nell'Infarto miocardico (GISSI) (a) 1986 Effectiveness of intravenous thrombolytic treatment in acute myocardial infarction. Lancet 1: 397–402 (b) 1987 Long-term effects of intravenous thrombolysis in acute myocardial infarction: final report of the GISSI study. Lancet 2: 871–874

11 806 patients were randomized within 12 hours of the onset of symptoms of myocardial infarction to receive either the same streptokinase regimen as in ISAM (1.5 million IU in one hour) or routine coronary care (i.e. no placebo was used). The use of all other therapy, including anticoagulants and antiplatelet agents, was optional. Overall, the mortality in hospital was 18% lower in the streptokinase

group (10.7% vs 13.0% control: 2P<0.001). Among patients randomized 1–3 hours after the onset of pain the apparent effect was only moderately favourable (9% vs 11%; NS), and the same was true among those entering 3–12 hours after the onset of pain (12% vs 14%; NS). In contrast, among the 10% of patients who entered within one hour, a very promising — and highly significant — difference was observed (8% vs 15%). But this early period was chosen for separate presentation only because the *apparent* effect was so extreme. Hence, the size of the benefit in the first hour may have been exaggerated by chance, and the real effect may be somewhat more moderate (perhaps as in the period 1–3 hours).

The exact assessment of side effects was complicated by the fact that no placebo was used, but three observations were still of interest. First, the excess incidence of stroke was about 1 or 2 per thousand (as suggested by the review of previous trials). Second, the incidence of pericarditis was reduced by streptokinase from 12% to 7%. Third, the incidence of non-fatal reinfarction was increased from 2% to 4%; this excess (and the reduction in mortality) was observed whether or not anticoagulants were given following fibrinolytic therapy. Later follow-up (to six months and to one year) indicates that these early differences in both mortality and reinfarction were maintained (though not significantly further increased).

The results of the G1SS1 II trial were presented at the annual meeting of the American College of Cardiology in March 1990. There was no significant difference in the mortality of patients receiving a streptokinase component from that of those receiving tissue plasminogen activator although side effects were less in the group receiving tissue plasminogen activator.

4. ISIS-2 (Second International Study of Infarct Survival) Collaborative Group 1988 Randomised trial of intravenous streptokinase, oral aspirin, both or neither among 17 187 cases of suspected acute myocardial infarction: ISIS-2. Lancet 2: 349–360

17 187 patients entering 417 hospitals up to 24 hours (median 5 hours) after the onset of suspected acute myocardial infarction were randomized, with placebo control, between: (i) a one-hour intravenous infusion of 1.5 million IU of streptokinase; (ii) one month of 160 mg daily enteric-coated aspirin; (iii) both active treatments; or (iv) neither. Each agent produced a highly significant reduction in 5-week vascular mortality: 791/8592 (9.2%) among patients allocated streptokinase infusion vs 1029/8595 (12.0%) among those allocated placebo infusion (odds reduction 25%±4%; 2P<0.0001); 804/8587 (9.4%) vascular deaths among patients allocated aspirin tablets vs 1016/8600 (11.8%) among those allocated placebo tablets (odds reduction; 23%±4%; 2P<0.00 001). The combination of streptokinase and aspirin was significantly (2P<0.0001) better than either agent alone, and their separate effects on mortality appeared to be additive: 343/4292 (8.0%) among patients allocated both active agents vs 568/4300 (13.2%) among those allocated neither (odds reduction: 42%±5%; 95% confidence limits 34–50%; 2P<0.0001). There was evidence of benefit from each agent even for patients treated late (odds reduction at 0–4, 5–12 and 13–24 hours: 35%±6%, 16%±7% and 21%±12% for streptokinase alone; 25%±7%, 21%±7% and 21%±12% for aspirin alone; and 53%±8%, 32%±9% and 38%±15% for the combination of streptokinase and aspirin). Streptokinase was associated with an excess of bleed requiring transfusion (0.5% vs 0.2%) and of confirmed cerebral haemorrhage (0.1% vs 0.01%), but with fewer other strokes (0.6% vs 0.8%). These 'other' strokes may have included a few undiagnosed cerebral haemorrhages but still there was no increase in total strokes (0.7% streptokinase vs 0.8% placebo infusion). Aspirin significantly reduced non-fatal reinfarction (1.0% vs 2.0%) and non-fatal stroke (0.3% vs 0.6%), and was not associated with any increase in cerebral haemorrhage or in bleeds requiring transfusion. An excess of non-fatal reinfarction was reported when streptokinase was used alone, but this was entirely avoided by the addition of aspirin. Those allocated the combination of streptokinase and aspirin had significantly fewer infarctions (1.8% vs 2.9%), strokes (0.6% vs 1.1%) and deaths (8% vs 13.2%) than those allocated neither. A median of 15 months follow-up showed that the differences in vascular and in total mortality produced by streptokinase and by aspirin persist long-term.

References

1. McClintock D K, Bell P H 1971 The mechanism of activation of human plasminogen by streptokinase. Biochemical and Biophysical Research Communications 43: 694–702
2. Reddy K N N, Markus G 1972 Mechanism of activation of human plasminogen by streptokinase. Journal of Biological Chemistry 247: 1683–1691
3. Brogden R N, Speight T M, Avery G S 1973 Streptokinase: a review of its clinical pharmacology, mechanism of action and therapeutic uses. Drugs 5: 357–445
4. Bell W R, Meek A G 1979 Guidelines for the use of thrombolytic agents. New England Journal of Medicine 301: 1266–1270
5. Kakkar V V, Scully M F 1978 Thrombolytic therapy. Medical Bulletin 34: 191–199
6. Marder V J, Soulen R L, Atichartakan V et al 1977 Quantitative venographic assessment of deep vein thrombosis in the evaluation of streptokinase and heparin therapy. Journal of Laboratory and Clinical Medicine 89: 1018–1029
7. Consensus Development 1980 Thrombolytic therapy and treatment. British Medical Journal 280: 1585–1587
8. Bachmann F 1968 Development of antibodies against perorally and rectally administered streptokinase in man. Journal of Laboratory and Clinical Medicine 72: 228–238
9. Flute P T 1973 The significance of streptokinase. Postgraduate Medical Journal 49 (suppl 5): 24–25
10. James D C O 1973 Anti-streptokinase levels in various hospital patient groups. Postgraduate Medical Journal 49 (suppl 5): 26–29
11. Laffel G L, Braunwald E 1984 Thrombolytic therapy. A new strategy for the treatment of acute myocardial infarction. New England Journal of Medicine 311: 710–717 and 770–776
12. Pfeifer G W, Doerr F, Brod K H 1969 Pharmacokinetics of ^{131}I-streptokinase in humans. Klinische Wochenschrift 47: 482–486
13. Fletcher A P, Alkjaersig N, Sherry S 1958 The clearance of heterologous protein from the circulation of normal and immunised man. Journal of Clinical Investigation 37: 1306–1315
14. Urokinase Pulmonary Embolism Trial: phase 1 results: a co-operative study 1970 Journal of the American Medical Association 214: 2163–2172
15. Siefring G E, Castellino F J 1976 Interaction of streptokinase with plasminogen. Journal of Biological Chemistry 251: 3913–3920
16. Walker M G, Dhall D P, Kasenally A T, Mowor G E 1973 The administration and stability of streptokinase. Postgraduate Medical Journal 49 (suppl 5): 33–34
17. ISIS-2 (Second International Study of Infarct Survival) Collaborative Group 1988 Randomised trial of intravenous streptokinase, oral aspirin, both or neither among 17 187 cases of suspected acute myocardial infarction: ISIS-2. Lancet 2: 349–360
18. Urokinase — Streptokinase Embolism Trial: phase 2 results 1974 Journal of the American Medical Association 229: 1606–1613
19. Tibbutt D A, Davies J A, Anderson J A et al 1974 Comparison by controlled clinical trial of streptokinase and heparin in treatment of life-threatening pulmonary embolism. British Medical Journal 1: 343–347
20. Miller G A H, Hall R J C, Paneth M 1977 Pulmonary embolectomy, heparin and streptokinase. Their place in the treatment of acute massive pulmonary embolism. American Heart Journal 93: 568–574
21. Goldhaber S Z, Buring J E, Lipnick R J, Hennekens C H 1984 Pooled analysis of randomized trials of streptokinase and heparin in phlebographically documented acute deep thrombosis. American Journal of Medicine 76: 393–397
22. Martin M, Fiebach O 1985 Ultra high streptokinase (UHSK) infusion in chronic arterial occlusions and acute venous thrombosis. Thrombosis and Haemostasis 54: 101
23. Kohner E M, Petit J E, Hamilton A M, Bulpitt C J, Dollery C T 1976 Streptokinase in central retinal vein occlusion: a controlled clinical trial. British Medical Journal 1: 550–553
24. Samama M, Conard J, Bilski-Pasquier G 1973 Streptokinase in peripheral arterial thrombo-embolism. Postgraduate Medical Journal 49 (suppl 5): 91–98
25. Arisz L, Tegzess A M, Donker A J M, Meijer S, Smit Sibinga C T, Van der Hem G K 1973 The use of streptokinase in obstructed arterio-venous shunts. Postgraduate Medical Journal 49 (suppl 5): 99–102
26. Witchitz S, Veyrat C, Moisson P, Scheinman N, Rozenstajn L 1980 Fibrinolytic treatment of thrombus on prosthetic heart valves. British Heart Journal 44: 545–554
27. Ledain L D, Ohayon J P, Lolle J P, Lorient-Roudaut F M, Roudaut J P, Besse P M 1986 Acute thrombotic obstruction with disc valve prostheses: diagnostic considerations and fibrinolytic treatment. Journal of the American College of Cardiology 7: 743–751
28. Gruppo Italiano per lo Studio della Streptochinasi nell'Infarto miocardico (GISSI) (a) 1986 Effectiveness of intravenous thrombolytic treatment in acute myocardial infarction. Lancet 1: 397–402 (b) 1987 Long-term effects of intravenous thrombolysis in acute myocardial infarction: final report of the GISSI study. Lancet 2: 871–874
29. Yusuf S, Collins R, Peto R et al 1985 Intravenous and intracoronary fibrinolytic therapy in acute mortality, reinfarction and side-effects from 33 randomised controlled trials. European Heart Journal 6: 556–585
30. The ISAM Group 1986 A prospective trial of intravenous streptokinase in acute myocardial infarction (ISAM). Mortality, morbidity, and infarct size at 21 days. New England Journal of Medicine 314: 1465–1471
31. ISIS (International Studies of Infarct Survival) Pilot Study Investigators 1987 Randomised factorial trial of high-dose intravenous streptokinase, of oral aspirin, and of intravenous heparin in acute myocardial infarction. European Heart Journal 8: 634–642
32. Hall R J C, Young C, Sutton G C, Campbell S 1972 Treatment of acute massive pulmonary embolism by streptokinase during labour and delivery. British Medical Journal 4: 647–649

S

Streptomycin

Streptomycin is an aminoglycoside antibiotic for the treatment of tuberculosis.

Chemistry

Streptomycin sulphate (or sulfate) (Solvo-strept S, Strycin, Darostrep, Novostrep, Dif-Estrepto E, Estrepto E, Estreptomade, Neodiestreptobap)

$C_{21}H_{39}N_7O_{12}$

0-2-Deoxy-2-methylamino-α-L-glucopyranosyl-(1→2)-0-5-deoxy-3-C-formyl-α-L-lyxofuranosyl-(1→4)-NN′-diamino-D-streptamine sulphate

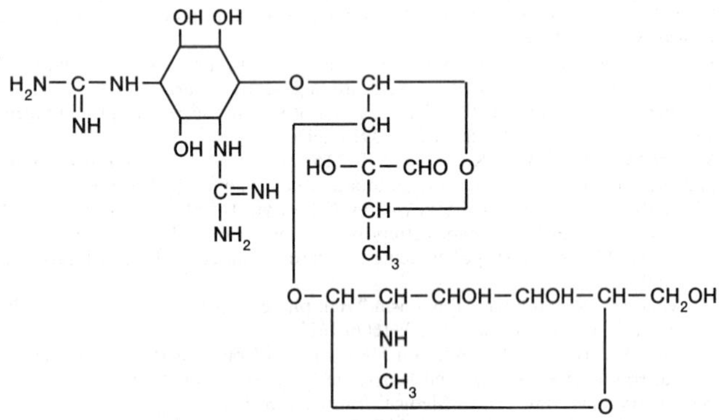

Molecular weight (free compound)	581.6
pKa	4.5–7.0[1]
Solubility	
in alcohol	practically insoluble
in water	most salts are highly soluble
Octanol/water partition coefficient	—

A white or almost white hygroscopic powder with a slightly bitter taste.[2] The base is produced by the growth of certain strains of *Streptomyces griseus*.[2]

Streptomycin is also a component in the drug combination product Streptotriad. It contains streptomycin sulphate, sulphadiazine, sulphadimidine, and sulphathiazole.

Pharmacology

Streptomycin is an antibiotic of the aminoglycoside group which is mainly used for the treatment of tuberculosis. Streptomycin, like other aminoglycosides, is actively transported across the bacterial cell membrane by an oxygen-dependent system. Factors determining the rate of intracellular accumulation include the concentration of divalent cations (Mg^{2+} and Ca^{2+}), environmental pH and oxygen tension. Streptomycin is inactive under anaerobic conditions. Streptomycin then binds to polysomes and inhibits the synthesis of proteins. The drug binds to the 30S subunit of the bacterial ribosome which consists of 21 proteins and a single 16S molecule of RNA. Changes in these proteins markedly affect the actions of streptomycin. A single amino acid substitution of asparagine for lysine at position 42 of one ribosomal protein (S_{12}) prevents binding of the drug and the mutant is totally resistant to the actions of streptomycin. Protein synthesis in bacteria is blocked by inhibiting the movement of the peptidyl-tRNA associated with translocation. In addition, streptomycin induces misreading of the genetic code due to an incorrect codon–anticodon interaction. The combined effects are bactericidal. Streptomycin is most active in an alkaline medium.[2–5]

Toxicology

Acute toxic effects in animals included clonic–tonic convulsions following intracisternal injections[6,7] and nausea, vomiting and ataxia following subcutaneous or intravenous injections.[6]

Chronic toxic effects in animals given subcutaneous, intravenous, or intramuscular injections included neurotoxicity, loss of appetite, proteinuria and the appearance of urinary casts.[6,8–10] Signs of neurotoxicity consist of changes in gait and posture, ataxia, progressive loss of rotational nystagmus and difficulty in performing unaccustomed skills such as swimming.[11] Streptomycin injected intracisternally or intrathecally caused difficulty in retaining normal posture, hyperexcitability, fast jerky movements in response to touch, muscular tremors, spontaneous nystagmus and epileptiform convulsions.[6] The time for neurotoxicity to develop varied with the size of the daily dose, the duration of administration (total dose), the animal species and the individual animal. At autopsy, kidneys from animals with evidence of renal toxicity showed albuminous deposits in subcapsular spaces, fatty change, and occasional tubular necrosis. Fatty change was seen in the liver of some monkeys.[10] It was considered likely that some chronic toxicity could have been caused by impurities rather than by streptomycin itself.[7,10] In several animals injected intramuscularly, areas of necrosis with evidence of repair were seen at sites of injection.[10]

There have been no teratogenicity tests in animals. In a review of reports of 203 women who were treated with the drug (usually in combination with isoniazid and p-aminosalicylic acid) during 206 pregnancies, 72 of whom were known to have been given the drug during the first 4 months of pregnancy, there were two spontaneous abortions, no premature or stillbirths, and no evidence of any teratogenic damage.[12] Short-term mutagenicity tests in bacteria and long-term carcinogenicity tests in animals have not been performed.

Clinical pharmacology

Streptomycin is active against a wide range of bacteria. It is active against *Mycobacterium tuberculosis*,[13] Gram-negative bacteria including *Escherichia coli*, *Klebsiella pneumoniae*, other *Enterobacteriaceae*,[14] *Brucella*, *Neisseria gonorrhoeae* and *N. meningitidis*,[15] *Yersinia pestis*,[16] *Haemophilus influenzae*, *Francisella tularensis*[17] and some species of *Proteus*, *Salmonella* and *Shigella*.[18] Streptomycin is the most effective antibiotic in the treatment of plague and tularaemia.[16,17] Streptomycin is also active against some Gram-positive organisms: a few strains of *Staphylococcus aureus* are sensitive to streptomycin as are some strains of *Actinomycetes*.[5] *Streptococcus faecalis* is usually resistant to streptomycin when given alone but benzylpenicillin and streptomycin act synergistically against most strains of *Streptococcus faecalis*.[3] Streptomycin is primarily used in the treatment of tuberculosis but is sometimes useful in the other conditions mentioned and in brucellosis. Severe cases of *Brucella melitensis* or *B. suis* are usually best treated with a combination of tetracycline and streptomycin. Streptomycin is also dramatically effective in the treatment of plague and tularaemia.

Pharmacokinetics

Many microbiological methods for measuring streptomycin concentrations have been reported.[19] The preferred method is by automated fluorescence polarization immunoassay.[20] With this method the lowest detectable concentration with 95% confidence is 0.6 $mg.l^{-1}$.

Absorption of streptomycin from the gastrointestinal tract is poor. When the drug is given orally, 60–100% can be recovered unchanged from the faeces.[21,22] The presystemic metabolism is zero. The mean plasma half life is 2.4–2.7 hours in adults less than 40 years of age, up to 9.0 hours in older adults, and 7.0 hours in premature and newborn infants. There is wide variation between patients and also in the same patient on repeat testing.[22] The apparent volume of distribution is 95.9 l ± 19.5 l (SE) in well-nourished patients, and 66.3 l ± 7.4 l (SE) in malnourished patients.[23]

About one-third of streptomycin is bound to plasma albumin and globulins, with about 20% bound in patients with kwashiorkor.[19,24,25] No significant amounts enter the red cells.[26] Streptomycin diffuses rapidly throughout the extracellular fluid[27] and crosses

Streptomycin

the placenta, concentrations in cord blood and amniotic fluid being about half those in maternal blood.[28,29] The drug can be found in the bile, kidney, lung, heart muscle, and trace amounts in the brain, CSF and liver.[27] It diffuses into the cerebrospinal fluid only when the meninges are inflamed,[30] but even then may fail to do so to a therapeutically significant extent.[31] Approximately 0.5% of the maternal dose is excreted in breast milk in 24 hours. The infant could thus ingest about 5 mg in 24 hours, the usual therapeutic dose for infants being 10–20 mg.kg^{-1}.[19]

Oral absorption	0–40%
Presystemic metabolism	nil
Plasma half life	
range	2.4–9.0 h
Volume of distribution	96 l.kg^{-1}
Plasma protein binding	33%

Concentration–effect relationship

Concentrations of 10 mg.l^{-1} and above are generally accepted as being therapeutically adequate,[19] but concentrations as low as 0.4 mg.l^{-1} can inhibit the growth of *M. tuberculosis*.[23,32] Most strains of *M. tuberculosis* are sensitive to less than 10 mg.l^{-1} streptomycin. Concentrations measured at 1, 2 and 3 hours after injection showed considerable variations in the same patient and were unhelpful with regard to the development of toxic effects. There is therefore no need to estimate peak levels. In contrast, there was a significant association between 24-hour levels and dizziness.[33] If streptomycin has to be given to patients with impaired renal function, including those on dialysis, it is not necessary to measure peak concentrations, but doses should be spaced such that the trough concentrations do not exceed 4 mg.l^{-1}.

Metabolism

Following parenteral administration, approximately 50% to 60% of the dose is excreted unchanged in the urine within 24 hours. The plasma half life is approximately 2.5 hours and this increases to approximately 100 hours when blood urea nitrogen concentrations are in the range of 100–150 mg per 100 ml.[34] A small proportion of the dose (about 1%) is excreted in the bile, this proportion falling when there is chronic hepatic dysfunction. Approximately 20% of a dose cannot be accounted for by urinary excretion, but no metabolites have yet been identified.[19] Following oral administration, 60–100% of the dose can be recovered unchanged from the faeces[35] but there is no evidence of enterohepatic circulation.

The structures of the metabolites are unknown and therefore pharmacological activity of the metabolites has not been determined.

Pharmaceutics

Streptomycin sulphate is presented as a white sterile powder for intramuscular injection, as an elixir and mixture for oral administration.

Oral dosage forms include:

Paediatric streptomycin elixir (BPC 1973). This contains streptomycin sulphate 157 mg, citric acid monohydrate 5 mg, sodium citrate 45 mg, methyl hydroxybenzoate 6.5 mg, amaranth solution 0.01 ml, sucrose 3.75 g, freshly boiled and cooled water to 5 ml. A dose of 5 ml is equivalent to 125 mg of streptomycin base.[2]

Streptomycin mixture CF (APF). Streptomycin elixir for infants. This contains streptomycin sulphate 157 mg, sodium citrate 45 mg, citric acid monohydrate 5 mg, methyl hydroxybenzoate 5 mg, syrup 4 ml, amaranth solution 0.01 ml, water to 5 ml. A dose of 5 ml is equivalent to 125 mg of streptomycin base.[2]

Parenteral dosage forms include:

Streptomycin sulphate injection (BP). Streptomycin sulphate is presented as a white sterile powder for preparation of streptomycin sulphate injection (BP) which is a sterile solution of the drug in water for injection, containing stabilizing agents and buffer (pH 5–6.5). The solution should be protected from light. It can be kept for up to 28 days in a refrigerator (below 4°C), and up to 7 days in a cool place (below 20°C). Solutions tend to discolour slightly on keeping, but their potency is not diminished. The powder should be protected from light and stored at a temperature not exceeding 20°C.

Therapeutic use

Indications

1. Tuberculosis
2. Plague and tularaemia
3. Other sensitive infections.

Contraindications

1. Ear disease
2. Pregnant women
3. Myasthenia gravis
4. Hypersensitivity to the drug
5. Impaired renal function.

Mode of use

In the treatment of tuberculosis in adults, the recommended dosage is 1.0 g or 0.75 g as a single deep intramuscular injection when given daily, but 1.0 g when given three times weekly, or twice weekly. Twice-weekly administration may continue for up to 12 months. The injection site should be changed frequently to avoid local necrosis. In patients over 40 years of age or in patients weighing less than 30 kg, 0.75 or 0.5 g per dose should be used, even if the patient's renal function is normal. In the treatment of tuberculosis in children, 20–40 mg.kg^{-1} should be given as a single daily or intermittent intramuscular injection to a maximum of 1.0 g. In newborn and premature infants the dosage should be 10–20 mg.kg^{-1}.

In the treatment of tuberculous meningitis, single daily intrathecal injections of 1 mg.kg^{-1} for up to 10 days may be given to a maximum of 50 mg daily in adults and children. With the use of modern regimens, however, it is unlikely that such treatment is necessary. Streptomycin for intrathecal injection should be dissolved in sodium chloride injection using 5 ml for infants and 10 ml for older children and adults. The concentration of the drug must not exceed 5 mg.ml^{-1}. After withdrawal of an equal volume of cerebrospinal fluid, the solution should be injected over a period of at least 10 minutes.

Whenever possible, streptomycin should be avoided in the treatment of patients with impaired renal function, because it is excreted unchanged by the kidneys. If it is necessary to use the drug in such circumstances, a normal dose should be given but at intervals such that the trough serum concentration does not exceed 4 mg.l^{-1}.[36] Hence, serum concentrations must be monitored.

The drug is removed only slowly by haemodialysis[37] and for patients on haemodialysis, 10 mg.kg^{-1} should be given every 5 to 7 days,[38] and the serum concentration should be monitored.

In the treatment of non-tuberculous infections the dose for adults is 1.0 g and for children 30 mg.kg^{-1} daily for 3 to 7 days by intramuscular injection. The dosage of Streptotriad in gastrointestinal infections is 2 tablets 3 times daily for adults for up to 4 days. One tablet contains 65 mg of streptomycin.

The highest intramuscular dosages used in the treatment of tuberculosis have been 2 g daily (divided) for 6 weeks, or 1 g twice daily for up to 8 weeks.[39,40] The highest intramuscular dosage used in the treatment of nontuberculous infections has been 2.4 g daily (divided) for up to 14 days.[40]

Indications

1. Tuberculosis

The use of streptomycin in primary chemotherapy in modern short-course treatment is decreasing in the technically advanced countries in particular, but may still be used in retreatment regimens, especially if the strain is resistant to other potent antituberculosis drugs.

In the treatment of tuberculosis, streptomycin should only be used in conjunction with other antituberculosis drugs. It is a moderately potent bactericidal drug, being particularly active against bacilli in a neutral or alkaline environment; it is highly effective in preventing the emergence of resistance to other antituberculosis drugs, but it adds little if anything to the bactericidal and sterilizing action of a combination of isoniazid, rifampicin, and pyrazinamide.[41–45] It is, however, an important component of regimens which contain only one other drug in addition to isoniazid, particularly if this is pyrazinamide or a bacteriostatic drug such as PAS, thiacetazone or

Streptomycin

ethambutol. It has the disadvantages that it has to be given by intramuscular injection, is relatively toxic, and frequently causes hypersensitivity reactions.

In the treatment of all forms of newly-diagnosed tuberculosis in both adults and children, the International Union Against Tuberculosis and Lung Disease recommends a daily regimen of isoniazid and rifampicin for 6 months with pyrazinamide in addition for the first 2 months.[46] The continuation phase of isoniazid and rifampicin may be given three times or twice a week. This has the advantage that the continuation phase can be administered on an outpatient basis under full supervision, every dose being given under the direct observation of outpatient health service staff or of a paramedical worker or lay person who has been taught to supervise chemotherapy. In programmes where chemotherapy is administered throughout under full supervision on an outpatient basis the regimen may be given 3 times a week from the start, but when this is done either streptomycin or ethambutol should be added for the first 2 months. Also, when there is a high rate of initial drug resistance, or if it is suspected that the patient's strain is resistant to isoniazid, either streptomycin or ethambutol should be added for the first 2 months, even when the regimen is given daily.

A number of alternative, less potent regimens, most of which are cheaper regimens suitable for some developing countries are also recommended, as follows:

1. Streptomycin, isoniazid, rifampicin and pyrazinamide daily for 2 months followed by isoniazid and thiacetazone daily for 6 months (total duration 8 months), isoniazid alone being acceptable in the continuation phase if there are problems with thiacetazone toxicity.
2. The same initial 2-month phase followed by streptomycin, isoniazid and pyrazinamide twice a week for 6 months under full supervision.
3. Isoniazid and rifampicin daily for 9 months, with or without streptomycin or ethambutol for the first 2 months.
4. Streptomycin, isoniazid, and thiacetacone (or ethambutol or para-amino salicylic acid, PAS) daily for 2 months followed by isoniazid and thiacetazone (or ethambutol or PAS) daily for 10 months.
5. Streptomycin, isoniazid and thiacetazone (or PAS) daily for 2 months, followed by streptomycin and isoniazid twice a week for 10 months under full supervision.

Regimens based on streptomycin, isoniazid, rifampicin, and pyrazinamide have the advantages of 1) sterilizing lesions rapidly so that defaulters stand a higher chance of cure than with previous regimens, 2) practically eliminating the risk of bacteriological failure due to the emergence of acquired resistance during treatment and 3) achieving excellent results in patients with strains of tubercle bacilli initially resistant to isoniazid, streptomycin, or both drugs.

2. Plague and tularaemia

In the treatment of plague, streptomycin 1.0 g should be given immediately, followed by 0.5 g 4-hourly until the fever subsides, followed by 0.5 g 6-hourly for a further 2 or 3 days.[47]

In the treatment of tularaemia, 30 $mg.kg^{-1}$ should be given daily (divided as 2 injections) for 2 weeks.[48]

Contraindications

Streptomycin is contraindicated in patients with ear disease (because of its ototoxicity), in pregnant women (because it crosses the placenta and can cause eighth nerve damage in the fetus),[49,50] in patients with myasthenia gravis (because it is a weak neuromuscular blocker)[51] and in patients who are known to be hypersensitive to the drug (because of the risk of a severe reaction which may include anaphylactic shock or exfoliative dermatitis). If possible it should be avoided in the treatment of patients with impaired renal function, because it is excreted unchanged by the kidneys and is also nephrotoxic.[36]

Adverse reactions

Potentially life-threatening effects

Anaphylactic shock may occur on rare occasions. Rarely severe and even fatal exfoliative dermatitis may occur.

Aplastic anaemia and agranulocytosis are rare occurrences which have been attributed to the drug.[52]

Acute overdosage

Acute haemolytic anaemia and renal failure were reported in a 45-year-old man after he injected himself with streptomycin and ampicillin. He had been injecting himself repeatedly with streptomycin for a period of 15 years.[53]

Severe or irreversible adverse effects

Haemolytic anaemia has been reported in a patient with glucose-6-phosphate dehydrogenase deficiency.[54]

Severe and persistent giddiness, vertigo, tinnitus, ataxia, and deafness can occur due to eighth nerve toxic damage and can become permanent.[55,56] The risks are higher in newborn infants and in patients aged more than 40 years, in whom recovery from ototoxicity is slower and less often complete than in older children and young adults. Serious and permanent toxic damage is uncommon with currently recommended dosages, provided that the drug dosage is reduced or the drug withdrawn when early symptoms and signs occur.

Evidence of minor renal tubular dysfunction, such as urinary casts and minor degrees of albuminuria, are not uncommon, but severe renal damage (proximal tubular necrosis) is rare.[55,57]

Symptomatic adverse effects

Cutaneous and generalized hypersensitivity reactions are common and, as mentioned earlier, can be severe (they can also affect nurses, pharmacists and others who handle the drug). The clinical manifestations are diverse,[58] but the commonest features are rash and fever.[59,60]

Streptomycin has a selectively toxic action on the eighth cranial nerve.[56,61] Vestibular damage is much commoner than auditory damage, which may include deafness, but both can occur together. These effects have been mentioned earlier. Transient giddiness and numbness, especially around the mouth, are common, particularly after a dose at the time of highest plasma concentrations.

When administered by intrathecal injection, streptomycin can cause root pain, pleocytosis in cerebrospinal fluid, and rarely evidence of brain stem irritation, such as neck pain, temporary retention of urine, and nystagmus.[55]

Interference with clinical pathology tests

There are no reports that the drug interferes with clinical pathology tests.

High risk groups

Neonates

Dosage should be 10–20 $mg.kg^{-1}$ to avoid eighth nerve toxicity.

Breast milk. The drug enters breast milk but not in sufficient quantities to harm the infant, but the risk of possible sensitization should be remembered.

Children

The drug may be given to children in appropriate doses.

Pregnant women

The drug should be avoided because of the risk of eighth nerve toxicity in the fetus.[49,50]

The elderly

Streptomycin should be used with caution in the elderly because of the risk of ototoxicity (see above).

Concurrent disease

The drug should be avoided in patients with impaired renal function or a normal dose (see above) should be given at intervals such that the trough serum concentration does not exceed 4 $mg.l^{-1}$.[36]

Drug interactions

Potentially hazardous interactions

Streptomycin is incompatible with acids and alkalis.[2]

Potentially useful interactions

Streptomycin and benzylpenicillin act synergistically against *Streptococcus faecalis*.[3] They should not be given together unless the preparation is freshly made, because the combination rapidly becomes less active on storage.

Streptomycin

References

1. British Pharmacopoeia 1980
2. Reynolds J E F, Prasad A B (eds) 1982 Martindale: the extra pharmacopoeia, 28th edn. The Pharmaceutical Press, London, pp 1083, 1213
3. Sapico F L, Keys T F, Hewitt W L 1972 Experimental enterococcal endocarditis II: a study of in vivo synergism of penicillin and streptomycin. American Journal of Medical Sciences 263: 128–135
4. Ruhen R N, Darrell J H 1973 Antibiotic synergism against Group D streptococci in the treatment of endocarditis. Medical Journal of Australia 2: 114–116
5. Mahgoub E S 1976 Medical management of mycetoma. Bulletin of the World Health Organization 54: 303–310
6. Molitor H, Kuna S 1947 The significance of neurotropic properties of commercial streptomycin. Archives Internationales de Pharmacodynamie et de Thérapie 74: 334–342
7. Molitor H 1949 The pharmacology of streptomycin. In: Waksman S A (ed) Streptomycin: nature and practical applications. Baillière, Tindall and Cox, London, ch 15, pp 254–275
8. Silber R H, Porter C C, Winburg M, Clark I 1947 The significance of impurities on the biochemical effects of streptomycin. Archives of Biochemistry 14: 349–360
9. Hinshaw H C, Feldman W H 1945 Streptomycin in treatment of clinical tuberculosis: a preliminary report. Proceedings of the Staff Meetings, Mayo Clinic 20: 313–318
10. Molitor H, Graessle O E, Kuna S, Mushett C W, Silber R H 1946 Some toxicological and pharmacological properties of streptomycin. Journal of Pharmacology and Experimental Therapeutics 86: 151–173
11. Caussé R, Gondet I, Vallancien B 1948 Action vestibulaire de la streptomycine chez la souris. Comptes rendus des séances de la Société de biologie 142: 747–749
12. Snider D E, Layde P M, Johnson M W, Lyle M A 1980 Treatment of tuberculosis during pregnancy. American Review of Respiratory Disease 122: 65–79
13. Schatz A, Waksman S A 1944 Effect of streptomycin and other antibiotic substances upon *Mycobacterium tuberculosis* and related organisms. Proceedings of the Society for Experimental Biology and Medicine 57: 244–249
14. Youmans G P, Fisher M W 1949 Action of streptomycin on microorganisms in vitro. In: Waksman S A (ed) Streptomycin: nature and practical applications. Baillière, Tindall and Cox, London, ch 7, pp 91–111
15. Miller C P, Bohnhoff M 1946 Streptomycin resistance of gonococci and meningococci. Journal of the American Medical Association 130: 485–488
16. Butler T, Mahmoud A A F, Warren K S 1977 Algorithms in the diagnosis and management of exotic diseases. XXV. Plague. Journal of Infectious Diseases 136: 317–320
17. Herrell W E 1968 Tularemia: recommended therapy. Clinical Medicine 75: 62
18. Jones D, Metzger H J, Schatz A, Waksman S A 1944 Control of gram-negative bacteria in experimental animals by streptomycin. Science 100: 103–105
19. Holdiness M R 1984 Clinical pharmacokinetics of the antituberculosis drugs. Clinical Pharmacokinetics 9: 511–544
20. Schwenzer K S, Anhalt J P 1983 Automated fluorescence polarization immunoassay for monitoring streptomycin. Antimicrobial Agents and Chemotherapy 23: 683–687
21. Stebbins R B, Graessle O E, Robinson H J 1945 Studies on the absorption and excretion of streptomycin in animals. Proceedings of the Society for Experimental Biology and Medicine 60: 68–72
22. Garrod L P, Lambert H P, O'Grady F 1973 Streptomycin. In: Lawrence P, Garrod M P (eds) Antibiotics and chemotherapy, 4th edn. Churchill Livingstone, Edinburgh, ch 6, pp 102–114
23. Prasad J S, Krishnaswami K 1978 Streptomycin pharmacokinetics in malnutrition. Chemotherapy 24: 333–337
24. Buchanan N 1977 Streptomycin and isoniazid metabolism in malnourished children. Acta Pediatrica Scandinavica 66: 663
25. Buchanan N, van der Walt L A 1977 The binding of antituberculosis drugs to normal and kwashiorkor serum. South African Medical Journal 52: 522–525
26. Rake G, Donovick R 1949 Absorption, distribution and excretion of streptomycin. In: Waksman S A (ed) Streptomycin: nature and practical applications. Baillière, Tindall and Cox, London, ch 14, pp 236–253
27. Adcock J D, Hettig R A 1946 Absorption, distribution and excretion of streptomycin. Archives of Internal Medicine 77: 179–195
28. Heilman D H, Heilman F R, Hinshaw H C, Nichols D R, Herrell W E 1945 Streptomycin: absorption, diffusion, excretion, and toxicity. American Journal of Medical Science 210: 576–584
29. Woltz J H E, Wiley M M 1945 Transmission of streptomycin from maternal blood to the fetal circulation and the amniotic fluid. Proceedings of the Society for Experimental Biology and Medicine 60: 106–107
30. Anderson D G, Jewell M 1945 The absorption, excretion and toxicity of streptomycin in man. New England Journal of Medicine 233: 485–491
31. Alexander H E, Leidy G, Rake G, Donovick R 1946 *Hemophilus influenzae* meningitis treated with streptomycin. Journal of the American Medical Association 132: 434–440
32. Bobrowitz I D 1971 Ethambutol compared to streptomycin in original treatment of advanced pulmonary tuberculosis. Chest 60: 14–21
33. Line D H, Poole G W, Waterworth P M 1970 Serum streptomycin levels and dizziness. Tubercle 51: 76–91
34. Garrod L P, O'Grady F (eds) 1971 Antibiotics and chemotherapy. Williams and Wilkins, Baltimore, p 105
35. Buggs C W, Pilling M A, Bronstein B, Hirschfeld J W, Worznik L, Key L J 1946 The absorption, distribution and excretion of streptomycin in man. Journal of Clinical Investigation 25: 94–102
36. Kunin C M 1967 A guide to use of antibiotics in patients with renal disease. A table of recommended doses and factors governing serum levels. Annals of Internal Medicine 67: 151–158
37. Edwards K D G, Whyte H M 1959 Streptomycin poisoning in renal failure: an indication for treatment with an artificial kidney. British Medical Journal 1: 752–754
38. Usada Y, Sekine O 1978 Chemotherapy of tuberculosis in patients on dialysis. In: Siegenthaler W, Lüthy R (eds) Current chemotherapy: proceedings of the 10th International Congress of Chemotherapy, Zurich, Switzerland, 1977. American Society for Microbiology, Washington DC, p 241
39. Keefer C S 1949 Clinical indications for streptomycin therapy. In: Waksman S A (ed) Streptomycin: nature and practical applications. Baillière, Tindall and Cox, London, ch 16, pp 279–281
40. Herrell W E 1949 Methods of administration and dosage. In: Waksman S A (ed) Streptomycin: nature and practical applications. Baillière, Tindall and Cox, London, ch 17, pp 282–290
41. East African/British Medical Research Councils 1966 Isoniazid with thiacetazone (thioacetazone) in the treatment of pulmonary tuberculosis in East Africa – Third investigation: the effect of an initial streptomycin supplement. Tubercle 47: 1–32
42. East African/British Medical Research Councils 1970 Isoniazid with thiacetazone (thioacetazone) in the treatment of pulmonary tuberculosis in East Africa – Second report of fifth investigation. Tubercle 51: 353–358
43. Mitchison D A 1979 Basic mechanisms of chemotherapy. Chest 76 (suppl): 771S–781S
44. Fox W 1983 Short-course chemotherapy for pulmonary tuberculosis. In: Saunders K B (ed) Advanced Medicine 19. Pitman, London, pp 307–326
45. Singapore Tuberculosis Service/British Medical Research Council 1985 Clinical trial of three 6-month regimens of chemotherapy given intermittently in the continuation phase in the treatment of pulmonary tuberculosis. American Review of Respiratory Disease 132: 374–378
46. International Union Against Tuberculosis and Lung Disease 1988 Antituberculosis regimens of chemotherapy: recommendations from the Committee on Treatment. Bulletin of the International Union Against Tuberculosis and Lung Disease 63 No. 2: 60–64
47. Christie A B 1987 Plague. In: Weatherall D J, Ledingham J G G, Warrell D A (eds) Oxford textbook of medicine, 2nd edn. Oxford University Press, Oxford, pp 5.246–5.251
48. Mitchell R G 1987 Tularaemia, glanders and meliodosis. In: Weatherall D J, Ledingham J G G, Warrell D A (eds) Oxford textbook of medicine, 2nd edn. Oxford University Press, Oxford, pp 5.242–5.244
49. Robinson G C, Cambon K G 1964 Hearing loss in infants of tuberculous mothers treated with streptomycin during pregnancy. New England Journal of Medicine 271: 949–951
50. Donald P R, Sellors S L 1981 Streptomycin ototoxicity in the newborn child. South African Medical Journal 60: 316–318
51. Hokkanen E 1964 Antibiotics in myasthenia gravis. British Medical Journal 1: 1111–1112
52. Deyke V F, Wallace J B 1948 Development of aplastic anaemia during the use of streptomycin: report of two cases. Journal of the American Medical Association 136: 1098
53. Letona J M L, Barbolla L, Frieyro E, Bouza E, Gilsanz F, Fernandez M N 1977 Immune haemolytic anaemia and renal failure induced by streptomycin. British Journal of Haematology 35: 561–571
54. Burka E R, Weaver Z, Marks P A 1966 Clinical spectrum of hemolytic anemia associated with glucose-6-phosphate dehydrogenase deficiency. Annals of Internal Medicine 64: 817–825
55. Bunn P A, Westlake R E 1949 Toxicity of streptomycin in the human. In: Waksman S A (ed) Streptomycin: nature and practical applications. Baillière, Tindall and Cox, London, ch 40, pp 524–545
56. Ballantyne J 1970 Iatrogenic deafness. Journal of Laryngology and Otology 84: 967–1000
57. Erlanson P, Lundgren A 1964 Ototoxic side effects following treatment with streptomycin, dihydrostreptomycin, and kanamycin. Acta Medica Scandinavica 176: 147–163
58. Hardie R A, Savin J A 1979 Drug induced diseases: drug-induced skin diseases. British Medical Journal 1: 935–937
59. Medical Research Council Tuberculosis Chemotherapy Trials Committee 1962 Long-term chemotherapy in the treatment of chronic pulmonary tuberculosis with cavitation. Tubercle 43: 201–267
60. British Medical Research Council 1973 Co-operative controlled trial of a standard regimen of streptomycin, PAS and isoniazid and three alternative regimens of chemotherapy in Britain. Tubercle 54: 99–129
61. Symonds J M 1978 Aminoglycoside ototoxicity. Journal of Antimicrobial Chemotherapy 4: 199–201

Streptozotocin

Streptozotocin is an antibiotic having selective toxicity for the β-cells of the islets of Langerhans.

Chemistry

Streptozotocin (Zanosar)
$C_8H_{15}N_3O_7$
2-Deoxy-2-[[(methylnitroso-amino)-carbonyl]amino]-d-glucopyranose

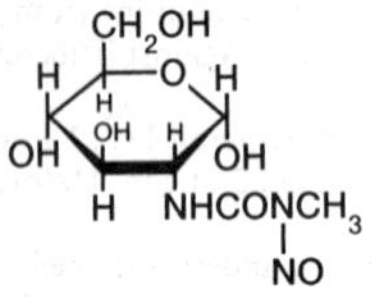

Molecular weight	265.2
pKa	—
Solubility	
in alcohol	soluble
in water	very soluble
Octanol/water partition coefficient	—

Streptozotocin is prepared as ivory-coloured, pointed platelets or prisms, m.p. 115°C. It rapidly degrades at 70°C, and is stable for 30 days at room temperature and for up to 6 months at 4°C.

Its pKa is not known as the determination method destroys the compound. Octanol/water partition coefficient is not known.

Streptozotocin was first isolated from cultures of *Streptomyces achromogenes*, variety 128, in 1959. Its structure was elucidated and it was synthesized in 1967.[1]

Pharmacology

Streptozotocin is an alkylating agent, and in addition depresses the intracellular handling of pyridine nucleotides. The drug is a nitrosourea, and it is unusual in this group in that the main antitumour action is methylation of proteins, and, in particular, nucleic acids. In this respect streptozotocin has the property that it is cytotoxic to cells in the G0 state as well as when the cell is dividing. In bacteria there is a specific alkylation of cytosine bases which leads to cell death. Streptozotocin had antileukaemic activity in mice[2] and was also found to have a selective toxicity for the β-cells of the islets of Langerhans, rendering experimental animals diabetic. Streptozotocin appears to alkylate DNA bases in the β-cell, causing breakage of the DNA strands. The particular action on the β-cells of the pancreas is probably secondary to the intracellular inhibition of nicotinamide adenine diphosphate nucleotide (NAD). No specific phase of the cell cycle is particularly sensitive to the lethal effects of streptozotocin.

Toxicology

Streptozotocin is teratogenic in the rat and abortifacient in the rabbit. Mutagenicity has been noted in animals and cultured mammalian cells, as well as in bacteria and plants. Carcinogenicity has been demonstrated in rats (pancreas, kidney and gonads), hamsters (liver) and mice (lung). An effect noted in the mouse is hyperglycaemia[3,4] but this effect is much less marked in rabbits[5] and is a result of a reduction in production of nicotinamide adenine diphosphate (NAD) synthesis and uptake in pancreatic cells.[6,7]

Clinical pharmacology

The same cytotoxic effect used to produce experimental diabetes in animals can be used to treat metastases from islet cell tumours, which may secrete active polypeptides. This may present as the WDHA syndrome of vasoactive intestinal polypeptide excess of gastrin producing tumours which give rise to persistent peptic ulceration.[8,9] There are no dose–response data in man and the precise mechanism of action is unknown. Regimes are empirical and largely due to Moertel (see refs 17–19). Streptozotocin has also been reported to cause regression of carcinoid tumour symptoms in 30% of patients,[10] although in this situation it appears to be relatively less effective as a palliative than somatostatin analogues.

Pharmacokinetics

The methods for assay of streptozotocin are HPLC to separate the two anomeric forms of streptozotocin, microbiological assay by disk inhibition which gives a lower limit of detection of 0.6 $g.l^{-1}$ for whole blood and 1.1 $g.l^{-1}$ for plasma, chemical assay by protein precipitation with 5% perchloric acid, and optical density measurement at 500 nm which gives a measure of the nitroso group of streptozotocin.

Streptozotocin must be given parenterally. Following intravenous injection, typical peak plasma concentrations are 30–40 $mg.l^{-1}$. The elimination from plasma is biphasic, with an initial half life of 15 minutes and a secondary half life of 35 minutes.[11] It readily crosses the blood–brain barrier. The major route of excretion is by the kidney and 70% of the administered dose can be recovered within 4 hours. The parent drug accounts for 10–20%, the rest being metabolites. At least three different metabolites can be distinguished but they have not been identified.[12] It is not known whether streptozotocin is excreted in milk, but it would be unwise to assume that it is not.

Oral absorption	nil
Presystemic metabolism	—
Plasma half life	
range	35–40 min
Volume of distribution	—
Plasma protein binding	—

Concentration–effect relationship

No data are available on this subject but it is unlikely that there will be a direct relationship between the plasma concentration of streptozotocin and its therapeutic effect.

Metabolism

Little is known of the detailed metabolism of streptozotocin in humans. Approximately 10–20% of the administered dose is recovered unchanged in the urine. Less than 1% of the administered dose is recovered from the faeces. Streptozotocin is a nitrosourea, and decomposes to generate isocyanates and chloroethyldiazohydroxide. The isocyanates are predominantly responsible for the toxic side effects of these compounds whereas the chloroethyl derivative has the antitumour activity.

Pharmaceutics

Synthetic streptozotocin is supplied by the Upjohn Company under the trade name Zanosar in 1 g vials. Unopened vials of zanosar should be stored at 2–8°C and protected from light. The product contains no preservatives and is not intended as a multiple-dose vial.

Streptozotocin is supplied for parenteral administration only. It is not absorbed orally and has no effect on gastrointestinal tumours when given by this route. It is supplied in vials containing 1 g of streptozotocin and 220 mg of anhydrous citric acid. This is made up in 9.5 ml of 5% dextrose or 0.9% saline for injection, with the operator wearing gloves to safeguard against inadvertent spillage being absorbed through the skin. (If spilled, the affected area should immediately be washed with soap and water.) The reconstituted solution is acidic (pH 3.5–4.5) and is stable in solution for up to 12 hours, but much less stable if the pH should rise. The resulting solution will contain 100 mg of streptozotocin and 22 mg of citric acid per ml. Where more dilute infusions are desirable, further dilution in the above vehicles is recommended.

Therapeutic use

The first report of the use of streptozotocin in human disease was by Murray-Lyons in 1968.[13] Apart from the indications listed below, streptozotocin has been tried in the palliation of cerebral tumours, but despite good CSF levels being obtained it is not effective.[14]

Situations in which streptozotocin has proved to be effective are:

Indications

1. Islet cell tumour of the pancreas

Functional, producing:
- Insulin
- Proinsulin
- ACTH
- Gastrin
- Glucagon
- Parathormone-like substance
- Alpha unit HCG
- Somatostatin
- Vasoactive intestinal polypeptide
- Diarrhoegenic hormones
- Calcitonin
- Serotonin

Non-functional.

2. Carcinoid syndrome

In addition, activity against adenocarcinoma of the pancreas and non-β-cell islet cell carcinoma has been claimed. Antiprotozoal action against *Trypanosoma rhodesiense* has been described in mouse models but the doses required to cure *T. rhodesiense* infection were toxic to the host.[15] There are no studies reported on this action in man.

Contraindications

There are no specific contraindications for use of the drug in advanced malignant disease, but as with other cytotoxic drugs the physician must assess the benefit against risk.

Renal function should be monitored as a precaution.

Mode of use

There are two commonly used regimes given for the administration of streptozotocin. The first is 500 mg.m^{-2} given intravenously for five consecutive days every six weeks until toxicity is observed or until markers of functional tumours have returned to normal. The second is 1 g.m^{-2} given intravenously in two doses, one week apart, with subsequent weekly doses up to 1.5 g.m^{-2} depending on response and toxicity. The dose may be limited by decline in renal function. Maximal response is usually achieved after 4 g.m^{-2} total dose. When administered on this schedule, the median time to onset of response is about 17 days and the median time to maximum response is about 35 days; the median total dose to onset of response is about 2000 mg.m^{-2} body surface area and the median total dose to maximum response is about 4000 mg.m^{-2} body surface area (data on file, Upjohn).

Nausea and vomiting are extremely common when using streptozotocin. More than 90% of patients will experience severe distress from these side effects which should be anticipated and antiemetic treatment given prophylactically. Often multiple antiemetic agents will be required to control these symptoms and it is said that methylprednisolone given 6 hours before the drug will ameliorate symptoms of nausea from cytotoxic agents.[16] There is some evidence from a preliminary study that, when given by a continuous infusion, nausea is reduced, but no clinical trials of efficacy have been performed. Mild glucose intolerance is reported in a few patients; the marked diabetogenic effect in small mammals such as mice only rarely occurs in humans at usual dosage.

Streptozotocin should not normally be used other than by experienced oncologists. Regular monitoring of renal function and full blood counts are advisable.

Renal damage[5] is not unusual, occurring in over 60% of cases[17] and is often the dose-limiting complication during a course of therapy. Initial fluid loading with forced diuresis, and the administration of the drug by slow infusion, will help to minimize the renal damage.

Hepatocellular necrosis has also been reported and there is often a dose-related liver injury with transiently elevated hepatic enzymes. The histological appearance is one of hepatocellular necrosis with centrilobular congestion. Bone marrow suppression, which may be selective, occurs in about 20% of patients, and may be marked with high-dose regimes (see also Adverse reactions below).

Gastrointestinal upset with diarrhoea is reported, as is CNS depression and confusion. Drug interactions are not common but they have been reported with phenytoin, where CNS depression may be marked. In addition there is evidence that phenytoin reduces the efficacy of streptozotocin. Combination of streptozotocin with 5-fluorouracil is superior in effect to either drug alone.[18,19]

Adverse reactions

Potentially life-threatening effects

Renal failure, bone marrow depression, acute hepatic failure, and perforation of the large intestine have been reported.

Renal dysfunction is dose-dependent and is observed in more than half the patients treated, damage being both glomerular and tubular, resulting in glycosuria, aminoaciduria, hypophosphataemia, acetonuria, hyperchloraemia, proteinuria and renal tubular acidosis.[5] If noted, renal toxicity is usually reversible on withdrawal of streptozotocin, but if administration is continued in the presence of renal dysfunction, irreversible renal failure may result. Marrow depression may occur in 20% of cases, and in 10% of patients leucopenia or thrombocytopenia will be noted.

One case of acute myeloblastic leukaemia has been reported in man following prolonged streptozotocin therapy.

Acute overdosage

There is no specific antidote to streptozotocin, and treatment is limited to supportive measures to support and maintain renal function and a normal blood picture, as well as blood glucose levels — which may, paradoxically, fall initially after acute overdosage.

Severe or irreversible adverse effects

These include gastrointestinal haemorrhage, confusion, pulmonary fibrosis, myocardial infarction, and increased intracranial pressure in the presence of a brain neoplasm.

Symptomatic adverse effects

The following symptomatic adverse effects have been reported: vomiting, diarrhoea, stomatitis, urticaria, fever, tremor, hypotension, limb paraesthesia, slurred speech, alopecia, thrombophlebitis, and ulceration of the skin. Nausea and vomiting occurs in over 90% of cases.

Other effects

Liver function tests may be abnormal in 25% of patients treated with streptozotocin.

Interference with clinical pathology tests

No interference with laboratory investigations has been reported.

High risk groups

Neonates

As no neonate appears to have developed malignant functional tumours of the pancreas, there are no data on special risks of administration of streptozotocin in this group.

Breast milk. There are no data on the excretion of streptozotocin in breast milk. Mothers being given the drug should not breast-feed.

Children

There are no data on the risks of streptozotocin in children.

Pregnant women

The use of such noxious agents, of teratogenic potential, in pregnancy is probably not justified, and in the presence of functional malignant tumour termination of pregnancy should be considered.

The elderly

The occurrence of severe nausea and vomiting require that supportive measures to prevent dehydration be undertaken prophylactically. There is no evidence that complications are more severe in the elderly, but their ability to withstand them is reduced. There are no data on comparison between the response to streptozotocin in the elderly and the young.

Concurrent disease
In a trial of 20 patients with Hodgkin's disease, there was no increase in efficacy when streptozotocin was added to the treatment regime, but the mortality was increased. Whether this was due to other cytotoxic drugs being administered coincidentally or to the Hodgkin's disease itself is not known.

Drug interactions

Potentially hazardous interactions

Phenytoin. Potentiation of the CNS-depressant effects of phenytoin has been reported along with a decrease in antitumour potency.

Cytotoxic drugs. Immunosuppression may be enhanced by the coincident administration of other cytotoxic compounds.

Adriamycin. Adriamycin elimination is decreased with the concurrent administration of streptozotocin; the excretory half life is increased from 49 hours to 100 hours.

Potentially useful interactions
5-Fluorouracil has antitumour synergy with streptozotocin.[19]

General review articles

Broder L E, Carter S K, Friedman M 1971 Streptozotocin and metastatic insulinoma. Annals of Internal Medicine 74: 445–446

Broder L E, Carter S K 1974 Chemotherapy of malignant insulinomas with streptozotocin. Excerpta Medica International Congress Series 312: 714–727

Herbai G, Lundin A 1976 Treatment of malignant metastatic pancreatic insulinoma with streptozotocin. Acta Medica Scandinavica 220: 447–452

Hughes C B 1986 Giving cancer drugs IV: some guidelines. American Journal of Nursing 86: 34–38

Mee A S 1985 The Zollinger–Ellison syndrome — diagnosis and management. South African Medical Journal 68: 499–501

Schein P, Kahn R, Gorden P, Wells S, Devita V T 1973 Streptozotocin for malignant insulinomas and carcinoid tumour. Archives of Internal Medicine 132: 555–561

Townsend C M, Thompson J C 1987 Up-to-date treatment of hypergastrinaemia. Advances in Surgery 20: 155–181

Wood S M, Bloom S R 1986 Hormone-producing tumours of the gut. Digestive Diseases 4(2): 57–71

Hall-Craggs 1982 Acute renal failure and renal tubular squamous metaplasia following treatment with streptozotocin. Human Pathology 13: 597

Tabor P A 1986 Drug-induced fever. Drug Intelligence and Clinical Pharmacy 20: 413–420

References

1. Herr R R, Eble T E, Bergy M E, Jahnke H K 1959 Isolation and characterization of streptozotocin. Antibiotic Annals 60: 236–240
2. Weiss R B 1982 Streptozotocin: a review of its pharmacology, efficacy and toxicity. Cancer Treatment Reports 66: 427–438
3. Evans J S, Gerritsen G C, Mann K M et al 1965 Antitumour and hyperglycaemic activity of streptozotocin (NSC-37 917) and its cofactor, U-15, 774. Cancer Chemotherapy Reports 48: 1–6
4. Rakieten N, Rakieten M L, Nadkarni M V 1963 Studies on the diabetogenic action of streptozotocin (NSC-37 917). Cancer Chemotherapy Reports 29: 91–98
5. Kushner B, Lazar M, Furman M et al 1969 Resistance of rabbits and guinea pigs to the diabetogenic effect of streptozotocin. Diabetes 18: 542–544
6. Dulin W E, Wyse B M 1967 Studies on the ability of compounds to block the diabetogenic activity of streptozotocin. Diabetes 18: 459–466
7. Schein P S, Cooney D A, McMenamin M G et al 1973 Streptozotocin diabetes, further studies on the mechanism of depression of nicotinamide adenine dinucleotide concentration in mouse pancreatic islets and liver. Biochemical Pharmacology 22: 2625–2631
8. Bloom S R, Polak J M 1984 Manifestations of pancreatic endocrine tumours. Excerpta Medica International Congress Series 655: 1095–1011
9. Wood S M, Bloom S R 1986 Hormone producing tumours of the gut. Digestive Diseases 4(2): 57–71
10. Schein P, Kahn R, Gorden P, Wells S, Devita V T 1973 Streptozotocin for malignant insulinomas and carcinoid tumour. Archives of Internal Medicine 132: 555–561
11. Clamon G, Riggs C, Stegink L 1986 Pharmacokinetic studies of Streptozotocin (STZ) by continuous infusion. Proceedings of the American Association of Cancer Research 27: 170
12. Zanosar Pharmacokinetic Profile, April 1983 Upjohn Ltd, Crawley, W Sussex. Personal communication
13. Murray-Lyons I M, Eddlestone A W R, Williams R 1968 Treatment of multiple-hormone-producing malignant islet-cell tumours with streptozotocin. Lancet 2: 895–898
14. Shapiro W R 1986 Therapy of adult malignant brain tumours: what have the clinical trials taught us? Seminars in Oncology 13: 38–45
15. Kinnamon K E, Steck E A, Rane D S 1979 Activity of antitumour drugs against African Trypanosomes. Antimicrobial Agents and Chemotherapy 15: 157
16. Rifai S, Aur R J A, Sackey K, Sabbah R S 1985 Control of nausea and vomiting in children and adolescents with cancer. Saudi Medical Journal 6: 605–615
17. Moertel C G, Reitmeier R J, Schutt A J, Hahn R G 1971 Phase 2 study of streptozotocin (NSC 85 998) in the treatment of advanced gastrointestinal cancer. Cancer Chemotherapy Reports 55: 303–307
18. Moertel C G 1975 Clinical management of advanced gastrointestinal cancer. Cancer 36: 675–682
19. Moertel C G, Hanley J A, Johnson L A 1980 Streptozotocin alone compared with Streptozotocin and fluorouracil in the treatment of advanced islet cell carcinoma. New England Journal of Medicine 303: 1189–1194
20. White F R 1963 Streptozotocin. Cancer Chemotherapy Reports 30: 49–53

Sucralfate

Sucralfate is a mucosal protectant used in the treatment of peptic ulceration.

Chemistry

Sucralfate (Antepsin, Sucralfin, Ulcar, Ulcermin)
$C_{12}H_{54}Al_{16}O_{75}S_8$
β-D-Fructofuranosyl-D-glucopyranoside octakis (hydrogen sulphate aluminium complex)

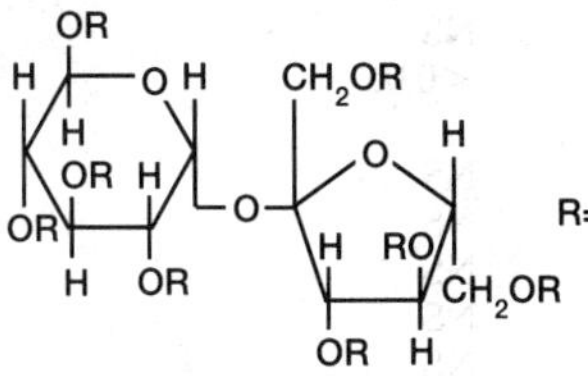

$R=SO_3[Al_2(OH)_5]$

A white to off-white granular powder with a chalky taste but little or no smell. It is prepared by reaction of sucrose octasulphate with aluminium hydroxide. It is not available in any combination.

Pharmacology

Sucralfate is a basic aluminium salt of sucrose octasulphate.[1] In vitro aluminium hydroxide ($Al_2(OH)_5$) ions dissociate in acid leaving negatively charged molecules of sucrose octasulphate which polymerize into a viscous paste, which is the active form of the drug.[2–6] This process takes place when the pH is below 4. When acid is added to sucralfate there is a pre-paste consumption of 0.0875 meq protons per meq drug, after which the paste is resistant to further attack of the acid until 90% (0.9 meq per meq sucralfate) of the hydrochloric acid required for complete dissolution has been added. Such acidic conditions are found in the empty human stomach for 3–6 hours after a 1 g tablet.

The negatively charged molecules of paste then bind to positively charged protein, mucosa and white cells in the ulcer base.[3–6] This adherent complex may be a barrier against acid, pepsin and bile salts. In animal studies, sucralfate adhered to the mucosa of gastric and duodenal ulcers for over 6 hours (but less than 24 hours), and adhered to ulcerated mucosa more than to normal mucosa.[7]

Sucralfate does not alter gastric acid secretion.[8] It is not an intraluminal antacid but might buffer hydrogen ions in an ulcer crater, thereby reducing peptic activity. Sucralfate in vitro at a pH of 2 inhibits pepsin activity both by absorption and by buffering hydrogen ions.[9] Sucralfate also produces a dose-related increase in bicarbonate secretion by gastric and duodenal mucosa.[69]

In vitro, sucralfate increases the viscosity of pig gastric mucus and decreases the penetration of the mucus by hydrogen ions.[10] Sucralfate also absorbs and/or depletes bile acid in the gastric lumen, especially at acidic pH. The absorption of glycocolic acid is comparable to that achieved by cholestyramine.[11,12] Sucralfate stimulates the luminal release of prostaglandins in the rat[13,14] and in the rabbit[15] an increase in prostaglandin E_2 secretion was noted in the gastric and duodenal mucosa.

Toxicology

Sucralfate has shown no toxicological effects in animals. There is no evidence of carcinogenicity in tests lasting up to 24 months in rats, and no evidence of teratological effects in mice, rats or rabbits.

Clinical pharmacology

Sucralfate is effective in the treatment of gastric and duodenal ulcers. It binds to the ulcer crater for greater than 6 hours after a single oral dose. Sucralfate paste binds more effectively to duodenal than to gastric ulcer craters, and binding is more marked to ulcerated mucosa than to normal mucosa.[16,17] Sucralfate inhibits pepsin activity in vivo[18] and causes an increased bicarbonate output from the stomach.[19]

In patients treated with sucralfate for 6 weeks an increase in the ratio of neutral to neutral plus acid mucoprotein complex was seen in the stomach.[20] Gastric transmucosal potential difference (PD) across the ulcerated mucosa of patients with gastric ulcer was significantly increased 2–4 hours after an oral dose of 0.5 g sucralfate. This was interpreted as an improvement in the diffusion barrier.[21] Sucralfate significantly increased the mucosal generation and luminal release of prostaglandin E_2, and 6-keto-PGF$_1\alpha$ and decreased that of thromboxane B_2 in healthy man.[8] The drug has no systemic effects in man and this is perhaps not surprising in view of the very poor absorption of the drug.

Pharmacokinetics

Tissue and blood concentrations of sucralfate have not been measured by any analytical methods.

Absorption of sucralfate from the gastrointestinal tract is minimal (3–5% of ^{14}C labelled dose in rats after 96 h). In six healthy men given a single 1 g of labelled drug, the total 4 day urinary excretion of radioactivity was 0.5–2.2%.[22]

Presystemic metabolism is unknown, as is the half life, the volume of distribution, plasma protein binding, entry into brain and other tissues, and excretion in human breast milk.

Concentration–effect relationship

The therapeutic action of sucralfate is topical and there is no evidence of any relationship to tissue or plasma concentrations.

Metabolism

Sucralfate is minimally (3–5%) absorbed, not metabolized, and is therefore excreted mainly in faeces, with no evidence of enterohepatic circulation.

Pharmaceutics

Sucralfate is available only in an oral formulation of tablets containing 1000 mg. Antepsin tablets (Ayerst, UK) are white/off-white, uncoated, oblong, biconvex with break bar and are marked 'Ayerst' with '1239' on reverse.

Carafate (Marion Labs, USA) are pale pink, uncoated, oblong tablets with a break bar and marked 'MARION' with '1712' on the reverse.

Sucralfate tablets are stable with no special storage conditions, have a shelf-life of 3 years, and carry a minimal risk of potentially allergenic substances.

Therapeutic use

Indications

1. Duodenal and gastric ulcers
2. Oesophagitis
3. Maintenance therapy for peptic ulcer disease.

Contraindications

None is known.

Mode of use

The tablets should be dispersed in 10–15 ml water. Administration before meals may prevent binding of sucralfate to proteins in food.[7]

Ulcer healing treatment is 4 g per day, either as 1 g one hour before meals three times a day, and at bedtime, or 2 g on rising and at bedtime, for 4–12 weeks.

Oesophagitis treatment is 4 g per day, as 1 g three times a day after meals and at bedtime for 4–12 weeks.

Maintenance treatment is 1 g twice daily. There is no official approval of this indication.

S

Indications

1. Healing of ulcers

Healing of gastric, pre-pyloric and duodenal ulcers by sucralfate is significantly higher than with placebo (see Tables 1 and 2) and is comparable with that after H_2-receptor antagonists with a similarly low incidence of side effects. Most trials have used 1 g four times a day: dosage with 2 g twice daily seemed equally effective in healing duodenal ulcers.

Peptic ulcers have a high recurrence rate, and it has been claimed that ulcers relapse less frequently and less fast after treatment with sucralfate than with H_2 receptor antagonists, but controlled trials have shown no significant differences (see Table 3).

Table 1 Controlled trials of sucralfate 1 g four times daily for healing duodenal ulcer

Trial	Weeks	Sucralfate		Control			P	C.I.	Ref.
		Healed	%		Healed	%			
DB	4	16/24	66	Placebo	17/30	56	NS		36
SB	6		80	Cimetidine 1 g		76	NS		37
PB	6	18/30	60	Placebo	7/29	24	<0.03		38
	12	23/30	82	Placebo	12/27	22	<0.05		
DB	4	11/16	69	Placebo	7/17	41	NS		39
DB	4	55/69	80	Placebo	33/55	60	<0.05		40
DB	2	11/33	33	Placebo	4/34	12			41
	4	27/33	92	Placebo	18/34	25			
DB	12	57/81	70	Placebo	42/78	54	<0.05		42
DB	4	9/15	60	Placebo	7/16	44	NS		43
	8	14/15	93	Placebo	5/16	31	<0.05		
DB	4		75			64			44
DB	4	11/13	85	Placebo	7/13	54	NS		45
DB	4		80	Cimetidine 1 g		76	NS		46
	8		90	Cimetidine 1 g		86	NS		
SB	4	23/35	66	Cimetidine 1 g	27/37	73	NS		47
	6	32/35	91		31/37	84	NS		
SB	4	22/31	71	Cimetidine 1 g	24/32	75	NS		48
	6	30/31	97		31/32	97	NS		
DB	4	24/33	73	Placebo	8/32	25	<0.001		49
DB	4	125/177	71	Cimetidine	149/194	72	NS	−15% +3%	50
	8	152/177	86		178/194	92	NS	−12% +5%	
SB	4	28/38	74	Sucralfate 2 g	28/36	78	NS		51
	8	32/38	84	twice daily	30/36	84	NS		

DB = double blind; SB = single blind; NS = not significant.

Table 2 Controlled trials of sucralfate for healing gastric ulcers: all sites, body, prepyloric (PP) and with duodenal ulcer (+DU)

Trial	Ulcer	Weeks	Sucralfate			Control			P	C.I.	Ref.
			Dose	Healed	%		Healed	%			
SB		6	1 g four times daily	17/27	63	Cimetidine	21/28	75	NS		37
		12		20/27	74		25/28	89	NS		
DB	all	4	1 g four times daily	8/13	62	Placebo	2/8	25	NS		39
DB	all	4	1 g four times daily	17/24	71		8/20	40	<0.005		40
DB	all	4	1.5 g three times daily	8/16	50	Placebo	2/12	17	NS		52
SB	all	4	1 g four times daily	17/36	47	Cimetidine	16/33	48	NS		53
		8		29/36	81		24/33	73	NS		
DB	all	4	1 g four times daily	6/12	50	Cimetidine	7/13	54	NS		54
		8		9/12	75		10/13	77	NS		
SB	all	4	1 g four times daily	10/28	36	Cimetidine	18/30	60	NS		48
		6		20/28	71		25/30	83	NS		
DB	Body	6	0.9 g four times daily	28/40	69	Placebo	10/31	33	<0.001		55
		8	granules	31/39	79	Placebo	13/31	41	<0.001		
	PP	6	granules	13/16	80	Placebo	4/16	25	<0.004		
		8	granules	15/16	93	Placebo	5/16	33	<0.001		
	+DU	6	granules	5/16	62	Placebo	9/16	56	NS		
		8	granules	12/15	78	Placebo	10/16	60	NS		
DB	pp	4	1 g four times daily	6	68			70	NS	−13, +17	56
		8			83			90	NS	−4, +19	
DB	Body	4	1 g four times daily	68	61	Cimetidine	66	69	NS	−23, +9	57
		8			94			94	NS	−8, +8	
		12			98			94	NS	+11, −2	

DB = double blind; SB = single blind; NS = nor significant.

2. Oesophagitis

There have been two controlled trials (Table 4). Symptomatic improvement has been as rapid as with placebo or with alginate/antacid. Endoscopic healing has been significantly higher than with placebo and comparable with an alginate/antacid mixture.

3. Maintenance therapy for peptic ulcer disease

Sucralfate has protected rats from developing duodenal ulcer induced by pentagastrin plus bethanechol,[23] and gastric erosions induced by alcohol.[24]

Maintenance dosage with sucralfate 1–3 g daily in patients with duodenal and gastric ulcer have significantly reduced their recurrence rates compared with placebo (Table 5). The efficacy and safety of maintenance therapy with sucralfate 1 g twice daily may be comparable with results with H_2-receptor antagonists, but in the absence of long-term toxicity data, treatment with sucralfate is still officially recommended only for up to 12 weeks.

4. Non-therapeutic clinical usage

Sucralfate labelled with ^{99m}Tc human serum albumin has been used to detect peptic ulceration by isotope scanning,[25] and also ulceration in inflammatory bowel disease (Crohn's and ulcerative colitis).[26]

Sucralfate

Adverse reactions

Potentially life-threatening effects

No life-threatening toxic effects have occurred in man due to this drug.

Acute overdosage

No cases of deliberate overdose have been reported.

Severe or irreversible adverse effects

When sucralfate was given 4 g daily to 17 patients with peptic ulcer for up to 10 weeks, plasma aluminium was not significantly different from controls,[27] but there was appreciable accumulation of aluminium in patients with renal failure.[28]

Symptomatic adverse effects

The most frequent effect of this kind noted since 1968 has been constipation in about 40% of patients, but this is not significantly more than after placebo or other ulcer-healing drugs.[29,30] A sucralfate bezoar has been reported.[31]

Other effects

Sucralfate is not known to modify any aspect of body biochemistry in healthy subjects.

Table 3 Relapse after initial ulcer-healing with sucralfate and H_2-receptor antagonists

Trial	Ulcer	Weeks	Initial treatment sucralfate		Initial treatment control			P	Ref.
			Relapse	%		Relapse	%		
Open	DU	26	9/29	31	Cimetidine	13/24	54	NS	58
Open	GU	26	9/18	50	Cimetidine	12/20	60	NS	58
	PU	40–48		48	Cimetidine		55	NS	59

NS = not significant.

Table 4 Controlled trials of sucralfate for oesophagitis

Trial	Weeks	Dose (g daily)	Sucralfate		Control			P	Sucralfate		Control			P	Ref.
			Improved	%		Improved	%		Healed	%		Healed	%		
DB	12	4			Placebo			NS	16/22	72	Placebo	10/25	40	<0.05	60
DB	6	6	25/36	69	Alginate/ antacid	21/32	66	NS	19/36	53	Alginate/ antacid	11/32	34	NS	61

DB = double blind; NS = not significant.

Table 5 Controlled trials of maintenance therapy with sucralfate for duodenal and gastric ulcers

Trial	Ulcer	Weeks	Dose (g daily)	Sucralfate		Control			P	Ref.
				Relapses	%		Relapses	%		
DB	DU	26	2	14/66	21	Placebo	30/60	50	<0.01	62
DB	DU	26	3	2/18	12	Placebo Cimetidine	13/22 6/24	59 33	<0.05	63
DB	DU	52	2.5	7/17	47	Placebo	12/15	80	<0.05	64
DB	DU	52	2	8/30	27	Placebo	25/31	81	<0.0001	65
DB	DU	52	2	10/24	42	Placebo	19/24	79	<0.003	66
SB	DU	52	1 2	7/15 6/19	47 32	Placebo	13/16	81	<0.05 <0.05	67
DB	GU	26	2	11/30	37	Placebo	11/25	44	NS	62
DB	GU	26	3	2/10	20	Placebo Cimetidine	3/9 5/11	33 45	NS	63
DB	GU	24	3	5/31	16	Placebo	21/30	70	<0.001	68

DB = double blind; SB = single blind; NS-not significant.

S

Interference with clinical pathology tests
No technical interferences of this kind are known.

High risk groups

Neonates
Safety and efficacy has not been established in neonates.

Breast milk. Excretion of sucralfate in breast milk of nursing mothers has not been studied.

Children
No data are available on the use of the drug in children.

Pregnant women
Safety and efficacy has not been established in pregnant women, who should be given sucralfate only for clear indications.

The elderly
No special dosage requirements of sucralfate in the elderly are known.

Concurrent disease

Renal failure. Sucralfate should be used with caution in patients with renal failure because of the possible absorption of aluminium and the effects of raised plasma aluminium on the kidney.[28]

Sucralfate binds phosphates so that these patients might develop hypophosphataemia.[32]

Drug interactions

Potentially hazardous interactions

Tetracyclines, phenytoin and digoxin. The bioavailability of these drugs may be reduced by sucralfate which should therefore not be given within 2 hours of any of them.[33]

Warfarin. Sucralfate may hinder the absorption of warfarin, so that caution should be exercised when these drugs are used together.

Sulpiride. The bioavailability of sulpiride was reduced by 40% when given together with sucralfate.[34]

Other significant interactions
None is known. In particular the bioavailability of ranitidine is not altered by sucralfate, so the two drugs may be given together.[35]

Potentially useful interactions
No interactions of this kind are known.

Major outcome trials

See Tables 1–5.

Reviews

Brogden R N, Heel R C, Speight T M, Avery G S 1984 Sucralfate. A review of its pharmacodynamic properties and therapeutic use in peptic ulcer disease. Drugs 27: 194–209

Garnett W R 1982 Drug reviews. Sucralfate — alternative therapy for peptic-ulcer disease. Clinical Pharmacy 1: 307–314

McGraw B F, Caldwell E G 1981 Sucralfate. Drug Intelligence and Clinical Pharmacy 15: 578–580

General review articles

Proceedings of the 1st international sucralfate symposium 1980 Journal of Clinical Gastroenterology 3 (suppl 2)

Caspary W F (ed) 1981 Duodenal ulcer, gastric ulcer: sucralfate, a new therapeutic concept. Ubran & Schwarzenberg, Munich

Lam S K, Misiewicz J J, Aarima M 1987 Proceedings of the fourth international sucralfate symposium, Sao Paolo 1986. Scandinavian Journal of Gastroenterology 22 (suppl 140)

Marks I N, Samloff I M, Aarima M, Siurala M (eds) 1983 Proceedings of the 2nd international sucralfate symposium, Stockholm 1982. Scandinavian Journal of Gastroenterology 18 (suppl 83)

Marks I N, Samloff I M (eds) 1985 Third international sucralfate symposium 1984 American Journal of Medicine 79 (2c)

Mistilis S P (ed) 1985 Current concepts in gastric cytoprotection. Medical Journal of Australia 142 (3)

References

1. Nagashima R 1981 Development and characteristics of sucralfate. Journal of Clinical Gastroenterology 3 (suppl 2): 103–110
2. Nagashima R 1981 Mechanisms of action of sucralfate. Journal of Clinical Gastroenterology 3 (suppl 2): 117–127
3. Nagashima R, Yoshida N 1979 Sucralfate, a basic aluminium salt of sucrose sulfate. I. Behaviors in gastroduodenal pH. Arzneimittelforschung 29: 1668–1676
4. Nagashima R, Hirano T 1980 Selective binding of sucralfate to ulcer lesions. I. Experiments in rats with acetic acid-induced gastric ulcer receiving unlabelled sucralfate. Arzneimittelforschung 30: 80–83
5. Nagashima R, Hinohara Y, Hirano T, Tohira Y, Kamiyama H 1980 Selective binding of sucralfate to ulcer lesion. II. Experiments in rats with gastric ulcer receiving ^{14}C sucralfate or potassium ^{14}C-sucrose sulfate. Arzneimittelforschung 30: 84–88
6. Nagashima R, Hinohara Y, Hirano T 1980 Selective binding of sucralfate to ulcer lesions. III. Experiments in rats with duodenal ulcer receiving ^{14}C-sucralfate. Arzneimittelforschung 30: 88–91
7. Giesing D H, Bighley L D, Iles R L 1981 Effect of food and antacid on binding of sucralfate to normal and ulcerated gastric and duodenal mucosa in rats. Journal of Clinical Gastroenterology 3 (suppl 2): 111– 116
8. Konturek S J, Kwiecien N, Obtulowicz W, Kopp B, Oleksy J 1986 Double-blind controlled study in the effect of sucralfate on gastric prostaglandin formation and microbleeding in normal and aspirin treated man. Gut 27: 1450–1456
9. Samloff I M, O'Dell C 1985 Inhibition of peptic activity by sucralfate. American Journal of Medicine 79 (suppl 2C): 15–18
10. Slomiany B L, Laszewicz W, Slomiany A 1986 Effect of sucralfate on the viscosity of gastric mucus and the permeability to hydrogen ion. Digestion 33: 146–151
11. Bruusgaard A, Elsborg L, Reinecke V 1981 Bile acid-'binding' properties of sucralfate. In: Caspary W F (ed) Duodenal ulcer, gastric ulcer: sucralfate, a new therapeutic concept. Urban & Schwarzenberg, Munich, pp 28–31
12. Graham D Y, Sackman J W, Giesing D H, Runser D J 1984 In vitro adsorption of bile salts and aspirin to sucralfate. Digestive Diseases and Sciences 29: 402–406
13. Hollander D, Tarnawski A, Gergely H, Zipser R D 1984 Sucralfate protection of the gastric mucosa against ethanol-induced injury: a prostaglandin-mediated process? Scandinavian Journal of Gastroenterology 19 (suppl 101): 97–102
14. Tarnawski A, Hollander D, Krause W J, Zipser R D, Stachura J, Gergely H 1986 Does sucralfate affect the normal gastric mucosa? Histologic ultrastructural and functional assessment in the rat. Gastroenterology 90: 893–905
15. Crampton J R, Gibbons L C, Rees W D W 1986 Sucralfate produces a dose dependent increase in PGE_2 synthesis by mammalian gastric and duodenal mucosa. Gut 27: A606
16. Nakasama S, Nagashima R, Samloff I M 1981 Selective binding of sucralfate to gastric ulcer in man. Digestive Diseases and Sciences 26: 297–300
17. Sasaki H, Hinohara Y, Tsunoda Y, Nagashima R 1983 Binding of sucralfate to duodenal ulcer in man. Scandinavian Journal of Gastroenterology 18 (suppl 83): 13–14
18. Garnett W R 1982 Sucralfate — alternative therapy for peptic-ulcer disease. Clinical Pharmacy 1: 307–314
19. Guslandi M 1985 Sucralfate and gastric bicarbonate. Pharmacology 31: 298–300
20. Guslandi M, Ballarin E, Tittobello A 1982 The ulcer-healing and mucosa-stimulating properties of sucralfate — a comparative study with cimetidine. Fortschritte der Medizin 100: 1778–1779
21. Mockel W, Hausding P 1981 Behavior of the transmural potential difference in the region of gastric ulcers in man under the influence of sucralfate. In: Caspary W F (ed) Duodenal ulcer, gastric ulcer: sucralfate, a new therapeutic concept. Urban & Schwarzenberg, Munich, pp 39–43
22. Giesing D H, Lanman R C, Runser D 1982 Absorption of sucralfate in man. Gastroenterology 82: A1066
23. Smolow C R, Bank S, Ackert G, Anfang C, Krantz V 1983 Prevention of experimental duodenal ulcer in the rat by sucralfate. Scandinavian Journal of Gastroenterology 18 (suppl 83): 15–16
24. Nagashima R, Hoshkino E, Hinohara Y, Sakai K, Hata S, Nakano H 1983 Effect of sucralfate on ethanol-induced gastric mucosal damage in the rat. Scandinavian Journal of Gastroenterology 18 (suppl 83): 17–20
25. Vasquez T E, Bridges R L, Braunstein P, Jansholt A L, Meshkenpour H 1983 Work in progress: gastrointestinal ulcerations — detection using a technetium-99m-labelled ulcer-avid drug. Radiology 148: 227–231
26. Dawson D J, Khan A N, Shreeve D R 1985 Technetium-99m–sucralfate isotope scanning. A new technique to detect active inflammatory bowel disease? Gut 26: A578
27. Kinoshita, Kumaki K, Nakano H et al 1982 Plasma aluminium levels of patients on long-term sucralfate therapy. Research Communications in Chemical Pathology and Pharmacology 35: 515–518
28. Leung A C T, Henderson I S, Halls D J, Dobbie J W 1983 Aluminium hydroxide as a phosphate binder in uremia. British Medical Journal 286: 1379–1381
29. Fisher R S 1981 Sucralfate: a review of drug tolerance and safety. Journal of Clinical Gastroenterology 3 (suppl 2): 181–184
30. Ishimori A 1981 Safety experience with sucralfate in Japan. Journal of Clinical Gastroenterology 3 (suppl 2): 169–173
31. Algozzine G J, Hill G, Sloggins W G, Marr M A 1983 Sucralfate bezoar. New England Journal of Medicine 309: 1387
32. Sherman R A, Hwang E R, Walker J A, Elsinger R P 1983 Reduction in serum phosphorus due to sucralfate. American Journal of Gastroenterology 78: 210–211
33. Giesing D H, Lanman R C, Dimmitt D C, Runsen D J 1983 Lack of effect of sucralfate in digoxin pharmacokinetics. Gastroenterology 85: 1165
34. Gouda M W, Hikal A H, Babhair S A, ElHofy S A, Mahrous G M 1984 Effect of sucralfate and antacids on the bioavailability of sulpiride in humans. International Journal of Pharmacy 257–263
35. Mullersman G, Gotz V P, Russell W P, Derendorf H 1986 Lack of clinically significant in vitro and in vivo interactions between ranitidine and sucralfate. Journal of Pharmaceutical Sciences 75: 95–998
36. Roufail W M 1978 Pilot trial of a sulfated polysaccharide in the treatment of duodenal ulcer disease. Southern Medical Journal 72: 262–264

Sucralfate

37. Marks I N, Wright J P, Denyer M, Garisck J A M, Lucke W 1980 Comparison of sucralfate with cimetidine in the short-term treatment of chronic peptic ulcers. South African Medical Journal 57: 567–573
38. Moshal M G, Spitaels J M, Khan F 1980 Sucralfate in the treatment of duodenal ulcers. A double-blind endoscopically controlled trial. South African Medical Journal 57: 742–744
39. Orchard R, Elliot C 1981 A double-blind placebo-controlled study of sucralfate in the treatment of gastric and duodenal ulcer. In: Caspary W F (ed) Duodenal ulcer, gastric ulcer: sucralfate, a new therapeutic concept. Urban & Schwarzenberg, Munich, pp 85–88
40. Fixa B, Komarova O 1980 Aluminium sucrose sulphate (sucralfate) in the treatment of peptic ulcer (double-blind study). In: Caspary W F (ed) Duodenal ulcer, gastric ulcer: sucralfate, a new therapeutic concept. Urban & Schwarzenberg, Munich, pp 80–84
41. Hollander D 1981 Efficacy of sucralfate for duodenal ulcers: a multicenter, double-blind trial. Journal of Clinical Gastroenterology 3 (suppl 2): 153–157
42. Ishimori A, Arakawa H 1981 A placebo-controlled, double-blind trial using sucralfate for the treatment of peptic ulcer. A multi-center Japanese study. In: Caspary W F (ed) Duodenal ulcer, gastric ulcer: sucralfate, a new therapeutic concept. Urban & Schwarzenberg, Munich, pp 93–101
43. Lahtinen J, Ala-Kaila K, Aukee S et al 1981 Sucralfate and antacid in the treatment of gastric and duodenal ulcer. The preliminary report of a multi-center double-blind trial. In: Caspar W F (ed) Duodenal ulcer, gastric ulcer: sucralfate, a new therapeutic concept. Urban & Schwarzenberg, Munich, pp 111–115
44. McHardy G G 1981 A multicenter double-blind trial of sucralfate and placebo in duodenal ulcer. Journal of Clinical Gastroenterology 3 (suppl 2): 147–162
45. Maier K, Sinn I, Topfer U, Feinauer B, von Gaisberg U, Heinkel K 1981 Clinical experience with sucralfate in the treatment of prepyloric and intraduodenal ulcers in a hospital setting. In: Caspary W F (ed) Duodenal ulcer, gastric ulcer: sucralfate, a new therapeutic concept. Urban & Schwarzenberg, Munich, pp 89–92
46. Martin F, Farley A, Gagnon M, Bensemana D 1982 A comparison of the healing capacities of sucralfate and cimetidine in the short-term treatment of duodenal ulcer: a double-blind randomised trial. Gastroenterology 82: 401–405
47. Hentschel E, Schutze K, Dufek W 1983 Controlled comparison of sucralfate and cimetidine in duodenal ulcer. Scandinavian Journal of Gastroenterology 18 (suppl 83): 31–35
48. Pop P, Nikkels R E, Thys O, Dorrestein G C M 1983 Comparison of sucralfate and cimetidine in the treatment of duodenal and gastric ulcers. A multicentre study. Scandinavian Journal of Gastroenterology 18 (suppl 83): 43–47
49. Sung J L, Yu J W, Wang T H, Wang C Y, Chew D S 1983 A placebo-controlled double-blind study of sucralfate in the short-term treatment of duodenal ulcer. Scandinavian Journal of Gastroenterologyerol 18 (suppl 83): 21–24
50. Glise H, Carlin G, Hallerback B et al 1986 Short-term treatment of duodenal ulcer. A comparison of sucralfate and cimetidine. Scandinavian Journal of Gastroenterology 21: 313–320
51. Brandstaetter G, Kratochvil P 1985 Comparison of two sucralfate dosages (2 g twice a day versus 1 g four times a day) in duodenal ulcer healing. American Journal of Medicine 79 (suppl 2C): 36–38
52. Rhodes J, Mayberry J F, Williams R A, Lawrie B W 1981 Clinical trial of sucralfate in the treatment of gastric ulcer. In: Caspary W F (ed) Duodenal ulcer, gastric ulcer: sucralfate, a new therapeutic concept. Urban & Schwarzenberg, Munich, pp 101–104
53. Lahtinen J, Aukee S, Miettinen P, Poikolainen E, Paakkonen M, Sandstrom R 1983 Sucralfate and cimetidine for gastric ulcer. Scandinavian Journal of Gastroenterology 18 (suppl 83): 49–51
54. Martin F, Farley A, Gagnon M, Poitras P, Bensemana D 1983 Short-term treatment with sucralfate or cimetidine in gastric ulcer: preliminary results of a controlled randomised trial. Scandinavian Journal of Gastroenterology 18 (suppl 83): 37–41
55. Lam S K, Lam W Y, Lai C L et al 1985 Efficacy of sucralfate in corpus, prepyloric and duodenal ulcer associated gastric ulcers. A double-blind, placebo-controlled study. American Journal of Medicine 79 (suppl 2C): 24–31
56. Svedberg L E, Carling L, Glise H et al 1985 Short-term treatment of prepyloric ulcer — a cytoprotective agent versus a histamine-2-antagonist. Gut 26: A559–560
57. Hallerback B, Anker-Hansen O, Carling L et al 1986 Short-term treatment of gastric ulcer: a comparison of sucralfate and cimetidine. Gut 27: 778–783
58. Marks I N, Wright J P, Lucke W, Girdwood A H 1983 Relapse rates following initial ulcer healing with sucralfate and cimetidine. Scandinavian Journal of Gastroenterology 18 (suppl 83): 53–56
59. Solhaug J H, Carling L, Glise H et al 1986 Ulcer relapse following initial healing with sucralfate or cimetidine. Digestive Diseases and Sciences 31 (suppl): 175
60. Weiss W, Brunner H, Buttner B R et al 1983 Therapie der Refluxösophagitis mit Sucralfat. Deutsche Medizinische Wochenschrift 108: 1706–1711
61. Laitinen S, Stahlberg M, Kairaluoma M I et al 1985 Sucralfate and alginate/antacid in reflux esophagitis. Scandinavian Journal of Gastroenterology 20: 229–232
62. Classen M et al 1983 Effect of sucralfate on peptic ulcer recurrence: a controlled double-blind multicenter study. Scandinavian Journal of Gastroenterology 18 (suppl 83): 61–68
63. Libeskind M 1983 Maintenance therapy of patients with healed peptic ulcer with sucralfate, placebo and cimetidine. Scandinavian Journal of Gastroenterology 18 (suppl 83): 69–70
64. Moshal M G, Spitaels J M, Mainion G L 1983 Double-blind placebo-controlled evaluation of one year therapy with sucralfate in healed duodenal ulcer. Scandinavian Journal of Gastroenterology 18 (suppl 83): 57–59
65. Behar J, Roufail W, Thomas E, Keller F, Dernbach W, Tesler M 1986 Efficacy of sucralfate in the prevention of recurrence of duodenal ulcer. Gastroenterology 90: 1343
66. Bolin T D, Davis A E, Duncombe V M, Billington B 1986 The role of maintenance sucralfate in prevention of duodenal ulcer recurrence. Digestive Diseases and Sciences 31: 2835
67. Marks I N, Girdwood A H 1985 Recurrence of duodenal ulceration in patients with maintenance sucralfate. South African Medical Journal 67: 626–628
68. Marks I N, Wright J P, Girdwood A H, Gilinsky N H, Lucke W 1985 Maintenance therapy with sucralfate reduces rate of gastric ulcer recurrence. American Journal of Medicine 79 (suppl 2C): 32–35
69. Crompton J R, Gibbons L C Reesh D W 1988 Stimulation of anphibian gastroduodenal bicarbonate secretion by sucralfate and aluminium: a role of local prostaglandin metabolism. Gut 29: 903–908

S

Sufentanil

Sufentanil is the most potent opioid (μ-receptor agonist) available for human clinical use, with a relatively rapid onset and short duration of effect which makes it particularly suitable for anaesthetic practice.

Chemistry

Sufentanil (Sufenta)
$C_{22}H_{30}N_2O_5S$
N[4-(methoxymethyl)-1-[2-(2-thienyl)ethyl]-4-piperidinyl]-N-phenyl propanamide

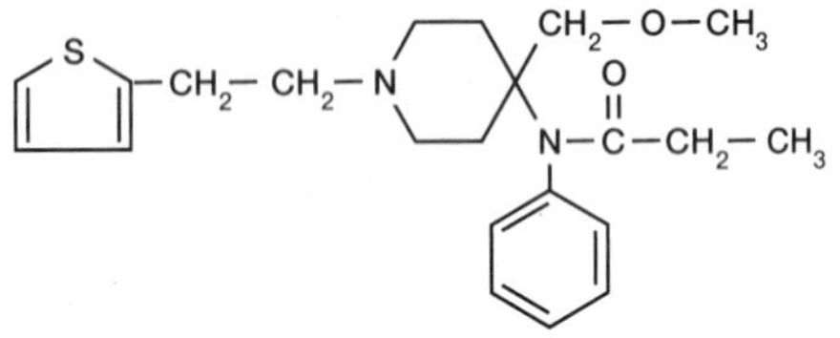

Molecular weight	578.7
pKa	8.01
Solubility	
in alcohol	—
in water	—
Octanol/water partition coefficient	1.75

Sufentanil is a synthetic opioid derived from fentanyl and is a crystalline compound.

Pharmacology

Sufentanil has typical opioid (μ-receptor) agonist effects, with an onset of maximum effect in approximately 5 minutes and a shorter duration of effect than equipotent doses of morphine or pethidine. Its duration of action is similar to that of fentanyl, but sufentanil is approximately 10 times more potent. It is, however, less cumulative than fentanyl, being eliminated faster.

Toxicology

Sufentanil does not have mutagenic potential and its animal testing failed to demonstrate mutagenic or carcinogenic effects. In high doses sufentanil causes death by respiratory depression. Severe bradycardia or asystole may occur in conjunction with vecuronium. In ventilated dogs extremely high doses cause convulsions and these have been associated rarely with its use in man.

Clinical pharmacology

Sufentanil produces dose-related analgesia in patients with postoperative pain, and also raises the threshold for experimental pain, in doses of 0.1–0.3 μg.kg^{-1}. The ability of sufentanil to inhibit transmission in pain-conducting nerve pathways led to its major use as a component of anaesthesia. Small doses (0.1 to 0.3 μg.kg^{-1}) may be used as a supplement in spontaneously breathing patients. Doses of 0.5 μg.kg^{-1} upwards will suppress somatic and autonomic nervous responses to surgery. Large doses (20 μg.kg^{-1} or more) may be used to induce and maintain anaesthesia for major surgery; sufentanil is regarded as the opioid with the most favourable properties for use in open heart surgery.

Sufentanil causes respiratory depression. Doses over 0.3 μg.kg^{-1} are unsuitable if spontaneous ventilation is required. The curve of respiratory response to arterial CO_2 is shifted to the right.

Muscle rigidity with 'stiff' chest is likely to occur with dosage over approximately 0.5 μg.kg^{-1}. Concurrent use of muscle relaxants is required for large doses.

Nausea and vomiting are adverse effects of sufentanil, like other opioids. Sufentanil, like morphine, decreases gastrointestinal motility.

The cardiovascular effects of sufentanil are an initial decrease in rate, with negligible inotropic activity. Reductions in systemic vascular resistance and arterial blood pressure are usual.

Sufentanil decreases metabolic activity and oxygen consumption. It reduces the metabolic responses to surgery.

Pharmacokinetics

The usual method of analysis is a radioimmunoassay that is sensitive, reliable and highly specific.[1] It is capable of assaying sufentanil in plasma down to a level of 0.06 μg.l^{-1}

Sufentanil is highly lipophilic with a n-octanol/water partition coefficient of 1.754. Tissue uptake is therefore extensive and membrane transfer rapid with fast onset of central nervous system effects. The distribution half life of 15 min and $t_{\frac{1}{2}}$ Keo of 6 min (time lag from achieving a plasma concentration to a set decrease of an EEG spectral edge) are similar to those of fentanyl. Placental transfer would be expected.

The plasma concentration profile following intravenous injection fits triexponentially, indicating the following mean parameters:[2] half life β 164 min, V_c 0.164 l.kg^{-1}, V_D 2.86 l.kg^{-1}, plasma clearance 12.66 ml.kg^{-1}.min^{-1}.

The volume of distribution is increased in obese patients, but the plasma clearance is similar[3] suggesting that a dose given on a mg.kg^{-1} basis would produce lower plasma concentrations and be eliminated more slowly. Distribution may be slower, however, so that dosage is better based on ideal weight, and slower elimination is only apparent when repeated doses or infusions are given.[4] As with other opioids the mean pharmacokinetics of sufentanil in the elderly are close to normal so that no special hazard is envisaged. A prolonged elimination half life may be seen in some elderly patients, however; supplementary doses may need to be reduced.[5] In small children, greater clearance suggests the requirement for more frequent dosing.[6]

Oral absorption	not relevant
Presystemic metabolism	—
Plasma half life	2–5 h
Volume of distribution	2.86 l.kg^{-1}
Plasma protein binding	92%

In patients with cirrhosis of the liver sufentanil might be expected to have a prolonged duration of effect, although no significant pharmacokinetic differences were found. Renal function plays no important part in the elimination of sufentanil so pharmacokinetic data show only an increased V_D.[7]

Concentration–effect relationship

Although dose–effect relations are clearly demonstrable there is inadequate documentation of concentration–effect relations. The t Keo (time lag between achieving a plasma concentration and its measured clinical effect, a particular level of decrease of EEG spectral edge) for sufentanil has been assessed at 5.8 minutes.[8]

Metabolism

Sufentanil undergoes oxidative N-dealkylation and O-demethylation in the liver, but metabolites have not been detected in the blood after administration of 3 μg.kg^{-1}. Desmethyl sufentanil has been detected in urine and has a pharmacological potency similar to that of fentanyl.[9] Whole-body rate of elimination is high, suggesting a high hepatic extraction ratio (0.8) and extensive presystemic metabolism after oral ingestion.

Pharmaceutics

Sufentanil (Sufenta; Janssen, US) is available in parenteral form as a clear solution of 5 μg.ml^{-1} sufentanil citrate in 2 ml and 10 ml ampoules, and 50 μg.ml^{-1} in 5 ml ampoules. The pH range is 3.5 to 6.0. The solution is stable when protected from light with a reasonable shelf-life, carrying no apparent risk from potentially allergenic substances.

Therapeutic use

Indications

1. As a component of anaesthesia
2. For opioid anaesthesia
3. As an analgesic.

Contraindications

1. Respiratory inadequacy
2. Hypovolaemia.

These are both relative contraindications.

Indications

1. As a component of anaesthesia
Sufentanil may be used in similar ways to fentanyl as an intravenous component of anaesthesia.

a. In a small dose (e.g. 0.1 μg.kg^{-1}) in spontaneously breathing patients to supplement an intravenous anaesthetic or N_2O/O_2 for maintenance of anaesthesia for minor surgery not involving skin incision, e.g. cystoscopy or dilatation and curettage of the uterus.[10]
b. In a small dose (e.g. 0.1 μg.kg^{-1}) in spontaneously breathing patients, or in a larger dose (e.g. 0.2 μg.kg^{-1}) in ventilated patients to decrease the requirement of volatile anaesthetic for maintenance of anaesthesia.
c. As a supplement to N_2O/O_2 maintenance of anaesthesia, to reduce or suppress somatic and autonomic nervous responses to surgery, in ventilated patients. Doses of 0.5–5 μg.kg^{-1} have been used; 1 μg.kg^{-1} is required for complete suppression of cardiovascular responses to tracheal intubation[10] and will usually control adequately cardiovascular responses to major surgery for approximately 45 minutes. The onset of effect is approximately 5 minutes. The effect may subsequently be extended by use of increments of 0.1 μg.kg^{-1}, which are less cumulative than those of fentanyl.[11] Larger initial doses may be used to give a longer duration of effect, but are usually used in an effort to reduce metabolic responses to surgery, such as increased plasma levels of adrenaline, noradrenaline, glucose, cortisol, etc. The duration of effect is approximately 1 hour per 1 μg.kg^{-1} sufentanil.

2. Opioid anaesthesia
Opioids are used as the basis of anaesthesia, together with O_2 and muscle relaxant in ventilated patients in order to avoid the cardiovascular depressant effects of intravenous anaesthetics, N_2O, and volatile anaesthetics. Sufentanil is probably the best opioid for this use, having little depressant effect on myocardial contractility and an appropriate rate of onset and duration of effect, similar to that of fentanyl but with faster elimination and less cumulation. Cardiac surgery is the main indication for such a technique which will invariably cause prolonged respiratory depression, usually treated by maintenance of artificial respiration in the postoperative period.

Doses in excess of 10 μg.kg^{-1} sufentanil are required for opioid analgesia but may fail to completely control cardiovascular responses to the greatest stimulation (e.g. sternal splitting) so that additional medication (e.g. sodium nitroprusside or a volatile anaesthetic) may be required at that time. Larger doses of sufentanil (up to 30 μg.kg^{-1}) may be used to improve suppression of both autonomic nervous and hormonal responses to surgery. The value of suppression of hormonal and metabolic responses to surgery is yet to be evaluated.

3. Analgesia
Sufentanil (20–50 μg) has been given epidurally for relief of postoperative or labour pains. Analgesia starts in approximately 5 minutes and lasts for about 5 hours.

Adverse reactions

Potentially life-threatening effects
Respiratory depression is the most consistent toxic effect of sufentanil. The drug should never be given unless full facilities for maintenance of oxygenation and ventilation (including endotracheal intubation) are to hand. During clinical anaesthesia, respiratory depression is normally of little consequence. The continuation of this effect into the postoperative period is usual and demands critical assessment and monitoring until the effect has passed. In patients with ventilatory insufficiency, respiratory depression may be life-threatening and even the use of artificial ventilation may cause severe problems. An opiate antagonist may be required. In patients with raised or potentially raised intracranial pressure (including head injuries) the rise in cerebral blood flow consequent on respiratory depression with increased $PaCO_2$ can be lethal and must be prevented.

Muscular rigidity may occur after sufentanil. It is dose-dependent and almost constant when dosages over 1 μg.kg^{-1} are used. Chest wall rigidity may make artificial ventilation impossible, thereby threatening life. Muscle relaxants must be available except when all but the smallest doses of sufentanil are used, together with facilities for tracheal intubation and artificial ventilation. Muscle relaxants should be given to work concomitantly with sufentanil in doses exceeding 0.5 μg.kg^{-1}.

Cardiovascular effects include reductions in cardiac rate and systemic vascular resistance, leading to a fall in arterial blood pressure. This is potentially life-threatening in hypovolaemic patients and in the presence of interacting drugs such as the volatile anaesthetics or muscle relaxants (particularly vecuronium).[12]

Acute overdosage
Sufentanil is usually given for therapeutic reasons in what constitutes an acute 'toxic overdose', that is, the patient would die from acute respiratory arrest if left without artificial ventilation. Maintenance of ventilation is all that is required for overdosage, although the use of a specific opioid antidote such as naloxone could be appropriate and is frequently used to reverse postoperative respiratory depression.

Severe or irreversible adverse effects
Tonic–clonic movements have been reported in two anaesthetized patients.[13]

Symptomatic adverse effects
Nausea and vomiting may occur after the use of sufentanil, as after other opioids.

High risk groups

Neonates
The neonate would be expected to be more sensitive to the respiratory depressant effects of sufentanil than older children, as is the case with other opioids.

Breast milk. Sufentanil should pass into milk but is subject to such extensive presystemic hepatic metabolism that an effect on the child is unlikely.

Children
In infants of less than 1 year only unpublished evaluations are known. For open-heart surgery doses of 5 or 10 μg.kg^{-1} were not completely effective in suppressing responses.

For children over this age the only published information relates to the use of sufentanil for opioid anaesthesia for cardiac surgery.[14] This supports the view (see, Pharmacokinetics) that children require relatively larger and more frequent doses.

Pregnant women
Sufentanil should readily pass the placental barrier (as it does in sheep) and might cause respiratory depression of the newborn if given during delivery, but specific evidence is lacking.

The elderly
No specific sensitivity exists in elderly patients.

Drug interactions

Potentially hazardous interactions
Muscle relaxants. The positive chronotropic effect of pancuronium makes it suitable for most uses with sufentanil. Vecuronium, suxamethonium and atracurium do not have this effect, and severe bradycardia may occur with these drugs. Asystole has been seen after sufentanil and vecuronium (with other drugs).[12] Curare and atracu-

rium may intensify the hypotension seen after sufentanil due to sympathetic ganglia blockade and/or histamine release.

Premedications. Phenothiazine medication will add to the reduction in systemic vascular resistance and to hypotension. Benzodiazepine medication will intensify the respiratory depression caused by sufentanil.

Other significant interactions

Anaesthetic agents. Sufentanil can be used to decrease the amount of volatile anaesthetic required during the maintenance of anaesthesia, and vice versa. Both reduce somatic and autonomic reflex responses to surgical stimulation. Both also depress respiration and simultaneous use will increase respiratory depression both during and after anaesthesia. A similar interaction occurs with intravenous anaesthetics; sufentanil reduces the dose of thiopentone required to induce anaesthesia.[15]

Potentially useful interactions

Some of the interactions described above may, when suitably controlled, be therapeutically useful.

Major outcome trials

Sufentanil is only used short-term, for the duration of anaesthesia.

Other trials

1. White P F, Sung M L, Doze V A 1985 Use of sufentanil in outpatient anaesthesia. Anesthesiology 63: A202

This was a dose-finding study in 80 women undergoing minor gynaecological surgery. Sufentanil 5, 10, 20 or 40 μg was given intravenously before methohexitone, N_2O and O_2. 5 μg was inadequate in suppressing the adverse effects of methohexitone and movement, whilst 40 μg induced too many sufentanil adverse effects, particularly apnoea and muscle rigidity. 10 or 20 μg were satisfactory.

2. Kay B, Rolly G 1977 Duration of action of anaesthetic supplements to anaesthesia: a double-blind comparison between morphine, fentanyl and sufentanil. Acta Anaesthesiologica Belgica 28: 25–32

Sufentanil 0.4 $\mu g.kg^{-1}$ was compared double-blind with fentanyl 4 $\mu g.kg^{-1}$ and morphine 4 $mg.kg^{-1}$ as the initial supplement to methohexitone, pancuronium, N_2O/O_2 anaesthesia, with increments of one-quarter of the initial dose given as required. The initial duration of effect of morphine (87 min) was twice that of fentanyl and sufentanil, which were similar. Fentanyl was more cumulative than sufentanil, so that in repeated dosage the requirement of fentanyl is approximately seven times that of sufentanil, a finding confirmed by a later comparison of sufentanil, fentanyl, morphine and pethidine.[16]

3. Bovill J G, Warren P J, Schuller J L, van Wezel H B, Hoeneveld M H 1984 Comparison of fentanyl, sufentanil, alfentanil anaesthesia in patients undergoing valvular heart surgery. Anaesthesia and Analgesia 63: 1081–1086

Fentanyl 75 $\mu g.kg^{-1}$, sufentanil 15 $\mu g.kg^{-1}$ and alfentanil 125 $\mu g.kg^{-1}$ were compared as anaesthetics for cardiac surgery, with pancuronium and O_2/air. Supplements of fentanyl 25 $\mu g.kg^{-1}$, sufentanil 5 $\mu g.kg^{-1}$ were used, alfentanil was given by infusion at 0.5 $mg.kg^{-1}.h^{-1}$. All three opioids gave similar, satisfactory results when given by this method.

References

1. Fahmy N R 1983 Sufentanil a review. In: Estafanous F G (ed) Opioids in anesthesia. Butterworth, Boston, pp 132–140
2. Bovill J G, Sebel P S, Blackburn C L, Oei-Lim V, Heykants J J 1984 The pharmacokinetics of sufentanil in surgical patients. Anesthesiology 61: 502–506
3. Schwartz A E, Matteo R S, Ornstein E, Young W L, Robinson S T 1986 Pharmacokinetics of sufentanil in the obese. Anesthesiology 65: A562
4. Vinik H R, Gelman S, Proctor J, Halpern N B 1986 Computerised infusion of sufentanil: a comparison of morbidly obese and non-obese patients. Anesthesia and Analgesia 65: S161
5. Matteo R S, Ornstein E, Young W L, Schwartz A E, Port M, Chang J 1986 Pharmacokinetics of sufentanil in the elderly. Anesthesia and Analgesia 65: S94
6. Davis P J, Robinson K A, Stiller R L, Cook D R 1985 Sufentanil kinetics in infants and children. Anesthesiology 63: A472
7. Fyman P, Avitable M, Moser F et al 1987 Sufentanil pharmacokinetics in patients undergoing renal transplantation. Anesthesia and Analgesia 66: S62

8. Cooke J E, Scott J C 1986 Do sufentanil and fentanyl have the same pharmacodynamics? Anesthesiology 65: A552
9. White P F, Sung M L, Doze V A 1985 Use of sufentanil in outpatient anaesthesia. Anesthesiology 63: A202
10. Kay B, Nolan D, Mayall R, Healy T E J 1987 The effect of sufentanil on cardiovascular responses to tracheal intubation. Anaesthesia 42: 382–386
11. Kay B, Rolly G 1977 Duration of action of anaesthetic supplements to anaesthesia: a double-blind comparison between morphine, fentanyl and sufentanil. Acta Anaesthesiologica Belgica 28: 25–32
12. Starr N J, Sethna D H, Estafanous F G 1986 Bradycardia and asystole following the rapid administration of sufentanil with vecuronium. Anesthesiology 64: 521–523
13. Molbegott L P, Flashburg M H, Karasic H L, Karlin B L 1987 Probable seizures after sufentanil. Anesthesia and Analgesia 66: 91–93
14. Moore R A, Yang S S, McNicholas K W, Gallacher J D, Clark D L 1985 Hemodynamic and anesthetic effects of sufentanil as the sole anesthetic for pediatric cardiovascular surgery. Anesthesiology 62: 725–731
15. Brizgys R V, Morales R, Owens B 1985 Low dose sufentanil. Anesthesiology 63: A377
16. Flacke J W, Bloor B C, Kripki B J et al 1985 Comparison of morphine, meperidine, fentanyl and sufentanil in balanced anaesthesia. Anesthesia and Analgesia 64: 897–910
17. Bovill J G, Warren P J, Schuller J L, van Wezel H B, Hoeneveld M H 1984 Comparison of fentanyl, sufentanil, alfentanil anaesthesia in patients undergoing valvular heart surgery. Anesthesia and Analgesia 63: 1081–1086

Sulfadoxine

Sulfadoxine is an ultra-long-acting sulphonamide, used in combination with pyrimethamine for the prophylaxis and treatment of malaria.

Chemistry

Sulfadoxine (Fanasil) was previously known by the generic name sulformethoxine.
$C_{12}H_{14}N_4O_4S$
N^1-(5,6-Dimethoxy-4-pyrimidinyl) sulfanilamide

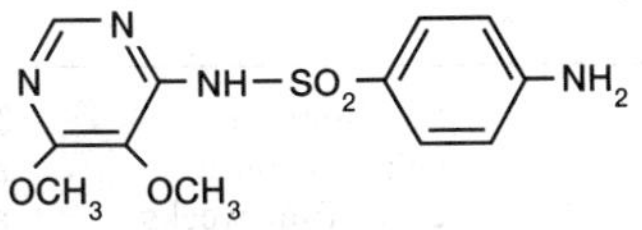

Molecular weight	310.3
pKa	6.3
Solubility	
in alcohol	slightly soluble
in water	very slightly soluble
Octanol/water partition coefficient	—

Sulfadoxine is a creamy-white, odourless crystalline compound prepared by chemical synthesis. It is available in the UK in combination with pyrimethamine as Fansidar.

Pharmacology

Sulfadoxine, like other sulphonamides, competitively inhibits the incorporation of para-aminobenzoic acid (PABA) into folic acid by bacteria. Sensitive bacteria are those that must synthesize their own folic acid. Sulfadoxine acts specifically as a competitive inhibitor of the enzyme dihydropteroate synthetase (EC 2.5.1.15) which is responsible for the incorporation of PABA into dihydropteroic acid. Pyrimethamine (combined with sulfadoxine in Fansidar) acts sequentially in the bacterial pathway of folic acid synthesis to inhibit the enzyme dihydrofolate reductase (EC 1.5.1.4), which converts dihydrofolate to tetrahydrofolate. Sulfadoxine and pyrimethamine do not affect mammalian cells since these cells are unable to synthesize folic acid themselves and require intact folic acid.

Toxicology

Injection of the 25% ampoule solution in rats and rabbits intravenously, intracutaneously and intramuscularly caused only mild to moderate local irritation.

In five- to six-week toxicity tests, rats tolerated 250 mg.kg^{-1}, rabbits 1000 mg.kg^{-1} and dogs 100 mg.kg^{-1} daily without harmful effects. In tests of longer duration, rats tolerated 120 mg.kg^{-1} daily for 18 months, dogs 50 mg.kg^{-1} daily for six months and 200 mg.kg^{-1} weekly for four months, without harmful effects except for the well-documented thyroid hyperplasia which usually occurs when high doses of sulphonamides are given for prolonged periods. Much higher doses caused bone marrow depression in a few growing rats, and in dogs some haemolysis and opacity of the ocular lenses occurred. Monkeys have completed a trial lasting 54 weeks when doses of 100 mg.kg^{-1} weekly and of 50 mg.kg^{-1} daily were given, without harmful effects. Special studies to discover any teratogenic effects in mice, rats and rabbits with daily doses occasionally 10–13 times higher than the weekly doses recommended for man, did not cause any abnormalities in the offspring.[1] No carcinogenic effects have been observed.

Clinical pharmacology

Sulfadoxine, like other sulphonamides, is active against a wide range of microorganisms. It is active against β-haemolytic streptococci, viridans streptococci, *Streptococcus pneumoniae*, *Clostridium tetani* and *Clostridium perfringens*. It is active against some strains of *Staphylococcus aureus*, *Bacillus anthracis*, *Bacillus cereus*, *Corynebacterium* spp., *Listeria monocytogenes*, *Neisseria meningitidis*, *Neisseria gonorrhoea*, *Haemophilus influenzae*, *Escherichia coli*, *Proteus* spp., *Klebsiella* spp., *Yersinia* spp., *Salmonella* spp., *Shigella* spp., *Vibrio* spp., *Nocardia asteroides*, *Actinomyces* spp., *Paracoccidioides braziliensis*, *Histoplasma capsulatum* and *Chlamydia trachomatis*. Sulfadoxine is most often used in combination with pyrimethamine for the prophylaxis or treatment of malaria. Sulfadoxine is active against the asexual blood forms of human malarial parasites but the action is a slow one. In combination with pyrimethamine the effect is enhanced.[2] There are no other known clinical pharmacological effects.

Pharmacokinetics

The preferred assay method is high performance liquid chromatography with ultraviolet detection, which has a quantitation limit of 50 μg.l^{-1}. Other commonly used antimalarials do not interfere with the assay.[3] Sulfadoxine can also be assayed by a microbiological method using *Bacillus subtilis* as the test organism, with a sensitivity[4] of 1 mg.l^{-1}. A simple urine test, a modification of the Bratton–Marshall reaction for sulphonamides, with a sensitivity of 5 mg.l^{-1} can be used under field conditions.[5]

Unlike many other long-acting drugs sulfadoxine is rapidly absorbed. Oral administration of 2 g sulfadoxine gives peak serum levels of 180–200 mg.l^{-1} within two to four hours. The serum half life is 150–200 hours (up to 340 hours in neonates). A week after a single oral dose of 1–2 g there is still more than 80 mg.l^{-1}, sufficient to be therapeutically active. On prolonged treatment with 0.5 g sulfadoxine a week the plasma concentration reaches a steady-state level of 98.4 mg.l^{-1} after about seven weeks. The sulphonamide and its metabolites are bound to plasma proteins to the extent of about 94%.

Penetration of sulfadoxine into erythrocytes is low in healthy volunteers, but it appears to be concentrated in malaria-infected erythrocytes.[6] Sulfadoxine enters the cerebrospinal fluid (the concentration is approximately 30–60% of that in the plasma), and the pleural, ascitic and synovial fluids (47–65% of plasma levels), crosses the placenta and is secreted in milk. Penetration into fatty tissue and skeletal musculature is poorer than into other tissues.

The elimination half life is 184 hours. Sulfadoxine is excreted by the kidneys, about 70% of a single dose being reabsorbed in the convoluted tubules, which accounts for its very long action. The small proportion of sulfadoxine which is metabolized and conjugated ($<9\%$) is excreted in the urine faster than unchanged drug so that of the urinary excreted material 30–60% is acetylated, up to 24% is conjugated with glucuronic acid and up to 6% is conjugated with sulphate.

Sulfadoxine is excreted into bile, but is mostly reabsorbed via the enterohepatic cycle.

Oral absorption	good
Presystemic metabolism	—
Plasma half life	
range	150–200 h
mean	177 h
Volume of distribution	0.13 l.kg^{-1}
Plasma protein binding	94%

Concentration–effect relationship

The in vitro efficacy of sulfadoxine against the malaria parasite is dependent upon culture conditions and no therapeutic range is established. There is no direct relationship between plasma concentration of sulfadoxine and therapeutic response in vivo.[7] Minimum inhibitory concentrations of microorganisms are in the range of 0.5–50 mg.l^{-1}.

Sulfadoxine

S

Metabolism

Only a small proportion is metabolized: about 5% to the N_4-acetyl derivative, 2–3% to the glucuronide, and 0.5% to the sulphate (Fig. 1).[8]

Fig. 1 Metabolism of sulfadoxine

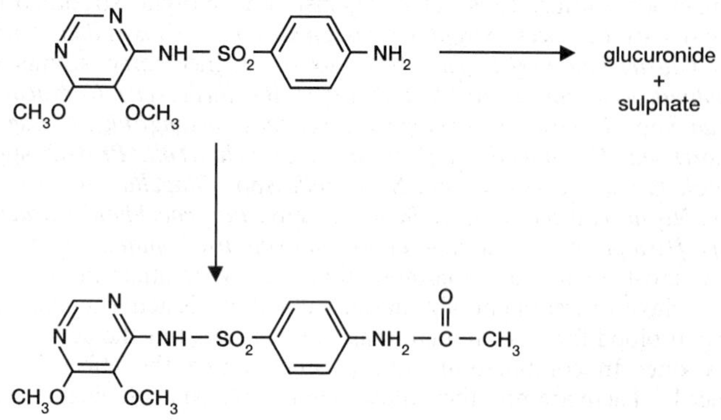

Pharmaceutics

Sulfadoxine (Fanasil) is available in some countries as scored 0.5 g tablets and ampoules containing 1 g in 4 ml for intramuscular use.

It is available in combination with pyrimethamine (Fansidar; Roche, UK/US) as round white tablets with 'ROCHE' and a hexagon imprinted on one face and two break bars on the other, containing 0.5 g sulfadoxine and 25 mg pyrimethamine. An ampoule solution, containing 0.5 g sulfadoxine and 25 mg pyrimethamine in 2.5 ml for deep intramuscular injection, is available in some countries.

No special storage precautions are required.

Therapeutic use

Indications

1. Treatment of malaria
2. Prophylaxis of malaria
3. Treatment of toxoplasmosis
4. Prophylaxis of *Pneumocystis carinii* pneumonia
5. To reduce transmission of cholera infection.

Contraindications

1. Known sulphonamide hypersensitivity
2. Severe renal or hepatic impairment
3. Blood dyscrasias
4. Premature and newborn infants
5. Early and late pregnancy
6. Nursing mothers
7. Glucose-6-phosphate dehydrogenase (G6PD) deficiency.

Mode of use

1. Treatment of malaria

Early studies showed that a combination of sulfadoxine with pyrimethamine enhanced the curative effect of either agent alone against resistant *Plasmodium falciparum*.[2]

Fansidar is active against all human pathogenic *Plasmodium*. It is indicated for *P. falciparum* strains that are resistant to antimalarial agents such as chloroquine or pyrimethamine alone,[9,10] such as are found in West and East Africa, Southeast Asia, Oceania and South America.[11–16] Less toxic and more effective therapy is available for other species of *Plasmodium*. [10,17–19]

Because of the slow action of pyrimethamine–sulfadoxine (Fansidar), a short course of quinine followed by a single dose of Fansidar is recommended.[11,20]

Table 1 shows the recommended dosage.

Table 1

	Single dose of Fansidar	
	Tablets	Ampoule solution (ml)
Adults	3	7.5
Children		
under 4 years (5–10 kg)	½	1.25
4–6 years (11–20 kg)	1	2.5
7–9 years (21–30 kg)	1½	3.75
10–14 years (31–45 kg)	2	5.0

Treatment with Fansidar does not result in 100% cure, even if the parasites are fully sensitive; 10–20% of individuals do not respond, either because vomiting or diarrhoea limit absorption or because of the way they metabolize or excrete sulphonamides.[21]

In certain malarious areas, however, particularly Southeast Asia, South America, Oceania, and West and East Africa, strains of *P. falciparum* may be encountered which have developed resistance to Fansidar,[22–30] due to resistance to both the sulfadoxine and pyrimethamine components.[31]

Precautions recommended by the manufacturer are that patients undergoing therapy should avoid excessive exposure to the sun, treatment must be discontinued immediately on the appearance of skin reactions, and sulfadoxine should only be prescribed in early pregnancy when absolutely necessary.

2. Prophylaxis of malaria

Fansidar is indicated for the prophylaxis of chloroquine-resistant falciparum malaria, but is not to be recommended for the other three species of human malaria.[32]

The recommended weekly doses are shown in Table 2.

Table 2

	Semi-immune subjects, once every four weeks	Non-immune subjects, once a week
Adults (according to bodyweight, higher dose for persons over 60 kg)	2 or 3 tablets	1 tablet
Children		
under 4 years (5–10 kg)	½ tablet	¼ tablet
4–8 years (11–29 kg)	1 tablet	½ tablet
9–14 years (30–45 kg)	2 tablets	¾ tablet

For malaria prophylaxis the first dose of Fansidar should be administered about one week before departure for an endemic area; administration should be continued during the stay and for six weeks on return.

Prophylaxis for up to 2 years has been well tolerated, but it is advised that leucocyte counts are performed every six months.

Failure of sulfadoxine–pyrimethamine prophylaxis has been reported in areas where Fansidar resistance is found.[33,34] Because of this and the reports of fatal reactions, Fansidar is no longer the prophylactic of choice.

3. Treatment of toxoplasmosis

Fansidar has been used in a dose of two tablets weekly for periods of 4–24 weeks in pregnant women with serological evidence of toxoplasmosis, with satisfactory outcome of pregnancy.[35] The treatment of choice, however, is pyrimethamine and sulphadiazine.

4. Prophylaxis of *Pneumocystis carinii* pneumonia

A combination of sulfadoxine and pyrimethamine has been found to be effective in a small trial to prevent *P. carinii* infection in an orphanage. A dose of 40 $mg.kg^{-1}$ (based on the sulfadoxine content) at least twice monthly was recommended for babies between the ages of two and six months at risk from this infection.[36,37]

Prophylaxis with Fansidar (one tablet weekly) has been used in AIDS patients. In nine patients it was well tolerated and there was no recurrence of *P. carinii*; in three patients it was discontinued when skin eruptions occurred and one of the patients had recurrent *P. carinii* pneumonia.[38]

5. To reduce transmission of cholera

In a placebo-controlled study sulfadoxine (0.5–2.0 g, depending on age) was given to family contacts of cholera patients within 24 h of the onset of symptoms in the index case. Isolation of *V. cholerae* from faeces in the following 15-day period was reduced from 42% in the placebo group to 19% in the sulfadoxine-treated group, and from days 3–6 was reduced from 8–9% in the placebo group to 1–2% in the sulfadoxine-treated group.[39] The recommended single oral dose of sulfadoxine for prophylaxis of cholera is shown in Table 3.[39,40]

Table 3

Adults	2 g
Children	
under 2 years	50 mg. kg^{-1}
2–4 years	0.5 g
5–8 years	1.0 g
9–14 years	1.5 g

Contraindications

1. Known sulphonamide hypersensitivity
There is usually cross-allergy between all the sulphonamides. There is no satisfactory test for sulphonamide allergy.

2. Severe renal or hepatic impairment
Crystalluria may occur in hypoproteinaemic patients, causing further renal damage. Hepatocellular jaundice due to hypersensitivity may exacerbate hepatic impairment.

3. Blood dyscrasias
Sulphonamides may cause acute agranulocytosis and, more rarely, aplastic anaemia, megaloblastic anaemia and thrombocytopenia.

4. Premature and newborn infants
Sulphonamides compete with bilirubin for albumin binding sites and can precipitate kernicterus.

5. Pregnancy
Fansidar has not been recommended in early pregnancy because of the possibility of teratogenicity. It is not recommended for use in the last two weeks of pregnancy because of the immaturity of the neonatal hepatic enzyme systems and the possibility of kernicterus. However, sulfadoxine has been used safely in pregnancy.[35]

6. Nursing mothers
There is a small risk of kernicterus, and of haemolysis in G6PD-deficient infants.

7. G6PD deficiency
Haemolytic anaemia may result from the administration of sulfadoxine.

Adverse reactions

Potentially life-threatening effects
Since 1982, 24 cases of erythema multiforme (Stevens–Johnson syndrome), a severe mucocutaneous reaction, with 7 fatalities, have been reported in the USA,[41,42] associated with multiple doses of Fansidar used for weekly malaria prophylaxis. The frequency of these reactions was estimated to be between 1/18 000 and 1/26 000 users. Severe cutaneous adverse reactions were reported to occur in 1 in 10 000 Swedish travellers.[43] There were 22 cases with three deaths among 149 000 persons in Mozambique following the use of sulfadoxine alone for mass prophylaxis in cholera, an incidence of 1 in 50 000.[40] There were 11 fatal cutaneous reactions among 109 485 persons who received one or more weekly doses of sulfadoxine as prophylaxis against meningococcal disease in Morocco, that is, one fatality per 10 000 users.[44] Three non-fatal cases of Stevens–Johnson syndrome were reported among 480 persons in South Africa given sulfadoxine as prophylaxis against *Streptococcus pneumoniae*.[45] Sulfadoxine appears to be responsible for the serious cutaneous reactions associated with pyrimethamine–sulfadoxine use.

Generalized toxic epidermolysis (Lyell's syndrome) has also been described, with an estimated mortality of 1 in 35 000 users.[43,46]

A case of fatal hepatic failure associated with Fansidar has been described.[47]

Acute overdosage
Possible symptoms are anorexia, nausea, vomiting, signs of excitation, convulsions, and haematological changes (megaloblastic anaemia, leucopenia, thrombocytopenia). Measures to be taken include gastric lavage and fluid replacement in acute intoxication; parenteral diazepam in cases of convulsions. Excretion of sulfadoxine may be accelerated by alkalization of the urine. Monitoring of renal function and repeated blood counts are recommended for up to four weeks after the overdosage. If haematological changes are found, folinic acid should be administered intramuscularly.

Severe or irreversible adverse effects
Two non-fatal cases of hypersensitivity pneumonitis have been described.[48,49]

Symptomatic adverse effects
Gastrointestinal reactions, such as a feeling of fullness, nausea, rarely vomiting, and stomatitis, and skin reactions, such as rash, erythroderma,[50] photosensitivity reactions,[46] pruritis and slight hair loss, have been described. There have been isolated reports of hepatitis and hepatic granulomata.[46,47,51,52] Leucopenia, thrombocytopenia, and megaloblastic anaemia have been observed rarely, and are almost always reversible.[9,46,53] Fatigue, headache, fever, and polyneuritis,[43,46] and orthostatic hypotension[16] have also been described.

Interference with clinical pathology tests
None has been reported.

High risk groups

Neonates
Fansidar is contraindicated in premature babies and during the first few weeks of life.

Breast milk. Sulfadoxine is excreted in breast milk. Nursing mothers should not take Fansidar.

Children
Fansidar can safely be used in children beyond the neonatal period.

Pregnant women
Fansidar is not contraindicated during pregnancy, but its use during early pregnancy should be avoided unless considered essential. A folate supplement should be given. Similarly, it should be avoided where possible in the last two weeks of pregnancy.

The elderly
Although no specific studies have been performed, Fansidar has been used extensively in the elderly and the dosage requirements and adverse effects appear to be similar to those of younger adults.

Concurrent disease
Repeated use of Fansidar is contraindicated in patients with severe renal insufficiency, marked liver parenchymal damage, or blood dyscrasias.

Sulphonamides can precipitate or aggravate porphyria.[54]

Drug interactions

Potentially hazardous interactions
Concurrent administration of trimethoprim or trimethoprim–sulphonamide combinations can result in increased impairment of folic acid metabolism and consequent haematological adverse effects.

Sulfadoxine potentiates the action of warfarin and thiopentone.

Other significant interactions
There may be an increase in incidence and severity of adverse reactions when chloroquine is used with Fansidar, as compared with the use of Fansidar alone.[55,56] There may be antagonism between mefloquine and Fansidar in some falciparum isolates.[57]

Potentially useful interactions
It has no hypoglycaemic effect and does not interfere with the action of antidiabetic agents.

Sequential blockade of folate synthesis by pyrimethamine potentiates the action of sulfadoxine in the treatment and prophylaxis of malaria.

Major outcome trials

1. Laing A B G 1964 Antimalarial effect of sulphorthodimethoxine (Fanasil). British Medical Journal 2: 1439–1440

In a six-week trial of sulphorthodimethoxine against pyrimethamine-resistant falciparum malaria in Tanganyika a weekly dose of 500 mg alone (191 children) or given with 25 mg pyrimethamine (208 children) eliminated parasitaemia, whereas 26% parasitaemia was seen in 192 children given 25 mg pyrimethamine alone.

2. Bartelloni P J, Sheehy T W, Tigertt W D 1967 Combined therapy for chloroquine-resistant *Plasmodium falciparum* infection. Journal of the American Medical Association 199: 141–177

S

Combined therapy of sulformethoxine and pyrimethamine with quinine was found to be superior to chloroquine–quinine therapy for treatment of *Plasmodium falciparum* infections in 115 non-immune patients in Vietnam (2% versus 41% of patients had reappearance of clinical disease).

3. Harinasuta T, Viravan C, Reid H A 1967 Sulphormethoxine in chloroquine-resistant falciparum malaria in Thailand. Lancet 1: 1117–1119

A single dose of 1000 or 1500 mg sulphormethoxine radically cured 61% of 18 patients with acute chloroquine-resistant falciparum malaria in Thailand. When combined with 50 mg pyrimethamine a single dose cured 90% of 19 patients and the response was more rapid (mean time to clearance of parasitaemia 2.9 versus 5.7 days).

4. Pape J W, Verdier R-I, Johnson W D 1989 Treatment and prophylaxis of *Isospora belli* infection in patients with the acquired immunodefficiency syndrome. New England Journal of Medicine 320: 1044–1047

Following a ten-day course of trimethoprim-sulphamethoxazole for treatment of symptomatic *Isospora belli*, all 12 patients who received sulfadoxine (500 mg)–pyrimethamine (25 mg) weekly remained asymptomatic and *Isospora belli* was not identified in the stools for a mean period of 16 months (range 7–29 months). In contrast, 5 of 10 who received placebo had recurrent, symptomatic isosporiasis over a mean period of 1.6 months (range 1–3.5 months).

Other trials

1. Laing A B G 1968 Hospital and field trials of sulformethoxine with pyrimethamine against Malaysian strains of *Plasmodium falciparum* and *P. vivax*. Medical Journal of Malaysia 23: 1–15
2. Lewis A N, Ponnampalam J T 1975 Suppression of malaria with monthly administration of combined sulfadoxine and pyrimethamine. Annals of Tropical Medicine and Parasitology 69: 1–12
3. Lucas A O, Hendrickse R G, Okubadejo O A, Richards W H G, Neal R A, Kofie B A K 1969 The suppression of malarial parasitemia by pyrimethamine in combination with dapsone or sulphormethoxine. Transactions of the Royal Society of Tropical Medicine and Hygiene 63: 216–229
4. O'Holohan D R, Hugoe-Matthews J 1971 Malaria suppression and prophylaxis on a Malaysian rubber estate. Sulformethoxine–pyrimethamine single monthly dose vs. chloroquine single weekly dose. Southeast Asian Journal of Tropical Medicine and Public Health 2: 164–168
5. Deb B C, Sen Gupta P G, De S P, Sil J, Sikdar S N, Pal S C 1976 Effect of sulphadoxine on transmission of *Vibrio cholerae* infection among family contacts of cholera patients in Calcutta. Bulletin of the World Health Organization 54: 171–175
6. Barbosa J C, Ferreira I 1978 Sulfadoxine–pyrimethamine (Fansidar) in pregnant women with *Toxoplasma* antibody titres. In: Siegenthaler W, Luthy R (eds) Current chemotherapy: proceedings of the 10th International Congress of Chemotherapy, Zurich, Switzerland. American Society for Microbiology, Washington DC, p 134

General review articles

Cook G C 1988 Prevention and treatment of malaria. Lancet 1: 32–37

Kucers A, Bennett N McK 1987 Sulphonamides. In: Kucers A (ed) The use of antibiotics: a comprehensive review with clinical emphasis, 4th edn. William Heinemann Medical Books, London, pp 1075–1117

References

1. Böhni E, Fust B, Rieder J, Schaerer K, Havas L 1969 Comparative toxicological, chemotherapeutic and pharmacokinetic studies with sulphormethoxine and other sulphonamides in animals and man. Chemotherapy 14: 195–226
2. Chin W, Contacos P G, Coatney G R, King H K 1966 The evaluation of sulfonamides, alone or in combination with pyrimethamine, in the treatment of multi-resistant falciparum malaria. American Journal of Tropical Medicine and Hygiene 15: 823–829
3. Edstein M 1984 Quantification of antimalarial drugs. I. Simultaneous measurement of sulfadoxine, N_4-acetylsulphadoxine and pyrimethamine in human plasma. Journal of Chromatography 305: 502–507
4. Weidekamm E, Plozza-Nottebrock H, Forgo I, Dubach U C 1982 Plasma concentrations of pyrimethamine and sulfadoxine and evaluation of pharmacokinetic data by computerised curve fitting. Bulletin of the World Health Organization 60: 115–122
5. de Almeida-Filho J, de Souza J M 1983 A simple urine test for sulfonamides. Bulletin of the World Health Organization 61: 167–168
6. Edstein M D 1987 Pharmacokinetics of sulfadoxine and pyrimethamine after Fansidar administration in man. Pharmacology 33: 229–233
7. Sarikabhuti B, Keschamrus N, Noeypatimanond S et al 1988 Plasma concentrations of sulfadoxine in healthy and malaria infected Thai subjects. Acta Tropica 45: 217–224
8. WHO Scientific Group 1984 Advances in malaria chemotherapy. World Health Organization Technical Report Series 711: 99
9. Lucas A O, Hendrickse R G, Okubadejo O A, Richards W H G, Neal R A, Kofie B A K 1969 The suppression of malarial parasitemia by pyrimethamine in combination with dapsone or sulphormethoxine. Transactions of the Royal Society of Tropical Medicine and Hygiene 63: 216–229
10. Laing A B G 1968 Hospital and field trials of sulformethoxine with pyrimethamine against Malaysian strains of *Plasmodium falciparum* and *P. vivax*. Medical Journal of Malaysia 23: 1–15
11. Hall A P, Doberstyn E B, Mettaprakong V, Sonkom P 1975 Falciparum malaria cured by quinine followed by sulfadoxine–pyrimethamine. British Medical Journal 2: 15
12. Hall A P, Doberstyn E B, Karncahnachetanee C et al 1977 Sequential treatment with quinine and mefloquine or quinine and pyrimethamine–sulfadoxine for falciparum malaria. British Medical Journal 1: 1626
13. World Health Organization 1984 Malaria risk in international travel. Reprinted from WHO Weekly Epidemiologic Record 29, 30, 31: 221–227, 229–235, 237–240
14. Strickland G T, Khaliq A A, Sarwar M, Hassan H, Pervez M, Fox E 1986 Effects of Fansidar on chloroquine-resistant *Plasmodium falciparum* in Pakistan. American Journal of Tropical Medicine and Hygiene 35: 61–65
15. Bjorkman A, Willcox M 1986 In vivo and in vitro susceptibility of *Plasmodium falciparum* to sulphadoxine/pyrimethamine in Liberia, West Africa. Transactions of the Royal Society of Tropical Medicine and Hygiene 80: 572–574
16. Ekue J M K, Phiri D E D, Sheth U K, Mukunyandela M 1987 A double-blind trial of a fixed combination of mefloquine plus sulfadoxine–pyrimethamine compared with sulfadoxine–pyrimethamine alone in symptomatic falciparum malaria. Bulletin of the World Health Organization 65: 369–373
17. Doberstyn E B, Teerakiartkamjorn C, Andre R G, Phintuyothin P, Noeypatimanondh S 1979 Treatment of vivax malaria with sulfadoxine–pyrimethamine and with pyrimethamine alone. Transactions of the Royal Society of Tropical Medicine and Hygiene 73: 15–17
18. Darlow B, Vrbova H, Gibney S, Jolley D, Stace J, Alpers M 1982 Sulfadoxine–pyrimethamine for the treatment of acute malaria in children in Papua New Guinea. II. *Plasmodium vivax*. American Journal of Tropical Medicine and Hygiene 31: 10–13
19. Ponnampalam J T, Frank H A 1983 Treatment of vivax malaria with a single dose of sulfadoxine and pyrimethamine (Fansidar). Singapore Medical Journal 24: 104–108
20. Doberstyn E B, Hall A P, Vetvutanapibul K, Sonkom P 1976 Single-dose therapy of falciparum malaria using pyrimethamine in combination with diformyldapsone or sulfadoxine. American Journal of Tropical Medicine and Hygiene 25: 14–19
21. WHO Scientific Group 1984 Advances in malaria chemotherapy. World Health Organization Technical Report Series 711: 29–30
22. Reacher M, Campbell C C, Freeman J, Doberstyn E B, Brandling-Bennett A D 1981 Drug therapy for *Plasmodium falciparum* malaria resistant to pyrimethamine–sulfadoxine (Fansidar). Lancet 2: 1066–1068
23. Dixon K E, Williams R G, Pongsupat T, Pitaktong U, Phintuyothin P 1982 A comparative trial of mefloquine and Fansidar in the treatment of falciparum malaria: failure of Fansidar. Transactions of the Royal Society of Tropical Medicine and Hygiene 76: 664–667
24. World Health Organization 1980 Synopsis of the world malaria situation (1980). WHO Weekly Epidemiological Report 57: 209–213, 258
25. Darlow B, Vrbova H, Gibney S, Jolley D, Stace J, Alpers M 1982 Sulfadoxine–pyrimethamine for the treatment of acute malaria in children in Papua New Guinea. I. *Plasmodium falciparum*. American Journal of Tropical Medicine and Hygiene 31: 1–9
26. Johnson D E, Roendej P, Williams R G 1982 Falciparum malaria acquired in the area of the Thai–Khmer border resistant to treatment with Fansidar. American Journal of Tropical Medicine and Hygiene 31: 907–912
27. Hess U, Timmermans P M, Jones M 1983 Combined chloroquine/Fansidar-resistant falciparum malaria appears in East Africa. American Journal of Tropical Medicine and Hygiene 32: 217–220
28. Win K, Thwe Y, Lwin T T, Win K 1985 Combination of mefloquine with sulfadoxine–pyrimethamine compared with two sulfadoxine–pyrimethamine combinations in malaria prophylaxis. Lancet 2: 694–695
29. Watt G, Padre L P, Tuazon L R, Laughlin L W 1987 Fansidar resistance in the Philippines. Transactions of the Royal Society of Tropical Medicine and Hygiene 81: 521
30. Gubler J 1988 Sulfadoxine–pyrimethamine resistant malaria from west or central Africa. British Medical Journal 296: 433
31. Childs G E, Sabchareon A, Chongsuphajaisiddi T, Wimonwattrawatee T, Ratharatorn B, Webster H K 1986 Analysis of resistance to pyrimethamine/sulphadoxine of isolates of *Plasmodium falciparum* from Eastern Thailand. Transactions of the Royal Society of Tropical Medicine and Hygiene 80: 66–68
32. Centers for Disease Control 1982 Problems encountered with using Fansidar as prophylaxis for malaria. Morbidity and Mortality Weekly Report 31: 232–234
33. Miller K D, Lobel H O, Pappaioanou M, Patchen L C, Churchill F C 1986 Failures of combined chloroquine and Fansidar prophylaxis in American travelers to East Africa. Journal of Infectious Diseases 154: 689–691

34. Lobel H O, Roberts J M, Somaini B, Steffen R 1987 Efficacy of malaria prophylaxis in American and Swiss travelers to Kenya. Journal of Infectious Diseases 155: 1205–1209
35. Barbosa J C, Ferreira I 1978 Sulfadoxine–pyrimethamine (Fansidar) in pregnant women with toxoplasma antibody titres. In: Siegenthaler W, Luthy R (eds) Current chemotherapy: proceedings of the 10th International Congress of Chemotherapy, Zurich, Switzerland. American Society for Microbiology, Washington DC, p 134
36. Post C, Fakouhi T, Dutz W et al 1971 Prophylaxis of epidemic infantile pneumocystosis with a sulfadoxine–pyrimethamine combination. Current Therapeutic Research 13: 273–280
37. Dutz W, Khodadad E J, Post C, Kohout E, Nazarian J, Esmaili H 1971 Marasmus and *Pneumocystis carinii* pneumonia in institutionalised infants. Zeitschrift fur Kinderheilkunde 117: 241–258
38. Gottlieb M S, Knight S, Mitsuyasu R, Weisman J, Roth M, Young L S 1984 Prophylaxis of *Pneumocystis carinii* infection with pyrimethamine–sulfadoxine. Lancet 2: 398–399
39. Deb B C, Sen Gupta P G, De S P, Sil J, Sikdar S N, Pal S C 1976 Effect of sulphadoxine on transmission of *Vibrio cholerae* infection among family contacts of cholera patients in Calcutta. Bulletin of the World Health Organization 54: 171–175
40. Hernborg A 1985 Stevens–Johnson syndrome after mass prophylaxis with sulfadoxine for cholera in Mozambique. Lancet 2: 1072–1073
41. Miller K D, Lobel H O, Satriale R F, Kuritsky J N, Stern R, Campbell C C 1986 Severe cutaneous reactions among American travelers using pyrimethamine–sulfadoxine (Fansidar) for malaria prophylaxis. American Journal of Tropical Medicine and Hygiene 35: 451–458
42. Centers for Disease Control 1985 Adverse reactions to Fansidar and updated recommendations for its use in the prevention of malaria. Morbidity and Mortality Weekly Report 8: 713–714
43. Hellgren U, Rombo L, Berg B, Carlson J, Wiholm B-E 1987 Adverse reactions to sulfadoxine–pyrimethamine in Swedish travellers: implications for prophylaxis. British Medical Journal 295: 365–366
44. Bergoend H, Loffler A, Amar R, Maleville J 1968 Reactions cutanees survenues au cours de la prophylaxie de masse de la meningite cerebro-spinale parun sulfamide long-retard (propos de 997 cas). Annales de Dermatologie et de Venereologie 95: 481–490
45. Taylor G M 1968 Stevens–Johnson syndrome following the use of an ultra long-acting sulphonamide. South African Medical Journal 42: 501–503
46. Olsen V V, Loft S, Christensen K D 1982 Serious reactions during malaria prophylaxis with pyrimethamine–sulfadoxine. Lancet 2: 994
47. Zitelli B J, Alexander J, Taylor S et al 1987 Fatal hepatic necrosis due to pyrimethamine–sulfadoxine (Fansidar). Annals of Internal Medicine 106: 393–395
48. McCormack D, Morgan W K C 1987 Fansidar hypersensitivity pneumonitis. British Journal of Diseases of the Chest 81: 194–196
49. Svanbom M, Rombo L, Gustafsson L 1984 Unusual pulmonary reaction during short term prophylaxis with pyrimethamine–sulfadoxine (Fansidar). British Medical Journal 1: 1876
50. Langtry J A A, Harper J I, Staughton R C D, Barrington P 1986 Erythroderma resembling Sezary syndrome after treatment with Fansidar and chloroquine. British Medical Journal 292: 1107–1108
51. Lazar H O, Murphy R L, Phair J P 1985 Fansidar and hepatic granulomas. Annals of Internal Medicine 102: 722
52. Wejstal R, Lindberg J, Malmvall B-E, Norkrans G 1986 Liver damage associated with Fansidar. Lancet 1: 854–855
53. Muto T, Ebiswa I, Mitsui G 1971 Malaria in Laos II Peripheral leucocyte counts during long term administration of combined folic acid inhibitors (pyrimethamine with sulformethoxine or sulfamonomethoxine). Japanese Journal of Experimental Medicine 41: 459–470
54. Peterkin G A G, Khan S A 1969 Iatrogenic skin disease. The Practitioner 202: 117 126
55. World Health Organization 1985 Malaria chemoprophylaxis. WHO Weekly Epidemiologic Record 60: 181–188
56. Bradley D J, Hall A P, Peters W 1985 Fansidar in malaria prophylaxis. British Medical Journal 291: 136
57. Hoffman S L, Rustama D, Dimpudus A J et al 1985 RII and RIII type resistance of *Plasmodium falciparum* to combination of mefloquine and sulfadoxine–pyrimethamine in Indonesia. Lancet 2: 1039–1040

Sulindac

Sulindac is a non-steroidal anti-inflammatory drug which is clinically similar to indomethacin. The pharmacological activity derives from the sulphide metabolite; the parent compound is therefore a pro-drug. Unlike most other non-steroidal drugs, sulindac has relatively little effect on prostaglandin synthesis in the kidney.

Chemistry

Sulindac (Clinoril)
$C_{20}H_{17}FO_3S$
(Z)-5-Fluoro-2-methyl-1-[[4-(methylsulphinyl)phenyl]methylene]-1H-indene-3-acetic acid

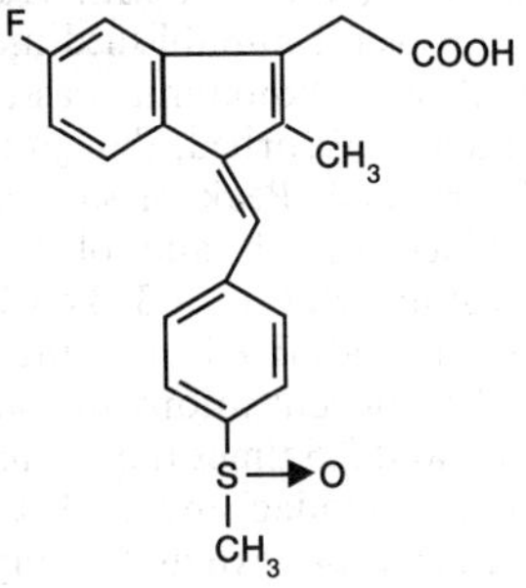

Molecular weight (sulphide)	356.42 (340.42)
pKa	4.7
Solubility	
in alcohol	1 in 30 to 1 in 100
in water	practically nil
Octanol/water partition coefficient (2.5°C)	0.28

Sulindac is a yellow, odourless, crystalline powder with a bitter taste. It is a substituted indene acetic acid, prepared by chemical synthesis. There are E and Z geometric isomers with comparable in vivo pharmacological activities and therefore the racemate is used as sulindac. There are no combination products.

Pharmacology

Sulindac is an antipyretic, an anti-inflammatory and an analgesic drug. It is a pro-drug which in vitro and in cellular systems is readily and reversibly converted to the active sulphide metabolite. The sulphide metabolite is some 500 times more active as an inhibitor of prostaglandin synthesis than the parent drug. The exact mode of action of sulindac is not certain. It seems that it inhibits cyclo-oxygenase in the prostaglandin synthesis pathway but has an effect on plasma and synovial fluid prostaglandin concentrations with some sparing of those in the gastric mucosa and kidney. This may be because the sulphide metabolite has less ready access to prostaglandins in the stomach and kidney. It influences other mediators of inflammation such as the lipoxygenase pathway, oxidant radicals, other lipid mediators and the chemotaxis and other functions of inflammatory cells. The relations between these actions and pharmacological effects is uncertain.

Toxicology

Treatment of rats for up to 1 year with 5–10 $mg.kg^{-1}$ daily caused a low incidence of gastrointestinal ulcers which were not seen in dogs. Teratogenicity testing in mouse, rat and rabbit showed no evidence of clinically relevant abnormalities. Carcinogenicity tests were also negative.

Clinical pharmacology

The sulphide metabolite of sulindac inhibits prostaglandin synthetase, inhibits human synoviocyte cyclic AMP-phosphodiesterase activity and modifies other mediators of inflammation. It has anti-inflammatory, analgesic and antipyretic actions and inhibits platelet aggregation.

The normal daily dose is either 200 or 400 mg. Although patients have been given 600–900 mg doses above 400 mg are not recommended by the manufacturer. The latter doses are not recommended by the manufacturers because the incidence of abnormal liver function tests rises with doses above 600 mg.

Sulindac does not have major effects on other body functions. It is proposed that because it is administered as a pro-drug and has relatively little effect on gastric and renal prostaglandins, it may be less likely than other non-steroidal drugs to adversely affect the gastric mucosa and the kidney. However, sulindac can still cause gastric irritation and adversely affect renal function in some patients.

Pharmacokinetics

A preferred method for assaying sulindac in plasma has not been agreed. A method involving titration with sodium hydroxide[1] has been used. In addition, several unpublished methods based on UV absorption, TLC, HPLC and radioimmunoassay are referred to.

About 90% of sulindac is absorbed, though its bioavailability has not been properly determined. Peak plasma concentrations of the parent drug are obtained in 1 h and of the major therapeutic metabolites, in 2 h in fasting subjects or 3–4 h when given with food.[2] Steady-state conditions are attained after the 11th dose on a 12-hourly regimen and the concentrations of parent compound and major metabolite are 1.5 and 2.5 times those after a single dose. Food delays the absorption of sulindac and peak concentrations of the parent compound and, to a lesser extent, the sulphide metabolites are lower. The plasma concentration curves suggest that the drug is eliminated in the bile and reabsorbed from the intestine. Its half life is 7.8 h and that of the sulphide metabolite 16.4 h.

There is little information on the distribution of sulindac and its metabolites in man. Animal data suggest that it is widely distributed.[3] It presumably penetrates into the joints but only small concentrations are attained in breast milk (10–20% plasma concentrations) and very little passes to the fetus. The degree of protein binding is high: parent compound 93.1%, sulphide 95.4% and sulphone 97.9%.

Liver disease may affect the levels of circulating metabolites and a reduction in dosage may be necessary.

Oral absorption	~90%
Presystemic metabolism	—
Plasma half life	7.8 h
(sulphide)	16.4 h
Volume of distribution	—
Plasma protein binding	93%

Concentration–effect relationship

There is no evidence of a direct relationship between the plasma concentration of sulindac and its therapeutic effect.

Metabolism

Sulindac is metabolized by oxidation to its sulphone and is reduced to the corresponding sulphide, which is the form which is therapeutically active (see Fig. 1). The excretion of sulindac and its metabolites is rather complicated. About 30% of the dose is excreted as the sulphone or its conjugate and 20% is excreted as sulindac or its conjugate in the urine. The urine also contains unidentified metabolites which may amount to 25% of the dose. The rest of the dose appears in the faeces and is the end result of unabsorbed drug, biliary excretion, enterohepatic circulation and bacterial degradation of the products reaching the colon.

Pharmaceutics

Sulindac, Clinoril (Merck, Sharpe and Dohme, UK/USA) is only available as tablets. They are brilliant yellow, scored, hexagonal biconvex tablets containing 200 mg and marked 'MSD 942', or 100 mg (UK) and marked 'MSD 943', or 150 mg (USA) and marked 'MSD 941'.

These tablets do not contain any allergenic substances. They should be stored in a cool place, protected from light and will then have a shelf-life of 5 years.

Therapeutic use

Indications

1. Rheumatoid arthritis
2. Osteoarthritis
3. Acute gout
4. Ankylosing spondylitis
5. Periarticular disorders.

Contraindications

1. Allergic reactions to aspirin or other NSAID
2. Active peptic ulceration
3. History of recent upper gastrointestinal bleed
4. Young children, pregnancy, lactation.

Mode of use

Sulindac is usually given in a dose of 100–200 mg twice daily and is taken with fluids or food. 400 mg per day is considered the normal dose and doses above 400 mg per day are not recommended.

Indications

1. Rheumatoid arthritis

Sulindac has been evaluated in much the same way as other non-steroidal drugs. Several short-term studies[4] have attempted to evaluate sulindac and compare it with aspirin. Although most studies involve too few patients, too many assessments and too short a follow-up to provide absolutely convincing evidence, overall a pat-

Fig. 1 The metabolism of sulindac

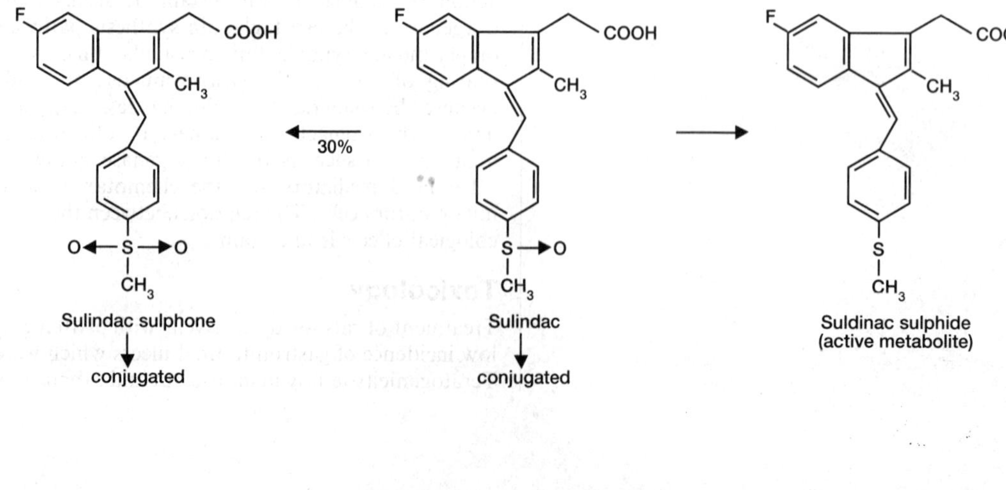

Sulindac

tern emerges of a drug which is at least as effective as aspirin and better tolerated. Sulindac therefore has a place in the symptomatic treatment of rheumatoid arthritis and because it is a pro-drug and therefore unlikely to have any effect on protective prostaglandins in the stomach, it might be expected to have a particular role in patients with a tendency to suffer from indigestion. The clinical trial data support the view that sulindac is better tolerated in the stomach than aspirin.[5]

2. Osteoarthritis
Relatively large numbers of patients have been recruited into the many trials of sulindac in degenerative joint disease.[4] Although it is possible to criticize trial design and objectivity of assessments in some instances, overall the conclusion that sulindac is more effective than placebo and at least as effective as aspirin or ibuprofen would be difficult to refute.[6]

3. Acute gout
The efficacy of sulindac has been assessed in a limited number of studies. It appears to be effective and it has been claimed that 400 mg sulindac is as successful as 600 mg phenylbutazone daily, but this needs to be confirmed. Therapy for seven days is usually adequate.

4. Ankylosing spondylitis
The role of sulindac in ankylosing spondylitis is not clearly defined. It appears to be more effective than placebo and may be comparable to phenylbutazone. However, there do not appear to be adequate studies to determine the relative merits of sulindac as compared with naproxyn, indomethacin and phenylbutazone.

5. Periarticular disorders
Sulindac has been given to a number of groups of patients with periarticular disorders. It appears to be reasonably effective and well tolerated.

Contraindications

1. Allergy to aspirin and other NSAIDs
This is a routine precaution, serious allergic reactions have not been a problem in patients on sulindac.

2. Active peptic ulceration
It is accepted that NSAIDs as a group may cause symptoms ascribed to gastric intolerance and said to be caused by their tendency to impair the formation of gastroprotective prostaglandins. Although gastrointestinal adverse effects are the most frequent side effects of sulindac and abdominal pain is the commonest of these, severe peptic ulcer type pains and upper gastrointestinal haemorrhage is relatively uncommon.

3. History of recent upper gastrointestinal bleed
Sulindac is contraindicated for the same reasons as in peptic ulcer.

4. Infancy, pregnancy and lactation
These are relative contraindications, as data on the safety of sulindac in these subgroups is insufficient to make it possible to recommend the drug with confidence.

Adverse reactions

Potentially life-threatening effects
Deaths due to sulindac are extremely rare and if attributable to the drug would be caused by gastrointestinal haemorrhage, blood dyscrasias, or a severe allergic reaction.

Acute overdosage
Accidental or suicidal overdoses with sulindac are extremely uncommon. The management might include the administration of activated charcoal, the production of an alkaline diuresis, maintenance of fluid and electrolyte balance, and full clinical support. There are no specific antidotes.

Severe or irreversible adverse effects
These are the same as the potentially life-threatening effects described above.

Symptomatic adverse effects
The most frequently reported adverse effects are those affecting the gastrointestinal tract. They include abdominal pain, nausea and constipation. In comparative studies, upper abdominal problems are less severe and less frequent than those caused by aspirin, and sulindac may be considered comparable to ibuprofen as a potential cause of gastrointestinal adverse effects.

Sulindac may also cause mild adverse effects on the central nervous system, such as drowsiness, dizziness and headache. These are rarely severe enough to prevent the patient from taking the drug.

Other adverse effects, such as rash, pruritis, and mild disturbances of liver function tests, have been reported but are infrequent and rarely serious.

Interference with clinical pathology tests
Significant elevations (three times upper normal) of AST(SGOT) or ALT(SGPT) occurred in trials in $< 1\%$ of patients. Clinical trials with sulindac 600 mg daily have been associated with increased incidence of mild liver function test abnormalities.

High risk groups

Neonates
The drug should not be used in neonates.

Breast milk. No information is available on the excretion of the drug in breast milk, so lactating mothers should not take it.

Children
The safety of the drug in children has not been established.

Pregnant women
The safety of the drug during pregnancy has not been established, so it should not be given.

The elderly
No special precautions are required, but it would seem prudent to use a lower dose (200 mg rather than 400 mg or 600 mg), at least initially, and to be more careful in those with overt renal impairment and definite or incipient cardiac failure.

Concurrent disease
The drug should be avoided in patients with known or suspected peptic ulcer. Sulindac metabolites have been identified in renal stores and caution should be used in giving the drug to patients with a history of renal lithiasis. Patients with liver disease should be monitored and the dose adjusted if necessary.

Drug interactions

Potentially hazardous interactions
No interactions of this type have been reported.

Other significant interactions
Before prescribing any NSAID it is advisable to remember that it may interact with anticoagulants, lithium, oral hypoglycaemic agents, and diuretics or other antihypertensive drugs.[7] However, in contrast to most other NSAIDs, sulindac does not reduce the efficacy of a variety of antihypertensive agents used to treat mild to moderate hypertension.[8,9] Ideally, the effects of such drugs if sulindac is added to the therapeutic regimen should be monitored, but a serious interaction would not be expected. Dimethylsulphoxide should not be used on concomitantly with sulindac.

Potentially useful interactions
No interactions of this kind are known.

Major outcome trials

There do not appear to have been any large-scale studies which have made a major impact on our understanding of the clinical role of sulindac.

Other trials

1. Calin A, Britton M 1979 Sulindac in ankylosing spondylitis. Journal of the American Medical Association 242: 1885–1886

A double-blind 6 months, parallel-groups study comparing indomethacin 75–150 mg daily with sulindac 200–400 mg daily. During the 6-month period the patients were assessed objectively and subjectively on eight occasions. The two drugs appeared to be equally effective but gastrointestinal problems were experienced twice as often on indomethacin.

2. Huskisson E C, Scott J 1978 Sulindac — trials of a new anti-inflammatory drug. Annals of the Rheumatic Diseases 37: 89–92

This paper reports three trials. One was a short, three-way, crossover trial in patients with rheumatoid arthritis comparing sulindac, aspirin and placebo in 24 out-patients. The second was an 8-week study in patients with osteoarthritis comparing aspirin with sulindac using an open design but with random allocation to parallel treatment groups. The third was a similar type of study over 10 weeks in patients with rheumatoid arthritis. Sulindac appeared to be as effective as aspirin, to have a simpler twice daily regimen, and to cause fewer gastric side effects, but it produced mild constipation in 20–30% of patients.

General review articles

Brogden R N, Heel R C, Speight T M, Avery G S 1978 Sulindac: a review of its pharmacological properties and therapeutic efficacy in rheumatic diseases. Drugs 16: 97–114

Rhymer A R 1979 Sulindac. Clinics in Rheumatic Diseases 5: 553–568

References

1. Duggan D E, Hare L E, Ditzler C A, Lei B W, Kwan K C 1977 Disposition of sulindac. Clinical Pharmacology and Therapeutics 21: 326–335
2. Verbeeck R K, Blackburn J L, Loewen G R 1982 Clinical pharmacokinetics of non-steroidal anti-inflammatory drugs. Clinical Pharmacokinetics 8: 297–331
3. Duggan D E, Hooke K F, Hwang S S 1980 Kinetics of the tissue distributions of sulindac and metabolites. Drug Metabolism and Disposition 8: 241–246
4. Brogden R N, Heel R C, Speight T M, Avery G S 1978 Sulindac: a review of its pharmacological properties and therapeutic efficacy in rheumatic diseases. Drugs 16: 97–114
5. Carusa I, Bianchi Porro G 1980 Gastroscopic evaluation of anti inflammatory agents. British Medical Journal 280: 75–78
6. Ghosh A K, Rastogi A K 1981 A randomised comparison between sulindac and ibuprofen in osteoarthritis of the aged. Current Medical Research and Opinion 7: 482–487
7. Day R O, Graham G G, Champion G D, Lee E 198 Antirheumatic drug interactions. Clinics in Rheumatic Diseases 10: 251–275
8. Lewis R V, Toner J M, Jackson P R, Ramsey L E 1986 Effects of indomethacin and sulindac on blood pressure of hypertensive patients. British Medical Journal 292: 934–935
9. Wong D G, Spence J D, Lamki L, Freeman D, McDonald J W D 1986 Effect of non-steroidal anti-inflammatory drugs on control of hypertension by beta-blockers and diuretics. Lancet 2: 997–1001

Sulphacetamide

Sulphacetamide is a bacteriostatic analogue of para-aminobenzoic acid which is nowadays used mainly for the treatment of ophthalmic infections.

Chemistry

Sulphacetamide sodium (Sulphacetamide eye-drops, Minims Sulfacetamide, Isopto Cetamide, Albucid, Ocusol)
$C_8H_9N_2NaO_3S.H_2O$
N[1]-Acetylsulphanilamide sodium

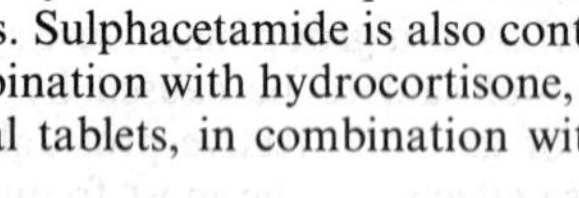

Molecular weight	254.2
pKa	5.78
Solubility	
in alcohol	1 in 30 to 1 in 100
in water	1 in 1.5
Octanol/water partition coefficient	Unknown

A white or yellowish-white, odourless, bitter-tasting, crystalline powder which slowly darkens on exposure to light, it is prepared by chemical synthesis. Sulphacetamide is also contained in Cortucid eye ointment, in combination with hydrocortisone, and in Sultrin vaginal cream and vaginal tablets, in combination with sulphathiazole and sulphabenzamide.

Pharmacology

Sulphacetamide is structurally similar to p-aminobenzoic acid (PABA) and therefore acts by competitive blockade of the enzyme dihydrofolic acid (DHF) synthetase.[1] DHF synthetase is required to convert PABA to dihydrofolic acid (DHF). Sulphacetamide therefore inhibits production of DHF, which is required for synthesis of tetrahydrofolic acid (THF), purines and, ultimately, DNA. (See Fig. 1.) Mammalian cells derive DHF from dietary folic acid and therefore bypass this part of the pathway.

Toxicology

No information is available.

Clinical pharmacology

The following organisms are usually sensitive to sulphacetamide: *Streptococcus pyogenes*, *Strep. pneumoniae*, *Strep. viridans*, *Staphylococcus aureus*, *Haemophilus influenzae* and *Chlamydia trachomatis*.

Enterobacter aerogenes, *Alcaligenes* spp., *Pseudomonas aeruginosa* and *Proteus* spp. may appear sensitive in vitro but infections due to these organisms seldom respond to sulphacetamide.

The spectrum of activity of sulphacetamide has been reduced by acquired bacterial resistance. Sulphacetamide resistance may be due to increased synthesis of PABA or to production of DHF synthetase with a lowered affinity for sulphacetamide. Resistance is common in *Escherichia coli*, *Neisseria gonorrhoeae* and *N. meningitidis*. Resistance in many Gram-negative organisms may be mediated by resistance plasmids (R plasmids).

Pharmacokinetics

Analytical methods used include the colorimetric assay[2] and a high pressure liquid chromatography[3] method. The latter method gives an average recovery of 100.9% for sulphacetamide in ophthalmic preparations.

If given orally, sulphacetamide is rapidly absorbed, reaching a peak serum concentration in 4–5 hours. The drug is metabolized by acetylation in the liver and is rapidly excreted in the urine. The plasma half life ranges from 7 to 13 hours. Up to 10% of blood sulphacetamide is present as the acetyl derivative. Sulphacetamide is approximately 80–85% bound to plasma albumin.

Concentrations of sulphacetamide in the cerebrospinal fluid are approximately 30–80% of plasma concentrations. In the urine, 30% of sulphacetamide is present as the acetyl derivative.

Originally used in the treatment of urinary tract infection,[4] it was found to have low activity in systemic infections. Because of its high solubility, neutrality, non-irritant properties and ready penetration into tissues,[5] sulphacetamide is now used mainly in the treatment of ophthalmic infections. It is less commonly used, in combination with other sulphonamides, in vaginal infections.

A study[6] into the penetration and distribution of topically applied 30% sulphacetamide solutions in the ocular tissues of rabbits showed that the concentration reached a peak in 15 minutes and was still adequate after 1 hour. At 15 minutes, the concentration of sulphacetamide in the cornea was 9.7 $g.l^{-1}$, in the conjunctiva 7.8 $g.l^{-1}$, in the aqueous humour 2.0 $g.l^{-1}$, in the sclera 1.2 $g.l^{-1}$ and in the iris 1.1 $g.l^{-1}$. Addition of a wetting agent[7] (Duponal, a detergent derived from technical lauryl alcohol) to sulphacetamide solution was found not only to increase the concentration of sulphacetamide in the anterior ocular tissues, but also to prolong the duration for which an effective chemotherapeutic concentration is maintained. When it is used to treat conjunctivitis, low concentrations of sulphacetamide may be found in the blood.

Oral absorption	Rapid
Presystemic metabolism	Acetylation
Plasma half life	
range	7–13 h
mean	9 h
Volume of distribution	Unknown
Plasma protein binding	80–85%

Concentration–effect relationship

There is no clear relationship between concentrations of sulphacetamide and its antimicrobial effect in man, since the drug is now only used topically.

Metabolism

If taken systemically, sulphacetamide is partially metabolized by acetylation to an inactive metabolite in the liver and is rapidly excreted in the urine, 70% in the unchanged form (Fig. 2).

Pharmaceutics

Sulphacetamide is available as eye drops, eye ointment, vaginal cream and vaginal tablets.

Eye drops contain 5%, 10%, 15%, 20% and 30% solutions of sodium sulphacetamide. Minims eye drops (Smith and Nephew, UK) are available as a clear, colourless, or sometimes slightly yellow, 10% solution in single-use units, each containing approximately 0.5 ml.

Fig. 1 Mode of action of sulphacetamide

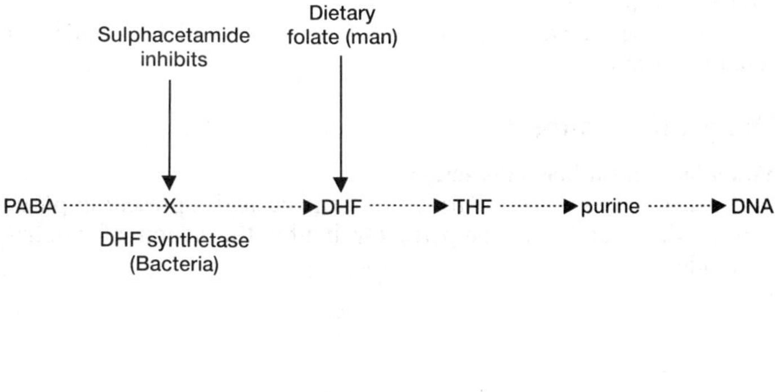

Sulphacetamide

Fig. 2 Metabolism of sulphacetamide

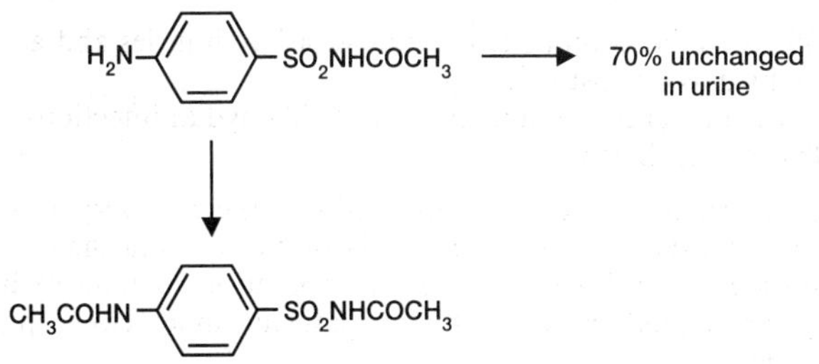

Isopto Cetamide eye drops (15%) (Alcon, UK) are contained in a 10 ml unbreakable, semi-rigid container which should be kept tightly closed. The clear, colourless solution also contains 0.5% hypromellose and preservatives (0.05% methylparaben and 0.01% propylparaben).

Albucid eye drops (Nicholas, UK) 10%, 20% and 30%, are contained in 10 ml opaque, white polythene bottles with green, brown and red caps, respectively.

Ocusol eye drops (Boots, UK) contain only 5% sodium sulphacetamide; however, together with 0.1% zinc sulphate and 0.01% cetrimide, they produce an antibacterial effect equivalent to that of a 30% solution of sulphacetamide.

Eye drops should be stored in a cool place and should not be exposed to strong light — discoloration will result. Single-use units should be discarded after each use. 10 ml containers should be discarded 1 month after opening. The shelf-life of unopened containers is 3 years.

Eye ointments (Albucid, Nicholas, UK) contain 2.5% and 6% sodium sulphacetamide in a greasy base and 10% sodium sulphacetamide in a water-miscible base including parabens, sodium sulamyd (Schering, US).

Cortucid eye cream (Nicholas, UK) is a bland cream containing 10% sodium sulphacetamide and 0.5% hydrocortisone in a water-miscible base. Sodium thiosulphate is present as a preservative.

Eye ointments should be stored in a cool, dry place. The shelf-life is 4 years.

Sultrin (Ortho-Cilag, UK/US) is a topical agent applied to the vagina as cream or tablets. Sultrin triple sulfa cream is a white non-staining cream. A plastic vaginal applicator (Ortho) can be used for application. Sultrin vaginal tablets are white, non-staining, water-dispersible, lozenge-shaped tablets engraved on one side with the Ortho shield design and on the obverse with C. Each tablet contains 143.75 mg sulphacetamide, 172.5 mg sulphathiazole and 184 mg sulphabenzamide in a rapidly disintegrating base.

Therapeutic use

Indications

1. Eye infections
a. Treatment
b. Prophylaxis
2. Non-specific vaginosis.

Contraindications

1. Sulphonamide hypersensitivity
2. Herpex simplex corneal infection (Cortucid)
3. Renal failure (Sultrin vaginal cream/tablets only).

Mode of use

Two to four sulphacetamide eye drops should be applied 2–4 hourly, or more frequently in severe infections. The same dose applies to neonates and children. The concentrations required are as follows:

10–15% for mild conjunctivitis, industrial eye industries and as prophylaxis against infection
20% for moderate conjunctivitis and ophthalmia neonatorum
30% for severe conjunctivitis and chlamydial infections
One Ocusol eye drop can be given four times daily.

Eye ointments are longer lasting and can be applied less frequently. Grease-based eye ointment should be applied to the eyelids at night.

Eye ointment in a miscible base should be applied two to four times daily. The concentrations required are as follows:

2.5% for mild conjunctivitis, industrial eye injuries and as prophylaxis against infection
6% for moderate conjunctivitis and chlamydial infections
10% for blepharitis.

Cortucid eye cream should be dropped into the eye every 3–6 hours for the first 2 days and less frequently thereafter until the condition has subsided for at least 2 days. This preparation contains hydrocortisone and should be used only in patients under close specialist supervision.

One applicatorful of Sultrin vaginal cream or one Sultrin vaginal tablet should be applied intravaginally twice daily for 10–14 days.

Indications

1. Eye infections

Treatment. Sodium sulphacetamide is most commonly used in the treatment of acute conjunctivitis[8] due to sensitive organisms. The 30% solution has been used, in conjunction with systemic cefuroxime, in the treatment of ophthalmia neonatorum caused by β-lactamase-producing *N. gonorrhoeae*.[9] However, many gonococci are now sulphacetamide-resistant.

Topical sodium sulphacetamide has been used in the treatment of *C. trachomatis* conjunctivitis[10,11] and trachoma although tetracycline eye ointment is now preferred, together with oral erythromycin or tetracycline.

Sodium sulphacetamide ointment can be applied to the lid margins in the treatment of staphylococcal blepharitis.

Prophylaxis. Sodium sulphacetamide can be used in the prophylaxis of eye infections after trauma, e.g. industrial injuries[12,13] and burns.

Sodium sulphacetamide has also been used in the prophylaxis of ophthalmia neonatorum.[14,15] It was found to be no more effective than silver nitrate in the prevention of gonococcal infections, although it produced less chemical conjunctivitis. With the present high proportion of sulphonamide-resistant *N. gonorrhoeae*, sulphacetamide is no longer used for this purpose.

2. Non-specific vaginosis

Topical vaginal Sultrin tablets or cream have been recommended in the treatment of non-specific vaginosis.[16] Treatment must be continued for 14 days. However, other investigators have found a lack of clinical response to these preparations and alternatives are preferable.[17] At present, oral metronidazole, 400 mg 12-hourly for 7 days or as a 2 g single dose, is recommended as first choice for the treatment of non-specific vaginosis.

Contraindications

1. Sulphonamide hypersensitivity

Hypersensitivity reactions in patients using topical sulphacetamide include skin rashes, Stevens–Johnson syndrome, conjunctivitis and vaginal irritation. Sulphacetamide eye or vaginal preparations should not be used in patients with a history of allergy to sulphonamides.

2. Herpes simplex corneal infection (Cortucid)

Cortucid contains hydrocortisone which aggravates herpetic eye infections to the extent that loss of vision or even loss of the eye may occur. 'Red eye' can be caused by herpes simplex infection, which may be difficult to distinguish from bacterial infection clinically. Therefore, this preparation should be used only on patients under close, specialist supervision.

3. Renal failure (Sultrin vaginal cream/tablets)

The main route of excretion of the sulphonamides contained in Sultrin vaginal cream/tablets is via the kidneys, and therefore these preparations should be avoided in patients with renal impairment.

Adverse reactions

Potentially life-threatening effects

The Stevens–Johnson syndrome, or severe erythema multiforme, may occur after the use of topical sodium sulphacetamide in the treatment of conjunctivitis.[18–20] The syndrome usually occurs 1–3 weeks after exposure to the drug but symptoms can occur within hours or days if the patient has previously been exposed to sulphonamides.

Acute overdosage

There have been no reports of overdose with sodium sulphacetamide eye drops. However, ingestion of a 10 ml solution does not present a toxicological hazard.

If ingestion of large quantities of Sultrin vaginal tablets or cream occurs then gastric lavage may be necessary. High fluid intake should be ensured and sodium bicarbonate should be given for alkalinization of the urine. These precautions will assist elimination of sulphonamides in the urine.

Severe or irreversible adverse effects

In patients with the dry-eye syndrome, concentration of sulphacetamide eye drops on the surface of the eye may result in the formation of white, elevated corneal plaques with damage to the superficial epithelial cells.[21] Contamination of multidose eye preparations may result in serious eye infections. Contamination should be avoided and the container should be discarded after 1 month. Alternatively, single-use containers can be used.

Hypersensitivity reactions to eye preparations are uncommon but include conjunctivitis,[22] skin rashes and the Stevens-Johnson syndrome.

Symptomatic adverse effects

Topical application of sulphacetamide eye drops or ointment may cause burning or stinging but this is rarely severe enough to warrant discontinuation of treatment. The irritation is usually transient and occurs especially with the higher concentrations. Ocusol eye drops containing 5% sulphacetamide, zinc sulphate and cetrimide have the antibacterial effect equivalent to that of a 30% solution of sulphacetamide but are less likely to cause local irritation.

Sulphacetamide eye ointment in the greasy base may cause blurring of vision and should therefore be used at night.

Sultrin vaginal preparations may cause vaginal irritation.

Other effects

No biochemical effects have been described as a result of the use of topical sulphacetamide.

Interference with clinical pathology tests

None of the sulphacetamide preparations currently available have been reported to interfere with clinical pathology tests.

High risk groups

Neonates

No special precautions are required.

Breast milk. No special precautions are required when breast-feeding.

Children

No special precautions are required for the use of eye drops or eye ointments.

Pregnant women

No special precautions required for the use of sodium sulphacetamide eye drops or ointments.

Cortucid should not be used in large amounts or for long periods. The corticosteroid component can cause fetal abnormalities in pregnant animals, although the relevance of this is not established in humans.

Sultrin vaginal cream and tablets should be used cautiously in pregnancy as the effects on the outcome of pregnancy are unknown.

The elderly

The dosage of eye drops or ointments should not be reduced in the elderly. Vaginal cream and tablets can be given providing the renal function is normal.

Concurrent disease

Renal impairment. Sultrin vaginal cream should be avoided in renal impairment.

Drug interactions

Potentially hazardous interactions

Purulent eye exudate. Para-aminobenzoic acid is present in purulent exudates and can competitively inhibit the action of sulphacetamide.

Sulphacetamide

Other significant reactions

Local anaesthetic agents. Amethocaine and oxybuprocaine are derivatives of p-aminobenzoic acid and therefore competitively inhibit the action of sulphacetamide, thus rendering it therapeutically inactive.[23] Therefore, these combinations should not be used.

Silver preparations. Sodium sulphacetamide solutions are incompatible with silver preparations.

Gentamicin. It has been found that high concentrations of sulphacetamide antagonize gentamicin's bactericidal effect. Although the mechanism is not known, the two drugs should not be used concurrently in the topical treatment of eye infections.

Potentially useful interactions

No interactions of this kind have been reported.

Major outcome trials

1. Mayer L L 1948 Sodium sulfacetamide in ophthalmology. Archives of Ophthalmology 39: 232–239

3000 eyes with acute and chronic conjunctivitis were treated with 30% sodium sulphacetamide solution. In many cases of bilateral infection, controls were carried out without medication or with various other agents including silver nitrate, nitromersol, ethyl hydrocupreine and hexylresorcinol. Average mean recovery periods were greatly shortened with the use of sodium sulphacetamide compared with other agents.

General review articles

Reynolds J E F (ed) 1982 Sulphonamides and trimethoprim. In: The extra pharmacopoeia (Martindale), 28th edn. The Pharmaceutical Press, London, pp 1457–1459, 1472–1473

Goodman L S, Gilman A G, Rall T W, Murad F (eds) 1985 Sulphonamides and trimethoprim-sulfamethoxazole. In: The pharmacological basis of therapeutics, 7th edn, ch 49, pp 1095–1114

Barker B M, Prescott F 1973 The sulphonamides. In: Antimicrobial agents in medicine. Blackwell Scientific Publications, Oxford, pp 76–90

Garrod L P, Lambert H P, O'Grady F 1981 Sulphonamides. In: Antibiotics and chemotherapy, 5th edn. Churchill Livingstone, Edinburgh, ch 1, pp 11–25

Today's Drugs 1964 Sulphonamides (1) and (2). British Medical Journal 1: 419–421 and 483–486

Today's Drugs 1968 Sulphonamides. British Medical Journal 2: 674–676

Kucers A, Bennett N McK 1989 Sulphonamides. In: The use of antibiotics: a comprehensive review with clinical emphasis, 4th edn. William Heinemann Medical Books Ltd, London, pp 1075–1117

Duke Elder S 1962 The sulphonamides. In: System of ophthalmology Vol VII. The foundations of ophthalmology, heredity, pathology, diagnosis and therapeutics. Henry Kimptom, London, pp 647–658

References

1. Woods D D 1962 The biochemical mode of action of the sulphonamide drugs. Journal of General Microbiology 29: 687–702
2. Reeves D S, Phillips I, Williams J D, Wise R (eds) 1978 Sulphonamides. In: Laboratory methods in antimicrobial chemotherapy. Churchill Livingstone, Edinburgh, ch 35, pp 222–226
3. Penner M H 1975 Assay of sulphacetamide sodium ophthalmic solutions by high-pressure liquid chromatography. Journal of Pharmaceutical Sciences 64: 1017–1019
4. Welebir F, Barnes R W 1941 The use of sulphacetamide in bacillary infections of the urinary tract. Journal of the American Medical Association 117: 2132–2135
5. Robson J M, Scott G I 1942 Local effectiveness of sodium sulphacetamide (Albucid soluble) in the treatment of experimental ulcers of the cornea. British Medical Journal 1: 5–8
6. Robson J M, Tebrich W 1942 Penetration and distribution of sodium sulphacetamide in ocular tissues of rabbits. British Medical Journal 1: 687–690
7. Ginsburg M, Robson J M 1945 The effect of detergent on the penetration of sodium sulphacetamide (Albucid soluble) into ocular tissues. British Journal of Ophthalmology 29: 185–193
8. Benedict W L, Henderson J W 1947 Sodium sulphacetamide. Its use in treatment of certain diseases of the eye. American Journal of Ophthalmology 30: 984–986
9. Dunlop E M C, Rodin P, Seth A D, Kolator B 1980 Ophthalmia neonatorum due to beta-lactamase-producing gonococci. British Medical Journal 281: 483
10. Johnson J E, Taraska S P, Rhodes K H, Kleinberg F, Smith T F 1976 Inclusion blenorrhea. A case report. Mayo Clinic Proceedings 51: 574–577
11. Csonka G W, Coufalik E D 1977 Chlamydial, gonococcal, and herpes virus infections in neonates. Postgraduate Medical Journal 53: 592–594
12. Dickson R M 1942 Traumatic ulcer of the cornea with special reference to coal miners. British Journal of Ophthalmology 26: 529–546
13. Dickson R M 1948 First aid treatment of industrial eye injuries. Archives of Ophthalmology 39: 544–548
14. Bickel J E 1950 Sodium sulfacetamide for the prophylaxis of gonorrheal ophthalmia neonatorum. Journal of Pediatrics 37: 854–857
15. Ormsby H L 1955 Ophthalmia neonatorum. Canadian Medical Association Journal 72: 576–580
16. Bhattacharyya M N 1981 Vaginitis revisited. British Medical Journal 283: 1126
17. Pheifer T A, Forsyth P S, Durfee M A, Pollock H M, Holmes K K 1978 Non-specific vaginitis. Role of *Haemophilus vaginalis* and treatment with metronidazole. New England Journal of Medicine 298: 1429–1434
18. Gottschalk H R, Stone O J 1976 Stevens–Johnson syndrome from ophthalmic sulfonamide. Archives of Dermatology 112: 513–514
19. Rubin Z 1977 Ophthalmic sulfonamide-induced Stevens–Johnson syndrome. Archives of Dermatology 113: 235–236
20. Genvert G I, Cohen E J, Donnenfield E D, Blecher M H 1985 Erythema multiforme after use of topical sulfacetamide. American Journal of Ophthalmology 99: 465–468
21. Tabbara K F, Veirs E R 1984 Corneal white plaques caused by sulfacetamide eyedrops. American Journal of Ophthalmology 98: 378–380
22. Duke Elder S 1965 Allergic kerato-conjunctivitis. In: System of ophthalmology Vol VIII. Diseases of the outer eye. Henry Kimptom, London, pp 453–454
23. Evans R A 1975 Treatment of eye injuries. British Medical Journal 2: 195
24. Burger L M, Sanford J P, Zweighaft T 1973 The effect of sulfonamides on the anti-pseudomonas activity of gentamicin in vitro. American Journal of Ophthalmology 75: 314–318

Sulphadiazine

Sulphadiazine is a short-acting bacteriostatic analogue of para-aminobenzoic acid.

Chemistry

Sulphadiazine (sulfadiazine)
$C_{10}H_{10}N_4O_2S$
N′-(Pyrimidin-2-yl)sulphanilamide

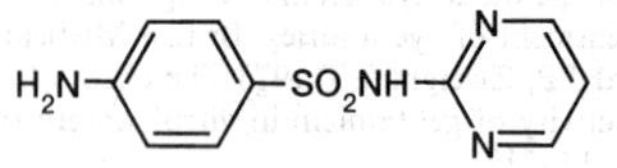

Molecular weight	250.3
pKa	6.4
Solubility	
in alcohol	slight
in water	1 in 13 000
Octanol/water partition coefficient	0.05

Sulphadiazine is a white or yellowish-white, odourless, almost tasteless powder which slowly darkens on exposure to light. The aqueous solubility is 1: 13 000. It is prepared by chemical synthesis. Sulphadiazine sodium is available for injection. Sulphadiazine is also contained in two oral combination products with streptomycin, sulphadimidine and sulphathiazole and with sulphamerazine and sulphathiazole. Silver sulphadiazine cream (Flamazine) is available for topical use.

Pharmacology

Sulphadiazine is structurally similar to *p*-aminobenzoic acid (PABA) and therefore acts by competitive blockade of the enzyme dihydrofolic acid (DHF) synthetase (Fig. 1).[1] DHF synthetase is required to convert PABA to dihydrofolic acid (DHF). Sulphadiazine, therefore, inhibits production of DHF which is required for synthesis of tetrahydrofolic acid (THF), purines and, ultimately, DNA. Mammalian cells derive DHF from dietary folic acid and therefore bypass this part of the pathway. Silver sulphadiazine is thought to act by binding to cell membranes and, to a lesser extent, to the bacterial cell wall. Thus, the drug has a different mode of action from sulphadiazine free base.

Toxicology

Epidemiological studies[2] have not demonstrated sulphadiazine teratogenicity in humans.

No carcinogenic or teratogenic effects have been reported with silver sulphadiazine in long-term toxicity studies in animals.

Clinical pharmacology

The following organisms are usually sensitive to sulphadiazine: *Streptococcus pyogenes*, *Strep. pneumoniae*, *Strep. viridans*, *Staphylococcus aureus*, *Bacillus anthracis* (some strains), *Clostridium perfringens*, *Corynebacterium diphtheriae*, *Haemophilus influenzae*, *H. ducreyi*, *Brucella* spp., *Calymmatobacterium granulomatis*, *Yersinia pestis*, *Vibrio cholerae*, *Nocardia* spp., *Actinomyces* spp. and *Chlamydia trachomatis*.

In combination with pyrimethamine, sulphadiazine is also active against malarial parasites, *Toxoplasma gondii* and *Pneumocystis carinii*.

Enterobacter aerogenes, *Alcaligenes* spp., *Pseudomonas aeruginosa* and *Proteus* spp. may appear sensitive in vitro but infections due to these organisms seldom respond to sulphadiazine.

As with other sulphonamides, the spectrum of activity of sulphadiazine has been reduced by acquired bacterial resistance. Sulphadiazine resistance may be due to increased synthesis of PABA or to production of DHF synthetase with a lowered affinity for sulphadiazine. *Streptococcus faecalis* is invariably resistant to sulphadiazine. Most strains of *Shigella* spp. are now resistant. Resistance is also common in *Escherichia coli*, *Neisseria gonorrhoeae* and *N. meningitidis*. Resistance in many Gram-negative organisms may be mediated by resistance plasmids (R plasmids).

Silver sulphadiazine is active against most staphylococci, streptococci (including enterococci), *Escherichia coli*, *Enterobacter* spp., *Klebsiella* spp., *Proteus* spp. and *Pseudomonas aeruginosa*. Some strains of *Candida albicans* are also sensitive. However, topical use of silver sulphadiazine in one burns unit resulted in a large increase in the proportion of sulphadiazine-resistant Gram-negative bacilli.[3]

Pharmacokinetics

The usual analytical method is a colorimetric method which measures free and total sulphadiazine separately.[4] Gas–liquid chromatography[5] and high performance liquid chromatography[6] methods have also been described and are more sensitive and specific. Microbiological assays are less accurate.[7]

Sulphadiazine is rapidly absorbed after oral administration, the main site of absorption being the small intestine. Peak plasma concentrations are reached in 3–4 hours after a single dose. The mean plasma half life is 10 hours with a range of 7–12 hours.[8] The half life of the N_4 acetylsulphadiazine metabolite is 8–18 hours.[8] Before reaching the tissues, sulphadiazine is partially acetylated in the liver (see 'Metabolism').

Sulphadiazine is widely distributed throughout the body with a volume of distribution of 0.36 $l.kg^{-1}$. Up to 15% of blood sulphadiazine is present as the acetyl derivative. Sulphadiazine is 20–55% bound to plasma albumin.

Therapeutic cerebrospinal fluid concentrations are attained within four hours of a single oral dose of 60 $mg.kg^{-1}$. Concentrations of sulphadiazine in the cerebrospinal fluid are approximately 70% of plasma concentrations. Sulphadiazine concentrations in other body fluids in relation to blood concentrations are: saliva, 25%; breast milk, 20%; prostatic fluid, 10%; and tears, 4%.[9] Although only small concentrations of sulphadiazine are present in breast milk, there is still a danger of precipitation of haemolysis in glucose-6-phosphate dehydrogenase-deficient babies.[10] Blood concentrations in the fetus are 50–90% of those in maternal blood.

Oral absorption	100%
Presystemic metabolism (acetylation)	13–38%
Plasma half life	
range	7–12 h
mean	10 h
Volume of distribution	0.36 $l.kg^{-1}$
Plasma protein binding	20–55%

Fig. 1

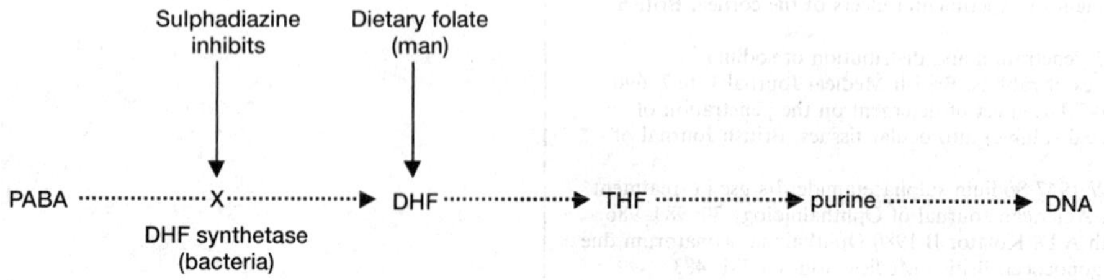

Sulphadiazine is excreted slowly, 50% of a single oral dose being excreted in 24 hours. Both sulphadiazine and its metabolic products are excreted mainly via the kidney, predominantly by glomerular filtration, although tubular secretion also occurs. This is followed by up to 70% tubular reabsorption. From 13 to 38% is excreted as the acetyl derivative, depending on whether the subject is a fast or slow acetylator of sulphadiazine.[8] The acetyl derivative is more water soluble and is less reabsorbed in the renal tubules. Sulphadiazine clearance is enhanced in alkaline urine which renders both the sulphadiazine and its acetylated derivative more soluble, resulting in less tubular reabsorption. Toxic levels may occur in impaired renal function.

Only small amounts of sulphadiazine are excreted in the bile.

Concentration–effect relationship

Minimum inhibitory concentrations (MIC) of sulphadiazine for most sensitive organisms are in the range of 0.5 to 20 mg.l^{-1}. In severe infections a blood concentration of 100–150 mg.l^{-1} is desirable. Therapeutic drug monitoring is not performed routinely. However, because of varying individual rates of acetylation, plasma concentrations of free sulphadiazine should be determined periodically when patients with severe infections are treated with large doses. Sulphadiazine should be avoided in patients with renal failure unless facilities for measuring the concentrations of sulphadiazine and its acetyl derivative are available.[11]

There are no published studies of a possible association between the in situ concentration of the two moieties during treatment of burns with silver sulphadiazine cream and the effect on the number of colonizing or infecting bacteria.

Metabolism

The major route of metabolism is acetylation in the liver. The acetyl group (CH_3CO) becomes attached to the free para-amino (NH_2) group of the sulphadiazine molecule to produce N_4-acetylsulphadiazine (Fig. 2).

The rate of acetylation is genetically determined and shows a bimodal character, individuals being classified as fast or slow acetylators. The same set of acetylating enzymes also acetylates isoniazid, therefore fast acetylators of sulphadiazine also inactivate isoniazid rapidly. N_4-acetylsulphadiazine has no antibacterial activity but retains the toxicity of the parent drug. The acetylated fraction increases considerably in renal failure, due to retention of the drug in the body. It decreases in hepatic failure.

When silver sulphadiazine is applied topically, absorbed sulphadiazine is metabolized in the liver by N_4-acetylation and by 5-hydroxylation. Absorbed silver, if any, may remain in the body, predominantly in the liver, for long periods of time, being slowly excreted via the bile.

Pharmaceutics

Sulphadiazine is available as generic oral, parenteral and topical forms.

1. Tablets containing 500 mg sulphadiazine are white, plain, round, uncoated and 12.5 mm in diameter.
2. Sulphadiazine is available for intravenous use as a colourless solution containing 1 g of sulphadiazine (as the more soluble sodium salt) in 4 ml ampoules (concentration 250 mg.ml^{-1}). This preparation is strongly alkaline and should be diluted with Water for Injections or added to saline for infusion. The undiluted solution may be administered by deep intramuscular injection. This preparation must never be given intrathecally or subcutaneously as it can cause necrosis.
3. Silver sulphadiazine (Flamazine (S&N, UK)/Flint SSD (Flint, USA)/Silvadene (Marion, USA) is available as a 1% w/w white hydrophilic cream for topical use. It is supplied in tubes of 50 g (Flamazine only) or jars of 250 g and 500 g. In Australia, a 1% cream supplemented with chlorhexidine gluconate 0.2% is available (Silvazine). Silver sulphadiazine cream should be applied with a sterile spatula or a hand covered with a sterile glove.

Fig. 2 Metabolism of Sulphadiazine

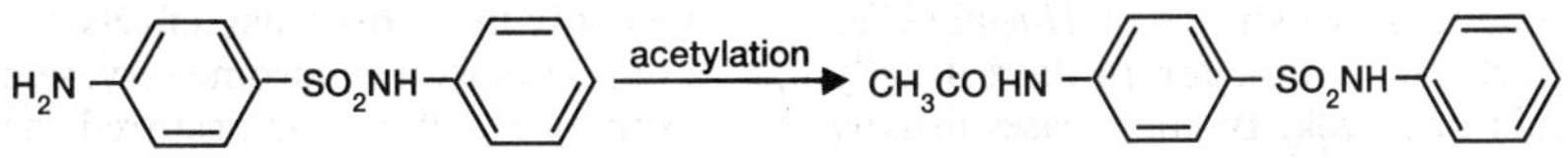

Sulphadiazine

S

All preparations should be stored in airtight containers in a cool place (4–8°C), protected from light. One container of silver sulphadiazine should be reserved for one patient.

The shelf-life for sulphadiazine tablets and injection is five years. Silver sulphadiazine cream is stable for three years.

Sulphadiazine may be allergenic. Some formulations of silver sulphadiazine contain cetyl alcohol and propylene alcohol.

Therapeutic use

Indications

1. Nocardiosis
2. Toxoplasmosis
3. Topical antibacterial agent for burns, ulcers and pressure sores (silver sulphadiazine)
4. Meningococcal infections: treatment and prophylaxis
5. Rheumatic fever prophylaxis
6. Urinary tract infections
7. Intestinal infections
8. Chancroid
9. Malaria
10. Pneumocystis pneumonia
11. Glanders
12. Lower respiratory tract infections.

Contraindications

1. Sulphonamide hypersensitivity
2. Renal failure
3. Hepatic failure
4. Infants under six weeks
5. The third trimester of pregnancy
6. Acute porphyria
7. Glucose-6-phosphate dehydrogenase deficiency.

Precautions

With oral or parenteral use of sulphadiazine, adequate fluid intake must be ensured, e.g. for adults an intake of 3–3.5 l in 24 hours should be maintained with a urinary output of not less than 1.4 l daily. In addition, agents such as sodium bicarbonate should be given to render the urine alkaline. These precautions reduce the risk of crystalluria.

Mode of use

Use of sulphadiazine has declined with the availability of new, more effective, less toxic antimicrobial agents and with the increase in sulphadiazine resistance of many organisms.

Indications

1. Nocardiosis

Sulphadiazine is the treatment of choice for nocardiosis.[12] The recommended dose is 4–6 g daily, with up to 8–9 g daily for severely ill patients. Treatment should be continued for several months to prevent relapse. Sulphadiazine may be combined with streptomycin or ampicillin for maximum effectiveness. When indicated, surgical drainage or resection is also advised.

2. Toxoplasmosis

If treatment is necessary, sulphadiazine (4 g loading dose followed by 1 g 6-hourly) should be given in combination with pyrimethamine (100 mg loading dose followed by 25 mg daily) for a total of six weeks. Folinic acid (6 mg daily) should also be given to prevent pyrimethamine-related bone marrow suppression. Peripheral blood cell and platelet counts should be performed twice weekly on patients on this regime.

3. Topical antibacterial agent
Silver sulphadiazine has been used effectively in the prevention and treatment of infection in patients with burns,[13] ulcers, pressure sores and wounds. The cream should be applied in a layer 3–5 mm thick using a sterile spatula or hand covered with a sterile glove. In the treatment of burns, silver sulphadiazine should be applied every 24 hours, after hydrotherapy and debridement to enhance removal of eschar. In leg ulcers, it should be applied at least three times a week after desloughing and cleansing. Care should be taken not to spread silver sulphadiazine on to non-ulcerated skin and it should not be used on very wet ulcers.

Silver sulphadiazine does not sterilize the wound but it suppresses the numbers and types of bacteria colonizing it. It can prevent the progression, due to infection, of partial-thickness burns to full-thickness wounds and can reduce the mortality and morbidity in patients with burns. Silver sulphadiazine is painless on application. It is easy to apply and remove and does not stain.

4. Meningococcal infections
Treatment. Approximately 30% of strains of *N. meningitidis* in England and Wales are now resistant to sulphadiazine.[14] In one UK outbreak,[15] 76% of 49 group B strains and 3 out of 7 group C strains were sulphonamide-resistant. If meningitis is known to be due to a sulphonamide-sensitive strain then intravenous sulphadiazine may be given. For adults, a loading dose of 2–3 g is followed by 1 g 4-hourly for 2 days, following which oral sulphadiazine 1 g 4–6 hourly should be continued until 2–3 days after clinical recovery. For children, 50 $mg.kg^{-1}$ body weight is given initially, followed by 100 $mg.kg^{-1}$ daily in four divided doses.

However, benzylpenicillin or chloramphenicol have higher and more reliable activity. Sulphadiazine is therefore no longer recommended as the treatment of choice for meningococcal infections.

Prophylaxis. Sulphadiazine may be given to close contacts of patients with meningococcal disease if the strain is known to be sensitive to sulphonamides. For adults, 1 g 12-hourly for 2 days is recommended. Children aged 1–12 years should be given half this dose. However, rifampicin is currently preferred for 'blind' prophylaxis.

5. Rheumatic fever prophylaxis
Oral sulphadiazine 1 g once daily has been used in continuous prophylaxis of rheumatic fever.[16] Doses of 500 mg daily should be given to patients weighing less than 30 kg. Sulphadiazine is more toxic and less effective than benzathine penicillin.[17] Sulphadiazine-resistant strains of *Strep. pyogenes* may arise. Sulphadiazine can be used in penicillin-allergic patients although erythromycin is a preferable alternative.[18]

Sulphadiazine is ineffective in the treatment of pharyngitis due to *Strep. pyogenes*.

6. Urinary tract infections
Sulphadiazine, 500 mg twice daily for adults or 4 $mg.kg^{-1}$ twice daily for children, can be used in the treatment of acute, uncomplicated urinary tract infections. However, sulphadiazine-resistant Enterobacteriaceae are now common, especially in hospitals; enterococci are invariably resistant; and *Staph. saprophyticus* infections may relapse after treatment. Sulphadiazine is not usually effective against chronic, recurrent, or nosocomial urinary tract infections.

7. Intestinal infections
Sulphadiazine is of no use in the treatment of salmonella infections. Most strains of *Shigella* spp. are now sulphonamide-resistant. Therefore, sulphadiazine is of little use in treatment of bacillary dysentery. Streptotriad, a combination of three sulphonamides and streptomycin, has been used in the treatment[19] and short-term prophylaxis[20] of travellers' diarrhoea. Prophylaxis is not recommended for casual holidays[21] as it encourages selection of multi-resistant organisms and carries a small risk of serious side effects. The traveller should be advised to avoid unsafe food and water. If necessary, trimethoprim can be taken at the first sign of symptoms by those on important, e.g. business or military, trips or by those with underlying disease, e.g. the immunocompromized or the elderly person with cardiovascular disease.

8. Chancroid
In chancroid due to sulphadiazine-sensitive strains of *Haemophilus ducreyi*, sulphadiazine, 1 g 6-hourly by mouth, for 14 days usually results in healing of lesions within one week. Bubonic cases usually require treatment with streptomycin as well as sulphadiazine and lymph node aspiration.[22] However, more than 15% of strains of *Haemophilus ducreyi* exhibit high level resistance to sulphonamides and more than 30% show moderate resistance.[23] Therefore, the treatment of choice, nowadays, is erythromycin or co-trimoxazole.

9. Malaria
The combination of pyrimethamine and sulphadiazine has been used successfully in the treatment of *Plasmodium falciparum* malaria.[24] However, the longer acting sulphonamide, sulphadoxine, in combination with pyrimethamine is, nowadays, preferred in the treatment of chloroquine-resistant malaria.

10. *Pneumocystis carinii* pneumonia
Although co-trimoxazole is presently the best choice for treatment and prophylaxis of *Pneumocystis carinii* pneumonia, the combination of pyrimethamine and sulphadiazine has been used successfully.[25] Doses of sulphadiazine, 1 g 6-hourly, and pyrimethamine, 25 mg twice daily, have been recommended, together with 6 mg folinic acid daily to avoid pyrimethamine-induced bone marrow suppression. However, experience with this combination has been limited. Peripheral blood cell and platelet counts should be performed twice weekly on patients on this regime.

11. Glanders
Sulphadiazine, 100 $mg.kg^{-1}$ in divided doses for 3 weeks, has been used successfully in combination with surgical drainage, or supportive measures, as appropriate.[26]

12. Lower respiratory tract infections
Although sulphadiazine has been used in the treatment of pneumococcal and other pneumonias, nowadays safer and more effective antimicrobial agents are available.

Contraindications

1. Sulphonamide hypersensitivity
Sulphadiazine is contraindicated in patients with a history of sulphonamide hypersensitivity. There is usually cross hypersensitivity between all the sulphonamides. Hypersensitivity reactions include skin rashes, Stevens–Johnson syndrome, serum sickness, drug fever, nephrotoxicity and hepatotoxicity. Anaphylactoid type reactions may occur in patients previously sensitized to sulphonamides.

2. Renal failure
Sulphadiazine is contraindicated in patients with any degree of renal failure unless facilities for regular monitoring of the concentrations of sulphadiazine and its acetyl derivative are available. The proportion of acetylated sulphadiazine increases considerably in renal impairment due to prolonged stay of the drug in the body.

3. Hepatic failure
Sulphadiazine should not be given to patients with impaired liver function. An alternative antimicrobial agent should be chosen.

4. Infants under six weeks
Sulphadiazine should not be used in the treatment of neonatal infections as it competes with bilirubin for albumin binding sites and may increase the risk of kernicterus. Recent work, however, suggests that sulphadiazine does not cause kernicterus.[2]

5. The third trimester of pregnancy
Sulphadiazine should not be used in the last trimester of pregnancy because of the risk of kernicterus in the neonate, although it may be doubtful whether there is indeed a risk.[2]

6. Acute porphyria
Sulphadiazine can precipitate or aggravate porphyria.[27]

7. Glucose-6-phosphate dehydrogenase deficiency
Sulphadiazine should be avoided in patients with glucose-6-phosphate dehydrogenase deficiency as it may precipitate haemolysis, resulting in haemoglobinuria and acute renal failure. Premature infants normally have low levels of this enzyme therefore sulphadiazine is contraindicated in these patients.

Adverse reactions

Potentially life-threatening effects
Stevens–Johnson syndrome (erythema multiforme), a serious hypersensitivity reaction, has occurred rarely with the use of sulphadiaz-

Sulphadiazine

ine.[28] The disease can be fatal in 25% of cases. For this reason, sulphadiazine should be discontinued immediately a skin rash appears.

Sulphadiazine-induced liver damage[29] is also rare, usually appearing 3–5 days after start of therapy. The patient develops fever, headache, nausea, hepatomegaly, jaundice and abnormal liver function tests. Death may occur. Hepatitis is not related to the dose of sulphadiazine or to pre-existing liver disease. The focal or diffuse necrosis which occurs may be due to direct drug toxicity or to hypersensitization. Liver damage may progress even after drug withdrawal.

Acute overdosage

Overdose of sulphadiazine causes crystalluria. Symptoms of crystalluria include loin pain and haematuria, and anuria if total obstruction of the renal pelvis or ureters occurs. In cases of recent overdose, the stomach should be emptied by gastric washout. Large volumes of fluids should be administered, by intravenous infusion if necessary. Sodium bicarbonate should be given to render the urine alkaline. These measures should reduce the risk of crystalluria. Heat should be applied to the loins for symptomatic relief. If the condition persists, cystoscopy and ureteric catheterization may be required with irrigation of warm 2.5% sodium bicarbonate solution. The catheters should be left in situ for 24–48 hours or until renal function has been restored.

Severe or irreversible adverse effects

It is generally considered that sulphonamides should not be given in late pregnancy because of the risk of kernicterus. However, recent work suggests that sulphadiazine does not cause kernicterus.[2]

Acute haemolytic anaemia is induced by sulphadiazine in patients with glucose-6-phosphate dehydrogenase deficiency. This enzyme normally combats the oxidization of haemoglobin by sulphadiazine. When the enzyme is deficient, as occurs in genetic defects or premature infants, the denatured haemoglobin accumulates in the red blood cells in the form of Heinz bodies. Intravascular haemolysis and haemoglobinuria then occurs. Therefore, sulphadiazine is contraindicated in patients with glucose-6-phosphate dehydrogenase deficiency.

Nephrotoxic effects of sulphadiazine[30] include crystalluria with obstructive nephropathy, hypersensitivity reactions, and acute renal failure secondary to haemolysis. Precipitation of sulphadiazine occurs in acid urine, especially in patients with poor urine output, for example in dehydration. Crystals are deposited in the renal parenchyma, calyces, pelves and ureters, resulting in obstruction. Loin pain, haematuria, anuria and progressive uraemia can result. Prevention of crystalluria requires a high fluid intake and large amounts of sodium bicarbonate (approximately 12 g per day) in order to maintain the urinary pH above 7.15. The risk of crystalluria is also reduced with sulphonamide combinations (e.g. Sulphatriad and Streptotriad).

Hypersensitivity reactions to sulphadiazine include allergic interstitial nephritis. Nephrotic syndrome has occurred after the use of topical silver sulphadiazine. Sulphadiazine-induced haemolysis in patients with glucose-6-phosphate dehydrogenase deficiency has resulted in haemoglobinuria and acute renal failure. Nephrotoxicity occurs more commonly with intravenous than with oral preparations.

A serum sickness type of reaction may occur after 3–17 days of sulphadiazine therapy and is characterized by fever, joint pains, urticarial rash, conjunctivitis, bronchospasm and leucopenia. Immediate reactions of the anaphylactoid type may occur in previously sensitized patients.

Granulocytopenia occurs in approximately 0.1% of patients on sulphadiazine. This may be due to a hypersensitivity reaction or to a direct toxic effect on the bone marrow. Sulphadiazine should be discontinued, whereupon spontaneous recovery usually occurs within one week, although it may be delayed for several weeks. Leucopenia has also been associated with the topical use of silver sulphadiazine.[31]

Systemic lupus erythematosus has rarely been associated with the use of sulphadiazine.[32]

Symptomatic adverse effects

Nausea and vomiting occur in 1–9% of patients treated with sulphadiazine. These side effects may be due to gastrointestinal irritation or to stimulation of the medullary emetic centre. If necessary, sulphadiazine can be continued while the nausea and vomiting are treated symptomatically.

Allergic rashes occur in 1.5% of patients,[33] usually 7–10 days after the start of treatment. The rash is usually maculopapular or urticarial and may appear earlier in previously sensitized patients. Fever, malaise and pruritus are often present simultaneously. Sulphadiazine should be discontinued immediately a rash appears because of the danger of severe reactions such as the Stevens–Johnson syndrome.

Drug fever occurs in 1.5–4% of patients. Fever usually occurs 7–10 days after the start of sulphadiazine but may appear earlier in patients previously sensitized. It should be differentiated from the fever associated with severe adverse effects such as granulocytopenia and acute haemolytic anaemia.

Headache and dizziness occurred in 2 out of 446 patients treated with sulphadiazine.[34] These symptoms resolved on discontinuation of the drug.

Interference with clinical pathology tests

Sulphadiazine can interfere technically with the Berthelot method for estimations of blood urea, producing falsely raised results.[35]

High risk groups

Neonates

Sulphadiazine is contraindicated in neonates as it competes with bilirubin for albumin binding sites and may increase the risk of kernicterus although recent results cast doubt upon this.[2]

Breast milk. Although only small concentrations of sulphadiazine are present in breast milk, there is still a danger of precipitation of haemolysis in glucose-6-phosphate dehydrogenase deficient babies.[10]

Children

The dosage of sulphadiazine should be reduced according to the manufacturer's recommendations.

Pregnant women

Epidemiological studies in humans have not revealed an association between sulphadiazine and fetal malformations.[2] However, the risk–benefit factors should be assessed before the use of sulphadiazine in pregnancy. Sulphadiazine is contraindicated in the last trimester of pregnancy because of the risk of kernicterus in the neonate however, recent work suggests that such a risk may not exist.[2] There is insufficient data regarding the safety of Streptotriad in pregnancy.

The elderly

No special precautions are required providing renal and hepatic function are normal.

Concurrent disease

Renal failure. Sulphadiazine is contraindicated in renal impairment.

Hepatic failure. Sulphadiazine is contraindicated in liver failure.

Drug interactions

Potentially hazardous interactions

Warfarin. The metabolism of warfarin by liver microsomal enzymes is inhibited by therapeutic doses of sulphadiazine. This may result in increased prothrombin time and bleeding problems unless the dose of warfarin is reduced.

Ascorbic acid. Ascorbic acid should be avoided in patients taking sulphadiazine as the likelihood of crystalluria and renal damage is increased when the urine is acid.

Hexamine. Hexamine should not be given with sulphadiazine as acidification of the urine increases the risks of crystalluria and renal damage.

Other significant interactions

Phenytoin. Sulphadiazine inhibits the metabolism of phenytoin by liver microsomal enzymes.[36] The increased levels of phenytoin may result in nystagmus and ataxia.

Tolbutamide/chlorpropamide. Therapeutic doses of sulphadiazine inhibit the metabolism of oral hypoglycaemic agents by liver microsomal enzymes. This may result in increased hypoglycaemic effect.

Para-aminobenzoic acid. The action of sulphadiazine may be competitively antagonized by *p*-aminobenzoic acid which should not be given concomitantly.

Methotrexate. Sulphadiazine displaces methotrexate from albumin binding sites and therefore increases the risk of methotrexate toxicity.

S

Potentially useful interactions

Pyrimethamine. The antibacterial action of the diaminopyrimidine derivative, pyrimethamine, is potentiated by sulphadiazine because of the sequential blockade of bacterial folic acid metabolism. This combination has been used in the treatment of toxoplasmosis, *Pneumocystis carinii* pneumonia and *Plasmodium falciparum* malaria.

Trimethoprim. Trimethoprim is another diaminopyrimidine derivative which produces a synergistic effect with sulphadiazine by sequential blockade of folic acid metabolism. This combination has been used in the form of Co-trimazine which contained 410 mg sulphadiazine and 90 mg trimethoprim in each 500 mg tablet. Co-trimazine had an antibacterial spectrum similar to that of co-trimoxazole and was used in the treatment of urinary tract infections. This combination is no longer commercially available in Great Britain.

Clinical Trials

1. Finland M, Strauss E, Peterson O L 1941 Sulfadiazine: therapeutic evaluation and toxic effects on four hundred and forty six patients. Journal of the American Medical Association 116: 2641–2647

Sulphadiazine was used in an uncontrolled trial in the treatment of 446 patients with various infections including meningococcal infection, urinary tract infections, and respiratory tract infections. It was not effective in the treatment of chronic urinary infections, chronic respiratory tract infections, endocarditis or chronic gonococcal arthritis.

Toxic effects from sulphadiazine were relatively mild and infrequent and included nausea and vomiting in 9.2%. Other toxic effects noted were leucopenia, morbilliform rashes, crystalluria, headache and dizziness. One patient developed ureteral colic, haematuria and anuria requiring ureteral catheterization.

A review of animal experiments, in vitro studies and pharmacokinetics is given.

General review articles

Reynolds J E F (ed) 1982 Sulphonamides and trimethoprim. In: The extra pharmacopoeia (Martindale), 28th edn. The Pharmaceutical Press, London, pp 1457–1459, 1473–1475

Goodman L S, Gilman A G, Rall T W, Murad F (eds) 1985 Sulphonamides and trimethoprim–sulfamethoxazole. In: The pharmacological basis of therapeutics, 7th edn. Macmillan, New York, ch 49, pp 1095–1114

Barker B M, Prescott F (eds) 1973 The sulphonamides. In: Antimicrobial agents in medicine. Blackwell Scientific Publications, Oxford, pp 76–90

Garrod L P, Lambert H P, O'Grady F (eds) 1981 Sulphonamides. In: Antibiotics and chemotherapy, 5th edn. Churchill Livingstone, Edinburgh, ch 1, pp 11–25

Today's Drugs 1964 Sulphonamides (1) and (2). British Medical Journal 1: 419–421 and 483–486

Today's Drugs 1968 Sulphonamides. British Medical Journal 2: 674– 676

Ballin J C 1974 Evaluation of a new topical agent for burn therapy: silver sulfadiazine (Silvadene). Journal of the American Medical Association 230: 1184–1185

Reese R E, Douglas R G (eds) 1983 A practical approach to infectious diseases. Little, Brown and Company, Boston/Toronto, pp 127–129

Kucers A, Bennett N McK (eds) 1989 Sulphonamides. In: The use of antibiotics: a comprehensive review with clinical emphasis, 4th edn. William Heinemann Medical Books, London, pp 1075–1117

References

1. Woods D D 1962 The biochemical mode of action of the sulphonamide drugs. Journal of General Microbiology 29: 687–702
2. Baskin C G, Law S, Wenger N K 1980 Sulphadiazine rheumatic fever prophylaxis during pregnancy: does it increase the risk of kernicterus in the newborn? Cardiology 65: 222–225
3. Bridges K, Lowbury E J L 1977 Drug resistance in relation to use of sulphadiazine cream in a burns unit. Journal of Clinical Pathology 30: 160–164
4. Bratton A C, Marshall E K 1939 A new coupling component for sulfanilamide determination. Journal of Biological Chemistry 128: 537–550
5. Gyllenhaal O, Ehrsson H 1975 Determination of sulphonamides by electron-capture gas chromatography. Journal of Chromatography 107: 327–333
6. Vree T B, Hekster Y A, Baars A M, Damsma J E, van der Kleijn E 1978 Determination of trimethoprim and sulfamethoxazole (co-trimoxazole) in body fluids of man by means of high-performance liquid chromatography. Journal of Chromatography 146: 103–112
7. Reeves D S, Phillips I, Williams J D, Wise R (eds) 1978 Sulphonamides. In: Laboratory methods in antimicrobial chemotherapy. Churchill Livingstone, Edinburgh, ch 35, pp 222– 226
8. Vree T B, O'Reilly W J, Hekster Y A, Damsma J E, van der Kleijn E 1980 Determination of the acetylator phenotype and pharmacokinetics of some sulphonamides in man. Clinical Pharmacokinetics 5: 274–294
9. Wilkinson P J, Reeves D S 1979 Tissue penetration of trimethoprim and sulphonamides. Journal of Antimicrobial Chemotherapy 5: 159–168
10. Anderson P D 1977 Drug intelligence. Drugs and breast feeding. Clinical Pharmacology 11: 208–223
11. Reeves D 1982 Sulphonamides and trimethoprim. In: Good antimicrobial prescribing. A Lancet review. Lancet, London, pp 63–74
12. Peabody J W, Seabury J H 1960 Actinomycosis and nocardiosis. A review of basic differences in therapy. American Journal of Medicine 28: 99–115
13. McDougall I A 1972 Use of silver sulphadiazine in the treatment of burns at Royal Perth Hospital. Medical Journal of Australia 1: 979–981
14. Abbott J D, Jones D M, Painter M J, Young S E J 1985 The epidemiology of meningococcal infections in England and Wales, 1912–1983. Journal of Infection 11: 241–257
15. Cartwright K A V, Stuart J M, Noah N D 1986 An outbreak of meningococcal disease in Gloucestershire. Lancet 2: 558–561
16. Kaplan E L, Bisno A, Derrick W et al 1977 AHA Committee Report. Prevention of rheumatic fever. Circulation 55: 1–4
17. Wood H F, Feinstein A R, Taranta A, Epstein J A, Simpson R 1964 Rheumatic fever in children and adolescents. A long term epidemiologic study of subsequent prophylaxis, streptococcal infections and clinical sequelae III. Comparative effectiveness of three prophylaxis regimens in preventing streptococcal infections and rheumatic recurrences. Annals of Internal Medicine 60: 31–46
18. Ginsburg C M, Eichenwald H F 1976 Erythromycin: a review of its uses in paediatric practice. The Journal of Paediatrics 89: 872–884
19. Thubron R S 1979 Hong Kong dog and the Tokyo trots. British Medical Journal 2: 1225
20. Turner A C 1967 Traveller's diarrhoea: a survey of symptoms, occurrence, and possible prophylaxis. British Medical Journal 4: 653–654
21. Higginson A G 1979 'Travellers' diarrhoea'. Practitioner 223: 529–538
22. Lykke-Olesen L, Larsen L, Pedersen T G, Gaarslev K 1979 Epidemic of chancroid in Greenland 1977–78. Lancet 1: 654–655
23. Nsanze H, Plummer F A, Ronald A R 1984 Haemophilus ducreyi. Clinical Microbiology Newsletter 6: 71–74
24. McGregor I A, Williams K, Goodwin L G 1963 Pyrimethamine and sulphadiazine in treatment of malaria. British Medical Journal 2: 728–729
25. Kirby H B, Kenamore B, Guckian J C 1971 Pneumocystis carinii pneumonia treated with pyrimethamine and sulfadiazine. Annals of Internal Medicine 75: 505–509
26. Mandell G L, Douglas R G, Bennett J E (eds) 1985 Pseudomonas species (including melidiosis and glanders). In: Principles and practice of infectious diseases, 2nd edn. John Wiley & Sons, New York, ch 179, pp 1250–1254
27. Peterkin G A G, Khan S A 1969 Iatrogenic skin disease. The Practitioner 202: 117–129
28. Cameron A J, Baron J H, Priestley B L 1966 Erythema multiforme, drugs and ulcerative colitis. British Medical Journal 2: 1174–1178
29. Dujovne C A, Chan C H, Zimmerman H J 1967 Sulfonamide liver injury: review of the literature and report of a case due to sulfamethoxazole. New England Journal of Medicine 277: 785–788
30. Appel G B, Neu H C 1977 The nephrotoxicity of antimicrobial agents (third of three parts). New England Journal of Medicine 296: 784–787
31. Caffee H H, Bingham H G 1982 Leukopenia and silver sulphadiazine. The Journal of Trauma 22: 586–587
32. Cohen P, Gardner F H 1966 Sulfonamide reactions in systemic lupus erythematosus. Journal of the American Medical Association 197: 817–819
33. Weinstein L, Madoff M A, Samet C M 1960 Medical progress. The sulfonamides (concluded). New England Journal of Medicine 263: 952–957
34. Finland M, Strauss E, Peterson O L 1941 Sulphadiazine. Journal of the American Medical Association 116: 2641–2647
35. Herxheiner A (ed) 1972 Interference of drugs with chemical diagnostic tests. Drugs and Therapeutics Bulletin 10: 69–72
36. Hansen J M, Siersbaek-Nielsen K, Skovsted L, Kampmann J P, Lumholtz B 1975 Potentiation of warfarin by co-trimoxazole. British Medical Journal 2: 684

Sulphadimidine

Sulphadimidine is an antibacterial sulphonamide.

Chemistry

Sulphadimidine (sulphamethazine, sulfamezathine, Diazil)
$C_{12}H_{14}N_4O_2$
N′-(4,6-Dimethylpyrimidin-2-yl)sulphanilamide

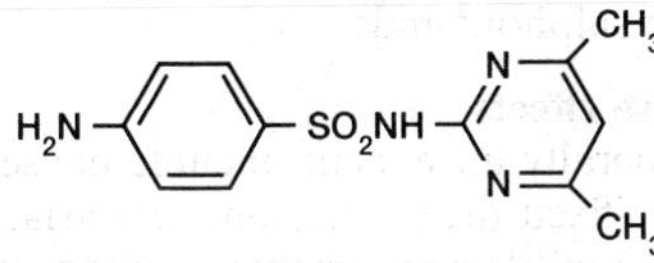

Molecular weight	278.3
pKa (sulphonamide group)	7.4
Solubility	
in alcohol	1 in 120
in water	1 in 650
Octanol/water partition coefficient	2.0

Sulphadimidine is a white, tasteless and odourless crystalline powder, prepared by chemical synthesis. It darkens and decomposes on exposure to light. Sulphadimidine sodium is available as Sulphamethazine.

Sulphadimidine is also found in an oral combination product with sulphadiazine, sulphathiazole and streptomycin sulphate (Streptotriad).

Pharmacology

Sulphadimidine competitively inhibits the incorporation of para-aminobenzoic acid into folic acid by bacteria. Sensitive bacteria are those that must synthesize their own folic acid. Sulphadimidine acts specifically as a competitive inhibitor of the enzyme responsible for the incorporation of para-aminobenzoic acid into dihydropteroic acid which is the immediate precursor of folic acid[1,2]. Sulphadimidine does not affect mammalian cells since these cells require intact folic acid and cannot synthesize it.

Toxicology

No tests of mutagenicity in bacteria or long-term carcinogenicity in animals have been carried out. There is no evidence of teratological effects in rats.

Clinical pharmacology

There is no pharmacological response to sulphadimidine other than cure of bacterial infection sensitive to sulphonamide treatment[3,4]. The recommended daily dose range (1.5–7.5 g) was decided partly from experimental data in mice and non-infected patients, and partly from empirical use in the treatment of susceptible infections.[5] Although early studies did not differentiate between acetylator phenotypes (see below), initial treatment in adults with 4 g orally, followed by 2 g orally every 6 hours generally results in blood sulphadimidine concentrations between 50 and 100 mg.l^{-1}, with similar concentrations during a regimen of 1 g every 4 hours.[6] Concentrations ranging between 38 and 298 (mean 165) mg.l^{-1} result from use of an age-adjusted regimen in children.[7] Apart from transient nausea and vomiting, no concentration-related symptoms of toxicity have been described following doses of up to 12 g daily.

Sulphadimidine is normally effective against *Streptococcus pyogenes*, *Streptococcus pneumoniae*, and some strains of *Haemophilus influenzae*, *Vibrio cholerae*, *Corynebacterium diphtheriae*, *Brucella* spp., *Actinomyces*, *Nocardia* and *Chlamydia trachomatis*.

Pharmacokinetics

The preferred analytical method is thin-layer chromatography, which will separate all the sulphonamides, and is sensitive[8] to 0.5 µg.l^{-1}. HPLC with UV detection has also been used, but the limit of sensitivity is poorer. Sulphadimidine is absorbed almost completely from the gastrointestinal tract and undergoes no presystemic metabolism. The plasma half life is dependent upon the rate of acetylation, mean 1.5 h in rapid acetylators, 5.5 h in slow acetylators.[9] (See below.) The apparent volume of distribution[10] is 0.61 l.kg^{-1}, similar to total body water. Sulphadimidine is highly bound (90%) to albumin in plasma.[11]

The concentration of sulphadimidine in the CSF exceeds 50% of the concentration in blood.[5]

Sulphadimidine readily crosses the placenta and equilibration between maternal and fetal blood is usually established in 3 hours. Concentrations in the fetus are sufficient to cause anti-bacterial and toxic effects (see Adverse reactions). Unbound sulphadimidine also diffuses into breast milk to achieve appreciable concentrations.

Oral absorption	>95%
Presystemic metabolism	nil
Plasma half life	
rapid acetylators	
range	1–5 h
mean	1.5 h
slow acetylators	
range	1–11 h
mean	5.5 h
Volume of distribution	0.61 l.kg^{-1}
Plasma protein binding	90%

Sulphadimidine undergoes extensive hepatic biotransformation to N^4-acetylsulphadimidine. This metabolic step exhibits genetic polymorphism, two phenotypes being evident: rapid acetylators, in whom only 1% of the dose is excreted unchanged; and slow acetylators, who excrete 13% of the dose as unchanged drug. In Europe and North America, only 40–45% of the population are rapid acetylators, but the 'dominant' phenotype (rapid) is much more common in Asians (80–90%) and in Eskimos (c. 100%).[12] The effects of hepatic disease upon metabolism have not been documented.

The renal clearance of sulphadimidine is dependent upon urinary pH, but this is of no clinical relevance, since the plasma half life is determined solely by the rate of metabolism.[13]

Investigations of the elimination of sulphadimidine in patients with renal disease have not always examined the effect of impaired renal function independently of acetylator phenotype and urinary pH. Impaired renal function reduces the excretion of N^4-acetylsulphadimidine to a much greater extent than that of unconjugated sulphadimidine, and accumulation of the latter seldom occurs.[14,15] Reduced renal clearance of drug and metabolite may compromise antibacterial effect in the treatment of urinary tract infection.[15]

Concentration–effect relationship

A therapeutic effect occurs when the concentration in blood exceeds the minimum inhibitory concentration (MIC) of the organism(s) responsible for the infection.

The MIC for *Chlamydia trachomatis* is about 0.1 mg.l^{-1} while for *Nocardia* it may need to be 100 mg.l^{-1}. The concentration of sulphadimidine needed in urine for the treatment of a urinary tract infection with *E. coli* varies between 4 and 64 mg.l^{-1} depending upon the strain.

Metabolism

Sulphadimidine is extensively metabolized in the liver by acetylation. More than 90% of the total dose is excreted in the urine as unchanged drug or metabolite. There is no evidence of enterohepatic circulation (see Fig. 1).

Sulphadimidine

Fig. 1 Metabolism of sulphadimidine

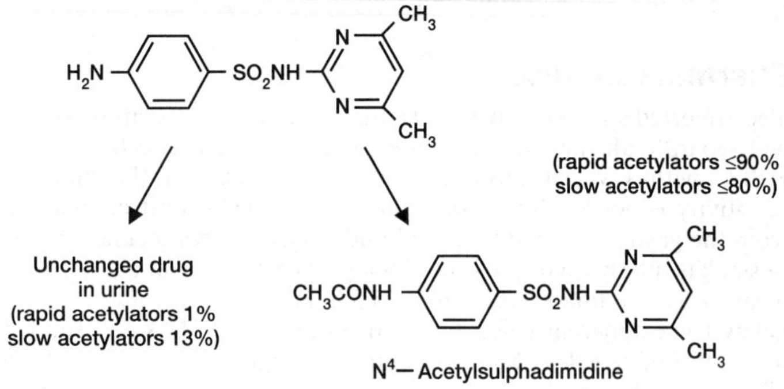

The metabolite is N^4-acetylsulphadimidine. It is less active, microbiologically, than the parent compound.

Pharmaceutics

Sulphadimidine is available in oral and parenteral forms:

1. Tablets containing 500 mg of sulphadimidine (BP) are available from Antigen (Eire). The tablets are white, biconvex and uncoated, and are scored on one side but otherwise unmarked. They should be protected from light and have a maximum shelf-life of 3 years.
2. Paediatric sulphadimidine mixture (BPC, 1973), containing sulphadimidine 500 mg in 5 ml, is available as a raspberry flavoured suspension.
3. Sulphadimidine injection (BP), containing a sterile aqueous solution of sulphadimidine sodium (1 g), is available for parenteral use in 3 ml ampoules.
4. Sulphamezathine injection (ICI, UK) contains sulphadimidine sodium 1 g in 3 ml ampoules.

Therapeutic use

Indications

1. Meningococcal meningitis
2. Urinary tract infection.

Contraindications

Previous hypersensitivity to sulphonamides.

Mode of use

For infections susceptible to treatment with sulphonamides, sulphadimidine is given by mouth in an initial dose of 3 g, followed by 1 g every 4 hours or 1.5 g every 6 hours. Urinary tract infection generally requires a lower initial dose (2 g) followed by 0.5–1 g every 6 or 8 hours. If oral administration is not possible, sulphadimidine may be given by deep intramuscular injection (which is painful), or intravenously, the dose being the same as the oral dose. Sulphadimidine should not be injected subcutaneously or intrathecally. Treatment is continued until the patient's condition has improved, or until an alternative antibacterial agent is substituted.

Indications

Although sulphadimidine has traditionally been part of the treatment of meningococcal meningitis, meningococcal resistance to sulphonamides has now become so prevalent that the use of sulphadimidine can no longer be recommended unless the causative organism is known to be sensitive. There is no evidence that combinations of penicillin, chloramphenicol and sulphonamides are any more effective than penicillin or chloramphenicol given alone. For the same reason, sulphadimidine is no longer the preferred drug for chemoprophylaxis in the prevention of meningococcal infection, unless the outbreak has undoubtedly been caused by a sulphonamide-sensitive organism. Only rifampicin or minocycline have proved consistently effective in eliminating meningococcal carriage.[16]

Adverse reactions[17,18]

Potentially life-threatening effects

Allergic reactions have been associated with sulphadimidine, as with all sulphonamides. In its most severe form, as the Stevens–Johnson syndrome, the reaction may rarely be life-threatening. No more useful indication of frequency can be given for an individual sulphonamide.

Acute overdosage

In cases of overdose, a greater proportion of the dose is excreted unchanged and the effect of urine pH upon renal clearance may be used to advantage. The urine should be rendered alkaline (target pH 7.5–8.5) by giving sodium bicarbonate 10 g by mouth every hour, or by a continuous intravenous infusion of molar sodium lactate (1.87%). Fluid intake should be sufficient to ensure a daily output of at least 1.5 litre.

Severe or irreversible adverse effects

Severe effects upon the skin (toxic epidermal necrolysis), eyes (iritis, retinal haemorrhage, optic neuropathy, extra-ocular muscle palsy), lungs (pulmonary eosinophilia), liver (acute hepatitis, cholestatic jaundice), pancreas (haemorrhagic/necrotizing pancreatitis), blood (haemolytic anaemia in G6PD-deficient subjects), blood-forming organs (agranulocytosis, aplastic anaemia, thrombocytopenia), and blood vessels (arteritis, acute vasculitis) can occasionally result from treatment with any sulphonamide.

Symptomatic adverse effects

Adverse effects, generally infrequent, include nausea, vomiting, cyanosis, fever, rashes (fixed drug eruption, urticaria, photosensitivity, purpura, erythema multiforme, erythema nodosum, bullous eruptions), leucopenia, crystalluria, haematuria and transient anuria. Sulphadimidine is one of the most soluble sulphonamides and is unlikely to cause crystalluria if fluid intake is maintained.

Interference with clinical pathology tests

None has been reported.

High risk groups

Neonates

Kernicterus may be precipitated by many sulphonamides, following the displacement of unconjugated bilirubin from plasma protein binding sites. Sulphadimidine should not be used in neonates.

Breast milk. Sulphonamides appear in breast milk in appreciable amounts and mothers taking the drug should not breast-feed their infants.

Children

Dosage should be reduced as follows: 6 months to 1 year — one-sixth of adult dose; 1 to 5 years — one-third of adult dose; 6 to 12 years — half of adult dose; 13 to 15 years — two-thirds of adult dose.

Pregnant women

Use in pregnancy should be avoided.

The elderly

No particular problems arise other than in connection with impaired renal function.

Concurrent disease

Renal failure. In severe renal failure the dose interval may be increased from 6 h to 12 h without loss of effect.[19] The drug should not be used to treat urinary tract infection in these circumstances.

Drug interactions

Potentially hazardous interactions

Sulphadimidine displaces sulphonylurea drugs from plasma protein binding sites, resulting in transient symptomatic hypoglycaemia.

Other significant reactions

The absorption of oral sulphadimidine is reduced by concurrent administration of antacids.

Potentially useful interactions

None is known.

Major outcome trials

So impressive were the results obtained by treating life-threatening pneumococcal[3,5] and meningococcal[7] infections with sulphonamides

Sulphadimidine

when these drugs first became available, compared with the previous lack of effective treatment, that controlled trials were unnecessary; open studies alone sufficed.

1. Brown P C C, Donaghy M C, Dootson P H, Titcombe D H M, McLaren D M 1971 Sulphadimidine and nalidixic acid therapy in urinary tract infections in general practice. Practitioner 207: 819–826

Sulphadimidine has been compared with nalidixic acid for the treatment of acute urinary tract infection. Urine culture in 354 patients in one general practice revealed bacterial infection in 177 (*E. coli* in 77%). Patients were randomized to treatment for 14 days with either sulphadimidine (1 g every 6 h after loading dose 2 g) or nalidixic acid (1 g every 6 h). After the course (completed by 93%), 16 of 86 in the sulphadimidine group (18.6%) and 5 of 85 in the nalidixic acid group (6.3%) still had infected urine, and this difference was statistically significant ($p<0.02$).

2. Ormonde N W H, Gray J A, Murdoch J McC et al 1969 Chronic bacteriuria due to Escherichia coli. I. Assessment of the value of combined short and long-term treatment with cycloserine, nitrofurantoin, and sulphadimidine. Journal of Infectious Diseases 120: 82–85

In patients with recurrent *E. coli* urinary tract infection, sulphadimidine has been compared with cycloserine and nitrofurantoin. 89 women with bacteriologically proven infection were randomized to treatment every 6 h for 10 days with either sulphadimidine (1 g), cycloserine (125 mg) or nitrofurantoin (100 mg). All three drugs eradicated infection to a similar extent in 80% of patients. Those with sterile urine then received one daily dose of the respective drug for 6 months, and urine samples were examined over a 12 month period. During the first 6 months, relapses were more common in those receiving sulphadimidine (23%) and cycloserine (16%) than in those receiving nitrofurantoin (5%), but the latter produced more unwanted effects. During the second 6 months, when no treatment was given, 36% of patients relapsed.

References

1. Woods D D 1940 The relation of p-aminobenzoic acid to the mechanism of the action of sulphanilamide. British Journal of Experimental Pathology 21: 74–90
2. Brown G M 1962 The biosynthesis of folic acid. II. Inhibition by sulfonamides. Journal of Biological Chemistry 237: 536–540
3. Pakenham-Walsh R 1943 Pneumococcal meningitis. Recovery with sulphamethazine. Lancet 1: 649–650
4. Burke J B 1956 Prophylactic sulphadimidine in children subject to recurrent infections of upper respiratory tract. British Medical Journal 1: 538–541
5. Macartney D W, Stewart-Smith G, Luxton R W, Ramsay W A, Goldman J 1942 Sulphamethazine: clinical trial of a new sulphonamide. Lancet 1: 639–641
6. Rose F L, Martin A R, Bevan H G L 1943 Sulphamethazine (2-4′-aminobenzenesulphonylamino-4:6-dimethylpyrimidine). A new heterocyclic derivative of sulphanilamide. Journal of Pharmacology and Experimental Therapeutics 77: 127–141
7. Jennings P A, Patterson W H 1942 Sulphamethazine: clinical trials in children. Lancet 2: 308–309
8. Thomas M H, Soroka K E, Simpson R M, Epstein R L 1981 Determination of sulfamethazine in swine tissue by quantitative thin-layer chromatography. Journal of Agricultural and Food Chemistry (Washington) 29: 621–624
9. Vree T B, O'Reilly W J, Hekster Y A, Damama J E, van der Kleijn E 1980 Determination of the acetylator phenotype and pharmacokinetics of some sulphonamides in man. Clinical Pharmacokinetics 5: 274–294
10. Avery G S (ed) 1980 Drug treatment, 2nd edn. ADIS Press, Sidney/Churchill-Livingstone, London, Appendix A
11. Reeves D S, Wilkinson P J 1979 The pharmacokinetics of trimethoprim and trimethoprim/sulphonamide combinations, including penetration into body tissues. Infection 7 (suppl 4): 330–341
12. Sjöqvist F, Borgä O, Orme M L'E 1980 Fundamentals of clinical pharmacology. In: Avery G S (ed) Drug treatment, 2nd edn. ADIS Press, Sidney, pp 1–61
13. Vree T B, Hekster Y A, Damsma J E, Tijhuis M, Friesen W T 1981 Pharmacokinetics and mechanism of renal excretion of short acting sulphonamides and N_4-acetylsulphonamide derivatives in man. Structural requirements of sulphonamides for active tubular secretion. European Journal of Clinical Pharmacology 20: 283–292
14. Williams D M, Wimpenny J, Asscher A W 1968 Renal clearance of sodium sulphadimidine in normal and uraemic subjects. Lancet 2: 1058–1060
15. Adam W R, Brown D J, Hales P, Dawborn J K 1973 The use of sulphadimidine (Sulphamezathine) in patients with renal failure. Medical Journal of Australia 1: 936–938
16. Greenwood B M 1987 Meningococcal infection. In: Weatherall D J, Ledingham J G G, Worrall D A (eds) Oxford Textbook of Medicine, 2nd edn. Oxford University Press, New York, pp 5: 199–208
17. Davies D M (ed) 1981 Textbook of adverse drug reactions 2nd edn. Oxford University Press, Oxford
18. Dukes M N G (ed) 1984 Meyler's side effects of drugs, 10th edn. Elsevier, Amsterdam–New York–Oxford
19. Sharpstone P 1977 Diseases of the urinary system. Prescribing for patients with renal failure. British Medical Journal 2: 36–37

S

Sulphamethoxazole

A lipid soluble antibacterial sulphonamide widely used in combination with trimethoprim.

Chemistry

Sulphamethoxazole (Sulfamethoxazole, Gantanol)
$C_{10}H_{11}N_3O_3S$
5-Methyl-3-sulphanilamido-isoxazole

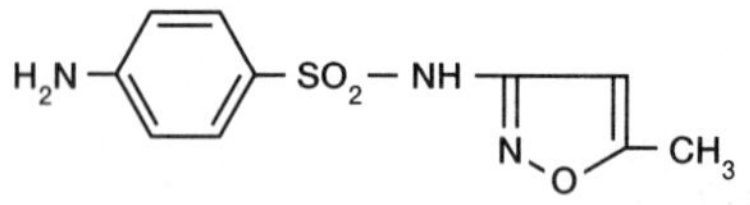

Molecular weight	253.3
pKa (sulphonamide group)	5.7
Solubility	
in alcohol	1 in 50
in water	1 in 3400
Octanol/water partition coefficient	—

Sulphamethoxazole is a white or yellowish-white, odourless or almost odourless, crystalline powder with a slight taste, and a bitter after-taste, prepared by chemical synthesis. Sulphamethoxazole is available in the UK and other countries in combination with trimethoprim as co-trimoxazole (Septrin, Bactrim).

Pharmacology

Sulphamethoxazole competes with para-aminobenzoic acid, to which it is structurally related, for the active site on dihydropteroate synthetase, a bacterial enzyme involved in the synthesis of folic acid. It also exerts a minor action on the enzyme dihydrofolate reductase, which is inhibited by trimethoprim. Sulphamethoxazole does not affect mammalian cells since these cells require intact folic acid and cannot synthesize it.

Toxicology

Prolonged administration of sulphamethoxazole in animals produces bone marrow hypoplasia, fatty liver, and changes in the thyroid and pituitary glands, the latter only in the rat.[1]

Teratogenicity attributed to sulphamethoxazole or co-trimoxazole has not been reported to date in humans, but the drugs are not used often during pregnancy. In rats, sulphamethoxazole at a dose of 600 $mg.kg^{-1}$ on days 8 to 16 of pregnancy caused cleft palate.[1] Maintenance of folate levels prevents the fetal defects caused by large doses of the drug.[1]

Clinical pharmacology

Sulphamethoxazole is active in vitro against a wide range of micro-organisms, both Gram-positive and Gram-negative. It is active against *Streptococcus pyogenes*, *Strep. pneumoniae*, *Escherichia coli*, *Strep. viridans*, *Neisseria meningitidis* and *Corynebacterium diphtheriae*. Some strains of *Bacillus anthracis*, *Haemophilus influenzae*, *Klebsiella* spp. and *Proteus* spp. are also sensitive to sulphamethoxazole. High concentrations (64 $mg.l^{-1}$) are often needed to be effective against *Brucella* spp. and *Nocardia*. The drug is usually inactive against *Providencia* spp., *Pseudomonas aeruginosa*, *Mycoplasmas*, *Leptospirae* and *Rickettsiae*. *Chlamydia trachomatis* is usually sensitive to low concentrations of sulphamethoxazole (0.1–0.5 $mg.l^{-1}$). The resistance of Gram-negative bacteria to sulphamethoxazole is commonly mediated by R-plasmids.

Pharmacokinetics

The preferred analytical method for sulphamethoxazole is high performance liquid chromatography.[2,3] The limits for detection of sulphamethoxazole were 0.5 $mg.l^{-1}$ and 1.0 $mg.l^{-1}$. The advantage of this method is that the drug is measured specifically and selectively.[2] Other analytical methods include estimation of the free aromatic amino group by absorption spectrophotometry[4] and fluorospectrometry.[5]

When administered alone or in combination with trimethoprim in cotrimoxazole, sulphamethoxazole exhibits first-order kinetics. Sulphamethoxazole is classed as a medium-acting sulphonamide, based on absorption and excretion patterns. The drug is almost 100% absorbed following oral administration;[6] peak plasma concentrations are achieved within 4 hours after a single dose and the levels are generally sustained at 8 hours.[7] The proportion of free, non-acetylated sulphamethoxazole is almost 100% of the total drug in the first hours, falling to 75 to 85% 8 hours after administration.[7] The mean plasma half life is 8.6 hours with a range of 7 to 12 hours.

Sulphamethoxazole and its acetylated derivatives are excreted by the kidneys, both by glomerular filtration and by tubular secretion, with urinary recovery within 24 hours of 25 to 50% of the dose, nearly two-thirds of which is unconjugated.[7] Within 72 hours, 85% of the dose is excreted non-acetylated. Some of the drug secreted by the tubules is reabsorbed.[8]

The pH and flow-rate of the urine influence the renal clearance of sulphamethoxazole.[8,9,10] Alkalinization above pH 7 increases the urinary recovery of non-acetylated drug, whereas acid loading has no effect.[9] Up to 25% of the dose is excreted unchanged, but this can increase to 40% when the urine is alkaline.

The volume of distribution[11] is 0.21 ± 0.02 $l.kg^{-1}$ and the drug, being lipid-soluble, is widely distributed throughout the body, particularly to extracellular fluids.[12] Sulphamethoxazole exhibits plasma protein binding of 65% but the binding of non-acetylated drug is consistently decreased in uraemic patients.[9]

Studies of the pharmacokinetics of sulphamethoxazole in patients with impaired renal function (creatinine clearance less than 30 $ml.min^{-1}$) have shown a prolonged serum half life and reduced quantitative urinary recovery.[9,13,14] Altered dose regimes according to glomerular filtration rate have been proposed.[15,16,17] The drug is readily removed by haemodialysis at rates similar to those observed in patients with normal kidneys,[9,16] but its use should be avoided in patients with severe renal failure.[17]

Oral absorption	100%
Presystemic metabolism	—
Plasma half life	
range	7–12 h
mean	8.6 h
Volume of distribution	0.21 ± 0.02 $l.kg^{-1}$
Plasma protein binding	65%

Concentration–effect relationship

Therapeutic success is achieved when the concentration of sulphamethoxazole exceeds the minimum bactericidal (inhibitory) concentration (MIC) of the drug for the infecting organism. A typical isolate of *E. coli* will have an MIC for sulphamethoxazole of 3 $mg.l^{-1}$.

Metabolism

Hepatic biotransformation of sulphamethoxazole produces inactive acetylated and conjugated derivatives. The rate of acetylation varies between individuals, with 'fast' and 'slow' acetylators. About 20% of all renal excretion of sulphamethoxazole occurs in the unaltered form[18] with the major urinary metabolite being N_4-acetylsulphamethoxazole (60 to 65% of the urinary product).[18] This metabolite has a much shorter half life (2 to 3.5 hours) than the parent drug.[19] The ring-N-glucuronide and the N_1-glucuronide account for about 15% of total urinary excretion.[18] Other minor metabolites include the 5-hydroxylated drug and further glucuronides (Fig. 1). All these derivatives are considered to be bacteriostatically inactive.

Pharmaceutics

Sulphamethoxazole is available only in the oral form, but this is no longer marketed in the UK. Gantanol (Roche, US) tablets contain 500 mg or 1 g sulphamethoxazole USP. The 500 mg tablet is a round, flat, bevelled, pale green, scored tablet, whilst the 1 g size is an orange, scored capsule-shaped tablet. They are imprinted 'GANTANOL' and 'GANTANOL DS' respectively together with the imprint 'ROCHE'. The drug is also available as an oral suspension containing 100 mg sulphamethoxazole USP in each millilitre. The suspension contains a carboxyvinyl polymer as suspending agent and should be stored in an airtight container and both preparations should be protected from light. The suspension is cherry flavoured with sodium benzoate as preservative.

The drug is available in fixed-dose combination with phenazopyridine hydrochloride, Azo Gantanol (Roche, US) as a urinary antiseptic and analgesic, and combined with trimethoprim in co-trimoxazole.

Therapeutic use

Indications

1. Treatment of infections caused by sulphamethoxazole-sensitive organisms, usually in the urinary tract
2. Treatment of lymphogranuloma venereum.

Sulphamethoxazole is active in vitro against a wide range of organisms, both Gram-positive and Gram-negative. It is not active against *Enterococcus faecalis*, *Providencia* spp., most strains of *Pseudomonas aeruginosa*, *Mycoplasmas*, *Treponemata*, *Leptospirae*, *Rickettsiae*, some non-tuberculous mycobacteria and *Chlamydia psittaci*. However, the types of *C. trachomatis* causing lymphogranuloma venereum are susceptible. The resistance of Gram-negative bacteria to sulphamethoxazole is commonly mediated by R-plasmids.

Contraindications

1. Hypersensitivity to sulphamethoxazole or other sulphonamides
2. Severe renal insufficiency (creatinine clearance less than 15 ml.min^{-1}) when repeated estimations of the plasma concentration of sulphamethoxazole cannot be made
3. Patients with severe liver parenchymal damage.

Mode of use

Sulphamethoxazole should not be used to treat infections caused by bacteria which are resistant to the drug. The dose of the antibiotic varies according to the therapeutic indication, age and renal function of the recipient.

The usual dose is 2 g initially, followed by 1 g twice daily. A total daily dose of 3 g should not be exceeded. A suggested dose for children is 50 to 60 mg.kg^{-1} body weight initially, followed by 25 to 30 mg.kg^{-1} twice daily (a maximum daily paediatric dose of 75 mg.kg^{-1} should not be exceeded). Regimes for adjustment of dose in renal failure have been suggested.[15,16,17]

Indications

1. Urinary tract infection

Sulphamethoxazole has been shown to be effective in the treatment of urinary tract infections at a dose of 50 mg.kg^{-1} body weight per day for 10 days.[20] Reports suggest a similar effect with sulphamethoxazole alone or co-trimoxazole in the therapy of urinary tract infection in children[20] and adults.[21]

2. Lymphogranuloma venereum

Sulphamethoxazole 1 g orally twice a day for at least 2 weeks has been recommended as an alternative treatment to doxycycline.[22]

Adverse reactions

Potentially life-threatening effects

The most serious form of hypersensitivity reaction to sulphonamides is the Stevens–Johnson syndrome, consisting of erythema multiforme and ulceration of the mucous membranes of the oropharynx, eyes and urethra. The severity of the disease varies, but it may be fatal. Cases of the Stevens–Johnson syndrome have been reported in elderly people during co-trimoxazole therapy, as have fatal cases of toxic epidermal necrolysis (Lyell's syndrome).[23] The skin reactions have been attributed to the sulphamethoxazole component.[24]

Acute overdosage

Symptoms of acute overdose are likely to be nausea, vomiting, abdominal pain, dizziness and confusion. Gastric lavage should be performed within 2 hours of ingestion. Overdose of sulphamethoxa-

Fig. 1 Metabolism of sulphamethoxazole

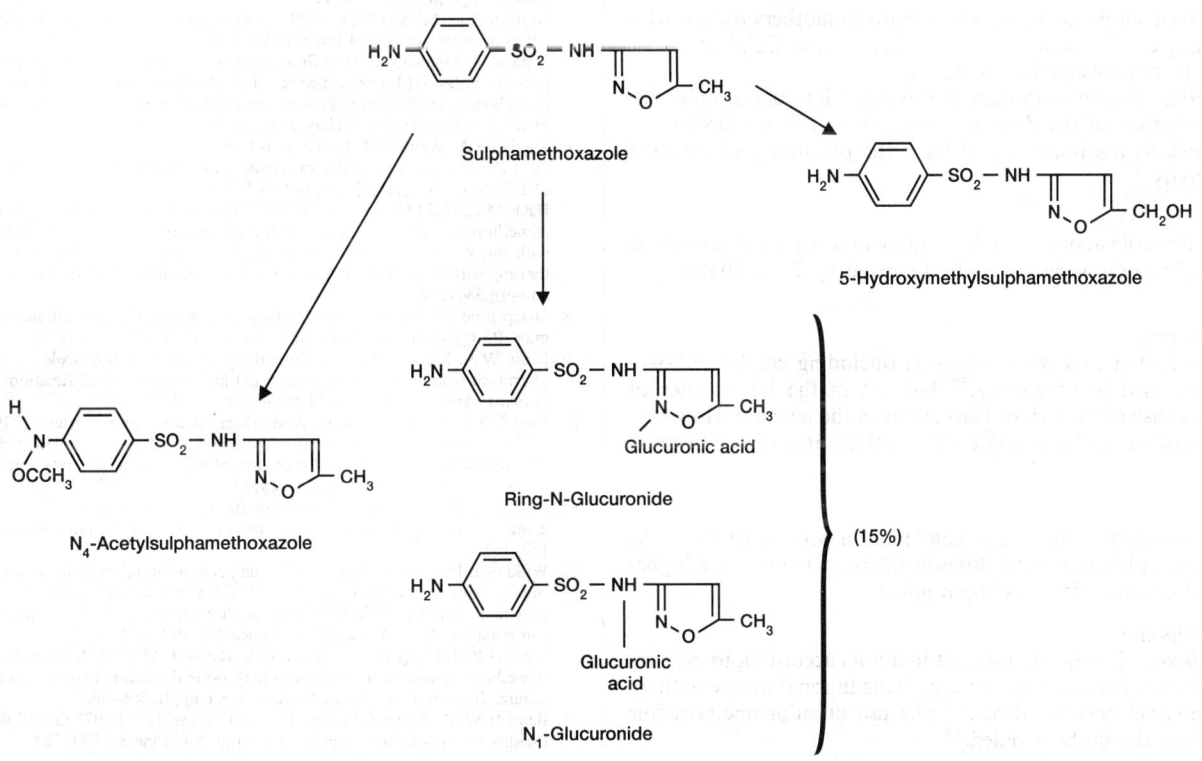

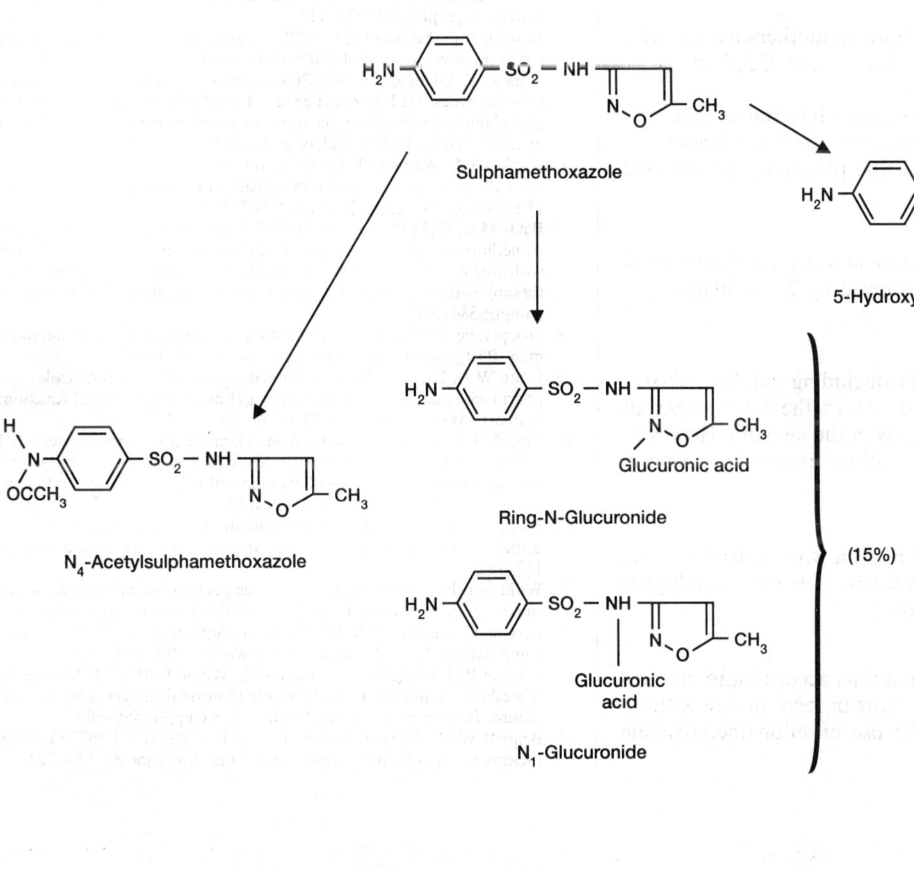

zole may be specifically treated by an increase in fluid intake and by alkalinization of the urine to above pH 7, which elevates urinary recovery of the drug and lowers serum levels.

Severe or irreversible adverse effects

Renal failure with crystalluria. In the presence of hypoalbuminaemia, therapy with sulphamethoxazole, in co-trimoxazole, has been associated with renal failure in patients with septicaemia.[25] In two cases described, most of the sulphamethoxazole was in the free form in the plasma and not protein bound. It is assumed that crystalluria was secondary to the increased load of free drug filtered by the kidneys.

Hepatic damage. Following sulphamethoxazole treatment, reversible hepatocellular jaundice has been reported in association with raised serum transaminases and cell necrosis on liver biopsy.[26,27,28] Subsequent challenge with sulphonamide reproduced the liver damage.

Symptomatic adverse effects

Rashes are a fairly frequent adverse effect of sulphamethoxazole therapy[29,30] and may be associated with a 'serum-sickness-like' syndrome with fever and headache.[31] Adverse effects occur frequently with the use of high-dose co-trimoxazole in AIDS patients and it has been suggested that high serum levels of sulphamethoxazole may be partially responsible.[32] Sulphamethoxazole has also been associated with gastrointestinal disturbance, including nausea, vomiting and abdominal pain.[30]

Haematological disturbances have been described during sulphamethoxazole therapy with reports of reversible agranulocytosis, suggesting an immunological reaction caused by the drug.[33] Other reported effects include aggravation of haemolysis in some Chinese people with glucose-6-phosphate dehydrogenase deficiency,[34] eosinophilia, haemolytic anaemia, thrombocytopenia and hypoprothrombinaemia.[30]

Individual case reports have also linked sulphamethoxazole with the syndrome of benign intracranial hypertension[35] and, in a patient with renal failure, to hypoglycaemia related to hypoinsulinaemia, probably induced by the drug.[36]

Interference with clinical pathology tests

In high quantities, sulphamethoxazole interferes with the measurement of serum theophylline levels by high performance liquid chromatography.[37]

High risk groups

Neonates

Neonates given sulphamethoxazole, or born to mothers treated with the drug, may develop jaundice or even kernicterus. Sulphonamides should not be administered to neonates.

Breast milk. Sulphamethoxazole is excreted into breast milk, but the administration of the drug to a lactating woman represents a negligible risk to the infant, apart from the possibility of inducing hypersensitivity.

Children

Sulphamethoxazole may be used in children at a suggested dose of 50 to 60 $mg.kg^{-1}$ body weight initially, followed by 25 to 30 $mg.kg^{-1}$ twice daily.

Pregnant women

It is now accepted that co-trimoxazole (including sulphamethoxazole) can be used in pregnancy,[38] but not in the later stages of gestation because of the risk of kernicterus in the neonate. However, manufacturers' prescribing advice still cautions against use in pregnancy.

The elderly

Sulphamethoxazole, alone and in combination with co-trimoxazole, has been used widely in normal doses in elderly patients, but a higher incidence of adverse effects has been noted.

Concurrent disease

Renal failure. Dosage adjustment in adults according to creatinine clearance has been suggested for patients in renal failure with an increased interval between doses.[17] The use of sulphamethoxazole during dialysis should be avoided.[17]

Hepatic disease. Sulphamethoxazole has been associated with hepatocellular necrosis[26,27,28] and should not be used in patients showing marked liver parenchymal damage.

Drug interactions

Potentially hazardous interactions

Warfarin. Studies[39,40] have shown that sulphamethoxazole, in co-trimoxazole, interacts with the anticoagulant warfarin and potentiates the hypoprothrombinaemic effect. Although often cited as an example of displacement from protein binding, inhibition of warfarin metabolism is a more probable explanation.[41]

Phenytoin. In patients receiving co-trimoxazole, the plasma half life of phenytoin has been shown to be increased.[42] This effect has not been reported with sulphamethoxazole alone, but has been demonstrated with other sulphonamides.[42]

Potentially useful interactions

Combination of sulphamethoxazole with trimethoprim in co-trimoxazole provides a therapeutically useful potentiation of antibacterial effect.

Major outcome trials

The availability of trimethoprim and co-trimoxazole has prompted a decline in the use of sulphamethoxazole as a single agent, and it is no longer available as such in the UK. Therefore, results of recent clinical trials with sulphamethoxazole alone are lacking and the reader is referred to the monograph on co-trimoxazole.

General review articles

Koch-Weser J, Rubin R H, Swartz M N 1980 Drug therapy: trimethoprim-sulphamethoxazole. New England Journal of Medicine 303: 426–432

Kucers A, Bennett N McK 1987 The use of antibiotics: a comprehensive review with clinical emphasis, 4th edn. William Heinemann, London, pp 1075–1117

References

1. Udall V 1969 Toxicology of sulphonamide–trimethoprim combinations. Postgraduate Medical Journal (suppl) 45: 42–45
2. Vree T B, Hekster Y A, Baars A M, Damsma J E, van der Kleijn E 1978 Determinations of trimethoprim and sulphamethoxazole (co-trimoxazole) in body fluids of man by means of high-performance liquid chromatography. Journal of Chromatography 146: 103–112
3. Bury R W, Mashford M L 1979 Analysis of trimethoprim and sulphamethoxazole in human plasma by high pressure liquid chromatography. Journal of Chromatography 163: 114–117
4. Bratton A C, Marshall E K 1939 A new coupling component for sulphanilamide determination. Journal of Biological Chemistry 128: 537
5. Amano T, Mizukami S 1965 Studies on the determination methods with polyaldehydes. III Fluorescence reaction of primary aromatic amines with phthalaldehyde and its application for the determination of sulfonamides. Journal of the Pharmacological Society of Japan 85: 1035–1041
6. Kaplan S A, Weinfeld R E, Abruzzo C W, McFaden K, Jack M L, Weissman L 1973 Pharmacokinetic profile of trimethoprim–sulphamethoxazole in man. Journal of Infectious Diseases 128 (suppl): 547–555
7. Bach M C, Gold O, Finland M 1973 Absorption and urinary excretion of trimethoprim, sulphamethoxazole and trimethoprim–sulphamethoxazole: results with single doses in normal young adults and preliminary observations during therapy with trimethoprim–sulphamethoxazole. Journal of Infectious Diseases 128 (suppl): 584–598
8. Sharpstone P 1969 The renal handling of trimethoprim and sulphamethoxazole in man. Postgraduate Medical Journal (suppl) 45: 38–42
9. Craig W A, Kunin C M 1973 Trimethoprim–sulphamethoxazole pharmacodynamic effects of urinary pH and impaired renal function: studies in humans. Annals of Internal Medicine 78: 491–497
10. Vree T B, Hekster Y A, Baars A M, Damsma J E, van der Kleijn E 1978 Pharmacokinetics of sulphamethoxazole in man: effects of urinary pH and urine flow on metabolism and renal excretion of sulphamethoxazole and its metabolite N_4-acetylsulphamethoxazole. Clinical Pharmacokinetics 3: 319–329
11. Morgan D J, Raymond K 1980 Evaluations of slow infusions of cotrimoxazole by using predictive pharmacokinetics. Antimicrobial Agents and Chemotherapy 17: 132–137
12. Wilkinson P J, Reeves D S 1979 Tissue penetration of trimethoprim and sulphonamides. Journal of Antimicrobial Chemotherapy 5 (suppl B): 159–167
13. Bergan T, Brodwall E K 1972 Human pharmacokinetics of a sulphamethoxazole combination. Acta Medica Scandinavica 192: 483–492
14. Welling P G, Craig W A, Amidon G L, Kunin C M 1973 Pharmacokinetics of trimethoprim and sulphamethoxazole in normal subjects and in patients with renal failure. Journal of Infectious Diseases 128 (suppl): 556–566
15. Bennett W M, Singer I, Golper T, Feig P, Coggins C J 1977 Guidelines for drug therapy in renal failure. Annals of Internal Medicine 86: 754–783

16. Bennett W M, Muther R S, Parker R A et al 1980 Drug therapy in renal failure: dosing and guidelines for adults. Part 1: Antimicrobial agents, analgesics. Annals of Internal Medicine 93: 62–89
17. Appel G B, Neu H C 1977 The nephrotoxicity of antimicrobial agents (first of three parts). New England Journal of Medicine 296: 663–670
18. Rieder J 1973 Metabolism and techniques for assay of trimethoprim and sulphamethoxazole. Journal of Infectious Diseases 128 (suppl): 567–573
19. Vree T B, Hekster Y A, Damsma J E, van der Kleijn E, O'Reilly W J 1979 Pharmacokinetics of N_1-acetyl- and N_4-acetyl sulphamethoxazole in man. Clinical Pharmacokinetics 4: 310–319
20. Howard J B, Howard J E 1978 Trimethoprim–sulphamethoxazole vs sulphamethoxazole for acute urinary tract infections in children. American Journal of Diseases in Childhood 132: 1085–1087
21. Bergan T, Skjerven O 1979 Comparison of sulphamethoxazole alone and combined with trimethoprim in urinary tract infections. Infection 7: 14–16
22. Centres for Disease Control 1985 1985 STD treatment guidelines. Morbidity and Mortality Weekly Review suppl 34/4S
23. Frisch J M 1973 Clinical experience with adverse reactions to trimethoprim–sulphamethoxazole. Journal of Infectious Diseases 128 (suppl): 607–611
24. Reusser P 1977 Side effects of co-trimoxazole. In: Viswanathan R, Jaggi O P (eds) Advances in chronic obstructive lung disease, Proceedings of the World Congress on Asthma, Bronchitis and Conditions Allied. The Asthma and Bronchitis Foundation, University of Delhi, pp 579–589
25. Buchanan N 1978 Sulphamethoxazole, hypoalbuminaemia, crystalluria, and renal failure. British Medical Journal 2: 172
26. Fries J, Siraganian R 1966 Sulfonamide hepatitis: report of a case due to sulfamethoxazole and sulfisoxazole. New England Journal of Medicine 274: 95–97
27. Macoul K L 1966 Brief recording: hepatitis attributed to sulfamethoxazole. New England Journal of Medicine 275: 39
28. Dujovne C A, Chan C H, Zimmerman H G 1967 Sulfonamide hepatic injury: review of the literature and report of a case due to sulfamethoxazole. New England Journal of Medicine 277: 785–788
29. Burton J P 1962 Rash with Gantanol. New England Journal of Medicine 266: 951
30. Koch-Weiser J, Sidel V W, Dexter M, Parish C, Finer D C, Kanarek P 1971 Adverse reactions to sulfisoxazole, sulfamethoxazole, and nitrofurantoin. Archives of Internal Medicine 128: 399–404
31. Clark A J L, Mouchizadeh J, Faunch R, McMichael H B 1980 Trimethoprim alone. Lancet 1: 1030
32. Bowden F J, Harman P J, Lucas C R 1986 Serum trimethoprim and sulphamethoxazole levels in AIDS. Lancet 1: 853
33. Palva I P, Koivisto O 1971 Agranulocytosis associated with trimethoprim–sulphamethoxazole. British Medical Journal 4: 301
34. Chan T K, Todd D, Tso S C 1976 Drug-induced haemolysis in glucose-6-phosphate dehydrogenase deficiency. British Medical Journal 2: 1227–1229
35. Ch'ien L T 1970 Intracranial hypertension and sulfamethoxazole. New England Journal of Medicine 283: 47
36. Arem R, Garber A J, Field J B 1983 Sulfonamide-induced hypoglycaemia in chronic renal failure. Archives of Internal Medicine 143: 827–829
37. McKenzie S A, Baillie E, Godfrey S 1978 Effect of practical timing of dosage on theophylline blood levels in asthmatic children treated with choline theophyllinate. Archives of Disease in Childhood 53: 167–168
38. Leading article 1983 Pyrimethamine combinations in pregnancy. Lancet 2: 1005–1007
39. Hassall C, Feetam C L, Leach R H, Meynell M J 1975 Potentiation of warfarin by co-trimoxazole. Lancet 2: 1155–1156
40. Tilstone W J, Gray J M B, Nimmo-Smith R H, Lawson D H 1977 Interaction between warfarin and sulphamethoxazole. Postgraduate Medical Journal 53: 388–390
41. O'Reilly R A, Motley C H 1979 Racemic warfarin and trimethoprim–sulfamethoxazole interaction in humans. Annals of Internal Medicine 91: 34–36
42. Hansen J M, Siersbaek-Nielsen K, Skovsted L, Kampmann J P, Lumholtz B 1975 Potentiation of warfarin by cotrimoxazole. British Medical Journal 2: 684

Sulphasalazine

Sulphasalazine is a first-choice drug in the long-term suppression of inflammation of inflammatory bowel disease. In some countries sulphasalazine is registered for the treatment of rheumatoid arthritis in patients who do not respond to non-steroidal anti-inflammatory agents.

Chemistry

Sulphasalazine (Sulfasalazine, salicylazosulphapyridine, Salazopyrin, Azulfidine, Azulfidina)
$C_{18}H_{14}N_4O_5S$
2-Hydroxy-4′-(2-pyridylsulphamoyl)azobenzene-3-carboxylic acid

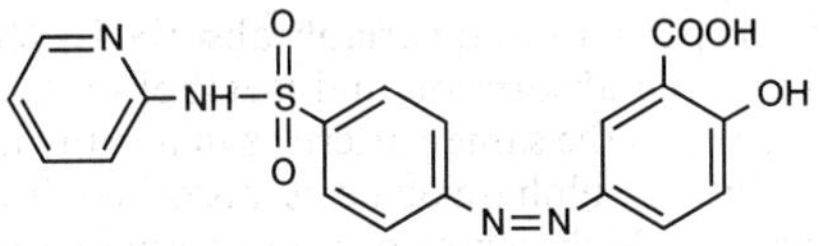

Molecular weight	398.39
pKa	2.4, 8.3 11.0
Solubility	
in alcohol	1 in 2900
in water	insoluble
Octanol/water partition coefficient	0.75

Sulphasalazine is a bright yellow to light brownish yellow, odourless, fine powder. It is prepared by chemical synthesis.

Pharmacology

Sulphasalazine is a drug that has anti-inflammatory, immunosuppressive and antibiotic actions. After oral administration about 80% of the drug passes into the colon where it is split by gut bacteria into its two component parts, sulphapyridine and 5-aminosalicylic acid. Most of the pharmacological effects of sulphasalazine are due to the two breakdown products rather than to sulphasalazine itself. Sulphapyridine is a sulphonamide antibiotic that kills bacteria by acting as a competitive antagonist for para-aminobenzoic acid (PABA), so that PABA is not incorporated into dihydropteroic acid. 5-aminosalicylic acid is an anti-inflammatory agent that, like aspirin, inhibits cyclo-oxygenase and so prevents the synthesis of prostaglandins. In vitro both sulphasalazine and sulphapyridine inhibit the natural killer-cell activity of peripheral mononuclear cells and also inhibit lymphocyte transformation. In animal models of rheumatoid arthritis sulphasalazine suppresses specific antibody production in the intestine and thus has effects on both the humoral and cellular components of the immune response.

Toxicology

Toxicological testing in animals has failed to demonstrate any results of potential clinical relevance, with the exception of a drug-induced and dose-related thyroid hyperplasia of a reversible type in the rat. There was a very modest hyperplasia of the thyroid gland at a dosage of 250 and 500 $mg.kg^{-1}$ body weight per day over six months in the dog. There was a slight influence on testicular epithelium at a dose level of 500 $mg.kg^{-1}$. No teratogenic abnormalities were found at 200 and 500 $mg.kg^{-1}$ body weight, whilst at 800 $mg.kg^{-1}$ body weight, abnormalities were found, reflecting general toxicity. No teratological abnormalities were found in the rabbit.

Sulphasalazine does not have mutagenic potential. No long-term carcinogenic tests have been performed in animals.

Clinical pharmacology

Sulphasalazine has been used for many years in the treatment of ulcerative colitis.[1] It was initially thought that the antibiotic effect of sulphapyridine was all important. Sulphapyridine is active against certain Gram-negative and Gram-positive organisms. It is also active against *Nocardia*, *Chlamydia* and some protozoa. However, recent evidence suggests that the anti-inflammatory actions of 5-aminosalicylic acid are at least as important as those of sulphapyridine. In contrast, in the treatment of rheumatoid arthritis,[2] it is sulphapyridine that possesses the antirheumatic activity and not 5-aminosalicyclic acid. In human studies sulphasalazine and sulphapyridine have been shown to reduce the number of activated monocytes and B-lymphocytes and to increase T-lymphocyte numbers.

Pharmacokinetics

The preferred analytical method for the drug and its metabolites is HPLC[3–5] which has a sensitivity of 500 $mg.l^{-1}$ using UV detection and fluorescence detection. The determination of sulphapyridine and N-acetylsulphapyridine is best done by the Owerbach's method.[4] The preferred method for the 5-amino-2-hydroxybenzoic acid and 5-acetylamino-2-hydroxy benzoic acid is the Hansen's method.[5]

Sulphasalazine is partially and variably absorbed after oral administration. The intestinal absorption and metabolism in patients with ulcerative colitis follows the same pattern as in healthy individuals.[6,7] 20–30% of the intact sulphasalazine is absorbed from the small intestine.[6,7] There is a high degree of protein binding of sulphasalazine (95%–99%).[8] It has a high affinity for connective tissue. High concentrations are found in peritoneal, pleural and synovial fluids.[9] The remainder of the sulphasalazine passes to the colon where it is split into its components by bacterial action (Fig. 1).[10]

Fig. 1 Metabolism of sulphasalazine by gut bacteria

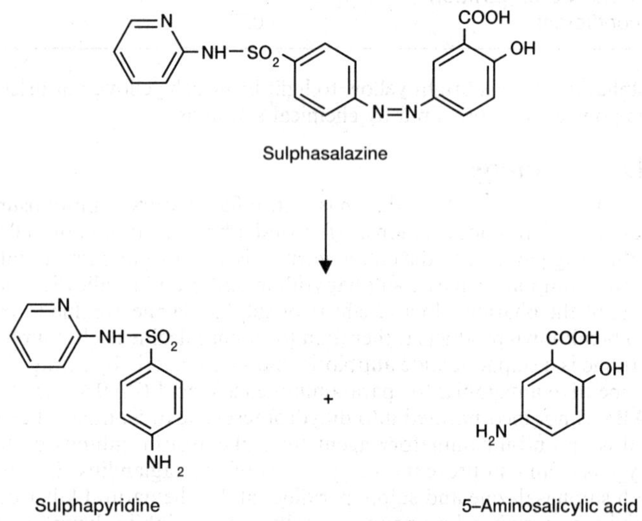

The two metabolites formed are sulphapyridine (SP) and 5-aminosalicylic acid (5-ASA). The possibility exists that the latter is acetylated to some extent presystemically in the intestinal wall.[11,12] No important differences in the disposition of sulphasalazine have been found, comparing patients with inflammatory bowel disease and control.[7]

Sulphasalazine plasma concentrations reach a peak within 3 to 5 hours after ingestion. Only 1–13% of the drug can be recovered in the urine during its first introduction and also during long therapy. There is some evidence that sulphasalazine is excreted in the bile.[13] Sulphapyridine and its metabolites are demonstrable in the serum 4 to 6 hours after the ingestion of the first dose of sulphasalazine.[7] As sulphapyridine itself is more or less completely absorbed from the small intestine,[14] this delay can be accounted for by the time taken for bacterial azo splitting of the drug in the colon and subsequent absorption of split products.[7] This finding is further confirmed by studies showing a failure to split sulphasalazine in patients with ileostomy.[15]

The products of bacterial hydrolysis, sulphapyridine and 5-aminosalicylic acid, are absorbed from the colon. Sulphapyridine is distributed throughout the whole body,[16] and undergoes acetylation in the liver, sharing the acetylation polymorphism of other such compounds.[17,18] The major routes of elimination of sulphapyridine from the body are shown in Fig. 2.

The majority of the 5-aminosalicylic acid (80%) is excreted in the stool,[9] although there is acetylation of 5-aminosalicylic acid in the colonic wall and in the liver.[11,12] The small proportion of 5-amino salicylic acid which is excreted in urine, is excreted as acetyl 5-ASA.[6] The overall metabolism is outlined in Fig. 3.

Although sulphasalazine is distributed throughout the body, autoradiographic studies have not demonstrated entry into the brain,[16] and only negligible amounts are excreted in breast milk. Sulphapyridine concentrations in breast milk are approximately 40% of serum concentrations. It is unlikely that there is excretion of 5-aminosalicylic acid into breast milk because of low serum concentrations.[19]

Oral absorption	20–30%
Presystemic metabolism	70–80%
Plasma half life	
range	3–11 h
mean	6 h
Plasma half life (sulphapyridine)	
range	6–17 h
mean	10 h
Plasma half life (acetyl-5-aminosalicyclic acid)	
range	4–10 h
mean	7 h
Volume of distribution	—
Plasma protein binding	95–99%

Concentration–effect relationship

No defined range of plasma concentration has been related to a therapeutic effect. A total serum sulphapyridine concentration of 20–50 $mg.l^{-1}$ appears to coincide with clinical improvement. No such therapeutic–concentration relationship could be shown with serum concentrations of sulphasalazine, individual sulphapyridine metabolites or 5-aminosalicylic acid. It may well be that the serum total sulphapyridine reflects the generation of 5-aminosalicylic acid in the colon and this latter is the effective agent in certain areas.[7] Limited reports of dose–response relationships have been documented.[20–22]

Metabolism

After the compound has been split into sulphapyridine and 5-aminosalicylic acid as described in Pharmacokinetics, these compounds are further metabolized. Sulphapyridine is subject to polymorphic acetylation in the liver, the proportions of free sulphapyridine and acetylsulphapyridine in the serum being dependent upon the acetylator phenotype of the subject.[18]

Sulphapyridine is also subjected to hydroxylation followed by conjugation to glucuronic acid and N-4 acetylation. 50% of the total recovery of sulphapyridine in the urine is in the form of the glucuronides, either sulphapyridine glucuronide or acetylsulphapyridine glucuronide (Fig. 3).

5-aminosalicylic acid appears to be substantially excreted in the stool with only a small proportion being excreted in urine. The 5-aminosalicylic acid excreted in the urine is more than 90% in the form of the acetylated aminosalicylic acid.[6,7]

Pharmaceutics

Sulphasalazine is available as Salazopyrin (Pharmacia, UK) Azasulfidine (Pharmacia, USA).

1. Salazopyrin tablets: orange, round, convex tablets containing 0.5 g of sulphasalazine

Sulphasalazine

2. Enteric-coated tablets: orange, eliptical, convex, film-coated tablets containing 0.5 g of sulphasalazine. In the USA this preparation is Azasulfidine EN and is debossed '102' with the Pharmacia logo
3. Salazopyrin suspension: orange-lemon flavoured yellow suspension containing 250 mg per 5 ml of sulphasalazine
4. Salazopyrin suppositories: yellow suppositories containing 0.5 g sulphasalazine. Unavailable in the USA
5. Salazopyrin enema: a yellow water suspension containing 3% sulphasalazine with particle size of the order of 10 μm. The density (20°C) is about 1.01 $g.ml^{-1}$. The enema is supplied in a transparent, plastic bottle equipped with a nozzle set and a one-way valve. The suspension settles quickly but is easily re-suspended. Unavailable in the USA

Preservatives which may cause allergy include methyl and propyl

Fig. 2 Metabolism of sulphapyridine

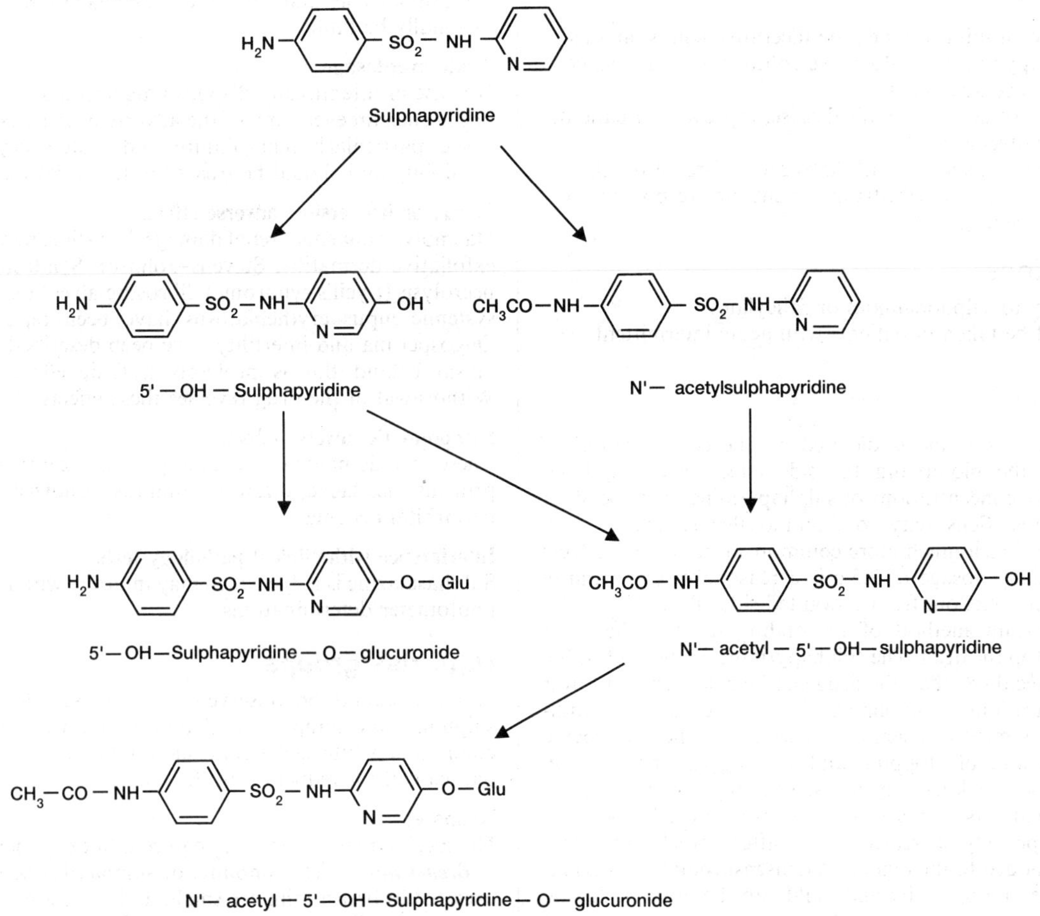

Fig. 3 The overall metabolic route of sulphasalazine

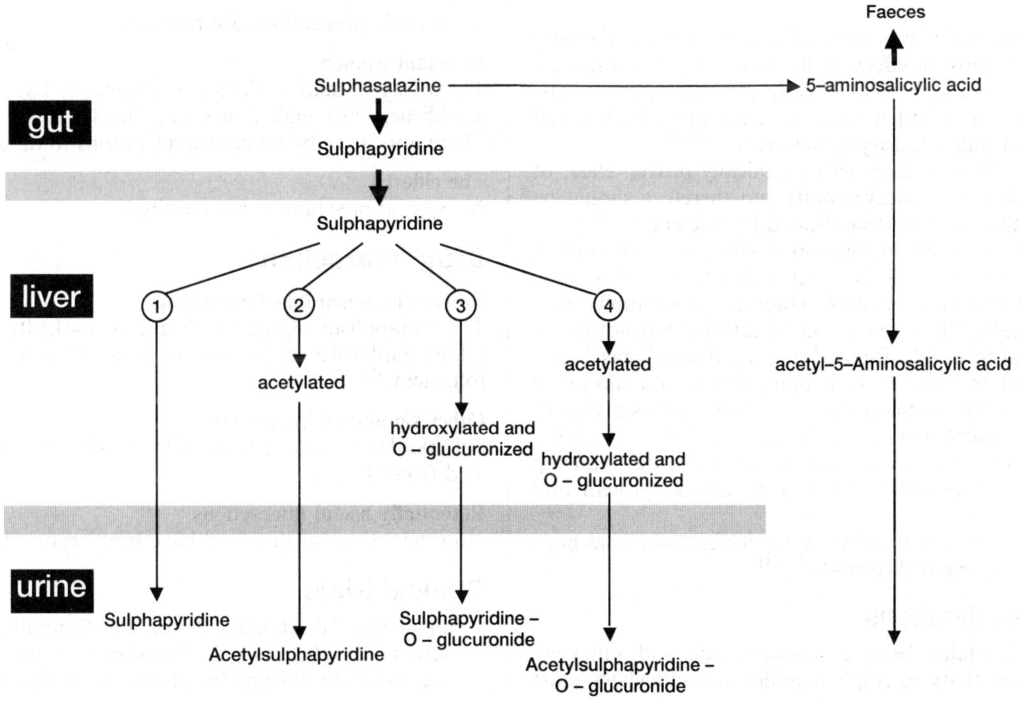

hydroxy benzoate in the enema preparation and sodium benzoate in the suspension.

Salazopyrin tablets should be stored at room temperature. The suppositories should be stored in a cool place (8–15°C). The enema should be stored at a temperature not exceeding 30°C and the suspension at room temperature. Shelf-life is 5 years for tablets and suppositories, 3 years for the enema and 2 years for the suspension.

Therapeutic use

Indications

1. In the treatment of mild to moderate ulcerative colitis, and as adjunctive therapy in severe ulcerative colitis; for maintenance of remission in ulcerative colitis
2. In the treatment of active Crohn's disease, especially in patients with colonic involvement
3. In some countries Salazopyrin EN-tabs are registered for the treatment of rheumatoid arthritis in patients not responding to NSAIDS (UK licence).

Contraindications

1. Hypersensitivity to sulphonamides or salicylates
2. Caution should be taken in patients with acute intermittent porphyria.

Mode of use

The dosage of sulphasalazine is dictated by the concentration of sulphapyridine in the blood and the side effects accruing from sulphapyridine. The concentrations of sulphapyridine are dependent on acetylator status. Sensitivity to 5-aminosalicylic acid is now becoming recognised as a much more common source of side effects than hitherto. A daily dosage of 2.5 g is a reasonable compromise between efficacy and freedom from unwanted side effects.[23]

The most important method of responding to side effects of Salazopyrin is to stop the drug. The sulphapyridine washes out of the body in two to three days, then the drug can be restarted at a lower dose. The concentrations of sulphapyridine can be measured indirectly by the development of haemolysis checked by the erythrocyte count. This procedure of stopping and starting can be used on patients with nausea, sickness, cyanosis, haemolysis and transient reticulocytosis.[24] Patients with a history of rash should be given an initial dose of 1 g per day, increasing to 2 g after a week. Antihistamines can also be added to the regime. A densensitising kit (Pharmacia) starts the dose at 1 mg daily and builds up the dose gradually. Such therapy is rarely necessary now there are alternative sources of 5-aminosalicylic acid.

Indications

Until recently sulphasalazine was singular insofar as it was the only drug with a clinically proven effect on inflammatory bowel disease that delivered 5-aminosalicylic acid directly into the lumen of the colon. Sulphasalazine is, together with corticosteroids, the basis of rational treatment of inflammatory bowel disease.[13,25]

Sulphasalazine is the only drug with a clinically proven effect of maintaining remission in ulcerative colitis and therefore should be continued indefinitely unless contraindicated by side effects.[26–29]

When Nanna Svartz tried to develop a compound combining sulphonamide and salicylic acid to treat patients with rheumatic polyarthritis, she found that the sulphanilamide preparations were active in what she called the septic forms of arthritis but not in the common rheumatoid form. She found, however, that sulphasalazine had a definite effect in patients with polyarthritis and ulcerative colitis.[30,31] More recently, sulphasalazine has been used as a second-line drug in the treatment of rheumatoid arthritis.[2] Recent studies indicate that sulphasalizine is a disease modifying drug, inducing decreases in inflammatory indices such as C-reactive protein and ESR.[32–33]

The value of sulphasalazine in active and quiescent colitis has been formally established by controlled trials,[34–36]

Specific contraindications

As sulphasalazine contains both a sulphonamide and salicylate component, hypersensitivity to sulphonamides and salicylates must be regarded as a contraindication. Individuals who are slow acetylators are more likely to develop side effects from the sulphonamide.

Due to inherited defects of certain enzyme systems, porphyria can be precipitated or aggravated by sulphonamides.[37]

Adverse reactions

Most adverse effects are dose-dependent and are usually related to the sulphonamide component.[7]

Potentially life-threatening effects
Agranulocytosis and thrombocytopenia occur rarely and may occasionally be fatal.

Acute overdosage
No case of intentional self-poisoning appears to have been reported, but in such an event any of the adverse effects described below might ensue, particularly renal failure, and acute salicylate poisoning is a possibility and should be treated in the usual way.

Severe or irreversible adverse effects
Haemolytic anaemia, renal damage, hepatitis, peripheral neuropathy, exfoliative dermatitis, Stevens–Johnson Syndrome, toxic epidermal necrolysis (Lyell's syndrome), fibrosing alveolitis, serum sickness and systemic lupus erythematosus have been reported. All are rare. Oligospermia and infertility have been described in man. The mechanism behind this is probably a toxic effect of sulphapyridine. Withdrawal of the drug reverses these effects.[38]

Symptomatic adverse effects
These include nausea, anorexia, pyrexia, exanthematous rashes, and pruritus, headache, dizziness, tinnitus, yellowish skin discoloration, periorbital oedema.

Interference with clinical pathology tests
Sulphasalazine is a dye which may interfere with non-specific spectrophotometer determinations.

High risk groups

Patients should be observed for adverse effects, because of the sulphonamide component. Careful monitoring of blood reticulocyte count and white cell count should be carried out. Symptoms of nausea call for reduction of dosage.

Neonates
No specific precautions are required, but experience is very limited.

Breast milk. The amounts of sulphasalazine and its metabolites excreted in breast milk are small, and there are no contraindications to breast-feeding in mothers taking the drug. No special precautions are required.

Children
No specific precautions are required.

Pregnant women
The safety of sulphasalazine in pregnancy has not been completely established, although it has been fairly widely used in pregnancy. There appear to be no contraindications to its use in pregnancy.

The elderly
No special precautions are required.

Drug interactions

Potentially hazardous interactions
The metabolism of sulphasalazine is markedly reduced in patients taking antibiotics, cholestyramine and possibly ferrous sulphate and folic acid.[39–42]

Other significant interactions
Sulphasalazine may interfere with the absorption of digoxin and folic acid from the gut.

Potentially useful interactions
No interactions of this kind have been reported.

Clinical trials

1. Misiewicz J J, Lennard-Jones J E, Connell A M, Baron J H, Jones F A 1965 Controlled trial of sulphasalazine in maintenance therapy for ulcerative colitis. Lancet 1: 185–188

80 out-patients with proctocolitis were randomly assigned under double-blind conditions to either sulphasalazine 0.5 g four times daily or placebo and followed up for a 12-month period. 13 patients withdrew, 8 from the sulphasalazine group and 5 from the placebo, either due to non-attendance or poor compliance. Of the 67 analysed patients (34 sulphasalazine, 33 placebo), 24 in the sulphasalazine group and 8 in the placebo group remained symptom-free; conversely, 24 in the placebo group and 7 in the sulphasalazine group relapsed. Side effects led to termination of treatment in three patients on sulphasalazine and one on placebo. The authors concluded that sulphasalazine given in a dose of 0.5 g four times daily for a year, reduces the number of relapses of ulcerative colitis.

2. Dissanayake A S, Truelove S C 1973 A controlled therapeutic trial of long term maintenance treatment of ulcerative colitis with sulphasalazine (Salazopyrin). Gut 14: 923–926

64 patients with proven ulcerative colitis who had been maintained on sulphasalazine as their sole form of treatment for a minimum period of one year were entered into a controlled trial of sulphasalazine versus dummy tablets for a period of six months. All the patients admitted were not only symptom-free but also showed no evidence of inflammation on sigmoidoscopy and rectal biopsy. A patient was judged to have relapsed when there was a recurrence of colitic symptoms accompanied by sigmoidoscopic and histological evidence of inflammation.

The patients who received dummy tablets had more than four times the relapse rate of those receiving sulphasalazine. The results were similar in patients who had been on maintenance treatment with sulphasalazine for less than three years before entry into the trial and in those who had been on this treatment for more than three years.

It is concluded that maintenance treatment of ulcerative colitis with sulphasalazine should be continued indefinitely unless contraindicated by side effects.

General review articles

Eastwood M A Pharmacokinetic patterns of sulphasalazine. Therapeutic Drug Monitoring 1: 149–152

van Hees P A M 1979 Clinical and pharmacological aspects of sulphasalazine Diss. XI International Congress of Gastroenterology, Azulfidine Salazopyrin Symposium. Zeitschrift für Gastroenterologie 1981 vol. XIX suppl.

Azad Khan A K 1976 The actions of sulphasalazine. In: Topics in Gastroenterology 4, Blackwell Scientific ch 24 2–16

Peppercorn M A 1983 Sulphasalazine update. The Advisory No. 2, vol. 3

Pullar T 1989 Sulphasalazine and related drugs in rheumatoid arthritis. Pharmacology and Therapeutics 42: 459–468

Truelove S C 1981 The treatment of ulcerative colitis. Schweizerische Medizinische Wochenschrift 111: 1342–1346

References

1. Campbell D 1981 Possible mode of action of azulphadine/ salazopyrin. Zeitschrift für Gastroenterology 19 (suppl) 14–19
2. Amos R S, Bax D E, Greaves M S 1986 Sulphasalazine for rheumatoid arthritis. Studies on dose, acetylator phenotype and efficacy. Drugs 32 (suppl 1): 58
3. Shaw P N et al 1983 Journal of Chromatography: Biomedical Applications 25: 393–397 274
4. Owerbach J, Johnson N F, Bates T R, Pieniaszek H J, Jusko W J 1978 High performance liquid chromatographic assay of sulphapyridine and acetylsulphapyridine in biological fluids. Journal of Pharmaceutical Sciences 67: 1250–1253
5. Hansen S H 1981 Assay of 5-aminosalicylate and its acetylated metabolites in biological fluids by high performance liquid chromatography on dynamically modified silica. Journal of Chromatography 226: 504–509
6. Schroder H, Campbell D E S 1972 Absorption, metabolism and excretion of salicylazosulfapyridine in man. Clinical Pharmacology and Therapeutics 13: 539–551
7. Das K M, Eastwood M A, McManus J P A, Sircus W 1973 The metabolism of salicylazosulphapyridine in ulcerative colitis. Gut 14: 631–641
8. Jansen J A 1977 Kinetics of the binding of salicylazosulfapyridine to human serum albumin. Acta Pharmacologica et Toxicologica 41: 401–416
9. Hanngren A, Hansson E, Svartz N, Ullberg S 1963 Distribution and metabolism of salicyl-azo-sulfapyridine. Part I. Acta Medica Scandinavica 173: 61–72
10. Peppercorn M A, Goldman P 1973 Distribution of studies of salicylazosulphapyridine and its metabolites. Gastroenterology 64: 240–245
11. Pieniaszek H J, Bates T R 1979 Metabolism of 5-aminosalicylic acid, a therapeutically active metabolite of sulfasalazine in rats. Journal of Pharmaceutical Science 68: 1323–1325
12. Haagen Nielsen O, Bondesen S 1983 Kinetics of 5-aminosalicylic acid after jejunal instillation in man. British Journal of Clinical Pharmacology 16: 738–740
13. Truelove S C 1981 The treatment of ulcerative colitis Schweizerische Medizinische Wochenschrift 111: 1342–1346
14. Das K M, Chowdhury J R, Zapp B, Fara J W 1979 Small bowel absorption of sulphasalazine and its hepatic metabolism in human beings, cats and rats. Gastroenterology 77: 280–284
15. Das K M, Eastwood M A, McManus J P A, Sircus W 1974 The role of the colon in the metabolism of salicylazosulphapyridine. Scandinavian Journal of Gastroenterology 9: 137–141
16. Hanngren A, Hansson E, Svartz N, Ullberg S 1963 Distribution and metabolism of salicylazosulphapyridine. Acta Medica Scandinavica 173: 61–72
17. Schroder H, Evans D A P 1972 Acetylator phenotype and adverse effects of sulphasalazine in healthy subjects. Gut 13: 278–284
18. Schroder H, Evans D A P 1972 The polymorphic acetylation of sulphapyridine in man. Journal of Medical Genetics 9: 168–175
19. Jarnerot G, Into-Malmberg N B 1979 Sulphasalazine treatment during breast feeding. Scandinavian Journal of Gastroenterology 14: 869–871
20. Azad Khan A K, Howes D T, Piris J, Truelove S C 1980 Optimum dose of sulphasalazine for maintenance treatment in ulcerative colitis. Gut 21: 232–240
21. Azad Khan A K, Nurazzaman M, Truelove S C 1983 The effect of the acetylator phenotype on the metabolism of sulphasalazine in man. Journal of Medical Genetics 20: 30–36
22. Azad Khan A K, Truelove S C 1980 Circulating levels of sulphasalazine and its metabolites and their relation to the clinical efficacy of the drug in ulcerative colitis. Gut 21: 706–710
23. Das K M, Eastwood M A, McManus J P A, Sircus W 1973 Adverse reactions during salicylazosulfapyridine therapy and the relation with drug metabolism and acetylator phenotype. New England Journal of Medicine 14: 631–641
24. Holdsworth C D 1982 Sulphasalazine desensitization. British Medical Journal 284: 118
25. van Hees P A M, Van Lier H J J, Van Elteren et al 1981 Effect of sulphasalazine in patients with active Crohn's disease: a controlled double-blind study. Gut 22: 404–409
26. Misiewicz J J, Lennard-Jones J E, Connell A M, Baron J H, Jones F A 1965 Controlled trial of sulphasalazine in maintenance therapy for ulcerative colitis. Lancet 1: 185–188
27. Dissanayake A S, Truelove S C 1973 A controlled therapeutic trial of long term maintenance treatment of ulcerative colitis with sulphasalazine (Salazopyrin), Gut 14: 923–926
28. Palmer K R, Goepel J R, Holdsworth C D 1981 Sulphasalazine retention enemas in ulcerative colitis: a double-blind trial. British Medical Journal 282: 1571–1573
29. Ashworth M, Arthur M, Turmer A D, Smith P R 1984 A comparison of serum concentration of sulphasalazine and some of its metabolites after therapy by the oral or rectal route. Pharmatherapeutica 3: 551–555
30. Svartz N 1942 Salazopyrin, a new sulfanilamide preparation. B Therapeutic results in ulcerative colitis. Acta Medica Scandinavica 110: 580–581
31. Svartz N 1948 The treatment of 124 cases of ulcerative colitis with Salazopyrin and attempts at desensitization in cases of hypersensitivity to sulfa. Acta Medica Scandinavica (suppl) 206: 465–471
32. Van der Heijde D M, Van Reid P L, Nuver-Zwart I H, Gribman F W and Van de Potte L B 1989 Effects of hydroxychloroquine and sulphazine on progression of joint damage in rheumatoid arthritis. Lancet 1: 1036–1038
33. Amos R S, Pullar T, Box D E, Situnayate D, Capell H H A, McConkey B 1986 Sulphasalazine for rheumatoid arthritis: toxicity in 774 patients monitored for one to 11 years British Medical Journal 293: 420–423
34. Barron J H, Connell A M, Lennard-Jones J E, Jones F A 1962 Sulphasalazine and salicylazosulphadimidine in ulcerative colitis Lancet 1: 1094
35. Moertel C G, Bargen J A 1959 A critical analysis of the use of salicylazosulphapyridine in chronic ulcerative colitis. Annals of Internal Medicine 51: 879
36. Dick A P, Grayson M J, Carpenter R G, Petrie A 1964 Control trial of sulphasalazine in the treatment of ulcerative colitis. Gut 5: 437
37. Grant Peterkin G A, Khan S A 1969 Iatrogenic skin disease. Practitioner 202: 117–126
38. Toovey S, Hudson E, Hendry F, Levi A J 1981 Sulphasalazine and male infertility: reversibility and possible mechanism. Gut 22: 445–451
39. Azad Khan A K, Truelove S C, Aronson J K 1982 The disposition and metabolism of sulphasalazine (salicylazosulphapyridine) in man. British Journal of Clinical Pharmacology 13: 523–528
40. Pieniaszek H J, Bates T R 1976 Cholestyramine-induced inhibition of salicylazosulfapyridine (sulphasalazine) metabolism by rat intestinal microflora. Journal of Pharmacology and Experimental Therapeutics 198: No. 1: 240–245
41. Das K M, Eastwood M A 1973 Effect of iron and calcium on salicylazosulphapyridine metabolism. Scottish Medical Journal 18: 45–50
42. Halsted C H, Gandhi G, Tamura T 1981 Sulfasalazine inhibits the absorption of folates in ulcerative colitis. New England Journal of Medicine 305: 1513–1517

S Sulphinpyrazone

Sulphinpyrazone is a uricosuric drug used in the treatment of gout.

Chemistry

Sulphinpyrazone (Anturan, Anturane)
$C_{23}H_{20}N_2O_3S$
1,2-Diphenyl-4-[2-(phenylsulphinyl)ethyl]-3,5-pyrazolidenedione

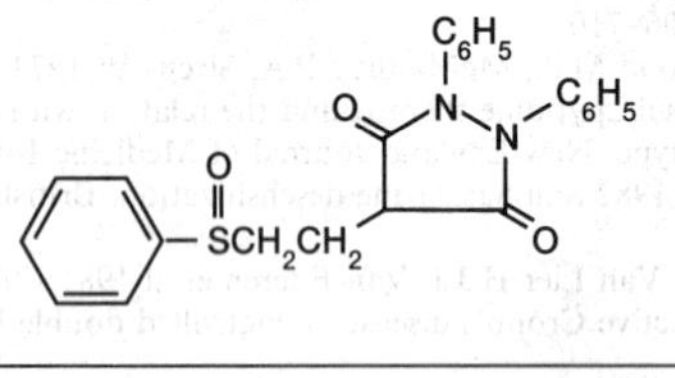

Molecular weight	404.5
pKa (of designated functional group)	2.8
Solubility	
in alcohol	1 in 40
in water	slightly soluble
Octanol/water partition coefficient	—

A crystalline solid, stable to light and air, it is prepared by chemical synthesis. It is chemically related to phenylbutazone.

Pharmacology

Sulphinpyrazone is a potent inhibitor of the renal tubular reabsorption of uric acid, although in common with other uricosuric drugs small doses can reduce uric acid excretion. It reduces renal tubular secretion of many organic anions (cf. probenecid). In a series of phenylbutazone congeners, uricosuric activity is related to pKa, suggesting that it acts in the ionic form to block reabsorption of uric acid by renal tubular cells.[1] Sulphinpyrazone inhibits cyclooxygenase, and inhibits a number of platelet functions. Its sulphide and sulphone metabolites are more potent than the parent compound with respect to inhibition of aggregation of human platelets in vitro[2] and the sulphide is about five times more active than the sulphone.[3] Despite its action on cyclooxygenase it has only modest anti-inflammatory effects, very slight analgesic effects and no anti-pyretic activity. This may reflect its low potency as an inhibitor of cyclooxygenase.

Toxicology

Median lethal doses ($mg.kg^{-1}$) in the mouse are 240 (intravenous) and 298 (oral); in the rat 154 (intravenous) and 375 (oral) and in the rabbit 195 (intravenous) In subchronic testing in rats dosed by stomach tube over 4 weeks a daily dose of 180 $mg.kg^{-1}$ (48% of the acute LD_{50}) caused no fatality during the test period. In animals dying during the acute toxicity test and in those in the chronic study that were subsequently dissected, the following pathological changes in the stomach and upper small intestine were found fairly consistently: hyperaemia of the stomach, petechial bleeding, and ulceration of the mucous membrane.[4]

Clinical pharmacology

Usual therapeutic doses of sulphinpyrazone are generally well tolerated. Oral doses above 100 mg increase urinary excretion of uric acid. Urate clearance may rise to seven times the initial value while inulin clearance remains unchanged, i.e. glomerular filtration is unaffected. There is an appreciable inhibition of para-aminohippuric acid (PAH) clearance, which is probably due to inhibition of tubular secretion of PAH rather than to reduction in renal blood flow. During chronic dosing of healthy volunteers with 200 mg four times daily for six days, there was increasing inhibition of ex vivo platelet aggregation induced by platelet-activating factor, but inhibition of arachidonic acid-induced aggregation did not increase cumulatively, and collagen-induced aggregation was not inhibited.[5] The same dose of sulphinpyrazone has been reported to cause a small (<2 min), but statistically significant prolongation of bleeding time.[6] The combination of aspirin and sulphinpyrazone has been shown to be similar to low dose heparin in preventing deep vein thrombosis in patients at risk.

Pharmacokinetics

Plasma concentrations of sulphinpyrazone and its sulphide and sulphone metabolites can be determined using reverse phase high performance liquid chromatography with ultraviolet detection at 254 nm.[7] Oral bioavailability is 90–100%[8,9] with a t_{max} of 1–2 hours. Volume of distribution[9] is about 0.06 $l.kg^{-1}$. Protein binding is 98–99%.[10] There is no information on distribution to breast milk, cerebrospinal fluid or across the placenta. The half life of sulphinpyrazone is 2–4 hours with a late (deep compartment) elimination phase of 6 h.[9] The $t_{\frac{1}{2}}$ of p-hydroxysulphinpyrazone is about 1 h, and that of the sulphone 3 h and of sulphide and p-hydroxysulphide 12–17 h.[7] During regular dosing of healthy volunteers (200 mg four times a day for six days) the plasma concentration of the sulphide metabolite rose slightly from 2.1 ± 0.8 $mg.l^{-1}$ 12 h after the fourth dose to 2.8 ± 0.8 $mg.l^{-1}$ 12 h after the 24th dose.[5]

Oral absorption	90–100%
Presystemic metabolism	—
Plasma half life	6 h
Volume of distribution	0.06 $l. kg^{-1}$
Plasma protein binding	98–99%

Concentration–effect relationship

The concentration–effect relationship of sulphinpyrazone on uric acid excretion has not been well defined, but this is of little practical importance since therapy can be individualized according to the plasma concentration of uric acid. Chronic dosing (200 mg four times daily) gave mean trough sulphinpyrazone concentrations of 7.2 ± 1.2 $mg.l^{-1}$ 12 h after the 24th dose, and of the sulphide metabolite of 2.8 ± 0.8 $mg.l^{-1}$ and of the sulphone metabolite of 1.6 ± 0.3 $mg.l^{-1}$, with corresponding peak concentrations of 15.6 ± 2.6 $mg.l^{-1}$, 3.9 ± 0.9 $mg.l^{-1}$ and 1.9 ± 0.7 $mg.l^{-1}$. These concentrations were associated with only a modest inhibition of thrombin-stimulated platelet thromboxane B_2 formation (average 55% inhibition) and of urinary excretion of a prostacyclin metabolite (63% inhibition).[5]

Metabolism

Of an oral dose of sulphinpyrazone 25–40% is excreted unchanged, and about 25% is excreted as a glucuronide conjugate.[8,11] Metabolites include p-hydroxysulphinpyrazone, the sulphone, the sulphide and its p-hydroxy derivative and are excreted mainly as glucuronide conjugates (Fig. 1). In humans the hind gut microflora are the principal agents responsible for the reduction of sulphinpyrazone to the sulphide metabolite active on platelets.[12,13]

Pharmaceutics

Sulphinpyrazone (Anturan; Geigy, UK) is available in oral form as 100 mg and 200 mg yellow sugar-coated tablets, marked 'GEIGY'. Anturane (CIBA, USA) is available as a 100 mg white round tablet coded '41' and as a 200 mg dark-green capsule coded 'CIBA 168' in white. These preparations should be protected from heat and moisture.

Therapeutic use

Indications

1. Prophylaxis of gout. Treatment of hyperuricaemia when clinically indicated.

Sulphinpyrazone

S

Sulphinpyrazone is no longer recommended for prevention of cardiac mortality following recent myocardial infarction.

Contraindications

Absolute or relative contraindications include:

1. History of hypersensitivity to sulphinpyrazone, phenylbutazone or related drugs
2. Active peptic ulceration
3. Severe hepatic disease
4. Acute gout within three weeks
5. Nephrolithiasis or renal failure
6. Concurrent salicylate treatment.

Mode of use

For prophylaxis of gout and treatment of hyperuricaemia, treatment is initiated with 100–200 mg daily in single or divided doses, with milk or after food, increasing over 2–3 weeks according to the plasma uric acid concentration to about 600–800 mg daily in divided doses and reducing subsequently for maintenance.

Adverse reactions

Potentially life-threatening effects

Blood dyscrasias (leucopenia, agranulocytosis, aplastic anaemia and thrombocytopenia) are rare, but serious, and may possibly reflect the chemical similarity of sulphinpyrazone to phenylbutazone.

Acute overdosage

There is no specific antidote for sulphinpyrazone and treatment is supportive. Immediate treatment of recent overdose may include forced emesis and/or gastric lavage to recover undigested tablets and supportive and symptomatic therapy as individually indicated.

Severe or irreversible adverse effects

As with other cyclooxygenase inhibitors sulphinpyrazone may predispose to peptic ulceration and cause bleeding from pre-existing ulcer disease. If used inappropriately to treat patients with uric acid calculi, it can cause further calculi, renal colic and haematuria. The risk of these complications is reduced by treating patients with a history of urinary calculi not with uricosuric drugs, but rather with allopurinol, and by initiating treatment with a low dose and encouraging high fluid intake and alkalinizing the urine. Polyneuritis has been reported, albeit very rarely.

Symptomatic adverse effects

Nausea and epigastric discomfort are the commonest unwanted symptoms. Skin rashes occur occasionally. At the onset of treatment, rapid mobilization of uric acid from the tissues can precipitate acute attacks of gout. This has been noted in around 4% of the patients during the first 2–6 weeks of treatment.[14,15] This problem can be minimized by using a low initial dose and using a non-steroidal drug such as indomethacin during the first 7–10 days of treatment or at the first hint of an acute attack during initial weeks of therapy.

Other effects

Sulphinpyrazone reduces serum uric acid by inhibiting renal tubular reabsorption of uric acid. It is a weak inhibitor of cyclooxygenase, thereby reducing serum thromboxane concentration and urinary prostaglandin metabolite excretion.[5]

Interference with clinical pathology tests

Sulphinpyrazone inhibits the tubular secretion of many organic anions, including para-aminohippuric acid (PAH). PAH clearance is therefore unreliable as a measure of renal blood flow in subjects receiving sulphinpyrazone. Tests involving phenolsulphthalein or other organic acids may also be invalidated.

High risk groups

Neonates

There is no experience with sulphinpyrazone in this age-group.

Breast milk. There is no information on the distribution of sulphinpyrazone to breast milk, so it is best for women taking the drug to avoid breast-feeding.

Children

Paediatric usage is not established. Gout is uncommon in children (Hippocrates). Children with hypoxanthine-guanine phosphoribosyltransferase deficiency (Lesch–Nyhan syndrome) should be treated with allopurinol because of the risk of uric acid nephropathy. They are usually extremely sensitive to allopurinol, although uricosuric agents such as sulphinpyrazone may occasionally be added in resistant cases with tophi.

Pregnant women

The usual precautions apply. Gout is uncommon in women of childbearing age, and experience is extremely limited.

The elderly

No specific problems of sulphinpyrazone use have been identified in this age-group. However, toxicity of other cyclooxygenase inhibitors has been particularly severe in this age-group, and caution (avoiding excessive dosage and careful biochemical monitoring) is appropriate.

Concurrent disease

Particular care should be exercised in patients with renal impairment (in whom the drug may in any case be ineffective), and in those with coexistent liver disease. Sulphinpyrazone should not be given to patients with uric acid nephropathy. Reduced formation of the sulphide metabolite occurs in patients with ileostomy,[13] so reduced anti-platelet effects are to be anticipated in such patients.

Drug interactions

Potentially hazardous interactions

Oral anticoagulants. Concurrent administration of sulphinpyrazone to patients stabilized on warfarin can result in prolongation of the prothrombin time, and bleeding. It was speculated that such an interaction might arise from competition with binding sites on plasma proteins, but since the effect is persistent rather than transient, it is unlikely that this is the sole explanation. The dose of warfarin should be reduced to about 50% of that previously established when sulphinpyrazone is introduced.

Hypoglycaemic agents. Sulphinpyrazone can prolong the half life of tolbutamide by reducing its metabolic clearance,[16] but clinically

Fig. 1 Metabolism of sulphinpyrazone

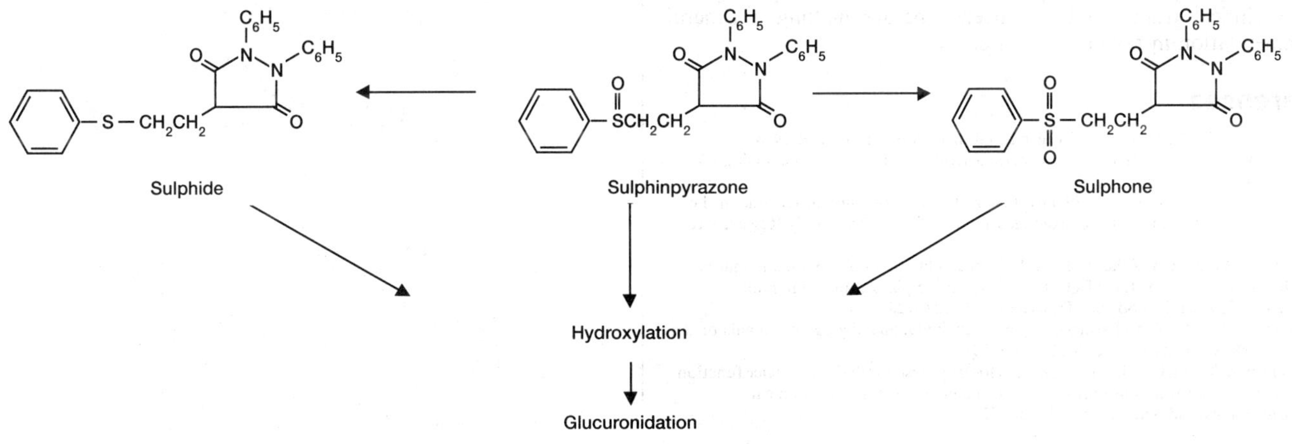

important hypoglycaemia is uncommon. It has been suggested that sulphinpyrazone can enhance insulin activity, thereby causing hypoglycaemia in insulin-requiring diabetics, but this appears to be uncommon.

Penicillin and other antibacterials. Sulphinpyrazone prolongs the half life of penicillin substantially, probably by competing for the renal tubular mechanism that secretes penicillin into the urine.[17] This interaction is likely to be clinically important only when massive doses of penicillin are being used, as in the treatment of pneumococcal meningitis or bacterial endocarditis. Conversely, penicillin and other antibacterials active against anaerobic organisms (e.g. metronidazole) may reduce the anti-platelet effect of sulphinpyrazone by reducing the resident anaerobic microflora in the hind gut that are normally principally responsible for the reduction of sulphinpyrazone to its biologically active sulphide metabolite.[13] Sulphonamides compete with sulphinpyrazone for plasma protein binding, but it is unlikely that this is of major clinical importance.

Phenytoin

Sulphinpyrazone prolongs the half life of phenytoin and reduces its clearance. Displacement from plasma protein binding sites occurs, but is of less relevance than inhibition of microsomal biotransformation. The effect is of such magnitude that clinically important changes could be expected to occur.[16]

Other significant interactions

Salicylate. Salicylate inhibits the uricosuric effect of sulphinpyrazone and vice versa.[18–20] These drugs should not be co-administered during treatment of gout.

Probenecid. Probenecid increases the plasma concentration of sulphinpyrazone and its p-hydroxy metabolite by competing for renal tubular secretion.

Potentially useful interactions

The combination of a uricosuric agent such as sulphinpyrazone with allopurinol, which inhibits uric acid synthesis, is useful in particularly resistant cases of hyperuricaemia associated with gout (e.g. with chronic tophi).

Major outcome trials

There are no large scale clinical trials on the use of sulphinpyrazone as a uricosuric agent, and indeed such studies appear to be unnecessary for this indication. Clinical trials have been performed on the use of sulphinpyrazone after myocardial infarction, but a completely consistent picture has not emerged. The original claims that sulphinpyrazone prevented sudden cardiac death after myocardial infarction[21] were not accepted by the American Food and Drug Administration.[22] An independent re-analysis of the data by a committee headed by Pitt produced results similar to, though somewhat less striking than, those originally reported,[23] and the effects were less impressive when analysed by intention to treat, as would be expected. In a smaller Italian study (727 patients) treatment with sulphinpyrazone did not affect either total mortality or sudden death rate, but did reduce the incidence of re-infarction (34 in placebo group, 15 in treated group) and also of all thromboembolic events over an average follow-up period of 19 months.[24] Since major outcome trials have now demonstrated the efficacy of β-blockers and of aspirin in reducing mortality after myocardial infarction, the evidence in favour of using sulphinpyrazone for this indication is not compelling and further clinical trials would be needed before making a general recommendation in favour of its use.

References

1. Burns J J, Yü T F, Dayton P, Burger L, Gutman A B, Brodie B B 1958 Relationship between pKa and uricosuric activity in phenylbutazone analogues. Nature 182: 1162–1163
2. Pedersen A K, Jakobsen P 1979 Two new metabolites of sulphinpyrazone in the rabbit: a possible cause of the prolonged in vivo effect. Thrombosis Research 16: 871–876
3. Pay G F, Wallis R B, Zelaschi D 1980 A metabolite of sulphinpyrazone that is largely responsible for the effect of the drug on the platelet prostaglandin pathway. Biochemical Society Transactions 8: 727–728
4. Domenjoz R 1960 The pharmacology of phenylbutazone analogues. Annals of the New York Academy of Sciences 86: 263–291
5. Pedersen A K, FitzGerald G A 1985 Cyclo-oxygenase inhibition, platelet function, and metabolite formation during chronic sulfinpyrazone dosing. Clinical Pharmacology and Therapeutics 37: 36–42

6. Weston M J, Rubin M H, Langley P G, Westaby S, Williams R 1977 Effects of sulphinpyrazone and dipyridamole on capillary bleeding time in man. Thrombosis Research 10: 833–840
7. Jakobsen P, Pedersen A K 1981 Simultaneous determination of sulphinpyrazone and four of its metabolites by high performance liquid chromatography. Journal of Chromatography 223: 460–465
8. Dieterle W, Fagle J W 1975 Biotransformation and pharmacokinetics of sulphinpyrazone (Anturan) in man. European Journal of Clinical Pharmacology 9: 135–145
9. Lecaillou J-B, Souppart C 1979 Sulphinpyrazone kinetics after intravenous and oral administration. Clinical Pharmacology and Therapeutics 26: 611–617
10. Perel J M, Snell M M 1964 A study of structure activity relationship in regard to species difference in the phenylbutazone series. Biochemical Pharmacology 13: 1305–1317
11. Senczuk W, Jodynis-Liebert J 1979 Studies on kinetics of anturan excretion in man. International Journal of Clinical Pharmacology and Biopharmaceutics 17: 303–306
12. Strong H A, Oates J, Sembi J, Renwick A G, George C F 1984 Role of the gut flora in the reduction of sulphinpyrazone in humans. Journal of Pharmacology and Experimental Therapeutics 230: 726–732
13. Renwick A G, Strong H A, George C F 1986 The role of the gut flora in the reduction of sulphoxide-containing drugs. Biochemical Pharmacology 35: 64
14. Unzell W C, Glover R P, Gibbs J O, Blair R A 1964 Effects of sulphinpyrazone on serum uric acid in gout. Geriatrics 19 (12): 894–909
15. Kersley G D, Gibbs A R 1960 Uricosuric agents in the treatment of gout. Annals of the Rheumatic Diseases 19: 351–355
16. Simonsen K, Bush G, Nierni G et al 1982 Influence of sulphinpyrazone on the metabolism of antipyrine, phenytoin and tolbutamide. Clinical Pharmacology and Therapeutics 13: 516–519
17. Kampmann J, Hansen J M, Siersback-Nielsen K, Laursen H 1972 Effect of some drugs on penicillin half life in blood. Clinical Pharmacology and Therapeutics 13: 516–519
18. Kersley G D, Cook E R, Tobey D C J 1958 Value of uricosuric agents and in particular of G28 315 in gout. Annals of the Rheumatic Diseases 17: 326–333
19. Seegmiller J E, Grayzel A I 1960 Use of the newer uricosuric agents in the management of gout. Journal of the American Medical Association 173: 1076–1080
20. Yü T F, Dayton P G, Gutman A B 1963 Mutual suppression of the uricosuric effects of sulphinpyrazone and salicylate. A study in interactions between drugs. Journal of Clinical Investigation 42: 1330–1339
21. The Anturane Reinfarction Trial Research Group 1978, 1980 Sulfinpyrazone in the prevention of cardiac death after myocardial infarction. New England Journal of Medicine 298: 289–295 and 302: 250–256
22. Temple R, Pledger G W 1980 The FDA's critique of the Anturane Reinfarction Trial. New England Journal of Medicine 303: 1488–1492
23. The Anturane Reinfarction Trial Policy Committee 1982 The Anturane Reinfarction Trial: re-evaluation of outcome. New England Journal of Medicine 306: 1005–1008
24. The Anturane Reinfarction Italian Study Group 1982 Sulphinpyrazone in post-myocardial infarction. Lancet 1: 237–242

Sulphur

Chemistry

Sulphur is an element, molecular weight 32. It is pale yellow to greenish yellow in colour, soft, odourless and tasteless, and usually used in the form of precipitated sulphur which is an amorphous or microcrystalline powder.

It melts at around 115°C to form a yellow liquid which becomes dark and viscous at around 160°C. It is insoluble in water and alcohol, and soluble in carbon disulphide, light petroleum and turpentine.[1]

Pharmacology

Sulphur has been used for centuries in dermatological practice. It is said to be useful against sepsis, parasites, acne and seborrhoea.[2] These properties may depend on disulphides and polython acids formed from the interaction of sulphur with organic substances.[2] It also has some antifungal properties. Sulphur must be converted to pentathionic acid ($H_2S_5O_6$) in order to exert a germicide effect.

Toxicology

No evidence exists for carcinogenic or mutagenic properties.

Clinical pharmacology

There has been little research into the basis of the effects attributed to sulphur, or mechanisms of action. Claims are made for keratolytic properties,[3,4] but it is more likely to act as an irritant producing scaling which has been interpreted as keratolysis.[5]

Pharmacokinetics

A sensitive liquid chromatography method is available for analysis of sulphur-containing amino acids in blood.[6] A method is also described for determining total as well as inorganic urinary sulphur.[7]

Little work has been done in the field of pharmacokinetics. There is no evidence available to suggest significant absorption through the skin. Of an oral load of methionine 80% of the sulphur content is reported to be converted to inorganic sulphur which appears in the urine.[8]

Concentration–effect relationship

Since sulphur is only used topically this section is not relevant.

Metabolism

Sulphur is essential to human metabolism.[8] Total body sulphur is approximately 100 g.[8,9] This is mainly present in the amino acids methionine, cysteine and cystine and the mucopolysaccharide chondroitin sulphate,[10] being predominantly localized to the skin, nails and hair.[8,9] Metabolic balance is maintained through its absorption in the gut, and by losses in urine, faeces and the integument.[8]

A decrease in urinary sulphur has been demonstrated in conditions of increased epidermal turnover such as severe psoriasis.[9]

Pharmaceutics

Sulphur is mixed with various vehicles depending on its intended use; these may contain up to 20% sulphur and be mixed with keratolytics such as salicylic acid, benzoyl peroxide and resorcinol.[2] The British National Formulary mentions a paste, cream, lotion and ointment[12] as well as proprietary preparations. Sulphur-containing shampoos are also available.[13] Other preparations mentioned include sulphur baths and lozenges.[1] Some abrasive cleanser formulations use sublimed sulphur rather than the more usual precipitated sulphur, which is free from grittiness.

Radiolabelled colloidal sulphur is used in diagnostic radiology.

Therapeutic use

Indications

1. The treatment of parasitic infections
2. The treatment of acne and seborrhoeic conditions
3. The treatment of skin sepsis
4. As a laxative
5. For the attachment of isotopes in diagnostic radiology.

Contraindications

None.

Mode of use

As a laxative, it is prepared in the form of lozenges.[1] It is used in colloidal form in diagnostic radiology.[21] Apart from these, its use on the skin is in various strengths and vehicles depending on the intended therapeutic effect.

Indications

1. Antiparasitic properties

Sulphur was widely used for centuries in the treatment of scabies, but was falling out of favour as long ago as 1890.[14] It was usually used in strengths from 2 to 15% in petrolatum. Mention has also been made of its successful use as a 20% cream during the Second World War[2] and its use in developing countries is suggested as an alternative where more modern preparations are not available or are too expensive.[15]

2. Acne and sebborhoea

The antiacne properties of sulphur have been questioned despite centuries of use. Work on the rabbit ear model suggested that sulphur-containing agents were comedogenic, when applied under occlusion.[16] Although this result has been disputed by further work,[17] the issue remains contentious and the use of the rabbit ear as a model for human disease has been questioned.[5]

Sulphur in various preparations has been used in hyperkeratotic skin disorders for its keratolytic properties[3,4,11] but there is little evidence for keratolysis and irritation when scaling is a more likely result.[5] More cosmetically acceptable alternative preparations are available under these circumstances.

Sulphur-containing shampoos have been used with considerable success[18] for seborrhoeic scalp disorders. There are also claims that a 10% sulphur cream is effective in the treatment of acne rosacea.[19]

3. Antisepsis

Sulphur-containing shampoos have been successfully used to treat tinea versicolor infections.[20,21] Sulphur is reported as having a mild antibacterial action[14] and sulphur-containing baths have been recommended.[1,11]

4. Laxative properties

When taken by mouth, sulphur is converted in the gut to alkali sulphides whose irritant action produces a mild laxative effect.[1]

5. Diagnostic radiology

Particles of colloidal sulphur ranging from 0.1 to 0.3 μm in diameter are radiolabelled with technetium. When injected intravenously these are selectively phagocytosed by reticuloendothelial cells in the liver, spleen and bone marrow enabling these organs to be outlined with a gamma camera.[21]

Contraindications

No specific contraindications are recorded.

Adverse reactions

Potentially life-threatening effects

None has been reported despite widespread use.

Severe or irreversible adverse effects

No reactions of this kind have been reported.

Symptomatic adverse effects

Mild irritation at the site of application may occasionally occur.

Interference with clinical pathology tests

No technical interferences of this kind appear to have been reported.

Sulphur

S

High risk groups

Neonates
The drug is unlikely to be used in neonates.

Breast milk. There appears to be no contraindication to the use of topically applied sulphur by lactating mothers.

Children
The drug may be used in children.

Pregnant women
There is no evidence that harm results from the use of local application of sulphur during pregnancy.

The elderly
The drug may be used in elderly patients.

Drug interactions

Potentially hazardous interactions
None has been described.

Other significant interactions
Sulphur is incompatible with iodine and mercury. When mixed with mercury, it forms a black precipitate. It is compatible when mixed with antibiotics, antihistamines, steroids and tars.[14]

Potentially useful interactions
In view of its reported mild antiseptic, anti-seborrhoeic and antiacne properties,[2] it is often mixed with more active agents in these areas as an adjunct to treatment.

Major outcome trials

1. Blom I, Hornmark A M 1984 Topical treatment with sulphur 10% for rosacea. Acta Dermato-Venereologica 64: 358–359

This was a prospective study of 40 patients randomly allocated either oral tetracyclines or topical sulphur treatment for acne rosacea. Follow-up at 4 weeks showed no difference in the two treated groups, and the sulphur was said to be well tolerated.

2. Bamford J T M 1983 Treatment of tinea versicolor with sulphur salicylic shampoo. Journal of the American Academy of Dermatology 8: 211–213

The author used a shampoo base containing 2% sulphur and 2% salicylic acid. 40 patients were randomly allocated to two groups using either the sulphur/salicylic acid mixture or placebo lotion. Review at 3 months with microscopic examination for residual fungi showed a cure rate of 19 out of 22 in the sulphur/salicylic treated group, 1 out of 17 in the placebo group.

References

1. Reynolds J E F (ed) 1982 Martindale: The extra pharmacopoeia, 28th edn. Pharmaceutical Press, London, p 504
2. Polano M K 1984 Topical skin therapeutics. Churchill Livingstone, Edinburgh, pp 90–91
3. Barry B W 1983 Dermatological formulations (Drugs and the therapeutic sciences), vol 18. Marcel Dekker, New York, p 28
4. Wilkinson J B (ed) 1973 Harry's cosmeticology, 6th edn. Leonard Hill, Edinburgh, p 558
5. Reisner R M 1984 Some controversial areas in the topical treatment of acne. In: Epstein E (ed) Controversies in dermatology. W B Saunders, Philadelphia, pp 271–272
6. Watanabe Y, Kazuhiro I 1984 Sensitive detection of amino acids in human serum and dried blood discs of 3mm diameter for diagnosis of inborn errors of metabolism. Journal of Chromatography 309: 279–286
7. Papadopoulu D B 1957 Urinary sulphur partition in normal men and cancer patients. Clinical Chemistry 3: 257–262
8. Roe B A 1969 Sulphur metabolism in relation to cutaneous disease. British Journal of Dermatology 81 (suppl 2): 49–60
9. Wilkinson J B (ed) 1973 Harry's cosmeticology, 6th edn. Leonard Hill, Edinburgh, p 345
10. Rook A, Wilkinson D S, Ebling F J G, Champion R H, Burton J L 1986 Textbook of dermatology 4th edn. Blackwell Scientific Publications, Oxford pp 2335
11. Sulzburger M B, Wolf J 1952 Practical dermatology. Yearbook Publishers, Chicago, p 842
12. British National Formulary, No. 19 1990 British Medical Association/The Pharmaceutical Society of Great Britain, London p 396
13. British National Formulary, No. 19 1990 British Medical Association/The Pharmaceutical Society of Great Britain, London p 399
14. Epstein E 1977 Traditional methods of treatment In: Orkin M, Maibach H I, Parish L C, Schwartzman R M (eds) Scabies and pediculosis. J B Lippincott, Philadelphia, pp 105–108
15. Shatin H 1975 Dermatoses caused by arthropods. In: Canizares O (ed) Clinical tropical dermatology. Blackwell Scientific Publications, Oxford, p 239
16. Mills O H, Kligman A M 1972 Is sulphur helpful or harmful in acne vulgaris. British Journal of Dermatology 86: 620–627
17. Strauss J S, Goldman P H, Nacht S, Gans E H 1978 A reexamination of the potential comedogenicity of sulfur. Archives of Dermatology 114: 1340–1342
18. Wilkinson J B (ed) 1973 Harry's cosmeticology, 6th edn. Leonard Hill, Edinburgh, p 372
19. Blom I, Hornmark A-M 1984 Topical treatment with sulfur: ten percent for rosacea. Acta Dermato-Venereologica 64: 358–359
20. Rook A, Wilkinson D S, Ebling F J G, Champion R H, Burton J L 1986 Textbook of dermatology, 4th edn. Blackwell Scientific Publications, Oxford, p 2544
21. Bamford J T M 1983 Treatment of tinea versicolor with sulfur–salicylic shampoo. Journal of the American Academy of Dermatology 8: 211–213
22. Sulzburger M G, Wolf J (eds) 1952 Practical dermatology. Yearbook Publishers Inc, Chicago, p 80

Sulpiride

Sulpiride is a selective antagonist at the dopamine-2 (D_2) receptor. It is a substituted benzamide neuroleptic used in the management of schizophrenia and certain types of depression.

Chemistry

Sulpiride (Dogmatil, Abilit, Aiglonyl, Championyl, Coolspan, Dixibon, Dolmatil, Eglonyl, Ekilid, Equilid, Guastil, Lisopride, Megotil, Metexal, Miradol, Mirbanil, Seeglu, Suprium, Synedil, Tepavil, Vipral)
$C_{15}H_{23}N_3O_4S$
N-(1-Ethylpyrrolidine-2-ylmethyl)-2-methoxy-5-sulphamoyl-benzamide)

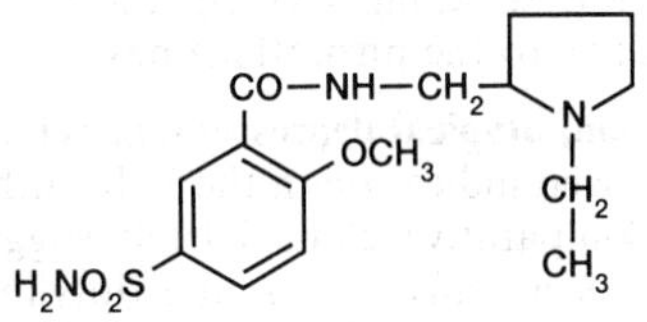

Molecular weight	341.4
pKa	8.9
Solubility	
in alcohol	weakly soluble
in water	practically insoluble
Octanol/water partition coefficient	2.9

It is a white odourless, amorphous or crystalline powder with a slightly bitter taste, produced by chemical synthesis. It is also available as the combination products Dogmatil, Avisonal, Milpiride, Sulpan, Tepazepam, Modulex, Gelmatil, Lexpiride and Dogmalex.

Pharmacology

Sulpiride selectively binds to both central and peripheral D_2 dopamine receptors.[1,2] No significant binding occurs at adenylate cyclase-dependent (D_1), histaminergic (H_1), serotonergic (5HT), adrenergic (α_1 and α_2), cholinergic (muscarinic) or GABAergic receptors.[3–8] Unlike conventional neuroleptic compounds, sulpiride binds to D_2 receptors in a sodium-dependent manner[1] and is selectively active on mesolimbic brain structures.[9,10] In addition, recent studies have demonstrated preferential blockade of auto- inhibitory presynaptic D_4 receptors situated on the terminals of corticostriatal glutamate fibres which would result in increased release of glutamate and a functional increase in dopamine.[11]

When administered at higher doses, sulpiride displays typical neuroleptic effects by inhibiting climbing behaviour in mice[12] and increasing cerebral dopamine turnover,[13] but in contrast to conventional neuroleptics, it is non-sedative[14] with virtually no cataleptogenic effect or ability to antagonize apomorphine-induced stereotyped behaviour.[15,16]

At low doses, sulpiride no longer acts as a neuroleptic but conversely produces an 'activating' effect, increasing spontaneous locomotor activity and potentiating apomorphine-induced motility in rodents, which may be explained by D_4 or presynaptic D_2 blockade.[11,17]

Chronic oral administration of sulpiride to rodents does not induce dopamine receptor hypersensitivity.[18] A single injection of sulpiride suppresses dyskinetic movements in monkeys with neuroleptic-induced 'tardive dyskinesia' without inducing the rebound dyskinesia which can be observed following administration of conventional high potency neuroleptics.[19]

Sulpiride inhibits apomorphine-induced emesis in dogs.[20] Serum prolactin levels are raised following administration to rodents. Haemodynamic effects are mild and limited to a reduction in peripheral vascular resistance.[21] Sulpiride increases gastric motility and blood flow;[22] the latter action may be responsible for the curative effect observed on gastric ulcers in rodents and primate models.[23]

Toxicology

Acute toxicological testing has been carried out in rats and mice. LD_{50} values in mice after intravenous and oral administration were 61–68, and 6500–7700 $mg.kg^{-1}$ respectively. Values for rats were 110 (intravenous), 200 (intramuscular), and > 6000 $mg.kg^{-1}$ (oral) (unpublished data).

Subchronic and chronic toxicity testing has not demonstrated particular toxicity related to administration of sulpiride. Cardiovascular, respiratory, liver and renal function are not affected by treatment. Neurological disturbances (somnolence, prostration, tremor in dogs) typical of neuroleptic compounds occur at higher dose levels. Endocrine disturbances and histological modifications of endocrine organs typical of this therapeutic class are also observed (unpublished data).

Mutagenicity studies including Ames test, human lymphocytes, micronucleus, CTA, mouse lymphoma, chromosomes, analysis of Chinese hamster bone marrow cells, and sister chromatid exchanges in Chinese hamster bone marrow cells have all been negative (unpublished data).

Clinical pharmacology

The clinical activity of sulpiride is dose-dependent. Antipsychotic effect occurs at doses generally ranging from 400 to 1800 mg daily,[24–26,35–37] with a maximal reported therapeutic daily dose of 3600 mg.[27] Negative symptoms of schizophrenia appear to respond best to doses less than 800 mg daily.[28] Alerting, antidepressant and anxiolytic activity is prevalent at lower doses. Doses of 50–300 mg daily are active for treatment of psychiatric disorders characterized by anxiety, depression, and psychosomatic or psychofunctional disturbances.[29]

Significant elevations of homovanillic acid (HVA) concentrations in CSF were observed in schizophrenics receiving 800 mg of oral sulpiride daily.[30] HVA levels were maximal after 1 and 2 weeks of therapy and slowly declined reaching normal levels by 8 weeks, but MOPEG and 5HIAA levels were unaffected by sulpiride treatment in keeping with the selective dopamine blockade observed in in vitro binding studies. Plasma prolactin levels increase after oral and intramuscular administration of sulpiride for oral doses as low as 50 mg. After oral administration of a single dose peak prolactin levels are reached within 30 min to 2 hours, returning to normal levels within 2–7 days.[31]

Learning, memory, and driving psychomotor skills were not diminished in healthy volunteers receiving 150 mg of oral sulpiride daily for 2 weeks.[32]

Pharmacokinetics

Sulpiride assays have been carried out using high performance liquid chromatography with fluorescent or electrochemical ultraviolet detection.[33–35] Sensitivity of the method ranges from 1 to 10 $\mu g.l^{-1}$. Reproducibility is good.

In man, sulpiride is moderately well absorbed from the gastrointestinal tract. The bioavailability of the oral form ranges from 25 to 40%.[36,37] The compound does not undergo presystemic metabolism. Peak plasma levels are obtained within 2–4 hours. The elimination half life ranges from approximately 6–8 hours.[37–41] The volume of distribution is 0.65–1.4 $l.kg^{-1}$. Binding to plasma protein is low (14%), but has been reported to be as high as 40% in schizophrenic patients.[36,42] Sulpiride crosses the blood–brain barrier. Drug concentration in cerebrospinal fluid is approximately 13% of plasma levels. The compound is excreted almost entirely as unchanged substance in urine; 80% of the compound is eliminated within 24 hours after oral administration and by 48 hours 95% of the compound is excreted.[37] Sulpiride is excreted into breast milk but concentrations are low. Maximal concentrations following a 50 mg oral dose were 135 μg.l^{-1}.[43]

Oral absorption	25–40%
Presystemic metabolism	nil
Plasma half life range	6–8 h
Volume of distribution	0.65–1.4 l.kg^{-1}
Plasma protein binding	14%

Concentration–effect relationship

Most studies to date have not found a correlation between sulpiride plasma concentration and antipsychotic effect.[26,44] Negative symptoms of schizophrenia, however, appear to respond better when plasma levels are reduced. In schizophrenic patients receiving a fixed dose of 800 mg of sulpiride daily, 'autistic' symptoms were improved in patients whose sulpiride plasma levels fell below the mean plasma level of 1.5 μmol.l^{-1} calculated for all patients in the sulpiride group.[44] A controlled trial comparing use of 150 or 1200 mg of sulpiride daily for treatment of chronic schizophrenics with predominantly negative symptoms demonstrated significant improvement only in patients receiving the lower dosage.[28] Mean plasma levels in the low-dose patient ranged from 39 to 141 μg.l^{-1}. Further studies using carefully selected patients and scales will be required to verify these results and possibly establish a therapeutic range.

Metabolism

Between 90 and 95% of sulpiride is excreted unchanged in urine. A very small fraction is eliminated in faeces. A single metabolite, 5-oxypyrrolidinyl sulpiride, which is pharmacologically inactive is produced and eliminated in urine (5%) (see Fig. 1).[34,38]

Pharmaceutics

Injectable solution: 2 ml ampoules, each containing 100 mg of sulpiride (50 mg.ml^{-1}); shelf-life, 3 years; optimal storage temperature, 2–30°C.

Tablets: white scored tablets each containing 200 mg of sulpiride; identifying marks: France and export countries, 'DOGMATIL 200'; Dolmatil (Bristol Myers Squibb, UK) marked, 'D200'; shelf-life, 5 years; optimal storage temperature, below 30°C.

Capsules: white opaque capsules each containing 50 mg of sulpiride, identifying mark, 'Dogmatil 50'; shelf-life, 5 years; optimal storage temperature: below 30°C.

Syrup: 200 ml bottle containing 1 g of sulpiride (5 mg.ml^{-1}). Transparent slightly amber syrup. Solution available in France contains sodium cyclamate. Syrups for export contain sodium saccharinate only. Shelf-life, 5 years; optimal storage temperature, 2–30°C.

Therapeutic use

Indications

1. Acute and chronic schizophrenia, chronic psychosis
2. Reactive depression, atypical depression, mixed anxiety–depression.

Contraindications

1. Phaeochromocytoma.

Mode of Use

The therapeutic dose is dependent on the nature of the presenting symptoms and the pharmacological profile of the drug with sedative affects predominating at higher doses and an alerting action at lower doses. Patients with positive symptoms such as hallucinations, delusions, formal thought disorders and incongruity of affect usually require oral doses in the range 800 to 1600 mg daily. The maximum oral dose which has been used in such patients is 2400 mg daily. In some countries, where an intramuscular formulation is marketed, doses of 400–800 mg intramuscularly daily in 2 to 3 divided doses have been used. In patients with predominantly negative symptoms such as anergia, apathy, flattening of affect or poverty of speech, a lower starting oral dose of 400 mg twice daily is sufficient and this can be reduced towards 200 mg twice daily as a response occurs. In patients with mixed positive and negative symptoms the usual oral dosage range is 400–600 mg twice daily.

Indications

1. Acute and chronic schizophrenia
This is the only indication approved in the U.K. Clinical improvement is often evident within one week of starting therapy and continues for several weeks. Autistic symptoms and lack of social contact are particularly likely to improve with sulpiride. It is free of autonomic side-effects due to adrenergic or cholinergic blockade compared with classical neuroleptics such as cholorpromazine and, at lower doses, it is less sedating. Extra-pyramidal side-effects occur with similar frequency to the phenothiazines.

2. Reactive depression, atypical depression, mixed anxiety-depression
This is not an approved indication in the U.K. although it is in some other countries. Comparative clinical trials suggest that sulpiride, 200–400 mg daily, is as effective as amitriptyline in the relief of neurotic depression and causes fewer autonomic side-effects.

Contraindications

Phaeochromocytoma is the only absolute contraindication to sulpiride treatment.

Adverse reactions

Potentially life-threatening effects
Hypertensive crisis may occur in patients with phaeochromocytoma.[45] This condition has consequently been considered as a contraindication to treatment. Malignant neuroleptic syndrome has been observed after administration of sulpiride.[46] Other neuroleptic compounds known to cause this syndrome, however, were concomitantly administered to all patients listed in the report.

Acute overdosage
The toxicity of sulpiride is low.[47–49] Coma has followed ingestion at sulpiride alone but patients have survived dose of upto 20 g. Overdose may result in restlessness, extrapyramidal symptoms, agitation, confusion and hypotension. The duration of intoxication is generally short with symptoms abating within several hours. No particular haematological or hepatic toxicity has been reported. Overdose should be treated with supportive measures and antiparkinson medication when indicated. Coma requires appropriate nursing in an intensive care unit.

Severe or irreversible adverse effects
Reports of tardive dyskinesia[50–52] have been extremely infrequent and include only one patient, an elderly woman, who had had no previous exposure to conventional neuroleptics. Documentation of

Fig. 1 Metabolism of sulpiride

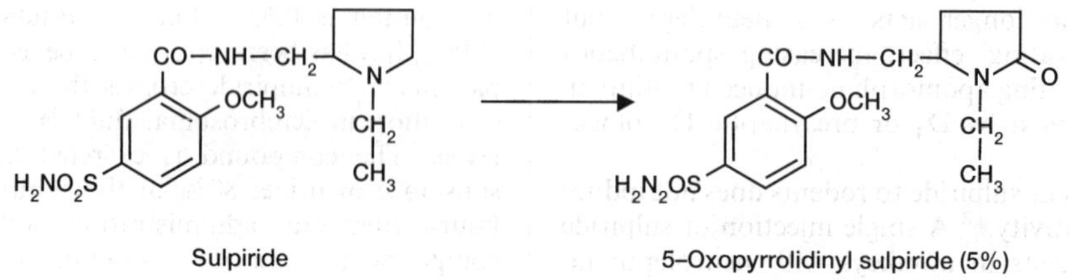

the five other reported cases was insufficient to reach any conclusions as to causal relationship with sulpiride.

Symptomatic adverse effects[53]
Extrapyramidal adverse effects, principally akathisia but including acute dystonia and parkinsonism, have been observed in a small number of patients. Motor agitation including excitability, irritability, anxiety and mood inversion have been reported following higher doses. Sulpiride is largely free of cholinergic side effects although there are a few reports of dry mouth, paralysis of accommodation and disturbance of micturition. Somnolence, lassitude and insomnia are recognised side-effects. Weight gain, galactorrhoea and amenorrhoea have also been reported. Serum prolactin levels are elevated but are reversible after cessation of treatment.[54] Other adverse effects reported infrequently include: disturbances of cardiac rhythm and modifications of ECG tracings (anomalies of repolarization and one case of left bundle branch block) and disturbance of sexual functioning both as increased and decreased libido. Leucopenia and elevated aminotransferase and alkaline phosphatase levels have been reported on occasion.

Interference with clinical pathology tests
The drug may interfere with tests for estimating glucose and cholesterol concentrations in serum.

High risk groups

Neonates
Sulpiride has no therapeutic indications in this age group.

Breast milk. Sulpiride is secreted in breast milk and consequently potential benefits of treatment must be balanced against possible ill effects on the infant when considering use of the drug.

Children
Experience in children under the age of 14 years is limited. The drug has been used in doses ranging between 5 mg/kg and 10 mg/kg to treat psychotic and psychoaffective disorders in children aged from 4 and 15 years[55–57] but there is insufficient data to make confident recommendations.

Pregnant women
Despite the negative results of teratogenicity testing and lack of teratogenic effects after long-term use, the manufacturer recommends avoiding use during pregnancy, particularly the first trimester. Consequently, potential benefits of treatment must be weighed against possible risks when considering the use of sulpiride in this patient group.

The elderly
In view of the reduced neuronal reserve of the elderly brain and the possibility of impaired renal function resulting in slower elimination of drug, lower dosage should be used in elderly patients.

Concurrent disease

Epileptics. Sulpiride may be prescribed in patients with stabilized epilepsy receiving anti-convulsant therapy. Dosage of the latter medication should remain unchanged.

Patients with renal insufficiency. Since sulpiride is mainly eliminated through the renal pathway, dosage should be decreased and frequency of administration eventually readjusted in patients suffering from this disorder.

Drug interactions

Potentially hazardous interactions
There are no clinical published or unpublished reports of specific potentially hazardous interactions between sulpiride and other drugs. As with other compounds in this therapeutic class, however, precautions include use with antihypertensive medication and CNS depressants, including hypnotics, tranquillizers, neuroleptics, anaesthetics and analgesics.

Potentially useful interactions
Combined use with tricyclic antidepressants (clomipramine, amitriptyline) has been described as being useful in treatment of severe depression.[58,59]

Major outcome trials

1. Harnryd C, Bjerkenstedt L, Bjork K, Gullberg B, Oxenstierna G 1984 Clinical evaluation of sulpiride in schizophrenic patients. A double blind comparison with chlorpromazine. Acta Psychiatrica Scandinavica 69 (suppl 311): 7–30

The authors carried out a double-blind randomized trial comparing sulpiride and chlorpromazine for treatment of acute psychotic episodes in 50 schizophrenic patients who received fixed doses of either 800 mg of sulpiride or 400 mg of chlorpromazine daily for 8 weeks. CPRS (Comprehensive Psychopathology Rating Scale) scores for global morbidity, psychotic and depressive symptoms and global NOSIE (Nursing Observation Scale for Inpatient Evaluation) ratings improved significantly for both groups of patients at all rating periods (1, 2, 4 and 8 weeks), although improvement at 1 week was significantly more pronounced with sulpiride. A significant reduction in the CPRS autistic symptoms score occurred at all rating periods for patients treated with sulpiride, but was noted only at week 4 in patients receiving chlorpromazine. Extrapyramidal adverse reactions occurred at similar frequency in both treatment groups. Autonomic adverse effects, however, tended to be lower with sulpiride. ALT serum levels significantly increased above normal levels in chlorpromazine-treated patients. Prolactin levels were elevated in both groups but were higher in patients receiving sulpiride. No women in either group complained of amenorrhoea. Lactation occurred in four of fifteen women treated with sulpiride.

2. Yura R, Kato Y, Shibahara Y et al 1976 A double-blind comparative study of the effects of sulpiride and imipramine on depression. Clinical Psychiatry 18 (5): 89–102

The authors conducted a comparative double-blind trial of sulpiride and imipramine in 149 out-patients, who in a majority of cases were diagnosed as having moderating severe neurotic depression. Medication was prescribed according to a flexible dosage schedule of 150–450 mg of sulpiride or 30–90 mg of imipramine daily for three weeks. Similar improvement in global severity scores occurred in both groups. Physician and patients ratings of depressed mood and depressive ideation were more markedly improved at 1 and 2 weeks in sulpiride patients. Adverse effects, notably vertigo, were observed more often in patients treated with imipramine.

3. Alfredsson G, Bjerkenstedt L, Edman G, Harnryd C, Oxenstierna G, Sedvall G, Wiesel F A 1984 Relationships between drug concentrations in serum and CSF, clinical effects and monoaminergic variables in schizophrenic patients treated with sulpiride or chlorpromazine. Acta Psychiatrica Scandinavica (Suppl) 311: 49–74

Schizophrenic patients were treated with fixed doses of sulpiride (800 mg) or chloropromazine (400 mg) during eight weeks using a double-blind design, in order to examine relationships between pharmacokinetic, clinical and biochemical parameters. During steady state, concentrations of sulpiride in serum varied fourfold between patients and CPZ twentyfold. Drug concentrations in serum and CSF were highly correlated in CPZ- but not in sulpiride-treated patients. In the sulpiride group, improvement of psychotic morbidity and HVA elevation in CSF tended to be negatively related to the drug concentrations in serum. In CPZ-treated patients, improvement of psychotic morbidity, HVA elevation and prolactin elevation all tended to be positively correlated to drug concentrations in serum and CSF. CPZ-treated patients with extrapyramidal side effects also had significantly higher CPZ concentrations in serum. In both treatment groups, the MOPEG reduction in CSF tended to be correlated to improvement of psychotic morbidity. In the schizophrenic patients studied and with the doses used, sulpiride concentrations tended to be maximal with regard to clinical and biochemical effects. For CPZ on the other hand, drug concentrations in some patients seemed to be too low to induce optimal effects.

4. Lepola U, Koskinen T, Romon R, Salo H, Gordin A 1989 Sulpiride and perphenazine in schizophrenia. A double-blind clinical trial. Acta Psychiatrica Scandinavica 80: 92–6

This was a randomized, double-blind parallel-group trial in 17 patients with acute and 30 with chronic schizophrenia. Patients were evaluated using the 16-item Brief Psychiatric Rating Scale (BPRS) prior to the onset of treatment and 1 and 2 weeks, and 1, 2, 3, and 4 months thereafter. In patients with acute schizophrenia, total BPRS scores declined significantly at the end of the trial compared with pretreatment values in sulpiride-treated patients but not in those treated with perphenazine but the differences was not statistically significant. A statistically significant decline was observed in total BPRS for patients suffering from chronic schizophrenia, in both treatment groups.

See references 25, 26, 60–64 for other clinical trials in schizophrenia, depression and psychosomatic and functional disorders.

References

1. Jenner P, Marsden C D 1981 Substituted benzamide drugs as selective neuroleptic. Neuropharmacology 20: 1285–1293
2. Kebabian J W, Calne D B 1979 Multiple receptors for dopamine. Nature 277: 93–96
3. Elliot P N C, Jenner P, Huizing G, Marsden C D, Miller R 1977 Substituted benzamides as cerebral dopamine antagonists in rodents. Neuropharmacology 16: 333–342
4. Scatton B 1982 Effects of dopamine agonists and neuroleptic agents on striatal acetylcholine transmission in the rat: evidence agonist dopamine receptor multiplicity. Journal of Pharmacology and Experimental Therapeutics 220: 197
5. Chang R S L, Tran V T, Snyder S H 1978 Histamine H1-receptors in brain labelled with ^{3}H-mépyramine. European Journal of Pharmacology 4: 463–464
6. Leyson J E 1981 In vitro binding of neuroleptic receptors. In: Usdin E, Dahl S G, Gram L F, Lingjaerde O (eds) Clinical pharmacology in psychiatry. Macmillan Publishers Ltd, London
7. Greenberg D A, U'Prichard D C, Snyder S H 1965 Alpha-noradrenergic receptor binding in mammalian brain: differential labelling of agonist and antagonist states. Life Sciences 19: 69–76
8. Laduron P M, Verwimp M, Leysen J E 1979 Stereospecific in vitro binding of ^{3}H-dexetimide to brain muscarinic receptors. Journal of Neurochemistry 32: 421–427
9. Westerink B H C 1978 Effects of centrally acting drugs on regional dopamine metabolism. Advances in Biochemical Psychopharmacology 19: 255–266
10. Yoshida M, Yokoo H, Kojima H, Suetake K, Anraku S, Ianaga K 1981 The acute effects of sulpiride on the central dopamine turnover in rats: a quantitative histochemical study. Experientia 37: 491–492
11. Sokoloff P, Martres M P, Schwartz J C 1980 Three classes of dopamine receptor (D2, D3, D4) identified by binding studies with ^{3}H apomorphine and ^{3}H domperidone. Naunyn Schmiedeberg's Archives of Pharmacology 315: 89–102
12. Protais P, Costentin J, Schwartz J L 1976 Climbing behavior induced by apomorphine in mice: a simple test for the study of dopamine receptors in striatum. Psychopharmacology 50: 1–6
13. Tagliamonte A, de Montis G, Glianas M, Vargiu L, Corsini G U, Gessa G L 1975 Selective increase of brain dopamine synthesis by sulpiride. Journal of Neurochemistry 24: 707–710
14. Laville C, Margarit J 1968 Influence du sulpiride sur l'activité et vigilance chez la souris. Pathologie Biologie 16; nos 11–12, pp 13–14
15. Honda F, Satoh Y, Shimomura K et al 1977 Dopamine receptor blocking activity of sulpiride in the central nervous system. Japanese Journal of Pharmacology 27: 397–411
16. Costall B, Naylor R 1977 Behavioural characterization of neuroleptic properties in the rodent. Proceedings of the Royal Society of Medicine 70 (suppl 10): 5–14
17. Boissier J R, Puech A J, Simon P 1977 Action of a classic and unusual neuroleptics on various behavioural apomorphine-induced effects. In: Costa E, Gessa G L (eds) Advances in biochemical psychopharmacology, vol 16. Raven Press, New York, pp 631–634
18. Jenner P, Davis A, Kilpatrick G, Rupniak N M, Chivers J K, Marsden C D 1985 Selective interactions of sulpiride with brain dopamine receptors. In: Schiff A A, Sir Martin Roth, Freeman H L (eds) Schizophrenia: new pharmacological and clinical developments. Royal Society of Medicine Services Limited, London, International Congress and Symposium Series, No 94, pp 51–64
19. Haggstrom J E 1984 Effects of sulpiride on persistent neuroleptic-induced dyskinesia in monkeys. Acta Psychiatrica Scandinavica 69 (suppl 311): 103–108
20. Laville C, Margarit J 1968 Activité antiémétique du sulpiride vis-à-vis des divers poisons émétisants chez le chien. Compte-rendus de la Société de Biologie 162: 869–874
21. Kobayashi T, Murayama S, Kuga T, Takemoto M, Sano K 1968 Pharmacological study on Dogmatil (sulpiride). Ve Congress on therapeutic research on new drugs, Tokyo, pp 59–66
22. Semba T, Fujii K, Ooya S 1968 Influence of Dogmatil (sulpiride) on gastric movement and gastric blood circulation. Ve Congress on therapeutic research on new drugs. Tokyo, pp 48–58
23. Strocchi P, Gandolfi O, Montanaro N 1976 Effect of single and repeated administration of sulpiride on the restraint ulcer in the rat. Arzneimittelforschung (Drug Research) 26: 419–421
24. Harnryd C, Bjerkenstedt L, Bjork K, Gullberg B, Oxenstierna G 1984 Clinical evaluation of sulpiride in schizophrenic patients. A double blind comparision with chlorpromazine. Acta Psychiatrica Scandinavica 69 (suppl 311): 7–30
25. Bratfos O, Haug J O 1979 Comparison of sulpiride and chlorpromazine in psychoses. A double blind multicenter study. Acta Psychiatrica Scandinavica 60: 1–9
26. Gerlach J, Behnke K, Heltberg J, Munk-Andersen E, Nielsen H 1985 Sulpiride and halperidol in schizophrenia: a double-blind cross-over study of therapeutic effect, side effects and plasma concentrations. British Journal of Psychiatry 147: 283–288
27. Sugano K, Yoshida S, Suzuki S, Sato S, Takaesu Y, Ichihashi H 1973 Clinical application of sulpiride for schizophrenics. Medical Consultation and New Remedies 10 (11): 52 pp
28. Zann M, Colonna L, Petit M, Lesieur P 1986 Etude contrôlée de l'effet désinhibiteur du sulpiride chez 18 patients hébéphrènes. Psychologie Médicale 18: 560–570
29. Yura R, Kato Y, Shibahara Y et al 1976 A double-blind comparative study of the effects of sulpiride and imipramine on depression. Clinical Psychiatry 18: 89–102
30. Harnryd C, Bjerkenstedt L, Gullberg B, Oxenstierna G, Sedvall G, Wiesel F A 1984 Time course for effects of sulpiride and chlorpromazine on monoamine metabolite and prolactin levels in cerebrospinal fluid from schizophrenic patients. Acta Psychiatrica Scandinavica 69 (suppl 311): 75–92
31. Sugnaux F 1983 Dose-dependent pharmacokinetics of sulpiride and sulpiride induced prolactin secretion in man. European Journal of Drug Metabolism and Pharmacokinetics 8: 189–190
32. Liljequist R, Linnoila M, Mattila M J, Sarrio I, Seppala C 1975 Effect of two weeks treatment with thloridazine, chlorpromazine, sulpiride and bromazepam, alone or in combination with alcohol, on learning and memory in man. Psychopharmacologia 44: 205–208
33. Wiesel F A, Alfredson G, Ehrnebo M, Sedvall G 1980 The pharmacokinetics of intravenous and oral sulpiride in healthy human subjects. European Journal of Clinical Pharmacology 17: 385–391
34. Sugnaux F 1982 Investigation of sulpiride and its metabolites in the hypophysis of rats. European Journal of Mass Spectrometry in Biochemical Medicine and Environmental Research 2: 1–12
35. Bressolle F, Bres J 1985 Dosage du sulpiride et du sultopride par chromatographie liquide à haute performance en vue de leur étude pharmacocinétique. Journal of Chromatography 341: 391–399
36. Alfredsson G, Bjerkenstedt L, Edman G et al 1982 Relationships between drug concentrations in serum and CSF, clinical effects and monoaminergic variables in schizophrenic patients treated with sulpiride or chlorpromazine. Acta Psychiatrica Scandinavica 69 (suppl 311): 49–74
37. Imondi A R, Alam A S, Brennan J J, Hagerman L M 1977 Sulpiride metabolism in rhesus monkeys and man. Federation Proceedings 36: Abstract No. 4005
38. Imondi A R, Alam A S, Brennan J J, Hagerman L M 1978 Metabolism of sulpiride in man and rhesus monkeys. Archives Internationale de Pharmacodynamie et de Thérapie 232: 79–91
39. Bressolle F, Bres J, Blanchin M D, Gomeni R 1984 Sulpiride: pharmacokinetics in humans after intramuscular administration at three dose levels. Journal of Pharmaceutical Sciences 73 (8): 1128–1136
40. Bressolle F, Bres J, Faure A 1984 Pharmacocinétiques phasmatique, érythrocytaire et urinaire du sulpiride chez l'Homme. In: Aiache J M, Hirtz J (eds) 2ème Congrès Européen de Biopharmacie et de Pharmacocinétique, Salamanque, Proceeding. Imprimerie de l'Université de Clermont-Ferrand vol 3, pp 287–304
41. Wiesel F A, Alfredsson G, Ehrnebo M, Sedvall G 1980 The pharmacokinetics of intravenous and oral sulpiride in healthy human subjects. European Journal of Clinical Pharmacology 17: 385–391
42. Alam A S, Imondi A R, Udinski J, Hagerman L M 1979 Bioavailability of ^{14}C-sulpiride in dogs. Archives Internationales de Pharmacodynamie 242: 4–13
43. Bertrand P, Gros R, Tandia L 1982 Dosage du sulpiride dans le lait maternel. Compte-rendu thérapeutique de pharmacie clinique 1: 27–31
44. Alfredsson G, Harnryd C, Wiesel F A 1985 Effects of sulpiride and chlorpromazine on autistic and positive psychotic symptoms in schizophrenic patients — relationship to drug concentrations. Psychopharmacology 85: 8–13
45. Plans C, Tallada N, Yetano V, Morera J 1977 Muerte subita en un caso de feocromocitoma latente desencadenada por sulpiride. Revista Clinical Espanola 152: 327–329
46. Shalev A, Munitz H 1986 The neuroleptic malignant syndrome: agent and host interaction. Acta Psychiatrica Scandinavica 73: 337–347
47. Frejaville J P, Jouglard J 1973 Les surdosages en sulpiride. XIIIéme Journée des Centres Anti-Poisons, Marseille, 1–2 octobre
48. Gaultier M, Frejaville J P 1973 A propos de 20 surdosages en sulpiride. Journal Européen de Toxicologie 6: 42–44
49. Gekiere F, Borenstein P 1981 Dépressions et benzamides. In: Dépression et suicide. Pergamon Press, pp 797–802
50. Bourgeois M, Graux C, Arrethche-Berthelot N 1976 Les dyskinésies tardives des neuroleptiques. Enquête sur 1660 malades d'hôpital psychiatrique. Annales Médicales Psychologiques 1: 737–746
51. Jouhet P, Jouhet D 1981 A propos de l'affinité des neuroleptiques pour les différents récepteurs dopaminergiques (pré- et post-synaptiques) et des éventuelles orientations thérapeutiques qui en découlent. Actualités Psychiatriques 11: 87–92
52. Pollak P, Gaio J M 1984 Synthèse sur les effets extrapyramidaux des neuroleptiques. Congrès de Psychiatrie et de Neurologie de Langue Francaise, LXXXIIème session — Luxembourg, Rapport de neurologie, Masson Editeur, Paris, pp 103–111
53. Alberts J L, Francois F, Josserand F 1985 Etudes des effets secondaires rapportés à l'occasion de traitements par Dogmatil. Semaine des Hôpitaux de Paris 61: 1351–1357
54. Mielke D H, Gallant D M, Kessler C 1977 An evaluation of a unique new antipsychotic agent, sulpiride: effects on serum prolactin and growth hormone levels. American Journal of Psychiatry 134: 1371–1375
55. Dubois B, Balmelle J, Fontaine G 1970 Intérêt du sulpiride en pédiatrie. Semaine des Hôpitaux de Paris 46: 87–92
56. Gil M 1973 Le sulpiride dans les troubles du caractère et du comportement de l'adolescent(e). Sciences Médicales 4: 409–416
57. Pallegoix J, Chavanne J 1973 Contribution à l'emploi du sulpiride dans un service de psychiatrie infantile. Revue de Neuropsychiatrie Infantile 21: 379–383
58. Bouvier C, Masquin A, Amieux M C 1971 Indications psychiatriques du sulpiride. A propos de 60 observations. Journal Médical Lyonnais 52: 519–533
59. Masquin A 1972 Association du Dogmatil et de l'anafranil dans le traitement des mélancolies. Information Psychiatrique 48: 218–219
60. Edwards J G, Alexander J R, Alexander M S, Gordon A, Zutchi T 1980 Controlled trial of sulpiride in chronic schizophrenic patients. British Journal of Psychiatry 137: 522–529

61. Viskanen P, Tamminen T, Viukari M 1975 Sulpiride versus amitriptyline in the treatment of depression. Current Therapeutic Research 17: 281
62. Aylward M, Maddock J, Dewland P M, Lewis P A 1981 Sulpiride in depressive illness. Advances in Biological Psychiatry 7: 154–165
64. Kawano M, Nozoe S, Yamanaka T et al 1975 Evaluation of sulpiride effects on neurosis and psychosomatic diseases by double-blind method. Japanese Journal of Clinical and Experimental Medicine 52: 304–316

Sumatriptan (succinate)

Sumatriptan is a 5-hydroxytryptamine 1-like (5-HT_1-like) receptor agonist used in the treatment of migraine.

Chemistry

Sumatriptan succinate (Imigran)
$C_{14}H_{21}N_3O_2S.C_4H_6O_4$
3-[2-(Dimethylamino)ethyl]-N-methyl-1H-indole-5-methane sulphonamide, butane-1,4-dioate (1:1)

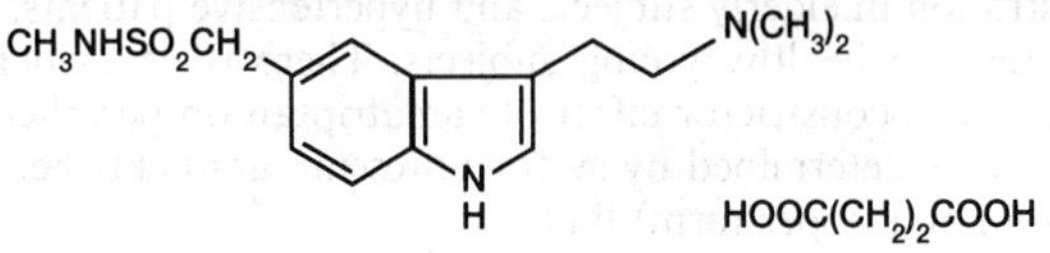

Molecular weight (free base)	413.5 (295.4)
pKa	—
Solubility	
in alcohol	—
in water (saline)	1 in 10
Octanol/water partition coefficient (pH 10.7)	12.0

Solubility in saline (0.9% w/v) approximately 109 $mg.ml^{-1}$ at 20°C (sumatriptan base).

Sumatriptan is a white to off-white powder prepared by chemical synthesis. It is not available in any combination products.

Pharmacology

Sumatriptan is a specific and selective 5-hydroxytryptamine 1-like (5HT_1-like) receptor agonist with little or no effect at a variety of other receptor types.[1] This receptor is found predominantly in cranial blood vessels and, in animals, sumatriptan selectively constricts the carotid arterial circulation which supplies blood to the extracranial and intracranial tissues such as the meninges. Thus, the main action of the drug is to produce a dose-related vasoconstriction in the cerebral circulation. However, there is a small degree of vasoconstriction in other territories such as the coronary arteries. Sumatriptan does not bind to α-adrenergic, β-adrenergic, muscarinic, dopaminergic or benzodiazepine receptors.

Toxicology

Sumatriptan has been administered to a variety of species by the intravenous, subcutaneous and oral routes. The results of the toxicity studies revealed nothing to contraindicate the use of sumatriptan in man.

Near life-time exposure to sumatriptan did not induce a treatment-related increase in the incidence of any tumour in either mice or rats.

Sumatriptan produced no detectable or reproducible increases in genotoxic activity in a range of studies using either prokaryotic or eukaryotic cell systems in vitro or in vivo in the rat.

Sumatriptan showed no adverse effects on any aspects of reproduction in animals.

Clinical pharmacology

The pathophysiology of migraine is poorly understood and, other than cerebral blood flow and gastric emptying, there are no objective pharmacodynamic parameters which might reflect the therapeutic efficacy of sumatriptan. The majority of the clinical pharmacology studies have therefore focused on the safety and tolerability of the drug, evaluating cardiovascular and central nervous system effects.

No conclusive effects of sumatriptan, on cerebral blood flow were seen in healthy subjects.

Sumatriptan caused a small but statistically significant delay in gastric emptying. This finding was unexpected and opposite to results obtained in animal studies. As relief of nausea and vomiting is evident in patient studies, this would suggest that effects on gastric emptying are not critical in the relief of migraine symptoms by sumatriptan.

Psychomotor tests performed after oral administration of sumatriptan to healthy subjects did not demonstrate any significant sedative effects.

Sumatriptan, after both subcutaneous and oral administration, resulted in an increase in systolic (SBP) and diastolic blood pressure (DBP). Increases were short-lasting and of rapid onset, after subcutaneous dosing, but with no clearly defined dose-response relationships.

After oral dosing, there is a less well defined vasopressor effect, of slower onset, with peak increases being smaller than after parenteral administration. Repeated subcutaneous treatment, for five days or oral dosing for seven days did not result in a cumulative effect on blood pressure. Increases in blood pressure after subcutaneous administration in elderly subjects and hypertensive patients, were no greater than in healthy young subjects. There is no evidence of a significant vasoconstrictor effect of sumatriptan on peripheral arteries in man, as determined by systolic pressure gradients between the lower (toe) and upper (arm) limbs.[2]

Dilatation of meningeal vessels with an accompanying localized inflammatory response is thought to be the underlying mechanism of migraine.[3] Sumatriptan has been shown to inhibit the localized inflammatory response in the meninges in response to activation of the trigeminal nerve.[4] Such activation may result from a localized vasoconstriction of dural blood vessels which has been demonstrated in human tissue.[5]

Pharmacokinetics

Sumatriptan and its principal metabolite (Fig. 1) are determined in plasma, urine and other biological fluids by reversed-phase high performance liquid chromatography (HPLC) with either electrochemical detection (sumatriptan) or U.V. detection (metabolite). A sensitivity of 1 $mg.l^{-1}$ is obtained using plasma samples.

Sumatriptan is rapidly absorbed after both subcutaneous and oral dosing; has a plasma half life of about 2 h; has approximately 100% subcutaneous bioavailability and approximately 14% oral bioavailability; is eliminated primarily by metabolism and has similar pharmacokinetics in healthy young subjects, healthy elderly subjects and migraine patients.

Sumatriptan is rapidly absorbed after subcutaneous dosing into the deltoid region of the arm, with maximum plasma concentrations (C_{max}) occurring 5–25 minutes after dosing. The mean subcutaneous absolute bioavailability is 96%, with a range of 68–134%. The pharmacokinetics of sumatriptan are linear over the subcutaneous dose range 1–16 mg. Subcutaneous administration of sumatriptan into the thigh results in a small decrease in rate but not extent of absorption of drug when compared to administration into the arm.

Sumatriptan is rapidly absorbed after oral dosing and frequently displays more than one peak plasma concentration. This 'multiple peaking' gives rise to considerable intersubject variability in time to C_{max} (0.5–5.0 hours).

However, it should be noted that mean values of between 70% and 80% of C_{max} are obtained at 30–45 minutes after dosing. Food has no effects on the absorption of sumatriptan. The mean absolute oral bioavailability of sumatriptan is 14%, with a range of 10–26%. This low systemic availability is due mainly to presystemic metabolism but is also due to incomplete absorption. With the exception of rate of absorption, the pharmacokinetics of sumatriptan are linear over the oral dose range 25–400 mg.

Plasma protein binding of sumatriptan is low (14–21%) and therefore displacement interactions with other drugs are unlikely to occur.

After parenteral administration, sumatriptan concentrations initially decline very rapidly in plasma, with a mean distribution half life of about 5 min. Sumatriptan has a mean apparent volume of distribution, once distribution equilibrium has been attained, of 170 l, suggesting that it has a greater affinity for tissue than for plasma. Once distribution is complete the mean plasma half life is about 2 h. Up to 12 h after oral dosing, the mean sumatriptan plasma half life is also about 2 h. However, at later times, a longer terminal half life is evident with a mean value of 7.3 h. This longer half life makes only a minor contribution to the disposition of the drug.

The mean total plasma clearance of sumatriptan is approximately 1.2 $l.min^{-1}$ and the mean renal plasma clearance is approximately 260 $ml.min^{-1}$ (ie. about 20% of the total). The renal clearance of sumatriptan is considerably greater than the glomerular filtration rate (120 $ml.min^{-1}$) indicating that sumatriptan undergoes active renal tubular secretion. The non-renal clearance accounts for about 80% of the total clearance, suggesting that sumatriptan is eliminated primarily by metabolism.

Oral absorption	rapid, incomplete
Presystemic metabolism	high
Plasma half life	
mean	2 h
Volume of distribution	170 l
Plasma protein binding	14–21%

No information is available on the excretion of sumatriptan in breast milk, though in animals such excretion does occur. It is not known whether the drug crosses the placenta. The pharmacokinetics of subcutaneous and oral sumatriptan in healthy elderly subjects are similar to those in healthy young subjects. Similarly, the pharmacokinetics of subcutaneous sumatriptan in mainly female migraine patients are similar to those in healthy male subjects. In comparison with administration of oral sumatriptan to patients during a pain-free period, administration of drug to patients during a migraine attack results in a slight decrease in the mean rate and extent of absorption of drug. The magnitude of this effect is small and, though consistent for each dose level, does not reach statistical significance for c_{max} or AUC and is not considered to be of any clinical consequence.

Although specific information is not available, it is possible that plasma concentrations of sumatriptan may be elevated in patients with severe hepatic impairment, whereas in those with renal dysfunction no marked change in the kinetics of drug are anticipated.

Concentration–effect relationship

There is no evidence concerning any correlation between the plasma concentration of sumatriptan (or its metabolites) and the therapeutic effect.

Metabolism

The major metabolite of sumatriptan is the indole acetic acid analogue (Fig. 1) which is excreted mainly in the urine, where it is present as both the free acid and as a glucuronide conjugate.

Fig. 1 Indole acetic acid analogue: the major metabolite of sumatriptan

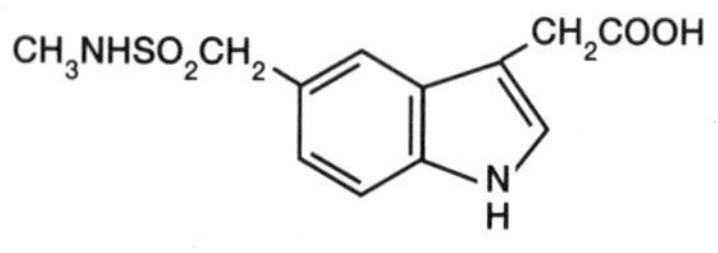

After oral dosing, plasma concentrations of the major metabolite are 6–7 times greater than those of parent drug. This is due, at least in part, to presystemic metabolism of sumatriptan. The major metabolite has a similar mean plasma half life to sumatriptan indicating that its clearance is greater than or equal to that of the parent drug. The indole acetic acid analogue of sumatriptan has no 5-HT_1 or 5-HT_2 activity when tested in vitro.

Pharmaceutics

Tablet: Tablets containing 100 mg sumatriptan as the succinate salt. Subcutaneous injection: Prefilled glass syringes containing 0.5 ml of an isotonic solution of 6 mg of sumatriptan as the succinate salt. These syringes may be used independently or with an autoinjector device.

Sumatriptan (succinate)

Therapeutic use

Indications

1. Acute treatment of migraine
2. Acute treatment of cluster headache.

Contraindications

1. Hypersensitivity to sumatriptan
   Relative:
2. Ischaemic heart disease
3. Hypertension.

Mode of use

The recommended adult dose of sumatriptan injection is 6 mg, injected subcutaneously. A second injection may be required in migraine headache during the next 24 h, but at least one hour should elapse before the second dose is administered. The maximum dose in 24 h is therefore two 6 mg injections (12 mg). The subcutaneous injection may be given by medical personnel or by the patient using an autoinjection device.

Oral treatment is usually initiated with a single 100 mg tablet, although further tablets may be given during the next 24 h to a total daily dose of 300 mg.

Sumatriptan is best given as early as possible after the onset of an attack or prodromal warning, although it can still be used with effect at a later stage in the attack.

Indications

1. Migraine

Sumatriptan is used as an acute treatment for migraine. It provides relief of both the headache and other symptoms such as nausea and photophobia. It may also relieve vomiting. When given subcutaneously, sumatriptan starts to act within 10 min and achieves its maximum effect at 90–120 min. A 6 mg dose is effective in more than 80% of patients. Oral administration leads to a slower onset of effect — with improvement detected at 30 min and maximum response at 2–4 h. Sumatriptan is intended to be used as an acute treatment for migraine — its efficacy as a prophylactic agent for the reduction of attack frequency has not been tested.

2. Cluster headache

Sumatriptan given subcutaneously as a 6 mg dose, will relieve the severe acute pain of a cluster headache attack. Pain relief and resolution of the associated ipsilateral conjunctival injection, occurs within 5–15 min of administration of the drug. There is no data available yet on the prevention of cluster attacks by repeat dosing with sumatriptan.

Contraindications

2. Ischaemic heart disease

In early clinical trials when sumatriptan was administered by intravenous injection, adverse events suggestive of myocardial ischaemia were seen in a small number of patients. In two cases these were associated with new ischaemic ECG changes, one of changes indicative of coronary vasospasm and the other of non-specific T-wave changes. No such cases have occurred after sumatriptan was given by the subcutaneous or oral routes. Sumatriptan should not therefore be given intravenously. In patients with a history of ischaemic heart disease, Prinzmetal or variant angina, sumatriptan should only be given if the potential benefits clearly outweigh the risks. In such patients the first 2–3 treatments should be given under continuous medical supervision with facilities for ECG monitoring.

3. Hypertension

Transient increases in blood pressure, have been observed in a small number of patients and healthy volunteers. Sumatriptan should therefore be administered with great caution to patients with severe hypertension.

Adverse reactions

Potentially life-threatening effects

There have been no deaths caused by sumatriptan. As discussed above, there have been two cases of myocardial ischaemia with associated ECG changes after intravenous administration.

Acute overdosage

Three cases of accidental overdosage with sumatriptan are known. However, the overdosage was minimal (up to twice the maximum recommended daily dose) and only 1 patient experienced an adverse event. This was severe burning on the forehead and it resolved spontaneously within 90 min.

There is no specific antidote for sumatriptan. In the case of significant overdosage, standard supportive treatment should be provided and the patient's blood pressure and ECG should be monitored for at least 10 h. Vasodilator therapy might be required.

Severe or irreversible adverse effects

One case of transient atrioventricular dissociation with bradycardia and possible syncope lasting one to two min, occurred shortly after subcutaneous administration of 3 mg sumatriptan to a patient with a history of stress-related syncope. No other conduction disturbance occurred more commonly after sumatriptan than after placebo.

A dystonic reaction has been reported though the sequence of events suggested tetany secondary to hyperventilation.

Symptomatic adverse effects

The most common symptomatic effect associated with treatment with sumatriptan administered subcutaneously is transient pain at the site of injection. Other adverse effects which have been reported include the following: sensations of tingling, heat, heaviness, pressure or tightness in any part of the body, flushing, dizziness and feelings of weakness. These are mostly mild to moderate in intensity and transient (resolved within 1 h). Fatigue and drowsiness have been reported. Nausea and vomiting occurred in some patients, but the relationship of sumatriptan is not clear. Transient increases in blood pressure arising soon after treatment have been recorded.

Although direct comparisons are not available, nausea, vomiting and fatigue appear to be less frequent with subcutaneous administration of sumatriptan than with tablets. Conversely, flushing and sensations of tingling, heat, pressure and heaviness may be more common after the injection.

Other effects

Sumatriptan does not cause clinically significant abnormalities in haematology, clinical chemistry, or urinalysis tests. Small, but statistically significant elevations in the mean values of liver function tests have occurred in a few trials, though most increases were within the normal range.

Interference with clinical pathology tests

No such interferences have been reported.

High risk groups

Neonates

There is no experience of use of the drug in neonates.

Breast milk. Sumatriptan is excreted in breast milk in animals. No data exist in humans, so it is best for mothers taking the drug not to breast-feed.

Children

There is no experience with sumatriptan use in children.

Pregnant women

Thirteen pregnancies have been reported in patients taking sumatriptan. No abnormalities have been seen in the babies delivered to date. Though sumatriptan is not teratogenic in rabbits or rats, its use in pregnancy should be considered only if the benefits are expected to outweigh the possible risks to the fetus.

The elderly

There is little experience with the use of sumatriptan in the elderly. As older patients are more likely to suffer from ischaemic heart disease this contraindication needs to be borne in mind. Use is therefore not recommended until further data becomes available.

Concurrent details

Hepatic impairment. Migraine patients treated with sumatriptan and who have hepatic impairment may be exposed to higher drug concentrations than those with normal hepatic function. Caution should therefore be exercised in treating such patients with this drug.

Renal impairment. The total plasma clearance of sumatriptan in anuric patients would be expected to be approximately 80% of that in patients with normal renal function and as a result, sumatriptan plasma concentrations should only increase by about 25% in total renal failure.

Ischaemic heart disease and hypertension. (see under Contraindications)

Drug interactions

Potentially hazardous interactions

As the drug has occasionally caused drowsiness, patients taking other drugs having this effect should be warned to take care when driving or using dangerous machinery.

Other significant interactions

Food. Food does not significantly affect the oral bioavailability of sumatriptan.

Alcohol. Alcohol does not significantly affect the pharmacokinetic or pharmacodynamic profile of sumatriptan.

Potentially useful interactions

None has been reported.

Clinical trials

Migraine

1. Byer J, Gutterman D L, Plachetka J R, Bhattacharyya H 1989 Dose response study for subcutaneous GR43 175 in the treatment of acute migraine. cephalalgia 9 suppl 10, 349–410

This was a placebo-controlled, double-blind, dose-ranging study of subcutaneous sumatriptan 1–8 mg in the acute treatment of migraine in 242 patients. All doses of sumatriptan gave better headache relief than placebo with a clear increase in response rate with increasing dose. A 6 mg injection was found to offer the best combination of efficacy and tolerability.

2. The Subcutaneous Sumatriptan International Study Group 1990 Effective treatment of migraine attacks with subcutaneous sumatriptan. (data on file Glaxo)

In this double-blind study in 639 patients, 6 mg, 6 mg + 6 mg, 8 mg and placebo were compared. The value of a 6 + 6 mg regimen with the doses given 1 hour apart was also compared to 6 mg + placebo. Significant headache relief was seen in 86 to 92% of the actively-treated patients, with between 59 and 72% pain free by two h. The additional benefits of a second dose, or a higher initial dose of 8 mg were minimal compared to a single 6 mg dose.

3. The Sumatriptan Autoinjector Study Group 1990 Self treatment of acute migraine with subcutaneous sumatriptan using an autoinjector. (data on file Glaxo)

235 patients treated a migraine attack at home with either 6 mg subcutaneous sumatriptan or placebo using an autoinjector device. The trial was randomized and double-blind. Efficacy rates were comparable to those seen in a clinic setting in other trials with 83% of the sumatriptan group having headache relief within 2 h. Self injection proved highly acceptable to the patients and no unexpected side effects occurred.

4. Dahlof C, Winter P, Ludlow S 1989 Oral GR43 175, a 5HT1-like agonist for treatment of the acute migraine attack: an international study — preliminary results. Cephalalgia 9 suppl 10: 351–352

This interim analysis was conducted on data from 624 patients of the 1188 recruited into the parallel-group, placebo-controlled comparison of 100 mg, 200 mg and 300 mg of oral sumatriptan. Headache relief was obtained in 67–75% of the sumatriptan-treated groups compared to 22% on placebo. There was no clear dose response relationship for efficacy though adverse events did increase with dose.

5. The S2BT25 Sumatriptan International Study Group 1990 A randomized double-blind comparison of sumatriptan and Cafergot in the acute treatment of migraine. (data on file Glaxo)

592 patients participated in this comparative trial of sumatriptan, 100 mg oral versus Cafergot. Sumatriptan gave significantly greater headache relief rates than Cafergot (66% of patients responding vs 48% $p<0.001$). Sumatriptan also gave significantly better improvement of nausea and photophobia than Cafergot. More adverse events were reported after sumatriptan than Cafergot but this excess was largely due to reports of bad taste due to the dispersible tablet used in the trial. This dispersible tablet has since been replaced by a film coated tablet with no taste.

Cluster headache

1. Sumatriptan Cluster Headache Study Group 1990 Acute treatment of cluster headache with subcutaneous sumatriptan. (data on file Glaxo)

49 patients participated in this double-blind cross over comparison of 6 mg sumatriptan and placebo. One cluster attack was treated with each treatment within 10 min of its onset. Sumatriptan gave a higher headache relief rate from 5 min onwards and this superiority achieved statistical significance at 10 min. By 15 min 74% of sumatriptan-treated attacks had improved compared to 26% after placebo. Ipsilateral conjunctival injection, one feature of the associated autonomic dysfunction of cluster headache, also resolved after sumatriptan treatment.

Other trials

Oral Sumatriptan and Aspirin plus Metoclopramide Comparative Study Group 1990 A study to compare oral sumatriptan with oral aspirin plus metoclopramide in the acute treatment of migraine (data on file Glaxo)

References

1. Peroutka S J, McCarthey B G 1989 Sumatriptan (GR43 175C) interacts selectively with $5HT_{1B}$ and $5HT_{1D}$ binding sites. European Journal of Pharmacology 163: 133–136
2. Nielson T H, Tfelt-Hansen P 1989 Lack of effect of GR43 175 on peripheral arteries in man. Cephalalgia (suppl 9): 93–95
3. Moskowitz M A 1984 The neurobiology of vascular head pain. Annals of Neurology 16: 157–168
4. Buzzi M G, Moskowitz M A 1990 The anti-migraine drug, sumatriptan (GR43 175), selectively blocks neurogenic plasma extravasation in dura mater. British Journal of Pharmacology 99: 202–206
5. Humphrey P P A, Feniuk W, Motevalian M, Parsons, Whalley A A 1991 The vasoconstrictor action of sumatriptan on human dura mater. Fozard J R and Saxena P R (ed) Proceedings of the second IUPHAR satellite meeting on serotonin. Birkhäuser, Basel
6. Scott A K, Walley T, Breckenridge A M, Lacey L F, Fowler P A 1990 Lack of effect of propranolol on sumatriptan pharmacokinetics. British Journal of Clinical Pharmacology 30 (2): 332P

Suramin

Suramin was first introduced in 1920 for the treatment of trypanosomiasis following the discovery of the trypanocidal effects of trypan blue. Suramin was later found to be effective as a macrofilaricidal drug in onchocerciasis and more recently has been tried in the treatment of AIDS.

Chemistry

Suramin (Bayer-205, 309F, Antrypol, Germanin, Fourneau 309, Moranyl, Naganol, Naganin, Naphuride sodium)
$C_{51}H_{34}N_6Na_6O_{23}S_6$
8,8'-[Carbonylbis(imino-3,1-phenylenecarbonylimino(4-methyl-3,1-phenylene)carbonylimino)]bis-1,3,5-naphthalenetrisulphonic acid hexasodium salt

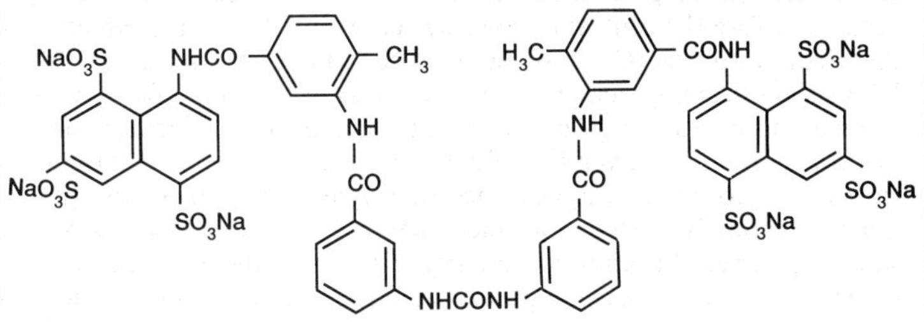

Molecular weight	1429
pKa	—
Solubility	
in alcohol	slight
in water	freely soluble
Octanol/water partition coefficient	—

Suramin is a white or slightly pink or cream-coloured powder with a slightly bitter taste prepared by chemical synthesis. It is hygroscopic. It is not available in any combination preparations.

Pharmacology

Suramin is potent inhibitor of enzymes and binds tightly to many different proteins in the body. The most sensitive enzymes examined seem to be hyalouronidase (inhibited at 10^{-6} M) and fumarase (10^{-7} M).[1] Suramin, following complexing with proteins, is taken up by lysosomes and stabilizes lysosomal membranes in the liver, kidney and placenta. Suramin also inhibits complement activation[2] and in high doses may inhibit the action of thrombin on fibrinogen. Suramin has been known to inhibit RNA polymerase for some years and this work has been re-examined in view of its potential as a treatment for AIDS. Suramin inhibits HTLV III reverse transcriptase activity but has similar activity against human DNA polymerase.[3] The mechanism of the action of suramin as an antifilarial or trypanocidal agent is not clear. However, in *Brugia pahangi* infected birds, suramin acted at the surface of the intestinal epithelium of the worms resulting in ultrastructural changes in the intestinal epilethelium.[4]

In trypanosomes, suramin progressively inhibits respiration and glycolysis by inhibition of glycerol-3-phosphate oxidase and glycerol-3-phosphate dehydrogenase.[5] In filariae, suramin does not cause inhibition of glycolysis.[4]

Toxicology

Acute toxicology testing of suramin has shown an LD_{50} in mice at 620 $mg.kg^{-1}$ after intravenous injection. The chief toxic effect is on the kidney in which it causes degeneration of the convoluted tubules.[1] In intravenous doses of 250 $mg.kg^{-1}$ to rats a state similar to mucopolysaccharidosis is induced with high concentrations of glycosaminoglycans in the liver.[6]

In chronic dosing studies using 152 mg daily for 36 days in a chimpanzee, the main toxic effects were of diarrhoea, emaciation, albuminuria and haemorrhage.

Suramin is very toxic to pregnant rats and 30 $mg.kg^{-1}$ for 12 days, which is similar to the human dose, killed 8% of mother rats. At higher doses the fetuses were killed and absorbed. Suramin is more an abortifacient in rats and does not cause malformations.[1] In mice, the fetuses are very susceptible to suramin, 60% dying after doses of 40–50 $mg.kg^{-1}$. Suramin does not cross the placenta but produces its effects by accumulating in the lysosomes of the phagocytic epithelial cells of the umbilical vesicle (which develops from the yolk sac) and this interferes with the nutrition of the embryo.[7] There is no evidence that suramin is teratogenic in man.

Clinical pharmacology

Suramin is poorly absorbed in man and is usually given by intravenous dosing. Usually a test dose of 100–200 mg is given initially followed by further intravenous doses. Suramin may cause severe nausea and vomiting though this is minimized by slow intravenous injection. Collapse, shock and sweating with loss of consciousness may occur and is more common in malnourished individuals. Collapse may occur in perhaps 1 in 2000 cases. The cause of these reactions is not known, but is probably non-specific due to the injection of a large polyanionic molecule. Fever is not unusual but consistent clinical pharmacological effects of suramin are not common. There is usually no direct effect on the cardiovascular or respiratory systems.

Pharmacokinetics

A variety of assays for suramin have been developed over the years but most of them are colorimetric assays and are insensitive and non-specific. Recently, attention has been focused on the pharmacokinetics of suramin and more modern methods of analysis have been developed. The analytical method of choice is by high performance liquid chromatography using ion pair extraction and ultraviolet detection.[8,9] The limit of detection is about 300–500 $\mu g.l^{-1}$.

Suramin is very poorly absorbed by mouth and since intramuscular or subcutaneous injections are intensely irritant suramin is practically always given by intravenous injection. After intravenous injection, suramin binds very tightly to serum proteins and 99.7% of suramin is bound in this way.[10] Suramin kinetics in plasma are best described by a two-compartment open model with an initial phase half life of between 2 and 6.5 days and a terminal half life of 36 to 60 days.[10–12] Total body clearance[10,11] is about 0.03–0.07 $l.h^{-1}$. The volume of distribution of suramin varies between 21 l.[12] and 89 l.[11] Suramin is slowly excreted unchanged by the kidney with a renal clearance[10] of 0.3 $ml.min^{-1}$. Initial concentrations of suramin in plasma are as high as 100 $mg.l^{-1}$ and remain above 20 $mg.l^{-1}$ for several weeks after a full course of therapy of 6.2 g suramin. After administration of radiolabelled suramin 12.0% of suramin was recovered in the urine over a 40-day period and 4.5% was recovered from the faeces.[11] Suramin is not concentrated in red blood cells or platelets and concentrations of suramin in cerebrospinal fluid are at most 1% of the corresponding plasma concentration.[12] Suramin does not cross the placenta but there are no data concerning its excretion in breast milk.

Oral absorption	very poor
Presystemic metabolism	not relevant
Plasma half life	
α-phase	2–6 d
β-phase	36–60 d
Volume of distribution	20–80 l
Plasma protein binding	99.7%

S

Concentration–effect relationship

There is no evidence that there is any relationship between the plasma concentration of suramin and its effect as an antifilarial or trypanocidal drug.[13] In the treatment of patients with AIDS-related complex, plasma concentrations of suramin were maintained at trough concentrations of 75–150 $mg.l^{-1}$ but there was no evidence of therapeutic efficacy or of plasma concentration relationship.[12]

Metabolism

There are very few studies of the metabolism of suramin. In the early literature it was suggested that suramin might undergo acid hydrolysis in the body but no evidence of this was seen in human studies using relatively crude methodology (by today's standards).[14] In animal studies, unidentified products of suramin from acid hydrolysis were detected but these were rapidly excreted in the urine.[15] In the more recent literature the metabolism of suramin was not studied. However in one study using ^{14}C-suramin in patients with onchocerciasis, plasma concentrations of ^{14}C were almost identical to concentrations of unchanged drug measured by high performance liquid chromatography.[11] This suggests that metabolites of suramin are not present in plasma. Metabolites of suramin could not be found in urine and excretion of suramin in urine was largely as unchanged drug.[10]

Pharmaceutics

Suramin is only available as ampoules for (intravenous) injection. Suramin injection (BPC 1973) is an ampoule of dry powder containing 1 g of suramin. It is dissolved in sterile water for injection. Although suramin is soluble in water the process of dissolution is a slow one. Manufacturers include Bayer, W. Germany (Germanin) and Specia, France (Moranyl).

The ampoules should be kept in a cool place and protected from light. In practice, the use of suramin in primitive conditions means that suramin can often not be stored in a cool place. A recent survey by a manufacturer of suramin ampoules stored in a variety of conditions (often above 40°C) for many years has revealed that there was surprisingly little deterioration of the drug on storage. This is contrary to the view which has been expressed by physicians working in the tropics that old suramin is more likely to cause adverse effects than recently prepared material.[16] It is only solutions of suramin that deteriorate rapidly on storage.

Therapeutic use

Indications

1. Treatment of onchocerciasis
2. Treatment of trypanosomiasis
3. ? Treatment of AIDS.

Contraindications

1. Renal disease
2. Severe debility.

The contraindications to the use of suramin are relative and depend on the initial indication. Adverse effects following the use of suramin in a fatal disease like trypanosomiasis are less important than with a non-fatal disease like onchocerciasis.

Mode of use

Suramin is given by intravenous injection with an initial test dose of 100–200 mg followed by weekly injections until the course is completed (see Indications).

Indications

1. Onchocerciasis

Suramin is a macrofilaricidal drug and is still the only recognized drug to kill the adult worm. Other drugs like diethylcarbamazine kill only the microfilariae, while ivermectin and benzimidazoles such as flubendazole seem to affect the release of microfilaria from the adult worm and may kill these microfilariae as well. Suramin also has some effects in lymphatic filariasis and may kill *Wuchereria bancrofti* but is almost never used for this condition. The standard regime for suramin is to give a single test dose of 100–200 mg intravenously and this is followed at weekly intervals with 1.0 g intravenous doses for 5–6 weeks.[17] Since suramin is so toxic, attempts have been made to reduce the total dose by following the initial dose of 0.2 g with weekly doses of 0.4, 0.6, 0.8 and 1.0 g in succeeding weeks to a total dose of 3.6 or 4.0 g[18] (doses for a 60 kg adult). The doses are reduced proportionately for patients weighing less than 60 kg (see Major outcome trial 2).

The effects of suramin are not immediate; killing of the adult worms may take some weeks to occur and may only be detected by removing a nodule of adult worms. The adult worms, following digestion of the nodule with collagenase, can be examined directly. Worms that have died some time previously will be calcified. Worms that have died recently show ultrastructural changes when examined with the electron microscope. Death of adult worms can be inferred by a gradual fall in the number of microfilariae found in skin snips. This fall will take place over a period of 3–12 months, and it may be 18 months before the snips are free of microfilariae. The test dose of suramin should always be given slowly (over 5 minutes), with adrenalin 1/1000, parenteral antihistamines and steroids at hand to deal with severe reactions. If more rapid demise of the microfilariae in the skin is required following the use of suramin, a course of diethylcarbamazine (or ivermectin) should be given. Suramin is considered too dangerous for large-scale use but it is of value in individual patients.

2. Trypanosomiasis

Suramin was for a long time the only effective treatment for Rhodesian sleeping sickness. Suramin is very effective in curing patients before the central nervous system is involved but passage of the drug into the CNS is poor. The course of treatment for Rhodesian sleeping sickness is a test dose of 200 mg followed by intravenous doses of 1 g on days 1, 3, 6, 14 and 21.[1,19] Further doses of 1 g weekly can be given for a further 5 weeks. Response to suramin can be judged by a disappearance of trypanosomes from the peripheral blood. If CNS involvement has occurred then melarsoprol should be given. Suramin is similarly effective in the early stages of infection with *Trypanosoma gambiense* but has no effect in infections with *Trypanosoma cruzi* (South American trypanosomiasis).

3. ? Treatment of AIDS

Since suramin is known to have an effect on DNA/RNA polymerase and on viral reverse transcriptase,[3] the drug has been tried in the treatment of patients with AIDS and related conditions. Although some changes in the viral patterns were seen, no significant effect of suramin on the disease process was noted[20,21] (see Major outcome trial 1). Suramin was also ineffective in chronic active hepatitis due to infection with viral hepatitis B.[22]

Suramin has in the past been used in the treatment of angioneurotic oedema. In this condition there is a lack of complement C1 esterase inhibitors and the scientific use of suramin is justified.[2] However its therapeutic benefit is very erratic.[1] Suramin has also been used in the treatment of pemphigus but there is little scientific rationale for this and more effective and less toxic remedies exist.[1]

Adverse reactions

Potentially life-threatening effects

Collapse, with nausea, vomiting, shock, sweating and loss of consciousness may occur. This usually occurs shortly after injection and is more dangerous in patients who are asthenic or malnourished. Although this reaction is not common, occurring perhaps in 1 in 2000, supplies of 1/1000 adrenaline, parenteral antihistamine and corticosteroids should be immediately available when an injection of suramin is given.

Acute overdosage

There is no literature on the effect of an overdose of suramin. It is most unlikely that an overdose would be self-administered.

Severe or irreversible adverse effects

Adverse effects can be divided into those that are due to death of the parasites and those that are due to the inherent toxicity of the drug. The former tend only to produce symptomatic effects.

Toxic effects due to the drug itself include nausea and vomiting, which is particularly common if the drug is injected rapidly. Fever,

Suramin

urticaria, photophobia, lachrymation, abdominal pain, and constipation may occur as part of a late reaction 3 to 24 hours after the injection.

Stomatitis and ulceration of the buccal, pharyngeal, and bronchial mucosae may occur. Bowel ulceration may lead to chronic diarrhoea and weight loss.

Kidney damage is the most important complication and albuminuria is common after suramin injection. The urine should be tested for protein before each injection of suramin. Only if proteinuria is heavy or casts are present in the urine should suramin therapy be stopped. Increased serum creatinine has been noted in 10% of patients (see Major outcome trial 1).

Jaundice may occur and death from liver damage has been recorded in two individuals with hepatitis B after being given suramin.[21]

Leucopenia, thrombocytopenia, and other bone marrow effects may be seen, with leucopenia in as many as 30% of patients (see Major outcome trial 1) although this may have been contributed to by the disease process itself.

Adrenal insufficiency is recorded[23] and may be seen in 25% of patients (Major outcome trial 1).

Severe reactions may occur which are related to the death of the parasite particularly in onchocerciasis. Eye lesions may progress following suramin therapy, and Fuglsang and Anderson[24] found aggravation of eye lesions in 41 out of 100 heavily infected patients when suramin was given. Such lesions may be posterior synechiae, corneal lesions, keratic precipitates, iridocyclitis, and, on occasion, blindness due to optic atrophy.[25]

Exfoliative dermatitis may occur and may be severe in the occasional patient.[24]

Symptomatic adverse effects

Suramin may cause symptomatic effects due to the death of worms. These effects include local urticaria, focal swelling at the site of nodules containing dying worms; skin eruptions; and a polyarthritis affecting the small joints of the hands, feet, wrists, ankle, and knees with occasional joint effusions.

Interference with clinical pathology tests

No technical interferences of this kind have been reported.

High risk groups

Neonates

Suramin would almost never be given to neonates.

Breast milk. There are no data on this subject, so it is probably best for women taking the drug to avoid breast-feeding.

Children

Suramin would rarely be given to children but on occasion the need may be there. No special problems in children are recorded.

Pregnant women

Suramin does not cross the placenta and apparently causes none of the problems seen in mice or rats. Suramin has been given to many pregnant women over the years and no case of infant malformation has been recorded.[26] Nevertheless, its use in pregnant women is not recommended unless the medical situation is urgent.

The elderly

There is no data on this topic. Although renal function is impaired in the elderly, the rate of excretion of suramin is very slow in people with normal renal function. It would be wise to watch renal function particularly carefully in the elderly patient.

Drug interactions

There is no data in the literature on any interaction between suramin and other drugs, whether harmful or beneficial.

Major outcome trials

1. Cheson B D, Levine A M, Mildvan D, Kaplan W, Wolfe P 1987 Suramin therapy in AIDS and related disorders — Report of the United States Suramin Working Group. Journal of the American Medical Association 258: 1347–1351

98 patients with AIDS, manifest as opportunistic infections, Kaposi's sarcoma or non-Hodgkins lymphoma were treated with suramin. After a dose of 200 mg intravenously they were given 0.5–1.5 g weekly for 6 weeks by intravenous injection. Only one patient out of 87 assessable individuals showed significant recovery; 7 patients had a minor response, 27 patients were considered stable over the period of follow up but the remaining 52 patients experienced progression of the disease. Side effects including fever, leucopenia, proteinuria and thrombocytopenia were common. Adrenal insufficiency was seen in 23% of patients.

2. Rougemont A, Hien M, Thylefors B, Prost A, Schulz-Key H, Rolland A 1984 Traitement de l'onchocercose par la suramine à faibles doses progressive dans les collectivités hyperéndemique d'Afrique occidental. II Résultas cliniques, parasitologiques et ophthalmologiques en zone de transmission interrompue. Bulletin of the World Health Organization 62: 261–269

78 adult patients with onchocerciasis in Upper Volta (now Burkino Fasu) were selected with a geometric mean microfilarial skin snip count of 250 per skin snip. Suramin was given in a dose of 0.2 g initially with subsequent weekly doses of 0.4 g, 0.6 g, 0.8 g, thereafter 1.0 g. Total doses varied between 3.0 and 4.0 g. The course of treatment was well tolerated and the worm burden was reduced by at least 90% at 3 months and remained stable for the 18 months of the trial. Visual acuity was usually increased and this dose regime seems preferable to the earlier higher-dose regime.

References

1. Hawking F 1978 Suramin: with special reference to Onchocerciasis. Advances in Pharmacology and Chemotherapy 15: 289–322
2. Eisen V, Loveday C 1973 Effects of suramin on complement, blood clotting, fibrinolysis and kinin formation. British Journal of Pharmacology 49: 678–687
3. Chandra P, Vogel A, Gerber T 1985 Inhibitors of retroviral DNA polymerase: Their implication in the treatment of AIDS. Cancer Research 45 (suppl 9): 4677s–4684s
4. Howells R E, Mendis A M, Bray P G 1983 The mode of action of suramin on the filarial worm *Brugia pahangi*. Parasitology 87: 29–48
5. Fairlamb A H, Bowman I B R 1980 Uptake of the trypanocidal drug suramin by blood stream forms of *Trypanosoma brucei* and its effect on respiration and growth rate in vivo. Molecular and Biochemical Parasitology 1: 315–333
6. Constantopoulos G, Rees S, Cragg B G, Barranger J A, Brady R O 1983 Suramin induced storage disease. Mucopolysaccharidosis. American Journal of Pathology 113: 266–268
7. Freeman J J, Lloyd J B 1986 Evidence that suramin and auro-thiomalate are teratogenic in rat by disturbing yolk sac-mediated embryonic protein nutrition. Chemico-Biological Interactions 58: 149–160
8. Edwards G, Rodick, C L, Ward, S A, Awadzi K, Orme M L'E, Breckenridge A M 1985 Determination of suramin in plasma by high-performance liquid chromatography. Journal of Chromatography 343: 224–228
9. Ruprecht R M, Lorsch J, Trites D H 1986 Analysis of suramin plasma levels by ion-pair high-performance liquid chromatography under isocratic conditions. Journal of Chromatography 378: 498–502
10. Collins J M, Klecker R W, Yarchoan R, Lane H C, Fauci A S 1986 Clinical pharmacokinetics of suramin in patients with HTLV III/LAV infection. Journal of Clinical Pharmacology 26: 22–26
11. Edwards G, Rodick C L, Ward S A, Awadzi K, Orme M L, Breckenridge A M 1986 Disposition of suramin in patients with onchocerciasis. Acta Pharmacologica et Toxicologica 59 (suppl 5 pt 2): 222
12. Van Boxtel C J, Schattenkerk E F K, Van Den Berg M, de Graaf Y P, Danner S A 1986 Therapeutic monitoring of suramin in patients with AIDS. Acta Pharmacologica et Toxicologica 59 (suppl 5 pt 2): 196
13. Leau O 1963 Relation entre concentration sanguine et activité therapeutique. Presse Medicale 71: 1969–1972
14. Spinks A 1948 Persistence in blood stream of some compounds related to suramin. Biochemical Journal 42: 109–116
15. Dewey H M, Wormall A 1946 Studies on suramin (antrypol: Bayer 205) Combination of drug with plasma and other proteins. Biochemical Journal 40: 119–124
16. Nnochiri E 1964 Observations on the treatment of onchocerciasis in an endemic area of Western Nigeria. Transactions of the Royal Society of Tropical Medicine and Hygiene 58: 413–418
17. Duke B O L 1968 The effects of drugs on *Onchocerca volvulus*. 3. Trials of suramin at different dosages and a comparison of the brands Antrypol, Moranyl and Naganol. Bulletin of the World Health Organization 39: 157–167
18. Rougemont A, Thylefors B, Duncan M, Prost A, Ranque Ph, Delmont J 1980 Traitement de l'onchocercose par la suramine à faible doses progressive dans les collectivités hypérendemiques d'Afrique de l'ouest. I. Résultas parasitologiques et surveillance ophthalmologique en zone de transmission non-interrompue. Bulletin of the World Health Organization 58: 917–922
19. Gutteridge W E 1985 Existing chemotherapy and its limitations. British Medical Bulletin 41: 162–170
20. Busch W, Brodt R, Ganser A, Helm E B, Stille W 1985 Suramin treatment for AIDS. Lancet 2: 1247
21. Kaplan L D, Wolfe P R, Volberding P A, Feorino P, Levy J A 1987 Lack of response to suramin in patients with AIDS and AIDS-related complex. American Journal of Medicine 82: 615–622

22. Loke R H, Anderson M G, Coleman J C, Tsiquake K N, Zuckerman A J 1987 Suramin treatment for chronic active hepatitis B — Toxic and ineffective. Journal of Medical Virology 21: 97–99
23. Py A, Dairou F, de Gennes J L 1987 Toxicité surrenale de la suramine. Presse Medicale 16: 1979
24. Fuglsang H, Anderson J 1974 Side effects of suramin. In: Research and control of onchocerciasis in the western hemisphere. PAHO Scientific Publication No 298: 54–57
25. Thylefors B, Rolland A 1979 The risk of optic atrophy following suramin treatment of ocular onchocerciasis. Bulletin of the World Health Organization 57: 479–480
26. Anderson J, Fuglsang H, Marshall T F de C 1976 Effects of suramin on ocular onchocerciasis. Tropenmedizin und Parasitologie 27: 279–296

Suxamethonium (chloride)

Suxamethonium is a short-acting depolarizing skeletal muscle relaxant.

Chemistry

Suxamethonium chloride (Anectine, Scoline, Succinylcholine)
$C_{14}H_{30}Cl_2N_2O_4$
2, 2′-[1,4 dioxo-1,4-butanediyl)bis(oxy)]bis[N, N,N-trimethylethanaminium] dichloride

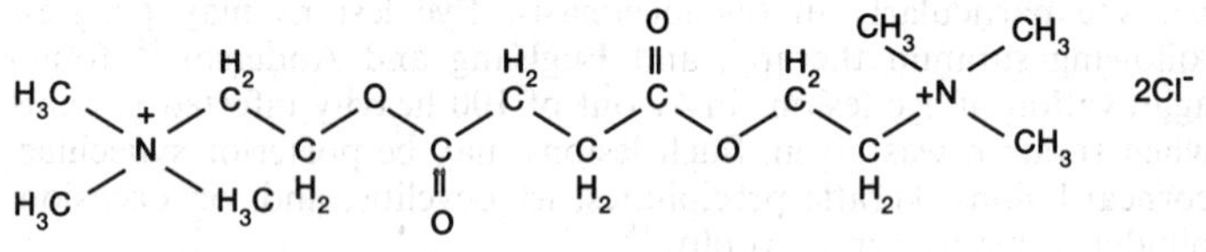

Molecular weight	361.3
pKa	not relevant
Solubility	
in alcohol	1 in 350
in water	1 in 1
Octanol/water partition coefficient	0

Suxamethonium is a white, odourless, slightly bitter powder and very soluble in water. The drug is unstable in alkaline solutions but relatively stable in acid solutions.

Pharmacology

Suxamethonium, an analogue of acetylcholine, depolarizes (activates) the cholinergic receptors of the skeletal muscle end-plate and produces a flaccid paralysis of the muscle.[1] Suxamethonium has no direct effect on the chemically insensitive voltage-dependent ion channels in the adjacent muscle membrane.

However, depolarization of the muscle end-plate establishes a voltage gradient between the two areas of the membrane opening the voltage-dependent ion channels of the muscle and leading in turn to transient contraction of the muscle. Although the end-plate remains depolarized, the muscle membrane accommodates to this depolarization and remains flaccid. If suxamethonium is kept continuously present during an infusion, the junctional membrane slowly regains its resting potential with the return of neuromuscular transmission; to maintain the effect, a higher infusion rate is required (tachyphylaxis). With continued infusion neuromuscular transmission will fail again (phase II block) even though the membrane potential of the end-plate remains unchanged and normal or near normal. A phase II block has clinical characteristics of a non-depolarizing block. The mechanism of this block is not known but channel blocking by penetration of suxamethonium into the sub-end-plate cytoplasm, intracellular accumulation of calcium and sodium, the loss of intracellular potassium, and activation of Na,K-ATPase all contribute.

Toxicology

Animal reproductive studies have not been conducted with suxamethonium.

Clinical pharmacology

The dosage of succinylcholine is essentially individualized and its administration should always be determined by the clinician after careful assessment of the patient. To avoid distress to the patient, succinylcholine should not be administered before unconsciousness has been induced. Succinylcholine should not be mixed with short-acting barbiturates in the same syringe or administered simultaneously during intravenous infusion through the same needle.

The average suxamethonium dose for relaxation of short duration is 0.5–1.0 $mg.kg^{-1}$ intravenously. Following administration of doses in this range, relaxation develops in about 1 minute; maximum muscular paralysis may persist for about 2 minutes, after which recovery takes place within 4 to 6 minutes. However, very large doses may result in more prolonged apnoea. An initial test dose of 0.1 $mg.kg^{-1}$ may be used to determine the sensitivity of the potential pseudocholinesterase-deficient patient and to minimize fasciculations.

Pharmacokinetics

There is no specific clinical assay for suxamethonium.

Although it is not known quantitatively how the plasma concentration of suxamethonium varies with time in humans, useful pharmacokinetic information can be realized by looking at the kinetics of the pharmacological effect. The kinetics of suxamethonium in humans can be approximated by a one compartment model with first order disappearance, to give the following expression:

$$C_0 = C\,e^{-Kt}$$

where C is concentration expressed as the dose or amount of drug D divided by the volume of distribution and K is the first order elimination rate constant.[2] If t is the duration of effect, D_d the dose, and D_0 the minimum effective dose then the above expression becomes:

$$D_0 = D_d\,e^{-K+d}$$

This equation can be solved for K to give:

$$K = 2.30/td\,(\log 10D_d - \log 10\,D_0)$$

Levy[3] applies this expression to data of Walts and Dillon[4] by plotting the duration of effect versus the log 10 of the dose and extrapolating the linear relationship to zero duration to obtain a value for D_0. He then calculated an elimination rate constant K of 0.20 min^{-1} or a $t\frac{1}{2}$ of 3.5 minutes. Others[5] applied the same treatment to the data of Holst-Larson[6] and obtained a $t\frac{1}{2}$ of 2.7 minutes. These half lives are in good agreement with the data of Eger.[2]

If the relationship between the intensity of pharmacological effect E and the dose D_0 is related log-linearly, then the following expression holds:[3]

$$E = m \log D_0 + q$$

where m and q are constants. Combining this with the expression for D_0 versus td gives the simple expression:

$$E = E_0 - km\,td/2.30$$

Here E_0 is the intercept at time zero and td is the time to whatever percentage blockade is selected. Levy[3] showed that this expression fits the data of Walts and Dillon[4] for suxamethonium, thus lending further support to a one compartment model.

The pharmacokinetic properties of suxamethonium have been studied in infants and children. Cook and Fischer[7] showed that equal doses of suxamethonium on a milligram per kilogram basis gave shorter durations of action in infants as compared with older children. For example, the intensity of neuromuscular blockade and the duration of blockade were similar for a dose of 1.0 $mg.kg^{-1}$ in infants as with a dose of 0.5 $mg.kg^{-1}$ in children. However, on a milligram per square metre basis the same linear relationship between effect and log dose held for both infants and children. Since body surface area reflects extracellular fluid volume more closely than does body weight, it appeared that the difference on a weight basis was due to the extracellular fluid volume being different with age. Thus, the volume of distribution would differ with age, assuming that plasma cholinesterase levels were near normal. Walts and Dillon[8] showed no difference between neonates and adults for the duration of effect following an injection of 40 $mg.m^{-2}$.

The kinetic calculations described earlier for suxamethonium in adults were extended to infants and children.[5] The elimination half lives for suxamethonium appeared to increase slightly from about 1.7–1.8 minutes in infants and children to 2.7–4.6 minutes in adults. The results include the data of Holst-Larson.[6] The rates of recovery of neuromuscular transmission, as calculated between 50 and 90% recovery, were highest for children and least for adults. In addition, the minimum effective doses to obtain selected levels of neuromuscular blockade were least in adults and highest in infants. These differences may be the result of changes in the volume of distribution or in plasma cholinesterase levels with age.

Suxamethonium (chloride)

S

Concentration–effect relationship

There is no evidence of a correlation between the plasma concentration of suxamethonium and its neuromuscular effects.

Metabolism

The short duration of action of suxamethonium has been attributed to its rapid disappearance from the blood. Most of this evidence comes from studies in dogs or in vitro measurements with human serum. Lack of a fast, suitable assay has prevented direct in vivo measurements of suxamethonium disappearance in humans. Most of the work with suxamethonium has been carried out with ^{14}C labelled substrates. Suxamethonium is rapidly hydrolysed in vitro by pseudocholinesterase (plasma cholinesterase) to the monocholine metabolite (Fig. 1). The latter has about $\frac{1}{80}$th the neuromuscular blocking action of suxamethonium and is slowly hydrolysed to succinate and choline.[9] At a typical zero order in vitro rate of hydrolysis of 27 mg suxamethonium per litre of normal human plasma per minute, a dose of 1.0 $mg.kg^{-1}$ would be hydrolysed within 1 minute in a 70 kg patient with 3.5 litres plasma volume.[10]

Fig. 1 The metabolism of suxamethonium

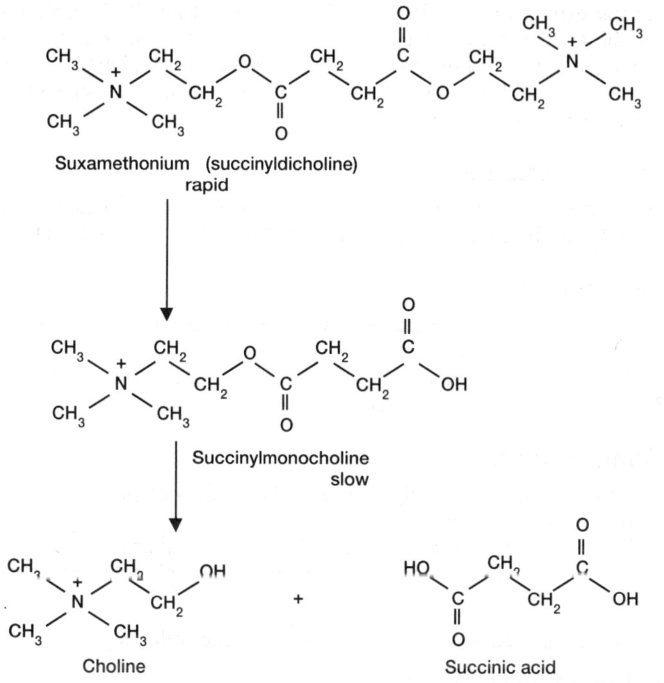

Recent in vivo studies in humans demonstrated suxamethonium in active form in the blood for over 3 minutes.[6] With circulation to the left arm occluded, suxamethonium was injected intravenously into the right hand and the twitch response of both arms monitored for neuromuscular blockade. Three minutes after injection, circulation was restored to the occluded arm and neuromuscular blockade was soon detected. Thus, the in vivo rate of hydrolysis of suxamethonium is probably as low as 3–7 $mg.l^{-1}.min^{-1}$.[6] Eger[2] found that a continuous infusion rate of 4 $mg.min^{-1}$ suxamethonium was required to maintain a 90% reduction in twitch height in humans. By assuming first order instead of zero order kinetics for the hydrolysis of suxamethonium, these infusion results are in general agreement with the results of Holst-Larson. Perhaps rapid redistribution of suxamethonium contributes to the clinically observed short duration of action.

Although the in vivo hydrolysis of suxamethonium by plasma cholinesterase is less rapid than previously assumed, it is still the main factor determining the rate of elimination. About one out of every 2800 humans has an atypical plasma cholinesterase which hydrolyses suxamethonium at a slower rate than normal.[11] In such cases the dose of suxamethonium must be reduced by as much as a factor of 10 or more.[12]

Suxamethonium (chloride)

S

Little information is available on the placental transfer of suxamethonium in humans. However, studies have been carried out using ^{14}C-suxamethonium in monkeys, where the placenta is similar to that of humans in terms of its functional anatomy. After injection of 2 mg.kg^{-1} into the maternal femoral vein, the fetal monkey concentration of suxamethonium reached a maximum in 5–10 minutes. The maximum fetal concentration was 4% of that of the maximum maternal concentration following injection into the maternal femoral vein and 12% after injection into the maternal abdominal aorta.[13] In another study, ^{14}C-suxamethonium was injected into the umbilical vein and the distribution of ^{14}C measured in the fetus.[14] The ^{14}C was rapidly distributed to the highly perfused organs with a large fraction associated with cartilaginous tissue. In both monkeys[13] and humans,[15] the plasma cholinesterase activity in fetal or premature infant blood was only about half that of adults. The differences appeared due to the quantity of enzyme rather than to enzyme binding properties. However, a dose of 1 mg.kg^{-1} during obstetric anaesthesia should not endanger the fetus in humans, provided repeated doses are not needed or atypical plasma cholinesterase is not encountered.

Pharmaceutics

Suxamethonium is available in the USA for intravenous use as a clear solution (20 mg.ml^{-1}) or as a powder (Anectine Flo-Pack; Burroughs-Wellcome) (500 or 1000 mg) for the preparation of intravenous drip solutions. In the UK both Anectine (Wellcome) and Scoline (Duncan Flockhart) are marketed as ampoules containing 100 mg suxamethonium in 2 ml. This equates to 36.5 mg of active cation per millilitre. Suxamethonium may be infused using either dextrose 5% or sodium chloride 0.9% as the vehicle.

Therapeutic use

Suxamethonium has no effect on consciousness or pain threshold and should only be used after general anaesthesia has been induced.

Indications

1. As an adjunct to general anaesthesia or sedation to facilitate endotracheal intubation
2. To provide skeletal muscle relaxation for surgical procedures
3. To facilitate control of ventilation (rarely).

Contraindications

1. Patients with genetically determined disorders of plasma pseudocholinesterase
2. Personal or family history of malignant hyperthermia
3. Myopathies associated with elevated creatine phosphokinase values.

It should be used with caution, if at all, in the following groups.

4. Patients with open-eye injuries
5. Neurological injuries, burns, and massive trauma.

Mode of use

The dose of succinylcholine administered by infusion depends upon the duration of the surgical procedure and the need for muscle relaxation. The average rate for an adult ranges between 35 and 100 μg.kg^{-1}.min^{-1}. Solutions containing from 0.1% to 0.2% (1–2 mg.ml^{-1}) succinylcholine have commonly been used for continuous intravenous drip. Solutions of 0.1% or 0.2% may conveniently be prepared by adding 1 g suxamethonium to 1000 or 500 ml of 5% dextrose solution or isotonic saline solution. The more dilute solution (0.1% or 1 mg.ml^{-1}) is probably preferable from the standpoint of ease of control of the rate of administration of the drug and, hence, of relaxation. This intravenous drip solution containing 1 mg per ml may be administered at a rate of 0.5 mg (0.5 ml) to 10 mg (10 ml) per minute but the usual recommended range is 2–5 mg.min^{-1}, to obtain the required amount of relaxation. The amount required per minute will depend upon the individual response as well as the degree of relaxation required. The 0.2% solution may be especially useful in those cases where it is desired to avoid overburdening the circulation with a large volume of fluid. It is recommended that neuromuscular function be carefully monitored with a peripheral nerve stimulator when using succinylcholine by infusion in order to avoid overdose and to detect a phase II block.

Adverse reactions

Potentially life-threatening effects

Profound, prolonged muscle relaxation with respiratory depression and apnoea are obvious manifestations of suxamethonium's pharmacological effects. Hypersensitivity to the drug may exist in rare cases. Suxamethonium can have profound cardiovascular effects;[16,17] increase intraocular,[18] intragastric,[19] or intracranial pressure;[20] and be associated with myalgias,[1] hyperkalaemia,[21,22] myotonia,[2] myoglobinaemia,[23,24] and malignant hyperthermia.[25]

Dysrhythmias

Suxamethonium exerts variable and seemingly paradoxical effects on the cardiovascular system. Typically, intravenous suxamethonium produces initial bradycardia and hypotension, followed after 15 to 30 seconds by tachycardia and hypertension. In the infant and small child profound sustained sinus bradycardia (rates of 50 to 60 per minute) is commonly observed; rarely asystole occurs. Nodal rhythm and ventricular ectopic beats are seen in about 80% of children given a single intravenous injection of suxamethonium; such dysrhythmias are rarely seen following intramuscular suxamethonium.

The incidence of bradycardia and other dysrhythmias is higher following a second dose of suxamethonium. Atropine (0.1 mg) appears to offer adequate protection against these bradyarrhythmias in all age groups. In infants, vagolytic doses of atropine (0.03 mg.kg^{-1}) are required for protection; in older children adequate protection is provided by doses of 0.005 mg.kg^{-1}.

Pulmonary oedema and pulmonary haemorrhage

Several young infants have developed fulminant pulmonary oedema or pulmonary haemorrhage following intramuscular (IM) suxamethonium (4 mg.kg^{-1}).[26] The pulmonary oedema occurred within minutes of the IM injection and responded to continuous positive pressure ventilation (CPAP). This may represent a haemodynamic form of pulmonary oedema from an acute elevation of systemic vascular resistance and an acute decrease in pulmonary vascular resistance. In addition, 'leaky' capillaries appear to be involved. Whether these cardiovascular changes are mediated by suxamethonium itself or some other vasoactive substance (e.g. histamine) is not known.

Hyperkalaemia and myoglobinaemia

In normal adults suxamethonium increases plasma levels of potassium by 0.3–0.5 mmol.l^{-1}. Even more modest increases are seen in children. Alarming levels of potassium, as high as 11 mmol.l^{-1}, along with cardiovascular collapse, have been reported with suxamethonium in a variety of situations, some of which include burns, massive trauma, stroke, and spinal cord injury. A common denominator appears to be either massive tissue destruction or CNS injury with muscle wasting. Strong fasciculations are not necessary to produce hyperkalaemia in susceptible patients. There are no data to suggest that the infant or small child is not vulnerable to massive potassium flux from the above conditions just as the adult.

Ryan et al.[23] noted a high incidence of myoglobinaemia (45%) following suxamethonium (1 mg.kg^{-1}) in prepubertal patients anaesthetized with halothane. A much lower incidence (8%) of the same degree of myoglobinaemia was noted by Harrington et al.,[2] although all of their children did have some myoglobin in their blood. Myoglobinuria was rare. Myoglobinaemia is rarely seen in adults following suxamethonium. Likewise, significant elevation of plasma levels of creatine phosphokinase (CPK), an indicator of muscle injury, has been demonstrated following suxamethonium in children. Myoglobinaemia and elevation of plasma levels of CPK were seen in the absence of strong fasciculations. The susceptibility of muscle in children to release myoglobin following depolarization with suxamethonium has no ready explanation. In the study by Harrington et al. there was no correlation between the occurrence of fasciculations, pretreatment with gallamine, dose (1 versus 2 mg.kg^{-1} of suxamethonium), or age and the degree of myoglobinaemia. However, all patients who developed myoglobinuria received 2 mg.kg^{-1} of suxamethonium. This study suggests that although myoglobinaemia may occur more often in children than in adults, it is of minimal clinical significance.

Tamoxifen citrate

Tamoxifen is a non-steroidal antioestrogen which inhibits competitively oestradiol binding to the high-affinity oestrogen receptor. Although it binds to this receptor it has no sustained oestrogenic effects.

Chemistry

Tamoxifen citrate (Noltam, Nolvadex, Tamofen)
$C_{26}H_{29}NO.C_6H_8O_7$
(Z)-2-(4-(1,2-Diphenylbut-1-enyl)phenoxy)-N,N-dimethylethylamine monocitrate

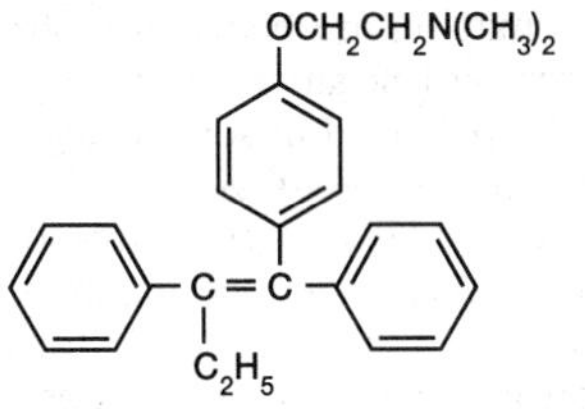

Molecular weight (free base)	563.6 (371.5)
pKa (in 50% aqueous acetone)	7.82
Solubility	
in alcohol	soluble
in water	slightly soluble
Octanol/water partition coefficient	—

Tamoxifen citrate is a white, odourless, fine crystalline powder, slightly soluble in water, and soluble in ethanol, methanol and acetone. It is prepared by chemical synthesis. Under normal storage conditions, protected from light and moisture, it is stable for at least 5 years. The citrate salt of the *trans* isomer of the triphenylethylene compound is used clinically. Tamoxifen is not a constituent of any combination products.

Pharmacology

Tamoxifen shows variable pharmacological properties. Depending upon the species studied it can act as either a pure oestrogen agonist, a partial agonist or an antagonist. In primates, including man, tamoxifen acts primarily as an oestrogen antagonist.

Tamoxifen binds to the high-affinity oestrogen receptor in the cytoplasm and the modified complex is then translocated to the nucleus. Tamoxifen competes for the binding sites with oestradiol and by occupying the receptor reduces the amount of receptor available for endogenous oestradiol. Tamoxifen prevents the normal feedback inhibition of oestrogen synthesis in the hypothalamus and in the pituitary. This usually results in increased secretion of LH–RH and gonadotrophins.

Toxicology

Acute toxicity is very low, values for the oral LD_{50} in mice ranging from 3 to 6 $g.kg^{-1}$ and in rats from 1.2 to 2.5 $g.kg^{-1}$. After chronic administration, the histopathological changes are confined chiefly to the reproductive tract and reflect the pharmacology of the drug in the species concerned.

As an antioestrogen, tamoxifen terminates pregnancy, but the maximum dose (up to 2 $mg.kg^{-1}$) which does not terminate pregnancy in rats or rabbits had no teratogenic effects, although a reversible deformation of the rib cage ('kinky ribs') has been observed in a small number of pups. The latter could be a consequence of placental hypertrophy, increasing the pressure on the fetal ribs. This anomaly is not seen in primates.

Tamoxifen was not mutagenic in a range of in vitro and in vivo mutagenicity tests. Gonadal tumours in mice and liver tumours in rats receiving tamoxifen have been reported in long-term studies. The clinical relevance of these findings has not been established.

Clinical pharmacology

The effects of tamoxifen are predominantly antioestrogenic. There are few good dose–response studies. In the only randomized study, 90 mg daily was no more effective than 30 mg in terms of tumour regression and duration of response.

The recommended daily doses range between 20 and 40 mg daily, the highest dose ever used being 160 mg twice daily, for periods in excess of 17 months.

Effects on gonadotrophins

In women with anovulatory infertility, tamoxifen 20 $mg.kg^{-1}$ daily caused LH and FSH to rise at about day eight of the cycle, in those who were ovulating. However, in another study serum concentrations of LH and FSH did not rise during five tamoxifen-induced conception cycles.[1–3]

In premenopausal women of reproductive age with normal ovarian function, tamoxifen in a dose of 20 mg daily does not cause any change in plasma gonadotrophin levels.[4] In postmenopausal women, however, in whom plasma oestrogen levels are low and both LH and FSH are elevated, tamoxifen, at a dose of 20–40 mg daily, results in a moderate decrease of gonadotrophin levels.[5–7]

In men, by displacing oestrogens from their hypothalamopituitary receptors, tamoxifen increases gonadotrophin secretion and plasma levels[8,9] with a secondary increase of testosterone and oestrogen levels. The gonadotrophin response to LH–RH is increased.[9]

Effects on prolactin

Tamoxifen, by its antioestrogenic effects, decreases prolactin levels in patients with hyperprolactinaemia,[10] but not in normal subjects,[11] and it reduces TRF-induced prolactin secretion.[10]

Effects on growth hormone

Secretion is not affected by tamoxifen, but there is a reduction in l-dopa-stimulated growth hormone secretion.

Effects on sex hormone binding globulin

In postmenopausal women[12] and in castrated men, tamoxifen, by its weak oestrogenic effect on the liver, increases sex hormone binding globulin, thyroxine binding globulin and transcortin[13] and, indirectly, cortisol levels.

Effects on plasma steroids

At doses above 10 mg daily, tamoxifen causes an increase in both oestradiol and progesterone concentration in women of reproductive age.[14] At a dose of 40 mg daily the rise in plasma oestradiol is about two-fold. A direct stimulatory effect on the ovaries seems possible.

Most authors agree that in postmenopausal women tamoxifen has no effect on plasma oestrogens.[15]

Clinical effects

At the endometrium tamoxifen acts as an antioestrogen and causes disappearance of cystic glandular hyperplasia. It reduces endometrial glandular development and suppresses withdrawal bleeding induced by ethinyloestradiol.[16] At the vagina in patients with anovulatory infertility, tamoxifen reduces the karyopyknotic index (KI).[17] In postmenopausal women tamoxifen increases KI in some women but fully cornified smears are not observed.[18]

Gynaecomastia, either at puberty or in oligozoospermic males, regresses under tamoxifen at a dose of 20 mg daily,[19] although the manufacturer does not recommend the drug for this use. It has been reported that tamoxifen inhibits lactation in puerperal women.[20,21]

Pharmacokinetics

Tamoxifen and its major metabolites, 4-hydroxytamoxifen and N-desmethyltamoxifen, may be assayed using thin-layer chromatography, high performance liquid chromatography[22] and gas chromatography–mass spectrometry.[23]

After oral administration, the compound is well absorbed and extensively metabolized. Elimination occurs, chiefly as conjugates, with practically no unchanged drug, principally through the faeces (50%), and to a lesser extent through the kidney (15%).[24]

Steady-state serum levels of tamoxifen of approximately 300 μg.l^{-1} were achieved after four weeks of therapy with 20 mg daily and an elimination half life of seven days was calculated. However, serum levels of desmethyltamoxifen were only reached after eight weeks of therapy and calculations suggested an elmination half life of 14 days for this metabolite.[25]

Tamoxifen circulates in plasma largely bound to albumin. Animal studies have shown that tamoxifen concentrations were higher in lung, liver, adrenals, kidney, pancreas, uterus and mammary tissues than in blood. In women, after administration of ^{14}C-tamoxifen before hysterectomy, Fromson and others[24] found radioactivity to be 2–3 times higher in the uterus than in blood.

There is evidence that tamoxifen crosses the blood–brain barrier.[26] No information on excretion in milk is available.

Oral absorption	extensive
Presystemic metabolism	—
Plasma half life	7 days
Volume of distribution	—
Plasma protein binding	high

Concentration–effect relationship

There is no evidence of a direct relationship between plasma concentration of tamoxifen and its various effects.

Metabolism

The major metabolic pathway, which is qualitatively similar for all species studied,[24,25] involves hydroxylation to 4-hydroxytamoxifen, N-demethylation to N-desmethyltamoxifen and subsequent conjugation.[24] Both these metabolites have antioestrogenic activity.

Pharmaceutics

Tamoxifen is available in tablet form for oral use.

1. Nolvadex (ICI, UK): white round, biconvex tablets containing 10 mg tamoxifen citrate. The tablet is marked 'Nolvadex 10' on the face and 'ICI' on the reverse. Nolvadex (ICI, USA) 10 mg is a biconvex white tablet debossed 'NOVALDEX 600' on one side with a debossed cameo on the reverse.
2. Nolvadex-D (ICI, UK): a white, octagonal, biconvex tablet containing 20 mg tamoxifen citrate, marked 'Nolvadex D' on one face and 'ICI' on the other.
3. Nolvadex-Forte (ICI, UK): a white, elongated, octagonal tablet with a bisection line, containing 40 mg tamoxifen in the form of citrate, marked 'Nolvadex forte' on one face and 'ICI' on the other.
4. Noltam (Lederle, UK): tablets contain either 10 mg or 20 mg tamofixen citrate.
5. Tamofen (Tillotts, UK): 10 mg, 20 mg and 40 mg tablets.

No sustained-release form is available. The formulations do not include any known potentially allergenic substance. Protected from heat and light, the shelf-life is 5 years for Nolvadex and 3 years for Nolvadex-D and Nolvadex-Forte.

Therapeutic use

Indications

1. Breast cancer
a. as an adjuvant immediately after surgery in patients with early disease
b. for advanced breast cancer
2. Infertility.

Contraindications

1. Pregnancy.

Mode of use

Numerous publications have proved the efficacy of tamoxifen in metastatic breast cancer but its use in early disease is still under study.

1. Breast cancer

a. Early disease

At the time of initial diagnosis microscopic metastases are probably present in many patients with breast cancer. Following surgical treatment with axillary clearance or sampling, adjuvant therapy with tamoxifen 10 mg twice daily for 2 years versus no treatment showed a significant advantage for tamoxifen over a mean period of 5½ years irrespective of menopausal status, stage, grade and oestrogen receptor status with a significant reduction in events and deaths. There does not appear to be any rebound increase in events of deaths on withdrawal of tamoxifen after 2 years.[27,28] In another study of tamoxifen 10 mg twice daily in node-negative breast cancer with oestrogen receptor positive tumours there was significant prolongation of disease-free survival among woman treated with tamoxifen as compared with placebo, in both those over and under 50 years of age.[29] A review of 61 randomised trials carried out before 1985 indicated that woman over 50 had a clear reduction in mortality with adjuvent tamoxifen (see Major outcome trials).

b. Advanced disease

Tamoxifen is now very widely used as endocrine therapy in advanced breast cancer. The usual dosage is 20–40 mg daily and an overall response rate of about 30% with complete remission in about 10% of cases is seen. As with all hormonal treatments, results in terms of complete or partial remission are better in oestrogen receptor-positive than in oestrogen receptor-negative mammary cancers. Particularly good responses may be predicted in some categories of patients. These are women over 70 years of age (47% objective response), those with mainly soft-tissue disease (48% objective response), those who have already benefited from other endocrine manipulations (55% objective response), or those who have oestrogen receptor-positive tumours.[28,29] However, the relationship between receptor-positive status and clinical response is not absolute. Half of all receptor-positive tumours fail to respond and 13% of receptor-negative tumours show some response. Clinical evidence suggests that about 30% of premenopausal women may also respond to tamoxifen. Soft-tissue metastases respond better than either bone or visceral metastases.[30]

Tamoxifen as sole therapy

Patients aged 60 or over with locally advanced breast cancer for whom surgery, irradiation or chemotherapy are unsuitable or unacceptable are candidates for treatment with tamoxifen. Response rates of 45–61% have been achieved.

2. Infertility

Female infertility

Before starting treatment with tamoxifen, pregnancy should be excluded. In women with anovulatory cycles the initial course of treatment consist of 10 mg twice daily on the second, third, fourth and fifth day of the cycle. If unsatisfactory basal therapeutic records or a poor preovulatory cervical mucus indicate an unsuccessful treatment course, the dose may be increased to 20 mg twice daily up to 40 mg twice daily.

Male infertility

The manufacturers do not recommend the use of the drug in male patients, although it has been studied in infertile males. In patients with idiopathic oligozoo(asthenoterato)spermia, tamoxifen in a dose of 10 mg twice daily given for 6 months or longer increases sperm density, without improving sperm motility[6,31] and in some patients may restore fertility. The rationale is that by blocking the oestrogen receptor at the hypothalamopituitary level, tamoxifen results in an increased LH and FSH secretion, leading to an increase of intratesticular testosterone and stimulation of Sertoli cell function.

Adverse reactions

Potentially life-threatening effects

A small number (~3% of cases treated) of patients with bone metastases of breast cancer may develop hypercalcaemia, which may be life-threatening and require withdrawal of the drug. There is still some debate as to whether the relationship between the drug and the hypercalcaemia is one of cause and effect.

There have been frequent reports of thromboembolytic events occurring during tamoxifen therapy. As an increased incidence of these events is known to occur in patients with malignant disease, a causal relationship with Novaldex has not been established.

Acute overdosage
No cases of deliberate overdosage appear to have been reported. On theoretical grounds an overdosage would be expected to cause enhancement of the antioestrogenic side effects mentioned above. Observations in animals show that extreme overdosage (100–200 times the recommended daily dosage) may produce oestrogenic effects.

There is no specific antidote to overdosage, and treatment must be symptomatic.

Severe or irreversible adverse effects
A small number of cases of corneal changes, cataract and retinopathy have been described, mainly in patients treated with high doses for long periods of time.

Cystic ovarian swellings have occasionally been observed in premenopausal women receiving tamoxifen.

A transient fall of thrombocytes, generally not lower than 80 000 mm^{-3}, has been reported in patients with breast cancer treated with tamoxifen but no haemorrhagic tendency has been reported, platelet counts recovered even when tamoxifen treatment was continued.

Symptomatic adverse effects
A relatively common complaint is gastrointestinal intolerance, as is transient dizziness. The antioestrogen effect may occasionally lead to vaginal bleeding and pruritis vulvae and (rarely) to fluid retention. Some patients may complain of hot flushes, vaginal (withdrawal) bleeding, pruritus vulvae and tumour-flare has occasionally occurred. Menstruation is suppressed in a proportion of premenopausal women receiving tamoxifen for the treatment of breast cancer.

Interference with clinical pathology tests
No technical interferences of this kind appear to have been reported.

High risk groups

Neonates
The drug should not be given to neonates.

Breast milk. Patients taking tamoxifen should not breast-feed.

Children
Use of the drug in children is not recommended.

Pregnant women
Use of the drug is contraindicated during pregnancy.

The elderly
No special precautions are necessary in older patients.

Drug Interactions

Potentially hazardous interactions
Tamoxifen has been reported to considerably increase the effect of warfarin, with possibly fatal results.[32,33]

Potentially useful interactions
None have been reported.

Major outcome trials

1. Ingle J N, Ahmann D L, Green S J et al 1981 Randomized clinical trial of diethylstilbestrol versus tamoxifen in postmenopausal women with advanced breast cancer. New England Journal of Medicine 304: 16–21

The trial involved 143 evaluable patients, of whom 94 had received no prior systemic therapy and 44 received previous chemotherapy. Regression rate was similar in patients treated with either DES or tamoxifen, but tamoxifen appeared to be associated with significantly less toxicity.

2. Cummings F S, Gray R, Davis T E et al 1985 Adjuvant tamoxifen treatment of elderly women with stage II breast cancer. A double blind comparison with placebo. Annals of Internal Medicine 103: 324–329

170 elderly women with stage II breast cancer stratified on the number of positive axillary nodes and oestrogen receptor status were randomly assigned to receive tamoxifen or placebo for 24 months in a prospective adjuvant trial. Benefit was seen in all six groups treated with tamoxifen, resulting in improved time to relapse, statistically fewer distant first recurrences and minimal toxicity; no improvement in overall survival has been seen yet.

3. Early Breast Cancer Trialists Collaborative Group 1988 Effects of adjuvant tomoxifen and of cyclotoxic therapy on mortality in early breast cancer. New England Journal of Medicine 319: 1681–1692

This is an overview of 61 randomised clinical trials involving a total of 28896 woman, which had begun before 1985, and included early breast cancer patients (with or without regional lymph-node involvement) who had received either adjuvent tamoxifen or cyclotoxic therapy. Reductions on mortality due to treatment were significant when tamoxifen was compared with no tamoxifen, when any chemotherapy was compared with no chemotherapy and when poly chemotherapy was compared with single agent chemotherapy. In the tamoxifen trials there was a clear reduction in mortality only among woman 50 or older whereas in the chemotherapy trials there was clear reduction in mortality only in woman under 50. The authors conclude that both tamoxifen and cyclotoxic can reduce five-year mortality.

General review articles

Furr B J and Jordan V C 1984 The pharmacology and clinic uses of tamoxifen. Pharmacology and Therapeutics 25: 127–205

Tucker M J, Adam H K and Patterson J S 1984 Tamoxifen In: safety testing of new drugs (ed Larcine D R, McLean A E and Weatherall M) Academic Press. London 614: 125–161

Lithland S and Jackson I M 1988 Antioestrogens in the management of hormone dependant cancer. Cancer Treatment Reviews 15: 183–194

References

1. Klopper A, Hall M 1971 New synthetic agent for the induction of ovulation. Preliminary trials in women. British Medical Journal 1: 152–154
2. Rose C, Thorpe S M, Mouridsen H T, Andersen J A, Brincker H, Andersen K W 1982 Antiestrogen treatment of postmenopausal women with primary high risk breast cancer: 36 months of life-table analysis and steroid hormone receptor status. Breast Cancer Research and Treatment 3: 77–84
3. Tsuiki A, Uehara S, Kyono K 1984 Induction of ovulation with an estrogen antagonist, tamoxifen (Clomid). Tohoku Journal of Experimental Medicine 144(1): 21–31
4. Groom C V, Griffiths K 1976 Effect of the antiestrogen tamoxifen on plasma levels of luteinizing hormone, follicle stimulating hormone, prolactin, oestradiol and progesterone in normal premenopausal women. Journal of Endocrinology 70: 421–428
5. Golder M P, Phillips M E A, Baum M et al 1975 Hormones in breast cancer patients on tamoxifen. British Journal of Cancer 32: 246–247
6. Willis K J, London D R, Butt W R 1976 Hormonal effects of tamoxifen in women with carcinoma of the breast. Journal of Endocrinology 69: 51P
7. Tajimia C, Fukushima T 1983 Endocrine profiles in tamoxifen-induced ovulatory cycles. Fertility and Sterility 40: 23–30
8. Willis K J, London D R, Bevis M A, Butt W R, Lynch S S, Holder G 1977 Hormonal effects of tamoxifen in oligospermic men. Journal of Endocrinology 73: 171–178
9. Vermeulen A, Comhaire F 1978 Hormonal effects of an antiestrogen, tamoxifen, in normal and oligospermic men. Fertility and Sterility 29: 320–327
10. Willis K J, London D R, Ward H W C, Butt W R, Lynch S S, Rudd B T 1977 Recurrent breast cancer treated with the antiestrogen tamoxifen: correlation between hormonal changes and clinical course. British Medical Journal 1: 425–428
11. Lerner H J, Band P R, Israel L, Leung B S 1976 Phase II study of tamoxifen: report of 74 patients with stage IV breast cancer. Cancer Treatment Reports 60: 1431–1435
12. Sakai F, Cheix F, Clavel M et al 1978 Increases in steroid binding globulin induced by tamoxifen in patients with carcinoma. Journal of Endocrinology 76: 219–226
13. Fex G, Adielsson G, Mattson W 1981 Oestrogen like effects of tamoxifen on the concentration of proteins in plasma. Acta Endocrinologica 97: 109–113
14. Manni A, Pearson O H 1982 Antiestrogens in tumour therapy. Clinical Oncology 1: 65–75
15. Manni A, Trujillo J E, Marshall J S, Brodkey S, Pearson O H 1974 Antihormone treatment of stage IV breast cancer. Cancer 43: 444–450
16. Masson G M, Klopper A 1971 In: Proceedings of a Workshop. ICI 46.474 — work in progress. ICI Ltd, Pharmaceutical Division, Macclesfield, p 40
17. Osmond Clark F, Murray M 1971 In: Proceedings of a Workshop. ICI 46.474 — work in progress. ICI Ltd, Pharmaceutical Division, Macclesfield, p 27
18. Ferrazzi E, Cartei G, Mattarazzo R, Fiorentino M 1977 Oestrogen-like effects of tamoxifen on vaginal epithelium. British Medical Journal 1: 1351–1352
19. Comhaire F 1976 Treatment of oligospermia with tamoxifen. International Journal of Fertility 21: 232–238

T

20. Shaaban M M 1975 Suppression of lactation by an antiestrogen, tamoxifen. European Journal of Obstetrics and Gynecological Reproductive Biology 4/5: 167–169
21. Masala A, Delitala G, Lo Dico G, Stoppelli I, Alagna S, Devilla L 1978 Inhibition of lactation and inhibition of prolactin release after mechanical breast stimulation in puerperal women given tamoxifen or placebo. British Journal of Obstetrics and Gynecology 85: 134–137
22. Golander Y, Sternson L A 1980 Paired ion chromatographic analysis of tamoxifen and two major metabolites in plasma. Journal of Chromatography 181: 41–49
23. Daniel P, Gaskell S J, Bishop H, Campbell Ch, Nicholson I 1981 Determination of tamoxifen and biologically active metabolites in human breast tumours and plasma. European Journal of Cancer and Clinical Oncology 17: 1183–1189
24. Fromson J M, Pearson S, Bramah J M 1973 The metabolism of tamoxifen (ICI 46.474) Part I: in laboratory animals. Xenobiotica 3: 693–710
25. Fromson J M, Pearson S, Bramah S M 1973 The metabolism of tamoxifen (ICI 46.474) Part II: in female patients. Xenobiotica 3: 711–714
26. Kurl R V, Morris I D 1978 Differential detection of cytoplasmic high affinity oestrogen receptors after the in vivo administration of the anti-oestrogens, clomifen, MER-25, tamoxifen. British Journal of Pharmacology 62 (4): 487–493
27. Controlled trial of tamoxifen as single adjuvant agent in management of early breast cancer: analysis at six years by Nolvadex Adjuvant Trial Organisation 1985 Lancet 1: 836–840
28. Pritchard K I, Thomason D B, Meakin J W et al 1981 The role of tamoxifen in premenopausal women with metastatic carcinoma of the breast. Proceedings of the American Society of Clinical Oncology 22: 436–439
29. Wada T, Koyama H, Terasawa T 1981 Effect of tamoxifen in premenopausal Japanese women with advanced breast cancer. Cancer Treatment Reports 65: 728–729
30. Cummings F J, Gray R, Davis T E et al 1985 Adjuvant tamoxifen treatment of elderly women with stage II breast cancer. Annals of Internal Medicine 103: 324–329
31. Buvat J, Buvat-Herbaut M, Marcolm G, Azdaens-Boutier K 1987 Antioestrogens as treatment of female and male infertility. Hormone Research 28: 219–229
32. Lodwick R, McConkey B, Brown A M, Beeley L 1987 Life-threatening interaction between tamoxifen and warfarin. British Medical Journal 295: 1141
33. Tenni P, Lalich D L, Byrne M J 1989 Life threatening interaction between tamoxifen and warfarin. British Medical Journal 298: 93

Temazepam

Temazepam is a member of the 1,4-benzodiazepine series.

Chemistry

Temazepam (3-hydroxydiazepam, Normison, Euhypnos, Euhypnos Forte, Euhypnos Elixir)
$C_{16}H_{13}O_2N_2Cl$
7-Chloro-1,3-dihydro-3-hydroxy-1-methyl-5-phenyl-2H-1,4-benzodiazepin-2-one

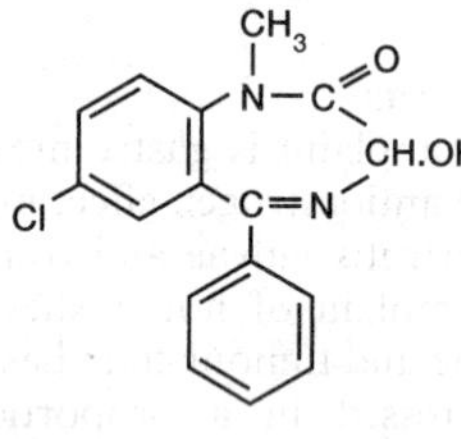

Molecular weight	300.7
pKa	1.6
Solubility	
in alcohol	1 in 10
in water	<1 in 10 000
Octanol/water partition coefficient	—

A white or off-white odourless, free flowing crystalline powder, it is prepared by chemical synthesis. C3 of the diazepine ring is asymmetric. There are no combination products including temazepam.

Pharmacology

Temazepam has similar pharmacological activity to oxazepam and diazepam, that is central nervous system sedation, anxiolysis and muscle relaxation. Animal studies show anticonvulsant activity.[1] These effects are likely to be due to potentiation of gamma-aminobutyric acid (GABA), although other neurotransmitters may also be affected.[2] Evidence suggests a close molecular association between the sites and action for GABA and the benzodiazepines.

Toxicology

Temazepam does not appear to have mutagenic potential and toxicological tests in beagles and rats, lasting 6 months at doses up to 120 $mg.kg^{-1}$, showed no significant toxic effects. There was no evidence of carcinogenicity in tests on rats lasting 2 years. Dysmorphogenic changes in rib formation have been observed in rats and rabbits receiving 240 $mg.kg^{-1}$ and 40 $mg.kg^{-1}$ respectively, but no such changes were seen with lower doses.[3] Fertility studies, however, on both male and female rats at doses up to 90 $mg.kg^{-1}$ showed no adverse effects on fertility.

Clinical pharmacology

In man temazepam has been shown to have both hypnotic/sedative and anxiolytic activity. In trials on healthy volunteers[4,5] bedtime doses of up to 30 mg significantly increased total sleep time and reduced wake time but effects on sleep onset latency were variable. Other trials have claimed decreased sleep onset latency.[6,7] Temazepam does not reduce the proportion of rapid eye movement (REM) sleep, but it does delay the onset of the first REM period and reduces stages 3 and 4 (slow wave) sleep.[4] Other studies using lower doses showed no effects on stage 3 and 4 (slow wave) sleep.[8,9] Temazepam has anxiolytic activity and has been used in man for the treatment of anxiety.[10] Temazepam also acts as a respiratory depressant particularly under hypoxic conditions. The recommended dose range by the manufacturers is 10–60 mg for insomnia, and 20–40 mg for premedication purposes. The highest dose known to have been used is 140 mg in a 'safety study in psychiatric disorders'.

Pharmacokinetics

The preferred analytical method for detecting the drug in plasma is by the original gas-chromatographic method of Belvedere et al,[11] with a sensitivity of 5 µg.l^{-1}. There are, however, now several high performance liquid chromatography (HPLC) methods for detecting the drug in plasma with sensitivities comparable to that of electron-capture gas chromatography.[12] With the newer formulations using a soft gelatin capsule, containing a solution of the drug in polyethylene glycol, absorption is rapid and nearly complete. Peak plasma concentrations are seen in less than one hour in fasting patients and 80% of the peak value is reached by about 20 minutes.[13,14]

Reported elimination half life values for temazepam after night time administration in young volunteers vary from 5.3–11.5 hours, depending on the study.[15,16] There is, however, an approximately 30% increase in the half life of temazepam when taken in the morning.[17] The mean elimination half life values in young volunteers after morning administration vary from 8.3–13.6 hours.[17–19] One study[19] with a mean of 8.3 hours has a range of 3.3–13.4 hours. In the elderly the half life may be longer with a mean value of about 15 hours having been reported.[20,3] The half life in elderly women may be longer than in elderly men.[21,22] First pass metabolism has not been investigated in man. It is suspected that by analogy with closely structurally related benzodiazepines e.g. lormetazepam,[23] that there is no significant first pass effect in humans. This view is supported by minimal intersubject variation in plasma levels.

Assuming complete oral bioavailability, the volume of distribution of temazepam[24] has been calculated as approximately 1.32–1.53 l.kg^{-1}. In vitro, temazepam was 76% bound to bovine serum albumin.[25] Another study[24] showed temazepam to be highly bound to plasma proteins with a mean free fraction of only 2–4%.

According to Wyeth, there are no studies in animals comparing the CSF and plasma or brain and plasma concentrations. There are no data available on the excretion of temazepam in human milk, but it is likely to be excreted in small amounts due to its similarity to other benzodiazepines which are excreted in milk.

Oral absorption	>95%
Presystemic metabolism	probably negligible
Plasma half life	5.3–11.5 h
Volume of distribution	1.3–1.5 l.kg^{-1}
Plasma protein binding	76–96%

Temazepam

Concentration–effect relationship

There is no information available on the relationship between plasma concentration and drug effects of temazepam.

Metabolism

Temazepam is extensively metabolized in the liver mainly by conjugation with glucuronic acid to inactive metabolites.[16] There is very little unchanged drug excreted. Excretion is mainly (80%) in the urine, with only about 12% appearing in the faeces.[16] The metabolic pathways are shown in Figure 1. They involve conjugation of the hydroxyl group, loss of the N-methyl group, and conjugation of the desmethyl derivative. All four compounds may be further metabolized to unidentified metabolites. A small amount of oxazepam is produced, but the amounts are insignificant. This is the only pharmacologically active metabolite. There is evidence of enterohepatic circulation in rats.[26]

Pharmaceutics

Temazepam is available in the UK as capsules and as an elixir.

Temazepam capsules (Wyeth, UK) are opaque, yellow soft gelatin capsules containing 10 mg or 20 mg temazepam. The 10 mg capsules are No 4 capsules printed with 'WYETH' in black lettering. The 20 mg capsules are No 10 capsules printed 'WYETH' on one side and '20' on the other in red lettering.

Normison capsules (Wyeth, UK) are opaque, yellow soft gelatin capsules containing 10 mg or 20 mg temazepam. The 10 mg capsules are No 4 capsules printed 'N10' in black lettering. The 20 mg capsules are No 10 capsules printed 'N20' in red lettering.

The 7.5 size has been replaced by No 10 capsules for both formulations.

Restoril (Sandoz, US) 15 mg capsules are maroon and pink and marked 'RESTORIL 15 mg' and '78-98'. 30 mg Restoril capsules are maroon and blue and marked 'RESTORIL 30 mg' and '78-99'. 15 mg and 30 mg capsules are also marketed by Barr Laboratories, USA.

Temazepam Gelthix capsules (Farmitalia, UK) are green soft gelatin capsules containing 10 mg, 15 mg, 20 mg or 30 mg of temazepam and marked with their respective strengths. The Gelthix capsules, which contain a semisolid gel, replace the original softgel capsules, which were subject to abuse by drug users.

Temazepam elixir (Farmitalia, UK) is a clear green lemon-mint flavoured elixir containing 10 mg of temazepam per 5 ml.

Temazepam tablets (Berk, UK) are available as green capsules of either 10 mg or 20 mg.

Temazepam capsules should be stored in a cool dry place and have a maximum shelf life of 2 years. There is no known risk from potentially allergenic substances. Temazepam elixir should be stored below 25°C and protected from light.

Fig. 1 Metabolic pathways of temazepam

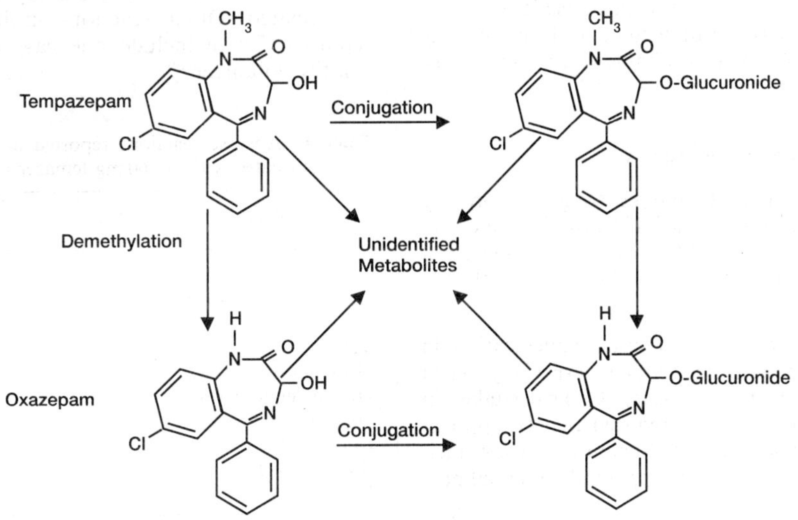

Therapeutic use

Indications

1. Short term treatment of insomnia
2. Premedication before minor surgery.

Contraindications

1. Previous history of sensitivity to benzodiazepines
2. Acute pulmonary insufficiency.

Mode of use

A dose of 10–30 mg half an hour before retiring is usually sufficient in the treatment of insomnia. The dose may be increased to 40–60 mg in patients who do not respond to the lower dosage schedule.

A dose of 20–40 mg may be given 30–60 minutes before surgical or other procedures as a premedication.

The manufacturers recommend lower doses in the elderly and suggest doses approximately half those given above. Like other benzodiazepines sudden withdrawal from very high doses may cause convulsions and even a toxic delirium. The evidence for physical dependence and a withdrawal syndrome with lower doses of benzodiazepines is increasingly accepted. There is increasing evidence to support a benzodiazepine withdrawal syndrome.[27] Withdrawal symptoms on stopping an excessive dosage of temazepam have been reported.[28]

Indications

1. Insomnia

Temazepam appears to be an effective hypnotic which increases total sleep time, although studies on sleep onset latency give variable results. [4–6,19] A study on insomniac outpatients[30] showed subjective improvement, however, in the time taken to fall asleep. Although a single dose has been shown to be an effective hypnotic[31] in the elderly, there is one study which suggests[32] that temazepam may be less effective in older age groups than in the young. There is, however, another study[33] which found that the response to 20 mg temazepam was greater and longer lasting in patients and healthy elderly volunteers than in younger controls. Its relatively short half life and simple one stage metabolism mean that it is largely free of residual 'morning after' effects such as hangover, drowsiness and dizziness. It should be noted that at doses of 30 mg some studies[34,35] showed residual effects on psychomotor performance the following day. These may, however, be less than with other hypnotics such as flurazepam.[4] It should also be remembered that the half life may be lengthened in the elderly,[20] accumulation has been reported[20] and impairment of psychomotor performance may occur.[36]

The manufacturers claim that rebound insomnia on stopping temazepam has not been reported. One sleep laboratory study[29] in insomniac patients given 30 mg daily for 5 weeks showed no evidence of tolerance or rebound insomnia on discontinuation.

Patients with insomnia unresponsive to lower doses have responded to doses of up to 60 mg of temazepam. Morning 'hangover' effects were reported to be fairly mild even at this dose level.[37]

The Royal College of Psychiatrists recommend that the prescribing of benzodiazepines such as temazepam is suitable when insomnia is:

i. Disabling
ii. Severe, or
iii. Subjecting the individual to extreme distress.

The underlying cause for insomnia should be sought before the prescription of drugs for symptomatic relief. If benzodiazepines are prescribed for insomnia, then this should be at a low dosage, not every night and normally for a maximum period of one month.[38]

2. Premedication

Temazepam is also suitable for use as an oral premedication in patients undergoing minor surgical procedures, especially when hospital admission is not considered necessary. Clinical studies in such patients, including the elderly, showed reduced anxiety, appreciable sedation, smoothness of anaesthetic induction and a low incidence of post operative sequelae. There was apparently minimal post operative sedation.[39,40]

Temazepam has recently been used as a premedicant in children either as the elixir[44] or as a small wafer consisting of a fast dissolving matrix (FDDF) which is tasteless.[42]

The study using FDDF temazepam (at a dose range of 0.25–0.33 $mg.kg^{-1}$ found it to be palatable, rapidly absorbed with a short predictable onset of optimal effect and a short duration of action. The study of Thomas[41] using higher dosages (0.5–1.5 $mg.kg^{-1}$) in comparison with trimeprazine tartrate found similar efficacy between the two drugs. Temazepam, however, was associated with more ectopic beats under anaesthesia, more post-operative vomiting, and more post-operative restlessness than trimeprazine tartrate.

Contraindications

1. Sensitivity to benzodiazepines

Hypersensitivity reactions to benzodiazepines are probably fairly rare but are an obvious contraindication to further use.

2. Acute pulmonary insufficiency

Like all benzodiazepines, temazepam acts as a central depressant and is not recommended in patients whose respiration is severely compromised.

Adverse reactions

Potentially life-threatening effects

No life threatening adverse effects have, apparently, been reported.

Acute overdosage

There is little data available on temazepam overdoses. One study[37] noted 13 cases of non-fatal overdose in a 12-week study of 10 057 patients. As with other benzodiazepines, overdosage should not present a threat to life, unless other drugs have been taken concurrently. However, two fatal self-poisonings have been reported with temazepam alone. These occurred in an elderly couple where suicide was the intent. Temazepam was the only drug detected and there was no involvement of alcohol.[43] Treatment is symptomatic and gastric lavage may prove useful if performed shortly after ingestion. The patient is likely to sleep and close observation with general supportive measures and maintenance of a clear airway are important.

Severe or irreversible effects

The manufacturers (Farmitalia Carlo Erba) report rare severe adverse effects including hypotension, blood dyscrasias and jaundice.

Symptomatic adverse effects

Temazepam is generally well tolerated, with adverse effects being mild and infrequent. The following table (table 1) has been compiled by the Wyeth company on the basis of 11 clinical trials [37,44–53] including 23 969 patients treated with 10–60 mg of temazepam for insomnia. Whether all these adverse effects are due to temazepam is open to debate. In a placebo-controlled study[30] most adverse effects occurred with similar frequency in drug-treated and placebo-treated groups, although a few instances of the more severe effects, such as depression, lethargy and nightmares, may have been drug-related. Other reactions in individual patients have been reported. These include one case of nystagmus in a physically healthy volunteer.[29]

Table 1 Adverse reactions reported in 11 clinical trials including 23 939 patients treated with 10–60 mg temazepam for insomnia

Adverse effect	Patients affected	
	No.	%
Gastrointestinal disturbances	366	1.5
Headache	336	1.4
Vertigo	224	0.9
Drowsiness/tiredness	215	0.9
Dreams/nightmares	196	0.8
Dry mouth/throat	76	0.3
Depression	59	0.2
Restless sleep	54	0.2
Skin rashes	30	0.1

Temazepam

Other effects

The manufacturers report that laboratory investigations carried out in humans treated for up to 5 months with temazepam showed no effects on haemopoetic, hepatic or renal systems.

Interference with clinical pathology test methods

There are no data available to suggest that temazepam interferes with clinical pathology tests.

High risk groups

Neonates

Temazepam has not been evaluated for any use in neonates and is not recommended by the manufacturers.

Breast milk. It is likely that temazepam is excreted in breast milk in small amounts, and may therefore exert effects on the infant.

Children

Temazepam is not recommended for the treatment of insomnia in children. It has now been successfully used as a premedication agent in children (see section on Premedication).

Pregnant women

The safety of temazepam has not been evaluated in human pregnancy and therefore its use should be avoided, especially in the first and last trimesters.

The elderly

Approximately half the usual dosages should be given because temazepam has a longer half life in the elderly and accumulation can occur[20]. Impairment of psychomotor performance in elderly subjects compared with younger controls, despite unaltered plasma concentrations, has been reported.[36] This increased sensitivity of the elderly may be due to a lower plasma protein binding measured in vitro[54] which might cause a higher free concentration in vivo. It may however be due to a central effect as benzodiazepine-induced increases in GABA binding and GABA-induced increases in neuronal inhibition are greater in aged animals.[55,56]

Drug interactions

Potentially hazardous interactions

In common with other benzodiazepines the concurrent use of general anaesthetic agents, narcotic analgesics and some antidepressants will result in an accentuation of their sedative effects.

Temazepam, like other benzodiazepines, will enhance the CNS effects of alcohol. This is potentially serious in the case of overdosage.

Potentially useful interactions

There is no information available.

Clinical trials

1. Heffron W A, Roth P 1979 Double-blind evaluation of the safety and hypnotic efficacy of temazepam in insomniac out patients. British Journal of Clinical Pharmacology 8: 69S–72S

This was a double-blind, parallel group design study involving 55 insomniac outpatients. Patients were randomly allocated to take either placebo at night (26 patients) or temazepam 30 mg at night (29 patients). Treatment was taken for four consecutive nights and sleep questionnaires were completed the following day. Patients reported that temazepam was more effective than placebo in reducing the difficulty in falling asleep and improving sleep maintenance. They also indicated that they awoke less often and were less disturbed by early morning awakenings. They reported as a group that average duration of sleep was increased by about one hour. Patients receiving temazepam reported feeling more alert in the morning and indeed throughout the rest of the day than the patients taking placebo.

Other trials

Mitler M M, Carskadon Mary A, et al 1979 Hypnotic efficacy of temazepam: a long term sleep laboratory evaluation. British Journal of Clinical Pharmacology 8: 63S–68S

Temazepam was evaluated in a strictly defined insomniac patient population. These were physically healthy volunteers with a history of chronic insomnia of at least six months duration not associated with significant psychopathology. Additionally, pre-study sleep laboratory findings revealed objective sleep latency of more than 15 minutes, objective sleep time of less than 6.5 hours and at least 30 minutes of objective wake time after sleep onset unless total sleep time was 5 hours or less. Two protocols were used; a short term (26 night) and a long term (54 night) evaluating the efficacy of 15 mg and 30 mg respectively of temazepam. The authors found temazepam to be both safe and effective at these doses. There was suppression of slow wave sleep with the higher dose but unlike other benzodiazepines there was no suppression of REM sleep. They also found no evidence of tolerance or rebound effects.

General review articles

Lader M H, Makin E J B, Nicholson A N 1979 Proceedings of a symposium on temazepam and related 1,4-benzodiazepines: effects on sleep and on performance October 1978. British Journal of Clinical Pharmacology 8 (suppl 1)

Greenblatt D J, Divoll M, Abernathy D R, Ochs H R, Shader R I 1983 Clinical pharmacokinetics of the newer benzodiazepines. Clinical Pharmacokinetics 8: 232–252

References

1. Hindmarch I 1975 A 1,4-benzodiazepine, temazepam (K 3917), its effects on some psychological parameters of sleep and behaviour. Arzneimittel Forschung 25: 1836–1839
2. Lader M H 1980 Introduction to psychopharmacology. Scope Publication (Upjohn) ch 8, p 98
3. Heel R C, Brogden R N, Speight T M, Avery G S 1981 Temazepam: a review of its pharmacological properties and therapeutic efficacy as an hypnotic. Drugs 21: 321–340
4. Roth T, Piccione P, Salis P, Kramer M, Kaffeman M 1979 Effects of temazepam, flurazepam and quinalbarbitone on sleep: psychomotor and cognitive function. British Journal of Clinical Pharmacology 8: 47S–54S
5. Nicholson A N, Stone B M 1979 Diazepam and 3 hydroxy-diazepam (temazepam) and sleep of middle age. British Journal of Clinical Pharmacology 7: 463–468
6. Wyeth In: Normison. Technical book. Wyeth Laboratories, p 3
7. Harry T V A, Latham A N 1980 Hypnotic and residual effects of temazepam in volunteers. British Journal of Clinical Pharmacology 9: 618–620
8. Nicholson A N, Stone B M et al 1976 Hypnotic and residual effects of temazepam in volunteers. British Journal of Clinical Pharmacology 3: 543–550
9. Beary M D, Lacey J H, Crutchfield M B, Bhat A V et al 1984 Psychosocial stress, insomnia and temazepam: a sleep laboratory evaluation in a 'general practice' sample. Psychopharmacology 83: 17–19
10. Sarteschi P, Cassano G B, Castrogiovanni P, Placidi G F, Sacchetti F 1972 Major and minor tranquillizers in the treatment of anxiety states. Arzneimittel Forschung 22: 93–97
11. Belvedere G, Tognoni G, Fugerio A, Morselli P L 1972 A specific, rapid and sensitive method for gas-chromatographic determination of methyl-oxazepam in small samples of blood. Analytical Letters 5 (8): 531–541
12. Patterson S E 1986 Determination of temazepam in plasma and urine by high-performance liquid chromatography using disposable solid-phase extraction columns. Journal of Pharmaceutical and Biomedical Analysis 4: 271–274
13. Fuccella L M, Bolcioni G, Tomassia V, Ferrario L, Tognoni G 1977 Human pharmacokinetics and bioavailability of temazepam administered in soft gelatin capsules. European Journal of Clinical Pharmacology 12: 383–386
14. Fuccella L M 1979 Bioavailability of temazepam in soft gelatin capsules. British Journal of Clinical Pharmacology 8: 31S–35S
15. Fuccella L M, Tosolini G, Moro E, Tamassia 1972 Study of physiological availability of temazepam in man. International Journal of Clinical Pharmacology 6: 303–309
16. Schwarz H J 1979 Pharmacokinetics and metabolism of temazepam in man and several animal species. British Journal of Clinical Pharmacology 8: 23S–29S
17. Fuccella L M 1979 Bioavailability of temazepam in soft gelatin capsules. British Journal of Clinical Pharmacology 8: 31S–35S
18. Salem S A M, Kinney C D, McDevitt D G et al 1981 Pharmacokinetics and psychomotor effects of nitrazepam and temazepam in young males and females. British Journal of Clinical Pharmacology 11: 412P–413P
19. Bittencourt P, Richens A, Toseland P A, Wicks J F C, Latham A N 1979 Pharmacokinetics of the hypnotic benzodiazepine, temazepam. British Journal of Clinical Pharmacology 8: 37S–38S
20. Cook P 1980 Change in benzodiazepine drug activity with ageing. In: Exton-Smith A N (ed) Current trends in therapeutics in the elderly. Oxford Medical Education Services, pp 23–32
21. Smith R B, Divoll M, Gillespie W R, Greenblatt D J 1983 Effect of subject age and gender on the pharmacokinetics of oral triazolam and temazepam. Journal of Clinical Psychopharmacology 3: 172–176
22. Cook P J 1986 Benzodiazepine hypnotics in the elderly. Acta Psychiatrica Scandinavica 74 (suppl 332): 149–158
23. Humpel M, Nieuweber B, Milins W, Hanke H, Wendt Kinetics and biotransformation of lormetazepam II. Radioimmunologic determination in plasma and urine of young and elderly subjects: first-pass effect. Clinical Pharmacology and Therapeutics 28: 673–679
24. Divoll M et al 1981 Effect of age and gender on the disposition of temazepam. Journal of Pharmaceutical Science 70: 1104–1107
25. Curry S H, Whelpton R 1979 Pharmacokinetics of related benzodiazepines. British Journal of Clinical Pharmacology 8: 15S–21S

26. Tse F L S, Ballard F, Jaffe J M 1982 A practical method for monitoring drug excretion and enterohepatic circulation in the rat. Journal of Pharmacological Methods 7: 139–144
27. Hallstrom C, Lader M H 1981 Benzodiazepine withdrawal phenomena. International Pharmacopsychiatry 16: 235–244
28. Ratna L 1981 Addiction to temazepam. British Medical Journal 282: 1837–1838
29. Mitler M M, Mary A, Carskadon B L et al 1979 Hypnotic efficacy of temazepam: a long term sleep laboratory evaluation. British Journal of Clinical Pharmacology 8: 63S–68S
30. Heffron W A, Roth P 1979 Double-blind evaluation of the safety and hypnotic efficacy of temazepam in insomniac out patients. British Journal of Clinical Pharmacology 8: 69S–72S
31. Briggs R S, Castleden C M, Kraft C A 1980 Improved hypnotic treatment using chlormethiazole and temazepam. British Medical Journal 280: 601–604
32. Stone B M 1979 Diazepam and its hydroxylated metabolites: studies on sleep in healthy man. British Journal of Clinical Pharmacology 8: 57S–63S
33. Swift C G, Haythorne J M, Clarke P, Stevenson I H 1981 The effect of ageing on measured responses to single doses of oral temazepam. British Journal of Clinical Pharmacology 11: 413P–414P
34. Nicholson A N 1979 Performance studies with diazepam and its hydroxylated metabolites. British Journal of Clinical Pharmacology 8: 39S–42S
35. Hindmarch I 1979 Effects of hypnotic and sleep inducing drugs on objective assessments of human psychomotor performance and subjective appraisals of sleep and early morning behaviour. British Journal of Clinical Pharmacology 8: 43S–46S
36. Swift C G 1982 Hypnotic drugs. In: Isaacs B (ed) Recent advances in geriatric medicine, vol II. Churchill Livingstone, Edinburgh
37. Fowler L K, Schiller M 1980 Euhypnos Forte, high dose temazepam for resistant insomnia: post marketing surveillance in 10 057 patients unresponsive to conventional hypnotic dosage. Journal of International Medical Research 8: 446–452
38. Priest R G, Montgomery S A 1988 Benzodiazepines and dependence: a college statement. Bulletin of Royal College of Psychiatry, vol 12, no 3
39. Beechey A P G, Eltringham R J, Studd C 1981 Temazepam as premedication in day surgery. Anaesthesia 36: 10–15
40. Clark G, Erwin D, Yate P, Burt D, Major E 1982 Temazepam as premedication in elderly patients. Anaesthesia 37: 421–425
41. Thomas D L, Vaughan R S, Vickers M D, Mapleson W W 1987 Comparison of temazepam elixir and trimeprazine syrup as premedication in children undergoing tonsillectomy and associated procedures. British Journal of Anaesthesia 59: 424–430
42. Shroeder H G 1986 The use of temazepam Expidet (FDDF) as a premedicant in children. Acta Psychiatrica Scandinavica 74 (suppl 332): 167–171
43. Martin C D, Chan S C 1986 Distribution of temazepam in body fluids and tissue in lethal overdose. Journal of Analytical Toxicology 10: 77–78
44. Fowler L K 1977 Temazepam (Euhypnos) as a hypnotic: a twelve week trial in general practice. Journal of International Medical Research 5: 295–296
45. Fowler L K 1980 Post marketing surveillance of Euhypnos (temazepam) a new hypnotic. Journal of International Medical Research 8: 295–299
46. Harry T V A, Johnson P A 1978 The effectiveness of temazepam as a hypnotic: an open, multicentre assessment in 804 patients with sleep disorders. Current Medical Research and Opinion 5: 476–483
47. Moon C A L, Schiller M 1979 Euhypnos Forte (temazepam) for resistant insomnia: a clinical trial. Journal of International Medical Research 7: 295–301
48. Sussman H S 1979 Euhypnos Forte (temazepam) in insomniac patients: a clinical trial in general practice. Journal of International Medical Research 7: 290–294
49. Cuanang H J R, Limos 1982 Treatment of insomnia with temazepam: double-blind placebo controlled evaluation. Clinical Therapeutics 4: 402
50. Priest R G, Rizvi Z A 1976 Nitrazepam and temazepam: a comparative trial of two hypnotics. Journal of International Research 4: 145–151
51. Frithz G, Groppi W 1981 Temazepam versus nitrazepam: a comparative trial in the treatment of sleep disturbances. Journal of International Medical Research 9: 338
52. Pines A, Nandi A R, Rahman M, Raafat H, Rooney J F F 1976 A clinical trial of temazepam, a sleep inducer, in hospital patients. Journal of International Medical Research 4: 132–137
53. Fowler L K 1977 Temazepam (Euhypnos) as a hypnotic: a multicentre trial in general practice. Journal of International Medical Research 5: 297
54. Divoll M, Greenblatt D J, Harmatz J S, Shader R I 1981 Effect of age and gender on disposition of temazepam. Journal of Pharmaceutical Sciences 70: 1104–1107
55. Calderini G, Bonetti A C, Aldinio A, Savoino G, Di Perri B, Biggio G, Toffano G 1981 Functional interaction between benzodiazepine and GABA recognition sites. Neurobiology of Ageing 2: 309–313
56. Lippa A S, Critchett D J, Ehlert F, Yamamura H I, Enna S J, Bartus R T 1981 Age related alterations in neurotransmitter receptors. An electrophysiological and biochemical analysis. Neurobiology of Ageing 2: 3–8

Terbutaline

Terbutaline is a selective β_2-adrenergic receptor agonist used in the treatment of asthma and premature labour.

Chemistry

Terbutaline sulphate (Bricanyl)
$C_{12}H_{19}NO_3.\frac{1}{2}H_2SO_4$
1-(3,5-Dihydroxy-phenyl)-2-(t-butylamino)ethanol sulphate

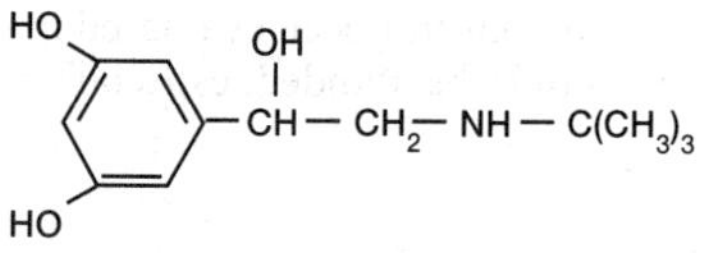

Molecular weight	274.3
pKa	8.8, 10.1, 11.2
Solubility	
in alcohol	1 in 500
in water	1 in 4
Octanol/water partition coefficient	—

A white to off white crystalline powder with a slightly bitter taste.

Pharmacology

Terbutaline is a selective β_2 adrenergic agonist with effects on smooth and skeletal muscle. These include bronchodilatation, relaxation of uterine muscle, vasodilatation and tremor. Smooth muscle relaxation is dose-dependent and is thought to occur via the adenyl cyclase — cyclic adenosine monophosphate (cAMP) system with binding of the drug to the β adrenergic receptor in the cell membrane causing conversion of ATP to cAMP which activates protein kinase. This leads to phosphorylation of proteins which ultimately increase bound intracellular calcium; the consequent reduced availability of ionized calcium inhibits actin-myosin linkage thus causing relaxation of smooth muscle.

β_2 agonists such as terbutaline also have an antiallergic effect on mast cells causing inhibition of release of bronchoconstrictor mediators including histamine and neutrophil chemotactic factor (NCF) following antigen provocation testing in vivo.[1,2] As with β receptors on bronchial smooth muscle, it is likely that the cAMP system acts as the 'second messenger' in regulating the mast cell response.

Toxicology

There is no evidence of teratogenicity in rabbits, rats or mice. In common with other β-agonists, terbutaline has been shown to induce benign mesovarian leiomyomas in the rat but there is no evidence of carcinogenicity.

Clinical pharmacology

Bronchodilatation occurs after administration of terbutaline in normal subjects and in those with asthma or chronic obstructive pulmonary disease (COPD). In normal subjects this effect is best demonstrated by measurements of airways resistance (or specific airways conductance) during panting or tidal breathing. In patients with airways obstruction simple tests of forced expiration suffice. Asthmatic subjects usually show the largest responses but the magnitude of effect depends on pretreatment airway calibre, dose, route and method of administration.[3]
Other actions on the respiratory system include enhanced mucociliary clearance.[4] and an antiallergic effect due to inhibition of mediator release.[1,2] The clinical relevance of these actions is not established.

Terbutaline

Terbutaline has a relaxant effect on smooth muscle at other sites including the myometrium, where its inhibitory effect is put to therapeutic use,[5] and peripheral blood vessels. Stimulation of β_2-receptors on vascular smooth muscle leads to vasodilatation and a reflex increase in heart rate and stroke volume.[6] The chronotropic effect of terbutaline is considerably less than that of a non-selective β-stimulant such as isoprenaline.

Stimulation of β_2-receptors results in widespread metabolic effects, including a fall in serum potassium concentration and rises in free fatty acid, glucose and insulin concentrations.[7] Terbutaline has also been shown to raise high-density lipoprotein–cholesterol levels.[8]

Studies of possible tolerance during long-term treatment with β_2-stimulants have produced conflicting results. Although tachyphylaxis is readily demonstrable in vitro and in non-airway β-receptors in vivo, the balance of evidence suggests that it is unlikely that a clinically important loss of therapeutic effect occurs in airway receptors in patients with asthma using regular conventional inhaled or oral doses.[9,10] A recent study[11] has, however, suggested a rebound increase in histamine-induced bronchial responsiveness 24 hours after cessation of regular inhaled treatment. The clinical relevance of this finding is uncertain.

Pharmacokinetics

Radioisotope labelling has been used for assaying terbutaline but the most commonly applied analytical methods involve gas chromatography and mass spectrometry.[12–14] An ionized derivative suitable for measurement is obtained either by chemical means or by electron impact. With the technique of Lefrink et al.[12] terbutaline concentrations as low as 0.1 μg.l^{-1} are detectable but under routine conditions a limit of 1 μg.l^{-1} with a coefficient of variation of 10% is more realistic.[12,15]

The interindividual variability in oral absorption is large, ranging between 25 and 80%;[16,17] presystemic metabolism is considerable but shows less interindividual variation, averaging about 60% of the absorbed dose.[16–19] The bioavailability of orally administered drug is consequently very variable (7–26%),[16] more because of differences in absorption than in presystemic conjugation. Food reduces the peak drug concentration and bioavailability. Plasma concentrations during pregnancy are lower than those achieved with the same dose in the non-pregnant state.[20] The sustained action of the slow-release formulation of terbutaline is due to slower absorption rather than to any difference in presystemic metabolism.[21] The site of presystemic metabolism is likely to include both the liver and intestinal wall but their relative importance is uncertain; the drug is conjugated, mainly to the sulphate and to a small extent to glucuronide.[22] The majority of an oral dose circulates as the sulphate conjugate which is pharmacologically inactive.

Oral absorption	25–80%
Presystemic metabolism	60%
Plasma half life	
range	14–18 h
terminal	14–18 h
Volume of distribution	1.6 l.kg^{-1}
Plasma protein binding	14–25%

When administered parenterally, most of the infused drug circulates unchanged; in the first hour after an intravenous dose of radio-labelled terbutaline it was shown that the unmetabolized drug accounts for more than 85% of the radioactivity.[19]

In general only about 10% or less of inhaled drug from a pressurized aerosol or nebulized solution is deposited in the airways. In the case of terbutaline inhaled by normal subjects from a pressurized aerosol, pulmonary absorption was shown to vary between 4 and 13% of the dose.[23] Unlike isoprenaline, no first pass pulmonary metabolism of terbutaline occurs.[24] Peak plasma concentrations after inhalation of a wet aerosol are approximately one-fifth of those after an identical oral dose and are achieved within 0.5–1 hour, compared with 2–3 hours after oral administration.[21] The lower plasma concentrations are associated with correspondingly less severe non-respiratory adverse effects.

The mean distribution volume averages 1.6 l.kg^{-1}.[16] The proportion protein bound is small (14–25%). The drug is very hydrophilic and only slowly enters the brain. It does cross the placenta and is excreted in breast milk in concentrations similar to plasma; levels in the suckling infant are however, undetectable.[26]

Concentration–effect relationship

Concentration-related rises in FEV_1 have been shown over the range 1–8 μg.l^{-1} after oral or subcutaneous terbutaline.[26,27] This is not relevant to administration by inhalation, where plasma levels for comparable efficacy are much lower. Assay in clinical practice is difficult and unnecessary. For a tocolytic effect plasma concentrations between 5 and 31.5 μg.l^{-1} have been reported.[20,28]

Metabolism

Unlike isoprenaline, terbutaline is not a substrate for catechol-O-methyltransferase or for monoamine oxidase.[29] Metabolism is by conjugation, predominantly to the sulphate with a small proportion of glucuronide (see Fig. 1).[22] A plasma half life of 2–5 hours is generally quoted but the terminal half life is considerably longer (14–18 h).[17] Approximately 90% of the drug is excreted by the kidneys with renal clearance close to the clearance of creatinine.[17] The proportion conjugated, however, depends heavily on the route of administration: after oral dosing about three-quarters is conjugated, while after parenteral administration the ratio is reversed with 16–35% conjugated.[16,30]

Fig. 1 Metabolism of terbutaline

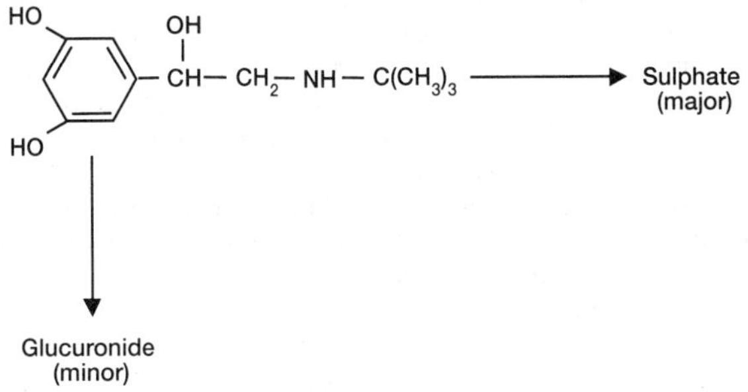

Pharmaceutics

Oral preparations include: Bricanyl, Bricanyl SA (Astra, UK), Monovent SA (Lagap).

5 mg off-white scored tablets, marked '5'.

7.5 mg white tablets in slow-release matrix (Bricanyl SA), marked 'A' and on opposite face 'BD'.

2.5 mg compound plain white tablets with 100 mg guaiaphenesin.

In the USA Bricanyl is licensed to laheside/Merrell Dow and is also marketed by Geigy as Brethine. Tablet strengths ar 2.5 mg and 5 mg.

300 μg.ml^{-1} in sorbitol-base for dilution with water (life of diluted syrup 14 days).

Expectorant: 300 μg.ml^{-1} plus 13.3 mg.ml^{-1} guaiaphenesin in sorbitol-based syrup.

Parenteral preparations include Bricanyl (Astra).

500 μg.ml^{-1} in 1 ml ampoules for subcutaneous, intramuscular or intravenous injection or infusion, 1 mg.ml^{-1} in the USA. Continuous infusion in glucose 5% of sodium chloride 0.9% over 8 hours.

Inhaled preparations include: Bricanyl (Astra). Brethaire (Geigy, USA)

Metered-dose aerosol: 250 μg per puff (refill canister available). The dose actually administered to the back of the mouth is 200 μg per puff.

Spacer inhaler: 250 μg per puff via collapsible 'spacer' extended mouthpiece (refill canister available). Canister may also be fitted into 'Nebuhaler'; a large biconical plastic device with one-way valve.

Breath-actuated dry powder inhaler ('Turbohaler'): 500 μg per inhalation.

Respirator solution: 2.5 mg.ml^{-1} in 2 ml ampoules (Respules) or 10 mg.ml^{-1} in 10 ml bottle for dilution with saline.

Terbutaline preparations are stable with a quoted shelf-life of 2 years for the respirator and injectable solutions and 3 years for pressurized aerosol, tablets and undiluted syrup. The respirator solution should be stored in a cool dark place. Respules and solutions for injection should be protected from light and stored at room temperature. None of the formulations contains tartrazine but the syrup and expectorant contain sodium benzoate.

T

Therapeutic use

Indications

1. Bronchodilator for use in asthma, chronic bronchitis, emphysema and other conditions associated with airways obstruction
2. In management of premature labour.

Contraindications

1. No absolute contraindications in the treatment of airways obstruction. Care is required in patients with thyrotoxicosis or ischaemic heart disease. Inhaled preparations are unlikely to cause problems unless large doses are used
2. In management of premature labour, antepartum haemorrhage or toxaemia of pregnancy are contraindications and caution is necessary in the presence of cardiac disease.

Mode of use

1. Bronchodilatation

Selective β_2-agonists given by inhalation are the bronchodilators of first choice in patients with asthma and other forms of airways obstruction. For the relief of occasional symptoms, one or two inhalations from a Turbohaler or metered dose aerosol as necessary may suffice. An inhaler may be used in similar fashion before exercise in subjects prone to exercise-induced asthma. In patients with asthma or COPD who have persistent symptomatic airways obstruction the drug should be inhaled regularly three or four times a day. The need for treatment and its effects should be monitored by measurements of PEF and/or FEV_1. The magnitude of improvement after inhalation helps in defining the optimal dose but a small or unrecordable increase on a single occasion does not necessarily imply the absence of a useful therapeutic effect. The clinical efficacy of the multidose powder inhaler is similar to that of the pressurized aerosol, provided that the individual can coordinate use of the latter.[31]

If regular inhaled treatment is insufficient to control chronic asthmatic symptoms the effect of an increased dose may be tried or alternative therapy added, e.g. inhaled steroid or slow-release theophylline. Troublesome nocturnal symptoms are usually improved by more regular daytime inhaled treatment (with or without the addition of an inhaled steroid) and can also be helped by the addition of a sustained-release oral preparation before retiring. A few asthmatic subjects with markedly variable airway function consistently show large increases in PEF or FEV_1 with large doses of β-stimulants; in these individuals the domiciliary use of a nebulizer and compressor pump with doses of terbutaline respirator solution up to 5 mg four times daily may be necessary to maintain symptomatic control. Such patients will almost inevitably also be taking inhaled or oral steroids, possibly together with a sustained-release theophylline preparation. Nebulizers are sometimes useful in small children who may be unable adequately to use a pressurized aerosol.

Other than the sustained-release tablets, oral preparations are indicated only for patients unable to use the inhaled route. Spacer devices are helpful in patients with poor coordination of metered dose aerosols and may give a longer therapeutic effect than the same dose via a metered dose inhaler.

In severe asthma a selective β-stimulant should be given by nebulization e.g. terbutaline respirator solution 5 mg two to four hourly, preferably driven by oxygen. Parenteral β-agonists are rarely used in the management of severe asthma as a similar degree of bronchodilatation can be obtained after nebulized drug with less severe tachycardia and the effect of nebulized drug is more prolonged.[33,34] Cardiac monitoring is advisable if parenteral treatment or large doses of nebulized terbutaline are given to a patient with ischaemic heart disease. Some patients with extremely variable ('brittle') asthma who are prone to life-threatening attacks have been treated with continuous subcutaneous infusion,[35] but the exact therapeutic role of such treatment has yet to be defined.

2. Prevention of premature labour

Terbutaline, like other selective β_2 stimulants, has an inhibitory effect on the myometrium and it decreases or abolishes uterine contractions in advanced labour in a dose-dependent manner. The drug is infused initially at 10 $\mu g.min^{-1}$, the rate being increased by 5 $\mu g.min^{-1}$ at intervals of 10 minutes until contractions cease. The infusion rate should not exceed 25 $\mu g.min^{-1}$. The maternal heart rate should be monitored and a rate exceeding 135 per minute should be avoided. Once the contractions have ceased the infusion rate is decreased by 5 $\mu g.min^{-1}$ at intervals of 30 minutes to the lowest rate producing continued suppression of uterine activity.[5] Treatment may be continued by subcutaneous or oral administration. This form of treatment is contraindicated after antepartum haemorrhage or in the presence of toxaemia of pregnancy.

Adverse reactions

Potentially life-threatening effects

Terbutaline is generally well tolerated and serious toxic effects are rare. Pulmonary oedema has been reported in pregnant women given β-stimulants to inhibit labour and very occasional reports have implicated terbutaline.[36] There has been one case report of a young woman in a similar setting who developed symptomatic and ECG evidence of cardiac ischaemia during terbutaline infusion.[37]

Acute overdosage

Deliberate overdose has been recorded rarely and is associated with extreme tachycardia, arrhythmias, and evidence of myocardial ischaemia, hyperglycaemia and hypokalaemia. In one non–fatal case a blood level of approximately 200 $\mu g.l^{-1}$ (i.e. 50 times the therapeutic level) was recorded 4 hours after ingestion of 100 5 mg tablets. Administration of a (cardioselective) β-sympathetic antagonist may be appropriate, but considerable care is necessary if the patient is asthmatic. A volume-expanding agent may be used if the patient is hypotensive, and in premature labour a loop diuretic should be given.

Severe or irreversible adverse effects

Oral terbutaline in normal therapeutic doses has been associated with increased ectopic activity and ventricular tachycardia in patients with pre-existing cardiac arrhythmias.[38] A sharp fall in plasma potassium caused by β_2 stimulation may be a contributory factor.

Symptomatic adverse effects

These are mainly predictable, dose-related and less likely with inhaled than with oral or parenteral preparations. They include tremor, anxiety, muscle cramps, headache, and palpitations. Tolerance develops to many of these effects with regular treatment.

Interference with clinical pathology tests

No interferences of this kind appear to have been reported.

High risk groups

Neonates

The drug is rarely used in the neonatal period.

Breast milk. Concentrations in breast milk produce undetectable levels in the child.[25]

Children

Children may have difficulty using pressurized aerosols, in which case syrup or nebulized solution is appropriate. Oral doses for children are 0.075 $mg.kg^{-1}$ three times daily. (0.075 mg is equivalent to 0.25 ml of undiluted syrup.)

Pregnant women

Oral treatment (20–40 mg daily) to prevent recurrent premature labour has been associated with impaired control of diabetes or of glucose tolerance.[40]

The elderly

Inability to use a pressurized aerosol is common in the elderly, and alternative inhalation devices, for example spacers or dry powder inhaler, may be needed. Oral or high-dose inhaled treatment may be more likely to provoke angina, cardiac arrhythmias or, in patients with prostatism, urinary retention.

Concurrent disease

Renal disease. Inhaled and oral doses are unchanged. It is recommended that the injected dose be reduced by half if the glomerular filtration rate is between 10 and 50 $ml.min^{-1}$. The intravenous preparation is contraindicated if GFR < 10 $ml.min^{-1}$.

Drug interactions

Food reduces the bioavailability of oral terbutaline. There are no significant adverse interactions with drugs other than β-antagonists.

Terbutaline

The theoretical synergism of β-stimulants and theophylline as bronchodilators is not borne out in practice; their effects are at best additive.

Major outcome trials

Numerous trials have shown the short-term efficacy of terbutaline as a bronchodilator. This effect precludes any long term placebo-controlled studies in patients with symptomatic airways obstruction. In an open study of long-term treatment with oral terbutaline, a steroid-sparing effect and reduced requirement for hospital admission was shown.[9] Evidence on β receptor tolerance after chronic treatment has been conflicting but, while tolerance is more readily demonstrable in other tissues, there is no good evidence for clinically significant tachyphylaxis of airway response in asthmatic subjects taking 'conventional' oral or inhaled doses.[9,10] Data on long-term effects are not yet available for large nebulized doses.

References

1. Martin G L, Atkins P C, Dunsky E H, Zweiman B 1980 Effects of theophylline, terbutaline and prednisolone on antigen-induced bronchospasm and mediator release. Journal of Allergy and Clinical Immunology 66: 204–212
2. Hegardt B, Pauwels R, Van der Straeten M 1981 Inhibitory effect of KWD2131, terbutaline and DSCG on the immediate and late allergen-induced bronchoconstriction. Allergy 36: 115–122
3. Thiringer G, Svedmyr N 1976 Comparison of infused and inhaled terbutaline in patients with asthma. Scandinavian Journal of Respiratory Disease 57: 17–24
4. Santa Cruz R, Landa J, Hirsch J, Sackner M A 1974 Tracheal mucus velocity in normal man and patients with obstructive lung disease: effects of terbutaline. American Review of Respiratory Disease 109: 458–463
5. Ingemarsson I 1976 Effect of terbutaline on premature labour. American Journal of Obstetric Gynecology 125: 520–524
6. Sackner M A, Dougherty R, Watson H, Wanner A 1975 Haemodynamic effects of epinephrine and terbutaline in normal man. Chest 68: 616–624
7. William-Olsson T, Fellenius E, Björntorp P, Smith U 1979 Differences in metabolic responses to beta adrenergic stimulation after propranolol or metoprolol administration. Acta Medica Scandinavica 205: 201–206
8. Hooper P L, Woo W, Visconti L, Pathak D R 1981 Terbutaline raises high density lipoprotein-cholesterol levels. New England Journal of Medicine 305: 1455–1457
9. Formgren H 1975 The therapeutic value of oral long-term treatment with terbutaline in asthma. Scandinavian Journal of Respiratory Disease 56: 321–328
10. Svedmyr N L V, Larsson S A, Thiringer G K 1976 Development of 'resistance' in beta adrenergic receptors of asthmatic patients. Chest 69: 479–483
11. Vathenen A S, Knox A J, Higgins B G, Britton J R, Tattersfield A E 1988 Rebound increaes in bronchial responsiveness after treatment with inhaled terbutaline. Lancet 1: 554–558
12. Leferink J G, Wagemaker-Engels I, Maes R A A, Lamont H, Pauwels R, Van der Straeten M 1977 Quantitative analysis of terbutaline in serum and urine at therapeutic levels using gas chromatography–mass spectrometry. Journal of Chromatography 143: 299–305
13. Clare R A, Davies D S, Baillie T A 1979 The analysis of terbutaline in biological fluids by gas chromatography electron impact mass spectrometry. Biomedical Mass Spectrometry 6: 31–37
14. Jacobsson S-E, Jönsson S, Lindberg C, Svensson L-A 1980 Determination of terbutaline in plasma by gas chromatography chemical ionization mass spectrometry. Biomedical Mass Spectrometry 7: 265–268
15. Leferink J G, Baillie T A, Lindberg C 1984 Quantitative analysis of terbutaline by gas chromatography–mass spectrometry. European Journal of Respiratory Disease 65 (suppl 134): 25–32
16. Davies D S 1984 Pharmacokinetics of terbutaline after oral administration. European Journal of Respiratory Disease 65 (suppl 134): 111–117
17. Nyberg L 1984 Pharmacokinetic parameters of terbutaline in healthy man. An overview. European Journal of Respiratory Disease 65 (suppl 134): 149–160
18. Nilsson M T, Persson K, Tegnér K 1972 The metabolism of terbutaline in man. Xenobiotica 2: 363–375
19. Davies D S, George C F, Blackwell E, Conolly M E, Dollery C T 1974 Metabolism of terbutaline in man and dog. British Journal of Clinical Pharmacology 1: 129–136
20. Lyrenäs S, Grahnén A, Lindberg B, Lindström, Lönnerholm G 1986 Pharmacokinetics of terbutaline during pregnancy. European Journal of Clinical Pharmacology 29: 619–623
21. Nyberg L, Kennedy B-M 1984 Pharmacokinetics of terbutaline given in slow release tablets. European Journal of Respiratory Disease 65 (suppl 134): 119–139
22. Hörnblad Y, Ripe E, Magnusson P O, Tegnér K 1976 The metabolism and clinical activity of terbutaline and its pro drug ibuterol. European Journal of Clinical Pharmacology 10: 9–18
23. Borgstrom L, Nilsson M 1990 A method for determination of the absolute pulmonary bioavailability of inhaled drugs: terbutaline. Pharmaceutical Research 7: 1068–1070
24. Briant R H, Blackwell E W, Williams F M, Davies D S, Dollery C T 1973 The metabolism of sympathomimetic bronchodilator drugs by the isolated perfused dog lung. Xenobiotica 3: 787–799
25. Lindberg C, Boreus L O, de Chateau P, Lindström B, Lönnerholm G, Nyberg L 1984 Transfer of terbutaline into breast milk. European Journal of Respiratory Disease 65 (suppl 134): 87–91
26. Van den Berg W, Leferink J G, Maes R A A, Fokkens J K, Kreukniet J, Bruynzeel P L B 1984 The effects of oral and subcutaneous administration of terbutaline in asthmatic patients. European Journal of Respiratory Disease 65 (suppl 134): 181–193
27. Billing B, Dahlqvist R, Garle M, Hörnblad Y, Ripe E 1984 Simultaneous treatment with terbutaline and theophylline. European Journal of Respiratory Disease 65 (suppl 134): 211–218
28. Berg G, Lindberg C, Ryden G 1984 Terbutaline in the treatment of premature labour. European Journal of Respiratory Disease 65 (suppl 134): 219–230
29. Persson K, Persson K 1972 The metabolism of terbutaline in vitro by rat and human liver O-methyltransferases and monoamine oxidases. Xenobiotica 2: 375–382
30. Tegnér K, Nilsson H T, Persson C G A, Persson K, Ryrfeldt A 1984 Elimination pathways of terbutaline. European Journal of Respiratory Disease 65 (suppl 134): 93–100
31. Newman S P, Moren F, Trofast E, Talaee N, Clarke S W 1989 Deposition and clinical efficacy of terbutaline sulphate from Turbuhaler, a new multi-dose powder inhaler. European Respiratory Journal 2: 247–252
32. O'Reilly J F, Gould G, Kendrick A H, Laszlo G 1986 Domiciliary comparison of terbutaline treatment by metered dose inhaler with and without conical spacer in severe and moderately severe chronic asthma. Thorax 41: 766–770
33. Lawford P, Jones B J M, Milledge J S 1978 Comparison of intravenous and nebulized salbutamol in initial treatment of severe asthma. British Medical Journal 1: 84
34. Hetzel M R, Clark T J H 1976 Comparison of intravenous and aerosol salbutamol. British Medical Journal 2: 919
35. O'Driscoll B R C, Ruffles S P, Ayres J G, Cochrane G M 1988 Long term treatment of severe asthma with subcutaneous terbutaline. British Journal of Diseases of the Chest 82: 360–367
36. Stubblefield P G 1978 Pulmonary oedema occurring after therapy with dexamethasone and terbutaline for premature labour: a case report. American Journal of Obstetrics and Gynecology 132: 341–342
37. Tye K-H, Desser K B, Benchimol A 1980 Angina pectoris associated with use of terbutaline for premature labour. Journal of the American Medical Association 244: 692–693
38. Banna A S, Sunderrajan E V, Agarwal M K, Addington W W 1979 Arrhythmogenic effects of orally administered bronchodilators. Archives of Internal Medicine 139: 434–437
39. Heath A, Hulten B-Å 1987 Terbutaline concentrations in self-poisoning: a case report. Human Toxicology 6: 525–526
40. Main E K, Main D M, Gabbe S G 1987 Chronic oral terbutaline tocolytic therapy is associated with maternal glucose intolerance. American Journal of Obstetrics and Gynecology 157: 644–647

Terfenadine

Terfenadine is an H_1 receptor antagonist with a very low incidence of CNS side effects. It does not belong to any group of classic H_1-antihistamines. It is structurally related to butyrophenone neuroleptics and to alkylamine H_1-antihistamines.

Chemistry

Terfenadine (Aldaban, Seldane, Teldane, Triludan)
$C_{32}H_{41}NO_2$
1-(4-*tert*-Butylphenyl)-4-[4-(α-hydroxybenzhydryl)piperidino]butan-1-ol

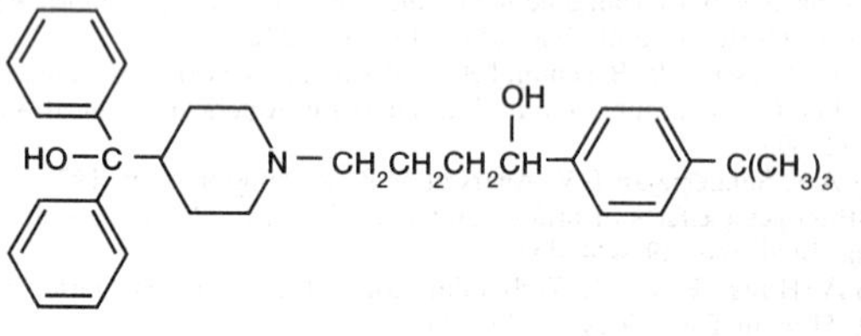

Molecular weight	471.7
pKa	8.58
Solubility	
in alcohol	1 in 59
in water	virtually insoluble
Octanol/water partition coefficient	10 000

Terfenadine is a crystalline solid prepared by chemical synthesis. It possesses a chiral centre.

Pharmacology

Terfenadine antagonizes dose dependently the effects of histamine on H_1-receptors in vitro (isolated guinea-pig ileum) and in vivo (skin weals).[1,2] The blockade in vitro is slow and long-lasting; it is competitive with moderate (30–100 $nmol.l^{-1}$), but unsurmountable with higher (300–1000 $nmol.l^{-1}$) concentrations of terfenadine. The non-competitive component of terfenadine action might contribute to its antihistamine effects in vivo.[2] The long duration of action may result from a slow dissociation of terfenadine from the H_1-receptors. With doses producing competitive inhibition, terfenadine is less potent (pA_2 8.2) than racemic chlorpheniramine (pA_2 9.2) on the guinea-pig ileum. In low to moderate concentrations, terfenadine exerts no H_2-antihistamine (gastric acid output from the perfused rat stomach), antiserotonin (serotonin weals in the rat), antimuscarine (guinea-pig ileum) or β- or α-antiadrenergic (rabbit's atria and aortic strips) effects, as compared with the respective antagonists. In non-competitive concentrations, terfenadine counteracts the contractions of the guinea-pig ileum induced by acetylcholine or barium chloride.

In the direct radioreceptor studies in vitro, terfenadine equally displaced ^{3}H-mepyramine from ileal and brain histamine H_1-receptors with IC_{50} values of 200–300 $nmol.l^{-1}$. In the experiments where terfenadine displaced labelled mepyramine with IC_{50} of 700 $nmol.l^{-1}$, it did not displace the radioligands for α_1, α_2 or β-adrenergic receptors, but it displaced the cholinergic radioligand QNB, the potency of terfenadine being about $\frac{1}{4}$ of its antihistamine potency. The respective ratio for dexchlorpheniramine was 1/50, suggesting that dexchlorpheniramine was more selective than terfenadine in its H_1-antihistamine actions.

When studied ex vivo, terfenadine did not displace labelled mepyramine from the brain of guinea-pigs pretreated with varying doses of terfenadine while dexchlorpheniramine did so.[3] Terfenadine penetrates poorly the blood–brain barrier, and it is free of the important central sedative action characteristic of older H_1-antihistamines. The lack of various central actions and interactions in animal tests[4] may result from terfenadine's poor penetration to the brain.

Toxicology

Terfenadine is a relatively non-toxic drug in animals, the acute oral LD_{50} being about 5 $g.kg^{-1}$. In chronic studies animals have tolerated well the doses of terfenadine considered to be 100-fold the clinically therapeutic doses.[5] The experimental data available on the carcinogenicity and mutagenicity of terfenadine indicate the lack of these ill effects.[5] Some embryotoxicity has been found in fertility tests with large doses of terfenadine; this is attributable to a direct toxic action on mothers and offspring rather than to developmental abnormalities in utero.

Clinical pharmacology

Like other H_1-antihistamines, terfenadine antagonizes various physiological and pathophysiological effects of histamine including increased capillary permeability and dilation, the formation of oedema, the 'flare' and 'itch' response, and the constriction of gastrointestinal and respiratory smooth muscle. The histamine-induced fall of blood pressure is partly mediated via H_2-receptors and is therefore incompletely blocked by terfenadine. The blockade of 'triple response' to intracutaneous injection of histamine has been used to document the presence of effective concentrations of H_1-antihistamines in man.

Oral single doses of 60–120 mg terfenadine produce nearly 100% suppression of this response. The onset of action is evident after 4 hours, and it lasts dose-dependently for 12 to 24 hours or even longer.[6–8] Healthy volunteers who received 60 mg terfenadine twice daily for two months showed no tolerance to terfenadine's weal and flare suppressant action at weekly tests.[9] Compared with astemizole, another non-sedative long acting H_1-antihistamine, terfenadine suppressed histamine weal more rapidly (2 hours vs. 3 days) but was shorter acting (1 day vs. 4 weeks).[10] Multiple dosing enhances terfenadine's weal suppressant effect, which in patient studies has proved qualitatively similar but quantitatively weaker than in healthy volunteers. In patients with allergic rhinitis, 300 mg twice daily produced significantly greater skin test suppression than the currently recommended 60 mg twice daily.[11]

Many laboratory studies have been done in healthy volunteers to document the alleged lack of central depressant effects on skilled performance after oral single or multiple doses of terfenadine. Briefly, terfenadine in doses up to 120 mg has not impaired skilled performance or produced subjective sedation, while the well known sedative antihistamines (chlorpheniramine, diphenhydramine, triprolidine, etc.) differed from placebo in this respect. The lack of impairment of performance has been confirmed during actual driving tests.[12,13] When tested for, terfenadine has not increased the detrimental effects of alcohol or diazepam on performance.[13,14] However, a large (240 mg) single dose of terfenadine has impaired performance, alone and in combination with alcohol (0.5 $g.kg^{-1}$).[15] This suggests that large therapeutic doses are not without central depressant potential.

In spite of the equivocal results from radioreceptor studies, terfenadine has no significant antimuscarine activity as evidenced by its failure to inhibit salivary secretion and pupil diameter in healthy subjects at standard therapeutic doses.[16,17] In asthmatic patients, terfenadine does not modify airway responsiveness to inhaled metacholine[18] but reduces the histamine-induced bronchoconstriction.[19]

Pharmacokinetics

The most specific analytical method is by gas chromatography–mass spectrometry. Quantification of terfenadine is also possible with specific and sensitive high pressure liquid chromatography (HPLC), or by radioimmunoassay[21] which has a limit of detection of < 1 $\mu g.l^{-1}$. This assay is less specific than GC–MS and HPLC but requires only small samples and is thus suitable for paediatric studies, etc. Concentrations of the active metabolite of terfenadine have been assayed with HPLC.[22] Clinically relevant human data about the disposition of terfenadine and its active metabolite are limited and partly unpublished.

Results with ^{14}C-terfenadine indicate that the drug is well absorbed from the gut, but less than 1% of plasma radioactivity represents unaltered terfenadine.[20] In animals, little radioactivity is detected in the brain and spinal cord.[23]

Following oral administration of terfenadine to fasting healthy subjects, it is almost completely absorbed. Mean peak plasma concentrations of terfenadine by radioimmunoassay (1.5–4.5 μg.l^{-1}) occur 1 to 2 hours after single oral doses (60–180 mg, respectively).[20] The respective AUC values were dose-related, too.[20] Peak plasma levels of unchanged terfenadine assayed by HPLC after single or multiple doses of up to 240 mg daily remain below 10 μg.l^{-1} (Merrell Dow Pharmaceuticals, data on file). The concentrations of its active metabolite measured by HPLC during maintenance (60 mg twice daily) with terfenadine showed minimum values of 30–70 μg.l^{-1} and peaks of 200–300 μg.l^{-1}, which are 50–100 fold the terfenadine concentrations after these doses. The concentrations of the metabolite remained stable over the two-month maintenance period.[9] similar peak plasma concentrations (mean 242 μg.l^{-1}) of the active metabolite were measured in children 2–3 h after intake of 1–2 mg.kg^{-1} of terfenadine.[22] The tissue distribution of terfenadine has not been investigated in human studies.

Terfenadine appears to undergo extensive first-pass metabolism, that can affect clinical response. There may be an enterohepatic circulation.[23] Excretion of unchanged terfenadine in urine is negligible.[20] Administration of the drug with food significantly decreases its bioavailability. With multiple dosing, steady-state plasma concentrations of unchanged drug are achieved within 1–2 weeks, as might be expected from its half life of 16–23 h.

Oral absorption	~100%
Presystemic metabolism	99%
Plasma half life	
range	16–23 h
metabolite I	4–5 h
Volume of distribution	—
Plasma protein binding	
(metabolite 1)	70%

Concentration–effect relationship

Effective antihistaminic concentrations of terfenadine on the isolated guinea-pig ileum are about 5–20 μg.l^{-1} (pA_2 8.2), and its potency is one-tenth that of (+)chlorpheniramine. In ex vivo and in vivo studies in guinea-pigs, oral doses of 1–2 mg.kg^{-1} of terfenadine antagonize histamine-induced bronchospasm and skin weal.[1,3] These doses refer to plasma concentrations of 5–10 μg.l^{-1}, assuming that guinea-pigs and humans handle terfenadine in roughly similar ways. In man, concentrations of 1.5–4.5 μg.l^{-1} of terfenadine have been measured over several hours in plasma after administration of antiallergic single doses of 60–180 mg of terfenadine. The peak effect (e.g. suppression of weal due to intradermal histamine) is measured 4–6 hours after drug intake, whereas plasma terfenadine peaks within 1–2 hours.[20] Peak plasma concentrations of the pharmacologically active metabolite I precede the maximum suppression of the histamine weal response.[9] This metabolite has an antihistamine potency of one-third that of terfenadine, it is moderately (70%) bound to human serum proteins, its AUC values after intake of terfenadine doses increase linearly with dose, but its plasma concentrations are uninfluenced by food (Merrell Dow Pharmaceuticals, data on file). According to the published data from prolonged treatment with terfenadine (60 mg twice daily), the mean elimination half life of the metabolite is 4–5 hours, and its plasma concentrations at least 50-fold those of terfenadine.[9] These concentrations provided a significant though not complete suppression of histamine weal and flare responses, with no development of tolerance. It seems that the active metabolite makes an important contribution to the clinical effects of terfenadine, the total H_1-antihistamine activity being raised to the levels which proved effective in animal experiments. The half life of the metabolite after the intake of 1 mg.kg^{-1} terfenadine (mean dose 69.6 mg) was 5–10 h in eight aged (mean 68 years) female volunteers. Five out of them reported sedation.[24]

Terfenadine

Metabolism

The metabolism of ^{14}C-terfenadine has been investigated in several species including man.[20,22] Several metabolites have been identified and quantified, and these account for 99.5% of the total dose. None of the metabolites is toxic and their excretion is mainly in the faeces in all species. The two major metabolic products (metabolites I and II) together account for about 70% of the radioactivity excreted in urine while metabolite I accounts for 50% of the radioactivity in faeces. Metabolite I is formed by oxidation at the tertiary butyl group to yield the respective carboxylic acid derivative, which probably contributes to terfenadine's clinical effects as discussed above. Metabolite II is pharmacologically inactive and formed, partly from the metabolite I, by oxidative dealkylation and splitting of the molecule to yield a piperidine carbinol derivative. With regular clinical doses of terfenadine its metabolism is not saturated. However, during intoxication (convulsions, cardiac dysrhythmias) with an unknown dose (240 mg per day or more) of terfenadine the peak plasma concentrations were 43 μg.l^{-1} for terfenadine and 504 μg.l^{-1} for metabolite I, respectively.[25] This ten-fold difference is less than the 50-fold difference found with low therapeutic doses of terfenadine[9,20] and suggests a restricted metabolism of terfenadine when it is given in very high doses.

Fig. 1 Major metabolites of terfenadine

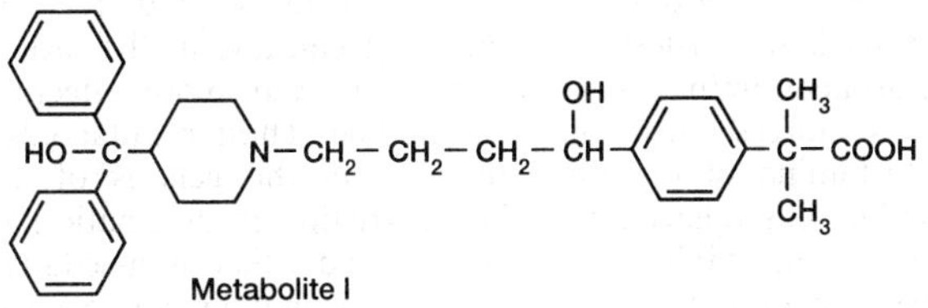

Metabolite I

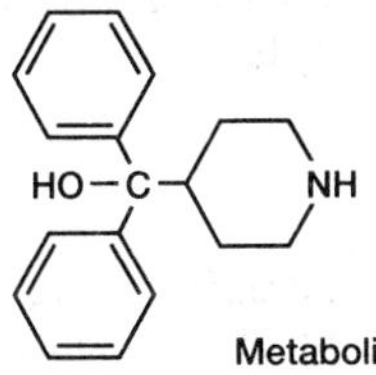

Metabolite II

Pharmaceutics

Terfenadine is available as for oral administration only.
tablets (60 mg) and suspension (6 mg.ml^{-1}).

1. Triludan tablets are white, scored, and marked 'O84' and 'M'. They contain 60 mg terfenadine.
2. Triludan Forte are white, elongated tablets, marked 'T'. They contain 120 mg terfenadine.
3. Triludan Suspension is a fruit-flavoured, sugar-free suspension containing 6 mg.ml^{-1} terfenadine.

The suspension when diluted should be kept refrigerated and has then a shelf-life of 14 days.

Terfenadine Triludan (Merrell Dow, UK) Seldane (Merrell Dow USA) has been licensed to Astra, Finland and Draco, Sweden.

Therapeutic use

Indications

1. Seasonal allergic rhinitis and conjunctivitis
2. Acute and chronic urticaria
3. Atopic dermatitis
4. Allergic asthma, angioedema
5. Other indications.

Contraindications

1. Known allergy to terfenadine
2. It is not recommended for use during pregnancy.

Mode of use

Like several other H_1-antihistamines, terfenadine has been shown to reduce various allergic symptoms, being most useful in acute exuda-

Terfenadine

tive types of allergy such as pollinosis and urticaria. The recommended adult dosage is 60 mg twice daily; recommendations for children are half to one-quarter of the adult dose.

The recommended oral adult dosing of 60 mg twice daily, shown to be equipotent to 120 mg once daily in seasonal allergic rhinitis,[26] might be only moderately effective, and several patients need daily doses of 240 mg or even more.[11] This concept tallies with the finding that responses to regular doses of terfenadine differ significantly but not fundamentally from a fairly high rate of placebo responses in some studies.[27,28] However, the necessity of using terfenadine at doses above 120 mg daily in patients with seasonal allergic rhinitis has been questioned.[29,56]

In controlled clinical trials, terfenadine has been compared with placebo, and sedative (brompheniramine, chlorpheniramine, clemastine, hydroxyzine) and non-sedative (acrivastine, astemizole, cetirizine, loratadine) H_1-antihistamines in seasonal and perennial allergic rhinitis and urticaria. In general, terfenadine (60 mg twice daily) has matched short-acting sedative antihistamines in efficacy whereas astemizole (10 mg once daily) has controlled the symptoms better, particularly if the trials have lasted for several weeks. Terfenadine, in turn, has a faster onset of therapeutic action.

The comparative doses of antihistamines selected may also modify the clinical results recorded, as shown by comparisons of terfenadine 60 mg twice daily with racemic chlorpheniramine 4 mg three times daily[30] or with dexchlorpheniramine 6 mg twice daily.[31] In the former trial, the drugs were similar in efficacy; in the latter trial, dexchlorpheniramine (a larger dose) proved more effective and definitely more sedative than terfenadine. Though autacoids other than histamine play prominent roles in the genesis of asthma, terfenadine has relieved bronchoconstriction in asthmatic patients, particularly in children. Terfenadine and other non-sedative H_1-antihistamines are partly effective in relieving itching associated with acute and chronic urticaria, whereas most chronic pruritic skin lesions remain unresponsive.[32] For extensive reviewing of comparative trials and references see McTavish et al 1990.

Indications

1. Allergic rhinitis and conjunctivitis

Controlled clinical trials in adults[27] and in children[22,28] have shown terfenadine to be effective in the management of seasonal allergic rhinitis in terms of the patients' symptom scores or/and reduced need of rescue antihistamines. Global improvement has been excellent in 60–85% of patients with terfenadine 60 mg twice daily (adults) or 15–30 mg twice daily (children). However, the placebo response rates were high (30–60%). The efficacy of terfenadine has been mostly, but not always, good in hay fever (50–70% control of symptoms), while it has proved less satisfactory in relieving perennial allergic rhinitis[33] and vasomotor rhinitis. Sympathomimetics may be useful adjuvants in the latter disorder. Generally, itching, sneezing, nasal rhinorrhoea and ocular symptoms have been relieved better than nasal congestion.[34] With regard to therapeutic efficacy in comparative trials, terfenadine has proved similar to sedative chlorpheniramine in seasonal[30] and perennial rhinitis, yet their responses in perennial rhinitis have been only modest.

When comparing terfenadine with non-sedative astemizole in patients with seasonal allergic rhinitis, the drugs have given similar results in two studies whereas terfenadide was ineffective in one trial of 8 weeks' duration. A comparative trial of terfenadine (60 mg twice daily) and astemizole (10 mg daily) for 4 weeks in patients with perennial allergic rhinitis showed astemizole to be more effective.[35] The time courses of drug effects, pharmacokinetic factors, and fluctuating environmental levels of allergens might modify the results in different trials. For other comparisons and details see McTavish et al, 1990.

2, 3. Allergic skin disorders

Itching is the main symptom to be relieved by using H_1-antihistamines in allergic dermatoses. Although itching is difficult to quantify, various antihistamines, terfenadine included, have a significant antipruritic effect in allergic skin disorders such as chronic urticaria[36] and atopic dermatitis in children.[37] The effects of non-sedative H_1-antihistamines in other types of pruritic skin disorders are less convincing. In suppression of pruritis linked with dermographism and urticaria, terfenadine has proved effective,[38] whereas sedative H_1-antihistamines may be more suitable for other pruritic skin conditions.[32] Controlled comparative trials with patients having chronic urticaria and treated with regular recommended doses of various H_1-antihistamines have shown that terfenadine matches brompheniramine and chlorpheniramine in efficacy, and is more effective than clemastine but less effective than astemizole (see McTavish et al, 1990). In recent studies, terfenadine 60 mg three times daily has reduced itching of adult patients with atopic eczema.[39]

4. Asthma

Oral terfenadine dose-dependently counteracts histamine-induced bronchoconstriction in asthmatic patients.[19] A large single dose (180 mg) of terfenadine given 3 hours before antigen provocation provides a 50% immediate protection against bronchoconstriction[40] Similarly, large single doses or prolonged dosing have protected against asthma attacks induced by exercise[41] or by hyperventilation.[42] Regular doses recommended for allergic seasonal rhinitis do not produce these effects consistently. Instead, terfenadine in dosages of 120 mg twice daily or 180 mg three times daily has reduced the intensity of symptoms of stable mild atopic asthma and the requirement of inhaled bronchodilators.[43,44] Since such large doses of terfenadine increase the potential of central side effects,[15,25] terfenadine is not the drug of first choice in the treatment of asthma and cannot replace the rational use of inhaled steroids or chromoglycate.

5. Other indications

There are few controlled studies to document the alleged beneficial symptomatic effect of terfenadine in the common cold. In one study[45] three consecutive doses of 60 mg terfenadine started within 6 to 48 hours after the onset of symptoms relieved the symptoms in 63% of recipients versus 40% of placebo recipients; nasal swelling, obstruction and redness were significantly reduced after terfenadine compared to placebo. In another study,[46] terfenadine 60 mg twice daily for 4 days failed to differ objectively or subjectively from placebo in modulating the symptomatology of the common cold.

Adverse reactions

Potentially life-threatening effects

In recommended therapeutic doses terfenadine does not exert severe toxic effects.

Acute overdosage

Terfenadine is probably less dangerous than most other H_1-antihistamines when taken in excessive doses accidentally (children) or intentionally. A retrospective analysis[47] of accidental terfenadine ingestion in children aged 1–5 years identified 28 cases. One child (2 years of age) who took 900 mg terfenadine received hospital treatment including activated charcoal and sorbitol; two children (2 years of age) who took 120–300 mg terfenadine received ipecac at home; 25 children (14 months to 4 years of age) who took 60–180 mg terfenadine received home management with observation alone. In all cases, followed-up children remained asymptomatic. The authors propose that children who ingest more than 120 mg, or who are less than one year old, should be referred to a health care facility for evaluation and treatment.[47]

Generalized convulsions and cardiac ventricular dysrhythmias have been reported in a 21-year-old woman who took terfenadine 240 mg a day plus an unknown amount.[25] At hospital admission, her plasma concentration of terfenadine was 43 $\mu g.l^{-1}$ and of its metabolite I 504 $\mu g.l^{-1}$, indicating an overdose. Nine hours later the respective concentrations were 26.5 and 389 $\mu g.l^{-1}$. The ECG parameters (prolongation of conduction time suggesting cardiotoxicity) returned to normal values over several days. In another case (Merrell Dow Pharmaceuticals, data on file) a severe ventricular arrhythmia developed 15 hours after the ingestion of 56 tablets/3360 mg of terfenadine plus other drugs. This progressed to ventricular fibrillation which responded well to defibrillation and lignocaine. These cases suggest that in high concentrations terfenadine can produce toxic effects characteristic of older antihistamines, and cardiac monitoring is recommended along with standard measures to remove any unabsorbed drug. It is not known if terfenadine is dialysable.

Severe or irreversible effects

Allergic hepatitis[48] is a rare adverse effect that may fall into this category.

Symptomatic adverse effects
The symptomatic adverse effects in therapeutic studies (120–400 mg daily) of terfenadine (mild drowsiness, fatigue, 'blurred thinking', depression) have been similar to respective symptoms reported after placebo.[49] These effects occur in 10–15% of patients, and the incidence is half that reported after chlorpheniramine 12 or 16 mg daily, dexchlorpheniramine 6 mg daily or clemastine 2 mg daily. Other novel non-sedative H_1-antihistamines (astemizole, loratadine, mequitazine) share this property of terfenadine. In general, the incidence of sedation does not increase with increased terfenadine doses (up to 600 mg daily)[50] or increased duration of treatment (for up to 12 weeks),[51] yet terfenadine can (rarely) produce nervous reactions from even standard recommended dose.[52] Anticholinergic effects are few, if any. Allergic sensitization to terfenadine is possible. Case reports of dermatological reactions (exacerbation of psoriasis, urticaria, rash), alopecia, angioedema, photosensitivity reactions and desquamation have been collected from patients receiving terfenadine. For a detailed list of side effects and respective references see McTavish et al. 1990.

Interference with clinical pathology tests
No technical interferences of this kind appear to have been reported.

High risk groups

Neonates
In principle, neonates might be a risk group since the LD_{50} value for terfenadine in newborn mice (438 mg.kg^{-1}) is one-tenth of that found in mature mice and rats (5 g.kg^{-1}).

Breast milk. Since the pharmacokinetics of terfenadine have been insufficiently investigated, there is no information about the presence of terfenadine or its metabolite I in breast milk.

Children
Children over one year of age have not shown particular sensitivity to moderately large doses of terfenadine.[22,47]

The elderly
Normal volunteers over 65 years of age (mean 68 years) have eliminated metabolite I somewhat more slowly than younger individuals, and half of them were sedated. It may be wise to avoid unnecessarily large doses in elderly patients.

Concurrent disease
Care should be taken if administering terfenadine to patients with severe renal or hepatic disease, since terfenadine is entirely cleared in the liver and its active metabolite I also excreted by the renal route.[20,22,48]

Drug interactions

Potentially hazardous interactions
No interactions of this kind have been reported with therapeutic doses.

Other significant interactions
The data available concerning the kinetic interactions of terfenadine are limited, yet it has been shown to stimulate hepatic microsomal enzymes. In human studies, an acute 60 mg dose of terfenadine[53] or maintenance with 120 mg twice daily of it for 16 days[54] have not significantly altered the kinetics of single doses of theophylline (250–400 mg) in healthy subjects. Similarly, one day or two weeks treatment with terfenadine 120 mg twice daily failed to modify the pharmacokinetics of phenytoin given as maintenance to epileptic patients.[55] There are no published human data to demonstrate possible alterations by other agents (drugs, smoking) in the pharmacokinetics of terfenadine.

Centrally acting H_1-antihistamines have an additive sedative effect with other antidepressants, for example psychotropic drugs. This was found with single doses of diphenhydramine (100 mg) but not with terfenadine (120 mg) when given in combination with 10 mg of diazepam.[14] The combinations of hypnotics and H_1-antihistamines are generally considered more dangerous than either agent alone. Such effects seem unlikely with terfenadine. MAO inhibitors may interact with conventional H_1-antihistamines, but there are no specific data available for terfenadine.

Terfenadine

Food may reduce the absorption of terfenadine. Pharmacodynamic interactions with alcohol (sedation, excitation) have not been found after single doses of terfenadine and alcohol (0.75 g.kg^{-1}) in combination[14] whereas 240 mg of terfenadine enhanced the effect of alcohol (0.5 g.kg^{-1}).[15] Thus, combinations of large doses of terfenadine and alcohol are not necessarily safe although specific reports are not available.

Potentially useful interactions
Terfenadine has been used together with other antiallergic agents such as inhaled corticosteroids or sodium cromoglycate. In a few comparative trials, the combined use of corticosteroid and terfenadine was relatively more effective on nasal than ocular symptoms in seasonal allergic rhinitis. The same applies to the combined use of terfenadine and nasally administered cromoglycate. Topical sympathomimetics may add to the modest effect of terfenadine on perennial allergic rhinitis; they are used together but the combined effects are not well documented. Histamine H_2-receptor blockers (for example, ranitidine) may add to terfenadine to relieve itching in acronic urticaria. For more detailed information and references see McTavish et al, 1990.

Clinical trials

Sorkin and Heel (1985) and McTavish et al (1990) have reviewed in detail the many clinical trials carried out with terfenadine. The therapeutic efficacy, in most trials, has been found to be superior to placebo and comparable with conventional H_1-antihistamines, but astemizole has proved better in perennial allergic rhinitis, and even in seasonal rhinitis if the trials have lasted for several weeks. The trials specifically quoted under Indications are important, the most extensive of which are on a multi-centre basis.

General review articles

McTavish D, Goa K L, Ferrill M 1990 Terfenadine, an updated review of its pharmacological properties and therapeutic efficacy. Drugs 39: 552–574

Paton D M, Webster D R 1985 Clinical pharmacokinetics of H_1-antagonists (the antihistamines). Clinical Pharmacokinetics 10: 477–497

Sorkin E M, Heel R C 1985 Terfenadine, a review of its pharmacodynamic properties and therapeutic efficacy. Drugs 29: 34–56

References

1. Cheng H C, Woodward J K 1982 Antihistaminic effect of terfenadine: a new piperidine-type antihistamine. Drug Development Research 2: 181–196
2. Cheng H C, Woodward J K 1982 A kinetic study of the antihistaminic effect of terfenadine. Arzneimittel-Forschung (Drug Research) 32: 1160–1166
3. Wiech N L, Martin J S 1982 Absence of an effect of terfenadine on guinea-pig brain histamine H_1-receptors in vivo determined by receptor binding techniques. Arzneimittel-Forschung (Drug Research) 32: 1167–1170
4. Niemegeers C J E, Awouters F H L, Janssen P A 1982 The in vivo pharmacological profile of histamine (H_1) antagonists in the rat. Drug Development Research 2: 559–566
5. Gibson J P, Huffmann K W, Newberne J W 1982 Preclinical safety studies with terfenadine. Arzneimittel-Forschung (Drug Research) 32: 1179–1184
6. Hüther K J, Renftle G, Barraud N, Burke J T, Koch-Weser J 1977 Inhibition effect of terfenadine on histamine-induced skin wheals in man. European Journal of Clinical Pharmacology 12: 195–199
7. Van Landeghem V H, Burke J T, Thebault J 1980 The use of a human bioassay in determining the bioequivalence of two formulations of the antihistamine terfenadine. Clinical Pharmacology and Therapeutics 27: 290–291
8. Shall L, Newcombe R G, Marks R 1988 Assessment of the duration of action of terfenadine in histamine-induced weals. British Journal of Dermatology 119: 525–531
9. Simons F E R, Watson W T A, Simons K J 1988 Lack of subsensitivity to terfenadine during long-term terfenadine treatment. Journal of Allergy and Clinical Immunology 82: 1068–1075
10. Työlahti H, Lahti A 1989 Start and end of the effects of terfenadine and astemizole on histamine-induced wheals in human skin. Acta Dermato-Venereologica 69: 269–271
11. Bantz E W, Dolen W K, Nelson H S 1987 A double-blind evaluation of skin test suppression produced by two doses of terfenadine. Journal of Allergy and Clinical Immunology 80: 99–103
12. Betts T, Markman D, Debenham S, Mortiboy D, McKevitt T 1984 Effects of two antihistamine drugs on actual driving performance. British Medical Journal 288: 281–282
13. O'Hanlon J F 1988 Antihistamines and driving safety. Cutis 42: 10–13
14. Moser L, Hüther K J, Koch-Weser J, Lundt P V 1978 Effects of terfenadine and diphenhydramine alone or in combination with diazepam or alcohol on psychomotor performance and subjective feelings. European Journal of Clinical Pharmacology 14: 417–423

Terfenadine

15. Bhatti J Z, Hindmarch I 1989 The effects of terfenadine with and without alcohol on an aspect of car driving performance. Clinical and Experimental Allergy 19: 609–611
16. Kulshrestha V K, Gupta P, Turner P, Wadsworth J 1978 Some clinical pharmacological studies with terfenadne, a new antihistamine drug. British Journal of Clinical Pharmacology 6: 25–29
17. Brion N, Beaumont D, Avenier C 1988 Evaluation of the antimuscarinic activity of atropine, terfenadine and mequitazine in healthy volunteers. British Journal of Clinical Pharmacology 25: 27–32
18. Patel K R 1987 Effect of terfenadine on methacholine-induced bronchoconstriction in asthma. Journal of Allergy and Clinical Immunology 79: 355–358
19. Rafferty P, Holgate S T 1987 Terfenadine (Seldane) is a potent and selective histamine H_1 receptor antagonist in asthmatic airways. American Review of Respiratory Disease 135: 181–184
20. Garteiz D A, Hook R H, Walker B J, Okerholm R A 1982 Pharmacokinetics and biotransformation studies of terfenadine in man. Arzneimittel-Forschung (Drug Research) 32: 1185–1190
21. Cook C E, Williams D L, Myers M et al 1981 Bioavailability of terfenadine in man. Biopharmaceutics and Drug Disposition 2: 185–190
22. Simons F E R, Watson W T A, Simons K J 1987 The pharmacokinetics and pharmacodynamics of terfenadine in children. Journal of Allergy and Clinical Immunology 80: 884–890
23. Leeson G A, Chan K Y, Knapp W C, Biedenbach S A, Wright G J, Okerholm R A 1982 Metabolic disposition of terfenadine in laboratory animals. Arzneimittel-Forschung 32: 1173–1178
24. Simons K J, Martin T J, Watson W T, Simons F E 1990 Pharmacokinetics and pharmacodynamics of terfenadine and chlorpheniramine in the elderly. Journal of Allergy and Clinical Immunology 85: 540–547
25. Davies A J, Harinda V, McEwan A, Ghose R R 1989 Cardiotoxic effects with convulsions in terfenadine overdose. British Medical Journal 298: 325
26. Henauer S, Hugonot L, Hugonot S et al 1987 Multi-centre double-blind comparison of terfenadine once daily versus twice daily in patients with hay fever. Journal of International Medical Research 15: 212–223
27. Kagan G, Dabrowicki E, Huddlestone L, Kapur T R, Wolstencroft P 1980 A double-blind trial of terfenadine and placebo in hay fever using a substitution technique for non-responders. Journal of International Medical Research 8: 404–407
28. Lockhart J D F, Maneksha G 1983 Children with allergies. Terfenadine suspension plus placebo. Practitioner 227: 1313–1315
29. Murphy-O'Connor J C, Renton R L, Westlake D M 1984 Comparative trial of two dose regimens of terfenadine in patients with hay fever. Journal of International Medical Research 12: 333–337
30. Kemp J P, Buckley C E, Gerschwin M E et al 1985 Multicenter, double-blind placebo-controlled trial of terfenadine in seasonal allergic rhinitis and conjunctivitis. Annals of Allergy 54: 502–509
31. Gutkowski A, Del Carpio J, Gelinas B, Schulz J, Turenne Y 1985 Comparative study of the efficacy, tolerance and side-effects of dexchlorpheniramine maleate 6 mg bid with terfenadine 60 mg bid. Journal of International Medical Research 13: 284–288
32. Krause L B, Shuster S 1983 Mechanism of action of antipruritic drugs. British Medical Journal 287: 1199–1200
33. Brostoff J, Lockhart J D F 1982 Controlled trial of terfenadine and chlorpheniramine maleate in perennial rhinitis. Postgraduate Medical Journal 58: 422–423
34. Rombaut N E I, Van Roy J P, Bracke E, Van den Bussche G 1986 Therapeutic effect of astemizole and terfenadine in students suffering from seasonal allergic rhinitis: a double-blind comparison. Drug Development Research 8: 79–85
35. Boland N 1988 A double-blind study of astemizole and terfenadine in the treatment of perennial rhinitis. Annals of Allergy 61: 18–24
36. Henauer S A, Adessi B, Allerga F et al 1989 Terfenadine once daily in chronic urticaria. Allergy 44: 447–452
37. Tholen St, Dieterich H A 1989 Terfenadine versus ketotifen in children with atopic dermatitis. Allergologie 12: 60–63
38. Krause L B, Shuster S 1984 The effect of terfenadine on dermographic wealing. British Journal of Dermatology 110: 73–79
39. Doherty V, Sylvester D G H, Kennedy C T C et al 1989 Treatment of itching in atopic eczema with antihistamines with a low sedative profile. British Medical Journal 298: 96
40. Rafferty P, Beasley R, Holgate S T 1987 The contribution of histamine to immediate bronchoconstriction provoked by allergen and adenosine 5'-monophosphate in atopic asthma. American Review of Respiratory Disease 136: 369–373
41. Patel K R 1984 Terfenadine in exercise-induced asthma. British Medical Journal 288: 1496–1497
42. Badier M, Beaumont D, Orehek J 1988 Attenuation of hyperventilation-induced bronchospasm by terfenadine: a new antihistamine. Journal of Allergy and Clinical Immunology 81: 437–440
43. Rafferty P, Jackson L, Smith R, Holgate S T 1988 Terfenadine in the treatment of grass pollen-sensitive asthmatics during the hay fever season. British Journal of Clinical Pharmacology 25: 623P–624P
44. Taytard A, Beaumont D, Pujet J C, Sapene M, Lewis P J 1987 Treatment of bronchial asthma with terfenadine: a randomised controlled trial. British Journal of Clinical Pharmacology 24: 743–746
45. Henauer S A, Glück U 1988 Efficacy of terfenadine in the treatment of common cold. A double-blind comparison with placebo. European Journal of Clinical Pharmacology 34: 35–40
46. Caffey M J, Kaiser D J, Hayden F G 1988 Ineffectiveness of oral terfenadine in natural colds: evidence against histamine as a mediator of common cold symptoms. Pediatric Infectious Disease Journal 7: 223–228
47. Spiller H A, Picciotti M, Perez E 1989 Accidental terfenadine ingestion in children. Veterinary and Human Toxicology 31: 154–156
48. Larrey D, Palazzo L, Benhamou J-P 1985 Terfenadine and hepatitis. Annals of Internal Medicine 103: 634
49. Barlow J L R, Beitman R E, Tsai T H 1982 Terfenadine, safety and tolerance in controlled clinical trials. Arzneimittel-Forschung (Drug Research) 32: 1215–1217
50. Brandon M L, Weiner M 1980 Clinical investigation of terfenadine, a non-sedating antihistamine. Annals of Allergy 44: 71–75
51. Gastpar H, Dieterich H A 1982 Comparative study of the efficacy and tolerance to terfenadine and clemastine in patients with seasonal allergic rhinitis. Arzneimittel-Forschung (Drug Research) 32: 1211–1213
52. Napke E, Biron P Nervous reactions after first dose of terfenadine in adults. Lancet 2: 615–616
53. Fitzsimmons W E, Luskin S S, MacLeod C M, Luskin A T 1989 Single-dose study of the effect of terfenadine on theophylline absorption and disposition. Annals of Allergy 62: 213–214
54. Brion N, Naline E, Beaumont D, Pays M, Advenier 1989 Lack of effect of terfenadine on theophylline pharmacokinetics and metabolism in normal subjects. British Journal of Clinical Pharmacology 27: 391–395
55. Coniglio A A, Garnett W R, Pellock J H et al 1989 Effect of acute and chronic terfenadine on free and total serum phenytoin concentrations in epileptic patients. Epilepsia 30: 611–616
56. Stern M A 1990 Comparative study of terfanadine at two dose levels in the management of hay fever. British Journal Clinical Practice 44: 359–363

Terodiline

Terodiline is a drug with combined anticholinergic and calcium channel blocking properties used to control the symptoms of urgency, urge incontinence and frequency of micturition from detrusor instability or hyperreflexia.

Chemistry

Terodiline hydrochloride (Micturin, Micturol, Mictrol)
$C_{20}H_{27}N.HCl$
N-tert-Butyl-1-methyl-3,3-diphenylpropylamine hydrochloride

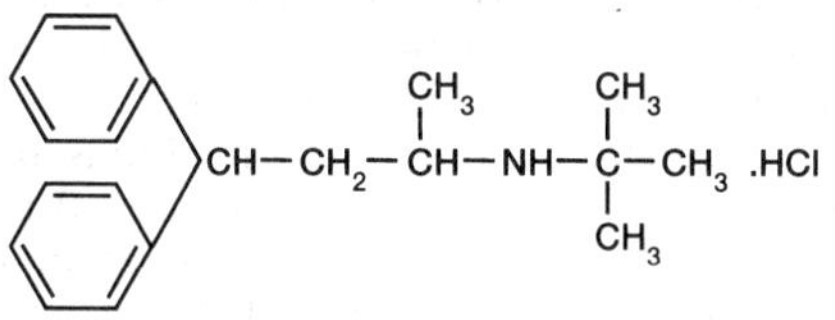

Molecular weight (free compound)	317.9 (262.4)
pKa	9.3
Solubility	
in alcohol	very soluble
in water	slightly soluble
Octanol/water partition coefficient	—

Terodiline hydrochloride is an almost odourless white crystalline powder prepared by chemical synthesis.

Pharmacology

Terodiline has both anticholinergic and calcium channel blocking properties effective within the same therapeutic dose range. The antimuscarinic and calcium antagonistic properties of terodiline have been confirmed by in vitro studies.[1,2] These effects both occur within the same therapeutic dosage range, but the anticholinergic effect predominates at lower concentrations and the calcium channel blocking effects at higher concentrations. Additionally it possesses local anaesthetic and spasmolytic effects.[3]

Toxicology

No evidence of mutagenicity or carcinogenicity has been found and animal studies have failed to demonstrate any results of potential clinical relevance.

Clinical pharmacology

In man, normal detrusor contraction seems to be mediated mainly by stimulation of muscarinic receptors. The atropine resistant part of the response to transmural stimulation in the normal human bladder has seldom been found to exceed 10% and its physiological importance has been questioned. However, in some patients with an unstable bladder a high degree of atropine resistance has been demonstrated.[4]

Calcium entry from the extracellular medium plays an important part in activation of the smooth muscle of the bladder. Calcium channel blockers (e.g. nifedipine) have been shown in vitro to block non-adrenergic non-cholinergic responses.[4] Clinically, good therapeutic effects have been obtained but at the expense of disturbing side effects.

In vitro, a combination of atropine and calcium channel blockers caused complete inhibition in isolated bladder preparations suggesting that this was attributable to the combined actions.[1]

A combination of anticholinergic and calcium channel blocking properties should be favourable, not only for increasing therapeutic action, but also for decreasing the side effects seen with effective doses of either calcium channel blockers or anticholinergics.[5-7]

Clinically, terodiline increases bladder capacity, reduces the frequency of micturition and reduces the incidence of incontinent episodes.[8,9] By titrating the dose terodiline has been proved superior to placebo in treating the symptoms of patients with detrusor instability, with no difference in the total number of side effects between the two groups. However, the incidence of anticholinergic side effects was greater in the drug-treated group.[10,11]

Pharmacokinetics

Terodiline was initially determined in urine and serum by gas chromatography and electron capture detection of benzopherone.[12] The sensitivity limit is about 2 μg.l^{-1}. More recently, gas chromatography with nitrogen detection has been used, giving more rapid analysis with similar sensitivity and precision as the earlier method.[13]

Terodiline is fully absorbed from the gastrointestinal tract in man[14] and has about 90% bioavailability. Peak plasma concentrations were found after about 4 h following a dose of 25 mg. In many subjects the serum concentrations were almost maximal after 1–2 hours with serum levels varying by less than 10% between 2 and 8 hours. The absorption half life varied from 0.3 to 1.5 hours (mean 0.7 ± 0.4 hours).

First-pass elimination is low.[10] The mean elimination half life is 60 h, hence steady-state serum concentrations and maximum therapeutic effect are not reached until 10–14 days of daily dosing.[14] Some enterohepatic circulation may occur and contribute to the shape of the serum concentration curve.[15] In general, the steady state serum levels are directly related to the dose of terodiline in humans.[8,16] Thus, after 3–4 weeks oral dosing (37.5 mg daily) the mean serum concentration was 0.4 mg.l^{-1} and at a higher dose (50 mg daily for one month)[16] it was 0.5 mg.l^{-1}. In a very few patients who were given doses of 75 mg or 150 mg daily for 2 weeks, steady-state levels reached 1.0 and 1.25 mg.l^{-1} respectively.[17]

Drug accumulation does not occur during long-term use of terodiline. The steady-state serum levels varied very little during long-term oral administration (25 mg twice daily for 3 months – 0.37 mg.l^{-1} for 6 months—0.40 mg.l^{-1}).

The steady-state serum levels were independent of age in the range 18–70 years. However, in older patients, serum levels are somewhat higher. In patients over 70 years (mean age 85) given 12.5 mg twice daily, the steady-state serum concentrations (0.5 mg.l^{-1}) were rather similar to those obtained after 25 mg twice daily in a middle-aged population.[18,19,26] In the frail elderly — usually hospitalized and over 75 years — the half life has been observed to increase to a mean of 130 hours.[18]

Renal clearance of the major metabolites exceeds that of the parent compound by at least 4-fold. Consequently, the concentration of terodiline metabolites falls below that of the parent drug. Since glucuronic acid conjugates are pharmacologically inactive and are rapidly cleared by the kidney, the presence of metabolites should not cause concern.[20] Renal clearance is mainly controlled by urinary pH and varies for unbound drug from 110 ml.min^{-1} at pH 5.8 to less than 10 ml.min^{-1} at pH 7.4.[21]

Terodiline is bound to serum proteins to about 85% over a wide range of plasma concentrations (12–2000 μg.l^{-1}). It binds to orosomucoid with a higher affinity than to serum albumin.

The apparent volume of distribution has been estimated at 480 l but a 4-fold variation has been demonstrated.[14] The distribution of labelled terodiline in the mouse, rat and rabbit has shown that brain and heart contained small concentrations of radioactivity compared with lung, intestines, liver and kidney. Whole body autoradiographic studies in mice demonstrated high activity in the adrenal medulla and pigmented tissues. There is no evidence for terodiline being toxic to melanin-bearing tissues.[22-24]

Oral absorption	100%
Presystemic metabolism	<10%
Plasma half life	
mean	60 h
Volume of distribution	~480 l
Plasma protein binding	85%

T

Testosterone (esters)

Testosterone is the major androgen secreted by the Leydig cells in the intertubular tissue of the testis and was first isolated in crystalline form in 1935.[1]

Chemistry

Testosterone (Andronaq, Hydrotest, Malogen, Oreton, Percutacrine Androgénique Forte, Testoral Sublings)
$C_{19}H_{28}O_2$
17β-Hydroxyandrost-4-en-3-one

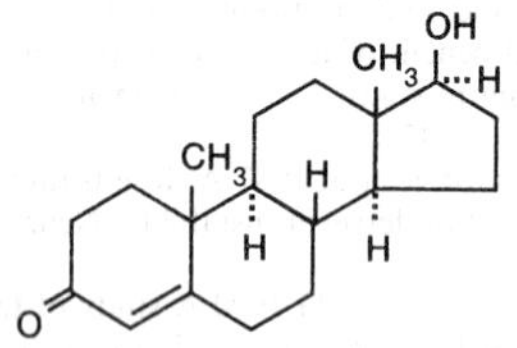

Molecular weight	288.4
pKa	—
Solubility	
in alcohol	1 in 6
in water	insoluble
Octanol/water partition coefficient	—

A white or creamy-white crystalline solid or crystalline powder. Testosterone is a naturally occurring steroid hormone. Since oral administration of testosterone leads to its rapid degradation by the liver, the 17β-hydroxyl group was chemically modified to create a series of esters of a number of carboxylic acids. The resultant decrease in polarity leads to increased solubility in oily vehicles, rendering absorption slower at the site of injection.

Testosterone compounds

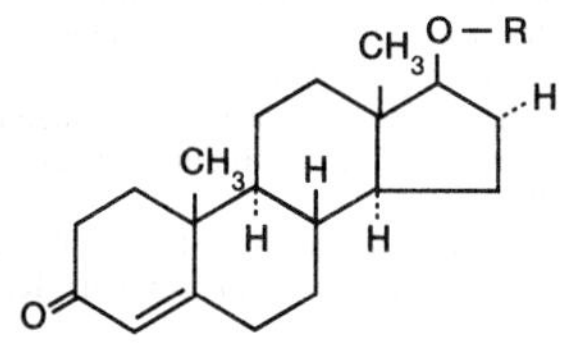

where R = $COCH_2CH_3$ in testosterone propionate
R = $CO(CH_2)_4CH_3$ in testosterone isocaproate
R = $CO(CH_2)_5CH_3$ in testosterone enanthate
R = $COCH_2CH_2C_5H_9$ in testosterone cypionate
R = $CO(CH_2)_4CH_3$ in testosterone decanoate
R = $CO(CH_2)_9CH_3$ in testosterone undecanoate

Testosterone propionate (Vivormone, Testoviron, Testex)
$C_{22}H_{32}O_3$
17β(1-Oxopropoxy)-androst-L-en-3-one

Molecular weight	344.5
pKa	—
Solubility	
in alcohol	1 in 6
in water	insoluble
Octanol/water partition coefficient	high

A colourless or yellowish-white crystalline solid, or a white or off-white crystalline powder. It is an ingredient of Mixogen, Testoviron Depot, and Sustanon (with other testosterone esters).

Testosterone isocaproate
$C_{25}H_{38}O_3$
17β-[(1-Oxohexyl)oxy]-androst-4-en-3-one

Molecular weight	386.6
pKa	—
Solubility	
in alcohol	>1 in 1
in water	insoluble
Octanol/water partition coefficient	high

White to creamy white crystals, or crystalline powder. It is an ingredient of Mixogen and Sustanon (with other testosterone esters).

Testosterone enanthate (Testostiron Depot, Primoteston Depot, Delatestryl)
$C_{26}H_{40}O_3$
17β-[(1-Oxoheptyl)oxy]-androst-4-en-one

Molecular weight	400.6
pKa	—
Solubility	
in alcohol	1 in 0.3
in water	insoluble
Octanol/water partition coefficient	high

It is a white to off-white crystalline powder. It is an ingredient of Testoviron Depot with other testosterone esters.

Testosterone cypionate (Andronate, Ciclosterone, Depot Testosterone)
$C_{27}H_{40}O_3$
17β-(3-Cyclopentyl-1-oxopropoxy)-androst-4-en-3-one

Molecular weight	412.6
pKa	—
Solubility	
in alcohol	>1 in 1
in water	insoluble
Octanol/water partition coefficient	high

A white or creamy white crystalline powder.

Testosterone decanoate
$C_{29}H_{46}O_3$
17β-[(1-Oxodecanyl)oxy]-androst-4-en-3-one

Molecular weight	442.7
pKa	—
Solubility	
in alcohol	high
in water	insoluble
Octanol/water partition coefficient	high

It is an ingredient of Sustanon, with other testosterone esters.

Testosterone undecanoate (Restandol, Andriol)
$C_{30}H_{48}O_3$
17β-[(1-Oxododecanyl)oxy]-androst-4-en-3-one

Molecular weight	458.7
pKa	—
Solubility	
in alcohol	high
in water	insoluble
Octanol/water partition coefficient	high

Testosterone (esters)

Pharmacology

Testosterone is a potent androgen that is secreted by the Leydig cells of the testis.[2] Two periods of secretory activity have been identified, one in fetal life, which is responsible, directly or indirectly via transformation to dihydrotestosterone, for masculinization of the indifferent external genitalia. The second phase, commencing at puberty, is responsible for inducing the male secondary sex characteristics.[3]

Testosterone action is mediated (i) through androgen receptors in the nuclei of sensitive tissues, (ii) by metabolism to dihydrotestosterone, which acts through specific receptors on target tissues, and (iii) by conversion by the action of the enzyme aromatase to oestradiol-17β, the latter acting through oestrogen receptors on target tissues.[4,5]

The receptors for androgen are found on target tissues, e.g. prostate, seminal vesicles, epididymis, etc. They are steroid-specific and of high affinity (K_D 10^{-9}–10^{-10}). The androgen–receptor complex binds to chromatin resulting in the increased transcription of specific structural genes, with subsequent mRNA and protein synthesis. The entire structure of the androgen receptor has been recently elucidated.[6]

Toxicology

Testosterone has been found to have no mutagenic activity, and similar data are available for its esters, particularly the recently introduced ester with undecanoic acid, which has been evaluated in the Ames *Salmonella* and rat micronucleus tests. Replacement or higher doses of testosterone or its esters will suppress gonadotrophic support of the testis resulting in suppression of spermatogenesis.[7] Even higher doses, when given to rats, will partially restore spermatogenesis, probably by partially restoring intratesticular testosterone concentrations. No adverse effects on liver function have been found with testosterone esters given in high doses.

Clinical pharmacology

In adult men, testosterone is secreted episodically, resulting from stimulation by episodic luteinizing hormone pulses from the anterior pituitary gland.[8] This testosterone secretion results in (i) growth of external genitalia, (ii) stimulation of spermatogenesis in conjunction with the gonadotrophic hormones, (iii) stimulation of the epididymis, vas deferens, prostate and seminal vesicles, (iv) skeletal growth whilst the epiphyses remain open, (v) increased muscle mass, (vi) lengthening of the vocal cords due to growth of laryngeal cartilages, (vii) stimulation of haemopoiesis by synergizing with erythropoietin, (viii) increased skin thickness and oiliness, the latter due to sebaceous gland stimulation, (ix) increased facial, body, axillary and pubic hair, and (x) ill-defined central nervous system changes resulting in stimulation of libido.

The adrenal gland is also a source of androgens in both males and females. Androstenedione and dehydroepiandrosterone produced by the adrenal cortex serve as substrates for peripheral conversion to testosterone in both men and women.[9] In men, this source of testosterone is insufficient to maintain spermatogenesis or secondary sexual characteristics. In women, adrenal and ovarian androgens contribute, by direct secretion and peripheral conversion, to the circulating levels of testosterone.

Testosterone administration orally is essentially ineffective since following absorption it is directly transported to the liver and inactivated, thereby decreasing levels prior to their accessibility to the peripheral circulation. Even intramuscular administration of testosterone results in a rapid decline in serum levels due to metabolism. Hence, androgen substitution therapy has required several modifications of the testosterone molecule since, even in the micronized form, extremely large doses produced limited effects.[10] These modifications have consisted of (i) alkylation at the 17α position and modification of the ring structure or (ii) esterification through the 17β-hydroxyl group with various carboxylic acids to provide a prolonged action.[11] The 17α-alkylated derivatives are considered in separate monographs and this monograph considers only the esters of testosterone.

Esterification of steroid hormones increases the duration of effect in relationship to the length of the aliphatic chain of the ester.[11] Furthermore, the esterification reduces the polarity of the molecule enabling testosterone esters to be formulated as injections using an oily vehicle, the duration of action being considerably prolonged. Once the esters reach the liver via the circulation, they are hydrolysed and the testosterone metabolized along pathways used by the natural hormone.[12] A number of carboxylic acids have been used for esterification, such as propionic, phenylpropionic, cypionic, isocaproic, decanoic and enanthic. Esters of testosterone with undecanoic acid appear to be preferentially absorbed and transported, via the lacteals, to the lymphatic system, thus bypassing the liver until they enter the circulation.[13]

Following hydrolysis of the ester, the circulating testosterone binds to receptors in target tissues and exerts its action through the same pathways as the naturally occurring hormone.

Pharmacokinetics

Testosterone esters are hydrolysed by the liver to yield the natural hormone, which can be measured in the circulation and tissues by specific radioimmunoassays, usually after extraction. Enzyme immunoassay has also been used. Following oral administration, testosterone is readily absorbed, but it is inactive due to extensive presystemic metabolism, which is reflected by a plasma clearance[14] of 0.8 $l.min^{-1}$. If dissolved in oil and administered intramuscularly, testosterone is rapidly absorbed and cleared. As described earlier, esterification delays absorption from the site of the injection; the length of the aliphatic chain progressively extends the duration of action due to slower release of the ester from the site of the injection. Thus, esters such as testosterone propionate have a duration of action of 24–48 hours. Others such as the enanthate and cypionate have almost identical patterns of absorption, the compounds being metabolized at the site of injection and after absorption. Levels of testosterone rise to reach a peak 4 to 5 days after the injection and slowly decline over the next 21 days.[15] This pattern can be modified if mixtures of esters are used such as the propionate, phenylpropionate, isocaproate and decanoate (as in Sustanon), peak plasma levels of testosterone being achieved 24–48 hours after administration and declining slowly over the subsequent 21 days.[16] Testosterone undecanoate is effective after oral administration due to absorption via the lymphatic system. Peak plasma testosterone levels occur 2–6 hours after the dose, and return to control levels 10–12 hours after administration.[16] Alternatively, if testosterone is administered subcutaneously as an implant, peak plasma levels are observed 2–10 weeks after implantation; the levels remain elevated for 16–18 weeks.

Once absorbed, testosterone circulates bound to testosterone oestradiol (or sex steroid) binding globulin (SSBG) and to albumin. Though albumin has a 1000-fold lower affinity for testosterone than sex steroid binding globulin, it has a 1000-fold greater capacity.[17] The proportion of testosterone bound to the two proteins varies between the sexes and in various physiological states: in the male 50% is bound to albumin and 44% to SSBG, whereas in females the proportions are 30% and 60%, respectively.[18] Approximately 2% circulates in the free form but recent studies indicate that in vivo the albumin-bound portion is also relatively easily exchangeable across the capillary membrane.[19] Changes in the concentration of both albumin and SSBG can occur in different physiological and pathological states, thereby altering the exchangeable testosterone concentration, its activity and clearance.

Testosterone is extensively metabolized in the liver, the main route of excretion being the urine (90% of dose) with much smaller amounts (6% of dose) in the faeces.

Concentration–effect relationship

The aim of effective treatment is to maintain stable testosterone levels in the normal male range (10–40 $nmol.l^{-1}$). There is evidence that increased levels will progressively increase such factors as prostate and seminal vesicle weight. These tissue responses were used as bioassays for androgens prior to the availability of more precise and less cumbersome methods of measurement. However, many of the subjective effects of testosterone such as those on libido and potency have not been closely related to the levels of this hormone in the normal or supranormal range. However, in a study using doses of testosterone enanthate of 100 mg or 400 mg given once per month, Davidson and colleagues[20] noted that sexual activity demonstrated a dose–response relationship. In general, attempts are made to achieve normal androgenic function using the minimal effective dose necessary, thereby avoiding potential problems of high-dose treatment such as prostatic hypertrophy.

Testosterone (esters)

Metabolism

Testosterone is inactivated to a large extent in the liver; this involves oxidation of the 17-hydroxyl group and reduction of ring A to form androstenedione.[12] Further reduction at the 3-keto position produces androsterone (see Fig. 1) or, alternatively, reduction of androstenedione at the 5β-position yields etiocholanolone. Of an administered dose of labelled testosterone, 90% appears in urine and 6% appears in the faeces, excreted via the biliary system. The labelled metabolites in urine consist of androsterone and etiocholanolone.

Fig. 1 Androsterone

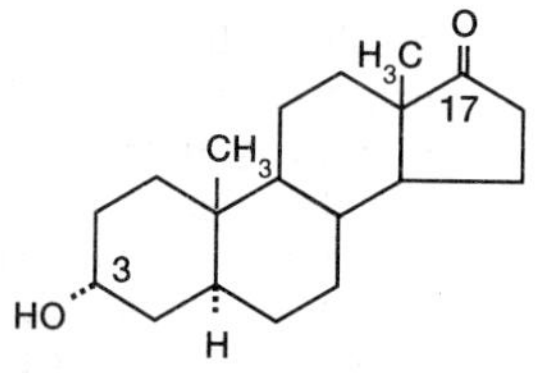

Some testosterone is also aromatized to form oestradiol. By the action of 5α-reductase, it is reduced to form dihydrotestosterone, an activity that is required for the expression of androgen action in some target tissues.[21]

Androstenedione has weak androgenic activity.

Pharmaceutics

Testosterone is available as an implant for subcutaneous administration, which may contain either 50, 100 or 200 mg of hormone. Testosterone is also available in esterified form predominantly for parenteral use but in one instance for oral administration as testosterone undecanoate (Andriol/Restandol, Organon) available as capsules of 40 mg dissolved in oleic acid. The esters for parenteral use are as follows:

1. Testosterone propionate (Vivormone; Paines & Byrne, UK) 25 or 50 mg in 1 ml oily solution.
2. Testosterone enanthate (Primoteston Depot; Schering, UK) 250 mg in 1 ml oily solution.
3. Testosterone cypionate (Depo Testosterone; Upjohn, USA). Doses of 100 and 200 mg are available in each 1 ml of cotton seed oil, benzyl benzoate and benzyl alcohol.
4. Mixed testosterone esters (Sustanon 100 mg; Organon, UK). This mixture contains testosterone propionate 20 mg, testosterone phenylpropionate 40 mg, and testosterone isocaproate 40 mg in 1 ml.
5. Mixed testosterone esters (Sustanon 250 mg; Organon, UK). This mixture contains testosterone propionate 30 mg, testosterone phenylpropionate 60 mg, testosterone isocaproate 60 mg, and testosterone decanoate 100 mg in 1 ml.

An aqueous injectable suspension (Legere Pharmaceuticals, USA) contains 100 mg testosterone in a 10 ml vial.

Therapeutic use

Indications

1. Substitution or replacement therapy for androgen deficiency
2. Therapy for micropenis
3. Stimulation of erythropoiesis
4. Muscle development
5. Infertility
6. Menopausal symptoms.

Contraindications

1. Known or suspected prostatic carcinoma
2. Overt cardiac failure.

Mode of use

There are several methods of achieving levels of testosterone that circulate in the normal range.

Short-acting esters of testosterone. These are required to be given as intramuscular injections every 24 to 72 hours. They are not recommended for long-term treatment in view of their relatively short duration of action.

Intermediate-acting esters of testosterone. These are given by deep intramuscular injections in a dose of 100 mg. The frequency of administration is determined according to clinical response. Usually one injection per 2 weeks will be adequate.

Long-acting esters of testosterone. These are given as intramuscular injections in a dose of 250 mg. The dosage should be adjusted to the individual response of the patient. Usually, one injection per 2 weeks will be adequate. The absorption results in peak levels 2–4 days after injection with a progressive fall over the ensuing 10–14 days.[14,16] The rapidity of the fall in testosterone levels varies between subjects and the interval between injections can be adjusted to suit the individual; the adequacy of action can be judged on the basis of measuring testosterone levels or on clinical responses, e.g. frequency of erections and adequacy of libido. In some patients the frequency of injections may need to be increased to once every 10 days whereas in others, intervals of up to 21 days may be adequate.

Orally active esters (testosterone undecanoate). This is used in doses of 80 mg twice daily but many men may not achieve adequate androgenization until daily doses of 240 mg are given.[16,22]

Testosterone implants. Between 4 to 6 (100 mg) implants are introduced subcutaneously under local anaesthesia using a trocar and cannula. Levels of testosterone should be monitored after 3 months to determine when the implants should be replaced. In a study using six 100 mg implants, testosterone levels fell below the normal range 16–18 weeks after their insertion.[16]

Indications

1. Substitution or replacement therapy in male hypogonadal disorders

Documentation of androgen deficiency requires the demonstration of low plasma testosterone levels in a patient with the clinical signs of androgen deficiency. These low testosterone levels are accompanied by elevated LH and FSH levels. In some patients, low normal testosterone levels are accompanied by significantly elevated LH levels suggesting a state of compensated Leydig cell failure. Often such patients manifest marginal symptoms of androgen deficiency and are significantly benefited by replacement therapy. Diagnosis of marginal androgen deficiency is complex and may require such documentation of an elevated LH rise to a single injection of LHRH and may require the patient keeping a diary of sexual function. Frequently, when questioned initially, the patient does not claim any sexual dysfunction as he may have never been fully androgenized.

In adolescents requiring substitution therapy, the dose of testosterone esters should be lowered to provide a gradual androgenization similar to that which occurs during puberty. This may avoid the rapid closure of epiphyses and prevent short stature occurring.

2. Treatment of micropenis

Use of testosterone in childhood to improve penile size is complicated by the problem of epiphyseal closure due to androgen. Small doses (25 mg) of long-acting esters of testosterone every 3–4 weeks for 3–4 months have been advocated.[23] Alternatively, topical administration of testosterone creams may be used though the action is unlikely to be due to the systemic absorption. However, the relative ease of application of creams compared to injections may offset the difficulties of erratic absorption.

3. Stimulation of erythropoiesis

The stimulation of haematocrit and haemoglobin noted during long-term therapy of patients with androgens has been applied to the treatment of patients with aplastic anaemia. The action is thought to occur through the stimulation of erythropoietin secretion.[24] Such treatment results in a response in approximately 50% of patients but there have been inadequate controlled randomized trials to determine the specificity of the response.[25,26] The availability of specific growth factors such as erythropoietin, GCSF, etc. may in time supersede this use.

4. Muscle development

In androgen-deficient patients, testosterone therapy results in positive nitrogen balance and increased muscle mass.[27] However, there is considerable controversy about whether adding androgens to those present in a normal man will result in improved muscle mass and performance. Conflicting results have been obtained in studies in athletes and body builders, most suggesting that it is the degree of training and high calorie intake that influence the increase of body muscle mass rather than the androgen treatment. Mostly oral synthetic androgens have been used instead of testosterone due to the ease of administration.[27–29] The problem is compounded in women by the effects of androgens causing virilization and masculinization.[30] Use of androgens for this purpose in athletes is banned by international sports organizations.

5. Male infertility
Testosterone esters will cause a suppression of FSH and LH levels leading to a decrease in sperm counts often to azoospermia.[7] This is a recognized complication of replacement therapy. However, in some studies, a three-month period of spermatogenic suppression was associated subsequently with a rebound to greater than pretreatment sperm counts.[31] Unfortunately, these studies have not been adequately controlled and this indication remains tenuous.

6. Menopausal symptoms
The symptoms of oestrogen deficiency occurring in association with the menopause are often relieved by oestrogen replacement therapy. However, loss of libido often persists and prospective studies indicate that low-dose androgen replacement results in improvement.[32,33]

Contraindications

1. Prostatic carcinoma
Prostatic carcinoma is known to be androgen-dependent in many instances and is therefore a contraindication to androgen therapy.

2. Overt cardiac failure
Since replacement doses of testosterone esters may cause sodium retention, especially in sensitive patients or those receiving high doses, overt cardiac failure should lead to caution in androgen administration. Other states that are potentially aggravated by sodium retention should also prompt care in androgen administration.

Adverse reactions

Potentially life-threatening effects
The development of hepatic carcinoma or peliosis hepatis (blood-filled cysts in the liver), which are complications of therapy with 17α-alkylated androgens, has not been reported with the use of testosterone or its esters.

Acute overdosage
This has not been a major problem. Higher than required doses may cause fluid retention or polycythaemia.

Severe or irreversible adverse effects
If given to prepubertal males or females for prolonged periods, testosterone or its esters will cause masculinization. Some of these features such as deepening of the voice due to lengthening of the vocal cords, clitoromegaly and male-pattern baldness may be irreversible. Similarly epiphyseal closure is also permanent and results in short stature.

Symptomatic adverse effects
Jaundice. This is a complication of the 17α-alkyl substitutions of testosterone and has not been noted with testosterone ester therapy.
Oedema. Replacement therapy does not usually result in sodium retention detectable as clinically evident oedema. Occasional sensitive patients or pubertal children given full adult doses of testosterone esters may show this complication, which ceases on dosage adjustment.
Polycythaemia. Some men on replacement doses of testosterone esters may have an elevation of their haematocrit to polycythaemic levels. It is uncertain why this effect is only seen in some men, but the explanation may lie in the results of recent studies which showed that replacement doses of androgens may be associated with the onset of sleep apnoea; the resultant anoxia may cause the polycythaemic response.[34] Should the increase in haematocrit reach significant levels, the frequency of injections can be decreased or alternatively the patient can be encouraged to donate blood.
Gynaecomastia. Some men develop breast enlargement when given testosterone esters. This usually is manifested by a small, tender disc of breast tissue and may be related to an active aromatase system converting the testosterone to oestradiol.

Testosterone (esters)

Decline in testis size and suppression of spermatogenesis. This will occur in many post-pubertal men with normal-sized testes given androgens.[35] It has, as its basis, the suppression of FSH and LH levels by testosterone, resulting in a decrease in spermatogenesis and a decline in seminiferous tubule diameter. Since the seminiferous tubules comprise over 90% of testis volume, a decline in testis size occurs.
Acne. Some subjects note an increase in acne associated with stimulation of sebaceous gland secretion.
Gastrointestinal problems. Some patients taking testosterone undecanoate orally develop nausea. It is probably related to the oily component contained in the capsules.[36]

Other effects
No changes in cholesterol or triglyceride levels in serum were noted in men during treatment with long-acting esters of testosterone.[7] No details are available concerning the action of testosterone on lipoprotein levels, but adverse changes have been noted during treatment with methyl testosterone. These include elevation in total cholesterol, raised LDL cholesterol and a fall in the HDL/LDL ratio.[37–40] These reports suggest that hypercholesterolaemia should be a contraindication to androgen therapy and that lipid levels should be measured prior to starting treatment.

Interference with clinical pathology tests
Testosterone interferes with some older urinary tests for aldosterone and 17-hydroxycorticosteroids, and plasma or serum tests for corticosteroids.

High risk groups

Neonates
There are no indications for the use of the drug in neonates.
Breast milk. Testosterone is contraindicated during breast-feeding.

Children
In pubertal or prepubertal children care should be taken to ensure careful selection of dose to prevent significant masculinization and closure of epiphyses until adequate growth has been achieved.

Pregnant women
The drug is contraindicated during pregnancy.

The elderly
Should androgens be used for replacement, care should be taken with dosage since the potential exists for growth in prostatic size and subsequent urinary difficulties.

Drug interactions

There are none of known significance.

Major outcome trials

1. Davidson J M, Cauargo C A, Smith E R 1979 Effects of androgen on sexual behaviour in hypogonadal men. Journal of Clinical Endocrinology and Metabolism 48: 955–959

This double-blind trial administered placebo or testosterone enanthate in two doses to hypogonadal men and demonstrated a dose-related response in the improvement of their sexual function.

2. Skakkebaek N E, Bancroft J, Davidson W D, Warner D 1981 Androgen replacement therapy with oral testosterone undecanoate in hypogonadal men: a double-blind controlled study. Clinical Endocrinology 14: 49–61

Significant androgenization was achieved with this form of oral testosterone when given to hypogonadal men.

Other trials

1. Nicholls D P, Anderson D C 1982 Clinical aspects of androgen deficiency in men. Andrologia 14: 379–388

This report describes the use of androgens in a variety of clinical conditions resulting in hypogonadism.

2. Cantrill J A, Dewis P, Large D M, Newman M, Anderson D C 1984 Which testosterone replacement therapy? Clinical Endocrinology 21: 97–107

This trial describes the comparison in terms of hormonal levels and clinical features of three forms of androgen replacement in hypogonadal men: i) intramuscular mixed testosterone esters 250 mg, (ii) fixed testosterone implants (6 × 100 mg) and (iii) testosterone undecanoate 80 mg twice daily. The authors conclude that the implants provided more stable long-term therapy for the maintenance of normal levels of testosterone.

References

1. David K, Dingemanse E, Freud J, Laqueur E 1935 Uber krystallinsches mannliches Hormon aus Hoden (Testosteron) Wirksamer als aus Harn oder aus Cholesterin bereitetes Androsteron. Hoppe-Seylers Zeitschrift fur Physiologische Chemie 233: 281–282
2. Christensen A K, Mason N R 1965 Comparative ability of seminiferous tubules and interstitial tissue of rat testes to synthesize androgen from progesterone-4-^{14}C in vitro. Endocrinology 76: 646–656
3. Lording D W, de Kretser D M 1972 Comparative ultrastructural and histochemical studies of the interstitial cells of the rat testis during fetal and postnatal development. Journal of Reproduction and Fertility 29: 261–269
4. Mainwaring W I P (ed) 1977 The mechanism of action of androgens. Monographs in Endocrinology, vol 10, pp 1–178
5. Ryan K J, Naftolin F, Reddy V, Flores F, Petro Z 1972 Estrogen formation in the brain. American Journal of Obstetrics and Gynecology 114: 454–460
6. Chang C, Kontis J, Liao S T 1988 Molecular cloning of human and cat complementary DNA encoding androgen receptors. Science 240: 324–326
7. Swerdloff R S, Campfield L A, Palacios A, McClure R D 1979 Suppression of human spermatogenesis by depot androgen: potential for male contraception. Journal of Steroid Biochemistry 11: 663–670
8. Naftolin F, Yen S S C, Tsai C C 1972 Rapid cycling of plasma gonadotrophins in normal men as demonstrated by frequent sampling. Nature New Biology 236: 92–93
9. Rosenfield R L 1972 Role of androgens in growth and development of the fetus, child and adolescent. Advanced Paediatrics 19: 172–213
10. Johnsen S G (ed) 1977 Long term androgen therapy with oral testosterone. In: Proceedings of hormonal control of male fertility, US Dept of Health Education and Welfare, Washington DC No NIH 78–1097, pp 123–143
11. Junkmann K 1957 Long-acting steroids in reproduction. Recent Progress in Hormone Research 13: 389–428
12. Murad F, Haynes R C 1985 Androgens. In: Goodman L S, Rall T W, Murad F (eds) The pharmacological basis of therapeutics, 7th edn. Macmillan, New York, pp 1440–1458
13. Horst H J, Holtje W J, Dennis M, Coert A, Geelen J, Voight K D 1976 Lymphatic absorption and metabolism of orally administered testosterone undecanoate in man. Klinische Wochenschrift 54: 875–879
14. Sokol R Z, Swerdloff R S 1986 Practical considerations in the use of androgen therapy. In: Santen R J, Swerdloff R S (eds) Male reproductive dysfunction. Marcel Dekker Inc, New York, pp 211–225
15. Sokol R Z, Palacios A, Campfield L A, Saul C, Swerdloff R S 1982 Comparison of the kinetics of injectable testosterone in eugonadal and hypogonadal men. Fertility and Sterility 37: 425–430
16. Cantrill J A, Dewis P, Large D M, Newman M, Anderson D C 1984 Which testosterone replacement therapy? Clinical Endocrinology 21: 97–107
17. Westphal U 1971 Steroid–protein interactions. Springer Verlag, New York
18. Dunn J F, Nisula B C, Rodbard D 1981 Transport of steroid hormones: binding of C21 endogenous steroids to both testosterone-binding globulin and corticosteroid-binding globulin in human plasma. Journal of Clinical Endocrinology and Metabolism 53: 58–67
19. Pardridge W M, Laidlaw E 1984 Tracer kinetic model of blood–brain barrier transport of plasma protein-bound ligands. Empiric testing of the free hormone hypothesis. Journal of Clinical Investigation 74: 745–752
20. Davidson J M, Camargo C A, Smith E R 1979 Effects of androgen on sexual behaviour in hypogonadal men. Journal of Clinical Endocrinology and Metabolism 48: 955–959
21. Griffin J E, Leshin M, Wilson J D 1982 Androgen resistance syndromes. American Journal of Physiology 243: E81–87
22. Skakkebaek N E, Bancroft J, Davidson D W, Warner P 1981 Androgen replacement with oral testosterone undecanoate in hypogonadal men: a double blind controlled study. Clinical Endocrinology 14: 49–61
23. Guthrie R D, Smith D W, Graham C B 1973 Testosterone treatment for micropenis during early childhood. Journal of Pediatrics 83: 247–252
24. Shahidi N T 1973 Androgens and erythropoiesis. New England Journal of Medicine 289: 73–80
25. Branda R F, Amsden T W, Jacob H S 1977 Randomized study of nandrolone therapy for anaemias due to bone marrow failure. Archives of Internal Medicine 137: 65–69
26. Camitta B M, Thomas E D, Nathan D G 1979 A prospective study of androgens and bone marrow transplantation for treatment of severe aplastic anaemia. Blood 53: 504–514
27. Kochakian C D 1956 The protein anabolic effects of steroid hormones. Vitamins and Hormones 4: 255–270
28. Hervey G R, Hutchinson I, Knibles A V, Burbunshaw L, Jones P R M, Morgan W G 1976 Anabolic effects of methandienone in men undergoing athletic training. Lancet 2: 699–702
29. Hervey G R, Knibles A V, Burbinshaw L et al 1981 Effects of methandienone on the performance and body composition of men undergoing athletic training. Clinical Science 60: 457–461
30. Fox E L 1984 Physiology of exercise and physical fitness. In: Strauss R H (ed) Sports medicine. W B Saunders, Philadelphia, pp 381–456
31. Wilson J D, Griffin J E 1982 The use and misuse of androgens. Metabolism 29: 1278–1294
32. Burger H G, Hailes J, Menelaus M, Nelson J, Hudson B, Balazs N 1984 The management of persistent menopausal symptoms with oestradiol–testosterone implants: clinical, lipid and hormonal results. Maturitas 6: 351–358
33. Fletcher C D, Farish E, Hart D M, Barlow D H, Gray C E, Conaghan C J 1986 Long-term hormone implant therapy — effects on lipoproteins and steroid levels in post menopausal women. Acta Endocrinologica 111: 419–423
34. Sandblom R E, Matsumoto A M, Schoene R B et al 1983 Obstructive sleep apnoea syndrome induced by testosterone administration. New England Journal of Medicine 308: 508–510
35. Heller C G, Nelson W O, Hill I C et al 1950 Improvement in spermatogenesis following depression of human testes with testosterone. Fertility and Sterility 1: 415–422
36. Maisey N M, Bingham J, Marks V, English J, Chakrabarty J 1981 Clinical efficacy of testosterone undecanoate in male hypogonadism. Clinical Endocrinology 14: 625–629
37. Oliver M F, Boyd G S 1956 Endocrine aspects of coronary sclerosis. Lancet 2: 1273
38. Herly B F, Seals D R, Hagberg J M et al 1984 High density lipoprotein cholesterol in body builders vs powerlifters: negative effects of androgen use. Journal of the American Medical Association 252: 507–513
39. Fahey T D 1984 HDL-C in five elite athletes using anabolic androgenic steroids. Physician and Sports Medicine 12: 120–130
40. Costill D L, Pearson D R, Fink W J 1984 Anabolic steroid use among athletes. Changes in HDL-C levels. Physician and Sports Medicine 12: 113–117

Tetracosactrin

Severe or irreversible adverse effects
Potentially severe effects may follow long-term administration of excessive doses of depot tetracosactrin and development of Cushing's syndrome. These effects include hypertension, diabetes mellitus, osteoporosis and growth retardation in children.

Symptomatic adverse effects
The development of pain and lumps at the site of injection has been reported in about 10% of patients.[13]

Symptoms of excess adrenocortical function resulting from tetracosactrin stimulation include hirsutism, acne, and menstrual disturbance, as well as skin atrophy and bruising. Skin pigmentation is a further well described adverse effect.

Other effects
Polymorphonuclear leucocytosis secondary to tetracosactrin therapy has been described.[17] Partially reversible macular degeneration has also been reported.[18]

The mineralocorticoid effects of prolonged tetracosactrin therapy may result in hypokalaemia. Elevated levels of a number of corticosteroid hormones, in both serum and urine, may follow injection of tetracosactrin; these include androgenic steroids as well as cortisol and its derivatives. A significant fall in plasma insulin concentration after a single injection of depot tetracosactrin has been described.[19]

Interference with clinical pathology tests
Tetracosactrin may interfere with radioimmunoassay of endogenous ACTH because of its structural similarity.

High risk groups

Neonates
Tetracosactrin depot should not be administered to neonates since poisoning may result from benzyl alcohol present in the preparation.

Breast milk. The use of tetracosactrin in lactating mothers has not been described, but it is probably best for them not to breast-feed while receiving the drug, although it is highly unlikely that appreciable amounts of the petide would appear in breast milk.

Children
A single dose of 250 µg 1.73 m^{-2} body surface area has been suggested as appropriate in the investigation of adrenocortical function. If tetracosactrin depot is administered for therapeutic purposes to children, the minimal effective dose should be given to reduce problems of growth retardation and symptoms of Cushing's syndrome. Recommended doses vary according to age from 250–1000 µg.day^{-1} initially, with similar doses every 2–8 days for maintenance therapy.

Pregnant women
The safety of tetracosactrin in pregnancy has not been established. The rise in plasma cortisol which follows administration of tetracosactrin depot is greater in pregnancy than in non-pregnant controls.[20]

The elderly
There is no evidence that different doses should be administered to elderly subjects.

Concurrent disease
Caution should be exercised in patients with untreated infections, heart failure and allergic conditions such as asthma when there may be increased likelihood of adverse reactions.

Drug interactions

Potentially hazardous interactions
Patients receiving treatment for diabetes mellitus or hypertension may require an increase in therapy because of the diabetogenic and sodium retaining characteristics of tetracosactrin.

Potentially useful interactions
No interactions of this kind have been reported.

Major outcome trials

Trials determining the therapeutic value of tetracosactrin in terms of long-term morbidity and mortality have not been reported.

General review articles

Burke C W 1985 Adrenocortical insufficiency. In: Besser G M, Rees L H (eds) The pituitary–adrenocortical axis. Clinics in endocrinology and metabolism. W B Saunders, London, pp 947–976

May M E, Carey R M 1985 Rapid adrenocorticotropic hormone test in practice. Retrospective review. American Journal of Medicine 79: 679–684

Weaver J A 1978 The therapeutic uses of long-acting ACTH. Scottish Medical Journal 23: 153–160

References

1. Shah R M 1977 Induction of cleft palate in hamster fetus following prenatal treatment with ACTH. Toxicology and Applied Pharmacology 42: 229–231
2. Besser G M, Butler P W P, Plumpton F S 1967 Adrenocorticotrophic action of long-acting tetracosactrin compared with corticotrophin gel. British Medical Journal 4: 391–394
3. Jeffcoate W J, Phenekos C, Ratcliffe J G, Williams S, Rees L, Besser G M 1977 Comparison of the pharmacokinetics in man of two synthetic ACTH analogues: α^{1-24} and substituted α^{1-18} ACTH. Clinical Endocrinology 7: 1–11
4. Besser G M, Orth D N, Nicholson W E, Bynny R L, Abe K, Woodham J P 1971 Dissociation of the disappearance of bioactive and radioimmunoreactive ACTH from plasma in man. Journal of Clinical Endocrinology and Metabolism 32: 595–602
5. May M E, Carey R M 1985 Rapid adrenocorticotropic hormone test in practice. Retrospective review. American Journal of Medicine 79: 679–684
6. Lindholm J, Kehlet H 1987 Re-evaluation of the clinical value of the 30 minute ACTH test in assessing hypothalamic–pituitary–adrenocortical function. Clinical Endocrinology 26: 53–59
7. Stewart P M, Corrie J, Seckl J R, Edwards C R W, Padfield P L 1988 A rational approach for assessing the hypothalamo–pituitary–adrenal axis. Lancet 1: 1208–1209
8. Breslin A B X 1979 Chronic asthma: which treatment? Drugs 18: 103–112
9. Weaver J A 1978 The therapeutic uses of long-acting ACTH. Scottish Medical Journal 23: 153–160
10. Nuki G, Jasani M K, Downie W W et al 1970 Clinico-pharmacological studies on depot tetracosactrin in patients with rheumatoid arthritis. Pharmacologica Clinica 2: 99–108
11. Norman A P, Sanders S S 1969 A study of the effect of corticotrophin on skeletal maturation and linear growth in six patients with severe asthma. Scandinavian Journal of Respiratory Diseases 68 (suppl): 49
12. Carter M E, James V H T 1970 Effect of corticotrophin therapy on pituitary adrenal function. Annals of Rheumatic Diseases 29: 73–80
13. Jensen N E, Sneddon I 1969 Allergic intolerance to tetracosactrin. British Medical Journal 2: 383–384
14. Patriarca G 1971 Allergy to tetracosactrin depot. Lancet 1: 138
15. Tan D B P 1972 Severe reaction from tetracosactrin. Medical Journal of Australia 1: 387
16. Plager J E, Cushman P 1962 Suppression of the pituitary-ACTH response in man by administration of ACTH or cortisol. Journal of Clinical Endocrinology and Metabolism 22: 147–154
17. Robinson A R 1972 Leucocytosis after tetracosactrin. British Medical Journal 4: 178
18. Williamson J, Nuki G 1970 Macular lesions during systemic therapy with depot tetracosactrin. British Journal of Ophthalmology 54: 405–409
19. Vince J D, Bremner F, Rooney P J et al 1973 The acute effect of tetracosactrin on carbohydrate, insulin, glucagon, gastrin and lipid metabolism in rheumatoid arthritis. Current Medical Research and Opinion 1: 379–384
20. Johnstone F, Campbell S 1975 Unbound plasma cortisol response to adrenal stimulation in pregnancy. Journal of Endocrinology 64: 185–186

T

Tetracycline (hydrochloride)

Tetracycline hydrochloride is a broad-spectrum antibiotic. It is active against a wide range of Gram-negative and Gram-positive bacteria.

Chemistry

Tetracycline hydrochloride (Achromycin V, Panmycin, Steclin, Tetrachel, Tetracyn, Sumycin)

$C_{22}H_{24}N_2O_8$.HCl

(4S,4aS,5aS,6S,12aS)-4-(Dimethylamino)-1,4,4a,5,5a,6,11,12a-octahydro-3,6,10,12,12a-pentahydroxy-6-methyl-1,11-dioxo-2-naphthacenecarboxamide monohydrochloride

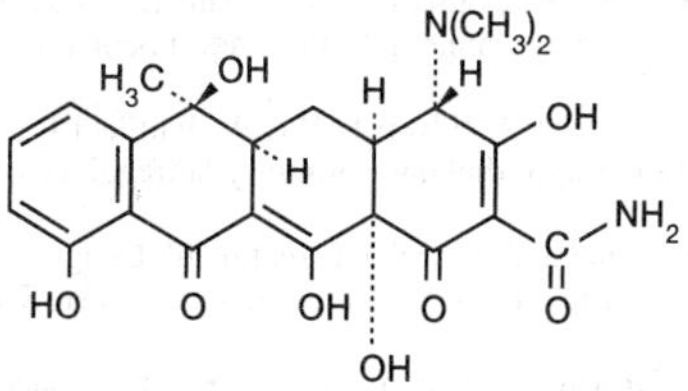

Molecular weight (free compound)	480.9 (444.4)
pKa	3.3, 7.7, 7.9
Solubility	
in alcohol (hydrochloride)	1 in 100
in water (hydrochloride)	1 in 10
Octanol/water partition coefficient	0.036

A yellow, odourless powder with a bitter taste, tetracycline is prepared by a fermentation process using *Streptomyces aureofaciens*.

Pharmacology

Tetracycline is a semi-synthetic tetracycline produced from chlortetracycline. Like other tetracyclines it has a wide spectrum of activity. In addition to its antibiotic activity it is also a chelating agent and will chelate Ca^{2+}, Mg^{3+} or Al^{3+} ions in the gut. Tetracycline has its main mechanism of action on protein synthesis, and an energy-dependent active transport system pumps the drug, like all tetracyclines, through the inner cytoplasmic membrane of bacteria. Once inside the bacterial cell, tetracycline inhibits protein synthesis by binding specifically to the 30S ribosomes. The drug appears to prevent access of aminoacyl tRNA to the acceptor site on the mRNA–ribosome complex.[1,2] This prevents the addition of amino acids to the growing peptide chain. Tetracycline will impair protein synthesis in mammalian cells if used at very high concentrations. However these cells lack the active transport system found in bacteria. There is also some evidence that tetracyclines may cause alterations in the cytoplasmic membrane thus allowing leakage of nucleotides from the cell. This would explain the rapid inhibition of DNA replication that ensues when cells are exposed to concentrations of tetracycline in excess of that required for inhibition of protein synthesis. Although tetracycline is often used on its own, there are specific situations where combining tetracycline with other antibiotics is helpful.[3–6]

Toxicology

Local injection of 100 mg doses of tetracycline into the gluteal muscles of the rabbit produced an area of necrosis surrounded by a zone of general inflammation. On microscopic examination, the necrotic area was found to be sharply demarcated from the viable tissue, and there was extravasation of red blood cells as well as leucocyte infiltration in the zone of inflammation. Inflammatory changes were found also in the sheath of the sciatic nerve, while repeated injections in the same site caused mild degenerative changes in the nerve bundles. These effects are comparable to those of intramuscular penicillin, streptomycin and sulphonamides, and are related to the surrounding inflammatory reaction.[7,8]

Acute systemic toxicity studies showed that the LD_{50} of tetracycline in mice and rats was approximately 160 $mg.kg^{-1}$ of body weight intravenously and about 2000 $mg.kg^{-1}$ orally.[9,10]

No teratogenicity was found in rats or sows given tetracycline.[11,12] The injection of 0.1–0.5 mg of the drug into chick embryos did not seriously impair growth, but there was a reduction in the size of the embryo.[13]

Clinical pharmacology

Tetracycline is primarily a bacteriostatic antibiotic and has a similar spectrum of activity to other tetracyclines.

Tetracycline is active against most strains of *Haemophilus influenzae* and is particularly useful for infections with *H. ducreyi*, *Actinomyces*, *Brucella* and *Vibrio cholerae*. Tetracycline is also active against *Nocardia*, *Chlamydia*, *Mycoplasma*, and a wide range of rickettsiae. Tetracycline is active against spirochaetes such as *Borrelia recurrentis*, *Treponema pallidum* and *T. pertenue*.

Tetracycline was initially useful for the treatment of Gram-positive infections but many strains are now resistant to the drug. The overall resistance in the UK of the pneumococci is about 10%. Tetracycline possesses some activity against *Staphylococcus aureus*, particularly for community-acquired infections, but in hospitals the prevalence of resistance to staphylococci is high. Many Gram-negative organisms have acquired resistance to tetracycline and for *E. coli* more than 50% of strains may be resistant. Tetracycline has no activity against *Pseudomonas aeruginosa* while most strains of *Campylobacter* are sensitive. Tetracycline is also active against anaerobic species of bacteria and since concentrations of the drug are quite high in the gastrointestinal contents, the enteric flora are usually altered by the drug.

Resistance to tetracyclines develops slowly and organisms that show resistance to one tetracycline frequently show resistance to others in the group (with some exceptions for minocycline and doxycycline). Most resistance is mediated by a plasmid and is an inducible trait, appearing only after exposure of the bacteria to the drug. Resistance seems to occur because the plasmid implants genetic material in the cell for a number of proteins and this affects penetration of the cell wall by tetracycline.

Pharmacokinetics

Tetracycline can be measured in urine or plasma by radioimmunoassay which has a detection limit[14] of 20 $\mu g.l^{-1}$ or by HPLC with a sensitivity[15] of 100 $\mu g.l^{-1}$.

Absorption of tetracycline occurs largely in the stomach and small intestine. After a single oral dose of 250 mg, serum concentrations of 2 $\mu g.ml^{-1}$ were achieved in 2–4 h.[16,17] The half life of tetracycline is 8.5 h[18] and its volume of distribution 1.3 $l.kg^{-1}$. The drug is 36–50% bound to plasma proteins.

Since urine is a main route of tetracycline excretion, impaired renal clearance causes accumulation of tetracycline in the blood.[19–22] The amount of tetracycline accumulated in the blood is in direct relationship to the degree of renal impairment.[23]

Oral absorption	irregular and incomplete
Presystemic metabolism	nil
Plasma half life	
mean	8.5 h
Volume of distribution	~1.3 $l.kg^{-1}$
Plasma protein binding	36–50%

Tetracyclines form highly insoluble complexes with calcium, magnesium, iron and aluminium ions. Thus, when present in the stomach from food, especially milk, these ions[24] reduce the absorption of tetracycline from the gastrointestinal tract. Tetracycline should be given before meals or at least two hours afterwards.

Tetracycline (hydrochloride)

Concentration–effect relationship

The therapeutic range will depend upon the minimum inhibitory concentration (MIC) of the antibiotic for the organism in question. Full susceptibility occurs when the MIC is less than 4.0 mg.l^{-1} and intermediate susceptibility is said to occur when the MIC is between 4.0 and 12.5 mg.l^{-1}. Concentrations greater than 25 mg.l^{-1} are usually required to inhibit most strains of group B and group D streptococci and strains of *Staphylococcus aureus*. The MIC for *Streptococcus pyogenes* is usually about 1.0 mg.l^{-1} and for the pneumococci it is often between 0.4 and 0.8 mg.l^{-1}.

Metabolism

In general, 24 hours after an oral dose[25] 56% of the tetracycline administered is excreted in the faeces and 30% in the urine. Of the tetracycline recovered from the urine and faeces, 95% is unchanged and 5% is in the form of 4-epitetracycline.[26] The kinetics of C4 epimerization in tetracyclines has been investigated.[27] The process of epimerization is shown in Fig. 1. The drug is excreted in bile and undergoes some enterohepatic circulation.

Fig. 1 Epimerization of tetracycline

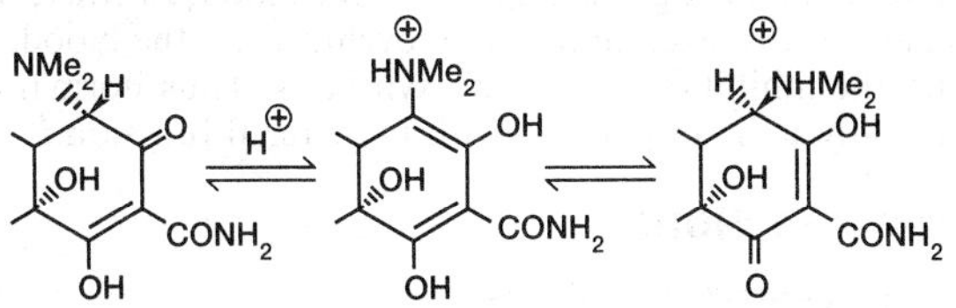

Pharmaceutics

Tetracycline is available in oral, intramuscular, intravenous and topical dosage forms.

Tetracycline hydrochloride (Achromycin V; Lederle, USA) is available for oral use as (i) 500 mg capsules that are two-piece, opaque, with a blue cap and yellow body printed with 'Lederle' over 'A5' on one half and 'Lederle' over '500 mg' on the other in grey ink and (ii) 250 mg two-piece, opaque capsules with a blue cap and yellow body, printed with 'Lederle' over 'A3' on one half and 'Lederle' over '250 mg' on the other in grey ink. In the UK, Achromycin V capsules are pink, 250 mg capsules marked 'Lederle 4885'. Achromycin tablets (Lederle, UK) are 250 mg, round, orange, film-coated tablets marked 'Lederle 4745'. An oral suspension is available which has a tetracycline equivalent of 125 mg per teaspoonful (5 ml); it is preserved with 0.12% of methylparaben and 0.03% propylparaben and is cherry-flavoured.

Tetracycline hydrochloride (Achromycin; Lederle, USA) is available for intramuscular use in both 100 mg and 250 mg vials. The 100 mg vial contains, in addition to the tetracycline hydrochloride, 40 mg of procaine hydrochloride, 46.84 mg of magnesium chloride and 250 mg of ascorbic acid. The 250 mg vial contains, in addition to the tetracycline hydrochloride, 40 mg of procaine hydrochloride, 46.84 mg of magnesium chloride and 275 mg of ascorbic acid.

Tetracycline hydrochloride (Achromycin; Lederle, USA) for intravenous use is available in vials containing 250 mg of antibiotic with 625 mg of ascorbic acid and vials containing 500 mg of drug with 1250 mg of ascorbic acid. Tetracycline hydrochloride (Achromycin) is also available as a 1% ophthalmic suspension and a 1% ophthalmic ointment.

The Achromycin V capsule has a maximum shelf-life of three years and the oral suspension two years. All formulations should be stored in a cool, dry place.

Therapeutic use

Indications

Tetracycline hydrochloride is indicated in infections caused by the following microorganisms:

1. Rickettsiae: (Rocky Mountain spotted fever, typhus fever and the typhus group, Q fever, rickettsialpox, tick fevers)
2. *Mycoplasma pneumoniae* (PPLO, Eaton agent)
3. Agents of psittacosis and ornithosis
4. Agents of lymphogranuloma venereum and granuloma inguinale
5. The spirochaetal agent of relapsing fever (*Borrelia recurrentis*)
6. In addition, infections caused by the following Gram-negative microorganisms can be treated with tetracycline:
   Haemophilus ducreyi (chancroid)
   Pasteurella pestis and *Pasteurella tularensis*
   Bartonella bacilliformis
   Bacteroides species
   Vibrio comma and *Vibrio fetus*
   Brucella species (in conjunction with streptomycin).
7. Because many strains of the following groups of microorganisms have been shown to be resistant to tetracyclines, culture and susceptibility testing are recommended. Tetracycline is indicated for treatment of infections caused by the following microorganisms, when bacteriologic testing indicates appropriate susceptibility to the drug:

   a) Gram-negative organisms
   Escherichia coli, *Enterobacter aerogenes* (formerly, *Aerobacter aerogenes*), *Shigella* species, *Mima* species and *Herellae* species, *Haemophilus influenzae* (respiratory infections), *Klebsiella* species (respiratory and urinary infections).
   b) Gram-positive organisms
   Streptococcus species: up to 44% of strains of *Streptococcus pyogenes* and 74% of *Streptococcus faecalis* have been found to be resistant to tetracycline drugs. Therefore, tetracyclines should not be used for streptococcal disease unless the organism has been demonstrated to be sensitive. For upper respiratory infections due to group A β-haemolytic streptococci, penicillin is the usual drug of choice, including prophylaxis of rheumatic fever.
   Diplococcus pneumoniae
   Staphylococcus aureus (skin and soft tissue infections). Tetracyclines are not the drug of choice in the treatment of any type of staphylococcal infection.
8. When penicillin is contraindicated, tetracyclines are alternative drugs in the treatment of infections due to:

   Neisseria gonorrhoea
   Treponema pallidum and *Treponema pertenue* (syphilus and yaws)
   Listeria monocytogenes
   Clostridium species
   Bacillus anthracis
   Fusobacterium fusiforme (Vincent's infection)
   Actinomyces species
9. In acute intestinal amoebiasis, the tetracyclines may be a useful adjunct to amoebicides.
10. Tetracycline therapy has been used successfully to treat patients with mild to moderately severe acne. Tetracyclines penetrate into the lipid-rich layers of the dermis and inhibit the primary organism responsible for acne. In severe acne, the tetracyclines may be useful adjunctive therapy.
11. Tetracycline hydrochloride is indicated in the treatment of trachoma, although the infectious agent is not always eliminated, as judged by immunofluorescence.
12. Inclusion conjunctivitis may be treated with oral tetracyclines or with a combination or oral and topical agents.
13. Tetracycline is indicated for the treatment of uncomplicated urethral, endocervical or rectal infections in adults caused by *Chlamydia trachomatis*.

Contraindications

1. Hypersensitivity to tetracyclines or any other ingredient in each presentation
2. Systemic lupus erythematosus
3. Because of tooth-staining in the fetus or child, tetracycline should not be given to children or pregnant women unless considered essential
4. Tetracycline should be used with caution in patients with renal or hepatic dysfunction, or in conjunction with other potentially hepatotoxic drugs.

Tetracycline (hydrochloride)

T

Mode of use[16]

The average adult dose of tetracycline is 250 mg four times daily, and this may be increased to 250 mg six or eight times daily for a severe infection. The recommended dosage for children above eight years is 25–50 mg.kg^{-1} of body weight per day in equally divided doses. The general rule is to continue therapy for one or two days after the symptoms have subsided.

Oral preparations should be taken one hour before or two hours after meals, and particular care should be taken to avoid food and medicines containing calcium.

The recommended dosage for intramuscular injection of tetracycline in adults is 250 mg administered once every 24 hours or 300 mg given in divided doses at 8- to 12-hour intervals. The dosage for infants and children above the age of eight years is 15–25 mg.kg^{-1} of body weight up to a maximum of 250 mg per single daily injection. The intramuscular preparation should be stored in the dry form until it is required. It is prepared for use by the addition of 2 ml of sterile water or sodium chloride injection USP to the vial of tetracycline. It will then remain stable for 24 hours, after which it must be discarded. The injection should be made deep into a large muscle mass, care being taken to avoid deposition close to a major nerve or leakage into the superficial tissues.

The usual adult dosage for intravenous use is 250–500 mg every 12 hours, and should not exceed 500 mg every 6 hours. For children above eight years of age, the usual intravenous dosage is 12 mg.kg^{-1} of body weight per day divided in two doses. The material for injection is prepared by adding 5 ml of sterile water to vials containing 250 mg and 10 ml to vials of 500 mg of tetracycline. In this solution, the preparation is stable for 12 hours. Before administration it should be diluted to at least 100 ml (up to 1000 ml) of fluid and used immediately. Suitable diluents are:

- Ringer's injection USP
- Sodium chloride injection USP
- Dextrose injection USP (5% dextrose in Sterile Water for Injection USP)
- Dextrose and sodium chloride injection, USP (5% in sodium chloride injection, USP)
- Lactated Ringer's injection USP
- Protein hydrolysate injection, low sodium, USP 5%, 5% with dextrose 5%, 5% with invert sugar 10%

The initial reconstituted solutions are stable at room temperature for 12 hours without significant loss of potency. The final dilution for administration should be administered immediately.

The use of solutions containing calcium should be avoided as these tend to form precipitates (especially in neutral to alkaline solution) and, therefore, should not be used unless necessary. However, Ringer's injection USP and lactated Ringer's injection USP can be used with caution since the calcium ion content in these diluents does not normally precipitate tetracycline in an acid media.

Indications

Some specific indications along with some information on dosage is given in Table 1.[16]

Contraindications

1. Hypersensitivity

As with any drug, tetracycline hydrochloride is contraindicated in persons who have shown hypersensitivity to any of the tetracyclines.

2. Systemic lupus erythematosus

Tetracyclines are thought to exacerbate this condition, probably because of the acquired photosensitivity, although the incidence is low.[34]

3. Yellow discoloration of teeth and enamel hypoplasia in the fetus or child

It is well known that after the first trimester of pregnancy tetracyclines may cause staining of a child's deciduous teeth. The teeth being calcified at the time of administration to the mother are affected. The permanent teeth are not calcified until after birth and this is generally completed by the age of seven or eight. Therefore, tetracycline should not be used in pregnant women or children under the age of eight unless it is considered essential.[35]

4. Renal or hepatic dysfunction

Tetracycline inhibits protein synthesis and subsequently amino acids are metabolized to urea and other nitrogenous end-products. When renal function is adequate the nitrogen is successfully excreted but in renal dysfunction nitrogen is retained in the blood. Further, the urine is the main route of excretion of tetracycline from the blood, thereby extending the inhibition of protein synthesis. Thus normal dosages are potentially toxic in patients with poor renal function.[36]

Adverse reactions

Potentially life-threatening effects

Anaphylaxis may occur on rare occasions.

Some cases of liver toxicity have occurred following the intravenous administration of tetracycline in high doses. Most reports have described a severe, acute hepatic dysfunction occurring in the course of intravenous tetracycline therapy for pyelonephritis in pregnancy.[37–41] In one instance, liver toxicity occurred in a postpartum patient who had undergone hysterectomy because of severe haemorrhage following a caesarean section.

It is recommended, therefore, that when intravenous administration is necessary, the total dosage should not exceed 2 g per day for adults or 10 mg.kg^{-1} for children above eight years old, and that oral administration be substituted as early as possible. In pregnancy and in patients with renal disease, the dosage should be lowered regardless of the route of administration. Mild, reversible hepatic toxicity has been demonstrated in one pregnant patient in whom renal infection was treated with normal oral doses of tetracycline.[42] In all such patients, it may be advisable to make regular determinations of the serum concentrations of the antibiotic during therapy, and it is suggested that the dosage be adjusted[43] to keep the serum level below 16 μg.ml^{-1}.

Acute overdosage

Apart from vomiting and diarrhoea, no ill effects are likely to result from a single overdose of the drug.

Severe or irreversible adverse effects

The antianabolic action of the tetracyclines may cause an increase in blood urea. While this is not a problem in those with normal renal

Table 1

Infection	Dosage and duration	Remarks
Acne vulgaris[28,29]	250 mg four times daily for 1 week; 125–250 mg for several weeks or months	Duration of therapy is determined by individual progress
Acute staphylococcal infections[4]	1–2 g daily in divided doses for 10–14 days	
Acute streptococcal infections	1–2 g daily in divided doses for 10 days	Prolonged therapy is needed to avoid risk of rheumatic fever or glomerulonephritis
Amoebiasis[30,31]	1 g daily in four divided doses for 7–10 days	Given in association with amoebicidal agents
Brucellosis[32]	500 mg four times daily plus 1 g streptomycin twice daily for 1 week; then 500 mg four times daily plus 1 g streptomycin daily for 1 week; than 500 mg four times daily (no streptomycin) for 1 week	Prolonged therapy is necessary to avoid relapse
Subacute bacterial endocarditis[33]	1–2 g daily in divided doses for 6 weeks	Usually given in combination with a bactericidal agent
Syphilis	Total 30–40 g given in divided doses over 10–15 days	Serology and spinal fluid examination should follow the administration of tetracycline

function, in patients with significantly impaired function, higher serum levels of tetracyclines may lead to azotaemia, hyperphosphataemia and acidosis.[44]

Symptomatic adverse effects
Gastrointestinal adverse effects are the most frequently reported, especially nausea and diarrhoea, though they are rarely severe enough to require complete cessation of therapy.[25,45]

As with other antibiotics, overgrowth of resistant organisms may occur to cause glossitis, stomatitis or vaginitis.

Skin reactions are rare with tetracycline but have been reported.[9] Enamel hypoplasia has occurred.[47] Increased intracranial pressure with bulging fontanelles has been associated with tetracycline therapy. The fontanelles returned to normal tension within a few hours of the antibiotic being withdrawn and there were no after-effects.[48,49] The mechanism of bulging fontanelles is unknown and no relationship was observed between dose or length of therapy and onset of this reaction.

Photosensitivity, manifested by an exaggerated sunburn reaction, has been observed in some individuals taking tetracyclines.[46] Fair-skinned patients likely to be exposed to direct sunlight or ultraviolet light should be advised that this reaction can occur with tetracycline drugs and treatment should be discontinued at the first evidence of skin erythema.

Other effects
It has been reported that there can be a decreased plasma prothrombin activity when tetracycline is administered, probably due to reduced vitamin K synthesis by gut bacteria; it may, therefore, be necessary to adjust the dosage of coumarin anticoagulants.[50]

Interference with clinical pathology tests
The tetracyclines in general may cause the following interference with some clinical laboratory tests:[51]

In pregnant women they may cause some elevation of serum amylase.

In those cases in which liver toxicity has occurred following intravenous administration, there may be increases in the bilirubin levels and serum alkaline phosphatase.

Tetracyclines may cause an increased fluorescence (false positive) in the Hingerty method for measuring urinary catecholamines.

With pre-existing renal impairment, tetracyclines may cause an increase in blood urea due to their antianabolic effect.

High risk groups

Neonates
Because of the risk of tooth staining, tetracyclines should not be given to neonates, unless absolutely essential.

Breast milk. There is probably negligible absorption of tetracyclines by breast-fed infants, because of chelation by the calcium in milk; but there is a remote possibility of tooth staining.

Children
What has been said above about neonates applies also to older children.

Pregnant women
The tetracyclines should be avoided in pregnant women, because of the risk of tooth staining and effect on bone growth in the fetus.

The elderly
Tetracyclines can be used in the elderly unless they have renal or hepatic dysfunction.

Drug interactions

Potentially hazardous interactions
It has been reported that tetracyclines in combination with methoxyfluorane have resulted in nephrotoxicity.[52] Milk and milk products as well as antacids containing calcium, aluminium or magnesium impair the absorption of tetracyclines and result in decreased serum levels.[17] Jawetz has reported an inhibition of the antimicrobial activity of penicillin when used in combination with tetracycline.[53]

Potentially useful interactions
No interactions of this kind appear to have been reported.

Tetracycline (hydrochloride)

T

General review articles

Sweeney W M, Dornbush A C, Hardy S M 1962 Demethychlortetracycline and tetracycline compared: relative in vitro activity and comparative serum concentrations during 7 days of continuous therapy. American Journal of Medical Science 243: 296–308

Sylvester J C (ed) 1964 Antimicrobial agents and chemotherapy, American Society for Microbiology, Ann Arbor, pp 477–484

Kunin C M 1962 Comparative serum building, distribution and excretion of tetracycline and a new analogue methacycline. Proceedings of the Society of Experimental Biology and Medicine 110: 311–315

Achromycin — Tetracycline HCl 1975 Current concepts. Medical Advisory Dept, Lederle Laboratories, Pearl River, New York

Hlavka J J, Boothe J H 1985 The tetracyclines. In: Handbook of experimental pharmacology 78, Springer-Verlag, Heidelberg

Conha B A, Comer J B 1982 The tetracyclines. Medical Clinics of North America 66: 294–302

Mitcher L A 1978 The chemistry of the tetracycline antibiotics. Medicinal Research Service 9: 1–45

Ory E M 1980 The tetracyclines. In: Antimicrobial therapy, 3rd edn. W B Saunders, Philadelphia, ch 9, pp 117–126

References

1. Hlavka J J, Boothe J H 1985 The tetracyclines. Handbook of experimental pharmacology 78. Springer-Verlag, Heidelberg, p 331
2. Hogenauer G, Turnowsky F 1972 The effects of streptomycin and tetracycline on codon–anticodon interactions. FEBS Letters 26: 185–188
3. Haggerty R J, Ziai M 1960 Acute bacterial meningitis in children. Pediatrics 25: 742–747
4. Dowling H F 1957 Mixtures of antibiotics. Journal of the American Medical Association 164: 44–48
5. Dowling H F 1958 When can combinations of antibiotics be used? Postgraduate Medicine 23: 594–597
6. Dowling H F 1963 How to combine antibiotics. Medical World News 4: 108
7. Hanson D J 1961 Local toxic effects of broad-spectrum antibiotics following injection. Antibiotics and Chemotherapy 11: 390–404
8. Hanson D J 1963 Intramuscular injuries and complications. General Practitioner 27: 109–115
9. Cronk G A, Naumann D E 1956–1957 The use of tetracycline in the treatment of nonbacterial pneumonias, infectious mononucleosis and acne. In: Welch H, Marti-Ibanez F (eds) Antibiotics annual. Medical Encyclopedia Inc, New York, pp 328–335
10. English A R, P'an S Y, McBride T J, Gardocki J F, Van Halsema G, Wright W A 1953–1954 Tetracycline — microbiologic, pharmacologic and clinical evaluation. In: Welch H, Marti-Ibane F (eds) Antibiotics annual. Medical Encyclopedia Inc, New York, pp 70–80
11. Hurley L S, Tuchmann-Dupleiss H 1963 Influence of tetracycline in the prenatal and postnatal development. Compte Rendus Academy of Science 257: 302–304
12. Dean B T, Tribble L F 1962 Effect of feeding therapeutic levels of antibiotic at breeding on reproductive performance of swine. Journal of Animal Science 21: 207–209
13. Bevelander G, Nakahara H, Rolle G K 1960 The effect of tetracycline on the development of the skeletal system of the chick embryo. Developmental Biology 2: 298–312
14. Faraf B A, Ali F M 1981 Development and application of a radioimmunoassay for tetracycline. Journal of Pharmacology and Experimental Therapeutics 217: 10–14
15. Hermansson J 1982 Rapid determination of tetracycline in human plasma. Journal of Chromatography 232: 385–393
16. Achromycin — tetracycline hydrochloride 1975 Current Concepts, Medical Advisory Department, Lederle Laboratories, Pearl River, New York
17. Neuvonen P J 1976 Interaction with the absorption of tetracyclines. Drugs 11: 45
18. Bergquist L M, Janzen C L, Simms N M, Searcy R L 1963 Formation of lipoprotein–tetracycline complexes in human serum. Antimicrobial Agents and Chemotherapy 3: 477–484
19. Farhat S M, Schelhart D L, Musselman M M 1958 Clinical toxicity of antibiotics correlated with animal studies. Archives of Surgery 76: 762–765
20. Farhat S M, Schelhart D L, Musselman M M 1958 Clinical observations on toxicity of tetracyclines in man with experimental studies in animals. In: Welsh H, Marti-Ibanez F (eds) Antibiotics annual 1957–1958. Medical Encyclopedia Inc, New York, pp 426–429
21. Shils M E 1962 Some metabolic aspects of tetracyclines. Clinical Pharmacology and Therapeutics 3: 321–338
22. Shils M E 1963 Renal disease and the metabolic effects of tetracycline. Annals of Internal Medicine 58: 389
23. Kunin C M, Rees S B, Merrill J P, Finland M 1959 Persistence of antibiotics in blood of patients with acute renal failure. Tetracycline and chlortetracycline. Journal of Clinical Investigation 38: 1487–1497
24. Steigbigel N H, Reed L W, Finland M 1968 Absorption and excretion of five tetracycline analogues in normal young men. American Journal of Medical Science 255: 296
25. Dowling H F 1955 Tetracycline. In: Antibiotic monographs no 3. Medical Encyclopedia Inc, New York
26. Kelly R G, Buyske D A 1960 Metabolism of tetracycline in the rat and the dog. Journal of Pharmacology and Experimental Therapeutics 130: 144–149

27. Remmers F G, Doerschuk 1963 Some observations on the kinetics of the C-4 epimerization of tetracycline. Journal of Pharmaceutical Sciences 52: 752–756
28. Schmitt C L 1963 Topical agents used in treatment of acne. Clinical Medicine 70: 1473–1476
29. Whyte H J 1964 Management of acne vulgaris in general practice. Postgraduate Medicine 35: 538–542
30. Kean B H 1960 Modern treatment of common parasitic diseases. Postgraduate Medicine 28: 35–41
31. Powell S J, Wilmot A J, Elsdon-Dew R 1960 Potentiating effect of quinolines on the action of tetracycline in amoebic dysentery. Lancet 1: 76–77
32. Bothwell P W 1963 Brucellosis. Practitioner 191: 577–587
33. Hewitt W L, Johnson B L 1963 Treatment of bacterial endocarditis. Disease of the Chest 43: 631–638
34. Doniz C A 1969 Tetracycline provocation in lupus erythematosus. Annals of Internal Medicine 50: 1217–1225
35. Cohlan S Q 1977 Tetracycline staining of teeth. Teratology 15: 127–131
36. Feingold D S 1963 Antimicrobial chemotherapeutic agents: The nature of their action and selective toxicity. New England Journal of Medicine 269: 957–964
37. Norman T D, Schultz J C, Hoke R D 1964 Fatal liver disease following the administration of tetracycline. Southern Medical Journal 57: 1038–1042
38. Kunelis C T, Peter J L, Edmondson H A 1965 Fatty liver of pregnancy and its relationship to tetracycline therapy. American Journal of Medicine 38: 359–377
39. Pulliam R, O'Leary J A 1964 Tetracycline-induced azotemia. Obstetrics and Gynecology 24: 509–511
40. Schultz J C, Adamson J S, Workman W W, Norman T D 1963 Fatal liver disease after intravenous administration of tetracycline in high dosage. New England Journal of Medicine 269: 999
41. Wruble L T 1965 Hepatotoxicity produced by tetracycline overdosage. Journal of the American Medical Association 192 (suppl 1): 92–94
42. Whalley R J, Adams R H, Combes B 1964 Tetracycline toxicity in pregnancy. Journal of the American Medical Association 189: 357–362
43. Dowling H F, Lepper M H 1964 Hepatic reactions to tetracycline. Journal of the American Medical Association 188: 307–309
44. Myelers Side Effects of Drugs 1980 ed 9 p 432–433 and 435–451. Published by Excerpta Medica
45. Pflug G R 1963 Toxicities associated with tetracycline therapy. American Journal of Pharmacy 135: 438–449
46. Post L F, Dougherty J 1962 Fixed drug eruption caused by tetracycline hydrochloride. Archives of Dermatology 86: 678–679
47. Bevelander G, Rolle G K, Cohlan S Q 1961 The effect of the administration of tetracycline on the development of teeth. Journal of Dental Research 40: 1020–1022
48. Benasayag L, Fiorini E 1962 Fontanelle hypertension induced by tetracycline. Revista del Hospital de Ninos 4: 230–231
49. Fields J P 1961 Bulging fontanelle; a complication of tetracycline therapy in infants. Journal of Pediatrics 58: 74–76
50. Searcy R L, Simms N M, Foreman J A, Bergquist L A 1964 Evaluation of the blood clotting mechanism in tetracycline treated patients. Antimicrobial Agents and Chemotherapy pp 179–183
51. Hansten P D 1971 Drug interactions. Lea and Febiger, Philadelphia
52. Kuzneu E Y 1970 Methoxyfluorane, tetracycline and renal failure. Journal of the American Medical Association 221: 62–64
53. Jawetz E 1968 The use of combinations of antimicrobial drugs. Annual Review of Pharmacology 8: 15

Theophylline

Theophylline is a naturally occurring alkaloid found in the leaves of *Camellia sinensis* (C. thea) which are widely used for making tea. Its main medical use is as a bronchodilator. Theophylline is an interesting example of a drug for which great efforts have been made to optimise its therapeutic efficacy based on a knowledge of pharmacokinetics and measurement of plasma concentrations (particularly in the United States).

Chemistry

Theophylline (Accurbron, Afonilum, Armophylline, Bronchonetard, Bronkodyl, Elixicon, LaBLO, Nuelin-SR, Phyppan, Rona-phyllin, Sto-Phyllin, Sustaine, Theocap, Theoclear, Theograd, Theosol, Theostat, Theovent, Uniphyllin)
$C_7H_8N_4O_2$
3,7-Dihydro-1,3-dimethylpurine-2,6(1H)-dione)

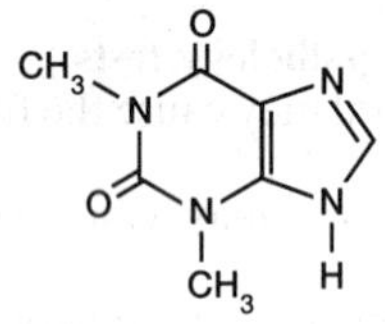

Molecular weight	180.2
pKa	8.8
Solubility	
in alcohol	1 in 80
in water	slightly soluble
Octanol/water partition coefficient	—

A white odourless, crystalline powder with a bitter taste. It is extracted from natural sources or prepared by chemical synthesis. Most pharmacopoeias allow either the anhydrous or monohydrate forms.

Theophylline forms organic complexes with compounds such as sodium or calcium salicylate and piperazine aminobenzoate. Such complexes are held together in solution by weak forces but are readily dissociable and are in equilibrium with free theophylline. Theophylline is also available as a number of salts or compounds which are completely dissociated in solution. Common theophylline salts are with choline, ethylenediamine, ethanolamine, lysine, sodium acetate, and sodium glycinate. Among the most widely used of these are choline theophyllinate and aminophylline.

Choline theophyllinate (Oxtriphylline, theophylline cholinate, Choledyl)
$C_{12}H_{21}N_5O_3$

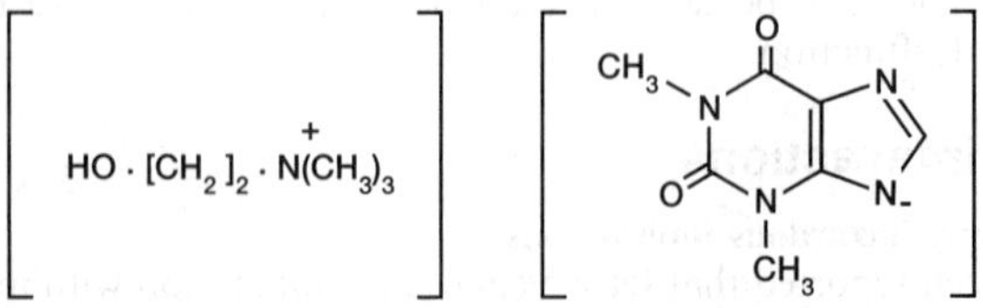

Molecular weight (theophylline)	283.3 (180.2)
pKa (acidic)	—
Solubility	
in alcohol	1 in 10
in water	1 in 1
Octanol/water partition coefficient	—

A 1:1 choline salt with theophylline containing 64% anhydrous theophylline.

Aminophylline (Phyllocontin and various generic formulations)
$(C_7H_8N_4O_2)_2,C_2H_4(NH_2)_2$

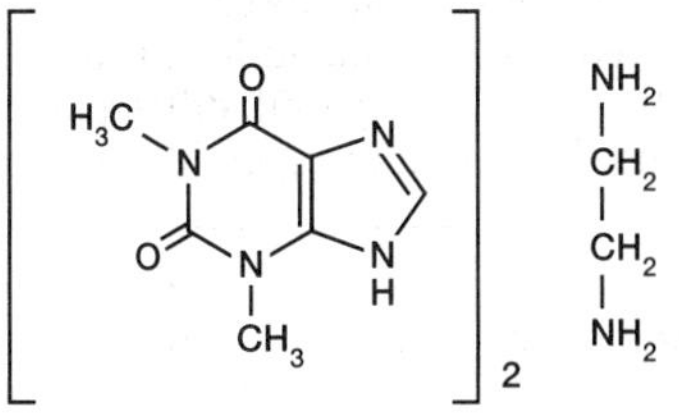

Molecular weight	
anhydrous	420.4
dihydrate	456.5
pKa	5.0
Solubility	
in alcohol	insoluble
in water	1 in 5
Octanol/water partition coefficient	
(theophylline)	0.955

A 2:1 compound with 1,2-ethylenediamine.

A number of N-7 and/or C-8 substituted derivatives of theophylline are available including bamifylline (8-benzyl-7-(2-(N-ethyl-N-2-hydroxyethylamino)ethyl)-theophylline), acepifylline piperazine (piperazine bis- theophylline-7-ylacetic acid), etophylline (7-(2-hydroxyethyl)-theophylline), diprophylline (7-(dihydroxy-propyl)-theophylline) and proxyphylline (7-(2-hydroxyproyl)-theophylline). These are often claimed to be theophylline derivatives containing an amount of theophylline equal to the molecular weight ratio between theophylline and the derivative. However, all are chemically stable N-7 substituted analogues of theophylline which are not converted to theophylline in vitro or in vivo. Most are far less potent than theophylline and relatively little is known about their pharmacology.[1] At least one product, acepifylline has negligible (<5%) bioavailability and any that is absorbed is eliminated with a half life of less than one hour.[2]

Pharmacology

A number of mechanisms have been proposed to account for the range of pharmacological effects of the methylxanthines. These include inhibition of cyclic nucleotide phosphodiesterase and alterations in intracellular translocation of calcium ions. However, the concentrations required for these actions are above the range of those producing pharmacological effects in vivo. Only 10–12% inhibition of the breakdown of the cyclic nucleotides AMP and GMP occurs at free theophylline concentrations of 20 to 50 μM which are found in the therapeutic range. Maximum phosphodiesterase inhibition producing measurable cyclic AMP increases require millimolar concentrations of the drug. Theophylline is a competitive antagonist of adenosine (A_1 and A_2 receptors) producing marked inhibition at concentrations ranging from 20 to 100 μM. Theophylline causes release of endogenous catecholamines at therapeutic concentrations. However, analogues such as 3-propylxanthine (enprofylline) are not adenosine antagonists but are potent bronchodilators. The mechanism of bronchodilation thus remains unclear. Recently, it has been suggested that an increase in the force of diaphragmatic contraction caused by methylxanthines contributes to their therapeutic effect in obstructive lung disease.

Toxicology

Most toxicological studies of the methylxanthines have been carried out with caffeine. Teratogenesis has been reported in mice at doses 30 times the usual human adult dose but this has not been confirmed by human epidemiological studies.[3] An association between caffeine ingestion and pancreatic cancer has been reported and a similar excess risk of pancreatic cancer was reported in US male veteran asthmatics treated with various bronchodilators including theophylline.[4] The significance of these studies is not yet clear. Initial reports of an association between caffeine consumption and increased risk of myocardial infarction were not confirmed by further studies.[4]

Theophylline

Clinical pharmacology

Theophylline given acutely in doses of 250–500 mg to normal subjects causes central nervous system stimulation, an increase in blood pressure, heart rate and force of contraction, an increase in gastric acid output, smooth muscle relaxation including bronchodilation, a transient diuresis, an increase in plasma free fatty acid concentrations and catecholamine release from the adrenal medulla.[1] Theophylline is primarily used as a bronchial smooth muscle relaxant in the treatment of asthma. Theophylline produces bronchodilation in a concentration-dependent manner.[5,6] In addition, theophylline inhibits the bronchoconstriction produced by exercise,[7] allergen,[8] histamine,[9] and adenosine[10] challenges. Continuous theophylline therapy significantly decreases the symptoms in chronic asthma,[11] reduces the requirement for 'as required' bronchodilators,[11] and reduces the steroid dosage requirement in steroid-dependent asthmatics.[12] Other actions that may be beneficial in the therapy of asthma and other pulmonary diseases include pulmonary vasodilation, stimulation of mucociliary clearance, and inhibition of mast cell mediator release.[13] Aubier and coworkers[14] found that theophylline improves diaphragmatic contractility before and after induction of diaphragmatic fatigue in normals and later confirmed that theophylline prevented diaphragmatic fatigue in patients with severe chronic obstructive pulmonary disease (COPD). Theophylline also improves cardiac output and right ventricular ejection fraction in patients with COPD.[15] Theophylline increases coronary blood flow and peripheral blood flow through vasodilation but produces cerebrovascular constriction and decreases cerebral blood flow.[16] Theophylline and other methylxanthines stimulate the medullary respiratory centre to increase minute ventilation in man.[16] This is primarily mediated through increasing the hypoxic ventilatory drive.[17] Theophylline significantly decreases or prevents apnoeic spells in premature infants.[18] It also reverses the respiratory depression produced by opioids and reduces Cheyne-Stokes respirations.[16]

Theophylline enhances the urinary excretion of water and electrolytes in a pattern similar to thiazide diuretics.[16] Enprofylline, an analogue which is not an adenosine antagonist retains bronchodilator activity and some cardiac effects, but seems to be devoid of the central nervous system stimulant, diuretic and metabolic effects of theophylline.[19]

Tolerance develops rapidly to the CNS stimulant, diuretic, metabolic and cardiovascular effects of theophylline and caffeine but not to the smooth muscle relaxant, and thus bronchodilator, effect.[20,21]

Pharmacokinetics

There are numerous analytical methods for quantitating theophylline including spectrophotometry, gas-liquid chromatography, high-performance liquid chromatography (HPLC), radioimmunoassay, and enzyme immunoassay.[22] For pharmacokinetic research, HPLC is considered the standard with a limit of sensitivity of $0.5\ mg.l^{-1}$. HPLC methods which separate theophylline from paraxanthine[23] are preferred to those that do not. Enzyme immunoassay techniques have gained wide popularity for routine clinical monitoring due to their ease of operation and rapid turn around time. The enzyme immunoassay techniques compare favourably to HPLC in sensitivity and specificity at theophylline concentrations found during routine clinical monitoring.[22] Commercial immunoassay methods include the Syva EMIT method (enzyme-multiplied immunoassay technique) and the Abbott TDX systems (fluorescence polarization immunoassay).

Theophylline and choline theophyllinate are well absorbed from the gastrointestinal tract. Peak levels occur 1–2 hours following administration of oral liquid preparation. The time to peak increases with increased dose. Food decreases the rate but not the completeness of absorption. Theophylline does not undergo first-pass hepatic metabolism. The dissolution rate appears to be the rate limiting step for absorption. The systemic bioavailability of good formulations is 90–100%.

Because of the relatively short plasma half life of theophylline many sustained release formulations have been developed. Most currently marketed sustained release formulations have bioavailabili-

Theophylline

ties in the range 80–100%. Food reduces the rate but not extent of absorption from most sustained release preparations available. Absorption of one formulation (Nuelin-SR, Riker) is more rapid when taken with antacid due to pH dependent dissolution of this product.[24] Nearly all sustained release theophylline products show a lower absorption rate during the night than during the day. In children, this results in evening predose (trough) concentrations that are lower than morning trough concentrations. The extent of this effect ranges from about 5% difference to nearly 300% but on average is around 20%.[25] The longer theophylline half life in adults makes the diurnal variation in absorption rate less important.

Medical and pharmaceutical experience demonstrate that different brands of sustained and slow release xanthines are not bioequivalent. Once patients are stabilized on one slow release preparation they should not be changed to another branded or generic slow or sustained release xanthine without retitration of dosage with careful monitoring of plasma theophylline levels to achieve optimum therapeutic levels with minimum toxicity.

Theophylline (from aminophylline) is rapidly distributed after intravenous administration. Following intravenous administration, the plasma theophylline concentration-over-time curve fits a 2-compartment open pharmacokinetic model. The early α-distribution phase is rapid and completed within 30 to 45 min. Theophylline readily distributes into all body compartments; it crosses the placenta and into breast milk. Theophylline is approximately 60% (50–70) bound to plasma proteins in normal volunteers and otherwise normal asthmatic and COPD patients. The volume of distribution is 0.3–0.7 $l.kg^{-1}$ with a mean value of 0.5 $l.kg^{-1}$.

The plasma protein binding is decreased in premature newborns (36%), patients with hepatic cirrhosis (32%), acidemia, and the elderly. This results in a corresponding increase in the volume of distribution for theophylline in these patients.[26,27] The volume of distribution is decreased (0.3 $l.kg^{-1}$) in obese patients.[28] The cerebral spinal fluid concentrations are approximately 90% of serum concentrations in premature neonates. Salivary concentrations are approximately 60% of the corresponding plasma concentration in children and adults[29] and 93% in premature newborns.[30] Salivary concentrations correlate with but are not identical to free concentrations of theophylline in the plasma. Due to the inter- and intra-patient variability in the saliva/plasma concentration ratio, salivary concentrations should not be used for monitoring theophylline therapy.[30]

In children and adults, theophylline is primarily eliminated by hepatic biotransformation with approximately 10% eliminated unchanged by the kidney.[31,32] In premature infants the urinary excretion of unchanged theophylline ranges from 90% to 50% depending on the age of the infant and then decreases as the patient grows older.[31,33] The metabolic pathways are capacity-limited. However, following single doses in man the renal excretion is initially increased due to diuresis giving an apparent linear elimination curve.[32] Nonlinear pharmacokinetics have been reported in children[33] and adults[34] with steady-state theophylline concentrations within the usual therapeutic range. Increases in plasma concentration can be up to twice that expected from the dose ratio.[35] Dose-dependent elimination has not been found consistently in all studies due to the considerable interindividual variability in metabolic capacity.[36]

Theophylline elimination kinetics have been extensively studied. The mean elimination half-life and ranges have been reported for the following age groups: premature neonates 30 hours, (12–57) 1–6 months 12 hours (5.7–29), 6 months–1 year 5.3 hours (2.2–10), 1–4 years 3.4 hours (1.9–5.5), 6–17 years 3.7 hours (1.4–7.9) and healthy adults 8.2 hours (3.6–12.8).[37,38] There is a wide interindividual variability in plasma theophylline clearance at all ages[39] necessitating the routine monitoring of plasma theophylline concentrations to achieve optimal benefit and prevent toxicity. Upton et al (1982)[40] demonstrated that individuals may commonly show fluctuations as large as 30% in theophylline clearance over a few weeks time.

A number of factors are known to affect the hepatic metabolism and thus the clearance of theophylline. A decreased theophylline clearance is associated with liver cirrhosis but not with acute hepatitis or cholestasis.[41] Severe congestive heart failure and cor pulmonale may produce a 40–70% reduction in theophylline clearance.[42] Viral infections particularly influenza B virus have been associated with increased steady-state theophylline plasma levels with toxicity.[43] Acute hypoxia may decrease theophylline clearance.[42] Elderly patients who are not otherwise compromised do not have an altered metabolic clearance of theophylline.[44] Renal failure has no discernible effect on theophylline elimination. Obesity does not alter theo phylline clearance.[29] Theophylline clearance is increased in cigarette and marijuana smokers and by rifampicin, sulphinpyrazone, phenobarbitone at full anticonvulsant doses, carbamazepine and phenytoin. Clearance is reduced by cimetidine, propranolol, erythromycin, troleandomycin disulfiram, verapamil, diltiazem, enoxacin, ciprofloxacin, pefloxacin, norfloxacin and pipemidic acid.

Oral absorption	90-100%
Presystemic metabolism	nil
Plasma half life	
range	1.4–12.8 h
mean: adult	8.2 h
children	3.7 h
Volume of distribution	0.5 $l.kg^{-1}$
Plasma protein binding	60%

Concentration–effect relationship

Theophylline is often thought of as a drug which has a particularly well defined therapeutic range with concentrations from 5 to 20 $mg.l^{-1}$ giving an optimum compromise between efficacy and toxicity. Although there is some truth in this belief the reality is more complex.

Bronchodilation

The linear increase in degree of human bronchial smooth muscle relaxation associated with logarithmic increases in theophylline concentration seen in vitro has been confirmed in vivo utilizing forced expiratory pulmonary function tests that measure resistance to airflow.[5,6] Mitenko and Ogilvie (1973) first reported the relationship in six asthmatic adults recovering from acute attacks of asthma. Their patients received intravenous aminophylline infusions in incremental dosages to achieve steady state concentrations of 5 $mg.l^{-1}$, 10 $mg.l^{-1}$, 20 $mg.l^{-1}$. The log plasma concentration-response curve has since been confirmed in asthmatics[6] and patients with chronic obstructive airway diseases.[45] In each of these studies some interpatient variability in the concentration-response curves was apparent. In contrast, studies in outpatient asthmatic children have demonstrated significant to complete improvement in pulmonary function tests with lower plasma theophylline concentrations (2-10 $mg.l^{-1}$).[45,46] More recently no significant bronchodilation within the first 24 hours was found in a group of patients hospitalized for acute obstruction[47], receiving intravenous aminophylline with mean plasma theophylline concentrations of 10 $mg.l^{-1}$. Aminophylline infusions producing mean plasma concentrations of 20 $mg.l^{-1}$ were required for a bronchodilator effect. These data indicate an interpatient variability and quite possibly an intra-patient variability in the bronchodilator concentration–response curves and a need for caution in interpreting plasma concentration data.

Prophylaxis of asthma symptoms

In a randomized double-blind crossover trial in 12 moderately severe asthmatic children, Weinberger and Bronsky (1974)[11] demonstrated that individualized oral theophylline regimens administered every 6 hours that produced mean peak plasma theophylline concentrations of 13 $mg.l^{-1}$ were significantly better than placebo in suppressing signs and symptoms of chronic asthma. Theophylline dosages that produced peak plasma concentrations of 6.5 $mg.l^{-1}$ were not significantly better than placebo. Each trial period was 1 week in duration. Similar results were reported with much lower peak serum theophylline concentrations (3–5 $mg.l^{-1}$) in a double-blind crossover trial utilizing a sustained-release theophylline preparation every 12 hours.[46] In a study of exercise-induced bronchospasm a significant number of patients demonstrated inhibition with plasma theophylline concentrations between 5 and 10 $mg.l^{-1}$. In addition, there were a few cases[7] who responded to concentrations less than 5 $mg.l^{-1}$ but not to concentrations greater than 15 $mg.l^{-1}$. In a trial with 8 asthmatic children, no correlation was found between plasma theophylline concentration and degree of inhibition of histamine- and methacholine-induced bronchospasm.[9]

The various sustained-release preparations exhibit differing disso-

Theophylline

lution rates that can result in significantly different plasma theophylline concentration fluctuations over the dosing interval particularly in young children with rapid clearance rates.[48,49] As yet, these pharmacokinetic differences have not been translated into significant therapeutic differences between products.[50]

The upper limit of the therapeutic range for theophylline has been defined by its toxicities. To evaluate the prevalence of toxicity at various plasma theophylline concentrations, data from 13 studies were pooled for a total population of 329 patients.[51] The prevalence of toxicity increased from 15% in patients with plasma theophylline concentrations from 15 to 19 $mg.l^{-1}$ to 62% from 20 to 29 $mg.l^{-1}$ and 85% from 30 to 39 $mg.l^{-1}$. Theophylline's narrow therapeutic index and wide interpatient variability in clearance make theophylline plasma concentration monitoring highly desirable, some would say mandatory, in order to achieve optimum results in patients treated with theophylline. However, arbitrary adjustments of the dosage to fit the patient into the 'usual' therapeutic range should be avoided. The plasma concentration which provides control of asthma symptoms with minimal or no toxicity is optimal for that patient.

Prevention of apnoea of prematurity

The therapeutic range of theophylline plasma concentrations for neonatal apnoea are still not well defined. Shannon et al (1975)[52] observed that plasma theophylline concentrations greater than 6 $mg.l^{-1}$ controlled apnoeic spells and that cardiovascular toxicity was associated with concentrations greater than 13 $mg.l^{-1}$. However, control of apnoea and bradycardia in low birth weight infants has been reported[53] with plasma theophylline concentrations as low as 2 to 4 $mg.l^{-1}$. In another study,[54] plasma theophylline concentrations between 5 and 12 $mg.l^{-1}$ were required to achieve a response with recurrence of apnoea in 15 patients when the plasma theophylline concentration fell below 5 $mg.l^{-1}$. Currently the generally accepted therapeutic range is 5 to 15 $mg.l^{-1}$. Any given plasma theophylline concentration represents more pharmacologically active drug in the neonate compared to children and adults due to the decreased serum protein binding. Another factor is methylation of theophylline to caffeine which occurs in neonates but not children or adults. Caffeine accumulates and exerts similar pharmacological effects to theophylline.

Adverse effects of theophylline, including nausea and vomiting, headache, insomnia and tachycardia, become increasingly frequent at plasma theophylline concentrations above 20 $mg.l^{-1}$. Severe toxicity (cardiac arrhythmias, convulsions)[55] are generally, but not always, associated with plasma concentrations above 35 to 40 $mg.l^{-1}$. In neonates, toxicity as defined by a heart rate greater than 180 beats per minute[56] often occurs at concentrations above 12 $mg.l^{-1}$.

Metabolism

Theophylline is extensively metabolized in the liver, with only about 10% being excreted unchanged in the urine.

There are three primary metabolic pathways:[57] 3-demethylation forming 1-methylxanthine, 1-demethylation forming 3-methylxanthine and 8-oxidation forming 1,3-dimethyluric acid (Fig. 1).

These reactions are carried out by the cytochrome P450 system in the liver. There is evidence for the involvement of at least two isoforms of cytochrome P450, one carrying out the 1-and 3-demethylations and the other the 8-oxidation.[35,58,59] 1-Methylxanthine undergoes rapid 8-oxidation by xanthine oxidase and is excreted as 1-methyluric acid. During concurrent allopurinol treatment, this secondary pathway is extensively inhibited, and 1-methylxanthine is excreted instead of 1-methyluric acid.[60] 3-Methylxanthine and 1,3-dimethyluric acid are excreted unchanged in the urine.

The active metabolite 3-methylxanthine is formed by N-demethylation. This metabolite is $\frac{1}{3}$ to $\frac{1}{5}$ as potent as theophylline. However, its excretion in the urine is more rapid than its hepatic formation so that it is unlikely to contribute to the pharmacological effect.[13] All three metabolic pathways are capacity limited.[32] Accumulation of the metabolites occurs in patients with renal dysfunction but dosage adjustments are not required.

In the premature infant, theophylline is primarily excreted unchanged in the urine and approximately 10% is methylated in the 7-position to produce caffeine which is also active in preventing neonatal apnoea.[33] Although this represents only a minor part of the theophylline dose, caffeine is very slowly eliminated, accumulates to plasma concentrations about one third those of theophylline, and contributes to the pharmacological effects. As such, a number of investigators recommend monitoring total methylxanthine plasma concentrations when using theophylline for neonatal apnoea. Theophylline clearance increases with postconceptional age primarily due to the development of the 8-hydroxylation pathway.[33] The N-demethylation pathway takes much longer to develop.

Pharmaceutics

Theophylline is available for oral, intravenous and rectal administration.

a. Intravenous formulations

The most common intravenous formulation is theophylline with ethylenediamine (aminophylline) which is 78% to 85% anhydrous theophylline and has a pH of 8.8 to 10.0. Common formulations contain 250 mg aminophylline (195 to 212 mg theophylline) per 10 ml). A preparation containing anhydrous theophylline (20 $mg.ml^{-1}$) is also available.

b. Oral formulations

A large number of oral formulations are available under a myriad of proprietary names.

Liquid formulations contain choline theophyllinate, aminophylline and anhydrous theophylline. Choline theophyllinate, which is 63.6% theophylline, is available as syrups (e.g. Choledyl syrup) or as tablets containing 100 mg and 200 mg choline theophyllinate (64 mg and 127 mg anhydrous theophylline). There are coated pink, biconvex with a debossed 'Choledyl 100' or coated yellow, biconvex with a debossed 'Choledyl 200' on one side. The oral liquid is an amber coloured, chocolate flavoured clear syrup. Each 5 ml contains 62.5 mg choline theophyllinate (40 mg anhydrous theophylline).

Aminophylline, which is 78% to 85% theophylline, is available as an oral liquid. Anhydrous theophylline is marketed as elixirs or as alcohol free syrups or suspensions. Liquid preparations containing theophylline sodium glycinate are also available.

Fig. 1 Metabolism of theophylline

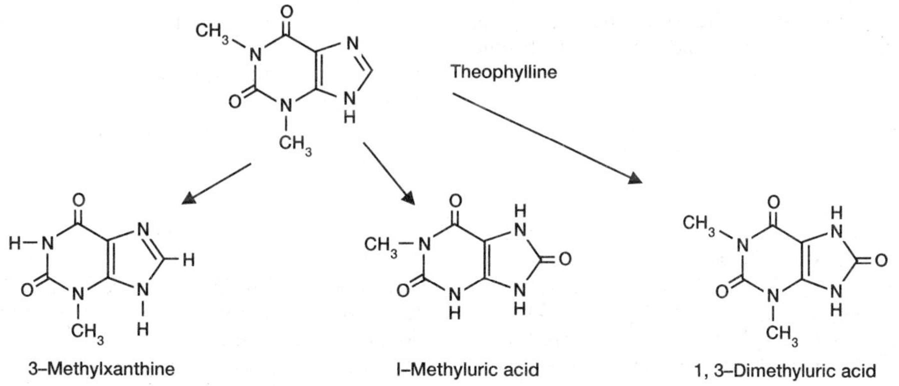

A large number of tablet, capsule and sprinkle formulations contain anhydrous theophylline (or theophylline monohydrate), aminophilline or choline theophyllinate. These are formulated to be rapidly absorbed (e.g. micronised crystals) or to give a sustained release of theophylline. Sustained release products are available as tablets, capsules containing coated beads, and as coated beads designed to be sprinkled onto food ('sprinkle' formulations). Because of the great variety of products, and the changes in proprietary names from country to country for the same product, local reference sources should be consulted regarding availability and description of theophylline formulations. It is important not to assume that the different oral formulations are bioequivalent. Clinicians should therefore familiarize themselves with the release profiles of one or two different sustained release formulations.

Some formulations are available for rectal administration either as enemas, solutions or suppositories. However, rectal absorption is unpredictable and these formulations are no longer used in many countries.

Common dosage sizes for rapidly absorbed tablets are 50, 100, 125, 200, 250 mg. Sustained release tablets contain between 60 and 500 mg theophylline but common dosage sizes are 100, 200, 300 mg and 400 mg. Some, but not all sustained release products are scored and can be halved without loss of sustained release characteristics (refer to product literature). Liquid formulations usually contain 30 to 50 mg theophylline per 5 ml. Some formulations give dosage sizes in terms of amount of theophylline salt and care must be taken to convert this to amount of anhydrous theophylline. All theophylline preparations should be stored in air tight containers and protected from light. Theophylline preparations are stable with a reasonable shelf life.

Therapeutic use

Indications

1. The control of acute asthma and acute exacerbation of chronic obstructive lung disease
2. The management of chronic asthma
3. The management of chronic obstructive lung disease
4. The control of apnoea of prematurity
5. Other proposed uses include (i) Prophylaxis of sudden infant death syndrome, (ii) Treatment of Cheyne-Stokes respiration.

Contraindications

1. Hypersensitivity to theophylline or other methylxanthines.

Mode of use

The clinical use of theophylline falls into two general categories, bronchodilation and respiratory stimulation. The use of theophylline as an antispasmodic for biliary colic or as a diuretic for congestive heart failure and pulmonary oedema has been discarded for more effective therapies.

a. Control of acute bronchospasm

Theophylline is a moderately potent bronchodilator in all disease states associated with acute bronchospasm. In suboptimal dosages, theophylline and β^2-agonists will produce additive bronchodilation. β^2-agonists will produce additional bronchodilation added to theophylline at maximum plasma theophylline concentrations. However, theophylline does not produce additional bronchodilation to maximally effective doses of β^2-agonists.[61] When used to treat acute airways obstruction (acute asthma, acute exacerbation of chronic obstructive lung disease) theophylline is administered intravenously as a loading dose followed by a continuous infusion.

i. Loading dose. The volume of distribution (V_D) of theophylline averages 0.5 $l.kg^{-1}$ so that the loading dose to achieve a plasma concentration of 12 $mg.l^{-1}$ is 6 $mg.kg^{-1}$ (loading dose = desired concentration × V_D). This should be administered as a loading infusion over 30 min to avoid toxicity (cardiac arrhythmias) due to initial high plasma concentrations before distribution occurs. As the actual range of V_D is about 0.3 to 0.7 $l.kg^{-1}$, this loading dose will give a range of concentrations from about 9 to 20 $mg.l^{-1}$. The V_D does not alter systematically with age, disease states or drug interactions. Where patients have had theophylline containing products in the previous 12 to 24 hours, or where there is a doubt, it is best not to administer a loading dose without determining the initial theophylline plasma concentration. If this is low, a desired increment in theophylline concentration can be achieved using a loading dose calculated by assuming that each $mg.kg^{-1}$ of theophylline will on average increase the plasma theophylline concentration by 2 $mg.l^{-1}$.

ii. Continuous infusion (maintenance dose). The maintenance dose rate is calculated from:
maintenance dose rate = desired plasma concentration × clearance.
The following initial maintenance infusion rates are based on clearance values found in various patient groups.[1]
young children (1–9 years) 0.8 $mg.kg^{-1}.h^{-1}$
older children (9–12 years) 0.7 $mg.kg^{-1}.h^{-1}$
adolescent smokers (12–16 years) 0.7 $mg.kg^{-1}.h^{-1}$
adolescent non-smokers (12–16 years) 0.5 $mg.kg^{-1}.h^{-1}$
adult smokers (16–50 years) 0.7 $mg.kg^{-1}.h^{-1}$
adult non-smokers (16–50 years) 0.4 $mg.kg^{-1}.h^{-1}$.
Patients above 16 years with liver dysfunction, cor pulmonale or cardiac failure (or combinations of these) 0.2 $mg.kg^{-1}.h^{-1}$.
Initial dose rates should not exceed 900 mg daily except in the last group where the maximum should be 400 mg daily.

Infants 6–52 weeks of age show a gradual increase in theophylline clearance with age due to slow maturation of the enzymes involved in theophylline metabolism. Initial infusion rates in this age group can be calculated[62] from:
initial dose rate = (0.008 × age in weeks) + 0.2 $l.mg^{-1}.kg^{-1}.h^{-1}$.

During intravenous theophylline administration, plasma concentration measurements should be made before the loading dose (for patients taking theophylline in the last 24 hours), after the loading dose, 12–24 hours after starting the maintenance infusion and then daily. For patients with short half lives (children, adult smokers) steady state will be approached in 16–36 hours but accumulation may continue for up to a week in patients with hepatic and/or cardiac dysfunction.

b. Apnoea of prematurity

Treatment is usually started by the intravenous route at a dose of 1 $mg.kg^{-1}$ twice daily for neonates less than 24 days old and at 1.5 $mg.kg^{-1}$ twice daily for neonates more than 24 days post natal. A loading dose of 3 to 5 $mg.kg^{-1}$ can be given.

At an appropriate time, dosing can be changed to the oral route using a liquid formulation. Oral and intravenous doses are the same. Giving oral doses with feeds slightly delays but does not alter the extent of absorption. Because of the long theophylline half life in these patients (24–64 hours), steady state may not be reached for a week or more. Caffeine (derived from theophylline) takes even longer to reach steady state. Plasma caffeine concentrations at steady state are about one third those of theophylline. Pre-dose plasma theophylline concentrations should be measured weekly during therapy and the dose adjusted to maintain pre-dose concentrations in the range 6 to 9 $mg.l^{-1}$.[56] Dose requirements gradually increase due to increase in size of the infant and maturation of the liver enzyme systems that metabolize theophylline.

c. Prophylactic (chronic) use in asthma and chronic obstructive airways disease

Around-the-clock theophylline therapy guided by plasma theophylline concentration monitoring decreases the symptoms in chronic asthma.[4,46] Chronic theophylline therapy will decrease symptoms in steroid-dependent asthmatics as well.[12] Sustained-release theophylline preparations are preferred for continuous therapy because of the greater ease of administration and improved patient compliance.[48–50] In short-term studies of 4 to 8 weeks, theophylline was as effective as cromoglycate therapy in preventing signs and symptoms of chronic asthma and the combination often provided further benefits.[63] Unlike cromoglycate, theophylline therapy did not seem to decrease bronchial hyperreactivity with long-term adminstration.[63]

Dosages are adjusted to maintain serum theophylline concentrations that provide optimal relief of symptoms with minimal side effects. Plasma theophylline concentrations greater than 20 $mg.l^{-1}$ should be avoided. Dosage increases should be followed with plasma concentration determinations because of the possibility of disproportionate increases in the steady-state concentrations.[34,37] Most of the sustained-release preparations may be administered every 12 hours in adults while administration every 8 hours may be necessary in some children with markedly rapid hepatic metabolism of theophylline.[49,50] Sustained-release tablets should not be chewed or crushed. The following are recommended dosages to achieve serum theophylline concentrations within the accepted therapeutic range:

Table 1

Age	Theophylline oral dose (mg.kg^{-1} daily)
1–6 months	10
6 months–1 year	15
1–9 years	24
10–16 years	18
Adults	10–15

Patients who have been stabilized on intravenous theophylline during an acute episode are changed directly to the same daily dose of an oral sustained release formulation, usually given 12-hourly. The daily dose for patients with cardiac failure or hepatic dysfunction should not exceed 400 mg daily without plasma concentration monitoring. Ideally body weights should be used in dosage calculations. To avoid initial side-effects, patients who have not previously been taking theophylline should be started on doses about half those given above, up to a maximum of 400 mg daily. The dose is then increased in 25% increments until the above median doses are reached or adverse effects occur. The final dosage adjustment is then made on the basis of a plasma theophylline concentration measured after at least 3 days on a stable dose with no missed or added doses. A pre-dose plasma concentration should be measured where possible for rapid release preparations as the variability in time of peak concentrations makes mid-dosage interval concentrations more difficult to interpret. Mid-dose measurements are effective for sustained release doses. Several studies have found theophylline disposition to be non-linear in at least a proportion of individuals. Dosage increases should therefore be made cautiously and in small increments.

In adult non-smokers, most sustained release preparations produce acceptably stable plasma concentrations when they are given 12-hourly. Patients with very short half lives (especially some children) may require 8-hourly dosing with some formulations to avoid excessive fluctuations in plasma theophylline concentrations.

For young children or patients who cannot swallow tablets, bead-filled capsules such as Slo-Phyllin Gyrocaps and Somophyllin-CRT can be opened and the beads sprinkled on soft food so long as the beads are not chewed. Theo-Dur Sprinkle is designed to be taken in this fashion but a large amount of food inhibits its absorption.

Indications

1. Acute asthma and acute exacerbation of chronic obstructive lung disease

Intravenous aminophylline produced significantly less bronchodilation than inhaled beta adrenergic agonists or subcutaneous adrenaline (epinephrine) in patients presenting to the emergency room with acute episodes of asthma.[64] In a study of 102 acutely ill patients treated in the emergency room for acute bronchospasm, there was no advantage found for intravenous aminophylline over oral theophylline.[65] In most cases, β-agonists are more potent bronchodilators and the first choice for reversing acute bronchospasm. The initial management of such episodes involves the administration of oxygen and nebulized β_2-selective adrenoceptor agonists such as salbutamol, terbutaline or fenoterol. Should this not be adequate, intravenous theophylline is given, usually in conjunction with intravenous hydrocortisone. Dosage regimens for theophylline are given under 'Mode of use' above.

2. Chronic asthma

Around-the-clock theophylline therapy guided by plasma theophylline concentration monitoring decreases the symptoms in chronic asthma.[11,46] Chronic theophylline therapy will decrease symptoms in steroid-dependent asthmatics as well.[12] Sustained-release theophylline preparations are preferred for continuous therapy because of the ease of administration and improved patient compliance.[48–50] In short-term studies of 4 to 8 weeks, theophylline was as effective as cromoglycate therapy in preventing signs and symptoms of chronic asthma and the combination often provided further benefits.[63]

Theophylline

Unlike cromoglycate, theophylline therapy did not seem to decrease bronchial hyperreactivity with long-term adminstration.[61]

Dosages are adjusted to maintain serum theophylline concentrations that provide optimal relief of symptoms with minimal side effects. Plasma theophylline concentrations greater than 20 mg.l^{-1} should be avoided. Dosage increases should be followed with plasma concentration determinations because of the possibility of disproportionate increases in the steady-state concentrations.[34,37] Most of the sustained-release preparations may be administered every 12 hours in adults while administration every 8 hours may be necessary in some children with markedly rapid hepatic metabolism of theophylline.[49,50] Sustained-release tablets should not be chewed or crushed. Theophylline remains effective for at least one year.[21]

3. Chronic obstructive lung disease

The reversibility of airways obstruction in chronic obstructive lung disease is relatively small, usually being of the order of 15% improvement in FEV_1, or FVC. Theophylline has repeatedly been shown to produce bronchodilation of this order, but it has been difficult to show subjective improvement in symptoms or improvement in work performance.[66] Some authors suggest that COPD patients may benefit from the cardiovascular[15] and diaphragmatic[14,67] activities of theophylline. Theophylline reduced the dyspnoea produced by exercise in patients with moderate to severe nonreversible airways obstruction without altering lung function tests.[68] It is recommended that adults be initially started on 300–400 mg daily and increased to 500–600 mg daily for nonsmokers or 800–900 mg daily for smokers.[69] Final adjustments should be guided by plasma theophylline concentration monitoring after at least 48 hours on the same dosage.

4. Apnoea of prematurity

Theophylline reduces or abolishes periodic breathing or apnoea in premature infants. This is accompanied by an increase in alveolar ventilation, an increased sensitivity to CO_2 and a shift of the CO_2 response curve to the left, but no alteration in lung mechanics.[70] These effects are consistent with a central respiratory stimulant effect of theophylline, an action also seen with caffeine. Adverse effects are infrequent if plasma theophylline concentrations are maintained below 12 mg.l^{-1}, and consist of tachycardia (>180 beats per minute), vomiting and hyponatraemia due to the initial diuretic effect of theophylline. As the patients grow older, their ability to metabolize theophylline improves and appropriate dosage adjustments may be required. Theophylline in similar doses is occasionally used to help wean neonates with respiratory distress syndrome from mechanical ventilation.[71]

5. Other uses

One study has suggested that theophylline may be effective in infants thought to be at risk of the Sudden Infant Death Syndrome due to recurrent apnoea and excessive periodic breathing.[71] Intravenous aminophylline in a dose of 250 mg has been shown to abolish periodic breathing and improve ventilation, lowering the arterial pCO_2.

Contraindications

The only contraindication to theophylline is hypersensitivity to methylxanthines. As most of the population is continuously exposed to these compounds from dietary sources, hypersensitivity is exceedingly rare. Allergy to ethylenediamine in aminophylline has been reported infrequently. Patients showing an allergic response to aminophylline can safely be changed to an anhydrous theophylline formulation.

Adverse reactions

Potentially life-threatening effects

Although it is uncommon, death associated with theophylline toxicity is well known. The first reports were associated with rapid intravenous infusions of aminophylline and were probably due to cardiac toxicity.[16,51] Most deaths from intentional or iatrogenic overdoses are associated with neurotoxicity and seizures produced by theophylline. The mortality rate associated with theophylline-induced seizures is high; a recent review of the reported cases in the literature found a 29% mortality rate.[51] There appears to be a correlation between age and mortality rate with patients 70 years and older having a mortality rate of 43% compared with 35% for children and adults and 11% for infants less than 2 years.

Theophylline-induced seizures are focal in onset but rapidly progress to become tonic-clonic in nature.[51] In elderly patients, the neurotoxicity may take on an encephalopathic picture with obtundation and periodic seizures. The electroencephalogram characteristically shows periodic lateralized epileptiform discharges. The mechanism for seizure induction is currently unknown but may involve focal hypoxia from cerebral vasoconstriction.[51] Increased guanosine monophosphate and inhibition of adenosine both predispose to epileptic discharges.[16,51] There is not a very close correlation between theophylline plasma concentration and seizure induction, although there is a significant increase in seizure frequency with theophylline plasma concentrations greater than 50 $mg.l^{-1}$ (42% of toxic patients versus 10% or less at concentrations less than 50% $mg.l^{-1}$).[51] The range of plasma concentrations that have been reported for theophylline-induced seizures is wide (25-180 $mg.l^{-1}$). Predisposing factors include severe underlying pulmonary disease with acidosis, hypoxaemia, and hypercarbia. Decreased serum albumin in hepatic disease or situations of decreased protein binding (i.e. elderly patients) may also predispose to seizures.[72]

Theophylline can produce life-threatening cardiac arrhythmias. A variety of cardiac arrhythmias have been described including premature atrial and ventricular contractions, atrial fibrillation, supraventricular tachycardia, and multifocal atrial tachycardia.[51]

Acute overdosage
Intentional and iatrogenic theophylline overdose resulting in death is well documented. The main clinical features of overdose include nausea, vomiting, gastrointestinal bleeding, metabolic acidosis, hypokalaemia, rhabdomyolysis, hypotension, cardiac arrhythmias and seizures, often ending in death.

The management of theophylline overdose is dependent on the plasma concentration. General measures include gastric lavage followed by the administration of activated charcoal by mouth. Frequent oral doses of activated charcoal with or without a laxative will significantly reduce the plasma theophylline[51] half life. Oral charcoal has the added advantage of inhibiting the absorption in oral overdoses. This is particularly important with the increased use of sustained-release theophylline preparations. The charcoal should be given as a slurry in a dose of 20–40 g every 2–4 hours orally or by nasogastric tube. An oral cathartic such as sodium sulphate or magnesium citrate may be used to prevent constipation. Haemoperfusion through charcoal columns is the most efficient method of removal but requires a high level of expertise. Haemodialysis and peritoneal dialysis have been used but are inefficient and cannot be recommended.[51,69] Plasma theophylline concentrations should be monitored frequently enough (every 4 hours) to assess efficacy of removal. Haemoperfusion should be considered for patients with severe symptoms unresponsive to supportive care or deterioration after 4–8 hours of oral charcoal therapy. A substantial proportion of young patients with plasma concentrations less than 80 to 100 $mg.l^{-1}$ as a result of acute theophylline ingestion do not develop serious problems.

Seizures are difficult to treat but may respond to intravenous diazepam, phenobarbital, or the combination,[51] but not to phenytoin.[51] Supraventricular tachycardias have responded to intravenous verapamil and the ventricular tachycardia and ectopic activity respond to propranolol or procainamide. Several cases have been reported where lignocaine was ineffective in controlling ectopic activity.[51]

Severe or irreversible adverse effects
Theophylline may increase the frequency of cardiac arrhythmias in COPD patients or patients with preexisting arrhythmias.[68] Of more recent concern is whether chronic therapy with the combination of theophylline with the β_2-adrenergics increase the risk of sudden death, presumably from cardiac toxicity.[74] Studies in acute asthma have not convincingly demonstrated an increase in arrhythmias from the combination.[61] The combination has been shown to increase the frequency but not the severity of cardiac arrhythmias. However, no increase in ectopic activity is seen in patients without preexisting cardiac disease.[61,68] Care should be exercised when prescribing these agents in patients with preexisting cardiac disease.

Symptomatic adverse effects
Theophylline produces a number of side effects with increasing frequency as the plasma theophylline concentration exceeds 15 $mg.l^{-1}$. The most frequent side effect is sinus tachycardia followed by anorexia, nausea and tremor.[51] Patients also complain of a number of CNS stimulatory effects including anxiety, headaches, nervousness, irritability, insomnia, and hyperactivity (in young children). There is increasing evidence of increased attention deficit in children who already have difficulty. Depression has also been reported in a few patients.[51] Allergic reactions to theophylline are extremely rare but have been noted with ethylenediamine. Urinary retention may occur in elderly males with preexisting partial urinary outflow obstruction.[51] Theophylline increases gastric acid secretion and decreases lower oesophageal sphincter pressure exacerbating gastrooesophageal reflux. Theophylline therapy may aggravate symptoms in women with fibrocystic breast disease.

Other effects
The methylxanthines cause transient elevations in free fatty acids. Theophylline lowers the serum potassium slightly, presumably secondary to endogenous catecholamine release.[51] Hyperglycaemia and metabolic acidosis are seen with overdoses.

Interference with clinical pathology tests
Theophylline may result in spurious elevations of serum uric acid as measured by the method of Bittner (automated by Lofland and Crouse). Intravenous aminophylline and oral theophylline produce a two to threefold increase in urinary catecholamine excretion.

High risk groups

Neonates
Theophylline elimination is impaired in neonates, and recommended doses for this group are correspondingly decreased.

Breast milk. Theophylline concentrations in breast milk are about 70% of those in maternal plasma[75] A nursing infant may receive as much as 10 to 15% of a mother's dose based on relative weight.[75] Especially for premature infants whose metabolism of theophylline may be impaired it is recommended that breast feeding is performed just before a dose of theophylline. Theophylline transfer to the infant can be minimized by maintaining the mother at the lower end of the theophylline therapeutic concentration range.

Children
Children metabolize theophylline more rapidly on a weight basis than adults.[76] Dosage requirements are increased and sustained release preparations are required due to the short elimination half life. In some children 8-hourly dosing is required with some sustained release preparations.[1]

Pregnant women
Theophylline crosses the placenta. Theophylline may inhibit labour and in some neonates of mothers taking theophylline tachycardia, jitteriness, irritability, gagging and vomiting have been reported. A recent very large study found no relationship between caffeine ingestion and excess of fetal abnormalities, low birthweight, or short gestation.[77] Theophylline can be considered safe in pregnancy.

The elderly
No special precautions are required unless congestive cardiac failure, pulmonary oedema, or hepatic dysfunction are present. Clearance is lower than in young adults and dose titration should therefore be cautious and controlled by plasma theophylline concentration measurements.

Concurrent disease
Theophylline clearance is reduced in severe congestive cardiac failure, pulmonary oedema, cor pulmonale, hepatic dysfunction, and hypoxaemic states. Dosages need to be reduced in these patients, sometime drastically, and theophylline clearance, and therefore dosage requirement, can change rapidly. Careful monitoring of plasma theophylline concentrations is required to avoid severe toxicity.

Theophylline clearance is reduced during acute respiratory viral illnesses and the dose may need to be adjusted to avoid toxicity. It is unclear whether this is due to the viral infection or to the fever.
Patients with hepatic disease may be more sensitive to any given plasma theophylline concentration due to a decreased plasma albumin level.[51] Protein binding may be half normal.[28] The plasma albumin level should be considered when interpreting the plasma theophylline concentration.

Theophylline

Drug interactions

Potentially hazardous interactions

Sympathomimetics. There is an increased risk of cardiac arrhythmias in patients with preexisting cardiac disease particularly with systemic sympathomimetics.

Pancuronium bromide. A severe sinus tachycardia has been reported with the concomitant use of aminophylline and pancuronium.

Anaesthetic agents. The risk of cardiac arrhythmias may increase particularly with halothane.

Propranolol. β-adrenoceptor blocking drugs are contraindicated in patients with asthma, allergic rhinitis, or chronic obstructive lung disease. Apart from the pharmacodynamic interaction, propranolol is a potent inhibitor of theophylline metabolism, reducing total body clearance by up to 60%.[59] Metoprolol does not alter theophylline clearance.

Cimetidine. The metabolism of theophylline is inhibited by cimetidine with a 20% to 40% decrease in theophylline clearance.[58] This interaction has been reported to cause severe theophylline toxicity, including vomiting, seizures, and death. Theophylline clearance is not affected by ranitidine.

Macrolide antibiotics. Erythromycin reduces theophylline clearance by 10% to 40% by inhibition of metabolism. The effect is time-dependent and is seen with erythromycin treatment lasting more than 5 days. It has been reported with erythromycin base, and with the ethylsuccinate and stearate. Theophylline dose should be reduced by 25% on beginning treatment with erythromycin. Triacetyloleandomycin is more potent than erythromycin, and a 50% reduction in theophylline dose is required. Josamycin and midecamycin do not appear to reduce theophylline clearance.[78]

Rifampicin. Rifampicin induces theophylline metabolism, increasing clearance by up to 80%. Theophylline dose should be increased by about 25% on starting rifampicin and reduced by half when rifampicin is stopped.[79] Careful monitoring of plasma theophylline concentrations is essential.

Anticonvulsants. Phenobarbitone at anticonvulsant doses (e.g. 90 mg daily for 28 days) increases theophylline clearance by about 30%. Lower doses have little or no effect. Phenytoin increases theophylline clearance by up to 70%, and carbamazepine has a similar effect. Patients taking these anticonvulsants are likely to require higher than usual theophylline doses, and plasma theophylline concentrations should be carefully monitored when anticonvulsant medications are changed.[80] It is not known whether therapeutic plasma theophylline concentrations compromise seizure control in epileptic patients.

Sulphinpyrazone. Usual doses of sulphinpyrazone enhance theophylline clearance by about 25%.[81]

Other significant interactions

Vaccination. Three studies in a total of 8 patients or volunteers found that influenza vaccination caused a 50% to 200% decrease in theophylline clearance 5 to 24 hours after vaccination. Six other studies, in a total of 48 patients, found no effect of influenza vaccine at times of 12 hours to 2 weeks after vaccination. There was no increase in adverse effects in 119 vaccinated nursing home patients taking theophylline.[80]

Allopurinol. Allopurinol in doses of 300 mg per day for 7 days does not alter theophylline clearance but higher doses (600 mg daily for 14 days) produced about a 20% decrease in clearance.

Antacids. Concomitant administration of antacids has no significant effect on the bioavailability or absorption characteristics of rapid release theophylline formulations nor on several sustained release preparations (Slo-Phyllin Gyrocaps, Rorer - USA; Theo-Dur, Key). The absorption rate, maximum concentration, and bioavailability of Theolair SR, Riker, after a single dose were all increased by antacid, by 24%, 39%, and 11% respectively.[24] In general, administration of antacids with theophylline does not produce a clinically significant problem.

Ephedrine. Chronic treatment with ephedrine and theophylline results in an increased incidence of adverse effects but efficacy is not enhanced.[82] Products containing various combinations of theophylline, barbiturates and/or indirectly acting sympathomimetics are irrational and should not be used.

Calcium channel blockers. Verapamil and diltiazem inhibit oxidative drug metabolism and produce mean decreases in theophylline clearance of 18% and 12% respectively.[84]

Quinolone antibiotics. A number of quinolone antibiotics inhibit theophylline clearance with differing potency.[85] The most significant interactions are with enoxacin and pipemidic acid (50% decrease in clearance) and pefloxacin and ciprofloxacin (20–30% decrease). Norfloxacin and ofloxacin produce only a minimal reduction in clearance of 5–10%.

Food. A number of dietary components have been reported to alter the metabolism and clearance of theophylline. A high protein diet increases theophylline clearance by about 30% compared with high carbohydrate or high fat diet, and a diet containing charcoal broiled meat increases theophylline clearance by about 20% compared with a control diet. These effects are not likely to be clinically important unless patients make sudden and drastic changes in their diet. Caffeine intake has little or no influence on theophylline disposition.

The extent of absorption of most theophylline formulations, both rapid and sustained release, is not affected by food. With individual preparations, either an increase (Theograd-250) or a decrease (Theo-Dur Sprinkle) in bioavailability has been found with particular types of food. The rate of absorption of most sustained release preparations is reduced by food but this is generally not of clinical importance.

Alcohol. Alcohol has not been reported to have any significant effect on theophylline.

Smoking. Smoking tobacco or marijuana increases theophylline total body clearance by 40 to 60% and reduces elimination half life by 20 to 50%.[83] The effect is small for patients who smoke less than 10 cigarettes per day but in general there is a poor relationship between number of cigarettes per day and theophylline clearance. The time required for disappearance of induction of theophylline metabolism after stopping smoking is uncertain, but it may be months or years. On average, higher maintenance theophylline doses are required in smokers, but loading doses are not altered.

Drugs that do not interact with theophylline

Adequate studies have shown no significant interaction of theophylline with corticosteroids, tetracycline, doxycycline, amoxycillin, cephalexin, cefaclor, and oral contraceptives.[80]

Potentially useful interactions

None has been described.

Clinical trials

Despite the extensive use of theophylline preparations in medicine there have been no well controlled outcome trials. Most published studies are of relatively short duration and were designed to asses the bronchodilator response.

1. Weinberger M M, Bronsky E A 1974 Evaluation of oral bronchodilator therapy in asthmatic children. Journal of Pediatrics 84: 421–427

This was a randomized double-blind crossover study of five drug regimens each given to 12 asthmatic children for one week. The treatments were; placebo, oral aminophylline, oral ephedrine, aminophylline plus ephedrine (high dose) and low dose combination of aminophylline and ephedrine. Theophylline, but not ephedrine, was highly effective in relieving the signs and symptoms of asthma. Addition of ephedrine to theophylline provided no added benefit.

2. Pedersen S, Nathan A 1983 Long-term treatment of children with sustained-release theophylline. European Journal of Respiratory Diseases 64: 564–570

This is a long-term study in 19 asthmatic children treated with sustained release theophylline. The severity of asthma was assessed prior to theophylline treatment and after one year's treatment when they participated in a placebo-controlled, randomized crossover study comparing 3 weeks on placebo or theophylline. Most parameters were improved in the placebo period compared to the pre-study period one year earlier. Despite this, theophylline still produced significant additional improvement in the mean values of the parameters studied demonstrating continued efficacy after treatment for a year.

3. Murciano D, Auclair M-H, Pariente R, Aubier M 1989 A randomised controlled trial of theophylline in patients with severe chronic obstructive pulmonary disease. New England Journal of Medicine 328: 1521–1525

T

In this double-blinded, placebo-controlled, crossover trial, 60 patients with COPD were studied before and after two months of placebo and two months of sustained-release theophylline. Theophylline therapy produced a significant reduction in dyspnea. Respiratory muscle function improved 2990 while forced expiratory volume in 1 sec increased 13%. Improvement in dyspnea was attributed to improved muscle performance.

Other trials

1. Jones R A K 1982 Apnoea of immaturity. 1. A controlled trial of theophylline and face mask continuous positive airways pressure. Archives of Disease in Childhood 57: 761–765

In this study 32 premature infants with recurrent apnoea were randomized to treatments with theophylline or continuous positive airways pressure (CPAP). All 18 infants on theophylline showed a fall in the rate of apnoeic episodes but CPAP treatment did not result in a significant fall in attack rate. Side effects of theophylline treatment were tachycardia and hyponatraemia, neither of which were serious.

2. Vozeh S, Kewitz G, Perruchoud A et al 1982 Theophylline serum concentration and therapeutic effect in severe bronchial obstruction: the optimal use of intravenously administered aminophylline. American Review of Respiratory Diseases 125: 181–184

In this double-blind study 20 patients with acute exacerbations of bronchial obstruction were randomly assigned to treatment at high (20 mg.l^{-1}) or low (10 mg.l^{-1}) serum theophylline concentrations maintained by aminophylline infusion. The high concentration group showed a significantly greater improvement in pulmonary function at 28 h, and required intravenous treatment for a shorter time than the low concentration group. The incidence of adverse effects in the two groups was similar.

General review articles

Aranda J V, Grondin D, Sasyniuk B I 1981 Pharmacologic considerations in the therapy of neonatal apnoea. Pediatric Clinics of North America 28: 113–133

Bukowskj M, Nakatsu K, Munt P W 1984 Theophylline reassessed. Annals of Internal Medicine 101: 63–73

Hendeles L, Weinberger M 1983 Theophylline: a 'state of the art' review. Pharmacotherapy 3: 2–44

Jonkman J H G, Upton R A 1984 Pharmacokinetic drug interactions with theophylline. Clinical Pharmacokinetics 9: 309–334

Svedmyr N (ed) 1980 Long term theophylline therapy. European Journal of Respiratory Disease 61 (suppl 109): 7–136

References

1. Hendeles L, Weinberger M 1983 Theophylline. A 'state of the art' review. Pharmacotherapy 3: 2–44
2. Zuidema J, Merkus F W H M 1979 Chemical and biopharmaceutical aspects of theophylline and its derivatives. Current Medical Research and Opinion 6 (suppl 6): 14–25
3. Ellinwood E H, Rockwell W J K 1984 Central nervous system stimulants and anorectic agents. In: Dukes M N G (ed) Meyler's side effects of drugs, 10th edn. Elsevier, Amsterdam, pp 1–23
4. Curatolo P W, Robertson D 1983 The health consequences of caffeine. Annals of Internal Medicine 98 (part 1): 641–653
5. Mitenko P A, Ogilvie R I 1973 Rational intravenous doses of theophylline. New England Journal of Medicine 289: 600–603
6. Racineux J L, Troussier J, Turcant A, Tuchais E, Allain P 1981 Comparison of bronchodilation effects of salbutamol and theophylline. Bulletin Europeen de Physiopathologie Respiratoire 17: 799–806
7. Pollock J, Kiechel F, Cooper D, Weinberger M 1977 Relationship of serum theophylline concentration to inhibition of exercise-induced bronchospasm and comparison with cromolyn. Pediatrics 60: 840–844
8. Pauwels R, Van Renterghem D, Van Der Straeten M, Johannesson N, Persson C G A 1985 The effect of theophylline and enprofylline on allergen-induced bronchoconstriction. Journal of Allergy and Clinical Immunology 76: 583–590
9. McWilliams B C, Menendez R, Kelly H W, Howick J 1984 Effects of theophylline on inhaled methacholine and histamine in asthmatic children. American Review of Respiratory Disease 130: 193–197
10. Cushley M J, Tattersfield A E, Holgate S T 1984 Adenosine-induced bronchoconstriction in asthma. American Review of Respiratory Disease 129: 380–384
11. Weinberger M M, Bronsky E A 1974 Evaluation of oral bronchodilator therapy in asthmatic children. Journal of Pediatrics 84: 421–427
12. Nassif E G, Weinberger M, Thompson R, Huntly W 1981 The value of maintenance theophylline in steroid-dependent asthma. New England Journal of Medicine 304: 71–75
13. Persson C G 1980 Some pharmacological aspects on xanthines in asthma. European Journal of Respiratory Diseases 61 (suppl 109): 7–16
14. Aubier M, De Troyer A, Sampson T, Macklem P T, Roussos C 1981 Aminophylline improves diaphragmatic contractility. New England Journal of Medicine 305: 249–252
15. Matthay R A, Berger H F, Loke J 1978 Effects of aminophylline on right and left ventricular performance in chronic obstructive pulmonary disease. American Journal of Medicine 65: 903–910
16. Rall T W 1985 Central nervous system stimulants: the methylxanthines. In: Gilman A G, Goodman L S, Rall T W, Murad F (eds) The pharmacological basis of therapeutics, 7th edn. Macmillan, New York, ch 25, pp 589–603
17. Sanders J S, Berman T M, Bartlett M M, Kronenberg R S 1980 Increased hypoxic ventilatory drive due to administration of aminophylline in normal men. Chest 78: 279–282
18. Dietrich J, Krauss A N, Reidenberg M, Drayer D E, Auld P A M 1978 Alterations in state in apneic preterm infants receiving theophylline. Clinical Pharmacology and Therapeutics 24: 474–478
19. Persson C G A, Erjefalt I, Edholm L E, Lamm C J 1982 Tracheal relaxant and cardiostimulant effects can be differentiated from diuretic and CNS-stimulant actions of xanthines. Role of adenosine antagonism? Life Sciences 31: 2673–2681
20. Hendeles L, Weinberger M 1980 Avoidance of adverse effects during chronic therapy with theophylline. European Journal of Respiratory Diseases 61 (suppl 109): 103–119
21. Pedersen S, Nathan E 1983 Long-term treatment of children with sustained-release theophylline. European Journal of Respiratory Diseases 64: 564–570
22. Thakker K D, Grady L T 1982 Theophylline. In: Florey K (ed) Analytical profiles of drug substances, vol 11. Academic Press, New York, pp 1–44
23. Miksic J R, Hodes B 1979 Theophylline analysis by reversed phase high-pressure liquid chromatography: elimination of interferences. Journal of Pharmaceutical Science 68: 1200–1202
24. Jonkman J H G 1984 Biopharmaceutical and pharmacokinetic drug interactions with theophylline. In: Jonkman J H G, Jenne J W, Simons F E R (eds) Sustained release theophylline in the treatment of chronic reversible airways obstruction. Excerpta Medica, Amsterdam, pp 98–110
25. Birkett D J, Coulthard K P, Lines D, Grgurinovich N 1984 Circadian variation in the absorption of three sustained release theophylline products in asthmatic children and the effect of food on absorption of somophyllin-CRT. British Journal of Clinical Practice 38 (suppl 35): 17–23
26. Scott P H, Tabachnik E, Macleod S M, Correia J, Newth C, Levison H 1981 Sustained-release theophylline for childhood asthma: evidence for circadian variation of theophylline pharmacokinetics. Journal of Pediatrics 99: 476–479
27. Aranda J V, Sitar D S, Parsons W D, Loughnan P M, Neims A H 1976 Pharmacokinetic aspects of theophylline in premature newborns. New England Journal of Medicine 295: 413–416
28. Mangione A, Imhoff T E, Lee R V, Shum L Y, Jusko W J 1978 Pharmacokinetics of theophylline in hepatic disease. Chest 73: 616–622
29. Gal P, Jusko W J, Yurchak A M, Franklin B A 1978 Theophylline disposition in obesity. Clinical Pharmacology and Therapeutics 23: 438–444
30. Knott C, Bateman M, Reynolds F 1984 Do saliva concentrations predict plasma unbound theophylline concentrations? A problem re-examined. British Journal of Clinical Pharmacology 17: 9–14
31. Toback J W, Gal P, Erkan N V, Roop C, Robinson H 1983 Usefulness of theophylline saliva levels in neonates. Therapeutic Drug Monitoring 5: 185–189
32. Grygiel J J, Birkett D J 1980 Effect of age on patterns of theophylline metabolism. Clinical Pharmacology and Therapeutics 28: 456–462
33. Tang-Liu D D S, Williams R L, Riegelman S 1982 Nonlinear theophylline elimination. Clinical Pharmacology and Therapeutics 31: 358–369
34. Weinberger M M, Ginchansky E 1977 Dose-dependent kinetics of theophylline disposition in asthmatic children. Journal of Pediatrics 91: 820–824
35. Dahlqvist R, Billing B, Miners J O, Birkett D J 1984 Nonlinear metabolic disposition of theophylline. Therapeutic Drug Monitoring 6: 290–297
36. Persson C G A, Andersson K E 1977 Respiratory and cardiovascular effects of 3-methylxanthine, a metabolite of theophylline. Acta Pharmacologica et Toxicologica 40: 529–536
37. Dahlqvist R, Billing B, Miners J O, Birkett D J 1984 Non-linear metabolic disposition of theophylline. Therapeutic Drug Monitoring 6: 290–297
38. Ogilvie R I 1978 Clinical pharmacokinetics of theophylline. Clinical Pharmacokinetics 3: 267–293
39. Gardner M J, Jusko W J 1982 Effect of age and sex on theophylline clearance in young subjects. Pediatrics Pharmacology 2: 157–169
40. Upton R A, Thiercelin J F, Guentert T W et al 1982 Intraindividual variability in 60 healthy young adults. Journal of Pharmacokinetics and Biopharmaceutics 10: 123–134
41. Staib A H, Schuppan D, Lissner R, Zilly W, Bomhard G V, Richter E 1980 Pharmacokinetics and metabolism of theophylline in patients with liver diseases. International Journal of Clinical Pharmacology, Therapy and Toxicology 18: 500–502
42. Jusko W J, Eaton M L 1982 Factors affecting theophylline disposition. In: MacLeod S M, Isles A (eds) Theophylline therapy update. Astra Pharmaceuticals Canada Ltd, Mississauga, Ontario, pp 19–29
43. Kraemer M J, Furukawa C T, Koup J R, Shapiro G G, Pierson W E, Bierman C W 1982 Altered theophylline clearance during an influenza B outbreak. Pediatrics 69: 476–480
44. Tserng K-Y, Takieddine F N, King K C 1983 Developmental aspects of theophylline metabolism in premature infants. Clinical Pharmacology and Therapeutics 33: 522–528
45. Levy G, Koysooko R 1975 Pharmacokinetic analysis of the effect of theophylline on pulmonary function in asthmatic children. Journal of Pediatrics 86: 789–793

46. Rachelefsky G S, Katz R M, Siegel S C 1978 A sustained-release theophylline preparation: efficacy in childhood asthma with low serum theophylline levels. Annals of Allergy 40: 252–257
47. Vozeh S, Kewitz G, Perruchoud A et al 1982 Theophylline serum concentration and therapeutic effect in severe acute bronchial obstruction: the optimal use of intravenously administered aminophylline. American Review of Respiratory Disease 125: 181–184
48. Tabachnik E, Scott P, Correia J et al 1982 Sustained-release theophylline: a significant advance in the treatment of childhood asthma. Journal of Pediatrics 100: 489–492
49. Weinberger M, Hendeles L 1983 Slow-release theophylline: rationale and basis for product selection. New England Journal of Medicine 308: 760–764
50. Menendez R, Kelly H W, Howick J, McWilliams B C 1983 Sustained-release theophylline: pharmacokinetic and therapeutic comparison of two preparations. American Journal of Diseases of Children 137: 469–473
51. Kelly H W 1987 Theophylline toxicity. In: Jenne J, Murphy S (eds) Drug therapy for asthma: research and clinical practice. Marcel Dekker, New York, pp 925–951
52. Shannon D C, Gotay F, Stein I M, Rogers M C, Todres I D, Moylan F M B 1975 Prevention of apnea and bradycardia in low birth-weight infants. Pediatrics 55: 589–594
53. Myers T F, Milsap R L, Krauss A N, Auld P A M, Reidenberg M M 1980 Low-dose theophylline therapy in idiopathic of prematurity. Journal of Pediatrics 96: 99–103
54. Jones R A K, Baille E 1979 Dosage schedule for intravenous aminophylline in apnoea of prematurity, based on pharmacokinetic studies. Archives of Disease in Childhood 54: 190–193
55. Zwillich C W, Sutton F D, Neff T A, Cohn W M, Matthay R A, Weinberger M M 1975 Theophylline-induced seizures in adults: correlation with serum concentrations. Annals of Internal Medicine 82: 784–787
56. Shannon D C, Gotay F, Stein I M, Rogers M C, Todres I D, Moylan F M B 1975 Prevention of apnea and bradycardia in low-birthweight infants. Pediatrics 55: 580–594
57. Grygiel J J, Wing L M H, Farkas J, Birkett D J 1974 Effects of allopurinol on theophylline metabolism and clearance. Clinical Pharmacology and Therapeutics 26: 660–667
58. Grygiel J J, Miners J O, Drew R, Birkett D J 1984 Differential effects of cimetidine on theophylline metabolic pathways. European Journal of Clinical Pharmacology 26: 335–340
59. Miners J O, Wing L M H W, Lillywhite K J, Robson R A 1985 Selectivity and dose-dependency of the inhibitory effect of propranolol on theophylline metabolism in man. British Journal of Clinical Pharmacology 20: 219–223
60. Birkett D J, Miners J O, Attwood J 1983 Secondary metabolism of theophylline biotransformation products in man — route of formation of 1-methyluric acid. British Journal of Clinical Pharmacology 15: 117–119
61. Kelly H W 1984 Controversies in asthma therapy with theophylline and β_2-adrenergic agonists. Clinical Pharmacy 3: 386–395
62. Nassif E G, Weinberger M 1981 Theophylline disposition in infancy. Journal of Pediatrics 98: 158–161
63. Godfrey S 1980 The relative merits of cromolyn sodium and high-dose theophylline therapy in childhood asthma. Journal of Allergy and Clinical Immunology 65: 97–104
64. Rossing T H, Fanta C H, Goldstein D H, Snapper J R, McFadden E R 1980 Emergency therapy of asthma: comparison of the acute effects of parenteral and inhaled sympathomimetics and infused aminophylline. American Review of Respiratory Disease 122: 365–371
65. Fanta C H, Rossing T H, McFadden E R 1982 Emergency room treatment of asthma: relationships among therapeutic combinations, severity of obstruction and time course of response. American Journal of Medicine 72: 416–422
66. Jenne J W 1984 Theophylline in chronic obstructive lung disease. In: Jonkman J H G, Jenne J W, Simons F E R (eds) Sustained release theophylline in the treatment of chronic reversible airways obstruction. Excerpta Medica, Amsterdam, pp 164–172
67. Murciano D, Aubier M, Lecocguic Y, Pariente R 1984 Effects of aminophylline on diaphragmatic strength and fatigue in patients with chronic obstructive pulmonary disease. New England Journal of Medicine 311: 349–353
68. Mahler D A, Matthaw R A, Snyder P E, Wells C K, Loke J 1985 Sustained-release theophylline reduces dyspnea in non reversible obstructive airway disease. American Review of Respiratory Disease 131: 22–25
69. Jenne J W 1984 Theophylline use in asthma: some current issues. Clinics in Chest Medicine 5: 645–658
70. Dave M J, Sankaran K, Simons K J, Simons F E R, Seshia M M, Rigatto H 1978 Physiologic changes induced by theophylline in the treatment of apnea in pre-term infants. Journal of Pediatrics 92: 91–95
71. Harris M C, Baumgart S, Rooklin A R, Fox W W 1983 Successful extubation of infants with respiratory distress syndrome using aminophylline. Journal of Pediatrics 103: 303–305
72. Kelly D H, Shannon D C 1985 Treatment of apnea and excessive periodic breathing in the full-term infant. Pediatrics 68: 183–186
73. Russo M E 1979 Management of theophylline intoxication with charcoal-column hemoperfusion. New England Journal of Medicine 300: 24–26
74. Wilson J D, Sutherland D C, Thomas A C 1981 Has the change to beta-agonists combined with oral theophylline increased cases of fatal asthma. Lancet 1: 1235–1237
75. Stec G P, Greenberger P, Ruo T I, Henthorn T, Morita J, Atkinson A J 1980 Kinetics of theophylline transfer to breast milk. Clinical Pharmacology and Therapeutics 28: 404–408
76. Grygiel J J, Ward H, Ogbourne M, Goldin A, Birkett D J 1983 Relationships between plasma theophylline clearance, liver volume and body weight in children and adults. European Journal of Clinical Pharmacology 24: 529–532
77. Babayan E A, Astahova A V, Lepakhin V K, Lopatin A S 1983 Central nervous system stimulants and anorectic agents. In: Dukes M N G (ed) Meyler's side effects of drugs annual 7. Excerpta Medica, Amsterdam, pp 1–15
78. Ludden T M 1985 Pharmacokinetic interactions of the macrolide antibiotics. Clinical Pharmacokinetics 10: 63–79
79. Robson R A, Miners J O, Wing L M H W, Birkett D J 1984 Theophylline–rifampicin interaction: non-selective induction of theophylline metabolic pathways. British Journal of Clinical Pharmacology 18: 445–448
80. Jonkman J H G, Upton R A 1984 Pharmacokinetic drug interactions with theophylline. Clinical Pharmacokinetics 9: 309–334
81. Birkett D J, Miners J O, Attwood J 1983 Evidence for a dual role of sulphinpyrazone on drug metabolism in man: theophylline–sulphinpyrazone interaction. British Journal of Clinical Pharmacology 15: 567–569
82. Weinberger M M, Bronsky E A 1975 Interaction of ephedrine and theophylline. Clinical Pharmacology and Therapeutics 17: 585–592
83. Grygiel J J, Birkett D J 1981 Cigarette smoking and theophylline clearance and metabolism. Clinical Pharmacology and Therapeutics 30: 491–496
84. Sirmans S M, Pieper J A, Lalonde R L, Smith D G, Self T H 1988 Effect of calcium channel blockers on theophylline disposition. Clinical Pharmacology and Therapeutics 44: 29–34
85. Edwards D J, Bowles S K, Svensson C K, Rybak M J 1988 Inhibition of drug metabolism by quinolone antibiotics. Clinical Pharmacokinetics 15: 194–204

T

Thiabendazole

Developed as a successful antiparasitic drug in veterinary medicine in the early 1960s, thiabendazole has variable activity against a wide range of helminths. It is the drug of choice for *Strongyloides stercoralis* (threadworm) and cutaneous larva migrans (creeping eruption) in man and is useful for mixed worm infestations.

Chemistry

Thiabendazole (Mintezol)
$C_{10}H_7N_3S$
2-(4′-Thiazolyl)-1H-benzimidazole

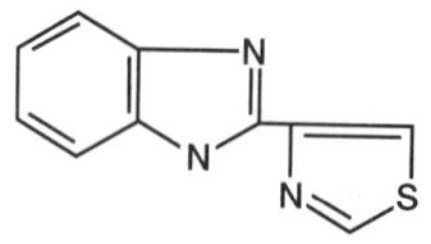

Molecular weight	201.3
pKa	4.7
Solubility	
in alcohol	1 in 50
in water	<1 in 10 000
Octanol/water partition coefficient	—

A stable white or cream-coloured, odourless, tasteless powder. Thiabendazole is not available in any compound preparations.

Pharmacology

Thiabendazole has a high degree of activity against many nematodes that infect the gut of man. It is also active against the larvae and eggs in vitro.[1,2] The main mechanism of action is probably by inhibiting the mitochondrial fumarate reductase system that is specific to helminths, by interacting with an endogenous quinone.[3] Thiabendazole affects *Strongyloides* by suppressing assembly of microtubules and also kills the larvae of *Trichinella spiralis* in muscle. The drug has anti-inflammatory, antipyretic and analgesic effects in laboratory animals. Thiabendazole also has some activity against fungi in vitro, particularly *Trichophyton* and *Microsporum*, but its use clinically in these infections has not been very successful.

Toxicology

The oral acute LD_{50} of thiabendazole (as base) for rats is around 3100 mg.kg^{-1}. Single oral doses of 200 mg.kg^{-1} or more cause vomiting in dogs. Up to 400 mg.kg^{-1} given daily for 180 days did not kill rats in a subacute study. No significant organ changes were found except those caused by inanition and weight loss.

Clinical pharmacology

Thiabendazole does not produce significant pharmacodynamic action on administration by the oral route in man. Although the drug is quite well absorbed in the dog, cat and man, it lacks specific action on respiratory, cardiovascular, and autonomic systems.

The primary effect of the drug is on *Strongyloides stercoralis* and larva migrans. Furthermore it has weaker antihelmintic properties on quite a number of nematodes such as *Ascaris*, *Oxyuris*, hookworm, *Trichuris*, *Trichostrongylus*, and *Trichinella* larvae. It also has strong larvicidal action and inhibits embryonic development of *Ascaris* eggs,[2] both in vitro. The beneficial clinical effects in *Trichinella spiralis* infection may be influenced by the analgesic and anti-inflammatory action of the drug. There have been a number of claims that the drug works in some fungal infections,[4,5] but clinical results are equivocal. Thiabendazole is not effective against filariasis.

Pharmacokinetics

Radiometric and spectrofluorometric assay methods[6] have been used for the analysis of thiabendazole and 5-hydroxythiabendazole in plasma, urine, milk, and tissue. Results obtained with chemical assay are in agreement with results obtained with the radiometric assay and the former is perhaps more convenient for pharmacokinetic work. The sensitivity of both methods is 0.1 mg.l^{-1} for plasma and tissue and 5 mg.l^{-1} for urine and faeces (precision of $95 \pm 6\%$). An HPLC method with fluorescence detection is also available.

Thiabendazole is rapidly and extensively absorbed after oral dosing. After a single oral dose of 11–15 mg.kg^{-1}, peak plasma levels of 2.1–6.2 mg.l^{-1} are obtained within 1–2 h,[7] and decline to almost zero in 24–48 hours. Thiabendazole is eliminated almost completely by metabolism in the liver. Within 48 hours, about 5% of the administered dose is recovered from the faeces and about 90% from the urine, with <1% excreted unchanged.

The pharmacokinetics of thiabendazole and its metabolites were determined after the first dose and during haemodialysis and haemoperfusion in an anephric female patient treated for a *Strongyloides* infection.[8] The half life, volume of distribution, and clearance for thiabendazole were 1.17 hours, 2.76 l.kg^{-1}, and 27.2 ml.min^{-1}, respectively. While thiabendazole and the 5-hydroxy metabolite did not accumulate during multiple dosing, the glucuronide and sulphate esters accumulated extensively despite haemodialysis and haemoperfusion.

It is not known whether thiabendazole crosses the placenta or is excreted in breast milk.

Oral absorption	>90%
Presystemic metabolism	—
Plasma half life	
mean	1.17 h
Volume of distribution	2.76 l.kg^{-1}
Plasma protein binding	—

Concentration–effect relationship

No measurement of drug plasma levels seem warranted in normal patients treated for helminth infections. In the case of renal failure the 5-hydroxy metabolites of the drug may accumulate as was shown in one anephric patient in whom these metabolites rose to six times their usual values.[9] The parent compound did not accumulate in this patient.

Metabolism

Thiabendazole is extensively metabolized in the liver, the major metabolite being the 5-hydroxy derivative. This is further metabolized by conjugation to the glucuronide and sulphate, which are eliminated in the urine. The 5-hydroxy metabolites are inactive.

Pharmaceutics

Thiabendazole (Mintezol) is available in 500 mg chewable tablets and as an oral suspension containing 500 mg per 5 ml. The original Merck, Sharp and Dohme tablet preparation is orange flavoured and marked 'MSD 907'. Containers should be tightly closed, protected from light and stored in a cool place. The round tablets are scored and coloured orange in the UK but are off-white in this US formulation.

Therapeutic use

Indications

Thiabendazole is most effective against *Strongyloides stercoralis* and cutaneous larva migrans, but less active against enterobiasis, trichostrongyliasis, trichinosis, ascariasis, trichuriasis and hookworm infection.

Contraindications

Known hypersensitivity to thiabendazole is a contraindication and if it occurs during treatment the drug should be immediately discontinued. There are no other absolute contraindications to the use of thiabendazole. Liver transaminases may increase during treatment and therefore it should be used with caution in patients with liver impairment. When used for the treatment of mixed infections with roundworms, *Ascaris* may migrate.

Mode of use

Thiabendazole is preferably given twice a day because if the daily dose is given as a single dose it gives rise to a higher incidence of adverse effects. The tablets or oral suspension should be given after meals to decrease gastric irritation. The tablets must be well chewed before swallowing. Dosage is more dependent on body weight rather than on the condition being treated. The standard daily dose is 50 $mg.kg^{-1}$ body weight for all roundworm infections. When given in two divided doses per day it may decrease the incidence of adverse effects. Dietary restrictions and purging are not necessary. Thiabendazole should not be used prophylactically.

Indications

1. *Strongyloides stercoralis*
Thiabendazole is the drug of choice for strongyloidiasis (threadworm infection). A dose of 25 $mg.kg^{-1}$ body weight is given twice a day for two successive days, after meals. The maximal daily dose is 3 g.

2. Cutaneous larva migrans
The drug is quite effective against this disease. A dose of 25 $mg.kg^{-1}$ body weight is given twice a day, for 2–4 consecutive days.[10,11]. About 50% of migrating larvae die spontaneously; the effect of thiabendazole is to kill over 90% and one study[9] claims to stop the activity of over 99% of the larvae on the first day of therapy. Corticosteroids have been found useful to decrease dermal irritation caused by the larvae.

3. *Trichinella spiralis*
The drug has been used in cases of larvae of *Trinchinella spiralis* migrating into the muscle. Marked clinical improvement has been claimed such as alleviation of symptoms and decrease in eosinophilia, but perhaps this is more due to the anti-inflammatory and analgesic effect of the drug. The effect on the migrating larvae itself is questionable. The dosage recommended is as described above for two to four consecutive days.

4. Other nematode infections
Enterobiasis (pinworm), *Necator americanus* and *Ancylostoma duodenale* (hookworm), or trichuriasis (whipworm) may be treated with thiabendazole if it forms multiple infections with *Strongyloides* or larva migrans. When *Ascaris* is present the possibility of migration into the oesophagus or bile duct should be taken into account. The cure rate in enterobiasis is about 90%; in ascariasis and hookworm infection the rate is less and more variable, while in trichuriasis the drug is least effective.

Adverse reactions

Potentially life-threatening effects
Hypersensitivity reactions may take the form of erythema multiforme, and in one case a Stevens–Johnson syndrome has resulted in death. Another case of severe cholestatic jaundice after prophylactic thiabendazole treatment occurred in a 32-year-old woman who died of a massive haemorrhage more than a month later.[12]

Acute overdosage
No cases of overdose have been reported. Should poisoning occur, the treatment should be symptomatic; no known antidote exists.

Severe or irreversible adverse effects
Known adverse effects are unlikely to be severe enough to cause disablement and irreversibility except for the rare hypersensitivity cases reported above.

Symptomatic adverse effects
Moderate adverse effects occur quite frequently, particularly with the higher doses of the drug, the most common being anorexia, nausea, vomiting, and dizziness. Gastrointestinal irritation may result in diarrhoea and epigastric pain. Other symptoms encountered less commonly include pruritus, headache, and drowsiness. Some patients may need to rest for a few hours to overcome the adverse reactions.

Thiabendazole

Other less common adverse effects are tinnitus, blurred vision, paraesthesia, icterus, increase in transaminase levels, and transient leucopenia.

Interference with clinical pathology tests
No interferences of this kind appear to have been reported.

High risk groups

Neonates
The drug is not used in this age group.
Breast milk. As it is not known whether the drug enters breast milk, mothers under treatment should not breast-feed.

Children
Children seem to tolerate the drug quite well, although there has not been enough experience in those weighing less than 15 kg. In a study of 132 ambulatory patients, 100 of whom were less than 15 years of age, one-third to one-half of the patients suffered from transient adverse effects. None was serious. The doses used in this study ranged from 25 $mg.kg^{-1}$ daily for 2 days to 50 $mg.kg^{-1}$ daily for 1 to 3 days.[13]

Pregnant women
Thiabendazole should not be used during pregnancy. Reports have suggested that it is teratogenic in mice, although reproduction studies in rabbits, rats, sheep and cattle have produced no fetal abnormalities attributable to the drug.

The elderly
There are no special problems in this age group.

Concurrent disease
Hepatic disease. Since the drug may occasionally cause jaundice, it should be used with extra caution in patients with liver disease.
Renal diesease. Renal function should be carefully monitored in patients with disorders of this organ.

Drug interactions

Potentially hazardous interactions
Thiabendazole may compete with other drugs for metabolism in the liver and thus increase the concentration of those drugs to potentially toxic levels, for instance, theophylline.

Potentially useful interactions
No interactions of this kind have been documented.

Major outcome trials

1. Most H, Yoeli M, Cambell W C, Cuckler A C 1965 The treatment of *Strongyloides* and *Enterobius* infections with thiabendazole. American Journal of Tropical Medicine and Hygiene 14: 379–382

This is a large-scale trial of mentally retarded children of various ages. Incidence of *Strongyloides* infections were 13% of 517 patients examined and *Enterobius* 56% of 735. Total doses of thiabendazole varied from 50 $mg.kg^{-1}$ to 100 $mg.kg^{-1}$ body weight given in either a single dose or twice daily, for one or two days.

The efficacy of thiabendazole is related to the amount of each dose as well as the total dosage given. For *Strongyloides*, 25 $mg.kg^{-1}$ body weight of the drug given as a single dose for two consecutive days gave a cure rate of 70%. The same dose given twice daily for two days gave 100% (17/17) cure. For enterobiasis the results were as follows: for a total dose of 50 $mg.kg^{-1}$, the cure rate was 55–81% and doubling the dose resulted in 95–100% cure rate. When the drug was given as divided doses per day the results were as mentioned at the lower range.

Adverse effects documentation were not regarded as trustworthy in this patient group.

2. Katz R, Ziegler J, Blank H 1965 The natural course of creeping eruption and treatment with thiabendazole. Archives of Dermatology 91: 420–424

A placebo-controlled trial on the efficacy of thiabendazole in 53 patients (28 treated) have been reported. Cutaneous changes disappeared in 81% of the total number of lesions in the placebo group in 4 weeks, but 99% disappeared in the treatment group. The placebo cure was unusually high in this trial compared to other studies.

T

Other trials

1. Franz K H 1963 Clinical trials with thiabendazole against human strongyloidiasis. American Journal of Tropical Medicine and Hygiene 12: 211–214

This study covered 88 Africans with various worm infections. Dosages of over 50 mg.kg^{-1} body weight gave higher rate of effectiveness against *Strongyloides*. Large particle formulations in capsules or small particle formulations in oral suspension gave equally good results but adverse effects such as nausea, vomiting, dizziness and drowsiness were more often encountered with the large particle formulation.

2. Kale O O 1977 A comparative trial of the anthelmintic efficacy of pyrantel pamoate (Combantrin) and thiabendazole (Mintezol). African Journal of Medical Science 6: 89–93

The efficacy of thiabendazole was compared against pyrantel pamoate to treat ascariasis, hookworm and trichuriasis. The doses were two doses of 25 mg.kg^{-1} body weight given on the same day for thiabendazole, and 10 mg.kg^{-1} body weight for pyrantel. Pyrantel gave cure rates of 93.8% and 29.1% for *Ascaris* and hookworm respectively, and 44.3% and 27.3% for thiabendazole. Both drugs were ineffective against *Trichuris*. The 135 patients were stratified on the basis of the intensity of hookworm infection and randomized.

General review articles

Cuckler A C, Mezey K C 1966 The therapeutic efficacy of thiabendazole for helminthic infections in man, a literature review. Arzneimittelforschung 16: 1–48

Arguedas J A G, Villarejos V M, Swartzwelder J C, Chavarria A P, Zeledon R, Kotcher E 1975 Community control of *Strongyloides stercoralis* by thiabendazole. Texas Reports on Biology and Medicine 33: 265–268

Hall W, McCabe W R 1967 Trichinosis, report of a small outbreak with observations of thiabendazole therapy. Archives of Internal Medicine 119: 65–68

Salunkhe D S, Gaitonde B B, Vakil B J 1964 Clinical evaluation of a new anthelmintic thiabendazole. Journal of Tropical Medicine and Hygiene 23: 412–416

Ishizaki T, Iijima T, Ito Y 1966 On a new treatment regimen with thiabendazole against *Ancylostoma duodenale*. Japanese Journal of Medical Science and Biology 19: 239–245

Fransz K H, Schneider W J, Pohlman M H 1965 Clinical trials with thiabendazole against intestinal nematodes infecting humans. American Journal of Tropical Medicine and Hygiene 14: 383–386

Stone O J, Stone C T, Mullins J F 1964 Thiabendazole, probable cure for trichinosis; report of first case. Journal of the American Medical Association 187: 536–538

Pelletier L L Jr 1984 Chronic strongyloidiasis in World War II Far East ex-prisoners of war. American Journal of Tropical Medicine and Hygiene 33: 55–61

Alcantara A K, Uylangco C V, Cross J H 1985 An obstinate case of intestinal capillariasis. Southeast Asian Journal of Tropical Medicine and Public Health 16: 410–413

References

1. Brown H D, Matzuk A R, Ilves I R et al 1961 Antiparasitic drugs. IV. 2-(4'-thiazolyl)-benzimidazole, a new anthelmintic. Journal of the American Chemical Society 83: 1964–1965
2. Egerton J R 1961 The effect of thiabendazole upon *Ascaris* and *Stephanurus* infections. Journal of Parasitology 47: section 2: 37
3. Kohler P, Bachmann R 1978 The effects of the antiparasitic drugs levamisole, thiabendazole, praziquantel and chloroquine on mitochondrial electron transport in muscle tissue from *Ascaris suum*. Molecular Pharmacology 14: 155–158
4. Upadhyay M P, West E P, Sharma A P 1980 Keratitis due to *Aspergillus flavus* successfully treated with thiabendazole. British Journal of Ophthalmology 64: 30–32
5. Battistini F, Bolivar C, Zaias N, Sierra R, Bolivar C, Rebell G 1974 Clinical antifungal activity of thiabendazole. Archives of Dermatology 109: 695–699
6. Tocco D J, Egerton J R, Bowers W, Christensen V, Rosenblum C 1965 Absorption, metabolism and elimination of thiabendazole in farm animals and a method for its estimation in biological materials. Journal of Pharmacology and Experimental Therapeutics 149: 263–271
7. Tocco D T, Rosenblum C, Martin C M, Robinson J H 1966 Absorption, metabolism and excretion of thiabendazole in man and laboratory animals. Toxicology and Applied Pharmacology 9: 31–39
8. Bauer L A, Raisys V A, Watts M T, Ballinger J 1982 The pharmacokinetics of thiabendazole and its metabolites in an anephric patient undergoing hemodialysis and hemoperfusion. Journal of Clinical Pharmacology 22: 276–280
9. Schumaker J D, Band J D, Lensmeyer G L, Craig W A 1978 Thiabendazole treatment of severe strongyloidiasis in a hemodialyzed patient. Annals of Internal Medicine 89: 644–645
10. Stone O J, Mullins J F M 1965 Thiabendazole effectiveness in creeping eruption. Archives of Dermatology 91: 427–429
11. Katz R, Ziegler J, Blank H 1965 The natural course of creeping eruption and treatment with thiabendazole. Archives of Dermatology 91: 420–424
12. Jalota R, Freston J W 1974 Severe intrahepatic cholestasis due to thiabendazole. American Journal of Tropical Medicine and Hygiene 23: 676–678
13. Botero D R 1965 Treatment of human intestinal helminthiasis with thiabendazole. American Journal of Tropical Medicine and Hygiene 14: 618–621

Thiacetazone

Thiacetazone is an antibacterial agent used in the chemotherapy of tuberculosis.

Chemistry

Thiacetazone (thioacetazone, TBI, Tibione, Contebin, Sdt 1041, RP 4207, Thizone, Novakol, Domakol, Aktivan, Ambathizon, Seroden, Benthiozone, Berkazon, Diasan, Ilbion, Tebalon, Siocarbzone, Tibicur, Tebethion, Panrone)
$C_{10}H_{12}N_4OS$
4-Acetylamidobenzaldehyde thiosemicarbazone

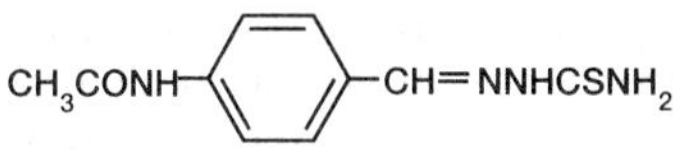

Molecular weight	236.3
pKa	—
Solubility	
in alcohol	1 in 500
in water	very slight
Octanol/water partition coefficient	—

Thiacetazone is a pale yellow, finely crystalline powder, melting with decomposition at 225–230°C. It is prepared by chemical synthesis by treating 4-acetamidobenzaldehyde with thiosemicarbazide in alcohol. It is available only in oral form, but is not available in any combined preparations.

Pharmacology

Thiacetazone, a thiosemicarbazone, is related to and derived from thiadiazole-containing sulphonamides, but is more effective and less toxic than the drugs from which it is derived. The drug is bacteriostatic primarily to mycobacteria. Although its mechanism of action is not totally understood it is believed to form copper complexes that interfere with the copper enzyme carriers within mycobacteria.

Toxicology

Thiacetazone has been found to be toxic to human embryo liver cells at concentrations of 25 mg.l^{-1} with complete necrosis of the cells at a concentration of 50 mg.l^{-1}.[1] This concentration, however, was at least 10–15 times that of the peak blood levels that were achieved in humans following ingestion of appropriate doses for treatment of tuberculosis. Few reports exist in the literature concerning the teratogenic effect of this agent upon the human fetus, especially in the light of the fact that it has always been used as a companion drug with other antituberculosis compounds. One study observed 19 children delivered to 18 mothers who received various combinations of thiacetazone with 4-aminosalicylic acid, isoniazid, streptomycin and pyrazinamide.[2] Only four minor aberrations were found suggesting, at least by this limited study, that this agent had little observed teratogenic effect upon the human fetus.

Clinical pharmacology

Thiacetazone is bacteriostatic to *Mycobacterium tuberculosis* at a minimum inhibitory concentration (MIC) of 0.4 mg.l^{-1}.[3] The drug is bacteriostatic to *Mycobacterium leprae* at an MIC of 0.2 mg.l^{-1}.[4] It is also active against *Mycobacterium bovis*. The sensitivity of these various mycobacteria to thiacetazone may vary in different strains throughout the world. There is usually no cross-resistance with isoniazid-resistant mycobacteria, but cross-resistance is seen between thiacetazone and ethionamide, thiocarlide or prothionamide. Resistance to thiacetazone will develop in about 30% of organisms after 4–6 months if the drug is used on its own.

In vivo studies of this drug, used in combination with 300 mg of isoniazid (daily), indicated that the minimal concentration of thiacetazone in the lesions necessary to prevent the emergence of isoniazid resistance appeared to be approximately 0.4 mg.l^{-1} serum. However, this number varies, depending upon the strain tested.[5] Slide sensitivity culture test demonstrated that 12 Kenyan patients were 100% inhibited, whereas 107 Hong Kong patient samples indicated only 77% inhibition at this concentration.[3]

Pharmacokinetics

The preferred analytical method is high performance liquid chromatography utilizing a reversed phase column packing with ultraviolet detection.[6] This method allows quantification of thiacetazone with a propionyl analogue internal standard (4-propionylaminobenzaldehyde thiosemicarbazone), with a limit of detection of 3 μg.l^{-1} in plasma or urine. Anti-infectious agents such as ethambutol, isoniazid, *p*-aminosalicylic acid, pyrazinamide, rifampicin, streptomycin, ethionamide, prothionamide, clofazimine and dapsone do not interfere with this assay. Other analytical methods are also available and have recently been described.[7]

The absorption of this compound is not well documented but appears to be slow. On oral administration of 150 mg, plasma concentrations of 1.6–3.2 mg.l^{-1} are found 4–5 hours following ingestion.[8,9] The mean plasma half life is 12.9 hours.

Unfortunately, no information is available from the literature concerning either the distribution of this agent into various tissues or its apparent volume of distribution. In normal plasma the drug appears to be 95% bound to proteins.[8] Likewise, no information is available from the literature concerning the penetration of this agent into CSF fluid.[10] Measurable quantities of thiacetazone have not been observed in either human breast milk or on placental transfer.[8]

Oral absorption	—
Presystemic metabolism	—
Plasma half life	
range	6–24 h
mean	12.9 h
Volume of distribution	—
Plasma protein binding	95%

Approximately 20% (range 9–43%), of unchanged thiacetazone is excreted into urine irrespective of the actual dose size in the range 150–600 mg.[3] One limited study indicated that 3.1% of the unchanged compound was excreted into the faeces over a 6 day period.[6] The effects of acute and chronic hepatic disease have not been documented. The urinary elimination of this compound is biphasic. In the first 24 hours the mean half life is 14 hours (range of 5–24 hours) and from 24 hours onward the apparent half life from the urinary excretion averaged 21.5 hours (range of 15.8–38.6 h).[9] Pharmacokinetics of this compound have not been reported in renal disease or in elderly patients.

Concentration–effect relationship

The bacterostatic effect of 150 mg of this agent administered orally may persist up to 24 hours after a single dose.[3] In this particular study the serum concentration at 24 hours was 0.6 mg.l^{-1}, which was above that for inhibition of most strains of *Mycobacterium tuberculosis*. The MIC for *Mycobacterium leprae* is usually 0.2 mg.l^{-1}.[2] and for *Mycobacterium tuberculosis* it is only 0.4 mg.l^{-1}.[3]

Metabolism

Limited information is available concerning the metabolism of this compound. Thus far, at least four metabolites have been identified: 4-aminobenzaldehyde thiosemicarbazone, 4-acetylaminobenzaldehyde, 4-aminobenzaldehyde and 4-acetylaminobenzoic acid (Fig. 1). Excretion of the free drug occurs mostly into the urine, with approximately 3.1% in the faeces. Less than 1% of a dose is excreted in the urine as

T

Holdiness M R 1985 Cerebrospinal fluid pharmacokinetics of the antituberculosis drugs. Clinical Pharmacokinetics 10: 532–534
Holdiness M R 1987 Teratogenicity of the antituberculosis drugs. Early Human Development 15: 61–74
Holdiness M R 1987 Neurological manifestations and toxicities of the antituberculosis drugs. Medical Toxicology 2: 33–51
Holdiness M R 1987 A review of iatrogenic nutritional deficiencies induced by antituberculosis drugs. Nutrition Research 7: 891–900
Holdiness M R 1987 A review of blood dyscrasias induced by antituberculosis drugs. Tubercle 68: 301–309

References

1. Holdiness M R 1987 Teratogenicity of the antituberculosis drugs. Early Human Development 15: 61–74
2. Marcus J C 1967 Nonteratogenicity of antituberculosis drugs. South African Medical Journal 41: 758–759
3. Ellard G A, Dickinson J M, Gammon P T, Mitchison D A 1974 Serum concentrations and antituberculosis activity of thiacetazone. Tubercle 55: 41–54
4. Colston M J, Hilson G R F, Lancaster R D 1980 Intermittent chemotherapy of experimental leprosy in mice. American Journal of Tropical Medicine and Hygiene 29: 103–108
5. Leat J L, Mares J 1970 Improvement of drug-sensitivity test on tubercle bacilli. Tubercle 51: 68–75
6. Jenner P J 1983 High performance liquid chromatographic determination of thiacetazone in body fluids. Journal of Chromatography Biomedical Applications 276: 463–470
7. Holdiness M R 1985 Chromatographic analysis of the antituberculosis drugs in biological samples. Journal of Chromatography Biomedical Applications 340: 321–359
8. Holdiness M R 1984 Clinical pharmacokinetics of the antituberculosis drugs. Clinical Pharmacokinetics 9: 511–544
9. Jenner P J, Ellard G A, Swai O B 1984 A study of thiacetazone blood levels and urinary excretion in man, using high performance liquid chromatography. Leprosy Review 55: 121–128
10. Holdiness M R 1985 Cerebrospinal pharmacokinetics of the antituberculosis drugs. Clinical Pharmacokinetics 10: 532–534
11. Joint IUAT/WHO Study Group 1982 Tuberculosis control. Tubercle 63: 157–169
12. Singapore Tuberculosis Services/Brompton Hospital/British Medical Research Council Investigation 1974 A controlled clinical trial of the role of thiacetazone containing regimens in the treatment of pulmonary tuberculosis in Singapore: second report. Tubercle 55: 251–260
13. East African/British Medical Research Council Fifth Thiacetazone Investigation — Third Report 1973 Isoniazid with thiacetazone in the treatment of pulmonary tuberculosis in East Africa. Third report of fifth investigation. Tubercle 54: 169–179
14. Fox W 1979 The current status of short-course chemotherapy. Tubercle 60: 177–190
15. Third East African/British Medical Research Council Study 1980 Controlled clinical trial for four short-course regimens of chemotherapy for two durations in the treatment of pulmonary tuberculosis. Tubercle 61: 59–69
16. Ellard G A 1984 The potential clinical significance of the isoniazid acetylator phenotype in the treatment of pulmonary tuberculosis. Tubercle 65: 211–227
17. Holdiness M R 1985 Adverse cutaneous reactions to antituberculosis drugs. International Journal of Dermatology 24: 280–285
18. Girling D J 1982 Adverse effects of antituberculosis drugs. Drugs 23: 56–74
19. Jopling W H 1983 Side effects of antileprosy drugs in common use. Leprosy Review 54: 261–270
20. Holdiness M R 1987 Neurological manifestations and toxicities of the antituberculosis drugs. Medical Toxicology 2: 33–51
21. Pearson C A 1978 Thiacetazone toxicity in the treatment of tuberculosis patients in Nigeria. Journal of Tropical Medicine and Hygiene 81: 238–242

Thiamine hydrochloride (Vitamin B_1)

Chemistry

Thiamine hydrochloride (vitamin B_1, Benerva, Betalin S, Betaxin, Bewon, Biamine)
$C_{12}H_{17}ClN_4OS.HCl$
3-(4-Amino-2-methylpyrimidin-5yl-methyl)-5-(2-hydroxyethyl)-4-methylthiazolium chloride hydrochloride

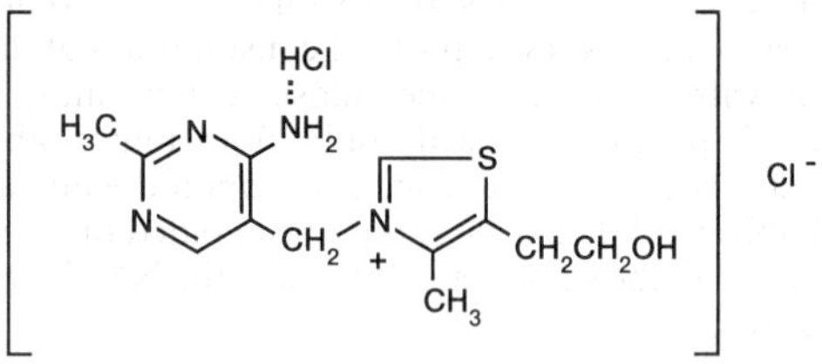

Molecular weight (free base)	337.3 (300.8)
pKa	4.8
Solubility	
in alcohol	1 in 100
in water	1 in 1
Octanol/water partition coefficient	—

Thiamine hydrochloride consists of colourless crystals, or a white crystalline powder, with a meat-like odour, and bitter taste. It is prepared by chemical synthesis.

Various multivitamin preparations (B-complex group) such as Neurobion and B-plex fort contain vitamin B_1 as an active ingredient, in tablets, capsules and injectable ampoules. They are also sold over the counter as nutritional supplements in the form of syrups and elixirs.

Pharmacology

Thiamine, in the form of thiamine pyrophosphate, is the coenzyme for decarboxylation of α-ketoglutaric acid. It also participates along with other coenzymes, i.e. lipoic acid, coenzyme A, FAD and NAD, in the oxidative decarboxylation of pyruvic acid, which leads to the formation of acetyl CoA.

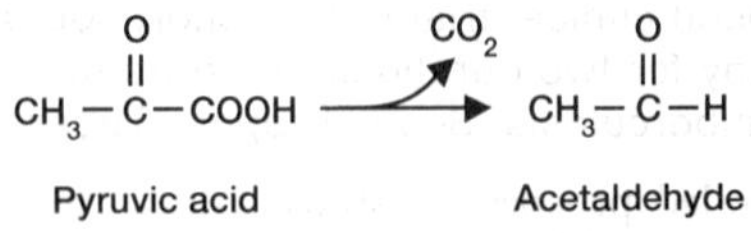

Thiamine pyrophosphate is also the coenzyme of transketolase. In thiamine deficiency, the hexose monophosphate pathway of glucose oxidation is retarded at the level of the transketolase, so pentose sugars accumulate to levels three times the normal.[1]

Thiamine deficiency affects the peripheral nervous system, the gastrointestinal tract, and the cardiovascular system. This vitamin is necessary for the optimal growth of infants and children. A heat-labile enzyme, thiaminase, present in raw fish destroys its activity. Chastek paralysis occurs in foxes fed a diet containing 10% or more of uncooked fish, due to the thiaminase in raw fish. Mild deficiencies of B_1 may occur even with apparently adequate diets, especially when energy needs are increased due to hyperthyroidism or increased carbohydrate intake.

Toxicology

There are no reports of teratogenic, mutagenic or carcinogenic effects of vitamin B_1.

Thiamine hydrochloride (Vitamin B_1)

Clinical pharmacology

Thiamine is not stored in the body, and is regularly lost from tissues during short periods of deficiency. In order to maintain normal health, an adequate amount of thiamine is required every day. Thiamine requirement is related to carbohydrate intake and the metabolic rate. A daily intake of 400 µg per 4200 kJ, i.e. 1000 kCal, is recommended. The total requirement increases during periods of active growth or heavy physical labour, during pregnancy and lactation, in pathological conditions such as fever and hyperthyroidism and in other conditions causing increased metabolism or diuresis.

In the body thiamine is converted to thiamine pyrophosphate, the main site of this reaction being the liver. Thiamine pyrophosphate acts as a coenzyme in the decarboxylation of α-keto acids such as pyruvate and α-ketoglutarate. In thiamine deficiency, pyruvic acid and lactic acid accumulate in tissues. Thiamine pyrophosphate also acts as the coenzyme of transketolase in the direct oxidative pathway of glucose metabolism. Deficiency of thiamine leads to fatigue, anorexia, gastrointestinal disturbance, tachycardia, irritability and neurological symptoms. Thiamine is devoid of pharmacodynamic action when given in usual therapeutic doses.

Beri-beri, a disease due to vitamin B_1 deficiency, is common in alcoholics, in pregnant women receiving an inadequate diet, and in people with malabsorption syndrome, prolonged diarrhoea and hepatic disease. Beri-beri is of two kinds:

(i) Chronic dry beri-beri, characterized by polyneuropathy
(ii) Acute wet beri-beri, in which oedema and serous effusions predominate.

Chronic dry beri-beri occurs in adults and is associated with malabsorption or multiple vitamin deficiencies. It may also occur in long-term dialysis and in patients on total parenteral feeding. In chronic alcoholism, Wernicke's encephalopathy may develop. This is characterized by ophthalmoplegia, ataxia, polyneuropathy, and mental deterioration, often accompanied by amnestic confabulatory psychosis. Immediate parenteral administration of vitamin B_1 is necessary in such situations to limit permanent damage to the CNS. Wet beri-beri is endemic in areas where polished rice forms a large part of the diet. It is associated with anorexia, muscle weakness, personality changes, severe circulatory disturbances, oedema, and heart failure. Severe deficiency in infants has been reported to be fatal. Oral administration of thiamine corrects most uncomplicated deficiencies but the parenteral route may be used in acute situations. In all individuals the absorptive capacity for thiamine is limited. The maximum individual oral dose absorbed is about 5 mg.

The clinical symptoms of deficiency are related to the amount of deprivation.[2] Encephalopathy and Korsakoff's syndrome result from severe deprivation and beri-beri and polyneuritis occur in milder conditions of deficiency. The commonest cause of B_1 deficiency is alcoholism. In this condition appetite is usually poor and food consumption drops, and a large portion of caloric intake is in the form of alcohol. Thiamine deficiency leads to polyneuritis with motor and sensory defects. Ophthalmoplegia, nystagmus, and ataxia, which respond rapidly to thiamine administration, are associated with Wernicke's syndrome. In Wernicke's encephalopathy, learning and memory are impaired. The other cognitive functions are intact. Korsakoff's psychosis is characterized by confabulations and is less likely to be reversible once established.[3] Thiamine stores of some patients with Wernicke's encephalopathy have an abnormality in the thiamine-dependent enzyme transketolase. The affinity of the enzyme for pyridoxal phosphate is reduced. Marginal deficiency of thiamine may be sufficient to produce serious neurological damage.[4] Chronic alcoholics with polyneuritis and motor or sensory defects have been given 40 mg of oral thiamine daily. Wernicke's syndrome is an emergency and is treated with daily doses of 100 mg of vitamin intravenously.

Infantile beri-beri occurs due to deficiency of thiamine in infancy. This is characterized by loss of appetite, vomiting and greenish stools, followed by paroxysmal attacks of muscular rigidity. Aphonia due to loss of laryngeal nerve function is a diagnostic feature. Signs of cardiac involvement are represented by rapid weak pulse, with face and neck veins being engorged due to cardiac failure. Death may occur within 12 to 24 hours unless vigorous treatment is instituted. Infants with a mild form of this condition respond to oral therapy with 10 mg of thiamine daily. If acute collapse occurs, doses of 25 mg intravenously are given but prognosis is very poor. Subacute necrotizing encephalopathy is a fatal disease of children which is represented by difficulty with feeding and swallowing, vomiting, hypotonia, external ophthalmoplegia and peripheral neuropathy.[5,6] Seizures are associated with this condition. Other inborn errors of thiamine metabolism have been described by Scriver.[7]

Gastrointestinal disorders such as ulcerative colitis, gastrointestinal hypotonia and chronic diarrhoea, have been found to be associated with beri-beri and thiamine is used as a therapeutic agent in such conditions.

During pregnancy thiamine requirement increases. Neuritis of pregnancy (due to thiamine deficiency) takes the form of multiple peripheral nerve involvement. The signs and symptoms resemble beri-beri. This problem occurs due to poor intake of thiamine or in patients with hyperemesis gravidarum. A dose of 5–10 mg (given parenterally) is recommended.

In thiamine deficiency the oxidation of α-keto acids is impaired and there is an increase in the pyruvate concentration in blood. This is used as one of the diagnostic signs of thiamine deficiency. A measure of transketolase activity in erythrocytes has also been used to monitor thiamine status.[1] Thiamine requirement is greatest when carbohydrate is the major energy source.

Thiamine is essential for metabolism of carbohydrates. Thiamine requirements are proportional to carbohydrate intake. Older people utilize thiamine less efficiently and a daily intake of 1 mg is recommended. During pregnancy and lactation an additional intake of 0.6 mg per 4200 kJ (1000 kcal) is recommended. Vitamin B_1 is not stored in the body. Hypermetabolic conditions increase the requirement for thiamine.

Pharmacokinetics

In early days the specific absorption as well as the analytical thiochrome procedure were used to assay this vitamin. Thiamine, along with other vitamins, is now estimated by high pressure liquid chromatography with fluorescence, which has a sensitivity[8,9] of 150 $mg.l^{-1}$.

Thiamine is well absorbed from the gastrointestinal tract and widely distributed throughout the body. At low or physiological thiamine concentrations, thiamine transport appears to be a saturable, active process. In contrast, at high or pharmacological doses transport is mainly by passive diffusion. Thiamine is rapidly absorbed from the upper small intestine. Thiamine is not stored in the body to any appreciable extent. Excess ingested thiamine appears in urine as intact thiamine or as pyrimidine which arises from degradation of the thiamine molecule.[10]

The plasma half life of thiamine is 24 h, whereas its half life in the body is 10–20 days. Normal levels of this vitamin in the blood are 0.2–0.4 $\mu g.l^{-1}$ in blood and 3.6 $\mu g.g^{-1}$ in brain. Human breast milk contains 230 $\mu g.l^{-1}$ of thiamine.

Oral absorption	high
Presystemic metabolism	—
Plasma half life	~24 h
Volume of distribution	—
Plasma protein binding	—

Concentration–effect relationship

The therapeutic dose depends upon the extent of deficiency. There is no evidence of any correlation between the plasma concentration of thiamine and its therapeutic effects.

Metabolism

Thiamine is not stored to any great extent in the body. Phosphorylated forms are present in all cells. Excess ingested vitamin is excreted in the urine as the free vitamin or a metabolite. Thiamine is phosphorylated to the active coenzyme, thiamine pyrophosphate (TPP), which functions as cocarboxylase for various reactions in carbohydrate metabolism, including the transketolase reaction in the direct oxidative pathway of glucose metabolism.

Thiamine hydrochloride (Vitamin B_1)

T

Pharmaceutics

Thiamine is prescribed as the pure vitamin, in a mixture of vitamins or in the form of vitamin-rich concentrates. Thiamine hydrochloride is a white crystalline powder.

Vitamin B_1 tablets are marketed containing 3 to 500 mg each of thiamine hydrochloride. Beneva tablets (Roche, UK) contain 25 mg, 50 mg, 100 mg or 300 mg of thiamine. An elixir containing 1 mg per 5 ml is available.

Thiamine hydrochloride injections contain 100 $mg.ml^{-1}$. Large parenteral doses are given in severe deficiency but there is no evidence that increased response occurs with doses larger than 300 mg daily. After symptoms of deficiency have been corrected, the dose required is not greater than the RDA. Intravenous doses should be administered slowly over at least 20 minutes to reduce the risk of idiosyncratic reactions.

On exposure to air of average humidity the vitamin absorbs a quantity of water corresponding to nearly one mole, forming a hydrate. Commercial vitamin contains about 4% water which is removable by drying at 100°C or in vacuum over sulphuric acid. In dry form the vitamin is stable. Heating at 100°C for 24 hours does not diminish potency. In aqueous solution, it can be sterilized at 110°C, but if the pH of the solution is above 5.5 it is destroyed rapidly. It should be stored in cool, dark, dry, non-metallic containers.

Therapeutic use

Indications

1. Treatment and prophylaxis of thiamine deficiency.

Contraindications

There are no absolute contraindications but the risk of anaphylaxis is increased by repeated parenteral administration.

Mode of use

The preferred route of administration is oral. However, intravenous and intramuscular preparations of vitamin B_1 are also available. Parenteral administration is unnecessary except in patients with impaired absorption or cardiac failure. Vitamin B_1 does not produce toxic effects when given orally and any excess is excreted rapidly in urine.

The recommended intake of thiamine is 400 μg per 4200 kJ (1000 kcal) of diet (Table 1).

Table 1 Recommended dietary intake of thiamine[11]

	Age	Dose per day (mg)
Infants	6 months	0.3
	6–12 months	0.5
Children	1–3 years	0.7
	4–6 years	0.9
	7–10 years	1.2
Males	11–18 years	1.4
	19–22 years	1.5
Females	11–22 years	1.1
	>23 years	1.0
Pregnancy		1.4
Lactation		1.5

With a vitamin B_1 dosage of more than 400 mg intravenously, subacute symptoms such as lethargy, somnolence, mild ataxia, heaviness in limbs, and diminution of gut tone were seen. Relief was achieved after 48 hours if vitamin B_1 was withheld.

Thiamine deficiency often occurs in association with deficiency of other vitamins, especially in severe malabsorption and malnutrition. Thiamine deficiency can also occur from consumption of raw fish containing thiaminase.[12,13] Thiamine deficiency is common in Thailand where fish is consumed fermented rather than cooked. Betal nut and tea leaves contain antithiamine compounds, i.e. caffeine and tannins.[14] Thiamine-rich foods include pork, offal, whole grains and enriched cereals, bread, legumes and nuts. Thiamine is stable in acidic solutions but is destroyed by heat in neutral or alkaline solutions.

Doses as large as 100 $mg.l^{-1}$ of parenteral fluid are used in severe thiamine deficiency. Once thiamine deficiency is corrected there is no need for parenteral administration or for the administration of amounts in excess of daily requirement. It is recommended that chronic alcoholics with polyneuritis and motor or sensory deficit receive 40 mg of oral thiamine daily. Infantile beri-beri is treated with 10 mg of thiamine daily.

Precautions

Allergic sensitivity may develop, especially after parenteral use. Intramuscular injections are painful. No untoward effects occur when thiamine is administered orally in amounts greater than the therapeutic dose. Anaphylactic reactions have been produced by injection of thiamine given alone. The risk of anaphylactic shock increases with repeated administration by the parenteral route.

Adverse reactions

Potentially life-threatening effects
Vitamin B_1 does not have adverse effects when given orally, but in a few fatal cases anaphylactic reactions have occurred after intravenous administration of large doses (400 mg) in sensitive patients, especially children, and in one case following an intramuscular dose of 125 mg.[15] The risk of such reactions increases with repeated administration of the drug by the parenteral route.

Acute overdosage
No cases of deliberate overdosage have been reported.

Severe or irreversible adverse effects
In patients with a history of sensitivity to vitamin B_1, pruritis, urticaria, weakness, sweating, nausea, restlessness, tightness of throat, angioneurotic oedema, cyanosis, pulmonary oedema, haemorrhage into the gastrointestinal tract and collapse have been reported.

Symptomatic adverse effects
Transient mild soreness may occur at the site of intramuscular or subcutaneous injection, and when the intravenous administration is given too rapidly. The patient may experience temporary faintness or dizziness. Intramuscular injections are painful. Following prolonged parenteral administration of large doses the following symptoms may occur: nausea, anorexia, lethargy, somnolence, mild ataxia, and heaviness in limbs. All symptoms subside within a few days when treatment is stopped.

Interference with clinical pathology tests
No interferences of this kind have been reported.

High risk groups

The drug may be given safely to neonates, children, pregnant and lactating women and elderly patients.

Drug interactions

Potentially hazardous interactions
No interactions of this kind have been reported.

Potentially useful interactions
Vitamin B_1 acts synergistically with other vitamins of the B-complex group and its potential for causing adverse effects is considerably reduced.

General review articles

Anderson W I, Morrow L A 1987 Thiamine deficiency encephalopathy with concurrent myocardial degeneration and polyradiculoneuropathy in a cat. Cornell Veterinarian 77: 251–257

Freeman G B, Nielsen P E, Gibson G E 1987 Effect of age on behavioural and enzymatic changes during thiamine deficiency. Neurobiology of Aging 8: 429–434

Le-Roche K, Riche D, Sara S J 1987 Persistence of habituation deficits after neurological recovery from severe thiamine deprivation. Behavioural Brain Research 26: 37–46

Patrini C, Reggiani C, Laforenza U, Rindi G 1988 Blood–brain transport of thiamine monophosphate in the rat: a kinetic study in vivo. Journal of Neurochemistry 50: 90–93

Sable H Z, Gubler C J (eds) 1982 Thiamine, twenty years of progress. Annals of New York Academy of Science. New York Academy of Science, vol 378
Thomas A D, Jeyasingham M D, Pratt D E, Shaw G K 1987 Nutrition and alcoholic encephalopathies. Acta Medica Scandinavica (suppl) 717: 55–65
Van-der Westhuyzen J, Davies R E, Icke G C, Jenkins T 1987 Thiamine status and biochemical indices of malnutrition and alcoholism in settled communities of Kung San. Journal of Tropical Medicine and Hygiene 90: 283–289
Van-Noort B A, Bos P J, Klopping C, Wilmink J M 1987 Optic neuropathy from thiamine deficiency in a patient with ulcerative colitis. Documenta Ophthalmologica 67: 45–51
Waldenlind L 1978 Studies on thiamine and neuromuscular transmission. Acta Physiologica Scandinavica (suppl 459): 1–35

References

1. Brin M 1968 Blood transketolase determination in the diagnosis of thiamine deficiency. Heart Bulletin 17: 86–89
2. McLaren D 1978 Metabolic disorders. In: Conn H F (ed) Current therapy. W B Saunders, Philadelphia, pp 409–410
3. Victor M, Adam R D, Collins G H 1971 The Wernicke–Korsakoff syndrome. F A Davis, Philadelphia, pp 1–206
4. Blass J P, Gibson G E 1977 Abnormality of thiamine requiring enzyme in patients with Wernicke–Korsakoff syndrome. New England Journal of Medicine 297: 1367–1376
5. Pincus J H, Cooper J R, Murphy J V, Rabe E F, Lansdale D, Dunn H G 1973 Thiamine derivatives in subacute necrotizing encephalopathy, a preliminary report. Pediatrics 51: 716–721
6. Pincus J H, Cooper J R, Piros K, Turner V 1974 Specificity of urine inhibitor test for Leigh's disease. Neurology (Minneap) 24: 885–890
7. Scriver C R 1973 Vitamin responsive inborn errors of metabolism. Metabolism 22: 1319–1344
8. Botticher B, Botticher D 1987 A new HPLC method for the simultaneous determination of B_1, B_2 and B_6 vitamers in serum and whole blood. International Journal of Vitamin and Nutrition Research 57: 273–278
9. Lavigne C, Zee I A, Simard R E, Gosselin C 1987 High performance liquid chromatographic diode array determination of ascorbic acid, thiamine and riboflavin in goat's milk. Journal of Chromatography 20: 410(1) 202–205
10. Yoyumpa A M 1982 Characterization of normal intestinal thiamine transport in animals and man. In: Sable H Z, Gubler C T (eds) Annals of the New York Academy of Sciences, vol 378, pp 337–346
11. 1980 Recommended dietary allowances, 9th edn. National Research Council, Washington
12. Murata K 1965 Thiaminase. In: Simazono N, Katsura E (eds) Review of Japanese literature on beri-beri and thiamine. Igaku Shoin Ltd, Tokyo, pp 220–254
13. Fugita A 1954 Thiaminase. Advances in Enzymology 15: 389–421
14. Vimakesant S L, Nakornchi S, Dhanamutta S, Hilker D M 1974 Effect of tea consumption on thiamine status in man. Nutrition Reports International 9: 371–374
15. Assem E S K 1973 Anaphylactic reaction to thiamine. Practitioner 211: 565

Thioguanine

Developed in the 1940s, 6-thioguanine is one of the original thiopurines and has been used widely in the treatment of acute leukaemia.

Chemistry

Thioguanine (6-thioguanine, 6TG, Lanvis)
$C_5H_5N_5S$
2-Aminopurino-6(1H)-thione

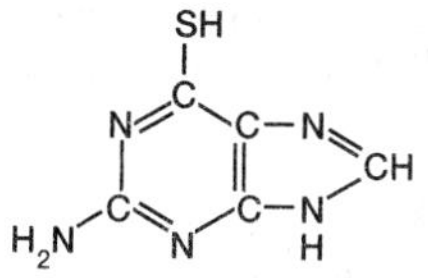

Molecular weight	167.2
pKa	8.1
Solubility	
in alcohol	practically insoluble
in water	practically insoluble
Octanol/water partition coefficient	high

A pale yellow, odourless or almost odourless crystalline powder, 6-thioguanine (6TG) is used clinically in tablet form. It is not available in combination with any other drugs. 6-Thioguanine is readily soluble in dilute alkaline solutions.

Pharmacology

6TG is an analogue of guanine and participates in many of the same cellular reactions as guanine. Guanine is converted to the nucleotide guanylic acid (guanine-ribose-phosphate, GRP) by the enzyme hypoxanthine guanine phosphoribosyl transferase (HGPRT). 6TG competes with guanine for this enzyme. Despite intensive study, it has not been possible to define every single main site of action. Cytotoxicity may be due to a series of effects caused by sequential blockade of purine nucleotide biosynthesis. Three major areas of interference have been identified experimentally.

1. Incorporation of thioguanine nucleotides into DNA and RNA. In some drug-resistant cell lines this uptake may be suppressed.
2. Thioguanylic acid (6TGRP) acts as a pseudo feedback inhibitor of de novo purine synthesis. 6TGRP thus inhibits phosphoribosyl pyrophosphate-amido transferase.
3. Inhibition of purine nucleotide interconversion.

Thus thioguanylate (6TGRP) inhibits two enzymes and 6TG is incorporated direct into DNA as the deoxynucleoside triphosphate. Supporting this latter mechanism of action as the major effect, arabinosyl cytosine (cytarabine — AraC), an inhibitor of DNA synthesis, protects mice against the toxicity of simultaneously administered 6TG. There is also incorporation of 6TG into RNA and it is possible that metabolic alterations result, thus contributing to its cytotoxicity.

Toxicology

The toxicology of the various thiopurines has been examined in mice, rats, cats and dogs. It has been concluded that there is no significant difference between the various thiopurines on the basis of a single dose but 6TG is ten times more toxic than 6-mercaptopurine on daily administration for 5 days. 6TG produces neutropenia, anaemia, thrombocytopenia and prolongation of clotting time, but all these effects are reversible after drug administration has been discontinued. Hepatic lesions typical of 6-mercaptopurine intoxication, however, were not seen with 6TG. 6TG also appears to cause protein catabolism in addition to its effect on bone marrow, thus probably contributing to the weight loss seen in tumour-bearing mice in controlled experiments. There is no evidence of its causing mutagenic effects in experimental animals.

Clinical pharmacology

Thioguanine is a cytotoxic drug primarily used for the induction of remissions in acute myelogenous leukaemia. 6TG is a cell cycle-specific drug and it kills cells exposed in G1 and S-phases. It has a self-limiting effect as it interferes with the progress of the cell cycle. In some systems, following a short exposure to 6TG, cells are able to undergo one or two divisions before cytotoxicity is seen. There is some improvement in the therapeutic ratio in mice for ascites tumour against normal tissue when 6TG is given over 24 hours instead of 12-hourly. However, because the S-phase in human leukaemia lasts for about 20 hours, there may be an advantage to 12-hourly, twice daily dosage. In man the cumulative effect of repeated doses leads to the induction of enzymes that anabolyse 6TG to 6TGRP as well as di- and triphosphates. Compared with a single dose, it has been shown that 6TG and 6TGRP may be increased 100-fold following five repeated doses.

Pharmacokinetics

The most successful analytical method for 6TG has been the measurement of the radioactivity levels of ^{35}S-labelled thioguanine in man. However, methods are now available utilizing spectrofluorimetry (sensitivity 5 $\mu g.l^{-1}$)[1] and HPLC with UV detection (sensitivity 130 $\mu g.l^{-1}$)[2] for measuring the unlabelled compound itself in plasma.

6TG is incompletely absorbed following oral administration and also shows considerable individual variation. The amount absorbed after oral administration is less than half the administered dose. Free thioguanine is undetectable in the blood after oral administration of unlabelled drug and little or no unchanged thioguanine is excreted in the urine. The inability to detect thioguanine, however, does not give any indication of cytotoxic effect and is not of prognostic significance since the drug is active intracellularly.

The half life of nucleotide derivatives in the tissues is very prolonged. The early studies on labelled drug showed maximum radioactivity between 8 and 12 hours following oral administration.[3] Following intravenous administration the mean plasma half life varies widely, with a median of 80 minutes. 6TG is eliminated primarily in the urine. The drug appears unchanged in the urine in the first two hours after intravenous dosage but thereafter only metabolites are excreted. Following oral administration, it is not possible to recover unchanged drug in the urine, but 24–46% of the administered dose can be recovered as the metabolites 6-methyl thioguanine, 6-thiouric acid and also desulphurated metabolites. 6TG is not extensively deaminated in contrast with 6-mercaptopurine and azathiopurine, so that only a small amount is converted to the 6-thiouric acid. 6TG distributes widely and rapidly throughout and after 20 hours all tissues except brain show a higher concentration of 6TG or 6TG metabolites than does the blood.

Oral absorption	24–46%
Presystemic metabolism	nil
Plasma half life	
range	3–6 h
Volume of distribution	—
Plasma protein binding	—

Concentration–effect relationship

The effect of 6TG on the target tissues in man is dose-dependent but also dependent upon the growth status of the tissue. Incorporation of DNA into marrow is usually very low after administration of a single dose of 6TG, but after five daily doses the DNA is largely occupied by 6TG.[4] This indicates that most marrow cells enter DNA synthesis during the 5-day period. Studies have been conducted examining 6TG at single daily doses of between 67.5 $mg.m^{-2}$ and 135 $mg.m^{-2}$. Incorporation of 6TG into DNA is roughly linear for 8 hours after an intravenous dose but this shortens to a 4-hour phase after an oral dose. All these data suggest that the concentration–effect relationship is strongly related to schedule rather than total dose employed.[5]

Metabolism and excretion

Before it is active, 6TG must be metabolized to the active metabolite thioguanylic acid (6TGRP). The cumulative effect of repeated doses leads to the induction of enzymes that metabolize 6TG to thioguanylic acid and its di and triphosphates (Fig. 1). Thioguanine is also metabolized to inactive compounds via two major routes: methylation to 2-amino-6-methylthiopurine[6] and deamination by guanase to 6-thioxanthine.[7] This metabolite is oxidized by xanthine oxidase to 6-thiouric acid. Allopurinol does not affect the toxicity or the antitumour activity of thioguanine. Although there may be a build up of 6-thioxanthine, the main reason that allopurinol does not potentiate the toxicity of 6-thioguanine is that the deamination pathway is weak. The major labelled urinary metabolites of ^{35}S-thioguanine are inorganic sulphate, 2-amino-6-methyl thiopurine and thiouric acid.

Pharmaceutics

6TG is available in oral form.

1. Lanvis (Wellcome, UK): pale yellow, round, biconvex tablets containing 40 mg of thioguanine. They are scored and marked as 'WELLCOME U3B'.
2. A 100 mg tablet is available from Burroughs Wellcome (USA). The tablets are pale yellow, round biconvex and impressed with the legend 'Wellcome USA'. 6TG is available for intravenous use as a clear solution containing 6TG 100 mg in 5 ml (available from the National Cancer Institute). 6TG preparations are stable with a reasonable shelf-life and carry a minimum risk from potentially allergenic substances. Preparations should be protected from light.

Therapeutic use

Indications

1. Induction of remission in acute myeloblastic leukaemia in children and in adults.

Contraindications

Pregnancy.

Mode of use

Clinical effect depends upon the induction of cytostasis in rapidly growing malignancies typified by acute myeloblastic leukaemia. Oral treatment is typically 100 $mg.m^{-2}$ twice daily over 3–5 days in current schedules in combination with other cytotoxic drugs. Thioguanine may be given once or twice daily under various regimes. It is almost never used in isolation and doses have to be modified for this reason in accordance with the effects of concomitantly administered cytotoxic drugs. Profound myelotoxicity is almost inevitable in acute leukaemias as it is important to obtain maximum incorporation of the drug into the tumour DNA.[8]

Indications

Acute myelogenous leukaemia

In 1966 Burchenall[9] suggested that there had been no evidence of cross-resistance between anti-pyrimidine and anti-purine substances in mouse tumour systems and a synergistic effect could be expected between cytosine arabinoside and thiopurines. Cytosine arabinoside had been shown to have potent activity in granulocytic leukaemias but discontinuation of therapy was often followed by relapse.[10] Improved survival rates were obtained in combination with purine analogues in the treatment of mouse L1210 leukaemias. Cytosine arabinoside/thioguanine was thereafter used in acute myeloblastic monocytic and myelomonocytic leukaemia (AML) and in occasional cases with lymphoblastic leukaemia (ALL). The combined and partial remission rates were for cytosine arabinoside alone around 17%; in combination with thioguanine increasing to 50%. Attempts to improve the therapeutic efficacy of cytosine arabinoside/thioguanine suggested that since thioguanine is rapidly absorbed from the bloodstream by the tissues and rapidly metabolized, it was logical to use the drug every 12 hours since it is converted into its active form, the nucleotide thioguanylic acid, only within the cell and the nucleotide cannot traverse the cell wall. Hence 12-hourly administration is likely to lead to greater cytocidal effects on myeloblastic tumour cells in cycle although possibly at the cost of increased toxicity. This resulted in a protocol using 12-hourly administration of cytosine arabinoside at 3 $mg.kg^{-1}$ intravenously and thioguanine at 2.5 $mg.kg^{-1}$ orally until over 90% of the leukaemic cells had been destroyed. Therapy was routinely discontinued after between 11 and 36 administrations because maximum bone marrow depressant effect was not seen until 10–14 days later. After 3 weeks respite, the treatment cycle was repeated.

6TG has been used for about 15 years in combination with daunomycin and cytosine arabinoside in the induction of acute myelogenous leukaemia in adults and children.[11,12] The first evaluation of 6TG with cytosine arabinoside (AraC) was in 40 unselected patients with AML and ALL. A remission lasting a mean of 6 months occurred in 21 out of 38 patients with AML.[13] Considerable support for the efficacy of this therapy came from studies from the CALGB Group in Boston. Modifications of this original regime were made altering the induction regime to 5 successive days on an intermittent schedule and giving the thioguanine 12-hourly.[14] Although some remissions occurred lasting in excess of 4 years, the majority of patients failed to enter permanent remission and a major change was produced only when a third drug, daunomycin, was added to the regime.[15] In initial studies, response rates increased to 82% mainly due to complete remissions using a 7-day course of arabinosyl cytosine 100 $mg.m^{-2}$ together with thioguanine at 100 $mg.m^{-2}$ 12-hourly and daunomycin at 60 $mg.m^{-2}$ added on days 5, 6 and 7. A long follow-up has been reported on 1127 patients with AML treated with this 'DAT' schedule, showing that 67% of all patients had complete remission using this induction schedule. The remission rates were poorer at 50% for those aged over 60 years compared with 74% for those aged less than 60 years. A marked effect of survival benefit was seen for those entering on this therapy later in the trial compared with those in the initial phase. This indicates the importance of excellent supportive therapy in influencing the survival benefit of treatments for acute leukaemia. The median survival for all patients is just 12 months but 18% of the population are alive and disease-free at 5 years, with an advantage for survival in children and young adults (less than 30 years of age). The early clinical trials of thioguanine carried out before multiple therapy was generally adopted indicated the optimum dosage was 2.5 $mg.kg^{-1}$ body weight per day. Remissions were seen in 4 of 5 patients with chronic myelocytic leukaemia, one remaining in remission fourteen months after treatment. Observations on 33 patients with chronic granulocytic leukaemia indicated that effective doses of this drug and other thiopurines were similar. Thioguanine could produce responses lasting between 2 and 69 months in 25 cases.

Contraindications

Pregnancy

This is a potentially teratogenic drug and should not be administered to women in the first trimester of pregnancy. However, a number of infants have been born to mothers who have received thioguanine during pregnancy. An apparently normal full-term infant was delivered to a mother with acute myeloblastic leukaemia treated with thioguanine starting on the 25th week of pregnancy. However, a second mother was treated with cytosine arabinoside and thioguanine at 2.5 $mg.kg^{-1}$ daily starting during the 20th week of pregnancy and was delivered of a stillborn infant by therapeutic abortion in the 24th week. Cultures of the chorionic tissue showed evidence of trisomy C and a very abnormal chromosome pattern.

Adverse reactions

Potentially life-threatening effects

A myelosuppressant cytotoxic drug, 6TG is capable of producing irreversible bone marrow depression. Apart from simple overdosage

Fig. 1 Metabolism of 6-thioguanine

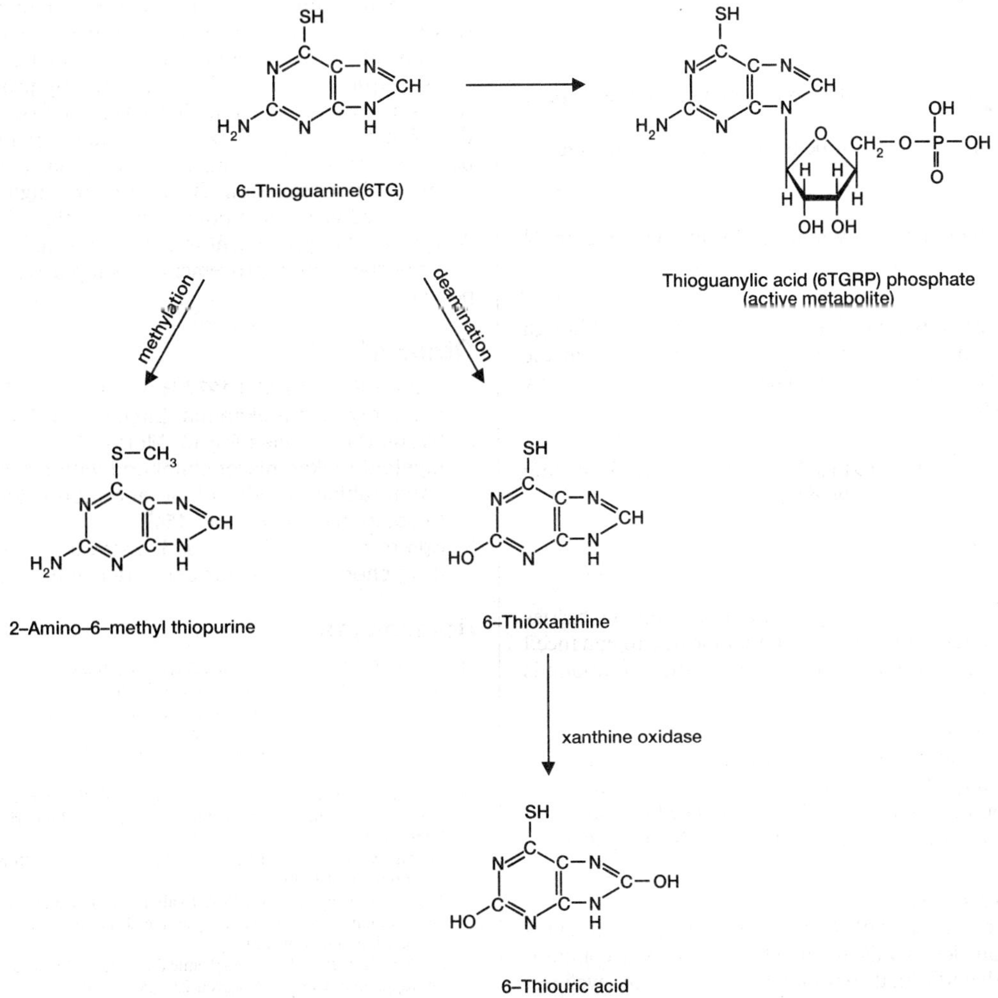

of the drug, these situations may occur (a) when the bone marrow reserve is impaired due to disease, such as infiltration by leukaemia, (b) when the patient has been irradiated in areas including the normal marrow, (c) when the drug is given together with concomitant bone marrow suppressive agents such as most other cytotoxic drugs.

Acute overdosage
Cases of deliberate overdose of 6TG have not been recorded. When excessive toxicity is recognized, the only useful therapy is supportive treatment with antibiotics to cover the problems of neutropenia, and platelet transfusions to cover the period of excessive thrombocytopenia. It is usual to reserve platelet transfusions for symptomatic bleeding rather than just to treat low counts.

Severe or irreversible adverse effects
The unwanted side effects of thioguanine are similar to those of other thiopurines. Prolonged administration at 2.5 mg.kg^{-1} daily can cause leucopenia, gastrointestinal upset and occasionally anaemia or prolongation of the clotting time. Leucopenic and thrombocytopenic effects can occur at therapeutic dosages and gastrointestinal disturbances are quite frequent. Leucopenia occurs on average within three to five weeks of treatment after 60 mg.kg^{-1} of thioguanine is taken, and to this extent it is probably less toxic dose for dose than 6-mercaptopurine. Because of its slightly reduced toxicity to the marrow, 6-thioguanine may be preferred to 6-mercaptopurine in multidrug regimes. Thioguanine exerts hepatotoxic effects due to biliary stasis but these effects are less severe than those seen with 6-mercaptopurine. Rarely veno-occlusive disease of the liver has been seen and in one case centrilobular necrosis.[16–20]

Symptomatic adverse effects
As mentioned earlier, gastrointestinal effects are common.

Other effects
Thioguanine may cause moderate elevation of the serum alkaline phosphatase and bilirubin because of its mild hepatotoxic effect.

Interference with clinical pathology tests
None has been reported.

High risk groups

Neonates
The drug is rarely used in neonates, but when used the dose is calculated on a mg:kg basis.

Breast milk. Children should not be breast-fed by women receiving cytotoxic drugs.

Children
Children receive the same dosage regimes as adults on a mg.kg.$^{-1}$ basis.

Pregnant women
This drug is mutagenic and is contraindicated in pregnancy, although successful pregnancies have been reported following therapy in the second and third trimesters with combinations of chemotherapy including thioguanine.

The elderly
No special precautions are required as doses are adjusted according to the direct myelotoxic effects of the drug.

Drug interactions

Potentially hazardous interactions
Any cytotoxic drug which has toxicity for the bone marrow carries the risk of a negative interaction with 6-thioguanine due to enhanced myelotoxicity. Other significant reactions with other compounds have not been reported.

Other significant reactions

Allopurinol. When allopurinol is administered, it has little effect on the efficacy and safety of thioguanine, as opposed to the effect on 6-mercaptopurine, the metabolism of which is reduced considerably by allopurinol, often requiring dose reductions by as much as 60–70%.

Potentially useful interactions
Arabinosyl cytosine combines with 6-thioguanine to produce cytotoxicity against human leukaemia in the clinic. This is a common combination now with additional compounds such as anthracyclines.

Other drug interactions have been shown recently, for example 6TG produces additive or greater than additive effects against human tumour cells in vitro when combined with α-interferon. Both 6TG and α_2-interferon are capable of inducing differentiation in HL60 cell lines and both suppress the production of Cmyc-mRNA by 98% at 48 hours. This seems to correlate with differentiation rather than cytotoxicity. Synergy has also been reported for thiopurines combined with alkylating agents by pretreating mice bearing human glioma xenografts. Thioguanine can potentiate nitrosoureas and procarbazine. The mechanism of the nitrosourea–thioguanine synergy remains uncertain although it may be that the incorporation of a thiol group into cellular DNA increases its susceptibility to alkylation.

Major outcome trials

1. Rees J K H, Gray R G, Swirsky D, Hayhoe F G J 1986 Principal results of the Medical Research Council's 8th Acute Myeloid Leukaemia Trial. Lancet 2:

Between 1978 and 1983, 1127 patients with acute myeloid leukaemia (AML) were entered into the MRC's 8th AML trial. All received the same induction therapy consisting of daunorubicin, cytarabine and 6-thioguanine (DAT 1+5). 67% of patients entered complete remission and were randomized to consolidation with two or six further courses of DAT. Adults aged less than 55 were randomized for CNS prophylaxis with intrathecal cytarabine and methotrexate. Finally, those still in remission after 1 year of cytarabine and thioguanine maintenance were randomized to receive either late intensification with cyclophosphamide, vincristine, cytarabine and prednisolone (COAP) or continued AT. The median survival for the whole group was 12 months, the median duration of first remission 15 months, with relapse-free survival at 5 years estimated at 18%. The factors most strongly associated with poor survival were poor performance status and advanced age at presentation, but even amongst patients over 60 years of age half went into remission. Six courses of DAT consolidation gave a small advantage compared with two courses, reducing the number of late relapses but there was no significant survival advantage. Late intensification showed a marginally significant advantage over continued AT maintenance. The incidence of CNS relapse was low and not affected by prophylaxis. The second remission rate varied from 10% when the first remission was shorter than 6 months to 61% when continued for more than 2 years. 40 patients received histocompatible allogeneic bone marrow transplantations in first remission. Because of the high initial death rate the transplanted group had poorer survival than those not transplanted. A significant improvement in the survival in later cohorts underlined the importance of improvements in supportive care over the five-year period.

Other trials

1. Gale R P, Cline M J 1977 High remission induction rate in acute myeloid leukaemia. Lancet 1: 497–499
2. Evans D I K, Jones P H M, Morley C J 1975 Treatment of acute myeloid leukaemia of childhood with cytosine arabinoside, daunorubicin, prednisolone and mercaptopurine or thioguanine. Cancer 36: 1547
3. Spiers A S D, Goldman J M, Catovsky D et al 1977 Multiple drug chemotherapy for acute leukaemia. Cancer 40: 20–29

References

1. Dooley T, Maddocks J L 1980 Assay of 6-thioguanine in human plasma British Journal of Clinical Pharmacology 9: 77–82
2. Andrews P A, Egoron M J, May M E, Bachur N R 1982 Revised phase high-performance liquid chromatography analysis of 6-thioguanine applicable to pharmacologic studies in humans Journal of Chromatography 227 Biomedical Applications 16: 83–91
3. Elion G B L, Callahan S W, Hitchings G W, Rundles R W, Laszlo J 1962 Experimental, clinical and metabolic studies of thiopurines. Cancer Chemotherapy Reports 16: 197–202
4. Le Page G A 1960 Incorporation of 6-thioguanine into nucleic acids. Cancer Research 20: 403–408
5. A M A Council on Drugs 1967 Evaluation of two anti-neoplastic agents, pipobroman (vercyte) and thioguanine. Journal of the American Medical Association 200: 139–140
6. Le Page G A 1963 Basic biochemical effects and mechanisms of actions of 6-thioguanine. Cancer Research 23: 1202–1206

7. Le Page G A, Whitecar J P Jr 1971 Pharmacology of 6-thioguanine in man. Cancer Research 31: 1627–1631
8. Beard M E J, Fairley G H 1974 Acute leukaemia in adults. Seminars in Haematology 11: 5–24
9. Burchenall J H 1956 Clinical effects of purines. Medical Clinics of North America 40: 935–949
10. Carey R W, Ribasmundo M, Ellison R R 1975 Comparative study of cytosine arabinoside therapy alone and combined with thioguanine, mercaptopurine or daunorubicin in acute myelocytic leukaemia. Cancer 36: 1560–1566
11. EORTC 1974 Joint Report. A second comparative trial in remission induction by cytosine arabinoside given every twelve hours or CAR and thioguanine or CAR and daunorubicin and maintenance therapy by CAR or methyl GAG in acute myeloid leukaemia. European Journal of Cancer 10: 413–418
12. MRC 1974 Joint Report. Treatment of acute myeloid leukaemia with daunorubicin, cytosine arabinoside, mercaptopurine, L-asparaginase, prednisolone and thioguanine — results of treatment with five multiple drug schedules. British Journal of Haematology 27: 373–389
13. Spiers A S D 1972 Multiple drug regimen for refractory acute leukaemias. British Journal of Haematology 23: 262–263
14. Spiers A S D, Gordon D H E, Cower J, Goldman J M 1975 Thioguanine as primary treatment for chronic myelocytic leukaemia. Lancet 1: 829–832
15. Spiers A S D, Roberts P D, Marsh G W et al 1975 Acute lymphoblastic leukaemia — clinical chemotherapy with three combinations of four drugs, COAP, POMP, CAR regimen. British Medical Journal 4: 614–617
16. Griner P F, Elbadawi A, Packman C H 1976 Veno-occlusive disease of the liver after chemotherapy of acute leukemia. Report of two cases Annals of Internal Medicine 85: 578–582
17. Gill R A, Orstad G R, Cardemon J M, Maneval D C, Sumner H W 1982 Hepatic veno-occlusive disease caused by 6-thioguanine Annals of Internal Medicine 96: 58–60
18. Krivoy N, Raz R, Carter A, Alroy G 1982 Reversible hepatic veno-occlusive disease and 6-thioguanine Annals of Internal Medicine 96: 788
19. Satti M B, Weinbren K, Gordon Smith E C 1982 6-Thioguanine as a cause of toxic veno-occlusive disease of the liver Journal of Clinical Pathology 35: 1086–1091
20. D'Cruz C A, Wimmer R S, Harcki H T, Huff D S, Naiman J L 1983 Veno-occlusive disease of the liver in children following chemotherapy for acute myclocytic leukemia Cancer 52: 298–304

Thiopentone (sodium)

Thiopentone was the first thiobarbiturate to be used as a rapidly acting intravenous anaesthetic. It still remains the most widely used drug for induction of general anaesthesia.

Chemistry

Thiopentone (Intraval, Pentothal, thiopental sodium)
$C_{11}H_{17}N_2S\ NaO_2$
Na salt of dl-5-ethyl-5'(1-methylbutyl)-2-thiobarbiturate.
4,6,(1H,5H)-Pyrimedinedione-5-ethyldihydro-5-(1-methylbutyl)-2-thioxo monosodium salt

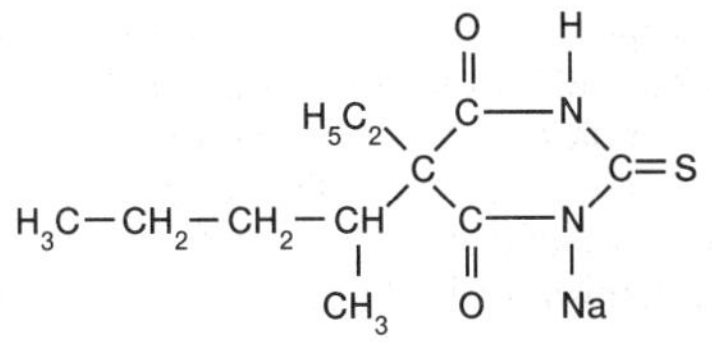

Molecular weight (free acid)	264.3 (242.3)
pKa	7.6
Solubility	
in alcohol	1 in 10–1 in 30
in water	1 in 1.5
Octanol/water partition coefficient	high

The sodium salt of thiopentone is a pale yellow to pale green hygroscopic powder, with a bitter taste, prepared from substituted derivatives of malonic acid and urea. It is freely soluble in water. Thiopentone is optically active, the racemate is used clinically. It is not present in any compound preperations.

Pharmacology

Thiopentone reversibly depresses the activity of all excitable tissues. The central nervous system (CNS) is particularly sensitive to its action and single anaesthetic induction doses have remarkably little effect on skeletal, cardiac or even smooth muscle. In healthy subjects it is only with large doses and/or prolonged administration that one encounters serious cardiovascular or respiratory depression and deleterious effects on other systems.

The exact mode of action of the barbiturates is not known, but a likely mechanism is a direct effect on the specialized portions of the neural membrane, modifying synaptic transmission. The ability of a number of agents to depress Na-dependent excitatory synaptic transmission can be correlated with hydrophobicity which, in turn, is strongly correlated with anaesthetic potency in vivo. Available evidence suggests that excitatory synaptic transmission is mainly depressed by barbiturates while inhibitory synaptic transmission is usually unaffected or enhanced. The site of action appears to be at a component of the ion channel control mechanism rather than on the associated receptor.

The effects of barbiturates on the various pathways and subsystems of the CNS represent the total effect of these complex and diverse actions of the drugs on many millions of individual neurones. For obvious reasons, pathways subserving the maintenance of consciousness and centripetal transfer of sensory information have been the main objects of study in investigations of barbiturate action. The spinal cord dorsal horn has an important modulatory role in the onward transfer of sensory information. Monosynaptic spinal reflexes are depressed by barbiturates as are spontaneous and evoked

Thiopentone (sodium)

T

activity in dorsal horn cells. Thus, action at spinal cord level contributes to the overall picture of barbiturate anaesthesia. In contrast, the classical sensory pathways of the spinal cord and brain stem, which contain only two or three synapses, appear to be relatively resistant to the effects of barbiturates.

However, information also travels cortically in the multisynaptic reticular formation. The demonstration[1] that stimulation of the reticular formation causes electroencephalographic (EEG) and behavioural arousal suggests that an action at this site might have a role in the production of the anaesthetic state. Pentobarbitone blocks sensory and auditory cortical evoked responses by a direct action on the reticular formation,[2] while EEG arousal in response to direct reticular stimulation is also blocked by barbiturates.[3] Analysis of the effects of thiopentone on the human sensory evoked response shows that the late component of the response, which is believed to be due to reticular stimulation, is blocked by anaesthetic doses of the drug, while the early, specific component remains intact.[4] These results suggest that reticular formation blockade is an essential component of the mechanism of barbiturate action on the brain. Depression by barbiturates of transmission through the ventrobasal thalamus has also been attributed to an effect on reticular tone.[5]

Functional denervation of the cortex, through increased inhibitory and decreased facilitatory reticular stimulation of the ventrobasal thalamus, may be a general mechanism of anaesthesia. However, there is no simple relationship between the concentration of a drug which produces anaesthesia and that which blocks cortical evoked responses.[6] Furthermore, the complex effects of barbiturates and other anaesthetics on synaptic transmission in isolated slices of cortex provide evidence of the probable importance of direct cortical effects, as well as of ascending systems, in the mechanism of barbiturate anaesthesia.

Toxicology

There are no relevant data on the chronic toxicology of thiopentone, including teratogenicity and carcinogenicity. This is not important as the drug is usually given only once over a very short period of time. Although hepatic dysfunction has been described following the use of large doses of thiopentone in animals, there are no clinical data to suggest that normal induction doses have a hepatotoxic effect, even in patients with an already damaged liver. It is, however, possible to demonstrate transient impairment of brain function tests following large doses and after infusions.[7]

Clinical pharmacology

Adequate doses of thiopentone will induce anaesthesia in one arm–brain circulation time and maximum depression of vital centres occurs within 1 min of administration. The loss of consciousness is usually smooth, although it is occasionally accompanied by slight spontaneous muscle movement, particularly in unpremedicated subjects. The plasma level necessary for anaesthesia in fit patients is around 40 $\mu g.l^{-1}$ with the free drug concentration for surgical anaesthesia in the region of 6 $\mu g.l^{-1}$.[8] The drug has no analgesic action and small doses may increase sensitivity to somatic pain. This hyperalgesia (antanalgesic) action limits its use as sole anaesthetic, and it has also been demonstrated in the postoperative period following large doses.

The EEG changes induced by thiopentone follow a constant pattern and can be correlated with the clinical depth of anaesthesia,[9] although it is difficult to relate them with plasma drug concentration in different patients.[10] Initially there is high amplitude, fast spike activity of mixed frequency (10–30 Hz). Amplitudes vary greatly; short runs of two to three waves with amplitude of 25–80 μV are interspersed with runs of lower amplitude. This is followed by a complex pattern of mixed frequency characterized by the presence of predominantly shortwave forms of irregular contour and random occurrence and with much variation in voltage. As anaesthesia deepens the EEG is characterized by a progressive suppression of cortical activity and increasing periods of relative quiescence separating groups of waves, which appear abruptly and consist of a short series of high voltage waves, with a frequency of 10 Hz, for about 1 s, followed immediately by two or more short waves (2 Hz) tailing off into the next suppression phase. In surgical anaesthesia the duration of cortical quiescence varies from 3 to 10 s and there is a reduction in the amplitude of the components which fall below 25 μV.

Thiopentone causes a reduction of cerebral metabolic rate, especially in areas of high activity. This is accompanied by a corresponding reduction of cerebral blood flow with cerebral vasoconstriction and reduction of intracranial pressure. Doses sufficient to produce light general anaesthesia reduce cerebral blood flow by about 30%, with a 50% fall in deep anaesthesia. However, the main effects of barbiturates on cerebral blood flow are secondary to those on blood pressure and cerebral blood flow shows a proportionate fall in acute hypotension.

Induction doses of thiopentone also have a marked anticonvulsant action.

With the barbiturates, more so than with other drugs used in anaesthesia, the clinical level of anaesthesia is related to the intensity of the surgical stimulus as well as to the degree of cerebral depression. After thiopentone an undisturbed patient with depressed respiration and abdominal and masseter relaxation might show a picture of moderately deep surgical anaesthesia, but on application of a surgical stimulus the respiration is stimulated, relaxation is lost and reflex movement of a limb may occur. If sufficient thiopentone is given to produce surgical anaesthesia in the presence of strong stimulation, a dangerous degree of respiratory depression may occur when the stimulation ceases. Pretreatment with opioids reduces the dose of thiopentone required to produce surgical anaesthesia but also depresses respiration sometimes for a long period; a similar state of affairs can be produced at the end of the operation. With the use of nitrous oxide–oxygen to supplement thiopentone it is possible to produce a pattern of anaesthesia somewhat similar to that observed with other drugs without excessive dosage and without causing dangerous and prolonged periods of depression of vital functions.

Acute tolerance is one aspect of the cerebral action of thiopentone which cannot be explained readily. With single doses, return of consciousness will occur at a higher plasma concentration than following smaller doses. Larger increments are required to maintain a constant level of anaesthesia after a large induction dose than is necessary after smaller ones. Equally baffling is the finding that with continuous administration the plasma levels at which certain signs occur increases with time. Subjects have been known to converse seemingly rationally with plasma levels in excess of those at which they were anaesthetized 6 h or so previously.[11] A pharmacokinetic explanation for this has been suggested but is far from proven.[12]

Pharmacokinetics

Thiopentone is extensively bound to plasma proteins, the degree of binding (50–80%) varying with plasma/tissue pH and with drug concentration. Because of its high lipid solubility the free unionized thiopentone rapidly crosses the blood–brain barrier and EEG changes can be detected in 15–18 s. The brain continues to take up the drug for a further 30–60 s and thereafter the concentration of drug in the efferent venous blood slightly exceeds the arterial inflow concentration and brain concentration falls.

In most subjects the distribution of the drug can be modelled with a two-compartment system but a three-compartment model is needed to fit the curve in some. The initial distribution is to highly perfused tissues (including brain) and the subsequent slower redistribution to lean tissues, with some contribution by fat; the final elimination phase involves metabolism of the drug and redistribution to poorly perfused fat. It is the redistribution to lean tissues that results in recovery from the drug.

The distribution half life is 8.5 min in the rapid phase and 63 min in the slow phase. Clearance is 3.4 $ml.kg^{-1}.min^{-1}$. The elimination half life is approximately 9 h. Conditions in which the plasma protein binding of the drug, in the blood pH or in the distribution of blood flow are altered may influence the concentration entering the CNS and the distribution half life.

Oral absorption	—
Presystemic metabolism	—
Plasma half life	
range	4–12 h
mean	9 h
Volume of distribution	2.5 $l.kg^{-1}$
Plasma protein binding	50–80%

Concentration–effect relationship

The plasma concentration needed for anaesthesia is around 40 μg.l^{-1} with a free concentration of about 6 μg.l^{-1}.[10]

Metabolism

Metabolism of thiopentone is mainly by the liver. It is slow but almost complete with oxidation of the 1-methyl butyl side-chain to a hypnotically inactive metabolite. Very little unchanged drug is excreted in the urine.

Pharmaceutics

Proprietary preparations: Intraval Sodium (Rhône Poulenc, UK; Rhône Poulenc, France); Min-i-mix Thiopentone Sodium (I.M.S., UK/USA); Pentothal (Abbott, USA); Trapenal (Germany).

Commercial preparations of thiopentone contain a mixture of 6 parts of anhydrous sodium carbonate and 100 parts (w/w) of the barbiturate with sufficient triple distilled water to make a 2.5% solution. Vials of powder containing 0.5 g and bottles containing 2.5 g for extemporaneous preparation with water for injections give a 2.5% solution.

Vials of 0.5 g, 1.0 g and bottles of 5 g may be used for the less common 5% solution. A sterile transfer device is supplied with each 2.5 g and 5 g bottle. Pre-filled injection devices (Min-I-Mix) are available from International Medication Systems (IMS) in a strength of 500 mg for a 20 ml volume.

Solutions are incompatible with acids, most analgesics, the phenothiazines, adrenaline and noradrenaline and some muscle relaxants including alcuronium. Although the precipitate which forms when thiopentone and suxamethonium are mixed dissolves in excess thiopentone, hydrolysis of the relaxant occurs leading to a 50% loss of potency in 1 h.

Therapeutic use

Indications

1. As an anticonvulsant
2. For induction of general anaesthesia
3. For maintenance of general anaesthesia either by intermittent administration or infusion in combination with an analgesic and muscle relaxant if needed.

Other uses

4. Possibly for the prevention and treatment of cerebral ischaemia.

Contraindications

1. Porphyria.

Relative contraindications

2. Known or suspected full stomach
3. Unavailability of means of resuscitation
4. Inadequate access to patient and airway
5. Lack of facilities for recovery or attendants to take home day-cases
6. Marked hypovolaemia including blood loss
7. Uraemia
8. History of severe asthma
9. Severe cardiac disease.

Mode of use

This is normally by single intravenous dose given into any suitable limb vein, but preferably avoiding the ulnar side of the antecubital fossa in case pulsations in an aberrant ulnar artery are either not detected or obliterated by a tight tourniquet. Injection can be directly into the vein or into a fast-running infusion. The speed of injection and dose will depend on the fitness of the patient, the role of thiopentone in the full anaesthetic and to some extent on the nature of the operation. It is a common practice, particularly in unfit patients, to inject a small initial test dose and, depending on the response, to follow this by an adequate amount to produce loss of consciousness. One has to allow for the arm–brain circulation time which can be quite prolonged in some patients. A bolus dose (over 10–15 s) is indicated as part of a 'crash' technique, otherwise the dose is given over 20–30 s. It is common practice to precede thiopentone with a small dose of a short-acting opioid and this not only reduces the 'induction' dose but improves the smoothness of the induction, although at the risk of inducing a period of apnoea.

Intermittent doses can be given as sole agent for very brief operations but for longer procedures this should be supplemented by nitrous oxide–oxygen or a parenteral opioid or both.

Thiopentone is not the ideal drug for infusion but it has been used in a dilute solution as an anticonvulsant or for prevention and treatment of cerebral ischaemia (see below).

Dosage

The induction dose varies with:

1. age of the patient
2. fitness of the patient
3. premedication
4. pretreatment with opioids immediately prior to induction.

Taking the normal induction dose as 4–5 mg.kg^{-1} this can be as high as 6–8 mg.kg^{-1} in children and as low as 2–2.5 mg.kg^{-1} in the elderly. There is a marked reduction in requirements over the age of 60, irrespective of physical fitness, and this appears to be mainly a true pharmacodynamic (in comparison with pharmacokinetic) effect. Any degree of 'unfitness' will reduce dosage requirements. Continuous intravenous infusion will maintain hypnosis if the concentration is between 0.2% and 0.4%. The rate is varied according to patient response.

Subjects with an acquired tolerance to sedatives, hypnotics, opioids or even alcohol, have increased requirements of thiopentone and this may occur in patients with a degree of cardiovascular or other disease which would engender sensitivity to the toxic effects of such doses. This situation is best dealt with by prior administration of a suitable dose of fentanyl or alfentanil.

4. Prevention and treatment of cerebral ischaemia

Since doses of barbiturates which render the EEG isoelectric reduce the cerebral metabolic rate by about half, with no further effects from larger doses[13] the value of continuous infusions of thiopentone in minimizing the sequelae from hypoxic episodes has been investigated. A recent study of the randomized application of prophylactic barbiturate coma in the treatment of severe head injury failed to demonstrate any beneficial effect from the therapy,[14] rather in some patients there was a deleterious effect from its hypotensive action. Earlier claims for a therapeutic effect were probably due to the intensive therapy to which their patients were subjected. Thiopentone can, however, be of value in patients with post-hypoxic convulsions. These seizures increase cerebral metabolic rate at a time when compensatory increases in cerebral blood may be limited.

The value of thiopentone in reducing intracranial pressure in neurosurgical operations is not questioned but similar effects can be produced by moderate hyperventilation. A second dose given immediately prior to tracheal intubation will prevent the increase in blood pressure and cerebrospinal pressure which often accompany this event.[15] Another similar indication for a supplementary dose of thiopentone is during carotid endarterectomy; 4–5 mg.kg^{-1} given just before internal carotid artery occlusion will result in around 5 min ECG burst suppression, which, although less than the total period of arterial occlusion, will be followed by local metabolic depression in the poorly perfused brain areas.

Contraindications

Most of these are relative and depend on the experience of the administrator, the urgency of the procedure and availability (or lack) of means for resuscitation.

The only absolute contraindication is in patients with a history of known or suspected porphyria.

In the relative contraindications listed above the drug can be given, but either in low dosage or with special precautions, its use depending on the experience of the administrator and availability of alternative techniques, including the suitability for local anaesthesia.

Adverse reactions

Potentially life-threatening effects

The most common serious adverse effects are due to depression of respiration or circulation but hypersensitivity reactions also occur.

Thiopentone is a powerful central depressant of respiration and a

Thiopentone (sodium)

transient apnoea (up to half a minute) usually occurs during induction. In normal doses in fit patients this is not a clinical problem except after heavy opioid premedication. As with most anaesthetics the sensitivity of the respiratory centre to carbon dioxide is depressed proportionately to the depth of anaesthesia. In deep anaesthesia the action of hypoxia on the carotid sinus plays an important part in the maintenance of respiration but the shift of control of respiration from carbon dioxide to hypoxia is accompanied by a decrease in minute volume. Carbon dioxide retention may be particularly difficult to detect since thiopentone may also reduce the usual rise in pressure which it causes.

Hypotension is more marked in the undisturbed patient and surgical stimulation or laryngoscopy and tracheal intubation usually results in a rise in pressure; in many instances a marked overshoot occurs. Lightening of anaesthesia does not necessarily reverse the hypotension, which may persist into the postoperative period and, if accompanied by respiratory depression, will lead to hypoxia.

Immediately on administration of thiopentone one sees marked vasodilatation, and measurements of intrathoracic blood volume suggest that blood has been shunted from the central pool to the periphery, resulting in a decreased venous return which in turn reduces cardiac output and arterial pressure. In normal doses, thiopentone causes minimal depression of the heart but marked depression occurs with large doses.[17] On repeat or prolonged administration there is a delay in recovery of arterial pressure, suggesting that direct myocardial depression is playing an important role. The degree of cardiovascular depression is related to both the rate of administration (more marked with rapid administration) and the total dose given. Even large doses given as an infusion may cause less hypotension than a small rapid injection. The response varies with the condition of the patient, particularly with regard to blood volume, acid–base balance and cardiovascular disease and hypertension: these relate mainly to the ability to compensate for the effects of peripheral vasodilatation. Concurrent or previous administration of drugs which themselves cause vasodilatation or reduce compensatory tachycardia also enhance the hypotensive effect of thiopentone. Thiopentone abolishes the compensatory vasoconstriction produced by an increase in intrathoracic pressure and persistent hypotension can accompany hyperventilation. In the absence of hypercarbia, arrhythmias are uncommon after thiopentone.

Hypersensitivity reactions. Transient erythema is a common occurrence after administration of thiopentone: this appears to be more frequent in women and occurs in the 'blushing' area.

More serious reactions are rare with thiopentone, although the incidence appears to be increasing in recent years. It is often difficult to distinguish between relative overdose ('normal' dose given to an unfit patient) and true hypersensitivity to thiopentone. The latter resembles the effects of histamine liberation and might involve this as an intermediary. A small number of thiopentone reactions occur in patients with previous exposure (Type 1) and involve the production of IgE antibodies. However, the majority are not antibody-mediated, occurring in patients with a history of atopy (hay fever or eczema or other sensitivity), involving non-immune mechanisms such as the direct release of histamine.[19,20]

The clinical picture is one of sudden onset of pallor, cardiovascular collapse (tachycardia and hypotension) and bronchospasm. The latter is most difficult to treat, but the hypotension due to sudden vasodilatation usually responds rapidly to rapid colloid infusion and vasopressors. There is also usually a slight delay in onset of action of the anaesthetic.

The majority of reactions have oedema of the eyelids as a feature and some have massive wheals. A 1 mm layer of subcutaneous fluid throughout the body can produce a circulatory loss of 1.5 litres. This is usually exceeded when visible oedema is present. Bronchospasm may in part be due to oedema. However, the most serious form is oedema of the glottis and when this occurs one must administer intravenous adrenaline.

It is estimated that hypersensitivity reactions to thiopentone occur in between 1 in 23 000[21] and 1 in 36 000[22] administrations. This may seem a negligible risk but even with aggressive treatment it causes a 50% mortality which is higher than with other intravenous anaesthetics. This may be because the drug remains in the body for a long time, but there is the additional factor of the toxic effects of thiopentone on the cardiovascular system, which are greater than those of methohexitone or etomidate.

Severe or irreversible adverse effects

The most serious toxic action of thiopentone is its ability to induce an acute attack in patients with latent porphyria. This is brought about by stimulation of ALA synthesase, the enzyme which catalyses the rate-limiting reaction of haem production. Not every type of porphyria is adversely affected by thiopentone[18] but the outcome is so serious following an acute attack that any suspicion of porphyria should be an absolute contraindication to its use.

Local effects due to accidental arterial injection. Pain on injection is uncommon with 2.5% thiopentone, even when small veins are used. Venous thrombosis is also a rare occurrence. The drug causes tissue damage if injected subcutaneously, particularly in large volumes and in elderly patients with a poor peripheral circulation or sparse subcutaneous tissue. Arterial injection can cause serous sequelae and care must be taken to avoid this. Intense pain, radiating into the fingers often, but not invariably, follows an intra-arterial injection. Pain usually disappears after a few minutes but with large amounts of drug it can persist for several hours. The radial pulse will usually disappear and there may be blanching of the limb. If the circulation is quickly re-established this may be followed by reactive hyperaemia. Oedema of the limb will occur when the muscles have been invaded by thiopentone. Depending on the degree of spasm of blood vessels and anatomical distribution of blood from affected vessels, sequelae can vary from transient hyperaesthesia of the affected area to loss of a digit or even a limb, but the latter has not been reported with a 2.5% solution.

Damage results from unrelieved vascular spasm, followed by thrombosis. Spasm may be related to the deposition of crystals of insoluble thiopentone acid in a blood stream of decreasing capacity: direct blockage is unlikely but release of ATP from damaged blood cells or platelets and an area of intimal damage at the puncture site could initiate the intravascular thrombosis.

Symptomatic adverse effects

Cough and hiccough are uncommon during induction with thiopentone, but there is some heightening of laryngeal reflexes, particularly in light anaesthesia, and a tendency to laryngospasm which may be induced by minor stimuli. Bronchospasm is a rare, but not unknown, complication with this drug, particularly in asthmatic subjects in whom thiopentone is best avoided. In many cases the term 'bronchospasm' is used to describe a complex situation involving spasm of intercostal and other muscles which can be reversed by the use of muscle relaxants.

In common with other anaesthetics, oliguria occurs during thiopentone anaesthesia — partly as a result of reduction in renal blood flow and partly from an increase in circulating antidiuretic hormone. This is of no clinical importance. In therapeutic doses thiopentone has no effect on the tone of the gravid uterus, but tone is reduced in deep anaesthesia.

Other effects

A mild hyperglycaemia occurs during anaesthesia, during which patients' ability to handle a glucose load is impaired. Hyperglycaemia may however be the normal response to stress rather than an effect of the drug on glucose metabolism.

Interference with clinical pathology tests

None reported.

High risk groups

Neonates and children

Provided appropriate dose adjustments are made there is no special hazard.

Breast milk. As the drug is used on a single occasion this is not a problem.

Pregnant women

There are no special problems other than the usual precautions required anaesthetizing a pregnant woman.

The elderly

Elderly patients require substantially lower doses of thiopentone and are more likely to have multisystem disease which makes them vulnerable to the effects of overdose.

Drug interactions

There is no obvious interaction between thiopentone and any of the commonly used myoneural-blocking drugs.

All barbiturates are inducers of hepatic microsomal drug metabolizing enzymes but this is not likely to be a problem with a single dose of thiopentone.[23] If thiopentone were to be used on a number of occasions over a short period of time then enzyme induction might occur and lead to the enhanced clearance (and diminished therapeutic effect) of drugs such as warfarin, phenytoin, tricyclic antidepressants and corticosteroids. Barbiturates have an additive effect with other CNS depressants (e.g. antihistamines) to cause severe depression but this is less likely to be a problem with thiopentone. Aspirin is known to displace thiopentone from its protein binding sites in plasma but this is not thought to give rise to any serious clinical problems,[24] although pretreatment with intravenous aspirin reduces the induction dose.

General review articles

Dundee J W, Wyant G M 1986 Intravenous anaesthesia, 2nd ed. Churchill Livingstone, Edinburgh

Dundee J W 1979 Intravenous anaesthetic agents. In: Current topics in anaesthesia. E J Arnold, London

References

1. Moruzzi G, Magoun H W 1949 Brain stem reticular formation and activation of the EEG. Electroencephalography and Clinical Neurophysiology 1: 455–473
2. French J D, Verzeano M, Magoun H W 1953 An extralemniscal sensory system in the brain. Archives of Neurology and Psychiatry 69: 505–518
3. Arduini A, Aruini M G 1954 Effect of drugs and metabolic alterations on brain stem arousal mechanism. Journal of Pharmacology and Experimental Therapeutics 110: 76–85
4. Abrahamian H A, Allison T, Goff W R, Rosner B S 1963 Effects of thiopental human cerebral evoked responses. Anesthesiology 24: 650–657
5. King E E, Naquet R, Magoun H W 1957 Alterations in somatic afferent transmission through thalamus by central mechanisms and barbiturates. Journal of Pharmacology and Experimental Therapeutics 119: 48–63
6. Clarke D L, Rosner B S 1973 Neurophysiologic effects of general anesthetics. I. The electroencephalogram and sensory evoked responses in man. Anesthesiology 38: 564–582
7. Kawar P, Briggs L P, Bahar M et al 1982 Liver enzyme studies with disoprofol (ICI 35 868) and midazolam. Anaesthesia 37: 305-308
8. Becker K E 1978 Plasma levels of thiopental necessary for anesthesia. Anesthesiology 49: 192–196
9. Kiersey D K, Bickford R G, Faulconer A 1951 EEG patterns produced by thiopental sodium during surgical operations: description and classification. British Journal of Anaesthesia 23: 141–152
10. Brand L, Mazzia V D B, van Poznak A, Burns J J, Mark L C 1961 Lack of correlation between encephalographic effects and plasma concentrations of thiopentone. British Journal of Anaesthesia 33: 92–96
11. Dundee J W, Price H L, Dripps R S 1956 Acute tolerance to thiopentone in man. British Journal of Anaesthesia 28: 344–352
12. Hudson R J, Stanski D R, Saidman L F, Meathe E 1983 A model for studying depth of anaesthesia and acute tolerance to thiopental. Anesthesiology 59: 301–308
13. Michenfelder J D 1974 The interdependency of cerebral functional and metabolic effects following massive doses of thiopental in the dog. Anesthesiology 41: 231–236
14. Ward J D, Becker D P, Miller J D et al 1985 Failure of prophylactic barbiturate coma in the treatment of severe head injury. Journal of Neurosurgery 62: 383–388
15. Unni V K N, Johnston R A, Young H S A, McBride R J 1984 Prevention of intracranial hypertension during laryngoscopy and endotracheal intubation: use of a second dose of thiopentone. British Journal of Anaesthesia 56: 1219-1223
16. Moffatt J A, McDougall M J, Brunet B et al 1983 Thiopentone bolus during carotid endartectomy — rational drug therapy. Canadian Anaesthetists Society Journal 30: 615–619
17. Chamberlian J H, Sede R G F L, Chung D C W 1977 Effect of thiopentone on myocardial function. British Journal of Anaesthesia 49: 865–870
18. Leading Article 1985 Latent acute hepatic porphyria. Lancet 1: 197–198
19. Dundee J W, Fee J P H, McDonald J R, Clarke R S J 1978 Frequency of atopy and allergy in an anaesthetic patient population. British Journal of Anaesthesia 50: 793–798
20. Fee J P H, McDonald J R, Dundee J W, Clarke R S J 1978 Frequency of previous anaesthesia in an anaesthetic patient population. British Journal of Anaesthesia 50: 917–920
21. Shaw H 1974 Anaesthetic complications. New Zealand Society of Anaesthetists Newsletter 21: 144
22. Beamish D, Brown D T 1981 Adverse responses to i.v. anaesthetics. British Journal of Anaesthesia 53: 55–58
23. Fee J P H, Dundee J W 1986 Antipyrine elimination is not increased by a single induction dose of thiopentone. British Journal of Clinical Pharmacology 22: 224P
24. Dundee J W, Halliday N J, McMurray T J 1986 Aspirin and probenecid pretreatment influences the potency of thiopentone and the onset of action of midazolam. European Journal of Anaesthesiology 3: 247–251

Thioridazine (hydrochloride)

Thioridazine hydrochloride is a neuroleptic phenothiazine drug used primarily for its antipsychotic actions.

Chemistry

Thioridazine hydrochloride (Melleril, Mellaril, Melleretten)
$C_{21}H_{26}N_2S_2.HCl$
10-[2-(1-Methyl-2-piperidyl)ethyl]-2-methylthiophenothiazine hydrochloride

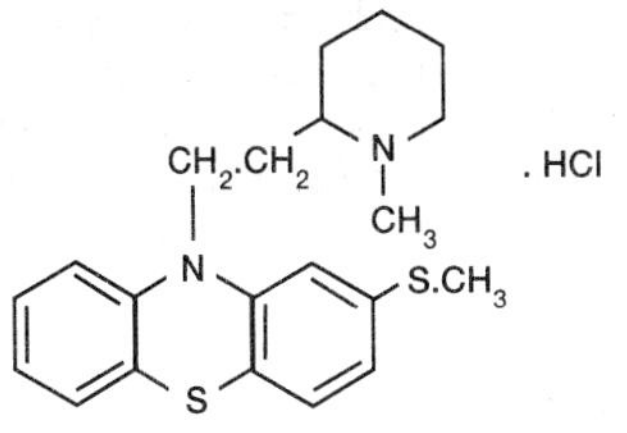

Molecular weight of hydrochloride (free base)	407.0 (370.6)
pKa (amino group)	9.5
Solubility	
in alcohol of hydrochloride (free base)	1 in 10 (1 in 6)
in water of hydrochloride (free base)	1 in 9 (insoluble)
Octanol/water partition coefficient (hydrochloride and free base)	5.66

Thioridazine hydrochloride is a white or cream, crystalline powder with a very bitter taste and faint odour. It is used in the formulation of tablets.

Thioridazine base is a white or slightly yellow crystalline powder which darkens on exposure to light. It is odourless or with a faint odour. It is used in the formulation of liquid oral dosage forms.

Thioridazine and its hydrochloride are prepared by chemical synthesis. Neither is available in any combination preparations.

Pharmacology

Thioridazine primarily acts as a neuroleptic drug. In this it suppresses complex behaviour and spontaneous movements but leaves untouched spinal reflexes and unconditioned nociceptive behaviour. These effects are due to the blocking action of thioridazine at the postsynaptic dopamine (D_2) receptors.[1,2] In the mesolimbic dopamine system of the brain, this action accounts for the antipsychotic actions of the drug, while similar actions in the nigrostriatal system may produce the extrapyramidal effects of parkinsonism.

Thioridazine has other effects on the central nervous system. In the chemoreceptor trigger zone, the dopamine blockade accounts for the weak antiemetic effect of the drug. It acts on the hypothalamus to increase prolactin secretion, and is also an antagonist at dopamine D_1 receptors, but the exact significance of this in the CNS is unclear. Thioridazine, like chlorpromazine has anticholinergic effects at muscarinic receptors and has more antimuscarinic activity than chlorpromazine.[3] Thioridazine acts to relax skeletal muscle, possibly by an action in the basal ganglia since the drug has no effect at the neuromuscular junction. Thioridazine is an antagonist at α_1-adrenoceptors and is also an antagonist at histamine (H_1) receptors, and 5-hydroxytryptamine receptors.

Toxicology

Thioridazine does not have mutagenic potential. Animal toxicology tests using high doses demonstrated drowsiness, dilation of pupils

T

and lack of appetite. Studies in rats and rabbits produced no evidence of teratogenic effects.

Clinical pharmacology

Thioridazine, like most phenothiazines, when given to normal subjects produces unpleasant sensations of sedation without sleep, restlessness and unclear thinking. In patients with psychotic symptoms the drug produces calmness and responsiveness. Aggressive behaviour diminishes and hallucinations and delusions gradually disappear.

The antipsychotic effects of thioridazine are thought to result from the blockade of dopamine receptors in the mesolimbic system of the brain. After 30 days treatment with thioridazine a 48% increase in homovanillic acid in the CSF of 14 schizophrenic patients was noted, indicating a blockade of central dopamine receptors.[1] Thioridazine is often classified as an atypical neuroleptic since it behaves differently from other neuroleptics in standard animal screening tests and a specific blockade of dopamine receptors within the mesolimbic system of human brain has been reported.[2] It is much less likely to produce acute extrapyramidal side effects than other neuroleptics. This is probably due to its potent anticholinergic action.[3] The anticholinergic action tends to be manifest as side effects such as dry mouth, blurred vision and urinary retention. The α_1-adrenergic blocking actions of thioridazine are partly responsible for postural hypotension which tends to occur with large initial doses or large increases in dosage. Thioridazine has almost no antiemetic or clinical antihistaminic effects.

Pharmacokinetics

The preferred analytical method for thioridazine and its major metabolites is high performance liquid chromatography with ultraviolet detection.[4] The minimum detectable amounts using 1 ml plasma samples are 10 $\mu g.l^{-1}$ for thioridazine, northioridazine, mesoridazine and sulphoridazine. This can be improved to 2 $\mu g.l^{-1}$ by using fluorescence detection.

Reports of thioridazine concentrations following intravenous dosing are lacking and hence it is not possible to give a definitive description of thioridazine pharmacokinetics. Following oral administration thioridazine is believed to be readily absorbed[5,6] with a systemic bioavailability of approximately 60%. Food does not appear to affect the plasma concentrations, though the time to peak may be delayed. Plasma concentrations of thioridazine show large interindividual variation, up to 20-fold;[7] intraindividual variation is considerably less.[8] Peak concentrations usually occur some 1–4 hours after oral dosing. The decline in plasma concentrations appears to be multiphasic with a terminal half life within the range 16–36 hours.

Thioridazine is widely distributed throughout the body with an apparent volume of distribution of approximately 10 $l.kg^{-1}$. Radioisotope studies in rats indicate rapid distribution with highest levels in lung, liver, brain, spleen, adrenal, kidney and small intestine.[9] Thioridazine is extensively metabolized with less than 1% of the dose appearing as unchanged drug in the urine. Elimination of thioridazine metabolites occurs mainly via the bile and with less than 10% of the dose appearing in urine.

Thioridazine is more than 95% bound in plasma principally to α_1-acid glycoprotein. The unbound concentration of thioridazine in CSF is approximately twice that in plasma.[11] Thioridazine is excreted in breast milk and crosses the placental barrier.

Thioridazine plasma concentrations tend to be lower and metabolite concentrations higher, in alcoholics than in non-alcoholics possibly due to alcohol-induced increased metabolic capacity.[10] Elderly alcoholics with signs of liver damage have higher than expected plasma concentrations.[12]

The elimination of thioridazine appears to be impaired in the elderly resulting in a longer half life and higher plasma concentrations.[13]

The elimination of thioridazine is likely to be impaired in hepatic dysfunction, although the consequences of this will be complicated by the fact that several of the metabolites normally produced are therapeutically active. Renal impairment is unlikely to alter the kinetics of the drug.

Total thioridazine concentrations correlate positively with α_1-acid glycoprotein levels[14] and hence are likely to be elevated during infections and in disease states where α_1-acid glycoprotein levels are increased.

Thioridazine inhibits the metabolism of, and its metabolism is inhibited by, tricyclic antidepressants and some β-adrenoceptor antagonists such as propranolol.

Alterations in the pharmacokinetics of thioridazine are only likely to be of clinical significance in patients receiving doses close to the recommended maximum dose.

Oral absorption	>60%
Presystemic metabolism	—
Plasma half life	16–36 h
range	—
mean	—
Volume of distribution	10 $l.kg^{-1}$
Plasma protein binding	96.5–99.3%

Concentration–effect relationship

There are a number of conflicting reports of relationships between blood levels and clinical response. This may be a reflection of the heterogeneous nature of psychosis and the presence of active metabolites of thioridazine. Optimal therapeutic response has been associated with thioridazine concentrations of 250–750 $\mu g.l^{-1}$ in patients over 40 years old and with total concentrations of thioridazine plus sulphoxidized metabolites greater than 750 $\mu g.l^{-1}$ in younger patients.[15] Conversely, a number of other reports [8,16–18] have failed to demonstrate a relationship between clinical improvement and, variously, plasma or red blood cell concentrations of thioridazine and its sulphoxidized metabolites. Concentrations of thioridazine in excess of 1 $mg.l^{-1}$ are associated with hypotension.

Metabolism

Thioridazine has a large number of potential metabolites arising from sulphoxidation, N-demethylation, hydroxylation and conjugation reactions in the liver. In man sulphoxidation is the predominant route with N-demethylation a minor route. Hydroxylation with subsequent conjugation is a major pathway in the rat[9] but hydroxylated metabolites have not been identified in man. Sulphoxidation occurs at both the side-chain, resulting in thioridazine-2-sulphoxide (mesoridazine) and thioridazine-2-sulphone (sulphoridazine), and at the ring to form thioridazine-5-sulphoxide (Fig. 1). Metabolites which are sulphoxidized at both the 2- and 5- positions have also been identified in urine from patients.[19] The 2- and 5-sulphoxide and 2-sulphone metabolites are found in significant concentrations in plasma, often higher than those of thioridazine. Unbound plasma concentration ratios of metabolite:parent drug have been reported as 24:1 for thioridazine-5-sulphoxide, 9:1 for thioridazine-2-sulphoxide and 2:1 for thioridazine-2-sulphone.[10] Thioridazine-5-sulphoxide has no psychoactive properties but may be responsible for the cardiac side effects associated with thioridazine therapy.[20,21] Thioridazine-2-sulphoxide (mesoridazine) and thioridazine-2-sulphone (sulphoridazine) are active metabolites, each being approximately 50% more potent than the parent drug.[7] They contribute to the antipsychotic effect of thioridazine.[7,22] Mesoridazine is available in the USA (Serentil) as an antipsychotic drug.

Excretion is largely in the bile and thence in the faeces; less than 10% of the dose is excreted in urine. Only trace amounts (<1%) of the dose are excreted as unchanged drug in urine, with slightly greater amounts of mesoridazine and sulphoridazine.

Pharmaceutics

Thioridazine is only available as the following oral dosage forms: tablets, suspension and syrup.

Melleril tablets (Sandoz, UK) are white, film-coated and with a bevel edge. They are available in four strengths, containing 10, 25, 50 and 100 mg of thioridazine hydrochloride BP. Melleril tablets are embossed 'MEL' on one face and the strength on the other. Mellaril tablets (Sandoz, USA) are formulated in seven strengths, the additional ones being 15 mg, 150 mg and 200 mg. Each bears the word 'MELLARIL' and the strength.

Thioridazine (hydrochloride)

The suspension is an opaque, creamy/white formulation of thioridazine base and is available in strengths of 25 and 100 mg in 5 ml (equivalent to 27.5 and 110 mg of thioridazine hydrochloride in 5 ml).

The syrup is a clear orange formulation containing 25 mg of thioridazine base (equivalent to 27.5 mg of the hydrochloride) in 5 ml.

The suspension formulations should not be diluted but may be blended to produce strengths between 25 and 100 mg of thioridazine base per 5 ml.

Thioridazine is prone to autoxidation and hence all preparations should be stored in airtight containers and protected from light. Melleril preparations are stable with shelf-lives of 3–5 years.

Allergic reactions to thioridazine, including skin rashes and jaundice, have been reported but are rare.

Therapeutic use

Indications

1. Schizophrenia, mania and hypomania
2. Moderate to severe psychomotor agitation
3. Anxiety, agitation and restlessness in the elderly
4. Behavioural disorders in epileptic children.

Contraindications

1. Comatose states
2. Severe depression of the CNS
3. A history of blood dyscrasias
4. Severe cardiovascular disorders.

Mode of use

1. Schizophrenia, mania and hypomania

Thioridazine is widely used in the control of schizophrenia, mania and hypomania. It is similar to chlorpromazine in respect of potency, sedative effect and incidence of orthostatic hypotension. However, in contrast to other neuroleptics thioridazine has little effect on the seizure threshold and may be preferred in patients with epilepsy. The recommended daily adult dose range is 150–600 mg of thioridazine hydrochloride. Doses up to 800 mg daily may be administered under specialist supervision to hospitalized patients for not more than 4 weeks. For maintenance therapy the dose should be reduced to the minimum effective level. There is no evidence that higher doses produce greater clinical effect and side effects including irreversible pigmentary retinopathy may occur at doses exceeding 800 mg daily.[23]

2. Moderate to severe psychomotor agitation

Thioridazine decreases agitation and is indicated at daily doses of 75–200 mg for the control of violent or dangerously impulsive behaviour. It may also be used as an adjunct in the short-term management of anxiety.

3. Anxiety, agitation and restlessness in the elderly

Thioridazine decreases restlessness and agitation in the elderly and results in a significant improvement in thought disorders. The recommended daily dose range for geriatric patients is 30–100 mg. Initial doses should be in the lower region of the range with gradual increases as necessary. In psychogeriatric patients thioridazine (25 mg) has been indicated as a suitable sleeping aid without causing daytime drowsiness or impairment of daily activities.[24] A number of reports[25,26] indicate that thioridazine is at least as effective as diazepam in relieving anxiety and agitation in the elderly.

4. Behavioural disorders in epileptic children

Unlike a number of other neuroleptics thioridazine has little effect on seizure threshold and is useful in the treatment of behavioural disorders in epileptic children. Its use is, however, restricted to patients with severe mental or behavioural problems such as aggressiveness, self-mutilation or senseless hyperactivity. The usual daily dose for children under 5 years of age is 1 mg.kg^{-1} body weight. The dose range for children 5 years and over is usually 75–150 mg daily increasing in severe cases to 300 mg daily.

Contraindications

1. Comatose states

Thioridazine is contraindicated in comatose states due to its CNS depressant effects and hypotensive and other actions on the cardiovascular and respiratory systems.

Fig. 1 Metabolism of thioridazine

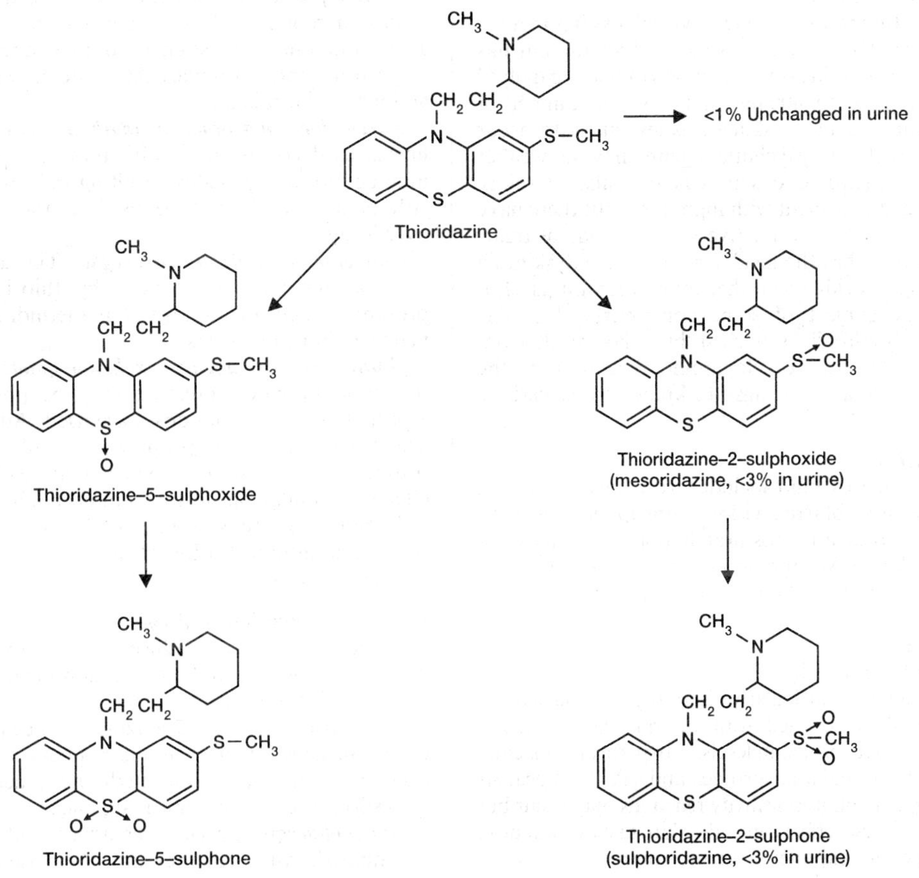

Thioridazine (hydrochloride)

2. Severe depression of the CNS
Thioridazine may enhance the CNS depressant effects of other drugs including anaesthetics, hypnotics, sedatives, narcotic analgesics and alcohol.

3. A history of blood dyscrasias or bone marrow depression
Blood dyscrasias, including transient leucopenia and very rarely agranulocytosis, have been reported during thioridazine treatment. These effects have most commonly been reported during the first three months of treatment but occasionally occur later. Regular blood counts should be performed during the first three months of treatment and whenever signs of persistent infection or other signs of blood dyscrasia occur.

4. Severe cardiovascular disorders
The administration of phenothiazine drugs is contraindicated in severe cardiovascular disease, as this may be exacerbated.

Adverse reactions

Potentially life-threatening effects
In isolated cases, neuroleptic malignant syndrome (muscular rigidity, hyperthermia, altered mental status, autonomic instability), a condition necessitating immediate discontinuation of the drug, has been observed.

Sudden and unexplained death, apparently due to arrhythmia or cardiac arrest,[27] has been reported in patients treated with tricyclic neuroleptic agents including thioridazine.[28] Agranulocytosis occurs but it is rare.

Acute overdosage
In cases of acute overdosage, coma with shallow breathing, hypotension and absence of reflexes usually results. Motor restlessness, hyperflexia, cardiac arrythmias and epileptiform convulsions may also occur. Deaths from overdosage, apparently due to cardiac arrhythmias, have been reported.[29] Treatment of overdosage should be initiated by gastric lavage and followed by general supportive measures with particular attention paid to the cardiac and respiratory systems. Acute hypotension should be treated with plasma expanders. Resistant cases may warrant a vasopressor, but adrenaline should not be used and careful monitoring, particularly of metabolic acidosis, cardiac function and delayed cardiac effects is required.

Severe or irreversible adverse effects
Irreversible pigmentary retinopathy, leading to visual loss has in most cases been associated with daily doses in excess of 1000 mg but has also been reported in patients taking doses in excess of 600 mg daily[23] and in one patient taking up to 400 mg daily over a number of years.[30] The development of acute dyskinesia is less likely to occur with thioridazine than with antipsychotic agents having weaker antimuscarinic properties. Tardive dyskinesias can also develop, usually following prolonged treatment with high doses but there have been occasional incidences following relative short periods of treatment. There is little evidence that the incidence of tardive dyskinesia is lower in patients taking thioridazine rather than other antipsychotics, although this is the subject of some controversy.[31,32] The pathogenesis of tardive dyskinesia is unclear but may result from supersensitivity and proliferation of dopamine receptors in the nigrostriatal system; antimuscarinic drugs are known to exacerbate the symptoms.

Symptomatic adverse effects
Common adverse effects of this kind include drowsiness, sedation, dry mouth, nasal congestion, blurred vision, constipation, urinary retention, tremor, tachycardia and postural hypotension, most of which tend to be dose-related. At high doses arrhythmias and ECG changes, including prolongation of the Q–T interval and abnormalities of the T-wave, may occur. In addition to the depressant effects on the central nervous system, paradoxical effects of excitement, agitation and insomnia have been noted.

Sexual dysfunction, manifest particularly as retrograde ejaculation and priapism, is commonly associated with thioridazine treatment. Thioridazine is known to elevate prolactin levels;[33] hyperprolactinaemia may result in oligomenorrhoea and amenorrhoea and galactorrhoea. At doses in excess of 400 mg daily photosensitivity reactions may occur but very rarely. Other rare adverse effects include skin rashes, jaundice, hepatitis and liver dysfunction and altered seizure control.

Interference with clinical pathology tests
Thioridazine may interfere with the Frings procedure for measuring urinary alkaloids and barbiturates, the Trinder method for measuring urinary salicylate, and some urinary tests for pregnancy.

High risk groups

Neonates
There is no specific information on doses used in neonates.

Breast milk. Thioridazine is excreted in breast milk and mothers taking the drug should not breast-feed.

Children
The recommended daily doses for children under 5 years is 1 mg.kg^{-1} and 75–300 mg daily for severe cases in children 5 years and over.

Pregnant women
The effects of thioridazine on the fetus are not known and it should not be used in pregnancy without compelling reasons. Phenothiazine drugs cross the placental barrier and the newborn of mothers taking thioridazine may show signs of lethargy, tremor or hyperactivity.

The elderly
The elderly tend to show impaired elimination of thioridazine and may be more susceptible to effects and particularly some adverse effects of the drug. As a consequence initial doses should be small then slowly increased and maintained at a minimum level. Hypotensive and hypothermic side effects, the latter much less likely than with chlorpromazine, are of particular concern in the elderly.

Concurrent disease
Thioridazine should be used with caution in patients with cardiac arrhythmias, cardiac disease, renal failure and liver dysfunction. The monitoring of liver function is essential in patients with liver disease. Thioridazine should also be used with caution in patients with Parkinson's disease, myasthenia gravis, epilepsy, severe respiratory disease, narrow angle glaucoma, phaeochromocytoma or prostatic hypertrophy.

Drug interactions

Potentially hazardous interactions

CNS depressants. The effect of CNS depressants (including hypnotics, narcotic analgesics, anaesthetics, and tricyclic antidepressants) and other adverse effects of these agents, including those on the respiratory and cardiovascular systems, may be potentiated by the actions of thioridazine.

Adrenaline (and other sympathomimetic agents). When adrenaline is used concurrently with thioridazine, its α-adrenergic effects may be blocked, possibly resulting in hypotension and tachycardia. Adrenaline should not be used in the treatment of thioridazine overdosage.

Guanethidine and related drugs. The antihypertensive effects of these agents may be reduced by thioridazine. Thioridazine will prevent the neuronal uptake of guanethidine and related sympathetic neurone-blocking drugs.

Antihypertensive agents (excluding guanethidine-like agents). The reduction in blood pressure may be potentiated by thioridazine especially if high initial doses are used. Additionally, the concurrent use of thioridazine and propranolol results in elevated blood concentrations of both drugs,[34] which may lead to additive hypotensive effects. A similar but less pronounced effect is seen with pindolol.[35]

Lithium. There is an increased risk of severe neurotoxicity from concurrent administration of lithium and thioridazine, although the incidence is rare.

Other significant interactions

Antacids. Antacids reduce the oral absorption of phenothiazine drugs and they should not be administered within two hours of dosing with thioridazine.

Anticonvulsants. Thioridazine has been reported to increase, decrease, or have no effect on plasma concentrations of phenytoin and other anticonvulsants, although the general consensus is that the alterations are not of clinical significance.[36]

Anticholinergic agents. The adverse effects of these drugs will be potentiated. Although they are often used in combination without

Thioridazine (hydrochloride)

complication, a report of constipation and adynamic ileus and reports of heat stroke with other phenothiazines have appeared. Anticholinergics will also exacerbate tardive dyskinesia.

Tricyclic antidepressants. Concurrent treatment with phenothiazines and tricyclics has led to increases in blood concentrations of both drugs. Excessive weight gain has been reported following several months treatment with thioridazine and amitriptyline.[37] It has also been suggested that tricyclics may be a contributory factor in the development of tardive dyskinesia.[38]

Quinidine. The inhibitory effect of quinidine on cardiac contractility may be potentiated by thioridazine.

Food. Food has not been reported to have any significant effect on plasma concentrations. A delay in the time to reach peak concentrations is likely.

Alcohol. The effects of alcohol on the CNS are potentiated by thioridazine.

Levodopa. Phenothiazines may reduce the antiparkinsonian effects of levodopa.

MAO inhibitors. Concurrent use with MAO inhibitors may prolong and intensify the sedative and antimuscarinic effects of phenothiazines.

Major outcome trials

1. Leger Y 1966 A four year appraisal of thioridazine. American Journal of Psychiatry 123: 728–732

This report is a four year survey of mainly chronic patients, treated with thioridazine for variable periods ranging from a few weeks but predominantly for periods of more than two years. 87% of the 768 schizophrenia inpatients were noted to show some degree of improvement and 37% were satisfactorily discharged. The side effects were reported to be mainly mild. Hypotension was minimized by increasing the dose gradually. It was concluded that thioridazine was highly effective and tolerated.

2. Herman E, Pleasure H 1963 Clinical evaluation of thioridazine and chlorpromazine in chronic schizophrenics. Diseases of the Nervous System 24: 54–59

This was a double-blind clinical evaluation of thioridazine and chlorpromazine in 24 female and 42 male patients suffering from chronic schizophrenia and who had been hospitalized for at least two years. The results indicated that thioridazine and chlorpromazine were similarly effective in treating chronic schizophrenia; the incidence of parkinsonism was much lower with thioridazine.

General review articles

Black J L 1985 Antipsychotic drugs: a clinical update. Mayo Clinic Proceedings 60: 777–789

Dahl S G 1986 Plasma level monitoring of antipsychotic drugs: Clinical utility. Clinical Pharmacokinetics 11: 36–61

Davis J M, Casper R 1977 Antipsychotic drugs: clinical pharmacology and therapeutic use. Drugs 14: 260–282

Jain A K, Kelwala S, Gershon S 1988 Antipsychotic drugs in schizophrenia: current issues. International Clinical Psychopharmacology 3: 1–30

Jorgensen A 1986 Metabolism and pharmacokinetics of antipsychotic drugs. In: Bridges J W, Chasseaud L F (eds) Progress in drug metabolism, vol 9. Taylor and Francis, London, ch 4, pp 132–135

References

1. Bowers M B 1975 Thioridazine: central dopamine turnover and clinical effects of antipsychotic drugs. Clinical Pharmacology and Therapeutics 17: 73–78
2. Borison R L, Fields J Z, Diamond B I 1981 Site-specific blockade of dopamine receptors by neuroleptic agents in human brain. Neuropharmacology 20: 1321–1322
3. Miller R J, Hiley D R 1974 Anti-muscarinic properties of neuroleptics and drug-induced parkinsonism. Nature 248: 596–597
4. Kilts C D, Patrick K S, Breese G R, Mailman R B 1982 Simultaneous determination of thioridazine and its S-oxidised and N-demethylated metabolites using high performance liquid chromatography on radially compressed silica. Journal of Chromatography 231: 377–391
5. Eiduson S, Geller E 1963 The excretion and metabolism of ^{35}S labelled thioridazine in urine, blood, bile and faeces. Biochemical Pharmacology 12: 1429–1435
6. Hammell M R, Martinez M N, Digle S V, Parkman T P 1987 Bioequivalence of thioridazine drug products — the FDA viewpoint. Drug Intelligence and Clinical Pharmacy 21: 362–369
7. Axelsson R 1977 On the serum concentrations and antipsychotic effects of thioridazine, side-chain sulfoxide and thioridazine side-chain sulfone, in chronic psychiatric patients. Current Therapeutic Research 21: 587–605
8. Ng C H, Crammer J L 1977 Measurement of thioridazine in blood and urine. British Journal of Clinical Pharmacology 4: 173–183
9. Zehnder K, Kalberer F, Reis W, Rutschmann J 1962 The metabolism of thioridazine and one of its pyrollidine analogues in the rat. Biochemical Pharmacology 11: 535–550
10. Nyberg G, Axelsson R, Martensson E 1981 Cerebrospinal fluid concentrations of thioridazine and its main metabolites in psychiatric patients. European Journal of Clinical Pharmacology 19: 139–148
11. Axelsson R, Martensson E, Alling C 1982 Serum concentrations and protein binding of thioridazine and its metabolites in patients with chronic alcoholism. European Journal of Clinical Pharmacology 23: 359–363
12. Axelsson R, Martensson E 1977 The concentration pattern of nonconjugated thioridazine metabolites in serum by thioridazine treatment and its relationship to physiological and clinical variables. Current Therapeutic Research 21: 561–586
13. Axelsson R 1976 On the pharmacokinetics of thioridazine. In: Sedvall G, Uvnas B, Zotterman Y (eds) Antipsychotic drugs: pharmacodynamics and pharmacokinetics. Pergamon Press, Oxford, pp 353–358
14. Nyberg G, Svensson C, Olofsson U, Axelsson R, Martensson E 1987 Total plasma concentrations, red blood cell concentrations, and radioreceptor assay values compared with unbound plasma concentrations of thioridazine and thioridazine metabolites in psychiatric patients. Therapeutic Drug Monitoring 9: 426–432
15. Axelsson R, Martensson E 1983 Clinical effects related to the serum concentrations of thioridazine and its metabolites. In: Gram L F et al (eds) Clinical pharmacology in psychiatry — bridging the experimental–therapeutic gap. Macmillan, London, pp 165–174
16. Papadopoulos A S, Chand T G, Crammer J L, Lader S 1980 A pilot study of thioridazine and metabolites in chronically treated patients. British Journal of Psychiatry 136: 591–596
17. Sajadi C, Smith R C, Shvartsburd A, Morton V, Mirabi M, Gordon J 1984 Neuroleptic blood levels in outpatient maintenance therapy of schizophrenia. Psychopharmacology Bulletin 20: 110–113
18. Smith R C, Baumgartner R, Ravichandran G K et al 1984 Plasma and red cell levels of thioridazine and clinical response in schizophrenia. Psychiatry Research 12: 287–296
19. Papadopoulos A S, Crammer J L 1986 Sulphoxide metabolites of thioridazine in man. Xenobiotica 16: 1097–1107
20. Gottschalk L, Dinovo E, Biener R, Nandi B 1978 Plasma concentrations of thioridazine metabolites and ECG abnormalities. Journal of Pharmaceutical Sciences 67: 155–157
21. Heath A, Svensson C, Martensson E 1985 Thioridazine toxicity — an experimental cardiovascular study of thioridazine and its major metabolites in overdosage. Veterinary and Human Toxicology 27: 100–105
22. Lewis M H, Mobilio J M, Rissmiller D J, Mailman R B 1984 Thioridazine pharmacodynamics: clinical effects may depend upon drug metabolism. Journal of the American Osteopathic Association 84 (suppl): 124–128
23. Hamilton J D 1985 Thioridazine retinopathy within the upper dosage limit. Psychosomatics 26: 823–824
24. Linnoila M, Viukari M 1976 Efficacy and side effects of nitrazepam and thioridazine as sleeping aids in psychogeriatric in-patients. British Journal of Psychiatry 128: 566–569
25. Covington J S 1975 Alleviating agitation, apprehension and related symptoms in geriatric patients. Southern Medical Journal 68: 719–724
26. Kirven L E, Montero E F 1973 Comparison of thioridazine and diazepam in the control of nonpsychotic symptoms associated with senility: Double blind study. Journal of the American Geriatrics Society 21: 546–551
27. Sydney M A 1973 Ventricular arrhythmias associated with use of thioridazine hydrochloride in alcohol withdrawal. British Medical Journal 4: 467
28. Newton R W 1973 Ventricular dysrhythmias and thioridazine in alcohol withdrawal. British Medical Journal 4: 738
29. Donion P T, Tupin J P 1977 Successful suicides with thioridazine and mesoridazine: A result of probable cardiotoxicity. Archives of General Psychiatry 34: 955–957
30. Lam R W 1985 Pigmentary retinopathy associated with low-dose thioridazine treatment. Canadian Medical Association Journal 132: 737
31. Ayd F J, Coyle J T, Hollister L E, Simpson G M 1984 Tardive dyskinesia and thioridazine. Archives of General Psychiatry 41: 414–415
32. Westlin W F 1984 Tardive dyskinesia and thioridazine: A reply. Archives of General Psychiatry 41: 416
33. Frantz A G, Sachar E J 1976 Prolactin and growth hormone levels in man. In: Sedvall G, Uvnas B, Zotterman Y (eds) Antipsychotic drugs: pharmacodynamics and pharmacokinetics. Pergamon Press, Oxford, pp 421–436
34. Silver J M, Yudofsky S C, Kogan M, Katz B L 1987 Elevation of thioridazine plasma concentrations by propranolol. American Journal of Psychiatry 143: 1290–1292
35. Greendyke R M, Gulya A 1988 Effect of pindolol administration on serum concentrations of thioridazine, haloperidol, phenytoin and phenobarbitone 49: 105–107
36. Kutt H 1982 Phenytoin interactions with other drugs. In: Woodbury D M, Penry J K, Pippenger C E (eds) Antiepileptic drugs. Raven Press, New York, pp 227–240
37. Pfister A K 1978 Weight gain from combined phenothiazine and tricyclic therapy. Journal of the American Medical Association 239: 1959
38. Ayd F J 1974 Pharmacokinetic interaction between tricyclic antidepressants and phenothiazine neuroleptics. International Drug Therapy Newsletter 9: 31

T

Thyroxine (sodium)

A naturally occuring hormone produced by the thyroid gland.

Chemistry

Thyroxine sodium (levothyroxine sodium, L-thyroxine sodium, Eltroxin. Levothroid, Synthroid)
$C_{15}H_{10}I_4N\ NaO_4 . \times H_2O$
Sodium 4-0-(4-hydroxy-3, 5-di-iodophenyl)-3,5-diiodo-L-tyrosine hydrate

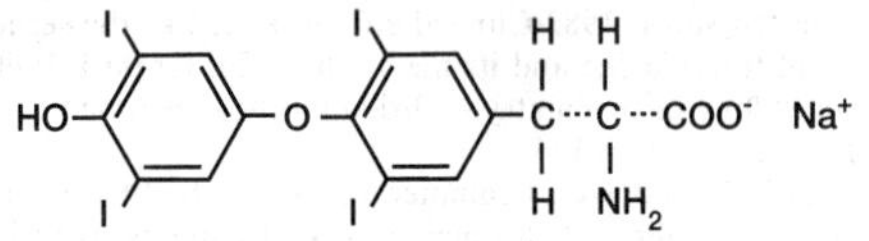

Molecular weight	
(anhydrous)	798.9
(free acid)	776.9
pKa (COOH, OH, NH_2)	2.2, 6.5, 10.1
Solubility	
in alcohol	1 in 300
in water	1 in 700
Octanol/water partition coefficient	—

An odourless almost white to pale brownish-yellow, tasteless, hygroscopic, amorphous or crystalline powder. It may develop a slight pink colour on exposure to light. It is prepared by chemical synthesis. The L-isomer is used clinically. It is soluble in solutions of alkali, but unstable. Thyroxine sodium is also available in combination with liothyronine sodium in a ratio of 4:1 (Liotrix tablets USP) but there is no advantage in this preparation over thyroxine per se. Thyroxine is often abbreviated to T4 in medical and biochemical reports.

Pharmacology

Thyroxine (T4) is a naturally occurring hormone produced by the thyroid gland and converted to the more active hormone triiodothyronine (T3) in peripheral tissues. Receptors for T3 are found on cell membranes, mitochondria and cell nuclei. The precise signals controlling the conversion of T4 to T3 within the cell are not known.[1] The thyroid hormones are required for normal growth and development particularly of the nervous system. They increase the resting or basal metabolic rate of the whole organism and have stimulatory effects on the heart, skeletal muscle, liver and kidney. Thyroid hormones enhance lipolysis and the utilization of carbohydrate.

Toxicology

Thyroxine sodium is not known to have either carcinogenic or teratogenic effects.

Clinical pharmacology

Doses in the range of 100 to 200 μg daily are usually sufficient to maintain a euthyroid state when treating patients for hypothyroidism. The dose required should be sufficient to render the patient clinically euthyroid and to restore circulating thyroid hormone and serum thyrotrophin (TSH) levels to the normal range. Rarely patients may require as much as 300 μg daily but a more typical replacement dose is 150 μg thyroxine daily.[2,3]

Correction of the hypothyroid state results in increased physical and mental well-being, weight reduction, improved tolerance of cold, relief of constipation, increased heart rate and peripheral vascular perfusion. Basal metabolic rate is increased and there is reduction of serum cholesterol and triglycerides with increased carbohydrate utilization.

Pharmacokinetics

The usual analytical method for measurement of thyroxine in serum or plasma is by radioimmunossay, which has a limit of sensitivity of $\sim 12\ nmol.l^{-1}$. Other, non-radioisotope methods are being developed which may shortly supersede radioimmunoassays. The normal physiological range for total thyroxine is $60–150\ nmol.l^{-1}$ and for free (unbound) T4 is $10–25\ pmol.l^{-1}$.

Thyroxine is incompletely and variably absorbed from the gastrointestinal tract. It has a half life of approximately seven days in a normal person, but this may be shortened in hyperthyroid states and prolonged in hypothyroid states, due to altered rate of metabolism of the hormone. Thyroxine is largely bound to plasma protein, mainly to thyroxine binding globulin (TBG) but also to prealbumin and less avidly to albumin. The unbound or free fraction, although only about 0.03% of total thyroxine, is of course the fraction available for peripheral action and conversion to the more active metabolite triiodothyronine (T3). Alterations to serum protein levels will affect the concentration of total but not free thyroxine; thus pregnancy or oestrogens increase TBG and nephrotic syndrome and other protein-losing states will lower TBG. Thyroxine is partly converted to T3 and other metabolites (see Metabolism) and conjugates with glucuronic and sulphuric acids are excreted in the bile. Some conjugated material is hydrolysed in the colon and 20–40% of thyroxine is excreted in the faeces. Some free thyroxine as well as deiodinated metabolites and conjugates are excreted in the urine.

Neither renal nor hepatic disease appears to have any marked effects on the disposition of thyroxine.

Placental transfer of thyroxine is believed not to occur except possibly in the earliest few weeks of gestation before fetal production of thyroxine develops. Thyroxine is secreted in breast milk but not in sufficient amounts to correct hypothyroidism in a breast-fed infant.[4]

Oral absorption	40–75%
Presystemic metabolism	—
Plasma half life	
mean	7 days
Volume of distribution	—
Plasma protein binding	99.97%

Concentration–effect relationship

Increasing concentrations of thyroxine beyond the normal physiological range (in the absence of any increase in binding proteins or other non-thyroid illness or interference by drugs such as oestrogens) produces increasing symptoms and signs of hyperthyroidism. Conversely, insufficient thyroxine produces symptoms and signs of hypothyroidism. The latter are non-specific and easily missed but can be confirmed biochemically by an elevated serum thyrotrophin (TSH) level as well as low thyroxine.

Metabolism

Thyroxine is extensively metabolized in the thyroid, liver, kidney and anterior pituitary. It is excreted in urine and faeces, partly as free drug and partly as conjugates and deiodinated metabolites (Fig. 1).

There are four main pathways of metabolism: deiodination to triiodothyronine (T3 or liothyronine) which is the principal active form of thyroxine (6–11% of dose in urine) or to reverse triiodothyronine (rT3) which is inactive. Further deiodination of T3 leads to the formation of thyroacetic acid (4-hydroxyphenoxyphenylacetic acid) (12–22% of dose in urine); deamination to the tetrone; conjugation to the glucuronide or sulphate; and ether bond cleavage to di-iodotyrosines.

Between 30 and 55% of the dose is excreted in the urine and 20–40% in the faeces. The most important pathway is deiodination to the active metabolite triiodothyronine (T3) and its mirror image, reverse T3 which is metabolically inactive (Fig. 1). Increased levels of rT3 may be found in severe non-thyroid illness of many kinds with

Thyroxine (sodium)

variable T4 levels and protects against excessive conversion to the active T3 in such circumstances.[5]

Pharmaceutics

Thyroxine is available in tablet form in three strengths, 25 µg, 50 µg and 100 µg. Eltroxin (Glaxo UK) is available as a 50 µg white scored tablet and a 100 µg white tablet both marked with tablet name, strength and 'Glaxo'. The tablets are all very small and easily confused with each other. Tablets should be protected from direct sunlight and they have a reasonable shelf-life when stored properly. In the USA tablet strengths range from 25 µg to 300 µg. Thyroxine may also be available as a solution containing 100 $\mu g.ml^{-1}$. Levothyroid injection (USV, US) and Synthroid injection (Flint, US) contains either 200 µg or 500 µg of thyroxine in a 10 ml vial. They are lyophilized with mannitol and contain a buffering agent. They should be reconstituted with sodium chloride 0.9% injection only and used immediately.

Therapeutic use

Indications

1. Treatment of hypothyroidism
   a. congenital
   b. acquired
      (i) primary thyroid failure
      (ii) autoimmune
      (iii) post surgery
      (iv) post radioiodine therapy
      (v) drug therapy
      (vi) in myxoedema coma
   c. secondary to pituitary/hypothalamic disease
2. Suppression of goitre
3. In conjunction with antithyroid drugs in treatment of thyrotoxicosis.

Contraindications

There are few contraindications but special precautions must be taken in patients with angina, heart failure, the elderly and in patients with adrenal failure (primary, or secondary to pituitary disease.)

Thyroid hormones should not be used in the treatment of obesity unless there is evidence of hypothyroidism confirmed biochemically.

Mode of use

All the clinical uses require that thyroxine be given in a dosage sufficient to maintain the patient in a euthyroid state. In adult patients without cardiac problems oral treatment is usually started with 50 µg daily and increased at two-week intervals to 100 µg then 150 µg daily and the patient's well-being and thyroid function tests are reassessed after 6–8 weeks. The daily dosage may then require further minor adjustment so as to ensure clinical and biochemical euthyroidism.[2,3]

In the elderly and in patients with angina a more cautious regime is advised starting with 25 µg daily and increasing the dose by 25 µg increments every two weeks until euthyroid. If there is an exacerbation of angina then the dose of thyroxine should be reduced by one step and propranolol or similar agent introduced. After the introduction of propranolol a further attempt could be made to increase the thyroxine dose but sometimes it is necessary to compromise by accepting a suboptimal replacement dosage in respect of the restoration of thyroid hormone levels to normal.[6] The appropriate dose for neonates and children is considered below (see Congential hypothyroidism).

In patients given thyroxine after thyroid ablation for differentiated thyroid cancer it is essential that the dose of thyroxine is sufficient (usually 150–200 µg T4) to suppress any TSH drive which might otherwise stimulate growth of residual TSH-sensitive tumour tissue.[7]

Indications

1. Treatment of hypothyroidism

Congenital hypothyroidism

Congenital hypothyroidism is detected by routine screening for raised TSH ± T4 at birth or five days later when the immediate postnatal surge in TSH has largely subsided. It occurs in 1:2500 to 1:3500 births in Europe and North America and may be due to congenitally complete absence of thyroid tissue or an inadequate source of thyroid hormones such as ectopic thyroid. Replacement therapy should be started as soon as the diagnosis is made to prevent the mental and physical retardation that would otherwise occur. Initial therapy consists of a recommended daily dose of T4 of 10 $\mu g.kg^{-1}$ for infants under 6 months of age then 8 $\mu g.kg^{-1}$ from 6 to 12 months, 6 $\mu g.kg^{-1}$ from 1 to 5 years and 4 $\mu g.kg^{-1}$ from 5 to 10 years. The dose of thyroxine should be sufficient to suppress the TSH level to normal and maintain T4 and T3 levels in the normal range. The initial diagnosis and cause can be reappraised when the infant is a year old and should be developing along normal growth patterns.

Acquired primary hypothyroidism

This is usually due to autoimmune thyroid disease and affects women approximately ten times more frequently than men. It is also commoner in older than younger women. Partial thyroidectomy or radioiodine therapy for thyroxtoxicosis commonly result in hypothyroidism (cumulative incidence of 30–50% after 10–15 years). Total thyroidectomy and ablative doses of radioiodine for differentiated thyroid cancer will inevitably result in hypothyroidism. Hypothyroidism may also occur as a result of drug therapy, e.g. lithium for depression and amiodarone for cardiac arrhythmias, and is reversible if the offending drug can be withdrawn.

The symptoms and signs of hypothyroidism are non-specific and may develop insidiously. The diagnosis of primary hypothyroidism is confirmed by an elevated serum TSH with a low serum thyroxine. Thyroxine replacement therapy should be sufficient to suppress the serum TSH and restore normal T4 levels as well as relieve the patient's symptoms. Caution is necessary with elderly patients and those with heart disease (see Mode of use).

Myxoedema coma is a rare, but often fatal condition, which usually occurs as a result of long-neglected hypothyroidism. The condition may be difficult to distinguish from hypothermia per se. Treatment is mainly supportive with maintenance of adequate respiration and circulation and gradual rewarming. Treatment with steroids is usually recommended because of the likelihood of adrenal

Fig. 1

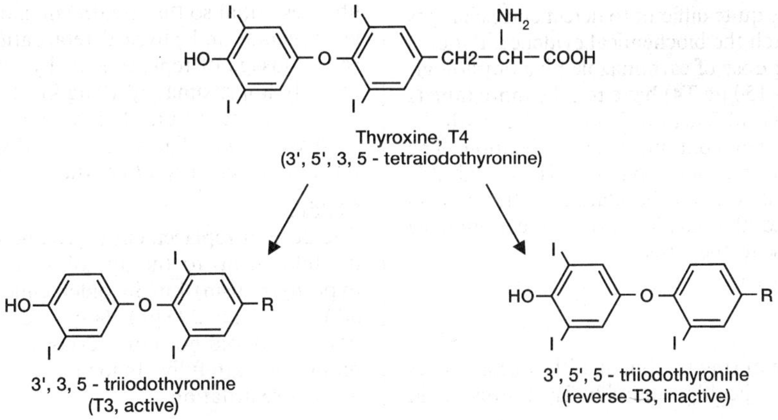

impairment. The choice of thyroid hormone replacement is empirical. Levothyroxine 200–500 μg intravenously has been advocated for initial treatment but small doses of triiodothyronine are also effective (see Triiodothyronine).[8]

Hypothyroidism secondary to pituitary/hypothalamic disease
Hypothyroidism may result from a pituitary tumour or craniopharyngioma or other rare lesions which destroy pituitary function. Secondary hypothyroidism is seldom an early manifestation of such diseases and deficiency of other pituitary hormones such as ACTH and gonadotrophins are likely to be present. The diagnosis of secondary hypothyroidism will depend on demonstration of low serum thyroxine and an undetectable TSH (in a sensitive assay) or absent TSH response to intravenous TRH (but the latter test often gives variable responses.)

It is important to correct any steroid deficiency first before initiating thyroxine replacement therapy, which might otherwise enhance metabolism and physical activities at a rate which could result in stress-induced adrenal insufficiency owing to the lack of ACTH reserves. Thyroxine replacement is then built up stepwise until the patient is clinically euthyroid with normal serum T4 levels.

2. Suppression of goitre
There are numerous causes of goitre and where possible treatment should be to correct the cause, e.g. iodine deficiency. When a goitre is associated with hypothyroidism confirmed by a raised TSH then thyroxine therapy is appropriate for replacement purposes irrespective of its effect on the size of the goitre. A so-called simple goitre may however occur in the absence of disturbed thyroid function due to growth factors which do not necessarily stimulate function. Such goitres may not need to be treated but if they are sufficiently large to distress the patient, but not so large as to cause pressure symptoms requiring surgical relief, then a trial of thyroxine therapy may be justified. The result of such a trial is difficult to predict for the individual as there have been wide differences in the degree of regression of goitre reported by experienced observers. Significant regression might be expected in one-third to a half of such cases.

A similar trial of thyroxine therapy in a dosage sufficient to suppress any endogenous TSH drive or hormone production (150–200 μg T4 daily) may be worth undertaking in a patient with a moderately enlarged multinodular goitre. It is necessary to have established that the patient is not hypothyroid and that the gland is not malignant. Shrinkage of the gland is less likely to occur with multinodular goitre than with simple goitre. Surgery may be needed if there is any pressure on the trachea or surrounding tissues. If surgery is undertaken for benign multinodular goitre then some authorities advocate the immediate institution of thyroxine therapy to prevent recurrence of nodules in the thyroid remnants, although long-term evidence that this is effective is lacking.

3. In conjunction with antithyroid drugs in the treatment of thyrotoxicosis
The medical treatment of thyrotoxicosis may be managed either by tailoring the dose of carbimazole or propylthiouracil (PTU) to the minimum required to maintain the patient euthyroid, or by using continually a large dose of carbimazole or PTU sufficient to totally block thyroid function and adding a physiological replacement dose of thyroxine to prevent hypothyroidism. Those who favour the former approach argue that the smallest dose of an antithyroid drug that is necessary is all that should be given. However, patients frequently escape from such treatment and may suffer a series of relapses or overtreatment as it is quite difficult to detect early changes clinically and they may not match the biochemical evidence. Patients treated with the larger blocking dose of carbimazole plus physiological thyroxine replacement (100–150 μg T4) have to take more tablets but avoid the fluctuations in thyroid function that can occur with the alternative regime, so long as they continue their medication. The combination regime of carbimazole plus thyroxine is not suitable during pregnancy as carbimazole crosses the placenta whereas thyroxine effectively does not and the smallest dose of carbimazole should be used to minimize risk to the fetus.

Adverse reactions

Potentially life-threatening effects
No reactions of this kind occur during treatment with normal doses in hypothyroid but otherwise healthy individuals; however, in patients who also have underlying heart disease there is always a danger of exacerbation of angina or dysrhythmias or potentially fatal myocardial infarction. Cautious initial replacement therapy is therefore advisable particularly in the elderly or anyone known to be suffering from ischaemic heart disease (see Mode of use).

The manifestations of toxicity due to thyroxine excess are those of thyrotoxicosis and in varying degree dependent on the dose and the rapidity of ingestion.

Acute overdosage
A massive acute overdose is fortunately uncommon but potentially lethal as it could produce a thyrotoxic crisis with cardiovascular collapse, hyperpyrexia and coma.[9] This might take a day or two to develop given the absorption characteristics of the drug. If the patient presents soon after ingestion of an acute overdose then gastric aspiration and lavage is indicated. Other treatment includes propranolol and supportive measures to maintain the circulation. Antithyroid drugs such as propylthiouracil or lithium might be of use but are not likely to be rapid enough in their action to prevent the thyrotoxic crisis developing.

Severe or irreversible adverse effects
Iatrogenic hyperthyroidism due to excessive thyroxine replacement therapy recommended by a doctor is not rare. If restoration of normal thyroid hormone levels is attempted too rapidly, or excessive levels achieved by too large a dose, the patient may develop tachycardia or arrhythmia, loose stools, diarrhoea, weight loss, heat intolerance, insomnia and agitation. A similar picture results from the surreptitious ingestion of excess thyroxine by a patient — thyrotoxicosis factitia. All these symptoms disappear within a month of withdrawal of the drug.[10]

Adverse effects due to idiosyncratic reactions to thyroxine tablets are extremely rare.

Symptomatic adverse effects
Apart from those already described there are no adverse effects of this kind.

Interference with clinical pathology tests
Thyroxine interfering with tests. Serum T4, T3 and TSH can be measured in patients taking thyroxine to determine optimum replacement dosage and compliance. To test endogenous thyroid function in a patient on thyroxine in whom the diagnosis of hypothyroidism is suspected to be wrong or unproven thyroxine will need to be discontinued for 3 to 4 weeks before repeating the tests. Thyroxine will also suppress radioiodine uptake in normal individuals.

Factors interfering with the measurement of thyroxine. Several factors may alter serum levels of thyroxine to give misleading results.[11] Increased binding to TBG during pregnancy and with oestrogen therapy will increase total (but not free) T4 levels. Loss of protein due to nephrotic syndrome or liver disease will lower total (but not free) T4 levels. Competitive binding to TBG by drugs such as phenylbutazone and phenytoin lowers total T4 levels, but TSH remains normal. Rarely the presence of an unusual protein may cause abnormal binding of thyroid hormones. Occasionally antibodies to thyroxine may develop in a patient's serum and these will interfere with any radioimmunoassay method of measuring T4.

High risk groups

Neonates
Early detection of hypothyroidism at birth or within the first week of life is essential so that treatment can be initiated promptly to prevent later mental and physical retardation (see Congenital hypothyroidism). Dosage of replacement thyroxine is adjusted for body weight. Initially approximately 10 $\mu g.kg^{-1}$. is needed to suppress TSH and restore normal serum thyroxine levels.

Breast milk. The amount of thyroxine in breast milk is variable but not sufficient to affect the normal infant.

Children
The dose of replacement thyroxine needed to correct hypothroidism in children up to the age of 10 is outlined above (see Congenital hypothyroidism) but in older children is similar to that needed in adults (100 μg–200 μg) daily and should be sufficient to maintain normal thyroid hormone levels. Growth and development should be monitored carefully. Inadequate replacement therapy will result in growth retardation.

Thyroxine (sodium)

Pregnant women
Women on maintenance thyroxine for hypothyroidism who become pregnant should not need to alter the dose because of the pregnancy so long as they are confirmed to be euthyroid initially, by normal TSH levels. Total serum thyroxine levels are increased in pregnancy (due to altered TBG binding) but free thyroxine levels decline with advancing pregnancy.

Patients on treatment for thyrotoxicosis with a combination of antithyroid drugs plus physiological replacement thyroxine are better treated by a small dose of carbimazole or propylthiouracil alone during pregnancy to minimize placental transfer of the latter. Thyroxine does not cross the placental barrier in the second and third trimester, although it may do so in early pregnancy.

The elderly
Caution is necessary when introducing thyroxine replacement therapy in the elderly because of the risk of exacerbating or precipitating arrhythmia, angina or heart failure. Small doses, 25 µg daily, are given at longer intervals between increments until euthyroidism is achieved unless angina is exacerbated (see Mode of use).[6]

Concurrent disease
Any severe non-thyroid illness may lower the levels of circulating thyroxine either by reduction of carrier proteins or even with normal proteins by interference with the conversion of T4 to T3 or reverse T3. Reduction of serum T4 below the defined normal range does not require additional treatment in such circumstances unless the patient becomes hypothyroid as evidenced by a raised TSH.

In patients already on thyroxine replacement therapy the development of renal failure or liver disease dose not usually necessitate any adjustment to the usual daily dose, although the tests of thyroid function may be affected (see above). The presence of arrhythmias, angina, or heart failure necessitates very cautious use of thyroxine if the hypothyroidism is to be treated (see Mode of use).

Drug interactions

Potentially hazardous interactions
Thyroxine, when given to hypothyroid patients who are already on anticoagulants, will potentiate the effect of warfarin and other dicoumarin anticoagulants necessitating a marked reduction (50%) in warfarin dosage to prevent excessive prolongation of the prothrombin time and partial thromboplastin time.[16]

The mechanism of action is uncertain but may be due to the increased catabolism, reducing platelet factors or reduction of serum lipids thereby reducing the amounts of vitamin K available to the liver.

Other significant interactions
Cholestyramine may reduce absorption of thyroxine.[12]
Phenylbutazone may cause a false low total serum thyroxine by competition for binding sites on TBG (but free thyroxine and TSH remain normal).

Carbamazepine and phenytoin may also interfere with protein binding of thyroxine and cause false low total serum thyroxine levels. Phenytoin can also lower free T4 levels by increased clearance.[13]

Amiodarone is widely used for cardiac arrhythmias and commonly produces elevated thyroxine levels, but triiodothyronine levels are usually normal, as the drug interferes with the conversion of T4 to T3. Serum T3 and TSH levels rather than T4 should be used to monitor the patient's thyroid status.[14,15]

Potentially useful interactions
No reactions of this kind have been reported.

References

1. Chopra I J 1986 Nature, source and biologic significance of thyroid circulating hormones. In: Ingbar S H, Braverman L E (eds) Werner's The thyroid, 5th edn. J B Lippincott Co, Philadelphia, ch 7, pp 136–153
2. Evered D A, Young E T, Ormston B J, Menzies R, Smith P A, Hall R 1973 Treatment of hypothyroidism: a reappraisal of thyroxine therapy. British Medical Journal 3: 131–134
3. Pearch C J, Himsworth R L 1984 Total and free thyroid hormone concentrations in patients receiving maintenance replacement treatment with thyroxine. British Medical Journal 288: 693–695
4. Bode H M, Vamjonack W J, Crawford J D 1978 Mitigation of cretinism by breast-feeding. Paediatrics 62: 13–16
5. Utiger R D 1980 Decreased extra thyroidal triiodothyronine production in non-thyroidal illness: benefit or harm? American Journal of Medicine 69: 807–810
6. Leading article 1981 Management of angina and hypothyroidism. British Medical Journal 282: 1818
7. Lamberg B A, Rantanen M, Saarinen P 1977 Choosing thyroxine dose after treatment of thyroid cancer. Lancet 2: 1290–1291 (letter)
8. Newmark S R, Himathongkam T, Shane J M 1974 Myxoedema coma. Journal of the American Medical Association 230: 884–885
9. Van Hofe S E, Young R L 1977 Thyrotoxicosis after a single ingestion of levothyroxine. Journal of the American Medical Association 237: 1361
10. Harvery R F 1973 Thyroxine 'addicts'. British Medical Journal 2: 35–36
11. Davies D M (ed) 1985 Endocrine disorders. In: Textbook of adverse drugs reactions, 3rd edn. Oxford University Press, Oxford, pp 336–339
12. Northcutt R C, Stiel J N, Hollifield J W, Stant E G 1969 The influence of cholestyramine on thyroxine absorption. Journal of the American Medical Association 208: 1857–1861
13. Yeo P P B, Bates D, Howe J G et al 1978 Anticonvulsants and thyroid function. British Medical Journal 1: 1581–1583
14. Burger A, Dinichert D, Nicod P, Jenny M, Lemarchand-Beraud T, Valloton M B 1976. The effect of amiodarone on serum T3, rT3, T4 and TSH: a drug influencing peripheral metabolism of thyroid hormones. Journal of Clinical Investigation 58: 255–259
15. Melmed S, Nademanee K, Allen K W, Henderickson J, Singh B N, Herhman J M 1981 Hyperthyroxinaemia with bradycardia and normal thyrotrophin secretion following chronic amiodarone administration. Journal of Clinical Endocrinology and Metabolism 53: 997–1001
16. Costigan D C, Freedman M H, Ehlich R M 1984 Potentiation of oral anticoagulant effect by L-thyroxine. Clinical Paediatrics 23: 172–174

T

Tiaprofenic acid

Tiaprofenic acid is a propionic acid derivative, a non-steroidal anti-inflammatory drug used in a variety of arthritic conditions.

Chemistry

Tiaprofenic acid (Surgam)
$C_{14}H_{12}O_3S$
S-Benzoyl-α-methyl-2-thiopheneacetic acid

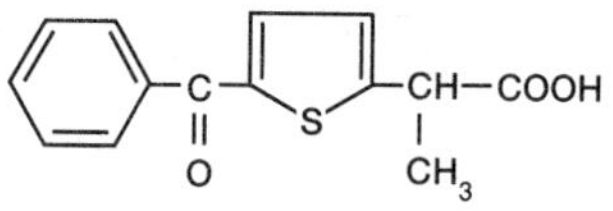

Molecular weight	260.3
pKa (carboxyl)	3.0
Solubility	
in alcohol	1 in 5
in water	sparingly soluble
Octanol/water partition coefficient	—

A white micro-crystalline material prepared by chemical synthesis. It is not available in drug combination.

Pharmacology

Tiaprofenic acid is a non-steroidal anti-inflammatory drug with analgesic and antipyretic activity. In animal models it has anti-inflammatory activity greater than that of aspirin or phenylbutazone. Tiaprofenic acid is a potent inhibitor of prostaglandin synthetase activity[1] (cyclooxygenase) and is more potent than indomethacin in this regard. The analgesic effect of tiaprofenic acid is greater than that of aspirin or phenylbutazone as measured in the rat inflamed paw model and has significant antipyretic activity.

It has been suggested that this drug shows some selectivity of inhibition of prostaglandin synthesis in some tissues more than others. However, the evidence relating to this is poor and is based on one preliminary observation and a second reference which showed that tiaprofenic acid suppressed the synthesis of plasma thromboxane and PGE_2 at concentrations that only partially affected the formation of renal prostaglandins. However, there was no suggestion that this was a specific action of tiaprofenic acid, as it applies to other NSAIDs.

Toxicology

Tiaprofenic acid does not have mutagenic potential and toxicological testing in animals failed to demonstrate any results of clinical significance apart from gastric erosions and prolongation of the bleeding time. No carcinogenic effect related to treatment was demonstrated in long-term administration to mice or rats. Teratogenic effects were not shown in either rats or rabbits. In mice, however, an increased fetal loss was shown at a daily oral dose of 100 $mg.kg^{-1}$.

Clinical pharmacology

Tiaprofenic acid is an effective anti-inflammatory and analgesic drug in clinical practice and is used in the treatment of rheumatoid arthritis and osteoarthritis. It is as effective as indomethacin or aspirin in clinical studies but may produce fewer side effects than these two agents. Tiaprofenic acid reduces joint swelling and relieves pain but has no long-term effect on the disease process. Tiaprofenic acid inhibits platelet adhesiveness and prolongs the bleeding time. By inhibiting prostaglandin synthesis in the uterus tiaprofenic acid may delay the onset of labour.

Tiaprofenic acid has little effect on renal function in normal individuals but can worsen renal function in patients who depend upon the action of prostaglandin E_2 to maintain renal blood flow. This may occur in hypertension, diabetes and a number of other conditions. Tiaprofenic acid may cause gastric erosions partly by directly irritating the gastric mucosa, and partly by inhibiting the synthesis of cytoprotective prostaglandins.

Pharmacokinetics

The preferred analytical method for drug analysis is HPLC with ultraviolet detection which can detect levels of 0.5 $\mu g.ml^{-1}$ and is rapid and specific.[2]

Tiaprofenic acid is rapidly absorbed from the gastrointestinal tract and peak plasma levels are seen 90 min after an oral dose[3] with a plasma half life of 1.5–2 h. Peak plasma concentrations recorded for different doses are: 20.5–32.2 $mg.l^{-1}$ for a 200 mg dose; 18.6–73.3 $mg.l^{-1}$ for a 300 mg dose; 19.5–34.9 $mg.l^{-1}$ for a 300 mg sustained-release capsule. These also give an indication of the interindividual variation. There is no presystemic metabolism.

Tiaprofenic acid has an apparent volume of distribution of 10% body weight. It enters the CNS only in trace amounts (<0.165% total dose per 100 g tissue) but has good penetration into synovial fluid[4] and high levels persist after the fall of serum levels; the concentrations of tiaprofenic acid ($mg.ml^{-1}$) in serum and synovial fluid (mean of six patients) following 200 mg study dose in patients taking 200 mg three times a day are showed in the table below.

Table 1

	Serum	SF
Time	1.9	2.4
Peak	26.0	5.3
Final sample (8 hours)	2.0	4.4

Tiaprofenic acid is highly protein bound.

Oral absorption	readily
Presystemic metabolism	nil
Plasma half life	1.5–2 h
Volume of distribution	—
Plasma protein binding	97–98%

Concentration–effect relationship

In common with other non-steroidal anti-inflammatory drugs clinical efficacy is not directly related to plasma levels. Consequently, there is no therapeutic range.

Metabolism

Tiaprofenic acid is excreted in the urine (60%) and bile (40%). Of that excreted in the urine only 10% is metabolized. There is no enterohepatic circulation.

The primary pathways of metabolism are reduction and hydroxylation; excretion of the parent compound and metabolites is mainly in the form of acylglucuronide conjugates. None of the metabolites is pharmacologically active.[5]

Pharmaceutics

Tiaprofenic acid is available as sustained-release capsules of 300 mg (Surgam SA; Roussel, UK) and as tablets of 200 mg or 300 mg, or as dispersible sachets of 300 mg. The tablets are white, convex and either 10 mm (200 mg) or 11 mm (300 mg) in diameter, marked on one side with 'Surgam' ('200' or '300') and on the other with the Roussel logo. The sustained-release formulation is a maroon–pink capsule containing the drug in white pellets. A 24 hour release is claimed.

Tiaprofenic acid does not contain tartrazine or other potentially allergenic substances. The tablets are stable with a 3 year shelf-life and should be stored in a cool place protected from light.

Therapeutic use

Indications

1. Rheumatoid arthritis
2. Osteoarthritis
3. Ankylosing spondylitis
4. Musculoskeletal disorders
5. Pain.

Contraindications

1. Peptic ulceration
2. Drug hypersensitivity
3. Severe renal impairment.

Mode of use

Tiaprofenic acid is used in a daily dose of 600 mg either as 200 mg three times daily or 300 mg twice daily to produce its anti-inflammatory and analgesic actions. Studies that directly compared 200 mg three times daily with 300 mg twice daily have shown no difference between the two regimens in terms of either side effects or efficacy. Because of the perceived advantage of less frequent dosage, 300 mg twice daily is the recommended mode of use.

Drug comparison studies have looked at the use of 600 mg as two 300 mg sustained-release capsules; the timing of morning or evening was unaffected by this. The majority of studies looking at flexible dosage did not include a comparison drug. There is no scientific evidence for the preferential use of this drug.

Indications

1. Rheumatoid arthritis
The few studies where tiaprofenic acid has been used as sole agent demonstrated a significant improvement over placebo in practically all criteria measured. Tiaprofenic acid has been found to be of comparable efficacy to aspirin, indomethacin, ibuprofen and naproxen in short-term studies.[6] No problems with sudden cessation of the drug have been reported.

2. Osteoarthritis
Studies in osteoarthritis[6] have shown tiaprofenic acid to be as useful as a variety of standard non-steroidal anti-inflammatory drugs such as aspirin, diclofenac, ibuprofen, and indomethacin.

3. Ankylosing spondylitis
Tiaprofenic acid has been shown to be an effective treatment for the symptoms of ankylosing spondylitis.[7]

4. Musculoskeletal disorders
In open studies tiaprofenic acid was shown to significantly improve patients with pain of discogenic origin, and significantly help patients with neuralgia and tendinitis.[8]

5. Pain
Controlled studies of patients with postoperative[9] or post-traumatic[10] pain showed tiaprofenic acid to be as effective as aspirin and indomethacin and more effective than placebo.

Contraindications

1. Peptic ulceration
Like all non-steroidal anti-inflammatory drugs tiaprofenic acid is contraindicated in active peptic ulceration; attempts should be made to use a non-ulcerogenic drug. Generally, it is well tolerated with about 10% of patients developing gastrointestinal tract symptoms.

2. Hypersensitivity
A previous allergic reaction to the drug is an absolute contraindication and caution should be exercised in patients with previous sensitivity to aspirin or other non-steroidal anti-inflammatory drugs.

3. Severe renal impairment
In patients with severe renal impairment the dosage should be reduced to 200 mg twice daily.

Adverse reactions

Potentially life-threatening effects
The potentially lethal effects are similar to those of other non-steroidal anti-inflammatory drugs, namely gastrointestinal tract haemorrhage, hypersensitivity, renal failure, hepatic failure, and agranulocytosis.

Acute overdosage
There are three case reports of overdosage with tiaprofenic acid. Patients suffered epigastric pain and nausea but did not lose consciousness; they were treated symptomatically with antacids. In one well-documented case, the patient took 2000 mg (i.e. 10 tablets) but did not exhibit any specific adverse effects apart from the gastrointestinal ones already mentioned.

Severe or irreversible adverse effects
Apart from those described above, none has been described.

Symptomatic adverse effects
These include heartburn, gastritis, nausea, vomiting, drowsiness, paraesthesiae, sweating and skin rash. In a long-term open study, 12% of patients developed adverse effects.[11]

Interference with clinical pathology tests
Tiaprofenic acid produces a falsely high reading in the Zimmerman reaction (used to determine urinary 17-oxosteroid levels.)[12]

High risk groups

Neonates
The drug is not recommended for use in neonates.

Breast milk. No adverse reactions have been noted in mothers or offspring when tiaprofenic acid has been administered during lactation[13] but experience is limited.

Children
The drug is not recommended for use in children.

Pregnant women
Tiaprofenic acid should not be administered in the first trimester.

The elderly
Dosage modifications may be required in the elderly.

Drug interactions

Potentially hazardous interactions
A recent study has indicated that neither indomethacin nor tiaprofenic acid affected the diuresis caused by frusemide. In addition, tiaprofenic acid did not have any effect on potassium or sodium excretion, whereas indomethacin increased the latter and decreased the former. Tiaprofenic acid may prolong the prothrombin time of patients controlled on anticoagulants.[15]

Potentially useful interactions
None has been described.

Major outcome trials

1. Meurice J 1983 Treatment of osteoarthritis: a 3 month comparison between tiaprofenic acid and indomethacin. Current Medical Research and Opinion 8: 295–301

60 elderly patients with osteoarthritis of the hip and the knee received either tiaprofenic acid or indomethacin for 3 months in a double-blind study. Patients who had received tiaprofenic acid continued with therapy for 11 months. Both drugs produced significant improvement in the measured parameters, but indomethacin produced more side effects. Of the 30 patients maintained on tiaprofenic acid for the further 11 months, there were no withdrawals due to side effects.

References

1. Jouquey S, Deraedt R 1976 Effect of tiaprofenic acid on biosynthesis of prostaglandins. Report on file, Cassenne Ltd
2. Ward G T, Stead J A, Freeman M 1982 A rapid and specific method for the determination of tiaprofenic acid in human plasma by HPLC. Journal of Liquid Chromatography 5: 165
3. Daymond T J, Herbert R 1983 Pharmacokinetic studies of a high dose of tiaprofenic acid in patients suffering from arthritis. British Journal of Clinical Pharmacology 15: 157
4. Daymond T J, Herbert R 1982 Simultaneous bioavailability of tiaprofenic acid in serum and synovial fluid in patients with rheumatoid arthritis. Rheumatology 7: 188–193
5. Pottier J, Cousty-Berlin D, Raynaud P 1977 Pharmacokinetics of the anti-inflammatory tiaprofenic acid in humans, mice, rabbits and dogs. Journal of Pharmaceutical Sciences 66: 1030–1036

T

6. Thompson M, Daymond T J, Essigman W K, Huskisson E C, Wojtulewski J A 1982 Short-term efficacy and tolerance of tiaprofenic acid in rheumatoid arthritis and osteoarthritis. Multi-centre, placebo controlled trials. Rheumatology 8: 215–223
7. Popert A J, Bedi S S, Lambert J, Nichol F, Pal B, Sweetman B J 1985 The treatment of ankylosing spondylitis with non-steroidal anti-inflammatory drugs. In: Berry H (ed) New trends in rheumatology 4. Excerpta Medica, Amsterdam, pp 62–66
8. Donald J F, Layes Molla A 1980 A comparative double-blind study of tiaprofenic acid and aspirin in treatment of muscular rheumatism, fibrositis, sprains, and soft tissue injuries in general practice. Journal of International Medical Research 8: 382–387
9. Ormiston M C, Vaughton K C, Thornton E J, LaCoste J J, Milroy E 1981 The comparative effectiveness of tiaprofenic acid and aspirin in the treatment of post-prostatectomy pain. British Journal of Clinical Practice 35: 360–362
10. Cutting C J, Thornton E J 1981 A comparative trial of tiaprofenic acid versus aspirin in the control of pain following injury. Pharmatherapeutica 2: 509–512
11. Wojtulewski J A, Daymond T J, Dimidtriadis P D et al 1983 Long-term efficacy and tolerance of tiaprofenic acid in rheumatoid arthritis and osteoarthritis. In: Berry H (ed) Proceedings of Moscow European Congress of Rheumatology. Excerpta Medica, Amsterdam, pp 116–124
12. Nahoul K 1979 Interference with Zimmerman Reactum. Journal of Steroid Biochemistry 10: 471
13. Jones R W, Freeman N 1986 Tiaprofenic acid in human plasma and breast milk. Acta Pharmacologica et Toxicologica 59 (suppl 5) Abs 521
14. Ishioka T 1987 Is tiaprofenic acid different from the other NSAIDs with regard to renal function in the elderly: In: Huskisson E C, Shiokaway (eds) New trends in rheumatology 5. Excerpta Medica, Amsterdam, pp 159–168
15. Whittaker S J, Jackson C W, Whorwell P J 1986 A severe, potentially fatal, interaction between tiaprofenic acid and nicoumalone. British Journal of Clinical Practice 40: 440

Ticarcillin (disodium)

A semi-synthetic penicillin with broad-spectrum activity against Gram-positive and Gram-negative bacteria, including *Pseudomonas aeruginosa.*

Chemistry

Ticarcillin disodium (Ticar)
$C_{15}H_{14}N_2O_6S_2Na_2$
The disodium salt of 6-{(R)-2-[Carboxy-2-(3-thienyl)-acetamido]} penicillanic acid

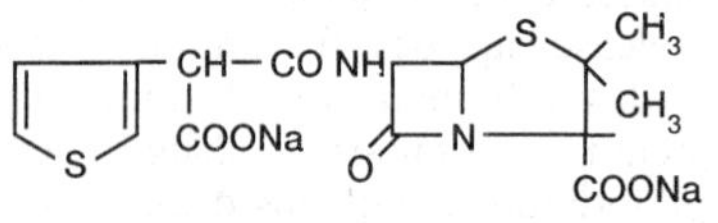

Molecular weight (free acid)	428.4 (384.4)
pKa	2.44, 3.64
Solubility	
in alcohol	1.5 in 100
in water	1 in 10
Octanol/water partition coefficient	very low

A semi-synthetic α-carboxypenicillin produced by the substitution of the phenyl group at the 6-position of the carbenicillin molecule with a 3-thienyl group. Supplied as the disodium salt, it is a white to pale yellow hygroscopic powder which is freely soluble in water. Each gram contains about 5.3 mmol of sodium. Ticarcillin is also available combined with the β-lactamase inhibitor clavulanic acid (as the potassium salt) as clavulanate-potentiated ticarcillin (Timentin). This is white to pale yellow in appearance; each gram contains approximately 0.3 mmol potassium and 5.0 mmol sodium.

Pharmacology

Ticarcillin inhibits bacterial cell wall synthesis by binding to penicillin-sensitive enzymes present in the cell wall (predominantly penicillin binding protein 3). It has a rapidly acting bactericidal effect both in vitro and in vivo. Although ticarcillin is relatively stable to certain β-lactamases with a predominant cephalosporinase activity, it is inactivated by many plasmid-mediated β-lactamases with penicillinase activity.[1] The addition of the β-lactamase inhibitor clavulanic acid renders susceptible many otherwise resistant β-lactamase-producing bacteria.

Toxicology

Animal studies have failed to demonstrate any significant toxigenic, carcinogenic or mutagenic potential. The LD_{50} in mice is 3000–3700 $mg.kg^{-1}$ when given intravenously. There is no evidence for teratological effects although studies are inadequate to completely exclude adverse effects on the fetus. The addition of clavulanic acid does not produce any measurable increase in toxicological effects in the various animal species studied.[2]

Clinical pharmacology

Ticarcillin is bactericidal against susceptible bacteria with a range of activity similar to that of carbenicillin.

Against Gram-positive bacteria, ticarcillin is less active than ampicillin, but this probably has no clinical relevance at the serum concentrations attained. Penicillin-sensitive staphylococci are inhib-

Ticarcillin (disodium)

ited by 2–4 mg.l^{-1}; however, ticarcillin is inactivated by staphylococcal β-lactamase and therefore such strains should be considered resistant (MIC 16 mg.l^{-1} or greater).[3–5] Activity against most streptococci is good; β-haemolytic streptococci (Lancefield groups A, B, C and G) are all susceptible to 2 mg.l^{-1} or less,[5] while other streptococci (including pneumococci) are susceptible to 4 mg.l^{-1} or less.[3,5] *Streptococcus faecalis*, however, is relatively resistant, with an MIC[5,6] usually greater than 32 mg.l^{-1}.

The activity in vitro of ticarcillin against the Enterobacteriaceae and *Ps. aeruginosa* is intermediate between that of carbenicillin and the ureidopenicillins (mezlocillin, azlocillin and piperacillin). Activity against *Escherichia coli* and *Proteus mirabilis* is similar to that of carbenicillin and ampicillin,[4,7] although ticarcillin is considerably more active than ampicillin against indole-positive *Proteus* spp.[4,7] Typical MICs for *E. coli* are 4 mg.l^{-1}, for *P. mirabilis* 1 mg.l^{-1}, and for *P. vulgaris* 16 mg.l^{-1}. Most *Enterobacter* are susceptible (MIC 8 mg.l^{-1}), including about 40% of strains resistant to ampicillin[6] but not strains resistant to carbenicillin. Salmonellae and shigellae are inhibited by low levels of ticarcillin, although clinical usefulness would not be expected. *Serratia* are relatively resistant, with MICs of 32–64 mg.l^{-1} or higher.[4,6] Ticarcillin has no significant activity against *Klebsiella* or *Citrobacter*.

Ticarcillin disodium is 2–4 times more active in vitro than carbenicillin against *Ps. aeruginosa* though less than azlocillin and piperacillin.[8] Typical MICs for sensitive strains[6] are 16 mg.l^{-1}. However, bactericidal activity may be greater for ticarcillin than for these other compounds, a property that has been demonstrated in animal infections.[9] Activity is much lower against other pseudomonads and also carbenicillin-resistant strains of *Ps. aeruginosa*.

Ticarcillin has good activity against *Haemophilus influenzae* (MIC 0.25 mg.l^{-1}), including some ampicillin-resistant strains.[5,10] Those producing β-lactamase, however, are resistant. Activity against *Neisseria* is excellent, MIC for *N. meningitidis* being 0.012 mg.l^{-1} (median) and for penicillin-sensitive gonococci less than 0.5 mg.l^{-1}. β-Lactamase-producing *N. gonorrhoeae* tend to be more resistant; MIC[10] 1–8 mg.l^{-1}.

Most penicillin-sensitive anaerobes are highly sensitive to ticarcillin, with the exception of the *Bacteroides fragilis* group, the majority of which are resistant by virtue of β-lactamase production (MIC 64 mg.l^{-1} or greater).[11] Other *Bacteroides, Clostridia, Fusobacteria* and anaerobic cocci are inhibited by 16 mg.l^{-1} or less of ticarcillin.[6,11]

Many bacteria are resistant to ticarcillin by virtue of β-lactamase production. The addition of the β-lactamase inhibitor clavulanic acid renders many of these bacteria susceptible. Clavulanate-potentiated ticarcillin has activity against most β-lactamase-producing *S. aureus, H. influenzae, N. gonorrhoeae* and *B. fragilis*.[12,13] It also has an extended spectrum amongst the Enterobacteriacae, including many ticarcillin resistant species, such as *Klebsiella*.[12,13] Most strains of *Acinetobacter, Enterobacter, Serratia* and *Pseudomonas* remain resistant to the combination due to the production of β-lactamases which are not inhibited by clavulanic acid.[13]

Pharmacokinetics

The preferred assay method is by high performance liquid chromatography,[1] with a sensitivity of 0.5 µg.ml^{-1}.

Ticarcillin is not absorbed from the gastrointestinal tract and so must be administered parenterally. Peak serum levels after either intramuscular or intravenous injection are dose-related. Ticarcillin is readily absorbed after intramuscular injection; peak serum levels of 25–30 mg.l^{-1} are attained 30–60 min after the administration of 1 g, falling to 5–8 mg.l^{-1} at 4 hours.[15,16] Serum levels after a given intravenous dose depend on the rapidity of injection. A 3 g dose given over 5 min produces a peak of 250 mg.l^{-1} at 20 min, falling to 30 mg.l^{-1} at 4 hours. The same dose over 120 min produces a delayed peak of 190 mg.l^{-1} at 2 hours, falling to a similar level by 4 hours.[15] Ticarcillin given by a constant infusion of 1–2 g.h^{-1} results in steady-state levels[17,18] of between 105 and 125 mg.l^{-1}.

The protein binding of ticarcillin is 45–65% and the apparent volume of distribution is 0.21 l.kg^{-1}, both values slightly higher than for carbenicillin. Distribution of ticarcillin in tissues is similar to that of carbenicillin. Interstitial fluid (skin window) concentrations of 11.7 mg.l^{-1} can be obtained after a 3 g intravenous dose.[19] Levels in muscle and fat after 5 g intravenously are 10–20% of those in serum.[20] High concentrations can be found in various body fluids; levels in pleural fluid are 30–66% of serum concentrations[21] and ascitic fluid levels average 34%.[22] Therapeutic levels may be obtained in bone provided high doses are used. Levels in sputum are low, being 3–5% of those in serum.[22,23] Ticarcillin does not readily cross the blood–brain barrier and therefore CSF levels are very low. Higher levels can be obtained in the presence of inflammation, though not sufficient to be reliably therapeutic.[21,22]

Ticarcillin readily crosses the placenta to give steady-state levels in cord serum and amniotic fluid of 70 and 50%, respectively, of those in serum.[24] Very little crosses into breast milk.

The plasma half life of ticarcillin in normal subjects is 67–76 min after intravenous administration[17,25] and, unlike the ureidopenicillins, is not dose-dependent.[18,26] Renal impairment produces a progressive reduction in the rate of clearance of ticarcillin, resulting in a prolonged half life of up to 15 hours when creatinine clearance[27,28] is below 10 ml.min^{-1}. This may be further prolonged in concomitant severe hepatic failure.[28] The half life is also prolonged in neonates; 3.5–5.6 hours in neonates under 7 days and weighing less than 2000 g, decreasing progressively with increasing age and body weight.[29]

Almost all (mean of 94%) of a 5 g intravenous dose of ticarcillin was excreted in the urine within 24 hours either as unchanged drug or penicilloic acid. A very small amount (3.5%) can be recovered from faeces.[25] Urinary concentrations are therefore very high and tend to remain high if there is renal impairment.[28] Renal excretion is by a combination of glomerular filtration and active renal tubular secretion, giving a renal clearance[15,17] of 106 ml.min^{-1}. Probenicid reduces urinary excretion by about 25%, resulting in raised serum levels and a longer half life.[17,28]

Ticarcillin is readily removed by haemodialysis, reducing the half life by 65–77%.[27,28] Peritoneal dialysis is much less efficient unless serum levels are very high.[27,28]

Oral absorption	negligible
Presystemic metabolism	not applicable
Plasma half life	
range	67–76 min
mean	70 min
Volume of distribution	0.21 l.kg^{-1}
Plasma protein binding	45–65%

Clavulanic acid has a very similar pharmacokinetic profile to that of ticarcillin, making it a suitable candidate for the combination. In addition, its presence does not significantly alter the pharmacokinetic parameters of ticarcillin.[2] Both drugs should therefore be present at the site of infection.

Concentration–effect relationship

The MIC values for typical organisms are shown in the Clinical pharmacology section.

Larger doses are recommended for severe infections and for less susceptible bacteria, particularly *Ps. aeruginosa*. In experimental infections due to *Ps. aeruginosa* in neutropenic mice, ticarcillin has been shown to be more effective at higher dosages than azlocillin which reaches a maximal effect, despite the latter's increased in vitro activity.[8] The relevance of this for clinical practice is uncertain.

Monitoring serum levels is not normally required provided due regard is taken of renal function.

Metabolism

Ticarcillin is metabolized in the liver to the inactive corresponding penicilloic acid derivative (Fig. 1) which is excreted in the urine. The proportion of penicilloic acid present increases with time such that urinary levels after 12 hours are 10–14% of the total dose recovered.[15,25] No other significant metabolites can be found.

Pharmaceutics

Ticarcillin, Ticar (SmithKline Beecham, UK/USA) is available for parenteral use only in vials containing 1 g, 3 g or 5 g ticarcillin sodium, or as a 5 g infusion bottle. Vials contain approximately 5.3 mmol, 16.0 mmol and 26.7 mmol, respectively, of sodium.

Fig. 1 Metabolism of ticarcillin

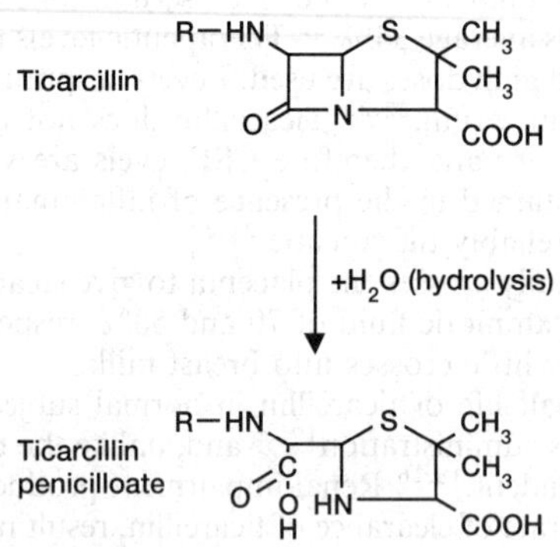

Vials of ticarcillin powder can be stored at room temperature, but once reconstituted should normally be used within 30 min. Aqueous solutions will retain activity for longer periods; 24 hours at room temperature and 72 hours at 5°C, although strict aseptic techniques must be used when reconstituting if solutions are to be kept.

Water for Injections BP is the preferred diluent for reconstitution, although ticarcillin is also compatible with glucose (5%) and 0.9% sodium chloride (not recommended due to the increased sodium load). It is incompatible with proteinaceous fluids, blood, plasma and intravenous lipids. Ticarcillin should not be mixed with an aminoglycoside due to possible inactivation of the latter.[30]

Ticarcillin is also available combined with clavulanic acid as Timentin (SmithKline Beecham UK/USA) in vials containing 3.2 g (3.0 g ticarcillin with 200 mg clavulanic acid), 1.6 g (1.5 g with 100 mg) and 800 mg (750 mg with 50 mg). General advice given above for ticarcillin regarding reconstitution, storage and compatibility of solutions is applicable to Timentin.

Therapeutic use

Indications

The treatment of severe infections due to susceptible bacteria of the genitourinary, respiratory, and gastrointestinal tracts, soft tissue and skin, bones and joints and cardiovascular system.

Contraindications

Hypersensitivity to penicillin-class antibiotics.

Mode of use

a. Ticarcillin

The recommended daily dosage is 15–20 g administered in divided doses at 4–8-hourly intervals. The higher dose should be used for serious infections, especially those in immunocompromised patients or when due to less sensitive organisms such as *Ps. aeruginosa.* A suggested maximum daily dosage of 24 g can be given under such circumstances. For uncomplicated urinary tract infections, a dosage of 3–4 g daily in divided doses is sufficient.

Intravenous administration can either be by slow injection over 3–4 min (to avoid vein irritation), or by infusion over 30–40 min. Longer periods of infusion are not recommended. The use of probenecid will achieve higher and more prolonged serum levels but it should not be used if renal function is impaired.

Intramuscular injections should not exceed 2 g per injection and should be given into a large muscle mass.

b. Clavulanate-potentiated ticarcillin

The usual dosage is 3.2 g given 6–8-hourly up to a maximum of 3.2 g 4-hourly for serious infections. Administration is by intermittent infusion over a 30–40 min period. Longer infusion times are not recommended since this may result in sub-therapeutic serum concentrations. Clavulanate-potentiated ticarcillin should not be given by direct intravenous or intramuscular injection.

Indications

The use of ticarcillin has declined following the introduction of the ureidopenicillins. However, when combined with clavulanic acid, a number of advantages are conferred which renders the combination therapeutically useful.

1. Urinary tract infection

The treatment of complicated urinary tract infection with ticarcillin, predominantly due to *Ps. aeruginosa*, results in eradication of bacteruria in over 90% of cases.[31] After long-term follow-up the overall success rate falls to 75%, due either to relapse or superinfection (often by *Klebsiella*). Failure is usually due to the presence of underlying renal calculi or an indwelling catheter.[22] Comparable results can be obtained using either ticarcillin or azlocillin.[31]

Clavulanate-potentiated ticarcillin also achieves 90% or greater bacteriological and clinical success in such infections.[32] Both drugs have the advantage of lacking nephrotoxicity.

2. Respiratory tract infections

The use of ticarcillin has been largely confined to patients with cystic fibrosis, when *Ps. aeruginosa* is often present, although exacerbations of chronic bronchitis and bronchiectasis have also been successfully treated.[22,33] In cystic fibrosis, ticarcillin both alone and combined with gentamicin or tobramycin has achieved 70% success.[23] Eradication of *Ps. aeruginosa* is not always achieved and is not a prerequisite for clinical improvement. Ticarcillin-resistant strains can often be isolated after therapy but may not be clinically relevant.

Clavulanate-potentiated ticarcillin is effective in severe hospital-acquired pneumonia,[34] but is unlikely to provide any additional advantage over ticarcillin in cystic fibrosis unless β-lactamase-producing bacteria such as *H. influenzae* or *S. aureus* are responsible for exacerbation of infection.

3. Septicaemia

Both ticarcillin and clavulanate-potentiated ticarcillin are effective in the treatment of known or suspected Gram-negative sepsis.[22,35] For empirical treatment, ticarcillin is usually combined with an aminoglycoside and if *Ps. aeruginosa* is suspected, the combination is also recommended. The extended spectrum of clavulanate-potentiated ticarcillin should make it an attractive single agent for the empirical therapy of suspected septicaemia, except in the immunocompromised host.

4. Infection in the immunocompromised host

The importance of early institution of empirical antibiotics in the treatment of febrile episodes in immunocompromised patients is well established. Ticarcillin alone produces a relatively low response rate in this group of patients but is effective when combined with an aminoglycoside. There is little to choose between the various aminoglycosides.[36] Amikacin plus ticarcillin has been endorsed by the European Organisation on Treatment of Cancer,[37] although more recently the use of azlocillin has given marginally better results.[38] The use of a second β-lactam agent in place of the aminoglycoside, such as moxalactam,[39] can give equally good results.

Clavulanate-potentiated ticarcillin combined with an aminoglycoside is at least as effective as other combinations for these patients[40] and does have some theoretical advantages with its activity against commonly encountered β-lactamase-producing bacteria. Another approach has been to use vancomycin in combination with ticarcillin together with an aminoglycoside when extra Gram-positive cover is required.[41]

5. Anaerobic infections

Although ticarcillin has been effective for treating anaerobic infections, including some due to *B. fragilis*,[42] it does not offer any benefits over other more appropriate agents. The activity of clavulanate-potentiated ticarcillin against β-lactamase-producing isolates, particularly *B. fragilis*, makes it an attractive choice for mixed aerobic and anaerobic infections.[43]

Adverse reactions

Potentially life-threatening effects

Severe and occasionally fatal anaphylactic reactions are a risk with the use of any penicillin-class antibiotic, but have rarely been noted following ticarcillin use. The addition of clavulanic acid does not affect the incidence of such reactions.

Acute overdosage

No cases appear to have been reported.

Ticarcillin (disodium)

Severe or irreversible adverse effects

Nephrotoxicity and, to a lesser extent, ototoxicity have both been reported in patients receiving ticarcillin in combination with aminoglycosides. However, there is no evidence that the ticarcillin contributes to such toxicity; indeed under experimental conditions it can provide a protective effect against aminoglycoside-induced nephrotoxicity.[44]

Neurotoxicity (generalized myoclonus, hyperreflexia, asterixis and stupor) has been reported in a patient with renal failure and very high serum levels.[45] Dosage was probably excessive in this patient. No such adverse effects have been noted with clavulanate-potentiated ticarcillin, probably because of the lower doses employed.

Ticarcillin in large doses causes platelet dysfunction (decreased platelet aggregation) and a prolonged bleeding time[21,46] but this does not result in a significant incidence of bleeding during therapy. The effect is dose-related and is aggravated if renal function is impaired. It is more commonly seen during carbenicillin use. Such effects should be less during clavulanate-potentiated ticarcillin use because of the lower doses employed. Any haemorrhagic manifestations reported have been associated with the underlying disease rather than with the drug. Other haematological effects, such as neutropenia, which may be life-threatening,[47] and thrombocytopenia, are rarely recorded.

Symptomatic adverse effects

Ticarcillin is well tolerated by most patients even in dosages of 24 g daily. Intramuscular administration may result in pain and induration at the injection site in a minority of patients but can be eliminated by using lignocaine. Phlebitis after intravenous injection has also been noted but is not common. For both ticarcillin and clavulanate-potentiated ticarcillin it is related to the concentration of the solution and the speed of injection.[42]

Other adverse effects occasionally seen with both drugs are diarrhoea, nausea, vomiting, oral moniliasis and glossitis, all of which are reversible on stopping therapy.

Other effects

Ticarcillin can cause a measurable increase in the bleeding time but other clotting indices (prothrombin time, activated partial thromboplastin time, thrombin time) remain unchanged.[46] A positive Coombs test may be recorded during clavulanate-potentiated ticarcillin use and is due to the clavulanic acid component.[48] Hypokalaemia is reported in a varying proportion of patients receiving ticarcillin[49] and is probably due to the drug acting as a non-resorbable anion in the distal renal tubule. It is readily corrected by potassium supplements.[22]

Other biochemical effects are unusual and transient, such as elevated serum transaminases and alkaline phosphatase, and hypernatraemia.

Interference with clinical pathology tests

No technical interferences of this kind have been reported.

High risk groups

Neonates

The half life of ticarcillin falls with increasing age and maturity.[29] For neonates under 2000 g, a suggested dose is 75 mg.kg^{-1} 12-hourly for the first week, then 8-hourly thereafter. Neonates over 2000 g can receive 75 mg.kg^{-1} 8-hourly for the first week followed by 100 mg.kg^{-1} 8-hourly. Clavulanate-potentiated ticarcillin can be given to premature and full term infants at a dosage of 80 mg.kg^{-1} every 12 hours, increasing to 8-hourly after the perinatal period.

Breast milk. Very little ticarcillin crosses into breast milk. However, due to the risk of sensitization, other methods of feeding should be considered if used during lactation.

Children

The usual dose of ticarcillin is 200–300 mg.kg^{-1} daily given in divided doses. A lower dose of 50–100 mg.kg^{-1} daily may be used for uncomplicated urinary tract infections. Clavulanate-potentiated ticarcillin is given in a dose of 80 mg.kg^{-1} every 6–8 hours.

Pregnant women

Animal studies have shown no teratogenic effects of ticarcillin alone or when combined with clavulanic acid. However, use in pregnancy should not be considered unless absolutely necessary.

The elderly

Other than observing dosage adjustments in renal failure, no special precautions are required.

Concurrent disease

Renal failure. The rate of clearance of ticarcillin from the circulation decreases progressively with decreasing renal function, resulting in a prolonged half life. Dosage adjustment therefore depends on the degree of renal impairment.[50]

Table 1

Creatinine clearance ml.min^{-1}	Ticarcillin	Clavulante-potentiated ticarcillin
<10	2 g 12-hourly	1.6 g 12-hourly
10–30	2 g 8-hourly	1.6 g 8-hourly
>30	2 g 4–6-hourly	3.2 g 8-hourly

Haemodialysis removes ticarcillin readily from the circulation and therefore a supplementary dose of 2–3 g ticarcillin or 1.6 g clavulanate-potentiated ticarcillin should be given midway during each dialysis period.

Peritoneal dialysis is less effective at removing ticarcillin; a dosage of 2 g 8-hourly or 1.6 g 8-hourly clavulanate-potentiated ticarcillin would be appropriate.

Hepatic failure. The presence of hepatic failure with concomitant severe renal dysfunction may further prolong the half life of ticarcillin and a further reduction in dosage may be required. Monitoring serum levels should also be considered.

Drug interactions

Potentially hazardous interactions

Aminoglycosides are inactivated by ticarcillin if mixed in vitro in direct proportion to the time of exposure and ticarcillin concentration.[30] A similar effect can also be demonstrated during clinical usage in patients with impaired renal function, possibly because serum levels are higher and maintained for longer in such patients.[51] Therefore ticarcillin and aminoglycosides should not be mixed together in the same infusion.

Cefoxitin can be shown to antagonize the action of several β-lactams (including ticarcillin) against certain Gram-negative bacteria, especially *Ps. aeruginosa, Enterobacter* and *Serratia*.[52] This combination is therefore best avoided in such situations.

Severe hypernatraemia has been reported following concomitant lithium and ticarcillin use. Lithium can provoke marked polyuria which may prove hazardous when combined with the high sodium load of ticarcillin in patients with impaired renal function or inadequate hydration.[53]

Other significant interactions

Various antineoplastic agents have been studied in vitro with ticarcillin. Only 5-fluorouracil has been shown to affect the MIC against some bacterial strains, producing a reduction of the MIC and thus implying a synergistic effect.

Potentially useful interactions

Ticarcillin exhibits a synergistic effect when administered with aminoglycosides against many strains of *Ps. aeruginosa* and a variable number of other Gram-negative bacteria.[54] However, synergy cannot be automatically assumed, since indifference or antagonism may also be demonstrated in vitro.

Major outcome trials

EORTC International Antimicrobial Therapy Project Group 1978 Three antibiotic regimens in the treatment of infection in febrile granulocytopenic patients with cancer. Journal of Infectious Diseases 137: 14–29

One of the first large-scale prospective randomized trials of empirical antibiotic therapy of febrile granulocytopenic patients with cancer. The antibiotics chosen initially were ticarcillin plus cephalothin, ticarcillin plus gentamicin and cephalothin plus gentamicin. However, supplies of ticarcillin were sufficient only to complete the first six

Ticarcillin (disodium)

T

months of the trial; carbenicillin then had to be substituted for the remaining 18 months.

A total of 625 febrile episodes were treated, with infection documented microbiologically in 269 (43%) and clinically in a further 127 (20%). Altogether 349 pathogens were isolated, the majority (61%) being Gram-negative bacilli (*E. coli* 83, *Klebsiella* 57, and *Ps. aeruginosa* 40) with *S. aureus* accounting for a further 16%. Of the 349 pathogens isolated, 48% were isolated from blood cultures.

The overall treatment success rate was 70%, there being no significant difference between the various antibiotic combinations, including comparisons between the ticarcillin and carbenicillin arms of the trial. Patients with documented Gram-negative bacteraemia tended to respond less frequently in all groups. Important factors in determining a favourable response were sensitivity of the organism isolated to one of the antibiotics used and a rise in peripheral granulocyte count during therapy. The combination of cephalothin plus gentamicin was significantly more nephrotoxic than the other combinations and was less effective in treating infections due to *Ps. aeruginosa.*

The combination of gentamicin plus carbenicillin or ticarcillin was considered to represent the best initial empirical therapy, taking into account efficacy and toxicity, for this group of patients. Such regimens (particularly using ticarcillin) have been used extensively in many centres and tend to be regarded as the standard against which other newer agents are compared.

Other studies

Parry M F, Neu H C 1978 A comparative study of ticarcillin plus tobramycin versus carbenicillin plus gentamicin for the treatment of serious infections due to Gram-negative bacilli. American Journal of Medicine 64: 961–966

This study compared the efficacy of two antibiotic combinations in 82 patients with documented serious systemic Gram-negative infection. The majority had pulmonary infections (63) mainly due to cystic fibrosis (51). *Ps. aeruginosa* was the predominant pathogen occurring in 76 (93%) of patients. Those with the ticarcillin combination responded more frequently (92%) than those receiving carbenicillin (71%). The difference was seen predominantly in those patients with pulmonary infection due to *Ps. aeruginosa.*

General review articles

Brogden R N, Heel R C, Speight T M, Avery G S 1980 Ticarcillin: a review of its pharmacological properties and therapeutic efficacy. Drugs 20: 325–352

Leigh D A, Phillips I, Wise R (eds) 1986 Timentin — ticarcillin plus clavulanic acid. A laboratory and clinical perspective. Journal of Antimicrobial Chemotherapy 17 (suppl C)

References

1. Labia R, Morand A, Peduzzi J 1986 Timentin and β-lactamases. Journal of Antimicrobial Chemotherapy 17 (suppl C): 17–26
2. Jackson D, Cockburn A, Cooper D L, Langley P F, Tasker T C G, White D J 1985 Clinical pharmacology and safety evaluation of Timentin. American Journal of Medicine 79 (suppl 5B): 44–55
3. Sutherland R, Burnett J, Rollinson G N 1970 α-carboxy-3-thienylmethylpenicillin (BRL 2288), a new semisynthetic penicillin: *in vitro* evaluation. Antimicrobial Agents and Chemotherapy: 390–395
4. Fuchs P C, Thornsberry C, Barry A L, Gavan T L, Gerlach E H, Aones R N 1977 Ticarcillin: a collaborative *in vitro* comparison with carbenicillin against over 9000 clinical bacterial isolates. American Journal of Medical Sciences 274: 255–263
5. Sanders C C 1981 Comparative activity of mezlocillin, penicillin, ampicillin, carbenicillin and ticarcillin against Gram-positive bacteria and *Haemophilus influenzae.* Antimicrobial Agents and Chemotherapy 20: 843–846
6. Monif R G, Clark P P, Shuster J J, Baer H 1978 Susceptibility of the anaerobic bacteria, group D streptococci, *Enterobacteriaceae,* and *Pseudomonas* to semisynthetic penicillins; carbenicillin, piperacillin and ticarcillin. Antimicrobial Agents and Chemotherapy 14: 737–742
7. Shah P P, Briedis D J, Robson H G, Conterato J P 1979 *In vitro* activity of piperacillin compared to that of carbenicillin, ticarcillin, ampicillin, cephalothin and cefamandole against *Pseudomonas aeruginosa* and *Enterobacteriaceae.* Antimicrobial Agents and Chemotherapy 15: 346–350
8. Harris R L, Smith N J, Dietrich J E et al 1984 *In vitro* bactericidal effect of azlocillin, mezlocillin, piperacillin and ticarcillin against gram-negative bacteria. Current Therapeutic Research 35: 633–642
9. van der Voet G B, Mattie H, van Furth R 1985 Comparison of the antibacterial activity of azlocillin and ticarcillin *in vitro* and in irradiated neutropenic mice. Journal of Antimicrobial Chemotherapy 16: 605–613
10. Baker C N, Thornsberry C, Jones R N 1980 *In vitro* antimicrobial activity of cefoperazone, cefotaxime, moxalactam (LY 127 935), azlocillin, mezlocillin and other β-lactam antibiotics against *Neisseria gonorrhoeae* and *Haemophilus influenzae,* including β-lactamase producing strains. Antimicrobial Agents and Chemotherapy 17: 757–761
11. Roy I, Bach V, Thadepalli H 1977 *In vitro* activity of ticarcillin against anaerobic bacteria compared with that of carbenicillin and penicillin. Antimicrobial Agents and Chemotherapy 11: 258–261
12. Fuchs P C, Barry A L, Thornsberry C, Jones R N 1984 *In vitro* activity of ticarcillin plus clavulanic acid against 632 clinical isolates. Antimicrobial Agents and Chemotherapy 25: 392–394
13. Sutherland R, Beale A S, Boon R J, Griffin K E, Slocombe B, Stokes D H, White A R 1985 Antibacterial activity of ticarcillin in the presence of clavulanate potassium. American Journal of Medicine 29 (suppl 5B): 13–24
14. Shull V H, Dick J D 1985 Determination of ticarcillin levels in serum by high-pressure liquid chromatography. Antimicrobial Agents and Chemotherapy 28: 597–600
15. Neu H C, Garvey G J 1975 Comparative *in vitro* activity and clinical pharmacology of ticarcillin and carbenicillin. Antimicrobial Agents and Chemotherapy 8: 457–462
16. Gouyette A, Kitzis M D, Guibert J, Acar J F 1982 Pharmacokinetics and bioavailability of intramuscular preparations of ticarcillin. Journal of Antimicrobial Chemotherapy 10: 419–425
17. Libke R D, Clarke J T, Ralph E D, Luthy R P, Kirby W M M 1975 Ticarcillin vs. carbenicillin: clinical pharmacokinetics. Clinical Pharmacology and Therapeutics 17: 441–446
18. Dalhoff A, Hoffler D 1977 Ticarcillin: pharmacokinetics in man according to different administration schedules. Journal of International Medical Research 5: 308–312
19. Tan J S, Salstrom S J 1977 Levels of carbenicillin, ticarcillin, cephalothin, cefazolin, cefamandole, gentamicin, tobramycin and amikacin in human serum and interstitial fluid. Antimicrobial Agents and Chemotherapy 11: 698–700
20. Daschner F D, Thoma G, Langmaack H, Dalhoff A 1980 Ticarcillin concentrations in serum, muscle and fat after a single intravenous injection. Antimicrobial Agents and Chemotherapy 17: 738–739
21. Ervin F R, Bullock W E 1976 Clinical and pharmacological studies of ticarcillin in gram-negative infections. Antimicrobial Agents and Chemotherapy 9: 94–101
22. Parry M F, Neu H C 1976 Ticarcillin for treatment of serious infections with gram-negative bacteria. Journal of Infectious Diseases 134: 476–485
23. Parry M F, Neu H C, Merlino M, Gaerian P F, Ores C N, Denning C R 1977 Treatment of pulmonary infections in patients with cystic fibrosis: a comparative study of ticarcillin and gentamicin. Journal of Pediatrics 90: 144–148
24. Hirsch H A 1980 Transfer of various antibiotics into the uterine compartments during steady state in the mother. International Journal of Biological Research in Pregnancy 1: 124–127
25. Davies B E, Humphrey M J, Langley P F, Lees L, Legg B, Wadds G A 1982 Pharmacokinetics of ticarcillin in man. European Journal of Clinical Pharmacology 23: 167–172
26. Guglielmo B J, Flaherty J F, Batman R, Barriere S L, Gambertoglio J G 1986 Comparative pharmacokinetics of low and high-dose ticarcillin. Antimicrobial Agents and Chemotherapy 30: 359–360
27. Kosmidis J, Charalambopoules D, Daikos G K 1978 Elimination kinetics of ticarcillin in renal failure and the influence of peritoneal dialysis and haemodialysis. In: Proceedings of an International Symposium on Ticarcillin. Excerpta Medica, Amsterdam, pp 39–44
28. Parry M F, Neu H C 1976 Pharmacokinetics of ticarcillin in patients with abnormal renal function. Journal of Infectious Diseases 133: 46–49
29. Nelson J D, Shelton S, Kusmiesz H 1975 Clinical pharmacology of ticarcillin in the newborn infant: relation to age, gestational age, and weight. Journal of Pediatrics 87: 474–479
30. Pickering L E, Gearhart P 1979 Effect of time and concentration upon interaction between gentamicin, tobramycin, netilmicin, or amikacin and carbenicillin or ticarcillin. Antimicrobial Agents and Chemotherapy 15: 592–596
31. Cox C E 1983 A comparison of azlocillin and ticarcillin in the treatment of complicated urinary tract infections. Journal of Antimicrobial Chemotherapy 11 (suppl B): 183–188
32. Westenfelder M, Pelz K, Hulla F W 1986 Clinical evaluation of Timentin in complicated urinary tract infection. Journal of Antimicrobial Chemotherapy 17 (suppl C): 97–102
33. Pines A, Khaja G, Raafat H, Sreedharan K S 1978 Clinical experience with ticarcillin (BRL 2288) in 130 patients treated for severe respiratory infections. In: Proceedings of an International Symposium on Ticarcillin. Excerpta Medica, Amsterdam, pp 93–96
34. Schwigon C D, Hulla F W, Schulze B, Maslak A 1986 Timentin in the treatment of nosocomial bronchopulmonary infections in intensive care units. Journal of Antimicrobial Chemotherapy 17 (suppl C): 115–122
35. Degener J E, Wagenvoort J H T, Dzoljic-Danilovic G, Michel M F, Brus-Weijer A 1986 The efficacy of the combination of Timentin and tobramycin in the treatment of patients with bacteraemia. Journal of Antimicrobial Chemotherapy 17 (suppl C): 141–148
36. Love L J, Schimpff S C, Hahn D M et al 1970 Randomized trial of empirical antibiotic therapy with ticarcillin in combination with gentamicin, amikacin or netilmicin in febrile patients with granulocytopenia and cancer. American Journal of Medicine 66: 603–610
37. EORTC International Antimicrobial Therapy Project Group 1983 Three antibiotic regimens in the treatment of infection in febrile granulocytopenic patients with cancer. Journal of Infectious Diseases 137: 14–29
38. Klastersky J, Glauser M P, Schimpff S C, Zinner S H, Gaya H 1986 Prospective randomized comparison of three antibiotic regimens for empirical theory of suspected bacteraemic infection in febrile granulocytopenia patients. Antimicrobial Agents and Chemotherapy 29: 263–270

39. Fainstein V, Bodey G P, Bolivar R, Elting L, McCredie K B, Keating M J 1984 Moxalactam plus ticarcillin or tobramycin for treatment of febrile episodes in neutropenic cancer patients. Archives of Internal Medicine 144: 1766–1770
40. Mackie M J, Reilly J T, Purohit S, Bartzokas C A 1986 A randomized trial of Timentin and tobramycin versus piperacillin and tobramycin in febrile neutropenic patients. Journal of Antimicrobial Chemotherapy 17 (suppl C): 219–224
41. Shenep J L, Hughes W T, Roberson P K et al 1988 Vancomycin, Ticaricillin and Amikacin compared with Ticarcillin–Clavulanate and Amikacin in the empirical treatment of febrile, neutropenic children with cancer. New England Journal of Medicine 319: 1053–1058
42. Webb D, Thadepalli H, Roy I, Bach V T 1978 Ticarcillin disodium in anaerobic infections. Archives of Internal Medicine 138: 1618–620
43. de Barbeyrac B, Quentin C, Bebbear C 1986 The activity of ticarcillin in combination with clavulanic acid against *Bacteroides* species: an *in vitro* comparison with other antibiotics. Journal of Antimicrobial Chemotherapy 17 (suppl C): 35–39
44. English J, Gilbert D N, Kohlhepp S et al 1985 Attenuation of experimental tobramycin nephrotoxicity by ticarcillin. Antimicrobial Agents and Chemotherapy 27: 897–902
45. Kallay M C, Tabechain H, Riley G R, Chessin L N 1979 Neurotoxicity due to ticarcillin in patient with renal failure. Lancet 1: 608–609
46. Brown C H, Natelson E A, Bradshaw W, Alfrey C P, Williams T W 1975 Study of the effects of ticarcillin on blood coagulation and platelet function. Antimicrobial Agents and Chemotherapy 7: 652–656
47. Gastineau D, Spector R, Philips D 1980 Severe neutropenia associated with ticarcillin therapy. Annals of Internal Medicine 94: 711–712
48. Williams M E, Thomas D, Harman C P, Mintz P D, Donowitz G R 1985 Positive direct antiglobulin tests due to clavulanic acid. Antimicrobial Agents and Chemotherapy 27: 125–127
49. Nanji A A, Lindsay J 1982 Ticarcillin associated hypokalaemia. Clinical Biochemistry 15: 118–119
50. Parry M F, Neu H C 1976 Pharmacokinetics of ticarcillin in 7 patients with abnormal renal function. Journal of Infectious Diseases 133: 46–49
51. Kradjan W A, Burger R 1980 *In vitro* inactivation of gentamicin by carbenicillin and ticarcillin. Archives of Internal Medicine 140: 1668–1670
52. Sanders C C, Sanders W E, Goering R V 1982 *In vitro* antagonism of β-lactam antibiotics by cefoxitin. Antimicrobial Agents and Chemotherapy 21: 968–975
53. Finch R A 1971 Hypernatraemia during lithium and ticarcillin therapy. Southern Medical Journal 74: 376–377
54. Comber K R, Basker M J, Osborne C D, Sutherland R 1977 Synergy between ticarcillin and tobramycin against *Pseudomonas aeruginosa* and *Enterobacteriaceae in vitro* and *in vivo*. Antimicrobial Agents and Chemotherapy 11: 956–964

Tienilic acid

Tienilic acid is a diuretic with uricosuric properties. It was withdrawn from most markets in 1980 because of suspected hepatotoxicity and is now available only in France.

Chemistry

Tienilic acid (Diflurex)
$C_{13}H_8Cl_2O_4S$
[2,3-Dichloro-4(2-thenoyl)phenoxy] acetic acid

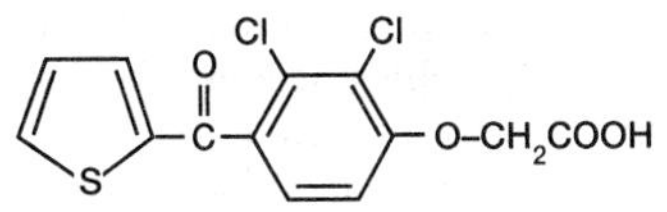

Molecular weight	331.2
pKa (carboxylic acid)	2.7
Solubility	
in alcohol	1 in 14
in water	slightly soluble
Octanol/water partition coefficient	—

Tienilic acid is a white crystalline powder prepared by chemical synthesis.

Pharmacology

Tienilic acid is an effective orally acting diuretic. It causes a moderate sodium and chloride diuresis with only a slight kaliuresis. It causes an increased osmotic clearance and a negative free water clearance with no effect on urine pH or bicarbonate excretion. It appears to act by inhibiting sodium reabsorption in the cortical diluting segment of the renal tubule.[1] Tienilic acid also in most species causes an increased excretion of uric acid in the urine and appears to be working in a similar way to probenecid.

Toxicology

Information on toxicology is not readily available. The drug is not an enzyme inducer and does not inhibit microsomal oxidation.

Clinical pharmacology

The natriuretic action of tienilic acid is comparable to that of hydrochlorothiazide, over doses of 0.05 to 2.5 $\mu.kg^{-1}$ when given intravenously.[1] The duration of activity appears to be about 12–14 hours. The natriuretic effect is greater in conditions of alkalosis than acidosis. The renal clearance of urate is increased five-fold at maximum.

The uricosuric action is only slightly less than that of probenecid, and a reduced serum uric acid is maintained during at least 6 months of treatment.[2] The uricosuric, but not the natriuretic, effect of tienilic acid is blocked by pyrazinamide, and the uricosuric effect of probenecid is enhanced by tienilic acid. This implies inhibited reabsorption of both filtered and secreted urate.[3] There appears to be competition between tienilic acid and para-amino-hippuric acid for urinary excretion, implying active secretion of tienilic acid by the tubules. Tienilic acid also lowers blood pressure and is similar in efficacy to thiazide diuretics. This effect is sustained and there is no rebound on stopping treatment.[2]

Pharmacokinetics

Tienilic acid and its metabolites have been measured by HPLC[4], with a detection limit of 200 $\mu g.l^{-1}$.

Following oral administration of 250 mg of the drug to normal subjects, absorption is good and peak plasma levels of around 11 mg.l^{-1} are observed after 3 hours; the plasma half lives of the active agent and metabolites are similar, at 2–3½ h.[5] Protein binding is of the order of 99.5% at therapeutic concentrations,[6] with one major binding site and several of lesser affinity.

Oral absorption	good
Presystemic metabolism	—
Plasma half life	
range	2–3.5 h
Volume of distribution	—
Plasma protein binding	99.5%

Concentration–effect relationship

There is no evidence of any correlation between the plasma concentration of tienilic acid and its biological effects.

Metabolism

The major metabolites are (2,3-dichloro-4-(α-hydroxyl-2-thienyl) phenoxy) acetic acid and a dihydroxylated metabolite. In plasma, the alcoholic and diacid metabolites account for less than 10% of the estimated tienilic acid. It was suggested that the poor recovery may be due to biliary excretion or perhaps other unknown metabolites.

Pharmaceutics

Tienilic acid is available for therapeutic use only in France, as white tablets containing 250 mg.

Therapeutic use

Indications

1. The treatment of hypertension with moderate elevation of serum urate
2. The treatment of sodium retention, accompanied by moderate elevation of serum uric acid; not recommended in the treatment of sodium retention due to hepatic or renal disease.

Contraindications

1. Liver damage
2. Sensitivity to the drug
3. Concurrent treatment with anticoagulants
4. Renal calculi.

Mode of use

Oral treatment is commenced with 250 mg of the drug daily. In this dosage, the hypotensive effect is similar to that of 50 mg of hydrochlorothiazide daily.[7] If necessary, the dose can be increased to a maximum of 500 mg daily. The hypotensive effect is maintained for at least 6 months. The drug can be given in association with propranolol, and the hypotensive effect of the combination suggests that the effects of the two drugs are additive.[8] With the exception of its action on serum uric acid, the effects of tienilic acid on blood chemistry are similar to those of thiazide diuretics: some hypokalaemia, possibly mild early elevation of creatinine, and increase in triglycerides.

In cardiac failure, tienilic acid is also about as effective as hydrochlorothiazide,[9] and has been used orally in doses up to 1000 mg daily.

Though the drug is not recommended by the makers for treatment of sodium retention in renal disease, there is some evidence of efficacy in patients with nephrotic syndrome, when given in a dose of 250–500 mg daily by mouth.[10]

Adverse reactions

Potentially life-threatening effects

The principal danger of tienilic acid is that of hepatotoxicity. The drug was withdrawn from most markets after reports of 363 cases of liver damage with 24 deaths. The role of tienilic acid in causing liver damage has been challenged[11] but the drug has remained off the market except in France.

Acute renal failure has been reported, generally in patients previously on other diuretics,[12] and possibly due to urate deposition in the renal tubules. In view of this it was recommended that other diuretics should be withdrawn 3 days before starting tienilic acid, and that adequate hydration should be ensured.[13]

Acute overdosage

In the case of recent ingestion, gastric lavage should be carried out. Treatment should be symptomatic and directed at fluid and electrolyte replacement, which should be monitored together with the blood pressure and renal function.

Severe or irreversible adverse effects

Hypokalaemia, usually reversible by potassium, transient elevation of creatinine, and increased triglycerides have also been noted.[14] Generalized dermatitis has been reported,[15] requiring withdrawal of the drug. Acute arthralgia was reported in two patients.[16] It was thought that this might have been gout, but proof was not obtained.

Interference with clinical pathology tests

No interferences of this kind appear to have been reported.

High risk groups

No information is available on the use of tienilic acid in neonates, children, pregnant or lactating women, or the elderly. The risks of giving the drug in the presence of certain concurrent diseases have been mentioned under Contraindications and Mode of use.

Drug interactions

Potentially hazardous interactions

Warfarin. Because of its high protein binding, it is likely that tienilic acid might displace coumarin anticoagulants from plasma protein binding sites although the effect would be quite small and transitory.[9]

Phenytoin. It was suspected that phenytoin toxicity developed in an epileptic patient given tienilic acid, but this was not substantiated.[8]

Other significant interactions

Salicylates. Aspirin interferes with the diuretic effect of tienilic acid, and tienilic acid inhibits the excretion of salicylate.[4]

Lithium. It is suspected that lithium levels may be affected by the administration of tienilic acid.

Potentially useful interactions

None have been reported.

References

1. Maass A R, Snow I B 1979 Renal pharmacology of tienilic acid. Postgraduate Medical Journal 55 (suppl 3): 37–46
2. Noble R E, Beg M A 1979 Longterm usage of tienilic acid in essential hypertension. Postgraduate Medical Journal 55 (suppl 3): 120–126
3. Lau K, Stote R M, Goldberg M, Agus Z S 1977 Mechanisms of the uricosuric effect of the diuretic tienilic acid (Ticrynafen) in man. Clinical Science and Molecular Medicine 53: 379–386
4. Kerremans A L M, Gribnau F W J, Tan Y, van Ginneken C A M 1982 Pharmacokinetic and pharmacodynamic studies of tienilic acid in healthy volunteers. European Journal of Clinical Pharmacology 22: 515–521
5. Dubb J W, Stote R M, Maass A R, Hwang B V, Familiar R G, Alexander F 1979 Tienilic acid: pharmacokinetics, salicylate interaction and creatinine secretion studies. Postgraduate Medical Journal 55 (suppl 3): 47–57
6. Wood A J, Bolli P, Waal-Manning H J, Simpson F O 1978 Ticrynafen: kinetics, protein binding and effects on serum and urinary uric acid. Clinical Pharmacology and Therapeutics 23: 697–702
7. Beg M A, Ragland R 1979 Longterm usage of tienilic acid in essential hypertension. Postgraduate Medical Journal 55 (suppl 3): 127–131
8. Pearson R M, Bulpitt C J, Havard G W H 1979 Propranolol and tienilic acid in essential hypertension. Postgraduate Medical Journal 55 (suppl 3): 115–119
9. Weber K T, Fishman A P 1979 Tienilic acid, a uricosuric diuretic, in the treatment of heart failure. Postgraduate Medical Journal 55 (suppl 3): 58–62
10. Morgan A, Birch H, Lee H A 1979 The use of tienilic acid in nephrotic syndrome; a clinical study. Postgraduate Medical Journal 55 (suppl 3): 63–67
11. Simpson F O, Waal-Manning H J 1980 Total ban on tienilic acid. Lancet 1: 978–979
12. Bennett W M, Van Zee B E, Hutchings R 1979 Acute renal failure from ticranyfen. New England Journal of Medicine 301: 1179–1180
13. Selby T 1979 Acute renal failure from ticranyfen. New England Journal of Medicine 301: 1180–1181
14. Fohlich E D, de Carvalho J G R, Dunn F G, Chrysant S G 1979 Antihypertensive and renal effects of tienilic acid. Postgraduate Medical Journal 55 (suppl 3): 98–102
15. Veterans Administration Co-operative Study Group on Antihypertensive Agents 1979 Comparative effects of Ticranyfen and Hydrochlorothiazide in the treatment of hypertension. New England Journal of Medicine 301: 293–297
16. King R M, Wichman B A 1979 Acute arthralgia (gout?) after Ticranyfen. New England Journal of Medicine 301: 1065

Timolol (maleate)

Timolol is a moderately lipophilic non-selective β-adrenoceptor blocking drug, devoid of partial agonist activity, or membrane activity.

Chemistry

Timolol maleate (Betim, Blocadren, Tenserin, Timacor, Timolate, Timophe, Timoptol, Timotre)

$C_{13}H_{24}N_4O_3S.C_4H_4O_4$

(−)-(S)-(1)-tert-Butylamino-3-(4-morpholinyl-1,2,5-thiadiazol-3-yloxy)propan-2-ol hydrogen maleate

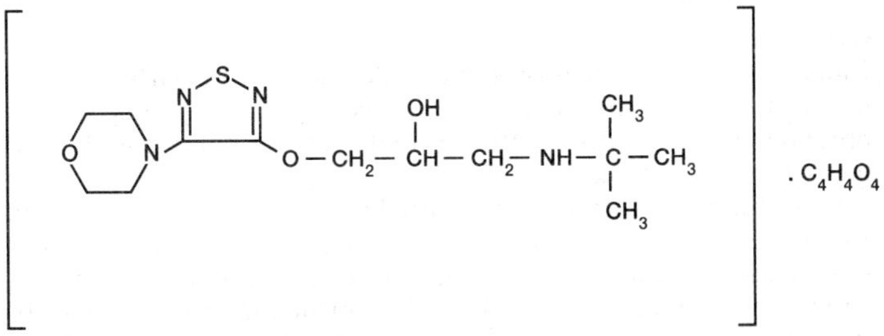

Molecular weight (free base)	432.5 (316.4)
pKa	—
Solubility	
in alcohol	soluble
in water	soluble
Octanol/water partition coefficient	1.16 at pH 7.4, 37°C

Timolol maleate is a white crystalline solid prepared by chemical synthesis. It is an ingredient of Moducren, Prestim and Timolide.

Pharmacology

Timolol is a competitive antagonist at both β_1- and β_2-adrenoceptors; it is therefore a non-selective β-blocking drug. It has minimal partial agonist activity and has no local anaesthetic activity. Timolol is five to ten times more potent than propranolol as a β-adrenoceptor antagonist. It is moderately lipophilic and has a half life of about 5 h.[1,2]

Toxicology

Timolol has low toxicity and animal tests have not demonstrated evidence of changes relevant to the dosage used in man. No fetal malformations were seen in mice or rabbits at a dose of 50 $mg.kg^{-1}$ a day, and the same was true in rats at the same dose, other than a delay in fetal ossification.

In a two-year study of timolol maleate in rats, there was a statistically significant ($p<0.05$) increase in the incidence of adrenal phaeochromocytomas in male rats given 300 times the maximum recommended human dose (1 $mg.kg^{-1}$ daily). Similar differences were not observed in rats given doses equivalent to 25 or 100 times the maximum recommended human dose. In a lifetime study in mice, there were statistically significant ($p<0.05$) increases in the incidence of benign and malignant pulmonary tumours and benign uterine polyps in female mice at 500 $mg.kg^{-1}$ daily, but not at 5 or 50 $mg.kg^{-1}$ per day. There was also a significant increase in mammary adenocarcinomas at the 500 $mg.kg^{-1}$ daily dose. This was associated with elevations in serum prolactin which occurred in female mice administered timolol at 500 $mg.kg^{-1}$, but not at doses of 5 or 50 $mg.kg^{-1}$ daily. An increased incidence of mammary adenocarcinomas in rodents has been associated with administration of several other therapeutic agents which elevate serum prolactin, but no correlation between serum prolactin levels and mammary tumours has been established in man. Furthermore, in adult human female subjects who received oral dosages of up to 60 mg of timolol maleate, the maximum recommended human oral dosage, there were no clinically meaningful changes in serum prolactin.

There was a statistically significant increase ($p<0.05$) in the overall incidence of neoplasms in female mice at the 500 $mg.kg^{-1}$ daily dosage level.

Timolol maleate was devoid of mutagenic potential when evaluated in vivo (mouse) in the micronucleus test and cytogenetic assay (doses up to 800 $mg.kg^{-1}$) and in vivo in a neoplastic cell transformation assay (up to 100 $\mu g.ml^{-1}$). In Ames tests the highest concentrations of timolol employed, 5000 or 10 000 µg per plate, were associated with statistically significant elevations ($p<0.05$) of revertants observed with tester strain TA100 (in seven replicate assays), but not in the remaining three strains. In the assays with tester strain TA100, no consistent dose–response relationship was observed, nor did the ratio of test to control revertants reach 2. A ratio of 2 is usually considered the criterion for a positive Ames test.

Reproduction and fertility studies in rats showed no adverse effect on male and female fertility at doses up to 150 times the maximum recommended human dose.

Clinical pharmacology

Timolol inhibits the effect of isoprenaline on the heart in man; 4 $\mu g.min^{-1}$ of isoprenaline gave a 20% increase in heart rate, whereas 1 h after timolol 5 mg no effect was seen from 8 $\mu g.min^{-1}$ isoprenaline. Thus it causes a reduction in heart rate which is particularly noticeable on exercise. A dose of 2.5 mg timolol gives about the same fall in heart rate as 40 mg of propranolol in the standing position. The effect on heart rate is maximal about 45–90 minutes after oral administration, then begins to decline after 3–4 hours.[1]

Timolol lowers blood pressure in both the standing and lying positions but the exact mechanism of this is unclear. It reduces cardiac output at rest and on exercise without lowering the glomerular filtration rate. Timolol increases peripheral resistance,[3] so reducing peripheral blood flow,[4,5] and thus may cause cold hands and feet. Oral timolol 30–60 mg daily in hypertensive patients reduced resting cardiac index from 3.62 $l.min^{-1}.m^{-2}$ to 2.89 $l.min^{-1}.m^{-2}$ heart rate fell from 85 to 63 beats per minute. The fall in cardiac index was similar to that found with equipotent doses of propranolol.[5]

Timolol decreases maximal exercise tolerance in normal individuals but in patients with angina, exercise tolerance is usually increased, due to a reduction in total myocardial oxygen consumption. The reduction in cardiac output[3] may not always be beneficial and cardiac failure may ensue in susceptible individuals — particularly those whose endogenous sympathetic tone is high. Timolol, in addition to lowering the heart rate, has antiarrhythmic effects due to the slowing of conduction in the atria and in the A-V node, and due to the decrease in spontaneous rate of depolarization of ectopic pacemakers.

Timolol probably has most of the haemodynamic and clinical pharmacological effects of propranolol, though few studies have been performed.[6] It may cause marked airways obstruction in patients with obstructive airways disease and this may even occur after the use of timolol eye drops.[6] Timolol reduces plasma renin levels, prolongs insulin-induced hypoglycaemia and reduces the HDL lipoprotein fraction in the plasma.[6]

Pharmacokinetics

Timolol has been estimated by gas–liquid chromatography, by radioisotope methods and by high performance liquid chromatography.[7] The lower limit for detection by HPLC in plasma[8] was found to be 27 $\mu g.l^{-1}$.

Timolol is virtually completely absorbed with a peak concentration 1–2 h after oral administration. There is considerable presystemic metabolism, between 50 and 70%, with consequent effects on systemic bioavailability. This first-pass metabolism is less than that seen with propranolol, but there is still reported variation in blood levels of between two- and seven-fold.

Timolol is largely metabolized in the liver but 20% is excreted unchanged by the kidney. An active metabolite has been described with one-seventh the β-blocking activity of timolol in dogs.[9] The half life is reported to be between 2 and 5 h but may be up to 8 h after prolonged oral treatment. Poor metabolizers of debrisoquine have been found to be poor metabolizers of timolol. Poor metabolizers have about twice the plasma timolol concentration of extensive metabolizers after single oral doses; pharmacodynamic differences were only significant at 12 and 24 h after administration.[10]

Timolol has a large volume of distribution; figures of 1.74 to 3.64 $l.kg^{-1}$ have been reported. Data on plasma protein binding are sparse; it has been reported to vary from 10 to 80%.[5] Animal work indicates that timolol is concentrated in liver, lungs and kidney, but, in spite of similar lipophilicity to metoprolol, brain penetration, at least in the rat, is low.[11] There is no information as to whether timolol crosses the placenta or enters breast milk, but its lipophilicity profile, in particular, might suggest it would do both.

Not surprisingly, as timolol is largely metabolized in the liver, there is no change in half life in patients with renal failure.[12] Pharmacokinetic data are not available in children and the elderly.

Ocular administration in rabbits results in peak concentration in the aqueous humour of about 13 times that in the plasma. Studies in man indicate that on occasion systemic concentrations of timolol after ocular administration may reach a β-blocking concentration.

Oral absorption	100%
Presystemic metabolism	50–70%
Plasma half life	
range	2–5 h
Volume of distribution	1.74–3.64 $l.kg^{-1}$
Plasma protein binding	10–88%

Concentration–effect relationship

An increasing inhibition of exercise tachycardia has been shown with dosages of timolol between 5 and 20 mg and a relationship between plasma concentration and exercise has been demonstrated.[13] However, there is no evidence of any correlation between the plasma concentration of timolol and its antihypertensive effect.

Metabolism

Timolol is extensively metabolized in the liver to various derivatives. One pathway is by cleavage of the morpholine ring.[7] About 20% of an administered dose is excreted unchanged in the urine.

Pharmaceutics

Timolol is available in oral form and as an ophthalmic solution.

1. Betim (Leo, UK). Timolol maleate 10 mg. White, flat tablets engraved with '102' on scored face with Assyrian lion on reverse.
2. Blocadren (MSD, USA). Timolol maleate 5 mg, 10 mg and 20 mg. Blue half-scored tablets marked respectively 'MSD 59', 'MSD 136', 'MSD 437' on one side, with or without 'Blocadren' on the other side. The 5 mg and 10 mg strengths are round, while the 20 mg strength is capsule shaped. Only the 10 mg strength is available in the UK.
3. Timoptol (MSD, UK)/Timoptic (MSD, USA): equivalent to 0.25% and 0.5% w/v ophthalmic solution of timolol, in 5 ml metered dose unit. The preservative is benzalkonium chloride.

Timolol is also available in combination tablets.

4. Moducren (MSD/Morson, UK): Timolol maleate 10 mg, hydrochlorothiazide 25 mg, amiloride 2.5 mg. Blue, square, scored tablets marked 'Moducren'.
5. Prestim (Leo, UK): Timolol maleate 10 mg, bendrofluazide 2.5 mg. White, flat, petal-shaped tablets, engraved with '132' on scored face, Assyrian lion on reverse.
6. Prestim Forte (Leo, UK): Timolol maleate 20 mg, bendrofluazide 5 mg. White, flat, petal-shaped tablets, engraved with '146' on scored face, Assyrian lion on reverse.
7. Timolide (MSD, USA): Timolol maleate 10 mg, hydrochlorothiazide 25 mg. Light-blue, flat, hexagonal tablets, marked 'MSD 67' on one side.

A shelf-life for Blocadren of 5 years is quoted, for Timoptol, 2 years. The tablets should be stored in a cool place and protected from light.

Therapeutic use

This would be expected to be similar to that of propranolol, but as investigations with timolol have not been so wide the approved indications are fewer.

Indications

1. Long-term management of essential hypertension
2. Angina pectoris
3. Secondary prevention of myocardial infarction in those patients who survive the acute phase
4. Prophylaxis of migraine
5. Glaucoma (Timoptol).

Contraindications

1. Obstructive airways disease
2. Cardiac insufficiency and cardiogenic shock
3. Heart block
4. Hypoglycaemia.

Mode of use

Oral

Clinical use is dependent on β-blockade, most particularly of receptors in the heart. Although both β_1-receptors and β_2-receptors are present in the heart, β_1-receptors mediate nerve impulses and thus β_1-block is more important.

Oral treatment with timolol is usually commenced at a dosage of 10 mg once daily or 5 mg twice daily in hypertension. The dose may be increased as required and dosages above 20 mg should be administered on a divided-dose schedule. Treatment for angina should be started at a dose of 5 mg two or three times a day; increments should not exceed 10 mg per day, or 15 mg per day after the first increment.

Exacerbations of ischaemia in patients at risk, increased angina and myocardial infarction have been reported after abrupt withdrawal of β-adrenoceptor-blocking drugs. Timolol, like other similar drugs, should not be abruptly stopped before anaesthesia. Although there is no evidence for timolol it is likely that, as has been reported with other non-agonist β-blocking drugs, there is an up-regulation of β-receptors during drug administration. Evidence from other β-blocking drugs suggests that no post-β-blockade hypersensitivity occurs provided that a very small dose (possibly 2.5 mg a day of timolol) is continued for two weeks.[14]

Ocular

One drop of a 0.25% solution is applied twice daily to the affected eye(s), increasing to one drop of 0.5% solution twice daily if response to the lower dose is insufficient. Intraocular pressure should be assessed after 4 weeks to allow sufficient time for the response to stabilize, pressure being best measured at different times in the day because of diurnal variation in intraocular pressure. Once-daily treatment may sometimes be satisfactory, but this should be checked by pressure measurements.

Indications

1. Hypertension

Timolol may be used as a first-choice drug for hypertension;[15] it controls a similar number of patients to propranolol.[1,16,17] In a multicentre study in which 129 patients received timolol 10–30 mg twice daily, average blood pressure was reduced from 154/103 to 145/94 mmHg, in 57% of patients being reduced to 90 mmHg diastolic or a reduction of 10 mmHg compared to 13% of the 174 patients who received placebo.[15] Left ventricular mass is reduced after 16 weeks of chronic timolol treatment.[18] Timolol has been shown to have an additive effect with a variety of agents, including diuretics,[19] nifedipine[20] and methyldopa.[21]

The usual initial dose for timolol is 10 mg a day. Most studies have used up to 40 mg a day, usually on a twice-daily basis, up to a recommended limit of 60 mg a day.

How timolol and other β-adrenoceptor-blocking drugs lower the blood pressure is not clear, although reduction of cardiac output without a full compensatory rise in peripheral resistance seems to be the main haemodynamic change.[6]

2. Angina pectoris

Timolol is an effective prophylactic in angina pectoris.[1,22] In one study timolol gave equal or greater than 50% reduction in angina attack rate in 78% of patients, reducing the average weekly attack rate from 6.1 on placebo to 2.5 per week on timolol.[22]

Dosage of timolol should be commenced at 5 mg twice daily and titrated up as required, initially with an increment totalling 10 mg a day then with amounts not exceeding 15 mg a day. The recommended dose range is 15–45 mg daily.

The optimum dose of a β-blocking drug in angina pectoris, provided that it is tolerated, generally is the dose that gives maximum inhibition of the exercising heart rate.

3. Secondary prevention of myocardial infarction

Timolol has been found to be effective in reducing the sudden death rate in patients who had experienced a myocardial infarction from 13.9% on placebo to 7.7% on timolol over 12 to 33 months of observation, a reduction of 44%. It also reduced the probability of a further myocardial infarction.[23]

Treatment is usually started 7–28 days postinfarction. Dosage should be started at 5 mg twice daily and if no untoward effect occurs increased to 10 mg twice daily after 2 days.

4. Migraine

Timolol is an effective prophylactic in migraine.[24,25]

5. Glaucoma

Timolol (Timoptol 0.25%, 0.5%) eye drops have been found to be an effective agent in lowering intraocular pressure in patients with glaucoma by about 26–38%, and are more effective than pilocarpine or adrenaline.[26] They act by both improving drainage and reducing production of aqueous humour.[26] In some patients there is an increase in intraocular pressure in spite of continuing treatment, but in the majority response to timolol is maintained.[6]

Systemic side effects can occur following the use of timolol eye drops and asthma has been reported.[27] In a follow-up of 489 patients 15.9% experienced side effects. A burning pain in the eyes may subside in a week but led to discontinuation of treatment in 2% of cases, and blurred vision also led to treatment being withdrawn in 2%. Dry eyes had an incidence of 10%.[27]

Contraindications

These are similar to those for all non-selective β-adrenoceptor-blocking drugs.[6]

1. Obstructive airways disease

Timolol is contraindicated in patients with asthma as a severe attack may be precipitated[28] due to the blocking action of timolol on the β_2-dilator action of adrenaline. There is a possibility that some patients with allergic rhinitis may experience bronchospasm, and patients with chronic obstructive airways disease may also be worsened. Patients who have received timolol will be unresponsive to normal doses of β_2-stimulant drugs. Bronchospasm has been reported after timolol eye drops.

2. Cardiac insufficiency and cardiogenic shock

A major compensatory mechanism in myocardial insufficiency, either left or right sided, is sympathetic stimulation leading to an increase in heart rate. Timolol, like other β-blocking drugs, will interfere with this compensatory mechanism, and may precipitate severe symptoms.

3. Heart block

Timolol should be avoided in second or third degree heart block and in patients with an already slow heart rate, 45–55 beats.min^{-1}. A slow heart rate in an asymptomatic patient who is otherwise well in sinus rhythm need not necessarily be a cause for concern.

4. Hypoglycaemia

Muscle glycogenolysis is β_2-receptor mediated, and hepatic glycogenolysis is also β-mediated, although here α-receptors also play a part. As might be expected, therefore, timolol prolongs insulin hypoglycaemia. The cardiovascular responses to hypoglycaemia would also be expected to be modified, the β-mediated vasodilator action of liberated adrenaline being inhibited leaving the α-vasoconstrictor action unopposed, and consequently there is an increased rise of blood pressure. It is for these reasons that some physicians do not give timolol to insulin-dependent diabetics although β-blocking drugs have been given to such patients on many occasions.

Adverse reactions

Potentially life-threatening effects

No specific toxicity has been reported. Dangerous reactions reported are consequent on β-blockade. A fatal asthma attack has been reported following the use of timolol eye drops.[29]

Timolol should not be withdrawn suddenly in patients with ischaemic heart disease, such as those with myocardial infarction or angina pectoris, in whom symptoms may be worsened.

Acute overdosage

Overdosage with timolol has not been reported. Haemodialysis might be expected to be of only limited value to reduce serum concentration, because of the large volume of distribution of timolol.

Any overdosage with timolol should be managed along the lines used for other β-blocking drugs.[30] Excessive bradycardia may be treated with intravenous atropine.

Isoprenaline, if given, should be administered as an infusion in graded doses increased rapidly (e.g. minute intervals) until heart rate increases to an adequate level. Impracticable dosage levels may be required, hospital supplies being inadequate. Glucagon may be a useful cardiac stimulant as the adenyl cyclase system is stimulated independent of the β-receptor. Digitalis and diuretics may be employed. Bronchospasm may be treated with aminophylline, or again, extremely large doses of isoprenaline or salbutamol (arrived at by a graded approach).

Severe or irreversible adverse effects

Severe side effects from timolol are most likely to be associated with poor patient selection and to occur at the beginning of treatment.

Asthma is likely to be dramatically worsened in an asthmatic, and heart failure may be worsened or precipitated in patients in or on the verge of heart failure.

Symptomatic adverse effects

The symptomatic effects of timolol are similar to those of other β-blocking drugs and seldom require withdrawal of treatment. Sometimes dosage reduction will relieve adverse effects without loss of therapeutic efficacy. Those reported infrequently include nausea, vomiting, bradycardia, fatigue, light-headedness, cold extremities, insomnia, depression and paraesthesia. Cardiac insufficiency, hypotension and A-V block have occurred on rare occasions.[6,23] Similar adverse effects have been described after ocular use.[31]

Other effects

The biochemical changes caused by timolol would be expected to be similar to those induced by other non-selective agents. There is a modest increase in serum potassium, and small increases in urate and creatinine.[6] Insulin hypoglycaemia can be prolonged.[32] Timolol, like propranolol, increases triglycerides and reduces HDL.[33] It is not clear whether these changes are clinically important.

Interference with clinical pathology tests

There are no known interferences of this kind.

High risk groups

Neonates

There are no data on the use of timolol in neonates.

Breast milk. Caution is required in nursing women as timolol is likely to appear in breast milk, though data are lacking. Discontinuation of timolol is advised.

Children

There are no data on timolol.

Pregnant women

The safety of timolol in pregnancy has not been established.

The elderly

In both angina pectoris and hypertension, dosage with timolol should be titrated gradually, say at one-week intervals, so no problem should arise.

Drug interactions

Potentially hazardous interactions

Adrenaline. As with other non-selective β-blockers, marked increases in blood pressure and bradycardia would be expected from the administration of adrenaline in the presence of timolol.

Anaesthetic agents. Heart rate and cardiac output may fall in anaesthesia to a greater degree in patients taking β-blockers. This can be counteracted by atropine 1–2 mg intravenously. Timolol should not be abruptly stopped before anaesthesia, as potentiation of the effects of any liberated catecholamines would be expected.

Clonidine. Rebound hypertension following abrupt withdrawal of clonidine may be potentiated by a β-blocker such as timolol.

Insulin. Care should be taken in giving timolol to insulin-dependent diabetics. The signs of hypoglycaemia will be masked and the rise of blood pressure associated with hypoglycaemia will be prolonged.

Other significant interactions

Food. Data are not available on the effect of food on timolol absorption. Food enhances absorption of propranolol and as timolol undergoes considerable first-pass metabolism food might also be expected to enhance its absorption.

Smoking. In view of its β_2-blocking action on the vasodilator component of the actions of adrenaline, timolol might be expected to enhance the rise of blood pressure that has been reported with smoking, particularly in combination with caffeine, although no data are available. Smoking may also induce its metabolism in the liver.

Other drugs. As there is considerable liver metabolism of timolol by liver microsomal enzymes it is possible that other drugs metabolized in this way may interact, giving increased blood levels. There have been few studies with timolol but it has been shown to inhibit the hepatic metabolism of lignocaine.[34]

Indomethacin. It is probable that the hypotensive action of timolol may be reduced by indomethacin.

Potentially useful interactions

Timolol would be expected to inhibit the tachycardia associated with some vasodilators such as minoxidil. It reduces thiazide-induced hypokalaemia.[35]

Major outcome trials

1. The Norwegian Multicenter Study Group 1981 Timolol induced reduction in mortality and reinfarction in patients surviving acute myocardial infarction. New England Journal of Medicine 304: 801–807

In a randomized, double-blind, multi-centre study, timolol 10 mg twice daily and placebo were compared in 1884 patients surviving acute myocardial infarction, with an average follow-up of 17 months, range 12–33 months. There was a sudden death rate of 13.9% in the placebo group, and 7.7% in the timolol group, a reduction of 44.6% ($p = 0.0001$). The reinfarction rate was 20.1% in the placebo group, and 14.4% in the timolol patients ($p < 0.0006$). Benefit was still present at six-years follow-up.[36] Most benefit was seen in the patients who stopped smoking.[37]

References

1. Brogden R N, Speight T M, Avery G S 1975 Timolol: a preliminary report of its pharmacological properties and therapeutic efficacy in angina and hypertension. Drugs 9: 164–177
2. Heel R C, Brogden R N, Speight T M, Avery G S 1979 Timolol: A review of its therapeutic efficacy in the topical treatment of glaucoma. Drugs 17: 38–55
3. Lund-Johansen P 1983 Hemodynamic effects of antihypertensive agents. Canadian Medical Association Journal 128(1): 21–23
4. Sugimoto K, Fujimura A, Hino N, Kumagai Y, Nakashima H, Ebihara A 1986 Clinical significance of β_1-selectivity in β-receptor blocking agents. Acta Pharmacologica et Toxicologica (suppl) 14: 805 (abstract)
5. Aronsown W S, Ferlinz J, Del Vicario M, Moorthy K, King J, Cassidy J 1976 Effect of timolol versus propranolol on hypertension and hemodynamics. Circulation 54: 47–51
6. Cruickshank J M, Prichard B N C 1988 β-Blockers in clinical practice. Churchill Livingstone, Edinburgh, p 1003
7. Tocco D J, Duncan A E W, Deluna F A, Hucker H B, Gruber V F, Vandenheuvel W J A 1975 Physiological disposition and metabolism of timolol in man and laboratory animals. Drug Metabolism and Disposition 3(5): 361–370
8. Tracqui A, Kintz P, Himber J, Lugnier A A J, Mangin P 1988 A specific HPLC method for determination of β-blockers topically used in ophthalmological diseases. Forensic Science International 38: 37–41
9. Wasson B K, Scheigetz J, Rooney C S et al 1980 Urinary metabolites of timolol from humans and laboratory animals. Syntheses and β-adrenergic blocking activities. Journal of Medicinal Chemistry 23(II): 1178–1184
10. Lennard M S, Tucker G T, Woods H F 1986 The polymorphic oxidation of β-adrenoceptor antagonists. Clinical pharmacokinetic considerations. Clinical Pharmacokinetics 11: 1–17
11. Tocco D J, Clineschmidt B V, Duncan A E W, deLuna F A, Baer J E 1980 Uptake of the β-adrenergic blocking agents propranolol and timolol by rodent brain: relationship to central pharmacological actions. Journal of Cardiovascular Pharmacology 2: 133–143
12. Lowenthal D T, Pitone J M, Affrime M B et al 1978 Timolol kinetics in chronic renal insufficiency. Clinical Pharmacology and Therapeutics 23(5): 606–615
13. Bobik A, Jennings G L, Ashley P, Korner P I 1979 Timolol pharmacokinetics and effects on heart rate and blood pressure after acute and chronic administration. European Journal of Clinical Pharmacology 16: 243–249
14. Prichard B N C, Walden R J, Tomlinson B, Liu J-B 1988 The cardiovascular effect of withdrawal of β-adrenoceptor blocking drugs. Current Opinion in Cardiology 3 (suppl 2): S19–S29
15. Rofman B A, Fulaga S F, Gabriel M A, Thiyagarajan B, Nancarrow J F, Abrams W B 1980 Multiclinic evaluation of timolol in the treatment of mild-to-moderate essential hypertension. Hypertension 2: 643–648
16. Aronow W S, Ferlinz J, Del Vicario M, Moorthy K, King J, Cassidy J 1976 Effect of timolol versus propranolol on hypertension and hemodynamics. Circulation 54(1): 47–51
17. Lohmoller G, Frohlich E D 1975 A comparison of timolol and propranolol in essential hypertension. American Heart Journal 89(4): 437–442
18. Rowlands D B, Glover D R, Stallard T J, Littler W A 1982 Control of blood pressure and reduction of echo-cardiographically assessed left ventricular mass with once-daily timolol. British Journal of Clinical Pharmacology 14: 89–95
19. Castenfors H 1977 Long-term effect of timolol and hydrochlorothiazide or hydrochlorothiazide and amiloride in essential hypertension. European Journal of Clinical Pharmacology 12: 97–103
20. Christensen C K, Pedersen O L, Mikkelsen E 1982 Renal effects of acute calcium blockade with nifedipine in hypertensive patients receiving β-adrenoceptor-blocking drugs. Clinical Pharmacology and Therapeutics 32(5): 572–576
21. Lubbe W F 1976 Antihypertensive therapy with timolol and α-methyldopa. South African Medical Journal 50: 279–285
22. Aronow W S, Turbow M, Van Camp S, Lurie M, Whittaker K 1980 The effect of timolol vs. placebo on angina pectoris. Circulation 61(1): 66–69
23. Norwegian Multicenter Study Group 1981. Timolol-induced reduction in mortality and reinfarction in patients surviving acute mycardial infarction. New England Journal of Medicine 304(14): 801–807
24. Stellar S, Ahrens S P, Meibohm A R, Reines S A 1984 Migraine prevention with timolol. Journal of the American Medical Association 252 (18): 2576–2580
25. Tfelt-Hansen P, Standnes B, Kangasneimi P, Hakkarainen H, Olesen J 1984 Timolol vs. propranolol vs. placebo in common migraine prophylaxis: a double-blind multicenter trial. Acta Neurologica Scandinavica 69: 1–8
26. Heel R C, Brogden R N, Speight T M, Avery G S 1979 Timolol: a review of its therapeutic efficacy in the topical treatment of glaucoma. Drugs 17: 38–55
27. Wilson R P, Spaeth G L, Poryzees E 1980 The place of timolol in the practice of ophthalmology. Ophthalmology 87: 451–454
28. Raine J M, Palazzo M G, Kerr J H, Sleight P 1981 Near-fatal bronchospasm after oral nadolol in a young asthmatic and response to ventilation with halothane. British Medical Journal 282: 548–549
29. Fraunfelder F T, Barker A F 1984 Respiratory effects of timolol. New England Journal of Medicine 311 (22): 1441
30. Prichard B N C, Battersby L A, Cruickshank J M 1984 Overdosage with β-adrenergic blocking agents. Adverse Drug Reaction and Accidental Poisoning Review 3: 91–111
31. Van Buskirk E M 1980 Adverse reactions from timolol administration. Ophthalmology 87: 477–450
32. Angelo-Nielson K 1980 Timolol topically and diabetes mellitus. Journal of the American Medical Association 244 (20): 2263
33. Gundersen T, Kjekshus J, Stokke O, Pedersen T 1985 Timolol maleate and HDL cholesterol after myocardial infarction. European Heart Journal 6: 840–844
34. Deacon C S, Lennard M S, Bax N D S, Woods H F, Tucker G T 1981 Inhibition of oxidative drug metabolism by β-adrenoceptor antagonists is related to their lipid solubility. British Journal of Clinical Pharmacology 12: 429–431
35. Hettiarachchi J, Ramsay L E, Davies D L, Fraser R, Watson W S 1977 Amelioraton of bendrofluazide-induced hypokalaemia by timolol. Clinical Pharmacology and Therapeutics 22 (19): 58–62
36. Pedersen T R for the Norwegian Multicenter Study Group 1985 Six-year follow-up of the Norwegian Multicenter Study on timolol after acute myocardial infarction. New England Journal of Medicine 313: 1055–1058
37. Ronnevik P K, Gundersen T, Abrahamsen A M 1985 Effect of smoking habits and timolol treatment on mortality and reinfarction in patients surviving acute myocardial infarction. British Heart Journal 54: 134–139

T

Tinidazole

Tinidazole is a nitroimidazole which has antimicrobial actions against the microaerophilic protozoa *Giardia lamblia*, *Entamoeba histolytica* and *Trichomonas vaginalis*, and against obligate anaerobic bacteria. Tinidazole is well absorbed from the gut and gives high serum levels which are well sustained because of its long half life.

Chemistry

Tinidazole (Fasigyn)
$C_8H_{13}N_3O_4S$
1-[2-(Ethylsuphonyl)ethyl]-2-methyl-5-nitroimidazole

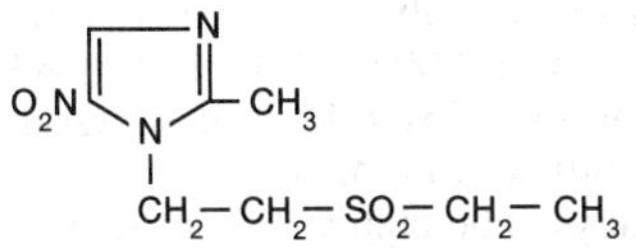

Molecular weight	247
pKa	1.81
Solubility	
in alcohol	—
in water	—
Lipid/water partition coefficient	1.4

Pharmacology

Tinidazole readily diffuses through the cell membranes of aerobic and anaerobic organisms. It is reduced at the 5-nitro position by nitroreductase in obligate anaerobes and the generation of reduced tinidazole allows more drug to diffuse into the organism. As a result high concentrations accumulate within target organisms. This occurs at the low redox potentials associated only with anaerobes. Amine and hydroxylamine derivatives of the reduced compound are thought to damage the macromolecules and deoxyribonucleic acid of anaerobic organisms.[1] Full details of the mechanisms are not understood, but reduced tinidazole probably causes a loss of the helical structure of DNA. In addition, strand breakage occurs and DNA function is impaired.

Toxicology

Acute toxicity studies showed an LD_{50} of >2000 mg.kg^{-1} in mice and rats for tinidazole given either orally or intraperitoneally.[2] Subacute toxicity tests showed no evidence of adverse effects in life or at post mortem from 150 mg.kg^{-1} twice daily for 30 days in rats and monkeys.[2] Up to 2500 mg.kg^{-1} (mice) and 2000 mg.kg^{-1} (rats) given intragastrically for 14 days caused no adverse reactions.[3] Pregnant rats and mice received 2000 mg.kg^{-1} and 2500 mg.kg^{-1} respectively for 6 days at the time of organ development. There were no fetal abnormalities in the mice but fetal mortality was increased in rats receiving 500 mg.kg^{-1} or more.[3]

Tinidazole has mutagenic potential shown by induction of mutation in *Salmonella typhimurium* in the Ames test. The reduced drug causes this effect. Eukaryotic cells contain little nitroreductase and so do not produce significant amounts of the mutagens. The effects of reduced drug produced within anaerobic organisms in a human host are not known. The mutagens may be ineffective because of binding to macromolecules in the anaerobes or conversion to inactive forms[1] so that they do not come into contact with human cells. Chromosomes from peripheral blood lymphocytes of patients taking metronidazole showed no evidence of damage.[1] The potential for mutagenic effects in man appears low.

There is no evidence that tinidazole has carcinogenic potential in experimental animals (manufacturer's data).

Clinical pharmacology

Tinidazole kills obligate anaerobic bacteria and the microaerophilic protozoan parasites. A range of anaerobic bacteria are susceptible with an MIC_{90} of 1.6 mg.l^{-1} in 114 strains from 9 species (see Table 1). These include *Bacteroides fragilis*, other *Bacteroides* species, *Fusobacterium* species and *Clostridium* species.[4] Tinidazole is also active against *Trichomonas vaginalis*, *Entamoeba hystolytica* and *Giardia lamblia*. Occasional resistant strains are encountered among *Peptostreptococcus*, *Peptococcus* and *Clostridium*. *Propionibacterium acnes* is uniformly resistant.

Tinidazole is used in the treatment of anaerobic sepsis involving the gums, sinuses and respiratory tract and in cases of peritonitis and intra-abdominal abscess. It can also be used in brain abscess where the importance of anaerobic bacteria is now well recognized.

Tinidazole has been used for the chemoprophylaxis of infection related to gastrointestinal and gynaecological surgery.

Pharmacokinetics

High performance liquid chromatography is used most often for measuring tinidazole concentrations[5] and will measure 0.3 mg.l^{-1} in serum. Other metabolites did not interfere with the assay nor did a wide range of antibiotics. Average recovery of tinidazole added to serum was 87% over concentrations from 0.2 to 20 mg.l^{-1}.

Tinidazole is rapidly absorbed from the gut with peak levels occurring 0.5 to 2 hours after ingestion. Systemic bioavailability is 100% with protein binding of about 12%. Serum levels were 43–58 mg.l^{-1} 2 hours after a 2.0 g single oral dose; 20–40 mg.l^{-1} at 6 hours; 15–20 mg.l^{-1} at 24 hours; and 2–5 mg.l^{-1} at 48 hours.[6] This is explained by the long half life of 12 to 14.7 hours. The serum levels after a 500 mg intravenous infusion were 14.5 mg.l^{-1} at 5 minutes; 9.7 mg.l^{-1} at 1.5 hours; 7.5 mg.l^{-1} at 6 hours; and 3.2 mg.l^{-1} at 24 hours.

The half life was prolonged to 15.1 hours in patients with chronic renal failure not on maintenance dialysis but was normal, 12.9 hours, immediately after dialysis in patients who did require maintenance dialysis.[7] A reduced half life, 4.9 hours, was found during dialysis.[7] The presence of renal failure does not require alterations in dosage regimens.

The drug is rapidly distributed through body tissues. Patients with appendicitis who received 500 mg intravenously prior to surgery had serum levels of 11.4 to 8.3 mg.l^{-1} from 10 to 120 minutes post-infusion. Concentrations in tissues over the same time period were: appendix 12.6 to 6.3 mg.l^{-1}; skeletal muscle 9.6 to 7.3 mg.l^{-1}; and fat 2.8 to 1.9 mg.l^{-1}.[8] The drug is moderately lipophilic but fat concentrations are low. Tissues of the male and female genital tracts show high levels.[9,10] There is good penetration into cerebrospinal fluid[11,12] with levels equal to those in serum. The apparent volume of distribution is 0.6–0.7 l.kg^{-1}. Tinidazole crosses the placenta and reaches the fetus.[12] It also is found in breast milk and the maximum potential dose to the infant was calculated at 0.1 mg.kg^{-1} after the mother received 1.6 g by infusion prior to caesarian section.[13] Salivary levels of the drug approximate to serum levels.

Oral absorption	100%
Presystemic metabolism	nil
Plasma half life	
range	12–14 h
mean	13.5 h
Volume of distribution	0.64 1.kg^{-1}
Plasma protein binding	12%

Tinidazole is excreted into the bile in concentrations just less than 50% of serum levels. The mechanisms involved in eliminating

Tinidazole

T

tinidazole from the body are incompletely understood. About 25% of the administered dose is excreted unchanged in the urine. Metabolites also appear in the urine and constitute a further 12%. There is also some faecal excretion of tinidazole. There are some variations in these figures from different authors but it appears that the fate of 60–70% of administered drug is not adequately explained but is presumably metabolized.

Concentration–effect relationship

Many species of obligate anaerobic bacteria are potentially pathogenic in man. *Bacteroides fragilis*, *B. melaninogenicus*, *Fusobacterium necrophorum* and *Peptostreptococcus anaerobius* are among the commonest pathogens in anerobic sepsis. The sensitivities of a range of organisms are shown in Table 1. Because of its low toxicity and the high serum and tissue levels obtained estimations of blood levels are not needed.

Metabolism

Metabolism of the drug produces a hydroxylated derivative which can be further modified to a glucuronide conjugate. Both of these appear in the urine. Two other metabolites of the drug excreted in the urine have not been characterized.

Pharmaceutics

Oral and parenteral preparations of tinidazole (Fasigyn; Pfizer, UK) are available. The white, film-coated tablet contains 500 mg of tinidazole. Some early studies used a 150 mg tablet but this is no longer produced. The tablets should be stored at temperatures below 25°C protected from light and moisture. The shelf-life is 60 months. A syrup preparation is not available. Infusions of the drug are available with either 800 mg in 400 ml or 1600 mg in 800 ml. The infusion should be stored below 25°C away from light. Any unused drug should be discarded after a dose has been withdrawn from the bottle. The shelf-life is 24 months.

Therapeutic use

Indications

1. Treatment of giardiasis
2. Treatment of amoebiasis
3. Treatment of trichomoniasis
4. Prophylaxis of anaerobic infection related to abdominal and pelvic surgery
5. Treatment of anaerobic infection.

Contraindications

1. Pregnancy.

Mode of use

The parasitic protozoa are treated with single doses of 1.5–2.0 g (50 $mg.kg^{-1}$ in children) taken with or just after food for 1 to 3 days (see below). Single oral doses of 2.0 g given 12 hours before surgery or 1600 mg given as an infusion just before surgery or 800 mg given before and repeated up to 12 hours after surgery are used in the prophylaxis of anaerobic sepsis. The doses given apply to adults. The manufacturers have no data on which to make recommendations for children under 12 years. For the treatment of established anaerobic sepsis 1.0 g may be given orally twice daily followed by 500 mg twice daily or 1.0 g as a single daily dose. Intravenous treatment is begun with an initial infusion of 800 mg followed by 800 mg per day either as a single dose or two doses 12 hourly. Oral therapy should be substituted for the intravenous as soon as possible. Treatment should continue for 5–7 days. The clinical response will determine if longer treatment is needed.

Indications

1. Giardiasis

The most convenient regimen is a single dose of 1.5 g taken with food.[22] Children are given 50 $mg.kg^{-1}$. The large 500 mg tablet may be difficult for small children to swallow. The cut surface of the tablet

Table 1

Reference	Organism (no. of strains)	MIC ($mg.l^{-1}$)
Reynolds et al.[14]	*Fusobacterium* (8)	⩽0.5
	Bacteroides fragilis (59)	⩽2.0
Wust[4]	*B. fragilis* (39)	⩽3.1
	B. melaninogenicus (2)	⩽0.1
	Fusobacterium (13)	⩽1.6
	Peptococcus and *Peptostreptococcus* spp. (24)	⩽3.1
	Propionibacterium acnes (7)	>100.0
Klastersky et al.[15]	*B. fragilis* (200)	⩽3.0
	B. melaninogenicus	⩽13.0 MIC_{50}
		⩽0.15 MIC_{50}
	Fusobacterium (54)	⩽1.5 MIC_{90}
	Clostridium (72)	⩽12.0 MIC_{100}
	Gram-positive cocci (30)	⩽0.15 MIC_{50}
Tannock[16]	*Bacteroides* spp. (46)	⩽4.0
	Fusobacterium (13)	⩽4.0
	Clostridium (7)	⩽4.0
Niederau et al.[17]	*B. melaninogenicus* (13)	⩽1.6 (11 out of 13)
Hoffler et al.[18]	*Propionibacterium acnes*	>100.0
Carmona et al.[19]	*Gardnerella vaginalis* (51)	⩽12.0
Shanker & Monro[20]	*G. vaginalis*	7.4 (tinidazole)
		0.58 (OH-tin*)
Bannatyne et al.[21]	*G. vaginalis* (510)	⩽4.44 MIC_{90}
Goodwin et al.[39]	*Helicobacter pylori* (20)	4.0 MIC_{90}

*OH-tin represents the hydroxy metabolite of tinidazole which appears to be much more potent than the parent compound. Bannatyne et al.[21] found the same for the hydroxy derivative of metronidazole.

has a very bitter taste and so it is difficult for children to take less than a whole tablet. This regimen gave a 90% cure rate in adults with relapses occurring up to 29 days after treatment. Not all relapses cause symptoms and so are only detected by follow-up stool microscopy 6–8 weeks after treatment. Serum levels and tinidazole half lives did not differ in those cured and those not cured.

2. Amoebiasis

Amoebic dysentery can be treated with single doses of 2.0 g (60 $mg.kg^{-1}$) for 3 days.

In amoebic liver abscess single high doses 2.0 g (60 $mg.kg^{-1}$) are given daily with food for 3 days. Scragg and Proctor[23] used the 60 $mg.kg^{-1}$ regimen in children and found good results with 5 or 3 days of medication. A satisfactory response was seen in 23 out of 25 children. In all cases therapeutic, percutaneous aspiration of the liver was undertaken at the outset and repeated as indicated. This has been the standard practice in all the studies of amoebic liver abscess undertaken by the Durban group. In adults treated in Durban, tinidazole or metronidazole (2.0 g as a single daily dose for 3 days) gave equally good results with rapid resolution of pain, fever and tenderness in similar times.[24] Reaspiration was needed in 5/21 (tinidazole) and 5/27 (metronidazole) and retreatment was needed in 4 of the tinidazole group and 3 of the metronidazole group.

3. Trichomoniasis

A single dose of 2.0 g will eradicate *T. vaginalis*. This dosage gives a 95% cure rate at 7 days.[25] The sexual partner of the patient should receive the same dose.

4. Chemoprophylaxis of anaerobic infection related to abdominal and pelvic surgery

Abdominal surgery

Tinidazole is well suited for use in the prophylaxis of infection after abdominal surgery because it is bactericidal and produces high and sustained serum and tissue levels after a single dose. Anaerobic organisms are the main pathogens causing sepsis after a range of abdominal surgical procedures. The use of tinidazole has been recommended before total and Polya gastrectomies, biliary tract surgery when the bile duct is to be explored and small bowel surgery when the gut is to be opened.[26] Gierksky and his colleagues[26,29] give tinidazole 1600 mg plus doxycycline 400 mg by intravenous infusion one hour before surgery, adding the doxycycline for its actions on aerobic, Gram-negative organisms.

A single dose of tinidazole 500 mg infused over 20 minutes immediately before emergency appendicectomy reduced the incidence of septic complications from nine episodes in 33 patients receiving placebo to one episode in 33 receiving tinidazole.[27] Giving tinidazole for three more days after surgery produced no extra benefit.

The value of chemoprophylaxis prior to colorectal surgery is now accepted and investigations continue to determine the choice of drug and the duration of administration. A single 2.0 g dose of tinidazole given orally with food 12 hours before elective colorectal surgery significantly reduced the incidence of wound infections to 3 out of 41 receiving tinidazole compared with 11 out of 31 receiving placebo.[28] Tinidazole 1600 mg plus doxycycline 400 mg given intravenously 2 hours before surgery was compared with half of these doses given daily for five days before surgery in a large multi-centre study.[29] Infection rates were low in both groups with regard to wound infections, intra-abdominal sepsis, perineal sepsis and septicaemia. Giving these antibiotics for several days before surgery was not beneficial nor was continued administration of tinidazole and doxycycline for three days after surgery.[30]

Pelvic surgery

Tinidazole 2.0 g orally 12 hours before and 48 hours after abdominal hysterectomy significantly reduced the rate of isolation of anaerobes from high vaginal swabs taken on the third and seventh postoperative days.[31] When anaerobes persisted their growth was not enhanced in those given tinidazole. In contrast, the growth of anaerobes was more profuse in patients given placebo. *Bacteroides melaninogenicus* in 83 out of 100 specimens was the most frequent isolate. Other *Bacteroides* were isolated from 71 specimens. Wound infection and pelvic cellulitis were less common in those receiving prophylaxis (6/50 against 25/50). This difference was not significant. Eight out of ten postoperative wound infections in those not receiving prophylaxis resolved spontaneously. The duration of hospital stay was not compared. Patients given 2.0 g of tinidazole 12 hours before surgery had significantly less pelvic sepsis than control patients and the hospital stay was prolonged in 17 infected control patients and in two treated patients.[32] The same regimen was effective in reducing the occurrence of local infection after vaginal hysterectomy[33] and 1600 mg tinidazole infused intravenously within the hour before vaginal hysterectomy reduced the occurrence of sepsis. Tinidazole prophylaxis before emergency caesarian section was effective in preventing postoperative endometritis and wound sepsis.[34]

5. The treatment of anaerobic infections

The rationale for using tinidazole in treating anaerobic infections follows from its similarity to metronidazole and the known efficacy of that drug in this clinical setting. Tinidazole need only be given once or twice daily and this may increase patient compliance among outpatients and reduce nursing time spent in drug administration in inpatients. Anaerobic bacteria are important in the pathogenesis of aspiration pneumonia and so the choice of antibiotics must take this into consideration. Penicillin is often used but tinidazole may be used as an alternative. When additional cover for aerobic Gram-negative organisms is needed a third generation cephalosporin can be added. Peritonitis, abdominal abscess and brain abscess are conditions in which anaerobic organisms are important constituents of the microflora and tinidazole may be used. Doses of 500 mg 12-hourly are usual and the duration of treatment depends on the response to treatment. Surgical treatment to drain or aspirate abscesses may be needed.

Gardnerella vaginalis is a cause of vaginitis which responds well to treatment with tinidazole. Single doses of 2.0 g are effective but 500 mg twice daily for 5 days can also be used.[19,35] The hydroxy metabolite is also active against this organism (Table 1[20])

Tinidazole produced good results in the treatment of wound infections in patients with cancer in a double-blind trial comparing it with clindamycin and doxycycline.[15] Clindamycin gave the best results but tinidazole was not significantly less good.

Helicobacter pylori (previously known as *Campylobacter pylori* and *Campylobacter pyloridis*) has been incriminated in the pathogenesis of antral gastritis and peptic ulceration. Recent studies have shown that reduced recurrence rates of gastritis and ulceration are associated with eradication of *Helicobacter*. The addition of tinidazole to cimetidine cleared organisms in 70% of patients allowing healing in 92% with relapse in 21% over the next 12 months.[40] Children with *Helicobacter pylori* antral gastritis and abdominal pain were treated with amoxycillin and tinidazole for 6 weeks. The organism was cleared in 30 out of 32 children and most became symptom free with tinidazole only. By 6 months 2 out of 12 had symptomatic relapse with organisms present.[41]

Contraindications

1. Pregnancy

This is because of the mutagenicity of the nitroimidazole compounds in bacteria and carcinogencity in some rodent studies (although this effect has not been reported with tinidazole)[1] so that the drug should be avoided during pregnancy. Tinidazole is present in breast milk in low concentration. The outcome of pregnancy was examined in 597 women who received metronidazole at various stages. No adverse effect was found.[36] No information is available for tinidazole so that the general rule applies that it should not be used in pregnancy or nursing mothers unless the benefits of its use outweigh the potential risks.

Adverse reactions

Potentially life-threatening effects

Severe reactions are uncommon, but generalized urticaria, facial and laryngeal oedema, hypotension, bronchospasm and dyspnoea have been reported. In six instances adrenaline was needed, but all the patients affected recovered. These episodes occurred after 2.0 g oral doses in 9 adults and a five-year-old child given 500 mg.[37]

Acute overdosage

No instances of deliberate or accidental overdose have been reported.

Severe or irreversible adverse effects

There are none apart from those noted above.

Symptomatic adverse effects
The usual symptomatic effects are a metallic taste in the mouth and mild nausea. Headache and vomiting have also been recorded. Rashes are uncommon. Thrombophlebitis may occur at the site of intravenous infusion.

Other effects
Leucopenia appears to be very uncommon and in one report which drew attention to its occurrence, the patient was also receiving cefuroxime and pivampicillin. Biochemical hepatitis followed administration of 625 mg (50 $mg.kg^{-1}$) once only. There were no other causes that could be defined and the abnormalities resolved completely.

Interference with clinical pathology tests
None has been reported for tinidazole though metronidazole interferes with plasma glucose measurements using the hexokinase method, resulting in a falsely high value especially in hepatic failure.

High risk groups

Neonates
There is little information on the effects and use of tinidazole in neonates.

Breast milk. Tinidazole should not be given to nursing mothers as it enters breast milk.

Children
Dosage regimens for children are 50–60 $mg.kg^{-1}$ as a single oral dose given for 1 day (giardiasis) or 3 days (invasive amoebiasis). There is no information on the use of tinidazole for the prophylaxis or treatment of anaerobic infections in children under 12 years.

Pregnant women
Tinidazole should not be used in pregnancy as a general rule because of the carcinogenic and mutagenic potential of this group of drugs (see above). Metronidazole used in low doses in pregnancy caused no adverse effect[36] but similar information is not available for tinidazole.

The elderly
No special recommendations are made.

Drug interactions

Potentially hazardous interactions
Metronidazole is reported to have a disulfiram-like interaction with alcohol causing nausea, vomiting, abdominal cramps and flushing. Patients taking tinidazole should not drink alcohol.

Potentially useful interactions
No useful interactions have been reported. An in vitro study[38] has shown synergism between tinidazole and ampicillin, doxycycline and co-trimoxazole. This synergism may contribute to the efficacy of the combination of tinidazole with doxycycline in chemoprophylaxis of anaerobic sepsis after abdominal surgery.

Major outcome trials

1. Gierksky K-I, Danielson S, Garberg O et al 1982 Single dose pre-operative antimicrobial prophylaxis in abdominal operations. Journal of Antimicrobial Chemotherapy 10 (suppl A): 123–128

This is a prospective, multi-centre controlled trial involving 661 patients. They were randomly allocated to receive tinidazole 1600 mg plus doxycycline 400 mg intravenously over 2 hours on the morning before elective abdominal surgery or no prophylaxis. A placebo was not given because nothing was available to produce a yellow-coloured solution like that of doxycycline. The types of surgery performed were similar in the two groups. Cases in which the colon was opened were excluded. There were significantly more oesophageal reconstructions and pancreatectomies in the prophylaxis group than in the control group. 296 patients received prophylaxis and 290 received no prophylaxis. Infective episodes were 11 in the former and 55 in the latter; most of these were wound abscesses (8 and 44 respectively). Hospital stay was shorter in those given prophylaxis (9.3 days against 11.5 days). Total additional antibiotic administration was less in the prophylaxis group and the total number of infective complications unrelated to the abdomen was less in those given prophylaxis. This study shows benefits for this antibiotic combination in the prophylaxis of abdominal sepsis in surgery involving opening the small intestine.

2. Viitanen J, Tunturi T, Auvinen O, Pessi T 1984 Tinidazole prophylaxis in appendicectomies: a controlled study of single dose versus 3 day therapy. Scandinavian Journal of Gastroenterology 19: 111–115

465 patients clinically diagnosed as acute appendicitis received either no medication or tinidazole 500 mg in 100 ml of saline over 20 minutes during the induction of anaesthesia or the same dose intravenously during induction of anaesthesia and 8 hourly for 3 days postoperatively by the intravenous or oral route according to the patient's condition. All operations were done by a standard technique without drainage of the peritoneal cavity. Infective complications were lower in those receiving antibiotics (7% single dose, 5% multi-dose) than in controls (12%). The major effect was in those with gangrenous appendicitis where infection rates were 3% (single dose) and 7% (multi-dose) compared with 27% in controls. When the appendix had perforated postoperative infective rates were high for all three groups: 32% (controls), 43% (single dose) and 46% (multi-dose). The result may have been brought about by not draining the peritoneal cavity. Single-dose tinidazole proved to be valuable in preventing postoperative sepsis.

3. Giercksky K E, Danielsen S, Garberg O et al 1982 A single dose tinidazole and doxycycline prophylaxis in elective surgery of colon and rectum. Annals of Surgery 195: 227–231
4. Karhunen M, Koskela O, Hannelin M 1980 Single dose tinidazole in prophylaxis of infections following hysterectomy. British Journal of Obstetrics and Gynaecology 87: 70–72
5. Karhumen M, Koskela O, Hällström K 1981 Single dose tinidazole in prophylaxis of infections following vaginal surgery. Journal of Antimicrobial Chemotherapy 8: 283–290
6. Karhunen M, Koskela O, Teisala K, Suikarri A-M, Mattila J 1985 Prophylaxis and treatment of anaerobic infections following Caesarian section with tinidazole. Chemotherapy 31: 228–236

Other trials

1. Jokipii L, Jokipii A M M 1979 Single dose metronidazole and tinidazole as therapy for giardiasis; success rates, side effects and drug absorption and elimination. Journal of Infectious Diseases 140: 984–988
2. Simjee A E, Gathiram V, Jackson T F H G, Khan B F Y 1985 A comparative trial of metronidazole against tinidazole in the treatment of amoebic liver abscess. South African Medical Journal 68: 923–924

References

1. Tully F P, Sullivan C E 1981 Metronidazole; in vitro activity, pharmacology and efficacy in anaerobic baterial infections. Pharmacotherapy 1: 28–32
2. Miller M W, Howes A L, English A R 1969 Tinidazole, a potent new anti-protozal agent. In: Hobby G L (ed) Antimicrobial Agents and Therapeutics. American Society of Microbiology, pp 257–260
3. Owaki Y, Momiyama H, Sakai T, Nabato I I 1974 Effects of tinidazole on the fetuses and their post-natal development in mice and rats. Pharmacometrics 8: 421
4. Wüst J 1977 Susceptibility of anaerobic bacteria to metronidazole, ornidazole and tinidazole and routine susceptibility testing by standardised methods. Antimicrobial Agents and Chemotherapy 11: 631–637
5. Nachbauer J, Joly H 1978 Rapid assay of tinidazole in plasma by high performance liquid chromatography. Journal of Chromatography 87: 491–497
6. Hunt P S, Davidson A J L, Alden J, Cheng B 1982 Bile and serum levels of tinidazole after a single oral dose. British Journal of Clinical Pharmacology 13: 233–234
7. Flourat B C, Imbert C, Dubois D M et al 1983 Pharmacokinetics of tinidazole in chronic renal failure and in patients on haemodialysis. British Journal of Clinical Pharmacology 15: 735–741
8. Viitanen J, Auvinen O, Tunturi T 1983 Serum and tissue tinidazole concentrations after intravenous infusion. Chemotherapy 29: 13–17
9. Viitanen J, Haataja H, Männistö P 1985 Concentrations of metronidazole and tinidazole in male genital tissues. Antimicrobial Agents and Chemotherapy 28: 812–814
10. Ripa T, Weström L, Mard L P-A, Andersson K E 1977 Concentrations of tinidazole in body fluids and tissues in gynaecological patients. Chemotherapy 23: 227–235
11. Jokipii A M M, Myllyla V V, Jokipii L 1977 Penetration of the blood brain barrier by metronidazole and tinidazole. Journal of Antimicrobial Chemotherapy 3: 239–245

12. Karhunen M 1984 Placental transfer of metronidazole and tinidazole in early human pregnancy after a single infusion. British Journal of Clinical Pharmacology 18: 254–257
13. Eraldson G R, Lindgren S, Nord C-E, Rave A T 1985 Tinidazole milk excretion and pharmacokinetics in lactating women. British Journal of Clinical Pharmacology 19: 503–507
14. Reynolds A V, Hamilton-Miller J M T, Brumfitt W 1975 A comparison of the in vitro activity of metronidazole, tinidazole and nimorazole against Gram-negative anaerobic bacilli. Journal of Clinical Pathology 28: 775–778
15. Klastersky J, Husson M, Weerts-Ruhl D, Davean D 1977 Anaerobic wound infections in cancer patients: comparative trial of clindamycin, tinidazole and doxycycline. Antimicrobial Agents and Chemotherapy 12: 563–570
16. Tannock G W 1979 Susceptibility of New Zealand isolates of anaerobic bacilli to tinidazole. New Zealand Medical Journal 90: 149–150
17. Niederau W, Höffler U, Pulverer G 1980 Susceptibility of *Bacteroides melaninogenicus* to 45 antibiotics. Chemotherapy 26: 121–127
18. Höffler U, Niederau W, Pulverer G 1980 Susceptibility of cutaneous propionibacteria to newer antibiotics. Chemotherapy 26: 7–11
19. Carmona O, Silva H, Acosta H 1983 Vaginitis due to *Gardnerella vaginalis*: treatment with tinidazole. Current Therapeutic Research 33: 898–904
20. Shanker S, Monro R 1982 The sensitivity of *Gardnerella vaginalis* to metabolites of tinidazole and tinidazole. Lancet 1: 167
21. Bannatyne R M, Jackowski J, Cheung R, Biers K 1987 Susceptibility of *Gardnerella vaginalis* to metronidazole, its bioactive metabolites and tinidazole. American Journal of Clinical Pathology 87: 640–641
22. Jokipii L, Jokipii A M M 1982 Treatment of giardiasis: comparative evaluation of ornidazole and tinidazole as a single dose. Gastroenterology 83: 394–404
23. Scragg J N, Proctor E M 1977 Tinidazole in treatment of amoebic liver abscess. Archives of Diseases in Childhood 52: 408–410
24. Simjee A E, Gathiram V, Jackson T F H G, Khan B F Y 1985 A comparative trial of metronidazole against tinidazole in the treatment of amoebic liver abscess. South African Medical Journal 68: 923–924
25. Swarz H 1977 International experience with a new single 2.0 g dose of tinidazole ('Fasigyn'). Current Medical Research and Opinion 2: 149–150
26. Giercksky C-E, Fuglesang J, Christiansen E, Johnson J A, Bergan T 1980 Short term chemotherapeutic prophylaxis in gastrointestinal operations. Surgery, Gynecology and Obstetrics 151: 349–352
27. Viitanen J, Tunturi T, Auvinen O, Pessi T 1984 Tinidazole prophylaxis in appendicectomies. A controlled study of single dose versus three day therapy. Scandinavian Journal of Gastroenterology 19: 111–115
28. Hunt P S, Francis P K, Peck G, Farrell K, Sali A 1979 Tinidazole in the prevention of wound infection after elective colorectal surgery. Medical Journal of Australia 1: 107–109
29. Giercksky K-E, Danielson S, Garberg O et al 1982 A single dose tinidazole and doxycycline prophylaxis in elective surgery of the colon and rectum. Annals of Surgery 195: 227–231
30. Ofstad E, Braband G, Helsinger N et al 1980. Tinidazole and doxycycline as antimicrobials in elective colorectal surgery: a randomised, multicentre trial. Scandinavian Journal of Gastroenterology 15 (suppl 59): 29–35
31. Applebaum P C, Moodley J, Chatterton S A, Cowden D B, Africa C W 1980 Tinidazole in the prophylaxis and treatment of anaerobic infection. Chemotherapy 26: 145–151
32. Karhunen M, Koskela O, Hannelin M 1980 Single dose tinidazole in prophylaxis of infection following hysterectomy. British Journal of Obstetrics and Gynaecology 87: 70–72
33. Karhunen M, Koskela O, Hällström K 1981 Single dose tinidazole in prophylaxis of infections following vaginal surgery. Journal of Antimicrobial Chemotherapy 8: 283–290
34. Karhunen M, Koskela O, Teisala K, Suikarri A -M, Mattila J 1985 Prophylaxis and treatment of anearobic infections following Caesarian section with tinidazole. Chemotherapy 31: 228–236
35. Piot P, Van Dyck E, Godts P, Vander Leyden J 1983 A placebo controlled, double blind comparison of tinidazole and triple sulphonamide cream for the treatment of non-specific vaginitis. American Journal of Obstetrics and Gynecology 147: 85–89
36. Morgan I 1978 Metronidazole treatment in pregnancy. Internation Journal of Gynaecology and Obstetrics 15: 501–502
37. McEwen J 1983 Hypersensitivity reactions to tinidazole. Medical Journal of Australia 1: 498–499
38. Bergan T, Potland M H 1984 In vitro interactions between metroniadazole or tinidazole and ampicillin, doxycyline and co-trimoxazole. Scandinavian Journal of Gastroenterology 19: (suppl 91): 95–101
39. Goodwin C S, Blake P, Blincow E 1986 The minimum inhibitory and bacteriocidal concentrations of antibiotics and anti-ulcer agents against Campylobacter pyloridis. Journal of Antimicrobial Chemotherapy 17: 309–314
40. Marshal B J, Goodwin C S, Warren J R et al 1988 Prospective double-blind trial of duodenal ulcer relapse after eradication of Campylobacter pylori. Lancet 2: 1437–1442
41. Oderda G, Vaira D, Holton J, Ainley C, Altare F, Ansaldi N 1989 Amoxycillin plus tinidazole for Campylobacter pylori gastritis in children: assessment by serum IgG antibody, pepsinogen 1, and gastrin levels. Lancet 1: 690–692

Tobramycin

Tobramycin is a bactericidal aminoglycoside antibiotic for parenteral administration. It was originally isolated from the fermentation broth of an actinomycete, *Streptomyces tenebrarius*. When grown in the proper fermentation medium, *S. tenebrarius* produces nebramycin, a complex of basic water-soluble factors that belong to the structurally related group of antibiotics called 'aminoglycosides'. Factor 6 of the nebramycin complex — tobramycin — demonstrated the highest specific activity and the widest antimicrobial spectrum and hence was chosen to be evaluated in the area of human chemotherapy. It is indicated for the treatment of serious bacterial infections caused by susceptible strains of microorganisms. Tobramycin is similar to most of the other aminoglycoside antibiotics in regard to physiologic distribution, pharmacologic properties and spectrum of activity, but it is more active in vitro against *Pseudomonas aeruginosa*, and, in comparison with gentamicin, is less likely to cause renal adverse reactions.

Chemistry

Tobramycin (nebramycin factor 6, Nebecin (e) (sulphate), Gernebcin (sulphate), Tobralex, Tobrex)
$C_{18}H_{37}N_5O_9$
6-O-(3-Amino-3-deoxy-α-D-glucopyranosyl)-2-deoxy-4-O-(2,6-diamino-2,3,6-trideoxy-α-D-ribo-hexopyranosyl)-D-streptamine

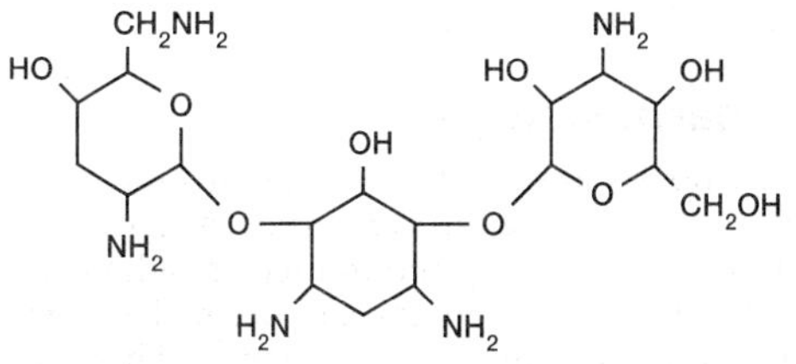

Molecular weight	467.5
pKa	6.7, 8.3, 9.9
Solubility	
in alcohol	1 in 2000
in water	1 in 1.5
Octanol/water partition coefficient	low

The British approved name is tobramycin sulphate. It is a white to off-white hygroscopic powder which is prepared to a pH of 5.5 to 6. It is highly soluble in water but only slightly soluble in alcohol and practically insoluble in organic solvents such as ethyl acetate and chloroform. A solution in water is dextrorotatory. Tobramycin is compatible with most intravenous fluids currently used throughout the world, but is not compatible with heparin solutions and can interact chemically with β-lactam compounds depending on the concentration and pH of both tobramycin and the β-lactam compound. There are no combination products in which tobramycin is a component.

Pharmacology

Tobramycin is active against a wide range of bacilli. The mode of action of tobramycin is almost certain to be the same as its more extensively investigated predecessor aminoglycosides which are first actively transported across the bacterial cell membrane by an oxygen-dependent system. Factors determining the rate of intracellular accumulation include the concentration of divalent cations (Mg^{2+}

Tobramycin

T

and Ca^{2+}), environmental pH and oxygen tension. Aminoglycosides are inactive under anaerobic conditions.

Aminoglycosides such as tobramycin bind irreversibly to the 30S subunit of the bacterial ribosome, blocking protein synthesis by inhibiting the movement of peptidyl-tRNA associated with translocation as well as increasing the frequency of misreading of the genetic code due to incorrect codon–anticodon interaction. The effect is bactericidal.

Toxicology

Toxicological and pharmacological studies in animals indicate that the effects produced by different aminoglycosides are similar in kind but that they differ in degree. The results of such studies are affected by the species of animal selected for study, the dose administered and the methodology. Hence, data from such studies may not always be directly applicable to clinical situations in man.

In comparative toxicology studies in animals, tobramycin demonstrated a subtle but consistent advantage over gentamicin.[1] The ototoxicity of tobramycin in experimental animals has been defined by several workers[2] and in all these studies, tobramycin was found to be less ototoxic than gentamicin. In rats, rabbits and dogs, the nephrotoxicity of tobramycin has been demonstrated but shown to be less than that of gentamicin.[3] However, the mechanism of renal damage appears to be the same as for other aminoglycosides. To evaluate the neuromuscular blocking activity of tobramycin, gentamicin and neomycin, the decrease in soleus twitch force following intravenous administration was determined in cats. Tobramycin had minimum depressant effects at 40 $mg.kg^{-1}$ and maximum effects at 60–100 $mg.kg^{-1}$. Comparable maximum effects were observed with 50 $mg.kg^{-1}$ of gentamicin and with 30 $mg.kg^{-1}$ of neomycin.

In teratogenicity tests a 25–100 $mg.kg^{-1}$ daily dose of tobramycin given to mice during organogenesis produced no embryocidal or teratogenic effects.[1] Tobramycin can cause ototoxicity in both pregnant animals and their offspring. The nature of these effects may very with the stage of pregnancy and in guinea pigs ototoxicity in the offspring was only observed if the agent was given in the terminal four weeks of gestation.[4] No mutagenicity or carcinogenicity tests have been carried out on the agent.

Clinical pharmacology

Tobramycin is poorly absorbed from the gastrointestinal tract, and is usually administered by the intravenous or intramuscular route. It is rapidly absorbed following intramuscular administration. Peak serum concentrations of tobramycin occur between 30 and 90 minutes after intramuscular administration.[5,6] Therapeutic levels are generally considered to range from 4 to 6 $mg.l^{-1}$. When tobramycin is administered by intravenous infusion over a one-hour period, the serum concentrations are similar to those obtained by intramuscular administration.

Tobramycin dosage needs to be reduced in patients with impaired renal function. In such patients a loading dose of 1 $mg.kg^{-1}$ is usually given and subsequent dosing can either be with reduced doses every 8 hours or normal doses given at prolonged intervals. The plasma concentrations of tobramycin should be monitored. Tobramycin, when given intravenously is best given by bolus dosing in 50 ml of intravenous fluid over 20 minutes rather than by continuous intravenous infusion. The largest dose of tobramycin known to have been used is 12 $mg.kg^{-1}$ daily.

Most aerobic and facultative Gram-negative bacilli are inhibited by 3–6 $mg.l^{-1}$ of tobramycin. Some strains of *Serratia*, *Providencia*, *Pseudomonas aeruginosa* and *Acinetobacter* are less sensitive but tobramycin is more active than gentamicin against *Pseudomonas aeruginosa*. Among Gram-positive bacteria, streptococci and *Listeria monocytogenes* are usually resistant and staphylococci, although sensitive in vitro, tend to be clinically resistant either because aminoglycosides do not enter macrophages or because of the development of resistant small-colony variants during therapy. Tobramycin is also active in vitro against diphtheroids, gonococci, meningococci, *Haemophilus* species, *Mycoplasma* and *Legionella pneumophila* although the clinical significance of these findings remains to be determined. Tobramycin has little useful activity against *Mycobacterium tuberculosis*, unlike most other aminoglycosides. Tobramycin has no activity against anaerobes.

Resistance to aminoglycosides is the consequence of bacterial inactivating enzymes, cell wall impermeability or changes in the 30S ribosomal proteins. Epidemic resistance amongst the Enterobacteriaceae results from plasmid-determined inactivating enzymes which acetylate, adenylate or phosphorylate the aminoglycoside substrate.

Variable degrees of antibacterial synergy can be demonstrated in vitro when aminoglycosides are combined with either β-lactam antibiotics (penicillins and cephalosporins) or vancomycin. Tobramycin acts synergistically with cephalosporins or semisynthetic penicillins against Enterobacteriaceae and *Pseudomonas aeruginosa*. However, unlike gentamicin, little useful synergy is seen between tobramycin and penicillin against *Streptococcus faecalis*.

Pharmacokinetics

As for gentamicin, a variety of techniques are available for the assay of tobramycin. The bioassay technique is still most widely used since it requires little technical expertise and is available in the laboratories of most hospitals.[7] Other assay methods available include EMIT assays, radioimmunoassays, fluorescent immunoassays and HPLC with fluorescence detection. These methods are highly sensitive and specific. The HPLC method has a limit of sensitivity of 200 $\mu g.l^{-1}$.[8] Tobramycin, like other aminoglycosides, is not absorbed from the gastrointestinal tract following oral administration and undergoes no presystemic metabolism. The plasma half life of a parenteral dose is 2–3 hours in adults with normal renal function.

Tobramycin is distributed in the extracellular fluids, and the apparent volumes of distribution of tobramycin and gentamicin are identical.[9] The apparent volume of distribution of tobramycin is approximately 30% of body weight in patients with normal renal function but decreases markedly to 12.4% in the anuric patient. Fewer studies of the levels of tobramycin in body fluids have been done than with kanamycin and gentamicin. However, on the basis of studies with these compounds, it can be surmised that the concentrations of tobramycin in bile are low, as they are in prostatic fluid. In contrast to this, adequate levels can be detected in the peritoneal, pleural and synovial fluids (in the presence of inflammation), and in interstitial fluid, renal lymph, bronchial secretions and peritoneal fluid.[10–13] Tobramycin diffuses poorly across the blood–brain barrier, and intrathecal instillation is probably necessary to achieve adequate levels. There is some evidence for tissue accumulation, and drug has been detected in serum and urine for several days after treatment was stopped. This has led to reports of a long terminal elimination phase of about 6 days. Tobramycin is excreted in breast milk in very low concentrations; a level of 0.6 $mg.l^{-1}$ was recorded in one patient one hour after an intramuscular injection of 80 mg. The drug can cross the placenta and accumulate in the fetal kidney.

The pharmacokinetics of tobramycin in newborns are similar to those of gentamicin. The half life of tobramycin is $>$8 h in infants weighing $<$1500 g, 6–8 h in infants weighing 1500–2500 g and 4 h in those weighing $>$2500 g. At a dose of 2 $mg.kg^{-1}$, peak serum levels of 4–6 $mg.l^{-1}$ are achieved and the drug can be given without accumulation every 12 h to infants weighing $<$2500 g and every 8 h to those weighing $>$2500 g.[14,15]

Binding of tobramycin to serum proteins is low and has been estimated to vary from 0 to 30%.[16]

Tobramycin is excreted unchanged in the urine, with up to 90% of the dose recovered in 24 h, most of this being excreted in the first 6 h. The elimination of the drug is reduced in renal failure and with deteriorating renal function with age.

Oral absorption	very poor
Presystemic metabolism	nil
Plasma half life	
range	2–3 h
Volume of distribution	0.3 $l.kg^{-1}$
Plasma protein binding	~10%

Concentration–effect relationship

In life-threatening infections, peak serum levels of at least 4–5 $mg.l^{-1}$ should be achieved. Some investigations suggest 8 $mg.l^{-1}$. It would seem that, as the use of serum levels becomes more widespread, predose (trough) levels should be obtained to avoid toxic reactions. These levels should not be above $2\,mg.l^{-1}$. Peak concentrations should be measured 30 minutes after intramuscular injection or after the completion of the intravenous dosing.

Metabolism

Following parenteral administration, little, if any, metabolic transformation occurs and tobramycin is eliminated almost exclusively by glomerular filtration. Renal clearance is similar to that of endogenous creatinine. In patients with normal renal function, up to 84% of the dose is recoverable from the urine in 8 hours and up to 93% in 24 hours. When renal function is impaired, excretion of tobramycin is slowed and accumulation of the drug may cause toxic blood levels. In patients undergoing dialysis, 25–75% of the administered dose may be removed, depending on the duration and type of dialysis. There is no evidence of enterohepatic circulation of the drug and the drug does not undergo any important metabolic reactions in man. No pharmacologically active metabolites are formed.

Pharmaceutics

No oral form of tobramycin is available. For intramuscular or intravenous administrations, the following preparations are available as Nebcin (Lilly, UK/US):

a) 1 ml glass vials containing $40\,mg.ml^{-1}$ of tobramycin sulphate (UK)
b) 2 ml glass vials containing 80 mg of tobramycin sulphate
c) Paediatric ampoules containing 20 mg in 2 ml of tobramycin sulphate
d) 60 mg in 1.5 ml or 80 mg in 2 ml pre-filled syringes (US)
e) 1.2 g in 40 ml multidose vial for hospital pharmacy admixture (US)

No slow-release form is available. All preparations can be stored at room temperature and the maximum shelf-life of the preparations is two years. Vials are not suitable for intrathecal use since they contain 0.5% w/v phenol as a preservative which is toxic to the central nervous system.

Therapeutic use

Indications

1. Septicaemia due to Gram-negative organisms
2. Paediatric sepsis
3. Respiratory infections
4. Urinary tract infections
5. Trauma and wound infections
6. CNS infections
7. *Pseudomonas* endocarditis
8. *Pseudomonas* eye infections.

Contraindications

Contraindications to the use of tobramycin include:

1. Hypersensitivity reactions to the agent, which are rare. Cross-hypersensitivity with other aminoglycoside exists.
2. A relative contraindication to its use is the presence of impaired renal function unless the dosage can be adjusted and regular blood level monitoring performed as described earlier.

Mode of use

The dose of tobramycin is calculated on the patient's body weight with appropriate adjustments for factors such as the severity of infection, the age of the patient and the patient's renal function.

In patients with normal renal function, except neonates, tobramycin administered every 8 hours does not accumulate in the serum. However, in those with reduced renal function and in neonates, the serum concentration of the antibiotic is usually higher and can be measured for longer periods of time than in normal adults. Dosage for such patients must, therefore, be adjusted accordingly.

When similar doses of gentamicin and tobramycin were given rapidly by bolus injection, they peaked at markedly higher concentrations in serum than did the same doses infused over a 30 minute to 2 hour period. Moreover, disappearance from the serum was faster than that reported for longer infusions.[17] These data suggest that when tobramycin (or gentamicin) is administered intravenously, consideration should be given both to the dose and the duration of infusion.

The recommended adult dosage of tobramycin for patients with serious infections is $3\,mg.kg^{-1}$ daily in three equal doses every 8 hours. In those with life-threatening infections, up to $5\,mg.kg^{-1}$ daily may be administered in three or four equal doses. The dosage should be reduced to $3\,mg.kg^{-1}$ daily as soon as clinically indicated. In such patients, serum levels must be monitored.

The dosage for children is $6–7.5\,mg.kg^{-1}$ daily in three or four equally divided doses and for neonates up to $4\,mg.kg^{-1}$ daily in two equal doses every 12 hours.

It is desirable to limit treatment to a short term. The usual duration of treatment is 7–10 days. A longer course of therapy may be necessary in difficult and complicated infections. In such cases, monitoring of renal, auditory and vestibular functions is advised, because toxicity is more likely to occur when treatment is extended longer than 10 days.

As for gentamicin, the maintenance dose varies considerably in different patients. Of particular importance are patients with impaired renal function. In such patients, following a loading dose of $1\,mg.kg^{-1}$ subsequent dosage must be adjusted either with reduced doses administered at 8-hour intervals or with normal doses given at prolonged intervals (as for gentamicin). Serum tobramycin concentrations should be monitored during therapy.

The highest dose of tobramycin known to have been used is $12\,mg.kg^{-1}$ daily.

Indications

1. Septicaemia and other severe infections due to aerobic Gram-negative bacilli

The experience published so far demonstrates that tobramycin is effective in treatment of such septicaemias due to sensitive organisms.[18–20] The organisms that have been treated are *E. coli*, *Klebsiella pneumoniae*, *Enterobacter*, *Pseudomonas aeruginosa* and *Acinetobacter*. However, most clinicians opt to use the more familiar gentamicin rather than tobramycin for the treatment of infections caused by the Enterobacteriaceae. Nevertheless, many patients treated with tobramycin have shown a satisfactory response.

2. Sepsis in paediatric patients

Tobramycin has been used to treat paediatric sepsis.[21,22] Many of these patients who failed to respond to tobramycin also failed to respond to other agents and most had severe underlying disease such as leukaemia and other malignancies or over 60% burns.[23]

3. Respiratory infections

Bendush and Weber[24] have noted an 80% satisfactory response rate among 156 patients treated for respiratory infections. Combination therapy of respiratory infections with tobramycin plus another agent has been studied in patients with cancer. Klastersky et al.[25] compared the efficacy of tobramycin–cephalothin, tobramycin–ticarcillin and ticarcillin–cephalothin. The highest rate of clinical success in treatment of pulmonary infections in these patients was with tobramycin–ticarcillin. The results of treatment of *Pseudomonas* pulmonary infections in patients with cystic fibrosis have been studied by a number of groups,[26–28] and the effects are encouraging.

4. Urinary tract infections

These have been successfully treated with tobramycin.[29–32] Different dosage programmes have been used by various authors and most studies comparing tobramycin and gentamicin have shown that the two agents are equally efficacious. Combined therapy of urinary tract infections with tobramycin and carbenicillin, or tobramycin and a cephalosporin has been used, but the results are not more favourable than those with tobramycin alone. Thus, tobramycin has been shown to be very effective in the treatment of urinary tract infections produced by susceptible Enterobacteriaceae or *Pseudomonas*. However, in the presence of significant structural abnormalities, or if an indwelling urethral catheter is present, the relapse rate is similar to that seen with other antibiotics.

5. Trauma and wound infections

Subcutaneous, postoperative and traumatic wound infections produced by tobramycin-susceptible *Pseudomonas*, *E. coli*, *Proteus* and *Klebsiella* have been successfully treated with tobramycin. Experience

Tobramycin

in infections of skin and soft tissue[24] reveals that infections due to *Pseudomonas* responded as well as infections produced by the Enterobacteriaceae and *Staphylococcus aureus*. Bone infections due to *Pseudomonas* have been successfully managed with tobramycin by several groups as have intra-abdominal infections.[33–35]

6. CNS infections
Paediatric and postoperative infections of the central nervous system have been successfully treated with systemic or intrathecal tobramycin in combination with other antibiotics such as carbenicillin or ampicillin.[15,23,36]

7. *Pseudomonas* endocarditis
Burch et al.[37] reported treatment of several patients with endocarditis due to *Pseudomonas*. One patient received tobramycin alone and was cured. Two other patients required surgery to effect a cure and this remains an important adjunct to therapy. However, the greater activity of tobramycin against *Pseudomonas* suggest that it is the antibiotic of choice. At the present time, only combined therapy with tobramycin and a β-lactam antibiotic with antipseudomonal activity can be advised for the treatment of *Pseudomonas* endocarditis.

8. Eye infections with *pseudomonas*
Experimental studies of tobramycin in corneal ulcers or *Pseudomonas* keratitis in animals have been performed[38,39] and it has been shown to be more effective than gentamicin in animal models. However, further studies are needed to clarify the role of tobramycin in human eye infections.

Adverse reactions

Potentially life-threatening effects
Tobramycin is selectively concentrated in renal cortical cells and it produces changes in the proximal tububles resembling those of gentamicin. The drug has the potential to cause renal impairment characterized by the excretion of casts, oliguria, proteinuria and a progressive rise in blood urea and serum creatinine levels. Retrospective surveys have indicated that nephrotoxicity is an infrequent side effect occurring in less than 4% of patients.

Nephrotoxicity has primarily occurred in patients receiving high doses for prolonged periods. Other predisposing factors include dehydration and endotoxaemia, and the concomitant use of other nephrotoxic agents. As with gentamicin, peak levels above 12 $\mu g.ml^{-1}$ and trough levels greater than 2 $\mu g.ml^{-1}$ may be associated with a higher incidence of toxicity but in animal studies tobramycin has demonstrated a lower level of nephrotoxicity.[40,41]

Acute overdosage
In the event of overdosage or toxic reactions with tobramycin, haemodialysis or peritoneal dialysis will reduce serum levels. Haemodialysis is preferable because it is more efficient.

Severe or irreversible adverse effects

Ototoxicity
Ototoxicity, manifested as either auditory or vestibular toxicity can occur with the use of tobramycin. The auditory changes are irreversible, usually bilateral and may be partial or total. Tobramycin-induced ototoxicity occurs in less than 2% of patients receiving the agent.[42] Eighth-nerve impairment may develop in patients with pre-existing renal damage and in those with normal renal function to whom aminoglycosides are administered for longer periods or in higher doses than those recommended. The risk of aminoglycoside-induced hearing loss increases with the degree of exposure to either high peak or high trough concentrations. Both eighth-nerve and renal function should be monitored during therapy and evidence of impairment in vestibular or auditory function requires discontinuation of the drug or dosage adjustment. Some data suggest that tobramycin may be less ototoxic than gentamicin.[42]

Neuromuscular blockade
As with other aminoglycosides, the possibility that prolonged or secondary apnoea may occur should be considered if tobramycin is administered to anaesthetized patients who are also receiving neuromuscular blocking agents. This effect may be reversed by the administration of calcium salts. Tobramycin should be administered with caution in patients with myasthenia gravis or parkinsonism because of its potential curare-like effect on neuromuscular function.

Symptomatic adverse effects
Local reactions such as pain at the site of injection, phlebitis and skin reactions may occur with parenteral tobramycin. Nausea and vomiting may also occur. Urticaria and maculopapular rashes have been reported in association with the use of tobramycin.

Other effects
Other drug-related reactions which have occurred with the use of tobramycin include changes in liver enzymes and changes in the haematocrit and haemoglobin values. These effects are uncommon.

Interference with clinical pathology tests
No technical interferences of this kind appear to have been reported.

High risk patient groups

Neonates
Dosage is required up to 4 $mg.kg^{-1}$ daily in two equal doses every 12 h. Tobramycin must be administered with caution in neonates due to their renal immaturity. It is desirable to limit treatment to short courses, the usual duration being 7–10 days.

Breast milk. Tobramycin is secreted in breast milk in very low concentrations, and as it is not absorbed in significant amounts it is unlikely to harm the infant, though the possibility of alteration in gut flora should be borne in mind.

Children
Children require higher doses than adults of 6–7.5 $mg.kg^{-1}$ daily in three or four equally divided doses.

Pregnant women
Tobramycin crosses the placenta and can accumulate in the fetal kidney. It is, therefore, not recommended unless the patient's condition justifies the risk.

The elderly
The dose should be reduced if renal function is impaired.

Concurrent disease
The most important systemic disease requiring dose modification with the use of tobramycin is renal failure. As for gentamicin, either reduced doses administered at 8-hour intervals or normal doses given at prolonged intervals may be administered. Nomograms are available to calculate the reduced dosage if 8-hour intervals are maintained. In either case, monitoring of serum levels is essential to maintain a safe, yet therapeutic serum level.

Drug interactions

Potentially hazardous interactions
Aminoglycosides should not be given concurrently with potent diuretics such as ethacrynic acid and frusemide since these enhance its nephrotoxicity. Concurrent or sequential use of other neurotoxic or nephrotoxic antibiotics such as other aminoglycosides, cephaloro-dine, polymyxin B, cisplatinin and vancomycin should be avoided where possible. The aminglycoside may potentiate the effect of neuromuscular blocking agents.

Other significant interactions
Tobramycin is physically incompatible with carbenicillin when the two are mixed together.

Potentially useful interactions
Tobramycin, as other aminoglycosides, may demonstrate synergy with various β-lactam antibiotics. This synergism can often be demonstrated in vitro and patients treated with such synergistic associations often exhibit a high bactericidal activity in their serum and respond more favourably to therapy.

Major outcome trials

Tobramycin has been extensively studied throughout the world and reports have appeared in the literature citing its efficacy and safety in a broad range of infections. Various published studies include reports of its use in paediatric patients, surgical patients, patients with urinary tract infections, lower respiratory tract infections, osteomyelitis, skin and soft tissue infections, and patients with septicaemia and endocarditis. Many of these studies have been referred to in the section under therapeutic indications.

Tobramycin

1. Bendush C L, Weber R 1976 Tobramycin sulphate: a summary of worldwide experience from clinical trials. Journal of Infectious Diseases 134 (suppl): 5219–5234

In this worldwide study of 3506 patients, the therapeutic effectiveness of tobramycin was evaluated by 156 investigators. Clinical safety was also assessed in this study.

Data from 746 patients demonstrated the effectiveness of tobramycin in treating pyelonephritis, cystitis and unspecified urinary tract infections. In 84% of these patients, the pathogen was eliminated without recurrence. It was also effective in the treatment of asymptomatic bacteriuria.

Of the 24 patients with genital infections, 21 responded satisfactorily to tobramycin. All three patients who did not respond adequately had complicating factors.

Of 214 patients with respiratory tract infections 78% showed an adequate response.

Of 134 cases with infections of the skin, soft tissue and bone, 79% showed a good response.

Of the 144 patients treated for proved or suspected septicaemia, 84% responded satisfactorily. 122 of the septicaemia patients received concomitant therapy with a second and sometimes a third antibiotic. Serious underlying disorders were present in almost all of the 41 patients treated for central nervous infection and 24 of them received additional therapy with another antibiotic. Of the 41 patients, 18 were considered to have demonstrated a satisfactory response.

Out of 39 patients with peritonitis, 29 responded satisfactorily, but in many cases operative intervention was also required.

In this study, the safety of tobramycin was also evaluated and a low rate of adverse reactions were found namely: kidney 1.5%, nervous system 0.6%, local reactions at the infection site 0.9%, and hypersensitivity and skin reactions 0.5%. Reactions were usually mild and reversible. No deaths or cases of acute renal failure were reported.

Other trials

Various studies have been undertaken to compare the incidence of nephrotoxicity and ototoxicity in similar groups of patients receiving gentamicin or tobramycin.[43–45] In general, they seem to support previously published clinical pharmacology studies which indicated that, on the basis of its pharmacokinetics, gentamicin may be more nephrotoxic and ototoxic than tobramycin.[1]

References

1. Welles J S, Emmerson J L, Gibson W R et al 1973 Preclinical toxicology studies with tobramycin. Toxicology and Applied Pharmacology 25: 398–409
2. Brummett R F, Himes D, Saine B 1972 A comparative study of the ototoxicity of tobramycin and gentamicin. Archives of Otolaryngology 96: 505–512
3. Luft F C, Kleit S A 1974 Renal parenchymal accumulation of aminoglycoside antibiotics in rats. Journal of Infectious Diseases 130: 656–659
4. Akiyoshi M 1978 Evaluation of ototoxicity and safety of tobramycin in guinea pigs. In: Current Chemotherapy, Proceedings of the 10th International Congress of Chemotherapy, Zurich September 18–23. American Society of Microbiology, Washington DC, p 911
5. Simon V K, Mosinger E U, Malerczy V 1973 Pharmacokinetic studies of tobramycin and gentamicin. Antimicrobial Agents and Chemotherapy 3: 445–450
6. Horikoshi N, Valdivieso M, Bodey G P 1974 Clinical pharmacology of tobramycin. American Journal of Medical Science 266: 453–458
7. Neu H C 1976 Tobramycin: An overview. The Journal of Infectious Diseases 134 (suppl): S3–S19
8. Haughey D B, Janicke D M, Adelman M, Schentag J J et al 1980 High-pressure liquid chromatography analysis and single-dose disposition of tobramycin in human volunteers. Antimicrobial Agents and Chemotherapy 17: 649–653
9. Regamey C, Gordon R C, Kirby W M M 1973 Comparative pharmacokinetics of tobramycin and gentamicin. Clinical Pharmacology and Therapeutics 14: 396–403
10. Chisholm G D, Waterworth P M, Calnan J S et al 1973 Concentrations of antibacterial agents in intestinal tissue fluid. British Medical Journal 1: 569–573
11. Szwed J J, Luft F CC, Black H R et al 1974 Comparison of the distribution of tobramycin and gentamicin in body fluids of dogs. Antimicrobial Agents and Chemotherapy 5: 444–446
12. Pennington J E, Reynolds H Y 1973 Tobramycin in bronchial secretions. Antimicrobial Agents and Chemotherapy 4: 299–301
13. Weinstein A J, Karchmer A W, Moellering R C Jr 1973 Tobramycin concentrations during peritoneal dialysis. Antimicrobial Agents and Chemotherapy 4: 432–434
14. Kaplan J M, McCracken G H, Thomas M L et al 1973 Clinical pharmacology of tobramycin in newborns. American Journal of Diseases of Children 125: 656–660
15. Kannan M N, Dalton H P, Escobar M R 1973 Tobramycin in the neonatal period. Virginia Medical Monthly 100: 1030–1034
16. Gordon R C, Regamey C, Kirby W M M 1972 Serum protein binding of the aminoglycoside antibiotics. Antimicrobial Agents and Chemotherapy 2: 214–216
17. Stratford B C, Dixson S 1974 Serum levels of gentamicin and tobramycin after slow intravenous bolus injection. Lancet 1: 378–379
18. Blair D C, Fekety F R Jr, Bruce B et al 1975 Therapy of *Pseudomonas aeruginosa* infections with tobramycin. Antimicrobial Agents and Chemotherapy 8: 22–29
19. Jaffe G, Ravreby W, Meyers B R et al 1974 Clinical study of the use of the new aminoglycoside tobramycin for therapy of infections due to Gram-negative bacteria. Antimicrobial Agents and Chemotherapy 5: 75–81
20. Helm E, Shah P M, Stille W 1974 Clinical experience with tobramycin. In: Tobramycin: selected proceedings from the Eighth International Congress of Chemotherapy, Athens 1973. Excerpta Medica, Amsterdam, pp 55–58
21. Rosaschino F 1974 First results on the employment of tobramycin in paediatrics. In: Tobramycin: selected proceedings from the Eighth International Congress of Chemotherapy, Athens 1973. Excerpta Medical, Amsterdam, pp 83–86
22. Cohen J D, Miale T D 1976 Tobramycin and cephalothin for treatment of suspected sepsis in neutropenic children with cancer. Journal of Infectious Diseases 134 (suppl): S175–S177
23. Raine P A M, Young D G, McAllister T A et al 1976 Tobramycin in paediatric use. Journal of Infectious Diseases 134 (suppl): S165–S169
24. Bendush C L, Weber R 1976 Tobramycin sulphate: a summary of worldwide experience from clinical trials. Journal of Infectious Diseases 134 (suppl): S219–S234
25. Klastersky J, Hensgens C, Debusscher L 1975 Empiric therapy for cancer patients: comparative study of ticarcillin–tobramycin, ticarcillin–cephalothin and cephalothin–tobramycin. Antimicrobial Agents and Chemotherapy 7: 640–645
26. McCrae W M, Raeburn J A, Hanson E J 1976 Tobramycin therapy of infections due to *Pseudomonas aeruginosa* in patients with cystic fibrosis: Effect of dosage and concentration of antibiotic in sputum. Journal of Infectious Diseases 134 (suppl): S191–S193
27. Crozier D N, Khan S R 1976 Tobramycin in treatment of infections due to *Pseudomonas aeruginosa* in patient with fibrosis. Journal of Infectious Diseases 134 (suppl): S187–S190
28. Parry M F, Neu H C 1976 Tobramycin and ticarcillin therapy for exacerbations of pulmonary disease in patients with cystic fibrosis. Journal of Infectious Diseases 134 (suppl): S194–S197
29. Altucci P, Abbate G F, Gattoni A et al 1976 Clinical evaluation of tobramycin in urinary tract infections. Journal of Infectious Diseases 134 (suppl): S139–S141
30. Walker B D, Gentry L O 1976 A randomized, comparative study of tobramycin and gentamicin in treatment of acute urinary tract infections. Journal of Infectious Diseases 134 (suppl): S146–S149
31. Ivan E, Nagy A E, Csatary K N 1976 Bacteriological, clinical and pharmacological investigations with tobramycin in patients with serious urinary tract infection. Journal of Infectious Diseases 134 (suppl): S153–S155
32. Bennett A H 1976 Evaluation of tobramycin in severe urinary tract infection. Journal of Infectious Diseases 134 (suppl): S156–S157
33. Helm E, Shah Pm, Stille W 1974 Clinical experience with tobramycin. In: Tobramycin: selected proceedings from the Eighth International Congress of Chemotherapy, Athens 1973. Excerpta Medica, Amsterdam, pp 55–58
34. Geddes A M, Goodall J A D, Spiers C F et al 1974 Clinical and pharmacological studies with tobramycin. In: Tobramycin: selected proceedings from the Eighth International Congress of Chemotherapy, Athens, 1973. Excerpta Medica, Amsterdam, pp 51–54
35. Ishiyama S, Nakayama I, Iwamoto H et al 1976 Clinical use of tobramycin in patients with surgical infections due to Gram-negative bacilli. Journal of Infectious Diseases 134 (suppl): S178–S181
36. Kaiser A B, McGee Z A 1975 Aminoglycoside therapy of Gram-negative bacillary meningitis. New England Journal of Medicine 293: 1215–1220
37. Burch K. Nichols R D, Quinn E L et al 1973 A clinical trial of tobramycin with pharmacological and microbiological studies. Henry Ford Hospital Medical Journal 21: 135–142
38. Sonolin G, Okumoto H, Wilson F M 1973 The effect of tobramycin on *Pseudomonas* keratitis. The American Journal of Cepthalmology 76: 555–560
39. Purnell W D, McPherson S D Jr 1974 An evaluation of tobramycin in experimental corneal ulcers. The American Journal of Cepthalmology 78: 318–320
40. Meyers B R, Hirschman S Z 1972 Pharmacologic studies on tobramycin and comparison with gentamicin. Journal of Clinical Pharmacology 12: 321–324
41. Smith C R, Lipsky J J, Laskin O L et al 1980 Double-blind comparison of the nephrotoxicity and auditory toxicity of gentamicin and tobramycin. New England Journal of Medicine 302: 1106–1109
42. Neu H C, Bendush C I 1976 Ototoxicity of tobramycin: a clinical overview. Journal of Infectious Diseases 134 (suppl): S206–S218
43. Kahlmeter G, Hallberg T, Kamme C 1978 Gentamicin and tobramycin in patients with various infections — nephrotoxicity. Journal of Antimicrobial Chemotherapy (suppl A) 4: 47–52
44. Schentag J J, Lsezkay G, Plaut M E et al 1978 Comparative tissue accumulation of gentamicin and tobramycin in patients. Journal of Antimicrobial Chemotherapy (suppl A) 4: 23–30
45. Fee W E Jr, Vierra V, Lathrop G R 1978 Clinical evaluation of aminoglycoside toxicity: tobramycin versus gentamicin, a preliminary report. Journal of Antimicrobial Chemotherapy (suppl A) 4: 31–36

T

Tocainide (hydrochloride)

Tocainide is an antiarrhythmic drug which is a primary amine analogue of lignocaine with similar electrophysiological, haemodynamic and antiarrhythmic effects.

Chemistry

Tocainide hydrochloride (Tonocard, Xylotocan)
$C_{11}H_{16}N_2O.HCl$
RS-N-(2,6-Dimethylphenyl)alaninamide hydrochloride
2-Amino-N-(2,6-dimethylphenyl) propanamide

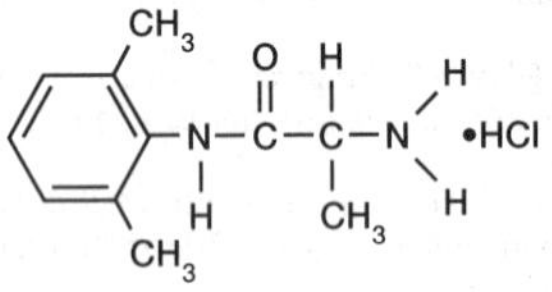

Molecular weight	228.7
pKa	7.7
Solubility	
in alcohol	freely soluble
in water	freely soluble
Octanol/water partition coefficient	2.5

A white odourless crystalline powder with a bitter taste. It is prepared by chemical synthesis and the racemate is used clinically. It is freely soluble in water.

Pharmacology

Tocainide produces dose-dependent decreases in sodium and potassium conductance thereby reducing the rate of rise of phase O of the action potential (membrane responsiveness). It is thus a Class I antiarrhythmic agent according to the classification of Vaughan Williams. It shortens the effective refractory period and action potential duration and increases the ratio of effective refractory period/action potential duration at 50% repolarization.[1] Tocainide also enhances the electrical stability of the ventricle by elevating the ventricular fibrillation threshold.[2]

Toxicology

Tocainide does not have mutagenic potential, and two-year carcinogenicity studies in rats and 18-month studies in mice showed no carcinogenic potential. There is no evidence of impaired fertility or teratogenicity in rats and rabbits. Maternal and fetal toxicity was observed at very high dose levels and fetal toxicity was considered to be secondary to maternal toxicity. Toxicity studies in monkeys have shown a deleterious effect on the central nervous system in oral daily doses of 100 $mg.kg^{-1}$ and greater.

Clinical pharmacology

Tocainide has similar electrophysiological properties in man to those of lignocaine.[3,4] The drug has no effects on sinus cycle length or tests of sinus node function. Cardiac conduction intervals are unchanged by tocainide although clinically insignificant increases in atrioventricular nodal conduction have been reported in man[3] and in animals.[1] The QT interval, as a measure of ventricular repolarization, tends to shorten. Although Anderson et al[3] reported significant decreases in the effective refractory periods of all components of the cardiac conduction system, other studies[4–6] have failed to show any consistent effect. Studies on patients with the Wolff–Parkinson–White syndrome are extremely limited[5] but suggest that the drug may prolong the effective refractory period of accessory pathways. Daily doses in the range 1200 to 2400 mg have been shown to be effective in suppressing simple ventricular premature beats, complex ventricular ectopy and ventricular tachycardia.[7–10] No definitive conclusions can be drawn concerning its use in junctional re-entrant tachyarrhythmias, although the limited data available[5] suggest it may be of use.

Investigation of the haemodynamic effects of tocainide in man have produced rather variable results. A study in healthy volunteers[6] showed no alteration of blood pressure or systemic vascular resistance at rest or on exercise. In a study in patients with coronary artery disease[11] the drug given intravenously produced small but significant increases in pulmonary and systemic vascular resistance, pulmonary and aortic arterial pressures and left and right ventricular end-diastolic pressures but overall cardiac function was not significantly depressed. Oral tocainide in patients with valvular heart disease[12] produced only a slight increase in mean systemic systolic blood pressure with no evident myocardial depressant effect. Although the haemodynamic changes that have been observed may have little clinical significance, it is suggested that tocainide be used with caution in patients with uncompensated left or right ventricular failure.

Pharmacokinetics

Tocainide can be assayed either using a gas chromatographic technique with the drug either as a Schiff base or in non-derivatized form[13] or by a high pressure liquid chromatographic technique.[13,14] The two methods appear to give coincident values and have the same limits of sensitivity.

Following oral administration of tocainide absorption occurs rapidly and bioavailability approaches 100%. Time to reach peak plasma levels after a single dose is approximately one hour in fasting subjects. Administration with food decreases peak levels and delays the rate of absorption but does not affect overall bioavailability.[15] Tocainide does not undergo significant hepatic first-pass metabolism. After intravenous infusion of the drug, the plasma profile can be described in most cases by a 2-compartment open model, with a rapid distribution phase of about 10 minutes.[16] The mean plasma half life is similar after both oral and intravenous administration with reported values ranging from 8.9 hours to 40.6 hours but predominantly 12 to 15 hours.

The apparent volume of distribution at steady state has been reported to vary from 1.46 $l.kg^{-1}$ to 3.2 $l.kg^{-1}$. Animal studies have shown that the drug enters cerebrospinal fluid with plasma/CSF ratios of 1.1 to 1.6 after intravenous administration. In mice the drug concentrates in the kidney, gastric mucosa, wall of the eye and choroid plexus and later in the wall of some major arteries. After 48 hours small amounts of the drug are found only in the kidney and the wall of major arteries. There is no information on its excretion in human breast milk.

Tocainide does not appear to be significantly bound to plasma proteins. One recent study has suggested that only 4–22% is bound to macromolecules,[17] whereas an earlier study suggested that 50% of the drug was protein bound.[15] Binding appears to be independent of plasma tocainide concentration. Binding is also unaffected by trauma when levels of the protein α_1-acid glycoprotein, an acute phase reactant, are high.[17] Free fractions of many other antiarrhythmic agents have been found to be strongly correlated with the plasma concentration of α_1-acid glycoprotein, but this does not appear to be so with tocainide.

Oral absorption	100%
Presystemic metabolism	nil
Plasma half life	
range	8.9–40.6 h
mean	12–15 h
Volume of distribution	1.46–3.2 $l.kg^{-1}$
Plasma protein binding	4–22%

Hepatic degradation is a major route of elimination of the drug. Between 39 and 52% of a dose of tocainide is excreted unchanged in the urine within the first 72 hours.[18,19] Approximately 30% of the dose is excreted in the urine in the form of one of the metabolites, the glucuronide of N-carboxytocainide[18] and small amounts of other metabolites, lactylxylidide and tocainide oxime have also been recovered in the urine.[19] Since hepatic degradation is important in the elimination of tocainide, the effects of hepatic enzyme inducers and inhibitors have been investigated.

Although animal studies have demonstrated a decreased elimination half life and an unchanged proportion excreted after pretreatment with the enzyme inducer phenobarbitone, no such alterations in the disposition of tocainide occurred in the only similar study done in man.[20] Similarly, recent studies have shown that tocainide elimination kinetics are not markedly altered in patients with chronic hepatic failure,[21] although it is recommended that the dosage should be reduced by 50% in patients with severe hepatic disease and plasma concentrations determined.

As would be expected the elimination of tocainide is impaired in patients with renal dysfunction. In patients with end-stage renal failure and a creatinine clearance of less than 5 ml.min^{-1} the plasma half life was significantly prolonged to about 27 hours (range 16.6 to 42.7 hours).[22] In the same study, in patients with creatinine clearances ranging from 10 ml.min^{-1} to 55 ml.min^{-1} the plasma half life was prolonged to 19.2 hours. During haemodialysis, in the patients with end-stage renal failure, the half life fell to 8.5 hours, corresponding to removal of 25% of the quantity of drug present at the start of the procedure. It is suggested that in patients with total renal failure, the dose of tocainide is reduced by 50% and a reduction of dose may also be necessary in patients with partial renal dysfunction, together with plasma level monitoring.

Concentration–effect relationship

In patients whose ventricular arrhythmias respond to tocainide there is a relationship between plasma drug concentration and antiarrhythmic response,[9,10] although this is a non-linear curve. In one study significant ventricular premature beat suppression (greater than 70%) occurred when the plasma concentration was above 6 mg.l^{-1}, with 90% arrhythmia suppression at concentrations[10] above 10 mg.l^{-1}. In general, a therapeutic range of 4 to 10 mg.l^{-1} is considered to be acceptable.

There appears to be a positive correlation between responsiveness to lignocaine given by a bolus infusion and subsequent responsiveness to tocainide.[9,23] Also the best response to tocainide tends to occur in those patients who are very sensitive to lignocaine.[9]

Metabolism

As already indicated approximately 40–50% of the drug is excreted unchanged in the urine and the remainder is metabolized (see Fig. 1). The drug undergoes carboxylation and conjugation to form the glucuronide of N-carboxytocainide. Approximately 30% of a dose of the drug is recovered in this form in the urine. Deamination of tocainide produces the metabolite, lactoxylidide. Since less than 2% of a tocainide dose can be accounted for by the lactoxylidide in the urine, it is likely that this metabolite undergoes further metabolism.[19] At steady state, lactoxylidide may be 20 to 90% of the tocainide serum level, because its elimination is slow. Small amounts of a third metabolite, tocainide oxime, have also been identified in urine. None of the metabolites appear to be pharmacologically active.

Pharmaceutics

Tocainide is available in oral and parenteral forms. Tablets contain either 400 mg or 600 mg of tocainide hydrochloride. The tablets are yellow, biconvex and film-coated: the 400 mg tablets are circular and coded 'A/TT' (Astra, UK) or oval and coded 'MSD 707' (MSD, USA), whilst the 600 mg tablets are circular and coded 'A/TC' (Astra, UK) or oblong and coded 'MSD 709' (MSD, USA).

The parenteral form is available in Europe as a clear aqueous sterile solution as an injection vial containing 15 ml, each ml containing 50 mg. It should be given by intermittent infusion in a volume of 50–100 ml of glucose 5% or sodium chloride 0.9% over 15–30 minutes.

No special storage conditions are required and the maximum shelf-life for all formulations is three years. None of the formulations include potentially allergenic substances.

Fig. 1 Metabolism of tocainide[6]

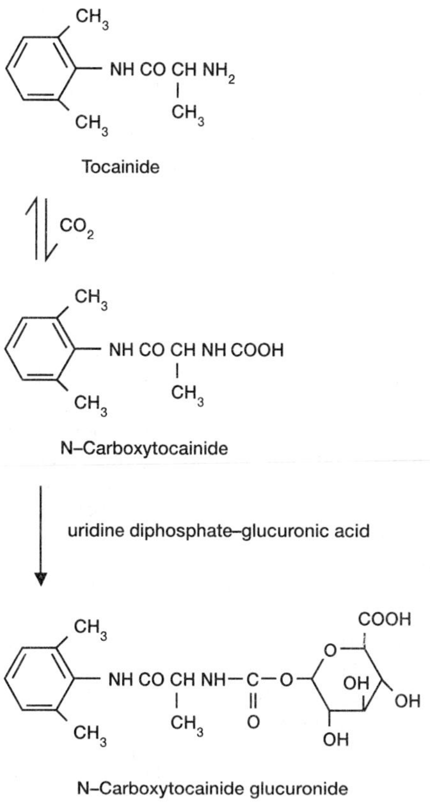

Therapeutic use

Indications

1. The treatment and prophylaxis of life-threatening acute and chronic ventricular arrhythmias, including those complicating myocardial infarction. Tocainide is not a first-choice drug because it causes a relatively high incidence of neutropenia.

Contraindications

1. Known hypersensitivity to amide drugs
2. Second or third degree atrioventricular block in the absence of an artificial ventricular pacemaker.

Mode of use

For the acute treatment of ventricular arrhythmias, including those following myocardial infarction, 500–750 mg of tocainide hydrochloride should be given by slow intravenous injection or by infusion given over 15–30 minutes followed immediately by 600–800 mg orally. Eight hours after the acute treatment, maintenance therapy can be commenced with 1200 mg daily divided into 2 or 3 oral doses. Using this regime therapeutic plasma levels are achieved within 15 minutes and remain within the therapeutic range during chronic oral therapy.[16] The oral daily dosage may be increased to 1800–2400 mg in divided doses if necessary. The highest dose known to have been used is 4000 mg.

Alternatively, oral tocainide may be given following a lignocaine infusion. Because of the shorter half life of intravenous lignocaine, in order to maintain therapeutic levels of lignocaine until the tocainide plasma level is in the therapeutic range, oral tocainide should be started in a regime of 600 mg 6 hourly. The lignocaine infusion can be stopped on administration of the second dose of tocainide and after the third dose of tocainide normal maintenance therapy with the drug (600 mg 12 hourly, see above) can be continued.[24]

Sudden withdrawal of tocainide does not result in any adverse effects attributable to the drug. Any risk associated with tocainide withdrawal is that due to the risk of non-treatment of ventricular arrhythmias in a patient in need of such treatment. In a study of the efficacy of tocainide in ventricular arrhythmias, withdrawal of tocain-

T

ide in 18 patients after several months treatment resulted in the reappearance of arrhythmias in 12 patients.[25]

Indications

1. The treatment and prophylaxis of acute and chronic ventricular arrhythmias, including those complicating myocardial infarction

Myocardial infarction. Tocainide has been shown to be effective and well tolerated as a prophylactic antiarrhythmic agent in patients following myocardial infarction.[26–28] Two of these[26,27] are short-term studies (24 to 48 hours) using oral therapy with tocainide. Both studies showed that in comparison to placebo tocainide therapy was associated with a highly significant reduction of ventricular arrhythmias, particularly of complex types which might be expected to produce haemodynamic upset during the in-hospital phase of acute myocardial infarction. In the study of Ryden et al,[28] intravenous tocainide followed by oral therapy was compared with placebo in patients with an acute myocardial infarction. The follow-up period was six months. Over the first 24 hours the tocainide-treated patients had significantly fewer ventricular premature beats and episodes of ventricular tachycardia than the placebo group, but during the six month follow-up there was no significant difference between the two groups. The mortality rate was low and was similar in the two groups, and tocainide did not appear to prevent ventricular fibrillation, symptomatic ventricular tachycardia or sudden death in these patients with acute myocardial infarction. However, in a similar study in patients with a recent (less than 10 days) myocardial infarction followed for 6 months,[29] oral tocainide significantly reduced the incidence of serious ventricular arrhythmias and the number of ventricular premature beats in comparison to placebo. The number of patients in this study was too small to draw conclusions regarding the mortality rate. The result of the above studies[26–29] would suggest that tocainide is more effective than placebo in the prophylaxis of ventricular arrhythmias following acute myocardial infarction.

Two studies[30,31] have been reported in patients with acute myocardial infarction and ventricular arrhythmias requiring antiarrhythmic therapy (i.e. not prophylaxis). Tocainide, given initially intravenously and then orally, was found to be as equally effective as a continuous lignocaine infusion.[30] In the second study,[31] all patients received intravenous tocainide and were then randomized to either oral tocainide or placebo. Although the intravenous tocainide significantly reduced ventricular arrhythmias, there was no difference between the two groups during the oral phase of the study.

Chronic ventricular arrhythmias. There are many reports attesting the efficacy of tocainide in the treatment of chronic ventricular arrhythmias.[7–10,23,24,32–34] The majority of these studies have involved the treatment of complex ventricular premature beats, ventricular tachycardia and ventricular fibrillation in patients who have proved resistant to a number of other conventional oral antiarrhythmic agents. In the largest of these studies,[7] a multi-centre open study, oral tocainide was administered to 628 patients with ventricular tachycardia or frequent and/or complex ventricular premature beats. Overall, 61% of the patients responded successfully to tocainide treatment. In the 252 patients with documented, severe, symptomatic arrhythmias, 71% responded and the majority (87%) showed a total abolition of symptomatic events. In the studies cited above, in patients with resistant recurrent ventricular tachycardia, a greater than 75% suppression occurred in about 63% of cases. In comparative trials with other antiarrhythmic agents tocainide has been found to be as equally effective as procainamide,[35] quinidine[36] and lignocaine.[30]

In chronic ventricular arrhythmias tocainide may be given 2 or 3 times daily. The use of a thrice-daily regimen enables a lower dose to be used at each administration and thus reduces the peak plasma levels and dose-related side effects. Dose-related and gastrointestinal tract side effects may also be reduced by giving tocainide with food as this reduces peak plasma levels without affecting bioavailability.[15]

Contraindications

1. Known hypersensitivity to amide drugs

This is extremely rare.

2. Second or third degree atrioventricular block in the absence of an artificial ventricular pacemaker

Because tocainide resembles lignocaine in that it reduces ventricular automaticity, there may be a risk of asystole in third degree, complete atrioventricular block.

Adverse reactions

Potentially life-threatening effects

Blood dyscrasias including aplastic anaemia, leucopenia, agranulocytosis, and thrombocytopenia, have been reported (0.3%) in patients receiving tocainide. These disorders usually occurred after 2–12 weeks of therapy and deaths have been reported. The manufacturer advises weekly blood counts for the first 12 weeks of treatment and frequently thereafter. Patients should be warned to report promptly bruising, bleeding, sore throat, fever etc.

Aggravation of pre-existing ventricular arrhythmias has been reported during initiation of treatment with tocainide but does not appear to be common — 1.1% of 369 patients with serious resistant ventricular arrhythmias in the study of Horn and others.[37] Two cases of ventricular fibrillation induced by tocainide have been reported.[38] Aggravation of pre-existing cardiac conduction disturbances has also been reported but a direct causal relationship with tocainide has not been proven. Bradycardia has been noted after both intravenous and oral tocainide.

Acute overdosage

Data on deliberate overdose are very limited. There has only been one reported case[39] and this had a fatal outcome. The patient developed convulsions and complete heart block followed by asystole. Anticipated results of overdose may include central nervous system excitation, including convulsions, respiratory depression and cardiovascular disturbances including atrioventricular block, bradycardia and hypotension. Treatment should be symptomatic and adequacy of ventilation must be assured immediately if convulsions or signs of respiratory depression occur. Should convulsions persist despite ventilation with oxygen, small increments of anticonvulsant agents may be given intravenously, e.g. benzodiazepine, an ultra-short-acting or short-acting barbiturate.

Severe or irreversible adverse effects

Interstitial pneumonitis, pulmonary fibrosis, fibrosing alveolitis, pulmonary oedema and pneumonia with characteristic clinical, radiological and pulmonary function changes, have been reported.[37,40] Withdrawal of tocainide, possibly with the addition of corticosteroids, generally leads to improvement.

In the report of Horn and others,[37] tocainide was reported to have possibly aggravated heart failure in 5 patients with severe pre-existing heart failure. On the other hand, however, a number of patients were unable to tolerate disopyramide or propranolol because of heart failure improved on tocainide.

The development of a lupus erythematosus-like illness has been described but the majority of reported cases[37] occurred either in patients taking other drugs or with a previous history of such symptoms.

Symptomatic adverse effects

Transient, minor symptomatic adverse reactions to tocainide are relatively common with tocainide but are generally well tolerated.

Table 1 The most frequent adverse effects seen in patients treated with tocainide

Adverse effect	Percentage of patients
Gastrointestinal	
Nausea	34
Vomiting	16
Anorexia	15
Central nervous system	
Dizziness	31
Lightheadedness	24
Tremors	22
Paraesthesia	16
Confusion	15
Nervousness	13
Other	
Palpitations	17
Shortness of breath	13
Rash	12

The majority of these are gastrointestinal or neurological in nature. In the study of Horn and colleagues,[37] 16% of patients had to discontinue therapy because of adverse effects and 80% of the withdrawals were due to neurological or gastrointestinal effects. Table 1 lists the percentage occurrence of the most frequent adverse effects in 369 patients treated with tocainide for up to 41.5 months.[37] Other adverse effects reported include visual hallucinations, convulsions, diarrhoea, headache and sweating. The development of hepatitis and elevation of liver enzymes have also been noted with tocainide.[41]

The majority of these adverse effects are mild, transient, dose-related and reversible with a reduction in dosage, by taking the drug with food, or by therapy discontinuation.

Other effects

Positive antinuclear factor titres have occasionally been reported during tocainide therapy.[37,41] Skin reactions include rash, Steven Johnson syndrome and exfoliative dermatitis.

Interference with clinical pathology tests

None documented.

High risk groups

Neonates

Safety and effectiveness have not been established.

Breast milk. It is not known whether tocainide is secreted in human breast milk. Either nursing or the drug should be discontinued, taking into account the importance of the drug to the mother.

Children

Safety and effectiveness not established.

Pregnant women

There are no adequate and well controlled studies in pregnant women. Tocainide should be used during pregnancy only if potential benefit justifies potential risk to fetus. Maternal and fetal toxicity have been shown in animal studies (see Toxicology).

The elderly

As already suggested (see Pharmacokinetics) the dose of tocainide should be reduced in renal or hepatic impairment, and hence caution is advised in the elderly because of the potential risk of accumulation since renal and/or hepatic elimination may be decreased.

Drug interactions

Hepatic enzyme inducers and enzyme inhibitors

Animal studies have shown that the metabolism of tocainide is affected by hepatic enzyme inducers and enzyme inhibitors. However, in the only study performed in man,[20] pretreatment with the enzyme inducer phenobarbitone or co-administration of a competitive substrate for the metabolizing enzyme system, such as clofibrate or salicylamide, were shown not to influence the elimination of tocainide.

Other antiarrhythmic drugs

Concurrent administration of digoxin and tocainide produces no significant differences in the response to tocainide or altered incidence of adverse effects compared with those patients given tocainide alone. Tocainide does not affect serum digoxin concentrations.[34]

The administration of metoprolol and tocainide to patients with heart disease, but free from sinus node disease or impaired atrioventricular conduction, results in a small depression of myocardial contractility which does not result in clinical sequelae.[42] However, in patients with the sick sinus syndrome and impaired atrioventricular conduction, significant depression of function occurs and the combined use of these drugs in these situations should be avoided.

Major outcome trials

The largest clinical trial of the use of tocainide in ventricular arrhythmias is that of Young et al.[7] This is a multi-centre, open study, the results of which have been detailed under Indications.

General review articles

Harrison D C (ed) 1980 Proceedings of the symposium on cardiac arrhythmias. A decade of progress - 1980. American Heart Journal 100 (No. 6, part 2)

Tocainide (hydrochloride)

Holmes B, Brogden R N, Heel R C, Speight T M, Avery G S 1983 Tocainide. A review of its pharmacological properties and therapeutic efficacy. Drugs 26: 93-123

Pottage A, Ryden L (eds) 1981 Workshop on tocainide. Proceedings of a conference held in Copenhagen. A B Hassle, Molndal, Sweden

T

References

1. Moore E N, Spear J F, Horowitz L N, Feldman H S, Moller R A 1978 Electrophysiologic properties of a new antiarrhythmic drug — tocainide. American Journal of Cardiology 41: 703–709
2. Schnittger I, Griffin J C, Hall R J, Meffin P J, Winkle R A 1978 Effects of tocainide on ventricular fibrillation threshold. Comparison with lidocaine. American Journal of Cardiology 42: 76–81
3. Anderson J L, Mason J W, Winkle R A et al 1978 Clinical electrophysiologic effects of tocainide. Circulation 57: 685–691
4. Horowitz L N, Josephson M E, Farshidi A 1978 Human electropharmacology of tocainide, a lidocaine congener. American Journal of Cardiology 42: 276–280
5. Waleffe A, Bruninx P, Mary-Rabine L, Kulbertus H E 1979 Effects of tocainide studied with programmed electrical stimulation of the heart in patients with re-entrant tachyarrhythmias. American Journal of Cardiology 43: 292–299
6. Swedberg K, Pehrson J, Ryden L 1978 Electrocardiographic and hemodynamic effects of tocainide (W-36095) in man. European Journal of Clinical Pharmacology 14: 15–19
7. Young M D, Hadidian Z, Horn H R, Johnson J L, Vassallo H G 1980 Treatment of ventricular arrhythmias with oral tocainide. American Heart Journal 100: 1041–1045
8. Sonnhag C 1980 Efficacy and tolerance of tocainide during acute and long-term treatment of chronic ventricular arrhythmias. European Journal of Clinical Pharmacology 18: 301–310
9. Woosley R L, McDevitt D G, Nies A S, Smith R F, Wilkinson G R, Oates J A 1977 Suppression of ventricular ectopic depolarizations by tocainide. Circulation 56: 980–984
10. Winkle R A, Meffin P J, Fitzgerald J W, Harrison D C 1976 Clinical efficacy and pharmacokinetics of a new orally effective antiarrhythmic, tocainide. Circulation 54: 884–889
11. Winkle R A, Anderson J L, Peters F, Meffin P J, Fowles R E, Harrison D C 1978 The hemodynamic effects of intravenous tocainide in patients with heart disease. Circulation 57: 787–792
12. Ryan W F, Karliner J S 1979 Effects of tocainide on left ventricular performance at rest and during acute alterations in heart rate and systemic arterial pressure: an echocardiographic study. British Heart Journal 41: 175–181
13. Persson B-A 1981 Tocainide — analytical methodology. In: Pottage A, Ryden L (eds) Workshop on tocainide. A B Hassle, Molndal, Sweden, pp 84–89
14. Meffin P J, Harapat S R, Harrison D C 1977 High-pressure liquid chromatographic analysis of drugs in biological fluids II: Determination of an antiarrhythmic drug, tocainide, as its dansyl derivative using a fluorescence detector. Journal of Pharmaceutical Sciences 66: 583–586
15. Lalka D, Meyer M B, Duce B R, Elvin A T 1976 Kinetics of the oral antiarrhythmic lidocaine congener, tocainide. Clinical Pharmacology and Therapeutics 19: 757–766
16. Graffner C, Conradson T-B, Hofvendahl S, Ryden L 1980 Tocainide kinetics after intravenous and oral administration in healthy subjects and in patients with acute myocardial infarction. Clinical Pharmacology and Therapeutics 27: 64–71
17. Elvin A T, Axelson J E, Lalka D 1982 Tocainide protein binding in normal volunteers and trauma patients. British Journal of Clinical Pharmacology 13: 872–874
18. Elvin A T, Keenaghan J B, Byrnes E W et al 1980 Tocainide conjugation in humans: Novel biotransformation pathway for a primary amine. Journal of Pharmaceutical Sciences 69: 47–49
19. Ronfeld R A, Wolshin E M, Block A J 1982 On the kinetics and dynamics of tocainide and its metabolites. Clinical Pharmacology and Therapeutics 31: 384–392
20. Elvin A T, Lalka D, Stoeckel K et al 1980 Tocainide kinetics and metabolism. Effects of phenobarbitone and substrates for glucuronyl transferase. Clinical Pharmacology and Therapeutics 28: 652–658
21. Barclay G, Finlayson N, Hayler A M, Holt D W, Johnston A 1983 A comparison of lignocaine and tocainide elimination in chronic liver disease. British Journal of Pharmacology 16: 579P
22. Wiegers U, Hanrath P, Kuck K H et al 1983 Pharmacokinetics of tocainide in patients with renal dysfunction and during haemodialysis. European Journal of Clinical Pharmacology 24: 503–507
23. Winkle R A, Mason J W, Harrison D C 1980 Tocainide for drug-resistant ventricular arrhythmias: Efficacy, side effects, and lidocaine responsiveness for predicting tocainide success. American Heart Journal 100: 1031–1036
24. Upward J W, Holt D, Emergy P, Akhras F, Jackson G 1983 The appropriate dosage regime for the transition from intravenous lignocaine to oral tocainide after acute myocardial infarction. European Journal of Clinical Pharmacology 25: 589–594
25. Engler R, Ryan W, LeWinter M, Bluestein H, Karliner J S 1979 Assessment of long-term antiarrhythmic therapy: studies on the long-term efficacy and toxicity of tocainide. American Journal of Cardiology 43: 612–618
26. Swedberg K, Holmberg S 1981 Antiarrhythmic effects and patient tolerance to tocainide in acute myocardial infarction — a randomized double-blind study lasting 48 hours. In: Pottage A, Ryden L (eds) Workshop on tocainide. A B Hassle, Molndal, Sweden, pp 190–193
27. Campbell R W F, Bryson L G, Bailey B J, Murray A, Julian D G 1981 Prophylactic administration of tocainide in acute myocardial infarction. In: Pottage A, Ryden L (eds) Workshop on tocainide. A B Hassle, Molndal, Sweden, pp 201–204

T

28. Ryden L, Arnman K, Conradson T-B, Hofvendahl S, Mortensen O, Smedgard P 1980 Prophylaxis of ventricular tachyarrhythmias with intravenous and oral tocainide in patients with and recovering from acute myocardial infarction. American Heart Journal 100: 1006–1012
29. Bastian B C, Macfarlane P W, McLauchlan J H et al 1980 A prospective randomized trial of tocainide in patients following myocardial infarction. American Heart Journal 100: 1017–1022
30. Rehnqvist N 1980 Comparison of tocainide and lidocaine in AMI. In: Pottage A, Ryden L (eds) Workshop on tocainide. A B Hassle, Molndal, Sweden pp 187–189
31. Nyquist O, Forssell G, Nordlander R, Schenck-Gustafsson K 1980 Hemodynamic and antiarrhythmic effects of tocainide in patients with acute myocardial infarction. American Heart Journal 100: 1000–1005
32. Haffajee C I, Alpert J S, Dalen J E 1980 Tocainide for refractory ventricular arrhythmias of myocardial infarction. American Heart Journal 100: 1013–1016
33. Maloney J D, Nissen R G, McColgan J M 1980 Open clinical studies at a referral center: Chronic maintenance tocainide therapy in patients with recurrent sustained ventricular tachycardia refractory to conventional antiarrhythmic agents. American Heart Journal 100: 1023–1030
34. Ryan W, Engler R, LeWinter M, Karliner J S 1979 Efficacy of a new oral agent (tocainide) in the acute treatment of refractory ventricular arrhythmias. American Journal of Cardiology 43: 285–291
35. Agnew M, Whitlock R M L 1980 A double blind crossover study of tocainide, procainamide durules and placebo in patients with chronic ventricular ectopic activity. New Zealand Medical Journal 91: 363
36. Morganroth N, Price B, Dreifus L S 1982 Comparative efficacy and tolerance of quinidine vs low dose tocainide. Circulation Research 30: 207A
37. Horn H R, Hadidian Z, Johnson J L, Vassallo H G, Williams J H, Young M D 1980 Safety evaluation of tocainide in the American Emergency Use Program. American Heart Journal 100: 1037–1040
38. Engler R L, LeWinter M 1981 Tocainide-induced ventricular fibrillation. American Heart Journal 101: 494–496
39. Clarke C W F, El-Mahdi E O 1984 Fatal oral tocainide overdosage. British Medical Journal 288: 760
40. Perlow G M, Jain B P, Pauker S G, Zarren H S, Wistran D C, Epstein R L 1981 Tocainide-associated interstitial pneumonitis. Annals of Internal Medicine 94: 489–490
41. Levin R I, Fox A 1982 Hepatitis in human subjects associated with tocainide administration. Clinical Research 30: 200A
42. Ikram H 1980 Hemodynamic and electrophysiologic interactions between antiarrhythmic drugs and beta blockers, with special reference to tocainide. American Heart Journal 100: 1076–1080

Tocopherol (vitamin E)

Tocopheryl acetate, is a synthetic preparation of a naturally occurring lipid, d-α-tocopherol or vitamin E. Its therapeutic use is principally for prevention and correction of vitamin E deficiency. Its main action is as an antioxidant, protecting other lipids principally in cell membranes, from oxidative and free radical damage.

Chemistry

dl-α-Tocopheryl acetate (vitamin E acetate, Ephynal, Vit-E (as d-isomer))

$C_{31}H_{52}O_3$

dl(2,5,7,8-Tetramethyl-2-(4',8',12'-trimethyltridecyl)-6-chromanol acetate

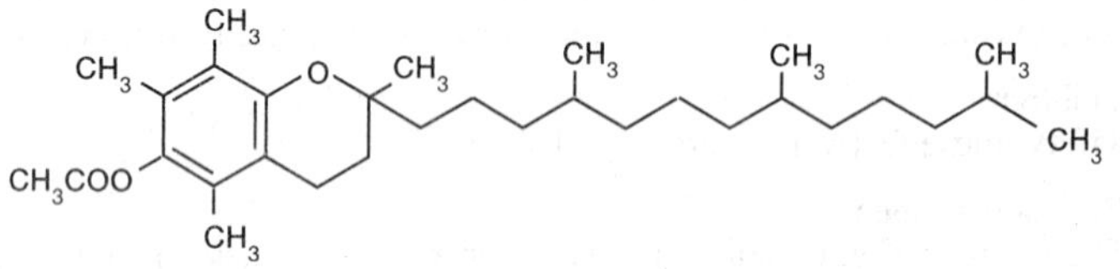

Molecular weight (free alcohol)	472.8 (430.8)
pKa	—
Solubility	
in alcohol	>1 in 2
in water	<1 in 10,000
Octanol/water partition coefficient	high

It is a clear, slightly greenish-yellow viscous oily liquid. Virtually unaffected by oxidising effects of air, light and ultraviolet light, unlike the free alcohol (vitamin E). α-Tocopheryl acetate is prepared chemically from naturally occuring α-tocopherol. It is present in a variety of multi-vitamin preparations, e.g. Concavit, Octavit.

Pharmacology

The main role of tocopherol seems to be as a defence against oxidative stress and lipid peroxidation. In most cell membranes there is one molecule of tocopherol for every 1000 lipid molecules. Tocopherol mops up peroxide radicals and then needs a supply of reduced hydrogen to restore the steady-state situation. This is usually supplied by ascorbic acid or reduced glutathione.

Toxicology

No information is available.

Clinical pharmacology

The main pharmacological action of tocopherol in man is its antioxidant effect, protecting polyunsaturated fatty acids from peroxidization. Little is known about any other pharmacological effects in man.

Pharmacokinetics

The preferred assay method involves HPLC with ultraviolet detection[1,2]. This method has a sensitivity of about 1 $mg.l^{-1}$ and coefficient of variation of 5.6% at a mean plasma concentration 58 $mg.l^{-1}$. About 70% of an oral dose is absorbed. It is widely distributed in all tissues in the lipid fraction, with some affinity for adipose tissue. It is transported in chylomicrons, redistributed freely into all lipoproteins — thus the bulk is in low-density

Tocopherol (vitamin E)

lipoproteins (LDL). Plasma tocopherol concentration correlates with total lipids and with LDL concentrations,[3] and thus also with age.

Concentration–effect relationship

No data are available.

Metabolism

A small proportion of tocopherol is excreted via the urine following hepatic metabolism to glucuronides of tocopheronic acid and its gamma lactone. The major route of elimination from the body is by slow excretion of these products in the bile.[2]

Pharmaceutics

Available as Ephynal (Roche, UK) suspension, 500 mg tocopherol acetate in 5 ml water-miscible suspension. Ephynal tablets in strengths of 3 mg, 10 mg, 50 mg and 200 mg. Also included in a large number of mixed vitamin preparations e.g. Octovit (10 mg as acetate), Ketovite (5 mg as acetate), Gevral (10 mg as acetate), Multibionta (5 mg as acetate). Ephynal suspension should be stored below 25°C and may be diluted with syrup BP for immediate use.

For parenteral administration during parenteral nutrition etc., α-tocopherol is available in a variety of proprietary multivitamin mixtures, e.g. Vitlipid-N (1 mg in 10 ml ampoule).

Whereas free tocopherol may be destroyed by oxidation, the acetate ester (and indeed the succinate ester which is also available) is very stable in light and air. The esters are rapidly hydrolysed in the small intestine. Aqueous dispersions are more readily absorbed and used when intestinal absorption may be impaired.

Therapeutic use

Indications

Tocopherol has been tried in a wide range of conditions in which lipid peroxidation or oxygen toxicity is believed to play a part. Few if any of these indications have been validated by properly designed controlled trials and therapeutic use of the drug is often based largely on unsubstantiated hypotheses about disease aetiology.

1. Replacement therapy in nutritional deficiency states
2. Heavy metal poisoning
3. Hepato-toxin poisoning
4. Haemolytic anaemia
5. Cardiovascular disease
6. Oxygen therapy
7. Miscellaneous conditions.

Contraindications

There are no absolute contraindications.

Indications

1. Replacement therapy in nutritional deficiency states

Vitamin E is widely distributed in foods, principally being found in association with vegetable oils and the products which are made from them. The recommended dietary allowance in the US is 8 mg per day for women, 10 mg daily for men.[4] The daily requirements of infants and young children are probably proportionally higher than in adults and deficiency is more worrying since it may affect development of the neurological system rather than simply the functioning of an old one. These daily amounts are met by most adults' diets but the absolute daily requirement is dependent to some degree on proportion of polyunsaturated fats in the diet, and on the exposure of the individual to toxins, which have a capacity to generate free radicals, including iron.[6] The dietary requirement may also be affected by impaired fat absorption.

Tocopherol is a lipid and its absorption from the small bowel will be reflected by other indices of lipid absorption. Vitamin E deficiency has been documented in a variety of intestinal and malabsorptive disorders as evidenced by low circulating concentrations. Usually, there are other nutritional deficiencies as well and it is difficult to be confident that vitamin E deficiency is leading to either symptoms or derangement of direct functional correlates such as red blood cell half life. The diagnosis is usually made on suspicion and this may be supported by a low plasma concentration which responds to supplementation. Reduced red blood cell survival usually improves after vitamin E supplementation and peroxide-induced haemolysis has been used as a functional correlate of vitamin E status.[5] Neuropathological and myopathic abnormalities have been observed in patients at risk for vitamin E deficiency and a neurological syndrome has been described in children with chronic cholestasis and biochemical evidence of vitamin E deficiency, which includes areflexia, gait disturbance, diminished proprioception and vibratory sense and ophthalmoplegia. Clinical conditions most likely to cause vitamin E malabsorption are those with severe deficiency of bile production or secretion (since this is essential to form mixed micelles for adequate tocopherol absorption), pancreatic insufficiency, particularly cystic fibrosis in children. Steatorrhoea and vitamin E malabsorption also occur in disease of the intestinal mucosa such as coeliac disease.[6] The principal transport protein for vitamin E is β-lipoprotein.[7] Abetalipoproteinaemia and also hypobetalipoproteinaemia in liver disease may precipitate vitamin E deficiency.[8]

For abetalipoproteinaemia a wide variety of dosages have been used ranging from 100 mg up to several grams daily. At present there is no evidence to indicate benefit in very high dosages and thus for adults 100–200 mg daily is adequate under most circumstances. When there is very severe malabsorption, such as in abetalipoproteinaemia, dosages as high as 100 $mg.kg^{-1}$ body weight daily may result in barely detectable increase in plasma concentration and parenteral administration is preferred. However, these massive doses have been shown to correct the abnormal in vitro red cell haemolysis and also to prevent the retinal and neurological complications.[9] When vitamin E is administered on suspicion of deficiency then a daily intake in the range 200–600 mg is considered safe.[3] The synthetic dl isomer contains 50% of active d-α-tocopherol.

2. Heavy metal poisoning

Animal studies show that additional vitamin E above the usual dietary intake can protect against tissue toxicity from metal poisoning including silver, mercury and lead. Supplementation may be considered in human patients, but it is not standard practice.

3. Hepato-toxin poisoning

Supplementing vitamin E may help reduce tissue damage in exposure to hepato-toxic compounds such as carbon tetrachloride, benzine,[10] paraquat[11] and the effect of some drugs.[12] Some of the cytotoxic antineoplastic drugs are believed to cause side effects by the production of free radicals and lipid peroxidation.[13,14] Vitamin E supplementation in patients treated with drugs such as adriamycin is reasonable on theoretical grounds,[14] but the evidence is conflicting, and damage may be aggravated in some cases.[15] A combination of vitamin E and testosterone, administered intraperitoneally in rats enhanced recovery of hepatic protein content (presumably synthesis) in animals irradiated experimentally to 5.5 Gy.[16]

Hepatic damage in iron overload is associated with tocopherol depletion, suggesting a therapeutic role for α-tocopherol in conditions such as haemochromatosis.[17]

4. Haemolytic anaemia

Vitamin E is probably the endogenous antioxidant protecting circulating red cells and there is a greater risk of haemolysis from a variety of causes with vitamin E deficiency. High dose supplementation has been examined as a means of protecting the red cells and has been found effective in a variety of haemolytic disorders including glucose-6-phosphate dehydrogenase (G-6-PD) deficiency,[18,19] glutathione synthetase,[18] β-thalassaemia major,[20] and sickle cell anaemia.[21] An inverse relationship between plasma α-tocopherol concentration and MCHC in sickle cell patients and their relatives suggests that relative deficiency of vitamin E may aggravate the condition,[22] and possibly that haemolysis contributes to vitamin E depletion.

In infancy, vitamin E supplementation has been investigated as a means of preventing or correcting haemolytic anaemia in the neonate. It has been suggested that haemolytic anaemia is more frequent in infants receiving a diet rich in linoleic acid and fortified with iron. Some commercial formulas in the past have contained low levels of vitamin E and this has been considered a causative factor. Commercial formula feeds for premature and neonatal infants now contain a higher or more appropriate concentration of vitamin E in relation to polyunsaturated fats, fatty acids and iron content.[23–25] Because of the relationship between neonatal haemolysis and jaundice, vitamin E has been used in attempts to reduce hyperbilirubinaemia. Routine administration of vitamin E does not seem warranted but there may be benefits for small preterm infants.[26–28]

5. Cardiovascular disease
Although the hypothesis that subclinical vitamin E deficiency may contribute to the development of ischaemic vascular disease remains tenable, treatment with vitamin E (even in massive doses) does not have unequivocal effects on traditional risk factors for ischaemic vascular disease[29–31] nor is there convincing evidence of the beneficial effects in any symptomatic cardiac condition.[32,33] In some patients with intermittent claudication there may be an improvement with prolonged vitamin E treatment in terms of walking distance.[34]

6. Oxygen therapy
High concentrations of oxygen as used in lung disease, and particularly in respiratory distress syndrome in infancy, is associated with toxic effects, in particular retrolental fibroplasia. Premature infants often have low circulating vitamin E and supplementation in pharmacological doses can protect against this toxicity and possibly even reverse established damage.[35–39] Hittner and others[38] carried out a double-blind prospective study comparing vitamin E 100 $mg.kg^{-1}$ daily against a control group receiving 5 $mg.kg^{-1}$ per day in preterm infants weighing 1500 g or less. The severity of retrolental fibroplasia was significantly reduced and the suggestion is that vitamin E supplementation should be started as early as possible, or preferably before oxygen therapy.

7. Miscellaneous conditions
Hypothermic cardiac surgery is followed by increased cardiac oxygen consumption, and depletion of myocardial α-tocopherol content associated with evidence of free-radical injury: preoperative therapy with α-tocopherol has been suggested.[40]

Long lists of medical conditions are sometimes found for which vitamin E has been recommended or suggested, but where there is no scientific rationale or evidence for efficacy,[3] or deeply conflicting evidence.[15] Most of these are conditions of an episodic or uncertain course, and often subjective nature. Farrell and Bieri[41] evaluated the voluntary ingestion of vitamin E in a group of 28 adults for a variety of sub-medical indications. No evidence of adverse effects was discovered on standard laboratory screening and it was concluded that subjective claims for beneficial effects were very variable.

Adverse reactions

Potentially life-threatening effects
Interference with anticoagulation therapy has been reported with high-dose vitamin E supplementation (1200 mg daily), with prolonged prothrombin time.[42] It is possible that this relates to interference in vitamin K absorption or function at the level of prothrombin formation.[43]

It has been suggested that premature infants treated with high-dose vitamin E may be more prone to necrotizing enterocolitis and sepsis.[28,44]

Acute overdosage
No cases of this kind appear to have been reported.

Severe or irreversible adverse effects
Apart from those described above, there are none.

Symptomatic adverse effects
Nausea, flatulence or diarrhoea may occur. High-dose vitamin E (mostly > 400 mg daily) has been associated with a variety of minor side effects, including hypertension, fatigue, diarrhoea, myopathy and thrombophlebitis.[45]

Interference with clinical pathology tests
No technical interferences of this kind have been reported.

High risk groups

Neonates
Caution is advised in premature infants with high-dose vitamin supplementation, because of reported risk of necrotizing enterocolitis.[44]

Breast milk. There appears to be no contraindication to breast-feeding by mothers taking the normally recommended dose.

Children
The drug may be used in children.

Pregnant women
The drug may be used in the normally recommended dose, but the safety of high-dose therapy has not been established.

The elderly
No special precautions are necessary in elderly patients.

Drug interactions

Potentially hazardous interactions
High doses of vitamin E can impair intestinal absorption of vitamins A and K. Vitamin E may impair vitamin K function at the level of prothrombin formation and thus potentiate the effect of warfarin.[43]

Potentially useful interactions
None has been described.

Major outcome trials

None has been reported.

General review articles

Aranda J V, Chemtob S, Laudignon N, Sasyniuk B I 1986 Furosemide and vitamin E — two problem drugs in neonatology. Pediatric Clinics of North America 33: 583–602

Bieri J G, Corash L, Hubbard V S 1983 Medical doses of vitamin E. New England Journal of Medicine 308: 1063–1071

Goss-Sampson M A, Muller D P R, Lloyd J K 1989 Clinical importance of vitamin E: a review. Journal of Human Nutrition and Diet 2/3: 145–150

References

1. Bieri J G, Tolliver T J, Catignani G L 1979 Simultaneous determination of alpha-tocopherol and retinol in plasma or red cells by high pressure liquid chromatography. American Journal of Clinical Nutrition 32: 2143–2149
2. Hatam L J, Kayden H J 1979 A high performance liquid chromatographic method for the determination of tocopherol in plasma and cellular elements of the blood. Journal of Lipid Research 20: 639–645
3. Bieri J G, Corash L, Hubbard V S 1983 Medical doses of vitamin E. New England Journal of Medicine 308: 1063–1071
4. Food and Nutrition Board, National Research Council 1980 Recommended dietary allowances, 9th revised edn. National Academy of Sciences, Washington, pp 66–68
5. Melhorn D K, Gross S, Lake G A, Leu J A 1971 The hydrogen peroxide fragility test and serum tocopherol level in anemias of various etiologies. Blood 37: 438–446
6. Goss-Sampson M A, Muller D P R, Lloyd J K 1989 Clinical importance of vitamin E: a review. Journal of Human Nutrition and Diet 2/3: 145–150
7. Goransson G, Norden A, Akesson B 1973 Low plasma tocopherol levels in patients with gastrointestinal disorders. Scandinavian Journal of Gastroenterology 8: 21–25
8. Azizi E, Zaidman J L, Eshchar J, Szeinberg A 1978 Abetalipoproteinemia treated with parenteral and oral vitamins A and E, and with medium chain triglycerides. Acta Paediatrica Scandinavica 67: 797–801
9. Muller D P R, Lloyd J K, Wolff O H 1983 Vitamin E and neurological function. Lancet 1: 225–228
10. Hove E L 1955 Anti-vitamin E stress factors as related to lipid peroxides. American Journal of Clinical Nutrition 3: 328–336
11. Kurisaki E 1989 Lung toxicity of paraquat. Eisei Kagaku 35: 261–272
12. Plaa G L, Witschi H 1976 Chemicals, drugs and lipid peroxidation. Annual Review of Pharmacology and Toxicology 16: 125–141
13. Goodman J, Hochstein P 1977 Generation of free radicals and lipid peroxidation by redox cycling of adriamycin and daunomycin. Biochemical and Biophysical Research Communications 77: 797–803
14. Bachur N R, Gordon S L, Gee M V 1978 A general mechanism for microsomal activation of quinone anticancer agents to free radicals. Cancer Research 38: 1745–1750
15. Shinozawa S, Gomita Y, Araki 1988 Effect of high dose alpha-tocopherol and alpha-tocopherol acetate pretreatment on adriamycin (doxorubicin)-induced toxicity and tissue distribution. Physiological Chemistry and Physics and Medical NMR 20: 329–335
16. El-Kashef H S, Saaqa H N 1988 A mixture of testosterone propionate and vitamin E for recovery from radiation-induced changes in the liver protein nitrogen of whole body gamma-irradiated rats. Isotope and Radiation Research 20: 121–139
17. McCarthy P T, Rice-Evans C, Hallinan T, Gor J, Green N, Diplock A T 1989 Iron overload, tocopherol levels and susceptibility to oxidative damage. Biochemical Society Transactions 17: 696–697
18. Spielberg S P, Boyer L A, Corash L M, Schulman J D 1979 Improved erythrocyte survival with high-dose vitamin E in chronic hemolyzing G6PD and glutathione synthetase deficiencies. Annals of Internal Medicine 90: 53–54
19. Corash L, Spielberg S, Bartsocas C et al 1980 Reduced chronic hemolysis during high-dose vitamin E administration in Mediterranean type glucose-6-phosphate dehydrogenase deficiency. New England Journal of Medicine 303: 416–420

20. Rachmilewitz E A, Shifter A, Kahane I 1979 Vitamin E deficiency in B-thalassemia major: changes in hematological and biochemical parameters after therapeutic trial with α-tocopherol. American Journal of Clinical Nutrition 32: 1850–1858
21. Natta C L, Machlin L J, Brin M 1980 A decrease in irreversibly sickled erythrocytes in sickle cell anemia patients given vitamin E. American Journal of Clinical Nutrition 33: 968–971
22. Jain S K, Ross J D, Izundu C, Masters G, Nance N 1989 Vitamin E in sickle cell disease patients. Annals of the New York Academy of Sciences 402–403
23. Williams M L, Shott R J, O'Neal P L, Oski F A 1975 Role of dietary iron and fat on vitamin E deficiency anemia of infancy. New England Journal of Medicine 292: 887–890
24. Ehrenkranz R A 1980 Vitamin E and the neonate. American Journal of Diseases of Children 134: 1157–1166
25. Bell E F, Filer L J Jr 1981 The role of vitamin E in the nutrition of premature infants. American Journal of Clinical Nutrition 34: 414–422
26. Gross S J, Landaw S A, Oski F A 1977 Vitamin E and neonatal hemolysis. Pediatrics 59: 995–997
27. Gross S J 1979 Vitamin E and neonatal bilirubinemia. Pediatrics 64: 321–323
28. Aranda J V, Chemtob S, Laudignon N, Sasyniuk B I 1986 Furosemide and vitamin E — two problem drugs in neonatology. Pediatric Clinics of North America 33: 583–602
29. Hermann W J Jr, Ward K, Faucett J 1979 The effect of tocopherol on high density lipoprotein cholesterol: a clinical observation. American Journal of Clinical Pathology 72: 848–852
30. Hatam L J, Kayden H J 1981 The failure of α-tocopherol supplementation to alter the distribution of lipoprotein cholesterol in normal and hyperlipoproteinemic persons. American Journal of Clinical Pathology 76: 122–124
31. Barboriak J J, El Ghatit A Z, Shetty K R, Kalbfleisch J H 1982 Vitamin E supplements and plasma high-density lipoprotein cholesterol. American Journal of Clinical Pathology 77: 371–372
32. Olson R E 1973 Vitamin E and its relation to heart disease. Circulation 43: 179–184
33. Farrell P M 1980 Deficiency states, pharmacological effects and nutrient requirements. In: Machlin L J (ed) Vitamin E: a comprehensive treatise. Marcel Dekker, New York, pp 520–620
34. Haeger K 1973 Walking distance and arterial flow during long term treatment of intermittent claudication with d-α-tocopherol. Vasa 2: 280–288
35. Ehrenkranz R A, Ablow R C, Warshaw J B 1979 Prevention of bronchopulmonary dysplasia with vitamin E administration during the acute stages of respiratory distress syndrome. Journal of Pediatrics 95: 873–878
36. Owens W C, Owens E U 1949 Retrolental fibroplasia in premature infants. II. Studies on the prophylaxis of the disease: the use of alpha tocopherol acetate. American Journal of Ophthalmology 32: 1631–1637
37. Johnson L, Schaffer D, Boggs T, Quinn G, Mathis M 1980 Vitamin E Rx of retrolental fibroplasia (RLF) Grade III or worse (Abstract). Pediatric Research 14: 601
38. Hittner H M, Godio L B, Rudolph A J et al 1981 Retrolental fibroplasia: efficacy of vitamin E in a double-blind clinical study of preterm infants. New England Journal of Medicine 305: 1365–1371
39. Phelps D L 1982 Vitamin E and retrolental fibroplasia in 1982. Pediatrics 70: 420–425
40. Weisel R D, Mickle D A G, Finkle C A, Tumati L C, Masonik M M, Ivanov J 1989 Myocardial free-radical injury after cardioplegia. Circulation (suppl): 14–18
41. Farrell P M, Bieri J G 1975 Megavitamin E supplementation in man. American Journal of Clinical Nutrition 28: 1381–1386
42. Corrigan J J Jr, Marcus Fl 1974 Coagulopathy associated with vitamin E ingestion. Journal of the American Medical Association 230: 1300–1301
43. Corrigan J J Jr 1982 The effect of vitamin E on warfarin-induced vitamin K deficiency. Annals of the New York Academy of Sciences 393: 361–367
44. Sobel S, Gueriguian J, Troendle G, Nevius E 1982 Vitamin E in retrolental fibroplasia. New England Journal of Medicine 306: 867
45. Roberts H J 1979 Thrombophlebitis associated with vitamin E therapy. Angiology 30: 169–177

T

Tolazoline (hydrochloride)

Tolazoline is an alpha-adrenergic receptor antagonist used as a systemic and pulmonary vasodilator.

Chemistry

Tolazoline hydrochloride (Priscol, Priscoline, Dilazol, Zoline, Vasodil, Prefaxil, Benzidazol, Vasimid, Kasimid, Artonil, Vasodilatan, Lambril, Olitensol)

$C_{10}H_{12}N_2.HCl$

2-Benzyl-2-imidazoline hydrochloride

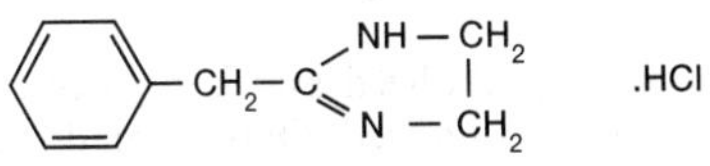

Molecular weight (free base)	196.7 (160.2)
pKa(-NH-)	10.4
Solubility	
in alcohol	1 in 2
in water	1 in 0.5
Octanol/water partition coefficient	—

A white or creamy white odourless crystalline powder with a bitter taste. Must be protected from light. Tolazoline is obtained by chemical synthesis. It is not available in any combination preparations.

Pharmacology

Tolazoline was originally thought to have vasodepressor activity but subsequent studies have shown that the drug has a number of pharmacological properties. The most important of these is alpha-adrenergic receptor antagonism, a property it shares with another 2-substituted imidazoline, phentolamine. It also has some parasympathomimetic activity e.g. gastrointestinal tract stimulation that is blocked by atropine. Tolazoline also has histamine like effects with activity primarily at H_2 receptors causing stimulation of gastric secretion.[1] Tolazoline causes relaxation of smooth muscle and is an antagonist at $5HT_1$ receptors.[2]

Toxicology

The acute toxicity (LD_{50}) of tolazoline administered orally is 400 $mg.kg^{-1}$ and 1200 $mg.kg^{-1}$ in mice and rats respectively.

Long-term carcinogenicity studies in animals have not been performed with tolazoline.

Clinical pharmacology

The clinical pharmacology of tolazoline is a combination of its various pharmacological effects. In usual clinical doses there is very little evidence of α adrenergic blocking activity and this effect is in any case transitory. Tolazoline given intravenously produces cardiac stimulation and tachycardia (mainly due to a sympathomimetic effect) and vasodilation due primarily to a direct effect on smooth muscle. Blood pressure is usually elevated by tolazoline. There is usually a reduction in peripheral resistance and an increase in venous capacitance. Pulmonary arterial pressure is usually reduced by tolazoline. The cardiac stimulatory effects of tolazoline may result in cardiac arrhythmias. Tolazoline usually causes mydriasis in man rather than miosis because the intrinsic eye muscles are relatively resistant to any α-blocking effects of the drug.

Histaminergic (H_2) stimulation may result in increased gastric secretion and contributes to peripheral and pulmonary vasodilation. In addition the parasympathetic effects of tolazoline may cause hyperperistalsis and diarrhoea which can be blocked by atropine. Abdominal discomfort is thus a common side effect of tolazoline therapy. In addition tolazoline may cause profuse sweating and salivation that may be due to parasympathomimetic effects. However direct effects of tolazoline may also be responsible for these latter effects since tolazoline is known to cause salivation in animals with denervated salivary glands.

Pharmacokinetics

Tolazoline in plasma can be assayed by high pressure liquid chromatography with UV detection[3]. The limit of detection is 200 $\mu g.l^{-1}$. Little is known about the fate of tolazoline in the body. Tolazoline is well absorbed after oral administration and intramuscular injection. After oral administration and intramuscular injection, the maximum vasodilator effects of tolazoline are produced after 45 – 100 minutes and 30 – 60 minutes respectively. After a single dose the effects last for several hours. It is not known how the drug is distributed in the body. There are no data on diffusion through the placenta, and on breast milk excretion. The drug should be used with caution in pregnant or nursing women. It is not known whether tolazoline penetrates the CNS. This strong organic base is 23% bound to plasma proteins.

Tolazoline is poorly metabolized and is rapidly excreted by filtration in the urine, largely unchanged. Only a small fraction is excreted by the renal tubular active transport system for organic bases.

In adults, renal elimination of the drug results in half life elimination of 90 – 120 minutes with 90% of a dose excreted unchanged into the urine within 12 hours.

In neonates, the half life of tolazoline varies enormously from 1.5 to 41 hours, depending on urine output.

Oral absorption	>90%
Presystemic metabolism	nil
Plasma half life	
range	90-120 min
Volume of distribution	—
Plasma protein binding	23%

Concentration–effect relationship

There is no evidence of any relationship between the plasma concentration of tolazoline and its therapeutic effects.

Metabolism

Tolazoline is excreted in the urine, essentially without metabolism.

Pharmaceutics

Tolazoline is available in oral, cutaneous and parenteral forms.
- Tablets contain 25 mg of tolazoline hydrochloride. Priscol (Ciba UK). Also available as Priscol in Australia, Germany, Spain, Switzerland.
- Tolazoline hydrochloride injection (USP): a sterile solution in water for injections. PH3 to 4. 4 ml ampoules each ml contains 25 mg of tolazoline hydrochloride. Store between 15°C and 30°C (59°F-86°F).
- Tolazoline hydrochloride (Priscoline CIBA, USA) in 10 ml multiple-dose vials (25 mg.ml).
- Unguentum Tolazolini. (Nord. P.). Tolazoline Ointment. Tolazoline hydrochloride 10 g, water 5 g, wool fat 17 g and white soft paraffin 68 g.

Therapeutic use

Indications

Tolazoline was once used extensively to treat vascular disorders but present day indications are few.
1. Pulmonary hypertension especially in neonates
2. Peripheral vascular disorders.

Contraindications

1. Hypersensitivity to tolazoline
2. Hypotension and shock
3. Angina pectoris and cardiac infarction
4. Mitral stenosis
5. Recent cerebrovascular accident
6. Gastroduodenal ulcers.

Mode of use

Tolazoline is not administered frequently and should be used only in a highly supervised setting such as intensive care units, at least for intravenous infusion.
In neonates and other patients an initial intravenous dose of 1 $mg.kg^{-1}$ over 45 to 120 seconds followed by an infusion of 1 to 2 $mg.kg^{-1}$ hourly is usually required. Response, if any, can be expected within 30 minutes after the initial dose.
In the treatment of peripheral vascular disorders, 10 to 50 mg, 4 to 6 times a day by either subcutaneous, intramuscular or intravenous route have been used. In the same line of indications intra-arterial administration 25 to 50 mg have been proposed once a day and then 2 to 3 times a week.

Indications

1. Pulmonary hypertension of the newborn
Tolazoline meets its main indication with the initial treatment of persistent pulmonary hypertension of the new born when systemic oxygenation is not controlled by usual supportive care.[4] It should be noted that there is very little experience with administrations lasting beyond 48 hours. Improvement in pulmonary perfusion is indirectly judged by an increase in aortic PaO_2. Despite the initial improvement in PaO_2 in about 60% of these infants, the overall survival rate ranged only from 44% to 57%.

2. Peripheral vascular disorders
The vasodilator properties of tolazoline were used more frequently in the past than today to improve blood flow in ischaemic extremities. There is considerable doubt about long term efficacy[5]

Contraindications

1. Hypersensitivity to tolazoline
Tolazoline is contraindicated in patients who already experienced an hypersensitivity to the drug.

2. Hypotension and shock
Vasodilators should not be used in such situations except in very rare, highly monitored cases.

3. Angina pectoris and cardiac infarction
Tolazoline may precipitate cardiac infarction because of its adverse effect on the heart filling pressure and arrhythmias.

4. Recent cerebrovascular accident
Tolazoline is contraindicated in patients after a thrombotic stroke.

5. Mitral stenosis
Tolazoline may produce rapid alterations in pulmonary arterial pressure and therefore must not be used in patients with mitral stenosis.

6. Gastroduodenal ulcers
Because of its parasympathomimetic and histaminergic properties, tolazoline stimulates gastric secretion and may activate gastroduodenal ulcers.

Adverse reactions

Potentially life-threatening effects
These include severe hypotension and shock due to excessive vasodilatation and precipitation of cardiac infarction and severe arrhythmias, mainly associated with the reflex hyperactivation of the sympathetic nervous system and with direct histaminergic stimulation.

Acute overdosage
Severe tolazoline-induced hypotension should be controlled by placing the patient in the supine position with the head down and by expanding the plasma volume. If despite these procedures a vasopressor drug remains necessary, then angiotensin should be preferred to other drugs. In such a condition, adrenaline or noradrenaline must not be used because of exacerbation of the hypotension by stimu-

lation of β-adrenoceptors while α-adrenoceptors are inhibited by tolazoline.

Severe or irreversible adverse effects
In addition to hypotension and cardiac arrhythmias, apprehension, shivering, sweating, nausea and vomiting may occur.
Tolazoline may precipitate stress ulcer and cause gastrointestinal bleeding, as well as pulmonary haemorrhage.
Leucopenia and thrombocytopenia have been described.
Rarely, tolazoline may paradoxically raise blood pressure and even cause hypertension.

Symptomatic adverse effects
Main effects of this kind include piloerection and flushing.
Intra-arterial administration of tolazoline may cause a feeling of warmth or burning in the injected limb.

Other effects
In addition to the stimulation of gastric secretions, tolazoline increases salivary, lacrimal and pancreatic secretions.

Interference with clinical pathology tests
No specific interference has yet been described.

High risk groups

Neonates
It is mandatory to monitor blood pressure carefully during administration of tolazoline to neonates, who are especially at risk of hypotension and consecutive renal failure.

Breast milk. No data are available, so it is probably best for breast feeding mothers to avoid the drug.

Children
The drug may be used in children.

Pregnant women
It is not known whether tolazoline can cause fetal harm when administered to pregnant women.

The elderly
The elderly are more at risk of cardiac arrhythmias, cardiac infarction and stroke if excessive doses of vasodilators such as tolazoline are used.

Drug interactions

Potentially hazardous interactions

Vasopressors. Tolazoline should not be used in combination with adrenaline or noradrenaline, as the combination may cause a paradoxical and aggravated fall in blood pressure.

Other significant interactions

Alcohol. Tolazoline may produce a disulfiram-like reaction after alcohol ingestion.

Potentially useful interactions
Tolazoline has been used intra-arterially prior to arteriography, to improve the visualization of the vasculature.

References

1. Yellin T O, Sperow J W, Buck S H 1975 Antagonism of tolazoline by histamine H2-receptor blockers. Nature 253: 561-563
2. Ward R M 1984 Pharmacology of tolazoline. Clinics in Perinatology 11: 703-713
3. Rovei V et al 1982 Journal of Chromatography 231; Biomed. Appl. 20: 210-215
4. Grover R F, Reeves J T, Blount S G 1961 Tolazoline hydrochloride (Priscoline). An effective pulmonary vasodilator. American Heart Journal 61: 5--15
5. Coffman J D 1979 Medical intelligence - drug therapy, vasodilator drugs in peripheral vascular disease. New England Journal of Medicine 300: 713–717

Tolbutamide

Tolbutamide is a sulphonyl urea oral hyoglycaemic agent which acts by increasing pancreatic insulin secretion, it is used in the treatment of non-insulin dependent diabetes.

Chemistry

Tolbutamide (Rastinon, Glyconon, Orinase, Oribetic, Pramidex)
$C_{12}H_{18}N_2O_3S$
1-Butyl-3-p-tolylsulphonylurea

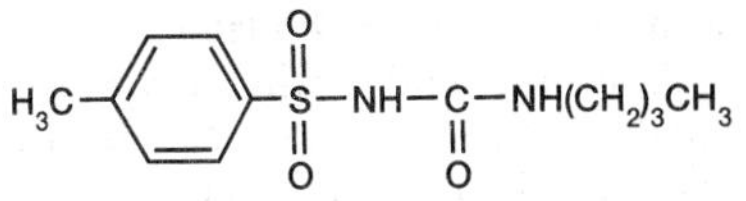

Molecular weight	270.4
pKa (Sulphonylurea)	5.3
Solubility	
in alcohol	1 in 10
in water	insoluble
Octanol/water partition coefficient	—

Tolbutamide is a white, crystalline powder, almost odourless with a slightly bitter taste, prepared by chemical synthesis.

Pharmacology

Tolbutamide is effective in reducing blood sugar and its main mechanism of action is by stimulation of the islet cells in the pancreas to secrete insulin. Tolbutamide administration causes degranulation of β-cells, which is usually associated with an increased rate of secretion of insulin, and the concentration of insulin in the blood has been shown to rise. Tolbutamide binds to receptors on the β-cell in the pancreas and the release of insulin is immediate. It appears to stimulate Ca^{++} influx into the islet cell,[1] and it is likely that the receptor is the ATP-sensitive K^+ channel itself.[2] Tolbutamide also increases the concentration of cyclic AMP in pancreatic islet cells, thus affecting adrenergic control of insulin release.

It is probable that tolbutamide also has extrapancreatic effects and causes peripheral tissues to become sensitive to insulin, thus leading to an overall decreased need for insulin synthesis.

Toxicology

Tolbutamide has not been shown to have mutagenic or carcinogenic potential. There are no toxicological studies in animals which show any clinically significant effects at doses close to those used in man. In animal experiments the acute and chronic toxicity of tolbutamide has been shown to be remarkably low. Teratogenicity testing in animals has shown fetocidal and teratogenic effects at doses of 1000–2500 $mg.kg^{-1}$ daily.

Clinical pharmacology

In healthy subjects oral and intravenous administration of tolbutamide causes a fall in blood sugar. Haupt and co-workers[3] found after oral administration of tolbutamide (25 $mg.kg^{-1}$) there was a 12% fall in blood glucose after 1 h which had reached a maximum (28%) after 3 h. At 5 h blood glucose concentrations were still 15% less than levels prior to drug administration. Other investigators[4] have noted a similar effect, with a fall in blood glucose of 18% at 1.5 h compared with initial fasting levels. In general the maximal fall in blood sugar occurs 30 min after intravenous injection. Tolbutamide has a relatively short duration of action and thus the drug is usually given in divided doses.

The average daily dose required is 0.5 to 1.5 g (1–3 tablets); depending on individual needs, dose increments are available up to 3 g daily. However, patients who do not respond to 2 g daily will not generally respond to higher doses.

There are several controversial studies on the effect of tolbutamide on plasma lipids.[5] In several cross-sectional studies[6,7] it has been shown that diabetics, treated with sulphonylureas have low HDL concentrations, but this may be related to inadequate glycaemic control rather than a direct effect. Prospective studies have produced inconsistent results and Melander et al[8] conclude in a review that it is unlikely that sulphonylureas have a direct effect on plasma lipids.

Several reports suggest sulphonylureas may reduce platelet adhesiveness and aggregation, however this is thought to be secondary to blood glucose reduction.[8]

Pharmacokinetics

The preferred analytical method is high performance liquid chromatography[9] which permits measurement of drug and metabolite at concentrations of 2 $mg.l^{-1}$.

Tolbutamide is readily absorbed after oral administration with peak plasma concentrations seen 3–4 h later. It is rapidly and widely distributed throughout the body, with a volume of distribution approximately equal to that of the extracellular fluid. The half life shows considerable individual variation, but is generally in the range of 4–8 h. The drug has been shown to enter the CSF, and can be detected in breast milk, but there is no evidence of accumulation in any specific organs. Tolbutamide is highly bound to plasma proteins (97%).

Oral absorption	>95%
Presystemic metabolism	—
Plasma half life	
range	4–12 h
mean	7 h
Volume of distribution	0.1–0.2 $l.kg^{-1}$
Plasma protein binding	97%

Concentration–effect relationship

Therapeutically effective serum levels are quoted as being 60–100 $mg.l^{-1}$, although in practice a wide range of levels is encountered and there is little clinical need to measure tolbutamide concentrations since the effect is so easy to measure.

Metabolism

Tolbutamide is metabolized in man, through oxidative metabolism to produce carboxytolbutamide and hydroxytolbutamide (Fig. 1). In

Fig. 1 The metabolism of tolbutamide

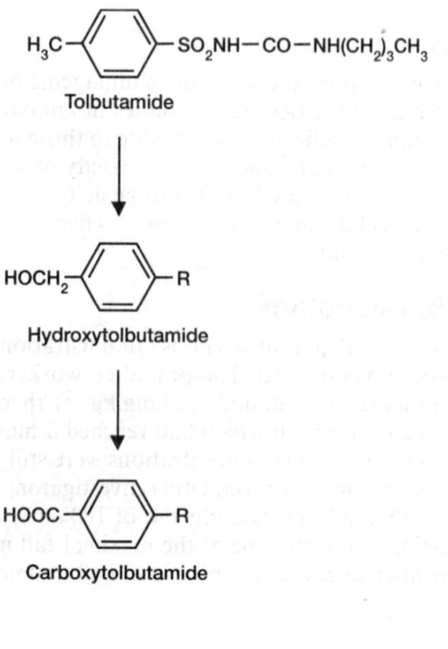

the oxidized form, about 90% of the drug is excreted in the urine within 48 h in the ratio of 2:1 of the above metabolites. Most of the remaining 10% is excreted in the bile, and only traces of unchanged tolbutamide can be found in the urine. After an intravenous dose the ratio of the carboxy derivative to the hydroxymethyl derivative rises to 4:1. None of the metabolites is active.

Pharmaceutics

Tolbutamide is available in 250 mg and 500 mg tablets.

1. Rastinon (Hoechst, UK) uncoated white, round, scored tablets containing 500 mg tolbutamide, one side impressed with the Hoechst insignia, the other bearing the marks 'Rastinon' and '0.5' on either side of the score mark.
2. Orinase tablets (Upjohn, USA) are round, white, uncoated, marked 'ORINASE 250' and coded '701' on the reverse (250 mg) or for the 500 mg strength marked 'ORINASE 500'.

Tolbutamide tablets should be kept in a cool dry place, protected from light and in containers similar to those of the manufacturers. The maximum shelf-life of Rastinon tablets is 5 years at room temperature, but this may vary with generic preparations.

Therapeutic use

Indications

1. The control of blood glucose in previously untreated non-insulin dependent diabetics
2. Treatment of diabetics when the blood glucose is unsatisfactory despite treatment with diet
3. In combination with metformin when the blood glucose is unsatisfactory despite treatment with diet and tolbutamide
4. Some non-insulin dependent diabetes previously treated with insulin
5. Substitution for another oral hypoglycaemic.

Contraindications

1. Diabetic ketoacidosis (absolute contraindication). Diabetics who develop ketoacidosis on withdrawal of insulin are generally unsuitable for oral therapy
2. Insulin-dependent diabetes mellitus
3. Serious impairment of renal, hepatic, adrenocortical or thyroid function (relative contraindication)
4. Circumstances of unusual stress, e.g. most surgical procedures
5. Pregnancy.

Mode of use

Tolbutamide depends on some residual β-cell function to be of any benefit. Stabilization can be achieved with two tablets daily. The subsequent dose must depend on an individual's response. The average daily dose is 500 mg to 1.5 g which should usually be taken in divided doses, but may be given in a single dose, despite the short half life. Doses above 2 g daily are unlikely to be of any benefit. Changeover from other oral hypoglycaemic agents to tolbutamide can be carried out without a break in therapy. Tolbutamide may also be withdrawn suddenly provided provision is made for the patient or doctor to monitor blood or urine glucose. Tolbutamide is of especial use in the elderly as it has little tendency to accumulate, unlike some other sulphonylureas.

Indications

1. Control of blood glucose in previously untreated diabetics

In broad terms there is only one indication for tolbutamide therapy and that is for the treatment of non-insulin dependent diabetes mellitus. Previously undiagnosed, often elderly diabetics may be treated with tolbutamide and diet. The starting dose is 0.5–1 g a day and this should be titrated according to the effect on blood sugar. Treatment should be aimed at keeping the urine free from glucose and/or maintaining blood glucose between 4 and 10 $mmol.l^{-1}$. The dosing and treatment rationale given in Mode of use also applies to the indications below.

Tolbutamide

2. Treatment of diabetics when the blood glucose is unsatisfactory despite treatment with diet
It is generally advisable on diagnosis to treat non-insulin dependent patients (especially the obese) with a six-week trial of diet. If, however, glycaemic control is not satisfactory tolbutamide may be added at this point.

3. In combination with metformin
Tolbutamide may be used in conjunction with metformin when either drug alone is failing to provide adequate glycaemic control.

4. Some non-insulin dependent diabetics
Tolbutamide may be used in non-insulin dependent diabetics who have been treated with insulin. On withdrawal of insulin tolbutamide may be started the same day, with careful monitoring for hyperglycaemia or ketonuria.

5. Substitution for another oral hypoglycaemic
On some occasions it is appropriate to change a diabetic treated with another sulphonylurea to tolbutamide. Patients with impaired renal function who are at risk from chlorpropamide accumulation and resultant hypoglycaemia are better treated with tolbutamide as almost all the drug is metabolized.

Contraindications

1. Diabetic ketoacidosis
This is an absolute contraindication for tolbutamide therapy as these patients require insulin.

2. Insulin-dependent diabetes mellitus
Although tolbutamide has been used in insulin-dependent diabetes these patients by definition require insulin.

3. Serious impairment of renal, hepatic, adrenocortical or thyroid function
In patients with serious impairment of renal or hepatic function tolbutamide may accumulate, leading to hypoglycaemia, and therefore should be avoided. In states of impaired hepatic function metabolism is reduced, prolonging duration of action as well as impairing counter-regulatory responses to hypoglycaemia. Thus these two effects can promote severe and prolonged hypoglycaemia. Renal impairment may also induce hypoglycaemia, not only by altering tolbutamide elimination but also by reducing endogenous insulin clearance. Tolbutamide is known to cause dilution hyponatraemia by inappropriate ADH secretion, which is especially undesirable in the face of impaired adrenocortical function. Although the clinical significance is controversial, tolbutamide has been implicated in impaired thyroid function and its use is best avoided in patients with serious pre-existing thyroid dysfunction.

4. Unusually stressful circumstances
In situations of severe stress, the hyperglycaemia due to increased secretion of the counter-regulatory hormones make insulin therapy preferable.

5. Pregnancy
There is overwhelming evidence that diabetes should be extremely well controlled in pregnancy and insulin therapy is recommended. Although tolbutamide is not a known teratogen its use in pregnancy has been associated with some harmful effects.

Adverse reactions

Potentially life-threatening effects
Hypoglycaemia is by far the most significant adverse reaction produced by tolbutamide and this is associated with a marked increase in circulating insulin levels. In severe cases, increasing cerebral impairment may be followed by coma and death. Most cases are a result of severe accidental overdose, or deliberate self-poisoning. Severe hepatic dysfunction resulting in death has been reported[1] and suspension of treatment at the first sign of hepatic injury is essential.

Acute overdosage
The patient usually presents with vomiting and dose-related hypoglycaemia. Very large ingestions (30 g or more) in combination with alcohol can result in death. The patient should be managed with sufficient intravenous glucose to normalize the blood sugar. Conscious patients may be treated with oral glucose repeated as necessary. If the patient is comatose, glucose should be administered by intravenous infusion with frequent monitoring of blood sugar. Bolus injection of glucose is not recommended because of the possibility of rebound hypoglycaemia. Alternatively, glucagon may be administered in a dose of 1 mg subcutaneously or intramuscularly to produce consciousness. If required, diazepam may be administered to reduce excitement (5 mg intravenously). For very severe cases, some authorities have recommended repeated injections of glucagon in addition to large amounts of glucose by intravenous infusion. General supportive treatment is indicated in the unconscious patient. Repeated oral administration of activated charcoal may be of benefit.

Severe or irreversible adverse effects
Severe hyponatraemia may rarely occur but is reversible on discontinuing treatment. Blood dyscrasias such as pancytopenia with hepatosplenomegally, thrombocytopenia and allergic thrombocytopenia rarely occur. Trauman et al[12] noted the development of pancytopenia after 3 years treatment. In this instance, when tolbutamide was discontinued and the usual treatment undertaken, the anaemia persisted whilst the leucopenia and thrombocytopenia were reversed. An increase in cardiovascular mortality has been reported but interpretation of the data is controversial (see Major outcome trials).

Symptomatic adverse effects
Mild gastrointestinal symptoms such as nausea, vomiting and dyspepsia can occur. Skin sensitivity reactions occur within the first 6 months to 2 years of treatment and range from generalized photosensitivity to mild maculopapular reactions. Sensitization from previous sulphonamide therapy is thought to be a factor. Mild symptomatic hypoglycaemia can occur when the dose is not tailored with due regard to the patient's dietary habits. Reduced food intake is responsible for 12–16% of severe hypoglycaemia.

Other effects
Transient abnormalities in liver function tests have been observed as well as possible impairment of thyroid function.

Interference with clinical pathology tests
On rare occasions, urine containing tolbutamide metabolites may give a false-positive reaction for albumin by the acidification-after-boiling test, since this procedure causes the metabolites to precipitate as flocculent particles. This may be circumvented using Albustix or similar tests.

High risk groups

Neonates
The drug is not recommended in neonates.

Breast milk. Small quantities of the drug can be detected in breast milk but the effects are not known.

Children
As non-insulin dependent diabetes is rare in childhood tolbutamide is not recommended.

Pregnant women
The use of tolbutamide is not recommended during pregnancy.

The elderly
Because of its complete metabolism and relatively short duration of action tolbutamide is recommended in the elderly non-insulin dependent diabetic.

Concurrent disease
In patients with serious impairment of renal or hepatic function, tolbutamide may accumulate leading to hypoglycaemia and therefore should be avoided. Renal impairment may also induce hypoglycaemia, not only by altering tolbutamide elimination but also by reducing endogenous insulin clearance.

Tolbutamide is known to cause dilutional hyponatraemia by inappropriate ADH secretion which is especially undesirable in the face of impaired adrenocortical function. Although the clinical significance is controversial, tolbutamide has been implicated in impaired thyroid function and its use is best avoided in patients with serious pre-existing thyroid dysfunction.

Theoretically, tolbutamide is potentiated by hypoalbuminaemia

Tolbutamide

T

due to its high degree of protein binding. In states of impaired hepatic function metabolism is reduced, prolonging duration of action as well as impairing counter-regulatory responses to hypoglycaemia. Thus, these two effects can promote severe and prolonged hypoglycaemia.

Drug interactions

Potentially hazardous interactions

The hypoglycaemic effect of tolbutamide may be enhanced by dicoumarol, salicylates, sulphonamides, phenylbutazone and clofibrate due to displacement of tolbutamide from binding proteins, thereby increasing the free concentration transiently. Beta-adrenergic blocking agents may also enhance the hypoglycaemic effect by blocking the adrenergic response to hypoglycaemia. Beta-blockade also tends to mask the symptoms of hypoglycaemia, except for sweating. Potentiation has also been reported with chloramphenicol and cyclophosphamide.

The hypoglycaemic effect of tolbutamide may be diminished by administration of counter-regulatory hormones such as corticosteroids, adrenaline and the oral contraceptives. Thiazide diuretics are known to impair glucose tolerance and thereby diminish the effect of tolbutamide.

Potentially useful interactions

The concurrent use of metformin may improve glycaemic control.

Major outcome trials

1. University Group Diabetes Program 1970 A study of the effects of hypoglycaemic agents in vascular complications in patients with adult onset diabetes. II. Mortality results. Diabetes 19 (suppl 20): 785–830

The UGDP reported an increased mortality from cardiovascular causes in newly diagnosed non-insulin dependent diabetics treated with a fixed dose of tolbutamide compared with placebo- or insulin-treated groups. The study was a collaborative, double-blind, prospective trial. A total of 823 newly diagnosed diabetics recruited from 12 participating centres were prescribed a diet designed to achieve and maintain ideal body weight. The treatments were placebo (205 patients), tolbutamide 1.5 g a day in divided doses (204 patients), fixed-dose insulin 10, 12, 14, or 16 units per day according to surface area (210 patients), or variable insulin dose altered in accordance with the blood glucose.

75% of these patients had been under follow-up for at least five years by the time the mortality in each group was analysed. There were 26 deaths in the tolbutamide group attributed to cardiovascular causes of which 10 were attributed to myocardial infarction, whereas there were only 10 cardiovascular deaths in the placebo group, none of which were attributed to myocardial infarction. The cardiovascular mortality in the insulin-treated groups was not significantly different from placebo. Overall mortality was slightly higher in the tolbutamide group but this was not statistically significant. The findings of this study proved to be highly controversial and were much criticized on methodological and statistical grounds, although the American Statistical Society endorsed the design and interpretation. Apart from the failure of the studies described below to show any increase in cardiovascular mortality in tolbutamide-treated patients when compared to placebo, the main criticisms of the UGDP study were:

1. Divergence from the admission criteria with regard to the diagnosis of diabetes; 7% of the subjects failed to meet the diagnostic criteria.
2. Failure to randomize risk factors for cardiovascular disease between the groups despite screening for such factors.
3. Substantial variation in mortality between the participating centres. 85% of the cardiovascular deaths in the tolbutamide-treated group were reported by 3 out of the 12 centres.
4. No deaths at all were attributed to myocardial infarction in the placebo group.

Shen et al[11] made statistical efforts to correct for the criticisms of UGDP and concluded that a significant increase in cardiovascular mortality in the tolbutamide group might still be present. However, despite many years of regulation, other prospective randomized studies and inclusion of a warning note on the package in the USA, the findings of the UGDP study have never been substantiated.

2. Paasikivi J 1970 Long term tolbutamide treatment after myocardial infarction. Acta Medica Scandinavica 507 (suppl): 1–82

Paasikivi studied 178 patients with impaired glucose tolerance or 'mild' diabetes following myocardial infarction. Of these, 95 patients were randomly assigned to receive tolbutamide (maintenance dose 500 mg twice daily) and the remaining 83 were assigned to placebo. After five years follow-up there was no increase in cardiovascular death in the tolbutamide-treated group.

3. 1971 Bedford study. Acta Diabetologica Latina 8 (suppl 1): 444

The Bedford study included 248 patients with 'borderline' diabetes (now classified as impaired glucose tolerance). Patients in this study were randomly assigned to placebo or tolbutamide (500 mg twice daily). There were 126 patients in the placebo group and 122 in the tolbutamide group. Cardiovascular deaths after over five years follow-up were reported as 8 in the tolbutamide group and 13 in the placebo group. These death rates were not significantly different.

General review articles

Melander A, Bitzen P, Ole Faber, Lief Groop 1989 Sulphonylurea antidiabetic drugs: an update of their clinical pharmacology and their general therapeutic use. Drugs 37: 58–72

Foy J M 1978 Oral hypoglycaemic agents. Pharmaceutical Journal 221: 94

Stowers J M, Borthwick L J 1977 Oral hypoglycaemic drugs. Drugs 14: 41

Cader Asmal, Marble A 1984 Hypoglycaemic agents: on update. Drugs 14: 62

Paice B J, Paterson K R, Lawson D H 1985 Undesired effects of the sulphonylurea drugs. Advances in Drug Reactions and Poisoning Reviews 1: 23–26

Reynolds 1987 Martindale. The extra pharmacopoeia, 25th edn. The Pharmaceutical Press, p 859

References

1. Lebrun P, Malaisse W J, Herchuelz A 1989 Modalities of glicazide-induced Ca^{++} influx into the pancreatic β cell. Diabetes 31: 1010–1015
2. Boyd A E 1988 Sulphonylurea receptors, ion channels and fruitflies. Diabetes 37: 847–850
3. Haupt E et al 1977 Proceedings of the first symposium on C-peptide, p 133
4. Greenfield M S, Reaven G M et al 1982 Lipid metabolism in non insulin dependent diabetes mellitus. Archives of Internal Medicine 142: 1948–1500
5. Taskinen M-R et al 1982 Lipoprotein lipase activity and serum lipoprotein in untreated Type 2 (insulin-independent) diabetes associated with obesity. Diabetologia 22: 46–50
6. Berry E M, Bar-On H 1981 Comparison of sulphonylurea and insulin treatment on lipid levels in maturity onset diabetic men and women. Israeli Journal of Medical Sciences 17: 384–387
7. Calvert G D, Mannik T et al 1978 Effects of therapy on plasma-high-density-lipoprotein-cholesterol concentration in diabetes mellitus. Lancet 2: 66–68
8. Melander, A, Bitzen P, Ole Faber, Lief Groop 1989 Sulphonylurea antidiabetic drugs: an update of their clinical pharmacology and their general therapeutic use: Drugs 37: 58–72
9. Ragolo G, Meyer M C 1981 High performance liquid chromatographic assay of tolbutamide and carboxy-tolbutamide in human plasma. Journal of Pharmaceutical Sciences 70: 1166–1168
10. Gregory D H et al 1967 A case of tolbutamide-induced fatal hepatic necrosis. Archives of Pathology 84: 194
11. Shen S, Bressler R 1977 Clinical pharmacology of oral antidiabetic agents. New England Journal of Medicine 507 (suppl) 1–82

Tolmetin (sodium)

Tolmetin is a pyrrole, acetic acid derivative, non-steroidal anti-inflammatory drug.

Chemistry

Tolmetin sodium (Tolectin, Tolectin DS, Midocil, Tolmex)
$C_{15}H_{14}NO_3.Na.2H_2O$
1-Methyl-5-(4-methylbenzoyl)-1H-pyrrole-2-acetic acid, sodium salt, dihydrate

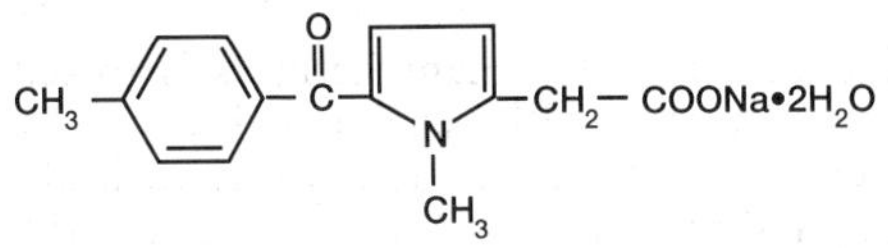

Molecular weight	315.3
(free acid, anhydrous)	(258.3, 279.3)
pKa	3.5
Solubility	
in alcohol	practically insoluble
in water	soluble
Octanol/water partition coefficient	0.8

A yellow crystalline powder prepared by chemical synthesis. There are no combination products.

Pharmacology

Tolmetin is a non-steroidal anti-inflammatory drug (NSAID) with analgesic and antipyretic actions. It inhibits cyclooxygenase activity with a reduction in the tissue production of prostaglandins such as $PGF_2\alpha$ and PGE_2. The anti-inflammatory activity is greater than that of aspirin but in animal studies is less than that of indomethacin or phenylbutazone.

Toxicology

Tolmetin does not have mutagenic potential and toxicological testing in animals failed to demonstrate any results of clinical relevance. There was no evidence of carcinogenicity in mice (up to 50 $mg.kg^{-1}$ daily) or in rats (75 $mg.kg^{-1}$ daily). Teratogenicity was not shown in rats or rabbits (up to 50 $mg.kg^{-1}$ daily). Tolmetin causes gastric erosions and prolongs the bleeding time. As with other prostaglandin inhibitors, effects on parturition and viability of rat offspring were noted with tolmetin.

Clinical pharmacology

Tolmetin is an effective anti-inflammatory[2] and analgesic drug[2] in clinical practice and is used in the treatment of rheumatoid arthritis and osteoarthritis. The usual daily dose is 600–1800 mg. Tolmetin exhibits a linear dose–response relationship over the therapeutic dose range. There is a modest increase in half life over a dose range of 200–800 mg; this is not clinically significant. It is as effective in clinical trials as indomethacin from both the efficacy and side effect points of view (see Major outcome trials). Tolmetin relieves joint swelling and pain in patients with rheumatoid arthritis but has no long-term effect on the disease process. Tolmetin inhibits platelet thromboxane production and prolongs bleeding time. By inhibiting prostaglandin synthesis in the uterus tolmetin delays the onset of labour.

Tolmetin has no effect on renal function in normal individuals but like other NSAIDs may worsen renal function in patients whose renal function depends on the production of prostaglandin E_2 (e.g. in renal failure, severe hypertension, diabetic nephropathy, cirrhosis of the liver). This inhibition of prostaglandin synthesis may explain the loss of hypotensive control or diuretic effect of many drugs when an NSAID is co-administered. Tolmetin may cause gastric erosions partly by directly irritating the gastric mucosa and partly by inhibiting the synthesis of cytoprotective prostaglandins.

Pharmacokinetics

The preferred analytical method for analysis of the drug is HPLC with ultraviolet detection which has a sensitivity[3] of 40 $\mu g.l^{-1}$. Tolmetin is rapidly and almost completely (99%) absorbed following oral administration,[4] with peak plasma concentrations being achieved within 0.25–1 h of dosing. Peak plasma concentration is approximately 30 $mg.l^{-1}$ after a dose of 300 mg. Presystemic metabolism is thought to be negligible. Its mean plasma half life is 6.8 h (range 5.5–8.5 h).[5] Tolmetin is highly bound to plasma proteins (99.7%), resulting in a volume of distribution of only 0.098 $l.kg^{-1}$ (range 0.064–0.168 $l.kg^{-1}$).[6] The free fraction of the drug is increased from 0.3% to 3.1% by salicylic acid at 400 $mg.l^{-1}$ and in patients with rheumatoid arthritis with uraemia (to 0.6% free drug).[7]

There is no information regarding brain/CSF levels, placental transfer or excretion in lactating humans. There is good penetration of tolmetin into synovial fluid where levels remain higher than in plasma for a wash-out period.[5] Tolmetin is extensively metabolized in the liver. Excretion is almost entirely in the urine with up to 15% as unchanged drug. It is possible that elimination of the drug will be impaired in hepatic disease. Renal failure and deteriorating renal function with age are unlikely to have a major effect on the kinetics of the drug.

Oral absorption	99%
Presystemic metabolism	minimal
Plasma half life	
range	5.5–8.5 h
mean	6.8 h
Volume of distribution	0.098 $l.kg^{-1}$
Plasma protein binding	99.7%

Concentration–effect relationship

In common with other non-steroidal anti-inflammatory drugs clinical efficacy is probably not directly related to plasma levels and no therapeutic range has been defined. In addition, there is a poor relationship between drug levels and clinical response.

Metabolism

Tolmetin is metabolized in the liver, with 99% of the dose excreted in the urine largely in the first 8 h.[4] There is no enterohepatic circulation.

The major pathway involves N-demethylation and oxidation. Dicarboxylic acid metabolites account for 73% of the drug with 12% excreted as glucuronide conjugates; 10% of the dose is excreted unchanged. Other metabolites account for 3%. None of the metabolites is pharmacologically active.

Pharmaceutics

Tolmetin is available in an oral form only as Tolectin 400 mg capsules, size 0 (all orange) and Tolectin 200 mg capsules, size 1 (orange–ivory) (Cilag, UK/McNeill, USA), printed T-400 and T-200 respectively.

The drug should be stored at room temperature and in dry conditions. If packed in high density polyethylene easy-open containers with metal closures, it has a shelf-life of 3 years.

Therapeutic use

Indications

1. Rheumatoid arthritis
2. Osteoarthritis
3. Ankylosing spondylitis
4. Peri-articular disorders.

Contraindications

1. Peptic ulcer
2. Drug hypersensitivity.

Mode of use

The usual adult dosage is 600–1800 mg daily given in 2, 3 or 4 divided doses depending on patient response and the severity of the disease. In juvenile rheumatoid arthritis the dosage is 20–25 $mg.kg^{-1}.day^{-1}$ in 3–4 divided doses. The maximum dose is 30 $mg.kg^{-1}.day^{-1}$ or 1800 $mg.day^{-1}$ whatever the body weight.

Indications

1. Rheumatoid arthritis

Double-blind studies have shown that tolmetin is significantly better than placebo and as effective as aspirin or indomethacin in producing improvement in patients with rheumatoid arthritis.[8]

Tolmetin, like other non-steroidal anti-inflammatory drugs, has an anti-inflammatory action which reduces the number of inflamed joints, reduces the duration of early morning stiffness and improves functional capacity.

2. Osteoarthritis

Osteoarthritic patients are helped by the anti-inflammatory and analgesic effects of tolmetin which result in an improved functional capacity, an increased walking distance and better grip strength. Tolmetin is comparable to aspirin in efficacy, but produces fewer adverse effects.[9]

3. Ankylosing spondylitis

Tolmetin has proved of comparable efficiency to other non-steroidal anti-inflammatory drugs in the treatment of this disorder.[10]

4. Peri-articular disorders

Tolmetin has been used in the treatment of these disorders.[11]

Contraindications

1. Peptic ulcer

Like all non-steroidal anti-inflammatory drugs, tolmetin is contraindicated in patients with active peptic ulceration in whom efforts should be made to treat with a non-ulcerogenic drug.

2. Drug hypersensitivity

A previous allergic reaction to the drug is an absolute contraindication to its use, and caution should be exercised in patients with a history of previous sensitivity to aspirin or other non-steroidal anti-inflammatory drugs.

Adverse reactions

Potentially life-threatening effects

The potentially lethal effects are similar to those of other non-steroidal anti-inflammatory drugs, namely gastrointestinal tract haemorrhage and anaphylaxis. The anaphylactic reactions are extremely rare and are no more common than with other anti-inflammatory drugs. Other possible problems include renal failure, hepatic failure and agranulocytosis. The most frequently reported severe adverse reaction has been allergic/anaphylactic, the precise frequency of which is unknown. As tolmetin increases extracellular fluid volume caution should be exercised in patients with cardiac failure.

Acute overdosage

Overdose with tolmetin has been treated symptomatically with gastric lavage and administration of activated charcoal, with subsequent monitoring of renal and hepatic function. A 4000 mg overdose was treated successfully; however, a 6000 mg overdose proved fatal and it appears that the main symptoms were associated with the gastrointestinal tract and the central nervous system.

Severe or irreversible adverse effects

Other than those described immediately above, none has been reported.

Symptomatic adverse effects

In a retrospective analysis of 1000 patients with rheumatoid arthritis the adverse effects encountered, in order of frequency, included nausea (11%), gastrointestinal distress, headache, weight gain, hypertension, diarrhoea, weight loss (5%), dizziness, flatulence, vomiting, rash, oedema, hearing loss, tinnitus and visual disturbance.

Interference with clinical pathology tests

Tolmetin metabolites give false positive results for proteinuria using tests which rely on acid precipitation.[13] No interference is seen in tests for proteinuria using dye-impregnated commercially available reagent strips.

High risk groups

Neonates

The drug is not recommended in neonates.

Breast milk. Tolmetin has been shown to be secreted in human milk. Mothers taking it should not breast-feed because of the possible adverse effects of prostaglandin-inhibiting drugs in neonates.

Children

The drug is not indicated for children younger than 2 years. In older children there are no specific problems.

Pregnant women

The drug is not recommended for use during pregnancy.

The elderly

The recommendation of the manufacturers is to reduce the dose in the elderly especially with renal impairment. As 10% of the drug is excreted unchanged this is unlikely to lead to significant accumulation, and the warnings for use in the elderly are probably more appropriately related to the symptoms in the gastrointestinal tract.

Drug interactions

Potentially hazardous interactions

Anticoagulants. The prothrombin time may be prolonged in patients on anticoagulant therapy.

Other significant interactions

None has been described.

Potentially useful interactions

Tolmetin has a potential steroid-sparing effect, and also an additive or synergistic effect with acetaminophen.

Major outcome trials

1. Caldwell J 1975 A double-blind comparison of efficacy and side-effect liability of tolmetin and indomethacin. In: Ward J R (ed) Tolmetin: a new non-steroidal anti-inflammatory agent. Excerpta Medica Foundation International Congress Series 372, pp 160–167

A double-blind multicentre comparison of tolmetin with indomethacin in 224 patients over a six month period. Tolmetin was given at a mean dosage of 1214 mg and indomethacin at 166 mg. Both groups produced a significant improvement in all measured parameters with little to choose between the drugs. Investigators adjudged both drugs to have produced a marked or moderate improvement in 62% of patients. 200 side effects were seen in 72 patients on tolmetin and 182 side effects in 77 patients on indomethacin. The major site of side effects for both drugs was gastrointestinal; indomethacin produced more CNS side effects.

2. Andelman S Y 1979 A double blind multicentre evaluation of tolmetin versus indomethacin in the management of osteoarthritis of the hip. Current Therapeutic Research 26: 144–154 and Data on file. Science Information Division, McNeil Pharmaceutical, McNeilab, Inc

A three to twelve month multicentre double-blind study in 243 patients with osteoarthritis of the hip. Tolmetin and indomethacin were shown to produce comparable improvement in virtually all assessments and produced equal numbers of side effects.

References

1. Wong S 1975 Pharmacology of tolmetin. In: Ward J R (ed) Tolmetin: a new non-steroidal anti-inflammatory agent. Excerpta Medica Foundation International Congress Series 372, pp 1–22

2. Wong S, Gardocki J F, Pruss T P 1973 Pharmacologic evaluation of Tolectin and McN 2891, two anti-inflammatory agents. Journal of Pharmacology and Experimental Therapeutics 185: 127–138
3. Desiraju R K, Sedbury D C, Ng K 1982 Simultaneous determination of tolmetin and its metabolites in biological fluids by HPLC. Journal of Chromatography 232: 119–128
4. Grindel J M, Migdalof B H, Plostnieks J 1979 Absorption and excretion of tolmetin in arthritic patients. Clinical Pharmacology and Therapeutics 26: 122–128
5. Dromgoole S H, Furst D E, Desiraju R K, Nayak R K, Kirschenbaum M A, Paulus H E 1982 Tolmetin kinetics and synovial fluid prostaglandin E levels in rheumatoid arthritis. Clinical Pharmacology and Therapeutics 32: 371–377
6. Selley M L, Glass J, Triggs E J, Thomas J 1975 Pharmacokinetic studies of tolmetin in man. Clinical Pharmacology and Therapeutics 17: 599–605
7. Pritchard J F, O'Neill P J, Affrime M B, Lowenthal D T 1984 Influence of uremia and hemodialysis on the plasma protein binding of tolmetin. Pharmacology 29: 312–319
8. Ward J R (ed) 1975 Tolmetin, a new non-steroidal anti-inflammatory agent. Excerpta Medica Foundation International Congress, Series 372
9. Salzman R, Kaplan S 1979 A double blind multicentre comparison on the treatment of osteoarthritis of the knee. Current Therapeutic Research 25: 508–518
10. Strandel W 1977 The question of drug treatment of ankylosing spondylitis. Therapiewoche 27: 2273
11. Maibach E 1977 The treatment of extra articular rheumatic diseases and fresh distortion with Tolectin. Therapiewoche 27: 2318
12. Ehrlich G E 1983 Long term therapy with tolmetin in rheumatoid arthritis. Journal of Clinical Pharmacology 23: 287–300
13. Ehrlich G E, Wortham G F 1975 Pseudoproteinuria in tolmetin treated patients. Clinical Pharmacology and Therapeutics 17: 467–468

Tranexamic acid

Antifibrinolytic agents are a new class of drugs of which ε-aminocaproic acid (EACA) (6-aminohexanoic acid) was the first synthetic representative. The relationship between the chemical structure and its antifibrinolytic properties is well established, based on its action as a lysine substitute.[1] The 5-carbon chain is important for its antifibrinolytic effect, which in principle is based on the same molecular interactions as for the other aminocarboxylic acids, tranexamic acid (AMCA) and p-aminomethylbenzoic acid (PAMBA). The antifibrinolytic potency of the aminocarboxylic acids depends on the presence of free amino and carboxylic groups and on the distance between the carboxylic group and the carbon atoms to which the amino group is attached.[2,3]

Clinical experience with PAMBA is very limited and only a limited number of controlled clinical trials were conducted with EACA. As tranexamic acid is 7 to 10 times more potent than ε-aminocaproic acid and has the same low toxicity, the latter drug is now little used and neither EACA nor PAMBA will be further discussed.

Chemistry

Tranexamic acid (Cyklokapron, Anvitoff, Exacyl, Frénolyse, Tranex, Transamin, Ugurol) is the trans-stereoisomer of 1,4-aminomethylcyclohexane carboxylic acid ($C_8H_{15}NO_2$) a synthetic amino acid. Initial investigations with the drug were performed using a preparation containing a mixture of two stereoisomers, but it was subsequently found[4–6] that only the trans-stereoisomer has antifibrinolytic activity

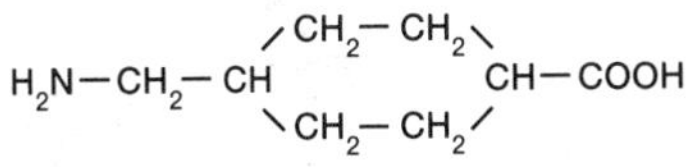

Molecular weight	157
pKa (carboxylic and amino group)	4.3, 10.6
Solubility	
in alcohol	1 in 1000–1 in 10 000
in water	1 in 6
Octanol/water partition coefficient	—

Tranexamic acid is a white odourless powder which forms white crystals, which are soluble in water, acids and alkalis, slightly in alcohol but remain insoluble in organic solvents.

Pharmacology

Tranexamic acid produces an antifibrinolytic effect by competitively inhibiting the activation of plasminogen to plasmin.[7,8] At high concentrations, it is also a weak non-competitive inhibitor of plasmin and it is now clear that this is not its main antifibrinolytic action. Human plasminogen contains structures, called lysine binding sites, which are of importance not only for its interaction with synthetic antifibrinolytic amino acids but also with α_2-antiplasmin and with fibrin.[11]

Native human plasminogen contains 1 lysine binding site with high affinity for tranexamic acid ($K_d = 1.1\ \mu mol.l^{-}$) and 4 or 5 with low affinity ($K_d = 750\ \mu mol.l^{-}$). The binding of plasminogen and of the heavy chain of plasmin to fibrin monomer is also mediated through the lysine binding sites of plasminogen to specific lysine residues of fibrin; this interaction is virtually completely blocked by the synthetic antifibrinolytic amino acids. It is primarily the high affinity lysine binding site of plasminogen which is involved in its binding to fibrin;

saturation of this binding site with tranexamic acid displaces plasminogen from the fibrin surface.[12] This results in retardation of fibrinolysis because no matter how rapidly plasmin is formed, it cannot bind to fibrinogen or fibrin monomers, thereby precluding the proteolytic action by the serine–histidine enzyme site. Conversely, when the lysine binding sites of plasmin are blocked by tranexamic acid, inactivation by α_2-antiplasmin is virtually impossible.

Fig. 1 Schematic representation of the interactions between fibrin(ogen), plasmin(ogen), α_2-antiplasmin and plasminogen activator. The size of the arrows is roughly proportional to the affinity between the different components

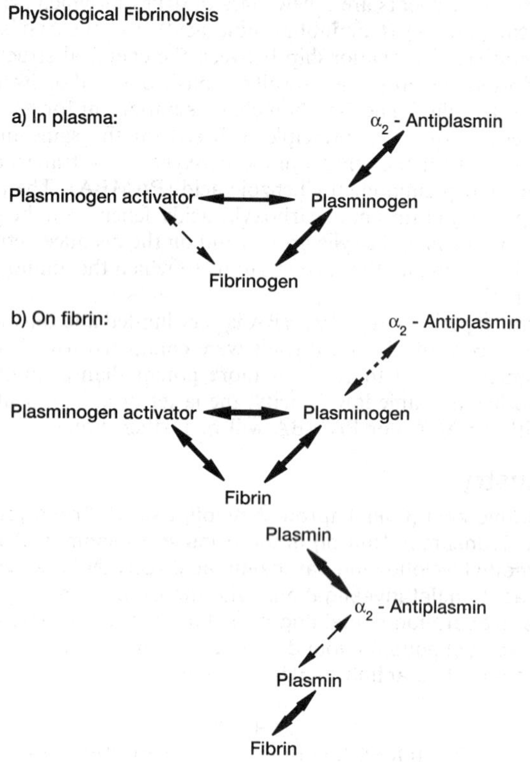

Toxicology

Tranexamic acid has a low acute and chronic toxicity after oral or parenteral administration; for example, the LD_{50} for mice is over 10 g.kg^{-1} after oral administration and 1 to 1.5 g.kg^{-1} after intravenous administration in five species.

In dogs, atrophy of the rod and cone layers in the anterior retina have been reported following oral administration over a period of a year of doses approximately 7 times higher (2 × 800 mg.kg^{-1} daily) than the maximum recommended for man per kilogram body weight per day. Intravenous doses (2 g.kg^{-1} daily) approximately 18 times the maximum recommended for man produced retinal damage in some dogs and cats over 7 days. Such changes were not observed in dogs receiving oral doses about 3.5 times the maximum recommended dose for humans for a year, nor in monkeys receiving approximately 18 times the maximum dose for man intravenously for 1 or 2 weeks. No retinal changes have been found in patients receiving tranexamic acid over periods ranging from several weeks to 6 years.[9]

Therapy with fibrinolytic inhibitors carries a theoretical risk of an increased tendency to thrombosis, and extravascular blood clots formed when the inhibitor is in the circulation may be resistant to physiological fibrinolysis. However, dogs fed 220 mg.kg^{-1} of tranexamic acid daily for 2 weeks showed no microscopic evidence of fibrin deposition in numerous body tissues. Faint signs of fibrin have been detected in renal tissue by electron microscopy.

In teratology studies in mice, rats and rabbits with doses up to 5 g.kg^{-1} daily no fetal abnormalities were found.[4] No adverse effects attributable to tranexamic acid were noted in perinatal and postnatal studies or in fertility studies in rats and the drug has no mutagenic properties.[10]

In one strain of rats receiving daily oral doses (3–5 g.kg^{-1} daily) approximately 27 times higher than the maximum dose recommended for humans, biliary hyperplasia and adenocarcinoma of the liver have been demonstrated after the administration of tranexamic acid for a period of 22 months, but not after 12 months. Such tumours did not occur in rats after oral administration of doses approximately 6 times higher than the maximum recommended for man.

Clinical pharmacology

The antifibrinolytic effect of tranexamic acid is related mainly to a reversible complex formation with a modified plasminogen and the associated conformational changes of this proenzyme.[11]

Defective fibrin formation or excessive rapid dissolution of fibrin results in excessive or recurrent bleeding. The untimely dissolution of haemostatic fibrin can be prevented by antifibrinolytic drugs which stabilize the fibrin structures. Furthermore, antifibrinolytic treatment increases collagen synthesis and tensile strength with granulation tissue, presumably by preserving the fibrin matrix.[13]

Tranexamic acid competitively inhibits the activation of enterokinase (5 × 10^{-2} M) and non-competitively inhibits the proteolytic activity of trypsin at 4-fold greater concentrations.[8] The effect of tranexamic acid on thrombin is still weaker (7 × 10^{-3} M).[7]

Pharmacokinetics

Tranexamic acid is determined in biological fluids by electron capture gas chromatography or by high voltage electrophoresis. The absorption of tranexamic acid from the gastrointestinal tract at a dose of 10 mg.kg^{-1} body weight produces serum levels of 2 to 3 µg.ml^{-1}, a level some 10% less than that found after the corresponding intravenous dose.[7,14] Food has no influence on the absorption of the drug in humans.[14]

Following intravenous administration of 10 mg.kg^{-1} body weight of tranexamic acid, plasma concentrations at 1, 3 and 5 hours after injection are 18, 10 and 5 mg.l^{-1} respectively. The apparent elimination half life has been reported to be 80–120 minutes.[15]

At therapeutic concentrations (5–10 mg.l^{-1}), tranexamic acid is very weakly protein bound, about 3%, and this seems fully accounted for by its binding to plasminogen which is saturated at very low concentrations.

Tranexamic acid displays in humans a considerably higher and more sustained antifibrinolytic activity in tissues than does ε-aminocaproic acid when measured in specimens from the large intestine, kidneys and prostate.[16] The drug also passes into seminal fluid and thereby inhibits its fibrinolytic activity but has no influence on sperm migration.[17] Tranexamic acid is able to cross the blood aqueous barrier in the eyes and the damaged blood–brain barrier as shown in patients with ruptured intracranial aneurysm[18] and rapidly diffuses to the joint fluid and the synovial membrane. It also passes through the placenta and its concentration in cord blood may reach that of the maternal blood.[19] The concentration in breast milk of lactating women one hour after the last dose of a 2-day treatment was about one-hundredth of the peak serum concentration.

Oral absorption	50%
Presystemic metabolism	
Plasma half life	1.4 h
Volume of distribution	1 l.kg^{-1}
Plasma protein binding	negligible

Concentration–effect relationship

The therapeutic concentration of tranexamic acid is 5–10 mg.l^{-1}; at this concentration the protein binding of the drug is very low (circa 3%).

Metabolism

In man, about 30% of the administered dose is recovered in the urine during the first hour after intravenous administration of 10 mg.kg^{-1}, a total of about 45% during the first 3 hours, and about 90% after 24 hours.[7,8] One can therefore conclude that little, if any, metabolism of the drug takes place. Mainly unchanged drug appears in the urine; however, a N-acetylated derivative and a deaminated decarboxylic acid were detected in small quantities. Comparison of the renal clearance of tranexamic acid with the glomerular filtration rate suggests a glomerular filtration without either tubular excretion or absorption.

Pharmaceutics

Tranexamic acid (Cyklokapron, Kabivitrum) is available for intravenous injection in 100 mg per ml solution (5 ml, 10 ml). The tablets contain 500 mg and are white, oblong (UK) or round (W. Germany), flat and stamped 'CY' with an arc above and below the lettering.

A syrup is available containing 500 mg per 5 ml. Diluted with syrup BP it is stable for 14 days.

Therapeutic use

Indications

1. Prevention of bleeding after surgery or trauma
   a. Tooth extraction in patients with haemophilia
   b. Cervical conization
   c. Tonsillectomy and adenoidectomy
   d. Prostatic surgery
   e. Ocular trauma
2. Prevention of rebleeding of subarachnoid haemorrhage
3. Prevention of spontaneous bleeding in haemophilia
4. Treatment of primary or IUD-induced menorrhagia
5. Treatment of gastric and intestinal haemorrhage
6. Treatment of recurrent epistaxis
7. Prevention of spontaneous or postoperative corneal oedema
8. Treatment of hereditary angioneurotic oedema.

Contraindications

1. Severe renal insufficiency
2. Haematuria
3. Disturbances in colour vision
4. High thrombotic risk.

Mode of use

The usual dose of tranexamic acid is 0.5–1 g (10–15 $mg.kg^{-1}$ body weight) given intravenously 2 to 3 times daily starting immediately after surgery and after a few days, 1–1.5 g orally 3 to 4 times daily. There is no need to start the treatment intravenously except in the first days after surgery.

Indications

1. Prevention of bleeding after surgery or trauma

a. Tooth extraction in patients with haemophilia

The oral mucosa and the salivary gland have been found to contain a high concentration of plasminogen activators. This may explain why haemorrhage after oral surgical procedures may be caused by local fibrinolytic activity. Bleeding may be particularly marked in patients with a haemorrhagic diathesis.[19,20]

Forbes et al[21] in a prospective randomized double-blind study found that tranexamic acid, 1 g 3 times a day for 5 days given in conjunction with factor VIII or IX, significantly reduced blood loss and transfusion requirements after dental extraction in patients with haemophilia. Before suturing the site is irrigated with 4.8% tranexamic acid and repeated mouth washes with the same solution for 2 minutes are recommended.[22] Further world wide experience has since confirmed the favourable conclusion of the initial reports. Prior to dental extraction, 25 $mg.kg^{-1}$ tranexamic acid is given intravenously together with a factor VIII or IX concentrate. After surgery, 25 $mg.kg^{-1}$ tranexamic acid is administered orally 3 to 4 times daily for 8 days. Usually, no further substitution therapy with coagulation factor concentrates is required after surgery. The use of tranexamic acid has reduced the need for factor VIII or IX concentrates by 80%, thereby avoiding potential hazards inherent to blood products.[23]

b. Cervical conization

Postoperative bleeding requiring extra measures occurs in about 14% of cases when using the open technique. Since the uterine cervix contains a high concentration of plasminogen activator, it is logical to treat these patients with fibrinolytic inhibitors. Two double-blind trials revealed a significant reduction in blood loss (average of 70%) in patients who received 1.5 g tranexamic acid daily for at least 12 days postoperatively.[24,25]

c. Tonsillectomy and adenoidectomy

In two double-blind trials comparing tranexamic acid (10 $mg.kg^{-1}$) with placebo injected intravenously half an hour before surgery, a significant reduction of blood loss (28%) during the procedure was obtained in the tranexamic group, with less late rebleeding (27% compared with 67%) in the control group.[26,27]

d. Prostatic surgery

Urine contains the plasminogen activator urokinase, which induces the breakdown of blood clots, thereby enhancing bleeding in the urinary tract. Moreover, prostatic tissue contains large amounts of plasminogen activator. These are two reasons for haemorrhages occurring following prostatectomy.

The effects of tranexamic acid on the frequency of haemorrhage in the first days after prostatectomy or in the following 4 weeks have been demonstrated in several controlled trials.[28–31] The incidence of secondary bleeding was reduced from 50% in the control group to 24% in the treatment group. For this indication, the recommended dose is 0.5–1 g (10–15 $mg.kg^{-1}$ body weight) intravenously 2 to 3 times daily starting immediately after surgery during the first 3 postoperative days, and thereafter 1 to 1.5 g orally 3 to 4 times daily until macroscopic haematuria is no longer present. One should be aware, however, that if bleeding is heavy, there is a risk of clot retention in the kidney (high bleeding site, e.g. in non-operated haemophiliacs) or in the ureter with subsequent urinary obstruction.

e. Ocular trauma

Ocular trauma, accidental or surgical, is often accompanied by haemorrhage in the anterior chamber of the eye. The most serious complication of traumatic hyphaema is secondary bleeding, usually occurring in the second to seventh post-traumatic day in some 38% of the patients. Impaired vision or blindness may be the disastrous consequence. The purpose of antifibrinolytic therapy is to prevent rebleeding in the anterior chamber and the vitrous body.

The results of two controlled trials show that tranexamic acid treatment (1 g three times daily) significantly reduces the frequency of secondary haemorrhage.[32,33] These findings support the favourable impression of 5 other trials with historical controls.[34–38]

It is reasonable to conclude that tranexamic acid protects the haemostatic plug from premature dissolution, sealing the damaged vessel and preventing secondary haemorrhage after traumatic hyphaema without having to confine the patient to bed rest. A disadvantage is that antifibrinolytic treatment delays dissolution of the primary clot and is therefore contraindicated in massive intraocular haemorrhage (filling more than half the anterior chamber).

2. Prevention of rebleeding in subarachnoid haemorrhage

Numerous isolated case reports and 13 uncontrolled clinical trials have provided data either in favour or against treatment with ε-aminocaproic acid or tranexamic acid.[39] In addition to an American cooperative study,[40] seven randomized controlled clinical trials using tranexamic acid in the management of ruptured cerebral aneurysm have been published. Four were in favour[41–44] while four others question the benefit of the drug in terms of rebleeding incidence.[45–48] This discrepancy may be due to multiple clinical and therapeutic variables and to flaws in methodology. As noted above, tranexamic acid passes the blood–brain barrier, and it suppresses fibrinolytic activity mainly in the leptomeninges. This treatment can be considered during the first 10 days and initial benefit appears sometimes to be lost due to delayed cerebral ischaemic deficits. The total mortality was recently shown not to be reduced at 3 months in the tranexamic acid treated group compared to the control, not because absence of reduced rebleeding (24% in the control group versus 9% in the tranexamic group, $P<0.001$) but as a result of increased incidence of ischaemic complications (15% in the control group, 24% in the tranexamic group, $P<0.01$).[44] Until some method can be found to minimize ischaemic complications, tranexamic acid is of no benefit in patients with subarachnoid haemorrhage.

There is a suggestion that low dose tranexamic acid (3 g daily) together with aprotinin (400 000 KIU daily) would be a more rational combination for lowering the rebleeding incidence without late ischaemic complications and post-subarachnoid haemorrhage.[49]

3. Prevention of spontaneous bleeding in haemophilia
Tranexamic acid has been used as prophylaxis against spontaneous bleeding episodes in haemophilia in a dose of 2 g daily. Home prophylaxis and treatment with factor VIII or IX concentrates is at present the preferred treatment.

4. Treatment of primary or IUD-induced menorrhagia
In a random population 9–11% of the women have menstrual blood loss in excess of 80 ml per period. This is the upper limit of normal because blood loss in excess of this frequently causes iron deficiency anaemia.[50] Antifibrinolytic drugs have been investigated in women with essential menorrhagia. The rationale for this treatment is that these patients have higher plasminogen activator levels in the endometrium on the first day of the period compared with women having normal menstrual blood loss.[51]

Four clinical trials, three of which were randomized, double-blind cross-over studies with tranexamic acid[52–54] showed, in terms of comparison between menstrual blood losses during a control period and treatment period, a dose-dependent reduction (35 to 51%) of menstrual blood loss in essential menorrhagia. The dose recommended for this indication is 1–1.5 g (12–25 $mg.kg^{-1}$ body weight) of tranexamic acid orally 3 to 4 times daily for 3 to 4 days. The treatment is started when the bleeding has become profuse.

A second situation frequently associated with excessive menstrual blood loss is the use of inert or, to a lesser degree, copper intrauterine devices. A comparative study showed that 51% of Lippes D users had menstrual blood losses above 80 ml, as did 25% of the Cu 7 users.[55] This increase may be due to a higher local fibrinolytic activity in the endometrium.[56,57] A well designed controlled trial in women with an inserted inert or copper releasing intrauterine device has demonstrated that 6 g of tranexamic acid daily reduced significantly the uterine blood loss[58] from 82.7% to 11.5%.

In another double-blind trial tranexamic acid and a prostaglandin synthesis inhibitor were compared in women with an intrauterine contraceptive device.[59] The mean menstrual blood loss before treatment was 135 ml and fell to 102 ml on the prostaglandin synthesis inhibitor and to 59 ml on tranexamic acid. More women on tranexamic acid complained of side effects but in none was the drug withdrawn.

5. Treatment of gastric and intestinal haemorrhage
In eight randomized, double-blind studies, the effect of tranexamic acid was evaluated in patients with bleeding in the upper gastrointestinal tract.[60–67] Bleeding was distal to oesophagogastric junction and presumably was most often due to diffuse gastritis and erosive gastroduodenitis. In the light of these studies, it would appear appropriate to give antifibrinolytic drugs in addition to customary forms of treatment in patients with gastroduodenal bleeding.

There is a preliminary evidence that tranexamic acid may be useful in patients with giant hypertrophic gastritis (Menetrier's disease).[68] Local fibrinolytic activity also occurs in the colon, more particularly around small submucosal vessels as noted in biopsy material of patients with active ulcerative colitis.[69,70] A group of such patients were treated with enemas containing 5 g tranexamic acid dissolved in 100 ml of warm water administered twice daily for 6 months;[69] in all patients with pathologically increased fibrinolytic activity in the mucosa, remission of the disorder was obtained. In addition to these uncontrolled trials, two double-blind trials have been reported, one with equivocal results.[71] The second was conducted in patients with ulcerative colitis in a stable phase and revealed that oral tranexamic acid (1.5 g thrice daily) resulted in a significant reduction of rectal haemorrhages but was without effect on stool frequency or consistency.[72]

6. Treatment of recurrent epistaxis
Diffuse bleeding from the anterior portion of the nose can easily be treated with a cotton wool pledget impregnated with decongestant nose drops. For persistent nose-bleeds, the cotton wool or Spongostan can be impregnated with tranexamic acid solution and left in place until it falls out by itself after a few days. Patients treated by packing could also be given tranexamic acid orally.[73]

7. Prevention of spontaneous or postoperative corneal oedema
Endothelial dystrophy is a degenerative disease of the cornea (Fuchs' disease) beginning in the central portion of the corneal endothelium causing pain and progressive impaired vision. Systemic treatment with tranexamic acid has been investigated in this condition.[74] Corneal oedema is also seen in connection with cataract extraction and trabeculectomy.

Two double-blind trials in postoperative corneal oedema after cataract operation[75] and trabeculectomy[76] revealed that tranexamic acid is effective in reducing corneal thickness and associated with improved visual activity.

8. Treatment of hereditary angioneurotic oedema
Hereditary angioneurotic oedema is an autosomal dominant disease and is due to a deficiency of C1-esterase inhibitor. A deficiency of this inhibitor may lead to an uncontrolled activation of the complement system and overproduction of fragments of C2, C3 and C5, many of which have vasoactive properties. C_1-esterase inhibitor also impedes the action of kallikrein on the kininogen conversion and neutralizes plasmin. This disease is characterized by recurrent, transient and non-itching oedema of the skin and of the mucosa of the gastrointestinal and upper respiratory tracts, associated with acute attacks of abdominal pain and risk of asphyxiation respectively.

The results of two randomized double-blind cross-over trials with tranexamic acid versus placebo revealed a reduction in the number and severity of the attacks of oedema.[77,78]

9. Prevention of bleeding in acute promyelocytic leukaemia
Patients with acute promyelocytic leukaemia often develop a bleeding diathesis during treatment which can be predicted by a decrease of α-2-antiplasmin below 30% of normal. Treatment with a fibrinolytic inhibitor was shown to be effective in an open study[79] but also in a double-blind trial.[80].

Contraindications

Care should be taken in patients with renal insufficiency due to risk of drug accumulation and in pronounced haematuria as renal or ureteric obstruction may develop due to clots resistant to spontaneous lysis because of the high content of tranexamic acid in the urine. The drug should probably not be given to patients with acquired disturbance of colour vision and in patients with a high risk of thrombosis.

Adverse reactions

Potentially life-threatening effects
There is a theoretical risk of an increased thrombotic tendency during treatment with fibrinolysis inhibitors.[81] A few patients have developed intracranial thrombosis during treatment with tranexamic acid. This association may be fortuitous, although further observations are needed to assess the reality of this suspected hazard.

Acute overdosage
No information on acute overdosage is available.

Severe or irreversible adverse effects
It is well known that extravascular blood clots formed when the inhibitor is in the circulation may be resistant to physiological fibrinolysis (e.g. thrombi in the renal pelvis or bladder in patients with haematuria) and this explains occasional pain and obstruction of urine flow. It should be mentioned that a few cases of acute renal failure and myopathy have been described but only with EACA and most probably this was an idiosyncratic response.[82]

Symptomatic adverse effects
Adverse effects of tranexamic acid are rare and mainly limited to nausea or diarrhoea, and occasionally an orthostatic reaction. These effects may occur more readily after rapid intravenous infusion. Purpuric rashes have been observed during treatment with EACA, but not with tranexamic acid.[83]

Interference with clinical pathology tests
No information is available on this subject.

High risk groups

Neonates
As mentioned above, it is not known whether reduction of the normally high fibrinolytic activity in the neonate is harmful.

Breast milk. Tranexamic acid is secreted in the mother's milk. This concentration is only a hundredth of the corresponding serum levels[84] and the drug may be given during lactation without risk to the child.

Tranexamic acid

Children

There is no contraindication to the use of the drug in children.

Pregnant women

Tranexamic acid crosses over to the fetus.[19] It is not known whether a reduction of the normally high fibrinolytic activity in the fetus and neonate is harmful.

The elderly

No special precautions are necessary in the elderly unless there is evidence of impaired renal function.

Concurrent disease

Renal disease. In patients with serum creatinine concentration of 120–150 μmol.l^{-1}, 10 mg.kg^{-1} tranexamic acid may be administered intravenously twice daily. In those with serum creatinine concentrations between 250 and 500 μmol.l^{-1}, the same dose may be given at 24-hour intervals, and in those with serum creatinine concentrations over 500 μmol.l^{-1} the same dose may be given at 48-hour intervals.[85]

Drug interactions

Potentially hazardous interactions

Tranexamic acid can be mixed with most solutions such as electrolyte, carbohydrate, amino acid and dextran solutions. It is compatible with heparin. The drug should not be mixed with transfusion blood or with infusion solutions containing penicillin.

Potentially useful interactions

No reactions of this kind appear to have been reported.

General review articles

Ogston D 1984 Antifibrinolytic drugs: chemistry, pharmacology, and clinical usage. John Caley and Son

Verstraete M 1977 Haemostatic drugs. A critical appraisal. Martinus Nijhoff Medical Division, The Hague

Verstraete M 1985 Clinical application of inhibitors of fibrinolysis. Drugs 29: 236–261

References

1. Okamoto S, Hijikata A 1975 Rational approach to proteinase inhibitors. Drug Design 6: 143–169
2. Sjoerdsma A, Nilsson I M 1960 Alipathic amino compounds as inhibitors of plasminogen activation. Proceedings of the Society of Experimental Biology and Medicine 103: 533–538
3. Stürzebrecher J, Markwardt F 1982 Synthetische Inhibitoren des Thrombosis und andere Gerinnungsenzyme. Struktur und Wirkung. Beitrage zur Wirkstofforschung 16: 1–92
4. Melander B, Gleneecki G, Grandstrand B, Hanshoff G 1965 Biochemistry and toxicology of Amikapron: the antifibrinolytic active isomer of AMCHA. Acta Pharmacologica et Toxicologica 22: 340–362
5. Okamoto S, Sato S, Takada Y, Okamoto U 1964 An active stereo isomer (trans form) of AMCHA and its fibrinolytic (antiplasminic) action in vitro and in vivo. Keio Journal of Medicine 13: 177–185
6. Markwardt F 1978 Synthetic inhibitors of fibrinolysis. In: Markwardt F (ed) Fibrinolytics and antifibrinolytics. Springer Verlag, Berlin, pp 511–577
7. Andersson L, Nilsson I M, Nilehn J E, Hedner U, Grandstrand B, Melander B 1965 Experimental and clinical studies on AMCA, the antifibrinolytic active isomer of p-aminomethyl cyclohexane carboxylic acid. Scandinavian Journal of Haematology 2: 230–247
8. Dubber A H, McNicol G P, Douglas A S 1965 Amino methyl cyclohexane carboxylic acid (AMCHA). A new synthetic fibrinolytic inhibitor. British Journal of Haematology 11: 237–245
9. Theil P L 1981 Ophtalmological examination of patients in long-term treatment with tranexamic acid. Acta Ophthalmologica 59: 237–241
10. Shimada H, Nagai E, Monta H, Akimoto T 1979 Mutagenicity studies of tranexamic acid. Oyo Yakuri 18: 165–172
11. Thorsen S 1975 Differences in the binding to fibrin of native plasminogen and plasminogen modified by proteolytic degradation. Influence of omega amino-carboxylic acid. Biochimica et Biophysica Acta 393: 55–65
12. Hoylaerts M, Lijnen H R, Collen D 1981 Studies on the mechanism of antifibrinolytic action of tranexamic acid. Biochimica et Biophysica Acta 673: 75–85
13. Kwaan H C, Astrup T 1969 Tissue repair in presence of locally applied inhibitors of fibrinolysis. Experimental and Molecular Pathology 11: 82–88
14. Eriksson O, Kjellman H, Schannong M 1971 The biological availability of Cyclokapron tablets compared with Cyklokapron solution administered orally. Data on file, Kabi AB, Stockholm
15. Kaller H 1967 Enterale Resorption, Verteilung und Elimination von 4-aminomethylcyclohexancarbonsäure (AMCHA) und ε-aminocapronsäure (EACS) bein Menschen. Naunyn-Schmiedebergs Archif für Pharmacologie und Experimentelle Pathologie 256: 160–168
16. Andersson L, Nilsson I M, Colleen S, Grandstrand B, Melander B 1968 Role of urokinase and tissue activator in sustaining bleeding and the management thereof with EACA and AMCA. Annals of the New York Academy of Sciences 146: 642–658
17. Liedholm P, Astedt B, Kullander S 1973 Passage of tranexamic acid (AMCA) to semen in man and its effect on the fibrinolytic activity and in migration of spermatozoa. Fertility and Sterility 24: 517–520
18. Tovi D, Thulin C A 1972 The ability of tranexamic acid to cross the blood–brain barrier and diffuse in patients with ruptured intracranial aneurysms. Acta Neurologica Scandinavica 48: 257
19. Walzman M, Bonnar J 1982 Effects of tranexamic acid on the coagulation and fibrinolytic systems in pregnancy complicated by placental bleeding. Archives of Toxicology 5 (Suppl): 214–220
20. Vinckier F, Vermylen J 1984 Wound healing following dental extraction in rabbits: effects of tranexamic acid, warfarin anticoagulation, and socket packing. Journal of Dental Research 63: 646–649
21. Forbes C D, Barr R D, Reed G et al 1972 Tranexamic acid in control of haemorrhage after dental extraction in haemophilia and christmas disease. British Medical Journal 2: 311–313
22. Sindet-Pedersen S, Ramström G, Bernvil S, Blombäck M 1989 Hemostatic effect of tranexamic acid mouthwash on anticoagulant-treated patients undergoing oral surgery. New England Journal of Medicine 320: 840–843
23. Evans B E, Aledort L M 1976 Hemophilia and dental treatment. Journal of the American Dental Association 96: 827–834
24. Landin L E, Weiner E 1975 Late bleeding after conization. The effect of tranexamic acid (Cyclokapron). Opuscular Medica 20: 280–284
25. Rybo G, Westerberg H 1976 The effect of tranexamic acid (AMCA) on postoperative bleeding after conization. Acta Obstetrica et Gynecologica Scandinavica 51: 347–350
26. Verstraete M, Tyberghein J, de Greef Y, Daems L, Van Hoof A 1977 Double-blind trials with ethamsylate, batroxobin or tranexamic acid on blood loss after adenotonsillectomy. Acta Clinica Belge 32: 136–141
27. Castelli G, Vogt E 1977 Der Erfol einer antifibrinolytische Behandlung mit Tranexamsaure zur Reduktion der Blutverlustes während und nach Tonsillektomien. Schweizerische Medizinische Wochenchrift 107: 780–784
28. Hedlung P O 1969 Antifibrinolytic therapy with Cyclokapron in connection with prostatectomy. Scandinavian Journal of Urology and Nephrology 3: 177–182
29. Kaufmann J, Siefker K 1969 Medikamentöse genkung postoperatiever Blutungen nach Prostatiktomien. Urologie 8: 57–59
30. Rö J S, Knutrud O, Stormorken H 1970 Antifibrinolytic treatment with tranexamic acid (AMCHA) in pediatric urinary tract surgery. Journal of Pediatric Surgery 5: 315–320
31. Gamba G, Fornasari P M, Grignani G, Dolci D, Colloi D 1979 Haemostasis during transverical prostatic adenectomy. Blut 39: 89–98
32. Jerndal T, Frisén M 1976 Tranexamic acid (AMCA) and late hyphaema. A double-blind study in cataract surgery. Acta Ophthalmologica 54: 417–429
33. Varnek L, Dalsgaard C, Hansen A, Klie F 1980 The effect of tranexamic acid on secondary haemorrhage after traumatic hyphaema. Acta Ophthalmologica 58: 787–793
34. Bramsen T 1976 Traumatic hyphaema treated with the antifibrinolytic drug tranexamic acid. I. Acta Ophthalmologica 54: 250–256
35. Bramsen T 1977 Traumatic hyphaema treated with the antifibrinolytic drug tranexamic acid. II. Acta Ophthalmologica 55: 616–620
36. Kamp Mortensen K, Sjölie A K 1978 Secondary haemorrhage following traumatic hyphaema. A comparative study of conservative and tranexamic treatment. Acta Ophthalmologica 56: 763–768
37. Missotten L, de Clippeleer L, Van Tornout I, Beenders P 1977 The value of tranexamic acid (Cyclokapron) in the prevention of secondary bleeding, a complication of traumatic hyphaema. Bulletin de la Société Belge d'Ophthalmologie 179: 47–52
38. Uusitalo R J, Saari M S, Aine E, Saair K M 1981 Tranexamic acid in the prevention of secondary haemorrhage after traumatic hyphaema. Acta Ophthalmologica 59: 539–545
39. Ramirez-Lassepas M 1981 Antifibrinolytic therapy in subarachnoid hemorrhage caused by ruptured intracranial bleeding. Neurology 31: 316–322
40. Nibblelink D W 1975 Cooperative aneurysm study: antihypertensive and antifibrinolytic therapy following subarachnoid haemorrhage from ruptured intracranial aneurysm. In: Whismant et al (eds) Cerebral vascular disease. Grune and Stratton, New York, pp 155–173
41. Chandra B 1978 Treatment of subarachnoid hemorrhage from ruptured intracranial aneurysm with tranexamic acid: a double blind clinical trial. Annals of Neurology 3: 502–504
42. Fodstad H, Liliequeist B, Shannong M, Thulin C A 1978 Tranexamic acid in the preoperative management of ruptured intracranial aneurisms. Surgical Neurology 10: 9–15
43. Maurice-Williams R C 1978 Prolonged antifibrinolytics: an effective non-surgical treatment for ruptured intracranial aneurysms? British Medical Journal 1: 945–947
44. Vermeulen M, Lindsay K W, Murray G D et al 1984 Antifibrinolytic treatment in subarachnoid hemorrhage. New England Journal of Medicine 311: 432–437
45. Fodstad H, Forsell A, Liliequeist B, Schannong M 1981 Antifibrinolysis with tranexamic acid in aneurysmal subarachnoid haemorrhage: a consecutive controlled trial. Neurosurgery 8: 158–165
46. Gelmers J H 1980 Prevention of recurrence of spontaneous subarachnoid haemorrhage by tranexamic acid. Acta Neurochirurgica 52: 45–50
47. Kaste M, Ramsay M 1969 Tranexamic acid in subarachnoid hemorrhage. A double-blind study. Stroke 10: 519–522
48. Van Rossum J, Wintzen A R, Endtz L J, Schoen J H R, Jorge H 1977 Effect of tranexamic acid on rebleeding after subarachnoid hemorrhage: a double-blind controlled clinical trial. Annals of Neurology 2: 238–242
49. Guidetti B, Spallone A 1976 The role of antifibrinolytic therapy in the preoperative management of recently ruptured intracranial aneurysms. Surgical Neurology 15: 239–248
50. Hallberg L, Högdahl A M, Nilsson L, Rybo G 1966 Menstrual blood loss – a population study. Acta Obstetrica et Gynecologica Scandinavica 45: 320–351
51. Rybo G 1966 Plasminogen activators in the endometrium II. Clinical aspects. Acta Obstetrica et Gynecologica Scandinavica 45: 429–450

52. Callender S T, Warner G T, Cope E 1970 Treatment of menorrhagia with tranexamic acid. A double blind trial. British Medical Journal 4: 214–216
53. Nilsson L, Rybo G 1967 Treatment of menorrhagia with an antifibrinolytic agent, tranexamic acid (AMCA). A double blind investigation. Acta Obstetrica et Gynecologica Scandinavica 46: 572–580
54. Vermylen J, Verhaege-Declercq M L, Verstraete M, Fierens F 1968 A double-blind study of the effect of tranexamic acid in essential menorrhagia. Thrombosis et Diathesis Haemorrhagica 20: 583–587
55. Guillebaud J, Bonnar J, Morehead J, Matthews A 1976 Menstrual blood-loss with intrauterine devices. Lancet 1: 387–390
56. Kasonde J M, Bonnar J 1976 Plasminogen activators in the endometrium of women using intrauterine contraceptive devices. British Journal of Obstetrics and Gynaecology 83: 315–319
57. Larsson B, Liedholm P, Astedt B 1975 Increased fibrinolytic activity in the endometrium of patients using copper IUD (Gravigard). International Journal of Fertility 20: 77–80
58. Weström L, Bengtsson L P 1970 Effect of tranexamic acid (AMCA) in menorrhagia with intrauterine contraceptive devices. Journal of Reproductive Medicine 5: 154–161
59. Ylkiorkala O, Viinikka L 1983 Comparison between antifibrinolytic and prostaglandin treatment in the reduction of increased menstrual blood loss in women with intrauterine contraceptive devices. British Journal of Obstetrics and Gynaecology 90: 78–83
60. Barer D, Ogilvie A, Coggon D, Henry D, Atkinson M, Langman M J S 1982 Cimetidine and tranexamic acid in the treatment of acute upper gastrointestinal bleeding. Unpublished data
61. Barer D, Ogilvie A, Henry D et al 1983 Cimetidine and tranexamic acid in the treatment of acute upper gastrointestinal tract bleeding. New England Journal of Medicine 308: 1571–1575
62. Bergqvist D, Dahlgren S, Hessman Y 1980 Local inhibition of the fibrinolytic system in patients with massive upper gastrointestinal hemorrhage. Uppsala Journal of Medical Science 85: 173–178
63. Biggs J C, Hugh T B, Dodds A J 1976 Tranexamic acid and upper gastrointestinal haemorrhage. A double blind trial. Gut 17: 729–734
64. Cormack F, Chakrabart R R, Jouhar A J, Fearnley G R 1973 Tranexamic acid in upper gastrointestinal haemorrhage. Lancet 1: 1207–1208
65. Engqvist A, Boström O, von Feilitzen F et al 1979 Tranexamic acid in massive haemorrhage from the upper gastrointestinal tract. A double-blind study. Scandinavian Journal of Gastroenterology 14: 839–844
66. Stael von Holstein C, Eriksson S B S, Källen R 1987 Tranexamic acid as an aid to reducing blood transfusion requirements in gastric and duodenal bleeding. British Medical Journal 294: 7–10
67. Henry D A, O'Connell D L 1989 Effects of fibrinolytic inhibitors on mortality from upper gastrointestinal haemorrhage. British Medical Journal 298: 1142–1146
68. Kondo M, Ibezaki M, Kato H, Masuda M 1978 Antifibrinolytic therapy of giant hypertrophic gastritis (Menetrier's disease). Scandinavian Journal of Gastroenterology 13: 851–856
69. Kondo M, Fukomoto K, Yoshikawa T et al 1981 Tissue fibrinolysis in the digestive mucosa. III. Treatment of ulcerative colitis by the direct administration of an antifibrinolytic agent as an enema. Nippon Shokakibyo Gakkai Zasshi 3: 653–657
70. Kwaan H C, Cocco A, Medenloff A I, Astrup T 1969 Fibrinolytic activity in the normal and inflamed rectal mucosa. Scandinavian Journal of Gastroenterology 4: 441–445
71. Mowat N A G, Douglas A S, Brunt P W, McIntosch J A R, King P C, Boddy K 1973 Epsilon aminocaproic acid therapy in ulcerative colitis. American Journal of Digestive Diseases 18: 959–965
72. Hollanders D, Thomson J M, Schofield P F 1983 Tranexamic acid therapy in ulcerative colitis. Postgraduate Medical Journal 58: 87–91
73. Petruson B 1974 A double-blind study to evaluate the effect of epistaxis with oral administration of the antifibrinolytic drug tranexamic acid (cyclokaptron) Acta Oto-Laryngologica (suppl 317): 57–61
74. Bramsen T, Ehlers N 1977 Bullous keratopathy (Fuchs' endothelial dystrophy) treated systemically with 4-trans-aminocyclohexano-carboxylic acid. Acta Ophthalmologica 55: 665–673
75. Bramsen T, Corydon L, Ehlers N 1978 A double-blind study of the influence of tranexamic acid on the central corneal thickness after cataract extraction. Acta Ophthalmologica 56: 121–126
76. Bramsen T 1978 A double-blind study on the influence of tranexamic acid on the intraocular pressure and the central corneal thickness after trabeculectomy for glaucoma simplex. Acta Ophthalmologica 56: 998–1005
77. Blohmé G 1972 Treatment of hereditary angioneurotic oedema with tranexamic acid. A random double-blind cross-over study. Acta Medica Scandinavica 192: 293–298
78. Scheffer A L, Austin K F, Rosen F S 1972 Tranexamic acid therapy in hereditary angioneurotic oedema. New England Journal of Medicine 287: 452–454
79. Schwartz B S, Williams E C, Conlan M G, Mosher D F 1986 Epsilon-amino-caproic acid in the treatment of patients with acute promyelocytic leukemia and acquired alpha-2-plasmin inhibitor deficiency Annals of Internal Medicine 105: 873–877
80. Arrisati G, Buller H R, Hn Cate J W, Mandelli F 1989 Tranexamic acid for control of haemorrhage in acute Promyelocytic leukaemia. The Lancet ii: 122–124
81. Markwardt F, Nowak G, Meerbach W, Rüdiger K D 1976 The influence of drugs on disseminated intravascular coagulation (DIC). I. Effects of antifibrinolytics and fibrinolytics on thrombin-induced DIC in rats. Thrombosis Research 9: 143–152
82. Biswas C K, Reid Milligan D A, Agte S D, Kenward D H, Tillex P J B 1980 Acute renal failure and myopathy after treatment with aminocaproic acid. British Medical Journal 2: 115–116
83. Chakrabarti A, Collet K A 1980 Purpuric rash due to epsilon-aminocaproic acid. British Medical Journal 2: 197–198

84. Eriksson O, Kjellman H, Nilsson L 1971 Tranexamic acid in human milk after oral administration of Cyklokapron[R] to lactating women. Data on file, Kabi A B, Stockholm
85. Andersson L, Erikson O, Hedlund P O, Kjellman H, Lindqvist B 1978 Special considerations with regard to the dosage of tranexamic acid in patients with chronic renal diseases. Urological Research 6: 83–88

Tranylcypromine (sulphate)

Tranylcypromine is the only non-hydrazine monoamine oxidase inhibitor currently in use in psychiatry. It has a molecular structure similar to that of amphetamine although its pharmacological effects are rather different.

Chemistry

Tranylcypromine (Parnate)
$C_9H_{11}N)_2.H_2SO_4$
(dl)-trans-2-Phenylcyclopropylamine sulphate

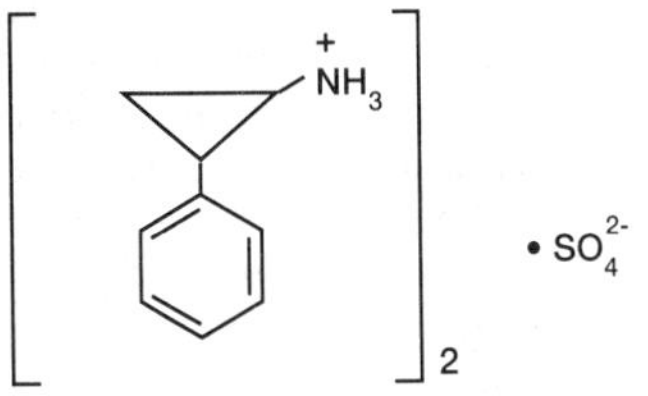

Molecular weight (free base)	364.5 (133.2)
pKa (amino group)	8.2
Solubility	
in alcohol	virtually insoluble
in water	1 in 25
Octanol/water partition coefficient	—

A white or almost white crystalline powder, odourless and with an acid taste. Tranylcypromine is also available in an oral combination product with trifluoperazine (Parstelin).

Pharmacology

Tranylcypromine produces inactivation of monoamine oxidase (MAO) subtypes A and B, and this is usually thought to be an irreversible step. It is thought that this involves a sulfhydryl group in the active centre of the enzyme reacting with an imine following the action of MAO. Maximal inhibition of the enzyme is achieved within a few days of giving tranylcypromine. A single dose has been shown to increase levels of noradrenaline, adrenaline, dopamine and 5-hydroxytryptamine in a variety of body tissues.[1] The drug is thought to act as an antidepressant by increasing synaptic concentrations of monoamines in the brain. Unlike amphetamine tranylcypromine does not have an immediate effect.

Toxicology

Studies on rats and rabbits have failed to show any evidence of teratogenicity, but no data is available on the possible mutagenic nature of this drug.

Clinical pharmacology

Two functional forms of monoamine oxidase have been demonstrated, subtypes A and B. Pargyline and clorgyline selectively block types A and B respectively. Tranylcypromine is not selective in its action, but its therapeutic effect is believed to be due to inhibition of subtype A.

Tranylcypromine also causes the release of dopamine and blocks its reuptake, probably causing its amphetamine-like properties, such as increased motor activity and hypersensitivity to external stimuli. Tranylcypromine is unlike amphetamine (in spite of structural similarities) in the sense that tolerance to its effects is rare. Tranylcypromine does not replace amphetamine in patients dependent on the latter drug.

MAO inhibitors are potent suppressors of REM sleep and this effect has been used therapeutically in narcolepsy. However, the effects on the EEG in man are slight.

Liver enzymes involved with the metabolism of barbiturates, opiates and hypoglycaemic agents are affected, with clinical consequences (see below).

Pharmacokinetics

High resolution gas chromatography with AFID detection is the analytical method of choice, with a limit of sensitivity of 2 μg.l^{-1}.[2]

Tranylcypromine is rapidly absorbed from the gastrointestinal tract following oral administration and distributed widely throughout the body, including the brain and liver.[3,4] Peak plasma concentrations occur within 1 hour of dosing. Its pharmacokinetics are poorly understood because its inactive metabolites are difficult to detect. There is evidence of presystemic elimination.[5]

The plasma half life is between 1.5 and 2.7 hours depending on the dosage schedule, urinary pH and enantiomer used.[6–8] No details are known about its binding to plasma protein or the effects of disease on this and other aspects of pharmacokinetics. Tranylcypromine has been detected in breast milk.

The drug is extensively metabolized, probably in the liver. Small amounts of the drug (usually < 2%) are excreted unchanged in the urine. Acidification of the urine can increase this to 8%.

Oral absorption	extensive
Presystemic metabolism	may occur
Plasma half life	
range	1.5–2.7 h
mean	2 h
Volume of distribution	—
Plasma protein binding	—

Concentration–effect relationship

The therapeutic effect is not related to the plasma concentration of tranylcypromine,[9–11] but to the extent of monoamine oxidase inhibition. Monoamine oxidase inhibition occurs throughout the body[12–14] and a therapeutic effect has been shown to require at least 80% inhibition of platelet monoamine oxidase. However, despite almost immediate enzyme inhibition following the start of tranylcypromine therapy, the clinical effect usually takes a week to become manifest and may be delayed for 2–3 weeks.

Metabolism

The metabolism of tranylcypromine, which occurs in the liver, is almost complete (90–95%) with only 5% of the drug being excreted unchanged in the urine.

Three main pathways of metabolism have been described: acetylation to N-acetyltranylcypromine, decyclization to hippuric acid, and glucuronic acid conjugation (Fig. 1).

These metabolites are pharmacologically inactive. Amphetamine, chemically similar to tranylcypromine, has been found in the blood after overdosage, but has not been found when a therapeutic dosage regime has been used.[15]

Although one of these pathways involves acetylation, there is no evidence to indicate that the acetylator status of a subject determines whether a high dose (40–60 mg) rather than a low dose (10–30 mg daily) influences clinical outcome in the way that has been observed with phenelzine.

Pharmaceutics

Tranylcypromine is only available in tablet form. Tablets contain 10 mg of tranylcypromine sulphate and are geranium-red, sugar-coated and marked 'SKF' (SmithKline Beecham, UK) or marked 'PARNATE SKF' (SmithKline Beecham, USA)

Tranylcypromine is also available as a combined preparation with trifluoperazine. These tablets contain 10 mg tranylcypromine as the sulphate and 1 mg trifluoperazine as the hydrochloride; they are green and marked 'SKF'.

Fig. 1 Metabolism of tranylcypromine

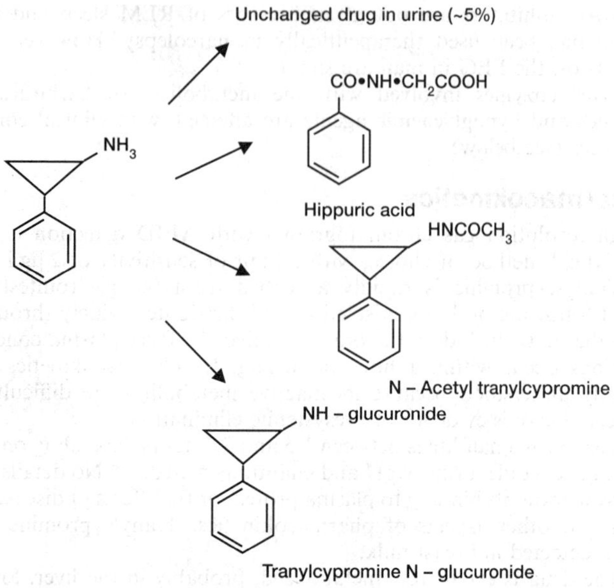

The tablets should be stored in a dry place; Parnate tablets are stable, with a shelf-life of 5 years and are said not to contain potentially allergenic substances; the shelf-life of Parstelin tablets is shorter. Tablets should be dispensed with a warning card informing of the dangers of interaction with other drugs and food containing tyramine (see below).

Therapeutic use

Indications

1. Depressive disorders both psychotic and neurotic.

Other uses

2. Anxiety/phobic states
3. Obsessional states.

Contraindications

1. Cerebrovascular disease
2. Severe cardiovascular disease
3. Liver disease
4. Blood dyscrasia
5. Phaeochromocytoma
6. Hyperthyroidism
7. Alcohol or drug abusers.

Mode of use

The usual starting dose is 10 mg twice daily and, because of the possible alerting nature of this drug, the second dose should be given in the early afternoon. The dose can be increased after one week to 30 mg daily, although some authors[16] recommend that up to 40–60 mg daily can be tried, particularly if the patient is unresponsive at a lower dose. The evidence for higher doses being more effective is slight and is based indirectly on studies involving phenelzine.

Tranylcypromine, possibly through its effect on the dopaminergic system, can produce a dramatic effect after only a few days, unlike other monoamine oxidase inhibitors. However, it is worth continuing treatment for four weeks, even if no clinical benefit is seen initially. Because of the delay in response and subsequent risk of poor compliance, short-term use of a benzodiazepine should be considered where symptoms of anxiety are prominent.

There are no clear guidelines as to the duration of treatment; when a therapeutic response has been obtained, the dosage can be reduced to a maintenance level of 10–20 mg daily.

In view of the possible risk of addiction and abuse,[17,18] the use of tranylcypromine should be closely monitored. Patients may experience difficulties in stopping this drug, but whether this is due to a withdrawal state or the re-emergence of the chronic mental disorder being treated is unclear.

Tranylcypromine (sulphate)

Indications

There are no conditions for which tranylcypromine is to be regarded as the primary drug of choice. Evidence for its effectiveness in treating anxiety and phobic states is based indirectly on studies using other monoamine oxidase inhibitors. It has more of a euphoric and antidepressant effect than other monoamine oxidase inhibitors, but no study has shown it to be more effective than tricyclic antidepressants in treating depressive disorder.

In view of the increased incidence of side effects and the dietary restrictions that have to be observed, it should be regarded as a second-line measure for treating patients who have not responded to a tricyclic antidepressant, unless a rapid response to treatment is desired or if there is evidence that tranylcypromine has previously proved effective.

1. Depression, both psychotic and neurotic

When discussing the effectiveness of tranylcypromine, one immediately runs into the problems of classification. This is still an area of controversy and numerous classifications and rating scales vie for universal acceptance. At the time of the early studies the type of depression was unspecified, but an idea of its severity can be had by considering whether the subjects were seen in hospital or outpatients. On the whole, inpatients were used and tranylcypromine was shown to be no more effective than placebo.[19,20] Tyrer[21] suggested that inadequate dosages may have been one reason for the earlier ineffectiveness and recommended that up to 60 mg be used per day.

For the purpose of this review, depression will be considered under the established headings of neurotic and psychotic and the reader will have to accept that some classifications, such as the DSM III with its diagnostic category of major depressive disorder, straddle both groups.

Psychotic depression

Tranylcypromine is not regarded as a first-line treatment for psychotic depression. The only exceptions would be in a patient where previous treatment with the same drug proved effective or where a first degree relative had responded to a similar drug in the past. The latter recommendation is based on work by Pare[22] but the problems of diagnosing an absent relative and assessing their response to treatment are considerable. Tranylcypromine has been used as the sole antidepressant or in combination with a tricyclic antidepressant.

Tranylcypromine alone. It has been compared with tricyclic antidepressants and been shown to be of similar efficacy, but not superior.[23,24] Shaw recommends that it be used as a second option if a tricyclic antidepressant fails. Tranylcypromine has been compared with placebo in 59 patients fulfilling the Research Diagnostic Criteria for major affective disorder and it was found to be particularly effective in a subgroup of patients where features of anergia and hypersomnia were prominent. Nolen[25] reports that patients with major depressive disorder by DSM III criteria who were resistant to various treatments, not including ECT, responded favourably to tranylcypromine in 58% of cases.

In combination with tricyclic antidepressants. The combination of a monoamine oxidase inhibitor and a tricyclic antidepressant has been considered dangerous and fatalities have been recorded. Other authors[26,27] maintain that provided certain precautions are taken, the risk is far less than was once believed. In fact, Pare[28] suggests that the use of a reuptake inhibitor, such as amitriptyline, would protect against the 'cheese reaction' by preventing the uptake of tyramine into noradrenaline storage sites. Later work by the same author has, however, cast some doubt on this finding. The combination of tranylcypromine and clomipramine is particularly dangerous.[29] If combination therapy is considered, then it is advisable to stop all medication for two weeks and then to start both drugs together. Even if combination therapy is considered, the evidence that it is more effective than either drug used alone is slim. Individual case reports[30–33] are equivocal and controlled studies have shown that combination therapy is no more effective than when both drugs are given individually. Better designed studies, however, will be necessary before this question can be fully resolved.

Neurotic depression (including atypical depression)

The problems of classifying mild states of depression or depression and anxiety are legion and this is of importance when considering possible indications for tranylcypromine. West and Dally[34] suggested

Tranylcypromine (sulphate)

that monoamine oxidase inhibitors were more effective in non-endogenous compared with endogenous depression. They showed this class of drugs to be more effective in patients with hysterical, phobic and anxiety symptoms and who did not have loss of energy or diurnal mood variation. They used the term 'atypical depression'; Sargeant[35] further developed the concept and when Lascelles[36] demonstrated the effect of monoamine oxidase inhibitors in atypical facial pain, the concept expanded further still to a chaotic mixture of depressive disorders, anxiety states, phobic states and personality disorders.

Tyrer[37] attempted to ease the chaos by extracting key symptoms which appeared to predict a good response. These were marked anxiety, rapid change in mood and other symptoms in response to circumstances and somatization of symptoms. A poor response occurred in those with prominent insomnia, guilt feelings and weight loss. Nies and Robinson[38] further expanded the symptom profile (see Table 1).

Table 1 Typical symptom profile of monoamine oxidase inhibitor responsive patients (from Pare 1985)

Psycopathological symptoms	Vegetative symptoms
mood reactivity retained	initial insomnia
irritability	hypersomnia
panic episodes	weight gain
agrophobia	hyperphagia
social fears	craving sweets
hypochondriasis	lethargy and fatigue
obsessive preoccupations	tremulousness
Interpersonal reactions	Historical features
self-pity/blaming others	personal loss before intensification
communicative suicidal actions	poor ECT response
rejection sensitive	liking amphetamines
vanity/applause-seeking	dysphoric tricyclic responses
histrionic personality	alcohol/sedative abuse

Further work needs to be done on patient groups with such profiles, testing their response to monoamine oxidase inhibitors. Few studies have been carried out using tranylcypromine, but one such double-blind trial on non-endogenous depression comparing tranylcypromine with nortriptyline showed both drugs to be more effective than placebo, but there was little difference between the two.

2. Anxiety/phobic states

Monoamine oxidase inhibitors are effective in anxiety states,[39] independent of their action on depressive symptoms. However, no specific trials that use tranylcypromine have been done.

Monoamine oxidase inhibitors have been shown to be effective in the treatment of agoraphobia and social phobia.[40] No well-conducted trials have been carried out using tranylcypromine, but one report has shown it to be effective against phobic symptoms in 32 patients.[41]

3. Obsessional states

Only single case reports are available.[42–44] Jenike[42] found a rapid response in two patients with severe obsessive/compulsive disorders, but both patients had prominent anxiety and phobic symptoms. It is questionable whether the response was primarily to their obsessions or accompanying anxiety symptoms.

Contraindications

1. Cerebrovascular disease

Tranylcypromine has slight epileptogenic properties and can cause increased cerebral blood flow, due to the increased blood pressure, during a sympathomimetic crisis. However, decreased cerebral blood flow is a more likely sequel due to the drug's hypotensive effect.

2. Cardiovascular disease

Although monoamine oxidase inhibitors have occasionally been used therapeutically to lower blood pressure, the use of tranylcypromine in patients with severe cardiovascular disease is contraindicated because of the danger of sympathomimetic crises and of atrial flutter. Postural hypotension may also occur.

3. Liver disease

Pare drew attention to the hepatotoxic effects of monoamine oxidase inhibitors, particularly iproniazid. The evidence that tranylcypromine can produce such effects is slim, but liver disease remains a relative contraindication.

4. Blood dyscrasia

There is a slight risk of blood dyscrasias.

5. Phaeochromocytoma

There can be an augmentation of the symptoms of a sympathomimetic crisis in patients who have a phaeochromocytoma.[49]

Adverse reactions

Potentially life-threatening effects

Marks[45] suggested that tranylcypromine is the most likely monoamine oxidase inhibitor to cause a severe sympathomimetic crisis resulting in death. However, in 1970 3.5 million patients were believed to be taking tranylcypromine worldwide and only 50 cerebrovascular accidents, resulting in 15 deaths, were recorded. In most of these the presence of non-drug-induced pathology was recognized as being of equal importance.

Acute overdosage

Deliberate overdoses have been reported with fatalitics occurring when over 150 mg of tranylcypromine were ingested. There may be a long lag period before symptoms appear and a prolonged period of observation is required before discharge from hospital is safe. Symptoms that have been reported include neuromuscular weakness, agitation, mental confusion, tachypnoea, hypertension, tachycardia, hyperthermia, involuntary movements, convulsions, headache, dizziness, chest pain, coma and death.

Symptomatic treatment to correct blood pressure, temperature and fluid balance is indicated. There is no specific antidote. Gastrointestinal motility is reduced and lavage is recommended for up to several hours post-ingestion. Tranylcypromine excretion is increased by acidification of the urine.[46] At 16 hours post-ingestion the average ratio of excretion of tranylcypromine at pH 5 compared to pH 8 is 7:1. Pancuronium (with mechanical ventilation) has been shown to help reverse muscle spasm and pyrexia.[50]

Severe or irreversible adverse effects

Liver dysfunction can occur and liver function tests should be monitored in those patients with a past history of liver disease or who are considered to be at risk of liver damage, for example heavy drinkers.

Dependence on tranylcypromine, with an escalation of dosage and a withdrawal syndrome, has been reported. If tranylcypromine has been used to treat a chronic illness however, the possibility of the re-emergence of this condition rather than a withdrawal state should be entertained. It is perhaps surprising that addiction to tranylcypromine is not more commonly reported and this may be due to the lag period between drug ingestion and therapeutic response.[37]

Symptomatic adverse effects

Mild headache, peripheral neuritis, drowsiness, weakness, palpitations, weight gain, nausea and transient restlessness and anticholinergic side effects such as dry mouth, blurred vision, postural hypotension, delayed ejaculation and difficulty in micturition can occur.

Anxiety, agitation and hypomania may occur, although the possibility that such mood swings are due to the bipolar nature of the illness being treated rather than to a drug effect must be considered.

Insomnia may occur, but can be countered by administering the final dose of the drug earlier in the day.

Other effects

A rise in central and peripheral catecholamine levels has been reported.

Interference with clinical pathology tests

No data available.

High risk groups

Neonates

There is no indication for the use of tranylcypromine in neonates and no studies are available on the possible dangers.

Breast milk. Tranylcypromine can pass into the milk of lactating dogs and in the absence of any evidence for its safety in neonates it should not be prescribed for nursing mothers.

T

Children
What has been said above about neonates also applies to older children.

Pregnant women
There is no available evidence as to the safety of tranylcypromine in human or animal pregnancies. Its use is not advised during pregnancy, especially in the first or third trimesters.

The elderly
As the elderly are more vulnerable to adverse effects, tranylcypromine should be used with caution.

Drug interactions

Potentially hazardous interactions
Food. Blackwell[47] first drew attention to the dangers of monoamine oxidase inhibitors interacting with pressure amines, such as tyramine. Elevated blood pressure, headache, sweating, pallor, stiff neck, chest pains, palpitations and even cerebral haemorrhage and death have been described. Because of this, all patients taking tranylcypromine should be issued with a card warning them of the dangers of certain foods and various drugs. Only foods high in dopamine and tyramine are absolutely contraindicated, e.g. pickled herrings, ripe cheese, broad bean pods, Marmite, Bovril, Oxo, drinks containing tyramine. There is great variation in the tyramine and dopamine content of many foods in the UK. The absence of foods which are absolutely contraindicated should not make too great an impact on the patient's diet. This is perhaps just as well, as in one study of 98 patients on tranylcypromine only 31% were found to be keeping to their dietary restrictions. If a hypertensive crisis occurs the most effective means of controlling the blood pressure is with intravenous injections of phentolamine.

Marks[45] believed that tranylcypromine was the monoamine oxidase inhibitor most likely to cause this reaction and it has been estimated that there is one death per 14 000 patient years. This is higher than the rate for tricyclics, but still much less than the mortality rate of untreated depression.

Sympathomimetics. Indirectly acting sympathomimetics, for example nasal decongestants such as pseudoephedrine, phenylephrine and ephedrine, bronchial dilators and appetite suppressants such as fenfluramine, may be dangerous because tranylcypromine may inhibit their metabolism and that of the noradrenaline they release, thus causing a hypertensive reaction.

Tricyclic antidepressants. The use of a tricyclic antidepressant within two weeks of stopping tranylcypromine is absolutely contraindicated and can be fatal.[29] The use of tranylcypromine within two weeks of stopping a tricyclic is theoretically contraindicated, but in practice seems to cause few problems. Tranylcypromine and clomipramine are a particularly hazardous combination and deaths have been reported.

Opiates. Tranylcypromine potentiates the effects of opiate analgesics, most probably through the inhibition of the liver enzymes responsible for their metabolism. Pethidine is absolutely contraindicated[48] and other opiates should first be given in 5–10% of their normal dosage to identify susceptible patients.

Carbamazepine. This drug has some pharmacological similarities to tricyclic antidepressants and the same cautions should be exercised.

Reserpine and methyldopa. Hyperactivity and excitation occur.

Other significant interactions
Antidiabetic drugs. The effect of oral hypoglycaemic agents and insulin can be potentiated by tranylcypromine.

Barbiturates. The action of barbiturates can be enhanced, presumably by enzyme inhibition.

Antihypertensives. There can be potentiation of the effects of hypotensive agents, with the exception of guanethidine whose action is antagonized.

Anticholinergics. There can be potentiation of the effects of anticholinergic agents by tranylcypromine.

Potentially useful interactions
There are no reports of tranylcypromine being used to utilize any of the interactions listed above.

Tranylcypromine (sulphate)

Major outcome trials

1. Himmelhoch J M, Fuchs C Z, Symons B J 1982 A double-blind study of tranylcypromine treatment of major anergic depression. Journal of Nervous and Mental Disease 170: 628–634

This was a prospective, double-blind, controlled study lasting six weeks that compared tranylcypromine against a placebo in a subgroup of outpatients with a diagnosis of major depressive disorder. 59 patients were selected who fulfilled this criterion, had a Raskin Depression Score of more than 7 and who in addition showed features of anergic depression, e.g. anergia, hypersomnia, weight gain, psychomotor retardation and loss of interest. 31 patients were given placebo and 28 tranylcypromine in unspecified dosage. During six weeks treatment there were dropouts in both groups. There was a significant improvement in a number of depressive symptoms in the tranylcypromine group compared with the placebo group, but unfortunately no comparison with a tricyclic antidepressant was made and despite these patients fulfilling the Research Diagnostic Criteria for major depressive disorder they were only moderately depressed as judged by their outpatient status.

2. White K et al 1984 Tranylcypromine vs. nortriptyline vs. placebo in depressed outpatients: a controlled trial. Psychopharmacology 82: 258–262

In a double-blind trial tranylcypromine, nortriptyline and a placebo were compared over a four-week period. Subjects received 30–60 mg of tranylcypromine and 75–150 mg of nortriptyline with average doses of 44.4 mg and 109.4 mg respectively. These patients fulfilled the Research Diagnostic Criteria for major depressive disorder, but could be regarded as having neurotic depression because of the absence of typical 'endogenous' features. Assessment showed both drugs to be more effective than placebo on the Zung Self Rating Scale and New Physicians Rating Scale, but not when compared on the Hamilton Depressive Rating Scale. There was no evidence to suggest that tranylcypromine was more effective than nortriptyline.

General review articles

Atkinson R, Ditman K 1965 Tranylcypromine: a review. Clinical Pharmacology and Therapeutics 6: 631–655
Morris J B, Beck A T 1974 The efficacy of anti-depressant drugs. Archives of General Psychiatry 30: 667–674
Pare C M B 1985 The present status of monoamine oxidase inhibitors. British Journal of Psychiatry 146: 576–584
Tollefson G 1983 Monoamine oxidase inhibitors: a review. Journal of Clinical Psychiatry 44: 280–288

References

1. Glowinski 1972 Monoamine oxidases — new vistas. In: Costa E, Sandler M (eds) Advances in biochemical psychopharmacology, vol 5. Raven Press, New York, pp 423–440
2. Bailey E, Barron E J 1980 Determinations of tranylcypromine in human plasma and urine. Journal of Chromatography 29: 154–157
3. Baselt R C 1977 Tranylcypromine concentrations and monoamine oxidase activity in tissues from a fatal poisoning. Journal of Analytical Toxicology 1: 168–170
4. Calverley D G 1981 A method for measurement of tranylcypromine in rat brain regions using gas chromatography with electron capture detection. Biochemical Pharmacology 30: 861–867
5. Weber H, Spahn H, Möhrke W, Mutschler E 1984 Pharmacokinetics of tranylcypromine enantiomers in healthy volunteers. Journal of Pharmacy and Pharmacology 36 (suppl): 50
6. Bailey E, Barron E J 1980 Determination of tranylcypromine in human plasma and urine. Journal of Chromatography 183: 25–31
7. Mutschler E, Möhrke W 1983 Kinetics of monoamine oxidase inhibitors. Modern Problems in Pharmacopsychiatry 19: 126–134
8. Turner P, Young J H, Paterson J et al 1967 Influence of urinary pH on the excretion of tranylcypromine. Nature 215: 881–882
9. Murphy D L 1983 Anti-depressants. In: Burrows G D (ed) Drugs in psychiatry, vol 1. Elsevier, Amsterdam, pp 209–227
10. Giller E, Lieb J 1980 Monoamine oxidase inhibitors and platelet monoamine oxidase inhibition. Communications in Psychopharmacology 4: 79–82
11. Pope H G, Hudson J I, Jonas J M et al 1984 Anti-depressant treatment. Preliminary experience and practical recommendations. Journal of Clinical Psychopharmacology 4: 173
12. Robinson D S, Nies A, Ravaris E L, Lamborn K R 1973 The monoamine oxidase inhibitor phenelzine in the treatment of depressive/anxiety states. Archives of General Psychiatry 29: 407–413
13. Robinson D S 1978 Clinical pharmacology of phenelzine. Archives of General Psychiatry 35: 629–635

14. Davidson J, McLeod M N, Blum R 1978 Acetylation phenotype: platelet monoamine oxidase inhibition and the effectiveness of phenelzine in depression. American Journal of Psychiatry 135: 467–469
15. Reynolds G P 1980 Effects of tranylcypromine stereoisomers on monoamine oxidase in man. British Journal of Clinical Pharmacology 9: 521–523
16. Tyrer P J 1982 Drugs in psychiatric practice. Butterworths, Sevenoaks, pp 258–260
17. Griffin N 1981 Addiction to tranylcypromine. British Medical Journal 283: 346
18. Morgan J H C 1981 Addiction to tranylcypromine. British Medical Journal 283: 618
19. Greenblatt M 1964 Differential response of hospitalized depressed patients to somatic therapy. American Journal of Psychiatry 120: 935–943
20. MRC 1965 Report of Clinical Psychiatry Committee. British Medical Journal 1: 881–886
21. Tyrer P J 1979 Clinical use of monoamine oxidase inhibitors. In: Paykel E S, Coppen A (eds) Psychopharmacology of affective disorder. Oxford University Press, Oxford, pp 159–178
22. Pare C M B, Mack S W 1971 Differentiation of two genetically specific types of depression by the response to anti-depressant drugs. Journal of Medical Genetics 8: 306–309
23. Hutchinson J T, Smedberg D 1963 Treatment of depression: a comparative study of E.C.T. and six drugs. British Journal of Psychiatry 109: 536–538
24. Spear F G, Hall P, Stirland J D 1964 A comparison of subjective responses to imipramine and tranylcypromine. British Journal of Psychiatry 110: 53–55
25. Nolen W 1984 Effects of oxoprotiline, fluroxamine, sleep deprivation 5-hydroxytryptamine and tranylcypromine in resistant depression. Abstract Collegium International, Neuro-psychopharmacolegium 14th CINP Congress, Florence, June 1984
26. Shuckit M, Robins E, Feighner J 1971 Tricyclic anti-depressants and monoamine oxidase inhibitors: combined therapy in the treatment of depression. Archives of General Psychiatry 24: 509
27. Sethna E R 1974 A study of refractory causes of depressive illness and their response to combined anti-depressant treatment. British Journal of Psychiatry 124: 265–272
28. Pare C M B, Kline N, Hallstrom C, Cooper T B 1982 Will amitriptyline prevent the 'cheese' reaction of monoamine oxidase inhibitors. Lancet 2: 183–186
29. Beaumont G 1973 Clomipramine (Anafranil) in the treatment of pain, enuresis and anorexia nervosa. Journal of International Medical Research 1: 435–437
30. Kline N S 1982 Amitriptyline protects patients on monoamine oxidase inhibitors from tyramine reactions. Journal of Clinical Psychopharmacology 2: 434–435
31. Razani J 1983 The safety and efficacy of combined amitriptyline and tranylcypromine anti-depressant treatment. Archives of General Psychiatry 40: 657–661
32. White K 1983 Electrocardiographic effects of tranylcypromine vs. amitriptyline. Journal of Clinical Psychiatry 44: 91–93
33. White K L 1981 Tranylcypromine. Psychopharmacology Bulletin 17: 157–159
34. West E D, Dally P J 1959 Effects of iproniazid in depressive syndromes. British Medical Journal 1: 1491–1494
35. Sargeant W 1961 Drugs in the treatment of depression. British Medical Journal 1: 225–227
36. Lascelles R G 1960 Atypical facial pain and depression. British Journal of Psychiatry 112: 651–659
37. Tyrer P J 1976 Towards rational therapy with monoamine oxidase inhibitors. British Journal of Psychiatry 128: 354–360
38. Nies A, Robinson M D 1982 Monoamine oxidase inhibitors. In: Paykel E S (ed) Handbook of affective disorders. Churchill Livingstone, Edinburgh
39. Tyrer P J, Candy J, Kelly D 1973 A study of the clinical effects of phenelzine and placebo in the treatment of phobic anxiety. Psychopharmacologica 32: 237–254
40. Tyrer P J 1979 Anxiety states. In: Granville-Grossman K L (ed) Recent advances in clinical psychiatry, vol 3. Churchill Livingstone, Edinburgh, pp 161–183
41. Lyons H A, Degerli M 1978 Indications for the use of tranylcypromine and trifluoperazine. Scottish Medical Journal 23: 307–309
42. Jenike M A 1981 Rapid response of severe obsessive-compulsive disorder to tranylcypromine. American Journal of Psychiatry 138: 1249–1250
43. Swinson R P 1984 Response to tranylcypromine and thought stopping in obsessional disorder. British Journal of Psychiatry 144: 425–427
44. Jenike M A 1983 Monoamine oxidase inhibitors in obsessive-compulsive disorders. Journal of Clinical Psychiatry 44: 131–132
45. Marks J 1965 Interactions involving drugs used in psychiatry. In: Marks J, Pare C M B (eds) The scientific basis of drug therapy in psychiatry. Pergamon Press, Oxford
46. Turner P, Young J H, Paterson J 1967 Influence of urinary pH on the excretion of tranylcypromine. Nature 215: 881–882
47. Blackwell B 1963 Hypertensive crisis due to monoamine oxidase inhibitors. Lancet 2: 849–851
48. Stockley I 1981 Drug interactions. Blackwell Scientific Publications, Oxford
49. Cook R F, Katritsis D 1990 Hypertensive crisis precipitated by a momoamine oxidase inhibitor in a patient with phaeochromocytoma. British Medical Journal 300: 614
50. Henry J, Volans G 1984 Psychoactive drugs. British Medical Journal 289: 1291–1294

Trazodone (hydrochloride)

Trazodone is a phenylpiperazine derivative of triazolopyridine and represents a clinically effective and chemically distinct antidepressant which appears to have considerable value in the treatment of depression.[1–6] It is the first triazolopyridine derivative to be used clinically, and it is unique among the major classes of anxiolytics and antipsychotic agents in respect of its chemical structure and pharmacology. It generally fails to produce typical effects in the usual laboratory tests used to evaluate antidepressant activity and, furthermore, it is neither a psychostimulant, a monoamine oxidase inhibitor, nor a tricyclic antidepressant, but has significant actions at serotonin receptors.[7]

Chemistry

Trazodone hydrochloride (Molipaxin, Desyrel, Manegan, Thombran, Trittico)
$C_{19}H_{22}ClN_5O.HCl$
2-(3-(4-(3-Chlorophenyl)piperazin-1-yl)propyl)-1-2-4-triazolo(4,3-*a*)pyridin-3(2*H*)one hydrochloride

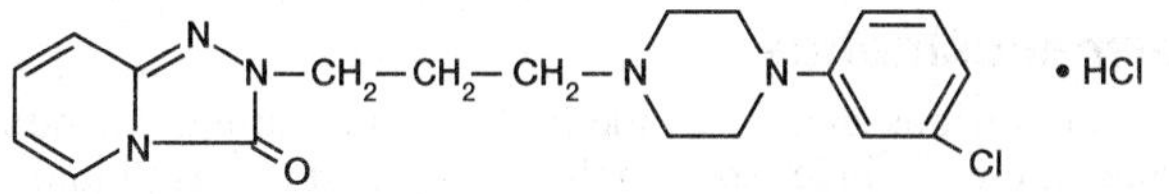

Molecular weight (free base)	408.3 (371.8)
pKa (amino group)	6.7
Solubility	
in alcohol	low
in water	freely soluble
Octanol/water partition coefficient	—

Trazodone hydrochloride is a white odourless crystalline substance with a bitter taste. It is freely soluble in water, sparingly soluble in alcohol and methyl alcohol, and soluble in chloroform and has a melting point of about 225°C.

Pharmacology

With respect to the classical animal models used to screen for antidepressant activity, trazodone has been found not to potentiate the behavioural effects of l-dopa, not to inhibit monoamine oxidase activity, and not to have anticholinergic effects.[8] It also fails to potentiate the behavioural effects of the serotonin precursor, 5-hydroxytryptophan, in pargyline-treated mice, a property shared with many antidepressant agents.[8,9]

In common with antipsychotic agents, trazodone reduces conditioned avoidance responses at doses that do not affect unconditioned responses, as well as protecting mice from amphetamine group toxicity. Trazodone also antagonizes α-adrenergic receptor agonists, and reduces self-stimulating behaviours, although it does not antagonize amphetamine- and apomorphine-induced stereotyped behaviours. Furthermore, trazodone lacks the cateleptogenic or hypothermic activity of other antipsychotic agents.[9]

In common with antianxiety agents, trazodone causes sedation; unlike the benzodiazepines, however, it suppresses rapid-eye-movement (REM) sleep, and lacks the anticonvulsant and muscle-relaxing properties of these drugs.[10] Thus, while it shares some pharmacological effects with all of the three major classes of psychopharmacological agents, it also has properties that distinguish it from any of these three classes. Like several other centrally acting agents, trazodone causes analgesia in many analgesic test systems in animals.

Trazodone (hydrochloride)

T

Trazodone inhibits synaptic serotonin reuptake, a property shared with imipramine, amitryptiline and clomipramine, although it is only one-fifteenth as potent in this regard as is clomipramine.[9] Its ability to inhibit synaptic serotonin uptake is 220–370 times that of noradrenaline or dopamine. Thus, while trazodone is weaker than clomipramine in inhibiting serotonin uptake, it is much more specific and selective in that it only slightly affects catecholamine uptake. It does not cause serotonin release, but inhibits fenfluramine-induced serotonin release and hyperthermia. Furthermore, trazodone is devoid of any muscarinic receptor affinity, thus accounting for its lack of anticholinergic side effects.[8,9] Trazodone binds to α-receptors and seems to act as an α_2-receptor antagonist, thus reversing the central cardiovascular effects of clonidine.

Toxicology

Studies in rats receiving trazodone in oral dosages of up to 300 mg.kg^{-1} daily for 18 months have shown no evidence of carcinogenesis.[1] (See also High risk groups: pregnant women.)

Clinical pharmacology

The mechanism of trazodone's antidepressant action in man is not fully understood. However, it seems likely that this is related to its action in inhibiting serotonin reuptake. It has little effect on catecholamine reuptake, and has no anticholinergic effect. It is effective as an antidepressant and as with most antidepressants this effect takes several days to become manifest. It has a sedative action, so like amitryptiline it may be best taken at night. Perhaps because of its lack of effects on catecholamine reuptake and on the muscarinic acetylcholine receptor, trazodone has few effects on the cardiovascular system. It is thus likely to be safer in patients who have recently had a myocardial infarction.

Pharmacokinetics

There are various analytical methods for measuring trazodone in plasma: these include spectrophotofluorimetry, gas–liquid chromatography with flame ionization, nitrogen selective or mass-fragmentographic detection or high performance liquid chromatography (HPLC). HPLC using an organosilane-modified silica column together with UV or electrochemical oxidation detection is the preferred method (sensitivity 2 µg.l^{-1}).

After oral administration, absorption of trazodone is rapid and complete, and plasma levels are essentially identical, regardless of the route of administration. Within two hours after it is taken by mouth, the drug reaches peak blood concentrations. Trazodone has a biphasic half life, with the first component having an elimination half life of 1 to 4.4 hours and the second component having an elimination half life of 7 to 13 hours. Plasma levels peak at 90 minutes in a fasting state and at 150 minutes in a non-fasting state, with a 30% reduction in peak levels in a non-fasting state. Because the time to steady state is a function of a drug's half life, trazodone's brief half life means steady state is usually achieved in a few days although the half life (and time to steady state) varies considerably from patient to patient.[1]

Oral absorption	100%
Presystemic metabolism	—
Plasma half life range	1.0–4.4 h
Volume of distribution	—
Plasma protein binding	89–95%

The concentrations of trazodone in rat brain were significantly higher than those in plasma. In this species, the highest uptake was in the liver followed by the kidneys, pancreas and adrenals. In the rabbit the highest uptake was in the kidney followed by the adrenals, lung and liver. In humans, 89–95% of the drug in plasma is bound to plasma protein, in vitro, at concentrations attained with therapeutic doses.[1]

Concentration–effect relationship

The available information relating trazodone blood concentrations to the antidepressant response is inadequate . Putzolu et al, not surprisingly, found no correlation between plasma concentrations and response after a single 25 mg dose.[11] However, by the 33rd day of treatment some evidence of an inverse correlation of plasma concentration and response was observed. Mann et al reported an eight-fold interindividual variation in trazodone blood concentrations resulting from the same dose.[5] These researchers could not detect any relationship between plasma concentrations and therapeutic effect.[5]

Metabolism

Trazodone is rapidly absorbed from the gastrointestinal tract and extensively metabolized. Very little unmetabolized drug appears in the urine. Trazodone is metabolized by hydroxylation, splitting of the pyridine ring and epoxidation followed by hydrolysis. 1-m-Chlorophenylpiperazine is a pharmacologically active metabolite. The majority of a trazodone dose (75%) is excreted by the kidney within 72 hours, predominantly as hydroxylated and carboxylic acid metabolites. The balance appears in the faeces but there is no evidence of enterohepatic circulation.

Pharmaceutics

Trazodone is supplied for oral administration as tablets, capsules or liquid.

1. Molipaxin (Roussel, UK) is available as a 150 mg tablet: salmon pink, film-coated, biconvex, approximately 11 mm in diameter with a white core. The tablet is embossed with 'Molipaxin 150' on one face, with a break line on the reverse.

Fig. 1 Metabolism of trazodone

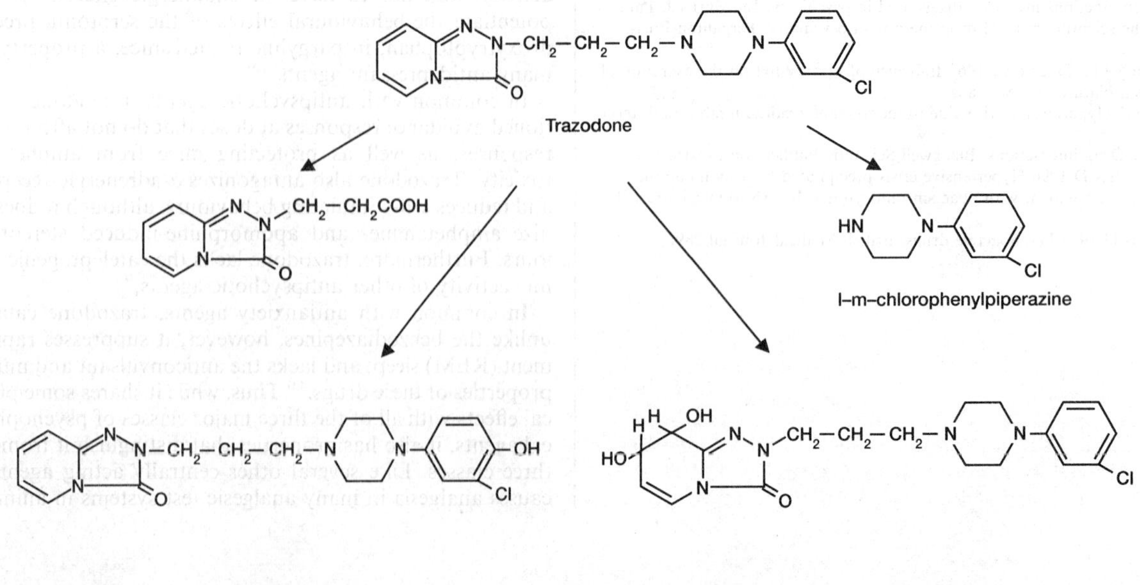

Trazodone (hydrochloride)

2. Molipaxin capsules contain 50 mg or 100 mg of trazodone hydrochloride. The 50 mg capsules are size No. 3, opaque violet–green, printed with the number 'R365B' and the Roussel logo. The 100 mg capsules are size No. 2 opaque violet–fawn, printed with the number 'R365C' and the Roussel logo.
3. Desyrel (Mead Johnson, USA): tablets in two strengths. The 50 mg tablets are round, orange/scored, film-sealed and imprinted with the MJ logo and '716'.
   The 100 mg tablets are round, white/scored, film-sealed and imprinted with the MJ logo.
4. There is also a Molipaxin liquid (Roussel, UK) which is a clear, colourless solution with an orange flavour.

The tablets should be stored at room temperature and should be protected from temperatures above 40°C. They should be dispensed in airtight, light-resistant containers. The liquid should also be protected from the light and stored at room temperature. The liquid has a maximum shelf-life of 2 years whereas the capsules have a maximum shelf-life of 5 years.

The capsule shells contain tartrazine which is a potentially allergenic substance.

Therapeutic use

Indications

1. Alleviating specific target symptoms of depression such as anxiety, somatization, psychomotor retardation, diurnal variation, and anergic, insomniac and depressed mood.

Contraindications

1. Hypersensitivity.

Mode of use

Trazodone is a trazolopyridine antidepressant whose mode of action in depression is not fully understood.

In the treatment of depression, trazodone is given by mouth as the hydrochloride in doses of 100 or 150 mg daily, initially, then increased according to severity up to a maximum of 600 mg daily in exceptionally severe depression.[1] Once the response is adequate the dose should be reduced gradually to the lowest effective level. The highest dose known to have been used is 800 mg daily. The daily dosage may be divided throughout the day after food or given as a single dose at night.

Symptomatic improvement may be seen within the first week of administration, and optimum improvement within the second week. Of those who eventually respond, 25% may require up to 4 weeks of continuous therapy for significant improvement to occur.

Indications

1. Alleviating specific target symptoms of depression

Trazodone is indicated for the treatment of depression. Symptoms of depression likely to respond in the first week of treatment include depressed mood, insomnia, anxiety, somatic symptoms and hypochondriasis.[1–6] The efficacy of trazodone has been demonstrated in both in-patient and out-patient settings and for depressed patients with and without prominent anxiety. The depressive illness of patients studied corresponds to the Major Depressive Episode Criteria of the American Psychiatric Association's Diagnostic and Statistical Manual, III. Major Depressive Episode implies a prominent and relatively persistent (nearly every day for at least two weeks) depressed or dysphoric mood that usually interferes with daily functioning, and includes at least four of the following eight symptoms: change in appetite, change in sleep, psychomotor agitation or retardation, loss of interest in usual activities or decrease in sexual drive, increased fatiguability, feelings of guilt or worthlessness, slowed thinking or impaired concentration, and suicidal thoughts or attempts.

Trazodone is devoid of anticholinergic activity. Consequently, troublesome side effects such as dry mouth, blurred vision and urinary hesitancy have occurred no more than in patients receiving placebo therapy. This may be important when treating depressed patients who are at risk from conditions such as glaucoma, urinary retention and prostatic hypertrophy. In animal studies trazodone has been shown to be less cardiotoxic than the tricyclic antidepressants and clinical studies suggest the drug may be less likely to cause cardiac arrhythmias in man.[1] Trazodone has had no effect on arterial blood pCO_2 or pO_2 levels in patients with respiratory insufficiency due to chronic bronchial or pulmonary disease.

Contraindications

1. Hypersensitivity

Trazodone is contraindicated in patients hypersensitive to trazodone.

Adverse reactions

Potentially life-threatening effects

There have been no reported deaths of patients taking trazodone alone. However, there have been two single case reports of life-threatening cardiac arrhythmias.

Acute overdosage

An increasing volume of data suggests that trazodone might be less hazardous than other antidepressants when ingested in overdose. Death from overdose has occurred in patients ingesting trazodone and other drugs concurrently (namely alcohol; alcohol + chloral hydrate + diazepam; amylobarbitone; chlordiazepoxide; or meprobamate).[1]

The most severe reactions reported to have occurred with an overdose of trazodone alone have been priapism, respiratory arrest, seizures and ECG changes.[12–15] The reactions reported most frequently have been drowsiness and vomiting. Overdosage may cause an increase in incidence or severity of any of the reported adverse reactions.

There is no specific antidote for trazodone. Treatment should be symptomatic and supportive in the case of hypotension or excessive sedation. Any patient suspected of having taken an overdose should be given syrup of ipecacuanha and activated charcoal as an adjunct to stomach emptying or gastric lavage.

Severe or irreversible adverse effects

Trazodone has been associated with the occurrence of priapism. In approximately one-third of the cases reported, surgical intervention was required and, in a portion of these cases, permanent impairment of erectile function or impotence resulted. Male patients with prolonged or inappropriate erections should immediately discontinue the drug and consult their physician.

Recent clinical studies in patients with pre-existing cardiac disease indicate that trazodone may be arrhythmogenic in some patients in that population.[13] Arrhythmias identified include isolated premature ventricular contractions (PVCs), ventricular couplets, and, in two patients, short episodes (3–4 beats) of ventricular tachycardia. Until the results of prospective studies are available, patients with pre-existing cardiac disease should be closely monitored, particularly for cardiac arrhythmias. There have also been reports of arrhythmias in patients treated with trazodone, some of whom did not have pre-existing cardiac disease. Other cardiovascular adverse effects of trazodone include disturbances of cardiac conduction, bradycardia, syncope, palpitations and weak inotropism.

Trazodone should also be used with caution in patients with epilepsy and hepatic or renal insufficiency. Patients with suicidal tendencies should be carefully supervised during treatment.

Symptomatic adverse effects

Adverse effects associated with trazodone and reported in $> 1\%$ of subjects include drowsiness, dizziness, headache, incoordination, decreased concentration, impaired memory, hypotension (including orthostatic hypotension and syncope), dyspepsia, nasal and sinus congestion, change in libido and impotence.

Other effects

Occasional low total white blood cell counts and neutropenia have been noted in patients receiving trazodone. These were not considered clinically significant and did not necessitate discontinuation of the drug; however, the drug should be discontinued in any patient whose white blood cell count or absolute neutrophil count falls below normal levels. White blood cell and differential counts are recommended for patients who develop fever and sore throat (or other signs of infection) during therapy.

There have been reports of a slight deficiency of human growth hormone and a drop in prolactin levels. There are also changes in liver enzyme activity.

Trazodone (hydrochloride)

Interference with clinical pathology tests
No technical interferences of this kind have been reported.

High risk groups

Neonates
Safety and effectiveness in children below the age of 18 have not been established.

Breast milk. Trazodone and/or its metabolites have been found in the milk of lactating rats, suggesting that the drug may be secreted in human milk. A recent study in humans has shown that the exposure of babies to trazodone via breast milk is very small.[16] However, caution should still be exercised when trazodone is administered to a nursing woman.

Children
Safety and effectiveness in children below the age of 18 have not been established.

Pregnant women
In two studies in the rat, trazodone has been shown to cause increased fetal resorption and other adverse effects on the fetus when given at dose levels approximately 30–50 times the proposed maximum human dose. There was also an increase in congenital abnormalities in one of three rabbit studies at approximately 15–50 times the maximum human dose. There are no adequate and well-controlled studies in pregnant women. Trazodone should be used during pregnancy only if the potential benefit justifies the potential risk to the fetus.

The elderly
In a double-blind controlled study in 60 depressed geriatric patients, trazodone in an initial dose of 100 mg increased to 400 mg daily was as effective as imipramine in an initial dose of 50 mg, increased to 200 mg daily, and both antidepressants were more effective than placebo in relieving depression.[17] Trazodone was much better tolerated, with fewer adverse effects, and may therefore possess an advantage in antidepressant treatment of certain patients in the older age groups.

Drug interactions

Potentially hazardous interactions

Electroshock therapy. Concurrent administration of trazodone with electroshock treatment should be avoided, because of the lack of experience in this area.

Alcohol. Trazodone may enhance the response to alcohol. The two drugs may have an additive effect in causing depression of the central nervous system.

Other significant interactions[1]

Tyramine. Trazodone 50 mg thrice daily has no effect on the blood pressure response to tyramine.

Noradrenaline. Trazodone may slightly decrease sensitivity to noradrenaline.

Clonidine. Trazodone could inhibit the hypotensive effects of clonidine.

Barbiturates. Volatile anaesthetics, suxamethonium and muscle relaxants. The effects of these can be potentiated by trazodone.

Antihypertensives. Trazodone might potentiate the hypotensive effects of antihypertensives but there are no specific studies.

Digoxin or phenytoin. Increased serum digoxin or phenytoin levels (up to 50% increase) have been reported to occur in patients receiving trazodone concurrently with either of these two drugs.

Monoamine oxidase inhibitors. Trazodone should not be administered concurrently with MAOI or within two weeks of terminating treatment with these compounds.

Food. It is recommended that trazodone be taken shortly after a meal or light snack. Within any individual patient, total drug absorption may be up to 20% higher when the drug is taken with food rather than on an empty stomach, resulting in a decrease in maximum concentration and a lengthening in the time to maximum concentration. Peak plasma levels occur approximately one hour after dosing when trazodone is taken on an empty stomach or two hours after dosing when taken with food. The risk of dizziness/lightheadedness may increase due to the higher peak plasma concentration when the drug is taken under fasting conditions.

Potentially useful interactions
None has been reported.

Major outcome trials

1. Gershon S, Mann J, Newton R, Gunther B J 1981 Evaluation of trazodone in the treatment of endogenous depression: results of a multicenter double-blind study. Journal of Clinical Psychopharmacology 1 (6) (suppl): 395–445

A multi-centre study indicates that trazodone appears to be effective in treating endogenous depression and to have significant advantages over the tricyclic antidepressant, imipramine, in terms of side effects (especially unwanted anticholinergic effects). Trazodone may also have a special therapeutic potential in the elderly, in schizophrenics with secondary depression, and possibly in the treatment and prophylaxis of depression in bipolar affective disorders not fully controlled by lithium.

Other trials

1. Goldberg H L, Rickels K, Finnerty R 1981 Treatment of neurotic depression with a new antidepressant. Journal of Clinical Psychopharmacology 1 (6)(suppl): 35S–38S

A placebo-controlled study was performed to compare the efficacy of trazodone with that of a standard tricyclic antidepressant, amitryptiline, in out-patients suffering from moderately severe to severe neurotic depression. The results of the various psychiatric rating scales and the physicians' overall evaluation of therapeutic response indicate that trazodone is a very effective antidepressant.

2. Feighner J P 1980 Trazodone, a triazolopyridine derivative, in primary depressive disorder. Journal of Clinical Psychiatry 41 (7): 250–255

A double-blind controlled study was conducted to compare the effects of imipramine and placebo with trazodone in 45 hospitalized patients with primary depression. After a three- to seven-day baseline period, patients were treated for four weeks. Response was assessed by the Hamilton Psychiatric Scale for Depression, Structured Clinical Interview, Clinical Global Impression, and Global Ward Behaviour Scale. The antidepressant effect of trazodone was evident within seven days of treatment and persisted throughout the study. Patients treated with imipramine also improved, but the response was not as great or as rapid as in the trazodone group.

3. Gerner R, Estabrook W, Steuer J, Jarvik L 1980 Treatment of geriatric depression with trazodone, imipramine, and placebo: a double-blind study. Journal of Clinical Psychiatry 41 (6): 216–220

60 unipolar depressed geriatric out-patients were subjects in a double-blind study of trazodone versus imipramine and placebo. Over the four-week study, patients in the two active medication groups improved significantly compared to placebo on both observer and self-ratings. Although imipramine and trazodone had similar therapeutic efficacy, trazodone was judged to have fewer side effects than imipramine, suggesting that trazodone may have particular clinical utility in the geriatric population which is especially vulnerable to cardiovascular and anticholinergic side effects.

4. Gershon S, Newton R 1980 Lack of anticholinergic side effects with a new antidepressant — trazodone. Journal of Clinical Psychiatry 41 (3): 100–104

An analysis was made of the occurrence of anticholinergic side effects in 15 multi-centre studies of 379 patients with endogenous depression who received either trazodone, imipramine or placebo. The incidence of four anticholinergic side effects was examined: dry mouth, blurred vision, bowel movement disturbance, and delayed urine flow. When the number of patients having each of the four symptoms was compared, there were no statistically significant differences in the incidence of side effects between the trazodone and placebo groups. However, comparisons between trazodone and imipramine indicated the incidence of side effects was significantly lower in the trazodone group.

5. Mungavin J M, Ankier S I 1983 Comparison of two dosage regimens of trazodone (Molipaxin) in the treatment of depression. Clinical Trials Journal (London) 20 (4): 181–188

195 patients with depression were treated orally with trazodone (Molipaxin) for four weeks in an open study. 97 patients received 50 mg three times daily, increasing after two weeks to 50 mg morning and noon plus 100 mg at night, while 98 patients received 100 mg at night, increasing after one week to 200 mg at night.

The results showed no statistical differences between the dosage regimens with regard to clinical efficacy or the incidence of side effects. The prescriber, therefore, has the flexibility to use either dosage regimen.

References

1. Brogden R N, Heel R C, Speight T M, Avery G S 1981 Trazodone: a review of its pharmacological properties and therapeutic use in depression and anxiety. Drugs 21: 401–476
2. Al-Yassiri M M, Ankier S I, Bridges P K 1981 Trazodone — a new antidepressant. Life Sciences 28: 2449–2458
3. Feighner J P 1980 Trazodone, a triazolopyridine derivative, in primary depressive disorder. Journal of Clinical Psychiatry 41 (7): 250–255
4. Davis J M, Vogel C 1981 Efficacy of trazodone: data from European and United States studies. Journal of Clinical Psychopharmacology 1 (6) (suppl): 27S–34S
5. Gershon S, Mann J, Newton R, Gunther B J 1981 Evaluation of trazodone in the treatment of endogenous depression: results of a multicenter double-blind study. Journal of Clinical Psychopharmacology 1 (6) (suppl): 39S–44S
6. Feighner J P, Merideth C H, Hendrickson G 1981 Maintenance antidepressant therapy: a double-blind comparison of trazodone and imipramine. Journal of Clinical Psychopharmacology 1 (6) (suppl): 45S–48S
7. Maj J, Palider W, Rawlow A 1979 Trazodone, a central serotonin antagonist and agonist. Journal of Neural Transmission 44: 237–248
8. Clements-Jewery S, Robson P A, Chidley L J 1980 Biochemical investigations into the mode of action of trazodone. Neuropharmacology 19: 1165–1173
9. Riblet L A, Taylor D P 1981 Pharmacology and neurochemistry of trazodone. Journal of Clinical Psychopharmacology 1 (6) (suppl): 17S–22S
10. Wheatley D 1984 Trazodone: alternative dose regimens and sleep. Pharmatherapeutica 3 (9): 607–612
11. Putzolu S, Pecknold J G, Baiocchi L et al 1976 Trazodone clinical and biochemical studies. II. Blood levels and therapeutic responsiveness. Psychopharmacology Bulletin 12: 40–41
12. Gomoll A W, Byrne J E 1981 Cardiovascular effects of trazodone in animals. Journal of Clinical Psychopharmacology 1 (6) (suppl): 70S–75S
13. Himmelhoch J M 1981 Cardiovascular effects of trazodone in humans. Journal of Clinical Psychopharmacology 1 (6) (suppl): 76S–81S
14. Branconnier R J, Cole J O 1981 Effects of acute administration of trazodone and amitriptyline on cognition, cardiovascular function, and salivation in the normal geriatric subject. Journal of Clinical Psychopharmacology 1 (6) (suppl): 82S–88S
15. Newton R 1981 The side effect profile of trazodone in comparison to an active control and placebo. Journal of Clinical Psychopharmacology 1 (6) (suppl): 89S–93S
16. Verbeeck R K, Ross S G, McKenna E A 1986 Excretion of trazodone in breast milk. British Journal of Clinical Pharmacology 22: 367–370
17. Gerner R, Estabrook W, Steuer J, Jarvik L 1980 Treatment of geriatric depression with trazodone, imipramine, and placebo: a double-blind study. Journal of Clinical Psychiatry 41 (6): 216–220
18. Goldberg H L, Rickels K, Finnerty R 1981 Treatment of neurotic depression with a new antidepressant. Journal of Clinical Psychopharmacology 1 (6) (suppl): 35S–38S
19. Gershon S, Newton R 1980 Lack of anticholinergic side effects with a new antidepressant — trazodone. Journal of Clinical Psychiatry 41 (3): 100–104
20. Mungavin J M, Ankier S I 1983 Comparison of two dosage regimens of trazodone (molipaxin) in the treatment of depression: a multicentre general practice study. Clinical Trials Journal (London) 20(4): 181–188

Treosulfan

Treosulfan is a cytotoxic alkylating agent used in the treatment of solid tumours.

Chemistry

Dihydroxybusulphan (Treosulfan Leo)

$C_6H_{14}O_8S_2$

L-Threitol 1,4-dimethanesulfonate

```
CHOH—CH2—O—SO2—CH3
|
CHOH—CH2—O—SO2—CH3
```

Molecular weight	278.3
pKa	not relevant
Solubility	
in alcohol	1 in 200
in water	1 in 14
Octanol/water partition coefficient	—

Treosulfan is a white, odourless crystalline powder prepared by chemical synthesis. It is supplied for clinical use as 250 mg capsules for oral administration and as powder for reconstitution for intravenous administration.

Pharmacology

Treosulfan is a non-cell cycle specific bifunctional alkylating agent belonging to the alkyl sulfonate group and is similar in structure to busulfan. Its cytotoxic capability arises from the ability to alkylate nucleic acids of DNA resulting in misreading of the DNA code, cross-linking of DNA and single- and double-strand breaks. It inhibits DNA, RNA and protein synthesis in rapidly dividing tissues.

The parent compound treosulfan is inactive. However in vivo it is transformed to the epoxide and diepoxide derivatives (Fig. 1).[1] The transformation is dependent on temperature and pH and is not enzymatically dependent. It is thought that the epoxy groups then alkylate with nucleophilic sites on nucleic acids in a similar way to the positively charged immonium ions derived from the classical alkylating agents such as nitrogen mustard. The most likely site of attack is the N^7 position of guanine and possibly the O^6 position of guanine and N^3 position of cytidine, as alteration of these latter two positions has more effect on the interference of accurate base-pairing. Other bifunctional alkylating agents can cause cross-linking of DNA and it is likely that treosulfan acts in a similar manner. Cross-strand covalent binding has been shown to correlate well with lethality.[2]

Toxicology

Treosulfan is mutagenic in animals and plants and has been found to be significantly carcinogenic in humans, acute myeloid leukaemia being the most common second malignancy occurring.[3–6] In animals and man the dose-limiting toxicity is myelosuppression, and at the LD_{50} dose in dogs and monkeys (approximately 190 $mg.kg^{-1}$ intravenously daily for 11 days) anorexia and weight loss were also observed.[4]

Clinical pharmacology

Treosulfan is an effective alkylating agent that is chiefly used in the treatment of ovarian carcinoma. Treosulfan, like busulphan, is toxic to all stem cell lines of the bone marrow with peak effects on granulopoiesis some 2–4 weeks after drug administration. Although nausea and vomiting occur in about 20% of patients, diarrhoea is unusual. There are no other known pharmacological effects of treosulfan in man but the drug is a known carcinogen.[3]

Pharmacokinetics

Treosulfan can be assayed by gas–liquid chromatography.[7] The compound is available as either an oral or intravenous preparation. The oral bioavailability is good and approaches that of intravenous treosulfan. After oral treosulfan the plasma half life ($t_{1/2}$) is 1.7 hours (range 1.5–1.9 h) and after intravenous injection 1.6 hours (range 1.4–1.8 h). The volume of distribution is approximately 66 litres but a wide range has been reported (44–88 l.). Treosulfan levels in tears and saliva closely follow plasma levels and although no studies have been performed in lactating animals or humans it is likely there will also be significant quantities secreted in breast milk. There are no known effects of age or disease on drug clearance. There are no data available on the degree of protein binding or the level of penetration into the CSF.

Oral absorption	good
Plasma half life	1.4–1.9 h
Volume of distribution	44–88 l
Plasma protein binding	—

Concentration–effect relationship

There are no data correlating therapeutic effect of treosulfan with plasma concentrations.

Metabolism

There are no data concerning the enzymatic metabolism of treosulfan. As discussed above, treosulfan undergoes non-enzymatic decomposition to the pharmacologically active monoepoxide and diepoxide with release of methane sulfonic acid (Fig. 1). 11– 21% of the administered dose is recovered from the urine over 24 hours, with most of this recovery occurring within 6 hours. There are no data on the amount of bile elimination.

Fig. 1 Conversion pathway of treosulfan to active products

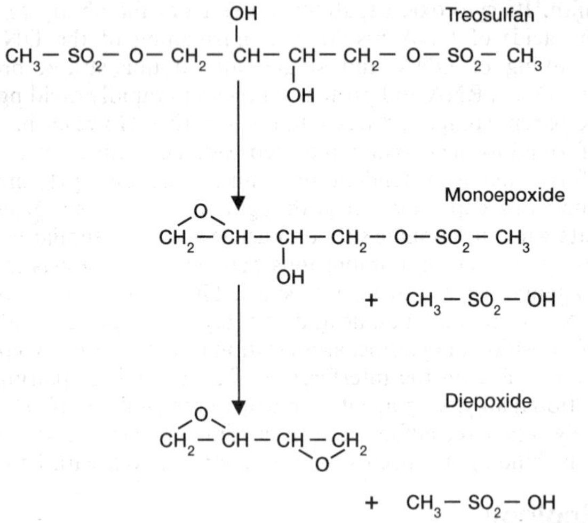

Pharmaceutics

Treosulfan (Leo, UK) is available in both oral and parenteral forms.

The oral form is a 250 mg capsule with a white opaque cap. For intravenous use treosulfan is supplied in glass infusion bottles containing 5 g of treosulfan as a white crystalline powder for reconstitution with 100 ml sterile water for injection using the transfer needle supplied. After reconstitution treosulfan should be administered immediately. Care must be taken during intravenous administration to ensure that extravasation does not occur, as treosulfan is a vesicant and leakage into the tissues will cause local pain and tissue damage. If this occurs the infusion must be stopped immediately and another vein used. Plastic containers should be avoided.

Treosulfan

Both the oral and parenteral formulations have a shelf life of 5 years.

Therapeutic use

Indications

1. Ovarian cancer

Contraindications

1. Pregnancy
2. Lactation.

Mode of use

There are several accepted treatment regimens using the oral capsules, the most commonly used being.[8,9]

1. 250 mg 4 times daily for 4 weeks, repeated after a 4 week break
2. 500 mg 3 times daily for 1 week given in a 4 week cycle.

The drug is not generally given as a dose per m^2 as there is a very wide interpatient variability with respect to haematological toxicity. Older and less fit patients should be commenced at 75% of the doses mentioned above. The timing and dose of drug used in subsequent courses is dependent on the severity and time course of the haematological toxicity. Treatment should not be recommenced unless the white blood count is greater than $3 \times 10^9.l^{-1}$ and platelet count greater than $100 \times 10^9.l^{-1}$ and if this means treatment has had to be delayed then consideration should be given to a dose reduction of 25%.

Intravenous treosulfan may also be used in those patients unable to tolerate the oral capsules. The recommended dose is 5–15 g intravenously every 1 to 3 weeks dependent on haematological toxicity, as for the oral regimens.[10]

If concurrent chemotherapy is also administered the dose of treosulfan given will need to be adjusted downward according to the myelotoxicity of the other drugs.

Indications

1. Ovarian carcinoma

The only currently accepted indication for treosulfan is in the treatment of ovarian cancer, where it may be used like any other alkylating agent. This may be either as first-line treatment for less-fit patients with advanced stage disease or as possible second-line therapy in fitter patients who receive platinum-based regimens as first-line therapy. Treosulfan is thought to cause more severe cumulative suppression than other oral alkylating agents, making further alternative therapy difficult.

Contraindications

1. Pregnancy

As treosulfan is mutagenic and carcinogenic its use in pregnancy is contraindicated although there are no case reports available on the incidence of malformed human infants.

2. Lactation

There is no information on the amount of treosulfan present in human breast milk but transfer into breast milk is likely to be significant and hence its use in this situation is strictly contraindicated.

Adverse reactions

Potentially life-threatening effects

There is no reported immediate life-threatening toxicity of treosulfan apart from bone marrow suppression. However, treosulfan is a carcinogen and Pedersen-Bjergaard et al[11] (1980) report 8 cases of acute myeloid leukaemia in 533 patients receiving long-term treatment with treosulfan and 5 of these patients had died by the time of the report.

Acute overdosage

As there is a marked inter-patient variability in the degree of myelosuppression induced by treosulfan, it is not uncommon to see patients showing the effects of overdose. There is no acute toxicity seen with overdose of either intravenous or oral treosulfan. However, as with all myelotoxic cytotoxic agents, overdose will be associated with a more severe and prolonged haematological nadir than usual. This is likely to occur after approximately two weeks. During this time patients must be watched closely for signs of infection which should be treated aggressively during the period of neutropenia. Platelet and blood transfusions may also be necessary should severe thrombocytopenia or anaemia develop.

Severe or irreversible adverse effects
The only severe adverse effects of treosulfan are associated with the severe myelosuppression seen especially in patients pretreated with myelosuppressive cytotoxic drugs and when treosulfan is used in conjunction with other cytotoxic drugs.

Symptomatic adverse effects
Nausea and vomiting occur in approximately 20% of patients receiving either the oral or intravenous forms of treosulfan. Nausea is usually easily controlled with antiemetic drugs such as metoclopramide or prochlorperazine. Approximately 25% of patients may experience generalized skin pigmentation and, although cases of Addisonian adrenal syndromes have been described, most patients with pigmentation have a normal serum cortisol.[12,13] Stomatitis may also occur in a small proportion of patients at the time of their neutropenic nadir.[9]

As mentioned above, treosulfan is toxic to all stem-cell lines of the bone marrow and symptoms from the effects of myelosuppression may be seen. The peak effect is likely to be seen around two weeks after drug administration. This may be manifested in the form of increased susceptibility to infection. Any patient who develops a fever of greater than 38°C should be considered for empirical intravenous broad-spectrum antibiotic therapy. Thrombocytopenia may also occur and render the patient susceptible to bruising or bleeding, and supportive care with platelet transfusions may be necessary should this occur in the presence of a low platelet count. When treosulfan is used concurrently with other drugs or in patients previously treated with cytotoxic drugs the effects on the bone marrow may be severe.

Interference with clinical pathology tests
There is no known interference by treosulfan with clinical pathology tests.

High risk groups

Neonates
There is no information on the use of treosulfan in neonates.

Breast milk. There is no information on the concentration of treosulfan in breast milk but it is likely to be present in high concentrations and is hence contraindicated in the lactating mother.

Children
There is no information on the use of treosulfan in children.

Pregnant women
Treosulfan is mutagenic and carcinogenic and although there is no reported experience of its use in pregnant women it is contraindicated for these reasons.

The elderly
There is no contraindication to the use of treosulfan in the elderly but a 25% dose reduction is recommended in elderly patients.

Drug interactions

Potentially hazardous interactions
Except for the additive myelosuppressive effects when other cytotoxic drugs are given concurrently, there are no known potentially hazardous drug interactions. When treosulfan is given with other myelosuppressive drugs appropriate dose reductions of all drugs should be made.

Potentially useful interactions
It has been shown[14] in animal tumour lines that combinations of cisplatin and treosulfan produce longer remissions than either agent alone. Clinical studies of the combination are few but Fennelly et al[9] (1983) suggest that response rate and duration of response may be prolonged compared to that achieved with either drug alone.

Treosulfan

Major outcome trials

1. Fennelly J J 1980 Treosulfan (hydroxybusulfan) in ovarian carcinoma. Curr Chemother Inf Dis Proc 11th ICC and 19th ICAAC American Society of Microbiology: 1683–1684

This study, although involving only 69 patients, is one of the largest studies reporting results of treosulfan in patients with previously untreated ovarian carcinoma. Patients with stages I to IV disease were treated with treosulfan orally 250 mg four times daily for 4 weeks on alternate months until either primary or secondary resistance developed. Of 47 evaluable patients with measurable disease as evaluated by clinical examination and ultrasound, 12 (25%) showed a complete response and 12 (25%) showed a partial response. Of the 47 evaluable patients 34 had advanced stage III and IV disease and of these 8 (23.5%) showed a complete response for a mean of 29 months and 10 (29.4%) showed a partial response for a mean of 5.8 months. 80% of patients had some degree of marrow suppression, particularly leucopenia, although in only two patients did the white blood cell count fall below $1 \times 10^9.l^{-1}$. 15 patients experienced thrombocytopenia and 9 of these had platelet counts below $50 \times 10^9.l^{-1}$. Pigmentation occurred in 2 patients, nausea in 5 and vomiting in 2. Survival was dependent on stage with 3 year survivals of 75%, 50%, 25% and 0% for patients with stages I, II, III and IV respectively. The author concluded that treosulfan had similar efficacy to other alkylating agents in ovarian carcinoma.

2. Masding J, Sarkar T, White W F et al 1990 Intravenous treosulfan versus treosulfan plus cisplatin in advanced ovarian carcinoma. British Journal of Obstetrics and Gynaecology 97: 342–351

This study is the largest study comparing the efficacy of intravenous treosulfan alone with intravenous treosulfan in combination with cisplatin in previously untreated ovarian carcinoma. 175 patients with all stages of disease were randomized postoperatively to receive either treosulfan 7 $g.m^{-2}$ intravenously every 3 weeks for 12 months (if responding) or the same dose of treosulfan in addition to cisplatin 50 $mg.m^{-2}$ intravenously every 3 weeks. 135 patients were evaluable for response. The combined treatment resulted in an overall response rate of 86.4% versus 71% ($p<0.05$) for the treosulfan alone. The combination was particularly superior with respect to response in those patients i) under 60 years of age, ii) with stage III and IV disease, iii) with poorly differentiated tumours, and iv) with residual disease postoperatively of greater than 2 cm. Median survival was not significantly different (86 and 134 weeks following treosulfan and combination chemotherapy, respectively) although it was significantly superior following combination therapy in the subgroups above. The authors conclude that those patients with minimal residual disease (<2 cm) and those with stages Ic and II disease can be safely treated with treosulfan alone whilst those with more advanced disease should receive cisplatin in addition.

General review articles

White W F 1978 Investigation of response to, and complications of, treosulfan in the treatment of malignant ovarian tumours. Current Chemotherapy 1978: 1311–1312

References

1. Feit P W, Rastrup-Andersen N, Matagne R 1970 Studies on epoxide formation from (2S,3S)-threitol 1,4-bismethanesulfonate. The preparation and biological activity of (2S,3S)-1,2-epoxy-3,4-butanediol 4-methanesulfonate. Journal of Medicinal Chemistry 13: 1173–1175
2. Kohn K W 1977 Interstrand cross-linking of DNA by 1,3-bis(2-chloroethyl)-1-nitrosourea and other 1-(2-haloethyl)-1-nitrosoureas. Cancer Research 37: 1450–1454
3. Mazue G, Combes M 1983 Carcinogenic activity of antineoplastic agents in laboratory animals. Bulletin du Cancer (Paris) 70: 26–30
4. IARC 1981 Treosulfan. IARC Monographs on the Evaluation of the Carcinogenic Risk of Chemicals to Humans 26: 341–347
5. Petrue E, Schmahl D 1986 Second neoplasms associated with cytotoxic chemotherapy of gynaecologic carcinomas. Tumor Diagnosis and Therapy 7: 99–107
6. Kaldor J M, Day N E, Pettersson F et al 1990 Leukemia following chemotherapy for ovarian cancer. New England Journal of Medicine 322: 1–6
7. Welsh J, Stuart J F B, Soukop M et al 1982 The pharmacokinetics of oral and IV treosulfan. British Journal of Cancer 46: 467
8. Fennelly J 1977 Treosulfan (dihydroxybusulphan) in the management of ovarian carcinoma. British Journal of Obstetrics and Gynaecology 84: 300–303

T

9. Fennelly J J, Jones M P, Cantwell B, Meagher D 1983 Role of second look procedures in evaluating combined treosulfan and cisplatin in ovarian carcinoma. In: Proceedings of the 13th International Congress of Chemotherapy, Vienna, Austria
10. Masding J, Sarkar T, White W F et al 1990 Intravenous treosulfan versus treosulfan plus cisplatin in advanced ovarian carcinoma. British Journal of Obstetrics and Gynaecology 97: 342–351
11. Pedersen-Bjergaard J, Nissen N I, Sorensen H M et al 1980 Acute non-lymphocytic leukaemia in patients with ovarian carcinoma following long-term treatment with treosulfan (=dihydroxybusulfan). Cancer 45: 19–29
12. Prior J, White I 1978 Addisonian syndrome associated with treosulfan. Lancet 2: 1207–1208
13. Whyte W F, Masding J E 1982 Treosulfan chemotherapy in advanced ovarian cancer: a long-term evaluation in previously untreated disease. British Journal of Cancer 46: 491
14. Preece A W, Wells-Wilson M 1982 Enhancement of response of a lymphoblastic tumour by combination of the cycle specific drugs cisplatin and treosulfan. British Journal of Cancer 46: 498

Tretinoin

Tretinoin is a Vitamin A derivative used in the treatment of acne vulgaris.

Chemistry

Tretinoin (Vitamin A acid, Retin HA gel, Retin HA lotion)
$C_{20}H_{28}O_2$
3,7-Dimethyl-9-(2,6,6-trimethyl-1-cyclohexen-1-yl)-2,4,6,8-nona-*all trans*-tetraenoic acid

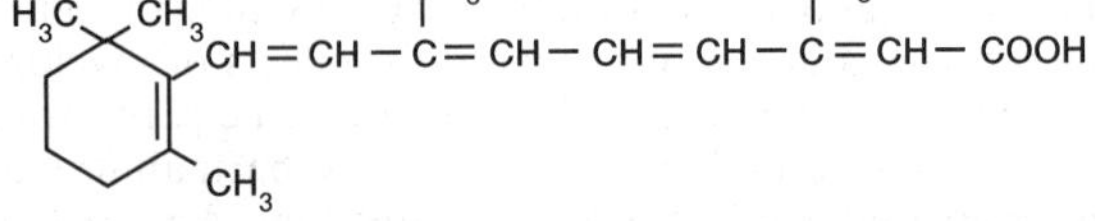

Molecular weight	300.4
pKa	—
Solubility	
in alcohol	slightly soluble
in water	insoluble
Octanol/water partition coefficient	log P 6.614

Tretinoin is a yellow to light orange crystalline powder prepared by chemical synthesis, the naturally occurring form is *all-trans*.

Pharmacology

The precise mechanism of action of topically applied tretinoin has not been determined but it has several actions on the epidermis and follicular epithelium of the pilosebaceous duct. Its action on epidermal structures may vary according to the concentration and the time for which the treatment is used.[1] Tretinoin inhibits the synthesis of tonofilaments and reduces the attachments between keratinized cells. This reduces the transit time of epithelial cells through the epidermis. In the acute phase of treatment, histological examination of the epidermis shows acanthosis and loss of the granular layer and inter and intracellular oedema, but with chronic use the granular layer returns.[1] Tretinoin provokes similar changes in the upper pilosebaceous duct but has no effect on the sebaceous gland.

Toxicology

Data on possible organ damage following what is limited systemic absorption in doses close to that used in humans are not available. Reproduction studies performed in rats and rabbits at dermal doses up to 50 times the human dose (assuming the human dose to be 500 mg of gel per day) have revealed no evidence of impaired fertility or harm to the fetus.[2] However, there was a slightly higher incidence of irregularly contoured or partially ossified skull bones in some rat and rabbit fetuses. There are no adequate and well controlled studies in pregnant women. Long-term animal studies to determine the carcinogenic potential of tretinoin have not been performed. Studies in hairless albino mice exposed to sunlight suggest that tretinoin may accelerate the tumorigenic potential of ultraviolet radiation. Although the significance to man is not clear, patients should avoid or minimize exposure to sun.

Clinical pharmacology

There are no studies designed to evaluate human tolerance, dose ranging and dose–response relationships.

Pharmacokinetics

Studies on the local metabolism of tretinoin are lacking.

Metabolism

There are virtually no data regarding the metabolism of tretinoin (VAA). Using radiolabelled VAA, it has been found that most of the VAA remains in the epidermis, especially the horny layer.[3] Apparently 80% of the drug remained on the surface, with 20% being absorbed into the epidermis and dermis. Measurements made 100 minutes after topical application showed a label equivalent of from 3.2 to 8.7 $\mu g.g^{-1}$ of tissue in the epidermis and of from 0.2 to 0.5 $\mu g.g^{-1}$ of tissue in the dermis.

Application of 6 g of 0.05% radiolabelled VAA gel did not produce measurable plasma levels in 12 hours, but there was urinary excretion of 0.1% of the applied dose in four human subjects. When 0.1% ointment (not tretinoin) was applied under occlusion to the back for 16 hours, 50% of the applied dose remained on the surface, and there was urinary excretion of 6% of the dose in 56 hours.

The sparse available data suggest that the absorption of VAA is not significant in humans and that urinary excretion is not important in the elimination of the drug. Studies of labelled VAA intravenously injected into rats showed that 60% is excreted in the bile and 20% in the urine. To summarize the limited absorption–metabolism information, it appears that the small amounts of VAA absorbed from topical application are metabolized by the liver.

Pharmaceutics

Tretinoin is available as Retin-A (Ortho-Cilag, UK/Ortho, USA) in the following formulations:

1. 0.025% w/w lotion (0.05% w/w in USA)
2. 0.025% w/w gel also 0.01% w/w (UK/USA)
3. 0.025% w/w cream (UK) 0.1 w/w (US only) and 0.05 w/w (UK, USA).

None of the preparations contains potentially allergenic substances and a true allergic contact dermatitis is very rare. As with other retinoids, tretinoin is light sensitive and in particular the lotion which is dispensed in amber bottles should be protected from light and stored in a cool place. The expiry date is as indicated on the container but is of the order of 36 months.

Therapeutic use

Indications

1. Acne vulgaris.

Other uses

2. Senile comedones
3. Trichostasis spinulosa
4. Of possible use in naevus comedonicus and pseudofolliculitis.

Contraindications

1. Known allergy
2. Pregnancy or suspected pregnancy.

Mode of use

Retin-A cream, gel or liquid should be applied once a day, before retiring, to the skin where lesions appear, using enough to cover the entire affected area lightly. The frequency and strength of application can be adjusted to obtain maximum clinical efficacy with minimal erythema and scaling.

Indications

1. Acne vulgaris

It has been shown that tretinoin is effective in the therapy of both open and closed comedones, papules and pustules: 88.8% of the patients showed a fair-to-excellent overall improvement with tretinoin alone, whereas 25% of the patients responded to placebo.[3] In a similar, double-blind, half-face study it was shown that 15.9% responded to a sulphur–resorcinol lotion, 31.9% responded to benzoyl peroxide, and 61.9% responded to tretinoin.[4] In long-term studies, good-to-excellent results were seen in 76% of patients using tretinoin, while only 31% of those who used benzoyl peroxide had similar results. However, in another study benzoyl peroxide was superior to tretinoin.[5]

Tretinoin does not decrease the skin surface free fatty acid production nor the *Propionibacterium* acnes population, but when the drug was used with demeclocycline, the combination was more therapeutically effective than either agent alone.[6,7] Within 12 weeks, tretinoin was effective on acne that varied from mild comedonal to severe cystic acne and had a 'tetracycline-sparing effect'. In severe cystic acne, the addition of benzoyl peroxide was also beneficial for patients who had tolerated tretinoin without significant inflammation.

A patient using tretinoin should wait 15 to 30 minutes after washing his face before applying the medication in order to decrease the erythema and stinging.[7] The corners of the nose, mouth, eyes and mucous membranes must be avoided because of the risk of irritation. Mild soap should be used, and the face should be washed no more than two or three times per day.

Most dermatologists in Europe use tretinoin alone in patients with mild or moderate acne, but in most patients with moderate and certainly severe acne, combined therapy using oral antibiotics such as tetracycline or erythromycin would be given. There are few studies to indicate whether the topical therapy increases the beneficial effect of oral antibiotics, but although controversial[8] limited evidence suggests that this is so.[6,7]

Other uses

2. Senile comedones

A 0.1% tretinoin solution has been shown to be successful in the treatment of senile comedones over a period of 6 to 8 weeks.[9] Subsequent treatment every 2 or 3 days kept the areas clear.

3. Trichostasis spinulosa

Some people have prominent nasal follicles due to the accumulation of cornified material and small hairs. Tretinoin works well in such patients.[10] After several weeks of daily treatment, therapy two or three times weekly only is required.

4. Naevus comedonicus and pseudofolliculitis

Tretinoin is of possible questionable benefit in these conditions.

Naevus comedonicus. This uncommon naevus can be treated with tretinoin: extrusion of the horny plugs occurs in 3 or 4 weeks with daily application. Subsequent treatment every 2 or 3 days kept the comedones from re-forming.

Pseudofolliculitis. In pseudofolliculitis, papules occur in the beard area of predominantly black males from the penetration of hair tips into the skin. A 0.05% solution of tretinoin applied daily can achieve good-to-excellent results but never complete clearing.[11] In older men with more severe disease, the response is less successful. Patients with good results were maintained on twice-weekly therapy. Tretinoin may provide satisfactory control of mild pseudofolliculitis when it is not practical for the patient to stop shaving — cession of shaving can be most beneficial.

Adverse reactions

Potentially life-threatening effects

None has been reported.

Acute overdosage

No cases have been encountered.

Severe or irreversible adverse effects

None has been reported.

Symptomatic adverse effects

True allergic contact dermatitis is rare but a primary irritant dermatitis, manifesting itself as irritation, erythema, peeling and sensation of warmth, is common. Slight stinging is common as a mild reaction in many people but settles usually with continuous use and/or reduction in frequency of application of the drug.[7]

Interference with clinical pathology tests

None is known.

High risk groups

Neonates

Tretinoin is not recommended for use in neonates.

T

Breast milk. The drug is best avoided by breast-feeding mothers.

Children
The drug can be used in young children with comedonal acne, initially the lowest concentration (0.01%) should be used, the dosage gradually being increased through to the 0.025%.

Pregnant women
The drug is contraindicated in this group.

The elderly
The drug can also be used in the elderly who develop senile comedones, as in all age groups an irritant dermatitis may occur but this can be well controlled by minimising or reducing the frequency and strength of the therapy.

Drug interactions

Potentially hazardous interactions
Particular caution should be exercised in using preparations containing peeling agents (i.e. sulphur, resorcinol, benzoyl peroxide or salicylic acid). Use of topical preparations with high concentrations of alcohol, menthol, spices or lime — such as shaving lotions, astringents and perfume — should be avoided, especially during initial therapy.

Potentially useful interactions
Since acne lesions are of two major types — the non-inflamed and the inflamed — then the combined topical use of tretinoin, which specifically deals with the non-inflamed lesions, and benzoyl peroxide, which has a greater effect on inflamed lesions, can be helpful. The benzoyl peroxide can be applied in the morning and the retinoic acid in the evening.[12] Similarly, topical tretinoin probably acts synergistically with oral tetracycline in the treatment of acne.[6,7]

References

1. Plewig G, Wolff H H, Braun-Falco O 1971 Topical treatment of normal and pathological human skin with Vitamin A acid. Clinical, histological and electron-microscopic studies. Arch. Klin. Exp. Derm. 239: 390–413
2. Juneja J S, Murthy S K, Ganguly J 1964 Effect of retinoic acid on the reproductive performances of male and female rats. Indian Journal of Experimental Biology 2 July 1964: 153–154
3. Pedace J, Stoughton R 1971 Topical retinoic acid in acne vulgaris. British Journal of Dermatology 84: 465–469
4. Gandola M, Argenziano G, Barba C et al 1976 Topical vitamin A acid in the treatment of acne vulgaris (a controlled multicenter trial). Archives of Dermatological Research 255: 129–138
5. Cunliffe W J 1985 Comparison of topical benzoyl peroxide and tretinoin. Data presented at the Canadian Dermatological Society June 1985
6. Mills H Jr, Marples R, Kligman 1972 Acne vulgaris. Oral therapy with tetracycline and topical therapy with vitamin A. Archives of Dermatology 106: 200–203
7. Leyden J J, Marples R R, Mills O H, Kligman A M 1974 Tretinoin and antibiotic therapy in acne vulgaris. Southern Medical Journal January 67 (1): 20–25
8. Gould D J, Ead R, Cunliffe W J 1978 Oral tetracycline and retinoic acid gel in acne. The Practitioner 221
9. Kligman A M, Mills O H 1971 Topically applied tretinoin for senile (solar) comedones. Archives of Dermatology 104: 420–421
10. Mills O H Jr, Kligman A M 1973 Topically applied tretinoin in the treatment of trichostasis spinulosa. Archives of Dermatology 108: 378–380
11. Kligman A M, Mills O H Jr 1973 Pseudofolliculitis of the beard and topically applied tretinoin. Archives of Dermatology 107: 551–552
12. Hurwitz S 1976 The combined effect of vitamin A acid and benzoyl peroxide in the treatment of acne. Cutis 17: 585–590

Triamcinolone

Triamcinolone is a potent synthetic glucocorticoid that is used to treat a number of autoimmune and allergic conditions. Triamcinolone acetonide was the first halogenated corticosteroid to be widely used topically and when first introduced was found to be dramatically more effective than any previous topical corticosteroid.[1,2] It was the first topical corticosteroid to have any therapeutic effect on psoriasis.

Chemistry

Triamcinolone (Adcortyl, Aristocort, Celeste, Delphicort, Kenacort, Ledercort, Omcilon, Orion, Tricortale, Volon)
$C_{21}H_{27}FO_6$
9α-Fluoro-11β,16α,17α,21-tetrahydroxypregna-1,4-diene-3,20-dione

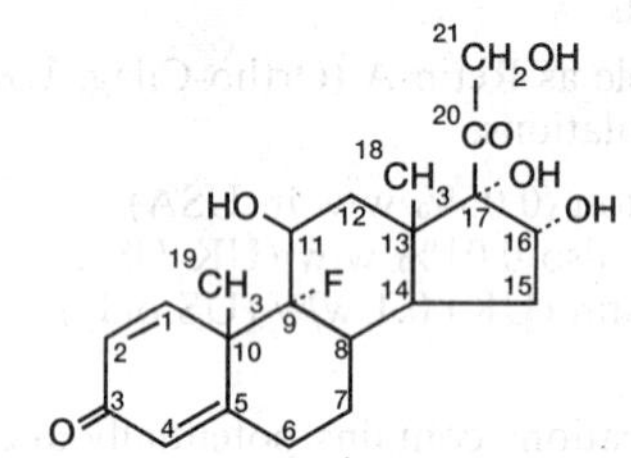

Molecular weight	394.4
pKa	—
Solubility	
in alcohol	1 in 40
in water	1 in 240
Octanol/water partition coefficient	—

Triamcinolone acetonide (Adcortyl, Aristoderm, Ftorocort, Kenacort-A, Kenalog, Kenaquart, Ledercort, Omcilon-A, Solodelf, Tramacin, Vetalog, Volon A, Volonimat)
$C_{24}H_{31}FO_6$
9α-Fluoro-11β,21-dihydroxy-16α,17[1-methylethylidenebis(oxy)] pregna-1,4-diene-3,20-dione;
9α-fluoro-11β,16α,17,21-tetrahydroxypregna-1,4-diene-3,20-dione cyclic 16,17-acetal with acetone

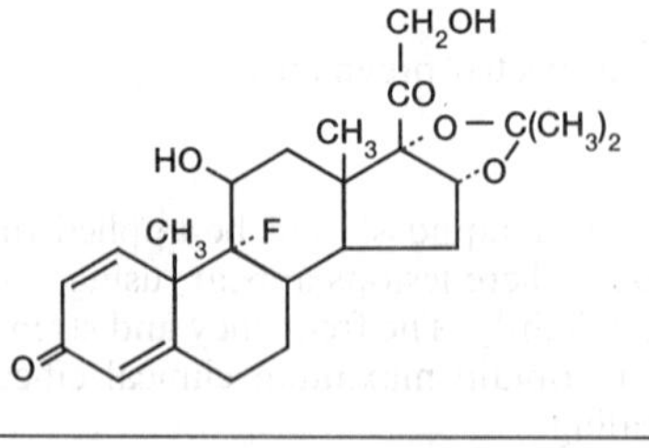

Molecular weight	434.5
pKa	—
Solubility	
in alcohol	1 in 150
in water	almost insoluble
Octanol/water partition coefficient	—

Triamcinolone hexacetonide (Aristospan, Lederspan)
$C_{30}H_{41}FO_7$
9α-Fluoro-11β,21-dihydroxy-16α,17α-isopropylidenedioxypregna-1,4-diene-3,20-dione,21-(3,3-dimethylbutyrate)

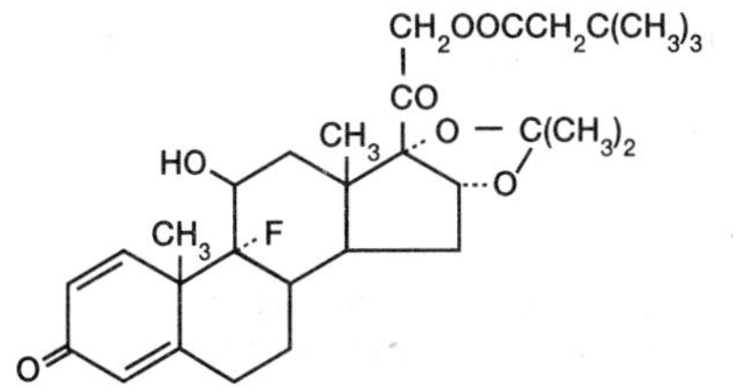

Molecular weight	532.6
pKa	—
Solubility	
in alcohol	slightly soluble
in water	almost insoluble
Octanol/partition coefficient	—

Triamcinolone is a white or almost white, crystalline powder. It is odourless or almost odourless and prepared by chemical synthesis.

Pharmacology

Triamcinolone is a synthetic fluorinated corticosteroid in which glucocorticoid activity is greatly increased and mineralocorticoid activity is much diminished compared with that of cortisol. It has the following actions.

(a) Carbohydrate metabolism. Gluconeogenesis is increased and liver glycogen stores are maintained. Peripheral utilization of glucose by transport across cell membranes is decreased due to insulin antagonism.

(b) Protein metabolism. Amino acids are mobilized from a number of tissues but mainly skeletal muscle, bone and skin, and in the liver are converted into glucose and are stored as glycogen. High doses may cause loss of tissue protein and negative nitrogen balance.

(c) Fat metabolism. Fat is mobilized and deposition on shoulders, face and abdomen is increased.

(d) Water and electrolyte balance. Corticosteroids with mineralocorticoid action cause sodium retention and potassium depletion but triamcinolone possesses little or no such activity.

(e) Anti-inflammatory actions. Corticosteroids suppress or prevent development of the signs of inflammation, i.e. local heat, redness, tenderness and swelling, regardless of its cause. The early microscopic features (capillary dilation, oedema, migration of leucocytes and phagocytes) and the later signs (proliferation of capillaries and fibroblasts, collagen deposition) are inhibited. Some of these features occur because of formation of the phospholipase inhibitor lipocortin which diminishes the supply of arachidonic acid available for synthesis of prostaglandins and leukotrienes.

(f) Blood cells and lymphoid tissue. Erythrocytes and neutrophil leucocytes are increased in number, eosinophil and basophil leucocytes and lymphocytes are decreased in number, as is the mass of lymphoid tissue, when corticosteroids are administered.

Toxicology

General effects of prolonged use are described below under Adverse reactions. Teratogenicity data on triamcinolone itself are lacking but those for corticosteroids in general are described in the monograph on Cortisone acetate.

Clinical pharmacology

The principal effects of triamcinolone in man relate to its glucocorticoid action and suppression of inflammatory responses. Glucocorticoid activity leads to increased gluconeogenesis and decreased utilization of glucose in the tissues.[3,4] Protein catabolism is accelerated and synthesis from dietary protein is decreased[5,6] although the overall effect on nitrogen balance depends on other factors including diet, dose and duration of treatment. At a clinically effective maintenance dose of up to 12 mg daily for short periods, nitrogen balance may be retained[7] but a negative balance may develop at doses between 12 and 24 mg daily.[5,8] Muscle wasting may be particularly marked with triamcinolone. Triamcinolone has negligible mineralocorticoid activity and indeed dose-related natriuresis occurred in healthy volunteers who received 4–64 mg daily for 4 days.[7,9–11] Potassium loss was observed in subjects who received triamcinolone 32–64 mg daily for 20 days[9] but not in those taking 16–32 mg daily.[11]

Corticosteroids prevent or suppress the initial phenomena of the inflammatory process, i.e. redness, tenderness, local heat, swelling and also the later sequelae that include proliferation of fibroblasts and deposition of collagen.

Pharmacokinetics

Triamcinolone may be assayed in nanogram quantities in body fluids by liquid chromatography[12–14] and by radioimmunoassay,[15] the detection limit by the latter method being 0.1 $\mu g.l^{-1}$.

Triamcinolone acetonide, administered intravenously in the form of its phosphate ester, in high (10 $mg.kg^{-1}$) and medium (80 mg) dose was rapidly hydrolysed to triamcinolone acetonide, the pharmacokinetics of which were subsequently analysed.[16] Non-linearity was shown by the finding of a significant difference in clearance, 45.2 $l.h^{-1}$ with the high and 69.5 $l.h^{-1}$ with the medium dose, whereas there was no significant difference in terminal half life, 88 and 87 min, or in apparent volume of distribution, 99.5 l and 148.0 l, respectively.

After intra-articular injection in doses of 10, 20 and 40 mg triamcinolone acetonide was detected in plasma for > 2 weeks.[19] The concentration–time curve declined in a tri-exponential manner and the half life of the terminal phase was 3.2–6.4 days compared with about 1.5 hours after intravenous dosing[16] indicating that continued absorption influences this phase after intra-articular administration. Total body clearance was 38.8–62.9 $l.h^{-1}$ compared to 69.5 $l.h^{-1}$ after intravenous administration and is compatible with complete absorption from the site of injection. The mean residence time at the site of administration was 3.2–4.3 days. The plasma concentrations of triamcinolone acetonide administered as the hexacetonide in doses of 20 and 40 mg were lower and declined in a bi-exponential manner with a terminal half life of 4.6 days, and the total body clearance was 75.0–67.5 $l.h^{-1}$ which also indicated complete absorption.

Binding of triamcinolone to plasma proteins is consistently less than that of cortisol and other corticosteroid analogues and at physiological concentrations there is at least five times more free triamcinolone than cortisol in plasma.[18]

Oral absorption	Not applicable
Presystemic metabolism	Not applicable
Plasma half life	
range	1.5–5 hours
Volume of distribution	99.5–148 litres
Plasma protein binding	Low

Topical triamcinolone acetonide is absorbed through the skin in varying proportions of the applied dose depending upon the severity of the damage to the stratum corneum barrier that has resulted from the skin disease being treated. It is probable that no more than 5% of the applied dose is absorbed.

Concentration–effect relationship

The relation between plasma cortisol and plasma triamcinolone acetonide was defined over a concentration range.[19] This indicated that there was a threshold plasma triamcinolone acetonide concentration of 3–4 $\mu g.l^{-1}$ that would cause the plasma cortisol to decline to < 50 $\mu g.l^{-1}$. A relationship between plasma concentration and therapeutic effect, e.g. suppression of inflammation, has not been established and there is no case for therapeutic drug monitoring.

Metabolism

Triamcinolone acetonide administered intravenously as its phosphate ester is rapidly and completely hydrolysed to triamcinolone acetonide. Renal clearance of the latter is low, less than 1% being recovered unchanged in the urine.[16] The major route of excretion in the rat, dog and monkey is the bile. The principal metabolite recovered in the urine from these species is 6β-hydroxytriamcinolone acetonide, lesser amounts appearing as the glucuronide and sulphate conjugates.[17] In man, 6β-hydroxytriamcinolone is the main urinary metabolite after triamcinolone by mouth.[20] Thus, unlike hydrocortisone and prednisolone which are subject to several well established metabolic conversions, triamcinolone is metabolized principally to the 6β-hydroxy derivative; this may result from inhibition of other pathways by the presence of the 9α-fluoro and the 16α-hydroxyl groups.

Pharmaceutics

Triamcinolone is available as tablets in the UK, in topical and injection forms in the UK and USA and only in the USA as an inhaler for obstructive airways disease.

1. Ledercort (Lederle, UK): Tablets 2 mg, which are blue, oblong, coded 'LL11' and contain triamcinolone 2 mg each. Ledercort Tablets 4 mg are white, oblong, coded 'LL4406' and contain triamcinolone 4 mg each. The tablets should be stored at 15–30°C.
2. Lederspan Injection (Lederle, UK): 20 $mg.ml^{-1}$ suspension for intra-articular and intrasynovial administration and 5 $mg.ml^{-1}$ suspension for intralesional and sublesional administration. These contain micronized triamcinolone hexacetonide which should be stored at room temperature and not frozen.
3. An intra-articular/intramuscular formulation is manufactured as Kenalog (Squibb, UK, USA) and as Aristocort Forte (Lederle, USA). Both are presented as sterile, aqueous suspensions of triamcinolone acetonide 40 $mg.ml^{-1}$. These preparations should be stored at room temperature and freezing should be avoided.
   10 $mg.ml^{-1}$ and 25 $mg.ml^{-1}$ formulations are marketed for intralesional use in the USA.
   The 10 $mg.ml^{-1}$ strength is available in the UK as Adcortyl Intra-articular/Intradermal.
4. Ledercort Cream 0.1% (Lederle, UK) is white and contains triamcinolone acetonide; it should be stored in a cool place and if diluted should not be used more than one month after issue. In the USA two other strengths of Aristocort cream (Lederle) are also marketed: 0.025% and 0.5%.
5. Ledercort Ointment 0.1% (Lederle, UK) is pale yellow and contains triamcinolone acetonide; it should be stored in a cool place. Aristocort 0.5% ointment is also available in the USA in addition to a 0.1% strength.
6. Kenalog (Squibb, USA) spray delivers 0.2 mg per 2 second spray of acetonide onto the skin.
7. Azmacort (Rorer, USA) inhaler delivers 100 μg traimcinolone acetonide per actuation.
8. Kenalog in Orabase (Squibb, USA) provides 1 mg (0.1%) triamcinolone as acetonide in a Plastibase dental gel. Adcortyl in Orabase (Squibb, UK) is a similar 0.1% preparation in an adhesive base of gelatine, pectin and sodium carboxymethylcellulose in a polyethylene and liquid paraffin base.

Therapeutic use

Indications

Triamcinolone

1. Rheumatoid, gouty and osteoarthritis
2. Rheumatic fever
3. Disseminated lupus erythematosus
4. Nephrotic syndrome
5. Bronchial asthma
6. Dermatoses
7. Haemolytic disorders.

Topical uses

8. Control of all forms of subacute or subsiding eczemas or as part of a regimen of slowly decreasing the potency of topical steroids being used in the management of chronic eczema
9. Flexural and facial psoriasis
10. Idiopathic and genital pruritis
11. Lichen planus
12. Aphthous ulcers and mucosal erosive erythema multiforme.

Contraindications (relative)

1. Active infection
2. Diabetes
3. Osteoporosis
4. Myopathy
5. Peptic ulcer
6. Psychosis
7. Tissue healing.

Topical use is contraindicated (relatively) in

8. Infective lesions such as impetigo, tinea corporis and herpes simplex
9. Neonates
10. Acne vulgaris
11. Rosacea
12. Gravitational ulceration.

Mode of use

1. Arthritis

Triamcinolone is now rarely used in the systemic treatment of rheumatoid arthritis but may be administered intra-articularly to relieve pain and inflammation due to rheumatoid and gouty arthritis and osteoarthritis.[21,22] Patients must be warned not to overuse joints when symptomatic benefit has been obtained and intra-articular injections repeated over a long period may cause severe joint destruction and bone necrosis. Triamcinolone may also be given locally to alleviate bursitis and tenosynovitis, care being taken to inject into the space between the tendon sheath and the tendon and not into the tendon itself as this may cause it subsequently to rupture.[23] The dose depends on the size of the joint or synovial space and the degree of inflammation. Normally 2–6 mg of the hexacetonide form will suffice for small joints and 10–30 mg for large joints every 3–4 weeks; the dose requirements for the acetonide form are approximately double these. It is mandatory to pay strict attention to asepsis during administration. Triamcinolone instilled into the pericardial sac prevents the accumulation of intractable effusion in uraemic patients.[24–26]

2–5. As an anti-inflammatory steroid

Triamcinolone may be administered orally as an anti-inflammatory steroid. It has been used in rheumatic fever (6–20 mg daily), disseminated lupus erythematosus (3–30 mg daily), nephrotic syndrome (16–20 mg daily, bronchial asthma (8–16 mg daily), dermatoses (8–16 mg daily) and autoimmune haemolytic anaemia when the initial dose is 12–24 mg daily. Alternatively, triamcinolone acetonide 40–100 mg may be given by deep intramuscular injection for depot effect repeated at intervals according to the patient's response, but usually every 3–4 weeks. This mode of administration may provide benefit, e.g. in asthma,[27] and be associated with fewer adverse effects of the type associated with chronic use of corticosteroids.

Triamcinolone acetonide may be administered by pressurized aerosol to treat bronchial asthma. Patients who cannot tolerate beclomethasone dipropionate as an aerosol due to cough or wheezing can inhale triamcinolone aerosol without difficulty.[28] Children who received triamcinolone by aerosol for 6 to 32 months did not exhibit significant adrenal suppression as judged by morning plasma cortisol concentrations.[29]

6. Skin lesions

Triamcinolone hexacetonide (0.5 mg or less per square inch of affected skin) may be injected into or under various cutaneous lesions and may benefit cystic acne, alopecia areata, nummular eczema, granuloma annulare, keloids,[30] lichen planus, discoid lupus erythematosus and pyoderma gangrenosum.[31]

Topical use

Triamcinolone acetonide topical preparations are applied to the skin in a thin film using the minimum quantity possible. They should not be used as emollients, which should be supplied as an additional prescription.

8. Eczema

Triamcinolone acetonide preparations are of value in subacute or subsiding eczemas of any type and may form part of a group of topical steroids of varying potency which are used in descending sequence as eczema comes under control.[32]

9. Psoriasis

Triamcinolone acetonide preparations are of great value in the treatment of facial and flexural psoriasis. As with all topical steroids

Triamcinolone

in these areas, they should be used for the shortest time possible with return to lower potency steroids when possible.

10. Ideopathic and genital pruritis
Triamcinolone acetonide can be used to treat idiopathic and genital pruritis when all organic causes have been excluded.

11. Lichen planus
In mild, not extensive, lichen planus, triamcinolone acetonide preparations are indicated. The preparation in an adhesive base is very useful in erosive mucosal lichen planus.

12. Apthous ulcers and erosive erythema multiforme
Aphthous ulceration and erosive erythema multiforme are usefully treated with triamcinolone in the adhesive base.
Topical use in children does not appear to cause significant adrenal suppression.[33]

Contraindications

Contraindications are relative and depend on the advantage to be expected, the intended duration of use and route of administration, e.g. systemic vs. topical.

1. Active infection
Corticosteroids impair response to infection and may activate or exacerbate local or systemic viral infection, systemic fungal infections or active infections not controlled by antimicrobial drugs, and latent or healed tuberculosis.

2. Diabetes
The dose of drugs used for diabetes may need to be increased and control of the disease may become more difficult.

3. Osteoporosis
With long-term use osteoporosis may become worse, particularly in the elderly, and there is danger of vertebral collapse.

4. Myopathy
Previous proximal myopathy with corticosteroid is a contraindication because of the special risk of this adverse effect with triamcinolone (see below).

5. Peptic ulcer
Peptic ulcer is weakly associated with corticosteroid use and there is a risk of haemorrhage or perforation. Patients who are also taking non-steroidal anti-inflammatory drugs are especially at risk.

6. Psychosis
Paranoia or depression with risk of suicide may be precipitated, especially in patients with a history of these illnesses.

7. Tissue healing
Delay in tissue healing may be important in a patient who has recently had an intestinal anastomosis.

Adverse reactions

Potentially life-threatening effects
Corticosteroids suppress the normal inflammatory responses and chronic use may activate latent infection, for example tubercular or fungal. The clinical signs of perforation of peptic ulcer may be masked. Prolonged systemic use of triamcinolone suppresses hypothalamic–pituitary–adrenal responsiveness and abrupt withdrawal of the steroid may lead to a hypoadrenal crisis. In some patients responsiveness is impaired by use of triamcinolone as an inhaled aerosol.[34]

The use of large amounts of triamcinolone acetonide preparations over very large areas of the body can lead to sufficient systemic absorption to produce adrenal suppression,[9] Cushings syndrome, diabetes, hypertension and growth suppression in children.

Acute overdosage
Accidental or intentional ingestion of a single excessive dose of a corticosteroid is unlikely to have serious results, but any symptoms that did occur would have to be treated symptomatically.

Severe or irreversible adverse effects
Prolonged use is associated with the development of characteristic cushingoid body changes including moon face, buffalo hump and distribution of fat on the torso rather than the limbs. In addition osteoporosis and spontaneous fractures may occur. Use in children may result in restriction of their growth.

There is a weak association between peptic ulcer and corticosteroid use, and a stronger association when a corticosteroid and a non-steroidal anti-inflammatory drug are used concurrently. A corticosteroid may also suppress symptoms and delay healing of an existing ulcer. Psychotic disturbance may be precipitated. Ocular effects include glaucoma, which may occur rarely after subconjunctival injection of triamcinolone,[36] and posterior subcapsular cataract. Myopathy may be associated with the use of systemic corticosteroids in general but it appears to be a particular problem with 9α-fluorinated derivatives such as triamcinolone. Atrophy develops gradually, painlessly and symmetrically, affecting principally the hip and to a lesser extent the shoulder muscles. When administration of the corticosteroid is stopped, the myopathy usually improves over a number of months. Children appear to be at greatest risk.

Minor degrees of adrenal suppression commonly occur following the use of triamcinolone acetonide preparations over even relatively small areas of the body under plastic occlusion. Serious adverse effects nearly always follow from uncontrolled repeat prescriptions and have been reported more frequently in psoriasis than in eczema due to the fact that the parakeratotic keratin of the psoriatic is more permeable than normal keratin.[37]

The local side effects of topical corticosteroids on the skin are atrophy, steroid purpura, striae and increased skin fragility. The use of topical triamcinolone acetonide on the face may result in perioral rosacea (perioral dermatitis). Striae may occur, especially in the flexures. The sudden withdrawal of topical triamcinolone acetonide or other high potency topical corticosteroids in patients with psoriasis, may result in generalized exfoliative or generalized pustular psoriasis. Topical triamcinolone acetonide applied to patients with acne vulgaris will exacerbate the condition, and tinea so treated will result in the condition of tinea incognito,[38] whilst if scabies is accidentally treated with topical high potency steroids, the infestation may be exaggerated or the diagnosis missed for a long period.[39]

Symptomatic adverse effects
Diabetes may become more difficult to treat, requiring a higher dose of insulin, and latent diabetes may become active. Acne, hirsutism, striae and purpura may appear. Menstrual irregularity may occur. As triamcinolone possesses little mineralocorticoid action, salt and water retention which may otherwise result from corticosteroid excess, are minimal. Local subcutaneous atrophy may develop after injection of triamcinolone (for example for bursitis),[40] as with other corticosteroids.

Interference with clinical pathology tests
No technical interferences of this kind have been reported.

High risk groups

Neonates
Systemic corticosteroid should be used with caution in view of possible growth retardation. Triamcinolone acetonide by intramuscular injection (Kenalog) is not recommended for children under 6 years.

Breast milk. There are no data on the passage of triamcinolone into breast milk.

Children
What has been said above about neonates also applies to older children.

Pregnant women
Although a teratogenic risk is not established, use of triamcinolone during pregnancy should be avoided.

Topical administration of corticosteroids to pregnant animals can cause fetal abnormalities. While the relevance of this finding to human subjects has not been established, the drug should not be used on large areas of skin or in large amounts for prolonged periods during pregnancy.

The elderly
Special observation is advised for the elderly who may be harbouring latent tuberculosis.

Concurrent disease
Enhanced effects may be encountered in patients with cirrhosis in whom inactivation of triamcinolone will be delayed.

T

Drug interactions

Potentially hazardous interactions

Combination of a corticosteroid with a non-steroidal anti-inflammatory drug increases the risk of developing peptic ulcer and gastrointestinal haemorrhage.

Other significant interactions

Corticosteroids have been reported to antagonize neuromuscular blockade caused by pancuronium.[41,42] The risk of hypokalaemia may be increased if triamcinolone is given concurrently with sympathomimetics and theophylline which lower plasma potassium and with potassium-losing diuretics; hypokalaemia may also potentiate the effects of cardiac glycosides. The diabetogenic effect of corticosteroids will impair blood glucose control with insulin and oral hypoglycaemic agents. Steady-state plasma concentration of salicylate is reduced by intra-articular injection of corticosteroids, including triamcinolone.[43] Oral candidiasis may complicate inhaled corticosteroid therapy but with triamcinolone acetonide aerosol the incidence appears to be low.[44,45]

Potentially useful interactions

No interactions of this kind have been reported.

Clinical trials

1. Grieco M H, Dwek J, Larsen, Rammohan G 1978 Clinical effect of aerosol triamcinolone acetonide in bronchial asthma. Archives of Internal Medicine 138: 1337–1341

In a double-blind, 12-week study of patients with reversible bronchial asthma dependent on oral corticosteroid, 20 of 31 patients (64.5%) who received triamcinolone acetonide aerosol 800 µg daily were able to discontinue steroid therapy compared to 3 of 29 (10.3%) treated with aerosol placebo. Forced expiratory volume in the first second, forced vital capacity and maximum mid-expiratory flow rate all improved significantly in the group that received triamcinolone. The mean oral dose of prednisolone equivalent decreased from 13.3 to 2.9 mg daily over the period of assessment and the mean 8 a.m. plasma cortisol rose from 5.3 to 8.6 $\mu g.dl^{-1}$ in these patients as is compatible with lessening of adrenal suppression. Significant oral candidiasis was noted in two patients.

2. Bird H A, Ring E F, Bacon P A 1979 A thermographic and clinical comparison of three intra-articular steroid preparations in rheumatoid arthritis. Annals of Rheumatic Diseases 38: 36–39

In a double-blind study of 30 patients with rheumatoid arthritis, prednisolone t-butyl acetate, methylprednisolone acetate or triamcinolone hexacetonide was injected into one knee joint. Thermographic improvement was recorded with all three drugs but was greatest initially and was most long-lasting with triamcinolone. No systemic improvement was seen with any drug after a single injection, although all three steroid preparations suppressed endogenous cortisol.

3. Petri M, Dobrow R, Neiman R, Whiting-O'Keefe Q, Seaman W E 1987 Randomised, double-blind, placebo-controlled study of the treatment of painful shoulder. Arthritis and Rheumatism 30: 1040–1045

The effect of injection of triamcinolone into the subacromial bursa was compared with that of naproxen by mouth in 100 patients with painful shoulder. The outcome was judged by the degree of active abduction, pain, limitation of function and a clinical index that combined weighted measures of all these. Both drugs were superior to placebo and triamcinolone was superior to naproxen for relief of pain and by the clinical index. Multiple linear regression analysis showed that drug treatment accounted for only 16% of the variation in outcome, and 44% was accounted for by the clinical index prior to treatment, i.e. those with most room for improvement were least likely to improve.

References

1. Vickers C F H, Tighe S M 1960 Topical triamcinolone in eczema. British Journal of Dermatology 72: 352–354
2. Cohen J, Baer R L 1961 Observations upon the use of topical triamcinolone acetonide preparations in different concentrations. Dermatologica 122: 116–119
3. Lerner L J 1966 Laboratory and clinical evaluation of long acting corticoids, triamcinolone acetonide. Clinical Medicine 73: 53–54

Triamcinolone

4. Lerner L J, Bianchi A, Turkheimer A R, Singer F M, Borman A 1964 Anti-inflammatory steroids; potency, duration and modification of activities. Annals of the New York Academy of Sciences 116: 1071–1077
5. Albanese A A, Lorenze E J, Orto L A 1962 Nutritional and metabolic effects of some newer steroids: 1. Oxandrolone and triamcinolone. New York Journal of Medicine 62: 1607–1613
6. Liddle G 1961 Clinical pharmacology of the anti-inflammatory steroids. Clinical Pharmacology and Therapeutics 2: 623–635
7. Hellman L, Zumoff B, Minsky A, Kretchmer N, Kramer B 1959 Treatment of the nephrotic syndrome with triamcinolone. Pediatrics 23: 686–689
8. Freyberg R H, Bernsten C A Jr, Hellman L 1958 Further experiences with 1,9 α fluoro, 16 hydroxyhydrocortisone (Triamcinolone) in treatment of patients with rheumatoid arthritis. Arthritis and Rheumatism 1: 215
9. Curd G W, Spurr C L 1958 Metabolic effects of 9-α-fluoro-16-α-hydroxyl-delta-1 hydrocortisone. American Journal of Medicine 25: 116–117
10. Hellman L, Zumoff B, Schwartz M K, Gallagher R F, Bernsten C A, Freyberg R H 1957 Antirheumatic and metabolic effects of a new synthetic steroid. Annals of Rheumatic Diseases 16: 141–144
11. McMahon F G, Gordon E S, Kenoyer W C, Keil P 1960 Renal and pituitary-inhibiting effects of exogenous corticosteroids in normal subjects. Metabolism 9: 511–527
12. Au D S, Runikis J O, Abbott F S, Burton R W 1981 GLC analysis of hydrocortisone, triamcinolone acetonide, and desonide in culture media of mouse and human dermal fibroblasts using flame-ionization detection. Journal of Pharmaceutical Sciences 70: 917–923
13. Schoneshofer M, Kage A, Weber B 1983 New 'on-line' sample pretreatment procedure for routine liquid-chromatographic assay of low-concentration compounds in body fluids, illustrated by triamcinolone assay. Clinical Chemistry 29: 1367–1371
14. Agabeyoglu I T, Wagner J G, Kay D R 1980 A sensitive high-pressure liquid chromatographic method for the determination of prednisone, prednisolone and hydrocortisone in plasma. Research Communications in Chemical Pathology and Pharmacology 28: 163–167
15. Haack D, Vecsei P 1982 Radioimmunologische Bestimmungen von Triamcinolonacetonid und ihre Andwendungin einer Studie zur Hudrolyse wasserloslicher Kortikoidester. Arzneimittel Forschung/Drug Research 32 (suppl 11) 832–834
16. Mollman H, Rohdewald P, Schmidt E W, Salomon V, Derendorf H 1985 Pharmacokinetics of triamcinolone and its phosphate ester. European Journal of Clinical Pharmacology 29: 85–89
17. Kripalani K J, Cohen A I, Weliky I, Schreiber E C 1975 Metabolism of triamcinolone-21-phosphate in dogs, monkeys and rats. Journal of Pharmaceutical Sciences 64: 1351–1359
18. Florini J R, Buyske D A 1961 Plasma protein binding of triamcinolone-H^3 and hydrocortisone-H^{14}. Journal of Biological Chemistry 236: 247–251
19. Derendorf H, Mollmann H, Gruner A, Haak D, Gyselby G 1986 Pharmacokinetics and pharmacodynamics of glucocorticoid suspensions after intra-articular administration. Clinical Pharmacology and Therapeutics 39: 313–317
20. Florini J R, Smith L L, Buyake D A 1961 Metabolic fate of a synthetic corticosteroid (triamcinolone) in the dog. Journal of Biological Chemistry 236: 1038–1042
21. Valtonen E J 1981 Clinical comparison of triamcinolone hexacetonide and betamethasone in the treatment of osteoarthritis of the knee-joint. Scandinavian Journal of Rheumatology 41 (suppl): 1–7
22. Allen R C, Gross K R, Laxer R M, Malleson P N, Beauchamp R D, Petty R E 1986 Intraarticular triamcinolone hexacetonide in the management of chronic arthritis in children. Arthritis and Rheumatism 29: 997–1001
23. Ford L T, DeBender J 1979 Tendon rupture after local steroid injection. Southern Medical Journal 72: 827–830
24. Fuller T J, Knochel J P, Brennen J P, Fetner C D, White M G 1976 Reversal of intractable uraemic pericarditis by triamcinolone hexacetonide. Archives of Internal Medicine 136: 979–982
25. Buselmeier T J, Davin T D, Simmons R L, Najarian J S, Kjellstrand C M 1978 Treatment of intractable pericardial effusion. Avoidance of pericardiectomy with local steroid instillation. Journal of the American Medical Association 240: 1358–1359
26. Quigg R J, Idelson B A, Yoburn D C, Hymes J L, Schick E C, Bernard D B 1985 Local steroid in dialysis-associated pericardial effusion. A single intrapericardial administration of triamcinolone. Archives of Internal Medicine 145: 2249–2250
27. Willey R F, Fergusson R J, Godden D J, Crompton G K, Grant I W 1984 Comparison of oral prednisolone and intramuscular depot triamcinolone in patients with severe chronic asthma. Thorax 39: 340–344
28. Shim C S, Williams M H Jr 1987 Cough and wheezing from beclomethasone diproprionate aerosol are absent after triamcinolone acetonide. Annals of Internal Medicine 106: 700–703
29. Sly R M, Imseis M, Frazer M, Joseph F 1978 Treatment of asthma in children with triamcinolone acetonide aerosol. Journal of Allergy and Clinical Immunology 62: 76–82
30. Kiil J 1977 Keloids treated with topical injections of triamcinolone acetonide (Kenalog). Immediate and long-term results. Scandinavian Journal of Plastic and Reconstructive Surgery 11: 169–172
31. Goldstein F, Krain R, Thornton J J 1985 Intralesional steroid therapy of pyoderma gangrenosum. Journal of Clinical Gastroenterology 7: 449–501
32. Vickers C F H, Charters S, McKean C D 1976 The use of topical steroids of differing potency in the management of the atopic child. British Journal of Dermatology 94 (suppl 12): 32–33
33. Rasmussen J E 1978 Percutaneous absorption of topically applied triamcinolone in children. Archives of Dermatology 114: 1165–1167
34. Droszcz W, Malunowicz E, Lech B, Krawczynska H, Madalinska M 1979 Assessment of adrenocortical function in asthmatic patients on long-term triamcinolone acetonide treatment. Annals of Allergy 42: 41–43

35. Munro D D 1979 Topical corticosteroid therapy and its effects on the hypthalmic pituitary axis. Dermatologica 152 (suppl): 173–180
36. Mills D W, Siebert L F, Climenhaga D B 1986 Depot triamcinolone-induced glaucoma. Canadian Journal of Ophthalmology 21: 150–152
37. Scoggins R B, Kligman B 1965 Percutaneous absorption of corticosteroids. New England Journal of Medicine 273: 831–836
38. Ives F A, Marks R 1968 Tinea incognito. British Medical Journal 111: 149–152
39. Clayton R, Farrow S 1975 Norwegian scabies following topical steroid therapy. Postgraduate Medical Journal 51: 657–659
40. Jacobs M B 1986 Local subcutaneous atrophy after corticosteroid injection. Postgraduate Medicine 80: 159–160
41. Meyers E F 1977 Partial recovery from pancuronium neuromuscular blockade following hydrocortisone administration. Anesthesiology 46: 148–150
42. Laflin M J 1977 Interaction of pancuronium and corticosteroids. Anesthesiology 47: 471–472
43. Edelman J, Potter J M, Hackett L P 1986 The effect of intra-articular steroid on plasma salicylate concentration. British Journal of Clinical Pharmacology 21: 301–307
44. Pingleton W W, Bone R C, Kerby G R, Ruth W E 1977 Oropharyngeal candidiasis in patients treated with triamcinolone acetonide aerosol. Journal of Allergy and Clinical Immunology 60: 254–258
45. Chervinsky P, Petraco A J 1979 Incidence of oral candidiasis during therapy with triamcinolone acetonide aerosol. Annals of Allergy 43: 80–83

Triamterene

Triamterene is a potassium-conserving diuretic.

Chemistry

Triamterene (Dytac, Dyrenium, Jariopur, Teriam)
$C_{12}H_{11}N_7$
2,4,7-Triamino-6-phenylpteridine

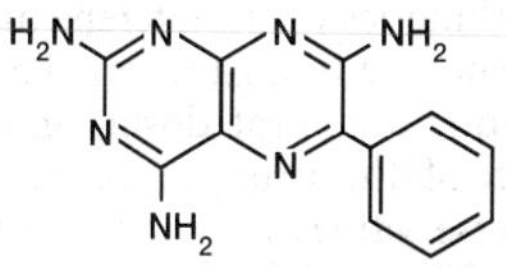

Molecular weight	253.3
pKa (amino)	6.2
Solubility	
in alcohol	1 in 3000
in water	1 in 1000
Octanol/water partition coefficient	—

Triamterene is a yellow, odourless crystalline powder, which is almost tasteless, having a slightly bitter after-taste. It is prepared by chemical synthesis.

Triamterene is available in oral combinations with hydrochlorothiazide (Dyazide), frusemide (Frusene), benzthiazide (Dytide) and chlorthalidone (Kalspare).

Pharmacology

Triamterene is a mild diuretic, acting primarily on the distal nephron. It increases the excretion of sodium and of chloride without increasing the excretion of potassium. The mechanism of action does not involve aldosterone antagonism.[1] The primary action seems to be to inhibit the electrogenic entry of sodium thus causing a fall in the electrical potential across the tubular epithelium. Since this potential is one of the main forces in the secretion of potassium this mechanism is likely to be the basis of the potassium sparing effect.

Toxicology

Toxicological studies have not demonstrated any specific problem of clinical relevance. Teratogenicity tests in the rat and rabbit have shown no evidence of fetal abnormality or effect on live birth index and litter size.

Clinical pharmacology

Triamterene is a mild diuretic and used alone causes a modest increase in the excretion of sodium and chloride by the kidney. When the excretion of potassium is increased by other diuretics (e.g. thiazides) triamterene causes a marked decrease in its excretion.[2] Triamterene has no significant pharmacological action other than that on the kidney. It does not cause an increase in plasma urate or perturb glucose homeostasis, unlike thiazide diuretics. Because of the dangers of hyperkalaemia, triamterene should not normally be prescribed with spironolactone or potassium supplements. Particular care is needed in patients with impairment of renal function.

Pharmacokinetics

The preferred assay method for triamterene in plasma is based on the extraction of the drug as the perchlorate ion pair from the plasma,

T

and high performance liquid chromatography (HPLC) of the extract coupled with fluorescence detection.[3] Linearity of this method is good to 2 μg.l^{-1}, the coefficient of variation is acceptable (< 10%) at 2 μg.l^{-1}, the limit of detection.

Variations in the fate of orally and intravenously administered triamterene have been observed in healthy adult males,[4] which reflect considerable inter-subject variability in absorption, plasma protein binding and elimination of the drug. Bioavailability in normal subjects after oral administration varied from 30 to 70%. The half life was 1.5–2.5 h and the peak plasma concentration was reached 2–4 h after dosing. A metabolite of the drug was detected in plasma only 30 minutes after the oral dose, and in the urine at 1.5 h, indicating a rapid and extensive metabolism of the drug. However, the assay method used was not able to distinguish all metabolites. In this same study, the binding of triamterene to albumin ranged from 43 to 53%. The apparent volume of distribution was 2.2–3.7 l.kg^{-1} in two subjects. Low concentrations of triamterene have been detected in the CNS of guinea-pigs and baboons and high concentrations in guinea-pig heart.[5]

Mutschler et al,[6] using an even more sensitive assay method, studied the pharmacokinetics of triamterene and its metabolites after both oral and intravenous administration. The comparison of AUC values after intravenous and oral dosing gave a bioavailability of 52%. The absorption of the drug appeared to be 83%. The large difference between these values may indicate substantial presyetemic metabolism. Between 30 and 70% of an oral dose is excreted in the urine with 1–10% of the dose as unchanged triamterene.

Oral absorption	30–83%
Presystemic metabolism	possibly 40%
Plasma half life range	1.5–2.5 h
Volume of distribution	2.2-3.7 l.kg^{-1}
Plasma protein binding	45–70%

The elimination of triamterene is reduced in renal failure and the drug is contraindicated in progressive renal failure. Hepatic disease markedly prolongs the duration of action of the drug and increases the plasma concentrations. It is likely that triamterene is excreted in breast milk and crosses the placenta, but the extent is not known.

Concentration–effect relationship

No experimental work has been done to show whether the therapeutic effect of triamterene occurs within a defined range of plasma concentrations. When taken on an empty stomach, the drug can act within 2 to 4 hours, with peak effects occurring in about 6 hours. The full effect may be delayed until after several days of treatment.

Metabolism

Triamterene is extensively metabolized and is mainly excreted as metabolites in the urine. The metabolic pathway involves the formation of *p*-hydroxytriamterene, which becomes conjugated with active sulphate to form *p*-hydroxytriamterene sulphate (Fig. 1). This metabolite has pharmacological activity equal to that of triamterene, as seen in experiments in the rat and dog. N-glucuronides of triamterene have been described, which are excreted in the bile.[7]

Pharmaceutics

Triamterene is available as tablets or capsules for oral administration. The leading brand, Dytac capsules (SmithKline Beecham, UK) or Dyrenium (SmithKline Beecham, USA), are opaque maroon-coloured capsules, marked 'SKF', each containing 50 mg triamterene as a yellow, granular powder. A 100 mg capsule of triamterene is available in the USA (SmithKline Beecham) in a larger maroon-coloured capsule. There are no parenteral or slow-release dosage forms available.

The capsules must be stored in a dry place, and under suitable conditions have a shelf-life of 5 years. Dytac capsules do not contain tartrazine or other azo dyes.

Triamterene is also available in combination with thiazide diuretics including benzthiazide, chlorthalidone and hydrochlorothiazide. A frusemide combination is also marketed.

Triamterene

Fig. 1 The metabolism of triamterene

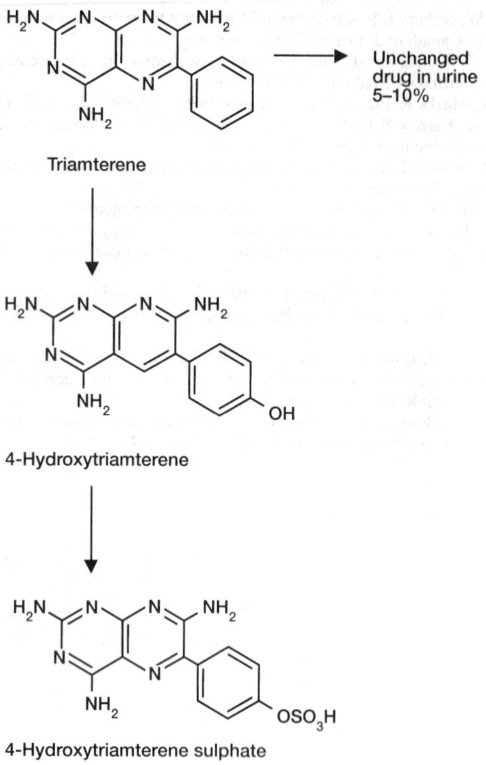

Therapeutic use

Indications

Triamterene is a potassium-conserving diuretic used in:

1. Control of oedema in cardiac failure
2. Control of oedema in cirrhosis of the liver or nephrotic syndrome
3. Drug-induced oedema
4. Premenstrual oedema.

In combination with hydrochlorothiazide, it is also indicated in:

5. Mild to moderate hypertension.

Contraindications

1. Hyperkalaemia
2. Progressive renal failure
3. Known hypersensitivity
4. Routine use of potassium supplements or other potassium conserving agents
5. Use with angiotensin converting enzyme inhibitors.

Mode of use

All clinical indications depend upon the diuresis induced by the action of triamterene on the distal renal tubule.

When given alone, the usual dosage range is from 150 mg to 250 mg triamterene a day. The optimal daily dosage is 200 mg a day, given in divided doses after breakfast and lunch. The maintenance dosage, which is usually initiated after one week, is 200 mg daily in divided doses on alternate days. This ensures satisfactory diuresis, without a concomitant increase in blood urea. Triamterene is often given in conjunction with another diuretic, such as hydrochlorothiazide, when lower doses of both agents must be used initially.

After the first week of dosing with triamterene, it is recommended that blood urea and serum potassium determinations are performed periodically.

Indications

1. Oedema in cardiac failure

Triamterene is used in combination with other diuretic drugs to control mild oedematous states arising from cardiac decompensation.

When used alone, the optimal dose is as stated above. In combination with thiazide diuretics, the optimum dose is generally 50 mg a day.

2. Oedema in cirrhosis of the liver or nephrotic syndrome
Triamterene is used in combination with saluretic drugs with kaliuretic properties to prevent hypokalaemia in patients with cirrhosis of the liver. In a study of a single oral dose of 200 mg triamterene in eight controls and seven patients with alcoholic cirrhosis, the effect on urine output, sodium and potassium excretion was determined over 72 hours.[8] In controls triamterene produced a rapid increase in these parameters, subsiding quickly 8 hours after dosing. In the cirrhotic patients, urine output and sodium and potassium excretions were lower at baseline, and the drug had much less effect. However, diuresis persisted for up to 48 hours after dosing, with a cumulative increase in sodium excretion over this period of 76 ± 33 mEq Na.

The pharmacokinetics of triamterene are altered by liver impairment.

Contraindications

1. Hyperkalaemia
The reduction in potassium excretion induced by triamterene may exacerbate hyperkalaemic states, resulting in dangerous hyperkalaemia. Serum electrolytes should be monitored during triamterene therapy.

2. Progressive renal failure
The excretion of triamterene and its ester metabolite is delayed by impaired renal function as measured by creatinine clearance rates.[9] Clearance rates below 25 $ml.min^{-1}$ are a contraindication to triamterene therapy as retention of the drug may lead to severe hyperkalaemia.

3. Known hypersensitivity
Fever and rigours resulting from a hypersensitivity reaction have been reported with triamterene therapy.

4. Routine use of potassium supplements or other potassium conserving agents
Potassium supplements or other potassium conserving agents such as spironolactone should not be given with triamterene because of the risk of causing hyperkalaemia.

5. With ACE inhibitors
Use of potassium retaining diuretics with angiotensin converting enzyme inhibitors has caused life-threatening hyperkalaemia. The mechanism appears to be a combination of reduced glomerular filtration causing drug retention and the mild hyperkalaemic effect of ACE inhibitors due to reduced angiotensin-II stimulated aldosterone release.

Adverse reactions

Potentially life-threatening effects
Hypovolaemia, hyperkalaemia and acute renal failure have all been reported with triamterene.[10] Seventeen cases of interstitial nephritis have been reported in the worldwide literature. In almost every case the patient was receiving concomitant thiazide therapy. The pathological lesion consists of a mononuclear infiltration of the cortical interstitium, with sparing of the glomeruli but marked degeneration of tubular epithelial cells. Immunofluorescence for immunoglobulins is negative, but non-necrotizing granulomas suggest delayed hypersensitivity.[11]

Acute overdosage
Symptoms of electrolyte imbalance, particularly hyperkalaemia, are found. Patients have gastrointestinal disturbances, muscular weakness and possible hypotension. Overdose is treated by the induction of vomiting and/or gastric lavage, correction of electrolyte imbalance and hypovolaemia and supportive measures.

Severe or irreversible adverse effects
Renal stones have been reported in patients on triamterene therapy, with the drug or its metabolite forming a part of the stone.[12] This may be exacerbated by the hyperuricaemia sometimes induced by triamterene. A case of nephrogenic diabetes insipidus has been reported in a patient taking a triamterene–hydrochlorothiazide combination.[13]

Triamterene

Thrombocytopenic purpura, megaloblastic anaemia and rashes have also been reported.

Symptomatic adverse effects
Nausea, vomiting, diarrhoea, headache, weakness and dry mouth have been reported. Correction of hyperkalaemia and hypovolaemia reverses many of these symptoms.

Other effects
Hyperkalaemia, hyperuricaemia and elevations in blood urea and serum creatinine have all been attributed to triamterene therapy.

Interference with clinical pathology tests
Triamterene may interfere with the fluorescence measurement of quinidine. Under certain light conditions it may cause a blue fluorescence.

High risk groups

Neonates
Triamterene is contraindicated in neonates.

Breast milk. There are no data on the excretion of triamterene into human breast milk. It is excreted into cow's milk.

Children
Triamterene is contraindicated in children.

Pregnant women
Triamterene crosses the placenta in animals. In a series of five infants exposed to the drug in the first trimester of pregnancy, no defects were observed.[14] No increase in malformations was noted in over 271 exposures when triamterene was used at any time during pregnancy.[15]

The elderly
The elderly may be more prone to the loss of potassium when taking diuretics, and so the administration of a potassium sparing agent is often recommended. However, blood urea and serum potassium levels should be monitored regularly in this group. The dosage of triamterene need not be adjusted, except in the case of renal impairment.

Drug interactions

Potentially hazardous interactions

Potassium supplements. There are a few case reports which have demonstrated an association between hyperkalaemia and the use of triamterene with potassium supplementation.[16] This is a well established interaction and the effects are more marked in patients with renal failure. Triamterene should only be used with potassium supplements in severe hypokalaemia and only then under close supervision.

ACE inhibitors. ACE inhibitors used with and potassium sparing diuretics can cause hyperkalaemia.[17]

Other significant interactions

Amantadine. There is some evidence that a triamterene–hydrochlorothiazide combination may reduce the renal excretion of amantadine.[18] In patients receiving amantadine, one should use triamterene with caution, and if necessary reduce the dosage of the former.

Indomethacin. It has been proposed that indomethacin inhibits the prostaglandins that are normally secreted to protect against triamterene-induced nephrotoxicity.[19] Thus renal function should be carefully monitored in patients receiving both drugs.

Potentially useful interactions
The reversal by triamterene of potassium loss caused by diuretics is the basis of the therapeutic usefulness of this compound.

Major outcome trials

There are no major trials reported with triamterene alone.

1. Amery A, Birkenhager W, Birxco P et al 1985 Mortality and morbidity from the European working party on high blood pressure in the elderly trial. Lancet 1: 1349–1354

Triamterene (50 mg) was used in combination with hydrochlorothiazide (25 mg), as one to two capsules per day in a double-blind placebo-controlled trial of 840 patients with diastolic blood pressure in the range 90–119 mmHg who were aged 60 or more. Analysis by intention to treat showed a significant reduction in cardiac mortality in the treated group of 47% in the double-blind part of the trial. Deaths from myocardial infarction were reduced by 60%. There was also a reduction in severe congestive heart failure and stroke.

Other trials

1. Papademetriou V, Burris J, Kukich S, De Freis E D 1985 Effectiveness of potassium chloride or triamterene in thiazide hypokalemia. Archives of Internal Medicine 145: 1986–1990

16 hypertensive patients with diuretic induced hypokalaemia were studied. Potassium chloride 24–96 mEq daily and triamterene 50–200 mg daily were given in an open non-randomized sequential crossover study. Eight of the 16 patients had normal serum potassium levels after potassium chloride treatment and 10 of 16 had normal serum potassium after triamterene therapy.

2. Hamdy R C, Davies A, Arnod K et al 1984 The short term effects of reducing blood pressure in elderly patients with propranolol and dyazide. Age and Ageing 13: 83–88

In this study, 38 patients aged over 69 years with blood pressures above 170/100 received either propranolol 40–80 mg daily or two tablets of a combination of hydrochlorothiazide 25 mg and triamterene 50 mg. Both therapeutic agents significantly reduced the blood pressure, but the triamterene-containing product resulted in a decrease in glomerular filtration rate and an increase in serum creatinine.

3. Jackson P R, Ramsey L E, Wakefield V 1982 Relative potency of spironolactone, triamterene and potassium chloride in thiazide induced hypokalaemia. British Journal of Clinical Pharmacology 14: 257–263

Nine hypertensive patients taking bendrofluazide 10 mg daily were studied in a randomized crossover trial of spironolactone 50 mg and 100 mg daily, triamterene 100 mg and 200 mg daily and potassium chloride 32 mmol and 64 mmol daily. Spironolactone and triamterene had significant and parallel dose–response curves in increasing serum potassium levels.

General review articles

Kosman M E 1974 Management of potassium problems during long-term diuretic therapy. Journal of the American Medical Association 230: 743

Spiekerman R E 1966 Potassium-sparing effects of triamterene in the treatment of hypertension. Circulation 34: 524

1972 Potassium sparing diuretics: spironolactone v triamterene and amiloride. Drug and Therapeutics Bulletin 10: 30–32

References

1. Baba W I, Tudhope G R, Wilson G M 1962 Triamterene, a new diuretic drug. I. Studies in normal men and in adrenalectomized rats. II. Clinical trial in oedematous patients. British Medical Journal 2: 756–764
2. Gatzy J T 1971 The effect of potassium-sparing diuretics on ion transport across excised toad bladder. Journal of Pharmacology and Experimental Therapeutics 176: 580–594
3. Sved S, Sertie J A A, McGilveray I J 1979 Rapid assay for triamterene in plasma. Journal of Chromatography 162: 474–479
4. Pruitt A W, Wirikel J S, Dayton P G 1977 Variations in the fate of triamterene. Clinical Pharmacology and Therapeutics 21: 610–619
5. Dayton P G, Pruitt A W, McNay J L, Steinhorst J 1972 Studies with triamterene, a substituted pteridine. Unusual brain to plasma ratio in mammals. Neuropharmacology II: 435–446
6. Mutschler E, Gilfrich H J, Knauf H, Mohrte W, Volger K D 1983 Pharmacokinetics of triamterene. Clinical and Experimental Hypertension 5: 259–269
7. Andrash H, Fink T, Schmid E 1971 Uber die Haraus scheidung des Antikaliuretikums Triamterene und seines phenolischen Metaboliten 2, 4, 7-Triamino-6-p-hydroxy-phenylpteridin bei Lebergesunden und Kranken mit Leberzirrhose. Zeitschrift für Gastroenterologie 9: 249–245
8. Villeneuve J P, Rocheleau F, Raymond G 1984 Triamterene kinetics and dynamics in cirrhosis. Clinical Pharmacology and Therapeutics 35: 831–837
9. Knauf H, Mohrke W, Mutschler E 1983 Delayed elimination of triamterene and its active metabolite in chronic renal failure. European Journal of Pharmacology 24: 453–456
10. Anonymous 1986 Triamterene and the kidney. The Lancet 1: 424
11. Magill A B, Ballon H S, Cameron E C, Rae A 1980 Acute interstitial nephritis associated with thiazide diuretics. American Journal of Medicine 69: 939–943
12. Ettinger B, Weil E, Mandel N S, Darling S 1979 Triamterene induced nephrolithiasis. Annals of Internal Medicine 91: 745–746
13. Macleod M D, Bell G M, Irvine W J 1981 Nephrogenic diabetes insipidus associated with Dyazide (triamterene–hydrochlorothiazide). British Medical Journal 283: 1155–1156

14. Heinonen O P, Slone D, Shapiro S 1977 In: Birth defects and drugs in pregnancy. Littleton Publishing Sciences Group, ch 28, p 372
15. Heinonen O P, Slone D, Shapiro S 1977 In: Birth defects and drugs in pregnancy. Littleton Publishing Sciences Group, ch 28, p 441
16. O'Reilly M V, Murnaghan D P, Williams M B 1974 Transvenous pacemaker failure induced by hypokalaemia. Journal of the American Medical Association 228: 336
17. Burnakis T G, Mioduch H J 1984 Archives of Internal Medicine 144: 2371–2372
18. Wilson T W, Rajput A J 1983 Amantadine–dyazide interaction. Canadian Medical Association Journal 129: 974
19. Favre L, Glasson P, Vallotton M B 1982 Reversible acute renal failure from combined triamterene and indomethacin: a study in healthy subjects. Annals of Internal Medicine 96: 317–320

Triazolam

Triazolam is a short acting benzodiazepine hypnotic.

Chemistry

Triazolam (Halcion)
$C_{17}H_{12}Cl_2N_4$
8-Chloro-6-(2-chlorophenyl)-1-methyl-4H[1,2,4]triazolo[4,3-a]-[1,4]-benzodiazepine

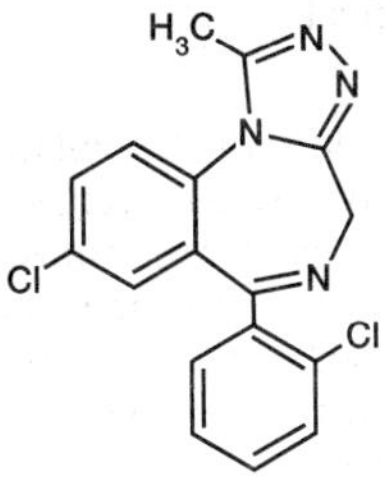

Triazolam

Molecular weight	343.2
pKa, benzodiazepine N –, triazole N –, open form amine	1.5–3.0, 1.2–5 6.5
Solubility	
in alcohol	1 in 150
in water	1 in 35 000
Octanol/water partition coefficient	237

Triazolam is a white crystalline powder or an off-white odourless transparent crystalline material. It is prepared by chemical synthesis and is not present in any combination preparations.

Pharmacology

Triazolam exhibits specific and high affinity binding to sites within the central nervous system (IC_{50} for displacement of diazepam binding to rat brain homogenate = 4.0 nM).[1] The binding of triazolam and other benzodiazepine compounds to these sites leads to profound but reversible alterations in the kinetics of a GABA-dependent transmembrane chloride channel, with the result that GABA-ergic synaptic inhibition within the CNS is enhanced. The 'endogenous' ligand for these receptors, if any, remains unknown, although there have been many candidates.[1,2] It is likely that binding of benzodiazepine compounds to such receptors is at least partly responsible for their clinical effects since there is broad agreement between the relative binding affinities of different benzodiazepines in vitro and their pharmacological potency in vitro.

Animal studies have shown triazolam to have significant hypnotic, muscle relaxant and anticonvulsant effects, with a potency on a weight for weight basis of between 4 and 34 times that of diazepam.[3] Triazolam has no anti-emetic or anti-parkinsonian activity.

Toxicology

The mean lethal dose of triazolam (LD_{50}) by mouth is greater than 5000 mg.kg^{-1} in rats, and greater than 1000 mg.kg^{-1} in mice.[4,5] Chronic administration to rats (30–100 mg.kg^{-1} daily for 90 days) and dogs (10–30 mg.kg^{-1} daily for 90 days) is not associated with any demonstrable toxic effects.[4,5] Administration of high doses of triazolam (30 mg.kg^{-1} daily) to pregnant mice, rats and rabbits has no teratogenic effect.[6]

Clinical pharmacology

All benzodiazepine compounds have hypnotic, antianxiety, anticonvulsant and muscle relaxant effects when administered to laboratory animals. Many short term double-blind crossover studies in patients with insomnia have shown that oral triazolam (0.5 mg) shortens the time to onset of sleep, increases total sleep duration, decreases the frequency of nocturnal awakening and improves the overall quality of sleep when compared to placebo.[7–10] Formal sleep laboratory studies have yielded similar results, and suggest that triazolam has no adverse effects on the duration of random eye movement (REM) sleep.[3] There are few data concerning the dose–response relationship for triazolam, but it is likely that doses above 0.25 mg have little added hypnotic effect and may be associated with an increased incidence of unwanted side effects, particularly daytime hangover.[11–14] The results of longer term studies suggest that there is no significant tendency for the development of tolerance to the hypnotic effects of triazolam.[15–17]

Interpreting the results of studies which compare the hypnotic efficacy of triazolam with that of other compounds is complicated by the problem of dose equivalence, but it appears that triazolam (0.5 mg) may be more effective than flurazepam (30 mg),[7,11] quinalbarbitone (100 mg),[9] chloral hydrate (500 mg)[12] and nitrazepam (5 mg),[13,18] and equivalent to midazolam (15 mg).[19] Triazolam (0.25 mg) and flunitrazepam (1 mg) appear to have equivalent hypnotic effects.[20] Comparisons with commonly used agents such as temazepam and dichloralphenazone are not available.

There are no human data concerning the anticonvulsant or muscle relaxant effects of triazolam. Anxiolytic effects have been reported in man, but only as a secondary consideration in trials of triazolam in the treatment of insomnia. Triazolam has no significant effects on respiratory rate, blood pressure or pulse rate when used in standard doses.

Pharmacokinetics

The preferred analytical method for measuring triazolam in human serum is high performance liquid chromatography (HPLC) with UV detection: the lower limit of detection is approximately 1 μg.l^{-1} in extracted serum, and known metabolites of triazolam do not interfere with the assay.[12]

Triazolam is at least 85% absorbed after oral administration and peak plasma concentrations are seen after 0.75–2.5 h in fasting individuals. Bioavailability after oral administration is approximately 0.61.[22,23] A small amount of triazolam is metabolized presystemically in the liver, around 25% of the dose. The apparent volume of distribution in man is approximately 1.0 l.kg^{-1} regardless of age or sex:[24,25] Animal studies indicate that the highest levels occur in the central nervous system, liver, kidneys, bladder and skin.

Triazolam crosses the placenta in pregnant rats and is excreted in the milk of lactating rats at concentrations 70% of those in maternal plasma.[26] Although comparable data are not available in man it is likely that both transplacental transfer and excretion in breast milk will occur.

Triazolam is 89% bound to human serum proteins as determined by binding studies performed at 37°C in vitro.[27] Studies performed using equilibrium dialysis, however, indicate that triazolam is only 10–25% bound to human plasma proteins in vivo. Approximately half is bound to human serum albumin, with most of the remainder bound to α_1 acid glycoprotein.

The mean elimination half life of triazolam has been quoted as between 2.3 and 3.7 hours,[28–31] and its clearance ranges from 6.2 to 8.8 ml.min^{-1}.kg^{-1} in normal subjects.[32]

The pharmacokinetics of oral triazolam are little altered in chronic dialysis patients, but absorption is enhanced by co-administration of oral aluminium hydroxide as a phosphate-binder. Triazolam is extensively biotransformed in the liver with approximately 90% of an oral dose excreted in the urine as metabolites with the remainder in the faeces. Only small amounts of triazolam are excreted unchanged. Mild liver disease appears to have little effect on the hepatic metabolism of triazolam , although with increasing hepatic dysfunction there is an increase in half life and reduced clearance of triazolam in patients with cirrhosis.[33,34]

Animal studies indicate that long-term triazolam therapy is not associated with hepatic enzyme induction.[35] Studies in man have confirmed the absence of clinically important induction by triazolam.[36]

T

Renal disease is unlikely to have any effect on the elimination of triazolam. In elderly patients the bioavailability of triazolam is increased, possibly due to decreased presystemic metabolism and clearance is such that some reduction in dose may be required.[37,38]

Oral absorption	85%
Presystemic metabolism	~25%
Plasma half life	
range	1.5–5.9 h
Volume of distribution	0.79–1.8 l.kg^{-1}
Plasma protein binding	10–25%

Concentration–effect relationship

Whilst there is a direct relationship between plasma triazolam concentration and impairment of psychomotor performance, there is wide scatter of the data.[25] Routine measurement of plasma triazolam concentration has no place in clinical practice.

Metabolism

Triazolam is extensively metabolized, with elimination highly dependent on hydroxylation of the parent compound and subsequent conjugation to the glucuronides. The major metabolites of triazolam in plasma are α-hydroxy- and 4-hydroxytriazolam, together with their respective glucuronides (Fig. 1). Following oral administration of ^{14}C labelled triazolam to healthy subjects, α-hydroxytriazolam and 4-hydroxytriazolam accounted for 69% and 11% of urinary radioactivity respectively, primarily as the glucuronides.[39]

Minor metabolites include α-4-dihydroxytriazolam, α-arylhydroxytriazolam and possibly also the benzophenone analogues; dichloro-3,5-dihydroxymethyltriazolyl-benzophenone, dichloro-3-hydroxymethyltriazolyl-benzophenone and dichloro-3-methyltriazolyl-benzophenone.

α-hydroxytriazolam inhibits binding of [^3H] flunitrazepam to rat brain membranes in vitro with a potency that is 74% of that for triazolam,[40] and has significant pharmacological activity (50–100% activity of triazolam) in mice in vivo.[41] α-4-Dihydroxytriazolam had 37% and 4-hydroxytriazolam had 18% of the activity of triazolam on inhibitory [3H] flunitrazepam binding,[40] but very low CNS activity in vivo in mice.[41] A study in six healthy subjects showed that intravenous α-hydroxytriazolam (1 mg) had a sedative effect that was weaker than intravenous triazolam (1 mg) but greater than intravenous triazolam (0.25 mg).[42] However, because it reaches a peak concentration of < 20% that of triazolam and is rapidly inactivated by glucuronidation, this metabolite is not thought to contribute to the activity of triazolam. The glucuronide and benzophenol metabolites have no pharmacological activity.[43]

Pharmaceutics

Triazolam, Halcion (Upjohn UK/USA) is only available in tablet form:

a) Powder blue, flat, oval tablets scored on one side and imprinted 'UPJOHN 17' on the other side (UK) or 'HALCION 0.25' (USA), containing 0.25 mg triazolam.

b) Pale lavender, flat, oval tablets scored on one side and imprinted 'UPJOHN 10' on the other side (UK) or 'HALCION 0.125' (USA), containing 0.125 mg triazolam (for geriatric use).

Both preparations should be kept in tightly sealed containers and protected from light.

Therapeutic use

Indications

1. Recurrent insomnia and poor sleeping habits
2. Oral premedication.

Contraindications

1. Known hypersensitivity to benzodiazepine compounds.

Mode of use

1. Insomnia

The recommended dose of triazolam in adults is 0.25 mg taken before retiring. There is little evidence that higher doses have a substantially greater hypnotic effect, and data from monitored release programmes in the UK suggest that only 5–10% of patients require triazolam 0.5 mg. Tablets containing 1 mg triazolam are available in some countries, but this dose has been particularly associated with substantial daytime hangover effects.

2. Oral premedication

The short plasma half life of triazolam makes this compound theoretically attractive for use as premedication in the practice of daycase surgery. Several small randomized, double-blind, placebo-controlled trials have been performed, and suggest that triazolam 0.25 mg has significant sedative, amnesic and probably anxiolytic effects in daycase surgical patients, with recovery from these effects occurring within six hours.[44–46]

Adverse reactions

As with other benzodiazepine compounds, triazolam has very few adverse effects that are entirely unrelated to its primary pharmacological effects. Virtually all adverse effects are dose-related.

Potentially life-threatening effects

There is one reported case of fatal intrahepatic cholestasis that was possibly associated with the use of triazolam in therapeutic doses over a period of six months.[47]

Acute overdosage

It is extremely difficult to commit suicide by deliberate overdosage of any benzodiazepine compound taken alone. It appears that recovery from benzodiazepine overdosage is rapid. The time course of this recovery appears to be temporally unrelated to the rate of elimination of the parent drug or any active metabolites, an observation which is poorly understood.[48]

The management of triazolam overdosage includes basic supportive measures combined with gastric lavage. Animal experiments suggest that haemodialysis and forced diuresis are of no therapeutic value.

Severe or irreversible adverse effects

A Dutch psychiatrist described what he termed a 'cluster syndrome' of severe psychological disturbance in 25 insomniac patients treated with triazolam.[49] Reported problems include depersonalization, severe anxiety, feelings of unreality, suicidal ideation, restlessness, paranoia, hyperacusis, parasthesiae, and altered sense of smell and taste. This report proved to be controversial, and the observations have not been

Fig. 1 Metabolism of triazolam

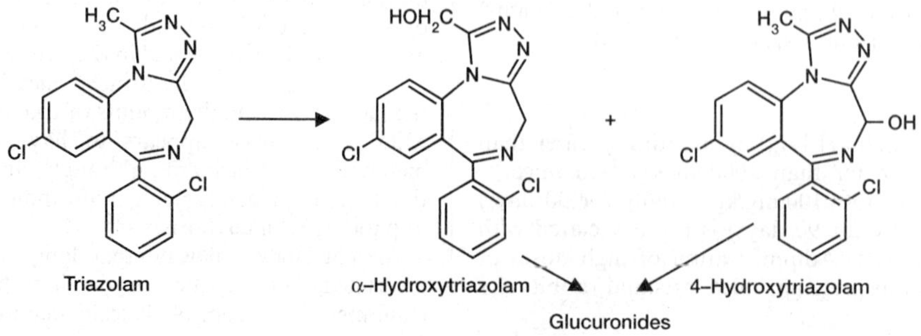

confirmed in any formal study of triazolam in the treatment of insomnia even when the highest (1 mg) doses were used.[15]

Symptomatic adverse effects
Pakes and others examined the results of several clinical trials of triazolam in the short-term management of insomnia.[3] The incidence of adverse effects with a dose of either 0.25 mg or 0.5 mg was generally no greater than that after placebo, with residual drowsiness (<5%), dizziness (<5%), dry mouth (<5%) and nervousness (<5%) being the commonest complaints. Daytime hangover effects become more prominent with the 1 mg dose.

Triazolam may produce mild anterograde amnesia, but only during the period of hypnotic effect. This property may be considered an advantage when triazolam is used as an oral premedication agent. Uncommon adverse effects include alterations in taste sensation, pruritus, skin rashes, blurred vision, hiccups, palpitations, epigastric discomfort, diarrhoea and burning eyes.

Rebound insomnia following withdrawal of hypnotic agents with a short half life, including triazolam, undoubtedly occurs, but is unlikely to prove a clinical problem unless high doses are administered.[50,51]

Interference with clinical pathology tests
No technical interferences of this kind have been reported.

High risk groups

Neonates
There is no clinical indication for the use of triazolam in neonates.

Breast milk. Following oral administration of triazolam 0.5 $mg.kg^{-1}$ to lactating rats, the peak concentration in milk was 70% of that in maternal plasma.[26] Comparable data in humans is not available, but it is recommended that triazolam should not be prescribed to nursing mothers.

Children
There is no clinical indication for the use of the drug in children.

Pregnant women
Following oral administration of triazolam 0.5 $mg.kg^{-1}$ to pregnant rats, fetal plasma concentrations were up to 52% of that found in maternal plasma at the same time.[26] It is therefore recommended that triazolam should not be prescribed during pregnancy.

The elderly
The systemic bioavailability of oral triazolam appears to increase substantially with advancing age, probably as a result of decreased presystemic metabolism in the liver.[37,38] Thus triazolam 0.125 mg appears to be an effective hypnotic in the elderly. Higher doses should be used with caution as there have been reports of unexpected psychomotor disturbance with triazolam 0.25 mg in the elderly.[52]

Drug interactions

Potentially hazardous interactions
In a randomized, two-way, crossover trial, triazolam 0.5 mg was administered with a vodka–water mixture and a tap water control to five healthy subjects.[53] Triazolam plasma concentrations were measured over 15 h post-dose. There were no significant differences between the two groups in peak triazolam concentration, time to peak, plasma half life, or apparent oral clearance. The effect of chronic alcohol consumption on triazolam pharmacokinetics has not been established in man. However, as far as pharmacodynamic interactions are concerned, despite lack of data on interaction between triazolam and alcohol, it should be assumed that alcohol (and other central nervous system defusants) has at least an additive effect, and patients should be warned of the possible dangers of such combinations when driving or operating dangerous machinery.

Other significant interactions

Smoking. Chronic cigarette smoking has no effect on the pharmacokinetics of a single oral dose of triazolam.[54]

Cimetidine, isoniazid, and erythromycin.[4] These compounds all increase the area under the plasma concentration/time curve (AUC), peak serum concentration and plasma half life of oral triazolam and decrease triazolam clearance: such findings are consistent with an inhibitory effect on triazolam metabolism,[44–47] but their clinical importance, if any, remains unknown.

Triazolam

Food. The administration of triazolam immediately after a meal rather than in the fasting state has no effect on the extent of triazolam absorption, but does reduce the rate thereof.

Potentially useful interactions
No interactions of this kind have been reported.

General review articles

Pakes G E, Brogden R N, Heal R C, Speight T M, Avery G S 1981 Triazolam: a review of its pharmacological properties and therapeutic efficacy in patients with insomnia. Drugs 22: 81–110

Kroboth P D, Juhl R P 1983 Triazolam (Halcion, the Upjohn Company). Drug Intelligence and Clinical Pharmacy 17: 495–500

Wood C, Rue Y (eds) 1983 Experience with triazolodiazepines as hypnotics. Royal Society of Medicine — Forum Series: Number 8

References

1. Haefely W, Kyburz E, Gerecke M, Mohler H 1985 Recent advances in the molecular pharmacology of benzodiazepine receptors and in the structure–activity relationships of their agonists and antagonists. In: Testa B (ed) Advances in Drug Research, vol 14. Academic Press, London, pp 165–322
2. Haefely W 1988 Endogenous ligands of the benzodiazepine receptor. Pharmacopsychiatry 21: 43–46
3. Pakes G E, Brogden R N, Heel R C, Speight T M, Avery G S 1981 Triazolam: a review of its pharmacological properties and therapeutic efficacy in patients with insomnia. Drugs 22: 81–110
4. Dharma A P 1979 Triazolam. Drugs of Today 15: 27–33
5. Hare S A 1975 A comparison of three benzodiazepine hypnotics as oral pre-anaesthetic medication. South African Medical Journal 49: 1883–1884
6. Tuchmann-Duplessis H 1976 Effect of the benzodiazepines on offspring. Revue de Medicine 37: 2013–2023
7. Sunshine A 1975 Comparison of the hypnotic activity of triazolam, flurazepam hydrochloride, and placebo. Clinical Pharmacology and Therapeutics 17: 573–577
8. Wang R I H, Stockdale S L 1973 The hypnotic effect of triazolam. Journal of International Medical Research 1: 600–607
9. Okawa K K, Allen G S 1978 A clinical comparison of triazolam with placebo and secobarbital in insomniac patients. Journal of Internal Medicine Research 6: 343–347
10. Rickels K, Gingrich R L, Morris R J, Rosenfeld H, Perloff M M, Clark E L, Schilling A 1975 Triazolam in insomniac family practice patients. Clinical Pharmacology and Therapeutics 18: 315–324
11. Bowen A J 1978 Comparative efficacy of triazolam, flurazepam and placebo in out-patient insomniacs. Journal of International Medical Research 6: 337–342
12. Fabre L F, McLendon D M, Harris R T 1976 Preference studies of triazolam with standard hypnotics in outpatients with insomnia. Journal of International Medical Research 4: 247–254
13. Cloos F, Cretaur R, Defesche C et al 1977 Randomized double-blind cross-over patient preference studies comparing triazolam versus nitrazepam in insomnia. Acta Therapeutica 3: 73–88
14. Chatwin J C, Johns W L 1977 Triazolam: an effective hypnotic in general practice. Current Therapeutic Research 21: 207–214
15. Deberdt R 1980 Triazolam, a benzodiazepine hypnotic used continuously for one year: further communication. Current Therapeutic Research 28: 31–33
16. Leibowitz M, Sunshine A 1978 Long-term efficacy and safety of triazolam and flurazepam. Journal of Clinical Pharmacology 18: 302–309
17. Singh A N, Saxena B Double-blind crossover comparison of triazolam and flurazepam in hospitalised psychiatric patients with insomnia. Current Therapeutic Research 27: 627–633
18. Puech A J, Dordain G, Hecquet S, Paturand J-P, Simon P 1978 Etude croisée en double avengle effectuée pan des omnipracticiens comparant triazolam et nitrazepam chez des insomniaques. Therapie 33: 287–292
19. Costa J A, Silva E, Aciola A, Naylor C, Jones da Silva C, Ferreira I 1983 Midazolam and triazolam in out-patients: a double-blind comparison of hypnotic efficacy. British Journal of Clinical Pharmacology 16: 179S–183S
20. Cordingley G J, Dean B C, Harris R I 1984 A double-blind comparison of two benzodiazepine hypnotics, flunitrazepam and triazolam, in general practice. Current Medical Research and Opinion 8: 714–719
21. Adams W J, Rykert U M, Bombardt P A 1980 High performance liquid chromatographic determination of triazolam in human serum. Analytical Letters 13: 149–161
22. Kroboth P D, Smith R B, Rosanke T et al 1986 Triazolam route of administration studies. I. Pharmacokinetics. Pharmacy Research 3 (suppl): 110S
23. Smith R B, Kroboth P D, McAuley J W et al 1986 Triazolam route of administration studies. II. Absorption from sublingual solution. Pharmacy Research 3 (suppl): Abstract 48
24. Dehlin O, Bjornson G, Borjesson L et al 1983 Pharmacokinetics of triazolam in geriatric patients. European Journal of Clinical Pharmacology 25: 91–94
25. Baktir M S, Fisch H U, Huguenin P, Bircher J 1983 Triazolam concentration–effect relationships in healthy subjects. Clinical Pharmacology and Therapeutics 34: 195–201
26. Kitigawa H, Esumi Y, Kurosawa S, Sekine S, Yokoshima T 1979 Metabolism of 8-chloro-6-(o-chlorophenyl)-1-methyl-4H-s-triazolo[4,3-a][1,4]benzodiazepine, triazolam, a new central depressant. I. Absorption, distribution and excretion in rats, dogs and monkeys. Xenobiotica 9: 415–428
27. Eberts F S, Philopoulos Y, Reineke L M, Vliek R W 1981 Triazolam disposition. Clinical Pharmacology and Therapeutics 29: 81–93
28. Smith R B Kroboth P D, Varner P D 1987 Pharmacokinetics of trazolam after intravenous administration Journal of Clinical Pharmacology 27: 971

29. Scavone Greenblatts D S, Friedmann H, Shoder R I et al 1986 Enhanced bioavailability of Triazolam following sublingual versus oral administration Journal of Clinical Pharmacology 26: 208
30. Friedman H, Greenblatt D J, Bursknn E S, Harmatz I S 1986 Population study of triazolam pharmacokinetics British Journal of Clinical Pharmacology 22: 639
31. Jochemsen et al 1983 British Journal of Clinical Pharmacology 16: 291S
32. Greenblatt D J, Divoll M, Abernathy D R 1983 Reduced clearance of triazolam in old age: relation to antipyrine oxidizing capacity. British Journal of Clinical Pharmacology 15: 303–309
33. Baktir G, Fisch H U, Karlaganis G, Bircher J 1984 Differential explanation for excessive and prolonged sedation due to triazolam in cirrhosis. Naunyn-Schmiedeberg's Archives of Pharmacology (suppl 325: R91
34. Kroboth P D, Smith R B, Van Thiel D H et al 1987 Nighttime dosing of triazolam in patients with liver disease and normal subjects: kinetics and daytime effects. Journal of Clinical Pharmacology 27: 555–560
35. Kitigawa H, Esumi Y, Kurosawa S, Sekine S, Yokoshima T 1979 Metabolism of 8-chloro-6-(o-chlorophenyl)-1-methyl-4H-s-triazolo-[4,3-a][1,4]benzodiazepine, triazolam, a new central depressant. II. Identification and determination of metabolites in rats and dogs. Xenobiotica 9: 429–439
36. Dehlin O, Bjornson G, Borjesson L et al 1983 Pharmacokinetics of triazolam in geriatric patients. European Journal of Clinical Pharmacology 25: 91–94
37. Smith R B, Divoll M, Gillespie W R, Greenblatt D J 1983 Effect of age and gender on the pharmacokinetics of oral triazolam and temazepam. Journal of Clinical Psychopharmacology 3: 172–176
38. Greenblatt D J, Divoll M, Abernathy D R 1983 Reduced clearance of triazolam in old age: relation to antipyrine oxidising capacity. British Journal of Clinical Pharmacology 15: 303–309
39. Eberts F S, Philopoulos Y, Reineke L M, Vliek R W 1981 Triazolam disposition. Clinical Pharmacology and Therapeutics 29: 81–93
40. Moschitto L J, Greenblatt D J 1983 Concentration-independent plasma protein binding of benzodiazepines. Journal of Pharmacy and Pharmacology 35: 179–180
41. Gall M, Kamdar B V, Collins R J 1978 Pharmacology of some metabolites of triazolam, alprazolam and diazepam prepared by simple, one-step oxidation of benzodiazepines. Journal of Medical Chemistry 21: 1290–1294
42. Ziegler W H, Schalch E, Leishman B, Eckert M 1983 Comparison of the effects of intravenously administered midazolam, triazolam and their hydroxymetabolites. British Journal of Clinical Pharmacology 16: 63S–69S
43. Fraser A D 1987 Urinary screening for alprazolam, triazolam, and their metabolites with the EMIT* d.a.u.* benzodiazepine metabolite assay. Journal of Analytical Toxicology 11: 263–266
44. Tipping T, Blogg C, Thomas D 1987 Triazolam premedication. Anaesthesia 42: 316–317
45. Thomas D, Tipping T, Halifax R, Blogg C E, Hollands M A 1986 Triazolam premedication. A comparison with lorazepam and placebo in gynaecological patients. Anaesthesia 41: 692–697
46. Pinnock C A, Fell D, Hunt P C W, Miller R, Smith G 1985 A comparison of triazolam and diazepam as premedication agents for minor gynaecological surgery. Anaesthesia 40: 324
47. Cobden I, Record C O, White R W B 1981 Fatal intrahepatic cholestasis associated with triazolam. Postgraduate Medical Journal 57: 730–731
48. Greenblatt D J, Woo E, Allen M D, Orsulak P J, Shader R I 1978 Rapid recovery from massive diazepam overdose. Journal of the American Medical Association 240: 1872–1874
49. van der Kroef C 1979 Reactions to triazolam. Lancet 2: 526
50. Nicholson A N 1980 Hypnotics: rebound insomnia and residual sequelae. British Journal of Clinical Pharmacology 9: 223–225
51. Wood C, Rue Y (eds) 1983 Experience with triazolodiazepines as hypnotics. Royal Society of Medicine — Forum Series: Number 8
52. Patterson J F 1987 Triazolam syndrome in the elderly. Southern Medical Journal 80: 1425–1426
53. Ochs H R, Greenblatt D J, Arendt R M 1984 Pharmacokinetic noninteraction of triazolam and ethanol. Journal of Clinical Psychopharmacology 4: 106–107
54. Ochs H R, Greenblatt D J, Burstein E S 1987 Lack of influence of smoking on triazolam pharmacokinetics. British Journal of Clinical Pharmacology 23: 759–763
55. Pourbaix S, Desager J P, Hulhoven R, Smith R B, Harvengt C 1985 Pharmacokinetic consequences of longterm coadministration of cimetidine and triazolobenzodiazepines, alprazolam and triazolam, in healthy subjects. International Journal of Clinical Pharmacology Therapeutics and Toxicology 23: 447–451
56. Abernethy D R, Greenblatt D J, Divoll M, Moschitto L J, Harmatz J S, Shader R I 1983 Interaction of cimetidine with the triazolobenzodiazepines alprazolam and triazolam. Psychopharmacology 80: 275–278
57. Ochs H R, Greenblatt D J, Knuchel M 1983 Differential effect of isoniazid on triazolam oxidation and oxazepam conjugation. British Journal of Clinical Pharmacology 16: 743–746
58. Phillips J P, Antal E J, Smith R B 1986 A pharmacokinetic interaction between erythromycin and triazolam. Journal of Clinical Psychopharmacology 6: 297–299

Trifluoperazine (hydrochloride)

Trifluoperazine hydrochloride is a neuroleptic phenothiazine drug used primarily for its antipsychotic actions.

Chemistry

Trifluoperazine hydrochloride (Stelazine)
$C_{21}H_{24}F_3N_3S.2HCl$
10-[3-(4-Methylpiperazin-1-yl)propyl]-2-trifluoromethyl-phenothiazine dihydrochloride

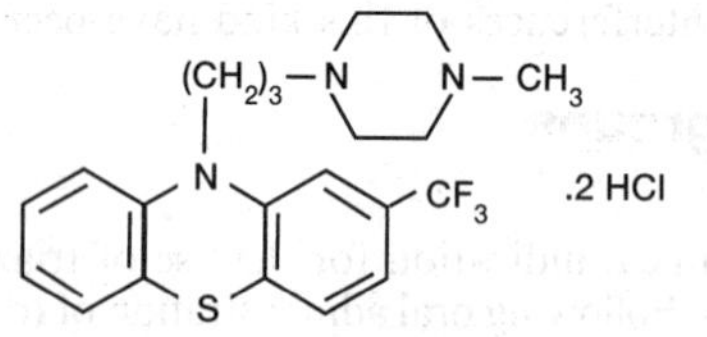

Molecular weight (free base)	480.4 (407.5)
pKa (piperazinyl group)	8.1
Solubility	
in alcohol	1 in 11
in water	1 in 2
Octanol/water partition coefficient	very high

Trifluoperazine hydrochloride is a white to pale yellow, hygroscopic, crystalline powder with a very bitter taste but practically odourless. It is prepared by chemical synthesis.

Pharmacology

Trifluoperazine primarily acts as a neuroleptic drug. In this it suppresses complex behaviour and spontaneous movements but leaves untouched spinal reflexes and unconditioned nociceptive behaviour. Trifluoperazine achieves these effects by mixed blockade of dopamine D_1 and dopamine D_2 receptors, although binding to D_2 receptors is more important. In the mesolimbic dopamine system of the brain, this action accounts for the antipsychotic actions of the drug, while similar actions in the nigrostriatal system may produce the extrapyramidal effects of parkinsonism. Central dopamine D_2 receptor occupancy has been reported to be approximately 80% in patients treated with trifluoperazine, compared to 65–84% with other antipsychotic agents.[1]

Trifluoperazine has other effects on the central nervous system. In the chemoreceptor trigger zone the dopamine blockade accounts for the antiemetic effect of the drug, and trifluoperazine acts on the hypothalamus to increase prolactin secretion. Trifluoperazine has weak anticholinergic effects at muscarinic receptors, and is also a weak antagonist at alpha$_1$-adrenoceptors and at histamine H_1 receptors. Trifluoperazine also binds weakly to $5HT_2$ receptors. Equilibrium dissociation constants (K_d) from receptors in human brain are respectively 2.6, 24, 63 and 667 nM for D_2, α_1, H_1 and muscarinic receptors.[2]

Toxicology

Trifluoperazine does not have mutagenic potential. Teratogenic effects have been reported to occur in rats but not in mice.[3] However, several studies have failed to show a teratogenic effect in humans.[4]

Clinical pharmacology

Trifluoperazine is a high potency neuroleptic and is generally regarded as being 20 times more potent than chlorpromazine (on a mg to mg basis). In patients with psychotic symptoms the drug produces calmness and responsiveness. Aggressive behaviour diminishes and hallucinations and delusions gradually disappear. Initiative is reduced, with slowness of response and drowsiness, but intellectual capabilities are not impaired. With trifluoperazine there is a generalized slowing of the EEG with an increase of θ waves. The seizure threshold may be lowered by trifluoperazine and fits can be induced in epileptic patients. In man the rise of prolactin in blood following the administration of trifluoperazine is well recognized, but the other endocrine effects are rarely a clinical problem. The antiemetic effects of trifluoperazine are well recognized due to an effect on the chemoreceptor trigger zone. Trifluoperazine may lower blood pressure and increase heart rate due to the α-adrenoceptor blocking effect, but this effect is less marked than with chlorpromazine. Trifluoperazine has relatively weak anticholinergic effects, but may cause blurring of vision, constipation, decreased sweating and occasional retention of urine. It has more marked extrapyramidal effects than chlorpromazine.

Pharmacokinetics

The preferred analytical method for trifluoperazine is gas chromatography with mass spectrometry,[5] with a minimum detectable plasma concentration of approximately 0.1 $\mu g.l^{-1}$. A reported radioimmunoassay (RIA)[6] may be more useful for routine clinical monitoring. Significant cross-reactivity with 7-hydroxytrifluoperazine and N-desmethyltrifluoperazine occurs and concentrations determined using RIA are markedly higher than those determined by GC–MS. This may, however, be advantageous since 7-hydroxylated and N-demethylated metabolites of other phenothiazines are known to be pharmacologically active. The minimum detectable amount using the RIA assay with 0.2 ml of plasma is 0.25 $\mu g.l^{-1}$.

Plasma concentrations of trifluoperazine have not been reported following intravenous dosing and hence it is not possible to give a definitive description of trifluoperazine pharmacokinetics. Additionally, there are no detailed reports of pharmacokinetic studies in patients.

Following oral administration, trifluoperazine is almost completely absorbed in the rat and subject to extensive presytemic metabolism.[7] In both patients and healthy volunteers peak concentrations of trifluoperazine occur some 1–6 hours after oral dosing.[8–10] Oral administration of 5 mg of trifluoperazine to volunteers results in peak plasma concentrations between 0.25 and 4 $\mu g.l^{-1}$.

Administration of a 20 mg oral dose to four patients resulted in similar peak concentrations.[8] The decline in plasma concentrations appears to be biphasic with a terminal half life in both patients and volunteers of approximately 14 hours. Wide variations in plasma concentrations of trifluoperazine occur after oral dosing, although neither race nor smoking habit are contributors to the variability.[10] Trifluoperazine is widely distributed throughout the body with much higher concentrations in lung, liver, kidney and brain than in blood. The apparent volume of distribution after oral dosing (V/F) is approximately 160 $l.kg^{-1}$. The oral plasma clearance (CL/F) of trifluoperazine is approximately 600 $l.h^{-1}$. Trifluoperazine is extensively metabolized, with less than 1% of the dose appearing as unchanged drug in the urine.[11] Elimination of trifluoperazine metabolites occurs via the bile and urine. The biliary route appears to be the predominant route in both rat and dog.[12,13]

Trifluoperazine is highly bound (>99%) in plasma, principally to α_1-acid glycoprotein. Trifluoperazine is excreted in breast milk and crosses the placental barrier.

Oral absorption	~100%
Presystemic metabolism	extensive
Plasma half life	
range	7–18 h
mean	14 h
Volume of distribution	
(oral administration)	160 $l.kg^{-1}$
Plasma protein binding	>99%

Concentration–effect relationship

Detailed studies of the relationship between trifluoperazine concentration and therapeutic effects have not been reported. A number of studies comparing high and low dose regimens, for example 80 and 15 mg daily,[14] 60 and 10 mg daily,[15] 600 and 60 mg daily,[16] indicate no greater therapeutic response at the high doses. Inverted U-shaped dose–response curves have been reported for other phenothiazine antipsychotics and a preliminary communication has reported a curvilinear relationship between trifluoperazine concentration and effect.[17]

Metabolism

Trifluoperazine is extensively metabolized and a large number of potential metabolites may result from sulphoxidation, N-oxidation, N-demethylation, hydroxylation, piperazine ring cleavage and conjugation (Fig. 1). In patients, less than 1% of the dose is excreted as unchanged trifluoperazine.[11] The sulphoxide metabolite has been identified in the plasma of volunteer subjects in concentrations approximately twice those of the parent compound[18] and 6% of the dose is excreted as the sulphoxide metabolite in the urine of patients.[11] Plasma concentrations of 7-hydroxytrifluoperazine are approximately half of those of the parent compound in volunteer subjects[19] and conjugates of 7-hydroxytrifluoperazine have also been identified in the urine of patients.[20]

Trifluoperazine-N^4-oxide has been identified in the plasma of volunteers in concentrations similar to those of trifluoperazine.[21] Metabolites resulting from piperazine-ring opening and dealkylation occur in rats and analogous metabolites have been found in humans with the related compound piperazine.[22]

Pharmaceutics

Trifluoperazine is available in the following oral dosage forms: tablets, capsules, syrup, concentrate and injection.

1. Stelazine tablets (SmithKline Beecham, UK/USA) are blue, sugar-coated with 'SKF' printed in black on one face. They are available in two strengths in the UK, containing the equivalent of 1 or 5 mg of trifluoperazine, presented as the hydrochloride. In the USA there are four strengths, each being a round, convex, sugar-coated, blue tablet: 1 mg coded 'S03', 2 mg coded 'S04', 5 mg coded 'S06' and 10 mg coded 'S07'.
2. Stelazine Spansule capsules (SmithKline Beecham, UK) have a clear, colourless body and an opaque yellow cap, filled with a mixture of light blue, dark blue and white pellets. They are available in three strengths, containing the equivalent of 2, 10 or 15 mg of trifluoperazine (as the hydrochloride). The capsules are marked '2', '10' or '15'. The capsule contents are formulated to release two-thirds of the trifluoperazine dose over a 6–8 hour period.
3. Stelazine syrup (SmithKline Beecham, UK) is a clear, pale yellow, peach-flavoured formulation containing 1 mg trifluoperazine (as the hydrochloride) in 5 ml.
4. Stelazine concentrate (SmithKline Beecham, UK) is a clear, pale yellow, peach-flavoured formulation containing 50 mg trifluoperazine (as the hydrochloride) in 5 ml. It has a bitter, numbing after-taste and must be diluted before administration.
5. Stelazine injection (SmithKline Beecham, UK) is presented as 1 ml ampoules containing 1 mg of trifluoperazine (as the hydrochloride). In the USA, Stelazine injection contains 2 mg trifluoperazine per ml. The formulation includes sodium tartrate, sodium diphosphate and sodium saccharine (together with 0.75% benzyl alcohol as preservative in US).

Trifluoperazine is prone to autoxidation and all preparations should be protected from light. The syrup, concentrate, dilutions of the concentrate and capsules should be stored below 30°C. The tablets and capsules should be stored in a dry place.

Stelazine preparations have reasonably long shelf-lives. Dilutions of the syrup have a shelf-life of 14 days and those of the concentrate 3 months, providing they are stored at less than 30°C and protected from light. Diluents must not contain sodium salts of hydroxybenzoate preservatives.

Allergic reactions to trifluoperazine, including jaundice and skin rashes, have been reported but are rare.

Therapeutic use

Indications

1. Schizophrenia and other psychoses
2. Severe psychomotor agitation

3. Anxiety
4. Nausea and vomiting.

Contraindications

1. Comatose states
2. Existing blood dyscrasias or bone marrow depression
3. Liver damage
4. Hypersensitivity to phenothiazines.

Mode of use

1. Schizophrenia and other psychoses

Trifluoperazine is widely used in the control of schizophrenia and in paranoid, but not depressive, psychoses. It is some 20 times more potent than chlorpromazine and is less likely to result in sedative or hypotensive side effects. The tendency to produce extrapyramidal side effects is, however, more pronounced.

The usual adult dose is 10–50 mg per day, given orally in divided doses or once daily as the delayed-release capsule. The recommended initial starting dose is 5 mg twice daily increasing after one week to 15 mg per day. Further increases of 5 mg per day, at intervals of not less than three days, may then be made. For maintenance therapy, the dose should be reduced to the minimum effective level.

In children up to 12 years an initial dose of up to 5 mg daily in divided doses is recommended. This may then be adjusted according to response, weight and age.

Trifluoperazine may be given by deep intramuscular injection for the treatment of acute symptoms in the doses described below. There is no evidence that very high doses produce greater clinical effect and side effects are likely to be more troublesome at high doses.[14–16] In common with other major tranquillizers, clinical improvement may not be evident for several weeks after commencing therapy and there may be a delay in the recurrence of symptoms after discontinuation of treatment. It is recommended that treatment is not stopped abruptly and that a gradual withdrawal from high dosage therapy is used.

2. Severe psychomotor agitation

Trifluoperazine is indicated in the treatment of severe agitation and dangerously impulsive behaviour in doses similar to those described above. A more rapid and intense effect may be achieved by deep intramuscular injection. The usual intramuscular dose for an adult is 1–3 mg per day, given in divided doses. The maximum recommended intramuscular dose is 6 mg per day. In children the recommended intramuscular dose is 50 $\mu g.kg^{-1}$ in divided doses.

3. Anxiety

Trifluoperazine is indicated for the short-term treatment of generalized non-psychotic anxiety. The adult dose is 2–4 mg per day given in divided doses, increasing to 6 mg per day if necessary. Doses in excess of 6 mg per day are more likely to be associated with extrapyramidal side effects in some patients. The maximum daily dose is 1 mg in children 3–5 years and 4 mg in children 6–12 years, taken in divided doses.

4. Nausea and vomiting

Trifluoperazine is effective in the symptomatic treatment of severe nausea and vomiting. The usual adult dose is 2–4 mg per day, given by mouth in divided doses or as a single daily dose of the delayed-release capsule. The maximum recommended daily doses are 6 mg per day in adults, 4 mg in children 6–12 years and 1 mg in children 3–5 years, all given orally in divided doses. Administration by deep intramuscular injection may also be indicated, in which case the

Fig. 1 Major pathways of trifluoperazine metabolism

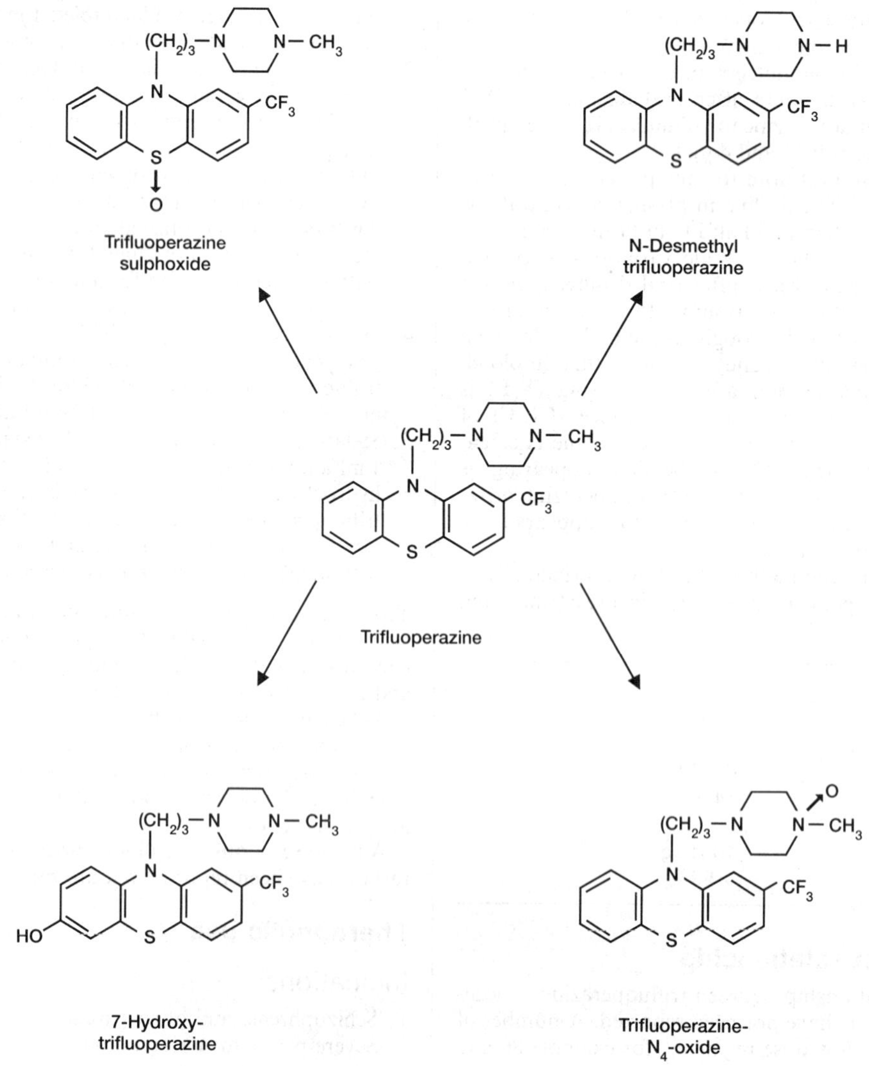

maximum dose is 1–3 mg for an adult and 50 μg.kg^{-1} for children, given in divided doses.

Contraindications

1. Comatose states
Trifluoperazine is contraindicated in comatose states due to its CNS depressant effects and hypotensive and other actions on the cardiovascular and respiratory systems.

2. Existing blood dyscrasias or bone marrow depression
Blood dyscrasias, including agranulocytosis, pancytopenia, leucopenia and thrombocytopenia have been reported very rarely during trifluoperazine treatment. Signs of persistent infection or other signs of blood dyscrasia should be investigated.

3. Liver damage
Trifluoperazine in common with other phenothiazine drugs has been associated with jaundice.[23] Whilst the incidence is very low, trifluoperazine is contraindicated in patients with known liver disease.

4. Hypersensitivity to phenothiazines
Hypersensitivity reactions to phenothiazines include agranulocytosis, leucopenia, leucocytosis, haemolytic anaemia, photosensitization, rashes, contact sensitization and jaundice. Whilst these have been reported only very rarely with trifluoperazine, it should not be used in patients with known hypersensitivity to other phenothiazines.

Adverse reactions

Potentially life-threatening effects
Deaths caused by trifluoperazine are rare.

Acute overdosage
The signs and symptoms of acute overdosage will be predominantly extrapyramidal. Akathisia and dystonic syndromes have been reported, including torticollis, protrusion of tongue, drooling with and without tremors and trismus. Hypotension and decreased consciousness may also occur. Treatment of overdosage should be initiated by gastric lavage but vomiting should not be induced. Oral activated charcoal (0.8 g.kg^{-1}) in combination with sorbitol (2 g.kg^{-1}) has been used in cases of minor overdosage.[24] These procedures should be followed by general supportive measures, with particular attention paid to the cardiac and respiratory systems. Due consideration should be given to the prolonged absorption from delayed-release capsule formulations. In a case report,[25] ECG abnormalities were successfully treated with physostigmine in a patient presenting with arrhythmias following overdosage with up to 3000 mg of trifluoperazine, resulting in a plasma level of 7 mg.l^{-1}. Hypotension should be treated with fluid replacement. Resistant or severe cases may warrant a vasopressor; noradrenaline may be considered but adrenaline is contraindicated.

Severe or irreversible adverse effects
The development of acute dyskinesias is more likely to occur with trifluoperazine than with certain less potent antipsychotic agents. Tardive dyskinesias may also develop, usually following prolonged treatment with high doses but occasionally following relatively short periods of treatment. There is little evidence that the incidence of tardive dyskinesia is any different in patients taking trifluoperazine than in those taking other antipsychotics. The pathogenesis of tardive dyskinesias is unclear but may result from supersensitivity and proliferation of dopamine receptors in the nigrostriatal system; antimuscarinic drugs are known to exacerbate the symptoms.

Symptomatic adverse effects
The most common of these effects include drowsiness, lassitude, dry mouth, blurred vision, dizziness, mild postural hypotension, motor restlessness, akathisia and acute dystonia or dyskinesia. Muscular weakness, anorexia, insomnia, skin reactions including photosensitization, oedema, weight gain, and confusion occur occasionally. Constipation, urinary hesitancy and retention and hyperpyrexia have been reported only very rarely. Most of the adverse effects tend to be dose-related and disappear with continuation of treatment. The extrapyramidal symptoms rarely occur at daily doses of less than 6 mg. At high doses, some other phenothiazines have been associated with arrhythmias and ECG changes including prolongation of the Q-T interval and abnormalities of the T wave; such effects are rare with trifluoperazine. In addition to the depressant effects on the central nervous system, paradoxical effects of agitation and insomnia have been noted, especially in some non-psychotic patients. Trifluoperazine may elevate prolactin levels which may result in oligomenorrhoea, amenorrhoea and galactorrhoea.

Other effects
Trifluoperazine is reported to elevate serum prolactin[26] and may elevate serum cholesterol.[27]

Interference with clinical pathology tests
Phenothiazines may interfere with certain determinations of urinary ketones and urobilinogen.

High risk groups

Neonates
There is no specific information on doses used in neonates.

Breast milk. Trifluoperazine is excreted in breast milk, but the amounts present are unlikely to markedly affect the infant.[28]

Children
In the treatment of nausea and vomiting or anxiety and agitation, the recommended maximum daily doses are 1 mg per day for children 3–5 years and 4 mg per day for children 6–12 years, given by mouth in divided doses. For the treatment of psychotic disorders, treatment should be initiated with a daily dose not exceeding 5 mg and should be increased with caution at intervals of not less than three days. Trifluoperazine has not been extensively given intramuscularly to children but an initial dose of 50 μg.kg^{-1}, given in divided doses, is suggested.

Pregnant women
Several studies have failed to demonstrate a teratogenic effect of trifluoperazine taken during pregnancy.[4] Nevertheless, trifluoperazine should be avoided in pregnancy, especially during the first trimester, unless essential. Phenothiazine drugs cross the placental barrier and the newborn of mothers taking trifluoperazine may show signs of lethargy, tremor or hyperactivity. However, no lasting behavioural or developmental effects on the child have been observed as a result of exposure to neuroleptics in later pregnancy.

The elderly
The elderly are likely to be more susceptible to the effects and particularly some side effects of trifluoperazine and may show impaired elimination of the drug. As a consequence, initial doses should be at most half of the standard adult dose, then slowly increased and maintained at a minimum level.

Concurrent disease
Trifluoperazine should be used cautiously in patients with cardiac arrhythmias, cardiac disease or renal failure. Trifluoperazine should also be used with caution in patients with Parkinson's disease or epilepsy. Although the anticholinergic activity of trifluoperazine is minimal, this should be considered when treating patients with myasthenia gravis, narrow-angle glaucoma or prostatic hypertrophy.

Drug interactions

Potentially hazardous interactions

Adrenaline. Adrenaline should not be used in the treatment of trifluoperazine overdosage. The vasopressor action of adrenaline may be antagonized by the α-adrenergic blocking action of trifluoperazine and the β-vasodilator effect then predominates.

Guanethidine and related drugs. The antihypertensive effects of these agents may be reversed by trifluoperazine. Other phenothiazines have been noted to prevent the neuronal uptake of guanethidine and related sympathetic neurone-blocking drugs, although this is less likely to occur with trifluoperazine.

Antihypertensive agents (excluding guanethidine-like agents). The reduction in blood pressure may be potentiated by trifluoperazine if high initial doses are used.

Alcohol. The CNS depressant effects of alcohol are potentiated by trifluoperazine.

Other significant interactions

CNS depressants. These drugs (including hypnotics, narcotic analgesics, anaesthetics, tricyclic antidepressants) may have their depressant effects on the nervous system potentiated by the actions of trifluoperazine.

Antacids. Antacids reduce the oral absorption of phenothiazine drugs and they should not be administered within two hours of dosing with trifluoperazine.

Tricyclic antidepressants. Concurrent treatment with phenothiazines and tricyclics has led to increases in blood concentrations of both drugs. It has also been suggested that tricyclics may be a contributory factor in the development of tardive dyskinesias.[29]

Levodopa. There is mutual antagonism between phenothiazines and levodopa. Extrapyramidal side effects of phenothiazines will be reduced with levodopa but there may also be some antagonism of the antipsychotic effects. Phenothiazines may antagonize the effects of levodopa and they are generally contraindicated in patients with Parkinson's disease.

Food. Food has not been reported to have any significant effect on plasma concentrations. A delay in the time to reach peak concentrations is, however, likely. Concern has been expressed over precipitation reactions occurring between phenothiazines and tea and coffee. However, it is generally accepted that ingestion of these beverages does not affect the absorption of phenothiazine drugs.

Tobacco. Cigarette smoking has been reported to have no effect on trifluoperazine concentrations.[10]

Potentially useful interactions

No interactions of this kind have been reported.

Clinical trials

1. Mendels J, Krajewski T F, Huffer V et al 1986 Effective short-term treatment of generalized anxiety disorder with trifluoperazine. Journal of Clinical Psychiatry 47: 170–174

This is a study of the efficacy of trifluoperazine in the short-term treatment of generalized anxiety disorder in 415 out-patients receiving 2–6 mg of trifluoperazine per day for four weeks. The multicentre trial was conducted double-blind and placebo-controlled. The out-patients were aged between 22 and 72 years and had a diagnosis of moderate to severe generalized anxiety disorder.

A number of psychiatric rating scales, including HAM-A, NPRL, Part 1 of the CGI and PSIR were used in the assessment. Significant improvements ($p<0.01$) in each of the anxiety rating scales were noted in trifluoperazine-treated patients compared with placebo controls by the end of the study The incidence of side effects was generally similar in both groups; however, drowsiness and related symptoms, and anticholinergic effects such as dry mouth and blurred vision, were reported more frequently by the trifluoperazine-treated group.

2. Simpson G M, Cuculic Z 1976 A double-blind comparison of loxapine succinate and trifluoperazine in newly admitted schizophrenics. Journal of Clinical Pharmacology 16: 60–65

This study was conducted in 43 newly admitted schizophrenic patients (27 male, 16 female; age range 16–61 years). After a drug-free period of three days the patients received either trifluoperazine ($n=19$) or loxapine ($n=24$) for four weeks. The initial dose of trifluoperazine was 10–20 mg per day and this was increased to between 20 and 50 mg per day by the end of the study. The dose of loxapine was initially 20–80 mg per day and this was increased to between 40 and 80 mg by the end of the study.

Using BPRS and CGI assessments, improvements were noted which were both significant and comparable for both groups. The most frequent side effects were extrapyramidal (reported in 68% of the trifluoperazine group), the incidence and severity of which were similar for both groups.

3. Edwards J G, Alexander J R, Alexander M S, Gordon A, Zutchi T 1980 Controlled trial of sulpiride in chronic schizophrenic patients. British Journal of Psychiatry 137: 522–529

This was a double-blind comparative study of sulpiride (600–1800 mg per day) and trifluoperazine (15–45 mg per day) in 38 chronic schizophrenics (19 in each group) aged between 25 and 74 years. Significant improvements were noted using the BPRS at 2, 4 and 6 weeks for both groups. Global assessments were also improved for both groups with a greater number of patients in the trifluoperazine group showing improvement at 2 weeks. No significant extrapyramidal effects were noted.

4. Lovett W C, Stokes D K, Taylor L B, Young M L, Free S M, Phelan D G 1987 Management of behavioural symptoms in disturbed elderly patients: comparison of trifluoperazine and haloperidol. Journal of Clinical Psychiatry 48: 234–236

This was a double-blind comparison of trifluoperazine with haloperidol in the treatment of behavioural symptoms associated with chronic brain syndromes and senile psychoses in 54 institutionalized elderly patients (mean age 82 years). The study was conducted over a six-week period with initial doses of 1 mg trifluoperazine or 0.5 mg haloperidol each given twice daily.

Using CGI scores some improvement was noted in 86% of the patients treated with haloperidol. Moderate improvements were observed in 27% of the trifluoperazine-treated patients. Marginally significant trends favouring trifluoperazine over haloperidol were noted in BPRS, NOSIE and SCAG scales. The type and incidence of adverse reactions were similar for the two treatments with sedation being the most frequent complaint. None of the patients developed extrapyramidal symptoms.

General review articles

Black J L 1985 Antipsychotic drugs: a clinical update. Mayo Clinic Proceedings 60: 777–789

Brill H (ed) 1958 Trifluoperazine: clinical and pharmacological aspects. Lea and Febiger, Philadelphia.

Davis J M, Casper R 1977 Antipsychotic drugs: Clinical pharmacology and therapeutic use. Drugs 14: 260–282

Jain A K, Kelwala S, Gershon S 1988 Antipsychotic drugs in schizophrenia: Current issues. International Clinical Psychopharmacology 3: 1–30

Jorgensen A 1986 Metabolism and pharmacokinetics of antipsychotic drugs. In: Bridges J W, Chasseaud L F (eds) Progress in drug metabolism, vol. 9. Taylor and Francis, London, ch 4, pp 132–135

Moyer J H (ed) 1959 Trifluoperazine: further clinical studies and laboratory studies. Lea and Febiger, Philadelphia

Post A, Warren R J, Zarembo J E 1980 Trifluoperazine hydrochloride. In: Analytical profiles of drug substances, Vol, 9, Academic Press, London, pp 543–580

References

1. Farde L, Wiesel F-A, Halldin C, Sedvall G 1988 Central D-2 receptor occupancy in schizophrenic patients treated with antipsychotic drugs. Archives of General Psychiatry 45: 71–76
2. Black J L 1985 Antipsychotic drugs: a clinical update. Mayo Clinic Proceedings 60: 777–789
3. Rodriquez Gonzalez M D, Friman Perez M 1985 Teratogenic effect of trifluoperazine in rats and mice. Acta Biologica Hungarica 36: 233–237
4. Brockington I F, Kumar R (eds) 1982 Motherhood and mental illness. Academic Press, London, p 249
5. Midha K K, Roscoe R M H, Hall K, Hawes E M, Cooper J K, McKay G, Shetty H U 1982 A gas chromatographic mass spectrometric assay for plasma trifluoperazine concentrations following single doses. Biomedical Mass Spectrometry 9: 186–190
6. Midha K K, Hubbard J W, Cooper J K, Hawes E M, Fouriner S, Yeung P 1981 Radioimmunoassay for trifluoperazine in human plasma. British Journal of Clinical Pharmacology 12: 189–193
7. Schmalzing G 1977 Metabolism and disposition of trifluoperazine in the rat II. Kinetics after oral and intravenous administration in acutely and chronically treated animals. Drug Metabolism and Disposition 5: 104–115
8. Gillespie T J, Sipes I G 1981 Sensitive gas chromatographic determination of trifluoperazine in human plasma. Journal of Chromatography 223: 95–102
9. Midha K K, Korchinski E D, Verbeeck R K, Roscoe R M H, Hawes E M, Cooper J K, McKay G 1983 Kinetics of oral trifluoperazine disposition in man. British Journal of Clinical Pharmacology 15: 380–382
10. Midha K K, Hawes E M, Hubbard J W, Korchinski E D, McKay G 1988 A pharmacokinetic study of trifluoperazine in two ethnic populations. Psychopharmacology 95: 333–338
11. West N R, Rosenblum M P, Sprince H, Gold S, Boehme D H, Vogel W H 1974 Assay procedures for thioridazine, trifluoperazine and their sulfoxides and determination of urinary excretion of these compounds in mental patients. Journal of Pharmaceutical Sciences 63: 417–420
12. Flanagan J L, Newman J H, Maas A R, Van Loon E J 1962 Excretion patterns of phenothiazine-^{35}S compounds in rats. Effect of change in structure on metabolism. Journal of Pharmaceutical Sciences 51: 996–999
13. Van Loon E J, Flanagan J L, Novick W J, Maas A R 1964 Hepatic secretion of and urinary excretion of three ^{35}S labelled phenothiazines in the dog. Journal of Pharmaceutical Sciences 53: 1211–1213

14. Prien R F, Levine J, Cole J O 1969 High dose trifluoperazine therapy in chronic schizophrenia. American Journal of Psychiatry 126: 305–313
15. Carscallen H B, Rochman H, Lovegrove T D 1969 High dosage trifluoperazine in schizophrenia. Canadian Psychiatric Association Journal 13: 459–461
16. Wijsenbeek H, Steiner M, Goldberg S C 1974 Trifluoperazine: a comparison between regular and high doses. Psychopharmacologica 36: 147–150
17. Sramek J J, Potkin J G, Hahn R 1988 Neuroleptic plasma concentrations and clinical response. In search of a therapeutic window. Drug Intelligence and Clinical Pharmacy 22: 373–380
18. Aravagiri M, Hawes E M, Midha K K 1984 Radioimmunoassay for the sulfoxide metabolite of trifluoperazine and its application to a kinetic study in humans. Journal of Pharmaceutical Sciences 73: 1383–1387
19. Aravagiri M, Hawes E M, Midha K K 1985 Radioimmunoassay for the 7-hydroxy metabolites of trifluoperazine and its application to a kinetic study in humans. Journal of Pharmaceutical Sciences 74: 1196–1202
20. Fagarasan M, Fagarasan E 1983 (Determination of 7-hydroxytrifluoperazine by mass spectrometry) Revista de Chimie (Bucharest) 34: 1133–1134
21. Aravagiri M, Hawes E M, Midha K K 1986 Development and application of a specific radioimmunoassay for trifluoperazine N^4-oxide to a kinetic study in humans. Journal of Pharmacology and Experimental Therapeutics 237: 615–622
22. Breyer U, Gaertner H J, Prox A 1974 Formation of identical metabolites from piperazine- and dimethylamino-substituted phenothiazine drugs in man, rat and dog. Biochemical Pharmacology 23: 313–322
23. Jones J K, Van de Carr S W, Zimmerman H, Leroy A 1983 Hepatotoxicity associated with phenothiazine. Psychopharmacology Bulletin 19: 24–27
24. Minocha A, Krenzelok E P, Spyker D A 1985 Dosage recommendations for activated charcoal–sorbitol treatment. Clinical Toxicology 23: 579–587
25. Weisdorf D, Kramer J, Goldberg A, Klawans H L 1978 Physostigmine for cardiac and neurological manifestations of phenothiazine poisoning. Clinical Pharmacology and Therapeutics 24: 663–667
26. Sachar E J (ed) 1976 Hormones, behaviour and psychopathology. Raven Press, New York, pp 161–176
27. Rheinhardt D J 1962 Serum cholesterol elevation with trifluoperazine (Stelazine) therapy. Delaware Medical Journal 34: 318
28. Goldberg H L, DiMascio A 1978 Psychotropic drugs in pregnancy. In: Lipton M A, DiMascio A, Killam K F (eds) Psychopharmacology: a generation of progress. Raven Press, New York, pp 1047–1055
29. Ayd F J 1974 Pharmacokinetic interaction between tricyclic antidepressants and phenothiazine neuroleptics. International Drug Therapy Newsletter 9: 31

Trimeprazine (tartrate)

A phenothiazine H_1-receptor antagonist with pharmacological activity intermediate between chlorpromazine and promethazine, used mainly on account of its central sedative actions in the treatment of pruritus and as an oral premedicant prior to general anaesthesia.

Chemistry

Trimeprazine tartrate (known as Alimemazine tartrate outside the UK, Vallergan, Nedeltran, Panectyl, Repeltin, Temaril, Theralene, Variargil)
$(C_{18}H_{22}N_2S)_2C_4H_6O_6$
10-[3-(Dimethylamino)-2-methylpropyl]phenothiazine tartrate

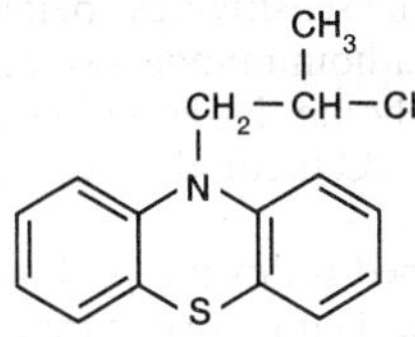

tartrate

Molecular weight of tartrate (free compound)	747.0 (298.4)
pKa	9.2
Solubility	
in alcohol	1 in 30
in water	1 in 4
Octanol/water partition coefficient	800

A white or slightly cream-coloured, odourless or almost odourless, non-hygroscopic, crystalline powder with a bitter taste. It is prepared by chemical synthesis and darkens in colour on exposure to light. It should be stored at a temperature of less than 40°C, preferably 15–30°C, and in airtight containers protected from light.

Pharmacology

Trimeprazine is a competitive antagonist of histamine at H_1-receptors. It is a phenothiazine type of compound and is more potent an antihistamine than promethazine. It has no action on histamine H_2-receptors. Trimeprazine readily crosses the blood–brain barrier and has sedative and antiemetic actions in the central nervous system. Trimeprazine also has anticholinergic, local anaesthetic and weak α_1-adrenoceptor antagonist actions.

Toxicology

In common with all H_1-receptor antagonists, trimeprazine would be expected to reduce uterine blood flow and thus, when used in the first trimester of pregnancy, be associated with an increased incidence of spontaneous abortion and hence a reduced fertility. Studies in rats fed 50 $mg.kg^{-1}$ (25 times the human therapeutic dose) confirm this effect but reveal no evidence of teratogenicity. There is no evidence of organ toxicity or carcinogenicity in chronic dosing studies in dogs.

Human studies reveal no consistent evidence of teratogenicity with first-trimester use of trimeprazine[1] or with H_1-antihistamines,[2] consistent with the animal data, and in one of these studies the incidence of fetal abnormalities was significantly less than in the control group.[2]

Clinical pharmacology

Trimeprazine has been less well studied for its clinical pharmacological effects than the more recently introduced antihistamines. It is an

T

antihistamine with both central and peripheral effects. Its peripheral actions have been utilized in the treatment of allergic rhinitis, but the non-sedating antihistamines are usually preferred for this indication. In a study to compare the effects of trimeprazine in allergic rhinitis with those of chlorpheniramine, hydroxycine, diphenhydramine and tripelennamine, trimeprazine produced fewer adverse effects in general but was least preferred by the patients overall.[3] In non-histamine-mediated itching, relief of itching is related to sedative effects in the CNS rather than to antihistamine properties.[4] Thus trimeprazine may be preferred here to non-sedative antihistamines such as terfenadine, astemizole, loratadine or cetirizine.

Trimeprazine is effective as a pre-anaesthetic sedative in children[5] and in doses of 4 $mg.kg^{-1}$ may also diminish post-anaesthetic vomiting because of its antiemetic effect.[6] Trimeprazine suppresses the histamine-evoked secretion of saliva and this effect is as much due to the anticholinergic effects of the drug as to its antihistamine effect. The anticholinergic effect of trimeprazine may thus cause dry mouth and blurred vision. The α-adrenoceptor-blocking effects of trimeprazine are weak and thus there are rarely any effects on pulse rate or blood pressure.

Pharmacokinetics

Both a radioimmunoassay[7] and a high performance liquid chromatographic (HPLC) method employing electrochemical detection[8] have recently been described with sensitivities below 0.4 $\mu g.l^{-1}$ and 0.2 $\mu g.l^{-1}$ respectively. The radioimmunoassay recognizes both trimeprazine and an active metabolite, N-desmethyltrimeprazine (49% cross-reactivity) while the HPLC method detects parent compound only.

Trimeprazine is well absorbed following oral administration with the bioavailability of the syrup being greater than that of the tablet formulation.[8] Following oral administration of 5 mg trimeprazine as either a syrup or a tablet the mean (±SEM) areas under the curve from time zero to the last point of positive detection are 7.87±2.11 $mg.l^{-1}.ml^{-1}$ (syrup) and 4.15±0.76 $mg.l^{-1}.ml^{-1}$ (tablet). Peak plasma levels occur 3.5–4.5 hours after administration[8,9] and there is a large volume of distribution consistent with a wide body tissue distribution. Trimeprazine is extensively (>90%) plasma protein bound.[8]

Over 70% of trimeprazine is renally excreted with only a 3% faecal recovery of radiolabelled trimeprazine being identified in five days following oral administration.[9] The rate of excretion would thus be expected to decrease with impaired renal function and a reduced dosage regime is recommended in the elderly. With normal renal function the half life of excretion of unchanged trimeprazine is 4.78±0.59 hours.[8] The half life of an active metabolite, N-desmethyltrimeprazine, may be longer.[7]

No measurements of cord blood levels have been made. Although trimeprazine is excreted in human milk, the levels are too low to exert clinical effects on the infant[10] and the American Academy of Pediatrics considers trimeprazine administration to be compatible with breast-feeding.[11]

Oral absorption	>80%
Presystemic metabolism	—
Plasma half life	3.6–7 h
mean	4.8 h
Volume of distribution	—
Plasma protein binding	>90%

Concentration–effect relationship

There is no evidence for any correlation between the plasma concentration of trimeprazine and its therapeutic effects.

Metabolism

Two primary pathways in metabolism have been described: sulphoxidation and N-dealkylation producing two major metabolites, trimeprazine sulphoxide and N-desmethyltrimeprazine (Fig. 1). Only the N-desalkyl metabolite is active as an H_1-receptor antagonist.

Trimeprazine (tartrate)

Fig. 1

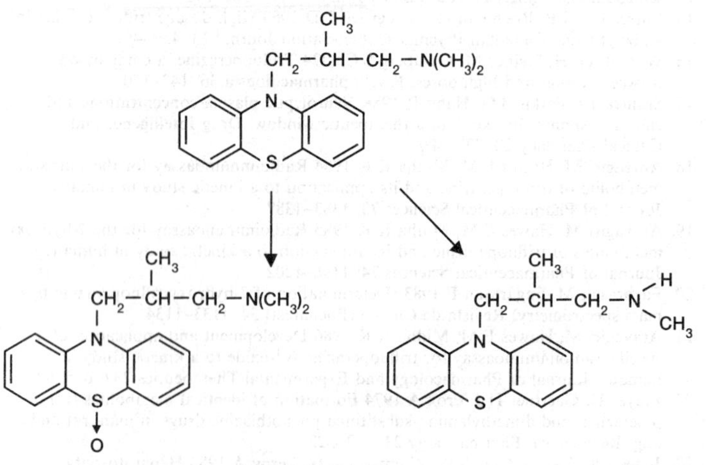

Trimeprazine sulphoxide — Desmethyltrimeprazine

Pharmaceutics

Trimeprazine, Temaril (Herbert, USA)/Vallergan (Rhone Poulenc, UK), is available as an oral medication in either solid dose forms or syrup formulations.

Temaril tablets containing 2.5 mg trimeprazine are round, grey, coated tablets.

Vallergan tablets are dark-blue, film-coated and imprinted 'V10', and contain 10 mg trimeprazine tartrate. Two strengths of Vallergan syrup exist, a 'standard syrup' containing 7.5 mg trimeprazine tartrate in 5 ml, which is a clear, bright, straw-coloured, syrupy, apricot-flavoured liquid, and a 'Forte syrup' which is a colourless to very pale yellow, syrupy, apricot-flavoured liquid containing 30 mg trimeprazine tartrate in each 5 ml. Temaril syrup contains 2.5 mg in 5 ml. It is a clear, red, raspberry–strawberry-flavoured liquid containing 5.7% alcohol. None of the preparations contains tartrazine. The syrups both contain sugars, sodium benzoate, and ethanol.

Temaril sustained-release capsules contain 5 mg trimeprazine. The cap is opaque grey and the body clear. Codings are 'HL' and 'T50'. The formulation includes benzyl alcohol and cetylpyridinium chloride.

The recommended shelf-life of the syrup formulations of trimeprazine is 2 years and for the film-coated tablets 5 years.

Therapeutic use

Indications

1. Urticaria and pruritus
2. Premedication for anaesthesia
3. Night sedation.

Contraindications

1. Hypersensitivity reactions to trimeprazine
2. Patients in charge of vehicles or machinery
3. Ventilatory impairment.

In addition to the absolute contraindications there are a number of situations in which caution for prescribing is necessary and can be considered as relative contraindications.

1. Pregnancy
2. Renal impairment
3. Concomitant use of sedatives, hypnotics or alcohol
4. Prostatic hypertrophy
5. Narrow-angle glaucoma
6. Epilepsy
7. Parkinson's disease
8. Myasthenia gravis
9. Hypersensitivity reactions to other phenothiazines
10. Elderly patients.

Mode of use

The use of trimeprazine is now limited to its central sedative H_1-receptor antagonistic action, other H_1-antihistamines having better pharmacological profiles for use in conditions in which peripheral H_1-receptor antagonism is the desired effect.

Trimeprazine tartrate is given by mouth for the relief of pruritus in doses of 10–40 mg daily for adults and 7.5–20 mg daily for children, in 3 or 4 divided doses. In severe cases in adults up to 100 mg daily has been administered. Reduced doses, 10 mg in the morning or twice daily, should be used in the elderly for this indication. When used as a premedicant prior to general anaesthesia in children the standard dose is 2 $mg.kg^{-1}$ body weight by mouth, as the forte syrup, administered 90–120 min prior to induction. When used for night sedation a recommended dose is 3 $mg.kg^{-1}$ as the syrup,[12] but up to 6 $mg.kg^{-1}$ has been suggested,[13] although this is not recommended by the manufacturer. Trimeprazine is now not advised for infants less than 2 years old.

Indications

1. Urticaria and pruritus

As histamine promotes vasodilatation and increases vascular permeability it will produce oedema formation. These effects are predominantly mediated via H_1-receptors and thus H_1-antihistamines have been used to prevent and treat skin weal formation in urticaria, as this is considered to be largely histamine-mediated. The patient acceptability and use of trimeprazine in this instance is, however, limited by its central sedative effects and it has been superseded by the newer non-sedative H_1-receptor antagonists for this indication.

The use of trimeprazine in the treatment of pruritus was established early in its clinical use[14,15] and has been found to be of benefit in relieving itch due to a variety of skin conditions, including atopic eczema, infantile eczema, lichen planus, lichen simplex, contact dermatitis, neurodermatitis, senile pruritus, plaster pruritus and anogenital pruritus.[16–21] This beneficial effect in pruritus is related to CNS sedation rather than peripheral H_1-receptor antagonism.[4]

2. Premedication for anaesthesia

Trimeprazine has been widely used as a premedicant in children, particularly prior to ENT operations, as it is available in a syrup formulation and has antiemetic and antisialogogic properties in addition to its sedative and calming effects. An early comparative study found trimeprazine 4 $mg.kg^{-1}$ administered 1.5 hours prior to induction superior to quinalbarbitone 6 $mg.kg^{-1}$, promethazine 0.8 $mg.kg^{-1}$ and chlorpromazine 0.8 $mg.kg^{-1}$, and atropine sulphate 0.9 mg.[22]

A comparison of two doses of trimeprazine, 2.2 $mg.kg^{-1}$ and 4.4 $mg.kg^{-1}$, found greater sedation with the larger dose in children <7 years old[23] and most subsequent studies have employed a 2–3 $mg.kg^{-1}$ dose. At this dose level, comparisons of trimeprazine with the benzodiazepines, diazepam,[6,24] temazepam[25,26] and lorazepam[24,27] have found equal sedative efficacy but more postoperative vomiting in the benzodiazepine-treated children, indicating a preference for trimeprazine. Trimeprazine has been administered with droperidol[28] and this combination is reported to produce less postoperative vomiting and a smoother general anaesthesia induction, although this has not been a consistent finding.[29] Due to its length of clinical effect, trimeprazine has proved unsuitable for day case surgery, as over 50% of children are reported to be too sleepy to be discharged.[30] On account of this a microdose (6–12 mg total dose) was tried in 101 children aged 2 to 12 in comparison with placebo. The placebo proved superior as a premedicant which was considered to be related to the CNS stimulation that has been reported with lower doses of trimeprazine in children.[31] This low dose is, however, not employed and at the standard dose clear benefit exists over placebo with respect to anaesthetic room behaviour, postoperative vomiting and the incidence of distressed behaviour at home following hospital discharge.[24,32] An additional advantage of trimeprazine as a premedicant is the lower dose of thiopentone subsequently required to induce general anaesthesia.[33]

3. Night sedation

Trimeprazine at a dose[12,34] of 3 $mg.kg^{-1}$ and a dose[13] of 6 $mg.kg^{-1}$ has been recommended by authors for sleeping problems in infants on a short-term basis to alter their sleep pattern. There have, however, been reports of respiratory depression in children following trimeprazine therapy[35] and it has been suggested that trimeprazine may be implicated in infant cot death syndrome,[36] although this suggestion was not supported by the European Commission following a review of the data.[37] Trimeprazine is not recommended for use in children less than 2 years old.

In adults, benzodiazepines are the preferred pharmacological treatment of insomnia.

Contraindications

The absolute contraindications are:

1. Hypersensitivity

Previous adverse effects related to trimeprazine due to hypersensitivity contraindicate subsequent use. Such reactions include reversible agranulocytosis,[38] respiratory depression,[35] malignant hyperthermia[39,40] and hypotension.[41,42]

2. Use of machinery or vehicles

As trimeprazine produces sedation, patients on this treatment should not take charge of vehicles, other means of transport, or machinery, as there is an increased risk of accidents occurring.[43] This is pertinent to all patients taking trimeprazine for the first time or who on previous administration have experienced disorientation, confusion or drowsiness.

3. Ventilatory impairment

Trimeprazine is a CNS sedative and has been reported to produce respiratory arrest requiring resuscitation.[35] It should therefore be avoided in patients with impaired ventilatory drive.

The relative contraindications are:

1. Pregnancy

The manufacturers recommend that trimeprazine should be avoided in early pregnancy, unless the physician considers it necessary. While there is a theoretical risk of embryotoxicity, several studies have identified no risk of teratogenicity and trimeprazine has been widely used for sedation and as an antiemetic without ill effects.

2. Renal impairment

As trimeprazine is predominantly renally excreted,[9] reduced clearance and elevated serum levels will occur in patients with impaired renal function. The prescribed dose should be reduced appropriately to the level of renal function or an alternative phenothiazine that undergoes hepatic clearance employed in its place.

3. Concomitant use of sedatives, hypnotics or alcohol

Trimeprazine is a CNS sedative and may be additive with or potentiate the CNS depressant effects of other centrally acting drugs, such as opiates, barbiturates, sedative antihistamines, tranquillizers or alcohol. Caution should be exhibited if such drugs are co-administered with trimeprazine.

4. Prostatic hypertrophy

Trimeprazine has anticholinergic activity and its use may precipitate acute urinary retention in men with prostatic hypertrophy, as anticholinergic agents relax the detrusor muscle and decrease bladder tone. Such a problem is more likely in the elderly and use of the drug should be cautious if there is a history indicative of prostatic hypertrophy.

5. Glaucoma

The anticholinergic action of trimeprazine may lead to an increase in intraocular pressure in patients with untreated narrow-angle glaucoma or a predisposition to the disease. Trimeprazine has no effects on intraocular pressure in the normal eye.

6. Epilepsy

Phenothiazine H_1-antihistamines have been reported to induce seizures at therapeutic doses in patients not known to have previously experienced epilepsy as well as in documented epilepsy.[44] Therefore, caution should be exerted with trimeprazine in patients with epilepsy or who are suffering from conditions known to predispose to an epilepsy tendency.

7. Parkinson's disease

Tremor, bradykinesia, gait difficulty and falls have been described in association with trimeprazine therapy[45] so its use should be cautious in the elderly and its effects monitored in this respect.

8. Myasthenia gravis
The anticholinergic actions of trimeprazine may interfere with the control of myasthenia gravis.

9. Hypersensitivity reactions to other phenothiazines
Phenothiazines may be associated with a number of hypersensitivity reactions including jaundice, dystonic reactions, the malignant hyperthermia syndrome and leucopenia. A non-phenothiazine H_1-antihistamine should be selected in preference to trimeprazine if an H_1-antihistamine is required in individuals previously experiencing such adverse reactions.

10. Elderly patients
Prostatic hypertrophy and glaucoma are more common in the elderly and will be exacerbated by the anticholinergic effects of trimeprazine, which may also lead through this mechanism to reduced bowel motility and constipation. The α-antagonistic properties of trimeprazine, although weak, may promote hypotension due to vasodilatation, an effect more prominent when standard doses of trimeprazine are used in the presence of impaired renal clearance. At extremes of temperature trimeprazine will increase the risk of hypothermia or hyperthermia.

Adverse reactions

Potentially life-threatening effects
Four fatalities due to trimeprazine have been reported to the UK Committee on Safety of Medicines, three from malignant hyperthermia and one from circulatory failure. The doses administered to children experiencing malignant hyperthermia[39,40] were 3 $mg.kg^{-1}$ and 6 $mg.kg^{-1}$. Hypotension is reported both in children at standard doses[41] of 2.7–4.2 $mg.kg^{-1}$ and in adults.[42] There have also been reports of respiratory arrests in two children requiring resuscitation[35] following oral administration of doses of 2.3 $mg.kg^{-1}$ and 2.5 $mg.kg^{-1}$. Respiratory depression due to phenothiazines has been implicated as a cause of cot deaths,[36] although the European Commission which reviewed the data felt the evidence available did not support such a link.[37] Despite this, trimeprazine, which has been used in infants and young children for the treatment of insomnia,[13,34] is not now recommended by the manufacturers in children under the age of 2 years.

Acute overdosage
Minor overdoses in adults may result in deep sleep. Cardiovascular effects, such as hypotension and tachycardia, are not marked, as trimeprazine's α-antagonistic actions are weak. The CNS effects may lead to hypoventilation and respiratory failure due to depression of the respiratory centre, epileptiform seizures, and extrapyramidal effects. The anticholinergic actions of trimeprazine cause dry mouth, blurred vision, dilated pupils, delirium, psychosis and, on occasions, pyrexia.

There is no specific antidote and treatment is symptomatic and supportive. Gastric lavage is of value soon after overdose but haemodialysis has no benefit in view of the large volume of distribution of trimeprazine. Analeptics should be avoided as they may induce seizures, so respiratory failure is best treated by mechanical ventilation. Hypotension, resulting from generalized vasodilatation, is managed with the patient horizontal and the legs elevated. In severe cases volume expansion may be required by intravenous infusion. If the hypotension is profound and fails to respond to standard therapy then positive inotropes such as dopamine may be of value. Adrenaline is ineffective in this situation and may even exacerbate the hypotension. All intravenous fluids should be warmed prior to administration so as not to aggravate hypothermia. The avoidance of hypothermia, by keeping the patient warm, limits the likelihood of arrhythmias. Severe dystonic reactions usually respond to orphenadrine (20–40 mg) or procyclidine (5–10 mg) administered intravenously or intramuscularly. Convulsions are best treated with intravenous diazepam. The neuroleptic malignant syndrome (hyperpyrexia) should be treated by cooling.

Severe or irreversible adverse effects
There is one report of spontaneous hypoglycaemia in a child receiving trimeprazine,[46] and reversible agranulocytosis has been reported.[38] Chronic therapy may be associated with a photosensitive dermatitis.

Symptomatic adverse effects
The most commonly reported symptomatic adverse effect with trimeprazine is drowsiness. With regular therapy ambulant patients may notice dizziness or incoordination. Other ill effects reported include dry mouth, disturbing dreams, nasal stuffiness, headache, elation, depression, abdominal discomfort, galactorrhoea and photosensitive dermatitis.

Interference with clinical pathology tests
There are no reports of trimeprazine interfering with clinical pharmacological tests. However, there is a report of trimeprazine, used for sedation in computerized tomographic head scanning in situations in which acute poisoning enters the differential diagnosis, interfering with subsequent toxicological investigations.[47] This is overcome by taking toxicological samples prior to trimeprazine administration.

High risk groups

Neonates
Trimeprazine tartrate is not advised in neonates in view of its marked CNS sedative effects. The lower age limit of use recommended by the manufacturer is 2 years.

Breast milk. Trimeprazine is excreted in breast milk, but at concentrations insufficient to adversely affect a suckling infant[10] and its use by the mother during breast-feeding is considered safe by the American Academy of Pediatrics.[11]

Children
Trimeprazine is widely used in children as a premedicant prior to anaesthesia at a dose of 2 $mg.kg^{-1}$.

Pregnant women
Caution is advised by the manufacturer with respect to the use of trimeprazine during pregnancy. Epidemiological studies, however, indicate that it is safe to use trimeprazine when considering teratogenicity. A collaborative perinatal project monitored 50 282 mother–child pairs of which 14 had first-trimester trimeprazine[1] and 140 used trimeprazine at some time during pregnancy.[48] No evidence of major teratogenic effects was found in this study.

The elderly
A reduced dose, 10 mg in the morning or twice daily, is recommended in the elderly as trimeprazine is renally excreted, and a reduced clearance and enhanced effect may be anticipated in the elderly as creatinine clearance is known to decline with age. In addition, the anticholinergic actions may, in men, induce acute urinary retention in the presence of prostatic hypertrophy and, in both sexes, worsen glaucoma or cause adynamic ileus.

Drug interactions

Potentially hazardous interactions
CNS sedatives. Concomitant use of trimeprazine with other CNS sedatives such as opiates, barbiturates, tranquillizers or sedative H_1-antihistamines may lead to an additive or potentiating effect.[49]

Alcohol. Alcohol enhances the CNS sedative effects of trimeprazine and the Committee on Safety of Medicines recommends that patients be warned not to take alcohol while on H_1-antihistamine therapy.

Anticholinesterases. The anticholinergic actions of trimeprazine will antagonize the effects of anticholinesterase agents such as neostigmine and pyridostigmine.

Other significant interactions
Tricyclic antidepressants. The use of tricyclic antidepressants which have anticholinergic actions concomitantly with trimeprazine will produce greater anticholinergic effects, such as dry mouth and blurred vision. In the elderly, the risk of urinary retention, glaucoma and adynamic ileus will be greater.

Potentially useful interactions
The antisialogogic effects of trimeprazine are enhanced if given with an anticholinergic agent prior to general anaesthesia.

Major outcome trials

1. Binning R, Walson W R, Samrah M, Martin E 1962 Premedication for adenotonsillectomy. British Journal of Anaesthesia 34: 812–816

The effects of four oral premedicant regimes were investigated in 456 children aged $2\frac{1}{2}$–8 years undergoing adenotonsillectomy. They either received quinalbarbitone (n = 121) 6 mg.kg^{-1}; promethazine and chlorpromazine (n = 120), each at 0.8 mg.kg^{-1}; trimeprazine tartrate (n = 135) 4 mg.kg^{-1}; or atropine (n = 80) 0.9 mg. The children's sedation on arrival in the anaesthetic room, and their degree of cooperation during induction and nasopharyngeal and bronchial secretions, were all assessed by the anaesthetist. Their postoperative restlessness and vomiting were both assessed by a ward sister. Trimeprazine was considered the best premedicant as the children were calm on arrival in the anaesthetic room, but not over-sedated (60% awake on arrival) and the anaesthetic was easy to induce. There was a low incidence of postoperative restlessness (12%) and postoperative vomiting (7%); both were significantly less ($p < 0.001$) than with the other premedicants. In addition, the trimeprazine syrup was recorded as being easy to administer and palatable.

Other trials

1. Krause L, Shuster S 1983 Mechanism of action of antipruritic drugs. British Medical Journal 287: 1199–1200

The effects on nocturnal itching of the non-sedative H_1-antihistamines astemizole (n = 6) and terfenadine (n = 6) were compared with the sedating H_1-receptor antagonist trimeprazine (n = 7) and the sedative benzodiazepine nitrazepam (n = 7) in 23 patients with itchy dermatosis (21 eczema, 2 psoriasis). The study was a parallel group study in two parts due to the slower onset of maximal effect with astemizole. Patients received either terfenadine 60 mg three times daily, trimeprazine tartrate 10 mg three times daily or nitrazepam 10 mg at night for days 3 and 4 of a six night study, or astemizole 10 mg every morning for a mean of 28 days (range 19 to 40). Their nocturnal itch was assessed by visual analogue scale and nocturnal scratching by objective monitoring of nocturnal limb movement. These recordings were made in hospital over 6 nights with treatment being taken as follows; days 1–2 no oral drug therapy, days 3–4 oral drug treatment and days 5–6 no oral medication, with the exception of astemizole-treated patients in which nights 1 and 2 were compared with two further nights after prolonged treatment.

The non-sedative H_1-antihistamines were ineffective in relieving either itching or scratching limb movement, whereas trimeprazine and nitrazepam had clinical benefit ($p < 0.05$). Three patients who had no benefit from terfenadine were subsequently tried on trimeprazine with clinical benefit. This trial concluded that in the treatment of itch not related to local histamine release (those other than urticaria and dermatographism) the beneficial effects of treatment are related to CNS sedation rather than peripheral H_1-receptor antagonism. Thus the non-sedating H_1-antihistamines have no role to play in the treatment of pruritus when local histamine release is not considered to be an aetiological factor.

General review articles

Pearlman D S 1976 Antihistamines: pharmacology and clinical use. Drugs 12: 258–273

Schuller D E, Turkewitz D 1986 Adverse effects of antihistamines. Postgraduate Medicine 79.2: 75–86

References

1. Heinonen O P, Slone D, Shapiro S 1977 Birth defects and drugs in pregnancy. Publishing Sciences Group, Littleton, pp 323–324
2. Nelson M M, Forfar J O 1971 Associations between drugs administered during pregnancy and congenital abnormalities. British Medical Journal 1: 523–527
3. von-Maur K 1985 Antihistamine selection in patients with allergic rhinitis. Annals of Allergy 55: 458–462
4. Krause L, Shuster S 1983 Mechanism of action of antipruritic drugs. British Medical Journal 287: 1199–1200
5. Burtles R, Astley B 1983 Lorazepam in children. A double-blind trial comparing lorazepam, diazepam, trimeprazine and placebo. British Journal of Anaesthesia 55: 275–279
6. Bramwell R G, Manford M L 1981 Premedication of children with trimeprazine tartrate. British Journal of Anaesthesia 53: 821–826
7. McKay G, Rauw G A, Stonkus M D et al 1984 Radioimmunoassay for trimeprazine in human plasma. Journal of Pharmacological Methods 12: 203–211
8. Hu O Y-P, Gfeller E, Perrin J H, Curry S H 1986 Relative bioavailability of trimeprazine tablets investigated in man using HPLC with electrochemical detection. Journal of Pharmacy and Pharmacology 38: 172–176
9. Johnson P C, Masters Y F 1962 Effect of sustained release on absorption and excretion of ^{35}S-labelled trimeprazine tartrate. Journal of Laboratory and Clinical Medicine 59: 993–999

10. O'Brien T E 1974 Excretion of drugs in human milk. American Journal of Hospital Pharmacy 31: 844–854
11. Committee on Drugs, American Academy of Pediatrics 1983 The transfer of drugs and other chemicals into human breast milk. Pediatrics 72: 375–383
12. Valman H B 1981 ABC of 1 to 7. Sleep problems. British Medical Journal 283: 422–423
13. Simonoff E A, Stores G 1987 Controlled trial of trimeprazine-tartrate for night waking. Archives of Disease in Childhood 62: 253–257
14. Callaway J L, Olansky S 1957 Trimeprazine an adjuvant in the management of itching dermatoses. North Carolina Medical Journal 18: 320–321
15. Anderson T E, Chalmers D 1959 A trial of trimeprazine in itching dermatoses. British Journal of Dermatology 71: 214–218
16. London I D 1959 Double-blind evaluation of trimeprazine. Archives of Dermatology 80: 220–222
17. Smith M A, Curwen M P 1961 Controlled trial of two oral antipruritic drugs, trimeprazine and methdilazine. British Journal of Dermatology 73: 351–358
18. Ingram J T 1962 Management of infantile eczema. British Medical Journal 2: 44–46
19. Trimpi N D 1960 Effective plan for control of pruritus ani. Diseases of the Colon and Rectum 3: 125
20. Hudson A L 1959 A new drug for control of itching — trimeprazine. Canadian Medical Association Journal 80: 125
21. Bell B T, Viek P, Santangelo S C 1960 Use of trimeprazine to control pruritus in orthopaedic surgery. Journal of the American Medical Association 174: 1976–1977
22. Binning R, Watson W R, Samrah M, Martin E 1962 Premedication for adenotonsillectomy. British Journal of Anaesthesia 34: 812–816
23. Davies D R, Doughty A 1966 Oral premedication in children with trimeprazine. British Journal of Anaesthesia 38: 878–885
24. Haq I U, Dundee J W 1968 Studies of drugs given before anaesthesia XVI: oral diazepam and trimeprazine for adenotonsillectomy. British Journal of Anaesthesia 40: 972–978
25. Thomas D L, Vaughan R S, Vickers M D, Mapleson W W 1987 Comparison of temazepam elixir and trimeprazine syrup as oral premedication in children undergoing tonsillectomy and associated procedures. British Journal of Anaesthesia 59: 424–430
26. Furness G, Boyle M M, Lee J P H 1986 Temazepam elixir for premedication in paediatric ENT operations. British Journal of Anaesthesia 58: 811P
27. Peters C G, Brunton J T 1982 Comparative study of lorazepam and trimeprazine for oral premedication in paediatric anaesthesia. British Journal of Anaesthesia 54: 623–628
28. Layfield D J, Walker A K Y 1984 Premedication for children with oral trimeprazine and droperidol. Anaesthesia 39: 32–34
29. Bullen C, Bramwell R G 1982 Oral premedication for children with a droperidol, trimeprazine and methadone mixture. Anaesthesia 37: 212–213
30. Johnson T W, Young P N 1986 Premedication for children. Anaesthesia 41: 1059
31. Kendall C 1981 Sleep problems in young children. British Medical Journal 283: 1265
32. Padfield N L, Twohig M M, Fraser A C 1986 Temazepam and trimeprazine compared with placebo as premedication in children. An investigation extended into the first 2 weeks at home. British Journal of Anaesthesia 58: 487–493
33. Duncan B B, Zaimi F, Newman G B, Jenkins J G, Aveling W 1984 Effect of premedication on the induction dose of thiopentone in children. Anaesthesia 39: 426–428
34. Richman N 1985 A double-blind drug trial of treatment in young children with waking problems. Journal of Child Psychology and Psychiatry 26: 591–598
35. Mann N P 1981 Trimeprazine and respiratory depression. Archives of Disease in Childhood 56: 481–482
36. Kahn A, Blum D 1982 Phenothiazines and sudden infant death syndrome. Pediatrics 70: 75–78
37. Scrip 1987 1182: 23
38. Brachman P S, McCreary T W, Florence R 1959 Agranulocytosis induced by trimeprazine. New England Journal of Medicine 260: 378–380
39. Moyes D G 1973 Malignant hyperpyrexia caused by trimeprazine. British Journal of Anaesthesia 45: 1163–1164
40. Peltz B, Carstens J 1975 An unusual case of malignant hyperpyrexia. Anaesthesia 30: 346–350
41. Loan W B, Cuthbert D 1985 Adverse cardiovascular response to oral trimeprazine in children. British Medical Journal 290: 1548–1549
42. Dundee J W, Moore J 1961 The effects of premedication with phenothiazine derivatives on the course of metholezilone anaesthesia. British Journal of Anaesthesia 33: 382–396
43. Skegg D C G, Richards S M, Doll R 1979 Minor tranquillisers and road accidents. British Medical Journal 1: 917–919
44. Adelman M H, Jacobson E, Lief P A, Miller S A 1959 Promethazine hydrochloride in surgery and obstetrics. Journal of the American Medical Association 169: 73–75
45. Stephen P J, Williamson J 1984 Drug induced parkinsonism in the elderly. Lancet 2: 1082–1083
46. Basheer S M 1971 Spontaneous hypoglycaemia in a child treated with trimeprazine. Journal of the Irish Medical Association 64: 189–190
47. Flanagan R J, Saynor D A, Raper S M 1980 Sedation for neurological investigations in children may interfere with toxicological analyses. Lancet 1: 830
48. Heinonen O P, Slone D, Shapiro S 1977 Birth defects and drugs in pregnancy. Publishing Sciences Group, Littleton, p 437
49. Winter C A 1948 Potentiating effect of antihistaminic drugs upon sedative action of barbiturates. Journal of Pharmacology and Experimental Therapeutics 94: 7–11

T

Trimetaphan (camsylate)

A short-acting ganglion blocking agent with a rapid onset of action.

Chemistry

Trimetaphan camsylate (trimethaphan camsylate, trimethaphan camphorsulphonate, Arfonad)
$C_{22}H_{25}N_2OS.C_{10}H_{15}O_4S$
1,3-Dibenzylperhydro-2-oxoimidazo[4,5-c]thieno[1,2-a]thiolium (+)-camphor-10-sulphonate

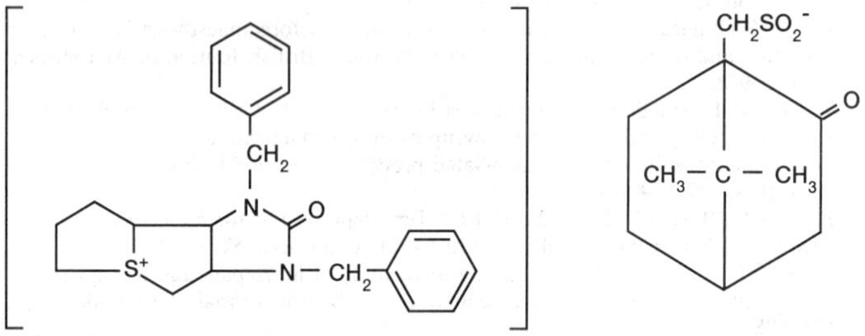

Molecular weight	596.8
pKa	—
Solubility	
in alcohol	1 in 2
in water	1 in 5
Octanol/water partition coefficient	—

White crystals or a white crystalline powder that is odourless with a bitter taste. It is prepared by chemical synthesis and is not present in any combined preparations.

Pharmacology

Trimetaphan is an antagonist at postsynaptic acetylcholine receptors within autonomic ganglia and a direct-acting vasodilator the mechanism of which is unknown. In addition, at high doses, it produces competitive blockade of α-adrenoceptors and neuromuscular blockade possibly by ion channel blockade. Trimetaphan is a potent inhibitor of pseudocholinesterase and causes release of histamine from mast cells by a direct effect.

Toxicology

There is no evidence that trimetaphan has any carcinogenic, mutagenic, teratogenic or embryotoxic effects.

Clinical pharmacology

Trimetaphan produces non-depolarizing blockade of autonomic ganglia by combination with postsynaptic acetylcholine receptors probably in a competitive manner.[1] The consequences of ganglion blockade are postural hypotension, urinary retention, constipation, cycloplegia, mydriasis, xerostomia, and anhydrosis. Intraocular pressure may be increased if aqueous drainage is impeded as a result of the mydriasis; however, if the blood pressure is allowed to fall intraocular pressure will fall markedly. This is thought to be due to a reduction in ciliary blood flow during hypotension since autoregulation does not occur in this vascular bed.[2] Cardiac output is reduced with corresponding falls in organ blood flow.

At higher concentrations trimetaphan has a direct vasodilator action and also α-adrenoceptor blocking properties.[3] The direct vasodilator effect is more pronounced in femoral and mesenteric vessels than in cerebral vessels and the mechanism is unknown. α-Adrenoceptor blockade is probably minimal with normal clinical doses. It appears to be competitive in nature as shown by a parallel right shift of the dose–response curve to noradrenaline and the ability to protect the receptor site from occupation with phenoxybenzamine in animal preparations.

The intravenous administration of trimetaphan produces an almost immediate fall in the arterial blood pressure, which is rapidly reversed by discontinuing administration, usually with return to normal or control levels within 10 minutes. However, delayed recovery lasting more than 30 minutes has been reported on several occasions.

In large doses trimetaphan produces clinically significant neuromuscular blockade by an action at the motor end-plate. The exact mechanism of this effect is not known but it does not appear to involve an interaction with acetylcholine receptors, as is the case with conventional neuromuscular blocking drugs, and may be due to blockade of end-plate ion channels.[4–6]

Trimetaphan is a potent inhibitor of pseudocholinesterase. The nature of this inhibition is unknown. It was originally believed that trimetaphan was metabolized by pseudocholinesterase but this is not now thought to occur.[7,8] Inhibition of pseudocholinesterase will affect the action of drugs that are metabolized by this enzyme and, for example, the plasma half life of suxamethonium is approximately double during infusions of trimetaphan. Trimetaphan is also a weak inhibitor of true cholinesterase with about one twenty-thousandth the potency of neostigmine but this effect is not clinically significant.[9]

Trimetaphan causes histamine release from mast cells and basophils probably by a direct effect on these cells. The amount of histamine release is related to the rate of administration and is greater following bolus doses than during infusions of the drug. It is not thought that histamine release is an important factor in the production of hypotension by trimetaphan.[10]

Pharmacokinetics

Trimetaphan has been measured in body fluids by a colorimetric method with methyl orange. This assay is relatively non-specific and insensitive. Therapeutic plasma levels have not been measured and the pharmacokinetic profile of the drug has never been determined.

In the kidney, in addition to glomerular filtration trimetaphan may also be actively secreted. It has been estimated that as much as 30% of an administered dose appears unchanged in the urine. It crosses the placenta and causes ganglion blockade in the fetus. Animal studies indicate that oral absorption is erratic and incomplete.

Concentration–effect relationship

Trimetaphan is a very short-acting drug and there is no evidence of any correlation between plasma concentration of the drug and its therapeutic effects.

Metabolism

The pathways involved in the metabolism of trimetaphan and the effects of renal and hepatic failure on its distribution and metabolism are unknown.

Pharmaceutics

Trimetaphan (Arfonad; Roche, UK/USA) is available only as an intravenous preparation. In the UK ampoules contain 250 mg in 5 ml of water with hydrochloric acid added to adjust the pH of the solution to 5.2. In the USA the strength is similar but the ampoule size is 10 ml. Ampoules should be stored at 6°C and should not be allowed to freeze.

The drug should be diluted prior to use in normal saline or dextrose saline and such solutions are stable for 14 days at 25°C. Trimetaphan solutions are physically incompatible with thiopentone, gallamine triethiodide, d-tubocurarine, iodides, bromides and strongly alkaline solutions. It is therefore recommended that trimetaphan solutions are not used as a vehicle for any other drugs and vice versa. It should be administered via a dedicated infusion system.

Therapeutic use

Indications

1. To induce hypotension during surgical procedures
2. Treatment of hypertensive crises
3. Modification of the stress response to surgery
4. Treatment of myocardial infarction
5. Predicting the potential hypotension produced by spinal anaesthesia.

Contraindications

1. Severe arteriosclerotic disease
2. Pyloric stenosis.

Mode of use

Trimetaphan is administered intravenously and while intermittent bolus doses are often used, a continuous infusion is by far the most common method of administration. Concentrations of 0.1% or 0.5% in normal saline or dextrose saline are used. The recommended starting rate of infusion is 0.5–2 $mg.min^{-1}$ and this is adjusted according to the response. Adequate hypotension is usually achieved by infusion rates of 0.5–6 $mg.min^{-1}$ but there is marked individual variation and careful observation of its effects is necessary so that direct arterial blood pressure monitoring is mandatory during its use in anaesthesia. Tachycardia is often seen but is not as troublesome as with other hypotensive agents such as sodium nitroprusside. Tachyphylaxis may occur with prolonged usage.

Indications

1. Production of induced hypotension during surgical procedures
This is the only licensed indication for the use of trimetaphan in the UK. Hypotension may be induced in a variety of surgical procedures to reduce blood loss or to improve operative conditions. Systolic blood pressures of 60–80 mmHg seem to be well tolerated by young patients with no history of atherosclerotic disease. As outlined above the hypotensive effect of trimetaphan is due to its ganglion blocking and direct vasodilating actions but their relative importance is unknown. The haemodynamic effects vary between species. In man moderate hypotension can be achieved without a fall in cardiac output.[11] Peripheral vascular resistance is decreased and a redistribution of cardiac output occurs away from the splanchnic, renal and cerebral vascular beds. If the venous return falls then cardiac output also falls. Cerebral blood flow is reduced and oxygen extraction by the brain is increased. The tissue oxygen tension in the cerebral cortex is better maintained during hypotension induced by trimetaphan than by haemorrhage.[12] Spinal cord blood flow is also decreased. Renal blood flow, urine output and creatinine clearance fall but it has been suggested that renal oxygenation is not impaired.[13,14] Moderate degrees of hypotension do not seem to greatly affect hepatic blood flow[15,16] but in experimental models hepatic failure is common following profound hypotension produced by trimetaphan.[17,18]

Despite trimetaphan being a direct coronary artery dilator[19] coronary blood flow falls during induced hypotension and increased oxygen extraction by the myocardium has been observed indicating that the fall in perfusion is greater than the reduction in myocardial work.[20] However, even in patients suffering from ischaemic heart disease, hypotension with trimetaphan does not produce signs or symptoms of myocardial ischaemia.[21]

The increase in intracranial pressure (ICP) seen on induction of hypotension with trimetaphan in animals has been ascribed to dilatation of the cerebral vasculature either as a result of the autoregulatory response to reduced systemic arterial blood pressure or, more likely, direct vasodilation by the drug.

The response in man is less marked with only 10% of cases exhibiting an increase in ICP when trimetaphan is used to induce hypotension.[22] The blood–brain barrier is reported to be better maintained during trimetaphan-induced hypotension than following sodium nitroprusside though the clinical significance of this is unknown.[23]

Trimetaphan has little if any effect on the pattern of spontaneous respiration during anaesthesia but it increases the ventilation perfusion mismatch within the lung as a result of the fall in pulmonary perfusion pressure.[24,25]

Trimetaphan has been largely superseded by sodium nitroprusside for the production of induced hypotension during surgical procedures because its duration of action is shorter and more predictable and also because of evidence that cerebral and coronary blood flows are better maintained. However, there have been no clinical trials demonstrating significant differences in outcome following hypotension with the two agents. Concern over the dangers of cyanide toxicity with nitroprusside have lead some workers to investigate the use of mixtures of ten parts by weight of trimetaphan to one part sodium nitroprusside and early reports are encouraging.[26]

2. The treatment of hypertensive crises
Trimetaphan is now rarely used in the management of hypertensive crises,[27] as there are better alternative agents available. The one indication remaining is the treatment of hypertension associated with dissecting aortic aneurysms where trimetaphan reduces the velocity of ventricular ejection and hence lowers the shearing forces applied to the aortic aneurysm.[28]

3. Modification of the stress response to surgery
Trimetaphan has been used to prevent hypertension during both cardiopulmonary bypass procedures and orthopaedic surgery. The hypertension is due to increased activity in sympathetic nerves which trimetaphan obtunds at sympathetic ganglia and the adrenal gland. As a result plasma adrenaline and noradrenaline levels show hardly any increase[29,30] and there is less activation of the renin/angiotensin system[31] compared with the use of sodium nitroprusside to produce the same reduction in arterial blood pressure, which causes a reflex increase in sympathoadrenal activity.

4. The treatment of myocardial infarction
Trimetaphan produces beneficial haemodynamic changes in patients following myocardial infarction. Preload, afterload and cardiac output are all reduced with a consequent reduction in myocardial work. Predicted infarct size has been shown to be reduced by 24% by controlling hypertension with trimetaphan.[32]

5. Predicting the hypotension produced by spinal anaesthesia
The degree of hypotension produced by a 3 mg intravenous bolus of trimetaphan has been used as a predictive test of the degree of hypotension likely to follow spinal anaesthesia but this test is now rarely used.[33]

Contraindications

1. Severe atherosclerotic disease
The risk of further reducing blood supply to vital organs already compromised by atherosclerotic disease is considered to be an absolute contraindication to the production of induced hypotension with trimetaphan in patients with known atheromatous vascular disease.

2. Pyloric stenosis
Ganglionic blockade will compromise the gastric outflow in patients with pyloric stenosis.

Adverse reactions

Potentially life-threatening effects
Deaths directly attributed to trimetaphan are rare. In large doses trimetaphan can produce clinically important muscle relaxation leading to respiratory arrest. One patient is reported to have died as a result of aspiration of gastric contents following respiratory arrest due to trimetaphan.[9,34]

Acute overdosage
There have been no cases of deliberate overdose with trimetaphan. Clinical overdosage will result in profound hypotension, which will respond to posture, volume expansion and vasopressors. Tachycardia and also respiratory depression from neuromuscular blockade may occur.

Severe or irreversible adverse effects
The histamine release produced by trimetaphan may induce asthmatic attacks in susceptible individuals.

Symptomatic adverse effects
All the side effects of ganglion blockade are produced during the administration of trimetaphan and like its hypotensive action they are short lived after withdrawal of the drug. Since most of the patients in whom trimetaphan is used are anaesthetized symptoms, do not occur.

Interference with clinical pathology tests
No technical interferences of this kind have been reported.

High risk groups

Neonates
The drug is contraindicated in this age group due to the risk of producing paralytic ileus or meconium ileus.

Breast milk. Although the drug has not been measured in breast milk, arguably its use in lactating mothers is contraindicated, because of the remote possibility of producing paralytic ileus in the breast-fed newborn infant.

Children
There is no contraindication for use of the drug in children.

Pregnant women
Trimetaphan is contraindicated in pregnancy due to the risk of producing paralytic ileus or meconium ileus in the newborn.

The elderly
The elderly are more susceptible to the hypotensive actions of trimetaphan and are more likely to have coexisting atherosclerotic disease. Greater care is therefore needed.

Concurrent disease
Patients with degenerative disease of the central nervous system, diabetes and patients with Addison's disease may be very sensitive to the hypotensive actions of trimetaphan.

Drug interactions

Potentially hazardous interactions
Anaesthetic agents. The hypotensive actions of the volatile anaesthetic agents and trimetaphan are additive.

Other significant interactions
Suxamethonium. The duration of action of suxamethonium is prolonged by trimetaphan inhibition of pseudocholinesterase. The reduced pseudocholinesterase activity seen in pregnant women near term may make this effect more pronounced.[35]

Non-depolarizing muscle relaxants. The neuromuscular blocking action of trimetaphan will enhance that of the non-depolarizing muscle relaxants.

Potentially useful interactions
None has been reported.

General review articles

Adams A P 1975 Techniques of vascular control for deliberate hypotension during anaesthesia. British Journal of Anaesthesia 47: 777–792

McDowall D G 1985 Induced hypotension and brain ischaemia. British Journal of Anaesthesia 57: 110–119

References

1. Large W A, Sim J A 1986 A comparison between mechanisms of actions of different nicotinic blocking agents on rat submandibular ganglia. British Journal of Pharmacology 89: 538–592
2. Dias P L, Andrew D S, Romanes G J 1982 Effect on the intraocular pressure of hyptensive anaesthesia with intravenous trimetaphan. British Journal of Ophthalmology 66: 721–724
3. Harioka T, Hatano Y, Mori K, Toda N 1984 Trimetaphan is a direct arterial vasodilator and an α adrenoceptor blocker. Anesthesia and Analgesia 63: 290–296
4. Deacock A R de C, Hargrove R L 1962 The influence of certain ganglionic blocking agents on neuromuscular transmission. British Journal of Anaesthesia 34: 357–362
5. Nakamura K, Hatano Y, Mori K 1988 The site of action of trimetaphan-induced neuromuscular blockade in isolated rat and frog muscle. Acta Anaesthesiologica Scandinavica 32: 125–130
6. Pollard B J, Van Der Speck A F L 1987 The neuromuscular blocking effect of trimetaphan alone and in combination with different non depolarizing muscle relaxants in the rat. Journal of Pharmacy and Pharmacology 39: 896–899
7. Sklar G S, Lanks K W 1977 Effects of trimetaphan and sodium nitroprusside on hydrolysis of succinylcholine in vitro. Anesthesiology 47: 31–33
8. Anton A H, Czinn S, Jazwa J, Tam L A, Amaranath L 1978 Trimetaphan camsylate (Arfonad) and human plasma cholinesterase. Research Communications in Chemical Pathology and Pharmacology 22: 375–383
9. Nakamura K, Koide M, Imanaga T, Ogasawara H, Takahashi M, Yoshikawa M 1980 Prolonged neuromuscular blockade following trimetaphan infusion. Anaesthesia 35: 1202–1207
10. Fahmy N R, Soter N A 1985 Effects of trimetaphan on arterial blood histamine and systemic hemodynamics in humans. Anesthesiology 62: 562–566
11. Scott D B, Stephan G W, Marshall R L, Jenkinson J L, MacRae W R 1972 Circulatory effects of controlled arterial hypotension with trimetaphan during nitrous oxide/halothane anaesthesia. British Journal of Anaesthesia 44: 523–527
12. Maekawa T, McDowall D G, Okuda Y 1977 Oxygen tension on the brain surface during hypotension induced by haemorrhage, trimetaphan or sodium nitroprusside. Acta Neurologica Scandinavica 56: 504–505
13. Behnia R, Koushanpour E, Goldstick T K, Linde H W, Osborn R 1984 Renal tissue oxygenation following induced hypotension in dogs. British Journal of Anaesthesia 56: 1037–1043
14. Behnia R, Martin A, Koushanpour E, Brunner E A 1982 Trimetaphan-induced hypotension: Effect on renal function. Canadian Anesthetists Society Journal 29: 581–586
15. Sivarajan M, Amory D W, McKenzie S M 1985 Regional blood flows during induced hypotension produced by nitroprusside or trimetaphan in the rhesus monkey. Anesthesia and Analgesia 64: 759–766
16. Gelman S 1986 Hepatic blood flow during controlled hypotension. Anesthesia and Analgesia 65: 423–424
17. Aguilar J A, Boldrey E B 1960 The effect of arfonad on the monkey. Anesthesiology 21: 3–12
18. Dong W K, Bledsoe S W, Eng D Y et al 1983 Profound arterial hypotension in dogs. Brain electrical activity and organ integrity. Anesthesiology 58: 61–71
19. Wang H H, Liu L P M, Katz R L 1977 A comparison of the cardiovascular effects of sodium nitroprusside and trimethaphan. Anesthesiology 46: 40–48
20. Rowe G G, Afonsa S, Lugo J E, Boake W C 1964 Systemic and coronary hemodynamic effects of trimetaphan camphorsulphonate (Arfonad) in the dog. Anesthesiology 25: 156–160
21. Nitter-Hauge S 1978 Circulatory effects of controlled arterial hypotension with trimethaphan (Arfonad). British Heart Journal 40: 401–405
22. Turner J M, Powell D, Gibson R M, McDowell D G 1977 Intracranial pressure changes in neurosurgical patients during hypotension induced with sodium nitroprusside or trimetaphan. British Journal of Anaesthesia 49: 419–425
23. Ishikawa T, Funatsu N, Okamoto K, Takeshita H, McDowall G 1983 Blood brain barrier function following drug-induced hypotension in the dog. Anesthesiology 59: 526–531
24. Hannhart B, Bertrand D, Peslin R, Bohadana A 1983 Effects of induced hypotension on breathing pattern in halothane-anaesthetized man. European Journal of Clinical Investigation 13: 379–382
25. Skene D S, Sullivan S F, Patterson R W 1978 Pulmonary shunting and lung volumes during hypotension induced with trimetaphan. British Journal of Anaesthesia 50: 339–343
26. Fahmy N R 1895 Nitroprusside versus a nitroprusside–trimethaphan mixture for induced hypotension: hemodynamic effects and cyanide release. Clinical Pharmacology and Therapeutics 37: 264–270
27. Vidt D G 1986 Treatment of hypertensive emergencies. American Heart Journal 111: 220–225
28. Palmer R F, Lasseter K C 1974 Nitroprusside and aortic dissecting aneurysm. New England Journal of Medicine 294: 1403–1404
29. Corr L, Grounds R M, Brown M J, Whitwam J G 1986 Plasma catecholamine changes during cardiopulmonary bypass: a randomised double-blind comparison of trimetaphan camsylate and sodium nitroprusside. British Heart Journal 56: 89–93
30. Hamaji M, Tashiro C, Oka N, Seki I, Kawashima Y, Yoshima I 1983 Plasma catecholamine response to hypotension induced by trimetaphan and by sodium nitroprusside during nitrous oxide-oxygen-fentanyl anesthesia. Medical Journal of Osaka University 34: 37–41
31. Knight P R, Lane G A, Hensinger R N, Bolles R S, Bjoraker D G 1983 Catecholamine and renin–angiotensin response during controlled hypotensive anesthesia induced by sodium nitroprusside or trimetaphan camsylate. Anesthesiology 59: 248–253
32. Shell W E, Sobel B E 1974 Protection of jeopardized ischemic myocardium by reduction of ventricular afterload. New England Journal of Medicine 291: 481–486
33. Lapides J, Schroeder K F, Bourne R B, Lanning R J 1967 Arfonad test for predicting blood rpessure response to spinal anesthesia. Journal of Urology 97: 758–762
34. Dale R C, Schroeder E T 1976 Respiratory paralysis during treatment of hypertension with trimethaphan camsylate. Archives of Internal Medicine 136: 816–818
35. Poulton T J, James F M, Lockridge O 1979 Prolonged apnea following trimethaphan and succinylcholine. Anesthesiology 50: 54–56

Trimethoprim

Trimethoprim is a folic acid antagonist originally used as an antimalarial but now used in respiratory and urinary infections.

Chemistry

Trimethoprim (Syraprim, Ipral, Monotrim, Trimogal, Trimopan)
$C_{14}H_{18}N_4O_3$
5-[(3,4,5-Trimethoxyphenyl)methyl]-2,4-pyrimidinediamine

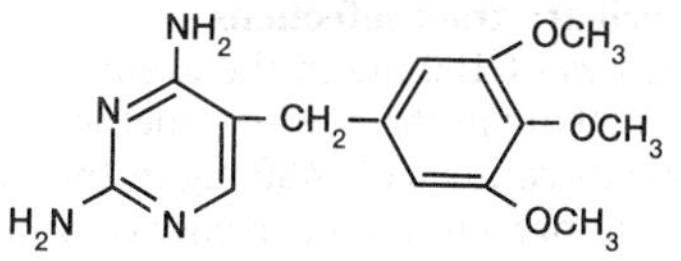

Molecular weight	290.3
pKa (amino)	7.3
Solubility	
in alcohol	1 in 300
in water	1 in 2300
Octanol/water partition coefficient	0.64

A white or yellowish-white, odourless or almost odourless crystalline powder or crystals with a very bitter taste, prepared by chemical synthesis. Trimethoprim is also available in combination with sulphamethoxazole as co-trimoxazole (Septrin, Bactrim)

Pharmacology

Trimethoprim is a structural analogue of the pteridine portion of dihydrofolic acid, and serves as a competitive inhibitor of the enzyme dihydrofolate reductase. Dihydrofolate reductase catalyses the reduction of dihydrofolic acid to the active form of folic acid, tetrahydrofolic acid. Trimethoprim inhibits the bacterial enzyme at concentrations far lower than those required to inhibit the mammalian enzyme and the drug also inhibits protozoal dihydrofolate reductase. The enzyme in *Escherichia coli* is inhibited by a 5 nM concentration of the enzyme compared to 260 000 nM for rat liver enzyme and 70 nM for *Plasmodium berghei* enzyme. Pyrimethamine is more effective at inhibiting the protozoal enzyme but about 500 times less effective at inhibiting dihydrofolate reductase in *E. coli.*[1]

Trimethoprim exerts a bactericidal effect in vitro in the presence of methionine, glycine and a purine and this allows inhibition of DNA synthesis without inhibition of protein synthesis. This results in cell elongation without division and leads eventually to cell death. The presence of thymidine renders trimethoprim merely bacteriostatic.

Toxicology

Trimethoprim does not exhibit mutagenic effects[2] and information on carcinogenicity is lacking. Fetal adverse effects including increased fetal death rate and a characteristic pattern of malformations have been observed in rats given high doses of trimethoprim (300 mg.kg^{-1} daily),[3] although no such effects have been observed in rabbits. Generalized depression of haemopoiesis was observed in monkeys after 14 days treatment with trimethoprim (300 mg.kg^{-1} daily).[3] Concurrent treatment with leucovorin improved survival in monkeys given this dosage of trimethoprim, proving that the toxic effects were due to folate inhibition.[4]

Clinical pharmacology

Trimethoprim is active against plasmodia but is not used now for that purpose since pyrimethamine is much more effective. Trimethoprim is active in vitro against a wide variety of Gram-positive and Gram-negative organisms. In particular, it is active against *Streptococcus pyogenes* and *Streptococcus pneumonia*, *Haemophilus influenzae*, *Corynebacterium diphtheriae* and *E. coli.* It has no activity against *Clostridium*, *Mycobacterium* or *Treponema* and is relatively inactive against *Brucella* sp. Trimethoprim is commonly used in combination with sulphamethoxazole but because of the side effects of the combination trimethoprim is increasingly used on its own.

Some authors have suggested that the use of trimethoprim alone has led to an increase in the incidence of resistance to this agent.[5] However, this has been disputed by the findings that increased resistance to trimethoprim was noticed before the drug became available as a single agent.[6] Resistance seems to be transferred by R-plasmids resistant to both components of the combination product co-trimoxazole.[7,8] However, resistance to *Staphylococcus aureus* appears to be determined by a chromosomal gene.

Pharmacokinetics

The most commonly used analytical method is a spectrofluorimetric assay.[9] Although sensitive enough to detect plasma levels of 50 µg.l^{-1} of trimethoprim, this method is not absolutely specific, as metabolites of trimethoprim may give rise to fluorescence. Other analytical methods include gas chromatography[10] and high performance liquid chromatography.[11] With electrochemical detection, the limit of sensitivity of the latter is 10 µg.l^{-1}.

Urinary recovery of labelled drug following an oral dose indicates that trimethoprim is rapidly and completely absorbed.[9] Peak plasma levels occur between 1 and 4 hours following a single dose and concentrations are linearly related to dose.[12,13] The mean plasma half life is 10 hours with a range of 8.6 to 17 hours. Trimethoprim is excreted chiefly by glomerular filtration and renal tubular secretion, some 50–60% of the dose being found in the urine within 24 hours;[13] 80% of drug recovered is in the unmetabolized form.[14] There is no evidence of first-pass metabolism. Rifampicin produces a slight shortening of trimethoprim half life during co-administration, but this is not thought to be of clinical significance.

The high apparent volume of distribution, 70–100 l, suggests that trimethoprim is widely distributed throughout the body. Concentrations in a number of body tissues and fluids, especially urine and bronchial secretions, are higher than corresponding plasma concentrations.[13–16] Trimethoprim exhibits moderate plasma protein binding, 42–46%, which is slightly reduced in the presence of sulphamethoxazole.[9]

The concentration of trimethoprim in the CSF is 20–60% of the plasma concentration. Trimethoprim is excreted in breast milk in concentrations which exceed those found in plasma by about 25%.[17] Drug levels measured in pregnancy show 75% of the maternal plasma concentration in amniotic fluid, 57% in the cord blood and 50% in fetal tissue.[18]

Oral absorption	>95%
Presystemic metabolism	negligible
Plasma half life	
range	8.6–17 h
mean	10 h
Volume of distribution	70–100 l
Plasma protein binding	42–46%

Trimethoprim undergoes some hepatic biotransformation with a small proportion of the dose being excreted into the bile. In patients with impaired liver function or decompensated liver disease the plasma concentration is lowered by an average factor of 1.5–2.0. The elimination half life is increased by up to twice that in healthy patients, although this is still within the range encountered in healthy patients.[33]

Investigations of the disposition of trimethoprim in renal patients has revealed an increase in the half life of the drug in patients with severe renal impairment (creatinine clearance < 10 ml.min^{-1}) leading to high steady-state plasma levels.[19,20] An altered dose regime for patients with impaired renal function has been suggested.[19]

T

Concentration–effect relationship

Therapeutic success is achieved when the concentration of trimethoprim exceeds the minimum bactericidal or minimum inhibitory concentration (MIC) for the infecting organism. Thus, with a typical isolate of *E. coli* the MIC for trimethoprim is 0.3 $mg.l^{-1}$ compared to 3 $mg.l^{-1}$ for sulphamethoxazole. When the two antibiotics are mixed in a 1:20 ratio the MIC for trimethoprim falls to 0.05 $mg.l^{-1}$.

Metabolism

Approximately 20% of an oral dose of trimethoprim is metabolized, the majority of the drug being excreted unchanged. Urinary excretion is increased in acid urine. Excretion is almost entirely in the urine and only 4% of the dose can be recovered from the faeces. Five metabolites have been identified: trimethoprim-1-oxide, trimethoprim-3-oxide, 4-hydroxytrimethoprim, 3-hydroxytrimethoprim and α-hydroxytrimethoprim (Fig. 1). Only the latter three metabolites have any antibacterial activity.

Pharmaceutics

Trimethoprim is available in both oral and parenteral forms.

Tablets contain 100 mg and 300 mg of trimethoprim BP. Syraprim tablets (Wellcome, UK) are white and scored and are coded 'Y3C' for 300 mg and 'O9A' for 100 mg. Proloprim (Burroughs Wellcome, USA) are similarly coded for the 100 mg strength. In the USA there is a 200 mg yellow tablet coded '200'. Both are imprinted with 'PROLOPRIM'. Trimpex (Roche, USA) is a white elliptical tablet containing 100 mg and imprinted 'TRIMPEX 100'.

Trimethoprim is also available as a white, sugar-free suspension containing 50 mg trimethoprim BP in each 5 ml. It is marketed as Ipral (Squibb, UK), Monotrim (Duphar, UK) and Trimopan (Beck, UK).

Trimethoprim is available for intravenous use as an aqueous solution of trimethoprim lactate equivalent to 20 mg of trimethoprim base in 1 ml of water. Each ampoule contains 5 ml. It is marketed as Monotrim (Duphar, UK) and Syraprim (Wellcome, UK).

All preparations should be stored below 25°C and be protected from light. Trimethoprim preparations are stable with a 5 year shelf-life and carry no risk from potentially allergenic substances, although these factors may vary between generic preparations.

Therapeutic use

Indications

1. Treatment of infections caused by trimethoprim-sensitive organisms, particularly those affecting the urinary and respiratory tracts
2. Long-term prophylaxis of recurrent, or suspension of chronic, urinary tract infections caused by sensitive organisms.

Contraindications

1. Hypersensitivity to trimethoprim
2. Severe impairment of renal function (creatinine clearance < 10 $ml.min^{-1}$) where repeated estimations of the plasma concentration, or haemodialysis, cannot be carried out
3. Severe haematological disorders.

Mode of use

Doses employed vary according to indication and the intravenous preparation is usually reserved for use in severe infections. No adverse reaction has been observed following abrupt cessation of the drug.

Indications

1. Urinary and respiratory tract infection

Trimethoprim has been shown to be effective in the treatment of acute urinary tract infection in doses ranging from 100 mg twice daily for 5 days[21] to 200 mg twice daily for 7 days.[22] Courses of 300 mg daily have proved as effective as amoxycillin 250 mg 3 times daily.[23] Single dose treatments of acute urinary tract infection using 400 mg of trimethoprim have compared favourably with single doses of 3 g amoxycillin or 1920 mg of co-trimoxazole.[24]

As trimethoprim has been shown to be concentrated in sputum as well as in urine, it is of particular use in respiratory tract infections. It has been shown to be equally as effective as co-trimoxazole in a variety of chest infections, with fewer side effects.[21] Another study has shown trimethoprim to be more effective than co-trimoxazole in the treatment of pneumonia.[25]

2. Prophylaxis of urinary tract infections

Trimethoprim in doses of 100 mg in the evening has been compared with nitrofurantoin 50 mg in the evening, methenamine hippurate 1 g in the evening and co-trimoxazole 480 mg in the evening, and found to be more effective at preventing recurrence of urinary tract infection with fewer side effects than the other treatments.[20]

Contraindications

1. Impaired renal function

Trimethoprim is chiefly excreted by glomerular filtration and renal tubular secretion. Impaired renal function (creatinine clearance < 10 $ml.min^{-1}$) leads to delayed elimination of the drug and greatly increased plasma levels. Risk of interference with haemopoiesis may be increased.

2. Haematological disorders

Although reported haematological side effects of trimethoprim are mild and rare, the possibility of megaloblastic changes due to folic acid inhibition exists. Patients deficient in folate should be given a folic acid supplement. Folinic acid may be useful in the treatment of trimethoprim-induced haemological problems.

Adverse reactions

Potentially life-threatening effects

None has been reported.

Acute overdosage

There is one report of a man with manic depressive psychosis who attempted suicide by taking 80 tablets of trimethoprim. His symptoms included vomiting, headache, swelling of the face and weakness. He was treated with activated charcoal and intravenous fluids, and his only complaint after 48 hours of observation was mild epigastric pain following gastric lavage.

Medical treatment is successful in the treatment of overdosage.

Fig. 1 Metabolites of trimethoprim

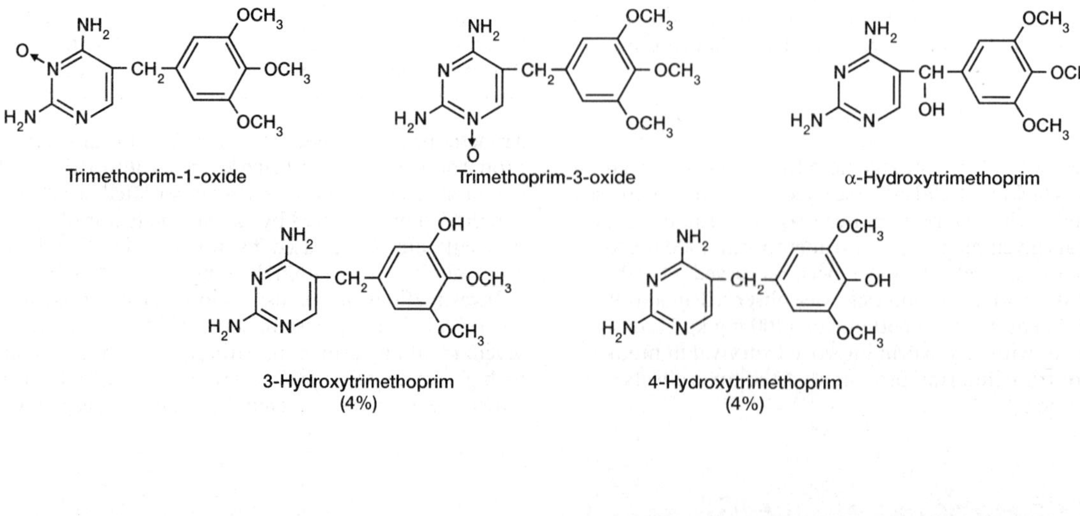

Acidification of the urine and promotion of diuresis will increase the elimination of trimethoprim. Calcium folinate in doses of 5–10 mg daily will counteract any adverse effects of trimethoprim on bone marrow, should such effects occur.

Severe or irreversible adverse effects
None has been reported.

Symptomatic adverse effects
Trimethoprim is generally well tolerated, although mild gastrointestinal disturbances such as nausea, vomiting, glossitis and sore mouth have been reported.[22] Rashes have been reported[20] but are generally mild and a rare occurrence unless larger doses are used (>400 mg daily) for long periods (>10 days).[26] Haematological abnormalities have been mild and of little clinical significance. Megaloblastic anaemia associated with trimethoprim has been reported but it is rare and usually mild, except in patients with pre-existing folate depletion.[27]

Other effects
Trimethoprim impairs phenylalanine metabolism, but this is of no significance in phenylketonuric patients on appropriate dietary restriction.[28]

Interference with clinical pathology tests
Trimethoprim may interfere with the estimation of serum/plasma creatinine when the alkaline picrate reaction is used. This may result in an overestimation of the order of 10%.[29]

High risk groups

Neonates
There is no recommended dose range for neonates but if trimethoprim is used, folate supplementation should be considered.

Breast milk. Trimethoprim is excreted in breast milk at concentrations which exceed the plasma concentration by some 25%. However, the dose received by the infant would be low and unlikely to cause toxic effects.

Children
Trimethoprim is used in children at a dose of 8 $mg.kg^{-1}$ daily, normally in two divided doses. Recommended doses for prophylaxis of urinary tract infections are 50 mg for children aged 6–12 years and 100 mg daily thereafter.

Pregnant women
The safety of trimethoprim in human pregnancy has not been established.

The elderly
Caution should be exercised when treating geriatric patients who may be prone to nutritional folate deficiency. Folate supplementation should be considered in such cases.

Drug interactions

Potentially hazardous interactions

Pyrimethamine. Megaloblastic anaemia has been associated with the concurrent administration of pyrimethamine and co-trimoxazole.[30] A similar interaction is likely to occur with trimethoprim.

Phenytoin. Trimethoprim has been reported to decrease the metabolic clearance rate of phenytoin leading to an increase in mean half life from 12 h to 18 h.[31]

Cyclosporin. A deterioration in renal function has been reported in kidney transplant patients to whom trimethoprim and cyclosporin have been administered concurrently.[32]

Potentially useful interactions
Potentiation of the antibacterial effects of trimethoprim by combination with sulphamethoxazole has been demonstrated in vitro and in vivo. This potentiation has been shown to be of benefit in the treatment of *Pneumocystis carinii* pneumonia, brucellosis, nocardiasis and gonococcal infections.

Major controlled trials

1. Lacey R W, Lord V L, Gunasekera H K W, Leiberman P J, Luxton D E A 1980 Comparison of trimethoprim alone with trimethoprim–sulphamethoxazole in the treatment of respiratory and urinary infections with particular reference to selection of trimethoprim resistance. Lancet 1: 1270–1273

This is a prospective, randomized, double-blind study of 279 patients with respiratory (229 patients) or urinary infections treated with co-trimoxazole or trimethoprim alone. Diagnoses of chest diseases comprised acute bronchitis, basal pneumonia, bronchopneumonia or acute exacerbations of chronic bronchitis, with sputum cultures being taken before treatment (day 0) and on days 7 and 14. Diagnosis of urinary tract infection was confirmed by two fresh mid-stream or catheter specimens of urine containing 10^5 bacteria of a single species per ml. Patients were evenly distributed between the two treatment regimens according to age, sex and severity of infection. Doses of 100 mg trimethoprim or 100 mg trimethoprim combined with 500 mg sulphamethoxazole were administered twice daily for 5 days. Trimethoprim was found to be as effective as co-trimoxazole in the treatment of respiratory and acute urinary tract infections, although a lower incidence of side effects was recorded with trimethoprim.

2. Brumfitt W, Pursell R 1972 Double-blind trial to compare ampicillin, cephalexin, co-trimoxazole and trimethoprim in treatment of urinary infection. British Medical Journal 2: 673–676

This is a double-blind trial involving 339 patients with urinary tract infections of varying severity in defined groups. The groups consisted of 83 patients with hospital-acquired infection; 96 patients with frequency and dysuria from domiciliary practice; and 149 pregnant women with asymptomatic infection, diagnosed at antenatal screening. Patients were randomly allocated to receive twice daily doses of ampicillin 1 g, cephalexin 1 g, co-trimoxazole 960 mg or trimethoprim 200 mg, for 7 days, regardless of the sensitivity of the infecting organism. Diagnosis of infection and criterion for cure were strictly defined, and a similar range of age and severity of infection was found between treatment groups.

Treatment successes, judged by urine culture at one week and at four to six weeks post treatment, were found to be 83% for co-trimoxazole and trimethoprim, 73% for ampicillin and 69% for cephalexin across the range of infections. In domiciliary infections, trimethoprim was found to be at least as effective as the other treatments with less than half the incidence of side-effects. In hospital-acquired infections, co-trimoxazole seemed superior to trimethoprim, although the difference was not statistically significant.

General review articles

Brogden R N, Carmine A A, Heel R C, Speight T M, Avery G S 1982 Trimethoprim: a review of its antibacterial activity, pharmacokinetics and therapeutic use in urinary tract infections. Drugs 23: 405–430

Finland M, Kass E H, Platt R (ed) 1982 Trimethoprim-sulfamethoxazole revisited. Review of Infectious Diseases 4: 196–618

Hitchings G H (ed) 1983 Inhibition of folate metabolism in chemotherapy. The origins and uses of co-trimoxazole. Springer-Verlag, Berlin

References

1. Ferone R, Burchall J J, Hitchings G H 1969 *Plasmodium berghei* dihydrofolate reductase — isolation, properties and inhibition by antifolates. Molecular Pharmacology 5: 49–59
2. Genther C S, Schoeny R S, Loper J C, Smith C C 1977 Mutagenic studies of folic acid antagonists. Antimicrobial Agents and Chemotherapy 12: 84–92
3. Fraser P 1968 Effects of trimethoprim, sulphamethoxazole and 1:2 and 1:4 mixtures of trimethoprim and sulphamethoxazole in pregnant animals. Wellcome Foundation Rep, Wellcome Foundation, Beckenham, UK, p 6155
4. Udall V 1969 Toxicology of sulphonamide–trimethoprim combinations. Postgraduate Medical Journal 45 (suppl): 42–45
5. Maskell R 1983 Trimethoprim resistance in Gram-negative urinary pathogens. British Medical Journal 286: 1182–1183
6. Brumfitt W, Hamilton-Miller J M T, Gooding A 1980 Resistance to trimethoprim. Lancet 1: 1409–1410
7. Brumfitt W, Hamilton-Miller J M T, Wood A 1983 Evidence for a slowing in trimethoprim resistance during 1981 — a comparison with earlier years. Journal of Antimicrobial Chemotherapy 2: 503–509
8. Pedler S J, Bint A J 1983 Trimethoprim resistance in Gram-negative urinary pathogens. British Medical Journal 286: 1514
9. Schwartz D E, Ziegler W H 1969 Assay and pharmacokinetics of trimethoprim in man and animals. Postgraduate Medical Journal 45: 32–37
10. Land D, Dean K, Bye A 1978 The gas–liquid chromatographic analysis of trimethoprim in plasma and urine. Journal of Chromatography 146: 143–147
11. Helboe P, Thomsen M 1977 High performance liquid chromatographic determination of trimethoprim and sulphonamide combinations in pharmaceuticals. Archives of Pharmacy and Chemical Science 5: 25–32

T

12. Nolte H, Büttner H 1973 Pharmacokinetics of trimethoprim and its combination with sulphamethoxazole in man after single and chronic oral administration. Chemotherapy 18: 274–284
13. Bach M C, Gold D, Finland M 1973 Absorption and urinary excretion of trimethoprim, sulfamethoxazole and trimethoprim–sulfamethoxazole: results with single doses in normal young adults and preliminary observations during therapy with trimethoprim–sulfamethoxazole. Journal of Infectious Diseases 128 (suppl): 584–599
14. Sigel C W, Grace M E, Nichol C A 1973 Metabolism of trimethoprim in man and measurement of a new metabolite: a new fluorescence assay. Journal of Infectious Diseases 128 (suppl): 580–583
15. Sattar M A, Cawley M I D, Holt J E, Sankey M G, Kaye C M 1983 The penetration of trimethoprim and sulphamethoxazole into synovial fluid. Journal of Antimicrobial Chemotherapy 12: 229–233
16. Dudley M N, Levitz R E, Quintiliani R, Hickingbotham J H, Nightingale C H 1984 Pharmacokinetics of trimethoprim and sulfamethoxazole in serum and cerebrospinal fluid of adult patients with normal meninges. 26: 811–814
17. Miller R D, Salter A J 1973 The passage of trimethoprim–sulphamethoxazole into breast milk and its significance. Proceedings of the 8th Congress of Chemotherapy Athens, vol 1, pp 687–691
18. Reid D W J, Caille G, Kaufmann N R 1975 Maternal and trans-placental kinetics of trimethoprim and sulfamethoxazole, separately, and in combination. Canadian Medical Association Journal 112: 67–72
19. Rieder J, Schwartz D E, Fernex M et al 1974 Pharmacokinetics of the antibacterial combination sulfamethoxazole plus trimethoprim in patients with normal or impaired kidney function. In: Schonfeld et al (eds) Antibiotics and Chemotherapy. Karger, Basel, 18, pp 148–198
20. Kasanen A, Anttila M, Elfving R et al 1978 Trimethoprim: pharmacology, antimicrobial activity and clinical use in urinary tract infections. Annals of Clinical Research 10 (suppl 22): 5–35
21. Lacey R W, Lord V L, Gunasekera H K W, Leiberman P J, Luxton D E A 1980 Comparison of trimethoprim alone with trimethoprim sulphamethoxazole in the treatment of respiratory and urinary infections with particular reference to selection of trimethoprim resistance. Lancet 1: 1270–1273
22. Brumfitt W, Pursell R 1972 Double-blind trial to compare ampicillin, cephalexin, co-trimoxazole and trimethoprim in the treatment of urinary tract infection. British Medical Journal 1: 673–676
23. Spencer R C, Fairclough D J, Cooper J 1981 Double-blind clinical trial of trimethoprim vs. amoxycillin in acute symptomatic urinary infection. Abstract of paper presented at the 12 International Congress of Chemotherapy, Florence
24. Harboard R B, Gruneberg R N 1981 Treatment of urinary tract infection with a single dose of amoxycillin, co-trimoxazole or trimethoprim. British Medical Journal 283: 1301–1302
25. Haataja M, Hanninen P, Platin L-H, Saarimaa H, Hajba A, Tala E 1985 Trimethoprim or co-trimoxazole in pneumonia. Current Therapeutic Research 37: 191–196
26. Iravani A, Richard G A, Baer H 1981 Treatment of uncomplicated urinary tract infections with trimethoprim vs. sulfisoxazole with special reference to antibody-coated bacteria and faecal flora. Antimicrobial Agents and Chemotherapy 19: 842
27. Koutts J, Van der Weyden M B, Cooper M 1973 Effect of trimethoprim on folate metabolism in human bone marrow. Australian and New Zealand Journal of Medicine 3: 245–250
28. England J M, Coles M 1972 Effect of co-trimoxazole on phenylalanine metabolism in man. Lancet 2: 1341–1343
29. Bye A 1976 Drug interference with creatinine assay. Clinical Chemistry 22: 283–284
30. Ansdell V E, Wright S G, Hutchinson D B A 1976 Megaloblastic anaemia associated with combined pyrimethamine and co-trimoxazole administration. Lancet 2: 1275
31. Hansen J M, Kampmann J P, Siersbaek-Nielsen K et al 1979 The effect of different sulphonamides on phenytoin metabolism in man. Acta Medica Scandinavica 624 (suppl): 106–110
32. Nyberg G, Gabel H, Althoff P, Bjork S, Herlitz H, Brynger H 1984 Adverse effect of trimethoprim on kidney function in renal transplant patients. Lancet 1: 394–395
33. Rieder J, Schwartz D E 1975 Comparison of the pharmacokinetics of the combination of trimethoprim and sulphamethoxazole in liver patients, and normal subjects. Drug Research 25: 656–666

Trimipramine (maleate)

Trimipramine is a tricyclic antidepressant in use since 1960.

Chemistry

Trimipramine maleate (Surmontil)
$C_{20}H_{26}N_2.C_4H_4O_4$
3-(10,11-Dihydro-5H-dibenz[b,f]azepin-5-yl)-2-methylpropyl-N,N-dimethylammonium hydrogen maleate

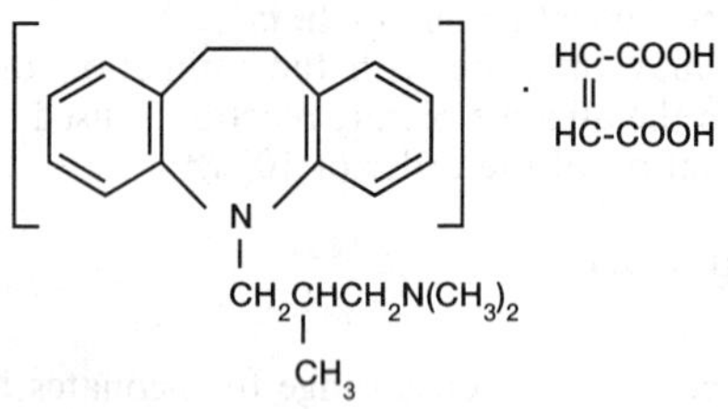

Molecular weight	410.5 (294.4)
pKa (amino group)	7.72
Solubility (maleate)	
in alcohol	1 in 1–1 in 10
in water	1 in 100–1 in 1000
Octanol/water partition coefficient	1.69

Trimipramine maleate is a white, odourless or almost odourless, crystalline powder with a bitter numbing taste. It is prepared by chemical synthesis and is used as the racemate.

Pharmacology

Trimipramine antagonizes the effect of reserpine-induced depression in animals. It also has potent antihistaminic activity and some anticholinergic activity and is a relatively weak noradrenaline and 5-HT reuptake blocker. It is a potent inhibitor of dopamine uptake and increases dopamine turnover. It desensitizes postsynaptic 5-HT receptors but has no effect on noradrenaline-stimulated adenylate cyclase activity or on β-adrenoceptors. It enhances cortical neuronal sensitivity to substance P after chronic administration.

Toxicology

Trimipramine has no mutagenic potential and there is no evidence from animal studies of a carcinogenic effect. There is some evidence of teratogenicity in the rabbit at high dosages but no effect on fertility.

Clinical pharmacology

Trimipramine has very similar properties to imipramine whose chemical structure is so similar. Trimipramine is primarily an antidepressant through its action on brain monoamines. The antidepressant effect takes 1–14 days to become manifest. It has relatively more sedative effects than imipramine and is thus useful for the treatment of patients whose depression is accompanied by sleep disorder. Trimipramine decreases the time spent in REM sleep and increases the amount of time spent in Stage 4 sleep.

Trimipramine has anticholinergic effects and dry mouth, tachycardia, constipation and difficulty with micturition may occur, especially in the early stages of treatment. In the cardiovascular system hypotension and cardiac arrhythmias may occur and care should be taken with the drug in elderly patients or patients with pre-existing heart disease. Trimipramine suppresses gastric secretion in addition to its constipating effect, perhaps due to its anticholinergic properties.

Pharmacokinetics

The preferred analytical method is gas–liquid chromatography with nitrogen–phosphorus detection[1], which has a sensitivity of 0.5 µg.l^{-1}.

Absorption following oral administration is about 80% with extensive first-pass hepatic clearance and bioavailability of 40%, but is variable. The mean plasma elimination half life is in the range 7 to 9 hours with a terminal value of 23 hours. The volume of distribution is 31 l.kg^{-1}. Trimipramine is highly bound (95%) to protein in plasma and free concentration of trimipramine is significantly raised in diseases which result in lower concentrations of plasma protein. Concentration of trimipramine in the CSF is unknown but entry into brain and other tissues is thought to be high.

Oral absorption	80%
Presystemic metabolism	extensive
Plasma half life	7–9 h
Volume of distribution	31 l.kg^{-1}
Plasma protein binding	95%

Concentration–effect relationship

There is no clear 'therapeutic window' of trimipramine plasma levels, though the therapeutic range[2] is probably 20 to 100 µg.l^{-1}.

Metabolism

Trimipramine is extensively metabolized in the liver. Two primary pathways of metabolism have been described: demethylation (to µ-desmethyltrimipramine) and hydroxylation (to 2-hydroxytrimipramine).

Desmethyltrimipramine is further hydroxylated, and 2-hydroxytrimipramine demethylated, to form 2-hydroxydesmethyltrimi pramine. Trimipramine is largely metabolized by demethylation prior to conjugation, yielding a glucuronide (see Fig. 1). It is unknown whether the major metabolite, desmethyltrimipramine, is pharmacologically active.

Fig. 1 Metabolism of trimipramine

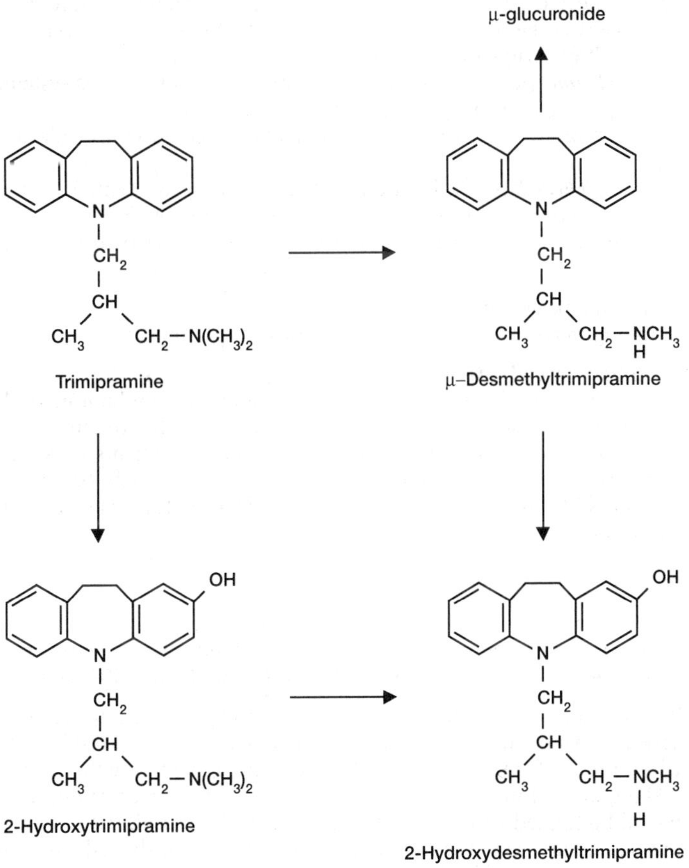

Pharmaceutics

Trimipramine is available only in oral forms:

1. Surmontil tablets (Rhone Poulenc, UK): contain 10 mg and 25 mg trimipramine (as maleate). The face is indented with the name and strength; the reverse is plain.
2. Surmontil capsules (Rhone Poulenc, UK): white opaque body and green cap, containing the equivalent of 50 mg trimipramine (as maleate). The capsules are printed 'M&B SU50'.
3. Surmontil (Wyeth, USA): capsules in three strengths. The 25 mg capsules are blue/yellow, coded '4132'; the 50 mg capsules are blue/orange, coded '4133'; the 100 mg capsules are blue/white, coded '4158'.

All preparations should be protected from light and stored in a dry place below 25°C. Preparations have a maximum shelf-life of 5 years.

Therapeutic use

Indications

1. Depressive illness particularly where a sedative effect is desirable
2. Preoperative night sedation
3. Reversal of weight loss secondary to functional digestive disorders
4. Peptic ulceration.

Contraindications

1. Recent myocardial infarction, cardiac arrhythmias, particularly heart block
2. Mania
3. Severe liver disease
4. Narrow-angle glaucoma.

Mode of use

Trimipramine is in routine clinical use only as an antidepressant. It is usually given in an initial dose of 50–75 mg daily and this is administered best as a single dose in the later evening. Dosages shown to be effective[2] have ranged between 75 and 400 mg and dosage should in general be increased until a therapeutic effect is seen or the maximum tolerated dose reached.[3] Since trimipramine has relatively weak anticholinergic effects, withdrawal symptoms following abrupt cessation of trimipramine are unlikely.

Indications

1. Depression

Trimipramine is used as a single agent in the treatment of mild and moderate depression. In common with other tricyclic antidepressants trimipramine is most likely to be effective in the presence of vegetative symptoms such as early morning waking, diurnal mood variation and weight loss but less likely to be effective in depression associated with delusions or hallucinations. The antidepressant effect is sometimes manifest within two to three weeks but may not occur until the maximum tolerated dose has been administered for four to six weeks. Relief of sleep disturbance and agitation precedes complete clinical response. Trimipramine has been used in combination with monoamine oxidase inhibitors in the treatment of resistant depression, and the trimipramine–monoamine oxidase inhibitor combination is safer than that of most tricyclic antidepressants with monoamine oxidase inhibitors.[4] Trimipramine is particularly useful in depression associated with marked sleep disturbance or agitation and may obviate the need for concurrent hypnotic or major tranquillizer use.[2]

Trimipramine is also useful in the continuation and maintenance therapy of depression. Continuing treatment for six to twelve months following remission has clearly been shown to reduce risk of relapse.[2] There is no clear evidence suggesting benefit from further maintenance treatment. The continuation dosage should where possible be the same as that which produced initial remission, but can be decreased cautiously if sedation proves excessive.

2. Preoperative sedation

Trimipramine has been used to relieve the anxiety associated with preoperative insomnia though the manufacturers are hesitant in endorsing this use in view of the class effect of tricyclic antidepressants on cardiac electrophysiology. In a study in which trimipramine was administered for three consecutive nights preoperatively, anxiety and tension were relieved and sleep restored in 94% of cases and no complications with surgery or anaesthesia were noted.[5]

3. Control of weight loss
Trimipramine, like amitriptyline, has some propensity to induce weight gain in both depressed patients and healthy volunteers. This has been used to advantage in treating emaciated patients with functional digestive disorders.[6]

4. Peptic ulceration
Trimipramine has some effect in promoting the healing of gastric and duodenal ulcers. It depresses the volume of pentagastrin-stimulated gastric secretion and reduces acid and pepsin output, with significant reduction of maximal acid output after three weeks of therapy in patients with endoscopically proven duodenal ulceration.[7]

Contraindications

1. Recent myocardial infarction, heart block and other cardiac arrhythmias
Trimipramine has the quinidine-like effect of decreasing contractility and tends to flatten T waves.

2. Mania
In common with other tricyclic antidepressants, trimipramine may be associated with a switch from depression to mania, particularly in patients with dipolar illnesses. The emergence of mania can be treated by discontinuing the trimipramine and adding a major tranquillizer.

3. Severe liver disease
Liver enzyme abnormalities during treatment with trimipramine are rare and usually transitory, but in common with other tricyclics, trimipramine should be used with caution in patients with severe hepatic disease.

4. Narrow-angle glaucoma
Because of its anticholinergic effects, trimipramine may increase intraocular pressure in patients with narrow-angle glaucoma.

Adverse reactions

Potentially life-threatening effects
Agranulocytosis, thrombocytopenia and jaundice occur rarely.[2]

Acute overdosage
Like other tricyclic antidepressants, trimipramine has been associated with a small number of fatalities, usually associated with suicidal overdose. Overdose is not usually fatal; reviews totalling 82 cases revealed no fatalities,[8,9] but five individual case reports of fatality have been published. Clinical features of overdose are drowsiness, sinus tachycardia, dry mouth, dilated pupils and increased reflexes. In severe cases cardiac and respiratory depressant actions predominate. Bizarre electrocardiographic changes may be seen, with increase in conduction time and in some cases heart block. Hypotension and reduced cardiac output may be seen and hypoxia due to respiratory depression may occur, as may coma and convulsions.

Severe or irreversible adverse effects
Trimipramine may, particularly in elderly patients, produce psychomotor agitation, leading to toxic confusion. Convulsions may occur, especially at high dosage. These effects may be associated either with sudden increases in dose of trimipramine or sudden trimipramine withdrawal.

Symptomatic adverse effects
The major effects are sedation, light-headedness, postural hypotension, and anticholinergic symptoms and signs particularly fine tremor and dry mouth. Other side effects include headache, rash, tingling, nausea, abdominal pain, dyspepsia, constipation, leg cramps, dreams, restlessness, insomnia and difficulty in concentration.

Though trimipramine is not associated with an increase in arrhythmias in normal doses, it may cause benign flattening of T waves in the ECG.

These adverse effects are largely dose-related and occur early in treatment. The risk of their occurrence can be minimized by adding increments gradually from a low starting dose. In most cases adverse effects abate with reduction or withdrawal of trimipramine, although such withdrawal should itself be gradual.

Interference with clinical pathology tests
No interference with such tests is known.

High risk groups

Neonates
Trimipramine is not recommended for use in neonates.

Breast milk. The extent to which trimipramine is excreted in breast milk is unknown although its high protein binding suggests that breast milk concentrations will be lower than those found in plasma. Nevertheless mothers taking this drug should not breast-feed.

Children
Trimipramine is not recommended for use in children.

Pregnant women
Trimipramine is not recommended for use in pregnancy.

The elderly
Trimipramine is not usually associated with significant problems in the elderly, though they are at relatively greater risk of agitation, confusion and postural hypotension. It is therefore advisable to administer lower doses of trimipramine more frequently in this group of patients.

Patients requiring anaesthesia
Anaesthetics given during trimipramine therapy may increase the risk of arrhythmias and hypotension. If surgery is necessary, the anaesthetist should be made aware that a patient is being so treated.

Drug interactions

Potentially hazardous interactions

Antihypertensives. The hypotensive effect of clonidine, reserpine, guanethidine, alpha-methyldopa, debrisoquine, and bethanidine may be impaired by trimipramine.

Sympathomimetics. Trimipramine may potentiate the hypertensive effects of phenylephrine, ephedrine, noradrenaline, adrenaline, phenylpropanolamine and methylphenidate.

Monoamine oxidase inhibitors. Like other tricyclic antidepressants, trimipramine may, when given with monoamine oxidase inhibitors, increase weight gain and the incidence of anticholinergic effects. Hyperthermia, hyperreflexia, convulsions and death have been reported. Trimipramine is, however, a relatively safe and effective tricyclic to give in combination with MAOIs. It is advisable to start both drugs together in relatively low dose.

Anticholinergics. The effects on the pupil, central nervous system, bowel and bladder may be additive.

Barbiturates. Hepatic enzyme induction may decrease plasma levels of trimipramine.

Methylphenedate. Inhibition of hydroxylating or demethylating enzymes may increase plasma levels of trimipramine.

Alcohol. Alcohol may enhance the sedative effect of trimipramine.

Other significant interactions
Smoking may decrease plasma levels of trimipramine.

Potentially useful interactions
Like other tricyclic antidepressants, trimipramine may be used with benefit in combination with phenothiazines in the treatment of delusional depression. The addition of lithium in patients in whom trimipramine alone has failed to produce a response may be beneficial, possibly by a direct effect on serotonin receptors sensitized by trimipramine.

Major outcome trials

1. Pecknold J C, McClure D J, Elie R, Appeltauer L, Wrzesinski L 1979 Trimipramine and amitriptyline: Comparison in anxiety depression. Current Therapeutic Research 26 (5): 497–504

This was a four-week double-blind controlled trial of 30 patients with severe anxiety and depression given 150 mg of amitriptyline or trimipramine for three weeks with the option of increasing the dose to 200 mg in the fourth week. Only 10 subjects treated with trimipramine and 6 treated with amitriptyline completed the trial. A significant antidepressant response was seen in both groups but the reduction in anxiety was significantly greater in the trimipramine-treated group. Significant global improvement was also seen only in the trimipramine-treated group.

2. Rifkin A, Saraf K, Kane J, Ross D, Klein D F 1980 Comparison of trimipramine and imipramine: a controlled study. Journal of Clinical Psychiatry 41 (4): 124–129

This was a double-blind comparison of the effect of trimipramine and imipramine in 30 hospitalized patients with endogenomorphic depression. The dose of each drug was gradually increased to 300 mg daily and the study lasted four weeks. The trimipramine group showed greater global improvement and reduction in insomnia as well as lower frequency of side effects, but the antidepressant response was similar in the two groups.

Other trials

Peptic ulceration

1. Mackay H P, Pickard W R, Mitchell K G, Crean G P 1984 A double-blind study of trimipramine in the treatment of active duodenal ulceration. Scandinavian Journal of Gastroenterology 19: 190–193

This was a study of 36 patients with endoscopically proven duodenal ulcer who entered a randomized double-blind trial of trimipramine versus placebo. Of these, 31 completed the trial, 15 having received trimipramine 50 mg nocte and 16 placebo for four weeks. At the end of the trial 11 out of 15 on trimipramine and 6 out of 16 on placebo showed ulcer healing ($P<0.05$). At eight-week follow up, 11 out of 15 on trimipramine and 7 out of 16 on placebo showed healing; this difference was no longer statistically significant. Antacid use was greater in the placebo group.

Sleep disturbance associated with depression

2. Goulton J, Baker P G, Wilkinson M A 1978 A multi-centre general practice study of 'Surmontil' (trimipramine maleate) in the treatment of endogenous depression with associated sleep disturbances. British Journal of Clinical Practice 32: 323–325

This was an open multi-centred general practice trial involving 89 patients with endogenous depression and sleep disturbance. They were treated with 50 to 100 mg trimipramine 2 hours before going to bed. 90% reported improvement in sleep within 12 days, most of the improvement occurring within the first week and usually preceding any antidepressant response. In some cases improvement in sleep occurred even where subsequent antidepressant response failed to occur.

General review articles

Settle E C, Ayd F J 1980 Trimipramine: 20 years' worldwide clinical experience. Journal of Clinical Psychiatry 41: 266–274

Blackwell B 1981 Adverse effects of antidepressant drugs. Part 1: Monoamine oxidase inhibitors and tricyclics. Drugs 21: 201–219

References

1. Abernethy D R, Greenblatt D J, Shader R I 1984 Trimipramine kinetics and absolute bioavailability: use of gas–liquid chromatography with nitrogen–phosphorus detection. Clinical Pharmacology and Therapeutics 35: 348–353
2. Settle E C, Ayd F J 1980 Trimipramine: twenty years' worldwide clinical experience. Journal of Clinical Psychiatry 41: 266–274
3. Katona C L E, Barnes T R E 1985 Pharmacological strategies in depression. British Journal of Hospital Medicine 34: 168–171
4. Lippmann S, Baldwin H, Manshadi M 1982 Combined trimipramine/phenelzine treatment of depression: case report. Journal of Clinical Psychiatry 43: 430–431
5. Paul A K, Ghosh B B G 1977 Trimipramine in pre-operative night sedation. India Pract 2: 485–488
6. Crismer R, Naomi F, DeFrance P et al 1966 Treatment of emaciation with trimipramine. (RP 7162) Archives Françaises des Maladies de l'Appareil Digestif 56: 355
7. MacKay H P, Pickard W R, Mitchell K G, Crean G P 1984 A double-blind trial of trimipramine in the treatment of active duodenal ulceration. Scandinavian Journal of Gastroenterology 19: 190–193
8. Starkey I R, Lawson A A H 1980 Poisoning with tricyclic and related antidepressants — a ten year review. Quarterly Journal of Medicine 49: 33–49
9. Crome P, Newman B 1979 Fatal tricyclic antidepressant poisoning. Journal of the Royal Society of Medicine 72: 649–653

Triprolidine

Triprolidine is a histamine one receptor antagonist.

Chemistry

Triprolidine hydrochloride monohydrate (Actidil, Actidilon, Actiphyll, Pro-Actidil, Pro-Actidilon)

$C_{19}H_{22}N_2.HCl.H_2O$

(E)-2-[1-(4-Methylphenyl)-3-(1-pyrrolidinyl)-1-propenyl]pyridine hydrochloride monohydrate

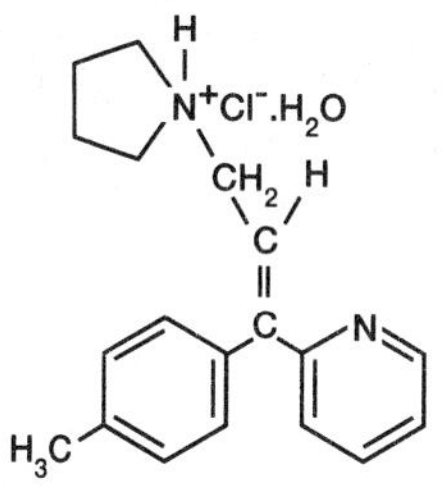

Molecular weight (free base)	332.9 (278.4)
pKa	3.6, 9.3
Solubility	
in alcohol	1 in 1.5
in water	1 in 2
Octanol/water partition coefficient	7900

Triprolidine is a white crystalline powder with a slightly unpleasant odour and bitter taste, prepared by chemical synthesis. It is used in combination in a variety of products: Actifed, Actigesic, Actilex, CoActifed, Emprazil, Linctifed, Trifedron and Tussifed.

Pharmacology

Triprolidine is a competitive histamine H_1-receptor antagonist. In the guinea-pig ileum preparation triprolidine is twice as active as mepyramine and chlorpheniramine. In protecting against histamine-induced bronchospasm in guinea-pigs the drug is five times more active than mepyramine.[1] Being an alkylamine the drug has less anticholinergic activity than the phenothiazines.

Toxicology

No toxicological results in animals have been observed which are of likely clinical relevance. In rats and rabbits there is no evidence of teratogenicity. The mutagenicity and carcinogenicity of triprolidine have not been evaluated.

Clinical pharmacology

Antagonism of H_1-receptors in vivo by triprolidine has been demonstrated by inhibition of the flare and weal response to intradermal histamine injection.[1] The flare component of this response is inhibited more effectively than the weal. The antagonistic activity after doses of 1.25–5 mg is relatively rapid in onset, maximal at 3 h after administration, and this parallels the time course of the CNS side effects of the drug.[3–5] However, there is no significant correlation between the degree of antagonism of peripheral H_1-receptors, measured in terms of the weal and flare response, and the actions on the CNS.[2] There is some evidence that the effects of triprolidine on REM sleep are due to effects other than histamine antagonism.[5] The principal CNS side effects include inability to concentrate, lassitude, dizziness, muscular weakness, incoordination and slight drowsiness to sleep. The sedative effects may decrease in severity after several days. The sedative effects of triprolidine have been the subject of extensive evaluation.[6–11]

Pharmacokinetics

Triprolidine may be measured in plasma by a thin-layer chromatographic method with fluorescence detection, sensitivity 800 mg.l^{-1}, or by specific radioimmunoassay.[12,13]

After a single oral tablet (of 2.5 mg), peak plasma concentrations of 5.5 ± 4.8 µg.l^{-1} are attained after 1.9 ± 0.6 h ($\pm$SD). Absorption is extensive but somewhat irregular. The mean plasma half life is 3.0 ± 1.5 h ($\pm$SD). No information is currently available concerning presystemic elimination for this compound.

Triprolidine is widely distributed throughout the body with an apparent volume of distribution of 8.7 ± 7.8 l.kg^{-1}. Complete tissue uptake and distribution data have not been reported, although unpublished studies show brain:plasma concentration ratios of 2.6 in rats and guinea pigs. Triprolidine is highly (90%) bound to plasma proteins, the major binding sites being on serum albumin and α_1-acid glycoprotein. It is estimated that after a single dose triprolidine is excreted in human breast milk such that an infant will receive 0.06–0.2% of the dose ingested by the mother.[14]
The plasma concentrations of triprolidine may be expected to show great variability in acute illness as one of the major binding proteins for the drug, α_1-acid glycoprotein, is an acute phase protein which may be present at elevated concentrations during illness. In view of the paucity of information regarding the human metabolism of triprolidine, it is not known whether the bioavailability and disposition of the drug are affected in hepatic or renal dysfunction.

Oral absorption	extensive
Presystemic metabolism	—
Plasma half life	
range	1.5–4.5 h
mean	3.0
Volume of distribution	8.7 ± 7.8 l.kg^{-1} ($\pm$SD)
Plasma protein binding	90%

Concentration–effect relationship

There is no evidence of a clear-cut relationship between the plasma concentration of triprolidine and its therapeutic effect.

Metabolism

The metabolic fate of triprolidine in man is not known, nor is there currently any information regarding its principal routes of elimination. One study has shown that in man only 1% of the dose administered is excreted in the urine as unchanged drug.[2] Metabolites formed by oxidative dealkylation and hydroxylation have been identified in guinea-pig liver. These compounds possess little or no antihistaminic activity.

Pharmaceutics

1. Triprolidine is available (Wellcome, UK) as tablets containing 2.5 mg triprolidine hydrochloride BP. The tablets are white, scored and coded 'Wellcome L2A'.
2. Slow-release tablets are also available (Pro-Actidil). Each tablet contains 10 mg triprolidine hydrochloride BP divided between three layers to produce a rapid onset of action followed by a prolonged therapeutic effect. These tablets are white, coded 'Wellcome M4A' and have a blue core and pink middle layer. The colouring dyes used are erythrocin lake dispersed and indigo carmine. These agents may be potential allergens in some patients.
3. The drug is also available as an orange coloured elixir (Actidil). Each 5 ml contains 2 mg triprolidine hydrochloride and has a mandarin orange flavour. This elixir preparation contains methylhydroxybenzoate as a preservative and the azo dye sunset yellow. These may be potential allergens in some patients.

All preparations of triprolidine should be protected from light. It is recommended that Actidil tablets and elixir be stored below 25°C. Pro-Actidil preparations should be stored below 15°C in a dry place.

Under these conditions Actidil tablets and elixir have a shelf-life of 4 years.

Therapeutic use

Indications

1. Symptomatic relief of allergic rhinitis
2. Allergic conjunctivitis
3. Urticaria
4. Angioedema (angioneurotic oedema).

Contraindications

1. Known hypersensitivity to triprolidine preparations
2. Use with alcohol intake or central sedation
3. Lack of information regarding human metabolism necessitates care when used in patients with hepatic or renal dysfunction. Use with care in patients with elevated intraocular pressure and patients with prostatic hypertrophy.

Mode of use

All clinical uses depend upon production of H_1-receptor antagonism. The recommended dose of Actidil in adults is 5–15 mg daily, given as divided doses. A daily dose of 30 mg is the highest dose known to have been used in man. In children aged between 3 months and 1 year, 1 mg should be administered three times daily. For the age range 1–6 years, 2 mg may be administered three times per day. In children aged 7–12 this can be increased to 3 mg three times daily. There are no reports of problems with the drug when used in the symptomatic relief of allergic rhinitis or urticaria, or if the drug is stopped suddenly.

As with most H_1-receptor antogonists the drug is most effective when used to relieve mild symptoms of upper respiratory tract allergies, e.g. sneezing, rhinorrhoea and pruritus of the nose, eyes and throat. Patients with seasonal allergic rhinitis are more responsive to therapy than those with vasomotor rhinitis.

For use in dermatological conditions the drug is more useful in alleviating acute as opposed to chronic urticarias.

Patients should be warned that triprolidine will enhance the sedative effects of other CNS depressants such as alcohol, hypnotics, sedatives and tranquillizers. For this reason, persons receiving medication should abstain from taking alcohol or sedatives whilst taking triprolidine. In view of the dulling of mental alertness caused by triprolidine alone, patients receiving medication should also be warned not to take charge of vehicles or machinery where loss of attention may lead to accidents.

Indications

1. Allergic rhinitis
Triprolidine is effective in relieving symptoms of seasonal allergic rhinitis[16] in a dose of 2.5 mg three times daily, but drowsiness is an unwanted side effect. One study[17] has evaluated a regimen of 1.25 mg three times daily in an attempt to avoid the unwanted effect. It was found that although this dose may be effective in some patients it cannot generally be recommended for the management of allergic rhinitis,[17] particularly since tolerance is known to develop to the central effects of triprolidine after treatment over several days.[4] Triprolidine acts initially to stop the sneezing in rhinitis, followed by diminution of the aqueous secretion and swelling of the mucous membrane of the nose.[18] Pro-Actidil has also been used to effect in allergic rhinitis, particularly as supportive therapy to allergen desensitization.[19]

2. Allergic conjunctivitis
Slow-release triprolidine (10 mg daily) has been used successfully for relief in allergic conjunctivitis,[20] as has a conventional release preparation.[21]

3. Urticaria
Slow-release triprolidine (10 mg daily) has been used successfully in urticaria with very good response after 2–3 days' treatment. Duration of treatment was directly related to the severity of the disease.[20,22]

Triprolidine

4. Angioedema

In an open study, Pro-Actidil (10 mg daily) was successful in the treatment of angioedema.[20] Doses of 5–10 mg per day of triprolidine (Actidil) have also been successfully employed.[21]

Symptomatic relief of the common cold

There have been suggestions that combined antihistamine and decongestant therapy provides some symptomatic relief of the common cold, although a well conducted Medical Research Council survey concluded that the benefit of this is not established.[23] One study has been conducted with triprolidine given alone, and in combination with pseudoephedrine.[24] There was no clear evidence of additional therapeutic benefit from the drug combination.

Adverse reactions

Potentially life-threatening effects

Life-threatening effects have not been reported for triprolidine hydrochloride.

Acute overdosage

There are two recorded cases of acute Actidil poisoning. Symptoms of acute toxicity include drowsiness, dizziness, incoordination, weakness, convulsions and respiratory depression. Necessary measures should be taken to maintain and support respiration. Gastric lavage should be performed if indicated and convulsions controlled with diazepam. A 5-year-old boy who ingested 60 ml of triprolidine pseudoephedrine linctus experienced hallucinations 5–18 hours after ingestion. Full recovery was made 24 hours after the incident.[25] There are *theoretical* grounds for believing that the elimination of triprolidine and its metabolites might be accelerated by dialysis.

Severe or irreversible adverse effects

None is known. However, very limited data from the Boston Collaborative Drug Surveillance Program have suggested that there may be an association between maternal antihistamine use in the first trimester of pregnancy and pyloric stenosis in neonates.[26,27]

Symptomatic adverse effects

In common with many other antihistamines, triprolidine may cause drowsiness and, in combination with alcohol, somnolence. Being a member of the alkylamine group, triprolidine has fewer anticholinergic and sedative properties than members of the phenothiazine group.

Triprolidine may also cause other side effects documented for other H_1-antihistamines. These include gastrointestinal disturbances (nausea, vomiting, diarrhoea, constipation, epigastric pain), headache, blurred vision and tinnitus. Although triprolidine exhibits fewer anticholinergic side effects than some other classes of antihistamine it may cause dryness of mouth and throat and should be used with care in conditions likely to be adversely affected by atropine (e.g. glaucoma, urinary retention).

There is a report of skin eruptions resembling poikiloderma of Civatte in two women after taking triprolidine. The eruptions reappeared on challenge and were exacerbated by ultraviolet radiation. The occurrence of this adverse effect is rare.

Interference with clinical pathology tests

No technical interferences of this kind are known.

High risk groups

Neonates

The drug should not be used in children under the age of 6 months.

Breast milk. There is evidence that following a single 2.5 mg dose 0.06–0.2% may be excreted in breast milk. This excretion may be higher in steady-state regimens. There are no published reports of adverse reactions in nursing infants.

Children

Children under 12 years should be prescribed triprolidine as an elixir preparation. The sustained-release preparation (e.g. Pro-Actidil) is not recommended for children under 12 years.

Pregnant women

No special precautions are required for triprolidine, but there is evidence that following a single 2.5 mg dose, 0.06–0.2% may be excreted in breast milk. This excretion may be higher in steady-state regimens. There are no published reports of adverse reactions in nursing infants.

The Boston Collaborative Drug Surveillance Program has provided very limited indication of a possible link between the use of antihistamines in the first trimester of pregnancy and neonatal pyloric stenosis. There is currently insufficient data to establish a firm link between these events, however.[27]

The elderly

No special precautions are required except in cases of renal or hepatic insufficiency in which the drug should be used initially at less than the recommended dose.

Concurrent disease

In severe hepatic or renal dysfunction triprolidine should be given initially at less than the usual recommended dose and the response to it used as a guide to the patient's requirement for further administration.

Drug interactions

Other than potentiation of the effects of alcohol, there are no known potentially hazardous or therapeutically useful interactions of triprolidine.

Major outcome trials

1. Wolfromm R, Liacopoulos P 1957 Etude clinique d'un nouvel anti-histaminique de synthese. La semaine des Hopitaux de Paris 33: 559–561

This is a study of the effect of triprolidine in patients with allergic disorders referred to an outpatient department. Triprolidine was practically without effect in allergic asthma (34 cases) or migraine (4 cases) when given as four 2.5 mg doses. In 36 cases of vasomotor rhinitis 27 patients received prompt relief for the duration of treatment, whereas 9 remained unchanged. Studies in dermatological conditions also showed the drug to be useful. Of 7 patients with urticaria only 2 cases were unimproved by the drug, and in 4 cases of angioneurotic oedema only 1 patient did not respond to this treatment. In all patient groups the secondary effects of somnolence, palpitations and nausea were mild and passed off quickly with reduction of dosage.

2. Bock S, Gartmann H 1967 Erfahrungen mit Pro-Actidil bei dermatosen mit pruritus. Therapeutische Umschau 24: 243–245

This is a study in 162 patients of the slow release preparation Pro-Actidil. The patients studied were suffering from pruritic dermatosis and received one tablet (10 mg) each evening. In 31% of the patients the drug was shown to eliminate the pruritus and diminish the urticae after administration of the first dose. In 29.5% the therapeutic effect was manifest after the second dose, whereas a further 21% showed improvement of symptoms after the third dose. In the remaining 18.5% there was little or no improvement with this treatment over a 7–14 day period. Minor side effects reported included tiredness (12.3%) and gastric disorders (2.5%).

Other trials

1. Yamamoto T, 1968 Clinical effects of Pro-Entra — a sustained release antihistamine agent. Rinsho no Ayumi 2: 30–31 (Japanese)

This is a study of the sustained-release preparations of triprolidine, Pro-Actidil, in 18 patients with either acute or chronic urticaria. Of these patients 22% showed no improvement whereas 11%, 56% and 11% showed beneficial effects rated as excellent, good and fair respectively.

2. Suzuiki A, Tuguchi K 1968 Clinical experiments of Pro-Entra in otolaryngology. Rinsho no Ayumi 2: 38-39 (Japanese)

This is a study employing a single daily dose of Pro-Actidil in allergic and acute eczematous otitis in 18 patients. An excellent response was seen in 44% of patients and a good response in the remaining 56% of the group.

References

1. Green A F 1953 The antagonism of histamine and the anaphylactic response by phenylpyridylallylamines. British Journal of Pharmacology 8: 171–176

2. Simmons K J, Singh M, Gillespie C A, Simons F E R 1986 An investigation of the H_1-receptor antagonist triprolidine: pharmacokinetics and antihistaminic effects. Journal of Allergy and Clinical Immunology 77: 326–330
3. Peck A W, Fowle A S E, Bye C 1975 A comparison of triprolidine and clemastine on histamine antagonism and performance tests in man. European Journal of Clinical Pharmacology 8: 455–463
4. Bye C E, Claridge R, Peck A W, Plowman F 1977 Evidence for tolerance to the central nervous effects of the histamine antagonist, triprolidine, in man. European Journal of Clinical Pharmacology 12: 181–186
5. Nicholson A N, Stone B M 1983 The H_1-antagonist mequitazine: studies on performance and visual function. European Journal of Clinical Pharmacology 25: 563–566
6. Cohen A F, Hamilton M, Strutt A, Philipson R, Peck A W 1984 A new H_1-receptor antagonist BW 825C: effects on tracking, reaction time and subjective ratings. British Journal of Clinical Pharmacology 17: 647P
7. Cohen A F, Hamilton M, Strutt A, Philipson R, Peck A W 1984 A new H_1-receptor antagonist BW 825C: effects on skin histamine rseponse, vigilance and autonomic variables. British Journal of Clinical Pharmacology 17: 647–648P
8. Nicholson A W, Stone B M 1984 The H_2 antagonists cimetidine and ranitidine: studies on performance. European Journal of Clinical Pharmacology 26: 579–582
9. Nicholson A W, Stone B M 1986 Antihistamines: impaired performance and the tendency to sleep. European Journal of Clinical Pharmacology 30: 27–32
10. Nicholson A W, Pascoe P A, Stone B M 1985 Histaminergic systems and sleep. Studies in man with H_1 and H_2 antagonists. Neuropharmacology 24: 245–250
11. Cohen A F, Hamilton M, Philipson R, Peck A W 1985 The acute effects of acrivastine (BW 825C), a new antihistamine, compared with triprolidine on measures of central nervous system performance and subjective effects. Clinical Pharmacology and Therapeutics 38: 381–386
12. DeAngelis R L, Kearney M F, Welch R M 1977 Determination of triprolidine in human plasma by quantitative TLC. Journal of Pharmaceutical Sciences 66: 841–843
13. Findlay J W A, Butz R F, Coker G G, DeAngelis R L, Welch R M 1984 Triprolidine radioimmunoassay: disposition in animals and humans. Journal of Pharmaceutical Sciences 73: 1339–1344
14. Findlay J W A, Butz R F, Sailstad J M, Warren J T, Welch R M 1984 Pseudoephedrine and triprolidine in plasma and breast milk of nursing mothers. British Journal of Clinical Pharmacology 18: 901–906
15. Williams B O, Liao S H T, Lai A A etal 1984 Bioavailability of pseudoephedrine and triprolidine from combination and single-ingredient products. Clinical Pharmacology 3: 638–643
16. Empey D W, Bye C, Hodder M, Hughes D T D 1975 A double-blind cross-over trial of pseudoephedrine and triprolidine, alone and in combination, for the treatment of allergic rhinitis. Annals of Allergy 34: 41–46
17. Britton M G, Empey D W, John G C, Hodder M, Hughes D T D 1979 Two doses of triprolidine for treatment of allergic rhinitis. Annals of Allergy 42: 330–332
18. Kaiser R, 1966. Uber die therapie nasaler allergien mit dem depot-antihistaminikum Pro-Actidil. Therapeutische Umschau 23: 323–326
19. Hussarek M 1963 Die moderne therapie der nasalen allergie. Wiener Medizinische Wochenschrift 113: 552–554
20. Young G C 1964 A sustained release antihistamine. The Practitioner 193: 664–667
21. Wolfromm R, Liacopoulos P 1957 Etude clinique d'un nouvel anti-histaminique de synthese. La semaine des Hopitaux de Paris 33: 559–561
22. Hirayama A, Tashiro R 1968 Effect of Pro-Entra on pruritic dermatoses. Rinsho no Ayumi 2: 37–41 (Japanese)
23. Medical Research Council Special Committee 1950. Clinical trials of antihistaminic drugs in the prevention and treatment of the common cold. British Medical Journal 2: 425–429
24. Bye C E, Cooper J, Empey D W et al 1980 Effects of pseudoephedrine and triprolidine, alone and in combination on symptoms of the common cold. British Medical Journal 281: 189–190
25. Ackland F M 1984 Hallucinations in a child after drinking triprolidine/pseudoephedrine linctus. Lancet 1: 1180
26. Eskenazi B, Bracken M B 1985 Pyloric stenosis and antihistamines (letter). American Journal of Epidemiology 122: 196–197
27. Aselton P, Jick H 1985 Re: pyloris stenosis and maternal antihistamine exposure at Group Health Cooperative (letter). American Journal of Epidemiology 122: 197
28. Bain J, Drennan P C, Miller M G 1984 Visual hallucinations in children receiving decongestants. British Medical Journal 288: 1688
29. Sankey R J, Nunn A J, Sills J A 1984 Visual hallucinations in children receiving decongestants. British Medical Journal 288: 1369
30. Sills J A, Nunn A J, Sankey R J 1984 Visual hallucinations in children receiving decongestants. British Medical Journal 288: 1912–1913

Tryptophan

Tryptophan is one of the essential amino acids. It is a nutrient which has been tried in the treatment of a variety of neuropsychiatric disorders.

Chemistry

Tryptophan (Optimax, Pacitron, Trofan, Tryptacin)
$C_{11}H_{12}N_2O_2$
L-2-Amino-3(indolyl)propionic acid

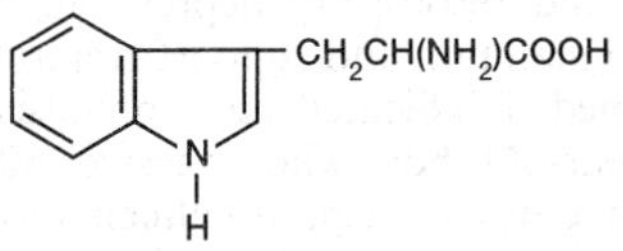

Molecular weight	204.2
pKa	2.4, 9.4
Solubility	
in alcohol	>1 in 10 000
in water	1 in 100
Octanol/water partition coefficient	low

Tryptophan can be isolated from casein which contains about 1.2% of the substance; or synthesized through a process starting with β-indolylaldehyde and hippuric acid. It is a very pale yellow solid. It is an ingredient of Optimax.

Pharmacology

Tryptophan is a natural amino acid that is the precursor of a number of important, biologically active molecules. It is oxidized by the tryptophan pyrrolase pathway to kynurenine and ultimately to NAD. It is decarboxylated to tryptamine and hydroxylated to 5-hydroxytryptophan and on to 5-HIAA. A combination of decarboxylation and hydroxylation leads to formation 5-hydroxytryptamine. Tryptophan is used as a drug because it acts as a 5-HT agonist. Tryptophan increases the synthesis of 5-HT because the rate-limiting enzyme of 5-HT synthesis, tryptophan hydroxylase, is not fully saturated with tryptophan. Since studies on the accumulation of 5-HT (in rat brain), after inhibition of aromatic amino acid decarboxylase, suggest that tryptophan hydroxylase is normally only about half saturated, tryptophan loading can double the rate of 5-HT synthesis.[1]

There are many other tryptophan metabolites besides 5-HT which may affect changes in brain function. Among them the most extensively studied is tryptamine, a substance which can modify the actions of 5-HT on various behaviours.[2]

It has also been noted that tryptophan administration enhances brain protein synthesis.[3]

Toxicology

Tryptophan is the most toxic of the common amino acids with an LD_{50} for adult male rats of 8 mmol.kg^{-1} body weight for the l-isomer, and 21 mmol.kg^{-1} for the d-isomer. The former dose represents more than 1500 mg of l-tryptophan per kg body weight, which, for an adult human, would be in the order of 80 000–120 000 mg. Given in such toxic doses to rabbits, tryptophan causes histopathological changes in the kidney tubules. The dog is even more sensitive to tryptophan than the rabbit. In similarly high doses, tryptophan provokes severe hyperglycaemia; and l-tryptophan causes marked glycosuria and loss of glycogen from skeletal muscle and liver.

Tryptophan

The dosages involved in producing toxic effects are far above the largest recommended doses for clinical use. The amino acid and its metabolites have not displayed intrinsic carcinogenic action. However, certain metabolites of tryptophan act, under certain experimental conditions, as procarcinogens in the production of tumours of the urinary bladder in mice, and recently dl-tryptophan has been shown to act similarly. With respect to cancer, probably the most important aspect is the carcinogenic potential of some of the products formed from tryptophan during the heat preparation of foods.

It is well established that tryptophan has a hyperglycaemic action. On the other hand, it is not known whether chronic use of large amounts could cause diabetes mellitus.

Tryptophan metabolites may cause scleroderma-like lesions in some patients. This might be explained by an altered flux of tryptophan along the kynurenine pathway and an increase in the 5-hydroxylation pathway.[4]

Clinical pharmacology

Tryptophan is effective, at least in the short term, as an antidepressant. This effect may also be accompanied by drowsiness.

Clinical pharmacological studies suggest that tryptophan pyrrolase may have a determining effect on tryptophan availability after tryptophan injection. Since large tryptophan loads induce the synthesis of increased amounts of tryptophan pyrrolase more than small loads, they do not lead to proportionately higher tryptophan levels. Accordingly, 50 mg.kg^{-1} of tryptophan in neurological patients caused a nine-fold increase in plasma tryptophan whereas 100 mg.kg^{-1} increased the value only 12-fold. Increasing doses also shorten the plasma half life of tryptophan in normal subjects and lead to only slightly higher peak values.[5] In normal subjects the administration of tryptophan in a dose of 90 mg.kg^{-1} resulted in drowsiness and euphoria,[6] whereas the considerably higher dose of 10 000 mg resulted in euphoria and light-headedness.[7] Further, it should be noted that after a single dose of 6000 mg of tryptophan, the plasma level had almost returned to normal after 12 h.[8]

Similar to higher doses, chronic treatment may lead to a progressive induction of tryptophan pyrrolase. In normal subjects who received daily doses of tryptophan for 7 days, the rise of plasma tryptophan after the last dose was less than that seen after an acute dose. Similar findings were reported in schizophrenic patients.

Pharmacokinetics

The preferred analytical methods for the detection of the substance in biological fluids are GLC with flame ionization detection and HPLC with spectroscopic assay. Sensitivity of both is 2–10 pmol.l^{-1}. Tryptophan is actively absorbed from the gut. The circulating tryptophan in the blood is distributed between two compartments; about 10–20% is free amino acid and the remainder is bound to serum albumin with some evidence of saturation at high concentrations of the drug.

Tryptophan is transported into the brain by an uptake system that it shares with other neutral amino acids. Brain tryptophan levels are regulated by plasma tryptophan levels, the nutritional state and the plasma concentrations of the other neutral amino acids, such as tyrosine, phenylalanine, leucine, isoleucine and valine.

The protein in almost all foods contains relatively small amounts of tryptophan in comparison to other amino acids. Since the same system that carries tryptophan from plasma to brain also transports the other neutral amino acids, a high protein meal retards the uptake of tryptophan into the brain by disproportionately increasing the plasma concentration of other amino acids that compete with tryptophan. Paradoxically, the single meal that most effectively elevates tryptophan levels in the brain is the one that completely lacks protein. This paradox led to the discovery that brain tryptophan content depends on the ratio of the plasma concentration of tryptophan to the sum of the concentrations of the other large neutral amino acids that compete with tryptophan for transport into the brain.

Insulin, administered exogenously or secreted in response to a high carbohydrate meal, also elevates plasma and brain tryptophan levels. The reason for this is that insulin markedly lowers serum non-esterified fatty acids (NEFA) — which compete with tryptophan for a common binding site on albumin molecules — and thereby allows more tryptophan to become bound to albumin. This increase in bound tryptophan causes total serum tryptophan levels to remain elevated at a time when the serum concentrations of other neutral amino acids are declining. Since the affinity of albumin for circulating tryptophan is less than that of the tryptophan-transport protein within the brain capillary endothelia, and its capacity for tryptophan is also very much lower, a major fraction of albumin-bound serum tryptophan is always available for brain uptake.[9]

The clearance of the drug shows evidence of saturation over the dose-range 10–50 mg.kg^{-1}. It is not known whether this is of systemic or presystemic clearance. The clearance of an oral dose of 10 mg.kg^{-1} is high, at greater than 30 ml.min^{-1}.kg^{-1}. The half life of tryptophan is relatively short, from 1.8–2.2 h, and this shows no change with dose.

Oral absorption	—
Presystemic metabolism	—
Plasma half life	
range	1.8–2.2 h
Volume of distribution	0.34–0.7 l.kg^{-1}
Plasma protein binding	~80%

Concentration–effect relationship

Amounts in the range 6000–8000 mg daily, given in divided doses, keep tryptophan hydroxylase reasonably close to saturation throughout the day. Higher doses presumably only increase the synthesis of tryptamine, induce tryptophan pyrrolase activity, and increase side effects, without having an appreciably greater effect on brain 5-HT.[8] There is no clear relationship between plasma concentrations of tryptophan and its therapeutic effects.

Metabolism

The main pathway for the metabolic breakdown of tryptophan begins with the conversion of the amino acid to kynurenine (see Fig. 1). The reaction is catalysed by the tryptophan pyrrolase system and consists of a direct transfer of molecular oxygen. In subsequent steps — through hydroxykynurenine, anthranilic acid, quinolinic acid, and nicotinic ribonucleotide — kynurenine is converted into NAD. It is estimated that about 1 mg of NAD arises from each 60 mg of tryptophan consumed.

Another pathway of tryptophan metabolism is decarboxylation. As a result, tryptamine is formed. In normal human urine, 5–18 mg of indole-3-acetic acid, the oxidation product of tryptamine, are excreted per day.[10]

A third pathway of tryptophan metabolism is hydroxylation. As a result, 5-hydroxytryptophan (5-HTP) is formed. The decarboxylation of 5-HTP yields 5-hydroxytryptamine (5-HT), also known as serotonin. In normal human urine, 2–8 mg of 5-hydroxyindoleacetic acid (5-HIAA), the oxidative deamination product of 5-HT, are excreted per day.

In the adult, only 10–20% of the dietary tryptophan can be accounted for in the urine. Of this, tryptophan itself represents about 40%; N-methyl-nicotinamide and its pyridone another 20%; anthranilic acid and indoleacetic acid 20%; kynurenine, acetylkynurenine and 3-hydroxykynurenine a little over 5%; and indican and the 5-hydroxy group of substances little less than 15%. A high proportion of the daily intake of tryptophan has an unknown fate and, unless some other pathway is discovered, it is likely that a considerable amount of the amino acid is metabolized to ammonia, water and carbon dioxide.[11]

Pharmaceutics

Proprietary brands of tryptophan were withdrawn from the market in 1990 after reports of eosinphilia and myalgia among those taking the drug. It is suspected that this may be due to an unidentified impurity in the tryptophan. Previously the drug had been available in the UK as Optimax WV (a yellow elongated tablet containing 500 mg; E. Merk) or as Pacitron (an oblong orange tablet; Rorer). Optimax also contained 5 mg pyridoxone and 10 mg ascorbic acid.

Tryptophan

A similar ratio was used for Optimax powder (a 6 g sachet). In the USA it was available as capsules containing 500 mg of tryptophan or tablets containing 500 mg and 1000 mg.[12] The drug may still be prescribed on a named-patient basis in the UK and USA.

Therapeutic use

Indications

There are no fully verified indications for the use of l-tryptophan. However, the substance has been successfully employed in the control of a variety of symptoms and in the treatment of a variety of disorders.

For the control of symptoms in:

1. Obesity
2. Insomnia
3. Pain
4. Aggression.

For the treatment of:

5. Affective disorder: depression
6. Affective disorder: mania
7. Obsessive-compulsive disorder
8. Levodopa-induced psychosis
9. Progressive myoclonus epilepsy.

Contraindications

There are no absolute contraindications for the use of l-tryptophan. However, the substance should be used with caution in patients with:

1. Cancer
2. Diabetes mellitus
3. Scleroderma
4. Achlorhydric states.

Mode of use

For all indications, i.e. control of symptoms and/or treatment of disorders, tryptophan is employed orally. Dosage and schedule of drug administration depend on indications. In the case of insomnia for example, a single dose of 1000 mg given before bedtime is appropriate.[13] To augment hypnotic effects the simultaneous administration of carbohydrate has been recommended.[14] The same also applies for the augmentation of analgesic[15] or anorectic[16] effects. On the other hand, in the treatment of depression, mania, aggression and/or obsessive-compulsive disorders, l-tryptophan has to be given on the basis of a divided dosage schedule, because of its relatively fast metabolism. An optimal therapeutic ratio might be obtained with a daily dose range of 6000 to 8000 mg which keeps tryptophan hydroxylase close to saturation point throughout the day.[8]

Indications

1. Obesity

Animal pharmacological findings suggest that an increase of 5-HT-mediated neurotransmission will decrease carbohydrate intake relative to protein. In keeping with this are the clinical observations that l-tryptophan in the dosage of 1000–3000 mg given approximately 45 minutes prior to food intake can decrease carbohydrate craving and calorie intake.[16,17] The hypothesis that l-tryptophan has anorectic effects and/or that l-tryptophan is indicated in the treatment of obesity still needs to be tested in properly designed and conducted clinical experiments.

2. Insomnia

In the dosage of 1000 mg, when given approximately 45 minutes before bedtime, l-tryptophan decreases sleep latency. In this dosage it was found to be effective in the treatment of mild cases of insomnia.[18] In the dosage of 2000 mg daily it was found to be effective in chronic and/or severe cases of insomnia.[19] Differential effectiveness in subjects with different sleep patterns has been reported.[20] The same applies to 'interval therapy',[21] i.e. the intermittent administration of l-tryptophan with an inactive placebo.

3. Pain

Increase in pain tolerance,[22] decrease in pain discriminability[15] and reduction in the subjective experience of pain[23] were reported with 2000–3000 mg of l-tryptophan administration in divided doses. These observations are in keeping with the animal pharmacological data

Fig. 1 The metabolism of tryptophan

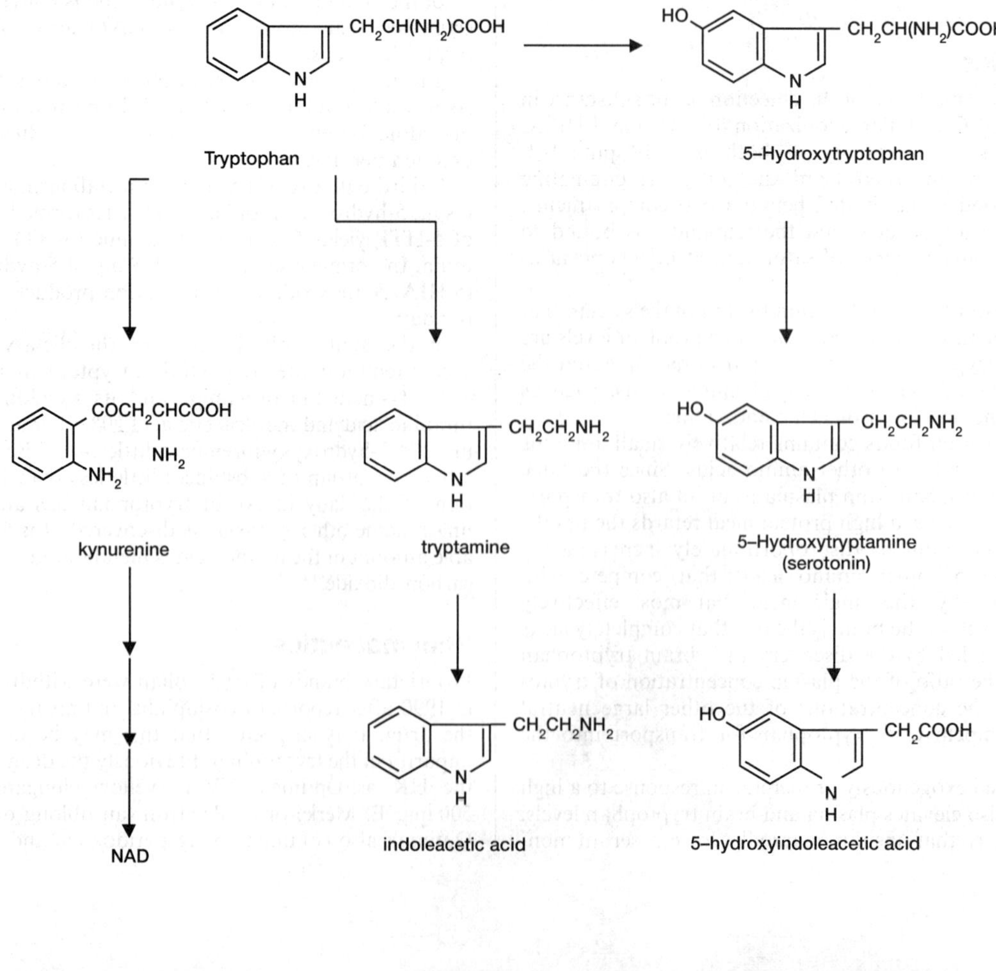

Tryptophan

that the neurotransmitter serotonin, the metabolic end-product of l-tryptophan, is involved in the modulation of pain perception.

4. Aggression
Animal pharmacological findings suggest that l-tryptophan reduces aggression. In keeping with this are the findings that in one clinical trial l-tryptophan in the daily dose range of 4000–8000 mg decreased aggression in schizophrenic patients.[24] The same, however, did not apply to normal subjects.

5. Affective disorder: depression
Results of clinical trials with l-tryptophan alone (1500–16 000 mg daily) in the treatment of depressive disorders are inconsistent.[8] To date, no l-tryptophan-responsive depressive subpopulation has been identified. On the other hand, there are some indications that patients with a low plasma ratio of tryptophan to other amino acids respond favourably to the drug.[25]

6. Affective disorder: mania
There are some indications that l-tryptophan in the daily dosage of 6000–12 000 mg may have therapeutic effects in manic patients. Clinical studies in this particular area of research have remained inconclusive because of their small sample size. Nevertheless, the findings that placebo substitution resulted in relapse in some patients[26] and interfered with improvement in a group of patients[27] suggest that this particular indication warrants further exploration.

7. Obsessive-compulsive disorder
In a small number of patients with obsessive-compulsive disorder, favourable therapeutic effects were seen with daily doses of 3000–9000 mg of l-tryptophan per day.[28] In spite of this no further exploratory work has been conducted in this particular diagnostic group.

8. Levo-Dopa-induced psychosis
In post-mortem studies tryptophan levels were found to be lower in levo-dopa-treated parkinsonian patients who displayed psychotic manifestations in the course of treatment than in patients without psychotic symptoms;[29] and l-tryptophan was found to be consistently effective in the alleviation of levo-dopa-induced psychopathological symptoms.[30–32]

9. Progressive myoclonus epilepsy
Treatment with l-tryptophan is indicated in patients with progressive myoclonus epilepsy, a disorder with a deficient intestinal absorption[33] and low 5-hydroxyindoleacetic acid levels.[34] To maintain therapeutic effects the substance has to be given in a dose of 100 $mg.kg^{-1}$ daily.[35]

Contraindications

1. Cancer
It is known that 2-acetylaminofluorane causes bladder tumours in rats only if the animals are given tryptophan; and that dogs develop a low degree of hyperplasia of the bladder epithelium with prolonged dietary supplementation of tryptophan. Three tryptophan metabolites, i.e. 5-hydroxykynurenine, 3-hydroxyanthranilic acid and anthranilic acid have some stimulating action on tumour formation in mice; and simultaneous administration of 3-hydroxykynurenine and iproniazid has produced an increase in tumour formation in the liver.[36] Furthermore, some patients with bladder cancer have shown an increase in the excretion of tryptophan metabolites when given a tryptophan load test. Because the same patients showed a greater recurrence of new tumours[37] treatment with l-tryptophan should be used with caution in patients with cancer or a history of cancer. To reduce the risk of bladder cancer it has been suggested that tryptophan should be supplemented when given in high doses with pyridoxine. Furthermore, tryptophan should be withheld in patients with a history of bladder cancer or with a source of physical irritation of the bladder.[8]

2. Diabetes mellitus
Tryptophan causes hyperglycaemia in both rats and man.[38] Because it also increases the half life of labelled glucose in the fasting rat and chronic treatment with nicotinic acid, a derivative of tryptophan metabolism, decreases glucose tolerance in man,[39] treatment with l-tryptophan should be used with caution in patients with diabetes mellitus or a history of diabetes.

3. Scleroderma
Some abnormalities of tryptophan metabolism have been indicated in patients with scleroderma-like lesions. Because patients with a carcinoid syndrome with high blood levels of serotonin may develop a scleroderma-like lesion[40] l-tryptophan administration should be used with caution in patients with scleroderma or a history of scleroderma-like conditions.

4. Achlorhydric states
3-Methylindole, even in small amounts, can cause pulmonary arterial hypertension followed by periods of irregular respiratory rate.[41] Since fermentive reactions might give rise to excessive amounts of 3-methylindole (skatole) or related metabolites of tryptophan, tryptophan administration is contraindicated in achlorhydric states, i.e. in patients with an excess of microorganisms in their intestinal flora.

Adverse reactions

Potentially life-threatening effects
Reports of eosinophilia and myalgia have led to the withdrawal of the drug from the market in 1990. It is suspected that this is due to an unidentified impurity.

Acute overdosage
Information on overdose with tryptophan is not available.

Severe or irreversible adverse effects
No severe or irreversible effects had been reported with l-tryptophan until 1989 (see above).

Symptomatic adverse effects
There are only a very few symptomatic adverse effects reported in patients treated with l-tryptophan. Most frequently encountered are nausea and sexual inhibition. Considerably less frequent are anorexia, dizziness, drowsiness and headache.[8]

Other effects
Large doses of tryptophan can cause lipogenesis with increased triglyceride levels in the liver but not in the blood.[43] Since such effects are seen only with excessive doses, they are of no clinical relevance.

Interference with clinical pathology tests
Information on interference with clinical pathology tests is not available for tryptophan.

High risk groups

Neonates
It has been observed that infants between 2 and 3 days old, fed with a formula containing tryptophan in 10% glucose, entered sleep sooner than infants fed with other formulas.[44]

Breast milk. There appears to be no contraindication to the use of tryptophan by lactating women.

Children
It has been reported that tryptophan was well tolerated in children with difficulties at school and disturbed relationships with parents.[45]

Pregnant women
Tryptophan has been safely employed in the daily dosage of 3000 mg in maternity blues.[45] Nevertheless, tryptophan should not be given in very high doses to pregnant women.[8]

The elderly
No special precautions are required. Daily doses as high as 6000 mg and single doses as high as 3000 mg were well tolerated in geriatric patients.[47,48]

Drug interactions

Potentially hazardous interactions
Monoamine oxidase inhibitors. Ethanol-like intoxication with drowsiness, hyper-reflexia, and clonus has been reported with the combined administration of tryptophan and an MAOI to hypertensive patients;[49] and hypomanic behaviour, ocular oscillation, ataxia, and myoclonus have been reported with this combination of drugs.[50]

Other significant interactions
Neuroleptics. Sexual disinhibition was noted with the combined administration of tryptophan and neuroleptics.

T

Monoamine oxidase inhibitors. Sexual disinhibition was noted with the combined administration of tryptophan and MAOIs.

Food. Carbohydrate can enhance tryptophan uptake in brain, whereas protein has the opposite effect.

Potentially useful interactions

Opiates. Tryptophan was noted to reverse tolerance to opiates in a small sample of patients.[51]

Antidepressants. Tryptophan was noted to potentiate the therapeutic effects of lithium, MAOIs, and cyclic antidepressants in some patients.

Major outcome trials

1. Demish K, Bauer J, Georgi K 1987 Treatment of severe chronic insomnia with l-tryptophan and varying sleeping times. Pharmacopsychiatry 20: 245–248

25 subjects suffering from severe chronic insomnia were treated for four weeks with 2000 mg of l-tryptophan in combination with a schedule of varying sleeping times which caused a sleep deficiency at the beginning of treatment. The clinical trial followed an intensive research design in which patients served as their own controls during a second four week period after withdrawal of medication. There was a markedly improved sleeping pattern in 19 (75%) of the 25 subjects during the first four weeks of active treatment; 10 (55%) of these 19 subjects, however, relapsed during the second four week control period. It was noted that during treatment with l-tryptophan a period of about one to two weeks is necessary before sleeping behaviour shows any obvious improvement.

2. Chouinard G, Young S N, Annable L 1985 A controlled clinical trial of l-tryptophan in acute mania. Biological Psychiatry 20: 546–557

In a modified double-blind, placebo-controlled clinical trial which followed a crossover design, 12 000 mg per day of l-tryptophan was given to 24 acutely manic patients for one week. During the second week the l-tryptophan was substituted by an inactive placebo in 12 patients. There was a favourable therapeutic response during the first week of active treatment which in general continued during the second week. It was noted, however, that during the placebo-controlled phase of the clinical trial, patients on l-tryptophan fared better than patients on placebo.

Other trials

Uncontrolled trials

1. Leino E, MacDonald E, Airaksinen M M, Riekkinen P J, Salott H 1981 L-tryptophan–carbidopa trial in patients with long-standing progressive myoclonus epilepsy. Acta Neurologica Scandinavica 64: 132–141

Controlled trials

2. Ayuso-Gutierez J L, Lopez-Ibor Alino J J 1971 Tryptophan and an MAOI (nialamide) in the treatment of depression: a double-blind study. International Pharmacopsychiatry 6: 92–97

General review articles

Baldessarini R J 1984 Treatment of depression by altering monoamine metabolism. Precursors and metabolic inhibitors. Psychopharmacology Bulletin 20: 224–239

Chouinard G, Young S N, Bradwein J, Annable L 1983 Tryptophan in the treatment of depression and mania. In: Mendlewicz J, van Praag H M (eds) Advances in biological psychiatry, vol 10. Karger, Basel, pp 47–66

d'Elia G, Hanson L, Raotmah 1978 L-tryptophan and 5-hydroxytryptophan in the treatment of depression: A review. Acta Psychiatrica Scandinavica 57: 239–252

Hartman E, Greenwald D 1984 Tryptophan and human sleep: an analysis of 43 studies. In: Schlossberger H G, Kochen W, Linzen B, Steinhard H (eds) Progress in tryptophan and serotonin research. Walter de Gruyter, Berlin, pp 297–304

References

1. Carlson J R, Lindquist M 1978 Dependence of 5-HT and catecholamine synthesis on concentrations of precursor amino-acids in rat brain. Naunyn-Schmiedebergs Archives of Pharmacology 303: 157–164
2. Jones R S G 1981 In vivo pharmacological studies on the interactions between tryptamine and 5-hydroxytryptamine. British Journal of Pharmacology 73: 485–493
3. Jorgensen A J F, Majumdar A P N 1976 Bilateral adrenalectomy: Effect of tryptophan force-feeding on amino acid incorporation into ferritin, transferrin, and mixed proteins of liver, brain and kidneys in vivo. Biochemical Medicine 16: 37–46
4. Sourkes T L 1983 Toxicology of serotonin precursors. Advances in Biological Psychiatry 10: 160–175
5. Green A R, Aronson J K, Curzon G, Woods H F 1980 Metabolism of an oral tryptophan load. I. Effects of dose and pretreatment with tryptophan. British Journal of Clinical Pharmacology 10: 603–610
6. Smith B, Prockop D J 1962 Central-nervous-system effects of injection of l-tryptophan by normal subjects. New England Journal of Medicine 269: 1338–1341
7. Olson R E, Gursey D, Vester J W 1960 Evidence for a defect in tryptophan metabolism in chronic alcoholism. New England Journal of Medicine 263: 1169–1174
8. Young S N 1986 The clinical pharmacology of tryptophan. In: Wurtman R J, Wurtman J J (eds) Nutrition and the brain, vol 7. Raven Press, New York
9. Growdon J H 1979 Neurotransmitter precursors in the diet: Their use in the treatment of brain disease. In: Wurtman J R, Wurtman J J (eds) Nutrition and the brain, vol 3. Raven Press, New York
10. Harper H A 1967 Review of physiological chemistry. Lange Medical Publications, Los Altos
11. Sourkes T L 1962 Biochemistry of mental disease. Harper and Row, New York
12. Physician's Desk Reference 1986 PRD 40 Edition. Medical Economics Co, Oradell
13. Hartmann E, Spinweber C L 1979 Sleep induced by l-tryptophan. Effects on dosages within the normal dietary intake. Journal of Nervous and Mental Disease 167: 497–499
14. Wurtman R J, Hefti F, Melamed E 1981 Precursor control of neurotransmitter synthesis. Pharmacological Reviews 32: 315–335
15. Lieberman H R, Corkin S, Spring B J, Growdon J H, Wurtman R J 1983 Mood, performance and pain sensitivity: Changes induced by food constituents. Journal of Psychiatric Research 17: 135–145
16. Wurtman J J, Wurtman R J, Growdon J H, Henry P, Lipscomb A, Zeisel S H 1981 Carbohydrate craving in obese people: Suppression by treatments affecting serotoninergic transmission. International Journal of Eating Disorders 1: 2–15
17. Hrboticky N, Leiter L A, Anderson G H 1985 Effects of l-tryptophan on short term food intake, subjective hunger and mood in healthy lean men. Nutrition Research 5: 595–607
18. Cole J O, Hartmann E, Brigham P 1980 l-tryptophan: Clinical studies. In: Cole J O (ed) Psychopharmacology update. The Collamore Press, Lexington, pp 119–148
19. Demisch K, Bauer J, Georgi K 1987 Treatment of severe chronic insomnia with l-tryptophan and varying sleeping times. Pharmacopsychiatry 20: 245–248
20. Lindsley J G, Hartmann E L, Mitchell W 1983 Selectivity in response to l-tryptophan among insomniac subjects: a preliminary report. Sleep 6: 247–256
21. Schneider-Helmert D 1981 Interval therapy with l-tryptophan in severe chronic insomniacs: A predictive laboratory study. International Pharmacopsychiatry 16: 162–173
22. Seltzer S, Stoch R, Marcus R, Jackson E 1982 Alteration of human pain thresholds by nutritional manipulation and l-tryptophan supplementation. Pain 13: 385–393
23. Seltzer S, Dewart D, Pollack R, Jackson E 1983 The effects of dietary tryptophan on chronic maxillofacial pain and experimental pain tolerance. Journal of Psychiatric Research 17: 181–186
24. Morand C, Young S N, Ervin F R 1983 Clinical response of aggressive schizophrenics to oral tryptophan. Biological Psychiatry 18: 575–578
25. Moller S E 1980 Evaluation of the relative potency of individual competing amino acids to tryptophan transport in endogenously depressed patients. Psychiatric Research 3: 141–150
26. Murphy D L, Baker M, Goodwin F K, Miller L, Kotin J, Bunney W E 1974 L-tryptophan in affective disorders: Indoleamine changes and differential clinical effects. Psychopharmacology 34: 11–20
27. Chouinard G, Young S N, Annable L 1985 A controlled clinical trial of l-tryptophan in acute mania. Biological Psychiatry 20: 546–557
28. Yaryura-Tobias J A, Bhagavan H M 1977 L-tryptophan in obsessive-compulsive disorders. American Journal of Psychiatry 134: 1298–1299
29. Birkmayer W, Danielczyk W, Neumayer E, Riederer P 1974 Nucleus ruber and L-DOPA psychosis. Biochemical post-mortem findings. Journal of Neural Transmission 35: 93–116
30. Birkmayer W, Neumayer E 1972 Die Behandlung der Dopa-Psychosen mit l-tryptophan. Nervenarzt 43: 76–78
31. Gehlen W, Muller J 1974 Zur Therapie der Dopa-Psychosen mit l-tryptophan. Deutsche Medizinische Wochenschrift 99: 457–463
32. Miller E M, Nieberg H A 1974 L-tryptophan in the treatment of levodopa-induced psychiatric disorders. Diseases of the Nervous System 35: 20–23
33. Koskiniemi M L 1980 Deficient intestinal absorption of l-tryptophan in progressive myoclonus epilepsy without lafora bodies. Journal of Neurological Science 47: 1–6
34. Leino E, MacDonald E, Airaksinen M M, Riekkinen P J 1980 Homovanillic acid and 5-hydroxyindoleacetic acid levels in cerebrospinal fluid of patients with progressive myoclonus epilepsy. Acta Neurologica Scandinavica 62: 45–54
35. Leino E, MacDonald E, Airaksinen M M, Riekkinen P J, Salott H 1981 L-tryptophan–carbidopa trial in patients with long-standing progressive myoclonus epilepsy. Acta Neurologica Scandinavica 64: 132–141
36. Fujii K, Watanabe M 1980 Comparative study of tumorigenicity in mice administered transplacentally or neonatally with metabolites of tryptophan and its related compounds. Journal of Cancer Research and Clinical Oncology 96: 163–168

37. Yoshida O, Brown R R, Bryan G T 1970 Relationship between tryptophan metabolism and heterotopic recurrences of human urinary bladder tumors. Cancer 25: 773–780
38. Hedo J A, Villanueva M L, Marco J 1977 Elevation of plasma glucose and glucagon after tryptophan ingestion in man. Metabolism 26: 1131–1134
39. Gaut Z N, Pocilenko R, Soloman H M, Thomas G B 1971 Oral glucose tolerance, plasma insulin, and uric acid excretion in man during chronic administration of nicotinic acid. Metabolism 20: 1131–1035
40. Fries J F, Lindgren J A 1973 Scleroderma-like lesions and the carcinoid syndrome. Archives of Internal Medicine 131: 550–553
41. Atkinson G, Bogan J A, Breeze R G, Selman I E 1977 Effects of 3-methylindole in cattle. British Journal of Pharmacology 61: 285–290
42. Silzer H 1990 British Medical Journal 300: 876
43. Fears R, Murrell E A 1980 Tryptophan and the control of triglyceride and carbohydrate metabolism in the rat. British Journal of Nutrition 43: 349–356
44. Yogman M W, Zeisel S H 1983 Diet and sleep patterns in newborn infant. New England Journal of Medicine 309: 1147–1149
45. Hoyes S 1982 Experiences with l-tryptophan in a child and family psychiatric department. Journal of International Medical Research 10: 157–159
46. Harris B 1980 Prospective trial of l-tryptophan in maternity blues. British Journal of Psychiatry 137: 233–235
47. Cooper A J, Datta S R 1980 A placebo controlled evaluation of l-tryptophan in depression in the elderly. Canadian Journal of Psychiatry 25: 386–390
48. Smith D F, Stromgren E, Petersen H N, Williams D G, Sheldon W 1984 Lack of effect of tryptophan treatment in demented gerontopsychiatric patients: A double-blind, crossover-controlled study. Acta Psychiatrica Scandinavica 70: 470–477
49. Oates J A, Sjoerdsma A 1960 Neurologic effects of tryptophan in patients receiving a monoamine oxidase inhibitor. Neurology 10: 1076–1078
50. Thomas J M, Rubin E H 1984 Case report of a toxic reaction from a combination of tryptophan and phenelzine. American Journal of Psychiatry 141: 281–283
51. Hosobuchi Y, Lamb S, Baskin D 1980 Tryptophan loading may reverse tolerance to opiate analgesics in humans. A preliminary report. Pain 9: 161–169

d-Tubocurarine chloride

d-Tubocurarine is a non-depolarizing skeletal muscle relaxant.

Chemistry

d-Tubocurarine chloride (Curarin, Intocostrin-T) pentahydrate is a mono-quaternary ammonium structure.[1]

$C_{37}H_{42}Cl_2N_2O_6$

d-7',12'-Dihydroxy-6,6'-dimethoxy-2,2',2'-trimethyltubocuranium dichloride

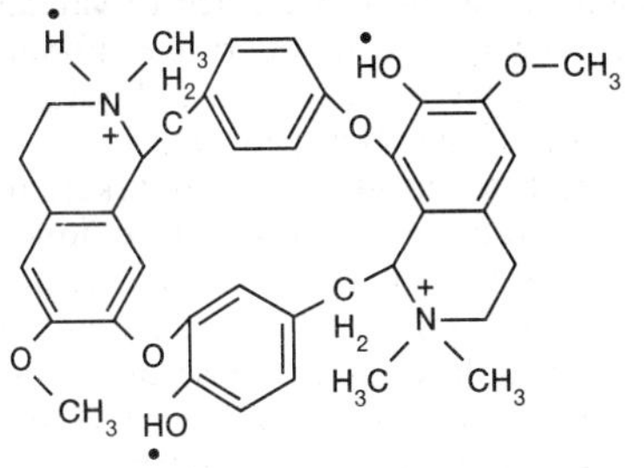

Molecular weight	681.7
pKa (amino group)	8.0
Solubility	
in alcohol	1 in 30
in water	1 in 20
Octanol/water partition coefficient	nil

d-Tubocurarine is a white crystalline compound, obtained from extracts of the stems of *Chondodendron tomentosum.*

Pharmacology

d-Tubocurarine has several effects at the neuromuscular junction.[2] It primarily acts as a competitive antagonist of acetylcholine at the postjunctional cholinergic receptor. Although d-tubocurarine is bound to the receptor for less than 1 ms this binding is long enough to prevent acetylcholine from causing the ion channel to open and depolarize the muscle. Flaccid paralysis results. At higher concentrations d-tubocurarine may enter the opened ion channel and add a non-competitive component to the block. In addition, d-tubocurarine may interfere with the synthesis and immobilization of acetylcholine, a prejunctional effect. d-Tubocurarine also causes histamine release from mast cells.

Toxicology

d-Tubocurarine has no known teratogenic or mutagenic effects. Poisoning from d-tubocurarine is almost always the result of clinical overdosage or injudicious use. Important untoward responses are prolonged apnoea and cardiovascular collapse from histamine release and ganglionic blockade.

Clinical pharmacology

d-Tubocurarine is usually administered intravenously but may rarely be given by the intramuscular route. d-Tubocurarine is virtually devoid of analgesic or other central nervous system effects. At clinically used doses, d-tubocurarine produces some blockade at autonomic ganglia, including the adrenal medulla and a small fall in blood pressure accompanied by slight tachycardia may be seen; on occasion a severe fall in blood pressure may occur. The release of histamine by d-tubocurarine is primarily seen following intracutaneous injection when a wheal and flare response is seen. Clinically excessive bronchial and salivary secretion may be seen which is thought to be due to histamine release.

Pharmacokinetics

Sensitive radioimmune or HPLC assays are now available (sensitivity 5 μg.l^{-1}).

Kalow[3] reported that 33% of a dose of d-tubocurarine appeared as unmetabolized drug in the urine in 10–15 hours after injection. This was later increased to 60–70% by collecting urine for 24 hours; however, no data have been presented to substantiate this claim.[4] The apparent major importance of renal function for excretion should be reflected in a prolonged duration of neuromuscular blockade in patients with renal failure given the same dose as administered to patients with normal renal function. In 6 patients with no renal function and undergoing abdominal surgery there was no prolongation of effects of d-tubocurarine after a dose of 0.42–0.95 mg.kg^{-1}.[5] However, cases of prolonged paralysis have been reported following use of large doses of d-tubocurarine in some other patients with renal failure.[6,7] Although some authors have claimed that d-tubocurarine is also eliminated through the bile, no experimental data from humans has been presented to validate this claim.[5] In dogs receiving 0.3 mg.kg^{-1} d-tubocurarine, about 11% of the injected dose was eliminated in the bile in 24 hours; this was increased to 39% with ligation of the renal pedicles.[8]

In a study in which blood samples were taken and assayed for d-tubocurarine by the radioimmunoassay technique, the duration of effect and the relationship between effect and serum concentration of the drug were about the same in 10 normal patients as compared with 10 others with renal failure after a dose of 0.3 or 0.5 mg.kg^{-1} d-tubocurarine.[9] The serum concentration of d-tubocurarine versus time curves were essentially parallel for normal subjects and patients with renal failure indicating that the clearance of d-tubocurarine occurred at the same rate in the two groups. In 5 patients with newly transplanted kidneys the ability to eliminate d-tubocurarine in the urine was markedly reduced. Thus, the data suggest that there is an alternative pathway for elimination of d-tubocurarine in humans following usual doses in renal failure, but that prolongation of blockade may occur after large or repeated doses.

d-Tubocurarine undergoes rapid distribution to plasma proteins, extracellular fluid and the tissue of major organs. After intravenous injection of 0.3 mg.kg^{-1}, the concentration of d-tubocurarine in muscle tissue reached a maximum within 5 minutes.[10] Similarly, significant levels of d-tubocurarine appeared in the lumbar cerebrospinal fluid within 15 minutes of a dose of 0.43–0.68 mg.kg^{-1}.[11] With a dose of 0.3 mg.kg^{-1}, the plasma or serum concentration of d-tubocurarine declined rapidly during the first 10 minutes due to the initial distribution to extracellular fluid, tissue and plasma proteins. This was followed by a period of about 60 minutes of combined redistribution and elimination; a third period of monoexponential disappearance from plasma with a half life of 150 minutes was also observed.[12] Although the serum or plasma d-tubocurarine concentration decay curves were essentially parallel among individual patients, the curves differed in their concentration at time zero.[9,12] This shift in initial concentration reflected differences in the apparent volume of distribution of d-tubocurarine among individuals.

At a plasma concentration of 5 mg.l^{-1} d-tubocurarine, about 44% is bound to plasma proteins, as determined by equilibrium dialysis, and 82–90% to gamma globulin, using electrophoresis.[13] In a more detailed study employing tritiated d-tubocurarine 15% of the drug was bound to gamma globulin and 24% to albumin using equilibrium dialysis, and 82–90% to gamma globulin using electrophoresis; the reason for this difference is not understood.[14]

A loose correlation between the required dose of d-tubocurarine and the serum level of gamma globulin was observed in 50 patients undergoing lower abdominal surgery for gynaecological cancer.[15] In related work d-tubocurarine dimethyl-^{14}C-ether iodide was about 40% bound to human plasma proteins over the concentration range of 0.006–8.8 mg.l^{-1} and was also bound in appreciable amounts to chondroitin sulphate and cartilage.[16] These connective type materials may also be a binding site for d-tubocurarine. It appears that at least 40–50% of d-tubocurarine is bound to plasma proteins at concentrations greater than those found clinically and that variations in the gamma globulin level may account for differences in the amount of drug bound among individual patients.

The apparent volume of distribution of d-tubocurarine is about 2.4–3.0 l.[17] Increased plasma protein binding of d-tubocurarine results in a larger total concentration at time zero, and therefore a smaller volume of distribution assuming that the concentration of unbound drug stays the same.

The importance of a different apparent volume of distribution in explaining interindividual variation in the duration of neuromuscular blockade was shown using computer simulations.[12,17,18] A rather wide range of recovery times can be expected for a given dose, depending on the apparent volume of distribution of d-tubocurarine in a particular patient. The time to decline to a particular serum concentration of d-tubocurarine is not directly proportional to the initial concentration. This is in agreement with clinical observations in that the duration of action is not proportional to the dose, particularly when booster injections are given during surgery.

An earlier pharmacokinetic model for d-tubocurarine was constructed assuming 42% of the drug was eliminated unchanged in the urine.[19] This model gave abnormally high recovery times for patients with renal failure.[20,21]

Oral absorption	
Presystemic metabolism	
Plasma half life	2–4 h
Volume of distribution	0.3–0.6 l.kg^{-1}
Plasma protein binding	40–50%

Concentration–effect relationship

Matteo et al.[18] used a very sensitive radioimmunoassay for d-tubocurarine and found a highly significant linear correlation between the degree of neuromuscular blockade in humans and the serum concentration of drug. In adults, a minimum concentration of 0.2 mg.l^{-1} was needed before any blockade developed and 0.7 mg.l^{-1} was needed for complete blockade. These concentrations agreed very closely with those calculated assuming a d-tubocurarine-receptor binding constant of 10^{-7} M and assuming 90% or 75% of the motor end-plate receptors were occupied by d-tubocurarine for essentially complete or minimum detectable blockade, respectively.[21]

Metabolism

Little or no metabolism of d-tubocurarine takes place.

Pharmaceutics

d-Tubocurarine Jexin (DF, UK) Tubarine (Calmic, UK) is marketed as a sterile solution containing 10 mg.ml^{-1} for intravenous use. In the USA the injection from Quad Pharmaceuticals contains 3 mg. ml^{-1}. The pH is 4 to 5 and d-tubocurarine is precipitated at high pH (e.g. sodium bicarbonate).

Solutions are sealed under nitrogen.

Therapeutic use

Indications

1. The primary use of d-tubocurarine is as an adjunct to surgical anaesthesia to facilitate endotracheal intubation.
2. To provide surgical relaxation, and to facilitate controlled ventilation. Occasionally, it may be used to facilitate controlled ventilation as a part of intensive respiratory care for patients with respiratory failure, tetanus, or status epilepticus.
3. Rarely, it may be used in the diagnosis of myasthenia gravis but there are better alternatives.

Contraindications

1. A previous history of an anaphylactoid reaction to d-tubocurarine
2. d-Tubocurarine should be used with *caution* in patients with myaesthenia gravis and other neuromuscular diseases, malignant hyperthermia, renal failure, or hypovolaemia. However, d-tubocurarine is not *absolutely* contraindicated in such patients.

d-Tubocurarine chloride

Mode of use

The dosage of tubocurarine chloride as an adjunct to surgical anaesthesia is essentially individualized. During nitrous oxide-narcotic anaesthesia (range 0.1–0.06 $mg.kg^{-1}$) the total initial dose is about 0.3 $mg.kg^{-1}$.[22,23] If potent inhalation anaesthetics are being used (i.e. halothane or isoflurane) the initial dose should be reduced by approximately one-third to one-half.[24,25] In obese patients the dose should be related to lean body mass. Administration in fractional dosage is advised to avoid overdosage. Subsequent fractional doses range from one-third to one-quarter the initial dose. The intensity and duration of action of the initial dose should be an indication of the amount required for repetitive doses.

The recommended dosage for tubocurarine in electroshock therapy is from 0.1 to 0.2 $mg.kg^{-1}$ body weight. When used in patients undergoing mechanical ventilation, the dosage must be individualized.

Patients with myasthenia gravis have such increased sensitivity to tubocurarine that doses ranging from one-fifth to one-hundredth of normal may produce profound muscle weakness. Antidotes and resuscitative equipment for performing artificial respiration should be immediately available if tubocurarine is being used as a diagnostic test for myasthenia gravis.

A typical adult dose of 0.3 mg d-tubocurarine produces complete non-depolarizing neuromuscular blockade, with a duration of about 50 minutes from intravenous injection to 50% recovery of neuromuscular transmission, and 75 minutes to 90% recovery.[26] The duration of blockade appears to depend simply on how long it takes the concentration of drug in the extracellular fluid to diminish to a particular value.

Adverse reactions

Potentially life-threatening effects

Poisoning from d-tubocurarine is almost always the result of clinical overdosage or injudicious use. Important untoward responses are prolonged apnoea and cardiovascular collapse from histamine release and ganglionic blockade.

Four cases of postoperative respiratory failure were reported in patients with renal failure following reversal of d-tubocurarine blockade by neostigmine.[27] Large doses of d-tubocurarine had been used (48–55 mg in total). Since no blood samples were taken, it was not clear whether the respiratory problems were due to elevated plasma levels of d-tubocurarine or to other complications present.

Acute overdosage

The effect of an acute overdose and its management are similar to those described immediately above.

Severe or irreversible adverse effects

A small number of patients may develop a serious anaphylactoid reaction to d-tubocurarine which may or may not involve presensitization.

Symptomatic adverse effects

d-Tubocurarine, like many organic bases, can liberate histamine from tissue mast cells and basophil leucocytes. Urticaria, itching, erythema at the site of injection, hypotension, and bronchoconstriction, all signs of histamine release, have been noted in patients. In patients anaesthetized with nitrous oxide–thiopental–fentanyl, the hypotensive property of d-tubocurarine given to facilitate endotracheal intubation correlates with four- to six-fold transient increases in serum histamine concentrations. Thus, the hypotension is brief; transient increases in heart rate may occur. d-Tubocurarine also blocks ganglionic nicotinic receptors, particularly parasympathetic ganglia, and produces some ganglionic blocks in a dose range similar to that required to produce neuromuscular blocks. Autonomic reflexes may be impaired. In addition, d-tubocurarine may have a direct cardiac depressant action. However, it seems clear that histamine following d-tubocurarine is responsible for the hypotension.

Interference with clinical pathology tests

No technical interferences of this kind have been reported.

High risk groups

Neonates

A dose of about 0.25 $mg.kg^{-1}$ can be used safely in neonates at birth up to 0.5 $mg.kg^{-1}$ at 28 days of age.[28] This agrees with other reports that newborns are more sensitive than children and adults to d-tubocurarine.[28,29] This greater sensitivity of newborns to d-tubocurarine does not appear due to differences in the serum albumin or serum globulin levels in 50 neonates aged 1–23 days.[30] Part of this difference in sensitivity to d-tubocurarine may be due to changes in the proportion of extracellular water or lean body mass with age; and some authors have suggested that d-tubocurarine doses should be based on body surface area instead of body weight.[31]

EMG studies demonstrated no increased sensitivity of hand muscles to d-tubocurarine in infants as compared with adults.[29,32] However, in infants respiratory depression parallels the neuromuscular blockade noted in the hands; in adults neuromuscular blockade of the hand occurs prior to respiratory depression. This important observation suggests that the respiratory muscles of the infant may be more sensitive to d-tubocurarine than those of the adult, or that the infant has less respiratory reserve than the adult. In actuality both may be true.

Fisher et al.[33] documented the sensitivity of the infant to d-tubocurarine as compared with older patients during equipotent nitrous oxide-halothane anaesthesia. Since the MAC of halothane is higher in infants than adults, infants received higher end-tidal concentrations of halothane. The volume of distribution for d-tubocurarine is quite high in the newborn infant as compared with the older child or adult, but plasma clearance of d-tubocurarine does not differ with age. The volume of distribution for d-tubocurarine appears relatively constant on a litres per square metre basis. More important, the plasma concentration associated with 50% neuromuscular block (Cpss) was age-related; Cpss in neonates was about one-third that noted for adults. The largest variability in elimination half life and volumes of distribution was seen in the data for the neonates. Likewise, Goudsouzian et al.[34] noted wide variations in the ED_{95} for d-tubocurarine in neonates during halothane anaesthesia. Some infants were paralysed with 0.18 $mg.kg^{-1}$ and others required 0.6 $mg.kg^{-1}$; the mean ED_{95} was similar to that of older children. This suggests that the neonate's response to non-depolarizing relaxants is quite unpredictable.

Breast milk. There are no data to suggest that d-tubocurarine accumulates in breast milk.

Children

In adults, Donlon et al.[22] have determined cumulative dose–response curves and noted recovery times for d-tubocurarine during nitrous oxide–oxygen–narcotic anaesthesia. At equipotent doses of these relaxants the recovery time from 95% block to 50% block averaged 45 minutes. Similar studies have been performed in children during halothane and balanced anaesthesia by other investigators.[34] The ED_{95} for these relaxants in children during balanced anaesthesia tended to be higher than that in adults and the recovery times tended to be shorter. The dose requirements (ED_{95}) of d-tubocurarine are reduced by halothane anaesthesia in children as in adults. During halothane-nitrous oxide anaesthesia there was little difference between the ED_{95} on a weight basis for the longer-acting muscle relaxants in infants and children.

Recently, Cook estimated the dose of d-tubocurarine, on a surface-area basis, that would be required to produce 95% twitch depression in infants, children, and adults during halothane anaesthesia.[35] In this estimate, one attempts to compensate for the wide variation in ECF that appears in infants, children, and adults. The ECF volume mirrors the volume of distribution for the non-depolarizing muscle relaxants. One is also comparing like anaesthetics — halothane with halothane — to produce 95% blockade. The adult and child require about 7–8 $mg.m^{-2}$ of d-tubocurarine; the 6- to 9-month-old infant requires 5–6 $mg.m^{-2}$; but the neonate requires about 4 $mg.m^{-2}$. This suggests that the neonate, and to a lesser degree the infant, is quite sensitive to d-tubocurarine when one compensates for the wide variation in volumes of distribution.

Pregnant women

d-Tubocurarine can be used during obstetrics and in neonates; although it does cross the placenta in small amounts. Within 10 minutes after maternal injection in humans the level of ^{14}C-dimethyltubocurarine in the umbilical vein reached 12% of the maternal venous level.[36]

d-Tubocurarine chloride

T

The elderly
d-Tubocurarine may have a prolonged effect in the elderly due to a decrease in clearance.[37]

Concurrent disease
d-Tubocurarine should be used with extreme caution in patients with myasthenia gravis or other neuromuscular diseases.

Drug interactions

Potentially hazardous interactions
None has been described.

Other significant interactions
A variety of other drugs may interact with d-tubocurarine at the nerve terminal, at the postsynaptic membrane, in the ion channel, or at a combination of sites. Aminoglycoside and polypeptide antibiotics can produce neuromuscular block in their own right and can augment the block from d-tubocurarine. In general, these antibiotics decrease acetylcholine release and affect postjunctional sensitivity to acetylcholine. Calcium channel blockers, magnesium, local anaesthetics, diazepam[38] and antiarrhythmics such as procainamide and quinidine, may have prejunctional and postjunctional effects that reduce the margin of safety of neuromuscular transmission.

Potentially useful interactions
Potent inhalation anaesthetics potentiate (augment) the neuromuscular block from d-tubocurarine in a concentration (dose)-related manner. At 1.25 MAC (minimum alveolar concentration) halothane reduces the dose of d-tubocurarine required for 95% paralysis by 50%; diethylether, enflurane, and isoflurane reduce the dose by about 65–70%; at higher multiples of MAC, the augmentation is greater. Similarly, if the dose of d-tubocurarine is kept constant (i.e. 1.5 $mg.m^{-2}$) the blocking effect increases as the concentration of potent anaesthetic increases. This augmentation is related to a drug interaction at the cholinergic receptor and by interfering with the open ion channel conductance.

References

1. Everett A J, Lowe L A, Wilkinson S 1970 Revision of the structure of (+)-tubocurarine chloride and (+)-chondrocurine. Chemical Communications 1970: 1020–1021
2. Standaert F G 1984 Pharmacology of the neuromuscular junction In: Brumback R A, Gerst J (eds) The neuromuscular junction. Futura Publishing Company Inc, Mt Kisco, New Jersey
3. Kalow W, Gunn D R 1953 Urinary excretion of d-tubocurarine in man. Journal of Pharmacology and Experimental Therapeutics 109: 74–82
4. Fleishli G, Cohen E N 1966 An analog computer simulation for the distribution of d-tubocurarine. Anesthesiology 27: 64–69
5. Churchill-Davidson H C, Way W L, deJong R H 1967 The muscle relaxants and renal excretion. Anesthesiology 28: 540–546
6. Homi J, Smith E R 1970 Anaesthetic management for renal transplantation. Some controversial aspects. In: Boulton, Bryce-Smith, Sykes et al (eds) Proceedings of the 4th World Congress of Anaesthesiologists. Excerpta Medica, Amsterdam, pp 679–684
7. Riordan D D, Gilbertson A A 1971 Prolonged curarization in a patient with renal failure. British Journal of Anaesthesia 43: 506–508
8. Cohen E N, Brewer H W, Smith D 1967 The metabolism and elimination of d-tubocurarine-H^3. Anesthesiology 23: 309–317
9. Miller R D, Matteo R D 1976 Renal failure and plasma concentrations of d-tubocurarine and its neuromuscular blockade in man. American Society of Anesthesiologists 181–182
10. Cohen E N, Corbascio A, Fleischli G 1965 The distribution and fate of d-tubocurarine. Journal of Pharmacology and Experimental Therapeutics 147: 120–129
11. Devasankaraiah G, Haranath P S R K, Krishnamurty A 1973 Passage of intravenously administered tubocurarine into the liquor space in man and dog. British Journal of Pharmacology 47: 787–798
12. Horowitz P E, Spector S 1973 Determination of serum d-tubocurarine concentration by radioimmunoassay. Journal of Pharmacology and Experimental Therapeutics 185: 94–100
13. Ghoneim M M, Kramer S E, Barrow R, Pandya H, Routh J I 1973 Binding of d-tubocurarine to plasma proteins in normal man and in patients with hepatic or renal disease. Anesthesiology 39: 410–415
14. Ghoneim M M, Pandya H 1975 Binding of tubocurarine to specific serum protein fractions. British Journal of Anaesthesia 47: 853–856
15. Stovner J, Theodorsen L, Bjelke E 1971 Sensitivity to tubocurarine and alcuronium with special reference to plasma protein pattern. British Journal of Anaesthesia 43: 385–391
16. Olsen G D, Chan E M, Riker W K 1975 Binding of d-tubocurarine di(methyl-^{14}C) ether iodide and other amines to cartilage, chondroitan sulfate and human plasma proteins. Journal of Pharmacology and Experimental Therapeutics 195. 242–250
17. Wingard L B, Cook D R 1976 Pharmacodynamics of tubocurarine in humans. British Journal of Anaesthesia 48: 839–845
18. Matteo R S, Spector S, Horowitz P E 1974 Relation of serum d-tubocurarine concentration to neuromuscular blockade in man. Anesthesiology 41: 440–443
19. Gibaldi M, Levy G, Hayton W L 1972 Kinetics of the elimination and neuromuscular blocking effect of d-tubocurarine in man. Anesthesiology 36: 213–218
20. Gibaldi M, Levy G, Hayton W L 1972 Tubocurarine and renal failure. British Journal of Anaesthesia 44: 163–165
21. Waud R E 1975 Serum d-tubocurarine concentration and twitch height. Anesthesiology 43: 381–382
22. Donlon J V Jr., Ali H H, Savarese J J 1974 A new approach to the study of four non-depolarizing relaxants in man. Anesthesia and Analgesia 53: 924–939
23. Donlon J V Jr, Savarese J J, Ali H H, Teplik R S 1980 Human dose–response curves for neuromuscular blocking drugs: a comparison of two methods of construction and analysis. Anesthesiology 53: 161–166
24. Miller R D, Eger E I II, Way W L, Stevens W C, Donlan W M 1971 Comparative neuromuscular effects of forane and halothane alone in combination with d–tubocurarine in man. Anesthesiology 35: 38–42
25. Waud B E, Waud D R 1979 Effects of volatile anesthetics on directly and indirectly stimulated skeletal muscle. Anesthesiology 41: 440–447
26. Walts L F, Dillon J B 1967 Clinical studies on succinylcholine chloride. Anesthesiology 28: 372–376
27. Miller R D, Cullen D J 1976 Renal failure and postoperative respiratory failure: recurarization? British Journal of Anaesthesia 48: 253–256
28. Walts L F, Dillon J B 1969 The response of newborns to succinylcholine and d-tubocurarine. Anesthesiology 31: 35–38
29. Long G, Bachman L 1974 Neuromuscular blockade by d-tubocurarine in children. Anesthesiology 28: 723–729
30. Vivori E, Vush G H, Ireland J T 1974 Tubocurarine requirements and plasma protein concentrations in the newborn infant. British Journal of Anaesthesia 46: 93–96
31. Wulfsohn N L 1972 d-Tubocurarine dosage based on lean body mass. Canadian Anaesthetists' Society Journal 19: 251–262
32. Churchill-Davidson H C, Wise R P 1964 The response of the newborn infant to muscle relaxants. Canadian Anaesthetists' Society Journal 11: 1–5
33. Fisher D M, O'Keeffe C, Stanski D R et al 1982 Pharmacokinetics and pharmacodynamics of d-tubocurarine in infants, children and adults. Anesthesiology 57: 203–208
34. Goudsouzian N G, Donlon J V Jr, Savarese J J, Ryan J F 1975 Re-evaluation of dosage and duration of action of d-tubocurarine in the pediatric age group. Anesthesiology 43: 416–425
35. Cook D R 1981 Sensitivity of the newborn to tubocurarine. British Journal of Anaesthesia 53: 320
36. Kivalo I, Saarikoski S 1976 Placental transfer of ^{14}C-dimethyltubocurarine during caesarean section. British Journal of Anaesthesia 48: 239–242
37. Matteo R S, Backus W W, McDaniel D D, Brotherton W P, Abraham R, Diaz J 1985 Pharmacokinetics and pharmacodynamics of d-tubocurarine and metocurine in the elderly. Anesthesia and Analgesia 64: 23–29
38. Wali F A 1985 Myorelaxant effects of diazepam: interactions with neuromuscular blocking agents and cholinergic drugs. Acta Anaesthesiologica Scandinavica 29: 785–789

Undecenoic acid

Undecenoic acid is a short chain fatty acid which is used in the topical treatment of dermatophyte infections of the skin.

Chemistry

10-Undecenoic acid (undecylenic acid)
$C_{11}H_{20}O_2$
Mainly as Undec-10-enoic acid CH_2:CH $[CH_2]_8$COOH

Molecular weight	184.3
pKa (carboxylate)	4.8
Solubility	
in alcohol	>1 in 10
in water	insoluble
Octanol/water partition coefficient	high

Undecenoic acid is a pale yellow liquid or a white to very pale yellow crystalline powder with a characteristic odour of perspiration. It is prepared by chemical synthesis. Creams and ointments are generally white with a characteristic mild odour. It is used in combination with its zinc salt (Compound Undecylenic acid ointment, Mycota), with phenylethylalcohol and cetrimide (Ceanel concentrate), with propylene glycol (Pomatum Undecylenici), as its methyl and propyl esters together with various salicylate derivatives and chlorbutol (Monphytol) or as its zinc salt with zinc napthenate (Tineafax) and with chlorophenoxyethanol and phenoxypropanol (Phytocil).

Pharmacology

Undecenoic acid, its esters and salts, are fungistatic to a wide variety of fungi including the common pathogens in the superficial mycoses.[1] At higher concentrations than those present in commercial preparations, the undecenoates are fungicidal.[2] They are also bacteriostatic and bacteriocidal. [3] Undecenoic acid is reputedly an effective insect repellant, but its unpleasant odour limits this clinical application.

Toxicology

Undecenoic acid is an irritant and if applied to abraded or broken skin may cause a transitory mild stinging. The use of undecenoic acid salts in the proprietary creams have reduced this irritant effect.

Contact allergic dermatitis to the acid or salts is rare[4,5] and may be restricted to a specific salt in an individual patient.[6] No toxicological testing for topical undecenoic acid has been performed in animals, but the LD_{50} orally in rats is 2.5 $g.kg^{-1}$. There is no information concerning any possible teratogenic or carcinogenic potential.

Clinical pharmacology

Undecenoic acid and its salts are antimicrobial and are active against certain pathogenic fungi — *Epidermophyton*, *Trichophyton* and *Microsporum* species. They are effective treatments of superficial fungal infections of the skin. The undecenoates also possess some antibacterial activity which may be important in mixed bacterial and fungal infections. The undecenoates have been largely superseded by the modern topical imidazole drugs.

Pharmacokinetics

There is no information about percutaneous absorption of undecenoic acid.

Concentration–effect relationship

Therapeutic effects of the undecenoates depend on local concentration not on systemic absorption. The undecenoates are particularly useful in superficial fungal infections of the skin as they are able to penetrate the lipid barrier of the stratum corneum and penetrate to fungal elements which have infiltrated the epidermis.

Metabolism

No information is available on the metabolism of undecenoic acid.

Pharmaceutics

Undecenoic acid (US approved name undecylenic acid) is an irritant to the skin, and is generally used in mixtures with its salts in antifungal preparations.

Undecenoates are available in the UK as a cream with zinc undecenoate 20% and undecenoic acid 5% (Mycota, Boots) as an ointment with zinc undecenoate 8% with zinc naphthenate solution 8% in a water base (Tineafax, Wellcome); as a paint of methyl undecenoate 5% and propyl undecenoate 1% with boric acid 2%, salicylic acid 31% and chlorbutol 3% (Monphytol, LAB); as a spray of undecenoic acid 2.5% and dichlorophen 0.25% (Mycota, Boots), as a dusting powder of zinc undecenoate 20% and undecenoic acid 2% (Mycota, Boots), zinc undecenoate 5.8%, 2-P-chloro phenoxyethanol 1%, 1-phenoxypropan-2-ol 2% (Phytocil, Rover), and zinc undecenoate 10% (Tineafax, Wellcome), as a shampoo of undecenoic acid 1%, cetrimide 10% and phenylethylalcohol 7.5% Ceanel concentrate, (Quinoderm). The only US formulation is a foot powder with aluminium chlorohydrate Breeze Mist (Peninol). Undecenoate preparations should be kept at temperatures not exceeding 30°C and should not be frozen. Preparations have a very long shelf-life.

Therapeutic use

Indications

1. The treatment of superficial fungal infections of the skin
2. The treatment of onychomycosis
3. As an insect repellant.

Contraindications

1. Contact allergy to undecenoic acid or its salts.

Mode of use

Creams, ointments, powders and sprays should be used after washing the area, once to twice daily for 2–4 weeks. The powders can be used after application of the cream, ointment or spray, or may be used by themselves in the prophylaxis of fungal infection of the feet or groin.

Indications

1. Superficial fungal infections of the skin

Undecenoic acid has strong in vivo and in vitro[7] antifungal properties, which provide the basis of its therapeutic use. The acid itself is irritant to the skin in concentration over 2%, and most preparations use the salts of undecenoic acid with or without the acid itself. The undecenoates are active against a large variety of fungi including the common dermatophyte pathogens *Epidermophyton*, *Trichophyton* and *Microsporum* species. The undecenoates are fungistatic at therapeutic levels but are fungicidal at higher concentrations.

Undecenoic acid is also bacteriostatic and has been shown to inhibit the growth of *Streptococcus pyogenes*, *Staphylococcus aureus*, *Pseudomonas aeruginosa* and *Candida albicans*. This may be of therapeutic importance in tinea pedis and tinea cruris where a concomitant bacterial infection may also be present.

2. Onychomycosis

A paint containing methyl or propyl esters of undecenoic acid with 31% salicylic acid and 2% boric acid (Monophytol) has been formulated for the treatment of tinea unguum. This is painted onto the nail bed four times daily following removal of as much of the infected nail as possible. Reported success with this paint has been published.[8] The use of 40% urea cream to chemically remove nails affected by onychomycosis with a topical imidazole will probably supersede this paint.

3. Insect repellant
Undecenoic acid is a very effective insect repellant, but its rancid smell limits its clinical use.

Contraindications

1. Contact allergy to the undecenoates
Although rare, contact allergy does occur to the undecenoates. This presents as an intensely itchy vesicular eruption following the use of the preparation. In a survey of 268 patients who were allergic to antifungal preparations, only 3% showed positive patch tests to undecenoic acid.[5] Selective allergy to only one undecenoate salt has been reported, with a patient showing positive patch tests to potassium undecenoate but not to the acid or other salts.[6]

Adverse reactions

Potentially life-threatening effects
No serious toxicity has been reported with the undecenoates.

Acute overdosage
Overdose by topical treatment has not been reported.

Severe or irreversible adverse effects
No effects of these kinds have been reported with the topical use of undecenoates.

Symptomatic adverse effects
Undecenoic acid is an irritant to the skin and even in the low concentration used in most preparations, may cause burning in inflamed or broken skin.

Interference with clinical pathology tests
No technical interferences of this type have been described.

High risk groups

Undecenoates can be safely used for superficial fungal infections of the skin in all age groups and during pregnancy.

Drug interactions

Potentially hazardous interactions
No adverse drug interactions of this kind have been reported.

Potentially useful interactions
No therapeutically useful interactions with other drugs have been reported.

Major outcome trials

1. Chretien J H, Esswein J G, Shape L M, Kiely J J, Lyddon F E 1980 Efficacy of undecenoic acid–zinc undecylenate powder in culture positive tinea pedis. International Journal of Dermatology 19: 51–54

151 patients with tinea pedis participated in a double-blind controlled study to investigate the efficacy of a powder preparation containing zinc undecylenate 20% and undecenoic acid 2% versus a placebo powder. KOH confirmation of fungus infection was an entry requirement. Erythema and scaling were significantly improved by therapy with the active preparation.

Other double blind studies

a. Smith E B, Powell R F, Graham J L, Ulrich J A 1977 Topical undecenoic acid in tinea pedis: a new look. International Journal of Dermatology 16: 52–56
b. Tschen E H, Becker L E, Ulrich J A, Hoge W H, Smith E B 1979 Comparison of over-the-counter agents for tinea pedis. Cutis 23: 696–698
c. Fuerst J F, Cox G F, Weaver S M, Duncan W C 1980 Comparison between undecylenic acid and tolnaftate in the treatment of tinea pedis. Cutis 25: 544–547

103 patients with tinea pedis were entered into a double-blind controlled study comparing undecylenic acid ointment (undecylenic acid 5%, zinc undecylenate 20%) with tolnaftate cream 1% and placebo (ointment base). Both agents were significantly superior to placebo, but not significantly different from each other. It would appear that there is a trend in favour of undecylenic acid preparation.

Undecenoic acid

Uncontrolled studies

1. Sulzberger M B, Kanot A 1946 Comparative evaluation of preparations for the prophylaxis and treatment of fungus infections of feet. US Navy Medical Bulletin 46: 822–833
2. Shapiro A L, Rothman S 1945 Undecylenic acid in the treatment of dermatomycosis. Arch Dermatol Syphilol 52: 166–171
3. Sullivan M, Fishbein H A 1948 Field trial of United States Army fungicidal ointment. Journal of Investigative Dermatology 10: 293–299

General review articles

Lyddon F E, Gundersen K, Malbach H 1980 Short chain fatty acids in the treatment of dermatophytoses. International Journal of Dermatology 19: 24–28

Muskatblit E 1947 Clinical evaluation of undecylenic acid as a fungicide. Arch Dermatol Syphilol 56: 256–263

Sulzberger M B, Karof A 1947 Undecylenic and propionic acids in the penetration and treatment of dermatophytosis. Arch Dermatol Syphilol 55: 391–395

Battistini F, Cordiro C, Urcuyo F G, Rojs R F, Ollague W, Zaias N 1983 The treatment of dermatophytoses of the skin: a comparison of undecylenic acid and its salt tolnoftate. International Journal of Dermatology 6: 388–389

References

1. Stedman R 1950 Antifungal agents and antimycotic therapy. Bulletin of the National Formulary Committee 18: 9–10
2. Wong E, Grant D 1984 Antifungal agents — uses in athletes foot. On Cont Pract 11: 2–6
3. Keeney E L, Lankford E, Ajello L 1945 The bacteriostatic and bacteriocidal effects of fatty acid salts on bacteria in broth culture. Bulletin of Johns Hopkins Hospital 77: 437–438
4. Gelfarb M, Leider M 1960 Allergic eczematous contact dermatitis. Arch Dermatol Syphilol 82: 642–643
5. Pankoke 1964 Iatrogene kartaktallergic geger antimycotica. Arch Klin Exp Dermatol 219: 555–557
6. Rogers S, Shatin H 1952 Dermatitis venenata due to potassium undecylenate. Archives of Dermatology 66: 289
7. Peck S M, Rosenfeld H 1958 The effects of hydrogen ion concentration, fatty acids and vitamin C on the growth of fungi. Journal of Investigative Dermatology 1: 237–265
8. Roberton J A 1973 Report on the use of 'Monphytal'. Chiropody Revue 34: 13–16

Urea (topical)

Urea is used as a topical treatment for dry skin and ichthyosis, and as a moisturizer of the skin.

Chemistry

Urea (carbonyldiamide, carbamide, ureum, Aquadrate, Calmurid, Nutraplus)
CH_4N_2O
Carbamide

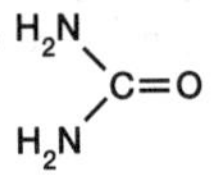

Molecular weight	60.06
pKa	0.2
Solubility	
in alcohol	1 in 10–12
in water	1 in 1
Octanol/water partition coefficient	low

Urea is a white, crystalline, odourless, stable and solid powder with a rather cool, flat taste. It is prepared by chemical synthesis. Creams containing urea are generally white to off-white with a characteristic mild odour. Urea is also available in a topical combination with 1% hydrocortisone (Alphaderm, Calmurid HC, Sential) and with dithranol 0.1%, 0.2% or 0.4% (Psoradate).

Pharmacology

Topical urea is bacteriostatic, bacteriocidal, fungistatic, proteolytic, hygroscopic and has mild local anaesthetic properties. These actions are dose dependent. Most of its therapeutic applications depend on its hygroscopic properties.

Toxicology

Topical urea is a well-established treatment in dermatology and has been used for decades without any reported toxicity. The irritant effect of some topical preparations has been ascribed to the low pH of the carrier medium.[1] There is no evidence of contact allergic reactions to urea.[2] Topical urea has been shown to have an effect on the cell kinetics of the skin by inhibiting division of the basal keratinocytes.[3] This effect is maximal within 6 weeks of starting treatment and leads to a thinning of the stratum corneum.[4] There is no evidence that this activity is progressive and there are no reported cases of skin atrophy following long-term use. No toxicological testing has been performed in animals and there is no information concerning any possible teratogenic or carcinogenic potential.

Clinical pharmacology

Topical urea is a potent hydrating agent in the skin, which provides the basis for its modern clinical use. This is mediated by its hygroscopic properties and its ability to cause configurational change in proteins in the stratum corneum. A 10% urea cream has been shown to increase the water-holding capacity of ichthyotic scale by 100% after 3 weeks treatment.[5,6]

At concentrations of 40%, urea is bacteriocidal and has historically been used extensively in the treatment of infected skin ulcers where it also acts as a debriding agent and a deodorizer for stinking foul lesions.[7] This application has been largely superceded by modern antibiotics and debriding agents. In concentrations of 10%, urea is bacteriostatic and fungistatic. This is probably of no therapeutic importance, but makes the addition of preservatives to urea-containing creams unnecessary.

At concentrations of 40%, urea is proteolytic and keratolytic.[8] The keratolytic effect remains the basis for the use of 40% urea creams in the chemical removal of nails in onychomycoses.[9]

48% urea is a very effective accelerant of skin penetration, probably by increasing the hydration of the stratum corneum.[10] This has been used as the rationale for combination creams, containing urea with 1% hydrocortisone or urea with dithranol. Urea has a mild local anaesthetic effect at concentrations of 20% to 40%, which is thought to explain its antipruritic properties.[11] In a double-blind study, 20% urea was found to be more effective than 0.5% hydrocortisone in suppressing trypsin-induced itch and was found to be clinically effective in patients with pruritus of various aetiologies.[12]

Pharmacokinetics

There is no information available about percutaneous absorption of urea.

Concentration–effect relationship

Therapeutic effects depend on local concentration, not on systemic absorption of the drug.

Metabolism

If absorbed, urea would be excreted unchanged in the urine.

Pharmaceutics

1. Aquadrate (Norwich Eaton, UK): 10% urea w/w in a specially formulated base which fulfils the functions of both an ointment and a cream.
2. Calmurid (Pharmacia, UK)/Carmol 20 (Syntex, USA): urea 10% and lactic acid 5% in a water-miscible base.
3. Nutraplus (Alcon, UK): urea 10% in a water-miscible base.
4. Ureacin-20, Ureacin-40 (Pedinol, USA): creams containing 20% and 40% urea. They are formulated in a vegetable oil base.

Combination creams are also available:

5. Alphaderm (Norwich Eaton, UK): urea 10% w/w and hydrocortisone 1% w/w in a specially formulated base which fulfils the functions of both an ointment and a cream.
6. Calmurid HC (Pharmacia, UK)/Carmol HC (Syntex, USA): urea 10% with lactic acid 5% and hydrocortisone 1% in a water-miscible base.
7. Psoradrate (Norwich Eaton, UK): urea 17% and dithranol 0.1%, 0.2% or 0.4% in a specially formulated base.
8. Amino-Cerv (Milex, USA): urea 8.34%. Methionine 0.83% and cystine 0.35% together with inositol, sodium proprionate and benzylalkonium chloride.
9. Carmol 10 (Syntex, USA)/Gly-Oxide (Marion, USA)/Ureacin (Pedinol, USA): a 10% lotion.
10. Debrox (Marion, USA): eardrops containing 6.5% carbamide peroxide.
11. Panafil (Rystam, USA): an ointment containing 10% urea and 10% papain.

Urea-based creams do not contain contact sensitiser.
Urea-based creams have a shelf-life of 2 years. Aquadrate should be stored at a temperature below 30°C; Alphaderm at below 25°C and Psoradate should be stored in a cool place, 6–15°C.

Therapeutic use

Indications

1. The treatment of ichthyosis and dry skin conditions
2. The management of eczemas
3. The management of psoriasis
4. The management of skin ulceration
5. The treatment of pruritus
6. The treatment of onychomycoses
7. The treatment of black hairy tongue.

Contraindications

1. Hypersensitivity
2. Bacterial, viral and fungal diseases (if urea is combined with a steroid).

Mode of use

Urea-containing creams are best used on optimally hydrated skin, and thus should be used after a bath. The creams should be liberally applied and allowed to dry into the skin rather than being rubbed into the skin. As the creams are very water soluble, creams should be reapplied after washing or water contact with the skin. Urea creams can be used several times a day, but a minimum of twice a day is necessary.

Combination creams containing hydrocortisone should be used twice daily in combination with an emollient, and avoiding broken skin. Combination creams containing dithranol should be used once daily taking care only to apply them to involved skin, and protecting clothing from contact with the cream, which could otherwise cause staining.

Indications

1. Ichthyosis and dry skin conditions
The modern therapeutic use of urea depends on its moisturizing effect on the skin. It is used in the treatment of dry skin conditions and the genetically determined ichthyoses. Urea 10% has been shown to be a very effective treatment of the milder ichthyoses, particularly the X-linked and dominant ichthyosis vulgaris,[5,13] and in these conditions has been shown to be as effective as 1% hydrocortisone[14] and more effective than simple emollients and salicylic acid BP.[13]

The use of urea creams in palmo-plantar hyperkeratosis is more controversial. Two studies have reported good therapeutic response using 10% urea creams in patients with hyperkeratosis of palms or feet,[15] and in a patient with congenital tylosis.[16] A double-blind study in 55 patients, however, failed to show that 10% urea (Calmurid) was any more effective than aqueous cream in the treatment of hyperkeratosis.[17]

2. Eczemas
Creams containing 10% urea have been shown to be very effective in controlling the ichthyotic stage of atopic dermatitis.[14]

Combination creams containing urea and hydrocortisone or 0.1% betamethasone valerate have been shown to be more effective than the steroid cream alone in the treatment of subacute and chronic eczemas.[16] Urea-containing creams may be irritant if applied to broken or exudative skin.

3. Psoriasis
Urea creams are of little therapeutic value in psoriasis, but combination creams containing urea and dithranol 0.1% or 0.2% are effective treatments. This is thought to be due to the increased penetration of the skin mediated by the increased hydration of the stratum corneum by the urea. A 0.4% cream is available for use in patients with a high tolerance to dithranol.

4. Skin ulceration
Historically, concentrated urea solutions have been used as soaks in the treatment of leg ulcers.[7] This relies on the antimicrobial activity of the solution and its proteolytic properties. It is particularly useful in 'dirty' ulcers, where it also deodorizes the ulcer. The effect of urea soaks on 'clean ulcers' is insignificant.

5. Pruritus
20% urea solutions have been shown to have an antipruritic action, probably mediated via its local anaesthetic properties. In trypsin-induced pruritus, 20% urea solution reduced itch duration by more than 20%, and was more effective than 0.5% hydrocortisone. Fifteen patients treated with 20% urea solution for generalized pruritus showed a good clinical response with relief of itch in all but one patient in whom urticaria was the underlying cause of the pruritus.[12]

6. Onychomycosis
The onychomycoses present a difficult therapeutic problem, as systemic treatment needs to continue for up to 2 years. The use of 40% urea by itself as a method of chemical evulsion of the nail, or in combination with a topical imidazole has been shown to be an effective treatment in these patients.[9] The urea is applied to the nail after painting the surrounding skin with Tinct Benz Co and a polythene occlusive dressing is placed over. The dressing is left in place for 1–2 weeks and then removed. The nail becomes soft and can be peeled off using artery forceps. Further treatment of the nail bed with a topical imidazole is recommended. The basis for this application is the keratolytic activity of the urea.

7. Black hairy tongue
A 40% urea solution applied to the tongue daily using a toothbrush daily, has been reported as being an effective treatment for black hairy tongue.[18]

Adverse reactions

Potentially life-threatening effects
No serious toxicity has been reported with topical urea. Historically it is considered a very safe drug.

Acute overdosage
Overdose by topical treatment has not been reported; and ingestion in large amounts is most unlikely.

Severe or irreversible adverse effects
No severe adverse effects have been reported with the use of topical urea.

Symptomatic adverse effects
Topical urea has been shown to cause burning and irritation if applied to inflamed, broken or exudative skin eruptions.

Interference with clinical pathology tests
No technical interferences of this kind have been reported.

High risk groups

Topical urea can be used in all age groups and during pregnancy and lactation, although few animal reproduction studies have been made.

Drug interactions

Potentially hazardous interactions
No drug interactions of this kind have been reported.

Potentially useful interactions
The addition of 10% urea to topical steroids and dithranol has been shown to enhance the action of these drugs. This is thought to be mediated by the increased hydration of the stratum corneum by the urea which aids percutaneous absorption of the drug.

Major outcome trials

1. Pope F M, Rees J K, Wells R S, Lewis K G S 1977 Outpatient treatment of ichthyosis: a double-blind trial of ointments. British Journal of Dermatology 86: 291–296

This double-blind controlled trial compared oily cream BP, salicylic acid ointment BP, urea cream (Calmurid) and Boots E45 cream in the treatment of ichthyosis vulgaris or X-linked ichthyosis. 84 patients were entered into the trial and were examined by three clinicians before and 2 weeks after treatment. Severity of disease was recorded and showed no bias in the urea-treated group.

Patient assessment showed no statistical difference between the ointments. Clinicians' assessment however showed a significantly better action of the urea cream in controlling the ichthyosis. No side effects for the urea cream were noted.

Other controlled trials

1. Grice K, Sattar H, Baker H 1973 Urea and retinoic acid in ichthyosis and their effect on transepidermal water loss and water holding capacity of stratum corneum. Acta Dermato-Venereologica 53: 114–118

This double-blind control trial compared a 10% urea cream (Calmurid) with its base, in the treatment of ichthyosis. 14 patients with ichthyosis vulgaris and X-linked ichthyosis were entered in the trial.

Patients were examined before and 3 weeks after treatment.

Significant clinical improvement was noted at sites treated with urea cream compared with those treated with base. No side effects were noted.

Examination of transepidermal water loss and water holding capacity of the stratum corneum before and after treatment showed a slight but significant reduction in the transepidermal water loss following treatment. However, urea caused a very highly significant increase in the water-holding capacity of the stratum corneum.

2. Fredrikson T, Gip L 1975 Urea cream in the treatment of dry skin and hand dermatitis. International Journal of Dermatology 14: 442–444

In this randomized double-blind control trial, two urea-containing creams of pH3 (Calmurid) and of pH6 (Aquacare) were compared in the treatment of 30 ichthyotic atopics and 30 hand eczemas. The creams were used twice daily and patients evaluated at 2 and 4 weeks. 13 patients treated with Calmurid complained of burning upon application. No patients treated with Aquacare reported side effects. Both creams proved effective treatments for both ichthyosis and hand dermatitis, but Aquacare showed statistically significantly better efficiency and patient preference compared with Calmurid.

Uncontrolled studies

1. Hindson T C 1971 Urea in the topical treatment of atopic eczema. Archives of Dermatology 104: 284–285
2. Rattner H 1943 Uses of urea in hand creams. Archives of Dermatology and Syphilology 48: 47–49

General review articles

Aaron H 1973 Urea for the treatment of dry skin. Medical Letters on Drugs and Therapeutics 15: 104

Ashton H, Frisk E, Stevenson C J 1971 Therapeutics XIII. Urea as a topical agent. British Journal of Dermatology 84: 194–196

Anon. 1971 Calmurid: a urea cream for the skin. Drugs and Therapeutics Bulletin 9: 29–30

Fisher A A 1977 Irritant reactions from topical urea preparations used for dry skin. Advantages of a urea-free 'Dead Sea Salt' cream. Cutis 18: 761–772

Rubin J 1976 Urea as a moisturiser. Cosmetic Toiletries 91: 59–60

Zuehlke R L 1974 Recent therapeutic advances for common cutaneous problems. American Family Physician 9: 70–74

Beare M J 1971 Advances in the treatment of diseases of the skin. Practitioner 207: 450–459

Swanbeck G 1972 Treatment of dry hyperkeratotic itchy skin with urea containing preparations. Dermatology Digest 11: 39–44

References

1. Fredrikson T, Grip L 1975 Urea creams in the treatment of dry skin and hand dermatitis. International Journal of Dermatology 14: 442–444
2. Rattner H 1943 Use of urea in hand creams. Archives of Dermatology and Syphilology 48: 47–49
3. Wohrab W, Schiemann S 1976 Untersuchungen zum mechanisms der Harnstoff Wirkung auf die Haut. Archives of Dermatological Research 255: 23–30
4. Blair C 1976 The action of urea–lactic acid ointment in ichthyosis. British Journal of Dermatology 94: 145–153
5. Grice K, Sattar H, Baker H 1973 Urea and retinoic acid in ichthyosis and their effect on transepidermal water loss and water-holding capacity of the stratum corneum. Acta Dermato-Venereologica 53: 114–118
6. Swanbeck G 1968 A new treatment of ichthyosis and other hyperkeratotic conditions. Acta Dermato-Venereologica 48: 123–127
7. Kligman A M 1957 Dermatologic uses of urea. Acta Dermato-Venereologica 37: 155–159
8. Ramsden W 1902 Some new properties of urea. Journal of Physiology (suppl) 28: 23–26
9. Nolting S 1984 Non-traumatic removal of the nail and simultaneous treatment of onycomycosis. Dermatologica 169 (suppl) 117
10. Allenby A C, Creasey N H, Edginton J A G, Fletcher J A, Schock C 1969 Mechanism of action of accelerants on skin penetration. British Journal of Dermatology 81 (suppl 4): 47–55
11. Bankoff G 1943 The practice of local anaesthesia. William Heinemann Medical Books Ltd, London, p 23
12. Swanbeck G, Rajka G 1970 Anti-pruritic effect of urea solution. Acta Dermato-Venereologica 50: 225–227
13. Pope F M, Rees J K, Wells R S, Lewis K G S 1977 Outpatient treatment of ichthyosis: a double blind trial of ointments. British Journal of Dermatology 86: 291–296
14. Stewart W D, Danto J C, Maddin W S 1969 Urea cream. Cutis 5: 1241–1242
15. Roston M 1970 The treatment of ichthyosis and hyperkeracotic conditions with urea. Australian Journal of Dermatology 11: 142–144

16. Hindson T C 1971 Urea in the topical treatment of atopic eczema. Archives of Dermatology 104: 284–285
17. General Practitioners Research Group 1973 Carbonide in hyperkeratosis. Practitioner 210: 294
18. Pegum J S 1971 Urea in the treatment of black hairy tongue. British Journal of Dermatology 84: 602

U

Urofollitrophin

Urofollitrophin is a preparation of gonadotrophin extracted from human menopausal urine, which possesses follicle stimulating hormone, but not luteinizing hormone, activity.

Chemistry

Urofollitrophin (Metrodin)

Follicle stimulating hormone is a glycopeptide and consists of two chains of amino acids. The α chain contains between 89 and 92 amino acids, and its functional part is shared by other glycopeptides (LH, TSH and HCG). The β chains differ in both amino acid and carbohydrate content and thus determine the action of the glycoprotein. The α and β chains are linked by disulphide bonds. The molecular weight of FSH is approximately 33 000, the β chain having a molecular weight of 14 000. The total molecular weight varies largely due to the carbohydrate moiety, although about 70 isoforms of FSH with slightly altered structure and amino acid sequences have been isolated from urine.

Each ampoule of urofollitrophin contains a white freeze-dried powder which requires reconstitution with sodium chloride prior to administration.

Pharmacology

Urofollitrophin acts directly on FSH receptors, which are found mainly in the ovary and the testis and thus influences gametogenesis and steroidogenesis. In sexually immature animals, preparations containing FSH have been shown to increase gonadal weight.[1] Urofollitrophin binds specifically to FSH receptors in the granulosa cells and Sertoli cells and activates adenylate cyclase which converts ATP to cyclic AMP and turns on protein kinases. These in turn control cholesterol ester turnover and cholesterol side-chain cleavage reaction. The drug has very little (<1%) LH activity.

Toxicology

Urofollitrophin has been shown to be devoid of acute toxicity and doses of up to 150 000 $i.u.kg^{-1}$ FSH body weight in mice have failed to demonstrate any teratogenic effects.

Clinical pharmacology

In daily doses, varying from 75 i.u. upwards, urofollitrophin has been demonstrated to produce follicular growth in the ovary in hypogonadotrophic individuals.[2] These changes stimulate steroidogenesis, with granulosa cell production of oestradiol-17β and the subsequent widespread action of this hormone. Increasing response is usual with increasing doses, and gonadal stimulation is most marked in the ovary. Receptor saturation leads to increased follicular recruitment and growth, a response used in superovulation associated with in vitro fertilization programmes.

Pharmacokinetics

Urofollitrophin can be assayed either by radioimmunoassay[3] or by radioligand-receptor assay. The sensitivity of the assay[4] is 0.3 $i.u.l^{-1}$. Urofollitrophin is administered by intramuscular injection and in a recent study, a mean half life of 24.6 hours was obtained after injecting healthy males with 150 i.u.[5] The drug is metabolized in the liver and the products are excreted in urine, although precise details of the metabolic processes are lacking. Urinary recovery of unchanged FSH using RRA is between 6.8 and 10.2%,[7] with the maximum recovery at 48 hours and all trace of FSH disappears by the 6th day. The renal clearance[8] has been determined at 0.57 $ml.min^{-1}$.

Concentration–effect relationship

There is no specific information about the relationship between plasma concentration and effect.

Metabolism

FSH is extensively metabolized by the liver with only a small proportion (6.8–10.2%) excreted unchanged in the urine. It is believed that after removal of the sialic acid (desialylation) in the liver[6] the drug is rapidly cleared from the circulation.

Pharmaceutics

Urofollitrophin (Serono UK, US) is available only in parenteral form for intramuscular injection.

The UK and US proprietary name is Metrodin. In Europe each ampoule contains 75 i.u. of FSH, less than 1 i.u. of LH and 10 mg of lactose, and is a freeze-dried white powder. Each ampoule is accompanied by an ampoule of solvent, sodium chloride injection BP which must be mixed with the urofollitrophin prior to administration. When reconstituted, it is stable for 20 days at less than 7°C and for 14.5 days at 25°C. In the freeze-dried form, the shelf-life is 2 years when stored below 25°C and protected from light and moisture.

Therapeutic use

Indications

1. Induction of ovulation in all WHO Group II patients including polycystic ovarian syndrome
2. Induction of superovulation in in-vitro fertilization programmes.

Contraindications

1. Ovarian dysgenesis
2. Ovarian failure
3. Presence of ovarian cysts.

Mode of use

Urofollitrophin therapy is designed to induce the development of a mature follicle which can be released by either an endogenous LH surge or the administration of human chorionic gonadotrophin (hCG). The therapy begins during the early follicular phase and continues until follicular growth is complete. The dose–response is very variable and must be individualized. However, few physicians would use more than 750 i.u. daily.

Indications

1. Induction of ovulation in all Group II patients including polycystic ovarian syndrome

It is uncertain as to the primary defect in polycystic ovarian syndrome, but the fault probably lies in the ovary. The defect seems to be in aromatase activity which is decreased and thus there is a low conversion rate of androgens to oestradiol. The elevated circulating androgens are therefore peripherally converted to oestrone which exerts a positive feedback on the hypothalamic–pituitary axis, decreasing FSH release and increasing LH secretion. The follicular growth is interfered with and follicles are unable to reach maturity.[9]

Therapy in the first instance is with clomiphene citrate and only those patients who fail to respond should be considered for urofollitrophin therapy. This may be administered by one of two regimes, both however, requiring intense patient monitoring.

The alternate day regime involves intramuscular injection of urofollitrophin on alternate days beginning on the third day of menstruation, at an initial dose of 225 i.u. This is continued for 3 doses and the response is judged by elevation of oestradiol and ultrasound examination of the ovaries. If the response has been suitable, hCG 10 000 i.u. is administered intramuscularly, 48 hours later, in the hope of releasing a mature oocyte. If the response has been inadequate, the dose should be increased by 75–150 i.u. and after a further 2 or 3 doses, the response reassessed. The dosage may be increased further if appropriate. Care must be taken to avoid hyperstimulation, and any signs should lead to cessation of therapy.

On the daily regime, therapy is commenced on day 3 of the menses, but at a much lower dose, 75–150 i.u. and after 5 days, the ovarian response assessed. A poor response may be countered by increasing the dose until the response is adequate, with the administration of HCG, 10 000 i.u. at the appropriate time.

The decision on the response varies but the recommendation is a maximum of 2 follicles and an oestradiol level between 1100 and 1500 $ng.l^{-1}$. It is usual to check the progesterone level 7 days after hCG injection to ensure an adequate luteal phase response.

The results of therapy have been summarized in Table 1.[10–20] None of the studies is large, or well controlled enough to reliably predict cumulative pregnancy rates.

Table 1 Summary of therapy results

Number of patients	142
Number of treatment cycles	304
Age range (years)	20–38
Previous therapy	all clomiphene failures
Dose regime	days 3–7, daily doses
(commencing day 3 of menses)	days 3–8, alternate days
Number of ovulatory cycles	245 (80.6%)
Number of pregnancies	51 (35.9%)

2. Induction of superovulation in IVF programmes
Human menopausal gonadotrophin has been used extensively to superovulate the ovaries to facilitate multiple oocyte maturation and retrieval. Urofollitrophin has also been used in this way and has been shown to be equally effective,[21] both in combination with clomiphene citrate and without, and also by intermittent chronic administration via a pump. The regimes are usually fixed at 150 i.u. daily with 50–100 mg of clomiphene citrate, for 5 days beginning on the 2nd or 3rd day of the cycle. Depending on the response after this dose, further increases may ensue to achieve the maximum response.

Contraindications

1. Ovarian dysgenesis
In conditions when there is anomalous development of the ovary, and no primordial follicles exist, there is no place for the administration of the drug.

2. Ovarian failure
Urofollitrophin has no value in those patients whose ovaries have prematurely failed and there are no remaining follicles.

3. Presence of ovarian cyst
As these may enlarge on FSH stimulation, urofollitrophin must not be administered in their presence.

Adverse reactions

Potentially life-threatening effects
Deaths have occurred from hyperstimulation syndrome following gonadotrophin therapy. This is a rare occurrence, and the main clinical features are ovarian enlargement, abdominal distension and weight gain. In severe cases, ascites, pleural effusion, electrolyte imbalance, hypovolaemia, hypotension and oliguria may develop. The basic problem is a shift of fluid from the intravascular into the abdominal cavity, the reason being unclear.

Treatment is conservative and empirical in a hospital environment. Pelvic and abdominal examination are contraindicated in view of the risk of ovarian rupture. The hyperstimulation syndrome usually regresses with time, approximately 7 days. The syndrome will not develop unless hCG has been given and therefore, high levels of oestradiol, in spite of the ultrasound findings is a contraindication to its administration.

The incidence of severe hyperstimulation syndrome in the reported series[10–20] was 2 in 287 cycles (0.7%), but mild–moderate hyperstimulation occurred in 54 of 287 cycles (19.1%).

Acute overdosage
The form of the preparation makes self-administered overdosage extremely unlikely, and no case has been reported.

Urofollitrophin

Severe or irreversible adverse effects
Only the hyperstimulation syndrome previously described is in any way serious.

Symptomatic adverse effects
These have been reported in less than 1 in 50 patients, and include gastrointestinal disturbances (nausea, vomiting, diarrhoea, colic and bloating), headache and breast tenderness. Febrile reactions have been reported with associated malaise and fatigue, and pain and tenderness at the site of injection. It is not clear whether these are pyogenic responses or possible allergic reactions. Dermatological sequelae such as dry skin, rash, hair loss and urticaria have been reported.

Other effects
No biochemical disturbance has been reported except in hyperstimulation syndrome. Here, there is a hypovolaemia which leads to decreased renal perfusion and increased sodium and water reabsorption. There is, therefore, a decrease in the exchange of hydrogen and potassium for sodium resulting in a hyperkalaemic acidosis. Elevated levels of urea also result.

Interference with clinical pathology tests
There is no effect on clinical assays.

High risk groups

Neonates
Not applicable.

Breast milk. Not applicable.

Children
Not applicable.

Pregnant women
Not applicable.

The elderly
Not applicable.

Drug interactions

There are no drug interactions reported.

Major clinical trials

1. Sallam H, Scammell G, Masson G et al 1986 Ovulation and pregnancy after 'pure' FSH in sclerocystic ovarian change. Presented at 11th World Congress of Gynecology, Berlin (W) Sept 15–20 1985

This was a prospective, multi-centre trial of 31 patients with polycystic ovarian syndrome who had failed to respond to clomiphene citrate or human menopausal gonadotrophin. Ovulation occurred in 91 out of 113 cycles and 10 women conceived. Mild hyperstimulation occurred in 12 cycles and moderate hyperstimulation in three. The previously elevated LH/FSH ratio fell during therapy.

The authors conclude that 'pure' FSH seems an effective and safe therapy for the induction of ovulation in women with polycystic ovarian syndrome, with a pregnancy rate of 30%.

2. Garcea N, Campo S, Panetta V et al 1985 Induction of ovulation with purified urinary follicle stimulating hormone in patients with polycystic ovarian syndrome. American Journal of Obstetrics and Gynecology 151: 635–640

Urofollitrophin was used in 18 patients with polycystic ovarian syndrome, and ovulation was induced in 39 of 43 treatment cycles. Hyperstimulation occurred in 9 cycles, and 9 patients conceived, giving a pregnancy rate of 50%. The authors again conclude that purified urinary follicle-stimulating hormone is a valid therapy for induction of ovulation in patients with polycystic ovaries, and with no increased risk of hyperstimulation over other gonadotrophin preparations.

3. Russell J B, Polan M L, DeCherney A H 1986 The use of pure follicle stimulating hormone for ovulation induction in normal ovulatory women in an in vitro fertilization program. Fertility and Sterility 45: 829–833

This was a prospective study to compare the use of urofollitrophin with human menopausal gonadotrophins (menotrophin). The study included 14 patients who were randomly allocated urofollitrophin and 9 patients on the menotrophin regime. Apart from these variables, the patient therapy was identical. The peak levels of oestradiol on the day of human chorionic gonadotrophin administration was similar and the oocyte recovery rate was similar (5.18: 5.00 per patient). There was no significant difference in fertilization rates but the rapid cleavage rate (26%: 4%) and the pregnancy rates (36%: 22%) were slightly higher in the urofollitrophin group. Although the numbers are small, the authors suggest that the use of urofollitrophin may be more physiological and could produce healthier oocytes and an improved pregnancy rate.

References

1. Rosenberg E, Coleman J, Gubree N, Maggillvaray W 1963 Clinical effect of urinary menopausal gonadotrophins. Journal of Clinical Endocrinology and Metabolism 23: 181–188
2. Braendle W, Sprotte C, Bettendorf G 1985 Gonadotrophin therapy in ovarian insufficiency: follicle stimulation with human urinary FSH. Geburtshilfe und Frauenheilkunde 45: 438–448
3. Diczfalusy E, Diczfalusy A 1969 Immunoassay of gonadotrophins. Acta Endocrinologica 63 (suppl 142)
4. Cheng K-W 1975 A radioreceptor assay for follicle stimulating hormone. Journal of Clinical Endocrinology and Metabolism 41: 581–585
5. Jockenhövel F, Fingscheidt S A, Khan S A, Behre H M, Nieschlag E 1990 Bio and immuno-activity of FSH in serum after intra-muscular injection of highly purified urinary human FSH in normal men. Clinical Endocrinology 33: 573–584
6. Ashwell G, Morell A G 1974 Role of surface carbohydrates in the hepatic recognition and transport of circulating glycoproteins. Advances in Enzymology 41: 99–104
7. Crooke A C, Morell M, Butt W R 1968 In: Rosenberg E (ed) Gonadotrophins. Los Altos
8. Kohler P O, Ross G T, Odell W D 1968 Metabolic clearance and production rate of human follicle stimulating hormone. Journal of Clinical Investigation 47: 38–45
9. Katz M 1981 Polycystic ovarian syndrome. Clinicals in Obstetrics and Gynaecology 8: 715–731
10. Venturoli S, Fabbri R, Paradisi R 1983 Induction of ovulation with human urinary follicle-stimulating hormone. European Journal of Obstetrics, Gynecology and Reproductive Biology 16: 135–145
11. Seibel M, McArdle C, Smith D, Taymor M 1985 Ovulation induction in polycystic ovarian syndrome with urinary follicle-stimulating hormone or human menopausal gonadotrophin. Fertility and Sterility 43: 703–706
12. Carlson J M, Siebel M, Thompson I, Berger M 1984 Chronic low-dose urinary FSH treatment for patients with polycystic ovarian disease. Fertility and Sterility 41: 668–671
13. Raj S G, Berger M, Grimes E, Taymor M 1977 The use of gonadotrophins for the induction of ovulation in women with polycystic ovarian disease. Fertility and Sterility 28: 1280–1284
14. Hoffman D, Lobo R, Campeau J et al 1985 Ovulation induction in clomiphene-resistant anovulatory women: differential follicular response to purified urinary follicle-stimulating hormone versus purifying urinary FSH and LH. Journal of Clinical Endocrinology and Metabolism 60: 922–927
15. Franks S, Polson D, Mason H 1985 Ovulation and pregnancy following low-dose pulsatile FSH in women with polycystic ovaries. Presented at American Endocrine Society Meeting 1985
16. Sallam H, Scammell G, Masson G et al 1986 Ovulation and pregnancy after 'pure' FSH in sclerocystic ovarian change. Presented at 11th World Congress of Gynecology, Berlin (W) Sept 15–20 1985
17. Gocial B, Wu C, Check J 1984 Urofollitrophin induction of ovulation in polycystic ovarian disease. Presented at 31st Annual Meeting of Society for Gynecologic Investigation, San Francisco, p 164
18. Dordoni D, Omodei U, Falsetti L, Scaglioni P, Zupi E 1984 Clomid negative polycystic ovarian syndrome: ovulation induction with pure FSH. Presented at 7th European Sterility Congress, Monte Carlo
19. Garcea N, Campo S, Panetta V et al 1985 Induction of ovulation with purified urinary follicle-stimulating hormone in patients with polycystic ovarian syndrome. American Journal of Obstetrics and Gynecology 151: 635–640
20. Flamigni C, Venturoli S, Paradisi R, Fabbri R, Porcu E, Magrini O 1985 Use of human urinary follicle-stimulating hormone in infertile women with polycystic ovaries. Journal of Reproductive Medicine 30: 184–188
21. Russell J B, Polan M L, DeCherney A H 1986 The use of pure follicle-stimulating hormone for ovulation induction in normal ovulatory women in an in-vitro fertilization program. Fertility and Sterility 45: 829–833

Urokinase

Urokinase is a plasminogen activator and is used as a thrombolytic agent. It appears to be as effective as streptokinase, but is more expensive and less widely used.

Chemistry

Urokinase (Abbokinase, Ukidan, Urokinase) is an enzyme obtained from human urine or from tissue cultures of human kidney cells. It is a polypeptide chain with two active forms of molecular weight 33 000 and 55 000. It is freely soluble in water.

Molecular weight	33 000, 55 000
pKa	—
Solubility	
in alcohol	—
in water	freely soluble
Octanol/water partition coefficient	low

Pharmacology

Urokinase is a proteolytic enzyme and its only known substrate is plasminogen. Unlike streptokinase, it acts directly on plasminogen by peptide bond cleavage at two different sites to produce the fibrinolytic enzyme plasmin.[1,2]

Toxicology

No information is available on the toxicology of this drug.

Clinical pharmacology

The administration of urokinase produces a fall in circulating plasminogen concentrations and an increase in circulating plasmin concentrations. High plasmin concentrations induce fibrinolysis and can also produce a coagulation defect, due partly to reduced levels of fibrinogen, factor V, and factor VIII, and partly to the presence of fibrin(ogen)-degradation products.[3,4]

One FIP (Féderation International Pharmaceutique) unit of urokinase hydrolyses 1 μmol of N-α-acetyl-glycyl-l-lysine methyl ester acetate per minute and is equivalent to 546 Ploug units. One Ploug unit is equivalent to 1.43 CTA (Committee on Thrombolytic Agents) units or 1.49 IU (International Units). In practice, the CTA and IU can be considered as equivalent to each other.

Although urokinase has not been studied to the same extent as streptokinase, there is no doubt that it is an effective thrombolytic agent. The extent and rate of thrombolysis that may be achieved depend on the structure, particularly the plasminogen content, of the thrombus as well as the intensity of the fibrinolytic state.[4] Older thrombi are more resistant to thrombolytic therapy.

Treatment with urokinase appears to be as effective as treatment with streptokinase. However, the two agents differ in three important respects. First, urokinase is approximately five times more expensive than streptokinase. Second, urokinase is not antigenic in man.[5] Accordingly, its use is not complicated by allergic phenomena or the presence of neutralizing antibody. This may have important implications for the treatment of patients in whom thrombolytic therapy has been used previously. Third, urokinase has a more direct mode of action.

The conventional regimen used to promote systemic thrombolysis with urokinase is a loading dose of 4400 IU.kg^{-1} given intravenously over a period of 10 minutes, followed by an infusion of 4400

$IU.kg^{-1}.h^{-1}$ for between 12 and 24 hours.[3] Urokinase may also be administered locally; for example, a thrombosed arteriovenous shunt may be reopened by instilling 5000 IU urokinase into the arterial limb of the shunt.[6]

Pharmacokinetics

Plasma concentrations of urokinase are seldom measured because if it is considered necessary to monitor the effects of treatment, it is easier and more appropriate to monitor indices such as the thrombin time, activated partial thromboplastin time, and plasma concentrations of plasminogen, plasmin, and fibrinogen.[4]

Peak fibrinolytic activity occurs approximately 2 hours after starting an infusion of urokinase.[7] After infusion urokinase is cleared from the circulation with a plasma half life of between 10 and 20 minutes.[8,9] A small proportion of the urokinase is excreted unchanged in the urine, while the majority appears to be degraded in the liver.[8,9]

Concentration–effect relationship

In contrast to streptokinase therapy, there appears to be a simple relationship between dose and effect during maintenance urokinase therapy. This is probably due to the direct mode of action of urokinase and the absence of neutralizing antibodies. Accordingly, a linear relationship[8] has been observed between plasma thrombolytic activity and the dose of urokinase for infusion rates ranging from 1000 $IU.kg^{-1}.h^{-1}$ to 10 000 $IU.kg^{-1}.h^{-1}$.

Many authorities advocate monitoring therapy by measuring the thrombin time, and trying to keep it between two and five times the normal value.[3] This will confirm activation of the fibrinolytic system, but cannot be used to predict clot lysis or haemorrhagic complications.[10] If the thrombin time becomes greatly prolonged, therapy can be discontinued until it returns to the normal range, when therapy can be restarted, perhaps at a lower dose.

Metabolism

The metabolism of urokinase, in man, is not fully understood. However, it appears that a small proportion is excreted unchanged in the urine,[8] while the majority is eliminated by hepatic metabolism.[9]

Pharmaceutics

1. Abbokinase (Abbott UK/USA): a sterile lyophilized powder obtained from tissue cultures of human kidney cells in vials of 250 000 IU with mannitol and sodium chloride.
2. Ukidan (Serono, UK): a sterile lyophilized powder obtained from human male urine in vials of 5000, 25 000 or 100 000 IU.
3. Urokinase (Leo, UK): a sterile lyophilized powder obtained from human male urine in vials containing 5000, 25 000 or 100 000 Ploug units (equivalent to approximately 7500, 37 500 or 150 000 IU, respectively).
4. A 5000 IU formulation for flushing catheters is also available as Abbokinase, Open-Cath (Abbott, USA).

Lyophilized urokinase is stable for up to 5 years at 4°C. The powder is freely soluble in water and may be reconstituted for infusion in water, 5% dextrose or physiological saline. Reconstituted material should be used within 24 hours.

Therapeutic use

Indications

1. Acute myocardial infarction
2. Acute pulmonary embolism
3. Acute deep vein thrombosis
4. Thrombosis on prosthetic materials (e.g. arterio-venous shunts, heart valves and vascular grafts)

Other uses

5. Other acute venous or arterial thrombosis
6. Vitreous haemorrhage
7. Hyphaema.

Relative contraindications

All contraindications are only relative, depending on the likely balance between benefit and risk.

Urokinase

1. Bleeding diathesis or other internal bleeding
2. Recent trauma (e.g. surgery, head injury, traumatic resuscitation)
3. Severe hypertension
4. Recent peptic ulcer
5. Recent stroke
6. Other conditions associated with an increased risk of bleeding
7. Severe renal or hepatic insufficiency.

Mode of use

All the clinical uses depend on the ability of urokinase to lyse thrombi. Several dosage regimens are in use. Urokinase may be given locally or systemically. When used systemically, thrombolysis is generally achieved by giving an intravenous loading dose followed by intravenous maintenance therapy for between 12 and 24 hours (for example, 4400 $IU.kg^{-1}$ in 10 minutes followed by 4400 $IU.kg^{-1}.h^{-1}$), although recently therapy using a single large intravenous dose (for example, 15 000 $IU.kg^{-1}$ in 10 minutes) has been reported.[11]

Indications

1. Acute myocardial infarction

Angiographic studies have shown that, in the acute phase of myocardial infarction, a substantial proportion of patients have coronary artery occlusion, and that recanalization can be achieved by using either intracoronary or intravenous thrombolytic agents. Intravenous therapy can be given far more easily — and perhaps an hour or some more promptly — than intracoronary therapy can. An overview of several trials of prolonged intravenous infusions and several large multi-centre trials of high-dose short-term infusions of different thrombolytic agents (see Major outcome trials and Streptokinase) has shown that intravenous thrombolytic therapy can reduce mortality. Although it has been suggested that, in order to prevent reocclusion, thrombolysis should be followed by some other intervention (such as anticoagulant or antiplatelet therapy, coronary angioplasty, or coronary artery bypass surgery), only antiplatelet therapy (with low-dose aspirin) has been shown to produce added benefit.[12]

2. Acute pulmonary embolism

Urokinase is used to treat patients suffering from life-threatening pulmonary embolism, with the aim of lysing clots in the pulmonary circulation (thereby reversing any haemodynamic disturbance) and lysing clots in the deep veins (thereby avoiding further embolism). Most authorities recommend an initial loading dose of 4400 $IU.kg^{-1}$ infused in 10 minutes, followed by an infusion of 4400 $IU.kg^{-1}.h^{-1}$ given into a peripheral vein or into the pulmonary artery via an indwelling catheter; both routes of administration have been shown to be effective.[13,14] Successful therapy is usually followed by a period of anticoagulation with heparin and/or warfarin. If therapy is not successful, embolectomy may be indicated.

Pulmonary angiography, right heart pressure studies, and radioisotope lung scanning have shown that, in massive embolism, the rate of dissolution of pulmonary emboli is greater in patients treated with streptokinase or urokinase than in patients treated with heparin alone.[13,15] There is no clear evidence, however, that thrombolytic therapy has any greater effect on mortality than does heparin. For, although it has been reported that patients in shock (systolic BP < 100 mmHg) have a lower mortality when treated with streptokinase, this result derives from a retrospective analysis of a non-randomized study.[16]

3. Acute deep-vein thrombosis

Reliable direct evidence about the effects of urokinase in deep-vein thrombosis is not available. But, a review of the six randomized trials comparing intravenous streptokinase with heparin in the treatment of phlebographically demonstrated acute proximal deep-vein thrombosis indicated that recanalization was achieved about four times more often with thrombolytic therapy (61.5% vs 17.6%; $2p < 0.0001$), while bleeds occurred significantly more frequently (14.0% vs 3.4%, $2p < 0.05$).[17] More recently, even better rates of thrombolysis have been reported in uncontrolled studies of an ultra high-dose streptokinase regimen, involving infusion of 6–9 million IU over six hours.[18]

4. Thrombosis on prosthetic materials
Local administration of between 5000 and 25 000 IU urokinase has been shown to be an effective method for relieving obstruction in arteriovenous shunts.[6,19] Systemic therapy with either streptokinase or urokinase has been used to treat patients with acute thrombotic obstruction of prosthetic heart valves with good results in approximately 70% of cases.[20,21]

Other uses

5. Other acute venous or arterial thrombosis
Thrombolytic therapy has been used in a wide variety of thromboembolic conditions (including central retinal vein occlusion, partial peripheral arterial occlusion, and thrombotic stroke) in which it may be of benefit. However, more information is required before these can be regarded as definite indications.

6. Vitreous haemorrhage
The intravitreal injection of between 5000 and 25 000 Ploug units of urokinase dissolved in a small (usually 0.3 ml) volume of sterile water or normal saline has been reported to produce marked objective improvement in the vision of some patients with longstanding vitreous haemorrhage.[22,23] However, some authors have reported disappointing results[24,25] and the drug's mode of action in this condition is not clear.[26]

7. Hyphaema
There is some evidence that irrigation of the anterior chamber of the eye with urokinase (5000 Ploug units dissolved in 2 ml dissolved water) may improve the outcome in some patients with traumatic hyphaema,[27,28] but this is not definitive.

Contraindications

Since urokinase therapy can induce a profound coagulation defect, it should generally be avoided in patients with a bleeding diathesis or active internal bleeding. For the same reason, conditions in which serious haemorrhagic complications may occur constitute a relative contraindication to thrombolytic therapy. These include recent trauma (e.g. surgery, head injury, traumatic cardiopulmonary resuscitation), severe hypertension, recent peptic ulceration, and recent stroke. Renal and/or hepatic insufficiency constitute a relative contraindication to urokinase therapy because the drug is excreted by these organs.

Adverse reactions

Potentially life-threatening effects
The unwanted effects of urokinase therapy are mainly due to bleeding. The incidence of bleeding appears to be similar to that following streptokinase therapy.[13] Minor bleeding (e.g. oozing from venepuncture site) is common, but serious haemorrhage (for example, bleeds requiring transfusion of more than 2 units of blood) following thrombolytic therapy is rare (perhaps just a few patients per thousand), particularly when traumatic arterial puncture is avoided.[12,13] In the event of serious haemorrhage, urokinase therapy should be stopped. Antifibrinolytic therapy (tranexamic acid, aminocaproic acid, or aprotinin) should be considered if there is evidence of persistent fibrinolytic activity in the blood. Transfusions of blood (preferably fresh) cryoprecipitate, or fresh frozen plasma may be necessary.[2,4]

There may also be an excess incidence of cerebral haemorrhage (perhaps 1–2 per 1000) in patients treated with systemic thrombolytic agents, but there does not appear to be an increase in total stroke, perhaps due to a reduction in thrombotic strokes.[12,29]

Acute overdosage
Any potentially life-threatening effects (in particular bleeding) should be dealt with as above).

Severe or irreversible adverse effects
These have been described above.

Symptomatic adverse effects
The only effect falling into this category is minor oozing of the blood from venepuncture sites.

Interference with clinical pathology tests
No technical interferences of this kind are known.

High risk groups

Neonates
The drug has rarely, if ever, been used in neonates.

Breast milk. No information is available on the presence of urokinase in breast milk.

Children
There is very little experience of urokinase therapy in children.

Pregnant women
Urokinase has been used, although pregnancy constitutes a relative contraindication.

The elderly
Although old age is often regarded as a relative contraindication to thrombolytic therapy, there is no good evidence to support this idea. Indeed, in patients with myocardial infarction the absolute benefit of thrombolytic therapy was greater in elderly subjects.[12,29]

Drug interactions

Anticoagulant therapy
Following thrombolysis, recanalized vessels (for example, coronary arteries) may be prone to reocclusion, particularly if a tight stenosis remains in the vessel. Hence, some authorities state that anticoagulant therapy should be used routinely after thrombolysis. But data from the randomized trials of thrombolytic therapy in acute myocardial infarction suggest that the effects of thrombolytic therapy on mortality and on reinfarction are about the same whether or not anticoagulant therapy is used.[12,29,30] Furthermore, anticoagulant therapy appears to increase the risk of haemorrhage following fibrinolytic therapy.[10,30,31] The benefits and risks of adding anticoagulant therapy to thrombolytic therapy are currently being assessed in several large randomized controlled trials (including G1SS1-2 and 1S1S-3).

Antiplatelet therapy
The efficacy of antiplatelet therapy, such as low-dose aspirin, following thrombolysis has recently been demonstrated.[12] Such therapy — which is far easier to give than anticoagulants (see above) — does not appear to be associated with an increased incidence of bleeding when used after thrombolytic therapy.[12,31]

Major outcome trials

1. Yusuf S, Collins R, Peto R et al 1985 Intravenous and intracoronary fibrinolytic therapy in acute myocardial infarction: overview of results on mortality, reinfarction and side effects from 33 randomised controlled trials. European Heart Journal 6: 556–585

During the past 25 years, 22 randomized trials of prolonged intravenous fibrinolytic treatment have been reported, involving a total of some 6000 patients in the acute phase of myocardial infarction. In the past two or three years, two small high-dose short-term intravenous trials and nine small intracoronary trials, involving a total of about 1000 patients have been reported. Because all these intravenous and intracoronary trials were small, their separate results appear contradictory and unreliable. But an overview of the data from these trials indicates that the prolonged intravenous regimen produces a highly significant ($22\% \pm 5\%$, $2p < 0.001$) reduction in the odds of death, and a frequency of side effects that is small in comparison with the absolute reduction in mortality. The apparent size of the reduction in mortality in the intravenous trials was similar whether anticoagulants were compulsory or optional, and, surprisingly, whether treatment was started early (<6 h from onset of symptoms) or late (generally 12–24 h). In addition, there was no evidence that urokinase was more effective than the less expensive streptokinase, or that, despite their technical complexity, the new intracoronary regimens were more effective than the intravenous regimens. But, these prolonged intravenous schedules were quite complex, which may partly explain why they are not widely used.

2. Gruppo Italiano per lo Studio della Streptochinasi nell'Infarto miocardico (GISSI)
   a) 1986 Effectiveness of intravenous thrombolytic treatment in acute myocardial infarction. Lancet i: 397–402
   b) 1987 Long-term effects of intravenous thrombolysis in acute myocardial infarction: final report of the GISSI study. Lancet ii: 871–874

Urokinase

11 806 patients were randomized within 12 hours of the onset of symptoms of myocardial infarction to receive either streptokinase (1.5 million IU in one hour) or routine coronary care (i.e. no placebo was used). The use of all other therapy, including anticoagulants and antiplatelet agents, was optional. Overall, the mortality in hospital was 18% lower in the streptokinase group (10.7% SK vs 13.0% control: $2p<0.001$). Among patients randomized 1–3 hours after the onset of pain the apparent effect was only moderately favourable (9% vs 11%; NS), and the same was true among those entering 3–12 hours after the onset of pain, 12% vs 14%; NS). In contrast, among the 10% of patients who entered within one hour, a very promising — and highly significant — difference was observed (8% vs 15%). But this early period was chosen for separate presentation only because the *apparent* effect was so extreme. Hence, the size of the benefit in the first hour may have been exaggerated by chance, and the real effect may be somewhat more moderate (perhaps as in the period 1–3 hours).

The exact assessment of side effects was complicated by the fact that no placebo was used, but three observations were still of interest. First, the excess incidence of stroke was about 1 or 2 per thousand (as suggested by the review of previous trials). Second, the incidence of pericarditis was reduced by streptokinase from 12% to 7%. Third, the incidence of non-fatal reinfarction was increased from 2% to 4%; this excess (and the reduction in mortality) was observed whether or not anticoagulants were given following fibrinolytic therapy. Later follow-up (to six months and to one year) indicates that these early differences in both mortality and reinfarction were maintained (though not significantly further increased).

3. ISIS-2 (Second International Study of Infarct Survival) Collaborative Group 1988 Randomised trial of intravenous streptokinase, oral aspirin, both or neither among 17 187 cases of suspected acute myocardial infarction: ISIS-2. Lancet ii: 349–360

17 187 patients entering 417 hospitals up to 24 hours (median 5 hours) after the onset of suspected acute myocardial infarction were randomized with placebo control, between: (i) a one-hour intravenous infusion of 1.5 million IU of streptokinase; (ii) one month of 160 mg daily enteric-coated aspirin; (iii) both active treatments; or (iv) neither. Each agent produced a highly significant reduction in 5-week vascular mortality: 791/8592 (9.2%) of patients allocated streptokinase infusion vs 1029/8595 (12.0%) of those allocated placebo infusion (odds reduction: $25\%\pm4\%$; $2p<0.0001$); 804/8587 (9.4%) vascular deaths among patients allocated aspirin tablets vs 1016/8600 (11.8%) among those allocated placebo tablets (odds reduction: $23\%\pm4\%$; $2p<0.00\,001$). The combination of streptokinase and aspirin was significantly ($2p<0.0001$) better than either agent alone. Their separate effects on mortality appeared to be additive: 343/4292 (8.0%) of patients allocated both active agents vs 568/4300 (13.2%) of those allocated neither (odds reduction: $42\%\pm5\%$; 95% confidence limits 34–50%; $2p<0.0001$). There was evidence of benefit from each agent even for patients treated late (odds reduction at 0–4, 5–12 and 13–24 hours: $35\pm6\%$, $16\pm7\%$ and $21\pm12\%$ for streptokinase alone; $25\pm7\%$, $21\pm7\%$ and $21\pm12\%$ for aspirin alone; and $53\pm8\%$, $32\pm9\%$ and $38\pm15\%$ for the combination of streptokinase and aspirin). Streptokinase was associated with excess bleeding requiring transfusion (0.5% vs 0.2%) and of confirmed cerebral haemorrhage (0.1% vs 0.01%), but with fewer other strokes (0.6% vs 0.8%). These other strokes may have included a few undiagnosed cerebral haemorrhages, but still there was no increase in total strokes (0.7% streptokinase vs 0.8% placebo infusion). Aspirin significantly reduced non-fatal reinfarction (1.0% vs 2.0%) and non-fatal stroke (0.3% vs 0.6%), and was not associated with any significant increase in cerebral haemorrhage or in bleeds requiring transfusion. An excess of non-fatal reinfarction was reported when streptokinase was used alone, but this was entirely avoided by the addition of aspirin. Those allocated the combination of streptokinase and aspirin had significantly fewer infarctions (1.8% vs 2.9%), strokes (0.6% vs 1.1%) and deaths (8.0% vs 13.2%) than those allocated neither. A median of 15 months follow up showed that the differences in vascular and in all cause mortality produced by streptokinase and by aspirin persist long term.

4. Urokinase pulmonary embolism trial. Phase 1 results: a cooperative study, 1970 Journal of the American Medical Association 214: 2163–2172

Intravenous urokinase (loading dose of 2000 CTA units per lb followed by 2000 CTA units per lb per hour given for 12 hours and followed by heparin therapy (loading dose of 75 IU per lb followed by 10 IU per lb per hour), was compared with heparin alone in a randomized trial of the treatment of acute pulmonary thromboembolism in 161 patients. At 24 hours, urokinase was associated with significantly better pulmonary angiograms (30 out of 57 patients allocated urokinase showed 'moderate' or greater improvements versus 5 of 57 patients allocated heparin alone; $2p<0.0001$), lung scans (22.1% improvement of the initial lesion vs 8.1%; $2p<0.005$), and right-sided pressure measurements. At 2 weeks, however, there were no significant differences in recurrence rates or in lung scan results. This trial was far too small to assess reliably the effect of urokinase on mortality. Bleeding was observed more frequently following urokinase, but in most cases this was not serious.

5. Urokinase–streptokinase embolism trial. Phase 2 results: a cooperative study 1974 Journal of the American Medical Association 229: 1606–1613

Intravenous urokinase (dose as in Phase 1), given for either 12 hours or for 24 hours, was compared with 24 hours of intravenous streptokinase in a randomized trial of the treatment of acute pulmonary thromboembolism in 167 patients. A control group given heparin only was not included. There were no clearly significant differences between the different urokinase regimens or between urokinase and streptokinase in terms of their effects on pulmonary angiograms, or on right-sided pressure measurements at 24 hours. Similarly, there were no significant differences in the lung scans at 24 hours (20% improvement of the initial lesion among patients allocated 12 hours of urokinase vs 29% with 24 hours of urokinase vs 19% with 24 hours of streptokinase), or at three and six months. The effects observed were of similar size to those found in Phase 1 (see above) among the urokinase-allocated patients and, hence, apparently better than heparin alone, although this provides only indirect evidence about the effects of 24-hour infusions of streptokinase and of urokinase relative to heparin.

Bleeding complications were observed with equal frequency (approximately 5%) in the three treatment groups (bleeds requiring transfusion of more than 2 units: 3/59 vs 4/54 vs 2/54). As with Phase 1 (see above), this study was too small to demonstrate reliably any differences in the effects of these treatments on mortality.

References

1. Kjeldgaard N O, Ploug J 1957 Urokinase as activator of plasminogen from human urine, II. Mechanism of plasminogen activation. Biochimica et Biophysica Acta 24: 283–289
2. Alkjaersig N, Fletcher A P, Sherry S 1958 The activation of human plasminogen: a kinetic study of activation with trypsin, urokinase, and streptokinase. Journal of Biological Chemistry 233: 86–90
3. Bell W R, Meek A G 1979 Guidelines for the use of thrombolytic agents. New England Journal of Medicine 301: 1266–1270
4. Kakkar V V, Scully M F 1978 Thrombolytic therapy. Medical Bulletin 34: 191–199
5. Genton E, Claman H N 1970 Urokinase: antigenic studies in patients following thrombolytic therapy. Journal of Laboratory and Clinical Medicine 75: 619–621
6. Hartley L C J, Ellis F G, Rendall M, Cameron J S, Ogg C S 1970 The use of urokinase in Scribner shunts. British Journal of Urology 42: 246–249
7. Marder V J, Donahue J F, Bell W R et al 1978 Changes in the plasma fibrinolytic system during urokinase therapy: comparison of tissue culture urokinase with urinary source urokinase in patients with pulmonary embolism. Journal of Laboratory and Clinical Medicine 92: 721–729
8. Fletcher A P, Alkjaersig N, Sherry S, Genton E, Hirsh J, Bachmann F 1965 The development of urokinase as a thrombolytic agent. Maintenance of a sustained thrombolytic state in man by its intravenous infusion. Journal of Laboratory and Clinical Medicine, 65: 713–731
9. Alkjaersig N, Fletcher A 1977 Metabolism or urokinase. In: Paoletti R, Sherry S (eds). Thrombosis and urokinase. Academic Press, London, pp 129–141
10. Urokinase pulmonary embolism trial. Phase 1 results: a co-operative study 1970 Journal of the American Medical Association 214: 2163–2172
11. Petitpretz P, Simmoneau G, Cerrina J et al 1984 Effect of a single bolus of urokinase in patients with life-threatening pulmonary emboli: a descriptive trial. Circulation 70: 861–866
12. ISIS-2 (Second International Study of Infarct Survival) Collaborative Group 1988 Randomized trial of intravenous streptokinase, oral aspirin, both or neither among 17 187 cases of suspected acute myocardial infarction: ISIS-2. Lancet 2: 349–360
13. Urokinase–Streptokinase Embolism Trial: Phase 2 results 1974 Journal of the American Medical Association 229: 1606–1613
14. Schwarz F, Stehr H, Zimmermann R, Manthey J, Kubler W 1985 Sustained improvement of pulmonary haemodynamics in patients at rest and during exercise after thrombolytic treatment of massive pulmonary embolism. Circulation 71: 119–123

U

15. Tibbutt D A, Davies J A, Anderson J A et al 1974 Comparison by controlled clinical trial of streptokinase and heparin in treatment of life-threatening pulmonary embolism. British Medical Journal 1: 343–347
16. Miller G A H, Hall R J C, Paneth M 1977 Pulmonary embolectomy, heparin and streptokinase. Their place in the treatment of acute massive pulmonary embolism. American Heart Journal 93: 568–574
17. Goldhaber S Z, Buring J E, Lipnick R J, Hennekens C H 1984 Pooled analysis of randomised trials of streptokinase and heparin in phlebographically documented acute deep vein thrombosis. American Journal of Medicine 76: 393–397
18. Martin M, Fiebach O 1985 Ultra high streptokinase (UHSK) infusion in chronic arterial occlusions and acute venous thrombosis. Thrombosis and Haemostasis 54: 101
19. Robinson P J, Glanville J N, Smith P H, Rosen S M 1970 Management of clotting in arteriovenous cannulae in patients on regular dialysis therapy. British Journal of Urology 42: 590–597
20. Witchitz S, Veyrat C, Moisson P, Scheinman N, Rozenstajn L 1980. Fibrinolytic treatment of thrombus on prosthetic heart valves. British Heart Journal 44: 545–554
21. Ledain L D, Ohayon J P, Lolle J P, Lorient-Roudaut F M, Roudaut R P, Besse P M 1986 Acute thrombotic obstruction with disc valve prostheses: diagnostic considerations and fibrinolytic treatment. Journal of the American College of Cardiology 7: 743–751
22. Forrester J V, Williamson J 1974 Lytic therapy in vitreous haemorrhage. Transactions of the Ophthalmological Society of the United Kingdom 94: 583–586
23. Chapman-Smith J S, Crock G W 1977 Urokinase in the management of vitreous haemorrhage. British Journal of Ophthalmology 61: 500–505
24. Cleary P E, Davies E W G, Shilling J S, Hamilton A M 1974 Intravitreal urokinase in the treatment of vitreous haemorrhage. Transactions of the Ophthalmological Society of the United Kingdom 94: 587–590
25. Holmes-Sellors P J, Kanski J J, Watson D M 1974 Intravitreal urokinase in the management of vitreous haemorrhage. Transactions of the Ophthalmological Society of the United Kingdom 94: 591–598
26. Editorial 1978 Vitreous haemorrhage. British Medical Journal 1: 940
27. Brodrick J D, Hall R D 1971 Management and prognosis of secondary hyphaema. Proceedings of the Royal Society of Medicine 64: 931–934
28. Rakusin W 1971 Urokinase in the management of traumatic hyphaema. British Journal of Ophthalmology 55: 826–832
29. Yusuf S, Collins R, Peto R et al 1985 Intravenous and intracoronary fibrinolytic therapy in acute myocardial infarction: overview of results on mortality, reinfarction and side-effects from 33 randomized controlled trials. European Heart Journal 6: 556–585
30. Gruppo Italiano per lo Studio della Streptochinasi nell' Infarto Miocardico (GISSI) 1986 Effectiveness of intravenous thrombolytic treatment in acute myocardial infarction. Lancet 1: 397–407 (and personal communication)
31. ISIS (International Studies of Infarct Survival) Pilot Study Investigators 1987 Randomized factorial trial of high-dose intravenous streptokinase, of oral aspirin, and of intravenous heparin in acute myocardial infarction. European Heart Journal 8: 634–642

Ursodeoxycholic acid

Chemistry

Ursodeoxycholic acid (Destolit, Ursofalk, URSO, Deursil, Ursocal)
$C_{24}H_{40}O_4$
3α-Hydroxy-7β-hydroxycholanoic acid

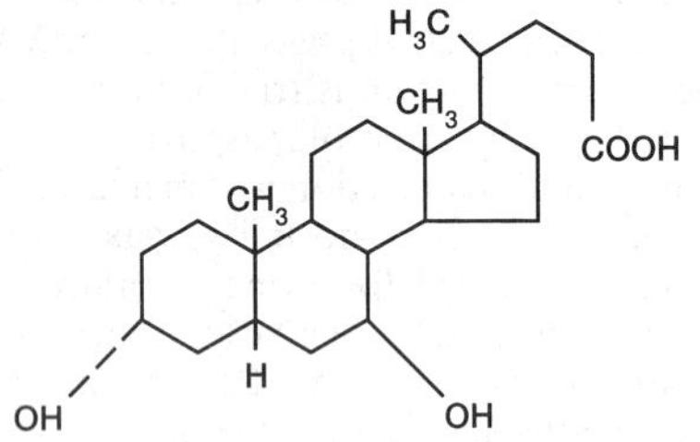

Molecular weight (free compound)	392.6
pKa (carboxylate)	5
Solubility	
in alcohol	freely soluble
in water	almost insoluble
Octanol/water partition coefficient	—

Ursodeoxycholic acid (UDCA) is a white, odourless, crystalline powder with a bitter taste; melting point 200–205°C.[1] Its pKa is 5 at infinite dilution. UDCA, the 7β epimer of chenodeoxycholic acid, is prepared chemically from chenodeoxycholic acid. Solubility of protonated UDCA is 53 μmol.l^{-1} at 37°C.[2] The solubility of UDCA increases markedly above pH 8. The critical micellar concentration (CMC) is 17 mmol.l^{-1} in water and 7 mmol.l^{-1} in 0.15 mol.l^{-1} Na^+.[3]

Pharmacology

The cholesterol saturation of bile is reduced by UDCA allowing gradual solubilization of cholesterol gallstones. Cholesterol secretion into bile is reduced and bile acid secretion rates increase during UDCA treatment[4] without a reduction in phospholipids. Total bile acid pool may be increased.[5] The rate controlling enzyme of hepatic cholesterol bile synthesis, 3-hydroxy-3-methyl glutaryl co-enzyme (HMG CoA-reductase activity) and the catabolic enzyme cholesterol 7α-hydroxylase are altered by UDCA therapy.

There is a 59% reduction in HMG. CoA-reductase activity and a 49% reduction in 7α-hydroxylase activity in vitro.[6] In clinical studies, two-fold increases to a 40% decrease in HMG CoA-reductase activity have been observed.[7,8]

It is probable that UDCA reduces cholesterol absorption[9] from the gastrointestinal tract.

Toxicology

UDCA does not have mutagenic potential and toxicological testing has demonstrated partially reversible hepatotoxicity in Rhesus monkeys in oral doses exceeding 100 mg.kg^{-1} daily.[10] Minor serum transaminase elevations in human studies are rare at pharmacological doses (less than 2% of cases).[11]

No evidence of alteration of hepatic structure has been demonstrated with UDCA either at light microscopy or at electromicrographic level.[12] Hepatotoxicity may be related to the ability of a species to sulphate the hepatotoxic metabolite, lithocholic acid.[11]

UDCA has no teratogenic effects in the mouse, rat and rabbit and does not appear to possess carcinogenetic or co-carcinogen properties.[13,14,15]

Clinical pharmacology

UDCA reduces the molar percentage of cholesterol in bile from about 9–10 mol% to 5–6 mol%. The reduction in cholesterol saturation index is dose-related.[16] Daily doses in the range 150–1000 mg have been used in early studies of gallstone dissolution, but it is now generally agreed that 8–10 mg.kg^{-1} daily taken as a single night time dosage is optimal in the non-obese patient.[11,17] Increased dosages up to 15 mg.kg^{-1} daily may be required in the obese patient. UDCA is usually prescribed in combination with chenodeoxycholic acid at a dose of 8.0 mg.kg^{-1} daily of each drug, thereby benefiting from the differing mechanism of gallstone dissolution of the two agents.

Other pharmacological effects of UDCA include a possible decrease in serum low density lipoprotein (LDL) cholesterol.[18] High density lipoprotein remains unchanged even in hyperlipidaemic patients.[11]

Pharmacokinetics

Serum concentrations of UDCA can be measured by either radioimmunoassay[19] or gas–liquid chromatography (GLC).[20] Because radioimmunoassay only measures conjugated bile salts and GLC cannot differentiate between conjugated and unconjugated bile salts, correlation between the two methods results in an underestimation of UDCA concentration by 30%, using radioimmunoassay.[21]

UDCA is passively and completely absorbed primarily in the upper intestine.[22] Time to peak serum concentration of UDCA varies from 30 minutes[23] to 150 minutes,[24] with the peak level attained being dose-related.[23] The proportion of UDCA in biliary bile acids increases linearly with dose even in patients on continuous UDCA therapy.[25]

The first-pass hepatic uptake of UDCA measured indirectly is reported as approximately 50%.[26] Direct measurements revealed an 85% recovery of a 100 mg dose in the bile of patients with total bile fistulas within 90 minutes, suggesting a first-pass clearance of 75%,[27] greater than the 50% estimated by indirect measurements.

Oral absorption	100%
Presystemic clearance (into bile)	50–75%
Plasma half life	—
Volume of distribution	—
Plasma protein binding	96–99%

The extracted UDCA is then conjugated to glycine and taurine in the liver prior to excretion in the bile, with a resultant decrease in the cholesterol saturation index. UDCA in a daily dosage of 250 mg becomes the predominant bile acid in bile.[11] Tissue distribution is limited to the enterohepatic organs and plasma. Elimination from the body occurs solely by the faecal route. Total bacterial transformation of UDCA occurs before elimination from the body. UDCA is 96–99% bound to protein in serum.[28]

No data are yet available on the excretion of UDCA in breast milk.

Concentration–effect relationship

Gallstone dissolution is unrelated to the concentrations of UDCA in peripheral blood. Biliary concentration of UDCA increases linearly with dosage to reach a plateau at 10 mg.kg^{-1} per 24 h, but there is no clear association between the observed biliary concentration of UDCA and the rate of gallstone dissolution.[11]

Metabolism

UDCA is fully conjugated with glycine (UDC-gly) or taurine (UDC-tau) by the hepatocytes prior to canalicular secretion. These N-acyl conjugates are often termed amidates. UDC-gly and UDC-tau undergo intestinal absorption, passage to the liver, and resecretion into the bile. UDCA and its conjugates are probably less readily absorbed than other bile acids and their conjugates, probably as a result of the greater hydrophilicity of the UDCA molecule. Unabsorbed UDCA and its conjugates pass into the large bowel and under the influence of bacterial enzymes, UDCA and its conjugates can undergo:

1. deconjugation to the free bile acid
2. dehydrogenation to 7-oxo derivatives
3. 7-dehydroxylation to form lithocholic acid.

Ursodeoxycholic acid

Lithocholic acid (LCA) is the principal metabolite of UDCA. LCA is partially absorbed, sulphated and conjugated with glycine or taurine in the liver prior to resecretion. It may also be sulphated in the terminal ileum.[11,28,29]

Elimination of UDCA and its metabolites occurs solely by the faecal route.

Fig. 1 Metabolism of ursodeoxycholic acid

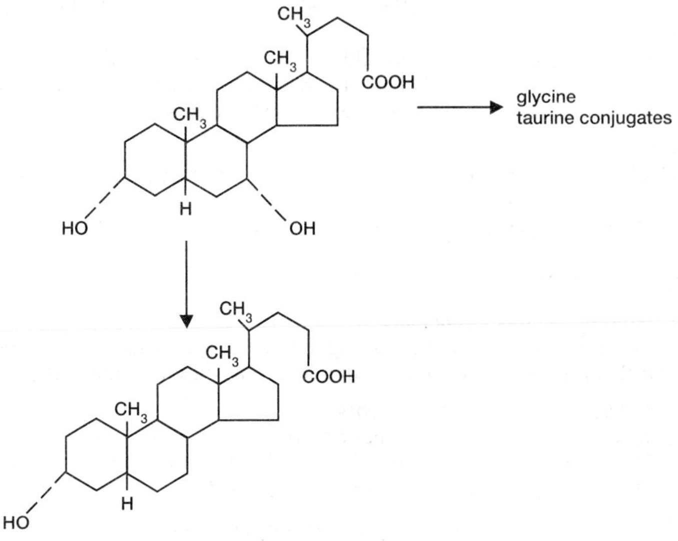

Lithocholic acid

Pharmaceutics

UDCA is available only in oral form:

1. Tablets, 150 mg Destolit (Merrell Dow, UK): the tablets are white, scored and marked with 'Destolit'.
2. Capsules, 250 mg, Ursofalk (Thames, UK): the capsules bear no distinguishing marks.

Preparations must be stored in well-closed containers in cool, dry conditions. UDCA is stable with a reasonable shelf-life.

Therapeutic use

Indications

1. The dissolution of cholesterol gallstones.

Contraindications

1. Non-functioning gallbladder
2. Calcified and pigment gallstones
3. Pregnancy and women who may become pregnant
4. Chronic liver disease
5. Inflammatory bowel disease.

Indications

1. Cholesterol gallstones

UDCA is usually used as a single night-time dosage of 8–12 mg.kg^{-1} and may be commenced immediately in suitable patients. At least one oral cholecystogram is necessary prior to commencing treatment to confirm the presence of both a functioning gallbladder and radiolucent stones (radiolucency suggests that the stones are mainly cholesterol in composition). A reduction in size of responsive gallstones usually occurs within six months. Small stones (less than 5 mm) undergo complete dissolution more readily than do large stones (greater than 10 mm) with complete dissolution rates at one year of 30% and 10% respectively.[30] If gallstones are completely radiolucent, small and smoothly rounded, they are almost certainly cholesterol stones.[31] The expected rate of dissolution would exceed 50% and may be as high as 80%.[30]

Gallstone calcification with consequent arrest of dissolution can occur after 6–12 months.[32]

Dissolution of gallstones may take up to 2–3 years. Complete dissolution is defined as the dissolution of gallstones in two consecutive oral cholecystograms three months apart plus a normal, real-time ultrasound examination of the gallbladder.

UDCA in combination with CDCA is used in the management of patients undergoing extracorporeal shock wave lithotripsy, treatment being maintained for three months after the disappearance of stones. Postdissolution recurrence rate is around 50% after 5 years, mainly within the first 2 years of stopping therapy and early reports suggest that prevention of recurrence may be enhanced by using a small postdissolution dosage of UDCA (100–150 mg daily).[33] Further trial results are awaited.

Relief of symptoms attributable to cholelithiasis are alleviated in 76% of patients with no apparent hepatic adverse effects in the form of transaminase changes being seen in 697 patients.[30]

Other uses
UDCA has also been used with some success in the treatment of pain and dyspepsia associated with different biliary tract disorders such as cholecystitis, gallstones and biliary dyskinesia.[34]

Contraindications

1. Non-functioning gallbladder
A non-functioning gallbladder suggests blockage of the cystic duct and this prevents entry of desaturated bile to dissolve gallstones.

2. Calcified and pigment gallstones
Calcified and pigment gallstones do not respond to UDCA therapy. Although pigment stones may be radiolucent, various radiological predictors can reduce the unwarranted use of UDCA.

3. Pregnancy and women who may become pregnant
As no information is available on the safety or effectiveness of UDCA either during pregnancy or in women who may become pregnant, UDCA is not recommended.

4. Chronic liver disease
Treatment with UDCA in conventional cholelitholytic doses has had no adverse effects in any patients with chronic active hepatitis.[35] However, because of the potential hepatotoxicity it is not advised in patients with chronic liver disease. The use of UDCA in primary biliary cirrhosis is being assessed.

5. Inflammatory bowel disease
There are no studies to suggest UDCA is harmful. However, the drug is not recommended.

Adverse reactions

Potentially life-threatening effects
There are no potentially lethal toxic side effects.

Acute overdosage
To date no deaths have been attributable to UDCA overdosage.

Severe or irreversible adverse effects
Since bile acids are thought to be one risk factor in the development of colonic carcinomas, UDCA treatment may be important. However, studies on the co-carcinogenicity of UDCA indicates it is the only bile acid with no co-carcinogenic effects.[36]

Symptomatic adverse effects
Diarrhoea is a rare side effect of UDCA, unlike other bile acid therapy.

Other effects
No increases of plasma aminotransferase activities have been reported with UDCA, unlike the situation with chenodeoxycholic acid. UDCA appears to have little or no effect on plasma lipids.

High risk groups

Neonates
The drug is not used in this age group.

Breast milk. No data are available, so breast feeding is best avoided.

Children
The drug is not used in children.

Pregnant women
The drug is best avoided during pregnancy, as no information as to its safety is available.

The elderly
No special precautions are necessary in the elderly.

Concurrent disease
The drug should not be given to patients with chronic liver disease or inflammatory bowel disease.

Drug interactions

Potentially useful interactions
UDCA in combination with chenodeoxycholic acid (CDCA) (10 $mg.kg^{-1}$ per 24 h CDCA, 10 $mg.kg^{-1}$ per 24 h UDCA) may be more effective in dissolving gallstones than either alone.[37] UDCA combined with a mixture of monoterpines (Rowachol) or a low cholesterol diet may enhance gallstone dissolution.

Other significant interactions
Any drugs that bind bile acids in vitro (for example cholestyramine, charcoal, colestipol and antacids) may interfere with the absorption of UDCA.

Major outcome trials

Tokyo Cooperative Gallstone Study Group 1980 Efficacy and indications of ursodeoxycholic acid treatment for dissolving gallstones. A multi-centre double-blind trial. Gastroenterology 78: 542–548

This was a double-blind study over one year on 151 subjects given placebo or two doses of UDCA either 150 mg daily or 600 mg daily for radiolucent stones.

Success as judged by partial or complete dissolution was 34.5% with 600 mg daily, 17.4% on 150 mg daily and 5% taking placebo.

Higher dissolution rates up to 83.3% were achieved when cases with non-calcified stones, stones less than 15 mm diameter and floating stones on 600 mg daily were analysed.

The drug was tolerated well, with few or no side effects. Although using a fixed dose, the outcome in the 600 mg per day group is close to the now recommended dose of 8–10 $mg.kg^{-1}$ daily of UDCA.

General review articles

Bouchier I A D 1980 The medical treatment of gallstones. Annual Review of Medicine 31: 59–77

Bachrach W, Hofmann A F 1982 Ursodeoxycholic acid in the treatment of cholesterol cholelithiasis. Digestive Diseases and Sciences 27(8): 737–761 and 27(9): 833–856

Dowling R H 1983 Cholelithiasis: medical treatment. Clinics in Gastroenterology 12: 125–178

Ward A, Brogden R N, Heel R C, Speight T M, Avery S S 1984 Ursodeoxycholic acid: a review of its pharmacological properties and therapeutic efficacy. Drugs 27(2): 95–131

References

1. Iida T, Toneja H R, Chang F C 1981 Potential bile acid metabolites. IV. Invasion of 7α-hydroxyl ursodeoxycholic acid. Lipids 16: 863
2. Igimi H, Carey M C 1980 pH-solubility relations of chenodeoxycholic acid and ursodeoxycholic acid: physical-chemical basis for dissimilar solution and membrane phenomena. Journal of Lipid Research 21: 72–79
3. Roda A, Hofmann A F, Mysels K J 1983 The influence of bile salt structure on self-association in aqueous solutions. Journal of Biological Chemistry 25: 258 (10): 6362–6370
4. Nilsell K, Angelin B, Leijd B, Einarsson K 1983 Comparative effects of ursodeoxycholic acid and chenodeoxycholic acid on bile acid kinetics and biliary lipid secretion in humans. Gastroenterology 85: 1248–1256
5. Bergmann K, Epple-Gutsfeld M, Leiss O 1984 Differences in the effects of chenodeoxycholic acid and ursodeoxycholic acid on biliary lipid secretion and bile acid synthesis in patients with gallstones. Gastroenterology 87: 136–143
6. Hirabayashi I N, Osugi T 1978 Effect of ursodeoxycholic acid on hepatic HMG-CoA reductase and cholesterol 7α-hydroxylase of rat in vitro. Pharmacometrics 15: 125–132
7. Angelin B, Ewerth S, Einorsson K 1983 Ursodeoxycholic acid treatment in cholesterol gallstone disease: effects on hepatic-3-hydroxy-3-methyl glutaryl coenzyme A reductase activity, biliary lipid composition and plasma lipid levels. Journal of Lipid Research 24: 461–468
8. Carulli N, Ponz de Leon M, Zironi F et al 1980 Hepatic cholesterol and bile acid metabolism in subjects with gallstones: comparative effects of short-term feeding of chenodeoxycholic acid and ursodeoxycholic acid. Journal of Lipid Research 21: 35–43
9. Ponz de Leon M, Carulli N, Loria P, Iori R, Zironi F 1980 Cholesterol absorption during bile acid feeding. Effect of ursodeoxycholic acid (UDCA) administration. Gastroenterology 78: 214–219

10. Sarva R P, Fromm H, Farivar S et al 1980 Comparison of the effects between ursodeoxycholic and chenodeoxycholic acids on liver function and structure and on bile acid composition in the Rhesus monkey. Gastroenterology 79: 629–636
11. Bachrach W, Hofmann A F 1982 Ursodeoxycholic acid in the treatment of cholesterol cholelithiasis, Part 1. Digestive Diseases and Sciences 27 (8): 737–761
12. Koch M M, Giampieri M P, Lorenzini I, Jezequel A M, Orlandi F 1980 Effect of ursodeoxycholic acid on liver structure in man. Quantitative data. Gastroenterologie Clinique et Biologique 4: 560–568
13. Takahashi H, Tozuka K, Miyashita T, Ushi K, Miyamota K 1975 Influence of ursodeoxycholic acid administered during pregnancy on the development of foetus and post natal growth in rats and mice. Kiso ro Rinsho (Clinical Reports) 9: 3223–3242
14. Toyoshima S, Fujita H, Sato R, Kashima M, Sato S 1978 Teratogenicity study of ursodeoxycholic acid in rabbits. Pharmacometrics 15: 1133–1140
15. Czygan P, Seizz H, Waldher R, Stiehl A, Ragdsch R 1983 Chenodeoxycholic acid but not ursodeoxycholic acid enhances colonic carcinogenesis in the rat. Gastroenterology 84: 1132
16. Meredith T J, Williams G U, Murphy G M, Saxton H M, Dowling R 1982 Retrospective comparison of 'Cheno' and 'URSO' in the medical treatment of gallstones. Gut 23: 382–389
17. Ward A, Brogden R N, Heel R C, Speight T M, Avery S S 1984 Ursodeoxycholic acid: a review of its pharmacological properties and therapeutic efficacy. Drugs 27 (2): 95–131
18. Thistle J L, Ott B J, Ellefson R D 1978 Serum lipoprotein cholesterol changes during bile acid ingestion for gallstone dissolution (Abstract). Gastroenterology 75: 990
19. Hill A, Ross P E, Bouchier I A D 1983 ^{125}I radioimmunoassay of serum ursodeoxycholyl conjugates. Clinica Chimica Acta 127: 327–336
20. Ross P E, Pennington C R, Bouchier I A D 1977 Gas–liquid chromatographic assay of serum bile acids. Analytical Biochemistry 80: 456–465
21. Ross P E 1982 Radioimmunoassay of serum bile acids. In: Colowich S, Kaplan N O (eds) Methods in Enzymology. Academic Press, vol 84, pp 321–349
22. Sama C, Morselli A M, Bazzoli F, Roda A, Roda E, Barbari L 1978 Bioavailability and pharmacology of UDCA in man. In: Dowling R H, Hofmann A F, Barbara L (eds) Workshop on Ursodeoxycholic Acid. MTP Press, Lancaster, p 88 (Abstract)
23. Tashro A 1979 Oral ursodeoxycholic acid tolerance test for patients with hepatobiliary disease. Acta Hepatologica Japan 20: 369–375
24. Matern S, Tietjen K G, Fackler O, Hinger K, Herz R, Gerok W 1979 Bioavailability of ursodeoxycholic acid in man: studies with a radioimmunoassay for ursodeoxycholic acid. In: Paumgartner G, Stiehl A, Gerok W (eds) Biological Effects of Bile Acids. MTP Press, Lancaster, pp 99–102
25. Bateson M C, Ross P E, Murison J C, Saunders J H B, Bouchier I A D 1980 Ursodeoxycholic acid therapy and biliary lipids: a dose – response study. Gut 21: 305–310
26. Marigold J H, Gilmore I T, Thompson R P H 1980 Direct hepatic extraction of bile acids in subjects with and without liver disease. VI International Bile Acid Meeting 'Bile acids and lipids', Frieburg, Germany, p 156 (Abstract)
27. Shinozaki K 1979 Pharmacokinetic study of oral ursodeoxycholic acid tolerance test. Acta Hepatologica Japan 20: 782–794
28. Hofmann A F 1983 Pharmacology of chenodeoxycholic and ursodeoxycholic acid in man. In: Paumgartner G, Steihl A, Gerok W (eds) Bile Acids and Cholesterol in Health and Disease. MTP Press, Lancaster, pp 301–336
29. Dew M J, Hawker P C, Nutter S, Allan R N 1980 Human intestinal sulfation of lithocholate: a new site for bile acid metabolism. Life Science 27: 317–323
30. Bachrach W H, Hofmann A 1982 Ursodeoxycholic acid in the treatment of cholesterol cholelithiasis, Part II. Digestive Diseases and Sciences 27 (9): 833–856
31. Bell G D, Dowling R H, Whitney B, Sutor D J 1975 The value of radiology in predicting gallstone type when selecting patients for medical treatment. Gut 16: 359–364
32. Bateson M C, Bouchier I A D, Trash D B, Maudgal D, Northfield T C 1981 Calcification of radiolucent gallstones with ursodeoxycholic acid. British Medical Journal 283: 645–646
33. Sugata F, Kobayashi A, Yamamura M, Shimizu M I 1980 Five year follow – up study on UDCA therapy for cholelithiasis with special reference to recurrence. XI International Congress of Gastroenterology. Hamburg, Germany, E.34.11 (Abstract)
34. Frigerio G 1979 Ursodeoxycholic acid (UDCA) in the treatment of dyspepsia: a report of a multi – centre controlled trial. Current Therapeutic Research 26: 214–224
35. Leuschner U, Leuschner M, Hubner K 1981 Gallstone dissolution in patients with chronic active hepatitis. Gastroenterology 80 (II): 1208
36. Stiehl A 1983 Side effects of chenodeoxycholic and ursodeoxycholic acid. In: Paumgartner G, Stiehl A, Gerok W (eds) Bile Acids and Cholesterol in Health and Disease. MTP Press, Lancaster, pp 387–392
37. Podda M, Zuin M, Dioguardi M L, Festorazzi S, Dioguardi N 1982 A combination of chenodeoxycholic acid and ursodeoxycholic acid is more effective than either alone in reducing biliary cholesterol saturation. Hepatology 2: 334–339

Vancomycin (hydrochloride)

This antibiotic was found in cultures of *Streptomyces orientalis* grown from a sample of Borneo soil whilst screening for anti-staphylococcal activity. After purification and partial characterization it was made generally available by Lilly in 1958.

Chemistry

Vancomycin hydrochloride (Vancocin)
$C_{66}H_{75}Cl_2N_9O_{24}.HCl$

Vancomycin is a complex glycopeptide. A disaccharide consisting of glucose and the aminosugar vancosamine is linked to the middle amino acid (phenylglycine) of a seven-membered peptide chain. This comprises three substituted phenylglycines, two chlorinated β-hydroxytyrosines, aspartic acid amide and N-methylleucine. Next-but-one-amino acids in the chain are linked (2 with 4, 4 with 6 and 5 with 7) through their aromatic side chains to form three large rings.[1] A semi-synthetic derivative of this structure is being evaluated.

The molecule contains numerous functional and ionizable groups (one carboxyl, three phenolic and two amine). Net molecular charge and solubility are least at neutral pH.

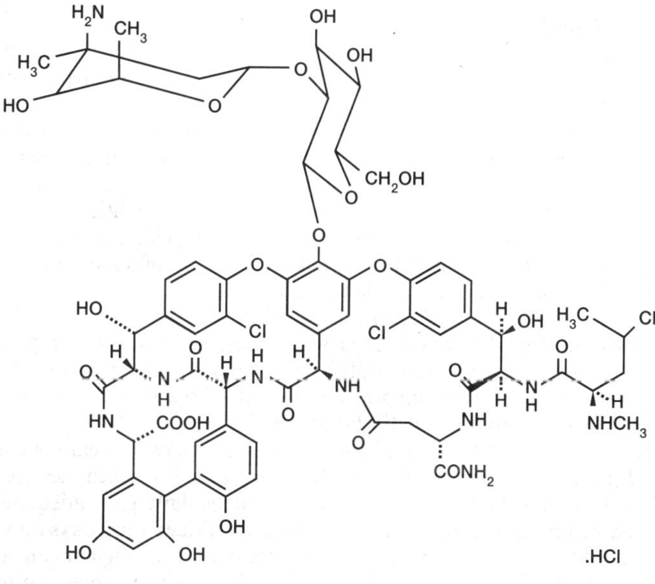

Molecular weight (free base)	1484.5 (1448)
pKa	—
Solubility	
in alcohol	1 in 700
in water (pH 7)	>1 in 10
Octanol/water partition coefficient	low

Vancomycin is a white odourless powder with a bitter taste. Purification of the fermentation product includes a series of ion-exchange resin and absorbent resin chromatography steps, and vancomycin precipitation.

Vancomycin is highly soluble in water at acid pH, soluble but unstable at alkaline pH. It is poorly soluble in organic solvents, except methanol.

Pharmacology

Vancomycin is bactericidal to Gram-positive cocci and certain Gram-positive bacilli. The mode of action is probably mixed; the permeability of the cell membrane may be altered and RNA synthesis may be impaired but the chief mode of action is inhibition of cell wall synthesis.[2] Precursors of peptidoglycan are believed to form a complex with vancomycin; the d-alanyl-d-alanine moiety of the former nestles in a cleft on the vancomycin surface where it is held by hydrogen bonding. Steric hindrance prevents further steps in the synthesis of peptidoglycan.[3]

In contrast to the β-lactam antibiotics, vancomycin seldom gives rise to L-phase vegetative forms even under experimental conditions. This may be a result of the multiple mode of action.[4] Unfortunately, and perhaps for similar reasons, vancomycin does not have the very high therapeutic index of the other cell wall-inhibiting antibiotics.

Toxicology

Early work with less pure material may have exaggerated toxicity. Hypotension (reduced by H_1 histamine-receptor antagonists), kidney damage and convulsions (in rodents given large doses intravenously) have been observed.[5] Ototoxicity has not been a consistent finding. Vancomycin intravenously failed to enhance the ototoxicity of intravenous ethacrynic acid in an animal model.[6]

Clinical pharmacology

The antibacterial actions are paramount.[7] Almost all strains of *Staphylococcus aureus* including producers of β-lactamase and *Staph. epidermidis* are sensitive;[8] resistance has not been observed amongst *Streptococcus pneumoniae* or *Strep. pyogenes*. Most strains of *Strep. viridans* and enterococci are sensitive and similarly most strains of *Clostridium* species including *Cl. difficile*. Median values for minimum inhibitory concentration (MIC) in vitro for all the species mentioned generally lie in the range 0.5–5 $mg.l^{-1}$; rarely does the MIC exceed 10 $mg.l^{-1}$. Relatively high MIC values are encountered more commonly amongst enterococci and staphylococci than amongst streptococci. The frequency of resistant strains within susceptible species has not increased since the early years of use.[9]

Pharmacokinetics

The assay of serum vancomycin concentration is usually by plate diffusion assay using *Bacillus subtilis*. The limit of detection is about 0.5 $mg.l^{-1}$ and the coefficient of variation about 10% in the concentration range 1–25 $mg.l^{-1}$.[10] Immunoassay and HPLC have been used.

After oral administration absorption is negligible. Small amounts can be detected in the urine of patients with normal renal function but serum concentrations are insignificant even in patients with severe renal insufficiency.[11]

Systemic administration is best by intravenous infusion in saline over not less than 1 hour. After cessation of infusion a triphasic decay is recognized. The initial 'distribution' half time is less than 10 min. The final 'elimination' phase half time is 5–11 h in healthy volunteers[12] and is substantially prolonged in renal insufficiency.

Estimates of steady-state distribution volume vary (0.47–0.9 $l.kg^{-1}$) and probably reflect binding to some tissue constituents. In plasma about 50% is protein bound. A variety of body fluids have been assayed. Generally (in ascitic, pericardial, pleural and synovial fluids) concentrations are of the same order as concurrent plasma concentrations. Bile concentrations are unexpectedly low and vancomycin is virtually undetectable in CSF unless the meninges are inflamed.[13]

Elimination is almost entirely by the kidney (<5% of dose in bile) and the renal clearance correlates well with creatinine clearance.[14] After correction for plasma protein binding the clearance of vancomycin from plasma water approximates to the glomerular filtration rate (GFR).

Some accumulation is to be expected when patients with normal renal function are given multiple dosage with an approximate 6 h interval. This is likely to be undetectable with a 12 h interval.

Patients with end-stage renal failure have a greatly prolonged elimination half time (mean 7.5 days) and dosage intervals of 7–14 days are recommended. Haemo- or peritoneal-dialysis have little influence on the rate of elimination or dosage requirements.[14]

Human data on placental transfer and secretion in breast milk are few. Transfer across the placenta does occur, however, and studies in the female cat have detected vancomycin in milk after systemic administration.

V

Oral absorption	very low
Presystemic metabolism	none
Plasma half life	
range	5–11 h
Volume of distribution	0.6 $l.kg^{-1}$
Plasma protein binding	50%

Concentration–effect relationship

Systemic therapy with vancomycin is reserved for serious or potentially serious infections with organisms which are resistant to other antibiotics. It is particularly important therefore that plasma concentrations should be adequate in relation to the sensitivity of the suspect pathogen. This requirement will commonly be met if the serum concentration exceeds 5 $mg.l^{-1}$ for a substantial part of the dosage interval. The conditions of the in vitro MIC determination are very different from those in vivo, however, and this statement can be no more than a general guide. Moellering and his colleagues[14] assumed a desirable mean plasma concentration of 15 $mg.l^{-1}$ in the construction of their dosage nomogram.

Deafness developed in a patient[15] exposed to 80–95 $mg.l^{-1}$ but when the concentration does not exceed 30 $mg.l^{-1}$ there is probably little risk of serious systemic toxicity. The maximum concentration attained, however, is an inverse function of the time over which the dose is infused. Since this has not been standardized, it is not possible to infer a maximum safe peak concentration from the literature.

The minimum bactericidal concentration (MBC) varies with the species. For many Gram-positive cocci it is close to the MIC,[8] whereas for most enterococci the MBC is unattainable.[16] It is therefore not possible to define an adequate therapeutic concentration in terms of MBC. Clinical microbiologists may choose to test serum taken an hour or two after dosage for its bactericidal activity in vitro against the isolated pathogen.

Metabolism

The persistence of vancomycin in the anephric patient implies that any elimination by biotransformation must be very slow. No metabolic derivatives have been identified. Following intravenous administration approximately 90% of the dose is excreted unchanged in the urine, 50% of the dose being excreted over the first 4 h.

Pharmaceutics

Vancomycin is available in formulations for oral and intravenous administration.

1. Vancocin Matrigel capsules (Lilly, UK) contain 125 mg or 250 mg vancomycin. The 125 mg capsules are dark blue/peach coded 'Lilly 3125'. The 250 mg ones are dark blue/grey coded 'Lilly 3126'.
2. Vancocin (Lilly, UK) for injection contains 500 mg vancomycin hydrochloride as a freeze-dried plug in a 10 ml rubber-stoppered vial. This is dissolved in 10 ml Water for Injections.

Intramuscular injection causes pain and tissue necrosis; similarly intravenous injection causes local thrombophlebitis.[7] Accordingly the dose should be diluted in 200 ml isotonic saline or dextrose solution (but not sodium bicarbonate) and infused intravenously over 1 hour minimum. Neutral or acid solutions are stable indefinitely at 0-6°C but should be used within 2 or 3 days to ensure sterility.

The contents of a vial for injection may be used for oral administration. Each dose may be reconstituted in 30 ml water and either drunk or administered by nasogastric tube. After reconstitution with water, this may be stored in a refrigerator (0°–6°C) for up to two weeks without significant loss of potency.

There are no combined formulations incorporating other antibiotics or drugs.

Therapeutic use

Indications

Oral administration

1. Antibiotic-associated colitis

Intravenous

Systemic use is limited to patients suffering from, or at risk of, life-threatening infections with vancomycin-sensitive bacteria which are resistant to safer antibiotics (for example, methicillin-resistant *Staph. aureus*). It may also be used in patients who suffer severe allergic responses to β-lactam antibiotics.

2. Endocarditis

other uses

3. Bacteraemia
4. Meningitis
5. Prophylaxis and treatment of infections in dialysis patients
6. Prophylaxis during cytotoxic drug therapy.

Contraindications

A history of allergy contraindicates systemic use. However, oral use, possibly with corticosteroid cover, may be justifiable in the patient with pseudomembranous colitis.

Mode of use

The oral formulation is usually given at a dose of 500 mg–1 g (children 44 $mg.kg^{-1}$) daily in three or four divided doses.

The intravenous formulation is given by infusion over 1 hour at a dose of 1–2 g (children 44 $mg.kg^{-1}$) daily in two or four divided doses. As described earlier the dose is diluted in 200 ml of isotonic fluid. The site of intravenous infusion should be changed frequently to minimize thrombophlebitis. In patients with reduced GFR the dosage rate is reduced by reducing dosage and/or prolonging the interval (see 'High risk groups'). Plasma concentration monitoring is required (British National Formulary, 1989).

Indications

1. Antibiotic-associated colitis

Although diarrhoea is a common side effect of antibiotic administration (parenteral as well as oral), only a small proportion of patients show colitis on sigmoidoscopy.

Superinfection with antibiotic-resistant *Staphylococcus aureus* was recognized early in the history of antibiotic therapy and associated particularly with the tetracyclines and other broad spectrum agents. More recently the syndrome of pseudomembranous colitis has been linked particularly with lincomycin and clindamycin. Stool culture yields *Clostridium difficile* in a high proportion of cases and its cytotoxic toxin is almost invariably detectable.

Oral vancomycin has been used effectively in staphylococcal enterocolitis for 20 years.[17] It is also effective against *Cl. difficile* superinfection (see 'Clinical trials'). Intravenous vancomycin is less effective than oral; the vancomycin content of the stool is low and variable and the toxin can still be detected.

The usual recommended course of oral vancomycin treatment is 0.5–1 g per 24 h over 7–10 days. Keighley and his colleagues (see 'Clinical trials') showed that 125 mg four times daily gave adequate concentrations in the faeces. This dose was continued for 5 days only. Modest dosage may have advantages since even vancomycin can so disrupt the bowel flora as to allow a *Clostridium difficile* infection to become established soon after the antibiotic is stopped.

2. Endocarditis

Before 1960 vancomycin was used to treat endocarditis caused by penicillin-resistant staphylcocci but with the advent of methicillin its use ceased. During recent years, however, there have been developments which have renewed the importance of vancomycin; these include methicillin-resistance amongst staphylococci, allergy to β-lactam antibiotics and increased importance of *Staph. epidermidis* infections in patients with prosthetic valves and in intravenous drug abusers. The topic has been reviewed recently.[16]

A course of vancomycin (2 g per 24 h or 44 $mg.kg^{-1}$ per 24 h in 2 or 4 divided doses) for 4–6 weeks is recommended in cases of staphylococcal endocarditis. The MBC is often higher than the MIC but is usually attainable in plasma in vivo so that vancomycin can be used alone.

Such a regime may be adequate against *Strep. viridans* but in order to attain bactericidal activity in appropriate dilutions of patient serum it may be necessary to add an aminoglycoside. The MBC

Vancomycin (hydrochloride)

against enterococci is unattainable in plasma in vivo and combination with an aminoglycoside is essential.[16]

3. Bacteraemia

The introduction of intravenous vancomycin to treat staphylococcal septicaemia reduced the previously high mortality to less than 30%. The development of the β-lactamase-resistant penicillins then enabled this cure rate to be maintained without the hazards of vancomycin toxicity. The advent of safer, more purified formulations of vancomycin and the increasing importance of methicillin-resistant strains of *Staph. aureus* have restored the importance of vancomycin during recent years.[7]

Soft tissue infections by methicillin-resistant staphylococci also respond well to vancomycin. In osteomyelitis, however, the need to prolong treatment for many months leads to a preference for anti-staphylococcal drugs which have a systemic effect by mouth.

4. Meningitis

Inflammation of the meninges has an important effect on the penetration of vancomycin into CSF. In its absence none was detected despite therapeutic concentrations (5–10 mg.l^{-1}) in plasma.[18] In children with infected ventriculocaval or ventriculoperitoneal shunts the ventricular CSF concentration averaged 18% (range 7–36.5) of the serum concentration.[19] Intrathecal and intraventricular routes have been used. In animals with experimentally induced staphylococcal meningitis the CSF/serum concentrations were higher for vancomycin than for β-lactam antibiotics.

Successful treatment of staphylococcal meningitis in adults[7] and in children[19] (with and without CSF shunts) has been reported with intravenous vancomycin. This application is not, however, included in the manufacturer's list of recommended uses.

5. Prophylaxis and treatment of infections in dialysis patients

Systemic vancomycin has been given over long periods to patients receiving chronic intermittent haemodialysis. The frequency of staphylococcal infections at shunt sites has been greatly reduced.[20] In view of the drug's persistence in functionally anephric patients it is sufficient to dose at intervals of 7–14 days.

Penetration from plasma into peritoneal dialysis fluid is not consistent. Therefore vancomycin is added directly to dialysis fluid for treatment of *Staph. aureus* or *epidermidis* peritonitis in patients treated by chronic peritoneal dialysis.[21] A concentration of 10 mg.l^{-1} in dialysis fluid is well above the MIC for most Gram-positive cocci.[8] Vancomycin at this concentration is stable in dialysis fluid for 24 hours or more at room temperature.

During peritoneal dialysis vancomycin passes slowly between peritoneal fluid and plasma; in view of the low peritoneal clearance (5–10 ml.min^{-1}) concurrent systemic dosage has been recommended.[22] It is questionable, however, whether this is needed in continuous ambulatory peritoneal dialysis when plasma vancomycin concentration will eventually plateau at the peritoneal fluid concentration.

6. Prophylaxis after cytotoxic drug therapy

Vancomycin has been used with other poorly absorbed antibiotics in oral and topical mixtures designed to reduce or even eliminate bacterial colonization of neutropenic patients. The addition of vancomycin to oral gentamicin and nystatin, for example, substantially reduced the anaerobes which could be cultured from the stool.[23] In another study also there was greater overall suppression of the bacterial flora of the gut but no corresponding reduction in the incidence of bacteraemia or total infective episodes (see 'Clinical trials').

Evaluation of antibiotic prophylaxis in neutropenic patients is complicated by the use of complex mixtures and by variation in the provision of protected environments.

Adverse reactions

Potentially life-threatening effects

These are probably limited to anaphylaxis[24] and possibly further kidney damage in the patient who has already suffered substantial renal impairment. Experience with the early formulations demonstrated proteinuria, microscopic haematuria, granular urinary casts and even uraemia. Recent experience suggests that nephrotoxicity is very uncommon.[25]

Acute overdosage

Severe acute overdosage has not been reported.

Severe or irreversible adverse effects

Ototoxicity is unknown with oral vancomycin,[26] even in patients with severe renal insufficiency.[11] Systemic treatment (1 g intravenously weekly for 6 weeks) with peak serum concentrations below 40 mg.l^{-1} produced no change in audiograms in a prospective study of patients with staphylococcal bacteraemia undergoing chronic haemodialysis,[27] but deafness has occurred in association with high plasma concentrations when uraemic patients have been given unmodified doses.[15] Similarly, systemic vancomycin possibly enhances the ototoxic effects of aminoglycosides. As with the aminoglycosides, acuity to high frequencies is most affected although there may be some reversibility.

Symptomatic adverse effects

Macular and urticarial skin rashes, red neck flushing, drug fever and eosinophilia are reported. Thrombophlebitis is a problem if the intravenous solution is diluted insufficiently or the site of infusion is not changed frequently. Rapid infusion leads to hypotension by histamine release as in experimental animals.[7]

Interference with clinical pathology tests

No significant interferences of this kind have been reported.

High risk groups

Neonates

The mean serum concentration half time is long (6–10 h) relative to older children and a reduced dose (15 mg.kg^{-1} initially, then 10 mg.kg^{-1} at intervals of 12 h) is recommended during the first week of life.[19,28]

Breast milk. Vancomycin is unlikely to enter the milk after oral dosage. The conditions for which intravenous drug is used (for example Gram-positive septicaemia) are scarcely compatible with breast feeding.

Children

Except in children known to have a reduced GFR, no dosage reductions are recommended. The mean serum concentration half time is generally shorter[28] (2–3 h) than in the adult.

Pregnant women

A 13-week-pregnant woman received 2 g intravenously daily for 28 days. No toxic effects were observed subsequently in the baby (Lilly, Information Department). However, use in pregnancy is not recommended.

The elderly

Pre-existing renal impairment and deafness are both likely in an elderly population. Serum concentration monitoring and audiometry are desirable when systemic treatment is indicated.

Concurrent disease

Renal disease. In patients with a reduced GFR from any cause it is desirable to reduce the dose proportionately. A nomogram has been constructed for this purpose.[14] Similarly there should be monitoring of serum vancomycin concentrations (perhaps twice weekly) and audiometry.[27]

The nomogram of Moellering and others[14] was based on a group of patients aged 12–78 years who covered the full range of kidney function. It appears with the vancomycin entry in the current ABPI Data Sheet Compendium. In patients with significant impairment of kidney function, who require systemic treatment by intravenous infusion, a loading dose of 15 mg.kg^{-1} but not exceeding 1000 mg is recommended. This is followed by a maintenance dose scaled according to creatinine clearance, obtained from a timed urine collection or calculated from the steady-state plasma concentration of creatinine. Table 1 gives a selection of doses obtained from the nomogram with some approximation. The dose of 250 mg every 48 hours corresponds in a 70 kg patient with the 1.9 mg.kg^{-1} per 24 h which is recommended for patients on dialysis.[14]

In a patient with normal renal function the plasma concentration may swing from 30 to 5 mg.l^{-1} twice a day. In the anephric patient, by contrast, the decline in concentration over 24 h will be barely perceptible even on a day of dialysis.

V

Table 1

Creatinine clearance (ml.min^{-1})	Maintenance dose (mg) and interval (h)
>100	500/8
70–100	500/12
35– 70	500/24
20– 35	250/24
10– 20	250/48

Drug interactions

Apart from the additive action of other nephrotoxic or ototoxic drugs, there are no specific interactions recognized.

Clinical trials

1. Keighley M R B, Burdon D W, Arabi Y et al 1978 Randomised controlled trial of vancomycin for pseudomembranous colitis and postoperative diarrhoea. British Medical Journal 2: 1667–1669

All 44 patients on one surgical ward who developed postoperative diarrhoea during a 6-month period in 1978 entered this study. They were allocated randomly to 5 days treatment with oral vancomycin (22) or placebo (22). The two groups were well balanced with respect to preoperative diagnosis. When the results of laboratory investigations became available, half the patients showed no evidence of pseudomembranous colitis.

In the vancomycin treatment group 12 patients showed evidence of pseudomembranous colitis; by the fifth day of treatment there was cure in (a) 11/12 as judged by eradication of *Cl. difficile*, (b) 8/9 as judged by disappearance of faecal toxin and (c) 6/7 as judged by loss of pseudomembrane on biopsy. One case only showed evidence of relapse: *Cl. difficile* was grown from an abscess during convalescence.

In the placebo group 9 patients showed evidence of pseudomembranous colitis; by the fifth day of treatment there was evidence of cure in (a) 1/9 as judged by eradication of *Cl. difficile*, (b) 1/6 as judged by disappearance of toxin and (c) 1/5 as judged by loss of pseudomembrane.

The p values for differences between treatments were respectively (a)<0.01, (b)<0.05 and (c) not given. The authors concluded that oral vancomycin was effective.

2. Bender J F, Schimpff S C, Young V M et al 1979 Role of vancomycin as a component of oral nonabsorbable antibiotics for microbial suppression in leukaemic patients. Antimicrobial Agents and Chemotherapy 15: 455–460

The authors compared the microbial flora (axilla, nose, mouth, rectum) and the incidence of infection in two groups of patients with acute leukaemia. The patients admitted (42) to the study all received vigorous antileukaemic chemotherapy and were at risk of granulocytopenia. A protected environment was not available but they were allocated randomly to alternative regimes of nonabsorbable antibiotics: (a) gentamicin and nystatin alone (GN) and (b) GN with vancomycin added (GVN).

The two groups were well balanced with respect to type of leukaemia. One patient died and three refused oral antibiotics; with these two losses from each group 18 received GVN and 20 GN.

Vancomycin made the regime less tolerable but produced greater overall suppression of the alimentary tract flora. Acquisition of potential pathogens was approximately equal in both groups. There was no difference in the numbers of patients who remained free from infections namely (a) 6/18 with GVN and (b) 6/20 with GN.

The authors concluded that under the conditions of their study vancomycin could safely be omitted from the GVN regime provided that bacteriological monitoring was performed to detect resistant organisms.

3. Shenep J K, Hughes W T, Roberson P K et al 1988 Vancomycin, ticarcillin, and amikacin compared with ticarcillin-clavulanate and amikacin in the empirical treatment of febrile, neutropenic children with cancer. New England Journal of Medicine 319: 1053–1058

Two antibiotic regimes (1. vancomycin, ticarcillin and amikacin (VTA); 2. placebo, ticarcillin with clavulanate and amikacin (TCA)) were compared in 101 children and young adults with fever and neutropenia. Treatments were allocated randomly with stratification for the presence of an intravascular catheter and for underlying disease (mainly acute leukaemias with some solid tumours). The design was double-blind and the two experimental groups were well balanced.

Treatment success (completion of 10 days treatment without fever or other complication) was more frequent in the VTA group (45/53 or 85%) than in the TCA group (30/48 or 62%; $P=0.010$). Similarly the appearance of a different organism in the blood (breakthrough bacteraemia) during the course of antibiotic treatment was significantly ($P=0.006$) less common in the presence of vancomycin (1/53 with VTA; 9/48 with TCA); responsible organisms were *Staph. epidermidis* and alpha-haemolytic streptococci. The greater incidence of breakthrough bacteraemia and one associated death in the TCA group led to the termination of this study at the point of interim analysis.

Despite the combination with an aminoglycoside there was no evidence of nephrotoxicity in the VTA group but a modest elevation of serum aminotransferases was found ($P=0.04$).

The authors conclude that vancomycin merits inclusion in the antibiotic combination used to treat febrile patients with neutropenia in clinical settings in which Gram-positive bacteraemias are a serious problem.

General review articles

Cooper G L, Given D B 1986 Vancomycin: a comprehensive review of 30 years of clinical experience. John Wiley, USA

Levine J F 1987 Vancomycin: a review. Medical Clinics of North America 71: 1135–1145

Newsom S W B 1982 Vancomycin. Journal of Antimicrobial Chemotherapy 10: 257–259

Wise R I, Kory M (eds) 1981 Reassessments of vancomycin — a potentially useful antibiotic. Reviews of Infectious Diseases 3 (suppl): S199–S300

References

1. Sheldrick G M, Jones P G, Kennard O, Williams D H, Smith G A 1978 Structure of vancomycin and its complex with acetyl-D-alanyl-D-alanine. Nature 271: 223–225
2. Jordan D C, Inniss W E 1961 Mode of action of vancomycin on Staphylococcus aureus. Antimicrobial Agents and Chemotherapy 218–225
3. Pfeiffer R R 1981 Structural features of vancomycin. Reviews of Infectious Diseases 3: S205–S209
4. Watanakunakorn C 1971 Vancomycin induction of L colonies of Staphylococcus aureus. Infection and Immunity 3: 709–710
5. Wold J S, Turnipseed S A 1981 Toxicology of vancomycin in laboratory animals. Reviews of Infectious Diseases 3: S224–S229
6. Brummett R E 1981 Effects of antibiotic–diuretic interactions in the guinea pig model of ototoxicity. Reviews of Infectious Diseases 3: S216–S223
7. Cook F V, Farrar W E 1978 Vancomycin revisited. Annals of Internal Medicine 88: 813–818
8. Cherubin C E, Corrado M L, Sierra M F, Gombert M E, Shulman M 1981 Susceptibility of Gram-positive cocci to various antibiotics including cefotaxime, moxalactam and N-formimidoyl thienamycin. Antimicrobial Agents and Chemotherapy 20: 553–555
9. Watanakunakorn C 1981 The antibacterial action of vancomycin. Reviews of Infectious Diseases 3: S210–S215
10. Walker C N 1980 Bioassay for determination of vancomycin in the presence of rifampicin or aminoglycosides. Antimicrobial Agents and Chemotherapy 17: 730–731
11. Bryan C S, White W L 1978 Safety of oral vancomycin in functionally anephric patients. Antimicrobial Agents and Chemotherapy 14: 634–635
12. Krogstad D J, Moellering R C Jr, Greenblatt D J 1980 Single dose kinetics of intravenous vancomycin. Journal of Clinical Pharmacology 20: 197–201
13. Moellering R C Jr, Krogstad D J, Greenblatt D J 1981 Pharmacokinetics of vancomycin in normal subjects and in patients with reduced renal function. Reviews of Infectious Diseases 3: S230–S235
14. Moellering R C Jr, Krogstad D J, Greenblatt D J 1981 Vancomycin therapy in patients with impaired renal function: a nomogram for dosage. Annals of Internal Medicine 94: 343–346
15. Geraci J E, Heilman F R, Nichols D R, Wellman W E 1958 Antibiotic therapy for bacterial endocarditis VII. Proceedings of the Staff Meetings of the Mayo Clinic 33: 172–181
16. Geraci J E, Wilson W R 1981 Vancomycin therapy for infective endocarditis. Reviews of Infectious Diseases 3: S250–S258
17. Khan M Y, Hall W H 1966 Staphylococcal enterocolitis — treatment with oral vancomycin. Annals of Internal Medicine 65: 1–8
18. Geraci J E, Heilman F R, Nichols D R, Wellman W E, Ross G T 1956 Some laboratory and clinical experiences with a new antibiotic, vancomycin. Proceedings of the Staff Meetings of the Mayo Clinic 31: 564–582

19. Schaad U B, Nelson J D, McCracken G H Jr 1981 Pharmacology and efficacy of vancomycin for staphylococcal infections in children. Reviews of Infectious Diseases 3: S282–S288
20. Morris A J, Bilinsky R T 1971 Prevention of staphylococcal shunt infections by continuous vancomycin prophylaxis. American Journal of the Medical Sciences 262: 87–92
21. Glew R H, Pavuk R A 1981 Stability of vancomycin and aminoglycoside antibiotics in peritoneal dialysis concentrate. Nephron 28: 241–243
22. Nielsen H E, Sórensen I, Hansen H E 1979 Peritoneal transport of vancomycin during peritoneal dialysis. Nephron 24: 274–277
23. Bodey G P 1981 Antibiotic prophylaxis in cancer patients: regimens of oral, nonabsorbable antibiotics for prevention of infection during induction of remission. Reviews of Infectious Diseases 3: S259–S268
24. Rothenberg H J 1959 Anaphylactoid reaction to vancomycin. Journal of the American Medical Association 171: 1101–1102
25. Appel G B, Neu H C 1977 The nephrotoxicity of antimicrobial agents. New England Journal of Medicine 296: 722–728
26. Kavanagh K T, McCabe B F 1983 Ototoxicity of oral neomycin and vancomycin. Laryngoscope 93: 649–653
27. Masur H, Francioli P, Ruddy M, Murray H W 1983 Vancomycin serum levels and toxicity in chronic hemodialysis patients with Staphylococcus aureus bacteraemia. Clinical Nephrology 20: 85–88
28. Schaad U B, McCracken G H Jr, Nelson J D 1980 Clinical pharmacology and efficacy of vancomycin in paediatric patients. Journal of Paediatrics 96: 119–126

Vecuronium (bromide)

Vecuronium bromide is a non-depolarizing neuromuscular blocking agent.

Chemistry

Vecuronium bromide (Norcuron)
$C_{34}H_{57}BrN_2O_4$
1-(3α,17β-Diacetoxy-2β-piperidino 5α androstan-16β-yl)-1-methylpiperidinium bromide

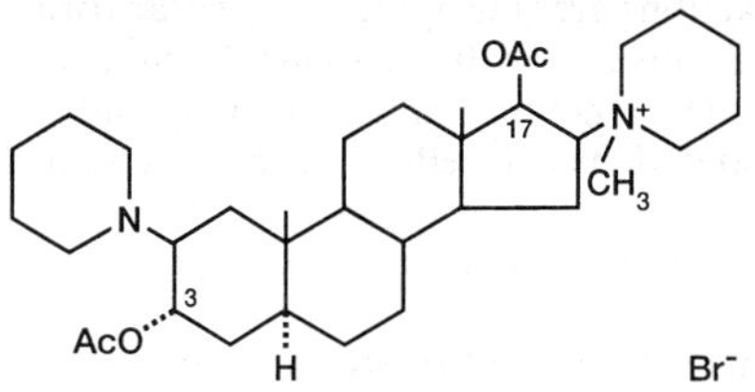

Molecular weight	637.7
pKa	8.97
Solubility	
in alcohol	1 in 44
in water	1 in 110
Octanol/water partition coefficient	—

It is prepared as white to off-white or slightly pink crystals or crystalline powder. Vercuronium bromide is prepared by chemical synthesis. It is not available in any combination products.

Pharmacology

Vecuronium is a potent non-depolarizing neuromuscular blocking agent with a high degree of selectivity for the receptors at the neuromuscular junction.[1] It is the 2β-monoquaternary analogue of pancuronium. The latter molecule contains two acetylcholine-like motifs built into the steroid nucleus. Due to the relative rigidity and asymmetry of this nucleus, the two acetylcholine motifs adopt very different three dimensional configurations. The motifs associated

Fig. 1 Vecuronium is the 2β-monoquaternary analogue of pancuronium

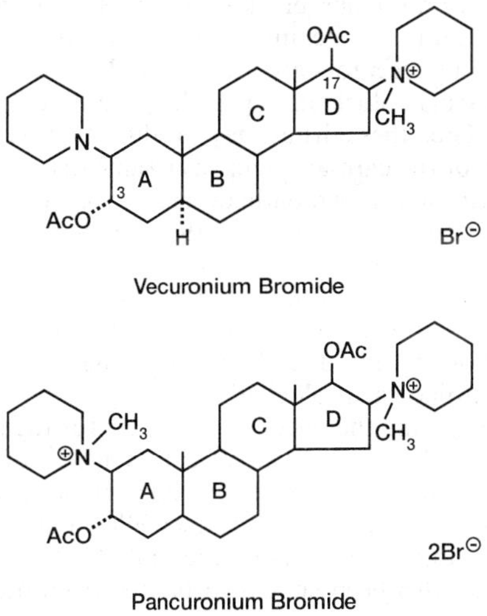

associated with the D-ring of the nucleus is always present in compounds of high neuromuscular blocking potency. Suggestions that the A-ring motif might be responsible for the cardiovascular side effects of pancuronium, particularly its vagolytic action, led to the synthesis of vecuronium, in which the N-methyl group on the A-ring motif is absent, effectively removing its acetylcholine-related properties (Fig. 1).

The mechanism of neuromuscular blockade by vecuronium at the neuromuscular junction is demonstrated by the following features:

a) it diminishes or abolishes the depolarization evoked by acetylcholine released either by nerve stimulation, iontophoresis or close intra-arterial injection
b) trains of nerve stimuli evoke a decreasing depolarization when vecuronium is present whereas repeated iontophoretic application does not. This argues for an additional action at pre-junctional nicotinic receptors.[2]
c) following nerve stimulation at tetanic rates, there is a potentiation of the subsequent depolarization or muscle contraction to slow frequency stimulation
d) the block produced by vecuronium may be antagonized by an anticholinesterase drug such as neostigmine or edrophoium.

Vecuronium's actions are thus typical of a curariform neuromuscular blocking drug. It acts mainly by blocking the effect of acetylcholine at the neuromuscular junction, rather than by preventing release of acetylcholine, and it has no effect on nerve conduction or muscle contractility.[3]

As with all muscle relaxants, vecuronium is more effective in decreasing the twitch response of fast limb muscles than of slow limb muscles in animals. Studies of the relative potency of vecuronium on the diaphragm (primarily slow fibres) and on adductor pollicis (fast fibres) indicates that the diaphragm requires about 40% more vecuronium for 95% depression of a single twitch response.[4]

Vecuronium has a relatively short to medium rate of onset and recovery non-depolarizing neuromuscular blocking action, with a rapid and minimal cumulation.[3] As a group, neuromuscular blocking drugs may cause histamine release, anticholinesterase activity, ganglion blockade and cardiovascular effects arising from various mechanisms; vecuronium produces minimal unwanted activity in these respects.

Vecuronium does not significantly alter plasma histamine levels.[5] It is more potent than pancuronium in inhibiting acetylcholinesterase but it is still too weak for this action to be evident at any concentration which might be achieved clinically. Vecuronium is about ten times less potent than pancuronium in inhibiting butyrylcholinesterase. Since the neuromuscular blocking potency of vecuronium in man is slightly greater than that of pancuronium, and since the antibutyrylcholinesterase activity of pancuronium is of little clinical relevance, the weak action of vecuronium in this respect has no consequences in man.[3]

Vecuronium exhibits only very weak ganglion-blocking activity: Durant and colleagues[6] found that doses of vecuronium 500 times greater than the neuromuscular blocking dose were required to depress contractions of the preganglionically-stimulated nictitating membrane of the cat.

Although neuromuscular blocking drugs do not generally block muscarinic receptors in the intestine, glands, bladder or eye, the cardiac muscarinic receptors are unusual in that they are sensitive to some neuromuscular blockers, especially gallamine, fazadinium and pancuronium. Thus these drugs may produce tachycardia by blocking the activity of the cardiac vagus. The same drugs may also block muscarinic receptors on sympathetic nerve endings that inhibit the release of noradrenaline, and thereby they can increase noradrenaline release. In addition, some neuromuscular blocking drugs block the neuronal re-uptake of noradrenaline (uptake 1), which results in the persistence of noradrenaline in the region of the receptors. The latter two actions involving noradrenaline would augment any tachycardia arising from cardiac vagal blockade.

Studies investigating the selectivity of drugs for the neuromuscular junction compared with cardiac receptors have found that, with vecuronium, the dose required to produce 50% vagal blockade is 60–80 times the dose required to product 50% neuromuscular block. Thus at clinical doses, vecuronium does not affect the cardiac vagus. Vecuronium has also been shown to be free from other muscarinic blocking actions, and it is 4.2 times less effective than pancuronium as a blocker of noradrenaline re-uptake at sympathetic nerve terminals.[7]

Toxicology

Long-term animal studies to determine the mutagenic and carcinogenic potentials of vecuronium bromide have not been performed to date.

Clinical Pharmacology

Vecuronium is administered by initial intravenous bolus followed by intravenous top-ups or infusion. It is a versatile non-depolarizing agent which can be used in all operative procedures requiring muscle relaxation.

The recommended initial bolus dose for tracheal intubation and subsequent surgical procedures is 80–100 μg.kg^{-1}.

This initial dose should produce good intubating conditions within 90–120 seconds, and may be expected to provide clinically acceptable muscle relaxation for a period of 20–30 minutes in adults;[8] 15–20 minutes in children and 30–40 minutes in infants. Incremental bolus doses of 30–50 μg.kg^{-1} may be given when required as assessed by neuromuscular response to train of four stimulation.

Onset of action of a neuromuscular blocking agent is usually defined as the time from completion of the intravenous injection to maximal depression of twitch response. Increasing the initial dose of vecuronium over 150 μg.kg^{-1} does not lead to a significantly faster onset of action,[9,10] although clinical studies have demonstrated that with halothane/nitrousoxide/fentanyl anaesthesia[11,12] the onset time decreases from 168 sec. at 100 μg.kg^{-1} to 92 sec at 250 μg.kg^{-1}. Agents used concomitantly with vecuronium to induce anaesthesia may influence the rate of onset of neuromuscular paralysis. For long surgical procedures, the initial dose may be increased to 150 μg.kg^{-1} or 250 μg.kg^{-1} with consequent longer duration of action: about 50 min and 80 min respectively.

The $ED_{90/95}$ in adults is 36–56 μg.kg^{-1} with nitrous oxide/opioid anaesthesia. There is no cumulative effect with repeated doses,[13] but considerable interindividual variations regarding duration of effect. Administration should be monitored by measuring the neuromuscular response to train of four nerve stimulation.

Spontaneous recovery from vecuronium blockade is both predictable and rapid. The average recovery index, ie time taken for recovery of twitch height from 25% to 75% for an intubating dose (80–100 μg.kg^{-1}) of vecuronium is about 10 min. Increasing the dose to 200 μg.kg^{-1} extends this to about 15 min, and 250 μg.kg^{-1} to about 30 min.

Vecuronium may also be administered by intravenous infusion. When the blockade produced by the initial bolus begins to lighten, an intravenous infusion of 50–80 μg.kg^{-1}.h^{-1} may be used to provide satisfactory clinical relaxation (90–95% depression of evoked twitch amplitude, one response to train of four stimulation) for as long as is required.

Infusions in children. The infusion rate of vecuronium to maintain 90–95% neuromuscular blockade during balanced anaesthesia is significantly dependent on age in paediatric patients;[14] for infants a rate of 62 μg.kg^{-1}.h^{-1}, and for children a rate of 154 μg.kg^{-1}.h^{-1} is recommended. Adolescent requirements approach those of adults, i.e. 50–80 μg.kg^{-1}.h^{-1}.

As with all neuromuscular blocking agents, wherever practical, monitoring of neuromuscular blockade should occur. The condition and age of the patient and concurrent drug treatment should be taken into consideration when determining the dose of vecuronium. Recovery from the relaxation produced by an infusion of vecuronium is usually rapid once the infusion is stopped.[15,16] Mean recovery times of 9–17 min. have been reported.[17,18] Vecuronium is virtually non-cumulative,[1,8,13,19,20] and reversal by anticholinesterases is easily achieved.[21] There should be some tangible evidence of returning neuromuscular transmission (e.g. first response to a train of four stimulation) prior to the administration of anticholinesterase in order to ensure a satisfactory prompt reversal.

Vecuronium is particularly useful in patients with cardiovascular disease as it has no clinically significant adverse cardiovascular effects,[22,23] either by histamine release or autonomic blockade.[6,8,9,10,22,24,25] It does not influence heart rate, or systolic or diastolic arterial blood pressure.

Vecuronium (bromide)

Pharmacokinetics

Vecuronium is not absorbed to any significant extent following oral administration.

Following a bolus intravenous injection, vecuronium is eliminated from the plasma tri-exponentially. Autoradiographic studies in animals reveal rapid initial distribution into the extracellular space, particularly muscle, heart and liver. Vecuronium does not cross the blood–brain barrier. The volume of distribution at steady state is of the order 0.3 $l.kg^{-1}$ in fit adults, total plasma clearance is 5.2 $ml.kg^{-1}.min^{-1}$ and the elimination half life is 71 min.[27] Vecuronium is not dependent on the kidney as its principle route of elimination, the major route of plasma clearance being via the liver.[28–30] In healthy patients, less than 25% of an injected dose is excreted via the kidney, 10% as the 3-OH metabolite. There is a high extraction of vecuronium by the liver, followed by excretion of unchanged and deacetylated drug via the bile into the intestine. 40–80% of an injected dose is excreted in bile, mainly in the unchanged form; only about 5% is excreted as the 3-OH (mono-deacetylated) metabolite. The rapid plasma clearance resulting from hepatic uptake is a major contributing factor to the short duration of vecuronium blockade.

The pharmacokinetics of vecuronium can be fitted best by a 3-compartment model. Following initial mixing in the plasma (central) compartment it distributes into the extracellular space. Vecuronium also diffuses rapidly into the third compartment (the liver) from the central compartment and is then excreted. This explains the brief duration and minimal accumulation of vecuronium.[31] About 60% of an administered dose is taken up into the third compartment within 20 minutes. Changes in the neuromuscular blocking effects of vecuronium with time correspond closely with changes in the amount of vecuronium in the second compartment, which approximates to the extracellular space. The concentration of vecuronium in this compartment at 50% effect is about 160 $\mu g.l^{-1}$.

Values quoted for plasma protein binding of vecuronium vary widely from 30%[32] to 90%[33] in healthy patients. This is probably due to the use of different techniques in determining the extent of protein binding.

Oral absorption	negligible
Presystemic metabolism	—
Plasma half life	71 min
Volume of distribution	0.3 $l.kg^{-1}$
Plasma protein binding	≤90%

Vecuronium is ionized in plasma and thus very little crosses the placenta. The extent to which vecuronium is excreted in breast milk is not known. However, given its polarity this is unlikely to be significant. Further, any that is ingested by a breast-feeding infant will not be absorbed from the gastrointestinal tract. The elimination of vecuronium is reduced in patients with liver dysfunction and some adjustment of dose in such patients is often required. There is a suggestion that the elimination of vecuronium may also be reduced in renal failure. There are also reports that the kinetics of the drug are altered in the elderly, requiring particular care in tailoring the dose in such patients.

Concentration–effect relationship

In adults, mean plasma vecuronium concentrations of 137 $\mu g.l^{-1}$ and 206 $\mu g.l^{-1}$ at steady state are associated with 50% and 90% neuromuscular blockade respectively.[34]

In an average adult, an intravenous bolus of 2.3 mg vecuronium gives a plasma concentration greater than 100 $\mu g.l^{-1}$ for about 12 min. Doubling the bolus dose gives 24 min, doubling again gives 40 min and doubling again 72 min. However there is a big interindividual variation with increasing variability of duration with increasing dose. Better control is achieved by giving a small initial bolus and then increments as required guided by train of four stimulation of the ulnar nerve.

Metabolism

The metabolism of vecuronium is relatively small[35,36] and it is primarily eliminated in the unchanged form in bile (~70%) and urine (10–20%). The potential metabolites of vecuronium, the 3-OH, 17-OH and 3,17-di-OH derivatives, closely resemble vecuronium in their pharmacological profiles but having reduced potency (see Fig. 2). They have not been detected in the plasma of normal patients. A small fraction of the injected dose appears in the bile and the urine as the 3-OH metabolite.

In the isolated rat phrenic nerve-hemidiaphragm preparation, vecuronium was 1.5 times more potent than the 3-deacetyl (3-OH) metabolite, 10.1 times more potent than the 17-deacetyl (17-OH) derivative and 17.6 times more potent than the 3,17-bisdeacetyl (3,17-di-OH) derivative.[8]

The neuromuscular and vagal blocking activities of these three potential metabolites have also been compared in anaesthetized cats and although the metabolites have greater vagal blocking potency than vecuronium, it is unlikely that sufficient is formed at neuromus-

Fig. 2 The metabolism of Vecuronium

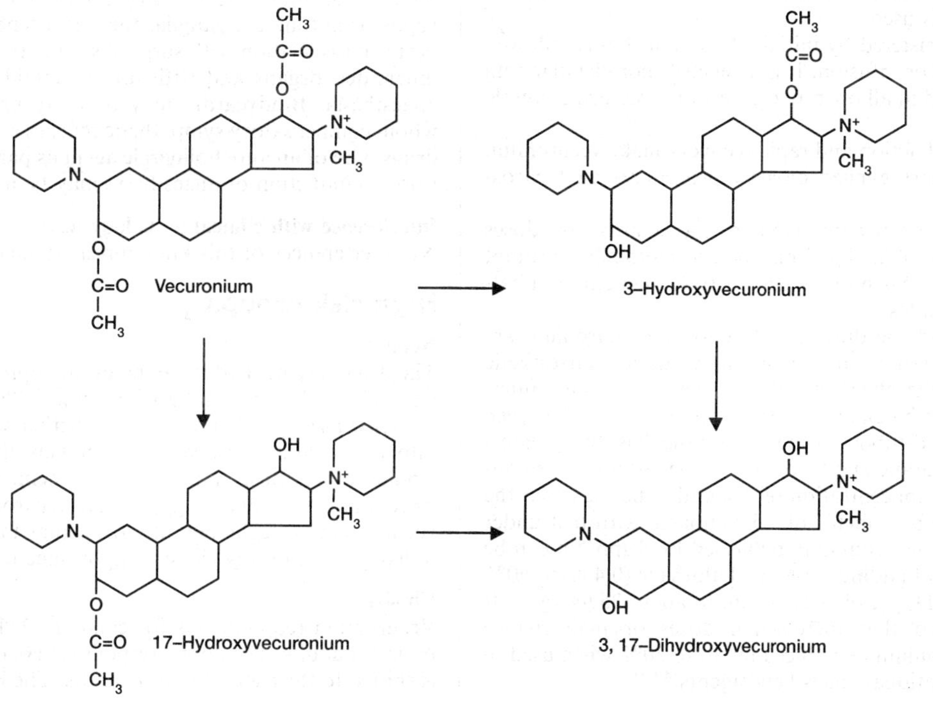

cular blocking doses of vecuronium to produce sufficient vagal block to lead to an increase in heart rate.[1]

Pharmaceutics

Vecuronium bromide (Norcuron; Organon Teknika, UK/Organon, USA) is available only as a preparation for intravenous use. It is not sufficiently stable for supply and storage in a ready made aqueous solution. it is presented in vials containing 10 mg vecuronium bromide, together with a 5 ml ampoule of Water for Injection, as a lyophilized powder to be reconstituted. In addition to the active compound, the lyophilized material contains citric acid, disodium phosphate buffers and mannitol as an osmoregulator. The reconstituted solution is clear, colourless and isotonic with a pH of 4. The lyophilized material remains stable for three years at room temperature, in the dark. Once reconstituted, vecuronium remains stable for only 24 h at room temperature.

Vecuronium may be diluted for use in infusions in the following fluids: 0.9% sodium chloride solution, 5.0% glucose solution, Ringer's solution and Ringer's glucose solution.

When used in dilute solutions, vecuronium must first be dissolved in Water for Injection and the resultant solution added to the infusion fluid. Under these conditions vecuronium will remain stable for up to 24 h at room temperature down to a concentration of 40 $mg.l^{-1}$. Vecuronium should not be mixed in the same syringe with other drugs, and any common administration line should be flushed with saline before use.

Therapeutic use

Indications

When neuromuscular blockade is required during general anaesthesia for surgical operations or to facilitate ventilation of the lungs in patients in the intensive care unit.

Contraindications

1. Known allergy to vecuronium
2. Patients at risk of aspiration of gastric contents, when a rapid sequence induction is required
3. Patients with upper airway obstruction, where the airway should be secured before administration of a long-acting neuromuscular blocking agent.

Mode of use

Vecuronium should only be used by individuals who are experienced in the use of neuromuscular blocking drugs and in the maintenance of an adequate airway and respiratory support. Facilities and personnel necessary for tracheal intubation, administration of oxygen and assisted or controlled ventilation should be immediately available whenever vecuronium is used.

Vecuronium is administered by initial intravenous bolus followed by intravenous top-ups or infusion. It is a versatile non-depolarizing agent which can be used in all operative procedures requiring muscle relaxation.

The short duration of action and rapid recovery make vecuronium especially useful in short gynaeocological procedures eg laparoscopy.[37,38]

For procedures of short duration (15 min) e.g. laparoscopy, doses of vecuronium as low as 60 $\mu g.kg^{-1}$ may be chosen to allow prompt antagonism of paralysis. Such doses demonstrate adequate intubating conditions at 3 minutes.

Both the potency and the duration of action of vecuronium are increased in the presence of potent inhalational anaesthetic agents,[39,40] although the effect of volatile agents on vecuronium-induced neuromuscular blockade is very much less than that seen with pancuronium or d-tubocurarine. Enflurane has the greatest effect, followed by isoflurane and halothane.[41] Nagashima[42] demonstrated that an inhaled concentration of 2% enflurane increased the potency of vecuronium by a factor of 1.5 compared with that under neurolept anaesthesia, and from data published by Rupp[24] it can be deduced that the effect of adding 0.6 MAC halothane (0.4%) to 60% N_2O is to reduce the $ED_{90/95}$ of vecuronium to about 25 $\mu g.kg^{-1}$. It has been recommended that incremental doses or maintenance infusion rates of vecuronium be reduced by up to 30% when used in conjunction with inhalational anaesthetic agents.[39]

There is no increase in intraocular[43,44] or intracranial pressure[45] associated with vecuronium administration so it may be used in ophthalmic surgery and neurosurgery. Low placental transfer means that it is also suitable for use in Caesarian deliveries. Vecuronium does not have any significant effect on lower oesophageal sphincter tone.[46]

Use in the intensive care unit

Intravenous infusion provides the most practical method for administration of muscle relaxant drugs to patients in the intensive care unit.[47] Advantages of vecuronium are its short duration of action, lack of cumulation, absence of histamine liberation or other adverse effects, and cardiovascular stability. Rapid recovery of neuromuscular function when the infusion is discontinued allows frequent and rapid assessment of neurological status and rapid progress to extubation. There is considerable interindividual variation in vecuronium requirements so infusion rates should be tailored to individual patient response. This is best achieved by monitoring neuromuscular blockade using a simple train of four nerve stimulator.

Precautions

Vecuronium infusions should be used with caution in patients with severe renal and hepatic dysfunction until more data on its use in these conditions are available. Reports in the recent literature would suggest that there is prolongation of the effect of vecuronium when given by intravenous infusion to patients with renal failure.[48,49]

Adverse reactions

Potentially life-threatening effects

No effects of this degree of severity appear to have been reported.

Acute overdosage

The spontaneous reversal of the neuromuscular blockade caused by vecuronium is rapid. In the event of overdosage, that is when administration of a cholinesterase-inhibiting agent fails to reverse the neuromuscular blocking effects, artificial ventilation of the patient's lungs must be continued until spontaneous breathing is restored.

As with other non-depolarizing neuromuscular blockers, vecuronium can cause a reduction in partial thromboplastin time and prothrombin time.

Severe or irreversible adverse effects

Over a period of 7 years, a total of 24 adverse reactions events have been documented. Those most frequently occurring include urticaria, bradyarrhythmias and bronchospasm. However, in all instances vecuronium had been administered concomitantly with other drugs and causality is difficult to establish.

Symptomatic adverse effects

Since vecuronium has virtually no blocking activity on the cardiac vagus or autonomic ganglia, there is a tendency for bradycardia to occur in association with surgical stimulation of parasympathetically innervated organs and with use of opioid analgesics or halothane anaesthesia. Bradycardia may be more pronounced in patients in whom compensatory sympathetic reflexes are impaired by β-blocking drugs. Use of an anticholinergic agent as part of the premedication or prior to induction of anaesthesia may be indicated.

Interference with clinical pathology tests

No interferences of this kind appear to have been reported.

High risk groups

Neonates

The drug may be used in neonates, in appropriate doses, if indicated (see below: Children and above Clinical Pharmacology).

Breast milk. It is not known whether vecuronium is distributed into breast milk; however it is unlikely that a significant amount would be present in milk due to its chemical structure. In addition, since animal studies suggest that gastrointestinal absorption of vecuronium is negligible, any drug that may be present in milk is unlikely to be of any clinical importance to the nursing infant.

Children

Vecuronium requirements for children (3–10 years) are higher than those for adults. The dose—response curve of vecuronium in children is shifted to the right of that in adults. The $ED_{90/95}$ is 55–64 $\mu g.kg^{-1}$

Vecuronium (bromide)

in children compared with 36–56 μg.kg^{-1} in adults.[50] The differences between children and adults could be the result of age-related differences in the pharmacokinetics and pharmacodynamics of vecuronium. The duration of action of vecuronium in children is short compared with that of other non-depolarizing agents in equivalent doses. The recovery index in children is shorter compared with adults; this could result from a higher plasma clearance in children compared with adults. There is no evidence of accumulation in children, and cardiovascular stability is maintained as in adults.

There are marked differences in the pharmacodynamics of vecuronium between infants and children.[51] The ED_{95} in neonates and infants is 40% smaller than that in children.[52] The lower ED_{95} in babies under one year may result from immaturity of neuromuscular transmission in these subjects. The onset of action is more rapid in infants than in children and adults. This may be because the relatively higher cardiac output during infancy causes more rapid delivery of vecuronium to the neuromuscular junction. The duration of effect of 100 μg.kg^{-1} is almost 60 minutes compared with less than 20 minutes in children, probably as a result of the larger volume of distribution leading to a longer elimination half life. In addition, the immature hepatic function in young infants might contribute to a lower plasma clearance of vecuronium. Vecuronium tends to have an effect in neonates and infants which is similar to that of a long-acting neuromuscular blocking agent.[53] The prolongation of effect and the reduced dose requirements in neonates and infants (see clinical pharmacology) appear to be features unique to vecuronium when compared with other neuromuscular blocking agents.

Pregnant women

Due to their ionized nature in plasma, neuromuscular blocking drugs do not readily cross the placental barrier. Vecuronium crosses the placenta to a very limited extent: its placental transfer is about 50% that of pancuronium. Due to ethical restrictions, there have been no studies investigating the use of vecuronium for non-obstetric surgery in pregnant women; however it is unlikely to cause any particular problems in this group. Vecuronium may be used for childbirth by Caesarean section without effect on the newborn child.[54]

The elderly

Vecuronium has a longer onset time,[55] lower plasma clearance and smaller volume of distribution at steady state in elderly compared with young adults, but similar distribution and elimination half lives and sensitivity of the neuromuscular junction.[56] Some studies have found reduced dosage requirements and a longer recovery time in older patients[57] compared with younger adults but others have found no such age-related effects.[58] The influence of age on neuromuscular blockade produced by vecuronium is less marked in comparison with that which occurs with pancuronium. Extra care should be taken in tailoring the dose of vecuronium to patient response in the elderly and consideration given to the potential for a prolonged recovery time.

Concurrent disease

Renal failure. Early studies investigating the use of vecuronium in patients with renal failure found that patients with this disorder had slightly delayed removal of vecuronium from the plasma, with only mild prolongation of effect and recovery.[59] In one study, renal failure was found to increase the plasma terminal half life of vecuronium by some 25%, although there was no significant clinical difference between the patients with impaired renal function and those without.[60] Another group[29] observed that pharmacokinetic analysis of the plasma concentration data of vecuronium in patients with and without renal function revealed no statistically significant differences in distribution and elimination half lives of the drug, and no difference in clearance or volume of distribution at steady state. Anephric patients who received 100 μg.kg^{-1} vecuronium had significantly higher plasma concentrations at 25% and 75% recovery than patients without renal failure. This surprising apparent tolerance to vecuronium in patients with renal failure was further supported by a tendency to a slower onset of action in these patients.[59]

In a recent combined pharmacodynamic and pharmacokinetic study,[61] changes in the pharmacokinetics of vecuronium were demonstrated in patients with renal failure during isoflurane anaesthesia. Vecuronium-induced neuromuscular blockade lasted longer in patients with renal failure than in those with normal renal function, and this might have been due to a lower plasma clearance and prolonged elimination half life of vecuronium in the renal failure group. There have also been reports[62–64] describing the accumulation of vecuronium in patients with renal failure and it should therefore only be used in these patients with careful monitoring of neuromuscular function.

Hepatic and/or biliary tract disease. In patients with cirrhosis it has been found[65] that recovery of the ratio A'/A of train of four (ratio of height of first twitch to control) is markedly prolonged when vecuronium 200 μg.kg^{-1} is given, but there is no effect with 150 μg.kg^{-1} compared with normals, and with 100 μg.kg^{-1} the activity of the drug seemed less in cirrhotics compared with normals. This significant and considerable prolongation of duration of action of vecuronium 200 μg.kg^{-1} in patients with slight impairment of hepatic function suggests that the duration of action might be very long in patients with more severe liver disease. A possible explanation for this effect is that hepatic uptake is a major determinant of vecuronium clearance. If higher doses saturate the hepatic uptake capacity of patients with liver disease, clearance would decrease. The clinical implication of dose-dependent clearance is that large or repeated doses may lead to accumulation of vecuronium in the plasma of patients with liver disease.[66]

The onset time of neuromuscular blockade following 100 μg.kg^{-1} is somewhat slower in cirrhotics compared with normal patients. This may be because cirrhotic patients have a larger central compartment volume of distribution; this would produce a lower concentration of drug in the central compartment during the first stage of distribution and thus cause slower onset of neuromuscular blockade. The more rapid recovery from a small dose in patients with cirrhosis is also consistent with an increase in the volume of distribution in this group.

Following vecuronium 150 μg.kg^{-1}, the rate of recovery in the cirrhotic patients was the same as that in normals. This may be due to a balance between the opposing tendencies noted, i.e. altered volume of distribution (tending to shorten duration of action) balanced by reduced hepatic clearance (tending to prolong action).[65]

In patients with cholestatic liver disease, the reduced plasma elimination results in an increased duration of action. The increased plasma concentration of bile salts in these patients reduces the liver uptake of vecuronium.

In hepatitis there is reduced plasma clearance leading to a longer duration of action.

Neuromuscular disease. Vecuronium has been successfully used in patients with myasthenia gravis, but very small doses must be used and it is mandatory that the extent of neuromuscular blockade be monitored throughout anaesthesia.[67,68] In cases of myopathy, neuromuscular disease and poliomyelitis, vecuronium should also be used with caution. Vecuronium has been used in patients susceptible to malignant hyperthermia without any problems,[69] and it has been used successfully in patients with muscular dystrophy.[70]

Hypothermia. In operations requiring hypothermia, the neuromuscular blocking activity of non-depolarizing drugs is decreased, and increases with rewarming of the patient.[71]

Burns. Burned patients (adults or children) are resistant to the neuromuscular blocking effects of non-depolarizing relaxants and the degree of resistance is related to the extent of the burn. In a study on burned children (0.5–17 years) it was found that the ED_{50} and ED_{95} were significantly increased in burned children compared with controls. There was a rightward shift of the dose–response curve related to magnitude of burn; that is as burn size increased the ED value increased proportionately.[72]

Hyperparathyroidism. As the calcium ion plays an important role in neuromuscular transmission, diseases such as hyperparathyroidism which alter calcium homeostasis may alter patient responses to neuromuscular blocking drugs. Patients with hyperparathyroidism demonstrate a shorter duration of action and reduced magnitude of twitch depression with vecuronium (30 μg.kg^{-1}).

Other conditions. Conditions which may potentiate the effect of vecuronium include hypokalaemia (e.g. after severe vomiting, diarrhoea, digitalization and diuretic therapy), hypermagnesaemia, hypocalcaemia, hypoproteinaemia, dehydration, respiratory[74] or metabolic acidosis and cachexia.

Respiratory or metabolic alkalosis may cause slight antagonism of neuromuscular blockade.

Drug interactions

Potentially hazardous interactions

Some of the interactions described below may, in some circumstances, be potentially hazardous.

Other significant interactions

Increased effect. Volatile anaesthetic agents including halothane, ether, enflurane, isoflurane, methoxyflurane and cyclopropane increase the neuromuscular blockade produced by vecuronium. This also occurs to a lesser extent with intravenous anaesthetic agents including thiopentone, propofol, methohexitone, ketamine, gammahydroxybutyrate and etomidate. Other drugs which increase the effect of vecuronium include fentanyl, other non-depolarizing muscle relaxants, prior administration of suxamethonium,[75,76] aminoglycoside antibiotics, tetracyclines, lincosamides, polymyxins, diuretics, β-adrenergic blocking agents, thiamine, monoamine oxidase inhibiting drugs, imidazole and calcium antagonists.[77]

Decreased effect. Drugs which decrease the effect of vecuronium include the anticholinesterases, prior chronic administration of corticosteroids, noradrenaline, azathioprine, theophylline, potassium chloride and calcium. Recovery of neuromuscular function is enhanced in the presence of phenytoin. Whether this is due to a pharmacokinetic or a pharmacodynamic mechanism is not known, but the latter is more likely.[78]

Variable effect. Depolarizing muscle relaxants given after the administration of vecuronium bromide may produce potentiation or attenuation of the neuromuscular blocking effect. The non-depolarizing drug increases resistance towards the neuromuscular blocking effect of the depolarizing drug, therefore high doses of a depolarizing drug are necessary before muscle relaxation can be obtained. These high doses of a depolarizing drug may cause endplate desensitization and prolonged postoperative apnoea. Recent evidence suggests that alkylating drugs should be considered a possible hazard when given to patients during anaesthesia involving the use of muscle relaxants.

Potentially useful interactions

Drug interactions are not necessarily disadvantageous. Interactions between anaesthetic agents and vecuronium are potentially useful as they produce a reduction in vecuronium requirements, and the interaction between anticholinesterase agents and vecuronium is used in daily clinical practice to reverse the neuromuscular blocking effects of vecuronium.

Clinical trials

1. Agoston S 1983 Clinical pharmacology of vecuronium: a preliminary report on a multicentre study in 800 patients. In: Agoston E (ed) Clinical experiences with Norcuron, CCP11. Exerpta Medica, Amsterdam, p 99

A multicentre trial carried out simultaneously in 15 different institutions in eleven countries investigating the clinical usability of vecuronium in patients under balanced anaesthesia or inhalational anaesthesia with enflurane or halothane. Points of interest were the comparison of the time course of neuromuscular blocking effects of vecuronium and pancuronium using comparable doses and criteria, and also a comparison of the results obtained from investigators using twitch height recording in their studies compared with those who relied upon clinical judgement alone. Three different protocols were used and each investigator studied a total of 50 patients: those who used balanced anaesthesia studied 25 patients receiving vecuronium 0.1 mg.kg^{-1} intravenously and 25 receiving the same dose of pancuronium (protocol A) or half the dose of either compound in groups of similar size following intubation with suxamethonium (protiol B). Investigators using additional anaesthesia (protocol C/D) used only vecuronium 0.1 mg.kg^{-1} intravenously under enflurane (25 patients) or halothane (25 patients) anaesthesia. Within each study patients were randomly allocated to one of the treatment groups. The maintenance dose of relaxant was always one fourth of the initial dose.

Onset times for both vecuronium and pancuronium were similar: 2–3 minutes after 0.1 mg.kg^{-1}. The clinical duration and total duration of action of vecuronium were 2–3 times shorter and spontaneous recovery 2–3 times faster compared with pancuronium. Under the experimental conditions of the study, there was no observable influence of enflurane or halothane on the time course of the effects of the initial dose of vecuronium or pancuronium. However with prolonged anaesthesia (2 hours) the total dosage requirement for vecuronium was reduced under enflurane anaesthesia. Vecuronium appeared to be free from cardiovascular or other side effects. There was no difference in the result obtained by twitch height recording and clinical judgement.

2. Mirakhur R K, Ferres C J, Clarke R S J, Bali I M, Dundee J W 1983 Clinical evaluation of Org NC45. British Journal of Anaesthesia 55: 119–124

Vecuronium was administered to 200 fit adult patients presenting for elective surgery in a dose of either 0.1 mg. kg^{-1}. 0.15 mg. kg^{-1} or 0.2 mg. kg^{-1}. Its effects were evaluated with regard to conditions for tracheal intubation time to onset of maximal block, duration of action and quality of reversal of blockade following administration of anticholinesterase.

Intubation could be satisfactorily carried out at around 90 sec in 90% of patients. The duration of clinical relaxation varied from 23 min with 0.1 mg. kg^{-1} and neuroleptanaesthesia to 71 min with 0.2 mg. kg^{-1} and anaesthesia with halothane or enflurane. There was no evidence of cumulation and the antagonism of residual block was prompt and easy following administration of neostigmine. There were no significant cardiovascular effects apparent on routine monitoring.

3. Wierda J M K H, Maestrone E, Bencini A F et al 1989 Haemodynamic effects of vecuronium. British Journal of Anaesthesia 62: 194–198

An open study in which 320 patients undergoing routine surgery were allocated to receive either a nitrous oxide-neurolept anaesthetic technique or nitrous oxide-halothane anaesthesia. 50% of patients in each anaesthetic group received atropine 7 µg. kg^{-1} with premedication, and 50% of each of these two groups received vecuronium. In this way, 8 groups were formed on a random basis. Heart rate, systolic and diastolic arterial blood pressure were measured before induction, immediately before (0 min) and at intervals following administration of vecuronium or saline for a total of 10 minutes. Ventilation of the lungs was maintained by facemask to avoid the effects of intubation on the cardiovascular system.

Vecuronium had no effect on heat rate or arterial blood pressure during nitrous oxide-neurolept anaesthesia nor nitrous oxide-halothane anaesthesia.

General review articles

Reilly C S, Nimmo W S 1987 New intravenous anaesthetics and neuromuscular blocking drugs. A review of their properties and clinical use. Drugs 34: 98–135

Miller R D, Rupp S M, Fisher D M, Cronnelly R, Fahey M R, Sohn Y J 1984 Clinical pharmacology of vecuronium and atracurium. Anesthesiology 61: 444–453

Miller R D 1984 Vecuronium: a new non-depolarizing neuromuscular-blocking agent. Pharmacotherapy 4: 238–247

Booij L H D J 1989 Muscle relaxants and medical status of patient. Current Opinion in Anaesthesiology 2: 488–492

Baird W L M, Savage D S 1985 Vecuronium — the first years. In: Clinics in Anesthesiology 3: 347–360

Bowman W C 1980 A new non-depolarizing neuromuscular blocking drug. Trends in pharmacological sciences 1: 263–266

References

1. Marshall I G, Agoston S, Booij L H D J, Durant N N, Foldes F F 1980 Pharmacology of ORG NC 45 compared with other non-depolarizing neuromuscular blocking drugs. British Journal of Anaesthesia 52: 11S–19S
2. Torda T A, Kiloh N, Myoneural actions of Org N C45 1982 British Journal of Anaesthesia 54: 1217–1221
3. Bowman W C 1983 Preclinical pharmacology of vecuronium bromide. In: Clinical experiences with Norcuron, CCP6, Ed. S Agoston, Exerpta Medica, Amsterdam pp 7–19
4. Lebrault C, Chauvin M, Guirimand F, Duvaldestin P 1989 Relative potency of vecuronium on the diaphragm and the adductor pollicis. British Journal of Anaesthesia 63: 389–392
5. Basta S A, Savarese J J 1983 Comparative histamine-releasing properties of vecuronium, atracurium, tubocurarine and metocurine,. In: Clinical experiences with Norcuron, CCP11, Ed. S Agoston, Exerpta Medica, Amsterdam p. 183

Vecuronium (bromide)

6. Durrant N N, Marshall I G, Savage D S, Nelson D N, Sleigh T, Carlyle I C 1979 The neuromuscular and autonomic blocking activities of pancuronium, Org NC 45, and other pancuronium analogues in the cat. Journal of Pharmacy and Pharmacology 31: 831–836
7. Salt P J, Barnes P K, Conway C M 1980 Inhibition of neuronal uptake of noradrenaline in the isolated perfused rat heart by pancuronium and its homologues Org 6368, Org 7268, and Org NC45. British Journal of Anaesthesia 52: 313–317
8. Agoston S 1983 Clinical pharmacology of vecuronium: a preliminary report on a multicentre study in 800 patients. In: Agoston S (ed) Clinical Experiences with Norcuron, CCP11. Exerpta Medica, Amsterdam, p. 99
9. Fahey M R, Morris R B, Miller R D, Sohn Y J, Cronnelly R, Gencarelli P 1981 Clinical pharmacology of Org NC45 (Norcuron): a new non-depolarizing muscle relaxant. Anesthesiology 55: 6–11
10. Mirakhur R K, Ferres C J, Clarke R S J, Bali I M, Dundee J W 1983 Clinical evaluation of Org NC45. British Journal of Anaesthesia 55: 119–124
11. Rorvik K, Husby P, Gramstad L, Vamnes J S, Bitsch-Larsen L, Koller M-E 1988 Comparison of large dose of vecuronium for prolonged muscular blockade. British Journal of Anaesthesia 61: 180–185
12. Ginsberg B, Glass P S, Quill T, Shafron D, Ossey K D 1989 Onset and duration of neuromuscular blockade following high dose vecuronium administration. Anaesthesiology 71: 201–205
13. Eriksson L I, Staun P, Cederholm I, Lennmarken C, Lofstrom J B 1988 Experience with vecuronium during long-lasting surgery. Acta Anaesthesiologica Scandinavica 32: 619–622
14. Meretoja O A 1989 Vecuronium infusion requirements in paediatric patients during fentanyl-N_{20-02} anaesthesia. Anesthesia and Analgesia 68: 20–24
15. Cannon J E, Fahey M R, Castagnoli K P et al 1987 Continuous infusion of vecuronium: The effect of anaesthetic agents. Anesthesiology 64: 503–506
16. Haraldsted V Y, Nielsen J W, Joensen F, Dilling-Hansen B, Hasselstrom L 1988 Infusion of vecuronium assessed by tactile evaluation of evoked thumb twitch. British Journal of Anaesthesia 61: 479–481
17. Agoston S, Salt P, Newton D, Bencini A, Boomsma P, Erdmann W 1980 The neuromuscular blocking action of Org NC45, a new pancuronium derivative, in anaesthetized patients. A pilot study. British Journal of Anaesthesia 52: 53S–59S
18. Buzello W, Noldge G 1982 Repetitive administration of pancuronium and vecuronium (Org NC45, Norcuron) in patients undergoing long-lasting operations. British Journal of Anaesthesia 54: 1151
19. Durant N N, Nguyen N, Lee C, Katz R L 1981 The cumulative effects of Norcuron and atracurium. Anesthesiology 55: A209
20. Fahey M R, Morris R B, Miller R D, Sohn Y J, Cronnelly R 1980 Comparative cumulative effects of Norcuron and pancuronium. Anesthesiology 53: S271
21. Mirakhur R K, Ferres C J 1984 Muscle relaxation with an infusion of vecuronium. European Journal of Anaesthesiology 1: 353–359
22. Lienhart A, Guggiari M, Maneglia R, Cousin M T, Viars P 1983 Cardiovascular effects of vecuronium in man. In: Agoston S (ed) Clinical experiences with Norcuron, CCP11. Exerpta medica, Amsterdam, p. 150–155
23. Morris R B, Cahalan M K, Miller R D, Wilkinson P L, Quasha A L, Robinson S L 1983 The cardiovascular effects of vecuronium (Org NC45) and pancuronium in patients undergoing coronary artery bypass grafting. Anesthesiology 58: 438–440
24. Rupp S M, Miller R D, Gencarelli P J 1984 Vecuronium-induced neuromuscular blockade during enflurane, isoflurane and halothane anaesthesia in humans. Anesthesiology 60: 102–105
25. Robertson E N, Booij L H D J, Fragen R J, Crul J F 1983 Clinical comparison of atracurium and vecuronium (Org NC45) British Journal of Anaesthesia 55: 125–129
26. Wierda J M K H, Maestrone E, Bencini A F et al 1989 Haemodynamic effects of vecuronium. British Journal of Anaesthesia 62: 194–198
27. Cronnelly R, Fisher D M, Miller R D, Gencarelli P, Nguyen-Gruenke L, Castagnoli N 1983 Pharmacokinetics and pharmacodynamics of vecuronium (Org NC45) and pancuronium in anaesthetized humans. Anesthesiology 58: 405–408
28. Sohn Y J, Bencini A, Scaf A H J, Kersten V W, Gregoretti S, Agoston S 1982 Pharmacokinetics of vecuronium in man. Anesthesiology 57: A256
29. Fahey M R, Morris R B, Miller R D, Nguyen T-L, Upton R A 1981 Pharmacokinetics of Org NC45 (Norcuron) in patients with and without renal failure. British Journal of Anaesthesia 53: 1049–1052
30. Bencini A F, Scaf A H J, Sohn Y J, Kersten-Kleef V W, Agoston S 1986 Hepatobiliary disposition of vecuronium bromide in man. British Journal of Anaesthesia 58: 988–995
31. Bencini A 1983 Clinical pharmacokinetics of vecuronium bromide. In: Clinical experiences with Norcuron, CCP6 Ed. S Agoston, Exerpta Medica, Amsterdam p. 25–37
32. Duvaldestin P, Henzel D 1982 Binding of tubocurarine, fazadinium, pancuronium and Org NC45 to serum proteins in normal man and in patients with cirrhosis. British Journal of Anaesthesia 54: 513–516
33. Foldes F F, Deery A 1983 Protein binding of atracurium and other short-acting neuromuscular blocking agents and their interaction with human cholinesterases. British Journal of Anaesthesia 55: 31S–34S
34. Van der Veen, Bencini A 1980 Pharmacokinetics and pharmacodynamics of Org NC45 in man. British Journal of Anaesthesia 52: 37S–41S
35. Marshall I G, Gibb A J, Durant N N 1983 Neuromuscular and vagal blocking actions of pancuronium bromide, its metabolites and vecuronium bromide (Org NC45) and its potential metabolites in the anaesthetized cat. British Journal of Anaesthesia 55: 703–714
36. Bencini A F, Houwertjes M C, Agoston S 1985 Effects of hepatic uptake of vecuronium and its putative metabolites upon their neuromuscular blocking actions on the cat. British Journal of Anaesthesia 57: 789–795
37. Fragen R J, Booij L H D J, Crul J F 1982 Vecuronium (Org NC45) for laparoscopy; clinical experience. Acta Anaesthesiologica Belgica 33: 177–181
38. Caldwell J E, Braidwood J M, Simpson D S 1985 Vecuronium bromide in anaesthesia for laparoscopic sterlization. British Journal of Anaesthesia 57: 765–769
39. Foldes F F, Nagashima H, Ohta Y, Ono K, Chaudhry I, Kaplan R, Nguyen H D 1983 Modification of the neuromuscular blocking effect of vecuronium by various anaesthetic agents. In: Agoston S (ed) Clinical experiences with Norcuron, CCP11. Exerpta Medica, Amsterdam, p. 132–139
40. Duncalf D, Nagashima H, Hollinger I, Badola R P, Kaplan R, Foldes F F 1981 Relaxation with Org NC45 during halothane anaesthesia. Anesthesiology 55: A203
41. Foldes F F, Bencini A, Newton D 1980 Influence of halothane and enflurane on the neuromuscular effects of Org NC45 in man. British Journal of Anaesthesia 52: 64S–65S
42. Nagashima H, Yun H, Radnay P A, Duncalf D, Kaplan R, Foldes F F 1981 Influence of anaesthesia on human dose-response of Org NC45. Anesthesiology 55: A202
43. Sia R L, Rashkovsky O M 1981 Org NC45 and intraocular pressure during anaesthesia. Acta Anaesthesiologica Scandinavica 25: 386–388
44. Jantzen J P, Hackett G H, Erdmann K, Earnshaw G 1986 Effect of vecuronium on intraocular pressure. British Journal of Anaesthesia 58: 433–436
45. Rosa G, Sanfilippo M, Vilardi V, Orfei P, Gasparetto A 1986 Effects of vecuronium bromide on intracranial pressure and cerebral perfusion pressure. British Journal of Anaesthesia 58: 437–440
46. Hunt P C W, Cotton B R, Smith G 1984 Barrier pressure and muscle relaxants. Anaesthesia 39: 412–415
47. Darrah W C, Johnston J R, Mirakhur R K 1989 Vecuronium infusions for prolonged muscle relaxation in the intensive care unit. Critical Care Medicine 17: 1297
48. Segredo V, Matthay M A, Sharma M L, Gruenke L D, Caldwell J E, Miller R D 1990 Prolonged neuromuscular blockade after long-term administration of vecuronium in two critically ill patients. Anesthesiology 72: 566–570
49. Smith C L, Hunter J M, Jones R S 1987 Vecuronium infusions in patients with renal failure in an ITU. Anaesthesia 42: 387–393
50. Meistelman C, Loose J P, Saint-Maurice C, Delleur M M, Da Silva G L 1986 Clinical pharmacology of vecuronium in children. British Journal of Anaesthesia 58: 996–1000
51. Fisher D M, Miller R D 1983 Neuromuscular effects of vecuronim (Org NC45) in infants and children during N_{20}, halothane anaesthesia. Anesthesiology 58: 519–523
52. Meretoja O A, Wirtavuori K, Neuvonen P J 1988 Age-dependence of the dose–response curve of vecuronium in paediatric patients during balanced anaesthesia. Anesthesia and Analgesia 67: 21–26
53. Meretoja O A 1989 Is vecuronium a long-acting neuromuscular blocking agent in neonates and infants? British Journal of Anaesthesia 62: 184–187
54. Dailey P A, Fisher D M, Shnider S M et al 1982 Pharmacokinetics, placental transfer and neonatal effects of vecuronium and pancuronium administered during caesarian section. Anesthesiology 60: 569
55. d'Hollander A, Barvais L, Massaut J, Duvaldestin P, Desmonts J M 1983 Vecuronium in geriatric patients. In: Agoston S (ed) Clinical experiences with Norcuron, CCP11. Exerpta Medica, Amsterdam, p. 171–174
56. Rupp S M, Castagnoli K P, Fisher D M, Miller R D 1987 Pancuronium and vecuronium pharmacokinetics and pharmacodynamics in younger and elderly adults. Anesthesiology 67: 45–49
57. d'Hollander AA, Massaux F, Nevelsteen M, Agoston S 1982 Age-dependent dose-response relationship of Org NC45 in anaesthetized patients. British Journal of Anaesthesia 54: 653
58. Rupp S M, Fisher D M, Miller R D, Castagnoli K 1983 Pharmacokinetics and pharmacodynamics of vecuronium in the elderly. Anesthesiology 59: A270
59. Bencini A F, Scaf A H J, Sohn Y J et al 1986 Disposition and urinary excretion of vecuronium bromide in anaesthetized patients with normal renal function or renal failure. Anesthesia and Analgesia 65: 245–251
60. Miller R D, Rupp S M, Fahey M R, Morris R B, Gencarelli P J, Sohn Y J 1983 Pharmacokinetics of vecuronium in patients with kidney disease. In: Agoston S (ed) Clinical experiences with Norcuron CCP11. Exerpta Medica, Amsterdam, p. 124–126
61. Lynam D P, Cronnelly R, Castagnoli K P et al 1988 The pharmacodynamics and pharmacokinetics of vecuronium in patients anaesthetized with isoflurane with normal renal function or with renal failure. Anesthesiology 69: 227–231
62. Starsnic M A, Goldberg M E, Ritter D E, Marr A T, Sosis M, Larijani G E 1989 Does vecuronium accumulate in the renal transplant patient? Canadian Journal of Anaesthesia 36: 35–39
63. Slater R M, Pollard B J, Doran B R H 1988 Prolonged neuromuscular blockade with vecuronium in renal failure. Anaesthesia 43: 250–251
64. Cody M W, Dorman F M 1987 Recurarization after vecuronium in a patient with renal failure. Anaesthesia 42: 993–995
65. Hunter J M, Parker C J R, Bell C F, Jones R S, Utting J E 1985 The use of different doses of vecuronium in patients with liver dysfunction. British Journal of Anaesthesia 57: 758–764
66. Arden J R, Lynam D P, Castagnoli K P, Canfell P C, Cannon J C, Miller R D 1988 Vecuronium in alcoholic liver disease: a pharmacokinetic and pharmacodynamic analysis. Anesthesiology 68: 771–776
67. Nilsson E, Meretoja O A 1990 Vecuronium dose-response and maintenance requirements in patients with myasthenia gravis. Anesthesiology 73: 28–32
68. Eisenkraft J B, Book W J, Papatestas A E 1990 Sensitivity to vecuronium in myasthenia gravis: a dose-response study. Canadian Journal of Anaesthesia 37: 301–306
69. Ording H, Fonsmark L 1988 Use of vecuronium and doxapram in patients susceptible to malignant hyperthermia. British Journal of Anaesthesia 60: 445–449
70. Buzello W, Huttarsch H 1988 Muscle relaxation in patients with Duchenne's muscular dystrophy. British Journal of Anaesthesia 60: 228–231
71. Denny N M, Kneeshaw J D 1986 Vecuronium and atracurium infusions during hypothermic cardiopulmonary bypass. Anaesthesia 41: 919–922
72. Mills A K, Martyn J A J 1989 Neuromuscular blockade with vecuronium in paediatric patients with burn injury. British Journal of Clinical Pharmacology 28: 155–159

V

73. Caldwell J E, Heier T, Miller R D. 1989 Hyperparathyroidism and vecuronium-induced neuromuscular blockade. Anesthesiology 71: A814
74. Gencarelli P J, Swen J, Koot H W J, Miller R D 1983 The effects of hypercarbia and hypocarbia on pancuronium and vecuronium neuromuscular blockades in anaesthetized humans. Anesthesiology 59: 376–380
75. Krieg N, Hendrickx H H L, Crul J F 1981 Influence of suxamethonium on potency of Org NC45 in anaesthetized patients. British Journal of Anaesthesia 53: 259–262
76. d'Hollander A A, Agoston S, DeVille A, Cuvelier F 1983 Clinical and pharmacological actions of a bolus injection of suxamethonium: two phenomena of distinct duration. British Journal of Anaesthesia 55: 131–134
77. Poorten J F, Dhasmana K M, Kuypers R S M, Erdmann W 1984 Verapamil and reversal of vecuronium neuromuscular blockade. Anesthesia and Analgesia 63: 155–157
78. Ornstein E, Matteo R S, Schwartz A E, Silverberg P A, Young W L, Diaz J 1987 The effect of phenytoin on the magnitude and duration of neuromuscular block following atracurium or vecuronium. Anaesthesiology 67: 191–196

Verapamil

Verapamil is a calcium antagonist that inhibits the inward movement of calcium into cardiomyocytes, smooth muscle cells and cells of the His-Purkinje system.

Chemistry

Verapamil hydrochloride (Securon, Cordilox, Univer, Berkatens, Isoptin)

$C_{27}H_{38}N_2O_4.HCl$

(dl)-5-(-(3,4-Dimethoxyphenethyl)-N-methylamino)-2-(3,4-dimethoxyphenyl)-2-isopropylvaleronitrile hydrochloride

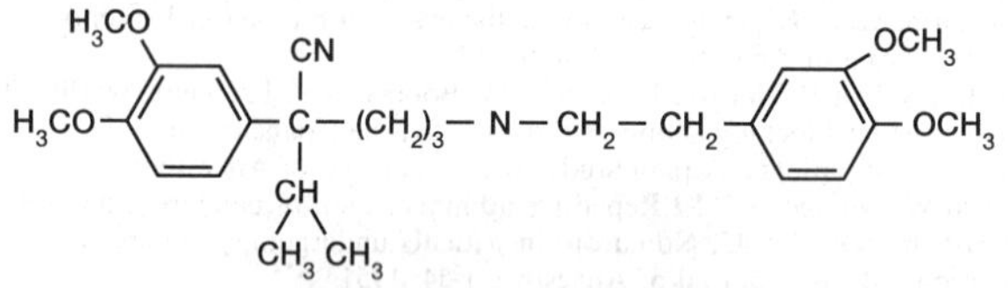

Molecular weight (free base)	491.9 (454.6)
pKa (amino group)	
Solubility	
in alcohol	1 in 25
in water	1 in 20
Octanol/water partition coefficient	—

Verapamil hydrochloride is a white, or almost white, colourless crystalline powder with a bitter taste. It is prepared by chemical synthesis as the racemic mixture, the (l)-isomer being more than 10 times as active as the (d)-isomer. A 5% solution in water has a pH of 4.5–6.5. It is sparingly soluble in alcohol, freely soluble in alcohol but practically insoluble in ether. Solutions are sterilized by autoclaving.

Pharmacology

Verapamil is a phenylalkylamine derivative that inhibits the entry of calcium into cardiac and smooth muscle cells and cells of the cardiac conduction system. Calcium for excitation contraction coupling can be derived from a number of sources. The extracellular fluid contains calcium and the sarcoplasmic reticulum also contains calcium bound to the cytosolic aspect of the cell membrane. Skeletal muscle is richly endowed with sarcoplasmic reticulum and this appears to be the major source of calcium ions involved in the contractile process. However, cardiac and smooth muscle have much less well developed sarcoplasmic reticulum and doubts remain as to the most important source of calcium ions in these tissues.

Modulation of intracellular calcium ions takes place by three major mechanisms. All membranes have calcium pump ATPase. It is a high affinity, low capacity system designed to eject calcium from the cells into the extracellular space or sarcoplasmic reticulum. The sodium/calcium exchange system is also probably present on all cell membranes. It is a low affinity, high capacity pumping system also designed to eject calcium from the cells but may also be a mechanism by which calcium enters the cell. Lastly, calcium ions may enter the cell via calcium channels which may exist at least in some tissues in high affinity and low affinity sub-types. Calcium channels are found predominantly, if not exclusively, on the sarcolemma and may be particularly dense in the t-tubules. Calcium channels have also been classified according to whether they are voltage or receptor dependent. Voltage-sensitive calcium channels have been divided into three classes depending on their conductance and sensitivity to voltage.[1]

They are designated, L, N and T types and only the L type is sensitive to the standard calcium channel blockers. L type channels are abundant in cardiac and smooth muscles and the differing properties of calcium channel blockers can in part be explained by differential binding to distinct sites on the L channel. Receptor mediated activation of the calcium channels is dependent upon activation of receptors, e.g. adrenergic or angiotensin II, which then cause a calcium dependent increase in contraction. Mixed but independent populations of voltage and receptor dependent channels exist in vascular smooth muscle, while in the myocardium voltage and receptor mediated calcium channel responses appear to interact on the same calcium channel.

The mechanisms by which calcium antagonists interact with the calcium channel are not fully elucidated. The calcium channel itself appears to exist in three main states, resting, open and inactive. Verapamil and diltiazem are ionized and water soluble and appear to bind to the cytosolic surface of the channel. The affinity of these drugs for their binding site increases with increased stimulation frequency of the cell and this may reflect the fact that these drugs can only reach their binding site when the calcium channel is in the open configuration. Dihydropyridine calcium channel antagonists may show a similar phenomenon but as they are less ionized, may bind to the channel after incorporation into the sarcolemma and therefore may be less dependent upon the calcium channel configuration for their action. Binding of the calcium channel inhibitors appears to be stereo-selective. At least three binding sites for calcium channel inhibitors exist but these appear to be allosterically linked and binding at one site will alter the affinity of the other sites for inhibitors.

Verapamil like other calcium channel blockers relaxes arterial smooth muscle but has little effect on most venous beds and thus cardiac preload is little affected. Verapamil slows atrioventricular conduction in the heart and depresses the rate of the sinus note pacemaker. These properties are not possessed by the dihydropyridine calcium antagonists (e.g. nifedipine) and this may be explained by the fact that verapamil (but not nifedipine) reduces the rate of recovery of the calcium channel.[2] Verapamil reduces the force of contraction of the myocardium.

Toxicology

There is no evidence of teratogenicity of carcinogenicity with verapamil.

Clinical pharmacology

Verapamil reduces vascular smooth muscle tone and hence peripheral vascular resistance. Verapamil has negative inotropic effects, hence cardiac output changes little in response to the reduction in vascular tone and blood pressure falls. Verapamil has only a mild depressant effect on sinus node automaticity, but a more prominent effect on atrioventricular nodal conduction, hence its use in controlling supraventricular arrhythmias. In common with many other agents which reduce blood pressure, verapamil may cause regression of left ventricular hypertrophy.

Verapamil is effective in the treatment of variant angina which is a direct result of a reduction in blood flow. However some reports suggest that verapamil is less effective than nifedipine.

Verapamil restores the sensitivity of the malaria parasite, *Plasmodium falciparum*, to antimalarial drugs such as chloroquine. It is thought that the calcium channel blocking activities of verapamil restore the penetration of chloroquine into *P. falciparum* infected red cells. The clinical value of this observation has not been fully elucidated.

Oral verapamil does not usually have a blood pressure lowering effect in normotensive subjects either at rest or during exercise.[3] However, in patients with cardiovascular disorders including hypertension, coronary artery disease and hypertrophic cardiomyopathy a blood pressure lowering effect has been noted. After a single oral dose of 160 mg verapamil to 24 hypertensive patients a maximal antihypertensive effect was seen around 2 hours with a blood pressure reduction up to 4 hours. A reduction in blood pressure during exercise has also been noted in hypertensive subjects. A reduction in resting heart rate of around 4–5 beats per min and a 10–20 mmHg reduction in systolic and diastolic blood pressure is to be expected at these doses. Exercise heart rate is reduced by 10–15 beats per min at peak exercise.[4]

Verapamil

Verapamil may have important effects on regional blood flow. Verapamil reduces coronary vascular resistance but as it reduces arterial pressure and myocardial oxygen consumption as well, there may be little change in coronary blood flow at rest. Verapamil does not appear to affect the glomerular filtration rate, while an increase in renal blood flow is disputed.[5] Reductions in hepatic vascular resistance and portal venous pressures after administration are also disputed.[6–8]

Pharmacokinetics

The preferred analytical method is high performance liquid chromatography (sensitivity 2 $\mu g.l^{-1}$) although gas liquid chromatography with mass spectrometry has been used extensively this method detects only one major metabolite norverapamil.

Over 90% of verapamil is absorbed following oral administration with peak plasma concentrations occurring between 1 and 2 hours. The sustained release preparations may have slightly reduced bioavailability and peak plasma concentrations occur between 4 and 8 hours. The absorption of the conventional verapamil does not seem to be affected markedly by food, but absorption of the sustained released preparation may be.[10]

Verapamil is subject to pre-systemic hepatic metabolism with up to 80% of the dose eliminated in this way. The bioavailability is thus 20–30%[11] Presystemic metabolism is stereospecific the (l)-isomer being preferentially eliminated. The more active (l)-isomer may be preferentially extracted in the liver, hence for a given plasma concentration intravenous verapamil appears to have two to three times the effect on the PR interval. The reason for preferential extraction of the (l)-isomer in the liver is not clear but could be related to the greater affinity of the (l)-isomer for calcium channels in the hepatic sinusoids.[12,13]

In patients with liver cirrhosis the bioavailability of verapamil is doubled and correlates well with antipyrine clearance.[14] Bioavailability is unchanged in chronic renal failure.

Verapamil is widely and rapidly distributed throughout the body with a distribution half-life of 15–30 minutes. Verapamil is 90% bound to plasma proteins, mainly to albumin and α_1 acid glycoprotein. This is independent of plasma concentration. Variation in the concentration of α_1 acid glycoprotein appears to contribute most to inter-individual protein binding of the drug. The (l) isomer has a higher unbound fraction approximately twice that of the (d) isomer resulting in a greater volume of distribution.[12] The volume of distribution after a single dose is between 4 and 7 l.kg−1, but in studies in essential hypertension values between 7 and 14 l.kg−1 have been reported after multiple dosing. The (l) isomer may have a larger volume of distribution than the (d)-isomer thus the volume of distribution is increased in liver[10] but not renal disease. Protein binding is reduced in liver disease but is not significantly altered in renal disease.

The half life of verapamil after a single oral or intravenous dose is between 2 and 7 h. However, after repeated administration it increases to 4.5 to 12 h, resulting in accumulation of the drug. The prolongation of the half life appears to be a consequence of both saturation of hepatic metabolism and changes in the haemodynamic effects of verapamil between single and multiple administration. Although the terminal half lives of the two isomers of verapamil are similar systemic clearance of the (l)-isomer is much greater than that of the (d)-isomer. The difference in the kinetics of the two isomers of verapamil results in much lower concentrations of the more potent (l)-isomer after oral dosing, thus explaining the apparent reduction in potency by this route.

The clearance of verapamil is reduced in hepatic disease, with increased bioavailability. Some adjustment of dosage may be required. Renal failure does not significantly alter the kinetics of the drug. The clearance is reduced and the half life prolonged in elderly subjects.

Verapamil is distributed to the cerebrospinal fluid. Verapamil crosses the placenta in small amounts[15] and is excreted in breast milk at concentrations between 23% and 100% of those found in the maternal plasma but is not detectable in the plasma of the infant.

Verapamil

V

Oral absorption	>90%
Presystemic metabolism	80%
Plasma half life range	2–7 h
Volume of distribution	4–7 l. kg^{-1}
Plasma protein binding	90%

There may be up to an 85% variation in oral clearance during long-term dosing in normal volunteers. 3% of the drug is excreted unchanged and 70% as metabolic products in the urine. 15% is excreted in the faeces.

Concentration–effect relationship

The peak plasma concentration of verapamil after a single 80 mg dose appears to be about 30 μg.l^{-1} and after three weeks of 80 mg three times daily, 110 μg.l^{-1} in normal volunteers. In patients plasma concentrations between 150 and 750 μg.l^{-1} are observed with repeated oral doses from 80 to 480 mg daily.[9] Sustained release preparations reduce the peak to trough ratio from about 10 down to 5, while achieving peak plasma concentrations between 100 and 300 μg.l^{-1} in doses of 240 to 480 mg daily. A relationship between peak plasma levels and drug effect is not clear. However, dose response relationships between administered dose and plasma concentration and administered dose and clinical effect have been observed. The anti-hypertensive effect may relate better to trough rather than peak drug concentration. Some studies of hypertensive patients have suggested a concentration–effect response (5.8 mmHg.100 μg.l^{-1} and 2.9 mmHg.100 μg.l^{-1} of verapamil for systolic and diastolic blood pressures respectively).[9,16]

A 10 mg intravenous bolus (over five minutes) of verapamil results in a peak plasma concentration of about 70 μg.l^{-1}.

Metabolism

The majority of verapamil is metabolized by O-demethylation and by N-dealkylation (25% and 40% respectively). Although the products of O-demethylation possess pharmacological activities similar to verapamil, they are rapidly metabolized to conjugates. N-Demethylation accounts for a further 10–15% of the metabolic products of verapamil (Fig 1). One of these products, norverapamil, has approximately 20% of the activity of the parent compound. This is detected only after oral administration of verapamil and is formed presumably during presystemic metabolism. Its half life may be slightly longer than that of verapamil and it will accumulate during chronic administration of the drug. It may then contribute to the clinical effect of verapamil.

Pharmaceutics

Verapamil is available as a non-proprietary preparation containing 40, 80, 120 or 160 mg of the drug.

Calan (Searle, US) ovoid tablets containing 80 mg (buff) and 120 mg (tan) imprinted with 'CALAN' and '80' or '120' injectable presentations include an ampoule or a vial containing 5 mg in 2 ml plus a vial containing 10 mg in 4 ml. The same strengths are available in pre-filled syringes.

Cordilox (Abbott, UK) tablets containing 40, 80, 120 or 160 mg of verapamil hydrochloride. Each tablet is yellow, biconvex, film-coated and imprinted with 'CORDILOX 40', '80', '120' or '160' respectively and the Abbott logo on the reverse. The yellow dyes used are E110 and E104.

There is also an intravenous preparation provided in colorless, labelled ampoules with 5 mg of verapamil hydrochloride in 2 ml of solution.

Isoptin (Knoll, US) dosage forms are similar to the Searle preparations listed above. The 80 mg tablets are biconvex yellow scored tablets marked 'ISOPTIN 80' on one side and 'KNOLL' on the reverse. The 120 mg tablets are biconvex white scored tablets marked 'ISOPTIN 120' on one side and 'KNOLL' on the reverse.

Securon (Knoll, US) tablets containing 40, 80, 120 or 160 mg of verapamil hydrochloride and lactose. Each tablet is white, film-coated and imprinted 'SECURON 40', '80', '120' or '160' respectively and the Knoll logo on the reverse.

A slow release preparation is also available as a pale green, oblong, film-coated tablet containing 240 mg of verapamil hydrochloride. It is scored on both sides and carries the Knoll logo on one side.

Univer (Rorer, UK) sustained released capsules are available containing 120, 180 or 240 mg of verapamil hydrochloride. The 120 mg and 240 mg capsules are yellow/dark blue and marked 'V120' or 'V240' respectively. The 180 mg capsule is yellow and marked 'V180'.

Fig. 1 The metabolism of verapamil

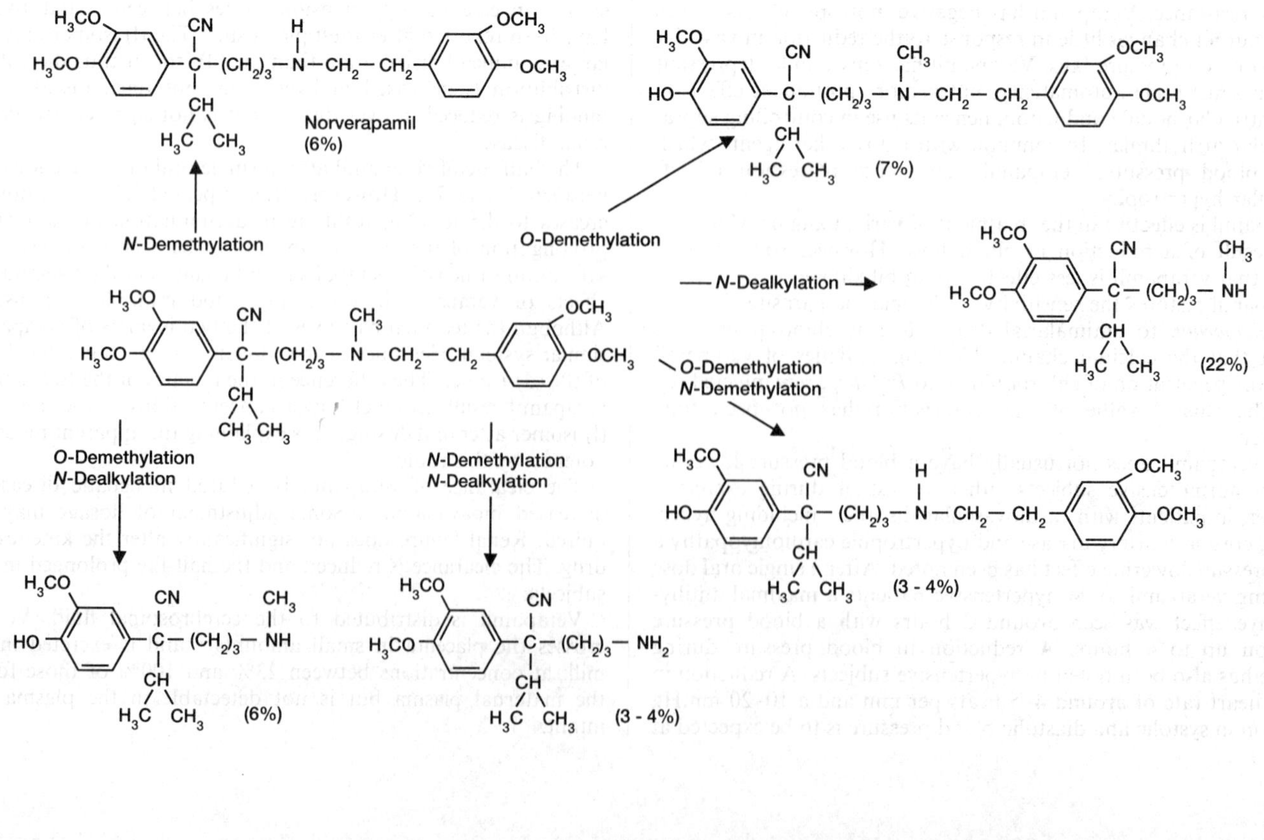

Verapamil

Therapeutic use

Indications

1. Supraventricular arrhythmias
2. Hypertension: essential; renal; pregnancy related; children; during coronary bypass surgery
3. Ischaemic heart disease; chronic stable angina pectoris; variant angina; unstable angina; myocardial infarction; post-infarction prophylaxis; anti-atherosclerotic effects
4. Miscellaneous; hypertrophic cardiomyopathy; pulmonary hypertension; neuroendocrine effects; respiratory effects; effect on platelets; migraine; psychiatric disorders; effects on the uterus; use in chloroquine resistant malaria.

Contraindications

1. Bradycardia or conduction defect
2. Hypotension
3. Heart failure
4. Combination with a β-blocker
5. Defective platelet function.

Indications

1. Supraventricular arrhythmias

Verapamil reduces sinus node rate, though the effect of oral doses in normal man is only slight at rest while it depresses the heart rate response to exercise. However, in patients with abnormal sinus node function, verapamil increases sinus node recovery time and may induce sino-atrial block or sinus arrest.[17]

Verapamil increases atrioventricular nodal conduction time after intravenous or oral therapy. This renders it of use for controlling the ventricular rate response in atrial fibrillation[18] and in the management of some cases of supraventricular tachycardia that involve the atrioventricular (a-v) node. Heart rate control during exercise appears to be superior to digoxin though it is not clear if this is translated into symptomatic improvement.[19] Oral therapy is of little use in atrial flutter when verapamil may temporarily increase the level of a-v block but leave the atrial tachycardia relatively unaffected.

Intravenous boluses of verapamil should always be given during electrocardiographic monitoring and rarely if ever given to a patient receiving a β-blocker. Careful monitoring of blood pressure is essential. Injection of 10 mg of verapamil in 30 seconds has a higher chance of therapeutic success, but a higher incidence of complications including complete heart block and cardiac standstill. Hypotension is also not infrequent and may be exacerbated by bradycardia or failure to control the tachycardia. Many physicians now inject 2.5 mg boluses at 30 second intervals monitoring the effects on conduction and blood pressure between. Calcium gluconate or chloride may be given cautiously to reverse hypotension and heart block if they occur. The success rates for conversion of atrioventricular nodal re-entry tachycardia is high (70–100%)[18] while conversion of atrial flutter (15–30% success) and atrial fibrillation (0–10% success) is much lower, and indeed some have suggested that the latter effect is coincidental.[18,19] Verapamil will often slow tachycardia rate even if it does not effect cardioversion.

Verapamil has little effect on intra-atrial or intra-ventricular conduction times. Consequently it has minimal effect on antegrade or retrograde conduction in the accessory pathway of the Wolff–Parkinson–White syndrome.[20] However, increasing the block in the a-v node will successfully terminate the arrhythmia in about two-thirds of patients.[18] Block of the a-v node may cause preferential conduction through the accessory pathway, which may even accelerate causing ventricular arrhythmias, especially in patients with associated atrial fibrillation.[18]

Verapamil may be of use in rare ventricular tachycardias that involve the His-Purkinje system. Use of verapamil in common forms of ventricular tachycardia may precipitate hypotension and cardiac arrest.

2. Hypertension

Essential hypertension. Doses of 160–480 mg day of standard formulation and sustained release verapamil have been employed. In placebo controlled studies diastolic pressure falls between 10 and 30 mmHg and is dose dependent.[21] Sustained release preparations seem as effective as standard therapy but may be administered once daily. Standard preparations of verapamil have been used twice daily with adequate blood pressure control.[22]

Comparative studies suggest that verapamil is at least as effective as other calcium antagonists, thiazide diuretics and ACE inhibitors. Verapamil is also as effective as a β-blocker, while it appears less likely to impair exercise performance,[23] may have greater patient acceptability[24] and may be superior in black patients.[25] Verapamil has been successfully combined with all the above, though caution is indicated when combining it with a beta-blocker as this may result in significant depression of cardiac function and a-v conduction disturbances.[26]

In common with other effective anti-hypertension agents verapamil may cause regression of left ventricular hypertrophy.

Verapamil may be especially effective in elderly patients and patients with low plasma renin activity, in contrast to β-blockers.[27]

Accelerated hypertension. Intravenous verapamil (5 mg) has been used to treat hypertensive crises,[28] though intravenous therapy is rarely required for this condition and may precipitate dangerous hypotension.

Renal hypertension. Verapamil is effective in hypertension with renal parenchymal disease and does not appear to reduce glomerular filtration despite a reduction in arterial pressure. Renal blood flow may increase.[29] Verapamil is also effective in renal vascular hypertension.[28]

Pregnancy-related hypertension. Intravenous verapamil has been used in a dose of 10 mg over two minutes followed by a 6.6 $\mu g.min^{-1}$ infusion to lower maternal blood pressure without affecting fetal heart rate.[30] In a study of 90 hypertensive pregnant women, efficacy was shown without adverse consequences to the fetus or neonate.[31]

Hypertension in children. Intravenous doses of 0.1 $mg.kg^{-1}$ followed by infusion (0.05 to 0.5 $mg.kg^{-1}$ hourly) have been used to treat severe renovascular hypertension.[32]

3. Ischaemic heart disease

Chronic stable angina pectoris. Verapamil 160–480 mg daily in divided doses or as a sustained release preparation is highly effective in the management of chronic stable angina.[33–38] Verapamil monotherapy appears superior to nifedipine for the control of angina[39] and is generally better tolerated.[39] Verapamil is as effective as diltiazem,[40] and superior to chronic oral nitrate therapy.[41] Verapamil in a dose of 160 mg daily appears as effective as 240 mg daily of propranolol[42] or 100 mg daily of atenolol[4] in the management of angina, though the reduction in exercise induced tachycardia is less marked, suggesting that the beneficial effects of verapamil are not merely mediated through heart rate reduction.

Caution should be exercised in combining verapamil with a β-blocker because, although it is a highly effective combination, it may markedly depress ventricular function and a-v conduction.[4,83]

Variant angina. Verapamil appears to be as effective as nifedipine in the management of variant angina.[43]

Unstable angina. Verapamil is effective for the management of patients with unstable angina,[44] and superior to oral nitrate therapy.[45]

Myocardial infarction. Ischaemia leads to an impairment of cellular calcium homeostasis leading to a high cytosolic calcium concentration and impairment of mitochondrial function. Verapamil has been shown to delay the onset of ischaemic damage and also to reduce the total infarct size in animal models.[46–57] However, an effect of verapamil on infarct size in man is disputed,[48,49] though infusion has been shown to reduce the frequency of ventricular arrhythmias including fibrillation.[50]

Post-infarction prophylaxis. In a study of 3498 patients verapamil 120 mg three times daily failed to reduce re-infarction (16% reduction) or mortality (15% reduction) significantly,[51] though a sub-analysis did show a reduction in late mortality and re-infarction (vide infra).

Post-coronary artery bypass surgery. Intravenous infusions of verapamil have been used to protect the heart from intraoperative and postoperative myocardial ischaemia during cardiac surgery.[49]

Anti-atherosclerotic effects. Experimental preparations have shown that verapamil markedly inhibits the development of atherosclerosis, reducing intracellular cholesterol and triglyceride levels and inhibiting cell proliferation in atherosclerotic plaque.[53,54] Encouraging retrospective data is available in man,[55] but studies with another calcium antagonist, nifedipine, have been disappointing. In general, verapamil has been found to have little effect on blood lipids.[56]

Verapamil

V

4. Miscellaneous uses

Hypertrophic cardiomyopathy. Verapamil can reduce the severity of left ventricular outflow obstruction, improve symptoms and increase exercise capacity in patients with hypertrophic cardiomyopathy.[57,58] Verapamil has also been reported to reduce left ventricular hypertrophy,[59] though this is now disputed.[60] Verapamil is not effective in controlling supraventricular or ventricular arrhythmias in this condition.[61] Occasional patients may develop serious problems, such as hypotension and cardiovascular collapse after verapamil, which are difficult to predict.[62] This may be due to peripheral vasodilatation, myocardial deppression or conduction disturbance.

Pulmonary hypertension. Verapamil can reduce pulmonary vascular resistance, but in the presence of severe pulmonary hypertension may cause a decline in right ventricular function resulting in the induction of heart failure.[63]

Neuroendocrine. Verapamil does not appear to impair glucose tolerance.[64] In hypertensive patients verapamil does not increase plasma levels of renin or aldosterone.[65]

Respiratory. In asthmatic patients verapamil has been reported to either have no effect[66] or to improve airways conductance.[67] Some investigators have reported that inhaled verapamil prevents methacholine induced bronchoconstriction.[67,68]

Platelet. In-vitro verapamil inhibits platelet aggregation, especially that caused by adrenaline.[69] This effect has also been observed in platelets obtained from subjects treated with 160 mg daily of verapamil.[69] Collagen-induced platelet aggregation is also inhibited at therapeutic concentrations.[70]

Migraine. Verapamil reduces the frequency of attacks.

Psychiatric disorders. Verapamil appears to have anti-manic effects but the usefulness of this action in therapy has not been established.

Uterine. Verapamil may cause relaxation of uterine muscle delaying or reversing the onset of labour.

Chloroquine resistant malaria. Verapamil is able to reverse the resistance to chloroquine in several strains of chloroquine resistant falciparum malaria. Verapamil inhibits a glycoprotein pump responsible for the drug resistance. However, the doses of racemic verapamil needed to reverse drug resistance are often toxic. It appears that the (d)-isomer which has little affinity for cardiovascular calcium channels mediates most of this effect.[71]

Contraindications

1. Bradycardia or conduction defect

Verapamil may cause an exacerbation of defective impulse formation or conduction in sino-atrial disease and cause minor conduction defects to progress to a higher degree of block. These effects are amplified in patients already receiving a β-blocker.[4] In patients with tri-fascicular block verapamil should be used with extreme caution if at all. Verapamil should not be administered intravenously in patients who have already received a β-blocker.

2. Hypotension

Verapamil should be avoided in patients with very low blood pressures. An intravenous dose of verapamil may cause hypotension, especially if the tachycardia for which it was given persists. Calcium, in the form of calcium gluconate or calcium chloride, given cautiously, can reverse hypotension (see Acute overdosage below). β-agonists such as isoprenaline have been used in certain cases, but should be avoided in patients with hypertrophic cardiomyopathy, when α-agonists such as phenylephrine are preferred.

3. Heart failure

Verapamil has a direct negative inotropic effect which is largely offset by its peripheral vasodilator actions. In patients with significant ventricular impairment and in those on β-blockers, the reduction in ventricular function can precipitate overt heart failure. In patients with aortic stenosis, in whom vasodilators do not reduce the ventricular afterload, verapamil may also be unwise.

4. Combination with a β-blocker

Combination with a β-blocker may precipitate atrial pauses, high-grade conduction block and symptoms and signs of heart failure. These effects are generally seen in those with prior underlying conduction defects or when higher doses of verapamil are given (120 mg three times daily or more).

5. Defective platelet function

Due to a reduction in platelet aggregation, defective platelet function or a reduced count are relative contra-indications to verapamil's use.

Adverse reactions

Potentially life-threatening effects

Verapamil can cause prolonged atrial pauses, high grade atrioventricular conduction block and rarely may exacerbate re-entry tachycardia of the Wolff–Parkinson–White syndrome. Difficulty in making the appropriate diagnosis may lead to patients with ventricular tachycardia receiving verapamil, which can lead to cardiovascular collapse.

Depression of cardiac function may induce heart failure in those with preceding significant underlying cardiac dysfunction. All of these effects may be exacerbated by combination with β-blockers. Intravenous verapamil should not be given to patients who have received a β-blocker. (See also under Contraindications above)

Acute overdosage

Patients present with hypotension, bradycardia and atrioventricular block. Calcium is a specific antidote which is successful in the majority of cases. Calcium gluconate should be administered as 10–20 ml of a 10% solution over 5–10 minutes. Calcium chloride may cause peripheral vasodilatation, hypotension and cardiac arrhythmias if administered rapidly and should be given as an infusion of 10–20 ml of a 10% solution diluted in 50–100 ml of 5% dextrose over 30–60 minutes. In selected cases, ventricular pacing and support with isoprenaline, dopamine, dobutamine and/or atropine may be required. 4-aminopyridine, a drug which enhances the influx of calcium into cells, has been employed in doses of 10 mg over five minutes and repeated once if needed, with some success.

Severe or irreversible adverse effects

The effects listed above under Potentially life-threatening effects are also relevant to this section. Large-scale reviews have suggested that about 1% of patients have to be withdrawn from treatment because of severe adverse effects.[71]

There are isolated reports of hepatic toxicity, mental confusion, myoclonic dystonia, hyperprolactinaemia and impotence.

Symptomatic adverse effects

The incidence of such effects is comparatively low when compared with other calcium antagonists, about 10–12%.[71,72] Constipation is most common, at around 10%, while headache, fatigue and dizziness occur in about 5%. Palpitation, flushing and nausea all occur in about 0.5% of cases. Rashes and arthalgia have also been reported. About 2–3% of patients stop treatment due to these milder adverse effects. Sustained-release preparations have a similar adverse effect profile.[73]

The incidence of constipation may have been underestimated in large-scale studies, as others have reported that up to 45% of patients may become constipated. Generally this can be overcome by increasing dietary fibre and fluid.

Other effects

Bradycardia is frequent but unless symptomatic or profound (ie. less than 35 beats per minute) requires only investigation to exclude atrioventricular block.

Interference with clinical pathology tests

None is known.

High risk groups

Neonates

Little information exists. Epstein has reported its use in infants as early as five days for supraventricular tachycardia at oral doses of 1–3 $mg.kg^{-1}$ three times daily. Caution is recommended, as cardiovascular collapse may occur.[74]

Breast milk. Verapamil has been used in pregnancy-related hypertension and enters the breast milk in high concentrations.[75] No adverse effects on the fetus or infant have been noted and infant blood levels of verapamil have been negligible. However, the manufacturers still recommend that mothers taking verapamil should not breast-feed.

Children

Intravenous verapamil has been used at doses of 0.1 $mg.kg^{-1}$ for

Verapamil

children with severe renovascular hypertension, followed by infusions of 0.05–0.5 mg.kg^{-1}.[24] Overall doses of around 10 mg.kg^{-1} daily are recommended for treatment in children.

Pregnant women
Both intravenous (up to 10 mg over 2 minutes) and oral (up to 480 mg daily in divided doses) verapamil have been used to manage pregnancy-related hypertension, without undue slowing of the fetal heart rate.[30,31]

The elderly
First-pass metabolism may be reduced in elderly patients, thereby increasing systemic bioavailability, but not all studies support this.[21,76] In older subjects a starting dose of 40 mg three times daily is recommended.

Concurrent disease
Patients with liver disease demonstrate reduced first-pass metabolism, delayed elimination and a raised fraction of verapamil unbound to plasma proteins.[14,77] In patients with liver disease a starting dose of 40 mg three times daily is recommended. Impaired renal function and haemodialysis appear to affect verapamil metabolism little. Verapamil is porphyrinogenic in animals.

Drug interactions

Potentially hazardous drug interactions

Digoxin. Verapamil increases plasma digoxin concentrations by 50% in normal volunteers and 70–100% in patients.[78,79] Verapamil appears to reduce the clearance (largely non-renal) of digoxin. Doses of digoxin should be reduced to prevent toxicity developing, especially high-grade atrioventricular block.

β-blockers. This combination may result in severe myocardial depression and high-grade atrioventricular block. Although the combination is highly effective in treating angina, it should only be given under expert supervision. Intravenous verapamil should not be given to patients on β-blockers (and vice versa) due to the risk of producing complete heart block.

Class I antiarrhythmics. This combination may result in profound cardiac depression and requires expert supervision.[80] Verapamil may reduce the clearance of quinidine.[81]

Other significant interactions
Drugs which induce hepatic enzymes, such as phenobarbitone and rifampicin increase the presystemic metabolism of orally administered verapamil. Verapamil increases free carbamazepine levels and may thereby induce neurotoxicity[82] within a few days.

Increased plasma levels of adriamycin, cyclosporin, theophylline and lithium have been reported. Verapamil may increase neuromuscular blockade due to vecuronium, cause bradycardia in association with halothane or neostigmine and myocardial depression in association with dantrolene.

Verapamil should not be injected into an intravenous line containing bicarbonate, as precipitation of verapamil hydrochloride will occur above pH 7.

Potentially useful interactions
As mentioned earlier, the combination of verapamil and a β-blocker is very effective in angina, the risks of myocardial depression make it necessary from this type of treatment to be given only under expert supervision.

Major outcome trials

Danish Study Group on Verapamil in Myocardial Infarction. Verapamil in acute myocardial infarction 1984 European Heart Journal 5: 516–528

A randomized, placebo-controlled multi-centre study which evaluated 7415 patients of whom 3498 were considered eligible for study and 1436 were subsequently proven to have a myocardial infarction as the cause of pain. 246 patients were withdrawn from placebo by six months mainly due to atrioventricular block, heart failure, refusal to continue or angina. 303 patients were withdrawn from verapamil, the excess being due to a two-fold increase in 2nd and 3rd degree heart block limited to the first week of therapy. The incidence of heart failure did not increase, but the incidence of angina was reduced. The one year mortality was 16.4% for placebo and 15.2% for verapamil (not significant). However, the incidence of late re-infarction was reduced by verapamil (3.9% versus 7%; $p<0.03$) and this was associated with a reduction in late mortality (3.7% v 6.4%; $p<0.05$). These data argue that there may be a role for verapamil in reducing the incidence of re-infarction in patients who have survived an infarct, but in whom beta-blockers are contraindicated.

Danish Study Group on Verapamil in Myocardial Infarction. Effect of verapamil on mortality and major events after acute myocardial infarction (The Danish Verapamil Infarction Trial II-DAVIT II) 1990 American Journal of Cardiology 66: 779–785

This is a randomized, placebo-controlled multicentre study which evaluated 4 481 patients with myocardial infarction. 490 patients died before randomization, while 2 216 were excluded (largely because of heart failure, conduction disturbances, prior treatment with beta-blockers or the fact that they did not wish to participate). 878 patients were randomized to treatment with verapamil and 897 to placebo between days 7 and 15 after admission. The groups were well matched. 344 patients randomized to verapamil and 309 randomized to placebo were withdrawn before completion of the study. The commonest cause of withdrawal before completion of the study. The commonest cause of withdrawal in both groups was angina pectoris, although this complaint was less prevalent in the group treated with verapamil. Constipation and conduction disturbances were more common in those treated with verapamil (3% and 1% respectively).

The 18-month mortality rates were 11.1% and 13.8% respectively in the verapamil and placebo groups (n.s.). However, when death and reinfarction were considered together, the major event rate was reduced from 21.6% to 18% by verapamil ($p=0.03$). In patients whose myocardial infarction was complicated by heart failure, verapamil appeared to exert no effect for good or ill. In contrast, subgroup analysis of those patients without heart failure suggested a reduction in mortality and morbidity with the use of verapamil.

The effects of verapamil after myocardial infarction seem broadly comparable to the beneficial effects of beta-blockers. This is in contrast with the trend to an adverse outcome with dihydropyridine calcium antagonists and the lack of effect of diltiazem. It is tempting to postulate that it is heart rate reduction, mediated by either verapamil or the beta-blocker, which leads to benefit, and this may be the reason for the worse outcome with dihydropyridine calcium antagonists.

Other trials

While well designed and controlled studies do exist for patients with angina and/or hypertension, they are not large. Large scale trials of verapamil's efficacy in angina or hypertension are probably unnecessary due to the potency of the drug.

1. Schamroth L 1980 The clinical use of intravenous verapamil. American Heart Journal 100: 1070–1075
   Schamroth L 1972 Immediate effects of intravenous verapamil on atrial fibrillation. Cardiovascular Research 5: 419

A review article and the author's personal experience rather than a study, but nonetheless one of the most useful papers in this area. The author indicates that for reciprocating (largely atrioventricular nodal re-entry) supraventricular tachycardia between 80 and 100% success rates can be expected. The success rates for atrial flutter were considerably less at around 15% and between 0 and 16% for atrial fibrillation. It is not clear if these latter conversion rates are any higher than the spontaneous conversion rate. Earlier reports of benefit for ventricular tachycardia were dismissed by the author.

2. Lewis G R J et al 1978 The treatment of hypertension with verapamil. New Zealand Medical Journal 87: 351–354

A randomized, double-blind, cross-over study of 23 hypertensive patients in whom beta-blockers were contraindicated. Dose dependent reductions in blood pressure occurred between 80 mg and 120 mg three times daily (188/106 to 173/93 mmHg to 161/84 mmHg respectively). Two patients failed to complete the trial due to dizziness, marked reduction in blood pressure occurred in these two patients when given verapamil. Six patients noted mild constipation. No other side effects were noted.

Verapamil

V

3. Findlay A N et al 1987 A double blind placebo controlled comparison of verapamil, atenolol, and their combination in patient with chronic stable angina pectoris. British Heart Journal 57: 336–343

A comparison of 120 mg three times daily of verapamil and 100 mg daily of atenolol in 15 patients with angina pectoris. Both treatments proved equally effective in reducing angina and improving indices. The anti-anginal effects of the combination proved even more powerful but several patients were withdrawn from the study due to the induction of heart failure, bradyarrhythmias, hypotension and lethargy. Only the combination caused a significant deterioration of ventricular function as assessed by radionuclide ventriculography. Combination therapy should be reserved for use only by those with a specialist interest.

General review articles

Schamroth L 1980 The clinical use of intravenous verapamil. American Heart Journal 100: 1070–1075

References

1. Schwartz A, McKenna E, Vaghy P L 1988 Receptors for calcium antagonists. American Journal of Cardiology 62: 3G–6G
2. Ehara T, Kauffman R 1988 The voltage- and time-dependent effects of (−)-verapamil on the slow inward current in isolated cat ventricular myocardium. Journal of Experimental Therapeutics 178: 49–55
3. Petri H, Arends B G, van Baak M A 1986 The effect of verapamil on cardiovascular and metabolic responses to exercise. European Journal of Applied Physiology 55: 499–502
4. Findlay A N, MacLeod K, Gillen G, Telliott A, Aitchison T, Dargie H J 1987 A double-blind placebo controlled comparison of verapamil, atenolol, and their combination in patients with chronic stable angina pectoris. British Heart Journal 57: 336–463
5. Sorensen S S, Thomsen O O, Danielsen H, Pedersen E B 1985 Effect of verapamil on renal plasma flow, glomerular filtration rate and plasma angiotensin II, aldosterone and arginine vasopressin in essential hypertension. European Journal of Clinical Pharmacology 29: 257–261
6. Freeman J G, Barton J R, Record C O 1985 Effect of isosorbide dinitrate, verapamil and labetalol on portal pressure in cirrhosis. British Medical Journal 291: 561–562
7. Kong C W, Lay C S, Tsai Y T et al 1986 The haemodynamic effect of verapamil on portal hypertension in patients with postnecrotic cirrhosis. Hepatology 6: 423–426
8. Lay C S, Tsai Y T, Kong C W et al 1988 Effects of verapamil on estimated hepatic blood flow in patients with HBsAg-positive cirrhosis. Hepato-gastroenterology 35: 121–124
9. Anderson P, Bondesson U, De Faire U 1986 Pharmacokinetics of verapamil in patients with hypertension. European Journal of Pharmacology 31: 155–163
10. Cubeddu L X, Feunmayor N T 1988 Comparative pharmacokinetics and pharmacodynamics of IR and SR verapamil in patients with hypertension: effects of food intake. Journal of Cardiovascular Pharmacology 12 (suppl 6): S188
11. Eichelbaum M, Somogyi A 1984 Inter- and intra-subject variation in the first-pass elimination of highly cleared drugs during chronic dosing studies with deuterated verapamil. European Journal of Pharmacology 26: 47–53
12. Eichelbaum M, Mikus G, Vogelgesang B 1984 Pharmacokinetics of (+)-, (+:-)-verapamil after intravenous administration. British Journal of Pharmacology 17: 453–458
13. McAllister R G, Kirsten E B 1982 The pharmacology of verapamil. IV Kinetic and dynamic effects after single intravenous and oral doses. Clinical Pharmacology and Therapeutics 31: 418–426
14. Somogyi A, Albrecht M, Kliems G, Schafer K, Eichelbaum M 1981 Pharmacokinetics, bioavailability and ECG response of verapamil in patients with liver cirrhosis. British Journal of Clinical Pharmacology 12: 51–60
15. Ferguson II J E, Siukola L V M, Albright G A 1988 Use of verapamil for paroxysmal supraventricular tachycardia during epidural anaesthesia for cesarean section. American Journal of Pharmacology 5: 128–130
16. Gonzalez-Gomez A, Cires Pujois M, Gamio Capestany F, Rodriguez de las Vega A, Garcia-Barreto D 1988 Relationships between verapamil plasma concentrations and its antihypertensive action. International Journal of Clinical Pharmacology, Therapy* Toxicology 26: 453–460
17. Carrasco H A, Feunmayor A, Barboza J S, Gonzalez G 1978 Effect of verapamil on normal sinoatrial node function and on sick sinus syndrome. American Heart Journal 96: 760–761
18. Rainkenberger R L, Prystowsky E N, Heger J J, Troup P J, Jackman W M, Zipes D P 1980 Effects of intravenous and chronic oral verapamil administration in patients with supraventricular tachycardia. Circulation 62: 996–1010
19. Schamroth L 1972 Immediate effects of intravenous verapamil on atrial fibrillation. Cardiovascular Research 5: 419
20. Spurrell R A J, Krikler D M, Sowton G E 1974 The effect of verapamil on the electrophysiological properties of the anomalous atrioventricular connections in Wolffe-Parkinson-White syndrome. British Heart Journal 36: 256–257
21. Cox J P, O'Boyle C A, Mee F, Kelly J, Aitkins N et al 1988 The anti-hypertensive efficacy of verapamil in the elderly evaluated by ambulatory blood pressure measurement. Journal of Human Hypertension 2: 41–47
22. Anderson P, Bondesson U, De Faire U, Forslund L, Hedback B et al 1987 Verapamil in hypertension: comparison of twice-and thrice-daily dosing on blood pressure and pharmacokinetics. Current Therapeutics Research 41: 773–784
23. Vanhees L, Fagard R, Amery A 1988 Effect of calcium channel blockade and β-adrenoceptor blockade on short graded and single level endurance exercise in normal men. European Journal of Applied Physiology 58: 87–91
24. Hawkins C M A, Fletcher A W, Bulpitt C J, Pike L A 1988 The effects of verapamil and propranolol on quality of life in hypertension. British Journal of Clinical Pharmacology 25: 98P–99P
25. Cubeddu L X, Aranda J, Singh B, Klein M, Brachfield J et al 1986 A comparison of verapamil and propranolol for the initial treatment of hypertension. Journal of the American Medical Association 256: 2214–2221
26. McInnes G T, Findlay I N, Murray G, Cleland J G F, Dargie H J 1985 Cardiovascular responses to verapamil and propranolol in hypertensive patients. Journal of Hypertension 3: S219–S221
27. Buhler F R, Hulthen U L, Kiowski W, Muller F B, Bolli P 1982 The place of the calcium antagonist verapamil in antihypertensive therapy. Journal of Cardiovascular Pharmacology 4 (suppl 3): S350–S357
28. Brittinger W D, Schwarezbeck A, Wittenmeier K W, Tuthenhoff W 1970 Klinisch-experimentelle untersuchungen uber die blutdrucksenkende wirkung von verapamil. Deutsche Medizinische Wochenschrift 95: 1871–1877
29. Boero R, Quarello F, Guarena C, Piccoli G 1986 Verapamil in arterial hypertension with renal disease. Nephron 44: 80
30. Serafini P C, Petracco A, Vicosa I M, Costa P L 1979 Antihypertensive effect of verapamil in severe pre-clampsia — a preliminary study. Arquivos Brasileiros de Cardiologia 32: 57–61
31. Orlandi C, Marlettini M G, Cassani A, Trabatti M, Agostini D et al 1986 Treatment of hypertension during pregnancy with the calcium antagonist verapamil. Current Therapeutic Research 39: 884–893
32. Scharer K, Alatas H, Bein G 1977 The treatment of renal hypertension with verapamil in childhood. Monatsschrift fur Kinderheilkunde 125: 706–712
33. Neumann M, Luisada A A 1966 Double-blind evaluation of orally administered iproveratril in patients with angina pectoris. American Journal of Medical Science 251: 552–556
34. Sandler G 1968 Clinical evaluation of verapamil in angina pectoris. British Medical Journal 2: 224–227
35. Livesley B, Catley P F, Campbell R C, Oram S 1973 Double-blind evaluation of verapamil, propranolol and isosorbide dinitrate against a placebo in the treatment of anginat pectoris. British Medical Journal 1: 375–378
36. Bala Subramanian V, Lahiri A, Siram P, Raftery E B 1980 Verapamil in chronic stable angina: a controlled study with computerized multistage treadmill exercise. Lancet 1: 841–844
37. Raftos J 1980 Verapamil in the long-term treatment of angina pectors. Medical Journal of Australia 2: 78–80
38. Kohli R S, Rodrigues E A, Hughes L O, Lahiri A, Raftery E B 1987 Sustained release verapamil, a once daily preparation: objective evaluation using exercise testing, ambulatory monitoring and blood levels in patients with stable angina. Journal of the American College of Cardiologists 9: 615–621
39. Dawson J R, Whitaker N H G, Sutton G C 1981 Calcium antagonists drugs in chronic stable angina: comparison of verapamil and nifedipine. British Heart Journal 46: 508–512
40. Khurmi N S, Raftery E 1987 Comparative effects of prolonged therapy with four calcium ion antagonists (diltiazem, nicardipine, tiapamil and verapamil) in patients with chronic stable angina pectoris. Cardiovascular Drugs and Therapy 1: 81–87
41. De Ponti C, Mauri F, Ciliberto G R, Caru B 1979 Comparative effects of nifedipine, verapamil, isosorbide dinitrate and propranolol on exercise-induced angina pectoris. European Journal of Cardiology 10: 47–58
42. Leon M B, Rosing D R, Bonow R O, Lipson L C, Epstein S E 1981 Clinical efficacy of verapamil alone and combined with propranolol in treating patients with chronic stable angina pectoris. American Journal of Cardiology 48: 131–139
43. Johnson S M, Mauritson D R, Willerson J F, Hills L D 1981 A comparison of verapamil and nifedipine in patients with Prinzmetal's variant angina pectoris. American Journal of Cardiology 47: 1295–1300
44. Parodi O, Maseri A, Simonetti I 1979 Management of unstable angina at rest by verapamil: a double-blind cross-over study in coronary care unit. British Heart Journal 41: 167–174
45. Rizzon P et al 1986 European Heart Journal 7: 67–76
46. Reimer et al 1977 Circulation 55: 581–587
47. Yellon D M et al 1983 American Journal of Cardiology 51: 1409–1413
48. Bussmann W D, Seher W, Gruengras M 1984 Reduction of creatine kinase and creatine kinase-MB indexes of infarct size by intravenous verapamil. American Journal of Cardiology 54: 1224–1230
49. Thuesen L, Jorgensen J R, Kvistgaard H J et al 1983 Effect of verapamil on enzyme release after early intravenous administration in acute myocardial infarction: double-blind randomized trial 286: 1107–1108
50. Beck O A, Hochrein H 1977 Treatment of ectopias and tachycardias in acute myocardial infarction. Deutsche Medizinische Wochenschrift 102: 201–204
51. Danish Study Group on Verapamil in Myocardial Infarction. 1984 Verapamil in acute myocardial infarction. European Heart Journal 5: 516–528
52. Hicks G L, DeWeese J A 1985 Verapamil potassium cardioplegia and cardiac conduction. Annals of Thoracic Surgery 39: 324–328
53. Orekhov A N, Baldenkov G N, Tertov V V et al 1988 Cardiovascular drugs and atherosclerosis: effects of calcium antagonists, β-blockers, and nitrates on atherosclerotic characteristics of human aortic cells. Journal of Cardiovascular Pharmacology 12 (suppl 6): S66–S68
54. Parmley W W, Blumlein S, Sievers R 1985 Modification of experimental atherosclerosis by calcium-channel blockers. American Journal of Cardiology 55: 165B–171B
55. Kober G, Nickelsen B, Jakobs B, Kaltenbach M 1986 The influence of long-term therapy with verapamil on the development of coronary artery stenosis. In: Rosenthal J (ed) Calcium antagonists and hypertension current status. Excerpta Medica, Amsterdam, pp 97–105
56. Midtbo K, Lauve O, Hals O 1988 No metabolic side effects of long-term treatment with verapamil in hypertension. Angiology 39: 1025–1059

57. Kaltenbach M, Hopf R, Kobere G, Bussman W D, Keller M, Peterson Y 1979 Treatment of hypertrophic obstructive cardiomyopathy with verapamil. British Heart Journal 42: 35–42
58. Bonow R D, Rosing D R, Bacharach S L et al 1982 Effects of verapamil on left ventricular systolic function and diastolic filling in patients with hypertrophic cardiomyopathy. Circulation 64: 787–796
59. Troesch M, Hirzel H O, Jenni R, Krayenbuhl H P 1979 Reduction in septal thickness following verapamil in patients with asymmetrical septal hypertrophy (abstract). Circulation 60: 155
60. Rosing D R, Condit J R, Maron B J et al 1981 Verapamil therapy: a new approach to the pharmacologic treatment of hypertrophic cardiomyopathy. III. Effects of long-term administration. American Journal of Cardiology 48: 545–553
61. McKenna W J, Harris L, Perez G, Krikler D M, Oakley C M, Goodwin J F 1981 Arrhythmia in hypertrophic cardiomyopathy: II. Comparisons of amiodarone and verapamil in treatment. British Heart Journal 46: 173–178
62. Epstein S E, Rosing D R 1981 Verapamil: its potential for causing serious complications in patients with hypertrophic cardiomyopathy. Circulation 64: 437–441
63. Packer M, Medina N, Yushak M, Wiener I 1984 Detrimental effects of verarpamil in patients with primary pulmonary hypertension. British Heart Journal 52: 106–111
64. Cruickshank J K, Anderson N McF, Wadsworth J, McHardy Young S, Jepson E 1988 Treating hypertension in black compared with white non-insulin dependent diabetics: a double-blind trial of verapamil and metoprolol. British Medical Journal 297: 1155–1159
65. Kubo S H, Cody R J, Covit A B, Feldschuh Laragh J H 1986 The effects of verapamil on renal blood flow, renal function and neurohormonal profiles in patients with moderate to severe hypertension. Journal of Clinical Hypertension 3: 38S–46S
66. Fish J E, Norman P S 1986 Effects of the calcium channel blocker, verapamil, on asthmatic airway responses to muscarinic, histaminergic and allergic stimuli. American Review of Respiratory Disease 133: 730–734
67. Sharma S K, Pande J N 1988 The effect of verapamil inhalation on pulmonary function in bronchial asthma. American Review of Respiratory Disease 137: 37
68. Boner A L, Vallone G, Andreoli A, Biancotto R, Warner J O 1987 Nebulized sodium cromoglycate and verapamil in methacholine induced asthma. Archives of Disease in Childhood 62: 264–268
69. Jones C R, Pasanisis F, Elliott H L, Reid J L 1985 Effects of verapamil and nisoldipine on human platelets: in vivo and in vitro studies. British Journal of Clinical Pharmacology 20: 191–196
70. Gotta A W, Capuano C, Hartung J, Sullivan C A 1988 Calcium entry blockers and human platelet aggregation. New York State Journal of Medicine 88: 132–133
71. Lewis J G 1983 Adverse reactions to calcium antagonists. Drugs 25: 196–222
72. Speders S, Sosna J, Schumacher A, Pfebbigsddorf G 1988 Efficacy and safety of Isoptin SR 240 mg in essential hypertension — results of a phase IV study under practice conditions. Hochdruck 8: 25–30
73. Zachariah P K, Sheps S G, Oshrain C, Schirger A, Stein W J 1987 Antihypertensive efficacy of sustained-release verapamil. Journal of Clinical Hypertension 3: 536–546
74. Epstein M L, Kiel E A, Victoria B E 1985 Cardiac decompensation following verapamil therapy in infants with supraventricular tachycardia. Pediatrics 75: 737–740
75. Inoue H, Unno N, Ou M-C, Iwama Y, Sugimoto T 1984 Level of verapamil in human milk. European Journal of Clinical Pharmacology 26: 657–658
76. Hosie J, Hosie G, Meredith P A 1989 The effects of age on the pharmacokinetics and pharmacodynamics of two formulations of verapamil. Journal of Cardiovascular Pharmacology 13 (suppl 4): S60–S62
77. Giacomini K M, Massoud N, Wong F M, Giacomini J C 1984 Decreased binding of verapamil to plasma proteins in patients with liver disease. Journal of Cardiovascular Pharmacology 6: 924–928
78. Rodin S M, Johnson B F, Wilson J, Ritchie P, Johnson J 1988 Comparative effects of verapamil and isradipine on steady-state digoxin kinetics. Clinical Pharmacology and Therapeutics 43: 668–672
79. Maragno I, Giannoti C, Tropeano P F, Rodighiero V, Gaion R M et al 1987 Verapamil-induced changes in digoxin kinetics in cirrhosis. European Journal of Clinical Pharmacology 32: 309–311
80. Holtzman J L, Finley D, Mottonen L et al 1987 Pharmacodynamic and pharmacokinetic interaction of flecainide and verapamil. Clinical Pharmacology and Therapeutics 41: 242
81. Edwards D J, Lavoie R, Beckman H, Blevins R, Rubenfire M 1987 The effects of co-administration of verapamil on the pharmacokinetics and metabolism of quinidine. Clinical Pharmacology and Therapeutics 41: 68–73
82. MacPhee G J A, McInnes G T, Thompson G G, Brodie M J 1986 Verapamil potentiates carbamazepine neurotoxicity: a clinically important inhibiting interaction. Lancet 1: 700–703
83. Bowles M J, Bala Subramanian V, Davies A B, Raftery E B 1981 Comparison of antianginal actions of verapamil and propranolol. British Medical Journal 182: 1754

Vidarabine (monohydrate)

Vidarabine was the first antiviral agent shown to have a sufficiently high therapeutic index to allow parenteral administration.

Chemistry

Vidarabine (adenine arabinoside, ara-A) monohydrate (Vira-A)
$C_{10}H_{13}N_5O_4.H_2O$
9-β-D-Arabinofuranosyladenine monohydrate

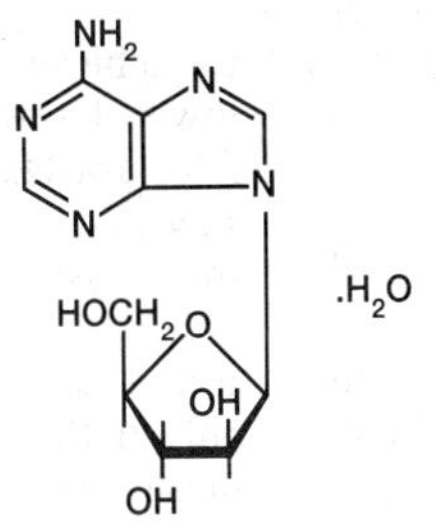

Molecular weight	285.3
pKa	—
Solubility	
in alcohol	—
in water	1 in 2000
Octanol/water partition coefficient	—

Vidarabine monohydrate is a white or off-white, crystalline powder that is obtained from fermentation cultures of *Streptomyces antibioticus*. It is poorly soluble in water (maximal solubility of 0.05%) but is more soluble (0.18%) in phosphate buffer.

Pharmacology

Vidarabine is an analogue of adenosine that is phosphorylated within the cell to arabinosyl ATP. This nucleotide can inhibit DNA polymerases by competing with dATP. Mammalian DNA synthesis is inhibited to a lesser extent than viral DNA. Vidarabine is also metabolized to hypoxanthine arabinoside (ara-Hx) which acts synergistically with its parent compound to inhibit the replication of large DNA viruses. The activity of this metabolite is only 10% of that of ara-A.

Toxicology

Vidarabine is teratogenic when given parenterally to several species (particularly rabbits) and also if applied in very high concentrations topically to the skin of rabbits. In contrast, animal studies did not indicate any evidence of mutagenicity. In carcinogenicity studies lasting up to 24 months there was a slightly increased incidence of liver and kidney neoplasms.[1] Toxicological testing did not demonstrate any results of major clinical relevance.

Clinical pharmacology

Vidarabine is active in vitro and in vivo against DNA viruses such as herpes simplex types 1 and 2, varicella-zoster, cytomegalovirus and vaccinia.[2,3] The activity against herpes simplex type 1 is greater than that against type 2. The drug is inactive against other DNA viruses such as adenoviruses and against RNA viruses. At effective antiviral concentrations there are no clinical effects on human cells.

Pharmacokinetics

The preferred analytical method is by high pressure liquid chromatography in a borate buffer system.[4] The limit of detection of this method is 0.2 mg.l^{-1}.

After oral administration vidarabine is rapidly deaminated the gastrointestinal tract and does not reach the systemic circulation. Following intravenous administration vidarabine is rapidly deaminated to arabinosyl hypoxanthine (ara-Hx) and widely distributed into tissues. The speed of deamination prevents the volume of distribution and protein binding from being determined. An infusion of 10–20 mg.kg^{-1} of vidarabine results in peak plasma levels of 3–10 mg.l^{-1} of total drug (mostly ara-Hx with barely detectable levels of ara-A). The ara-Hx levels do not accumulate with time and reflect the rate of infusion. The mean half life is 3.3 hours. Of the daily dose 41–53% is recovered in the urine as ara-Hx and 2% as ara-A.[5,6] There is no evidence of extracellular drug accumulation but studies have shown that vidarabine or its metabolites accumulate within erythrocytes over 5 to 7 days and persist for several weeks.

The kidney is the primary route of excretion. Patients with renal impairment have higher plasma levels and a slower rate of excretion of ara-Hx and the dosage of vidarabine may need to be adjusted by 25% in severe renal impairment.[6,7]

Vidarabine has been found to achieve highest tissue levels in kidney, liver and spleen with lower levels in muscle and brain. Vidarabine distributes to the CSF (as ara-Hx) reaching levels of one-third of that in plasma, which may persist for up to 10 days after therapy. It is likely that vidarabine crosses the placenta, though no data are available.

Following ocular administration, trace amounts of ara-Hx are found in the aqueous humour only if the cornea is severely damaged.[8,9] Systemic absorption should not occur following ocular administration.

Oral absorption	nil
Presystemic metabolism	—
Plasma half life (ara-A)	15 min
Plasma half life (ara-Hx)	
range	2–4.5 h
mean	3.3 h
Volume of distribution	—
Plasma protein binding	—

Concentration–effect relationships

There is no evidence of a correlation between the plasma concentration of vidarabine and its antiviral effect.

Metabolism

Vidarabine is rapidly deaminated to arabinosyl hypoxanthine by adenine deaminase in serum and in cells. This is then excreted in the urine together with a small amount of ara-A.

Fig. 1 The metabolism of vidarabine

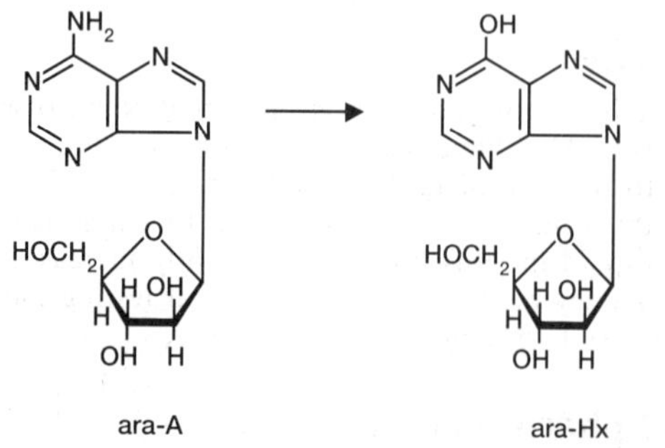

Pharmaceutics

Vidarabine is available under the name Vira-A (Parke-Davis, UK/USA) as a solution for intravenous administration and as an ophthalmic ointment:

1. Vials of 5 ml contain 200 mg.ml^{-1} vidarabine monohydrate, equivalent to 187.4 mg of vidarabine. Each ml contains benzethonium chloride (not more than 0.1 mg) as a preservative, and sodium dihydrogenphosphate and disodium hydrogenphosphate as buffering agents. The injection should be given diluted in a large volume of diluent (see Mode of use).
2. The ophthalmic ointment contains 3% vidarabine in a sterile inert base.

Therapeutic use

Indications

1. Varicella-zoster infection in the immunosuppressed patient
2. Herpes simplex encephalitis
3. Severe mucocutaneous herpes simplex (including neonatal herpes simplex)
4. Herpetic keratoconjunctivitis.

Contraindications

1. Patients who develop intolerance should not be given parenteral or topical vidarabine
2. Vidarabine should not be given by the intramuscular or subcutaneous route.

Mode of use

All the clinical uses depend upon the antiviral effects of the drug. The parenteral preparation should only be given to patients with serious infections where the benefits outweigh the risks. Doses of 10–15 mg.kg^{-1} are usually given as a 12-hourly infusion each day. Doses up to 30 mg.kg^{-1} have been used but no increased benefit has been documented and toxicity may be increased.

The contents of the vial must be diluted before administration and the solubility of vidarabine in intravenous infusion fluids is limited. Each 1 mg of vidarabine requires 2.22 ml of fluid for complete solubilization and 1 litre of infusion fluid will solubilize a maximum of 450 mg of vidarabine. Suitable infusion fluids are 5% dextrose or mixtures of 5% dextrose and sodium chloride. It is important that the vial is well shaken before transferring to the infusion fluid and that the resulting mixture is thoroughly agitated until it is completely clear. Final filtration with an in-line membrane filter is recommended.

Vidarabine must not be administered by the intramuscular or subcutaneous route and rapid or bolus intravenous injections must be avoided.

The volume of intravenous fluid necessitates special care when giving vidarabine to patients susceptible to fluid overloading or cerebral oedema.

The correct way to administer the ophthalmic ointment is to extrude one half inch of ointment into the conjunctival sac five times daily until corneal re-epithelialization has occurred. The treatment can then be reduced to twice daily for a further 7 days.

Indications

1. Varicella zoster

In immunocompromised patients both chickenpox and herpes zoster can be severe and even life-threatening if visceral involvement occurs. Vidarabine has been shown to be of benefit in both conditions.[10–12] Using aseptic technique 10 mg.kg^{-1} should be infused at a constant rate over a 12 to 24 hour period, each day for at least five days.

2. Herpes encephalitis

Therapy of herpes encephalitis with vidarabine decreases mortality and improves morbidity,[13,14] although there is evidence that acyclovir may be more beneficial.[15,16] Vidarabine treatment should be given at 15 mg.kg^{-1} daily for 10 days. It is important to start therapy as soon as the diagnosis is made and there is debate as to the necessity for pretherapy confirmation of the diagnosis by brain biopsy.

3. Mucocutaneous and neonatal herpes simplex

In mucocutaneous herpes simplex in the immunocompromised host the benefits of vidarabine are limited to older patients[17] and acyclovir is now the drug of choice. Vidarabine has shown indications of efficacy in neonatal herpes simplex infection[18] but, again, acyclovir has now been shown to be at least as effective and easier to administer. The established dose is 15 mg.kg^{-1} as a daily 12-hourly infusion for 10 days. A higher dose of 30 mg.kg^{-1} daily confirmed the efficacy but showed no further beneficial effect on decreasing mortality or improving morbidity. There is no evidence that vidarabine prevents the development of more severe disease, as equal numbers of drug and placebo-treated patients progressed during the study.

4. Herpes keratoconjunctivitis
Vidarabine is effective against dendritic keratitis or geographical ulcers due to herpes simplex virus,[19] including those lesions that have not responded to idoxuridine. In previously untreated lesions an average of seven days therapy is needed to achieve corneal re-epithelialization and 90% will heal within three weeks. If there is no response within seven days other forms of therapy are indicated. Topical vidarabine is less effective against stromal keratitis and uveitis but intravenous administration of 20 mg.kg^{-1} daily for seven days has given positive results.[20] There is evidence in animals that vidarabine treatment leads to a better quality of corneal epithelial regeneration than idoxuridine.[21] It is important to recognize that vidarabine does not influence viral latency and therefore recurrences of herpetic eye disease may be problematic.

Adverse reactions

Potentially life-threatening effects
No side effects of this kind have been described.

Acute overdosage
Acute massive overdosage of the intravenous form has not been reported, but as doses of vidarabine two to three times the antiviral dosage can produce haematopoietic depression, principally thrombocytopenia, if an overdose did occur the haematological, renal and liver function should be monitored. Acute massive oral overdosage of the solution or the ointment should not be toxic because drug absorption from the gastrointestinal tract is minimal.

Severe or irreversible adverse effects
Little toxicity is seen at doses of 5–15 mg.kg^{-1} per day but at 20 mg.kg^{-1} megaloblastic changes have been seen in the erythroid precursors in the bone marrow,[22] probably evidence of interference by vidarabine with human DNA synthesis. At higher doses thrombocytopenia and leucopenia may be induced.

The syndrome of inappropriate ADH secretion has been recorded during vidarabine therapy.[23] It resolved when vidarabine was discontinued.

Symptomatic adverse effects
The principal side effects of the parenteral solution involve the gastrointestinal tract: anorexia, nausea, vomiting and diarrhoea.[2] These reactions occur in about 14% of patients given 10–15 mg.kg^{-1} daily and seldom require termination of the drug.

CNS disturbances such as tremor, dizziness, hallucinations, confusion, ataxia and psychosis are rarely seen at therapeutic doses and are usually readily reversible. Other symptoms reported are weight loss, malaise, pruritus and rash. Many of these could be symptoms of the underlying disease.

The ophthalmic ointment may induce lacrimation, conjunctival infection, burning, irritation, superficial punctate keratitis, pain, photophobia, punctal occlusion and sensitivity in 10–15% of patients.

Other effects
Haematological changes noted are a fall in haemoglobin (16.5%), white cell count (6.8%), and platelet count (6.9%), possibly related to the high fluid load administered. Elevation of AST, SGOT and bilirubin elevations are sometimes seen.

Interference with clinical pathology tests
None has been recorded.

High risk groups

Neonates
There is no evidence of toxicity in neonates treated for severe herpes infections. The serum concentrations and half life of ara-Hx in full-term infants is the same as in adults,[24] but the renal clearance is considerably less, possibly due to a physiologically lower GFR. There was some evidence of higher serum levels and a larger volume of distribution of ara-Hx in premature infants.

Breast milk. It is not known whether vidarabine is excreted in human milk and although it is advised that mothers should not nurse their infants while receiving vidarabine, it is unlikely that nursing infants would absorb appreciable amounts of drug as it is rapidly deaminated in the gastrointestinal tract.

Children
There do not appear to be any particular problems of vidarabine administration to children.

Pregnant women
A safe dose for the human embryo has not been established and vidarabine should only be used in pregnancy for life-threatening illnesses when the possible benefits outweigh the risks.

The elderly
The drug has been used in a number of elderly patients with herpes encephalitis and herpes zoster and there are no particular problems recorded.

Drug interactions

Potentially hazardous interactions
There is some evidence that when vidarabine is given in conjunction with interferon for the treatment of hepatitis B infections, increased toxicity is noted.[25]

The concurrent administration of allopurinol increases the toxicity of vidarabine by interfering with metabolism of the drug.[26]

Major outcome trials

1. Whitley R J, Soong S J, Dolin R, Galasso G J, Ch'ien L T, Alford C A Jr and the NIAID Collaborative Antiviral Study Group 1977 Adenine arabinoside therapy of biopsy-proved herpes simplex encephalitis. New England Journal of Medicine 297: 287–294

This is a multi-centre, double-blind, randomized, placebo-controlled study carried out by the National Institute for Allergy and Infectious Diseases Collaborative Antiviral Study Group. Of 54 patients recruited, herpetic encephalitis was confirmed in only 28 patients. Of this 28, 18 received vidarabine intravenously at 15 mg.kg^{-1} daily for 10 days while the other 10 patients were given a placebo. A statistically significant difference in the mortality between the two groups was noted: 70% of the placebo group died compared with only 28% of the vidarabine-treated group. Many of the survivors were however left with severe sequelae and the authors point out that the major determinant of a satisfactory outcome is drug therapy initiated early in the course of the disease, i.e. before coma develops.

2. Whitley R J, Hilty M, Haynes R et al and the NIAID Collaborative Antiviral Study Group 1982 Vidarabine therapy of varicella in immunosuppressed patients. Journal of Pediatrics 101: 125–131

This was a NIH supported study of hospitalized immunocompromised patients with varicella of less than 72 h duration. 19 were given 10 mg.kg^{-1} vidarabine daily for 5 days and 14 placebo. Vidarabine accelerated the resolution of fever and decreased the development of visceral complications, especially pneumonitis, the incidence of which was reduced from 27% to 5%: all with little or no toxicity.

3. Whitley R J, Nahmias A J, Soong S J, Galasso G J, Flemming C L, Alford C A Jr and the NIAID Collaborative Antiviral Study Group 1980 Vidarabine therapy of neonatal herpes simplex virus infection. Pediatrics 66: 495–501

This was a NIH initiated multi-centre, double-blind placebo-controlled study of 63 newborns — 31 given vidarabine 15 mg.kg^{-1} daily for 10 days and 32 placebo. Mortality was decreased in babies with CNS or disseminated disease from 74% to 38% but this was chiefly due to an effect on those with CNS disease alone. The long-term morbidity was only marginally affected by therapy. With less severe initial disease there was a greater improvement in mortality and morbidity after vidarabine therapy.

Other controlled trials

1. Whitley R J, Ch'ien T, Dolin R et al 1977 Adenine arabinoside therapy of herpes zoster in the immunosuppressed. New England Journal of Medicine 294: 1193–1199

2. Whitley R J, Spruance S, Hayden F G et al and the NIAID Collaborative Antiviral Study Group 1984 Vidarabine therapy for mucocutaneous herpes simplex virus infections in the immunocompromised host. Journal of Infectious Diseases 149: 1–8

General review articles

Pavan-Langston D, Buchanan R A, Alford C A Jr (eds) 1975 Adenine arabinoside: an antiviral agent. Raven Press, New York

Pavan-Langston D 1977 Use of vidarabine in ophthalmology: a review. Annals of Ophthalmology 835–839

Whitley R J, Alford C A 1979 Developmental aspects of adenine arabinoside for parenteral therapy of human herpes virus infections. Advances in Ophthalmology 38: 288–296

Collier L H, Oxford J (eds) 1980 Developments in antiviral therapy. Academic Press, London

Hirsch M S, Schooley R T 1983 Treatment of herpes virus infections. New England Journal of Medicine 309: 963–970, 1034–1039

Nicholson K G 1984 Antiviral therapy. Lancet 2: 617–621, 677–682, 736–739

Wood M J, Geddes A M 1987 Antiviral therapy. Lancet 2: 1189–1193

References

1. Kurtz S M 1975 Toxicology of adenine arabinoside. In: Pavan-Langston D, Buchanan R A, Alford C A (eds) Adenine arabinoside: an antiviral agent. Raven Press, New York, pp 145–157
2. Buchanan R A, Hess F 1980 Vidarabine: pharmacology and clinical experience. Pharmacology and Therapeutics 8: 143–171
3. Schabel F M 1968 The antiviral activity of 9-B-D-arabino-furanosyladenine (ara-A). Chemotherapy 13: 321–338
4. Schneider H G, Glazko A J 1977 High-performance liquid chromatography of adenine and hypoxanthine arabinosides. Journal of Chromatography 139: 370–375
5. LePage G A, Khaliq A, Gottlieb J A 1973 Studies of 9-B-D-arabinofuranosyladenine in man. Drug Metabolism and Disposition 1: 756–759
6. Kinkel A W, Buchanan R A 1975 Human pharmacology. In: Pavan-Langston D, Buchanan R A, Alford C A (eds) Adenine arabinoside: an antiviral agent. Raven Press, New York, pp 197–204
7. Aranoff G R, Szwed J J, Nelson R L, Marcus E L, Kleit S A 1980 Hypoxanthine–arabinoside pharmacokinetics after adenine arabinoside administration to a patient with renal failure. Antimicrobial Agents and Chemotherapy 18: 212–214
8. Pavan-Langston D, Dohlman C H, Geary P, Sulzewski D 1973 Intraocular penetration of ara-A and IDU — therapeutic implications in clinical herpetic uveitis. Transactions of the American Academy of Ophthalmology and Otolaryngology 77: 455–466
9. Poirier R H, Kinkel A W, Ellison A C, Lewis R 1975 Intraocular penetration of topical 3 per cent adenine arabinoside. In: Pavan-Langston D, Buchanan R A, Alford C A (eds) Adenine arabinoside: an antiviral agent. Raven Press, New York, pp 307–312
10. Whitley R J, Hilty M, Haynes R, Bryson Y, Connor J D, Soong S J, Alford C A Jr and the NIAID Collaborative Antiviral Study Group 1982 Vidarabine therapy of varicella in immunosuppressed patients. Journal of Pediatrics 101: 125–131
11. Whitley R J, Ch'ien L T, Dolin R, Galasso G J, Alford C A Jr and the Collaborative Antiviral Study Group 1976 Adenine arabinoside therapy of herpes zoster in the immunosuppressed. New England Journal of Medicine 294: 1193–1199
12. Whitley R J, Soong S-J, Dolin R, Betts R, Linnemann C Jr, Alford C A Jr and the NIAID Collaborative Antiviral Study Group 1982 Early vidarabine therapy to control the complications of herpes zoster in immunosuppressed patients. New England Journal of Medicine 307: 971–975
13. Whitley R J, Soong S-J, Dolin R, Galasso G J, Ch'ien L T, Alford C A Jr and the NIAID Collaborative Antiviral Study Group 1977 Adenine arabinoside therapy of biopsy-proved herpes simplex encephalitis. New England Journal of Medicine 297: 287–294
14. Whitley R J, Soong S J, Hirsch M S et al and the NIAID Collaborative Antiviral Study Group 1981 Herpes simplex encephalitis: vidarabine therapy and diagnostic problems. New England Journal of Medicine 304: 313–318
15. Whitley R J, Alford C A, Hirsch M S et al and the NIAID Collaborative Antiviral Study Group 1986 Vidarabine versus acyclovir therapy in herpes simplex encephalitis. New England Journal of Medicine 314: 144–149
16. Skoldenberg B, Forsgren M, Alestig K et al 1984 Acyclovir versus vidarabine in herpes simplex encephalitis. Lancet 2: 707–711
17. Whitley R J, Spruance S, Hayden F G, Overall J, Alford C A Jr, Gwaltney J M Jr, Soong S-J and the NIAID Collaborative Antiviral Study Group 1984 Vidarabine therapy for mucocutaneous herpes simplex virus infections in the immunocompromised host. Journal of Infectious Diseases 149: 1–8
18. Whitley R J, Nahmias A J, Soong S J, Galasso G J, Flemming C L, Alford C A Jr and the NIAID Collaborative Antiviral Study Group 1980 Vidarabine therapy of neonatal herpes simplex virus infection. Pediatrics 66: 495–501

19. Pavan-Langston D, Dohlman C H 1972 A double blind study of adenine arabinoside therapy of viral keratoconjunctivitis. American Journal of Ophthalmology 74: 81–88
20. Abel R Jr, Kaufman H E, Sugar J 1975 Effect of intravenous adenine arabinoside on herpes simplex keratouveitis in humans. In: Pavan-Langston D, Buchanan R A, Alford C A (eds) Adenine arabinoside: an antiviral agent. Raven Press, New York, pp 393–400
21. Langston R H S, Pavan-Langston D, Dohlman C H 1974 Antiviral medication and corneal wound healing. Archives of Ophthalmology 92: 509–513
22. Ross A H, Julia A, Balakrishnan C 1976 Toxicity of adenine arabinoside in humans. Journal of Infectious Diseases 133 (suppl): A192–A198
23. Ramos E, Timmons R F, Schempf S S 1979 Inappropriate antidiuretic hormone following adenine arabinoside administration. Antimicrobial Agents and Chemotherapy 15: 142–145
24. Shope T C, Kauffman R E, Bowman D, Marcus E L 1983 Pharmacokinetics of vidarabine in the treatment of infants and children with infections due to herpes viruses. Journal of Infectious Diseases 148: 721–725
25. Sacks S L, Scullard G H, Pollard R B, Gregory P B, Robinson W S, Merigan T C 1982 Antiviral treatment of chronic hepatitis B virus infection: pharmacokinetics and side effects of interferon and adenine arabinoside alone and in combination. Antimicrobial Agents and Chemotherapy 21: 93–100
26. Friedman H M, Grasela T 1981 Adenine arabinoside and allopurinol: possible adverse drug interaction. New England Journal of Medicine 304: 423

Vigabatrin

This novel antiepileptic agent is a synthetic amino acid acting through enzyme inhibition of GABA aminotransferase.

Chemistry

Vigabatrin (Sabril)
$C_6H_{11}NO_2$
(RS)-4-Amino-5-hexenoic acid

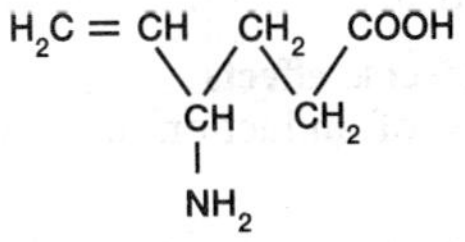

Molecular weight	129.6
pKa (carboxy, amino group)	4.02, 9.72
Solubility	
in alcohol	1 in 10
in water	1 in 3
Octanol/water partition coefficient	low

Vigabatrin is made as a racemic mixture of its two enantiomers. Only the S(+) enantiomer is active pharmacologically. It is a white to off-white odourless crystalline powder prepared by chemical synthesis.

Pharmacology

Vigabatrin is an enzyme-activated, irreversible inhibitor of aminobutyrate aminotransferase. It is thought to bind covalently to the active site of the enzyme as it undergoes catalytic conversion. A stable adduct is formed, however, resulting in irreversible inhibition. It does not inhibit GABA transferase from non-mammalian sources, glutamic acid decarboxylase or aspartate transaminase but alanine transaminase is slowly inhibited. Repeated dosing causes a more profound and sustained elevation of GABA concentration.[1] The anticonvulsant properties in animals are variable. It has an inhibitory effect on audiogenic and strychnine-induced seizures in rodents and photogenic seizures in primates.[2]

Seizure induction by the GABA receptor antagonists bicuculline and picrotoxin is blocked to a lesser extent. Electroshock seizures[3] and amygdala-kindled seizures[4] in the rat, but not pentylenetetrazol seizures, are also inhibited by vigabatrin. The timing of this protective function corresponds better to the increase in synaptosomal GABA concentration rather than whole brain GABA. Such anticonvulsant effects are brought about by the active enantiomer only.[5]

Other pharmacological effects mediated through an increase in brain GABA levels include a reduction in locomotor activity, general sedation, hypothermia and moderate analgesia.[6]

Toxicology

Studies of acute toxicological effects in rodents indicate that vigabatrin can cause CNS depression and convulsions in high doses. Alopecia and weight loss were seen in rodents on repeated administration. There are also reports of anorexia, anaemia and weight loss in dogs, and diarrhoea in monkeys when vigabatrin was administered in high doses.

Vigabatrin does not appear to have mutagenic or carcinogenic potential in animals.[6] Reproduction studies have shown only a low incidence of cleft palate in the rabbit.

A significant histological finding in chronic animal studies is the appearance of microvacuoles within myelinated tracts, particularly in the cerebellum, reticular formation, optic tract, anterior commissure, colliculus and hippocampus. Separation of the outer lamellar sheaths of myelinated fibres seems to be the primary microscopic change. In dogs this histological aberration was associated with abnormally slow somatosensory, but not auditory, potentials.[7] These histological changes are mostly reversible on stopping vigabatrin. Apart from the changes in evoked potentials, no other neurological changes have been associated with this lesion. So far, there is no evidence that it occurs in man.

Clinical pharmacology

Vigabatrin is well tolerated when taken by mouth and only the S(+) enantiomer is pharmacologically active. After oral dosing, vigabatrin produces dose-related increases in the cerebrospinal fluid concentrations of free and total GABA, homocarnosine (the GABA-histidine dipeptide) and α-alanine. These changes are all consistent with an inhibition of GABA transaminase activity in human brain. Similar changes can be seen in human platelets and measurement of platelet GABA transaminase may be a useful index of what is happening in the brain.

Vigabatrin is effective as supplementary therapy in the treatment of drug-resistant epilepsy, particularly involving complex partial seizures with or without secondary generalization. Less favourable responses have been seen in other types of seizures although these findings await more comprehensive evaluation. Vigabatrin occasionally causes agitation and insomnia in children while in some adults somnolence is the commonest side effect. The drug has been reported to provoke psychosis in some patients.

Pharmacokinetics

The analytical methods for measuring vigabatrin include ion-exchange high performance liquid chromatography with post-column derivatization and fluorescence detection of the dansylated derivative of the drug which has a sensitivity[8] of 100 μg.l^{-1}. At present this is an ideal practical method because of its ability to measure the two enantiomers separately.

Vigabatrin is rapidly absorbed, with peak plasma concentration occurring within 2 hours of dosing,[9] and this is not affected by food intake.[10] At least 80% of an oral dose is recovered in the urine irrespective of the dose administered, indicating minimal metabolism. Being hydrophilic, it is distributed in total body water; and its penetration into the CSF[11] is dose dependent. The bioavailability of the inactive enantiomer is probably better than that of the pharmacologically active one.

Elimination occurs principally through urinary excretion, biotransformation accounting for less than 20% of the dose. The terminal elimination half lives of the two enantiomers are similar at about 7–8 hours, giving a renal clearance of 1.3 ml.min^{-1}.kg^{-1}. The co-administration of the R(−) enantiomer has no influence on the pharmacokinetics of the S(+) enantiomer.[9] The active enantiomer is not converted to the inactive one in vivo.

About 50% of an oral dose of the S(+) enantiomer and 65% of the R(−) enantiomer is excreted in the urine in the first 48 hours. The clearance of both enantiomers correlates well with creatinine clearance.

Oral absorption	>80%
Presystemic metabolism	negligible
Plasma half life	7–8 h
Volume of distribution	0.85 ± 16 l.kg^{-1}
Plasma protein binding	negligible

Plasma concentrations of the drug are likely to be elevated in patients with renal dysfunction and in old age where there is a reduction in renal function. Some adjustment of the dose may be necessary.

Concentration–effect relationship

There is no correlation between therapeutic response and either plasma or CSF levels of vigabatrin, although there is significant evidence for dose-related anticonvulsive effects.[12] There are suggestions that inhibition of the enzyme GABA transaminase in platelets by vigabatrin corresponds well to the inhibition of the same enzyme in the CNS and therefore can serve as a measure of the pharmacodynamic effects of vigabatrin in man.[13]

Metabolism

As vigabatrin does not undergo any significant metabolic processes it is eliminated largely in the urine as unchanged parent compound.

Pharmaceutics

500 mg tablets of vigabatrin (Sabril, Merrell Dow, UK) are white, oval and are scored on one side with 'SABRIL' on the other side. They have been assigned a shelf-life of 3 years.

Therapeutic use

Indications

1. Epilepsy
2. Uses in other neurological disorders are under investigation, e.g. tardive dyskinesia, skeletal muscle spasticity and blepharospasm.

Contraindications

1. Use in pregnancy and lactation.

Mode of use

Studies so far have shown significant evidence for a dose-related antiepileptic effect. The majority of adult patients require a dose of 1.5 g daily. However, a significant number had optimal control with a dose of 2 g daily.[14] Doses of up to 4 g daily have been used with therapeutic advantage in some patients.[15] Children tolerate doses of 40–80 $mg.kg^{-1}$ daily while higher doses (above 100 $mg.kg^{-1}$ daily) were not associated with higher efficacy.[16]

It is recommended that the dose of vigabatrin should be titrated up gradually against seizure frequency until therapeutic benefit is achieved or limitation by adverse effects occurs. More favourable results are achieved with vigabatrin in patients taking one or two other antiepileptic agents, compared with those taking three or more drugs, irrespective of the nature of these drugs.

The present practice is to administer the drug on a twice-daily basis. As previously discussed, serum or CSF levels are not useful for monitoring therapeutic benefit except perhaps for checking compliance.

Indications

1. Epilepsy

Results of clinical studies in the treatment of resistant epilepsy have been encouraging. Vigabatrin appears to be particularly effective in the control of complex partial seizures[17] with or without secondary generalization. There is an indication that approximately 50% of patients with refractory partial seizures experience a 50% or more reduction in seizure frequency. Less impressive results are seen in the case of generalized epileptic disorders,[18,19] and in children suffering from Lennox–Gastaut and West syndromes.[16] Subjects with ten or fewer seizures per week, those without severe brain dysfunction, and those not receiving psychoactive drugs seem to fare better.

2. Other indications

Other possible therapeutic potentials for vigabatrin include the control of tardive dyskinesia, skeletal muscle spasticity, and blepharospasm. It has also shown some promise in the management of schizophrenia, particularly catatonic and/or hebephrenic. However, until large-scale randomized controlled trials have been carried out its use in these conditions is premature.

Special considerations

Psychomotor assessment of patients receiving vigabatrin revealed no adverse effects on learning, concentration and memory.[20] Vigabatrin does not seem to induce microsomal hepatic enzymes; therefore it is unlikely to be associated with failure of oral contraception.

Contraindications and precautions

To date there are no clear contraindications for treatment with vigabatrin but there is as yet inadequate evidence of safety in pregnancy. However, care should be taken when treating patients with renal failure. In such patients accumulation of the drug is likely because of impaired renal excretion, particularly if high doses are used.

Adverse reactions

Adverse reactions have been infrequent with vigabatrin therapy. Only 1.5–6% of patients receiving vigabatrin had to discontinue the drug because of adverse effects.

Potentially life-threatening effects

No effects of this kind have been reported.

Acute overdosage

Two cases[25] of accidental and suicidal overdose have been reported. Vertigo and tremor were prominent in the first case, in which the patient took 14 g daily for 3 days. Recovery in this case was uneventful. The second patient developed coma after 30 g of vigabatrin and 250 mg dipotassium clorazepate and had to be ventilated for 24 hours. Complete recovery occurred after 4 days. It is more likely that the deep loss of consciousness was caused by the clorazepate rather than the vigabatrin.

Severe or irreversible adverse effects

There are few reports of induction of psychosis, depression or confusion.

Symptomatic adverse effects

Somnolence is the most common adverse effect reported by 13–28% of patients. Fatigue is the second commonest, with an incidence of 5–9%. These effects were particularly noted when a maintenance dose of 2 g or more daily was started abruptly. Other adverse effects reported include dizziness, headache, ataxia, diplopia, nervousness and irritability, particularly in children. The incidence of these latter effects appeared to diminish upon continued use. Reductions in haematocrit and red cell count have been seen in a few patients. These were children treated with high doses of 250–600 $mg.kg^{-1}$ daily. These changes reversed within a few weeks of stopping the medication. No other haematological changes were seen.

There have been occasional suggestions of weight gain in long-term studies. It is not certain, however, if the latter is a pharmacological effect of vigabatrin.

There is doubt whether the intramyelenic oedema and white matter microvacuolation observed in animals occur in humans. The available data from studies of evoked potentials,[21,22] CT scanning, and magnetic resonance imaging have failed to show any significant abnormalities. Post-mortem examination of the limited number of human brain specimens available so far has not demonstrated any evidence of such histopathological changes.[23,24]

Other effects

Reduction in serum transaminases levels, particularly SGPT (ALT), has been observed in many patients, but this was not thought to indicate hepatotoxicity. There are no significant alterations in GGT activity and no consistent effect on alkaline phosphatase. There is no interference with any haematological parameter and no firm evidence of any urinary abnormalities.

Interference with clinical pathology tests

No interferences of this kind have been reported.

High risk groups

Neonates

The drug is unlikely to be used in neonates.

Breast milk. No information is available on the presence or absence of the drug in breast milk, so patients taking the drug should not breast-feed.

Children

Regular review of haematological parameters is advisable during the initial few months of starting therapy, especially in patients receiving a high dose. The dose of vigabatrin should be reduced or the drug stopped if significant falls in haemoglobin, PCV or red cell count are recorded. Attention should also be given to detect adverse changes in behaviour that may be associated with vigabatrin therapy. At the present stage of uncertainty it may also be advisable to screen for changes in evoked potentials by conducting pre- and post-therapy measurements.

Vigabatrin

Pregnant women

Animal studies have failed to show any significant teratogenic effects, with minimal effects on fertility and fetal development. In humans, knowledge is limited to 5 cases[25] of pregnant women who continued treatment throughout pregnancy. None of the newborns had any serious or significant abnormalities that could be linked with vigabatrin therapy. However, it is recommended that this medication should be withdrawn prior to contemplated conception and proper contraception procedures should be adopted prior to administration of vigabatrin to women of child-bearing potential.

The elderly

Adjustments to the vigabatrin dosage may be necessary because of an increase in the terminal half life due to reduced renal excretion. These dose adaptations should be based on creatinine clearance.

Drug interactions

The risk of potential interactions with other antiepileptic medications is reduced by the fact that vigabatrin is not protein-bound or metabolized by hepatic microsomal enzymes; nor does it induce drug metabolism. However, the following interactions have been identified:

Potentially hazardous interactions

Phenytoin. When vigabatrin is given to patients on phenytoin, there is a 20–40% reduction in steady-state serum levels of phenytoin. The explanation for this is obscure,[26] and is apparently not accounted for by an increased rate of metabolism.

Phenobarbitone and primidone. Smaller reductions in barbiturate levels, perhaps in the region of 7–10%, have been seen on addition of vigabatrin.[21] The reason for this is not clear.

Carbamazepine and valproate. No significant changes in plasma levels have been demonstrated on adding vigabatrin.

Potentially useful interactions

No interactions of this type have been described.

Major outcome trials

1. Rimmer E, Richens A 1984 Double-blind study of gamma-vinyl GABA in patients with refractory epilepsy. Lancet 1: 189–190

Vigabatrin in a dose of 3 g daily was added to existing therapy in a double-blind placebo-controlled cross over randomized study. Twenty-four patients were recruited of whom only 21 completed the study. One was withdrawn because of confusional state related to vigabatrin therapy, and two for non-compliance. Improvement was noted in all but one patient whilst on vigabatrin compared to placebo. Fourteen patients had >50% decrease in seizure frequency, and six of these recorded 75% fewer seizures. Beneficial therapeutic effect was greatest in the control of complex partial attacks compared to tonic–clonic convulsions. Adverse side effects were minimal.

2. Gram L, Klosterskov P, Dam M 1985 Gamma-vinyl-GABA: a double blind placebo-controlled trial in partial epilepsy. Annals of Neurology 17: 262–266

In this paper vigabatrin was used as an add-on therapy in a double-blind, crossover fixed-dose study, in which 21 patients with drug-resistant epilepsy took part. Eighteen patients completed the study; three patients (17%) had 75% reduction in seizure frequency and in eight patients (44%) seizures were reduced by 50%. Three patients got worse on vigabatrin. Except for two patients who were withdrawn because of adverse effects, the participants tolerated the drug well.

3. Loiseau P, Hardenberg J P, Pestre M, Guyot M, Schechter P J, Tell G P 1986 Double blind placebo controlled study of Vigabatrin (gamma-vinyl GABA) in drug resistant epilepsy. Epilepsia 27: 115–120

In this double-blind randomized crossover study, vigabatrin and placebo were compared as add-on therapy in 23 patients with refractory epilepsy. The majority had complex partial seizures and half of these patients had secondary generalization. The dose of vigabatrin used was 3 g per day. Nineteen patients completed the study and four dropped out: two due to increased seizures on changing from vigabatrin to placebo, one due to intolerance to vigabatrin therapy, and one due to poor seizure record. The results of the study were significantly in favour of vigabatrin treatment. Eleven out of the 19 patients had >50% reduction in weekly seizure frequency, two had 25–50% reductions, 4 remained unchanged and 2 deteriorated. Adverse effects were minimal.

Other trials

1. Pedersen S A, Klosterkov P, Gram L, Dam M 1985 Long-term study of gamma-vinyl GABA in the treatment of epilepsy. Acta Neurologica Scandinavica 72: 295–298
2. Tartari A, Manni R, Galimberti C A, Hardenberg J, Orwin J, Perucca A 1986 Vigabatrin in the treatment of epilepsy: A double-blind, placebo-controlled study. Epilepsia 27: 717–723

General review articles

Schechter P J, Tranier Y 1978 The pharmacology of enzyme activated inhibitors of GABA transaminase. In: Seiler N, Jung M J, Koch-Weser J (eds) Enzyme-activated irreversible inhibitors. Amsterdam, Elsevier, pp 149–162

Iadarola M J, Gale K 1981 Cellular compartments of GABA in brain and their relationship to anticonvulsant activities. Molecular and Cellular Biochemistry 39: 305–330

Meldrum B 1982 Pharmacology of GABA. Clinical Neuropharmacology 5: 293–316

Meldrum B S 1989 GABAergic mechanisms in the pathogenesis and treatment of epilepsy. British Journal of Clinical Pharmacology 27: 3S–11S

Graham D J 1988 Neuropathology of vigabatrin. British Journal of Clinical Pharmacology 27: 43S–45S

Lewis P J, Richens A (eds) 1989 Vigabatrin: a new anti-epileptic. British Journal of Clinical Pharmacology 27: 1S–130S

Mumford J P 1988 A profile of vigabatrin. British Journal of Clinical Practice 42 (suppl 61): 7–9

Richens A 1989 Potential antiepileptic drugs: Vigabatrin. In: Levy R H, Dreifuss F E, Mattson R H, Meldrum B, Penry J K (eds) Antiepileptic Drugs, 3rd edn. Raven Press, New York, pp 937–946

References

1. Persson L I, Ronnback L, Ben-Menachem E 1989 Changes in CSF and brain soluble proteins following vigabatrin treatment in rats. British Journal of Clinical Pharmacology 27: 735–775
2. Meldrum B, Horton R 1978 Blockade of epileptic responses in the photosensitive baboon, Papio papio, by two irreversible inhibitors of GABA-transaminase, gamma acetylenic GABA (4-amino-hex-5-ynoic) and gamma-vinyl GABA (4-amino-hex-5-enoic acid). Psychopharmacology (Berlin) 59: 47–50
3. Iadarola M J, Gale K 1982 Substantia nigra: site of anticonvulsant activity mediated by gamma-aminobutyric acid. Science 218: 1237–1240
4. Kalichman M W, Burnham W M, Livingstone K E 1982 Pharmacological investigation of gamma-aminobutyric acid (GABA) and fully developed seizures in the amygdala-kindled rat. Neuropharmacology 21: 127–131
5. Meldrum B S, Murugaiah K 1983 Anticonvulsant action in mice with sound-induced seizures of the optical isomers of gamma-vinyl GABA. European Journal of Pharmacology 89: 149–152
6. Palfryman M G, Schechter P J, Buckett W R, Tell G P, Koch-Weser J 1981 The pharmacology of GABA-transaminase inhibitors. Biochemical Pharmacology 30: 817–824
7. Arezzo J C, Schroeder C E, Litwak M S, Steward D L 1989 Effects of vigabatrin on evoked potentials in dogs. British Journal of Clinical Pharmacology 27: 535–605
8. Smithers J A, Lang J F, Okerholm R A 1985 Quantitative analysis of vigabatrin in plasma and urine by reversed phase high-performance liquid chromatography. Journal of Chromatography 341: 232–238
9. Haegle K D, Schechter P J 1986 Kinetics of the evaluation of vigabatrin after an oral dose of the racemate or the active S-enantiomer. Clinical Pharmacology and Therapeutics 40: 581–586
10. Frisk-Holmberg M, Kerth P, Meyer Ph 1989 Effect of food on the absorption of vigabatrin. British Journal of Clinical Pharmacology 27: 235–255
11. Schechter P J, Hanke N F J, Grove J, Heubert N, Sjoerdsma A 1984 Biochemical and clinical effects of gamma-vinyl GABA in patients with epilepsy. Neurology 34: 182–186
12. Gram L, Lyon B B, Dam M 1983 Gamma-vinyl GABA: a single blind trial in patients with epilepsy. Acta Neurologica Scandinavica 68: 34–39
13. Rimmer E, Kongola G, Richens A 1988 Inhibition of the enzyme, GABA-aminotransferase, in human platelets by vigabatrin, a potential antiepileptic drug. British Journal of Clinical Pharmacology 25: 251–259
14. Sivenius M R J, Ylinen A, Murros K, Matilainen R, Riekkinen P 1987 Double blind dose reduction study of vigabatrin in complex partial epilepsy. Epilepsia 28: 688–692
15. Browne T R, Mattson R H, Penry J K et al 1987 Vigabatrin for refractory complex partial seizures: multicentre single-blind study with long term follow up. Neurology 37: 184–189

16. Livingston J H, Beaumont D, Arzimanoglou A, Aicardi J 1989 Vigabatrin in the treatment of epilepsy in children. British Journal of Clinical Pharmacology 27: 1095–1125
17. Reynolds E H, Ring H, Heller A 1988 A controlled trial of gamma-vinyl GABA (vigabatrin) in drug resistant epilepsy. British Journal of Clinical Practice 42 (suppl 61): 33
18. Tassinari C A, Michaelucci R, Ambrosetto G, Salvi F 1987 Double-blind study of vigabatrin in the treatment of drug resistant epilepsy. Archives of Neurology 44: 907–910
19. Remy C, Favel P, Tell G, Hardenberg J, Schechter P J 1986 Double-blind, placebo-controlled, crossover study of vigabatrin in drug-resistant epilepsy of the adult. Bollettino Lega Italiana contro Epilessia 54/55: 241-243
20. Saletu B, Grunberger J, Linzmayer L, Scwartz J-J, Haegle K D, Schechter P J 1986 Psychophysiological and psychometric studies after manipulating the GABA system by vigabatrin, a GABA-transaminase inhibitor. International Journal of Psychophysiology 4: 63–80
21. Cosi V, Callieco R, Galimberti C A 1988 Effect of vigabatrin (gamma-vinyl GABA) on visual, brain stem auditory and somatosensory evoked potentials in epileptic patients. European Neurology 28: 42–46
22. Hammond E J, Ranger R J, Wilder B J 1988 Evoked potentials monitoring of vigabatrin patients. British Journal of Clinical Practice 42 symp. (suppl 61): 16–23
23. Hauw J J, Trottier S, Boutry J M, Sun P, Sazpovitch V, Duyckaerts C 1988 The neuropathology of vigabatrin. British Journal of Clinical Practice 42 (suppl 61): 10–13
24. Pedersen B, Hojgaard K, Dam M 1987 Vigabatrin: no microvacuoles in a human brain. Epilepsy Research 1: 74–76
25. Clinical Investigator Brochure 1988 Vigabatrin (GABA transaminase inhibitor) Merrell Dow Research Institute. Merrell Dow Pharmaceuticals Inc. Cincinnati, Ohio
26. Rimmer E M, Richens A 1989 Interaction between vigabatrin and phenytoin. British Journal of Clinical Pharmacology 27: 275–335

Vinblastine (sulphate)

The vinca alkaloids comprise three drugs commonly used in the management of malignant disease, with particular emphasis on the lymphomata, Hodgkin's disease and the leukaemias. Vinblastine is a natural alkaloid isolated from the periwinkle plant, *Vinca rosea* (*Catharanthus roseus*).

Chemistry

Vinblastine sulphate (vincaleuko-blastine sulphate, Velbe)
$C_{46}H_{58}N_4O_9H_2SO_4$

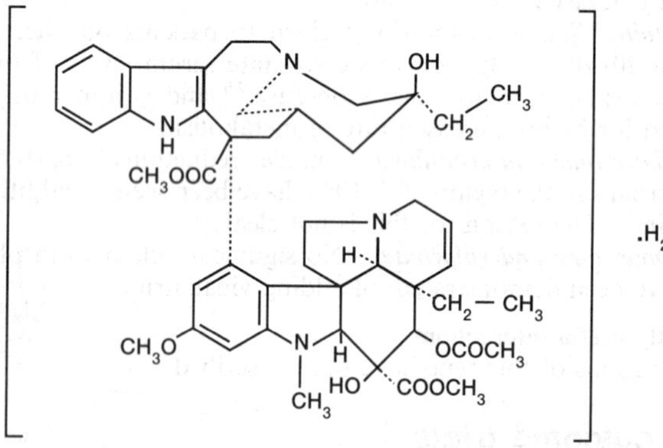

Molecular weight (free base)	909.1 (811.0)
pKa	5.4, 7.4
Solubility	
in alcohol	1 in 1200
in water	1 in 10
Octanol/water partition coefficient	high

The common structure of the vinca alkaloids is two multi-ring units of vindoline and catharanthine linked by a carbon–carbon bridge. Vinblastine differs from vincristine only by the exchange of a methyl group for a formyl group.

Vinblastine is an odourless, very hygroscopic white to slightly yellow amorphous crystalline powder. It is not present in any combination preparations.

Pharmacology

Vinblastine, like the other vinca alkaloids, exerts its biological effects by binding specifically with the protein tubulin.[1] Tubulin normally polymerizes to form microtubules, and, in the presence of vinblastine, there is inhibition in the assembly of tubulin into microtubules with resultant dissolution of the mitotic spindle. Cell division is thus arrested in metaphase and in the absence of an intact mitotic spindle, the chromosomes disperse throughout the cytoplasm, or are aggregated together in unusual formations such as stars. The inability of chromosomes to segregate correctly leads to cell death.

Vinblastine shares a common binding site on each tubulin dimer with the other vinca alkaloids, but this binding site is different from that occupied by other tubulin-binding alkaloids such as colchicine and podophyllotoxin. Only minute concentrations (less than 0.1 μm) are required for inhibition of the assembly of tubulin.[2]

Toxicology

Standard toxicology studies are not normally carried out for cytotoxic drugs because of the toxicity inherent in their mechanism of action, in particular to the haemapoetic stem cell system and gastrointestinal tract. Predicted toxic effects therefore are bone marrow depression, dystrophic gastrointestinal mucosal changes, neurotoxicity and vomiting. Vinblastine is teratogenic in the mouse, rat and monkey. In sensitive animal species neurotoxicity is manifested by damage to myelin and axon degeneration.[3] Treatment over a period of 7 months has been shown to decrease the number of neuronal microtubules in the peripheral nerves of cats.[4] The mutagenic tendency for vinblastine is unknown, although high concentrations will produce structural chromosome aberrations and chromosomal breaks at doses[5] of 2 mg.kg^{-1}. In patients who have received successful therapy with vinca alkaloids alone, or in combination, some successful pregnancies have occurred and, to date, there has been no evidence of increased fetal damage. However, a long-term registry will be necessary to establish the real incidence of potential malformations in patients bearing children having undergone successful therapy.

Clinical pharmacology

Vinblastine is generally administered by intravenous bolus injection, in combination with other cytotoxic agents in the treatment of malignant disease, for example the treatment of metastatic testicular tumours (with bleomycin and cisplatin). In spite of the similar structure of the vinca alkaloids, vinblastine shows little cross-resistance with vincristine. Vinblastine is also effective in the treatment of Hogkin's disease, other lymphomas, and breast tumours. Vinblastine is more likely to produce bone marrow depression than vincristine. The leucopenia following vinblastine therapy is usually most obvious 4–10 days after therapy is given and recovery occurs over the next 7–14 days. Vinblastine penetrates the central nervous system and after an intravenous injection in primates, concentrations of 1 nM are maintained for more than 72 h.[6] However, in human use, concentrations of vinblastine are likely to be lower.[7] Vinblastine may thus cause CNS toxicity. Peripheral neuropathy is the commonest sign of CNS toxicity and depression of the ankle jerk the earliest sign. Thereafter, a wide variety of manifestations may occur including muscular weakness, ataxia, tremors, convulsions and coma. However, CNS toxicity is less common following vinblastine therapy than with vincristine. Constipation, unlike with vincristine, is unusual and diarrhoea with vomiting and anorexia may occur following vinblastine use.

Resistance to vinblastine

There is a surprising lack of cross-resistance between the various vinca alkaloids, given their structural similarities. However, some tumour cells develop overexpression of the multidrug resistance (MDR) gene which produces high levels of the membrane pump protein, p-glycoprotein (P-170) leading to resistance to a wide range of cytotoxic agents (pleiotropic drug resistance), including vinca alkaloids, and anthracyclines. There seems to be some specificity in the molecular form of P-170 induced by each vinca alkaloid, in that cells selected for resistance to vinblastine may not share complete cross-resistance to vincristine.[8] Chromosomal abnormalities consistent with gene amplification have been seen in some of these cases. There have been suggestions that resistance to vinblastine can be overcome by the use of calcium channel blockers such as verapamil. Resistance to vinblastine may result from mutations in tubulin, which lead to decreased drug binding.

Pharmacokinetics

The preferred analytical method is by radioimmunoassay. This assay is not specific for parent drug and cannot differentiate among vinblastine, vincristine and vindesine separately. Sensitivity[9,10] is 2 µg.l^{-1}. Vinblastine is poorly absorbed after oral administration. Thus, administration is generally by intravenous injection, usually as a bolus. After injection, serum levels of vinblastine exhibit a triphasic decay, and whilst the half lives for the first two phases (0.06 h and 1.6 h) are similar amongst the vinca alkaloids, the terminal phase is longer for vinblastine at 20 h. The drug is widely distributed throughout the body and the volume of distribution at steady state ranges[11] from 8 to 27 l.kg^{-1}. The volume of the central compartment is 70% of body weight, significantly greater than that of vindesine which is only 5% of body weight or roughly the blood volume. Vinblastine is concentrated in platelets but the binding is easily reversible. Plasma protein binding is 99%. Vinblastine is rapidly cleared from the blood and distributed to the tissues with a clearance of vinblastine of 12 ml.min^{-1}.kg^{-1}. CSF penetration of vinblastine is minimal.[7]

It is not known whether vinblastine is excreted in breast milk. The drug is believed to cross the placenta.

In view of the role of the liver in the metabolism and excretion of vinblastine it is possible that some dosage reduction will be necessary in hepatic impairment.[12] There is no evidence that the elimination of the drug is altered in renal dysfunction.

Oral absorption	poor
Presystemic metabolism	negligible
Plasma half life	
mean	20 h
Volume of distribution	8–27 l.kg^{-1}
Plasma protein binding	99%

Concentration–effect relationship

There is little evidence of any relationship between the plasma concentration of vinblastine and its therapeutic effect. It is known that concentrations of 10^{-8} M are required in vitro to inhibit completely a lymphoblastoid cell line[12] and yet peak concentrations of vinblastine after standard doses are about 0.4 µM. It is probable that normal and tumour cells have different sensitivities to vinblastine. Following therapy with vinblastine, the nadir in the granulocyte count may be expected to occur five to ten days after administration, with recovery usually rapid thereafter reflecting the duration of action. For malignant cells the duration of action is variable and dependent on the usual parameters of cell sensitivity and repair characteristics and the emergence of drug-resistant sub-populations.[13]

Metabolism

The metabolism of vinblastine is complex and poorly understood. Very few of the metabolites, which are produced primarily in the liver, have been identified.[14] At least one of these, desacetylvinblastine, is active. Vinblastine is excreted in the urine ($\leqslant$14% of dose in 72 h) and faeces ($\leqslant$10% of dose in 72 h) but the metabolites may not be measured by the radioimmunoassay used in this study.[15]

Pharmaceutics

Vinblastine, Velban (Lilly, USA)/Velbe (Lilly, UK), is available only for intravenous injection, 10 mg in the form of lyophilized drug supplied in a combination package with an accompanying diluent of 10 ml sodium chloride 0.9% with benzyl alcohol as preservative. The pH of the reconstituted solution is 3.5 to 5. The solution may be injected via the drip tubing if an infusion of sodium chloride 0.9% is being administered.

Great care should be exercised during intravenous administration. If extravasation should occur the injection should be discontinued immediately and any remaining proportion of the dose should then be introduced into another vein. Local injection of hyaluronidase and the application of moderate heat to the area of leakage help to disperse the drug and may minimize any resultant cellulitis. Care should also be taken during the reconstitution and the appropriate protective clothing, gloves, mask and protective glasses should be used.

Therapeutic use

Vinblastine has now gained an accepted place in the routine management of certain malignancies generally in combination with other cytotoxic drugs. It is occasionally used as a single agent. Although similar in structure to the other vinca alkaloids there are differences in therapeutic effect which are reflected in the disease groups treated.

Indications

1. Generalized Hodgkin's disease
2. Non-Hodgkin's lymphoma
3. Histiocytosis X
4. Testicular cancer
5. Kaposi's sarcoma
6. Other solid tumours.

Contraindications

1. Intrathecal administration.

Precautions

2. Pregnancy
3. Reduced bone marrow reserve
4. Jaundice
5. The elderly.

Indications

1. Generalized Hodgkin's disease
Vinblastine is used as combination therapy for the management of generalized Hodgkin's disease. Vincristine was the first drug introduced into combination therapy and remains the choice in the United States in combination[16] but British groups have adopted vinblastine because of reduced neurotoxicity.[17] The combination consists of mechlorethamine, procarbazine, prednisolone, and vinblastine, given over a two-week period at intervals of six weeks. Therapy is normally repeated to six or to eight courses and 70% of patients can expect cure with this combination. Recent attention has been directed to giving alternating chemotherapy using both vinblastine and vincristine in a particular combination and there is some evidence to suggest that this approach may be more effective than the more traditional management.[18] However, it is too early to draw definite conclusions from the data. The usual doses of vinblastine are either 0.1 $mg.kg^{-1}$ or 6 $mg.m^{-2}$.

2. Non-Hodgkin's lymphoma
Vinblastine is included in combinations used when patients relapse but no definitive schedule can be recommended. The usual dose is 6 $mg.m^{-2}$.

3. Histiocytosis X
This is a localized disease but there are occasions when dissemination occurs, particularly to the lung. Vinblastine as a single agent is the preferred treatment.

4. Testicular cancer
Patients with metastatic teratoma may be treated with vinblastine in combination with cisplatinum, with or without bleomycin.[19] This particular combination is curative for the vast majority of patients with small volume disease although vinblastine has largely been replaced by etoposide. For those patients with bulky tumours more intensive therapy is necessary but even so approximately 6 out of 10 patients will achieve complete remission and this will be long-lasting. The usual dose is 0.2 $mg.kg^{-1}$ on each of two consecutive days every three weeks.

For seminoma the optimum regime has yet to evolve but the combination of vinblastine, cisplatinum and bleomycin is effective initially, but there is doubt as to whether some remissions will be sustained.

5. Kaposi's sarcoma
Vinblastine may be used in the treatment of Kaposi's sarcoma. A dose of 4 mg weekly, adjusted so that the leucocyte count remains above 2500 mm^{-3}, has been used with benefit in AIDS-related Kaposi's sarcoma.[20]

6. Other solid tumours
Other solid tumours including breast cancer have been treated with temporary palliative benefit. A 5-day infusion of vinblastine has been suggested by some workers.[21]

Contraindications

1. Accidental intrathecal administration
Accidental intrathecal administration is fatal. Should this occur there is no antidote that is effective.

Precautions

3. Reduced bone marrow reserve
In those patients where marrow reserve has been reduced by previous radiotherapy or by previous chemotherapy caution should be exercised during administration with conventional doses.

4. Impaired liver function
As the primary route of elimination is via the bile, caution should be exercised in the presence of the jaundiced patient. Vincristine would be the preferred drug in this situation, being less myelosuppressive than vinblastine although at a risk of a greater incidence of peripheral neuropathy. Administration to those patients in whom the bilirubin is normal, but in whom the liver enzymes are elevated, is not associated with increased myelosuppression. A raised serum alkaline phosphatase may be an indicator of the potential neurotoxicity at a later date.

5. Elderly patients
Patients over 60 are more prone to develop neurological complications, than younger patients, though this is less than with vincristine. Care should therefore be taken during treatment and dose reduction by 50% may be necessary.

Adverse reactions

Potentially life-threatening effects
All vinca alkaloids produce myelosuppression and this is related to both dose and frequency of administration. With usual doses myelosuppression is not normally severe but if there is any evidence of myelosuppression, the next treatment should be delayed until there has been complete recovery. Vinblastine is more myelosuppressive than vincristine and therefore if bone marrow function is compromised vincristine can be substituted as an alternative drug.

Acute overdosage
Accidental overdose can produce fatal myelosuppression and neurotoxicity. There is no specific antidote although the use of folinic acid has been suggested. Supportive care should include a) prevention of the adverse effects that result from the syndrome of inappropriate secretion of antidiuretic hormone; b) administration of an anticonvulsant; c) prevention and treatment of ileus; d) monitoring the patient's cardiovascular system and haematological monitoring and support.

Severe or irreversible adverse effects
Neurotoxicity. This is the most common adverse effect with this class of drug and indeed is characteristic of the group. The earliest manifestation of neurotoxicity is suppression of the Achilles tendon reflex. Maximal depression occurs about 17 days after a single dose and may take up to 1 to 3 months to return to normal.[22] If treatment is continued then paraesthaesiae affecting both feet and hands develop and this may be associated with severe pains in the region of the throat and, occasionally, the chest. With high-dose vinblastine the pain can be of such severity as to mimic a myocardial infarction. Peripheral nerve involvement is the most disabling manifestation and this is characterized by weakness of the toes and ankles and extension of the fingers and wrists. Non-myelinated nerves may be the most sensitive to vincristine, explaining the early onset of loss of the deep tendon reflex.[23] Cranial nerves may also be affected with ptosis and diplopia being the most common manifestation. Autononic dysfunction may also occur with gastrointestinal problems and postural hypotension. There is no known treatment other than discontinuing medication. Therapy with thiamine and vitamin B12 has been ineffective. Convulsions have been reported.

No additive neurotoxicity occurs when used in combination with other cytotoxic drugs with the exception of etoposide. This is also a tubulin-binding agent and there is therefore potential for a drug interaction. Vinblastine produces a similar spectrum of neurotoxicity to that of vincristine but is seen much less commonly probably because myelosuppression is the dose-limiting factor for this drug. However, when used in high dose then neurological complications will ensue.

Gastrointestinal toxicity. Adverse gastrointestinal reactions are usually mild (see below), but occasionally paralytic ileus and perforated peptic ulcers have been reported.

In patients with liver dysfunction neurotoxic reactions can be severe after routine doses. There is some speculative evidence that vincristine neurotoxicity is related to serum alkaline phosphatase. Desai et al observed a statistically significant relationship between AUC and degree of toxicity.[24] This was related both to the dose and to elevation of serum alkaline phosphatase, suggesting that elimina-

Vinblastine (sulphate)

tion of the drug is impaired when this enzyme is elevated. Dose reduction in this situation therefore may reduce toxicity.

Symptomatic adverse effects
Gastrointestinal side effects are common. Constipation, abdominal cramps, paralytic ileus, vomiting and diarrhoea have all been reported. This is more likely to occur with vinblastine and particularly if used in high dose for the management of testicular cancer. Constipation is the rule for those patients on induction chemotherapy for non-Hodgkin's lymphoma of unfavourable histology. Routine appropriate treatment is normally all that is required.

A number of miscellaneous adverse effects have been reported, including weight loss, fever, headache, alopecia, general malaise and dizziness. These effects are, however, uncommon. The syndrome of inappropriate ADH secretion has been reported for vinblastine.[24]

Interference with clinical pathology tests
No technical interferences of this kind have been reported.

High risk groups

Neonates
Experience is limited and the drug would only rarely be indicated.

Breast milk. It is not known whether vinblastine is excreted in human milk. However, in view of the potential for serious adverse reactions breast-feeding is best avoided.

Children
The drug has been used in children in appropriate doses.

Pregnant women
Teratogenic effects occur in animals and are likely to occur if vinblastine is administered during the first trimester of pregnancy. Should treatment be imperative then termination of pregnancy should be considered. Women of child-bearing age should be advised to avoid becoming pregnant.

The elderly
Patients over 60 are more prone to develop neurological complications than younger patients. Care should therefore be taken during treatment and dose reduction by 50% may be necessary.

Drug interactions

Potentially hazardous interactions
Acute bronchospasm and respiratory distress has been reported following administration of vinblastine in combination with mitomycin C.[26]

Potentially useful interactions
None is known.

General review articles

Bender R A, Chabner C A 1982 Tubulin binding agents. In: Chabner B A (ed) Pharmacologic principles of cancer treatment. W B Saunders, ch 2, pp 256–262

References

1. Creasy W A 1975 Vinca alkaloids and colchicine. In: Sartorelli A C, Johns D G (eds) Handbook of experimental pharmacology 38. Springer, Berlin, p 670
2. Owellen R J, Hartke C A, Dickerson R M, Hains F Q 1976 Inhibition of tubulin-microtubule polymerization by drugs of the vinca alkaloid class. Cancer Research 36: 1499–1502
3. Bradley W G, Lassman L P, Peerce G W 1970 The neuro-myopathy of vincristine in man: clinical, electro-physiologic and pathologic studies. Journal of Neurological Sciences 10: 107
4. Todd G C, Griffing W J, Gibson W R, Morton D M 1979 Animal models for the comparative assessment of neurotoxicity following repeated administration of vinca alkaloids. Cancer Treatment Reports 63: 35–41
5. Gebhart E, Schwanitz G, Hartwich H 1969 Zytogenetische Wirkung von Vincristin auf menschliche Leukozyten in vivo und *in vitro*. Medizinische Klinik 64: 2366–2371
6. Jackson D V, Castle M C, Poplack D G, Bender R A 1980 Pharmacokinetics of vincristine in the cerebrospinal fluid of sub-human primates. Cancer Research 40: 722–724
7. Jackson D V, Sethi V S, Spurr C L, McWhorter J M 1981 Pharmacokinetics of vincristine in the cerebrospinal fluid of humans. Cancer Research 41: 1466
8. Conter V, Beck W T 1984 Acquisition of multi-drug resistance by CCRF-CEM cells selected for different degrees of resistance to vincristine. Cancer Treatment Reports 68: 831–836
9. Root M A, Gerzon K, Dyke R W 1975 A radioimmunoassay for vinblastine and vincristine. Federation of Analytical Chemistry and Spectroscopy Societies: 125
10. Sethi V S, Burton S S, Jackson D V 1980 A sensitive RIA for vincristine and vinblastine. Cancer Chemotherapy and Pharmacology 4: 183
11. Nelson R L, Dyke R W, Root M S 1980 Comparative pharmacokinetics of vindesine, vincristine and vinblastine in patients with cancer. Cancer Treatment Reviews 8: 17
12. Schrek R 1974 Cytotoxicity of vincristine to normal and leukemic cells. American Journal of Clinical Pathology 62: 1–7
13. Don Jackson D V, Bender R A 1979 Cytotoxic thresholds of vincristine in L1210 murine leukemia and a human lymphoblastic cell line in vitro. Cancer Research 39: 4346–4349
14. Jackson D V, Castle M C, Bender R A 1978 Biliary excretion of vincristine. Clinical Pharmacology and Therapeutics 24: 101–107
15. Owellen R J, Hartke C A, Hains F O 1977 Pharmacokinetics and metabolism and vinblastine in humans. Cancer Research 37: 2597–2602
16. DeVita V T Jr, Lewis B J, Rozencweig M, Muggia F M 1978 The chemotherapy of Hodgkin's disease: past experiences and future directions. Cancer 42: 979–990
17. Sutcliffe S B, Wrigley P F M, Peto J et al 1978 MVPP chemotherapy regimen for advanced Hodgkin's disease. British Medical Journal 1: 679
18. Santoro A, Bonadonna G, Valagussa P et al 1987 Long-term results of combined chemotherapy-radiotherapy approach in Hodgkin's disease: superiority of AB & D plus radiotherapy versus MOPP plus radiotherapy Journal of Clinical Oncology 5: 27–37
19. Wilkinson P M 1985 Chemotherapy for non-seminomatous germ-cell tumours. Journal of the Royal Society of Medicine 78: 43–47
20. Volberding P A Abrams D I, Conant M et al 1985 Vinblastine therapy for kaposis sarcoma in the acquired deficiency syndrome Annals of Internal Medicine 103: 333–338
21. Yap H Y, Blumenschein G R, Keating M J, Hortobagyi G N, Tashima C K, Loo T L 1980 Vinblastine given as a continuous five-day infusion in the treatment of refractory-advanced breast cancer. Cancer Treatment Reports 64: 279–283
22. Weiss H D, Walker M D, Wiernik P H 1974 Neurotoxicity of commonly used anti neoplastic agents. New England Journal of Medicine: 127–134
23. Donoso J A, Green L S, Heller-Bettinger I E, Samson F E 1977 Action of the vinca alkaloids vincristine, vinblastine and desacetyl vinblastine amide on axonal fibrillar organelles in vitro. Cancer Research 37: 1401–1407
24. Stahel R A, Oelz O 1982 Syndrome of inappropriate ADH secretion secondary to vinblastine. Cancer Chemotherapy and Pharmacology 8: 253–254

V

Vincristine (sulphate)

One of three vinca alkaloids commonly used in the management of malignant disease, with particular emphasis on the lymphomata, Hodgkin's disease and the leukaemias. Vincristine is a natural alkaloid isolated from the periwinkle plant, *Vinca rosea* (*Catharanthus roseus*).

Chemistry

Vincristine sulphate (leurocristine sulphate, Oncovin)
$C_{46}H_{56}N_4O_{10}.H_2SO_4$
22-Oxovincaleukoblastine sulphate

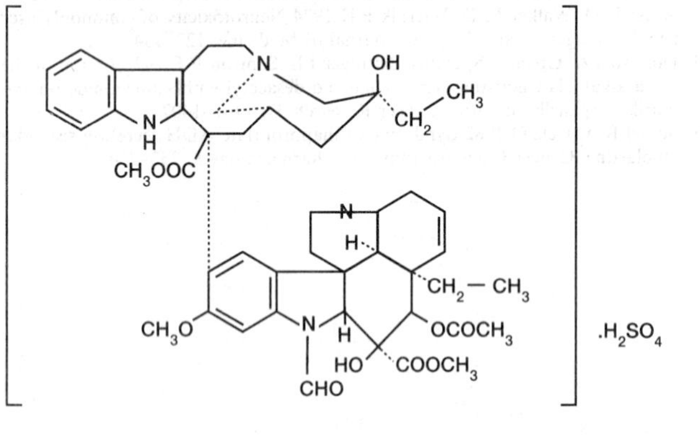

Molecular weight (free base)	923.0 (825.0)
pKa	5.0, 7.4
Solubility	
in alcohol	1 in 600
in water	1 in 2
Octanol/water partition coefficient	2.15

The common structure of the vinca alkaloids is two multi-ring units of vindoline and catharanthine linked by a carbon–carbon bridge. Vincristine differs from vinblastine only by the exchange of a methyl group for a formyl group.

Vincristine is an odourless, hygroscopic, white to yellow substance. It is not present in any combination preparations.

Pharmacology

Vincristine, like the other vinca alkaloids, exerts its biological effects by binding specifically to the protein tubulin.[1] Tubulin normally polymerizes to form microtubules, and, in the presence of vincristine, there is inhibition in the assembly of tubulin into microtubules with resultant dissolution of the mitotic spindle. Cell division is thus arrested in metaphase and in the absence of an intact mitotic spindle, the chromosomes disperse throughout the cytoplasm, or are aggregated together in unusual formations such as stars. The inability of chromosomes to segregate correctly leads to cell death.

Vincristine shares a common binding site on each tubulin dimer with the other vinca alkaloids, but this binding site is different from that occupied by other tubulin binding alkaloids such as colchicine and podophyllotoxin. Only minute concentrations (less than 0.1 micromolar) are required for inhibition of the assembly of tubulin.[2]

Toxicology

Standard toxicology studies are not normally carried out for cytotoxic drugs because of the toxicity inherent in their mechanism of action, in particular to the haemopoetic stem cell system and gastrointestinal tract. Predicted toxic effects therefore are bone marrow depression, dystrophic gastrointestinal mucosal changes, neurotoxicity and vomiting. In sensitive animal species neurotoxicity is manifested by damage to myelin and axon degeneration.[3] Treatment over a period of 7 months has been shown to decrease the number of neuronal microtubules in the peripheral nerves of cats.[4]

Vincristine is teratogenic in the mouse, rat and monkey. The mutagenic tendency for vincristine is unknown although high concentrations will produce structural chromosome aberrations and chromosomal breaks at doses[5] of 2 $mg.kg^{-1}$.

Clinical pharmacology

Vincristine is generally administered by intravenous bolus injection in combination with other cytotoxic agents in the treatment of malignant disease. In spite of the similar structure of the vinca alkaloids, vincristine shows little cross-resistance with vinblastine. Vincristine is more effective than vinblastine in lymphocytic leukaemia, and in acute leukaemia in children. Vincristine is less likely to produce bone marrow depression than vinblastine; however, hair loss appears to be more common with vincristine than with vinblastine.

The duration of action of vincristine is variable and dependent on the usual parameters of cell sensitivity and repair characteristics and the emergence of drug-resistant sub-populations.

Resistance to vincristine

There is a surprising lack of cross-resistance between the various vinca alkaloids, given their structural similarities. However some tumour cells develop overexpression of the multidrug-resistance (MDR) gene which produces high levels of the membrane pump protein, p-glycoprotein (P-170) leading to resistance to a wide range of cytotoxic agents (pleiotropic drug resistance), including vinca alkaloids and anthracyclines. There seems to be some specificity in the molecular form of P-170 induced by each vinca alkaloid, in that cells selected for resistance to vincristine may not show complete cross-resistance to vinblastine.[6] Chromosomal abnormalities consistent with gene amplification have been seen in some of these cases. Cross-resistance to adriamycin is not unusual and the fact that both vincristine and adriamycin are used commonly in the treatment of lymphomas may be of therapeutic relevance.[3] There have been suggestions that resistance to vincristine can be overcome by the use of calcium channel blockers such as verapamil. Resistance to vincristine may result from mutations in tubulin which lead to decreased drug binding.

Pharmacokinetics

The preferred analytical method is by radioimmunoassay. This assay is not specific for the parent drug and it cannot differentiate among vinblastine, vincristine and vindesine. The limit of sensitivity[7,8] is at least 0.5 $\mu g.l^{-1}$.

Vincristine is very poorly absorbed after oral administration. Hence, the drug is generally given by intravenous injection, usually as a bolus. After injection, serum levels of vincristine exhibit a triphasic decay. Whilst the half lives for the first two phases are similar to those for the other two vinca alkaloids, 0.08 h and 2.3 h, respectively, that for the terminal phase is much longer for vincristine, at 85 h. The drug disappears rapidly from the blood but binds extensively to tissues. It is widely distributed throughout the body with a volume of distribution at steady state[9] of 8.4 $l.kg^{-1}$. The volume of the central compartment is 33% of body weight, reflecting the extensive binding of the drug to the formed elements of the blood. This reflects the extensive binding of vincristine to formed elements of blood resulting in the long terminal half life and its low clearance. This suggests that an interval of 1 week between treatment periods is the minimum required to avoid cumulative toxicity.

Vincristine is concentrated in platelets with lesser proportions in the white cells than in erythrocytes. The uptake of vincristine into platelets has led to the use of vincristine in idiopathic thrombocytopenic purpura. Vincristine penetrates the central nervous system and after an intravenous injection in primates, concentrations of 1 nM are maintained for more than 72 hours.[10] However, in human use, concentrations of vincristine are likely to be lower.[11] Vincrisstine may thus cause CNS toxicity. The earliest sign of CNS toxicity is depression of the ankle jerk and thereafter a wide variety of manifestations may occur including muscular weakness, ataxia, tremors, convulsions and coma although peripheral neuropathy is the commonest sign of CNS toxicity. Constipation may occur with vincristine and is more common than after vinblastine therapy.

Vincristine crosses the placenta and although it is not known whether vincristine is excreted in breast milk, the possibility of adverse reactions in the nursing infant must be considered.

Vincristine is biotransformed in the liver and extensively excreted in the bile with 70% of the dose eliminated by this route in 72 h.[12] Much smaller amounts, approximately 12% of the dose, are excreted in urine over this period. Renal impairment and old age are unlikely to affect the elimination of the drug, although dosage reduction in the latter group may be required for other reasons. The half life of vincristine is likely to be prolonged in patients with hepatic dysfunction, particularly when there is jaundice.

Oral absorption	very poor
Presystemic metabolism	negligible
Plasma half life	
mean (terminal phase)	85 h
Volume of distribution	$8.4\ l.kg^{-1}$
Plasma protein binding	—

Concentration–effect relationship

There is little evidence of any relationship between the plasma concentration of vincristine and its therapeutic effect. It is known that concentrations of 10^{-8} M are required in vitro to inhibit completely a lymphoblastoid cell line[13] and yet peak concentrations of vincristine after standard doses are about 0.4 μM. It is probable that normal and tumour cells have different sensitivities because higher concentrations are required to affect normal lymphocytes than diseased lymphocytes and this may explain the sensitivity of lymphomatous disease to vincristine.[14]

Metabolism

Vincristine is metabolized, primarily in the liver, to a number of as yet unidentified metabolites.[12] The principal route of elimination is via the bile in the faeces, probably in the form of unidentified metabolites together with decomposition products. About 12% of the administered dose is excreted in the urine over 72 h, with 70% in the faeces.

Pharmaceutics

Vincristine, Oncovin (Lilly, UK/USA), is available in a lyophilized form in vials containing 1 mg, 2 mg and 5 mg each supplied in a combination package with a vial of diluting solution of 10 ml sodium chloride 0.9% with benzyl alcohol as preservative. It is also available as 1 ml containing 1 mg and 2 ml containing 2 mg for injection and including mannitol and parabens. The pH of vincristine is in the range 3.5 to 5. The solutions may be injected into the drip tubing of a running sodium chloride 0.9% infusion.

Great care should be exercised during intravenous administration. If extravasation should occur the injection should be discontinued immediately and any remaining proportion of the dose should then be introduced into another vein. Local injection of hyaluronidase or hydrocortisone and the application of moderate heat to the area of leakage help to disperse the drug and may minimize any resultant cellulitis. Care should also be taken during the reconstitution and the appropriate protective clothing, gloves, mask and protective glasses used.

Therapeutic use

Vincristine has now gained an accepted place in the routine management of certain malignancies generally in combination with other cytotoxic drugs. It is occasionally used as a single agent. Although very similar in structure to other vinca alkaloids there are differences in therapeutic effect which are reflected in the diseases treated.

Indications

1. Acute leukaemia, lymphoid and myeloid
2. Generalized Hodgkin's disease
3. Non-Hodgkin's lymphoma
4. Neuroblastoma
5. Wilms' tumour
6. Rhabdomyosarcoma
7. Breast cancer
8. Other solid tumours.

Contraindications

1. Intrathecal administration.

Precautions

2. Pregnancy
3. Patients with the demyelinating form of Charcot-Marie Tooth syndrome
4. Reduced bone marrow reserve
5. Jaundice
6. The elderly
7. Vincristine should not be readministered following acute bronchospasm.

Indications

1. Acute leukaemia

Vincristine is commonly employed as induction treatment for both acute lymphocytic and acute non-lymphocytic leukaemia.[15,16] Whilst vincristine in combination with prednisolone is effective for the treatment for acute lymphoblastic leukaemia in childhood, additional drugs are needed for both adult forms of leukaemia. About 75% of children with acute lymphoblastic leukaemia can expect cure with combination chemotherapy. The results are considerably less favourable in non-lymphocytic leukaemia and in adults. The recommended dose is 1.4 to $1.5\ mg.m^{-2}$ up to a maximum weekly dose of 2 mg.

2. Generalized Hodgkin's disease

Both vincristine and vinblastine are used as combination therapy for the management of generalized Hodgkin's disease. Vincristine was the first drug introduced into combination therapy and remains the choice in combination in the United States[17] but British groups have adopted vinblastine because of reduced neurotoxicity.[18] The combination consists of mechlorethamine, procarbazine, prednisolone, and vinblastine, given over a two-week period at intervals of six weeks. Therapy normally is repeated to six or to eight courses and 70% of patients can expect to achieve long-term cure with this combination. Recent attention has been directed to giving alternating chemotherapy using both vincristine and vinblastine in a particular combination and there is some evidence to suggest that this approach may be more effective than the more traditional management.[19] However, it is too early to draw definitive conclusions from the data. Both agents are also employed in combinations should patients relapse.

3. Non-Hodgkin's lymphoma

Vincristine may be used either singly or in combination for the management of patients with non-Hodgkin's lymphoma of favourable histology.[20] Long-lasting complete remissions can be achieved in 60–80% of patients when used in combination, generally with cyclophosphamide and prednisolone. Recent evidence suggests however that this is no more effective than chlorambucil as a single agent.[21] For patients with generalized lymphoma of unfavourable histology, again vincristine is the preferred drug generally used in combination with adriamycin and prednisolone.[22,23] Such combinations will induce complete remissions in 60–70% of treated patients and approximately half will remain in complete remission. Both drugs (vincristine and vinblastine) again form a part of combinations used when patients relapse but no definitive schedule can be recommended.

4. Neuroblastoma

Neuroblastoma is generally not particularly responsive to chemotherapy but vincristine or vinblastine in combination with other cytotoxic agents is generally the preferred treatment.

5. Wilms' tumour

The treatment depends on whether the patient has small or large volume disease. For patients with small volume disease the treatment of choice is the use of vincristine and actinomycin D given on a cyclical basis in combination with irradiation.[24] If the patient has bulk disease then cyclophosphamide or other drugs are added in combination which may improve the response rate.

6. Rhabdomyosarcoma
Vincristine is the preferred drug generally used in combination with other agents.[25]

7. Breast cancer
Vincristine is used as treatment for breast cancer generally again in combination with other drugs. The contribution to other cytotoxic drugs is disputed[26] and vincristine is not usually considered as a first-line drug in this condition. However, there have been recent studies suggesting that continuous infusion may be of benefit.[27]

8. Other solid tumours
Vincristine is commonly incorporated into combination chemotherapy regimens for head and neck cancer, multiple myeloma, sarcomas and small cell lung cancer. With the exception of myeloma there is little or no evidence that vincristine contributes significantly to the regimen.

Contraindications

1. Intrathecal administration
Accidental intrathecal administration is usually fatal. Should this occur the physician is referred to the data sheet for details of possible salvage procedure.

Precautions
2. Pregnancy
Teratogenic effects are likely to occur if administered during the first trimester of pregnancy. Should treatment be imperative then termination of pregnancy should be considered.

4. Reduced bone marrow reserve
In those patients where marrow reserve has been reduced by previous radiotherapy or by previous chemotherapy caution should be exercised during administration with conventional doses.

5. Impaired liver function
As the primary route of elimination is via the bile caution should be exercised in the presence of the jaundiced patient. Vincristine would be the preferred drug in this situation being less myelosuppressive than vinblastine although at a risk of a greater incidence of peripheral neuropathy. Administration to those patients in whom the bilirubin is normal but in whom the liver enzymes are elevated is not associated with increased myelosuppression. A raised serum alkaline phosphatase may be an indicator of the potential neurotoxicity at a later date.

6. Elderly patients
Patients over 60 are more prone to develop neurological complications with vincristine than younger patients. Care should therefore be taken during treatment and dose reduction by 50% may be necessary.

Adverse reactions

Potentially life-threatening effects
All vinca alkaloids produce some myelosuppression and this is related to both dose and frequency of administration. However, with conventional doses myelosuppression is not normally severe but if there is evidence of myelosuppression before the next treatment, delay should be considered until there has been complete recovery. Vincristine is less myelosuppressive than vinblastine and therefore if bone marrow function is compromised vincristine can be substituted as an alternative drug to vinblastine.

Acute overdosage
Accidental overdose can produce fatal myelosuppression and neurotoxicity. There is no specific antidote although the use of folinic acid has been suggested. Supportive care should include a) prevention of the adverse effects that result from the syndrome of inappropriate secretion of antidiuretic hormone; b) administration of an anticonvulsant; c) prevention and treatment of ileus; d) monitoring the patient's cardiovascular system; e) haematological monitoring and support.

Severe or irreversible adverse effects
Neurotoxicity. This is the most common adverse effect with this class of drug and, indeed, is characteristic of the group. It is most common with vincristine and is the dose-limiting factor. The earliest manifestation of neurotoxicity is suppression of the Achilles tendon reflex. Maximal depression occurs about 17 days after a single dose and may take up to 1 to 3 months for return to normal.[28] If treatment is continued then paraesthaesiae affecting both feet and hands develop and this may be associated with severe pains in the region of the throat and occasionally the chest. Peripheral nerve involvement is the most disabling manifestation and this is characterized by weakness of the toes and ankles and extension of the fingers and wrists. Non-myelinated nerves may be the most sensitive to vincristine explaining the early onset of loss of the deep tendon reflex.[29] Cranial nerves may also be affected with ptosis and diplopia being the most common manifestations. Autonomic dysfunction may also occur with gastrointestinal problems and postural hypotension. There is no known treatment other than discontinuing medication. Therapy with thiamine and vitamin B12 have been ineffective. Convulsions have also been reported.

In patients with liver dysfunction neurotoxic reactions can be severe after routine doses. There is some speculative evidence that vincristine neurotoxicity is related to serum alkaline phosphatase. Desai et al observed a statistically significant relationship beween AUC and degree of toxicity.[30] This was related both to the dose and to elevation of serum alkaline phosphatase suggesting that elimination of the drug is impaired when this enzyme is elevated. Dose reduction in this situation therefore may reduce toxicity.

Gastrointestinal toxicity. Adverse gastrointestinal reactions are usually mild (see below), but occasionally paralytic ileus and perforated peptic ulcer have occurred.

Symptomatic adverse effects
Gastrointestinal side effects are common. Constipation, abdominal cramps, paralytic ileus, vomiting and diarrhoea have all been reported. Constipation is the rule for those patients on induction chemotherapy for non-Hodgkin's lymphoma of unfavourable histology. Routine appropriate treatment is normally all that is required.

A number of miscellaneous adverse effects have been reported, including weight loss, fever, headache, alopecia, general malaise and dizziness. These effects are, however, uncommon. The syndrome of inappropriate ADH secretion has been reported with vincristine.[31]

Interference with clinical pathology tests
No technical interferences of this kind have been reported.

High risk groups

Neonates
The drug is unlikely to be used in this age-group.

Breast milk. It is not known whether vincristine is excreted in breast milk. However, in view of the potential for serious adverse reactions, breast-feeding is best avoided.

Children
The drug has been used in this group in appropriate doses.

Pregnant women
Vincristine is teratogenic in animals. In patients who have received successful therapy with vinca alkaloids alone or in combination some successful pregnancies have occurred and to date there has been no evidence of increased fetal damage. However, a long-term registry will be necessary to establish the real incidence of malformations in patients bearing children having undergone successful therapy.

The elderly
Older patients are more likely to develop neurological complications with vincristine. Dose reduction may be necessary and patients should be monitored carefully.

Concurrent disease
See above: Contraindications.

Drug interactions

Potentially hazardous interactions
Acute bronchospasm and shortness of breath have been reported following the use of vincristine in combination with or following mitomycin C.

Potentially useful interactions
Vincristine prevents the cellular exit of methotrexate in vitro and

Vincristine (sulphate)

there is therefore the potential synergistic effect of combining the two drugs in treatment. However, schedules of experimental treatment that employ vincristine with methotrexate have not shown therapeutic synergism.[32]

General review articles

Bender R A, Chabner C A 1982 Tubulin binding agents. In: Chabner B A (ed) Pharmacologic principles of cancer treatment. W B Saunders, ch 2, pp 256–262

References

1. Creasy W A 1975 Vinca alkaloids and colchicine. In: Sartorelli A C, Johns D G (eds) Handbook of experimental pharmacology 38. Springer, Berlin, p 670
2. Owellen R J, Hartke C A, Dickerson R M, Hains F Q 1976 Inhibition of tubulin-microtubule polymerization by drugs of the vinca alkaloid class. Cancer Research 36: 1499–1502
3. Bradley W G, Lassman L P, Peerce G W 1970 The neuro-myopathy of vincristine in man: clinical, electro-physiologic and pathologic studies. Journal of Neurological Sciences 10: 107
4. Todd G C, Griffing W J, Gibson W R, Morton D M 1979 Animal models for the comparative assessment of neurotoxicity following repeated administration of vinca alkaloids. Cancer Treatment Reports 63: 35–41
5. Gebhart E, Schwanitz G, Hartwich H 1969 Zytogenetische Wirkung von Vincristin auf menschliche Leukozyten in vivo und *in vitro*. Medizinische Klinik 64: 2366–2371
6. Conter V, Beck W T 1984 Acquisition of multidrug resistance by CCRF-CEM cells selected for different degrees of resistance to vincristine. Cancer Treatment Reports 68: 831–836
7. Root M A, Gerzon K, Dyke R W 1975 A radioimmunoassay for vinblastine and vincristine. Federation of Analytical Chemistry and Spectroscopy Societies: 125
8. Sethi V S, Burton S S, Jackson D V 1980 A sensitive RIA for vincristine and vinblastine. Cancer Chemotherapy and Pharmacology 4: 183
9. Nelson R L, Dyke R W, Root M S 1980 Comparative pharmacokinetics of vindesine, vincristine and vinblastine in patients with cancer. Cancer Treatment Reviews 8: 17
10. Jackson D V, Castle M C, Poplack D G, Bender R A 1980 Pharmacokinetics of vincristine in the cerebrospinal fluid of sub-human primates. Cancer Research 40: 722–724
11. Jackson D V, Sethi V S, Spurr C L, McWhorter J M 1981 Pharmacokinetics of vincristine in the cerebrospinal fluid of humans. Cancer Research 41: 1466
12. Jackson D V, Castle M C, Bender R A 1978 Biliary excretion of vincristine. Clinical Pharmacology and Therapeutics 24: 101–107
13. Schrek R 1974 Cytotoxicity of vincristine to normal and leukemic cells. American Journal of Clinical Pathology 62: 1–7
14. Don Jackson D V, Bender R A 1979 Cytotoxic thresholds of vincristine in L1210 murine leukemia and a human lymphoblastic cell line in vitro. Cancer Research 39: 4346–4349
15. Pinkel D 1976 Treatment of acute leukemia. Pediatric Clinics of North America 23/1: 117
16. Frei III E, Sallan S E 1978 Acute lymphoblastic leukemia: treatment. Cancer (Philad.) 42: 828
17. DeVita V T Jr, Lewis B J, Rozencweig M, Muggia F M 1978 The chemotherapy of Hodgkin's disease: past experiences and future directions. Cancer 42: 979–990
18. Sutcliffe S B, Wrigley P F M, Peto J et al 1978 MVPP chemotherapy regimen for advanced Hodgkin's disease. British Medical Journal 1: 679
19. Santoro A, Bonnadonna G, Valagussa P et al 1987 Long-term results of combined chemotherapy and radiotherapy approach in Hodgkin's Disease. Superiority of ABVD plus radiotherapy versus MOPP plus radiotherapy. Journal of Clinical Oncology 5: 27–37
20. Rosenberg S A 1979 Current concepts in cancer: non-Hodgkin's lymphoma — selection of treatment on the basis of histologic type. New England Journal of Medicine 301: 924–928
21. Lister T A, Cullen M H, Beard M E J et al 1978 Comparison of combined and single agent chemotherapy in non-Hodgkin's lymphoma of favourable histological type. British Medical Journal 1: 573
22. Bagley C M Jr, De Vita V T Jr, Berard C W, Canellos G P 1972 Advanced lymphosarcoma: intensive cyclical combination chemotherapy with cyclophosphamide, vincristine and prednisone. Annals of Internal Medicine 76: 227–234
23. Blackledge G, Bush H, Chang J et al 1980 Intensive combination chemotherapy with vincristine, adriamycin and prednisolone (VAP) in the treatment of diffuse histology non-Hodgkin's lymphoma (a report of 89 cases with extensive disease from the Manchester Lymphoma Group). European Journal of Cancer 16: 1439–1468
24. D'Angio G J 1976 The treatment of Wilm's tumour: results of the National Wilms' Tumour Study. Cancer 38: 633–346
25. Bramwell V H C, Crowther D, Deakin D P, Swindell R, Harris M 1985 Combined modality management of local and disseminated adult soft tissue sarcomas: a review of 257 cases seen over 10 years at the Christie Hospital and Holt Radium Institute, Manchester. British Journal of Cancer 51: 301–318
26. Steiner R, Stewart J F, Cartwell B M J, Minton M J, Knight R R, Rubens R I 1983 Adriamycin alone or in combination with vincristine in the treatment of advanced breast cancer. European Journal of Clinical Oncology 19: 1553–1557
27. Jackson D V, Sethi V S, Spurr C L et al 1981 Pharmacokinetics of vincristine infusion. Cancer Treatment Reports 65: 1043–1048
28. Weiss H D, Walker M D, Wiernik P H 1974 Neurotoxicity of commonly used anti neoplastic agents. New England Journal of Medicine 291: 127–134
29. Donoso J A, Green L S, Heller-Bettinger I E, Samson F E 1977 Action of the vinca alkaloids vincristine, vinblastine and desacetyl vinblastine amide on axonal fibrillar organelles in vitro. Cancer Research 37: 1401–1407
30. Dessai Z R, Van den Berg H W, Bridges J M, Shanks R G 1982 Can severe vincristine neurotoxicity be prevented? Cancer Chemotherapy and Pharmacology 8: 211–214
31. Robertson G L, Bhoopalam N, Zelkowitz L J 1973 Vincristine neurotoxicity and abnormal secretion of anti-diuretic hormone. Archives of Internal Medicine 132: 717
32. Bender R A, Nichols A P, Norton L, Simon R M 1978 Lack of therapeutic synergism of vincristine and methotrexate in L1210 murine leukemia in vivo. Cancer Treatment Reports 62: 997–1003

V

Vitamin K

Vitamin K is available in three forms — phytomenadione (vitamin K_1), its synthetic analogue menadiol sodium diphosphate and menadione (vitamin K_3), which does not possess a phytyl side-chain. Phytomenadione is most widely used. Information on menadiol is limited and will not be considered in detail.

Chemistry

Vitamin K (phytomenadione, Konakion, Phytonadone)
$C_{31}H_{46}O_2$
2-Methyl-3-phytyl-1,4-naphthoquinone
(The synthetic form exists as *trans* and *cis* isomers in a ratio of about 4:1. The *trans* form is biologically active.)

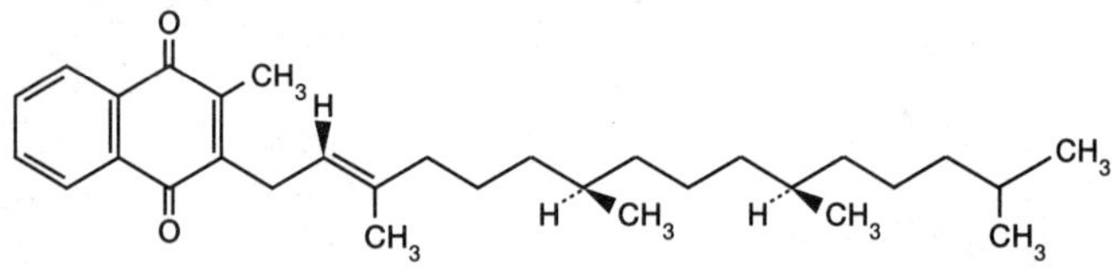

Molecular weight	450.7
pKa	not ionizable
Solubility	
in alcohol	1 in 70
in water	<1 in 10 000
Octanol/water partition coefficient	high

Phytomenadione is a golden yellow viscous oil which is unstable in sunlight and under alkaline conditions.

Menadiol has molecular weight 530.2 and is very soluble in water.

Pharmacology

Vitamin K is a co-factor for γ-carboxylation in the postribosomal synthesis of clotting factors II, VII, IX and X.[1] Vitamin K is also involved in γ-carboxylation of other proteins such as osteocalcin.[2]

Toxicology

There are no known teratogenic, mutagenic or carcinogenic effects of relevance in man.

Clinical pharmacology

Vitamin K is essential for normal coagulation. The active vitamin K-dependent clotting factors (II, VII, IX and X) are formed from precursors in the liver. The reaction responsible for activation is γ-carboxylation of glutamyl residues[1] on these protein precursors. The main use of vitamin K is in the reversal of excessive anticoagulant effect. The onset of action is delayed until the activated clotting factor concentrations in blood reach an effective level — usually within 4–6 hours.

Dose range for most patients is 5–20 mg initially, though 10 mg is the usual starting dose. This may require to be repeated, depending on the severity of the haemorrhage and type of anticoagulant.[3,4]

The role of vitamin K and its therapeutic effect in bone disease requires further evaluation.[2,5]

Pharmacokinetics

The preferred analytical method is by high performance liquid chromatography[21] the limit of detection is 100 ng.l^{-1}. One suitable method uses a normal phase Partisil column with 0.2% acetonitrile in hexane as the mobile phase.[7] Detection is by UV spectrophotometer at 254 nm. Extraction from plasma uses hexane after protein precipitation by methanol. This method separates *cis* vitamin K_1, *trans* vitamin K_1, K_1 epoxide and menaquinone (MK4) as internal standard.

Vitamin K_1 is normally given parenterally in the treatment of haemorrhage. After oral administration, absorption is said to be 80%.[8] There is wide inter and intra-individual variation. A recent study in normal volunteers found bioavailability ranging from 10 to 63% with peak concentrations occurring 3–5 hours after dosing.[4] Absorption is thought to take place by an energy-dependent saturable process in the proximal small intestine in the presence of bile salts.[8,9]

Vitamin K is rapidly distributed with a distribution half life of 0.20–0.22 hours. It is extensively bound to β-lipoproteins. Volume of distribution varies widely from 2 to 9 litres with a mean of 3.5 l.

Daily requirements for vitamin K are low (<1 μg.kg^{-1})[10] because of the existence of an efficient conservation mechanism — the vitamin K-epoxide cycle (see Metabolism). Following pharmacological doses, vitamin K is rapidly eliminated. After intravenous administration vitamin K concentrations decline biexponentially. Terminal elimination half life ranges from 1.2 to 3.5 hours with a mean value of around 2.2 hours.[4,11,12] Metabolites are mainly excreted in the bile.[13] Vitamin K pharmacokinetic parameters in anticoagulated patients are similar to values found in healthy volunteers.[14]

Oral absorption	10–63%
Presystemic metabolism	—
Plasma half life	
range	1.2–3.5 h
mean	2.2 h
Volume of distribution	3.5 l
Plasma protein binding	extensive

Concentration–effect relationship

There is no clear concentration–effect relationship in non-anticoagulated patients. Plasma levels of vitamin K are very low and the estimated total body pool[15] is about 100 μg.kg^{-1}. However, in the absence of coumarin anticoagulants, vitamin K for clotting factor synthesis is conserved in the vitamin K-epoxide cycle.

In patients treated with vitamin K because of anticoagulant overdose, the concentration of vitamin K must be high enough to overcome the inhibitory coumarin effect. In animals under maximum vitamin K inhibition, concentrations of 1.0 mg.l^{-1} are necessary to drive clotting factor synthesis.[4]

In man, vitamin K inhibition is usually submaximal unless a massive overdose of anticoagulant has been ingested. It is probable that a vitamin K concentration of around 0.5 mg.l^{-1} is necessary to drive clotting factor synthesis in most clinical situations.[4] This is relevant for treatment, as enough vitamin K must be administered to achieve the minimum effective concentration.

Metabolism

Vitamin K_1 is oxidized to vitamin K_1-2,3-epoxide (biologically inactive) during the carboxylation reaction.[16] The epoxide is reduced back to active vitamin K by a microsomal epoxide reductase.[16,17]

Detailed information on the other metabolic pathways is not available. The major route of elimination is thought to be oxidation in the mitochondria[18] followed by conjugation with glucuronic acid in the endoplasmic reticulum and excretion in the bile.[13]

Pharmaceutics

Vitamin K is available in oral and parenteral forms:

1. Konakion (Roche, UK): tablets containing 10 mg phytomenadione. The tablets are white, sugar-coated, printed 'Roche' in black across one face.
2. SynKavit (Roche, UK): tablets containing 12.63 mg of menadiol sodium diphosphate. The tablets are round, white with 'Synkavit' imprinted on one face and a single break bar across the other. In the USA SynaKayvite tablets (Roche) contain 5 mg and are round, white and imprinted 'SYNKAYVITE 5'. Mephyton tablets (MSD, USA) are 5 mg round, yellow, scored tablets coded 'MSD 43'.

3. Phytomenadione is available for intravenous use as an opalescent greenish-yellow solution in ampoules containing 1 mg in 0.5 ml and 10 mg in 1 ml. Konakion (Roche, UK/USA) Aquamephyton (MSD, UK) contains polyethoxylated caster oil which may be responsible for the adverse effects of the injectable form. The Aquamephyton formulation may be diluted with dextrose and saline solutions.
   Menadiol is also available for intravenous use but is less effective than phytomenadione in treating anticoagulant overdose. SynKayvite injectable (Roche, USA) is available as 5 mg in 1 ml, 10 mg in 1 ml and 75 mg in 2 ml.
   A new formulation of Konakion based on mixed micelles has recently been developed. This appears to avoid the problems due to the castor oil formulation. However, it is not yet widely available.

Tablets should be protected from light and stored in a cool place. Ampoules should be protected from light and not allowed to freeze.

Therapeutic use

Indications

1. Haemorrhage or threatened haemorrhage due to excessive dosing with oral anticoagulants
2. Prevention and treatment of neonatal haemorrhage
3. Vitamin K deficiency likely to predispose to haemorrhage, e.g. obstructive jaundice, malabsorption, dietary deficiency.

Contraindications

The main concern is to avoid use of parenteral vitamin K in patients who are hypersensitive to the constituents of the formulation. The causative agent is thought to be the polyethoxylated castor oil. Patients with an atopic history should not be given intravenous vitamin K except for severe haemorrhage. The new mixed micelle formulation may avoid the problem.

Mode of use

Ampoules

Phytomenadione solution may be administered by intravenous or intramuscular injection. Intramuscular injection is best avoided in the presence of haemorrhage because of the risk of a haematoma developing at the injection site. Intravenous injection should be slow, to minimize side effects due to histamine release. Dilution of the vitamin K solution in 20 ml of saline with infusion over 15 minutes reduces this risk and has caused no problems in a series of volunteer studies.[4,14] The new mixed micellar formulation appears to be safe without dilution, but evidence is limited at present.

The initial dose depends on the severity of haemorrhage. In severe haemorrhage up to 50 mg vitamin K may be given initially.[19] Vitamin K has a short duration of action and in the situation of massive anticoagulant overdose should be administered in a dose of 10 mg, 3–5 times daily until the plasma anticoagulant concentration is low (<2 mg.l^{-1} for warfarin).[19,20]

Prothrombin time must be monitored regularly and vitamin K administered to lower the INR below 1.5. The onset of effect usually occurs within 6 hours with maximum at around 24 hours after dosing. If 2NR begins to rise again further vitamin K should be given.

Tablets

Tablets should be chewed or allowed to dissolve slowly in the mouth. Tablets should not be used in the treatment of haemorrhage because large doses are necessary to achieve a plasma concentration which will drive clotting factor synthesis.[4]

The wide inter-individual variation in bioavailability makes it essential to titrate the dose for each patient to achieve a normal prothrombin time.

Indications

1. Anticoagulant overdose

a. Therapeutic overdose

In patients with prolonged prothrombin time but no haemorrhage, vitamin K should not be given unless there is a significant risk of bleeding.

In most patients with mild to moderate haemorrhage, a single dose of 10 mg vitamin K intravenously is sufficient but further doses can be given if necessary. Lower doses (1–2 mg) may be given if it is essential to avoid excessive lowering of the prothrombin time (i.e. where there is a high risk of thrombosis or embolism). Blood replacement may also be required.

Severe haemorrhage requires more aggressive therapy with infusion of fresh-frozen plasma and fresh whole blood as necessary. Vitamin K should be administered intravenously in an initial dose of 10–30 mg with further doses as necessary.

b. Massive overdose

In deliberate or accidental massive overdose with oral anticoagulants steps should be taken to minimize drug absorption by gastric lavage. If a high dose of anticoagulant is absorbed this will require antago-

Fig. 1 The metabolism of vitamin K_1

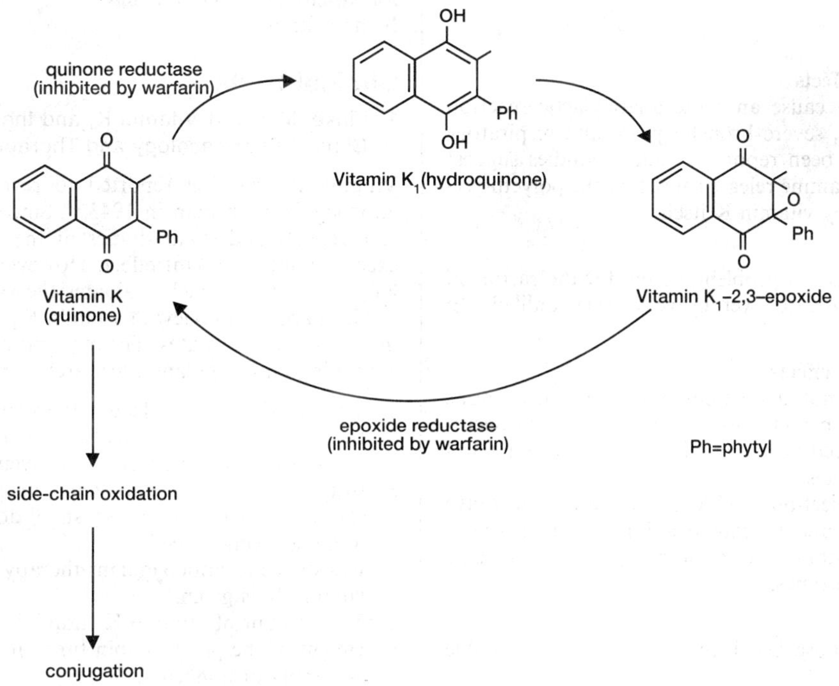

nism with large doses of vitamin K. In severe cases up to 50 mg should be administered intravenously as an initial dose.[19] Smaller doses of 10 mg should be repeated 3–5 times daily until the anticoagulant level returns to therapeutic values (<2 mg.l^{-1} for warfarin).

Hangover effect
Despite the short plasma half life of vitamin K there is a clinical impression that anticoagulated patients given vitamin K take some time to become sensitive again to the effect of warfarin. A recent study has confirmed that there is a 'hangover' effect which may last up to 2 weeks in some patients.[14]

Vitamin K has a short duration of effect in heavily overanticoagulated patients with a need for repeated doses in this situation or when one of the longer acting rodenticides has been ingested.[3] However, in mildly overdosed patients, vitamin K is stored in the liver and has a long duration of action.

2. Neonatal haemorrhage
All newborn babies have low concentrations of the vitamin K-dependent clotting factors which fall over the first 2–3 days of life and rise when feeding is established. If the level of K-dependent clotting factors is very low, spontaneous haemorrhage may occur. A late haemorrhagic syndrome may occur after 4–8 weeks, especially in breast-fed babies. Newborn babies have low levels of vitamin K in cord plasma, suggesting that vitamin K does not readily cross the placenta or that uptake is low because of low levels of binding lipoproteins.[21] Vitamin K_1 (1 mg by intramuscular injection) is given routinely to all premature or low birth weight babies. More widespread use has been controversial. However, babies at risk of neonatal haemorrhage cannot be predicted with certainty and many centres now administer vitamin K to all babies.

If babies are to be breast-fed, the vitamin K level in human milk can be increased by giving the mother 20 mg orally twice weekly.[20] The value of this in preventing haemorrhage requires evaluation.

Haemorrhage in neonates requires administration of 1 mg vitamin K by intramuscular injection with blood and plasma as necessary.

3. Vitamin K deficiency
Vitamin K deficiency may be treated with oral vitamin K (10–20 mg) in most cases. If there is severe malabsorption or bile salt deficiency, intramuscular administration may be required. Oral menadiol may be preferred in this situation. The dose should be titrated to maintain a normal prothrombin clotting time.

4. Radiosensitizer in treatment of cancer
Vitamin K has been suggested for use as a radiosensitizer in the treatment of cancer. However, evidence of its value is inconclusive and more potent radiosensitizers are now available. There has also been debate on the role of disturbed vitamin K physiology as a cause of malignancy.[22]

Adverse reactions

Potentially life-threatening effects
Intravenous vitamin K may cause an acute anaphylactic reaction with cardiovascular collapse, severe bronchospasm and respiratory failure. Several deaths have been reported. Animal studies suggest that this might be due to histamine release caused by the polyethoxylated castor oil rather than by vitamin K itself.

Acute overdosage
There is no evidence that this is a problem, except for the castor oil problem noted above. Deliberate overdosage is very unlikely to occur.

Severe or irreversible adverse effects
Flushing and sweating are not uncommon following intravenous injection. Bronchoconstriction and chest tightness may also occur. The symptoms may be reduced or avoided by diluting in saline and infusing slowly over 15 minutes.

Repeated intramuscular injections (>270 mg vitamin K) may give rise to local cutaneous and subcutaneous reactions in patients with liver disease.[23] Local haematoma formation may occur in patients with prolonged prothrombin times.

Symptomatic adverse effects
There are none to add to those listed under severe or irreversible effects.

Other effects
The polyethoxylated castor oil may also cause abnormal lipoprotein patterns, alteration of blood viscosity and erythrocyte aggregation. The clinical significance of this is uncertain. Two patients with inflammatory bowel disease developed cerebral arterial thrombosis after being given vitamin K parenterally.[24] One possible explanation is an increase in blood viscosity and erythrocyte aggregation.

Interference with clinical pathology tests
No intereferences of this kind have been reported.

High risk groups

Neonates
Reduced dose of 1 mg vitamin K is administered as described above.

Breast milk. Vitamin K is present in breast milk. This is more of an advantage than a hazard to the infant.

Children
There is no additional risk to this group.

Pregnant women
There is no additional risk to this group.

The elderly
Anticoagulated elderly patients show a greater response to injected vitamin K than young patients.[25] However, the standard dose of 10 mg vitamin K should be administered as in younger patients. It should rarely be necessary to use more than 20 mg initially.

Concurrent disease

Liver disease. Patients with liver disease may be more susceptible to local skin reactions on treatment with repeated intramuscular vitamin K. Liver function may be further depressed by high doses of vitamin K.

Drug interactions

Potentially hazardous interactions

Oral anticoagulants. The main source of interaction is between vitamin K and its antagonists such as warfarin. This may cause problems with anticoagulant control if a patient is taking a diet high in vitamin K (see Warfarin). Clearly the importance of this interaction is in reversing the effect of warfarin and other anticoagulants.

Enzyme-inducing drugs. Babies born to mothers taking anticonvulsants, such as phenobarbitone and phenytoin, during pregnancy are more at risk of developing haemorrhagic disease of the newborn. This was thought to be due to increased vitamin K metabolism. Recent studies in volunteers have found no significant effect of phenytoin or phenobarbitone on vitamin K elimination.[11,12]

Potentially useful interactions
None is known.

Clinical trials

1. Finkel M J 1961 Vitamin K_1 and the vitamin K analogues. Clinical Pharmacology and Therapeutics 2: 794–814

Vitamin K was first reported to reverse the effects of coumarin anticoagulants in man in 1943.[26] Since then there have been many case reports and small studies of the use of vitamin K to reverse excessive anticoagulant effect. However, there is no well-conducted large-scale study which evaluates the value of vitamin K treatment.

This paper is a review of vitamin K_1 and the vitamin K analogues in various clinical states. The main points on the use of vitamin K in correcting anticoagulant effect are:

1. Vitamin $K_1$is more effective than vitamin K analogues.
2. In the presence of serious haemorrhage at least 10–20 mg vitamin K_1 should be given intravenously.
3. In the absence of haemorrhage, prolonged prothrombin time should be treated with very small doses (<2.5 mg) of vitamin K to avoid over-correction.
4. Resistance to anticoagulant therapy may occur if too much vitamin K is given.
5. The amount of vitamin K_1 administered depends on:
a. Height of the prothrombin time and rate at which it is becoming prolonged

b. Presence and severity of haemorrhage
c. Amount and time since administration of anticoagulant
d. State of vitamin K stores in the body (clinically unknown!).

2. Owen G M, Nelsen C E, Baker G L, Connor W E, Jacobs J P 1977 Use of vitamin K_1 in pregnancy. American Journal of Obstetrics and Gynecology 99: 368–373

This was a large double-blind study of the effect of vitamin K (5 mg daily by mouth) or placebo administered prenatally on the relative prothrombin deficiency in the newborn. 500 women entered the study but only 204 were suitable for analysis. The others were excluded because of birth problems, lack of blood samples or inadvertent administration of vitamin K after birth. The infants in the two groups were well balanced in terms of parity, sex, birth weight, maternal age, feeding and days of vitamin K or placebo pre-treatment. Infants born to mothers receiving placebo had lower prothrombin times than those treated with vitamin K. There was no evidence of haemorrhage in either group. Serum bilirubin levels were similar in the two groups.

This alternative approach to giving all newborn babies 1 mg vitamin K_1 by intramuscular injection requires further evaluation. However, it is easier from an administrative point of view, to give a single injection than to ensure each mother takes vitamin K for the last 12 days of pregnancy. The large interindividual variation in vitamin K bioavailability may make the oral route unreliable in some patients.

References

1. Stenflo J, Suttie J W 1977 Vitamin K-dependent formation of γ-carboxyglutamic acid. Annual Review of Biochemistry 46: 154–172
2. Keith D A, Gundberg C M, Japour A, Aronoff J, Alvarez N, Gallop P M 1983 Vitamin K-dependent proteins and anticonvulsant medication. Clinical Pharmacology and Therapeutics 34: 529–532
3. Barlow A M, Gay A L, Park B K 1982 Difenacoum (Neosorexa) poisoning. British Medical Journal 285: 541
4. Park B K, Scott A K, Wilson A C, Haynes B P, Breckenridge A M 1984 Plasma disposition of vitamin K_1 in relation to anticoagulant poisoning. British Journal of Clinical Pharmacology 18: 655–662
5. Hart J P, Catterall A, Dodds R A et al 1984 Circulating vitamin K_1 levels in fractured neck of femur. Lancet 2: 283
6. Shearer M J 1983 High performance liquid chromatography of K vitamins and their antagonists. Advances in Chromatography 21: 243–301
7. Wilson A C, Park B K 1983 Quantitative analysis of pharmacological levels of vitamin K_1-2, 3-epoxide in rabbit plasma by high performance liquid chromatography. Journal of Chromatography 277: 292–299
8. Shearer M J, McBurney A, Barkham P 1974 Studies on the absorption and metabolism of phylloquinone (vitamin K_1) in man. Vitamins and Hormones 32: 513–524
9. Hollander D 1973 Vitamin K_1 absorption by everted intestinal sacs of the rat. American Journal of Physiology 225: 360–364
10. Frick P G, Reidler G, Brogli H 1967 Dose response and minimal daily requirement of vitamin K in man. Journal of Applied Physiology 23: 387–389
11. Park B K, Wilson A C, Kaatz G, Ohnhaus E E 1984 Enzyme induction by phenobarbitone and vitamin K_1 elimination. British Journal of Clinical Pharmacology 18: 94–97
12. Scott A K, Haynes B P, Park B K 1985 Hepatic enzyme induction by anticonvulsants and vitamin K_1 elimination. British Journal of Clinical Pharmacology 20: 301
13. Shearer M J, Mallinson C N, Webster G R, Barkhan P 1972 Clearance from plasma and excretion in urine, faeces and bile of an intravenous dose of titrated vitamin K in man. British Journal of Haematology 22: 579–588
14. Choonara I A, Scott A K, Haynes B P, Cholerton S, Breckenridge A M, Park B K 1985 Vitamin K_1 metabolism in relation to pharmacodynamic response in anticoagulated patients. British Journal of Clinical Pharmacology 20: 643–648
15. Duello T J, Matschiner J T 1972 Characterisation of vitamin K from human liver. Journal of Nutrition 10: 331–336
16. Willingham A K, Matschiner J T 1974 Changes in phylloquinone epoxide activity related to prothrombin synthesis and microsomal clotting activity in the rat. Biochemical Journal 140: 435–441
17. Bell R G 1978 Metabolism of vitamin K and prothrombin synthesis: anticoagulants and the vitamin K-epoxide cycle. Federation Proceedings 37: 2599–2604
18. McBurney A, Shearer M J, Barkhan P 1980 Preparative isolation and characterization of the urinary aglycones of vitamin K_1 (phylloquinone) in man. Biochemical Medicine 24: 250–267
19. Bjornsson T D, Blaschke T T 1978 Vitamin K_1 disposition and therapy of warfarin overdose. Lancet 2: 846–847
20. Shearer M J, Barkhan P 1979 Vitamin K_1 and therapy of massive warfarin overdose. Lancet 1: 266–267
21. Shearer M J, Rahim S, Barkhan P, Stimmler L 1982 Plasma vitamin K_1 in mothers and their newborn babies. Lancet 2: 460–463
22. Egilsson V 1977 Cancer and vitamin K. Lancet 2: 254–255
23. Bullen A W, Miller J P, Cunliffe W J, Losowsky M S 1978 Skin reactions caused by vitamin K in patients with liver disease. British Journal of Dermatology 98: 561–565

Vitamin K

24. Florholmen J, Waldum H, Norday A 1980 Cerebral thrombosis in two patients with malabsorption syndrome treated with vitamin K. British Medical Journal 281: 541
25. Shepherd A M M, Wilson N M, Stevenson I H 1977 Vitamin K pharmacokinetics: response in young and elderly patients. Clinical Pharmacology and Therapeutics 21: 117
26. Shapiro S, Redish M H, Campbell H A 1943 Prothrombin studies: III. Effect of vitamin K upon hypothrombinemia induced by dicoumarol in man. Proceedings of the Society for Experimental Biology and Medicine 52: 12–15

Warfarin (sodium)

Warfarin is the most widely used oral anticoagulant in the UK.

Chemistry

Warfarin sodium (Marevan)
$C_{19}H_{15}NaO_4$
(RS)-4-hydroxy-3-(3-oxo-l-phenylbutyl)coumarin sodium

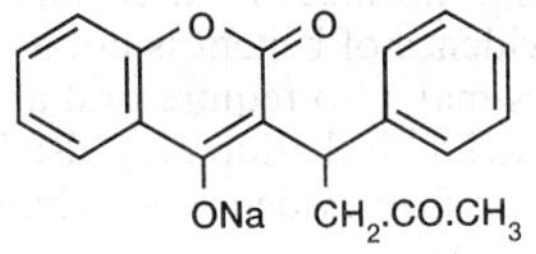

Molecular weight	330.3
pKa (OH)	5.0
Solubility	
in alcohol	>1 in 1
in water	>1 in 1
Octanol/water partition coefficient	1

Warfarin sodium is a white, odourless, amorphous or crystalline powder with a slightly bitter taste. It is discoloured by light. The racemate is used clinically.

Pharmacology

Warfarin is an indirect antagonist of vitamin K. Vitamin K is converted to vitamin K_1, 2,3-epoxide during the activation of clotting factor precursors.[1] The epoxide is metabolized by the enzyme vitamin K epoxide reductase to regenerate active vitamin K.[2] Warfarin inhibits epoxide reductase, thus reducing the amount of vitamin K available for clotting factor synthesis.[3] Clotting factor synthesis is reduced since vitamin K is required for γ-carboxylation of the coagulation proteins.

Toxicology

Warfarin has been shown to be teratogenic in animal studies and has been suspected of causing abnormalities and fetal death when administered during human pregnancy.

Clinical pharmacology

Warfarin reduces the synthesis of the vitamin K-dependent clotting factors (II, VII, IX and X protein) by the liver.[1] The onset of action is delayed until existing clotting factors have been catabolized. The rate-limiting step is degradation of factor VII which has the shortest half life. The aim of treatment is to achieve a partial inhibition of clotting factor synthesis such that the prothrombin time is prolonged by a factor of 2–3 times the normal value. In most patients this is achieved with a dose in the range 3–12 mg daily. However, daily requirements may range from 0.5 to 30 mg, with occasional resistant patients requiring very high doses (>100 mg).[5]

Pharmacokinetics

The preferred analytical method utilizes high performance liquid chromatography.[6,7] It separates warfarin from the hydroxy and alcohol metabolites but does not separate the R and S enantiomers. Using a micro method (100 μl plasma) with methyl tert-butyl ether extraction at acid pH, sensitivity is 50 $\mu g.l^{-1}$. If increased sensitivity is necessary (rarely) the method may be scaled up.

The HPLC method is technically easier than gas–liquid chromatography. Older spectrophotometric methods lack specificity and should not be used. The R and S enantiomers may also be separated by specialized HPLC,[8] or a radioimmunoassay may be used.

Warfarin is almost completely absorbed after oral administration with a systemic bioavailability of >95%.[9,10] Peak plasma concentrations are achieved 3–9 hours post-dosing. Volume of distribution ranges from 8 to 27% of body weight and roughly equates with that of albumin.[11,12] Warfarin is highly protein (albumin) bound with values ranging from 97 to 99.5%.[7,13] There may also be binding within the liver. Warfarin is not distributed into breast milk.[14] Warfarin binding is reduced in renal failure due to the presence of an endogenous protein-binding inhibitor[15] and in hypoalbuminaemic states.[16]

Elimination of warfarin is by hepatic metabolism with elimination of the metabolites in bile and urine. Elimination half lives range from 10 to 45 hours for total warfarin.[10] However, the more active S enantiomer has a shorter half life of 18–35 hours compared with 20–60 hours for the R enantiomer.[17] Total plasma warfarin clearance ranges from 2.5 to 6.4 $ml.h^{-1}.kg^{-1}$.

Oral absorption	>95%
Presystemic metabolism	minimal
Plasma half life	
range	10–45 h
mean	36 h
Volume of distribution	0.08–0.27 $l.kg^{-1}$
Plasma protein binding	97–99.5%

Concentration–effect relationship

The effect of warfarin on coagulation is controlled by measurement of the prothrombin time (PT) under standard conditions. Most centres report a control range of 2.0–3.0 times normal though others use a range of 1.8 up to 3.5. The range used should depend on the specific disease being treated. There is no direct relationship between plasma warfarin concentration and prothrombin time measurement, because the measured PT reflects a balance between the rate of clotting factor synthesis (R_{syn}) and the rate of degradation. Warfarin affects only the rate of synthesis which can be calculated from a knowledge of the PT and by making an assumption regarding the rate of degradation.[18,19] The logarithm of plasma warfarin concentration correlates well with inhibition of R_{syn}.[18]

There is no value in routine measurement of plasma warfarin concentrations because a dynamic end-point can be determined (PT). Measurement of warfarin concentration is of value in occasional patients who appear not to respond to normal doses of warfarin. This helps to differentiate non-compliance (common) from genuine resistance (rare). Therapeutic plasma concentrations at steady state are of the order of 300 $\mu g.l^{-1}$ to 3 $mg.l^{-1}$ with wide interindividual variation. Measurement of plasma warfarin concentrations is sometimes of use in the investigation of patients with prolonged prothrombin times.

Metabolism

Warfarin is extensively metabolised in the liver. The R and S enantiomers of warfarin are metabolized by different metabolic pathways. R-warfarin is predominantly reduced by soluble enzymes to RS-warfarin alcohol.[20] A small percentage is converted to hydroxy metabolites particularly at the 6-positron. S-warfarin is mainly metabolized to 7-hydroxywarfarin by a cytochrome-P-450-dependent, mixed function oxidase.[21,22] Small amounts of other hydroxy metabolites and a warfarin alcohol are also formed.

The warfarin alcohols and hydroxy metabolites are excreted in the urine and in bile. There is an enterohepatic recirculation. 85% of a dose may be recovered as metabolites in urine with less than 1% as the unchanged drug. The warfarin alcohols have some anticoagulant activity but are considerably less potent than the parent drug.

Pharmaceutics

Warfarin is available in tablet form containing warfarin sodium BP in many strengths. Colour conventions (Table 1) can be misleading, since shades may vary from batch to batch.

1. Marevan tablets (DF, UK) are engraved 'DF/M1' (1 mg), 'DF/M3' (3 mg) and 'DF/M5' (5 mg).

Table 1

Strength	Tablet colour
1 mg (UK)	brown
2 mg (USA)	lavender
2.5 mg (USA)	orange
3 mg (UK)	blue
5 mg (UK/USA)	pink (UK), peach (USA)
7.5 mg (USA)	yellow
10 mg (USA)	white

2. Warfarin WBP (Boehringer Ingelheim, UK) compressed tablets are impressed with the letters 'WBP/W' on one side.
3. Panwarfin tablets (Abbott, USA) are coded 'LM' (2 mg), 'LN' (2.5 mg), 'LO' (5 mg), 'LR' (7.5 mg) and 'LF' (10 mg).
4. Coumadin tablets (Du Pont, USA) are available in the same strengths and are embossed with the strength, as are the 2 mg, 2.5 mg and 5 mg tablets from Lemmon (USA).

Tablets should ideally be protected from heat, light and moisture for optimum stability.

Therapeutic use

Indications

1. Deep venous thrombosis/pulmonary embolism
2. Valvular heart disease and atrial fibrillation
3. Prevention of recurrent myocardial infarction
4. Systemic embolism
5. Transient ischaemic attacks
6. Reconstructive artery surgery.

Contraindications

1. Active haemorrhage or significant risk of haemorrhage
2. Severe hepatic or renal disease
3. Allergy.

Mode of use

The anticoagulant effect of warfarin depends on producing a reduction in clotting factor synthesis. Onset of anticoagulant effect is delayed until the existing clotting factors have been catabolized. Heparin is often used to achieve an immediate response until the warfarin effect occurs. The dose of warfarin is titrated on an individual basis to achieve a prothrombin time which is 2–3 times a control value. This requires careful standardization and is usually expressed as the International Normalized Ratio (INR).

The exact therapeutic range for each different indication has not been accurately determined in large controlled studies. Evidence for use of a lower range in treating venous thromboembolism will be discussed later.

The existence of hypercoagulability following warfarin withdrawal has been debated. Most evidence points to no increased risk when warfarin is stopped. However, if the underlying cause of embolism has not been removed (e.g. mitral valve disease with atrial fibrillation) the patient may still be at risk.

A baseline prothrombin time should be obtained and warfarin started in a dose of 10 mg daily for most patients, although some authorities prefer to start with 5 mg daily. Prothrombin time should be monitored daily during the stabilization period and the dose of warfarin titrated to achieve the desired effect. A tailored loading dose schedule has been published to aid this process.[23] The loading dose should be reduced in the presence of conditions which reduce warfarin requirements, for example, old age, hyperthyroidism and liver disease.

Once stabilization has been achieved the prothrombin time should be monitored regularly at intervals of 1 week up to 2 months, depending on individual patient factors.

Indications

1. Deep venous thrombosis/pulmonary embolism
Treatment is aimed at preventing deep venous thrombosis (DVT) and pulmonary embolism (PE) and early treatment of DVT/PE to reduce mortality from this condition.

Primary prevention. Warfarin should be used after orthopaedic surgery or for long-term prophylaxis in medical patients with a low risk of haemorrhage.[24] In other situations, alternative treatments (subcutaneous heparin, dextran, antiplatelet drugs) are preferred because of a lower risk of haemorrhage.

Established DVT. The aim is to prevent thrombosis extension and embolism. Accurate diagnosis by venography should be considered for most patients. Treatment is generally continued for 3 months for a single episode, but lifelong therapy may be necessary for recurrent episodes.

Established PE. The aim of treatment is to reduce mortality but firm proof of the value of oral anticoagulants is lacking.[23] Despite this, treatment with warfarin is recommended to continue for 3–6 months for a single episode.

2. Valvular heart disease and atrial fibrillation
Treatment aims to reduce the risk of systemic emboli. High risk patients with a combination of mitral stenosis, large left atrium and atrial fibrillation should be treated with lifelong therapy. Warfarin is also recommended for secondary prevention in patients with mitral valve disease or atrial fibrillation after an episode of systemic embolism, but firm evidence of benefit is not available. Patients with prosthetic heart valves may also require oral anticoagulants. Hyperthyroid patients with atrial fibrillation may also benefit from warfarin treatment, though again firm evidence is lacking.

3. Prevention of recurrent myocardial infarction
The use of oral anticoagulants following myocardial infarction remains controversial. The results from the Sixty Plus Reinfarction Study Research Group showing a significant reduction in death rate (7.6% in treated group; 13.4% in placebo group) by oral anticoagulants has rekindled interest in their use.[26]

4. Systemic embolism
Most arterial emboli originate from the heart and there is a high risk of recurrence. Lifelong anticoagulation should be considered. If the embolus results from an acute myocardial infarct, warfarin may be stopped after 6 months because the incidence of recurrence in that situation is low.

5. Transient ischaemic attack
Antiplatelet drugs are preferred, but occasional patients may benefit from the use of warfarin.

6. Reconstructive artery surgery
There is no definite evidence of benefit from the use of warfarin to improve long-term graft patency. Further large-scale trials are necessary.

Contraindications

1. Haemorrhage
The risks of withholding treatment must be balanced against the risks of warfarin treatment. The main adverse effect of warfarin is haemorrhage. Any condition which is likely to result in bleeding is therefore a contraindication to the use of warfarin, for example, active peptic ulcer, oesophageal varices, aneurysm, recent undiagnosed stroke, severe hypertension, acute pericarditis.

The safe use of warfarin requires good patient education and compliance. If the patient is unable to take warfarin reliably and it is not possible to supervise tablet administration, then it may be safer to avoid long-term use of oral anticoagulants.

2. Severe hepatic or renal disease
The presence of significant hepatic or renal disease increases the risk of adverse effects. Warfarin should rarely be used in these conditions but if anticoagulants are necessary frequent monitoring is essential.

3. Allergy
Known allergy to warfarin is rare, but an absolute contraindication to its use.

Adverse reactions

Potentially life-threatening effects
Haemorrhage due to excessive anticoagulant effect is the most important adverse reaction to warfarin. The incidence of haemorrhage can be greatly reduced by regular monitoring of prothrombin

Warfarin (sodium)

time to keep the INR below 2.5. Higher BCR values within the therapeutic range are not necessary in most patients (see Major outcome trials). The most common sites of bleeding are the gastrointestinal tract and brain, but any organ or tissue may be affected.

Acute overdosage

Warfarin overdose results in complete inhibition of vitamin K_1-dependent clotting factor synthesis. If the patient presents soon after taking the overdose, the anticoagulant effect can be reversed by giving intravenous vitamin K_1. A dose of 5 mg of vitamin K_1 intravenously may suffice in mild cases of overdosage. Re-anticoagulation may then be possible 48–72 hours later. More severe cases will need 10–20 mg vitamin K_1, given by slow intravenous injection, and the dose may need to be repeated. Later presentation with haemorrhage requires more aggressive intervention with infusion of fresh frozen plasma, whole blood as necessary and intravenous vitamin K_1. Gastrointestinal and cerebral haemorrhage are the most common causes of death in warfarin overdose.

Severe or irreversible adverse effects

Adverse effects other than haemorrhage are rare. Occasional skin necrosis occurs within 10 days of starting treatment. Alopecia and the purple toes syndrome have been described.

Symptomatic adverse effects

Nausea, vomiting, diarrhoea, hypersensitivity (skin rash) and fever have been reported.

High risk groups

Neonates

The drug is unlikely to be used in neonates.

Breast milk. Warfarin does not pose a major risk to the breast-fed infant. Warfarin was not detected in the serum of seven infants studied and had no effect on bleeding time in three infants studied.[14]

Children

The drug may be used in children when indicated.

Pregnant women

Warfarin should be avoided during the first trimester of pregnancy because of the risk of teratogenicity. The main abnormalities are chondrodysplasia punctata with first-trimester exposure and optic atrophy and microcephaly with later exposure. The risk of warfarin embryopathy is low — 16 in 418 pregnancies.[4] Warfarin should also be avoided during the last 4 weeks because it crosses the placenta and may cause haemorrhage at birth. A normal, full-term infant would be expected in 70% of pregnancies in which warfarin is administered.[27] Some authors consider that warfarin should not be used for thromboembolism in pregnancy but is necessary in pregnant patients with mitral valve disease or artificial heart valves.[28]

The elderly

Older patients require smaller doses of warfarin than young adults. The initial dose should be 7–8 mg with adjustment depending on prothrombin time. The reduced dose requirement is related to a pharmacodynamic change as there is no alteration in warfarin kinetics with age.[29,30]

Concurrent disease

Hyperthyroidism. Hyperthyroid patients require lower doses of warfarin than euthyroid patients. The initial dose should be 7–8 mg with adjustment depending on prothrombin time. Regular monitoring is important to avoid underdosing as the patient becomes euthyroid with treatment. The increased warfarin sensitivity is said to be due to increased degradation of clotting factors.[4] Hypothyroid patients require higher doses of warfarin than when they are euthyroid.

Drug interactions

Potentially hazardous interactions

A large number of reports of drug interactions with warfarin has been published. Most of these are based on isolated case reports which have not been studied in detail. Warfarin has a narrow therapeutic index. If a new drug is added to an anticoagulated patient's treatment, it is essential to monitor the prothrombin time closely for the first month unless the added drug is known *not* to interact.

Many reviews of warfarin interactions have been published.[31–34] The more important and well-documented interactions are summarized below.

Pharmacodynamic

Antiplatelet drugs. Drugs affecting platelet function may potentiate warfarin by an effect on haemostasis. High-dose aspirin decreases prothrombin synthesis.

Diuretics. Spironolactone may reduce the effect of warfarin by increasing the concentration of clotting factors. Bumetanide and frusemide had no effect in an acute dosing study.

Clofibrate. Clofibrate potentiates warfarin action by altering receptor sensitivity.

Antibiotics. Broad-spectrum antibiotics may suppress production of vitamin K_1 by the bowel flora. This may potentiate the warfarin effect in patients with reduced dietary intake of vitamin K. Some of the newer cephalosporins may potentiate warfarin effect by an unknown mechanism.

Drugs causing potential bleeding sites. Drugs which cause peptic ulceration or gastric erosions may precipitate haemorrhage in patients taking warfarin. Some of the interacting drugs (e.g. aspirin) also affect anticoagulants by other mechanisms.

Vitamin K. A high vitamin K diet, including some enteral feeds, will reduce the warfarin effect.

Pharmacokinetic

Increased warfarin effect

H_2-receptor antagonists. Cimetidine inhibits warfarin metabolism and potentiates its effect. Ranitidine does not have a significant effect on warfarin.

Analgesics and non-steroidal anti-inflammatory drugs (NSAID). Phenylbutazone is a well-documented example of a drug which stereoselectively inhibits warfarin metabolism.[21,22] The restricted use of phenylbutazone greatly reduces the chance of this potentially fatal interaction being observed. Some other NSAIDs (meclofenamic acid, mefenamic acid, piroxicam and azapropazone) also potentiate the anticoagulant effect. Dextropropoxyphene may inhibit warfarin metabolism. The commonly used Distalgesic (dextropropoxyphene plus paracetamol) may potentiate the effect of warfarin. Paracetamol has been considered to be safe in patients taking warfarin, but one study has shown potentiation of effect in a few patients after treatment for 3 weeks.

Sulphinpyrazone. Sulphinpyrazone enhances the warfarin effect by a stereoselective inhibition of the metabolism of the S-warfarin enantiomer.

Antibiotics. Co-trimoxazole and metronidazole also stereoselectively inhibit the metabolism of S-warfarin. Ketoconazole inhibits drug metabolism in vitro and there are case reports of potentiation of warfarin effect. Similarly, erythromycin may enhance the effect of warfarin.

Amiodarone. Amiodarone inhibits warfarin metabolism and potentiates the anticoagulant effect.

Other drugs. Lipid-soluble β-blockers (e.g. propranolol) and vaccination may inhibit drug metabolism. There are case reports of haemorrhage following the addition of β-blockers or influenza vaccination in patients taking warfarin. Formal studies have shown only a small effect with propranolol and no effect with influenza vaccination.

Oral contraceptives increase clotting factor concentrations and inhibit warfarin metabolism. The net effect depends on the balance between these factors. Oral contraceptives are contraindicated in most patients taking warfarin because of their thrombogenic effect.

Reduced warfarin effect

Enzyme induction. Hepatic microsomal enzyme-inducing drugs increase warfarin elimination and reduce the anticoagulant effect. Examples are carbamazepine, phenobarbitone and rifampicin. Phenytoin has a more complex interaction with warfarin and the end result is variable.

Cholestyramine. Cholestyramine reduces the anticoagulant effect of warfarin by impairing warfarin absorption and interrupting its enterohepatic recirculation.

Uncertain mechanisms

An interaction between warfarin and tamoxifen has been reported, resulting in an increased warfarin effect and (theoretically) a decreased effect of tamoxifen.[36]

W

Potentially useful interactions

None has been described.

Major outcome trials

Established pulmonary embolism

1. Egermayer P 1981 Value of anticoagulants in the treatment of pulmonary embolism: a discussion paper. Journal of the Royal Society of Medicine 74: 675–681

This paper is a critical review of the value of anticoagulants in the treatment of pulmonary embolism. There is no evidence from a large, well-conducted, double-blind clinical trial to support or refute the benefit from anticoagulants in PE. Use of warfarin appears to be based on anecdotal reports and a prospective study which was abandoned after five out of 19 untreated patients died, with no deaths in the treated group.[19] Other studies are criticized because of design faults.

Established deep venous thrombosis

2. Hull R et al (a) 1979 Warfarin sodium versus low-dose heparin in the long-term treatment of venous thrombosis. New England Journal of Medicine 301: 855–858; (b) 1982 Adjusted subcutaneous heparin versus warfarin sodium in the long-term treatment of venous thrombosis. New England Journal of Medicine 306: 189–194; (c) 1982 Different intensities of oral anticoagulant therapy in the treatment of proximal vein thrombosis. New England Journal of Medicine 307: 1676–1681

This series of papers reports on three randomized trials of the use of anticoagulants in prevention of recurrent venous thromboembolism. The diagnosis of DVT was established by venography.

The first study found that low-dose heparin was ineffective but that adjusted high-dose warfarin was highly effective at a cost of an appreciable risk of haemorrhage. The second report suggested that adjusted-dose subcutaneous heparin was an effective alternative to the use of warfarin, with less risk of bleeding. The final paper demonstrated that less intensive warfarin therapy was associated with a low risk of recurrent thromboembolism and also a low risk of haemorrhage. Less intensive warfarin dosing (prothrombin time twice control value) would appear to be the treatment of first choice, as it avoids repeated injections.

Myocardial infarction

3. International Anticoagulant Review Group 1970 Collaborative analysis of long term anticoagulant administration after acute myocardial infarction. Lancet 1: 203–209

An international group reviewed several studies of satisfactory design. They concluded that use of oral anticoagulants for 1–2 years resulted in a 20% reduction in mortality in males aged under 55 years with previous angina or myocardial infarction.

4. Sixty Plus Reinfarction Study Research Group 1980 A double-blind trial to assess long-term oral anticoagulant therapy in elderly patients after myocardial infarction. Lancet 2: 989–993

This study reopened the debate on the use of oral anticoagulants following myocardial infarction. A randomized double-blind multi-centre study of the use of oral anticoagulants following a myocardial infarction was carried out in 878 patients over 60 years of age. All patients were treated for 6 months then randomized to oral anticoagulant or placebo. The treated group had a significantly lower death rate (7.6 vs. 13.4%) and lower incidence of recurrent MI (5.7 vs. 15.9). Major haemorrhage occurred in 27 treated patients. There were no fatal extracranial haemorrhages. Intracranial events (haemorrhagic plus non-haemorrhagic) were less common in the treated group.

Atrial fibrillation

5. Petersen P. et al 1989 Placebo-controlled, randomized trial of warfarin and aspirin for prevention of thromboembolic complications in chronic atrial fibrillation. Lancet 1: 175–178

This was a well-designed trial of 1007 patients with non-rheumatic atrial fibrillation. Patients were treated with warfarin, aspirin or placebo and followed up for at least 2 years. Thromboembolic complications occurred in 5 patients in the warfarin group compared with 20 on aspirin and 21 on placebo. Significantly less vascular deaths occurred in the warfarin group. However, over one-third of the patients randomized to warfarin withdrew from the study and unwanted effects were three times more common in patients taking warfarin.

General review articles

Kelly J G, O'Malley K 1979 Clinical pharmacokinetics of oral anticoagulants. Clinical Pharmacokinetics 4: 1–15

O'Reilly R A, Aggeler P M 1970 Determinants of the response to oral anticoagulant drugs in man. Pharmacological Reviews 22: 35–96

Poller L 1985 Therapeutic ranges in anticoagulant administration. British Medical Journal 290: 1683–1686

Scott A K 1985 Anticoagulants in the treatment of cardiovascular disease. In: Breckenridge A (ed) Drugs in the management of heart disease. MTP Press, Lancaster, pp 199–222

References

1. Stenflo J, Suttie J W 1977 Vitamin K-dependent formation of γ-carboxyglutamic acid. Annual Review of Biochemistry 46: 154–172
2. Bell R G 1978 Metabolism of vitamin K and prothrombin synthesis — anticoagulants and the vitamin K-epoxide cycle. Federation Proceedings 37: 2599–2604
3. Park B K, Leck J B, Wilson A C, Serlin M J, Breckenridge A M 1979 A study of the effect of anticoagulants on [^{3}H]-vitamin K_1 metabolism and prothrombin complex activity in the rabbit. Biochemical Pharmacology 28: 1323–1329
4. Chang M K, Harvey D, de Swiet M 1984 Follow up study of children whose mothers were treated with warfarin during pregnancy. British Journal of Obstetrics and Gynaecology 91: 1070–1073
5. Breckenridge A M 1977 Interindividual differences in the response to oral anticoagulants. Drugs 14: 367–375
6. Shearer M J 1983 High performance liquid chromatography of K vitamins and their antagonists. Advances in Chromatography 21: 243–301
7. Scott A K, Park B K, Breckenridge A M 1984 Interaction between warfarin and propanolol. British Journal of Clinical Pharmacology 17: 559–564
8. Banfield C, Rowland M 1983 Stereospecific fluorescent high pressure liquid chromatographic analysis of warfarin and its metabolites in plasma and urine. Journal of Pharmaceutical Sciences 72: 921–924
9. O'Reilly R A, Aggeler P M, Leong L S 1963 Studies on the coumarin anticoagulant drugs: the pharmacodynamics of warfarin in man. Journal of Clinical Investigation 42: 1542–1551
10. Breckenridge A, Orme M 1973 Measurement of plasma warfarin concentration in clinical practice. In: Davies D S, Prichard B N C (eds) Biological effects of drugs in relation to their plasma concentrations. Macmillan, London, pp 145–151
11. O'Reilly R A 1974 Studies on the optical enantiomers of warfarin in man. Clinical Pharmacology and Therapeutics 16: 348–354
12. Hewick D S, McEwan J 1973 Plasma half-lives, plasma metabolites and anticoagulant efficacies of the enantiomers of warfarin in man. Journal of Pharmacy and Pharmacology 25: 458–465
13. O'Reilly R A 1973 The binding of sodium warfarin to plasma albumin and its displacement by phenylbutazone. Annals of the New York Academy of Sciences 226: 293–308
14. Orme M L'E, Lewis P J, de Swiet M et al 1977 May mothers given warfarin breast feed their infants. British Medical Journal 1: 1564–1565
15. Bachmann K, Shapiro R, Mackiewicz J 1977 Warfarin elimination and responsiveness in patients with renal dysfunction. Journal of Clinical Pharmacology 17: 292–299
16. Piroli R J, Passananti T, Shively C A, Vesell E S 1981 Antipyrine and warfarin disposition in a patient with idiopathic hypoalbuminaemia. Clinical Pharmacology and Therapeutics 30: 810–816
17. Hignite C, Uetrecht J, Tschanz C, Azarnoff P 1980 Kinetics of R and S warfarin enantiomers. Clinical Pharmacology and Therapeutics 28: 99–105
18. Nagashima R, O'Reilly R A, Levy G 1969 Kinetics of pharmacologic effects in man: the anticoagulant action of warfarin. Clinical Pharmacology and Therapeutics 10: 22–35
19. Choonara I A, Scott A K, Haynes B P, Cholerton S, Breckenridge A M, Park B K 1985 Vitamin K_1 metabolism in relation to pharmacodynamic response in anticoagulated patients. British Journal of Clinical Pharmacology 20 (6): 643–648
20. Hewick D S, Moreland T A 1975 An NADPH dependent warfarin reductase in human and rat liver and kidney soluble fraction. British Journal of Pharmacology 53: 441
21. Lewis R J, Trager W F, Chan K K et al 1974 Warfarin: stereochemical aspects of its metabolism and the interaction with phenylbutazone. Journal of Clinical Investigation 53: 1607–1617
22. Banfield C, O'Reilly R, Chan E, Rowland M 1983 Phenylbutazone–warfarin interaction in man: further stereochemical and metabolic considerations. British Journal of Clinical Pharmacology 16: 669–675
23. Fennerty A, Dolben J, Thomas P et al 1984 Flexible induction dose regimen for warfarin and prediction of maintenance dose. British Medical Journal 288: 1268–1270
24. Gallus A S 1983 Indications for oral anticoagulant treatment. Drugs 26: 543–549
25. Egermayer P 1981 Value of anticoagulants in the treatment of pulmonary embolism: a discussion paper. Journal of the Royal Society of Medicine 74: 675–681

26. Sixty Plus Reinfarction Study Research Group 1980 A double-blind trial to assess long-term oral anticoagulant therapy in elderly patients after myocardial infarction. Lancet 2: 989–993
27. Briggs G G, Bodendorfer T W, Freeman R K, Yaffe S J 1983 Drugs in pregnancy and lactation. A reference guide to fetal and neonatal risk. Williams and Wilkins, Baltimore, pp 89–92
28. de Swiet M 1984 Thromboembolism in medical disorders in obstetric practice. Blackwell Scientific Publications, Oxford, pp 95–115
29. Routledge P A, Chapman P H, Davies D M, Rawlins M D 1979 Pharmacokinetics and pharmacodynamics of warfarin at steady state. British Journal of Clinical Pharmacology 8: 243–247
30. Shepherd A M M, Hewick D S, Moreland T A, Stevenson I H 1977 Age as a determinant of sensitivity to warfarin. British Journal of Clinical Pharmacology 4: 315–320
31. Koch-Weser J, Sellers E M 1971 Drug interactions with coumarin anticoagulants. New England Journal of Medicine 285: 487–498 and 547–558
32. Serlin M J, Breckenridge A M 1983 Drug interactions with warfarin. Drugs 25: 610–620
33. Standing advisory committee for haematology of the Royal College of Pathologists 1982 Drug interaction with coumarin derivative anticoagulants. British Medical Journal 285: 274–275
34. Scott A K, Orme M C L'E 1983 Drug interactions with warfarin — current views. Adverse Drug Reaction Bulletin 103: 380–383
35. Barritt D W, Jordan S C 1960 Anticoagulant drugs in the treatment of pulmonary embolism. A controlled trial. Lancet 1: 1309–1312
36. Tenni P, Lalich D L, Byrne M J 1989 Life-threatening interaction between tamoxifen and warfarin. British Medical Journal 298: 93

Xamoterol (fumarate)

Xamoterol was the first β_1-adrenoceptor partial agonist to be approved for the treatment of heart failure.

Chemistry

Xamoterol (Corwin, Carwin, Xamtol, Corwil)
$C_{16}H_{25}N_3O_5$
dl-N-[2-[2-Hydroxy-3-(4-hydroxyphenoxy) propylamino]ethylmorpholine-4-carboxamide

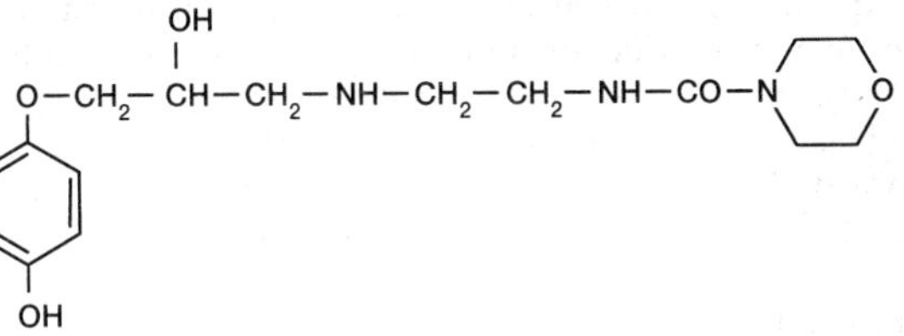

Molecular weight of fumarate (free base)	794 (339)
pKa	8.2
Solubility	
in alcohol	1 in 5000
in water	1 in 20
Octanol/water partition coefficient	1.1

A white to off-white powder, odourless but with a slightly bitter taste. It is prepared by chemical synthesis and marketed as a racemic mixture of two enantiomers.

It is not available in any combination preparations.

Pharmacology

Xamoterol is a selective β_1-adrenoceptor partial agonist (ratio of selectivity β_1:β_2-receptors is 18). It has no agonist activity at β_2-adrenoceptors and its partial agonist activity or intrinsic sympathomimetic activity (ISA) at the β_1-adrenoceptors is estimated at 43% of the activity of a full agonist (such as isoprenaline) when myocardial contractility or heart rate changes are used as end-points to evaluate the ISA.[2,4,7] As a partial agonist, xamoterol occupies the same receptors as isoprenaline, but elicits less response.[4] The occupation of β_1-adrenoceptors by xamoterol prevents access by the full agonists and reduces their effects. At rest or during mild exercise, when sympathetic tone is low, xamoterol binds to β_1-adrenoceptors to produce a mild stimulant effect.[3] As sympathetic neurotransmitter release increases, xamoterol reduces heart rate and minimizes stimulation of the heart by endogenous catecholamines.[2,4,5,8,9,11] During submaximal exercise (up to 50% of maximal load), the left ventricular filling pressure, the indices of myocardial contractility and relaxation as well as the relationship between stroke work index and filling pressure remained significantly improved.[5,8] At maximal exercise, the main significant difference is a reduction in heart rate without changes in cardiac output[8,9] (see also Virk et al, in Major outcome trials). Stroke volume is therefore increased during maximal exercise with xamoterol and the pulmonary capillary wedge pressure is reduced by 10 to 15%[8,9] (see also Virk et al, in Major outcome trials). Prolonged stimulation of β-adrenoceptors sometimes leads to tachyphylaxis but there is no evidence of down-regulation of β_1-adrenoceptors during prolonged xamoterol therapy.[10] If endogenous sympathetic tone is very high (e.g. at maximum exercise or in severe heart failure) xamoterol, by occupying the β_1-adrenoceptors, acts mainly as a β_1-adrenoceptor antagonist; thus heart failure may be exacerbated in patients with severe heart failure.[28]

Toxicology

Toxicological testing in animals failed to demonstrate any results of potential clinical relevance. When high doses of xamoterol were given to rats and rabbits during the second half of pregnancy, the cardiovascular effects of the drug led to deformations. Xamoterol has been evaluated in the Ames mutagenicity test and cytogenetic tests, and no adverse effects were found. At 2 years, no oncogenic effects were observed in rats and mice. Survival rates were increased by xamoterol in both species.

Clinical pharmacology

Xamoterol has been studied extensively in normal volunteers, in patients with mild to moderate heart failure (new York Heart Classification II–III) and in elderly patients;[4–6,8,9,11–14,31–33] (see also the German and Austrian Xamoterol Study Group 1988, and Rousseau M F et al 1983 in Major outcome trials). Intravenous doses of 0.5–200 $\mu g.kg^{-1}$ produced a dose-dependent decrease in left ventricular end-diastolic pressure and a dose-dependent increase in left ventricular contractility.[32] At rest, in patients with mild to moderate heart failure, cardiac index and myocardial contractility ($LVdP/dt_{max}$) are increased, while left ventricular filling pressure, left ventricular end-diastolic pressure and diastolic wall stress are all decreased. Changes in coronary blood flow are small. On submaximal exercise there is little change in cardiac index; however, myocardial contractility is increased[5] while maximum heart rate and left ventricular filling pressure are both reduced. The EC_{50} of xamoterol was identical in middle-aged and elderly patients and was not dependent on the baseline left ventricular function.[31–33] The other potential metabolic and endocrine effects of xamoterol are less well known, but it has been established that prolonged xamoterol therapy does not affect the plasma lipid profile. The recommended effective oral dose is 200 mg twice daily and with this dose regimen plasma levels provide 75%–90% of the maximum response attainable with xamoterol.[33] In patients with severe renal function impairment ($GFR < 35\ ml.min^{-1}\ 1.73\ m^{-2}$) a dose of 200 mg once daily is recommended.

Pharmacokinetics

The preferred analytical method for xamoterol is radioimmunossay (limit of detection 0.5 $\mu g.l^{-1}$; coefficient of variation < 10%).[1] Only approximately 9% of an oral dose of xamoterol is absorbed from the gastrointestinal tract, due to the hydrophilic nature of the compound which limits diffusion across the gastrointestinal wall into the blood.[15] The only route of metabolism that xamoterol appears to undergo is sulphate conjugation. From studies in the dog the gut wall may be a site of this conjugation after oral administration. Some sulphate conjugation may also occur in the liver.

The bioavailability of xamoterol after oral administration is approximately 5% (3.1–6.6%)[1,15,16] suggesting that there might be some presystemic metabolism (equivalent to 44% of the amount absorbed, or 4% of the dose), possibly by gut wall sulphation.

The time to achieve peak plasma concentrations is 1.1 hours in young subjects, but is significantly longer in elderly subjects (2.1 h).

Following oral administration, the maximum plasma concentration of xamoterol is proportional to dose, over the range 200–600 mg.

The plasma half life of xamoterol in healthy volunteers is about 16 h.[1]

The drug is distributed throughout the body, with a steady-state volume of distribution of 48–60 l, approximately 0.64 $l.kg^{-1}$, both in healthy volunteers and in patients with heart failure.[1,16] Plasma protein binding of xamoterol is negligible (3%). The volume of distribution is close to that of total body water, consistent with the hydrophilic nature of xamoterol and its low binding to plasma proteins.

Because of its hydrophilicity, xamoterol does not readily cross the blood–brain barrier. Xamoterol is secreted in the breast milk of lactating rats. Women should avoid the drug when breast-feeding.

The majority of drug absorbed is excreted in the urine, 94% after intravenous administration and 8.3% after oral administration, over 5 days. The only metabolite is the sulphate ester, which is also excreted in the urine, accounting for 56% of the drug absorbed after oral administration (4.7% of the dose).

ʻiver disease will have any effects on the kinetics patients the renal clearance of xamoterol is to 6.9 l.h^{-1} with a corresponding increase in ιo 27 h. Some dosage adjustment in such patients ɹ. It is likely that renal impairment reduces the prolongs the half life of the drug. On the contrary, it is ɹt hepatic dysfunction will affect the kinetics of xamoterol ι any dosage adjustment would be necessary.

ɹatients with heart failure the half life of xamoterol is increased ɹ1 h.[16,17]

The effects of cardiac failure on the kinetics of the drug are not significant.

Oral absorption	9%
Bioavailability	5%
Plasma half life	
mean	16 h
Volume of distribution	0.64 l.kg^{-1}
Plasma protein binding	3%

Concentration–effect relationship

Measurement of an index of left ventricular contractility (dP/dt at a developed pressure of 40 mmHg and normalized for this value) after xamoterol administration showed near-maximal effect at a plasma concentration of 150 µg.l^{-1} (EC_{90}) and 75% of maximum at a plasma concentration of 39 µg.l^{-1} (EC_{75}). The peak plasma concentration in heart failure patients receiving 200 mg of drug twice daily has been measured as 168 µg.l^{-1}; the trough concentration (12 hours after dosing) was 56 µg.l^{-1}. These concentrations could be predicted to produce positive inotropic responses of approximately 90% and 75% respectively.[29,32] Thus a heart failure patient at rest receiving 200 mg xamoterol twice daily can be expected to maintain an inotropic response of between 90% and 75% of the maximum over each 12-hour dosing interval. Because xamoterol is a partial agonist with only 43% of the agonist activity of a full agonist such as isoprenaline, even the maximum effect of xamoterol is only half that of a full agonist.

Metabolism

Absorbed xamoterol is eliminated from the body by renal excretion. Some tubular secretion may be involved.[16] The only metabolism of xamoterol is by sulphate conjugation of the 4-hydroxy group, occurring in the gut wall primarily, and also in the liver (Fig. 1). The sulphate conjugate is pharmacologically inactive, and comprises 56% of material in the urine after oral dosing (4.7% of the dose). The remainder of the absorbed drug (3.6% of the dose) is excreted unchanged in the urine. There is no evidence of enterohepatic circulation. Following intravenous administration 94% of the dose is excreted in urine.

Fig. 1 Metabolism of xamoterol

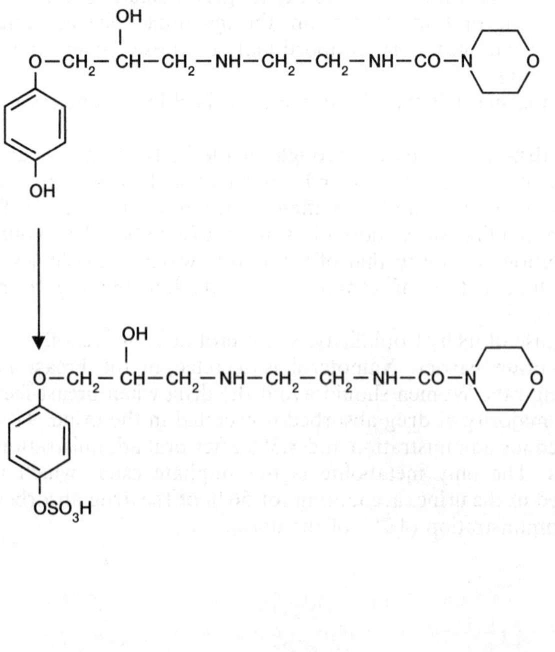

Pharmaceutics

The only available formulation of xamoterol, Corwin (ICI, UK), is a 200 mg tablet (round, biconvex, dark yellow, film-coated, impressed with 'Corwin' 200 on one face and a logo on the reverse) containing xamoterol as the fumarate. The formulation does not contain tartrazine or potentially allergenic substances. Corwin tablets should be stored at room temperature. The shelf-life of the 200 mg tablet is 5 years.

Therapeutic use

Indications

Xamoterol is indicated in patients with mild chronic heart failure. Xamoterol should be initiated after detailed assessment of the patients' heart failure status. Suitable patients should exhibit the following features:

be symptomatic (e.g. short of breath and/or fatigued) on normal activity but not symptomatic at rest.

be without evidence of congestion of cardiac origin (e.g. pulmonary oedema, peripheral oedema, raised jugular venous pressure, etc).

not requiring diuretics or with clinical signs controlled on low-dose diuretics (e.g. a thiazide, or no more than 80 mg frusemide a day or equivalent). Many heart failure patients suffer from concomitant ischaemic heart disease. In patients with angina pectoris, a reduction in myocardial ischaemia on exercise has been demonstrated with xamoterol at the dose levels recommended for heart failure.

Contraindications

Xamoterol is contraindicated in patients with moderate or severe heart failure.

Mode of use

Xamoterol can be used in patients with mild heart failure either alone or in addition to digoxin, diuretics and nitrates. The recommended effective dose is 200 mg twice daily.

Four multicentre safety and efficacy studies included 917 patients with mild-to-moderate heart failure (New York Heart Association [NYHA] class II–III) who were randomized to three months of treatment with either xamoterol 200 mg twice daily (n=617) or the placebo (n=300). Demographic details and concurrent treatment distribution were similar in the placebo and xamoterol-treatment groups. Most patients (70%) were in NYHA class II, and 17% were in class III the remainder were in Class I. Ischaemic heart disease was the most common cause of cardiac failure, and occurred in 79% of patients. Heart failure associated with hypertension, valvular disease, or cardiomyopathy was less common. Breathlessness was a symptom in 94% of patients, fatigue in 76%, angina pectoris in 54%, and peripheral oedema in 26%. The distribution of these symptoms was similar between the placebo and xamoterol-treatment groups, as was the distribution of physical signs of heart failure.

Xamoterol significantly increased exercise capacity by 19% over the placebo (37% vs 18%), a difference equivalent to 2.98 kJ ($p<0.0001$). Maximum exercise heart rate was significantly reduced by xamoterol as compared with the placebo (118 vs 130 beats/min, $p<0.0001$), although resting heart rate was unaffected. Xamoterol significantly improved the cardinal symptoms of heart failure, breathlessness and fatigue, as compared with the placebo, and as demonstrated by both visual analogue scale (VAS) and Likert scale measurements — that is breathlessness (VAS, $p<0.01$; Likert, $p<0.0001$) and fatigue (VAS, $p<0.01$; Likert, p=NS).

Treatment with xamoterol as compared with treatment with placebo ($p<0.001$) also improved quality of life. The incidences of withdrawal because of adverse experiences were similar in both the xamoterol and placebo groups (approximately 10%). Xamoterol treatment was not associated with adverse effects on haematological or biochemical variables.

The improved ventricular relaxation and filling caused by xamoterol results in a significant reduction in the abnormally high left ventricular filling pressure characteristic of heart failure. The improved diastolic performance can be especially important in older patients, in whom the relation between reduced effort tolerance and impaired ventricular relaxation was the subject of speculation several

Xamoterol (fumarate)

decades ago. The beneficial partial agonist effect of xamoterol on diastolic function, together with the attenuation of the tachycardia during maximum exercise (which reflects the antagonist action against excessive catecholamine levels during periods of high sympathetic drive), can allow better filling and prevent ischaemia. Thus, xamoterol can be particularly useful in patients with heart failure of ischaemic aetiology, in whom regional or global diastolic dysfunction is an important contributory factor to the impaired effort tolerance and symptoms.

Contraindications

1. Patients with moderate or severe heart failure
This includes patients who, for example, are dyspnoeic at rest, have peripheral or pulmonary oedema, raised jugular venous pressure, a large heart etc. Some such patients have shown serious deterioration on xamoterol.

As some patients, who by symptomatic criteria were assessed to have NYHA III–IV heart failure despite intensive treatment with diuretics and ACE inhibitors, showed deterioration,[34] and because the determination of severity of disease cannot always be precise, xamoterol is not recommended for use in moderate heart failure. On the basis of available data, xamoterol should therefore not be used in the following patients:

- those who are short of breath or fatigued at rest or severely limited on minimal exercise
- those who have a resting sinus tachycardia (>90 beats per minute) or hypotension (systolic BP<100 mmHg)
- those patients who are clinically unstable, i.e. who present with acute pulmonary oedema or who have a history of repeated episodes of acute pulmonary oedema
- those who have peripheral oedema, a raised jugular venous pressure, an enlarged liver, pulmonary oedema or a third heart sound
- those who require treatment with high doses of a loop diuretic (frusemide more than 80 mg per day or equivalent)
- those who already require both a loop diuretic and further therapy, such as an ACE inhibitor, to control their symptoms.

Xamoterol should be withdrawn from patients whose heart failure deteriorates whilst on the drug, for example if the patient develops worsening symptoms (e.g. shortness of breath and/or fatigue), or diminishing effort tolerance.

The value of the drug is now in doubt because of adverse reactions in moderate and severe cases and the greater safety of ACE inhibitors.

Adverse reactions

Potentially life-threatening effects
Some patients with severe heart failure have shown serious deterioration on xamoterol. Rarely, bronchospasm or hypotension have occurred.

Acute overdosage
Because of its pharmacological profile, the acute effects are unlikely to be life-threatening. As the binding of xamoterol to receptors is competitive, management with β_1 full agonists should control the situation if features of beta blockade predominate, but high doses might be needed.

Severe or irreversible adverse effects
Other than worsening of heart failure no effects of this kind have been reported. See comments above on severe heart failure, bronchospasm and hypotension.

Symptomatic adverse effects
From large double-blind, placebo-controlled studies, xamoterol when used as indicated is well-tolerated and adverse experiences are uncommon. Adverse effects in controlled studies showed a small excess in incidence over placebo of gastrointestinal complaints, headache and dizziness. Although in these studies there was also an apparent excess of angina/chest pain, such events are not uncommon and are to be expected in heart failure patients. Other controlled studies with xamoterol in patients with angina pectoris showed a reduced incidence of myocardial ischaemia during exercise. Rash, palpitations and muscle cramp were also reported.

In published reports, the type and frequency of adverse experiences in patients treated with xamoterol are similar to those in placebo groups;[18–20,30] (see also the German and Austrian Xamoterol Study Group 1988 and Waller D G et al in Major outcome trials).

Interference with clinical pathology tests
No interference with clinical pathology test methods has been reported.

High risk groups

Neonates
There is no paediatric experience with xamoterol and for this reason it is not recommended for use in neonates.

Breast milk. The drug is secreted in the milk of experimental animals and its use should be avoided in women when breast-feeding.

Children
What has been stated about neonates above also applies to older children.

Pregnant women
There is no evidence for the safety of the drug in human pregnancy. When high doses of xamoterol were given to rats and rabbits during the second half of pregnancy, the cardiovascular effects of the drug led to deformations. It is recommended, therefore, that administration of the drug is avoided in pregnancy unless the condition itself carries sufficient risks to the mother and fetus to warrant its use.

The elderly
No specific dosage reduction is necessary, except in those with suspected or established renal impairment.

Concurrent disease

Renal disease. Since xamoterol is excreted by the kidneys, dosage should be adjusted in cases of severe impairment of renal function. No significant accumulation of xamoterol occurs at a GFR greater than 35 $ml.min^{-1}$ per 1.73 m^{-2}. Significant accumulation of xamoterol occurs only when GFR decreases to below 35 $ml.min^{-1}$ 1.73 m^{-2}. This level of renal impairment is usually clinically evident and approximates to doubling of the serum creatinine (e.g. greater than 250 $\mu mol.l^{-1}$ or 3 $mg.dl^{-1}$). It is therefore recommended that the dose of xamoterol is reduced to one tablet (200 mg) daily when clinical evidence indicates suspected or established renal impairment (approximate doubling of serum creatinine value or a GFR of 15–35 $ml.min^{-1}$ 1.73 m^{-2}).

Liver disease. The pharmacokinetics of single oral and intravenous doses of xamoterol in patients with chronic liver disease (primarily alcoholic cirrhosis) have been found not to differ from that of healthy volunteers.[34] This finding is not unexpected, as xamoterol does not undergo hepatic phase 1 metabolism; renal clearance is the major elimination pathway and sulphate conjugation occurs mainly in the gut wall. There is therefore no need to modify xamoterol dosage in patients with impaired hepatic function.

Respiratory disease. Xamoterol should be used with great caution in patients with co-existing mild obstructive airways disease. Due to the β-adrenoceptor antagonist effect of xamoterol, an increase in airways resistance may occasionally be provoked in asthmatic patients. If bronchospasm does occur, xamoterol should be withdrawn, and the bronchospasm may be reversed by the use of inhaled bronchodilator preparations.[21,22]

Drug interactions

Potentially hazardous interactions
There are none.

Potentially useful interactions
Xamoterol has been co-administered without evidence of incompatibility with a wide range of other drugs, including thiazide and potassium-sparing diuretics, cardiac glycosides, warfarin, antiplatelet drugs and non-steroidal anti-inflammatory drugs.

The mode of action of xamoterol differs from that of other current heart failure treatments, such as diuretics, ACE inhibitors, nitrates and other vasodilators. Xamoterol may, therefore, logically be co-administered with other therapy where appropriate. In patients with atrial fibrillation, the addition of xamoterol to digoxin generally results in improved control of ventricular rate.

trials

1. ustrian Xamoterol Study Group 1988 ebo-controlled comparison of digoxin and ronic heart failure. Lancet 1: 489–493

ndomized, double-blind, multicentre, parallel group 3 patients with mild to moderate heart failure (NYHA II) of whom 23% were receiving diuretic therapy. Xamot- 0 mg twice daily was compared with digoxin 0.125 mg twice y and placebo over a period of 3 months. Exercise duration and work done was significantly improved on xamoterol compared with digoxin and placebo. Symptoms significantly improved on xamoterol compared with placebo, and clinical signs were ameliorated. In conclusion, this study conducted in a large number of patients demonstrated that xamoterol was more effective than digoxin or placebo in improving exercise capacity, signs and symptoms of heart failure. Additionally xamoterol was well tolerated.

2. Waller D G, Webster J, Sykes C A, Bhalla K K, Wray R 1989 Clinical efficacy of xamoterol, a β_1-adrenoceptor partial agonist, in mild to moderate heart failure. European Heart Journal 10: 1003–1010

This was a randomized, double-blind, multicentre, parallel group study in 240 patients with mild to moderate heart failure designed to compare xamoterol 200 mg twice daily, and placebo over a period of 3 months. Exercise duration was increased by xamoterol compared to placebo, and peak exercise heart rate was significantly reduced. Subjective improvements occurred in breathlessness, but not in fatigue, compared with placebo. In conclusion, xamoterol led to a sustained improvement in symptoms and exercise duration in patients with mild to moderate heart failure.

3. Virk S J S, Anfilogoff N H, Lawson N et al 1989 The acute effects of intravenous xamoterol (Corwin, ICI 118 587) on resting and exercise haemodynamics in patients with mild to moderate heart failure. European Heart Journal 10: 227–234

This study investigated the effects of intravenous xamoterol (0.2 mg.kg^{-1}), at rest and on exercise, on the haemodynamic variables of 30 patients with mild to moderate cardiac failure. Significant improvements in resting cardiac index, stroke volume and stroke work index occurred following xamoterol, as well as reductions in systemic vascular resistance and double product. On exercise, xamoterol attenuated the heart rate response to exercise, without impairing cardiac index, due to a significant increase in stroke volume.

Thus, xamoterol leads to significant improvements in cardiac performance following acute dosing both at rest and on exercise.

4. Rousseau M F, Pouleur H, Vincent M F 1983 Effects of a cardioselective β_1 partial agonist (Corwin) on left ventricular function and myocardial metabolism in patients with previous myocardial infarction. American Journal of Cardiology 51: 1267–1274

This open study set out to assess the effects of xamoterol on left ventricular systolic and diastolic function and myocardial metabolism in 25 patients with coronary artery disease and a previous myocardial infarction. Following a single acute intravenous dose of xamoterol (0.1 mg.kg^{-1}) contractility improved by 35%, global ejection fraction increased significantly, mean systolic and diastolic wall stress decreased significantly and the rate of relaxation improved. In this group of patients, myocardial oxygen consumption was unaffected by xamoterol, and no significant changes in myocardial lactate extraction or consumption were seen.

These data indicate that xamoterol increases cardiac efficiency by improving left ventricular systolic and diastolic function in patients with coronary artery disease and left ventricular dysfunction.

5. Vigholt-Sorensen E, Faergeman O, 1990 Ischaemic left ventricular failure: evidence of sustained benefit after 18 months' treatment with xamoterol. British Heart Journal 64: 186–189

Following a 7–14-day placebo run-in, xamoterol or placebo was administered in a double-blind crossover comparison of one-month treatment periods. Xamoterol 200 mg twice daily was subsequently given to all patients for 18 months, and a further randomized,

given to all patients for 18 months, and a further randomized,

double-blind crossover comparison was made. All 14 patients had mild to moderate heart failure. At both one and 18 months, xamoterol significantly increased the duration of exercise and work done compared with placebo. Improvements were sustained over the 18-month period. In conclusion, xamoterol given to mild to moderate heart failure patients long-term is both safe and effective, with benefits maintained over at least 18 months.

6. The Xamoterol in Severe Heart Failure Study Group 1990 Xamoterol in severe heart failure. Lancet 336: 1–6

516 patients with NYHA grade III or IV heart failure despite treatment with diuretics and ACE inhibitors were randomized to xamoterol 200 mg daily (n = 352) or placebo (n = 164). Breathlessness was less severe on xamoterol but there was no difference in exercise duration. On intention-to-treat analysis 32 (9.1%) patients in the xamoterol group and 6 (3.7%) in the placebo group died (p = 0.02). The authors conclude that xamoterol should be avoided in patients with severe heart failure.

References

1. Bastain W, Boyce M J, Stafford L E, Morton P B, Clarke D A, Marlow H F 1988 Pharmacokinetics of xamoterol after intravenous and oral administration to volunteers. European Journal of Clinical Pharmacology 34: 469–473
2. Nuttall A, Snow H M 1982 The cardiovascular effects of ICI 118,587: a β1-adrenoceptor partial agonist. British Journal of Pharmacology 77: 381–388
3. Pouleur H, Van Mechelen H, Balasim H, Rousseau M F, Charlier A 1984 Comparisons of the inotropic effects of the β1-adrenoceptor partial agonist SL 75.177.10 and ICI 118.587 with digoxin in the intact canine heart. Journal of Cardiovascular Pharmacology 6: 720–726
4. Furlong R, Brogden R N 1988 Xamoterol: a preliminary review of its pharmacodynamic and pharmacokinetic properties and therapeutic use. Drugs 36: 455–474
5. de Feyter P J, Serruys P W, Suryapranatah (1990) Improvement of the left ventricular contractility and relaxation with the β_1-adrenergic partial agonist xamoterol at rest and during exercise in patients with postinfarction left ventricular dysfunction: a placebo-controlled randomized trial. Circulation 81: III.99–III.106
6. Jennings G, Bobik A, Oddie C, Restall R 1984 Cardioselectivity, kinetics, haemodynamics and metabolic effects of xamoterol. Clinical Pharmacology and Therapeutics 35: 594–603
7. Malta E, Mian M A, Raper C 1985 The in vitro pharmacology of xamoterol (ICI 118,587). British Journal of Pharmacology 85: 179–187
8. Sato H, Inoue M, Matsuyama R, Ozaki H, Shimazu T, Takeda H, Ishida Y, Kamada T 1987 Haemodynamic effects of β1-adrenoceptor partial agonist xamoterol in relation to plasma norepinephrine levels during exercise in patients with left ventricular dysfunction. Circulation 75: 213–220
9. Detry J M, Decoster P M, Brasseur L A 1983 Hemodynamic effects of 'Corwin' (ICI 118,587) a new cardioselective β-adrenoceptor partial agonist. European Heart Journal 4: 584–591
10. Kowalski M T, Haworth D, Lu X, Thomson D S, Barnett D B 1990 Comparison of the effects of xamoterol and isoprenaline on rat cardiac β-adrenoceptors: studies of function and regulation. British Journal of Pharmacology 99: 27–30
11. Harry J D, Marlow H F, Wardleworth A G, Young J 1981 The action of ICI 118,587 (a β-adrenoceptor partial agonist) on the heart rate response to exercise in man. British Journal of Clinical Pharmacology 12: 266P
12. Pouleur H, van Eyll C, Cheron P, Hanet C, Charlier A A, Rousseau M F 1986 Changes in left ventricular filling dynamics after long-term xamoterol therapy in ischemic left ventricular dysfunction. Heart Failure 2: 176–184
13. Marlow H F, Wardleworth A G, Booth L M 1983 The hemodynamic effects of oral doses of ICI 118,587, a β-adrenoceptor partial agonist, in healthy volunteers. British Journal of Clinical Pharmacology 13: 269P–270P
14. Molajo A O, Bennett D H, Marlow H F, Snow H M, Bastain W 1987 The effects and dose–response relationship of xamoterol in patients with ischaemic heart disease. British Journal of Clinical Pharmacology 24: 373–379
15. Marten T R, Bourne G R, Miles G S, Shuker B, Rankine H D, Dutka V N 1984 The metabolism of ICI 118,587, a partial agonist of β1-adrenoceptors, in mice, rats, rabbits, dogs and humans. Drug Metabolism and Disposition 12: 652–660
16. Vigholt Sorensen E, Faergeman O, Day M, Bastain W 1988 Pharmacokinetics of xamoterol after intravenous and oral administration to patients with chronic heart failure. European Journal of Clinical Pharmacology 35: 183–185
17. Scott A K, Webster J, Petrie J C, Bastain W 1988 The effect of age and cardiac failure on xamoterol pharmacokinetics. British Journal of Clinical Pharmacology 25: 165–168
18. Blackwood R, Marlow H F 1988 Xamoterol in the management of patients with exertional breathlessness and fatigue due to cardiac disease. Journal of the American College of Cardiologists: 11 143A
19. Wray R and the European 'Corwin' Study Group 1988 The efficacy of xamoterol ('Corwin') in elderly patients with heart failure. European Heart Journal 9 (suppl A): 171
20. Timewell R M, Stark R D, Marlow H F and the European 'Corwin' Study Group 1988 Xamoterol monotherapy in heart failure. European Heart Journal 9 (suppl A): 301, 1708
21. Lofdahl C G, Svedmyr N 1984 Effects of xamoterol (ICI 118,587) in asthmatic patients. British Journal of Clinical Pharmacology 18: 597–601
22. Lammers J W, Muller M E, Folgering H R, Van Herwaarden C L 1986 A comparative study on the ventilatory and hemodynamic effects of xamoterol and atenolol in asthmatic patients. British Journal of Clinical Pharmacology 22: 595–602

23. Amende I, Simon R, Hood W P, Lichtlen P R 1986 Die akute Wirkung des Kardioselectiven β_1-partiellen Agonisten, Corwin, auf die Ventrikel funktion und den Myokardialen Sauerstoffverbrauch bei Patienten mit dilativer Kardiomyopathie. Z Kardiol 75: 291–295
24. Lemoine H, Bilski A, Kaumann A J 1989 Xamoterol activates β_1 but not β_2 adrenoceptors in mammalian myocardium: comparison of its affinity for β_1 and β_2 adrenoceptors coupled to the adenylate cyclase in feline and human ventricle with positive inotropic effects. Journal of Cardiovascular Pharmacology 13: 105–117
25. Molajo A O, Bennett D G 1985 Effect of xamoterol (ICI 118 587), a new β_1-adrenoceptor partial agonist, on resting haemodynamic variables and exercise tolerance in patients with left ventricular dysfunction. British Heart Journal 54: 17–21
26. Kayanakis J G, Snow M 1987 One year of Corwin therapy in cardiac failure. Cardiovascular Drugs Therapy 1: 256
27. Ikäheimo M J, Takkunen J T 1984 The effects of β_1-adrenoceptor partial agonist ICI 118,587 on left ventricular function in patients with coronary heart disease. International Journal of Cardiology 5: 339–349
28. Simonsen S 1984 Haemodynamic effects of ICI 118.587 in cardiomyopathy. British Heart Journal 51: 654–657
29. James M A, Papouchado M, Channer K S et al 1990 The effects of oral dosing of xamoterol on systolic time intervals in man and xamoterol plasma concentrations in heart failure patients. British Journal of Clinical Pharmacology 29: 447–453
30. Detry J M, Kayanakis J G, Bounhoure J P, Drury V W M for the European Xamoterol Study Group 1989 Xamoterol in patients with heart failure. European Heart Journal 10: abstract suppl, 385
31. Pouleur H, Rousseau M F, Hanet C, Marlow H F, Charlier A A 1987 Left ventricular sensitivity to β-adrenoceptor stimulating drugs in patients with ischemic heart disease and varying degrees of ventricular dysfunction. Circulation Research 61: 191–195
32. Marlow H F, Green F L, Snow H M, Pouleur H, Rousseau M F 1990 Relationship between positive inotropic responses and plasma concentrations of xamoterol in middle-aged and elderly patients. British Journal of Clinical Pharmacology 29: 511–518
33. Pouleur H, Etienne J, Van Mechelen H, Gurné O, Rousseau M F 1990 Effects of the β_1-adrenoceptor partial agonist xamoterol on the left ventricular diastolic function: an evaluation after 1 to 6 years of oral therapy. Circulation 81: I1187–I1192
34. Nicholls D P, Taggart A J, McCann J P, Bastain W, Shanks R G 1989 The pharmacokinetics of Xamoterol in liver disease. British Journal of Clinical Pharmacology 28: 718–721

Xipamide

Xipamide is a mono-sulphonamide derivative related to the benzothiadiazine or 'thiazide' diuretics. It was synthesized by Beiersdorf laboratories in Hamburg, Germany and introduced into clinical medicine in 1971.

Chemistry

Xipamide (Diurexan, Aquaphor, Aquaphoril, Altinol, Acturin, Diurex, Demiax, Lumitens, Chronexan, Xipamid, Hypotensin)
$C_{15}H_{15}ClN_2O_4S$
4-Chloro-5-sulphamoyl-2′,6′-salicyloxylidide

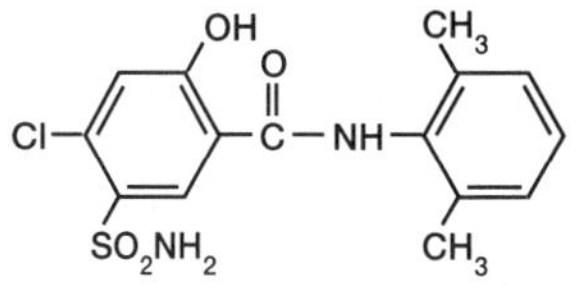

Molecular weight	354.8
pKa (phenol, sulphonamide)	4.8, 10.0
Solubility	
in alcohol	1:10–1:30
in water	insoluble
Octanol/water partition coefficient	21

Xipamide is a lipophilic substance which is stable in acid and also in basic solutions at room temperature. It is prepared by chemical synthesis. In the presence of strong alkaline conditions, the molecule is hydrolysed to form 2,6-xylidine.[1]

Commercially available combinations of xipamide include: xipamide, 4 mg/reserpine 0.1 mg (Durotan, FRG); xipamide, 10 mg/triamterene 30 mg (Neotri, FRG; Epitens, Egypt); and xipamide, 10 mg/propranolol 40 mg (Beta-Xipamide, India).

Xipamide is a xylidine derivative of hydroxy-chlorsulphonamide and differs from the benzothiadiazine diuretics in containing only one sulphamoyl radical and no benzothiadiazine heterocycle. Its closest chemical relative is clopamide, which differs only in the additional presence of a hydroxyl (OH) group at position 6 of the sulphonamide-containing ring and the second ring being xylidine in xipamide and piperidine in clopamide.

Pharmacology

Dose–response studies over the range 0.001–200 $mg.kg^{-1}$ in the rat, and over the range 0.04–10.00 $mg.kg^{-1}$ in the beagle, have shown that xipamide is an effective saluretic in these species. The saluretic responses occur with insignificant changes in urinary pH or glomerular filtration rate as measured by inulin clearance.[2]

In rats with experimental renal hypertension, significant lowering of blood pressure was seen with xipamide at doses of 1.0 and 5.0 $mg.kg^{-1}$.

Micropuncture studies in the rat have localized the site of action of xipamide within the nephron to the early part of the distal tubule.[3] The I_{50} for inhibition of carbonic anhydrase is 1.1×10^{-5}M, a concentration of similar magnitude to that found with classical benzothiadiazines.[4]

Studies of ion fluxes in human red cells have shown that xipamide has little affinity for the bumetanide-sensitive Na,Cl,K — co-transport system characteristically inhibited by loop diuretics. Xipamide, however, inhibits substantially at low concentrations the HCO_3^-/Cl^- anion exchanger ($IC_{50} = 17 \pm 5$ $\mu mol.l^{-1}$).[5] It is thus

Xipamide

possible that the molecular action of xipamide in the early part of the distal nephron may involve the inhibition of such a parallel anion exchanger system.

Toxicology

There are no published reports of toxicological findings in animals given xipamide acutely and long-term, that have potential clinical relevance. The oral LD_{50} for the mouse, rat and dog[2], was found to lie between 1500 and 1810 $mg.kg^{-1}$.

No teratogenic effects have been noted in rats or rabbits.

Clinical pharmacology

Saluretic action

Acute dose–response studies[6] over the range 0.035–0.750 $mg.kg^{-1}$ have shown a progressive saluresis which tends to plateau at a dose level of about 0.125 $mg.kg^{-1}$. The maximum saluretic effect occurred within the first 12 hours, with a pattern of ion excretion that resembles that of classical benzothiadiazines.[4] In a multiple dose–response study where xipamide was given in repeated doses daily over 15-day periods in randomized fashion, maximal saluresis was achieved at the 5 mg dose; higher doses up to 40 mg daily were associated with no further augmentation of the saluretic response but caused significant development of hypokalaemic alkalosis. All doses caused a significant elevation of total blood cholesterol, but left serum triglycerides unchanged.[7]

In a single-dose comparative study, 10 mg xipamide gave equivalent saluretic responses to 50 mg hydrochlorothiazide when both drugs were studied in a group of 10 healthy human subjects.[8] In another study where both 5 and 10 mg doses of xipamide were studied, both doses yielded similar saluretic responses to 50 mg hydrochlorothiazide.[9]

Despite these indications that maximal saluresis in healthy subjects is achieved at about the 5 mg dosage, the recommended daily dosage for oedema is 20–80 mg daily with a starting dose of 40 mg daily. There have been several published studies reporting clinical uses of 40 and 80 mg daily in treatment of oedema.[10]

Clearance experiments in man under conditions of maximal water diuresis and also in hydropenia have confirmed a site of action for xipamide in the early distal nephron.[11]

Antihypertensive action

Dose–response studies in hypertension have shown that, as with conventional benzothiadiazines, the relationship is flat, with occurrence of a plateau at about the 10–20 mg daily dose level.[6,12,13] The availability of only a 20 mg tablet as the lowest commercially available dose of xipamide has been criticized,[13] since it appears that lower doses may be equally efficacious in lowering blood pressure but may lack the propensity for producing adverse metabolic sequelae. Even with a daily dose of 20 mg xipamide, significant hypokalaemia has been noted in chronic treatment.[14]

Continued treatment with the higher doses of xipamide is associated with reduced urinary excretion of calcium, a feature common to all benzothiadiazines.[6] The higher dose schedules usually result in occurrence of hypokalaemic alkalosis, though there have been reports from some countries where chronic therapy with 40 mg daily has not caused significant hypokalaemia.[15]

Pharmacokinetics

The pharmacokinetics of xipamide have been studied using ^{32}S-labelled drug[18] and also using a densito-fluorimetric method where xipamide is complexed with a fluorescent aromatic reagent to form a benzylpyran-benzylsulphonamide derivative.[19] In addition, HPLC techniques for assaying xipamide have been developed and validated[20,21,22] and these are the currently preferred analytical methods; limit of assay is 100 $\mu g.l^{-1}$.

After 80 mg oral dosing, xipamide is rapidly absorbed with maximal plasma concentrations being attained in 30–60 min and a C_{max} of 15–20 $mg.l^{-1}$. By 48 h, approximately 80% of the oral dose is excreted unchanged in the urine. The mean plasma half life after intravenous administration of ^{35}S-xipamide has been reported as 5.0 h and a similar value has been obtained after 20 mg xipamide given orally in healthy volunteers;[18,20] in two patients with renal failure, the mean plasma half life of the drug was 22.2 h.[18]

Comparison of the AUC after oral and intravenous administration of xipamide, 20 mg in healthy volunteers has yielded a bioavailability estimate for the drug of 73%.[23] Estimates of V_d range from 15 to 21 litres;[18,23] the drug is 99% bound to plasma protein.

Oral absorption	73%
Presystemic metabolism	—
Plasma half life	
range	5.0±0.5 h
Volume of distribution	15–21 l
Plasma protein binding	99%

Concentration–effect relationship

There is no evidence for any correlation between the plasma concentration of xipamide and its therapeutic effects.

Metabolism

Xipamide is conjugated to form a more polar xipamide-O-glucuronide metabolite. During the first 48 h after dosing, approximately 50% of an oral dose is excreted as unchanged xipamide and approximately 30% as conjugated glucuronide (Fig. 1).

Fig. 1 The metabolism of xipamide

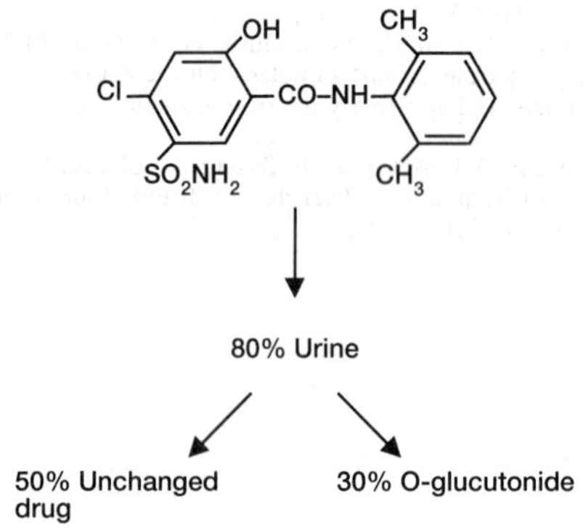

Pharmaceutics

Xipamide is only available in the oral form. There is no parenteral dosage form. The tablet, which contains 20 mg xipamide, is white, round with bisecting score on one side and debossed 'A' on the other side; diameter is 6 mm. It is stable for 5 years and there are no special storage conditions.

Therapeutic use

Indications

1. Hypertension
2. Treatment of oedema.

Contraindications

1. Hypersensitivity to drugs of sulphonamide structure
2. Severe renal failure
3. Severe hepatic failure
4. Use in pregnancy should be avoided.

Precautions

Despite the absence of any animal evidence of teratogenicity, xipamide should be avoided in pregnancy. In any event, hypovolaemia and increased plasma viscosity secondary to sustained saluretic effects may jeopardize placental function.

Mode of use

Xipamide should be taken by mouth after breakfast with some fluid.

Indications

1. Hypertension

Xipamide is an effective antihypertensive diuretic with a flat dose response curve. The manufacturers recommend 20 mg daily as the usual antihypertensive dose. From the published evidence of comparative efficacy of different doses of xipamide, it would appear that 10 mg daily is just as effective as 20 mg or higher dosage. The few studies that have been carried out of lower doses of 5 mg daily have suggested that these may be inadequate for clinical purposes.[6] In a study employing ambulatory intra-arterial monitoring of blood pressure, it has been shown that once-daily dosing with xipamide produced effective control of blood pressure throughout the 24 hour period.[14] Reyes and Leary (1981) carried out a mathematical analysis of the time sequence of response to initiation of xipamide therapy in a group of hypertensive patients treated over 4 months with a mean dose of approximately 24 mg xipamide daily. The analysis showed that xipamide, in the doses used, caused a rapid initial fall in systemic blood pressure followed by a more gradual degree of sustained reduction in blood pressure thereafter. This mathematical modelling of response was found to differ from the more gradual initiation of antihypertensive action and subsequent linear decline in blood pressure seen with classical benzothiadiazines such as hydrochlorothiazide or cyclothiazide.[16,17] Detailed discussion of individual published clinical trials of xipamide is to be found in the review article by Prichard and Brodgen (1985).

Addition of xipamide, 20–40 mg daily, to existing antihypertensive regimens consisting of β-blockers where the latter treatment was proving inadequate, has resulted in significant further falls in supine and standing blood pressure.[24,25] However, there appears to be no special advantage of xipamide over a small dose of, for example, 5 mg bendrofluazide.[23] In a double-blind, placebo-controlled study in eight subjects given 40 mg xipamide over 12 weeks superimposed on pre-existing therapy ranging from β blockade, the antihypertensive efficacy of xipamide was confirmed and a significant incidence of hypokalaemia was reported.[27]

The antihypertensive efficacy of xipamide, 20 mg, was found to be equivalent to indapamide, 2.5 mg, when given in single daily dosage in a double-blind randomized study of 3 months' duration in a group of 44 hypertensive patients.[28] An open multicentre study in general practice, including over 4000 patients, has shown effective antihypertensive activity and good patient tolerance of xipamide in a daily dose of 20 mg given as monotherapy or in combined use with either methyldopa or β-blockers over a period of 2 months.[29]

2. Oedema

As with all benzothiadiazine and thiazide-like drugs, xipamide is unsuitable for treatment of acute left ventricular failure and pulmonary oedema. In all other forms of oedema, xipamide can effect a sustained diuresis which may persist for 12 h or longer. The manufacturers recommend 40 mg daily as an initial dose in oedema, and, depending on the response, suggest that the dose can be subsequently lowered to 20 mg daily as maintenance therapy. In the continued management of mild to moderate cardiac failure, it is important not to precipitate powerful and sustained diuresis which merely leads to excessive neurohumoral responses of a compensatory nature. These compensatory changes mainly involve the renin–angiotensin–aldosterone (RAA) system and encourage substantial renal losses of potassium.

A more appropriate method of using such diuretics as xipamide is by the introduction of much smaller doses, e.g. 10 mg daily, to which could be added a small dose of an ACE inhibitor under carefully controlled conditions. This approach avoids reliance on progressive increase in the diuretic dose on its own as a primary means of controlling cardiac failure. It also minimizes or blocks the compensatory responses of the RAA system and prevents the occurrence of adverse electrolyte disturbances.

Adverse reactions

Potentially life-threatening effects

The most commonly noted metabolic derangement that has been noted has been hypokalaemia, and the variation in extent to which this has been a problem seems to have depended on the dosage of xipamide used, the length of therapy and the geographical location of the study, the last possibly reflecting differences in dietary intake of potassium.

The extent of the hypokalaemia has in some cases been very striking — 13 out of 14 hypertensive patients treated by MacGregor et al (1982)[13] with xipamide, 20 mg daily for 6 weeks, had a plasma potassium of less than 3.5 mmol.l^{-1}. In the absence of greater antihypertensive or saluretic efficacy at higher dosages, this evidence has been used to argue for greater use of lower dosages of xipamide in routine clinical practice. The mechanisms involved in causation of the metabolic sequelae of xipamide therapy are the same as those generated by other thiazide-like agents. The carbohydrate intolerance has been linked to decreased insulin secretion by the pancreatic beta cells and decreased tissue sensitivity to insulin; these effects may be due to direct action of the diuretic molecule or occur through diuretic-induced potassium depletion.[32] Several studies have shown dose-related worsening of hypokalaemia with increasing doses of xipamide. These electrolyte changes have occurred without any concomitant increase in the antihypertensive efficacy of the drug, supporting the view that as with all thiazide-like agents, xipamide should be used in the lowest effective dose in order to minimize occurrence of adverse biochemical changes. Hyperuricaemia, like hypokalaemia, appears to relate to the intensity of renal sodium loss evoked by xipamide. Whether the inconsistent lipid changes are also dose-related is unclear, but findings with subsaluretic dosages of other thiazide diuretics seem to indicate that this is the case.[33]

Acute overdosage

There are no reported instances of deliberate overdosage with xipamide.

Severe or irreversible adverse effects

Magnesium wastage, disturbed glucose tolerance and hyperuricaemia, have all been reported with long-term use of xipamide.[26]

Symptomatic adverse effects

Xipamide, like all thiazide-like saluretics, is a well-tolerated drug. The subjective adverse effects that have been reported include dizziness and vertigo which are likely to relate to the extent of the induced fall in blood pressure. In most instances, such symptoms have been mild and have not necessitated withdrawal of therapy. The importance of including placebo responses when assessing the significance of alleged drug-related symptoms is highlighted in the multicentre study reported by Weber et al (1977), who noted that headache occurred in 10 patients receiving placebo; in five patients treated with xipamide (20 mg daily) and in six patients treated with xipamide in the higher dose of 40 mg daily.[12] Nocturia can be a troublesome feature of long-acting thiazide therapy and occurs with xipamide. It is not often reported in published papers, but was noted in a significant proportion of hypertensive patients treated with xipamide, 20 mg daily, in a comparative trial with another long-acting thiazide-like agent, chlorthalidone, 50 mg daily.[30]

Other effects

Changes in plasma lipids have been followed in very few published studies and where they have, the findings have not always been consistent. In a study of 12 hypertensive patients given increasing doses of xipamide up to a maximum of 40 mg daily, Owens et al (1989) reported significant increases in plasma VLDL and also triglycerides at the maximum dose level of diuretic used.[6]

Interference with clinical pathology tests

No technical interferences of this kind appear to have been reported.

High risk groups

Neonates

No information is available on the use of the drug in neonates.

Breast milk. It is not known if xipamide enters breast milk, so it is best avoided by nursing mothers.

Children

No information is available on the use of the drug in children.

Pregnant women

Xipamide is best avoided in the management of hypertension or oedema of pregnancy (see Contraindications above).

The elderly

Diuretics in low dose are effective and relatively safe in managing hypertension and cardiac failure in the elderly. With xipamide, the lowest dose that is available for use is 10 mg (i.e. $\frac{1}{2} \times 20$ mg). This daily dose should not be exceeded in elderly patients, particularly since the dietary intake of potassium is often deficient in this age group.

Drug interactions

Potentially hazardous interactions
The propensity of high-dose xipamide to cause hypokalaemia has particular relevance to patients stabilized on a cardiac glycoside, since the actions of the latter are exaggerated in these circumstances. Patients on corticosteroids will be more vulnerable to xipamide-induced hypokalaemia.

Potentially useful interactions
These and other clinically relevant interactions common to all thiazide-like agents also have applicability to xipamide.

Clinical trials

The review articles by Prichard and Brogden (1985) and Kramer and Risler (1988) both give detailed analyses of the various clinical trials that have been carried out with xipamide.

A number of key studies are summarized below:

1. Weber J C P, Bird H, Cosh J et al 1977 Once daily treatment of mild to moderate hypertension with xipamide: a controlled study. British Journal of Clinical Pharmacology 4: 283–288

This is a double-blind, placebo-controlled, crossover trial of xipamide, 20 and 40 mg, compared with each other and with a placebo. 48 patients (mean age, 50 y) were studied, with DBP between 95 and 120 mmHg at point of entry. Each treatment period was 4 weeks in duration.

Results showed that both doses of xipamide produced falls in blood pressure that were statistically significant when compared to placebo but there was no significant differences between the effects of the two doses of xipamide. No serious side effects were seen, but xipamide at both doses caused hypokalaemia.

2. Leary W P, Asmal A C, Williams P C, Herron M 1978 Treatment of uncomplicated essential hypertension with xipamide. Current Therapeutic Research 24: 884–888

This is a double-blind study in 200 patients (mean age, 40 y) comparing the effects of xipamide, 20–40 mg, with those of placebo over a period of 6 months. DBP at entry to the study was 90–120 mmHg.

Results showed a significant fall in systolic and diastolic blood pressure. Changes in plasma urate, potassium and glucose were slight but consistent with those encountered with thiazide diuretics.

3. MacGregor G A, Banks R A, Markandu N D, Roulston J 1982 Xipamide and cyclopenthiazide in essential hypertension — comparative effects on blood pressure and plasma potassium. British Journal of Clinical Pharmacology 13: 859–863

This is a randomized crossover trial of xipamide and cyclopenthiazide in a group of 14 patients (mean age, 47 y) with supine DBP on entry of 97–130 mmHg who were treated for periods of 6 weeks with each diuretic.

Results showed that xipamide, either 10 or 20 mg, once daily, was as effective in lowering supine blood pressure as was daily cyclopenthiazide, 0.5 mg. By the sixth week of treatment, 13/14 patients on xipamide but only 6/14 patients on cyclopenthiazide had plasma potassium concentrations of 3.5 $mmol.l^{-1}$ or less.

4. Baehre M, Mimran A, Orsetti A, Mion C 1989 Double-blind, randomized, multicenter study of the safety and antihypertensive efficacy of xipamide vs indapamide. Current Therapeutic Research 46: 484–494

This is a double-blind randomized trial comparing xipamide, 20 mg per day, with indapamide, 2.5 mg per day. Three alternating month treatments followed a 1-month placebo run-in period. 52 patients (mean age, 56 y) were studied with blood pressure at entry equal or greater than 160/90 mmHg.

Results showed that the antihypertensive effect of xipamide was comparable to that of indapamide; clinical tolerability of both drugs was good. The results of the detailed biochemical monitoring undertaken are not reported, but four patients on xipamide and three on indapamide developed a significant hypokalaemia.

General review articles

1. 1975 Pharmacodynamic actions and toxicology of xipamide, 4-chlor-5-sulfamoyl-2',6'-salicyloxylidid. A series of original articles in German, each with a short English summary. Arzneimittelforschung 25 (2): 245–255
2. 1977 Chemistry and pharmacokinetics of xipamide, a two-part original article in German with a short English summary. Arzneimittelforschung 27 (11): 2140–2151
3. Prichard B N C, Brogden R N 1985 Xipamide: a review of its pharmacodynamic and pharmacokinetic properties and therapeutic efficacy. Drugs 30: 313–332
4. Kramer B K, Risler T 1988 Xipamide. Cardiovascular Drug Reviews 6: 141–154. A review article covering all the major publications on xipamide and including a detailed tabulated analysis of all clinical trials with the drug in hypertension and oedema.

References

1. Hempelmann F W 1977 Untersuchungen mit Xipamid (4-chlor-5-sulfamoyl-2',6'-salicyloxylidid). Teil I: Physikalisch-chemische und chemische Eigenschaften. Arzneimittelforschung 27: 2140–2143
2. Leuschner F, Neumann W, Bahrmann H 1975 Pharmakologische und toxikologische Eigneschaften des Saluretikums Xipamid (4-chlor-5-sulfamoyl-2',6'-salicyloxylidid). Arzneimittelforschung 25: 245–251
3. Deetjen P, Hardt K, Haberle D, Silbernagel S, Lingelbach W, Kuschinsky W 1968 Mikropunktionsuntersuchungen zur Wirkung des Saluretikums Xipamid. In: Proceedings of the Travemunde Symposium on: Klinische Pharmakologie der Diuretika. Urban & Schwarzenberg, Berlin, pp 208–212
4. Hempelmann F W, Leuschner F, Liebenow W 1975 die saluretische Wirkung von Xipamid (4-chlor-5-sulfamoyl-2',6'-salicyloxylidid) bei gesunden Probanden. Arzneimittelforschung 25: 252–255
5. Diez J, Esparza H, Arrazola A 1990 Molecular actions of not carboxylic acid loop diuretics. In: Diuretics III — Chemistry, Pharmacology and Clinical Applications. Eds: J B Puschett and A Greenberg. Elsevier, New York, pp 218–219
6. Owens C W I, Tomlinson B, Liu J-B et al 1989 A log-dose–response study of xipamide and its effect on metabolic parameters. Journal of Hypertension 7 (suppl 6): S320–S321
7. Knauf H, Haase W, Mutschler E 1980 Dosis-Wirkungs-Beziehungen von Xipamid bei gesunden Probanden. Arzneimittelforschung 30: 1599–1607
8. Henness D M, Weng T S 1979 Single-dose evaluations of xipamide: a comparison study with furosemide and hydrochlorothiazide. Clinical Therapeutics 2: 277–286
9. Leary W P, Asmal A C 1978 Xipamide: diuretic effects of low dosage in healthy adults. Current Therapeutic Research 24: 656–661
10. Piyasena K H G, Havard C W H, Weber J C P 1975 Xipamid, a potent new diuretic. Current Medical Research and Opinion 3: 121–125
11. Gold C H, Viljoen M 1979 Site of renal action of xipamide. Clinical Pharmacology and Therapeutics 25: 522–527
12. Weber J C P, Bird H, Cosh J et al 1977 British Journal of Clinical Pharmacology 4: 283–288
13. MacGregor G A, Banks R A, Markandu N D, Roulston J 1982 Xipamide and cyclopenthiazide in essential hypertension — comparative effects on blood pressure and plasma potassium. British Journal of Clinical Pharmacology 13: 859–863
14. Raftery E B, Melville D I, Gould B A, Mann S, Whittington J R 1981 A study of the antihypertensive action of xipamide using ambulatory intra-arterial monitoring. British Journal of Clinical Pharmacology 12: 381–385
15. Ktenas J A, Aravanis C 1980 Antihypertensive action of a new compound, xipamid. Current Therapeutic Research 28: 543–548
16. Reyes A J, Leary W P 1981 A formal method for the therapeutic classification of antihypertensive diuretics. Current Therapeutic Research 30: 1073–1088
17. Reyes A J, Acosta-Barrios T N, Leary W P 1981 The effects of xipamide upon high blood pressure in geriatric hypertensives: a mathematical description. Current Therapeutic Research 30: 1089–1095
18. Hempelmann F W, Dicker P 1977 Untersuchungen mit Xipamid (4-chlor-5-sulfamoyl-2',6'-salicyloxyldid). Teil II: Pharmakokinetik beim Menschen. Arzneimittelforschung 27: 2143–2151
19. Sobel M, Mutschler E 1980 Fluorimetrische Bestimmung von Xipamid in biologischem Material mit einem neuen Fluoreszenzreagenz. Journal of Chromatography 183: 124–130
20. Diembeck W, Dies R, Heinz N 1982 Pharmacokinetik von Xipamid und Triamteren bei gesunden Probanden. Arzneimittelforschung 32: 1482–1485
21. Sanz R T, Sadana G S, Bhounsule G J, Gaonkar M V, Nadkani A D, Nayak V G 1986 High-performance liquid chromatographic determination of xipamide and clopamide in pharmaceuticals. Journal of Chromatography 356: 468–472
22. Dadgar D, Kelly M 1988 High-performance liquid chromatographic determination of xipamide in human plasma. Analyst 113: 229–231
23. Knauf H, Mutschler E 1984 Pharmacodynamics and pharmacokinetics of xipamide in patients with normal and impaired kidney function. European Journal of Clinical Pharmacology 26: 513–520
24. Davies P S, Prichard B N C 1975 A dose–response study of xipamid in hypertension used in combination with other anti-hypertensive drugs. Journal of International Medical Research 3: 389–394
25. Dean S, Kendall M J, Potter S, Thompson M H, Jackson D A 1984 Nadolol in combination with indapamide and xipamide in resistant hypertensives. European Journal of Clinical Pharmacology 28: 29–33

26. Ramsay L E, Freestone S 1984 Xipamide: no advantage over bendrofluazide in hypertension. British Journal of Clinical Pharmacology 18: 616–618
27. Harding R D, Kalos A, Weber J C P, Dixon A St J 1974 Treatment of hypertension with xipamid — a new diuretic. Clinical Trials Journal (London) 11: 45–48
28. Baehre M, Mimran A, Orsetti A, Mion C 1989 Double-blind, randomized, multicenter study of the safety and antihypertensive efficacy of xipamide vs indapamide. Current Therapeutic Research 46: 484–494
29. Baehre M, Grimshaw J J 1988 The use of xipamide in antihypertensive therapy in general practice: a large multicenter study. Current Therapeutic Research 44: 737–743
30. Dies R, Heinz N 1978 Therapie der essentiellen Hypertonie mit Xipamid und Chlorthalidon. Klinikartz 7: 571–576
31. Heimsoth V H 1977 Studies covering combined treatments with xipamide. Results of a long-term antihypertensive treatment. International Journal of Clinical Pharmacology 15: 260–266
32. Helderman H J, Elahi D, Anderson D K 1983 Prevention of the glucose intolerance of thiazide diuretics by maintenance of body potassium. Diabetes 32: 106
33. Carlsen J E, Kóber L, Torp-Pedersen C, Johansen P 1990 Relation between dose of bendrofluazide, antihypertensive effect, and adverse biochemical effects. British Medical Journal 300: 975–978

Xylitol

Xylitol is a polyalcohol present as a natural substance in some berries and fruit. It is used as a carbohydrate source for parenteral nutrition in continental Europe, especially West Germany, but is not used clinically in the UK, USA or Australia. Its properties and its clinical use after trauma have been the subject of an extensive review.[1]

Chemistry

Xylitol
$C_5H_{12}O_5$

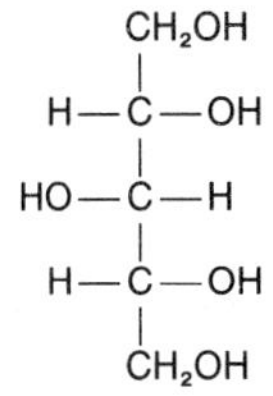

Molecular weight	152.1
pKa	13.7
Solubility	
in alcohol	1 in 83
in water	soluble
Octanol/water partition coefficient	—

Xylitol is an odourless, white hygroscopic crystalline powder.

Xylitol is a five-carbon polyalcohol which yields 4.06 kcal.g^{-1}. A 4.56% solution is physiologically isotonic. It has about the same sweetening power as sucrose, and is a common additive to foods. It is naturally present in fruit and vegetables including plums, strawberries, raspberries and cauliflower.

Pharmacokinetics

Xylitol can be measured in biological fluids by a colorimetric method employing sorbitol dehydrogenase,[3] or, after silylation, by gas chromatography.[2]

About 20% of an orally administered dose of xylitol is absorbed. Absorbtion is slow and the majority of the dose reaches the large intestine where it is extensively metabolized by the intestinal microflora. About 5–15 g are synthesized daily by humans. Premature infants are said to be able to metabolize it.[1]

Metabolism

Xylitol is metabolized mainly in the liver (70–80%) via xylulose and the pentose monophosphate and glucuronic acid pathways of carbohydrate metabolism. (See Fig.1.) Alternative routes of metabolism have been suggested based on a proposed overload of the transketolase reaction during infusions of 0.25 g.kg^{-1} body weight per hour.[4]

At this rate of infusion over a period of 20 hours, xylitol administration results in a rise in urinary excretion of glycolate by two or three orders of magnitude, but neither hyperoxalaemia nor hyperoxaluria was observed in patients without renal failure.[4] In rats, more than 85% of ^{14}C-xylitol appears as glucose within 30 minutes.[5]

Therapeutic use

Clinical use of xylitol has declined because of reports of renal failure, lactic acidosis, liver injury, changes in the level of consciousness with focal neurological signs and hyperuricaemia during clinical usage at dose levels of above 2.1 mmol.kg^{-1}.h^{-1} and especially above 3 mmol.kg^{-1}.h^{-1}

Fig. 1 The metabolism of xylitol

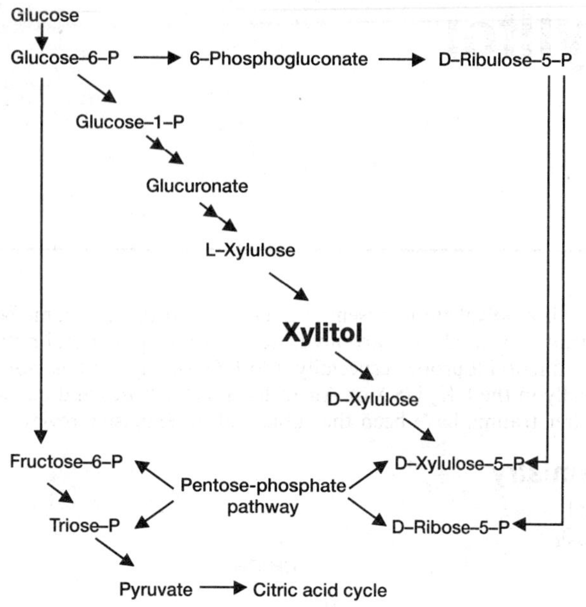

(315 to 456 mg.kg^{-1}.h^{-1}). Calcium oxalate crystals were found in renal tubules and in the wall of an artery in the midbrain.[6,7]

Continued clinical intravenous use[1,8,9] is principally in low dosage (250 mg.kg^{-1}.h^{-1}) combined with other sugars, particularly glucose and fructose. Proponents of its use justify such regimens in the post-traumatic period, when there is insulin resistance, on the basis that they give rise to less hyperglycaemia and hyperinsulinaemia.

(See also Glucose monograph).

General review articles

Ritzel G, Brubacher G (eds) 1976 Monosaccharides and polyalcohols in nutrition, therapy and dietetics. International Journal for Vitamin and Nutrition Research 15

Counsell J N (ed) 1978 Xylitol. Applied Science Publishers Ltd, London

Makinen K K 1978 Biochemical principles of the use of xylitol in medicine and nutrition with special consideration of dental aspects. Experientia (suppl) 30:

Bar A, Ritzel G (eds) 1985 Xyliton and oxalate. International Journal for Vitamin and Nutrition Research, suppl 28

Bar A, 1986 Xylitol. In: Alternative Sweeteners. Nabors L O, Gelhard R C (eds) Marcel Dekker, NewYork. pp 185 – 215

Bar A, 1991 Xylitol in Alternative Sweeteners (2nd Edition) Nabors L O, Gelard R C (eds) Marcel Dekker. New York

References

1. Georgieff M, Moldawer L L, Bistrian B R, Blackburn G L 1985 Xylitol and energy source for intravenous nutrition after trauma. Journal of Parenteral and Enteral Nutrition 9: 199–209
2. Mäkinen K K, Ylikahri R, Soderling E, Scheinin A, Mäkinen P L 1982 Turku sugar studies XXII. A re-examination of the subjects. International Journal for Vitamin and Nutrition Research (suppl 22): 9–27
3. Elphick M D, Dougall A J, Wilkinson A W 1972 The utilization of solutions of glucose and xylitol administered by intravenous infusion to neonatal surgical patients. In: Wilkinson A W (ed) Parenteral nutrition. Churchill Livingstone, Edinburgh
4. Hauschildt S, Chalmers R A, Lawson A M, Schultis K, Watts R W E 1976 Metabolic investigations after xylitol infusion in human subjects. American Journal of Clinical Nutrition 29: 258–273
5. Bassler K H, Bickel H 1972 The use of carbohydrates alone and in combination in parenteral nutrition. In: Wilkinson, A W (ed) Parenteral nutrition. Churchill Livingstone, Edinburgh
6. Thomas D W, Edwards J B, Gilligan J E, Lawrence J R, Edwards R G 1972 Complications following intravenous administration of solutions containing xylitol. Medical Journal of Australia 1: 1238–1246
7. Thomas D W, Gilligan J E, Edwards J B, Edwards R G 1972 Lactic acidosis and osmotic diuresis produced by xylitol infusion. Medical Journal of Australia 1: 1246–1248
8. Leutenegger A F, Goschke J, Stutz K et al 1977 Comparison between glucose and a combination of glucose, fructose and xylitol as carbohydrates for total parenteral nutrition of surgical intensive care patients. American Journal of Surgery 133: 199–205
9. Ladefoged K, Berthelsen P, Brockner-Nielsen, Jarnum S, Larsen V 1982 Fructose, xylitol and glucose in total parenteral nutrition. Intensive Care Medicine 8: 19–23

Xylometazoline hydrochloride

Xylometazoline is a nasal decongestant.

Chemistry

Xylometazoline hydrochloride (Otrix, Otrivine, Sinex Long Acting, 4-way, Long Acting Synephrine)

$C_{16}H_{24}N_2.HCl$

2-(4-tert-Butyl-2,6-dimethylbenzyl)-2-imidazoline hydrochloride

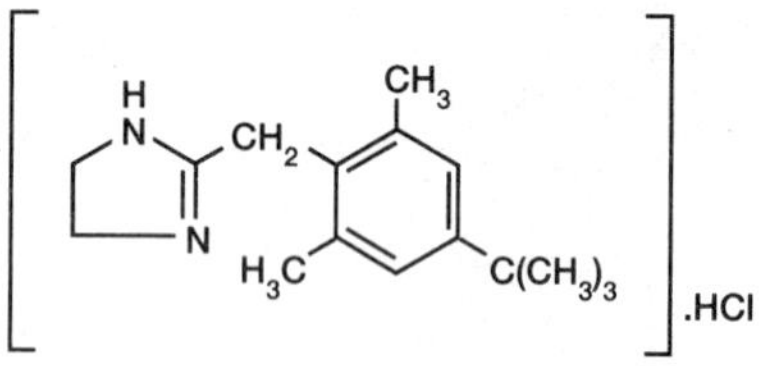

Molecular weight	280.8 (244.4)
pKa	—
Solubility	
in alcohol	1 in 4
in water	1 in 12
Octanol/water partition coefficient	—

Xylometazoline hydrochloride is a white or almost white, odourless, crystalline powder prepared by chemical synthesis. It is also available in combination with sodium cromoglycate as Rynacrom Compound.

Pharmacology

Xylometazoline is a sympathomimetic amine of the imidazoline class.[1,2] It is a direct agonist at α_2-adrenoceptors and has no action on β-adrenoceptors. Xylometazoline has no action on the uptake mechanism for catecholamines. Unlike phenylephrine, xylometazoline does not cause mydriasis. Given systemically xylometazoline, like other α_2-adrenergic agonists such as clonidine, causes CNS effects including sedation, dryness of the mouth and sweating, but these are rarely seen since the drug in practice is only used topically.

Toxicology

When administered systemically (e.g. experimentally in animals), the adverse effects are those of sympathetic stimulation including hypertension and tachycardia, mydriasis and pilomotor excitation, which persist for a prolonged period.

Xylometazoline use in excess also causes sedation, especially in infants.

A quarter of the acute lethal dose in rabbits given experimentally was fatal in half the animals within 16 days but, in the same period, one tenth of the lethal dose was well-tolerated in experimental animals.

No carcinogenicity or teratogenicity tests have been reported.

Clinical pharmacology

Xylometazoline is used for its vasoconstrictor properties, acting as an α_2-agonist. It produces a rapid and prolonged vasoconstriction lasting for up to 8–12 h.[3] It is used as a topical agent on the nasal mucosa, to produce nasal decongestion. Prolonged use of xylometazoline on the nasal mucosa may produce rebound vasodilation (drug-induced rhinitis). This may be due to inhibition of the release of noradrenaline from vasomotor adrenergic nerve endings through an action on the presynaptic α-receptors. Given topically in small doses,

Xylometazoline hydrochloride

xylometazoline has no systemic effects in adults, although it is noteworthy that the hypotensive effect of clonidine, which has a similar action, was first noted when the drug was under trial as a nasal decongestant.

Pharmacokinetics

Local vasoconstriction is normally achieved within 5 to 10 minutes of intranasal administration. The effect persists for some time, variously quoted as 5 to 6 h.

When xylometazoline in solution is correctly instilled in the nose there is normally no significant systemic absorption; one reason for this is the vasoconstriction induced by the drug. Incorrect or excessive intranasal application may, however, lead to some of the drug being absorbed from the nasal mucosa or the gastrointestinal tract (after swallowing). Ingestion can provoke systemic effects, especially in young children and the elderly.

Little information is available at present concerning the distribution, metabolism and excretion of xylometazoline in man.

Concentration–effect relationship

There is no evidence of any correlation between the plasma concentration of xylometazoline and its therapeutic effects and this would be unlikely with a topically applied agent.

Metabolism

Nothing is known about the metabolism of xylometazoline.

Pharmaceutics

Xylometazoline is marketed under the trade name of Otrivine by Ciba-Geigy (UK/USA). Otrivine nasal drops and spray contain 0.1%; Otrivine paediatric nasal drops contain 0.05%.

Xylometazoline hydrochloride is found in combination with sodium cromoglycate as Rynacrom Compound (Fisons, UK) in a 0.025% concentration.

A 5% solution in water has a pH of 5 to 6.6; a 4.8% solution in water is iso-osmotic with serum.

Solutions of xylometazoline should be stored in airtight containers and protected from light. The remains of an opened packet should be discarded at the end of a course of treatment. Because of the risk of cross infection, two people should not share the same dropper or spray.

The maximum shelf-life for each formulation is 5 years.

Therapeutic use

Indications

1. As a nasal decongestant in allergic rhinitis: used with or without the addition of sodium cromoglycate
2. As a nasal decongestant in sinusitis where there is evidence of obstruction of the ostia of the sinuses
3. As a nasal decongestant in otitis media where there is evidence of obstruction of either eustachian tube, especially in acute serous otitis media ('glue ear') and otitic barotrauma
4. It may also be used as a decongestant in an infective rhinitis (e.g. an acute viral upper respiratory infection); but where there is a secondary bacterial infection there is no evidence of benefit
5. As an ocular decongestant in allergic conjunctivitis, whether associated with seasonal (hay-fever) or perennial allergy
6. To 'whiten' an inflamed ('red') eye caused by a local irritant such as dust following the removal of the foreign body.

Contraindications

Before xylometazoline drops are used in the eye it is essential to exclude any ocular pathology (e.g. infection or glaucoma) which may indicate the need for specific treatment.

1. The presence of narrow-angle glaucoma is an absolute contraindication
2. The use of xylometazoline should be avoided whilst the patient is being treated with monoamine oxidase inhibitors and for 14 days thereafter
3. The use of xylometazoline should be avoided in patients with vasomotor rhinitis because of the temptation to continue its use beyond two weeks
4. Its use is also not recommended in atrophic rhinitis and where there is a hypersensitivity to the drug
5. Because of the risk of some of the solution being swallowed, xylometazoline nasal drops and spray should not normally be used in patients for whom the systemic administration of α-sympathomimetic drugs may be contraindicated (e.g. coronary artery diseases, hypertension and diabetes mellitus).
6. Though no adverse effects have been reported, xylometazoline has not yet been shown to be safe in pregnancy. Similarly, in lactating mothers no adverse effects have been reported in the baby.

Mode of use

Dosage

Adults, including children over the age of 12 years: 2 to 3 drops or 2 to 3 squirts (of the spray) of either 0.05% of 0.1% solution in each nostril, repeated at intervals of 8 to 12 h if needed, never more than once in 4 h or thrice daily.

Children aged six months to 12 years: 2 to 3 drops of 0.05% solution. (The spray is not available in this strength, even if older children could use it.) The dose may be repeated at intervals of approximately 8 to 12 h.

Infants under the age of 6 months: one drop of the 0.05% solution in each nostril, usually administered 5 to 10 minutes before a feed.

Because of the rebound phenomenon, treatment at any age should normally not exceed 3 to 5 days. It should never continue for more than two weeks.

Method of administration

Drops. The nose should be cleared by blowing and the head inclined back as far as possible. 2 or 3 drops of the solution should be dropped into each nostril. The head and shoulders should then be brought forward slowly and moved from side to side. (If the patient is inexperienced in the use of nose drops, it is an advantage to have a second person apply the drops.)

Only the 0.05% drops should be used in children. The method of administration is otherwise the same as for adults.

Nasal sprays. These should not be used in children under the age of 12 (because it is only available in the 0.1% strength).

In adults the nose should first be cleaned. Then with the head tipped slightly forwards, the nebulizer should be inserted into each nostril in turn and squeezed. As the bottle is squeezed, the patient should be instructed to give a quick sniff.

Metered-dose spray. This may be used for xylometazoline with sodium cromoglycate, and may be used in children or adults. The manufacturers' recommended dose (at all ages) is one squeeze to each nostril 4 times a day. However, the action of xylometazoline lasts for 8–12 h; that of sodium cromoglycate is much shorter.

Dosage is not precise, particularly with the drops: some may be wasted by trickling out of the nose. The spray is too large to be used in small children as their nostrils are small.

Local vasoconstriction is normally achieved within 5 to 10 minutes of intranasal administration. The full effect lasts for 5 to 6 h and subsides gradually over the course of the next 6 h.

If some of the solution used as nasal drops is swallowed it could be absorbed in the gastrointestinal tract and may produce systemic sympathomimetic effects.

Adverse reactions

Potentially life-threatening effects

None is known.

Acute overdosage

Used correctly (i.e. as an intranasal application) the local vasoconstriction produced by the drug slows absorption and a systemic action is unlikely. If, however, some of the drops are swallowed they can be absorbed from the gastrointestinal tract and the systemic actions of a sympathomimetic drug can be produced.[4] This is most likely in children and has been reported most frequently in this age group.

An overdose, if swallowed and absorbed, has been reported to cause sedation.

Severe or irreversible adverse effects

Overuse is associated with a more persistent rhinitis related to the rebound phenomenon — the condition known as 'rhinitis medicamentosa'[5] (often spoken of as 'nose-drop nose' or 'Fenox-nose', so called after one of the more popular nasal decongestants).

It is claimed by the manufacturer of xylometazoline that, because of its more prolonged action, it is less likely to cause rebound congestion than other decongestants.

Symptomatic adverse effects

Stinging, discomfort or a dryness locally in the nose or eye are encountered infrequently. If these symptoms persist, the discomfort from the use of the drops probably outweighs any advantage they may confer.

Headache has been reported, albeit infrequently, as has tachycardia in children.

High risk groups

Because of the rebound phenomenon, treatment at any age should not normally exceed 3 to 5 days, and never more than 2 weeks.

Neonates

The drug should not be used in this age group.

Breast milk. No adverse effects have been reported in the baby as a result of a breast-feeding mother taking the drug.

Children

Most of the reported major adverse effects from xylometazoline have been in children, among whom, it is assumed, there is a greater risk of swallowing the solution.

Pregnant women

Though no adverse effects have been reported, the safety of use in pregnancy has not been fully established and administration of xylometazoline during that time should be avoided unless absolutely essential.

The elderly

The drug may be used in elderly patients.

Drugs interactions

None have been reported.

References

1. Messek H 1962 Clinical experience with the vasoconstrictor Otrivine. Wiener Klinische Wochenschrift 74: 287
2. Aschan G, Drettner B 1964 An objective investigation of the decongestive effect of xylometazoline. Svenska Pktan 61: 378
3. Schuman K 1973 Uber die Wirksamkeit von Otriven auf Nasenschleimhäute Therapiewoche 23 (37): 3304
4. Soderman P, Sahlberg D, Wiholm B-D 1984 (letter). Lancet 1: 573
5. Black M J, Remsen K A 1980 Rhinitis medicamentosa. Canadian Medical Association Journal 122–881

Zidovudine

Zidovudine was the first drug licenced for treatment of infection with the human immunodeficiency virus type 1 (HIV1).

Chemistry

Zidovudine (Retrovir, formerly called azidothymidine or AZT)
$C_{10}H_{13}N_5O_4$
3′-azido-3′-deoxythymidine

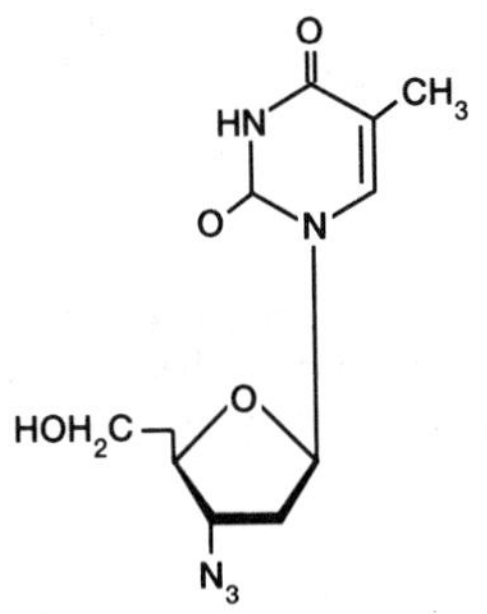

Molecular weight	267.2
pKa	9.68
Solubility	
in alcohol	1 in 14
in water	1 in 40
Octanol/water partition coefficient	1

Zidovudine is a white to off-white, odourless, crystalline solid. It is not present in any combination products. It is prepared by chemical synthesis.

Pharmacology

Zidovudine is a thymidine analogue in which the 3′hydroxy (OH) group is replaced by an azido (-N_3) group. Zidovudine is phosphorylated to the monophosphate by cellular thymidine kinase and thence by thymidylate kinase to the diphosphate form. Further phosphorylation then occurs to the triphosphate; it is zidovudine triphosphate which is the active inhibitor of HIV replication.

HIV replication involves the formation of a viral DNA transcript which becomes integrated into the host cell DNA. The formation of this transcript is mediated by reverse transcriptase (RNA-dependent DNA polymerase) and this enzyme is inhibited by zidovudine triphosphate. Other normal cellular DNA polymerases are inhibited only to a much lesser extent. Zidovudine triphosphate becomes incorporated into the growing chains of DNA via the DNA transcript and this leads to premature chain termination of the viral DNA. The HIV virus is thus unable to replicate.

Toxicology

Subchronic and chronic dosing

Early studies indicated that the cynomolgus monkey metabolised the drug most similarly to man and it was selected for subchronic and chronic dosing studies. A 3-month, 6-month and 12-month study in cynomolgus monkeys at doses up to 300 mg.kg^{-1} daily orally revealed a dose-related reversible macrocytic anaemia. The severity of anaemia at the termination of dosing was generally similar in all three studies. In the 12-month study the red cell changes had maximised by week 4 to 26 of treatment, and the severity of anaemia was not significantly affected by a further 6 months of treatment.

In rats, 3-month and 6-month studies at doses up to 500 mg.kg^{-1} daily and a 12-month study up to 450 mg.kg^{-1} daily revealed a reversible macrocytic anaemia at the highest dose in the 6-month and 12-month studies. The severity of anaemia at termination of dosing in both studies was similar.

Mutagenicity

No evidence of mutagenicity was observed in the Ames test. However, zidovudine was weakly mutagenic in a mouse lymphoma cell assay and was positive in an in vitro cell transformation assay. Clastogenic effects (chromosome damage) were observed in an in vitro study in human lymphocytes and in in vivo oral repeat dose micronucleus studies in rats and mice. An in vivo cytogenetic study in rats did not show chromosomal damage. The clinical significance of these findings is unclear.

Carcinogenicity

Zidovudine was administered orally at three dosage levels to separate groups of mice and rats (60 females and 60 males in each group). Initial single daily doses were 30, 60 and 120 mg.kg^{-1} daily and 80, 220 and 600 mg.kg^{-1} daily in mice and rats, respectively. The doses in mice were reduced to 20, 30 and 40 mh.kg^{-1} daily after Day 90 because of treatment related anaemia, whereas in rats only the high dose was reduced (to 450 and then 300 mg.kg^{-1} daily on Days 91 and 279, respectively).

In mice, seven late-appearing (after 19 months) vaginal neoplasms (5 squamous cell carcinomas, one squamous cell papilloma and one squamous polyp) occurred at the highest dose. One late-appearing squamous cell papilloma occurred in the vagina of a middle-dose animal. No vaginal tumours were found at the lowest dose.

In rats, two late-appearing (after 20 months) vaginal squamous cell carcinomas occurred in animals given the highest dose. No vaginal tumours occurred at the middle or low doses in rats.

There were no other drug-related tumours observed in either sex of either species.

Clinical pharmacology

Zidovudine triphosphate inhibits both HIV viral RNA-dependant DNA polymerase (reverse transcriptase) and human DNA polymerase, but the latter is only inhibited at concentrations 100 fold higher than those required for suppression of viral replication. Cell culture studies have demonstrated that incorporation of zidovudine by cellular DNA polymerase may occur, but only to a limited extent, and that chain termination has not been observed. Human T cell lymphotropic virus (HTLVI) is also inhibited by zidovudine triphosphate, but no antiviral activity has been demonstrated against Herpes simplex virus, Varicella zoster virus, influenza type A virus, measles virus or yellow fever virus.

Pharmacokinetics

The preferred analytical method is high performance liquid chromatography; either a solid-phase or reverse-phase column may be used.[1] The lower limit of detection is approximately 0.1 μmol.l^{-1} (25 μg.l^{-1}).

Zidovudine is almost completely absorbed by the oral route and peak plasma concentrations are seen between 0.5 to 1.5 h after dosing. About 25–40% of the dose is subject to pre-systemic metabolism, most likely in the liver. Systemic bioavailability is approximately 65% (range 52–75%). The mean plasma half life is approximately one hour (range 0.78–1.93 hours). Dose-independent kinetics have been observed over the dosage ranges used in man. The major route of metabolism is by hepatic glucuronidation ($\leqslant$80% of the dose), but following an intravenous dose 18% is excreted unchanged in the urine. Zidovudine is rapidly distributed throughout the body, with a volume of distribution of 1.6 ± 0.6 l.kg^{-1} (mean$\pm$SD). Zidovudine penetrates the blood–brain barrier.[3] Following intravenous administration of zidovudine, the cerebrospinal fluid–plasma ratio is 0.53 (range 0.2–0.73). The ratio after oral administration was 1.35 and 0.15 in the two patients studied. The wide variation in ratio is presumed to be due to variation in the blood–brain barrier. Zidovudine appears to be concentrated in semen,[4] and the ratio of semen: serum zidovudine levels ranged from

Zidovudine

Z

1.3–20.4 in the six patients studied. Zidovudine is 34–38% bound to plasma proteins.

Oral absorption	>90%
Presystemic metabolism	25–40%
Plasma half life	
range	0.78–1.93h
mean	1h
Volume of distribution	1.6 l.kg^{-1}
Plasma protein binding	34–38%

There are limited pharmacokinetic data in patients with renal or liver failure (see Contraindications). No data are available on the pharmacokinetics of zidovudine in the elderly.

It is not known whether zidovudine is excreted in human breast milk. Limited data indicates that it crosses the placenta.

Concentration–effect relationship

The relationships between in vitro susceptibility of HIV to zidovudine and clinical response to therapy remain under investigation. In vitro sensitivity testing has not been standardised and results may therefore vary according to methodological factors. Representative assays suggest that at a concentration of 0.013 mg.l^{-1} produces a 50% reduction in supernatant reverse transcriptase activity in H9 cells and peripheral blood lymphocytes. At a concentration of 0.13 mg.l^{-1} there is a 90% reduction in detectable HIV replication when the drug is added shortly after the susceptible cells have been infected. Concentrations approximately 100 times higher (range 8.8–13.3 mg.l^{-1}) are required to inhibit viral replication in chronically HIV-infected cells.

There are limited in-vitro data on the development of resistance to zidovudine. Reduced in-vitro sensitivity to zidovudine has been reported for HIV isolates from patients receiving prolonged courses of zidovudine.[4] The limited information so far available indicates that resistance probably develops more slowly in those with asymptomatic or early HIV disease.[5]

Metabolism

Zidovudine is metabolized predominantly in the liver, by glucuronidation. Approximately 18% of an oral dose of zidovudine is excreted unchanged in the urine. The only identified metabolite is 3′-azido-3′-deoxy-5′-β-D-glucopyranuronosylthymidine (GAZT zidovudine-5′-O-glucuronide), which is inactive and has a half life of one hour. Between 50 and 80% of an oral dose is excreted in urine as this conjugate.

Pharmaceutics

Zidovudine Retrovir (Burroughs Wellcome, UK/US) is presented in gelatin capsules containing 100 mg or 250 mg of zidovudine, together with inactive ingredients (corn starch, magnesium stearate, microcrystalline cellulose and sodium starch glycolate). The 100 mg capsules are opaque white with a dark blue band. 'Wellcome' and a unicorn logo are printed on the cap and 'Y9C' and '100' on the body. The 250 mg capsule is opaque white and opaque light blue with a dark blue band. 'Wellcome' and a unicorn logo are printed on the cap and 'H2F' and '250' on the body. Zidovudine capsules should be stored at 15–25°C and protected from light.

Therapeutic use

Indications

The management of the serious manifestations of HIV infection in patients with:

1. Acquired immunodeficiency syndrome (AIDS)
2. AIDS-related complex (ARC)
3. Early symptomatic and asymptomatic HIV infection
4. Other stages of HIV disease.

Contraindications

There are no absolute contraindications other than life-threatening allergic responses to any of the components of the capsules. Relative contraindications include:

1. Anaemia, neutropenia
2. Renal failure
3. Liver failure.

Mode of use

Clinical use is dependant on the anti-retroviral properties of zidovudine. Current data suggest that the host cannot eliminate HIV infection and that treatment with zidovudine needs to be lifelong, or continued until toxicity prevents further use. Although some of the initial studies with zidovudine have included administration of the drug intravenously, it is only available for general use by the oral route. Because of the short half life of zidovudine the initial studies have all employed a frequent dosage schedule; at present, the recommended starting dose is 200 mg every four hours (1200 mg, daily), for a 70 kg patient. The optimum dosage regimen remains to be determined and may vary from patient to patient. Dosages generally between 500 and 1500 mg daily have been used in clinical trials, and many centres are prescribing less frequent or lower doses (250 mg every six hours or 250–300 mg every 12 h). The selection of lower dosages may be related to patient factors such as stage of disease, bone marrow reserve or bodyweight. The efficacy of dosing at intervals longer than 6-hourly remains to be confirmed. The effectiveness of lower dosages against HIV-associated neurological dysfunction of malignancies is unknown.

Indications

1. Acquired immunodeficiency syndrome (AIDS)

Zidovudine is the only drug that has been shown in a controlled study to improve life expectancy and symptoms in patients with AIDS.[6] Best results are seen in those patients who have presented with their first opportunistic infection, usually *Pneumocystis carinii* pneumonia (group IV C1 of the HIV disease classification.)[7] Treatment is commenced as soon as the presenting illness has been treated, and is continued indefinitely at the same dose of 200 mg every four hours unless, or until, toxicity occurs (see below). Although there is clear evidence of improved survival in AIDS patients treated with zidovudine, there is as yet no data on the longer term use of the drug. The clinical impression of many physicians prescribing zidovudine is that, following initial improvement, many patients will ultimately develop progressive HIV disease. This appears to be confirmed by a recent French study, in which the average follow-up was seven months[8] compared with four months in the original American placebo-controlled study.[6] Patients in the latter study were switched to open-label treatment after termination of the placebo phase. Further follow-up suggests continuing survival benefit for at least 21 months which was the duration of study.[9]

When a patient presents with advanced HIV disease, frequently with a history of multiple opportunistic infections and a life expectancy of only a few weeks, zidovudine is of little benefit.

Progressive neurological disease is frequently seen in patients with AIDS (group IV B), and, although there are no controlled studies of the use of zidovudine, there is evidence that a trial of therapy is worthwhile[10,11], there may be improvement in neuropsychological function in patients with AIDS following treatment with zidovudine.[12] and an epidemiological study from Holland indicated a marked decline in the incidence of AIDS dementia complex following the introduction of zidovudine in 1987.[13]

2. AIDS-related complex (ARC)

Patients with ARC (groups IV A and IV C2) were included in the original American placebo-controlled study,[6] and the results were stratified according to their absolute T4 (CD4) count. The greatest benefit was seen in those with a low T4 count (<100 mm^{-3}), but improved survival and a reduced rate of opportunistic infection were seen in all ARC patients with longer follow up. Thus, all patients with ARC should be offered treatment with zidovudine. In some patients, in addition to improving their sense of well-being and overall survival, there will be resolution of their indicator infection, such as oral candida or hairy leukoplakia.

3. Early symptomatic and asymptomatic HIV infection

Zidovudine has recently been licenced for use in earlier stages of HIV disease. It may be used in those with early symptomatic disease or in individuals who are asymptomatic with markers of disease progression. The main marker of disease progression is a persistently reduced T4 lymphocyte count (CD4) of less than 200 mm^{-3} or of a count between 200 and 500 mm^{-3} that is falling rapidly.[14,15] There are no data of long-term efficacy and safety in asymptomatic individuals. Further trials are under way and the role of zidovudine in early HIV infection is as yet uncertain.[16,17]

4. Other stages of HIV disease

There is evidence that zidovudine may benefit some patients with HIV-related thrombocytopenia[18] or severe skin disease.[19,20]

It has been suggested that zidovudine should be given following occupational needle-stick injury to health care personnel, but there is as yet no evidence to support this.

Zidovudine has been shown to reduce serum and cerebrospinal fluid HIV antigen levels in both those with AIDS[21,22] and serum HIV antigen levels in symptomless HIV-positive individuals.[23] However, this has not yet been shown to improve clinical outcome, and HIV antigen levels may rise again despite continuing zidovudine.[24]

Contraindications

1. Anaemia, neutropenia

Anaemia, and or neutropenia whether as a result of HIV disease or of other drug therapy, are relative contraindications to the use of zidovudine. Zidovudine should not be given to patients with haemoglobin levels of less than 7.5 $g.dl^{-1}$ or with neutrophil counts of less than 0.75×10^9 per litre. Particular care should be taken in patients with haemoglobin levels of less than 9 $g.dl^{-1}$ or neutrophil counts less than 1×10^9 per litre, and lower daily dosages are usually appropriate from the start of treatment, with further adjustment according to subsequent haematological monitoring (see also Adverse reactions).

2. Renal failure

Limited data in patients with renal impairment do not suggest a particular need for dosage adjustment since zidovudine levels are not notably increased. However, accumulation of the glucuronide metabolite can be expected with renal impairment, although the effects of this accumulation are unknown.[25] Monitoring of plasma zidovudine (and its glucuride) levels, in conjunction with haematological parameters, may indicate the need for future dosage adjustment. Haemodialysis appears to have a limited effect on the elimination of zidovudine but enhances the elimination of the glucuronide metabolite. A 50% dose reduction has been suggested for patients receiving dialysis.[26]

3. Liver failure

Limited data in patients with cirrhosis suggest that accumulation of zidovudine may occur in patients with hepatic impairment because of decreased glucuronidation.[27] Dosage adjustments may be necessary but recommendations cannot be given at present. If monitoring of plasma zidovudine levels is not feasible other signs of intolerance may indicate that dosage reduction is needed.

Adverse reactions

Potentially life-threatening effects

The most serious adverse effects of zidovudine are those seen on the bone marrow and include anaemia (which may require transfusion), neutropenia and leucopenia.[28] These are more likely to occur in patients with more advanced disease and with the lowest T4 (CD4) cell counts prior to beginning treatment particularly with the high dosages of 1200 to 1500 mg daily. There is an almost universal increase in the mean corpuscular volume, thought to be due to impaired erythrocyte maturation, but this is not predictive of further marrow toxicity. Severe anaemia (haemoglobin less than 7.5 $g.dl^{-1}$) or neutropenia (neutrophil count less than 0.75×10^9 per litre) occurs in about 30% of patients with advanced disease and in about 5% or less of asymptomatic individuals receiving zidovudine. Anaemia or neutropenia usually occur after the first six weeks of therapy but occasionally earlier.

Treatment with zidovudine should be interrupted if the haemoglobin falls below 7.5 $g.dl^{-1}$, or the neutrophil count falls below 0.75×10^9/litre. For less severe myelosuppression (haemoglobin below 9 $g.dl^{-1}$ or neutrophil count below 1.0×10^9 per litre) dosage reduction such as halving the daily dose may be adequate or marrow recovery may be more rapid by a brief (2–4 weeks) interruption of therapy. When there is evidence of marrow recovery, a gradual reintroduction or increase in dose may be considered. In patients with significant anaemia, dose modification does not always eliminate the need for transfusions. Many physicians will maintain full dosage providing transfusion is not required more than once per month but there is no data to confirm that this is the correct course of action. Similarly, when dose reduction is made there is no data to indicate whether the dose should be reduced but the frequency of administration maintained (i.e. 100 mg every four hours) or whether the dose should be maintained with reduced frequency of administration (i.e. 200 mg every eight hours). Clearly, the latter schedule is more convenient for the patients although it's efficacy is not established. In some patients, particularly those with advanced disease requiring treatment with other myelosuppressive drugs, zidovudine may have to be discontinued indefinitely. There is often an initial rise in the platelet count after starting zidovudine, particularly if this was initially low, but this may be followed by a recurrence of thrombocytopenia. This is rarely severe enough to require alteration in the dosage of zidovudine.

Acute overdosage

There are limited case reports of zidovudine overdosage. Up to 200×100 mg tablets have been taken, with resulting serum zidovudine levels of up to 185 $\mu mol.l.^{-1}$ Clinical recovery from these overdoses was complete.[29,30]

Severe or irreversible adverse effects

A severe polymyositis may develop during treatment with zidovudine.[31] In some individuals the symptoms are mild and may be controlled by the use of a non-steroidal anti-inflammatory drug whilst in others symptoms can be severe enough to require cessation of therapy and recovery is slow. There are no data as to whether the drug can be reintroduced at a later date. Myalgia and myopathy are more frequent in patients with AIDS taking zidovudine but are less common in those with early disease[32,33] and may occur in patients not taking zidovudine.[34] The CPK is unreliable and zidovudine may need to be discontinued to see if the effects are drug-related. Recent data suggests that myopathy is due to depletion of muscle mitochondrial DNA by zidovudine.[35]

Dose reduction or cessation of treatment with zidovudine may rarely lead to an encephalitis.[36] The mechanism is unknown.

Symptomatic adverse effects

Nausea, headache and insomnia occur relatively commonly but treatment can usually be continued. In the longer follow-up provided by the French study of zidovudine, 21 out of 365 patients receiving the drug had therapy interrupted for non-haematological toxicity.[8]

Interference with clinical pathology tests

No technical interferences of this kind have been reported.

High risk groups

Neonates

There are no data on the use of zidovudine in neonates.

Breast milk. It is not known if zidovudine is excreted in breast milk. In view of this, and of the unknown effects of zidovudine on neonates, mothers who continue to receive zidovudine are usually advised not to breast feed.

Children

Zidovudine is only licensed for use in adults but open labelled studies of zidovudine in children give results consistent with experience in adults. Clinical benefits include weight gain, decrease in disease related symptoms, improvements in immunological indices and also in neurological function. In one study of 21 children given zidovudine by intravenous infusion for nearly a year, there was marked improvement in neurological disease.[37] Similarly, there was apparent clinical improvement in children given initial treatment with zidovudine intravenously and then continued on oral zidovudine at a dose of 100 $mg.m^{-2}$ every six hours.[38]

Pregnant women

Zidovudine crosses the placenta[39] but there are no data as to either the teratogenicity or the effects on fertility of zidovudine. Nevertheless, it may be appropriate to continue the drug during pregnancy providing the mother understands that no assurances as to the effect on the child can be given.

The elderly

There are no known specific precautions for the use of zidovudine in the elderly, since few such patients have received the drug. However, in view of the age-associated decrease in renal function a lower dosage regimen is probably appropriate.

Drug interactions

Potentially hazardous interactions

There are few data on drug interactions with zidovudine.

Hepatic enzyme inhibition. Concomitant use of drugs which inhibit hepatic glucuronidation (e.g. paracetamol, aspirin, indomethacin) might be expected to lead to an increase in toxicity. Paracetamol was shown to be associated with a higher incidence of neutropenia in the American controlled study[28] although limited data do not support a pharmacokinetic interaction.[40]

Probenecid. Probenecid may both inhibit glucuronidation and reduce renal excretion of zidovudine. There appears to be an increased incidence of rash when probenecid is given with zidovudine.[41]

Other drugs. Clearly, any drug with myelosuppressive actions will increase the toxicity of zidovudine and should be avoided if possible. Many patients have received other drugs, such as co-trimoxazole, ketoconazole or acyclovir, to prevent opportunistic infections at the same time as receiving zidovudine. There is no obvious increase in toxicity to zidovudine whilst receiving these drugs, although neurotoxicity in a patient receiving acyclovir and zidovudine has been reported.[42]

In vitro studies suggest synergistic activity between zidovudine and mismatched double-stranded RNA,[43] recombinant α-interferon[34] and granulocyte-macrophage-stimulating factor,[44] and inhibition by ribavirin.[45]

Potentially useful interactions

No interactions of this kind have been described.

Major outcome trials

1. Fischl M A, Richman M D, Grieco M H et al 1987 The efficacy of azidothymidine (AZT) in the treatment of patients with AIDS and AIDS-related complex. New England Journal of Medicine 317: 185–191

This is the only placebo-controlled trial of zidovudine in AIDS or ARC. The trial was begun in February 1986 at 12 participating centres in the United States, and included 281 patients. There were 160 patients with AIDS who had recovered from their first attack of *Pneumocystis carinii* pneumonia within the previous four months, and 121 patients with ARC and evidence of disease progression. The trial was due to last for 24 weeks but was ended in September 1986, after a mean of 17 weeks in the trial, because there was a significant reduction in mortality among the patients receiving zidovudine. Zidovudine was given at a dose of 250 mg every four hours around the clock. There were 19 deaths in the placebo group and only one in the zidovudine group ($p<0.001$).

After six weeks treatment with zidovudine, patients were significantly less likely to suffer opportunistic infections. Among the treated patients there was an improvement in the Karnefsky performance score, body weight and severity of symptoms. In addition, there was an initial improvement in the T4 (CD4) cell count but this was not sustained. Toxicity due to bone marrow suppression was common, with 34% of patients receiving zidovudine requiring dosage changes or discontinuation of the drug.

At the end of the placebo-controlled trial, all participating patients were offered zidovudine at a dose of 200 mg every four hours and further data was obtained from following these 227 patients (100 had previously received placebo and 127 had previously received zidovudine) for up to five months.

2. Dournon E, Matheron S, Rozenbaum W et al 1988 Effects of zidovudine in 365 consecutive patients with AIDS or AIDS-related complex. Lancet 2: 1297–1302

This study included 285 patients with AIDS and 80 with ARC who were treated with zidovudine 200 mg every 4 hours, unless modified by toxicity, and followed for a mean of 31 weeks (range 2–52 weeks). As in the initial American study, this study showed an initial improvement in weight, Karnefsky score and T4 (CD4) cell count. By six months of follow up these parameters had returned to their pretreatment levels. Unlike the American study, this study included AIDS patients with a broader spread of opportunistic infections. Only 97 patients (36.7%) had *Pneumocystis carinii* pneumonia (PCP) alone as their indicator of AIDS, and 31.6% of AIDS patients had had two or more opportunistic infections. Thus, many patients included in this study had more advanced disease than was the case among the patients included in the American study. Toxicity of zidovudine was again predominantly haematological, and treatment was interrupted or discontinued in 58.6% of patients. During the study, 53 of the 285 AIDS patients died (18.6%). Among the patients with post-PCP AIDS, and excluding the first six weeks of therapy, 9 out of 85 patients (10.6%) died, and 33 (33.8%) had a further opportunistic infection, after a mean follow up of 35 weeks.

The results of this study are disappointing since, although the initial benefit of zidovudine is confirmed, it is clear that for many patients this benefit is limited to months rather than years.

3. Fischl M A, Richman D D, Hansen N et al 1990 The safety and efficacy of zidovudine (AZT) in the treatment of subjects with midly symptomatic Human Immunodeficiency Virus Type 1 (HIV) infection. Annals of Internal Medicine 112: 727–737.

This 2-arm multicentre study enrolled 713 subjects with mildly symptomatic HIV infection, and compared zidovudine 1200 mg daily with placebo. The trial was terminated when, among the 505 subjects with less than 500 T4 cells on entry, the rate of progression to AIDS or ARC in zidovudine treated patients was observed to be roughly one-third that in placebo recipients. Among the 198 subjects with more than 500 T4 cells on entry, very few progressions were observed.

4. Volberding P A, Lagakos S W, Koch N A et al 1990 Zidovudine in asymptomatic human immunodeficiency virus infection. New England Journal of Medicine 322: 1000–1002

This was a 3-arm multi-centre study that included 3200 people with HIV infection. The study compared zidovudine 1500 mg daily with 500 mg daily or placebo. 1300 of the participants had fewer than 500 T4 cells upon entry and amongst those of this group on active treatment the rate of progression to AIDS or severe AIDS-related complex was roughly half of that seen in those receiving placebo. There appears to have been no difference between the response to the two dose levels of zidovudine. The trial has been terminated for patients with less than 500 T4 cells, but the trial continues for those with more than 500 T4 cells.

Controlled trials

1. Fischl M A, Parker C B, Pettinelli C et al 1990 A randomized controlled trial of a reduced daily dose of zidovudine in patients with acquired immunodeficiency syndrome. New England Journal of Medicine 323: 1009–1014

524 patients with HIV infection who had suffered a first episode of pneumocystis carinii infection were randomized to a high dose of zidovudine (250 mg every 4 hours) or a dose of 200 mg every 4 hours for 4 weeks followed by 100 mg every 4 hours.

At 24 months the survival was 27% for the high dose group and 34% for the low maintenance dose group ($P=0.033$). The haemoglobin level declined to less than 80 $g.l^{-1}$ in 101 of 262 in the high dose groups and 77 of 262 in the low maintenance dose group ($P=0.0009$). The decline in neutrophil count was also significantly less in the low dose group. The authors concluded that the reduced dose regime was at least as effective and less toxic than the high dose.

General review articles

Richman D D, Andrews J 1988 Results of continued monitoring of participants in the placebo-controlled trial of zidovudine for serious human immunodeficiency virus infection. American Journal of Medicine 85 (suppl 2A): 208–213

Hirsch M S 1988 Antiviral drug development for the treatment of human immunodeficiency virus infection. American Journal of Medicine 85 (suppl 2A): 182–185

Furman P A, Barry D W 1988 Spectrum of antiviral activity and mechanism of action of zidovudine. American Journal of Medicine 85 (suppl 2A): 176–181

Jackson G G, Paul D A, Falk L A et al 1988 Human immunodeficiency virus (HIV) antigenaemia (p24) in the acquired immunodeficiency syndrome (AIDS) and the effect of treatment of zidovudine (AZT). Annals of Internal Medicine 108: 175–180
Richman D D 1988 The treatment of HIV infection. AIDS 2 (suppl 1): S137–S142
Mitsuya H, Broder S 1987 Strategies for antiviral therapy in AIDS. Nature 325: 773–778
State of the art conference on azidothymidine therapy for early HIV infection 1990. American Journal of Medicine 89: 335–344
NIH conference. Antiretroviral therapy in AIDS 1990. Annals of Internal Medicine 113: 604–618

References

1. Blum M R, Liao S H T, Good S S, De Miranda P 1988 Pharmacokinetics and bioavailability of zidovudine in humans. American Journal of Medicine 85 (suppl 2A): 189–194
2. Klecker R W, Collins J M, Yarchoan R et al 1987 Plasma and cerebrospinal fluid pharmacokinetics of 3'-azido-3'deoxythymidine: a novel pyrimidine analog with potential application for the treatment of AIDS and related diseases. Clinical Pharmacology and Therapeutics 41: 407–412
3. Henry K, Chinnock B J, Quinn R P, Fletcher C V, De Miranda P, Balfour H H 1988 Concurrent zidovudine levels in semen and serum determined by radioimmunoassay in patients with AIDS or AIDS-related complex. Journal of the American Medical Association 259: 3023–3026
4. Larder B A, Darby G & Richman D D 1989 HIV with reduced sensitivity to zidovudine (AZT) isolated during prolonged therapy. Science 243: 1731–1734
5. Richman D D, Grimes J M & Lagakos S W 1990 Effects of stage of disease and drug dose on zidovudine susceptibilities of isolates of Human Immunolodeficiency Virus. Journal of Acquired Immune Deficiency Syndromes 3: 743–746
6. Fischl M A, Richman M D, Grieco M H et al 1987 The efficacy of azidothymidine (AZT) in the treatment of patients with AIDS and AIDS-related complex. New England Journal of Medicine 317: 185–191
7. 1986 Morbidity and Mortality Weekly Review 35 (20): 334–339
8. Dournon E, Matheron S, Rozenbaum W et al 1988 Effects of zidovudine in 365 consecutive patients with AIDS or AIDS-related complex. Lancet 2: 1297–1302
9. Stambuk D, Farthing C, Hawkins D, Youle M, Lawrence A, Gazzard B 1989 The efficacy and toxicity of azidothymidine (AZT) in the treatment of patients with AIDS and AIDS related complex (ARC): an open uncontrolled treatment study. Quarterly Journal of Medicine 70: 161–174
10. Yarchoan R, Klecker R W, Weinhold K J et al 1986 Administration of 3'-azido-3'deoxythymidine an inhibitor of HTLV-III/LAV replication to patients with AIDS or AIDS-related complex. Lancet 1: 575–580
11. Yarchoan R, Berg G, Brouwers P et al 1987 Response of human immunodeficiency virus associated neurological disease to 3'-azido-3'deoxythymidine. Lancet 1: 132–135
12. Schmitt F A, Bigley J W, McKinnis R, Logue P E, Evans R W, Drucker J L 1988 Neuropsychological outcome of zidovudine (AZT) treatment of patients with AIDS and AIDS-related complex. New England Journal of Medicine 319: 1573–1578
13. Portegies P, de Gans J, Lange J M A et al 1989 Declining incidence of AIDS dementia complex after introduction of zidovudine treatment. British Medical Journal 299: 819–821
14. Fischl M A, Richman D D, Hansen N et al 1990 The safety and efficacy of zidovudine (AZT) in the treatment of subjects with mildly symptomatic human immunodeficiency virus type I (HIV) infection. Annals of Internal Medicine 112: 727–737
15. Volberding P A, Lagakos S W, Koch N A et al 1990 Zidovudine in asymptomatic human immunodeficiency virus infection. New England Journal of Medicine 323: 1009–1014
16. Swart A M, Weller I, Darbyshire J H 1990 Early HIV infection: to treat or not to treat? British Medical Journal 301: 825–826
17. Friedland G H 1990 Early treatment for HIV. New England Journal of Medicine 322: 1000–1002
18. Hymes K B, Greene J B, Karpatkin S 1988 The effect of zidovudine on HIV-related thrombocytopenia. New England Journal of Medicine 318: 516–517
19. Duvic M, Rios A, Brewton G W 1987 Remission of AIDS-associated psoriasis with zidovudine. Lancet 2: 627
20. Ruzicka T, Froschl M, Hohenleutner U, Holzman H, Braun-Falco O 1987 Treatment of HIV-induced retinoid-resistant psoriasis with zidovudine. Lancet 2: 1469–1470
21. Chaisson R E, Allain J P, Leuther M, Volberding P A 1986 Significant changes in HIV antigen level in the serum of patients treated with zidovudine. New England Journal of Medicine 315: 1610–1611
22. De Gans J, Lange J M A, Derix M M A et al 1988 Decline of HIV antigen levels in cerebrospinal fluid during treatment with low-dose zidovudine. AIDS 2: 37–40
23. De Wolf F, Lange J M A, Goudsmit J et al 1988 Effect of zidovudine on serum immunodeficiency virus antigen levels in symptom-free subjects. Lancet 1: 373–376
24. Reiss P, Lange J M A, Boucher C A, Danner S A, Goudsmit J 1988 Resumption of HIV antigen production during continuous zidovudine treatment. Lancet 1: 421
25. Singlas E, Pioger J C, Taburet A M et al 1989 Zidovudine disposition in patients with severe renal impairment: influence of haemodialysis. Clinical Pharmacology and Therapeutics 46: 190–197
26. Deray G, Diquet B, Martinez F, Vidal A M, Petitclerc T, Ben Hmida M, Land G, Jacobs C 1988 Pharmacokinetics of zidovudine in a patient on maintenance hemodialysis. The New England Journal of Medicine 319: 1606–1607
27. Taburet A M, Navean S, Zorza G et al 1990 Pharmokinetics of zidovudine in patients with liver cirrhosis. Clinical Pharmacology and Therapeutics 47: 731–739
28. Richman D D, Fischl M A, Grieco M H et al 1987 The toxicity of azidothymidine (AZT) in the treatment of patients with AIDS and AIDS-related complex. New England Journal of Medicine 317: 192–197
29. Hargreaves M, Fuller G, Costello C, Gazzard B 1988 Zidovudine overdose. Lancet 2: 509
30. Pickus O B 1988 Overdose of zidovudine. New England Journal of Medicine 318: 1206
31. Bessen L J, Greene J B, Louie E, Seitzman P, Weinberg H 1988 Severe polymyositis-like syndrome associated with zidovudine therapy of AIDS and ARC. New England Journal of Medicine 318: 708
32. Gorard D A, Henry K, Guiloff R J 1988 Necrotising myopathy and zidovudine. Lancet 1: 1050
33. Dalakas M C, Illa I, Pezeshkpour G H et al 1990 Mitochondrial myopathy cause by longterm zidovudine therapy. New England Journal of Medicine 322: 1098–1105
34. Till M and McDonnell K M 1990 Myopathy with Human Immunodeficiency Virus Type 1 (HIV-1) infection: HIV-1 or zidovudine? Annals of Internal Medicine 113: 492–494
35. Arnaudo E, Dalakas M, Shanske S, Moraes C T, Dimauro S, Schon E A 1991 Depletion of muscle mitochondrial DNA in AIDS patients with zidovudine induced myopathy. Lancet 337: 508–510
36. Helbert M, Robinson D, Peddle B, Forster S, Kocsis A, Jeffries D, Pinching A J 1988 Acute meningo-encephalitis on dose reduction of zidovudine. Lancet 1: 1249–1252
37. Pizzo P A, Eddie J, Falloon J et al 1988 Effect of continuous intravenous infusion of zidovudine (AZT) in children with symptomatic HIV infection. New England Journal of Medicine 319: 889–896
38. Blanche S, Caniglia M, Fischer A et al 1988 Zidovudine therapy in children with Acquired Immunodeficiency Syndrome. American Journal of Medicine 85 (suppl 2A): 203–207
39. Gillet J Y, Garraffo R, Abrar D et al 1989 Fetoplacental passage of zidovudine. Lancet ii: 269–270
40. Steffe E M, King J H, Inciardi J F et al 1990 The effect of acetamonophen on zidovudine metabolism in HIV-infected patients. Journal of Acquired Immune Deficiency Syndromes 3: 691–694
41. Petty B G, Kornhauser D M, Lietman P S 1990 Zidovudine with probenecid — a warning. Lancet 335: 1044–1045
42. Bach M C 1987 Possible drug interaction during therapy with azidothymidine and acyclovir for AIDS. New England Journal of Medicine 316: 547
43. Mitchell W M, Montefiori D C, Robinson W E, Strayer D R, Carter W A 1987 Mismatched double-stranded RNA (Ampligen) reduces concentrations of zidovudine (Azidothymidine) required for in vitro inhibition of human immunodeficiency virus. Lancet 1: 890–892
44. Hartshorn K L, Vogt M W, Chou T C et al 1987 Synergistic inhibition of human immunodeficiency virus in vitro by azidothymidine and recombinant alpha A interferon. Antimicrobial Agents and Chemotherapy 31: 168–172
45. Hammer S M, Gillis J M 1987 Synergistic activity of Granulocyte-Macrophage Colony Stimulating Factor and 3'-Azido-3'-Deoxythymidine against Human Immunodeficiency Virus in vitro. Antimicrobial Agents and Chemotherapy 31: 1046–1050
46. Vogt M W, Harthorn K L, Furman P A et al 1987 Ribavirin antagonizes the effect of azidothymidine on HIV replication. Science 235: 1376–1379

Zopiclone

Zopiclone is a hypnotic agent belonging to a new chemical group, the cyclopyrrolones, a new class of psychotherapeutic agents. It is an original molecule, chemically unrelated to any other known hypnotic.

Chemistry

Zopiclone (Imovane, Zimovane, Amoban)
$C_{17}H_{17}ClN_6O_3$
6-(5-chloropyrid-2-yl)-5-(4-methylpiperazin-1-yl)-carbonyloxy-7-oxo-6,7-dihydro-5H-pyrrolo-(3,4-b)-pyrazine-5-one

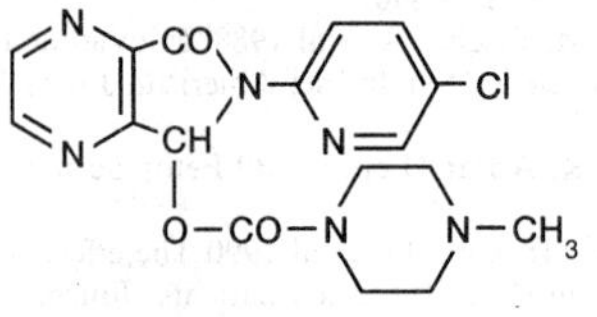

Molecular weight	388.8
pKa	6.7
Solubility	
in alcohol	practically insoluble
in water	practically insoluble
Octanol/water partition coefficient	—

Zopiclone is a fine, white, odourless and non-hygroscopic powder prepared by chemical synthesis.

Pharmacology

Zopiclone exhibits anticonvulsant, muscle relaxant and hypnosedative properties in animals.[1,2] Zopiclone recognizes specifically, and with high affinity, binding sites which belong to the $GABA_A$–benzodiazepine chloride channel macromolecular receptor complex. These results were first obtained by binding techniques using benzodiazepines as ligands. However, further in-depth studies using a cyclopyrrolone as ligand and biochemical modifications of the receptor, such as GABA shift or photoshift, reveal that zopiclone either acts on a site distinct from that of benzodiazepines or induces conformational changes different from those induced by benzodiazepines.[1,2]

Toxicology

There are no reports from toxicological studies in animals that are of potential clinical relevance. Zopiclone does not have mutagenic or teratogenic potential. Oncogenic studies show that for patients receiving long-term medication with zopiclone at the recommended dose range no carcinogenic potential exists.

Clinical pharmacology

In laboratory studies zopiclone improved sleep variables in healthy volunteers in a dose-dependent way. At doses higher than 5 mg, zopiclone shortened sleep onset latency, decreased the number of awakenings and improved duration and quality of sleep.[3,4]

At doses from 3.75 to 15 mg investigations in patients confirmed the hypnotic efficiency of zopiclone and established 7.5 mg as the optimum dose in those suffering from chronic or transient insomnia, and in the elderly.[5–10] At 7.5 mg zopiclone improves sleep parameters in healthy volunteers and insomniacs to a degree comparable with that found following the usual clinical doses of nitrazepam, flurazepam, temazepam, triazolam and flunitrazepam.[11–17] The effects of zopiclone on sleep stages have been studied both in healthy volunteers and in patients with sleep-related disturbance for treatment periods from 1 to 182 days. Zopiclone shortened the onset of stage 1 (at variance with what is known for barbiturate and benzodiazepine hypnotics) and had no consistent effect on stage 2. There was a tendency for an increase in slow wave sleep (stage 3 and 4) without any effect on REM sleep.[18–25]

The hypnosedative activity of zopiclone leads to an impairment of psychomotor functions which is maximal 1 hour after administration but disappears after 6–8 hours. As a consequence the carry-over effects of zopiclone the morning after nocturnal dosing are minimal for doses lower than 10 mg, both in adults and geriatric subjects.[3,4,9,17,23,24,26–28] The residual effects of zopiclone 7.5 mg on tests of psychomotor function were minimal and less pronounced than those following reference drugs (flurazepam 15 and 30 mg and flunitrazepam 1 and 2 mg).[20,24,26,27] Doses of 3.75 and 7.5 mg of zopiclone did not differ from placebo when the Multiple Sleep Latency Test was used to assess vigilance during the day.[17]

In studies assessing drug effects on memory, zopiclone 7.5 and 15 mg cause amnesia 1–2 hours after administration but no 'morning after' memory loss has been observed.[28]

Rebound effects and withdrawal symptoms were specifically investigated in 25 trials both in healthy volunteers and in sleep-disturbed patients (n = 832 subjects). No worsening of sleep variables with respect to baseline scores nor any significant modification of sleep stages were observed on discontinuation of continuous nocturnal treatment with zopiclone for periods up to 6 months.

No changes in heart rate, blood pressure or respiration have been noted during therapy with zopiclone.[16] There is no evidence in man of the anticonvulsant and muscle relaxant activity of zopiclone reported in animal studies.

Pharmacokinetics

Using 'cold' compounds the concentration of zopiclone and its two major urinary metabolites, the N-oxide and the N-desmethyl derivatives, were determined by high performance liquid chromatography (HPLC) in animal studies, and in the main kinetic studies in the human (the sensitivity threshold in plasma was 2 $\mu g.l^{-1}$ and in urine was 200 $\mu g.l^{-1}$).

Zopiclone 7.5 mg given orally is rapidly absorbed, producing peak plasma concentrations of 60–70 $\mu g.l^{-1}$ at 0.5–1.5 hours. One hour after administration, more than 95% of absorption is complete.

The bioavailability of zopiclone, expressed as a ratio of oral to intravenous values, is about 80% in man, suggesting the absence of significant presystemic metabolism. Total bioavailability appears to be independent of dose; a linear relationship exists between plasma concentration and doses in the range of 5–15 mg.

Zopiclone exhibits first-order kinetics. As confirmed by intravenous dosing with radioactive zopiclone in man, the drug is distributed rapidly into body tissues including the brain. After an intravenous dose and increasing oral doses of zopiclone, the volume of distribution of zopiclone was about 100 l, and the drug was 45% bound to plasma protein.

In lactating women given zopiclone 7.5 mg the milk/plasma ratio of the AUC was 0.51, with the milk concentration curve mimicking that seen in plasma. The elimination half life of zopiclone and its active N-oxide metabolite ranges from 3.5 to 6 hours. After intravenous administration zopiclone undergoes biphasic elimination with an elimination half life of 5 hours. Multiple-dose regimens in humans did not significantly change kinetic parameters and no differences were seen between males and females. Mild to moderate renal insufficiency does not alter the kinetics of zopiclone, and patients with end-stage renal disease have shown only slight changes in AUC, elimination half life and the time to maximum plasma concentrations. In elderly patients a slight increase in half life was observed, which is more pronounced in patients aged over 80 years.[30,31]

Oral absorption	>95%
Presystemic metabolism	—
Plasma half life	
range	3.5–6 h
Volume of distribution	100 l
Plasma protein binding	45%

Zopiclone

Concentration–effect relationship

No data are available at present.

Metabolism

Zopiclone is very extensively metabolized by three major pathways; only 4–5% of a dose is excreted unchanged in the urine. The side-chain undergoes oxidation to the less active N-oxide derivative which accounts for 11% of the dose, and demethylation to the inactive N-desmethyl zopiclone (15%): both these compounds are renally excreted (Fig. 1). Ester hydrolysis involving oxidative decarboxylation of 50% of a dose produces inactive metabolites partly eliminated via the lung as carbon dioxide; within 24 to 48 hours after a final dose virtually 100% of zopiclone and its two major metabolites is eliminated.

Pharmaceutics

Zopiclone (Zimovane; Rhone-Poulenc, UK) is available in oral tablet form. Tablets contain 7.5 mg of zopiclone, have to be protected from light and stored in a dry place below 30°C. Tablets are white, film-coated, elliptical with a break-line on one face, the reverse plain. In the UK they are marked 'ZM'.

Therapeutic use

Indications

1. In the treatment of transient, situational and chronic insomnia
2. Insomnia secondary to psychiatric disorders including difficulty in falling asleep, nocturnal awakenings and early wakening.

Contraindications

There are few contraindications apart from patients suffering from decompensated respiratory insufficiency. However, in a study to assess the effects of zopiclone on respiratory functions[36] no detrimental effects were observed. The use of zopiclone in patients suffering from myasthenia gravis is not recommended.

Mode of use

Zopiclone, at a dose of 7.5 mg, can significantly shorten sleep onset and improve duration and quality of sleep. At this dose no, or minimal, 'carry-over' effects exist and daytime functioning is preserved. In the case of situational transient insomnia such as in shift workers, short-term treatment (3–7 days) will be sufficient to re-establish normal sleep. Insomnia due to more persisting life stress or psychological distress can demand longer treatment, but in this case patients need to be periodically assessed for their insomnia and treatment should not be prolonged if not necessary.

Patients treated with zopiclone 7.5 mg for periods longer than 6 months showed no tolerance to the hypnotic effect and there was no need to increase the dose over time.

For all indications the suggested dose is 7.5 mg by oral administration shortly before retiring. The dose may be increased to 15 mg for patients who do not respond to lower doses because of severe or persistent insomnia.

Abuse and dependency potential was examined in a series of specific studies in alcoholics and drug addicts: patients did not desire or crave zopiclone,[32–34] and after continuous nocturnal treatment for 3–4 weeks there were no 'withdrawal reactions' even though the dose was not tapered.[35]

In patients previously on long-term treatment with benzodiazepines (6 months or more) it is advisable to taper the dose of benzodiazepines over a period of 1–2 weeks at the same time as using zopiclone at the suggested therapeutic dose.

Adverse reactions

Potentially life-threatening effects

No effects of this kind have been reported so far.

Acute overdosage

So far a few cases of overdose of up to 450 mg have been reported. All patients recovered uneventfully. Drowsiness, lethargy and ataxia were the principal effects reported and no particular medical treatment was necessary, apart from induced emesis and clinical monitoring of vital functions.

Severe or irreversible adverse effects

No effects of this kind have been observed so far. However, because of experience with long-term dependence upon benzodiazepines originally prescribed as hypnotics caution is warranted until wider experience with zopiclone is available.

Symptomatic adverse effects

The most commonly recorded adverse effect during controlled clinical trials is a mild metallic or bitter after-taste. Less commonly, mild gastrointestinal disturbances including nausea and vomiting or minor mental disturbances such as irritability, confusion and depressed mood have occurred. Allergic and allied manifestations (urticaria and various rashes) have only very rarely been observed.

Interference with clinical pathology tests

No interferences of this type appear to have been observed.

High risk groups

Neonates

No studies have been carried out in neonates, and consequently the administration of zopiclone in children is not recommended.

Breast milk. Zopiclone and/or its metabolites are excreted in breast milk. Use in nursing mothers is not recommended.

Children

What has been said above about neonates also applies to older children.

Fig. 1 The metabolism of zopiclone

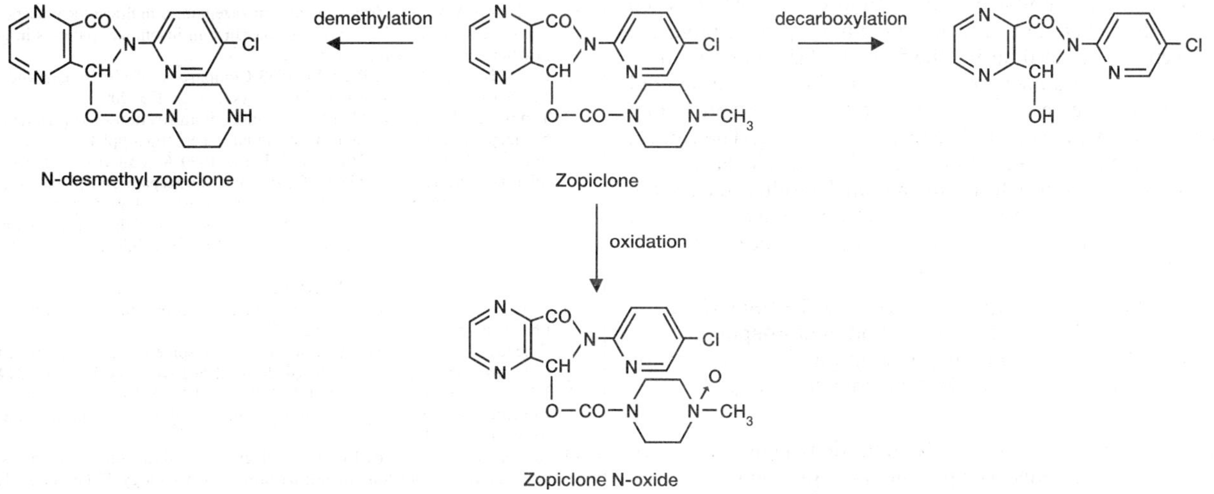

Pregnant women
No teratogenic or embryopathic effects have been demonstrated in animal experiments. Nevertheless, the established medical principle of not prescribing medications during pregnancy except only when absolutely necessary should be observed.

The elderly
A dose of 3.75 mg may be advisable initially but 7.5 mg is well tolerated and effective in these patients.

Concurrent disease
Severe hepatic insufficiency (serum albumin less than 30 $g.l^{-1}$ or presence of gross oedema) may significantly interfere with the elimination of zopiclone and the lower dosage level (3.75 mg) is recommended in such patients. The standard dose (7.5 mg) may be cautiously prescribed to patients with moderate (compensated) hepatic or renal insufficiency, but higher doses are not recommended in these patients. The product is removed by dialysis.

Drug interactions

Potentially hazardous interactions
No interactions of this kind have been reported. No impairment of psychomotor skills was found in healthy volunteers given alcohol one hour after zopiclone ingestion or the morning after. Alcohol did not influence the plasma concentration of zopiclone.[37–39]

Other significant interactions
Zopiclone plasma concentrations were increased by an intravenous administration of metoclopramide and decreased by atropine in 12 volunteers.[40] Subjects experienced less sedation with zopiclone plus atropine; hence, drugs which affect gastric emptying may influence the hypnotic activity of zopiclone. In contrast, pretreatment of surgical patients with oral ranitidine 150 mg 2 hours prior to zopiclone did not alter sedation.[41]

The pharmacokinetics of trimipramine 50 mg and zopiclone 7.5 mg in volunteers given simultaneous oral doses remain unchanged. However, a trend was seen toward a decreased AUC which might lead to a lessened antidepressant effect of trimipramine. The clinical importance of this interaction remains undetermined.

Potentially useful interactions
No interactions of this kind have been observed.

Clinical trials

1. Nicholson A N, Stone B M 1983 Zopiclone: sleep and performance studies in healthy man. Pharmacology 27 (suppl 2): 92–97

The effects of 2.5, 5.0, 7.5 and 20.0 mg zopiclone on sleep and on performance the next day were studied in 6 healthy adult males aged between 21 and 33 years. The experiment was double-blind and placebo-controlled. Doses of 5 and 10 mg zopiclone decreased the amount of awake activity and drowsy (stage 1) sleep over the first 6 h of sleep, but this effect was only present for the whole sleep period with the 10 mg dose. The duration and percentage of stage 3 sleep were increased with 7.5 mg. The 7.5 and 10 mg doses increased the combined duration of stages 2, 3 and 4 sleep over the first 6 h and over the whole night. The first period of rapid eye movement sleep was delayed with 7.5 mg, and with 10 mg the time spent in rapid eye movement sleep was reduced during the first 6 h of sleep but not over the whole night. The number of substitutions in the digit symbol substitution test was decreased 9 h after ingestion of 7.5 and 10 mg, and the number of symbols copied reduced after 10 mg. The clinical dose range of zopiclone is likely to be up to 7.5 mg. The latter dose provides a useful hypnotic effect with minimal residual effects the next day, whilst 5.0 mg is appropriate for those involved in skilled tasks where even the most minor changes in performance during the early part of the next day must be avoided.

2. Dehlin O, Rundgren A, Borjesson L et al 1983 Zopiclone to geriatric patients. A parallel double-blind dose-response clinical trial of zopiclone as a hypnotic to geriatric patients — a study in a geriatric hospital. Pharmacology 27 (suppl 2): 173–178

Zopiclone was given for 14 nights to 68 geriatric patients (mean age 81 years) with sleep problems. The patients were randomly allocated to four treatment groups: 3.75, 5, 7.5, or 10 mg of zopiclone. Sleep quantity and quality, side effects, and influence on psychomotor performance (digit symbol substitution and letter cancellation test) were studied before treatment, during active treatment and after withdrawal of the drug. All patients slept better on zopiclone compared to placebo. There were only slight differences between different dose levels as regards quantity and quality. No influence on psychomotor performance could be shown. The side effects were few. Zopiclone showed a good hypnotic efficacy, and 7.5 mg was thought to be the best dose for elderly patients.

3. Billiard M, Besset A, Lustrac de C, Brissaud L 1987 Dose-response effects of zopiclone on night sleep and on nighttime and daytime functions. Sleep 10 (suppl 1): 27–34
4. Anderson A A 1987 Zopiclone and nitrazepam: a multicentre placebo controlled comparative study of efficacy and tolerance in insomniac patients in general practice. Sleep 10 (suppl 1): 54–62
5. Subhan Z, Hindmarch I 1984 Effects of zopiclone and benzodiazepine hypnotics on search in short-term memory. Neuropsychobiology 12: 244–248
6. Autret E, Maillard F, Autret A 1987 Comparison of the clinical hypnotic effects of zopiclone and triazolam. European Journal of Clinical Pharmacology 31: 621–623
7. Monchesky T C, Phillips R, Billings B J 1986 Zopiclone: a new nonbenzodiazepine hypnotic used in general practice. Clinical Therapeutics 8: 283–291

General review articles

Goa L K, Heel R C 1986 Zopiclone: a review of its pharmacodynamic and pharmacokinetic properties and therapeutic efficacy as an hypnotic. Drugs 32: 48–65
Hindmarch I, Musch B 1990 Zopiclone in clinical practice. International Clinical Psychopharmacology 5 (suppl 2): 1–158

References

1. Blanchard J C, Boireau A, Julou L 1983 Brain receptors and zopiclone. Pharmacology 27 (suppl 2): 59–69
2. Julou L, Bardone M C, Blanchard J C, Garret C, Stutzmann J M 1983 Pharmacological studies on zopiclone. Pharmacology 27 (suppl 2): 46–58
3. Broadhurst A, Cushnaghan R C 1987 Residual effects of zopiclone (Imovane). Sleep 10 (suppl 1): 48–53
4. Lader M, Denney S C 1983 A double-blind study to establish the residual effects of zopiclone on performance in healthy volunteers. Pharmacology 27 (suppl 2): 98–108
5. Duriez R, Barthelemy C, Rives H, Courjaret J, Gregoire J 1979 Traitement des troubles du sommeil par la zopiclone: essais cliniques en double insu contre placebo. Therapie 34: 317–325
6. Monchesky T C, Billings B J, Phillips R 1986 Zopiclone: a new nonbenzodiazepine hypnotic used in general practice. Clinical Therapeutics 8: 283–291
7. Momose T 1983 Effectiveness of zopiclone. Pharmacology 27 (suppl 2): 196–204
8. Giercksky K E, Wickstrom E 1980 A dose-response study with zopiclone, a new tranquillizer. Clinical Therapeutics 3: 21–27
9. Dehlin O, Rundgren A, Borjesson L et al 1983 Zopiclone to geriatric patients: a parallel double-blind dose-response clinical trial of zopiclone as a hypnotic — a study in a geriatric hospital. Pharmacology 27 (suppl 2): 173–178
10. Elie R, Deschenes J-P 1983 Efficacy and tolerance of zopiclone in patients. Pharmacology 27 (suppl 2): 179–187
11. Anderson A A 1987 Zopiclone and nitrazepam: a multicenter placebo controlled comparative study of efficacy and tolerance in insomniac patients in general practice. Sleep 10 (suppl 1): 54–62
12. Pull C B, Dreyfus J F, Brun J P 1983 Comparison of nitrazepam and zopiclone in psychiatric patients. Pharmacology 27 (suppl 2): 205–209
13. Tamminen T, Hansen P P 1987 Chronic administration of zopiclone and nitrazepam in the treatment of insomnia. Sleep 10 (suppl 1): 63–72
14. Ponciano E, Freitas F, Hindmarch I et al 1990 A comparison of the efficacy, tolerance and residual effects of zopiclone, flurazepam and placebo in insomniac out patients. International Clinical Psychopharmacology 5 (suppl 2): 69–78
15. Autret E, Maillard F, Autret A 1987 Comparison of the clinical hypnotic effects of zopiclone and triazolam. European Journal of Clinical Pharmacology 31: 621–623
16. Wickstrom E, Barbo S E, Dreyfus J F et al 1983 A comparative study of zopiclone and flunitrazepam in insomniacs seen by general practitioners. Pharmacology 27 (suppl 2): 165–172
17. Wheatley D 1985 Zopiclone a non-benzodiazepine hypnotic controlled comparison to temazepam in insomnia. British Journal of Psychiatry 146: 312–314
18. Billiard M, Besset A, Lustrac De C, Brissaud L 1987 Dose-response effects of zopiclone on night sleep and on nighttime and daytime functioning. Sleep 10 (suppl 1): 27–34
19. Jovanovic U J, Dreyfus J F 1983 Polygraphical sleep recordings in insomniac patients under zopiclone or nitrazepam. Pharmacology 27 (suppl 2): 136–145

20. Mamelak M, Scima A, Price V 1983 Effects of zopiclone on the sleep of chronic insomniacs. Pharmacology 27 (suppl 2): 156–164
21. Mouret J, Ruel D, Maillard F, Bianchi M 1990 Comparative effects of zopiclone and triazolam on sleep in aged insomniacs. International Clinical Psychopharmacology 5 (suppl 2): 47–55
22. Nicholson A N, Stone B M 1987 Efficacy of zopiclone in middle age. Sleep 10 (suppl 1): 35–39
23. Nicholson A N, Stone B M 1983 Zopiclone: sleep and performance studies in healthy man. Pharmacology 27 (suppl 2): 92–97
24. Quadens O P, Hoffman G, Buytaert G 1983 Effects of zopiclone as compared to flurazepam on sleep in women over 40 years of age. Pharmacology 27 (suppl 2): 146–155
25. Tiberge M, Calvet U, Hayin K, Delahaye C, Arbus L 1988 Comparaison des effets de la zopiclone et du triazolam sur le sommeil du sujet sain. L'Encephale XIV: 319–324
26. Harrison C, Subhan Z, Hindmarch I 1985 Residual effects of zopiclone and benzodiazepine hypnotics on psychomotor performance related to car driving. Drugs under Experimental and Clinical Research 11: 823–829
27. Subhan Z 1983 The effects of benzodiazepines on short-term memory capacity. In: Benzodiazepines, sleep and daytime performance. The Medicine Publishing Foundation, Oxford, pp 29–41
28. Subhan Z, Hindmarch I 1984 Effects of zopiclone and benzodiazepine hypnotics on search in short-term memory. Neuropsychobiology 12: 244–248
29. Musch B, Bianchi M 1990 Lack of rebound effects and withdrawal symptoms with zopiclone: a review of 25 clinical studies. International Clinical Psychopharmacology 5 (suppl 2): 139–145
30. Gaillot J, Heusse D, Houghton G W, Marc Aurele J, Dreyfus J F 1983 Pharmacokinetics and metabolism of zopiclone. Pharmacology 27 (suppl 2): 76–91
31. Gaillot J, Roux Le Y, Houghton G W, Dreyfus J F 1987 Critical factors for pharmacokinetics of zopiclone in the elderly and in patients with liver and renal insufficiency. Sleep 10 (suppl 1): 7–21
32. Bechelli L P de C, Navas F, Pierangelo S A 1983 Comparison of the reinforcing properties of zopiclone and triazolam in former alcoholics. Pharmacology 27 (suppl 2): 235–241
33. Dorian P, Sellers E M, Kaplan H, Hamilton C 1983 Evaluation of zopiclone physical dependence liability in normal volunteers. Pharmacology 27 (suppl 2): 228–234
34. Boissl K, Dreyfus J F, Delmotte M 1983 Studies on the dependence-inducing potential of zopiclone and triazolam. Pharmacology 27 (suppl 2): 242–247
35. Lader M, Frcka G 1987 Subjective effects during administration and on discontinuation of zopiclone and temazepam in normal subjects. Pharmacopsychiatry 20: 67–71
36. Ranlov P J, Nielsen S P 1987 Effects of zopiclone and diazepam on ventilatory response in normal human subjects. Sleep 10 (suppl 1): 40–47
37. Mamelak M, Buck L, Csima A, Price V, Smiley A 1987 Effects of flurazepam and zopiclone on the performance of chronic insomniac patients: a study of ethanol–drug interaction. Sleep 10 (suppl 1): 79–87
38. Seppala T, Nuotto E, Dreyfus J F 1983 Drug–alcohol interactions on psychomotor skills: zopiclone and flunitrazepam. Pharmacology 27 (suppl 2): 127–135
39. Hindmarch I 1990 Immediate and overnight effects of zopiclone 7.5 mg and nitrazepam 5 mg with ethanol, on psychomotor performance and memory in healthy volunteers. International Clinical Psychopharmacology 5 (suppl 2): 105–113
40. Elliot P, Chestnutt W N, Elwood R J, Dundee J W 1983 Effect of atropine and metoclopramide on the plasma concentrations of orally administered zopiclone. British Journal of Anaesthesia 55: 159–160
41. Dundee J W, Elwood R J, Hildebrand P J, Singleton M 1983 Dose-finding and premedication studies with zopiclone. Pharmacology 27 (suppl 2): 210–215

Zuclopenthixol

Zuclopenthixol was the second thioxanthine antipsychotic drug to achieve wide therapeutic use.

Chemistry

Zuclopenthixol hydrochloride (Clopixol, Clopenthixol, Cisordinol)
$C_{22}H_{25}ClN_2OS.2HCl$
cis(Z)-2-(4-(3-(2-Chlorothioxanthenylid-9-ene)propyl)piperazin-1-yl) ethanol dihydrochloride
Zuclopenthixol decanoate
(Clopixol Depot, Clopixol Conc, Cisordinol Depot)
cis(Z)-2-(4-(3-(2-Chlorothioxanthenylid-9-ene)propyl)piperazin-1-yl)ethanol decanoate

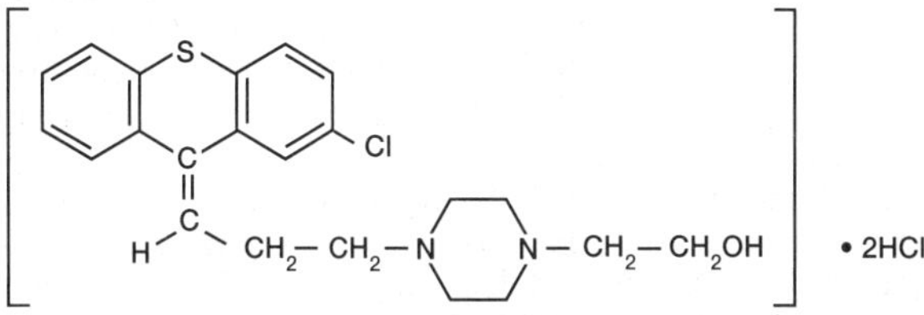

	Hydrochloride	*Decanoate*
Molecular weight	473.9	555.2
(free base)	(401.0)	
pKa	3.4, 6.1	
Solubility		
in alcohol	slight	—
in water	high	very low
Octanol/water partition coefficient	log p > 4.4	—

Zuclopenthixol hydrochloride is an off-white, granular powder, prepared by chemical synthesis, having no more than a slight odour and a bitter taste. It is very soluble in water.

Zuclopenthixol decanoate is a yellow, viscous oil with a slight odour, very sparingly soluble in water.

Pharmacology

Zuclopenthixol primarily acts as a neuroleptic drug. In this it suppresses complex behaviour and spontaneous movements but leaves untouched spinal reflexes and unconditioned nociceptive behaviour. Zuclopenthixol has high affinity for both dopamine D_1 and dopamine D_2 receptors.[1] In the mesolimbic dopamine system of the brain, these actions account for the antipsychotic actions of the drug, while similar actions in the nigrostriatal system may produce the extrapyramidal effects of parkinsonism.

Zuclopenthixol has other effects on the central nervous system. In the chemoreceptor trigger zone, the dopamine blockade accounts for the antiemetic effect of the drug. Zuclopenthixol acts on the hypothalamus to increase prolactin secretion. It has a weak anticholinergic effect at muscarinic receptors. Zuclopenthixol is an antagonist at α_1-adrenoceptors and is also an antagonist at histamine (H_1) receptors, and 5-hydroxytryptamine (5-HT_2) receptors.

Repeated-dose studies in animals suggest that supersensitivity, tolerance and cross-tolerance are less than with other classes of antipsychotic drug,[2] and that when compared with antipsychotic drugs from other chemical groups, the acute dopamine receptor-blocking effect of zuclopenthixol remains relatively unchanged by concomitant treatment with anticholinergic agents, benzodiazepines, or GABA-agonists.[3] However, there are no clinical data to support these claims.

Toxicology

Zuclopenthixol does not have carcinogenic or mutagenic potential, and toxicological testing in rats and dogs has failed to demonstrate any results of potential clinical relevance. There is no evidence of teratological potential in mice, rats and rabbits. Data from a perinatal study in rats shows that zuclopenthixol does not cause toxic effects in late pregnancy or during lactation.

Clinical pharmacology

Zuclopenthixol when given to normal subjects produces effects that are perceived as unpleasant even when given in small (2 mg) doses. Sedation without sleep, restlessness and unclear thinking are common effects. In patients with psychotic symptoms the drug produces calmness and responsiveness. Aggressive behaviour diminishes and the hallucinations and delusions gradually disappear. Initiative is reduced, with slowness of response and drowsiness, but intellectual capabilities are not impaired. With zuclopenthixol there is a generalized slowing of the EEG with an increase of theta waves. The seizure threshold is lowered by zuclopenthixol and fits may be induced in epileptic patients.

Clopenthixol has two stereoisomers, a *cis* and a *trans* form. The *cis*(Z)-isomer (known as zuclopenthixol) has been shown to possess antipsychotic activity, whereas the *trans*(E)-isomer is relatively inactive.[4] *Cis*(Z)-clopenthixol is a potent antagonist at both dopamine D_1 and D_2 receptors, whereas *trans*(E)-clopenthixol has relatively low activity at both D_1 and D_2 receptors.[5] Thus, dose for dose, *cis*(Z)-clopenthixol has twice the antipsychotic effect of the original racemic preparation of clopenthixol.[6] All marketed forms of the drug now contain only the *cis*(Z)-isomer.

The recommended dose is 2–80 mg daily orally. The highest dose known to have been used was 350 mg a day. For the depot preparation the recommended dose range is 100–750 mg intramuscularly every 2 to 4 weeks. The highest dose used was 1600 mg as a single dose.

In addition to its pronounced antipsychotic effect, zuclopenthixol possesses significant sedative effects. There is an immediate, transient and dose-dependent degree of sedation, which can be an advantage in the acute treatment phase of psychosis. Tolerance to this effect develops rapidly, but some residual sedation remains which can be particularly useful in the treatment of patients who are agitated, hostile or aggressive.

The antiemetic effects of zuclopenthixol are well recognized and are due to an effect on the chemoreceptor trigger zone. Zuclopenthixol may lower blood pressure and increases heart rate primarily due to the α-adrenoceptor blocking effect. Postural hypotension may be a risk in the elderly or in thin, frail individuals.

Zuclopenthixol has relatively weak anticholinergic effects but may cause blurring of vision, constipation, decreased sweating and occasional retention of urine. Zuclopenthixol lowers body temperature if the ambient temperature is lowered and this effect applies in both pyrexial and apyrexial individuals.

Pharmacokinetics

The preferred analytical method is high performance liquid chromatography.[7] The lower limit of sensitivity is about 0.5 $\mu g.l^{-1}$. The assay is not affected by the tricyclic antidepressants, amitriptyline, nortriptyline and imipramine, and the antiparkinson drugs orphenadrine, procyclidine and biperiden. However, the benzodiazepines do interfere with the assay.

Zuclopenthixol is rapidly absorbed from the gastrointestinal tract, with maximum serum concentrations occurring about 4 hours (2–12 hours) after a single oral dose.[7] The absorption seems to be complete but direct evidence is not available. There is moderately high presystemic metabolism and over 40% of an oral dose is eliminated in this way.

The maximum serum concentration of zuclopenthixol is reached 5 to 7 days after the depot injection.[7–9] The serum concentration then declines exponentially with a half life of 19 days, reflecting the rate of release from the depot. Zuclopenthixol decanoate is hydrolysed to the active substance, zuclopenthixol, when it reaches the body water phase. Significant serum levels of zuclopenthixol are maintained when the interval between depot injections is 4 weeks.[8]

Zuclopenthixol acetate is released from the oil vehicle by diffusion. The ester bond is then rapidly hydrolysed to release the active drug, zuclopenthixol. The increase in serum concentration is relatively fast, with the maximum serum concentration being reached after about 36 hours. This then slowly decreases so that 72 hours after the injection the serum level is about one third of the peak level[10].

Zuclopenthixol is distributed throughout the body in the same way as other antipsychotics, with highest concentrations of drug and metabolites in the liver, lungs, intestines and kidneys, and lower concen trations in the heart, spleen, brain and blood. The kinetics are linear since highly significant correlations exist between the dose and serum level and between the dose and the area under the serum concentration curve.[8,9,14,16] A regular daily dose of 20 mg zuclopenthixol orally will produce a mean steady-state serum level of about 13 $\mu g.l^{-1}$. The average serum level of zuclopenthixol corresponding to a 100 mg dose of zuclopenthixol decanoate every 2 weeks is about 8 $\mu g.l^{-1}$. Pharmacokinetically, a dose of 200 mg every 2 weeks has been calculated to be equivalent to a daily oral dose of 25 mg. Zuclopenthixol is excreted in human breast milk and the ratio of milk concentration to serum concentration[11] is on average 3 to 10. Although there is no specific evidence, it is likely that severe hepatic failure will result in reduced metabolism and hence reduced elimination of the drug. The effect of renal failure is more uncertain since only about 0.1% of unchanged drug is excreted in the urine. However, severe renal failure may lead to some accumulation of metabolites and could result in altered protein binding.

Oral absorption	>95%
Presystemic metabolism	44%
Plasma half life	
range	13–23 h
mean	20 h
Volume of distribution	20 $l.kg^{-1}$
Plasma protein binding	98%

The mean half life for the depot preparation is 19 days, which refers to rate of release from oil depot, not elimination of the drug.

Concentration–effect relationship

The lower limit for antipsychotic effect in moderately psychotic patients suffering from paranoid psychosis was found to be a serum concentration of 3–4 $\mu g.l^{-1}$, and 5–8 $\mu g.l^{-1}$ in severely psychotic patients.[12] In acute mania, serum levels in the range 5–8 $\mu g.l^{-1}$ were effective, but levels less than 5 $\mu g.l^{-1}$ were not.[13] A study of zuclopenthixol decanoate in schizophrenia[14] showed that high serum

Fig. 1 The metabolism of zuclopenthixol

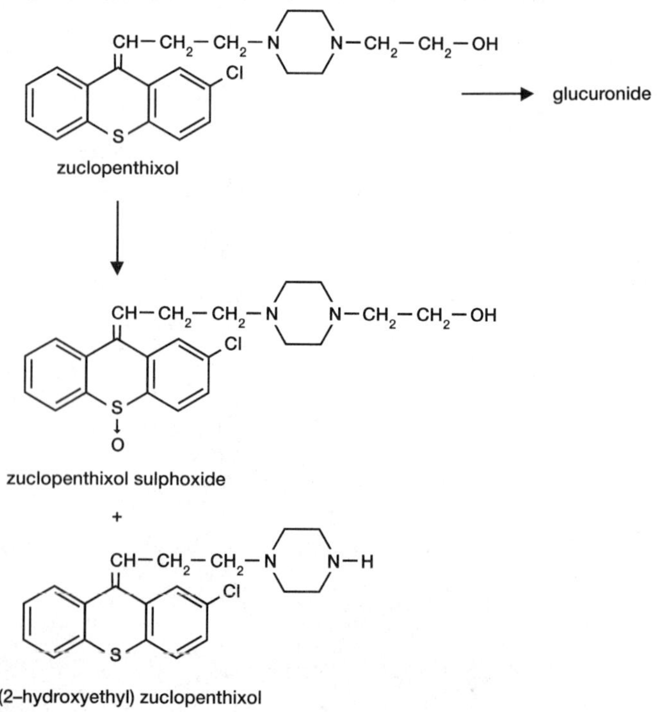

concentrations were associated with poor control of psychotic symptoms, and there were more side effects than with more modest doses. This may partly reflect the common clinical practice of using high doses when the antipsychotic response is unsatisfactory. This study also found that when moderately ill patients were each treated with their optimum dose of drug, those patients experiencing side effects had significantly higher serum concentrations than those without side effects. Despite such findings, therapeutic drug monitoring is used infrequently in normal clinical practice.

Metabolism

The drug is excreted mainly in the faeces but also to some degree in the urine. There is evidence of enterohepatic circulation. The excretion of the drug and metabolites in urine amounts to some 10–20% of the dose administered.

Zuclopenthixol is extensively metabolized in the liver.[15] The firstreaction is sulphoxidation, the second is side-chain N-dealkylation, and the third is glucuronic acid conjugation. The following metabolites have been identified:
clopenthixol glucuronide, clopenthixol sulphoxide, des(2-hydroxyethyl) clopenthixol and its sulphoxide metabolite.
None of the metabolites is pharmacologically active.

Pharmaceutics

Zuclopenthixol, Clopixol (Lundbeck, UK), is available in oral and parenteral forms and all forms contain only the *cis*(Z)-isomer of clopenthixol.

1. Tablets contain 2 mg (pink), 10 mg (light red-brown) and 25 mg (red-brown). The tablets are round, biconvex and film-coated.
2. Zuclopenthixol decanoate is an oily injection fluid with a duration of action of 2 to 4 weeks. 1 ml contains 200 mg (Clopixol Injection) or 500 mg (Clopixol Conc. Injection) zucopenthixol decanoate in Viscoleo, a clear yellow vegetable oil. Zuclopenthixol is converted to the highly lipophilic substance, zuclopenthixol decanoate, by esterification of zuclopenthixol with decanoic acid. When dissolved in oil and injected intramuscularly, zuclopenthixol decanoate diffuses very slowly into the surrounding body water, where it undergoes enzymatic breakdown to release the active component, zuclopenthixol.
3. Zuclopenthixol acetate is an oily injection fluid with a duration of action of 2 to 3 days. 1 ml contains 50 mg (Clopixol Acuphase Injection) zuclopenthixol acetate in Viscoleo. It is obtained by esterification of zuclopenthixol with acetic acid. When injected intramuscularly it diffuses slowly into surrounding body water where it undergoes enzymatic breakdown to release the active component, zuclopenthixol.

The depot formulations and zuclopenthixol acetate should be protected from light and has a maximal shelf life of 2 years. The tablets have a shelf life of 3 years. Zuclopenthixol drops, mixture and aqueous injection are not available in the UK.

Therapeutic use

Indications

1. Control of psychotic symptoms in schizophrenia and other psychoses
2. Maintenance therapy in schizophrenia to prevent relapse
3. Control of manic symptoms in the manic phase of manic-depressive psychosis.

Limited indications

4. Mental handicap with behavioural problems
5. Dementia with behavioural problems.

Contraindications

1. Acute alcohol, barbiturate and opiate intoxications
2. Comatose states
3. Advanced renal, hepatic or cardiovascular disease.

Relative contraindications

4. Psychoses with prominent apathy or withdrawal
5. Parkinson's disease.

Zuclopenthixol

Mode of use

Oral dosage should be individually adjusted according to the patient's condition. In general, small doses should be used initially and increased to the optimal effective level as rapidly as possible, based on therapeutic response.

Zuclopenthixol decanoate in normal and concentrated forms is administered by intramuscular injection. Local tolerance is good. Both dosage and the interval between dose should be individually adjusted according to therapeutic response.

A dose range of 10–50 mg a day is usual for oral treatment, normally given in divided doses, twice daily. For the control of symptoms in acute psychosis, an initial dose of about 20 mg a day would be appropriate. This could be increased, if necessary, by 10–20 mg every 2 to 3 days to 75 mg or more daily. For the maintenance treatment of chronic schizophrenia and other chronic psychoses the oral dose range is usually 20–40 mg a day. The maintenance treatment dose for zuclopenthixol decanoate would normally be 200–400 mg (1–2 ml) every 2 to 4 weeks.

A few patients may require higher doses or shorter intervals between doses. If doses over 250 mg every 1 to 4 weeks are thought to be indicated, then to avoid large volumes of the standard preparation, the more concentrated solution, zuclopenthixol decanoate (500 mg in 1 ml) is available.

If the clinician wishes to change the medication from oral zuclopenthixol to an equivalent dose of zuclopenthixol decanoate to be administered as maintenance treatment every two weeks, the dose of the depot may be calculated as approximately eight times the daily oral dose. Oral zuclopenthixol should be continued during the first week after the injection but in diminishing dosage. Patients being transferred from other depot injections should receive a dose in the ratio of 200 mg zuclopenthixol decanoate to 40 mg flupenthixol decanoate or to 25 mg fluphenazine decanoate.

Zuclopenthixol acetate has a dose range of 50–150 mg as a single injection which may be repeated, but preferably with an interval of 48 to 72 hours between injections. Some patients may need an additional injection between one and two days after the first injection. Zuclopenthixol acetate is not intended for long-term use and duration of treatment should not be more than two weeks. The maximum accumulated dosage in a course should not exceed 400 mg and the number of injections should not exceed four. Treatment may be continued with the same drug in oral or depot form. To introduce zuclopenthixol tablets, start two or three days after the last injection with 20–60 mg a day in divided doses, which if necessary can be increased by 10–20 mg each day. In order to substitute zuclopenthixol decanoate for zuclopenthixol acetate, give 200–400 mg concomitantly with the last injection of zuclopenthixol acetate. Zuclopenthixol acetate has much potential in the treatment of acutely disturbed psychotic patients who refuse oral antipsychotics,[17,18,19] as aqueous injections need to be repeated several times a day and long-acting depot medication is too inflexible in the initial stage of treatment. Zuclopenthixol acetate results in a fairly slow rise of zuclopenthixol, reaching a maximum concentration in about 36 hours, and this novel pharmacokinetic profile might be one of the explanations for the low frequency of side effects. Dystonia may occasionally be a problem in young men with acute psychosis[18]. Sedation is an effect which is useful in the treatment of acutely disturbed psychotic patients. The onset of sedation is rapid, becoming evident within 2 hours of the injection, and is maximal about 8 hours after injection which is more than 24 hours earlier than the maximum serum level is reached and thus the risk of over sedation, even after a second injection, is low.

Aside from the eventual relapse into the psychotic state there are no problems when zuclopenthixol is suddenly stopped.

For the control of agitation in mentally handicapped adult patients oral zuclopenthixol has been used in doses from 6 to 20 mg a day. If necessary, this can be increased to 25–40 mg a day.

In the control of agitation and confusion in patients with dementia, oral treatment in the range of 2–6 mg a day can be used. This should preferably be given late in the day. If necessary the dose can be increased to 10–20 mg a day.

Indications

1. Control of psychotic symptoms in schizophrenia and other psychoses

A double-blind study comparing oral clopenthixol with chlorproma-

Zuclopenthixol

zine[20] found both drugs equally effective in acute schizophrenia, but extrapyramidal side effects and drowsiness were commoner with clopenthixol. Sedation may have been worse because clopenthixol then comprised a racemic mixture of its two isomers. The *trans*(E)-isomer is associated more with sedation,[2] but is not present in zuclopenthixol as currently marketed. It was suggested that oversedation was a transient phenomenon and could be minimized by making dose increases gradually.

Open studies[21–26] also support claims that zuclopenthixol is an effective treatment in schizophrenia with few side effects. Extrapyramidal side effects and oversedation are commonly reported, especially in the first week of treatment, but tend to diminish thereafter.

Double-blind studies with zuclopenthixol decanoate have compared it with perphenazine enanthate[27] and fluphenazine decanoate (see Major outcome trials). These studies found zuclopenthixol to be as effective an antipsychotic drug and as well tolerated as the comparison drug. Compared with perphenazine enanthate there was significantly greater reduction in hostility, suspiciousness, and uncooperativeness. Neither study produced evidence of significant difference in liability to cause side effects.

However, in another double-blind comparison,[28] akathisia was found to be significantly more severe with fluphenazine decanoate, but autonomic side effects were significantly more severe with zuclopenthixol decanoate.

Open studies[29–31] of zuclopenthixol decanoate also testify to its effectiveness in the control of psychotic symptoms in schizophrenia and liability to cause sedation and extrapyramidal side effects.

Zuclopenthixol may be particularly suitable for schizophrenic patients manifesting aggression or excitement.[27,28]

2. Maintenance therapy in schizophrenia

A one-year, open study[30] found no difference in the rate of relapse requiring rehospitalization compared with the previous year on other antipsychotic maintenance medication. An open five-year follow-up study[31] reported that zuclopenthixol decanoate was an adequate long-term maintenance treatment, that it appeared to have a better calming effect than flupenthixol decanoate but at higher doses caused drowsiness and subdued hostility and aggression. Another open study[32] reported good maintenance treatment results with zuclopenthixol decanoate.

A one-year, double-blind study[33] compared zuclopenthixol decanoate with flupenthixol palmitate in 60 outpatients, who had not relapsed for at least 15 months. Outcome was similar in terms of improved symptomatic control, number of dropouts, and side effects, including extrapyramidal symptoms and oversedation. One significant difference found was reduction of hostility with zuclopenthixol, but not with flupenthixol. This was also reported in the double-blind comparison with perphenazine enanthate.[27]

Longer-term, double-blind comparisons of zuclopenthixol decanoate and standard depot drugs are needed to assess any advantage zuclopenthixol may have in maintenance treatment for schizophrenia.

3. Control of manic symptoms

There are no double-blind comparisons of zuclopenthixol with standard treatment, but there have been open trials[22–26] in which manic patients were included as part of heterogeneous samples. These studies suggest that zuclopenthixol dihydrochloride is effective in mania, but do not identify any particular advantages for it over standard antipsychotic treatment. Being a sedative antipsychotic may confer advantages to zuclopenthixol in certain clinical situations, such as the management of the aggressive or hostile, manic patient.

In a study[34] comparing the *trans* and *cis* isomers of zuclopenthixol, the dopamine blockade produced by the *cis* isomer was necessary for the antimanic effect, whereas the *trans* isomer was ineffective despite its pronounced sedative action. This suggests that zuclopenthixol should only be used in mania when not only an antimanic (antidopaminergic) effect is desired, but also a strong sedative effect to control disturbed behaviour.

Limited indications

4. Mental handicap with behavioural problems

When psychomotor excitation, agitation, violence and other manifestations of disturbed behaviour are seen in the setting of mental handicap in an adult, an assessment of causal factors should be made. In addition to social and psychological treatment, drug treatment to control these symptoms may be needed. Antipsychotic drugs are used for this purpose and there is evidence suggesting oral zuclopenthixol is more effective than haloperidol.[35] In an open trial[36] of patients with mental handicap there were indications that zuclopenthixol decanoate could be useful in reducing aggressive and disruptive behaviour. It was generally felt that the patients who responded well were those whose episodes of aggression occurred against a background of a chronic state of high arousal.

5. Dementia with behavioural problems

In dementia, disturbance of behaviour, especially when this includes persistent and severe agitation or aggression, can be an indication for antipsychotic medication. In comparison with haloperidol in dementia,[37] an advantage for oral zuclopenthixol was found in that agitation was significantly improved and side effects were not a problem. Reviews of the use of antipsychotic drugs in dementia[38–40] report that sedation is associated with increased incontinence, falls, confusion and social withdrawal. The most drug-responsive symptoms are agitation, insomnia and psychotic symptoms such as hallucinations. There is insufficient evidence to recommend any specific antipsychotic in dementia, and the strong sedative properties of zuclopenthixol which confer therapeutic advantages also predispose to potentially dangerous side effects.

Contraindications

Absolute

1. Acute alcohol, barbiturate and opiate intoxications

The accurate assessment and monitoring of any state of intoxication, or coma, can be impaired by the use of antipsychotic drugs. Being sedative, zuclopenthixol is particularly liable to exacerbate respiratory depression. Also, in common with all antipsychotics, it reduces the threshold for epileptic seizures, making seizures more likely.

2. Comatose states

(See states of intoxication above.)

3. Advanced renal, hepatic or cardiovascular disease

This can impair metabolism of the drug, leading to accumulation of the drug and toxic effects.

Relative

1. Psychoses with prominent apathy or withdrawal

Sedative antipsychotic drugs like zuclopenthixol can exacerbate apathy and withdrawal. In these situations an antipsychotic drug with less sedative properties may be preferable.

2. Parkinson's disease

The dopamine-blocking action of zuclopenthixol will exacerbate Parkinson's disease. Anticholinergic activity might benefit the condition but as zuclopenthixol possesses little anticholinergic activity it is not a good choice if an antipsychotic drug is necessary in a patient with Parkinson's disease.

Adverse reactions

Potentially life-threatening effects

Patients exposed to antipsychotic drugs may very occasionally develop the neuroleptic malignant syndrome. Core features are hyperthermia, hypertonicity of skeletal muscles, and fluctuating consciousness, along with instability of the autonomic nervous system (blood pressure instability, tachycardia, cardiac dysrhythmias). Aside from immediate cessation of antipsychotic drug treatment, the use of general supportive measures is vital. Administration of the directly acting muscle relaxant, dantrolene, or the dopaminergic agonist, bromocriptine, may be helpful. The syndrome may persist for more than a week after oral antipsychotics are discontinued and two or three times longer when associated with depot antipsychotics. After recovery, antipsychotic treatment can be resumed, but it is prudent to use a different antipsychotic drug.

By July 1986 the Committee on Safety of Medicines had received reports of 17 cases of this syndrome, 5 of which were fatal.[41] Zuclopenthixol was not implicated in any of these cases, but that may simply reflect how often it is prescribed, rather than a lower likelihood of its causing this syndrome.

Zuclopenthixol

Acute overdosage
The main clinical features of overdose include: somnolence, coma, extrapyramidal symptoms, convulsions, shock and hyperthermia or hypothermia. Treatment is symptomatic and supportive. Gastric lavage should be carried out immediately after oral ingestion and activated charcoal may be useful to prevent absorption. Measures aimed at supporting the cardiovascular and respiratory systems should be instituted.

Adrenaline must not be used in these patients. There is no specific antidote.

Severe or irreversible adverse effects
Like other antipsychotic drugs, zuclopenthixol should be used with caution in patients with epilepsy or advanced hepatic, renal or cardiovascular disease. Some of the symptomatic adverse effects can be severe or irreversible at times.

Symptomatic adverse effects
The frequency of unwanted effects is generally low and the severity of the symptoms is most often mild. The frequency and severity are most pronounced in the early phase of treatment and decline during continued treatment. After a few months of treatment the majority of patients are only slightly or not at all troubled with the side effects most often recorded.[21–30] With zuclopenthixol decanoate these effects occur especially during the first few days after the depot injection has been given.

Parkinsonism and acute dystonia are movement disorders associated with all antipsychotic drugs. They can usually be controlled by reduction of the antipsychotic dosage or the administration of anticholinergic drugs. For akathisia, benzodiazepines or low-dose propranolol may be useful.

Tardive dyskinesia, comprising oro-facial movements and choreiform movements of the trunk and limbs, may occur in older patients on long-term therapy. There is no effective drug treatment. Reduction or discontinuation of antipsychotic therapy may be beneficial.

Cardiovascular side effects, due to α_1-adrenoceptor blockade, include orthostatic hypotension and tachycardia.

Autonomic adverse effects include reduced salivation, disturbance of accommodation, urinary retention and constipation. However, as anticholinergic activity is low, these side effects are infrequent.

Sexual dysfunctions such as loss of libido and erectile dysfunction are recognized adverse effects of antipsychotic drugs,[42] and may therefore occur with zuclopenthixol.

Endocrine effects include weight change, menstrual disturbance, and transient galactorrhoea.

Temporary, slight alterations in liver function tests may occur, and rarely, transient benign leucopenia has been reported.

Other effects
Like other antipsychotic drugs, zuclopenthixol causes an increase in the prolactin level, which may result in breast engorgement, galactorrhoea and menstrual disturbance.

Interference with clinical pathology tests
None is known.

High risk groups

Neonates
The drug is not used in neonates.

Breast milk. As zuclopenthixol is found in breast milk only in very low concentrations it is not likely to affect the infant when therapeutic doses are used. However, zuclopenthixol should only be given with caution when breast-feeding.

Children
The use of zuclopenthixol in children is not recommended.

Pregnant women
Zuclopenthixol should not be administered during pregnancy unless the expected benefit to the patient outweighs the potential risk to the fetus. Animal studies have not shown an increased incidence of fetal damage or other deleterious effects on reproduction.

The elderly
In this group lower doses are often effective. The drug should be started at about half the normal adult dose and cautiously increased as required, monitoring carefully for adverse effects.

Concurrent disease
As mentioned earlier, the drug should be used with caution in patients with epilepsy or advanced hepatic, renal or cardiovascular disease.

Drug interactions

Potentially hazardous interactions

Alcohol. Zuclopenthixol enhances the CNS effects of alcohol.

Adrenergic-neurone-blocking drugs. Guanethidine and similarly acting drugs may have their antihypertensive effect blocked by antipsychotic drugs.

Other significant reactions

Tricyclic antidepressants. When these are given with antipsychotic drugs, the two drugs inhibit each other's metabolism, resulting in higher serum levels for both drugs.

Levodopa. The beneficial effect of this drug may be reduced.

Metoclopramide and prochlorperazine. Concomitant use of these drugs increases the risk of extrapyramidal symptoms.

Potentially useful interactions
None is known.

Major outcome trials

1. Heikkila L, Laitinen J, Vartiainen H 1981 Cis(Z)-clopenthixol and haloperidol in chronic schizophrenic patients — a double-blind clinical multicentre investigation. Acta Psychiatrica Scandinavica 64 (suppl 294): 30–38

This double-blind study compared *cis*(Z)-clopenthixol with haloperidol in 63 chronic schizophrenic in-patients over 12 weeks. Statistically significant reduction of Brief Psychiatric Rating Scale (BPRS) score occurred with both drugs from the second week onwards. The only statistically significant difference was a larger reduction of thinking disturbance in the *cis*(Z)-clopenthixol group. There was also a trend for less side effects, especially extrapyramidal side effects with *cis*(Z)-clopenthixol. Overall, *cis*(Z)-clopenthixol compared well with a standard antipsychotic drug.

2. Walker C A 1983 A double-blind comparative trial of the decanoates of clopenthixol and fluphenazine in the treatment of chronic schizophrenic outpatients. Pharmatherapeutica 3: 289–293

45 chronic schizophrenic out-patients who met Feighner's criteria were entered into a 24-week double-blind study. No differences were detected between the therapeutic effect of the drugs on the Manchester Scale or the Brief Psychiatric Rating Scale (BPRS). There were no differences detected between the drugs in liability to cause side effects.

General review articles

No comprehensive English language review article specifically covering thioxanthines or zuclopenthixol is available. However, these drugs are discussed in the context of a review of other antipsychotic drugs in:

Mackay A V P 1982 Antischizophrenic drugs. In: Tyrer P J (ed) Drugs in psychiatric practice. Butterworths, London, ch 4, pp 42–81

Bradley P B 1986 Pharmacology of antipsychotic drugs. In: Bradley P B, Hirsch S R (eds) The psychopharmacology and treatment of schizophrenia. Oxford University Press, Oxford, ch 2, pp 27–70

References

1. Hytell J, Larsen J-J, Christensen A V, Arnt J 1985 Receptor-binding profiles of neuroleptics. In: Casey, Chase, Christensen, Gerlach (eds) Dyskinesia — Research and treatment (Psychopharmacology Supplementum 2), Springer-Verlag, Berlin, ch 2, pp 9–18
2. Christensen A V, Arnt J, Hyttel J, Svendsen O 1984 Behavioural correlates to dopamine D-1 and dopamine D-2 antagonists. Polish Journal of Pharmacological Pharmacology 36: 249–264
3. Hyttel J, Christensen A V 1983 Biochemical and pharmacological differentiation of neuroleptic effect on dopamine D-1 and D-2 receptors. Journal of Neural Transmission (suppl 18): 157–164

4. Gravem A, Engstrand E, Guleng R J 1978 Cis(Z)-clopenthixol and clopenthixol in chronic psychotic patients. A double-blind clinical investigation. Acta Psychiatrica Scandinavica 58: 384–388
5. Hyttel J 1985 Dopamine D-1 and D-2 receptors. Characterization and differential effects of neuroleptics. Acta Pharmaceutica Suecica (suppl 1) 1: 426–439
6. Heikkila L, Kartsen D, Valli K 1981 A double-blind clinical investigation of cis(Z)-clopenthixol and clopenthixol in chronic schizophrenic patients. Acta Psychiatrica Scandinavica 64 (suppl 294): 25–29
7. Aaes-Jorgensen T 1980 Specific high-performance chromatographic method for estimation of the cis(Z)- and trans(E)-isomers of clopenthixol and a N-dealkyl metabolite. Journal of Chromatography 183: 239–245
8. Jorgensen A, Jorgensen K, Overo O 1980 Clopenthixol and flupenthixol depot preparations in outpatient schizophrenics. III Serum levels. Acta Psychiatrica Scandinavica 61 (suppl 279): 41–45
9. Viala A, Hou N, Ba B, Durand A, Dufour H, D'Agostino N, Berda C, Jorgensen A 1984 Blood and plasma kinetics of cis(Z)-clopenthixol and fluphenazine in psychiatric patients after intramuscular injection of their decanoic esters. Psychopharmacology 83: 147–150
10. Amdisen A, Aaes-Jorgensen T, Thompsen N J, Madsen V T, Nielsen M S 1986 Serum concentrations and clinical effect of zuclopenthixol in acutely disturbed, psychotic patients treated with zuclopenthixol acetate in Viscoleo. Psychopharmacology 90: 412–416
11. Aaes-Jorgensen T, Bjorndal F, Bartels U 1986 Zuclopenthixol levels in serum and breast milk. Psychopharmacology 90: 417–418
12. Bjorndal F, Aaes-Jorgensen T 1984 Serumkoncentrationer ved akutte paranoide psykoser behandlet med cis(Z)-clopenthixol. Nordisk Psykiatrisk Tidsskrift 38: 229–233
13. Bjorndal F, Aaes-Jorgensen T 1982 Manibehandling med cis(Z)-clopenthixol. Nordisk Psykiatrisk Tidsskrrift 36: 321–324
14. Jorgensen A, Aaes-Jorgensen T, Gravem A et al 1985 Zuclopenthixol decanoate in schizophrenia: serum levels and clinical state. Psychopharmacology 87: 364–367
15. Khan A R 1969 Some aspects of clopenthixol metabolism in rats and humans. Acta Pharmacologica et Toxicologica 27: 202–212
16. Aaes-Jorgensen T, Kirk L, Peterson E, Danneskiold-Samsoe P, Jorgensen A 1983 Serum concentrations of the isomers of clopenthixol and a metabolite in patients given cis(Z)-clopenthixol in Viscoleo. Psychopharmacology 81: 68–72
17. Amdisen A, Nielsen M S, Deneker S J et al 1987 Zuclopenthixol acetate in viscoleo — a new drug formulation. Acta Psychiatrica Scandinavica 75: 99–107
18. Lowert A C, Rasmussen E M, Holm R et al 1989 Acute psychotic disorders treated with 5% zuclopenthixol acetate in 'Viscoleo' ('Cisordinol-Acutard'), a global assessment of the clinical effect: an open multi-centre study. Pharmatherapeutica 5: 380–386
19. Chakravarti S K, Muthu A, Muthu P K, Naik P, Pinto R T 1990 Zuclopenthixol acetate (5% in Viscoleo): Single dose treatment for acutely disturbed psychotic patients. Current Medical Research and Opinion 12: 58–65
20. Kingstone E, Kolivakis T, Kossatz I 1971 Double-blind study of clopenthixol and chlorpromazine in acute hospitalized schizophrenics. International Journal of Clinical Pharmacology, Therapy and Toxicology 1/70: 41–45
21. Sechter D, Caillard V, Cuche H, Deniker D 1981 Open clinical study of cis(Z)-clopenthixol. Acta Psychiatrica Scandinavica 64 (suppl 294): 20–24
22. Mann B S, Moslehuddin K S, Owen R T et al 1985 A clinical assessment of zuclopenthixol dihydrochloride (Clopixol tablets) in the treatment of psychotic illness. Pharmatherapeutica 4: 387–392
23. Konig P, Seifert T, Eberhardt G 1986 Findings with cis(Z)-clopenthixol in the treatment of acute mania and schizophrenia. Pharmacopsychiatry 19: 424–428
24. Bobon D, Troisfontaines B, Kempeneers J et al 1986 Open multicentre trial of zuclopenthixol in mania and schizophrenia based on AMDP scales. Acta Psychiatrica Belgica 86: 152–176
25. Bereen F, Harte F B, Maguire J, Singh A N 1987 The use of oral zuclopenthixol in the treatment of functional psychotic illness. Pharmatherapeutica 5: 62–68
26. Bhattachaaryya S N, Ghoshal J, Sharma S K et al 1987 Acute functional psychoses: treatment with zuclopenthixol dihydrochloride (Clopixol) tablets. Pharmatherapeutica 5: 1–8
27. Ahlfors U G, Dencker S J, Gravem A, Remvig J 1980 Clopenthixol decanoate and perphenazine enanthate in schizophrenic patients — a double-blind Nordic Multicentre trial. Acta Psychiatrica Scandinavica 61 (suppl 279): 77–91
28. Tegler J 1985 A comparative trial of cis(Z)-clopenthixol decanoate and fluphenazine decanoate. Pharmacopsychiatry 18: 78–79
29. Viswanathan R, Rajhkowa S 1982 Clopenthixol decanoate in the treatment of chronic schizophrenic inpatients. Pharmatherapeutica 3: 93–99
30. Swestka J, Nahunek K, Ceskova E, Rysanek R 1984 Therapeutic effects of one year of clopenthixol decanoate in schizophrenia. Activitas Nervosa Superior (Praha) 26: 21–22
31. Carney M W P 1984 A five year follow-up study of chronic schizophrenics treated with clopenthixol decanoate. Pharmatherapeutica 4: 57–63
32. Borsetti G, Rocco P, Spilimbergo P G et al 1984 Long-term treatment of chronic schizophrenics with clopenthixol decanoate. Pharmatherapeutica 4: 53–56
33. Dencker S J, Lepp M, Malm U 1980 Clopenthixol and flupenthixol depot preparations in outpatient schizophrenics. Acta Psychiatrica Scandinavica 61: 10–28
34. Nolen W A 1983 Dopamine and mania — the effects of trans- and cis-clopenthixol in a double-blind pilot study. Journal of Affective Disorders 5: 91–96
35. Karsten D, Kivimaki T, Linna S, Pollari L, Turunen S 1981 Neuroleptic treatment of oligophrenic patients. A double-blind clinical multicentre trial of cis(Z)-clopenthixol and haloperidol. Acta Psychiatrica Scandinavica 64 (suppl 294): 39–45
36. Mlele T J J, Wiley Y V 1986 Clopenthixol decanoate in the management of aggressive mentally-handicapped patients. British Journal of Psychiatry 149: 373–376
37. Gotestam K G, Ljunghall S, Olsson B 1981 A double-blind comparison of the effects of haloperidol and cis(Z)-clopenthixol in senile dementia. Acta Psychiatrica Scandinavica 64 (suppl 294): 46–53

Zuclopenthixol

38. Helms M 1985 Efficacy of antipsychotics in the treatment of the behavioural complications of dementia: a review of the literature. Journal of the American Geriatric Society 33: 206–209
39. Risse S C, Barnes R 1986 Pharmacological treatment of agitation associated with dementia. Journal of the American Geriatric Society 34: 368–376
40. Murphy E 1987 Drug treatment of behaviour problems in the elderly. Prescribers' Journal 27: 20–25
41. Committee on Safety of Medicines, 1986 Current problems. Neuroleptic malignant syndrome — an underdiagnosed condition? WHO Drug Information no. 18: 2
42. Barnes T R E 1984 Drugs and sexual dysfunction. In: Gaind R N, Fawzy F I, Hudson B L, Pasnau R O (eds) Current Themes in Psychiatry, vol 3. Spectrum Publications, New York, ch 4, pp 51–92

Name index

Entries in bold type are references to monographs, which are to be found in alphabetic order. *Denotes that the drug is on the World Health Organisation list of essential drugs (information taken by permission from The use of essential drugs (sixth list), fourth report of the WHO Expert Committee, Geneva, World Health Organisation, 1990 (WHO Technical Report Series No. 796)). Some proprietary names are of combination products and more than one monograph may be referenced.

A

D

E

F

G

H

I

J

K

N

O

P

Q

R

S

T

U

V

W

X

Y

Z

Therapeutic use index

ABORTION
Progesterone antagonist
Mifepristone
Prostaglandins
Dinoprost (prostaglandin F)
Dinoprostone
Gemeprost

ABORTION PREVENTION
Progesterone
Hydroxyprogesterone

ACIDOSIS
Sodium bicarbonate

ACNE
Isotretinoin
Tretinoin
Tetracycline (hydrochloride)

ACUTE RENAL FAILURE
Dopamine agonist
Dopamine (hydrochloride)
Osmotic diuretic
Mannitol

ADRENAL INSUFFICIENCY
Glucocorticoid
Cortisone acetate
Hydrocortisone
Prednisolone and prednisone
Mineralocorticoid
Fludrocortisone acetate

AGITATION
Dopamine-D_2 agonist
Chlorpromazine (hydrochloride)
Promazine (hydrochloride)
Benzodiazepines see ANXIETY

ALCOHOL DEPENDENCE
Disulfiram

ALCOHOL WITHDRAWAL
Chlormethiazole (edisylate)

ALLERGY
Histamine-H1 antagonists
Astemizole
Azatadine (moleate)
Brompheniramine (maleate)
Chlorpheniramine (maleate)
Cyproheptadine (hydrochloride)
Diphenhydramine
Loratadine
Mebhydroline
Mequitazine
Pheniramine (maleate)
Promethazine (hydrochloride)
Terfenadine
Trimeprazine (tartrate)
Triprolidine
See also ASTHMA, Anti-allergic

ANABOLIC STEROID
Danazol
Nandrolone decanoate

ANAEMIA
Iron deficiency
Iron salts, iron dextran complex and iron-sorbitol citrate
Megaloblastic
Folic acid
Uraemia
Epoetin
Vitamin-B_{12} deficiency
Cyanocobalamin
Hydroxocobalamin

ANAESTHESIA
Anticholinergic
Atropine (sulphate)
Injectable
Etomidate
Ketamine (hydrochloride)
Methohexitone (sodium)
Pentobarbitone (sodium)
Propofol
Thiopentone (sodium)
Volatile agents
Enflurane
Ether
Halothane
Isoflurane
Nitrous oxide

ANDROGEN DEFICIENCY
Testosterone (esters)

ANGINA
Adrenergic-beta-1 blockade
Acebutolol (hydrochloride)
Atenolol
Betaxolol (hydrochloride)
Metoprolol (tartrate)
Adrenergic beta blockade, non selective
Nadolol
Oxprenolol (hydrochloride)
Pindolol
Propranolol (hydrochloride)
Timolol (maleate)
Calcium L-channel blockade
Amlodipine (besylate)
Diltiazem
Felodipine
Isradipine
Nicardipine
Nifedipine
Verapamil
EDRF (NO) agonists
Glyceryl trinitrate
Isosorbide dinitrate
Isosorbide 5-mononitrate
Molsidomine

ANGIOEDEMA
Adrenergic agonist
Adrenaline
Androgen
Stanozol

ANTICOAGULANT
Coumarins
Nicoumalone
Phenindione
Warfarin
Coumarin antagonist
Vitamin K
Heparins
Heparin sodium and heparin calcium
Heparin antagonist
Protamine (sulphate)
Prostacyclin agonist
Epoprostenol sodium (prostacyclin sodium salt)
Iloprost

ANTISEPTIC
Benzalkonium chloride
Cetrimide
Chlorhexidine
Hexachlorophane
Iodine compounds
Noxythiolin
Potassium permanganate

ANXIETY
Benzodiazepines
Chlordiazepoxide (hydrochloride)
Clobazam
Clorazepate potassium
Diazepam
Ketazolam
Lorazepam
Medazepam
Midazolam (hydrochloride)
Oxazepam
Prazepam
Triazolam
Serotonin 5-HT_{1A}
Buspirone (hydrochloride)
Other
Meprobamate

ASTHMA
Anti-allergic
Nedocromil sodium
Sodium cromoglycate
Beta adrenergic agonists
Adrenaline
Isoprenaline (hydrochloride and sulphate)
Beta-2 selective
Fenoterol (hydrobromide)
Isoetharine and salts
Orciprenaline (sulphate)
Rimiterol hydrobromide
Salbutamol
Terbutaline
Cholinergic antagonist
Ipratropium bromide
Glucocorticoid, inhaled
Beclomethasone dipropionate
Betamethasone (valerate)
Budesonide
Histamine-1 antagonist
Ketotifen (fumerate)
Phosphodiesterase inhibitor
Theophylline

ATTENTION DEFICIT DISORDERS
Dexamphetamine (sulphate)
Methylphenidate

BACTERIAL INFECTIONS
Adjunctive drugs
Dehydropeptidase-I inhibitor
Imipenem/cilastatin
Beta-lactamase inhibitor
Clavulanic acid
Aminoglycosides
Amikacin (sulphate)
Gentamicin (sulphate)
Kanamycin (acid sulphate)
Neomycin (sulphate)
Netilmicin (sulphate)
Streptomycin
Tobramycin
Antibiotics used in tuberculosis and leprosy
Clofazimine
Dapsone
Ethambutol (hydrochloride)
Ethionamide
Isoniazid
Prothionamide
Pyrazinamide
Rifampicin
Streptomycin
Thiacetazone
Beta lactams, penicillins and cephalosporin bacterial transpeptidase inhibitors
Amoxycillin
Ampicillin
Azlocillin (sodium)
Aztreonam
Benzathine penicillin
Benzylpenicillin (sodium or potassium)
Carbenicillin (sodium)
Carfecillin (sodium)
Cefaclor (monohydrate)
Cefamandole (sodium)
Cefixime
Cefotaxime (sodium)
Cefotetan
Cefoxitin
Cefsulodin (sodium)
Ceftazidime
Ceftizoxime sodium
Ceftriaxone (sodium)
Cefuroxime (sodium and axetil)
Cephalexin (monohydrate)
Cephaloridine
Cephalothin (sodium)
Cephazolin
Cephradine
Cloxacillin (sodium)
Flucloxacillin (sodium)
Imipenem
Latamoxef disodium
Mecillinam
Mezlocillin
Phenoxymethylpenicillin (potassium)
Piperacillin (sodium)
Pivmecillinam (hydrochloride)
Procaine penicillin
Ticarcillin (disodium)
Dihydrofolate reductase inhibitor
Trimethoprim
Lincomycin derivatives
Clindamycin (hydrochloride)
Lincomycin hydrochloride
Macrolide
Erythromycin
5-Nitro-imidazoles
Metronidazole
Tinidazole
Polymyxins
Colistin (sulphate and sulphomethate sodium)
Polymyxin B (sulphate)
Quinolone, bacterial DNA gyrase inhibitors
Cinoxacin
Ciprofloxacin (hydrochloride)
Enoxacin
Nalidixic acid
Norfloxacin
Ofloxacin
Sulphonamides
Silver sulphadiazine
(Co-trimoxazole)
Sulfadoxine
Sulphacetamide

Sulphadiazine
Sulphadimidine
Sulphamethoxazole
Tetracyclines
Chlortetracycline (hydrochloride)
Demeclocycline (hydrochloride)
Doxycycline (hydrochloride)
Lymecycline
Methacycline (hydrochloride)
Minocycline (hydrochloride)
Oxytetracycline (dihydrate)
Tetracycline (hydrochloride)
Other antibiotics
Bacitracin
Chloramphenicol
Framycetin sulphate
Fusidic acid
Gramicidin
Mupirocin
Nitrofurantoin
Pentamidine
Spectinomycin (hydrochloride)
Spiramycin
Vancomycin (hydrochloride)

BONE (PAGET'S) DISEASE
Bisphosphonates
Clodronate
Etidronate (disodium)
Pamidronate (disodium pentahydrate)
Calcitonin agonist
Calcitonin

CARDIAC ARRHYTHMIA
Adrenergic-beta-1 blockade
Acebutolol (hydrochloride)
Atenolol
Betaxolol (hydrochloride)
Metoprolol
Practolol
Adrenergic, non-selective beta blockade
Nadolol
Oxprenolol (hydrochloride)
Pindolol
Propranolol (hydrochloride)
Timolol (maleate)
Adrenergic neurone blockade
Bretylium (tosylate)
Class 1
Disopyramide
Encainide (hydrochloride)
Flecainide acetate
Lignocaine (hydrochloride)
Mexiletine (hydrochloride)
Procainamide (hydrochloride)
Propafenone (hydrochloride)
Quinidine (bisulphate and sulphate)
Tocainide (hydrochloride)
Class III
Amiodarone (hydrochloride)
(Sotalol)
Digitalis glycosides
Digoxin
Digitoxin
Ouabin

CEREBRAL OEDEMA
Dexamethasone
Mannitol

CNS STIMULANT
Caffeine

CONSTIPATION
Bisacodyl
Cascara
Ispaghula
Lactulose
Methylcellulose
Sennosides

CONTRACEPTION
Desogestrel
Ethinyloestradiol
Ethynodiol diacetate
Levonorgestrel
Lynoestrenol
Medroxyprogesterone acetate
Mestranol
Norethisterone (acetate, heptanoate)

COUGH
Mucolytic
Carbocisteine
Opiate
Codeine
Dextromethorphan (hydrobromide)
Pholcodine

CUSHING'S SYNDROME
Aminoglutethemide
Metyrapone

DECONGESTANT
Ephedrine
Oxymetazoline hydrochloride
Phenylephrine (hydrochloride)
Phenylpropanolamine (hydrochloride)
Pseudoephedrine hydrochloride
Xylometazoline hydrochloride

DENTAL CARIES
Fluorides

DEPRESSION
Amine uptake inhibitors
Dopamine
Trimipramine (maleate)
Noradrenaline, mainly
Desipramine (hydrochloride)
Doxepin (hydrochloride)
Imipramine hydrochloride
Lofepramine (hydrochloride)
Maprotiline hydrochloride
Mianserin
Protriptyline (hydrochloride)
Noradrenaline/serotonin
Amitriptyline (hydrochloride)
Dothiepin (hydrochloride)
Nortriptyline (hydrochloride)
Serotonin
Clomipramine (hydrochloride)
Fluoxetine (hydrochloride)
Fluvoxamine maleate
Trazodone (hydrochloride)
Monoamine oxidase inhibitor
Isocarboxazid
Phenelzine
Tranylcypromine (sulphate)
Serotonin precursor
Tryptophan

DERMATOLOGICALS
Anti-dandruff
Selenium sulphide
Antiperspirant
Aluminium acetate and chloride
Application
Ichthammol
Sulphur
Burns
Silver nitrate
Silver sulphadiazine
Glucocorticoid
Beclomethasone dipropionate (topical)
Clobetasol propionate
Clobetasone butyrate
Fluocinolone acetonide (topical)
Fluocinonide (topical)
Hydrocortisone
Moisturiser
Urea (topical)
Skin lotion
Calamine
Viral warts
Formaldehyde
Glutaraldehyde
Podophyllum

DIABETES INSIPIDUS
Argipressin
Desmopressin (acetate)
see also HYPERTENSION: Thiazide diuretics

DIABETES MELLITUS
Alpha-glycoside hydrolase inhibitor
Acarbose
Biguanide
Metformin (hydrochloride)
Insulin
Bovine insulin
Human insulin
Porcine insulin
Sulphonylurea
Chlorpropamide
Glibenclamide
Glibornuride
Gliclazide
Glipizide
Gliquidone
Glymidine
Tolbutamide

DIAGNOSTIC (ADRENAL CORTEX)
Tetracosactrin

DIARRHOEA
Opiate
Diphenoxylate (hydrochloride)
Loperamide (hydrochloride)
Oral rehydration
Oral rehydration salts

DYSFUNCTIONAL UTERINE BLEEDING
Progesterone

DYSMENORRHOEA
Dydrogesterone
see also PAIN: cyclo-oxygenase inhibitors

ENERGY SOURCE
Glucose

EPILEPSY
Beclamide
Carbamazepine
Ethosuximide
Phenobarbitone
Phenytoin
Primidone
Sodium valproate
GABA operated chloride channel
Clonazepam
Diazepam
GABA transaminase inhibitor
Vigabatrin

EUPHORIANT
Cocaine

FOLLICLE,
Maturation
Chorionic gonadotrophin
Stimulation
Menotrophin

FUNGAL INFECTION
Flucytosine
Griseofulvin
Polyene antifungal
Amphotericin B
Nystatin
Imidazole
Clotrimazole
Econazole (nitrate)
Itraconazole
Ketoconazole
Miconazole (nitrate)
Topical
Undecenoic acid

GALL STONES
Chenodeoxycholic acid
Ursodeoxycholic acid

GLAUCOMA
Anti-cholinergic
Pilocarpine (hydrochloride, nitrate)
Beta adrenergic blockade
Betaxolol (hydrochloride)
Timolol (maleate)
Carbonic anhydrase inhibitor
Acetazolamide (sodium)

GONADAL SUPPRESSION
Buserelin (acetate)

GOUT
Anti-mitotic
Colchicine
Cyclo-oxygenase inhibitors
Indomethacin
Others see PAIN: Cyclo-oxygenase inhibitors
Xanthine oxidase inhibitor
Allopurinol

GROWTH HORMONE DEFICIENCY
Somatropin

HAEMOPHILIA
Factor VIII

HALLUCINOGEN
Cannabis

HEART FAILURE
Sodium-potassium ATPase inhibitors
Digitoxin
Digoxin
Angiotensin converting enzyme inhbitor
Captopril
Enalapril (maleate)
Lisinopril
Ramipril
Diuretics
Loop
Bumetanide
Frusemide
Potassium conserving
Amiloride (hydrochloride)
Triamterene
Thiazide
Bendrofluazide
Chlorothiazide
Chlorthalidone
Clopamide
Cyclopenthiazide
Hydrochlorothiazide
Hydroflumethiazide
Indapamide
Mefruside
Methyclothiazide
Metolazone
Polythiazide
Xipamide

Inotropes (with additional actions)
Dopamine (hydrochloride)
Dobutamine (hydrochloride)
Xamoterol (fumerate)
Opiates see PAIN: opiates

HELMINTH INFECTION
Nematode
(Ascaris)
Bephenium hydroxynaphthoate
Piperazine
(Ascaris/ancylostoma/necator)
Pyrantel embonate
(Wucheria)
Diethylcarbamazine (citrate)
(Onchocerciasis)
Ivermectin
(Onchocerciasis/ trypanosomiasis)
Suramin
Nematode and cestode
(Ancyclostoma/strongyloides/ trichuris/taenia)
Albendazole
(Ancyclostoma/strongyloides/ trichuris)
Mebendazole
(Strongyloides)
Thiabendazole
Cestode
(Taenia)
Albendazole
Niclosamide
Trematode infection
(Schistosomiasis/cysticercosis)
Metriphonate
(Schistosomiasis/ paragonimiasis/fasciola)
Praziquantel

HEPARIN OVERDOSE
Protamine (sulphate)

HORMONE REPLACEMENT THERAPY
Dienoestiol
Ethinyloestradiol
Levonorgestrel
Oestradiol

HYPERALDOSTERONISM
Potassium canrenoate
Spironolactone

HYPERCALCAEMIA
Chelating agent
Disodium edetate (dihydrate)
Bisphosphonates
Clodronate
Etidronate (disodium)
Pamidronate (disodium pentahydrate)

HYPERCHOLESTEROLAEMIA
Anion exchange resin
Cholestyramine
Colestipol
HMG-CoA-reductase inhibitor
Lovastatin
Pravastatin (sodium)
Simvastatin
Fibrates
Bezafibrate
Clofibrate
Gemfibrozil
Other
Nicotinic acid
Probucol

HYPER-PROLACTINAEMIA
Bromocriptine
Cabergoline
Lisuride

HYPERTENSION
Adrenergic
Alpha-1 blockade
Doxazosin (mesylate)
Indoramin (hydrochloride)
Prazosin
Alpha-2 agonist
Clonidine (hydrochloride)
Methyldopa
Beta blockade, non selective
Nadolol
Oxprenolol (hydrochloride)
Pindolol
Propranolol (hydrochloride)
Sotalol
Timolol (maleate)
Beta-1 blockade
Acebutolol (hydrochloride)
Atenolol
Betaxolol (hydrochloride)
Bisoprolol
Metoprolol (tartrate)
Alpha plus beta blockade
Labetalol (hydrochloride)
Neurone blockade
Bethanidine (sulphate)
Debrisoquine (sulphate)
Guanethidine (monosulphate)
Amine depletion
Rauwolfia-reserpine
Angiotensin converting enzyme inhibitor
Captopril
Enalapril (maleate)
Lisinopril
Ramipril
Calcium L-channel blockade
Amlodipine (besylate)
Diltiazem (hydrochloride)
Felodipine
Isradipine
Nicardipine
Nifedipine
Verapamil
Diuretics
Loop
Bumetanide
Frusemide
Potassium conserving
Amiloride (hydrochloride)
Triamterene
Thiazide, and related
Bendrofluazide
Chlorothiazide
Chlorthalidone
Clopamide
Cyclopenthiazide
Hydrochlorothiazide
Hydroflumethiazide
Indapamide
Mefruside
Methyclothiazide
Metolazone
Polythiazide
Xipamide
Uricosuric
Tienilic acid
EDRF (NO) release
Sodium nitroprusside
Potassium channel (ATP sensitive) opener
Diazoxide
Minoxidil
Pinacidil monohydrate
Serotonin $5\text{-}HT_2$ (plus alpha adrenergic) blockade
Ketanserin (tartrate)
Vasodilators
Hydralazine (hydrochloride)

HYPERTHYROIDISM
Carbimazole
Iodine
Methimazole
Propylthiouracil
see also HYPERTENSION: Non-selective beta adrenergic blockade

HYPERURICAEMIA
Renal tubular anion exchange blockade
Probenecid
Sulphinpyrazone
Xanthine oxidase inhibitor
Allopurinol

HYPNOTIC
Barbiturate
Hexobarbitone (sodium)
Pentobarbitone
Quinalbarbitone (sodium)
Benzodiazepine
Flurazepam (hydrochloride)
Nitrazepam
Temazepam
Non-benzodiazepine GABA operated chloride channel
Zopiclone
Other
Chloral hydrate and chloral betaine
Methyprylone

HYPOCALCAEMIA
Calcium gluconate
see also VITAMIN DEFICIENCY, Vitamin D

HYPOTHYROIDISM
Thyroxine (sodium)
Liothyronine sodium

HYPOVOLAEMIA
Human albumin
Dextrans
Gelatin plasma substitutes

HYPOXAEMIA
Oxygen

ILEUS
Bethanecol
Distigmine (bromide)
Neostigmine
Pyridostigmine

IMMUNOSUPPRESSIVE
Antibody
Antilymphocyte globulin
Glucorticoid
Cortisone Acetate
Dexamethasone
Hydrocortisone
Methylprednisolone (sodium succinate)
Prednisolone and prednisone
Triamcinolone
IL2 synthesis inhibitor
Cyclosporin-A
Purine antimetabolite
Azathioprine

INDUCE HYPOTENSION
Trimetaphan (camsylate)

INDUCTION OF LABOUR
Oxytocin

INDUCTION OF OVULATION
Urofollitrophin

INDUCTION OF VOMITING
Ipecacuanha

INFERTILITY
Clomiphene (citrate)
Gonadorelin (hydrochloride)

LOCAL ANAESTHETIC
Amethocaine (hydrochloride)
Bupivacaine (hydrochloride)
Lignocaine (hydrochloride)
Prilocaine (hydrochloride)

MANIA
Lithium salts

MENIERES DISEASE
Betahistine (hydrochloride)

METHAEMOGLOBINAEMIA
Methylene blue

MIGRAINE
Alpha-2 adrenergic agonist
Clonidine
Beta adrenergic blocking drug
Acebutolol (hydrochloride)
Metoprolol (tartrate)
Nadolol
Propranolol (hydrochloride)
Timolol (maleate)
Ergot alkaloid
Dihydroergotamine (mesylate)
Ergotamine (tartrate)
Serotonin $5\text{-}HT_1$ agonist
Sumatriptan succinate
Serotonin 5-HT agonist
Methysergide (hydrogen maleate)
Pizotifen (hydrogen maleate)

MOTION SICKNESS
Promethazine

MULTIPLE CARBOXYLASE DEFICIENCY
Biotin

MYASTHENIA GRAVIS
Edrophonium (chloride)
Neostigmine (bromide and methylsulphate)
Physostigmine
Pyridostigmine (bromide)

MYDRIATIC
Homatropine hydrobromide

MYOCARDIAL INFARCTION
Adrenergic blockade
Non-selective beta
Nadolol
Oxprenolol (hydrochloride)
Pindolol
Propranolol (hydrochloride)
Timolol (maleate)
Beta-1
Acebutolol (hydrochloride)
Atenolol
Betaxolol (hydrochloride)
Metoprolol (tartrate)
Antiplatelet
Cyclo-oxygenase inhibitor
Aspirin (acetylsalicylic acid)
Coumarins
Nicoumalone
Phenindione
Warfarin (sodium)
Heparin
Heparin sodium and heparin calcium
Plasminogen activator
Alteplase
Anistreplase
Streptokinase
Urokinase

NAUSEA AND VOMITING
Dopamine-D_2
Chlorpromazine
Metoclopramide (hydrochloride)
Perphenazine
Prochlorperazine
Histamine-H_1 antagonist
Buclizine (hydrochloride)
Serotonin-$5HT_3$
Ondasetron (hydrochloride)

NEUROMUSCULAR BLOCKADE
Alcuronium chloride
Atracurium (besylate)
Pancuronium bromide
Suxamethonium (chloride)
d-Tubocurarine chloride
Vecuronium (bromide)

NEUTROPENIA
Filgrastim
Granulocyte-macrophage colony-stimulating factor

NON-STEROIDAL ANTINFLAMMATORY DRUGS (NSAIDS)
Aspirin (acetylsalicylic acid)
Benorylate
Benoxaprofen
Choline magnesium trisalicylate
Diclofenac sodium
Diflunisal
Etodolac
Fenbufen
Fenoprofen (calcium)
Flurbiprofen
Ibuprofen
Indomethacin
Ketoprofen
Mefenamic acid
Nabumetone
Naproxen
Phenylbutazone
Piroxicam
Salicylic acid
Sodium salicylate
Sulindac
Tiaprofenic acid
Tolmetin (sodium)

OBESITY
Dexfenfluramine (hydrochloride)
Diethylpropion (hydrochloride)
Fenfluramine (hydrochloride)

OEDEMA
Diuretics
Loop
Bumetanide
Ethacrynic acid
Frusemide
Potassium conserving
Amiloride (hydrochloride)
Triamterene
Thiazide, and related
Bendrofluazide
Chlorothiazide
Chlorthalidone
Clopamide
Cyclopenthiazide
Hydrochlorothiazide
Hydroflumethiazide
Indapamide
Mefruside
Metolazone
Polythiazide
Xipamide

OESTROGEN DEFICIENCY
Dienoestrol
Ethinyloestradiol

ONCOLOGY
Alpha interferon receptor agonist
Interferon alpha
Anthracyclines
Aclarubicin (hydrochloride)
Daunorubicin
Doxorubicin hydrochloride
Dihydrofolate reductase inhibitor
Methotrexate
DNA alkylation
Busulphan
Carmustine
Chlorambucil
Cyclophosphamide
Dacarbazine
Ifosfamide
Melphalan
Treosulphan
DNA intercalation, cross-linkage and strand breakage
Actinomycin D
Amsacrine
Bleomycins
Etoposide
Mitomycin C
Mitozantrone (hydrochloride)
Procarbazine hydrochloride
Hormone producing and sensitive tumours
Androgen agonist
Drostanolone propionate
Androgen antagonist
Cyproterone acetate
Flutamide
DNA strand breakage
Streptozotocin
LH-RH agonist
Goseralin (acetate)
Oestrogen agonist
Fosfestrol
Stilboestrol
Oestrogen antagonist
Tamoxifen citrate
Progesterone agonist
Megestrol acetate
Somatostatin agonist
Octreotide (acetate)
Methotrexate rescue
Folinic acid
Platinium derivatives
Carboplatin
Cisplatin
Purine and pyrimidine antimetabolites
Azacytidine
Cytarabine
Mercaptopurine monohydrate
Thioguanine
Ribonucleoside
Hydroxyurea
Sulphdryl uroprotective agent
Mesna
Thymidylate kinase inhibitor
Fluorouracil
Vinca alakaloids
Vinblastine (sulphate)
Vincristine (sulphate)

OPTHALMOLOGY
Fluorescein

PAIN
Cyclo-oxygenase inhibitors
Aspirin (acetylsalicylic acid)
Benorylate
Benoxaprofen
Choline magnesium trisalicylate
Diclofenac sodium
Diflunisal
Etodolac
Fenbufen
Fenoprofen (calcium)
Flurbiprofen
Ibuprofen
Indomethacin
Ketoprofen
Mefenamic acid
Nabumetone
Naproxen
Paracetamol
Phenylbutazone
Piroxicam
Salicylic acid
Sodium salicylate
Sulindac
Tiaprofenic acid
Tolmetin (sodium)
Opiates
Alfentanil (hydrochloride)
Buprenorphine (hydrochloride)
Codeine phosphate
Dextromoramide (tartrate)
Dextropropoxyphene (hydrochloride and napsylate)
Diamorphine hydrochloride
Dihydrocodeine (tartrate)
Dipipanone (hydrochloride)
Fentanyl (citrate)
Levorphanol (tartrate)
Meptazinol (hydrochloride)
Methadone (hydrochloride)
Morphine
Nalbuphine (hydrochloride)
Papaveretum
Pentazocine (hydrochloride)
Pethidine (hydrochloride)
Phenazocine (hydrochloride)
Phenoperidine hydrochloride
Sufentanil
Other
Nefopam (hydrochloride)

PANCREATITIS
Aprotinin

PARASITE INFECTION, EXTERNAL
Lice
Carbaryl
Lindane
Malathion
Scabies
Benzyl benzoate
Lindane
Malathion

PARENTERAL NUTRITION
L-Amino acids
Amino acid solutions for parenteral feeding
Carbohydrates
Fructose
Sorbitol
Xylitol
Fat
Lipid supplements

PARKINSONISM
Antimuscarinics
Benzhexol hydrochloride
Benztropine (mesylate)
Biperiden (hydrochloride)
Orphenadrine hydrochloride
Procyclidine (hydrochloride)
Dopamine agonists
Bromocriptine (mesylate)
Cabergoline
Levodopa
Lisururide (hydrogen maleate)
L-Amino acid decarboxylase inhibitors
Benserazide (hydrochloride)
Carbidopa
Monoamine oxidase-B inhibitor
Selegiline (hydrochloride)

PATENCY OF DUCTUS ARTERIOSUS
Alprostadil

PEPTIC ULCER
Antacid
Aluminium hydroxide and oxide
Calcium carbonate
Magnesium salts, oxides and hydroxide
Antisecretory muscarinic antagonists
Pirenzepine (dihydrochloride)
Poldine (methylsulphate)
Propantheline bromide
Histamine-H_2 antagonists
Cimetidine (hydrochloride)
Famotidine
Nizatidine
Ranitidine
Physical barrier
Alginic acid
Prostaglandin-E_2 agonist
Misoprostol
Proton pump inhibitor
Omeprazole
Surafce tension lowering
Dimethicone
Other drugs
Bismuth salts
Carbenoxolone (sodium)
Sucralfate

PERIPHERAL VASCULAR DISEASE
Alpha adrenergic antagonist
Tolazoline
Prostacyclin agonist
Iloprost
Vasodilator
Naftidofuryl oxalate
Oxpentifyline

PERITONEAL DIALYSIS
Peritoneal dialysis fluid

PHAEOCHROMOCTYOMA
Alpha-adrenergic blockade
Phenoxybenzamine (hydrochloride)
Phentolamine (mesylate)

POISONING
Absorbent
Charcoal (activated)
Kaolin
Antidotes, excretion enhancers
Benzodiazepine
Flumazenil
Cyanide
Dicobalt edetate
Sodium nitrite
Sodium thiosulphate
Iron
Desferrioxamine (mesylate)
Lead
Sodium calciumedetate
Lewiste
Dimercaprol
Methanol
Ethyl alcohol
Nerve gas
Atropine (sulphate)
Pralidoxime
Pyridostigmine (bromide)
Opiate
Naloxone (hydrochloride)
Naltrexone
Organophosphorus
Pralidoxime
Paracetamol
N-Acetylcysteine
Methionine

POSTPARTUUM HAEMORRHAGE
Ergometrine (maleate)
Methylergometrine (maleate)

POTASSIUM DEFICIENCY
Potassium salts

PREMATURE LABOUR
Isoxsuprine (hydrochloride)
Ritodrine (hydrochloride)

PREVENTION OF BLEEDING
Tranexamic acid

PROTOZOA INFECTION
Amoeba
Chloroquine
Dehydroemetine (hydrochloride)
Diloxanide furoate
Emetine (hydrochloride)
Metronidazole
Tinidazole
Giardia
Metronidazole
Tinidazole
Plasmodium
Amodiaquine
Chloroquine
Hydroxychloroquine (sulphate)
Mefloquine (hydrochloride)
Primaquine (phosphate)
Proguanil (hydrochloride)
Quinine
Pyrimethamine
Sulfadoxine
Trypanosome infection
Melarsoprol
Nifurtimox
Leishmania
Sodium stibogluconate

PSORIASIS
Coal tar
Dithranol
Etretinate

PSYCHOSIS
Benzamide
Sulpiride
Butyrophenones
Benperidol
Droperidol
Haloperidol
Dibenzodiazepines
Clozapine
Diphenylbutylpiperidine
Pimozide
Phenothiazines
Chlorpromazine
Fluphenazine
Methotrimeprazine (hydrochloride and maleate)
Perphenazine
Pipothiazine
Prochlorperazine
Thioridazine (hydrochloride)
Trifluoperazine (hydrochloride)
Trimeprazine (tartrate)
Thioxanthene
Chlorprothixene
Flupenthixol (hydrochloride and decanoate)
Zuclopenthixol

RADIOLOGICAL CONTRAST AGENT
Barium sulphate
Diatrizoate meglumine, diatrizoate sodium
Iohexol
Iopanoic acid
Iotroxate (meglumine idroxate)
Propyliodone

REFLUX OESOPHAGITIS
Cholinergic muscarinic agonist
Bethanecol
Histamine H_2 antagonists
Cimetidine
Famotidine
Nizatidine
Ranitidine
Physical barrier
Alginic acid
Proton pump inhibitor
Omeprazole
Surface tension lowering
Dimethicone

RESPIRATORY FAILURE
Doxapram hydrochloride

RHESUS HAEMOLYTIC DISEASE
Human anti-D (Rho) immunoglobulin

RHEUMATOID ARTHRITIS
Disease modifiers
Penicillamine
Gold compounds
Auranofin
Aurothiomalate
Pain, cyclo-oxygenase inhibitors
Aspirin (acetylsalicylic acid)
Benorylate
Benoxaprofen
Choline magnesium trisalicyclate
Diclofenac sodium
Diflunisal
Etodolac
Fenbufen
Fenoprofen (calcium)
Flurbiprofen
Ibuprofen
Indomethacin
Ketoprofen
Mefenamic acid
Nabumetone
Naproxen
Phenylbutazone
Piroxicam
Salicylic acid
Sodium salicylate
Sulindac
Tiaprofenic acid
Tolmetin (sodium)

SALT DEPLETION
Sodium chloride

SCHISTOSOMIASIS
Antihelminthic
Metriphonate
Oxaminiquine
Praziquantel

SCLEROSING AGENT
Phenol

SEDATIVE
Dopamine-D_2
Methotrimeprazine (hydrochloride and maleate)
see also ANXIETY, PSYCHOSIS

SHOCK
Dobutamine (hydrochloride)
Dopamine (hydrochloride)
Metaraminol (bitartrate)
Noradrenaline (acid tartrate)

SPASM SMOOTH MUSCLE
Clonazepam
Dicyclomine (hydrochloride)
Hyoscine butylbromide
Ketazolam
Mebeverine

SPASTICITY
Baclofen
Dantrolene sodium
Medezpam

SPREADING AGENT
Hyaluronidase

SUBARACHNOID HAEMORRHAGE
Nimodipine

THROMBOSIS
Antiplatelet
Cyclo-oxygenase inhihibitor
Aspirin (acetylsalicylic acid)
Phosphodiesterase inhibitor
Dipyridamole
Plasminogen activator
Alteplase
Anistreplase
Streptokinase
Urokinase

TOBACCO WITHDRAWAL
Nicotine

ULCERATIVE COLITIS
Mesalazine
Olsalazine (sodium)
Sulphasalazine

URGENCY AND INCONTINENCE
Dicyclomine
Hyoseine
Propantheline
Terolidine

URINARY RETENTION (ADYNAMIC BLADDER)
Bethanecol chloride
Neostigmine
Pyridostigmine

VASODILATOR
Papaverine (hydrochloride)
Tolazoline (hydrochloride)
see also PERIPHERAL VASCULAR DISEASE

VERTIGO
Betahistine
Cinnarizine
Prochlorperazine

VIRAL INFECTION
Interferon alpha
CMV
Foscarnet (sodium)
Ganciclovir (sodium)
Herpes
Acyclovir
Idoxuridine
Vidarabine (monohydrate)
HIV
Zidovudine
Influenza
Amantadine (hydrochloride)
RSV
Ribavarin

VITAMIN DEFICIENCY
A
Retinol
B
Calcium pantothenate
Nicotinamide
Pyridoxine (hydrochloride)
Riboflavin (vitamin B_2)
Thiamine hydrochloride (vitamin B_1)
B_{12}
Cyanocobalamin
Hydroxocobalamin
C
Ascorbic acid
D
Alfacalcidol
Calcifediol
Calciferol
Calcitriol
Other
Folic acid
Tocopherol (vitamin E)

WILSON'S DISEASE
Penicillamine